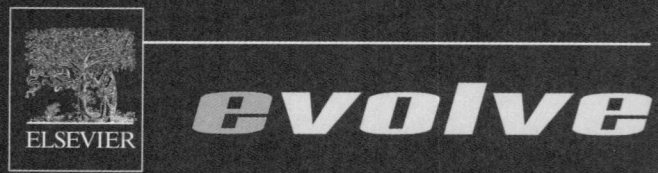

Medical-Surgical Nursing

Assessment and Nagement of Clinical Problems

Make the MOST out of your study time...
Get these companion resources today!

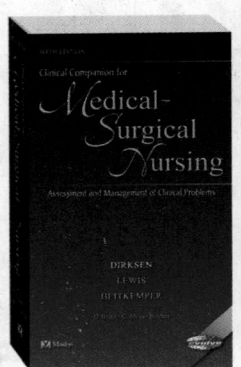

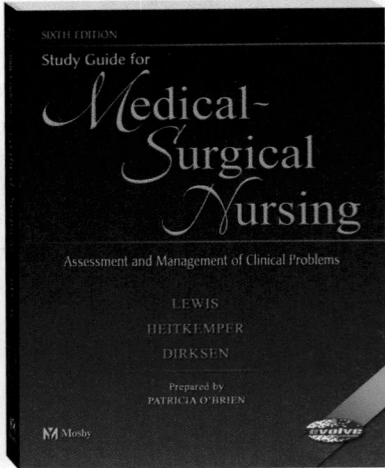

Cal Companion
f Medical-Surgical Nursing

Sh n Ruff Dirksen, RN, PhD; Sharon Mantik Lewis, RN, PhAAN; and Margaret McLean Heitkemper, RN, PhD, FA

Th ghly revised, this best-selling reference includes ap imately 200 medical-surgical conditions and pr ures in a concise, alphabetical format. This reference co s the information nurses need to know – in a format th asy to use in clinical settings.

20 832pp. • 0-323-01896-3

Als available on PDA.
So te includes BONUS material:
- lossary of key terms and definitions
- nergency Management information
- rbal Therapies content
- ormal Laboratory Values Guide
- Electronic Calculators

200 CD-ROM • 0-323-03199-4

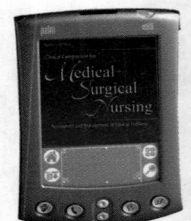

Stu Guide
for edical-Surgical Nursing

Patri Graber O'Brien, RN, CS, BSN, MSN, MA

Tho hly revised to reflect the new 6th edition of the t the study guide includes a wide variety of exer s and activities – including fill-in-the-blank worke ts, anatomy and physiology review, true-false quest s, critical thinking activities, crossword puzzles, case lies, matching, word scrambles, and multi-choice questions.

2004 688 pp. • 0-323-01855-6

Your success is "virtually" guaranteed with VCE!

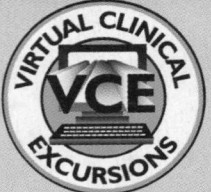

Virtual Clinical Excursions for Lewis: Medical-Surgical Nursing: Assessment and Management of Clinical Problems, 6th Edition

Have a real-world hospital experience without leaving the classroom or computer! These groundbreaking, new workbooks and CD-ROMs bring learning to life in two different multi-floor "virtual" hospital settings! Each virtual hospital visit allows you to access realistic information resources essential to patient care and contains built-in testing of clinical knowledge with NCLEX-RN-type questions.

*Now you can choose between **two different hospital settings** — both with a wide range of patients and disorders!*

VCE Version 1.0
2004 • Workbook and CD-ROM for Windows™ and Macintosh© • 0-323-02693-1

VCE Version 2.0
2004• Workbook and CD-ROM for Windows™ and Macintosh© • 0-323-02692-3

There' othing like it in your Nursing Education!

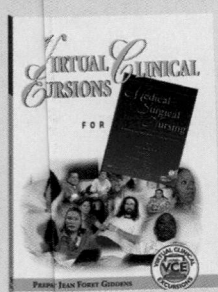

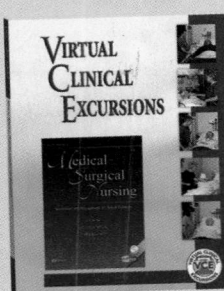

For more information
or to order....

Visit y ur local health sciences bookstore.
Call t -free 1-800-545-2522.
Visit o r website at www.elsevierhealth.com

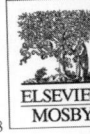

NMX-578

Medical-Surgical Nursing

Assessment and Management of Clinical Problems

SHARON MANTIK LEWIS, RN, PhD, FAAN
Professor, Schools of Nursing and Medicine
Castella Distinguished Professor of Nursing
University of Texas Health Science Center;
Clinical Nurse Scientist
Geriatric Research, Education, and Clinical Center
South Texas Veterans Health Care System
San Antonio, Texas

MARGARET McLEAN HEITKEMPER, RN, PhD, FAAN
Professor, Biobehavioral Nursing and Health Systems
Corbally Professor for Public Service, School of Nursing;
Adjunct Professor, Division of Gastroenterology
School of Medicine
University of Washington
Seattle, Washington

SHANNON RUFF DIRKSEN, RN, PhD
Associate Professor
College of Nursing
Arizona State University
Tempe, Arizona

SECTION EDITORS

Patricia Graber O'Brien, RNCS, MA, MSN
Instructor, College of Nursing
University of New Mexico;
Clinical Research Coordinator
Lovelace Scientific Resources
Albuquerque, New Mexico

Jean Foret Giddens, RN, PhD, CS
Associate Professor
College of Nursing
University of New Mexico
Albuquerque, New Mexico

Linda Bucher, RN, DNSc
Associate Professor
College of Health and Nursing Sciences
University of Delaware
Newark, Delaware

M Mosby
An Affiliate of Elsevier

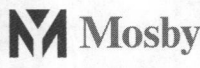

An Affiliate of Elsevier

11830 Westline Industrial Drive
St. Louis, Missouri 63146

MEDICAL-SURGICAL NURSING: ASSESSMENT
AND MANAGEMENT OF CLINICAL PROBLEMS,
6th edition

ISBN 0-323-01610-3

NOTICE

Nursing is an ever-changing field. Standard safety precautions must be followed, but as new research and
clinical experience broaden our knowledge, changes in treatment and drug therapy may become necessary
or appropriate. Readers are advised to check the most current product information provided by the manufacturer of each drug to be administered to verify the recommended dose, the method and duration of administration, and contraindications. It is the responsibility of the licensed prescriber, relying on experience
and knowledge of the patient, to determine dosages and the best treatment for each individual patient. Neither the publisher nor the editor assumes any liability for any injury and/or damage to persons or property
arising from this publication.

Previous editions copyrighted 1983, 1987, 1992, 1996, 2000

International Standard Book Number
0-323-01610-3

Executive Vice President, Nursing and Health Professions: Sally Schrefer
Executive Publisher: Robin Carter
Senior Developmental Editor: Kristin Geen
Editorial Assistant: Jamie Randall
Publishing Services Manager: Catherine Albright Jackson
Senior Project Manager: Mary Stueck
Design Coordinator: Teresa McBryan Breckwoldt
Cover Art: Studio Montage

Printed in the United States of America

Last digit is the print number: 9 8 7 6 5 4 3

About the Authors

SHARON MANTIK LEWIS, RN, PhD, FAAN

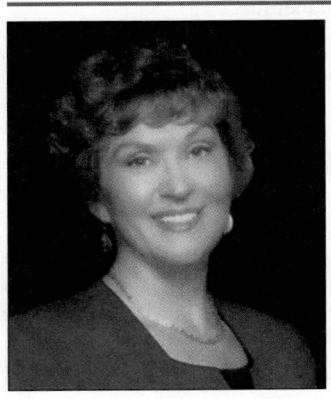

Sharon Lewis received her Bachelor of Science in nursing from the University of Wisconsin-Madison, Master of Science in nursing with a minor in biological sciences from the University of Colorado-Denver, and PhD in immunology from the Department of Pathology at the University of New Mexico School of Medicine. She had a 2-year postdoctoral fellowship from the National Kidney Foundation. Her more than 30 years of teaching experience include inservice education and teaching in associate degree, baccalaureate, master's degree, and doctoral programs in Maryland, Illinois, Wisconsin, New Mexico, and Texas. Favorite teaching areas are pathophysiology, immunology, and renal failure. She has been actively involved in clinical research for the past 20 years, investigating altered immune responses in various disorders. Her current research focus is on the newly emerging field of psychoneuroimmunology. At this time she is using biofeedback and immune parameters to study the effects of relaxation therapy for caregivers of Alzheimer's patients. Her free time is spent playing tennis, landscaping, and gardening.

MARGARET McLEAN HEITKEMPER, RN, PhD, FAAN

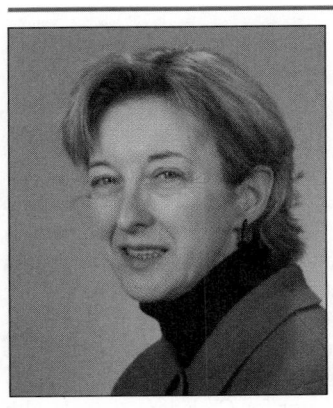

Margaret Heitkemper is Professor and Chairperson, Department of Biobehavioral Nursing and Health Systems, and Adjunct Professor, Division of Gastroenterology, at the School of Medicine at the University of Washington. She is also Director of the National Institutes of Health–National Institute for Nursing Research–funded Center for Women's Health Research at the University of Washington. In the spring of 2001, Dr. Heitkemper was appointed the John and Marguerite Corbally Endowed Professor for Public Service. Dr. Heitkemper received her Bachelor of Science in nursing from Seattle University, her Master of Science in gerontologic nursing from the University of Washington, and her doctorate in Physiology and Biophysics from the University of Illinois at the Medical Center, Chicago. She has been on faculty at the University of Washington since 1981 and has been the recipient of three School of Nursing and one university-wide Excellence in Teaching awards. In addition, she has served as a Scientific Advisory Board member for two pharmaceutical companies and the Medical Advisory Board of *Woman's Day* magazine, and in 2002 received the Distinguished Nutrition Support Nurse Award from the American Society for Parenteral and Enteral Nutrition (ASPEN).

SHANNON RUFF DIRKSEN, RN, PhD

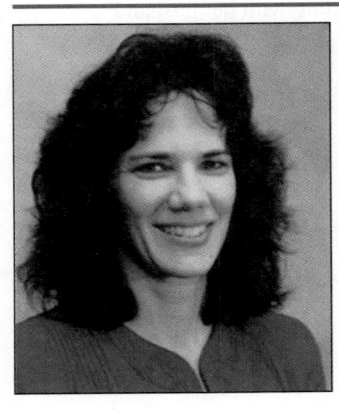

Shannon Dirksen received her Bachelor of Science in nursing from Arizona State University and her Master of Science and doctorate in nursing from the University of Arizona. In her 16 years of teaching at the graduate and undergraduate levels, she has taught at Edith Cowan University (Western Australia), Intercollegiate College of Nursing–Washington State University, University of New Mexico, and Arizona State University. She currently teaches nursing research and management and leadership. For the past 18 years, she has been actively involved in oncology research, focusing on survivorship well-being in white and Hispanic patients who have melanoma and breast cancer. She is the primary author of the *Clinical Companion to Medical-Surgical Nursing,* which companies this book.

PATRICIA GRABER O'BRIEN, RNCS, MA, MSN

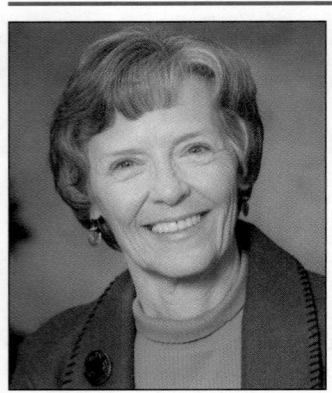

Patricia O'Brien received her Bachelor of Science in nursing from the University of Kansas, Master of Arts in adult education from the University of New Mexico, and Master of Science in nursing with majors in medical-surgical nursing and nursing administration from the University of Texas at El Paso. During her nursing career, she has worked in medical-surgical nursing and home health care, but most of her experience is in nursing education. She is a certified clinical nurse specialist in medical-surgical nursing. She has directed and taught in nursing programs of all levels of basic nursing preparation for more than 30 years. Her primary interests in teaching include nursing process, pharmacology, and metabolic problems. She formally retired from Albuquerque Technical-Vocational Institute, a community college, in 1993, and continues to teach part-time in the College of Nursing at the University of New Mexico. She is also employed part-time as a clinical research coordinator at Lovelace Scientific Resources in Albuquerque.

JEAN FORET GIDDENS, RN, PhD, CS

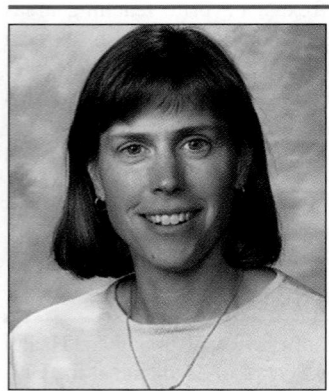

Jean Giddens received a Bachelor of Science in nursing from the University of Kansas, a Master of Science in nursing from the University of Texas at El Paso, and a PhD in Education and Human Resource Studies from Colorado State University. She is a certified clinical specialist in medical-surgical nursing. She has been involved in nursing education since 1984. She currently teaches nursing at the University of New Mexico, and also has taught in several other nursing programs, including Mesa State College in Grand Junction, Colorado, the University of Texas at El Paso, and Eastern New Mexico University at Roswell. Her content areas in nursing education include medical-surgical nursing, health assessment, nursing process, nursing fundamentals, and nursing pharmacology.

LINDA BUCHER, RN, DNSc

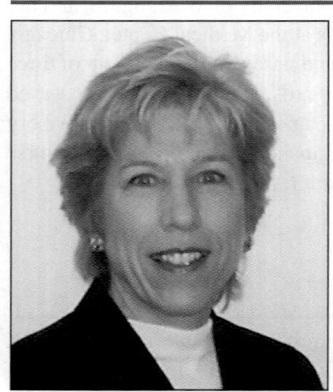

Linda Bucher received her Bachelor of Science in nursing from Thomas Jefferson University in Philadelphia, her Master of Science in adult health and illness from the University of Pennsylvania in Philadelphia, and her DNSc in nursing from Widener University in Chester, Pennsylvania. Her 22 years of teaching experience has spanned inservice and patient education, and teaching in associate, baccalaureate, and graduate nursing programs in New Jersey, Pennsylvania, and Delaware. Her preferred teaching areas include cardiopulmonary and emergency nursing and research. Currently, she holds a joint appointment as a Nursing Research Facilitator for Christiana Care Health Services and associate professor at the University of Delaware, both in Newark, Delaware. She maintains her practice by working per diem as an emergency nurse, is an active member of the American Association of Critical Care Nurses, and enjoys working as a volunteer nurse for Operation Smile. In her free time, she enjoys traveling in Europe and skiing with her husband.

Contributors

Richard B. Arbour, RN, MSN, CCRN, CNRN
Staff Nurse, Medical Intensive Care Unit
Albert Einstein Medical Center
Philadelphia, Pennsylvania

Elizabeth A. Ayello, RN, PhD, CS, CWOCN, FAAN
Clinical Associate Professor and Director of Adult Nursing
    Science
Senior Advisor, The John A. Hartford Institute for Geriatric
    Nursing
The Steinhardt School of Education
Division of Nursing, New York University
New York, New York

Catherine M. Bender, RN, PhD
Assistant Professor, School of Nursing
University of Pittsburgh
Pittsburgh, Pennsylvania

Donna Zimmaro Bliss, RN, PhD, CCRN, FAAN
Associate Professor, School of Nursing
University of Minnesota
Minneapolis, Minnesota

Lucy Bradley-Springer, RN, PhD, ACRN
Director, Mountain Plains AIDS Education and Training
    Center;
Associate Professor of Medicine
University of Colorado Health Sciences Center
Denver, Colorado

Catherine E. Brown, RN, CRNH
Education and Research Associate
Hospice of the Valley
Phoenix, Arizona

Linda Bucher, RN, DNSc
Associate Professor, College of Health and Nursing Sciences
University of Delaware
Newark, Delaware

Maria A. Connolly, RN, DNSc, CCRN
Dean, College of Nursing and Allied Health
University of St. Francis
Joliet, Illinois

Elizabeth A. Crago, RN, MSN
Project Director, Research Associate
University of Pittsburgh School of Nursing
Pittsburgh, Pennsylvania

Janet T. Crimlisk, RNCS, MS, ANP
Clinical Nurse Specialist
Boston Medical Center
Boston, Massachusetts

Anne Croghan, RN, MN, ARNP
Nurse Practitioner
VA Puget Sound Health Care System
Seattle, Washington

Shannon Ruff Dirksen, RN, PhD
Associate Professor, College of Nursing
Arizona State University
Tempe, Arizona

Laura Dulski, RNC, MSN, CS
Senior Clinical Nurse
New Life Family Center
Rush Presbyterian–St. Luke's Medical Center
Chicago, Illinois

Sheila A. Dunn, RN, MSN, C-ANP
Adult Nurse Practitioner, Primary Care
Belleville Veterans Clinic
Belleville, Illinois

Mary Ersek, RN, PhD
Research Scientist, Pain Research Department
Swedish Medical Center
Seattle, Washington

Hatice Y. Foell, RN, ARNP, MSN
Congestive Heart Failure Disease Management Program
Health First Heart Institute
Melbourne, Florida

Jean Foret Giddens, RN, PhD, CS
Associate Professor, College of Nursing
University of New Mexico
Albuquerque, New Mexico

Nancy J. Girard, RN, PhD, FAAN
Associate Professor and Chair
Acute Nursing Care Department
University of Texas Health Science Center
San Antonio, Texas

D. Patricia Gray, RN, PhD
Associate Professor and Chair
Department of Adult Health
Virginia Commonwealth University
Richmond, Virginia

Mikel Gray, RN, PhD, CUNP, CCCN, FAAN
Professor and Nurse Practitioner
Department of Urology
University of Virginia
Charlottesville, Virginia

Peggi Guenter, RN, PhD, CNSN
Managing Editor for Special Projects
American Society for Parenteral and Enteral Nutrition
Havertown, PA

Debra A. Hagler, RN, MS, CS, CCRN
Clinical Associate Professor, College of Nursing
Arizona State University
Tempe, Arizona

Lissi Hansen, RN, PhD
Postdoctoral Fellow, John A. Hartford Foundation
Department of Biobehavioral Nursing and Health Systems
University of Washington
Seattle, Washington

Margaret McLean Heitkemper, RN, PhD, FAAN
Professor, Biobehavioral Nursing and Health Systems
School of Nursing;
Adjunct Professor, Division of Gastroenterology
School of Medicine
University of Washington
Seattle, Washington

Marcia J. Hill, RN, MSN
Senior Research Nurse
M.D. Anderson Cancer Center
Houston, Texas

Mary Jo Holechek, RN, MS, CRNP, CNN
Transplant Nurse Practitioner, Transplant Office
Johns Hopkins Hospital
Baltimore, Maryland

Mary Ann House-Fancher, RN, MSN, ARNP
Nurse Practitioner, Department of Cardiothoracic Surgery
Health First Heart Institute
Melbourne, Florida

Carolyn I. Johns, RN, MS, CANP
Adult Nurse Practitioner, Cardiology
Lovelace Health Systems
Albuquerque, New Mexico

Kathleen J. Jones, RN, MS, ANP
Adult Nurse Practitioner
Hematology-Oncology Clinic
Walter Reed Army Medical Center
Washington, D.C.

Duck-Hee Kang, RN, PhD
Associate Professor, School of Nursing
University of Alabama at Birmingham
Birmingham, Alabama

Mary E. Kerr, RN, PhD, FAAN
Associate Professor, School of Nursing
Director for Center for Nursing Research
University of Pittsburgh
Pittsburgh, Pennsylvania

Catherine Kirkness, RN, PhD, CNN(C)
Research Assistant Professor
Department of Biobehavioral Nursing and Health Systems
University of Washington
Seattle, Washington

Cynthia J. Knipe, RN
Administrative Director
Wishard Health Services
Indianapolis, Indiana

Cathleen E. Kunkler, RN, BSN, ONC, CNA
Clinical Faculty Practical Nursing Program
Northern Tier Career Center
Towanda, Pennsylvania

Nancy Stoetzner Kupper, RN, MSN
Associate Professor
Tarrant County Junior College
Fort Worth, Texas

Barbara S. Levine, RN, PhD, CRNP, CS
Gerontological Nurse Consultant
BSL Consulting Services
Wayne, Pennsylvania

Sharon Mantik Lewis, RN, PhD, FAAN
Professor, Schools of Nursing and Medicine
University of Texas Health Science Center;
Clinical Nurse Scientist
Geriatric Research, Education, and Clinical Center
South Texas Veterans Health Care System
San Antonio, Texas

Carol O. Long, RN, PhD
Director of Professional Services
Carrigan's Health Care Services
Phoenix, Arizona;
Faculty Associate, Gerontology Program
Arizona State University
Tempe, Arizona

Kathleen T. Lucke, RN, PhD
Assistant Professor, School of Nursing
University of Texas Health Science Center
San Antonio, Texas

Nancy J. MacMullen, RN, APN, CCNS, PhD
University Professor
Governors State University
University Park, Illinois

Lisa B. Malick, RNC, MS, OCN
Assistant Professor
The Community College of Baltimore County
Baltimore, Maryland

Linda Griego Martinez, RN, MSN, CS, CCRN
Cardiology Care Manager
Presbyterian Heart Group
Albuquerque, New Mexico

De Ann F. Mitchell, RN, PhD
Professor, Nursing Department
Tarrant County College
Fort Worth, Texas

Patricia Graber O'Brien, RNCS, MA, MSN
Instructor, College of Nursing
University of New Mexico;
Clinical Research Coordinator
Lovelace Scientific Resources
Albuquerque, New Mexico

Judith M. Ozuna, RN, MN, ARNP, CNRN
Clinical Nurse Specialist in Neurology
VA Puget Sound Health Care System
Seattle, Washington

JoAnne K. Phillips, RN, MSN, CCRN, CCNS
Clinical Nurse Specialist, Surgical Critical Care
Hospital of the University of Pennsylvania
Philadelphia, Pennsylvania

Carmencita M. Poe, RN, EdD
Clinical Nurse Manager, Oncology/Medical-Surgical Nursing
Bon Secours De Paul Medical Center
Norfolk, Virginia

Kathleen A. Pollard, RN, MSN, CHPN
Education and Research Associate
Hospice of the Valley
Phoenix, Arizona

Anita Ralstin, RN, MS, CS, CNP
New Mexico Heart Institute
Albuquerque, New Mexico

Kathleen Rich, RN, MS, CCNS
Critical Care Clinical Specialist
The Methodist Hospitals, Inc.
Gary, Indiana

Dottie Roberts, RN, C, MSN, MACI, ONC
Medical-Surgical Clinical Nurse Specialist
Palmetto Health Baptist Medical Center
Columbia, South Carolina

Margaret Rosenzweig, RN, PhD, CRNP, AOCN
Assistant Professor, School of Nursing
University of Pittsburgh
Pittsburgh, Pennsylvania

Lynda Sawchuk, RN, ARNP, CWOCN
Enterostomal Therapy Nurse
Virginia Mason Medical Center
Seattle, Washington

Susan Semb, RN, MSN, CDE
Health Educator
Kaiser Permanente Health Education Department
San Diego, California

Anita Shoup, RN, MSN, CNOR
Clinical Nurse Consultant
Regent Medical
Edmonds, Washington

Debra J. Smith, RN, MSN, CCRN
Instructor, College of Nursing
University of New Mexico
Albuquerque, New Mexico

Sarah C. Smith, RN, MA, CRNO
Educational Associate
University of Iowa Health Care
Iowa City, Iowa

Cheryl Ross Staats, RN, MSN, CS
Assistant Professor, School of Nursing
University of Texas Health Science Center
San Antonio, Texas

Kathleen R. Stevens, RN, EdD, FAAN
Professor and Director
Academic Center of Evidence-Based Practice
University of Texas Health Science Center
San Antonio, Texas

Barbara Van de Castle, RN, APRN, MSN, BC
Instructor
Johns Hopkins University School of Nursing
Baltimore, Maryland

Catherine Warms, RN, PhD
Postdoctoral Research Fellow
Department of Biobehavioral Nursing and Health Care Systems
University of Washington
Seattle, Washington

Barbara G. White, RN, MS
Clinical Associate Professor, College of Nursing
Arizona State University
Tempe, Arizona

Mary E. Wilbur, RN, MSN
Continuum of Care Manager
Medical University of South Carolina
Charleston, South Carolina

Deidre D. Wipke-Tevis, RNC, PhD
Assistant Professor, Sinclair School of Nursing
University of Missouri
Columbia, Missouri

Linda Witek-Janusek, RN, PhD
Professor of Nursing, Marcella Niehoff School of Nursing
Loyola University of Chicago
Maywood, Illinois

Reviewers

Elizabeth Alden, RNC, BSN, CDE
Albuquerque, New Mexico

Margaret M. Andrews, RN, PhD, CTN
Rochester, New York

Anne M. Aquila, RN, MSN, CS
New Haven, Connecticut

Mary S. Baird, RN, MN, CNRN, ARNP
Olympia, Washington

Valerie O'Toole Baker, RN, MSN, CS
Erie, Pennsylvania

Christine A. Balt, RN, MS, CS, ACRN
Indianapolis, Indiana

Ellen Barker, RN, MSN, CNRN
Greenville, Delaware

Joanne M. Bartram, RN, MS, CFNP
Albuquerque, New Mexico

Mary Ellen Beebe, RN, MSN, CEN
Cleveland, Wisconsin

Viola G. Benavente, RN, MSN, CNS
San Antonio, Texas

Jean K. Berry, RN, PhD, CS
Chicago, Illinois

Patricia A. Blissitt, RN, PhD, CCRN, CNRN, CCM, CS
Seattle, Washington

Peter Bonner, MA, MS
Placitas, New Mexico

Heather Boyd-Monk, SRN, BSN, CRNO
Philadelphia, Pennsylvania

Elisabeth G. Bradley, RN, APN, CCRN
Newark, Delaware

Elizabeth J. Bridges, RN, PhD, CCNS
San Antonio, Texas

Vanessa Briones, RN, BSN
San Antonio, Texas

Karen R. Bruni, RN, MSN, NP, CVN
Albany, New York

Erica Camarillo, RN, BSN
San Antonio, Texas

Janis L. Carelock, RN, MSN, CCRN, CNS
Austin, Texas

Sharon G. Childs, RN, MS, CRNP-CS, CEN, ONC
Baltimore, Maryland

Phyllis Christiansen, RN, MN, ARNP
Seattle, Washington

Terry Cicero, RN, MN, CCRN
Seattle, Washington

Dorothy Hendel Clough, RN, PhD
Albuquerque, New Mexico

Margaret F. Cramer, RN, MSN
Manheim, Pennsylvania

Rebecca Crane-Okada, RN, PhD, AOCN
Santa Monica, California

Karen A. Crisfulla, RN, MSN, CCRN
Mount Laurel, New Jersey

Anne Croghan, RN, MN, ARNP
Seattle, Washington

Patricia Cryer, RN, MS, MSN, CENP
Tyler, Texas

Barbara I. Damron, RN, PhD
Santa Fe, New Mexico

Yvonne M. D'Arcy, RN, ARNP, MS, C-CS
Baltimore, Maryland

Angela J. DiSabatino, RN, MS
Newark, Delaware

Sheila A. Dunn, RN, MSN, C-ANP
Belleville, Illinois

Brenda Elliff, RN, MPA, ONC, CCM, LNCC
Coeur d'Alene, Idaho

Rebecca Fix, RN, CNP
Grand Rapids, Minnesota

John J. Gallagher, RN, MSN, CCNS, CCRN, CEN, RRT
Upland, Pennsylvania

Beverly Gay, RN, MSN, CCRN
Richmond, Virginia

Nancy J. Girard, RN, PhD, FAAN
San Antonio, Texas

Susan K. Goebel, RNC, MS, WHNP, SANE
Grand Junction, Colorado

Karen Goff, RN, BSN
Atlanta, Georgia

Judy L. Goodhart, RN, MSN
Grand Junction, Colorado

Rebecca B. Griffin, RN, MS
Waco, Texas

M. Susan Grinslade, RN, PhD(c)
San Antonio, Texas

Catherine M. Harris, RNCS, PhD
San Antonio, Texas

Sherry Garrett Hendrickson, RN, PhD, CNS
Austin, Texas

Marcia J. Hill, RN, MSN
Houston, Texas

Roxana Huebscher, RN, PhD, FNPC, HNC, CMT
Oshkosh, Wisconsin

Monica Jarrett, RN, PhD
Seattle, Washington

Janene Council Jeffery, RN, MSN, CDE
Austin, Texas

Vicki Y. Johnson, RN, PhD, FN, CUCNS
Birmingham, Alabama

Karla Jones, RN, MS
Ontario, Oregon

Duck-Hee Kang, RN, PhD
Birmingham, Alabama

Tamara M. Kear, RN, MSN, CNN
Wilmington, Delaware

Michelle Kelly, RN, BSc, MN
Sydney, Australia

Mary Jean Klein, RN, MS
Houston, Texas

Judy A. Knighton, RN, MScN
Sharon, Ontario, Canada

JoAnne Konick-McMahan, RN, MSN, CCRN
Philadelphia, Pennsylvania

Cathleen E. Kunkler, RN, BSN, ONC, CNA
Towanda, Pennsylvania

Ann L. Lambeth, RN, MSN
Grand Junction, Colorado

Helen L. Lamothe, RN, BSN, PHN, ONC
Golden, Colorado

Linda Laskowski-Jones, RN, MS, CS, CCRN, CEN
Newark, Delaware

Natasha Leskovsek, RN, MBA, JD
Washington, D.C.

Barbara S. Levine, RN, PhD, CRNP, CS
Wayne, Pennsylvania

Patricia A. Loflin, RN, MSN, FNP
Albuquerque, New Mexico

Kathy Lopez-Bushnell, EdD, MPH, RNC (FNP), COHNS
Albuquerque, New Mexico

Kathleen T. Lucke, RN, PhD
San Antonio, Texas

Jane A. Madden, RN, MSN
St. Louis, Missouri

Lisa B. Malick, RNC, MS, OCN
Baltimore, Maryland

Linda Griego Martinez, RN, MSN, CS, CCRN
Albuquerque, New Mexico

Katheryn Ellen McCash, RNC, MSN
Albuquerque, New Mexico

Holly Fadness McFarland, RN, MSN, CNN
Greenville, North Carolina

Lora McGuire, RN, MS
Joliet, Illinois

Laura Wild McIntosh, RN, MSN, CRNA
New Brunswick, New Jersey

Mary Ann Siciliano McLaughlin, RN, MSN
Magnolia, New Jersey

To the profession of nursing
and
to the important people in our lives

Preface

The sixth edition of *Medical-Surgical Nursing: Assessment and Management of Clinical Problems* has been thoroughly revised to incorporate the most recent medical-surgical nursing information in an attractive, easy-to-use format. More than just a textbook, this is a comprehensive resource containing essential information that students need to prepare for lectures, classroom activities, examinations, clinical assignments, and comprehensive care of patients. In addition to the readable writing style and full-color illustrations, the text includes many special features to help students learn the medical-surgical nursing content, including patient and family teaching, gerontology, collaborative care, cultural and ethnic considerations, nutrition, home care, evidence-based practice, nursing research, and much more.

The comprehensive and accurate content, special features, attractive layout, and student-friendly writing style combine to make this the number one medical-surgical nursing textbook used in more nursing schools around the country than any other medical-surgical nursing textbook.

The strengths of the first five editions have been retained, including the use of the nursing process as an organizational theme for nursing management. Numerous new features have been added to address some of the rapid changes in practice. Contributors have been selected for their acknowledged excellence in specific content areas; one or more specialists in the subject area have thoroughly reviewed each chapter to increase accuracy. The editors have undertaken final rewriting and editing to achieve internal consistency. All efforts were directed toward building on the strengths of the previous edition while preparing an even more effective new edition.

ORGANIZATION

Content is organized into two major divisions. The first division, Section One (Chapters 1 through 11), discusses general concepts related to adult patients. The second division, Sections Two through Twelve (Chapters 12 through 67), presents nursing assessment and nursing management of medical-surgical problems.

The various body systems are grouped to reflect their interrelated functions. Each section is organized around two central themes: assessment and management. Chapters dealing with assessment of a body system include a discussion of the following:

1. A brief review of anatomy and physiology, focusing on information that will promote understanding of nursing care
2. Health history and noninvasive physical assessment skills to expand the knowledge base on which decisions are made
3. Common diagnostic studies, expected results, and related nursing responsibilities to provide easily accessible information

Management chapters focus on the pathophysiology, clinical manifestations, diagnostic study results, collaborative care, and nursing management of various diseases and disorders. The nursing management sections are organized into assessment, nursing diagnoses, planning, implementation, and evaluation. To emphasize the importance of patient care in various clinical settings, nursing implementation of all major health problems is organized by the following levels of care:

1. Health Promotion
2. Acute Intervention
3. Ambulatory and Home Care

CLASSIC FEATURES

- **Patient and family teaching** is an ongoing theme throughout the text. Coverage includes a separate chapter (Chapter 4: Patient and Family Teaching) and more than 75 Patient and Family Teaching Guides throughout the text.
- **Home care/community-based care** is also emphasized in this edition. Coverage includes a separate chapter (Chapter 6: Community-Based Nursing and Home Care) and special Ambulatory and Home Care headings in Nursing Implementation sections.
- **Collaborative care** is highlighted in special Collaborative Care sections in all management chapters and more than 85 Collaborative Care tables throughout the text.
- **Gerontology coverage** includes Chapter 5: Older Adults, and appears throughout the text under Gerontologic Considerations headings and in Gerontologic Differences in Assessment and Effects of Aging tables.
- **Nutrition** is highlighted throughout the book. Nutritional Therapy tables summarize nutritional interventions for patients with various health problems.
- **Nursing management** is presented in a consistent and comprehensive format, with headings for Health Promotion, Acute Intervention, and Ambulatory and Home Care. In addition, **more than 60 Nursing Care Plans** appear in management chapters. These are thoroughly updated to incorporate current NANDA nursing diagnoses and defining characteristics, expected patient outcomes, specific nursing interventions with rationales, and collaborative problems.
- A separate chapter on **complementary and alternative therapy** addresses timely issues in today's health care settings related to nontraditional therapies.
- **Nursing research** encourages application of research into clinical practice. Nursing Research boxes appear throughout the text. Nursing Research Issues at the end of management chapters present possible research questions to be used for research studies.
- **Cultural and ethnic considerations** information is integrated into the text and appears in special boxes highlighting risk factors and other important issues related to the nursing care of various ethnic groups.

- **Ethical Dilemmas boxes** promote critical thinking for timely and sensitive issues that nursing students may deal with in clinical practice.
- **Emergency Management tables** outline the emergency treatment of health problems most likely to require emergency intervention.
- **Common Assessment Abnormalities tables** in assessment chapters alert the nurse to frequently encountered abnormalities and their possible etiologies.
- **Nursing Assessment tables** summarize the key subjective and objective data related to common diseases. Subjective data are organized by functional health patterns.
- **Health History tables** in assessment chapters present key questions to ask patients related to a specific disease or disorder.
- Student-friendly pedagogy includes:
  - **Learning Objectives** and **Key Terms** at the beginning of each chapter help students identify the key content for that body system or disorder.
  - **Review Questions** at the end of each chapter, which are matched to the learning objectives, help students learn the important points in the chapter. Answers are provided in an appendix so that the review questions serve as a self-study tool.
  - **Critical Thinking Exercises** appearing at the end of nursing management chapters include Case Studies with Critical Thinking Questions for clinical application as well as Nursing Research Issues.
  - **Resources** at the end of each chapter contain information about nursing and health care organizations that provide patient teaching and disease and disorder information. Resources include Internet sites to help students find current information online.

NEW FEATURES

- **Six new and expanded chapters:**
  - Culturally Competent Care (Chapter 2)
  - End-of-Life Care (Chapter 10)
  - Addictive Behaviors (Chapter 11)
  - Genetics and Altered Immune Responses (Chapter 13)
  - Nursing Management: Alzheimer's Disease and Dementia (Chapter 58)
  - Nursing Management: Musculoskeletal Trauma and Orthopedic Surgery (Chapter 61)
- **Complementary and Alternative Therapies boxes** expand on the information presented in Chapter 7, and summarize what nurses need to know about nontraditional therapies such as herbal remedies, acupuncture, and biofeedback.
- Selected nursing care plans incorporate **NIC (Nursing Interventions Classification) and NOC (Nursing Outcomes Classification)** to show how NIC, NOC, and NANDA nursing diagnoses can be linked.
- **Evidence-Based Practice boxes** present the use of evidence (results from research) to improve patient outcomes and the implications for nursing practice.
- A special **Culturally Competent Care heading** in selected Nursing Management sections highlights expanded cultural and ethnic content as it relates to specific diseases and disorders.
- **Genetics in Clinical Practice boxes** highlight the genetic basis, genetic testing, and clinical implications for genetic disorders that affect adults.

ANCILLARY PACKAGE

Learning Supplements for the Student

- The **Student CD-ROM** packaged with this text contains the following valuable learning aids:
  - **Forty disorder monographs,** including disorder overview, case study, and a variety of interactive learning activities, provide immediate feedback. This special icon 🔵 appears in the text to designate content areas where students are encouraged to use their CD-ROM for further self-study.
  - **Glossary** of key terms and definitions, available as one comprehensive glossary and organized by chapter
  - **Patient and Family Instruction handouts** in both English and Spanish to be printed and distributed to patients
- The **Virtual Clinical Excursions** CD-ROM and workbook to accompany this text is an exciting learning tool that sends students into the virtual clinical setting to "visit" patients, access charts, make assessments, monitor daily changes, formulate nursing diagnoses, plan interventions, and much more. This "hands-on" approach is ideal for learning communication, documentation, assessment, critical thinking, and other essential skills.
- The *Clinical Companion to Medical-Surgical Nursing,* **3rd edition,** presents approximately 200 common medical-surgical conditions and procedures in a concise, alphabetical format for quick clinical reference. Designed for portability, this popular reference includes the essential, need-to-know information for medical-surgical nursing practice. An attractive and functional two-color design highlights key information for quick, easy reference. This edition features expanded patient and family teaching content, as well as additional illustrations and tables to enhance usefulness and visual appeal.
- The **Study Guide** contains extensive review and testing material that has been thoroughly updated to reflect the revision of the textbook. It features a wide variety of clinically relevant exercises and activities, including fill-in-the-blank worksheets, anatomy identification review, true-false questions, critical thinking activities, crossword puzzles, case studies, matching exercises, word scrambles, and multiple-choice questions in NCLEX format. Answers to all questions are included in the back to provide students with immediate feedback as they study.
- The **Evolve website** 🌐 is available at *http://evolve.elsevier.com/Lewis/medsurg/* and features the following valuable learning aids:
  - Concept map creator and examples of concept maps
  - Glossary of key terms and definitions, available as one comprehensive glossary and organized by chapter
  - Patient and Family Instruction handouts in both English and Spanish that can be printed and distributed to patients
  - Content updates from the authors
  - WebLinks for each chapter
  - Chapter summaries
  - Case studies from the text with questions and the capability for students to submit answers to instructors online

Teaching Supplements for the Instructor

- The **Instructor's Resource Kit** remains the most comprehensive set of instructor's materials available, containing:
  - Suggested lecture strategies for each chapter, including teaching/learning objectives, chapter outlines, classroom strategies, and

collaborative/active learning activities with critical thinking questions

- A test bank with approximately 1500 questions with coded answers and text references (also available on CD-ROM in computerized format)
- The **Electronic Image Collection** contains more than 400 full-color images from the text for use in lectures and to import into PowerPoint.
- New to this edition are over 1600 **PowerPoint text slides** organized by diseases and disorders.

ACKNOWLEDGMENTS

The editors are especially grateful to many people at Elsevier who assisted with this major revision effort. In particular, we wish to thank the team of Robin Carter, Kristin Geen, Catherine Albright Jackson, Mary Stueck, and Teresa McBryan Breckwoldt. In addition, we want to thank the marketing team of Janet Blanner, Bob Boehringer, and Angel Magasano.

Our persevering typists have earned our special thanks and include Erica Camarillo, Vanessa Briones, and Jennifer Hale. Alissa Stanley and Barbara Owens worked diligently as research assistants. Barbara Van de Castle provided invaluable assistance as a consultant on nursing diagnoses and revision of the nursing care plans. Kathy Lucke assisted with a major revision of the ethical dilemmas boxes. Pat O'Brien's creative and conscientious work on the Study Guide, Student CD-ROM, Test Bank, Instructor's Resource Kit, and Evolve website was a tremendous asset. A special thanks goes to Peter Bonner who assisted with many details related to the production of the book.

We are particularly indebted to the nurses and student nurses who have put their faith in our book to assist them on their path to excellence. The increasing use of this book throughout the United States, Canada, Australia, and other parts of the world has been gratifying. We appreciate the many users who have shared their comments and suggestions on the previous editions.

We also wish to thank our contributors and reviewers for their assistance with the revision process. We sincerely hope that this book will assist both students and clinicians in practicing truly professional nursing.

Sharon Lewis
Margaret Heitkemper
Shannon Dirksen
Patricia O'Brien
Jean Giddens
Linda Bucher

Table of Contents for Student CD-ROM

The Student CD-ROM provided with this text contains the following features:

- **Glossary** of key terms and definitions
- **40 Case Studies** followed by interactive learning activities
- **40 Patient and Family Instruction guides** in both English and Spanish
- **List of nursing diagnoses**
- **Laboratory values reference**

This special icon 🖭 appears in the text to designate related study content on the CD-ROM.

CASE STUDIES

PATIENT AND FAMILY INSTRUCTION GUIDES

Detailed Contents

 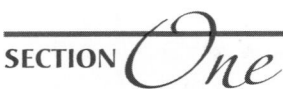

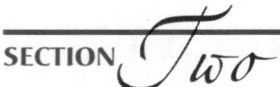

SECTION *Two*

Pathophysiologic Mechanisms of Disease

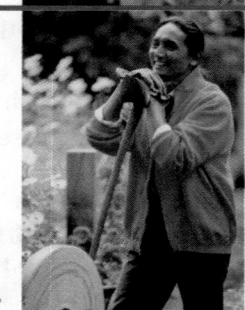

SECTION *Three*

Perioperative Care

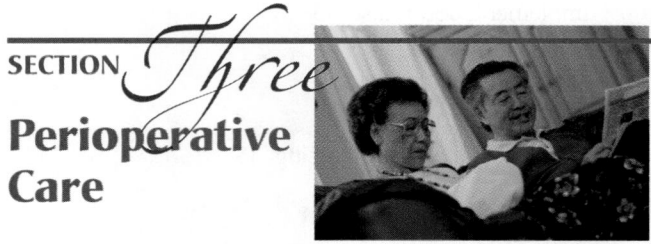

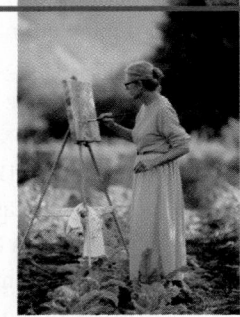
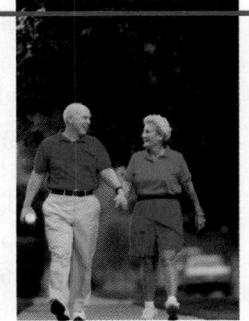

SECTION *Six*
Problems of Oxygenation: Transport

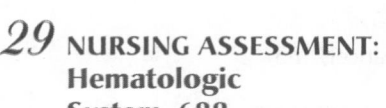

SECTION *Seven*
Problems of Oxygenation: Perfusion

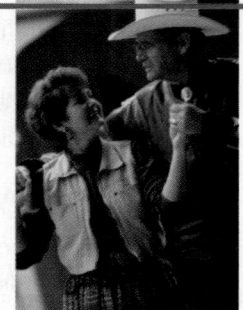

SECTION *Eight*
Problems of Ingestion, Digestion, Absorption, and Elimination

SECTION *Nine*
Problems of Urinary Function

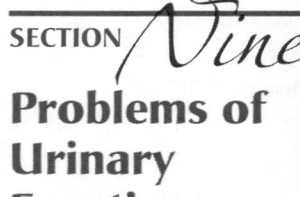
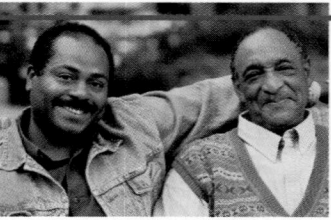

SECTION *Ten*
Problems Related to Regulatory Mechanisms

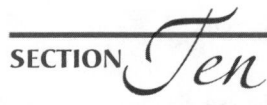
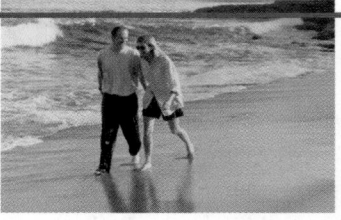

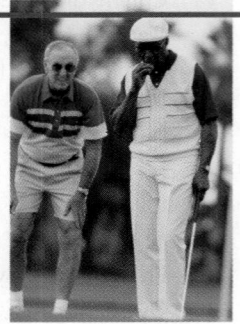

SECTION Eleven
Problems Related to Movement and Coordination

SECTION *Twelve*

Nursing Care in Specialized Settings

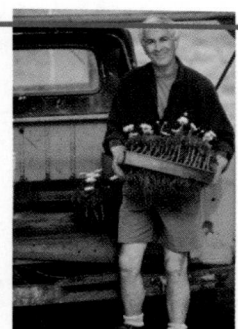

Concepts in Nursing Practice

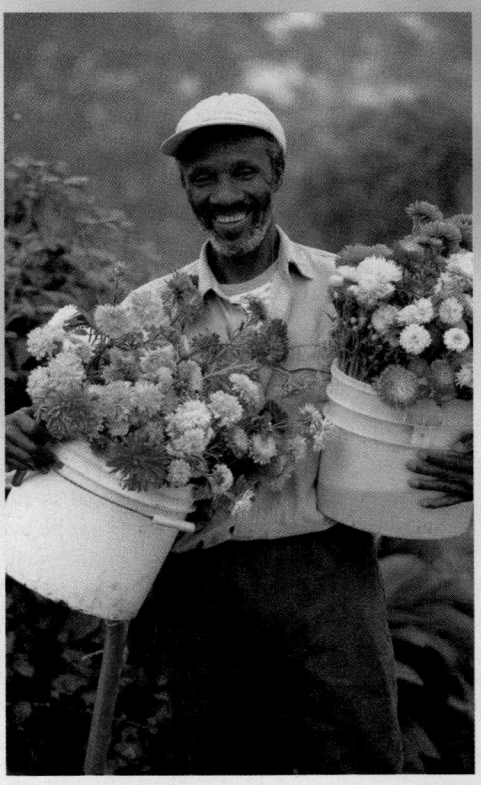

CHAPTER 1

Critical Thinking in the Nursing Process

Patricia Graber O'Brien

LEARNING OBJECTIVES

1. Describe the basic focus of the domain of nursing.
2. Describe what constitutes evidence-based practice.
3. Identify the benefits of using standardized nursing languages.
4. Describe the five phases of the nursing process.
5. Distinguish among the independent, dependent, and collaborative functions of nursing practice.
6. Differentiate between the process of making a nursing diagnosis and a nursing diagnosis as a form of diagnostic nomenclature.
7. Describe the process of writing and selecting patient outcomes.
8. Identify the criteria for selecting nursing interventions.
9. Describe how standardized nursing languages for nursing diagnoses, patient outcomes, and nursing interventions can be linked to plan patient care.
10. Identify the places in the nursing process where evaluation is appropriate.
11. Describe how computerized documentation can enhance nursing practice and improve patient care.

KEY TERMS

advanced practice nursing, p. 3
assessment, p. 6
case management, p. 4
clinical (critical) pathway, p. 13
collaborative problems, p. 9
computerized documentation, p. 14
defining characteristics, p. 9
evaluation, p. 7
evidence-based practice, p. 4
expected patient outcomes, p. 10

implementation, p. 7
managed care, p. 4
nursing, p. 2
nursing diagnosis, p. 8
nursing informatics, p. 15
nursing intervention, p. 11
nursing process, p. 6
planning, p. 7
standardized nursing languages, p. 6

NURSING YESTERDAY, TODAY, AND TOMORROW

There was a time when there was no distinction between nursing and medicine. The sick and injured were merely cared for by those with nurturant instincts.[1] Today there is a clearer delineation between nursing and medical practice.

Nurses deal with "the diagnosis and treatment of human responses to actual or potential health problems,"[2] whereas medicine is primarily concerned with the diagnosis and treatment of illness or injury. The unique nursing focus is on the response of an individual or group to an actual or potential health problem rather than on the disease process itself. For example, in caring for a person with a fractured hip, the nurse focuses on the self-care restrictions and the effects of immobility and pain. The surgeon is primarily concerned with the type of surgery and prosthesis to use in doing the surgical repair.

Many modern theorists, such as Neuman, Orem, and Rodgers, have attempted to precisely define nursing's domain.[3] Although

much work is needed in testing nursing theories, many of the current issues in nursing today were concerns of Florence Nightingale. In 1893 she addressed holistic health when she emphasized that one must nurse the whole person rather than the disease.[4] Current emphases in nursing practice, such as health promotion, patient and family teaching, family and community nursing, establishment of trust, use of good communication skills, and stress reduction techniques, were all an integral part of nursing as defined by Florence Nightingale.

Definitions of Nursing

A basic question revolves around how the profession of nursing views itself. Several well-known definitions of **nursing** indicate that a basic theme of health, illness, and caring has existed since Florence Nightingale. Following are two such examples:

The unique function of the nurse is to assist the individual, sick or well, in the performance of those activities contributing to health or its recovery (or to peaceful death) that he would perform unaided if he had the necessary strength, will, or knowledge. And to do this in such a way as to help him gain independence as rapidly as possible.[5]

Nursing is putting the patient in the best condition for nature to act.[4]

In this textbook the American Nurses Association's definition of nursing is used:

Nursing is the diagnosis and treatment of human responses to actual and potential health problems.[2]

Nursing's View of Humanity

Nursing's view of humanity must be considered when describing nursing. Although different terms have been used, there is widespread agreement among nursing theorists that an individual has physiologic (or biophysical), psychologic (or emotional), sociocultural (or interpersonal), spiritual, and environmental components or dimensions. In this text the human

Reviewed by Katheryn Ellen McCash, RNC, MSN, Professor Emeritus, College of Nursing, University of New Mexico, Albuquerque, N.M.

Selected material in this chapter was provided by Barbara Van de Castle, APRN, MSN, BC.

individual is considered "a biopsychosocial being in constant interaction with a changing environment."[6] The individual is composed of dimensions that are interrelated and not separate entities. Thus a problem in one dimension generally affects one or more of the other dimensions. Psychologic anxiety, for instance, affects the autonomic nervous system, a part of the biophysical dimension.

No two individuals are exactly alike. No one individual remains the same from moment to moment. Therefore each individual has value as an irreplaceable member of humanity. Inherent in this individuality is the right to develop one's unique potential according to a personal value system to the extent that the exercise of this right does not deny it to others.

The behavior of the individual is meaningful and oriented toward fulfilling needs and coping with environmental stresses. At times, however, an individual needs assistance to meet these needs and to cope successfully.

Advanced Practice Nursing

While entry-level nurses with associate or baccalaureate degree education function as generalists providing direct health care and focusing on ensuring coordinated and comprehensive care, additional education prepares nurses for advanced roles in specialty areas of practice.[7] **Advanced practice nursing** roles emphasize health assessment, diagnosis, and treatment of conditions previously considered only within the physician's domain (Fig. 1-1). Examples of advanced practice nurses are clinical specialists, nurse practitioners, nurse midwives, and nurse anes-

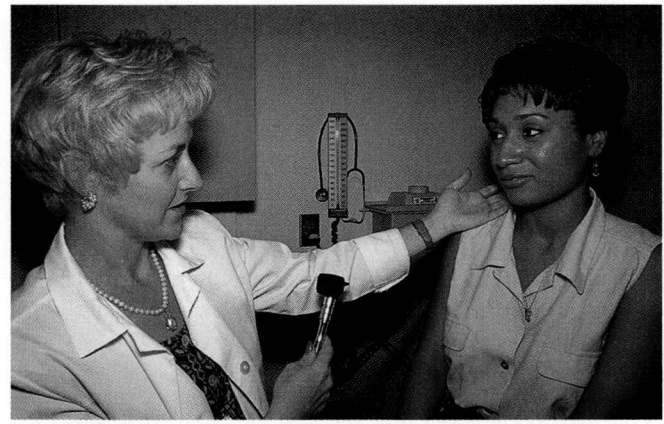

FIG. 1-1   Advanced practice nurses play an important role in primary care delivery.

thetists. In addition to managing and delivering direct patient care, advanced practice nurses have roles in health promotion, case management, administration, research, and multidisciplinary systems. Table 1-1 identifies some of the types, roles, and practice settings of advanced practice nurses.

Although there has been a lack of standardization of education, qualifications, and practice competencies of advanced practice nurses, there is a movement proposing a uniform national certification standard. A national standard would help the public

TABLE 1-1	Examples of Advanced Practice Nurses (APNs)	
TYPE OF APN	**PRACTICE ROLES**	**PRACTICE SETTINGS**
Nurse practitioner Family (FNP) Neonatal (NNP) Pediatrics (PNP) Adult (ANP) Gerontology (GNP) Acute care (ACNP) Psychiatry/mental health (PMHNP)	Management of primary care and health promotion for a wide variety of health problems in various specialties; roles include physical examination, diagnosis, treatment of health problems, patient/family education, and counseling	Primary care Ambulatory care Long-term care Hospitals Community care
Clinical nurse specialist Community health Gerontology Home health Medical-surgical Pediatrics Adult and/or child and adolescent Psychiatry and mental health	Management of complex patient care problems in various clinical specialty areas; roles include direct care, consultation, research, education, case management, and administration	Hospitals Ambulatory care Home health care Community care Rehabilitation
Certified nurse midwife (CNM)	Management of women's health care; focus on pregnancy, childbirth, postpartum period, care of the newborn, family planning, and gynecologic needs of women; consultation, collaborative management, or referral as indicated by the health status of the patient	Hospitals Homes Birthing centers Ambulatory care
Nurse anesthetist	Preoperative assessment, prescription of preoperative drugs, administration of anesthesia, monitoring of patients during anesthesia, and supervision of postanesthesia recovery	Hospital operating rooms Outpatient surgical centers Ambulatory care

Sources: *Certification and regulation of advanced practice nurses*, 2001, American Association of Colleges of Nursing, One Dupont Circle NW, Suite 530, Washington, DC 20036. Available at *www.aacn.nche.edu/Publications/positions/cerreg.htm* (accessed Nov 1, 2001); *List of credentials*, American Nurses Credentialing Center, 600 Maryland Avenue, SW, Suite 100 West, Washington, DC 20024. Available at *www.nursingworld.org/ancc/certify/cert/list.htm* (accessed Nov 1, 2002).

understand the advanced practitioner's scope of practice and ensure qualifications for advanced practice. The American Association of Colleges of Nursing has asserted that such a standard should require a graduate degree in nursing with a curriculum that incorporates professional standards and clearly defined core competencies.[8] In addition to advanced education, national credentialing examinations provided by the American Nurses Credentialing Center and nursing specialty organizations would be required.

Although advanced practice nurses may be certified through national standards, their scope of practice and any Medicaid reimbursement of their practice are ultimately determined by state statutes regulating nursing practice. Although most states recognize nurse practitioners, not all states recognize clinical nurse specialists, nor is prescriptive authority universal for all advanced practice nurses.[9] Individual states may also require additional standards for nurses to be certified or licensed for advanced practice within that state.

Delivery of Nursing Care

Historically, nursing care has been delivered using a variety of models. Team nursing was the model of care used in the 1960s and 1970s. Primary nursing was the model of the 1970s and 1980s. In this model there was a primary nurse who ensured that all the basic needs of the patient were met. **Managed care** is the current health care delivery concept that evolved from the health care reform movement of the 1990s. Interdisciplinary or collaborative care, as well as renewed appreciation of the joint contributions of various disciplines, is a component of managed care. Managed care involves **case management,** an approach that coordinates and links health care services to patients and their families. As a member of the interdisciplinary health care team, the nurse case manager coordinates the clinical care of the patient across care settings, from admission through discharge from the hospital, through other community agencies as needed, and back home in an effort to achieve optimal outcomes. (Case management is discussed in Chapter 6.)

Expanding Knowledge and Technology

Rapidly changing technologies and dramatically expanding knowledge affect all areas of health care. Today nurses use advanced assessment skills to determine the health status of their patients, increasing the database on which they make sound judgments. An increased understanding of pathophysiology, psychopathology, and pharmacology enables nurses to understand the scientific basis of assessment findings that indicate various levels of health or disease. Incorporation of sciences and humanities into nursing education has also expanded the knowledge base of nursing practice. As scientific knowledge continues to increase, nurses will continue to be challenged to keep current with new developments. In addition, the growth of knowledge in genetics is increasingly posing ethical dilemmas that nurses must be able to address both personally and with patients and families.

Federal Initiatives

The federal initiatives, *Healthy People 2000*[10] and *Healthy People 2010,*[11] indicate that major changes in access to and delivery of health care will occur through expanded coverage of broad segments of the population. The emphasis on health promotion, disease prevention, screening, and immunization in these initiatives is moving nurses from acute care centers into the community to address the nation's heath needs. In meeting the goals of these initiatives, nurses must address developments in health care delivery, nursing practice, research outcomes, and new technologies. *Nursing Education's Agenda for the 21st Century* notes that nurses need the following essential cognitive and interpersonal abilities for meaningful roles in future health care systems:[7]

- Critical thinking
- Ethical decision making
- Information seeking, sorting, and selection
- Establishing and maintaining nurse-patient relationships
- Therapeutic communication, including teaching and advocacy
- Design, management, and coordination of care
- Interdisciplinary team participation
- Sensitivity to socioeconomic level, religious lifestyle, and cultural diversity
- Critical self-assessment
- Health promotion and maintenance
- Economics and health care
- Ethical and legal principles
- Political and social action strategies
- Socioeconomic factors affecting health
- Information and health care technologies

Evidence-Based Practice*

Evidence-based practice (EBP) is the use of evidence (results from research) to improve quality and outcomes of health care (Table 1-2). The quality of health care improves when research results are used to guide clinical practice. EBP uses the best scientific evidence from research to obtain the best outcomes for patients and their families. The best evidence must be used as the scientific basis to guide nursing interventions with patients and their families.[12]

EBP should not be used as a synonym for research utilization and research practice. The more accurate view of EBP is that research use and research-based practice are subsets within the broader context of EBP. When research results are implemented and sustained, they result in EBP.

EBP is a rather recent concept that has grown out of the demand for high-quality, cost-effective care and the availability of rapidly expanding knowledge. EBP sprang from evidence-based medicine, which was first introduced about 25 years ago. The EBP trend quickly expanded from medicine to all health care professions and is now considered to be an interdisciplinary approach to health care.[13]

EBP combines the concepts of effectiveness and efficiency (Table 1-3). Nursing care based on evidence produces better outcomes in the most effective and efficient way. Application of EBP results in more accurate diagnoses, maximally effective and efficient interventions, and the most favorable patient outcomes.

The most distinguishing feature of EBP is that the new scientific base for practice is built through a summary of studies on a topic. These summaries are called evidence synthesis, systematic

---

*Material provided by Kathleen R. Stevens, RN, EdD, FAAN.

TABLE 1-2   Evidence-Based Practice Definitions

TERM	DEFINITION
Evidence-based medicine	Conscientious, explicit, and judicious use of current best evidence in making decisions about the care of individual patients. The practice of evidence-based medicine means integrating individual clinical expertise with the best available external clinical evidence from systematic research.* The integration of best research evidence with clinical expertise and patient values.†
Evidence-based practice	The transformation of scientific evidence from research results through the stages of (a) evidence summary, (b) translation into clinical recommendations, (c) implementation as best clinical practice, and (d) evaluation of outcome.‡
Evidence-based nursing practice	Conscientious, explicit, and judicious use of theory-derived, research-based information in making decisions about care delivery to individuals of groups of patients and in consideration of individuals' needs and preferences.§

*Sackett DL et al: Evidence-based medicine: what it is and what it isn't, *BMJ* 312:71, 1996.
†Sackett DL et al: *Evidence-based medicine: how to practice and teach EBM,* London, 2000, Churchill Livingstone.
‡Stevens KR: ACE Star model: cycle of knowledge transformation. Academic Center for Evidence-Based Practice. Available at *www.acestar.uthscsa.edu* (accessed 2002).
§Ingersoll GL: Evidence-based nursing: what it is and what is isn't, *Nursing Outlook* 48:151, 2000.

TABLE 1-3   Evidence-Based Practice (EBP)

What Is Evidence-Based Practice?
A process of
- Synthesizing research evidence
- Designing clinical practice guidelines
- Implementing practice changes
- Evaluating outcomes

Why Do We Need Evidence-Based Practice?
- Rapid increase in amount of information
- Rapid increase in health care costs
- Determination of efficient and effective health care practices
- Increased emphasis on performance and outcome standards

Where Is Evidence Found?
- Published research
- Systematic reviews (e.g., Cochrane Collaboration; available at *www.cochrane.org/*)*
- Special collections of EBP resources (e.g., Agency for Health-care Research and Quality [AHRQ]; available at *www.ahcpr.gov*)

*Descriptions can be found at this site, but access to systemic reviews is by subscription only.

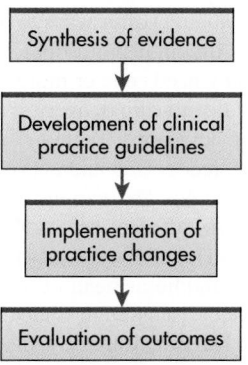

FIG. 1-2   Process of evidence-based practice.

reviews, or integrative reviews, depending on which organization produced them. The evidence synthesis summarizes all research results into a single conclusion about the state of the science. From this point, the clinician translates the knowledge into a clinical practice guideline, implements it through individual and organizational practice changes, and evaluates it in terms of effectiveness and efficiency of producing intended health care outcomes (Fig. 1-2). Clinical practice guidelines can take the form of protocols, clinical pathways, practice guidelines, policy statements, computer-based protocols, or algorithms.

To implement EBP, nurses must continuously seek scientific evidence that supports the care they provide. The incorporation of evidence should be balanced with clinical expertise and should take into account the patient's unique circumstances. EBP closes the gap between research and practice, providing more reliable and predictable care than that which is based on tradition, opinion, and trial and error. It provides nurses with a mechanism to manage the explosion of new literature, introduction of new technologies, concern about health care costs, and increasing emphasis on quality and patient outcomes.[14]

Throughout this book, EBP boxes are presented that relate to specific clinical problems for which summarized evidence exists, the evidence (best clinical practice), and the source of the evidence. In some cases, the evidence supports current practice and increases confidence that the nursing care will produce the desired outcome. In other cases, the evidence points to a change in practice. In either case, it is important for the nurse to be aware of the scientific basis for the care given.

Nursing Languages

The demands of the current health care system are also challenging nursing to define its practice and the impact it has on the health and health care of individuals, families, and communities. The nursing profession is asking questions such as what is it that nurses do, how do they do it, and does it make a measurable difference in the health of those they care for? How can nurses document care to identify what they do and what happens as a result of their care?

In response to these questions, nursing has moved toward standardizing nursing languages. **Standardized nursing languages** are used to clearly define and evaluate nursing care. They can promote continuity of patient care and provide data that can support the credibility of the profession. Instead of using a wide variety of words and methods to describe the same patient problems and nursing care, a readily understood common language can improve communication among nurses.[15] Standardized languages help identify the most effective nursing interventions as well. Do the patient problems of pressure ulcer, decubitus ulcer, and skin breakdown all mean the same thing? Does turning the patient every 2 hours mean the same thing as repositioning the patient every 2 hours? And if the patient is turned or repositioned every 2 hours, what happens as a result? How are the results described? If a patient was placed on an air mattress, were the results different from one who was placed on a standard mattress and only turned? How do nurses know what works best? Using standardized languages, nurses can easily collect and analyze nursing data to identify the effectiveness of nursing interventions.

Standardized languages (also called *nomenclatures, classification systems,* and *taxonomies*) offer ways to organize and describe nursing phenomena. Although philosophical debates exist concerning whether nursing needs one or more taxonomies considering the complexity of health care delivery, a number of classification systems are being developed. Table 1-4 lists the languages, or classification systems, recognized and approved by the American Nurses Association (ANA). The variety of languages that have been developed address different areas of nursing. The Omaha System and the Home Health Care Classification have been developed for long-term and home health care nursing. The Perioperative Nursing Dataset (discussed in Chapter 18) is used by perioperative nurses. The Nursing Management Minimum Data Set is available for use by nurse managers and administrators.

Three of the nursing languages recognized by the ANA are now available to consistently describe patient responses, nursing interventions, and patient outcomes. These include the North American Nursing Diagnosis Association (NANDA) Nursing Diagnoses Classification, Nursing Interventions Classification (NIC), and Nursing Outcomes Classification (NOC). Each of these classification systems focuses on one component of the nursing process. Patients' responses or problems can be labeled using the nursing diagnoses classified and defined by NANDA.[16] Nursing interventions, or treatments, can be selected and implemented from NIC developed by McCloskey and Bulechek at the University of Iowa College of Nursing.[17] Patient outcomes of nursing care can be identified and evaluated by selecting appropriate NOC outcomes and indicators identified and classified by Johnson, Maas, and Moorhead, also at the University of Iowa College of Nursing.[18] The use of these three classification systems in the nursing process and documentation are further described in this chapter and used throughout the text.

NURSING PROCESS

Nursing accomplishes its goal of assisting others to resolve actual or potential problems by the use of the nursing process. The **nursing process** is an assertive, problem-solving approach to the identification and treatment of patient problems. It provides an organizing framework for the knowledge, judgments, and actions that nurses bring to patient care.[19] Using the nursing process, the nurse can focus on the unique responses of patients to actual or potential health problems. The nursing process requires cognitive (thinking, reasoning), psychomotor (doing), and affective (feelings, values) skills and abilities of the nurse.

Phases of the Nursing Process

The nursing process consists of five phases: assessment, diagnosis, planning, implementation, and evaluation (Fig. 1-3). However, numerous other terms or phrases are used in nursing to describe the steps of the nursing process (Table 1-5). **Assessment** involves collecting subjective and objective information about the

---

TABLE 1-4	Nursing Languages

North American Nursing Diagnosis Association (NANDA)
  Nursing Diagnoses Definitions and Classifications
Nursing Interventions Classifications (NIC)
Nursing Outcomes Classification (NOC)
The Omaha System
Home Health Care Classification (HHCC)
Patient Care Data Set (PCDS)
Nursing Minimum Data Sets (NMDS)
Nursing Management Minimum Data Set (NMMDS)
Perioperative Nursing Dataset (PNDS)
Systematized Nomenclature of Medicine Reference Terminology
  (SNOMED RT)
International Classification for Nursing Practice (ICPN)
Alternative Link

Source: American Nurses Association: *Nursing information and data set evaluation center, recognized languages for nursing,* Washington, DC, 2000, American Nurses Association. Available at *www.nursingworld.org/nidsec/class1st.htm.*

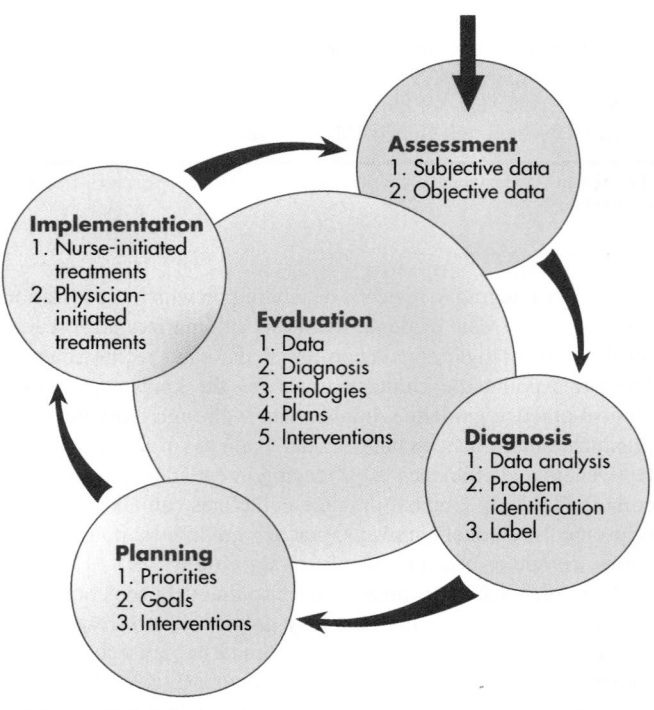

FIG. 1-3 Nursing process.

TABLE 1-5	Terms Used for Components of the Nursing Process

Assessment Phase
Data collection
Data gathering
Assessment
Collection of information
History and physical examination

Diagnosis Phase
Step I
Data analysis
Judgment
Decision making
Clustering information
Determination of strengths and weaknesses
Determination of unmet needs
Determination of assets and limitations
Step II
Nursing diagnosis
Problem identification
Etiology determination
Labeling the problem
Naming the problem

Planning Phase
Step I
Priority setting
Step II
Expected outcomes
Goal setting
Objective setting, subgoals
Desired behaviors
Outcome criteria
Step III
Planning interventions
Planning nursing actions
Nursing orders
Planning strategies of care

Implementation
Application
Intervention
Nursing care
Implementation
Treatment

Evaluation
Reassessment
Audit

TABLE 1-6	Comparison of Primary Goals: Nursing and Medicine

NURSING	MEDICINE
Determines responses to health problems, level of wellness, and need for assistance	Determines etiology of illness or injury
Provides physical care, emotional care, teaching, guidance, and counseling	Provides medical treatments and surgery
Interventions aimed at prevention and assisting the patient to meet his or her own needs	Interventions aimed at preventing and curing injury or illness

Interrelatedness of Phases

The five phases of the nursing process do not occur in isolation from one another. For example, nurses may gather data about the wound condition (assessment) as they change the soiled dressing (implementation). There is, however, a basic order to the nursing process, beginning with assessment. This provides the data on which to base the plan. A judgment about the nature of the assessment data usually follows immediately. A plan based on the nursing diagnosis then directs the nursing interventions implemented with the patient. Evaluation continues throughout the cycle. This continuous evaluation provides feedback on the effectiveness of the plan or the need for revision. Revision may be needed in the data collection method, the diagnosis, the expected outcomes/goals, the plan, or the intervention method. Once begun, the nursing process is not only continuous but also cyclic in nature. There is no limit to the number of times the cycle can be reinitiated. Application of the nursing process requires sound knowledge of the physical and behavioral sciences and a repertoire of intellectual, interpersonal, and technical skills.

The nursing profession and the medical profession use a problem-solving process in caring for a patient. The uniqueness of nursing's problem-solving approach stems from the goals of nursing and the means of accomplishing these goals. A comparison of the goals of medicine and nursing is made in Table 1-6.

Independent and Collaborative Functions

Nursing practice has independent, dependent, and collaborative functions. As the profession becomes more autonomous, nurse-initiated *(independent)* interventions, such as health teaching and counseling, are carried out to manage the nursing diagnosis.[17]

The nurse functions *dependently* when carrying out medical orders. Physician-initiated nursing functions may include administering medications, performing or assisting with certain medical treatments, and assisting with diagnostic tests and procedures. The exact roles of the nurse are often determined by state and agency policies. The nurse's role in most cases is one of "interdependence and coparticipation" with the patient and other health team members.

In the *collaborative* nursing role, the nurse is primarily responsible for monitoring for possible or actual complications and for treating the patient to prevent or manage the complication. In

patient. The nursing diagnosis phase involves analyzing the assessment data, drawing conclusions from the information, and labeling the human response. **Planning** consists of setting goals and expected outcomes with the patient and family, when feasible, and determining strategies for accomplishing the goals. **Implementation** involves the use of nursing interventions to activate the plan. In **evaluation** the nurse first determines if the identified outcomes have been met. Then the overall accuracy of the assessment, diagnosis, and implementation phases is evaluated.

this role the nurse may use either physician-prescribed or nurse-prescribed interventions. The collaborative role is frequently demonstrated in the intensive care unit as the nurse monitors patients for complications of acute illness, administers intravenous fluids and medications per physician orders, and implements nursing interventions such as providing emotional support or teaching about specific procedures.

ASSESSMENT PHASE

Data Collection

A sound database is the foundation for the entire nursing process. Collection of data is a prerequisite to diagnosis, planning, and intervention (Fig. 1-4). A human being as a biopsychosocial being has needs and problems in all dimensions: biophysical, psychologic, sociocultural, spiritual, and environmental. A nursing diagnosis made without supporting data in all dimensions can lead to incorrect conclusions and depersonalized care. For example, a hospitalized patient who does not sleep all night may be mistakenly diagnosed as having a disturbed sleep pattern. In fact the patient may have worked nights his entire adult life, and it is normal for him to be awake at night. Information concerning his sleeping habits is necessary to individualize his care so that he does not routinely receive a sleep medication at 10 PM. The importance of assessment in the process of clinical decision making cannot be overemphasized. The use of a nursing database (discussed in Chapter 3) is recommended to facilitate the collection of data.

Because nursing interventions are only as sound as the database on which they are formulated, it is critical that the database be accurate and complete. When possible, information gained from sources such as the patient's record, other health care workers, the patient's family, and the nurse's observations should be validated with the patient. Likewise, when possible, questionable statements by the patient should be validated by a knowledgeable person.

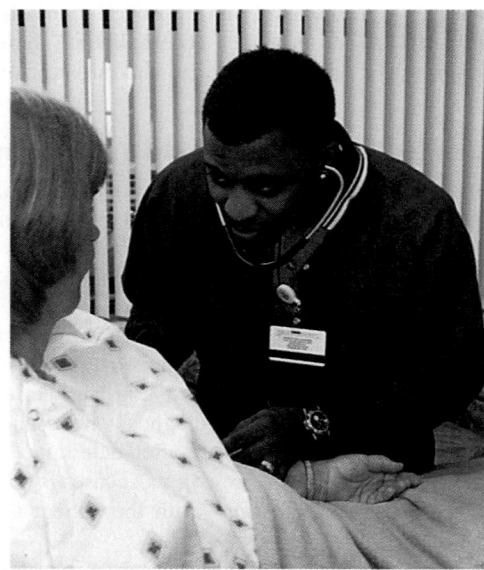

FIG. 1-4   Collection of data is a prerequisite to diagnosis, planning, and intervention.

DIAGNOSIS PHASE

Data Analysis and Problem Identification

The diagnosis phase begins with the clustering of information and ends with an evaluative judgment about a patient's health status. This evaluative judgment is reached after analysis of the assessment data. Analysis involves sorting through and organizing or clustering the information and determining unmet needs, as well as patient strengths. The findings are then compared with documented norms to determine whether anything is interfering or could interfere with the patient's needs or ability to maintain his or her usual health pattern.

After a thorough analysis of all available information, one of two possible conclusions results. Either there are no problems that require nursing intervention or the patient needs nursing assistance to solve a potential or actual problem. The statements of final conclusions about the problems are the nursing diagnoses.

Nursing Diagnosis

The term *nursing diagnosis* has many different meanings. To some it merely connotes the identification of a health problem. More commonly, a nursing diagnosis is viewed as the conclusion about an identified cluster of signs and symptoms. The diagnosis is generally expressed as concisely as possible according to specific guidelines.

Nursing diagnosis is the act of identifying and labeling human responses to actual or potential health problems. Throughout this book, the term *nursing diagnosis* will mean (1) the process of identifying actual and potential health problems and (2) the label or concise statement that describes "a clinical judgment about an individual, family, or community response to actual or potential health problems/life processes. A nursing diagnosis provides the basis for the selection of nursing interventions to achieve outcomes for which the nurse is accountable."[16] The human responses identified frequently result from a disease process. For example, a patient may have the medical diagnosis of chronic obstructive pulmonary disease (COPD). In this case the nursing diagnosis would focus on how the COPD affects daily functioning. Examples of patient responses to COPD might be anxiety, activity intolerance, or an inability to maintain a home.

A number of other terms or situations are not nursing diagnoses but are often mislabeled as such.[20] These include the following:

- Medical pathologic conditions (coronary artery disease)
- Diagnostic tests or studies (upper gastrointestinal series)
- Equipment (nasogastric tube)
- Signs (restlessness)
- Surgical procedures (hysterectomy)
- Treatments (pressure ulcer care)
- Therapeutic goals (perform own oral care)
- Nursing problems (difficult to turn)
- Therapeutic needs (needs more rest)
- Staff problems (Mr. Jones is too demanding)

NANDA Nursing Diagnoses. The North America Nursing Diagnosis Association (NANDA) is a nursing organization that has been developing a standardized nursing language for identifying, defining, and classifying patients' actual or potential responses to health problems since 1973. The two main purposes of NANDA are to develop a diagnostic classification system (taxonomy) and to identify and accept nursing diagnoses. In selecting a nursing diagnosis for a patient from the NANDA list, the nurse labels the patient's responses in a language that specifically identifies and defines the patient's problem for other nurses and health care providers. In addition, the use of the standardized language of nursing diagnoses documents the analysis, synthesis, and accuracy required in making a nursing diagnosis. It verifies nursing's contribution to cost-effective, efficient, quality health care.

Currently NANDA has accepted more than 150 nursing diagnoses for clinical testing (see Appendix A). Each nursing diagnosis has an assigned code number facilitating its use in computerized documentation. The nursing diagnoses used in this textbook are NANDA approved. However, it is acceptable to use non–NANDA approved nursing diagnoses when a new label is identified. The NANDA list is continually evolving as research results are interpreted and as nurses identify new human responses. Therefore the nurse may encounter diagnoses in clinical practice that are not cited on the list. Revisions of accepted nursing diagnoses and new diagnoses may be submitted to NANDA by individual nurses or nursing groups. For information on submitting diagnostic material contact NANDA, 1211 Locust St., Philadelphia, Pennsylvania, 19107; 800-647-9002; *www.nanda.org.*

Diagnostic Process

The diagnostic process involves analysis and synthesis of the data collected during assessment of the patient. Data that indicate dysfunctional or risk patterns are clustered, and a judgment about the data is made. It is important to remember that not all conclusions resulting from data analysis lead to nursing diagnoses. Nursing diagnoses describe health states that nurses can legally diagnose and treat. Data may also point to collaborative problems that nurses treat with other health care providers. During the diagnostic process the nurse identifies both nursing diagnoses and collaborative problems that necessitate nursing intervention.

Nursing diagnostic statements are acceptable when written as two-part or three-part statements. A two-part statement is acceptable if the signs and symptoms data are easily accessible to other nurses caring for the patient through such means as the nursing history or progress note. *Risk* nursing diagnoses are also two-part statements because signs and symptoms are not present. Use of a three-part statement is recommended during the learning process. When written as a three-part statement, the problem–etiology–signs and symptoms (PES) format is used.[20,21]

Problem (P): a brief statement of the patient's potential or actual health problem (e.g., pain)

Etiology (E): a brief description of the probable cause of the problem; contributing or related factors (e.g., related to surgical incision, localized pressure, edema)

Signs and symptoms (S): a list of the cluster of the objective and subjective data that lead the nurse to pinpoint the problem; critical, major, or minor defining characteristics (e.g., as manifested by verbalization of pain, isolation, withdrawal)

It is important to remember that gathering the "S" comes first in the diagnostic process, even though the format has been described as PES.

Identifying the Problem. The NANDA list of accepted nursing diagnoses has been organized using a modification of Gordon's functional health patterns (see Appendix A). This framework is useful when analyzing the data for actual, risk, and possible nursing diagnoses. Clinically relevant cues are clustered

into the functional health patterns. (The 11 functional health patterns are discussed in Chapter 3.) The process of making a nursing diagnosis from clustered cues begins with the recognition of dysfunctional patterns. Checking the definition of nursing diagnoses classified in the functional pattern areas helps to identify the appropriate label for the problem. Before final selection of any nursing diagnosis for the patient, the nurse verifies the diagnostic statement with the defining characteristics listed with the diagnosis.[16,20,22] The most accurate nursing diagnosis is based on the individual patient's data.

Etiology. The etiology of a nursing diagnosis is identified in the diagnostic statement. Taking time to refine the problem with its proper etiology directs the nurse to the correct interventions. Interventions are planned to manage the problem by directing nursing efforts toward the etiology. The etiology can be a pathophysiologic, maturational, situational, or treatment-related factor.[20] The etiology is written after the diagnostic label. These two components are separated by the phrase "related to." For example, in NCP 1-1 the nursing diagnosis is "Activity intolerance *related to* fatigue. secondary to cardiac insufficiency and pulmonary congestion." The etiology directs the nurse to select the appropriate interventions to modify the factor of fatigue. When the etiology is not included in the diagnosis, the nurse is not able to plan the correct intervention to treat the specific cause of the problem. When possible, the etiology should be validated with the patient. When the etiology is unknown, the statement reads "related to unknown etiology." When identifying risk nursing diagnoses, the specific risk factors present in the patient's situation are identified as the etiology.

Multiple etiologies become more common as expertise in the use of nursing diagnoses increases. There is often no single cause of a problem. Many nursing diagnoses presented in the nursing care plans of this book contain multiple etiologies. They can be used as a checklist of possible related factors to be considered when determining the nursing diagnosis specific to an individual patient.

Signs and Symptoms. Signs and symptoms, also called **defining characteristics,** are the clinical cues that, in a cluster, point to the nursing diagnosis.[16] *Critical* defining characteristics must be present in the database to make an accurate nursing diagnosis. *Major* defining characteristics are those signs or symptoms that are usually present when the diagnosis exists. At least one critical defining characteristic or one major defining characteristic must be present to have an actual nursing diagnosis. *Minor* defining characteristics have also been identified and are evidence of a possible nursing diagnosis. The signs and symptoms are included in the diagnostic statement using the phrase "as manifested by." The complete nursing diagnostic statement in NCP 1-1 is, "Activity intolerance *related to* fatigue secondary to cardiac insufficiency and pulmonary congestion *as manifested by* dyspnea, shortness of breath, weakness, increase in heart rate on exertion, and patient's statement, 'I feel too weak to do anything.'"

Collaborative Problems

Collaborative problems are potential or actual complications of disease or treatment that nurses treat with other health care providers, most frequently physicians.[20] A look at the primary goals of nursing helps in differentiating between nursing and medical diagnoses (see Table 1-6). During the diagnosis phase of the nursing process, the nurse identifies these risks for

NURSING CARE PLAN 1-1

Patient with Congestive Heart Failure*

NURSING DIAGNOSIS   **Activity intolerance** *related to* fatigue secondary to cardiac insufficiency and pulmonary congestion *as manifested by* dyspnea, shortness of breath, weakness, increase in heart rate on exertion, and patient's statement "I feel too weak to do anything."

OUTCOMES—NOC	INTERVENTIONS—NIC and *RATIONALES*
Activity Tolerance (0005)	*Energy Management (0180)*
▪ O₂ saturation IER in response to activity _____	▪ Encourage alternate rest and activity periods *to reduce cardiac work-load.*
▪ Heart rate IER in response to activity _____	▪ Provide emotional and physical rest *to reduce oxygen consumption and to relieve dyspnea and fatigue.*
▪ Respiratory rate IER in response to activity _____	▪ Monitor cardiorespiratory response to activity *to determine level of activity that can be performed.*
▪ ECG WNL _____	
▪ Skin color WNL _____	▪ Teach patient and significant other techniques of self-care *to minimize oxygen consumption.*
▪ Reported activities of ADLs performance _____	
▪ Systolic BP IER in response to activity _____	*Activity Therapy (4310)*
▪ Diastolic BP IER in response to activity _____	▪ Assist to choose activities consistent with physical, psychologic, and social capabilities *to determine level of activity that can be performed.*
Outcome Scale	▪ Collaborate with occupational, physical, and/or recreational therapists *to plan and monitor activity program.*
1 = extremely compromised	
2 = substantially compromised	▪ Determine patient's commitment to ↑ frequency and/or range of activity *to provide patient with obtainable goals.*
3 = moderately compromised	
4 = mildly compromised	
5 = not compromised	

ADLs, Activities of daily living; *BP,* blood pressure; *ECG,* electrocardiogram; *IER,* in expected range; *NIC,* Nursing Interventions Classification; *NOC,* Nursing Outcomes Classification; *WNL,* within normal limits.

*The complete nursing care plan for congestive heart failure is NCP 34-1 on pp. 850-851.

physiologic complications in addition to nursing diagnoses. Identification of collaborative problems requires knowledge of pathophysiology and possible complications of medical treatment. For example, collaborative problems for the patient with congestive heart failure in NCP 1-1 could include pulmonary edema, hypoxemia, arrhythmias, and/or cardiogenic shock.[20] In the interdependent role, nurses use both physician-prescribed and nursing-prescribed interventions to prevent, detect, and manage collaborative problems.

Collaborative problem statements are usually written as "potential complication: _____" (e.g., potential complication: pulmonary edema) without a "related to" statement. When potential complications are used in this textbook, "related to" statements have been added to increase understanding and relate the potential complication to possible causes.

PLANNING PHASE

Priority Setting

After the nursing diagnoses and collaborative problems are identified, the nurse must determine the urgency of the identified problems. Diagnoses of the highest priority require immediate intervention. Those of lower priority can be addressed at a later time. When setting priorities, the nurse should first intervene for life-threatening problems involving airway, breathing, or circulation.

Maslow's hierarchy of needs also acts as a useful guide in determining priorities. These needs include physical, safety, love and belonging, esteem, and self-actualization.[22] Lower-level needs must be reached before a higher level can be attained.

Another guideline in setting priorities is to determine the patient's perception of what is important. When the patient's prior-

ities are not congruent with the actual situation, the nurse may need to give explanations or do some teaching to help the patient understand the need to do one thing before another. Often it is more efficient to meet the patient's priority need before moving on to other priorities.

An additional suggestion is to identify nursing diagnoses that may be managed simultaneously. For example, the nurse may assess the condition of a pressure ulcer (impaired skin integrity) while giving morning care (bathing/hygiene self-care deficit).

Identified priorities change as a patient's level of wellness fluctuates. For example, the patient's highest priority in the morning may be a need for information about diabetes mellitus because she is going home and must care for herself. During the teaching session, the patient shows signs of a hypoglycemic reaction. The nurse would interrupt the teaching session to provide a glass of orange juice to avoid a progression of the hypoglycemia to a dangerous level. In this instance risk problems may have a higher priority than existing (actual) problems.

Identifying Outcomes

After priorities are established, expected outcomes or goals for the patient are identified. *Outcomes* are simply the results of care. **Expected patient outcomes** are *goals* that identify what is *desired* or *expected* as a result of care. The terms *goals* and *expected outcomes* are often used interchangeably, but either term refers to describing to what degree the patient's response identified in the nursing diagnosis should be prevented or changed as a result of nursing care. Expected outcomes should be set with the patient, if feasible, just as priorities of interventions are considered with the patient when possible. Although the ultimate goal for the patient is to maintain or attain a state of dynamic equilibrium at the highest possible level of wellness, the setting of more specific expected outcomes, both short term and long term, is necessary for systematic evaluation of the patient's progress. Expected patient outcomes identified in the planning stage specify the criteria to be used in the evaluation phase of the nursing process.

The nurse identifies both *long-term* and *short-term* goals by writing specific expected patient outcomes in terms of desired, realistic, measurable patient behaviors to be accomplished by a specific date. For example, a short-term expected outcome for the patient in NCP 1-1 might be, "The patient will maintain normal vital signs in response to activity in 2 days," whereas a long-term expected outcome might be "The patient will identify a realistic activity level to achieve or maintain by discharge." These outcomes would be evaluated in 2 days and at discharge, and the care plan should be revised as necessary if the outcomes were not met. However, these statements provide no criteria by which to evaluate the patient's degree of progress from admission to discharge. Goals or expected outcomes vary in their degree of specificity, and if the goal is not met, the nurse has no way of knowing how close or how far the patient was from achieving the goal. In addition, goals or outcomes written by individual nurses create nonstandardized data that cannot be used in research to determine what nursing interventions are most effective in reaching desired outcomes.[18]

Nursing Outcomes Classification (NOC). A research-based, standardized language for nursing outcomes, *Nursing Outcomes Classification (NOC),* has been developed to evaluate the effects of nursing interventions. NOC is a list of "concepts, definitions, and measures that describe patient outcomes influenced by nursing interventions."[18] Currently 260 coded outcomes have been organized into 7 domains and 29 classes *(www.nursing.uiowa.edu/noc/).* Each outcome has a label, a definition, a set of specific indicators to be used in rating the outcomes, and a five-point scale for rating the specific indicators.

For example, in NCP 1-1 the NOC *label* is activity tolerance (0005) and is *defined* as responses to energy-consuming body movements involved in required or desired activities.[18] The *indicators* describe the specific status of the patient in relation to the outcome. By choosing specific indicators that are listed with a given outcome the nurse selects the criteria for evaluating the outcome and the effects of nursing interventions. The five-point Likert-type measurement scale to rate the outcome is as follows: 1 = extremely compromised, 2 = substantially compromised, 3 = moderately compromised, 4 = mildly compromised, 5 = not compromised.

The measurement scale included with each outcome is constructed so that the fifth point of the scale is the most desirable condition relative to that outcome. The NOC system uses different measurements scales for various outcomes to rate patient progress. Each outcome is provided with an appropriate scale. Using the measurement scale, the nurse can rate each indicator for a particular patient at any given period of time. This enables the nurse to monitor the overall progression of the patient in relation to the outcome over time. By going back after the interventions are applied and rating each indicator on the scale of 1 through 5, the nurse can evaluate the effect of the intervention on the outcome.

It is important to understand that NOC outcomes are *not* prescriptive. Because they are neutral labels, they are not expected patient outcomes. However, they can be individualized for a patient and translated into expected patient outcomes by identifying a desired state on the measurement scale. An example of a short-term expected outcome using NOC for the patient in NCP 1-1 might be, "Patient will have activity tolerance at a level of 3, moderately compromised, on all selected indicators in 2 days." A long-term expected outcome might be, "Patient will have activity tolerance at a level of 4, mildly compromised, on all selected indicators by discharge."

NOC outcomes should be selected during the planning phase of the nursing process after nursing diagnoses have been identified and priorities established. An initial rating of the indicators should also be done to establish the patient's baseline. Expected patient outcomes can then be set with the patient by determining a realistic rating of the indicators to be achieved by the patient within a specified period of time.

Determining Interventions

After patient outcomes are identified, nursing interventions to accomplish the desired status of the patient should be planned. A **nursing intervention** is any treatment, based on clinical judgment and knowledge, that a nurse performs to enhance patient outcomes.[17] Nursing interventions include both direct and indirect care; nurse-initiated treatments resulting from nursing diagnoses; physician-initiated treatments resulting from medical diagnoses; and daily, essential activities that the patient cannot perform independently (Table 1-7). When choosing an intervention the nurse considers the following:[17]

1. Desired patient outcomes
2. Characteristics of the nursing diagnosis
3. Research base associated with the intervention
4. Feasibility of successfully implementing the intervention
5. Acceptability to the patient
6. Capability of the nurse

Sound knowledge, good judgment, and decision-making ability are required to effectively choose the interventions that the nurse will use (Fig. 1-5). Although many variables may influence outcomes, nursing interventions should always be chosen to influence the outcomes of care. In addition, the interventions that are selected should be directed toward altering the etiologic factors of the nursing diagnoses. The nurse should foster the use of a research-based approach to interventions. Clinical nursing research that establishes a base for evidence-based practice and that identifies the effectiveness of nursing interventions is being conducted and reported at an increasing rate. In the absence of a nursing research base, scientific principles from the behavioral and biologic sciences should guide the selection of interventions.

TABLE 1-7	Examples of Nursing Activities to Treat Health Care Problems
INTERVENTION	**NURSING ACTIVITIES**
Nurse-initiated treatments	Encourage patient to cough and deep breathe
Physician-initiated treatments	Administer medications
Essential activity patient cannot perform independently	Provide range-of-motion exercise

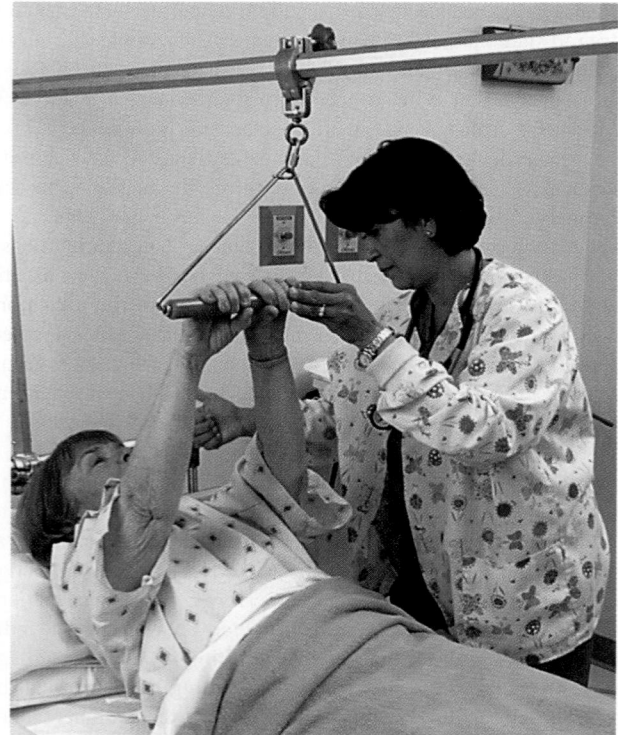

FIG. 1-5 Cooperation between the patient and the nurse is necessary in setting goals.

In addition, the nurse must use ingenuity, intuition, creativity, and past experience when tailoring a plan to meet a patient's needs. Factors such as availability of help, equipment, time, money, and other resources must also be considered. The nurse must also have the knowledge and skill to be able to carry out the interventions selected. As in the case of the determination of expected outcomes, the final selection of interventions remains the choice of the patient when the patient is able. The patient or the patient's family often has a wealth of information about measures that were successful or unsuccessful in the past. Significant time and effort are saved by asking the patient what has been tried and discarded as ineffective.

Nursing Interventions Classification (NIC). The third research-based standardized nursing language that focuses on the nursing process is *Nursing Interventions Classification (NIC)*. This classification includes the interventions that nurses do on behalf of patients, both independent and collaborative interventions, both direct and indirect care.[17] It includes treatments that nurses perform in all settings and in all specialties. NIC identifies both physiologic and psychosocial interventions, as well as interventions for illness treatment, illness prevention, and health promotion. It provides a common language for communication among nurses. Because each intervention has a coded number, the use of NIC interventions facilitates computer collection of standardized nursing data to evaluate the effectiveness of the interventions.

NIC includes 486 interventions with a label name, a definition, and a set of activities for the nurse to choose from in order to carry out the intervention. The interventions are grouped into 7 domains and 30 classes *(www.nursing.uiowa.edu/nic/)*. Although 486 interventions may seem overwhelming, nurses soon discover those interventions that are used most often in their particular specialty or with their patient population.[17] In creating a care plan for a patient, the nurse chooses specific interventions from the domain or class that is appropriate for the patient based on the nursing diagnosis and patient outcomes. A group of activities is listed for each intervention, and the nurse can select the appropriate activities from the list to implement the intervention.

For example, in NCP 1-1 the *labels* of energy management (0180) and activity therapy (4310) are used to describe the interventions selected for the patient. Energy management is *defined* as regulating energy use to treat or prevent fatigue and optimize function. Activity therapy is *defined* as prescription of and assistance with specific physical, cognitive, social, and spiritual activities to increase the range, frequency, or duration of an individual's activity. From a set of 30 activities, 4 have been chosen to implement the intervention of energy management. From a set of 27 activities, 3 have been chosen to implement the intervention of activity therapy.

NIC does *not* prescribe interventions for specific situations. The nurse is responsible for making the important decision of when to use an intervention and for whom. Nurses need to select the appropriate intervention based on their knowledge of the patient and the patient's condition.

NANDA–NOC–NIC Linkages

NANDA diagnoses, NOC outcomes, and NIC interventions can be linked to illustrate how the three distinct nursing languages can be connected and used together when planning care for patients.[23] The decision-making process used to determine a nursing diagnosis, project a desired outcome, and select interventions to achieve the desired outcome may be assisted by use of the linkages. An example of a NANDA-NOC-NIC linkage is found in Table 1-8.

The linkages that have been developed are only guides for planning care. They do not alter the critical-thinking skills that nurses must use in making decisions about patient care. The nurse must continually evaluate the situation and revise the diagnoses,

NURSING DIAGNOSIS

TABLE 1-8		Example of NANDA-NOC-NIC Linkage
NANDA Nursing Diagnosis: Impaired skin integrity (00046): A state in which the individual has altered epidermis and/or dermis		
NANDA-RELATED FACTORS	**NOC OUTCOMES**	**NIC INTERVENTIONS**
Pressure	Tissue integrity: Skin and mucous membranes (1101)	Pressure management (3500) Skin surveillance (3590)
Nutritional deficit	Nutritional status: Food and fluid intake (1008)	Nutrition monitoring (1160) Nutrition therapy (1120)
Knowledge deficit	Knowledge: Illness care (1824)	Teaching: Disease process (5602)

NANDA, North American Nursing Diagnosis Association; *NIC,* Nursing Interventions Classification; *NOC,* Nursing Outcomes Classification.

outcomes, and interventions to fit each patient's unique needs. Various nursing care plans throughout the text illustrate NANDA-NOC-NIC linkages. These include Nursing Care Plans 27-1, 28-1, 33-1, 34-1, 44-1, 47-1, 52-1, 56-1, 58-1, 61-2, and 63-1.

IMPLEMENTATION PHASE

Carrying out the specific, individualized plan constitutes the implementation phase of the nursing process. The nurse performs the activities of interventions or may designate and supervise others who are qualified to intervene. Throughout the implementation phase the nurse must evaluate the effectiveness of the method chosen to implement the plan. For example, the nurse may determine that the nursing assistant caring for a patient with a mastectomy should not continue to be the person who implements the patient's exercise plan. Perhaps the patient is more depressed than anticipated and would benefit from contact with a nurse who is knowledgeable about changes in body image and sensitive to patient cues that may indicate body image disturbance. The exercise plan might essentially remain the same, but the person implementing the plan would be different and would use different skills to carry out the plan. Referrals to other professionals may also be made when the nurse anticipates that expertise in specialized areas is required to help the patient.

EVALUATION PHASE

The diagram of the nursing process (see Fig. 1-3) indicates that all phases must be evaluated. Evaluation not only occurs after implementation of the plan but continues throughout the process.

The nurse evaluates whether sufficient assessment data have been obtained to allow a nursing diagnosis to be made. The diagnosis is, in turn, evaluated for accuracy. For example, was the pain actually related to the wound itself or related to pressure from a constricting dressing?

Next the nurse evaluates whether the expected patient outcomes and interventions are realistic and achievable. If not, a new plan should be formulated. This may involve revision of expected patient outcomes and interventions. Consideration must be given to whether the plan should be maintained, modified, totally revised, or discontinued in light of the patient's status.

The effectiveness of each intervention and its contribution to progress toward the expected patient outcome are also evaluated. In addition, the nurse considers whether a different method of implementation of the same plan will provide better results.

NURSING CARE PLANS

When the nurse has determined the nursing diagnoses, outcomes, and interventions for a patient, it is important that the plan be recorded to ensure continuity of care by other nurses and health professionals. The plan should contain specific directions for carrying out the planned interventions, including how, when, how long, how often, where, by whom, and with what resources the activities should be performed. For example, in NCP 1-1, the nurse may want to specify how the activity of "encourage alternate rest and activity periods" should be implemented—that the patient should rest for 30 minutes following bathing, eating, ambulating to the bathroom, or having visitors. The nurse may also want to specify who should monitor the patient's cardiorespiratory response to activity, what signs should be monitored, and when they should be monitored.

Various methods and formats are used to record the nursing care plan. One of the important factors influencing a choice of care plan format has to do with whether NANDA, NOC, and NIC are used in the particular agency. Care plans are usually written on a specific form adopted by an institution, but they may also be entered into a computer that is programmed to organize nursing data. Such a computer program enables all nurses caring for the patient to easily print and update the plan as necessary. Every nurse who cares for the patient must be able to have access to the plan, whether hand written or computer generated, to provide the planned care. The care plan is part of the patient's legal medical record, and when hand written, the nurse must document the patient's nursing care requirements, changes that are made as the plan is implemented, and the outcomes of the nursing interventions. Not every activity that the nurse implements with the patient will be recorded on the care plan. Routine procedures, such as drug and intravenous fluid administration, assessment of vital signs, and other activities prescribed by institutional policies or protocols, may be documented on a variety of other forms.

The format used in NCP 1-1 is only one of many formats used to record the care plan. This example shows the incorporation of NANDA, NOC, and NIC with blanks to evaluate the indicators with the rating scale. This example illustrates the plan for only one nursing diagnosis. Patients will often have several nursing diagnoses.

Standardized care plans are often used as guides for routine nursing care and as a basis for developing individualized care plans. When standardized care plans are used, they should be personalized and specific to the unique needs and problems of each patient.

The nursing care plans presented throughout this book are in two formats. One format uses the NANDA-approved nursing diagnoses with NOC outcomes and NIC interventions with their appropriate codes. These nursing care plans are indicated in the list of nursing care plans (inside back cover) and are designated as NNN nursing care plans. The other format of nursing care plans used in this book is a standardized form that includes NANDA-approved nursing diagnoses and interventions and outcomes that are applicable to any number of patients having the identified nursing diagnosis. These care plans do not use NOC and NIC. When these care plans are used, they should be individualized for a specific patient.

Clinical (Critical) Pathways

Care related to common health problems experienced by many patients is delineated using clinical (critical) pathways. A **clinical (critical) pathway** directs the entire health care team in the daily care goals for select health care problems. It includes a nursing care plan, interventions specific for each day of hospitalization, and a documentation tool.[24]

The clinical pathway is part of a case management system that organizes and sequences the caregiving process at the patient level to better achieve quality and cost outcomes. It is a cyclic process organized for specific case types by all related health care departments. The case types selected for clinical pathways are usually those that occur in high volume and are highly predictable, such as myocardial infarction, stroke, and angina.

The clinical pathway describes the patient care required at specific times in the treatment. A multidisciplinary approach moves the patient toward desired outcomes within an estimated length of stay. The exact content and format of clinical pathways vary among institutions.

If clinical pathways are used by an institution, they are usually specifically developed and used by that institution. In the clinical pathway, the nursing care plan is documented with the use of nursing diagnoses and evaluation of expected outcomes. Nurse-initiated and physician-initiated interventions designed to achieve the patient outcomes are identified throughout the pathway. The multidisciplinary approach can be seen in the referral to and consultation with other health professionals.

DOCUMENTATION

It is critical that the patient's progress be documented in a systematic way. Many documentation methods and formats are used, depending on personal preference, agency policy, and regulatory standards such as those maintained by the Joint Commission on Accreditation of Healthcare Organizations (JCAHO). Patient progress may be documented by nurses with the use of flow sheets, narrative notes, subjective-objective assessment plan (SOAP) charting, clinical pathways, and computer-based charting. Every method or combination of methods is designed to document the assessment of patient status, the implementation of interventions, and the outcome of interventions.

Problem Lists

JCAHO requires that a multidisciplinary problem list be developed for each patient. Nurses, physicians, social workers, dietitians, and other health care professionals are encouraged to contribute to the list. A comprehensive view of the patient's problems is achieved by having many different disciplines contribute to the list.

Nurses can easily use the problem list as a basis for identifying nursing diagnoses. For example, if one of the identified problems on the list for a patient with a stroke is hemiparesis, appropriate nursing diagnoses for the nurse to consider may be risk for impaired skin integrity and impaired physical mobility.

The problem list is an inherent component of the problem-oriented record, a multidisciplinary patient documentation method. A prescribed method of charting, called SOAP charting, is used with this record.

SOAP Charting

One method of evaluating and recording patient progress is the problem-oriented record, referred to as the subjective-objective assessment plan (SOAP) method.[25] This type of progress note is problem specific and incorporates the components described in Table 1-9. Because the problem list and the record are multidisciplinary, data associated with any identified problem may be recorded by any health care provider. In some institutions, however, nurses write SOAP notes in reference to a list of nursing diagnoses. The process of SOAP documentation is as follows:

1. Additional subjective and objective data are gathered related to the area of concern.
2. Based on old and new data, an assessment of the patient's progress toward the expected patient outcome and the effectiveness of each intervention is made.
3. Based on the reassessment of the situation, the initial plan is maintained, revised, or discontinued.

The following is an example of SOAP charting for the nursing diagnosis "risk for infection *related to* traumatized tissue secondary to surgery:"
S: Wound is more painful today
O: Temperature of 103° F, facial grimacing in response to movement, dressing saturated with purulent drainage
A: Risk for wound infection
P: Notify surgeon, take temperature q2h, reinforce dressing, obtain wound culture

Computerized Documentation

The use of computers to document patient care, or **computerized documentation,** is becoming more common in health care settings. Computer documentation systems are called Electronic Patient Record (EPR), Computerized Patient Record (CPR), or Electronic Health Record (EHR). These records are the patient's official chart. Data are entered into the health record, making charting easier, faster, and generally more available to health care providers.[25] Software programs allow nurses to quickly enter specific assessment data one time, and the information is automatically transferred to different reports. Instead of writing lengthy nursing notes, nurses can select choices on a screen that are used to build a comprehensive patient record. Before computerized charting, it was difficult to extract nursing information from the health record because it had to be obtained from paper charts by hand. Now that there are computerized records, errors can be reduced and reporting on patient care data is much easier.

As information is entered into the record, either a Diagnosis Related Group (DRG) or Current Procedure Terminology (CPT) code with information about the medical diagnosis is assigned. Easy retrieval of this type of data helps administration reduce billing costs and report on length of stay.

Approved medical terminology, such as the Unified Medical Language System (UMLS) developed with the National Library of Medicine (NLM) and the Agency for Healthcare Research and Quality (AHRQ), is used in computer systems. However, nursing diagnoses, nursing interventions, and nursing outcomes cannot be recorded on most computerized patient records because software companies have not included nursing classifications in their systems. By using classifications such as NANDA, NOC, and NIC it is possible to follow the links between diagnosis, interventions, and outcomes that will greatly advance evidence-based practice (EBP). For example, when choosing the NANDA diagnosis of *fatigue* on a computer, the code 00093 would be selected and entered into a database. Then the nurse would select a NOC outcome of *endurance* and the code 0001 would be incorporated into the database. The nurse would select the NIC interventions of *energy management (0180)* and *exercise promotion (0200)* and these codes would also be incorporated. The coded data can be separated from the patient's name, thus providing for the patient's anonymity and confidentiality.

TABLE 1-9	Components of a Problem-Oriented Progress Note
SOAP	**EXPLANATION**
Subjective (S)	Information supplied by patient or knowledgeable other
Objective (O)	Information obtained by nurse directly by observation or measurement, from patient records, or through diagnostic studies
Assessment (A)	Nursing diagnosis or problem based on subjective data and objective data
Plan (P)	Specific interventions related to a diagnostic or problem considering diagnostic, therapeutic, and patient education needs

Each piece of data that gets entered into the record can be tracked and reported on for many purposes. If nursing languages, or taxonomies, are used in information systems for documentation of nursing practice, nurses can track and report on the benefits of nursing care and just what it is that nurses do for patients. This would serve not only to improve practice guidelines, but also facilitate nursing research and easily demonstrate the effectiveness of nursing interventions. This will make nursing care visible while providing a continuing evaluation of nursing's efficacy.

Nursing Informatics. A nursing specialization called **nursing informatics** is a nursing specialty integrating nursing science, computer science, and information science in identifying, collecting, processing, and managing data and information to support nursing practice, administration, education, research, and the expansion of knowledge.[26] This specialization in nursing allows for nurses to work within the information systems (IS) department so that nursing issues can be integrated at the beginning of computer projects rather than just evaluating the problems for nursing when a project is complete. Nursing informatics studies the structure and processing of nursing information to arrive at clinical decisions and to build systems to support and automate that processing. An informatics nurse has a diverse role that ranges from designing, developing, marketing, and testing to implementation, training, use, maintenance, evaluation, and enhancement of computer systems.

FUTURE CHALLENGES OF NURSING

Nursing roles continually evolve as our society changes and we learn to apply new technology. Although nursing is defined in different ways, past and current definitions of nursing have commonalities of health, illness, and caring. It is important that these concepts are carried into future definitions of nursing as greater demands are placed on the profession. Future use of the nursing process will continue to require the use of reasoning, analytic thinking skills, and synthesis of rapidly expanding knowledge to assist others to maintain or attain optimal health.

During the past 25 years, the nursing profession made great advances in classifying nursing knowledge through the ongoing classification of nursing diagnoses, outcomes, and interventions. Expansion of all nursing languages will continue. Computerized documentation of nursing practice in nursing's own languages will be critical to the advancement of nursing practice.

An increasing emphasis on accountability, assertiveness, persistence, risk taking, and decision making is essential if nursing is to "get somewhere else." In its attempt to keep pace, nursing would do well to remember what the Queen in *Through the Looking Glass* said to Alice: "Now here, you see, it takes all the running you can do to keep in the same place. If you want to get somewhere else, you must run at least twice as fast as that."[27] This appears to be the future of nursing.

REVIEW QUESTIONS

The number of the question corresponds to the same-numbered objective at the beginning of the chapter.

1. An example of a nursing activity that reflects the American Nurses Association's definition of nursing is
   a. establishing that the patient with jaundice has hepatitis.
   b. determining the cause of hemorrhage in a postoperative patient based on vital signs.
   c. identifying and treating arrhythmias that occur in a patient in the coronary care unit.
   d. diagnosing that a patient with pneumonia cannot effectively cough up pulmonary secretions.

2. When using evidence-based practice, the nurse
   a. must use clinical practice guidelines developed by national health agencies.
   b. should use findings from randomized clinical trials to plan care for all patient problems.
   c. uses clinical decision making and judgment to determine what evidence is appropriate for a specific clinical situation.
   d. statistically analyzes the relationship of nursing interventions to patient outcomes to establish evidence that interventions are appropriate for the patient.

3. Standardized nursing languages benefit patient care in that
   a. patient problems and nursing care are clearly defined.
   b. nurses use the same terminology as physicians in delivery of patient care.
   c. a consistent, universal format is used to assess patient responses to health problems.
   d. established prescriptions for nursing care eliminate the need for time-consuming nursing care planning.

4. When the nurse determines that the patient's anxiety needs to be relieved before effective teaching can be implemented, the phase of the nursing process being used is
   a. assessment.
   b. diagnosis.
   c. planning.
   d. evaluation.

5. An example of an independent nursing intervention is
   a. administering blood.
   b. starting an intravenous fluid.
   c. teaching a patient about the effects of prescribed drugs.
   d. administering emergency drugs according to institutional protocols.

6. The process of making a nursing diagnosis differs from a diagnostic statement in that the diagnostic process involves
   a. stating what needs the patient has.
   b. identifying factors related to the pathology of a disease process.
   c. identifying the diagnosis, related factors, and signs and symptoms.
   d. analyzing assessment data to identify responses to health problems.

7. The nurse identifies the nursing diagnosis of constipation related to laxative abuse for a patient. The most appropriate expected patient outcome related to this nursing diagnosis is that
   a. the patient will stop the use of laxatives.
   b. the patient ingests adequate fluid and fiber.
   c. the patient passes normal stools without aids.
   d. the patient's stool is free of blood and mucus.

Continued

REVIEW QUESTIONS—cont'd

8. A patient has a nursing diagnosis of stress urinary incontinence related to overdistention between voidings. An appropriate nursing intervention for this patient related to this nursing diagnosis is to
   a. provide privacy for toileting.
   b. monitor color, odor, and clarity of urine.
   c. teach the patient to void at 2-hour intervals.
   d. provide the patient with perineal pads to absorb urine leakage.

9. Linkages of NANDA nursing diagnoses, NOC patient outcomes, and NIC nursing interventions can be used to
   a. evaluate patient outcomes.
   b. provide guides for planning care.
   c. predict the results of nursing care.
   d. shorten written care plans for individual patients.

10. The primary purpose of the evaluation phase of the nursing process is to
    a. assess the patient's strengths.
    b. describe new nursing diagnoses.
    c. implement new nursing strategies.
    d. identify patient progress toward outcomes.

11. The use of computers to document nursing practice with nursing languages
    a. protects patient anonymity and confidentiality.
    b. establishes that high standards of care are met.
    c. assists in the evaluation of the effectiveness of nursing interventions.
    d. promotes communication of the patient's progress to the health care team.

REFERENCES

1. Goodnow M: *Outlines of nursing history,* ed 6, Philadelphia, 1938, WB Saunders.
2. American Nurses Association: *Nursing: a social policy statement,* Washington, DC, 1995, The Association.
3. Fawcett J: *Analysis and evaluation of contemporary nursing knowledge: nursing models and theories,* Philadelphia, 2000, FA Davis.
4. Nightingale F: *Notes on nursing: what it is and what it is not, facsimile edition,* Philadelphia, 1946, Lippincott.
5. Henderson V: *The nature of nursing,* New York, 1966, Macmillan.
6. Roy S, Andrews H: *The Roy adaptation model,* ed 2, Stamford, Conn, 1999, Appleton & Lange.
7. American Association of Colleges of Nursing: *Nursing education's agenda for the 21st century,* Washington, DC, 2001, The Association. Available at *www.aacn.nche.edu/Publications/positions/nrsgedag.htm* (accessed Dec 31, 2001).
8. American Association of Colleges of Nursing: *Certification and regulation of advanced practice nurses,* Washington, DC, 2001, The Association. Available at *www.aanc.nche.edu/Publications/position/cerreg.htm* (accessed Dec 31, 2001).
9. American Nurses Association: *ANA analysis and comparison chart: analysis and comparison of advanced practice recognition with Medicaid reimbursement and insurance reimbursement laws 2000 chart,* Washington, DC, 2000, The Association. Available at *www.nursingworld.org/gova/charts/medicaid.htm* (accessed Dec 31, 2001).
10. US Department of Health and Human Services: *Healthy people 2000,* Washington, DC, 1991, US Department of Health and Human Services.
11. US Department of Health and Human Services: *Healthy people 2010,* Washington, DC, 2000, US Department of Health and Human Services.
12. Jennings BM, Loan LA: Misconceptions among nurses about evidence-based practice, *Journal of Nursing Scholarship* 33:122, 2001.
13. Stevens KR, Pugh JA: Evidence-based practice and perioperative nursing, *Seminars in Perioperative Nursing* 8:155, 1999.
14. Ingersoll GL: Evidence-based nursing: what it is and what it isn't, *Nursing Outlook* 48:151, 2000.
15. Aquilino M, Keenan G: Having our say: nursing's standardized nomenclatures, *Am J Nurs* 100:33, 2000.
16. North American Nursing Diagnosis Association: *Nursing diagnoses: definitions and classification 2001-2002,* Philadelphia, 2001, The Association.
17. McCloskey J, Bulechek G: *Nursing interventions classification (NIC),* ed 3, St Louis, 2000, Mosby.
18. Johnson M, Maas M, Moorhead S: *Nursing outcomes classification (NOC),* ed 2, St Louis, 2000, Mosby.
19. Wilkinson J: *Nursing process and critical thinking,* ed 3, Upper Saddle River, NJ, 2001, Prentice Hall.
20. Carpenito L: *Nursing diagnosis: application to clinical practice,* ed 8, Philadelphia, 2000, Lippincott.
21. Gordon M: *Manual of nursing diagnosis,* ed 9, St Louis, 2000, Mosby.
22. Maslow A: *Motivation and personality,* New York, 1954, Harper & Row.
23. Johnson M et al: *Nursing diagnoses, outcomes, and interventions: NANDA, NOC, and NIC linkages,* St Louis, 2001, Mosby.
24. Birdsall C, Sperry S: *Clinical paths in medical-surgical practice,* St Louis, 1997, Mosby.
25. Iyer PW, Camp NH: *Nursing documentation: a nursing process approach,* ed 3, St Louis, 1999, Mosby.
26. American Nurses Association: *The scope of practice for nursing informatics,* Washington, DC, 1994, The Association.
27. Carroll L: *Alice's adventures in wonderland and through the looking glass,* New York, 1973, Collier Books.

RESOURCES

American Nurses Association
600 Maryland Avenue SW, Suite 100 West
Washington, DC 20024
202-651-7000
800-274-4ANA
www.nursingworld.org

American Nursing Informatics Association (ANIA)
PMB 105
10808 Foothill Blvd., Suite 160
Ranch Cucamonga, CA 91730
909-985-2811
www.ania.org

Canadian Nurses Association
50 Driveway, Ottawa, ON
CANADA K2P 1E2
613-237-2133
800-361-8404
Fax: 613-237-3520
www.cna-nurses.ca/

Center for Nursing Classification
Room 407 NB
College of Nursing
University of Iowa
Iowa City, IA 52242-1121
319-353-5414
www.nursing.uiowa.edu/cnc

National Association of Hispanic Nurses
1501 16th Street NW
Washington, DC 20036
202-387-2477
Fax: 202-483-7183
E-mail: TheHispanicNurses@earthlink.net
www.thehispanicnurses.org/

National Black Nurses' Association, Inc.
8630 Fenton Street, Suite 330
Silver Spring, MD 20910-3803
301-589-3200
Fax: 301-589-3223

National Student Nurses' Association
45 Main Street, Suite 606
Brooklyn, NY 11201
718-210-0705
www.nsna.org

North American Nursing Diagnosis Association (NANDA)
1211 Locust Street
Philadelphia, PA 19107
215-545-8105
800-647-9002
Fax: 215-545-8107
E-mail: info@nanda.org
www.nanda.org

Sigma Theta Tau International
550 West North Street
Indianapolis, IN 46202
317-634-8171
888-634-7575
Fax: 317-634-8188
www.nursingsociety.org/

For additional Internet resources, see the website for this book at
http://evolve.elsevier.com/Lewis/medsurg/.

CHAPTER **2**

Culturally Competent Care
Barbara G. White

LEARNING OBJECTIVES

1. Define the terms culture, subculture, acculturation, assimilation, ethnicity, race, ethnocentrism, cultural imposition, values, transcultural nursing, culture-bound syndrome, explanatory model, and cultural competency.
2. Describe the potential effects of immigration on an individual's health.
3. Explain aspects of culture and ethnicity that may affect a person's health.
4. Describe strategies for successfully communicating with a person who speaks a language that the nurse does not understand.

5. Identify physiologic aspects of culture and ethnicity to consider when providing nursing care.
6. Identify ways that the nurse's own cultural background may influence nursing care when working with patients from different cultural and ethnic groups.
7. Identify strategies for incorporating cultural information in the nursing process when providing care for patients from different cultural and ethnic groups.

KEY TERMS

acculturation, p. 19	ethnocentrism, p. 19
assimilation, p. 19	explanatory model, p. 20
cultural competence, p. 19	race, p. 19
cultural imposition, p. 19	stereotyping, p. 19
culture, p. 18	subcultures, p. 18
culture-bound syndrome, p. 26	transcultural nursing, p. 19
ethnicity, p. 19	values, p. 18

In today's increasingly multicultural environment nurses will come in contact with individuals from many different cultures during their professional careers. They will find themselves in patient care situations that require an understanding of the patient's cultural beliefs if they are to effectively participate in planning and providing culturally competent care. Because of the changing demographic and cultural composition of the United States and other countries, it is important for nurses to be aware of cultural differences in health care practices and of the potential differences in expectations of patients and health care providers. The nurse needs to acknowledge and accept the influence of the patient's cultural beliefs and customs to prevent conflict from occurring between the goals of nursing and the practices based on the patient's cultural background.

Who are the nurses providing care for this diverse population? Registered nurses, who make up the largest portion of health care providers, are 90% white/Caucasians, 4% African Americans, 3.4% Asian/Pacific Islanders, 1.4% Hispanics, and 0.4% American Indian/Alaska Natives.[1] Although these nurses represent diversity in the workplace, their proportions do not match the patient population. These nurses may well find it challenging to provide care for patients from multiethnic populations. Even if nurses provide care for patients from their own cultural back-

ground, the nurse may be from a different subculture than the patient. For example, it would be inappropriate to assume that a Native American nurse can give culturally appropriate care to a Native American patient, especially if the patient and nurse are from different tribes of the more than 500 in the U.S. population.

CULTURE

There are many definitions of culture. In general, **culture** encompasses the knowledge, values, beliefs, art, morals, law, customs, and habits of the members of a society. Culture also includes the systems of technology and political practices. Cultural patterns of behavior develop over time and are shared by members of the same cultural group.[2] Culture affects ways of perceiving, behaving, and evaluating the world, and serves as a guide for people's values, beliefs, and practices, including those related to health and illness.[3]

Values are the sets of rules by which individuals, families, groups, and communities live. They are the principles and standards that serve as the basis for beliefs, attitudes, and behaviors. Although all cultures have values, the types and expressions of those values differ from one culture to another. These cultural values develop over time, guide decision making and actions, and may affect a person's self-esteem. Cultural values are often unconsciously developed as a child is assimilated into the culture, learning what is acceptable and unacceptable behavior. The extent to which a person's cultural values are internalized influences that person's tendency toward judging other cultures, while using his or her own culture as the accepted standard.[2,4-6]

Although individuals within a cultural group will have many similarities through their shared values, beliefs, and practices, there is also much diversity within groups. Each person is culturally unique. Such diversity may result from different perspectives and interpretations of situations. These differences may be based on age, gender, marital status, family structure, income, education level, religious views, and life experiences.

Within any cultural group there are smaller **subcultures** that may not hold all of the values of the dominant culture. These subcultures, including ethnic groups, have experiences that differ from the dominant group. These differences may be related to eth-

Reviewed by Viola G. Benavente, RN, MSN, CNS, Clinical Instructor, Department of Chronic Nursing Care, University of Texas at San Antonio, School of Nursing, San Antonio, Tex.

TABLE 2-1	**Basic Characteristics of Culture**

- *Learned* through the processes of language acquisition and socialization
- *Shared* by all members of the same cultural group
- *Adapted* to specific conditions such as environmental factors
- *Dynamic* and ever-changing

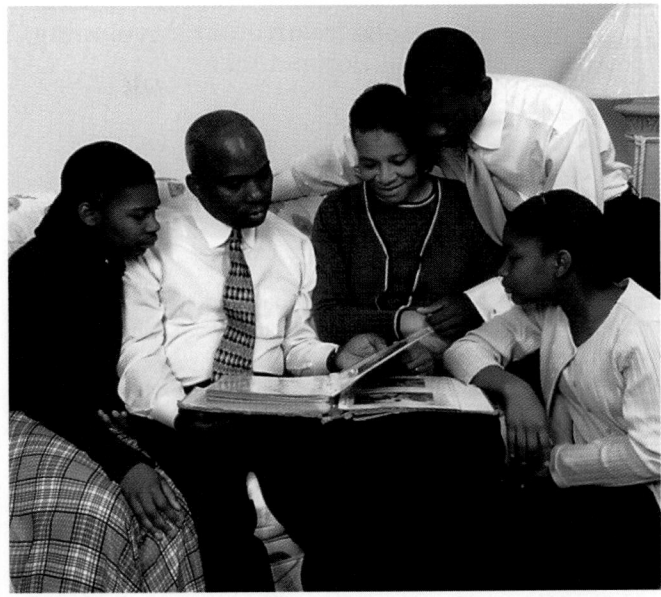

FIG. 2-1   Members of this family share a common heritage.

nic background, residence, religion, occupation, health-related characteristics, age, gender, education, or other factors that unite the group. Members of a subculture share certain aspects of culture that are different from the overall cultural group. Religious subcultures include Catholics, Jews, Muslims, and other members of any of the 1200 recognized religions. Ethnic subcultures include groups who share common traits such as ancestry, language, or physical characteristics. These include African Americans, Hispanics, and Native Americans.

It is important to understand certain aspects of culture if the nurse is to understand the impact of culture and how cultural practices may affect the way people take care of their health or treat illnesses. The four basic characteristics of culture are described in Table 2-1.[5]

Cultural practices change over time through active or passive processes, including acculturation and assimilation. **Acculturation** occurs when people modify their own culture as a result of contact with another culture.[6] This process may be a gradual change that results in increased similarities between the two cultures. **Assimilation** involves a generally one-way process where people lose their own cultural identity as they gradually adopt and incorporate characteristics of the prevailing culture.[6] Both acculturation and assimilation may be voluntary or, in some instances, involuntary (e.g., as a result of war or involuntary relocation).

The meaning of the terms *ethnicity* and *race* continues to evolve and be debated. **Ethnicity** refers to groups whose members share a common social and cultural heritage. This heritage is passed on through the generations and involves identification with that group (Fig. 2-1). Members of an ethnic group may share a common language, history, education, lifestyle, and religion. They share a sense of identity, loyalty, and social belonging.[4,7] Ethnic groups do not exist in isolation. They exist because of differences that separate them from other ethnic groups. The term **race** refers to divisions of humankind and is more closely related to people who share a common ancestry and physical characteristics such as skin color, bone structure, or blood group. *Ethnicity* is considered to be a more global and less discriminating term than *race* and is used in this book.

Stereotyping is the viewing of members of a specific culture, race, or ethnic group as being alike and sharing the same values and beliefs. This oversimplified approach does not take into account the individual differences that exist within a culture. In health care (as well as most other) settings, being a member of a particular ethnic group should not be considered to make the person an expert on other members of that same group. Such stereotyping can lead to false assumptions and affect a patient's care. For example, it would be inappropriate to assume that just because a nurse is Hispanic, she would know how a Hispanic patient's beliefs may affect his health care practices. The nurse may

have been born and raised in a large city and assimilated a different culture than the elderly male patient who was born and raised in a rural area of Mexico and has traditional beliefs about the causes and treatment of illness.

Ethnocentrism is the tendency to subconsciously view others using one's own customs as the standard.[3] When considering one's own ways of thinking, acting, and believing to be the only right and natural ways, there is a danger of seeing other's beliefs as unusual and bizarre, and therefore wrong.[6] Comparing others' ways to one's own can lead to seeing others as different or inferior. To avoid ethnocentrism, it is necessary to maintain an objective and nonjudgmental view of the values, beliefs, and practices of others. Failure to do this can result in ethnic stereotyping or cultural imposition.

Cultural imposition results when one's own cultural beliefs and practices are imposed on another person or group of people. In health care it can result in disregarding or trivializing a patient's health care beliefs or practices. Cultural imposition may result when a health care provider is not aware of another person's beliefs and moves forward with planning and providing care without taking into account the cultural beliefs of the patient.

CULTURAL COMPETENCE

The term **transcultural nursing** was coined by Madeleine Leininger in the 1950s. Transcultural nursing has developed into a specialty that focuses on the comparative study and analysis of cultures and subcultures. The goal of transcultural nursing is the discovery of culturally relevant facts that can guide the nurse in providing culturally appropriate and competent care.[4,8]

Cultural competence involves the complex integration of knowledge, attitudes, and skills that enable the nurse to provide culturally appropriate health care.[3,5,9] Developing cultural competence requires (1) cultural awareness, (2) cultural knowledge, (3) cultural skills, and (4) cultural encounter (Table 2-2).

TABLE 2-2	Processes Involved in Developing Cultural Competence

Cultural Awareness
- Identify one's own cultural background, values, and beliefs, especially as related to health and health care.
- Examine one's own cultural biases toward people whose cultures differ from one's own culture.

Cultural Knowledge
- Learn basic general information about predominant cultural groups in one's geographic area. Cultural pocket guides can be a good resource.
- Assess for presence or absence of cultural phenomena based on the understanding of generalizations about a cultural group.
- Do not make assumptions based on cultural background because the degree of acculturation varies among individuals.
- Read research studies that describe cultural differences.
- Read ethnic newspaper articles and novels.
- View documentaries about cultural groups.

Cultural Skills
- Be alert for unexpected responses with patients, especially as related to cultural issues.
- Become aware of cultural differences in predominant ethnic groups.
- Develop assessment skills to do a competent cultural assessment for any patient.
- Learn assessment skills for different cultural groups, including cultural beliefs and practices.

Cultural Encounter
- Create opportunities to interact with predominant cultural groups.
- Visit cultural events, such as religious ceremonies, significant life passage rituals, social events, and demonstrations of cultural practices.
- Visit markets and restaurants in ethnic neighborhoods.
- Explore ethnic neighborhoods, listen to different types of ethnic music, and learn games of various ethnic groups.
- Visit or volunteer at health fairs in local ethnic neighborhoods.
- Learn about prominent cultural beliefs and practices, and incorporate this knowledge into planning nursing care.

Cultural Awareness

Cultural awareness is a conscious learning process in which individuals become appreciative of and sensitive to the cultures of other people. Every person is a cultural being. Therefore any nurse-patient interaction will be affected by the culture of both the nurse and the patient. The nurse is influenced not only by his or her cultural background, but by the nursing profession and the culture of the health care setting in which the interaction occurs.[3] One of the first steps in developing cultural awareness is for the nurse to examine his or her own cultural biases toward people from different cultures. The nurse's biases may interfere with providing culturally appropriate health care because they have the potential to affect behavior toward members of other cultural groups.[10] Cultural awareness is an important step in providing culturally appropriate care and avoiding ethnocentrism and cultural imposition.

Cultural Knowledge

Cultural knowledge involves the process of understanding the key aspects of a group's culture, especially as it relates to health and health care practices. Different cultural groups have different beliefs about the cause of illnesses and the appropriateness of various treatments. It is important for the nurse to try to determine the patient's **explanatory model** (what causes the disease or illness and the potential methods the patient believes would best treat the condition). It is also important to determine how patients' different experiences and beliefs might affect their health and health care. Patients may be using culturally appropriate remedies that may affect the treatment prescribed by the health care provider. In addition to asking patients about the medications they may be taking, they also need to be asked about "natural" or herbal substances they take or actions they have taken to prevent or treat their condition. For example, a Chinese patient may be taking herbal remedies for diabetes, or a woman of Eastern European descent may take St. John's wort for depression. Either of these substances could interact with prescription drugs and cause untoward effects.

Lack of cultural competence can lead to misdiagnosis and mistreatment of patients.[3] When the patient's natural expression of pain or emotions or traditional health care practices are misinterpreted, the consequences can range from minor to serious. For example, the traditional Southeast Asian treatment of *cupping* uses glass cups that are heated to create a vacuum when placed on a patient's skin. This treatment is used for many illnesses, especially for increasing local circulation and treating lung congestion. Another treatment is *coining*, which involves placing a menthol oil or ointment on the skin and then rubbing or scraping the area with a coin. This treatment is used for pain, colds, heat exhaustion, vomiting, or headache and leaves marks that can look like a strap mark. If either of these treatments were used and the health care provider did not know what was being done, the results might appear to be from physical abuse.[3,11]

Cultural Skills

Cultural skills is the ability to collect relevant cultural data regarding health histories and performing culturally specific assessments. Skills based on cultural knowledge can be used to create a safe environment so that patients will share information about their health-related cultural practices. Specific information is presented throughout this book to assist with developing an awareness of cultural differences and learning assessment skills for different cultural groups. Table 2-3 presents a cultural assessment instrument.

Delivery of culturally appropriate care can prevent unnecessary conflicts between the nurse and patients who are from different cultural backgrounds. Providing culturally appropriate care also increases patient satisfaction and may assist the patient to follow through on the regimen that has been agreed on with the nurse.

Cultural Encounter

Cultural encounter is the process that encourages individuals to engage directly in cross-cultural interactions with people from culturally diverse backgrounds (Fig. 2-2). Cultural competence

TABLE 2-3   Cultural Assessment

Brief History of the Cultural Group with Which the Person Identifies

- With what cultural group(s) does the person affiliate (e.g., Hispanic, Polish, Navajo, or combination)? To what degree does the person identify with the cultural group (e.g., "we" concept of solidarity or a fringe member)?
- What is the person's reported racial affiliation (e.g., African American, Native American, Asian American, and so on)?
- Where was the person born?
- Where has the person lived (country, city) and when (during what years)? NOTE: If a recent relocation to the United States, knowledge of prevalent diseases in country of origin may be helpful.

Values Orientation

- What are the person's attitudes, values, and beliefs about birth, death, health, illness, health care providers?
- How does the person view work, leisure, education?
- How does the person perceive change?

Cultural Sanctions and Restrictions

- How does the person's cultural group regard expression of emotion and feelings, spirituality, and religious beliefs? How are dying, death, and grieving expressed in a culturally appropriate manner?
- How is modesty expressed by men and women? Are there culturally defined expectations about male-female relationships, including the health care relationship?
- Does the person have any restrictions related to sexuality, exposure of body parts, certain types of surgery (e.g., amputation, vasectomy, hysterectomy)?
- Are there any restrictions against discussion of dead relatives or fears related to the unknown?

Communication

- What language does the person speak at home? What other languages does the person speak or read? In what language would the person prefer to communicate with you?
- Does the person need an interpreter? If so, is there a relative or friend whom he or she would like to interpret? Is there anyone whom the person would prefer did not interpret (e.g., member of the opposite sex, a person younger/older than the person, member of a rival tribe or nation)?
- How does the person feel about health care providers who are not of the same cultural background (e.g., African American, middle-class nurse and Hispanic of a different social class)? Does the person prefer to receive care from a nurse or doctor of the same cultural background, gender, and/or age?

Health-Related Beliefs and Practices

- To what cause(s) does the person attribute illness and disease (e.g., divine wrath, imbalance in hot/cold or yin/yang, punishment for moral transgressions, hex, soul loss)?
- What does the person believe promotes health (eating certain foods, wearing amulets to bring good luck, exercise, prayer, rituals to ancestors, saints, or intermediate deities)?
- What is the person's religious affiliation (e.g., Judaism, Islam, Pentecostalism, West African voodooism, Seventh-Day Adventism, Catholicism, Mormonism)?
- Does the person rely on cultural healers (e.g., curandero, shaman, spiritualist, priest, minister, monk)? Who determines when the person is sick and when he or she is healthy? Who determines the type of healer and treatment that should be sought?
- In what types of cultural healing practices does the person engage (use of herbal remedies, potions, massage, wearing of talismans or charms to discourage evil spirits, healing rituals, incantations, prayers)?
- How are biomedical/scientific health care providers perceived? How does the person and his or her family perceive nurses or physicians? What are the expectations of nurses and nursing care?
- What is appropriate "sick role" behavior? Who determines what symptoms constitute disease/illness? Who decides when the person is no longer sick? Who cares for the person at home?
- How does the person's cultural group view mental disorders? Are there differences in acceptable behaviors for physical versus psychologic illnesses?

Nutrition

- What is the meaning of food and eating to the person? With whom does the person usually eat? What types of food are eaten? What does the person define as food? What does the person believe composes a "healthy" versus an "unhealthy" diet?
- How are foods prepared at home (type of food preparation, cooking oil(s) used, length of time foods are cooked, especially vegetables, amount and type of seasoning added to various foods during preparation)?
- Do religious beliefs and practices influence the person's diet (e.g., amount, type, preparation or delineation of acceptable food combinations, such as kosher diets)? Does the person abstain from certain foods at regular intervals, on specific dates determined by the religious calendar, or at other times?
- If the person's religion mandates or encourages fasting, what does the term "fast" mean (e.g., refraining from certain types or quantities of foods, eating only during certain times of the day)? For what period of time is the person expected to fast?
- During fasting, does the person refrain from liquids/beverages? Does the religion allow exemption from fasting during illness? If so, does the person believe that an exemption applies to him or her?

Socioeconomic Considerations

- Who composes the person's social network (family, peers, and cultural healers)? How do they influence the person's health or illness status?
- How do members of the person's social support network define caring (e.g., being continuously present, doing things for the person, looking after the person's family)? What are the roles of various family members during health and illness?
- How does the person's family participate in the nursing care (e.g., bathing, feeding, touching, being present)?
- Does the cultural family structure influence the person's response to health or illness (e.g., beliefs, strengths, weaknesses, and social class)? Is there a key family member whose role is significant in health-related decisions (e.g., grandmother in many African American families, eldest adult son in Asian families)?
- Who is the principal wage earner in the person's family? What is the total annual income? (NOTE: This is a potentially sensitive question that should be asked only if necessary.) Is there more than one wage earner? Are there other sources of financial support (extended family, investments)?

Data for spiritual considerations from Andrews MM, Hanson PA: Religion, culture, and nursing. In Andrews MM, Boyle JS, editors: *Transcultural concepts in nursing care,* ed 4, Philadelphia, 2003, JB Lippincott Williams & Wilkins. From Jarvis C: *Physical examination and health assessment,* ed 4, Philadelphia, 2004, WB Saunders.

Continued

TABLE 2-3	Cultural Assessment—cont'd

Socioeconomic Considerations—cont'd

- What impact does economic status have on lifestyle, place of residence, living conditions, ability to obtain health care, discharge planning?

Organizations Providing Cultural Support

- What influence do ethnic/cultural organizations have on the person's receiving health care (e.g., Organization of Migrant Workers, National Association for the Advancement of Colored People (NAACP), Black Political Caucus, churches, schools, Urban League, community-based health care programs and clinics)?

Educational Background

- What is the person's highest educational level obtained?
- Can the person read and write English, or is another language preferred? If English is the second language, are materials available in the primary language?
- What learning style is most comfortable/familiar? Does the person prefer to learn through written materials, oral explanation, or demonstration?

Religious Affiliation

- What is the role of religious beliefs and practices during health and illness?
- Are there healing rituals or practices that the person believes can promote well-being or hasten recovery from illness? If so, who performs these?

- What is the role of significant religious representatives during health and illness? Are there recognized healers (e.g., Islamic imams, Christian Scientist practitioners or nurses, Catholic priests, Mormon elders, Buddhist monks)?

Spiritual Considerations

- Does the person have religious objects in the environment?
- Does the person wear outer- or undergarments having religious significance?
- Are get-well greeting cards religious in nature or from a religious representative?
- Does the person appear to pray at certain times of the day or before meals?
- Does the person make special dietary requests (e.g., Kosher diet; vegetarian diet; diet free from caffeine, pork, shellfish, or other specific food items)?
- Does the person read religious magazines or books?
- Does the person mention God (Allah, Buddha, Yahweh, or a synonym), prayer, faith, or other religious topics?
- Is a request made for a visit by a member of the clergy or other religious representative?
- Is there an expression of anxiety or fear about pain, suffering, death?
- Does the person prefer to interact with others or to remain alone?

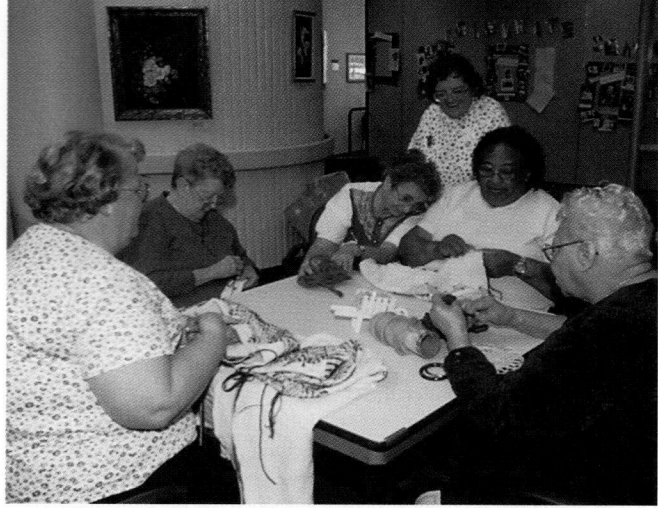

FIG. 2-2 The cultural encounter process encourages individuals to engage in cross-cultural interactions with people from culturally diverse backgrounds.

requires the experience of working with persons from different cultures and learning how their cultural beliefs and practices affect their health and health care practices. Through experience with members of a culture, the nurse can become more competent in caring for them.

CULTURAL FACTORS AFFECTING HEALTH AND HEALTH CARE

Many culture-related factors affect the patient's health and health care. Several potential factors are presented in Table 2-4.

Spirituality/Religion

Spirituality and religion are aspects of culture that may affect a person's beliefs about health and illness. They may also play a role in nutrition and decisions related to health and ways that a person responds to or treats an illness.

Spirituality refers to a person's effort to find purpose and meaning in life.[12] It is influenced by a person's unique life experiences and reflects one's personal understanding of life's mysteries. Spirituality relates to the soul or spirit more than to the body, and it may provide hope and strength for an individual during an illness.[13]

Religion is a more formal and organized system of beliefs, including belief in or worship of God or gods. Religious beliefs include the cause, nature, and purpose of the universe and involve prayer and ritual(s). Religion is based on beliefs about life, death, good and evil, and pain and suffering.[5]

The nurse can use many interventions to meet a patient's spiritual needs. These interventions may include prayer, scripture, listening, and referral.[12] Many patients find that rituals help them during times of illness.[13] Rituals help a person make sense of his or her life experiences and may take the form of prayer, meditation, or other rituals that the patient may create. The nurse needs to include spiritual assessment in the complete assessment of the patient and plan care based on that assessment.

TABLE 2-4	Cultural Factors Affecting Health and Health Care

Time Orientation
- For some cultures it is more important to attend to a social role than to arrive on time for an appointment with a health care provider.
- Some cultures are future oriented; others are past or present oriented.

Language and Communication
- Patients may not speak English and may not be able to communicate with the health care provider.
- Even with interpreters, there may be difficulties with communication.

Economic Factors
- Patients may not get health care because they cannot pay for it or the costs associated with travel for health care.
- Refugee or illegal immigrant status may deter some patients from using the health care system.
- Patients may lack health insurance.

Health Care System
- Patients may not make or keep appointments because of the time lag between the onset of an illness and an available appointment.
- Hours of operation of health care facilities may not accommodate patients' need to work or use public transportation.
- Cumbersome requirements to access some types of care may discourage some patients from taking the steps to qualify for health care or health care payment assistance.
- Some patients have a general distrust of health care professionals and health systems.
- Lack of ethnic-specific health care programs.

- Transportation may be a problem for patients who have to travel long distances for health care.
- Patients may not have a primary health care provider and may use emergency departments or urgent care centers for health care.
- Shortages of health care providers from specific ethnic groups may deter some people from seeking health care.
- Patients may have a lack of knowledge about the availability of existing health care resources.
- Facility policies may not be culturally sensitive (e.g., hospital policy may limit the number of visitors, which is problematic for cultures that value having many family members present).

Beliefs and Practices
- Care provided in established health care programs may not be perceived as culturally relevant.
- Religious reasons, beliefs, or practices may affect a person's decision to seek (or not seek) health care.
- Patients may delay seeking care because of fear or dependence on folk medicine and herbal remedies.
- Patients may stop treatment or discontinue visits for health care because the symptoms are no longer present, and there is the perception that further care is not required.
- Some patients associate hospitals and extended care facilities with death.
- Patient may have had a previous negative experience with culturally insensitive health care providers or discriminatory practices.
- Some people mistrust the majority population and institutions dominated by them.
- Some patients may feel apprehensive about unfamiliar diagnostic processes and treatment options.

Communication

Communication style is influenced by culture and may be verbal or nonverbal. Verbal communication includes not only the language or dialect, but also the voice tone, volume, timing, and one's willingness to share thoughts and feelings.[6] Nonverbal communication may take the form of writing, gestures, body movements, posture, and facial expressions. Nonverbal communication also includes eye contact, use of touch, body language, style of greeting, and spatial distancing.[14] Culture influences the ways that feelings are expressed, as well as what verbal and nonverbal expressions are appropriate in given situations.[4]

Silence is interpreted based on cultural experiences. Some people are comfortable with silence, whereas others become uncomfortable and may speak to decrease the silent times. Many Native Americans are comfortable with silence and interpret silence as essential for thinking and carefully considering a response. In these interactions, silence shows respect for the other person and demonstrates the importance of the remarks. In traditional Japanese and Chinese cultures, the speaker may stop talking and leave a period of silence for the listener to think about what has been said before continuing. Silence may be intended to show respect for the speaker's privacy, whereas in some cultures (e.g., French, Spanish, and Russian) the person may interpret silence as meaning agreement. In two very different approaches, Asian Americans may use silence to demonstrate respect for el-

ders, whereas African Americans may use silence as a response to what is perceived to be an inappropriate question.

Eye contact varies greatly among cultures. Although the nurse has probably been taught to maintain direct eye contact, patients who are Asian, Arab, or Native American may avoid direct eye contact and consider direct contact as disrespectful or aggressive. Hispanic patients may expect the nurse to look directly at them, but would not return that direct gaze. Other variables to consider include the role of gender, age, status, or position on what is considered to be appropriate eye contact. For example, Muslim-Arab women exhibit modesty when avoiding eye contact with men other than their husbands and when in public situations.

Family Roles and Relationships

Family roles differ from one culture to another (Fig. 2-3). For this reason it is important for the nurse to determine who should be involved in communication and decision making related to health care. In some cultural groups there is an emphasis on interdependence rather than independence. For instance, in the United States and Canada there are strong beliefs related to autonomy. In those countries an individual is expected to sign consent forms when receiving health care, whereas in some cultural groups it is another family member who is expected to make health care decisions. For some, there is a valuing of affiliation rather than confrontation, and cooperation rather than

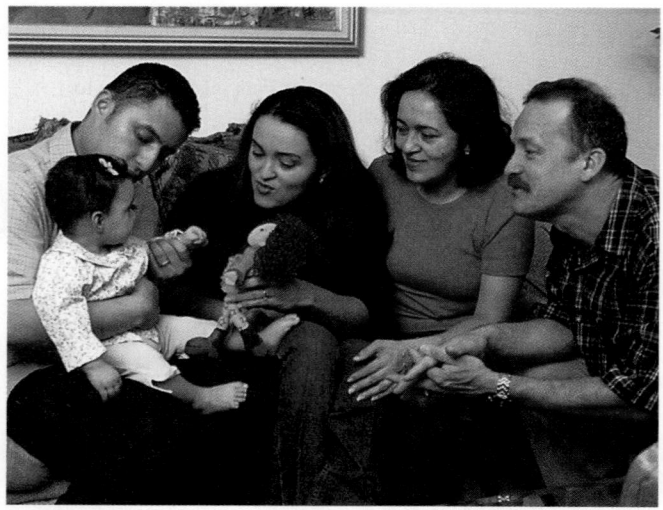

FIG. 2-3 Family roles and relationships differ from one culture to another.

competition. When the nurse encounters a family that values collectivity over individualism, there may be conflicts on how decisions are made. There may be a delay in treatment while the patient waits for significant family members to arrive before giving consent for a procedure or treatment. In other instances, the patient may make a decision that is best for the family but may have negative or adverse consequences for the patient. Being aware of such values will better prepare the nurse to advocate for the patient.

Another factor that is important in family roles is the expectation of who provides care. In some cultures, it is expected that family members will provide care for the patient even in the hospital. The patient may expect that the family or health care providers will provide all care. This expectation is the opposite of the predominant Western expectation that the patient will assume self-care as quickly as possible. There is an expectation that the patient will be discharged home where family members are expected to provide care. In some cultures, there is an expectation that the patient will have all care provided by the nurse or other professional caregiver.

The nurse needs to ask about culturally relevant male-female relationships for a particular culture and observe behaviors of persons from this culture when possible. This is preferable to violating a cultural norm and perhaps undermining the therapeutic relationship. For example, in some cultures it is not appropriate for a man to be alone with a woman other than his wife. This would need to be taken into account when providing care.

Personal Space

Personal space zones were identified by Hall.[15] The *intimate distance* ranges from 0 to 18 inches, and the *personal distance* ranges from 1.5 to 4 feet. The personal distance is the one experienced with friends. Social distance ranges from 4 to 12 feet, and public distance is 12 feet or more. Nurses often interact with their patients in the intimate or personal zones, which might be uncomfortable for the patient.

There is wide variation in the perception of appropriate distances when considering various cultural groups. Whereas an American nurse of European descent may be comfortable with a certain distance, a person from a Hispanic or Middle Eastern background may feel that the distance is too far and will move closer, perhaps causing the nurse to feel uncomfortable. If the nurse then moves away to a more comfortable distance, this may cause the other person to feel that the nurse is unfriendly, or the person may be offended. Personal space distance also varies within cultures. Americans, Canadians, and the British require more personal space than Latin Americans, Japanese, and Arabs.[3]

Touch

Physical contact with patients conveys various meanings depending on the culture. To do a comprehensive assessment, touching a patient is necessary. In some cultures, such as the Arab culture, male health care providers may be prohibited from touching a female patient. Touch is an important aspect of cultural practices, and the nurse needs to be sensitive to this aspect of culture.

Many Asians believe that touching a person's head is a sign of disrespect, especially because the head is believed to be the source of one's strength. *Mal ojo*, or the evil eye, is believed by many people in the world. In this culture-bound syndrome it is believed that the person (usually a child or woman) may become ill as a result of excessive admiration by another person. In some cultures the proper way to ward against the evil eye is to touch the head. In other cultures this would be unacceptable. It is important for the nurse to ask permission before touching anyone, particularly if it is necessary to touch the person's head.

Nutrition

Food is an important part of cultural practices, including both the foods that are eaten and rituals and practices associated with food. Patients may be asked to make major changes in their diets because of health problems. It is important that the health care provider take into account ethnic and cultural practices and habits when helping a patient plan changes. Food pyramids have been developed for many different ethnic groups. They take into account food preferences of those cultures, while still indicating healthy nutritional practices.

When individuals and families immigrate to an area that is very different from their country of origin, they may be faced with unfamiliar foods, food-storage systems, and food-buying habits. They also may be arriving from countries that have limited food supplies because of poverty, wars, and poor sanitation. They may arrive with conditions such as general poor nutrition, hypertension, diarrhea, or other problems such as dental caries. Other problems may develop after the person arrives in the new country. For example, Japanese immigrants to the United States often change their diets to include more saturated fats and cholesterol, leading to increased risks of colon and breast cancer compared with Japanese who live in Japan.[16,17]

Disease Occurrence and Susceptibility to Disease

Differences in occurrence of diseases in different racial and ethnic populations exist in the United States and Canada. African Americans, Hispanics, Native Americans, and certain Pacific Islanders have higher incidences of diabetes than whites.[18] Deaths from diabetes and related complications are higher among Native Americans and African Americans than among whites. Diabetes-associated renal failure is higher among Native Americans than among whites.

Cancer rates also differ by ethnic groups.[18] African Americans are more likely to die of cancer than are whites, Asian Americans, Pacific Islanders, Native Americans, or Hispanics. African American women are more likely to die of breast and colorectal cancers than are women of any other racial and ethnic group. African American men have high death rates for colon, rectum, lung, and prostate cancers. African American males have higher lung cancer death rates than white males. Hispanics have higher rates of cervical, esophageal, gallbladder, and stomach cancers than other population groups in the United States. Asian Americans have higher rates of stomach and liver cancers, and Alaska Natives have higher rates of colorectal cancer. For most cancers, certain racial and ethnic groups have lower survival rates than whites. The rate of breast and lung cancers among Hispanic women is increasing. Hispanic and African American women are diagnosed with these diseases at later stages and have lower survival rates than whites.

Differences among ethnic groups represent both a challenge to understand the reasons and an opportunity to reduce illness and death and to improve survival rates. Disparities in health among ethnic groups is discussed on the *Healthy People 2010* website *(www.health.gov/healthypeople/Document/tableofcontents.htm#partb)*. This site gives the baseline incidences of several diseases and discusses reasons that these disparities may exist. Individual chapters in this book discuss specific ethnic and cultural variations in disease and responses to treatment.

Immigration

Recent immigrants may be at risk for health problems for many reasons. These individuals may be at risk because of preexisting conditions that they have when immigrating, or they may be at increased risk after arriving in a new area. Relocation is associated with many losses and can cause stress and mental distress (Fig. 2-4). Elderly immigrants are especially affected by changes in role and social position and may be more depressed.[3]

Another potential problem is tuberculosis (TB). Asians who have immigrated recently from areas that have a high endemic

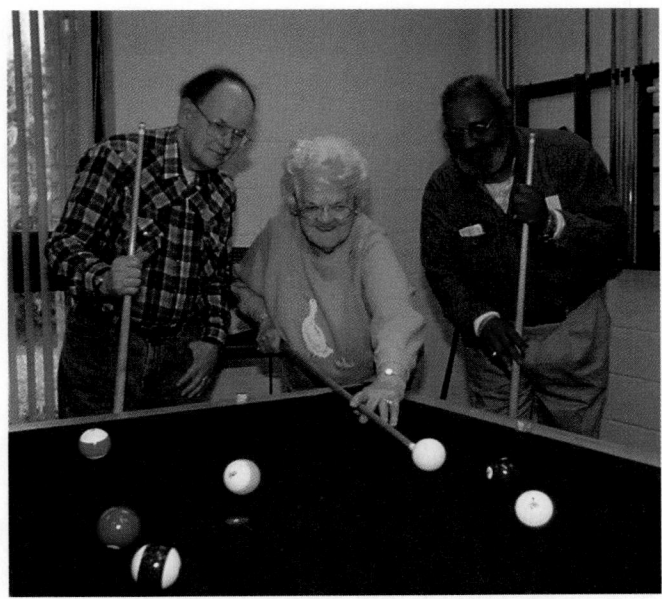

FIG. 2-4   Recently arrived immigrants participate in a common bonding experience.

rate of TB are more likely to have TB. Compared with the general population of the United States, the TB rate is 112 times greater for newly arrived Vietnamese, 60 times greater for Filipinos, 37 times greater for mainland Chinese, and 28 times greater for Koreans.[5]

Medications

Ethnic groups respond differently to some medications (Table 2-5). Compared with whites, Chinese are more sensitive to the effects of β-adrenergic blockers (e.g., propranolol [Inderal]). African Americans are less responsive than whites to the β-adrenergic blockers, especially propanolol, nadolol

TABLE 2-5	Ethnic Differences in Response to Drugs That Affect the Central Nervous System	
COMPARISON GROUPS	**DRUG CLASS EXAMPLE**	**CLINICAL RESPONSE**
Chinese/whites	Benzodiazepines (diazepam [Valium], alprazolam [Xanax])	Chinese require lower doses; more sensitive to sedative effects
Chinese/whites and Hispanics/whites	Antidepressants (imipramine [Tofranil], desipramine [Norpramin], amitriptyline [Elavil])	Chinese and Hispanics require lower doses; side effects greater in Hispanics
Asians/whites	Neuroleptics (e.g., haloperidol [Haldol])	Asians require lower doses
Asian Indians/whites	Analgesics (e.g., acetaminophen, codeine)	Asian Indians have greater clearance rates
Chinese/whites	Analgesics (e.g., codeine)	Chinese less able to metabolize and require increased doses to achieve therapeutic effects
Chinese/whites	Analgesics (e.g., morphine)	Chinese less sensitive to cardiovascular and respiratory effects and more sensitive to gastrointestinal effects
Asians/whites	Alcohol	Asians more sensitive to side effects
Native Americans/whites	Alcohol	Native Americans have faster metabolism and less tolerance

From Levy RA: *Ethnic and racial differences in response to medicines: preserving individualized therapy in managed care pharmaceutical programs*, Reston, Va, 1993, National Pharmaceutical Council.

(Corgard), and atenolol (Tenormin). Chinese may have sensitivity to atropine and increased responses to antidepressants and antiseizure drugs.[3] A small number of Arabs may poorly metabolize antiarrhythmics, antidepressants, β-adrenergic blockers, and opioids (e.g., codeine.) People from different cultural groups experience variations in the response to mydriatic drugs. A person with light-colored eyes may experience wider dilation when given mydriatic drugs than a person with dark eyes. Such variations in physiologic responses require astute assessment and evaluation.

Regardless of their cultural origins, many people use both cultural remedies and prescription drugs to treat their illnesses. Problems can result from interactions of these substances. For example, Chinese Americans who take ginseng as a tonic stimulant and an antihypertensive drug may overmedicate themselves.[2] Some Mexican Americans may treat gastrointestinal problems with preparations that contain lead. Many people now self-treat their depression with St. John's wort, which can result in an overdose if prescription antidepressants are also taken.

Patients may seek care from their traditional cultural healers. They may avoid standard Western medicine until herbal and other remedies are ineffective or the illness becomes acute. The challenge for the nurse is to try to accommodate the patient's need for traditional aspects of care while also using scientific approaches as appropriate and as acceptable to the patient. Evaluating the safety of the traditional cultural healing therapies is an important part of this process.

Psychologic Factors

Symptoms are interpreted through a person's cultural norms and may vary from the recognized allopathic interpretations of Western medicine. All symptoms have meaning, and the meanings may vary from one culture to another. People experience symptoms based on their explanatory models.

Culture-bound syndromes are illnesses or afflictions that are recognized within a cultural group. The symptoms, course of the illness, and people's reactions to the illness are limited to specific cultures. Culture-bound syndromes have their origins in psychosocial characteristics of that culture. For instance, Hispanics may experience *empacho,* a condition described as food forming into a ball that clings to the stomach or intestines, causing pain and cramping. Empacho is treated by folk remedies such as strong massage over the stomach, use of medications, or gently pinching and rubbing the spine.[11] Anorexia nervosa and bulimia have been described as Western culture-bound syndromes because they are predominantly found in those cultures.[3] Another culture-bound syndrome is *susto,* which is found throughout Latin America. Susto, sometimes referred to as "fright sickness" or "soul loss," is a traumatic anxiety-depressive state that may result from a frightening experience, such as a loud sound or some threat. Susto can cause anxiety, insomnia, listlessness, loss of appetite, and social withdrawal.[2] One treatment for susto is to have the affected person lie on the floor. The healer then sweeps indigenous herbs over the patient's body. See Table 2-6 for descriptions of other culture-bound syndromes.

Dermatologic Variations

Differences in skin color require the nurse to be astute in assessment skills. In addition to differences in assessing dark and light skin for signs of jaundice or cyanosis, the nurse should be

TABLE 2-6	Culture-Bound Syndromes
SYNDROME	**DESCRIPTION**
Bilis or colera	Caused by strongly experienced anger or rage. Many Latino groups believe that anger affects the body balance of hot and cold. Symptoms include acute nervous tension, headache, trembling, screaming, stomach disturbances, and, in severe cases, loss of consciousness.
Brain fag	West African term describing brain "fatigue" caused by the challenges of school. Symptoms include difficulties in concentrating, remembering, and thinking.
Falling out	Characterized by a sudden collapse, which may sometimes be preceded by dizziness or "swimming" in the head. The person can hear but is unable to move. Occurs primarily in southern United States and Caribbean groups.
Ghost sickness	Among Native Americans this condition is sometimes associated with witchcraft and a preoccupation with death. Symptoms include bad dreams, weakness, feelings of fear, danger, futility, dizziness, and a sense of suffocation.
Nervios	Many cultures have conditions involving "nerves." In the Latino population nervios may be brought on by difficult life experiences. Symptoms may include headaches or "brain aches," irritability, stomach and sleep disturbances, and an inability to concentrate.
Shenjing shuairuo	In China this condition is characterized by physical and mental fatigue, headaches and other pains, dizziness, sleep disturbances, and concentration difficulties.

aware of conditions that are specific to different ethnic groups. For instance, *keloids* (an overgrowth of scar tissue) may be present in dark-skinned people. The mongolian spot is a common hyperpigmentation among African American, Asian American, Native American, and Hispanic newborns.[5] Specific information related to skin assessment for different populations is discussed in Chapter 22.

Pain

Each culture has its own beliefs and ways of defining, expressing, and managing pain. Some people perceive pain as a sign of illness or disease. Some cultural groups have beliefs that pain and suffering are inevitable and should be endured. This is true for some African Americans and Hispanics. Filipinos may consider the acceptance of pain as living an honorable life. Consequently, they may not ask for pain medications. They may perceive the health care providers to be busy and would not want to add to their work by asking for medications. Individuals from other groups (e.g., Arabs) believe that pain is something to be controlled, and they would expect immediate relief. Chinese patients may describe their pain in terms that are different from those used by European Americans. Their description may be more diffuse and use terms such as *dull* rather than *stabbing*. They may also tend to treat pain externally using oils and massage. They may describe the pain and its causes based on imbalances of yin and yang.

NURSING MANAGEMENT
CULTURALLY COMPETENT CARE

■ Nurse's Self-Assessment

The first step in providing culturally competent care is for nurses to assess their own cultural background, values, and beliefs, especially those related to health and health care.[19] Many tools are available to assist in this process. Table 2-2 suggests ways to improve cultural competence. This information can help the nurse to better understand patients and provide more culturally competent and relevant care. Many other important aspects of culture related to health care are included in the Culturally Competent Care sections throughout this book.

■ Patient Assessment

A cultural assessment should be included in the nursing process. In some institutions, this assessment may involve a specific cultural assessment guide. An example of a cultural assessment guide is included in Table 2-3. It is important to determine (1) the patient's health beliefs and health care practices and (2) the patient's perspective of the meaning, cause, and preferred treatment of illness. When this is done, it will increase the likelihood of successful outcomes for both the nurse and the patient.

How is the nurse to be aware of the differences among ethnic groups? Using guides to cultural assessment will facilitate the nursing process when working with patients, families, or other groups who are from different cultures. Although pocket guides can assist in this process, nurses must be careful not to stereotype using these tools. Guides can be used to explore the degree to which patients share commonalities with the cultural information generally attributed to their cultural group.[18] Ultimately, it is most important to identify potential similarities and differences that can assist the nurse to deliver culturally relevant health care.

■ Nursing Implementation

Communication. Effective communication is most likely to occur when meanings are mutually understood, whether that communication is through gestures, spoken words, or voice tones. To show respect for the patient, any communication should take into account the patient's usual communication style. For instance, a health history should start out in an unhurried manner, and it should include acceptable social and cultural amenities appropriate for the culture. In some cultures it is best to start with general rather than direct questions. For some cultures it is most effective to engage in "small talk," with the discussion including answers that may seem to be unrelated to the questions. If the nurse appears to be "too busy," communication may be impaired.

When meeting a patient or family members, it is appropriate for nurses to introduce themselves and indicate how the patient should address them. Indicate if the patient should use first names, Mr., Ms., or Mrs., or a title, such as nurse. Ask the patient how he or she prefers to be addressed also. This shows respect and will assist the nurse to begin the relationship in a culturally appropriate manner.

If the nurse needs to gather personal information, it is important to understand the most effective approach to use. For instance, when talking with people from some cultural groups, it is imperative that the nurse takes time to establish trust and listen to the patient's responses to questions. There may be long (by American standards) silences as the person thinks about the question, taking time to show respect by giving the question the appropriate consideration before answering. In some cultures (Ojibwa and Western Apache) it would be acceptable to take a few days or weeks to properly answer a question. Clearly, most health care situations do not facilitate such answers. However, the nurse can take the time to listen and help establish trust.

Silence has many meanings, and it is important for the nurse to understand the nature of the meaning of silence for different cultural groups. It is important to clarify what silence means in an interaction with a patient. Patients will sometimes nod their head, or say "yes" as if agreeing with the nurse or to indicate they understand, when actually they are doing this out of their culturally acceptable manner of showing respect, and may not understand at all.

Some cultures, such as the Hmong, rely primarily on oral communication. When working with patients who are from an oral culture, it would be important to include oral instructions during the teaching-learning process.[4]

Learning to speak the language of patients is an important way to improve interactions. The nurse must be cautious and not try to serve as an interpreter if he or she does not have a command of the language, because this could lead to misunderstandings. When the nurse cannot speak the patient's primary language, it is important to enlist the assistance of a person who is qualified to do medical interpretation (Table 2-7). Table 2-8 provides guidelines for communicating when no interpreter is avail-

---

TABLE 2-7	Using a Medical Interpreter

Choosing an Interpreter
- Use an agency interpreter if possible.
- Interpreter should be a trained medical interpreter who knows how to interpret, has a health care background, understands patient's rights, and can help with advice about the cultural relevance or appropriateness of the health care plan and instructions.
- Use a family member if necessary. Be aware that there may be limitations if the family member does not understand medical terms, is younger or a different gender than the patient, or is not aware of the health care procedures or medical ethics.
- Interpreter should be able to do the following:
  - Translate the nonverbal as well as the literal translation.
  - Translate the message into understandable terms.
  - Act as a patient advocate to represent the patient's needs to the nurse.
- Be culturally sensitive and understand how to provide teaching instructions.

Strategies for Working with an Interpreter
- If possible, the interpreter should meet with the patient ahead of time to establish rapport before the interpreting begins.
- Use simple language, using as few medical terms as possible.
- Speak in one to two sentences to allow for easier translation.
- Obtain feedback to be sure the patient understands.

TABLE 2-8   Guidelines for Communicating when No Interpreter Is Available

1. Be polite and formal.
2. Pronounce name correctly. Use proper titles of respect, such as "Mr.," "Mrs.," "Ms.," "Dr." Greet the person using the last or complete name.
   Gesture to yourself and say your name.
   Offer a handshake or nod. Smile.
3. Proceed in an unhurried manner. Pay attention to any effort by the patient or family to communicate.
4. Speak in a low, moderate voice. Avoid talking loudly. Remember that there is a tendency to raise the volume and pitch of your voice when the listener appears not to understand. The listener may perceive that you are shouting and/or angry.
5. Use any words that you might know in the person's language. This indicates that you are aware of and respect his or her culture.
6. Use simple words, such as "pain" instead of "discomfort." Avoid medical jargon, idioms, and slang. Avoid using contractions (e.g., don't, can't, won't). Use nouns repeatedly instead of pronouns.
   Example:
   Do not say: "He has been taking his medicine, hasn't he?"
   Do say: "Does Juan take medicine?"
7. Pantomime words and simple actions while you verbalize them.
8. Give instructions in the proper sequence.
   Example:
   Do not say: "Before you rinse the bottle, sterilize it."
   Do say: "First wash the bottle. Second, rinse the bottle."
9. Discuss one topic at a time. Avoid using conjunctions.
   Example:
   Do not say: "Are you cold and in pain?"
   Do say: "Are you cold (while pantomiming)? Are you in pain?"
10. Validate if the person understands by having him or her repeat instructions, demonstrate the procedure, or act out the meaning.
11. Write out several short sentences in English and determine the person's ability to read them.
12. Try a third language. Many Indochinese speak French. Europeans often know two or more languages. Try Latin words or phrases.
13. Ask who among the person's family and friends could serve as an interpreter.
14. Obtain phrase books from a library or bookstore, make or purchase flash cards, contact hospitals for a list of interpreters, and use both a formal and an informal network to locate a suitable interpreter.

From Jarvis C: *Physical examination and health assessment*, ed 4, Philadelphia, 2004, WB Saunders.

able. With the large number of immigrants and the many different cultural groups in the United States and Canada, it is highly likely that the nurse will encounter patients who do not speak the dominant language.

Using a dictionary that translates from both the nurse's language and the patient's language is helpful (e.g., Spanish-English and English-Spanish dictionary). The nurse can look up ques-

tions and potential answers in several different languages using these types of dictionaries. One helpful approach would be to have these types of resources for those cultural groups who frequently use the health care facility. This would be especially beneficial for those instances when a qualified medical interpreter is not readily available and nurses need to learn important phrases in another language.

REVIEW QUESTIONS

The number of the question corresponds to the same-numbered objective at the beginning of the chapter.

1. Forcing one's own cultural beliefs and practices on another person is an example of
   a. stereotyping.
   b. ethnocentrism.
   c. cultural relativity.
   d. cultural imposition.
2. Immigration may potentially affect an individual's health in all of the following instances *except*
   a. The nurse might misinterpret silences during a nurse-patient interaction.
   b. Immigrants may be faced with unfamiliar foods, food-storage systems, and food-buying habits.
   c. Traditional health care practices such as cupping or coining may be misinterpreted as physical abuse.
   d. Immigrants are rarely affected by changes when they move to an area that has a different physical environment.

3. Which of the following most accurately describes cultural factors that may affect health?
   a. Diabetes and cancer rates differ by cultural/ethnic groups.
   b. Most patients find that religious rituals help them during times of illness.
   c. There is limited ethnic variation in physiologic responses to medications.
   d. Silence during a nurse-patient interaction usually means that the patient understands the instructions.
4. When communicating with a patient who speaks a language that the nurse does not understand, it is important to first attempt to
   a. have a family member translate.
   b. use a trained medical interpreter.
   c. use specific medical terminology so there will be no mistakes.
   d. focus on the translation rather than nonverbal communication.

Continued

REVIEW QUESTIONS—cont'd

5. Which of the following accurately reflects a physiologic aspect of culture/ethnicity to consider when providing nursing care?
   a. Mongolian spots seldom occur in the African American population.
   b. Chinese Americans may have increased responses to antidepressants and neuroleptics.
   c. There are no differences between death rates from diabetes and related complications for African Americans and whites.
   d. When mydriatic medications are used, a person with dark-colored eyes is likely to have wider pupil dilation than a person with light-colored eyes.

6. Which of the following is the first step in developing cultural competence?
   a. explore the patient's explanatory model
   b. create opportunities to interact with a variety of cultural groups
   c. examine one's own cultural background, values, and beliefs about health and health care
   d. learn assessment skills for different cultural groups, including cultural beliefs and practices and physical assessments

7. As part of the nursing process, cultural assessment is best accomplished by
   a. using a cultural assessment guide as part of the nursing process.
   b. seeking guidance from a nurse from the patient's cultural background.
   c. consulting a cultural pocket guide for general information about a specific culture.
   d. relying on the nurse's previous experience with patients from that cultural group.

REFERENCES

1. American Nurses Association: *Today's registered nurse—numbers and demographics,* 1997. Available at *www.ana.org/readroom/fsdemogr.htm.* (accessed March 21, 2002).
2. Giger JN, Davidhizar RE: *Transcultural nursing: assessment and intervention,* ed 3, St Louis, 1999, Mosby.
3. Andrews MM, Boyle JS: *Transcultural concepts in nursing care,* ed 3, Philadelphia, 1999, Lippincott.
4. Davidhizar RE, Giger JN: *Canadian transcultural nursing: assessment and intervention,* St Louis, 1999, Mosby.
5. Jarvis C: *Physical examination and health assessment,* ed 3, Philadelphia, 2000, WB Saunders.
6. Purnell LD, Paulanka BJ: *Transcultural health care: a culturally competent approach,* Philadelphia, 1998, FA Davis.
7. Huff RM, Kline MV: *Promoting health in multicultural populations: a handbook for practitioners,* Thousand Oaks, Calif, 1999, Sage Publications.
8. Leininger MM: *Transcultural nursing: concepts, theories, research, and practices,* New York, 1995, McGraw-Hill.
9. Campinha-Bacote J: The quest for cultural competence in nursing care, *Nurs Forum* 30:19, 1995.
10. Wells MI: Beyond cultural competence: a model for individual and institutional cultural development, *J Community Health Nurs* 17:189, 2000.
11. Spector RE: *Cultural diversity in health and illness,* ed 5, Upper Saddle River, NJ, 2000, Prentice Hall Health.
*12. Emblen JD, Halstead L: Spiritual needs and interventions: comparing the views of patients, nurses, and chaplains, *Clin Nurse Spec* 7:175, 1993.
13. Taylor EJ: *Spiritual care: nursing theory, research, and practice,* Upper Saddle River, NJ, 2002, Prentice Hall.
14. Lapierre ED, Padgett J: How can we become more aware of culturally specific body language and use this awareness therapeutically? *J Psychosoc Nurs* 29:38, 1991.
15. Hall E: Proxemics: the study of man's spatial relationships. In Gladstone I, editor: *Man's image in medicine and anthropology,* New York, 1963, New York International University Press.
16. Hunter J, Willett WC: Nutrition and breast cancer, *Cancer Causes Control* 7:56, 1996.
17. Potter JD: Nutrition and colorectal cancer, *Cancer Causes Control* 7:127, 1996.
18. Geissler EM: *Mosby's pocket guide to cultural assessment,* ed 2, St Louis, 1999, Mosby.
19. Campinha-Bacote J: A model and instrument for addressing cultural competence in health care, *J Nurs Educ* 38:203, 1999.

RESOURCES

EthnoMed
Harborview Medical Center
University of Washington
325 Ninth Avenue
Seattle, WA 98104
206-731-3000
www.ethnomed.org

Office of Minority Health Resource Center
P.O. Box 37337
Washington, DC 20013-7337
800-444-6472
Fax: 301-230-7198
www.omhrc.gov/

Transcultural Nursing Society
36600 Schoolcraft Road
Livonia, MI 48150-1173
734-432-5470
888-432-5470
Fax: 734-432-5463
www.tcns.org/

For additional Internet resources, see the website for this book at *http://evolve.elsevier.com/Lewis/medsurg/.*

---

*Nursing research–based reference.

CHAPTER *3*

Health History and Physical Examination

Sheila A. Dunn

LEARNING OBJECTIVES

1. Explain the purpose, components, and techniques related to a patient's health history and physical examination.
2. Obtain a nursing history using a functional health pattern format.
3. Describe the appropriate use and techniques of inspection, palpation, percussion, and auscultation.
4. Identify the equipment needed to perform a physical examination.
5. Describe the indications, purposes, and components of the branching or regional examination.
6. Record a nursing history and physical examination using a standard format.

KEY TERMS

auscultation, p. 37
branching (regional) examination, p. 36
database, p. 30
functional health patterns, p. 32
general survey statement, p. 36
inspection, p. 37
medical history, p. 30
negative finding, p. 36

nursing history, p. 30
objective data, p. 31
palpation, p. 37
percussion, p. 37
physical examination, p. 36
positive finding, p. 36
screening physical examination, p. 36
subjective data, p. 30

Obtaining a patient's health history and performing a physical examination are activities completed by the nurse during the assessment phase of the nursing process. The information obtained during this phase contributes to a database that identifies the patient's current and past health state and provides a baseline against which future changes can be evaluated. The purpose of the nursing assessment is to enable the nurse to make a judgment or diagnosis about the patient's health state.[1] Although assessment is identified as the first step of the nursing process, it is performed continuously throughout the nursing process to validate diagnoses, evaluate the patient's response to nursing interventions, and determine the extent to which patient outcomes and goals have been met.

DATA COLLECTION

Collection of data about the patient is not solely the nurse's responsibility. The **database** is all the health information about a patient. It includes the nursing history and physical examination, the physician's history and physical examination, results of laboratory and diagnostic tests, and information contributed by other health professionals. Numerous approaches and formats exist for gathering information about the patient in various health care settings. The purpose for which the information is to be used determines the methods of data collection. The nurse and physician

both perform a patient history and physical examination, but they use different formats and analyze the data differently because of each discipline's focus.

Medical Focus

A **medical history** is a standard format designed to collect data to be used primarily by the physician to determine risk for disease and diagnose a medical condition (Table 3-1). The medical history is usually collected by a member of the medical team (physician, resident, physician's assistant, or medical student) or a nurse practitioner. The physician's physical examination and laboratory and diagnostic tests assist in establishing a medical diagnosis and evaluating specific medical therapy. The information collected and reported by the physician is also used by nurses and other health care providers, but within the focus of their care. For example, the abnormal results of a neurologic examination by a physician may assist in the diagnosis of a brain lesion, but the nurse may use those same results to identify a nursing diagnosis of risk for falls. The physical therapist may also use the results to plan therapy involving exercise, splints, or ambulatory aids.

Nursing Focus

The focus of nursing care is the diagnosis and treatment of human responses to actual or potential health problems. The information obtained from the **nursing history** and physical examination is used to determine what responses the patient is exhibiting or could potentially exhibit as a result of a health problem. The nurse is interested in the functional capabilities of the patient. In the patient with a medical diagnosis of congestive heart failure, the patient's response may be anxiety or a lack of energy to carry out normal daily activities. These are human responses to the heart failure that can be diagnosed and treated by nurses. During the nursing history interview and physical examination the nurse obtains the necessary data to support the identification of nursing diagnoses.

Types of Data

The database includes both subjective and objective data. **Subjective data** are collected by interviewing the patient during the nursing history. It includes information that can only be de-

---

Reviewed by Joanne M. Bartram, RN, MS, CFNP, Family Nurse Practitioner, Lovelace Health Systems, Albuquerque, N.M.

TABLE 3-1	Medical History Format
Demographic data
Chief complaint
History of present illness
Past health history
Family health history
Review of systems

scribed or verified by the patient. It is what the person tells the nurse about himself or herself either as spontaneously offered information or as a response to direct questioning. Subjective data are also referred to as *symptoms*. Knowledgeable others, such as family members and caregivers, can also contribute subjective data about the patient.

Objective data are data that can be observed and measured. These types of data are obtained using inspection, palpation, percussion, and auscultation during the physical examination. Objective data are also provided by other health care providers and diagnostic testing. Objective data are also called *signs*. Although subjective data are usually obtained by interview and objective data are obtained by physical examination, it is common for the patient to provide subjective data while the nurse is performing the physical examination, and it is also common for the nurse to observe objective signs while interviewing the patient during the history.

Interviewing Considerations

The purpose of the patient interview is to obtain subjective data about the patient's past and present health state. Collection of data assists the nurse and the patient in identifying health problems, as well as patient strengths and resources. The nurse can use the data to identify areas where the patient may be unable to meet personal needs and therefore requires nursing assistance. The patient perceives this encounter as an indication of how the health care system will provide assistance.

Effective communication is a key factor in the interview process. Creating a climate of trust and respect is critical to establishing a therapeutic relationship.[2] The nurse must communicate acceptance of the patient as an individual by using an open, responsive, nonjudgmental approach. Individuals communicate not only through language but also in their manner of dress, gestures, and body language. Modes of communication are learned through one's culture, influencing not only the words, gestures, and posture one uses, but also the nature of information that is shared with others (see Chapter 2). In addition to understanding the principles of effective communication, each nurse must develop a personal style of relating to patients. Although no single style fits all people, wording specific questions in certain ways will increase the probability of eliciting the needed information. Ease at asking questions, particularly those related to sensitive areas such as sexual functioning and economic status, comes with experience. Videotaping interviews (with the patient's permission) and reviewing the interviews is an effective method to use to evaluate one's communication techniques and identify areas needing improvement.

The amount of time needed to complete a nursing history may vary with the format used and the experience of the nurse. It may be completed in one or several sessions, depending on the setting and the patient. In the case of an older adult patient with a low energy level, several short sessions may need to be scheduled. Allowing time for the patient to volunteer information about particular areas of concern enables the nurse to work with the patient to identify existing and potential health problems. When a patient is unable to provide the necessary data (e.g., is unconscious or aphasic), the nurse should ask the person who has assumed responsibility for the patient's welfare to provide as much information as possible.

Before beginning the nursing history, the nurse should explain to the patient that the purpose of a detailed history is to collect information that will provide a health profile for comprehensive health care, including health promotion. This detailed information is collected during entry into the health care system, and subsequently, only updates are needed. The nurse should explain that personal and social data are needed to individualize the plan of care. This explanation is necessary because the patient may not be accustomed to sharing personal information and may need to know the purpose of such questioning. The nurse should assure the patient that all information will be kept confidential.

To obtain factual, easily categorized information a direct interview technique can be used. Closed questions such as "Have you had surgery before?" that require brief, specific responses are used. When asking sensitive personal and social questions, the nurse can communicate the acceptance or normalcy of behaviors by prefacing questions with phrases such as "most people" or "frequently." For example, stating, "Most people have sexual concerns; do you have any you would like to discuss?" shows the patient that a particular situation may not be unique to that patient. Another method of putting the patient at ease is to word the question so that an affirmative answer appears expected. An example of this technique is to ask, "What do you like to drink at a party?" instead of, "Do you drink?" "How often do you drink alcohol?" is another way of obtaining information related to alcohol intake. These questions are open ended, encouraging the patient to discuss the issue in the patient's own words and at his or her own pace.[3]

The nurse must judge the reliability of the patient as a historian. An older adult may give a false impression about his or her mental status because of a prolonged response time or visual and hearing impairment. The complexity and long duration of health problems may also make it difficult for an older adult to be an accurate, orderly historian.

It is important that the nurse determine the patient's priority concerns and expectations from the present encounter. Often there is a lack of congruency between the priorities of the patient and the nurse. For example, the priority for the nurse might be to get a consent form signed, whereas the patient is interested only in getting relief from pain. Until the patient's priority need is met, the nurse will probably be unsuccessful in meeting the priority goal.

The amount of information that should be collected on initial contact with the patient is a nursing judgment based on the patient, the problem, and the setting. Interviews with older adult patients, patients with long-term chronic disease, and emergency department admissions are examples of situations in which the nurse must use this judgment. The nurse may choose to ask only those questions that are pertinent to a specific problem and to defer the complete history interview until a more appropriate time.

Symptom Investigation

At any time during assessment the patient may relate a symptom such as pain, fatigue, or weakness. Because symptoms are directly experienced by the patient and not observable to the nurse, the symptom must be investigated. Table 3-2 lists eight areas that should be investigated if a symptom is present. The information that is obtained may help determine the cause of the symptom. For example, if a patient states that he has "pain in his leg at times," the nurse would obtain and record the following information:

> Has right midcalf pain (location), described as "like being stabbed with a knife" (quality). Pain is so severe that it is not possible for the patient to continue walking (quantity). Onset is abrupt, lasting for 1 to 2 minutes; it occurs once or twice daily, and it last occurred on 5/5/03 (chronology). Generally occurs at work when climbing stairs after lunch, but last occurred when cutting lawn (setting). Pain is alleviated by rest for 2 to 3 minutes. The patient has been salting his food "more heavily" than he used to, but "it doesn't help" (alleviating factor). Leg pain is at times accompanied by chest pain that causes some nausea (associated manifestations). The patient has not altered his lifestyle because of the intermittent pain. He thinks it is caused by "muscle cramps from lack of salt" (personal meaning).

NURSING HISTORY: SUBJECTIVE DATA

The format used in this text for obtaining a nursing history includes an initial collection of important health information followed by assessment of the patient's **functional health patterns** (Table 3-3). Gordon has described an assessment format in which subjective data are collected during assessment of specific functional areas.[1] The format is designed to promote systematic data collection to determine the presence of problems amenable to nursing diagnosis and treatment. Analysis of the data collected with assessment of each functional health pattern facilitates the nursing diagnosis process.

Important Health Information

Important health information provides an overview of past and present medical conditions and treatments. Past health history, medications, and surgery or other treatments are included in this part of the history.

Past Health History. The past health history provides information about the patient's prior state of health. The patient is specifically asked about major childhood and adult illnesses, injuries, hospitalizations, operations, therapeutic regimens, travel, habits, and the use of supportive devices. Specific questioning is more effective than simply asking if the patient has had any illness or health problems in the past.

Medications. Specific details related to past or present medications are obtained. This includes the use of prescription drugs, over-the-counter drugs, vitamins, herbal products, and dietary supplements. Patients frequently do not consider herbal products and dietary supplements as drugs. Because they can interact adversely with existing medications, it is important to specifically ask about their use. (See Complementary and Alternative Therapies box on p. 34.) Examples of specific prescription and over-the-counter medications to ask about include corticosteroids, birth control pills, antibiotics, diuretics, aspirin, antacids, and laxatives. Older adult patients, in particular, should be questioned about medication routines. Changes in absorption, metabolism, reaction to drugs, and elimination of drugs, as well as surgery and concurrent disease, make drug-related concerns a serious potential problem for older adults.[4]

Surgery or Other Treatments. All injuries, hospitalizations, and surgeries are recorded along with the date of the event, the treatment, and the outcome (whether the problem was completely resolved). Blood transfusions received by the patient also are noted.

TABLE 3-2	Investigation of a Symptom
Location	
Ask	"Where do you feel it? Where is it located?"
Record	Region of the body Local or radiating, superficial or deep
Quality	
Ask	"What does it (feel, look) like?"
Record	The patient's analogy (e.g., "Like being burned")
Quantity	
Ask	"How often do you have this feeling? How bad is it? How much is it? How big is it?"
Record	Frequency (mild, moderate, severe), volume, size, extent, number
Chronology	
Ask	"When was the first time it occurred? Any particular time of day, week, month, or year?"
Record	Time of onset, duration, periodicity and frequency, course of symptoms
Setting	
Ask	"Where are you when this occurs? What are you doing?"
Record	Where patient is when symptom occurs, what patient is doing, if symptom is related to anything
Aggravating or Alleviating Factors	
Ask	"What makes it better? Worse? Is there any activity that seems to cause it? What have you done for it? Did it help? Was there some reason you didn't do anything about it?"
Record	Influence of physical and emotional activities, patient's attempts to alleviate (or treat) the symptom
Associated Manifestations	
Ask	"What other things do you see or feel when it occurs? Has it affected your appetite? Elimination? Sleeping?"
Record	Other symptoms
Meaning of the Symptom to the Patient	
Ask	"How has it affected your life? Why have you sought care now? What do you think may be the cause?"
Record	Patient's statements about the effect of the symptom and the cause of the symptom

TABLE 3-3	Nursing History: Functional Health Pattern Format

Demographic Data
Name, address, age, occupation
Culture and ethnicity

Important Health Information
Past health history
Medications
Surgery or other treatments

Functional Health Patterns
Health Perception–Health Management Pattern
1. Reason for visit?
2. General state of health?
3. Any colds in past year?
4. Most important things done to keep healthy? Breast self-examination? Testicular self-examination? Other routine screening?
5. Health compliance problems?
6. Cause of illness? Action taken? Results?
7. Things important to you while here?
8. Family health history?
9. Illness and injury risk factors: use of cigarettes, alcohol, drugs?
10. Allergies? Immunizations?

Nutritional-Metabolic Pattern
1. Typical daily food intake (describe)? Supplements?
2. Typical daily fluid intake (describe)?
3. Weight loss or gain (amount, time span)?
4. Desired weight?
5. Appetite?
6. Food or eating: Discomfort? Diet restrictions?
7. Appetite?
8. Heal well or poorly?
9. Skin problems: Lesions? Dryness?
10. Dental problems?
11. Change in appetite with anxiety?
12. Food preferences?
13. Food allergies?

Elimination Pattern
1. Bowel elimination pattern (describe): Frequency? Character? Discomfort? Laxatives? Enemas?
2. Urinary elimination pattern (describe): Frequency? Problem in control? Diuretics?
3. Any external devices?
4. Excess perspiration? Odor problems? Itching?

Activity-Exercise Pattern
1. Sufficient energy for desired or required activities?
2. Exercise pattern? Type? Regularity?
3. Spare time (leisure) activities?
4. Dyspnea? Chest pain? Palpitations? Stiffness? Aching? Weakness?
5. Perceived ability for (code for level):

    Feeding _____   Cooking _____   Grooming _____
    Bed mobility _____ Bathing _____   Dressing _____
    Toileting _____   Shopping _____   General mobility _____

Functional Levels Code
Level 0: Full self-care
Level I: Requires use of equipment or device
Level II: Requires assistance or supervision from another person
Level III: Is dependent and does not participate

Sleep-Rest Pattern
1. Generally rested and ready for daily activities after sleep?
2. Sleep onset problems? Aids? Dreams (nightmares)? Early awakening?
3. Usual sleep rituals?
4. Usual sleep pattern?

Cognitive-Perceptual Pattern
1. Hearing difficulty? Hearing aids?
2. Vision? Wear glasses? Last checked?
3. Any change in taste? Any change in smell?
4. Any recent change in memory?
5. Easiest way to learn things?
6. Any discomfort? Pain? How managed?
7. Ability to communicate?
8. Understanding of illness?
9. Understanding of treatments?

Self-Perception–Self-Concept Pattern
1. Self-description? Self-perception?
2. Effect of illness on self-image?
3. Relieving factors?

Role-Relationship Pattern
1. Live alone? Family? Family structure diagram?
2. Difficult family problems?
3. Family problem solving?
4. Family dependence on you for things? How managing?
5. Family's and others' feelings about illness/hospitalization?*
6. Problems with children? Difficulty handling?*
7. Belong to social groups? Have close friends? Feel lonely (frequency)?
8. Work satisfaction (school)? Income sufficient for needs?*
9. Feel part of or isolated from neighborhood where living?

Sexuality-Reproductive Pattern
1. Any changes or problems in sexual relations?*
2. Effect of illness?
3. Use of contraceptives? Problems?
4. When menstruation started? Last menstrual period? Menstrual problems? Gravida? Para?†
5. Effect of present condition or treatment on sexuality?
6. Sexually transmitted diseases?

Coping–Stress Tolerance Pattern
1. Tense a lot of the time? What helps? Use any medicines, drugs, alcohol?
2. Have someone to confide in? Available to you now?
3. Recent life changes?
4. Problem-solving techniques? Effective?

Value-Belief Pattern
1. Satisfied with life?
2. Religion important in your life?
3. Conflict between treatment and beliefs?

Other
1. Other important issues?
2. Questions?

Modified from Fuller J, Schaller-Ayers J: *Health assessment: a nursing approach*, ed 3, Philadelphia, 1999, Lippincott.
*If appropriate.
†For women.

COMPLEMENTARY & ALTERNATIVE THERAPIES
Assessment of Use of Herbal Products and Dietary Supplements

- Herbal products and dietary supplements may have side effects and/or may interact adversely with existing medications.
- Most patients do not tell health care providers that they are using herbal preparations and dietary supplements. They may fear health care professionals will disapprove of their use.
- Available forms include pills, capsules, tinctures, powders, teas, ointments, and suppositories.
- Patients at high risk for drug–herb interactions include those taking anticoagulant, antihypertensive, or immune–regulating therapy and patients receiving anesthesia for surgery.
- Nurses should create an accepting and nonjudgmental environment when assessing use of or interest in herbal products or dietary supplements.
- Use open-ended questions such as "What types of herbs, vitamins, or supplements do you take?" and "What effects have you noticed from using them?"
- Respond to patients with comments that invite an open-minded discussion.
- Avoid using the term "alternative therapy" because they may not consider what they are doing to be alternative.
- Many herbal preparations contain a variety of ingredients. Therefore the nurse may need to ask the patient or family members to bring labeled containers to the health care site to determine the composition of the products.
- Documentation of any herbal product(s) or dietary supplements used should be recorded in the patient database.

Functional Health Patterns

The nurse assesses the patient's functional health patterns to identify patient strengths in function and to determine if dysfunctional health patterns and/or potential dysfunctional patterns exist. Dysfunctional health patterns result in nursing diagnoses, and potential dysfunctional patterns identify risk conditions for problems. Use of the functional health pattern framework for assessment assists the nurse in differentiating between areas for independent nursing intervention and areas requiring collaboration or referral. Table 3-4 presents an overview of the content usually included in each functional health pattern.

Health Perception–Health Management Pattern. Assessment of the health perception–health management functional health pattern focuses on the patient's perceived level of health and well-being and on personal practices for maintaining health. This includes preventive screening activities, such as breast and testicular examinations; colorectal cancer, hypertension, and cardiac risk factor screening; Papanicolaou (Pap) test; and immunizations such as tetanus, pneumonia, and flu vaccines. The nurse should ask about the type of health care provider that the patient uses. Culture may play a role in who is the patient's primary health care provider. For example, if the patient is Native American, a medicine man may be considered as the primary health care provider. If the patient is of Hispanic origin, a curandero (Hispanic healer who uses folk medicine, herbal products, and/or magic to treat patients) may be the primary health care provider.

The questions for this pattern also seek to identify risk factors by obtaining a family history, history of health habits (e.g., smoking, alcohol, drug use), and exposure to environmental hazards.

There are several ways to identify the patient's perceived level of health and well-being. First, when questioning the patient, the nurse determines the patient's feelings of effectiveness at staying healthy by asking what helps and what hinders.

Next, the patient is asked to describe personal health and any concerns about it. This information should be recorded in the patient's own words. It often is useful to determine whether the patient considers his or her health to be excellent, good, fair, or poor.

In addition, the patient is asked about a family history of major problems, such as cardiovascular disease, hypertension, cancer, diabetes mellitus, psychiatric illness, and genetic disorders. Information about sexual abuse, violence, and drug and alcohol use/abuse should also be obtained. One of the objectives in this pattern is to identify any preventive measures used by the patient to promote personal health.

If the patient is hospitalized, expectations of this hospitalization should be determined. A description of the patient's understanding of the current health problem, including a description of its onset, course, and treatment, should be obtained. Determining what the patient does when ill is important. These questions elicit information about a patient's knowledge of the health problem, awareness of what should be done, and ability to use appropriate resources to manage the problem.

Nutritional-Metabolic Pattern. The processes of ingestion, digestion, absorption, and metabolism are assessed in this pattern. A 24-hour dietary recall should be obtained from the patient. From this information the nurse can evaluate the quantity and quality of foods and fluids consumed. If a problem is identified, the nurse may request that the patient keep a 3-day food diary for a more careful analysis of dietary intake. Food frequency questionnaires based on weekly intake are also available to obtain information from the person. Metabolism is evaluated by questioning the patient regarding weight gain, weight loss, energy level, and skin lesions or dryness.

The impact of psychologic factors such as depression, anxiety, and self-concept on nutrition is assessed. For example, "How is your appetite affected by anxiety?" is an appropriate question. Sociocultural factors such as food budget, who prepares the meals, and food preferences are also assessed.

Determining how the patient's present condition has interfered with eating and appetite is important. If the patient's present condition has produced symptoms such as nausea, gas, or pain, the effect of these symptoms on appetite should be determined. Food allergies and the need for a special or restricted diet should be noted. Additional information about the person's nutritional status can be determined by asking specific questions such as the following:

"How many fruits and vegetables do you eat a day?"
"Give me an example of your usual intake of meat."
"How well do you heal from a wound?"

Elimination Pattern. The nurse assesses bowel, bladder, and skin function in this pattern. The nurse asks about the frequency of bowel and bladder activity. A description of consistency, amount, color, and unusual odor should be elicited. The patient should be asked if loss of control or pain is associated with defecating or urinating. If laxatives or enemas are used, the

TABLE 3-4   Overview of Functional Health Patterns

Health Perception–Health Management Pattern
Description of health (usual); description of present illness (onset, course, treatment)
Relevance of health to activities
Preventive measures, general health care behavior
Previous hospitalizations, expectations of this hospitalization
Potential self-care problems

Nutritional-Metabolic Pattern
Usual food and fluid intake; appetite
Daily eating times
Recent weight change and reason
Food restrictions or preferences, food supplements
Swallowing, chewing, eating problems, food allergies
Skin lesions and general ability to heal
Condition of skin, hair, nails, mucous membranes, and teeth
Temperature, pulse, respiration, height, weight

Elimination Pattern
Bowel
Usual time, frequency, color, consistency
Assistive devices (laxatives, suppositories, enemas)
Constipation, diarrhea
Bladder
Usual frequency
Problems with dysuria or polyuria
Assistive devices
Skin Condition
Color, temperature
Turgor, lesions, edema, pruritus

Activity-Exercise Pattern
Exercise, activity, leisure, and recreation patterns
Limitations in activities of daily living

Sleep-Rest Pattern
Usual sleep routine, sleep pattern
Perception of quality and quantity of sleep

Cognitive-Perceptual Pattern
Sensory adequacy—hearing, sight, smell, touch, taste
Prosthetic devices (glasses, hearing aids)
Pain
Problems with vertigo
Heat or cold sensitivity
Language, understanding, memory abilities

Self-Perception–Self-Concept Pattern
Self-description
Effects of illness on self
Perception, body image, identity, self-esteem
Posture, eye contact, voice and speech patterns

Role-Relationship Pattern
Life roles and responsibilities
Satisfaction or dissatisfaction in family, work, and social relationships

Sexuality-Reproductive Pattern
Sexuality patterns; satisfaction or dissatisfaction with sexuality patterns
Adequacy of sexual knowledge
Reproductive state (female—premenopausal or postmenopausal)

Coping–Stress Tolerance Pattern
General coping strategies
Stress tolerance, stress reduction behaviors
Support systems
Ability to manage situations

Value-Belief Pattern
Values, goals, beliefs that are basis for decisions
Value or belief conflict
Spiritual practices

---

frequency, type, and results should be noted. If any collecting devices are used, such as catheter or colostomy equipment, the nurse asks about their use and care.

The skin is assessed again in the elimination pattern in terms of its excretory function. The patient should be asked about the condition of his or her skin and whether edema, pruritus, or excessive perspiration is problematic.

Activity-Exercise Pattern. The patient's usual pattern of exercise, activity, leisure, and recreation is assessed by the nurse. The patient should be questioned about his or her ability to perform activities of daily living. Table 3-3 includes the grading scale for self-care abilities under the activity-exercise pattern. If the patient is unable to perform activities of daily living, such as toileting, eating, and moving independently, the specific problems that limit an activity should be noted. Chest pain, dyspnea, dizziness, intermittent claudication, musculoskeletal pain, fatigue, and weakness are problems that commonly result in some degree of self-care deficit.

Sleep-Rest Pattern. This pattern describes the patient's pattern of sleep, rest, and relaxation in a 24-hour period. The individual's perception of the effectiveness of sleep and relaxation is pertinent. This information can be elicited by asking, "Do you feel rested when you wake up?" Most people take sleep for granted unless they have a problem with sleeping.

The patient's usual activities related to bedtime and the usual sleep pattern should be determined. Particular routines, position, medications, and environmental factors used to foster sleep should also be elicited.

Cognitive-Perceptual Pattern. Assessment of this pattern involves a description of all senses (vision, hearing, taste, touch, and smell) and the cognitive functions such as communication, memory, and decision making. The patient should be asked about any sensory deficits that affect the ability to perform activities of daily living. Routine eye care, including the date of the last examination, should be elicited. Ways in which the patient compensates for any sensory-perceptual problems should be discussed and noted. Patients should be asked how they communicate best and about their understanding of their illness and treatment. This information is used by the nurse in planning patient teaching.

In addition, pain is assessed in this pattern. (See Chapter 9 for details on pain assessment.)

Self-Perception–Self-Concept Pattern. This pattern describes the patient's self-concept, which is critical in determining the way the person interacts with others. Included are attitudes about self, perception of personal abilities, body image, and general sense of worth.[5]

The nurse should ask the patient for a self-description and how the health condition affects self-attitude. Nurses should avoid making value judgments about how people perceive themselves. What concerns the patient about a personal situation may differ from what concerns the nurse. For example, the patient may feel cheated by the system when denied disability benefits. The nurse may think the patient was not eligible for the benefit.

Role-Relationship Pattern. This pattern describes the roles and relationships of the patient, including major responsibilities. It also examines the patient's self-evaluation of his or her performance of the expected behaviors related to these roles.

The patient should be asked to describe family, social, and work relationships. The nurse should determine if patterns in these relationships are satisfactory or if strain is evident. The nurse should note the patient's feelings about his or her role in these relationships and the effect the present condition has on his or her role and relationship.

Sexuality-Reproductive Pattern. This pattern describes satisfaction or dissatisfaction with personal sexuality and describes the reproductive pattern. Assessing this pattern is important because many illnesses, surgical procedures, and medications affect sexual function. A patient's sexual and reproductive concerns may be expressed, teaching needs and treatable problems may be identified, and normal growth and development may be monitored through information obtained in this pattern.

The interview should be appropriate to the sex, age, and developmental stage of the patient. For example, a 40-year-old widowed female patient might be asked if she has any problems related to her genital area, such as vaginal discharge. She also should be asked whether she is sexually active and if so whether she practices safe sex. A 25-year-old male patient might be asked about his knowledge and use of condoms.

Obtaining information related to sexuality often is difficult for the nurse. However, it is important to take a health history and screen for sexual function and dysfunction. Based on the complexity of the problem, the nurse may be able to provide limited information or refer the patient to a more experienced professional.

Specifically, the nurse should determine if there is a lack of knowledge in relation to sexuality and reproduction. Whether the patient perceives a problem in the area of sexuality should also be determined. The effect of the patient's present condition or treatment on personal sexuality should be noted.

Coping–Stress Tolerance Pattern. This pattern describes the general coping pattern and the effectiveness of the coping mechanisms. Assessment of this pattern involves analyzing the specific stressors or problems that confront the patient, the patient's perception of the stressor, and the patient's response to the stressor.

The major losses or changes experienced by the patient in the previous year are important to document. Current major stressors confronting the patient are also important. The strategies used by the patient to deal with stressors and relieve tension should be noted. Individuals and groups who make up the patient's social support networks should be recorded.

Value-Belief Pattern. This pattern describes the values, goals, and beliefs (including spiritual) that guide health-related choices.[1] The patient's ethnic background and the effects of culture and beliefs about health and illness on health practices should be documented. The patient's wishes about continuation of religious practices and the use of religious articles should be noted and honored. The possibility of a conflict in values or beliefs can be determined by asking a question such as, "Does your plan of care cause any conflict in your value or belief system?"

PHYSICAL EXAMINATION: OBJECTIVE DATA

General Survey

Following the nursing history, a **general survey statement** is made. The general survey is a statement of the provider's general impression of a patient, including behavioral observations. This initial survey is considered a scanning procedure and begins with the provider's first encounter with the patient and continues during the health history interview.

Although the provider may include other data that seem pertinent, the major areas usually included in the general survey statement are (1) body features, (2) state of consciousness and arousal, (3) speech, (4) body movements, (5) obvious physical signs, (6) nutritional status, and (7) behavior. Vital signs, height, and weight are often included in the general survey statement. Observations of these areas provide the data for the general survey statement. The following is a sample of a general survey statement:

> Mrs. H. is a 34-year-old Hispanic woman, BP 130/84, P 88, R 18. No distinguishing body features. Alert but anxious. Speech rapid with trailing thoughts. Wringing hands and shuffling feet during interview. Skin flushed, hands clammy. Overweight relative to height. Sits with eyes downcast and shoulders slumped and avoids eye contact.

Physical Examination

The **physical examination** is the systematic assessment of the physical and mental status of a patient, and findings are considered objective data. Throughout the physical examination, any positive findings are explored using the same criteria as the investigation of a symptom during the nursing history (see Table 3-2). A **positive finding** indicates that the patient has or had the particular problem or sign under discussion. For example, if the patient with jaundice has an enlarged liver, it is a positive finding. Relevant information about this problem should then be gathered.

Negative findings may also be significant. A **negative finding** is the absence of a sign or symptom usually associated with a problem. For example, peripheral edema is common with congestive heart failure. If edema is not present in a patient with congestive heart failure, this should be specifically noted as "no peripheral edema."

Types. There are two types of physical examinations: the screening physical examination and the branching (regional) examination. The **screening physical examination** is performed for screening situations, health surveillance, and health maintenance purposes. It is an organized, purposeful check of major body systems to detect any possible problems. If a problem is detected in the course of the screening physical examination, a more detailed branching examination of the involved system should be done.

A **branching (regional) examination** is a more detailed assessment of a particular body system. The patient's clinical manifestations should alert the nurse to the appropriate branching examination. For example, abdominal pain indicates the need to do a branching examination of the abdomen. Some problems neces-

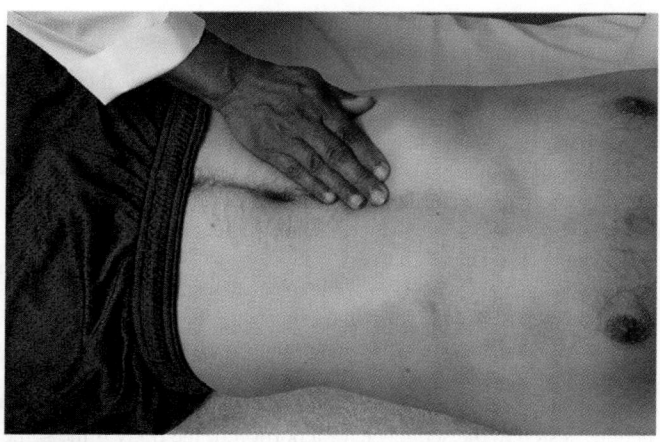

FIG. 3-1   Palpation is the examination of the body through the use of touch.

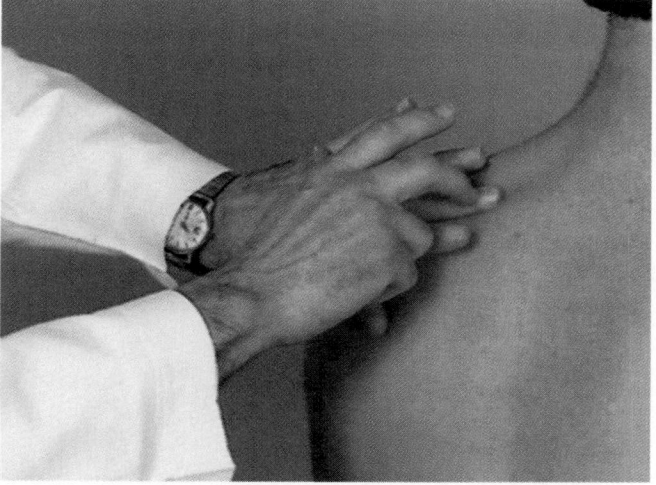

FIG. 3-2   Percussion technique: tapping the interphalangeal joint. Only the middle finger of the nondominant hand should be in contact with the skin surface.

sitate more than one branching examination. A complaint of headache may indicate the need to do musculoskeletal, neurologic, and head and neck examinations.

Techniques. Four major techniques are used in performing the physical examination: inspection, palpation, percussion, and auscultation.

Inspection. **Inspection** is the visual examination of a part or region of the body to assess normal conditions or deviations from normal. Inspection is more than just looking. This technique is deliberate, systematic, and focused. The nurse needs to compare what is seen with the known, generally visible characteristics of the body part being inspected. For example, most 30-year-old men have hair on their legs. Absence of hair may indicate a vascular problem and signals the need for further investigation, or it may be normal for a patient of a particular ethnicity. For example, Native American men have very little body hair.

Palpation. **Palpation** is the examination of the body through the use of touch. The use of light and deep palpation can yield information related to masses, pulsations, organ enlargement, tenderness or pain, swelling, muscular spasm or rigidity, elasticity, vibration of voice sounds, crepitus, moisture, and differences in texture.[6] The nurse will learn that different parts of the hand are more sensitive for specific assessments. For example, the tips of the fingers are used to palpate lymph nodes, the dorsa of hands and fingers are used to assess temperatures, and the palmar surface is best suited for feeling vibrations (Fig. 3-1).

Percussion. **Percussion** is an assessment technique involving the production of sound to obtain information about the underlying area. The percussion sound may be produced directly or indirectly. Direct percussion is performed by directly tapping the body with one or two fingers to elicit a sound. Indirect, or mediated, percussion is the more common percussion technique. The middle finger (pleximeter) of the nondominant hand is placed firmly against the body surface. The tip of the middle finger of the dominant hand (plexor) strikes the distal phalanx or the distal interphalangeal joint of the pleximeter finger (Fig. 3-2). A relaxed wrist and rapid strike produce the best sounds. The sounds and the vibrations produced are evaluated relative to the underlying structures. Deviation from an expected sound may indicate a problem. For example, the usual percussion sound in the right lower quadrant of the abdomen is tympany. Dullness in this area

may indicate a problem that should be investigated. (Specific percussion sounds of various body parts and regions are discussed in the appropriate assessment chapters.)

Auscultation. **Auscultation** is listening to sounds produced by the body to assess normal conditions and deviations from normal. Auscultation is usually indirect, using a stethoscope to clarify sounds by blocking out extraneous sounds (Fig. 3-3). The bell of the stethoscope is more sensitive to low-pitched sounds. The diaphragm of the stethoscope is more sensitive to high-pitched sounds. Auscultation is particularly useful in evaluating sounds from the heart, lungs, abdomen, and vascular system. (Specific auscultatory sounds and techniques are discussed in the appropriate assessment chapters.)

Not all assessment techniques are appropriate for all body parts and systems. The nurse will learn which techniques to use to elicit the most information. The physical assessment techniques are usually performed in the sequence of inspection, palpation, percussion, and auscultation. The only exception to this sequence is for the abdominal examination. In this situation the sequence is inspection, auscultation, percussion, and palpation.

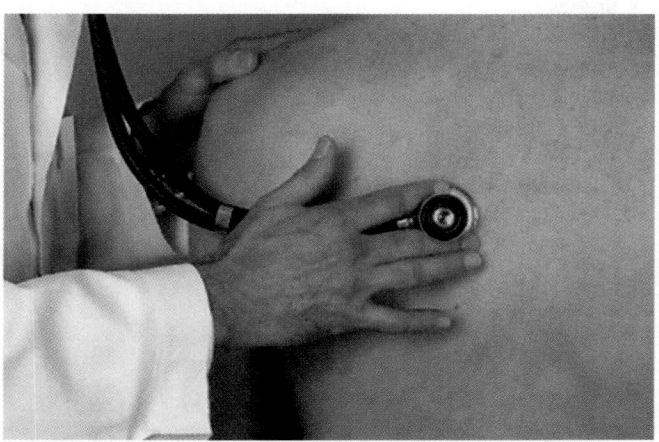

FIG. 3-3   Auscultation is listening to sounds produced by the body to assess normal conditions and deviations from normal.

TABLE 3-5   Equipment for Screening Physical Examination

Stethoscope (with bell and diaphragm, tubing 15-18 in [38-46 cm])
Wristwatch (with second hand or digitalized)
Blood pressure cuff
Ophthalmoscope/otoscope set
Eye chart (wall chart or Snellen pocket eye card)
Pocket flashlight
Tongue blades
Cotton balls
Percussion hammer
Tuning fork
Alcohol swabs
Patient gown
Paper cup with water
Examining table or bed

Palpation and percussion of the abdomen before auscultation can alter bowel sounds and produce false findings.

Equipment. The equipment needed for the physical examination should be easily accessible during the examination (Table 3-5). Organizing equipment before the examination saves the time and energy of the patient and the nurse. Lack of organization can discourage the patient and lead to lack of trust and confidence in the nurse. (The uses of specific pieces of equipment are discussed in the appropriate assessment chapters.)

Developing a System. The physical examination should be performed systematically and efficiently. Explanations should be given to the patient as the examination proceeds. The factors to be considered are the nurse's efficiency and the patient's comfort, safety, and privacy. The examiner is less likely to forget a procedure, a step in the sequence, or a portion of the body if the same sequence is followed every time. Table 3-6 presents an outline for the screening physical examination that is organized, logical, and

TABLE 3-6   Outline for Screening Physical Examination

1. General Survey
Observe general state of health (patient is seated):
- Body features
- State of consciousness and arousal
- Speech
- Body movements
- Physical signs
- Nutritional status
- Stature

2. Vital Signs
Record vital signs:
- Blood pressure
- Radial pulse
- Respiration
- Temperature
Record height and weight

3. Integument
Inspect and palpate skin for the following:
- Color
- Lesions
- Scars
- Bruises
- Edema
- Moisture
- Texture
- Temperature
- Turgor
- Vascularity
Inspect and palpate nails for the following:
- Color
- Lesions
- Size
- Flexibility
- Shape
- Angle

4. Head and Neck
Inspect and palpate head for the following:
- Shape and symmetry of skull
- Masses
- Tenderness
- Hair
- Scalp
- Skin
- Temporal arteries
- Temporomandibular joint
- Sensory (CN V, light touch, pain)
- Motor (CN VII, shows teeth, purses lips, raises eyebrows)
- Looks up, wrinkles forehead (CN VII)
- Raises shoulders against resistance (CN XI)
Inspect and palpate (occasionally auscultate) neck for the following:
- Skin (vascularity and visible pulsations)
- Symmetry
- Postural alignment
- Range of motion
- Pulses and bruits (carotid)
- Midline structure (trachea, thyroid gland, cartilage)
- Lymph nodes (preauricular, postauricular, occipital, mandibular, tonsillar, submental, anterior and posterior cervical, infraclavicular, supraclavicular)
Inspect and palpate eyes for the following:
- Visual acuity
- Eyebrows
- Position and movement of eyelids (CN VII)
- Visual fields
- Extraocular movements (CN III, IV, VI)
- Cornea, sclera, conjunctiva
- Pupillary response (CN III)
- Red reflex
- Eyeball tension
Inspect and palpate nose and sinuses for the following:
- External nose—shape; blockage
- Internal nose—patency of nasal passages; shape; turbinates or polyps; discharge
- Frontal and maxillary sinuses

AP, Anteroposterior; *CN,* cranial nerve; *CVA,* costovertebral angle; *PMI,* point of maximal impulse; *RML,* right middle lobe; *S₁ and S₂* heart sounds.

TABLE 3-6   Outline for Screening Physical Examination—cont'd

4. Head and Neck—cont'd

Inspect and palpate ears for the following:
- Placement
- Pinna
- Auditory acuity (Weber's or Rinne, whispered voice, ticking watch) (CN VIII)
- Mastoid process
- Auditory canal
- Tympanic membrane

Inspect and palpate mouth for the following:
- Lips (symmetry, lesions, color)
- Buccal mucosa (Stensen's and Wharton's ducts)
- Teeth (absence, state of repair, color)
- Gums
- Tongue for strength (asymmetry, ability to stick out tongue, side to side, fasciculations) (CN XII)
- Palates
- Tonsils and pillars
- Uvular elevation (CN IX)
- Posterior pharynx
- Gag reflex (CN IX and X)
- Jaw strength (CN V)
- Moisture
- Color
- Floor of mouth

5. Extremities

Observe size and shape, symmetry and deformity, involuntary movements

Inspect and palpate arms, fingers, wrists, elbows, shoulders for the following:
- Strength
- Range of motion
- Crepitus
- Joint pain
- Swelling
- Fluid

Test reflexes:
- Biceps
- Triceps
- Brachioradialis
- Patellar
- Achilles
- Plantar

Inspect and palpate legs for the following:
- Strength of hips
- Edema
- Hair distribution
- Pulses (dorsalis pedis, posterior tibialis)

6. Posterior Thorax

Inspect for muscular development, respiratory movement, approximation of AP diameter
- Palpate for symmetry of respiratory movement, tenderness of CVA, spinous processes, tumors or swelling, tactile fremitus
- Percuss for pulmonary resonance
- Auscultate for breath sounds

7. Anterior Thorax

Assess breasts for configuration, symmetry, dimpling of skin
Assess nipples for rash, direction, inversion, retraction
Initiate teaching or review of breast self-examination
Inspect for PMI, other precordial pulsations
Palpate for thrills, lifts, heaves, tenderness over precordium
Inspect neck for venous distention, pulsations, waves
Palpate axillae
Palpate breasts
Auscultate for rate and rhythm, character of S_1 and S_2 in the aortic, pulmonic, Erb's point, tricuspid, mitral areas; bruits at carotid, epigastrium; breath sounds at RML

8. Abdomen

Inspect for scars, shape, symmetry, bulging, muscular position and condition of umbilicus, movements (respiratory, pulsations, presence of peristaltic waves)
Auscultate for peristalsis, bruits
Percuss border of liver, four abdominal quadrants
Palpate to confirm positive findings; check liver (size, surface contour, tenderness); spleen; kidney (size, contour, consistency, tenderness); urinary bladder (distention); femoral pulses; inguinofemoral nodes

9. Completion of Examinations of Extremities

Observe the following:
- Range of motion of hips, knees, ankles, feet
- Crepitus
- Joint pain
- Swelling
- Fluid
- Muscle development
- Coordination (heel to shin)
- Homans' sign
- Proprioception (position sense of great toe)

10. Neurologic

Motor status observations:
- Gait
- Toe walk
- Heel walk
- Drift

Coordination:
- Finger to nose
- Romberg sign

Spine (scoliosis)

11. Genitalia*

Male External Genitalia

Inspect penis, noting hair distribution, prepuce, glans, urethral meatus, scars, ulcers, eruptions, structural alterations
Inspect epidermis of perineum, rectum
Inspect skin of scrotum; palpate for descended testes, masses, pain

Female External Genitalia

Inspect hair distribution; mons pubis, labia (minora and majora); urethral meatus; Bartholin's, urethral, Skene's glands (may also be palpated, if indicated); introitus
Assess for presence of cystocele, prolapse
Inspect perineum, rectum

*If the nurse has the appropriate training, the speculum and bimanual examination of women and the prostate gland examination of men should be performed after this inspection.

complete. Adaptations of the physical examination often are useful for the older adult patient, who may have age-related problems such as decreased mobility, limited energy, and perceptual changes.[7] An outline listing some of the useful adaptations is found in Table 3-7.

Recording the Screening Physical Examination. Only abnormal findings should be recorded during the actual examination. This prevents needless interruptions in the examination to write lengthy normal findings. At the conclusion of the examination, the nurse should combine the normal and abnormal findings in a carefully recorded physical examination. Table 3-8 is an example of how to record a screening physical on a healthy adult. See Chapter 5, Table 5-4, and the age-related assessment findings in each assessment chapter for helpful references in recording age-related assessment differences.

TABLE 3-7	*Gerontologic* Differences in Assessment — Adaptations in Physical Assessment Techniques

General Approach
Keep patient warm and comfortable, because loss of subcutaneous fat decreases ability to stay warm. Adapt positioning to physical limitations. Avoid unnecessary changes in position. Perform as many activities as possible in the position of comfort for the patient.

Skin
Handle with care because of fragility and loss of subcutaneous fat.

Head and Neck
Provide a quiet environment free from distraction because of patient's sensory deficits (e.g., decreased vision, touch, hearing).

Extremities
Use nonvigorous movements and reinforcement techniques. Avoid having patient hop on one foot or perform deep knee bends because of patient's limited range of motion of the extremities, decreased reflexes, and diminished sense of balance.

Thorax
Adapt examination for changes due to decrease in force of expiration, weakened cough reflex, and shortness of breath.

Abdomen
Be cautious in palpating patient's liver because it is easily palpated because of a thinner, softer abdominal wall. The older adult patient may have diminished pain perception in abdominal wall.

Genitalia
Use a well-lubricated, smaller speculum for vaginal examination because dryness and atrophy of the female genitalia may cause discomfort.

TABLE 3-8	Recording a Screening Physical Examination

Patient's Name _____

Age _____

General Status
Well-nourished, well-hydrated, well-developed white (woman) or (man) in NAD, appears stated age, looks pleasant, smiles readily, speech clear and evenly paced; is alert and oriented × 3; cooperative, calm

Skin
Clear $\bar{s}$ lesions, warm and dry, trunk warmer than extremities, turgor returns quickly, no ↑ vascularity, no varicose veins

Nails
Well-groomed, round 160-degree angle $\bar{s}$ lesions, nail beds pink, nails flexible

Hair
Thick, brown, shiny, normal (male, female) distribution

Head
Normocephalic, sinuses nontender

AC>BC, Air conduction greater than bone conduction; *BUS,* Bartholin's gland, urethral meatus, Skene's duct; *coord,* coordination; *EOM,* extraocular movements; *FN,* finger to nose; *LM,* landmarks; *LR,* light reflex; *MCL,* midclavicular line; *NAD,* no acute distress; *PERRLA,* pupils equal, round, reactive to light and accommodation; *prop,* proprioception; *ROM,* range of motion; *$\bar{s}$,* without; *TM,* tympanic membrane; *VA,* visual acuity.

TABLE 3-8	Recording a Screening Physical Examination—cont'd

Eyes
Visual fields intact on gross confrontation
VA: OD 20/20
    OS 20/20
    OU 20/20
    s̄ glasses
EOM: Intact on all gazes s̄ ptosis, nystagmus
Fundi: Red reflex present bilat no opacities, fundi: optic disc has clear margins and appropriate cup size, vessels taper with no indentation or displacement
Pupils: PERRLA, negative cover and uncover tests, negative Hirschberg test

Ears
Pinna intact, in proper alignment; external canal patent; small amount cerumen present; TMs intact; pearly gray LM, LR visible, not bulging; Rinne: AC>BC; Weber's: does not lateralize, whisper heard at 3 ft

Nose
Patent bilaterally; turbinates pink, no swelling

Mouth
Moist and pink, soft and hard palates intact, uvula rises midline on "ahh," 24 teeth present and in good repair

Throat
Tonsils surgically removed, no redness

Tongue
Moist, pink, size appropriate for mouth

Neck
Supple, s̄ masses, s̄ bruits, lymph nodes nonpalpable and non-tender
Thyroid: Palpable, smooth, not enlarged
ROM: Full, intact strong
Trachea: Midline, nontender

Breasts
Soft, nonpendulous, s̄ venous pattern, s̄ dimpling, puckering
Nipples: s̄ inversion, point in same direction, areola dark and symmetric, no discharge, no masses, nontender

Axilla
Hair present, shaved, no lesions, nontender

Lungs
No increase in AP diameter, resp rate 18, reg rhythm, no ↑ in tactile fremitus, no tenderness, lungs resonant throughout, diaphragmatic excursion 4 cm bilaterally, lung fields clear throughout

Heart
Rate 82, reg rate and rhythm; no lifts, heaves
PMI: 5th ICS at MCL; no palpable thrills; S_1, S_2 louder, softer in appropriate locations; no S_3, S_4; no murmurs, rubs, clicks
Carotid, femoral, pedal, and radial pulses present; equal, 2+ bilaterally

Abdomen
No pulsations visible, rounded, active bowel sounds, no bruits or CVA tenderness, no palpable masses

Liver
Lower border percussed at costal margin, smooth, nontender; approx 9 cm span

Spleen
Nonpalpable, nontender

Neurologic System
Cranial nerves I–XII intact
Motor (drift, toe stand) intact
Coord (FN, Romberg) intact
Reflexes: See diagram

Grading Scale	
0	No response
1+	Diminished
2+	Normal
3+	Increased
4+	Hyperactive

Sensation (touch, vibration, prop) intact

Musculoskeletal System
Well developed, no muscle wasting; s̄ crepitus, nodules, swelling
ROM: Full, intact, and equal bilaterally; no scoliosis
Strength: Equal, strong bilaterally
Gait: Walks erect 2-foot steps, arms swinging at side s̄ staggering

Female Genitalia*
External genitalia: No swelling, redness, tenderness in BUS; normal hair distribution, no cysts
Vagina: No lesions, discharge; bulging, pink
Cervix: Os closed; pink, no lesions, erosions, nontender
Uterus: Small, firm, nontender
Adnexa: No enlargement; nontender
Rectovaginal: Sphincter intact; confirms above findings

Male Genitalia
Normal male hair distribution, negative inguinal hernia
Penis: Urethral opening patent; no redness, swelling, discharge; no lesions, structural alterations
Scrotum: Testes descended; no redness, masses, tenderness
Rectal: No lesions, redness; sphincter intact; prostate small, nontender

Psychologic Status
Affect appropriate; eye contact
Orientation: Oriented × 3
Mood: Pleasant, appropriate
Thought content: Intelligent, coherent
Memory: Remote and recent intact
Serial sevens: Not done or intact

Signature _____

*Some of these data would be obtained from a pelvic examination if the nurse has the appropriate training.

PROBLEM IDENTIFICATION AND NURSING DIAGNOSES

After completing the history and physical examination, the nurse clusters and analyzes the data to develop a list of nursing diagnoses and collaborative problems. Fig. 3-4 illustrates the problem identification phase of the nursing process. Nursing diagnoses are health-related problems that are managed primarily by nursing care. (Chapter 1 explains the process of establishing nursing diagnoses.)

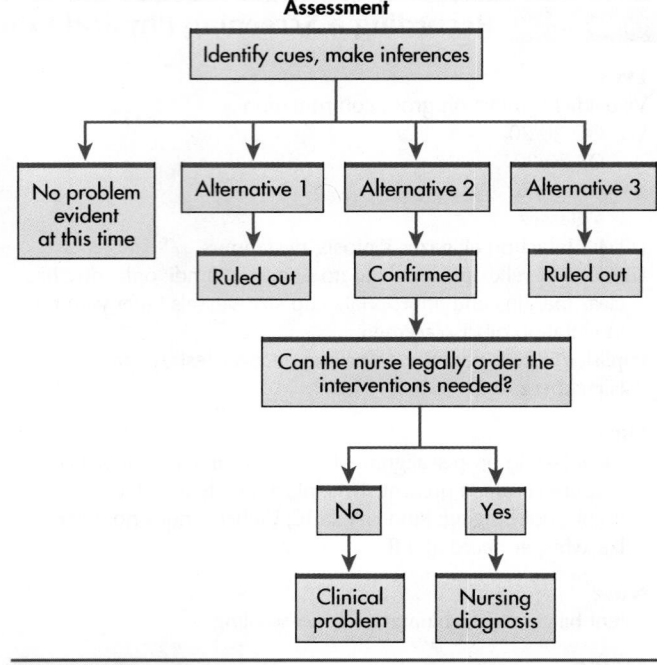

FIG. 3-4   Problem identification phase of the nursing process.

REVIEW QUESTIONS

The number of the question corresponds to the same-numbered objective at the beginning of the chapter.

1. The nursing history provides information to assist the nurse primarily in
   a. diagnosing a medical problem.
   b. investigating patient's symptoms.
   c. classifying subjective and objective data.
   d. supporting identification of nursing diagnoses.

2. The nurse would place information that the patient revealed about his concern that his illness is threatening his job security in which of the following functional health patterns?
   a. role-relationship
   b. cognitive-perceptual
   c. coping–stress tolerance
   d. health perception–health management

3. To examine the skin of a patient who has a full-thickness burn, the nurse primarily uses the technique of
   a. inspection.
   b. palpation.
   c. percussion.
   d. auscultation.

4. The piece of examination equipment that is used during auscultation is a/an
   a. stethoscope.
   b. blood pressure cuff.
   c. watch with a second hand.
   d. ophthalmoscope/otoscope.

5. A branching examination is performed when
   a. the patient denies a health problem.
   b. a baseline health maintenance examination is required.
   c. a specific problem is identified during physical examination.
   d. the medical diagnosis directs attention to a specific problem area.

6. After performing a screening history and physical, the first information the nurse records is the
   a. general survey.
   b. health history.
   c. patient symptoms.
   d. abnormal findings.

REFERENCES

1. Gordon M: *Manual of nursing diagnosis,* ed 10, St Louis, 2002, Mosby.
2. Barkauskas V, Baumann L, Darling-Fisher C: *Health and physical assessment,* ed 3, St Louis, 2002, Mosby.
3. Wilson S, Giddens J: *Health assessment for nursing practice,* ed 2, St Louis, 2000, Mosby.
4. Eliopoulos C: *Gerontological nursing,* ed 5, Philadelphia, 2000, Lippincott.
5. Fuller J, Schaller-Ayers J: *Health assessment: a nursing approach,* ed 3, Philadelphia, 1999, Lippincott.
6. Weber J, Kelley J: *Health assessment in nursing,* Philadelphia, 1998, Lippincott.
7. Seidel H et al: *Mosby's guide to physical examination,* ed 5, St Louis, 2003, Mosby.

CHAPTER *4*

Patient and Family Teaching

Patricia Graber O'Brien

LEARNING OBJECTIVES

1. Identify four specific goals of patient and family teaching.
2. Describe teaching implications related to adult learning principles.
3. Describe specific skills that enhance the nurse's role as teacher.
4. Identify strategies to manage the stresses of the nurse-teacher.
5. Discuss the role of the family in patient teaching.
6. Explain the basic steps in the teaching-learning process.
7. Identify physical, psychologic, and sociocultural characteristics of the patient that affect the teaching-learning process.
8. Describe the components of a correctly written learning objective.
9. Identify the advantages, disadvantages, and uses of various teaching strategies.
10. Describe common methods of short- and long-term evaluation.

KEY TERMS

androgogy, p. 44	self-efficacy, p. 48
empathy, p. 46	stages of behavioral change, p. 45
facilitator, p. 52	
learning, p. 43	teaching, p. 44
learning objectives, p. 50	teaching plan, p. 43
peer teaching, p. 52	teaching process, p. 47
reinforcement, p. 45	

ROLE OF PATIENT AND FAMILY TEACHING

Patient and family teaching is a critical part of nursing care and is one of the most challenging roles that nurses have today. In spite of mandates from the Joint Commission on Accreditation of Healthcare Organizations (JCAHO)[1] and institutional regulations that nurses offer patient and family education, constraints on time and resources and shortened lengths of inpatient hospitalization affect the nurse's ability to provide education. Unfortunately, teaching is frequently a neglected nursing intervention and this has devastating consequences for the patient. However, teaching patients about their health care can be a nursing intervention that most often makes a difference in a patient's quality of life.

Nurses provide patient and family education to help patients and their families maintain health and cope with acute and chronic health problems. More specific teaching goals include maintenance of health, prevention of disease, management of illness, and appropriate selection and use of treatment options. Primary health education can promote health and prevent disease, facilitating a high level of wellness throughout the lifespan. Teaching can help people make informed decisions about health practices and treatment choices. In patients with acute health problems, teaching can prevent complications and promote recovery. For those patients with chronic illnesses, teaching can promote self-care and independence. Seventy percent of the deaths in the United States are due to chronic illnesses with which patients often live for many years.[2] Whether patients adequately manage their chronic illnesses and maintain quality of life depends primarily on what they are taught and learn about their conditions.

Teaching may occur wherever nurses work, including the community, schools, industry, ambulatory care centers, hospitals, long-term care facilities, and homes. Although institutions may employ clinical nurse specialists and patient educators to establish and oversee patient education programs, all nurses in any setting are responsible for patient and family teaching. Every interaction the nurse has with patients or family members is an opportunity to provide teaching that can dramatically affect their lives.

Much patient teaching in inpatient facilities is incidental and is incorporated into nursing interventions that prevent complications and promote physiologic function. Teaching a patient to effectively cough and deep breathe following surgery to prevent atelectasis or teaching a patient how to use a patient-controlled analgesia (PCA) machine do not require formal teaching plans. However, when a patient has specific learning needs about health promotion, risk reduction, or management of a health problem, a teaching plan should be developed and implemented with the patient. A **teaching plan** includes assessment of the patient's ability, need, and readiness to learn with identification of problems that can be resolved with teaching. The nurse then determines objectives with the patient, delivers educational interventions, and evaluates the effectiveness of the teaching. This chapter describes the steps involved in providing patient and family education and discusses factors that contribute to successful educational experiences.

TEACHING-LEARNING PROCESS

Teaching is not just imparting information. Learning is not just listening to instruction. **Learning** occurs when there is an internal mental change characterized by rearrangement of neural paths. It can result in a persistent change in behavior. Observa-

Reviewed by Dorothy Hendel Clough, RN, PhD, Professor Emeritus, College of Nursing, University of New Mexico, Albuquerque, N.M.; and Elaine A. Slabinski, RN, MS, Director, Nursing Learning Resource Center, Department of Nursing, Wilkes University, Wilkes-Barre, Pa.

TABLE 4-1	Principles of Adult Education Applied to Patient Teaching
PRINCIPLES	**TEACHING IMPLICATIONS FOR THE NURSE**
Adults are independent learners.	• Teacher is a facilitator to direct the patient to resources, not the source of all information. • Patients expect to make decisions about their own lives and learning experiences and take responsibility for those decisions. • Respect for the patient's independence can be reflected in statements such as, "What do you think you need to learn about this topic?"
Readiness to learn arises from life's changes.	• Patients see life processes as problems to be solved. • Readiness and motivation to learn are high when facing new tasks. • Crises in health are "teachable moments."
Past experiences are resources for learning.	• Patients have had many life experiences and have engaged in informal learning for years. • Motivation is increased when patients feel that they already know something about the subject from past experiences. • Identification of past knowledge and experiences can help find familiar ground to increase patients' confidence.
Adults learn best when the topic is of immediate value.	• Patients need to apply learning immediately. • Long-term goals may have little appeal. • Short-term, realistic goals should be provided. • Focus education on information that the patient views as being needed right now.
Adults approach learning as problem solving.	• Patients seek out various resources for specific learning to help them deal with a problem. • Information that is not relevant to the problem is not readily learned. • When relevancy is not recognized by the patient, explanations of why they need to learn something should be offered. • Teaching should target the specific problem or circumstance.
Adults see themselves as doers.	• Patients learn better by doing. • Demonstrations, computer activities, and practice of skills should be offered when appropriate.
Adults resist learning when conditions are incongruent with their self-concepts.	• Patients do not learn when they are treated as children and told what they must do. • Patients need control and self-direction to maintain their sense of self-worth.

tion of this behavior is an indication that learning has occurred.[3] Learning may also result in a potential or capability to change behavior. This is seen in a patient who understands the instruction and is fully informed, but chooses not to change behavior. In this case, teaching gives the patient the capability to make a decision to change behaviors, but the decision is the patient's. The patient learns the necessary information to make an informed choice, and the choosing is the behavior that is observed.[4]

Teaching is a process of deliberately arranging external conditions to promote the internal change that results in a change in behavior. It can be a planned or incidental experience that uses a combination of methods such as instruction, counseling, and behavior modification to influence the patient's knowledge and behavior. The teacher is the one who plans and manages the external conditions to promote learning.[5] The challenge for the nurse is to identify and use strategies to help patients change behaviors that are beneficial for their health.

In patient education, the teaching-learning process involves the patient, the nurse, and the patient's family and/or social support system. The complex nature of each of these variables must be taken into account when planning and implementing the education process.

Adult Learner

Adult Learning Principles. Understanding how and why adults learn is important for the nurse to effectively teach patients. Educational research and theory development specifically about adults have identified adult learning principles and charac-

teristics that differentiate adult education from that of children. These concepts provide a foundation for effective teaching of adults. Many of the theories of adult learning have risen from the work of Malcolm Knowles, who identified seven principles of **androgogy** (adult learning) that are essential for the nurse to consider when teaching adults.[6] These principles and implications for patient teaching are presented in Table 4-1.

Characteristics of Adult Learners. Adult learners have certain characteristics that influence their learning and distinguish them from children learners[7] (Table 4-2).

Motivation of Adult Learners. Motivation for learning and readiness to learn depend on multiple factors, such as need, attitude, beliefs, stimulation, and reinforcement.[7] No one theory explains all motives for learning and changing behavior. Theorists continue to research why people behave as they do. When teaching adults, it is important to identify what is valued

TABLE 4-2	Adult Learner Characteristics

- Adjusts less easily to distractions.
- Suffers more from being deprived of success.
- Has greater difficulty in remembering isolated facts.
- Requires more light of better quality for study tasks.
- Is more rigid in thinking and has a set pattern of behavior.
- Requires a longer time to perform learning tasks although capacity to learn is unchanged.

TABLE 4-3	Stages of Change in the Transtheoretical Model	
STAGE	**PATIENT BEHAVIOR**	**NURSING IMPLICATIONS**
1. Precontemplation	Is not considering a change; is not ready to learn	Provide support, increase awareness of condition; describe benefits of change and risks of not changing
2. Contemplation	Thinks about a change; may verbalize recognition of need to change; says "I know I should" but identifies barriers	Introduce what is involved in changing the behavior; reinforce the stated need to change
3. Preparation	Starts planning the change, gathers information, sets a date to initiate change, shares decision to change with others	Reinforce the positive outcomes of change, provide information and encouragement, develop a plan, help set priorities, and identify sources of support
4. Action	Begins to change behavior through practice; tentative and may experience relapses	Reinforce behavior with reward, encourage self-reward, discuss choices to help minimize relapses and regain focus, help patient plan to deal with potential relapses
5. Maintenance	Practices the behavior regularly; able to sustain the change	Continue to reinforce behavior; provide additional education on the need to maintain change
6. Termination	Change has become part of lifestyle; behavior no longer considered a change	Evaluate effectiveness of the new behavior; no further intervention needed

Adapted from Prochaska J, Velicer W: The transtheoretical model of health behavior change, *Am J Health Promot* 12:38, 1997.

by the person to enhance motivation. If the person perceives a need for information to enhance health or avoid illness, or has a belief that a behavior change has health value, motivation to learn is increased. Humans also seek out stimulating experiences that increase their activity and desire to learn. Therefore learning activities must be stimulating to maintain a desire to reach a goal.

Reinforcement is a strong motivational factor for maintaining behavior. Reinforcement involves rewarding a desired behavior with a positive stimulus to increase its occurrence. Behavior may be strengthened by negative reinforcement when the behavior removes a negative consequence, such as pain or illness symptoms.[7]

When a change in health behaviors is recommended, patients and their families may progress through a series of steps before they are willing or able to accept a change in health behaviors. Six stages of change have been identified in the Transtheoretical Model of Health Behavior Change developed by Prochaska and Velicer.[8] The **stages of behavioral change** and the implications for patient teaching are described in Table 4-3. It is important to note that individuals progress through these stages at their own pace and that progression through the stages is often nonlinear and cyclic, going through periods of relapse and restarting the process. Assessment of the patient's stage of change will help the nurse guide the patient through one stage to the next.

Nurse as Teacher
Required Skills
Knowledge of subject matter. The scope and setting of nursing practice is large and diverse. Although it is impossible to be expert in all areas, the nurse can develop confidence as a teacher by developing a thorough knowledge of the subject that is to be taught. Additional study of health risks, diseases, and appropriate self-care in textbooks, journals, and other resources may be necessary if the nurse has limited experience with or knowledge of the subject. For example, if a nurse is teaching a patient about management of hypertension, the nurse must be able to explain what hypertension is, why it is important to control the disease, and what the patient needs to know about exercise, diet, and ex-

pected and untoward effects of medication. The nurse should be able to teach the patient to use blood pressure equipment to monitor the blood pressure and to identify situations that should be reported to health care providers. In addition, the nurse should provide the patient with sources of additional information, such as appropriate websites and support organizations (e.g., American Heart Association).

It is not unusual for the patient to ask questions the nurse may not be able to answer. If the nurse is not sure of an answer, the patient should be told and the nurse should follow through by seeking additional information to answer the question.

Communication skills. Patient education is an interactive process (Fig. 4-1). It is dependent on communication between the nurse and the patient or family member. During the teaching process the nurse should use basic communication skills as de-

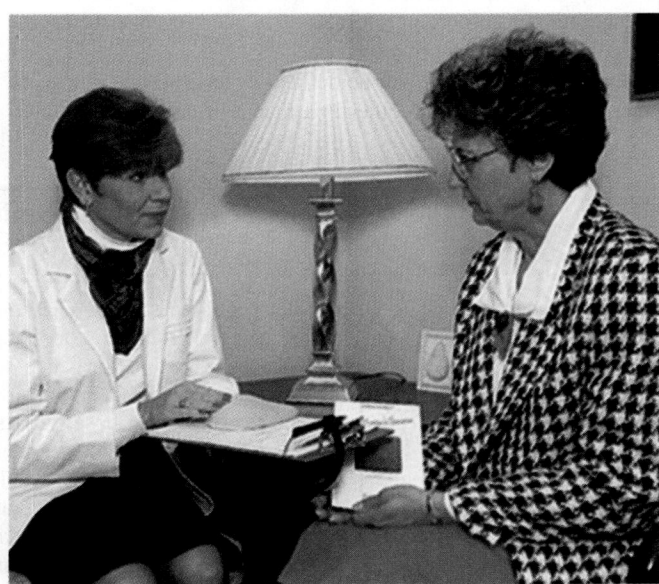

FIG. 4-1 Cooperation between the patient and the nurse is necessary for effective patient learning.

scribed in the patient interview in Chapter 3. Some additional communication skills that are particularly important in teaching are discussed in this chapter.

Medical jargon is inherently intimidating and frightening to most patients and their families. Patients can feel alienated when large, complex medical terms are used in their presence without an understanding of what the terms mean. The nurse should begin by defining the medical words or terms that are necessary to understanding the content to be taught. For example, if a patient is told that he has idiopathic dilated cardiomyopathy, he most likely will need the nurse to interpret this diagnosis in words that mean something to him. The nurse can explain that the term *idiopathic* is a scientific way of saying "for an unknown reason," *dilated* means enlarged, and *cardiomyopathy* describes a heart muscle not pumping with full force. Therefore the patient has an enlarged heart that is not working properly for an unknown reason. With this one-sentence interpretation, the nurse has enhanced the education process, but the patient should always be asked if words are understood or if there are other questions.

The importance of nonverbal communication in the teaching process should be considered. To provide positive nonverbal messages it is important for the nurse to sit facing the patient. If possible, the nurse should raise the bed or sit in a chair so that the nurse's and patient's eyes are level. Open body gestures communicate interest and a willingness to share. If time is limited, the nurse should tell the patient at the beginning of the interaction how much time the nurse can devote to the session. This will allow both the patient and nurse to set priorities on what needs to be taught during the allotted time.

It is also important for the nurse to develop the art of active listening. This means paying attention to what is said as well as observing the patient's nonverbal cues. The nurse must be prepared both physically and mentally to listen. This includes sitting directly in front of the patient, getting rid of distractions, and trying to dismiss personal worries. The nurse concentrates on the patient as a communicator of vital information and allows the patient full hearing by not interrupting. To allow time for listening without appearing in a hurry requires thoughtful organization and planning on the part of the nurse. Attentive listening allows for the obtaining of important information needed for the assessment phase of the teaching process.

Empathy. **Empathy** can be defined as having the courage to enter into the world of another in a manner that does not judge, sympathize, or correct, but in a manner where the goal is creative understanding. Empathy means putting aside one's own self for a moment and stepping into the shoes of the patient. With regard to patient teaching, empathy means assessing the patient's needs before implementing teaching. For example, the nurse who is working in a rural outpatient clinic is asked to teach a newly diagnosed diabetic patient the symptoms of hypoglycemia. The nurse enters the room with the packet of written information and finds the patient sitting very still, with gaze fixed and mouth slightly ajar. The empathetic approach to this situation may include entering the room, sitting down in a chair next to the patient, and discussing the feelings that the patient may be experiencing before starting the discussion of educational materials.

Stressors Related to Teaching. Lack of time is a major stressor for the nurse that detracts from the effectiveness of the teaching effort. Teaching often is not as instantly rewarding to the nurse as other interventions and therefore may not be given priority when time is limited and the environment does not value patient teaching. It is critical that the nurse identify the patient's learning needs so that important teaching can be done during any contact with the patient or family.

A second stressor is insecurity about knowledge and competence. This stressor many impair the nurse's ability to teach effectively and is described in this chapter in the discussion of the skills required of the nurse as a teacher. A third potential stressor is disagreement between nurse and patient regarding the expectations of teaching. The nurse must accept that some patients or families may not be willing to talk about the health problem or its implications. The patient or family may be in denial or hold ideas and values that are in conflict with conventional health care. The nurse may face hostility or resentment but must respect the patient's response to the health problem.

Another important stressor for the nurse who is attempting to provide patient education is the current health care system. Shortened lengths of hospitalizations have resulted in patients being discharged into the community with only the basic elements of educational plans established. At the same time health care is offering more and complex treatment options, increasing the educational needs of the patient and family. Patients and families also have more difficulty using resources as the complexity of the health care system increases. Strategies that can be used to help manage or overcome these stressors are presented in Table 4-4.

TABLE 4-4	Suggested Approaches to Overcoming Nurse-Teacher Stressors	
STRESSOR	**APPROACHES**
Lack of time	Preplan. Set realistic goals. Use time with patient efficiently, using all possible opportunities for teaching, such as when bathing or changing a dressing. Break teaching and practice into small time periods. Advocate for time for patient teaching. Carefully document what was taught and the time spent teaching in order to emphasize that it is a primary role of nursing and that it takes time.
Lack of knowledge	Broaden knowledge base. Read, study, ask questions. Screen teaching materials, participate in other teaching sessions, observe more experienced nurse-teachers, attend classes.
Disagreement with patient	Establish agreed-on, written goals. Develop a plan and discuss with patient before teaching begins. Introduce a role model to help illustrate therapeutic expectations. Enlist the aid of family and significant others. Revise expectations; learn to be satisfied with small achievements.
Powerlessness, frustration	Recognize personal reaction to stress. Develop a support system. Rely on friends and family for positive encouragement. Network with other nurses, health professionals, and community leaders to change the situation. Become proactive in legislative processes affecting health care delivery.

Family and Social Support

Support provided by the family is important to a patient's sense of physical, psychologic, and spiritual well-being.[9-11] Family members who learn what is needed for home care can promote the patient's self-care and prevent future hospitalizations.[12,13] It is important for the nurse to identify and include family members in the teaching plans for the patient.

In the family support model (Fig. 4-2) the patient's ultimate well-being is composed of his or her ability to perform self-care activities in and through both formal and informal support systems.[14] In this model no part of the system is an independent agent because the well-being of the individual depends on support from family, community resources, and the medical care system.[14] The support provided by the family unit greatly affects a patient's health. A recent study has demonstrated that the quality of the patient's marriage can affect the prediction of mortality from congestive heart failure.[15] Identifying patients with minimal support and working collaboratively with other health care professionals to develop networks for these patients may improve the patients' long-term outcomes.

Patients and families may have different educational needs. For example, the first priority of an elderly diabetic patient with a large ulcer on the back of his leg may be to learn how to rise from a chair in the least painful manner. On the other hand, family members may be most concerned about learning the technique for dressing changes. Both the patient's and the family's learning needs are important. The patient and family may also have differing or conflicting views of the illness and of treatment options. Frequently the health problem has effects on family roles and functions. Developing a successful teaching plan requires the nurse to view the patient's needs within the context of the family's needs. For example, the nurse may teach a patient with right-sided *paresis* (weakness) self-feeding techniques with special implements, but at a home visit the nurse finds the patient being fed by the spouse. On questioning, the spouse reveals that it is too difficult to watch the patient struggle with feeding, it takes too long, and it is easier to do it for the patient. This is an example of a situation where both the patient and the spouse need additional teaching about the goals of self-care.

PROCESS OF PATIENT EDUCATION

Many different models and approaches are used in the process of patient education. The nurse may find that specific institutions or programs may adopt specific models. Examples include the ASSURE model,[16] empowerment approach,[17] and Leventhal's self-regulation model.[18] However, the approach used most frequently by nurses is actually a parallel of the nursing process. The **teaching process** and the nursing process both involve development of a plan that includes assessment, diagnosis, setting patient outcomes or objectives, intervention, and evaluation. The teaching process, like the nursing process, may not always flow in sequential order, but the steps serve as checkpoints to ensure that the relevant variables that affect the teaching-learning activity have been considered.[5]

Assessment

During the general nursing assessment the nurse gathers data that determine if the patient has learning needs that teaching can meet. For example, what does the patient know about the health problem and how does he or she perceive the present problem? If a learning need is identified, a more refined assessment of need is made and that problem is addressed with the teaching process.[5] The general nursing assessment also identifies many variables that affect the teaching-learning process, such as the patient's physical and mental state of health and sociocultural characteristics. Assessment can also include the family members or caregivers to determine their abilities to care for the patient at home. The assessment that is performed for the purpose of developing a teaching plan includes physical, psychologic, and sociocultural characteristics that specifically affect learning and the patient's characteristics related to the teaching-learning process. Key questions addressing each of these areas are included in Table 4-5.

Physical Characteristics. The age of the patient is an important factor to consider in the teaching plan. The patient's experiences, rate of learning, and ability to retain information are affected by age. Barriers to effective learning such as impairment of vision, hearing, manual dexterity, or cognitive ability may be identified. The effects of aging are not the only factors to consider. For example, a man in his twenties who has never thought about his own mortality may be unable to grasp the long-term implications of an unhealthy behavior, such as smoking.

Sensory impairments, such as hearing or vision loss, decrease sensory input and can alter learning. Magnifying glasses and bright lighting may help the patient with impaired vision read teaching materials. Hearing loss can be helped with hearing aids and teaching techniques that use more visual stimuli. Central nervous system (CNS) function may be affected by disorders of the nervous system, such as stroke and head trauma, but also by other diseases, such as renal disease, liver impairment, and cardiovascular failure. Patients with alterations in CNS function have difficulty learning and may require small amounts of information repeated frequently. Manual dexterity is needed to perform procedures such as self-administration of injections or blood pressure monitoring. Problems performing manual procedures might be resolved by using adaptive equipment.

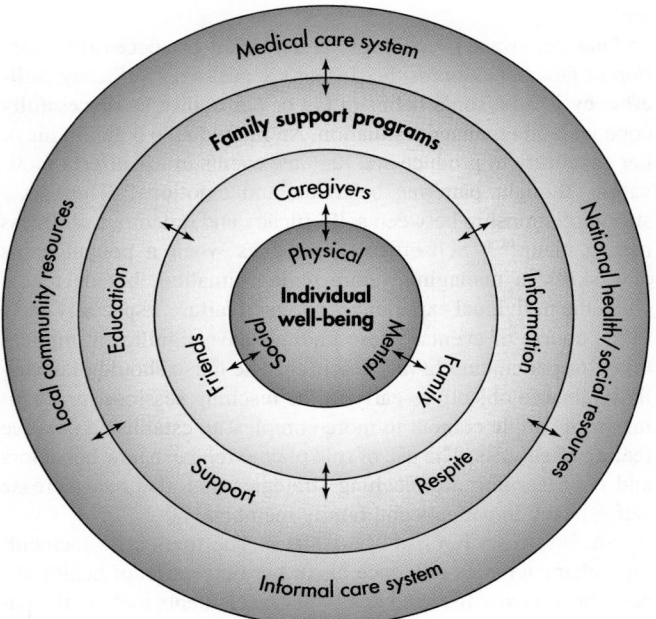

FIG. 4-2 Family support model.

TABLE 4-5	Assessment of Characteristics That Affect Patient Teaching

CHARACTERISTICS AND KEY QUESTIONS

Physical
- What is the patient's age and sex?
- Is the patient acutely ill?
- Is the patient fatigued? In pain?
- What is the primary diagnosis?
- Are there additional diagnoses?
- What is the patient's current mental status?
- What is the patient's hearing ability? Visual ability? Motor ability?
- What drugs does the patient take? Do they affect learning?

Psychologic
- Does the patient appear anxious, afraid, depressed, defensive?
- Is the patient in a state of denial?
- What is the patient's level of self-efficacy?

Sociocultural
- Is the patient employed?
- What is the patient's present or past occupation?
- How does the patient describe his or her financial status?
- What is the patient's educational experience and reading ability?
- What is the patient's living arrangement?
- Does the patient have family or close friends?
- What are the patient's beliefs regarding his or her illness or treatment?
- What is the patient's cultural/ethnic identity?
- Is proposed teaching consistent with the patient's cultural values?

Educational
- What does the patient already know?
- What does the patient think is most important to learn first?
- What prior learning experiences establish a frame of reference for current learning needs?
- What has the patient's health care provider told the patient about the health problem?
- Is the patient ready to change behavior or learn?
- Can the patient identify behaviors/habits that would make the problem better or worse?
- How does the patient learn best? Through reading, listening, doing things?
- In what kind of environment does the patient learn best? Formal classroom? Informal setting, such as home or office? Alone or among peers?

Pain, fatigue, and certain medications also influence the patient's ability to learn. No one can learn effectively when in severe pain. When the patient is experiencing pain, the nurse should provide only brief explanations and follow up with more detailed instruction when the pain has been managed. A fatigued and weakened patient cannot learn effectively because of the inability to concentrate. Sleep disruption is common during hospitalization, and patients are frequently exhausted at the time of discharge. Drugs that cause CNS depression, such as opioids and tranquiliz-

ers, cause a general decrease in mental alertness. Many chemotherapeutic agents cause nausea, vomiting, and headaches that also affect the patient's ability to assimilate new information. The nurse must adjust the teaching plan to accommodate these factors by setting high-priority goals that are need-based and realistic in expectations. Teaching methods should also be adjusted to accommodate for limitations in the patient's ability to learn at any given time. The patient may need follow-up teaching and referral to someone who can answer questions that arise after discharge.

Psychologic Characteristics. Psychologic factors have a major influence in the patient's ability to learn. Anxiety and depression are common reactions to illness. Although mild anxiety increases the learner's perceptual and learning abilities, moderate and severe anxiety limit learning. The nurse must use measures to decrease anxiety before the patient can learn. Both anxiety and depression can negatively affect the patient's motivation and readiness to learn. For example, the newly diagnosed diabetic patient who is depressed about the diagnosis may not listen or respond to instructions about blood glucose testing. Discussions with the patient about these concerns or referring the patient to an appropriate support group may enable the patient to learn that management of diabetes is possible.

Patients also respond to the stress of illness with a variety of defense mechanisms, such as denial, rationalization, or even humor. A patient who denies having cancer will not be receptive to information related to treatment options. A patient using rationalization will imagine any number of reasons for avoiding change or for rejecting instruction. For example, a patient with cardiovascular disease who does not want to change dietary habits will relate stories of persons who have eaten bacon and eggs every morning for years and lived to be 100 years of age. Humor is also used by some patients to filter reality or decrease anxiety. Laughter may be used to escape from the experience of facing threatening situations. A common example of the use of humor is seen when patients assign a name and personality characteristics to an intestinal stoma or even a drainage device. Humor in the teaching process is important and useful, but the nurse must determine when humor is used excessively to avoid reality.

One important psychologic determinant of successful adoption of new behaviors is the patient's sense of self-efficacy. **Self-efficacy** is a person's belief in his or her ability to successfully cope with and manage a situation. An individual's belief in his or her capability to produce and regulate events in life affects motivation, thought patterns, behavior, and emotions.[5] There is a strong relationship between self-efficacy and outcomes of illness management.[19,20] Self-efficacy increases when a person gains new skills in managing a threatening situation, but decreases when the individual experiences repeated failure, especially early in the course of events. These findings have significant implications for patient and family teaching. The nurse should plan easily attainable objectives early in the teaching sessions, proceeding from simple content to more complex, to establish a positive feeling of success. The use of role play to rehearse new behaviors and peer learning are teaching strategies that also can increase self-efficacy in patients and family members.

Sociocultural Characteristics. The patient's sociocultural characteristics influence his or her perception of health, illness, health care, life, and death. Social elements include the patient's lifestyle, status within a family, occupation, income, education, housing arrangement, and living location. Cultural elements include dietary and sleep patterns, exercise, sexuality, language, values, and beliefs.

Occupation and income.   Knowing the patient's present or past occupation may assist the nurse in determining the vocabulary to use during teaching. For example, an auto mechanic might understand the volume overload associated with heart failure as flooding of an engine. An engineer may understand the principles of physics associated with gravity and pressures when discussing vascular problems. This technique of teaching requires creativity but can promote a patient's understanding of pathophysiologic processes.

The patient's occupation will also give the nurse an idea about the patient's income or financial status. Management of chronic health problems is very expensive and the cost of care should be addressed with the patient or family. The nurse may need to use different teaching resources or improvise materials based on the patient's ability to afford supplies and equipment.

Education and reading ability.   The patient's level of formal education may be helpful in determining appropriate written materials and vocabulary to use when teaching the patient. However, the nurse cannot assume that patients read or comprehend at the level of their formal education. One study of patient education materials found that the mean education level of the patients was twelfth grade, but the mean reading level of the patients was seventh to eighth grade.[21]

Printed educational materials are extensively used for the purpose of teaching patients and families. The Joint Commission on Accreditation of Healthcare Organizations (JCAHO)[1] standards and the American Hospital Association's Patient's Bill of Rights[22] both mandate that a patient obtain current information concerning his or her diagnosis, treatment, and prognosis in terms that the patient can reasonably be expected to understand. This means that written materials must be appropriate for the patient's reading level. In the United States, the average reading level is eighth to ninth grade.[23] In addition, recent studies have shown that almost one quarter of the adult population in the United States and Canada is functionally illiterate (read below fifth-grade level); an additional one quarter has poor reading and comprehension skills.[24,25] People who are functionally illiterate could have difficulty identifying the correct amount of medicine to give based on the information found on the package. In the United States, this would be between 40 and 44 million people.

The low literacy level in North America is more prevalent than is generally recognized and has major implications for patient education. Low-literacy patients hide their deficiency well, and it is not always feasible to formally evaluate a patient's reading level. As a result it is now recommended that all patient education materials be written at the eighth-grade level, or even preferably at the sixth-grade level. Evaluations of current patient education materials have found the reading level of many materials to be at the tenth-grade level or higher.[21,26] This is well above the recommended and preferred levels. Nurses must be involved as health care organizations currently evaluate and revise the reading level of their educational materials.

Housing arrangement and living location.   The patient should be asked about living arrangements that can affect the teaching-learning process. Whether the patient lives alone, with friends, or with family will influence who else is included in the teaching process. If the patient lives in another city or a rural area at a distance from the site of teaching, the nurse may need to make arrangements for continued teaching in those areas. Modifications of instructions may need to be made if the patient does not have access to electricity, phones, or modern plumbing. An example of a patient needing consideration of living arrangements could be an Native American patient who lives on a reservation in a home with a dirt floor and must drive 100 miles each way three times a week for hemodialysis treatment.

Cultural considerations.   Learning is closely related to the wider culture and the subculture to which a patient belongs. Health practices, beliefs, and behavior vary by religious, ethnic, and family group. Many factors affecting patient teaching are included in the cultural assessment in Table 2-3. To prevent stereotyping patients according to cultural group, it is important to simply ask if there is a cultural group or practice with which the patient identifies. Patients may also be asked to describe their beliefs regarding health and illness.

One cultural element that specifically affects the teaching-learning process is a conflict between the patient's cultural beliefs and values and the behaviors promoted by teaching. For example, a patient who values a trim figure can be taught to diet and exercise to retain that figure while at the same time improving blood pressure control. However, in another patient's culture, being heavy is valued as a sign of financial success and sexuality. This patient may have more difficulty accepting the need for diet and exercise unless the importance of blood pressure control is understood.

The nurse must also assess the patient's use of cultural remedies and healers. For teaching to be effective, cultural health practices must be incorporated into the teaching plan. In addition, it is important to know who has authority in the patient's culture. The patient may defer to the authority, such as an elder or a spiritual leader or healer, for decisions. In this case, the nurse will also need to identify and work with the decision makers in the patient's culture.

Educational Characteristics.   Finally, the nurse should assess those patient characteristics that are directly related to the development of the teaching plan. These factors include the patient's learning needs, readiness to learn, and learning style.

Learning needs.   The assessment of learning needs should first determine what the patient already knows, if the patient has misinformation, and any history of past experiences with health problems. Patients with long-standing health problems have different learning needs than those patients with newly diagnosed health problems. The nurse then identifies the information, behaviors, or skills known to improve patient outcomes that should be included in the teaching plan. For example, patients who have had myocardial infarctions should be given information regarding the condition, risk factors, medications, diet, psychologic concerns, activities, stress management, and symptoms so that they can manage their condition and make informed decisions about potential lifestyle changes.[27]

It may appear on the surface that it is obvious what a patient should learn about managing an illness or what behaviors should be changed to promote health. However, there is often a significant difference between what health care professionals think is important for patients to learn and what patients want to know.[27,28] Remembering that adults learn best when teaching provides information that they view as being needed immediately, the nurse should prioritize what patients see as the most critical information when developing the teaching plan.

To individualize learning needs for a particular patient, the nurse may give the patient a list of the recommended topics and ask that the patient number the topics in order of importance. Another method includes writing each topic in question format on a single card and asking the patient to sort the cards in priority. Examples of the questions on the cards for a patient with congestive heart failure include, "What are the side effects of my medications?" and "How will I know when I should call my doctor?"[28] Blank cards could also be provided so the patient could identify any other needs. By allowing a patient to prioritize his or her own learning needs, the nurse can begin with the patient's most important needs and end with the least important. When information regarding life-threatening complications is a factor, the nurse can promote the patient's priority of learning this content by explaining why the information is a "need to know." Individualization of learning needs helps ensure that the most important topics are addressed when time limits the comprehensive discussion of all topics.

Readiness to learn. Before implementing the teaching plan the nurse should determine where the patient is in the stages of change process (see Table 4-3). If the patient is only in the precontemplation stage, the nurse may just provide support and increase the patient's awareness of the problem until the patient is ready to consider a change in behavior. Nurses in outpatient settings and home health care may continue to evaluate the patient's readiness to learn and implement the teaching plan as the patient moves through the stages of change.

Learning style. Each person has a distinct style of learning, as individual as his or her personality. The three learning styles are (1) visual (reading), (2) auditory (listening), and (3) physical (doing things). People often use more than one learning style. To assess a patient's learning style the nurse might ask how the patient learns best, if reading or listening is the preferred method to gain information, and how the patient has learned in the past. During assessment of the patient's learning style the nurse may be able to identify the patient who does not read. For example, the patient may tell the nurse that he or she does not read much, but likes to learn from television programs, the radio, or illustrations. Auditory methods should always be used when patients specifically identify them as learning styles.

Diagnosis

Information obtained from the assessment related to what the patient knows, believes, and is able to do is compared with what the patient wants to know, needs to know, and needs to be able to do. Identifying the gap between the known and unknown helps determine the nursing diagnosis, or the deficiency that can be corrected with teaching. A common nursing diagnosis for learning needs is that of deficient knowledge. This refers to the state in which the individual experiences an absence or a deficiency of cognitive knowledge related to a specific topic. Another nursing diagnosis commonly identified when patients have learning needs is that of ineffective health maintenance. This diagnosis

refers to an inability to identify, manage, and/or seek out help to maintain health.

If deficient knowledge is identified, it is important to specify the exact nature of the deficit so that the objectives, strategies, implementation, and evaluation relate to the identified problem. For example, the nursing diagnosis of deficient knowledge related to inability to recognize symptoms of drug toxicity provides the nurse with a clear direction for the teaching-learning process.

Planning

Following the assessment and the identification of a nursing diagnosis, the next step in the education process is setting goals, determining objectives for the learner, and planning the learning experience. The patient and nurse mutually prioritize the patient's learning needs and agree on learning objectives. Fig. 4-3 shows a nurse working with a patient to develop a teaching plan. If the physical or psychologic condition of the patient interferes with his or her participation, the patient's family or significant other can assist the nurse in the planning phase.

Writing clear, specific, and measurable learning objectives is important. Learning objectives describe the intended result of the learning process, guide the selection of teaching strategies and materials, and help evaluate patient and teacher progress. Learning objectives are parallel to patient outcomes in the nursing care plan and are written using the same criteria. Objectives should be in writing and made readily available to all members of the health care team, including the patient and family.

Writing Specific Learning Objectives. **Learning objectives** are written statements that define exactly how patients demonstrate their mastery of the content. The objectives contain the following four elements:

1. Who will perform the activity or acquire the desired behavior?

> Examples: I (the patient) will…
> I (the spouse) will…
> We (the patient's family) will…

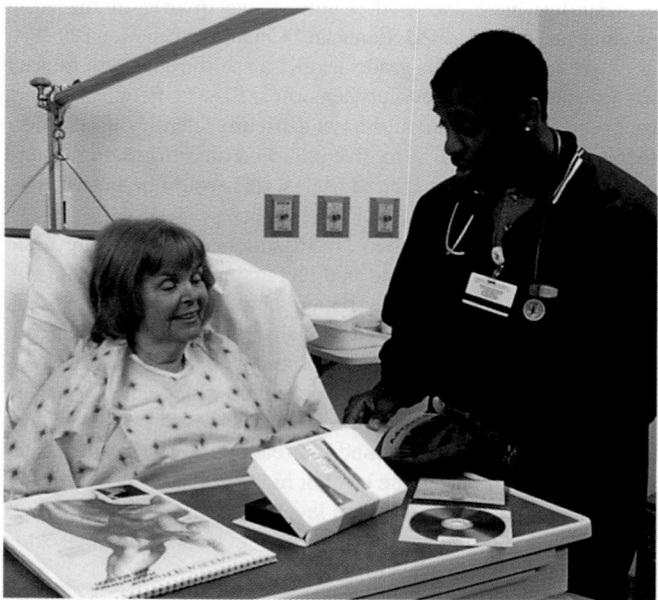

FIG. 4-3 Developing a teaching plan with the patient.

2. The actual behavior that the learner will exhibit to demonstrate mastery of the objective.

Examples: List the symptoms
              Self-administer an insulin injection
              Identify from a hospital menu

3. The conditions under which the behavior is to be demonstrated.

Examples: In front of the nurse
              Select from a random list
              Choose from a restaurant menu

4. The specific criteria that will be used to measure the patient's success, such as time and degree of accuracy.

Examples: With 100% accuracy
              Using correct technique
              Within 3 minutes

Note that well-written learning objectives have precise descriptions using terms with few interpretations. When writing objectives the nurse uses verbs such as "identify," "list," "describe," "demonstrate," "name," "recognize," and "compare and contrast." Vague, ambiguous terms, such as "appreciate," "learn," "understand," "enjoy," "feel," or "value," cannot be measured and should be avoided.

An example of a poorly written learning objective is, "The patient will appreciate the importance of foot care." In this objective it is not clear how the patient will demonstrate that he "appreciates" the importance of foot care, when and to whom he will demonstrate this behavior, or what criteria will be used to determine whether the objective has been met.

The following are examples of well-written learning objectives:

▪ The patient will be able to demonstrate to the nurse the correct technique for changing his colostomy bag.

▪ In front of the nurse, the patient will administer a subcutaneous injection of insulin to herself using correct technique.

▪ The patient will select breakfast, lunch, and dinner menus keeping within a 2000 mg sodium diet for 3 consecutive days with 90% accuracy.

▪ Given a list of symptoms of heart failure, the patient will identify the early symptoms of heart failure with 80% accuracy before discharge from the hospital.

When learning objectives are clear and specific and when they are written down and available in the patient record, all members of the health care team can work together to accomplish the same objectives. Once the objectives are clearly stated, the nurse, patient, and patient's family should choose the strategy or strategies that are most appropriate to meet the objectives of the learning process.

Selecting Teaching Strategies. Selecting a particular strategy is determined by at least three factors: (1) patient characteristics (e.g., age, educational background, degree of illness, culture); (2) subject matter; and (3) available resources. A discussion of some teaching strategies that can be employed to achieve learning objectives follows. Each has advantages and disadvantages that make it more or less suitable to a particular patient and learning situation (Fig. 4-4).

Lecture. The lecture format is an efficient, versatile, and economical teaching strategy that can be used when the amount of time is limited or when a group of patients and family members can benefit from a core of basic information. The nurse presents a series of related ideas or facts to one person or to a group. Usually, the lecture is short, from 15 to 20 minutes, and some visual reinforcement, such as an outline or illustration, emphasizes key points. It is important to remember that the average adult learner can remember five to seven points at a time. Disadvantages of the lecture format are that it often has negative "school learning" connotations, and individual learning is difficult to evaluate. The nurse is active, but the patients are passive unless they are allowed to participate or ask questions.

Lecture-discussion. The lecture-discussion can overcome some of the disadvantages of the lecture only. With this strategy, the nurse presents specific information by using the lecture technique, followed by a period during which patients and their families ask questions and exchange points of view with the nurse. This strategy assists the patient in becoming an active participant in the learning process and creates a more informal give-and-take learning environment.

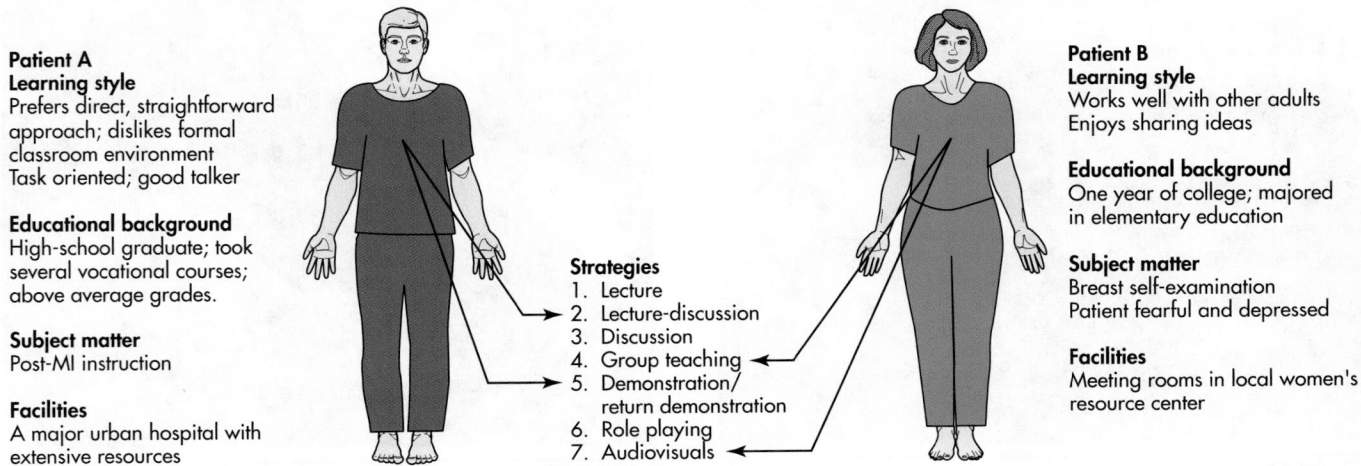

Patient A
Learning style
Prefers direct, straightforward approach; dislikes formal classroom environment
Task oriented; good talker

Educational background
High-school graduate; took several vocational courses; above average grades.

Subject matter
Post-MI instruction

Facilities
A major urban hospital with extensive resources

Strategies
1. Lecture
2. Lecture-discussion
3. Discussion
4. Group teaching
5. Demonstration/return demonstration
6. Role playing
7. Audiovisuals

Patient B
Learning style
Works well with other adults
Enjoys sharing ideas

Educational background
One year of college; majored in elementary education

Subject matter
Breast self-examination
Patient fearful and depressed

Facilities
Meeting rooms in local women's resource center

FIG. 4-4   Selecting teaching strategies. *MI*, Myocardial infarction.

Discussion. The purpose of discussion may be to exchange points of view concerning a topic or to arrive at a decision or conclusion. The nurse can discuss content with an individual or with a group, keeping the specific learning objectives in mind and clarifying information as needed. Participants' questions can also help the nurse identify and correct inaccurate information. This strategy is a good choice when the patient or patients have previous experience with a subject and have information to share, such as smoking cessation, post–coronary artery bypass surgery, or preoperative teaching classes. The discussion allows the patient or family members to actively participate and to apply their own experiences and observations to the learning process. The informal sharing and nonthreatening environment of discussions are positive factors, but this format usually requires more time depending on the topic and the number of participants.

Group teaching. There are two kinds of group teaching. In the first, the nurse acts as a **facilitator,** or helper, for group sharing about a common problem. Fig. 4-5 shows the nurse acting as a facilitator in small group discussion. As a facilitator, the nurse participates by keeping information moving among all group members. The nurse may introduce the patient to an existing group or may form a group of patients with similar problems, such as women who are caregivers.

A second kind of group teaching involves **peer teaching** as found in support groups. A support group is a self-help organization that can provide continuing information, shared experiences, acceptance, understanding, and useful suggestions about a problem or concern. Patients with problems such as impotence, cancer, alcoholism, Parkinson's disease, compulsive overeating, diabetes, or heart surgery can benefit from peer teaching. The nurse should actively look for opportunities to refer a patient or family to a support group. This action should be taken in addition to, not instead of, the nurse's planned teaching sessions.

Demonstration/return demonstration. The demonstration/return demonstration is a common strategy used by the nurse. The purpose is to show how to perform a motor skill, such as a dressing change, injection, or blood pressure measurement (Fig. 4-6). The focus is on correct procedure and application. To handle this strategy correctly, the nurse tells the patient the pur-

pose of the demonstration and makes sure that the patient can see and hear clearly. Then the nurse presents the demonstration in an informal manner, defines unfamiliar terms, and watches for signs of confusion from the patient. The nurse clarifies and repeats as needed, and then the patient returns the demonstration with the nurse as observer. The entire process should last no more than 15 to 20 minutes. Motor skills take practice to achieve, and the procedure should be practiced by the patient between teaching sessions.

Role play. Role play is another strategy that the nurse might employ depending on teaching objectives. This format is most often used when patients need to examine their attitudes and behaviors, when they need to understand the viewpoints and attitudes of others, or when they need to practice carrying out thoughts, ideas, or decisions. This strategy is challenging for the nurse because he or she is responsible for defining the problems, determining the goals, setting the climate, and determining the situation and roles to be played. The nurse gives information and clear instructions to role players and observers and provides time for feedback and evaluation. Role playing requires maturity, confidence, and flexibility on the part of the participants. It is important to remember that some patients may feel uncomfortable and inhibited with this method. Role playing takes time, which must be factored into the teaching plan. An example of the use of role playing is a wife who needs to rehearse how to talk with her husband about his need to quit smoking. In this case, "play acting" or practicing the discussion with the nurse ahead of time may be a helpful strategy.

Audiovisual materials. Audiovisual materials, including videotapes, slides, posters, computer-based programs, charts, audiotapes, or simple transparencies, are commonly used to supplement other teaching strategies. This strategy can enhance the presentation of information because it promotes learning through both visual and auditory stimulation. To use this strategy, the nurse must know what materials are available within the facility, from support agencies, and from professional groups. These materials must be previewed and evaluated for accuracy, completeness, and appropriateness to the learning objectives before being shown to the patient and family. Audio-

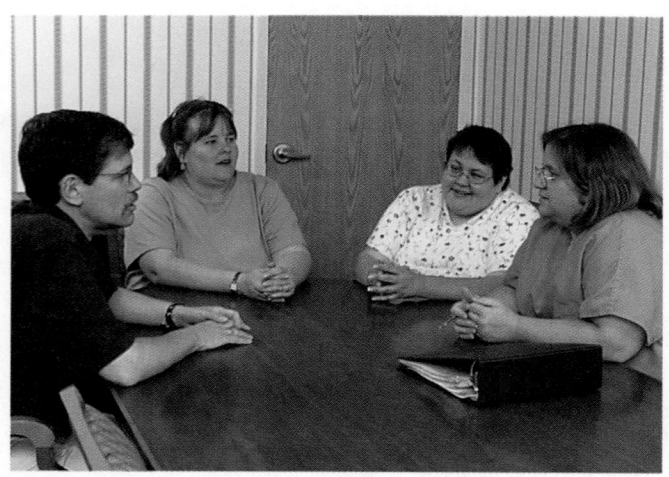

FIG. 4-5 Nurse acts as a facilitator in a small group discussion.

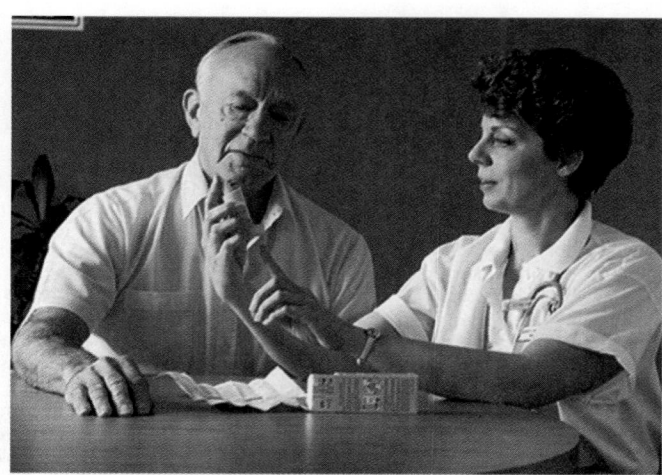

FIG. 4-6 Careful teaching using demonstration and return demonstration increases the possibility of successful learning by the patient.

tapes are relatively easy to use and can be inexpensive. The use of audiovisual materials can be extremely beneficial, particularly when teaching content that is largely visual, such as the steps and processes of procedures (e.g., dressing changes, injections, hemodialysis).

Internet. The use of the Internet and the World Wide Web for self-education by patients is increasing at a phenomenal rate. Many patients use their own computers or those available at public libraries to access health information on the Internet. The Internet also offers established education programs designed for specific learners. One nurse-designed, Internet-based information and support system for patients who have undergone coronary artery bypass graft surgery offers continuing contact with nurses and supplements the discharge education process.[29] However, use of the Internet as a source of information is a double-edged sword. It offers a large number of high-quality health resources and poses seemingly unlimited opportunities to inform, teach, and connect health professionals and patients alike. On the other hand, much Internet information is incomplete, misleading, or inaccurate.[30]

Not surprisingly, older patients use the Internet less frequently for health information than younger patients.[31] However, several computer education programs for older adults have been developed. Organizations dedicated to improving the quality of life for older adults are promoting user-friendly websites and publishing guides to help older adults evaluate health information on the Internet (available at *www.nlm.nih.gov/pubs/checklist.pdf*).[32]

The nurse is challenged by several factors when using the Internet as a teaching strategy. The nurse must have adequate computer competency to review and evaluate information and programs available on the Internet. Personal computer competency is also necessary to teach patients and families unfamiliar with computers how to access information, especially older adults. All patients who use the Internet must also be taught how to identify reliable and accurate information. The nurse should encourage patients to use sites established by the government, universities, or reputable medical or health-related associations (e.g., American Medical Association, American Diabetes Association, American Heart Association, National Institutes of Health, National Academies of Science, or U.S. Food and Drug Administration). Resources at the end of the chapter identify selected reliable patient education websites for the nurse to review and use for patient referral.

Printed materials. A wealth of printed health-related material is available for patient education. Printed materials are most often used in combination with previously presented teaching strategies. For instance, following a lecture on the physiologic effects of smoking, the nurse might distribute a pamphlet from the American Cancer Society that reviews and reinforces the topic. Or the nurse might select a book or magazine article written by a woman who has had a mastectomy and suggest that the patient read this material to prepare for other teaching sessions. Written materials are always recommended for patients whose preferred learning style is reading.

Written material must be appropriate for the reading level of the patient, as discussed earlier. Before written materials are used with patients, the nurse should evaluate the readability level if it is not indicated on the materials. Many different formulas have been developed to assess the readability of written materials, but one that is easy to use and has been used for many

years is the SMOG formula.[33] The steps to use the SMOG formula are as follows:[34]

1. Choose 10 consecutive sentences at the beginning, middle, and end of the document (30 total sentences).
2. Count every word in these sentences that has three or more syllables. If a word is repeated, count the repetition. Proper nouns with three or more syllables should be counted. Hyphenated words are considered one word.
3. Calculate the square root of the total number of words with three or more syllables.
4. Add 3 to the square root.
5. The result is the SMOG readability level.

For example, if there are 94 words with three or more syllables in the 30 sentences, the square root of 94 is 9.7, plus 3, equals a reading level of 12.7. This is too high for the average adult in the United States, who reads at the eighth-grade level, and is out of reach for those who are functionally illiterate.

When writing teaching materials the nurse can use several techniques to reduce the reading level, including the following: (1) give key information first using bold or italics; (2) use short, common words of one or two syllables; (3) define medical words in simple language if they must be used; (4) keep sentences under 10 words if possible, and 15 at the most; (5) use pictures or drawings; and (6) use an active voice in the manner you would say something.[23,34]

Major resources for acquiring relevant printed material include the hospital or care facility library, pharmacy, public library, federal and state agencies, universities, voluntary organizations, and research centers. Written materials, including computer-based programs, should be reviewed by the nurse before being used. In addition to reading level, the following criteria for review are suggested: (1) accuracy, (2) completeness, (3) whether the material meets specific learning goals, (4) use of pictures and diagrams to stimulate interest, (5) use of one main idea or concept per pamphlet or program, (6) whether the material contains information the patient would like to know, and (7) whether the material is culture and gender sensitive and appropriate.[5] In addition, materials that promote specific commercial or proprietary products should be avoided.

Implementation

During the implementation phase the nurse uses the planned strategies to present information and demonstrations. Verbal and nonverbal communication skills, active listening, and empathy are incorporated into the process. Based on the assessment of the patient's physical and psychologic condition, the nurse can determine how much active participation the patient can assume.

In implementing the teaching plan the nurse should remember the principles and characteristics of the adult learner. Reinforcement and reward are important, but the nurse should be aware that phrases such as "very good" or "aren't you doing well?" in the tone one would use with a child can be very condescending to adult learners. Techniques to enhance the teaching process with adults are presented in Table 4-6.

Evaluation

Evaluation is the final step in the learning process and is a measure of the degree to which the patient has mastered the learning objectives. The nurse monitors the performance level of the patient so that changes can be made as needed. The nurse may find that the patient has achieved the goals. However, if cer-

TABLE 4-6	Techniques to Enhance Patient Learning

- Keep the physical environment relaxed and nonthreatening.
- Maintain a respectful, warm, and enthusiastic attitude.
- Let the patient's expressed needs direct what information is provided.
- Focus on "must-know" information, saving "nice-to-know" information if time allows.
- Involve the patient and family in the process; emphasize active participation.
- Be aware of and take into consideration the patient's previous experiences.
- Emphasize the relevancy of the information to the patient's lifestyle and suggest how it may provide an immediate solution to a problem.
- Schedule and pace learning experiences according to the patient's needs and abilities.
- Individualize the teaching plan, even if standardized plans are used.
- Emphasize helping the patient to learn and not just transmitting subject matter.
- Review written materials with the patient.
- Remember that simple is best.
- Ask for frequent feedback.
- Affirm progress with rewards valued by the patient to reinforce desired behaviors.

tain goals are not reached, the nurse may need to reassess the patient and alter the teaching plan. If the patient has developed new needs, the nurse then plans new goals, content, and strategies.

For example, an elderly man with diabetes mellitus entered the hospital with a blood glucose level of 550 mg/dl (30.53 mmol/L). When the student nurse began to prepare his insulin injection, the nurse asked, "Are you going to have him give his own insulin and observe his technique?" "Oh, no," replied the student nurse, "He has been a diabetic for 20 years!" The assumption was that a patient with diabetes would know how to perform this task correctly. The two nurses returned to the patient's room and asked him to prepare an insulin injection. The patient filled the syringe with 20 units of insulin and 20 units of air, instead of 40 units of insulin. After correcting the dosage and questioning the patient more fully, the nurses concluded that the patient could not accurately see the markings on the syringe and that the patient may have been administering insufficient insulin to himself for a long period of time. The patient's vision was not as good as it had been 20 years ago, and special equipment was now necessary for him to safely and accurately administer the insulin.

Evaluation techniques may be short term or long term. Short-term evaluation techniques are used to quickly evaluate the patient's mastery of a concept, skill, or behavior change and can be accomplished in the following ways:

1. *Observe the patient directly.* "Show me how you will change your dressing." "Let me see how you administer your injection." By observation, the nurse determines if a task has been mastered, if further instruction is needed, or if the patient is ready for new or additional content. If a task is mastered, it is vital that the nurse affirms the patient's newly acquired skill. Affirmation presented in an appropriate manner for an adult is a strong motivating factor for continued learning.

2. *Observe verbal and nonverbal cues.* If the patient asks the nurse to repeat instructions, asks questions, shakes his or her head, loses eye contact, slumps or droops in the chair or bed, becomes restless and fidgety, or otherwise expresses doubt about understanding, the patient may be indicating that further instruction is needed or an alternative approach should be taken. The nurse must be alert to the patient's nonverbal as well as verbal cues.

3. *Ask direct questions.* "What are the major food groups?" "How often must you change your dressing?" "What should you do if you develop chest pain after returning home?" Open-ended questions will provide more information about the patient's understanding than questions that require a "yes" or "no" answer.

4. *Use a written measurement tool, graded for accuracy.* Paper-and-pencil tests may increase anxiety in patients. Adults may "freeze" when given a test, or "go blank" when asked to write something that will be graded. Assess the patient's comfort and learning style before using this method of evaluation.

5. *Talk with a member of the patient's family or support system.* "Is he eating regularly?" "How is he handling the walker?" "When is she taking her medications?" Because the nurse cannot be with the patient 24 hours a day, use other people who have contact with the patient.

6. *Seek the patient's self-evaluation of progress.* What evidence does the patient have that the objectives are being met? Is the patient confident or unsure? Is the patient ready to go forward with new material? It is important to remember that self-direction is important in adult learning. By seeking out a patient's opinion the nurse is allowing patient input into the evaluation process.

These short-term evaluation techniques can be used frequently and interchangeably to keep informed of the patient's progress and assess changing needs.

Long-term evaluation requires follow-up by the nurse, outpatient clinic, or outside agency. The nurse's role is to explain to the patient the positive outcomes associated with regular reevaluation by someone familiar with the patient's needs. The nurse should set up a schedule of visits for the patient before the patient leaves the hospital or clinic or refer the patient to the proper agencies. The nurse keeps written documentation of follow-up telephone calls or mailed, written reminders to urge the patient to maintain the follow-up schedule. The patient's family or support person should be familiar with the follow-up plan, so that everyone is involved in the patient's long-term progress.

The nurse takes the initiative in contacting persons or agencies involved in the patient's long-term follow-up. The nurse should telephone, visit, or write these health professionals and supply them with the education plan, including learning objectives, teaching plan, and short-term evaluation measures. These data are charted in the patient's medical records for further use.

Documentation is an essential component of the entire learning transaction. The nurse records everything from the assessment through short- and long-term plans for evaluation. As mentioned, the documentation should be forwarded to the agency or health professional providing long-term follow-up. Because many different members of the health care team will use these records in different places and for different reasons, the teaching objectives, content, strategies, and evaluation results should be written clearly and completely.

Standardized teaching plans are often included in care maps and clinical pathways and have become an accepted method of developing a teaching plan. Standardized teaching plans contain widely accepted knowledge and skills that a patient and family need to know concerning a specific health problem or procedure. However, the nurse should always individualize these plans to meet the patient's specific needs.

CRITICAL THINKING EXERCISES

Case Study
Example of the Teaching Process

Jane is admitted to the hospital for preliminary testing and preparation for a hysterectomy. The nurse is aware that a patient undergoing a hysterectomy is often deeply concerned about her self-concept as a woman. The nurse also knows that such patients need to express their feelings in an atmosphere of support and understanding. Therefore the nurse has sought to listen attentively and ask questions carefully in order to assess the patient's feelings about and knowledge of her surgical procedure. The nurse has asked open-ended questions, such as "How do you feel about having the surgery?" and "What concerns do you have about undergoing a hysterectomy?" By establishing a climate of trust and a counseling relationship, the nurse has completed the following assessment:

Biophysical Dimension

Age 44, white female, high school English teacher and coaches girls' varsity basketball team; good general health. Height and weight proportional and average for age. Patient reports that she jogs five evenings a week. No sensory impairment; vision, hearing, and reaction time seem normal.

Psychologic Dimension

Patient appears mildly anxious about surgery and worried about her husband's acceptance of her sexuality. She is also worried about missing work and leaving her classes to a substitute teacher. She states that she does not "let physical problems get me down," and that she dislikes "pills and hospitals." She states that she is used to "teaching" and not being "taught," and she tries to dominate any conversation or input from the nurse.

Sociocultural Dimension

Married with one child (son) age 23. Mother had a mastectomy at age 51; father healthy. Two younger sisters; both experienced difficult pregnancies but are otherwise healthy. Patient describes family communication as very good. She describes her lifestyle as work oriented and that her friends are primarily teaching associates. Her Norwegian and Lutheran heritage places a high priority on work and family. One of her close friends has previously undergone this procedure.

Learning Style

Responds well to formal lectures. Enjoys reading and group discussions.

Determine Objectives

After a brief period of rest and adjustment to the unfamiliar hospital environment, Jane states that she would like to learn more about the details of the upcoming planned surgical procedure. Together Jane and the nurse identify the following objectives:

Following the teaching session, I (Jane) will be able to:
1. Describe to the nurse the surgical procedure (hysterectomy).
2. Express to the nurse and my husband my feelings about maintaining an active and fulfilling sex life.
3. Complete arrangements with my family and school principal for convalescence and return to normal activities.
4. List the general recovery experiences that are expected and under what circumstances to seek medical advice.
5. Discuss "old wives' tales" regarding hysterectomy and verbalize concerns regarding undergoing the hysterectomy.
6. Identify ways to avoid constipation, weight gain, and potential periods and depression during the recovery period.
7. Identify ways to comfortably return to baseline sexual activities.

REVIEW QUESTIONS

The number of the question corresponds to the same-numbered objective at the beginning of the chapter.

1. The nurse is teaching a middle-aged Hispanic woman in a clinic about various methods to relieve the patient's symptoms of menopause. The goal of this teaching would be to
   a. prevent disease.
   b. maintain health.
   c. alter the patient's cultural belief regarding the use of herbs.
   d. provide information for selection and use of treatment options.

2. When planning teaching with consideration of adult learning principles, the nurse would
   a. present material in an efficient, lecture format.
   b. recognize that adults enjoy learning regardless of the relevance to their personal lives.
   c. provide opportunities for the patient to learn from other adults with similar experiences.
   d. postpone practice of new skills until the patient can independently practice the skill at home.

Continued

REVIEW QUESTIONS—cont'd

3. A necessary skill of the nurse in the role of teacher is the ability to
   a. determine when patients are too distressed physically or psychologically to learn.
   b. assure the patient that the nurse understands what is necessary for the patient to learn.
   c. develop standardized teaching plans for use with all patients to save time and overcome time constraints.
   d. present information in medical language to increase the patient's vocabulary and understanding of pathophysiology.

4. When the nurse is feeling stressed about the limited time available for patient teaching, a strategy that might be used is
   a. setting realistic goals that have high priority for the patient.
   b. referring the patient to a nurse educator in private practice for teaching.
   c. observing more experienced nurse-teachers to learn how to teach faster and more efficiently.
   d. providing reading materials for the patient instead of discussing information the patient needs to learn.

5. The nurse includes family members in patient teaching primarily because
   a. they provide most of the care for patients.
   b. patients have been shown to have better outcomes when families are involved.
   c. the patient may be too ill or too stressed by the situation to understand teaching.
   d. they might feel rejected and unimportant if they are not included in the teaching.

6. When the nurse, the patient, and the patient's family decide together what strategies would be best to meet the learning objectives, the step of the teaching process that is involved is
   a. planning.
   b. evaluation.
   c. assessment.
   d. implementation.

7. A patient characteristic that enhances the teaching-learning process is
   a. high anxiety.
   b. high self-efficacy.
   c. being in the precontemplative stage of change.
   d. being able to laugh about the health problem that is present.

8. An example of a correctly written learning objective is
   a. The patient will lose 25 pounds in 6 weeks.
   b. The patient should understand the implications of the condition.
   c. The patient will read two pamphlets on the subject of breast self-examination.
   d. The patient's spouse will demonstrate to the nurse how to correctly change a gastrostomy bag before discharge.

9. A patient tells the nurse that she enjoys talking with others and sharing experiences, but easily falls asleep when reading. In planning teaching strategies with the patient, the nurse recognizes that the patient would probably learn best with
   a. role play.
   b. group teaching.
   c. lecture-discussion.
   d. discussion supplemented with computer programs.

10. Short-term evaluation of teaching effectiveness includes
    a. observing the patient and asking direct questions.
    b. following the patient for 3 to 6 months after the teaching.
    c. monitoring for the behavior change for up to 6 weeks following discharge.
    d. asking the patient what he or she found helpful about the teaching experience.

REFERENCES

1. Joint Commission on Accreditation of Healthcare Organizations: *Comprehensive accreditation manual for hospitals: the official handbook,* Oakbrook Terrace, Ill, 2001, The Commission.
2. National Center for Chronic Disease Prevention and Health Promotion: *Chronic diseases and their risk factors: the nation's leading causes of death, 1999,* Washington, DC, 2001, Centers for Disease Control and Prevention.
3. Campbell KN: Adult education: helping adults begin the process of learning, *AAOHN J* 47:31, 1999.
4. Walker EA: Characteristics of the adult learner, *Diabetes Educ (Suppl)* 26:16, 1999.
5. Redman BK: *The practice of patient education,* ed 9, St Louis, 2001, Mosby.
6. Knowles M: *The adult learner: a neglected species,* ed 4, Houston, 1990, Gulf Publishing.
7. Phillips LD: Patient education: understanding the process to maximize time and outcomes, *J Intravenous Nurs* 22:19, 1999.
8. Prochaska JO, Velicer WF: The transtheoretical model of health behavior change, *Am J Health Promot* 12:38, 1997.
9. Parkerson GR, Gutman RA: Health-related quality of life predictors of survival and hospital utilization, *Health Care Financ Rev* 21:171, 2000.
10. Waller MA: Gay men with AIDS: perceptions of social support and adaptational outcome, *J Homosex* 41:99, 2001.
*11. Saleh US, Brockopp DY: Hope among patients with cancer hospitalized for bone marrow transplantation: a phenomenologic study, *Cancer Nurs* 24:308, 2001.
12. Gerstle JF, Varenne H, Contento I: Post-diagnosis family adaptation influences glycemic control in women with type 2 diabetes mellitus, *J Am Diet Assoc* 101:918, 2001.
13. Marcantonio ER et al: Factors associated with unplanned hospital readmission among patients 65 years of age and older in a Medicare managed care plan, *Am J Med* 107:13, 1999.
14. Boise L, Heagerty B, Eskenazi C: Facing chronic illness: the family support model and its benefits, *Patient Educ Couns* 27:75, 1996.
15. Coyne JC et al: Prognostic importance of marital quality for survival of congestive heart failure, *Am J Cardiol* 88:526, 2001.

*Nursing research–based reference.

16. Heinich F, Molenda M, Russell JD: *Instructional media and the new technologies of instruction,* ed 4, New York, 1992, Macmillan.

17. Feste C, Anderson RM: Empowerment: from philosophy to practice, *Patient Educ Couns* 26:139, 1995.

18. Leventhal H, Meyer D, Nerenz D: The common sense representation of illness danger. In Rachman S, editor: *Contributions to medical psychology,* New York, 1980, Permagon.

19. Edwards R et al: Self-efficacy as a predictor of adult adjustment to sickle cell disease: one year outcomes, *Psychosom Med* 63:850, 2001.

20. Mancuso CA et al: Self-efficacy, depressive symptoms, and patients' expectations predict outcomes in asthma, *Med Care* 39:1326, 2001.

21. Murphy PW et al: Neurology patient education materials: do our educational aids fit our patient needs? *J Neurosci Nurs* 33:99, 2001.

22. American Hospital Association: *Patient's bill of rights,* Chicago, 1992, The Association.

23. D'Alessandro DM, Kingsley P, Johnson-West J: The readability of pediatric patient education materials on the World Wide Web, *Arch Pediatr Adolesc Med* 155:807, 2001.

24. US Department of Education, National Center for Education Statistics: *Adult literacy, 1999,* Washington, DC, 1999, US Department of Education. Available at *http://nces.ed.gov/fastfacts/display.asp?id=69* (accessed Jan 10, 2002).

25. Human Resources Development Canada and the National Literacy Secretariat: *Reading the future: a portrait of literacy in Canada,* Ottawa, 1996, Human Resources Development Canada and the National Literacy Secretariat. Available at *www.nald.ca/nls/ials/introduct.htm* (accessed Jan 10, 2002).

26. Duffy MM, Snyder K: Can ED patients read your patient education materials? *J Emerg Nurs* 25:294, 1999.

*27. Turton J: Importance of information following myocardial infarction: a study of the self-perceived information needs of patients and their spouse/partner compared with the perceptions of nursing staff, *J Adv Nurs* 27:770, 1998.

28. Luniewski M, Reigle J, White B: Card sort: an assessment tool for the educational needs of patients with heart failure, *Am J Crit Care* 8:297, 1999.

29. Brennan PF et al: HeartCare: an Internet-based information and support system for patient home recovery after coronary artery bypass graft (CABG) surgery, *J Adv Nurs* 35:699, 2001.

30. Silberg WM, Lundberg GD, Musacchio RA: Assessing, controlling, and assuring the quality of medical information on the Internet, *JAMA* 277:1244, 1997.

31. Hendrix CC: Computer use among elderly people, *Comput Nurs* 18:62, 2000.

32. Vastag B: Easing the elderly online in search of health information, *JAMA* 285:1563, 2001.

33. McLaughlin GH: SMOG grading—a new readability formula, *J Reading* 12:639, 1969.

34. Winslow EH: Patient education materials: can patients read them, or are they ending up in the trash? *Am J Nurs* 101:33, 2001.

*Nursing research–based reference.

RESOURCES

Clinical and Patient Education
Medical University of South Carolina
(Reading grade level [RL] indicated on material)
www.musc.edu/medcenter/education/cpeducation/

HealthAnswers
Attn: HA Information
1140 Welsh Road, Suite 210
North Wales, PA 19454
215-412-3900
Fax: 215-412-5674
www.healthanswers.com/

Healthfinder
Office of Disease Prevention and Health Promotion
U.S. Department of Health and Human Resources
www.healthfinder.gov/

Medline Plus Health Information
U.S. National Library of Medicine
8600 Rockville Pike
Bethesda, MD 20984
www.nlm.nih.gov/medlineplus/

Health Information On-Line
(Sources of reliable Internet health information)
U.S. Food and Drug Administration
www.fda.gov/fdac/features/596_info.html

InteliHealth
960C Harvest Drive
Blue Bell, PA 19422
www.intelihealth.com

MedExplorer
Health/Medical Search Engine
www.medexplorer.com/

MedicineNet.com
www.medicinenet.com

Meducation World Wide Web Medical Education Resource
www.meducation.com/patient.html

Office of Disease Prevention and Health Promotion
Office of Public Health and Science, Office of the Secretary
200 Independence Avenue SW, Room 738G
Washington, DC 20201
202-401-6295
Fax: 202-205-9478
www.odphp.osophs.dhhs.gov

For additional Internet resources, see the website for this book at *http://evolve.elsevier.com/Lewis/medsurg/*.

CHAPTER **5**

Older Adults

Margaret McLean Heitkemper

LEARNING OBJECTIVES

1. Describe the impact of older adults on the health care system.
2. Describe the effects of ageism on care of older adults.
3. List the major concepts in adult developmental theories proposed by Erikson, Peck, Havighurst, and Levinson.
4. List the major biologic theories of aging and describe clinical manifestations related to specific age-related physiologic changes.
5. Describe the needs of special populations of older adults.
6. Identify differences in health status and disease manifestation between older and younger adults.
7. Identify the role of the nurse in health screening and promotion and disease prevention for older adults.
8. Describe nursing interventions to assist chronically ill older adults.
9. Describe common problems of older adults related to hospitalization and acute illness and the role of the nurse in assisting them with selected care problems.
10. Describe challenges and concerns related to the caregiving role.
11. Identify care alternatives to meet patient-specific needs of older adults.
12. Identify the legal and ethical issues related to older adults.

KEY TERMS

adult development, p. 59	gerontologic nursing, p. 58
ageism, p. 59	Medicare, p. 77
caregiver, p. 76	nonstochastic theory, p. 61
delirium, p. 72	old-old adult, p. 58
elder abuse, p. 76	polypharmacy, p. 73
ethno-geriatrics, p. 68	stochastic theory, p. 61
frail elderly, p. 67	young-old adult, p. 58

Gerontologic nursing is the care of older adults based on the specialty body of knowledge of gerontology. The nurse approaches the older adult patient with a whole-person (physical, psychologic, socioeconomic) perspective. This chapter presents specific information about older adults that will assist the nurse in providing care to individuals or groups. Care of older adults presents challenges to nurses that require skilled assessment and creative adaptations of nursing interventions.

DEMOGRAPHICS OF AGING

In the last three decades the older adult population (those 65 years of age and older) has grown twice as fast as the rest of the population. The U.S. Census done in 2000 found that approximately 35 million persons, or 12.4% of the population, were age 65 or older.[1] Similarly, in Canada approximately 12% of the population is over age 65. In 1999 in the United States, 16.1% of persons over age 65 were minorities, including 8.1% African Americans, 2.3% Asians or Pacific Islanders, and less than 1% American Indians or Native Alaskans. Persons of Hispanic origin (who may be of any race) represented 5.3% of the older population. Several factors have led to the overall increase in the older population. The large post–World War II immigrant population has now grown older. Common diseases of the early 1900s that killed many older adults, such as influenza and diarrhea, are now less common, and people are living longer. Drug therapies, including antibiotics and chemotherapy, and earlier detection of diseases have contributed to the increase in life span.

This growth in our older population is expected to continue into the next century, and by 2030 there will be 70 million older adults representing 20% of the population (Fig. 5-1). Within the next 10 years the "baby boomers" will begin to turn 65, placing greater demands on health care. Minority populations are projected to represent 25.4% of the elderly population by 2030. A child born in the United States in 1998 could expect to live 76.9 years, about 29 years longer than a child born in 1900. The U.S. Census Bureau predicts life expectancy to continue to increase for both men and women. In 1998 persons reaching age 65 had an average life expectancy of an additional 17.8 years (19.2 years for females and 16.0 years for males).[2,3] For Canadians a female child born in 1997 has a life expectancy of 81.4 years and a male child 75.8 years.[4]

The most rapidly increasing age-group is composed of those persons 75 years of age and older. Since the 1960s this group has increased 250%. The terms **young-old adult** (55 to 75 years of age) and **old-old adult** (75 years of age and older) were introduced in 1978. These two groups represent chronologic ranges that often present different characteristics and needs. The old-old adult is usually a widowed woman dependent on family or kinship support. Many have outlived children, spouses, and siblings. The old-old adult is often characterized as a hardy, elite survivor. Because the old-old adult has lived so long, she may have become the family icon, the symbol of family tradition and legacy. Approximately 20% of individuals 85 or older live in nursing homes or other institutions.[1] The term *frail elderly* has been suggested to represent those 75 years of age and older with a variety of ongoing and accumulating health concerns.[5] (Frail older adults are discussed later in this chapter.)

Reviewed by Barbara S. Levine, RN, PhD, CRNP, CS, Advanced Registered Nurse Practitioner, BSL Consulting Services, Wayne, Pa.

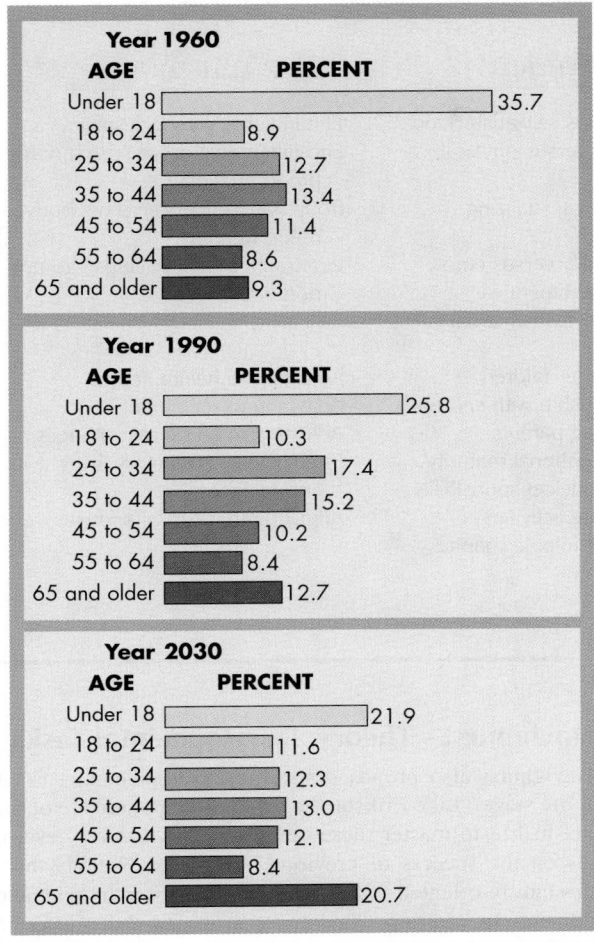

Year 1960

AGE	PERCENT
Under 18	35.7
18 to 24	8.9
25 to 34	12.7
35 to 44	13.4
45 to 54	11.4
55 to 64	8.6
65 and older	9.3

Year 1990

AGE	PERCENT
Under 18	25.8
18 to 24	10.3
25 to 34	17.4
35 to 44	15.2
45 to 54	10.2
55 to 64	8.4
65 and older	12.7

Year 2030

AGE	PERCENT
Under 18	21.9
18 to 24	11.6
25 to 34	12.3
35 to 44	13.0
45 to 54	12.1
55 to 64	8.4
65 and older	20.7

FIG. 5-1   Age distribution of total U.S. population.

ATTITUDES TOWARD AGING

Who is old? The answer to this question often depends on the age and attitude of the respondent. It is important that the nurse maintains the position that aging is normal and is not related to disease. Age is a date in time and is influenced by many factors, including emotional and physical health, developmental stage, socioeconomic status, culture, and ethnicity.

As people age, they are exposed to more and different life experiences. The accumulation of these differences makes older adults more diverse than any other age-group. As the nurse assesses the older adult, it is important to consider this diversity. The nurse should assess the patient for perceptions of age. Older adults with poor health report a higher perceived age and lower sense of psychologic well-being as compared with healthy older adults.[6] Age is important, but it may not be the most relevant data for determining appropriate care of an individual older adult patient.

Myths and stereotypes about aging, found throughout society, are supported by media reports of needy, problematic older adults. Myths and stereotypes regarding aging provide the basis of commonly held misconceptions that may lead to errors in assessments and unnecessary limitations to interventions. For example, if the nurse thinks all old people are rigid, new ideas will not be presented to the patient.

Ageism is a negative attitude based on age. It leads to discrimination in the care given to the older adult. The nurse who demonstrates negative attitudes may fear his or her own aging process or be misinformed about aging and the health care needs of the older adult. The nurse may benefit from gaining knowledge about normal aging and increasing contact with the healthy, independent older adult.

ADULT DEVELOPMENT

Adult development has been approached in several ways. Despite rigorous attempts no single theory has been universally accepted to explain the process. In fact, there is no way to isolate physical, sociocultural, and psychologic factors to study adult development. Adulthood reflects the interrelationship of all factors. Therefore the best approach toward holistic care incorporates the psychologic, biologic, and spiritual aspects of the unique person.

Theorists have explained **adult development** based on the following premises:
1. Adult development continues to occur in definable, predictable, and sequential patterns.
2. Critical periods occur throughout the life span when physical growth and psychosocial growth undergo reorganization.
3. In each stage of development, there are certain normative activities or tasks to be accomplished.
4. Mastering the tasks of preceding stages is fundamental to transition and mastery of tasks in future stages.

The adult development models of Erikson, Peck, Levinson, and Havighurst are summarized in Table 5-1 and are briefly described below.

Erikson's Theory: Psychosocial Developmental Conflicts

Erikson views personality development as resulting from the confrontations between ego and social milieu.[7] He identifies points in the life cycle when specific developmental conflicts become paramount because a person's capacities or experiences dictate that a major self-adjustment and adjustment to the environment must be made. In the process of making this adjustment, the individual moves toward one of two opposing positions, such as toward intimacy or toward isolation. When a person successfully masters a core conflict (such as intimacy), the negative sense (isolation) remains as a dynamic counterpart and may be demonstrated in new situations in which this conflict must be mastered again at a higher level. Although critical times for mastery of each core conflict exist, all conflicts are present throughout the life span.

Intimacy versus Isolation. In Erikson's model, the young adult task is intimacy. This involves fusing self-identity with the identities of others in friendships, for causes or creative efforts, or in close personal relationships, including sexual union. Intimacy requires a degree of commitment that necessitates sacrifice, compromise, and self-abandonment for the benefit of others. The young adult who avoids making this commitment to others, fearing the loss of self-identity, will experience a sense of isolation and consequently self-absorption.

Generativity versus Stagnation. During middle adulthood, the primary task is generativity. Generative adults are concerned with establishing the next generation by nurturing and guiding either their children or other young people. A sense

TABLE 5-1	Adult Developmental Stage Theories		
THEORIST	**YOUNG ADULTHOOD**	**MIDDLE ADULTHOOD**	**OLDER ADULTHOOD**
• Erikson	Intimacy versus isolation	Generativity versus self-absorption	Ego integrity versus despair
• Peck		Valuing wisdom versus physical power	Ego differentiation versus work role preoccupation
		Socializing versus sexualizing relationships	Body transcendence versus body preoccupation
		Emotional flexibility versus emotional impoverishment	Ego transcendence versus ego preoccupation
		Mental flexibility versus mental rigidity	
• Havighurst	Mate selection and marriage adjustments	Launching teenage children	Adjusting to health decline
	Establishing family and child rearing	Maturing relationship with spouse	Adjusting to retirement
	Home management	Adjusting to aging parents	Adjusting to social role changes
	Occupation launching	Career and occupational maturity	Establishing satisfactory living arrangements
	Beginning civic responsibility	Adult social and civic responsibility	Adjusting to death of spouse
• Levinson	Early adult transition	Developing leisure activities	
	Entering the adult world	Adjusting to physiologic changes	
	Thirties transition	Midlife transition	
	Settling down	Payoff years	

of productivity in work and creativity in living are also important components of this task. This core conflict probably arises out of an altruistic need to leave some mark that will make the world a better place in which to live. If generativity does not occur, adults experience a sense of stagnation and turn inward, becoming self-preoccupied and overly concerned with physical and psychologic health needs. The focus of self-absorbed people on physical changes of middle age may result in either invalidism or inappropriate youthfulness in an attempt to stay young.

Ego Integrity versus Despair. Older adulthood is a time for reviewing the past and rearranging the "photo album of life." This bringing together of all the previous life stages should result in a sense of wholeness, purpose, and a life well lived, or a sense of ego integrity, according to Erikson. When a person accepts and approves of a unique life, death also can be accepted as a meaningful part of life. However, if the life review is laden with opportunities missed or wrong directions taken, a sense of despair arises. Death is faced with anxiety. In this last stage of ego integrity versus despair, each person must face adjustments and come to a final conflict resolution that is the product of all previous developmental conflict resolutions.

Peck's Theory: Developmental Tasks

Based on Erikson's work, Peck further defined psychosocial tasks of middle and older adulthood.[8] With a general decline in physical and sexual functioning, the middle-aged adult's self-esteem can suffer if it is heavily based on such changes. However, judgmental abilities tend to increase with experience, so valuing the use of one's "head" becomes a positive alternative for maintaining self-esteem. People need flexibility to shift attachments and reinvest emotions in other people and pursuits. People also need the mental flexibility to allow for new solutions to life problems, rather than being dogmatic and governed by past experiences.

Havighurst's Theory: Developmental Tasks

Havighurst also proposed specific developmental tasks for each life stage.[9] Like Erikson, he contends that there are optimal points in life to master these tasks, and the mastery level depends on the success of previous life stages. Notably, he includes family-oriented tasks that are significant to individual development. In addition, Havighurst proposed that "successful achievement of [a task] leads to happiness and to success with later tasks, while failure leads to unhappiness in the individual, disapproval by the society, and difficulty with later tasks."[9]

Levinson's Theory: Evolution of Life Structures

Levinson's theory describes the evolution of life structures. Although men and women go through similar stages of development, women may have more difficulty planning a life course if the themes of family and career are viewed as mutually exclusive choices. Levinson's basic concept, individual life structure, is the pattern of a given life at any point in time. Any change in the person's self-system (e.g., judgments, motives, values) and his or her interactions with other systems (e.g., social and cultural context of life within the family, ethnicity, religion, occupation, and social events), and the particular set of roles he or she assumes, will disrupt the components. Such disruptions call for reorganizing of the life structure.[10]

Life structure is dynamic with predictable changes occurring as individuals move through life. The four major periods in adult life are early adulthood (ages 21 through 40), middle adulthood (ages 41 through 60), late adulthood (ages 61 through 80), and late-late adulthood (beyond 80). Within each of the four stages in adult life, individuals face transitions and stability. Transitions are a time to make changes and redirect growth toward personal goals and objective. Stable times present opportunities to build and maintain the intact life structures necessary to pursue those goals and objectives.

Other Theories of Adult Development

Other theorists have used life event and transition perspectives to describe adult development. To these theorists major life events are more important than chronologic age in assessing and understanding adult behaviors.[11] Activities within one's life such as being newly married, starting a job, middle-age parenting, divorce, retirement, illness, job-related pressures, adolescent children, and parenting one's parents provide stresses of varying degrees, not always associated with a specific age.[11] Another component of development is the individual's perception of and reaction to the expected or unexpected timing of life events and the aging process. In this model one's life experiences are viewed within the appropriate time context: historical time (calendar time), life time (chronologic age), and socially defined time (as related to age norms and expectations).[12]

Courtenay reviewed adult development models and found four characteristics that are common to all models.[13] All models focus on self-identity and growth through developmental tasks. An individual's psychologic identity is closely related to personal growth and the achievement of tasks that extend his or her capabilities. Another characteristic common among the models is that individuals move through hierarchic stages that range from the simple to the complex, from rigidity to flexibility, and from narrow to comprehensive perspectives.[13] The belief that human development occurs throughout the life span is a third characteristic. The vast variety and complexity of proficiencies faced by adults require constant evolution and lifelong pursuit. Today's increasing life span offers adults multiple opportunities for continued development. The fourth characteristic of these models is that the ultimate goal of adult development is to achieve autonomy, separateness, and independence.

BIOLOGIC AGING THEORIES

From a biologic view, *aging* is defined as the progressive loss of function. This age-related decrease occurs along with decreasing fertility and increased mortality. The exact etiology or cause of biologic aging remains to be determined. Biologic aging is clearly a multifactorial process involving genetics, oxidative stress, diet, and environment. Research efforts are directed at increasing both the average life span and the quality of life of older adults. It is hoped that new antiaging therapies will be developed to slow down or reverse age-related changes that result in chronic illness and disability. Based on numerous laboratory studies in rodents, caloric restriction (reducing dietary intake by 25% to 50%) has been most consistently shown to significantly extend the life span.[14] Caloric restriction in rodents results in a decrease in metabolic activity, but whether this accounts for the increase in longevity is not known. It is not feasible or ethical to conduct similar studies in humans. Thus whether this is applicable to humans remains to be determined. Some of the antiaging strategies that are currently under investigation are presented in Table 5-2.

There has long been an interest in slowing down or reversing the effects of aging. A number of nutrients have been examined and tested for their potential benefits in reducing the impact of aging. Examples include vitamin A (retinol), β-carotene, selenium, ginkgo, and chromium.[14] However, much more research is needed before it is determined whether any of these substances will delay aging or enhance the functional ability of older adults.

TABLE 5-2	Current Strategies for Slowing or Reversing Aging
ANTIAGING STRATEGIES	**SCIENTIFIC BASIS AND EXAMPLES OF FINDINGS**
Caloric restriction	• Increase in mean and maximum life span and delay in appearance of biologic aging markers in laboratory rodents (mice, rats) and nonhuman primates on >25% calorie-restricted diets. • Humans who have low caloric intake or low body mass index have lower overall mortality rates. • Unknown mechanism but may be related to decreased rate of cell division and/or decreased free radical production.
Cell-based therapies	• Studies done using cell transplantation techniques. • Include clinical procedures such as stem cell transplants used in the treatment of diseases. • Potential to help with age-related diseases (e.g., Parkinson's disease) is under investigation. • Unknown effect on mean life span.
Hormone therapy	• Hormones with anabolic effects decrease aging. • Women treated with hormone therapy during the postmenopausal period have decreased incidence of osteoporosis. • Results from clinical trials with androgens and growth hormone to determine effects on muscle mass and physical stamina are inconclusive at this time.
Genetic manipulation	• Laboratory studies to identify the "aging" genes, as well as age-related changes in DNA and RNA. • Potential ability to manipulate select genes to prolong life span or decrease incidence of age-related diseases.

Adapted from Vojta CL et al: Antiaging therapy: an overview, *Hosp Pract* 36:43, 2001.

Several theories regarding biologic aging are currently proposed. One way to categorize theories related to biologic aging is to designate those that propose that aging is due to chance (a **stochastic theory**) and those that propose that aging is not related to chance (nonstochastic). A **nonstochastic theory** hypothesizes that age-related molecular and cellular events are programmed by genes. Proposed theories of aging are shown in Table 5-3.

Stochastic Theories

The somatic mutation and intrinsic mutagenesis theories postulate that aging is a result of lifelong genetic damage. This damage may include the progressive accumulation of faulty copying in dividing cells or the accumulation of errors in information-containing molecules. According to *somatic mutation theory*, body cells develop spontaneous mutations in the same way germ cells do. Subsequent cell divisions perpetuate the mutations until organs be-

TABLE 5-3	Summary of Biologic Theories of Aging
THEORY	**DYNAMICS**
Stochastic Theories	
Error	Faulty synthesis of DNA, RNA, or both.
Somatic	Alteration in RNA/DNA; protein or enzyme synthesis causes defective structure or function.
Transcription	Failure of transcription or translation between cells; malfunctions of RNA or related enzymes.
Free Radical	Oxidation of fats, proteins, and carbohydrates creates free electrons that attach to other molecules, altering cellular function.
Cross-link	Lipids, proteins, carbohydrates, and nucleic acid react with chemicals or radiation to form bonds that cause an increase in cell rigidity and instability.
Nonstochastic Theories	
Programmed	Biologic clock triggers specific cell behavior at specific time. Organism capable of specific number of cell divisions and specific life span.
Neuroendocrine	Control mechanisms (pituitary and hypothalamus) regulate interplay between various organs and tissues; efficiency of signals between mechanisms is altered or lost.
Immunologic/autoimmune	Alteration of B and T cells leads to loss of capacity for self-regulation; normal or age-related cells recognized as foreign matter; system reacts by forming antibodies to destroy these cells.
Telomere-telomerase hypothesis	With aging there is a loss of telomeres (repeated sequences at the ends of DNA). This loss limits the number of times cells can divide.

come inefficient and ultimately fail. The *intrinsic mutagenesis theory* suggests that the increase in mutational cells occurs because of a breakdown of genetic regulatory mechanisms. The basic premise is that the regulatory capacity of the human genetic constitution diminishes throughout life. Thus more mutations occur with aging that will ultimately result in functional failure. Although both theories are attractive, little evidence exists to support or deny them.

The *free radical theory* was initially proposed in 1956 by Harman but in recent years has become the focus of new research.[15] A free radical is a highly reactive atom or molecule that carries an unpaired electron and thus seeks to combine with another molecule, causing an oxidative process. This process, also called oxidative stress, can ultimately disrupt cell membranes and alter DNA and protein synthesis. Common diseases such as atherosclerosis and cancer are associated with oxidative stress.[16] Cellular integrity, function, and regeneration mechanisms are injured. Free radicals are natural by-products of many normal cellular processes and are also created by such environmental factors as smog, tobacco smoke, and radiation. There are numerous natural protective mechanisms in place to prevent oxidative damage. Recent research has focused on the roles of various antioxidants, including vitamins C and E, β-carotene, and selenium, to slow down the oxidative process and ultimately the aging process.[17] However, optimal doses of these substances have not been established. These substances are being investigated for their usefulness in preventing diseases related to aging, such as oral, esophageal, and reproductive cancers; coronary artery disease; and cataracts.

Another stochastic theory is the *cross-link theory*, which postulates that over time and as a result of exposure to chemicals and radiation in the environment, cross-links form between lipids, proteins, and carbohydrates, as well as nucleic acids. These cross-links result in decreased flexibility and elasticity, and this increases rigidity in tissues (e.g., blood vessels). Such changes in cell structure may explain the observable cosmetic changes associated with aging, such as wrinkles of the skin, and decreased

distensibility of arterial blood vessels. However, it is unlikely that such changes account for all of the detrimental physical events associated with aging.

Nonstochastic Theories

For many years it was believed that cells had the capability to reproduce for an infinite amount of time. However, in the 1950s Hayflick in a series of classic experiments demonstrated that culture skin fibroblasts would reproduce or divide a finite number of times. From these observations rose the *programmed theory of cell death*. In this theory it is proposed that there is an impairment in the ability of the cell to continue dividing. A more recent theory of aging is the *telomere-telomerase hypothesis*.[18] Telomeres are specialized repeated sequences that are present at the ends of DNA strands. Telomerase is the enzyme that synthesizes these repeat sequences.[19] With aging there is loss of these strands and a decrease in telomerase activity, both of which affect the number of times a cell can divide.[18,19]

The *neuroendocrine theory* proposes that aging occurs because of functional decrements in neurons and associated hormones.[16,20] It suggests that neural and endocrine changes may be pacemakers for many cellular and physiologic aspects of aging. This approach relates aging to the organism's loss of responsiveness of neuroendocrine tissue to various signals. In some cases this is a result of a loss of receptors, but in others, it is caused by changes in neurotransmission beyond the receptors. An important focus of this theory is the functional changes of the hypothalamic-pituitary system. These changes are accompanied by a decline in functional capacity in other endocrine organs, such as the adrenal and thyroid glands, ovaries, and testes.[20]

The *immunologic theory* proposes declining functional capacity of the immune system as the basis for the aging process.[16] It suggests that aging is not a passive wearing out of systems but an active self-destruction mediated by the immune system. This theory is based on observing an age-associated decline in T cell functioning, accompanied by a decrease in resistance and an increase in autoimmune diseases with aging.[21] Whether the immunologic changes are genetically determined, regulated by environment, or influenced by endocrine factors remains to be defined. However, some studies of cell division suggest that the cells of the immune system become more diversified with age and demonstrate a progressive loss of self-regulatory patterns. The result is an autoimmune phenomenon in which cells normal to the body are mistaken as foreign and are attacked by the person's own immune system.

AGE-RELATED PHYSIOLOGIC CHANGES

Age-related changes affect every body system. These changes are normal and occur as people age. However, the age at which specific changes become evident differs from person to person and within the same person. For instance, a person may have gray hair at age 45 but relatively unwrinkled skin at age 80. The nurse should assess for these age-related changes. Table 5-4 presents gerontologic differences in assessment based on age-related physiologic changes and associated clinical manifestations.

TABLE 5-4   *G*erontologic Differences in Assessment — Age-Related Changes and Associated Clinical Manifestations

SYSTEM	EXPECTED AGING CHANGES	CLINICAL MANIFESTATIONS
Cardiovascular		
• Cardiac output	Force of contraction decreased	Myocardial oxygen demand increased
	Fat and collagen increased	Stroke volume and CO decreased
	Heart muscle decreased	Fatigue, shortness of breath, tachycardia occur
	Ventricular wall thickened	Blood flow to vital organs and periphery decreased
• Cardiac rate and rhythm	Dependence of atrial contraction increased	HR slow to increase with stress
	Loss of fibers from bundle of His	Decrease in maximum HR (e.g., 80-year-old
	Mitral valve stretching	person, 120 bpm; 20-year-old person, 200 bpm)
	Ventricles slow to relax	Possible AV block
	Sinus node pacemaker cells decreased	Recovery time from tachycardia prolonged
		Premature beats increased
• Structural changes	Aortic valves sclerotic and calcified	Diastolic murmur present in 50% of older patients
	Baroreceptor sensitivity decreased	Heart position landmarks change
	Mild fibrosis and calcification of valves	
• Arterial circulation	Elastin and smooth muscle reduced	Modest increase in systolic BP
	Vessel rigidity increased	Rigid arteries contribute to coronary artery and pe-
	Vascular resistance increased	ripheral vascular disease
	Aorta becomes dilated	
• Venous circulation	Tortuosity increased	Inflamed, painful, or cordlike varicosities
• Peripheral pulses	Arteries rigid	Pulses weaker but equal
		Circulation slowed to periphery
		Cold feet and hands
Respiratory		
• Structures	Cartilage degeneration	Kyphosis
	Vertebrae rigid	Anterior-posterior diameter increased
	Strength of muscles decreased	Use of accessory muscles decreased
	Respiratory muscles atrophy	Chest rigid and barrel-shaped
	Thoracic wall increased ridigity	Respiratory excursion decreased
	Ciliary action decreased	Cough and deep breathing diminished
• Change in ventilation and perfusion	Pulmonary vascular bed decreased	Lung compliance decreased
	Alveoli decreased	Total lung volume not changed
	Thickened alveolar walls	Vital capacity decreased
	Elastic recoil decreased	Residual lung volume increased
		Mucus thickens
		PaO_2 and O_2 saturation decreased
		Hyperresonance
• Ventilation control	Response to hypoxia and hypercarbia decreased	Ability to maintain acid-base balance decreased
		Respiratory rate 12-24/min

AV, Atrioventricular; *BP*, blood pressure; *bpm*, beats per minute; *CO*, cardiac output; *HR*, heart rate.

Continued

TABLE
5-4   *Gerontologic Differences in Assessment*
Age-Related Changes and Associated Clinical Manifestations—cont'd

SYSTEM	EXPECTED AGING CHANGES	CLINICAL MANIFESTATIONS
Integumentary		
▪ Skin	Collagen and subcutaneous fat decreased	Skin less elastic
	Sweat glands decreased	Wrinkles and folds increased
	Epidermal cell turnover slowed	Extremity fat lost; fat on trunk increased
	Skin tissue fluid decreased	Skin heals slowly
	Capillary fragility increased	Skin dry
	Pigment cells decreased	Skin tears and bruises easily
	Sebaceous gland activity decreased	Skin color uneven
	Sensory receptors decreased	Normal skin lesions increased
	Thresholds for touch, vibration, heat, pain increased	Ability to respond to heat and cold decreased
		Ability to feel light touch decreased
		Cutaneous pain sensitivity declines
▪ Hair	Melanin decreased	Gray or white hair
	Germ center and hair follicle decreased	Hair quantity decreased and thinner
		Scalp, pubic, axillary hair decreased
		Facial hair on men decreased
		Facial hair on women increased
▪ Nails	Blood supply to nail bed decreased	Growth slowed
	Longitudinal striations increased	Nails thickened and brittle
		Split easily
		Potential for fungal infection increased
Urinary		
▪ Kidney	Renal mass decreased	Protein in urine increased
	Number of functioning nephrons decreased	Potential for dehydration increased
	Glomerular filtration rate decreased	Creatinine clearance decreased
	Renal plasma flow decreased	Serum creatinine and BUN increased
		Excretion of toxins and drugs decreased
		Nocturia increased
▪ Bladder	Bladder smooth muscle and elastic tissue decreased	Capacity decreased
		Less control; stress incontinence
▪ Micturition	Sphincter control decreased	Frequency, urgency, and nocturia increased
Reproductive		
▪ Male structures	Prostatic enlargement	Sexual response less intense
	Testicular volume decreased	Longer to achieve erection
	Sperm count decreased	Erection maintained without ejaculation
	Seminal vesicles atrophy	Force of ejaculation decreased
	Serum testosterone constant	
	Estrogen level increased	
▪ Female structures	Estradiol, prolactin, progesterone diminished	Responses to changing hormone levels altered
	Size of ovaries, uterus, cervix, fallopian tubes, labia decreased	Cervical, vaginal secretions decreased
	Associated glands and epithelium atrophied	Intensity of sexual response gradually deceased
	Elasticity in the pelvic area decreased	Potential for vaginal infections increased
	Breast tissue decreased	Potential for vaginal and uterine prolapse increased
	Vaginal pH becomes alkaline	
Gastrointestinal		
▪ Oral cavity	Dentine decreased	Taste changes
	Gingival retraction	Potential loss of teeth
	Bone density lost	Gingivitis
	Papillae of tongue decreased	Bleeding gums and dry mouth
	Taste threshold for salt and sugar increased	Oral mucosa dry
	Salivary secretions decreased	
▪ Esophagus	Lower esophageal sphincter pressure decreased	Epigastric distress
	Motility decreased	Dysphagia
		Potential for hiatal hernia and aspiration

BUN, Blood urea nitrogen.

TABLE 5-4 Gerontologic Differences in Assessment
Age-Related Changes and Associated Clinical Manifestations—cont'd

SYSTEM	EXPECTED AGING CHANGES	CLINICAL MANIFESTATIONS
Gastrointestinal—cont'd		
▪ Stomach	Gastric mucosa atrophy	Decreased gastric emptying
	Blood flow decreased	
▪ Small intestine	Intestinal villae decreased	Slowed intestinal transit
	Enzyme secretions decreased	Absorption of fat-soluble vitamins delayed
	Motility decreased	
▪ Large intestine	Blood flow decreased	Potential for constipation and fecal impaction
	Motility decreased	
	Sensation to defecation decreased	
▪ Pancreas	Pancreatic ducts distend	Impaired fat absorption
	Lipase production decreased	Decreased glucose tolerance
	Pancreatic reserve impaired	
▪ Liver	Number and size of cells decreased	Lower border extends past costal margin
	Hepatic protein synthesis impaired	Decreased drug metabolism
	Ability to regenerate decreased	
Musculosketal		
▪ Skeleton	Intervertebral disk narrowed	Height diminished 1-4 in (2.5-10 cm)
	Cartilage of nose and ears increased	Nose and ears lengthen
		Kyphosis
		Pelvis wider
▪ Bone	Cortical and trabecular bone decreased	Bone resorption exceeds bone formation
		Potential for osteoporotic fractures
▪ Muscles	Number of muscle fibers decreased	Strength decreased
	Muscle fibers atrophy	Agility decreased
	Muscle regeneration slowed	Rigidity in neck, shoulders, hips, and knees increased
	Contraction time and latency period prolonged	Potential restless legs syndrome
	Flexion of joints increased	
	Ligaments stiffening	
	Sclerosis of tendons	
	Tendon flexor reflexes decreased	
▪ Joints	Cartilage erosion	Mobility decreased
	Calcium deposits increased	ROM limited
	Water in cartilage decreased	Osteoarthritis
Nervous		
▪ Structure	Loss of neurons in brain and spinal cord	Conduction of nerve impulses slowed
	Brain size decreased	Peripheral nerve function lost
	Dendrites atrophy	Reaction time decreased
	Major neurotransmitters decreased	Response time slowed
	Size of ventricles increased	Potential for altered balance, vertigo, syncope
		Postural hypotension increased
		Proprioception diminished
		Sensory input decreased
		EEG alpha waves decreased
▪ Sleep	Deep sleep decreased	Difficulty falling asleep
	REM sleep decreased in old-old adults	Period of wakefulness increased
		Sleep time averages 6 hr
Visual		
▪ Eye structure	Orbital fat lost	Eyes sunken
	Eyebrows and eyelashes gray	Eyes dry
	Elasticity of eyelid muscles decreased	Potential ectropion and entropion
	Tear production decreased	Potential conjunctivitis
▪ Cornea	Corneal sensitivity decreased	Potential corneal abrasion
	Corneal reflex decreased	
	Arcus senilis	

EEG, Electroencephalogram; *REM*, rapid eye movement; *ROM*, range of motion.

Continued

TABLE 5-4 *Gerontologic Differences in Assessment*
Age-Related Changes and Associated Clinical Manifestations—cont'd

SYSTEM	EXPECTED AGING CHANGES	CLINICAL MANIFESTATIONS
Visual—cont'd		
▪ Ciliary	Aqueous humor secretion decreased	Ability of lens to accommodate declines
	Ciliary muscle atrophy	Presbyopia
		Peripheral vision decreased
▪ Lens	Less elastic, more dense	Lens yellow and opaque
		Less ability to adapt to light and dark
		Tolerance to glare decreased
		Incidence of cataracts increased
		Night vision impaired
▪ Iris and pupil	Pigment lost	Visual acuity decreased
	Smaller pupil	Pupils appear constricted
	Vitreous gel debris increased	Floaters
Auditory		
▪ Structure	Hairs in external auditory canals of men increased	Potential conductive hearing loss
	Ceruminal glands decreased	Cerumen more dry
▪ Middle ear	Middle ear bone joints degenerate	Sound conduction decreased
	Ear drum thickens	
▪ Inner ear	Vestibular structures decline	Sensitivity to high tones: "s," "t," "f," "g" decreased
	Hair cells lost	Understanding of speech decreased
	Cochlea atrophies	Discrimination of background voice decreased
	Organ of Corti atrophies	Equilibrium-balance deficits
		Potential for tinnitus
Immune System		
	Secretory immunoglobulin (IgA) declines	Potential increase for infection on mucosal surfaces
	Thymus gland involuted	Impaired cell-mediated immune response
	Lymphoid tissue decreased	Malignancy incidence increased
	Antibody production impaired	Response to acute infection reduced
	Decreased proliferative response of T and B cells	Potential recurrence of latent herpes zoster and tuberculosis
	Autoantibodies increased	Autoimmune disease increased

TABLE 5-5	Factors Negatively Affecting Health of Older Women

- A disproportionately higher number of women than men live in poverty.
- Minority women have the highest poverty rates.
- Lack of formal work experience of older women leads to low incomes.
- More older women rely on social security as a major source of income than men.
- Older women more frequently live alone than men.
- Traditional caregiving and homemaking roles increase women's economic insecurity.
- Older women have less access to health insurance.
- Older women have a higher incidence of chronic health problems, such as arthritis, hypertension, strokes, and diabetes.
- Older women who are married are likely to be caregivers for ill husbands.

Compiled from Hooyman NR, Kiyak HA: *Social gerontology: a multidisciplinary perspective*, ed 5, Boston, 1999, Allyn & Bacon.

SPECIAL OLDER ADULT POPULATIONS

Older Adult Women

For the aging woman, the impact of an aging body and being a woman is considered a double jeopardy.[22] Women are often discriminated against for being older and female. By age 78 loss of a spouse is more common for women (63%) than for men (21%).[1] Table 5-5 lists numerous factors that have had a significant negative impact on the health of the older woman. Gender-based inequities in health care can be seen in the emphasis on (1) high out-of-pocket costs for depression, arthritis, and hypertension, which occur more often in women; (2) less research on diseases or syndromes that more commonly affect women such as fibromyalgia, irritable bowel syndrome, and headache; and (3) less aggressive diagnostic workup for anxiety, depression, and cardiac disease in women.[23]

The nurse is in an excellent position to be an advocate for equity for the older woman in the health care system and federal funding of research. Advocacy organizations, such as the Older Women's League (OWL) and the Society for Women's Health Research, can be helpful in this process.

TABLE 5-6	$\mathcal{G}$erontologic Differences in Assessment **Effects of Aging on Adult Mental Functioning**
FUNCTION	**EFFECT OF AGING**
Fluid intelligence	Declines during middle age
Crystallized intelligence	Improves
Vocabulary and verbal	Improves reasoning
Spatial perception	Constant or improves
Synthesis of new information	Declines during middle age
Mental performance speed	Declines during middle age
Short-term recall memory	Declines during old age
Long-term recall memory	Constant

Cognitively Impaired Older Adults

For the majority of healthy older adults, there is no noticeable decline in mental abilities. The older adult may experience a memory lapse or benign forgetfulness that is significantly different from cognitive impairment. This is often referred to as age-associated memory impairment. Table 5-6 presents the effects of aging on adult mental functioning.

The older adult who is forgetful should be encouraged to use memory aids to attempt recall in a calm and quiet environment, and actively engage in memory improvement techniques. Memory aids include clocks, calendars, notes, marked pillboxes, safety alarms on stoves, and identity necklaces or bracelets. Memory techniques include word association, mental imaging, and mnemonics.

Declining physical health is an important factor that influences cognitive impairment. The older adult who experiences sensory loss, cerebrovascular disease, or hypertension may show a decline in cognitive functioning. An appropriate cognitive assessment includes functional ability, memory recall, orientation, use of judgment, and appropriate emotional state. Standard mental status examinations and behavioral descriptions provide data for determining cognitive status. Cognitive impairment and dementia are discussed in Chapter 58.

Rural Older Adults

Persons over age 65 are less likely to live in metropolitan areas than younger persons. Approximately 50% of older persons live in the suburbs and 27% live in central cities. The remaining 23% live in nonmetropolitan areas.[1]

Rural older adults face special challenges. Because of geographic isolation and a higher poverty level, the rural older adult is often stressed by changing financial resources and declining self-care abilities.[24] Although the rural older adult fears dependence on others, symptoms of ill health are greater than those found in urban peers. These concerns may be related to two factors: the rural older adult is less likely to engage in health-promoting activities, and the rural community is underserved by health care workers.[24]

The nurse working with the rural older adult must clearly define the lifestyle values and practices of rural life (Fig. 5-2). Health care providers should consider transportation as a possible barrier to service. Alternative service approaches such as computer-based Internet sources and chat rooms, videotapes, ra-

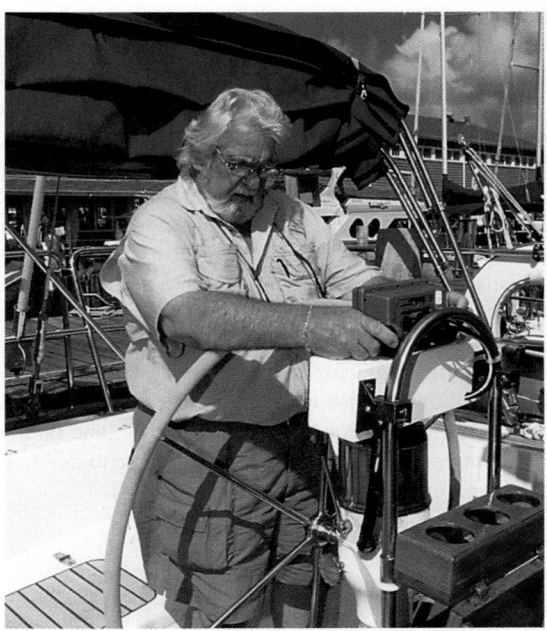

FIG. 5-2   Many older adults enjoy outdoor activities.

dio, and church social events should be used to promote healthful practices or to conduct health screening. Innovative models of nursing practice must be developed to assist the rural older adult.

Homeless Older Adults

In areas where homelessness is increasing, the older adult is at additional risk because many aging network services are not designed to reach out to homeless persons. It is estimated that between 14% and 50% of homeless persons are older adults.[25] The older homeless person is less likely to use shelters or meal sites. The low-income older adult often becomes homeless because of a lack of affordable housing. Key factors that are associated with homelessness include (1) having a low income, (2) reduced cognitive capacity, and (3) living alone. Nursing home placement is often an alternative to homelessness. Fear of institutionalization may explain the reason the older homeless adult does not use shelter and meal site services.

The older homeless person needs affordable housing. When cognitively impaired and alone, the older person needs financial management assistance. Solutions to the problem of homelessness among the elderly require more research and intervention studies.

Frail Older Adults

The **frail elderly** is a term used to identify those older adults who, because of declining physical health and resources, are most vulnerable. Frailty is not directly related to age per se, although age is a risk factor. Old age is just one element of frailty. Other risk factors include disability, multiple chronic illnesses, and the presence of geriatric syndromes. The old-old population (75 years of age and older) are the most at risk for frailty, although many in this age-group remain healthy and robust.

The frail older adult has difficulty coping with declining functional abilities and decreasing daily energy. When stressful life events (e.g., the death of a pet) and daily strain (e.g., caring for an ill spouse) occur, the frail individual often cannot cope with the effects of stress and, as a result, may become ill. Common health problems of the frail older adult include mobility limitations, sensory impairment, cognitive decline, falls, and increasing frailty.

The frail older adult is at particular risk for malnutrition and problems with hydration status. Malnutrition and dehydration are related to sociopsychologic factors such as living alone, depression, and low income. Physical factors such as declining cognitive status, inadequate dental care, sensory decreases, physical fatigue, and limited mobility also add to the risks of malnutrition and dehydration. Because many frail older adults have therapeutic diets and multiple drug regimens, their nutritional state may be altered. It is important for the nurse to monitor the frail older adult for adequate calorie, protein, iron, calcium, vitamin D, and fluid intake.

The acronym SCALES can remind the nurse to assess important nutritional indicators:

Sadness, or mood change
Cholesterol, high
Albumin, low
Loss or gain of weight
Eating problems
Shopping and food preparation problems

Once the older adult's nutritional needs are identified, common interventions include home-delivered meals, dietary supplements, food stamps, dental referrals, and vitamin supplements.

The nurse should remember that the frail older adult tires easily, has little physical reserve, and is at risk for disability, elder abuse, and institutionalization. This older adult is dependent on a network of family, individual, and social support that should be respected and supported.

Chronically Ill Older Adults

Although the U.S. health care system is dominated by an acute illness focus, daily living with chronic illness is a reality for many older adults. Although persons of all ages have chronic health problems, chronic illness is most common in the older adult.[1] The incidence of chronic illness triples after age 45. Eighty percent of persons 65 years of age and older have at least one chronic condition.[1] The most common chronic conditions present in the older adult are arthritis, visual impairment, diabetes, cardiovascular disease (including high blood pressure), deafness and hearing impairment, Alzheimer's disease, osteoporosis, hip fractures, urinary incontinence, stroke, Parkinson's disease, and depression.[5]

Often, chronic illness is composed of multiple health problems that have a protracted, unpredictable course. Diagnosis and the acute phase of a chronic illness are often managed in a hospital. All other phases of a chronic illness are usually managed at home. The management of a chronic illness can profoundly affect the lives and identities of the patient, caregiver, and family.

Although health status refers to acute and chronic illness, it also includes an individual's level of daily functioning. Functional health includes activities of daily living (ADLs), such as bathing, dressing, eating, toileting, and transfer. Instrumental ADLs (IADLs), such as using a telephone, shopping, preparing food, housekeeping, doing laundry, arranging transportation, taking medications, and handling finances, are also included in a functional health assessment.

As age increases, a pattern of declining functional health and increasing disability is seen. The nurse caring for the older adult

can advocate accurate, comprehensive assessment in which health and disease states are diagnosed accurately and can actively teach health promotion strategies.

Disease in the older adult is often difficult to accurately diagnose. The older adult tends to underreport symptoms and to treat these symptoms by altering functional status. The older adult eats less, sleeps more, or "waits it out." The older adult often attributes a new symptom to "old age" and will ignore it.

Disease in the older adult may vary greatly. As one disease is treated, another may be affected. For example, the use of a drug with anticholinergic properties such as a tricyclic antidepressant may cause urinary retention. In the older adult, disease symptoms are atypical, and complaints of "aching in the joint" may actually be a broken hip. Silent asymptomatic pathology frequently occurs. Cardiac disease may be diagnosed when the patient is being treated for a urinary tract infection. Pathologies with similar symptoms are often confused. Depression may be mistreated as dementia. A *cascade disease pattern* may occur. An example of cascade disease pattern would occur when the patient who experiences insomnia treats the condition with a hypnotic medication, becomes lethargic and confused, falls, breaks a hip, and subsequently develops pneumonia.

Tasks required for daily living with chronic illness include (1) preventing and managing crisis, (2) carrying out prescribed regimens, (3) controlling symptoms, (4) managing time, (5) adjusting to changes in the course of the disease, (6) preventing social isolation, and (7) attempting to normalize interactions with others. Both the patient and the nurse must practice behaviors different from those required of patients with an acute illness if the older adult is to accomplish the tasks associated with a chronic disease.

■ Culturally Competent Care: Older Adults

The term **ethno-geriatrics** is used to describe the specialty area of providing culturally competent care to ethnic elders.[5] The older adult who identifies with a certain ethnic group presents a particular challenge to the nurse (Fig. 5-3). Ethnic identity can be determined by asking the following questions:

1. Does this person identify with an ethnic or racial group?
2. Do others identify this person with an ethnic or racial group?
3. Does this person show behavioral patterns that are unique to the ethnic group?

Ethnic identity is often found in certain religious groups, nations, and minorities. As American society changes, ethnic institutions and neighborhoods may be altered. For the older adult with strong ethnic roots, the loss of friends who speak the "mother tongue," the loss of the church that supports social ethnic activities, and the loss of stores that carry desired ethnic foods may present situational crises that emphasize and diminish a sense of self-worth and personhood. This loss of self is increased when children and others deny or ignore ethnic practices and behaviors. Support for the ethnic older adult is most frequently found in family, religious practices, and isolated geographic or community ethnic clusters. In the old-old population, ethnic group members often live with extended family and often continue to speak their native language.

The ethnic older adult is faced with specific problems. Because the ethnic older adult often lives in older neighborhoods, physical security and personal safety related to crime become a concern. Because the individual with an ethnic identity often has

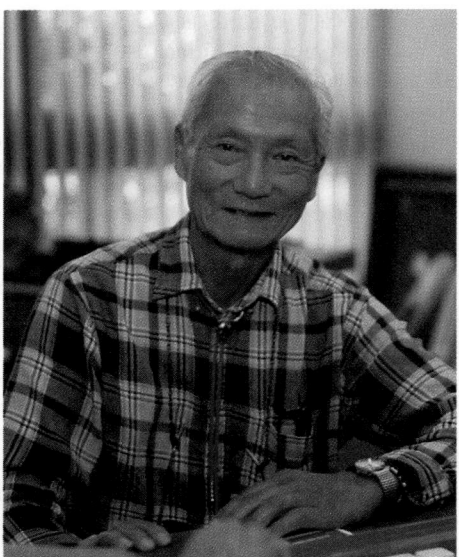

FIG. 5-3   Ethnic elders need special consideration.

TABLE 5-7	**Meeting the Needs of Ethnic Older Adults**

- Identify health practices, rituals, and food patterns that are central to an ethnic identity.
- Identify stereotypic attitudes in the ethnic older adult that interfere with multiethnic group participation.
- Inform ethnic older adult about services available.
- Support the ethnic older adult who is fearful about traveling outside the accepted neighborhood for services.
- Advocate for ethnic older adult to receive services that provide special attention to language limitations and cultural health practices.
- Use strategies specific to an ethnic group. For example, African Americans may respond to themes such as "do it for your loved ones." Asians may respond to fear of dependency themes.
- Learn about services and programs that focus on specific ethnic groups. Examples include home-meal services that serve ethnic foods or nursing homes that include specific ethnic or religious preferences.

a disproportionately low income, Medicare deductibles or drugs needed to treat chronic illnesses may not be affordable. Perceptions of health also differ by ethnic group. In 1999, 26.1% of older persons assessed their heath as fair or poor (compared with 9.2% for all persons). In the older adult group, over 40% of older African Americans and 35% of Hispanics rated their health as fair or poor as compared with 26% of older white adults.[1]

For the nurse to be effective with the ethnic older adult, a sense of respect and clear communication is critical. The nurse must identify self-behaviors that could be interpreted as noncaring or disrespectful, such as a refusal to allow a patient to display an item considered important for healing. Nursing interventions to assist in meeting the needs of the ethnic older adult are described in Table 5-7. Questions to ask the ethnic older adult about health-related practices include the following:

1. What makes people ill?
2. When do you know someone is sick?
3. What helps people get better?
4. Who can assist people to get well?
5. Do you believe this will help you get well?

American culture is changing. For some older adults, ethnic identity is also changing. The nurse should not assume that ethnic identity is or is not of value to the patient and the patient's family. The nurse must assess each older adult's ethnic orientation.[5] ■

NURSING MANAGEMENT
OLDER ADULTS

■ Nursing Assessment

As with all age-groups, assessment of the older adult provides the database for the rest of the nursing process. It is important to remember that the older adult may face a health problem with fear and anxiety. Health care workers may be perceived as helpful, but institutions may be perceived as negative, potentially harmful places. The nurse can communicate a sense of concern and care by careful use of direct and simple statements, appropriate eye contact, direct touch, and gentle humor. These actions assist the older adult to relax in this stressful situation.

Before beginning the assessment process the nurse should attend to primary needs first, ensuring that the patient is pain free and does not need to urinate. All assistive devices such as glasses and hearing aids should be in place. The interview should be short so the patient is not fatigued. The interviewer should allow adequate time to give information, as well as to respond to questions. The older adult and caregiver should be interviewed separately, unless the patient is cognitively impaired or specifically requests the caregiver's presence. Medical history may be lengthy. The nurse must determine what is relevant information. Old medical records should be obtained and available for review.

The focus of a comprehensive geriatric assessment is to determine appropriate interventions to maintain and enhance the functional abilities of the older adult. The comprehensive geriatric assessment is interdisciplinary and at a minimum includes the medical history, physical examination, functional abilities assessment, and social resources. The comprehensive geriatric assessment is often conducted at a geriatric evaluation unit (GEU) by an interdisciplinary geriatric assessment team. The interdisciplinary team may include many disciplines, but the minimum components include the nurse, the physician, and the social worker. After the assessment is complete, the interdisciplinary team meets with the patient and family to present the team's findings and recommendations. These assessment centers are often affiliated with large medical complexes.

Elements in a comprehensive nursing assessment include a history using a functional health pattern format (see Chapter 3), physical assessment, assessment of ADLs and IADLs, mental status evaluation, and a social-environmental assessment. Evaluation of mental status is particularly important for the older adult because results of this evaluation often determine the patient's potential for independent living. Evaluation of the results of a comprehensive nursing assessment helps determine the service and placement needs of the older adult patient. A good match between needs and services should be the goal of the assessment.

The comprehensive nursing assessment should be based on instruments specific to the older adult population (Table 5-8). Interpretation of laboratory results can be problematic because many values change with age, and parameters are not well defined for the older adult, particularly the old-old patient. The healthy adult may have age-related changes that may be considered abnormal in a younger population but are normal for an older adult. An appropriate reference book should be consulted for the correct ranges of laboratory values for the older adult. The nurse is in an important position to recognize and correct inaccurate interpretation of laboratory tests. Cure is often not possible because of the complexity and chronicity of the health problems that commonly affect the older adult. Consequently, the nurse directs the planning and implementation of those actions that assist the older adult in remaining as functionally independent as possible.

■ Nursing Diagnoses

With few exceptions the same nursing diagnoses apply to the older adult as to a younger person. Often, however, the etiology and defining characteristics are related to age and unique to the older adult. Table 5-9 lists nursing diagnoses that are seen in older adults as a result of age-related changes. The identification and management of nursing diagnoses result in improved patient function and quality patient care for the older adult.

■ Planning

When setting goals with the older adult, it is helpful to identify the strengths and abilities that the patient demonstrates. Personal characteristics such as hardiness, persistence, and the ability to laugh and learn are positive factors in goal setting. Caregivers should be included in goal development. The older adult who perceives increasing dependence and learned helplessness as an appropriate response may be resistant to self-care. Priority goals for the older adult may be gaining a sense of control, feeling safe, and reducing stress.

■ Nursing Implementation

When carrying out a plan of action, the nurse may need to modify the approach and techniques used on the basis of the physical and mental status of the elderly patient. Small body size, common in the frail older adult, may necessitate the use of pediatric equipment. Bone and joint changes often require transfer assistance, altered positioning, and use of gait belts and lift devices. The older adult with declining energy reserves requires extra rest periods alternated with short periods of exertion. A slower approach, restricted scheduling, and the use of a bedside commode or other adaptive equipment may be necessary.

Cognitive impairment, if present, requires the nurse to offer careful explanations and a calm approach to avoid producing anxiety and resistance in the patient. Depression can result in apathy and poor cooperation with the treatment plan.

Health Promotion. Health promotion and prevention of health problems in the older adult are focused on three areas: reduction in diseases and problems, increased participation in health promotion activities (Fig. 5-4), and increased targeted services that reduce health hazards. These goals are central to

---

TABLE 5-8   *Gerontologic Differences in Assessment*
Geriatric Assessment Instruments

AREA OF CONCERN	EXAMPLE OF ASSESSMENT INSTRUMENT	WHAT IS TESTED
Mental status	Folstein Mini-Mental State[1]	Tests orientation, memory, attention, language, recall Low score = cognitive impairment—general
Mood state	Geriatric Depression Scale[2]	30 affective items test for depression
Functional ability	Katz Index of Activities of Daily Living[3]	Tests bathing, dressing, toileting, transfer, continence, feeding Coded as: Independent—Assistance—Dependent
Functional ability	Lawton Instrumental Activities of Daily Living[4]	Tests telephone usage, traveling, shopping, meal preparation, housework, medication, money Coded as: Independent—Assistance—Dependent
Dementia indicators	Set Test[5]	Tests ability to name up to 10 items in 4 sets: *Fruit, Animals, Colors, Towns* (FACT) Score maximum = 40
Social support	Zarit Burden Interview[6]	Tests for feelings of burden in caregiving
Alcohol usage	CAGE[7]	Tests for alcohol abuse 4 items; response of yes in 2 or more = problem
	Michigan Alcohol[8] Screening Test—Geriatric Version	Tests for alcohol use
Falls assessment	Get Up and Go Test[9]	Tests balance and sway as risk for fall

[1]Folstein MF, Folstein SE, McHugh PR: Mini-mental state: a practical method for grading the cognitive state of patients for the clinician, *J Psychiatr Res* 12:189, 1975.
[2]Yesavage JA, Brink TL: Development and validation of a geriatric depression screening scale: a preliminary paper, *J Psychiatr Res* 17:41, 1983.
[3]Katz S et al: Studies of illness in the aged. The index of ADL: a standardized measure of biological and psychological function, *JAMA* 185:914, 1963.
[4]Lawton H, Brody E: Assessment of older people: self-maintaining and instrumental activities of daily living, *Gerontologist* 9:179, 1969.
[5]Isaacs B, Kennie AT: The Set Test as an aid to the detection of dementia in old people, *Br J Psychiatry* 123:467, 1973.
[6]Zarit SH: Relatives of impaired elderly: correlates of feelings of burden, *Gerontologist* 20:699, 1980.
[7]Mayfield D, Mcleod G, Hall P: The CAGE questionnaire: validation of a new alcoholism screening instrument, *Am J Psychiatry* 131:10, 1974.
[8]Gurnedi AM: *Older adults' measure of alcohol, medicines, and other drugs,* New York, 1997, Springer.
[9]Mathias S, Nayok U, Isaacs B: Balance in elderly patients: the "get up and go" test, *Arch Phys Med Rehabil* 67:387, 1986.

four major health initiatives currently guiding services for the older adult: (1) the *Healthy People 2010* national health objectives, (2) recommendations of the U.S. Preventive Services Task Force Guide to Clinical Preventive Services, (3) *Dietary Guidelines for Americans,* and (4) the Nutrition Screening Initiative.[26,27]

The nurse places a high value on health promotion and positive health behaviors. Programs have been successfully developed for screening for chronic health conditions, smoking cessation, geriatric foot care, vision and hearing screening, stress reduction, exercise programs, drug usage, crime prevention, and home hazards assessment. The nurse can carry out and teach the older adult about the need for specific preventive services.

NURSING DIAGNOSES & COLLABORATIVE PROBLEMS

TABLE 5-9	Nursing Diagnoses Associated with Age-Related Physiologic Changes

Cardiovascular System
Activity intolerance
Decreased cardiac output
Fatigue

Respiratory System
Impaired gas exchange
Ineffective airway clearance
Ineffective breathing pattern
Risk for aspiration
Risk for infection

Integumentary System
Impaired skin integrity

Urinary System
Deficient fluid volume
Impaired urinary elimination

Reproductive System
Disturbed body image
Ineffective sexuality patterns
Sexual dysfunction

Gastrointestinal System
Constipation
Imbalanced nutrition
Impaired oral mucous membrane

Musculoskeletal System
Impaired physical mobility
Chronic pain
Risk for injury
Self-care deficit

Nervous System
Disturbed thought processes
Disturbed sensory perception
Disturbed sleep pattern
Hyperthermia
Hypothermia

Senses
Disturbed body image
Impaired verbal communication
Social isolation

Immune System
Risk for infection

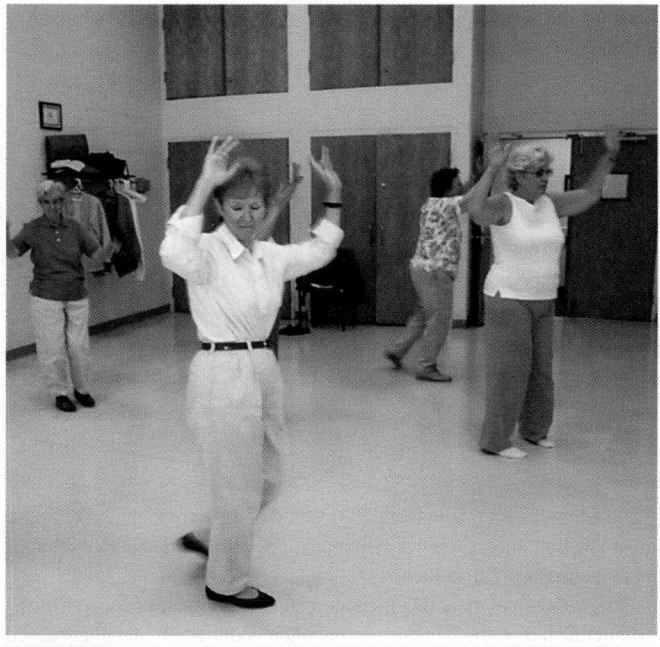

FIG. 5-4 Dancing is an example of a health promotion activity.

Health promotion and prevention can be included in nursing interventions at any location or level where the nurse and the older adult interact. The nurse can use health promotion activities to strengthen self-care, increase personal responsibility for health, and increase independent functioning that will enhance the well-being of the older adult. The nurse interested in older adult health promotion can contact the Health Promotion Institute or the National Institute on Aging (see Resources at end of chapter).

Teaching older adults. The nurse is involved in teaching the older adult self-care practices to enhance health and modify disease processes. The older adult presents the following challenges to learning: (1) time needed to learn is increased, (2) new learning must relate to the patient's actual experience, (3) anxiety and distractions decrease learning, (4) lack of risk taking and cautiousness decrease motivation to learn, and (5) sensory-perceptual deficits and cognitive decline require modified teaching techniques.

Specific approaches that increase the level of learning in the older adult include the following: (1) present material at a slower rate; (2) use visual aids when possible; (3) use peer educators when appropriate; (4) encourage participation of a spouse or family member; (5) use simple phrases or sentences and provide for repetition; and (6) support of the belief that change in behavior is both helpful and worth the effort of increased learning.[28] (Patient teaching is discussed in Chapter 4.)

Acute Care. Frequently the hospital is the first point of contact for the older adult and the formal health care system. Older adults account for over 35% of all hospital admissions and 48% of all days of hospital care.[1] The hospitalized older adult is often experiencing multisystem failure. Illnesses that most commonly result in hospitalization include arrhythmias, heart failure, stroke, fluid and electrolyte imbalances (e.g., hyponatremia, dehydration), pneumonia, and hip fractures. The complexity of the acute situation often results in a loss of the whole-person perspective and focuses care on the diseased part. Because the nurse provides an integrated approach, care that is individualized and helpful to the older adult can be reestablished.

When caring for the hospitalized older adult, both patient and caregivers are assisted when the nurse performs the following:

1. Identifies the frail and old-old patients at risk for the iatrogenic effects of hospitalization
2. Considers discharge needs early in the hospital stay, especially assistance with ADLs, IADLs, and medications
3. Encourages the development and use of interdisciplinary teams, special care units, and individuals who focus on the special needs of gerontologic patients
4. Develops standard protocols to screen for at-risk conditions commonly present in the hospitalized older adult patient, such as urinary tract infection and delirium
5. Advocates for referral of the patient to appropriate community-based services (see Chapter 6)

The outcome of hospitalization for the older adult varies. Of particular concern are the problems of high surgical risk, acute confusional state, nosocomial infection, and premature discharge with an unstable condition.

High surgical risk. Age-related body changes, chronic illness, and declining physical reserve place the older adult at an increased surgical risk. Other key factors that increase surgical risk include age older than 75 years, emergency operations, use of spinal anesthesia, and thrombolytic complications.[29] Age is an important risk factor for surgery-related mortality. Patients 80 years of age and older are more than twice as likely as patients 65 to 69 years of age to experience adverse outcomes following elective surgery.[29] The risk of surgery should be balanced against the benefit and appropriateness of surgery for the older adult patient. (See Chapters 17, 18, and 19 for additional surgical considerations for the older adult.)

Acute confusional state. The sudden onset of an acute confusional state (delirium) occurs in 18% to 38% of hospitalized older adults.[30] **Delirium** is usually a transient condition characterized by disorganized thinking, difficulty concentrating, and sensory misperceptions that lasts from 1 to 7 days. However, some delirium symptoms may persist up to and after discharge. Delirium has a rather rapid onset and a course that fluctuates over time. Risk factors include fluid, metabolic, and nutritional imbalances; medications; and infection. Delirium is one of the most frequent consequences of unscheduled surgery because the older adult has not been stabilized physically or prepared emotionally. The patient who experiences delirium will exhibit a decline in ability to perform ADLs.

Nosocomial infections. *Nosocomial* (hospital-acquired) infections occur at higher rates in older adults. For the old-old patient, the rate is two to five times the rate of a younger person. Age-related changes of decreased immunocompetence, the presence of pathologic conditions, and an increase in disability all contribute to higher infection rates. Infections common to the older adult include pneumonia, urinary tract infections, and skin infections.[5] Tuberculosis is disproportionately high in the older adult population. These infections often have atypical presentations showing cognitive and behavioral changes before alterations occur in laboratory values or temperature.[31] In addition, age-related changes in immune function, underlying diseases, increased frequency of adverse drug reactions, and institutionalization can all complicate the management of the older adult with infection.

Hospital discharge. At the time of hospital discharge, many older adults are considered to be in an unstable condition. The frail older adult and the old-old patient are particularly vulnerable. Most of these patients are discharged under Medicare regulations that require a registered nurse or qualified person to develop a plan for discharge. The discharge plan should be periodically reassessed, and caregivers and patients must be counseled to prepare the patient for posthospital care.

The nurse can use screening inventories to identify high risk patients. The postdischarge assistance needed by high risk patients includes bathing, taking medications, housekeeping, shopping, preparing meals, and making satisfactory transportation arrangements. Risk of unstable discharge increases in the patient who experiences greater length of stay and who is dependent on others for meals. Early hospital discharge is most successful when patients have had little change in functional status or are returning to a place with a high level of assistance, such as a long-term care facility.

Geriatric rehabilitation. Geriatric rehabilitation interventions are focused on adapting to or recovering from disability. With proper training, assistive equipment, and attendant personal care, the patient with disabilities can often live an independent life. For the younger disabled adult, the approach of personal attendant care with a focus on independent living stimulated the 1990 Americans with Disabilities Act. Advocates suggest that the elimination of environmental barriers allows the disabled to function normally in society. The older adult, primarily through Medicare reimbursement, can receive rehabilitative assistance through postincident, inpatient rehabilitation (limited days), and home care programs.

The nurse needs to understand physical disability in the older adult. The older person with cerebrovascular disease, arthritis, and coronary artery disease has a risk of becoming functionally limited. Hip fracture, amputation, and stroke occur at higher rates in the older adult population. These disabilities lead to increased mortality rates, decreased life span, and increased rates of institutionalization. Reducing residual disability through geriatric rehabilitation is important to the quality of life of the older adult.

Often the older adult has specific fears and anxieties related to falling and fatigue. The older adult is limited in the rehabilitation process by sensory-perceptual deficits, other disease states, slowed cognition, poor nutrition, and funding problems. Nurse and caregiver encouragement, support, and acceptance assist the older adult in remaining motivated for the hard work of rehabilitation.

Rehabilitation of the older adult is influenced by several factors. First, the older patient shows greater initial variability in functional capacity than an adult at any other age. Preexisting problems associated with reaction time, visual acuity, fine motor ability, physical strength, cognitive function, and motivation affect the rehabilitation potential of the older adult.

Second, the older adult often loses functioning because of inactivity and immobility. This deconditioning can occur as a result of unstable acute medical conditions, environmental barriers that limit mobility, and a lack of motivation to stay in condition. The effect of inactivity clearly leads to "use it or lose it" consequences. The older adult can improve flexibility, strength, and aerobic capacity even into very old age. The nurse must use passive and active range-of-motion exercises with all older adults to prevent deconditioning and subsequent functional decline.

Last, the goal of geriatric rehabilitation is to strive for maximal function and physical capabilities considering the individual's current health status. When a patient demonstrates suboptimal health, the nurse screens and evaluates for risk behaviors. For example, a woman with a history of osteoporosis should be given a fall-risk appraisal. The older adult patient with diabetes should receive a geriatric foot assessment and appropriate follow-up care.

Assistive devices. The use of assistive devices should be considered as an intervention for the older adult. Using appropriate assistive devices such as dentures, glasses, hearing aids, walkers, wheelchairs, adult briefs or protectors, adaptive utensils, elevated toilet seats, and skin protective devices can diminish disability. These tools and devices should be included in the patient's care plan when appropriate. Both the nurse and caregivers are critical to the success of these modifications.

Computer technology will continue to affect the evaluation and care of older adults. Electronic monitoring equipment can be used to monitor heart rhythms and blood pressure, as well as to locate the wandering patient in the home or long-term care facility. Computerized assistive devices can be used to help patients with speech difficulties following stroke, and pocket-sized devices can serve as memory aids.

Safety. Environmental safety is crucial in the health maintenance of the older person. With normal sensory changes, slowed reaction time, decreased thermal and pain sensitivity, changes in gait and balance, and medication effects, the older adult is prone to accidents. Most accidents occur in or around the home. Falls, motor vehicle accidents, and fires are the common causes of accidental death in older adults. Another environmental problem arises from the older person's impaired thermoregulating system that cannot adapt to extremes in environmental temperatures. The body of an older adult can neither conserve nor dissipate heat as efficiently as younger adults. Therefore both hypothermia and heat prostration occur more readily. This age-group accounts for the majority of deaths during severe cold spells and heat waves.

The nurse can provide valuable counsel regarding environmental changes, which may improve safety for the older adult. Measures such as stronger lighting, colored step strips, tub and toilet grab bars, and stairway handrails can be effective in "safety-proofing" the living quarters of the older adult. The nurse can also advocate for home fire and security alarms. Uncluttered floor space, railings, increased lighting and night-lights, and clearly marked stair edges are some of the easiest and most practical adaptations.

The older adult in an inpatient or long-term care setting needs a thorough orientation to the environment. The nurse should repeatedly reassure the patient that he or she is safe and attempt to answer all questions. The unit should foster patient orientation by displaying large-print clocks, avoiding complex or visually confusing wall designs, clearly designating doors, and using simple bed and nurse-call controls. Lighting should be adequate while avoiding glare. Beds should be close to the floor with four side rails that can be modified to individual needs and to prevent serious injury from falling. Environments that provide consistent caregivers and an established daily routine assist the older adult patient.

Pain management. Pain is common in older adults. Approximately 85% of adults over 65 experience pain at least once a year and almost 60% have multiple pain complaints.[32] Because of cognitive impairment, the elderly adult may not ask for pain relief. When pain is a known complication of a particular condition, the nurse should offer pain-relieving medications at regular intervals. Pain assessment in the elderly may be complicated by cognitive decline, sensory-perceptual deficits, and age-related changes. The use of verbal and visual pain scales can assist in correct assessment of pain. It is estimated that 25% to 50% of community-dwelling older adults also experience pain that inter-

feres with their ADLs. For the patient with ongoing pain, a pain diary may be helpful in identifying activities that relieve or increase pain. Because the older adult may believe that pain is something that must be endured, creative methods may be developed to deal with it. The nurse should ask the patient to describe techniques used to reduce pain.[33] Change in body position, heat, exercise, distraction, and rest may help alleviate pain. Mental imaging, positive thinking, and prayer and other spiritual interventions are also used. Poor pain management may lead to reduced socialization, limited mobility, impaired posture, sleep disturbances, depression, anxiety, constipation, and increased health care utilization.[34] (See Chapter 9 for an additional discussion of pain.)

Medication use. Medication use in the older adult requires thorough and regular assessment and care planning. The use and abuse of medication by the older adult is supported by the following facts:

1. On average a 70-year-old takes seven different medications.[35,36]
2. Individuals age 85 and over take an average of 12 prescribed drugs.
3. The frequency of adverse drug reactions increases as the number of prescribed drugs increases.
4. Twelve percent of older adult hospital admissions occur because of drug reactions.
5. After discharge from a hospital, even one unnecessary medication may put the older adult at risk for an adverse drug reaction.

Age-related changes alter the pharmacodynamics and pharmacokinetics of drugs. Drug-drug, drug-food, and drug-disease interactions all influence the absorption, distribution, metabolism, and excretion of drugs. Fig. 5-5 illustrates the effects of aging on drug metabolism. The most dramatic changes with aging are related to drug metabolism and clearance. Overall, by age 75 to 80 there is a 50% decline in the renal clearance of drugs. Hepatic blood flow decreases markedly with aging, and the enzymes largely responsible for drug metabolism are decreased as well. Thus the drug half-life is increased in the older as compared with younger patient.[36]

In addition to changes in the metabolism of drugs, the older adult may have difficulty as a result of cognitive decline, altered sensory perceptions, limited hand mobility, and the high cost of many prescriptions. Common reasons for drug errors made by the older adult are listed in Table 5-10. **Polypharmacy** (the use of multiple medications by one patient who has more than one health problem), overdose, and addiction to prescription drugs are recognized as major causes of illness in the older adult.[36]

To accurately assess drug use and knowledge, many nurses ask their older adult patients to bring to the health care appointment all medications (both over-the-counter and prescription) that they take regularly or occasionally. The nurse can then accurately assess all medications the older adult is taking, including drugs that the patient may have omitted or thought unimportant. Additional nursing interventions to assist the older adult in following a safe medication routine are listed in Table 5-11.

Depression. Approximately 15% of the community-dwelling older population has symptoms of depression. Depression is the most common mood disorder in older adults.[37] Rates of depressive symptoms in institutionalized older adults are high. Depression is associated with being female, being divorced or separated, low socioeconomic status, poor social support, and a recent adverse and unexpected event.[37] Depression in the older adult tends

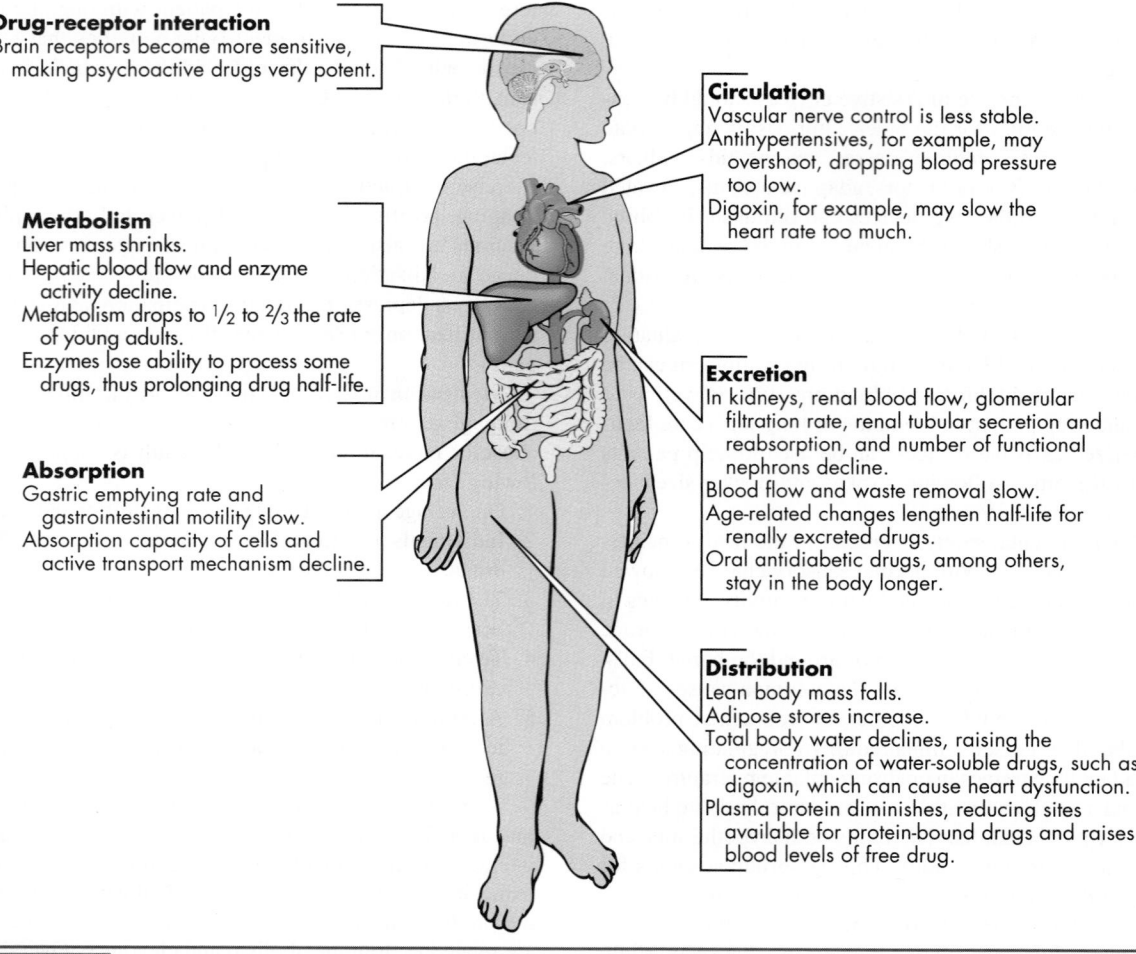

Drug-receptor interaction
Brain receptors become more sensitive, making psychoactive drugs very potent.

Metabolism
Liver mass shrinks.
Hepatic blood flow and enzyme activity decline.
Metabolism drops to $\frac{1}{2}$ to $\frac{2}{3}$ the rate of young adults.
Enzymes lose ability to process some drugs, thus prolonging drug half-life.

Absorption
Gastric emptying rate and gastrointestinal motility slow.
Absorption capacity of cells and active transport mechanism decline.

Circulation
Vascular nerve control is less stable.
Antihypertensives, for example, may overshoot, dropping blood pressure too low.
Digoxin, for example, may slow the heart rate too much.

Excretion
In kidneys, renal blood flow, glomerular filtration rate, renal tubular secretion and reabsorption, and number of functional nephrons decline.
Blood flow and waste removal slow.
Age-related changes lengthen half-life for renally excreted drugs.
Oral antidiabetic drugs, among others, stay in the body longer.

Distribution
Lean body mass falls.
Adipose stores increase.
Total body water declines, raising the concentration of water-soluble drugs, such as digoxin, which can cause heart dysfunction.
Plasma protein diminishes, reducing sites available for protein-bound drugs and raises blood levels of free drug.

FIG. 5-5   The effects of aging on drug metabolism.

TABLE 5-10   Common Causes of Medication Errors by Older Adults

- Poor eyesight
- Forget to take drugs
- Use of nonprescription over-the-counter drugs
- Use of medications prescribed for someone else
- Use of medications that are out of date (expired)
- Failure to understand instructions or the importance of drug treatment
- Refusal to take medication because of undesirable side effects such as nausea and impotence

TABLE 5-11   Drug Therapy   Medication Use by Older Adults

1. Emphasize medications that are essential.
2. Attempt to reduce medication use that is not essential for minor symptoms.
3. Screen medication use using a standard assessment tool—including over-the-counter drugs, eyedrops and eardrops, antihistamines, and cough syrups.
4. Assess alcohol use.
5. Encourage the use of written or medication-reminder systems.
6. Monitor drug dosage strength; normally the strength should be 30% to 50% less than that of the younger person.
7. Encourage the use of one pharmacy.
8. Work with health care providers and pharmacists to establish routine drug profiles on all older adult patients.
9. Advocate (with drug companies) for low-income prescription support services and dosage routines that are simple once-a-day time-release forms.

to arise from a loss of self-esteem and may be related to life situations such as retirement or loss of a spouse. Problems such as hypochondriac complaints, insomnia, lethargy, agitation, decreased memory, and inability to concentrate are common. Depression is an underrecognized problem for many older adults.

Late-life depression often occurs together with medical illness such as heart disease, stroke, diabetes, and cancer. Depression can exacerbate medical conditions by affecting compliance with diet, exercise, or drug regimens. It is important that assessment include physical examination and laboratory testing for physical disorders that may have symptoms similar to depression. Diseases of concern are thyroid disorders and vitamin deficiencies.

The older adult who exhibits depressive symptoms should be encouraged to seek treatment. Because a patient often feels unworthy and may withdraw and become isolated, the nurse may need to seek the support of the family to assist in helping the older adult seek treatment. The depressed older adult who is involved in caregiving should seek respite and reevaluate the caregiving role.

Of all suicides, older adults commit 20.6% in the United States and 12.4% in Canada.[38,39] The nurse should take seriously comments such as "ending this life." Suicide precautions should be followed. The low-income older man who is divorced or widowed with a history of substance abuse is at greatest risk for suicide. White men over age 65 are at five times higher risk to commit suicide than the general population.[38,39]

Nutritional therapy. Maintaining adequate nutrition can be a problem for the older adult for physical and social reasons. It is estimated that 30% to 40% of men and women over age 75 are at least 10% below ideal body weight. Physiologically, food may be less appealing with the decline in taste and smell, resulting in anorexia or loss of appetite.[40] Chewing is more difficult with dentures or loss of teeth. Swallowing and digestive problems may also result because of a decrease in saliva, gastric motility, and enzyme production. Socially, if a person eats alone, snacking on fast foods is easier than preparing meals. The lack of transportation or access to a grocery store, inability to see the merchandise, and poverty may be additional factors in poor nutrition. However, obesity may be a problem for some older adults. Normally this problem has arisen earlier in adulthood and continues because of difficulty in changing lifelong eating patterns. Problems with urinary incontinence can result in decreased intake of oral liquids, leading to dehydration.

The nurse can have the patient keep a 3-day dietary history. Analysis of this record is helpful in determining dietary adequacy. When appropriate the nurse can arrange for transportation to a senior meal site or delivery of home meals. Attention to and correction of the many reasons for poor nutrition in the elderly person is an important nursing responsibility. Management of nutritional problems is presented in Chapter 39.

Sleep. Adequacy of sleep is often a concern of the older adult because of changed sleep patterns. Older people experience a marked decrease in stage IV deep sleep and are easily aroused. In individuals over 75, the percent of sleep time spent in rapid eye movement (REM) sleep decreases. Older adults have difficulty maintaining prolonged sleep. Although the demand for sleep decreases with age, older adults may be disturbed by insomnia and complain that they spend more time in bed but still feel tired. Frequently, the older person prefers to spread sleep throughout 24 hours with short naps that provide adequate rest. Often, assurance from the nurse that this type of sleep pattern is adequate and normal for the patient's age will relieve anxiety concerning sleep. Many times a later bedtime will promote a better night's sleep and a feeling of being refreshed on awakening.

Behavioral management. When patient behaviors such as agitation, resisting care, and wandering become problematic, the nurse must plan interventions carefully. Initially the patient's phys-

ical status must be assessed. The patient is checked for changes in vital signs and urinary and bowel patterns that could account for behavioral problems. Disruptive behaviors can be interrupted and redirected by encouraging participation in activities such as singing, playing music, exercising, or walking with the nurse.

When the patient is agitated by the environment, either the patient or the stimulus should be moved. The patient can be assisted to call family members if this is reassuring. When a patient resists or pulls tubes or dressings, these items can be covered with stretch tube gauze or removed from the visual field. The older adult with behavioral problems should be reassured that the nurse is present to keep him or her safe. Reality orientation can be used to orient to time, place, and person. The confused or agitated patient should not be asked challenging "why" questions. If the patient cannot verbalize distress, his or her mood should be validated. The patient's emotional state should be closely observed. The patient's statement can be rephrased to validate its meaning.

When dealing with the difficult patient, the nurse's frustration should be acknowledged. The nurse should not threaten to restrain the patient or threaten to call the physician. A calming family member can be requested to stay with the patient until the person becomes calmer. The patient should be monitored frequently, and all interventions should be documented. The use of positive nurse actions can reduce the use of physical and chemical (drug therapy) restraints.

Use of restraints. Physical restraints are devices, materials, and equipment that physically prevent the individual from moving freely (by choice) in the environment.[5] This includes preventing the person from walking, standing, lying, transferring, or sitting. Common devices include seat belts, "geri-chairs," and jacket vests. The device cannot be removed by the individual who is being physically restrained. The Omnibus Budget Reconciliation Act (OBRA) of 1987 stated that restraints could be used only to ensure the person's safety or the safety of others. Furthermore, there must be a written order from a physician for physical restraints to be applied to long-term care patients. Since the passing of this act there has been a marked reduction in the use of physical restraints. Chemical and physical restraints should be a last resort in the care of the older patient. If a physical restraint device is to be used in the hospital or long-term care setting, it requires a physician or an independent licensed nurse practitioner to make the recommendation. There are additional regulatory requirements for restraint use, including time limit, care during restraint, and restraint-alternatives used.

The nurse should clearly document restraint use and the behaviors that require this intervention. It is not appropriate to use restraints on a patient whom the nurse assumes will fall or on the patient who demonstrates irritating behaviors such as calling out. The use of restraints makes care more time consuming and complex. Restraints do not reduce falls but do increase potential patient confusion and the severity of injury when falls occur. Restraint alternatives require vigilant, creative nursing care. Restraint alternatives include wedge cushions, low beds, body props, and electronic devices (bed alarm signaling). The nurse can avoid chemical restraint by using early interventions as discussed in the section on behavioral management. The use of restraints must follow rigid and explicit criteria. Long-term care regulations and the Joint Commission on Accreditation of

TABLE 5-12	Evaluating Nursing Care for Older Adults

Evaluation questions may include the following:
1. Is there an identifiable change in ADLs, IADLs, mental status, or disease signs and symptoms?
2. Does the patient identify a better health state?
3. Does the patient think the treatment is helpful?
4. Do the patient and caregiver think the care is worth the time and cost?
5. Can the nurse document positive changes that support interventions?
6. Does change adequately meet the required mandates for reimbursement?

ADLs, Activities of daily living; *IADLs,* instrumental activities of daily living.

Healthcare Organizations set standards for restraint usage. The movement to "restraint-free" environments is supporting restraint use decline.

■ Evaluation

The evaluation phase of the nursing process is similar for all patients. Evaluation is ongoing throughout the nursing process. The results of evaluation direct the nurse to continue the plan of care or revise as indicated. Often the change in health status is not as dramatic in the older adult as it is in the younger patient. Because of this, the nurse needs to be cautious in changing plans prematurely.

When evaluating nursing care with the older adult, the nurse should focus on functional improvement rather than cure. Useful questions to consider when evaluating the plan of care for an older adult are included in Table 5-12.

SOCIAL SUPPORT AND THE OLDER ADULT

Social support for the older adult occurs at three levels. Family and kinship relations are the first and preferred providers of social support. Second, a semiformal level of support is found in clubs, churches, neighborhoods, and senior citizen centers. Last, the older adult may be linked to a formal system of social welfare agencies, health facilities, and government support. Generally the nurse is part of the formal support system.

Caregivers

More than 80% of care is provided by a family caregiver who lives with the patient. A **caregiver** is someone who provides supervision, provides direct care, and coordinates services. The tasks of caregiving include (1) assisting with ADLs and IADLs, (2) providing emotional and social support, and (3) managing health care. A caregiver is usually a married woman who is often old herself, has chronic diseases and disabilities, and is often poor. Ethnic background influences the type of caregiving network. Italian American, Polish American, Irish American, Asian American, and African American people most commonly use extended family networks for caregiving.

Caregiver concerns change as the intensity of the caregiving role changes. For example, a caregiver may need to adjust work schedules to accommodate patient health care appointments, or the caregiver may need to be available to monitor the cognitively impaired patient's safety 24 hours a day.

Common problems facing the caregiver include the following: (1) a lack of understanding of the time and energy needed for caregiving; (2) a lack of information about specific tasks of caregiving, such as bathing or drug administration; (3) a lack of respite or relief from caregiving; (4) an inability to meet personal self-care needs, such as socialization and rest; (5) conflict in the family unit related to decisions about caregiving; and (6) financial depletion of resources as a result of a caregiver's inability to work and the increased cost of health care.

The intensity and complexity of caregiving places the caregiver at risk for high levels of stress. The caregiver may develop a sense of being overwhelmed with feelings of inadequacy, powerlessness, and depression.[41,42] Although most older adults deny loneliness even when they spend much time alone, the caregiver often lacks sufficient social interaction. The primary caregiver is often at risk for social isolation. The burden of caregiving separates the individual from others who provide social, emotional, and interactional involvement. Time commitments, fatigue, and, at times, socially inappropriate behaviors of the dependent older adult contribute to social isolation. The socially isolated caregiver needs to be identified, and plans should be designed to meet the needs for social support and exchange.

The burden of caregiving may result in the nursing diagnosis of caregiver role strain. The escalating incidence of caregiving sets the stage for increased incidences of elder abuse. Physical, financial, psychologic, or sexual abuse and neglect may occur in families ill equipped to handle caregiving. The nurse should assess the caregiver and the patient for the possibility of caregiver role strain and elder abuse.

Many family members involved in direct caregiving activities also identify rewards associated with this role. Positive aspects of caregiving include (1) knowing that their loved one is receiving good care (often in a home environment), (2) learning and mastering new tasks, and (3) finding opportunities for intimacy. At the same time the tasks involved in caregiving often provide opportunities for family members to gain greater insights into each other and strengthen their relationships.

The stress of caregiving may result in emotional problems such as depression, anger, resentment, and feelings of hopelessness and powerlessness.[43,44] The nurse should consider the caregiver as a patient and plan behaviors to reduce caregiver role strain. The nurse should communicate a sense of empathy to the caregiver while allowing discussion about the burdens and joys of caregiving. The caregiver can be taught about age-related changes and diseases and specific caregiving techniques. Attendance at a support group should be encouraged by the nurse. The nurse can also assist the caregiver in seeking help from the formal social support system regarding matters such as respite care, housing, health coverage, and finances. Finally, the nurse should monitor the caregiver for indications of declining health, emotional distress, and caregiver role strain.

Elder Abuse

The term **elder abuse** is used to describe the experience of physical harm (battering), verbal abuse, exploitation, denial of rights, forced restraint, and neglected needs usually by an individual responsible for the care of an older adult.[5,45] Elder abuse occurs in approximately 2% to 3% of the general older adult population.[41,42] The abuse is seldom reported to authorities even though it shows a repetitive pattern. The typical victim is an older

TABLE 5-13 Types of Elder Abuse

TYPE	EXAMPLE
Violation of individual rights	Lack of privacy; unwanted visitors
Exploitation	Taking a social security check or property
Physical abuse	Shaking or hitting
Psychologic neglect	Isolating or locking the person in a room
Psychologic abuse	Swearing at person; displaying threatening behavior
Physical neglect	Not providing correct medications or proper physical care

woman with at least one limitation in ADLs. Most of these women are widowed, Caucasian, poor, and dependent on the abuser for some aspect of care. Elder abuse is often associated with substance abuse, caregiver strain, and depression. The lack of reporting abuse may be related to the older adult's feeling of vulnerability, lack of self-worth, impaired cognitive functioning, and sense of isolation.

Elder abuse can occur in a variety of forms (Table 5-13). Self-neglect is also a form of elder abuse when the older adult is no longer competent to perform self-care or when the older adult has severe psychologic impairments. In assessing elder abuse the nurse must understand the legal limits of practice within state mandates. Physical assessment should include physical examination, including scrutiny of the musculoskeletal and genitourinary systems; neurologic and cognitive testing; and detailed social and sexual histories.[41,42] Signs and/or symptoms that cannot be explained medically may signal elder abuse. To intervene clinicians must be familiar with state laws governing reporting procedures and patient privacy. With a competent older adult victim, the nurse may be limited in intervention because of patient resistance. In some situations health care workers are seen as interferences and opportunists. There are several elder abuse assessment instruments that include basic information, signs of maltreatment, severity of signs, and response of abuser.[41] If the nurse suspects abuse, an appropriate assessment protocol should be carried out, and consultation should be obtained based on agency policy. Follow-up actions for the nurse may include consultation with adult protective services and potential court testimony. In most situations, nurses are mandated to report abuse.

SOCIAL SERVICES FOR THE OLDER ADULT

A network of services supports the older adult both in the community and in health care facilities. Most older adults are involved in at least one social or governmental service. This is true in both Canada and the United States. To understand the older adult situation, the nurse should know the government structures that fund and regulate the older adult programs.

In the United States the Department of Health and Human Services is the responsible federal agency for many older adult programs. In 1958 interest in the older citizen inspired the formation of the President's Council on Aging. From this beginning the Administration on Aging (AOA) has evolved. The general goal of AOA is to include older people wherever programs exist by cooperating and consulting with other agencies or organizations. There are several major grant programs under AOA. Title III of the Older Americans Act funds comprehensive, community-based service systems. Title IV funds the training of persons who are employed or preparing for employment in the field of aging. Funding from the AOA is funneled to state and local area agencies on aging.

In Canada the Department of National Health and Welfare is the responsible federal agency for many older adult programs. The policies of the federal and provincial governments cannot be easily separated. Policy often results in an intermingling of activities through shared jurisdiction and cost sharing. This shared role has been changing during the last 50 years. Before 1950 the provincial government's responsibility ended with assistance to the aged poor. Since that time a wide range of federal and provincial programs have evolved. The role of the government has changed from that of regulator to provider.

MEDICARE

Almost all U.S. citizens older than 65 years of age have Medicare coverage. **Medicare** is a health insurance program for people 65 years of age and older, as well as for some people with disabilities under age 65 and for people with end-stage renal disease requiring dialysis or a transplant. Medicare is designed for acute illness care. Reimbursement is based on daily documentation that indicates a patient is improving in function. This nursing documentation process is complex and critical for adequate reimbursement.

Medicare is composed of two parts, A and B. Part A covers inpatient hospital care. Medicare A pays reasonable charges on the basis of the diagnosis, not on the length of stay. Skilled nursing facility care in a hospital or long-term care facility is paid if the stay results in an improved or rehabilitated condition. These skilled nursing benefit days are limited. The percentage of coverage changes each year. Medicare A pays for home care if it requires skilled nursing or rehabilitation intervention and is needed on a part-time basis. The patient must be homebound. Durable medical equipment used daily is covered, but home safety equipment is not. Hospice care is covered under Medicare A. When hospice care is elected, the patient no longer qualifies for the condition to be treated in the standard Medicare program.

Part B covers outpatient treatment and physician's services. Medicare B is voluntary and has a monthly premium and an annual deductible before payment begins.

Medicare does not cover long-term nursing home care, custodial ADLs or IADLs care, dental care or dentures, preventive health care, prescription drugs, routine foot care, hearing aids, or eyeglasses. These costs plus the Medicare deductible costs account for the fact that most older adults pay for 50% of all acquired health care costs yearly. Analysis of chronic health care needs in the United States continues to indicate widespread unmet needs.

CARE ALTERNATIVES FOR OLDER ADULTS

Housing

Many older adults stay in their place of residence and do not move to a different home or geographic location (Fig. 5-6). Most do not move or return to the geographic location of childhood

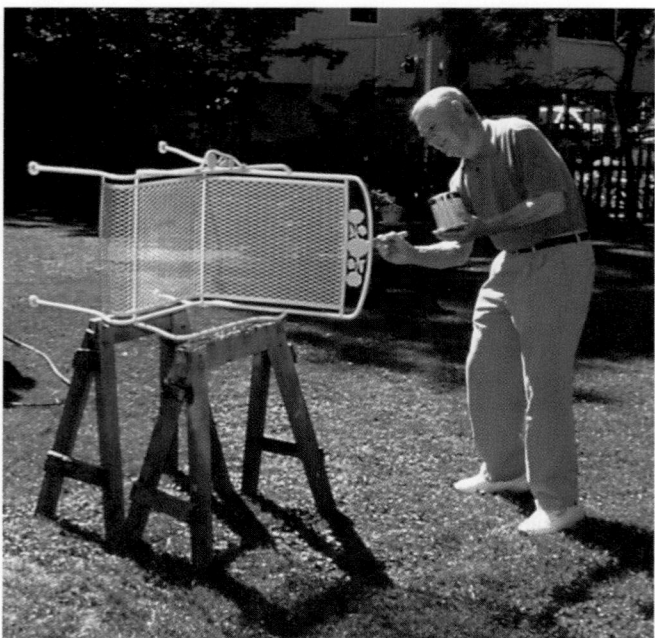

FIG. 5-6 Home maintenance is part of an older adult's independent lifestyle.

when health becomes frail. The community becomes important to the older adult as an environment that is safe from crime and accidents. The older adult needs privacy and companionship, as well as a sense of belonging. The community should be accessible. The older adult may need housing assistance through property tax relief, assistance with home repair, and fuel payment. A variety of subsidized, low-income housing arrangements are available for older adults in many areas.

For the older adult who chooses to remain in the home as functional abilities decline, home adaptations and modifications can be made. Homes can be made wheelchair accessible. Lighting can be increased and adjusted. Safety devices can be installed in bathrooms and kitchens. Alarms and assistive listening devices can be used.

Retirement communities may be an option for some older adults. These communities are age-segregated, self-contained developments and provide social activities, security, and recreational facilities. When retirement communities offer expanded health care and social support services, including long-term care, they become *continuing care retirement communities* (CCRCs). The CCRCs require an entrance fee and monthly fees for continuing care. (See Chapter 6 for discussion of community-based care settings.)

Congregate housing provides services to the older adult at two levels: independent and assisted living. Independent living facilities provide housing and congregate meals but no supervision. Other home maintenance and care services can be purchased from these facilities. Board and care homes provide housing and meals in small congregate home environments.

Assisted-living facilities are designed to provide housing and personalized health care. Because over half of community-based older adults require assistance with ADLs or IADLs, this is the most rapidly developing area of long-term care. Services vary from state to state. Nurses provide care to or manage assisted-living facilities and services. Nurses working in this area are challenged by questions related to regulations, use of unlicensed assistive workers, assessment to ensure safe "fit of resident to facility," and shared resident decision making.

Creative housing options are being developed by home sharing, the use of "granny flats," and apartment rentals in established older homes. The nurse can play a role in meeting the housing needs of older adults by identifying housing preferences and by advocating community housing changes that create a safe, livable community.

Community-Based Older Adults with Special Needs

Older adults with special care needs include homeless persons, persons who need constant assistance with ADLs, persons who are homebound, and persons who can no longer live at home. The older adult may be served by adult day care, home health care, and nursing home care.

Adult Day Care Programs. *Adult day care (ADC) programs* provide daily supervision, social activities, and ADLs assistance for two major groups of older adults—persons who are cognitively impaired and persons who have problems with ADLs. The services offered in the ADC programs are based on patient needs. Restorative programs for persons with problems of ADLs offer health monitoring, therapeutic activities, one-to-one ADLs training, individualized care planning, and personal care services. Programs designed for the cognitively impaired offer therapeutic recreation, support for family, family counseling, and social involvement. Patient characteristics in the cognitively impaired group include a high number of persons with Alzheimer's disease. In this group, incontinence is a common problem. Patient characteristics in the restorative care group include a large number of wheelchair users, problems with incontinence, and some depression.

Day care centers provide relief to the caregiver, allow continued employment for the caregiver, and delay institutionalization for the patient. Centers are regulated and standards are set by the state. Costs are not covered by Medicare. Adult day care is tax deductible as dependent care. Appropriate placement in a day care program that matches the patient's needs is important. The nurse can assist by knowing the available day care services and assessing the needs of the patient. The nurse is then in a position to aid the patient and family in making a good placement decision. The caregiver and the patient are often uninformed about day care and its services as an alternative care option.

Home Health Care. Home health care can be a cost-effective care alternative for the older adult patient who is homebound, has health needs that are intermittent or acute, and has supportive caregiver involvement. Home health care is not an alternative for the patient in need of 24-hour ADLs assistance or continuous safety supervision. Home health care services require physician recommendation and skilled nursing care for Medicare reimbursement. Unless these requirements are met, assistance by a home health aide for ADLs management or assistance by a homemaker for IADLs management will not be paid by Medicare. (Home health care is discussed in Chapter 6.)

Long-Term Care Facilities

Long-term care facilities are a placement alternative for the older adult who can no longer live alone, who needs continuous supervision, who has three or more ADLs disabilities, or who is

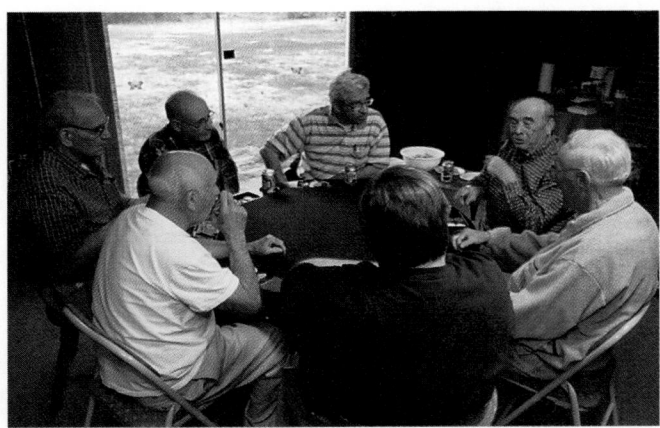

FIG. 5-7 Social interaction and acceptance is important for older adults.

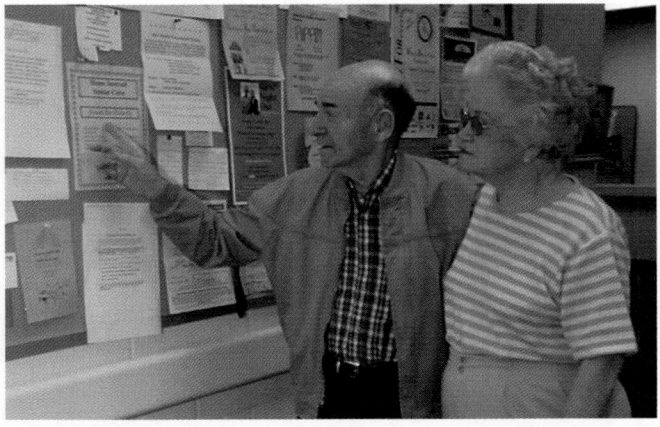

FIG. 5-8 Bulletin board at a senior center showing times that legal help is available.

frail. The cost of long-term care facilities is high. These costs are paid privately for 50% of all patients and by state-funded public assistance programs (Medicaid) for 40% of all patients. When patients receive Medicaid, they contribute all their personal income to pay their expenses, except for a small amount per month kept as a personal needs allowance. (Long-term care is discussed in Chapter 6.)

Three factors appear to precipitate placement in a long-term care facility: (1) rapid patient deterioration, (2) caregiver inability to continue care as a result of "burnout"—too much and too long, and (3) an alteration in or loss of family support system. Physical changes of confusion, incontinence, or a major health event (e.g., stroke) can accelerate placement.

The conflicts and fears faced by the family and patient make placement a transition time. Common caregiver concerns include the following: (1) process of admission will be resisted by the patient; (2) level of care given by staff will be insufficient; (3) patient will be lonely; and (4) financing of nursing care will not be adequate.

This time of disruption is increased by the physical relocation of the patient. The process of physical relocation results in adverse health effects for the older adult.[46] The crisis of *relocation syndrome* should be anticipated by the nurse, and appropriate interventions to reduce the effects of relocation should be used. Whenever possible the older adult should be involved in the decision to move and should be fully informed about the location. The caregiver can share information, pictures, or a videotape of the new location. New health personnel can send a welcome message. On arrival the new resident can be greeted by a staff member to orient the older adult. To bridge the relocation the new resident can be "buddied" with a seasoned resident.

The satisfied resident in a long-term care facility tends to show a variety of behaviors indicating adjustment (Fig. 5-7). The resident is assertive and self-reliant; keeps active, follows a routine, keeps mentally involved, and is sociable; maintains family interaction; and shows a level of acceptance. The satisfied resident also expresses a determined, positive perspective. The satisfied resident uses coping strategies that increase control and management of her or his life. The nurse can encourage and enable the use of these strategies.

Case Management

Matching older adult social support services to the needs of the older adult is complex. For family members who live out of town and cannot provide direct caregiving, the use of a case manager may be helpful. This is a new and developing role that the nurse is well suited to assume. The case manager supervises and manages care to ensure continuity of care for the older adult. The process of locating and organizing older adult services is time consuming. A written directory of nationwide services (*A National Eldercare Directory of Information and Referral*) is available from the National Association of Area Agencies on Aging (see Resources at end of chapter).

LEGAL AND ETHICAL ISSUES

Legal assistance is a concern for many older adults. Legal concerns center on advance directives, estate planning, taxation issues, and appeals for denied services. Legal aid is available to the low-income older adult by contacting a local multipurpose senior center (Fig. 5-8). This service is supported by funds authorized through Title III of the Older Americans Act.

Advance directives are mandated on admission to a health care facility by the Patient Self-Determination Act of 1991. There are primarily two types: a living will and a durable power of attorney for health. A *living will* is a directive that permits an individual to direct his or her health care in the event of a terminal or irreversible condition. Most living wills direct that in the event of a terminal illness, extraordinary medical care should not be initiated or should be withdrawn so that the process of dying will not be artificially prolonged. A living will is directive but not legally binding. A *durable power of attorney for health* is another form of advance directive that designates another person to voice health care decisions when the patient is unable to do so personally. A durable power of attorney for health is directive and legally binding. In most states it includes the naming of an individual to carry out directives when the patient cannot make choices. (Advance directives are discussed in Chapter 10 and Table 10-4.) Discussion of estate planning, taxation issues, and appeals for denied services is beyond the scope of this text.

The nurse who works with the older adult identifies areas of ethical concern that influence practice. This nurse identifies that these issues include the following: (1) to restrain or not restrain and (2) to evaluate the patient's ability to make decisions. Other ethical concerns related to (1) resuscitation, (2) treatment of infections, (3) issues of nutrition and hydration, and (4) transfer to more intensive treatment units are all a part of long-term care.

These situations are often complex and emotionally charged. The nurse can assist the patient, family, and other health care workers by acknowledging when an ethical dilemma is present, by keeping current on the ethical implications of new biotechnology, and by advocating for an institutional ethics committee to help in the decision-making process.

REVIEW QUESTIONS

The number of the question corresponds to the same-numbered objective at the beginning of the chapter.

1. The impact that older adults have on the health care system is illustrated by the fact that
   a. the aging population is growing faster than any other age-group.
   b. all persons over age 65 have at least two chronic diseases requiring medical care.
   c. older adults have a lower rate of hospitalization, home care, and physician visits than any other group.
   d. older adults tend to overreport symptoms and cannot distinguish normal changes of aging from symptoms of disease.

2. Ageism is characterized by
   a. denial of negative stereotypes regarding aging.
   b. positive attitudes toward the elderly based on age.
   c. negative attitudes toward the elderly based on age.
   d. negative attitudes toward the elderly based on physical disability.

3. A 45-year-old patient newly diagnosed with diabetes responds by telling the nurse that she must reevaluate what things in life are most important to her and focus her activities around these priorities. This response is most consistent with
   a. Peck's middle-age task of valuing wisdom versus physical power.
   b. the adjustment to declining health reflective of Havighurst's developmental tasks.
   c. a sense of wholeness and purpose to life described by Erikson's sense of ego integrity.
   d. Levinson's midlife transition, which involves the changing of life structures toward identified values.

4. When evaluating the blood pressure of an older adult, the nurse needs to know that
   a. systolic blood pressure decreases and diastolic pressure increases with aging.
   b. blood pressure should decrease with age because of decreased heart rate and cardiac output.
   c. the systolic blood pressure tends to rise with aging because of loss of elasticity of the arteries.
   d. dilation of the aorta and rigid arterial pulses make the blood pressure more difficult to measure accurately.

5. An ethnic older adult may experience a loss of self-worth when the nurse
   a. informs the patient about ethnic support services.
   b. allows a patient to rely on ethnic health beliefs and practices.
   c. has to use an interpreter to provide explanations and teaching.
   d. emphasizes that a therapeutic diet does not allow ethnic foods.

6. When older adults become ill they are more likely than younger adults to
   a. complain about the symptoms of their problems.
   b. refuse to carry out lifestyle changes to promote recovery.
   c. seek medical attention because of limitations on their lifestyle.
   d. alter their daily living activities to accommodate new symptoms.

7. Nursing interventions directed at health promotion in the older adult are primarily focused on
   a. disease management.
   b. controlling symptoms of illness.
   c. teaching positive health behaviors.
   d. providing a sense of control over health problems.

8. An important nursing action helpful to a chronically ill older adult is to
   a. avoid discussing future lifestyle changes.
   b. assure the patient that the condition is stable.
   c. treat the patient as a competent manager of the disease.
   d. encourage the patient to "fight" the disease as long as possible.

9. Delirium can be defined as
   a. an acute confusional state with a sudden onset.
   b. a prolonged state of confusion related to dementia.
   c. a confusional state that lasts only minutes to hours.
   d. a condition that is directly related to drug use.

10. An important fact for the nurse to know about caregivers is that they
    a. can often share the burden of caregiving with other family members.
    b. frequently require nurses to assist them in reducing caregiver strain.
    c. are usually trained health care workers who do not live with the patient.
    d. are generally strong and healthy but need teaching to carry out care activities.

11. An appropriate care choice for an older adult living with an employed daughter, but who requires constant assistance with activities of daily living, is
    a. adult day care.
    b. nursing home care.
    c. a retirement center.
    d. an assisted-living home.

12. A living will is an advance directive that
    a. is legally binding.
    b. encourages the use of artificial means to prolong life.
    c. allows a person to direct his or her health care in the event of terminal illness.
    d. designates who can act for the patient when the patient is unable to do so personally.

REFERENCES

1. Administration on Aging: *Profile of older Americans: 2000.* Available at *www.aoa.dhhs.gov/aoa/STATS/profile.* (accessed July 21, 2002).
2. *Projections of the total resident population by 5 year age groups, race, and Hispanic origin with special age categories: middle series, 1999 to 2000,* US Census Internet release date Jan 13, 2000. (accessed July 21, 2002).
3. *An aging world 2001.* US Census Bureau *www.census.gov/prod/1/pop* (accessed July 22, 2002).
4. Health statistics Canada. Available at *www.canoe.ca/HealthReference/statscan_9.html* (accessed July 22, 2002).
5. Ebersole P, Hess P: *Geriatric nursing and healthy aging,* St Louis, 2001, Mosby.
6. Shmuely Y et al: Predictors of improvement in health-related quality of life among elderly patients with depression, *Int Psychogeriatr* 13:63, 2001.
7. Erikson EH: *Childhood and society,* ed 2, New York, 1963, Norton.
8. Peck TA: Women's self-definition in adulthood: from a different model, *Psychology Women Quarterly* 10:274, 1986.
9. Havighurst RJ: *Developmental tasks and education,* ed 3, New York, 1972, McKay.
10. Levinson DH et al: *The seasons of a man's life,* New York, 1978, Knopf.
11. Lowenthal MF, Thurnher M, Chiriboga D: *Four stages of life,* San Francisco, 1975, Jossey-Bass.
12. Neugarten B: Adaptation and the life cycle, *Counseling Psychologist* 6:16, 1976.
13. Courtenay B: Are psychological models of adult development still important? *Adult Education Quarterly* 44:145, 1994.
14. Vojta CL et al: Antiaging therapy: an overview, *Hosp Pract* 36:43, 2001.
15. Finkel T, Holbrook NJ: Oxidants, oxidative stress and the biology of aging, *Nature* 408:239, 2000.
16. Knight JA: The biochemistry of aging, *Adv Clin Chem* 35:1, 2000.
17. Ames BN: Micronutrients prevent cancer and delay aging, *Toxicol Lett* 102-103:5, 1998.
18. DePinho RA: The age of cancer, *Nature* 408:248, 2000.
19. Ostler EL et al: Telomerase and the cellular lifespan: implications of the aging process, *J Pediatr Endocrinol Metab* 13(Suppl 6):1467, 2000.
20. Hermann M, Berger P: Hormonal changes in aging men: a therapeutic indication? *Exp Gerontol* 36:1075, 2001.
21. Meyer KC: The role of immunity in susceptibility to respiratory infection in the aging lung, *Respir Physiol* 128:23, 2001.
22. Cummings SM, Kropf NP, DeWeaver KL: Knowledge of and attitudes toward aging among non-elders: gender and race differences, *J Women Aging* 12:77, 2000.
23. McCandless NJ, Conner FP: Older women and the health care system: a time for change, *J Women Aging* 11:13, 1999.
24. Magilvy JK, Congdon JG: The crisis nature of health care transitions for rural older adults, *Public Health Nurs* 17:336, 2000.
25. Hwang SW: Mortality among men using homeless shelters in Toronto, Ontario, *JAMA* 283:2152, 2000.
26. Marwick C: *Healthy People 2010* initiative launched, *JAMA* 283:9890, 2000.
27. Quinn C: The nutritional screening initiative: meeting the nutritional needs of elders, *Orthop Nurs* 16:13, 1997.
28. Rankin S, Stallings P: *Patient education: principles and practice,* ed 4, Philadelphia, 2001, Lippincott.
29. Finlayson EV, Birkmeyer JD: Operative mortality with elective surgery in older adults, *Eff Clin Pract* 4:172, 2001.
30. Rizzo JA et al: Multicomponent targeted intervention to prevent delirium in hospitalized older patients: what is the economic value? *Med Care* 39:740, 2001.
31. Rajagopalan S: Tuberculosis and aging: a global health problem, *Clin Infect Dis* 33:1034, 2001.
32. Wallace M: Pain in older adults, *Ann Long-Term Care* 9:50, 2001.
33. Epps C: Recognizing pain in the institutionalized elder with dementia, *Geriatr Nurs* 22:71, 2001.
34. Gloth FM: Pain management in older adults: prevention and treatment, *J Am Geriatr Soc* 49:188, 2001.
35. Hujer ME, Mann AE, Mion LC: Substance abuse and the hospitalized elderly, *Orthop Nurs* 18:27, 1999.
36. Beers MH: Age-related changes as a risk factor for medication-related problems, *Generations* 24:22, 2000.
37. Alexopoulos G: Mood disorders. In Kaplan H, Sadock B, editors: *Kaplan and Sadock's comprehensive textbook of psychiatry,* Philadelphia, 2000, Lippincott Williams & Wilkins.
38. Lantz MS: Suicide in late life. Identifying and managing at-risk older patients, *Geriatrics* 56:47, 2001.
39. Brown GK, Bruce ML, Pearson JL: High-risk management guidelines for elderly suicidal patients in primary care settings, *J Geriatr Psychiatry* 16:593, 2001.
40. Thomas DR, Morley JE: Assessing and treating undernutrition in older medical outpatients, part III, *Clinical Geriatrics* 1(Suppl):46, 2001.
41. Ortmann C et al: Elder abuse. Using clinical tools to identify clues of mistreatment, *Geriatrics* 55:42, 2000.
42. Hajjar I, Duthie E: Prevalence of elder abuse in the United States: a comparative report between the national and Wisconsin data, *Wis Med J* 100:22, 2001.
43. Bookwala J, Schulz R: A comparison of primary stressors, secondary stressors, and depressive symptoms between elderly caregiving husbands and wives: the Caregiver Health Effects Study, *Psychol Aging* 15:607, 2000.
44. McKee KJ et al: The willingness to continue caring in family supporters of older people, *Health Soc Care Community* 7:100, 1999.
45. Reay AM, Browne KD: Fatal neglect of the elderly, *Int J Legal Med* 114:191, 2001.
46. Castle NG: Relocation of the elderly, *Med Care Res Rev* 58:291, 2001.

RESOURCES

Administration on Aging
330 Independence Avenue SW
Washington, DC 20201
800-677-1116 (Eldercare Locator—to find services for an older person in his or her locality)
202-619-0556 (AoA National Aging Information Center for technical information and public inquiries)
202-401-4541 (Office of the Assistant Secretary for Aging)
Fax: 202-260-1012
www.aoa.dhhs.gov

Alliance for Retired Americans
888 16th Street, NW
Washington, DC 20006
888-373-6497
Fax: 301-578-8911
www.retiredamericans.org/contact.htm

American Association of Homes and Services for the Aging
2519 Connecticut Avenue, NW
Washington, DC 20008-1520
202-738-2242
Fax: 202-783-2255
www.aahsa.org

American Association for International Aging
1900 L Street NW, Suite 512
Washington, DC 20036-5002
202-833-8893
Fax: 202-833-8762
www.unm.edu/~aging/AAIAInf.html

American Association of Retired Persons (AARP)
601 E Street NW
Washington, DC 20049
800-424-3410
www.aarp.org/index.html

American Geriatrics Society
The Empire State Building
350 Fifth Avenue, Suite 801
New York, NY 10118
212-308-1414
800-247-4779
Fax: 212-832-8646
www.americangeriatrics.org

American Society on Aging
833 Market Street, Suite 511
San Francisco, CA 94103-1824
415-974-9600
Fax: 415-974-0300
E-mail: info@asaging.org
www.asaging.org/

Canadian Association on Gerontology
100-824 Meath Street
Ottawa, ON
K1Z 6E8 Canada
613-728-9347
Fax: 613-728-8913
E-mail: info@cagacg.ca
www.cagacg.ca/

Centers for Medicare and Medicaid Services
7500 Security Boulevard
Baltimore, MD 21244-1850
410-786-3000
www.hcfa.gov

ElderWeb
1305 Chadwick Drive
Normal, IL 61761
309-451-3319
Fax: 866-422-8995
E-mail: ksb@elderweb.com
www.elderweb.com

Gerontological Society of America
1030 15th Street NW, Suite 250
Washington, DC 20005
202-842-1275
www.geron.org

Geroweb
Institute of Gerontology
Wayne State University
87 East Ferry Street
Detroit, MI 48202
313-577-2297
Fax: 313-875-0127
www.iog.wayne.edu/IOGlinks.html

Health Promotion Institute
National Council on the Aging
409 Third Street SW
Washington, DC 20024
www.ncoa.org

International Federation on Aging
Secretariat—Canada
380 Antoine Street W, Suite 3200
Montreal, Quebec
CANADA H2Y 3X7
514-287-9679
Fax: 514-987-1567

International Senior Citizens Association, Inc.
255 S Hill Street, Suite 409
Los Angeles, CA 90012
213-625-5008
Fax: 213-625-7115

Meals on Wheels America
1414 Prince Street, Suite 302
Alexandria, VA 22314
703-548-5558
www.projectmeal.org

National Advisory Council on Aging (NACA)
Ottawa, ON
Postal Locator: 1908A1
K1A 1B4 Canada
613-957-1968
Fax: 613-957-9938
E-mail:seniors@hc-sc.gc.ca
www.hc-sc.gc.ca/seniors-aines/seniors/english/naca/naca.htm

National Association of Area Agencies on Aging
927 15th Street NW, 6th Floor
Washington, DC 20005
202-296-8130
Fax: 202-296-8134
www.n4a.org

National Association for Hispanic Elderly
Asociacion Nacional por Personas Mayores
234 East Colorado Boulevard, Suite 300
Pasadena, CA 91101
626-564-1988
Fax: 656-564-2659
www.aoa.gov/directory/139.html

National Caucus and Center on Black Aged
1200 L Street NW, Suite 800
Washington, DC 20005
202-637-8400
Fax: 202-347-0895
www.ncba-blackaged.org/

National Council on the Aging, Inc.
409 Third Street SW, Suite 200
Washington, DC 20024
202-479-1200
Fax: 202-479-0735
www.ncoa.org/

National Gerontological Nursing Association
7794 Grow Drive
Pensacola, FL 32514
850-473-1174
800-723-0560
Fax: 850-484-8762
E-mail: ngna@puetzamc.com
www.ngna.org/

National Hispanic Council on Aging
2713 Ontario Road NW
Washington, DC 20009
202-265-1288
Fax: 202-745-2522
www.nhcoa.org/

National Indian Council on Aging
10501 Montgomery Blvd. NE, Suite 210
Albuquerque, NM 87111-3846
505-292-2001
www.nicoa.org/

National Institute on Aging
Building 31, Room 5C27
31 Center Drive, MSC 2292
Bethesda, MD 20892
301-496-1752
www.nia.nih.gov

Older Women's League (OWL)
666 11th Street NW, Suite 700
Washington, DC 20001
202-783-6686
800-825-3695
Fax: 202-638-2356
www.owl-national.org/

For additional Internet resources, see the website for this book at
http://evolve.elsevier.com/Lewis/medsurg/.

Carol O. Long

CHAPTER 6

Community-Based Nursing and Home Care

LEARNING OBJECTIVES

1. Describe how the factors changing the health care delivery system are influencing the shift of patient care from hospitals to community-based and home care settings.
2. Differentiate community-based nursing from community-oriented nursing.
3. Compare community-based patient care settings and the services provided in these settings.
4. Describe the roles and challenges of nurses working in community-based and home care settings.

KEY TERMS

acute rehabilitation, p. 86
ambulatory care, p. 85
case management, p. 84
community-based nursing, p. 83
community-oriented nursing, p. 83
continuing care retirement community, p. 86
health maintenance organizations (HMOs), p. 83
home health care, p. 87

intermediate care facility, p. 86
long-term acute care, p. 86
long-term care, p. 86
preferred provider organizations (PPOs), p. 84
residential care facilities, p. 87
skilled nursing facilities, p. 86
subacute care, p. 86
televisiting, p. 91
transitional care, p. 85

Major changes in nursing practice and patient care are occurring as a result of numerous factors affecting the health care system. Social, economic, technologic, and health factors are driving the delivery of health care from hospitals to community-based and home care settings. In response to these factors, the practice of professional nursing is also evolving. Nurses are providing patient care in a wide variety of health care settings outside of the hospital, allowing for increased diversity in nursing practice. For many years the vast majority of nurses have been employed in hospitals. However, it is now predicted that by 2010, 70% of nursing care will be provided in the community.[1]

Community-based nursing practice is different from community-oriented nursing. The focus of **community-based nursing** is illness-oriented care of individuals and families throughout the life span. Its goal is to help individuals and families manage acute or chronic health conditions in community and home settings. **Community-oriented nursing** includes *public health nursing,* which focuses on the health care of the community, and *community health nursing,* which has as its primary focus

the health care of individuals, families, and groups in a community. Community-oriented nursing is a nursing specialty, but community-based nursing is a philosophy of practice for all nursing specialties.[2]

This chapter presents an overview of the changing health care system and discusses nursing care in community-based settings and the home. Although long-term care and rehabilitation facilities are not typically considered community-based settings, they are included in this chapter.

CHANGING HEALTH CARE SYSTEM

Factors Influencing Change

Socioeconomic Considerations. The changes in health care have been largely initiated by the continued efforts of the government, employers, insurance companies, and regulating agencies to provide health care in the most cost-effective manner. Historically, the most notable event related to changing reimbursement patterns was the institution of prospective payment systems and the use of Diagnosis Related Groups (DRGs) in the Medicare program.[3] With these changes, hospitals were no longer reimbursed for all costs. Instead, payment for hospital services to Medicare patients was based on flat fees per admission based on DRGs. In many instances the implementation of DRGs has shifted patient care from acute care settings to community and home settings. The prospective payment system has been and continues to be one of the most significant factors affecting health care. These policies and recent advances in technology allow nurses to care for increasingly complex patients in community and home settings.

Private and other public health care systems eventually followed the prospective payment system established by the Medicare program. **Health maintenance organizations**

Reviewed by Leslie Neal, RN, C, PhD, CCRN, Assistant Professor, Marymount University, Arlington, Virginia; and Geoff F. Shuster, RN, DNSc, Associate Professor, College of Nursing, University of New Mexico, Albuquerque, N.M.

---

*An HMO consists of an association of health care professionals and facilities that provide a specified package of health care for a fixed sum of money paid in advance for a specified period of time. The HMO contracts with health care professionals and facilities to provide the specified care. Generally a patient cannot seek care outside of the health care provider and/or hospitals under contract with the HMO.

(HMOs)* and **preferred provider organizations (PPOs)*** evolved as a means of managing the expense of health care delivery.[3] In these managed care systems, charges are negotiated in advance of the delivery of care using predetermined reimbursement rates or capitation fees for medical care, hospitalization, and other health care services. Like the Medicare program, these organizations have caused a shift in the delivery of care from the acute care hospital setting to less expensive community settings.

Changing Demographics. The average age of people in the United States is increasing. The number of Americans over age 65 is increasing more rapidly than the general population.[4] As a result, health care needs and demands have changed. Our aging population is demanding more health care and straining the financial resources that fund it, such as the Medicare program. Aging Americans have disabilities that may compromise their ability to remain functional in their own homes without supportive community or professional help. The elderly also have complex medical and health care needs, often experiencing multiple chronic conditions that compromise their ability to remain independent. Physical and functional problems, dementia, fixed incomes, and limited family or community support put the elderly at an increased need for social and health care assistance.

Nature and Prevalence of Illness. The expanded life expectancy of the population and lifestyle factors contribute to increases in the number, severity, and duration of chronic conditions. Chronic diseases are responsible for 70% of the deaths in the United States. The four leading causes of death from chronic diseases—cardiovascular disease, cancer, diabetes, and chronic obstructive pulmonary disease—are in large part related to lifestyle behaviors.[5] Tobacco use, lack of physical activity, and poor nutrition (including obesity) are the major contributors to cardiovascular disease and cancer.[5] The focus of health care is now shifting from intervention in the acute phase of diseases toward early screening, detection, and prevention. Nursing practice directed toward the prevention and management of chronic illness occurs in community-based settings through (1) promotion of regular screening and use of positive health behaviors and (2) assisting individuals and families to manage chronic illness in the home.

Technology. Surgical innovations, such as advances in cardiac surgery, and medical interventions, such as new drugs for cystic fibrosis, have allowed individuals to live longer, shifting both acute and long-term care to community-based settings and the home. New technology has improved diagnostic procedures and management of patient care. Computers, lifesaving drugs, and telehealth interventions have simplified diagnosis and treatment and shortened hospital stays.

Patient care has moved to outpatient settings such as surgical centers, providing services that have been traditionally delivered only in hospitals. Complex patient care treatments, such as intravenous (IV) antibiotic therapy and total parenteral therapy, are increasingly being delivered in the home. Evolving technology, the focus on reducing rapidly increasing health care costs, and patient preference to be at home have stimulated the movement to provide health care in the community and home settings.

---

*A PPO is a group of health care professionals and/or hospitals who contract with an employer, insurance company, or third-party payer to provide medical care to a specified group of potential patients. The services offered are not prepaid or fixed. There is typically more choice in a PPO than in an HMO, and thus it is more costly.

Increasing Consumerism. Health care is becoming a more consumer-focused business. Patients are becoming more interested in their health care. As a result they are becoming active participants. Many patients eagerly seek out information about their health from the media and Internet sources. They also expect that information will be provided so that they may collaborate with health care providers in making the right decisions about their health care. In addition, the public has come to view health care as an entitlement or a human right. Health care legislation emphasizes equal access to health care services, regardless of the ability to pay. As increasing demands are made on scarce and costly health care resources, nurses are becoming more active partners with patients in promoting self-care through education and advocacy.

Case Management

Case management is a method used to coordinate and link health care services to patients and their families in the changing health care environment. Although health care agencies or organizations may define and practice case management in various ways, the concept of case management involves the coordination of patient care during the entire episode of illness across every setting where the patient receives care.[6] The goals of case management are to provide quality care along a continuum, decrease fragmentation of care across many settings, enhance the patient's quality of life, and contain costs. Case managers are an extremely important part of managed care and community-based nursing and home health care.

The case manager is accountable for short- and long-term outcomes, as well as overall financial outcomes.[7] The case manager establishes a plan of care with the patient and family, coordinates multidisciplinary teams, updates the patient and family on progress of care, and facilitates selection of appropriate health care resources. For example, a patient with severe coronary artery disease may be assigned a nurse as a case manager in an outpatient clinic. When the patient is hospitalized for coronary bypass surgery, the same case manager coordinates care so that all health care providers understand the patient's unique needs. When the patient is discharged, the case manager determines whether home health care or other services are necessary for the patient. The case manager may visit the patient in other settings to ensure that appropriate health care measures are being implemented.[8]

COMMUNITY-BASED CARE

Continuum of Patient Care

Depending on an individual's health status and the cost of care required, patients can move among different health care settings. There is a continuum of care whereby different settings accommodate the varying needs of the patient. Within this continuum, many persons today are cared for in community-based settings. For example, a person may be hospitalized in a trauma unit following a motor vehicle accident. After the person is stabilized, he or she may be transferred to a general medical-surgical unit and then to an acute rehabilitation facility. After a period of rehabilitation, the person may be discharged to his or her home to continue with outpatient rehabilitation and to be followed by home health care nurses and/or cared for in an outpatient clinic.

The continuum of care does not always include hospitalization. Most patients receive community-based care without experiencing an acute problem requiring hospitalization. Health problems may be identified in a variety of outpatient settings. In addition, individuals or families may seek specific assistance from health care resources in the community.

For example, a patient may be screened for diabetes mellitus in a community-based screening program and, when indicated, referred to a clinic where a diagnosis of diabetes can be established. A diabetes clinical nurse specialist may function as a case manager to coordinate the diabetes management team consisting of diabetic educators, nurses, dietitians, pharmacists, physicians, and other health care professionals. Services may include care and education at a variety of settings, as well as follow-up by home health care nurses.

Patients can be treated in a multitude of settings, opting for the one most appropriate for their health care needs but within the constraints of health care insurance plans and the cost of care. Today health care is increasingly constrained by third-party payer cost containment efforts. At the same time third-party payers are demanding outcome-based quality care. Although the hospital remains the mainstay for acute care interventions, settings such as extended care facilities, assisted living centers, and home health care offer patients the opportunity to live or recover in settings that maximize their independence and preserve human dignity.

Community-Based Nurses

Nurses practicing in community-based settings care for acutely or chronically ill individuals where they reside, work, or go to school.[9] Nursing roles include home health care nurses, school nurses, occupational nurses, and nurses working in outpatient clinics and ambulatory care centers. Nurses in nurse-managed clinics provide direct care to patients in an ambulatory setting. Parish, or congregational, nurses practice holistic health care within a faith community, emphasizing the relationship between spiritual faith and health. Parish nurses complement the work of other health care workers, acting as a liaison with congregational and community resources.[10]

The following sections provide an overview of selected patient care settings in the community where community-based nursing is provided. Table 6-1 compares these care settings with each other and with acute care provided in hospitals. As noted at the beginning of the chapter, some of these settings are not typically considered community-based settings. However, they do include areas where nurses practice outside of the hospital and constitute many of the less expensive community settings used in managed care.

Ambulatory Care

The delivery of health care primarily occurs in **ambulatory care** settings where health care services are provided on an outpatient basis. Patients may be seen in physician and nurse practitioner offices, nurse-managed clinics, emergency departments, community health centers, freestanding surgical centers, schools, churches, adult day care centers, and a multitude of public and proprietary clinics serving general or specific populations.

Nurses in ambulatory care settings may assist a physician in practice or, with additional training, assume nurse practitioner or advanced practice roles. Nurses in ambulatory care settings assess patients' problems, evaluate the need for resources and information, and provide the appropriate interventions that allow patients to care for themselves. Patient teaching and telephone follow-up are routine practices in ambulatory care settings. Nurses in freestanding surgical centers may assist with the preoperative and postoperative care for patients who will be discharged to home the same day.

Transitional Care

Transitional care refers to intermediary care between the acute care setting and the home. Patients who have recently been admitted to the acute care hospital but who cannot take care of

TABLE 6-1	Comparison of Patient Care Settings			
SETTING	EXAMPLES	EMPHASIS	FINANCING	PATIENT CARE
Acute care	Hospital	Cure, lifesaving surgical care	All payers	Acute care, short length of stay
Transitional care	Subacute care, acute rehabilitation, long-term acute care	Stabilization, rehabilitation	Medicare	Short- to long-term care
Long-term care	Skilled nursing facilities, intermediate care facility, retirement communities, residential care facilities	Restoration, support	Medicaid, out of pocket	Long-term care
Home health care	Formal and informal, primarily in the home	Teaching, rehabilitation, independence	Medicare, Medicaid, commercial insurance, charity	Short- to long-term care, part time, intermittent
Hospice	Home, inpatient	Care of the dying	Medicare, Medicaid, commercial insurance, charity	Until death
Ambulatory care	Physician or nurse practitioner in office, surgicenter, clinic, schools, work	Diagnosis, outpatient surgery, prevention, maintenance, treatment	All payers	Episodic

themselves may be placed for a short time in a transitional care setting.[11] Transitional care may take place in a distinct part of a hospital or a long-term care facility or in a separate, freestanding facility. Different levels of transitional care that exist in health care settings are described.

Subacute Care. **Subacute care** is postacute care designed for patients who need a greater intensity of care than that generally provided in a skilled nursing facility but no longer require acute care. Typical patients requiring subacute care are chronically ill, ventilator dependent, or those needing specialized monitoring, equipment, and nursing care. Many of the patients who require subacute care have exhausted their inpatient DRG days. Subacute care settings may exist in a distinct section of a hospital or in long-term care facilities. Nurses working in subacute care need to be familiar with tracheostomy care, ventilators, complex wound management, and care of the terminally ill. Although subacute patients are usually medically stable, they require multiple and complex treatments. Short-term acute care is designed to return the patient to the community or transition the patient to a lower level of care.[12]

Acute Rehabilitation. **Acute rehabilitation** is a postacute level of care specializing in therapies for patients with neurologic or physical injuries, such as those with head trauma, spinal cord injury, or stroke. Acute rehabilitation settings may be in separate units of a hospital or in freestanding facilities in the community. The patient in acute rehabilitation may receive several hours of exercise and other rehabilitative training or therapy daily. Patients learn to use assistive devices and need time and encouragement to perform activities of daily living and other aspects of self-care. Patients may need weeks to months of rehabilitative care before they can return home.

Long-Term Acute Care. **Long-term acute care** settings are distinct units of a hospital or may be a separate facility designed to care for patients who require acute care that may extend to 30 days. These individuals may be ventilator dependent or require extensive and complicated dressing changes or combinations of multiple medical and nursing interventions. Discharge planning is focused on discharge to home or long-term care settings.

Long-Term Care

Long-term care refers to the care of patients for a time period greater than 30 days. Long-term care may be required for individuals who are severely developmentally disabled, are mentally impaired, or have physical deficits requiring continuous medical or nursing management, such as those who are ventilator dependent or those with Alzheimer's disease.

Long-term care facilities include skilled nursing facilities, intermediate care facilities, retirement communities, and residential care facilities.[13] Each one of these areas is reviewed.

Skilled Nursing Facilities. **Skilled nursing facilities** provide care for patients who require 24-hour nursing supervision, many of whom are confined to bed for some portion of the day or are incontinent. These facilities offer treatment under the supervision of licensed practical nurses and at least one registered nurse who must be on duty during the day. Like other long-term care settings, skilled nursing facilities are licensed by state licensing authorities and Medicare pays for a small portion of this care.

Skilled nursing facilities offer a transitional level of postacute care in which the patient requires specified nursing skills and

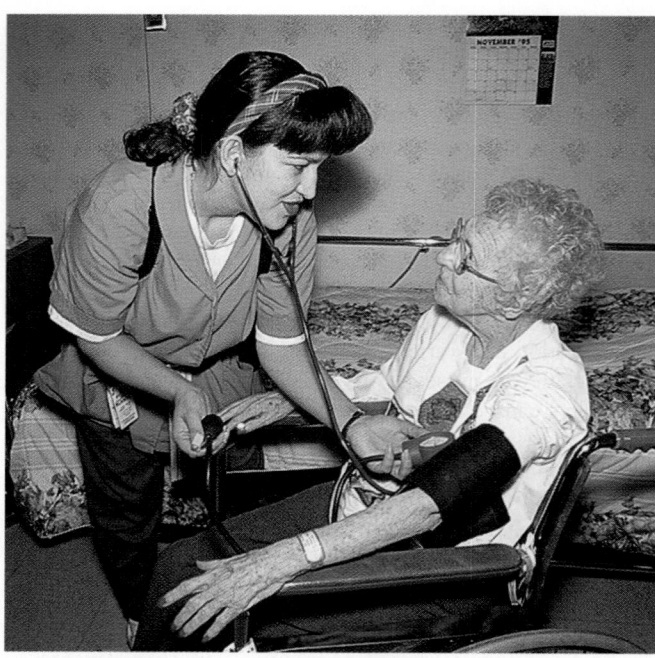

FIG. 6-1   Nurse taking blood pressure for patient in an intermediate care facility.

therapeutic support. Skilled nursing facilities provide an emphasis on rehabilitative therapies for convalescing patients. These patients may be too weak or ill to tolerate rapid rehabilitation. Patients in skilled care may need IV drugs, aggressive anticoagulant therapy, renal dialysis, or pain management (Fig. 6-1). Some patients are terminally ill or disabled to the degree that continuous nursing support is required.

Intermediate Care Facilities. An **intermediate care facility** provides convalescent care and regular medical, nursing, social, and rehabilitative services in addition to room and board for people not capable of independent living. These facilities offer a mix of medical care, nursing and rehabilitative care, and personal and residential care services.[14]

Residents in these facilities require less intensive nursing care than that provided by skilled nursing facilities (Fig. 6-2). Intermediate care can be temporary care for individuals recovering from an acute illness or injury, and often for those who have been discharged from the hospital. Residents may receive care in intermediate care facilities for several weeks to years or from youth to old age, making these facilities a permanent home and staff a second family. Common goals of these facilities are to assess what individuals are capable of doing and to help them achieve their potential by teaching and training them to achieve maximum independence.

Retirement Communities. Some long-term care settings may include the entire spectrum of care. Residents may reside in a **continuing care retirement community** (CCRC), which is a blend of several options, including housing complex, activity center, and health care system. CCRCs differ from other retirement options by providing a continuum of housing, services, and health care. There is a written agreement or contract between the resident and the CCRC that is generally intended to last the resident's lifetime or for a specific period of time.[15]

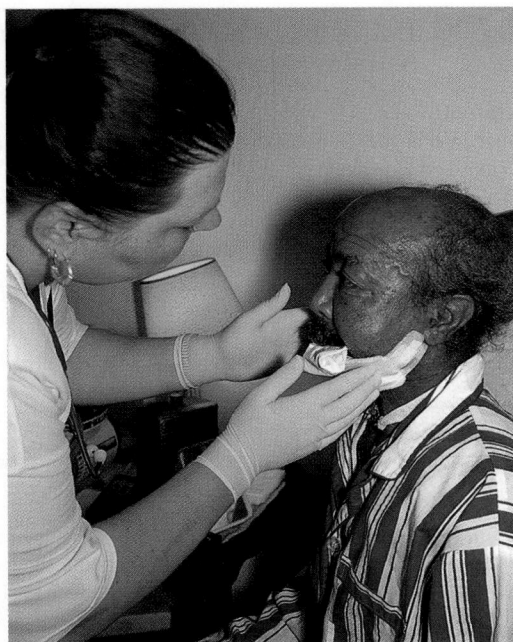

FIG. 6-2   Nurse providing care in a skilled nursing care facility.

TABLE 6-2	**Funding Mechanisms for Home Health Care**

1. Title programs under the Social Security Act of 1965
   - Medicare or Title XVIII
   - Medicaid or Title XIX
2. Title program under the Social Services Amendment of the Social Security Act of 1975
   - Title XX for homemaking and chore service for low-income persons
3. Older Americans Act of 1965
   - Title III, governed by the Area Agencies on Aging, for homemaker services, home health aide, nutrition, home-delivered meals, legal services
   - Title IV, research and demonstration projects for frail elderly who are at risk for institutionalization
4. Title V provides maternal, child health, and crippled children services
5. Private or commercial insurance
6. Managed care arrangements, such as through preferred provider organizations (PPOs) or health maintenance organizations (HMOs)
7. Veterans benefits through the Veterans Administration
8. Private payment or out-of-pocket payment
9. No-fault insurance
10. Charity organizations and foundations, such as the United Way

Residential Care Facilities. **Residential care facilities** may be referred to as supervisory care homes or assisted living arrangements.[13,15] Both settings are generally licensed by the state to ensure that quality living, safety, and health care standards are met. Residents generally must be able to care for themselves and move about without the help of another person. Residents often live in these care homes to obtain additional assistance for their activities of daily living, such as grooming and meal preparation, or supervision with their medications. Many of these facilities also have a skilled nursing facility. This enables residents who temporarily need skilled nursing care to receive it until they can return to their own residence.

Special Care Units. Some individuals with cognitive impairments may require special assistance in their long-term care. With increasing numbers of residents with Alzheimer's disease (AD) and other forms of dementia, special care units have been developed to address the unique needs of these individuals.[16] A segregated, low-stimulus environment and specially trained nurses guide residents, who have few physical problems, with special activity programming. Although these units are appropriate for early- to middle-stage AD, they may not be appropriate for those who have reached the advanced stages of dementia.

HOME HEALTH CARE

Home health care refers to health care delivered in the home setting. The National Association for Home Care (NAHC) defines *home care* as the broad spectrum of health care and social services provided in the home environment to recovering, disabled, or chronically ill patients.[17] Home health care may include health maintenance, education, illness prevention, diagnosis and treatment of disease, palliative care, and rehabilitation. Care may be delivered in assisted living situations when no other skilled nursing professionals are available for patient care needs. Pa-

tients receiving home health care may require intermittent services or full-time, 24-hours-a-day assistance.

Home health care has its roots in community health nursing.[18] In fact, until hospitals became the predominant source of health care, nurses often made visits to the patient's home to teach and provide care. At one time, home health care was one aspect of public health nursing, along with other community health services. It was not until the mid-1960s that home health care became established on its own. With the inception of Medicare (Title XVIII of the Social Security Act) and Medicaid (Title XIX), provisions were made for the federal government to reimburse home health care services through fiscal intermediaries. Over the years other forms of insurance have become available for the payment of home health care (Table 6-2).

In the past decade there has been an explosive growth in home health care services, coupled with a steady decline in hospital bed occupancy and length of hospital stay. The growth in home health care has been stimulated by DRGs, the increase in managed care, and the patient's preference to be cared for at home. Home health care is one of the most rapidly growing segments in health care today, with the primary motivation being to shift health care to less costly services.[19] However, the Balanced Budget Act of 1997 (P.L. 105-33) affecting Medicare reimbursement for home health care has created a financial crisis in many home health care agencies. This is a direct result of several factors, including a reduction in the reimbursement for visits; the implementation of additional, mandated monitoring and outcomes documentation; and limitations on what was considered as reimbursable skilled nursing. In 2000 prospective payment for Medicare home health care patients was instituted, and in 2001 further reductions in Medicare reimbursements were made.[17,20] This restrictive legislation has resulted in serious consequences for home health care agencies and their ability to provide patient care in the home. Home health agencies may be licensed by state licensing bureaus and certified to receive reimbursement for care to Medicare beneficiaries.[21]

Nurses and home health aides provide most home health care services.[22] Registered nurses are the coordinators of patient care, being accountable both for the supervision of personal care services by home health aides and for case management services, including all aspects of care in the home.

Patient Care in the Home

The most common diagnoses for home care patients are diabetes mellitus, hypertension, heart failure, osteoarthritis, stroke, chronic skin ulcers, chronic obstructive pulmonary disease, and heart disease.[22] Skilled nursing care may include observation, assessment, management, evaluation, teaching, training, administration of medications, wound care (Fig. 6-3), tube feedings, catheter care, and behavioral health interventions (Table 6-3). Commonly performed treatments in the home include administration of infusion therapy (i.e., antibiotic administration), patient-controlled analgesia for pain control, enteral feedings, parenteral nutrition, chemotherapy, and hydration therapy. The nurse and a rehabilitation team member may also provide medical equipment in the home to facilitate medical treatment and safety. These may include electrical beds, wheelchairs, commodes, walkers, and other assistive devices.

Patients have benefited from sophisticated technology in the home care setting. The miniaturization of infusion pumps makes it possible for patients to go to work while receiving antibiotics or total parenteral nutrition. The use of central venous catheter devices and peripherally inserted central catheters has eliminated many problems associated with short-term and less reliable IV therapy. Tabletop ventilators allow patients who are dependent on mechanical ventilation to be cared for in the home setting, allowing for even greater mobility when the equipment is strapped to the back of a wheelchair. Oxygen delivery in a variety of forms is also frequently provided in the home (see Chapter 28).

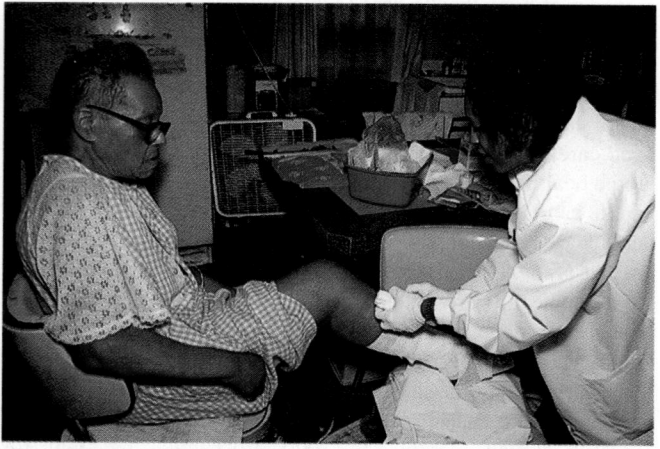

FIG. 6-3 Nurse providing wound care in the home.

TABLE 6-3	**Examples of Home Health Care Nursing Activities**

Assessment
Performance of in-depth holistic assessment of patient, family, and home environment.
Assessment of community services as a source of referral for patient/caregiver needs. Ongoing evaluation of patient's progress.

Wound Care
Dressing changes. Observation, assessment, and culture of wounds. Debridement and irrigation of wounds. Instructing patients and families in wound care.

Respiratory Care
Management of oxygen therapy, mechanical ventilation, chest physiotherapy. Suctioning and care of tracheostomies.

Vital Signs
Monitoring blood pressure and cardiopulmonary status. Teaching patients and families in taking of blood pressure and pulse.

Elimination
Assistance with colostomy irrigation and skin care procedures. Insertion of urinary catheters, irrigation, and observation for infection. Instruction of family in intermittent catheterization. Insertion, replacement, and sterile irrigation of urethral and suprapubic catheters. Bowel and bladder training.

Nutrition
Assessment of nutrition and hydration status. Teaching about prescribed diet. Administration of nasogastric and percutaneous tube feedings, including gastrostomy and jejunostomy tubes, and teaching families about tube feedings. Placement and replacement of tubes and ongoing management and evaluation.

Rehabilitation
Teaching patients and families to use assistive devices, range-of-motion exercises, ambulation, and transfer techniques.

Medications
Teaching patients and families about administration and side effects of medications. Monitoring compliance and effectiveness of prescribed drugs. Administration of and teaching about insulin injections.

Intravenous Therapy
Assessment and management of dehydration. Giving antibiotic drugs, parenteral nutrition, blood products, and analgesic and chemotherapeutic agents. Use of peripheral and central lines.

Pain Management
Assessment of pain, including location, characteristics, precipitating factors, and impact on life. Teaching patient and family about nonpharmacologic techniques (e.g., relaxation, imagery) for pain management. Providing optimal pain relief with prescribed analgesics.

Selected Laboratory Studies
Drawing blood for studies related to monitoring disease processes or therapy.

TABLE 6-4	Concerns of Patients Requiring Home Health Care Organized by Functional Health Patterns

Health Perception–Health Management Pattern
Self-care capability
Maintenance of safety
Adherence to prescribed therapy

Nutritional-Metabolic Pattern
Suitability of diet
Integrity of skin
Energy for daily activities

Elimination Pattern
Bowel control
Bladder control
Use of medications

Activity-Exercise Pattern
Endurance during activities
Impairments in mobility
Home maintenance management

Sleep-Rest Pattern
Decreased daytime alertness
Interference with sleep; interrupted sleep
Sleep/activity asynchrony

Cognitive-Perceptual Pattern
Capacity to learn
Acute pain and chronic pain
Sensory impairments
Complaints or discomforts

Self-Perception–Self-Concept Pattern
Body image disturbances
Feelings of self-worth
Feelings of powerlessness

Role-Relationship Pattern
Altered family or living arrangements
Capability for vocation/employment
Social contact and involvement
Altered family roles

Sexuality-Reproductive Pattern
Methods of contraception
Facilitation of conception
Alternative means of sexual activity

Coping–Stress Tolerance Pattern
Perception of intense stressors
Dealing with change and loss
Exhaustion of adaptive abilities
Management of stress
Sources of formal and informal support

Value-Belief Pattern
Maintenance of the human spirit
Holistic well-being
Worth of life and health
Desire to maintain independence

Adapted from Potter PA, Perry AG: *Fundamentals of nursing: concepts, process, and practice,* ed 4, St Louis, 1997, Mosby.

NURSING DIAGNOSES & COLLABORATIVE PROBLEMS

TABLE 6-5	Patients Requiring Home Health Care*

Acute pain *related to* disease process, therapy, decreased joint mobility

Caregiver role strain *related to* assuming total care of patient

Chronic pain *related to* chronic physical/psychosocial disability

Constipation *related to* decreased fluid intake, lack of mobility, narcotic analgesics

Deficient fluid volume *related to* inadequate nutrition and hydration, dysphasia, and confusion

Fatigue *related to* disease process and therapy

Imbalanced nutrition: less than body requirements *related to* inability to ingest or digest food, inability to absorb nutrients

Impaired home maintenance *related to* decreased mobility, decreased endurance

Impaired skin integrity *related to* physical immobility, radiation, pressure

Risk for aspiration *related to* enteral tube feedings, impaired gag reflex or swallowing, inability to expectorate sputum

Risk for infection *related to* inadequate primary or secondary defenses, impaired immune status, malnutrition

Risk for injury *related to* altered mobility, confusion, fatigue

Self-care deficit (any combination of the following): **bathing/hygiene, dressing/grooming, feeding, or toileting** *related to* pain, musculoskeletal impairment, decreased endurance

Social isolation *related to* physical immobility, alteration in physical appearance

*The nursing diagnoses in this table are examples of possible nursing diagnoses for a patient receiving home health care.

Concerns of patients requiring home health care are presented in Table 6-4. Examples of nursing diagnoses for patients requiring home health care are presented in Table 6-5.

Although the patient is the center of care and visit reimbursement is based on what is done for the patient, nursing care in the home must be family centered. An illness experienced by one family member will affect the entire family and alter family interactions. Families often provide care for ill members and assist in decision making about the type and extent of care provided. Care provided by health professionals is usually episodic, leaving the family with the burden of care day in and day out. In some situations, an elderly patient may be cared for by a spouse of similar age with chronic illnesses. In other situations an elderly parent needing care may live with a busy middle-aged family with dependent children. In any home care situation it is common for caregivers to become physically, emotionally, and economically overwhelmed with the responsibilities and demands of caring for a family member. The home health nurse needs to help family members understand and cope with changing roles, responsibilities, and stresses. Referral to various support groups in the community or on the Internet is one way the nurse can help family members cope with the experience of providing home care.

Teaching needs to involve both the patient and the family. Family members who are providing care should learn how to administer treatments and manage equipment. For example, diet modification is a cornerstone of diabetes management. Although an elderly diabetic person may be the patient, it may be the patient's spouse or daughter who does the grocery shopping and cooking. Dietary teaching that does not include the family may not be as successful.

Nursing in the home involves a very different set of dynamics than that of care provided in the hospital. In the hospital, the health care team has the dominant role and the environment is controlled. In the home, the family and/or the patient play the dominant role, and the nurse is a visitor in the health care setting. Home health care is delivered within the context of the family's and the patient's cultural values and beliefs. In the home, the nurse is more likely to encounter the patient's use of healing practices arising from cultural beliefs and the use of home remedies and complementary and alternative therapies. The home care nurse must be knowledgeable about cultural practices and alternative therapies to guide the patient and family in their safe and effective use. (Culture is discussed in Chapter 2, and complementary and alternative therapies are discussed in Chapter 7.)

Patients seen by home health care nurses are most often discharged from hospital settings. However, they may also be referred directly from a physician's office or nursing care facilities, or the patient may request this service. Coverage for home health care varies depending on whether the patient is covered by Medicare, an HMO, or other types of insurance.[23] In general, to qualify for coverage, patients have to be confined to the home, known as "homebound status," and in need of professional skilled care such as nursing.[24] Depending on the needs of the patient, home health visits may be as frequent as twice daily or as infrequent as once a month. Visits may be extensive and require significant time, such as the initial visit, or they may be shorter in length, such as visits to check a healing wound. These visits may be characterized by a predetermined routine or treatment regimen, such as insulin administration and blood glucose monitoring or wound care and dressing changes.

Home Health Care Team

The home health care team includes many members, including the patient, family, nurses, physician, social worker, physical therapist, occupational therapist, speech therapist, home health aide, pharmacist, respiratory therapist, and dietitian. Nursing care is one of the primary services in the home setting (Fig. 6-4). Skilled nursing care in the home requires the knowledge, assessment, execution of clinical skills, and judgment to evaluate the process and outcome of care on the basis of nursing intervention.[25]

Physical conditions or diagnoses that may trigger a referral to a *physical therapist* include orthopedic conditions, such as hip or knee surgeries or neuromuscular deterioration commonly seen with multiple sclerosis, amyotrophic lateral sclerosis, and stroke. The physical therapist will work with patients on strengthening and endurance, gait training, transfer training, and developing a patient education program. *Occupational therapists* may assist the patient with fine motor coordination, performance of the activities of daily living, cognitive-perceptual skills, sensory testing, and the construction or use of assistive or adaptive equipment. *Speech therapists* focus on various speech pathologies for those who have suffered speech or swallowing disorders seen in patients with stroke, laryngectomy, or progressive neuromuscular diseases. The *social worker* assists patients with coping skills,

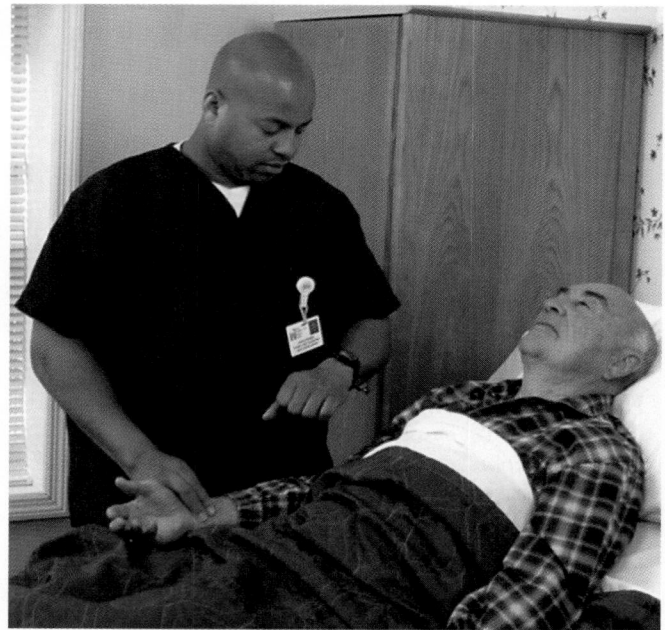

FIG. 6-4   Nursing care can be effectively provided in a home setting.

caregiver concerns, securing adequate financial resources or housing assistance, or making referrals to social service or volunteer agencies. *Home health aides* assist patients with their personal care needs, such as bathing, dressing, hair washing, or some homemaking activities, such as meal preparation or light housekeeping.

Other members of the home health care team may include *pharmacists*, who are involved in the preparation of infusion products; *respiratory therapists*, who may assist in oxygen therapy in the home; and *dietitians* for dietary consultation. The members of the home health care team work collaboratively with the home health care nurse to plan and evaluate the patient's progress on a regular basis with a significant emphasis placed on home education programs.

Home Health Nursing Roles

Home care nurses must have expert organizational skills, be able to make independent decisions, and know how to set priorities and respond to problems promptly.[26] They must adapt to a variety of circumstances that challenge their assessment, planning, and intervention abilities. For example, the nurse may need to modify the technique for dressing changes for a patient with limited manual dexterity and no running water in his or her home. Nurses who work in home care require additional skills in time and case management, communication, assessment and diagnosis, community resource identification, teaching, and discharge planning. Attributes of home health care nurses include flexibility, empathy, patient advocacy, and the ability to function independently in the home setting. Nurses need to balance administrative and agency demands and productivity standards with patient care needs.

Documentation is the key to continuing services in the patient's home. Reimbursement for nursing visits is retroactive based on documentation. Nurses must use concise and accurate documentation to ensure both legal and professional accountability. Documentation is the only way to substantiate recommendations about the patient's needs, the care provided, and the patient's response. These are all necessary to meet reimbursement criteria for the services rendered.[26]

The use of computerized patient records in home care is a growing trend. Some home care nurses document care as it is delivered using laptop computers. If computer patient records are fully integrated, the patient record can be retrieved by modem at many different sites simultaneously. The record is accessible to the nurse and others at the patient's home, home care office, physician's office, billing office, and hospital. In the patient's home the nurse can review the patient's history and plan of care and update the record as care is given. The accessibility of computerized records leads to better continuity of care and reduced documentation time. It also helps create a database for developing protocols for treating specific outcomes and the use of critical pathways.[27]

Another technologic innovation used in home health care and other community-based sites is televisiting, or telehealth. **Televisiting** allows the nurse to do triage and provide advice, counseling, and referral for a patient's health problem using the phone or computers with cameras.[8] The patient may be at home and the nurse at a different site, or the nurse may be in the patient's home and contact another member of the home health care team for consultation. The home health care nurse has a definite role in using advanced information technology in the delivery of care to the patient and family.

Home health care nurses must also be knowledgeable in the adaptive equipment or assistive devices used in the patient's home to promote independent functioning. Understanding rehabilitation terminology is helpful in collaborating with therapists and evaluating the patient's plan of care. Medical supplies provided through most home health care agencies include urinary catheters, wound care products, and IV therapy supplies.

Continuous quality improvement is a mandate for home health care agencies and nurses.[28] Infection control rates, readmissions to hospitals, and other facets of clinical care are monitored and evaluated with respect to quality care and patient outcomes. With the influx of managed care in home health care, nurses are expected to provide the maximum amount of quality care in a shorter period of time.

Federal regulations have been implemented to require patient outcome monitoring by home health care agencies with the use of the Outcome Assessment Information Set (OASIS). OASIS data are linked to how home health agencies receive reimbursement under the newly implemented Prospective Payment System (PPS), which was mandated by the Balanced Budget Act of 1997 and subsequent legislation.[29]

A holistic, nonjudgmental, and family-centered philosophy is essential for the nurse in the home. In addition to drawing on distinct knowledge, home care nursing also calls for a different process of decision making. Home care nurses focus on empowering the patient and family to meet their own needs so they can feel in control of their lives. Goals aim for long-term rather than short-term results. Decision making and priority setting become shared activities among the patient, family, and nurse.

Hospice

Hospice exists to provide support and care for persons in the last phases of incurable diseases so that they might live as fully and as comfortably as possible. Hospice is not a place but a concept of care that provides compassion, concern, and support for the dying.[30] Hospice care represents a return to previous times when dying individuals were helped to remain at home and to die at home, if possible, surrounded by familiar sights, sounds, and smells and by the love of those who care.

Many people choose to die at home in the comfort of their own home and surrounded by family and friends. Terminally ill patients may die in dignity at home without the heroic measures commonly seen in acute care settings. (Hospice and palliative care are discussed in Chapter 10.)

SUMMARY

Many changes are occurring in the health care delivery system. Patient care settings are becoming highly diversified. The evolving structure of health care is in flux, but it is becoming more focused on providing patient care in the community and home. The increasing number of home health care settings allows patients to receive technical nursing care, education, and support in the home environment.

Nursing is diversifying, adapting, and moving into a variety of patient care settings. As the nurses' roles expand, patients are expecting advanced clinical skills and complex health care within a variety of environments, including the community and home settings. Nurses are called on to maintain clinical proficiency and critical thinking skills and to become proficient in problem solving, teaching, management, and promoting wellness for patients in all settings along the continuum of patient care.

CRITICAL THINKING EXERCISES

Case Study
Home Health Care for Cardiac Patient

Patient Profile. José, 72 years old, is a Hispanic man who was discharged from the hospital 4 days after a myocardial infarction. He and his wife live in an apartment 5 miles from the hospital. His case manager at the hospital referred him to the home health care agency for follow-up care. Neither he nor his wife is able to drive. He is presently homebound because of weakness and shortness of breath. He is now unable to attend weekly church services because of his debilitated state and is depressed over his current condition.

Subjective Data
- Has history of hypertension
- Had heart attack 3 years ago
- Cannot walk one block without getting short of breath
- Has swollen feet and cannot wear shoes
- Had fractured hip that was surgically repaired 6 months ago

Continued

CRITICAL THINKING EXERCISES—cont'd

Collaborative Care
- O₂ at 3 L/min
- furosemide (Lasix) 40 mg bid
- captopril (Capoten) 50 mg bid
- 2 g sodium diet
- Assessment of home environment
- Patient education program

CRITICAL THINKING QUESTIONS

1. What are the initial priorities for the home health nurse?
2. What other members of the home health team should be involved in the care of José? What are their roles and responsibilities?

3. What type of patient education program should be implemented? What are the priority teaching goals?
4. What should the nurse consider in the nutrition assessment? How will the nurse address the cultural considerations related to his diet?
5. How can the nurse address José's coping skills and utilize community resources to intervene with his depression?
6. What types of medical equipment will José need? What teaching should accompany the use of this equipment?
7. José's wife inquires about an outpatient cardiac rehabilitation program. What would be an appropriate response from the home health nurse?
8. What are the long-term expected outcomes for José?

REVIEW QUESTIONS

The number of the question corresponds to the same-numbered objective at the beginning of the chapter.

1. Recent changes in the health care delivery system are most largely attributed to
   a. changing demographics and an aging society.
   b. more insurance payments for health care services.
   c. desires of patients to be in more restrictive settings.
   d. diagnosis-related groups (DRGs) and the influx of managed care.
2. In providing community-based patient care, nurses
   a. assess the needs of the community for illness prevention programs.
   b. determine how the health status of individuals and groups affect the community as a whole.
   c. provide coordinated and continuous care for ill patients and their families where they are in the community.
   d. deliver personal health services to individuals, families, and groups to promote and maintain the health of the community.

3. Patients may move among different care settings to
   a. maintain psychologic integrity.
   b. adhere to physician orders for treatment.
   c. maximize dependence on health care providers.
   d. ensure that physical, emotional, and psychosocial needs are met.
4. Nurses working in community-based and home care settings
   a. function autonomously in meeting patient needs.
   b. focus only on patient needs specific to the setting.
   c. use the same skills as in acute care or critical care settings.
   d. use case management skills along the continuum of care.

REFERENCES

1. Price CR, Capers ES: Associate degree nursing education: challenging premonitions with resourcefulness, *Nursing Forum* 30:26, 1995.
2. Williams CA: Community-oriented nursing and community-based nursing. In Stanhope M, Lancaster J, editors: *Foundations of community health nursing: community-oriented practice,* St Louis, 2002, Mosby.
3. Williams SJ: *Essential of health services,* ed 2, Australia, 2001, Delmar.
4. US Bureau of the Census. *Resident population of the United States: Middle series projections, 1996-2000, by age and sex. Current Population Reports, series P25-1130. Population projections of the United States by age, sex, race, and Hispanic origin: 1995 to 2050.* Available at *www.census.gov/population/projections/nation/nas/npas9600.txt* (accessed Nov 10, 2001).
5. National Center for Chronic Disease Prevention and Health Promotion: *Chronic diseases and their risk factors: the nation's leading causes of death, 1999,* Washington, DC, 2001, Centers for Disease Control and Prevention. Available at *www.cdc.gov/nccdphp/statbook/preface.htm* (accessed Nov 10, 2001).
6. Rossi P: *Case management in healthcare: a practical guide,* Philadelphia, 1999, WB Saunders.
7. American Nurses Association: *American Nurses Association nursing facts, 1994. Managed care: challenges and opportunities.* Available at *www.nursingworld.org/readroom* (accessed Nov 10, 2001).
8. Cary AH: Case management. In Stanhope M, Lancaster J, editors: *Foundations of community health nursing: community-oriented practice,* St Louis, 2002, Mosby.
9. Stanhope M, Lancaster J: *Community and public health nursing,* ed 5, St Louis, 2000, Mosby.
10. Biddix V, Brown H: Establishing a parish nursing program, *Nursing and Health Care Perspectives* 20:72, 1999.
11. Jones AM, Foster N: Transitional care: bridging the gap, *Medsurg Nurs* 6:32, 1997.
12. National Subacute Care Association: *FAQ: what is the definition of subacute care?* National Subacute Care Association, 2001. Available at *www.nsca.net/faq* (accessed Aug 8, 2001).
13. Ignatavicius DD: *Introduction to long-term care nursing: principles and practice,* Philadelphia, 1998, FA Davis.
14. American Health Care Association: *A consumer's guide to nursing facilities,* Washington, DC, 2000, American Health Care Association.
15. American Association of Homes and Services for the Aging: *Consumer information, 1998.* Available at *www.aahsa.org* (accessed Nov 10, 2001).
16. Kovach CR: *Late-stage dementia care,* Washington, DC, 1997, Taylor & Francis.
17. National Association for Home Care: *Basic statistics about home care 2000.* Available at *www.nahc.org* (accessed Nov 10, 2001).
18. American Nurses Association: *Scope and standards of home health nursing practice,* pub no 9905 HH, Washington, DC, 1999, American Nurses Association.
19. Schroeder MA, Long CO: Impact of home health care on clinical practice and education. In Chaska NL, editor: *The nursing profession, tomorrow and beyond,* Thousand Oaks, Calif, 2001, Sage Publications.

20. Balanced Budget Act of 1997 (PL 105-33): *HR3426—Medicare and Medicaid Health Insurance Act. US Statutes at Large,* vol III, pp 251-788, Washington, DC, Aug 1997, US Government Printing Office.

21. Long CO: Health care delivery services. In Neal L, Harris MD, editors: *Core curriculum for home health nursing. Section 1. Program management,* Washington, DC, 2001, Home Care University.

22. United States Department of Health and Human Services, Health Care Financing Administration: *A profile of Medicare home health chart book,* pub no HCFA-10138, 1999. Available at *www.hcfa.gov/stats/cbookhha.pdf* (accessed Nov 30, 2001).

23. Turner CH, Floyd LM: Reimbursement. In Neal L, Harris MD, editors: *Core curriculum for home health nursing. Section 1. Program management,* Washington, DC, 2001, Home Care University.

24. Stoker J: Defining homebound status, *Home Healthc Nurse* 17:119, 1999.

25. Long CO: Home health care nurse as case manager. In Neal L, Harris MD, editors: *Core curriculum for home health nursing. Section 1. Program management,* Washington, DC, 2001, Home Care University.

26. Monks KM: *Pocket guide to home healthcare,* Philadelphia, 2000, WB Saunders.

27. Oldham R, Meyer-Tulledge P: Psychiatric and home care documentation. In Iyer PW, Camp NH, editors: *Nursing documentation: a nursing process approach,* ed 3, St Louis, 1999, Mosby.

28. Macdonald BJ: Continuous quality improvement/quality assurance. In Neal L, Harris MD, editors: *Core curriculum for home health nursing. Section 1. Program management,* Washington, DC, 2001, Home Care University.

29. Health Care Financing Administration: Medicare program: prospective payment system and consolidated billing for skilled nursing facilities, *Federal Register* 63(91):26252-26316, 1998.

30. National Hospice and Palliative Care Organization: *Facts and figures on hospice care in America, 2001.* Available at *www.nhcpo.org* (accessed Nov 10, 2001).

RESOURCES

Accreditation Association for Ambulatory Health Care, Inc.
3201 Old Glenview Road, Suite 300
Wilmette, IL 60091-2992
847-853-6060
Fax: 847-853-9028
www.aaahc.org/

American Academy of Ambulatory Care Nursing
East Holly Avenue, Box 56
Pitman, NJ 08071-0056
856-256-2350
Fax: 856-589-7463
www.aaacn.inurse.com/

American Association of Homes and Services for the Aging
2519 Connecticut Avenue, NW
Washington, DC 20008-1520
202-783-2242
Fax: 202-783-2255
www.aahsa.org

American Association of Managed Care Nurses, Inc.
PO Box 4975
Glen Allen, VA 23058-4975
804-747-9698
Fax: 804-747-5316
www.aamcn.org/

American Association of Occupational Health Nurses, Inc.
2920 Brandywine Road, Suite 100
Atlanta, GA 30341
770-455-7757
Fax: 770-455-7271
www.aaohn.org/

American Long Term and Sub Acute Care Nurses Association
PO Box 1304
Toms River, NJ 08753
Fax: 732-573-0839
www.alsna.com

Association of Rehabilitation Nurses
4700 W. Lake Avenue
Glenview, IL 60025-1485
800-229-7530
847-375-4710
Fax: 877-734-9384
www.rehabnurse.org/

Canadian Gerontological Nurses Association
101-1001 West Broadway
Vancouver, BC
Canada V6H 4E4
www.cgna.net/

Canadian Home Care Association
17 York Street, Suite 40
Ottawa, Ontario
Canada K1N9J6
613-569-1585
Fax: 613-569-1604
www.cdnhomecare.on.ca/

Home Healthcare Nurses Association
228 Seventh Street, SE
Washington, DC 20003
202-546-4754
www.hhna.org

National Association for Home Care
228 Seventh Street SE
Washington, DC 20003
202-547-7424
Fax: 292-547-3540
www.nahc.org

National Gerontological Nursing Association
7794 Grow Drive
Pensacola, FL 32514
850-473-1174
800-723-0560
Fax: 850-484-8762
www.ngna.org/

For additional Internet resources, see the website for this book at *http://evolve.elsevier.com/Lewis/medsurg/.*

CHAPTER 7

Complementary and Alternative Therapies

D. Patricia Gray

LEARNING OBJECTIVES

1. Define complementary and alternative therapies.
2. Describe the National Center for Complementary and Alternative Medicine classification system for types of complementary and alternative therapies.
3. Discuss ways in which traditional Chinese medicine (TCM) differs from the practice of conventional medicine in North America.
4. Identify the types, principles, and effectiveness of mind-body interventions.

5. Discuss the general types of herbal therapy.
6. Describe the process of therapeutic touch.
7. Explain the scope of practice of chiropractic therapy.
8. Identify roles of the nurse regarding complementary and alternative therapies.
9. Describe a process for assessing patients' use of complementary and alternative therapies.

KEY TERMS

acupoints, p. 98	moxibustion, p. 98
acupressure, p. 96	Qi, p. 97
acupuncture, p. 98	Qigong, p. 96
bioelectromagnetics, p. 106	Reiki, p. 97
chiropractic therapy, p. 105	Tai Chi, p. 100
complementary and alternative therapies, p. 94	therapeutic touch, p. 106
	traditional Chinese medicine, p. 97
Feldenkrais method, p. 97	yin and yang, p. 97
homeopathy, p. 95	

The general health of North American people is steadily improving as evidenced by lower mortality rates and increased life expectancies. Biomedical and technologic advances have contributed to these improvements. However, conventional therapy has been less helpful in alleviating some chronic illnesses such as chronic back pain, fatigue, anxiety, arthritis, insomnia, and headaches. Additionally, conventional (allopathic, Western, mainstream) approaches to health care tend to be depersonalized and often fail to take into consideration all aspects of an individual, including body, mind, and spirit. Increasing access to global perspectives has resulted in greater exposure to healing philosophies from many cultures, suggesting many new ideas about health and healing to consumers and health care professionals.[1]

A variety of terms have been used to describe health-related approaches that are considered outside the mainstream of the dominant system of health care. The terms currently used in Western cultures to describe such approaches include *alternative, complementary, integrative, nontraditional, unconventional, holistic, natural,* and *unorthodox.* Currently, the most frequently used term to refer to such modalities and practices is *complementary and alternative therapies.* **Complementary and alter-**

native therapies are defined as a "broad domain of healing resources that encompasses all health system, modalities, and practices and their accompanying theories and beliefs, other than those intrinsic to the politically dominant health system of a particular society or culture in a given historical period."[2] The definition highlights that what might be considered "complementary and alternative" in one country or at one period of history might be considered "conventional" in another place or time. Notably, most of these therapies were developed outside the mainstream of conventional biomedical approaches and are generally available without medical authorization. Furthermore, many of these modalities are similar to autonomous nursing interventions such as touch, massage, stress management, and activities to facilitate coping.

People have increasingly sought alternatives to conventional approaches. In one survey 42% of Americans reported using at least one alternative therapy, and the total number of visits to alternative practitioners was also estimated to have increased. The most common therapies for which Americans visited an alternative practitioner included massage, chiropractic, hypnosis, biofeedback, and acupuncture.[3] The percentage of Canadians who saw an alternative therapy practitioner was estimated at 15%,[4] and 49% of Australians reported using alternative approaches.[5]

Complementary and alternative therapies are harmonious with many of the values of nursing. These include a view of humans as holistic beings, an emphasis on healing, recognition that the provider-patient relationship should be a partnership, and a focus on health promotion and illness prevention. Nursing's interest in complementary and alternative perspectives is reflected in the formation of specialty nursing groups. For example, in 1980 the American Holistic Nurses' Association was established to facilitate care for the "whole" patient and significant others through focusing on holistic principles of health, preventive education, and the integration of caring-healing modalities.[6]

Health care professionals have raised important questions about the effectiveness and safety of complementary and alternative approaches in the face of their increased use by consumers. In response to this need, the National Center for Complementary

Reviewed by Barbara Owens, RN, PhD(c), Doctoral student, School of Nursing, University of Texas Health Science Center, San Antonio, Tex.

and Alternative Medicine (NCCAM) as part of the National Institutes of Health (NIH) was established. The goals of NCCAM are to (1) conduct and support basic and applied research and research training on complementary and alternative approaches and (2) disseminate scientifically based information on complementary and alternative research, practice, and findings to health care providers and consumers (see the NCCAM website at *www.nccam.nih.gov*). In collaboration with NCCAM, the Cochrane Collaboration established a focus area on complementary and alternative approaches, providing a valuable source for synthesized evidence on this topic.[7]

NCCAM has proposed a classification system for complementary and alternative therapies that includes five major categories with various types of approaches under each category: (1) alternative medical systems, (2) mind-body interventions, (3) biologic-based therapies, (4) manipulative and body-based methods, and (5) energy therapies. Table 7-1 includes descriptions of major categories and selected approaches within each category. The list continually changes as practices proven safe and effective become accepted as "mainstream" health care practices. This chapter discusses complementary and alternative therapies using NCCAM's major categories.

TABLE 7-1	NCCAM Categories of Complementary and Alternative Therapies
CATEGORY AND EXAMPLES	**DESCRIPTION**

Alternative Medical Systems

	Complete theoretic and practice systems that have generally evolved or developed within a specific culture or within a specific, complex, and comprehensive theoretic framework.
Ayurveda	Developed in India, this is one of the world's oldest and most complete medical systems. Focus is on the balance of mind, body, and spirit. Disease is viewed as an imbalance between a person's life force (*prana*) and basic metabolic condition (*dosha*). Interventions used include diet, medicinal herbs, detoxification, breathing exercises, meditation, and yoga (Fig. 7-1).
Traditional Chinese medicine (TCM)	One of the world's oldest and most complete medical systems. TCM focuses comprehensively on restoring and maintaining the balanced flow of vital energy (Qi). Interventions used include acupressure, acupuncture, Chinese herbology, diet, meditation, Tai Chi, and Qigong.
Homeopathy	Developed in the 1700s by a German physician, Samuel Hannemann, homeopathy uses two main principles, "like cures like" and "healing occurs from the inside out." Following diagnosis, specific homeopathic remedies are prescribed. These consist of very small doses of specially prepared plant and mineral extracts and assist in the body's innate healing processes. Specific conditions for which homeopathy has been shown effective include asthma, rheumatoid arthritis, migraine, diarrhea, fibromyalgia, and allergic rhinitis.
Naturopathy	Developed in the United States, naturopathy emphasizes the restoration and maintenance of overall health rather than symptom management. Focus is on enhancing the body's natural healing responses using a variety of individualized interventions such as clinical nutrition, herbology, hydrotherapy, homeopathy, acupuncture, physical therapies, and counseling and psychotherapy. Naturopathic medicine has been effective in treating ear infections, female reproductive problems, infectious diseases, and respiratory conditions.
Environmental medicine	Dedicated to the diagnosis, treatment, and prevention of environmentally triggered illnesses. Substances in the environment and diet are viewed as potential stressors with the ability to destabilize the overall homeodynamic functioning of the body, thus leading to disease. The emphasis is on preventing the harmful effects of environmental toxins, including chemicals, air and water pollution, radiation, and communicable diseases. Interventions include patient teaching, therapeutic customized diets, detoxification, immunotherapy, counseling, and environmental protocols designed to reduce exposure to toxins.

Mind-Body Interventions

	Based on the belief that thoughts, attitudes, beliefs, and emotions affect physical functioning. Interventions are generally designed to enhance control of physical functions through mental processes and to manage thinking processes so that negative beliefs are replaced with positive attitudes.
	Many mind-body interventions are considered "mainstream" based on their well-established record of effectiveness and their inclusion in traditional medical training programs. These include biofeedback, hypnosis, relaxation therapy, patient education approaches, and cognitive-behavioral approaches.

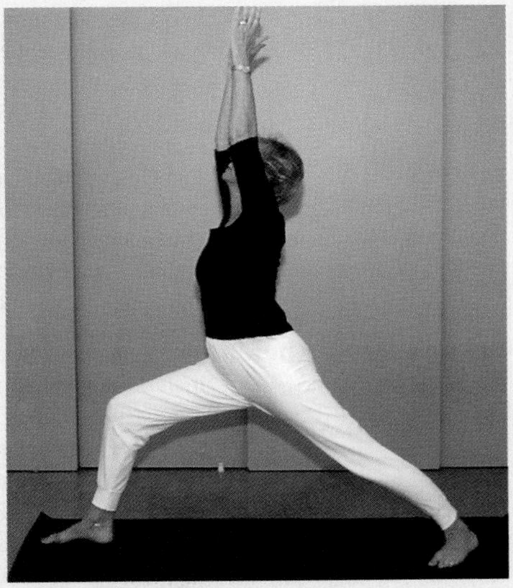

FIG. 7-1 Yoga.

Continued

TABLE 7-1	NCCAM Categories of Complementary and Alternative Therapies—cont'd
CATEGORY AND EXAMPLES	**DESCRIPTION**

Mind-Body Interventions—cont'd

Meditation (Fig. 7-2)	Self-directed practice for focusing, centering, and relaxing the mind and body. Frequently used for stress management and health promotion. Shown to reduce heart rate, respiratory rate, and blood pressure; decrease muscle tension and chronic pain, improve memory, and improve immune response; and enhance a peaceful state of mind.
Music therapy	Refers to the listening of music for therapeutic purposes (e.g., reducing stress or pain). Patient preferences about the type of music affect the effectiveness of the intervention (see box on p. 382).
Qigong	Similar to Tai Chi (see p. 100), Qigong is an ancient system of exercise focusing on breathing, visualization, and movement. Focuses on creating balance and enhancing self-regulation in the body. Whereas Tai Chi places emphasis on physical movement, Qigong focuses on developing skills in the appreciation and manipulation of internal energetic movement. Many systems and traditions of Qigong exist, ranging from simple calisthenics to complex autoregulatory exercises.
Art therapy	Involves creative expression through a variety of artistic mediums to facilitate expression of emotions, memories, and conscious and unconscious concerns and issues. The overall goal is to promote recovery or healing from past distress or trauma.
Prayer and mental healing	Includes a variety of intercessory approaches, often used at a distance from the person toward whom the intervention is directed, incorporating the use of compassion, caring, love, or empathy.

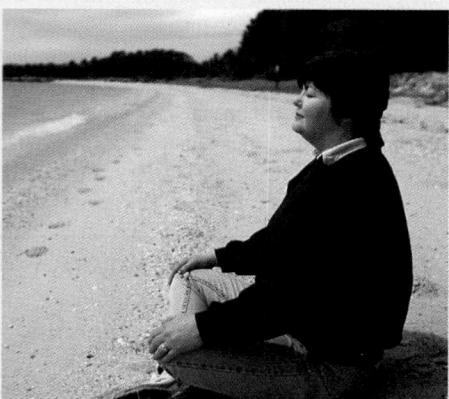

FIG. 7-2 Meditation can be used to relax the body and calm the mind.

Biologic-Based Therapies

	Include natural and biologic-derived products, interventions, and practices.
Aromatherapy	Involves the use of plant extracts known as essential oils to promote and maintain overall health. Oils may be applied topically or may be used in inhalation therapies. In general, these therapies are nontoxic. They should not be taken internally without proper medical supervision.
Herbal therapies	Examples of herbal medicines that have been well studied in the West include ginkgo biloba, echinacea, milk thistle, phytoestrogens, and saw palmetto. *Chinese herbal* remedies are derived from over 50,000 medicinal plant species and have been used for thousands of years. Most are of plant origin and a few are derived from mineral or animal sources. Examples include panax ginseng, fresh ginger, and Chinese foxglove root. *Ayurvedic herbs* have also been used extensively over the past 2000 years. They are categorized according to their metabolic effects (dosha). Examples include eclipta alba, commophora mukul, and picrorhiza kurroa.
Macrobiotic diet	Used within an overall approach to living focused on achieving harmonious and healthy interactions among an individual and his or her diet, lifestyle, and living environment. Dietary modifications are individualized based on geographic location, but generally include a diet high in whole cereal grains (50% by weight), vegetables (20%-30%), beans and sea vegetables (5%-10%), and vegetarian soups (5%-10%). Fish and seafood are recommended for occasional use. Foods that are eliminated include meat, animal fat, eggs, poultry, dairy products, simple sugars, and all artificially produced foods.
Orthomolecular therapy	Based on the premise that each individual has unique needs for various nutrients based in part on environmental pollution and food adulteration. The focus is on achieving nutritional balance and may involve administration of substances such as vitamins, essential amino acids, essential fats, and minerals, often in excess of generally recommended amounts.

Manipulative and Body-Based Methods

	Include interventions that involve manipulation or movement of the body by a therapist.
Acupressure	Pressure point technique involving the use of applied finger and hand pressure on specific areas of the body (usually acupoints defined by charts of energy meridians) to improve energy flow, relieve pain, and stimulate the body's innate healing abilities. Other pressure point techniques include shiatsu, reflexology, myotherapy, and jin shin do.

TABLE 7-1	NCCAM Categories of Complementary and Alternative Therapies—cont'd
CATEGORY AND EXAMPLES	**DESCRIPTION**

Manipulative and Body-Based Methods

Alexander technique	Type of movement reeducation therapy. Focuses first on developing awareness of unhealthy movement patterns, with a particular emphasis on alignment of the head, neck, and spine, and then on relearning basic movements such as walking, sitting, and getting up from a chair. The intended goal is to achieve a more balanced, graceful, coordinated, and relaxed style of moving. Other types of movement reeducation techniques include educational kinesiology, the **Feldenkrais method**, and the Trager approach.
Chiropractic therapy	Designed to restore and maintain health by properly aligning the spine using a variety of adjustment and manipulation techniques. Correct spinal alignment reduces interference from the nervous system and facilitates self-healing and improved health and well-being.
Rolfing (structural integration)	Type of structural bodywork based on the assumption that the fascia of the body has become thickened or tightened as a result of chronic stress, injury, or emotional trauma. Involves a set of prescribed sessions in which the therapist manipulates and realigns the fascia through a systematic process of deep tissue work. The goal is to improve freedom of movement and alignment of the head, neck, shoulders, thorax, pelvis, and legs.
Therapeutic massage (Fig. 7-3)	Process of soft tissue manipulation designed to reduce pain and stress and promote relaxation. It involves use of stroking, kneading, and friction techniques.

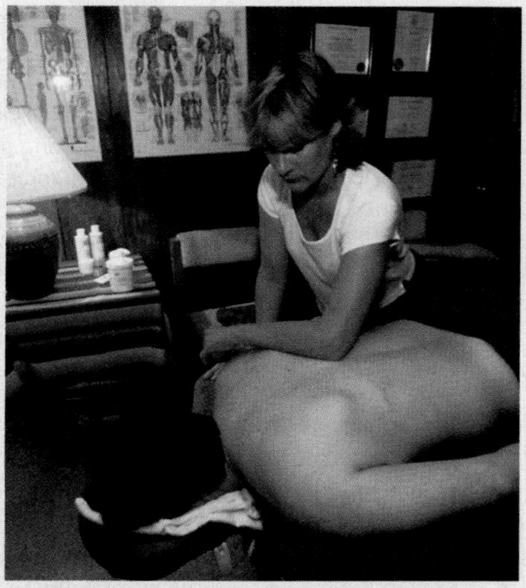

FIG. 7-3 Massage therapy can be effectively used to relieve tension.

Energy Therapies

	Energy therapies include those that focus on energy originating within the body (biofields) or on energy from other sources (electromagnetic fields). Biofield therapies assume the existence of energy that surrounds and permeates a person. Therapies are designed to manipulate and balance such fields to stimulate the body's innate healing abilities and to balance energetic flow. Bioelectromagnetic therapies involve the use of electromagnetic fields to treat a variety of problems, including pain, migraine headaches, asthma, and cancer.
Therapeutic touch	A biofield therapy, therapeutic touch involves the use of the hands to direct or modulate human energy fields. Outcomes include an improved sense of well-being and reduced sense of stress and discomfort. Other types of biofield therapies include healing touch, quantum touch, **Reiki**, and pranic healing.
Magnetic therapy	External application of magnets and magnetic energy in a variety of configurations, magnetic therapy is designed to improve blood flow and reduce pain.

ALTERNATIVE MEDICAL SYSTEMS

Alternative medical systems involve complete methods of health-related theory and practice that have been developed outside of the Western biomedical model. Many are traditional systems that are practiced by individual cultures throughout the world. Traditional Chinese medicine and acupuncture are one of the subcategories that NCCAM has identified (see Table 7-1).

Traditional Chinese Medicine

Traditional Chinese medicine (TCM) is one of the world's oldest and most comprehensive medical systems. Over the past several thousand years, it has evolved based on cultural and philosophic developments, as well as extensive clinical observation and testing. Several major concepts constitute Chinese medicine. The principle of **yin and yang** (Fig. 7-4) is a core tenet of Chinese art, philosophy, and science, as well as TCM. Yin and yang are viewed as dynamic, interacting, and interdependent energies, neither of which can exist without the other, each containing some part of the other within it. These energies are a part of everything in nature and must be maintained in a harmonious state of balance to achieve optimal health. Various states are associated with yin (cold, heavy, moist, negative) and yang (hot, dry, light, positive) energies. Imbalance is associated with illness. Causes of imbalance include situations such as excessive wetness, dryness, cold, heat, and emotional states, and other factors, such as dietary irregularities, imbalanced living habits, hereditary conditions, and social forces. In the case of imbalance, yang treatments are used to restore balance to excessive or deficient yin conditions and vice versa.[8]

Practitioners of TCM view human beings in terms of five inseparable dimensions. These include **Qi** (energy or the primal life force resulting from the interaction of yin and yang), *Jing* (genetic material of the physical body), *Shen* (spirit or all aspects of the mind, including mental, emotional, spiritual, and creative ac-

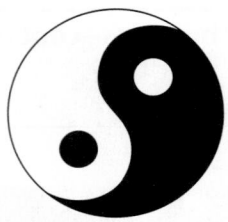

FIG. 7-4 Yin–yang symbol. The circle representing the whole is divided into yin (black) and yang (white). The small circles of opposite shading illustrate that within the yin there is yang and within the yang there is yin. The dynamic curve dividing them indicates that yin and yang are continuously merging. Thus yin and yang create each other, control each other, and transform into each other. When yin and yang are in balance, Qi (pronounced "chee"), or the fundamental life force, flows evenly through the body, leading to good health.

tivity), blood (considered the physical manifestation of Qi), and *Jin Ye* fluids (responsible for lubricating and moistening the organs). In addition, the Five Element Theory addresses various cyclic transformations that occur in nature. The five elements (wood, fire, earth, metal, water) correspond to the five energetic organ networks (liver/gallbladder, heart/small intestine, spleen/stomach, lung/large intestines, kidney/urinary bladder). These networks include not only physical but also psychologic and spiritual functions. Additionally, the body is believed to contain a series of energetic pathways, known as the *meridian systems,* through which Qi and other life energies flow, nourishing the body. TCM recognizes 12 major meridian pathways. Specific sites along the pathways, referred to as **acupoints,** allow access to the meridian system. There are several hundred acupoints, each corresponding to particular organs and their functions.[8]

Treatment modalities used in TCM include acupuncture, Chinese herbal medicines, diet, physical therapy, exercise (Tai Chi or Qigong), and meditation. The most well known of these in the Western hemisphere is acupuncture. In **acupuncture,** Qi is accessed and modified by stimulating specific acupoints (Fig. 7-5). Small (30- to 36-gauge) needles are used and, once inserted in a painless process, are left in place for 20 to 40 minutes. A process known as **moxibustion** may be used to warm the needles after they are inserted, thus increasing Qi and blood flow. Electrical stimulation may also be used and is helpful for persistent pain and numbness.[8] Findings from research conducted from the perspective of Western biomedicine indicate that acupuncture can cause multiple biologic responses.

These include the release of endorphins, activation of the hypothalamus and pituitary gland, alterations in immune function, and alterations in the levels of neurotransmitters and neurohormones.[9]

Clinical Applications of Acupuncture. Acupuncture is the primary treatment modality used by physicians of Chinese medicine. Acupuncture is the most common complementary therapy recommended by U.S. physicians and the second most commonly covered benefit by health insurance in the United States. Many allopathic physicians and health care professionals are also being trained and certified in acupuncture. However, in the United States, MDs may perform acupuncture without any formal training.

The World Health Organization (WHO) lists over 40 disorders that may benefit from acupuncture[10] (Table 7-2). An NIH Consensus Panel concluded that although additional research is needed, clinical studies have indicated that acupuncture is clearly effective in treating adult postoperative and chemotherapy-associated nausea and vomiting, as well as postoperative dental pain. Other conditions for which acupuncture may be useful include addiction, stroke rehabilitation, menstrual cramps, fibromyalgia, and myofascial pain.[9] Reports of two different meta-analyses reached different conclusions about the effectiveness of acupuncture for low back pain. One indicated that acupuncture was superior to control interventions,[11] and the other stated that there was no convincing evidence that it was effective in managing acute or chronic low back pain.[12]

Patients should insist on sterile disposable needles and should check to ensure that an MD acupuncturist is a qualified acupuncturist *(www.medicalacupuncture.org)* or verify that a non-MD acupuncturist has received training and has passed the

TABLE 7-2	Conditions That May Benefit from Acupuncture
Neurologic Disorders	
Meniere's disease	
Migraine headaches	
Peripheral neuropathy	
Trigeminal neuralgia	
Gastrointestinal Disorders	
Colitis	
Constipation	
Diarrhea	
Gastritis	
Hiccups	
Ulcers	
Respiratory Conditions	
Asthma	
Bronchitis	
Rhinitis	
Sinusitis	
Eye Disorders	
Central retinitis	
Conjunctivitis	
Myopia	
Musculoskeletal Disorders	
Carpal tunnel syndrome	
Osteoarthritis	
Sciatica	
Tennis elbow	

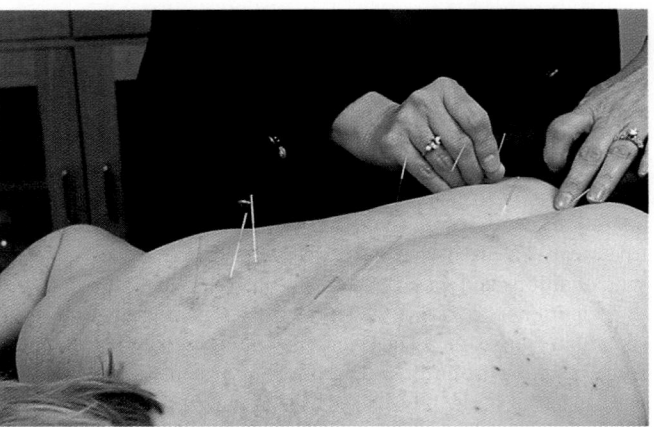

FIG. 7-5 Acupuncture.

National Commission of the Certification of Acupuncture (NCCA) examination.

Limitations of Acupuncture. Acupuncture is considered a safe therapy when (1) the practitioner has been appropriately trained and (2) the practitioner uses sterilized or disposable needles. Although complications have been noted, they are rare if appropriate steps are taken to ensure the safety of equipment and the patient. Acupuncture should be used with caution in those who have a history of seizures; are carriers of hepatitis B or have chronic hepatitis C; or have human immunodeficiency viral infection, bleeding disorders, thrombocytopenia, or skin infections.[13]

MIND-BODY INTERVENTIONS

Mind-body interventions include a variety of techniques designed to facilitate the mind's capacity to affect bodily function. These include behavioral, psychologic, social, and spiritual approaches to health. Specific examples of therapies and approaches are included in Table 7-1. It should be noted that behavioral approaches such as psychotherapy, certain uses of hypnosis, biofeedback, patient education, and support groups are considered by NCCAM as "mainstream" within the category of mind-body methods. Nurses frequently use many of these biobehavioral approaches (Table 7-3).

TABLE 7-3	Mind-Body Interventions That Can Be Used by Nurses

Meditation (see Fig. 7-2)
- Variety of techniques designed to create a sustained period of time in which one focuses attention and increases self-awareness.
- May include passive meditation (sitting meditation) or more active forms of meditation (walking meditation).
- Health benefits include increased oxygen uptake; reduction in blood pressure, heart rate, muscle tension; and enhanced pain tolerance and immune response.
- No known adverse effects.
- Once learned (and it can be self-taught) it is an appropriate self-care technique.

Relaxation
- Variety of relaxation techniques can be used to create a state of physical and mental calmness, peacefulness, and well-being, or the "relaxation response."
- Assists people in increasing self-awareness of their stress level and its physical manifestations.
- Most relaxation techniques focus on some aspect of the physical body (e.g., breathing, muscle tension).
- Used to reduce blood pressure and to decrease heart, respiratory, and metabolic rates, as well as in the treatment of pain, anxiety, depression, and other conditions related to stress.
- No known adverse effects.
- Once learned (and it can be self-taught), relaxation is appropriately practiced as a part of self-care.

Imagery
- Process of using mental images to create a desired state.
- Desired states may include relaxation, enhanced sports performance, pain relief, or immune modulation.
- Should be individualized, using an individual's dominant sensory mode (e.g., visual, auditory, kinesthetic) and avoiding images that are individually distressing.
- Once learned (and it can be self-taught), the use of imagery is well suited as a self-care technique.

Biofeedback (Fig. 7-6)
- Biofeedback training involves the use of various monitoring devices that help people become more aware of and able to control their own physiologic responses such as heart rate, body temperature, muscle tension, and brain waves.
- During biofeedback training, people use information (e.g., electroencephalogram, electrocardiogram, electromyogram, galvanic skin response, skin temperature) to recognize normal or desirable physiologic states and then use techniques such as imagery or relaxation training to achieve those states.
- Desirable states include normal heart rate, slow deep breathing, warm skin, and decreased galvanic skin response.
- Biofeedback training requires specialized training for both practitioners and patients. After such training, patients can appropriately use the techniques as part of self-care.
- After the individual is able to achieve the desired states, biofeedback is no longer needed.

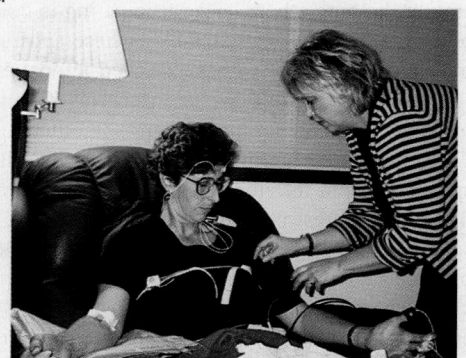

FIG. 7-6 Biofeedback monitoring. Electrodes are placed on the frontalis and trapezius muscles, as well as the fingers on the left hand. Pneumograph measurements are also made.

Psychotherapy
- Most popular forms include classical or Freudian, Jungian, cognitive/behavioral, humanistic/existential, solution-focused, and family.
- Emphasis is generally on an exploration of psychologic issues, although each of these approaches has its own unique approaches and outcomes.
- Has been shown to be effective in addressing a variety of mental and emotional problems and may also contribute to positive physical changes.
- Use of psychotherapy requires advanced specialized training, supervision by mentors, and, in most U.S. states, licensure to practice.

Tai Chi

Tai Chi is an ancient system of exercise that incorporates slow and graceful movement integrated with focused breathing and visualization to stimulate the flow of Qi (energy) throughout the body. The improved flow of Qi leads to increased self-awareness, vitality, oxygenation of the blood, resistance to disease, and improved sleep. Tai Chi developed within the context of traditional Chinese medicine and reflects its concern with the regulation of balance within the mind, body, and spirit. Tai Chi consists of a sequence of standardized movements, each known as a "form." When properly performed, the movements are precise and synchronized with breathing. The movements are low impact and low velocity. After the basic forms are learned, Tai Chi can be practiced in any location without special clothing or equipment.[8]

Clinical Applications of Tai Chi. Tai Chi is a gentle movement process. It is recommended for the reduction of muscular stress and tension, promotion of relaxation, increase in flexibility, improvement of posture, and overall health enhancement. Tai Chi appears to be effective in reducing pain and functional disability in persons with fibromyalgia.[14] Use of Tai Chi has been shown to increase balance, decrease falls,[15,16] and reduce fears of falling,[17] as well as increase the flexibility and sense of well-being in older adults.[18] When comparing a group of elderly Tai Chi practitioners to sedentary controls, the Tai Chi group had higher oxygen uptake, lower body fat, and better spine flexibility.[19,20]

Limitations of Tai Chi. There are few if any limitations to the use of Tai Chi. No adverse consequences have been reported. Future research should consider the psychologic, emotional, and spiritual benefits of the practice of Tai Chi.

Spirituality

Spirituality includes prayer and other unifying practices that (1) help people have a connection with something beyond themselves, (2) help give a sense of purpose and meaning to life, and (3) facilitate personal transcendence beyond the present context of reality.[21] Prayer is an intervention that is widely used to promote health and alleviate illness. *Intercessory* prayer is an organized and regular form of prayer in which someone communicates with his or her higher power on behalf of another who is in need.

Other spiritual practices include meditation, appreciating nature, connecting with friends and family, reading inspirational literature, helping others, and participating in community religious practices in places of worship.[22] These spiritual practices common in North America have derived almost exclusively from a Judeo-Christian tradition[23] and may fail to consider perspectives on spirituality inherent in Islam[24] or other religious traditions. There are long-standing debates about the relationship between spirituality and religion. Religion can be viewed as one but not the only way that people can access, develop, and practice their spirituality. The benefits associated with a developed spiritual practice include an improved sense of well-being and lower levels of depression.[25] During times of illness, effective spiritual coping strategies may help an individual find meaning in the illness and lead to increased coping abilities and decreased emotional distress.

Clinical Applications of Spirituality. Frequently used nursing interventions to address spirituality include referral to ministers or chaplains, prayer, active listening, facilitating and validating of patients' thoughts and feelings, conveying acceptance, and instilling hope.[26] Several randomized clinical trials have been conducted to evaluate the effectiveness of intercessory prayer for a variety of illnesses. A meta-analysis of these clinical trials concluded that although there were positive effects in some studies, overall the data were inconclusive to make definitive statements about the effectiveness of intercessory prayer.[27] However, additional research is needed to further clarify the relationships between intercessory prayer and health outcomes.

Nurses must assess patients' usual spiritual coping strategies and develop a plan to support and augment those strategies as needed. Nurses should also expect to work in collaboration with others, particularly ministers, pastors, and chaplains, to meet the complex spiritual needs of all patients. Nurses who are specifically interested in a practice focused on spiritual interventions can explore parish nursing, a specialty that emphasizes the relationship between spirituality and health.[28]

Limitations of Spirituality. No adverse effects have been documented because of spiritual interventions. A potential problem may occur when the nurse and the patient have differing views of spirituality. For example, the nurse needs to examine carefully the ethics of praying for a patient who has indicated no interest in spiritual interventions. If a patient asks for assistance with a particular spiritual intervention inconsistent with the nurse's beliefs, assistance from another nurse or a chaplain may be needed.

BIOLOGIC-BASED THERAPIES

Biologic-based therapies include herbal therapies (phytotherapy), special diet therapies, and orthomolecular medicine (see Table 7-1).

Herbal Therapies

Herbal therapies use individual herbs or mixtures of herbs for therapeutic value (Fig. 7-7). An herb is a plant or plant part (bark, roots, leaves, seeds, flowers, fruit) that produces and contains chemical substances that act on the body. It is esti-

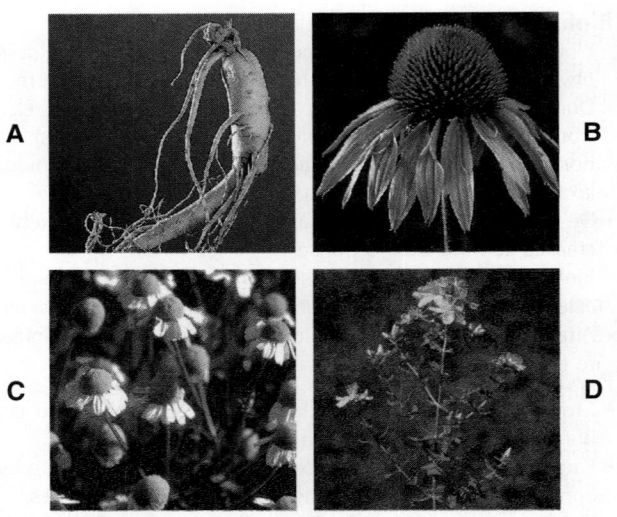

FIG. 7-7 Herbs. **A,** Ginseng. **B,** Echinacea. **C,** Chamomile. **D,** St. John's wort.

mated that approximately 25,000 plant species are used medicinally throughout the world and approximately 30% of modern prescription drugs are derived from plants. Botanical medicine is the oldest known form of medicine; archaeologic evidence suggests that Neanderthals used plant-based remedies 60,000 years ago. Use of herbal therapy gained widespread popularity in many countries as early as 3000 BC but began to decline with the development of modern scientific medicine in the early eighteenth century. However, approximately 80% of the world's population currently relies extensively on plant-derived remedies.

Over the past 30 years, a resurgence of interest in herbal therapies has occurred in countries whose health care is dominated by conventional medicine. Interest in herbal products is related to several factors, including the high cost and the potential for severe side effects associated with pharmaceutical drugs. Herbal remedies are considered "natural" and therefore may be viewed as healthier and safer. They are available directly to consumers and appeal to people who desire personal control and autonomy over their health, as well as to people who have limited access to conventional health care.[29]

Over 30% of Americans use herbal remedies, with the highest use among the well educated, the affluent, and women. Commonly used herbs in the United States include echinacea, garlic, goldenseal, saw palmetto, aloe, Ma Huang, cranberry, ginseng, St. John's wort, valerian, and feverfew.[30,31]

Regulating agencies in Germany, France, the United Kingdom, and Canada enforce standards of quality and safety assessments on manufacturers. In contrast, in the United States herbal products for their medicinal value are classified as dietary supplements. As such, they lie outside the jurisdiction of many of the safety and regulatory rules covering foods and drugs. *Dietary supplements* are defined by the U.S. Dietary Supplement Health and Education Act of 1994 to include vitamins, minerals, herbs, botanicals, amino acids, and any other dietary substances used to supplement the diet. This law specifically states that dietary supplements can be marketed without proven safety or efficacy and set no standards for quality control.

The practice of phytotherapy is regulated in many parts of the world. For example, in France all phytotherapists are also credentialed physicians, and in Germany 70% of all general medical practitioners prescribe herbal remedies to their patients. Prescribed herbals are covered under insurance programs. The governments of China and Japan officially support herbal therapies within their national health care system. However, in the United States information about herbal remedies is most often obtained at health food stores; through informal word of mouth; and from books, magazines, and the Internet.

Clinical Applications of Herbal Therapy. Medicinal plants work in much the same way as drugs; both are absorbed and trigger biologic effects that can be therapeutic. Many have more than one physiologic effect and thus have more than one condition for which they can be used. The range of action of herbs is extensive. A number of Internet resources provide information on herbal therapies (see Resources at end of chapter), providing information to health care providers and consumers. Internet sites that provide information should be evaluated carefully. Information used in evaluation should include the sponsoring organization and its credibility, the frequency of updates, the

COMPLEMENTARY & ALTERNATIVE THERAPIES

Information related to various complementary and alternative therapies can be found in the following boxes throughout the book.

Title	Chapter	Page
Acupuncture	62	1703
Bilberry	21	449
Biofeedback	44	1197
Echinacea	26	571
Garlic	33	809
Ginger	40	1005
Ginkgo biloba	58	1591
Ginseng	8	123
Glucosamine	63	1718
Goldenseal	26	572
Guided imagery	50	1377
Herbs and supplements that affect blood clotting	37	934
Herbs and supplements that affect blood glucose levels	47	1290
Herbs and supplements used for menopause	52	1412
Herbs and surgical patients	17	364
Herbs that affect healing	12	218
Kava	8	125
Lipid-lowering agents	33	809
Milk thistle	42	1145
Music therapy	18	382
St. John's wort	8	124
Saw palmetto	53	1438
Valerian	52	1412
Yoga	8	124
Zinc	26	573

types of supporting evidence that are included, and whether advertising for specific products is used.

A number of herbs have been determined to be safe and effective for a variety of conditions. These herbs, as well as the most frequently used herbal remedies, are included in Table 7-4. Herb boxes related to specific diseases are found throughout the book (see the box above).

Limitations of Herbal Therapy. Although herbal therapies have been shown to provide beneficial effects for a variety of conditions, side effects and interactions with prescription drugs have been described. There is concern that side effects resulting from the use of herbal remedies are underreported, thus promoting the impression that herbal remedies are completely safe to use. Because people tend not to share their use of herbal remedies and dietary supplements with their primary care provider, herb-drug interactions may also be underreported. For example, patients who are scheduled for surgery should be advised to stop taking herbal remedies 2 to 3 weeks before surgery.[32] Herbal products that interfere with surgical procedures are discussed in the box in Chapter 17. Patients who are being treated with conventional drug therapy should be advised to discontinue herbal remedies with similar pharmacologic effects, because the combination may lead to

TABLE 7-4	Commonly Used Herbs and Supplements*		
NAME	**EFFECTS**	**EXAMPLES OF COMMON USES**	**COMMENTS**
Aloe	• Antiinflammatory • Antimicrobial • Acceleration of wound healing • Alkalinization of gastric juices	• Minor burns • Wound healing • GI disorders (e.g., ulcers, nausea, constipation) • Menstrual cramps • Premenstrual syndrome	Internal use produces cathartic action. Not to be used on deep, vertical surgical wounds.
Angelica†	• Antispasmodic • Vasodilation • Balancing effects of estrogen • Mild sedative effect	• Menstrual irregularities • Hot flashes • Vaginal dryness • Abdominal cramps	Inhibits platelet aggregation. Prolongs bleeding time. May cause skin rashes and photosensitivity. Some of herb's components increase the risk for cancer.
Bilberry†	• Improvement of microcirculation in eyes • Mild antiinflammatory	• Myopia • Retinal problems • Inflammation of mouth and pharynx • GI disorders (e.g., diarrhea, ulcers, hemorrhoids) • Varicose veins	Has antiplatelet activity.
Black cohosh	• Estrogen-like effects	• Menopause • Menstrual cramps • Diarrhea	Large amounts can cause toxicity.
Cat's claw	• Stimulant of immune system • Antioxidant • Antiinflammatory • Lowering of blood pressure	• Cancer • GI disorders • Hypertension • Viral infections • Arthritis	Should not be used concurrently with immunosuppressants. Individuals with an autoimmune disease should not use.
Chamomile†	• Antiinflammatory • Antispasmodic • Antiinfective • Mild sedative effect	• Inflammatory diseases of GI and upper respiratory tracts • Inflammation of skin and mucous membranes • Topical use for wounds, rashes, and ulcers • Motion sickness • GI spasms • Restlessness, insomnia	Should not be used by people allergic to ragweed or individuals with allergic rhinitis or asthma. May affect coagulation.
Dehydroepiandrosterone (DHEA)	• Most abundant hormone produced by adrenal glands • Easily converted to potent androgens (e.g., testosterone) and estrogen	• Slow effects of aging • Erectile dysfunction • Memory improvement • Depression • Osteoporosis • Atherosclerosis	Little is known about safety of long-term DHEA use. Should not be used in people with benign prostatic hyperplasia, prostate cancer, breast or uterine cancer.
Echinacea	• Stimulant of immune system • Antibacterial • Antiinflammatory	• Upper respiratory and urinary tract infections • Allergic rhinitis • Wound healing	Should not be taken for more than 8 weeks. Therapy for 10-14 days is probably long enough. Patients with HIV, MS, or autoimmune diseases should not use. Should not use with corticosteroids. May be used in conjunction with antibiotics.

ACTH, Adrenocorticotropic hormone; *GI,* gastrointestinal; *HIV,* human immunodeficiency virus; *MS,* multiple sclerosis.

*Health care provider should be consulted before taking any herb or supplement.

†These herbs and supplements interfere with blood clotting in various ways. They should be used with caution or not at all in patients with bleeding or clotting disorders or those taking anticoagulant and antiplatelet aggregating drugs (e.g., warfarin [Coumadin], heparin, aspirin, ticlopidine [Ticlid], clopidogrel [Plavix]).

TABLE 7-4	Commonly Used Herbs and Supplements—cont'd		
NAME	**EFFECTS**	**EXAMPLES OF COMMON USES**	**COMMENTS**
Evening primrose[†]	• May have therapeutic effect on body's metabolism of fatty acid	• Premenstrual syndrome • Wound healing • Breast pain • Eczema	May cause immunosuppression. Promotes anticoagulation. Should not be used in individuals with seizure disorders.
Feverfew[†]	• Antiinflammatory • Inhibition of serotonin, prostaglandins, and histamine	• Migraine headaches • Arthritis • Fever	Inhibits platelet aggregation
Garlic[†]	• Antioxidant • Lowering of lipids • Inhibition of platelet aggregation • Antibacterial/antimycotic	• Elevated cholesterol levels • Atherosclerosis • Hypertension • Upper respiratory tract infection	Inhibits platelet aggregation. May cause mild increase in serum insulin levels so it should not be used with hypoglycemic agents without consulting health care provider.
Ginger[†]	• Antiemetic • Antiinflammatory	• Nausea and vomiting • Motion sickness	Interferes with coagulation.
Ginkgo biloba[†]	• Memory improvement • Increased blood flow to brain • Antioxidant • Increased metabolism efficiency	• Alzheimer's disease • Dementia • Depression • Asthma • Retinal disease • Heart disease • Peripheral arterial occlusive disease • Varicose veins • Premenstrual syndrome • Tinnitus	Takes 1-3 months for full therapeutic effect. Inhibits platelet aggregation. Possible drug interactions with anticoagulants. Used cautiously in people with risk for bleeding.
Ginseng[†] (Asian [panax] ginseng, Siberian ginseng)	• Increased physical endurance and stamina • Adaptogen: "balancing" of body • Stimulates pituitary secretion of ACTH and thus increases serum cortisol • Increased ability to cope with stress • Improved concentration and memory	• Fatigue • Stress • Mild depression • Decreased libido	Most famous Chinese herb. May decrease blood glucose levels. Inhibits platelet aggregation. May cause elevated blood pressure. Should not be used for more than 3 continuous months without 1-2 weeks between courses.
Glucosamine	• Amino acid that has a role in synthesis of cartilage	• Arthritis • Joint injury	Should be used cautiously in people with hypertension or cardiac disease.
Goldenseal[†]	• Antiinflammatory • Antimicrobial • Immune stimulation	• Respiratory and GI infections • Gallbladder inflammation • Cirrhosis of liver • Externally on wounds • Diarrhea	May cause GI upset. Commonly combined with echinacea and used as "over-the-counter" antimicrobial. May be used in conjunction with antibiotics. Has anticoagulation effects.
Hawthorn	• Mild angiotensin converting enzyme (ACE) inhibitor • Positive inotropic properties	• Mild hypertension • Heart failure • High cholesterol • Atherosclerosis • Tachycardia	Relatively safe herb. May take 2-4 weeks to get results. Large amounts may cause arrhythmias.

Continued

TABLE 7-4	Commonly Used Herbs and Supplements—cont'd		
NAME	**EFFECTS**	**EXAMPLES OF COMMON USES**	**COMMENTS**
Kava	• Antianxiety • Sedative • Skeletal muscle relaxant	• Anxiety/nervousness • Restlessness • Fibromyalgia • Tension headaches • Insomnia	Frequent use can cause skin dryness and itching. Possible liver toxicity, especially with high doses.
Melatonin	• Hormone that regulates sleep	• Insomnia • Jet lag	Use cautiously with other drugs that promote sleep and relaxation.
Milk thistle	• Stimulation of production of new liver cells • Reduction of liver inflammation • Protection of liver from damage • Antioxidant	• Liver and gallbladder disease • Hepatitis • Dyspepsia • Liver transplant recovery	Can have mild laxative effect. Health care provider should be consulted before using if person has a liver disease.
Peppermint oil	• Antispasmodic	• Irritable bowel syndrome • Topically for itching and rash	Need enteric-coated capsules. Do not use on an open skin wound.
St. John's wort	• Inhibition of monoamine oxidase (MAO) and serotonin reuptake • Antiviral against herpes viruses • Antibacterial	• Mild-to-moderate depression • Anxiety • Wound healing • Viral infections	Photosensitivity may occur in susceptible people. Used with caution in people taking selective serotonin reuptake inhibitors (SSRIs). Should not be used in HIV patients taking antiretroviral therapy, especially protease inhibitors.
Saw palmetto	• Prevents intraprostatic conversion of testosterone to dihydrotestosterone (needed for prostate cell multiplication) • Antiestrogen activity	• Benign prostatic hyperplasia • Urinary infections	Well tolerated. Does not affect prostate-specific antigen (PSA) levels. Have PSA levels done before use.
Valerian	• Sedative • Anxiolytic • Sleep promoting • Muscle relaxant	• Sleeping disorders • Nervousness/anxiety • Restlessness • Irritable bowel syndrome	Should not be taken with sleeping pills. May react negatively with antianxiety and antidepressant drugs.
Zinc	• Prevents replication of viruses • Stimulates immune system	• Upper respiratory tract infections • Wound healing • Herpes simplex • Acne • Dermatitis	Should not be used in patients with glaucoma.

an excessive reaction or to unknown interaction effects. General patient teaching guidelines related to herbal therapy use are presented in Table 7-5.

Some herbs, even in small amounts, are toxic. For example, germander, used in some weight loss programs, has been associated with cases of fatal fulminant hepatitis. Some herbs have also been found to contain toxic products that can cause cancer. For example, comfrey has been widely used for its wound-healing properties, and comfrey leaf continues to be sold in ointment form for topical application. However, comfrey root has especially high concentrations of certain pyrrolizidine alkaloids that are highly carcinogenic. Comfrey should not be used internally. However, ointments containing comfrey leaf are considered safe when applied to intact skin for limited amounts of time.[33]

Patients should be advised that if they take herbal therapies, they should adhere to the suggested dosage. If herbal preparations are taken in high doses, they can be toxic. The potency of a particular herbal remedy can vary widely because of factors such as where and how it was grown, as well as harvesting and processing methods. Patients who take herbal remedies should be

TABLE 7-5	$\mathcal{P}$atient & Family Teaching Guide
	Herbal Therapies

- Ask the patient about use of herbal therapies. Take a complete history of herbal use, including amounts, brand names, and frequency of use (see box on p. 34). Ask the patient about allergies.
- Investigate whether herbs are used instead of or in addition to traditional medical treatments. Find out whether herbal therapies are used to prevent disease or to treat an existing problem.
- Instruct the patient to inform health care provider before taking any herbal treatments.
- Make the patient aware of the risks and benefits associated with herbal use, including drug reactions when taken in combination with other drugs.
- Advise the patient using herbal therapies to be aware of any side effects while taking herbal treatments and to immediately report them to health care provider.

- Advise patients to avoid using herbs for serious medical conditions (e.g., heart disease, bleeding conditions).
- Make the patient aware that moisture, sunlight, and heat may alter the components of herbal treatments.
- Inform the patient of the need to be aware of the reputation of the manufacturers of herbal products and the safety of the product before buying herbal treatments.
- Encourage the patient to read labels of herbal therapies carefully. Advise the patient not to take more of an herb than is recommended.
- Inform the patient that most herbal therapies should be discontinued at least 2-3 weeks before surgery.
- Inform the patient that the employees of health food stores are not trained health care professionals.

advised to be cautious when changing brands of herbal products used. Contamination of herbal product with other herbs, or substances such as pesticides or heavy metals (e.g., arsenic, lead, mercury) used in processing, has been documented. A major source of many of these problems is the lack of control and standardization in the manufacture of the herbal preparation. For this reason, herbal medicine should be purchased only from reputable manufacturers. In addition, labels on herbal products should contain the scientific name of the herbs, name and address of the actual manufacturer, batch or lot number, date of manufacture, and expiration date. An independent testing company has begun testing brand name herbal products and publishing the names of those products that pass quality testing on their website (*www.ConsumerLab.com*).

An ongoing concern expressed by practitioners of conventional medicine is that the use of herbs may cause patients to forego potentially curative conventional care. Another concern is that patients will treat themselves for diseases not recommended for self-treatment (e.g., clinical depression or human immunodeficiency virus disease).

Because of the potential for adverse effects, herbal products should be used with caution in pregnant women, nursing mothers, and older adults with liver or cardiovascular disease. Much is still unknown about herbal remedies. Research efforts are focused on identifying the biologically active component of herbal remedies, documenting their biologic effects, and evaluating their effectiveness when compared to either placebo or traditional drug therapy. Use of whole herb products and examination of subtle effects on biologic and emotional functioning must also be studied before a complete understanding of the effects of herbal therapy can be achieved.

MANIPULATIVE AND BODY-BASED METHODS

Manipulative and body-based methods include interventions and approaches to health care that are based on manipulation or movement of the body. Examples include chiropractic therapy,

massage and body work, and unconventional physical therapies such as hydrotherapy.

Chiropractic Therapy

Chiropractic therapy, a manual healing art, was developed in 1895 in Iowa, although spinal and soft tissue manipulation has been practiced since early recorded history. The primary aim of chiropractic therapy is to restore and maintain health by properly aligning the spine. Correct spinal alignment reduces interference from the nervous system, facilitates self-healing, and improves health and well-being. Incorrect spinal alignment, termed *subluxation,* can result from mechanical, physical, or psychologic factors, as well as from illness, poor diet, or exposure to environmental toxins. After a thorough diagnostic workup, chiropractors use various adjustment and manipulation techniques to facilitate spinal alignment based on the patient's particular problem. Chiropractic care may be acute, corrective, or preventive. Chiropractic practice does not typically include drug therapy or surgery but may include suggestions for improved nutritional intake.

Clinical Applications of Chiropractic Therapy. Chiropractic is best known for its effectiveness in treating back pain. In 1994 the U.S. Agency for Health Care Policy and Research (now known as the Agency for Healthcare Research and Quality) issued guidelines for the treatment of low back pain. It recommended that the most conservative forms of care should be sought first and stated that spinal manipulation is the only safe and effective form of drugless care. Subsequent studies have validated this recommendation.[34] Chiropractic interventions are used to treat musculoskeletal abnormalities, headaches, dysmenorrhea, dizziness, tinnitus, and visual disorders.

Limitations of Chiropractic Therapy. Several diseases or joint conditions should not be treated with manipulation. If a malignancy is suspected or determined through diagnostic testing, the patient should be referred to a medical physician for further evaluation and treatment. Bone and joint infections also require pharmacologic or surgical intervention. Contraindications for chiropractic therapy include acute myelopathy, fractures, dislocations, and rheumatoid arthritis. Nerve damage and paralysis are extremely rare complications of chiropractic intervention.

ENERGY THERAPIES

Energy therapies are those that involve the manipulation of energy fields. They focus on energy fields originating within the body (biofields) or those from other sources (electromagnetic fields). Examples of biofield therapies include therapeutic touch, healing touch, and Reiki. Biofield healing therapies (see Table 7-1) are based on the theory that energy systems in the body need to be balanced in an effort to enhance healing. Some forms of energy therapy manipulate biofields by applying pressure and/or manipulating the body by placing the hands in, or through, these fields.

Therapeutic Touch

Therapeutic touch (TT) is method of detecting and balancing human energy (Fig. 7-8). It is a contemporary interpretation of several ancient healing practices. The structure of its current practice was developed in the early 1970s. A slightly modified version of TT has been promoted within nursing under the name "healing touch" for which a certification program has been developed.[35] TT assumes that a human being is an open energy system, that a balanced flow of energy underlies good health, that illness is a reflection of an imbalance in an individual's energy field, and that human beings have the innate capacity to transform and transcend their current state of being. Additionally, practitioners assume that anyone can learn TT as long as they have a desire to learn, a willingness to help, and a sense of compassion for others.[36,37] TT is believed to help restore balance in the human energy field, leading to an opportunity for healing that incorporates the whole person.

Therapeutic touch involves the conscious use of the hands to direct or modulate human energy fields. Energy imbalances can be identified by the practitioner. During the actual treatment, the practitioner directs and modulates the energy, attempting to rebalance the energy flow and achieve symmetry throughout the

energy field. This remodulation of energy is achieved either by the practitioner lightly touching the body or maintaining the hands in a position a few inches away from the body and consciously directing the flow of energy.

Clinical Applications of Therapeutic Touch. The North American Nursing Diagnosis Association has accepted the nursing diagnosis "energy field disturbance," for which TT is the only identified intervention. Research has been conducted on the effectiveness of TT for a wide range of conditions, including wound healing, sleep promotion, enhancement of immune functioning, and the reduction of anxiety, agitation, postoperative pain, tension headache, and stress.[38-41] Reviews of research on TT indicate that findings are inconsistent but clinically important and indicate that further research is warranted.

Limitations of Therapeutic Touch. Although there is great enthusiasm in nursing about the use of TT, its research base needs further development. Scientifically acceptable methods for detecting human energy fields are currently lacking, contributing to a great deal of controversy about the basic assumptions underlying TT.[42] There is concern that literature reviews about TT may overestimate its effectiveness.[43] Researchers widely cite the need for additional well-controlled studies that use consistent definitions of *therapeutic touch,* consistent intervention practices, and larger sample sizes before scientifically sound decisions can be reached about the clinical effectiveness of TT.

Although documentation of adverse consequences to TT is absent in the research literature, it may be contraindicated in certain patient populations. For example, persons who are sensitive to human interaction and touch (e.g., those who have been physically abused or have psychiatric disorders) may misinterpret the intent of the treatment and may feel threatened. Other patients who may be sensitive to energy repatterning should not be exposed to energy-based interventions. Examples of such patients include older or debilitated people and those in critical or unstable conditions.[44]

Bioelectromagnetic-Based Therapies

Bioelectromagnetics refers to the unconventional use of electromagnetic fields for medical purposes. Magnets have been used to enhance health for thousands of years. Currently, magnetic therapy is widely accepted in China, Japan, Korea, Germany, Switzerland, and Russia. In North America, magnetic therapy is becoming more popular, especially with athletes.

Numerous mechanisms have been proposed to explain the effects of magnetic therapy. These include (1) increasing endorphin levels or blocking pain signals to the brain, thus reducing pain; (2) increasing blood flow, thus enhancing cellular and tissue healing; (3) facilitating the movement of calcium away from arthritic joints and toward needed areas in the body; (4) enhancing enzyme functioning and thus overall functioning of the body; and (5) increasing serotonin levels, thus enhancing a sense of well being. The changes induced by magnetic therapy may be so subtle that they are difficult to assess and measure with current technology.[45,46]

Permanent magnets are used in a variety of configurations, including the placement of magnets directly over pain sites or specific acupuncture meridians. People may sleep on magnetic pads and mattresses or wear magnetic insoles in their shoes. Magnetized drinking water is also available. Magnetic therapy is also

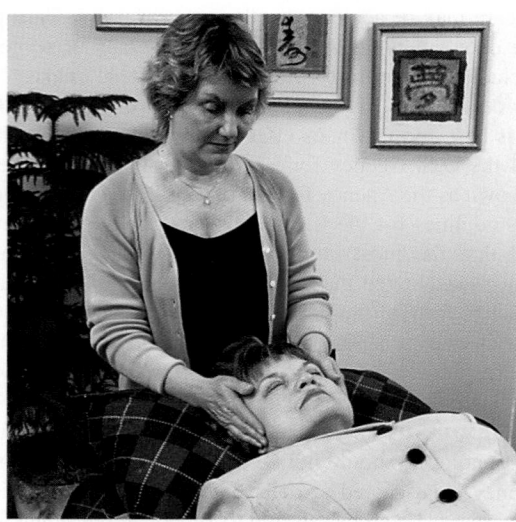

FIG. 7-8 In therapeutic touch, the practitioner directs her own interpersonal energy to help or heal another.

provided as a pulsed electromagnetic field (PEMF) and is used to stimulate the growth of bone and cartilage with potential for the treatment of arthritis.[46]

Clinical Use of Magnetic Therapy. Therapeutic permanent magnets are used most frequently for low back pain and are popular for a variety of other musculoskeletal complaints, although results of studies on the effectiveness of magnet therapy are inconsistent.[45] Findings may be inconsistent because the optimal length of treatment time and the optimal strength of the magnetic force have not been determined.

Limitations of Magnetic Therapy. There have been no documented adverse consequences from the use of magnetic therapy. People with metal plates and screws and with implanted devices, such as defibrillators and pacemakers, should avoid exposure to magnetic fields. People with seizure disorders and bleeding disorders are also advised to avoid using magnet therapy without proper medical supervision.

NURSING MANAGEMENT
COMPLEMENTARY AND ALTERNATIVE THERAPIES

The role of the nurse with respect to complementary and alternative therapies is evolving. Roles of the nurse may include (1) assessing patients' use of complementary and alternative therapies and their risk for complications or adverse interactions with conventional therapies; (2) serving as a resource about complementary or alternative therapies, including teaching patients about complementary and alternative options, providing information about evidence concerning effectiveness, and making referrals to qualified practitioners; (3) serving as a provider of therapies for which the nurse obtains training and certification, such as therapeutic touch or acupuncture; and (4) conducting research about complementary and alternative approaches.

■ Assessment

It has been reported that between 60% and 70% of patients fail to reveal to their primary care provider their use of alternative approaches.[47] Among 44% of Americans who reported regularly taking prescription drugs, almost one quarter indicated that they also take at least one herbal product, a high-dose vitamin, or both. Extrapolation to the entire U.S. population suggests that up to 15 million Americans may be at risk for prescription drug–herb interactions.[3] In addition to assessment of drug-herb interactions, it is important to assess patients' risk for untoward effects and to document the effectiveness of those interventions being used. The incorporation of complementary and alternative approaches in the plan of care may also be appropriate, given the patient's current use or interest in use of these strategies.

In assessing the use of complementary and alternative therapies, the degree of use must first be determined. Patients with a desire to be actively involved in their health care or who desire an approach to health care that includes emotional and spiritual aspects are likely to use complementary or alternative approaches.[48] Specific problems for which patients use complementary and alternative approaches include addiction problems, anxiety, chronic pain, chronic fatigue syndrome, chronic urinary tract infections, headaches, and sprains or mus-

cle strains.[49] These problems are often resistant to treatment with conventional therapies. Assessment questions to ask include the following:

1. What are you doing to maintain or improve your health and well-being?
2. How involved are you in planning and carrying out your health-related care?
3. What is your view of the ideal relationship between yourself and your primary health care provider?
4. Do you have any conditions that have not responded to conventional medicine? If so, have you tried any other approaches?
5. Are you using any vitamin, mineral, dietary, or herbal supplements?
6. Are you interested in obtaining information about alternative or complementary approaches?

Asking these questions in a way that conveys respect for the patient and genuine interest in his or her answers will be most effective in eliciting information. (For additional information on assessment of the use of complementary and alternative therapies, see the box in Chapter 3 on p. 34.)

The patient's responses to these questions allow a patient to be categorized as a nonuser, an occasional user, or a primary user. Nonusers may need additional assessment to determine why they are nonusers. Patients who are open to alternative approaches but have not yet used them may need further information. Nurses work closely with their patients and are in the unique position of becoming familiar with the patient's spiritual and cultural values and beliefs. Nurses may be able to determine which complementary and alternative therapies would be more appropriate with these values and beliefs and offer recommendations accordingly.

Patients who are identified as occasional or primary users should have their knowledge assessed regarding the therapies they are using. This includes determining the extent of knowledge, as well as the sources of information. The nurse should determine whether the patient is adequately informed and has reliable sources of information. Additionally, the nurse should document the effectiveness and any unexpected or adverse consequences of the intervention.

Patients who are occasional or primary users should also be assessed for risk related to the use of these therapies. Known high-risk therapies include unsafe herbs in addition to potential adverse interactions with concurrent herb and prescribed drug use (see Table 7-4). Surgery may create short-term risks related to interactions of herbal therapies. Other high-risk therapies include those that are high cost but provide low to uncertain benefits, as well as those that mask potentially life-threatening conditions or substitute for effective conventional therapies in life-threatening conditions.

Patients identified as being at high risk for complications related to use of complementary and alternative therapies must have a specific plan developed to inform them and other health care providers of their risk status. While recognizing that patients have the ultimate responsibility for decisions on the use of therapies, they need to be clearly and fully informed about potential adverse consequences of the current use of complementary and alternative therapies. Documentation of high-risk status must be included in patient records and communicated to other health care providers.

■ Serving as a Resource

To serve as a resource for patients, nurses must first develop their own knowledge base. Even if specific information about complementary and alternative therapies is not provided in basic nursing programs, nurses are educated as critical thinkers and problem solvers. Thus nurses are prepared to seek ongoing education regarding complementary and alternative therapies and to continue to read and critique research conducted on such therapies.[50] Resources for complementary and alternative approaches have dramatically increased with the development of the Internet. Examples of Internet and print resources are included at the end of this chapter. Nurses should also be prepared to assist patients in differentiating between Internet sites that promote untested approaches and those that include systematically reviewed information. Knowledge of Internet sites or other listings that include information about local practitioners of various therapies who are certified, registered, or licensed is also useful.

■ Serving as a Provider

Nursing has a long history of providing therapies that have been considered complementary and alternative within the context of contemporary biomedical approaches to health. These include massage, relaxation therapy, music therapy, and therapeutic touch, as well as other strategies to promote comfort, reduce stress, improve coping, and promote symptom relief. These and other complementary therapies are generally included within the scope of nursing practice, though they are not specifically addressed in most U.S. state nursing practice acts.[51] Similarly, practice acts in the United Kingdom and Australia address nurses' accountability for their own actions and their responsibility to know their limitations and function within those limits.[52] The requirements for use of a specific complementary or alternative therapy are not different than for the use of other nursing interventions. The nurse should have specific training in the use of the therapy and should be aware of the evidence base that addresses the conditions for which the therapy is indicated, the effectiveness of the therapy, and the potential for adverse outcomes or synergistic effects. As nurses seek to include complementary and alternative approaches into their practice, questions that must be addressed include the following:

1. What institutional or workplace policies must be in place to support the use of complementary and alternative approaches?
2. What consent or permission of patients is necessary before complementary or alternative approaches are used?
3. What monitoring or evaluation systems should be instituted to document the use and effectiveness of such interventions?

■ Involvement in Research

Nurses are responsible for critiquing and applying relevant research findings to their practice, as well as participating in the identification of researchable problems. Using summaries of research evidence on complementary and alternative therapies, such as those found in the Cochrane Collection, is one strategy for developing evidence-based approaches. Participating on teams whose focus is to develop evidence-based protocols that address appropriate use of complementary and alternative therapies is another effective approach. Practicing with a questioning mind can facilitate identification of research questions that can be investigated with research-trained health care professionals. Types of research questions that can be posed include describing the extent of patients' use of specific therapies, exploring patients' experiences of using various complementary and alternative therapies, and documenting the effectiveness of therapies commonly used by nurses.

Patient interest and participation in complementary and alternative therapies is increasing. Therefore it is important for nurses to be knowledgeable of the multiple therapies available and to develop effective strategies to document the use of these therapies. It is also important for nurses to keep abreast of the current research being done in this area to provide accurate information to both patients and other health care professionals.

CRITICAL THINKING EXERCISES

Case Study
College Student with Abdominal Distress
Patient Profile. Jane, a 21-year-old college student, was seen in the student health center for increasing episodes of abdominal fullness and discomfort with alternating diarrhea and constipation.

Subjective Data
- Reports being diagnosed with irritable bowel syndrome several years ago
- Was told to eat more fiber, but nothing has seemed to be effective in reducing her abdominal distress
- Is taking a heavy course load this semester
- Has to work 20 hours each week for her work-study contract
- Eats mainly fast foods and drinks several colas daily

CRITICAL THINKING QUESTIONS
1. Explain the psychologic stressors that may be contributing to Jane's abdominal discomfort.
2. Describe how her current diet may be affecting her both physiologically and psychologically.
3. What complementary or alternative therapy (or therapies) would be appropriate for Jane?
4. How would you recommend complementary therapies to her physician? What arguments could you use to support their use?

REVIEW QUESTIONS

The number of the question corresponds to the same-numbered objective at the beginning of the chapter.

1. One of the primary differences between complementary and alternative therapies and conventional therapies is that
   a. complementary and alternative therapies do not usually require medical authorization.
   b. complementary and alternative therapies should be used only in addition to conventional therapy and never as a primary treatment.
   c. conventional therapies are considered safe whereas complementary and alternative therapies are not considered safe.
   d. conventional therapies have proven effectiveness in treating chronic illnesses whereas complementary and alternative therapies have not.

2. Which of the following categories is not part of NCCAM's classification system?
   a. energy therapies
   b. exercise therapies
   c. biologic-based therapies
   d. alternative medical systems

3. The basis of traditional Chinese medicine differs from conventional medicine. This is shown in acupuncture, where the critical components include all of the following except
   a. Qi.
   b. yin and yang.
   c. channels or meridians.
   d. muscular manipulation.

4. Which of the following is considered a mind-body intervention?
   a. Qigong
   b. Ayurveda
   c. Therapeutic touch
   d. Feldenkrais method

5. A common complication of the use of garlic, ginkgo, ginseng, and ginger is
   a. allergic reactions.
   b. clotting alterations.
   c. skin photosensitivity.
   d. increased blood pressure.

6. The basis for therapeutic touch involves the
   a. acquisition of the relaxation response.
   b. stimulation of peripheral nerves to reduce pain.
   c. emission of vital energy by a trained practitioner for the purpose of healing another person.
   d. remodulation of energy by a trained practitioner in an attempt to rebalance the patient's energy field.

7. The primary goal of chiropractic therapy focuses on
   a. increasing spinal flexibility and muscle tone.
   b. reducing muscle tension that produces spinal instability.
   c. restoring the structural and functional vertebral imbalances that cause pain.
   d. combining vertebral manipulation and drug therapy for the treatment of chronic back pain.

8. The roles of the nurse regarding complementary and alternative therapies would include
   a. prescribing the appropriate herbal therapies for a patient.
   b. educating patients about the herbal products that they use or are interested in using.
   c. assessing the perspective of the patient's family about the patient's use of acupuncture.
   d. discouraging a patient with heart disease from using any form of bioelectromagnetic therapy.

9. In assessing a patient's use of complementary and alternative therapies, it is important that the nurse include all of the following except
   a. assess the patient's use and frequency of use of these therapies.
   b. determine the patient's knowledge of the therapies that he or she is using.
   c. use the term "alternative therapies" when assessing the patient's use of these therapies.
   d. create an open and nonjudgmental environment where the patient will be free to provide information.

REFERENCES

1. Engebretson J: Alternative and complementary healing: implications for nursing, *J Prof Nurs* 15:214, 1999.
2. Panel on Definition and Description: Defining and describing complementary and alternative medicine, *Alternative Therapies* 3:2, 1997.
3. Eisenberg D et al: Trends in alternative medicine use in the United States, 1990-1997: results of a follow up national survey, *JAMA* 280:1569, 1998.
4. Millar WJ: Use of alternative health care practitioners by Canadians, *Can J Public Health* 88:154, 1998.
5. MacLennan AH et al: Prevalence and cost of alternative medicine in Australia, *Lancet* 347:569, 1996.
6. Frisch et al: *AHNA standards for holistic nursing practice: guidelines for caring and healing,* Gaithersburg, Md, 2000, Aspen.
7. Ezzo J et al: Complementary medicine and the Cochrane Collaboration, *JAMA* 280:1628, 1998.
8. Trivieri L: *The American holistic medical association guide to holistic health,* New York, 2001, Wiley.
9. NIH consensus conference on acupuncture, *JAMA* 280:1518, 1998.

10. Bannerman RH: *The World Health Organization viewpoint on acupuncture,* Geneva, Switzerland, 1979, World Health Organization.

11. Ernst E: Acupuncture for low back pain: a meta-analysis of randomized clinical trials, *Arch Intern Med* 158:2235, 1998.

12. van Tulder MW et al: The effectiveness of acupuncture in the management of acute and chronic low back pain, *Spine* 24:113, 1999.

13. Ernst E, White A. *Acupuncture: a scientific appraisal,* Oxford, 1999, Butterworth-Heinemann.

14. Hadhazy V et al: Mind and body therapy for fibromyalgia (protocol). In *The Cochrane Library,* Oxford, 2001.

15. Wolf SL et al: Reducing frailty and falls in older persons: an investigation of Tai Chi and computerized balance training, *J Am Geriatric Soc* 44:489, 1996.

16. Beghe C: Meta-analysis: several strategies prevent falls and subsequent injury in older persons, *Evidence Based Medicine* 1:169, 1996.

17. Wolf SL et al: The effect of Tai Chi Chuan and computerized balance training on postural stability in older subjects, *Phys Ther* 77:371, 1997.

18. Wolf SL et al: Exploring the basis for Tai Chi Chuan as a therapeutic exercise approach, *Arch Phys Med Rehabil* 78:886, 1997.

19. Lan C et al: Cardiorespiratory function, flexibility, and body composition among geriatric Tai Chi Chaun practitioners, *Arch Phys Med Rehabil* 77:612, 1996.

20. Fontana JA: The energy costs of a modified form on T'ai Chi exercise, *Nurs Res* 49:91, 2000.

21. Sowell R et al: Spiritual activities as a resistance resource for women with HIV, *Nurs Res* 49:73, 2000.

22. Baldacchino D, Draper P: Spiritual coping strategies: a review of the nursing research literature, *J Adv Nurs* 34:833, 2001.

23. Narayanasamy A: A review of spirituality as applied to nursing, *Int J Nurs Stud* 36:117, 1999.

24. Rassol GH: The crescent and Islam: healing nursing and the spiritual dimension, *J Adv Nurs* 32:1476, 2000.

25. Holt-Ashley M: Nurses pray: use of prayer and spirituality as a complementary therapy in the ICU, *AACN Clinical Issues* 11:60, 2000.

26. Sellers SC, Haag BA: Spiritual nursing interventions, *J Holistic Nurs* 16:338, 1998.

27. Roberts L et al: Intercessory prayer for the alleviation of ill health (Cochrane review). In *The Cochrane Library,* Oxford, 2001.

28. Tuck I et al: Spirituality and spiritual care provided by parish nurses, *West J Nurs Res* 23:441, 2001.

29. Bauer BA: Herbal therapy: what a clinician needs to know to counsel patients effectively, *Mayo Clinic Proc* 75:835, 2000.

30. Ernst E: Harmless herbs? A review of the recent literature, *Am J Med* 104:170, 1998.

31. Winslow LS, Kroll DJ: Herbs as medicine, *Arch Intern Med* 158:2192, 1998.

32. Ang-Lee MK et al: Herbal medicines and perioperative care, *JAMA* 286:208, 2001.

33. *PDR for nonprescription drugs and dietary supplements,* New York, 2000, Medical Economics.

34. Mohseni-Bandpei MA et al: Spinal manipulation in the treatment of low back pain: a review of the literature with particular emphasis on randomized clinical trials, *Phys Ther Rev* 3:185, 1998.

35. Mentgen J: Healing touch, *Nurs Clin North Am* 36:43, 2001.

36. Krieger D: *Therapeutic touch: how to use your hands to help or heal,* New York, 1979, Prentice Hall.

37. Krieger D: *Therapeutic touch inner workbook: ventures in transpersonal healing,* Santa Fe, 1997, Bear.

38. Peters R: The effectiveness of therapeutic touch: a meta-analytic review, *Nurs Sci Q* 12:52, 1999.

39. Winsted-Fry P, Kijek J: An integrative review and meta-analysis of therapeutic touch research, *Alternative Therapies* 5:38, 1999.

40. O'Mathuna D: Therapeutic touch for healing acute wounds (protocol for a Cochrane review). In *The Cochrane Library* 3, 2001.

41. Daley B: Therapeutic touch, nursing practice, and contemporary wound healing research, *J Adv Nurs* 25:1123, 1997.

42. Rosa L et al: A close look at therapeutic touch, *JAMA* 279:1005, 1998.

43. O'Mathuna D: Evidence-based practice and reviews of therapeutic touch, *Journal of Nursing Scholarship* 32:279, 2000.

44. Mulloney SS, Wells-Federman C: Therapeutic touch: a healing modality, *J Cardiovasc Nurs* 10:27, 1996.

45. Collacott EA et al: Bipolar permanent magnets for the treatment of chronic low back pain, *JAMA* 283:1322, 2000.

46. Trock DH: Electromagnetic fields and magnets: investigational treatment for musculoskeletal disorders, *Rheum Dis Clin North Am* 26:51, 2000.

47. Eisenberg D et al: Talking with patients about their use of alternative therapies, *Prim Care* 24:699, 1997.

48. Eisenberg D: Advising patients who seek alternative medical therapies, *Ann Intern Med* 127, 1997.

49. Ullrich S, Hodge P: The Ullrich-Hodge alternative therapy assessment model, *Nurse Educ* 24:19, 1999.

50. Breda KL, Schulze MW: Teaching complementary healing therapies to nurses, *J Nurs Educ* 37:394, 1998.

51. Geddes N, Henry JK: Nursing and alternative medicine: legal and practice issues, *J Holistic Nurs* 15:271, 1997.

52. Ching M: Complementary therapies: research, education and practice in nursing, *Contemp Nurse* 7:173, 1998.

RESOURCES

Acupuncture.com
www.acupuncture.com

American Academy of Medical Acupuncture (AAMA)
5820 Wiltshire Blvd., Suite 428
Los Angeles, CA 90010
323-937-5514
E-mail: JDOWDEN@prodigy.net
www.medicalacupuncture.org/aama.htm

American Alliance of Aromatherapy
PO Box 309
Depoe Bay, OR 97341
800-809-9850

American Association of Naturopathic Physicians
8201 Greensboro Drive, Suite 300
McLean, VA 22102
703-610-9037
877-969-2267
Fax: 703-610-9005
www.naturopathic.org

American Association of Oriental Medicine
433 Front Street
Catasauqua, PA 18032
610-266-1433
888-500-7999
Fax: 610-264-2768
E-mail: aaom1@aol.com
www.aaom.org

American Chiropractic Association
1701 Clarendon Blvd.
Arlington, VA 22209
703-276-8800
Fax: 703-243-2593
www.amerchiro.org/

American Herbalists Guild
1931 Gaddis Road
Canton, GA 30115
770-751-6021
Fax: 770-751-7472
E-mail: ahgoffice@earthlink.net
www.americanherbalistsguild.com/

American Holistic Nurses' Association
PO Box 2130
Flagstaff, AZ 86003-2130
800-278-AHNA
www.ahna.org

American Institute of Hypnotherapy
    2002 East McFadden Avenue
    Santa Ana, CA 92705-4706
    714-261-6400
American Massage Therapy Association
    820 Davis Street, Suite 100
    Evanston, IL 60201
    847-864-0123
    Fax: 847-864-1178
    www.amtamassage.org
Association for Applied Psychophysiology and Biofeedback
    102000 West 44th Avenue, Suite 304
    Wheat Ridge, CO 80033-2840
    303-422-8436
    Fax: 303-422-8894
    E-mail: AAPB@resourcenter.com
    www.aapb.org
Ayurvedic Institute
    11311 Menaul NE, Suite A
    Albuquerque, NM 87112
    505-291-9698
    Fax: 505-294-7572
    E-mail: info@ayurveda.com
    www.ayurveda.com
Council of Colleges of Acupuncture and Oriental Medicine
    7501 Greenway Center Drive, Suite 820
    Greenbelt, MD 20770
    301-313-0868
    Fax: 301-313-0869
    www.ccaom.org/
Feldenkrais Guild of North America
    3611 SW Hood Avenue, Suite 100
    Portland, OR 97201
    503-221-6612
    800-775-2118
    Fax: 503-221-6616
    E-mail: guild@feldenkrais.com
    www.feldenkrais.com
Healing Touch International
    12477 West Cedar Drive, Suite 202
    Lakewood, Colorado 80228
    303-989-7982
    Fax-303-980-8683
    E-mail: htiheal@aol.com
    www.healingtouch.net

HerbMed
    Sponsoring agency: Alternative Medicine Foundation
    www.herbmed.org
Herb Research Foundation
    1007 Pearl Street
    Boulder, CO 80302
    303-449-2265
    800-748-2617
    Fax: 303-449-7849
    www.herbs.org/index.html
Holistic Alliance of Professional Practitioners, Entrepreneurs, Networkers, Inc. (HAPPEN)
    1031 NW 6th Street, Suite F-1
    Gainesville, FL 32601
    888-8HAPPEN
    Fax: 352-379-3055
    E-mail: happeninc@aol.com
    www.toolcity.net/kauffeld/happen
National Center for Complementary and Alternative Medicine
    NCCAM Clearinghouse
    PO Box 7923
    Gaithersburg, MD 20898
    301-519-3153
    888-644-6226
    Fax: 866-464-3616
    E-mail: info@nccam.nih.gov
    nccam.nih.gov
National Center for Homeopathy
    801 North Fairfax, Suite 306
    Alexandria, VA 22314
    703-548-7790
    877-624-0613
    Fax: 703-548-7792
    www.healthy.net/nch
National Certification Commission for Acupuncture and Oriental Medicine
    11 Canal Center Plaza, Suite 300
    Alexandria, VA 22314
    703-548-9004
    Fax: 703-548-9079
    www.nccaom.org/

For additional Internet resources, see the website for this book at *http://evolve.elsevier.com/Lewis/medsurg/*.

CHAPTER 8

Stress

Linda Witek-Janusek

LEARNING OBJECTIVES

1. Define the terms stressor, stress, demands, primary appraisal, secondary appraisal, coping, adaptation, and allostasis.
2. Describe the three stages of Selye's general adaptation syndrome.
3. Understand the role of cognitive appraisal and coping in the stress process.
4. Describe the role of the nervous and endocrine systems in the stress process.
5. Describe the effects of stress on the immune system.
6. Describe the effects of stress on health and illness.
7. Describe the coping strategies that can be used by a patient experiencing stress.
8. List the variables that may influence an individual's response to stress.
9. Describe the nursing assessment and management of a patient experiencing stress.

KEY TERMS

alarm reaction, p. 112	psychoneuroimmunology, p. 119
allostasis, p. 121	resilience, p. 115
appraisal, p. 116	reticular activating system, p. 117
coping, p. 122	sense of coherence, p. 115
emotion-focused coping, p. 123	stage of exhaustion, p. 114
eustress, p. 114	stage of resistance, p. 114
general adaptation syndrome, p. 112	stress, p. 112
	stressors, p. 112
problem-focused coping, p. 122	

THEORIES OF STRESS

Interest in the study of stress has intensified as investigators have begun to identify its role in relation to physical and emotional health. Three different but complementary stress theories have influenced most contemporary approaches to the study of stress. The first theory conceptualizes stress as a response to an environmental demand or stressor. This theory was first proposed by Selye, who identified stress as a nonspecific response of the body to any demand made on it.[1] Selye referred to these stress-inducing demands as **stressors.** Stressors can be physical or emotional and pleasant or unpleasant, as long as they require the individual to adapt (Table 8-1). In response to either physical (e.g., burns) or psychologic (e.g., death of a loved one) stressors, a series of physiologic changes occur. Selye called this pattern of responses the general adaptation syndrome (GAS).

A second stress theory views stress as a stimulus that causes a response. This theory originated with Holmes, Rahe, and Masuda, who developed a tool to assess the effects of life changes on health (Table 8-2).[2,3] *Life changes* are defined as conditions ranging from minor violations of the law to death of a loved one. The major assumption of this theory is that frequent life changes make people more vulnerable to illness. Using the life events tool (Table 8-2), 6-month totals of greater than or equal to 300, or 1-year totals equal to or greater than 500, are considered indicative of high recent life stress.

A third stress theory focuses on the person-environment transactions and is referred to as the transaction or interaction theory.[4] A proponent of this theory is Lazarus, who emphasized the role of cognitive appraisal in assessing stressful situations and selecting coping options. Lazarus and Folkman[5] defined psychologic **stress** as a particular relationship between the person and the environment that is appraised by the person as taxing or exceeding his or her resources and endangering his or her well-being. These three stress theories are discussed in more detail later in this chapter.

STRESS AS A RESPONSE

Historically, Selye's early research using animals supported his theory that stressors from different sources produce a similar physical response pattern. He termed these physical responses to stress the **general adaptation syndrome** (GAS). The GAS is composed of three stages: alarm reaction, stage of resistance, and stage of exhaustion. Once the environmental event or stressor stimulates the central nervous system, multiple responses occur because of activation of the hypothalamic-pituitary-adrenal axis and the autonomic nervous system. The nature of these responses, in which the stressor successively causes changes in the nervous, endocrine, and immune systems, is fundamental to understanding the physiologic and behavioral changes that occur in an individual experiencing stress.

Stage of Alarm Reaction

The first stage of the stress response is the **alarm reaction** of the GAS, in which the individual perceives a stressor physically or mentally and the *fight-or-flight response* is initiated. When the

TABLE 8-1	Examples of Stressors	
PHYSICAL	**EMOTIONAL**	
Burns	Diagnosis of cancer	
Hypothermia	Divorce	
Hypoxia	Failing an examination	
Infectious diseases	Financial loss	
Noise	Grieving loss of a family member	
Pain	Prolonged period of caregiving	
Running a marathon	Winning an athletic event	

Reviewed by Monica Jarrett, RN, PhD, Associate Professor, School of Nursing, University of Washington, Seattle, Wash.

TABLE 8-2   Social Readjustment Rating Scale*

LIFE CHANGE EVENT	LIFE CHANGE UNIT	LIFE CHANGE EVENT	LIFE CHANGE UNIT
Health		**Home and Family—cont'd**	
An injury or illness that		Change in arguments with spouse	50
Kept you in bed a week or more, or sent you to	74	In-law problems	38
the hospital		Change in the marital status of your parents	
Was less serious than above	44	Divorce	59
Major dental work	26	Remarriage	50
Major change in eating habits	27	Separation from spouse	
Major change in sleeping habits	26	Because of work	53
Major change in your usual type and/or amount of	28	Because of marital problems	76
recreation		Divorce	96
		Birth of grandchild	43
Work		Death of spouse	119
Change to a new type of work	51	Death of other family member	
Change in your work hours or conditions	35	Child	123
Change in your responsibilities at work		Brother or sister	102
More responsibilities	29	Parent	100
Fewer responsibilities	21		
Promotion	31	**Personal and Social**	
Demotion	42	Change in personal habits	26
Transfer	32	Beginning or ending school or college	38
Troubles at work		Change of school or college	35
With your boss	29	Change in political beliefs	24
With co-workers	35	Change in religious beliefs	29
With persons under your supervision	35	Change in social activities	27
Other work troubles	28	Vacation	24
Major business adjustment	60	New, close, personal relationship	37
Retirement	52	Engagement to marry	45
Loss of job		Girlfriend or boyfriend problems	39
Laid off from work	68	Sexual differences	44
Fired from work	79	"Falling out" of a close personal relationship	47
Correspondence course to help you in your work	18	An accident	48
		Minor violation of the law	20
Home and Family		Being held in jail	75
Major change in living conditions	42	Death of a close friend	70
Change in residence		Major decision regarding your immediate future	51
Move within the same town or city	25	Major personal achievement	36
Move to a different town, city, or state	47		
Change in family get-togethers	25	**Financial**	
Major change in health or behavior of family	55	Major change in finances	
member		Increased income	38
Marriage	50	Decreased income	60
Pregnancy	67	Investment and/or credit difficulties	56
Miscarriage or abortion	65	Loss or damage of personal property	43
Gain of a new family member		Moderate purchase	20
Birth of a child	66	Major purchase	37
Adoption of a child	65	Foreclosure on a mortgage or loan	58
A relative moving in with you	59		
Spouse beginning or ending work	46		
Child leaving home			
To attend college	41		
Because of marriage	41		
For other reasons	45		

From Miller MA, Rahe RH: Life changes scaling for the 1990s, *J Psychosom Res* 43:279, 1997.
*Six-month totals ≥300 LCU, or 1-year totals ≥500 LCU, are considered indications of high recent life stress.

stressor is of sufficient intensity to threaten the steady state or homeostasis of the individual, it leads to a series of physiologic changes that promote adaptation. This temporarily decreases the individual's resistance and may even result in disease or death if the stress is prolonged and severe.

Physical signs and symptoms of the alarm reaction are generally those of sympathetic nervous system stimulation. These signs include increased blood pressure, increased heart and respiratory rate, decreased gastrointestinal (GI) motility, pupil dilation, and increased perspiration. The patient may complain of such symptoms as increased anxiety, rapid heart rate, nausea, and anorexia.

Stage of Resistance

Ideally the individual quickly moves from the alarm reaction to the **stage of resistance,** in which physiologic reserves are mobilized to increase the resistance to stress. At this time adaptation may occur. The amount of resistance to the stressor varies among individuals, depending on the level of physical functioning, coping abilities, and total number and intensity of stressors experienced. For example, a person who has been exercising regularly and is physically fit will have greater ability to adapt to the stress of emergency surgery than a person who is deconditioned and leads a sedentary lifestyle.

Although few overt physical signs and symptoms occur in this stage as compared with the alarm stage, the person is expending energy in an attempt to adapt. The resources available to the individual limit this adaptive energy. These resources include not only the individual's internal physical and psychologic reserves, but also external resources such as social support from family, friends, and health care workers. When resources are adequate, the individual may successfully recover from a stressor such as surgery and return to his or her baseline (presurgery) state. If adaptation does not occur, the person may move to the next phase of the GAS, which is the stage of exhaustion.

Stage of Exhaustion

The **stage of exhaustion** is the final stage of the GAS. It occurs when all the energy for adaptation has been expended. Physical symptoms of the alarm reaction may briefly reappear in a final effort by the body to survive. A terminally ill person who becomes alert and has stronger vital signs shortly before death exemplifies this. The individual in the stage of exhaustion usually becomes ill and may die if assistance from outside sources is not available. This stage can often be reversed by external sources of adaptive energy, such as medication or psychotherapy.

Refinements in Selye's Stress Theory

Selye's work addressed the importance of conditioning factors that may affect the stress response. These conditioning factors include age, genetic makeup, previous experience with stressors, nutrition, and diet.[6] Selye coined the term **eustress** to refer to stress associated with positive events such as winning a tennis match. However, he never fully explained the health consequences of eustress versus stress. This relationship is currently under investigation by others, as exemplified by studies in which not only "daily hassles" but also positive events or "uplifts" experienced by an individual are measured.

Selye's description of stress focuses on the physiologic changes of the nervous, immune, gastrointestinal, and endocrine

TABLE 8-3	**Examples of Disorders and Diseases of Adaptation**
Angina	Hypertension
Asthma	Impotence
Carpal tunnel syndrome	Insomnia
Depression	Irritable bowel syndrome
Dyspepsia	Low back pain
Eating disorders	Myocardial infarction
Fatigue	Peptic ulcer disease
Fibromyalgia	Rheumatoid arthritis
Headaches	Sexual dysfunction

systems that occur as an organism responds to a specific stressor. His work indicates that there is a predictable uniform pattern in the physiologic response to various stressors. This emphasis is due in part to the fact that Selye used animal models that were not capable of representing complex psychologic processing of a stressor.

In humans there can be great variability among individuals in response to the same stressor. Stress perception, stress appraisal, and personal meaning attached to a stressor influence the way an individual responds to a stressor. There are also gender differences in the physiologic response to stress. In addition, the sympathetic nervous system response to stress varies with the different phases of the menstrual cycle.[7,8] These individual differences are not only observed in the cardiovascular response to stress, but also in the immune response to psychologic stress.[9] Thus stressors are likely to produce complex and varying profiles of hormonal and immunologic changes in different individuals. This may help explain why a variety of disorders and diseases of adaptation exist (Table 8-3) and also why there are individual differences in susceptibility to stress-related disease.

Additionally, there are differences in the behavioral and physiologic adaptive responses to a stressor based on duration of a stressor (acute or chronic) and intensity of a stressor (mild, moderate, or severe).[10] For example, an individual dealing with the chronic stress of caring for a loved one may also be exposed to a multitude of acute episodic stressors. Therefore the duration or chronicity of exposure to a stressor is an important variable that can influence an individual's adaptive response.

STRESS AS A STIMULUS

Life Events

Another approach to the study of stress is to view stress as a stimulus or event that disturbs an individual's homeostatic balance. Stress defined in this way is similar to Selye's definition of a stressor, and "life events" become the stressor to which a person responds. Questionnaires have been developed to measure stress in terms of life changes or life events.[2,3] Two such questionnaires are the Social Readjustment Rating Scale (SRRS) (see Table 8-2) and the Schedule of Recent Experiences (SRE). Life events questionnaires such as the SRRS and the SRE were developed in an attempt to numerically weight the impact (stress) of various life changes (e.g., death of a spouse, financial changes). A life event is regarded as stressful if it leads to some adaptive or coping behavior on the part of the involved individual.[3] Each event, whether desirable or not, is indicative of the amount of change it produces in the ongoing life patterns of the individual. Importantly, life events or life changes do not consistently affect people to the same degree. With this in mind, the Life Experiences Survey (LES) was developed. The LES not only assesses if the event is desirable or not but also measures the degree of impact the event had on the person's life.[11]

It was originally theorized that the more stressful life events occurring throughout a specific period of time, the greater the vulnerability to illness. Of particular interest was the research that reported an association between the number and intensity of life events and the resulting probability of physical and emotional illness following the events.[12] Although several studies have shown statistically significant relationships between stressful life events and illness onset, these relationships are often weak. Life events scaling has raised methodologic issues regarding additional factors (e.g., age, perception, previous experiences, health) that must be taken into account when considering life events. Furthermore, stressful life events may prove to have a greater impact on illness progression as opposed to illness onset.

Refinements in the Stress as a Stimulus Theory

Factors that affect an individual's response to life events include cultural influences, personality characteristics, clustering of events, biologic variables, socioeconomic status, timing, and support systems. These factors indicate the importance of using a holistic approach when assessing the impact of stress on an individual.

Hardiness, Sense of Coherence, and Resilience. Interestingly, some individuals experience significant adverse life events but do not succumb to illness. In attempting to understand why some individuals are shielded from the negative consequences of stress, researchers have identified key personal characteristics, such as hardiness, sense of coherence, and resilience, as possible modulators that buffer the impact of stress on health outcomes. Hardiness is believed to be a mediating factor in the stress-illness relationship.[13] The hardy person has (1) a clear sense of personal values and goals, (2) a strong tendency toward interaction with the environment, (3) a sense of meaningfulness, and (4) an internal rather than external locus of control. An internal locus of control means that the hardy person perceives that her or his life is self-determined, as opposed to being directed by outside or external events.

Sense of coherence (SOC), a concept closely related to hardiness, has been defined and developed by Antonovsky.[14] SOC is believed to be a more powerful mediator of stress and illness than hardiness and is a key determinant of health.[15] In general, SOC refers to how an individual sees the world and one's life in it. It is a personality characteristic or coping style rather than a response to a specific situation. The three components of SOC are comprehensibility (stimuli derived from one's internal and external environments are structured, predictable, and explorable), manageability (resources are available to meet the demands posed by these stimuli), and meaningfulness (demands are challenges worthy of investment and engagement). An individual with a strong SOC has an enduring tendency to see one's life as ordered, predictable, and manageable. On the other hand, individuals with a weaker SOC are more likely to interpret stressors as threatening or anxiety provoking.[16]

Resilience is another characteristic that is believed to moderate or buffer the negative effects of stress. **Resilience** is defined as being resourceful, being flexible, and having an available source of problem-solving strategies. Individuals who possess a high degree of resilience are not as likely to perceive an event as stressful or taxing.[17]

Characteristics such as hardiness, sense of coherence, and resilience may help explain why some people remain healthy despite enduring significant stress in their lives. Individuals who are hardy, are resilient, and have a strong sense of coherence are more likely to effectively cope with life's stressors.

Hassles, Uplifts, and Positive Emotions. Some would debate that it is not the number of major negative life events that produce wear and tear on the body but rather the day-to-day experience of minor life events or hassles that lead to stress-related illness. *Daily hassles* are experiences and conditions of daily living that are viewed as irritating, frustrating, and distressing. Hassles are appraised as harmful or threatening to an individual's well-being.[18] The frequency and intensity of daily hassles have a stronger relationship with somatic illness than life events.[5] Scales have been developed to measure daily hassles, and the items addressed reflect the content areas of work, family, social activities, environment, practical considerations, finances, and health (Table 8-4).[18] Health-related outcomes that have been found to be related to an increase in daily hassles include the onset of migraine headaches,[19] increase in symptoms of irritable bowel syndrome,[20] and increase in symptoms of genital herpes.[21]

As an adjunct to hassles, *uplifts* are defined as positive experiences or temporary joys that are likely to occur in everyday life.[5] This concept seems comparable with the term *eustress* described earlier by Selye. Uplifts may modify the negative effects of daily hassles. Although studies of the effects of negative experiences (hassles or life events) are more plentiful, scientists are beginning to evaluate the effect of positive emotional states and experiences on health outcomes. In general, positive emotional states or "emotional assets" are believed to be associated with healthier physiologic functioning, especially with respect to the cardiovascular and immune systems.[22]

One's dispositional style, be it optimism, pessimism, or hostility, modulates one's reactivity to stress, and this, in turn, likely affects health outcomes. Norman Cousins, the well-known journalist, reported that 10 minutes of laughter alleviated the pain he suffered from the chronic debilitating disease of ankylosing

TABLE 8-4	Examples of Daily Hassles
Caring for disabled child	
Chronic pain	
Concerns about job security	
Deadlines	
Difficulties with friends	
Inadequate financial resources	
Inconsiderate smokers	
Job dissatisfaction	
Marital problems	
Misplacing or losing things	
Planning meals	
Traffic	
Waiting	

spondylitis.[23] Laughter and humor may play a role in enhancing the immune system.[24] Research is currently evaluating the effects of positive emotions, such as laughter, on the stress response and health outcomes.

STRESS AS A TRANSACTION

Appraisal

In contrast to theories of stress as a response or stimulus, Lazarus's theory focuses on the person-environment transaction and the cognitive appraisal of demands and coping options.[5] When a person encounters an environmental demand, a multitude of internal and external data are received at the neurocognitive level. Lazarus proposed that these data are interpreted during the process of cognitive appraisal. **Appraisal** is a judgment or evaluative process that includes recognizing the degree of demands, or stressors, placed on the individual (Fig. 8-1). The appraisal process also involves the recognition of available resources or options that help one to deal with potential or actual demands.

During *primary appraisal,* demands are assessed according to the possible impact on the individual's well-being (i.e., what is at stake). A person decides if the situation is worthy of attention and perhaps mobilization of adaptive resources. Demands can be judged as irrelevant, benign-positive, or stressful. If demands are appraised as stressful, they can be classified as representing harm or loss, threat, or challenge. Harm or loss demands involve actual damage, and threat demands involve anticipated harm or loss. Challenge demands differ from threat and harm or loss demands because they are viewed as a potential for personal gain or growth. For example, hiking in the wilderness may place demands on the individual that will provide an opportunity to test and exhibit strength and endurance. Therefore stress is a situation in which demands exceed the individual's adaptive resources. If

an adaptive response to these demands does not occur, negative consequences will result.[5]

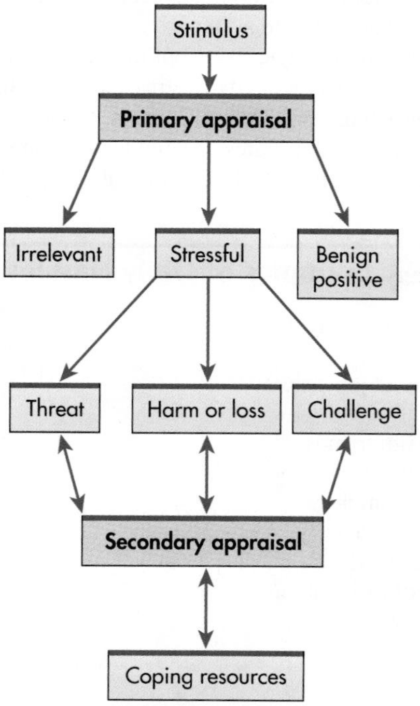

Secondary appraisal refers to the process of recognizing and evaluating the coping resources and options that are available. The costs and benefits of acting versus not acting are considered. Primary and secondary appraisals often occur simultaneously and interact with each other in determining stress. *Cognitive reappraisal* is the process of continuously relabeling cognitive appraisals. Certain factors influence the labeling of appraisals.[5] Situational factors include the intensity of the external demands, the immediacy of the expected impact, and ambiguity. Person-related factors include motivational characteristics, belief systems, and intellectual resources and skills.

Emotions are an integral component of Lazarus's person-environment transactional model. According to Lazarus, without emotions an individual would not be challenged or threatened. The primary and secondary appraisals of a threat and the meaning attached to the event give rise to a pattern of stress-related emotions.[24] Some stress-related emotions include anger, anxiety, guilt, fright, and sadness. For example, if a person appraised a situation as being dangerous and if that person believes he or she cannot cope, the emotions of anxiety or fright will arise. Emotions "depend on appraisals, which arise from and facilitate our struggles to survive and flourish in the world."[25]

Theoretic Summary

The role of *perception* is the key to understanding the difference between the three major stress theories presented. In Selye's stress response theory, all demands are stressors with the capacity to elicit a nonspecific adaptive response (i.e., GAS). Conditioning factors in individuals influence the stress response. In the life-change theory, perceived stressfulness of the event is not considered because each individual receives the same score for a certain stressor. In the Lazarus transaction theory, the cognitive appraisal process determines whether the demands will be assessed as stressful. Through cognitive appraisal, individuals experience different outcomes in dealing with demands, not only because of conditioning factors, but also as a result of how the demand is perceived and what personal meaning is attached to the demand. An event that is stressful to one individual may not be stressful to another.

PHYSIOLOGIC RESPONSE TO STRESS

To simplify the description of the physiologic response to stress, the following discussion is divided into the roles of the nervous system, the endocrine system, and the immune system. However, these systems are interrelated, and thus the ultimate response of the person to stress reflects the integration of the three systems (Fig. 8-2). Further, stress activation of these systems affects other physiologic systems, such as the cardiovascular, respiratory, gastrointestinal, renal, and reproductive systems. As a result, an individual's response to stress has the potential to lead to diseases of adaptation in any system. Understanding the physiologic changes associated with stress will help provide the foundation for the assessment of the patient experiencing stress and the implications for health outcomes.

Nervous System

Stressors, or demands, may be physical, psychologic, or social. The body will respond physiologically to both actual and potential stressors. The complex process by which an event is

FIG. 8-1 Cognitive appraisal process.

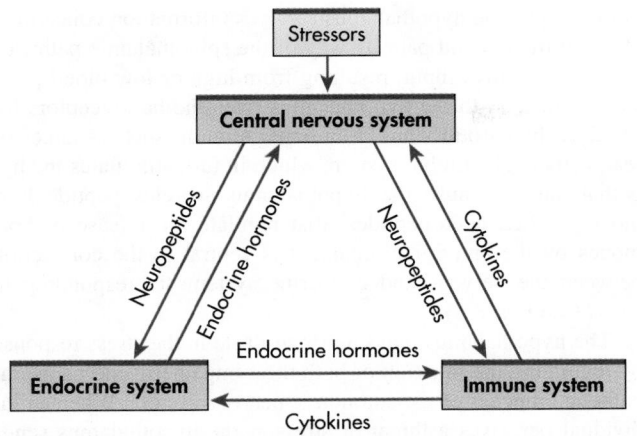

FIG. 8-2 Neurochemical links among the nervous, endocrine, and immune systems. The communication among these three systems is bidirectional.

perceived as a stressor and by which the body responds is not fully understood. The hypothalamus participates in both the emotional and physiologic responses to stressors. This control is significant because most stressors precipitate an emotional reaction. In addition to the hypothalamus, other parts of the central nervous system, including the cerebral cortex, limbic system, and reticular formation, are involved in the neural control of emotions and the physiologic response to stress (Figs. 8-3 and 8-4). The functions of these structures are closely interrelated.

Cerebral Cortex. After an external event has occurred, input is sent to the cerebral cortex via sensory impulses from the peripheral nervous system, including the eyes and the ears. For example, the pressure of a restraint on an arm or leg that is applied too tightly will act as a stressor. Afferent impulses that travel to the cortex from the periphery via the spinal cord (spinothalamic pathways) also activate the reticular formation in the area of the brainstem. The reticular formation then re-

lays input to the thalamus and from the thalamus to the cerebral cortex. This network of neurons, which is involved with arousal and consciousness, is called the **reticular activating system** (RAS). The RAS functions to maintain wakefulness and alertness.

The somatic, auditory, and visual associative areas of the cerebral cortex receive input from the peripheral sensory fibers and then interpret it. The prefrontal area serves to reduce the speed of the associative functions so that the person has time to evaluate the information in light of past experiences and future consequences (primary and secondary appraisal) and to plan a course of action. All these functions are involved in the perception of a stressor.

The temporal lobes of the cerebral cortex contain the auditory association areas, which, when stimulated, produce the sensation of fear. Stimulation of the temporal lobes can result in sounds that seem louder or softer, visual displays that seem nearer or farther, and experiences that seem familiar or strange. These effects modify the perception of stress.

Limbic System. The *limbic system*, which lies in the inner midportion of the brain near the base, includes the septum, cingulate gyrus, amygdala, hippocampus, and anterior nuclei of the thalamus. (Although the hypothalamus is located in the center of these structures it is not considered a part of the limbic system.) The limbic system is an important mediator of emotions and behavior. When these structures are stimulated, emotions, feelings, and behaviors can occur that ensure survival and self-preservation, such

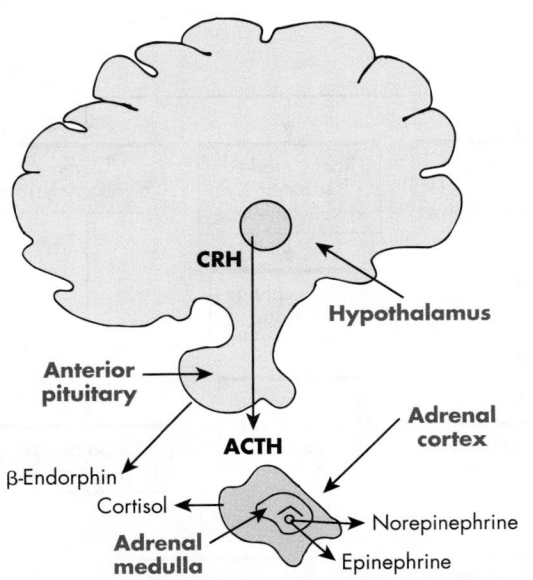

FIG. 8-3 Hypothalamic–pituitary–adrenal axis. *ACTH,* Adrenocorticotropic hormone; *CRH,* corticotropin-releasing hormone.

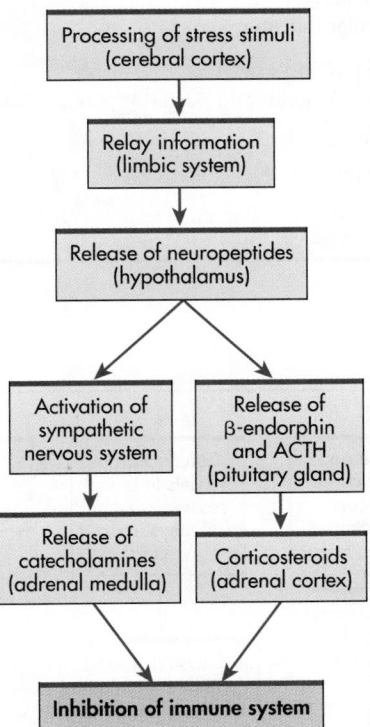

FIG. 8-4 The cerebral cortex processes stressful stimuli and relays the information via the limbic system to the hypothalamus. Corticotropin-releasing hormone (CRH) stimulates the release of adrenocorticotropic hormone (ACTH) from the pituitary gland. ACTH stimulates the adrenal cortex to release corticosteroids. The sympathetic nervous system is also stimulated, resulting in the release of epinephrine and norepinephrine.

as feeding, sociability, and sexuality. The cerebral cortex and limbic system interact to serve the experiential and executive functions of emotion. Endorphins are found in structures of the limbic system and in the thalamus, brain, and spinal cord. They are known to reduce the perception of painful stimuli. Endogenous opioids have also been shown to increase in response to stress in the absence of pain.

Reticular Formation. The *reticular formation* is located between the lower end of the brainstem and the thalamus. It contains the RAS, which sends impulses contributing to alertness to the limbic system and to the cerebral cortex and thalamus. In addition to receiving input from the periphery, the RAS also receives impulses from the hypothalamus. When the RAS is stimulated, it increases its output of impulses, leading to wakefulness. Both physiologic stress and perceived stress usually increase the degree of wakefulness and can lead to sleep disturbances.

Hypothalamus. The hypothalamus, which lies at the base of the brain just above the pituitary gland, has many functions that assist in adaptation to real and potential threats (Table 8-5).

TABLE 8-5 **Hypothalamic Functions**
Coordinates Impulses
• Autonomic nervous system
• Body temperature regulation
• Food intake
• Water balance
• Urine formation
• Cardiovascular function
Secretes Releasing Factors
• Regulation of anterior and posterior pituitary hormones
Affects Behavior
• Sexual functioning
• Emotion
• Alertness

For example, the hypothalamus receives information concerning physical trauma and pain by way of the spinothalamic pathway. Pressure-sensitive input, resulting from high or low blood pressure, is relayed to the hypothalamus from the baroreceptors located in the carotid sinus. Emotional stimuli, such as anger or fear, activate the limbic system, which in turn stimulates the hypothalamus. Because the hypothalamus secretes peptide hormones (called neuropeptides) that regulate the release of hormones by the anterior pituitary, it is central to the connection between the nervous and endocrine systems in responding to stress (see Fig. 8-3).

The hypothalamus plays a primary role in the stress response by regulating the function of both the sympathetic and parasympathetic branches of the autonomic nervous system. When an individual perceives a threat or stressor, the hypothalamus sends signals that initiate both the neural and endocrine responses to the stressor. It does this primarily by sending signals via nerve fibers to arouse the sympathetic nervous system and by releasing corticotropin-releasing hormone (CRH), which stimulates the pituitary to release adrenocorticotropic hormone (ACTH) (see Chapters 46 and 48). In response to certain stress conditions, the parasympathetic nervous system is stimulated. This may be manifested as increased GI motility, flushing, or bronchial constriction. In susceptible individuals, stress-induced parasympathetic nervous activation may exacerbate certain condition such as irritable bowel syndrome or asthma.

Endocrine System

Once the hypothalamus is activated in response to stress, the endocrine system becomes involved. The sympathetic nervous system stimulates the adrenal medulla to release epinephrine and norepinephrine (catecholamines). The effect of catecholamines and the sympathetic nervous system, including the adrenal medulla, is referred to as the sympathoadrenal response. Epinephrine and norepinephrine prepare the body for the *fight-or-flight response* (Fig. 8-5). This response is activated by physical stressors such as hypovolemia and hypoxia and emotional states, particularly anger, excitement, and fear.

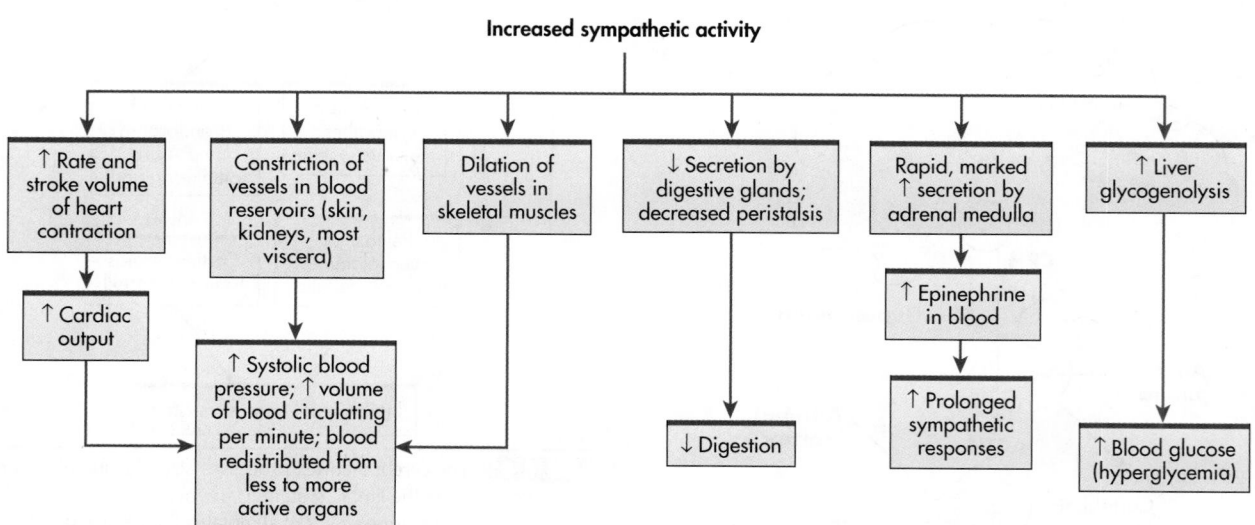

FIG. 8-5   Alarm reaction responses resulting from increased sympathetic activity. Note that these are the responses commonly referred to as the "fight-or-flight" reaction.

Both acute situational stress and chronic stress activate the hypothalamic-pituitary-adrenal (HPA) axis. The HPA axis is especially sensitive to situations marked by novelty, uncertainty, frustration, conflict, and lack of control. In response to perceived stress, the hypothalamus releases CRH, which stimulates the anterior pituitary to release proopiomelanocortin (POMC). Both ACTH (a hormone) and β-endorphin (a neuropeptide) are derived from POMC. Endorphins have analgesic-like effects and blunt pain perception during stress situations involving pain stimuli. ACTH, in turn, stimulates the adrenal cortex to synthesize and secrete corticosteroids (e.g., cortisol) and, to a lesser degree, aldosterone.

Corticosteroids are essential for the stress response. Cortisol produces a number of physiologic effects that include increasing blood glucose levels, potentiating the action of catecholamines on blood vessels, and inhibiting the inflammatory response. Corticosteroids play an important role in "turning off" or blunting aspects of the stress response, which if uncontrolled can become self-destructive. This is best exemplified by the ability of corticosteroids to suppress the release of proinflammatory mediators, such as the cytokines tumor necrosis factor (TNF) and interleukin-1 (IL-1). The persistent release of such mediators is believed to initiate organ dysfunction in conditions such as sepsis. Hence, corticosteroids act not only to support the adaptive response of the body to a stressor, but also act to suppress an overzealous and potentially self-destructive response.

Cortisol is commonly assessed in studies of stress and can be measured in plasma, urine, or saliva. Aldosterone acts to increase sodium reabsorption in the kidney tubules and, as a result, increases extracellular fluid (ECF). During stress, stimulation of the posterior pituitary results in the secretion of antidiuretic hormone (ADH), which promotes water reabsorption by the distal and collecting tubules of the kidney.

The secretion of adrenal androgens (dehydroepiandrosterone [DHEA]) and testicular androgens is typically decreased during stress. It has been shown that testosterone levels in men dramatically decrease during physical stressors, such as surgery, and also in response to psychologic stressors, such as anticipation of parachute jumping.[26] Stress effects on female reproductive hormones are more difficult to study because of their cyclic secretion. However, intense stress in females can delay ovulation and at times lead to amenorrhea.[27]

Stimulation of both the adrenal medulla and cortex results in an increased blood glucose level. This elevation provides the additional fuel for the increased metabolism needed for the fight-or-flight response. The increased cardiac output (resulting from the increased heart rate and increased ECF), increased blood glucose levels, increased oxygen consumption, and increased metabolic rate make the physical responses possible. In addition, dilation of skeletal muscle blood vessels increases blood supply to the large muscles and provides for quick movement; increased cerebral blood flow increases mental alertness. The increased blood volume (from increased ECF and the shunting of blood away from the GI system) and increased clotting time function to help maintain adequate circulation to vital organs in case of traumatic blood loss. These responses to stress illustrate the complexity and interrelated nature of the processes involved (Fig. 8-6).

The physiologic responses to stressors seem better suited to persons living in a primitive society than in the industrialized societies of today. Because of social conventions, many of the physiologic responses to stress are internalized and produce wear and tear on the body. As a result, many diseases (the diseases of adaptation) experienced by modern people are considered maladaptations to stress (see Table 8-3). For example, long-term exposure to catecholamines resulting from excessive activation of the sympathetic nervous system may increase risk of cardiovascular disease such as atherosclerosis and hypertension. Other conditions that are either precipitated or aggravated by stress include migraine headaches, irritable bowel syndrome, and peptic ulcers. Control of metabolic conditions, such as diabetes mellitus, is also affected by stress. Behavioral interventions aimed at stress reduction and relaxation have been successful in managing these diseases.

Immune System

Stress has a potential impact on the immune system.[28] **Psychoneuroimmunology** (PNI) is an interdisciplinary science that seeks to understand the interactions among psychologic, neurologic, and immune responses. Because it is now known that the brain is connected to the immune system by neuroanatomic and neuroendocrine pathways, stressors have the potential to lead to alterations in immune function (see Fig. 8-4). Nerve fibers extend from the autonomic nervous system and synapse on cells and tissues (i.e., spleen, lymph nodes) of the immune system. In turn, the cells of the immune system are equipped with receptors for many neuropeptides and hormones, which permit them to respond to nervous and neuroendocrine signals. As a result, the mediation of stress by the central nervous system leads to corresponding changes in immune cell activity. Multiple studies have shown that both acute and chronic stress can affect immune function, including decreased number and function of natural killer cells; altered lymphocyte proliferation; decreased production of cytokines (soluble factors secreted by white blood cells), such as interferon and interleukins; and decreased phagocytosis by neutrophils and monocytes.[28-30] Most of these studies have shown that stress induces immunosuppression. (Natural killer cells, lymphocytes, and cytokines are discussed in Chapter 13.)

Importantly, the network that links the brain and immune system is bidirectional (see Fig. 8-2). Signals from these systems travel back and forth.[28] This allows for reciprocal communication between these systems. Consequently, not only do emotions modify the immune response, but products of immune cells send signals back to the brain and alter its activity. Many of the communication signals sent from the immune system to the brain are mediated by cytokines, which are central to the coordination of the immune response. For example, cytokines act on the temperature regulatory center of the hypothalamus and initiate the febrile response to infectious pathogens. Moreover, the sickness behavior that accompanies infectious illness (e.g., lethargy, loss of appetite) is due to cytokines. This immune-brain communication network has led some scientists to view the immune system as a "sensory organ" that alerts the brain to invasion by microbial pathogens.[28]

Just as the brain and immune system share mutual communication pathways, so do the endocrine and immune systems. As a result, the immune system also affects the endocrine system, and hormones of the endocrine system interact with the immune system, thus altering its function (see Fig. 8-2). Both adrenal corticosteroids and catecholamines are known to suppress immune function. Interleukin-1 is a cytokine released by activated

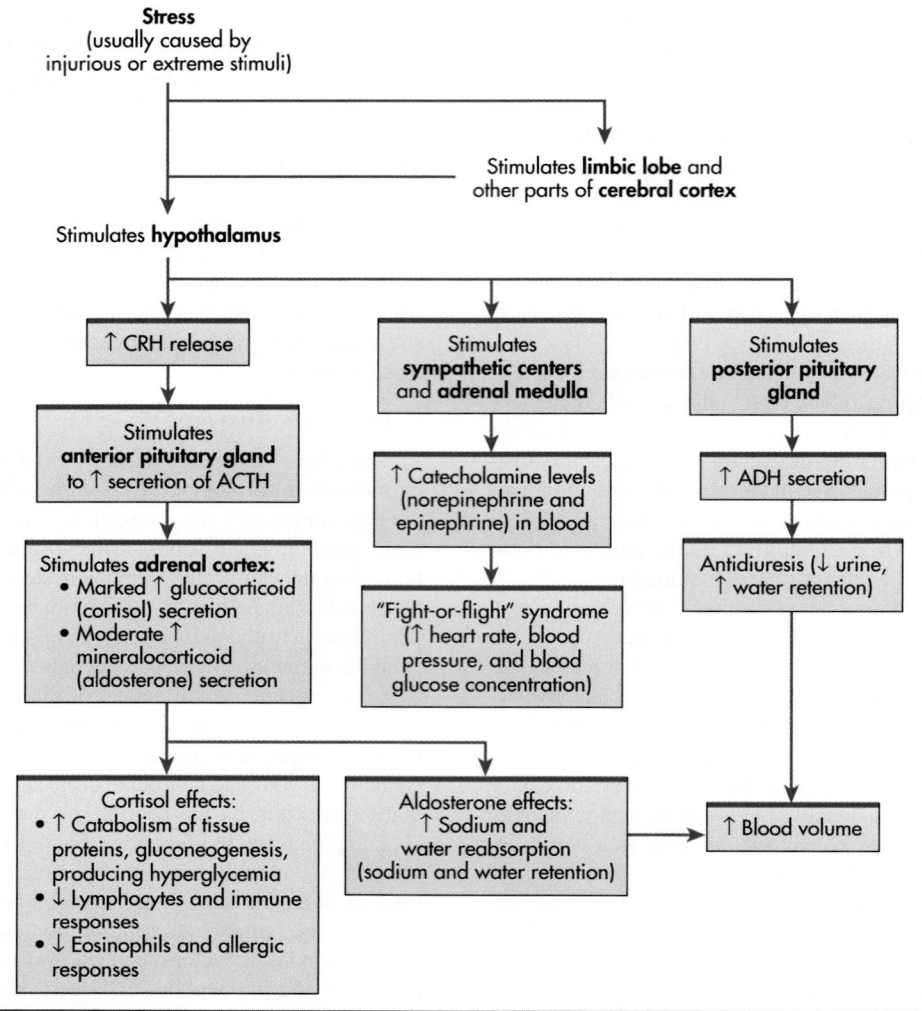

Stress
(usually caused by
injurious or extreme stimuli)

Stimulates **limbic lobe** and
other parts of **cerebral cortex**

Stimulates **hypothalamus**

↑ CRH release

Stimulates
sympathetic centers
and **adrenal medulla**

Stimulates
**posterior pituitary
gland**

Stimulates
anterior pituitary gland
to ↑ secretion of ACTH

↑ Catecholamine levels
(norepinephrine and
epinephrine) in blood

↑ ADH secretion

Stimulates **adrenal cortex:**
• Marked ↑ glucocorticoid
(cortisol) secretion
• Moderate ↑
mineralocorticoid
(aldosterone) secretion

"Fight-or-flight" syndrome
(↑ heart rate, blood
pressure, and blood
glucose concentration)

Antidiuresis (↓ urine,
↑ water retention)

Cortisol effects:
• ↑ Catabolism of tissue
proteins, gluconeogenesis,
producing hyperglycemia
• ↓ Lymphocytes and immune
responses
• ↓ Eosinophils and allergic
responses

Aldosterone effects:
↑ Sodium and
water reabsorption
(sodium and water retention)

↑ Blood volume

FIG. 8-6   Current concepts of the stress syndrome. *ACTH,* Adrenocorticotropic hormone; *ADH,*
antidiuretic hormone; *CRH,* corticotropin-releasing hormone.

macrophages that has been shown to directly stimulate the release of ACTH, thus indirectly initiating the neuroendocrine
stress response. It is now known that other hormonal systems interact with the immune system. Besides the adrenocortical hormones, other hormones such as endorphins, thyroid hormones,
reproductive hormones, growth hormone, and prolactin all modulate immune function. Although most stress hormones suppress
the immune system, some, such as prolactin, stimulate certain aspects of immunity.[28]

Because of the multiple biologic links between areas of the
brain concerned with stress mediation and emotions, there is the
possibility that stress may play a role in immune-based illness. It
is hypothesized that stress-induced immunosuppression may increase the risk of progression of immune-based diseases such as
multiple sclerosis, asthma, rheumatoid arthritis, and cancer.[28-30]
The stress of inadequately treated postoperative pain has been
shown to impair the immune system's surveillance of tumor
cells. It is believed that surgical manipulation of tumors may lead
to dissemination of tumor cells in the body and increase the risk
for postoperative tumor spread. Therefore adequate reduction of
postoperative pain and stress is important for cancer control.[31]

Stress may also alter immune function in such a manner that
an individual is more susceptible to infection. For example, psychologic stress may increase risk for developing the common
cold.[32] In a landmark study, healthy volunteers were inoculated
intranasally with low doses of upper respiratory tract viruses. The
subjects underwent psychologic testing to determine the occurrence of stressful events in their lives and their reactions to such
stresses. The results showed that both the rates of viral infection
and clinical colds increased with the degree of psychologic
stress. In this study social support buffered the harmful effects of
stress. The link between stress and susceptibility to infectious
disease has also been demonstrated in a study of elderly individuals caring for a spouse with Alzheimer's disease.[33] The chronic
stress of caregiver burden in these individuals was associated
with an impaired immune response to influenza vaccine. The results of this study suggest that chronic stress may increase an elderly person's vulnerability to influenza.

Many questions about stress and the immune response remain
unanswered. For example, it is not known how much stress is
needed to cause these changes or how much of an alteration in the
immune system is necessary before disease susceptibility occurs.

The current task of researchers in the field of PNI is to link stress-induced immune changes to illness and health outcomes.[28-30]

Behavioral strategies to enhance immunocompetence have been studied, and results are promising.[34] These strategies include relaxation and imagery techniques, biofeedback-assisted relaxation strategies, humor, exercise, mindfulness-based meditation, and social support.[35] An important study in this area showed that patients with metastatic breast cancer who were involved in a weekly support group lived longer (an average of 18 months) than patients in the control group.[36] These investigators made a final evaluation of the subjects from this study and showed that the difference in survival could not be explained by a difference in medical treatment between the two groups, thus further strengthening the importance of their findings.[37]

Effects of Chronic Stress on Brain Structure and Function

Stress leads to physiologic changes that are important to the adaptive survival of the individual. However, if stress is excessive, these same physiologic responses can be maladaptive and lead to harm and disease. Intriguing scientific evidence suggests that chronic and intense stress may in fact produce structural changes in the hippocampus.[38] The hippocampus plays an important role in long-term memory and is also important for cognitive functions, such as spatial learning. Animal models have shown that repeated stress (restraint or psychosocial stress) produces structural changes in the hippocampus.

The release of corticosteroids in response to stress appears to act in concert with certain neurotransmitters to produce stress-induced hippocampal damage. In humans, magnetic resonance imaging (MRI) studies of the brain have also shown that individuals who have endured prolonged stress (3 to 4 years) or have experienced traumatic events (violence, rape, war, natural disasters) also have selective atrophy of the hippocampus. These changes are accompanied by memory impairments.[38] Future studies are needed to address the neurochemical mechanisms that underlie stress-induced hippocampal damage and determine when and under what circumstances such hippocampal damage becomes irreversible.

Allostasis and Allostatic Load

A new way of viewing the physiologic adaptive response to stress has been proposed by neuroscientist Bruce McEwen, who has introduced the term *allostasis* to stress theory. **Allostasis** is defined as "the means by which the body reestablishes homeostasis in the face of a challenge."[39] Environmental challenges typically cause physiologic systems to operate at higher or lower levels of function than the average in an attempt to maintain homeostasis. For example, the physiologic response to low blood pressure consists of an increase in neural and endocrine functions aimed at elevating blood pressure. As a result, there is an increase in sympathetic drive, which produces peripheral vasoconstriction and increases in heart rate and contractility. In addition, there is an increase in hormones (e.g., aldosterone, ADH) needed to retain salt and water. It is important to note that these are some of the same physiologic responses that occur with any stress, including psychosocial stress.

These physiologic responses to stress are adaptive. However, if these adaptive responses persist they can accelerate pathologic processes leading to high blood pressure or development of atherosclerosis. Therefore the adaptive mechanisms are designed to "turn off" when no longer needed. If these allostatic responses do not terminate when no longer needed, over time they can produce excess "wear and tear" on the body, which McEwen terms *allostatic load*. Allostatic load is manifested as hypertension, atherosclerosis, abdominal obesity, bone demineralization, brain cell atrophy, and immune dysregulation. These responses may initiate disease in susceptible individuals or intensify existing disease. Such wear and tear or allostatic load can occur when the stress response is not properly shut off when it is no longer needed or when stress occurs too frequently (i.e., chronic stress). This modern view of the negative consequences of the stress response may increase our understanding of why intense or chronic stress contributes to illness and disease.

Stress, Health, and Illness

The preceding examination of the theoretic development of the field of stress research, and our current understanding of the biobehavioral response to environmental demands or stressors, has many implications for health and illness. Society today is filled with numerous psychosocial and economic stressors that produce the same behavioral and physiologic responses as in prehistoric times, when the physical stress of fighting a predator required the intense physiologic activation that occurs with the stress response. Because of the psychosocial nature of today's demands, such an intense physiologic response is probably unnecessary, but nevertheless it occurs. Over time, the stress response takes its toll and is believed to play a role in the development and/or progression of the so-called diseases of adaptation, or stress-related illnesses. For example, stress has been identified to contribute to a wide range of diseases, including: cardiovascular disease,[40] cancer,[41] arthritis,[42] multiple sclerosis,[43] irritable bowel syndrome,[44] fibromyalgia,[45] colds,[33] and asthma.[46]

There is much to learn about how stress affects health. Within the health care system, nurses are in a prime position to assess the level of stress in their patients, to assist them to identify high-risk periods, and to integrate stress-management programs and self-care approaches that can prevent the negative consequences of stress on health.

IDENTIFYING STRESSORS OR DEMANDS

Work-Related Stressors

The nurse should become familiar with the types of stressors experienced by various populations and individuals in particular circumstances (Fig. 8-7). For example, work-related stressors are common. Some demands are intrinsic to the job, such as poor working conditions, work overload, and time pressures. Other demands stem from the individual's role in the organization (role conflict), career development (overpromotion or underpromotion), relationships at work (difficulties in delegating responsibilities), and the organizational climate (restrictions on behavior). The extensive research on these factors and their effects validates inclusion of occupation and work experience as essential factors in assessment.

Nurses and student nurses have been extensively studied as groups experiencing high levels of stress and burnout. Stressors such as heavy workload, lack of adequate rewards, and lack of

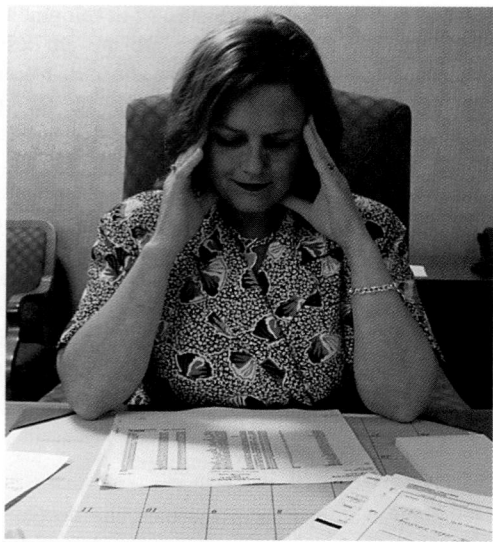

FIG. 8-7 Stress occurs every day in the lives of people.

participation in decision making have been identified in various practice settings. Knowledge of these stressors is important if nurses do not want to become victims of stress and burnout in the work environment.

Illness-Related Stressors

Another major source of stress relates to illness experienced by a patient, which often causes stress for family members as well as the patient. The nurse should assess what aspects of the illness are the most stressful for the patient. These may include such factors as physical health, job responsibilities, finances, and children. This information is valuable because it gives the nurse the patient's perspective on stressors. Although the nurse and patient generally agree on what stressors are experienced by the patient, the nurse typically rates all items as significantly more stressful than the patient does. These findings emphasize the need for understanding the patient's perception of the situation.

Results of a recent study found that at 2 weeks after discharge, intensive care unit (ICU) patients who recalled delusions, which were not counterbalanced by recall of factual memories of the ICU experience, were at greater risk for posttraumatic stress disorder.[47] Providing information, control, and reassurance are important nursing interventions that can have a significant impact on decreasing a patient's perception of stress and preventing psychologic disorders after discharge.[48] Another study identified hospital stressors of patients with acquired immunodeficiency syndrome (AIDS). Major stressors for this group of patients were loss of independence, separation from significant others, and medication problems.[49] Bone marrow transplant recipients report that their peak of emotional distress occurs after hospital admission but before bone marrow infusion and is especially marked in individuals who perceive little personal control. These results illustrate the importance of using stress-reducing strategies for patients anticipating a stressful procedure, especially for individuals who experience a lack of control.[50] Knowledge of stressors, the feelings these stressors invoke, and the psychologic sequelae they can produce will assist nurses to identify potential and ac-

tual sources of stress, as well as the impact these stressors have on the patient.

COPING

Coping is defined as the constantly changing cognitive and behavioral efforts to manage specific external or internal demands that are appraised as taxing or exceeding the resources of the person.[5] Defense processes, such as denial, may also be included as coping processes, because both defensive and coping processes intertwine and are intrinsic to the psychologic integrity of the individual. *Coping resources,* defined as characteristics or actions drawn on to manage stress (Table 8-6), include factors in the person or environment that encompass categories such as (1) health, energy, and morale; (2) positive beliefs; (3) problem-solving skills; (4) social skills; (5) social networks; and (6) financial resources.

Coping strategies function broadly in two ways: as problem-focused or emotion-focused efforts (Table 8-7). As an individual attempts to deal with demands (internal or environmental) or obstacles that create the demands, the person is said to be using **problem-focused coping** efforts. When the individual's effort is

---

TABLE 8-6   **Examples of Coping Resources**

Coping Resources in the Person

Health, Energy, Morale	*Problem-Solving Skills*
Robust health	Collection of information
High energy level	Identification of problem
High morale	Generation of alternatives
Positive Beliefs	*Social Skills*
Self-efficacy	Communication skills
Spiritual faith	Compatibility

Coping Resources in the Environment

Social Networks	*Utilitarian Resources*
Family members	Finances
Co-workers	Instructional manuals
Social contacts	Social agencies

TABLE 8-7   **Examples of Demands and Coping**

DEMANDS	COPING
Being diagnosed with diabetes	Attending diabetic education classes (P-F)
	Taking a short vacation (E-F)
Failing an examination	Obtaining a tutor (P-F)
	Having dinner with friends (E-F)
Being told that more work will be required as part of the job	Learning to use a word processor (P-F)
	Venting negative feelings about paperwork to spouse (E-F)
Being notified of an appointment for an IRS audit	Reviewing tax records with accountant (P-F)
	Practicing deep breathing exercises (E-F)
Giving a public speech for the first time	Practicing in front of family members (P-F)
	Jogging the morning of the speech (E-F)

E-F, Emotion-focused; *P-F,* problem-focused.

concentrated on methods of regulating the emotional response to the problem, the person is using **emotion-focused coping** efforts. For example, a patient with diabetes mellitus who learns to give injections is engaged in problem-focused coping. This patient is using emotion-focused coping when the distress of being diagnosed with diabetes is lessened by the thought that it would be worse if the diagnosis had been cancer. Combinations of emotion-focused and problem-focused coping can be used in dealing with the same stressor. An individual who has flexibility in coping or the ability to change coping strategies over time and across different stressful conditions is better equipped to handle stressful circumstances.

As an individual begins to deal with a stressor, modes of coping may include the following:

1. Information seeking (gathering data about the problem and possible solutions to the problem)
2. Direct actions (performing concrete acts to alter self or environment)
3. Inhibition of action (refraining from any action)
4. Intrapsychic processes (reappraising the situation; initiating cognitive activity aimed at improving feelings)
5. Turning to others (obtaining social support)
6. Escaping or avoiding

The choice of coping strategies depends on various factors. Factors that affect an individual's choice of coping strategies include degrees of uncertainty, threat, or helplessness and the presence of conflict.[4,25] If uncertainty is high, direct action is less likely to be selected as a coping strategy. If the degree of appraised threat is severe, more primitive coping modes such as panic are more likely to occur. In the presence of conflict, an individual may not be able to take direct actions. Helplessness promotes immobilization. The strategy chosen may also be influenced by the outcome of the cognitive appraisal that categorizes the stressor as harm, loss, threat, or challenge.

Individuals who experience the threat and uncertainty that accompany illness or disease use a variety of coping activities. Individuals who endure chronic pain and limited mobility pain from rheumatoid arthritis report that optimistic coping strategies were perceived to be most effective.[51] The way one responds to the experience of illness changes over time, and, in many, adaptation after an illness may lead to a reassessment of values, personal growth, and positive lifestyle changes. For example, individuals who have survived a myocardial infarction report that their illness motivated them to adopt a healthy lifestyle, and many women who have survived breast cancer report that their cancer experience improved close relationships.[52]

Spirituality has been found to be beneficial for individuals dealing with acute and chronic illness. In a study of elderly people coping with cancer, spiritual well-being was associated with hope and positive mood states.[53] Spirituality can relieve anxiety, provide a sense of purpose, and help cope with illness and approaching death. Nurses can assess the importance of spirituality and, if appropriate, support this method of coping. Additionally, hope has been found to offset feelings of despair and can empower an individual to cope with stress, chronic illness, and pain. Indeed, feelings of hopelessness and helplessness often characterize individuals overwhelmed by stress and lack of control.

Most of the health-related research has focused on types of coping strategies. Findings about which coping strategies are the most beneficial or adaptive are inconclusive and are probably in-

COMPLEMENTARY & ALTERNATIVE THERAPIES
Ginseng

Clinical Uses
Improve stamina, memory, concentration, and ability to cope with stress; enhance physical and mental performance; antioxidant and lipid-lowering agent.

Effects
Relieves stress and the effects of aging; increases energy. Can affect blood coagulation and platelet adhesion. Can decrease blood glucose levels. May cause increased blood pressure, headache, tremors, nervousness, or gastrointestinal distress. Concurrent use with monoamine oxidase (MAO) inhibitors can result in a manic-like state. Massive overdoses can result in ginseng abuse syndrome, which is characterized by hypertension, insomnia, and edema.

Nursing Implications
Should not be used in people with hypertension or cardiac disorders. Should be used with caution or not at all in patients taking anticoagulants, insulin or oral hypoglycemic agents, antihypertensive drugs, or MAO inhibitors. Should not be used for more than 3 continuous months without a 1- to 2-week break between courses.

dividualized and dependent on the context. Under certain conditions some coping mechanisms, such as denial, can be harmful. For example, a person who uses denial when experiencing symptoms suggestive of a myocardial infarction may not seek prompt medical intervention. On the other hand, when nothing can be done about a difficult situation and it is too emotionally painful to confront, denial may be a powerful way to control destructive emotions.[25] Continual assessment of stress and the strategies used to ameliorate its effects is needed, as both appraisal of and adaptation to the event change over time.

NURSING MANAGEMENT
STRESS

■ Nursing Assessment

The patient faces an array of potential stressors, or demands, that can have health consequences. The nurse must be aware of situations that are likely to result in stress and must also assess the patient's appraisal of the situation. In addition to the stressor itself, specific coping mechanisms have health consequences and therefore must be included in the assessment.

Although the manifestations of stress may vary from person to person, the nurse should assess the patient for the signs and symptoms of the stress response that occur as a result of changes in the nervous, endocrine, and immune systems. Three major areas are important in assessment of stress: demands, human responses to stress, and coping. These areas provide the nurse with a useful guide in the assessment process.

Demands. Stressors, or demands, on the patient may include major life changes, events, or situations, such as changes in family constellation or daily hassles the patient is experiencing. Demands may be categorized as *external* (environmental) or *internal* (e.g., perceived tasks, goals, commitments). Internal demands may also include physical demands resulting from disease or injury. In addition, the number of simultaneous demands, the duration of these demands, and previous experience with similar

COMPLEMENTARY & ALTERNATIVE THERAPIES
St. John's Wort

Clinical Uses
Anxiety, mild-to-moderate depression, infections, wound healing, pain.

Effects
Inhibits monoamine oxidase (MAO) and serotonin reuptake. May need to be taken for 2 to 4 weeks before an antidepressant effect is felt. Can increase memory and concentration. Also has antiinflammatory, antibacterial, and antiviral actions. Makes the skin more light sensitive.

Nursing Implications
Should not be taken with antiretroviral drugs used to treat human immunodeficiency virus (HIV) infection or immunosuppressive drugs. Must be discontinued before elective surgery due to possible MAO inhibitor effects because it may cause sedative-hypnotic intoxication. Should not be used with other psychoactive medications, MAO inhibitors, selective serotonin reuptake inhibitors (SSRIs), or tricyclic antidepressants. Should not be used unless health care provider is consulted if also taking decongestants, antihistamines, serotonin agonists, β-adrenergic blockers, and calcium channel blockers. Persons with fair skin should avoid exposure to strong sunlight and other sources of ultraviolet light, such as tanning beds.

COMPLEMENTARY & ALTERNATIVE THERAPIES
Yoga

Yoga includes a set of practices that include gentle stretches, posture, breathing practices, progressive deep relaxation, and meditation. The goal of yoga is attainment of physical and mental well-being through mastery of the body achieved through exercise, holding of postures, proper breathing, and meditation.

Clinical Uses
Yoga's primary emphasis is on general well-being. Although yoga has been shown to be beneficial in a variety of conditions, it is not considered a therapy for specific diseases. Rather, yoga employs a broad holistic approach that focuses on teaching people a new lifestyle and way of thinking. In the process, it is also found to have healing effects.

Effects
Yoga gives elasticity to the spine, firms up the skin, removes tension from the body, strengthens muscles, and corrects poor posture. Other benefits include decreasing nervousness and irritability and improving depression and mental fatigue.

Nursing Implications
Yoga can provide benefits to people at many different levels. It is important to assess why an individual is interested in yoga and provide information on the different types of yoga. Regardless of the type of yoga, deep abdominal relaxation breathing is a main component and helps one to focus on the inner self and promotes the relaxation response. Additional information on yoga can be found at *www.yogasite.com.*

demands should be assessed. Specific assessment guides for particular types of patients are also available.

Primary appraisal or perception of the demands is useful to assess. Demands may be categorized as representing harm or loss, threat, or challenge. An assessment of the personal meaning attached to the stressful situation will provide useful insight for planning interventions and self-management strategies with the patient. Family responses to demands on the patient should also be assessed.

Human Responses to Stress. Physiologic effects of demands that are appraised as stressful are mediated primarily via the sympathetic nervous system and the hypothalamic-pituitary-adrenal system. Responses such as increased heart rate, increased blood pressure, loss of appetite, hyperventilation, sweating, and dilated pupils are included. Symptomatic experiences may include headache, musculoskeletal pain, gastrointestinal upset, skin disorders, insomnia, and chronic fatigue. In addition, the patient may exhibit some of the stress-related illnesses or diseases of adaptation (see Table 8-3).

Behavioral human responses include observable actions and cognitions of the patient. Behavioral effects may include responses such as inability to concentrate, accident proneness, impaired speech, anxiety, crying, frustration, and shouting. Behavior in other aspects of life such as occupation may include absenteeism or tardiness at work, lowered productivity, and job dissatisfaction. Observable cognitive responses include self-reports of excessive demand, inability to make decisions, and forgetfulness. Some of these responses may also be apparent in significant others.

Coping. Secondary appraisal by the patient, or the patient's evaluation of coping resources and options, is important to assess. Resources such as supportive family members, adequate finances, and the ability to solve problems are examples of positive resources (see Table 8-6). Knowledge of the patient's resources will assist the nurse in supporting existing resources

and developing strategies to expand the patient's sources of support to include family, friends, and community resources. Positive social support and possessing a larger social network (relatives, friends, church groups, support groups) have been shown to exert powerful effects on the negative distress associated with illness. Conversely, aversive support (punishing, demanding, distancing relationships) may add to life stress and intensify the illness-associated pain and distress.

Coping strategies include cognitive and behavioral efforts to meet demands. The use and effectiveness of problem-focused and emotion-focused coping efforts should be addressed (see Table 8-7). These efforts may be categorized as direct action, avoidance of action, seeking information, defense mechanisms, and seeking assistance of others. The probability that a certain coping strategy will bring about the desired result is another important aspect to be assessed. Effective coping skills can be taught, and nurses are in a prime position to teach these skills.

■ Nursing Diagnoses

The importance of stress and coping to the nurse is shown by the amount of attention these concepts have received related to nursing diagnoses. A coping–stress tolerance pattern has been identified as 1 of 11 functional health patterns.[54] This pattern includes the diagnoses presented in Table 8-8. Assessment of the health pattern results in a description of the coping–stress tolerance patterns of a patient. Stressors can be identified at the individual, family, or community level.

NURSING DIAGNOSES

TABLE 8-8   Coping–Stress Tolerance Pattern

Caregiver role strain
Compromised family coping
Defensive coping
Disabled family coping
Impaired adjustment
Ineffective community coping
Ineffective coping
Ineffective denial
Post-trauma syndrome
Rape-trauma syndrome
Readiness for enhanced family coping
Relocation stress syndrome
Risk for caregiver role strain
Risk for other-directed violence
Risk for self-directed violence
Risk for self-mutilation

TABLE 8-9   Factors Affecting an Individual's Response to Stressors

Age
Cultural influences
Financial resources
Genetic makeup
Health status
Nutritional status
Personality characteristics
Previous experiences with stressors
Sleep status
Social support
Socioeconomic status

Two specific nursing diagnoses have been identified related to stress: ineffective coping and compromised family coping. *Ineffective coping* is defined as the inability to form a valid appraisal of the stressors, inadequate choices of practiced responses, and/or inability to use available resources. Potential etiologies include inadequate level of confidence in ability to cope, uncertainty, inadequate social support, inadequate resources, and high degree of threat. *Compromised family coping* refers to the usually supportive primary person (family member or close friend) providing insufficient, ineffective, or compromised support, comfort, assistance, or encouragement, which may be needed by the patient to manage or master adaptive tasks related to health challenge.[54]

■ Nursing Implementation

The first step in managing stress is to become aware of its presence. This includes identifying and expressing stressful feelings. The role of the nurse is to facilitate and enhance the processes of coping and adaptation. Nursing interventions depend on the severity of the stress experience or demand. In the person with multiple trauma, the person expends energy in an attempt to physically survive. The nurse's efforts are directed to life-supporting interventions and to the inclusion of approaches aimed at the reduction of additional stressors to the patient. For example, an individual who has endured multiple trauma is much less likely to adapt or recover if faced with additional stressors such as sleep deprivation or an infection.

The importance of cognitive appraisal in the stress experience should prompt the nurse to assess if changes in the way a person perceives and labels particular events or situations (cognitive reappraisal) are possible. Some experts also propose that the nurse consider the positive effects that result from successfully meeting stressful demands. Greater emphasis should also be placed on the part of cultural values and beliefs enhancing or constraining various coping options.

Because dealing with physical, social, and psychologic demands is an integral part of daily experiences, the coping behaviors that are used should be adaptive and should not be a source of additional stress to the individual. Generalizing about which coping strategies are the most adaptive is not yet possible. However, in evaluating coping behaviors, the nurse should look at the

short-term outcomes (i.e., the impact of the strategy on the reduction or mastery of the demands and the regulation of the emotional response) and the long-term outcomes that relate to health, morale, and social and psychologic functioning.

Various factors affect an individual's response to stressors (Table 8-9). Resistance to stress can be increased with a healthy lifestyle. Some behaviors are thought to promote and maintain health. These include the following:
1. Sleeping regularly 7 to 8 hours per night
2. Eating breakfast
3. Eating regular, well-balanced meals with minimal, healthy snacking
4. Eating moderately to maintain an ideal weight
5. Exercising moderately
6. Enjoying recreational and relaxing activities with friends
7. Drinking alcohol in moderation or not at all
8. Not smoking (best if have never smoked)
9. Learning to successfully handle life's stressors and hassles

These behaviors help people maintain good health regardless of sex, age, and economic status. These behaviors are also cumulative; that is, the greater the number of these factors habitually practiced by the individual, the better the health.

COMPLEMENTARY & ALTERNATIVE THERAPIES
Kava

Clinical Uses
Anxiety, nervousness, stress, restlessness, insomnia, tension headaches.

Effects
Antianxiety, sedative, and skeletal muscle relaxation. Side effects may include mild gastrointestinal disturbances. Frequent use can cause skin dryness, rash, and itching. Although liver toxicity is rare, it has been reported.

Nursing Implications
Contraindicated in people who are depressed or taking drugs or substances that act on the central nervous system, such as alcohol, barbiturates, antidepressants, and benzodiazepines. May increase the sedative-hypnotic effects of anesthetic agents. It should be discontinued at least 24 hours before surgery. People who have liver disease, or who are taking drugs that may affect the liver, should consult a health care provider before using kava-containing products.

NURSING RESEARCH
Stress and Hypertension

Citation

Boutain DMJ: Discourses of worry, stress, and high blood pressure in rural south Louisiana, *J Nurs Scholarship* 33:225, 2001.

Rationale

Hypertension is a significant health care problem among African Americans. Stress and worry may activate the sympathetic division of the autonomic nervous system, resulting in an increase in catecholamines. Catecholamines may further contribute to the hypertension via vasoconstriction of peripheral arterioles.

Purpose

The purpose of this study was to examine the concepts of worry and stress in relationship to high blood pressure in a rural African American sample.

Methods

Study participants included 15 African American women and 15 African American men with high blood pressure living in rural

Louisiana. A qualitative data collection approach was used. Each subject was interviewed twice over a 4-month period. In addition, the investigator conducted field experiences in the community.

Results and Conclusions

With regard to worry, the participants expressed concerns about themselves, their children, their family, and their community. Stress was expressed as associated with performing multiple tasks and confronting prejudices in the workplace and surrounding community.

Implications for Nursing Practice

Worry and stress are important health-related concepts in this vulnerable population. Nursing interventions should be focused on addressing these issues to reduce their potential impact on blood pressure management and compliance with therapy.

Good mental health practices are important for good health as well. These practices primarily result in a realistic, positive self-conception and the ability to solve problems. Teaching problem-solving skills can equip individuals to better handle present and future encounters with stressful circumstances.

Stress-reducing activities can be incorporated into nursing practice. The activities provide mechanisms whereby an individual is able to develop a sense of control of the situation. As stress-reducing practices are incorporated into daily activities, the individual is able to increase his or her confidence and self-reliance

and limit the emotional response to the stressful circumstances. Possessing a sense of control is an important characteristic that can deter the harmful effects inherent in the stress response.

The nurse can assume a primary role in planning stress-reducing interventions. Specific stress-reducing activities within the scope of nursing practice (some of which may require additional training) include relaxation training, guided imagery, cognitive reappraisal, music therapy, exercise, time management, decisional control, assertiveness training, massage, meditation, and humor (Table 8-10). Specific relaxation strategies are presented in Table 8-11.

TABLE 8-10   Examples of Stress Management Techniques

TECHNIQUE	DESCRIPTION
Progressive muscle relaxation	Self-taught or instructor-directed exercise that involves learning to contract and relax muscles in a systematic way, beginning with the face and ending with the feet. The exercise may be combined with breathing exercises.
Guided imagery	Purposeful use of one's imagination to achieve relaxation and control. An individual concentrates on images and mentally pictures oneself in the scene.
Thought stopping	Self-directed behavioral approach used to gain control of self-defeating thoughts. When these thoughts occur, the individual stops the thought process and focuses on conscious relaxation.
Exercise	Regular exercise, especially aerobic movement, results in improved circulation, increased release of endorphins, and an enhanced sense of well-being.
Humor	Humor in the form of laughter, cartoons, funny movies, riddles, audiocassettes, comic books, and joke books can be used for both the nurse and the patient.
Assertive behavior	Open, honest sharing of feelings, desires, and opinions in a controlled way. The individual who has control over her or his life is less subject to stress.
Social support	This may take the form of organized support and self-help groups, relationships with family and friends, and professional help.
Music	Music can move an individual from a negative mood state to one that is conducive to relaxation and positive affect.
Journaling	Individual expresses self in written form. This may include such things as personal events, thoughts, feelings, memories, and perceptions. May allow individual to increase self-awareness and coping.
Meditation	Meditative technique (e.g., transcendental meditation, mindfulness meditation) leads to a decrease in the psychologic and physiologic response to stress.
Biofeedback	Therapeutic modality that enables individuals to monitor skin temperature, muscle tension, heart rate, brain waves, and/or skin conductance to learn to control these physiologic responses to stressful or challenging events (see Chapter 7).
Massage	Systematic manipulation of the soft tissues of the body to reduce tension and enhance health and healing.

A number of nurse researchers have provided evidence for the effectiveness of stress management interventions in a variety of ill populations.[55-57] Nurses are in an ideal situation to take the lead in integrating stress management in their practice. Nurses are also well equipped to develop and test the effectiveness of new approaches to manage stress and promote positive health outcomes. However, it is important for the nurse to recognize when the patient or family needs to be referred to a professional with advanced training in counseling.

TABLE 8-11   **Relaxation Strategies**

Rhythmic Breathing*
1. Provide a quiet environment.
2. Help the patient get comfortable by elevating the legs with the knees bent (relaxing the leg, back, and abdominal muscles) or supporting the neck with a pillow. Check to see that arms and legs are not crossed.
3. Instruct patient to close eyes and to breathe in and out slowly, saying, "Breathe in, 2, 3, 4; breathe out, 2, 3, 4."
4. Once rhythmic breathing is established, instruct patient to listen to your voice, and with a low and steady voice, instruct patient to do the following:
   Breathe in and out slowly and deeply.
   Try to breathe from the abdomen.
   Feel more relaxed with each exhalation.
   Try to identify your own special feeling of relaxation (e.g., light and weightless or very heavy).
   While you are breathing, let your imagination take you to a place you remember as peaceful and pleasant; look around, listen to the sounds, feel the air, notice the smells.
   When you are ready to end this relaxation exercise, count silently from 1 to 3; on 1, move your lower body; on 2, move your upper body; on 3, breathe in deeply, open your eyes, and while breathing out slowly, say silently: "I am relaxed and alert." Stretch as if just waking up.

Progressive Relaxation*
1. Follow steps 1, 2, and 3 of rhythmic breathing.
2. Once the patient is breathing slowly and comfortably, instruct patient to tighten and relax an ordered succession of muscle groups, tensing and then relaxing them, while *feeling* the part relax.
3. Instruct patient to tense and then relax the calves, knees, and so on.

Relaxation by Sensory Pacing
1. Follow steps 1 and 2 of rhythmic breathing.
2. Instruct patient to slowly repeat and finish either in a low voice or to self each of the following sentences:
   Now I am aware of seeing . . .
   Now I am aware of feeling . . .
   Now I am aware of hearing . . .
   Instruct patient to repeat and complete each sentence 4 times, then 3 times, then twice, and finally once.
3. Instruct patient to allow the eyes to close when they feel heavy.

Relaxation by Color Exchange
1. Follow steps 1, 2, and 3 of rhythmic breathing.
2. Instruct patient to notice any tension, tightness, aches, or pains in the body and to give that sensation the first color that comes to mind.
3. Instruct patient to breathe in pure white light from the universe and send the light to the tense or painful place in the body, letting the white light surround the color of the discomfort.
4. Instruct patient to exhale the color of the discomfort and let the white light take its place.
5. Instruct patient to continue breathing in the white light and exhaling the color of the discomfort, allowing the white light to fill the entire body and bring about a sense of peace, well-being, and energy.

Modified Autogenic Relaxation
1. Follow steps 1, 2, and 3 of rhythmic breathing.
2. Instruct patient to repeat each of the following phrases to self 4 times, saying the first part of the phrase while breathing in for 2 to 3 sec, holding the breath for 2 to 3 sec, then saying the last part of the phrase while breathing out for 2 to 3 sec:

Breathing in	Breathing out
I am	relaxed
My arm and legs	are heavy and warm
My heartbeat	is calm and regular
My breathing	is free and easy
My abdomen	is loose and warm
My forehead	is cool
My mind	is quiet and still

Relaxing with Music
1. Provide patient with a tape recorder and headset.
2. Ask patient to select a favorite cassette of slow, quiet music.
3. Instruct patient to get into a comfortable position (either sitting or lying down but with arms and legs uncrossed) and to close eyes and listen to the music through the headset.
4. Instruct patient to imagine floating or drifting with the music while listening.

Rhythmic Massage
1. Massage near the area of tension in a circular, firm manner.
2. Avoid tender, red, or swollen areas.

*In conditioning of a relaxation response, a "signal breath" involving deep inhalation through the nose and forceful exhalation through the mouth is the key. The signal breath precedes and follows each run through the exercise.

CRITICAL THINKING EXERCISES

Case Study
Stress Associated with Cancer Diagnosis and Treatment

Patient Profile. Mrs. Zyskowski, a Polish immigrant, was diagnosed with stage II breast cancer at age 44. Her treatment plan included lumpectomy followed by a regimen of chemotherapy and then radiation therapy. She attributed her breast cancer to her depression, which developed while she cared for her mother, who suffered from Alzheimer's disease. Her mother passed away 6 months before her breast cancer diagnosis.

After completion of her lengthy breast cancer therapy, Mrs. Zyskowski's depression worsened. She no longer had her frequent visits to the breast cancer center, and she missed the interaction with the nurses and other patients. In addition, Mrs. Zyskowski feared that her cancer would recur and she worried that she would "pass it on" to her two teenage daughters. She would not discuss her fears with her husband or daughters because she did not want to burden them. She began to lose weight and constantly felt fatigued. She felt "alone" with her cancer and lost interest in other aspects of her life. She thought about joining a cancer support group but was embarrassed by her Polish accent.

CRITICAL THINKING QUESTIONS

1. Consider Mrs. Zyskowski's situation and describe the physiologic and psychologic stressors that she is dealing with. Describe the possible effects of these stressors on her health status.
2. What specific nursing interventions can be included in Mrs. Zyskowski's management that will enhance her adaptability?
3. Based on Mrs. Zyskowski's profile, what resources are available to Mrs. Zyskowski to help her cope with her cancer diagnosis and treatment?
4. Should Mrs. Zyskowski join a cancer support group? If so, how might this benefit her?
5. Review the assessment data provided, and write two or more nursing diagnoses. Are there any collaborative problems?

Nursing Research Issues

1. Will the incorporation of stress management strategies for newly diagnosed cancer patients improve adaptation to a cancer diagnosis and its associated treatment?
2. What is the relationship among stressful life events, stress appraisal, and adjustment to coronary artery disease?
3. Does a nursing intervention focused on stress reduction enhance wound healing in patients following surgery?

REVIEW QUESTIONS

The number of the question corresponds to the same-numbered objective at the beginning of the chapter.

1. According to Selye, *stress* is defined as
   a. any stimulus that causes a response in an individual.
   b. a response of an individual to environmental demands.
   c. a physical or psychologic adaptation to internal or external demands.
   d. the result of a relationship between an individual and the environment that exceeds the individual's resources.
2. A patient who has undergone extensive surgery for multiple injuries has a period of increasing blood pressure, heart rate, and alertness. The nurse recognizes that these changes are most typical of
   a. the resistance state of GAS.
   b. the alarm reaction of the GAS.
   c. the stage of exhaustion of GAS.
   d. an individual response stereotype.
3. The nurse recognizes that cognitive appraisal is most evident when a patient facing surgery says,
   a. "I don't think I'm strong enough to undergo surgery tomorrow."
   b. "I'm just going to trust the surgeon and put my life in his hands."
   c. "I have too many changes in my life to deal with surgery right now."
   d. "I am so anxious about this my heart is about to leap out of my chest."

4. The nurse would expect which of the following findings in a patient as a result of the physiologic effect of stress on the limbic system?
   a. an episode of diarrhea while awaiting painful dressing changes
   b. refusing to communicate with nurses while awaiting a cardiac catheterization
   c. inability to sleep the night before beginning to self-administer insulin injections
   d. increased blood pressure, decreased urine output, and hyperglycemia following a car accident
5. The nurse utilizes knowledge of the effects of stress on the immune system by encouraging patients to
   a. sleep for 10 to 12 hours per day.
   b. receive regular immunizations when they are stressed.
   c. use emotion-focused rather than problem-focused coping strategies.
   d. avoid exposure to upper respiratory infections when physically stressed.
6. The nurse recognizes that a person who is subjected to chronic stress and/or daily hassles could be at higher risk for
   a. osteoporosis.
   b. colds and flu.
   c. low blood pressure.
   d. high serum cholesterol.

REVIEW QUESTIONS—cont'd

7. The nurse recognizes that a patient with newly diagnosed cancer of the breast is using an emotion-focused coping process when she
   a. joins a support group for women with breast cancer.
   b. considers the pros and cons of the various treatment options.
   c. delays treatment until her family can take a weekend trip together.
   d. tells the nurse that she has a good prognosis because the tumor is small.

8. During assessment, the nurse recognizes that a patient is more likely to have a greater response when stressed when the patient
   a. feels that the situation is directing his life.
   b. sees the situation as a challenge to be addressed.
   c. has a clear understanding of his values and goals.
   d. uses more problem-focused than emotion-focused coping strategies.

9. An appropriate nursing intervention for a patient who has a nursing diagnosis of ineffective coping related to inadequate psychologic resources is
   a. controlling the environment to prevent sensory overload and promote sleep.
   b. encouraging the patient's family to offer emotional support by frequent visiting.
   c. arranging for the patient to phone family and friends to maintain emotional bonds.
   d. asking the patient to describe previous stressful situations and how she managed to resolve them.

REFERENCES

1. Selye H: The stress concept: past, present, and future. In Cooper CL, editor: *Stress research: issues for the eighties,* New York, 1983, Wiley.
2. Holmes T, Masuda M: Magnitude estimations of social readjustments, *J Psychosom Res* 11:219, 1966.
3. Miller MA, Rahe RH: Life changes scaling for the 1990s, *J Psychosom Res* 43:279, 1997.
4. Lyon BL: Stress, coping, and health: a conceptual overview. In Rice VH, editor: *Handbook of stress, coping, and health,* Thousand Oaks, Calif, 2000, Sage Publications.
5. Lazarus R, Folkman S: *Stress, appraisal, and coping,* New York, 1984, Springer.
6. Selye H: *The stress of life,* New York, 1956, McGraw-Hill.
7. Lacey JI, Lacey BC: Verification and extension of the principle of autonomic response stereotype, *Am J Psychol* 71:50, 1958.
8. McFetridge JA, Sherwood A: Hemodynamic and sympathetic nervous system responses to stress during the menstrual cycle, *AACN Clinical Issues* 11:158, 2000.
9. Kenney ME, Laudenslager ML: Beyond stress: the role of individual difference factors in psychoneuroimmunology, *Brain Behav Immun* 13:73, 1999.
10. O'Keefe MK, Baum A: Conceptual and methodological issues in the study of chronic stress, *Stress Med* 6:105, 1990.
11. Sarason, IG, Johnson, JH, Siegel JM: Assessing the impact of life changes: developing a life experiences survey, *J Consul Clin Psychol* 6:932, 1978.
12. Holmes TH, Masuda M: Life change and illness susceptibility. In Dohrenwend BA, Dohrenwend BP, editors: *Stressful life events: their nature and effects,* New York, 1974, Wiley.
13. Ford-Gilboe M, Cohen JA: Hardiness: a model of commitment, challenge, and control. In Rice VH, editor: *Stress, coping, and health,* Thousand Oaks, Calif, 2000, Sage Publications.
14. Antonovsky AA: *Unraveling the mystery of health: how people manage stress and stay well,* San Francisco, 1987, Jossey-Bass.
15. Williams SJ: The relationship among stress, hardiness, sense of coherence, and illness in critical care nurses, *Medical Psychotherapy* 3:171, 1990.
16. Wolff AC, Ratner PA: Stress, social support, and sense of coherence, *West J Nurs Res* 21:182, 1999.
17. Wagnild GM, Young HM: Development and psychometric evaluation of the resilience scale, *J Nurs Meas* 1:165, 1993.
18. Kanner AD et al: Comparison of two modes of stress measurement: daily hassles and uplifts versus major life events, *J Behav Med* 4:1, 1981.
19. Sorbi MJ, Maassen GH, Spierings EL: A time series analysis of daily hassles and mood changes in the 3 days before the migraine attack, *Behav Med* 22:103, 1996.
20. Dancey CP et al: The relationship between hassles, uplifts, and irritable bowel syndrome: a preliminary study, *J Psychosom Res* 39:827, 1995.
21. Swanson JM, Dibble SJ, Chenitz WC: Clinical features and psychosocial factors in young adults with genital herpes, *J Nurs Scholarship* 27:16, 1995.
22. Salovey P et al: Emotional states and physical health, *Am Psychol* 55:110, 2000.
23. Cousins N: *Anatomy of an illness,* New York, 1991, Bantam Doubleday Dell.
24. Kimata H: Effect of humor on allergen-induced wheal reactions, *J Am Med Assoc* 285:738, 2001.
25. Lazarus RS: Evolution of a model of stress, coping, and discrete emotions. In Rice VH, editor: *Stress, coping, and health,* Thousand Oaks, Calif, 2000, Sage Publications.
26. Chatterton RT et al: Hormonal responses to psychological stress in men preparing for skydiving, *J Clin Endocrinol Metab* 82:2503, 1997.
27. Magiakou MA et al: The hypothalamic-pituitary-adrenal axis and the female reproductive system, *Ann N Y Acad Sci* 816:42, 1997.
28. Witek-Janusek L, Mathews HL: Stress, immunity, and health outcomes. In Rice VH, editor: *Stress, coping, and health,* Thousand Oaks, Calif, 2000, Sage Publications.
29. Kiecolt-Glaser JK, Glaser R: Psychoneuroimmunology and health consequences: data and shared mechanisms, *Psychosom Med* 57:269, 1995.
30. Cohen S, Herbert TB: Health psychology: psychological factors and physical disease from the perspective of human psychoneuroimmunology, *Annu Rev Psychol* 47:113, 1996.
31. Page GG, Ben-Eliyahu S: The immune-suppressive nature of pain, *Semin Oncol Nurs* 13:10, 1997.
32. Cohen S et al: Types of stressors that increase susceptibility to the common cold in healthy adults, *Health Psychol* 17:214, 1998.
33. Kiecolt-Glaser JK et al: Chronic stress alters the immune response to influenza virus vaccine in older adults, *Proc Natl Acad Sci U S A* 93:3043, 1996.
34. Ironson G, Antoni M, Lutgendorf S: Can psychological interventions affect immunity and survival? Present findings and suggested targets with a focus on cancer and human immunodeficiency virus, *Mind/Body Med* 1:85, 1995.
35. Robinson FP, Mathews HL, Witek-Janusek L: Stress reduction and HIV disease: a review of intervention studies using a psychoneuroimmunology framework, *J Assoc Nurses AIDS Care* 11:87, 2000.
36. Spiegel D et al: Effect of psychosocial treatment on survival of patients with metastatic breast cancer, *Lancet* 2:881, 1989.
37. Kogon MM et al: Effects of medical and psychotherapeutic treatment on the survival of women with metastatic breast carcinoma, *Cancer* 80:225, 1997.
38. McEwen BS: Effects of adverse experiences for brain structure and function, *Biol Psychiatry* 48:721, 2000.

39. McEwen BS: Protective and damaging effects of stress mediators: central role of the brain, *Prog Brain Res* 122:25, 2000.

40. Benschop RJ et al: Cardiovascular and immune responses to acute psychological stress in young and old women: a meta-analysis, *Psychosom Med* 60:290, 1998.

41. Cohen S, Rabin BS: Psychologic stress, immunity, and cancer, *J Natl Cancer Inst* 90:30, 1998.

42. Crofford LJ, Jacobson J, Young E: Modeling the involvement of the hypothalamic-pituitary-adrenal and hypothalmic-pituitary-gonadal axes in autoimmune and stress-related rheumatic syndromes in women, *J Womens Health* 8:203, 1999.

43. Prat A, Antel JP: Neuroendocrine influences on autoimmune disease: multiple sclerosis. In Ader R, Cohen N, editors: *Psychoneuroimmunology,* New York, 2001, Academic Press.

44. Bennett EJ et al: Level of chronic life stress predicts clinical outcome in irritable bowel syndrome, *Gut* 43:256, 1998.

45. Shaver JLF et al: Sleep, psychological distress, and stress arousal in women with fibromyalgia, *Res Nurs Health* 20:247, 1997.

46. Wright RJ, Rodriquez M, Cohen S: Review of psychosocial stress and asthma: an integrated biopsychosocial approach, *Thorax* 53:1066, 1998.

47. Jones C et al: Memory, delusions, and the development of acute post-traumatic stress disorder–related symptoms after intensive care, *Crit Care Med* 29:573, 2001.

48. Kenny DT et al: *Stress and health: research and clinical applications,* Amsterdam, 2000, Harwood Academic.

49. Van Servellen G, Lewis CE, Leake B: The stresses of hospitalization among AIDS patients on integrated and special care units, *Int J Nurs Stud* 27:235, 1990.

50. Fife BL et al: Longitudinal study of adaptation to the stress of bone marrow transplantation, *J Clin Oncol* 18:1539, 2000.

51. Mahat G: Perceived stressors and coping strategies among individuals with rheumatoid arthritis, *J Adv Nurs Sci* 25:1144, 1997.

52. Petrie KJ et al: Positive effects of illness reported by myocardial infarction and breast cancer patients, *J Psychosom Res* 47:537, 1999.

53. Fehring RJ, Miller JF, Snow C: Spiritual well-being, religiosity, hope, depression, and other mood states in elderly people coping with cancer, *Oncol Nurs Forum* 24:663, 1997.

54. The Association: *Nursing diagnoses: definitions and classifications 2001-2002,* Philadelphia, 2001, North American Nursing Diagnoses Association.

55. Kolcaba K, Fox C: The effects of guided imagery on comfort of women with early stage breast cancer undergoing radiation therapy, *Oncol Nurs Forum* 26:67, 1999.

56. Mock V et al: Effects of exercise on fatigue, physical functioning, and emotional distress during radiation therapy for breast cancer, *Oncol Nurs Forum* 24:991, 1997.

57. Houston S, Jesurum J: The quick relaxation technique: effect on pain associated with chest tube removal, *Appl Nurs Res* 12:196, 1999.

RESOURCES

American Institute of Stress
124 Park Avenue
Yonkers, NY 10703
914-963-1200
Fax: 914-965-6267
E-mail: stress124@earthlink.net
www.stress.org/

Job Stress Help
www.jobstresshelp.com/

National Institute for Occupational Safety and Health (NIOSH) Stress at Work
800-35-NIOSH
www.cdc.gov/niosh/stresshp.html

Sidran Traumatic Stress Institute
200 East Joppa Road, Suite 207
Towson, MD 21286
410-825-8888
Fax: 410-337-0747
www.sidran.org/

Stress Information Website
McKinley Health Center
University of Illinois at Urbana-Champaign
www.uiuc.edu/departments/mckinley/health-info/stress.html

Stress Links—Michigan Electronic Library
www.mel.lib.mi.us/health/health-stress.html

Stress Management Resources
www.mentalhealth.about.com/cs/stressmanagement/

Stress Management Website
Indiana University Health Center
600 North Jordan
Bloomington, IN 47405
812-855-4011
www.indiana.edu/~health/stres.html

University of Wisconsin at Stevens Point Stress Assess Tool
http://wellness.uwsp.edu/Health_Service/Services/stress.htm

For additional Internet resources, see the website for this book at *http://evolve.elsevier.com/Lewis/medsurg/.*

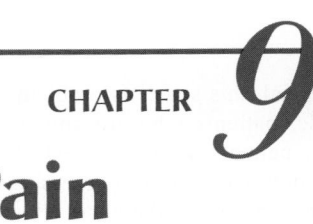

CHAPTER 9

Pain

Mary Ersek
Carmencita M. Poe

LEARNING OBJECTIVES

1. Define pain.
2. Describe the neural mechanisms of pain and pain modulation.
3. Differentiate between nociceptive and neuropathic types of pain.
4. Explain the physical and psychologic effects of unrelieved pain.
5. Interpret the subjective and objective data that are obtained from a comprehensive pain assessment.
6. Describe effective multidisciplinary pain management techniques.

7. Describe pharmacologic and nonpharmacologic methods of pain relief.
8. Explain the nurse's role and responsibility in pain management.
9. Discuss ethical and legal issues related to pain and pain management.
10. Evaluate the influence of one's own knowledge, beliefs, and attitudes about pain assessment and management.

KEY TERMS

analgesic ceiling, p. 143
breakthrough pain, p. 138
ceiling effect, p. 142
dermatomes, p. 134
equianalgesic dose, p. 141
modulation, p. 135
neuropathic pain, p. 133, 137
nociception, p. 132
nociceptive pain, p. 133, 136
pain, p. 132

patient-controlled analgesia, p. 149
perception, p. 135
physical dependence, p. 152
suffering, p. 132
titration, p. 141
transduction, p. 133
transmission, p. 134
trigger point, p. 150

PAIN

Pain is a complex, multidimensional experience. For some, it is a minor inconvenience. For others, it is a major problem that causes suffering and reduces quality of life. Pain is one of the major reasons that people seek health care. A thorough understanding of the physiologic and psychosocial dimensions of the pain is important for effective assessment and management of patients with pain.

Many health care professionals are involved in the management of the patient's pain. Pain management occurs in all clinical settings and among many different groups of patients. Nurses have a central role in pain assessment and management. Components of the nursing role include (1) assessing pain and communicating this information to other health care providers, (2) ensuring the initiation of adequate pain relief measures, and (3) evaluating the effectiveness of these interventions. This chapter presents current knowledge about pain and pain management to enable the nurse to assess and manage pain successfully in collaboration with other health care providers.

MAGNITUDE OF THE PAIN PROBLEM

Each year 15% to 20% of Americans have acute pain caused by injury or surgery. Persistent pain from conditions such as arthritis is estimated to afflict 25% to 30% of the population. Frequent back pain is experienced by over 26 million Americans between ages 20 and 64 and is the leading cause of disability in Americans under 45 years of age.[1] Over 25 million people in the

United States suffer from migraine headaches, and 9 out of 10 people report having nonmigraine headaches each year. Twenty million Americans experience jaw and lower facial pain annually. Almost 4 million people in the United States, mostly women, suffer from fibromyalgia, a condition characterized by widespread pain and other symptoms.[1] In Canada, an estimated 80% of physician visits are due to a pain-related condition. Approximately 3.9 million Canadians (17%) over age 15 have chronic pain.[2]

Despite the high prevalence of acute and chronic pain, many studies document inadequate pain management across care settings and patient populations. For example, nearly 40% of hospitalized seriously ill and older patients who died in university hospitals experienced moderate to severe pain during the last days of life despite planned interventions by nurses to encourage physicians to manage the patient's pain.[3] Studies of terminally ill patients reveal that unrelieved pain exists during the last month of life.[4] It is estimated that only 30% of cancer patients receive adequate pain relief.[5] Chronic, inadequately treated pain also is a problem among institutionalized elderly.[6-8] Consequences of untreated pain include unnecessary suffering, physical and psychosocial dysfunction, impaired recovery from acute illness and surgery, immunosuppression, and sleep disturbances.[9-11] In the acutely ill patient, unrelieved pain can result in increased morbidity as a result of respiratory dysfunction, increased heart rate and cardiac workload, increased muscular contraction and spasm, decreased gastrointestinal (GI) motility and transit, and increased catabolism[12] (Table 9-1).

The financial impact of pain is staggering. Unrelieved and inadequate management of pain costs an estimated $100 billion each year as a result of longer hospital stays, rehospitalizations, and visits to outpatient clinics and emergency rooms.[13,14] A significant number of people with pain are disabled by their pain, resulting in a serious economic problem in society, as well as a major health problem. Lost workdays because of pain add up to over 50 million dollars a year.

The reasons for the undertreatment of pain are varied. Among health care professionals, frequently cited reasons include (1) a lack of knowledge and skills to adequately assess and treat pain,[15] (2) a lack of access to practical treatment protocols, and (3) inaccurate and inadequate information regarding addiction, toler-

TABLE 9-1	Harmful Effects of Unrelieved Pain
SYSTEM	**RESPONSES**
Endocrine	↑ Adrenocorticotropic hormone (ACTH), ↑ cortisol, ↑ antidiuretic hormone (ADH), ↑ epinephrine, ↑ norepinephrine, ↑ growth hormone, ↑ renin, ↑ aldosterone, ↓ insulin, ↓ testosterone
Metabolic	Gluconeogenesis, glycogenolysis, hyperglycemia, glucose intolerance, insulin resistance, muscle protein catabolism, ↑ lipolysis
Cardiovascular	↑ Heart rate, ↑ cardiac output, ↑ peripheral vascular resistance, hypertension, ↑ myocardial oxygen consumption, ↑ coagulation
Respiratory	↓ Tidal volume, atelectasis, shunting, hypoxemia, ↓ cough, sputum retention, infection
Genitourinary	↓ Urinary output, urinary retention
Gastrointestinal	↓ Gastric and bowel motility
Musculoskeletal	Muscle spasm, impaired muscle function, fatigue, immobility
Neurologic	Reduction in cognitive functions, mental confusion
Immunologic	↓ Immune response

Modified from McCaffery M, Pasero C: *Pain: clinical manual,* ed 2, St Louis, 1999, Mosby.

ance, respiratory depression, and other side effects of opioids. In addition, some health care providers fear that aggressive pain management may hasten or cause death.[16] Nurses tend to routinely administer the smallest prescribed analgesic dose when a range of doses is prescribed.[17] Such practices do little to provide relief from unremitting pain and are not consistent with current pain management guidelines.[18-20]

Among patients, attitudes toward pain and opioids play a major role in the underreporting and undertreatment of pain.[21,22] Fear of addiction, tolerance, and side effects often makes patients reluctant to report pain or comply with a regimen that involves opioid drugs. Other hindrances include the belief that pain is inevitable and a result of worsening disease and the expectation that the drugs will not relieve pain. Fatalism and the desire to be a "good" patient who does not complain were also cited as patient-related reasons. Such attitudes are particularly common among older adults.[21]

DEFINITIONS OF PAIN

Pain is defined as whatever the person experiencing the pain says it is, existing whenever the person says it does.[23] It is a personal experience that is influenced by genetic, psychosocial, and cultural factors. The International Association for the Study of Pain (IASP) defines *pain* as an unpleasant sensory and emotional experience associated with actual or potential tissue damage, or described in terms of such damage.[24] Note that these definitions emphasize the subjective nature of pain, in which the patient's self-report is the most valid means of assessment. Although understanding the patient's experience and relying on

his or her self-report is essential, this stance is problematic in many patients. For example, patients who are comatose or who suffer from dementia, patients who are mentally disabled, and patients with expressive aphasia possess varying ability to report pain. In these instances, the nurse should incorporate nonverbal information such as behaviors into their assessment of pain.

In considering the IASP definition, it is useful to recognize that not all potentially tissue-damaging (noxious) stimuli result in pain. It is important for the nurse to differentiate pain from nociception. **Nociception** is the activation of the primary afferent nerves with peripheral terminals (free nerve endings) that respond differently to noxious (tissue-damaging) stimuli. *Nociceptors* function primarily to sense and transmit pain signals. Nociception may or may not be perceived as pain, however, depending on a complex interaction within the nociceptive pathways. If nociceptive stimuli are blocked, pain is not perceived.

Pain is not synonymous with suffering, although pain can cause substantial suffering. **Suffering** has been defined as the state of severe distress associated with events that threaten the intactness of the person.[25] Suffering can occur in the presence or absence of pain. Pain can also occur with or without suffering. For example, the woman awaiting breast biopsy may suffer because of anticipated loss of her breast. After the biopsy, she may have pain without suffering if the biopsy is negative, or pain with suffering if the biopsy is positive for malignancy. Interventions aimed at relieving pain and suffering may have some commonalities. However, some interventions for suffering will be inadequate for pain, just as some interventions for pain are inadequate for suffering.

DIMENSIONS OF PAIN AND THE PAIN PROCESS

As a multidimensional phenomenon, pain consists of five dimensions (Fig. 9-1): the *physiologic, sensory* (i.e., the perception of pain by the individual that addresses the pain location, intensity, pattern, and quality), *affective, behavioral,* and *cognitive* dimensions. The pain experience results from complex interactions among these dimensions. The following discussion describes each dimension and the ways in which different dimensions influence pain.

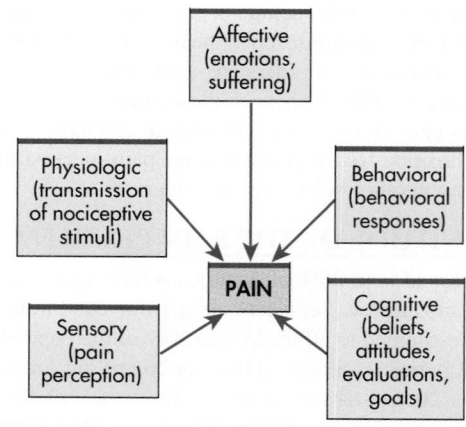

FIG. 9-1 The five dimensions of pain.

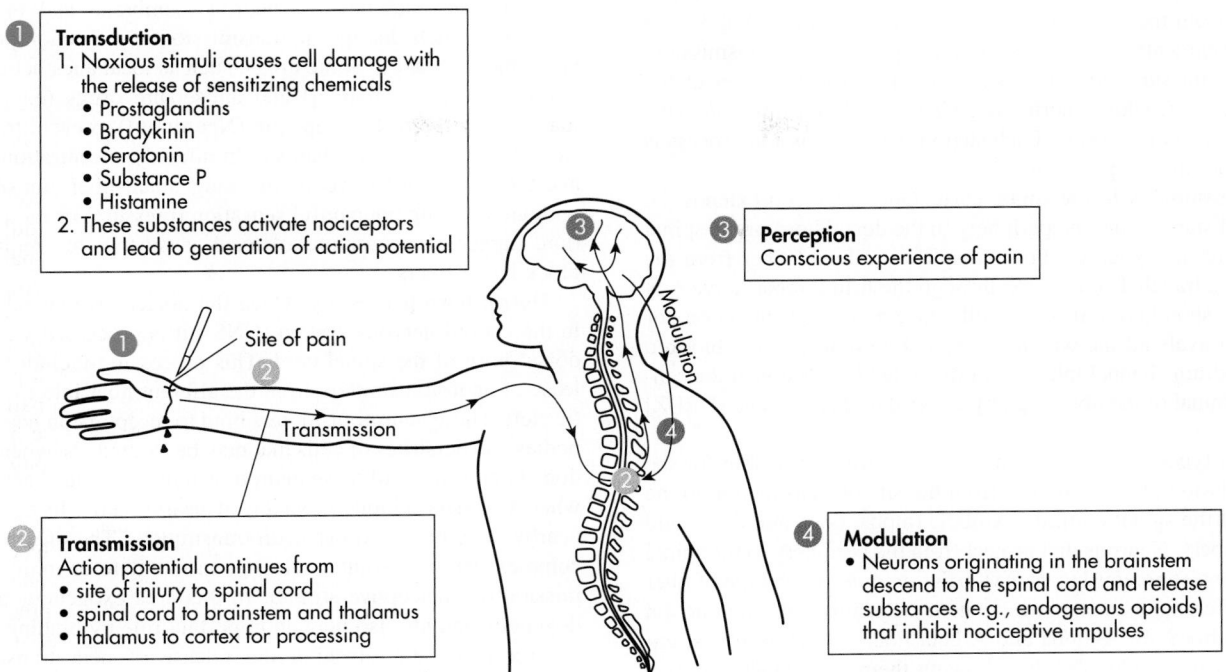

FIG. 9-2 Nociceptive pain originates when the tissue is injured. *1,* Transduction occurs when there is release of chemical mediators. *2,* Transmission involves the conduct of the action potential from the periphery (injury site) to the spinal cord and then to the brainstem, thalamus, and cerebral cortex. *3,* Perception is the conscious awareness of pain. *4,* Modulation involves signals from the brain going back down the spinal cord to modify incoming impulses.

Physiologic Dimension of Pain

Understanding the physiologic dimension of pain requires knowledge of neural anatomy and physiology. The neural mechanism by which pain is perceived consists of four major steps: (1) transduction, (2) transmission, (3) perception, and (4) modulation. Fig. 9-2 outlines these four steps.

Transduction. **Transduction** is the conversion of a mechanical, thermal, or chemical stimulus into a neuronal action potential. Transduction occurs at the level of the peripheral nerves, in particular the free nerve endings, or nociceptors. Noxious (tissue-damaging) stimuli (e.g., pressure), thermal damage (e.g., sunburn), mechanical damage (e.g., surgical incision), or chemical damage (toxic substances) cause the release of numerous chemicals into the area around the peripheral afferent nociceptor (PAN). Some of these chemicals (e.g., bradykinin, serotonin, histamine, potassium, norepinephrine) activate or sensitize the PAN to excitation. If the PAN is activated or excited, it will fire an action potential to the spinal cord.

An action potential is necessary to convert the pain stimulus to an impulse and move from the periphery to the spinal cord. The pain action potential results from two sources: (1) a release of the sensitizing and activating chemicals (**nociceptive pain**) and (2) abnormal processing of stimuli by the nervous system (**neuropathic pain),** both producing a change in the charge along the neuronal membrane. In other words, when the PAN terminal is transduced, the PAN membrane becomes depolarized, and sodium enters the cell. Potassium exits the cell, thereby generating an action potential. The action potential is then transmitted along the entire length of the neuron to cells in the spinal cord.

Understanding the chemical milieu surrounding the PAN is important to understanding the transduction of chemical, thermal, or mechanical stimuli into a neural impulse (action potential). Inflammation and the subsequent release of chemical mediators increase the likelihood of transduction. This increased susceptibility is called *sensitization.* For example, a sunburn in which there is inflammation secondary to thermal injury can result in the sensation of pain or discomfort when the affected skin is lightly touched. Several chemicals such as leukotrienes, prostaglandins, and substance P are probably involved in this process of sensitization. It is known that the release of substance P, a chemical stored in the distal terminals of the PAN, will sensitize the PAN and dilate nearby blood vessels, with subsequent production of edema and release of histamine from mast cells.[26]

Therapies directed at altering either the PAN environment or sensitivity of the PAN are used to prevent the transduction and initiation of an action potential. Decreasing the effects of chemicals released at the periphery is the basis of several pharmacologic approaches to pain relief. For example, nonsteroidal antiinflammatory drugs (NSAIDs), such as ibuprofen (Advil, Motrin) and naproxen (Naprosyn, Aleve), and corticosteroids, such as dexamethasone (Decadron), exert their analgesic effects by blocking pain-producing chemicals. NSAIDs block the action of cyclooxygenase, and corticosteroids block the action of phospholipase, thereby interfering with the production of prostaglandins (see Fig. 9-9).

Transmission. Transmission is the movement of pain impulses from the site of transduction to the brain (see Fig. 9-2).[10] Three segments are involved in nociceptive signal transmission: (1) transmission along the nociceptor fibers to the level of the spinal cord, (2) dorsal horn processing, and (3) transmission to the thalamus and the cortex. Each step in the transmission process is important in pain perception.

Transmission to the spinal cord. One nerve cell extends the entire distance from the periphery to the dorsal horn of the spinal cord with no synapses. For example, an afferent fiber from the great toe travels from the toe through the fifth lumbar nerve root into the spinal cord; it is one cell. Once generated, an action potential travels all the way to the spinal cord unless it is blocked by a sodium channel inhibitor or disrupted by a lesion at the central terminal of the fiber (e.g., by a dorsal root entry zone [DREZ] lesion).

Two types of peripheral nerve fibers are responsible for the transmission of pain impulse from the site of transduction to the level of the spinal cord: the A fibers (alpha, beta, and delta) and the C fibers. Neurons that project from the periphery to the spinal cord are also referred to as *first-order neurons*. Each type of fiber has different characteristics, which determines its conduction rate (Table 9-2). A-alpha and A-beta fibers are large fibers, enclosed with myelin sheaths, allowing them to conduct impulses at a rapid rate. A-delta fibers are smaller fibers also with myelin sheaths. Because of their smaller size, however, they conduct at a slower rate than the larger A-alpha and A-beta fibers. C fibers are the smallest fibers and are unmyelinated. They conduct at the slowest rate. The conduction rates have important implications for the modulation of noxious information from A-delta and C fibers.

Stimulation of different fibers results in different sensations. Stimulation of A-delta fibers results in pain described as pricking, sharp, well localized, and short in duration. C fiber activation pain is described as dull, aching, burning sensations and is characterized by its diffuse nature, slow onset, and relatively long duration. The A-alpha (sensory muscle) and A-beta (sensory skin) fibers typically transmit nonpainful sensations such as light pressure to deep muscles, soft touch to skin, and vibration. All of these fibers extend from the peripheral tissues through the dorsal root ganglia to the dorsal horn of the spinal cord. The manner in which nerve fibers enter the spinal cord is central to the notion of spinal dermatomes. **Dermatomes** are areas on the skin that are innervated primarily by a single spinal cord segment. Fig. 9-3 illustrates different dermatomes and their innervations.

TABLE 9-2	Characteristics of Peripheral Nerve Fibers		
TYPE OF FIBER	**SIZE**	**MYELINIZATION**	**CONDUCTION VELOCITY***
A–alpha	Large	Myelinated	Rapid
A–beta	Large	Myelinated	Rapid
A–delta	Small	Myelinated	Medium
C	Smallest	Not myelinated	Slow

*The conduction rates are important because information carried to the spinal cord by the more rapid nerve fibers will communicate with dorsal horn cells sooner than information carried by the slower fibers.

Drugs that stabilize the neuron membrane and inactivate sodium channels disrupt the transmission of the action potential along the PAN axon. Some drugs, such as local anesthetics (e.g., bupivacaine [Sensorcaine]) and antiseizure drugs (e.g., carbamazepine [Tegretol], gabapentin [Neurontin]), prevent transmission via this type of mechanism. In diluted concentrations, local anesthetics are effective in blocking small-fiber transmission without affecting nonpainful sensation (pressure) or motor function. Larger concentrations of local anesthetics are required to block larger fibers.

Dorsal horn processing. Once the nociceptive signal arrives in the central nervous system (CNS), it is processed within the dorsal horn of the spinal cord. This processing includes the release of neurotransmitters from the afferent fiber into the synaptic cleft. These neurotransmitters bind to receptors on nearby cell bodies and dendrites of cells that may be located elsewhere in the dorsal horn. Some of these neurotransmitters produce activation, whereas others inhibit activation of nearby cells. In turn, these nearby cells release other neurotransmitters. The effects of the complex neurotransmitter release can facilitate or inhibit transmission of nociceptive stimuli. In this area exogenous and endogenous opioids also play an important role by binding to opioid receptors and blocking the release of neurotransmitters, particularly substance P. Endogenous opioids, which include the

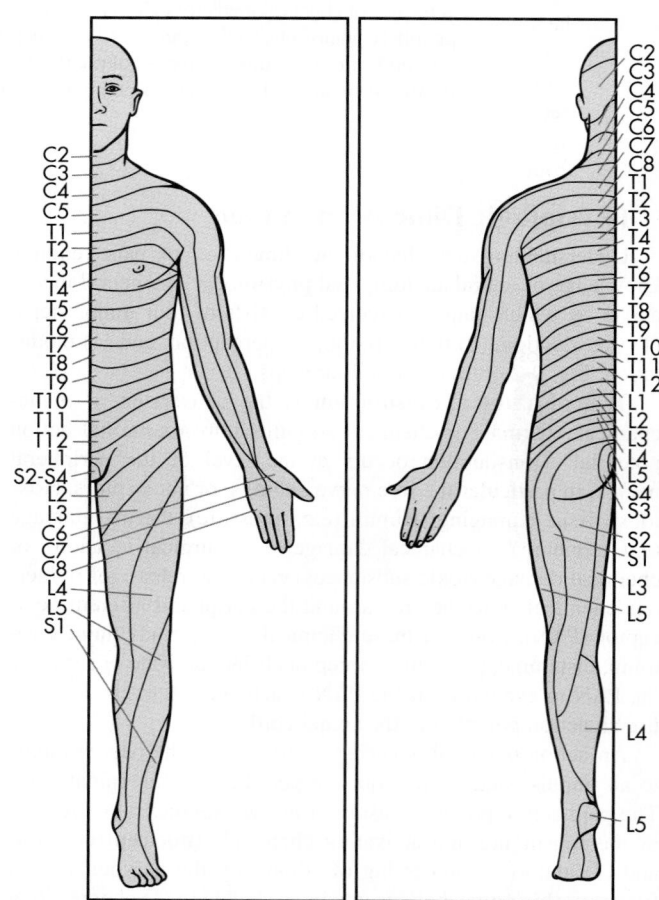

FIG. 9-3 Spinal dermatomes representing organized sensory input carried via specific spinal nerve roots. *C,* Cervical; *L,* lumbar; *S,* sacral; *T,* thoracic.

enkephalins and β-endorphin, are chemicals that are synthesized and secreted by the body. They are capable of producing effects that are similar to those of exogenous opioids such as morphine.

The dorsal horn of the spinal cord contains specialized cells called wide dynamic range (WDR) neurons. These neurons receive input from noxious stimuli primarily carried by A-delta and C fiber afferents (especially from viscera), nonnoxious stimuli from A-beta fibers, and indirect input from dendritic projections.[26] The discovery that WDR neurons receive input from noxious as well as innocuous stimuli from distant areas provides a neural explanation for referred pain. Inputs from nociceptive fibers and A-beta fibers converge on the WDR neuron, and, when the message is transmitted to the brain, the originating area of the body is poorly localized. Pain is therefore perceived in the body part presumably innervated by the A-beta fiber rather than from the visceral A-delta or C fibers. The concept of referred pain must be considered when interpreting the location of pain reported by the person with injury to or disease involving visceral organs. The location of a tumor may be distant from the pain location reported by the patient (Fig. 9-4). For example, pain from liver disease is located in the right upper abdominal quadrant, but it frequently is referred to the anterior and posterior neck region and to a posterior flank area. If referred pain is not considered when evaluating a pain location report, diagnostic tests and therapy could be misdirected.

Sensitization or enhanced excitability can also occur at the level of the spinal cord. As a variety of input is received and neurotransmitters, especially substance P and glutamate, are released, neurons in the spinal cord may respond in a prolonged or exaggerated fashion. Glutamate, an excitatory neurotransmitter, acts through N-methyl-D-aspartate (NMDA) receptors. These receptors produce alterations in neural processing of afferent stimuli that can persist for long periods. Chronic activation of the NMDA receptors can cause neural remodeling, thereby increasing the number of areas activated in response to peripheral input.

For this reason, an important goal of therapy is to prevent pain and avoid sensitization. The most commonly used NMDA antagonist currently is the anesthetic agent ketamine (Ketalar). Unfortunately, intolerable side effects, such as hallucinations, limit its usefulness. Development of newer NMDA antagonist drugs is an active area of research.

Transmission to the thalamus and the cortex. From the dorsal horn, nociceptive stimuli are communicated to the *third-order neuron,* primarily in the thalamus, and several other areas of the brain. Fibers of dorsal horn projection cells enter the brain through several pathways, including the spinothalamic tract (STT) and spinoreticular tract (SRT). Distinct thalamic nuclei receive nociceptive input from the spinal cord and have projections to several regions in the cerebral cortex, where the perception of pain is believed to occur.

Perception. **Perception** occurs when pain is recognized, defined, and responded to by the individual experiencing the pain. In the brain, nociceptive input is perceived as pain. There is no single, precise location where pain perception occurs. Instead, pain perception involves several brain structures. For example, it is believed that the reticular activating system is responsible for the autonomic response of warning the individual to attend to the pain stimulus; the somatosensory system is responsible for localization and characterization of pain; and the limbic system is responsible for the emotional and behavioral responses to pain. The cortical structures also are thought to be crucial to constructing the meaning of the pain. Therefore behavioral strategies such as distraction, relaxation, and imagery are effective pain-reducing therapies for many people. Directing attention away from the pain sensation, patients can reduce the sensory and affective components of pain.

It is known that the brain is necessary for pain perception; hence no brain, no pain. Until it is understood clearly where pain is perceived, prudent nursing practice involves treatment of any noxious stimulus as potentially painful, even in the comatose patient who may not respond behaviorally to noxious stimuli. In other words, lack of a behavioral response does not indicate that the person lacks pain perception.

Modulation. **Modulation** involves the activation of descending pathways that exert inhibitory or facilitatory effects on the transmission of pain. Depending on the type and degree of modulation, the nociceptive stimuli may or may not be perceived as pain. Modulation of pain signals can occur at the level of the periphery, spinal cord, brainstem, and cerebral cortex. Descending modulatory fibers release chemicals such as serotonin, norepinephrine, gamma-aminobutyric acid (GABA), and endogenous opioids that can inhibit pain transmission.

A number of pain management drugs exert their effects through the modulatory systems. For example, tricyclic antidepressants, such as amitriptyline (Elavil), are used in the management of chronic nonmalignant and cancer pain. These agents interfere with the reuptake of serotonin and norepinephrine, thereby increasing their availability to inhibit noxious stimuli and produce analgesia. Baclofen (Lioresal), an analog of the inhibitory neurotransmitter GABA, can interfere with the transmission of nociceptive impulses, producing analgesia for many chronic conditions, particularly those accompanied by muscle spasms. Table 9-3 presents a brief summary of how pain-relieving drugs can affect pain transduction, transmission, perception, and modulation.

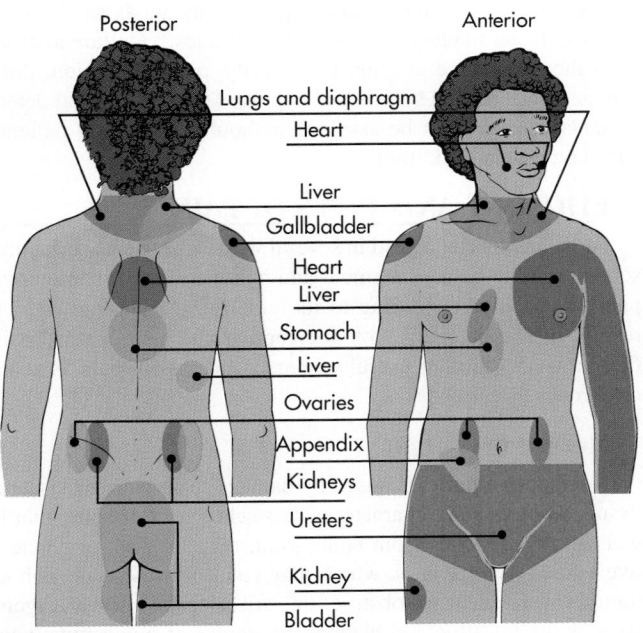

Posterior   Anterior

Lungs and diaphragm
Heart
Liver
Gallbladder
Heart
Liver
Stomach
Liver
Ovaries
Appendix
Kidneys
Ureters
Kidney
Bladder

FIG. 9-4 Typical areas of referred pain.

TABLE 9-3 Drug Therapy — Interrupting the Pain Pathway

PAIN MECHANISM	MECHANISM OF ACTION
Transduction	
Nonsteroidal antiinflammatory drugs (NSAIDs)	Block prostaglandin production
Local anesthetics	Block action potential initiation
Antiseizure agents (e.g., gabapentin [Neurontin])	Block action potential initiation
Corticosteroids	Block action potential initiation
Transmission	
Opioids	Block release of substance P
Perception	
Opioids	Decrease conscious experience of pain
NSAIDs	
Adjuvants (e.g., antidepressants)	
Modulation	
Tricyclic antidepressants (e.g., amitriptyline [Elavil])	Interfere with reuptake of serotonin and norepinephrine

Sensory, Affective, Behavioral, Cognitive, and Sociocultural Dimensions of Pain

Pain is a subjective experience that varies from person to person. Because of the complex neural mechanisms of nociceptive processing, pain is perceived as a multidimensional sensory and affective experience to which there are cognitive, behavioral, and sociocultural responses.

The *sensory* component of pain is the recognition of the sensation as painful. Sensory-pain elements include pattern, area, intensity, and nature (PAIN). Information about these elements and knowledge about the pain process are indispensable to clinical decision making and appropriate pain therapy.

The *affective* component of pain refers to the emotional responses to the pain experience. These affective responses include anger, fear, depression, and anxiety. Negative emotions impair the patient's quality of life. They become part of a vicious cycle in which pain leads to negative emotions such as depression, which in turn intensifies pain perception, leading to more depression and impaired function. It is important for nurses to recognize this cycle and intervene quickly and effectively to stop it.

The *behavioral* component of pain refers to the observable actions used to express or control the pain. For example, facial expressions such as grimacing may reflect pain or discomfort. Posturing may be used to decrease pain associated with specific movements. A person often adjusts his or her daily physical and social activities in response to the pain. In this way, pain, especially chronic pain, has profound effects on functioning.[9]

Behaviors involved with taking medications also greatly influence the pain experience. For example, a person who is reluctant to take an opioid because of the fear of addiction will likely experience distress and unrelieved pain.[21] On the other hand, a person with chronic pain may, over time, develop an elaborate regimen of drug taking and nondrug strategies to manage pain.[27]

The *cognitive* component of pain refers to beliefs, attitudes, memories, and meaning attributed to the pain. The meaning of the pain to the patient can be particularly important. For example, a woman in labor may experience severe pain, but can manage it without analgesics because for her it is associated with a joyful event; moreover, she may feel control over her pain because of the training she received in prenatal classes and the knowledge that the pain is self-limited. In contrast, a woman with chronic, undefined musculoskeletal pain may be plagued by thoughts that her pain is "not real," is uncontrollable, or is caused by her own actions.[28] These cognitions will influence the ways in which a person responds to the pain and must be incorporated into the comprehensive treatment plan.

The cognitive dimension also includes pain-related beliefs and the cognitive coping strategies that people use. For example, some people cope with pain by distracting themselves, whereas others convince themselves that the pain is permanent, untreatable, and overwhelming. Not surprisingly, people with the latter thoughts have poorer outcomes.[29]

Cognitions about the pain also determine a patient's goal for and expectations about pain relief and treatment outcomes. Moreover, factors that affect cognition, such as sedation, dementia, delirium, and mental disability, alter the pain experience and responses to pain.

Finally, the *sociocultural* dimension of pain encompasses factors such as demographics (e.g., age, gender, education, socioeconomic status), support systems, social roles, and culture. Age, gender, and education have been found to influence pain beliefs and coping strategies.[21,30,31] Age and gender also influence nociceptive processes and responses to opioids.[32,33] Families and caregivers influence the patient's response to pain through their beliefs and behaviors. For example, families may discourage the patient from taking opioids because they fear the patient will become addicted. For patients who are unable to care for themselves, family or professional caregivers may act as gatekeepers and administer inadequate doses of analgesics.[34] Culture also affects the experience of pain, specifically, pain expression, drug use, and pain-related beliefs and coping. Thus the cultural determinants of pain must be assessed without stereotyping patients based on ethnic background.

ETIOLOGY AND TYPES OF PAIN

Pain can be categorized in several ways. These categorization schemes aid in pain assessment and treatment. Most commonly, pain is classified according to its underlying pathology, which results in the categories of nociceptive and neuropathic pain (Table 9-4).[23] Another useful scheme is to classify pain as acute or chronic (Table 9-5).

Nociceptive Pain

Nociceptive pain is caused by damage to somatic or visceral tissue. *Somatic pain,* characterized as aching or throbbing that is well localized, arises from bone, joint, muscle, skin, or connective tissue. *Visceral pain,* which may result from stimuli such as tumor involvement or obstruction, arises from internal organs such as the intestine and bladder. Examples of nociceptive pain include pain from a surgical incision or a broken bone, arthritis,

TABLE 9-4	Comparison of Nociceptive and Neuropathic Pain	
	NOCICEPTIVE PAIN	**NEUROPATHIC PAIN**
Definition	Normal processing of stimuli that damages normal tissue or has the potential to do so if prolonged; usually responsive to nonopioids and/or opioids.	Abnormal processing of sensory input by the peripheral or central nervous system; treatment usually includes adjuvant analgesics.
Types	*Somatic Pain:* Arises from bone, joint, muscle, skin, or connective tissue; usually aching or throbbing in quality and is well localized.	*Centrally Generated Pain:*
	Visceral Pain: Arises from visceral organs, such as the GI tract and bladder. Can be further subdivided into the following:	• Deafferentation pain. Injury to either the peripheral or central nervous system (e.g., phantom pain may reflect injury to peripheral nerve).
	• Tumor involvement of the organ capsule that causes aching and fairly well-localized pain.	• Sympathetically maintained pain. Associated with dysregulation of the autonomic nervous system (e.g., reflex sympathetic dystrophy).
	• Obstruction of hollow organ that causes intermittent cramping and poorly localized pain.	*Peripherally Generated Pain:*
		• Painful polyneuropathies. Pain is felt along the distribution of many peripheral nerves (e.g., diabetic neuropathy, alcohol-nutritional neuropathy, Guillain-Barré syndrome).
		• Painful mononeuropathies. Usually associated with a known peripheral nerve injury, and pain is felt at least partly along the distribution of the damaged nerve (e.g., nerve root compression, trigeminal neuralgia).

Adapted from McCaffery M, Pasero C: *Pain: clinical manual,* ed 2, St Louis, 1999, Mosby.

TABLE 9-5	Differences between Acute and Chronic Pain	
	ACUTE PAIN	**CHRONIC PAIN**
Onset	Sudden	Gradual or sudden
Duration	<3 months or as long as it takes for normal healing to occur	>3 months; may start as acute injury or event but continues past the normal time for recovery
Severity	Mild to severe	Mild to severe
Cause of pain	Generally can identify a precipitating event or illness (e.g., illness, surgery)	May not be known; original cause of pain may differ from mechanisms that maintain the pain
Course of pain	↓ Over time and goes away as recovery occurs	Typically pain does not go away; characterized by periods of waxing and waning
Typical physical and behavioral manifestations	Manifestations reflect sympathetic nervous system activation: • ↑ Heart rate • ↑ Respiratory rate • ↑ Blood pressure • Diaphoresis/pallor • Anxiety, agitation, confusion • Urine retention	Predominantly behavioral manifestations: • Flat affect • ↓ Physical movement/activity • Fatigue • Withdrawal from others and social interaction
Usual goals of treatment	Pain control with eventual elimination	Pain control to the extent possible; focus on enhancing function and quality of life

or cardiac ischemia. Nociceptive pain is usually responsive to nonopioids as well as opioids. A comparison of nociceptive and neuropathic pain is provided in Table 9-4.

Neuropathic Pain

Neuropathic pain is caused by damage to nerve cells or changes in spinal cord processing. Typically described as burning, shooting, stabbing, or electrical in nature, neuropathic pain can be sudden, intense, short-lived, or lingering. Neuropathic pain is not well controlled by opioid analgesics alone, and treatment often includes the use of adjuvant analgesics, including tricyclic antidepressants (amitriptyline [Elavil]). Neuropathic pain can either be centrally or peripherally generated. *Deafferentation pain* (injury to either the peripheral or central nervous system) and *sympathetically maintained pain* (associated with dysregulation of the autonomic nervous system) are considered centrally generated pain. Painful peripheral neuropathies (pain felt along the distribution of multiple peripheral nerves) and painful mononeuropathies (pain felt at least partly along the distribution of the damaged nerve) are considered peripherally generated pain. Examples of neuropathic pain include postherpetic neuralgia, phantom limb pain, diabetic neuropathies, and trigeminal neuralgia.

Table 9-5 shows the classification of pain as acute or chronic. Acute and chronic pain are different as reflected in their cause, course, manifestations, and treatment. Examples of *acute pain* include postoperative pain, labor pain, pain from trauma (e.g., lacerations, fractures, sprains) and infection (e.g., dysuria), and angina. For acute pain, treatment includes analgesics for symptom control and treatment of the underlying cause (e.g., splinting for a fracture, antibiotic therapy for an infection). Normally, acute pain diminishes over time as healing occurs. *Chronic pain* persists for longer periods, often defined as longer than 3 months or past the time when healing would be expected to occur. Chronic pain can be disabling and often is accompanied by anxiety and depression.[35] Sometimes, chronic pain is further subdivided into malignant, or cancer, and nonmalignant pain. Chronic cancer-related pain arises from many causes, including disease progression, diagnostic procedures, anticancer therapies, and infection.[36] Cancer pain often is considered separately because its cause can be determined, its course differs from nonmalignant pain (cancer pain often worsens with documented disease progression), and the use of opioids in treating cancer pain is more widely accepted than for the treatment of noncancer pain.[19,37]

PAIN ASSESSMENT

The goals of a nursing pain assessment are to describe the patient's sensory, affective, behavioral, cognitive, and sociocultural pain experience for the purpose of implementing pain management techniques and to identify the patient's goal for therapy and resources for self-management. Often it is the nurse who is responsible for gathering and documenting assessment data and for making collaborative decisions with the patient and other health care providers about pain management. The following sections describe key components in pain assessment.

Sensory Component

The sensory component of every pain assessment should include pattern, area, intensity, and nature (PAIN) of the pain. These elements are essential in identifying appropriate therapy based on the type and severity of the pain.

Before beginning any assessment, the nurse needs to recognize that patients may use words other than "pain." For example, older adults may deny that they have pain, but respond positively when asked if they have soreness or aching.[38] The words need to be documented that the patient uses in describing pain, and the patient should be consistently asked about pain using those words.

Pattern of Pain. Pain onset (when it starts) and duration (how long it lasts) are components of the pain pattern. Acute pain typically increases during wound care, ambulation, coughing, and deep breathing. Acute pain associated with surgery or injury tends to diminish over time with recovery as tissues heal. In contrast, chronic pain usually waxes and wanes over time. For example, a person with chronic osteoarthritis pain may experience increased stiffness and pain on arising in the morning. As the joint is gently mobilized, the pain often decreases.

A patient may have pain all the time (constant, around-the-clock pain), as well as discrete periods of intermittent pain.

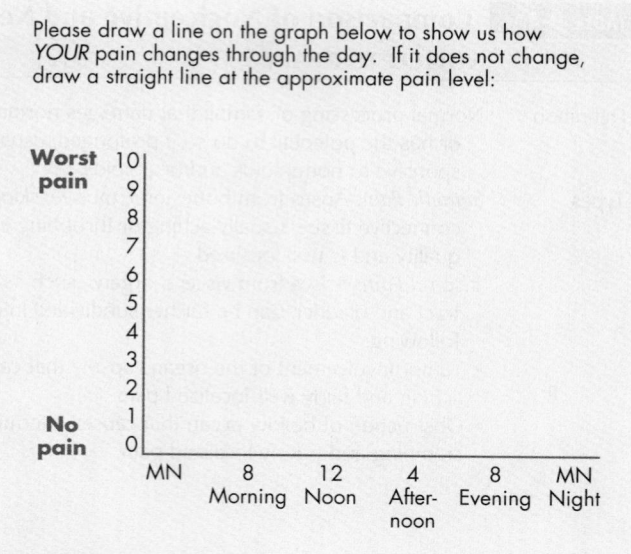

Please draw a line on the graph below to show us how *YOUR* pain changes through the day. If it does not change, draw a straight line at the approximate pain level:

FIG. 9-5   A method of tracking pain over time.

Breakthrough pain is a transient, moderate to severe pain that occurs above the pain treated by current analgesics. Many patients with cancer experience breakthrough pain. It is usually rapid in onset, brief in duration, with highly variable intensity and frequency of occurrence. Episodic, procedural, or incident pain is a transient increase in pain that is caused by a specific activity or event that precipitates the pain. Examples include dressing changes, movement, eating, position changes, and certain procedures such as catheterization.

Fig. 9-5 shows one method for the patient to document the pain pattern. This method allows the patient to report how the intensity of the pain changes with time. A similar method could be used to document the changes in the area or nature of the pain.

Area of Pain. The area or location of pain assists in identifying possible causes of the pain and in determining treatment. Some patients may be able to specify the precise location(s) of their pain, whereas others may describe very general areas, or comment that they "hurt all over." The location of the pain may also be *referred* from its origin to another site (see Fig. 9-4), as described earlier in the chapter. Pain may also *radiate* from its origin to another site. For example, angina pectoris is known to radiate from the chest to the jaw or down the left arm. *Sciatica* is pain that originates from compression or damage to the sciatic nerve or its roots within the spinal cord. The pain is projected along the course of the peripheral nerve, causing painful shooting sensations down the back of the thigh and inside of the leg.

Typically, information about the location of pain is elicited by asking the patient to (1) describe the site(s) of pain, (2) point to painful areas on the body, or (3) mark painful areas on a pain map (Fig. 9-6). Because many patients have more than one site of pain, it is important to make certain that the patient describes every location.

Intensity of Pain. Assessing the severity, or *intensity*, of pain provides a reliable measurement that is used in determining the type of treatment, as well as evaluating the effectiveness of therapy. Pain scales are useful tools to help the patient communicate the intensity of pain and to guide treatment. Scales must

Initial Pain Assessment Tool

Date _____

Patient's Name _____   Age _____   Room _____

Diagnosis _____   Physician _____

Nurse _____

1. LOCATION: Patient or nurse mark drawing.

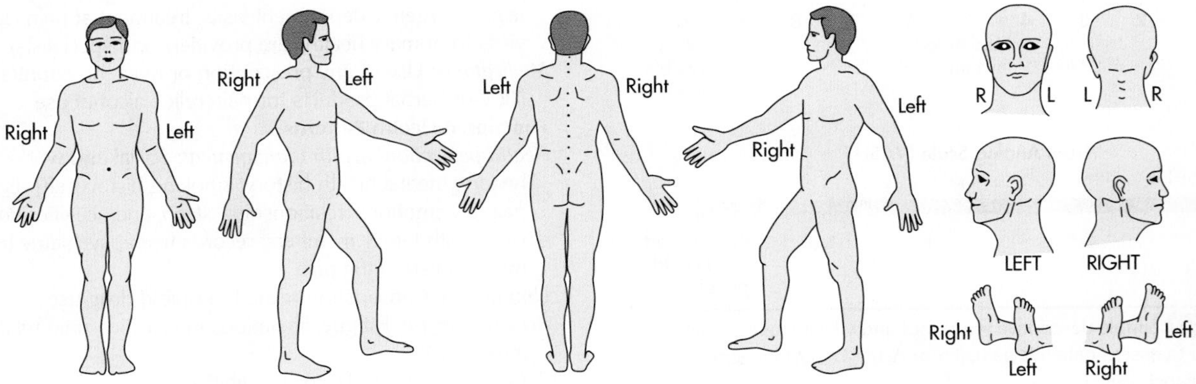

2. INTENSITY: Patient rates the pain. Scale used _____

   Present: _____
   Worst pain gets: _____
   Best pain gets: _____
   Acceptable level of pain: _____

3. QUALITY: (Use patient's own words, e.g., prick, ache, burn, throb, pull, sharp) _____
   _____

4. ONSET, DURATION, VARIATIONS, RHYTHMS: _____
   _____

5. MANNER OF EXPRESSING PAIN: _____
   _____
   _____

6. WHAT RELIEVES THE PAIN? _____
   _____
   _____

7. WHAT CAUSES OR INCREASES THE PAIN? _____
   _____
   _____

8. EFFECTS OF PAIN: (Note decreased function, decreased quality of life.)
   Accompanying symptoms (e.g., nausea) _____
   Sleep _____
   Appetite _____
   Physical activity _____
   Relationship with others (e.g., irritability) _____
   Emotions (e.g., anger, suicidal, crying) _____
   Concentration _____
   Other _____

9. OTHER COMMENTS: _____
   _____

10. PLAN: _____
   _____

FIG. 9-6 Initial pain assessment tool. (May be duplicated for use in clinical practice. From McCaffery M, Pasero C: *Pain: clinical manual*, ed 2, St Louis, 1999, Mosby, p 60. Copyright © 1999, Mosby.)

Simple Descriptive Pain Intensity Scale[1]

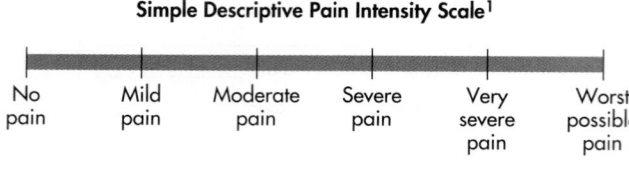

| No pain | Mild pain | Moderate pain | Severe pain | Very severe pain | Worst possible pain |

0–10 Numeric Pain Intensity Scale[1]

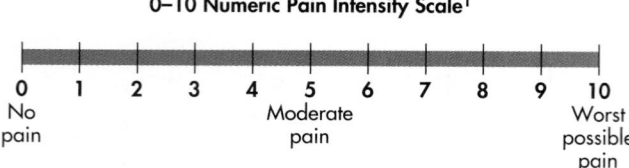

| 0 No pain | 1 | 2 | 3 | 4 | 5 Moderate pain | 6 | 7 | 8 | 9 | 10 Worst possible pain |

Visual Analog Scale (VAS)[2]

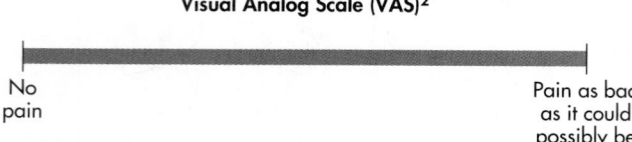

| No pain | | Pain as bad as it could possibly be |

FIG. 9-7   Simple descriptive word tool and visual analog scale (VAS) used to assess patient's pain. (From Acute Pain Management Guideline Panel, 1992.)

[1]If used as a graphic rating scale, a 10-cm baseline is recommended.
[2]A 10-cm baseline is recommended for VAS scales.

be adjusted to age and cognitive development. Numeric scales (e.g., 0 = no pain and 10 = the worst pain), verbal descriptor scales (e.g., none, a little, moderate, and severe), or visual analog scales (a 10-cm line with one end labeled "no pain" and the other end labeled "worst possible pain") can be used by most adults to rate the intensity of their pain (Fig. 9-7). For those patients unable to respond to other pain intensity scales, a series of faces ranging from "smiling" to "crying" can be used. These scales have been investigated for use in a variety of patient populations, including young children and older adults. Results indicate that they provide valid and reliable assessment data.[39,40]

Nature of Pain. The *pain nature* refers to the quality or characteristics of the pain. Many commonly used words to describe the nature of pain are included in the McGill Pain Questionnaire. This instrument captures the qualitative and affective components of pain. It also assists in identifying the type of pain. For example, patients typically describe neuropathic pain as a burning, cold, shooting, stabbing, or itchy sensation. Nociceptive pain may be described as sharp, aching, throbbing, and cramping. Recent studies indicate that different types of pain are more responsive to some therapies than others. For example, the antiseizure drug gabapentin (Neurontin) has been found to be more effective in multiple sclerosis pain described as throbbing, pricking, and cramping than for pain that has a dull or aching quality.[41]

Affective, Behavioral, Cognitive, and Sociocultural Components

Comprehensive pain assessment includes evaluation of all pain dimensions and should be completed at admission to a facility or service. This thorough evaluation should be repeated at appropriate intervals to assess the effectiveness of treatment. In an acute care setting, time limitations may dictate an abbreviated assessment of the affective, behavioral, cognitive, and sociocultural di-

TABLE 9-6	Nursing Assessment Pain

Subjective Data
Important Health Information
Past health history: Pain history includes onset, location, intensity, quality, patterns, and expression of pain; coping strategies; past treatments and their effectiveness; pain triggers; review of health care utilization related to the pain problem (e.g., emergency department visits, treatment at pain clinics, visits to primary health care providers and specialists)
Medications: Use of any prescription or over-the-counter, illicit, or herbal products for pain relief; alcohol use
Functional Health Patterns
Health perception–health management: Social and work history; mental health history; smoking history; effects of pain on emotions, relationships, sleep, and activities; interviews with family members; records from psychiatric treatment related to the pain
Elimination: Constipation related to opioid drug use
Activity-exercise: Fatigue, limitations in activities, pain related to muscle use
Sexual-reproductive: Decreased libido
Coping–stress tolerance: Psychologic evaluation using standardized measures to examine coping style, depression, anxiety
Objective Data
Complete physical examination, including evaluation of functional limitations
Psychosocial evaluation

mensions of pain. At a minimum, the effects of the pain on the patient's sleep and daily activities, relationships with others, physical activity, and emotional well-being should be assessed. In addition, the ways in which the patient expresses the pain and the strategies that the patient has used to control the pain should be included.

In some clinical settings, additional assessment information is necessary to ensure effective treatment. This is particularly true when working with chronic nonmalignant pain patients. Initial evaluation for this patient population typically includes items shown in Table 9-6. This comprehensive assessment often involves the entire multidisciplinary pain team, including physicians, nurses, psychologists, and physical and occupational therapists.

PAIN TREATMENT

Basic Principles

All pain treatment is guided by the same underlying principles. Although treatment regimens range from the relatively simple, short-term management of postoperative pain to the multimodal, long-term therapy required for many chronic pain syndromes, all treatment should follow the same basic standards.

First, the patient must always be believed. This principle reflects the basic definition of pain as a subjective experience. The patient is not only the best judge of his or her own pain, but also is the expert on the effectiveness of each pain treatment.

Second, every patient deserves adequate pain management. This principle is embodied in the recent pain management guidelines established by the Joint Commission on Accreditation of

Healthcare Organizations (JCAHO).[42] Unfortunately, many patient populations, including racial minorities,[8,33] the elderly,[43] and people with past or current substance abuse,[23] are at high risk for inadequate pain management. Health care providers need to be aware of their own biases and ensure that all patients are treated respectfully.

Third, treatment must be based on the patient's goals. Discussion about the patient's and family's goals for pain treatment should occur at the initial pain assessment. Sometimes this goal can be described in terms of pain intensity (e.g., the desire for average pain to decrease from an "8/10" to a "3/10"). Other patients may describe a functional goal (e.g., a person may want the pain to be relieved to an extent that allows him or her to perform daily activities). Over the course of prolonged therapy, these goals should be reassessed, and progress toward meeting them should be documented. If the patient has unrealistic goals for therapy, such as wanting to be completely rid of all chronic arthritis pain, the nurse should work with the patient to establish a more workable goal.

Fourth, treatment plans should use a combination of drug and nondrug therapies. Although medications are often considered the mainstay of therapy, particularly for moderate to severe pain, nondrug therapies should be incorporated to increase the overall effectiveness of therapy and to allow for the reduction of drug dosages to minimize adverse drug effects.[9,18]

Fifth, a multidisciplinary approach is necessary to address all dimensions of pain. Pain management clinics generally incorporate the expertise of many health care professionals. However, even in situations that do not involve a specialized pain team, multiple perspectives and knowledge should be used.

Sixth, all therapies must be evaluated to ensure that they are meeting the patient's goals. Therapy must be individualized for each patient, and often achievement of an effective treatment plan requires trial and error. Adjustments in drug, dosage, or route are common to achieve maximal benefit while minimizing adverse effects. This trial-and-error process can become frustrating for the patient and family. They need to be reassured that pain relief is possible and that the health care team will continue to work with them to achieve adequate pain relief.

Seventh, drug side effects must be prevented and/or managed.[9,18,19] Side effects are a major reason for treatment failure and nonadherence.[27] Side effects are managed in one of several ways as described in Table 9-7.[19] The nurse plays a key role in

TABLE 9-7 Drug Therapy: Managing Side Effects of Pain Medications

- Changing the dosing regimen to maintain relatively constant blood levels
- Changing to a different medication in the same class
- Adding a drug to counteract the adverse effect of the analgesic (e.g., opioid-induced sedation can be managed by administering a stimulant such as dextroamphetamine [Dexedrine] or methylphenidate [Ritalin])
- Using an administration route that minimizes drug concentrations at the site of the side effect (e.g., intraspinal administration of opioids is sometimes used to minimize high drug levels that produce sedation, nausea, and vomiting)

monitoring for and treating side effects, as well as patient and family teaching to minimize adverse effects.

Finally, patient and family teaching should be a cornerstone to the treatment plan. Content should include information about the cause(s) of the pain, pain assessment methods, treatment goals and options, expectations of pain management, instruction regarding the proper use of drugs, side effect management, and nondrug and self-help pain relief measures.[18] Teaching should be documented, and patient and family comprehension of the teaching should be evaluated.

DRUG THERAPY FOR PAIN

Although a physician or nurse practitioner prescribes the drugs, it is usually the nurse's responsibility to evaluate the effectiveness and side effects of prescribed drugs. It is also a nursing responsibility to communicate the outcomes of analgesic therapy to the health care provider and suggest changes when appropriate. As the nurse implements these roles, knowledge and skill related to several pharmacologic concepts are used. These include calculating equianalgesic doses, scheduling analgesic doses, titrating opioids, and selecting from the prescribed analgesic drugs.

Equianalgesic Dose

The term **equianalgesic dose** refers to a dose of one analgesic that is equivalent in pain-relieving effects compared with another analgesic. This equivalence permits substitution of analgesics in the event that a particular drug is ineffective or causes intolerable side effects. Generally, equianalgesic doses are provided for opioids and are important because there is no upper dosage limit for many of these drugs. Equianalgesic charts and conversion programs are widely available in textbooks, in clinical guidelines, in health care facility pain protocols, and on the Internet. They are useful tools, but health care providers need to understand their limitations. Equianalgesic dosages are approximate, and some are based on small, single-dose studies.[19,23] The data for equianalgesic dosing in long-term opioid therapy is particularly limited. In addition, discrepancies exist among different published charts.[44] All changes in opioid therapy must be carefully monitored and adjusted for the individual patient. When possible, health care providers should use equianalgesic conversions that have been approved for their facility or clinic and should consult a pharmacist before making changes.

Scheduling Analgesics

Appropriate analgesic scheduling should focus on preventive or ongoing control of pain rather than providing analgesics only after the patient's pain has become severe. A patient should be premedicated before painful procedures and activities that are expected to produce pain. Similarly, a patient with constant pain should receive analgesics around the clock rather than on an "as needed" (prn) basis. These strategies control pain before it starts and usually result in lower analgesic requirements. Fast-acting drugs should be used for incident or breakthrough pain, whereas long-acting analgesics are more effective for constant pain. Examples of fast-acting and sustained-release analgesics are described later in this section.

Titration. Analgesic **titration** is dose adjustment based on assessment of the adequacy of analgesic effect versus the side effects produced. There is wide variability in the amount of analgesic needed to manage pain, and titration is an important strategy in addressing this variability. An analgesic can be titrated upward or downward, depending on the situation. For example, in a postoperative patient the dose of analgesic generally decreases over time as the acute pain resolves. On the other hand, opioids for chronic, severe cancer pain may be titrated upward many times over the course of therapy to maintain adequate pain control. The goal of titration is to use the smallest dose of analgesic that provides effective pain control with the fewest side effects.[23]

Analgesic Ladder

Several national and international groups have published practice guidelines recommending a systematic plan for using analgesic drugs.[18-20] One widely used system is the analgesic ladder proposed by the World Health Organization (WHO) (Fig. 9-8).[20] The WHO treatment plan calls for concurrent treatment of the cause of the pain when possible and use of a three-step ladder approach. Step 1 drugs are used for mild pain, step 2 for mild to moderate pain, and step 3 for moderate to severe pain. If pain persists or increases, drugs from the next higher step are used to control the pain. For chronic nonmalignant pain and cancer pain, drug use is recommended from the bottom of the ladder to the top (i.e., up the ladder from step 1 to step 2 to step 3). For acute pain, the steps can be reversed in order from the top step to the bottom step (i.e., down the ladder from step 3 to step 2 to step 1) as recovery occurs and pain decreases.

Drug Therapy for Mild Pain. When pain is mild (1 to 3 on a scale of 0 to 10), nonopioid analgesics (aspirin and other salicylates, other nonsteroidal antiinflammatory drugs [NSAIDs], and acetaminophen) are used (Table 9-8). These agents are characterized by the following: (1) there is a **ceiling effect** to their analgesic properties; that is, increasing the dose beyond an upper limit provides no greater analgesia; (2) they do not produce tolerance or physical dependence; and (3) many are available without a prescription. It is important to monitor over-the-counter (OTC) analgesic use to avoid serious problems related to drug interactions, side effects, and overdose.

A number of nonopioid analgesics such as acetylsalicylic acid (ASA, aspirin) and NSAIDs inhibit the chemicals that activate the PAN (Fig. 9-9). Thus when these agents are used, the PAN is transduced less often or a larger stimulus is needed to produce transduction.

Aspirin is effective for mild pain but its use is limited by its common side effects, including gastric upset and bleeding. Other salicylates such as choline magnesium trisalicylate cause fewer GI disturbances and bleeding abnormalities. Like aspirin, acetaminophen (Tylenol) has analgesic and antipyretic effects, but it has no antiplatelet or antiinflammatory effects. Although acetaminophen is well tolerated, doses of greater than 4000 mg/day, acute overdose, or use by patients with alcoholism or liver disease can result in severe hepatotoxicity.

The NSAIDs represent a broad class of drugs with varying efficacy and side effects. Some NSAIDs possess equal analgesic efficacy as aspirin, whereas others have somewhat higher efficacy.[19] Patients vary greatly in their responses to a specific NSAID, so when one NSAID does not provide relief, another should be tried. Side effects can be serious and include bleeding tendencies secondary to decreased platelet aggregation, GI problems ranging from dyspepsia to ulceration and hemorrhage, renal insufficiency, and occasionally CNS dysfunction. NSAIDs that selectively inhibit cyclooxygenase-2 (COX-2) include celecoxib (Celebrex) and rofecoxib (Vioxx). There is some evidence that because of their selective inhibition, this class of NSAIDs has less GI toxicity. However, they cost considerably more than other NSAIDs.[45]

Drug Therapy for Mild to Moderate Pain. When pain is moderate in intensity (4 to 6 on a scale of 0 to 10) or mild but persistent despite nonopioid therapy, step 2 drugs are indicated.

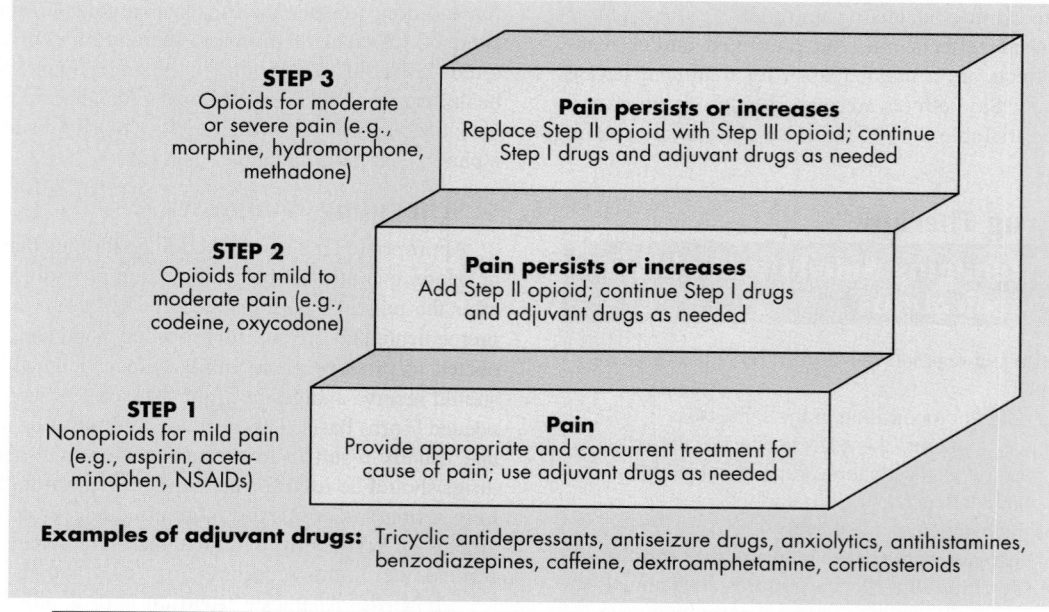

STEP 3
Opioids for moderate or severe pain (e.g., morphine, hydromorphone, methadone)

Pain persists or increases
Replace Step II opioid with Step III opioid; continue Step I drugs and adjuvant drugs as needed

STEP 2
Opioids for mild to moderate pain (e.g., codeine, oxycodone)

Pain persists or increases
Add Step II opioid; continue Step I drugs and adjuvant drugs as needed

STEP 1
Nonopioids for mild pain (e.g., aspirin, acetaminophen, NSAIDs)

Pain
Provide appropriate and concurrent treatment for cause of pain; use adjuvant drugs as needed

Examples of adjuvant drugs: Tricyclic antidepressants, antiseizure drugs, anxiolytics, antihistamines, benzodiazepines, caffeine, dextroamphetamine, corticosteroids

FIG. 9-8 The analgesic ladder proposed by the World Health Organization. *NSAIDs,* Nonsteroidal antiinflammatory drugs (e.g., ibuprofen, naproxen, ketorolac).

TABLE 9-8 Drug Therapy

Comparison of Selected Nonopioid Analgesics

DRUG	ANALGESIC EFFICACY COMPARED TO STANDARDS	NURSING CONSIDERATIONS
acetaminophen (Tylenol)	Comparable to aspirin	Rectal suppository available; sustained-release preparations available; maximum daily dose of 4 g
Salicylates		
aspirin	Standard for comparison	Rectal suppository available; sustained-release preparations available. Possibility of upper GI bleeding
choline magnesium trisalicylate (Trilisate)	Longer duration than aspirin	Unlike aspirin and NSAIDs, does not increase bleeding time
Nonsteroidal Antiinflammatory Drugs (NSAIDs)		
ibuprofen (Motrin, Nuprin, Advil)	Superior at 200 mg to aspirin 650 mg	Concern regarding the potential for upper GI bleeding
indomethacin (Indocin)	25 mg comparable to aspirin 650 mg	Not routinely used because of high incidence of side effects; rectal, IV, and sustained-release oral forms available
ketorolac (Toradol)	30-60 mg equivalent to 6-12 mg morphine	Limit treatment to 5 days; may precipitate renal failure in dehydrated patients
mefenamic acid (Ponstel)	250 mg comparable to aspirin 650 mg	Limit treatment to 1 week
diclofenac K (Cataflam)	50 mg superior in efficacy and analgesic duration to aspirin 650 mg	Available in oral, ophthalmic, topical preparations
Cyclooxygenase-2 (COX-2) Inhibitors		
celecoxib (Celebrex) rofecoxib (Vioxx)	Similar to other NSAIDs	Cause fewer GI side effects, including bleeding, than other NSAIDs but risk still present; are more costly than other NSAIDs

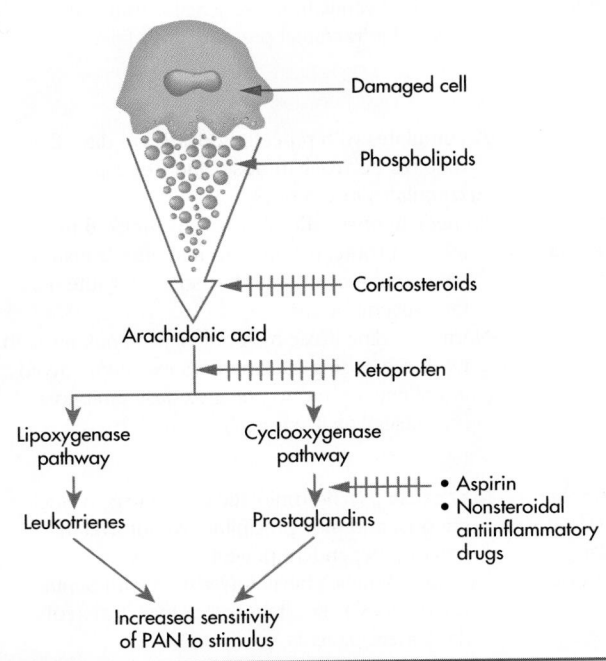

FIG. 9-9 Schematic representation of two pathways that lead to the production of chemicals that cause the peripheral afferent nociceptors (PAN) to be more easily excited. Drugs that block the synthesis of these chemicals are also shown.

Commonly used drugs for mild to moderate pain are listed in Table 9-9.

One class of step 2 drugs is opioids. Opioids include many drugs (Tables 9-9 and 9-10) that produce their effects by binding to receptors. Opioid receptors are found in the central nervous system, on the terminals of sensory nerves, and on the surface of immune cells.[37] There are three major opioid receptors: mu (μ), kappa (κ), and delta (δ). Recently, the receptors have been reclassified as OP1 (delta), OP2 (kappa), and OP3 (mu).[37] Most clinically useful opioids bind to the mu receptors. Mu agonists include morphine, oxycodone, hydromorphone, and methadone. Opioid *agonists* (e.g., morphine) bind to the receptors and cause analgesia. *Antagonists* (e.g., naloxone [Narcan]) bind to the receptors but do not produce analgesia; they also block other effects of opioid receptor activation, such as sedation and respiratory depression. Mixed *agonist-antagonists* (e.g., pentazocine [Talwin], butorphanol [Stadol]) bind as agonists on the kappa receptor and as weak antagonists or partial agonists on the mu receptor (Fig. 9-10). Because of this difference in binding, mixed agonist-antagonists produce less respiratory depression than pure mu agonists.

However, they also cause more dysphoria and agitation. In addition, opioid agonist-antagonists have an **analgesic ceiling** (a dose at which no additional analgesia is produced regardless of further dose increases) and can precipitate withdrawal if used in

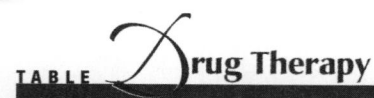

TABLE 9-9

Opioid Analgesics Commonly Used for Mild to Moderate Pain

DRUG	COMMENTS	NURSING CONSIDERATIONS
Morphine-like Agonists		
codeine	Many preparations include combination with nonnarcotic analgesics; codeine metabolized to morphine in the body	Many preparations of codeine and other opioids are limited by the dose of nonnarcotic analgesic (e.g., the maximum dose of acetaminophen is 4 g/day)
oxycodone (OxyContin)	Same as for codeine	Same as for codeine
hydrocodone (Vicodin)	Same as for codeine	Same as for codeine
tramadol (Ultram)	Maximum dose is 400 mg/day	May cause seizures, although rare
Mixed Agonist-Antagonist		
pentazocine (Talwin)	Formulated in combination with acetaminophen, aspirin, ibuprofen; some preparations include naloxone to discourage parenteral abuse	May cause psychotomimetic effects; may precipitate withdrawal in narcotic-dependent patients
butorphanol (Stadol)	Not available orally; not scheduled under Controlled Substance Act; butorphanol nasal spray used to treat migraine headaches	Psychotomimetic effects lower than with pentazocine (Talwin); may precipitate withdrawal in narcotic-dependent patients
Partial Agonist		
buprenorphine (Buprenex)	Lower abuse potential than morphine; does not produce psychotomimetic effects	May precipitate withdrawal in narcotic-dependent patients; not readily reversed by naloxone (Narcan)

Adapted from the American Pain Society: *Principles of analgesic use in the treatment of acute pain and chronic cancer pain,* ed 4, Skokie, Ill, 1999, American Pain Society.

TABLE 9-10

Opioid Analgesics Commonly Used for Severe Pain

DRUG	COMMENTS	NURSING CONSIDERATIONS
Morphine	Standard comparison for opioid analgesics; sustained-release preparation (MS Contin); once-a-day formulation (Kadian)	For all opioids, use with caution in patients with impaired ventilation, bronchial asthma, increased intracranial pressure, liver failure
Morphine-like Agonists		
hydromorphone (Dilaudid)	Slightly shorter duration than morphine	
methadone (Dolophine)	Good oral potency; 24–36 hr half-life	Accumulates with repeated dosing; on days 2–5 requires decrease in dose, and frequency
levorphanol (Levo-Dromoran)	Plasma half-life 12–16 hr	Accumulates in 2–3 days
fentanyl (Sublimaze, Duragesic, Actiq)	Available as injection (Sublimaze) or transdermal fentanyl (Duragesic); oral transmucosal fentanyl citrate (Actiq) now available for breakthrough cancer pain	Immediate onset after IV route; within 7–8 min after IM route; within 5–15 min after transmucosal route; onset after transdermal route may take several hours
meperidine (Demerol)	Slightly shorter acting than morphine	Normeperidine (toxic metabolite) accumulates with repetitive dosing causing CNS excitation; avoid in patients on monoamine oxidase inhibitors (e.g., selegiline [Deprenyl])
Mixed Agonist-Antagonists		
pentazocine (Talwin)	Formulated in combination with acetaminophen, aspirin, ibuprofen; some preparations include naloxone to discourage parenteral abuse	May cause psychotomimetic effects (e.g., hallucinations) and may precipitate withdrawal in narcotic-dependent patients
butorphanol (Stadol)	Not available orally; not scheduled under Controlled Substance Act	Psychotomimetic effects lower than with pentazocine; may precipitate withdrawal in narcotic-dependent patients
Partial Agonist		
buprenorphine (Buprenex)	Lower abuse potential than morphine; does not produce psychotomimetic effects	May precipitate withdrawal in narcotic-dependent patients; not readily reversed by naloxone

Adapted from the American Pain Society: *Principles of analgesic use in the treatment of acute pain and chronic cancer pain,* ed 4, Skokie, Ill, 1999, American Pain Society.

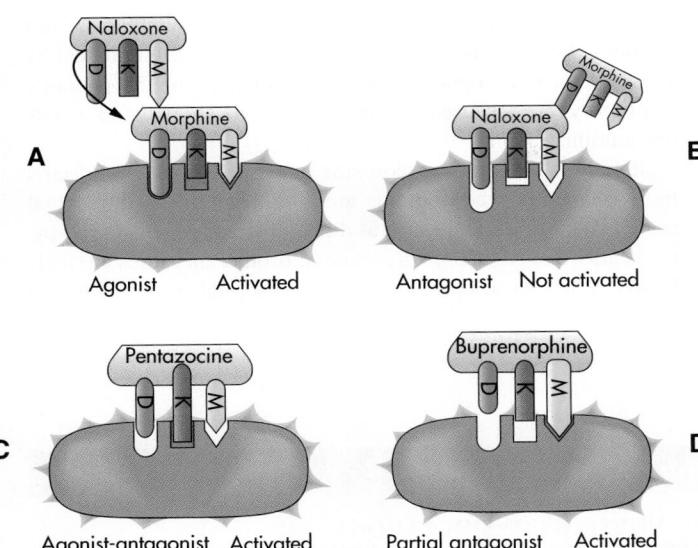

A   Agonist   Activated
B   Antagonist   Not activated
C   Agonist-antagonist   Activated
D   Partial antagonist   Activated

FIG. 9-10 Opioid receptor subtypes. *A,* Agonist action. *B,* Antagonist action. *C,* Agonist-antagonist action. *D,* Partial agonist action. *M,* Mu receptor; *K,* kappa receptor; *D,* delta receptor.

a patient who is physically dependent on agonist drugs. Partial opioid agonists (e.g., buprenorphine [Buprenex]) bind weakly to mu and kappa receptors, which decreases their analgesic efficacy. Partial opioid agonists currently have limited availability and clinical value in pain management.[19,23]

At step 2, commonly used opioids include codeine, hydrocodone, and oxycodone. These drugs usually are prescribed in products combining an opioid with a nonopioid analgesic (e.g., codeine plus acetaminophen [Tylenol #3], hydrocodone plus acetaminophen [Vicodin]), thereby limiting the opioid dose that can be given. One opioid, propoxyphene (Darvon), is often included as a step 2 drug. However, it is only as effective as 600 mg of aspirin and produces a toxic metabolite that can cause seizures. Thus it generally is not recommended in analgesic guidelines.[23]

A third type of medication available for mild to moderate pain is tramadol (Ultram). Tramadol is a weak mu-agonist and also inhibits the reuptake of norepinephrine and serotonin. It has approximately the same efficacy as Tylenol #3. The most common side effects are similar to those of other opioids, including nausea, constipation, dizziness, and sedation. Tolerance, physical dependence, and addiction do not appear to occur with tramadol, although use of this drug is being closely monitored in the United States to identify risks of addiction.[19,46]

Drug Therapy for Moderate to Severe Pain. Step 3 drugs are recommended for moderate to severe pain (7 to 10 on a scale of 0 to 10) or when step 2 drugs do not produce effective pain relief. Most commonly used step 3 analgesics are mu-agonists, although these drugs also bind with the other receptors. These drugs are effective for moderate to severe pain because they are potent, have no analgesic ceiling, and can be delivered via many routes of administration. Step 3 drugs are presented in Table 9-10.

Morphine is the standard of comparison for all other opioid analgesics. Equianalgesic charts generally present dosages in equivalent morphine doses. Morphine is one of the most commonly prescribed opioids for moderate to severe pain, although fentanyl (Duragesic), hydromorphone (Dilaudid), methadone

(Dolophine), and oxycodone (Percocet) also are used extensively. A long-acting morphine (Avinza) is available for the treatment of moderate to sever chronic pain in patients that require continuous, around-the-clock therapy for an extended period of time. A once-daily dose of Avinza in the extended-release capsule formulation provides relief from pain for 24 hours.

Meperidine (Demerol, Pethidine) is a potent mu-agonist used for severe pain, but its use is limited by the high incidence of neurotoxicity (e.g., seizures) associated with the accumulation of its metabolite, normeperidine. Thus meperidine is contraindicated for patients with acute pain lasting more than 2 days and for those in whom large doses (more than 600 mg per 24 hours) are needed.[19] It should not be used in treating chronic pain. A hyperpyrexic syndrome with delirium, which can cause death, can occur if meperidine is given to patients taking monoamine oxidase inhibitors.[19]

Although step 3 opioids have no analgesic ceiling, many patients experience dose-limiting side effects. In opioid-naive patients, side effects include constipation, nausea and vomiting, sedation, respiratory depression, and pruritus. With continued use, many side effects diminish; the exception is constipation. Less common side effects include urinary retention, myoclonus, dizziness, confusion, and hallucinations.

Constipation is the most common opioid side effect. Because tolerance to opioid-induced constipation does not occur, a bowel regimen should be instituted at the beginning of opioid therapy and continue for as long as the person takes opioids. Although dietary roughage, fluids, and exercise should be encouraged to the extent possible, these measures rarely are sufficient by themselves. Thus most patients should begin immediately on a gentle stimulant laxative (e.g., senna) plus a stool softener (e.g., docusate sodium [Colace]). Other agents (e.g., milk of magnesia, bisacodyl [Dulcolax], and lactulose) can be added if necessary. Left untreated, constipation can lead to impaction and paralytic ileus that can be difficult to differentiate from obstruction.

Nausea often is a problem in opioid-naive patients. The use of antiemetics such as metoclopramide (Reglan), transdermal scopolamine (Transderm-Scop), hydroxyzine (Vistaril), or a phenothiazine (e.g., prochlorperazine [Compazine]) can prevent or minimize opioid-related nausea and vomiting until tolerance develops, which usually occurs within 1 week. Metoclopramide is particularly effective when a patient complains of gastric fullness. Opioids delay gastric emptying, and this effect can be reversed by metoclopramide. If nausea and vomiting are severe and persistent, changing to a different opioid may be necessary.

Concerns about sedation and respiratory depression are two of the most common fears associated with opioids. Sedation usually is seen in opioid-naive patients. However, for most patients sedation resolves with the development of tolerance. Persistent sedation with chronic opioid use can be effectively treated with psychostimulants (e.g., caffeine, dextroamphetamine [Dexedrine], methylphenidate [Ritalin]), which may also improve the analgesic effects of opioids.

Respiratory depression is rare in opioid-tolerant patients and when opioids are titrated to analgesic effect. Patients at risk for respiratory depression include opioid-naive patients, elderly patients, or patients with underlying lung disease. Patients are also at higher risk when they are asleep. For this reason, it is important to observe the rate and depth of respirations of the sleeping patient for 3 to 4 hours past the expected time for peak blood concentrations based on the route of administration.[19] Clinically significant respiratory depression cannot occur in patients who are awake. Thus level of consciousness should be monitored in addition to the respiratory rate.[19]

If severe respiratory depression occurs and stimulation of the patient (calling and shaking patient) does not reverse the somnolence or increase the respiratory rate and depth, naloxone (Narcan, 0.4 mg in 10 ml saline), an opioid antagonist, can be administered intravenously or subcutaneously in 0.5 ml increments every 2 minutes. However, if the patient has been taking opioids regularly for more than a few days, naloxone should be used judiciously and titrated carefully because its use can precipitate se-

vere, agonizing pain, profound withdrawal symptoms, and seizures. Because naloxone's half-life (60 to 90 minutes) is shorter than most opiates, nurses should monitor the patient's respiratory rate because it can drop again 1 to 2 hours after naloxone administration.[19,23]

Itching is another common side effect of opioids and occurs most frequently when opioids are administered via intraspinal routes. An antihistamine such as diphenhydramine (Benadryl) often is effective but causes drowsiness. If other measures are ineffective, a low-dose opioid antagonist (e.g., naloxone) or mixed

TABLE 9-11 Drug Therapy — Adjuvant Drugs Used for Pain Management

DRUG	SPECIFIC INDICATION	NURSING CONSIDERATIONS
Corticosteroids	Inflammation	Avoid high dose for long-term use
Antidepressants amitriptyline (Elavil) doxepin (Sinequan) imipramine (Tofranil-PM) nortriptyline (Pamelor)	Neuropathic pain	Monitor for anticholinergic adverse effects
Antiseizure clonazepam (Klonopin) gabapentin (Neurontin) carbamazepine (Tegretol)	Neuropathic pain	Start with low doses, increase slowly; *clonazapam and carbamazepine*: check liver function tests, renal function, and blood counts at baseline and then at 2 and then 6 wk; *gabapentin*: monitor for idiosyncratic side effects (e.g., ankle swelling, ataxia)
Muscle Relaxant baclofen (Lioresal)	Neuropathic pain, muscle spasms	Monitor for weakness, urinary dysfunction; avoid abrupt discontinuation because of CNS irritability
α_2-Adrenergic Agonist clonidine (Duraclon)	Particularly useful for neuropathic pain	Side effects include sedation, orthostatic hypotension, dry mouth; often combined with anesthetics (e.g., bupivacaine [Sensorcaine])
Anesthetics: Systemic or Oral mexiletine (Mexitil)	Diabetic neuropathy; neuropathic pain	Monitor for side effects, including dizziness, perioral numbness, paresthesias, tremor; can cause seizures, arrhythmias, and myocardial depression at high doses; avoid in patients with preexisting cardiac disease
Anesthetics: Local Topical EMLA (eutectic mixture of local anesthetics): lidocaine 2.5% + prilocaine 2.5%	Local skin analgesic before venipuncture, incision; possibly effective for postherpetic neuralgia	Must be applied under an occlusive dressing (e.g., Tegaderm, DuoDerm, or on an anesthetic disk); absorption from the genital mucosa more rapid and onset time shorter (5-10 min) than after application to intact skin; common adverse effects include mild erythema, edema, skin blanching
capsaicin (Zostrix)	Pain associated with arthritis, postherpetic neuralgia, diabetic neuropathy	Apply sparingly, rub well into affected area; wash hands with soap and water after application; side effects include skin irritation (burning, stinging) at the application site; cough
Psychostimulants dextroamphetamine (Dexedrine) methylphenidate (Ritalin)	Manage opioid-induced sedation	Side effect is insomnia; avoid dosing late in the day; usually well tolerated at low doses

agonist-antagonist can be used, but the patient must be carefully assessed for reversal of analgesia and withdrawal.[23]

Adjuvant Analgesic Therapy. Adjuvant analgesic therapies are drugs used in conjunction with opioid and nonopioid analgesics. Adjuvants are sometimes referred to as coanalgesics. They include drugs that enhance pain therapy through one of three mechanisms: (1) enhancing the effects of opioids and nonopioids, (2) possessing analgesic properties of their own, or (3) counteracting the side effects of other analgesics. Commonly used analgesic adjuvants are listed in Table 9-11. Fig. 9-11 shows the sites of actions of pharmacologic and nonpharmacologic therapies for pain. Adjuvant drugs are used at every step in the WHO ladder.

Antidepressants. Tricyclic antidepressants enhance the descending inhibitory system by preventing the cellular reuptake of serotonin and norepinephrine. Higher levels of serotonin and norepinephrine in the synaptic cleft inhibit the transmission of nociceptive signals in the CNS. Tricyclic antidepressants have been shown to be effective for a variety of pain syndromes, especially those involving neuropathic pain. Doses required for pain relief often are lower than those necessary for depression. Unfortunately, anticholinergic side effects such as dry mouth, urinary retention, sedation, and orthostatic hypotension decrease patient acceptance and adherence. The usefulness of selective serotonin reuptake inhibitors (e.g., paroxetine [Paxil], sertraline [Zoloft], and fluoxetine [Prozac]) in treating pain has been mixed.[23]

Antiseizure agents. Antiseizure drugs such as gabapentin (Neurontin), carbamazepine (Tegretol), and clonazepam (Klonopin) stabilize the membrane of the neuron and prevent transmission. These agents are effective for neuropathic pain and prophylactic treatment of headaches.[19]

α_2-Adrenergic agonists. Currently, clonidine (Catapres) is the most widely used α_2-adrenergic agonist. The mechanisms by which this agent works to reduce pain are not fully understood, but it may affect modulation and transmission. It is effective against chronic headache and neuropathic pain. Common side effects are sedation, dry mouth, and orthostatic hypotension.

Corticosteroids. These drugs, which include dexamethasone (Decadron) and methylprednisolone (Medrol), are used for several pain problems, including acute and chronic cancer pain, pain secondary to spinal cord compression, and some neuropathic pain syndromes. Mechanisms of action are unknown but may involve the ability of corticosteroids to decrease edema and inflammation, and in some cases to shrink tumors. Corticosteroids have many side effects, especially when given chronically in high doses. Adverse effects include hyperglycemia, fluid retention, dyspepsia and GI bleeding, impaired healing, muscle wasting, osteoporosis, and susceptibility to infection.

Local anesthetics. Oral, parenteral, and topical applications of local anesthetics are used to interrupt transmission of pain signals to the brain. Local anesthetics are used for acute pain resulting from surgery or trauma. Chronic neuropathic pain also can be controlled with local anesthetics. Side effects can include dizziness, paresthesias, and seizures (at high doses). Incidence and severity of side effects depend on dose and route of administration. These agents also affect cardiac conductivity, thereby causing arrhythmias and myocardial depression.[47]

Administration Routes. Opioids and other analgesic agents can be delivered via many routes. This flexibility allows the health care provider to (1) target a particular anatomic source of the pain, (2) achieve therapeutic blood levels rapidly when necessary, (3) avoid certain side effects through localized administration, and (4) provide analgesia when patients are unable to swallow. The following discussion highlights the uses and nursing considerations for analgesics deliverered through a variety of routes.

Oral. Generally, oral administration is the route of choice for the person with a functioning GI system.[18,19] Oral drugs are usually less expensive than those delivered by other routes. In cancer pain management, federal guidelines recommend that other routes be used only when oral administration is not possible.[18]

Many opioids are available in oral preparations, such as liquid and tablet formulations. To obtain equivalent analgesia as doses administered intramuscularly or intravenously, larger oral doses are needed. For example, 10 mg of parenteral morphine is equivalent to approximately 30 mg of oral morphine.[19] The reason larger doses are required is related to the *first-pass effect* of hepatic metabolism. This means that oral opioids are absorbed from the GI tract into the portal circulation and shunted to the liver. Partial metabolism in the liver occurs before the drug enters systemic circulation and becomes available to peripheral receptors or can cross the blood-brain barrier and access CNS opioid receptors, which is necessary to produce analgesia. Oral opioids are as effective as parenteral opioids if the dose administered is large enough to compensate for the first-pass metabolism.

Oral preparations also are available in short-acting and long-acting preparations. For example, morphine is available in immediate-release solutions or tablets. These products are effec-

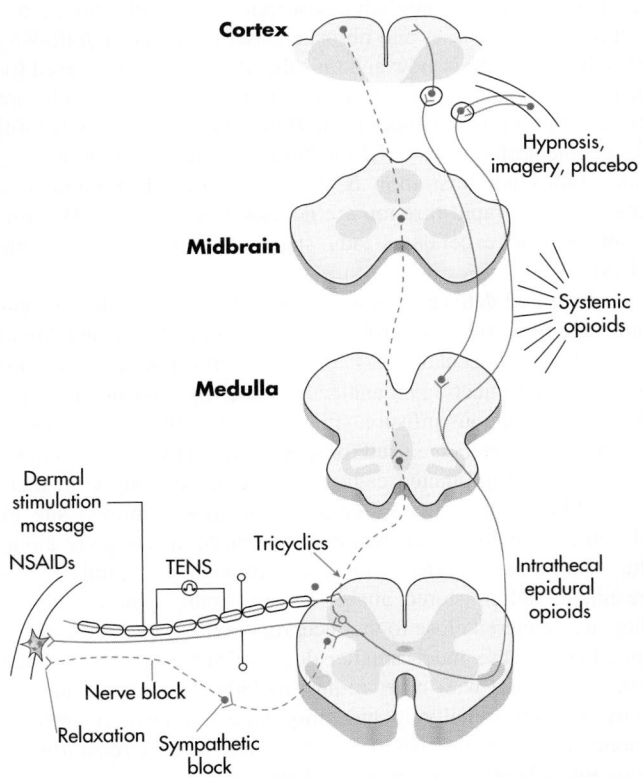

FIG. 9-11 The sites of commonly used pharmacologic and nonpharmacologic analgesic therapies. *NSAIDs,* Nonsteroidal antiinflammatory drugs; *TENS,* transcutaneous electrical nerve stimulation.

Labels in figure: Cortex; Hypnosis, imagery, placebo; Midbrain; Systemic opioids; Medulla; Dermal stimulation massage; NSAIDs; TENS; Tricyclics; Intrathecal epidural opioids; Nerve block; Relaxation; Sympathetic block

tive in providing rapid, short-term pain relief. Sustained-release oral morphine tablets are administered every 8 to 12 hours and include two proprietary products: Oramorph-SR and MS Contin. As with other sustained-release preparations, these products should not be crushed, broken, or chewed. Kadian is a sustained-release morphine product that is administered every 24 hours. Because Kadian is in a specialized, capsule form, the capsule can be opened and the contents sprinkled on applesauce. Oxycodone also comes in a sustained-release tablet (OxyContin). Sustained-release formulations for hydrocodone and hydromorphone are under development.

Sublingual and buccal. Opioids administered under the tongue or held in the mouth and absorbed into systemic circulation are exempt from the first-pass effect. Although morphine is commonly administered to persons with cancer pain via the sublingual route, little of the drug is absorbed from the sublingual tissue. Instead, much of the drug is dissolved in saliva and swallowed, making its metabolism similar to oral morphine.

Fentanyl citrate (Actiq) is administered orally using the oral transmucosal system (OTS) for drug delivery. The fentanyl dose is embedded in a flavored lozenge on a stick. The drug is absorbed by the permeable buccal mucosa after being rubbed actively over it (not sucked as a lollipop), allowing for the drug to enter the bloodstream and travel directly to the CNS. Pain relief typically occurs within 5 to 7 minutes after administration. Duration of action ranges from 2.5 to 5 hours. Actiq is approved for use before surgery and procedures, although it must be used cautiously in opioid-naive patients. The drug also is effective for the treatment of cancer-related breakthrough pain.[48]

Intranasal. Intranasal administration allows delivery of medication to highly vascular mucosa and avoids the first-pass effect. Butorphanol (Stadol) is one of the few intranasal analgesics that is available in the United States; it is not available in Canada. This drug is indicated for acute headache and other intense, recurrent types of pain. Several intranasal opioid agents are being investigated.

Rectal. The rectal route is often overlooked but is particularly useful when the patient cannot take an analgesic by mouth. Rectal suppositories that are effective for pain relief include hydromorphone (Dilaudid), oxymorphone (Numorphan), and morphine.

Transdermal. Fentanyl (Duragesic) is available as a transdermal patch system for application to nonhairy skin. This delivery system is useful for the patient who cannot tolerate oral analgesic drugs. Absorption from the patch is slow. Therefore transdermal fentanyl is not suitable for rapid dose titration but can be effective if the patient's pain is stable and the dose required to control it is known. Patches may need to be changed every 48 hours rather than the recommended 72 hours based on individual patient responses.

A new product for postherpetic neuralgia is a 5% lidocaine-impregnated transdermal patch (Lidoderm patch). The patch, placed directly on the intact skin in the area of postherpetic pain, is left in place for up to 12 hours. It should not be left in place for 24 hours continuously because toxic accumulations can occur. Special precaution should be given to persons receiving class I antiarrhythmic drugs or products containing local anesthetic agents because their effect will be additive and may induce toxicity.[49]

Currently, creams and lotions containing 10% trolamine salicylate (Aspercreme, Myoflex cream) are available. These agents have been recommended by the manufacturers for joint and muscle pain. This aspirin-like substance is absorbed locally. This route of administration avoids gastric irritation, but the other side effects of high-dose salicylate are not necessarily prevented.

Ointments, lotions, gels, liniments, and balms (most of which are OTC products), are sometimes applied to the skin to achieve pain relief. Common ingredients include methyl salicylate combined with camphor and/or menthol. On application, these agents usually produce a strong hot or cold sensation and should not be used after massage or a heat treatment when blood vessels are already dilated. Skin testing is advisable when the patient has not used the particular agent before because the strengths of the agents vary and different intensities of sensation are produced. These products are indicated for arthralgia, bursitis, myalgia, and tendinitis.

Other topical analgesic agents, such as capsaicin (e.g., Icy-Hot, Zostrix) and prilocaine plus lidocaine (EMLA), also provide analgesia. Derived from red chili pepper, capsaicin depletes and prevents reaccumulation of substance P in the peripheral sensory neurons. It can control pain associated with postherpetic neuralgia, diabetic neuropathy, and arthritis. EMLA is useful for control of pain associated with venipunctures, ulcer debridement, and possibly postherpetic neuralgia. The area to which EMLA is applied should be covered with a plastic wrap for 30 to 60 minutes before beginning a painful procedure.

Parenteral routes. The parenteral route includes subcutaneous (SC), intramuscular (IM), and intravenous (IV) administration. Single, repeated, or continuous dosing (SC or IV) is possible via parenteral routes. Although it is frequently used, the IM route is not recommended because these injections cause significant pain, result in unreliable absorption, and with chronic use can result in abscesses and fibrosis. Onset of analgesia following SC administration is slow and thus the SC route rarely is used for acute pain management. However, continuous SC infusions are effective for chronic cancer pain. This route is especially helpful for people with abnormal GI function and limited venous access. Intravenous administration is the best route when immediate analgesia and rapid titration are necessary. Continuous IV infusions provide excellent steady state analgesia through stable blood levels.

Intraspinal delivery. Intraspinal (epidural or intrathecal) opioid therapy involves inserting a catheter into the subarachnoid space (for intrathecal delivery) or the epidural space (for epidural delivery) and injecting an analgesic, either by intermittent bolus doses or continuous infusion (Fig. 9-12). Percutaneously placed temporary catheters are used for short-term therapy (2 to 4 days), and surgically implanted catheters are used for long-term therapy. Although the lumbar region is the most common site of placement, epidural catheters may be placed at any point along the neuroaxis (cervical, thoracic, lumbar, or caudal). Intraspinally administered analgesics are highly potent because they are delivered close to the receptors in the dorsal horn of the spinal cord. Thus much smaller doses of analgesics are needed when compared with other routes, including IV. Drugs that are delivered intraspinally include morphine, fentanyl, hydromorphone, and clonidine. Nausea, itching, and urinary retention are common side effects of intraspinal opioids.

Complications of intraspinal analgesia include catheter displacement and migration, infusions of neurotoxic agents, and infection. Clinical manifestations of catheter displacement or mi-

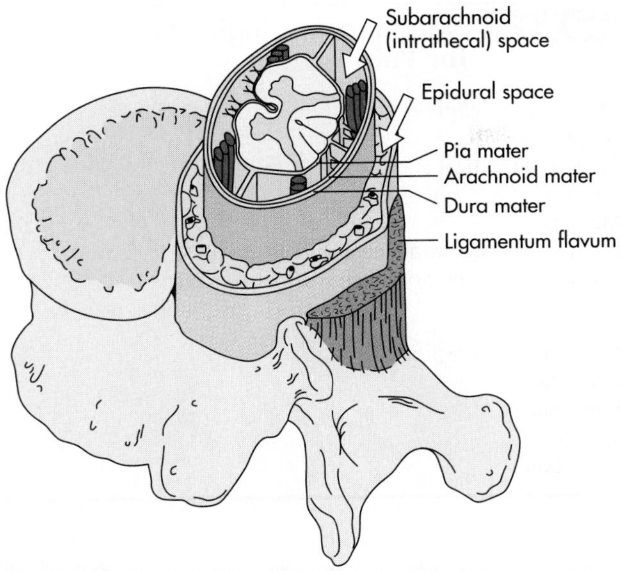
Subarachnoid (intrathecal) space
Epidural space
Pia mater
Arachnoid mater
Dura mater
Ligamentum flavum

FIG. 9-12 Spinal anatomy. The spinal cord extends from the foramen magnum to the first or second lumbar vertebral space. The subarachnoid space (intrathecal space) is filled with cerebrospinal fluid that continually circulates and bathes the spinal cord. The epidural space is a potential space filled with blood vessels, fat, and a network of nerve extensions.

gration depend on catheter location. A catheter that moves out of the intrathecal or epidural space will cause a decrease in pain relief with no improvement even with additional analgesia. Correct placement of an intrathecal catheter can be checked by aspirating cerebrospinal fluid. Migration of a catheter into a blood vessel causes an increase in drug side effects because of systemic drug distribution. A number of drugs and chemicals are highly neurotoxic when administered intraspinally. These include many preservatives such as alcohol and phenol, antibiotics, potassium, and total parenteral nutrition. To avoid inadvertent injection of IV drugs into an intraspinal catheter, the catheter should be clearly marked as an intraspinal access device, and only preservative-free drugs should be injected.

Infection is a rare complication of intraspinal analgesia. However, it is a serious complication that can be difficult to detect. The skin around the exit site should be carefully assessed for inflammation, drainage, or pain. Signs and symptoms of an intraspinal infection include diffuse back pain, pain or paresthesias during bolus injection, and unexplained sensory or motor deficits. Fever may or may not be present. Acute bacterial infection (meningitis) is manifested by fever, headache, and altered mental status. Infection is avoided by providing regular, meticulous wound care and using sterile technique when caring for the catheter and injecting drugs.

Patient-controlled analgesia. A specific type of SC, IV, or intraspinal delivery system is **patient-controlled analgesia** (PCA), or demand analgesia. With PCA, a dose of opioid is delivered when the patient decides a dose is needed. PCA uses an infusion system in which the patient pushes a button to receive a bolus infusion of an analgesic. PCA is used widely for the management of acute pain, including postoperative pain and cancer pain. The addition of a continuous infusion to a PCA regimen will improve nighttime pain relief and promote sleep.

Use of PCA begins with patient teaching. The patient needs to understand the mechanics of getting a drug dose and how to titrate the drug to achieve good pain relief. The patient should be encouraged to self-administer the analgesic before pain intensity is greater than the patient's desired pain intensity goal. The patient also needs to be assured that he or she cannot "overdose" because the pump is programmed to deliver a maximum number of doses per hour. Pressing the button after the maximum dose is administered will not result in additional analgesic. If the maximum doses are inadequate to relieve pain, the pump can be reprogrammed to increase the amount or frequency of dosing. In addition, bolus doses can be given by the nurse if they are included in the physician's orders. To make a smooth transition from infusion PCA to oral drugs, the patient should receive increasing doses of oral drug as the PCA analgesic is tapered.

SURGICAL THERAPY

Nerve Blocks

Nerve blocks are used to reduce pain by temporarily or permanently interrupting transmission of nociceptive input by application of local anesthetics or neurolytic agents (e.g., alcohol, phenol). Neural blockade with local anesthetics is sometimes used for perioperative pain. For intractable chronic pain, nerve blocks are used when more conservative therapies fail. Nerve blocks have been a successful pain management technique for more localized chronic pain states, such as peripheral vascular disease, trigeminal neuralgia, causalgia, and some cancer pain. A nerve block was formerly considered advantageous in managing localized pain caused by malignancy and in debilitated patients who could not withstand a surgical procedure for pain relief. This use is currently being reevaluated in view of the increasing life expectancy of persons being treated for malignancies and the availability of other therapeutic modalities.

Surgical Interventions

Neurosurgical interventions are performed for severe pain that is unresponsive to all other therapies. It is estimated that these procedures are required in less than 10% of cancer patients to achieve adequate pain control.[18] Neurosurgical interventions for pain encompass three groups of procedures: implantation of drug-infusion systems (e.g., permanent epidural and intrathecal catheters), neuroablation, and neuroaugmentation. *Neuroablative techniques* destroy nerves, thereby interrupting pain transmission. Destruction is accomplished by surgical resection or thermocoagulation, including radiofrequency coagulation. Neuroablative interventions that destroy the sensory division of a peripheral or spinal nerve are classified as neurectomies, rhizotomies, and sympathectomies. Neurosurgical procedures that ablate the lateral spinothalamic tract are classified as cordotomies if the tract is interrupted in the spinal cord, or tractotomies if the interruption is in the medulla or the midbrain of the brainstem. Fig. 9-13 identifies the sites of neurosurgical procedures for pain relief. Both cordotomy and tractotomy can be performed with the aid of local anesthesia by a percutaneous technique in which the pain fibers are isolated by fluoroscopy and a radiofrequency lesion is created.

Neuroaugmentation involves electrical stimulation of the brain and the spinal cord. Spinal cord stimulation (SCS) is performed much more often than deep brain stimulation. One of the

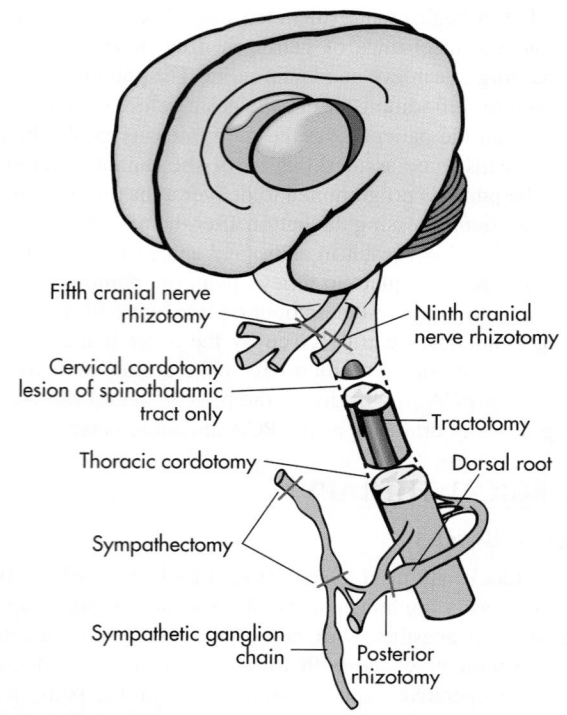

Fifth cranial nerve rhizotomy

Ninth cranial nerve rhizotomy

Cervical cordotomy lesion of spinothalamic tract only

Tractotomy

Thoracic cordotomy

Dorsal root

Sympathectomy

Sympathetic ganglion chain

Posterior rhizotomy

FIG. 9-13 Sites of neurosurgical procedures for pain relief.

TABLE 9-12 Nonpharmacologic Therapies for Pain

Physical Therapies
Acupuncture
Application of heat and cold
Exercise
Massage
Percutaneous electrical nerve stimulation (PENS)
Transcutaneous electrical nerve stimulation (TENS)
Vibration

Cognitive Therapies
Distraction
Hypnosis
Imagery
Relaxation

most common uses of SCS is for "failed back surgery syndrome." It also has been shown to be effective in peripheral neuropathy, peripheral vascular disease, and other neuropathic disease states.[50] Potential complications include surgical complications such as bleeding and infection, migration of the battery (which usually is implanted in the abdomen), and nerve damage. Stimulation of deep brain structures (e.g., thalamus) was performed in the 1970s and 1980s to achieve pain control but rarely is done today. Instead, brain surface stimulation, particularly in areas of the motor cortex, is actively being studied.[50]

NONPHARMACOLOGIC THERAPY FOR PAIN

Nonpharmacologic pain management strategies can reduce the dose of an analgesic required to control pain and thereby minimize side effects of drug therapy. Some strategies are believed to alter ascending nociceptive input or stimulate descending pain modulation mechanisms. Nonpharmacologic pain relief methods can be categorized as physical or cognitive strategies (Table 9-12).

Physical Pain Relief Strategies

Massage. Massage is a common therapy for pain, and many massage techniques exist. Examples include moving the hands or fingers over the skin slowly or briskly with long strokes or in circles (superficial massage) or applying firm pressure to the skin to maintain contact while massaging the underlying tissues (deep massage). Specific massage techniques include acupressure and trigger point massage. A **trigger point** is a circumscribed hypersensitive area within a tight band of muscle that is caused by acute or chronic muscle strain. Several common trigger points have been identified on the neck, back, and arms. Trigger point massage is performed either by applying strong, sustained digital pressure, deep massage, or gentler massage with ice followed by muscle heating.

Vibration. Vibration is thought to provide pain relief by activating mechanoreceptors in the muscles. Clinical trials have shown that vibration can alleviate nociceptive pain, orofacial pain, phantom limb pain, and musculoskeletal pain.[51] Some vibration devices can be purchased without a prescription and used by the patient. Several types of vibration therapy also are used by physical therapists.

Transcutaneous Electrical Nerve Stimulation. *Transcutaneous electrical nerve stimulation* (TENS) involves the delivery of an electric current through electrodes applied to the skin surface over the painful region, at trigger points, or over a peripheral nerve. A TENS system consists of two or more electrodes connected by lead wires to a small, battery-operated stimulator (Fig. 9-14). Usually, a physical therapist is responsible for administering TENS therapy, although nurses also can be trained in the technique.

TENS has been enthusiastically embraced by some pain health care providers, although there is little scientific evidence from well-designed clinical trials to support its effectiveness.[51] The strongest evidence in favor of TENS comes from studies of

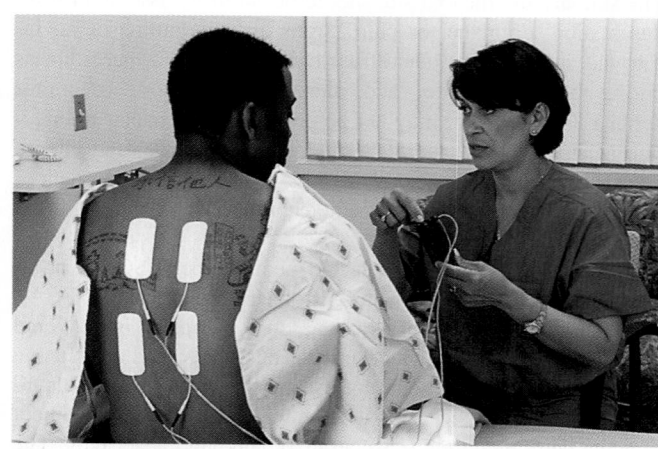

FIG. 9-14 Initial TENS treatment being given by a physical therapist to assess value in pain relief.

patients with dysmenorrhea or angina pectoris and some groups of neuropathic pain patients.[51]

Percutaneous Electrical Nerve Stimulation. *Percutaneous electrical nerve stimulation* (PENS) stimulates deeper peripheral tissues through the insertion of a needle to which a stimulator is attached near a large peripheral or spinal nerve. The amount of electric current is regulated to provide maximum pain relief. If the percutaneous stimulation successfully reduces the patient's pain, a permanent peripheral nerve stimulator is surgically implanted. PENS is a relatively new therapy but has been shown to be effective in the treatment of headaches, diabetic peripheral neuropathy, and low back pain.[52]

Acupuncture. Acupuncture is a technique of traditional Chinese medicine in which very thin needles are inserted into the body at designated points. Acupuncture is applied to many, varied pain problems, including musculoskeletal conditions, repetitive strain disorders, myofascial pain patterns, postsurgical pain, postherpetic neuralgia, peripheral neuropathic pain, and headaches.[53] Many patients receive acupuncture for pain. It is important to point out that although acupuncture is generally considered a safe procedure, it is not without risks and complications may occur, including infection, pneumothorax, and bleeding (acupuncture is discussed in Chapter 7).

Heat Therapy. Heat therapy is the application of either moist or dry heat to the skin. Heat therapy can be either superficial or deep. Superficial heat can be applied using an electric heating pad (dry or moist), a hot pack, hot moist compresses, or a hot water bottle. For exposure to large areas of the body, patients can immerse themselves in a hot bath, shower, or whirlpool. Physical therapy departments provide deep-heat therapy through such techniques as short-wave diathermy, microwave diathermy, and ultrasound therapy. Patient teaching regarding heat therapy is described in Table 9-13.

Cold Therapy. Cold therapy involves the application of either moist or dry cold to the skin. Dry cold can be applied by means of an ice bag, moist cold by means of towels soaked in ice water, cold hydrocollator packs, or immersion in a bath or under running cold water. Icing with ice cubes or blocks of ice made to resemble Popsicles is another technique used for pain relief.

Cold therapy is believed to be more effective than heat for a variety of painful conditions, including acute pain from trauma or surgery, acute flare-ups of arthritis, muscle spasms, and headache. Evidence suggests that cold therapy relieves more pain than heat therapy, works faster than heat, and provides longer-lasting pain relief than heat.[23]

Exercise. Exercise is a critical part of the treatment plan for a patient with chronic nonmalignant pain. Many chronic pain patients become physically deconditioned as a result of their pain, which in turn leads to more pain. Exercise acts via many mechanisms to relieve pain. It enhances circulation and cardiovascular fitness, reduces edema, increases muscle strength and flexibility, and enhances physical and psychosocial functioning. An exercise program should be tailored to the physical needs and lifestyle of the patient and should include aerobic exercise, stretching, and strengthening exercises. The program also should be supervised by medically trained personnel (e.g., exercise physiologist, physical therapist).

Cognitive Therapies

Techniques to alter the affective, cognitive, and behavioral components of pain include a variety of cognitive strategies and behavioral approaches. Some of these techniques require little training and often are adopted independently by the patient. For others, a trained therapist is necessary.

Distraction. Distraction involves redirection of attention on something and away from the pain. It is a simple but powerful strategy to relieve pain. Distraction can be achieved by engaging the patient in any activity that can hold his or her attention (e.g., watching TV, conversing, listening to music, playing a game). It is important to match the activity with the patient's energy level and ability to concentrate. For example, having a patient perform complex calculations will not work if he or she is "mathphobic" or very fatigued.

Imagery is a structured distraction technique that uses the patient's own imagination to develop sensory images that divert focus away from the pain sensation and emphasize other sensory experiences and pleasant memories. Like other distraction techniques, guided imagery provides a mental substitute for the pain (imagery is discussed in Chapter 7).

Hypnosis. Hypnotic therapy is a structured technique that enables a patient to achieve a state of heightened awareness and focused concentration that can be used to alter the patient's pain perception.[18] There is strong scientific support for the effectiveness of hypnosis for acute and cancer pain.[54]

Relaxation. Relaxation techniques are varied, but their goal is the same: to reach a state that is free from anxiety and muscle tension.[18] Relaxation reduces stress, decreases acute anxiety, distracts from the pain, alleviates skeletal muscle tension, combats fatigue, facilitates sleep, and enhances the effectiveness of other pain-relief measures.[18,55] Elicitation of the relaxation response requires a quiet environment, a comfortable position, and a mental device as a focus of concentration (e.g., a word, a sound, the heartbeat, or the person's breathing). Relaxation strategies include deep-breathing regimens, heartbeat breathing, music, slow and rhythmic breathing, and progressive relaxation exercises with a trainer. These strategies are described in Chapters 7 and 8.

TABLE 9-13

Patient & Family Teaching Guide
Heat and Cold Therapy

When patients use superficial heating techniques, they should be taught the following:
- Do not use heat on an area that is being treated with radiation therapy, is bleeding, has decreased sensation, or has been injured in the past 24 hours.
- Do not use any menthol-containing products (e.g., Ben-Gay, Vicks, Icy Hot) with heat applications because this may cause burns.
- Cover the heat source with a towel or cloth to prevent burns.

When patients use superficial cold techniques, they should be taught the following:
- Cover the cold source with a cloth or towel.
- Do not apply cold to areas that are being treated with radiation therapy, have open wounds, or have poor circulation.
- If it is not possible to apply the cold directly to the painful site, try applying it right above or below the painful site, or on the opposite side of the body on the corresponding site (e.g., left elbow if the right elbow hurts).

NURSING and COLLABORATIVE MANAGEMENT
PAIN

The nurse is an important member of the multidisciplinary pain management team. The nurse acts as planner, educator, patient advocate, interpreter, and supporter of the patient in pain and the patient's family. Because pain can be present in any patient in a wide variety of care settings (e.g., home, hospital, clinic), the nurse must be knowledgeable about current therapies and flexible in trying new approaches to pain management. The extent of the nurse's involvement depends on the unique factors associated with the patient, the setting, and the cause of the pain. Many nursing roles have been described earlier: conducting pain assessments, administering therapies, monitoring for side effects, and teaching patients and families. However, the success of these actions depends on the nurse's ability to establish a trusting relationship with the patient and family and to address the concerns that they have regarding pain and its treatment.

■ Effective Communication

Because pain is a subjective experience, patients need to feel confident that their reporting of pain will be believed and will not be perceived as "complaining." The patient and the family also need to know that the nurse considers the pain significant and understands that pain may totally disrupt a person's life. The nurse needs to communicate concern about the patient and assure the patient that he or she is committed to helping the patient obtain pain relief and cope with any unrelieved pain. Pharmacologic and nonpharmacologic interventions should be incorporated into the treatment plan, and the patient should be supported through the period of trial and error that may be necessary to implement an effective therapeutic plan. It also is important to clarify responsibilities in pain relief. The nurse should help the patient understand the role of the members of the health care team, as well as the roles and expectations of the patient.

In addition to addressing specific aspects of pain assessment and treatment, the nurse evaluates the total impact that the pain may have on the lives of the patient and family. Thus other possible nursing diagnoses must be considered. Table 9-14 lists possible nursing diagnoses that may be appropriate for the patient in

NURSING DIAGNOSES

TABLE 9-14	Pain

Activity intolerance
Acute pain
Anxiety
Chronic pain
Constipation
Disturbed sleep pattern
Disturbed thought processes
Fatigue
Fear
Hopelessness
Ineffective coping
Ineffective role performance
Interrupted family processes
Powerlessness
Risk for self-mutilation
Social isolation

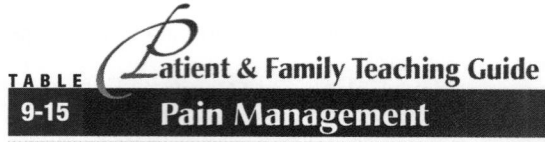

TABLE 9-15	Patient & Family Teaching Guide — Pain Management

The goals of teaching related to pain management include that the patient and family member understand the following:
- Need to maintain a record of pain level and effectiveness of treatment.
- No need to wait until pain becomes severe to take drugs or use nondrug therapies for pain relief.
- Medication will stop working after it is taken for a period of time, and dosages may need to be adjusted.
- Potential side effects and complications associated with therapy/therapies. Side effects can include nausea and vomiting, constipation, sedation and drowsiness, itching, urinary retention, sweating.
- Need to report when pain is not relieved to tolerable levels.

pain. Table 9-15 addresses teaching needs of patients and families related to pain management.

■ Barriers to Effective Pain Management

Pain is a complex, subjective experience, and its management is influenced greatly by psychosocial, sociocultural, and legal-ethical factors. These factors include emotions, behaviors, beliefs, and attitudes of patients and family members about pain and use of pain therapies. Achieving effective pain management requires careful consideration of these factors.

Concerns regarding tolerance, dependence, and addiction are common barriers. Patients, family members, and health care providers often share these concerns. It is important for the nurse to understand and to be able to explain the differences among these various concepts.[56]

Tolerance. *Tolerance* occurs with chronic exposure to a variety of drugs. In the case of opioids, tolerance is characterized by the need for an increased opioid dose to maintain the same degree of analgesia. Tolerance is not a significant determinant in long-term opioid dosage requirements for either cancer patients or chronic nonmalignant pain patients.[57] If dosage needs do increase in cancer patients, it usually is the result of disease progression rather than tolerance.[57] Although tolerance is not as common as once thought, it is essential to assess for increased analgesic needs in patients on chronic therapy. The first sign of tolerance may be that the patient begins to experience regular end-of-dose failure.[19] If manifestations of possible tolerance appear, appropriate evaluations should be made to rule out other causes of increased analgesic needs, such as disease progression or infection. Approaches to managing tolerance are to (1) increase the dose of the analgesic, (2) substitute another drug in the same class (e.g., changing from morphine to oxycodone), or (3) add a drug from a different drug class to augment pain relief without increasing side effects. It is important to note that there is no ceiling effect for opioid-agonist drugs. Thus there is no upper limit to the dose of opioids. Some patients are successfully maintained on hundreds of milligrams per hour of an opioid.

Physical Dependence. Like tolerance, **physical dependence** is an expected physiologic response to ongoing exposure to pharmacologic agents that is manifested by a withdrawal syndrome

TABLE 9-16	Manifestations of Withdrawal from Short-Acting Opioids	
	EARLY RESPONSE (6-12 HR)	**LATE RESPONSE (48-72 HR)**
Psychosocial Secretions	Anxiety Lacrimation Rhinorrhea Diaphoresis	Excitation Diarrhea
Other	Yawning Piloerection Shaking chills Dilated pupils Anorexia Tremor	Restlessness Fever Nausea and vomiting Abdominal cramping pain Hypertension Tachycardia Insomnia

that occurs when blood levels of the drug are abruptly decreased.[56] Symptoms of opioid withdrawal are listed in Table 9-16. When opioids are no longer needed to provide pain relief, a tapering schedule should be used in conjunction with careful monitoring. A typical tapering schedule begins with calculating the 24-hour dose used by the patient and dividing by 2. Of this decreased amount, 25% is given every 6 hours. After 2 days, the daily dose is reduced by an additional 25% every 2 days until the 24-hour oral dose is 30 mg (morphine equivalent) per day. After 2 days on this minimum dose, the opioid is then discontinued.[19] Despite this slow weaning schedule, the nurse should assess carefully for signs and symptoms of opioid withdrawal. In addition to assessing and preventing opioid withdrawal, it is also important to recognize that other commonly prescribed drugs for pain also cause physical dependence and therefore must be slowly tapered. These include benzodiazepines and muscle relaxants.[23]

Addiction. Addiction is a complex neurobiologic condition characterized by a drive to obtain and take substances for other than the prescribed therapeutic value (see Chapter 11). Tolerance and physical dependence are not indicators of addiction. Rather they are normal physiologic responses to chronic exposure to certain drugs, including opioids.

Opioid addiction in acute care patients with no history of substance abuse is a risk estimated at less than 1%. However, this low risk often has been applied erroneously to other patient populations, such as those on long-term opioid therapy for chronic noncancer pain or patients with a history of addiction. In these populations the risk of addiction is likely to be higher.[58] A realistic approach to pain management must acknowledge that the possibility of opioid addiction is not 0%.[58] That does not mean, however, that opioid therapy should be avoided.[23] Instead, expectations of the health care team and the patient need to be discussed openly and documented. Signs and symptoms of possible addiction must be monitored and interventions promptly initiated.

In addition to the fears about addiction, physical dependence, and tolerance, other barriers hinder effective pain management. These include concern about side effects, difficulties remembering to take drugs, desire to be stoic about pain, and not wanting to distract the health care provider from treating the disease.

NURSING RESEARCH
Pain Medication Adherence

Citation

Miaskowski C et al: Lack of adherence with the analgesic regimen: a significant barrier to effective cancer pain management, *J Clin Oncol* 19:4275, 2001.

Purpose

Little information is available on how well cancer outpatients who experience cancer-related pain adhere to their analgesic regimen on a long-term basis. The purpose of this study was to evaluate oncology outpatients' level of adherence to their analgesic regimen during a 5-week period.

Methods

Sixty-five adult oncology patients were recruited from seven outpatient settings. Patients had an average pain intensity score of 2.5 (out of 10) and had radiographic evidence of bone metastasis. Patients completed a demographic questionnaire, the Karnofsky performance status rating, a daily pain diary, and a daily pain drug diary. To obtain information on the duration of pain, patients were asked to indicate how many hours of the day the pain lasted.

Results and Conclusions

Adherence rates were higher when patients were prescribed opioid analgesics on an around-the-clock (ATC) basis. Over the 5 weeks, patients took an average of 88.9% of their ATC dose. In contrast, oncology outpatients who were prescribed prn opioid analgesics took only 24.7% of the prescribed dose. There were no significant differences during the 5 weeks of the study in the percentage of the ATC or prn patients who reported severe pain (i.e., worst pain intensity score of 7).

Implications for Nursing Practice

Oncology outpatients demonstrated a low level of adherence to analgesic pain regimen, especially prn dosing. Further research is needed to determine what factors contribute to patients' decision-making processes regarding analgesic intake and what additional factors influence patients' level of adherence with an analgesic regimen.

Table 9-17 lists these and other barriers and includes strategies to address the barriers.

INSTITUTIONALIZING PAIN EDUCATION AND MANAGEMENT

Besides patient and family barriers, other major barriers to effective pain management are inadequate health care provider education and lack of organizational support. Traditionally, medical and nursing school curricula have spent little time teaching future physicians and nurses about pain and symptom management. This lack of emphasis contributed to the problem that health care providers lacked the knowledge and skills to treat pain adequately. Moreover, pain assessment and treatment were not priorities in clinical practice. Health care providers also were likely to have misconceptions about pain. Similar to patients, many physicians and nurses confused physical dependence, tolerance, and addiction and were more likely to assess pain by observing behaviors rather than accepting a patient's report.[59]

TABLE 9-17   Patient & Family Teaching Guide

Reducing Barriers to Pain Management

BARRIER	NURSING CONSIDERATIONS
Fear of addiction	• Provide accurate definition of addiction. • Explain that addiction is uncommon in patients taking opioids.
Fear of tolerance	• Provide accurate definition of tolerance. • Teach that tolerance is normal physiologic response to chronic opioid therapy. If tolerance does develop, the drug may need to be changed (e.g., morphine in place of oxycodone). • Teach that there is no upper limit to pure opioid agonists (e.g., morphine). Dosages can be increased indefinitely, and patient should not save drugs for when their pain is worse. • Teach that tolerance develops more slowly to analgesic effects of opioids than to many side effects (e.g., sedation, respiratory depression). Tolerance does not develop to constipation; thus a regular bowel program should be started early.
Concern about side effects	• Teach methods to prevent and to treat common side effects. • Emphasize that side effects such as sedation and nausea decrease with time. • Explain that different drugs have unique side effects and other pain drugs can be tried to reduce the specific side effect. • Teach nondrug therapies to minimize the dose of drug needed to control pain.
Fear of injections	• Explain that oral medicines are preferred. • Emphasize that even if oral route becomes unusable, transdermal or indwelling parenteral routes can be used rather than injections.
Desire to be a "good" patient	• Explain that patients are partners in their care and that the partnership requires open communication of both the patient and nurse. • Emphasize to patients that they have a responsibility to keep the nurse informed about their pain.
Desire to be stoic	• Explain that although stoicism is a valued behavior in many cultures, failure to report pain can result in undertreatment and severe, unrelieved pain.
Forgetting to take analgesic	• Provide and teach use of pill containers. • Provide methods of record keeping for drug use. • Recruit family members as appropriate to assist with the analgesic regimen.
Fear of distracting the health care provider from treating the disease	• Explain that reporting pain is important in treating both the disease and its symptoms.
Concern that pain signifies disease progression	• Explain that increased pain or analgesic needs may reflect tolerance. • Emphasize that new pain may come from a non–life-threatening source (e.g., muscle spasm, urinary tract infection). • Institute pharmacologic and nonpharmacologic strategies to reduce anxiety. • Ensure that the patient and family members have current, accurate, comprehensive information about the disease and prognosis. • Provide psychologic support.
Sense of fatalism	• Explain that research has shown that pain can be managed in most patients. • Explain that most therapies require a period of trial and error. • Emphasize that side effects can be managed.
Ineffective medication	• Teach that there are multiple options within each category of medication (e.g., opioid, NSAIDs) and another medication from the same category may provide better relief. • Emphasize that finding the best treatment regimen often requires trial and error. • Incorporate nondrug approaches in treatment plan.

Adapted from Ersek M: Enhancing effective pain management by addressing patient barriers to analgesic use, *J Hospice Palliat Nurs* 1:87, 1999.
NSAIDs, Nonsteroidal antiinflammatory drugs.

Over the past decade, some improvements have been made in overcoming these barriers. Medical and nursing schools now devote more time to addressing pain, and many educational programs have enhanced professional expertise in varied clinical settings.[60,61] In addition, the International Association of the Study of Pain has published a core curriculum on pain that was developed for different groups of health care providers. Although progress has been made, there is still room for improving knowledge and expertise.[5]

Health care institutions also have been remiss in their support of pain management. In the past decade, researchers and health care providers have documented the central role that institutional commitment and practices have in changing clinical practice; without institutional support, pain outcomes are unlikely to change.[62] One major step in institutionalizing pain management is the development and adoption of the Joint Commission on Accreditation of Healthcare Organizations (JCAHO) guideline on pain.[42] JCAHO is the accrediting body for most U.S. health care facilities (hospitals, nursing homes, health care clinics). Under the new standards, health care facilities are required to (1) recognize the patient's rights to appropriate assessment and management of pain; (2) identify pain in patients during their initial assessment and as needed, during ongoing, periodic reassessments; (3) educate health care providers in pain assessment and management and ensure competency; and (4) educate patients and their families about pain management. As a result of these guidelines, institutions have now implemented the practice of assessing every patient's pain regularly from the time of admission as a *fifth vital sign.*[42,62,63]

ETHICAL ISSUES IN PAIN MANAGEMENT

Fear of Hastening Death by Administering Analgesics

It is common for the health professional, patient, and family members to be concerned that providing sufficient drug to relieve pain will precipitate the death of a terminally ill person.[64] This fear persists despite the American Nurses Association's (ANA's) stance that nurses should not hesitate to treat pain aggressively, even if it may hasten the death of a terminally ill person. The ethical justification for administering analgesics despite the possibility of hastening death follows the bioethical principle of the *rule of double effect.* This rule states that if an unwanted consequence (i.e., hastened death) occurs as a result of an action taken to achieve a moral good (i.e., pain relief), the action is justified because the nurse's intent is to relieve pain and not to hasten death.[65]

Requests for Assisted Suicide

Unrelieved pain is one reason that patients make requests for assisted suicide; aggressive pain management may decrease the number of requests. Assisted suicide is a complex issue that extends beyond pain and pain management. The ANA has carefully described the role of nurses in providing end-of-life care and symptom management. This role does not include active participation in assisted suicide or euthanasia.[66] Currently, Oregon is the only place in North America where assisted suicide is legal. To address the legal and ethical issues confronting nurses in this unique situation, the Oregon Nurses Association prepared a position paper on this topic.[67]

Use of Placebos in Pain Assessment and Treatment

Although their use has declined recently, placebos still are sometimes used to assess and to treat pain. Using a placebo involves deceiving patients by making them believe that they are receiving an analgesic (usually an opioid) when in fact they are typically receiving an inert substance such as saline. Health care providers have defended the use of placebos by arguing that a placebo will help distinguish patients who have "real pain" from patients who are malingering, or will decrease the incidence of side effects. However, placebos may be used more frequently in "difficult" patients who frustrate staff. Many professional organizations have published statements condemning the use of placebos.[23] To protect patients from the unethical use of placebos, it is recommended that each health care facility have a written policy about placebo use.[23]

■ Gerontologic Considerations: Pain

Chronic nonmalignant pain is a common problem in the elderly and is often associated with significant physical disability and psychosocial problems.[9,33,43] Estimates of the prevalence of chronic pain problems among community-dwelling older adults have ranged from 58% to 70%.[9] Among the elderly living in nursing homes, the estimated prevalence is 45% to 80%.[9] The most common painful conditions among older adults are musculoskeletal conditions such as osteoarthritis, low back pain, and previous fracture sites. Chronic pain often results in depression, sleep disturbance, decreased mobility, increased health care utilization, and physical and social role dysfunction.[9] Despite its high prevalence, pain in the elderly often is inadequately assessed and treated.[7-9]

There are several barriers to pain assessment in the older patient. In general, the barriers discussed earlier in the chapter are more prevalent among elderly patients. Thus older patients often believe that pain is a normal, inevitable part of aging. They may also believe that nothing can be done to relieve the pain. Older adults may not report pain for fear of being a "burden" or a "bad patient." They may have greater fears of taking opioids than other age-groups.[21,37] Also, older patients are more likely to use words such as "aching," "soreness," or "discomfort" rather than "pain."[9] Despite their reluctance to report pain, current research indicates that pain tolerance actually decreases with age.[33] For all these reasons, nurses must be persistent in asking older adults about pain. The assessment process should be carried out in an unhurried, supportive manner.

Another barrier to pain assessment in older adults is the relatively high prevalence of cognitive, sensory-perceptual, and motor problems that interfere with a person's ability to process information and to communicate.[38] Examples of these problems include dementia and delirium, post-stroke aphasia and paraplegia, and language barriers. Also, hearing and vision deficits may complicate assessment. Therefore pain assessment tools may need to be adapted for older adults. For example, it may be necessary to use a large-print pain intensity scale. Although there is some concern that older adults have difficulty using pain scales, it has been documented that many older adults, even those with mild-to-moderate cognitive impairment, can use quantitative scales accurately and reliably. There is some evidence that older adults prefer numeric rating scales and verbal descriptor scales[38] (see Fig. 9-7).

As for other patients with chronic pain, a thorough physical examination and history should be performed to identify causes of pain, possible therapies, and potential problems.[9] Because depression and functional impairments are common among elderly persons with pain, these also must be assessed.[9]

Although recommendations for older persons with pain are similar to those for other age-groups,[9,18,19] treatment of pain in the elderly is complicated by several factors. First, older adults metabolize drugs more slowly than younger patients and thus are at greater risk for higher blood levels and adverse effects. For this reason, the adage "start low and go slow" is applied to analgesic therapy in this age-group. Second, the use of NSAIDs in the elderly is associated with a high frequency of serious GI bleeding. For this reason, acetaminophen should be used whenever possible. Third, older people often are taking many drugs for one or more chronic conditions. The addition of analgesics can result in dangerous drug interactions and increased side effects. Fourth, cognitive impairment and ataxia can be exacerbated when analgesics such as opioids, antidepressants, and antiseizure drugs are used, again requiring health care providers to titrate drugs slowly and monitor carefully for side effects.

Treatment regimens for older adults must incorporate nondrug modalities. Exercise and patient teaching are particularly important nonpharmacologic interventions for older adults with chronic pain. Family and paid caregivers also should be included in the treatment plan. ■

SPECIAL POPULATIONS

Cognitively Impaired Individuals

Although patient self-report is the gold standard of pain assessment, severe cognitive impairment often prevents patients from communicating clearly regarding their pain. For these persons, behavioral and physiologic changes may be the only indicators that they are in pain. Therefore the nurse must be astute at recognizing behavioral symptoms of pain.

Several scales have been developed to assess pain in cognitively impaired elders.[68-71] Typically, these scales assess pain based on common behavioral indicators such as the following:

- Vocalization: moans, grunts, cries, sighing
- Facial expressions: grimacing, wincing, frowning, clenched teeth
- Breathing: noisy, labored
- Body movements: restlessness, rocking, pacing
- Body tension: clenched fist, resistance to movement
- Consolability: inability to be consoled or distracted

Because it is not possible to validate the meaning of the behaviors, nurses should rely on their own knowledge of the patient's usual behavior. If the nurse does not know the patient's baseline behaviors, she or he should obtain this information from other caregivers, including family members. When pain behaviors are present, they should be carefully reassessed following administration of a pain therapy.

Patients with Substance Abuse Problems

Currently, nearly 14 million Americans (1 of every 13 adults) abuse alcohol or are alcoholic. Several million more adults engage in risky drinking patterns that could lead to alcohol problems. In addition, about 14.8 million Americans (age 12 and older) are current users of illicit drugs. Of these, about 3.5 million are dependent on illicit drugs, and an additional 8.2 million are dependent on alcohol. Substance abuse among nonmalignant pain patients has been estimated at 3% to 19%.[72] Given these statistics, the nurse is faced with the challenge of assessing and providing pain relief to individuals with the dual diagnosis of pain and substance abuse disorder.

Individuals with a past or current substance abuse disorder have the right to receive effective pain management. A comprehensive pain assessment is imperative, including a detailed history, physical examination, psychosocial assessment, and diagnostic workup to determine the cause of the pain. The goal of the pain assessment is to facilitate the establishment of a treatment plan that will relieve the individual's pain effectively, as well as prevent and minimize withdrawal symptoms.

Opioids may be used effectively and safely in patients with substance dependence when indicated for pain control. Withholding opioids from chemically dependent patients with pain has not been shown to increase the likelihood of recovery from addiction. Opioid agonists-antagonists (e.g., pentazocine [Talwin], butorphanol [Stadol]) should not be used in this population because they may precipitate withdrawal. The use of "potentiators" and psychoactive drugs that do not have analgesic properties should be avoided.[23] In individuals who are tolerant to CNS depressants, larger doses of opioids or increased frequency of drug administration is necessary to achieve pain relief.

Pain management for people with addiction is challenging and usually requires a multidisciplinary team approach. Team members need to be aware of their own attitudes and misconceptions about people with substance abuse problems, which may result in undertreatment of pain.[23]

CRITICAL THINKING EXERCISES

Case Study
Pain

Patient Profile. Mrs. C. is a 280 lb (112 kg) 48-year-old African American woman admitted for an incision and drainage of a right renal abscess.

Subjective Data
- RN for 20 years
- Lives alone
- Desires 0 pain during therapy but will accept 1 to 2 on a scale of 0 to 10
- Reports incision area pain as a 2 or 3 between dressing changes and as a 10 during dressing changes
- States sharp, pulling pain persists 1 to 2 hr after dressing change
- Reports pain between dressing changes controlled by two Percocet tablets
- Reports morphine 2 mg IV barely touches pain during dressing changes

Objective Data
- Requires qid dry-to-dry dressing changes for 1 week
- Morphine 4 to 15 mg IV every 1 to 2 hours

CRITICAL THINKING QUESTIONS

1. Initially, what dose of IV morphine should be given?
2. Describe the assessment data that supports the dose selected in question 1.
3. How long should the nurse wait after the IV morphine dose to begin the dressing change?
4. If an initial dose of 6 mg IV morphine reduces the pain to a 6 during the dressing change, what nursing action is indicated?
5. What dose should be administered for subsequent dressing changes?
6. What additional pain therapies might the nurse plan to help Mrs. C. through the dressing change?
7. When Mrs. C. is discharged needing dressing changes for 3 days at home, how would the home care nurse organize her care? The nurse knows that Mrs. C. has obtained adequate pain relief with 8 mg IV morphine.
8. Based on the data presented, write one or more appropriate nursing diagnosis. Are there any collaborative problems?

CRITICAL THINKING EXERCISES—cont'd

Nursing Research Issues

1. Does a person with acute, chronic nonmalignant, or cancer pain spontaneously tell others about the pain?
2. What information (location, intensity, quality, pattern) does the patient with pain tell others?
3. What is the most effective and efficient way to overcome misconceptions the patient has about addiction, dependence, and tolerance to opioid drugs?
4. Based on the patient's usual methods of coping with pain, what nonpharmacologic pain-management strategies are most effective in promoting pain relief?
5. What is the onset of action, peak action, and duration of action for specific nonpharmacologic pain-management strategies?

REVIEW QUESTIONS

The number of the question corresponds to the same-numbered objective at the beginning of the chapter.

1. Pain is best described as
   a. a creation of a person's imagination.
   b. an unpleasant, subjective experience.
   c. a maladaptive response to a stimulus.
   d. a neurologic event resulting from activation of nociceptors.
2. A neurotransmitter known for its involvement in pain modulation is
   a. dopamine.
   b. acetylcholine.
   c. prostaglandin.
   d. norepinephrine.
3. Which of the following words is most likely to be used to describe neuropathic pain?
   a. dull
   b. mild
   c. aching
   d. burning
4. Unrelieved pain is
   a. to be expected after major surgery.
   b. to be expected in a person with cancer.
   c. dangerous and can lead to many physical and psychologic complications.
   d. an annoying sensation, but it is not as important as other physical care needs.
5. During the initial pain assessment process, the nurse should
   a. assess critical sensory components.
   b. teach the patient about pain therapies.
   c. conduct a comprehensive pain assessment.
   d. provide appropriate treatment and evaluate its effect.
6. An example of distraction to provide pain relief is
   a. TENS.
   b. music.
   c. exercise.
   d. biofeedback.
7. An appropriate nonopioid analgesic for mild pain is
   a. oxycodone.
   b. ibuprofen (Advil).
   c. lorazepam (Ativan).
   d. cyclobenzaprine (Flexeril).
8. An important nursing responsibility related to pain is to
   a. leave the patient alone to rest.
   b. help the patient appear to not be in pain.
   c. believe what the patient says about the pain.
   d. assume responsibility for eliminating the patient's pain.
9. A nurse administering a prescribed dose of an IV opioid that was titrated for a person with severe pain related to a terminal illness would be considered to be participating in
   a. euthanasia.
   b. assisted suicide.
   c. the patient's addiction.
   d. palliative pain management.
10. A nurse believes that patients with the same type of tissue injury should have the same amount of pain. This statement reflects
    a. a belief that will contribute to appropriate pain management.
    b. an accurate statement about pain mechanisms and an expected goal of pain therapy.
    c. a premise that the nurse's belief will have no effect on the type of care provided to people in pain.
    d. the nurse's lack of knowledge about pain mechanisms, which is likely to contribute to poor pain management.

REFERENCES

1. American Pain Foundation. Available at *www.painfoundation.org/page_ fastfacts.asp* (accessed Feb 2, 2002).
2. Canadian Pain Society. Available at *www.medicine.dal.ca/cps/* (accessed Feb 2, 2002).
3. SUPPORT Principal Investigators: A controlled trial to improve care for seriously ill hospitalized patients: the study to understand prognoses and preferences for outcomes and risk of treatments (SUPPORT), *JAMA* 274:1591, 1995.
4. Desbiens NA, Wu AW: Pain and suffering in seriously ill hospitalized patients, *J Am Geriatr Soc* 48:S183, 2000.
5. Phillips DM: JCAHO pain management standards are unveiled, *JAMA* 284:428, 2000.

*6. Ferrell BA, Ferrell BR, Rivera L: Pain in cognitively impaired nursing home patients, *J Pain Symptom Manage* 10:591, 1995.
7. Won A et al: Correlates and management of nonmalignant pain in the nursing home, *J Am Geriatr Soc* 47:936, 1999.
8. Bernabei R et al: Management of pain in elderly patients with cancer, *JAMA* 279:1877, 1998.
9. American Geriatrics Society Panel on Chronic Pain in Older Persons: The management of chronic pain in older persons, *J Am Geriatr Soc* 46:635, 1998.
10. Pasero C, Paice JA, McCaffery M: Basic mechanisms underlying the causes and effects of pain. In McCaffery M, Pasero C, editors: *Pain: clinical manual,* ed 2, St Louis, 1999, Mosby.

*Nursing research–based reference.

11. Page GG, Eliyahu S: The immune-suppressive nature of pain, *Semin Oncol Nurs* 13:10, 1997.

12. Cousins M, Power I: Acute and postoperative pain. In Wall PD, Melzack R, editors: *Textbook of pain,* ed 4, Edinburgh, 1999, Churchill Livingstone.

*13. Grant M et al: Unscheduled readmissions for uncontrolled symptoms: a health care challenge for nurses, *Nurs Clin North Am* 30:673, 1995.

14. Sheehan J et al: What cost chronic pain? *Irish Med J* 89:218, 1996.

15. McMillan SC et al: Management of pain and pain-related symptoms in hospitalized veterans with cancer, *Cancer Nurs* 23:327, 2000.

16. Pargeon KL, Hailey BJ: Barriers to effective cancer pain management: a review of literature, *J Pain Symptom Manage* 18: 358, 1999.

*17. Erkes EB et al: An examination of critical care nurses' knowledge and attitudes regarding pain management in hospitalized patients, *Pain Manage Nurs* 2:47, 2001.

18. Agency for Health Care Policy and Research: *Clinical practice guideline: management of cancer pain,* Rockville, Md, 1994, US Department of Health and Human Services.

19. American Pain Society: *Principles of analgesic use in the treatment of acute pain and chronic cancer pain,* ed 4, Skokie, Ill, 1999, American Pain Society.

20. World Health Organization: *Cancer pain relief,* ed 2, Geneva, 1996, World Health Organization.

*21. Ward SE et al: The impact on quality of life of patient-related barriers to pain management, *Res Nurs Health* 21:405, 1998.

*22. Ersek M, Kraybill BM, Du Pen AR: Factors hindering patients' use of medication for cancer pain, *Cancer Pract* 7:226, 1999.

23. McCaffery M, Pasero C: *Pain: a clinical manual for nursing practice,* ed 2, St Louis, 1999, Mosby.

24. International Association for the Study of Pain: *IASP pain terminology, 1994.* Available at *www.iasp_pain/org/terms-p.html* (accessed Feb 8, 2002).

25. Cassell EJ: The nature of suffering and the goals of medicine, *N Engl J Med* 306:639, 1982.

26. Willis WD, Westlund KN: Neuroanatomy of the pain system and of the pathways that modulate pain, *J Clin Neurophysiol* 14:2, 1997.

*27. Ersek M: Enhancing effective pain management by addressing patient barriers to analgesic use, *J Hosp Palliat Nurs* 1:87, 1999.

28. Johansson EE et al: The meanings of pain: an exploration of women's descriptions of symptoms, *Soc Sci Med* 48:1791, 1999.

29. Geisser ME et al: Catastrophizing, depression and the sensory, affective and evaluative aspects of chronic pain, *Pain* 59:79, 1994.

30. Watkins KW et al: Age, pain and coping with rheumatoid arthritis, *Pain* 82:217, 1999.

31. Keefe FJ et al: The relationship of gender to pain, pain behavior, and disability in osteoarthritis patients: the role of catastrophizing, *Pain* 87:325, 2000.

32. Vallerand AH, Polomano RC: The relationship of gender to pain, *Pain Manage Nurs* 1:8, 2000.

33. Gagliese L, Katz J, Melzack R: Pain in the elderly. In Wall PD, Melzack R, editors: *Textbook of pain,* ed 4, Edinburgh, 1999, Churchill Livingstone.

34. Ferrell BR: Pain observed: the experience of pain from the family caregiver's perspective, *Clin Geriatr Med* 17:595, 2001.

35. Gonzales VA, Martelli MF, Baker JM: Psychological assessment of persons with chronic pain, *Neurorehabilitation* 4:69, 2001.

36. Cherny NL: Cancer pain: principles of assessment and syndromes. In Berger AM, Portenoy RK, Weissman DE, editors: *Principles and practice of supportive oncology,* Philadelphia, 1998, Lippincott-Raven.

37. Twycross RG: Opioids. In Wall PD, Melzack R, editors: *Textbook of pain,* ed 4, Edinburgh, 1999, Churchill Livingstone.

38. Herr K, Garrand L: Assessment and measurement of pain in older adults, *Clin Geriatr Med* 17:457, 2001.

*39. Herr KA et al: Evaluation of the faces pain scale for use with the elderly, *Clin J Pain* 14:29, 1998.

40. Hicks CL et al: The faces pain scale—revised: toward a common metric in pediatric pain measurement, *Pain* 93:173, 2001.

41. Mao J, Chen LL: Gabapentin in pain management, *Anesth Analg* 91:680, 2000.

42. Joint Commission on Accreditation of Healthcare Organizations: *JCAHO pain standards for 2001.* Available at *www.jcaho.org/standard/pain management.html* (accessed Feb. 8, 2002).

43. Leo RJ, Singh A: Pain management in the elderly: use of psychopharmacologic agents, *Ann Long-Term Care* 10:37, 2002.

44. Pereira J et al: Equianalgesic dose ratios for opioids. a critical review and proposals for long-term dosing, *J Pain Symptom Manage* 22:672, 2001.

45. Schnitzer TJ: Osteoarthritis management: the role of cyclooxygenase-2-selective inhibitors, *Clin Ther* 23:313, 2001.

46. Preston KL, Jasinski DR, Testa M: Abuse potential and pharmacological comparison of tramadol and morphine, *Drug Alcohol Depend* 27:7, 1991.

47. Berde CB, Strichartz GR: Local anesthetics. In Miller RD, editor: *Anesthesia,* ed 5, Philadelphia, 2000, Churchill Livingstone.

48. Payne R et al: Long-term safety of oral transmucosal fentanyl citrate for breakthrough cancer pain, *J Pain Symptom Manage* 22:575, 2001.

49. Anderson C: What's new in pain management? *Home Healthc Nurse* 18:648, 2000.

50. Simpson BA: Spinal cord and brain stimulation. In Wall PD, Melzack R, editors: *Textbook of pain,* ed 4, Edinburgh, 1999, Churchill Livingstone.

51. Hansson P, Lundeberg T: Transcutaneous electrical nerve stimulation, vibration and acupuncture as pain-relieving measures. In Wall PD, Melzack R, editors: *Textbook of pain,* ed 4, Edinburgh, 1999, Churchill Livingstone.

52. Hamza MA et al: Percutaneous electrical nerve stimulation: a novel analgesic therapy for diabetic neuropathic pain, *Diabetes Care* 23:365, 2000.

53. Carlsson CPO, Sjolund BH: Acupuncture for chronic low back pain: a randomized placebo-controlled study with long-term follow-up, *Clin J Pain* 17:296, 2001.

54. Sellick SM, Zaza C: Critical review of 5 nonpharmacologic strategies for managing cancer pain, *Cancer Prev Control* 2:7, 1998.

*55. Good M et al: Relaxation and music to reduce postoperative pain, *J Adv Nurs* 33:208, 2001.

56. Consensus document from the American Academy of Pain Medicine, the American Pain Society, and the American Society of Addiction Medicine: *Definitions related to the use of opioids for the treatment of pain,* 2001. Available at *www.ampainsoc.org/advocacy/opioids2.htm* (accessed July 26, 2002).

57. South SM, Smith MT: Analgesic tolerance to opioids, *Pain Clinical Updates* 9:1, 2001.

58. Passick SD: Responding rationally to recent reports of abuse/diversion of OxyContin®, *Pain Symptom Manage* 21:359, 2001.

59. Glajchen M: Chronic pain: treatment barriers and strategies for clinical practice, *J Am Board Fam Pract* 14:211, 2001.

60. Meekin SA et al: Development of a palliative education assessment tool for medical student education, *Acad Med* 75:986, 2000.

61. Weissman DE et al: Improving pain management in long-term care facilities, *J Palliat Med* 4:567, 2001.

62. Pasero C, McCaffery M, Gordon DB: Build institutional commitment to improving pain management, *Nurs Manage* 30:27, 1999.

63. Gordon DB, Berry PH, Dahl JL: JCAHO's new focus on pain: implications for hospice and palliative nurses, *J Hospice Palliat Nurs* 2:135, 2000.

64. Stanley KJ, Zoloth-Dorfman L: Ethical considerations. In Ferrell BR, Coyle N, editors: *Textbook of palliative nursing,* New York, 2001, Oxford University Press.

65. Beauchamp TL, Childress JF: *Principles of biomedical ethics,* ed 5, New York, 2001, Oxford University Press.

66. American Nurses Association: ANA's position on assisted suicide, *Am Nurse* 28:9, 1996.

67. Oregon Nurses Association: *Position paper on the death with dignity act, 1995.* Available at *www.oregonrn.org/services-whitepapers-0001.php* (accessed Feb 8, 2002).

*68. Feldt KS: The checklist of nonverbal pain indicators (CNPI), *Pain Manage Nurs* 1:13, 2000.

*69. Hurley AC et al: Assessment of discomfort in advanced Alzheimer patients, *Res Nurs Health* 15:369, 1992.

*70. Kovach CR et al: Assessment and treatment of discomfort for people with late-stage dementia, *J Pain Symptom Manage* 18:412, 1999.

*71. Kovach CR et al: Use of the assessment of discomfort in dementia protocol, *Appl Nurs Res* 14:193, 2001.

72. National Institute on Drug Abuse: *Pain medications and other prescription drugs, 2001.* Available at *www.drugabuse.gov/Infofax/PainMed.htmlm* (accessed Feb 8, 2002).

---

*Nursing research–based reference.

RESOURCES

Agency for Healthcare Research and Quality
2101 E. Jefferson Street, Suite 501
Rockville, MD 20852
301-594-1364
E-mail: info@ahrq.gov
www.ahcpr.gov

American Academy of Orofacial Pain
19 Mantua Road
Mount Royal, NJ 08061
856-423-3629
Fax: 856-423-3420
www.aaop.org/

American Academy of Pain Management (ACPM)
13947 Mono Way #A
Sonora, CA 95370
209-533-9744
www.aapainmanage.org/

American Academy of Pain Medicine (AAPM)
4700 West Lake Avenue
Glenview, IL 60025-1485
847-375-4731
Fax: 877-734-8750
E-mail: aapm@amctec.com
www.painmed.org/

American Chronic Pain Association
PO Box 850
Rocklin, CA 95677
916-632-0922
Fax: 916-632-3208
www.theacpa.org/

American Headache Society
19 Mantua Road
Mount Royal, NJ 08061
856-423-0043
Fax: 856-423-0082
E-mail: ahshq@talley.com
www.ahsnet.org

American Pain Society
4700 West Lake Avenue
Glenview, IL 60025-1485
847-375-4715
Fax: 877-734-8758
E-mail: info@ampainsoc.org
www.ampainsoc.org/

American Society of Addiction Medicine
4601 North Park Avenue, Arcade Suite 101
Chevy Chase, MD 20815
301-656-3920
Fax: 301-656-3815
E-mail: email@asam.org
www.asam.org/

American Society of Pain Management Nursing
7794 Grow Drive
Pensacola, FL 32514
888-342-7766
Fax: 850-484-8762
www.aspmn.org/

American Society for Psychosocial and Behavioral Oncology/AIDS (ASPBOA) and International Psycho-Oncology Society (IPOS)
www.ipos-aspboa.org/

American Society of Regional Anesthesia and Pain Medicine
PO Box 11086
Richmond, VA 23230-1086
804-282-0010
Fax: 804-282-0090
www.asra.com/welcome.htm

Association for Applied Psychophysiology and Biofeedback
10200 West 44th Avenue, Suite 304
Wheat Ridge, CO 80033-2840
800-477-8892
303-422-8436
Fax: 303-422-8894
www.aapb.org/

City of Hope Pain/Palliative Care Resource Center
c/o City of Hope National Medical Center
Nursing Research and Education
1500 East Duarte Road
Duarte, CA 91010
E-mail: prc@coh.org
www.cityofhope.org/prc/web/

Hospice and Palliative Nurses Association
Penn Center West One, Suite 229
Pittsburgh, PA 15276
412-787-9301
Fax: 412-787-9305
E-mail: HPNA@hpna.org
www.hpna.org/index.asp

International Association for the Study of Pain (IASP)
909 NE 43rd Street, Suite 306
Seattle, WA 98105-6020
206-547-6409
Fax: 206-547-1703
E-mail: IASP@locke.hs.washington.edu
www.halcyon.com/iasp/

Joint Commission on Accreditation of Healthcare Organizations (JCAHO) Pain Standards, 2001
JCAHO accreditation standards on pain assessment and management, approved July 31, 1999
www.jcaho.org/standard/stds2001_mpfrm.html

Last Acts Web Site
Ms. Karen Long, Professional Outreach
Stewart Communications, Ltd.
325 West Huron, Suite 300
Chicago, IL 60610
312-751-1297
Fax: 312-751-1372
E-mail: karenl@stewcommltd.com
www.lastacts.org

National Committee on Treatment of Intractable Pain
PO Box 9553
Friendship Station
Washington, DC 20016
202-965-6717
Fax: 202-293-4827

North American Chronic Pain Association of Canada
60 Lorne Avenue
Dartmouth, NS
Canada B2Y 3E7
866-470 PAIN (7246)
Fax: 905-793-8781
www.chronicpaincanada.org/

OncoLink: Pain Management
www.oncolink.com/

Pain.com
www.pain.com/

PainLink
www.edc.org/PainLink/

Pediatric Pain Research Lab
c/o Dalhouise University
Halifax, NS
Canada B3H 4R2
902-494-2211
http://is.dal.ca/~pedpain

University of Iowa College of Nursing
Patient educational resources on pain for adults and kids
www.nursing.uiowa.edu/sites/pedspain/resources/inform.htm

University of Wisconsin Pain and Policy Studies Group
www.medsch.wisc.edu/painpolicy/

For additional Internet resources, see the website for this book at *http://evolve.elsevier.com/Lewis/medsurg/*.

CHAPTER *10*

End-of-Life Care

Cheryl Ross Staats
Kathleen A. Pollard
Catherine E. Brown

LEARNING OBJECTIVES

1. Describe the physical manifestations at the end of life.
2. Relate the common psychologic manifestations at the end of life.
3. Explain the process of grief at the end of life.
4. Examine the cultural and spiritual issues related to end-of-life care.
5. Discuss ethical and legal issues in end-of-life care.

6. Discuss the purpose of palliative care and hospice.
7. Describe the nursing management for the dying patient.
8. Explore the special needs of family caregivers in end-of-life care.
9. Discuss the special needs of the nurse who cares for dying patients and their families.

KEY TERMS

advance directives, p. 164	death rattle, p. 161
bereavement, p. 162	end-of-life care, p. 160
brain death, p. 161	grief, p. 162
Cheyne-Stokes respiration, p. 161	hospice, p. 165
death, p. 160	palliative care, p. 165

Life and death have intrigued humankind throughout history. Artists, writers, philosophers, scientists, religious leaders, and many others have pondered the meaning of life and death. Mortality and the death experience are difficult and awkward topics to discuss and accept in Western society. However, death is as real a part of life as birth.

The concepts of death and dying were rarely discussed or studied in the West before the 1960s. Many times patients who were not expected to survive were placed in isolated hospital areas, were given less than quality care, and died without appropriate medical care. Family members, faith communities, or both were usually the care providers.

Today, with the reality of the "graying of America" and the increasing number of persons with chronic diseases, terminal illness and dying are not viewed as the taboo topics that they once were. The special needs of the dying and the terminally ill are now acknowledged and integrated into care. Death and dying are researched by scientists, health care professionals, theologians, and laypersons. Information concerning death and dying can be found in both popular and professional literature.

End-of-life care (EOL care) is the term currently used for issues related to death and dying. The Institute of Medicine defines *end of life* as the concluding phase of a normal life span, although life can end at any age.[1] The time from diagnosis of a terminal illness to death varies considerably depending on the patient's diagnosis and extent of disease. EOL care focuses on physical and psychosocial needs at the end of life for the patient and the patient's family. The goals for EOL care are to (1) provide comfort and supportive care during the dying process, (2) improve the quality of the remaining life, and (3) help ensure a dignified death (Fig. 10-1).

PHYSICAL MANIFESTATIONS AT END OF LIFE

Death occurs when all vital organs and systems cease to function. **Death** is the irreversible cessation of circulatory and respiratory function or the irreversible cessation of all functions of the entire brain, including the brainstem. Trauma and disease processes can affect physical manifestations at the end of life. As death approaches, metabolism is reduced and the body gradually slows down until all function ends. Generally, respirations cease first. Then the heart stops beating within a few minutes. Physical manifestations of approaching death are listed in Table 10-1.

Sensory Changes

With decreased oxygenation and circulation to the brain, there are alterations in the interpretation of sensory input. Sensory changes can include blurred vision, decreased sense of taste and smell, and decreased pain and touch perception. The blink reflex

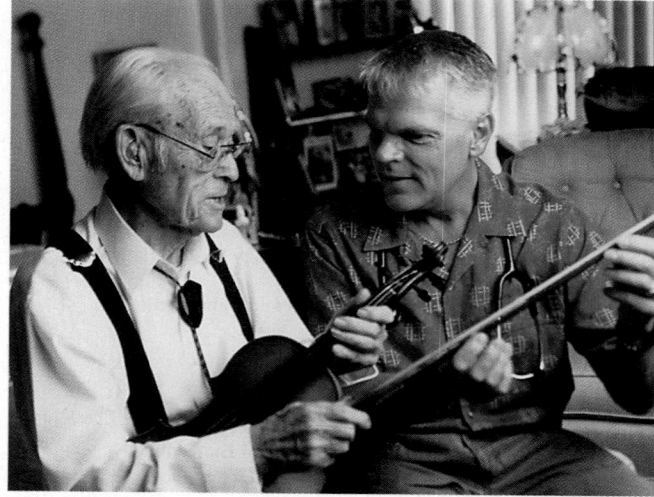

FIG. 10-1 One goal of end-of-life care is to improve the quality of the patient's remaining life.

Reviewed by Janene Council Jeffery, RN, MSN, CDE, Professor, Austin Community College, Associate Degree Nursing Program, Austin, Tex; and Patsy Ruppert Rider, RN, MSN, CNS, Clinical Instructor in Nursing, University of Texas at Austin, Austin, Tex.

TABLE 10-1	Physical Manifestations of Approaching Death		
SYSTEM	**MANIFESTATIONS**	**SYSTEM**	**MANIFESTATIONS**
Sensory system 　Hearing 　Touch 　Taste and smell 　Sight	• Usually last sense to disappear • Decreased sensation • Decreased perception of pain and touch • Decreased with disease progression • Blurring of vision • Sinking and glazing of eyes • Blink reflex absent • Eyelids remain half-open	Gastrointestinal system	• Slowing of digestive tract and possible cessation of function (may be enhanced by pain-relieving drugs) • Accumulation of gas • Distention and nausea • Loss of sphincter control may produce incontinence • Bowel movement may occur before imminent death or at time of death
Integumentary system	• Mottling on hands, feet, arms, and legs • Cold, clammy skin • Cyanosis on nose, nail beds, knees • "Waxlike" skin when very near death	Musculoskeletal system	• Gradual loss of ability to move • Sagging of jaw resulting from loss of facial muscle tone • Difficulty speaking • Swallowing can become more difficult • Difficulty maintaining body posture and alignment • Loss of gag reflex • Jerking seen in patients on large amounts of opioids
Respiratory system	• Increased respiratory rate • Cheyne-Stokes respiration (abnormal pattern of respiration characterized by alternating periods of apnea and deep, rapid breathing) • Inability to cough or clear secretions resulting in grunting, gurgling, or noisy congested breathing (death rattle) • Irregular breathing, gradually slowing down to terminal gasps (may be described as guppy breathing)	Cardiovascular system	• Increased heart rate; later slowing and weakening of pulse • Irregular rhythm • Decrease in blood pressure • Delayed absorption of drugs administered intramuscularly or subcutaneously
Urinary system	• Gradual decrease in urinary output • Incontinent of urine • Unable to urinate		

is eventually lost, and the patient appears to stare. The sense of touch decreases first in the lower extremities because of circulatory alterations. Hearing is commonly believed to be the last sense to remain intact at the end of life.

Circulatory and Respiratory Changes

With decreased oxygenation and altered circulation causing metabolic changes, the heart rate slows and weakens and the blood pressure falls progressively. Body temperature may be elevated related to a disease process and changes in hypothalamic function. Respirations may be rapid or slow, shallow, and irregular. Breath sounds may become wet and noisy, both audibly and on auscultation. Noisy, wet-sounding respirations, termed the **death rattle,** are due to mouth breathing and accumulation of mucus in the airways. **Cheyne-Stokes respiration** is an abnormal pattern of breathing characterized by alternating periods of apnea and deep, rapid breathing. This type of breathing is usually seen as a person nears death.

There is decreased circulation, especially noticeable on the skin. The extremities become pale, mottled, and cyanotic. The skin feels cool to the touch, first in the feet and legs, then progressing to the hands and arms, and finally progressing to the torso. The skin may feel warm because of an elevated body temperature related to an underlying disease process.

Loss of Muscle Tone

As death becomes imminent, metabolic changes cause the muscular system to gradually weaken, leading to sluggish functional abilities. Facial muscles lose tone, causing the jaw to sag. Decreased muscle coordination leads to difficulty in speaking. Swallowing becomes increasingly difficult, and the gag reflex is eventually lost. Gastrointestinal motility and peristalsis diminish, leading to constipation, gas accumulation, distention, and nausea. Pain-relieving drugs may exacerbate these gastrointestinal manifestations. The ability of the urinary system to function and produce urine decreases. Loss of sphincter control can lead to fecal and urinary incontinence.

Brain Death

The diagnosis of death is based on brain or cerebral death. **Brain death** occurs when the cerebral cortex stops functioning or is irreversibly destroyed. The cerebral cortex, or the higher brain, is responsible for voluntary movement and actions, as well as for cognitive functioning.[2]

Since the development of technology that assists in supporting life, controversies have arisen related to an exact definition of death. Questions and discussions have developed around whether brain or cerebral death occurs when the whole brain (cortex and brainstem) ceases activity or when cortical function alone stops.

In 1995 the Quality Standards Subcommittee of the American Academy of Neurology recommended diagnostic criteria guidelines for clinical diagnosis of brain death in adults. These criteria for brain death include coma or unresponsiveness, absence of brainstem reflexes, and apnea. Specific assessments by a physician are required to validate each of the criteria.[3]

Currently, legal and medical standards require that all brain function must cease for brain death to be pronounced and life support to be disconnected by the physician. Diagnosis of brain death is of particular importance when organ donation is an option. In some states, under specific circumstances registered nurses are legally permitted to pronounce death. Policies and procedures may vary from state to state, among the Board of Nurse Examiners for Registered Nurses in each state, and among institutions.[4]

PSYCHOSOCIAL MANIFESTATIONS AT END OF LIFE

A variety of feelings and emotions affect the dying patient and family at the end of life. Specific psychosocial manifestations are listed in Table 10-2. Most patients and families struggle with a terminal diagnosis and the realization that there is no cure. Time may be needed to process the impending death and to formulate emotional responses. The patient and the family feel overwhelmed, fearful, powerless, and fatigued. The patient's needs and wishes must be respected. Patients need time to ponder their thoughts and express their feelings. Response time to questions may be sluggish because of fatigue, weakness, and confusion.

GRIEF

Grief is the emotional and behavioral response to loss. It is an emotional reaction that is necessary to maintain quality in both emotional and physical well-being. The grieving process involves a total individual experience associated with thoughts, feelings, and behaviors. Grieving related to loss from death is a complex and intense emotional experience.

Grief is manifested in a variety of ways. Every loss is as different as each person is unique. There are no guidelines to predict grief reactions. Individuals experience different aspects of the grieving process at different times. The individual's cultural beliefs, religious influences or spiritual beliefs, and value system influence grief reactions. The intensity of grief is driven by an individual's personality, the nature of the relationship with the dying person, concurrent life crises, coping resources, and the availability of support systems.[5]

Kübler-Ross, Martocchio, and Rando have each identified stages of grief.[6-8] A comparison among the three is listed in Table 10-3. Kübler-Ross identified denial, anger, bargaining, depression, and acceptance as the five stages of grieving.[6] Martocchio presented five clusters of grief to include (1) shock and disbelief; (2) yearning and protest; (3) anguish, disorganization, and despair; (4) identification of bereavement; and (5) reorganization and resolution.[7] Rando refined three phases of responses to grieving that were identified as avoidance, confrontation, and accommodation.[8]

In conjunction with grief, significant others who survive respond to the loss of the loved one through bereavement. **Bereavement** is an individual's response to the loss of a significant person. It is important to note that bereavement for the family and significant others may begin before the death occurs. Working through the grief process helps the dying person and significant others adapt to the loss.

The process of resolution in normal grief may take months to years. *Pathologic grief* can manifest as chronic grief when the intensity does not wane after the first year. The bereaved person becomes "bogged down" in the grieving process. Grief can manifest as *conflicted grief* when the bereaved person has not resolved ambivalent feelings toward the deceased. Grief can manifest as *absent grief* when the bereaved person appears to be coping and carrying on as if nothing has happened.

Grief that is prolonged, unresolved, or disruptive may be termed *maladaptive* or *dysfunctional grief*. Grief that is delayed or exaggerated may be identified as dysfunctional. Dysfunctional grieving may relate to a real loss or a perceived loss. It may oc-

---

TABLE 10-2	Psychosocial Manifestations of Approaching Death

- Altered decision making
- Anxiety about unfinished business
- Decreased socialization
- Fear of loneliness
- Fear of meaninglessness
- Fear of pain
- Helplessness
- Life review
- Peacefulness
- Restlessness
- Saying goodbyes
- Unusual communication
- Vision-like experiences
- Withdrawal

TABLE 10-3	Comparison of Stages of Grieving	
KÜBLER-ROSS (1969)[6]	**MARTOCCHIO (1985)[7]**	**RANDO (1993)[8]**
Denial	Shock and disbelief	Avoidance
Anger/bargaining	Yearning and protest	Confrontation
Depression	Anguish, disorganization, and despair	
	Identification of bereavement	
Acceptance	Reorganization and restoration	Accommodation

> A nurse does not strive only to alleviate physical pain or render physical care—she ministers to the person. The nurse cares for the individual, not a body part. The existence of suffering whether physical, mental, or spiritual is the proper concern of the nurse.

From Allen-Shelly J, Fish S: *Spiritual care: the nurse's role*, ed 3, Downers Grove, Ill, 1988, InterVarsity Press.

cur when grief is not resolved from a prior experience or when the expression of grief is blocked in some way. With dysfunctional grief, feelings and behaviors may become exaggerated and disruptive to a person's usual lifestyle.

Grief that is helpful or that assists the person in accepting the reality of death is called *adaptive grief.* Adaptive grief is a healthy response. It may be associated with grieving before a death actually occurs or when the reality that death is inevitable is known.

The grief process takes time, energy, and work. Goals for the grieving process include resolving emotions, reflecting on the dying person, expressing feelings of loss and sadness, and valuing what has been shared.

VARIABLES AFFECTING END-OF-LIFE CARE

People experiencing the inevitability of death are in need of caregivers who are knowledgeable about personal issues and attitudes that affect the EOL experience. The attitudes of the dying person, family and significant others, and nurses affect the death experience.

Health care professionals must be aware of cultural differences as they care for patients and families[9] (Fig. 10-2). An adequate understanding of cultural, religious, and familial influences is beneficial when focusing on the dying person's and family's needs, wants, and fears. Although there may be influences from culture, religion, and family, the uniqueness of each person will lead to varied responses.

Culture and religious beliefs affect a person's understanding of and reaction to death or loss. Frequently, beliefs and attitudes are interrelated between culture and religion. The Western work ethic is closely related to the American ethic, which emphasizes independence, self-reliance, hard work, and rugged individualism. With these attitudes many people believe that privacy is imperative. Death and dying tend to be private matters shared only with significant others. Often feelings are repressed or internalized. People who believe in "toughing it out" or "being strong" may not express themselves when they are experiencing a tragic loss.

Some cultural groups, such as African Americans and Hispanic Americans, may express their feelings more easily. In some predominantly African American churches, expressing emotions plays an important role. Kinship tends to be very strong in the Hispanic American culture. Family members, both immediate and extended, provide support for one another. Expressing feelings of loss is encouraged and accepted easily. (Culturally competent care is discussed in Chapter 2.)

Assessment of spiritual needs in EOL care is a key consideration (Fig. 10-3). Spiritual needs do not necessarily equate to religion. A person may be of no particular faith but have a deep spirituality. Many times at the end of life, patients question their beliefs about a higher power, their own journey through life, religion, and an afterlife. Some patients may choose to pursue a spiritual path. Some may not. Their individual choice needs to be respected.

Deep-seated religious beliefs may surface for some patients when they deal with their terminal diagnosis and related issues. Spiritual distress may occur with a challenge to and questioning of beliefs and values surrounding the past, present, and future.[10]

Some dying patients are secure in their faith about the future. It is common to observe patients relinquishing material values of life and focusing on values they believe will lead them on to another place. Patients whose spiritual lives appear to be in order have a more peaceful death.[11]

Differences among cultural, religious, and spiritual beliefs and values are innumerable. Nursing assessments of beliefs and preferences should be completed on an individual basis to avoid stereotyping individuals with particular behaviors and belief systems. (Culture is discussed in Chapter 2.)

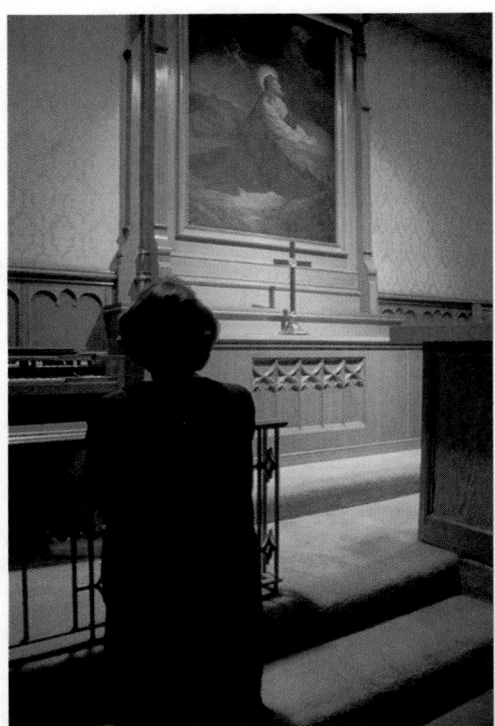

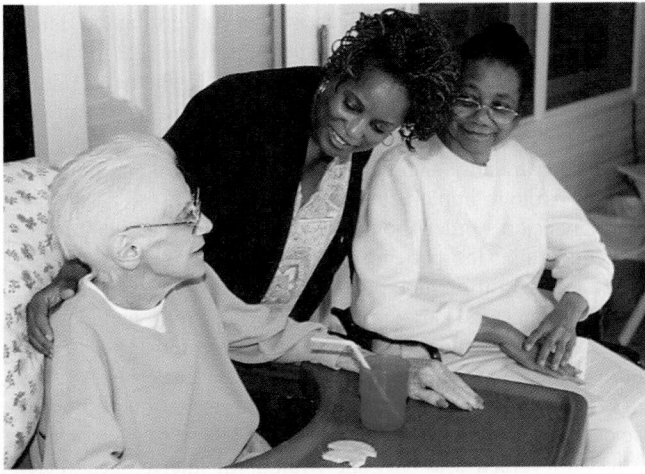

FIG. 10-2 Health care professionals must be aware of cultural differences as they care for patients and families.

FIG. 10-3 Spiritual needs are an important consideration in end-of-life care.

LEGAL AND ETHICAL ISSUES AFFECTING END-OF-LIFE CARE

Patients and families struggle with many decisions during the terminal illness and dying experience. Many people decide that the outcomes related to their care should be based on their own wishes. The decisions may involve the choice for (1) organ and tissue donations, (2) advance directives (e.g., medical power of attorney, living wills), and (3) resuscitation.

Persons who are legally competent may choose organ donation. Any body part or the entire body may be donated. The decision to donate organs or to provide anatomic gifts may be made by a person before death. The decision to donate organs may be made by immediate family members following death. Family permission must be obtained at the time of donation.

Some people carry donor cards. Some states allow for organ donation to be marked on drivers' licenses. The names of agencies that handle organ donation will vary by locale. Common names for such an agency might be the organ bank, organ-sharing network, and organ sharing alliance. Both organ and tissue donations follow specific legal guidelines. Legal requirements and facility policies for organ or tissue donation must be followed. The physician must be notified immediately when organ donation is intended because some tissues must be used within hours after death.[12]

Legal Documents Used in End-of-Life Care

In 1991 the Omnibus Reconciliation Act of 1990 became effective. It is frequently known as the Patient Self-Determination Act.[13] This act requires all institutions that participate in Medicare to provide written information to patients concerning their right to accept or refuse treatment. This information should include the right to initiate advance directives. **Advance directives** are written statements of a person's wishes regarding medical care. The first advance directive was known by laypersons as a *living will*. It was developed by the Euthanasia Education Council, which is now known as the Partnership for Caring.

Most states have replaced the idea of living wills with *natural death acts*. Within many of these acts are specific aspects related to the individual's wishes. *Directives to physicians* (DTP), *durable power of attorney for health care* (DPAHC), and *medical power of attorney* (MPOA) may be included in the natural death acts. Under the natural death acts an individual can tell the physician exactly what treatment is or is not desired. Each state has its own unique requirements.[14] Table 10-4 identifies common legal and ethical documents used in EOL care.

Copies of state-specific forms can be obtained from local medical associations and the Internet. However, a person may write his or her wishes without special forms. Verbal directives may be given to physicians with specific instructions in the presence of two witnesses. Attorneys and notaries may not necessarily be required. In the event that the person is not capable of communicating his or her wishes, the family and the physician can agree on what measures will or will not be taken. The physician should record the family's decision.

In the past 30 years cardiopulmonary resuscitation (CPR) has become common practice in health care. Patients who suffered respiratory or cardiac arrest have been given CPR unless a *do-not-resuscitate (DNR) order* was given by the physician. Many times patients and families have had no choice as to whether CPR was used.

In recent years, much has been written concerning the right to die and the right to choose. Many people believe that the patient or the patient's family has the right to decide whether CPR will be used. It is no longer the sole decision of the physician. The American Nurses Association (ANA) supports the patient's right to self-determination and believes that nurses will and must play a primary role in implementation of the law.[15]

A physician's order should be written to include the information concerning the patient's or family's wishes for the use of CPR. Several different types of CPR decisions can be made. Complete and total heroic measures, which may include CPR, drugs, and mechanical ventilation, can be referred to as a *full code*. Some people choose variations of the full code. A *chemical code* involves the use of drugs for resuscitation without the use of CPR. A "no code" or a DNR order allows the person to die with comfort measures only and without the interference of technology. Some states have implemented a form called *out-of-hospital DNR* for use by terminally ill patients who wish to have

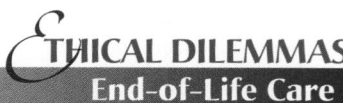

ETHICAL DILEMMAS
End-of-Life Care

Situation
A terminally ill 50-year-old woman with metastatic breast cancer has developed severe bone pain that is not adequately controlled by her present dose of IV morphine. She moans at rest and verbalizes severe pain from any movement to reposition her. Even though she appears to sleep at intervals, she requests pain medicine frequently and her family is demanding additional pain medicine for her. At the team conference the nurses have discussed the need for more effective pain control, but are concerned that additional pain medicine could hasten her death.

Important Points for Consideration
- Adequate pain relief is an important outcome for all patients but in particular for patients who are terminally ill. The *principle of beneficence* means that care is provided to benefit patients.
- When the goal of treatment of the terminally ill is providing adequate pain control to alleviate suffering, the goal is based on the *principle of nonmaleficence:* preventing or reducing harm to the patient. The secondary effect of hastening the patient's death is ethically justified.
- *Euthanasia,* the deliberate act of hastening death, is not morally acceptable.
- Adequate pain relief at the end of life continues to be a major concern of health care professionals and consumers.

Critical Thinking Questions
1. What type of discussions should occur among members of the health care team, patient, and family as this phase of care is approached in the terminally ill?
2. Distinguish between assisted suicide and euthanasia, and between promotion of comfort and relief of pain in dying patients. (Use the ANA position statements.)

TABLE 10-4   Common Documents Used in End-of-Life Care

DOCUMENT	DESCRIPTION	SPECIAL CONSIDERATIONS
Advance directive	A general term used to describe documents that give instructions about future medical care and treatments	• Specific measures to be used or withheld can or may be specified.
Directive to physicians	A written document specifying the patient's wish to be allowed to die without heroic or extraordinary measures	• Specific measures to be used or withheld can be specified.
Do not resuscitate (DNR)	A written physician's order instructing health care providers not to attempt CPR; often requested by family; must be signed by a physician to be valid	• Any specific measures to be used or withheld must be specified.
Durable power of attorney for health care	A term used by some states to describe a document used for listing the person or persons to make health care decisions should a patient become unable to make informed decisions for self	• May be the same as medical power of attorney. • Specific measures to be used or withheld can be specified.
Living will	A lay term used frequently to describe any number of documents that give instructions about future medical care and treatments or the wish to be allowed to die without heroic or extraordinary measures should the patient be unable to communicate for self	• Specific documents must be identified.
Medical power of attorney	A term used by some states to describe a document used for listing the person or persons to make health care decisions should a patient become unable to make informed decisions for self	• May be the same as durable power of attorney for health care, health care proxy, or appointment of a health care agent or surrogate. Specific measures to be used or withheld can be specified. • Person appointed may be called a health care agent, surrogate, attorney-in-fact, or proxy.

no heroic measures used to prolong life after they leave an acute care facility.[16,17]

A new term being used to replace "no code" or DNR is the term *allow natural death (AND).* This term more accurately conveys what actually happens. It is also sometimes referred to as "comfort code" status, meaning that all comfort measures associated with pain control and symptom management are carried out. However, the natural physiologic progression to death is not delayed or interrupted.

Withholding or withdrawing treatments must be included in an advance directive. What is to be done and what is not to be done must be included in clear terms. The ANA position statements on foregoing nutrition and hydration and active euthanasia from 1992 and 1994, respectively, recognize that honoring the refusal of treatments that a patient does not desire, are disproportionately burdensome to the patient, or will not benefit the patient can be ethically and legally permissible. Additionally, the decision to withhold artificial nutrition and hydration should be made by the patient or surrogate with the health care team.[18,19]

The nurse needs to be aware of legal issues and the wishes of the patient.[20] Advance directives and organ donor information should be located in the medical record and identified on the patient's record and/or the nursing care plan. All caregivers responsible for the patient need to know the patient's wishes. Additionally, the nurse is responsible for becoming familiar with state, local, and agency procedures in EOL documentation.

PALLIATIVE CARE AND HOSPICE

Palliative care is health care aimed at symptom management rather than curative treatment for diseases that no longer respond to treatment. Palliative care is focused on caring interventions rather than toward curative treatments. The trend toward palliative care focuses health care toward allowing natural death in a pain-controlled and symptom-controlled environment with psychosocial support.

Palliative care is the framework for hospice care. Palliative care can start much earlier in a disease process, whereas hospice traditionally is limited to the projected last 6 months of life.

Hospice is a concept of care that provides compassion, concern, and support for the dying (Fig. 10-4). Hospice and palliative care are frequently used interchangeably. Hospice exists to provide support and care for persons in the last phases of incurable diseases so that they might live as fully and as comfortably as possible. Hospice care ensures that patient and family needs are the focus of any intervention.

During the 1970s the concept of hospice was integrated into health care in the United States, and by the end of the decade,

> You matter because you are you and you matter to the last moment of your life. We will do all we can not only to help you die peacefully, but to live until you die.

From Clark D: *Cicely Saunders, founder of the modern-day hospice movement,* New York, 2002, Oxford University Press.

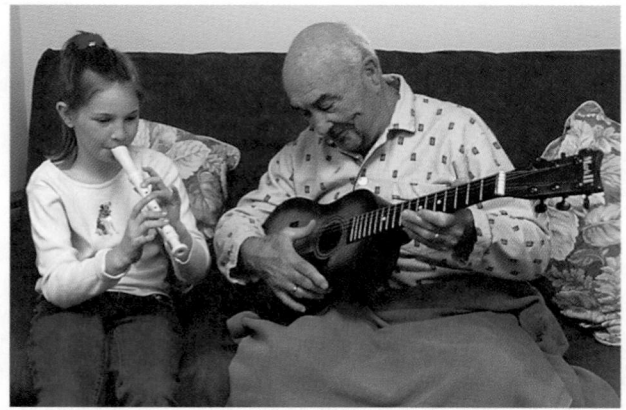

FIG. 10-4 Hospice care is designed to provide compassion, concern, and support for the dying.

every state had existing hospice programs. Currently there are approximately 3100 hospice programs.[21] Like home health care, hospice programs are organized under a variety of models. Some are hospital based, others are part of existing home health care agencies, and others are freestanding or community-based, volunteer-intensive programs.[21] However, regardless of their organization, all hospices emphasize palliative rather than curative care.

Hospice care is generally provided in the home with inpatient care reserved for acute pain management or respite care for families or caregivers in need of a break. Home care is provided on a part-time, intermittent, on-call, regularly scheduled, or continuous basis. Hospice services are available 24 hours a day and 7 days a week to provide help to patients and families in their homes. The inpatient hospice settings have been deinstitutionalized to make the atmosphere as relaxed and homelike as possible (Fig. 10-5). Staff and volunteers are available to the patient and family. A multidisciplinary team approach often provides holistic health care.

A medically supervised interdisciplinary team of professionals and volunteers provides hospice services. The hospice nurse is an integral part and plays a pivotal role in coordination of the hospice team. Hospice nurses work collaboratively with hospice

physicians, pharmacists, dietitians, physical therapists, social workers, certified nursing assistants, clergy, and volunteers to provide care and support to the patient and family members. Hospice nurses are educated in pain control and symptom management. As with home health care, hospice care requires excellent teaching skills, compassion, flexibility, and adaptability to patient needs.

The decision to begin hospice care is difficult. Several reasons for this exist. Patients, families, and physicians may lack information about hospice care. Physicians may be reluctant to give referrals because they sometimes view a patient's decline as their personal failure. Some patients or family members see it as giving up.

Admission to a hospice program has two criteria. First, the patient must desire the services; second, a physician must certify that the patient has 6 months or less to live. Studies are being conducted to determine if these criteria meet the needs of chronically ill and dying patients. Patients with terminal conditions such as cancer, acquired immunodeficiency syndrome, chronic obstructive pulmonary disease, and end-stage cardiovascular or renal disease may qualify for hospice care.[22] In addition, patients with disease processes such as Alzheimer's disease and other dementias, amyotrophic lateral sclerosis (ALS), Parkinson's disease, and liver disease may qualify for hospice care.

Bereavement counseling is an important aspect of hospice programs. The objective of a bereavement program is to provide support and to assist survivors in the transition to a life without the deceased person. Grief support is incorporated into the plan of care for family members and significant others during the patient's illness, as well as after the death.

NURSING MANAGEMENT END OF LIFE

Nursing care of terminally ill and dying patients is holistic and encompasses all aspects of psychosocial and physical needs. Nursing care focuses on the psychosocial manifestations and the grieving process, as well as the physical changes that are associated with dying. The patient and the family need to be the focus of nursing care. Respect, dignity, and comfort are important for the patient and for the family. In addition, nurses and other care providers must recognize their own needs when dealing with grief and dying.

■ Nursing Assessment

Assessment of the terminally ill or dying patient varies with the patient's condition and proximity of approaching death. In general, the assessment is limited to essential data. The nurse documents the specific event or change that brought the patient into the health care agency. The patient's medical diagnoses, medication profile, and allergies are recorded. If the patient is alert, a brief review of the body systems to detect important signs and symptoms should be completed. Discomfort, pain, nausea, and dyspnea are carefully assessed so prompt interventions can be implemented.

The functional assessment of activities of daily living elicits information about the patient's abilities, food and fluid intake, patterns of sleep and rest, and response to the stress of terminal illness. Coping abilities of the patient and family should also be assessed.

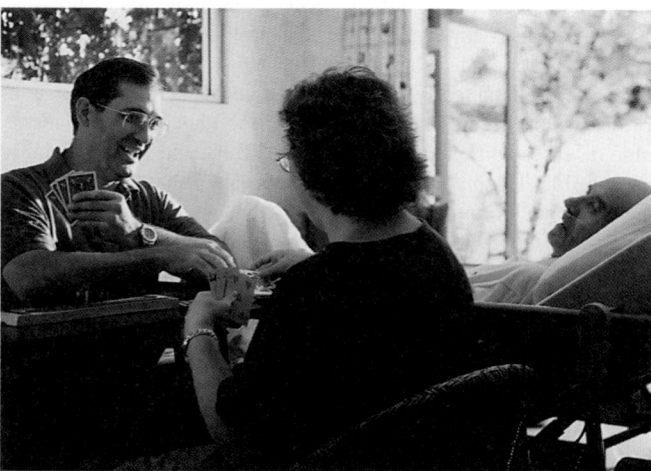

FIG. 10-5 Inpatient hospice settings have been deinstitutionalized to make the atmosphere as relaxed and homelike as possible.

The physical assessment is abbreviated and focuses on changes that accompany terminal illness and the specific disease process. The frequency of assessment depends on the patient's stability but is done at least every 8 hours. As changes occur, assessment and documentation need to be done more frequently.

As death approaches, neurologic assessment is especially important and includes level of consciousness, presence of reflexes, and pupil responses. Evaluation of vital signs, skin color, and temperature indicates changes in circulation. Respiratory status, character and pattern of respirations, and the characteristics of breath sounds are monitored and described. Monitoring nutritional and fluid intake, urinary output, and bowel function provides assessment data for renal and gastrointestinal functioning. Skin condition must be assessed on an ongoing basis because skin becomes fragile and may easily break down.

It is important to be sensitive and not to impose repeated, unnecessary assessments on the dying patient. Health history data that are available in the chart should be used when available rather than tiring the patient with an interview. However, it is important to assess the patient's status frequently.

■ Nursing Diagnoses

Several nursing diagnoses dealing with psychosocial manifestations (Table 10-5) and physical manifestations (Table 10-6) are associated with EOL care.

■ Planning

Planning for EOL care entails a holistic approach. Coordination of care must focus on both the patient's needs and the needs of the family members and significant others. Education, counseling, advocacy, and support for the patient and the family are priorities. Psychosocially, nursing goals center on the patient's abilities to express and share feelings with others. Nursing care

NURSING DIAGNOSES

TABLE 10-5	Psychosocial Manifestations at the End of Life

- Acute confusion
- Anticipatory grieving
- Chronic confusion
- Chronic sorrow
- Compromised family coping
- Death anxiety
- Disturbed sleep pattern
- Disturbed thought processes
- Dysfunctional grieving
- Fear
- Hopelessness
- Impaired adjustment
- Impaired social interaction
- Impaired verbal communication
- Ineffective coping
- Ineffective denial
- Interrupted family processes
- Readiness for enhanced spiritual well-being
- Risk for loneliness
- Social isolation
- Spiritual distress

NURSING DIAGNOSES

TABLE 10-6	Physical Care at the End of Life

- Acute pain
- Bowel incontinence
- Chronic pain
- Constipation
- Decreased cardiac output
- Diarrhea
- Fatigue
- Imbalanced nutrition: Less than body requirements
- Impaired bed mobility
- Impaired comfort
- Impaired gas exchange
- Impaired oral mucous membrane
- Impaired physical mobility
- Impaired skin integrity
- Impaired swallowing
- Impaired tissue integrity
- Impaired urinary elimination
- Ineffective airway clearance
- Ineffective breathing pattern
- Ineffective thermoregulation
- Ineffective tissue perfusion
- Nausea
- Risk for aspiration
- Risk for infection
- Risk for injury
- Self-care deficit
- Total urinary incontinence

goals during the last stages of life involve comfort measures and physical maintenance care.

Education of both the patient and family is an important part of the nurse's planning in EOL care. Families need ongoing information on the disease, the dying process, and any care that will be provided. They need information on how to cope with many issues during this period of their lives. Denial and grieving may be barriers to learning and understanding at the end of life for both the patient and family members. Nurses must take the time to develop a comprehensive plan to support, educate, and evaluate patients and families in EOL care issues.

■ Nursing Implementation

Nursing interventions for the dying patient focus on comfort and improving the quality of life. Psychosocial care and physical care are interrelated for both the dying patient and the family members or significant others.

Psychosocial Care

Anxiety and depression. Anxiety is an uneasy feeling caused by a source that is not easily identified. Anxiety is frequently related to fear. Patients often exhibit signs of anxiety and depression during the EOL period. Causes of depression and anxiety may include pain that is out of control, psychosocial factors related to the disease process or impending death, altered physiologic states, and drugs used in high doses. Encouragement, support, and education decrease some of the anxiety. Management of anxiety may include both pharmacologic and nonpharmacologic interventions.

Fear. Fear is a typical feeling associated with dying. The nurse frequently assists the dying person to cope with fears. Three specific fears associated with dying are fear of pain, fear of loneliness and abandonment, and fear of meaninglessness.

- *Fear of pain.* There is a tendency to associate death with pain. Common sayings such as "on pain of death" or "a violent death" have influenced the way that death is perceived. A dying person who has lost a loved one to a painful death may expect the same type of experience. Subsequently many people assume that pain always accompanies death. Physiologically, there is no absolute indication that death is always painful. Psychologically, pain may occur based on the anxieties and separations related to dying. Terminally ill patients who do experience physical pain should have pain-relieving drugs available. The patient and the family need assurance that drugs will be given promptly when needed and that side effects of drugs can and will be managed. Patients can participate in their own pain relief by discussing pain relief measures and their effects. Most patients want their pain relieved without the side effects of grogginess or sleepiness. Pain relief measures such as drugs need not deprive the patient of the ability to interact with others.

- *Fear of loneliness and abandonment.* Most terminally ill and dying people do not want to be alone and fear loneliness. Many dying patients are afraid that loved ones who are unable to cope with the patient's imminent death will abandon them. Dying patients typically want someone whom they know and trust to stay with them (Fig. 10-6). It may be a loved one or a caregiver. The simple presence of someone provides support and comfort. Neither words nor actions are necessary unless the patient requires something. Holding hands, touching, and listening are considered to be high-quality nursing responses. Simply providing companionship allows the dying person a sense of security.

- *Fear of meaninglessness.* Fear of meaninglessness leads most people to review their lives. They review their intentions during life, examining actions and expressing regrets about what might have been. Life review helps patients recognize the value that their lives have held. Patients need to look at positive aspects of their lives. Nurses and family members can help patients review their lives. The worth of the dying person needs to be expressed. The nurse can assist patients and their families in identifying the positive qualities of the patient's life. The shar-

ing of thoughts and feelings may provide comfort for the patient. The nurse needs to respect and accept the practices and rituals associated with the patient's life review while remaining nonjudgmental.

Communication. Therapeutic communication is an important nursing intervention used to assist the dying patient and family (Fig. 10-7). Empathy and active listening are essential communication components in EOL care. *Empathy* is the identification with and understanding of another's situation, feelings, and/or motives. Listening is an active process required in the development of empathy toward another's feelings.

Patients and families need to be allowed time to express their feelings and thoughts. Making time to listen and interact in a sensitive way enhances the relationship among the nurse, patient, and family. Listening is essential. There may be silence. Frequently silence is related to the overwhelming feelings experienced at the end of life. Silence can also allow time to gather thoughts. Listening to the silence sends a message of acceptance and comfort.

Unusual communication by the patient may take place at the end of life. Frequently, near the end of life, the patient's communication may become what is oftentimes identified as confused, disoriented, or garbled. Patients may speak to or about family members or others who have predeceased them, give instructions to those who will survive them, or speak of projects yet to be completed.[23] Active, careful listening allows for the identification of specific patterns in the dying person's communication and decreases the risk for inappropriate labeling of behaviors.

Grief. Resolution of grief is the primary focus for anticipatory and dysfunctional grieving. Interventions are similar for these two types of grieving, and therefore they are addressed together. Specific interventions are planned for the specific stage of the grief process or the specific feelings expressed by the patient or family. Goals for grief resolution include patient expression of feelings related to grief, acknowledgment of the impending loss, and demonstrations of behaviors that reflect progress in grief resolution.

Priority interventions for grief must focus on providing an environment that allows the patient to express feelings. Open discussion of feelings helps both the patient and family work toward resolution of the grief process. The patient should be free to express feelings of anger, fear, or guilt without judgment on the part

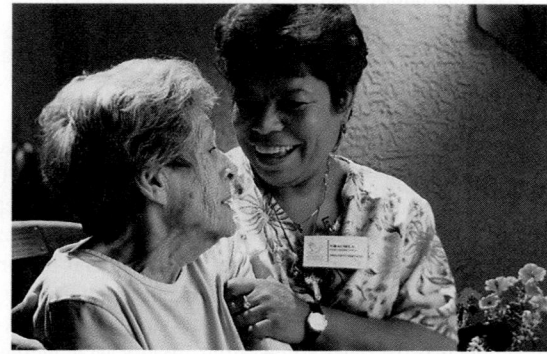

FIG. 10-6 Dying patients typically want someone whom they know and trust to stay with them.

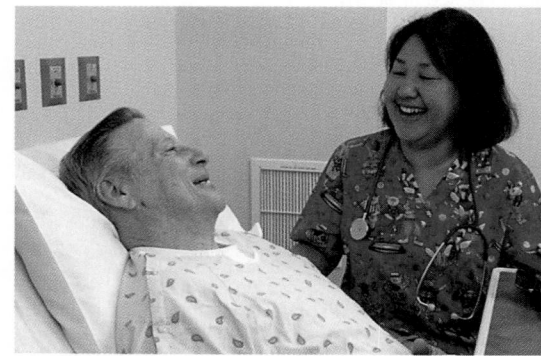

FIG. 10-7 Therapeutic communication is an important aspect of end-of-life nursing care.

of the nurse. The patient and family need to know that the grief reaction is normal. Respect for the patient's privacy and need or desire to talk (or not to talk) is important. Honesty in answering questions and giving information is essential. Families and patients need encouragement to continue their usual activities as much as possible. They need to discuss their activities and maintain some control over their lives. At times it helps to discuss what can and cannot change. Assistance with planning for the future or for the funeral may be needed based on the patient's or family's coping abilities.

Anger is a common and normal response to grief. It is important to understand that the grieving person cannot be forced to accept the loss. The surviving family members may be angry at the dying loved one who is leaving them. There is a need to acknowledge and encourage the expression of feelings but at the same time realize how difficult it is to come to terms with grief. Nurses are sometimes the target of the anger, and must understand what is happening and not react on a personal level.

Feelings of hopelessness and powerlessness are common at the end of life. The nurse needs to encourage realistic hope within the limits of the situation. The patient and the family should be allowed to identify and to deal with what is within their control and to recognize what is beyond their control. Patient-identified goals can be encouraged to restore some sense of power. Decision making about care can also foster a sense of power and control for the patient.

Evaluation of the specific coping skills demonstrated and expressed by the patient or the family will assist in planning care. Outcome criteria for goal achievement include verbalization of specific feelings, expression that the loss is real, and identification of specific progress in the grief work. The criteria are evaluated based on specific behaviors and verbalizations exhibited by the patient or the significant others.

As death approaches, the nurse should encourage the family to respond appropriately to the psychosocial manifestations at the end of life. Table 10-7 discusses management of psychosocial manifestations near death.

▪ Physical Care

Nursing management related to physical care at the end of life deals with symptom management and caring rather than treatments for curing a particular disease or disorder.[24] Meeting the patient's physiologic and safety needs is the priority. Physical care focuses on the needs for oxygen, nutrition, pain relief, mobility, elimination, and skin care. People who are dying deserve and require the same physical care as people who are expected to recover. Nursing management at the end of life focuses on symptom management. Table 10-8 delineates the physical care at the end of life.

Postmortem Care. After the patient is pronounced dead, the nurse prepares or delegates preparation of the body for immediate viewing by the family with consideration for cultural customs and in accord with state law and agency policies and procedures. In general, the nurse closes the patient's eyes, replaces dentures, washes the body as needed (placing pads under the perineum to absorb urine and feces), and may remove tubes and dressings. The body should be straightened, leaving the pillow to support the head and prevent pooling of blood and discoloration of the face. The family should then be allowed privacy and as much time as they need with the deceased person. In the case of an unexpected or unanticipated death, preparation of the body for viewing or release to a funeral home depends on state law and agency policies and procedures.

SPECIAL NEEDS OF CAREGIVERS IN END-OF-LIFE CARE

Special Needs of Family Caregivers

The dying process of a loved one can be a long and arduous journey. Being present during a family member's dying process can be highly stressful. The role of caregiver includes working

TABLE 10-7 Nursing Management: Psychosocial Care at End of Life	
CHARACTERISTIC	**NURSING MANAGEMENT**
Withdrawal Patient near death may seem to be withdrawn from the physical environment, maintaining the ability to hear while not able to respond.	▪ Converse as if the patient is alert, using a soft voice and gentle touch.
Unusual Communication Patient may become restless and agitated or perform repetitive tasks. Unusual communication may indicate that an unresolved issue is preventing the dying person from letting go.	▪ Encourage the family to tell the dying person, "It's okay to go. I will be fine."
Vision-like Experiences Patient may talk to persons who are not there or see places and objects not visible. Vision-like experiences assist the dying person in coming to terms with meaning in life and transition from it.	▪ Affirm the dying person's experience as a part of transition from this life.
Saying Goodbyes It is important for the patient and family members to acknowledge their sadness, mutually forgive one another, and say goodbye.	▪ Encourage the dying person and family members to verbalize their feelings of sadness, loss, forgiveness; to touch, hug, cry. ▪ Allow the patient and family privacy to express their feelings and comfort one another.

TABLE 10-8	Nursing Management: Physical Care at End of Life
CHARACTERISTIC	**NURSING MANAGEMENT**

Pain

- Pain may be a major symptom associated with terminal illness and the one most feared.
- Pain can be acute or chronic.
- Physical and emotional irritations can aggravate pain.

- Assess pain thoroughly and regularly to determine the quality, intensity, location, and contributing factors.
- Minimize possible irritants such as skin irritations from wetness, heat or cold, and pressure.
- Administer medications around the clock in a timely manner and on a regular basis to provide constant relief rather than waiting until the pain is unbearable and then trying to relieve it.
- Provide complementary and alternative therapies such as guided imagery, massage, acupressure, heat and cold, therapeutic touch, distraction, and relaxation techniques as needed.
- Evaluate effectiveness of pain relief measures frequently to ensure that the patient is on a correct, adequate drug regimen.
- Do not delay or deny pain relief measures to a terminally ill patient.

Delirium

- A state characterized by confusion, disorientation, restlessness, clouding of consciousness, incoherence, fear, anxiety, excitement, and often hallucinations.
- May be misidentified as depression, psychosis, anger, or anxiety.
- Use of opioids and/or corticosteroids in end-of-life care may cause delirium.
- Underlying disease process may contribute to delirium.
- Generally considered a reversible process.

- Perform a thorough assessment for reversible causes of delirium, including pain, constipation, and urinary retention.
- Provide a room that is quiet, well lighted, and familiar to reduce the effects of delirium.
- Reorient the dying person to person, place, and time with each encounter.
- Administer ordered benzodiazepines and sedatives as needed.
- Stay physically close to frightened patient. Reassure in a calm, soft voice with touch and slow strokes of the skin.
- Provide family members with emotional support and encouragement in their efforts to cope with the behaviors associated with delirium.
- Encourage the family to participate in the care for the patient.

Restlessness

- May occur as death approaches and cerebral metabolism slows.

- Assess for spiritual distress as a cause for restlessness and agitation.
- Do not restrain.
- Use soothing music; slow, soft touch and voice.
- Limit the number of persons at the bedside.

Dysphagia

- May occur because of extreme weakness and changes in level of consciousness.

- Identify the least invasive alternative routes of administration for drugs needed for symptom management.
- Suction orally as needed.

Dehydration

- May occur during the last days of life.
- Hunger and thirst are rare in the last days of life.
- As the end of life approaches, patients tend to take in less food and fluid.

- Assess condition of mucous membranes frequently to prevent excessive dryness, which can lead to discomfort.
- Maintain complete, regular oral care to provide for comfort and hydration of mucous membranes.
- Do not force the patient to eat or drink.
- Encourage consumption of ice chips and sips of fluids or use moist cloths to provide moisture to the mouth.
- Use moist cloths and swabs for unconscious patients to avoid aspiration.
- Apply lubricant to the lips and oral mucous membranes as needed.
- Reassure family that cessation of food and fluid intake is a natural part of the process of dying.

Dyspnea

- Subjective symptom.
- Accompanied by fear of suffocation and anxiety.
- Underlying disease process can exacerbate dyspnea.
- Coughing and expectorating secretions become difficult.

- Assess respiratory status regularly.
- Elevate the head and/or position on side to improve chest expansion.
- Use a fan or air conditioner to facilitate movement of cool air.
- Administer supplemental oxygen as ordered.
- Administer drugs such as narcotics, sedatives, diuretics, antibiotics, corticosteroids, and bronchodilators as ordered to relieve congestion and coughing and to decrease apprehension.
- Suction as needed to remove accumulation of mucus from the airways.

TABLE 10-8   Nursing Management: Physical Care at End of Life—cont'd

CHARACTERISTIC	NURSING MANAGEMENT
Weakness and Fatigue • Expected at the end of life. • Metabolic demands related to disease process contribute to weakness and fatigue.	• Assess the patient's tolerance for activities. • Time nursing interventions to conserve energy. • Assist the patient to identify and complete valued or desired activities. • Provide support as needed to maintain positions in bed or chair. • Provide frequent rest periods.
Myoclonus • Mild to severe jerking or twitching sometimes associated with high use of opioids. • Patient may complain of involuntary twitching of upper and lower extremities.	• Assess for the initial onset, the duration, and any discomfort or distress experienced by patient. • If myoclonus is distressing or becoming more severe, discuss possible drug therapy modifications with the physician. • Changes in opioid medication may alleviate or decrease myoclonus.
Skin Breakdown • Skin integrity is difficult to maintain at the end of life. • Immobility, urinary and bowel incontinence, dry skin, nutritional deficits, anemia, friction, and shearing forces lead to a high risk for skin breakdown. • Disease and other processes may impair skin integrity. • As death approaches, circulation to the extremities decreases and they become cool, mottled, and cyanotic.	• Assess the skin for signs of breakdown. • Implement protocols to prevent skin breakdown by controlling drainage and odor and keeping the skin and any wound areas clean. • Perform wound assessments as needed. • Follow appropriate nursing management protocol for dressing wounds. • Follow appropriate nursing management protocol for a patient who is immobile, but consider realistic outcomes of skin integrity vs. maintenance of comfort. • Follow appropriate nursing management to prevent skin irritations and breakdown from urinary and bowel incontinence. • Use blankets to cover for warmth; never apply heat. • Prevent the effects of shearing forces.
Bowel Patterns • Constipation can be caused by immobility, use of opioid medications, lack of fiber in the diet, and dehydration. • Diarrhea may occur as muscles relax or from a fecal impaction related to the use of opioids and immobility.	• Assess bowel function. • Assess for and remove fecal impactions. • Encourage movement and physical activities as tolerated. • Encourage fiber in the diet if appropriate. • Encourage fluids if appropriate. • Use suppositories, laxatives, or enemas if ordered.
Urinary Incontinence • May result from disease progression or changes in the level of consciousness. • As death becomes imminent, the perineal muscles relax.	• Assess urinary function. • Use absorbent pads for urinary incontinence. • Follow the appropriate nursing protocol for the consideration and use of indwelling or external catheters. • Follow appropriate nursing management to prevent skin irritations and breakdown from urinary incontinence.
Anorexia, Nausea, and Vomiting • May be caused by complications of disease process. • Drugs contribute to nausea. • Constipation, impaction, and bowel obstruction can cause anorexia, nausea, and vomiting.	• Assess the patient for complaints of nausea and/or vomiting. • Assess possible contributing causes for nausea or vomiting. • Have family members provide the patient's favorite foods. • Discuss modifications to the drug regimen with the health care provider. • Provide antiemetics before meals if ordered. • Offer and provide frequent meals with small portions of favorite foods. • Offer culturally appropriate foods. • Provide frequent mouth care, especially after vomiting.

> The loss of a loved person is one of the most intensely
> painful experiences any human being can suffer.

From John Bowlby: *Notes on symptom control in hospice and palliative care,* rev ed, Essex, 2000, Hospice Education Institute.

and communicating with the patient, supporting the patient's concerns, helping the patient resolve any unfinished business, working with other family members and friends, and dealing with the caregiver's own needs and feelings. An understanding of the grieving process as it affects both the patient and the family caregivers is of great importance.

Recognizing signs and behaviors among family members who may be at risk for abnormal grief reactions is an important nursing intervention. These may include dependency and negative feelings about the dying person, inability to express feelings, concurrent life crises, a history of depression, difficult reactions to previous losses, perceived lack of social or family support, low self-esteem, multiple previous bereavements, alcoholism, and/or substance abuse.

Family caregivers and other family members need encouragement to continue their usual activities as much as possible. They need to discuss their activities and maintain some control over their lives. At times it helps to discuss what can and cannot change.

Grieving relatives, friends, and significant others can provide emotional support for one another. Health care providers need to be sensitive to the importance of significant others who are not necessarily relatives. Resources such as community counseling and local support may assist some people in working through their grief. Generally, simply allowing the involved people to express their feelings helps to resolve the grief. Caregivers should be encouraged to facilitate the building of a support system of extended family members, friends, faith community, and clergy. The caregivers should have access to people whom they can call on at any time to express any feelings that they are experiencing. Caregivers and family members should also allow time to be alone.[25]

Family caregivers need to be encouraged to take care of themselves. Keeping a journal can help the caregiver express feelings that may be difficult to express verbally. Eating a balanced diet at regular times will provide for the caregiver's well-being. Nourishing the spirit as well as the body is important for the caregiver to consider. Physical contact with others provides emotional support and acknowledgement of the caregiver's own need for physical comfort. Exercise often relieves stress. Maintenance of regular activities and interests is also important to help the caregiver. Humor is important, and its use from time to time in some situations can provide distraction and relieve stress-filled situations.

Special Needs of Nurses

Many nurses who care for dying patients do so because they are passionate about providing quality EOL care. However, caring for dying patients is intense and emotionally charged. A bond or connection develops among the patient, family, and nurse. Nurses need to be aware of how grief affects them personally. The nurse who is responsible for the care of terminally ill or dying patients is not immune to feelings of loss. It is common for nurses to feel helpless and powerless when dealing with death. Feelings of sorrow, guilt, and frustration need to be expressed.

There are interventions that help to ease physical and emotional stress for the nurse. It is necessary for the nurse to recognize and acknowledge what can and cannot be controlled. Recognizing personal feelings allows openness in exchanging feelings with the patient and family. Realizing that it is okay to cry with the patient or family during the grief process is essential to the nurse's well-being.

Interventions focusing on personal needs will assist in alleviating stress for the nurse. Involvement in hobbies or other interests, scheduling time for oneself, maintaining a peer support system, and developing a support system beyond the workplace will benefit the nurse. Crises and grief result in varying forms of stress for nurses. Hospice agencies can provide care of their team members with professionally assisted groups, informal discussion sessions, and flexible time schedules.

Terminal illness and dying are extremely personal events that affect the patient, the family, and health care providers. Providing care for patients and their families at the end of life is a challenging and rewarding experience. EOL care offers an opportunity to apply the skills and personal commitments that nurses bring to their profession.

REVIEW QUESTIONS

The number of the question corresponds to the same-numbered objective at the beginning of the chapter.

1. Mr. Garcia is in the terminal stages of lung cancer. On assessment it is noted that he has rapid, audibly noisy respirations with an associated grunting sound. The correct terminology to use in documenting the assessment data would be to specify that he is experiencing
   a. tachypnea.
   b. death rattle.
   c. guppy breathing.
   d. Cheyne-Stokes respirations.

2. Mrs. Johnson has inoperable pancreatic cancer. Until recently she has been very active in her neighborhood association. Her husband is concerned because his wife is "not herself." Which common EOL psychologic manifestation is she demonstrating?
   a. decreased socialization
   b. decreased disease progression
   c. decreased sense of helplessness
   d. decreased perception of pain and touch

REVIEW QUESTIONS—cont'd

3. Tom has repeatedly asked his mother to donate his deceased father's belongings to charity, but his mother has refused. She sits in the bedroom closet, crying and talking to her long-dead husband. What type of grief is Tom's mother experiencing?
   a. adaptive
   b. disruptive
   c. anticipatory
   d. dysfunctional
4. While caring for his dying wife, Mr. Smith states that his wife is a devout Roman Catholic but he is a Baptist. Who is considered the most reliable source for spiritual preferences concerning EOL care for Mrs. Smith?
   a. a priest
   b. Mr. Smith
   c. Mrs. Smith
   d. hospice staff
5. The family attorney informed Mr. Wilson's adult children and wife that he did not have an advance directive after he suffered a serious stroke. Who is responsible for identifying EOL measures to be instituted when the patient cannot communicate his or her specific wishes?
   a. adult children
   b. notary and attorney
   c. physician and family
   d. physician and nursing staff
6. The primary purpose of hospice is to
   a. allow patients to die at home.
   b. provide better quality of care than the family can.
   c. coordinate care for dying patients and their families.
   d. provide comfort, support, and care of dying patients and their families.
7. Mrs. Alejandro, who has end-stage cardiac disease and is not a candidate for a heart transplant, is medicated with morphine. Recently she has been having chest pain and expressing concern that she may have another heart attack and die in pain. The nurse can decrease the psychosocial impact of physical symptoms of such pain by
   a. referring Mrs. Alejandro to a community agency.
   b. encouraging pain relief measures that cause sleepiness.
   c. evaluating the side effects of Mrs. Alejandro's drugs.
   d. evaluating the pain relief and the effects of the relief measures.
8. When Mr. Washington was diagnosed with renal failure, his new wife asked his children from a previous marriage to help with their father's care. Each of the children refused to help. Mrs. Washington cared for her husband without help until his death. The behaviors of the children indicate that they may be at risk for abnormal grief reactions related to
   a. maintenance of negative feelings.
   b. development of new relationships.
   c. maintenance of current relationships.
   d. development of independent behaviors.
9. Sue Vale has been working full time as a nurse with terminally ill patients for 3 years. She has been experiencing irritability and mixed emotions when expressing sadness since four of her patients died on the same day. To optimize the quality of her nursing care she should examine her own
   a. full-time work schedule.
   b. past feelings toward death.
   c. patterns for dealing with grief.
   d. demands for involvement in care.

REFERENCES

1. Field M, Cassel C: *Approaching death: improving care at the end of life,* Washington, DC, 1997, National Academy Press.
2. Wijdicks EFM: Current concepts: the diagnosis of brain death, *N Engl J Med* 344:1215, 2001.
3. Capron AM: Brain death—well settled yet still unresolved, *N Engl J Med* 344:1244, 2001.
4. Banks G: Verifying a death, *Nurs Stand* 14:22, 2000.
5. Waller A, Caroline NL: *Handbook of palliative care in cancer,* ed 2, Boston, 2000, Butterworth & Heinemann.
6. Kübler-Ross E: *On death and dying,* New York, 1969, MacMillan.
7. Martocchio BC: Grief and bereavement healing through hurt, *Nurs Clin North Am* 20:327, 1985.
8. Rando TA: *Treatment of complicated mourning,* Champaign, Ill, 1993, Research Press.
9. Kastenbaum RJ: *Death, society, and human experience,* ed 6, Boston, 1998, Allyn & Bacon.
10. Kaye P: *Notes on symptom control in hospice and palliative care,* rev ed, Essex, 2000, Hospice Education Institute.
11. Highfield MEF: Providing spiritual care to patients with cancer, *Clin J Oncol Nurs* 4:115, 2000.
12. Roark DC: Overhauling the organ donation system, *Am J Nurs* 200:44, 2000.
13. Omnibus Reconciliation Act, Title IV §4206, 1990, *Cong Rec* 12638.
14. Partnership for Caring, Inc. (nd). Available at *www.partnershipforcaring. org/* (accessed Nov. 7, 2002).
15. American Nurses Association, ANA Position Statements: *Nursing and the Patient Self-Determination Act,* Washington, DC, 1991 American Nurses Association.
16. American Nurses Association, ANA Position Statements: *Nursing care and do-not-resuscitate decisions,* Washington, DC, 1992 American Nurses Association.
17. Forbes S, Bern-King M, Gessert C: End-of-life decision making for nursing home residents with dementia, *Image J Nurs Sch* 32:251, 2000.
18. American Nurses Association, ANA Position Statements: *Foregoing nutrition and hydration,* Washington, DC, 1992 American Nurses Association.
19. American Nurses Association, ANA Position Statements: *Active euthanasia,* Washington, DC, 1994 American Nurses Association.
20. Basile CM: Advance directives and advocacy in end-of-life decisions, *Nurse Pract* 23:44, 1998.
21. National Hospice and Palliative Care Organization. Available at *http://www.nhpco.org/public/.*
22. Ferrell BR, Coyle N: *Textbook of palliative nursing,* Oxford, 2001, Oxford University Press.
23. Callanan M, Kelley P: *Final gifts: understanding the special awareness, needs, and communication of the dying,* New York, 1993, Bantam-Doubleday-Dell.
24. Lynn J, Schuster JL, Kabcenell A: *Improving care for the end of life,* New York, 1998, Oxford University Press.
25. Lynn J, Harrold J: *Handbook for mortals: guidance for people facing serious illness,* New York, 1999, Oxford University Press.

RESOURCES

Americans for Better Care of the Dying
4125 Albermarle Street NW, Suite 210
Washington, DC 20016
202-895-9485
Fax: 202-895-9484
www.abcd-caring.org

Association for Death Education and Counseling
342 North Main Street
West Hartford, CT 06117-2507
860-586-7503
Fax: 860-586-7550
www.adec.org

Coalition on Donation
1100 Boulders Parkway, Suite 700
Richmond, VA 23225-8770
804-330-3620
Fax: 804-323-7343
http://shareyourlife.org

Compassion in Dying Federation
6312 SW Capitol Hwy., Suite 415
Portland, OR 97201
503-221-9556
www.compassionindying.org

Foundation for Hospice and Home Care
513 C Street NE
Washington, DC 20002
202-547-6586
202-546-8968
www.aoa.dhhs.gov/aoa/dir/100.html

Hospice Association of America
519 C Street NE
Washington, DC 20002
202-546-4759
Fax: 202-546-9312
www.nahc.org/HAA/consumer.html

Hospice Education Institute
190 Westbrook Road
Essex, CT 06426
800-331-1620

Hospice Foundation of America
2001 S. Street NW, Suite 300
Washington, DC 20009
202-638-5419
Fax: 202-638-5312
www.hospicefoundation.org/page3.htm

Hospice Nurses' Association
Medical Center East, Suite 375
211 North Whitfield Street
Pittsburgh, PA 15206-3031
412-361-2470
Fax: 412-361-2425
www.roxane.com/hpna.org

Last Acts Campaign
Stewart Communications, Ltd.
325 W. Huron, Suite 300
Chicago, IL 60610
312-751-1297
Fax: 312-751-1372
www.lastacts.org

Last Acts Coalition (Robert Wood Johnson Foundation)
325 W. Huron, Suite 300
Chicago, IL 60610
312-751-1297
www.lastacts.org

Last Acts National Program Office
Ms. Karen Orloff Kaplan, President and CEO
Partnership for Caring, Inc.
1620 Eye Street NW, Suite 202
Washington, DC 20006
202-296-8071
Fax: 202-296-8352
www.lastacts.org

National Hospice and Palliative Care Organization
1700 Diagonal Road, Suite 625
Alexandria, VA 22314
703-837-1500
Fax: 703-837-1233
www.nhpco.org

National Hospice Organization (NHO)
1901 North Moore Street, Suite 901
Arlington, VA 22209
800-658-8898
www.nho.org

Palliative Care Nursing
Kathleen Hartman Sabatier, MS, RN
Director, The Institute for Johns Hopkins Nursing
525 N. Wolfe Street, Suite 533
Baltimore, MD 21205
410-614-3160
Fax: 410-614-8972
www.palliativecarenursing.net/

Partnership for Caring, Inc.
National Office
1620 Eye Street NW, Suite 202
Washington, DC 20006
202-296-8071
Fax: 202-296-8352
www.partnershipforcaring.org

For additional Internet resources, see the website for this book at
http://evolve.elsevier.com/Lewis/medsurg/.

Addictive Behaviors

Patricia Graber O'Brien

LEARNING OBJECTIVES

1. Define addiction, addictive behavior, substance misuse, substance abuse, dependence, tolerance, withdrawal, craving, abstinence, and detoxification.
2. Describe the neurophysiology of addiction.
3. Identify the major health complications of substance abuse.
4. Recognize the effects of the use of stimulants, depressants, hallucinogens, and inhalants.
5. Identify nursing interventions for tobacco and smoking cessation.
6. Describe the nursing management of patients who experience intoxication, overdose, or withdrawal from stimulants, depressants, or hallucinogens.
7. Describe nursing management of the surgical patient who abuses drugs.
8. Discuss the nursing management of pain in the patient who is dependent on central nervous system depressants.
9. Describe the use of motivational interviewing to initiate behavior change in patients with addictions.
10. Discuss substance abuse problems of the older adult.

KEY TERMS

addiction, p. 175	opioids, p. 187
addictive behaviors, p. 175	physiologic dependence, p. 177
brain reward system, p. 176	potentiation, p. 185
craving, p. 176	psychologic dependence, p. 177
cross-tolerance, p. 185	relapse, p. 176
cue-induced craving, p. 176	substance abuse, p. 175
dependence, p. 175	substance dependence, p. 175
detoxification, p. 185	tolerance, p. 176
Korsakoff's psychosis, p. 194	transtheoretical model of change, p. 197
motivational interviewing, p. 197	
opiates, p. 187	Wernicke's encephalopathy, p. 194

Addiction and substance abuse are serious problems affecting the health care system and society today. Addictions that create social and health problems include abuse of chemical substances. In addition, addictions include some compulsive behaviors such as eating disorders, gambling, computer gaming and interacting, and even strenuous exercising. Illicit (illegal) drugs most commonly used in the United States include, in descending order, marijuana, cocaine, heroin, methamphetamines, inhalants, and hallucinogens.[1] Alcohol, tobacco, food, sex, and gambling addictions, however, are responsible for more illness and death than are illicit drugs. Substance abuse and misuse may also occur with drugs prescribed for therapeutic uses. It is estimated that about 14.8 million Americans use illicit drugs, with 3.5 million dependent on illicit drugs and an additional 8.2 million dependent on alcohol.[1] Substance abuse also represents a major social and health problem in Canada. Although prevalence of drug use varies by region in Canada, smoking and alcohol use are major causes of death.[2,3]

Individuals who abuse substances use the health care system more than those who do not abuse substances. All nurses care for patients dependent on substances, whether they are identified as dependent or not, simply because of the prevalence of substance abuse and its high relationship with health problems. In every health care setting the nurse has a responsibility to identify and intervene with patients who are abusing or addicted to substances.

Substance abuse and **substance dependence** (defined in Table 11-1) are specific psychiatric diagnoses.[4] Comprehensive discussions of addictive behaviors and substance abuse are provided in psychiatric references. Long-term management of addiction is most often provided in specialized treatment facilities and mental health clinics that provide both pharmacologic and behavioral therapies. This chapter is limited to addressing the nursing role in identifying and managing the addicted or substance-abusing patient in the general ambulatory or acute care setting. Eating disorders are discussed in Chapter 39, and health problems related to addictive behaviors are discussed throughout the text.

OVERVIEW OF ADDICTIVE BEHAVIORS

Terminology of Addictive Behavior

A lack of standard terminology for addiction and substance abuse problems makes defining various terms difficult. Different psychiatric, social, and philosophic viewpoints lead to preference of one term over another by professional groups and laypeople. In this chapter, **addiction** is defined as a compulsive, uncontrollable **dependence** on a substance, habit, or practice to such a degree that cessation causes severe emotional, mental, or physiologic reactions. Those behaviors that are associated with maintaining an addiction are referred to as **addictive behaviors.** These and additional terms used in describing abuse of substances are presented in Table 11-1.

Neurophysiology of Addiction

Addiction is a complex disorder that is a treatable, chronic, relapsing disease of the brain. Current research is providing detailed knowledge of the effect of addictive drugs on an individual's brain and behavior. Most addictive drugs, and possibly

Reviewed by Kathy Lopez-Bushnell, EdD, MPH, RNC (FNP), COHNS, Clinical Nurse Researcher, University of New Mexico Hospital, Albuquerque, N.M.

TABLE 11-1	Terminology of Substance Abuse
TERM	**DEFINITION**
Abstinence	Avoidance of substance use.
Addiction	Compulsive, uncontrollable dependence on a substance, habit, or practice to such a degree that cessation causes severe emotional, mental, or physiologic reactions.
Addictive behavior	Behavior associated with maintaining an addiction.
Craving	Subjective need for a substance, usually experienced after decreased use or abstinence. Cue-induced craving is stimulated in the presence of experiences previously associated with drug taking.
Dependence	Reliance on a substance that has reached the level that absence of it will cause an impairment in function.
• Physical	Altered physiologic state from prolonged substance use; regular use is necessary to prevent withdrawal.
• Psychologic	Compulsive need to experience pleasurable response from the substance.
Detoxification	Process of removing the substance and its effects from the individual's body.
Relapse	Return to substance use during abstinence.
Substance	Drug, chemical, or biologic entity that is self-administered.
Substance abuse	Overindulgence in and dependence on a substance that has a negative impact on psychologic, physiologic, and social functioning of an individual. *Substance abuse* is synonymous with *chemical dependence*.
Substance misuse	Use of a drug for purposes other than those for which it is intended.
Tolerance	Decreased effect of a substance that results from repeated exposure. It is possible to develop cross-tolerance to other substances in the same category.
Withdrawal	Constellation of physiologic and psychologic responses that occur when there is abrupt cessation or reduced intake of a substance on which an individual is dependent or when the effect is counteracted by a specific antagonist.

certain compulsive behaviors, appear to increase the availability of dopamine in the "pleasure" area of the mesolimbic system of the brain. This area has been identified as the **brain reward system** and is a system that creates the sensation of pleasure for certain behaviors necessary for survival, such as eating and sexual behavior.[5]

Normally dopamine is released at a slow rate by neurons in the mesolimbic system, producing normal affect or mood. Both endogenous and exogenous opiates have been found to increase the firing rate of dopaminergic neurons. Cocaine has been shown to decrease the reuptake of dopamine at the synapse, thereby decreasing its breakdown and increasing the amount of available dopamine. Nicotine, alcohol, marijuana, amphetamines, and caffeine also increase dopaminergic neuron activity at the synapse. The resulting increase in mesolimbic dopamine leads to mood elevation and euphoria, factors that provide strong motivation to repeat the experience. Many addictive drugs also increase the availability of other neurotransmitters, such as serotonin and gamma-aminobutyric acid (GABA), but dopamine's effect on the reward system appears to be pivotal to the addictive process.[6]

Addiction results from the prolonged effects of addictive drugs or behaviors on the brain. Repeated use of addictive drugs changes the neural circuitry involving dopamine cells and reduces the responsiveness of dopamine receptors. This decreased responsiveness leads to **tolerance,** the need for a larger dose of a drug to obtain the original euphoria, and also reduces the sense of pleasure from experiences that previously resulted in positive feelings. Without the substance or behavior the individual experiences depression, anxiety, and irritability. To even feel normal, the individual must take the drug or perform the behavior.[7]

Drug **craving** is another characteristic of addiction. An important type of craving experienced by addicts, **cue-induced craving,** occurs in the presence of people, places, or things that

they have previously associated with drug taking. Cue-induced craving may occur after long periods of abstinence and is a common cause of **relapse** (see Table 11-1 for definitions of these terms). Current research indicates that cue-induced craving is accompanied by heightened activity in key brain areas involved in mood and memory. Although neurotransmitter activity is no doubt involved, it is yet to be determined what specific processes in the brain link drug abusers' memories so strongly to the desire to take drugs.[8]

Contributing Factors to Addiction

It is important that addiction not be perceived simply as a physical disease but as a biobehavioral disorder. It is a disease that is expressed in behavioral ways and within a social context. Once addiction occurs, it changes the brain, perpetuating itself. But it starts with the voluntary act of taking drugs, and if drugs are never used, addiction does not occur. No single factor has been identified to determine whether an individual might abuse a substance, nor is it understood why some people become addicted and others do not. Some contributing factors include those typically associated with drug abuse: drug availability, peer influences (Fig. 11-1), environment, psychiatric illnesses, adverse social conditions, and cultural influences. However, there is increasing evidence that genetics plays a significant role in alcoholism and nicotine use and that there are significant gender differences in drug abuse risks.[9]

Research supported by the National Institute on Drug Abuse has shown that men are more likely than women to have opportunities to use drugs, but when given an opportunity to use drugs for the first time, men and women are equally likely to do so and to progress from initial use to addiction. Men and women are equally likely to become addicted to or dependent on cocaine, heroin, hallucinogens, tobacco, and inhalants. However, women are more likely than men to abuse sedatives and tranquilizers and

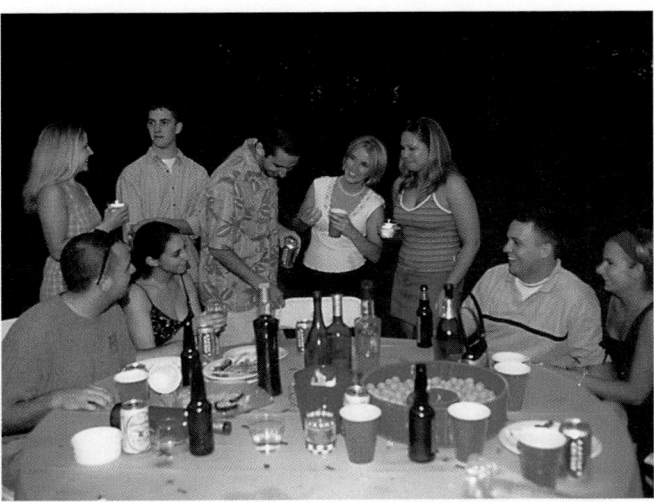

FIG. 11-1   Peer influence can contribute to alcohol abuse in young adults.

are less likely to abuse alcohol and marijuana.[10] Researchers have also identified the presence of a natural genetic mutation that inhibits nicotine metabolism in the brain. Men with this mutation are less likely to become addicted to nicotine and find it easier to quit smoking. However, the presence or absence of the defective gene does not affect women's smoking.[9]

Cultural factors also affect the incidence of substance abuse and are often related to other factors such as unemployment, poverty, or adverse social conditions. Although the rates of drug use are similar among white, African American, and Hispanic populations, much higher rates of alcoholism are present in Native Americans.[11,12] The alcoholism death rate for Native Americans is 440% higher than for the U.S. population in general.[12] All minority groups have a higher incidence of health problems associated with substance abuse, especially minority women. Drug-related acquired immunodeficiency syndrome (AIDS) has been the leading cause of death since 1993 in African American women, and more Native American women die from alcoholism than other women in the United States.[11,13] A major concern for all ethnic minorities is that current assessment and treatment of addictions in minority populations must become more culturally sensitive, addressing cultural values and practices, to reduce the use of drugs and their related health problems.

Health Complications of Substance Abuse

In spite of the extent of social disruptions caused by addiction, drug abuse–related health problems constitute the most immediate, extensive, and long-lasting problems caused by addictions. Almost every drug of abuse harms some tissue or organ in addition to the brain. Some health problems are caused by the effects of specific drugs, such as liver damage related to alcohol use and emphysema related to smoking. Other health problems result from the behaviors of addiction, such as injecting drugs and neglecting nutrition. Hepatitis C and human immunodeficiency virus (HIV) infection are associated with injected drug abuse. Drug abuse is nearly twice as likely to be directly or indirectly associated with AIDS in women as in men.[10,14] Common health complications of substance abuse are identified in Table 11-2.

Stimulants

NICOTINE

Characteristics

The addictive behavior that the nurse is most likely to encounter in a patient is nicotine dependence. Nicotine is the alkaloid in tobacco that causes dependence and is the most rapidly addicting of the drugs of abuse. It is estimated that 66.8 million Americans (30.2%) age 12 and older use a tobacco product and that about 6 million Canadians (24%) age 15 and older smoke cigarettes.[1,15] Cigarette smoking is the predominant form of tobacco abuse in North Americans.

Effects of Use

Nicotine is rapidly absorbed into the blood through the lungs in smoking, and more slowly through the buccal mucosa in chewing and through the nasal mucosa in snuffing. When absorbed, it produces a wide range of effects in the peripheral and central nervous systems through action at nicotinic receptors. Responses include increased blood pressure, heart rate, cardiac output, coronary blood flow, and cutaneous vasoconstriction. These effects result in stimulation of the cardiovascular system and increased myocardial oxygen consumption. In the brain the action of nicotine on nicotinic receptors causes general central nervous system (CNS) stimulation with increased alertness and arousal. In the gastrointestinal (GI) tract, stimulation of nicotinic receptors increases GI motility and secretion. Through both peripheral and central nervous system effects, nicotine also causes changes in the endocrine system, including release of prolactin, growth hormone, vasopressin, endorphins, and adrenocorticotropic hormone (ACTH) with a subsequent increase in cortisol.[5] Although nicotine abusers report that nicotine use causes a depressant effect with relaxation and relief of anxiety, it is thought that these effects actually occur when periodic nicotine withdrawal is relieved by further nicotine.[16] The effects of nicotine are listed in Table 11-3.

The strong **psychologic dependence** (see Table 11-1) associated with nicotine use is supported by the fact that it rapidly acts on the pleasure-producing mesolimbic area of the brain. **Physiologic dependence** (see Table 11-1) occurs with regular heavy use and is evidenced by increased tolerance and withdrawal symptoms following attempts to stop smoking. Withdrawal symptoms may occur within the first few hours after stopping, peak in 24 to 48 hours, and may last from a few weeks to several months. Symptoms include craving, restlessness, and hyperirritability.[17] Additional symptoms of withdrawal are presented in Table 11-3. After withdrawal subsides, cue-induced craving may cause smoking relapse.

Complications

The complications of nicotine abuse are related to the dose and the method of ingestion. Smoking cigarettes is the most deleterious method of nicotine use. Cigarette smoke contains more than 4000 chemicals and gases, including at least 45 cancer-causing or tumor-promoting agents and a number of hydrocarbons or solvents. Although nicotine is not believed to be carcinogenic, it is the addictive substance and has no therapeutic value.

The chronic respiratory irritation caused by cigarette smoke is the most important risk factor in the development of lung can-

TABLE 11-2	Common Health Problems Related to Substance Abuse
SUBSTANCE	**HEALTH PROBLEMS***
Nicotine and smoking	Chronic obstructive pulmonary disease (COPD)
	Cancers of the lung, mouth, larynx, esophagus, stomach, pancreas, bladder, prostate, cervix
	Coronary artery disease, peripheral artery disease
	Peptic ulcer disease, gastroesophageal reflux disease (GERD)
Cocaine	Nasal sores, septal necrosis or perforation
	Chronic sinusitis
	"Crack lung" pneumonia
	Cardiac arrhythmias, myocardial ischemia and infarction
	Stroke
	Psychosis
Amphetamines	Cardiac arrhythmias, myocardial ischemia and infarction
	Death of brain cells
	Syndrome of uncontrollable tremors
Caffeine	Gastrointestinal irritation, peptic ulcer disease, gastroesophageal reflux disease (GERD)
	Anxiety, sleep disruption
	Elevated blood pressure
Alcohol (see Table 11-7)	Gastritis, peptic ulcer disease
	Cirrhosis of the liver, pancreatitis
	Cancers of esophagus, stomach, head and neck, lung
	Dementias
	Decreased bone density
	Hypertension
Sedative-hypnotics	Possible memory impairment
	Respiratory depression
	Risk for falls and fractures
Opioids	Sexual dysfunction
	Gastric ulcers
	Glomerulonephritis
Cannabis	Bronchitis, chronic sinusitis
	Memory impairment
	Impaired immune function
	Reproductive dysfunction
BEHAVIORS	**HEALTH PROBLEMS**
Injecting drugs	Blood clots, phlebitis, skin infections
	Hepatitis B and C
	HIV/AIDS
	Other infections: endocarditis, tuberculosis, pneumonia, meningitis, tetanus, bone and joint infections, lung abscesses
Snorting drugs	Nasal sores, septal necrosis or perforation
	Chronic sinusitis
Risky sexual behavior	HIV/AIDS
	Hepatitis B and C
	Other sexually transmitted diseases
Personal neglect	Malnutrition, impaired immunity
	Accidental injuries

Sources: Shuckit MA: *Drug and alcohol abuse: a clinical guide to diagnosis and treatment,* ed 5, New York, 2000, Kluwer Academic/Plenum; Dogen CE: *Substance abuse disorders: assessment and treatment,* San Diego, 2000, Academic Press.
HIV/AIDS, Human immunodeficiency virus/acquired immunodeficiency syndrome.
*The health problems related to substance abuse are discussed in the appropriate chapters throughout the text where addictive behaviors are identified as risk factors for these problems.

TABLE 11-3   Effects of Frequently Abused Substances

SUBSTANCE	PHYSIOLOGIC AND PSYCHOLOGIC EFFECTS	EFFECTS OF OVERDOSE	WITHDRAWAL SYMPTOMS
Stimulants			
Nicotine	Increased arousal and alertness; performance enhancement; increased heart rate, cardiac output, and blood pressure; cutaneous vasoconstriction; fine tremor, decreased appetite; antidiuretic effect; increased gastric motility	Rare: nausea, abdominal pain, diarrhea, vomiting, dizziness, weakness, confusion, decreased respirations, seizures, death from respiratory failure	Craving, restlessness, depression, hyperirritability, headache, insomnia, decreased blood pressure and heart rate, increased appetite
Cocaine Amphetamines: amphetamine (Benzedrine), chlorphentermine (Pre-Sate), dextroamphetamine (Dexedrine), methamphetamine (Desoxyn), methylphenidate (Ritalin), phenmetrazine (Preludin)	Euphoria, grandiosity, mood swings, hyperactivity, hyperalertness, restlessness, anorexia, insomnia, hypertension, tachycardia, marked vasoconstriction, tremor, arrhythmias, seizures, sexual arousal, dilated pupils, diaphoresis	Agitation; increased temperature, pulse, respiratory rate, blood pressure; cardiac arrhythmias, myocardial infarction, hallucinations, seizures, possible death	Severe craving, severely depressed mood, exhaustion, prolonged sleep, apathy, irritability, disorientation
Caffeine	Mood elevation, increased alertness, nervousness, jitteriness, irritability, insomnia; increased respirations, heart rate, and force of myocardial contraction; relaxation of smooth muscle, diuresis	Rare: Hyperstimulation, nervousness, confusion, psychomotor agitation, anxiety, dizziness, tinnitus, muscle twitching, elevated blood pressure, tachycardia, extrasystoles, increased respiratory rate	Headache, irritability, drowsiness, fatigue
Depressants Alcohol Sedative-hypnotics • Barbiturates: secobarbital (Seconal), phenobarbital (Luminal), pentobarbital (Nembutal), amobarbital (Amytal) • Benzodiazepines: diazepam (Valium), chlordiazepoxide (Librium), alprazolam (Xanax) • Nonbarbiturates-nonbenzodiazepines: methaqualone (Quaalude), chloral hydrate (Noctec)	Initial relaxation, emotional lability, decreased inhibitions, drowsiness, lack of coordination, impaired judgment, slurred speech, hypotension, bradycardia, bradypnea, constricted pupils	Shallow respirations; cold, clammy skin; weak, rapid pulse; hyporeflexia, coma, possible death	Anxiety, agitation, insomnia, diaphoresis, tremors, delirium, seizures, possible death
Opioids heroin morphine opium codeine fentanyl (Sublimaze) meperidine (Demerol) hydromorphone (Dilaudid) propoxyphene (Darvon) pentazocine (Talwin) oxycodone (Percodan) methadone (Dolophine)	Analgesia, euphoria, drowsiness, detachment from environment, relaxation, constricted pupils, constipation, nausea, decreased respiratory rate, slurred speech, impaired judgment, decreased sexual and aggressive drives	Slow, shallow respirations; clammy skin; constricted pupils; coma; possible death	Watery eyes, dilated pupils, runny nose, yawning, tremors, pain, chills, fever, diaphoresis, nausea, vomiting, diarrhea, abdominal cramps

Continued

TABLE 11-3	Effects of Frequently Abused Substances—cont'd		
SUBSTANCE	**PHYSIOLOGIC AND PSYCHOLOGIC EFFECTS**	**EFFECTS OF OVERDOSE**	**WITHDRAWAL SYMPTOMS**
Cannabis Marijuana Hashish	Relaxation, euphoria, lack of motivation, slowed time sensation, sexual arousal, abrupt mood changes, impaired memory and attention, impaired judgment, reddened eyes, dry mouth, lack of coordination, tachycardia, increased appetite	Fatigue, paranoia, panic reactions, hallucinogen-like psychotic states	None except for rare insomnia, hyperactivity
Hallucinogens Lysergic acid diethylamide (LSD) Psilocybin (mushrooms) Dimethyltryptamine (DMT) Diethyltryptamine (DET) 3,4 Methylenedioxy-amphetamine (MDA) Mescaline (peyote) Phencyclidine (PCP)	Perceptual distortions, hallucinations, delusions (PCP), depersonalization, heightened sensory perception, euphoria, mood swings, suspiciousness, panic, impaired judgment, increased body temperature, hypertension, flushed face, tremor, dilated pupils, constricted pupils (PCP), nystagmus (PCP), violence (PCP)	Prolonged effects and episodes, anxiety, panic, confusion, blurred vision, increases in blood pressure and temperature	None
Inhalants Aerosol propellants Fluorinated hydrocarbons Nitrous oxide (in deodorants, hair spray, pesticide, whipped cream spray, spray paint, cookware coating products) Solvents (gasoline, kerosene, nail polish remover, typewriter correction fluid, cleaning solutions, lighter fluid, paint, paint thinner, glue) Anesthetic agents (nitrous oxide, chloroform) Nitrites (amyl nitrite, butyl nitrite)	Euphoria, decreased inhibitions, giddiness, slurred speech, illusions, drowsiness, clouded sensorium, tinnitis, nystagmus, arrhythmias, cough, nausea, vomiting, diarrhea; irritation to eyes, nose, mouth	Anxiety, respiratory depression, cardiac arrhythmias, loss of consciousness, sudden death	None

cer and chronic obstructive pulmonary disease (COPD). The toxic gases inhaled in cigarette smoke constrict the bronchi, paralyze the cilia, thicken the mucus-secreting membranes, dilate the distal airways, and destroy the alveolar walls. Tar in cigarette smoke contains several hundred chemicals, some of which are carcinogenic.[17]

Chronic irritation from smoking also is a factor in the increased incidence of cancer of the mouth, larynx, and esophagus in those who smoke tobacco in any form. Carcinogens absorbed into the blood from tobacco smoke may be responsible for the increased incidence in smokers of cancers of the bladder, prostate, and pancreas.

Carbon monoxide is also a component of cigarette smoke. Its effects, combined with those of nicotine, increase the risk for coronary artery disease. Carbon monoxide has a high affinity for hemoglobin and combines with it more readily than oxygen, reducing oxygen carrying capacity. Smokers also inhale less oxygen when smoking, adding to the decreased available oxygen. Together with the increased myocardial oxygen consumption

that nicotine causes, carbon monoxide significantly decreases the oxygen available to the myocardium. The result is an even greater increase in heart rate and myocardial oxygen consumption that may lead to myocardial ischemia.

Passive, or involuntary, smoking occurs under conditions of heavy smoking and poor ventilation when nonsmokers are exposed to cigarette smoke. Children whose parents smoke have a higher prevalence of respiratory symptoms and respiratory disease. In adults, involuntary, or secondhand, smoking is associated with decreased pulmonary function, increased risk for lung cancer, and increased mortality rates from coronary artery disease.[5]

Women appear to be at greater risk than men for smoking-related diseases. Women who smoke have almost double the risk of myocardial infarction than men and may also have nearly double the risk of lung cancer as men. Smoking in women is associated with greater menstrual bleeding and duration of dysmenorrhea, as well as greater variability in menstrual cycle length. In addition, there is also some evidence that breast and cervical cancer risk may be increased among women who smoke.[18]

Although those who use smokeless tobacco (snuff, plug, and leaf) have less risk of lung disease compared with smokers, the use of smokeless tobacco is not without complications. Holding tobacco in the mouth increases the risk of cancer of the mouth, cheek, tongue, and gingiva nearly fiftyfold.[17] Smokeless tobacco users also experience the wide systemic effects of nicotine.

All users of nicotine in any form may develop complications that are directly related to the effects of nicotine itself. Such complications may include an increased risk for peripheral arterial disease, delayed wound healing, reproductive disorders, peptic ulcer disease, and gastroesophageal reflux disease (GERD).[17] Common health problems associated with tobacco use are presented in Table 11-2.

Collaborative Care

A combination of medications, behavioral approaches, and support is believed to be most effective in long-term tobacco cessation. A variety of nicotine replacement systems in the form of gum (nicotine polacrilex [Nicorette]), transdermal patches (Habitrol, Nicoderm), nasal spray, and nicotine inhalers can be used to reduce the amount of the craving and withdrawal symptoms associated with tobacco cessation. These agents enable a smoker to reduce nicotine previously obtained from cigarettes with a system that provides slower delivery of the drug and elimination of the carcinogens and gases associated with tobacco smoke. Bupropion (Zyban), an antidepressant that does not contain nicotine, decreases the symptoms of withdrawal and has been approved for tobacco cessation.

Participation in tobacco cessation programs can help tobacco users focus on other aspects of quitting while they receive some relief from nicotine withdrawal symptoms with the use of replacement systems. Behavioral approaches can teach patients to avoid high-risk situations for smoking relapse, such as those that promote cue-induced craving. Tobacco cessation programs also promote development of other coping skills, such as cigarette refusal skills, assertiveness, alternative activities to cope with stress, and use of peer support systems.[9,19]

Women are less successful than men in quitting smoking. Some of the reasons include concern about weight gain, less responsiveness to nicotine replacement therapy, variability in mood and withdrawal as a function of the menstrual cycle, inadequate emotional support from others, and the possibility that smoking-associated environmental cues may be more influential in smoking behavior in women than men.[18] The identification of factors that contribute to women's poorer success in quitting smoking has led to study of better smoking cessation approaches for women.

COCAINE

Characteristics

Today cocaine is the most abused major stimulant in the United States and Canada. Although the use of cocaine is not as high today as at its peak in 1983, the annual number of new users of any form of cocaine is increasing in youths ages 12 to 17 years.[1,3] "Crack," a cocaine alkaloid that gets its name from the popping sound the crystals make when heated, is also popular because it is less expensive, is readily available, is easy to use, and has an increased purity over cocaine.

Effects of Use

Cocaine is the most potent of the abused stimulants. Its effects have been extensively studied, and it serves as the prototype of an addictive stimulant substance. All stimulants work in part by increasing the amount of dopamine in the brain, producing euphoria and increasing energy and alertness. This action on the brain reward system magnifies pleasure and leads to rapid dependence. In addition to stimulation of the CNS, cocaine and other stimulants also affect the peripheral nervous system and the cardiovascular system. Effects include adrenaline-like actions that lead to increased heart rate, blood pressure, and body temperature; arrhythmias; marked vasoconstriction; tremors of the hands; nausea or vomiting; and diminished appetite. Additional physical and psychologic effects are presented in Tables 11-3 and 11-4. Chronic use may lead to impairment of concentration and memory, irritability and mood swings, paranoia, and depression.[5,16]

The most common method of administration of cocaine is intranasal (snorting), but it may be smoked as "crack" cocaine or in "freebase" form, injected intravenously, taken orally, or absorbed through mucous membranes. Smoking and intravenous

TABLE 11-4	Effects of Cocaine and Amphetamine Use	
	EARLY EFFECTS	**LONG-TERM EFFECTS**
Central nervous system	Excitation, euphoria, restlessness, talkativeness	Depression, hallucinations, tremors, visual disturbances, seizures, headache, insomnia, stroke
Cardiovascular system	Tachycardia, hypertension, angina, arrhythmias, palpitations	Arrhythmias, hypotension, congestive heart failure, myocardial infarction, cardiomyopathy
Respiratory system	Increased respiratory rate, dyspnea, chest pain, epistaxis	Chronic cough, inflamed throat, congestion of lungs, brown/black sputum production, pneumonia, respiratory distress and/or arrest, pulmonary edema, rhinorrhea, rhinitis, erosion and perforation of the nasal septum
Reproductive system	Heightened sexual desire, delayed orgasm and ejaculation; women may have difficulty achieving orgasm	Difficulty in maintaining erection and ejaculation; loss of interest in sexual activity; women may develop aberrant sexual behavior
Gastrointestinal system	Decreased appetite	Dehydration, weight loss, nausea; intestinal ischemia may cause gangrenous bowel
Psychologic	Behavior changes or mood swings	Depression or suicidal thoughts

(IV) methods result in the fastest absorption and the highest "rush." Peak blood levels develop within 5 to 30 minutes with most methods of administration, and the longest effects occur following intranasal ingestion.[20]

Although cocaine withdrawal is not accompanied by obvious physical signs, there may be subtle muscular aches and pains, and there is an intense psychologic response. In the first 9 hours to 14 days, withdrawal is characterized by intense craving and cocaine-seeking behavior. There is marked agitation, feelings of depression, exhaustion, and a need to sleep (see Table 11-3). Eventually mood becomes more normal, but a desire to return to the drug, especially prompted by cue-induced craving, remains for an indefinite period of time.[5]

Complications

Complications are directly related to the route of administration, type of cocaine, dose, and individual vulnerabilities (see Table 11-2). Intravenous administration may result in collapse and scarring of the veins at the injection site, cellulitis, wound abscess, endocarditis, hepatitis B and C, and HIV infection. With intranasal use, the nasal septum and mucosa may be damaged, and frequent sniffing and rhinitis are common signs of chronic intranasal use. Pulmonary damage from smoking crack may be evident with black or dark brown sputum and a pneumonia known as "crack lung." Bilateral loss of eyebrow and eyelash hair may occur during "freebasing," a process of heating cocaine with a volatile substance such as ether to make crack.

A *stimulant psychosis* may occur with the chronic use of any stimulant. A cocaine psychosis usually progresses from paranoid delusions to visual hallucinations of "snow lights" (colored lights when cocaine is administered) and tactile hallucinations of bugs crawling under the skin. Skin excoriations from scratching; needle marks; and elevated blood pressure, heart rate, and tempera-ture are findings that help differentiate a stimulant psychosis from schizophrenia.[5]

Acute cocaine toxicity may be manifested by cardiac palpitations, tachycardia, increased respiratory rate, and fever. At high levels of overdose, seizures, hypertension, and arrhythmias or myocardial ischemia can occur. The patient experiences restlessness, paranoia, agitated delirium, confusion, and repetitive stereotyped behaviors. Death is often related to stroke, fatal arrhythmias, or myocardial infarction.[5]

Collaborative Care

An individual who is addicted to cocaine frequently does not seek treatment for drug abuse but rather for problems with sleep, appetite, depression, sinusitis, respiratory infections, chest pain, or headaches. The nurse should have a high degree of suspicion of stimulant drug abuse in any patient seeking health care who has dilated pupils, tachycardia, hyperactivity, fever, or behavioral abnormalities.

Emergency management of cocaine intoxication will depend on the patient findings at the time of treatment and may be complicated by the possibility that the patient has combined the use of cocaine with heroin, alcohol, or phencyclidine hydrochloride (PCP). Emergency management of cocaine toxicity is presented in Table 11-5.

AMPHETAMINES

Characteristics

Amphetamine is a synthetic drug and, with its derivatives and similar stimulants, is strictly regulated. Specific drugs classified as amphetamines are identified in Table 11-3. Because amphetamines may be prescribed for treatment of narcolepsy, attention deficit disorders, and weight control, abuse may occur from

---

TABLE 11-5   *E*mergency Management

Cocaine and Amphetamine Toxicity

ETIOLOGY	ASSESSMENT FINDINGS	INTERVENTIONS
Intranasal, inhalation, parenteral, oral, vaginal, rectal, or sublingual administration of cocaine; oral or parenteral administration of amphetamines	**Cardiovascular** ▪ Palpitations ▪ Tachycardia ▪ Hypertension ▪ Arrhythmias ▪ Myocardial ischemia or infarction **Central Nervous System** ▪ Feeling of impending doom ▪ Euphoria ▪ Agitation ▪ Combativeness ▪ Seizures ▪ Hallucinations ▪ Confusion ▪ Paranoia ▪ Fever **Other** ▪ Track marks ▪ Consumption of bags of cocaine	**Initial** ▪ Ensure patent airway ▪ Anticipate need for intubation if respiratory distress evident ▪ Establish IV access and initiate fluid replacement as appropriate ▪ Obtain a 12-lead ECG ▪ Treat ventricular arrhythmias as appropriate with lidocaine, bretylium (Bretylol), or procainamide (Pronestyl) ▪ Administer IV haloperidol (Haldol) for psychosis ▪ Administer IV diazepam (Valium) or lorazepam (Ativan) for seizures ▪ Naloxone (Narcan) IV should be given if CNS depression is present and concurrent opiate use is suspected ▪ Anticipate the need for propranolol (Inderal) or labetalol (Normodyne) for hypertension and tachycardia **Ongoing** ▪ Monitor vital signs, level of consciousness, cardiac rhythm ▪ Use restraints only if needed to protect the patient and staff

CNS, Central nervous system; *ECG,* electrocardiogram; *IV,* intravenous.

slowly increasing the prescribed dose. However, they are also initially used as the "poor man's cocaine," and methamphetamine (crank) and smokable methamphetamine crystals (crystal, ice) are produced illegally in clandestine laboratories and are in great demand on the black market.

Effects of Use

Amphetamines are similar to cocaine and stimulate the central and peripheral nervous systems and the cardiovascular system to produce euphoria, hyperactivity, and increased heart rate and blood pressure. Initial use results in increased alertness, improved performance, relief of fatigue, and anorexia. As with cocaine use, amphetamines used over time may lead to irritability, anxiety, paranoia, and hostile and violent behaviors (see Table 11-3).

Amphetamines are usually taken orally. Rapid effects are obtained by smoking, snorting, or IV injection. Amphetamines have a longer half-life than cocaine and, because they are more often taken orally, have a longer effect. Withdrawal symptoms of amphetamines are similar to those of cocaine use and are presented in Table 11-3.[20]

Complications

Toxic reactions to amphetamines are similar to those of cocaine. Increased levels of stimulation, sometimes described as "overamping," may result in amphetamine psychosis, paranoia, seizures, and death (see Table 11-3). Without medical intervention, death may occur as a result of arrhythmias, myocardial infarction, hyperthermia, or cerebral hemorrhage.

Collaborative Care

Patients often seek treatment for complications of amphetamine abuse such as panic reactions or temporary psychosis related to intoxication, overdose, or withdrawal. Emergency management of amphetamine toxicity is the same as that for cocaine and is presented in Table 11-4.

CAFFEINE

Characteristics

Caffeine is the most widely used psychoactive substance in the world, and its use to promote alertness and alleviate fatigue is safe in most people. Although weaker than other stimulant drugs, caffeine shares characteristics of intoxication, tolerance, and withdrawal symptoms in some individuals. Approximately 80% of adults in North America report a regular intake of caffeine, and 20% of those using caffeine consume doses larger than 350 mg, enough to cause clinical symptoms and dependence. One cup of coffee contains approximately 90 to 150 mg of caffeine, with drip preparation yielding the highest amount of caffeine. A cup of tea averages 30 to 100 mg of caffeine depending on the brewing method. Traditional cola soft drinks average 25 to 50 mg of caffeine.[5] In addition to beverages, caffeine is found in numerous prescription and over-the-counter analgesics, stimulants, appetite suppressants, and cold and flu preparations.

Effects of Use

Caffeine is a relatively weak CNS stimulant. It is a diuretic and a myocardial stimulant. It relaxes smooth muscles, promotes vasodilation, constricts cerebral arteries, increases gastric acid secretion, and enhances contraction of skeletal muscles. Oral doses of 200 mg (two cups of coffee) can elevate mood, produce insomnia, increase irritability, cause anxiety, and offset fatigue. Chronic or heavy intake of 500 mg or more per day is known to cause intoxication manifested by nervousness, insomnia, gastric hyperacidity, muscle twitching, confusion, tachycardia or cardiac arrhythmias, and psychomotor agitation. Ingestion of a lethal dose is extremely rare but could occur with caffeine-containing drugs or the oral ingestion of 10 g (70 to 100 cups of coffee).[5] The effects of caffeine are presented in Table 11-3.

Physical and psychologic dependence on caffeine has been found with chronic use of more than 500 mg/day. However, dependence may occur in some individuals at lower doses. The most commonly reported withdrawal symptoms are headache, irritability, drowsiness, and fatigue that occur within 12 to 24 hours following abstinence (see Table 11-3). Caffeine withdrawal may be responsible for some cases of headache that occur after general anesthesia. It is thought that weekend headaches may be related to caffeine withdrawal because caffeine consumption in many individuals is higher at work than at home.[21]

Complications

Chronic and heavy use of caffeine may cause GI upset, including abdominal pain, diarrhea, and heartburn. Habitual users are reported to have slightly higher blood pressure, heart rates, and basal metabolic rates (see Table 11-2). Because symptoms of chronic use develop gradually, most people with caffeine dependence do not link sleep disruption, anxiety, and other symptoms with caffeine intake. In toxic doses, caffeine influences behavior patterns and may precipitate panic states.

Collaborative Care

Management of the patient with symptoms of caffeine dependence includes assisting the patient to gradually reduce or stop the intake of caffeine. A list of caffeinated products with their dosages may be helpful to the patient who quits coffee only to substitute other foods and beverages containing caffeine. Substituting decaffeinated beverages may also help. Decaffeinated coffee and tea contain 2 to 4 mg of caffeine per cup. Toxic reactions to caffeine and lethal doses of caffeine are managed symptomatically, with attention to maintaining respirations and controlling hypertension, arrhythmias, and seizures.

Depressants

Drugs classified as depressants have common physiologic and psychologic effects. Drugs in this category include alcohol, sedative-hypnotics, and opioid narcotics. With the exception of alcohol and some federally regulated drugs, most CNS depressants are medically useful. These drugs are also widely recognized for their abuse potential, which leads to rapid tolerance, dependence, and medical emergencies involving overdose and withdrawal.

ALCOHOL

Characteristics

Alcohol is the most widely consumed substance of abuse in the United States. Almost half of Americans ages 12 and older report current drinking of alcohol.[1] In Canada, 72% of the population age 15 or older drink alcohol.[2] Alcoholism, or alcohol dependence, is estimated at 10% in both countries. The use of alcohol, whether by occasional drinkers or by those who are alcohol dependent, causes significant negative consequences, in-

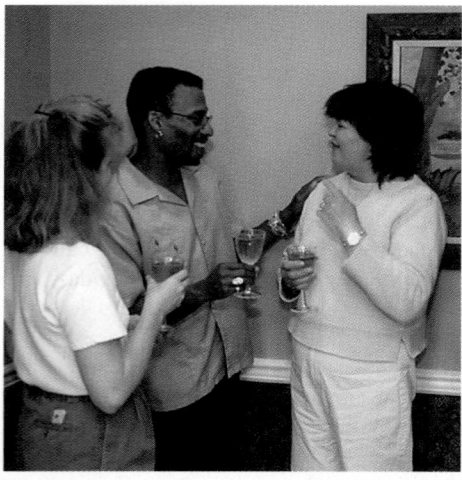

FIG. 11-2 Alcohol abuse is not easy to identify in our society.

TABLE 11-6   Blood Alcohol Concentration (BAC) and Related Effects

BAC* MG/DL (MG%)	PSYCHOPHYSIOLOGIC EFFECT
20 (0.02)	Light and moderate drinkers begin to feel some effects. Approximate BAC is reached after one drink.[†]
40 (0.04)	Most people begin to feel relaxed.
60 (0.06)	Judgment is mildly impaired. People are less able to make rational decisions about their capabilities (e.g., driving skills).
80 (0.08)	Definite impairment of muscle coordination and driving skills occurs. Person is legally intoxicated in some states.
100 (0.10)	Clear deterioration of reaction time and control is observed. Person is legally intoxicated in most states.
120 (0.12)	Vomiting occurs unless this level is reached slowly.
150 (0.15)	Balance and movement are impaired. Equivalent of one-half pint of whiskey is circulating in the bloodstream.
300 (0.30)	Many people lose consciousness.
400 (0.40)	Most people lose consciousness, and some die.
450 (0.45)	Breathing stops; person eventually dies.

*Blood alcohol concentration (BAC) is generally recorded in milligrams of alcohol per deciliter (mg/dl) of blood or milligrams percent (mg%). Percentage is used for legal definitions of intoxication. BAC is dependent on how much alcohol is consumed, how fast it is consumed, and the person's weight.
[†]One drink is 12 oz beer, 5 oz wine, or 1 oz distilled spirits, all of which provide the same amount of alcohol.

cluding automobile accidents, arrests, violence, occupational injuries, and poor job performance.

Alcoholism is currently viewed as a chronic, progressive, potentially fatal disease if left untreated. Numerous factors appear to be interrelated in the development of alcohol dependence and may include genetic and biologic factors, psychosocial factors, and cultural-environmental background. Alcohol dependence generally occurs over a period of years and may be preceded by heavy social drinking (Fig. 11-2).

Effects of Use

Alcohol affects almost all cells of the body and has complex effects on the neurons in the CNS. Alcohol, like other addictive substances, causes increased levels of dopamine and also depresses all areas and functions of the CNS. Alcohol is absorbed directly from the stomach and small intestine. Absorption is slower in the presence of water or food, especially proteins and fats. Faster absorption occurs when alcohol is mixed with carbonated liquids. Metabolism of alcohol in the liver occurs at a rate of approximately one drink (7 g of alcohol) per hour.[16] One drink is equal to 12 ounces of beer, 5 ounces of wine, or 1 ounce of distilled spirits.

The effects of alcohol are related to the concentration of alcohol and individual susceptibility to the drug. The concentration of alcohol in the body can be determined by assessing the blood alcohol concentration (BAC). Alcohol may be measured in the blood within 15 to 20 minutes of ingestion, peaks in 60 to 90 minutes, and is excreted in 12 to 24 hours. BAC is affected by the amount consumed, drinking rate, body size and composition, drink concentration, and hormones. For the nonalcoholic drinker, the BAC is generally predictable of alcohol's effects (Table 11-6). The relationship between BAC and behavior is different in a person who has developed tolerance to alcohol and its effects. This individual is commonly able to drink large amounts without obvious impairment and perform complex tasks without problems at BAC levels several times higher than levels that would produce obvious impairment in the nontolerant drinker.

Intoxication is evidenced with increasing BAC and results in behavioral and physical changes (see Table 11-3). Behavioral effects may include relaxation, sedation, loss of inhibitions, aggression, impaired judgment, irritability, euphoria, depression, and emotional lability. Physical signs include slurred speech,

lack of motor coordination, nystagmus, and flushing resulting from dilation of peripheral blood vessels. Disturbances in memory and blackouts may occur in dependent drinkers.

After excessive drinking, individuals may experience hangovers manifested by malaise, nausea, headache, thirst, and a general feeling of fatigue. In alcoholics, sudden withdrawal may have life-threatening effects. Withdrawal should be anticipated if the individual reports consumption of over 10 drinks every day for a period of 2 weeks. Four characteristic signs of withdrawal are gross tremors, seizures, hallucinations, and delirium tremens (DTs).[5]

Most alcoholics experience a minor withdrawal syndrome in the first 10 to 12 hours after the last drink, which peaks at 24 to 28 hours and may last up to 5 days. Characteristic symptoms include tremulousness, anxiety, increased heart rate, increased blood pressure, sweating, nausea, hyperreflexia, and insomnia (see Table 11-3). Seizures are most likely to occur 7 to 48 hours after the last drink. Alcohol withdrawal delirium, or DTs, is a serious complication that may occur from 30 to 120 hours after the last drink. Delirium components include disorientation, visual or auditory hallucinations, and increased hyperactivity without seizures. Death may be caused by hyperthermia, peripheral vascular collapse, or cardiac failure.[22]

Complications

Acute alcohol toxicity may occur with binge drinking or the use of alcohol with other CNS depressants. Alcohol-induced CNS depression leads to respiratory and circulatory failure manifested by depressed respirations, hypotension, hypothermia, and a decreased level of consciousness (see Table 11-3).

Individuals who abuse alcohol have many health problems. Physical complications of chronic alcohol abuse are outlined in Table 11-7 and are frequently the reasons that alcohol-dependent individuals seek health care. Complications may also arise from the interaction of alcohol with commonly prescribed or over-the-counter drugs. Drugs that interact with alcohol in an additive manner include antihypertensives, antihistamines, antianginals, and salicylates (aspirin). Alcohol taken with aspirin may cause or exacerbate GI bleeding. Alcohol taken with acetaminophen may increase the risk of liver damage. Potentiation and cross-tolerance with other CNS depressants also may occur. **Potentiation** occurs when an additional CNS depressant is taken with alcohol, increasing the effect. **Cross-tolerance,** requiring an increased dose for effect, occurs when an alcohol-dependent individual is alcohol free and receives other CNS depressants.[5]

Collaborative Care

Initial treatment of alcoholism is aimed at **detoxification** (defined in Table 11-1) as necessary and stabilization of the patient's condition. In toxic reactions, naloxone (Narcan), an opiate antagonist, may be given if opioids have been used with alcohol. Supportive measures are used to promote ventilation and circulation until the alcohol is metabolized. The patient who is intoxicated with rising BACs should not be given other depressants because of their additive effects.

Management of alcohol withdrawal frequently includes the use of medications to decrease symptoms, increase level of comfort, and decrease the risk of seizures and DTs. Table 11-8 presents the clinical manifestations of alcohol withdrawal and suggested drug treatment.

Although cessation of drinking is the short-term goal that is accomplished through detoxification, rehabilitation and sustained abstinence are the primary long-term goals. Patients

TABLE 11-8	Clinical Manifestations of Alcohol Withdrawal and Suggested Drug Treatment

Clinical Manifestations

Gross tremors
Seizures
Hallucinations
Delirium tremens (DTs)
Minor withdrawal syndrome:
- Tremulousness, anxiety
- Increased heart rate
- Increased blood pressure
- Sweating
- Nausea
- Hyperreflexia
- Insomnia

Major withdrawal (DTs):
- Disorientation
- Visual/auditory hallucinations
- Increased hyperactivity without seizures

Drug Treatment

Benzodiazepines (e.g., chlordiazepoxide [Librium])
Thiamine (prevents Wernicke's encephalopathy)
Multivitamins (folic acid, B vitamins)
Phenytoin (Dilantin) for seizures or past history of seizures
Magnesium sulfate (if serum magnesium is low)
Temazepam (Restoril) for sedation
Haloperidol (Haldol) for hallucinations
For DTs: may need IV fluids (do not overhydrate), cooling blanket, well-lit quiet room, consistent staff, frequent vital signs, check for hypoglycemia, assessment of any other health problems

TABLE 11-7	Effects of Chronic Alcohol Abuse

BODY SYSTEM	EFFECTS
Central nervous system	Alcoholic dementia; Wernicke's syndrome (confusion, nystagmus, paralysis of ocular muscles, ataxia); Korsakoff's syndrome (confabulation, amnesic disorder); impairment of cognitive function, psychomotor skills, abstract thinking, and memory; depression, attention deficit, labile moods, seizures, sleep disturbances
Peripheral nervous system	Peripheral neuropathy including pain, paresthesias, weakness
Immune system	Increased risk for tuberculosis and viral infections; increased risk for cancer of oral cavity, pharynx, esophagus, liver, colon, rectum, and possibly breast
Hematologic system	Bone marrow depression, anemia, leukopenia, thrombocytopenia, blood clotting abnormalities
Musculoskeletal system	Painful, tender, swelling of large muscle groups; painless progressive muscle weakness and wasting; osteoporosis
Cardiovascular system	Elevated pulse and blood pressure; decreased exercise tolerance; cardiomyopathy (irreversible); increased risk for hemorrhagic stroke, coronary artery disease, hypertension, sudden cardiac death
Hepatic system	Steatosis (reversible)—nausea, vomiting, hepatomegaly
	Alcoholic hepatitis (reversible)—anorexia, nausea, vomiting, fever, chills, abdominal pain, cirrhosis; cancer
Gastrointestinal system	Gastritis, peptic ulcer, esophagitis, esophageal varices, enteritis, colitis, Mallory-Weiss tear, pancreatitis
Nutrition	Decreased appetite, indigestion, malabsorption, vitamin deficiencies
Urinary system	Diuretic effect from inhibition of antidiuretic hormone
Endocrine and reproductive system	Altered gonadal function, testicular atrophy, decreased beard growth, decreased libido, diminished sperm count, gynecomastia, glucose intolerance
Integumentary system	Palmar erythema, spider angiomas, rosacea, rhinophyma

should be referred to inpatient or intensive outpatient programs for treatment. Treatment includes behavioral therapy and may also include drugs that block the desired effects of alcohol, such as naltrexone (Trexan), or agents that prevent drinking by causing aversive consequences when alcohol is consumed, such as disulfiram (Antabuse).

SEDATIVE-HYPNOTICS

Characteristics

Sedative-hypnotic agents that are commonly abused include barbiturates, benzodiazepines, and barbiturate-like drugs. Benzodiazepines have largely replaced barbiturates for medical treatment of anxiety and insomnia because they are safer in terms of risk of overdose and toxicity. Barbiturates are preferred as recreational drugs because they more frequently produce euphoric effects.

Two patterns of abuse and dependence have been recognized with sedative-hypnotic drugs. The first pattern begins with prescription use of the drug for the treatment of anxiety or insomnia. Subsequently, the patient may become tolerant to the effects and increase the dose and frequency of use without medical advice or indication. The second and more common pattern involves illegal sources, which often begins with intermittent use by teenagers or young adults at parties and leads to daily use to achieve effects.

Effects of Use

Sedative-hypnotic drugs act primarily on the CNS, causing sedation at low doses and sleep at high doses. Excessive amounts produce an initial euphoria and an intoxication that includes impaired judgment, slurred speech, and loss of inhibitions and motor coordination. Although benzodiazepines are believed to have a wide margin of safety, they are not without adverse reactions, including *rebound anxiety* and insomnia with short-acting drugs and confusion and memory loss with long-acting drugs. The drugs are usually taken orally, but barbiturates may be injected intravenously.[5] The effects of sedative-hypnotics are presented in Table 11-3.

Tolerance develops rapidly to the sedative effects, requiring higher doses to achieve euphoria. Tolerance may not develop to the brainstem-depressant effects so an increased dose may trigger hypotension and respiratory depression, resulting in death.

Withdrawal from sedative-hypnotics can be very serious. The patient may develop anxiety, tremors, weakness, nausea and/or vomiting, muscle cramps, and increased reflexes. After 24 hours the patient is craving the drug and may experience delirium, seizures, and respiratory and cardiac arrest (see Table 11-3). Symptoms of withdrawal peak on the second or third day for short-acting drugs (e.g., alprazolam [Xanax], secobarbital [Seconal], pentobarbital [Nembutal]) and on the seventh or eighth day for long-acting drugs (e.g., diazepam [Valium], chlordiazepoxide [Librium], phenobarbital [Luminal]).[20]

Complications

An overdose of a sedative-hypnotic may cause death as a result of respiratory depression. Symptoms of overdose are listed in Table 11-3. Complications associated with IV use of the drugs can also occur. These may include cellulitis, vascular complications, hepatitis B and C, endocarditis, bacterial infections, and HIV infection.

Collaborative Care

Overdoses of benzodiazepines are treated with flumazenil (Romazicon), a specific benzodiazepine antagonist. There are no known antagonists to counteract the effects of other sedative-hypnotic drugs. Emergency life support measures must be taken in cases of overdose. Table 11-9 presents emergency management of CNS depressants. Treatment of an individual dependent on a sedative-hypnotic requires gradual withdrawal of the drug.

TABLE 11-9   Emergency Management
Overdose of Depressant Drug

ETIOLOGY	ASSESSMENT FINDINGS	INTERVENTIONS
Ingestion, inhalation, or injection of CNS depressants—accidental or intentional	• Aggressive behavior • Agitation • Confusion • Lethargy • Stupor • Hallucinations • Depression • Slurred speech • Pinpoint pupils • Nystagmus • Seizures • Needle tracks • Cold, clammy skin • Rapid, weak pulse • Slow or rapid shallow respirations • Decreased O_2 saturation • Hypotension • Arrhythmia • ECG changes • Cardiac or respiratory arrest	**Initial** • Ensure patent airway • Anticipate intubation if respiratory distress evident • Establish IV access • Obtain temperature • Obtain 12-lead ECG • Obtain information about substance (name, route, when taken, amount) • Obtain specific drug levels or comprehensive toxicology screen • Obtain a health history including drug use and allergies • Administer antidotes as appropriate • Perform gastric lavage if necessary • Administer activated charcoal and cathartics as appropriate **Ongoing** • Monitor vital signs, temperature, level of consciousness, O_2 saturation, cardiac rhythm

CNS, Central nervous system; *ECG,* electrocardiogram; *IV,* intravenous.

Hospitalization is recommended during drug withdrawal for individuals who have been abusing large amounts of the drugs to safely manage their symptoms.

OPIOIDS

Characteristics

Opiates are natural substances, such as morphine and codeine, that are directly derived from opium. **Opioids** include the opiates in addition to the many semisynthetic and synthetic narcotic agents used as analgesics. Commonly abused opioids are identified in Table 11-3. Narcotic antagonists include naloxone (Narcan) and nalorphine (Nalline).

Individuals dependent on opioids include those who use illegal drugs sold on the street and those who misuse opioids in a medical setting. Street use usually involves the use of heroin or fentanyl (Sublimaze) and is found in younger people who often began their substance problems with tobacco and alcohol and then progressed to marijuana and other drugs of abuse. In a medical setting, some people misuse prescribed analgesics. These individuals tend to be middle-class and older than those using street drugs. A significant group in the medical setting includes health care professionals, who may have the highest rate of opioid abuse and dependence of any middle-class population.[5] Ready availability of drugs, stresses of caring for other people's problems, and long hours that interfere with family life are considered contributing factors in health care professionals.

Although the rates of opioid use are lower than for other illegal drugs, their use is associated with high levels of crime, violence, HIV infection, and death from overdose. Approximately 5% of the U.S. population uses an opioid drug in a manner other than prescribed, and about 0.1% of the U.S. population currently uses heroin.[1] Abuse of opioids is low in Canada, with only 0.5% of Canadians reporting the use of heroin at some time during their lives.[2]

Effects of Use

By acting on opiate receptors and neurotransmitter systems in the CNS, opioids cause CNS depression and a major effect on the brain reward system. As drugs of abuse, they are taken orally, sniffed, smoked, or injected subcutaneously ("skin-popping") or intravenously ("mainlining").

The primary effects include analgesia, drowsiness, slurred speech, detachment from the environment, and decreased respiratory rate, GI peristalsis, and pupil size. Intravenous use usually causes a "rush" of feelings in the lower abdomen, along with warm skin flushing, and a strong sense of euphoria (see Table 11-3). Opioids lead to rapid tolerance and physical dependence after short-term use. Cross-tolerance among the drugs is common.

Signs of overdose of opioids include pinpoint pupils, clammy skin, depressed respiration, coma, and death, if not treated. Unintentional overdose frequently occurs with recreational use of the drugs because of the unpredictability in potency and purity. Signs of overdose are presented in Table 11-3.

Withdrawal from opioids occurs with decreased amounts or cessation of the drug after prolonged moderate to heavy use. The administration of a narcotic antagonist, such as naloxone (Narcan), will cause withdrawal symptoms in dependent individuals. Symptoms may include craving, abdominal cramps, diarrhea, nausea, and vomiting. Additional symptoms are presented in Table 11-3.

Complications

The most common serious medical complication associated with heroin use, which is usually injected intravenously, is HIV infection. HIV infection has been detected in as many as 60% of IV drug users in certain localities. In addition, it has been estimated that 55% of men and women who were infected by heterosexual activity acquired their disease through sex partners who were IV drug users. Drug abuse by any route of administration increases the risk of contracting HIV because of the tendency of substance abusers to engage in risky sexual behaviors in exchange for drugs or money or because of lack of inhibition.[5]

Hepatitis C is also a serious problem. It is estimated to affect 80% of the drug-injecting population of the United States, and young adults who inject drugs have the highest rate of new infections. Although hepatitis B is also a significant problem, it is currently outpaced by the incidence of hepatitis C.[23]

Other complications occur as a consequence of injecting drugs or neglect of health and hygiene. These include a variety of infections, as well as damage to the kidneys, electrolyte abnormalities, and arrhythmias. Health problems associated with opioid use are presented in Table 11-2.

Collaborative Care

Overdose of opioids can precipitate a medical emergency. Table 11-9 outlines interventions for overdose of depressant drugs. A toxicologic blood or urine screen may be helpful to identify the specific drug. A narcotic antagonist such as naloxone (Narcan) should be given as soon as life support is instituted. The patient should be monitored closely because narcotic antagonists have a shorter duration of action than most opioids. It is also possible the patient may have a mixed drug ingestion that does not respond to narcotic antagonists.

Treatment of withdrawal is symptom based and does not always require the use of medications. Withdrawal symptoms are acutely uncomfortable but not as life threatening as withdrawal from other CNS depressants. Methadone in decreasing doses may be used during detoxification to decrease symptoms and may also be used for maintenance treatment.

Methadone maintenance programs combined with education, counseling, and vocational training programs are the most effective method of decreasing the risk of heroin use and the most promising available treatment for IV opioid users. Antagonist therapy that seeks to eliminate drug use by blocking the drug's effects is a less successful treatment of dependence. Antagonist therapy includes the use of naltrexone (Trexan), an oral narcotic antagonist that must be voluntarily taken daily.

Hallucinogens

Hallucinogens are a variety of psychoactive substances that act to produce a change in level of consciousness, alter mood, and induce hallucinations. Table 11-3 identifies common hallucinogens and their effects.

CANNABIS

Characteristics

Cannabis, or marijuana, is the most widely used illicit drug in North America. It is currently used by about 11 million Americans ages 12 and older and by approximately 7.4% of the population in

Canada.[1,2] It is usually the first illegal drug used by young people, and its use is more common in adolescents and young adults. Patterns of use are similar to alcohol in that there is occasional use, misuse resulting in temporary problems, and abuse or dependence associated with a high potential for future problems.

In North America cannabis is usually sold as marijuana or hashish. The key active ingredient in cannabis responsible for most of the psychoactive effects is tetrahydrocannabinol (THC). Marijuana, which is derived from the dried leaves and flowering tops of the cannabis plant, is a less potent source of THC than hashish, which is a resinous secretion of the plant. Although a number of potential benefits of THC have been reported, the only demonstrated benefits are for control of drug-resistant glaucoma and nausea resulting from cancer chemotherapy.[5]

Effects of Use

At low to moderate doses, THC produces fewer physiologic and psychologic alterations than do other classes of psychoactive drugs, including alcohol. Although its mechanism of action is uncertain, THC affects dopamine and other neurotransmitter activity and a variety of receptors in the brain. When marijuana is smoked, effects usually occur in about 20 to 30 minutes and may last up to 7 hours. Because it is stored in body fat, it is eliminated slowly, resulting in a half-life of 2 to 7 days.[20] Tolerance of many effects occurs, but physiologic dependence does not usually develop even with long-term heavy use. Marijuana has low toxicity, and there is no known level of lethal dose.

The most commonly affected organs are the brain and the cardiovascular and respiratory systems. Most changes are reversible. Signs of intoxication are presented in Table 11-3. Problems of habitual users include impaired short-term memory, decreased motor coordination, tremors, increased heart and respiratory rates, and depression.[5]

Complications

Complications of marijuana use are generally mild and transient. Heavy use may cause bronchitis, increased rates of precancerous lesions in the lungs, sinusitis, pharyngitis, acute memory impairment, depression of the immune system, and alterations in the reproductive and endocrine systems (see Table 11-2). Complications may also be seen when marijuana is used with other drugs such as heroin and cocaine. It may precipitate seizures in persons with epilepsy, psychotic episodes in persons with schizophrenia, and ketoacidosis in persons with diabetes mellitus, and it may complicate preexisting conditions in persons with heart disease.[5]

Collaborative Care

Acute reactions, including intoxication and withdrawal, are usually mild and time limited. An individual may be treated for toxic reactions to a combination of drugs that includes marijuana or may seek treatment for panic reactions. Treatment is directed toward relief of symptoms, and the administration of drugs is avoided if possible.

INHALANTS

Inhalation is the major route of ingestion for a number of common household and industrial volatile substances. Forms of use include sniffing, huffing, bagging, and spraying. Because inhalants are readily accessible, are inexpensive, and produce a rapid high, their use among preadolescents and adolescents is high.

There are four main classes of inhalants: volatile solvents, aerosols, anesthetic agents, and nitrites. They act as CNS depressants but are also extremely damaging to the cardiovascular and respiratory systems. Common agents and their effects are presented in Table 11-3. Users may develop peripheral neuropathies and exhibit tremors and weakness. Sudden death may result from direct toxic effects, aspiration of gastric contents, trauma, and/or suffocation.[20]

NURSING MANAGEMENT
ADDICTIVE BEHAVIORS

■ Nursing Assessment

It is not an easy task to identify drug-dependent individuals who seek health care for problems other than treatment of the addiction. Yet early recognition and identification of a patient with substance dependence is crucial to successful treatment outcomes for any health problem. Possible behaviors and physical complaints suggesting substance dependence are listed in Table 11-10, but these behaviors are not all-inclusive. Because the nurse may fail to recognize signs and symptoms of abuse in a patient who does not fit the stereotype of an "addict" and because most patients will underreport or deny substance abuse, an assessment of drug and alcohol use should be performed for all patients. The history should include all substances, including prescribed medications, over-the-counter drugs, caffeine, tobacco, alcohol, and recreational drugs. During the assessment the nurse should be aware of patient behaviors that influence history taking such as denial, avoidance, underreporting or minimizing substance use, or giving inaccurate information. Although open-ended questions that ask the patient to describe substance use can provide some information, two specific questions that have better predictive value for detecting alcohol dependence are as follows: "Have you ever

---

TABLE 11-10   Symptoms and Behaviors That May Suggest Dependence on Substances

- Trauma secondary to falls, auto accidents, fights, or burns
- Fatigue
- Insomnia
- Headaches
- Vague physical complaints
- Sexual dysfunction, decreased libido, erectile dysfunction
- Anorexia, weight loss
- Seizure disorder
- Appearing older than stated age, unkempt appearance
- Problems in areas of life function (e.g., frequent job changes; marital conflict, separation, and/or divorce; work-related accidents, tardiness, absenteeism; legal problems, including arrest; social isolation, estrangement from friends and/or family)
- Driving while intoxicated (more than one citation suggests dependence)
- Leisure activities that involve alcohol and/or other drugs
- Financial problems, including those related to spending for substances
- Failure of standard doses of sedatives to have a therapeutic effect
- Changes in mood
- Overabundant use of mouthwash or toiletries
- Frequent references to alcohol or alcohol use indicating preoccupation with and importance of alcohol in the person's life

had a drinking problem?" and "When was your last drink?"[22] Using questions in a way that lets the patient know that you find a behavior normal or at least understandable is also helpful. The nurse might ask, "Given your situation, I wonder if you have been using anything to help relieve your stress?"[24]

Although a variety of screening tools are available, one culturally sensitive tool that is easily used by nurses to identify alcohol dependence is the Alcohol Use Disorders Identification Test (AUDIT) (Table 11-11). A score of 8 points or less is considered nonalcoholic, whereas 9 points or above indicates alco-

---

TABLE 11-11 **Alcohol Use Disorders Identification Test (AUDIT)**

Please answer each question by checking one of the circles in the second column.

		SCORE
1. How often do you have a drink containing alcohol?	• Never	(0)
	• Monthly or less	(1)
	• 2–4 times per month	(2)
	• 2–4 times per week	(3)
	• 4+ times per week	(4)
2. How many drinks containing alcohol do you have on a typical day when you are drinking?	• 1 or 2	(0)
	• 3 or 4	(1)
	• 5 or 6	(2)
	• 7 to 9	(3)
	• 10 or more	(4)
3. How often do you have six or more drinks on one occasion?	• Never	(0)
	• Less than monthly	(1)
	• Monthly	(2)
	• Weekly	(3)
	• Daily or almost daily	(4)
4. How often during the last year have you found that you were not able to stop drinking once you had started?	• Never	(0)
	• Less than monthly	(1)
	• Monthly	(2)
	• Weekly	(3)
	• Daily or almost daily	(4)
5. How often in the last year have you failed to do what was normally expected of you because you were drinking?	• Never	(0)
	• Less than monthly	(1)
	• Monthly	(2)
	• Weekly	(3)
	• Daily or almost daily	(4)
6. How often during the last year have you needed a first drink in the morning to get yourself going after a heavy drinking session?	• Never	(0)
	• Less than monthly	(1)
	• Monthly	(2)
	• Weekly	(3)
	• Daily or almost daily	(4)
7. How often during the last year have you had a feeling of guilt or remorse about drinking?	• Never	(0)
	• Less than monthly	(1)
	• Monthly	(2)
	• Weekly	(3)
	• Daily or almost daily	(4)
8. How often during the last year have you been unable to remember what happened the night before because you had been drinking?	• Never	(0)
	• Less than monthly	(1)
	• Monthly	(2)
	• Weekly	(3)
	• Daily or almost daily	(4)
9. Have you or someone else been injured as a result of your drinking?	• No	(0)
	• Yes, but not in the last year	(2)
	• Yes, during the last year	(4)
10. Has a relative, friend, doctor, or other health worker been concerned about your drinking or suggested that you cut down?	• No	(0)
	• Yes, but not in the last year	(2)
	• Yes, during the last year	(4)

Scoring for AUDIT: Questions 1 through 8 are scored 0, 1, 2, 3, or 4. Questions 9 and 10 are scored 0, 2, or 4 only. The minimum score (nondrinkers) is 0 and the maximum possible score is 40. A score of 9 or more indicates hazardous or harmful alcohol consumption.

Source: Saunders JB et al: Development of the Alcohol Use Disorders Screening Test (AUDIT), WHO collaborative project on early detection of persons with harmful alcohol consumption. II, *Addiction* 88:791, 1993. Available at *www.niaaa.nih.gov/publications/audit.htm.*

TABLE 11-12   CAGE Questionnaire Adapted to Include Drugs (CAGEAID)

Have you felt you ought to cut down on your drinking (*or drug use*)?

_____Yes   _____No

Have people annoyed you by criticizing your drinking (*or drug use*)?

_____Yes   _____No

Have you felt bad or guilty about your drinking (*or drug use*)?

_____Yes   _____No

Have you ever had a drink (*or used drugs*) first thing in the morning to steady your nerves or get rid of a hangover (*or to get the day started*)?

_____Yes   _____No

From Fleming MF, Barry KL: *Addictive disorders*, St Louis, 1992, Mosby; and Ewing JA: Detecting alcoholism: the CAGE questionnaire, *JAMA* 252:1905, 1984. NOTE: **Boldface** text shows the original CAGE question; ***boldface italic*** text shows modifications of CAGE questions used to screen for drug disorders. In general population, two or more positive answers indicate a need for a more in-depth assessment.

holism. Another instrument frequently used is the CAGE questionnaire (Table 11-12). In addition, if the patient provides information concerning drug use that is inconsistent with assessment findings, the nurse should question the patient further.

Physical assessment also reveals clues about substance abuse. The nurse must be alert to signs and symptoms of the many health problems associated with addictive behaviors that may be apparent during the physical examination. Assessment of the patient's general appearance and nutritional status and examination of the abdomen, skin, and the cardiovascular, respiratory, and neurologic systems often reflect problems associated with substance abuse.[25]

Even if a patient does not admit to substance abuse or dependence, if there is any indication of alcohol or other CNS depressant use when a patient is hospitalized, the nurse should always question when the patient last used the substance. This information will help the nurse anticipate drug interactions or the time of possible onset of withdrawal symptoms if the patient is indeed dependent on a substance.

During assessment, several other approaches promote accurate information of drug use by a substance-abusing patient. The history should be taken in a setting that ensures privacy and avoids interruption. The patient is unlikely to discuss any substance abuse in the presence of accompanying family members or friends from whom it is hidden. It is also important for the nurse to explain why the information is needed and how it will be used to provide appropriate care. Telling the patient that complete honesty is necessary to avoid drug interactions or manage withdrawal symptoms is critical. The substance-abusing patient may also be afraid of losing control of drug administration and may be concerned that substance use will be reported to legal authorities. The patient should be informed that the federal Confidentiality Law (42 U.S.C. §290dd-2) prohibits nurses or other health care providers from disclosing any treatment of substance abuse without the specific written consent of the patient. The nurse should reassure the patient that all information will remain confidential and will be used only to provide safe care.

A critical factor in obtaining accurate information from the patient during assessment is the ability of the nurse to promote open and nonjudgmental communication with the patient. The nurse must be aware of personal feelings and attitudes about substance abuse and be able to express concern for the patient without criticism or rejection.

■ Nursing Diagnoses

Nursing diagnoses for the patient in alcohol withdrawal may include, but are not limited to, those presented in NCP 11-1. In addition, other nursing diagnoses for an individual with substance abuse may include, but are not limited to, the following:

- Ineffective denial *related to* refusal to acknowledge substance abuse or dependence
- Disturbed thought processes *related to* drug or alcohol ingestion
- Risk for infection *related to* increased environmental exposure to pathogens and risk-taking behavior
- Imbalanced nutrition: less than body requirements *related to* lack of nutritional intake
- Ineffective health maintenance *related to* lack of knowledge of progression of substance abuse and its effects
- Ineffective coping *related to* lack of knowledge of problem-solving and assertiveness skills
- Disabled family coping *related to* substance abuse by significant member

■ Planning

The overall goals are that the patient with addictive behaviors will (1) have normal physiologic functioning, (2) acknowledge a substance abuse problem, (3) explain the psychologic and physiologic effects of substance use, (4) abstain from the use of addicting substances, and (5) cooperate with a proposed treatment plan.

■ Nursing Implementation

Health Promotion. Prevention of substance abuse problems and addictive behaviors includes primary, secondary, and tertiary prevention. Primary prevention targets primarily adolescents and young adults with education about effects, negative outcomes, and effects of continued use of addictive substances. Secondary prevention focuses on early detection of substance abuse, interventions through peer or employee assistance programs, and continuing education about substance-free alternatives and stress management techniques. Tertiary prevention occurs when individuals have established dependence and includes motivating individuals to enter addiction treatment and referral to treatment and relapse prevention programs.

Prevention of tobacco use. Prevention of tobacco use in children and adolescents is the emphasis of primary and secondary prevention of substance abuse. Most current adult smokers began daily smoking by age 16, and it is estimated that 3000 minors in the United States begin smoking each day. Recently there has been a general decline in tobacco use after age 25, but smoking and the use of smokeless tobacco among young people age 12 and older have escalated, increasing by nearly one third in the past several years.[26] Because nicotine abuse is highly correlated with illicit drug and alcohol use, especially in adolescents, if tobacco use is not started and maintained during childhood and adolescence, there is a much better chance that other drugs will not be abused as this population ages. Programs developed to help children explore the external influences (e.g., peer pressure) that may cause one to start smoking and that help them identify alternative behaviors make it less likely for these children to start smoking. An emphasis on the health hazards of tobacco use, as

NURSING CARE PLAN 11-1

Patient in Alcohol Withdrawal

EXPECTED PATIENT OUTCOMES	NURSING INTERVENTIONS and *RATIONALES*
NURSING DIAGNOSIS	**Risk for injury** *related to* sensorimotor deficits, seizure activity, and confusion.
• No falls or injuries • Decrease in tremors and psychomotor activity • No seizures • Able to verbalize risk for injury associated with alcohol use before discharge	• Assess for risk factors such as impaired mobility (e.g., unsteady gait), sensory deficits, tremors, impaired judgment, confusion, seizure activity *to plan appropriate preventive measures.* • Assess for signs of injury such as lacerations, bruises, or burns *to treat appropriately.* • Monitor vital signs frequently, especially heart rate, *because prompt recognition of extreme autonomic nervous system response is necessary for early intervention to prevent progression of symptoms.* • Administer benzodiazepines as ordered *to control hyperactivity,* thiamine *to reduce neurologic complications (e.g., Wernicke's encephalopathy),* and antiseizure medications as ordered *to prevent seizures.* • Use protective devices or restraints if necessary *to prevent injury of patient or others.* • Use seizure precautions *to prevent injury.* • Encourage verbalization of consequences of alcohol use *to prevent relapse and further injury.*
NURSING DIAGNOSIS	**Disturbed sensory perception (auditory and/or visual)** *related to* sensory overload *as manifested by* inaccurate interpretation of environmental stimuli, disorientation, hallucinations.
• No hallucinations • Oriented to person, place, and time	• Assess patient's orientation to reality *to determine appropriate interventions.* • Provide quiet, nonstimulating, well-lit environment *to reduce external stimuli and calm overactive CNS.* • Orient to nurse and environment with each contact; use calm, matter-of-fact approach; provide consistent staff; explain procedures and what is expected *to assist in reality orientation and decrease anxiety.* • Do not reinforce fears or hallucinations by agreeing or disagreeing *because this does not promote reality orientation.* • Administer benzodiazepines as ordered *to reduce CNS stimulation.* • Administer antipsychotic medication (e.g., haloperidol [Haldol]) if ordered *to decrease severity of hallucinations.*
NURSING DIAGNOSIS	**Ineffective breathing pattern** *related to* alcohol toxicity and/or airway obstruction as manifested by rapid respirations, dyspnea, use of accessory muscles.
• Maintenance of effective breathing • No indications of hypoxia	• Monitor respiratory rate, depth, and pattern *so appropriate interventions may be taken.* • Position patient on side and in semi-Fowler's position *to reduce possibility of aspiration and to enhance lung expansion by lowering diaphragm.* • Monitor effects of medications given for withdrawal *to detect respiratory depression.* • Encourage coughing and deep breathing *to prevent complications of hypoventilation.* • Administer supplemental oxygen *to treat hypoxia.*
NURSING DIAGNOSIS	**Risk for other-directed violence** *related to* hallucinations and altered thought processes.
• No destructive or violent behavior • Control over behavior and psychomotor activity	• Assess level of risk as evidenced by feelings of fear, hallucinations, environmental misperceptions, poor impulse control, panic *to ensure early recognition of violent behavior and plan appropriate interventions.* • Provide safe environment on the basis of risk level *to prevent injury to self or others.* • Use medications or restraints as necessary *to prevent escalation of threatening behavior.* • Communicate expectation of need to maintain control of behavior in clear, simple language and contract for "no harm" *so patient can accept responsibility to maintain control of behavior at expected level.*

CNS, Central nervous system.

well as on those of other addictive behaviors, should be part of the total curriculum beginning in elementary schools.

Tobacco use cessation. Cigarette smoking is the single most preventable cause of death in the United States, and nicotine has the highest dependence rate of any other substance of abuse.[27] Promotion of smoking and tobacco cessation is one intervention in which every nurse has a professional role. Unfortunately, it is a role that has been largely ignored. It has been reported that

70% of smokers say they would like to quit, but only half of those are encouraged to do so by health care providers.[28] Because fewer than 5% of smokers are successful on their first attempt at quitting and the average smoker requires multiple attempts before being successful, some health care providers have become cynical with regard to counseling their patients to abstain from tobacco use. However, smoking a few cigarettes during a cessation attempt (a *slip*) is much different than resuming the full smoking habit (a *relapse*). To help put an end to the thousands of unnecessary cases of chronic illness and death, the nurse must be proactive, identifying and talking with tobacco users to provide them with information on ways to stop the use of tobacco.

The Agency for Healthcare Research and Quality (AHRQ) has developed the *Clinical Practice Guideline: Treating Tobacco Use and Dependence* for use by clinicians, including nurses, to aggressively motivate smokers and other tobacco users to quit.[28] The guideline identifies the "five *As*" of brief clinical interventions that should be used at each patient encounter. These inter-

ventions are designed to identify tobacco users, encourage them to quit, determine their willingness to quit, assist them in quitting, and arrange for follow-up to prevent relapse. If a tobacco user is unwilling to quit, a motivational intervention using the "five *Rs*" provides the nurse an opportunity to educate, reassure, and motivate tobacco users to quit at each contact. These interventions are presented in Table 11-13. A patient and family teaching guide (Table 11-14) expands on the fourth brief strategy, "Assist—aid the patient in quitting," with specific information about nicotine replacement and interventions using behavioral approaches and social support.

TABLE 11-13   Clinical Practice Guideline: Treating Tobacco Use and Dependence (Brief Clinical Interventions)

THE FIVE *As* FOR INDIVIDUALS WHO DESIRE TO QUIT	THE FIVE *Rs* FOR INDIVIDUALS UNWILLING TO QUIT
1 **Ask**—identify all tobacco users at every contact 2. **Advise**—strongly urge all tobacco users to quit 3. **Assess**—determine willingness to make a quit attempt 4. **Assist**—aid the patient in developing a plan to quit 5. **Arrange**—schedule follow-up contact	1. **Relevance**—ask the patient to indicate why quitting is personally relevant (e.g., family, health) 2. **Risks**—ask the patient to identify negative consequences of tobacco use (e.g., cough, shortness of breath) 3. **Rewards**—ask the patient to identify potential benefits of stopping tobacco use (e.g., saving money, feel better) 4. **Roadblocks**—ask patient to identify barriers or impediments to quitting (e.g., weight gain, partner smokes) 5. **Repetition**—repeat process every clinic visit

Source: US Department of Health and Human Services: *Clinical practice guideline: treating tobacco use and dependence*, Washington, DC, 2000, US Public Health Service.

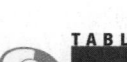

TABLE 11-14   Patient & Family Teaching Guide
Smoking and Tobacco Use Cessation

The following interventions are methods that work for quitting tobacco use. Patients have the best chance of quitting if they use more than one method.

Develop a Quit Plan
- Set a quit date, ideally within 2 weeks.
- Tell family, friends, and co-workers about quitting and request understanding and support.
- Anticipate withdrawal symptoms and challenges when quitting.
- Before quitting avoid smoking in places where you spend a lot of time (work, car, home).
- Throw away all tobacco products on the quit date.
- Do not take even a single puff or dip after the quit date. Total abstinence is essential.

Use Approved Nicotine Replacement Systems
Do not use other forms of tobacco when using nicotine replacement systems.

Nicotine Patch
- Trade names for the nicotine patch include Nicoderm, Nicotrol, Habitrol, and Prostep. Nicoderm and Nicotrol are available as over-the-counter agents. Store brands of the nicotine patch are also available.
- Patches should be replaced every day (preferably in morning) and placed in a hairless location on the body between the neck and waist.

- Most smokers should start using a full-strength patch (15 to 22 mg of nicotine) daily for 4 weeks and then use a weaker patch for another 4 weeks (5 to 14 mg of nicotine).
- Side effects may include minor skin irritation, which is why it is important to apply the patch in a different place each day.

Nicotine Gum
- Nicotine gum (marketed as Nicorette) is sold over the counter in 2 mg and 4 mg strengths.
- One piece of 2 mg gum has the same amount of nicotine as one cigarette.
- 2 mg pieces are used when 20 or fewer cigarettes a day are smoked; 4 mg should be used when more than 20 cigarettes a day are smoked.
- 2 mg pieces may be substituted for cigars, pipe smoking, or oral tobacco at a rate at which these products are used.
- Gum should be chewed until a "peppery" taste is felt and then "parked" between the cheek and gum.
- Each piece of gum should be used for about 30 minutes.
- Side effects include heartburn and indigestion that may be eased by drinking water when it occurs.
- Acidic beverages (coffee, juice, soda) interfere with oral absorption.

Nicotine Nasal Spray
- Nicotine in a nasal spray (marketed as Nicotrol NS) is sprayed directly into each nostril.

Sources: US Department of Health and Human Services: *Clinical practice guideline: treating tobacco use and dependence*, Washington, DC, 2000, US Public Health Service; *You can quit smoking: consumer guide*, June 2000, US Public Health Service. Available at *www.surgeongeneral.gov/tobacco/consquits.htm; What are the benefits of quitting smoking?* New York, July 2001, American Lung Association. Available at *www.lungusa.org/tobacco/quit_ben.html; You can quit smoking: tips for the first week*, March 2001, US Public Health Service. Available at *www.surgeongeneral.gov/tobacco/1stweek.htm.*

TABLE
11-14 | *Patient & Family Teaching Guide*
Smoking and Tobacco Use Cessation—cont'd

Nicotine Nasal Spray—cont'd
- Should be used in anticipation of or at the beginning of urge to smoke.
- 1 spray (0.5 mg) in each nostril, 5 times per hour not to exceed maximum of 40 times per day.
- Do not sniff or inhale when administering the dose because this increases the irritation effect; tilt the head back when delivering the nasal spray.
- Side effects include watery eyes and nose, burning sensation in nose, throat irritation, and sneezing or coughing.

Nicotine Inhaler
- Available in cartridge (Nicotrol inhaler) with 4 mg nicotine over 80 inhalations. Available by prescription.
- Delivers one third the nicotine of one cigarette.
- 1 cartridge equals 2 cigarettes; start at 6 cartridges per day for 20 minute each use.
- Best effect achieved by frequent puffing on inhaler.
- Puffing on inhaler releases nicotine vapor into mouth.

Nonnicotine Therapy
- Bupropion (Zyban), available by prescription, increases dopamine and epinephrine levels in the brain, which are also stimulated by nicotine and give a person energy and a sense of well-being.
- Start 1 to 2 weeks before quit date: 150 mg every morning, then increased to twice a day for 7 to 12 weeks after quitting. Maintenance therapy may be initiated for up to 6 months.
- Side effects include headache, dry mouth, insomnia, and drowsiness.
- Alcohol should be avoided or used only in moderation.

Dealing with Urges to Use Tobacco
- Be aware of things that may cause you to want to smoke or use other tobacco, such as being around other smokers, being under time pressure, getting into an argument, feeling sad or frustrated, and drinking alcohol (alcohol should be avoided or used only in moderation).
- Avoid difficult situations while you are trying to quit. Try to lower your stress level.
- Exercise, such as walking, jogging, or bicycling, can help.
- Distract yourself from thoughts of smoking and the urge to use tobacco by talking to someone, getting busy with a task, or reading a book.
- Drink lots of water.

Support and Encouragement
- If you have tried to stop using tobacco before, identify what helped and what hurt in previous quit attempts.
- Counseling can help you learn how to live life as a nonuser. You may want to join a quit-tobacco program.
- If you get the urge for tobacco, call someone to help talk you out of it—preferably an ex-user.
- Do not be afraid to talk about how you feel while quitting, especially fears of not being able to quit for good. Ask your spouse/partner, friends, and co-workers to support you. Self-help materials and hot lines are also available:
  - American Lung Association: 800-586-4872; *www.lungusa.org*
  - American Cancer Society: 800-227-2345; *www.cancer.org/tobacco*

- Cancer Information Service: 800-422-6237; *www.nci.nih.gov*
- Smoking Cessation Consumer Tool Kit: 800-358-9295; *www.ahrq.gov*
- Smoking, Tobacco, and Health: 800-CDC-1311; *www.cdc.gov/tobacco*
- Try To Stop, Massachusetts Department of Public Health: 800-TRY TO STOP; *www.trytostop.org*

Avoiding Relapse
Most relapses occur within the first 3 months after quitting. Do not be discouraged if you start using tobacco again. Remember, most people try several times before they finally quit. Explore different ways to break habits. You may have to deal with some of the following triggers that cause relapse.
- *Change your environment.* Get rid of cigarettes, tobacco (in any form), and ashtrays in your home, car, and place of work. Get rid of the smell of cigarettes in your car and home.
- *Alcohol.* Consider limiting or stopping alcohol use while you are quitting tobacco.
- *Other smokers at home.* Encourage housemates to quit with you. Work out a plan to cope with others who smoke, and avoid being around them.
- *Weight gain.* Tackle one problem at a time. Work on quitting tobacco first. You will not necessarily gain weight, and increased appetite is often temporary.
- *Negative mood or depression.* If these symptoms persist, talk to your health care provider. You may need treatment for depression.
- *Severe withdrawal symptoms.* Your body will go through many changes when you quit tobacco. You may have a dry mouth, cough, or scratchy throat, and you may feel irritable. The patch or gum may help with cravings.
- *Thoughts.* Get your mind off tobacco. Exercise and do things you enjoy.
- *Keep a list.* Keep a list of "slips" and near-slips, what caused them, and what you can learn from them.
- *Focus on the benefits of quitting:*
  1. At 20 minutes after you quit, blood pressure decreases, pulse rate drops, and the body temperature of your hands and feet increases.
  2. At 8 hours, the carbon monoxide level in your blood drops to normal and the oxygen level in your blood increases to normal.
  3. At 24 hours, your chance of a heart attack decreases.
  4. At 48 hours, nerve endings start regrowing and the ability to smell and taste is enhanced.
  5. At 2 weeks to 3 months, your circulation improves; walking becomes easier; lung function increases; and coughing, sinus congestion, fatigue, and shortness of breath decrease.
  6. At 1 year, your risk of heart disease is decreased to half that of a smoker.
  7. By 10 to 15 years, risk of stroke, lung and other cancers, and early death returns to nearly the level of people who have never smoked.

Research into tobacco use behaviors and successful strategies to promote tobacco cessation is ongoing. Many factors are recognized as being important in the initiation and continuation of tobacco use, such as peer pressure, rebelliousness, curiosity, self-image, environmental cues, and psychologic needs. One cessation program is not necessarily the best for every tobacco user. Other methods offered in tobacco cessation programs may involve hypnosis, acupuncture, behavioral interventions, aversion therapy, group support programs, individual therapy, and self-help options. Except in special circumstances, nicotine replacement therapy is recommended for all tobacco users in addition to other approaches. Research has found that clinical advice alone will help only 2% of patients quit smoking, whereas the addition of nicotine replacement therapy results in a quit rate of 11% in 1 year.[28] Nicotine replacement therapy is not generally recommended for pregnant women and persons who have recently experienced an acute myocardial infarction, have unstable angina, or have life-threatening arrhythmias.

The advice and motivation of health care professionals can be a powerful force in smoking cessation. The nurse who smokes or uses tobacco is in a difficult position to help the patient change tobacco use habits. The nurse as a role model can do much to facilitate or harm educational attempts with persons in the community, as well as in the hospital. A nurse who uses tobacco must try to stop before serving as a role model for the patient. A smoker turned nonsmoker may be in a good position to suggest strategies for success.

The nurse must have a thorough knowledge of the physiologic changes that are encountered with tobacco cessation and consistently provide facts and support to help a tobacco user actually quit, forever. The nurse also needs to be aware of resources in the community to assist the individual who is motivated to quit. Local chapters of the American Lung Association and the American Cancer Society have information on available programs.

Acute Intervention. Acute care situations precipitated by substance abuse involve acute intoxication, overdose, or withdrawal (see Table 11-3). Intoxication responses usually last less than 24 hours and are directly related to the ingestion of psychoactive drugs. Intoxication effects are generally dose related, and symptoms often include the desired effects of using the drug. Overdose leads to toxic reactions that may include respiratory and circulatory arrest and other life-threatening complications. Overdose occurs with the ingestion of an excessive dose of one drug or when a combination of similarly acting drugs is used. The nurse should be aware that intoxication and overdose may occur in a hospitalized patient dependent on substances if visitors provide sources of substances. Table 11-15 provides a timeline of commonly abused substances and routes to assist in anticipating intoxication, overdose, and withdrawal manifestations.

Alcohol intoxication. Acute alcohol intoxication may manifest as an emergency primarily because of the narrow range between the intoxicating, the anesthetic, and the lethal doses of this drug. It is important to obtain as accurate a history as possible, using collateral information as necessary, and assess for injuries, trauma, diseases, and hypoglycemia. The basic principles of airway, breathing, and circulation (the ABCs) must be implemented. Vital signs and level of consciousness should be monitored. Generally the heart rate is normal in uncomplicated intoxication but elevated in withdrawal.

Patients with chronic alcoholism may experience **Wernicke's encephalopathy,** an inflammatory, hemorrhagic, degenerative condition of the brain resulting from a deficiency of thiamine. The patient should be assessed for ocular abnormalities, including nystagmus and paralysis of the lateral rectus muscles, as well as ataxia and a global confusion state. Untreated or progressive Wernicke's encephalopathy may lead to **Korsakoff's psychosis,** a form of amnesia characterized by loss of short-term memory and an inability to learn. Because symptoms of encephalopathy may be difficult to distinguish from intoxication or withdrawal and because Wernicke's encephalopathy is potentially reversible, IV thiamine is often administered to intoxicated patients. Patients with alcohol intoxication may also be hypoglycemic from a lack of food intake. Glucose solutions may precipitate Wernicke's encephalopathy in a previously unaffected patient. For this reason, thiamine should be started before treatment with IV glucose solution in all patients with alcoholism and continued until the patient resumes a normal diet.

The nurse should stay with the patient as much as possible, orienting to reality as necessary. Agitation and anxiety are common, and the patient should be assessed for increasing belligerence and a potential for violence. The patient is also at high risk for injury because of lack of coordination and impaired judgment, and protective measures should be used. It is critical to continue assessment and interventions until the BAC has decreased to at least 100 mg/dl (0.10 mg%) and until any associated disorders or injuries have been ruled out. A BAC of 100 mg/dl is usually reached within 6 to 10 hours.[20]

Cannabis intoxication. In acute marijuana intoxication, the nurse should perform a physical examination, a toxicology screen, and a thorough history. The approach is basically the same for treating panic, flashbacks, and toxic reactions related to the use of marijuana or other hallucinogens. An individual with cannabis intoxication or other acute problems related to cannabis use is seldom hospitalized. The main interventions are to provide a quiet environment and to support and reassure the patient by explaining what is happening. The patient should understand that

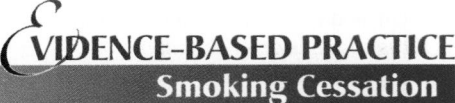

EVIDENCE-BASED PRACTICE
Smoking Cessation

Clinical Problem
Are nursing interventions effective for smoking cessation?

Best Clinical Practice
- Strong evidence suggests that nursing interventions are effective in reducing smoking.
- Every patient who uses tobacco should be offered at least brief treatment.

Implications for Nursing Practice
- The standard of care is to ask every patient, "Do you smoke?" and "Do you want to quit?"
- If the answer is yes, the nurse needs to provide information on how to stop smoking (see Tables 11-13 and 11-14).

References for Evidence
Rice VH, Stead LF: Nursing interventions for smoking cessation, *Cochrane Tobacco Addiction Group Cochrane Database of Systematic Reviews* issue 2, 2001.
US Public Health Service: Treating tobacco use and dependence. Summary, June 2000. US Public Health Service. Available at *www.surgeongeneral.gov/tobacco/smokesum.htm.*

TABLE 11-15	Onset, Peak, Duration, and Withdrawal Onset of Abused Substances			
SUBSTANCE/ROUTE	ONSET	PEAK	DURATION	ONSET OF WITHDRAWAL SYMPTOMS
Inhaled				
Nicotine	Immediate	5 min	5-15 min	3-4 hr
Marijuana	5-20 min	30-60 min	3-7 hr	–
Cocaine	Immediate	5-30 min	60 min	9 hr
Inhalants	Immediate	10-15 min	20-45 min	–
Intravenous				
Cocaine	Immediate	10-20 min	20-30 min	2 hr
Opioids	Immediate	60-90 min	2-4 hr	8-10 hr
Amphetamines	Immediate	10-20 min	20-30 min	2 hr
Oral				
Alcohol	15-20 min	60-90 min	12-14 hr	10-12 hr
Amphetamines	10-30 min	60-90 min	2-4 hr	8-10 hr
Sedative-hypnotics	15-30 min	2-4 hr	4-12 hr	12-16 hr
Caffeine	10-20 min	30 min	3-7 hr	12-24 hr
Opioids	30 min	2 hr	4-8 hr	8-10 hr
Intranasal				
Cocaine	3-5 min	5-30 min	2-4 hr	4 hr
Amphetamines	3-5 min	5-20 min	45 min	2 hr
Buccal				
Nicotine	10-15 min	20-30 min	30-60 min	1-2 hr

the level of intoxication may fluctuate over several days as metabolites are released.

Overdose. A drug overdose is an emergency situation, and management is based on the type of substance involved. Drug overdose can be accidental or intentional. If multiple substances have been ingested, a complex and potentially confusing clinical picture can result. The first priority of care in overdose is always the patient's ABCs. Continuous monitoring of neurologic status, including level of consciousness, and respiratory and cardiovascular function is critical until the patient is stable. Vital signs and intake and output should be monitored. Emergency management of overdose and toxicity of CNS stimulants and CNS depressants is presented in Tables 11-5 and 11-9.

Pharmacologic agents are administered as ordered to counteract toxic effects of drugs. Naloxone (Narcan) and flumazenil (Romazicon) may be administered when a depressant effect is present but the ingested drug is unknown. Naloxone rapidly reverses the effects of opioids, and flumazenil reverses the effects of benzodiazepine overdose. The effects of these antagonists require frequent monitoring because these drugs have a short half-life and may need to be repeated after the initial reversal of toxic effects. Specific antagonists are not available for other drugs of abuse, but a variety of other medications may be used to control symptoms.

The patient who has overdosed on sedative-hypnotics other than benzodiazepines must be treated aggressively and may require dialysis to decrease the drug level and to prevent irreversible CNS depressant effects and death. Gastric lavage and administration of activated charcoal may be instituted if the drug was taken orally within 4 to 6 hours. Central nervous system stimulants are not used in the treatment of depressant drug overdose.

As soon as the patient is stable, a thorough history and physical examination must be completed. When the patient is unwilling or unable to give a history, a collateral history should be obtained from the patient's significant others. Recent drug and alcohol use, including the type, amount, and time of use, and the presence of any chronic illnesses are important in the continuing treatment of the patient. A patient who intentionally overdosed should not be allowed to return home until seen by a psychiatric professional.

Withdrawal. In general, withdrawal signs and symptoms are opposite in nature from the direct effects of the drug (Table 11-3). Because abused substances are psychoactive, changes are consistently noted in the neurologic system. These changes often manifest as acute anxiety and protracted depression. Withdrawal from CNS depressants, including alcohol, is the most dangerous withdrawal syndrome and may be life threatening. The nurse must be alert to the possibility of withdrawal in any patient who has a history of substance abuse. The nurse should also suspect substance dependence in patients who discharge themselves against medical advice (AMA). This may occur when patients are not being treated appropriately and need the substance to prevent withdrawal symptoms. In withdrawal from all abused substances, nursing management includes monitoring physiologic function, ensuring safety and comfort, preventing the progression of symptoms, providing reassurance and orientation, and motivating the patient to engage in long-term treatment.[16]

Alcohol withdrawal. A patient with alcohol dependence who is hospitalized for other illnesses, health conditions, or trauma often develops alcohol withdrawal when the ingestion of alcohol is abruptly stopped. The signs and symptoms of alcohol withdrawal generally begin 10 to 12 hours after the patient's last drink and may last for 3 to 5 days (see Table 11-15). The most common severe manifestations are hallucinations and seizures. The progression of early symptoms to DTs can be prevented by administration of benzodiazepines, such as lorazepam (Ativan). Thiamine and multiple vitamins are important to prevent development of Wernicke's encephalopathy and Korsakoff's psychosis. A quiet, calm environment is important to prevent exacerbation of symptoms. The use of restraints and IV lines should be avoided whenever possible.[29] Supportive care is needed to ensure adequate rest and nutrition. The nursing care plan for the patient in alcohol withdrawal is presented in NCP 11-1.

Withdrawal from other CNS depressants. Withdrawal from sedative-hypnotics can be highly variable, and the severity and onset of symptoms depend on many factors, including the drug, the pattern of use, the dose and duration of use, and the presence of concurrent alcohol use. Symptoms may begin 12 hours after cessation of a short-acting drug and more than 100 hours after cessation of a long-acting drug. Withdrawal from high doses is potentially life threatening and requires close monitoring in an inpatient setting. Management of withdrawal from sedative-hypnotic agents is symptomatic and includes a gradual reduction in drug dosage. Long-acting agents such as diazepam (Valium), chlordiazepoxide (Librium), clonazepam (Klonopin), or phenobarbital may be substituted for the drug and tapered after stabilization. Mild to moderate symptoms can persist for 2 to 3 weeks after a 3- to 5-day period of acute symptoms.[30]

Although withdrawal from opioids is not life threatening, symptoms are dramatic, temporarily disabling, and painful. Symptoms result from rebound excitability in those organs that were previously depressed by the use of opioids, and their onset and intensity depend on the pattern of use and the duration of the drug (see Table 11-15). Specific nursing approaches include careful monitoring of symptoms and providing comfort, nutrition, and hygiene. Methadone or other opioids may be administered in decreasing amounts over a period of 2 weeks to control withdrawal symptoms. Nonopioids such as benzodiazepines or clonidine (Catapres) may also be administered to reduce opioid withdrawal symptoms.[30]

Stimulant withdrawal. Withdrawal from cocaine and amphetamines does not usually cause obvious physical symptoms, but psychologic and behavioral manifestations do occur. Craving for the drug is intense during the first hours to days of drug cessation and may continue for weeks (see Table 11-15). It is unusual for an individual dependent on stimulants to be hospitalized for management of withdrawal symptoms. However, the nurse may identify withdrawal symptoms in a patient dependent on cocaine or amphetamines who is hospitalized for management of other health problems. Nursing management of withdrawal symptoms is supportive and includes measures to decrease agitation and restlessness in the early phase and allowing the patient to sleep and eat as needed in later phases. Mild symptoms of stimulant withdrawal can also be experienced by the patient dependent on caffeine when meals and fluids are withheld before diagnostic testing or during a surgical experience. Withdrawal symptoms are also experienced by patients dependent on nicotine when smoking restrictions are applied. A nicotine replacement system should be provided for tobacco users to control symptoms of withdrawal when they are hospitalized.

Perioperative care. An individual who abuses substances is more likely to have accidents and injuries that require surgery. All trauma victims must be carefully assessed for signs and symptoms of substance overdose and withdrawal that could lead to adverse drug interactions with analgesics or anesthetics. During elective surgery in both inpatient and outpatient surgical settings, the patient dependent on substances is at high risk for postoperative complications and death. Preoperative assessment must include a thorough health history and assessment of substance use, including questions related to nicotine and caffeine use. Respiratory changes in smokers make introduction of endotracheal and suction tubes more difficult and increase the risk for postoperative respiratory problems. Postoperative headaches may be caused by caffeine withdrawal in heavy users. During the patient's surgical recovery period, the nurse should be alert for signs and symptoms of drug interactions with pain medications or anesthesia or for signs of withdrawal. Special nursing considerations for the substance-abusing patient undergoing surgery are presented in Table 11-16.

Special precautions must be taken for the patient who is intoxicated or alcohol dependent and requires surgery. Alcohol use may be overlooked in an accident victim if there are injuries that cause CNS depression, and many persons are undiagnosed as alcoholics at the time of admission for elective surgery. Optimally, health problems such as malnutrition, dehydration, and infection should be treated before surgery is performed. The patient who is alcohol dependent but is not currently drinking usually requires an increased level of anesthesia because of cross-tolerance. The intoxicated individual needs a decreased level of anesthesia because of the synergistic effect of the alcohol.

Whenever possible, surgery is postponed in intoxicated individuals until the BAC is less than 200 mg/dl. Synergistic effects occur with anesthesia when BAC is over 150 mg/dl, and a patient with a BAC over 250 mg/dl has a significantly increased surgical risk and mortality rate. Acute withdrawal and DTs may be triggered by surgery and the cessation of alcohol consumption. Surgery should be delayed for at least 48 to 72 hours, if possible, or IV alcohol may be given to avoid withdrawal if immediate surgery is required. Alcohol interferes with pulmonary function, decreased liver function affects metabolism of many drugs, and the medical problems associated with alcohol use may affect the outcome of surgery. Vital signs, including body temperature, must be closely monitored to identify signs of withdrawal, possible infections, and respiratory or cardiac problems. Anesthetics and pain medications used in the acute period can delay withdrawal symptoms for up to 5 days postoperatively.[31]

TABLE 11-16 Considerations for Substance-Abusing Patients Undergoing Surgery

- Standard amounts of anesthetic and analgesic drugs may not be sufficient if patient is cross-tolerant.
- Increased doses of pain medications may be required if patient is cross-tolerant.
- Anesthetic agents may have a prolonged sedative effect if the patient has liver dysfunction. This situation requires an extended observation period.
- Patients have an increased susceptibility to cardiac and respiratory depression.
- Patients have an increased risk for bleeding, postoperative complications, and infection.
- Withdrawal symptoms from substances may be delayed for up to 5 days because of effects of anesthetics and pain medications.
- Dosage of pain medications must be reduced gradually.

ETHICAL DILEMMAS
Impaired Health Care Providers

Situation

The nurses on the surgical unit know that one of their colleagues has undergone treatment for prescription drug addiction. She seemed to be doing well until recently, when she became totally focused on her separation and subsequent divorce. Her colleagues suspect that she is using drugs again and worry that it will affect her patient care.

Important Points for Consideration

- Nurses have an ethical obligation to prevent harm from coming to patients.
- Nurses are responsible for documenting the observed behaviors, possibly confronting their colleague and reporting their observations to their supervisor and to the state board of nursing.
- In most states, mandatory reporting of substance abuse is required and whistle-blowing protection is provided under the nurse practice act.
- Greater benefit may also result for the nurse suspected of substance abuse when the opportunity for treatment is provided under provisions of the state nurse practice act, rather than ignoring the problem.

Critical Thinking Questions

1. How should the nurses handle this situation?
2. What are the provisions of your state's nurse practice act regarding impaired nurses?

Pain management. Although nurses and physicians have historically been reluctant to administer opioids to substance-abusing patients for fear of promoting or enhancing addictions, there is no evidence that providing opioid analgesia to these patients in any way worsens their addictive disease. When addicted patients experience any type of acute pain, the goal is to treat the pain. Addiction treatment is not the priority while the patient is in pain.

If the patient acknowledges opioid use, it is important to determine the types and amounts of drugs used. It is best to avoid exposing the patient to the drug of abuse, and effective equianalgesic doses of other opioids may be determined if daily drug doses are known. If a history of drug abuse is unknown, or if the patient does not acknowledge substance abuse, the nurse should suspect abuse when normal doses of analgesics do not relieve the patient's pain. Aggressive behavior patterns and signs of withdrawal may also occur. Withdrawal symptoms can exacerbate pain and lead to drug-seeking behavior or illicit drug use. Toxicology screens may be helpful in determining recently used drugs. Discussing these findings with the patient may help gain the patient's cooperation in pain control.

Severe pain should be treated with opioids, and at much higher doses than those used with drug-naive patients. The use of one opioid is preferred. A mixed opioid agonist-antagonist such as butorphanol (Stadol) or a partial agonist such as buprenorphine (Buprenex) should be avoided because these may precipitate withdrawal symptoms. Nonopioid and adjuvant analgesics and nonpharmacologic pain relief measures may also be used as appropriate. To maintain opioid blood levels and prevent withdrawal symptoms, analgesics should be provided around the clock. Supplemental doses should be used to treat breakthrough pain. Although controversial for treating addicted patients, patient-controlled analgesia (PCA) may improve pain control and reduce drug-seeking behavior.[32]

A written agreement or treatment plan that describes the pain management should be shared with the patient. The plan should ensure that pain will be treated based on the patient's perception and report of pain, but also clearly outline the gradual tapering of the analgesic dose, eventual substitution of parenteral analgesics with long-acting oral preparations, and possibly cessation of opioids by the time of discharge.[33]

As pain is controlled, the issue of treatment of the patient's substance abuse can be discussed with the patient. If the patient can be motivated to enter treatment and rehabilitation, the nurse should have treatment referral references available.

Motivational interviewing for addictive behaviors. The nurse is in a unique position to motivate and facilitate addictive behavior change while caring for patients in primary and acute care settings. When patients seek care for health problems related to substance abuse or when hospitalization interferes with the patient's normal use of substances, the patient's awareness of problems associated with addictive behaviors is increased. Intervention by nurses at this time can be a crucial factor in promoting behavior change.

A current Treatment Improvement Protocol (TIP), *Enhancing Motivation for Change in Substance Abuse Treatment,* is a best practice guideline provided by the Substance Abuse and Mental Health Services Administration's Center for Substance Abuse Treatment.[34] This protocol describes the use of motivational interviewing developed by Miller and Rollnick.[35] **Motivational interviewing** uses nonconfrontational interpersonal communication techniques to motivate patients to change behavior. The techniques are linked to the stages of change as identified by Prochaska and DiClemente in the transtheoretical model of change.[36] The stages of change identified in the **transtheoretical model of change** include precontemplation, contemplation, preparation, action, maintenance, and termination, as described in Chapter 4. The first five stages are applied in motivational interviewing. The stages are not viewed as linear, but rather as a cycle through which patients move back and forth. During the process of change, relapse and recycling is an expected finding. Patients who do not change behaviors or who return to substance use after a period of cessation are often labeled "noncompliant" and "unmotivated." However, this may reflect a normal relapse or may indicate that the interventions used do not consider the patient's stage of change.[37] Therefore it is important for the nurse to identify the patient's current stage of readiness for change and the stage to which the patient is moving. Patients who are in the early stages of change need and use different kinds of motivational support than patients at later stages of change.

Motivational interviewing includes the use of any intervention that enhances the patient's motivation for change. The interventions are those that respect the patient's autonomy and establish a nonjudgmental, collaborative relationship.[34] The key aspects of successful motivational interviewing are presented in Table 11-17.

A substance-abusing patient who seeks care for a medical problem or is hospitalized is often in the *precontemplation* or *contemplation* stage of change. In the precontemplation stage patients are not concerned about their substance use and are not considering changing their behavior. An example is when a patient is asked if he thinks his smoking contributes to his shortness of breath and he replies that he does not think so because he has never had it before during years of smoking. During this stage it is most important for the nurse to help the patient increase aware-

TABLE 11-17   Key Aspects of Successful Motivational Interviewing

- Express empathy through reflective listening.
- Compliment rather than denigrate.
- Listen rather than tell.
- Gently persuade, with the understanding that change is up to the patient.
- Develop discrepancy between patient's goals or values and current behavior, helping the patient recognize the discrepancies between where he or she is and where he or she hopes to be.
- Avoid argument and direct confrontation, which can cause defensiveness and a power struggle.
- Adjust to, rather than oppose, patient resistance.
- Focus on the patient's strengths to support the hope and optimism needed to make changes.

ness of risks and problems related to the current behavior and to create doubt about the use of substances.[34] Asking the patient what he or she thinks could happen if the behavior is continued, providing evidence of the problem such as abnormal laboratory values, and offering factual information about the risks of substance abuse are indicated.[38] Although patients may not be ready to change behavior while experiencing an acute health problem, the seeds of doubt can be sown. In other cases, such as when a patient experiences a life-threatening condition, there may be an immediate awareness of the problem and motivation to change.

A patient in the *contemplation* stage of change often experiences ambivalence. The patient understands that the behavior is a problem and that change is necessary, yet feels that change is too difficult or that the pleasures of using the behavior are worth the risks. This can be seen in the patient who says, "I know that I have to stop drinking. This car accident almost killed me. And one more traffic ticket while I'm intoxicated means I'll lose my license. But all my friends drink, and it is the only way I can relax. I don't think I can do it." During this stage of change the nurse should help the patient thoughtfully consider the positive and negative aspects of his or her substance use, gently trying to tip the balance in favor of beneficial behavior. Helping the patient discover internal motivators in addition to those external motivators (e.g., accidents, traffic tickets, legal and health problems, costs) that push the patient toward change can move the patient from contemplating change to preparation and action. Summarizing the patient's concerns and affirming the patient's ambivalence are useful techniques. Throughout this process, the patient's personal choices and responsibilities for change should be emphasized.[34]

As the patient moves from contemplation to *preparation,* a commitment to change can be strengthened by helping the patient develop self-efficacy. *Self-efficacy* in this case is the patient's optimism that substance-use behaviors can be changed, and the nurse should support even the smallest effort to change. Movement through action and maintenance stages of change requires continued support to increase the patient's involvement and participation in treatment. A comprehensive discussion of motivational interviewing throughout the entire change process is presented in the Treatment Improvement Protocol available at *http://hstat.nlm.nih.gov/hq/Hquestfws/T/db/local.tip.tip35/screen/Browse/s/47724/action/GetText/linek/15.*

The resolution of acute health problems or discharge from the hospital often occurs before the patient moves to the preparation and action stages of change. It is critical that, as the patient develops readiness to change in the contemplative stage of change, support of the change process be continued by referral to appropriate community and outpatient resources.

Ambulatory and Home Care. Before treatment and rehabilitation for addiction are considered, acute health problems must be resolved. Many of the patients with substance abuse problems that the nurse encounters in hospitals and primary care centers seek care because of health problems associated with substance abuse, not to receive care for the addiction. It is the nurse's responsibility, in collaboration with physicians, social workers, and addiction specialists, to address the patient's substance problem and motivate the patient to change behaviors and seek treatment for the addiction. Although the nurse working in the medical-surgical setting is not usually involved in long-term treatment of patients with addictive behaviors, it is the nurse's responsibility to identify the problem, increase the patient's awareness of the problem, and be able to refer the patient to inpatient and outpatient programs in the community that provide treatment and rehabilitation. Failure to confront the patient's addiction, thus enabling the patient's addictive behavior, is a breach of professional responsibility.

■ Gerontologic Considerations: Addictive Behaviors

Substance misuse and substance abuse in older adults are much less likely to be recognized by nurses and other health care providers than in younger adults. Older adults do not fit the image that most people in today's society have of those who abuse substances. In addition, patterns of substance use in older adults are considerably different from those in younger and middle-age adults. Because alcohol and substance abuse among older adults is often mistaken for other conditions (e.g., neuropathy, anemia, mental status changes) associated with the aging process, the problem is often undiagnosed and untreated.

In addition, denial of the problem is frequent and older adults do not typically seek help voluntarily. Estimates of alcohol abuse in the older population range from 4% to 20% in the community and up to 25% among hospitalized older adults.[39] These numbers are expected to increase dramatically in the future as the baby boomer generation ages because, as a group, they have more accepting attitudes and use more alcohol and drugs than earlier generations.

Although illicit drug use is minimal in older adults except for long-term addicts, older adults have the highest use of over-the-counter (OTC) and prescription drugs. The prescription drugs used by older adults are primarily psychoactive in nature, including sedative, hypnotic, anxiolytic, and opioid agents. Older women are more likely than men to become dependent on prescription drugs, especially benzodiazepines.[40] The simultaneous use of OTC drugs, prescription drugs, and alcohol occurs in many older adults. This presents a pattern of drug misuse and abuse that is not commonly seen in younger populations.

The effects of alcohol and other psychoactive substances increase with aging. Age-related decreases in circulation, metabolism, and excretion slow the body's detoxification of drugs, potentiate tolerance, and accelerate physical dependence on addictive substances. Physiologic changes that accompany aging may lead to intoxication at levels that may not have been a problem earlier in life. A 75-year-old can achieve a blood alcohol level of about 0.08% after 1.5 ounces of distilled liquor, 5 ounces of wine, or 12 ounces of beer.[41]

The adverse effects of interaction of alcohol and other drugs also increase with aging. When taken with alcohol, sedative-hypnotic drugs, minor tranquilizers, and CNS depressants have additive and synergistic effects. Misuse and abuse of psychoactive agents, either alone or in combination, by older adults may cause confusion, disorientation, delirium, memory loss, and neuromuscular impairment. The effects of alcohol and drug use can also be mistaken for medical or psychiatric conditions common among older adults, such as insomnia, depression, poor nutrition, congestive heart failure, and frequent falls. Withdrawal symptoms also occur in the older adult when alcohol, opioids, or sedative-hypnotics are abruptly stopped and may be more severe than in younger individuals.[39] Because of the high incidence of alcohol use in older adults, the nurse should always consider that changes in the older patient may be caused by alcohol use or withdrawal.

Identification of substance misuse and abuse in the older patient presents a challenge. Family members who are concerned about a patient's possible problem are important sources of information. Evidence of addictive disorders is not always obvious in the older adult, and manifestations may be similar to those caused by common health problems of the elderly. As with all patients, it is important for the nurse to discuss all drug and alcohol use with older patients, including OTC drug use. The patient's knowledge of medications that are currently being taken should be assessed.

Questionnaires customarily used to screen for alcoholism may be inappropriate for the older adult, who may not exhibit the social, legal, and occupational consequences of alcohol abuse generally used to diagnose problem drinkers. A simple tool for identifying alcohol problems in older adults is *HEAT* (how, excess, anyone else, trouble): *How* do you use alcohol? Have you ever thought you used alcohol to *excess*? Has *anyone else* ever thought you used too much? Have you ever had any *trouble* resulting from your use? Positive responses to any question should be further explored.[42] Screening for warning signs such as unexplained falls; neglect of personal hygiene; and complaints of mood, sleep, or memory problems is important.

Patient education for the older adult includes teaching about the desired effects, possible side effects, and appropriate use of prescribed and OTC drugs. The nurse should recommend that the patient use only one pharmacy because many pharmacies maintain a drug profile that may prevent problems with drug interactions. Patients should be advised not to drink alcohol when using prescribed and OTC drugs. Where there is no medical condition or possible drug interactions that would preclude the use of alcohol, older patients should be advised to limit their alcohol intake to one drink per day.[43]

Developmental, physical, and psychosocial changes that occur with aging contribute to the late-onset abuse of alcohol and other drugs by older adults. The older adult may have difficulty coping with losses that occur with increasing age, such as retirement, death of family and friends, relocation, social isolation, and poor health.

Knowing that older people may respond to the stresses of age with alcohol or drug use, the nurse should monitor people who are experiencing losses and identify those who are having difficulty coping. When risks are noted, these individuals can be taught coping skills and introduced to support services. Home visits by a nurse provide a good source of assessment of the problems and also provide valuable support. When the nurse suspects an alcohol or substance dependence in the older patient, the nurse should refer the patient for treatment. It is a mistaken belief that older persons have little to gain from alcohol and drug dependence treatment. The rewards of treatment can lead to greater quality and quantity of life for older adults. ■

CRITICAL THINKING EXERCISES

Case Study
Substance Misuse and Abuse
Patient Profile. Mrs. Carla Miller, a 78-year-old white woman, is admitted to the emergency department after falling and injuring her right shoulder and arm. She has been widowed for 4 years and lives alone. Recently her best friend died. Her only family is a daughter who lives out of town. When the nurse contacts the daughter by phone, she tells the nurse that her mother has appeared to be more disoriented and confused over the past year when she has talked to her on the phone.

Subjective Data
- Is complaining of severe pain in her right shoulder and upper arm
- Admits she had some wine in the late afternoon to stimulate her appetite
- Has experienced several falls in the past 2 months
- Reports that she fell after taking her sleeping pill prescribed by her physician because she does not sleep well
- Speech is hesitant and slurred
- Says she smokes about one-half pack of cigarettes a day

Objective Data
Physical Examination
- Oriented to person and place, but not time
- Blood pressure 162/94, pulse 92, respirations 24
- Bruising and edema of right upper arm
- Tremors of hands

Diagnostic Tests
- X-ray reveals comminuted fracture of the proximal humerus requiring surgical repair
- Blood alcohol concentration (BAC) 120 mg/dl (0.12 mg%)
- Complete blood count: hemoglobin 10.6 g/dl, hematocrit 38%

CRITICAL THINKING QUESTIONS
1. What other information is needed to assess Mrs. Miller's condition?
2. How should questions regarding these areas be addressed?
3. What factors may contribute to Mrs. Miller's use of psychoactive substances?
4. What nursing interventions are appropriate during Mrs. Miller's preoperative period?
5. What possible complications and other health problems may become apparent during Mrs. Miller's postoperative recovery?
6. What nursing interventions are appropriate following Mrs. Miller's surgery?
7. Based on the assessment data presented, write one or more nursing diagnoses. Are there any collaborative problems?

REVIEW QUESTIONS

The number of the question corresponds to the same-numbered objective at the beginning of the chapter.

1. A person who injects heroin to experience the euphoria it causes is demonstrating
   a. abuse.
   b. addiction.
   c. tolerance.
   d. addictive behavior.

2. The effects of long-term addictive substances on the brain leads to
   a. increased availability of dopamine.
   b. destruction of the mesolimbic system.
   c. loss of pleasure from experiences that previously resulted in enjoyment.
   d. potentiation of effects of similar drugs taken when the individual is drug free.

3. A major public health problem related to the behaviors of substance abuse is the prevalence of
   a. hepatitis C.
   b. malnutrition.
   c. infective endocarditis.
   d. respiratory depression and arrest.

4. The nurse would suspect cocaine overdose in the patient who is experiencing
   a. craving, restlessness, and irritability.
   b. agitation, cardiac arrhythmia, and seizures.
   c. diarrhea, nausea and vomiting, and confusion.
   d. slow, shallow respirations, hyporeflexia, and blurred vision.

5. The most appropriate nursing intervention for a patient who is seen at the clinic for increasing shortness of breath but who is not interested in quitting smoking is to
   a. accept the patient's decision and not intervene until the patient expresses a desire to quit.
   b. realize that some smokers will never quit, and trying to assist them only increases the patient's and the nurse's frustration.
   c. increase the patient's motivation to quit by explaining that continued smoking will only increase the breathing problems.
   d. ask the patient at every clinic visit to identify the relevance, risks, and benefits of quitting and what barriers to quitting are present.

6. While caring for a patient who is experiencing alcohol withdrawal the nurse should
   a. provide a quiet, nonstimulating, dimly lit environment.
   b. orient the patient to the environment and personnel with each contact.
   c. assist the patient to ambulate frequently to increase the metabolism of alcohol.
   d. provide stimulant beverages such as coffee or tea to counteract the effects of alcohol.

7. A patient who is dependent on intravenous barbiturates is scheduled for surgery following an automobile accident. The nurse recognizes that this patient
   a. may need less pain medication during the postoperative period.
   b. should be provided with tapering doses of barbiturates following surgery.
   c. may have an immediate onset of withdrawal symptoms when given anesthetic and analgesic agents.
   d. has a low risk for physical withdrawal symptoms but is likely to experience craving and drug-seeking behavior during the postoperative period.

8. Pain management of patients dependent on opioids or other CNS depressants requires that the nurse
   a. avoid giving narcotics.
   b. provide patient-controlled analgesia.
   c. insist the patient stop all drugs of abuse.
   d. treat the patient's report of pain with opioids.

9. During motivational interviewing with a patient, the nurse should
   a. insist that the patient maintain abstinence while undergoing therapy.
   b. relate motivational techniques to the patient's stage of behavior change.
   c. use any method of communication that will make the patient change behavior.
   d. ask a prescribed set of questions to increase the patient's awareness of addiction behaviors.

10. Substance abuse problems in older adults are most commonly related to
    a. use of drugs and alcohol as a social activity.
    b. misuse of prescribed and over-the-counter drugs and alcohol.
    c. continuing the use of illegal drugs initiated during middle age.
    d. a pattern of binge drinking for weeks or months with periods of sobriety.

REFERENCES

1. *1999 national household survey on drug abuse,* Washington, DC, 2000, Substance Abuse and Mental Health Services Administration (SAMHSA), Office of Applied Studies, US Department of Health and Human Services.
2. Poulin C, Single E, Fralick P: *Canadian Community Epidemiology Network on Drug Use (CCENDU): second national report, 1999,* Ottawa, 1999, Canadian Community Epidemiology Network on Drug Use. Available at *www.ccsa.ca/ccendu/Reports/1999national.htm* (accessed Jan 2, 2002).
3. Canadian Center on Substance Abuse: *Canadian profile of 1999 illicit drugs,* Toronto, Ontario, 1999, Canadian Center on Substance Abuse. Available at *www.ccsa.ca/cp99ill.htm* (accessed Feb 15, 2002).
4. American Psychiatric Association: *The diagnostic and statistical manual of mental disorders,* ed 4, Washington, DC, 1994, American Psychiatric Press.
5. Shuckit MA: *Drug and alcohol abuse: a clinical guide to diagnosis and treatment,* ed 5, New York, 2000, Kluwer Academic/Plenum.
6. Addiction Research Unit, Department of Psychology, State University of New York at Buffalo: The biological basis of addiction. In *Primer on drug addiction,* Buffalo, NY, 2000. Available at *http://wings.buffalo.edu/aru* (accessed Jan 2, 2002).
7. Begley S: The brain: the origins of dependence, *Newsweek,* p. 40, Feb 13, 2001.
8. Zickler P: Cue-induced craving linked to brain regions involved in decisionmaking and behavior, *NIDA Notes* 15:6, 2000.

9. NIDA: Update on nicotine addiction and tobacco research, *NIDA Notes* 15:5, 2000.

10. NIDA: Gender differences in drug abuse risks and treatment, *NIDA Notes* 15:4, 2000.

11. Francis HL: The medical consequences of drug use in minority populations. In *Bridging science and culture to improve drug abuse research in communities*, Bethesda, Md, 2001, National Institute on Drug Abuse, National Institutes of Health. Available at *http://165.11278.61/Meetings/Bridging/BridgeAbs1.html* (accessed Feb 15, 2002).

12. Indian Health Service: *Comprehensive health care program for American Indians and Alaska Natives*, Washington, DC, 1999, Indian Health Service, US Department of Health and Human Services. Available at *www.his.gov/nonmedicalprograms/profiles/profileaccomp.asp* (accessed Feb 15, 2002).

13. The National Women's Health Information Center: *Native American women's health*, Washington, DC, 1999, National Women's Health Information Center, US Department of Health and Human Services. Available at *www.4woman.gov/faq/easyread/native_american-etr.htm* (accessed Feb 15, 2002).

14. Leshner AI: Addressing the medical consequences of drug abuse, *NIDA Notes* 15:1, 2000.

15. Health Canada: *Trends in smoking, 2000: how many smokers in Canada?* Ottawa, 2000, Tobacco Control Programme, Health Canada. Available at *www.hc-sc.gc.ca/hppb/tobacco* (accessed Feb 15, 2002).

16. Naegle MA, D'Avanizo CE: *Addictions and substance abuse: strategies for advanced practice nursing*, Upper Saddle River, NJ, 2000, Prentice Hall.

17. Ruppert RA: The last smoke, *Am J Nurs* 99:26, 1999.

18. Cody MM: Is there help for a smoker? Understanding nicotine replacement therapy, *Am J Nurse Pract* 5:32, 2001.

19. Perkins KA: Smoking cessation in women: special considerations, *CNS Drugs* 15:391, 2001.

20. Dogen CE, Shea WM: *Substance use disorders: assessment and treatment*, San Diego, 2000, Academic Press.

21. Lane JD, Phillips-Bate BG: Caffeine deprivation affects vigilance, performance, and mood, *Physiol Behav* 65:171, 1998.

22. Powell AH: Alcohol withdrawal in critical care, *Dimens Crit Care Nurs* 18:24, 1999.

23. NIDA News Release: *The makings of a public health epidemic: drug abuse, HIV/AIDS and hepatitis C*, Bethesda, Md, May 9, 2000, National Institute on Drug Abuse, National Institutes of Health.

24. Henderson-Martin B: No more surprises: screening patients for alcohol abuse, *Am J Nurs* 100:26, 2000.

25. Crigger N: Defying denial: clues to detecting alcohol abuse, *Am J Nurs* 98:20, 1998.

26. Hanson MJ: Which straw will break the camel's back? *Am J Nurs* 99:63, 1999.

27. Satcher D: *Reducing tobacco use: a report of the surgeon general—2000*, Washington, DC, 2000, US Department of Health and Human Services.

28. US Department of Health and Human Services: *Clinical practice guideline: treating tobacco use and dependence*, Washington, DC, 2000, US Public Health Service.

29. Sachse DS: Delirium tremens, *Am J Nurs* 100:41, 2000.

30. Haack MR: Treating acute withdrawal from alcohol and other drugs, *Nurs Clin North Am* 33:75, 1998.

31. Stewart KB, Richards AB: Recognizing and managing your patient's alcohol abuse, *Nursing* 30:57, 2000.

32. Compton P, McCaffery M: Treating acute pain in addicted patients, *Nursing* 31:17, 2001.

33. Brown J et al: A question of pain, *Nursing* 29:50, 1999.

34. Miller WR: *Enhancing motivation for change in substance abuse treatment: treatment improvement protocol (TIP) series 35*, DHHS pub no (SMA) 99-3354, Rockville, Md, 1999, US Department of Health and Human Services. Available at *http://hstat.nlm.nih.gov/hp/Hquest/db/local.tip.tip35/screen/TocDisplay/da/1/s/36610/action/Toc* (accessed Feb 15, 2002).

35. Miller RW, Rollnick S: *Preparing people to change addictive behavior*, New York, 1991, Guilford Press.

36. Prochaska JO, DiClemente CC: *The transtheoretical approach: crossing traditional boundaries of therapy*, Homewood, Ill, 1984, Dow Jones-Irwin.

37. Shinitzky HE, Kub J: The art of motivating behavior change: the use of motivational interviewing to promote health, *Public Health Nurs* 18:178, 2001.

38. Compton P, Monahan G, Simmons-Cody H: Motivational interviewing: an effective brief intervention for alcohol and drug abuse patients, *Nurse Pract* 24:27, 1999.

39. Ondus KA et al: Substance abuse and the hospitalized elderly, *Orthop Nurs* 18:27, 1999.

40. Scott CM, Popovich DJ: Undiagnosed alcoholism and prescription drug misuse among the elderly, *Caring* 20:20, 2001.

41. Lantz MS: Alcohol abuse in the older adult, *Clinical Geriatrics* 10:40, 2002.

42. Gurnack AM, editor: *Older adults' misuse of alcohol, medicines, and other drugs*, New York, 1997, Springer.

43. National Institute on Alcohol Abuse and Alcoholism: *Alcohol and aging. Alcohol alert no. 40*, Rockville, Md, 1998, National Institute on Alcohol Abuse and Alcoholism.

RESOURCES

Alcoholics Anonymous
AA World Services, Inc.
PO Box 459
New York, NY 10163
212-870-3400
www.alcoholics-anonymous.org/

American Lung Association
1740 Broadway
New York, NY 10019
212-315-8700
www.lungusa.org

American Psychiatric Nurses Association
Colonial Place Three
2107 Wilson Blvd, Suite 300-A
Arlington, VA 22201-3042
703-243-2443
Fax: 703-243-3390
E-mail: info@apna.org
www.apna.org

American Society of Addiction Medicine
4601 North Park Avenue, Arcade Suite 101
Chevy Chase, MD 20815
301-656-3920
Fax: 301-656-3815
E-mail: Email@asam.org
www.asam.org

International Nurses Society on Addictions
PO Box 10752
Raleigh, NC 27605
919-821-1292
Fax: 919-833-5743
www.intnsa.org

Narcotics Anonymous
World Service Office
PO Box 9999
Van Nuys, CA 91409
818-773-9999
Fax: 818-700-0700
www.na.org/

National Clearinghouse for Alcohol and Drug Information
PO Box 2345
Rockville, MD 20847-2345
301-468-2600
800-729-6686
Fax: 301-468-6433
E-mail: info@health.org
www.health.org/about/

National Council on Alcoholism and Drug Dependence, Inc.
20 Exchange Place, Suite 2902
New York, NY 10005
212-269-7797
Fax: 212-269-7510
Hope Line: 800-NCA-CALL
E-mail: national@ncadd.org
www.ncadd.org

National Institute on Drug Abuse
National Institutes of Health
6001 Executive Blvd., Room 5213
Bethesda, MD 20892
301-443-1124
www.nida.nih.gov

Tobacco Information and Prevention Source (TIPS)
National Center for Chronic Disease Prevention and Health Promotion
404-488-5705
E-mail: tobaccoinfo@cdc.gov
www.cdc.gov/tobacco

For additional Internet resources, see the website for this book at
http://evolve.elsevier.com/Lewis/medsurg/.

Pathophysiologic Mechanisms of Disease

SECTION OUTLINE

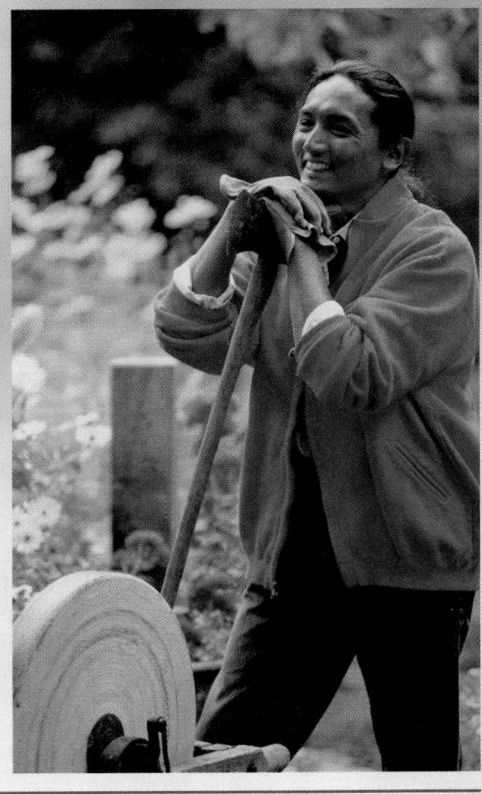

CHAPTER *12*

Inflammation, Infection, and Healing

Sharon Mantik Lewis
Elizabeth A. Ayello

LEARNING OBJECTIVES

1. Explain the cellular adaptive mechanisms to sublethal injury.
2. Describe the causes and mechanisms of lethal cell injury.
3. Differentiate among types of cell necrosis.
4. Describe the components and functions of the mononuclear phagocyte system.
5. Describe the inflammatory response, including vascular and cellular responses and exudate formation.
6. Explain local and systemic manifestations of inflammation and their physiologic bases.
7. Describe the pharmacologic, dietary, and nursing management of inflammation.
8. Differentiate among healing by primary, secondary, and tertiary intention.
9. Describe the factors that delay wound healing and common complications of wound healing.
10. Describe a patient risk assessment for pressure ulcers.
11. Discuss measures to prevent the development of pressure ulcers.
12. Explain the etiology and clinical manifestations of pressure ulcers.
13. Discuss collaborative and nursing management of a patient with pressure ulcers.

KEY TERMS

adhesions, p. 216	inflammatory response, p. 207
anaplasia, p. 205	lethal injury, p. 204
atrophy, p. 204	metaplasia, p. 205
dehiscence, p. 215	necrosis, p. 206
dysplasia, p. 205	pressure ulcer, p. 225
evisceration, p. 216	regeneration, p. 212
fibroblasts, p. 213	repair, p. 212
hyperplasia, p. 204	shearing force, p. 225
hypertrophic scar, p. 215	sublethal injury, p. 204
hypertrophy, p. 204	

This chapter focuses on cell injury, inflammation, and healing. The problem of antibiotic-resistant organisms is discussed, and current recommendations for infection control are presented. Assessment for pressure ulcer risk and interventions to prevent and treat pressure ulcer are described.

CELL INJURY

Cell injury can be sublethal or lethal. **Sublethal injury** alters function without causing cell death. The changes caused by this type of injury are potentially reversible if the injurious stimulus is removed. **Lethal injury** is an irreversible process that causes cell death.

Cell Adaptation to Sublethal Injury

Cell adaptations to sublethal injuries are common and are part of many physiologic and disease processes. For example, prolonged exposure to sunlight stimulates melanin production

and thus provides protection of deeper skin layers by tanning the skin. Lack of muscular activity can lead to atrophy and decreased muscle tone. Adaptive processes of the cell include hypertrophy, hyperplasia, atrophy, and metaplasia (Fig. 12-1). Other responses that are considered maladaptive are dysplasia and anaplasia.

Hypertrophy. Hypertrophy is an increase in the size of cells without cell division. For example, the uterus during pregnancy enlarges from hormonal stimulation. The heart of a person with severe hypertension enlarges to compensate for the increased resistance to its pumping action. Removal of one kidney results in an increase in the size of the remaining kidney because of the increased work demand. Muscle hypertrophy results from an increase in the size of muscle fibers in response to an increase in cellular protein, as would occur in an individual who does weight training.

Hyperplasia. Hyperplasia is an increase in the number of cells resulting from increased cellular division. This process is reversible when the stimulus is removed. Compensatory hyperplasia is an adaptive process whereby cells of certain organs regenerate. For example, if portions of the liver are removed, the remaining cells will undergo increased mitosis to compensate for the cells removed. Hormonal hyperplasia occurs primarily in organs responsive to estrogen, such as the breast and uterus. For example, the uterus undergoes hyperplasia during pregnancy and the female breast experiences hyperplasia during lactation.

Atrophy. Atrophy is a decrease in the size of a tissue or organ caused by a decreased number of cells or reduction in the size of the individual cells. It frequently occurs as a result of disease (e.g., musculoskeletal disease), lack of blood supply (e.g., thrombus formation), natural aging process (e.g., decreased breast size after menopause), inactivity (e.g., decreased muscle size), and nutritional deficiency.

Reviewed by Alissa D. Stanley, RN, BSN, Graduate Student, School of Nursing, University of Texas Health Science Center at San Antonio, San Antonio, Tex.; and Duck-Hee Kang, RN, PhD, Associate Professor, School of Nursing, University of Alabama, Birmingham, Ala.

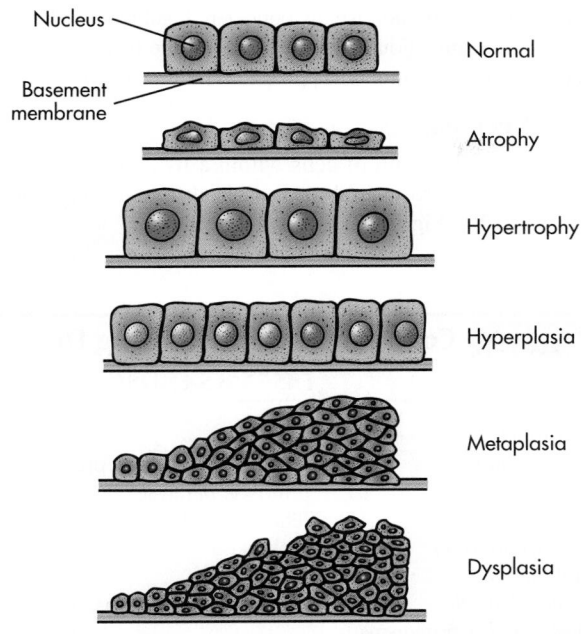

Nucleus

Basement membrane

Normal

Atrophy

Hypertrophy

Hyperplasia

Metaplasia

Dysplasia

FIG. 12-1 Adaptive and maladaptive alterations in simple cuboidal epithelial cells.

Metaplasia. **Metaplasia** is the reversible transformation of one cell type into another. An example of physiologic metaplasia is when circulating monocytes change to macrophages as they migrate into inflamed tissues. An example of pathophysiologic metaplasia is when the normal pseudostratified columnar epithelium of the bronchi changes to squamous epithelium in response to chronic cigarette smoking. If the irritating stimulus (the cigarette smoke) is removed, the bronchial metaplasia may be reversible.

Dysplasia. **Dysplasia** is an abnormal differentiation of dividing cells resulting in changes in the size, shape, and appearance of the cells. Minor dysplasia is found in some areas of inflammation. Dysplasia is potentially reversible if the stimulus is removed. Frequently, dysplasia can be a precursor of malignancy, such as in cervical dysplasia.

Anaplasia. **Anaplasia** is cell differentiation to a more immature or embryonic form. Malignant tumors are often characterized by anaplastic cell growth.

Causes of Lethal Cell Injury

Many different agents and factors can cause lethal cell injury (Table 12-1). The mechanism of actual cell death varies. Examples include deterioration of the nucleus, such as *pyknosis* (nu-

TABLE 12-1	Causes of Lethal Cell Injury
CAUSE	**EFFECT ON CELL**
Physical Agents	
▪ Heat	Denaturation of protein, acceleration of metabolic reactions
▪ Cold	Decreased blood flow from vasoconstriction, slowed metabolic reactions, thrombosis of blood vessels, freezing of cell content that forms crystals and can burst cell
▪ Radiation	Alteration of cell structure and activity, alteration of enzyme systems, mutations
▪ Electrothermal injury	Interruption of neural conduction, fibrillation of cardiac muscle, coagulative necrosis of skin and skeletal muscle
▪ Mechanical trauma	Transfer of excess kinetic energy to cells causing rupture of cells, blood vessels, tissue; examples include:
	Abrasion: scraping of skin or mucous membrane
	Laceration: severing of vessels and tissue
	Contusion (bruise): crushing of tissue cells causing hemorrhage into skin
	Puncture: piercing of body structure or organ
	Incision: surgical cutting
Chemical Injury	Alteration of cell metabolism, interference with normal enzymatic action within cells
Microbial Injury	
▪ Viruses	Taking over of cell metabolism and synthesis of new particles that may cause cell rupture, cumulative effect possibly producing clinical disease
▪ Bacteria*	Destruction of cell membrane or cell nucleus, production of lethal toxins
Ischemic Injury	Compromised cell metabolism, acute or gradual cell death
Immunologic†	
▪ Antigen-antibody response	Release of substances (histamine, complement) that can injure and damage cells
▪ Autoimmune	Activation of complement, which destroys normal cells and produces inflammation
Neoplastic Growth	Cell destruction from abnormal and uncontrolled cell growth
Normal Substances (e.g., digestive enzymes, uric acid)	Release into abdomen causing peritonitis, crystallization of excess accumulation in joints and renal tissue

*Bacteria are commonly classified as gram-negative or gram-positive bacteria.
†See Chapter 13 for a more detailed discussion.

clear condensation and shrinking) and *karyolysis* (dissolution of nucleus and contents), disruption of cell metabolism, and rupture of the cell membrane.

Microbial invasion frequently, but not always, results in cell injury and death. Infection occurs when *pathogens* (microorganisms capable of producing disease) invade and multiply in body tissues.[1] (Common viruses and bacteria that cause diseases in humans are listed in Tables 12-2 and 12-3.) *Opportunistic organisms* are mi-croorganisms that are not usually considered pathogens. However, they may cause infection if the resistance of the host is decreased from events such as immunosuppression, trauma, or illness.

Cell Necrosis

Necrosis is the death of cells within a living organism. Different types of necrosis tend to occur in different organs or tissues (Table 12-4, Fig. 12-2).

TABLE 12-2	**Common Viruses Causing Disease**
TYPE	**DISEASES CAUSED**
• Adenoviruses	Upper respiratory tract infection, pneumonia
• Arbovirus	Syndrome of fever, malaise, headache, myalgia; aseptic meningitis; encephalitis
• Coronavirus	Upper respiratory tract infection
• Coxsackieviruses A and B	Upper respiratory tract infection, gastroenteritis, acute myocarditis, aseptic meningitis
• Echoviruses	Upper respiratory tract infection, gastroenteritis, aseptic meningitis
• Hepatitis	
A	Viral hepatitis
B	Viral hepatitis
C	Viral hepatitis
• Herpesviruses	
Cytomegalovirus (CMV)	Pneumonia in immunosup-pressed individuals, infectious mononucleosis–like syndrome
Epstein-Barr	Mononucleosis, Burkitt's lymphoma (possibly)
Herpes simplex	
Type 1	Herpes labialis ("fever blisters"), genital herpes infection
Type 2	Genital herpes infection
Varicella-zoster	Chickenpox; shingles
• Human immuno-deficiency virus (HIV)	HIV infection, acquired immuno-deficiency syndrome (AIDS)
• Influenza A and B	Upper respiratory tract infection
• Mumps	Parotitis, orchitis in postpubertal males
• Papovavirus	Warts
• Parainfluenza 1–4	Upper respiratory tract infection
• Parvovirus	Gastroenteritis
• Poliovirus	Poliomyelitis
• Pox viruses	Smallpox
• Reoviruses 1, 2, 3	Upper respiratory tract infection
• Respiratory syncytial virus	Gastroenteritis, respiratory tract infection
• Rhabdovirus	Rabies
• Rhinovirus	Upper respiratory tract infection, pneumonia
• Rotaviruses	Gastroenteritis
• Rubella	German measles
• Rubeola	Measles
• West Nile virus	Flu-like symptoms, meningitis, encephalitis

TABLE 12-3	**Common Bacteria Causing Disease**
TYPE	**DISEASES CAUSED**
• Clostridia	
C. botulinum	Food poisoning with progressive muscle paralysis
C. tetani	Tetanus (lockjaw)
• Corynebacterium diphtheriae	Diphtheria
• Escherichia coli	Urinary tract infections, peritonitis
• Haemophilus organisms	
H. influenzae	Nasopharyngitis, meningitis, pneumonia
H. pertussis	Whooping cough
• Helicobacter pylori	Peptic ulcers
• Klebsiella-Enterobacter organisms	Urinary tract infections, peritonitis, pneumonia
• Legionella pneumophila	Pneumonia (Legionnaires' disease)
• Mycobacteria	
M. leprae	Leprosy (Hansen's disease)
M. tuberculosis	Tuberculosis
• Neisseriae	
N. gonorrhoeae	Gonorrhea, pelvic inflammatory disease
N. meningitidis	Meningococcemia, meningitis
• Proteus species	Urinary tract infections, peritonitis
• Pseudomonas aeruginosa	Urinary tract infections, meningitis
• Salmonella species	
S. typhi	Typhoid fever
Other Salmonella organisms	Food poisoning, gastroenteritis
• Shigella species	Shigellosis, diarrhea with abdominal pain and fever (dysentery)
• Staphylococcus aureus	Skin infections, pneumonia, urinary tract infections, acute osteomyelitis, toxic shock syndrome
• Streptococci	
S. faecalis	Genitourinary infection, infection of surgical wounds
S. pneumoniae	Pneumococcal pneumonia
S. pyogenes (group A β-hemolytic streptococci)	Pharyngitis, scarlet fever, rheumatic fever, acute glomerulonephritis, erysipelas, pneumonia
S. pyogenes (group B β-hemolytic streptococci)	Urinary tract infections
S. viridans	Bacterial endocarditis
• Treponema pallidum	Syphilis

TABLE 12-4	Types of Necrosis
TYPE	DESCRIPTION
Coagulative necrosis	Necrotic cells maintain their outline. Lytic enzymes are somewhat inhibited. Proteins are denatured. Enzymes lose their function. Commonly caused by a lack of blood supply.
Liquefactive necrosis	Necrotic cells rapidly disappear as lytic enzymes digest tissues. Commonly occurs in the brain where the supply of lytic enzymes is abundant.
Caseous necrosis	Necrotic cells disintegrate, but cell fragments remain for long periods of time. Called caseous (cheeselike) necrosis because of its crumbly appearance. Frequently found in tuberculosis of the lung.
Gangrenous necrosis	Necrotic cells result from severe hypoxia and subsequent ischemic injury, which is common after impaired circulation in the lower legs. Dry gangrene refers to the dry, shriveled, darkened area (see Fig. 12-2), and wet gangrene refers to the liquefied underlying necrotic tissue.

TABLE 12-5	Location and Name of Macrophages*
LOCATION	NAME
Connective tissue	Histiocytes
Liver	Kupffer cells
Lung	Alveolar macrophages
Spleen	Free and fixed macrophages
Bone marrow	Fixed macrophages
Lymph nodes	Free and fixed macrophages
Bone tissue	Osteoclasts
Central nervous system	Microglial cells
Peritoneal cavity	Peritoneal macrophages
Pleural cavity	Pleural macrophages
Skin	Histiocyte, Langerhans' cells
Synovium	Type A cells

*In addition, monocytes become macrophages once they leave the blood and enter the tissues.

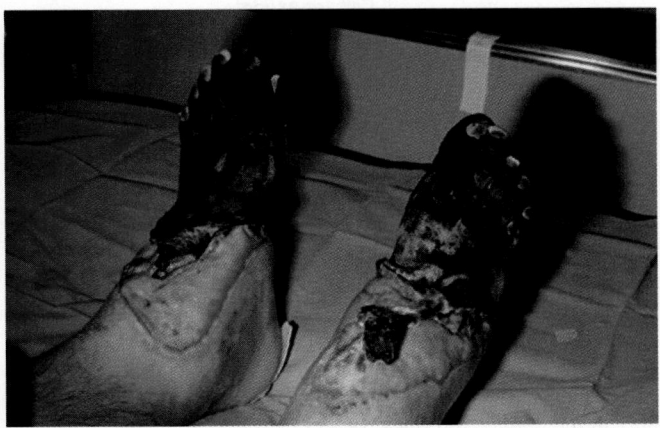

FIG. 12-2   Gangrene of the toes.

DEFENSE AGAINST INJURY

To protect against injury and infection, the body has various defense mechanisms. These defense mechanisms are (1) the skin and mucous membranes, which are the first lines of defense (see Chapter 22); (2) the mononuclear phagocyte system; (3) the inflammatory response; and (4) the immune system (see Chapter 13).

Mononuclear Phagocyte System

The *mononuclear phagocyte system* (MPS) consists of monocytes and macrophages and their precursor cells. In the past, the MPS system was called the reticuloendothelial system (RES). However, it is not a body system with distinctly defined tissues and organs. Rather, it consists of phagocytic cells located in various tissues and organs (Table 12-5). The phagocytic cells are either fixed or free (mobile). The macrophages of the liver, spleen, bone marrow, lungs, lymph nodes, and nervous system (microglial cells) are fixed phagocytes. The monocytes (in blood) and the macrophages found in connective tissue, termed *histiocytes,* are mobile, or wandering, phagocytes.

Monocytes and macrophages originate in the bone marrow. Monocytes spend a few days in the blood and then enter tissues and change into macrophages. Tissue macrophages are larger and more phagocytic than monocytes.

The functions of the macrophage system include recognition and phagocytosis of foreign material such as microorganisms, removal of old or damaged cells from circulation, and participation in the immune response (see Chapter 13).

Inflammatory Response

The **inflammatory response** is a sequential reaction to cell injury. It neutralizes and dilutes the inflammatory agent, removes necrotic materials, and establishes an environment suitable for healing and repair. The term *inflammation* is often but incorrectly used as a synonym for the term *infection*. Inflammation is always present with infection, but infection is not always present with inflammation. However, a person who is neutropenic may not be able to mount an inflammatory response. An infection involves invasion of tissues or cells by microorganisms such as bacteria, fungi, and viruses. In contrast, inflammation can also be caused by nonliving agents such as heat, radiation, trauma, and allergens (see Table 12-1). If infection is also present, it is from a superimposed invasion of microorganisms.

The mechanism of inflammation is basically the same regardless of the injuring agent. The intensity of the response depends on the extent and severity of injury and on the reactive capacity of the injured person. The inflammatory response can be divided into a vascular response, a cellular response, formation of exudate, and healing.

Vascular Response. After cell injury, arterioles in the area briefly undergo transient vasoconstriction. After release of histamine and other chemicals by the injured cells, the vessels dilate. This vasodilation results in *hyperemia* (increased blood flow in the area), which raises filtration pressure. Vasodilation and chemical mediators cause endothelial cell retraction, which increases capillary permeability. Movement of fluid from capillaries into tissue spaces is thus facilitated. Initially composed of serous fluid, this inflammatory exudate later contains plasma proteins, primarily albumin. The proteins exert oncotic pressure that fur-

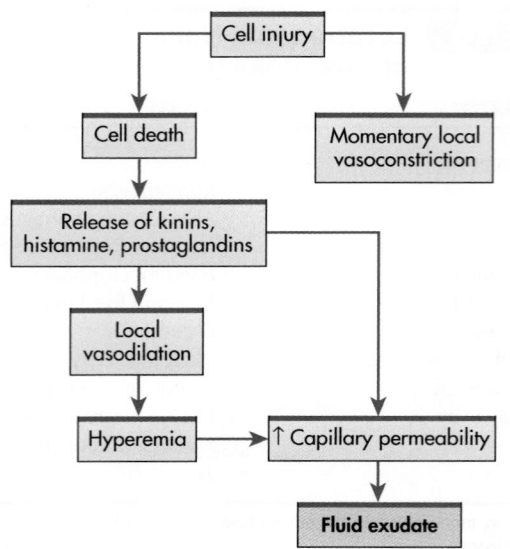

FIG. 12-3 Vascular response in inflammation.

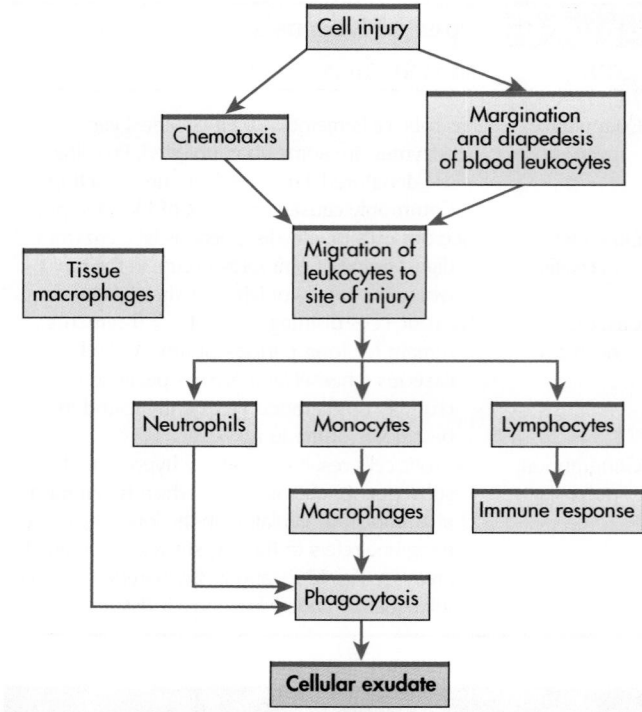

FIG. 12-4 Cellular response in inflammation.

ther draws fluid from blood vessels. The tissue becomes edematous. This response is illustrated in Fig. 12-3.

As the plasma protein fibrinogen leaves the blood, it is activated to fibrin by the products of the injured cells. Fibrin strengthens a blood clot formed by platelets. In tissue the clot functions to trap bacteria, to prevent their spread, and to serve as a framework for the healing process.

Cellular Response. The cellular response to injury is illustrated in Fig. 12-4. The blood flow through capillaries in the area slows as fluid is lost and viscosity increases. Neutrophils and monocytes move to the inner surface of the capillaries (margination) and then, in ameboid fashion, through the capillary wall (*diapedesis*) to the site of injury (Fig. 12-5).

Chemotaxis is the directional migration of white blood cells (WBCs) along a concentration gradient of chemotactic factors, which are substances that attract leukocytes to the site of inflammation. Chemotaxis is the mechanism for ensuring accumulation of neutrophils and monocytes at the focus of injury. Chemotactic factors include bacterial-derived chemotactic factors, complement-derived chemotactic factor (C5a), lipid-derived chemotactic factors (leukotriene B$_4$, 5-HPETE, platelet-activating factor), platelet-derived chemotactic factors, and coagulation-related chemotactic factors.

Neutrophils. Neutrophils are the first leukocytes to arrive (usually within 6 to 12 hours). They phagocytize (engulf) bacteria, other foreign material, and damaged cells. With their short life span (24 to 48 hours), dead neutrophils soon accumulate. In time a mixture of dead neutrophils, digested bacteria, and other cell debris accumulates as a creamy substance termed *pus*.

To keep up with the demand for neutrophils, the bone marrow releases more neutrophils into circulation. This results in an elevated WBC count, especially the neutrophil count. Sometimes the demand for neutrophils increases to the extent that the bone marrow releases immature forms of neutrophils (bands) into circulation. (Mature neutrophils are called segmented neutrophils.) The finding of increased numbers of band neutrophils in circulation is called a *shift to the left,* which is commonly found in patients with acute bacterial infections. (See Chapter 29 for a discussion on neutrophils.)

Monocytes. Monocytes are the second type of phagocytic cells that migrate from circulating blood. They are attracted to the site by chemotactic factors and usually arrive at the site within 3 to 7 days after the onset of inflammation. On entering the tissue spaces, monocytes transform into macrophages. Together with the tissue macrophages, these macrophages assist in phagocytosis of the inflammatory debris. The macrophage role is important in cleaning the area before healing can occur. Macrophages have a long life span; they can multiply and may stay in the damaged tissues for weeks. These long-lived cells are important in orchestrating the healing process.

In some cases, macrophages perform tasks other than phagocytosis. They may accumulate and fuse to form a *multinucleated*

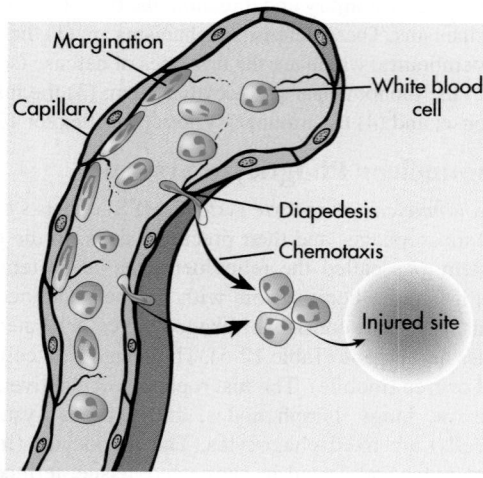

FIG. 12-5 Margination, diapedesis, and chemotaxis of white blood cells.

TABLE 12-6 Mediators of Inflammation

MEDIATOR	SOURCE	MECHANISMS OF ACTION
Histamine	Stored in granules of basophils, mast cells, platelets	Causes vasodilation and increased vascular permeability by stimulating contraction of endothelial cells and creating widened gaps between cells
Serotonin	Stored in platelets, mast cells, enterochromaffin cells of GI tract	Causes vasodilation and increased vascular permeability by stimulating contraction of endothelial cells and creating widened gaps between cells; stimulates smooth muscle contraction
Kinins (e.g., bradykinin)	Produced from precursor factor kininogen as a result of activation of Hageman factor (XII) of clotting system	Cause contraction of smooth muscle and dilation of blood vessels; result in stimulation of pain
Complement components (C3a, C4a, C5a)	Anaphylatoxic agents generated from complement pathway activation	Stimulate histamine release; stimulate chemotaxis
Fibrinopeptides	Produced from activation of the clotting system	Increase vascular permeability; stimulate chemotaxis for neutrophils and monocytes
Prostaglandins and leukotrienes	Produced from arachidonic acid (see Fig. 12-7)	PGE_1 and PGE_2 cause vasodilation; LTB_4 stimulates chemotaxis
Cytokines	For information on cytokines, see Table 13-5	

LT, Leukotrienes; *PG*, prostaglandin.

giant cell. The giant cell attempts to phagocytize particles too large for macrophages. The giant cell is then encapsulated by collagen, leading to the formation of a granuloma. A classic example of this process occurs with the tubercle bacillus in the lung. While the bacillus is walled off, a chronic state of inflammation exists. The granuloma formed is a cavity of necrotic tissue.

Lymphocytes. Lymphocytes arrive later at the site of injury. Their primary role is related to humoral and cell-mediated immunity (see Chapter 13).

Eosinophils and basophils. Eosinophils and basophils have a more selective role in inflammation. Eosinophils are released in large quantities during an allergic reaction. They release chemicals that act to control the effects of histamine and serotonin. They are also involved in phagocytosis of the allergen-antibody complex. Eosinophils also contain highly caustic chemicals that are capable of destroying a parasite's cell surfaces. The histamine and heparin that basophils carry in their granules are released during inflammation.

Chemical Mediators. Mediators of the inflammatory response are presented in Table 12-6.

Complement system. The complement system is a major mediator of the inflammatory response. Major functions of the complement system are enhanced phagocytosis, increased vascular permeability, chemotaxis, and cellular lysis. All of these activities are important in the inflammatory response.

When activated, the components occur in the sequential order of C1, C4, C2, C3, C5, C6, C7, C8, and C9 (Fig. 12-6). The num-

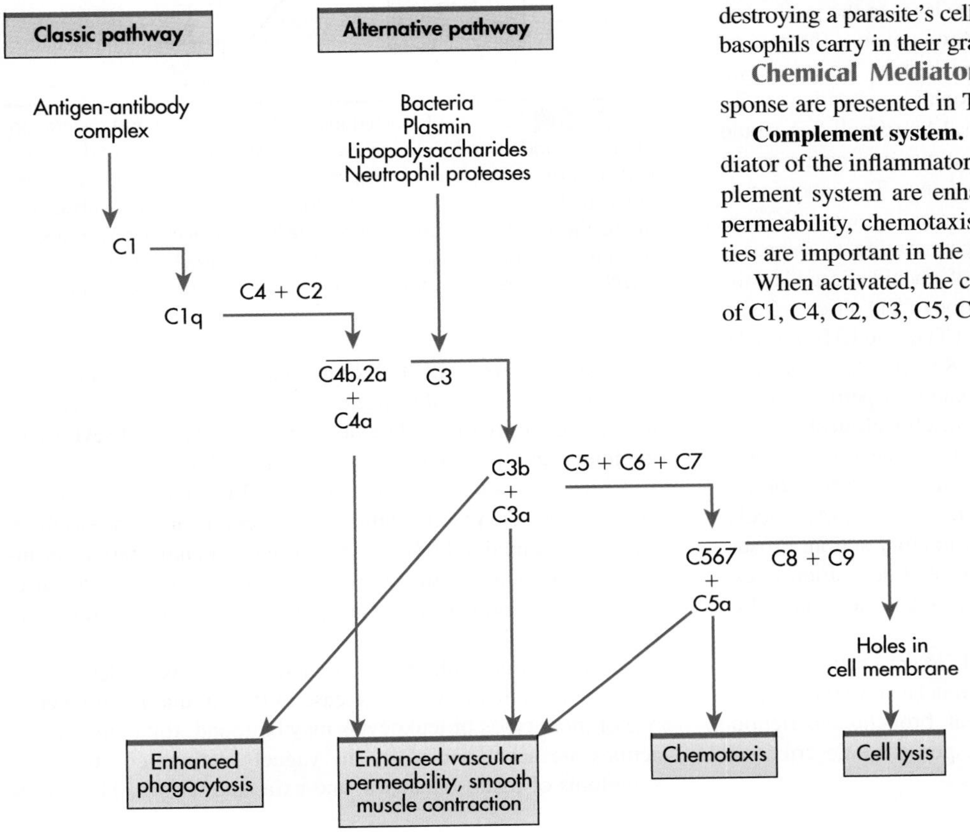

FIG. 12-6 Sequential activation and biologic effects of the complement system.

bering reflects the order of their discovery. Some components have subparts designated by lowercase letters, such as C3a, C3b, and C5a. The primary pathway for activation of the complement system is through fixation of component C1 to an antigen-antibody complex. The immunoglobulins IgG and IgM are responsible for fixing complement. Each activated complex can act on the next component, creating a cascade effect.

An alternative pathway exists in which C3 is activated without prior antigen-antibody fixation. Bacterial products, lipopolysaccharides, and neutrophil proteases can stimulate the complement sequence at the C3 level with activation of C5 through C9.

Complement activation increases phagocytosis through opsonization and chemotaxis. *Opsonization* occurs when the antigen, in combination with complement factor C3b and immunoglobulin, sticks to the surface of phagocytic cells. This leads to more rapid phagocytosis. In addition, complement component C5a promotes chemotaxis.

The components C3a, C5a, and C4a are termed *anaphylatoxins* and bind to receptors on mast cells and basophils, thus triggering histamine release. Histamine causes smooth muscle contraction, vasodilation, and an increase in vascular permeability.

The entire complement sequence of C1 to C9 must be activated for cell lysis to occur. The final components (C8, C9) act on the cell surface, causing rupture of the cell membrane and lysis. Bacteria, red blood cells (RBCs), and nucleated cells are susceptible to the lysis.

Prostaglandins and leukotrienes. *Prostaglandins* (PGs) are substances that can be synthesized from the phospholipids of cell membranes of most body tissues, including blood cells. On stimulation by chemotactic factors or phagocytosis or after cell injury, phospholipids can be converted to arachidonic acid (a 20-carbon polyunsaturated fatty acid), which is then oxidized by two different pathways (Fig. 12-7).

The *cyclooxygenase metabolic pathway* leads to the production of PGs of the D, E, F, and I series and thromboxanes (formed on activation of platelets). PGs of the E and I series are potent vasodilators and inhibit platelet and neutrophil aggregation. PGE_2 can also sensitize pain receptors to arousal by stimuli that would normally be painless. PGE_2 is also a potent pyrogen, acting on the temperature-regulating area of the hypothalamus. Thromboxane A_2 is a potent vasoconstrictor and platelet-aggregating agent. PGs are generally considered proinflammatory, contributing to increased blood flow, edema, and pain. Metabolism of arachidonic acid by the *lipoxygenase pathway* leads to the production of leukotrienes (LTs). LTB_4 is a potent chemotactic factor. LTC_4, LTD_4, and LTE_4 form the slow-reacting substance of anaphylaxis (SRS-A), which constricts smooth muscles of bronchi and increases capillary permeability.

Drugs that inhibit PG synthesis are useful clinically. Nonsteroidal antiinflammatory drugs (NSAIDs), one type of these drugs, are a prototype drug treatment for many acute and chronic inflammatory conditions. Acetylsalicylic acid (ASA) blocks platelet aggregation; it also has antiinflammatory action. Prostacyclin (PGI_2) has been used to prevent platelet deposition in extracorporeal systems, such as hemodialysis and heart-lung bypass oxygenators.

Another group of drugs that inhibit PGs are corticosteroids. They are valuable in the treatment of asthma because they inhibit leukotriene production and thus prevent bronchoconstriction. (Other mediators of the inflammatory response are described in Table 12-6.)

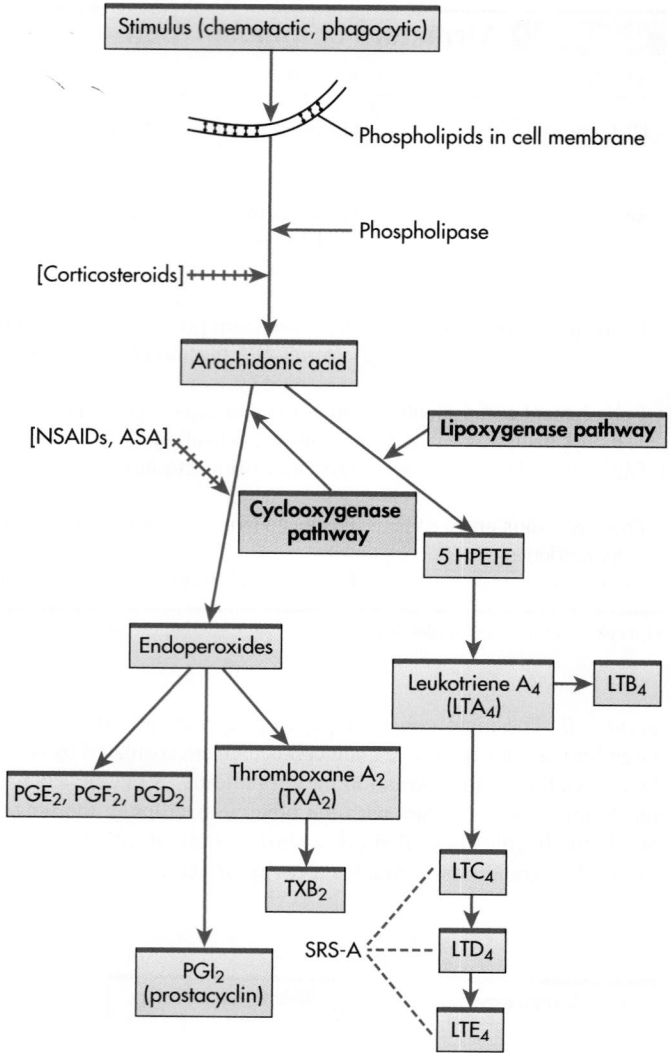

FIG. 12-7 Pathway of arachidonic acid oxygenation and generation of prostaglandins and leukotrienes. Corticosteroids, nonsteroidal anti-inflammatory drugs, and acetylsalicylic acid act to inhibit various steps in this pathway. LTC_4, LTD_4, and LTE_4 form the slow-reacting substance of anaphylaxis (SRS–A), an important mediator of allergic responses, by causing bronchoconstriction and increased vascular permeability. *5-HPETE*, 5-hydroperoxyeicosatetraenoic acid; *PG*, prostaglandins.

Exudate Formation. Exudate consists of fluid and leukocytes that move from the circulation to the site of injury. The nature and quantity of exudate depend on the type and severity of the injury and the tissues involved (Table 12-7).

Clinical Manifestations. The local response to inflammation includes the manifestations of redness, heat, pain, swelling, and loss of function (Table 12-8). Systemic manifestations of inflammation include leukocytosis with a shift to the left, malaise, nausea and anorexia, increased pulse and respiratory rate, and fever.

Leukocytosis results from the increased release of leukocytes from the bone marrow. An increase in the circulating number of one or more types of leukocytes may be found. Inflammatory reactions are accompanied by the vaguely defined constitutional symptoms of malaise, nausea, anorexia, and fatigue. The causes

TABLE 12-7   Types of Inflammatory Exudate

TYPE	DESCRIPTION	EXAMPLES
Serous	Serous exudate results from outpouring of fluid that has low cell and protein content; it is seen in early stages of inflammation or when injury is mild.	Skin blisters, pleural effusion
Catarrhal	Catarrhal exudate is found in tissues where cells produce mucus. Mucus production is accelerated by inflammatory response.	Runny nose associated with upper respiratory tract infection
Fibrinous	Fibrinous exudate occurs with increasing vascular permeability and fibrinogen leakage into interstitial spaces. Excessive amounts of fibrin coating tissue surfaces may cause them to adhere.	Adhesions
Purulent (pus)	Purulent exudate consists of WBCs, microorganisms (dead and alive), liquefied dead cells, and other debris.	Furuncle (boil), abscess, cellulitis (diffuse inflammation in connective tissue)
Hemorrhagic	Hemorrhagic exudate results from rupture or necrosis of blood vessel walls; it consists of RBCs that escape into tissue.	Hematoma

RBCs, Red blood cells; *WBCs,* white blood cells.

TABLE 12-8   Local Manifestations of Inflammation

MANIFESTATIONS	CAUSE
Redness (rubor)	Hyperemia from vasodilation
Heat (color)	Increased metabolism at inflammatory site
Pain (dolor)	Change in pH; change in local ionic concentration; nerve stimulation by chemicals (e.g., histamine, prostaglandins); pressure from fluid exudate
Swelling (tumor)	Fluid shift to interstitial spaces; fluid exudate accumulation
Loss of function (functio laesa)	Swelling and pain

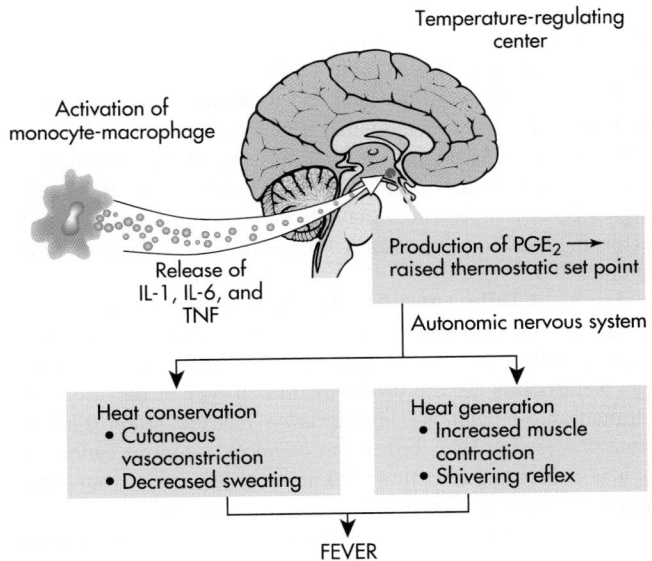

FIG. 12-8 Production of fever. When monocytes/macrophages are activated, they secrete cytokines such as interleukin-1 (IL-1), interleukin-6 (IL-6), and tumor necrosis factor (TNF), which reach the hypothalamic temperature-regulating center. These cytokines promote the synthesis and secretion of prostaglandin E_2 (PGE$_2$) in the anterior hypothalamus. PGE$_2$ increases the thermostatic set point, and the autonomic nervous system is stimulated, resulting in shivering, muscle contraction, and peripheral vasoconstriction.

of these systemic changes are poorly understood but are probably due to complement activation and the release of *cytokines* (soluble factors secreted by WBCs that act as intercellular messengers) from stimulated WBCs. Three of these cytokines, interleukin-1 (IL-1), interleukin-6 (IL-6), and tumor necrosis factor (TNF), are important in causing the constitutional manifestations of inflammation, as well as inducing the production of fever. An increase in pulse and respiration follows the rise in metabolism as a result of an increase in body temperature. (Cytokines are discussed in Chapter 13.)

Fever. The onset of fever is triggered by the release of cytokines. The most potent of these cytokines are IL-1, IL-6, and TNF (released from mononuclear phagocyte cells). α-Interferon (α-IFN), β-interferon (β-IFN), and γ-interferon (γ-IFN) are also cytokines that can stimulate the responses to cause a fever.[2] These cytokines cause fever by their ability to initiate metabolic changes in the temperature-regulating center (Fig. 12-8). The synthesis of prostaglandin E_2 (PGE$_2$) is the most critical metabolic change. PGE$_2$ acts directly to increase the thermostatic set point. The hypothalamus then activates the sympathetic branch of the autonomic nervous system to stimulate increased muscle tone and shivering and decreased perspiration and blood flow to

the periphery. Epinephrine released from the adrenal medulla increases the metabolic rate. The net result is fever.

With the physiologic thermostat fixed at a higher-than-normal temperature, the rate of heat production is increased until the body temperature reaches the new set point. As the set point is raised, the hypothalamus signals an increase in heat production and conservation to raise the body temperature to the new level. At this point the individual feels chilled and shivers. The shivering response is the body's method of raising the body's temperature until the new set point is attained. This seeming paradox is dramatic: the body is hot yet an individual piles on blankets and may go to bed to get warm. When the circulating body temperature reaches the set point of the core body temperature, the chills

TABLE 12-9   Stages of the Febrile Response

STAGE	CHARACTERISTICS
Prodromal	Nonspecific complaints such as mild headache, fatigue, general malaise, muscle aches
Chill	Cutaneous vasoconstriction, "goose pimples," pale skin; feeling of being cold; generalized, shaking chill; shivering causing body to reach new temperature set by control center in hypothalamus
Flush	Sensation of warmth throughout body; cutaneous vasodilation; warming and flushing of skin
Defervescence	Sweating; decrease in body temperature

TABLE 12-10   Regenerative Ability of Different Types of Tissues

TISSUE TYPE	REGENERATIVE ABILITY
Epithelial	
Skin, linings of blood vessels, mucous membranes	Cells readily divide and regenerate
Connective Tissue	
Bone	Active tissue heals rapidly
Cartilage	Regeneration possible but slow
Tendons and ligaments	Regeneration possible but slow
Blood	Cells actively regenerate
Muscle	
Smooth	Regeneration usually possible (particularly in GI tract)
Cardiac	Damaged muscle replaced by connective tissue
Skeletal	Connective tissue replaces severely damaged muscle; some regeneration in moderately damaged muscle occurs
Nerve	
Neuron	Generally nonmitotic; do not replicate and replace themselves if irreversibly damaged
Glial	Cells regenerate; scar tissue often forms when neurons are damaged

GI, Gastrointestinal.

and warmth-seeking behavior cease.[3] The febrile response is classified into four stages (Table 12-9).

The released cytokines and the fever they trigger activate the body's defense mechanisms. Beneficial aspects of fever include increased killing of microorganisms, increased phagocytosis by neutrophils, and increased proliferation of T cells. Higher body temperatures may also enhance the activity of interferon, the body's natural virus-fighting substance (see Chapter 13).

Types of Inflammation. The basic types of inflammation are acute, subacute, and chronic. In *acute inflammation* the healing occurs in 2 to 3 weeks and usually leaves no residual damage. Neutrophils are the predominant cell type at the site of inflammation. A *subacute inflammation* has the features of the acute process but lasts longer. For example, infective endocarditis is a smoldering infection with acute inflammation, but it persists throughout weeks or months (see Chapter 36).

Chronic inflammation lasts for weeks, months, or even years. The injurious agent persists or repeatedly injures tissue. The predominant cell types present at the site of inflammation are lymphocytes and macrophages. Examples of chronic inflammation include rheumatoid arthritis and tuberculosis. Tuberculosis is a type of chronic granulomatous inflammation. A chronic inflammatory process is debilitating and can be devastating. The prolongation and chronicity of any inflammation may be the result of an alteration in the immune response.

HEALING PROCESS

The final phase of the inflammatory response is healing. Healing includes the two major components of regeneration and repair. **Regeneration** is the replacement of lost cells and tissues with cells of the same type. **Repair** is healing as a result of lost cells being replaced by connective tissue. Repair is the more common type of healing and usually results in scar formation.

Regeneration

The ability of cells to regenerate depends on the cell type (Table 12-10). Labile cells, such as cells of the skin, lymphoid organs, bone marrow, and mucous membranes of the gastrointestinal (GI), urinary, and reproductive tracts, divide constantly. Injury to these organs is followed by rapid regeneration.

Stable cells retain their ability to regenerate but do so only if the organ is injured. Examples of stable cells are liver, pancreas, kidney, and bone cells.

Permanent cells do not regenerate. Examples of these cells are neurons of the central nervous system (CNS) and cardiac muscle cells. Damage to CNS neurons or heart muscle can lead to permanent loss. Healing will occur by repair with scar tissue.

Repair

Repair is a more complex process than regeneration. Most injuries heal by connective tissue repair. Repair healing occurs by primary, secondary, or tertiary intention (Fig. 12-9).

Primary Intention. *Primary intention* healing takes place when wound margins are neatly approximated, such as in a surgical incision or a paper cut. A continuum of processes is associated with primary healing (Table 12-11). These processes include three phases.

Initial phase. The initial phase lasts for 3 to 5 days. The edges of the incision are first aligned and sutured (or stapled) in place. The incision area fills with blood from the cut blood vessels, and blood clots form. This forms a provisional matrix for WBC mi-

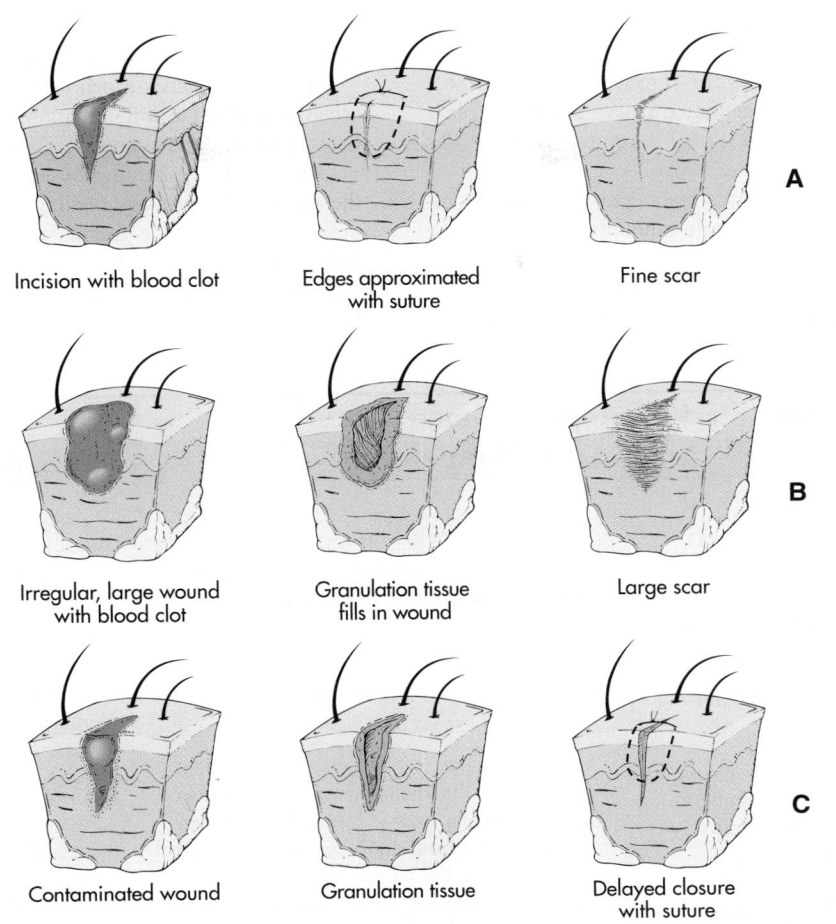

FIG. 12-9   Types of wound healing. **A,** Primary intention. **B,** Secondary intention. **C,** Tertiary intention.

Incision with blood clot   Edges approximated with suture   Fine scar   **A**

Irregular, large wound with blood clot   Granulation tissue fills in wound   Large scar   **B**

Contaminated wound   Granulation tissue   Delayed closure with suture   **C**

TABLE 12-11	**Phases in Primary Intention Healing**
PHASE	**ACTIVITY**
Initial (3 to 5 days)	Approximation of incision edges; migration of epithelial cells; clot serving as meshwork for starting capillary growth
Granulation (5 days to 4 weeks)	Migration of fibroblasts; secretion of collagen; abundance of capillary buds; fragility of wound
Scar contracture (7 days to several months)	Remodeling of collagen; strengthening of scar

gration. An acute inflammatory reaction occurs. The area of injury is composed of fibrin clots, erythrocytes, neutrophils (both dead and dying), and other debris. Macrophages ingest and digest cellular debris, fibrin fragments, and RBCs. Extracellular enzymes derived from macrophages and neutrophils help digest fibrin. As the wound debris is removed, the fibrin clot serves as a meshwork for future capillary growth and migration of epithelial cells.

Granulation phase. The *granulation (fibroblastic, proliferative, reconstructive)* phase is the second step and lasts from 5 days to 3 weeks. The components of granulation tissue include proliferating fibroblasts; proliferating capillary sprouts (angioblasts); various types of WBCs; exudate; and loose, semifluid, ground substance.

Fibroblasts are immature connective tissue cells that migrate into the healing site and secrete collagen. In time the collagen is organized and restructured to strengthen the healing site. At this stage it is termed *fibrous* or *scar tissue.*

During the granulation phase the wound is pink and vascular. Numerous red granules (young budding capillaries) are present. At this point the wound is friable, at risk for dehiscence, and resistant to infection.

Surface epithelium at the wound edges begins to regenerate. In a few days a thin layer of epithelium migrates across the wound surface. The epithelium thickens and begins to mature, and the wound now closely resembles the adjacent skin. In a superficial wound, reepithelialization may take 3 to 5 days.

Maturation phase and scar contraction. The maturation phase where scar contraction occurs overlaps with the granulation phase. It may begin 7 days after the injury and continue for several months or years. Collagen fibers are further organized, and the remodeling process occurs. Fibroblasts disappear as the wound becomes stronger. The active movement of the myofibroblasts causes contraction of the healing area, helping to close the defect and bring the skin edges closer together. A mature scar is then formed. In contrast to granulation tissue, a mature scar is virtually avascular and pale, and it may be more painful at this phase than in the granulation phase.

Secondary Intention. Wounds that occur from trauma, ulceration, and infection and have large amounts of exudate and wide, irregular wound margins with extensive tissue loss may not have edges that can be approximated. The inflammatory reaction may be greater than in primary healing. This results in more debris, cells, and exudate. The debris may have to be cleaned away (debrided) before healing can take place.

In some instances a primary incision may become infected, creating additional inflammation. The wound may reopen, and healing by secondary intention takes place.

The process of healing by secondary intention is essentially the same as by primary healing. The major differences are the greater defect and the gaping wound edges. Healing and granulation take place from the edges inward and from the bottom of the wound upward until the defect is filled. There is more granulation tissue, and the result is a much larger scar.

TABLE 12-12 Red-Yellow-Black Concept of Wound Care		
RED WOUND	**YELLOW WOUND**	**BLACK WOUND**
Characteristics		
Traumatic or surgical wound, possible presence of serosanguineous drainage, pink to bright or dark red healing or chronic wounds with granulating tissue	Presence of slough or soft necrotic tissue; liquid to semiliquid slough with exudate ranging from creamy ivory to yellow-green	Black, gray, or brown adherent necrotic tissue; possible presence of pus
Purpose of Treatment		
Protection and gentle atraumatic cleansing	Wound cleansing to remove nonviable tissue and absorb excess drainage	Debridement of eschar and nonviable tissue
Dressings and Therapy		
Transparent film dressing (e.g., Tegaderm, Opsite), hydrocolloid dressing (e.g., Duoderm), hydrogels (e.g., Vigilon), gauze dressing with antimicrobial ointment or solution, Telfa dressing with antibiotic ointment	Wound irrigations, hydrotherapy in conjunction with wet-to-dry dressing, moist gauze dressing with or without antibiotic or antimicrobial agent, hydrocolloidal dressing, hydrogel covered with gauze, absorption dressing (e.g., Debrisan beads, paste)	Topical enzyme debridement, surgical debridement, hydrotherapy, chemical debridement (e.g., Dakin's solution), moist gauze dressing, hydrogel covered with gauze, absorption dressing covered with gauze

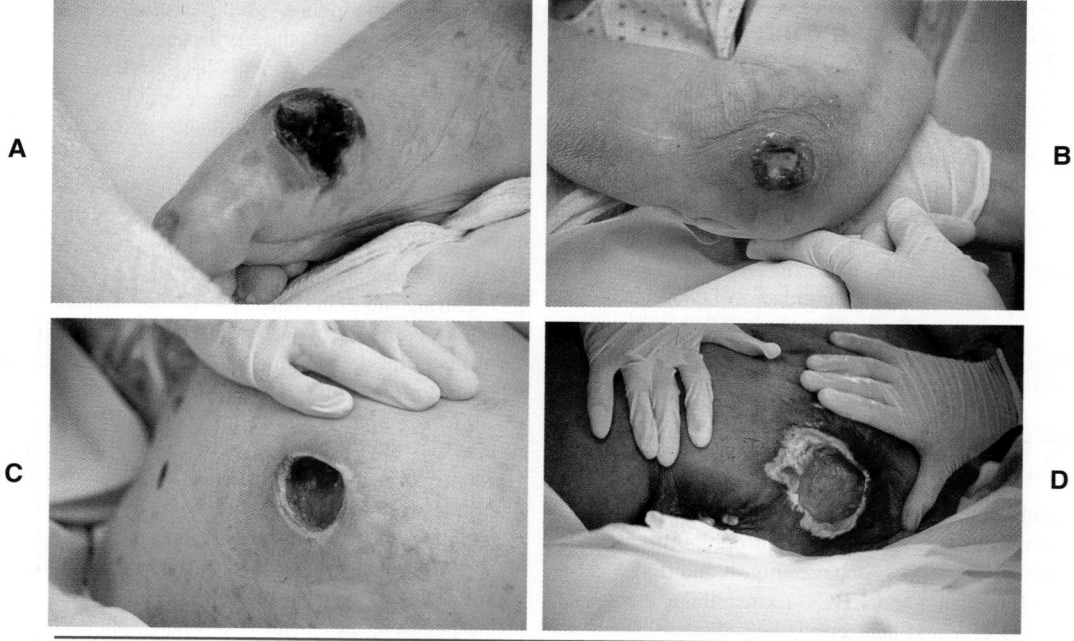

FIG. 12-10 Wounds classified by color assessment. **A**, A black wound. **B**, A yellow wound. **C**, A red wound. **D**, A mixed-color wound.

Wound classification. Identifying the etiology of a wound is essential to classifying the wound properly. Wounds can be classified by their cause (surgical or nonsurgical; acute or chronic) or depth of tissue affected (superficial, partial thickness, or full thickness).[4] A superficial wound involves only the epidermis. Partial-thickness wounds extend into the dermis. Full-thickness wounds have the deepest layer of tissue destruction because they involve the subcutaneous tissue and sometimes even extend into the fascia and underlying structures such as the muscle, tendon, or bone (see Fig. 24-3).

Another system that is sometimes used clinically to classify open wounds is based on the color of the wound (red, yellow, black) rather than on the depth of tissue destruction (Table 12-12, Fig. 12-10). It can be applied to any wound allowed to heal by secondary intention, including surgically induced wounds left to heal without skin closure because of a risk for infection. A wound may have two or three colors at the same time. In this situation the wound is classified according to the least-desirable color present.

Tertiary Intention. *Tertiary intention* (delayed primary intention) healing occurs with delayed suturing of a wound in which two layers of granulation tissue are sutured together. This occurs when a contaminated wound is left open and sutured closed after the infection is controlled. It also occurs when a primary wound becomes infected, is opened, is allowed to granulate, and is then sutured. Tertiary intention usually results in a larger and deeper scar than primary or secondary intention.

Delay of Healing

In a healthy person, wounds heal at a normal, predictable rate. Little can be done to accelerate this process. However, some factors delay wound healing. These are summarized in Table 12-13.

Complications of Healing

The shape and location of the wound determine how well the wound will heal. Complications result from interference with wound healing. These factors may include malnutrition, obesity, decreased blood supply, tissue trauma, denervation, wound debris such as necrotic tissue, and infection. Complications that may result include hypertrophic scars and keloids, contracture, dehiscence, excess granulation tissue, adhesions, and major organ dysfunction.

Hypertrophic Scars and Keloid Formation. Hypertrophic scars and keloid formation occur when the body produces excess collagen tissue. A **hypertrophic scar** is inappropriately large, red, raised, and hard. However, it remains confined to the wound edges and regresses in time. In contrast, a keloid is an even greater protrusion of scar tissue that extends beyond the wound edges and may form tumorlike masses (Fig. 12-11). In addition, keloids are permanent, without any tendency to subside. The patient with keloids often complains of tenderness, pain, and hyperesthesia, particularly in the early stages of development. A predisposition to keloid formation is thought to be hereditary and occurs more often in dark-skinned people, particularly African Americans. Neither complication is life threatening, but both can have serious cosmetic implications.

Contracture. Wound contraction is necessary for healing. This process may become abnormal when there is excessive contraction resulting in deformity or contracture. A shortening of muscle or scar tissue results from excessive fibrous formation, especially if the wound is near a joint (see Fig. 24-13). Contracture frequently occurs in burns in which a great loss of skin and subcutaneous tissue occurs (see Chapter 24).

Dehiscence. Dehiscence is the separation and disruption of previously joined wound edges. It usually occurs when a primary healing site bursts open. There are three possible contributing

TABLE 12-13   Factors Delaying Wound Healing

FACTOR	EFFECT ON WOUND HEALING
Nutritional deficiencies	
Vitamin C	Delays formation of collagen fibers and capillary development
Protein	Decreases supply of amino acids for tissue repair
Zinc	Impairs epithelialization
Inadequate blood supply	Decreases supply of nutrients to injured area, decreases removal of exudative debris, inhibits inflammatory response
Corticosteroid drugs	Impair phagocytosis by WBCs, inhibit fibroblast proliferation and function, depress formation of granulation tissue, inhibit wound contraction
Infection	Increases inflammatory response and tissue destruction
Mechanical friction on wound	Destroys granulation tissue, prevents apposition of wound edges
Advanced age	Slows collagen synthesis by fibroblasts, impairs circulation, requires longer time for epithelialization of skin, alters phagocytic and immune responses
Obesity	Decreases blood supply in fatty tissue
Diabetes mellitus	Decreases collagen synthesis, retards early capillary growth, impairs phagocytosis (result of hyperglycemia), reduces supply of O_2 and nutrients secondary to vascular disease
Poor general health	Causes generalized absence of factors necessary to promote wound healing
Anemia	Supplies less oxygen at tissue level

WBCs, White blood cells.

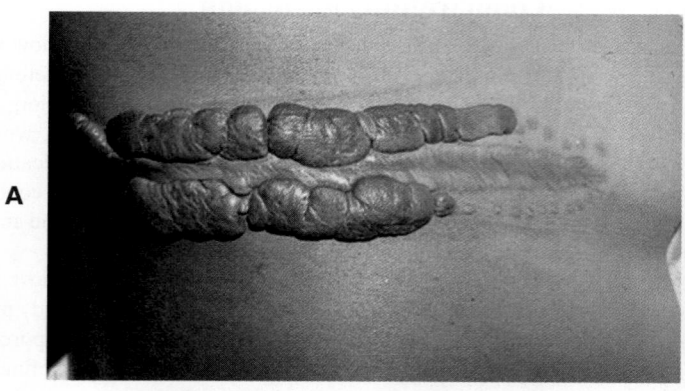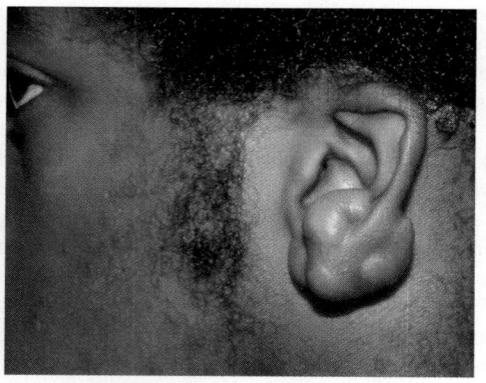

FIG. 12-11   A, Keloid formation resulting from suture mark. B, Large keloid scar in African American male.

causes of dehiscence. First, an infection may cause an inflammatory process. Second, the granulation tissue may not be strong enough to withstand the forces imposed on the wound. For example, during the granulation phase of wound healing, the patient is at risk for wound dehiscence. Third, obese individuals are at a high risk for dehiscence because adipose tissue interferes with healing. **Evisceration** occurs when wound edges separate to the extent that intestines protrude through the wound.

Excess Granulation Tissue. Excess granulation tissue ("proud flesh") may protrude above the surface of the healing wound. If the granulation tissue is cauterized or cut off, healing continues in a normal manner.

Adhesions. **Adhesions** are bands of scar tissue between or around organs. Adhesions may occur in the abdominal cavity or between the lungs and pleura. Adhesions in the abdomen may cause an intestinal obstruction. Adhesions between the lungs and pleura require decortication, or stripping of pleura, to permit normal ventilation.

Collaborative Care

Collaborative care related to inflammation and infection is highly variable. It depends on the causative agent, the degree of injury, and the patient's condition. Superficial skin injuries may only need cleansing. Adhesive strips may be used instead of sutures. The treatment plan can include covering these wounds with a film dressing to provide a moist healing environment and wound protection from trauma. Deeper skin wounds can be closed by suturing the edges together. If the wound is contaminated, it must be converted into a clean wound before healing can occur normally. Debridement of a wound that has multiple fragments or devitalized tissue may be necessary. If the source of inflammation is an internal organ (e.g., appendix, ruptured spleen), surgical removal of the organ is the treatment of choice.

Drug Therapy. Drugs are used to decrease the inflammatory response (Table 12-14). Antihistamine drugs may also be used to inhibit the action of histamine. (Antihistamines are discussed in Chapters 13 and 26.)

Antibiotic-resistant organisms. Organisms that have become resistant to antibiotics are becoming an ever-increasing problem in the treatment of infections. Organisms that consistently had been susceptible to all antimicrobial agents for years now have developed resistance not only to the classic agents but

also to newer agents. Methicillin-resistant *Staphylococcus aureus* (MRSA), vancomycin-resistant enterococci (VRE), and penicillin-resistant *Streptococcus pneumoniae* (PRSP) are three of the most troublesome bacterial strains of present concern (Table 12-15). Approximately 2 million nosocomial (hospital-acquired) infections occur in the United States each year, one half of which are caused by antibiotic-resistant organisms. More than 50% of all hospital-acquired *S. aureus* infections are methicillin resistant. (Resistance to *Mycobacterium tuberculosis* is discussed in Chapter 27.)[5]

These bacteria are highly adaptable organisms that have acquired resistance through clever mechanisms to evade pharmacologic innovations. Bacteria have evolved genetic and biochemical ways of resisting antimicrobial actions. Genetic mechanisms include mutation and acquisition of new DNA. Biochemically the bacteria resist antibiotics by producing enzymes that destroy or inactivate the drugs, altering drug target sites so the antibiotic cannot bind to the bacteria, and changing their cell walls to keep drugs out.[5]

Inappropriate antibiotic use has been one of the major factors contributing to the development of drug-resistant organisms. Health care providers often administer antibiotics for viral infections, are pressured by the patient to provide unnecessary antibiotic therapy, inadequately treat bacterial infections, and use broad-spectrum or combination agents for infections that should be treated with first-line antibiotics.

MRSA is spread primarily by direct contact with the hands of health care workers. The organism can remain viable for days on environmental surfaces and clothing. Hospital patients most at risk include those who are immunosuppressed (e.g., receiving chemotherapy, taking immunosuppressive therapy), have invasive devices (e.g., indwelling catheters), and/or have breaks in the skin barrier (e.g., surgical wound).

VRE is hardier than MRSA and can remain viable on environmental surfaces for weeks. An antiseptic soap such as chlorhexidine (Hibiclens) is needed to kill these bacteria.

As the magnitude of the problem continues to increase, nurses must become familiar with ways in which the emergence of resistance in bacteria can be prevented or minimized. Hand washing remains the first line of defense in preventing the spread of nosocomial bacteria. Patients and their families should be taught the proper use of antibiotics (Table 12-16). Appropriate use of

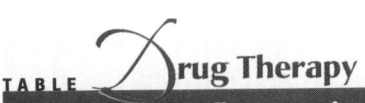

TABLE 12-14   Drug Therapy
Inflammation and Healing

DRUG	MECHANISMS OF ACTION
Antipyretic Drugs	
Salicylates (aspirin)	Lower temperature by action on heat-regulating center in hypothalamus, resulting in peripheral dilation and heat loss; interfere with formation and release of PGs; selectively depress CNS
acetaminophen (Tylenol)	Lowers temperature by action on heat-regulating center in hypothalamus
NSAIDs (e.g., ibuprofen [Motrin, Advil])	Inhibit synthesis of PGs
Antiinflammatory Drugs	
Salicylates	Inhibit synthesis of PGs, reduce capillary permeability
Corticosteroids	Interfere with tissue granulation, induce immunosuppressive effects (decreased synthesis of lymphocytes), prevent liberation of lysosomes
NSAIDs (e.g., ibuprofen [Motrin], piroxicam [Feldene])	Inhibit synthesis of PGs (see Fig. 12-7)
Vitamins	
Vitamin A	Accelerates epithelializatin
Vitamin B complex	Acts as coenzymes
Vitamin C	Assists in synthesis of collagen and new capillaries
Vitamin D	Facilitates calcium absorption

CNS, Central nervous system; *NSAIDs,* nonsteroidal antiinflammatory drugs; *PABA,* paraaminobenzoic acid; *PGs,* prostaglandins.

TABLE 12-15   Antibiotic-Resistant Organisms

	METHICILLIN-RESISTANT *STAPHYLOCOCCUS AUREUS* (MRSA)	VANCOMYCIN-RESISTANT ENTEROCOCCI (VRE)	PENICILLIN-RESISTANT *STREPTOCOCCUS PNEUMONIAE* (PRSP)
Location	Nasal secretions, skin	GI tract, female genital tract	Respiratory tract
Mode of transmission	Contact; person to person, contact with contaminated surfaces	Contact; person to person, contact with contaminated equipment	Droplets from respiratory tract
Nursing considerations	Wash hands with antiseptic soap Wear gloves for patient contact Isolate patient in private room Wear gown if soiling is likely	Wash hands with antiseptic soap Wear gloves for patient contact Isolate patient in private room Wear gown if soiling is likely Wear gown for patient contact	Wash hands with antiseptic soap Wear mask if coming in close contact with patient Isolate patient in private room

antibiotics is crucial to treatment success and reduction in the emergence of resistant pathogens.

Nutritional Therapy. There are special nutritional measures to consider to facilitate wound healing. A high fluid intake is needed to replace fluid loss from perspiration and exudate formation. An increased metabolic rate intensifies water loss. There is a 7% increase in metabolism for every 1° F increase in temperature above 100° F (37.8° C) or a 13% increase for every 1° C increase.

A diet high in protein, carbohydrate, and vitamins with moderate fat intake is necessary to promote healing. Protein is needed to correct the negative nitrogen balance resulting from the increased metabolic rate. Protein is also necessary for synthesis of

immune factors, leukocytes, fibroblasts, and collagen. Carbohydrate is needed for the increased metabolic energy required in inflammation and healing. If there is a carbohydrate deficit, the body will break down protein for the needed energy. Fats are also a necessary component in the diet to help in the synthesis of fatty acids and triglycerides, which are part of the cellular membrane. Vitamin C is needed for capillary synthesis, capillary formation, and resistance to infection. The B-complex vitamins are necessary as coenzymes for many metabolic reactions. If a vitamin B deficiency develops, a disruption of protein, fat, and carbohydrate metabolism will occur. Vitamin A is also needed in healing because it aids in the process of epithelialization. It increases col-

TABLE 12-16

Patient & Family Teaching Guide

Reduce Risk for Antibiotic–Resistant Infection

1. **Do not take antibiotics to prevent illness.** Doing this increases your risk for developing resistant infection. Exceptions include taking antibiotics before certain surgeries and taking antibiotics before dental work if you have a heart valve disorder.

2. **Wash your hands frequently.** Hand washing is the single most important thing you can do to prevent an infection.

3. **Follow directions.** Not taking your antibiotic as prescribed or skipping doses can encourage the development of antibiotic-resistant bacteria.

4. **Finish your antibiotic.** Do not stop taking your antibiotic as soon as you feel better. By stopping your antibiotic early, the hardiest bacteria survive and multiply. Eventually you could develop an infection resistant to many antibiotics.

5. **Do not request an antibiotic for flu or colds.** If your health care provider says that you do not need an antibiotic, chances are you do not. Antibiotics are effective against bacterial infections but not viruses, which cause colds and flus.

6. **Do not take leftover antibiotics.** People often save unfinished antibiotics for later use or borrow leftover drugs from family or friends. This is dangerous because (1) the leftover antibiotic may not be appropriate for you, (2) your illness may not be a bacterial infection, and (3) old antibiotics can lose their effectiveness and in some cases can even be fatal.

Adapted from September 1997 *Mayo Clinic Health Letter* with permission of Mayo Foundation for Medical Education and Research, Rochester, Minn.

COMPLEMENTARY & ALTERNATIVE THERAPIES
Herbs Used for Healing

Clinical Uses
The following herbs have been used topically for treating minor wounds, including sunburns, cuts, and abrasions: aloe, chamomile, echinacea, evening primrose, goldenseal, St. John's wort.

Effects
Although there is little scientific evidence, these herbs may have antiinflammatory actions.

Nursing Implications
These herbs should not be used on deep wounds. If used, they should be used after the wound has begun to heal. Aloe can safely be used on recent sunburns, minor burns, and superficial cuts and abrasions.

---

lagen synthesis and tensile strength of the healing wound. Patients are sometimes given vitamin A to counteract the effects of steroids on wound healing.

If the patient is unable to eat, enteral feedings and supplements should be the first choice if the GI tract is functional. Parenteral nutrition is indicated when enteral feedings are contraindicated or not tolerated. (Enteral and parenteral nutrition are discussed in Chapter 39.)

NURSING MANAGEMENT
INFLAMMATION, INFECTION, AND HEALING

■ Nursing Implementation

Health Promotion. The best management of inflammation is the prevention of infection, trauma, surgery, and contact with potentially harmful agents. This is not always possible. A simple mosquito bite causes an inflammatory response. Because occasional injury is inevitable, concerted efforts to minimize inflammation and infection are needed.

Adequate nutrition is essential so that the body has the necessary factors to promote healing when injury occurs. Individuals at risk for wound-healing problems are those with malabsorption problems (e.g., Crohn's disease, GI surgery, liver disease), defi-

cient intake or high energy demands (e.g., malignancy, major trauma or surgery, sepsis, fever), and diabetes. An individual should always be considered at risk for wound-healing problems if the following have occurred: (1) loss of 20% or more of total body weight in the preceding 6 months or (2) 10% loss of total body weight in the preceding 2 months.

Early recognition of the manifestations of inflammation and infection is necessary so that appropriate treatment can begin. This may be rest, drug therapy, or specific treatment of the injured site. Immediate treatment may prevent the extension and complications of inflammation.

Acute Intervention

Observation and vital signs. The ability to recognize the clinical manifestations of inflammation is important. In the individual who is immunosuppressed (e.g., taking corticosteroids or receiving chemotherapy), the classical manifestations of inflammation may be masked. In this individual, early symptoms of inflammation may be malaise or "just not feeling well."

Observation and recording of wound characteristics are essential. The consistency, color, and odor of any drainage should be recorded and reported if abnormal for the situation. *Staphylococcus* and *Pseudomonas* species are common organisms that cause purulent, draining wounds.

Vital signs are important to note with any inflammation and especially when an infectious process is present. When infection is present, temperature may rise, and pulse and respiration rates may increase. If a wound infection develops in a postoperative patient, vital signs will show a change within 3 to 5 days after surgery.

Fever. The most important aspect of fever management should be determining its cause. Although fever is usually regarded as harmful, an increase in body temperature is an important host defense mechanism. In the seventeenth century, Thomas Sydenham noted that "fever is a mighty engine which nature brings into the world for the conquest of her enemies."[6] Steps are frequently taken to lower body temperature to relieve the anxiety of the patient and medical personnel. Because mild to moderate fever usually does little harm, imposes no great discomfort, and may benefit host defense mechanisms, antipyretic drugs are rarely essential to patient welfare. Moderate fevers (up to 103° F [39.5° C]) usually produce few problems in most patients. However, if the patient is very young or very old, is extremely uncomfortable, or has a significant medical problem (e.g., severe cardiopulmonary disease, brain injury), the use of antipyretics should be considered. Fever in the immunosuppressed patient should be treated rapidly and antibiotic therapy begun because infections can rapidly progress to septicemia.

Fever (especially if greater than 104° F [40° C]) can be damaging to body cells, and delirium and seizures can occur. At temperatures greater than 105.8° F (41° C), regulation by the hypothalamic temperature control center becomes impaired, and damage can occur to many cells, including those in the brain.

Older adults have a blunted febrile response to infection.[3] The body temperature may not rise to the level expected for a younger adult or may be delayed in its onset. The blunted response can delay diagnosis and treatment. By the time fever (as defined for younger adults) is present, the illness may be more severe.

Several drugs are commonly used to lower the body temperature set point in the hypothalamus. Aspirin specifically blocks PG synthesis in the hypothalamus and elsewhere in the body. Acetaminophen acts on the heat-regulating center in the hypothalamus. Some NSAIDs (e.g., ibuprofen [Motrin, Advil]) have antipyretic effects (see Fig. 12-7). Corticosteroids are antipyretic through the dual mechanisms of inhibiting IL-1 production and preventing PG synthesis. The action of these drugs results in dilation of superficial blood vessels, increased skin temperature, and sweating.

Antipyretics should be given around the clock to prevent acute swings in temperature. Chills may be evoked or perpetuated by the intermittent administration of antipyretics. These agents cause a sharp decrease in temperature. When the antipyretic wears off, the body may initiate a compensatory involuntary muscular contraction (i.e., chill) to raise the body temperature back up to its previous level. This unpleasant side effect of antipyretic drugs can be prevented by administering these agents regularly and frequently at 2- to 4-hour intervals. Although sponge baths increase evaporative heat loss, there is no evidence that they decrease the body temperature unless antipyretic drugs have been given to lower the set point; otherwise, the body will initiate compensatory mechanisms (e.g., shivering) to restore body heat. The same principle applies to the use of cooling blankets; they are most effective in lowering body temperature when the set point has also been lowered. The nursing care of the patient with a fever is presented in NCP 12-1.

Rest and immobilization. Rest and immobilization of the inflamed area promote healing by decreasing the inflammatory process, assisting in the repair process, and decreasing metabolic needs. Immobilization with a cast, splint, or bandage lessens wound debris and the possibility of hemorrhage. The repair process is facilitated by allowing fibrin and collagen to form across the wound edges with little disruption. Rest helps the body better use its nutrients and oxygen for the healing process.

Elevation. Elevating the injured extremity will reduce the edema at the inflammatory site and increase venous return. Elevation helps reduce pain and improve the circulation of blood, which provides the oxygen and nutrients needed for healing.

NURSING CARE PLAN 12-1

Patient with a Fever

EXPECTED PATIENT OUTCOMES	NURSING INTERVENTIONS and *RATIONALES*
NURSING DIAGNOSIS	**Hyperthermia** *related to* infection *as manifested by* increased body temperature and increased heart and respiratory rate.
▪ Body temperature below 100° F (37.8° C)	▪ Assess patient's temperature every 2-4 hr *to monitor temperature.* ▪ Administer antipyretic drugs q3-4hr if ordered. ▪ Keep environmental temperature at 70° F (21.1° C). ▪ Avoid heavy layers of clothing or bed covers *to aid in lowering body temperature.* ▪ Change linen frequently if patient is diaphoretic *to prevent shivering and subsequent rise in body temperature from muscular activity.*
NURSING DIAGNOSIS	**Risk for deficient fluid volume** *related to* increased metabolic rate, diaphoresis, and decreased oral intake.
▪ No signs of dehydration	▪ Assess for rapid respirations and pulse; damp skin, clothing, and bed clothes; unwillingness or inability to ingest fluids; signs of dehydration such as dry lips and tongue, poor skin turgor, sunken eyes *to determine risk for or presence of fluid volume deficit.* ▪ Encourage fluid intake of 3-4 L/day if tolerated *to replace fluid lost as a result of fever and diaphoresis.* ▪ Monitor vital signs q2-4hr *because increasing pulse and respirations and decreasing blood pressure can indicate hypovolemia.* ▪ Administer IV fluids if necessary *to replace fluid loss if oral intake is inadequate.* ▪ Monitor intake and output accurately and carefully estimate insensible losses *to evaluate need for replacement.*

Oxygenation. Adequate oxygenation of the inflamed area is essential because oxygen promotes the differentiation of fibroblasts and collagen synthesis. Oxygen is also essential for cell growth and division. A person with arterial disease, hypovolemia, or hypotension is at great risk for infection and may benefit from oxygen administration.

Heat and cold. Applications of heat and cold are somewhat controversial interventions. Cold application is usually appropriate at the time of the initial trauma to cause vasoconstriction and decrease swelling, pain, and congestion from increased metabolism in the area of inflammation. Heat may be used later (e.g., after 24 to 48 hours) and when swelling has subsided to promote healing by increasing the circulation to the inflamed site and subsequent removal of debris. Heat is also used to localize the inflammatory agents. Warm, moist heat may help debride the wound site if necrotic material is present.

Normothermic wound therapy. Normotheric wound therapy (Warm-up Active Wound Therapy) is a specialized system that provides warm, moist wound healing. The system uses a noncontact, radiant-heat bandage. The device consists of a noncontact, domed wound cover into which a flexible infrared heating card is inserted. A battery pack powers the device and warms the wound to a predetermined temperature. The inside of the wound cover contains a foam ring, which acts as a wick to drain away exudate. This type of wound therapy is used in various types of chronic wounds.

Wound management. The type of wound management and dressings required depend on the type, extent, and characteristics of the wound.[7] The purposes of wound management include (1) cleaning a wound to remove any dirt and debris from the wound bed, (2) treating infection to prepare the wound for healing, and (3) protecting a clean wound from trauma so it can heal normally. Emergency care of the patient with a skin wound is presented in Table 23-6. Pressure ulcers are discussed in more detail later in this chapter.

Sutures and fibrin sealant are used to facilitate wound closure and create an optimal setting for wound healing. Most commonly sutures are used to close wounds because suture material provides the mechanical support necessary to sustain closure. A wide variety of suturing materials are available. In contrast, fibrin sealant is a biologic tissue adhesive that can function as a useful adjunct to sutures. Fibrin sealant can be used in conjunction with sutures or tape to promote optimal wound integrity, or it can be used independently to seal wound sites where sutures cannot control bleeding or would aggravate bleeding. This adhesive can effectively seal tissue and eliminate potential spaces. The use of fibrin sealant has resulted in a low rate of infection and has promoted healing. Further study is needed to determine the best fibrin sealant mixtures both to achieve hemostasis and to encourage healing.[8]

For wounds that heal by primary intention, it is common to cover the incision with a dry, sterile dressing that is removed as soon as the drainage stops or in 2 to 3 days. Medicated sprays that form a transparent film on the skin may be used for dressings on a clean incision or injury. Transparent film dressings are also commonly used (Fig. 12-12). Sometimes a surgeon will leave a surgical wound uncovered.

Wound healing management by secondary intention depends on the wound etiology and type of tissue in the wound. This type of management can be described as the red-yellow-black concept of wound care (see Table 12-12 and Fig. 12-10). Examples of types of wound dressings are presented in Table 12-17.

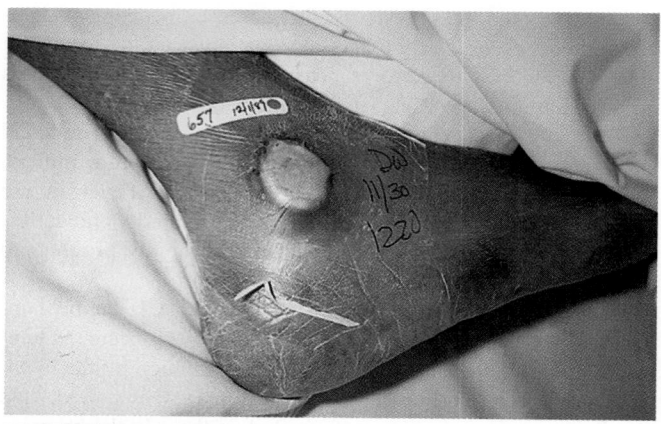

FIG. 12-12 Transparent film dressing.

Red wound. A *red wound* can be a superficial or deep wound if it is clean and pink in appearance. Examples include skin tears, pressure ulcers (stage II), partial-thickness or second-degree burns, and wounds created surgically that are allowed to heal by secondary intention. The purpose of treatment is protection of the wound and gentle cleansing (if indicated). Clean wounds that are granulating and reepithelializing should be kept slightly moist and protected from further trauma until they heal naturally. A dressing material that keeps the wound surface clean and slightly moist is optimal to promote epithelialization. Transparent film or adhesive semipermeable dressings (e.g., Opsite, Tegaderm) are occlusive dressings that are permeable to oxygen. Antimicrobials such as bacitracin, neomycin, and povidone-iodine ointment can be used if there is a wound infection; the wound is then usually covered with a sterile dressing. Unnecessary manipulation during dressing changes may destroy new granulation tissue and break down fibrin formation.

Yellow wound. A *yellow wound* has nonviable necrotic tissue, which creates an ideal situation for bacterial growth and therefore must be removed. The purpose of treatment is continual cleansing to remove nonviable tissue and to absorb excessive drainage. A type of dressing used in yellow wounds is an absorption dressing (e.g., calcium alginate, foam, hydrogel), which absorbs exudate and cleanses the wound surface. Absorption dressings work by drawing excess drainage from the wound surface. After these preparations are saturated with exudate, they should be removed by washing with sterile saline or water. The amount of wound secretions determines the number of dressing changes.

Hydrocolloid dressings such as Duoderm are also used to treat yellow wounds. The inner part of these dressings interacts with the exudate, forming a hydrated gel over the wound. When the dressing is removed, the gel separates and stays over the wound. The wound must be cleansed gently to prevent damage to newly formed tissue. These types of dressings are designed to be left in place for up to 7 days or until leakage occurs around the dressing.

Black wound. A *black wound* is covered with thick, dry, black necrotic tissue called *eschar.* Examples of black wounds include full-thickness or third-degree burns, pressure ulcers (stages III and IV), and gangrenous ulcers. The risk of wound infection increases in proportion to the amount of necrotic tissue present. The immediate treatment is debridement of the nonviable, eschar

TABLE 12-17 Types of Wound Dressings

TYPE	DESCRIPTION	EXAMPLES
Gauze	Provides absorption of exudates. Supports debridement if applied and kept moist. Can be used to maintain moist wound surface. Can be used as filler dressings in sinus tracts.	Numerous products available
Nonadherent dressings	Woven or nonwoven dressings may be impregnated with saline, petrolatum, or antimicrobials. Are minimally absorbent. Used mainly on minor wounds or as a second dressing.	Adaptic, Vaseline gauze, Xeroform
Transparent polyurethane films	Semipermeable membrane that permits gaseous exchange between wound bed and environment. Minimally absorbent so fluid environment is created in presence of exudate. Bacteria do not penetrate membrane. Used for dry noninfected wounds or wounds with minimal drainage.	Biocclusive, BlisterFilm, OpSite, Polyskin, Tegaderm, Transeal
Hydrocolloid	Presently comes in many forms. Occlusive dressing does not allow O_2 to diffuse from atmosphere to wound bed. Occlusion does not interfere with wound healing. Supports debridement and prevents secondary infections. Used for superficial and partial-thickness wounds with light to moderate drainage.	Comfeel, DuoDerm, IntraSite, Restore, Tegasorb
Polyurethane foams	Moderate to heavy amounts of exudates can be absorbed. Can be used on infected wounds. Used for partial- or full-thickness wounds or infected wounds.	Allevyn, Hydrasorb, Lyofoam
Absorption dressing	Large volumes of exudates can be absorbed. Supports debridement. Maintains moist wound surface. Placed into wounds and can obliterate dead space. For partial- or full-thickness wounds or infected wounds.	Debrisan, Kaltostat, Sorbsan
Hydrogel	Debridement because of moisturizing effects. Maintains moist wound surface. Provides limited absorption of exudates. Available as sheet, gel, and gauze. Most require a secondary dressing. Can dry out wounds. Used for partial- or full-thickness wounds, deep wounds with minimal drainage, and necrotic wounds. Has a cooling effect on the wound so is effective in managing painful wounds.	Aquasorb, ClearSite, Elastogel, Geliperm, IntraSite, Vigilon
Alginates	Highly absorbent dressing made from seaweed material. Available in rope and sheet forms. Dressing forms a gel-like substance which causes gentle debridement. Can dry out wounds. Used for wounds with moderate to heavy exudates. Requires a second dressing.	AlgiDERM, SeaSorb, Sorbsan, Mesalt, Kalfostat
Antimicrobial	Dressing is layered with crystalline silver, which has antibacterial and antifungal properties. Used for partial- to full-thickness wounds.	Acticoat

tissue. The debridement method used depends on the amount of debris and the condition of the wound tissue. There are several approaches to debridement:

1. *Surgical debridement.* This quickest method of debridement is indicated when large amounts of nonviable tissue are present and the patient is septic.
2. *Mechanical debridement.* This method is used when minimal debris is present. A common form of mechanical debridement is wet-to-dry dressings in which open-mesh gauze is moistened with normal saline, packed on or into the wound surface, and allowed to dry. Wound debris adheres to the dressing. When the dressing is removed, the coarse debris is entrapped in the gauze. One disadvantage to this method is that it is nonselective and will also debride some healthy tissue. This method of mechanical debridement is painful, and the patient should receive appropriate pain management before the removal of a wet-to-dry dressing.

Topical antimicrobials and antibactericidals (e.g., povidone-iodine [Betadine], Dakin's solution [sodium hypochlorite], hydrogen peroxide [H_2O_2], and chlorhexidine [Hibiclens]) should be used with caution in wound care because they can damage the new epithelium of healing tissue. Therefore they should never be used in a clean granulating wound.

Another method of mechanical debridement is wound irrigation. It is important to make sure that bacteria are not accidentally driven into the wound. Whirlpool is another method of mechanical debridement. Mechanical debridement should not be used in a clean granulating wound.

3. *Autolytic debridement.* Semiocclusive or occlusive dressings (see Table 12-17) may be used to promote softening of dry eschar by autolysis. These types of dressings are used in open wounds with necrotic debris and no infection. The area around the wound must be assessed for maceration when these dressings are used.
4. *Enzymatic debridement.* This method uses drugs that are applied topically to the necrotic tissue in the wound and then covered with moist dressing such as saline-moistened gauze. Examples of these drugs include collagenase and papain-urea. The manufacturer's directions must be followed because these products are different in terms of the pH range of use, frequency of application, and type of cleaning solutions to avoid.

Negative-pressure wound therapy. Negative-pressure wound therapy (vacuum-assisted wound closure) is a new type of therapy that uses suction to remove drainage and speed wound healing.[9] In this therapy the wound is cleaned, and a special dressing consisting of sponges packed with tubing and a transparent adhesive dressing is used. Sponges are placed into the wound to absorb drainage. Tubing from the wound is then attached to a pump, which creates a negative pressure in the wound bed. Wound types suitable for this therapy include acute or traumatic wounds, surgical wounds that have dehisced, pressure ulcers, and chronic ulcers.

Hyperbaric oxygen therapy. Hyberbaric O_2 therapy is the systemic delivery of O_2 at increased atmospheric pressures.[10] The patient is placed in an enclosed chamber where 100% O_2 is administered at 1.5 to 3 times the normal atmospheric pressure. This form of therapy accelerates granulation tissue formation and wound closure.

Infection prevention and control. The nurse and the patient must scrupulously follow aseptic procedures for keeping the wound free from infection. The patient should not be allowed to touch a recently injured area. The patient's environment should be as free as possible from contamination from items introduced by roommates and visitors. Antibiotics may be administered prophylactically to some patients. If an infection develops, a culture and sensitivity test should be done to determine the organism and the most effective antibiotic for that specific organism. The culture should be taken before the first dose of antibiotic is given.

Occupational Safety and Health Administration guidelines. The Occupational Safety and Health Administration (OSHA) standard for preventing occupational transmission of bloodborne pathogens was revised in 2001.[11] This standard mandated that any employer whose employees are potentially exposed to blood from needles and other sharps must implement sharps safety devices wherever feasible. In addition, employees at risk need to be provided appropriate personal protective equipment (PPE). The nurse needs to minimize or eliminate exposure to infectious material. When that is not possible, appropriate PPE must be selected. These include gloves, clothing, and facial protection (Table 12-18). Appropriate PPE will vary depending on the situation.

Infection precautions. If the patient develops an infection that is considered a risk to others, infection precautions may be needed. The purpose of these precautions is to prevent the transmission of organisms from patients to health care providers, from health care providers to patients, and from one patient to another. Four precaution systems were commonly used until recently: (1) category-specific precautions, (2) disease-specific precautions, (3) universal precautions, and (4) body substance isolation.

Category-specific precautions are recommended to prevent transmission of the most infectious diseases in each category (e.g., respiratory isolation, enteric isolation). This system frequently means more isolation precautions than necessary are required to prevent transmission of a certain organism.

Disease-specific precautions handle each infectious disease or condition separately. With this system, it is possible to list only those precautions necessary to interrupt transmission of the specific organism.

Universal precautions recommend that blood and body fluid precautions be consistently used for all patients, regardless of blood-borne infection status. Universal precautions are intended to prevent parenteral, mucous membrane, and nonintact skin exposure of health care workers to blood-borne pathogens. In addition, immunization with hepatitis B vaccine is recommended as an important adjunct to universal precautions for health care workers who are exposed to blood and blood products.[12]

The *body substance isolation* (BSI) system is intended to reduce nosocomial transmission of infectious agents among patients and to reduce the risk of transmission of infectious agents to health care personnel.

The Centers for Disease Control and Prevention (CDC) revised the guidelines for isolation precautions to incorporate features of all of these systems into a single easy-to-understand system.[13] The 1996 guidelines contain two levels of precautions (Table 12-19): *standard precautions*, which are designed for the care of all patients in hospitals and health care facilities regardless of their diagnosis or presumed infection status; and *transmission-based precautions*, which are used for patients known to be or suspected of being infected with epidemiologically important pathogens that can be transmitted by airborne or

---

TABLE 12-18 | **Occupational Safety and Health Administration (OSHA) Requirements for Personal Protective Apparel to Minimize Exposure to Blood-Borne Pathogens***

EQUIPMENT	INDICATIONS FOR USE
Gloves	Must be used when it can be reasonably anticipated that the employee may have contact with blood or other potentially infectious materials, when performing vascular access procedures,* and when handling or touching contaminated items or surfaces. Gloves must be replaced if torn, punctured, or contaminated or their ability to function as a barrier is compromised.
Clothing (gowns, aprons, caps, boots)	Need to be used when occupational exposure is anticipated. The type and characteristic will depend on the task and degree of exposure anticipated.
Facial protection (mask with glasses with solid side shields or a chin-length face shield)	Must be used when splashes, sprays, spatters, or droplets of blood or other potentially infectious materials pose a hazard to the eyes, nose, or mouth.

NOTE: Employers must provide, make accessible, and require the use of personal protective equipment (PPE) at no cost to the employee. PPE also must be provided in appropriate sizes. Hypoallergenic gloves or other similar alternatives must be made available to employees who have an allergic sensitivity to gloves.
*Some exceptions are made for voluntary blood donation centers.

TABLE 12-19   CDC Recommendations for Isolation Precautions in Health Care Facilities*

	STANDARD PRECAUTIONS	TRANSMISSION-BASED PRECAUTIONS: AIRBORNE	TRANSMISSION-BASED PRECAUTIONS: DROPLET	TRANSMISSION-BASED PRECAUTIONS: CONTACT
When to use	All patients	Use in addition to standard precautions for patients known to be or suspected of being infected with microorganisms transmitted by airborne droplet (e.g., measles, varicella, tuberculosis).	Use in addition to standard precautions for patient known to be or suspected of being infected with microorganisms transmitted by droplets (e.g., *Haemophilus influenzae, Neisseria meningitidis, Streptococcus pneumoniae, Mycoplasma pneumoniae*).	Use in addition to standard precautions for specified patients known to be or suspected of being infected with epidemiologically important microorganisms that can be transmitted by direct contact with patient (e.g., enteric pathogens, multidrug–resistant bacteria, *Staphylococcus aureus, Clostridium difficile,* herpes simplex) or in direct contact with environmental surface or patient care items in the patient's environment.
Hand washing	Wash hands after touching blood, body fluids, secretions, excretions, and contaminated items, regardless of whether gloves are worn; wash hands immediately after gloves are removed, between patient contacts, and to prevent transfer of microorganisms to other patients or environments.	Same as standard precautions.	Same as standard precautions.	Same as standard precautions.
Gloves	Wear nonsterile gloves when touching blood, body fluids, secretions, excretions, and contaminated items; put on clean gloves just before touching mucous membranes and nonintact skin; remove gloves promptly after use, before touching noncontaminated items, environmental surfaces, or going to another patient.	Same as standard precautions.	Same as standard precautions.	In addition to glove use as described in standard precautions, wear gloves when entering the room whenever providing direct patient care or having hand contact with potentially contaminated surfaces or items in patient's environment.
Mask, eye protection, face shield	Wear mask and eye protection or face shield to protect mucous membranes of eyes, nose, and mouth during procedures and patient care activities likely to generate splashes or sprays of blood, body fluids, secretions, and excretions.	In addition to standard precautions, wear respiratory protection when entering room of patient known to have or suspected of having tuberculosis.	In addition to standard precautions, wear a mask when working within 3 ft of patient.	Same as standard precautions.

*A complete listing of recommendations is published in Garner J: Guidelines for isolation precautions in hospitals, *Infect Control Hosp Epidemiol* 17:53, 1996. CDC, Centers for Disease Control and Prevention.

Continued

TABLE 12-19　CDC Recommendations for Isolation Precautions in Health Care Facilities—cont'd

	STANDARD PRECAUTIONS	TRANSMISSION-BASED PRECAUTIONS: AIRBORNE	TRANSMISSION-BASED PRECAUTIONS: DROPLET	TRANSMISSION-BASED PRECAUTIONS: CONTACT
Gown	Wear clean, nonsterile gown to protect skin and prevent soiling of clothing during procedures and patient care activities likely to generate splashes or sprays of blood, body fluids, secretions, or excretions or likely to cause soiling of clothing; remove gown promptly when tasks are completed; wash hands.	Same as standard precautions.	Same as standard precautions.	Wear clean, nonsterile gown if substantial contact is anticipated with patient, surfaces, or items in environment; wear gown if patient is incontinent or has diarrhea, an ileostomy, a colostomy, or uncontained wound drainage; remove gown carefully when tasks are completed; wash hands.
Linen	Handle, transport, and process used linen in manner that prevents skin and mucous membrane exposure, contamination of clothing, and environmental soiling.	Same as standard precautions.	Same as standard precautions.	Same as standard precautions.
Patient transport		Limit movement and transport of patient from room to essential purposes only; if transport or movement is necessary, minimize patient dispersal of droplet nuclei by placing surgical mask on patient, if possible.	Limit movement and transport of patient from room to essential purposes only; if transport or movement is necessary, minimize patient dispersal of droplet nuclei by masking patient, if possible.	Limit movement and transport of patient from room to essential purposes only; if transport is necessary, ensure that precautions are maintained to minimize contamination of environmental surfaces or equipment.

droplet transmission or by contact with dry skin or contaminated surfaces.[14,15]

The 1996 standard precautions system synthesizes the major features of universal precautions and BSI and applies to (1) blood; (2) all body fluids, secretions, and excretions regardless of whether they contain visible blood; (3) nonintact skin; and (4) mucous membranes. Standard precautions are designed to reduce the risk of transmission of microorganisms from both recognized and unrecognized sources of infection in hospitals. Standard precautions should be applied to all patients regardless of diagnosis or infection status.

Transmission-based precautions are designed for patients suspected or documented of being infected with highly transmissible or epidemiologically important pathogens for which additional precautions beyond standard precautions are needed to interrupt transmission in hospitals. The three types of transmission-based precautions are *airborne precautions, droplet precautions,* and *contact precautions.* They may be combined together for diseases that have multiple routes of transmission. When used either by themselves or in combination these precautions are used in addition to standard precautions.

All hospitals are encouraged to review and consider adoption of standard precautions and transmission-based precautions and dis-

continue use of the older forms of isolation precautions. The CDC offers hospitals the option of modifying the recommendations according to their needs and circumstances and as directed by federal, state, or local regulations. For example, OSHA's requirements are still operable, and all facilities are required to comply with these provisions. The CDC's 1996 standard precautions incorporate all requirements of OSHA's blood-borne pathogens standard.

Protective isolation. A low WBC count and depressed immune responses (e.g., in patient undergoing cancer chemotherapy, patient with neutropenia, or patient with leukemia or lymphoma) may in some facilities be placed on another type of isolation termed *protective (reverse) isolation.* The purpose of protective isolation is to protect the vulnerable patient from environmental sources of infection. However, some studies have not definitively proven that protective isolation is of value, and the use of this form of isolation is controversial. Institutional policies related to protective isolation vary considerably, and if they exist, they should be followed when the patient's condition warrants this intervention. (Protective isolation is discussed in Chapter 30.)

Psychologic implications. The patient may be distressed at the thought or sight of an incision or wound because of fear of scarring or disfigurement. Drainage from a wound often causes increased alarm. The patient needs to understand the healing process and the normal changes that occur as the wound heals. When a nurse is changing a dressing, inappropriate facial expressions can alert the patient to problems with the wound or the nurse's ability to care for it. Wrinkling of the nose by the nurse may convey disgust to the patient. A nurse should also be careful not to focus on the wound to the extent that the patient is not treated as a total person.

Ambulatory and Home Care. Because patients are being discharged earlier after surgery and many have surgery as outpatients, it is important that the patient, the family, or both know how to care for the wound and perform dressing changes. Wound healing may not be complete for 4 to 6 weeks or longer. Adequate rest and good nutrition should be continued throughout this time. Physical and emotional stress should be minimal. Observing the wound for complications such as contractures, adhesions, and secondary infection is important. The patient should understand the signs and symptoms of infection. The patient should note changes in wound color and the amount of drainage. The health care provider should be notified of any signs of abnormal wound healing.

Drugs will often be taken for a period of time after recovery from the acute infection. Drug-specific side effects and adverse effects should be reviewed with the patient; the patient should be instructed to contact the health care provider if any of these effects occur. Awareness of the necessity to continue the drugs for the specified time is an important point to teach the patient. For example, a patient who is instructed to take an antibiotic for 10 days may stop taking the drug after 5 days because of decreased or absent symptoms. However, the organism may not be entirely eliminated, and it may also become resistant to the antibiotic if the drug is not continued (see Table 12-16).

PRESSURE ULCERS*

Etiology and Pathophysiology

A **pressure ulcer** is a localized area (usually over a bony prominence) of tissue necrosis caused by unrelieved pressure that occludes blood flow to the tissues.[16] The most common site for pressure ulcers is the sacrum, with heels being second.[17] Factors that influence the development of pressure ulcers include the amount of pressure (intensity), the length of time the pressure is exerted on the skin (duration), and the ability of the patient's tissue to tolerate the externally applied pressure. It has yet to be determined whether pressure ulcers are formed because the tissue destruction occurs from the bone outward to the skin or from the epidermis inward toward the deeper tissue layers surrounding the bony prominence.[16] Besides pressure, **shearing force** (pressure exerted on the skin when it adheres to the bed and the skin layers slide in the direction of body movement), *friction* (two surfaces rubbing against each other), and *excessive moisture* contribute to pressure ulcer formation.[18] Factors that put a patient at risk for the development of pressure ulcers are presented in Table 12-20.

Clinical Manifestations

The clinical manifestations of pressure ulcers depend on the extent of the tissue that is involved. Pressure ulcers are graded or staged according to their deepest level of tissue damage or "wounding." Table 12-21 illustrates the four pressure ulcer stages

---
*This section written by Elizabeth A. Ayello.

TABLE 12-20   Risk Factors for Pressure Ulcers
• Advanced age
• Anemia
• Contractures
• Diabetes mellitus
• Elevated body temperature
• Immobility
• Impaired circulation
• Incontinence
• Low diastolic blood pressure (<60 mm Hg)
• Mental deterioration
• Neurologic disorders
• Obesity
• Pain
• Prolonged surgery
• Vascular disease

based on the National Pressure Ulcer Advisory Panel (NPUAP) guidelines.[19-21] When eschar is present, accurate staging of the pressure ulcer is not possible until the eschar is removed by debridement and the ulcer bed can be seen.[17]

If the pressure ulcer becomes infected, the patient may display signs of infection, such as leukocytosis and fever. In addition, the pressure ulcer may increase in size, odor, and drainage; have necrotic tissue; and be indurated, warm, and painful. The most common complication of a pressure ulcer is recurrence. Therefore it is important to note the location of previously healed pressure ulcers on an initial admission assessment of a patient.

NURSING *and* COLLABORATIVE MANAGEMENT
PRESSURE ULCERS

Care of a patient with a pressure ulcer requires local care of the wound and support measures of the whole person such as adequate nutrition, pain management, control of other medical conditions, and pressure relief. The current trend is to keep a pressure ulcer slightly moist, rather than dry, to enhance reepithelialization. In addition to the nurse, other members of the health team, such as the plastic surgeon, the dietitian, the physical therapist, and the occupational therapist, can provide valuable input into the complex treatment necessary to prevent and treat pressure ulcers. Both conservative and surgical strategies are used in the treatment of pressure ulcers, depending on the stage and condition of the ulcer. Therapeutic and nursing management are discussed together because the activities are interrelated.

■ Nursing Assessment

Patients should be assessed for pressure ulcer risk initially on admission and at periodic intervals based on the patient's condition and care setting.[22] For example, in acute care a patient should be reassessed every 48 hours; in long-term care, a resident should be reassessed weekly for the first 4 weeks after admission and then minimally monthly or quarterly; in home care a person should be reassessed every nurse visit.

Risk assessment should be done using a validated assessment tool such as the Braden scale[23] (Table 12-22). To obtain a patient's pressure ulcer risk assessment score on the Braden scale,

TABLE 12-21	**Staging of Pressure Ulcers**	
DEFINITION/DESCRIPTION	**DIAGRAM**	**CLINICAL PRESENTATION**

Stage I

A stage I pressure ulcer is an observable pressure-related alteration of intact skin whose indicators, as compared to an adjacent or opposite area on the body, may include changes in one or more of the following:

Skin temperature (warmth or coolness)

Tissue consistency (firm or boggy feel)

Sensation (pain, itching)

The ulcer appears as a defined area of persistent redness in lightly pigmented skin, whereas in darker skin tones, the ulcer may appear with persistent red, blue, or purple hues.

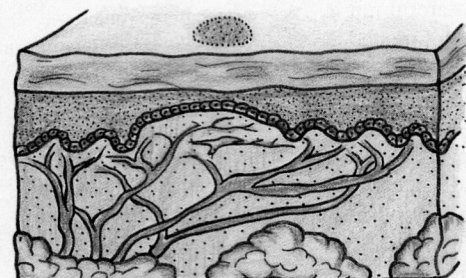 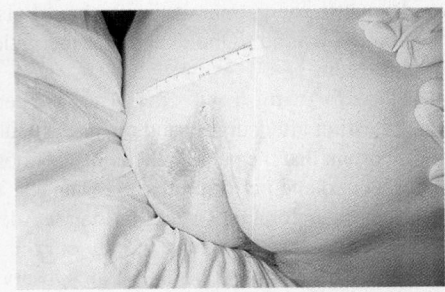

Stage II

Partial-thickness skin loss involving epidermis, dermis, or both. The ulcer is superficial and presents clinically as an abrasion, blister, or shallow crater.

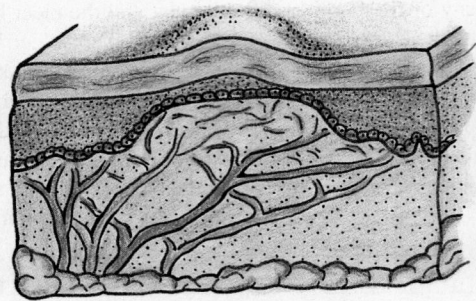 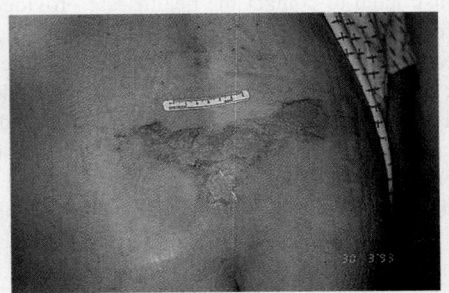

Stage III

Full-thickness skin loss involving damage to or necrosis of subcutaneous tissue that may extend down to, but not through, underlying fascia. The ulcer presents clinically as a deep crater with or without undermining of adjacent tissue.

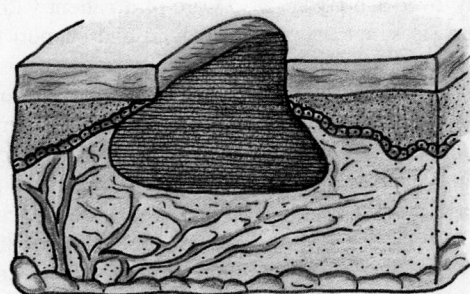 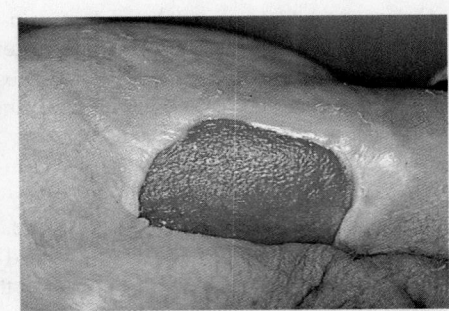

Stage IV

Full-thickness skin loss with extensive destruction, tissue necrosis, or damage to muscle, bone, or supporting structures (e.g., tendon, joint capsule). Undermining and sinus tracts may also be associated with stage IV pressure ulcers.

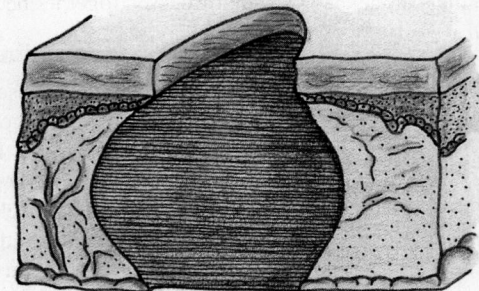 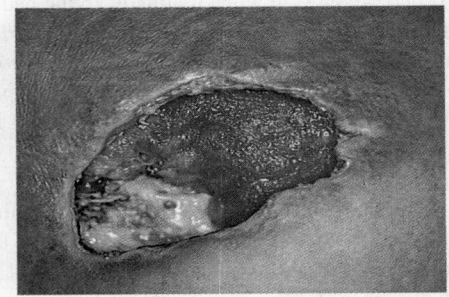

Source: Fifth National NPUAP Conference: Task Force on Darkly Pigmented Skin and Stage I Pressure Ulcers, approved Feb 1998, National Pressure Ulcer Advisory Panel.

TABLE 12-22   Braden Scale for Predicting Pressure Sore Risk

PATIENT'S NAME _____   EVALUATOR'S NAME _____

DATE OF ASSESSMENT _____

	POINT VALUE				SCORE
	1	2	3	4	

Sensory Perception—Ability to respond meaningfully to pressure-related discomfort

Completely limited: unresponsive (does not moan, flinch, or grasp) to painful stimuli, due to diminished level of consciousness or sedation or limited ability to feel pain over most of body	**Very limited:** responds only to painful stimuli; cannot communicate discomfort except by moaning or restlessness or has a sensory impairment that limits the ability to feel pain or discomfort over half of body	**Slightly limited:** responds to verbal commands, but cannot always communicate discomfort or the need to be turned or has some sensory impairment that limits ability to feel pain or discomfort in one or two extremities	**No impairment:** responds to verbal commands; has no sensory deficit that would limit ability to feel or to voice pain or discomfort	

Moisture—Degree to which skin is exposed to moisture

Constantly moist: skin is kept moist almost constantly by perspiration, urine, etc.; dampness is detected every time patient is moved or turned	**Very moist:** skin is often, but not always, moist; linen must be changed at least once per shift	**Occasionally moist:** skin is occasionally moist, requiring an extra linen change approximately once per day	**Rarely moist:** skin is usually dry, linen only requires changing at routine intervals	

Activity—Degree of physical activity

Bedfast: confined to bed	**Chairfast:** ability to walk severely limited or non-existent; cannot bear own weight and/or must be assisted into chair or wheelchair	**Walks occasionally:** walks occasionally during day, but for very short distances, with or without assistance; spends most of each shift in bed or chair	**Walks frequently:** walks outside room at least twice per day and inside room at least once every 2 hours during waking hours	

Mobility—Ability to change and control body position

Completely immobile: does not make even slight changes in body or extremity position without assistance	**Very limited:** makes occasional slight changes in body or extremity position but unable to make frequent or significant changes independently	**Slightly limited:** makes frequent though slight changes in body or extremity position independently	**No limitation:** makes major and frequent changes in position without assistance	

Nutrition—Usual food intake pattern

Very poor: never eats a complete meal; rarely eats more than ½ of any food offered; eats two servings or less of protein (meat or dairy products) per day; takes fluids poorly; does not take a liquid dietary supplement or is NPO and/or maintained on clear liquids or IVs for more than 5 days	**Probably inadequate:** rarely eats a complete meal and generally eats only about ½ of any food offered; protein intake includes only three servings of meat or dairy products per day; occasionally will take a dietary supplement or receives less than optimum amount of liquid diet or tube feeding	**Adequate:** eats over half of most meals; eats four servings of protein (meat or dairy products) per day; occasionally will refuse a meal, but will usually take a supplement when offered or is on a tube feeding or total parenteral nutrition regimen that probably meets most of nutritional needs	**Excellent:** eats most of every meal; never refuses a meal; eats four or more servings of protein (meat or dairy products); occasionally eats between meals; does not require supplementation	

Friction and Shear

Problem: requires moderate to maximum assistance in moving; complete lifting without sliding against sheets is impossible; frequently slides down in bed or chair, requiring frequent repositioning with maximum assistance; spasticity, contractures, or agitation lead to almost constant friction	**Potential problem:** moves feebly or requires minimum assistance; during a move skin probably slides to some extent against sheets, chair, restraints, or other devices; maintains relatively good position in chair or bed most of the time but occasionally slides down	**No apparent problem:** moves in bed and in chair independently and has sufficient muscle strength to lift up completely during move; maintains good position in bed or chair		

From Braden B, Bergstrom N: Predictive validity of the Braden scale for pressure sore risk in a nursing home population, *Res Nurs Health* 17:459, 1994. Copyright © Barbara Braden and Nancy Bergstrom. All rights reserved.

add the numeric scores for the factors in each of the six subscales (sensory perception, moisture, activity, mobility, nutrition, and friction and shear) to obtain the total score. Scores can range from 6 to 23. The lower the numeric score on the Braden scale, the higher the patient's predicted risk of developing a pressure ulcer. Incremental changes in the score indicate the level of risk: no risk (19 to 23), at risk (15 to 18), moderate risk (13 to 14), high risk (10 to 12), very high risk (9 or below). Knowing the level of risk can determine how aggressive preventive measures should be.

Identification of stage I pressure ulcers may be difficult for patients with dark skin.[24,25] Table 12-23 presents techniques to help assess darker skin. Subjective and objective data that should be obtained from a person with a pressure ulcer are presented in Table 12-24.

■ Nursing Diagnoses

Nursing diagnoses for the patient with a pressure ulcer may include, but are not limited to, these presented in NCP 12-2.

■ Planning

The overall goals are that the patient with a pressure ulcer will (1) have no deterioration of the ulcer stage, (2) reduce or eliminate the factors that lead to pressure ulcers, (3) not develop an infection in the pressure ulcer, (4) have healing of pressure ulcers, and (5) have no recurrence.

■ Nursing Implementation

Health Promotion. A primary nursing responsibility is the identification of patients at risk for the development of pressure ulcers (see Tables 12-20 and 12-22) and implementing pressure ulcer prevention strategies for those identified as being at risk. Prevention remains the best treatment for pressure ulcers. Devices such as alternating pressure mattresses, foam mattresses with adequate stiffness and thickness, wheelchair cushions, padded commode seats, foam boots, and lift sheets are useful in reducing pressure and shearing force. However, they are not adequate substitutes for frequent repositioning. Once a person has been identified as being at risk for pressure ulcer development, prevention strategies should be implemented (Table 12-25).

Acute intervention. Once a pressure ulcer has developed, the nurse should initiate interventions based on the ulcer characteristics (e.g., stage, size, location, amount of exudate, type of wound, presence of infection or pain) and the patient's general status (e.g., nutritional state, level of mobility). Careful documentation should be made of the size of the pressure ulcer. A wound-measuring card or tape can be used to note the ulcer's maximum length and width in centimeters. To find the depth of the ulcer, gently place a sterile cotton-tipped applicator into the deepest part of the ulcer. The length of the portion of the applicator that probed the ulcer can then be measured. Documentation of the healing wound can be done by using several available pressure ulcer healing tools such as the NPUAP Pressure Ulcer Scale of Healing (PUSH) tool[26,27] (see Fig. 23-12) and the Pressure Sore Status Tool (PSST).[28] Some agencies require that pictures of the pressure ulcer be taken initially and at regular intervals during the course of treatment.

Local care of the pressure ulcer may involve debridement, wound cleaning, application of a dressing, and relief of pressure. It is important to select the appropriate pressure-relieving technique (e.g., pad, overlay, mattress, specialty bed) to relieve pressure and

---

TABLE 12-23   Assessing Patients with Dark Skin
• Look for changes in skin color, such as skin that is darker (purplish, brownish, bluish) than surrounding skin.
• Use natural or halogen light source to accurately assess the skin color. Fluorescent light casts blue color, which can make skin assessment difficult.
• Assess the area for the skin temperature using your hand. The area may feel initially warm, then cooler.
• Touch the skin to feel its consistency. Boggy or edematous feel may indicate a stage I pressure ulcer.
• Ask the patient if he or she has any pain or itchy sensation.

TABLE 12-24   Nursing Assessment — Pressure Ulcers
Subjective Data
Important Health Information
Past health history: Stroke, spinal cord injury; prolonged bed rest or immobility; circulatory impairment; poor nutrition; altered level of consciousness; prior history of pressure ulcer; immunologic abnormalities; advanced age; diabetes; anemia; trauma
Medications: Use of narcotics, hypnotics, systemic corticosteroids
Surgery or other treatments: Recent surgery
Functional Health Patterns
Nutritional-metabolic: Obesity, emaciation; decreased fluid, calorie, or protein intake; vitamin or mineral deficiencies; clinically significant malnutrition as indicated by low serum albumin, decreased total lymphocyte count, and decreased body weight (15% less than ideal body weight)
Elimination: Incontinence of urine, feces, or both
Activity-exercise: Weakness, debilitation, inability to turn and position body; contractures
Cognitive-perceptual: Pain or altered cutaneous sensation in pressure ulcer area; decreased awareness of pressure on body areas; capacity to follow treatment plan
Objective Data
General
Fever
Integumentary
Diaphoresis, edema, and discoloration, especially over bony areas such as sacrum, hips, elbows, heels, knees, ankles, shoulders, and ear rims, progressing to increased tissue damage characteristic of ulcer stages*
Possible Findings
Leukocytosis, positive cultures for microorganisms from pressure ulcer

*See Table 12-21.

NURSING CARE PLAN 12–2

Patient with a Pressure Ulcer

EXPECTED PATIENT OUTCOMES	NURSING INTERVENTIONS and *RATIONALES*
NURSING DIAGNOSIS	**Impaired skin integrity** *related to* pressure and inadequate circulation *as manifested by* evidence of pressure ulcer.
• Intact skin • Healing of skin wound without complications	• Assess causative factors such as activity, mobility, presence or absence of sensory deficits, nutrition and hydration status, circulation and oxygenation, skin moisture status *to reduce or eliminate factors that contribute to development or progression of the pressure ulcer.* • Assess stage and document wound characteristics on a regular basis in relation to location, length, width and depth of wound, amount of granulation tissue visible and/or epithelialization, necrotic tissue, local or systemic infection, presence and character of exudate, including volume, color, consistency, and odor *to provide baseline and ongoing data for monitoring pressure ulcer.* • Use pressure relief devices (e.g., foam boots, wheelchair cushions). • Institute and document position change schedule q2hr *to avoid prolonged pressure in one area.* • Keep heels off of bed. Keep head of bed at or below 30-degree angle and flat when not contraindicated *to avoid sacral, buttock, and heel pressure.* • Use assistive devices (e.g., trapeze, turning sheets, lifts) to aid patient movement. • Protect patient's skin from excess moisture *to prevent maceration.* • Institute 2000 to 3000 calories/day (more if increased metabolic demands), 2000 ml/day of fluid *to provide calories, protein, and fluids necessary for tissue repair.* • Offer vitamin and mineral supplements if there are deficiencies. • Initiate prescribed treatment based on pressure ulcer characteristics and in accordance with AHCPR 1994 guidelines.* • Assess the psychosocial impact of pressure ulcer on the patient and caregivers and provide support or make referrals to other health care providers as indicated. • Teach patient and family about cause, prevention, and treatment of pressure ulcer *to prevent recurrence* (see Table 12-25).

*Pressure ulcer treatment: clinical practice guideline, no 95-0653, Dec 1994, Agency for Health Care Policy and Research, US Department of Health and Human Services.

Patient & Family Teaching Guide

TABLE 12-25   Pressure Ulcer

1. Identify and explain risk factors and etiology of pressure ulcers to patient and family.
2. Assess all at-risk patients at time of first hospital and/or home visit or whenever the patient's condition changes. Thereafter at regular intervals based on care setting (48 hours for acute care or every visit in home care).
3. Teach family care techniques for incontinence. If incontinence occurs, cleanse skin at time of soiling, use topical moisture barriers, and use pads or briefs that are absorbent.
4. Demonstrate correct positioning to decrease risk of skin breakdown. Instruct family to reposition bed-bound patient at least every 2 hours, chair-bound patient every hour. NEVER position the patient directly on the pressure ulcer.
5. Assess resources (i.e., adequacy of caregiver availability and skill, finances, and equipment) of patients requiring pressure ulcer care at home. When selecting ulcer care dressing, consider cost and amount of caregiver time.
6. Teach patient and/or caregiver to use clean dressings over sterile dressings using "no touch" technique when changing dressings. Instruct family on disposal of contaminated dressings.
7. Teach patient and family to inspect skin daily. Assess and document pressure ulcer status at least weekly; may require help from patient and family.
8. Evaluate program effectiveness.

keep the patient off of the pressure ulcer. A pressure ulcer that has necrotic tissue or eschar (except for dry, stable necrotic heels) must have the tissue removed by either surgical, mechanical, enzymatic, or autolytic debridement methods.[29] Once the pressure ulcer has been successfully debrided and has a clean granulating base, the goal is to provide an appropriate wound environment that supports moist wound healing and prevents disruption of the newly formed granulation tissue. Reconstruction of the pressure ulcer site by operative repair, including skin grafting, skin flaps, musculocutaneous flaps, or free flaps, may be necessary.

Pressure ulcers should be cleaned with noncytotoxic solutions that do not kill or damage cells, especially fibroblasts. Solutions such as Dakin's solution (sodium hypochlorite solution), acetic acid, povidone iodine, and hydrogen peroxide (H_2O_2) are cytotoxic and therefore should not be used to clean pressure ulcers.[29] It is also important to use enough irrigation pressure to adequately clean the pressure ulcer (4 to 15 psi) without causing trauma or damage to the wound.[29]

After the pressure ulcer has been cleansed, it should be covered with an appropriate dressing. Some factors to consider when selecting a dressing are maintenance of a moist environment, prevention of wound desiccation (drying out), ability to absorb the wound drainage, location of the wound, amount of caregiver time, cost of the dressing, presence of infection, clean versus sterile dressings, and care delivery setting.[29] A wet-to-dry dressing should never be used on a clean granulating pressure ulcer; this type of dressing should be used only for mechanical debridement of the wound. (Dressings are discussed in Table 12-17.)

Stage II through IV pressure ulcers are considered to be contaminated or colonized with bacteria. It is important to remember that in persons who have chronic wounds or who are immunocompromised, the clinical signs of infection (purulent exudate, odor, erythema, warmth, tenderness, edema, pain, fever, and elevated white cell count) may not be present even though the pressure ulcer is infected.

The maintenance of adequate nutrition is an important nursing responsibility for the patient with a pressure ulcer.[30] Often, the patient is debilitated and has a poor appetite secondary to inactivity. The 1994 Agency for Health Care Policy and Research (AHCPR) (now Agency for Healthcare Research and Quality [AHRQ]) Treatment Clinical Guidelines define clinically significant malnutrition as a serum albumin less than 3.0 g/dl, total lymphocyte count less than 1800/μl, or body weight decrease of more than 15%. Oral feedings must be adequate in calories, proteins, fluids, vitamins, and minerals to meet the patient's nutritional requirements. The caloric intake needed to correct and maintain a nutritional balance may be 30 to 35 calories per kilogram per day and 1.25 to 1.50 grams of protein per kilogram per day. Nasogastric feedings can be used to supplement the oral feedings. If necessary, parenteral nutrition consisting of amino acid and glucose solutions is used when oral and nasogastric feedings are inadequate. (Parenteral and enteral nutrition are discussed in Chapter 39.) NCP 12-2 outlines the care for the patient with a pressure ulcer.

Ambulatory and home care. Pressure ulcers affect the quality of life of patients and their caregivers. Because the recurrence of pressure ulcers is common, the education of both the patient and the care provider in prevention techniques is extremely important (see Table

---

EVIDENCE-BASED PRACTICE
Prevention and Treatment of Pressure Ulcers

Clinical Problem
Are pressure-relieving beds, mattresses, and cushions (support surfaces) effective for preventing and treating pressure ulcers?

Best Clinical Practice
- *Prevention.* There is good evidence of the effectiveness of high-specification foam over standard hospital foam. Pressure-relieving mattresses in the operating room reduce the incidence of pressure sores postoperatively.
- *Treatment.* There is good evidence that fluidized and low air loss beds improve healing. Seat cushions have not been adequately evaluated.

Implications for Nursing Practice
- Special products designed to prevent or assist in healing pressure ulcers, such as beds, mattresses, and cushions, are effective.
- Nurses need to identify patients at risk for the development of pressure ulcers and implement preventive measures, including pressure-relieving devices.
- When a pressure ulcer is being treated, pressure-relieving devices need to be used to assist in optimally treating the patient.

Reference for Evidence
Cullum N et al: Beds, mattresses, and cushions for pressure sore prevention and treatment, *Cochrane Database of Systematic Reviews* issue 1, 2002.

NURSING RESEARCH
Patient's Perspective of Having a Pressure Ulcer

Citation
Langemo DK et al: The lived experience of having a pressure ulcer, *Adv Skin Wound Care* 13:225, 2000.

Purpose
To explore the experience of living with a pressure ulcer

Methods
This qualitative, phenomenologic study explored the meaning of having a stage II, III, or IV pressure ulcer by eight respondents who ranged in age from 27 to 52 years. Unstructured interviews were held with four adults who currently had a pressure ulcer and four adults whose previous pressure ulcers had healed at least 6 months before the study. The seven men and one woman responded verbally to the following statement: "Please describe your experience of having a pressure ulcer. Share all the thoughts, perceptions, and feelings you can recall until you have no more to say about this experience."

Results and Conclusions
Pressure ulcers had a significant effect on the physical, social, and financial status of the respondents. Analysis of the verbatim interview transcripts resulted in the following seven major themes: perceived etiology of the pressure ulcer; life impact and changes; psychospiritual impact; extreme painfulness associated with the pressure ulcer; need for knowledge and understanding; need for and effect of numerous, stressful treatments; and the grieving process.

Implications for Nursing Practice
Although pressure ulcers are serious chronic wounds, little research has looked at the impact of having a pressure ulcer from the patient's perspective. By attempting to understand pressure ulcers from a patient's perspective, the nurse can provide empathetic, holistic care to the person who literally and figuratively has a "breakdown of self." Some of the patient issues that nurses need to assess and provide care for are body image changes, loss of independence, and loss of control.

12-25). (A sixth-grade level version of the patient guide to pressure ulcer prevention is available on the NPUAP website for use in patient teaching.) The care provider needs to know the etiology of pressure ulcers, prevention techniques, early signs, nutritional support, and care techniques for actual pressure ulcers. Because the patient with a pressure ulcer often requires extensive care for other health problems, it is important that the nurse support the caregiver through the added responsibility of pressure ulcer treatment.

■ Evaluation

Expected outcomes for the patient with a pressure ulcer are presented in NCP 12-2.

CRITICAL THINKING EXERCISES

Case Study
Inflammation and Infection

Patient Profile. Roger, a 75-year-old African American man, was admitted to the hospital emergency department with partial-thickness burns that involved his face, neck, and upper trunk. He also had a lacerated right leg. His injuries occurred about 24 hours earlier when he fell out of a tree onto his gas grill (which was lit) while trying to get his cat.

Subjective Data
- Complains of slightly hoarse voice and irritated throat
- States that he tried to treat himself because he does not have health insurance
- Has been coughing up sooty sputum
- Complains of severe pain in left hip

Objective Data
Physical Examination
- Leg wound is gaping and looks infected, temperature 101.1° F (38.4° C)
- X-rays reveal a fractured right tibia and fractured left hip

Laboratory Studies
- WBC count 26,400/μl (26.4 × 10^9/L) with 80% neutrophils (10% bands)

Collaborative Care
- Surgery is performed to repair the left hip

CRITICAL THINKING QUESTIONS
1. What clinical manifestations of inflammation did Roger exhibit, and what are their pathophysiologic mechanisms?
2. What type of exudate formation did he develop?
3. What is the basis for the development of the temperature?
4. What is the significance of his WBC count and differential?
5. Because his wound was deep, primary tissue healing was not possible. How would you expect healing to take place? What complications could he develop?
6. What risk factors does Roger have to develop a pressure ulcer?
7. Based on the assessment data provided, write one or more appropriate nursing diagnoses. Are there any collaborative problems?

REVIEW QUESTIONS

The number of the question corresponds to the same-numbered objective at the beginning of the chapter.

1. Physiologic hyperplasia is commonly found in
   a. a distended urinary bladder.
   b. the female breast during lactation.
   c. the bronchi of a chronic cigarette smoker.
   d. an enlarged myocardium in congestive heart failure.
2. When radiation therapy is used in the treatment of cancer, the desired effect is death of cancer cells by
   a. altering cellular metabolism and activity.
   b. producing mutations that interfere only with cancer cell function.
   c. accelerating metabolic reactions to reduce the normal life span of cells.
   d. stimulating synthesis of new particles that cause cell rupture and death.
3. A common cause of coagulation necrosis is
   a. autophagocytosis.
   b. pulmonary embolus.
   c. malignant brain tumor.
   d. peripheral vascular disease.
4. A patient with an impaired mononuclear phagocyte system will have
   a. increased circulation of histamine.
   b. decreased susceptibility to infection.
   c. decreased vascular response to cell injury.
   d. decreased surveillance for damaged or mutated cells.
5. The role of the complement system in opsonization affects which response of the inflammatory process?
   a. healing
   b. cellular
   c. vascular
   d. formation of exudate
6. Fever that accompanies inflammation is most likely caused by
   a. activation of the complement system.
   b. release of IL-1, IL-6, and TNF from monocytes.
   c. increased production and activity of neutrophils.
   d. massive vasodilation during the vascular response.
7. A patient has an open, infected surgical wound that is treated with irrigations and moist gauze dressings. The nurse expects that this wound
   a. is classified as a black wound.
   b. has to heal by tertiary intention.
   c. heals by regeneration of epithelial cells.
   d. heals by the same processes as an uninfected deep wound.
8. Contractures frequently occur after burn healing because of
   a. secondary infection.
   b. lack of adequate blood supply.
   c. weakness of connective tissue.
   d. excess fibrous tissue formation.

Continued

REVIEW QUESTIONS—cont'd

9. Rest and immobilization are important measures of acute care for wound healing because they
   a. decrease the inflammatory response.
   b. increase the circulation to the affected area.
   c. increase the body's production of corticosteroids.
   d. are known mechanisms to increase cytokine production.

10. An 85-year-old patient is assessed to have a score of 15 on the Braden scale. This means that the patient
    a. has an existing stage I pressure ulcer.
    b. is at risk for developing a pressure ulcer.
    c. is in need of a daily pressure ulcer risk assessment.
    d. is not at risk for developing a pressure ulcer at this time.

11. A 65-year-old stroke patient who is confined to bed is assessed to be at risk for the development of a pressure ulcer. Based on this information, the nurse should
    a. implement a q2hr turning schedule.
    b. have the patient maintain a high-fat diet.
    c. keep head of bed elevated to 90 degrees at all times.
    d. vigorously massage reddened bony prominences daily.

12. An 82-year-old man who is being cared for at home by his family has a 1 cm wide by 2 cm long pressure ulcer. The wound is shallow, measuring 0.5 cm in depth, and pink tissue is completely visible on the wound bed. This pressure ulcer should be documented as
    a. stage I.
    b. stage II.
    c. stage III.
    d. stage IV.

13. Which one of the following orders should a nurse question as part of the plan of care for a patient with a stage III pressure ulcer?
    a. pack the ulcer with foam dressing
    b. turn and position the patient every 2 hours
    c. clean the ulcer every shift with Dakin's solution
    d. assess for pain and medicate before dressing change

REFERENCES

1. Jackson M, Rickman LS, Pugliese G: Emerging infectious diseases, *Am J Nurs* 100:66, 2000.
2. Dinarello CA: Thermoregulation and the pathogenesis of fever, *Infect Dis Clin North Am* 10:433, 1996.
3. Nicoll LH: Heat in motion: evaluating and managing temperature, *Nursing* 32(suppl):1, 2002.
4. Van Rijswijk L: Wound assessment and documentation. In Krasner DL, Rodeheaver GT, Sibbald RG, editors: *Chronic wound care: a clinical source book for healthcare professionals*, ed 3, Wayne, Pa, 2001, HMP Communications.
5. Sheff B: Taking aim at antibiotic-resistant bacteria, *Nursing* 31:63, 2001.
6. Atkins E: Fever: its history, cause, and function, *Yale J Biol Med* 55:283, 1982.
7. Bello YM, Phillips TJ: Chronic leg ulcers: types and treatment, *Hosp Pract* 24:101, 2000.
8. Spotnitz WD, Falstrom JK, Rodeheaver GT: The role of sutures and fibrin sealant in wound healing, *Surg Clin North Am* 77:651, 1997.
9. Mendez-Eastman S: New treatment for an old problem: negative-pressure wound therapy, *Nursing* 32:58, 2002.
10. Boykin JV: How hyperbaric oxygen therapy helps heal chronic wounds, *Nursing* 32:24, 2002.
11. Occupational Safety and Health Administration: Occupational exposure to bloodborne pathogens: needlesticks and other sharps injuries, final rule, 29 CFR part 1910, *Federal Register* 66:5318, 2001.
12. Perry J: The bloodborne pathogens standard 2001, *Nursing* 31:32hn16, 2001.
13. Garner J: Guidelines for isolation precautions in hospitals, *Infect Control Hosp Epidemiol* 17:53, 1996.
14. Borton D: Isolation precautions, part 1: how to protect your patients and yourself, *Nursing* 31:14, 2001.
15. Borton D: Isolation precautions, part 2: matching conditions to precautions, *Nursing* 31:18, 2001.
16. Maklebust J, Sieggreen M: *Pressure ulcers—guidelines for prevention and nursing management*, ed 3, Springhouse, Pa, 2001, Springhouse.
17. Morison MJ: *The prevention and treatment of pressure ulcers*, St Louis, 2001, Mosby.
18. Bryant RA: *Acute and chronic wounds—nursing management*, ed 2, St Louis, 2000, Mosby.
19. National Pressure Ulcer Advisory Panel, Cuddigan J, Ayello EA, Sussman C, editors: *Pressure ulcers in America: prevalence, incidence, and implications for the future*, Reston, Va, 2001, NPUAP.
20. AHCPR Panel for the Prediction and Prevention of Pressure Ulcers in Adults: *Pressure ulcers in adults: prediction and prevention. Clinical practice guideline, number 3*, AHCPR pub no 92-0047, Rockville, Md, May 1992, Agency for Health Care Policy and Research, Public Health Service, US Department of Health and Human Services.
21. National Pressure Ulcer Advisory Panel Board of Directors, Cuddigan J, Berlowitz DR, Ayello EA, editors: Pressure ulcers in America: prevalence, incidence, and implications for the future—an executive summary of the National Pressure Ulcer Advisory Panel monograph, *Adv Skin Wound Care* 14:208, 2001.
22. Ayello EA, Braden B: Why is pressure ulcer risk assessment so important? *Nursing* 31:75, 2001.
23. Krasner DL, Rodeheaver GT, Sibbald RG, editors: *Chronic wound care: a clinical source book for healthcare professionals*, ed 3, Wayne, Pa, 2001, Health Management Communications.
24. Henderson CT et al: Draft definition of stage I pressure ulcers: inclusion of persons with darkly pigmented skin, *Adv Wound Care* 10:16, 1997.
*25. Lyder CH et al: The Braden scale for pressure ulcer risk: evaluating the predictive validity in black and Latino/Hispanic elders, *Appl Nurs Res* 12:60, 1999.
26. National Pressure Ulcer Advisory Panel: PUSH tool information and registration form. Available at *www.npuap.org*.
27. PUSH Task Force, Thomas DR et al: Pressure ulcer scale for healing: derivation and validation of the PUSH tool, *Adv Wound Care* 10:96, 1997.
*28. NPUAP PUSH Task Force, Stotts NA et al: An instrument to measure healing in pressure ulcers: development and validation of the pressure ulcer scale for healing (PUSH), *J Gerontol* 56:M795, 2001.
29. Bergstrom N et al: *Treatment of pressure ulcers. Clinical practice guideline, number 15*, AHCPR pub no 95-0652, Rockville, Md, 1994, US Department of Health and Human Services, Public Health Service, Agency for Health Care Policy and Research.
30. Ferguson M et al: Pressure ulcer management: the importance of nutrition, *Medsurg Nurs* 9:163, 2000.

*Nursing research–based reference.

RESOURCES

Advances in Skin and Wound Care
www.woundcarenet.com
American Society for Microbiology
1752 North Street NW
Washington, DC 20036
202-737-3600
www.asmusa.org
Association for Professionals in Infection Control and Epidemiology, Inc.
1275 K Street, NW, Suite 1000
Washington, DC 20005-4006
202-789-1890
Fax: 202-789-1899
www.apic.org/
Infection Control and Hospital Epidemiology
www.slackinc.com/general/iche/ichehome.htm
Infectious Diseases Society of America (IDSA)
66 Canal Center Plaza, Suite 600
Alexandria, VA 22314
703-299-0200
Fax: 703-299-0204
www.IDSociety.org
Johns Hopkins Healthcare Epidemiology and Infection Control
www.hopkins-heic.org/
National Center for Infectious Diseases, Antimicrobial Resistance
www.cdc.gov/drugresistance/
National Foundation for Infectious Diseases
4733 Bethesda Avenue, Suite 750
Bethesda, MD 20814
301-656-0003
Fax: 301-907-0878
www.NFID.org

National Pressure Ulcer Advisory Panel
11250 Roger Bacon Drive, Suite 8
Reston, VA 20190-5202
703-464-4849
Fax: 703-435-4390
www.npuap.org
Society for Healthcare Epidemiology of America, Inc. (SHEA)
19 Mantua Road
Mount Royal, NJ 08061
856-423-0087
Fax: 856-423-3420
www.shea-online.org/
World Health Organization
Regional Office for the Americas/Pan American Health Organization
525 23rd Street NW
Washington, DC 20037
202-974-3000
Fax: 202-974-3663
www.who.int/
Wound, Ostomy and Continence Nurses Society
WOCN National Office
4700 West Lake Avenue
Glenview, IL 60025
888-224-WOCN or 866-615-8560
Fax: 866-615-8560
www.wocn.org

For additional Internet resources, see the website for this book at *http://evolve.elsevier.com/Lewis/medsurg/*.

CHAPTER *13*

Genetics and Altered Immune Responses

Sharon Mantik Lewis
Duck-Hee Kang

LEARNING OBJECTIVES

1. Define common terms related to genetics and genetic disorders: autosome, carrier, heterozygous, homozygous, mutation, recessive, and sex-linked.
2. Compare and contrast the most common classifications of genetic disorders.
3. Describe the functions and components of the immune system.
4. Compare and contrast humoral and cell-mediated immunity regarding lymphocytes involved, types of reactions, and effects on antigens.
5. Identify the five types of immunoglobulins and their characteristics.
6. Differentiate among the four types of hypersensitivity reactions in terms of immunologic mechanisms and resulting alterations.
7. Identify the clinical manifestations and emergency management of a systemic anaphylactic reaction.

8. Describe the assessment and collaborative care of a patient with chronic allergies.
9. Describe the etiologic factors, clinical manifestations, and treatment modalities of autoimmune diseases.
10. Explain the relationship between the human leukocyte antigen system and certain diseases.
11. Describe the etiologic factors and categories of immunodeficiency disorders.
12. Identify the types and side effects of immunosuppressive therapy.
13. Describe new technologies in immunology, including hybridoma technology, recombinant DNA technology, and gene therapy.

KEY TERMS

anergy, p. 245	humoral immunity, p. 242
antigen, p. 239	hypersensitivity reaction, p. 245
autoimmunity, p. 254	immunocompetence, p. 245
cell-mediated immunity, p. 242	immunodeficiency, p. 256
cytokines, p. 242	immunosuppressive therapy, p. 257
human leukocyte antigens, p. 249	monoclonal antibodies, p. 259

GENETICS

Genetics has a profound impact on health and disease. The study of genetics has become increasingly important for health care professionals. The identification of a genetic basis for many diseases has affected the study of genetics and its relevance to nurses. This has directly influenced the care of patients at risk for or diagnosed with a disease that has a genetic basis.[1] Nurses need to know the basic principles of genetics, be familiar with the impact that genetics has on health and disease, and be prepared to assist the patient and family in dealing with genetic issues.[2]

Basic Principles of Genetics

In the 1860s, a monk named Gregor Mendel discovered how traits are transmitted from parents to offspring while experimenting with pea plants. This discovery led to the study of *genetics*, also known as the study of inheritance. (Common terms used in the study of genetics are listed and defined in Table 13-1.)

Genes. *Genes* are the basic units of heredity. There are approximately 30,000 to 40,000 genes in each person's genetic

makeup, or *genome*. The Human Genome Project is an effort to map all of the human genome (see Genetics in Clinical Practice box). Any change in gene structure leads to a *mutation* that may alter the type and amount of protein produced.

Genes are arranged in a specific linear formation along a chromosome. Each gene has a specific location on a chromosome, termed a *locus*. An *allele* is one of two or more alternative forms of a gene that occupy corresponding loci on homologous chromosomes. Each allele codes for a specific inherited characteristic. When two gene pairs are different alleles, the allele that is fully expressed is the *dominant allele*. The other allele that lacks the ability to express itself in the presence of a dominant allele is the *recessive allele*. Physical traits expressed by a person are termed *phenotype*, and the actual genetic makeup of the person is termed *genotype*.

Chromosomes. *Chromosomes* are contained in the nucleus of a cell and occur in pairs. There are 23 pairs of chromosomes; 22 of the 23 pairs of chromosomes are said to be *homologous* and are termed *autosomes*. Autosomes are the same in both males and females. The sex chromosomes make up the twenty-third pair of chromosomes. A female has two X chromosomes, and a male has one X and one Y chromosome. One chromosome of each pair is inherited from the mother and one from the father. One half of each child's chromosomes (and therefore the genetic makeup) comes from his or her father and one half from his or her mother.

DNA. Genes are made up of a nucleic acid called *deoxyribonucleic acid* (DNA). DNA stores genetic information and encodes the instructions for synthesizing specific proteins needed to maintain life. DNA also dictates the rate at which proteins will be made. The DNA molecule is double stranded and is identified as a double helix. Each DNA molecule is made up of many smaller molecules including sugar, nitrogenous bases, and phos-

---

Reviewed by Alissa D. Stanley, RN, BSN, Graduate Student, School of Nursing, University of Texas Health Science Center, San Antonio, Tex.

GENETICS in CLINICAL PRACTICE
Genetics in Clinical Practice Boxes

GENETIC DISORDER	LOCATION OF GENETICS BOX	
	CHAPTER	PAGE
α_1–Antitrypsin	28	660
Alzheimer's disease	58	1586
Ankylosing spondylitis	63	1734
Breast cancer	50	1367
Cystic fibrosis	28	681
Duchenne muscular dystrophy	62	1698
Familial adenomatous polyposis (FAP)	41	1082
Familial hypercholesterolemia	33	802
Hemachromatosis	30	720
Hemophilia A and B	30	726
Hereditary nonpolyposis colorectal cancer (HNPCC)	41	1083
Human genome project	13	235
Huntington's disease	57	1578
Ovarian cancer	52	1424
Polycystic kidney disease	44	1192
Sickle cell disease	30	716
Types 1 and 2 diabetes mellitus	47	1270

GENETICS in CLINICAL PRACTICE
Human Genome Project

The Human Genome Project (HGP), which was initiated in 1990, is an international effort to map all 30,000 to 40,000 human genes (the human genome) and determine the complete sequence of more than 3 billion DNA bases. It involves more than 2000 scientists from 20 institutions in 6 countries. The legal, social, and ethical issues that may arise from the project are also being addressed. The U.S. HGP is sponsored by the Department of Energy (DOE) and the National Institutes of Health (NIH).

The HGP will help improve the diagnosis of disease, allow for earlier detection of genetic predisposition to disease, and play a critical role in determining risk assessment for genetic-related diseases. In addition, the results of the HGP will assist in helping health care professionals match organ donors with recipients in transplant programs.

Websites covering the topic of the HGP include *Human Genome Project Information* at *www.ornl.gov/hgmis* and *NIH National Human Genome Research Institute* at *www.nhgri.nih.gov.*

TABLE 13-1   Glossary of Genetic Terms

TERM	DEFINITION
Allele	One of two or more alternative forms of a gene that can occupy a particular chromosomal locus
Autosome	Any chromosome that is not a sex chromosome
Carrier	Individual who carries a copy of a mutated gene for a recessive disorder
Chromosome	Gene-carrying structure in the nucleus of all human cells consisting of DNA and protein
Codominance	Two dominant versions of a trait that are both expressed in the same individual
Congenital	Condition present at birth
Dominant allele	Gene that is expressed in the phenotype of a heterozygous individual
Gene	Unit of hereditary information located on a specific part of a chromosome
Genetics	Study of inheritance
Genome	Complete genetic information of an organism
Hereditary	Transmission of a disease or condition from parent to offspring
Heterozygous	Having two different alleles for one given gene
Homozygous	Having two identical alleles for one given gene
Locus	Position of a gene on a chromosome
Mutation	Change in the DNA sequence of a gene affecting the original expression of the gene
Oncogene	Gene that is able to initiate and contribute to the conversion of normal cells to cancer cells
Pedigree	Family tree that contains the genetic characteristics and disorders of that particular family
Phenotype	Clinically expressed traits of an individual
Protooncogene	Normal cellular genes that are important regulators of normal cellular processes; mutations can activate them to become oncogenes
Recessive allele	Allele that has no noticeable effect on the phenotype in a heterozygous individual
Sex-linked gene	Gene located on a sex chromosome
Trait	Physical characteristic that one inherits, such as hair and eye color

phate units. The four nitrogenous bases making up DNA are adenine, thymine, guanine, and cytosine.

RNA. *Ribonucleic acid* (RNA) is very similar to DNA. Although they are very similar, there are some significant differences. Like DNA, RNA contains the nitrogenous bases adenine, guanine, and cytosine. However, RNA lacks the nitrogenous base thymine and instead contains uracil. RNA is single stranded and contains ribose instead of deoxyribose sugar. RNA transfers the genetic information obtained from DNA to the proper location for protein synthesis and plays a critical role during the synthesis of proteins (Fig. 13-1).

Protein Synthesis. *Protein synthesis,* or the making of proteins, occurs in two steps: *transcription* and *translation* (see

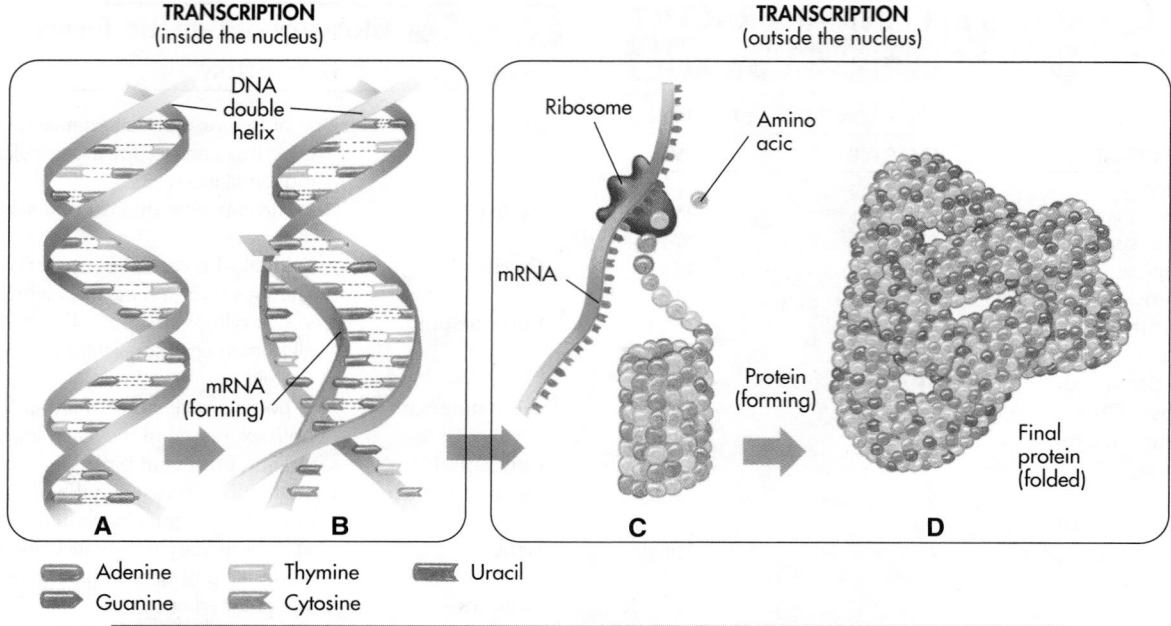

TRANSCRIPTION
(inside the nucleus)

DNA double helix

mRNA (forming)

A   B

TRANSCRIPTION
(outside the nucleus)

Ribosome

Amino acic

mRNA

Protein (forming)

Final protein (folded)

C   D

Adenine   Thymine   Uracil
Guanine   Cytosine

FIG. 13-1   A, The DNA molecule contains a sequence of genes. B, During transcription, the DNA code is transcribed as mRNA. C, During translation, the mRNA code is translated at the ribosome and the proper sequence of amino acids is assembled. The amino acid strand coils or folds as it is formed. D, The coiled amino acid strand folds again to form a protein molecule with a specific, complex shape.

Fig. 13-1). Transcription occurs inside the nucleus of the cell. A specialized type of RNA called messenger RNA (mRNA) enters the nucleus and makes an exact copy of the information needed from DNA. The mRNA then exits the nucleus of the cell and enters the cytoplasm where translation occurs. The mRNA becomes attached to a ribosome where another specialized type of RNA, transfer RNA (tRNA), arranges the amino acids in the correct sequence to assemble the protein. Once the protein is made, it is released from the ribosome and is able to perform its specific function.

Mitosis. *Mitosis* is a type of cell division that results in the formation of genetically identical daughter cells. The chromosomes of each cell duplicate. As a result of the division, two cells (daughter cells) form. These daughter cells contain identical sets of chromosomes, which are also identical to the cell that divided, or the parent cell.

Meiosis. *Meiosis* occurs only in sexual reproductive cells. In meiosis, the number of chromosomes is reduced, resulting in half of the usual number of chromosomes. Therefore oocytes and sperm contain only a single copy of each chromosome, whereas all other body cells contain duplicates of each chromosome.

In meiosis, a process known as crossing over may occur. *Crossing over* is when genetic material is exchanged between the two chromosomes in the cell. Because one chromosome is from the mother and the other from the father, the recombination from the process of crossing over creates a greater amount of diversity in the genetic makeup of the oocytes and sperm. During meiosis, a pair of chromosomes normally separates. However, sometimes this does not completely occur. *Nondisjunction,* the failure of the two chromosomes to separate during meiosis, causes an abnormal number of chromosomes. The result is an oocyte or sperm with two copies of the same chromosome, or sometimes a copy of a chromosome is missing. Examples of disorders caused by

chromosome abnormalities include Down syndrome and Turner syndrome. These disorders are characterized by physical and/or mental defects.

Inheritance Patterns

Genetic disorders can be categorized into autosomal dominant, autosomal recessive, or sex-linked (X-linked) recessive disorders (Table 13-2). If the mutant gene is located on an autosome, the genetic disorder is called *autosomal.* If the mutant gene is on the X chromosome, the genetic disorder is called *X-linked.*

Autosomal dominant disorders are caused by a mutation of a single gene pair (heterozygous) on a chromosome. Autosomal dominant disorders show variable expression. *Variable expression* means that the symptoms expressed by the individuals with the mutated gene vary from person to person even though they have the same mutated gene. Although autosomal dominant disorders have a high probability of occurring in families, sometimes these disorders cause a new mutation or skip a generation. This is termed *incomplete penetrance.*

Autosomal recessive disorders are caused by mutations of two gene pairs (homozygous) on a chromosome. *X-linked recessive disorders* are caused by a mutation on the X chromosome. Usually only men are affected by this disorder because women who carry the mutated gene on one X chromosome have another X chromosome to compensate for the mutation. However, women who carry the mutated gene can transmit the mutated gene to their offspring.

Multifactorial inherited conditions are caused by a combination of genetic and environmental factors. These disorders run in families but do not show the same inherited characteristics as the single-gene mutation conditions. Multifactorial conditions are poorly understood but include diabetes mellitus, obesity, hypertension, cancer, and coronary artery disease.

TABLE 13-2 | **Comparison of Genetic Disorders**

GENETIC DISORDER	CHARACTERISTICS	EXAMPLES
Autosomal dominant	Males and females are affected* equally More common than recessive disorders and usually less severe Affected individuals show variable expression Incomplete penetrance in some conditions Affected individuals will have an affected parent Children of a heterozygous (affected) parent will have a 50% chance of being affected Individuals affected in successive generations	Huntington's disease Familial hypercholesterolemia Neurofibromatosis Breast and ovarian cancer related to BRCA genes Marfan syndrome Hereditary nonpolyposis colorectal cancer
Autosomal recessive	Males and females affected equally Heterozygotes are carriers and usually asymptomatic Affected individuals will have unaffected† parents who are heterozygous for trait 25% chance offspring of heterozygous parents will be affected; 50% chance offspring will be carriers Usually there is a negative family history of disease	Cystic fibrosis Tay-Sachs disease Phenylketonuria Sickle-cell disease Thalassemia
X-linked recessive	Most affected individuals will have unaffected parents Affected individuals are usually males Daughters of affected male are carriers Sons of affected male are unaffected	Hemophilia Duchenne muscular dystrophy Wiskott-Aldrich syndrome

*Have the disease.
†Do not have the disease.

Genetic Testing

Genetic testing includes any procedure done to analyze chromosomes, genes, or any gene product that can determine a mutation or a predisposition to a condition. A blood sample or buccal smear is frequently used to obtain samples for genetic testing. Prenatal genetic testing can involve an amniocentesis or chorionic villus sampling (CVS) to obtain fetal cells. In an amniocentesis a small amount of amniotic fluid is removed. CVS involves the removal of a small amount of tissue from the placenta. The tissue has the same genetic makeup as the fetus.

Genetic tests include direct DNA testing, linkage testing, biochemical testing, and karyotyping.[3] Direct DNA testing examines either the DNA or RNA of the gene for any mutations. Linkage testing looks for gene markers that cause disease in family members from at least two generations. Biochemical testing includes analyzing gene products such as enzymes and proteins. Karyotyping investigates the number, form, size, and arrangement of the chromosomes.

Gene Therapy

Gene therapy can be used to replace or repair defective or missing genes with normal genes. A normal gene can be inserted into a human chromosome to counteract the effects of a missing or abnormal gene using recombinant DNA technology (see p. 260).

The first approved gene therapy trials involved children with severe combined immunodeficiency disease caused by adenosine deaminase deficiency. T lymphocytes from these children were obtained, and the missing gene was inserted into these T cells (Fig. 13-2). The new T cells were then reinjected into the children's bloodstreams. The gene signaled the cells to produce the

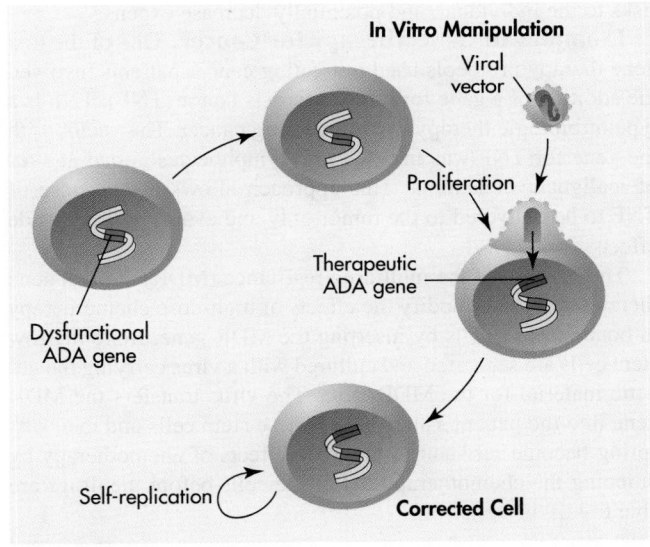

FIG. 13-2 Gene therapy for adenosine deaminase (ADA) deficiency attempts to correct this immunodeficiency state. The viral vector containing the therapeutic ADA gene is inserted into the patient's lymphocytes. These cells can then make the ADA enzyme.

missing enzyme, and these children were capable of developing a functioning immune system.

Gene therapy has been used for a variety of other genetic disorders, including cystic fibrosis, Gaucher's disease, familial hypercholesterolemia, α_1-antitrypsin deficiency, and Fanconi's anemia. Gene therapy is also being investigated in different types of cancer, including melanoma, renal cell, and hematologic malignancies.

Gene therapy is also being used in viral infections, including human immunodeficiency virus and hepatitis B and C.

Gene therapy has promise for treating a wide array of problems that do not respond to conventional methods of intervention. Although gene therapy is still experimental, the impact of adding another treatment option has created excitement and hope.

Methods of Gene Delivery. One of the major hurdles in gene therapy is finding a way to insert the gene into the body. This is done using *vectors* (gene carriers). The most common vectors are attenuated or modified versions of viruses. The modified viruses cannot replicate in the person, but are able to deliver genetic material.

Gene therapy can be done using ex vivo or in vivo methods. The ex vivo method, which is used most commonly, involves removal of target cells from the body to be altered genetically and then reinfused. This method has been used with lymphocytes, hepatocytes, skin keratinocytes, fibroblasts, and bone marrow cells. The disadvantage of this method is that nondividing cells (e.g., kidney, brain cells) are not easily grown in vitro. In this approach a vector virus carries the desired therapeutic gene into the human cell. The transduced cells are then reinfused back into the patient. Nonviral methods can also be used and usually involve physical transfection of the genetic material. One method involves direct microinjection of DNA into cells by particle acceleration.

In the in vivo method the altered gene and its vector are directly instilled into the patient. This approach allows more promise for its potential to directly affect disease sites, minimize risks to the individual, and potentially decrease expense.

Examples of Gene Therapy for Cancer. One of the first gene therapy protocols used in treating cancer patients involved the addition of a gene for tumor necrosis factor (TNF). TNF is a type of biologic therapy used in treating cancer. The vector with the gene for TNF was inserted into lymphocytes aimed at sites of malignant melanoma. This approach allows a high dose of TNF to be delivered to the tumor only and avoids systemic side effects.

The purpose of the multidrug resistance (MDR) clinical gene therapy trials is to modify the effects of high-dose chemotherapy in bone marrow cells by inserting the MDR gene. Bone marrow stem cells are separated and cultured with a virus carrying the genetic material for the MDR gene. The virus transfers the MDR gene into the patient's stem cells. These stem cells and their offspring become resistant to the toxic effects of chemotherapy by pumping the chemotherapy out of the cells before the drugs are able to kill the cells.

NURSING MANAGEMENT
GENETICS

It is imperative that nurses be knowledgeable about the fundamentals of genetics. By understanding the profound influence that genetics has on health and disease, the nurse can assist the patient and family in making critical decisions related to genetic issues, such as genetic testing. In addition, the nurse is responsible for referring patients, when necessary, for genetic counseling. The nurse should be able to give patients and their families accurate information pertaining to genetics, genetic diseases, and probabilities of genetic disorders. Inheritance patterns can be assessed by the nurse and explained to the patient and family

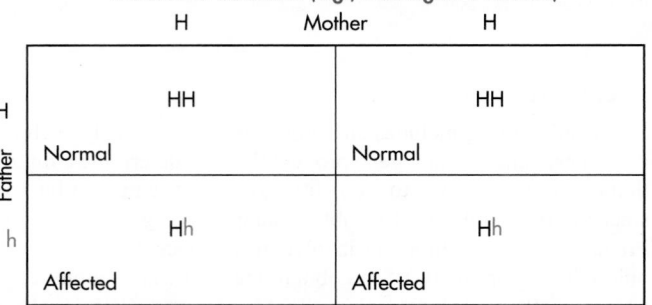

FIG. 13-3 Punnett squares can be used to determine inheritance possibilities. **A**, If the mother and father are both carriers for cystic fibrosis, there is a 25% chance that offspring will have cystic fibrosis. **B**, If the mother is a carrier for the hemophilia gene and the father has a normal genotype, there is a 50% chance that any male offspring will have hemophilia. There is a 50% chance that any female offspring will be a carrier. **C**, If the mother has a normal genotype and the father has Huntington's disease, there is a 50% chance that offspring will have the disease.

through the use of Punnett squares (Fig. 13-3) and/or family pedigrees.[4] Maintaining patient confidentiality and respecting the patient's values and beliefs is critical in upholding the professional role of the nurse.

Genetic testing may raise many psychologic issues.[5] Knowledge of a carrier status of a genetic disorder may influence a person's career plans and decisions for marriage and childbearing. It may also affect significant others in grappling with serious life and health care issues. Furthermore, there are ethical concerns. Who should know the result of a genetic test? How should the society or government protect individuals' privacy of test results and prevent individuals from discrimination? Genetic information should not be misused to stigmatize individuals or particular

(see Fig. 13-3)

ETHICAL DILEMMAS
Genetic Testing

Situation

A 30-year-old woman informs you that she is 3 months pregnant. She has two children with her current husband. This pregnancy was unplanned, and her youngest child has cystic fibrosis (CF). She expresses concern regarding the possibility of having another child with CF. She mentions that she would like to have genetic testing on her fetus. Her husband asks you if they will have another child with CF.

Important Points for Consideration

- With complete and accurate information, the woman and her husband can make a decision on their own without coercion from others.
- With genetic testing, the patient and her family can find out whether or not their child will have cystic fibrosis.
- Genetic counseling is a requirement before and after obtaining genetic testing because of the complexity of the information and the emotional issues involved.
- The nurse, knowing that cystic fibrosis is an autosomal recessive condition, can use Punnett squares (see Fig. 13-3) to show the woman and her husband the probability of having another child with CF.

Critical Thinking Questions

1. What information would you give the patient regarding genetic testing in order for her and her husband to make a decision?
2. What would you advise this couple to do?
3. How would you assist this couple in making a decision about possibly terminating the pregnancy if the results of the genetic testing show that the fetus tested positive for the CF gene?

TABLE 13-3   Types of Acquired Specific Immunity

Active
Natural
Natural contact with antigen through clinical infection (e.g., recovery from chickenpox, measles, mumps)
Artificial
Immunization with antigen (e.g., immunization with live or killed vaccines)

Passive
Natural
Transplacental and colostrum transfer from mother to child (e.g., maternal immunoglobulins in neonate)
Artificial
Injection of serum from immune human (e.g., injection of human γ-globulin)

immune to some of the infectious agents that cause illnesses in other species. *Acquired immunity* is the development of immunity, either actively or passively (Table 13-3).

Active Acquired Immunity. *Active acquired immunity* results from the invasion of the body by foreign substances such as microorganisms and subsequent development of antibodies and sensitized lymphocytes. With each reinvasion of the microorganisms, the body responds more rapidly and vigorously to fight off the invader. Active acquired immunity may result naturally from a disease or artificially through inoculation of a less virulent antigen (e.g., immunizations). Because antibodies are synthesized, immunity takes time to develop but is long lasting.

Passive Acquired Immunity. *Passive acquired immunity* implies that the host receives antibodies to an antigen rather than synthesizing them. This may take place naturally through the transfer of immunoglobulins across the placental membrane from mother to fetus. Artificial passive acquired immunity occurs through injection with γ-globulin (serum antibodies). The benefit of this immunity is its immediate effect. Unfortunately, passive immunity is short lived, because the host did not synthesize the antibodies and consequently does not retain memory cells for the antigen.

Antigens

An **antigen** is a substance that elicits an immune response. Most antigens are composed of protein. However, other substances such as large-size polysaccharides, lipoproteins, and nucleic acids can act as antigens. All of the body's cells have antigens on their surface that are unique to that person and enable the body to recognize self. The immune system becomes "tolerant" to the body's own molecules and therefore is nonresponsive to self.

Lymphoid Organs

The lymphoid system is composed of central (or primary) and peripheral lymphoid organs. The *central lymphoid organs* are the thymus gland and bone marrow. The *peripheral lymphoid organs* are the tonsils; gut-, genital-, bronchial-, and skin-associated lymphoid tissues; lymph nodes; and spleen (Fig. 13-4).

ethnic groups. Attention must be paid to better understand psychosocial needs of individuals and societal responses and health care policy related to genetic testing.

NORMAL IMMUNE RESPONSE

Immunity is a state of responsiveness to foreign substances such as microorganisms and tumor proteins. Immune responses serve three functions:[6,7]

1. *Defense.* The body protects against invasions by microorganisms and prevents the development of infection by attacking foreign antigens and pathogens.
2. *Homeostasis.* Damaged cellular substances are digested and removed. Through this mechanism the body's different cell types remain uniform and unchanged.
3. *Surveillance.* Mutations continually arise in the body but are normally recognized as foreign cells and destroyed.

Types of Immunity

Immunity is classified as innate (natural) or acquired. *Innate immunity* exists in a person without prior contact with an antigen. This type of immunity involves a nonspecific response, and neutrophils and monocytes are the primary white blood cells (WBCs) involved. One type of innate immunity present at birth is species specificity of infectious agents.[8] Humans are naturally

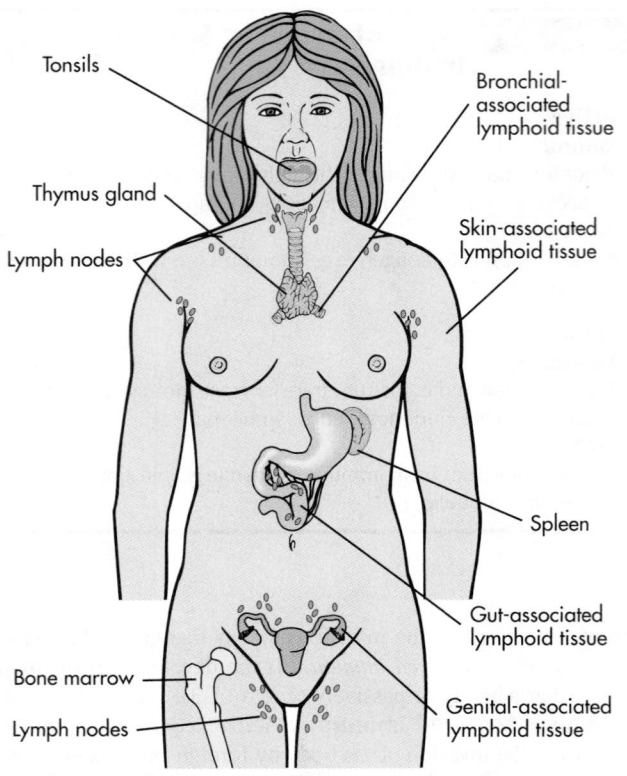

FIG. 13-4 Organs of the immune system.

Lymphocytes are produced in the bone marrow and eventually migrate to the peripheral organs. The thymus is important in the differentiation and maturation of T lymphocytes and is therefore essential for a cell-mediated immune response. During childhood the gland is large. The gland shrinks with age and is a collection of reticular fibers, lymphocytes, and connective tissue in older persons.

Lymphoid tissue is found in the submucosa of the respiratory (bronchial-associated), genitourinary (genital-associated), and gastrointestinal (gut-associated) tracts. This tissue protects the body surface from external microorganisms. The tonsils are a typical example of lymphoid tissue.

The skin-associated lymph tissue primarily consists of lymphocytes and Langerhans' cells (a type of resident macrophage) found in the epidermis of skin. When Langerhans' cells are depleted, the skin can neither initiate an immune response nor support a skin-localized delayed hypersensitivity response.

When antigens are introduced into the body, they may be carried by the bloodstream or lymph channels to regional lymph nodes. The antigens interact with B and T lymphocytes and macrophages in the lymph node. The two important functions of lymph nodes are (1) filtration of foreign material brought to the site and (2) circulation of lymphocytes.

The spleen is important as the primary site for filtering foreign substances from the blood. It consists of two kinds of tissue: white pulp containing B and T lymphocytes and red pulp containing erythrocytes. Macrophages line the pulp and sinuses of the spleen. The spleen is the major site of immune responses to blood-borne antigens. If the spleen is removed in children, it can predispose them to life-threatening septicemia.

Cells Involved in Immune Response

Mononuclear Phagocytes. The *mononuclear phagocyte system* includes monocytes in the blood and macrophages found throughout the body. (See Chapter 12 for a more complete description of macrophages.) Mononuclear phagocytes have a critical role in the immune system. They are responsible for capturing, processing, and presenting the antigen to the lymphocytes. This stimulates a humoral or cell-mediated immune response. Capturing is accomplished through phagocytosis. The macrophage-bound antigen, which is highly immunogenic, is presented to circulating T or B lymphocytes and thus triggers an immune response (Fig. 13-5).

Lymphocytes. Lymphocytes are produced in the bone marrow (Fig. 13-6). Lymphocytes differentiate into B and T lymphocytes.

B lymphocytes. In birds, *B lymphocytes* (bursa-equivalent lymphocytes) mature under the influence of the bursa of Fabricius. However, this lymphoid organ does not exist in humans. The bursa-equivalent tissue in humans is the bone marrow. B cells differentiate into *plasma cells* when activated. Plasma cells produce antibodies (immunoglobulins) (Table 13-4).

T lymphocytes. Cells that migrate from the bone marrow to the thymus differentiate into *T lymphocytes* (thymus-dependent cells). The thymus secretes hormones, including thymosin, that stimulate the maturation and differentiation of T lymphocytes. T cells compose 70% to 80% of the circulating lymphocytes and are primarily responsible for immunity to intracellular viruses, tumor cells, and fungi. T cells live from a few months to the life span of an individual and account for long-term immunity.

T lymphocytes can be categorized into T cytotoxic, T helper, and T suppressor cells. Antigenic characteristics of WBCs have now been classified using monoclonal antibodies. These antigens are classified as *clusters of differentiation* or *CD antigens*. Many types of WBCs, especially lymphocytes, are referred to by their CD designations. All mature T cells have the CD3 antigen.[7]

T cytotoxic cells. T cytotoxic cells are involved in attacking antigens on the cell membrane of foreign pathogens and releasing cytolytic substances that destroy the pathogen. These cells have antigen specificity and are sensitized by exposure to the antigen.[9] Similar to B lymphocytes, some sensitized T cells do not attack the antigen but remain as memory T cells. As in the humoral immune response, a second exposure to the antigen will result in a more intense and rapid cell-mediated immune response.

T helper and T suppressor cells. T helper (CD4) cells and T suppressor (CD8) cells are involved in the regulation of cell-mediated immunity and the humoral antibody response. These two cell types are often referred to as immunoregulatory cells. With many autoimmune diseases the number of T suppressor cells decreases in proportion to the number of T helper cells, thus resulting in an overaggressive immune response. The human immunodeficiency virus (HIV) invades T helper cells, thus decreasing their number and function. Therefore individuals with HIV infection do not mount an aggressive immune response and are at an increased risk for opportunistic infections and malignancies.

Natural killer cells. Natural killer (NK) cells are also involved in cell-mediated immunity. These cells are not T or B cells, but are large lymphocytes with numerous granules in the cytoplasm. NK cells do not require prior sensitization for their generation. These cells are involved in recognition and killing of virus-infected cells, tumor cells, and transplanted grafts. The mechanism of recognition is not fully understood. NK cells have a significant role in immune surveillance for malignant cell changes.

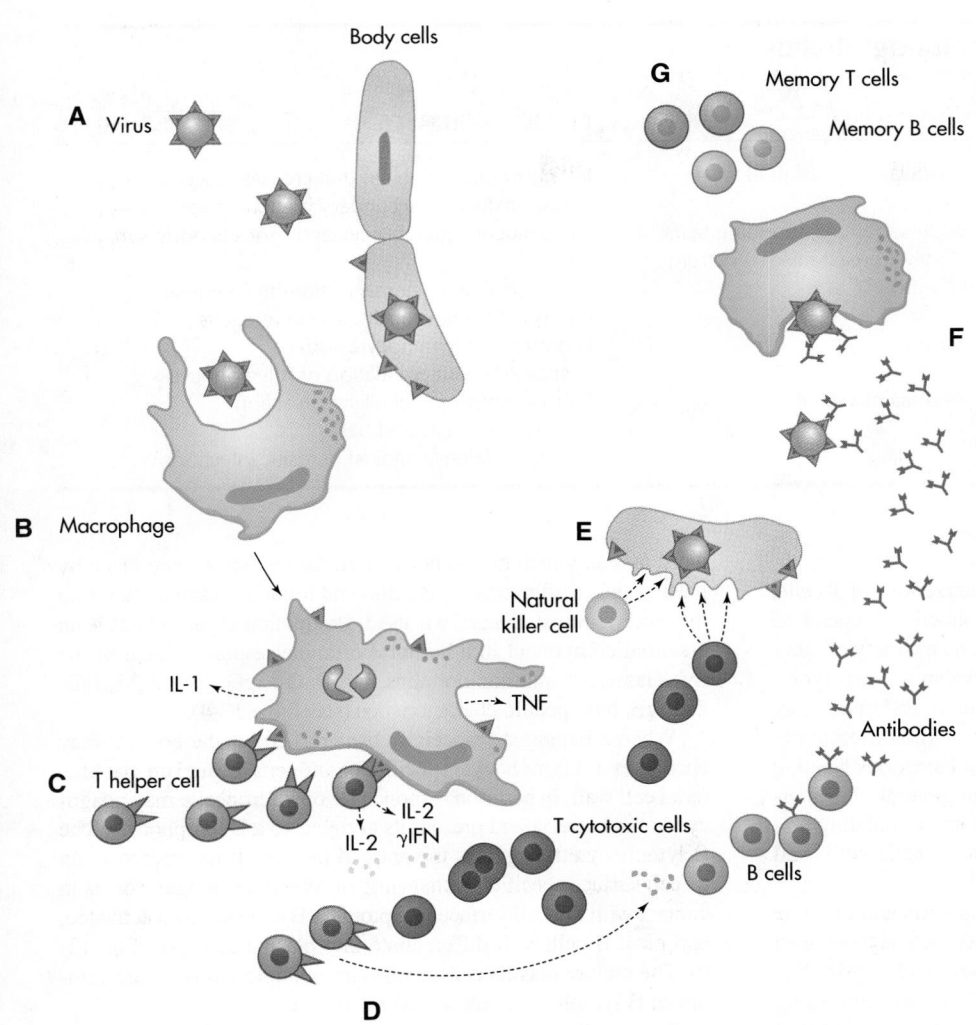

FIG. 13-5 The immune response to a virus. **A,** A virus invades the body through a break in the skin or another portal of entry. The virus must make its way inside a cell in order to replicate itself. **B,** A macrophage recognizes the antigens on the surface of the virus. The macrophage digests the virus and displays pieces of the virus (antigens) on its surface. **C,** A T helper cell recognizes the antigen displayed and binds to the macrophage. This binding stimulates the production of cytokines (interleukin-1 [IL-1] and tumor necrosis factor [TNF]) by the macrophage and interleukin-2 (IL-2) and γ-interferon (γIFN) by the T cell. These cytokines are intercellular messengers that provide communication among the cells. **D,** IL-2 instructs other T helper cells and T cytotoxic cells to proliferate (multiply). T helper cells release cytokines, causing B cells to multiply and produce antibodies. **E,** T cytotoxic cells and natural killer cells destroy infected body cells. **F,** The antibodies bind to the virus and mark it for macrophage destruction. **G,** Once the virus is gone, activated T and B cells are turned off by suppressor T cells. Memory B and T cells remain behind to respond quickly if the same virus attacks again.

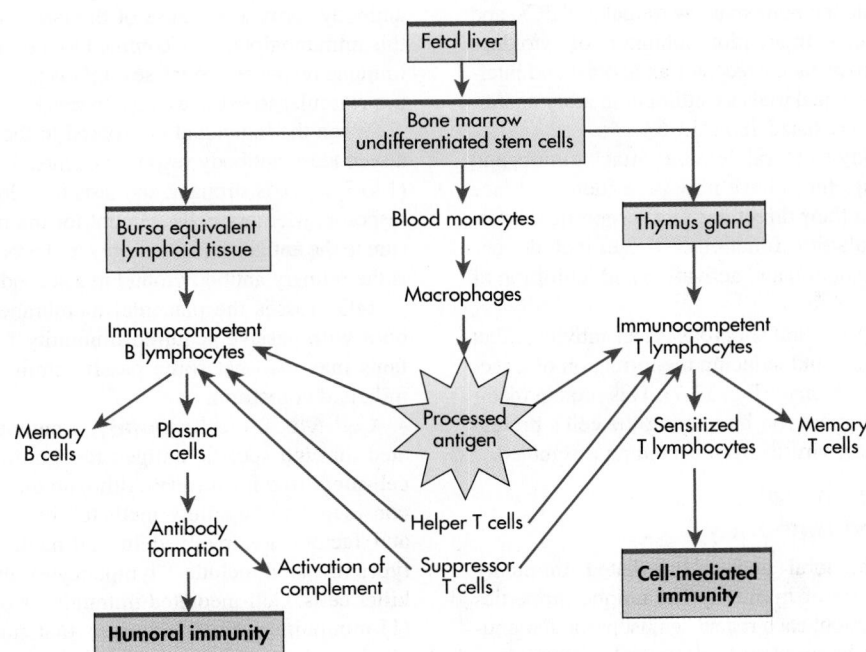

FIG. 13-6 Relationships and functions of macrophages, B lymphocytes, and T lymphocytes in an immune response.

TABLE 13-4   Characteristics of Immunoglobulins

CLASS	RELATIVE SERUM CONCENTRATION (%)	LOCATION	CHARACTERISTICS
IgG	76	Plasma, interstitial fluid	Is only immunoglobulin that crosses placenta Is responsible for secondary immune response
IgA	15	Body secretions, including tears, saliva, breast milk, colostrum	Lines mucous membranes and protects body surfaces
IgM	8	Plasma	Is responsible for primary immune response Forms antibodies to ABO blood antigens
IgD	1	Plasma	Is present on lymphocyte surface Assists in the differentiation of B lymphocytes
IgE	0.002	Plasma, interstitial fluids	Causes symptoms of allergic reactions Fixes to mast cells and basophils Assists in defense against parasitic infections

Cytokines

The immune response involves complex interactions of T cells, B cells, monocytes, and neutrophils. These interactions depend on **cytokines** (soluble factors secreted by WBCs and a variety of other cells in the body) that act as messengers between the cell types. Cytokines instruct cells to alter their proliferation, differentiation, secretion, or activity. There are currently at least 100 different cytokines, and they can be classified into distinct categories.[10] Some of these cytokines are listed in Table 13-5. In general, the interleukins act as immunomodulatory factors, colony-stimulating factors act as growth-regulating factors for hematopoietic cells, and interferons are antiviral and immunomodulatory.

Cytokines have a beneficial role in hematopoiesis and immune function. They can also have detrimental effects such as those seen in chronic inflammation, autoimmune diseases, and sepsis. Cytokines such as erythropoietin (see Chapter 45), colony-stimulating factors (see Chapters 15 and 30), interferons (see Chapter 15), and interleukin-2 (see Chapter 15) are used clinically to (1) stimulate hematopoiesis, (2) stimulate the bone marrow to make WBCs, and (3) treat various malignancies. In addition, inhibitors of cytokines such as soluble tumor necrosis factor receptor antagonist and interleukin-1 are being used in clinical trials as antiinflammatory agents. (Clinical uses of cytokines are listed Table 13-6.)

Interferon helps the body's natural defenses attack tumors and viruses. Three types of interferon have now been identified (see Table 13-4). In addition to their direct antiviral properties, interferons have immunoregulatory functions. These include enhancement of NK cell production and activation and inhibition of tumor cell growth.

Interferon is not directly antiviral but produces an antiviral effect in cells by reacting with them and inducing the formation of a second protein termed *antiviral protein* (Fig. 13-7). This protein mediates the antiviral action of interferon by altering the cell's protein synthesis and preventing new viruses from becoming assembled.

Comparison of Humoral and Cell-Mediated Immunity

Humans need both humoral and cell-mediated immunity to remain healthy. Each type of immunity has unique properties and different methods of action; each reacts against particular antigens. Table 13-7 compares humoral and cell-mediated immunity.

Humoral Immunity. **Humoral immunity** consists of antibody-mediated immunity. The term *humoral* comes from the Greek word *humor,* which means body fluid. Antibodies are produced by plasma cells (differentiated B cells) and found in plasma; therefore the term *humoral immunity* is used. Production of antibodies is an essential component in a humoral immune response. Each of the five classes of immunoglobulins, which are IgG, IgA, IgM, IgD, and IgE, has specific characteristics (see Table 13-4).

When a pathogen (especially bacteria) enters the body, it may encounter a B lymphocyte specific for antigens located on that bacterial cell wall. In addition, a monocyte or macrophage may phagocytize the bacteria and present its antigens to a B lymphocyte. The B lymphocyte recognizes the antigen because it has receptors on its cell surface specific for that antigen. When the antigen comes in contact with the cell surface receptor, the B cell becomes activated, and most B cells will differentiate into plasma cells (see Fig. 13-6). The mature plasma cell secretes immunoglobulins. Some stimulated B lymphocytes remain as memory cells.

The primary immune response is evident 4 to 8 days after the initial exposure to the antigen (Fig. 13-8). IgM is the first type of antibody formed. Because of the large size of the IgM molecule, this immunoglobulin is confined to the intravascular space. As the immune response progresses, IgG is produced and can move from intravascular to extravascular spaces.

When the individual is exposed to the antigen the second time, a secondary antibody response occurs. This response occurs faster (1 to 3 days), is stronger, and lasts for a longer time than a primary response. Memory cells account for the memory of the first exposure to the antigen and the more rapid production of antibodies. IgG is the primary antibody found in a secondary immune response.

IgG crosses the placental membrane and provides the newborn with passive acquired immunity for at least 3 months. Infants may also get some passive immunity from IgA in breast milk and colostrum.

Cell-Mediated Immunity. Immune responses that are initiated through specific antigen recognition by T cells are termed **cell-mediated immunity.** Although these reactions were initially considered to be solely mediated by T cells, several cell types and factors are involved in cell-mediated immunity. The cell types involved include T lymphocytes, macrophages, and natural killer cells. Cell-mediated immunity is of primary importance in (1) immunity against pathogens that survive inside of cells, including viruses and some bacteria (e.g., *Mycobacterium*); (2) fungal infections; (3) rejection of transplanted tissues; (4) contact hypersensitivity reactions; and (5) tumor immunity.

TABLE 13-5   Types and Functions of Cytokines

TYPE	PRIMARY FUNCTIONS
Interleukins (ILs)	
IL-1	Augments the immune response; inflammatory mediator; promotes maturation and clonal expansion of B cells; enhances activity of NK cells; activates T cells, activates macrophages
IL-2	Induces proliferation and differentiation of T cells; activation of T cells, NK cells, and macrophages; stimulates release of other cytokines (α-IFN, TNF, IL-1, IL-6)
IL-3 (multicolony-stimulating factor)	Hematopoietic growth factor for hematopoietic precursor cells
IL-4	B cell growth factor; stimulates proliferation and differentiation of B cells; induces proliferation of T cells; stimulates growth of mast cells
IL-5	B cell growth and differentiation; promotes growth and differentiation of eosinophils
IL-6	Enhances the inflammatory response; B cell stimulation; promotes differentiation of B cells into plasma cells; stimulates antibody secretion; induces fever; synergistic effects with IL-1 and TNF
IL-7	Promotes growth of T and B cells; increases expression of IL-2 and its receptor
IL-8	Chemotaxis of neutrophils and T cells; stimulates superoxide and granule release
IL-9	Acts as mitogen, supporting proliferation in absence of antigen; enhances T cell survival; mast cell activation
IL-10	Inhibits cytokine production by T and NK cells; promotes B cell proliferation and antibody responses; potent suppressor of macrophage function
IL-11	Is a multifunctional regulator of hematopoiesis and lymphopoiesis; osteoclast formation; elevates platelet count; inhibits proinflammatory cytokine production
IL-12	Promotes α-IFN production; induction of T helper cells; activates NK cells; stimulates proliferation of activated T and NK cells
IL-13	B cell growth and differentiation; inhibits proinflammatory cytokine production
IL-14	Stimulates proliferation of activated B cells
IL-15	Mimics IL-2 effects; stimulates proliferation of T cells and NK cells
IL-16	Proinflammatory cytokine; chemoattractant of T cells, eosinophils, and monocytes
IL-17	Promotes release of IL-6, IL-8, G-CSF; enhances expression of adhesion molecules
IL-18	Induces α-IFN, IL-2, and GM-CSF production; important role in development of T_h cells; enhances NK activity; inhibits production of IL-10
IL-19	Similar to IL-10
IL-20	Similar to IL-10
IL-21	Similar to IL-2, IL-4, and IL-5
IL-22	Similar to IL-10
IL-23	Similar functions to IL-12; promotes memory T cell proliferation
IL-24	Similar to IL-10
Interferons (IFNs)	
α-Interferon (α-IFN) β-Interferon (β-IFN)	Inhibit viral replication; activate NK cells and macrophages; antiproliferative effects on tumor cells
γ-Interferon (γ-IFN)	Activates macrophages, neutrophils, and NK cells; promotes B cell differentiation; inhibits viral replication
Tumor Necrosis Factor (TNF)	Activates macrophages and granulocytes; promotes the immune and inflammatory responses; kills tumor cells; is responsible for extensive weight loss associated with chronic inflammation and cancer
Colony-Stimulating Factors (CSFs)	
Granulocyte colony–stimulating factor (G-CSF)	Stimulates proliferation and differentiation of neutrophils; enhances functional activity of mature PMN
Granulocyte-macrophage colony–stimulating factor (GM-CSF)	Stimulates proliferation and differentiation of PMN and monocytes
Macrophage colony–stimulating factor (M-CSF)	Promotes the proliferation, differentiation, and activation of monocytes and macrophages
Erythropoietin	Stimulates erythroid progenitor cells in bone marrow to produce red blood cells

NK, Natural killer; *PMN*, polymorphonuclear neutrophils.

TABLE 13-6   Clinical Uses of Cytokines

CYTOKINE	CLINICAL USES
α-Interferon Roferon-A Intron A	• Hepatitis B and C • Kaposi's sarcoma • Hairy cell leukemia • Lymphomas • Leukemias • Melanoma • Renal cell carcinoma • Multiple myeloma
β-Interferon β-Interferon-1b (Betaseron) β-Interferon-1a (Avonex, Refib)	• Multiple sclerosis
Colony-Stimulating Factors **G-CSF** filgrastim (Neupogen) **GM-CSF** sargramostim (Leukine, Prokine)	• Neutropenia • Neutropenia
Soluble TNF Receptor etanercept (Enbrel) (Soluble TNF receptor)	• Rheumatoid arthritis
Interleukin-2 aldesleukin (Proleukin)	• Renal cell carcinoma • Malignant melanoma • Lymphoma • Acute myelocytic leukemia
Erythropoietin Epogen, Procrit	• Anemia
IL-1 Receptor Antagonist anakinra (Kineret)	• Rheumatoid arthritis

G-CSF, Granulocyte colony–stimulating factor; *GM-CSF,* granulocyte-macrophage colony–stimulating factor; *IL,* interleukin; *TNF,* tumor necrosis factor.

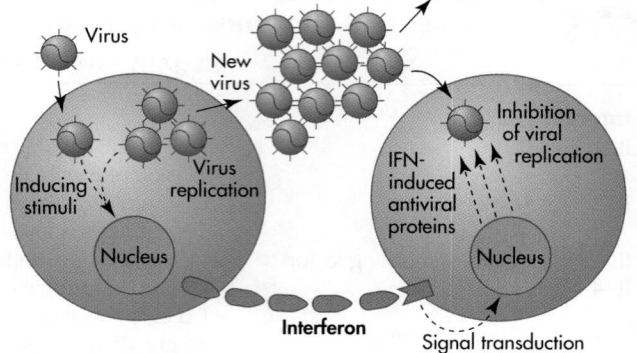

FIG. 13-7 Mechanism of action of interferon. Virus A attacks a cell. The cell begins to synthesize viral DNA and interferon. Interferon serves as an intercellular messenger. Interferon induces the production of antiviral proteins. Virus A is not able to replicate in the cell.

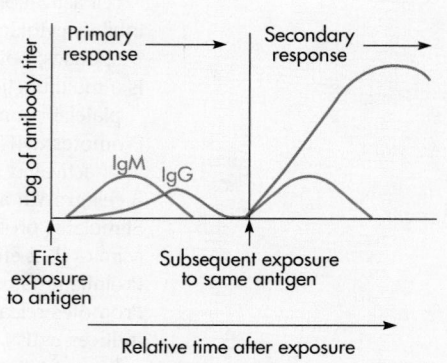

FIG. 13-8 Primary and secondary immune responses. The introduction of antigen induces a response dominated by two classes of immunoglobulins, IgM and IgG. IgM predominates in the primary response, with some IgG appearing later. After the host's immune system is primed, another challenge with the same antigen induces the secondary response, in which some IgM and large amounts of IgG are produced.

TABLE 13-7   Comparison of Humoral Immunity and Cell-Mediated Immunity

CHARACTERISTICS	HUMORAL IMMUNITY	CELL-MEDIATED IMMUNITY
Cells involved	B lymphocytes	T lymphocytes, macrophages
Products	Antibodies	Sensitized T cells, lymphokines
Memory cells	Present	Present
Protection	Bacteria Viruses (extracellular) Respiratory and gastrointestinal pathogens	Fungus Viruses (intracellular) Chronic infectious agents Tumor cells
Examples	Anaphylactic shock Atopic diseases Transfusion reaction Bacterial infections	Tuberculosis Fungal infections Contact dermatitis Graft rejection Destruction of cancer cells

■ Gerontologic Considerations: Effects of Aging on the Immune System

With advancing age there is a decline in the immune system[11] (Table 13-8). The primary clinical evidence for this *immunosenescence* is the high incidence of tumors in older adults. A greater susceptibility also occurs to infections (e.g., influenza, pneumonia) from pathogens that an older person had been relatively immunocompetent against earlier in life.

Aging does not affect all aspects of the immune system. The bone marrow is relatively unaffected by increasing age. However, aging has a pronounced effect on the thymus, which decreases in size and activity with aging. These changes in the thymus are probably a primary cause of immunosenescence. Both T and B cells show deficiencies in activation, transit time through the cell cycle, and subsequent differentiation. However, the most significant alterations involve T cells. As thymic output of T cells diminishes, the differentiation of T cells increases. Consequently, there is an accumulation of memory cells rather than new precursor cells responsive to previously unencountered antigens.

Delayed hypersensitivity response, as determined by skin testing with injected antigens, is frequently decreased or absent in older adults. This altered response reflects **anergy** (immunodeficient condition characterized by lack of or diminished reaction to an antigen or a group of antigens). The clinical consequences of a decline in cell-mediated immunity are evident. ■

ALTERED IMMUNE RESPONSE

Immunocompetence exists when the body's immune system can identify and inactivate or destroy foreign substances. When the immune system is incompetent or underresponsive, severe infections, immunodeficiency diseases, and malignancies may occur. When the immune system overreacts, hypersensitivity disorders such as allergies and autoimmune diseases may occur.

Hypersensitivity Reactions

Sometimes the immune response is overreactive against foreign antigens or fails to maintain self-tolerance, and this results in tissue damage. This is termed a **hypersensitivity reaction.** A type of hypersensitivity response occurs when the body fails to recognize self-proteins and reacts against its own protein. The diseases that occur as a result of immune responses against self-antigens are termed *autoimmune diseases.*

Classification of hypersensitivity reactions may be done according to the source of the antigen, the time sequence (immediate or delayed), or the basic immunologic mechanisms causing the injury. Basically, four types of hypersensitivity reactions exist. Types I, II, and III are immediate and are examples of humoral immunity. Type IV is a delayed hypersensitivity reaction and is related to cell-mediated immunity. Table 13-9 presents a summary of the four types of hypersensitivity reactions.

TABLE 13-8	*Gerontologic Differences in Assessment* **Effects of Aging on the Immune System**

- Thymic involution
- ↓ Cell-mediated immunity
- ↓ Delayed hypersensitivity response
- ↓ IL-1 and IL-2 synthesis
- ↓ Expression of IL-2 receptors
- ↓ Proliferative response of T and B cells
- ↓ Primary and secondary antibody responses
- ↓ Autoantibodies

IL, Interleukin.

TABLE 13-9   Types of Hypersensitivity Reactions

	TYPE I: ANAPHYLACTIC REACTIONS	TYPE II: CYTOTOXIC REACTIONS	TYPE III: IMMUNE-COMPLEX REACTIONS	TYPE IV: DELAYED HYPERSENSITIVITY REACTIONS
Antigen	Exogenous pollen, food, drugs, dust	Cell surface of RBC Basement membrane	Extracellular fungal, viral, bacterial	Intracellular or extracellular
Antibody involved	IgE	IgG IgM	IgG IgM	None
Complement involved	No	Yes	Yes	No
Mediators of injury	Histamine SRS-A	Complement lysis Neutrophils	Neutrophils Complement lysis	Cytokines T cytotoxic cells Monocytes/macrophages Lysosomal enzymes
Examples	Allergic rhinitis Asthma	Transfusion reaction Goodpasture syndrome	Serum sickness Systemic lupus erythematosus Rheumatoid arthritis	Contact dermatitis Tumor rejection Transplant rejection
Skin test	Wheal and flare	None	Erythema and edema in 3 to 8 hours	Erythema and edema in 24 to 48 hours (e.g., TB test)

RBC, Red blood cells; *SRS-A,* slow-reacting substance of anaphylaxis; *TB,* tuberculosis.

Type I: Anaphylactic Reactions. *Anaphylactic reactions* are type I reactions that occur only in susceptible persons who are highly sensitized to specific allergens. IgE antibodies, produced in response to the allergen, have a characteristic property of attaching to mast cells and basophils (Fig. 13-9) (see Chapter 28, Fig. 28-2). Within these cells are granules containing potent chemical mediators (histamine, serotonin, slow-reacting substance of anaphylaxis [SRS-A], eosinophil chemotactic factor of anaphylaxis [ECF-A], kinins, and bradykinin). (Leukotriene components [LTC$_4$, LTD$_4$, and LTE$_4$] of SRS-A are discussed in Chapters 12 and 28 and Fig. 12-7.) On the first exposure to the allergen, IgE antibodies are produced and bind to mast cells and basophils. On any subsequent exposures, the allergen links with the IgE bound to mast cells or basophils and triggers degranulation of the cells and the release of chemical mediators from the granules.[12] In this process, the mediators that are released attack target organs, causing clinical allergy symptoms.[13] These effects include smooth muscle contraction, increased vascular permeability, vasodilation, hypotension, increased secretion of mucus, and itching. Fortunately, the mediators are short acting and their effects are reversible. (The mediators and their effects are summarized in Table 13-10.)

A genetic predisposition to the development of allergic diseases exists. The capacity to become sensitized to an allergen appears to be the inherited trait rather than the specific allergic disorder. For example, a father with asthma may have a son who has allergic rhinitis.

The clinical manifestations of an anaphylactic reaction depend on whether the mediators remain local or become systemic or whether they affect particular organs. When the mediators remain localized, a cutaneous response termed the *wheal-and-flare reaction* occurs. This reaction is characterized by a pale wheal containing edematous fluid surrounded by a red flare from the hyperemia. The reaction occurs in minutes or hours and is usually not dangerous. A classic example of a wheal-and-flare reaction is the mosquito bite. The wheal-and-flare reaction serves a diagnostic purpose as a means of demonstrating allergic reactions to specific allergens during skin tests.

Common allergic reactions include anaphylaxis and atopic reactions.

Anaphylaxis. *Anaphylaxis* can occur when mediators are released systemically (e.g., after injection of a drug, after an insect sting). The reaction occurs within minutes and can be life threatening because of bronchial constriction and subsequent airway obstruction and vascular collapse.[14] The target organs affected are seen in Fig. 13-10. Initial symptoms include edema and itching at the site of the exposure to the allergen. Shock can occur rapidly and is manifested by rapid, weak pulse; hypotension; di-

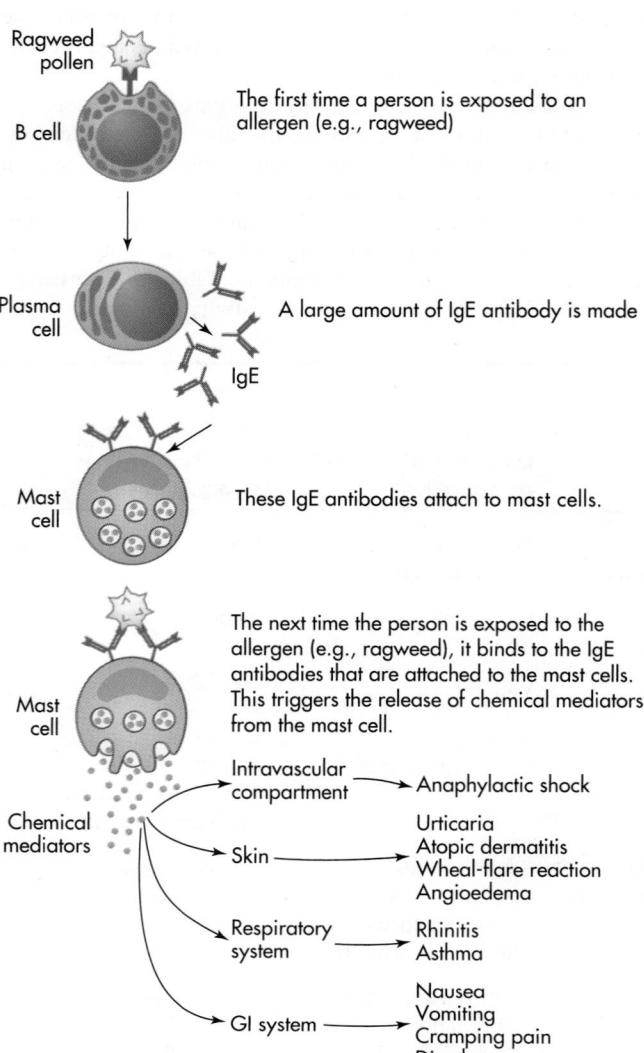

FIG. 13-9 Steps in a type I allergic reaction.

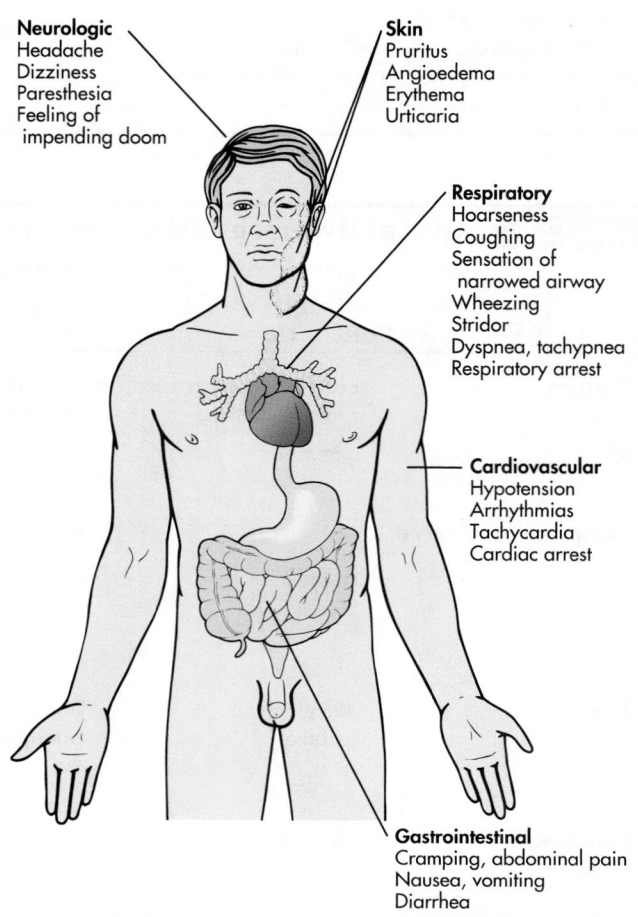

FIG. 13-10 Clinical manifestations of a systemic anaphylactic reaction.

TABLE 13-10 Mediators of Allergic Response

TYPE AND SOURCE	BIOLOGIC ACTIVITY	CLINICAL OUTCOMES
Histamine Mast cell and basophil granules	Increases vascular permeability; constricts smooth muscle; stimulates irritant receptors	Edema of airways and larynx; bronchial constriction; urticaria, angioedema, pruritus; nausea, vomiting, diarrhea; shock
Leukotrienes Metabolites of arachidonic acid by lipoxygenase pathway*	Constrict bronchial smooth muscle; increase vascular permeability	Bronchial constriction; enhanced effect of histamine on smooth muscle
Prostaglandins Metabolites of arachidonic acid by cyclooxygenase pathway*	Stimulate vasodilation; constrict smooth muscle	Wheal-and-flare reaction on skin; hypotension; bronchospasm
Platelet-Activating Factor Mast cell	Aggregates platelets; stimulates vasodilation	Increase in pulmonary artery pressure; systemic hypotension
Kinins Kininogen	Stimulate slow, sustained smooth muscle contraction; increase vascular permeability; stimulate secretion of mucus; stimulate pain receptors	Angioedema with painful swelling; bronchial constriction
Serotonin Platelets	Increases vascular permeability; stimulates smooth muscle contraction	Mucosal edema; bronchial constriction
Anaphylatoxins C3a, C4a, C5a from complement activation	Stimulate histamine release	Same as for histamine

*See Chapter 12, Fig. 12-7.

lated pupils; dyspnea; and possibly cyanosis. This is compounded by bronchial edema and angioedema. Death will occur if emergency treatment is not initiated.[15,16] Some of the important allergens leading to anaphylactic shock in hypersensitive persons are listed in Table 13-11.

Atopic reactions. An estimated 20% of the population is *atopic*, an inherited tendency to become sensitive to environmental allergens. The atopic diseases that can result are allergic rhinitis, asthma, atopic dermatitis, urticaria, and angioedema.

Allergic rhinitis, or hay fever, is the most common type I hypersensitivity reaction. It may occur year-round (perennial allergic rhinitis), or it may be seasonal (seasonal allergic rhinitis). Airborne substances such as pollens, dust, or molds are the primary cause of allergic rhinitis. Perennial allergic rhinitis may be caused by dust, molds, and animal dander. Seasonal allergic rhinitis is commonly caused by pollens from trees, weeds, or grasses. The target areas affected are the conjunctiva of the eyes and the mucosa of the upper respiratory tract. Symptoms include nasal discharge, sneezing, lacrimation, mucosal swelling with airway obstruction, and pruritus around the eyes, nose, throat, and mouth. (Treatment of allergic rhinitis is discussed in Chapter 26.)

Many patients with *asthma* have an allergic component to their disease. These patients frequently have a history of atopic disorders (e.g., infantile eczema, allergic rhinitis, food intolerances). In asthma, SRS-A and histamine are primarily responsible for action on the bronchioles (see Chapter 28, Fig. 28-2). These mediators produce bronchial smooth muscle constriction, excessive secretion of viscoid mucus, edema of the mucous membranes of the bronchi, and decreased lung compliance. Because of these physi-

TABLE 13-11 Allergens Causing Anaphylactic Shock

Drugs

Penicillins	Sulfonamides
Insulins	Aspirin
Tetracycline	Local anesthetics
Chemotherapeutic agents	Cephalosporins
Nonsteroidal antiinflammatory drugs	

Insect Venoms
Hymenoptera*

Foods

Eggs	Milk
Nuts	Peanuts
Shellfish	Fish
Chocolate	Strawberries

Animal Serums

Tetanus antitoxin	Rabies antitoxin
Diphtheria antitoxin	Snake venom antitoxin

Treatment Measures

Blood products (whole blood and components)	Iodine-contrast media for IVP or angiogram test
Allergenic extracts in hyposensitization therapy	

*Wasps, hornets, yellow jackets, bumblebees, and ants.
IVP, Intravenous pyelogram.

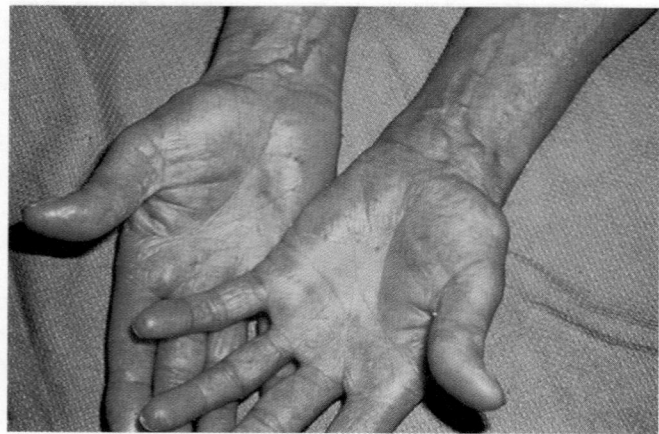

FIG. 13-11 Chronic lesions of atopic dermatitis on the hands of a woman; erythema, crusts, and cracks are evident.

ologic alterations, patients manifest dyspnea, wheezing, coughing, tightness in the chest, and thick sputum. (Pathophysiology and management of asthma are discussed in Chapter 28.)

Atopic dermatitis is a chronic, inherited skin disorder characterized by exacerbations and remissions. It is caused by several environmental allergens that are difficult to identify. Although patients with atopic dermatitis have elevated IgE levels and positive skin tests, the histopathologic features do not represent the typical, localized wheal-and-flare type I reactions. The skin lesions are more generalized and involve vasodilation of blood vessels, resulting in interstitial edema with vesicle formation (Fig. 13-11). (Dermatitis is discussed in Chapter 23.)

Urticaria (hives) is a cutaneous reaction against systemic allergens occurring in atopic persons. It is characterized by transient wheals (pink, raised, edematous, pruritic areas) that vary in size and shape and may occur throughout the body. Urticaria develops rapidly after exposure to an allergen and may last minutes or hours. Histamine causes localized vasodilation (erythema), transudation of fluid (wheal), and flaring. Flaring is due to blood vessels on the edge of the wheal dilating in response to a reaction augmented by the sympathetic nervous system. Histamine is responsible for the pruritus associated with the lesions. (Urticaria is discussed in Chapter 23.)

Angioedema is a localized cutaneous lesion similar to urticaria but involving deeper layers of the skin and the submucosa. The principal areas of involvement include the eyelids, lips, tongue, larynx, hands, feet, gastrointestinal (GI) tract, and genitalia. Swelling usually begins in the face and then progresses to the airways and other parts of the body. Dilation and engorgement of the capillaries secondary to release of histamine cause the diffuse swelling. Welts are not apparent as in urticaria; the outer skin appears normal or has a reddish hue. The lesions may burn, sting, or itch and can cause acute abdominal pain if in the GI tract. The swelling may occur suddenly or over several hours and usually lasts for 24 hours.

Type II: Cytotoxic and Cytolytic Reactions. Cytotoxic and cytolytic reactions are type II hypersensitivity reactions involving the direct binding of IgG or IgM antibodies to an antigen on the cell surface. Antigen-antibody complexes activate the complement system, which mediates the reaction. Cellular tissue is destroyed in one of two ways: (1) activation of the complement cascade resulting in cytolysis and (2) enhanced phagocytosis.

Target cells frequently destroyed in type II reactions are erythrocytes, platelets, and leukocytes. Some of the antigens involved are the ABO blood group, Rh factor, and drugs. Pathophysiologic disorders characteristic of type II reactions include ABO incompatibility transfusion reaction, Rh incompatibility transfusion reaction, autoimmune and drug-related hemolytic anemias, leukopenias, thrombocytopenias, erythroblastosis fetalis (hemolytic disease of the newborn), and Goodpasture syndrome. The tissue damage usually occurs rapidly.

Hemolytic transfusion reactions. A classic type II reaction occurs when a recipient receives ABO-incompatible blood from a donor. Naturally acquired antibodies to antigens of the ABO blood group are in the recipient's serum but are not present on the erythrocyte membranes (see Chapter 29, Table 29-10). For example, a person with type A blood has anti-B antibodies, a person with type B blood has anti-A antibodies, a person with type AB blood has no antibodies, and a person with type O blood has both anti-A and anti-B antibodies.

If the recipient is transfused with incompatible blood, antibodies immediately coat the foreign erythrocytes, causing *agglutination* (clumping). The clumping of cells blocks small blood vessels in the body, uses existing clotting factors, and depletes them, leading to bleeding. Within hours, neutrophils and macrophages phagocytize the agglutinated cells. As complement is fixed to the antigen, cytolysis occurs. Cellular lysis causes the release of hemoglobin into the urine and plasma. In addition, a cytotoxic reaction causes vascular spasms in the kidney that further block the renal tubules. Acute renal failure can result from the hemoglobinuria. (Blood transfusions are discussed in Chapter 30.)

Goodpasture syndrome. *Goodpasture syndrome* is a rare disorder involving the lungs and kidneys. An antibody-mediated autoimmune reaction occurs involving the glomerular and alveolar basement membranes. The circulating antibodies combine with tissue antigen to activate complement, which causes deposits of IgG to form along the basement membranes of the lungs or kidneys. This reaction may result in pulmonary hemorrhage and glomerulonephritis. The disease is usually rapidly progressive. Corticosteroids, immunosuppressive drugs (e.g., cyclophosphamide [Cytoxan]), and plasmapheresis have been used effectively to slow the progression of the disease. (Goodpasture syndrome is discussed in Chapter 44.)

Type III: Immune-Complex Reactions. Tissue damage in immune-complex reactions, which are type III reactions, occurs secondary to antigen-antibody complexes. Soluble antigens combine with immunoglobulins of the IgG and IgM classes to form complexes that are too small to be effectively removed by the mononuclear phagocyte system. Therefore the complexes deposit in tissue or small blood vessels. They cause the fixation of complement and the release of chemotactic factors that lead to inflammation and destruction of the involved tissue.

Type III reactions may be local or systemic and immediate or delayed. The clinical manifestations depend on the number of complexes and the location in the body. Common sites for deposit are the kidneys, skin, joints, blood vessels, and lungs. Severe type III reactions are associated with autoimmune disorders such as systemic lupus erythematosus (SLE), acute glomerulonephritis, and rheumatoid arthritis (RA). (SLE and RA are discussed in Chapter 63, and acute glomerulonephritis is discussed in Chapter 44.)

Type IV: Delayed Hypersensitivity Reactions. A *delayed hypersensitivity reaction*—a type IV reaction—is also termed a *cell-mediated immune response.* Although cell-mediated responses are usually protective mechanisms, tissue damage occurs in delayed hypersensitivity reactions.

The tissue damage in a type IV reaction does not occur in the presence of antibodies or complement. Rather, sensitized T lymphocytes attack antigens or release cytokines. Some of these cytokines attract macrophages into the area. The macrophages and enzymes released by them are responsible for most of the tissue destruction. The delayed hypersensitivity response takes 24 to 48 hours for a reaction to occur.

Clinical examples of a delayed hypersensitivity reaction include contact dermatitis (Fig. 13-12); hypersensitivity reactions to bacterial, fungal, and viral infections; and transplant rejections. Some drug sensitivity reactions also fit this category.

Contact dermatitis. *Allergic contact dermatitis* is an example of a delayed hypersensitivity reaction involving the skin. The reaction occurs when the skin is exposed to substances that easily penetrate the skin to combine with epidermal proteins. The substance then becomes antigenic. Over a period of 7 to 14 days, memory cells form to the antigen. On subsequent exposure to the substance, a sensitized person develops eczematous skin lesions within 48 hours. The most common potentially antigenic substances encountered are metal compounds (e.g., nickel, mercury); rubber compounds; catechols present in poison ivy, poison oak, and sumac; cosmetics; and some dyes.

In acute contact dermatitis the skin lesions appear erythematous and edematous and are covered with papules, vesicles, and bullae. The involved area is very pruritic but may also burn or sting. When contact dermatitis becomes chronic, the lesions resemble atopic dermatitis because they are thickened, scaly, and lichenified. The main difference between contact dermatitis and atopic dermatitis is that contact dermatitis is localized and restricted to the area exposed to the allergens, whereas atopic dermatitis is usually widespread.

Microbial hypersensitivity reactions. The classic example of a microbial cell-mediated immune reaction is the body's defense against the tubercle bacillus. Tuberculosis results from invasion of lung tissue by the highly resistant tubercle bacillus. The organism itself does not directly damage the lung tissue. However, antigenic material released from the tubercle bacilli reacts with T lymphocytes, initiating a cell-mediated immune response. The resulting response causes extensive caseous necrosis of the lung.

After the initial cell-mediated reaction, memory cells persist, so subsequent contact with the tubercle bacillus or an extract of purified protein from the organism causes a delayed hypersensitivity reaction. This is the basis for the purified protein derivative (PPD) tuberculosis skin test read 48 to 72 hours after the injection. (Tuberculosis is discussed in Chapter 27.)

Transplant rejection. Rejection of organs occurs by cell-mediated immunity if the donor organ does not perfectly match the recipient's **human leukocyte antigens** (HLAs), also termed *histocompatibility antigens.* The rejection can be prevented by closely matching ABO, Rh, and HLAs between donor and recipient. Unfortunately, many different HLAs exist, and a perfect match is nearly impossible unless the tissue is from oneself or an identical twin.

Graft rejection is a complicated process that involves sensitized T lymphocytes (see Chapter 45, Fig. 45-19). If the tissue is mismatched, sensitized T lymphocytes arrive at regional lymph nodes within 6 to 10 days. The clinical signs of rejection appear in about 14 days when sensitized T lymphocytes attack the graft. At this time the vascularization stops and the tissue becomes necrosed. (Transplant rejection is discussed in Chapter 45.)

ALLERGIC DISORDERS

Although an alteration of the immune system may be manifested in many ways, allergies or type I hypersensitivity reactions are seen most frequently.

Assessment

For a thorough assessment of a patient with allergies, a complete database must be obtained. This consists of a comprehensive patient history, physical examination, diagnostic workup, and skin testing for allergens.

Health History. A comprehensive history that covers family allergies, past and present allergies, and social and environmental factors is essential. The information may be obtained from the patient or the patient's caregiver.

Family history, including information about atopic reactions in relatives, is especially important in identifying at-risk patients. The specific disorder, clinical manifestations, and treatments prescribed should be assessed.

Past and present allergies must be noted. Identifying the allergens that may have triggered a reaction is essential to control allergic reactions. Determination of the time of year that an allergic reaction occurs can be a clue to a seasonal allergen. Information should also be obtained about any over-the-counter or prescription medications used to treat the allergies.

In addition to identification of the allergen, information about the clinical manifestations and course of allergic reaction should be obtained. If the patient is a woman, assessment of symptoms during pregnancy, menstruation, or menopause may be important. Social and environmental factors, especially the physical environment, are important. Questions about pets, trees, and plants on property; pollutants in the air; and floor coverings, house plants, and cooling and heating systems in the home and workplace can provide valuable information about allergens. In addition, a daily or weekly food diary with a description of any untoward reactions is important. Of particular interest is a screening for any reaction to medication. Finally, questions about the patient's lifestyle and stress level should be reviewed in connection with the appearance of allergic symptoms.

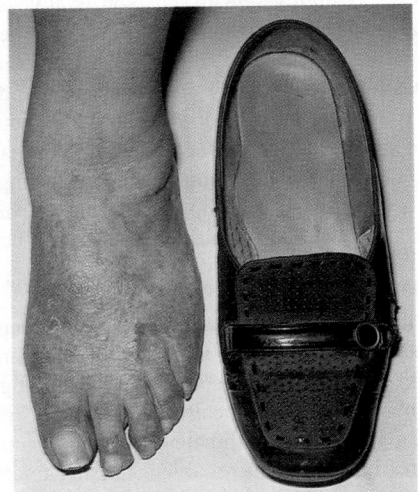

FIG. 13-12 Contact dermatitis. The distribution of the dermatitis gives an obvious clue to its cause.

TABLE 13-12	Nursing Assessment Allergies

Subjective Data

Important Health Information

Past health history: Recurrent respiratory problems, seasonal exacerbations; unusual reactions to insect bites or stings; past and present allergies

Medications: Unusual reactions to any medications; use of over-the-counter drugs, use of medications for allergies

Functional Health Patterns

Health perception–health management: Family history of allergies; malaise

Nutritional-metabolic: Food intolerances; vomiting

Elimination: Abdominal cramps, diarrhea

Activity-exercise: Fatigue; hoarseness, cough, dyspnea

Cognitive-perceptual: Itching, burning, stinging of eyes, nose, throat, or skin; chest tightness

Role-relationship: Altered home and work environment, presence of pets

Objective Data

Integumentary

Rashes, including urticaria, wheal and flare, papules, vesicles, bullae; dryness, scaliness, scratches, irritation

Eyes, Ears, Nose, and Throat

Eyes: Conjunctivitis; lacrimation; rubbing or excessive blinking; dark circles under the eyes ("allergic shiner")

Ears: Diminished hearing; immobile or scarred tympanic membranes; recurrent ear infections

Nose: Nasal polyps; nasal voice; nose twitching; itchy nose; rhinitis; pale, boggy mucous membranes; sniffling; repeated sneezing; swollen nasal passages; recurrent, unexplained nosebleeds; crease across the bridge of nose ("allergic salute")

Throat: Continual throat clearing; swollen lips or tongue; red throat; palpable neck lymph nodes

Respiratory

Wheezing, stridor; thick sputum

Possible Findings

Eosinophilia of serum, sputum, or nasal and bronchial secretions; ↑ serum IgE levels; positive skin tests; abnormal chest and sinus x-rays

Physical Examination. A comprehensive head-to-toe physical examination should be given to a patient with allergies, with particular attention focused on the site of the allergic manifestations. A comprehensive assessment that includes subjective and objective data should be obtained from the patient (Table 13-12).

Diagnostic Studies

Many specialized immunologic techniques can be performed to detect abnormalities of lymphocytes, eosinophils, and immunoglobulins. A complete blood count (CBC) and serology tests are commonly done.

A CBC with WBC differential is required with an absolute lymphocyte count and eosinophil count. Cellular immunodeficiency is diagnosed if the lymphocyte count is below $1200/\mu l$ $(1.2 \times 10^9/L)$. T cell and B cell quantification is used to diagnose specific immunodeficiency syndromes. The eosinophil count is elevated with type I hypersensitivity reactions involving IgE im-

munoglobulins. Serum IgE level is also generally elevated in type I hypersensitivity reactions and serves as a diagnostic indicator of atopic diseases.

Radioallergosorbent test (RAST) is an in vitro diagnostic test for IgE antibodies to specific allergens. Although expensive, it is safe but less sensitive and takes longer than skin tests for detecting allergens. RAST is helpful in confirming reactivity to various foods or drugs in individuals with a history of severe anaphylactic reactions.

Sputum, nasal, and bronchial secretions also may be tested for the presence of eosinophils. If asthma is suspected, pulmonary function tests for vital capacity, forced expiratory volume, and maximum midexpiratory flow rates are helpful.

Skin Tests. Skin testing is generally used to confirm specific sensitivity in patients with atopic disease after the history has suggested possible allergens for testing.

Procedure. Skin testing may be done by one of two methods: (1) a cutaneous scratch or prick or (2) an intracutaneous injection. The areas of the body usually used in testing are the arms and back. Allergen extracts are applied to the skin in rows with a corresponding control site opposite the test site. Saline or another diluent is applied to the control site. In the scratch test the epidermal skin layer is scratched with a lancet and the allergen extract is applied at the site. The prick test involves placing a drop of allergen extract on the skin and then piercing the underlying epidermis with a needle. In the intracutaneous method the allergen extract is injected intradermally in rows. Because the allergic reaction is more severe with this method, the test is used only for persons who did not react to cutaneous methods.

Results. If the person is hypersensitive to the allergen, a positive reaction will occur within minutes after insertion in the skin and may last for 8 to 12 hours. A positive reaction is manifested by a local wheal-and-flare response. The size of the positive reaction does not always correlate with the severity of allergy symptoms. False-positive and false-negative results may occur. Negative results from skin testing do not necessarily mean the person does not have an allergic disorder, and positive results do not necessarily mean that the allergen was causing the clinical manifestations. Positive results imply that the person is sensitized to that allergen. Therefore correlating skin test results with the patient's history is important.

Precautions. A highly sensitive person is always at risk for developing an anaphylactic reaction to skin tests. Therefore a patient should never be left alone during the testing period. Sometimes skin testing is completely contraindicated and the RAST test is used. If a severe reaction does occur with a cutaneous test, the extract is immediately removed and antiinflammatory topical cream is applied to the site. For intracutaneous testing, the arm is used so that a tourniquet can be applied during a severe reaction. A subcutaneous injection of epinephrine may also be necessary.

Collaborative Care

After an allergic disorder is diagnosed, the therapeutic treatment is aimed at reducing exposure to the offending allergen, treating the symptoms, and if necessary desensitizing the person through immunotherapy. All health care workers must be prepared for the rare but life-threatening anaphylactic reaction, which requires immediate medical and nursing interventions. It is extremely important that all of a patient's allergies be listed on the chart, the nursing care plan, and the medication record.

TABLE 13-13   Emergency Management
Anaphylactic Shock

ETIOLOGY	ASSESSMENT FINDINGS	INTERVENTIONS
• Injection of, inhalation of, ingestion of, or topical exposure to substance that produces profound allergic response • See Table 13-11 for more complete listing	See Fig. 13-10	**Initial** • Ensure patent airway. • Remove insect stinger if present. • Epinephrine 1:1000, 0.2-0.5 ml SQ for mild symptoms; repeat at 20-minute intervals. • Epinephrine 1:10,000, 0.5 ml IV at 5- to 10-minute intervals for severe reaction. • Administer high-flow oxygen via non-rebreather mask. • Place recumbent and elevate legs. • Keep warm. • Administer diphenhydramine (Benadryl) IM or IV. • Administer histamine H_2 blockers such as cimetidine (Tagamet). • Maintain blood pressure with fluids, volume expanders, vasopressors (e.g., dopamine [Intropin], norepinephrine bitartrate [Levophed]). **Ongoing Monitoring** • Monitor vital signs, respiratory effort, oxygen saturation, level of consciousness, and cardiac rhythm. • Anticipate intubation with severe respiratory distress. • Anticipate cricothyrotomy or tracheostomy with severe laryngeal edema.

IM, Intramuscular; *IV*, intravenous; *SQ*, subcutaneous.

Anaphylaxis. Anaphylactic reactions occur suddenly in hypersensitive patients after exposure to the offending allergen. They may occur following parenteral injection of drugs (especially antibiotics), blood products, and insect stings. The cardinal principle in therapeutic management is speed in (1) recognition of signs and symptoms of an anaphylactic reaction, (2) maintenance of a patent airway, (3) prevention of spread of the allergen by using a tourniquet, (4) administration of drugs, and (5) treatment for shock.[16] Table 13-13 summarizes the emergency treatment of anaphylactic shock.

Mild symptoms such as pruritus and urticaria can be controlled by administration of 0.2 to 0.5 ml of epinephrine, diluted 1:1000, given subcutaneously every 20 minutes according to the health care provider's orders or a hospital emergency drug protocol. An intravenous infusion should be initiated to provide a route for administration of 0.5 ml of epinephrine, diluted 1:10,000, at 5- to 10-minute intervals; volume expanders; and vasopressor agents such as dopamine (Intropin) if intractable hypotension occurs.

Oxygen via a non-rebreather mask should be administered. Endotracheal intubation or a tracheostomy is mandatory for O_2 delivery if progressive hypoxia exists. Other agents are used, including an antihistamine such as diphenhydramine (Benadryl) intravenously or intramuscularly for urticaria and angioedema.

In more severe cases of anaphylaxis, hypovolemic shock may occur because of the loss of intravascular fluid into interstitial spaces that occurs secondary to increased capillary permeability. Peripheral vasoconstriction and stimulation of the sympathetic nervous system occur to compensate for the fluid shift. However, unless shock is treated early, the body will no longer be able to compensate, and irreversible tissue damage will occur, leading to death. (Hypovolemic shock is discussed in Chapter 65.)

Chronic Allergies. Most allergic reactions are chronic and are characterized by remissions and exacerbations of symptoms. Treatment focuses on identification and control of allergens, relief of symptoms through drug therapy, and hyposensitization of a patient to an offending allergen.

Allergen recognition and control. The nurse plays an important role in helping the patient make lifestyle adjustments so that there is minimal exposure to offending allergens. The nurse must reinforce that, even with drug therapy and immunotherapy, the patient will never be desensitized or completely symptom free. The nurse can initiate various preventive measures that will help control the allergic symptoms.

Of primary importance is the need to identify the offending allergen. Sometimes this is done through skin testing. In the case of food allergies, an elimination diet is sometimes valuable. If an allergic reaction occurs, all food eaten should be eliminated and gradually reintroduced one at a time until the offending food is detected.

Many allergic reactions, especially asthma and urticaria, may be aggravated by fatigue and emotional stress. The nurse can be instrumental in initiating a stress management program with the patient. Relaxation techniques can be practiced when the patient comes for frequent immunotherapy treatments.

Sometimes control of allergic symptoms requires environmental control, including changing an occupation, moving to a different climate, or giving up a favorite pet. In the case of airborne allergens, sleeping in an air-conditioned room, damp dusting daily, covering mattresses and pillows with hypoallergenic covers, and wearing a mask outdoors may be helpful.

If the allergen is a drug, the patient should be instructed to avoid the drug. The patient also has the responsibility to make the drug intolerance well known to all health care providers. The patient should wear a Medic Alert bracelet listing the particular drug allergy and have the offending drug listed on all medical and dental records.

For a patient allergic to insect stings, commercial bee-sting kits containing preinjectable epinephrine and a tourniquet are available. The nurse has the responsibility to instruct the patient about the technique of applying the tourniquet and self-injecting the subcutaneous epinephrine. This patient also should wear a Medic Alert bracelet and carry a bee-sting kit whenever going outdoors.

Drug Therapy.   The major categories of drugs used for symptomatic relief of chronic allergic disorders include antihistamines, sympathomimetic/decongestant drugs, corticosteroids, antipruritic drugs, and mast cell–stabilizing drugs. Many of these drugs may be obtained over the counter and are often misused by patients.

Antihistamines.   Antihistamines are the best drugs for treatment of allergic rhinitis and urticaria (see Chapter 26, Table 26-2). They are less effective for severe allergic reactions. They act by competing with histamine for H_1-receptor sites and thus blocking the effect of histamine. Best results are achieved if they are taken as soon as allergy signs and symptoms appear. Antihistamines can be used effectively to treat edema and pruritus but are relatively ineffective in preventing bronchoconstriction. With seasonal rhinitis, antihistamines should be taken during peak pollen seasons. (Antihistamines are discussed in Chapter 26.)

Sympathomimetic/decongestant drugs.   The major sympathomimetic drug is epinephrine (Adrenalin), which is the drug of choice to treat an anaphylactic reaction. Epinephrine is a hormone produced by the adrenal medulla that stimulates α- and β-adrenergic receptors. Stimulation of the α-adrenergic receptors causes vasoconstriction of peripheral blood vessels. β-Receptor stimulation relaxes bronchial smooth muscles. Epinephrine also acts directly on mast cells to stabilize them against further degranulation. The action of epinephrine lasts only a few minutes. For the treatment of anaphylaxis the drug must be given parenterally (usually subcutaneously).

Several specific, minor sympathomimetic drugs differ from epinephrine because they can be taken orally or nasally and last for several hours. Included in this category are phenylephrine (Neo-Synephrine) and pseudoephedrine (Sudafed). The minor sympathomimetic drugs are used primarily to treat allergic rhinitis.

Corticosteroids.   Nasal corticosteroid sprays are very effective in relieving the symptoms of allergic rhinitis (see Chapter 26 and Table 26-2). Occasionally patients have such severe manifestations of allergies that they are truly incapacitated. In these situations, a brief course of oral corticosteroids can be used.

Antipruritic drugs.   Topically applied antipruritic drugs are most effective when the skin is not broken. These drugs protect the skin and provide relief from itching. Common over-the-counter drugs include calamine lotion, coal tar solutions, and camphor. Menthol and phenol may be added to other lotions to produce an antipruritic effect. Some more potent drugs that require a prescription include methdilazine (Tacaryl) and trimeprazine (Temaril). These drugs should be used with great caution because of the associated risk of agranulocytosis.

Mast cell–stabilizing drugs.   Cromolyn (Intal, Nasalcrom, Rynacrom) and nedocromil (Tilade) are mast cell–stabilizing agents that inhibit the release of histamines, leukotrienes, and other agents from the mast cell after antigen-IgE interaction. They are available as an inhalant nebulizer solution, a nasal spray, or an oral pill. They

are used in the management of asthma (see Chapter 28) and in the treatment of allergic rhinitis (see Chapter 26). An important feature of these drugs is a very low incidence of side effects.

Immunotherapy.   Immunotherapy is the recommended treatment for control of allergic symptoms when the allergen cannot be avoided and drug therapy is not effective. Relatively few patients with allergies have symptoms so intolerable that they require allergy immunotherapy. Immunotherapy is absolutely indicated only in individuals with anaphylactic reactions to insect venom. It involves administration of small titers of an allergen extract in increasing strengths until hyposensitivity to the specific allergen is achieved. For best results the patient should continue to avoid the offending allergen whenever possible because complete desensitization is impossible.

Mechanism of action.   IgE immunoglobulin level is elevated in atopic individuals. When IgE combines with an allergen in a hypersensitive person, a reaction occurs, releasing histamine in various body tissues. Allergens more readily combine with IgG immunoglobulin than with other immunoglobulins. Therefore immunotherapy involves injecting allergen extracts that will stimulate increased IgG levels. The binding of IgG to allergen-reactive sites interferes with allergen binding to mast cell–bound IgE, preventing mast cell degranulation, and thus reduces the number of reactions that cause tissue damage. The goal of long-term immunotherapy is to keep "blocking" IgG levels high. In addition, allergen-specific T suppressor cells develop in individuals receiving immunotherapy.

Method of administration.   The allergens included in immunotherapy are chosen on the basis of the results of skin testing with a panel of allergens found in the local geographic area. Immunotherapy involves the subcutaneous injection of titrated amounts of allergen extracts biweekly or weekly. The dose is small at first and is increased slowly until a maintenance dosage is reached. Generally it takes 1 to 2 years of immunotherapy to reach the maximal therapeutic effect. Therapy may be continued for about 5 years. After that, consideration is given to discontinuing therapy. In many patients a decrease in symptoms is sustained after the treatment is discontinued. For patients with severe allergies or sensitivity to insect stings, maintenance therapy is continued indefinitely. Best results are achieved when immunotherapy is administered throughout the year.

NURSING MANAGEMENT IMMUNOTHERAPY

The nurse is often primarily responsible for giving immunotherapy. Adverse reactions should always be anticipated, especially when using a new-strength dose, after a previous reaction, or after a missed dose. Early signs and symptoms indicative of a systemic reaction include pruritus, urticaria, sneezing, laryngeal edema, and hypotension. Emergency measures for anaphylactic shock should be initiated immediately. A local reaction should be described according to the degree of redness and swelling at the injection site. If the area is greater than the size of a quarter in an adult, the reaction should be reported to the health care provider so that the allergen dosage may be decreased.

Immunotherapy always carries the risk of a severe anaphylactic reaction. Therefore a health care provider, emergency equipment, and essential drugs should be available whenever injections are given.

Record keeping must be accurate and can be invaluable in preventing an adverse reaction to the allergen extract. Before giving an injection, the nurse should check the patient's name with the name on the vial. Next, the vial strength, amount of last dose, date of last dose, and any reaction information should be screened.

The nurse should always administer the allergen extract in an extremity away from a joint so that a tourniquet can be applied for a severe reaction. The site should be rotated for each injection. The nurse must aspirate for blood before giving an injection to ensure that the allergen extract is not injected into a blood vessel. An injection directly into the bloodstream can potentiate an anaphylactic reaction. After the injection is given, the patient should be carefully observed for 20 minutes because systemic reactions are most likely to occur immediately. However, the patient should be warned that a delayed reaction can occur as long as 24 hours later.

Latex Allergies

Allergies to latex products have become a problem of increasing proportion, affecting both patients and health care professionals. The increase in allergic reactions has coincided with the sharp increase in glove use related to the introduction of universal precautions against infectious diseases in 1987.[17] It is estimated that 8% to 17% of health care workers regularly exposed to latex are sensitized. The more frequent and prolonged the exposure to latex, the greater the likelihood of developing a latex allergy.[18] In addition to gloves, many latex-containing products are used in health care, such as blood pressure cuffs, stethoscopes, tourniquets, intravenous (IV) tubing, syringes, electrode pads, O_2 masks, tracheal tubes, colostomy and ileostomy pouches, urinary catheters, anesthetic masks, and adhesive tape. Latex proteins can become aerosolized through powder on gloves and can result in serious reactions when inhaled by sensitized individuals.

Types of Latex Allergies. Two types of latex allergies that can occur are type IV allergic contact dermatitis and type I allergic reactions. Type IV contact dermatitis is caused by the chemicals used in the manufacturing process of latex gloves. It is a delayed reaction that occurs within 6 to 48 hours. Typically the person first has dryness, pruritus, fissuring, and cracking of the skin, followed by redness, swelling, and crusting at 24 to 48 hours. Chronic exposure can lead to lichenification, scaling, and hyperpigmentation. The dermatitis may extend beyond the area of physical contact with the allergen.

A type I allergic reaction is a response to the natural rubber latex proteins and occurs within minutes of contact with the proteins. These types of allergic reactions can manifest as various reactions ranging from skin redness, urticaria, rhinitis, conjunctivitis, or asthma to full-blown anaphylactic shock. Systemic reactions to latex may result from exposure to latex protein via various routes, including the skin, mucous membranes, inhalation, or blood.

NURSING *and* COLLABORATIVE MANAGEMENT LATEX ALLERGIES

The identification of patients and health care workers sensitive to latex is crucial in the prevention of adverse reactions. A thorough health history and history of any allergies should be collected, especially on patients with any complaints of latex contact symptoms. Not all latex-sensitive individuals can be identified, even with a careful and thorough history. Risk factors include long-term multiple exposures to latex products (e.g., health care personnel, individuals who have had multiple surgeries, rubber industry workers). Additional risk factors include a patient history of hay fever, asthma, and allergies to certain foods (e.g., avocados, guava, kiwi, bananas, water chestnuts, hazelnuts, tomatoes, potatoes, peaches, grapes, apricots).

The National Institute for Occupational Safety and Health (NIOSH) has published recommendations for preventing allergic reactions to latex in the workplace. This free publication (no. 97-135) can be obtained from NIOSH (800-356-4674 or *www.cdc.gov/niosh*). In summary they include the following:

1. Use nonlatex gloves for activities that are not likely to involve contact with infectious materials (e.g., food preparation, housekeeping).
2. Use powder-free gloves with reduced protein content.
3. Do not use oil-based hand creams or lotions when wearing gloves.
4. After removing gloves, wash hands with mild soap and dry thoroughly.
5. Frequently clean work areas that are contaminated with latex-containing dust.
6. Know the symptoms of latex allergy, including skin rash; hives; flushing; itching; nasal, eye, or sinus symptoms; asthma; and shock.
7. If symptoms of latex allergy develop, avoid direct contact with latex gloves and products.
8. Wear a medical alert bracelet and carry an epinephrine pen.

Latex precaution protocols should be used for those patients identified as having a positive latex allergy test or a history of signs and symptoms related to latex exposure. Many health care facilities have created latex-free product carts that can be used for patients with latex allergies.

Multiple Chemical Sensitivities

Multiple chemical sensitivities (MCS), also known as *idiopathic environmental intolerances* (IEI), is an acquired disorder in which certain people exposed to various chemicals and food in the environment have many symptoms related to multiple body systems. These symptoms are usually subjective and are not found during physical examination. The patient experiences wide-ranging symptoms, but evidence of pathology or physiologic dysfunction is lacking.

Primarily, IEI is found in women. Symptoms include fatigue, headache, nausea, pain, dizziness, mouth irritation, disorientation, and cough. Almost any chemical can initiate the symptoms of IEI. Food additives, drugs, and naturally occurring food, including drinking water, often cause sensitivity. However, odor seems to be the principal trigger. Gas exhaust, perfumes, cigarette smoke, plastics, pesticides, and industrial solvents are some of the most common odors associated with IEI. The uniqueness of IEI is that symptoms occur at levels below the established guidelines of toxic levels and concentrations.

The causes of IEI are thought to be from immunologic, psychologic, toxicologic, and sociologic factors. Diagnosis is usually made based on a patient's health history. There is no established test used to diagnose IEI. Diagnostic tests that are used include provocation-neutralization and immunologic testing (e.g., CBC, lymphocyte subsets, antibody titers). Immunologic testing, however, has not been widely accepted as a diagnostic test. The provocation-neutralization test is done by exposing the patient to certain environmental substances to produce symptoms and then at higher and lower doses to initiate the disappearance of symptoms.

Treatment includes minimizing exposure to known irritants, elimination of foods causing sensitivity, and exercising regularly. Physical therapy, massage, prayer, and meditation are also recommended.

AUTOIMMUNITY

Autoimmunity is an inappropriate reaction to self-proteins; the immune system no longer differentiates self from nonself with respect to these substances. For some unknown reason, immune cells that are normally unresponsive (tolerant to self-antigens) are activated. Both T cells and B cells have the ability for tolerance to self-antigens. Therefore an alteration in T cells alone or in both B cells and T cells can produce autoantibodies and autosensitized T cells to cause pathophysiologic tissue damage. The particular autoimmune disease manifested depends on which self-antigen is involved.[19]

Autoimmune diseases tend to cluster so that a given person may have more than one autoimmune disease (e.g., rheumatoid arthritis, Addison's disease), or the same or related autoimmune diseases may be found in other members of the same family. This observation has led to the concept of genetic predisposition to autoimmune disease.

Theories of Causation

The cause of autoimmune diseases is still unknown.[20] Age is thought to play some role, because the number of circulating autoantibodies increases in persons over age 50. It appears that no one theory is conclusive. A combination of etiologic factors may be involved.

Genetic Susceptibility. Most autoimmune diseases have a genetic basis. Most of the research work in this area correlates certain HLA types with an autoimmune condition. (HLA and disease association are discussed later in this chapter.)

Initiation of Autoreactivity. Even in a genetically predisposed person, some trigger is required for the initiation of autoreactivity. This may include infectious agents such as a virus.[20] Viral infections can cause an alteration of cells or tissues that are not normally antigenic. The virally induced changes can make the cells or tissues antigenic. There is some evidence that viruses may be involved in the development of multiple sclerosis and type 1 diabetes mellitus. Rheumatic fever and rheumatic heart disease are autoimmune responses triggered by streptococcal infection and mediated by antibodies against group A β-hemolytic streptococci that cross-react with heart muscles and valves and synovial membranes.

Drugs can also be precipitating factors in autoimmune disease. Hemolytic anemia can result from methyldopa (Aldomet) administration. Procainamide (Pronestyl) can induce the formation of antinuclear antibodies and cause a lupus-like syndrome.

Hormones also have a role in autoimmune disease. More women than men have autoimmune disease. During pregnancy many autoimmune diseases get better. Following delivery, the woman with an autoimmune disease frequently has an exacerbation.

Autoimmune Diseases

Generally, autoimmune diseases are grouped according to organ-specific and systemic diseases. (See Table 13-14 for examples of autoimmune diseases.) Systemic lupus erythematosus (SLE) is a classic example of a systemic autoimmune disease characterized by damage to multiple organs. It occurs most frequently in women ages 20 to 40 years. The etiology is unknown, but there appears to be a loss of self-tolerance for the body's own DNA antigens.

In SLE, tissue injury appears to be the result of the formation of antinuclear antibodies. For some reason (possibly a viral infection), the cell membrane is damaged and DNA is released into the systemic circulation where it is viewed as nonself. This DNA is normally sequestered inside the nucleus of cells. On release into circulation the DNA antigen reacts with an antibody. Some antibodies are involved in immune complex formation, and others may cause damage directly. Once the complexes are deposited, complement is activated and further damages the tissue, especially the renal glomerulus. (Systemic lupus erythematosus is discussed in Chapter 63.)

Apheresis

Apheresis has been effectively used to treat autoimmune diseases and other diseases and disorders. *Apheresis* is the use of a procedure to separate components of the blood followed by the removal of one or more of these components. Compound words are often used to describe any particular apheresis procedure, depending on the blood components being collected. *Cytapheresis*

TABLE 13-14 Examples of Autoimmune Diseases*

Systemic Diseases
Systemic lupus erythematosus
Rheumatoid arthritis
Progressive systemic sclerosis (scleroderma)
Mixed connective tissue disease

Organ-Specific Diseases
Blood
Autoimmune hemolytic anemia
Immune thrombocytopenic purpura
Central Nervous System
Multiple sclerosis
Guillain-Barré syndrome
Muscle
Myasthenia gravis
Heart
Rheumatic fever
Endocrine System
Addison's disease
Thyroiditis
Hypothyroidism
Type 1 diabetes mellitus
Gastrointestinal System
Pernicious anemia
Ulcerative colitis
Kidney
Goodpasture syndrome
Glomerulonephritis
Liver
Primary biliary cirrhosis
Autoimmune hepatitis
Eye
Uveitis

*These diseases are discussed in chapters throughout the book.

is a general term for cell separation and removal. *Plateletpheresis* is the removal of platelets, usually for collection from normal individuals to infuse into patients with low platelet counts (e.g., patients taking chemotherapy who develop thrombocytopenia). *Leukocytapheresis* is a general term indicating the removal of WBCs and is used in chronic myelogenous leukemia to remove high numbers of leukemic cells. *Lymphocytapheresis* is used to decrease high lymphocyte counts such as in individuals with chronic lymphocytic leukemia.

Plasmapheresis. *Plasmapheresis* is the removal of plasma containing components causing or thought to cause disease. When plasma is removed, it is replaced by substitution fluids such as saline or albumin. Therefore the term *plasma exchange* more accurately describes this procedure.

Plasmapheresis has been used to treat autoimmune diseases such SLE, glomerulonephritis, Goodpasture syndrome, myasthenia gravis, thrombocytopenic purpura, rheumatoid arthritis, and Guillain-Barré syndrome. Apheresis procedures are also done on healthy donors to obtain plasma and selected blood components to administer as replacement therapy for patients.

The rationale for performing therapeutic plasmapheresis in autoimmune disorders is to remove pathologic substances present in plasma. Many disorders for which plasmapheresis is being used are characterized by circulating autoantibodies (usually of the IgG class) and antigen-antibody complexes. Immunosuppressive therapy has been used to prevent recovery of IgG production, and plasmapheresis has been used to prevent antibody rebound.

In addition to removing antibodies and antigen-antibody complexes, plasmapheresis may also remove inflammatory mediators (e.g., complement) that are responsible for tissue damage. In the treatment of SLE, plasmapheresis is usually reserved for the patient in an acute attack who is unresponsive to conventional therapy.

Plasmapheresis involves the removal of whole blood through a needle inserted in one arm and circulation of the blood through a cell separator. Inside the separator the blood is divided into plasma and its cellular components by centrifugation or membrane filtration. A needle is inserted into the opposite arm for return of the blood to the patient. Plasma, platelets, WBCs, or RBCs can be separated selectively. The undesirable component is removed, and the remainder is returned to the patient. The plasma is generally replaced with normal saline, lactated Ringer's solution, fresh frozen plasma, plasma protein fractions, or albumin. When blood is manually removed, only 500 ml may be taken at one time. However, with the use of apheresis procedures, over 4 L of plasma can be pheresed in 2 to 3 hours.

As with administration of other blood products, nurses must be aware of side effects associated with plasmapheresis. The most common complications are hypotension and citrate toxicity. Hypotension is usually the result of vasovagal reaction or transient volume changes. Citrate is used as an anticoagulant and may cause hypocalcemia, which may manifest as headache, paresthesias, and dizziness.

HISTOCOMPATIBILITY

Human Leukocyte Antigen System

The HLA system consists of a series of linked genes that occur together on the sixth chromosome in humans.[21,22] The products of these genes include the cell membrane antigens of the HLA series.

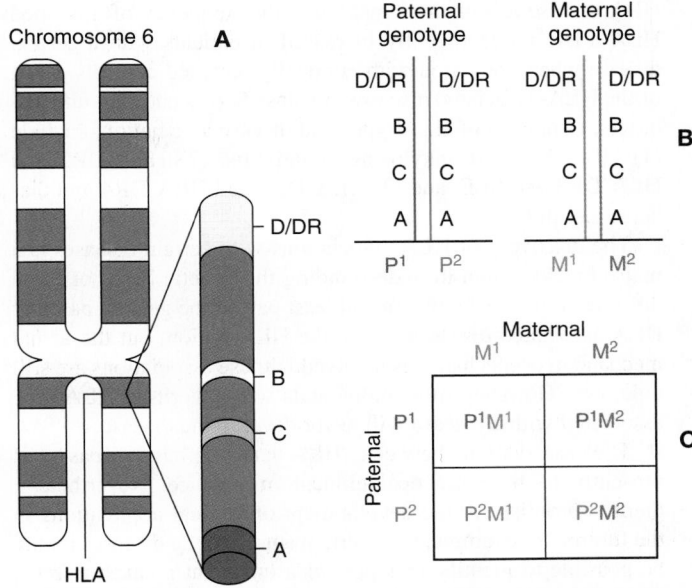

FIG. 13-13 Patterns of HLA inheritance. **A,** HLA genes are located on chromosome 6. **B,** The two haplotypes of the father are labeled P^1 and P^2 and the haplotypes of the mother are labeled M^1 and M^2. Each child inherits two haplotypes, one from each parent. **C,** Therefore only four combinations—P^{1}M^1, P^{1}M^2, P^{2}M^1, P^{2}M^2—are possible, and 25% of the offspring will have identical HLA haplotypes.

Because of its importance in the study of tissue matching, the chromosomal region incorporating the HLA genes is termed the *major histocompatibility complex*. The genes determining the products recognized as the HLA-A, HLA-B, HLA-C, HLA-D, and HLA-DR antigens are clustered together (Fig. 13-13). HLA antigens are present on all nucleated cells and platelets.

An important characteristic of HLA genes is that they are highly polymorphic. Each HLA locus can have many different possible alleles. The specific allele is identified by a number. For example, a person could be A6, B7, C8, D1, DR7. With many alleles possible at each HLA locus, many combinations exist. Each person has two antigens for each locus, one inherited from each parent. Both antigens of a locus are expressed independently (i.e., they are codominant). The entire set of A, B, C, D, and DR antigens located on one chromosome is termed a *haplotype*. A complete set of antigens located on a chromosome is inherited as a unit (haplotype). One haplotype is inherited from each parent (see Fig. 13-13).

Because of the polymorphic nature of the HLA system, it is an ideal marker for genetic studies. This characteristic also makes it a useful tool in settling paternity disputes. The frequencies of HLAs vary considerably among different races. For example, HLA-B8 is relatively high in American whites, but it is very low in Native American and Japanese persons.

Human Leukocyte Antigen and Disease Associations

The early interest in HLA was stimulated by its potential role in matching donors and recipients of organ transplants. During the last few years, interest in the association between HLA and disease has grown. Strong associations between HLA type and susceptibility to certain diseases have been demonstrated.[21,22]

HLA disease associations mean that the frequency of a defined HLA allele is significantly increased in patients with a certain disease when compared with ethnically matched controls. Most of the HLA-associated diseases are classified as autoimmune disorders. Examples of HLA types and disease associations include (1) HLA-B27 and ankylosing spondylitis, (2) HLA-DR2 and HLA-DR3 and SLE, and (3) HLA-DR3 and HLA-DR4 and diabetes mellitus.

The discovery of HLA associations with certain diseases is a major breakthrough in understanding the genetic bases of these diseases. It is now known that at least part of the genetic bases of HLA-associated diseases lies in the HLA region, but the actual mechanism or mechanisms involved in these associations are still unknown. However, most individuals who inherit an HLA type associated with a disease will never develop the disease.

The association between HLA and certain diseases is presently of little practical clinical importance. Nevertheless, there is promise for the development of clinical applications in the future. For example, with certain autoimmune diseases it may be possible to identify members of a family at greatest risk for developing the same or a related autoimmune disease. These persons would need close medical supervision, preventive measures implemented (if possible), and early diagnosis and treatment instituted to prevent chronic complications.

Histocompatibility Studies

The purpose of histocompatibility testing is to identify the HLA antigens for both donors and potential recipients. A serologic test is used to type for the antigens at all five loci (A, B, C, D, and DR). Lymphocytes are isolated from peripheral blood and then combined with serum that contains antibodies to HLAs. Currently only the A, B, and DR antigens are thought to be clinically significant for transplantation. Because there are two antigens at each locus, a total of six antigens are identified. The total time required for HLA typing is about 4 to 6 hours. In cadaveric transplantation an attempt is made to match as many antigens as possible between the HLA-A, HLA-B, and HLA-DR loci. Antigen matches of five and six antigens and certain four-antigen matches have been found to have better clinical outcomes (i.e., the patient is less likely to reject the transplanted organ).

Another test done is called a *crossmatch*. This is done at the time a living donor is being evaluated and just before surgery for cadaver donors. A crossmatch uses serum from the recipient mixed with donor lymphocytes to test for any preformed cytotoxic (anti-HLA) antibodies to the potential donor organ. A positive crossmatch indicates that the recipient has cytotoxic antibodies to the donor and is an absolute contraindication to transplantation. The potential recipient may have been exposed to antigens similar to those of the donor by means of previous blood transfusions, pregnancy, or a previous organ transplant. If transplanted, the organ would undergo hyperacute rejection. This procedure takes about 3 to 5 hours. A negative crossmatch indicates that no preformed antibodies are present and it is safe to proceed with transplantation.

Crossmatching is also performed to detect preformed cytotoxic antibodies in the recipient serum to HLAs on lymphocytes from random donors. In this situation, rather than using specific donor lymphocytes, the recipient serum is mixed with a randomly selected panel of donor lymphocytes to determine reactivity. This is called the panel of reactive antibodies (PRA) and indicates the recipient's sensitivity to various HLAs. The results are calculated in percentages. A high PRA indicates that the person has a large number of cytotoxic antibodies, which means that there is a poor chance of finding a crossmatch-negative donor. In patients awaiting transplantation, a PRA panel is usually done on a regular basis.

IMMUNODEFICIENCY DISORDERS

When the immune system does not adequately protect the body, **immunodeficiency** exists. Immunodeficiency disorders involve an impairment of one or more immune mechanisms, which include (1) phagocytosis, (2) humoral response, (3) cell-mediated response, (4) complement, and (5) a combined humoral and cell-mediated deficiency. Immunodeficiency disorders are *primary* if the immune cells are improperly developed or absent and *secondary* if the deficiency is caused by illnesses or treatment. Primary immunodeficiency disorders are rare and often serious, whereas secondary disorders are more common and less severe.

Primary Immunodeficiency Disorders

The basic categories of primary immunodeficiency disorders are (1) phagocytic defects, (2) B cell deficiency, (3) T cell deficiency, and (4) a combined B cell and T cell deficiency[23] (Table 13-15).

TABLE 13-15   Primary Immunodeficiency Disorders

DISORDER	AFFECTED CELLS	GENETIC BASIS
Chronic granulomatous disease	PMN, monocytes	Sex-linked
Job syndrome	PMN, monocytes	
Bruton's X-linked hypogammaglobulinemia	B	Sex-linked
Common variable hypogammaglobulinemia	B	
Selective IgA, IgM, or IgG deficiency	B	Some sex-linked
DiGeorge syndrome (thymic hypoplasia)	T	
Severe combined immunodeficiency disease	Stem, B, T	Sex-linked or autosomal recessive
Ataxia telangiectasia	B, T	Autosomal recessive
Wiskott-Aldrich syndrome	B, T	Sex-linked
Graft-versus-host disease	B, T	

Secondary Immunodeficiency Disorders

Some of the important factors that may cause secondary immunodeficiency disorders are listed in Table 13-16. Drug-induced immunosuppression is the most common. Immunosuppressive therapy is prescribed for patients to treat autoimmune disorders and to prevent transplant rejection. In addition, immunosuppression is a serious side effect of drugs used in cancer chemotherapy. Generalized leukopenia often results, leading to a decreased humoral and cell-mediated response. Therefore secondary infections are common in immunosuppressed patients.

Stress may alter the immune response. This response involves interrelationships among the nervous, endocrine, and immune systems (see Chapter 8).

A hypofunctional state of the immune system exists in young children and older adults. Laboratory studies have demonstrated that immunoglobulin levels decrease with age and therefore lead to a suppressed humoral immune response in older adults. Thymic involution occurs with aging along with decreased numbers of T cells. The incidence of malignancies and autoimmune diseases increases with aging and may be related to immunologic alterations.

Malnutrition alters cell-mediated immune responses. When protein is deficient over a prolonged period, atrophy of the thymus gland occurs and lymphoid tissue decreases. In addition, an increased susceptibility to infections always exists.

Radiation destroys lymphocytes either directly or through depletion of stem cells. As the radiation dose is increased, more bone marrow atrophies, leading to severe pancytopenia and suppression of immune function.

Surgical removal of lymph nodes, thymus, or spleen can suppress the immune response. Splenectomy in children is especially dangerous and may lead to septicemia from simple respiratory infections.

Hodgkin's disease greatly impairs the cell-mediated immune response, and patients may die from severe viral or fungal infections. (Hodgkin's disease is discussed in Chapter 30.) Viruses, especially rubella, may cause immunodeficiency by direct cytotoxic damage to lymphoid cells. Systemic infections can place such a demand on the immune system that resistance to a secondary or subsequent infection is impaired.

Graft-versus-Host Disease

Graft-versus-host (GVH) disease occurs when an immunoincompetent (immunodeficient) patient is transfused or transplanted with immunocompetent cells. A GVH response may result from the infusion of any blood product containing viable lymphocytes, such as in therapeutic blood transfusions, and from the transplantation of fetal thymus, fetal liver, or bone marrow. In most transplantation situations, the biggest concern is the host's rejection of the graft. However, in GVH disease the graft rejects the host or recipient tissue.

The GVH response may have its onset 7 to 30 days after transplant. Once the reaction is started, little can be done to modify its course. The exact mechanism involved in this reaction is not completely understood. However, it involves donor T cells attacking and destroying vulnerable host cells.

The target organs for the GVH phenomenon are the skin, GI tract, and liver. The skin disease may be a maculopapular rash, which may be pruritic or painful. It initially involves the palms and soles of the feet but can progress to a generalized erythema with bullous formation and desquamation. The liver disease may manifest as mild jaundice with elevated liver enzymes ranging to hepatic coma. The intestinal disease may be manifested by mild to severe diarrhea, severe abdominal pain, GI bleeding, and malabsorption. The biggest problem with GVH disease is infection, with different types of infections seen in different periods. Bacterial and fungal infections predominate immediately after transplantation when granulocytopenia exists. The development of interstitial pneumonitis is the predominant later problem.

There is no adequate treatment of GVH disease once it is established. Although corticosteroids are often used, they enhance the susceptibility to infection. The use of immunosuppressive agents (e.g., methotrexate, cyclosporine) has been most effective as a preventive rather than a treatment measure. Radiation of blood products before they are administered is another measure to prevent T cell replication.

IMMUNOSUPPRESSIVE THERAPY*

The goal of **immunosuppressive therapy** is to adequately suppress the immune response to prevent rejection of the transplanted organ while maintaining sufficient immunity to prevent overwhelming infection. Many of the medications used to achieve immunosuppression have adverse effects. By using a combination of medications that work in different phases of the immune response, lower doses of each drug produce effective immunosuppression while minimizing side effects.[24] Immunosuppressive protocols are highly variable among transplant cen-

---

TABLE 13-16   Causes of Secondary Immunodeficiency

- Drug-induced immunodeficiency
  Chemotherapy drugs
  Corticosteroids
- Stress
- Age
  Infants
  Older adults
- Malnutrition
  Dietary deficiency
  Cirrhosis
  Cachexia
- Radiation
- Surgery
- Anesthesia
- Trauma
- Burns
- Diseases
  Acquired immunodeficiency syndrome (AIDS)
  Alcoholic cirrhosis
  Chronic renal disease
  Diabetes mellitus
  Malignancies
  Systemic lupus erythematosus

*The material in this section was contributed by Mary Jo Holecheck, RN, MS, CRNP, CNN.

ters, with different combinations of medications used. Most patients are initially on triple therapy. The standard triple therapy usually includes a calcineurin inhibitor, a corticosteroid, and mycophenolate mofetil (CellCept). Doses of some immunosuppressant drugs may be decreased over time. Some patients can be weaned off corticosteroids (prednisone) after 1.5 to 2 years.

The major immunosuppressive agents are (1) calcineurin inhibitors, including cyclosporine (Sandimmune, Neoral, Gengraf) and tacrolimus (Prograf, FK506); (2) corticosteroids (prednisone, methylprednisolone [Solu-Medrol] IV); (3) mycophenolate mofetil (CellCept); and (4) sirolimus (Rapamune). Azathioprine (Imuran) and cyclophosphamide (Cytoxan) have been used in the past, but are rarely used now because they have been replaced with safer, more effective drugs. Antithymocyte globulin

(ATG), antilymphocyte globulin (ALG), and muromonab-CD3 are IV medications used for short periods to prevent early rejection (induction therapy) or reverse acute rejection. The most common drugs, route of administration, mechanism of action, and adverse side effects are presented in Table 13-17.

Calcineurin Inhibitors

This group of drugs includes tacrolimus and cyclosporine. The mechanism of action of these drugs is to prevent the production and release of interleukin-2 (IL-2), interleukin-4 (IL-4), and γ-interferon by interfering with calcineurin binding. These cytokines are needed to promote T cell proliferation and activation. Therefore these drugs prevent a cell-mediated attack against the transplanted organ (see Chapter 45, Fig. 45-19). These drugs

TABLE 13-17 Drug Therapy — Immunosuppressive Therapy

AGENT	ROUTE	MECHANISM OF ACTION	SIDE EFFECTS
Corticosteroids prednisone, methylprednisolone (Solu-Medrol)	PO, IV	Suppress inflammatory response; inhibit cytokine production and T cell activation	Peptic ulcers, hypertension, GI bleeding, osteoporosis, aseptic necrosis, Na^+ and H_2O retention, acne, muscle weakness, easy bruising, delayed healing, hyperglycemia, increased appetite, mood alterations, leukopenia, cataracts, hyperlipidemia, ↓ resistance to infection
tacrolimus (Prograf, FK 506)	PO, IV	Calcineurin inhibitor; prevents production and release of IL-2, IL-4, and α-interferon; inhibits production of T cytotoxic lymphocytes	Nephrotoxicity, neurotoxicity, seizures, tremors, nausea and vomiting, hyperglycemia, hypertension, alopecia, lymphoma, ↓ resistance to infection
cyclosporine (Sandimmune) (Neoral, Gengraf) (Neoral and Gengraf are microemulsions with better absorption than Sandimmune)	PO, IV PO	Calcineurin inhibitor; prevents production and release of IL-2, IL-4, and α-interferon; inhibits production of T cytotoxic lymphocytes	Nephrotoxicity, neurotoxicity, headaches, seizures, tremors, hyperglycemia, hypertension, nausea and vomiting, hyperlipidemia, gingival hyperplasia, hirsutism, hepatotoxicity, lymphoma, ↓ resistance to infection
mycophenolate mofetil (CellCept)	PO, IV	Antimetabolite that inhibits purine synthesis; suppresses proliferation of T and B cells	Diarrhea, nausea and vomiting, leukopenia, thrombocytopenia, resistance to infection, ↑ incidence of malignancies
sirolimus (Rapamune)	PO	Suppresses lymphocyte proliferation; inhibits B cells from synthesizing antibodies	Diarrhea, hyperlipidemia, hypercholesterolemia, arthralgias, delayed wound healing, thrombocytopenia, resistance to infection, ↑ incidence of malignancies
Muromonab-CD3 (OKT3)	IV push	Monoclonal antibody that binds to CD3 receptors on lymphocytes, causing cell lysis; inhibits function of cytotoxic T cells	Fever, chills, tachycardia, pulmonary edema, muscle and joint pain, diarrhea, hypertension or hypotension, aseptic meningitis, ↓ resistance to infection, ↑ incidence of malignancies
daclizumab (Zenapax)	IV	Monoclonal antibody that acts as IL-2 receptor antagonist by inhibiting the binding of IL-2; inhibits T cell activation and proliferation	Generally no side effects
basiliximab (Simulect)	IV	Same as daclizumab	Same as daclizumab
Polyclonal antibody serums: ATG, ALG (Thymoglobulin, ATGAM)	IV	Polyclonal antibodies directed against lymphocytes; particularly deplete T cells	Serum sickness (fever, chills, muscle and joint pain), tachycardia, back pain, shortness of breath, hypotension, anaphylaxis, leukopenia, thrombocytopenia, rash, resistance to infection, ↑ incidence of malignancies

ALG, Antilymphocyte globulin; *ATG*, antithymocyte globulin; *IL*, interleukin.

do not cause bone marrow suppression or alterations of the normal inflammatory response. They are generally used in combination with corticosteroids and mycophenolate mofetil. Many of the side effects of calcineurin inhibitors are dose related. These drugs are nephrotoxic. Drug levels are followed closely to prevent toxicity. Neoral and Gengraf, microemulsions of cyclosporine, are replacing Sandimmune because of better and more consistent absorption.[25] Neoral and Sandimmune are not biocompatible and should never be interchanged for one another.

Tacrolimus is 100 times more potent than cyclosporine, allowing for smaller doses to be given. It does not cause hirsutism or gingival hyperplasia as does cyclosporine. Its most significant side effects include neurotoxicities, such as tremor and altered mental status, and diabetes. Tacrolimus is the most often prescribed calcineurin inhibitor.

Sirolimus

Sirolimus is a new immunosuppressive agent with structural similarities to tacrolimus, but a different mechanism of action. Sirolimus suppresses lymphocyte proliferation and inhibits B cells from synthesizing antibodies.[25] At relatively low doses, it has a synergistic effect with cyclosporine, corticosteroids, or both. It is also used in combination with tacrolimus. Everolimus (Certican) is similar to sirolimus. It is currently undergoing clinical testing.

Mycophenolate Mofetil

Mycophenolate mofetil (CellCept) is a lymphocyte-specific inhibitor of purine synthesis with suppressive effects on both T and B lymphocytes. This drug appears to be most effective when used in combination with tacrolimus or cyclosporine. Its effects are additive because it acts later in the lymphocyte activation pathway by a different mechanism. It is used in place of azathioprine at many transplant centers because of its lymphocyte-specific effects. It has also been shown to decrease the incidence of late graft loss. The major limitation of this drug is its GI toxicities, including nausea, vomiting, and diarrhea. In many cases the side effects can be diminished by lowering the dose or giving smaller doses more frequently. Myfortic is an enteric-coated form of mycophenolate mofetil. It is currently undergoing clinical testing.

Polyclonal Antibodies (Antithymocyte Globulin and Antilymphocyte Globulin)

Antilymphocyte globulin (ALG) and antithymocyte globulin (ATG) are used as induction therapy or to treat acute rejection. The purpose of induction therapy is to severely immunosuppress an individual immediately after transplantation to prevent early rejection. These agents are prepared by immunizing horses or rabbits with human lymphoid material (thymocytes, lymph nodes, or spleen cells). The antibody made against the human lymphocytes is then purified and administered intravenously. The actual mechanism of action of ATG and ALG is not clear, but they induce lymphopenia and decrease the proliferative response of T lymphocytes, possibly as a result of the generation of T suppressor lymphocytes.

Allergic reactions to the foreign proteins from the host animal, manifested by fever, arthralgias, and tachycardia, are common but usually not severe enough to preclude use. These side effects can be attenuated by administering the preparation slowly, over 4 to 6 hours, and premedicating patients with acetaminophen (Tylenol), diphenhydramine (Benadryl), and methylprednisolone (Solu-Medrol). The main toxicities of polyclonal antibodies are lymphopenia and thrombocytopenia caused by antibody contaminants that are not completely removed during preparation of the antibodies.

Monoclonal Antibodies

Monoclonal antibodies are used for preventing and treating acute rejection episodes. (Monoclonal antibodies are discussed later in this chapter.) Muromonab-CD3 was the first of these monoclonal antibodies to be used in clinical transplantation. It is a mouse monoclonal antibody that binds with the CD3 antigen found on the surface of human thymocytes and mature T cells. It is an anti–antigen receptor antibody that interferes with the function of the T lymphocyte, the pivotal cell in the response to graft rejection. It is administered via IV push daily for 7 to 14 days. All T cells are affected rather than just the subset active in graft rejection. Within minutes after the initial infusion of muromonab-CD3, the number of circulating T cells decreases significantly.

A flulike syndrome occurs during the first few days of treatment, due to cytokine release. Side effects include fever, rigors, headache, myalgias, and various GI disturbances. To reduce the expected side effects of muromonab-CD3, patients should receive acetaminophen, diphenhydramine, and IV corticosteroids before administering the dose.

Newer-generation monoclonal antibodies include daclizumab (Zenapax) and basiliximab (Simulect).[26] These monoclonal antibodies are a hybrid of mouse and human antibodies and have fewer side effects than muromonab-CD3 because they have been humanized by replacing large parts of the molecule with human IgG.

New Immunosuppressive Therapy

The search continues to find immunosuppressants that specifically target the cells responsible for rejection while limiting drug toxicities. FTY 720 interferes with the ability of lymphocytes to respond to stimulation. It lowers the number of T and B cells in the peripheral blood, but increases the number in the lymph nodes and Peyer's patches. It suppresses lymphocyte infiltration into transplanted grafts and prolongs lymphopenia. It is currently in clinical trials.

HuM291 is a humanized form of OKT3, currently in clinical trials, that has few side effects because it does not stimulate cytokine release. OKT4A is another monoclonal antibody being tested. There is also ongoing research into T cell blockade and immunomodulation.[24]

NEW TECHNOLOGIES IN IMMUNOLOGY

Hybridoma Technology: Monoclonal Antibodies

Monoclonal antibodies are homogeneous populations of identical antibody molecules produced by specialized tissue cell culture lines. The procedure uses cell fusion techniques and standard in vitro tissue culture systems (Fig. 13-14). The two essential biologic components are immunized mice or rats and myeloma tumor cell lines, which are of lymphoid origin. Single antibody-forming cells (lymphocytes) from rodents previously immunized with antigen are fused with myeloma cells to create hybrid cells with properties of both parent cell types. The hybrids have an unlimited capacity to grow, similar to that of the myeloma parent cell. The hybrids produce the single type of antibody molecule that they inherited from the normal, antibody-forming parent cell. Hybrid cells derived in this way can produce unlimited quantities of specific antibodies. With appropriate selection techniques, producing monoclonal antibodies to virtually any antigen is possible. Because the monoclonal antibodies are a completely homogeneous population, their use incurs fewer problems than conventional polyclonal antisera.

Monoclonal antibodies are finding wide application in many areas of medicine and biologic science. Thousands of monoclonal antibodies have been made against many different types of antigens. Monoclonal antibodies have begun to replace conventional antibodies in blood banking and are used in the identification of organisms in the bacteriology laboratory. Monoclonal antibodies have also been extensively used in radioimmunoassays to measure serum levels of various substances (e.g., parathyroid hormone). They have been useful in quantitating types of WBCs and subtypes of lymphocytes. They are also used in the diagnosis of leukemia. More recently, monoclonal antibodies have been used

in the treatment of malignancies (see Chapter 15). They have been used to treat transplant rejection episodes, purge bone marrow of tumor cells in bone marrow transplants, and remove mature T cells that cause GVH disease in bone marrow transplants.

A major limitation of monoclonal antibodies used for humans is that they are mouse antibodies and therefore can elicit an antibody response by the host against the foreign agent. Recently, human hybridomas have been produced using human myelomas. These hybrids synthesize human monoclonals and are therefore advantageous for in vivo use in diagnosis and therapy.

Recombinant DNA Technology

Recombinant DNA technology, a form of genetic engineering, involves taking segments of DNA from one type of organism and combining them with genes from a second organism (Fig. 13-15). When the cell divides, the DNA is transcribed and a specific protein coded by the DNA is made. In this way relatively simple organisms such as *Escherichia coli,* yeast, or mammalian tissue culture cells can be used to make large quantities of human proteins. This process is used to make human insulin and cytokines (e.g., α-interferon, interleukin-2), as well as many other substances.

Polymerase Chain Reaction

When rapid genetic diagnosis is necessary, *polymerase chain reaction* (PCR) can provide a way to make many copies of a DNA or RNA sequence in only a few hours. PCR involves the artificial replication of a DNA or RNA sequence. The DNA or RNA strands can be separated to form new templates that are used for replication. PCR requires only small amounts of sample

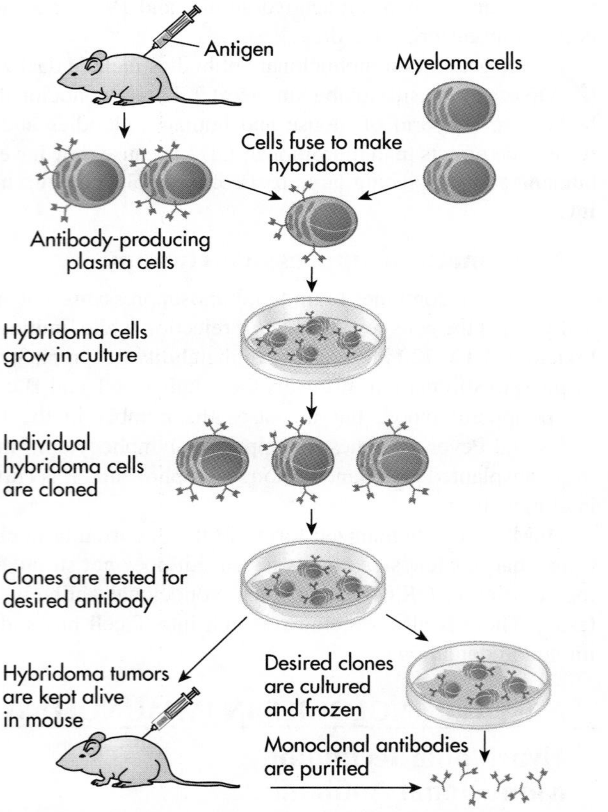

FIG. 13-14 Monoclonal antibodies are identical antibodies made by clones of a single antibody-producing cell. The target antigen is injected into a mouse. Plasma cells are harvested from the spleen of the mouse and fused with myeloma cells. The fused cells, or hybridomas, are then cloned. A clone can secrete monoclonal antibodies over a long period of time.

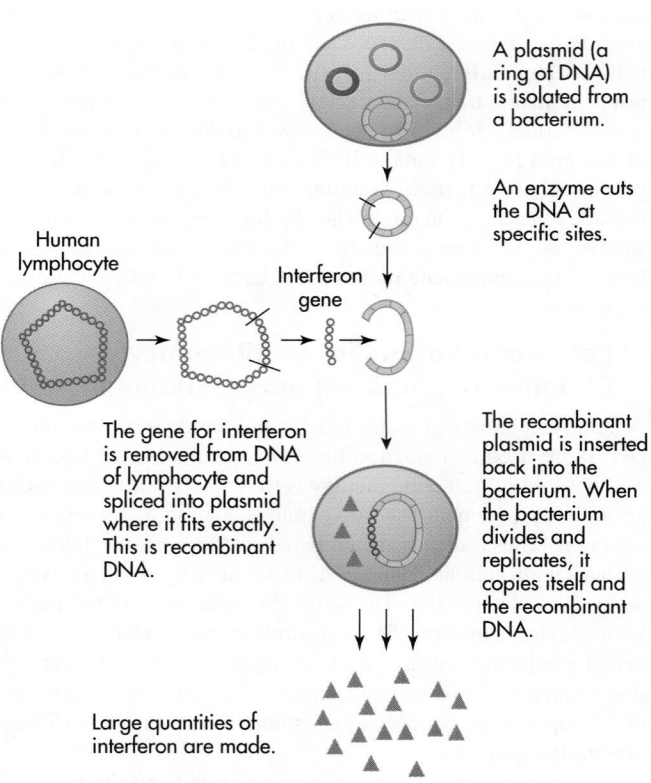

FIG. 13-15 Mass production of interferon by recombinant gene technology.

(e.g., blood, buccal swabs, secretions) in contrast to other laboratory assays. PCR is used extensively in forensic medicine to identify DNA of criminal suspects by using samples from blood, hair, and semen. PCR can also be used as a confirmatory test in HIV testing. This is especially important when an infant of a mother who is HIV-antibody positive also tests HIV positive. In this situation it is not known whether the antibodies from the infant's blood are from the baby or the mother. PCR techniques can be used on the baby's lymphocytes to determine whether the baby is infected with HIV.

REVIEW QUESTIONS

The number of the question corresponds to the same-numbered objective at the beginning of the chapter.

1. If a person is heterozygous for a given gene, it means that the person
   a. is a carrier for a genetic disorder.
   b. is affected by the genetic disorder.
   c. has two identical alleles for the gene.
   d. has two different alleles for the gene.

2. A father who has a sex-linked recessive disorder and a wife with a normal genotype will
   a. pass the carrier state to his male children.
   b. pass the carrier state to all of his children.
   c. pass the carrier state to his female children.
   d. not pass on the genetic mutation to any of his children.

3. The function of monocytes in immunity is related to their ability to
   a. stimulate the production of T and B lymphocytes.
   b. produce antibodies on exposure to foreign substances.
   c. bind antigens and stimulate natural killer cell activation.
   d. capture antigens by phagocytosis and present them to lymphocytes.

4. One function of cell-mediated immunity is
   a. formation of antibodies.
   b. activation of the complement system.
   c. surveillance for malignant cell changes.
   d. opsonization of antigens to allow phagocytosis by neutrophils.

5. The reason newborns are protected for the first 6 months of life from bacterial infections is because of the maternal transmission of
   a. IgG.
   b. IgA.
   c. IgM.
   d. IgE.

6. In a type I hypersensitivity reaction, the primary immunologic disorder appears to be
   a. binding of IgG to an antigen on a cell surface.
   b. deposit of antigen-antibody complexes in small vessels.
   c. release of lymphokines to interact with specific antigens.
   d. release of chemical mediators from IgE-bound mast cells and basophils.

7. The nurse is alerted to possible anaphylactic shock immediately after a patient has received intramuscular penicillin by the development of
   a. edema and itching at the injection site.
   b. sneezing and itching of the nose and eyes.
   c. a wheal-and-flare reaction at the injection site.
   d. chest tightness and production of thick sputum.

8. The nurse advises a friend who asks him to administer his allergy shots that
   a. it is illegal for nurses to administer injections outside of a medical setting.
   b. he is qualified to do it if the friend has epinephrine in an injectible syringe provided with his extract.
   c. avoiding the allergens is a more effective way of controlling allergies and allergy shots are not usually effective.
   d. immunotherapy should only be administered in a setting where emergency equipment and drugs are available.

9. A patient is undergoing plasmapheresis for treatment of systemic lupus erythematosus. The nurse explains that plasmapheresis is used in her treatment to
   a. remove T lymphocytes in her blood that are producing antinuclear antibodies.
   b. remove normal particles in her blood that are being damaged by autoantibodies.
   c. exchange her plasma that contains antinuclear antibodies with a substitute fluid.
   d. replace viral-damaged cellular components of her blood with replacement whole blood.

10. Association between HLA antigens and diseases is most commonly found in what disease conditions?
    a. malignancies
    b. infectious diseases
    c. neurologic diseases
    d. autoimmune disorders

11. The most common cause of secondary immunodeficiencies is
    a. drugs.
    b. stress.
    c. malnutrition.
    d. human immunodeficiency virus.

12. If a person is having an acute rejection of a transplanted organ, which of the following drugs would most likely be used?
    a. tacrolimus
    b. cyclosporine
    c. muromonab-CD3
    d. mycophenolate mofetil

13. Which of the following techniques can be used to modify an individual's genetic structure?
    a. gene therapy
    b. polymerase chain reaction
    c. recombinant RNA technology
    d. monoclonal antibody production

REFERENCES

1. Maher AB, Salmond SW, Pellino TA: *Orthopaedic nursing,* ed 3, St Louis, 2002, WB Saunders.
2. Lea DH: Ahead to the past: how genetics is changing your practice, *Nursing* 32:48, 2002.
3. Lea DH, Williams JK: Genetic testing and screening, *Am J Nurs* 102:36, 2002.
4. Sahis J: Human genetics: constructing a family pedigree, *Am J Nurs* 102:44, 2002.
5. Mahowald MB et al: *Genetics in the clinic,* St Louis, 2001, Mosby.
6. Delves PJ, Roitt D: The immune system: part 1, *N Engl J Med* 343:37, 2000.
7. Delves PJ, Roitt D: The immune system: part 2, *N Engl J Med* 343:108, 2000.
8. Medzhitov R, Janeway C Jr: Innate immunity, *N Engl J Med* 343:338, 2000.
9. von Andrian UH, Mackay CR: T-cell functions and migration, two sides of the same coin, *N Engl J Med* 343:1020, 2000.
10. O'Shea JJ, Ma A, Lipsky P: Cytokines and autoimmunity: nature reviews, *Immunology* 2:37, 2002.
11. Yung RL: Changes in immune function with age, *Rheum Dis Clin North Am* 26: 455, 2000.
12. Kay AB: Allergy and allergic diseases: part 1, *N Engl J Med* 344:30, 2001.
13. Kay AB: Allergy and allergic diseases: part 2, allergic diseases and their treatment, *N Engl J Med* 344:109, 2001.
14. Kleinpell R: Taking the shock out of anaphylaxis, *Nursing* 32:1, 1998.
15. Jurewicz MA: Anaphylaxis: when the body overreacts, *Nursing* 30:58, 2000.
16. Rusznak C, Peebles RS Jr: Anaphylaxis and anaphylactoid reactions: a guide to prevention, recognition, and emergent treatment, *Postgrad Med* 111:101, 2002.
17. Lenehan G: Latex allergy: separating fact from fiction, *Nursing* 32:59, 2002.
18. Becker HS: An analysis of the epidemiology of latex allergy: implications for primary prevention, *Medsurg Nurs* 9:135, 2000.
19. Davidson A, Diamond B: Autoimmune diseases, *N Engl J Med* 345:340, 2001.
20. Albert LJ, Inman RD: Molecular mimicry and autoimmunity, *N Engl J Med* 341:2068, 1999.
21. Klein J, Sato A: The HLA system: part 1, *N Engl J Med* 343:702, 2000.
22. Klein J, Sato A: The HLA system: part 2, *N Engl J Med* 343:782, 2000.
23. Buckley R: Primary immunodeficiency diseases due to defects in lymphocytes, *N Engl J Med* 343:1313, 2000.
24. Huizinga R: Update on immunosuppression, *Nephrology Nursing Journal* 29:261, 2002.
25. Danovitch G: Immunosuppressive medications and protocols for kidney transplantation. In Danovitch G, editor: *Handbook of kidney transplantation,* ed 3, Philadelphia, 2001, Lippincott Williams & Wilkins.
26. Bell J, Colaneri J: Basiliximab (Simulect): simplifying induction therapy, *Nephrology Nursing Journal* 27:243, 2000.

RESOURCES

American Academy of Allergy, Asthma, and Immunology (AAAAI)
611 East Wells Street
Milwaukee, WI 53202
800-822-2762 or 414-272-6071
www.aaaai.org/
American Association of Immunologists
9650 Rockville Pike
Bethesda, MD 20814-3994
301-530-7178
Fax: 301-571-1816
http://mercury.faseb.org/aai/
American College of Medical Genetics
9650 Rockville Pike
Bethesda, MD 20814-3998
301-530-7127
Fax: 301-571-0677
www.acmg.net/

American Public Health Association
800 I Street NW
Washington, DC 20001-3710
202-777-APHA (2742)
Fax: 202-777-2534
www.apha.org/
American Society for Microbiology
1752 North Street NW
Washington, DC 20036
202-737-3600
www.asmusa.org/
American Society of Human Genetics
9650 Rockville Pike
Bethesda, MD 20814-3998
866-HUMGENE (486-4363)
301-571-1825
Fax: 301-530-7079
http://ns1.faseb.org/genetics/ashg/ashgmenu.htm
Asthma and Allergy Foundation of America (AAFA)
1123 20th Street NW, Suite 402
Washington, DC 20036
202-466-7643
Fax: 202-466-8940
www.aafa.org
Centers for Disease Control and Prevention, Office of Genomics and Disease Prevention
4770 Buford Hwy., Mailstop K28
Atlanta, GA, 30341-3724
770-488-3235
Fax: 770-488-3236
www.cdc.gov/genomics
Gene Clinics
www.geneclinics.org
Genetic Alliance
4301 Connecticut Avenue NW, Suite 404
Washington, DC 20008-2304
202-966-5557
Fax: 202-966-8553
www.geneticalliance.org/
Genetics Program for Nursing Faculty
Cincinnati Children's Hospital Medical Center
3333 Burnet Avenue
Cincinnati, OH 45229-3039
800-344-2462 or 513-636-7963
www.cincinnatichildrens.org/traininged/training/gpnf
Human Genome Program of the U.S. Department of Energy
www.ornl.gov/hgmis/
International Society of Nurses in Genetics (ISONG)
http://nursing.creighton.edu/isong
National Allergy Bureau
611 East Wells Street
Milwaukee, WI 53202
414-272-6071
Fax: 414-272-6070
www.aaaai.org/nab/
National Center for Infectious Diseases
Centers for Disease Control and Prevention
1600 Clifton Road, Mailstop C-14
Atlanta, GA 30333
404-639-3311
www.cdc.gov/ncidod/index.htm
National Coalition for Health Professional Education in Genetics (NCHPEG)
2360 West Joppa Road, Suite 320
Lutherville, MD 21093
410-583-0600
Fax: 410-583-0520
www.nchpeg.org/

National Foundation for Infectious Diseases
  4733 Bethesda Avenue, Suite 750
  Bethesda, MD 20814
  301-656-0003
  Fax: 301-907-0878
  www.nfid.org/

National Human Genome Research Institute
  National Institutes of Health
  Building 31, Room 4B09
  31 Center Drive, MSC 2152
  9000 Rockville Pike
  Bethesda, MD 20892-2152
  301-402-0911
  Fax: 301-402-2218
  www.nhgri.nih.gov/

National Institute for Allergy and Infectious Diseases
  Building 31, Room 7A-50
  31 Center Drive MSC 2520
  Bethesda, MD 20892-2520
  301-496-2263
  www.niaid.nih.gov

National Institute of Nursing Research, Division of Intramural Research (NINR)
  301-496-0207
  www.nih.gov/ninr/research/dir.htm

Understanding Gene Testing
  www.accessexcellence.org/AE/AEPC/NIH/

For additional Internet resources, see the website for this book at *http://evolve.elsevier.com/Lewis/medsurg/.*

CHAPTER *14*

Human Immunodeficiency Virus Infection

Lucy Bradley-Springer

LEARNING OBJECTIVES

1. List the modes and variables involved in the transmission of the human immunodeficiency virus (HIV).
2. Describe the pathophysiology of HIV infection.
3. Outline HIV disease progression in the spectrum of untreated HIV infection.
4. List the diagnostic criteria for acquired immunodeficiency syndrome (AIDS).
5. Explain the methods of testing for HIV infection.
6. Discuss the collaborative management of HIV infection.

7. Explain the characteristics of opportunistic diseases associated with AIDS.
8. Discuss the long-term consequences of HIV infection and/or treatment of HIV infection.
9. Compare and contrast the methods of HIV prevention that eliminate risk and those that decrease risk.
10. Describe the nursing management of HIV-infected patients and HIV-at-risk patients.

KEY TERMS

acquired immunodeficiency syndrome (AIDS), p. 268
acute retroviral syndrome, p. 268
AIDS-dementia complex, p. 285
clades, p. 273
fusion indicator, p. 273
human immunodeficiency virus (HIV), p. 266
Kaposi's sarcoma (KS), p. 284
nonnucleoside reverse transcriptase inhibitors, p. 273
nucleoside reverse transcriptase inhibitors, p. 273

nucleotide reverse transcriptase inhibitors, p. 273
opportunistic diseases, p. 267
oral hairy leukoplakia, p. 268
postexposure prophylaxis, p. 280
protease inhibitors, p. 273
retrovirus, p. 266
reverse transcriptase, p. 266
viral load, p. 264
viremia, p. 267
window period, p. 270

several important advances have been made, including the development of laboratory tests to assess the number of HIV particles in the blood **(viral load)**, the production of new drugs, combination drug therapy, the ability to test for antiretroviral drug resistance, and treatment to decrease the risk of transmission from mother to baby.[1] In developed countries around the world, these advances have led to decreases in the number of HIV-related deaths, improved quality of life, and decreases in the number of children born with HIV.[2] Unfortunately, these advances are not effective or available for all those who need them. Although great progress has been made, the HIV epidemic is not over. Nursing care for patients with HIV infection continues to be a critical need that must change as new findings and treatment advances emerge.

Human Immunodeficiency Virus Infection

The history of the human immunodeficiency virus (HIV) epidemic in the United States and Canada has unfolded over the last two decades. Although HIV obviously had been present for a number of years before 1981, it was not until that year that public health officials documented the presence of a new disease that would become known as the acquired immunodeficiency syndrome (AIDS). By 1985 the causative agent, HIV, had been identified, and AIDS was determined to be the end stage of chronic HIV infection. In addition, an antibody test was developed and routes of transmission were determined. Drug therapy to treat the infection became available in 1987 with the release of zidovudine (ZDV, AZT, Retrovir) and has since expanded. Since 1994

Significance of Problem

By the end of December 2001, over 816,000 cases of AIDS had been diagnosed and over 467,000 AIDS-related deaths had been reported in the United States and its territories.[2] In North America, an estimated 900,000 people are living with HIV. Approximately 45,000 new infections occur each year, and women and adolescents are being infected at increasing rates. In addition, 10% of people with AIDS in the United States are 50 years of age or older. HIV in the United States is an increasing problem for people of color, people who live in poverty, people who live in rural areas, and people who deal with violence in their lives.[2] HIV infection patterns in Canada and Western Europe resemble those in the United States.

Globally, HIV is even more devastating, with an estimated 42 million people, including 3.2 million children, living with HIV. Some countries suffer a higher burden related to HIV. Since the beginning of the epidemic, sub-Saharan Africa has been the most devastated, but Asia, Russia, Central America, and South America also have rampant epidemics. In developing countries the major mode of transmission is through heterosexual sex, and women

Reviewed by Christine A. Balt, RN, MS, CS, ACRN, Nurse Practitioner, Division of Infectious Disease, Wishord Memorial Hospital, Indianapolis, Ind.

and children bear a large part of the burden of illness. Industrialized countries have fared better, but have not been able to eliminate the infection or provide appropriate care to all HIV-infected individuals.[3] For the most part, HIV remains a disease of marginalized individuals: those who are disenfranchised by virtue of gender, race, sexual orientation, poverty, drug use, or lack of access to health care.[4,5]

Transmission of HIV

HIV is a fragile virus. It can only be transmitted under specific conditions that allow contact with infected body fluids, including blood, semen, vaginal secretions, and breast milk. Transmission of HIV occurs through sexual intercourse with an infected partner, exposure to HIV-infected blood or blood products, and perinatal transmission during pregnancy, at the time of delivery, or through breastfeeding.[6]

HIV-infected individuals can transmit HIV to others within a few days after becoming infected. After that, the ability to transmit HIV is lifelong. Transmission of HIV is subject to the same requirements as other microorganisms: a large enough amount of the virus must enter the body of a susceptible host. Duration and frequency of contact, volume of fluid, virulence and concentration of the organism, and host immune status all affect whether infection actually occurs after an exposure. The viral load in the blood, semen, vaginal secretions, or breast milk of the "donor" is an important variable. In HIV infection large amounts of virus can be found in the blood during the first 2 to 6 months after infection and again during the late stages of the disease (Fig. 14-1). Unprotected sexual or blood exposure to an infected individual is more risky during these periods, although HIV can be transmitted during all phases of the disease.[7]

HIV is not spread casually. The virus cannot be transmitted through hugging, dry kissing, shaking hands, sharing eating utensils, using toilet seats, or attending school or working with an HIV-infected person. It is not transmitted through tears, saliva, urine, emesis, sputum, feces, or sweat. Repeated studies have failed to demonstrate transmission of the virus by respiratory droplets, enteric routes, or casual encounters in any setting.[7]

Health care workers have a very low risk of acquiring HIV at work, even after a needle-stick injury.[7,8]

Sexual Transmission. Sexual contact with an HIV-infected partner is the most common mode of transmission. Sexual activity provides an opportunity for contact with semen, vaginal secretions, and/or blood, all of which have lymphocytes that may contain HIV.

Although men who have sex with men (MSM) still account for most cases of HIV in the United States and Canada, heterosexual transmission is becoming more prevalent and is now the most common method of infection for women. The most risky form of sexual intercourse is unprotected anal intercourse.[2,9] During any form of sexual intercourse (anal, vaginal, or oral), the risk of infection is greater for the partner who receives the semen, although infection can also be transmitted to an inserting partner. This increased risk occurs because the receiver has prolonged contact with the semen. This helps explain why women are more easily infected than men during heterosexual intercourse. Sexual activities that involve blood, such as during menstruation or as a result of trauma to tissues, also increase the risk of transmission. In addition, the presence of genital lesions caused by other sexually transmitted diseases (STDs) (e.g., herpes, syphilis) increases the likelihood of infection.[9]

Contact with Blood and Blood Products. HIV is transmitted by exposure to contaminated blood through the accidental or intended sharing of injection equipment. Sharing equipment to inject illegal drugs is a major means of transmission in many large metropolitan areas and is becoming more common in smaller cities and rural areas. Equipment used to inject any drug, whether prescribed or not, is contaminated after use. Used equipment is potentially contaminated with HIV and/or other blood-borne organisms, and sharing that equipment can result in disease transmission.[7,9]

In the United States, transfusion of infected blood and blood products has caused only 1% of adult AIDS cases.[2] In 1985 routine screening of blood donors to identify at-risk individuals and testing donated blood for the presence of HIV were implemented, thereby improving the safety of the blood supply. HIV infection as a result of blood transfusions is now unlikely, but still possible because blood donated during the first few months of infection will not test positive for HIV antibodies (see Fig. 14-1).[10] No new cases of HIV related to the use of clotting factors by people with hemophilia are expected because these products are now treated with heat or chemicals that kill HIV and other blood-borne viruses.

By the end of February 2002, 57 health care workers (including 24 nurses) in the United States had been determined to have been infected with HIV after an occupational exposure. The Centers for Disease Control and Prevention (CDC) was following 137 more who may have been infected at work.[11] The greatest risk for work-related transmission of HIV occurs through puncture wounds. The risk of infection after a needle-stick exposure to HIV-infected blood is 0.3% to 0.4%. The risk is higher if the exposure is caused by blood from a patient with a high viral load, the puncture wound is deep, the needle has a hollow bore and visible blood, the device provided venous or arterial access, or the patient dies within 60 days. Splash exposures of blood on skin with an open lesion also present some risk, although the risk is much lower than from a puncture wound.[8]

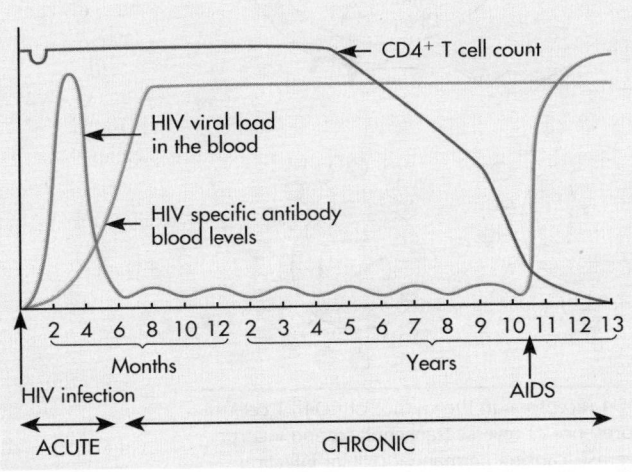

FIG. 14-1 Viral load in the blood and CD4+ T cell counts over the spectrum of untreated human immunodeficiency virus (HIV) infection.

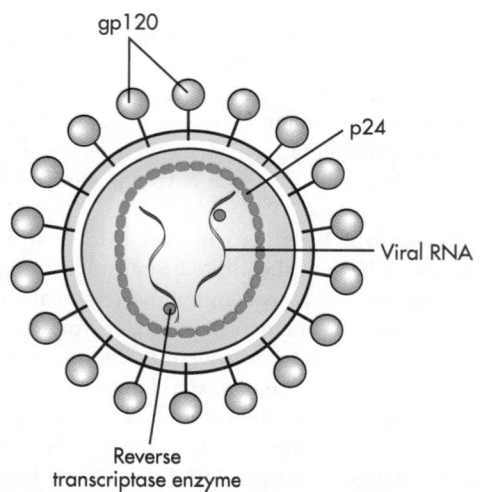

FIG. 14-2 HIV is surrounded by an envelope made up of proteins (including gp120) and contains a core of viral RNA and proteins (including p24).

Perinatal Transmission. Perinatal transmission is the most common route of infection for children. Transmission from an HIV-infected mother to her infant can occur during pregnancy, at the time of delivery, or after birth through breastfeeding. On average, 25% of infants born to untreated HIV-infected women will be born with HIV. This means that 75% of these infants would not be infected even without treatment.[12]

Pathophysiology

Human immunodeficiency virus (HIV) is a ribonucleic acid (RNA) virus that was discovered in 1983. RNA viruses are called **retroviruses** because they replicate in a "backward" manner (going from RNA to deoxyribonucleic acid [DNA]). Like all viruses, HIV cannot replicate unless it is inside a living cell. HIV can enter a cell when the gp120 "knobs" (Fig. 14-2) on the viral envelope bind to specific CD4 receptor sites on the cell's surface (Fig. 14-3). Once bound, viral genetic material enters the cell. In the cell, viral RNA is transcribed into a single strand of viral DNA with the assistance of **reverse transcriptase,** an enzyme made by HIV and other retroviruses. This strand copies itself, becoming double-stranded viral

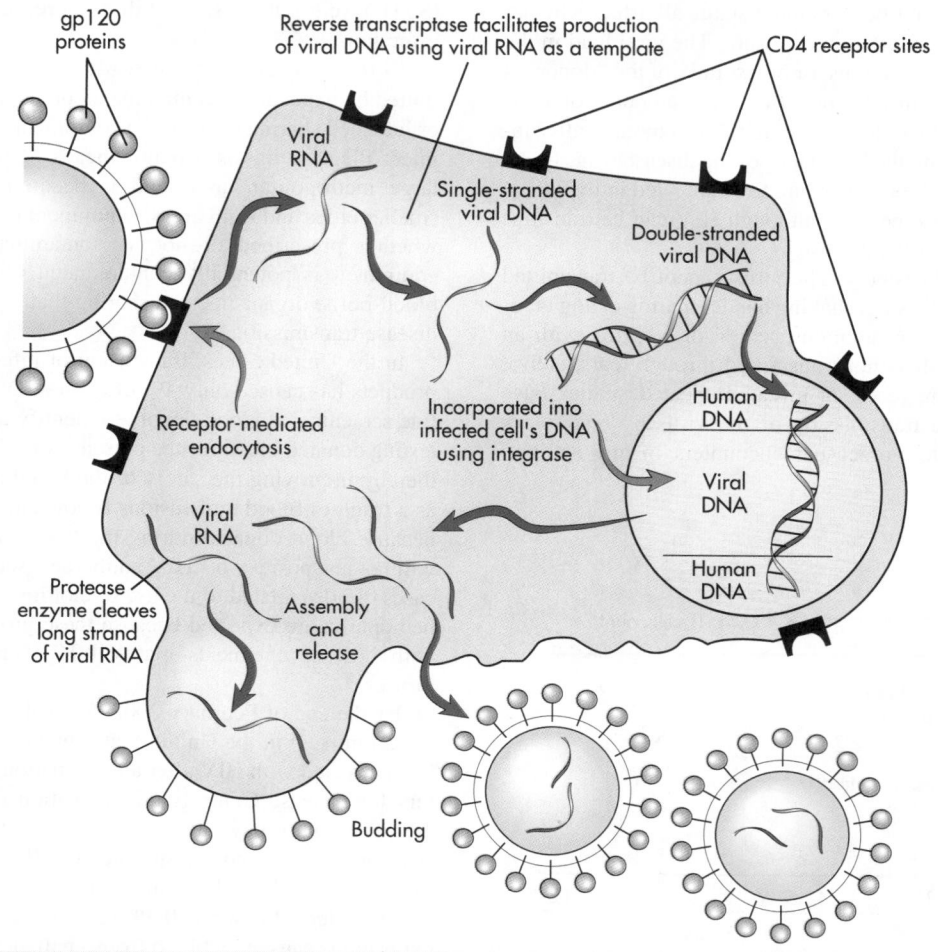

FIG. 14-3 HIV has gp120 proteins that attach to the CD4 receptors on the surface of CD4+ T cells. Viral RNA then enters the cell, produces viral DNA in the presence of reverse transcriptase, and incorporates itself into the cellular genome in the presence of integrase, causing permanent cellular infection and the production of new virions. New viral RNA develops initially in long strands that are cut in the presence of protease and leave the cell through a budding process that ultimately contributes to cellular destruction.

DNA. At this point, viral DNA can enter the cell's nucleus and, using an enzyme called *integrase*, splice itself into the genome, becoming a permanent part of the cell's genetic structure. There are two consequences of this action: (1) because all genetic material is replicated during cellular division, all daughter cells from the infected cell will also be infected; and (2) because the genome now contains viral DNA, the cell's genetic codes can direct the cell to make HIV. Production of HIV within the cell is a complicated process that results in long strands of HIV RNA. These are cut into appropriate lengths with the assistance of the enzyme *protease*.[10]

Initial infection with HIV results in **viremia** (large amounts of virus in the blood). This is followed within a few weeks by a prolonged period during which HIV levels in the blood remain low even without treatment (see Fig. 14-1). During this time, which may last for 10 to 12 years, there are few clinical symptoms.[13] It was initially thought that this phase represented a latency period during which very little viral activity occurred. It is now known that HIV replication occurs at rapid and constant rates in the blood and lymph tissues from early in the infection. A steady-state viral load can be maintained in the body of infected individuals for many years. To do this, 10^8 to 10^9 new viruses are produced each day.[14] A major consequence of rapid replication is that copy errors are made, causing mutations that contribute to difficulties in treatment and vaccine development.[15]

In a normal immune response, foreign antigens interact with B cells and T cells. In the initial stages of HIV infection these cells respond and function normally. B cells make HIV-specific antibodies that are effective in reducing viral loads in the blood, and activated T cells mount a cellular immune response to viruses trapped in the lymph nodes.[10]

HIV infects human cells that have CD4 receptors on their surfaces. These include lymphocytes, monocytes/macrophages, astrocytes, and oligodendrocytes. Immune dysfunction in HIV disease is caused predominantly by damage to and destruction of CD4$^+$ T cells (also known as T helper cells or CD4$^+$ T lymphocytes). These cells are targeted because they have more CD4 receptors on their surfaces than other CD4 receptor–bearing cells. This is unfortunate because CD4$^+$ T cells play a key role in the ability of the immune system to recognize and defend against pathogens. Adults normally have 800 to 1200 CD4$^+$ T cells per microliter (μl) of blood. The normal life span of a CD4$^+$ T cell is about 100 days, but HIV-infected CD4$^+$ T cells will die after an average life span of only 2 days.[10,16]

Viral activity destroys about 1 billion CD4$^+$ T cells every day. Fortunately, the bone marrow and thymus are able to produce enough CD4$^+$ T cells to replace the destroyed cells for many years. Eventually, however, the ability of HIV to destroy CD4$^+$ T cells exceeds the body's ability to replace the cells. The result is a decline in the CD4$^+$ T cell count and a decrease in immune capability. Generally the immune system will remain healthy with greater than 500 CD4$^+$ T cells/μl. Immune problems start to occur when the count drops to 200 to 499 CD4$^+$ T cells/μl. Severe problems develop with less than 200 CD4$^+$ T cells/μl. In HIV infection, a point is eventually reached where so many CD4$^+$ T cells are destroyed that not enough remain to regulate immune responses (see Fig. 14-1). The major concern related to immune suppression is the development of **opportunistic diseases** (infections and cancers that occur in immunosuppressed patients that can lead to disability, disease, and death).[10]

Activated CD4$^+$ T cells provide an ideal target for HIV. These cells are attracted to the site of concentrated infection in the lymph nodes where they are exposed to HIV. Once infected, activated cells support viral replication and assist in spreading infection throughout the body. Lymphoid tissue becomes an early and persistent reservoir for HIV; reservoirs protect the virus from contact with drugs and support continued viral replication. Eventually HIV causes significant damage to the lymph system. This allows the virus to spill over into the blood (a factor in disease progression) and causes significant impairment of the immune system.[17]

HIV can destroy CD4$^+$ T cells in a number of ways. Viral replication includes a process of budding (see Fig. 14-3). Budding leaves small holes in the cell's membrane. These holes allow the contents of the cells to leak out and the cell dies. A second method of destruction involves infected cells that can also fuse with other cells. This fusion process continues until many cells, some of which are not infected, combine into a mass called a syncytium that destroys all affected cells. A third process of destruction is initiated by the infected person's immune system and the antibodies that are produced against HIV. These antibodies bind to the surface of infected cells and activate the complement system, which ultimately destroys the infected cells.[16]

HIV can also infect monocytes by attaching to CD4$^+$ receptors on monocytes or by *phagocytic ingestion*. Infected monocytes move into body tissues where they differentiate into macrophages. Although HIV replicates in infected macrophages, no external budding occurs. This allows the cell to remain intact while becoming an "HIV factory." A local inflammation may cause infected macrophages to rupture, distributing HIV into surrounding tissues. Skin, lymph node, lung, central nervous system, and possibly bone marrow tissues have been directly infected in this manner.[10]

Clinical Manifestations and Complications

The typical course of untreated HIV infection follows the pattern shown in Fig. 14-4. However, it is important to remember that HIV is highly individualized. The information depicted in Fig. 14-4 represents data from large groups of people and should not be used to predict an individual's life span after HIV infection.

Acute Infection. Development of HIV-specific antibodies (*seroconversion*) is frequently accompanied by a flulike syndrome

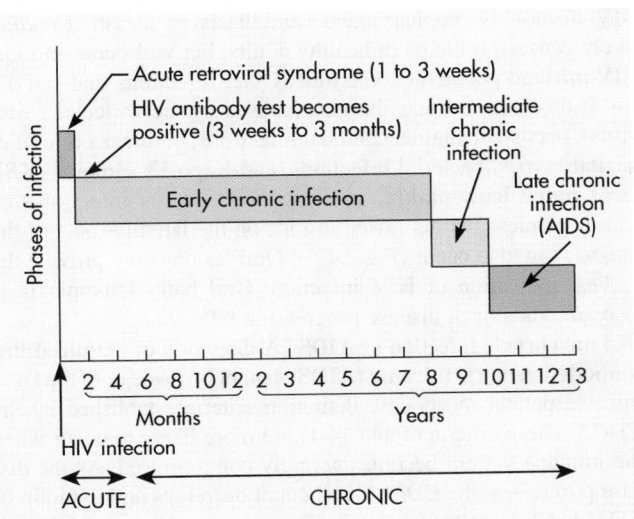

FIG. 14-4 Timeline for the spectrum of untreated HIV infection. The timeline represents the course of the illness from the time of infection to clinical manifestations of disease.

of fever, swollen lymph glands, sore throat, headache, malaise, nausea, muscle and joint pain, diarrhea, and/or a diffuse rash. These symptoms, called **acute retroviral syndrome,** generally occur 1 to 3 weeks after the initial infection and last for 1 to 2 weeks, although some of the symptoms may continue for several months. During this time a high level of HIV in the blood is noted and CD4+ T cell counts fall temporarily but quickly return to baseline (see Fig. 14-1). In most people, acute retroviral symptoms are moderate and may be mistaken for a cold or flu. In some people neurologic complications, such as aseptic meningitis, peripheral neuropathy, facial palsy, or Guillain-Barré syndrome, have developed.[13]

Chronic HIV Infection

Early chronic infection. The median interval between untreated HIV infection and a diagnosis of AIDS is about 10 years. During this time CD4+ T lymphocyte counts remain above 500 cells/μl (normal or slightly decreased) and the viral load in the blood will be low. This phase has been referred to as asymptomatic disease, but fatigue, headache, low-grade fever, night sweats, persistent generalized lymphadenopathy (PGL), and other symptoms often occur.[10,13]

Because most of the symptoms during early infection are vague and nonspecific for HIV, people may not be aware that they are infected. During this time, infected people continue activities that may include high-risk sexual and drug-using behaviors, creating a public health problem because infected people can transmit HIV to others even if they have no symptoms. Personal health is also affected because people who do not know they are infected have no motivation to seek treatment or to make changes in health habits that could beneficially alter the quality and quantity of their lives.[18]

Intermediate chronic infection. When the CD4+ T cell count drops to 200 to 500 cells/μl, the viral load rises and HIV advances to a more active stage. Symptoms seen in earlier phases tend to become worse, causing persistent fever, frequent drenching night sweats, chronic diarrhea, recurrent headaches, and fatigue severe enough to interrupt normal routines. Other problems that may occur at this time include localized infections, lymphadenopathy, and nervous system manifestations.[10,13]

The most common infection associated with this phase of HIV disease is oropharyngeal candidiasis or thrush. *Candida* rarely causes problems in healthy adults, but will occur in most HIV-infected people at some time. Other infections that can occur at this time include shingles (caused by the varicella zoster virus), persistent vaginal candidal infections, outbreaks of oral or genital herpes, bacterial infections, and Kaposi's sarcoma (KS). **Oral hairy leukoplakia,** an Epstein-Barr virus infection that causes painless, white, raised lesions on the lateral aspect of the tongue, can also occur (Fig. 14-5). Oral lesions may provide the earliest indication of HIV infection. Oral hairy leukoplakia is also an indicator of disease progression.[10,13]

Late chronic infection or AIDS. A diagnosis of **acquired immunodeficiency syndrome (AIDS)** cannot be made until the HIV-infected patient meets case definition criteria established by the CDC.[19] These criteria (Table 14-1) are more likely to occur when the immune system becomes severely compromised. As the disease progresses, the CD4+ T cell count decreases and the ratio of CD4+ to CD8+ cells (T helper to T suppressor cells), which is usually about 2:1, gradually reverses. The amount of HIV that can be detected in the blood is increased. Decreases in the absolute number of lymphocytes, as well as the percent of lymphocytes, may oc-

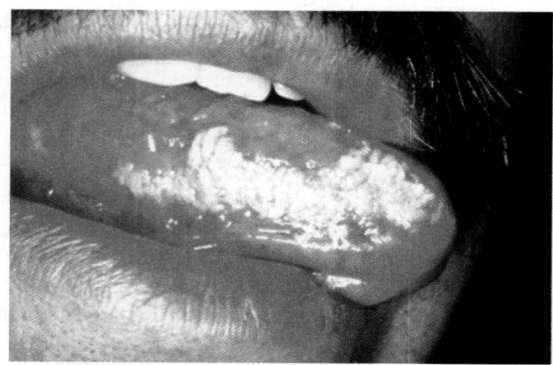

FIG. 14-5 Oral hairy leukoplakia on the tongue.

cur. All of these factors further compromise the immune system, increasing the risk of developing one or more of the opportunistic diseases that contribute to disability and death.[10,13]

Opportunistic diseases, commonly a reactivation of a prior infection, generally do not occur in the presence of a functioning immune system. Numerous infections, a variety of malignancies, wasting, and dementia can result from HIV-related immune impairment. Organisms that do not usually cause disease in people with functioning immune systems can cause severe, debilitating, disseminated, and life-threatening infections during the advanced stage of chronic HIV infection (Table 14-2). Unfortunately, sev-

TABLE 14-1   Diagnostic Criteria for AIDS

AIDS is diagnosed when an individual with HIV develops at least one of these conditions:
1. CD4+ T cell count drops below 200 cells/μl.
2. Development of one of the following opportunistic infections (OIs):
   - *Fungal*: candidiasis of bronchi, trachea, lungs, or esophagus; *Pneumocystis carinii* pneumonia (PCP); disseminated or extrapulmonary histoplasmosis
   - *Viral*: cytomegalovirus (CMV) disease other than liver, spleen, or nodes; CMV retinitis (with loss of vision); herpes simplex with chronic ulcer(s) or bronchitis, pneumonitis, or esophagitis; progressive multifocal leukoencephalopathy (PML); extrapulmonary cryptococcosis
   - *Protozoal*: disseminated or extrapulmonary coccidioidomycosis, toxoplasmosis of the brain, chronic intestinal isosporiasis; chronic intestinal cryptosporidiosis
   - *Bacterial*: *Mycobacterium tuberculosis* (any site); any disseminated or extrapulmonary *Mycobacterium*, including *M. avium* complex or *M. kansasii*; recurrent pneumonia; recurrent *Salmonella* septicemia
3. Development of one of the following opportunistic cancers:
   - Invasive cervical cancer, Kaposi's sarcoma (KS), Burkitt's lymphoma, immunoblastic lymphoma, or primary lymphoma of the brain
4. Wasting syndrome occurs. *Wasting* is defined as a loss of 10% or more of ideal body mass.
5. Dementia develops.

Modified from Centers for Disease Control and Prevention (CDC): Recommendations and reports: 1993 revised classification system for HIV infection and expanded surveillance case definition for AIDS among adolescents and adults, *MMWR* 41(RR-17):1, 1992.

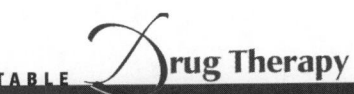

TABLE
14-2

Drug Therapy
Common Opportunistic Diseases Associated with AIDS*

ORGANISM/DISEASE	CLINICAL MANIFESTATIONS	DIAGNOSTIC TESTS	TREATMENT
Respiratory System			
Pneumocystis carinii pneumonia (PCP)	Nonproductive cough, hypoxemia, progressive shortness of breath, fever, night sweats, fatigue	Chest x-ray, induced sputum for culture, bronchoalveolar lavage specimen collection for cytology	trimethoprim-sulfamethoxazole (Bactrim), pentamidine (NebuPent), dapsone + trimethoprim, clindamycin (Cleocin) + primaquine, atovaquone (Mepron), trimetrexate (Neutrexin) + folinic acid + corticosteroids
Histoplasma capsulatum	Pneumonia, fever, cough, weight loss; disseminated disease	Sputum culture, serum or urine antigen assay	amphotericin B (Fungizone), itraconazole (Sporanox), fluconazole (Diflucan)
Mycobacterium tuberculosis	Productive cough, fever, night sweats, weight loss	Chest x-ray, sputum for AFB stain and culture	isoniazid (INH), ethambutol (Myambutol), rifampin (Rifadin), pyrazinamide (Pyrazinamide), streptomycin
Coccidioides immitis	Fever, weight loss, cough	Sputum culture, serology	amphotericin B (Fungizone), fluconazole (Diflucan), itraconazole (Sporanox)
Kaposi's sarcoma (KS)	Dyspnea, respiratory failure	Chest x-ray, biopsy	Cancer chemotherapy, α–interferon, radiation
Integumentary System			
Herpes simplex type 1 (HSV1) and type 2 (HSV2)	Mouth and nasal mucocutaneous ulcerative lesions (type 1), genital and perianal mucocutaneous ulcerative lesions (type 2)	Viral culture	acyclovir (Zovirax), famciclovir (Famvir), valacyclovir (Valtrex), foscarnet (Foscavir)
Varicella zoster virus (VZV)	Shingles, erythematous maculopapular rash along dermatomal planes, pain, pruritis	Viral culture	acyclovir (Zovirax), famciclovir (Famvir), valacyclovir (Valtrex), foscarnet (Foscavir)
Kaposi's sarcoma (KS)	Firm, flat, raised or nodular, hyperpigmented, multicentric lesions	Biopsy of lesions	Cancer chemotherapy, α–interferon, radiation of lesions, liquid nitrogen/cryotherapy for skin lesions
Bacillary angiomatosis	Erythematous vascular papules, subcutaneous nodules	Biopsy of lesions	erythromycin, doxycycline
Eye			
Cytomegalovirus (CMV) retinitis	Lesions on the retina, blurred vision, loss of vision	Ophthalmoscopic examination	ganciclovir (Cytovene), foscarnet (Foscavir), cidofovir (Vistide); valganciclovir (Valcyte), ganciclovir ocular implant (Vitrisert)
Herpes virus type 1 (HSV1)	Blurred vision, corneal lesions, retinal necrosis	Ophthalmoscopic examination	acyclovir (Zovirax), famciclovir (Famvir), valacyclovir (Valtrex), foscarnet (Foscavir)
Varicella zoster virus (VZV)	Progressive outer retinal necrosis (PORN), vision loss	Ophthalmoscopic examination	acyclovir (Zovirax), famciclovir (Famvir), valacyclovir (Valtrex), foscarnet (Foscavir)
Gastrointestinal System			
Cryptosporidium muris	Watery diarrhea, abdominal pain, weight loss, nausea	Stool examination, small bowel or colon biopsy	Antidiarrheals, paromomycin (Humatin), azithromycin (Zithromax), atovaquone (Mepron), octreotide (Sandostatin)
Cytomegalovirus (CMV)	Stomatitis, esophagitis, gastritis, colitis, bloody diarrhea, pain, weight loss	Endoscopic visualization, culture, biopsy, rule out other causes	ganciclovir (Cytovene), foscarnet (Foscavir), cidofovir (Vistide)
Herpes simplex type 1 (HSV1)	Vesicular eruptions on tongue, buccal, pharyngeal, or perioral esophageal mucosa	Viral culture	acyclovir (Zovirax), famciclovir (Famvir), valacyclovir (Valtrex), foscarnet (Foscavir)

Source: Bartlett JG, Gallant JE: *2001-2002 Medical management of HIV infection*, Baltimore, 2001, Johns Hopkins University.
AFB, Acid-fast bacilli; *CNS,* central nervous system; *CSF,* cerebrospinal fluid; *CT,* computed tomography; *GI,* gastrointestinal; *MRI,* magnetic resonance imaging.
*Opportunistic diseases are reported in this table by systems frequently affected. However, it is important to note that in HIV infection dissemination is common.

Continued

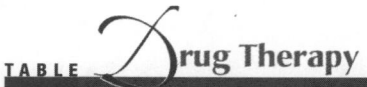

TABLE
14-2

Drug Therapy

Common Opportunistic Diseases Associated with AIDS—cont'd

ORGANISM/DISEASE	CLINICAL MANIFESTATIONS	DIAGNOSTIC TESTS	TREATMENT
Gastrointestinal System—cont'd			
Candida albicans	Whitish-yellow patches in mouth, esophagus, GI tract	Microscopic examination of scraping from lesion, culture	fluconazole (Diflucan), clotrimazole (Lotrimin), itraconazole (Sporanox), amphotericin B (Fungizone)
Mycobacterium avium complex (MAC)	Watery diarrhea, weight loss	Small bowel biopsy with AFB stain and culture	clarithromycin (Biaxin), rifampin (Rifadin), ciprofloxacin (Cipro), rifabutin (Mycobutin), amikacin, azithromycin (Zithromax)
Isospora belli	Diarrhea, weight loss, nausea, abdominal pain	Stool examination, bowel biopsy	trimethoprim-sulfamethoxazole (Bactrim), pyrimethamine + folinic acid
Salmonella	Gastroenteritis, fever, diarrhea	Blood and stool culture	ciprofloxacin (Cipro), ampicillin, amoxicillin, trimethoprim-sulfamethoxazole (Bactrim)
Kaposi's sarcoma (KS)	Diarrhea, hyperpigmented lesions of mouth and GI tract	GI series, biopsy	Cancer chemotherapy, α-interferon, radiation
Non-Hodgkin's lymphoma	Abdominal pain, fever, night sweats, weight loss	Lymph node biopsy	Chemotherapy
Neurologic System			
Toxoplasma gondii	Cognitive dysfunction, motor impairment, fever, altered mental status, headache, seizures, sensory abnormalities	MRI, CT scan, toxoplasma serology, brain biopsy (usually deferred)	pyrimethamine + folinic acid + sulfadiazine, clindamycin (Cleocin), azithromycin (Zithromax), clarithromycin (Biaxin)
JC papovavirus	Progressive multifocal leukoencephalopathy (PML), mental and motor declines	MRI, CT scan, brain biopsy	Effective antiretroviral therapy may help
Cryptococcal meningitis	Cognitive impairment, motor dysfunction, fever, seizures, headache	CT scan, serum antigen test, CSF analysis	amphotericin B (Fungizone), fluconazole (Diflucan), itraconazole (Sporanox), flucytosine (Ancobon)
CNS lymphomas	Cognitive dysfunction, motor impairment, aphasia, seizures, personality changes, headache	MRI, CT scan	Radiation, chemotherapy
AIDS-dementia complex (ADC)	Insidious onset of progressive dementia	CT scan	Effective antiretroviral therapy may help

eral opportunistic diseases are likely to occur at the same time, further compounding the difficulties of diagnosis and treatment.[13] The good news is that advances in treatment have led to significant decreases in the rates of opportunistic diseases. This is because successful treatment of HIV helps maintain the functioning immune system, which can prevent opportunistic disease.[20]

Diagnostic Studies

Diagnosis of HIV Infection. The most useful screening tests for HIV are those that detect HIV-specific antibodies. The major problem with these tests is that there is a median delay of 2 months after infection before antibodies can be detected (see Fig. 14-1). This creates a **window period** during which an infected individual will not test HIV-antibody positive. HIV-antibody screening is generally done in the sequence shown in Table 14-3. This process produces highly accurate results. HIV antibody testing can now be done on oral fluids and urine.[13,21] Newer tests allow rapid (20-minute) blood tests for HIV that can be done in an office setting. The tests are highly reliable and provide immediate feedback to patients who can then be counseled about treatment and prevention.

Diagnosis of HIV in newborns can be problematic. All infants born to HIV-infected mothers will be positive on the HIV-antibody test because maternal antibodies cross the placental barrier. These antibodies remain present in the infant for up to 18 months. For that reason, early detection of HIV infection in infants depends on testing for HIV antigen through the use of HIV DNA polymerase chain reaction (PCR), HIV RNA PCR, or viral culture (PCR is discussed in Chapter 13). These tests can definitively diagnose HIV in infected infants by 4 weeks of age.[12]

Laboratory Studies in HIV Infection. The progression of HIV infection is monitored by CD4+ T cell counts. As the disease progresses, there is usually a decrease in the number of CD4+ T cells, a marker for decreased immune function (see Fig. 14-1). However, CD4+ T cell counts, although extremely important, reveal only part of the clinical picture. Laboratory tests that measure viral activity allow better assessment of clinical status and disease progression. *Viral load* (also referred to

| TABLE 14-3 | HIV Antibody Test Screening Process |

The following steps are used in the process of testing blood for antibodies to HIV:

1. A highly sensitive enzyme immunoassay (EIA) is done to detect serum antibodies that bind to HIV antigens on test plates. Blood samples that are negative on this test are reported as negative.
   - Posttest counseling should include an assessment of risk behaviors, especially looking for recent risks.
   - If recent risks are found, encourage retesting at 3 weeks, 6 weeks, and 3 months.
2. If the blood is EIA positive, the test is repeated.
3. If the blood is repeatedly EIA positive, a more specific confirming test, such as the Western blot (WB) or immunofluorescence assay (IFA), is done.
   - WB testing uses purified HIV antigens electrophoresed on gels. These are incubated with serum samples. If antibody in the serum is present, it can be detected.
   - IFA is used to identify HIV in infected cells. Blood is treated with a fluorescent antibody against p17 or p24 antigen and then examined using a fluorescent microscope.
4. Blood that is reactive in all of the first three steps is reported as HIV-antibody positive.
5. If the results are indeterminant, the following steps are taken:
   - If in-depth risk assessment reveals that the individual does not have a history of high-risk activities, reassure the patient that she or he is extremely unlikely to be infected with HIV and suggest retesting in 3 months.
   - If in-depth risk assessment reveals that the individual does have a history of high-risk activities, repeat antibody test at 1, 2, and 6 months; discuss harm reduction measures to protect partners from infection; consider tests for HIV antigen detection.

as viral burden) counts the number of viral particles in a sample of blood. Viral loads can be determined with HIV RNA PCR or branched-chain DNA (bDNA) tests. These tests provide information that helps determine when to initiate therapy, the efficacy of therapy, and whether clinical goals are being met.[13,20,21]

A variety of abnormal laboratory tests of the blood are common in untreated HIV infection and may be caused by HIV, opportunistic diseases, or complications of drug or radiation therapy. A decreased white blood cell (WBC) count, especially low neutrophil counts (neutropenia), is often seen; low platelet counts (thrombocytopenia) may be caused by antiplatelet antibodies or drug therapy; and anemia is associated with the chronic disease process, as well as with common adverse effects of some of the antiretroviral agents.[13] Altered liver function tests are common. These may be caused by disease processes or drug therapy and may be more common with newer drug therapy. Early identification of coinfection with hepatitis B virus (HBV) and/or hepatitis C virus (HCV) is important because these infections may have a more serious course in the patient with HIV infection and may ultimately limit options for antiretroviral drug therapy (ART).[13]

As mentioned previously, it is now possible to test for resistance to antiretroviral drugs in people being treated for HIV infection. Two types of assays are used: genotype and phenotype. The *genotype assay* detects drug-resistant viral mutations that are present in the reverse transcriptase and protease genes. The *phenotype assay* measures the growth of the virus in various concentrations of antiretroviral drugs (much like bacteria-antibiotic sensitivity tests). These assays are especially useful in making decisions about new drug combinations in patients who are not responding to their current therapies.[20]

Collaborative Care

Collaborative management of the HIV-infected patient focuses on monitoring HIV disease progression and immune function, initiating and monitoring ART, preventing the development of opportunistic diseases, detecting and treating opportunistic diseases, managing symptoms, and preventing or decreasing the complications of treatment. Ongoing assessment and health care provider–patient interactions are required to accomplish these objectives.

The initial visit provides an opportunity to gather baseline data and to establish rapport. A complete history and physical examination, including an immunization history and psychosocial and dietary evaluations, should be conducted. Findings from the history, assessment, and laboratory tests help determine the patient's needs. This is a good time to initiate patient education related to the spectrum of HIV disease, treatment, preventing transmission to others, improving health, and family planning. Patient input should be used to develop a plan of care, and necessary referrals can be made. It is important to remember that a newly diagnosed patient may be in a state of shock or denial and unable to retain or understand information.[18] The nurse should be prepared to repeat and clarify information over the course of several months. If case reports are required by the state health department, they should be completed at this time.

Drug Therapy for HIV Infection. The goals of drug therapy in HIV infection are to (1) decrease HIV RNA levels to less than 50 copies/μl (undetectable HIV RNA levels are possible and preferred), (2) maintain or raise CD4$^+$ T cell counts to greater than 200 cells/μl (a range of 800 to 1200 cells/μl is preferred), which is known as *immune reconstitution;* and (3) delay the development of HIV-related symptoms, including a wide range of opportunistic diseases. A variety of drug therapies are now available to help patients meet these goals. Because of the rapidity with which new therapies are evolving, there has been considerable confusion about how and when to initiate therapy and what to use. The National Institutes of Health (NIH) has published a report on the principles of therapy (Table 14-4). Guidelines on the use of antiretroviral agents have also been published.[20] Recommendations for starting therapy in the chronically infected patient are summarized in Table 14-5. A major goal of these recommendations is to prevent development of viral resistance to the drugs. Resistance can happen rapidly when patients miss or delay doses of their drugs. For this reason, strict adherence to treatment protocols is extremely important.

In general, drugs used to treat HIV are antiretroviral drugs that work at various points in the HIV replication cycle (Table 14-6). Research is progressing rapidly to develop new drugs. No drug or combination of drugs can cure HIV, but therapy can decrease viral replication and delay progression of disease in

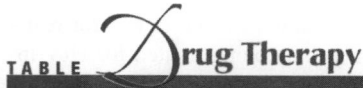

TABLE

TABLE 14-4

Summary of Principles of Drug Therapy for HIV Infection

1. Ongoing HIV replication leads to immune system damage and progression to AIDS. HIV infection is always harmful, and clinically significant immune dysfunction is common.
2. Plasma HIV RNA levels indicate the magnitude of HIV replication and its associated rate of CD4$^+$ T cell destruction; CD4$^+$ T cell counts indicate the extent of HIV-induced immune damage already suffered. Regular, periodic measurements of plasma HIV RNA levels and CD4$^+$ T cell counts are necessary to determine the risk of disease progression in an HIV-infected individual and to determine when to initiate or modify ART regimens.
3. Because rates of disease progression differ among individuals, treatment decisions should be individualized by level of risk indicated by plasma HIV RNA levels and CD4$^+$ T cell counts and based on patient's desires for therapy.
4. The use of potent combination ART to suppress HIV replication limits the potential for selection of antiretroviral-resistant HIV variants, the major factor limiting the ability of antiretroviral drugs to inhibit virus replication and delay disease progression. Maximum achievable suppression of HIV replication should be the goal of therapy.
5. The most effective means to accomplish durable suppression of HIV replication is the simultaneous initiation of combinations of effective anti-HIV drugs with which the patient has not been previously treated and that are not cross-resistant with antiretroviral agents with which the patient has been previously treated.
6. Antiretroviral drugs used in combination therapy regimens should always be used according to optimum schedules and dosages.
7. The available effective antiretroviral drugs are limited in number and mechanism of action, and cross-resistance between specific drugs has been documented. Therefore any change in ART can decrease future therapeutic options.
8. Women should receive optimal ART regardless of pregnancy status.
9. Acute primary HIV infections should be treated with combination ART to suppress virus replication to levels below the limit of detection.
10. HIV-infected persons, even those with viral loads below detectable limits and those on effective ART, should be considered infectious and should be counseled to avoid sexual and drug-use behaviors that are associated with transmission or acquisition of HIV and other infectious pathogens.

Revised from *Report of the NIH Panel to define principles of therapy of HIV infection,* 1997, National Institutes of Health.
ART, Antiretroviral therapy.

TABLE 14-5

Indications for the Initiation of Antiretroviral Therapy in the Chronically HIV-Infected Patient

CLINICAL CATEGORY	CD4$^+$ T CELL COUNT	PLASMA HIV RNA	RECOMMENDATION
Symptomatic (AIDS, severe symptoms)	Any value	Any value	Treat
Asymptomatic, AIDS	<200/μl	Any value	Treat
Asymptomatic	200/μl–350/μl	Any value	Treatment should generally be offered, though controversy exists*
Asymptomatic	<350/μl	>30,000 (bDNA) or >55,000 (RT-PCR)	Some experts would recommend initiating therapy, recognizing that the 3-year risk of developing AIDS in untreated patients is >30%. In the absence of very high levels of plasma HIV RNA, some would defer therapy and monitor the CD4$^+$ T cell count and level of plasma HIV RNA more frequently. Clinical outcome data after initiating therapy are lacking.
Asymptomatic	<350/μl	<30,000 (bDNA) or <55,000 (RT-PCR)	Many experts would defer therapy and observe, recognizing that the 3-year risk of developing AIDS in untreated patients is <15%.

Revised from *Guidelines for the use of antiretroviral agents in HIV-infected adults and adolescents,* 2001, Department of Health and Human Services.
bDNA, Branched-chain deoxyribonucleic acid; *PCR,* polymerase chain reaction; *RT,* reverse transcriptase.
*Clinical benefit has been demonstrated in controlled trials only for patients with CD4$^+$ T cells <200/μl. However, most experts would offer therapy at a CD4$^+$ T cell threshold <350/μl. All decisions to initiate therapy should be based on prognosis for disease-free survival in the absence of treatment, as determined by the CD4$^+$ T cell count and level of plasma HIV RNA, the potential risks and benefits of therapy, and the willingness of the patient to accept therapy.

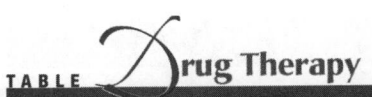

TABLE 14-6	Drug Therapy — Mechanisms of Action of Drugs Used to Treat HIV Infection

DRUG CLASSIFICATION	MECHANISM OF ACTION
Nonnucleoside reverse transcriptase inhibitors (NNRTIs)	Combine with reverse transcriptase enzyme to block the process needed to convert HIV RNA into HIV DNA
Nucleoside reverse transcriptase inhibitors (NRTIs)	Insert a bit of protein (a nucleoside) into the developing HIV DNA chain, blocking further development of the chain and leaving the production of the new strand of HIV DNA incomplete
Nucleotide reverse transcriptase inhibitors	Inhibit the action of reverse transcriptase
Protease inhibitors (PIs)	Prevent the protease enzyme from cutting HIV proteins into the proper lengths needed to allow viable virions to assemble and bud out from the cell membrane
Fusion inhibitors (entry inhibitors)	Prevent binding of HIV to cells, thus preventing entry of HIV into healthy cells

many patients. The major advantage of having antiretroviral drugs from different drug groups is that combination therapy can attack viral replication in several different ways, making it more difficult for the virus to recover and decreasing the likelihood of drug resistance. An additional advantage is that alternatives now exist for those patients who do not respond to a specific drug regimen.[20,22]

Currently approved drugs include three groups that inhibit the ability of HIV to make a DNA copy early in replication, one group that inhibits the ability of the virus to reproduce in the late stages of replication, and one group that prevents entry of HIV into the cell (Table 14-7). **Nucleoside reverse transcriptase inhibitors** (NRTIs), **nonnucleoside reverse transcriptase inhibitors** (NNRTIs), and **nucleotide reverse transcriptase inhibitors** work by inhibiting the activity of reverse transcriptase, while **protease inhibitors** (PIs) work by interfering with the activity of the enzyme protease. **Fusion inhibitors** work by inhibiting the binding of HIV to cells. A major problem with most drugs used in ART is that resistance develops rapidly when they are used alone or taken in inadequate doses. For that reason combinations of three or more antiretroviral drugs, prescribed at full strength, should be used. PIs and NNRTIs also have a number of dangerous and potentially lethal interactions with other commonly used drugs, including over-the-counter drugs and herbal therapies.[20,23,24] For example, St. John's wort can interfere with ART. Some herbs (e.g., echinacea, astragalus) should not be used because they can enhance the replication of HIV.

Although treatment protocols can reduce the viral loads by 90% to 99% in many cases, there are some problems.[20] Up to 50% of patients with HIV will not experience a dramatic response to ART, causing feelings of guilt, despair, and futility. In addition, many patients will not be able to use combination therapies because of the expense, side effects, or inability to adhere to required schedules and dietary changes. Expense is an important concern for many. Combination ART is more cost effective than the cost of advancing disease, but the drugs are still not universally available.[25]

Drug Therapy for Opportunistic Diseases. Management of HIV is complicated by the many opportunistic diseases that can develop as the immune system deteriorates (see Table 14-2). Although it is usually not possible to eradicate opportunistic diseases, treatments that can control them are available. Advances in the diagnosis and treatment of opportunistic diseases have con-

tributed significantly to increased life expectancy.[13,26] Table 14-2 lists treatments for common opportunistic diseases in HIV-infected individuals.

A preferred approach to opportunistic diseases is to prevent their occurrence. A number of opportunistic diseases associated with HIV can be delayed or prevented through the use of adequate ART (resulting in immune reconstitution) and disease-specific prevention measures. Prophylaxis contributes significantly to the decreased morbidity and mortality associated with HIV infection and is recommended according to established criteria (Table 14-8).[13,26]

Vaccination. Early in the HIV epidemic there was optimism that a vaccine would be quickly developed. Despite considerable research, a vaccine still eludes scientists. The problems that impede HIV vaccine development are numerous.[21] HIV lives inside cells where it can hide from circulating immune factors. HIV also mutates rapidly, so that infected individuals develop HIV variants that may not all respond to a simple vaccine. In addition, two strains of HIV (HIV-1 and HIV-2) cause AIDS and at least nine **clades** (or families) of HIV-1 exist around the world. Development of an effective vaccine for clade B (the predominant group in the Americas and Western Europe) may not prove effective in developing countries, where the need is even greater. A major problem for vaccine development is that it is not known how to measure protective immunity for HIV. Antibody development after vaccination usually indicates immunity, but HIV-infected patients already produce antibodies that do not prevent disease or confer immunity.[27,28]

There are also social, ethical, and economic issues related to vaccination. Because no known animal model for HIV exists, vaccine efficacy can be established only through human testing. There are many questions related to HIV vaccines. How will volunteers be recruited? How will true protection be determined? Will volunteers be exposed to HIV after immunization to test immunity? Because HIV is a global problem, with developing countries bearing the brunt of the epidemic, is it possible to develop a vaccine that can be widely distributed in a short amount of time at an acceptable cost? Despite the overwhelming nature of these issues, considerable research is in progress. Vaccines in various stages of development have been tested in animals, and a few have progressed to human trials. Some vaccines are even being tested in HIV-infected patients to determine if their use can boost an infected person's immune response. The development of

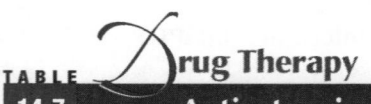
DRUG/ADMINISTRATION	ADVERSE EFFECTS
Nucleoside Reverse Transcriptase Inhibitors (NRTIs)	Lactic acidosis with hepatic steatosis is a rare but potentially life-threatening problem; lipodystrophy, especially fat atrophy and mitochondrial toxicity are associated with NRTIs
zidovudine (AZT, ZDV, Retrovir)	Nausea, vomiting, anemia, leukopenia, myopathy, fatigue, headache
didanosine (ddI, Videx)—dose of 2 tablets ensures adequate buffer for absorption; must be chewed or dissolved to release buffer; also available in a time-released formulation as Videx EC	Nausea, diarrhea, peripheral neuropathy (dose related and reversible), pancreatitis
zalcitabine (ddC, Hivid)	Oral ulcers, peripheral neuropathy (dose related and reversible), pancreatitis
stavudine (d4T, Zerit), stavudine XR (extended release)	Peripheral neuropathy, pancreatitis
lamivudine (3TC, Epivir)	Minimal toxicities, nausea, nasal congestion
abacavir (Ziagen)	Nausea; hypersensitivity reaction, including fever, nausea, vomiting, diarrhea, lethargy, malaise, sore throat, shortness of breath, cough, rash; may produce life-threatening event if hypersensitivity is rechallenged
emtricitabine (Emtriva, FTC)-take with or without food	Headache, diarrhea, nausea, rash, skin discoloration, lactic acidosis with hepatic steatosis, lipodystrophy
Combivir (lamivudine and zidovudine combination)	Combines side effects of lamivudine and zidovudine
Trizivir (lamivudine, zidovudine, and abacavir combination)	Combines side effects of lamivudine, zidovudine, and abacavir
Nucleotide Reverse Transcriptase Inhibitor	
tenofovir DF (Viread)	Nausea, vomiting, vaginal irritation, renal impairment
Nonnucleoside Reverse Transcriptase Inhibitors (NNRTIs)	
nevirapine (Viramune)	Rash, Stevens-Johnson syndrome, hepatitis, increased transaminase levels
delavirdine (Rescriptor)—mix tablets in 3 oz or more of water to produce a slurry; separate from antacid intake by 1 hour	Rash, liver function changes, pruritis
efavirenz (Sustiva)—take at bedtime to help with side effects	Rash, dizziness, trouble concentrating, unusual dreams, confusion, encephalopathy; false-positive cannaboid test
Protease Inhibitors (PIs)	Common adverse affects include hyperglycemia, hyperlipidemia, and lipodystrophy
saquinavir (Fortovase)—refrigerate capsules; OK at room temperature for 90 days	Diarrhea, nausea, headache
indinavir (Crixivan)—ensure adequate hydration during therapy; patient should drink 2-4 L of fluid a day; do not take with grapefruit juice	Nausea, diarrhea, asymptomatic hyperbilirubinemia, interstitial nephritis, kidney stones
ritonavir (Norvir)—refrigerate capsules; OK at room temperature for 30 days; frequently used in low doses with other PIs to boost the effect	Nausea, diarrhea, vomiting, taste perversion, circumoral and perioral paresthesias, hepatitis
nelfinavir (Viracept)	Diarrhea, flatulence, nausea
amprenavir (Agenerase)—oral solution and capsule doses are not interchangeable (mg to mg)	Nausea, vomiting, headache, taste perversion, perioral paresthesia, severe skin rashes, increased liver functions; oral solution contains an alcohol that can interact with metronidazole (Flagyl) and cause feelings of inebriation
Kaletra (lopinavir and ritonivir combination)—refrigerate capsules; OK at room temperature for 60 days	Nausea, diarrhea, taste perversion, rash, perioral and circumoral paresthesia, hepatitis
atazanavir (Reyataz)—take with a meal or snack	Nausea, diarrhea, hyperbilirubinemia
Fusion Inhibitor (Entry Inhibitor)	
enfuvirtide (Fuzeon)—inject subcutaneously bid; instructions for reconstitution, refrigeration, and injection site rotation must be followed	Skin irritation at injection site, fatigue, nausea, insomnia, peripheral neuropathy

Sources: Bartlett J, Gallant JE: *2001-2002 Medical management of HIV infection,* Baltimore, 2001, Johns Hopkins University; CDC: *Guidelines for the use of antiretroviral agents in HIV-infected adults and adolescents,* 2001; and Wolbach J et al: *A pharmacist's guide to antiretroviral medications for HIV-infected adults and adolescents,* Denver, 2001, Mountain Plains AIDS Education and Training Center.

*Current recommendations for therapy require combinations of three or more of these drugs. Treatment with only one drug (monotherapy) is acceptable only in unique and rare circumstances.

†Many of these drugs, especially the NNRTIs and PIs, cause serious and potentially fatal interactions when used in combination with other commonly used drugs, some of which are available over the counter.

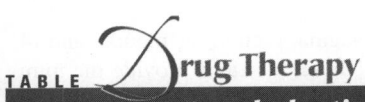

TABLE 14-8   Drug Therapy
Prophylactic Interventions for Patients with HIV

INFECTION	PROPHYLACTIC INTERVENTIONS	COMMENTS
Pneumocystis carinii pneumonia (PCP)	trimethoprim-sulfamethoxazole (TMP-SMX) (preferred) or dapsone, dapsone with pyrimethamine + folinic acid, aerosolized pentamidine, atovaquone; prophylaxis may be discontinued if immune reconstitution evidenced by a CD4+ T cell count of >200/μl is documented for 3 mo or more; restart if CD4+ T cell count falls < 200/μl	Initiate when CD4+ T cells <200/μl. Offer to any patient with a history of PCP, fever of undetermined origin for 2 wk or more, or oropharyngeal candidiasis regardless of CD4+ T cell count. Oral drugs that provide systemic effects are preferred. Side effects of TMP-SMX and dapsone, especially rash, fever, and anemia, are common and may limit use. Dapsone should not be used in patients with G6PD deficiency (can lead to hemolytic anemia).
Mycobacterium tuberculosis (TB)	Treat if PPD is ≥ 0.5 mm reactive, after high-risk exposure, or if prior positive PPD without treatment; isoniazid (INH) + pyridoxine for 9-12 mo; consider directly observed therapy	Rule out active disease, extrapulmonary disease, or drug-resistant strain, all of which require multidrug therapy. Negative PPD in the presence of HIV does not exclude a diagnosis of TB. Provide ongoing assessment and intervention.
Toxoplasmosis	trimethoprim-sulfamethoxazole (TMP-SMX) or dapsone with pyrimethamine + folinic acid or atovaquone ± pyrimethamine + folinic acid; prophylaxis may be discontinued if immune reconstitution evidenced by a CD4+ T cell count of >200/μl is documented for 3 mo or more; restart if CD4+ T cell count falls <100/μl	Initiate with positive toxoplasmosis IgG titer when CD4+ T cells <100/μl; cross protective for PCP.
Mycobacterium avium complex (MAC)	clarithromycin (Biaxin) or azithromycin (Zithromax), rifabutin (Mycobutin); prophylaxis may be discontinued if immune reconstitution evidenced by a CD4+ T cell count of >100/μl is documented for 6-12 mo; restart if CD4+ T cell count falls <50/μl	Initiate when CD4+ T cells <50/μl. Rule out disseminated disease or tuberculosis. Rifabutin has caused dose-related uveitis (>600 mg/day) that is reversible with drug withdrawal or dose reduction.
Varicella zoster virus (VZV)	varicella zoster immune globulin (VZIG) administered within 96 hr after an exposure, preferably within 48 hr	Only after significant exposure to chicken pox or shingles for patients with no history of disease or negative on a VZV antibody test.
Pneumococcal pneumonia	Pneumococcal vaccine	Provide as soon as possible during course of infection. Antibody response is optimal when CD4+ T cells are at least 350/μl.
Influenza virus	Whole or split virus influenza vaccine	Provide annually, before influenza virus season; revaccinate if initial vaccine was given when CD4+ T cell was <200/μl.
Hepatitis B virus (HBV)	Hepatitis B vaccine series; screen and vaccinate those who show no evidence of previous HBV infection	Provide as soon as possible during course of infection. Encourage vaccine in injecting drug users, sexually active gay men, sexual partners or household contacts of HBV-infected individuals, and those with hepatitis C virus (HCV).
Hepatitis A virus (HAV)	Hepatitis A vaccine series; screen and vaccinate those without evidence of previous HAV infection	Provide as soon as possible during course of infection. Offer to those with HCV.

Sources: Bartlett J, Gallant JE: *2001-2002 Medical management of HIV infection,* Baltimore, 2001, Johns Hopkins University; Kirton CA: Immunizations in HIV care. In Kirton CS, Talotta D, Zwolski K, editors: *Handbook of HIV/AIDS nursing,* St Louis, 2001, Mosby.
G6PD, Glucose-6-phosphate dehydrogenase; *PPD,* purified protein derivative (tuberculin).

a successful vaccine will not replace current prevention methods that decrease risk behaviors, because no vaccine is likely to be 100% effective.[27]

NURSING MANAGEMENT
HIV INFECTION

■ Nursing Assessment

Nursing assessment for individuals not known to be infected with HIV should focus on behaviors that could put the person at risk for HIV infection and other sexually transmitted and blood-borne diseases. Nurses can help individuals assess risks by asking four basic questions: (1) Have you ever had a blood transfusion or used clotting factors? If so, was it before 1985? (2) Have you ever shared needles, syringes, or other injecting equipment with another person? (3) Have you ever had a sexual experience in which your penis, vagina, rectum, or mouth came into contact with another person's penis, vagina, rectum, or mouth? and (4) Have you ever had an STD? These questions provide the minimum data needed to initiate a risk assessment. A positive response to any of these questions requires an in-depth exploration of the issues specific to the identified risk.[18]

Further assessment is needed when an individual has been diagnosed with HIV infection. Subjective and objective data that should be obtained are presented in Table 14-9. Ongoing nursing assessments are essential because early recognition and treatment of problems can decrease the progression of HIV infection. A complete history and thorough systems review can help the nurse identify problems in a timely manner.

■ Nursing Diagnoses

Nursing diagnoses related to HIV infection are dictated by several variables: the stage (e.g., is prevention of HIV infection the issue? Are there concerns related to ongoing infection? Is the

---

TABLE 14-9 Nursing Assessment
HIV-Infected Patient

Subjective Data

Important Health Information

Past health history: Route of infection; hepatitis; other STDs; tuberculosis; foreign travel; frequent viral, fungal, and/or bacterial infections

Medications: Use of immunosuppressive drugs

Functional Health Patterns

Health perception–health management: Perception of illness; alcohol and drug use; malaise

Nutritional-metabolic: Weight loss, anorexia, nausea, vomiting; lesions, bleeding, or ulcerations of lips, mouth, gums, tongue, or throat; sensitivity to acidic, salty, or spicy foods; difficulty swallowing; abdominal cramping; skin rashes, lesions, or color changes; nonhealing wounds

Elimination: Persistent diarrhea, change in character of stools; painful urination

Activity-exercise: Chronic fatigue, muscle weakness, difficulty walking; cough, shortness of breath

Sleep-rest: Insomnia; night sweats, fatigue

Cognitive-perceptual: Headaches, stiff neck, chest pain, rectal pain, retrosternal pain; blurred vision, photophobia, diplopia, loss of vision; hearing impairment; confusion, forgetfulness, attention deficit, changes in mental status, memory loss, personality changes; paresthesias, hypersensitivity in feet, pruritis

Role-relationship: Support system, financial resources

Sexuality-reproductive: Lesions on genitalia (internal or external), pruritis or burning in vagina, painful sexual intercourse, changes in menstruation, vaginal or penile discharge; use of birth control measures, pregnancies, desire for future children

Coping–stress tolerance: Stress levels, previous losses, coping patterns, self-concept

Objective Data

General

Lethargy, persistent fever, lymphadenopathy, peripheral wasting, fat deposits in truncal areas and upper back; social withdrawal

Integumentary

Decreased skin turgor, dry skin, or diaphoresis; pallor, cyanosis; lesions, eruptions, discolorations, or bruises of skin and mucous membranes; vaginal or perianal excoriation; alopecia, delayed wound healing

Eyes

Presence of exudate; retinal lesions or hemorrhage; papilledema

Respiratory

Tachypnea, dyspnea, intercostal retractions; crackles, wheezing, productive or nonproductive cough

Cardiovascular

Pericardial friction rub, murmur, bradycardia, tachycardia

Gastrointestinal

Mouth lesions, including blisters (HSV), white–gray patches *(Candida)*, painless white lesions on lateral aspect of the tongue (hairy leukoplakia), discolorations (KS); gingivitis, tooth decay or loosening; redness or white patchy lesions of throat; vomiting, diarrhea, incontinence; rectal lesions; hyperactive bowel sounds, abdominal masses, hepatosplenomegaly

Musculoskeletal

Muscle wasting

Neurologic

Ataxia, tremors, lack of coordination; sensory loss; slurred speech, aphasia; memory loss, apathy, agitation, depression, inappropriate behavior; decreasing levels of consciousness, seizures, paralysis, coma

Reproductive

Genital lesions or discharge, abdominal tenderness secondary to pelvic inflammatory disease (PID)

Possible Findings

Positive HIV antibody assay (EIA or ELISA, confirmed by WB or IFA); detectable viral load levels by bDNA or PCR, ↓ CD4$^+$ lymphocytes, reversal of CD4:CD8 ratio; ↓ WBC count, lymphopenia, anemia, thrombocytopenia; electrolyte imbalances; abnormal liver function tests; ↑ cholesterol, triglycerides, and blood glucose.

EIA, Enzyme immunoassay; *ELISA,* enzyme-linked immunosorbent assay; *HSV,* herpes simplex virus; *IFA,* immunofluorescence assay; *KS,* Kaposi's sarcoma; *PCR,* polymerase chain reaction; *STDs,* sexually transmitted diseases; *WB,* Western blot; *WBC,* white blood cell.

patient in terminal phases of the disease?); presence of specific etiologic problems (e.g., respiratory distress, depression, wasting); and social factors (e.g., issues related to self-esteem, sexuality, family interactions, finances). Because HIV infection is a complex and individually experienced disease, a broad spectrum of nursing diagnoses may include, but not limited to, those presented in Table 14-10.

■ Planning

Prevention of HIV infection presents a number of challenges for the patient, many of which are related to the difficulties of behavior change. Nurses can be instrumental in this process. Nursing interventions to prevent disease transmission depend on assessment of the patient's individual risk behaviors, knowledge, and skill deficits. Nursing orders based on these assessments will encourage the patient to learn safer, healthier, and less risky behaviors.[29]

Infection with HIV affects the entire range of a person's life from physical health to social, emotional, economic, and spiritual well-being. Once infected, treatment cannot eliminate HIV from the body. The overriding goals of therapy, therefore, are to keep the viral load as low as possible for as long as possible; to maintain or restore a functioning immune system; to improve the patient's quality of life; and to reduce HIV-related disease, disability, and death.[20] Nursing interventions can assist the patient to (1) adhere to drug regimens, (2) promote a healthy lifestyle, (3) prevent opportunistic disease, (4) protect others from HIV, (5) maintain or develop healthy, supportive relationships, (6) maintain activities and productivity, and (7) come to terms with issues related to disease, death, disability, and spirituality. Goals are individualized and change as new treatment protocols develop and/or as HIV disease progresses.[30]

■ Nursing Implementation

The complexity of HIV disease is related to its chronic nature. As with most chronic and infectious diseases, primary prevention and health promotion are the most effective health care strategies.[30] When prevention fails, however, disease results. HIV has no cure, continues for life, causes increasing physical disability, contributes to impaired health, and ultimately causes death.[31,32]

Nursing interventions at every stage of HIV disease can be instrumental in improving the quality and quantity of the patient's life. Nurses who emphasize a holistic and individualized approach to care are well suited to and capable of providing optimal care to these patients. Table 14-11 presents a synopsis of nursing goals, assessments, and interventions at each stage of HIV infection.

Health Promotion. A major goal of health promotion is to prevent disease. Even with recent successes in the treatment of HIV, prevention is crucial for control of the epidemic. Another goal of health promotion is to detect disease early so that, if primary prevention has failed, early intervention can be implemented.[33]

Prevention of HIV infection. HIV infection is preventable. At this time, education and behavior change are the most effective prevention tools. Educational messages should be specific to the patient's need, culturally sensitive, language appropriate, and age specific. Nurses are excellent resources for this type of education, but nurses must be comfortable with and know how to talk about sensitive topics such as sexuality and drug use.[29,34,35]

Prevention behaviors have been known and recommended since the mid-1980s. It is important to remember that a range of activities can reduce the risk of HIV infection and that individuals will choose different techniques. The goal is for the person to develop safer, healthier, and less risky behaviors than are currently being used. These techniques can be divided into *safe activities* (those that eliminate risk) and *risk-reducing activities* (those that decrease risk, but do not eliminate it). The more consistently and correctly prevention methods are used, the more effective they are in preventing HIV infection.[29,30]

Decreasing risks related to sexual intercourse. Safe sexual activities eliminate the risk of exposure to HIV in semen and vaginal secretions. Abstaining from all sexual activity is the most effective way to accomplish this goal, but there are safe options for those who cannot or do not wish to abstain. *Outercourse* (limiting sexual behavior to activities in which the mouth, penis, vagina, or rectum does not come into contact with a partner's mouth, penis, vagina, or rectum) is safe because there is no contact with blood, semen, or vaginal secretions. Outercourse includes massage, masturbation, mutual masturbation ("hand job"), telephone sex, and other activities that meet the "no contact" requirements. *Insertive sex* between partners who are not infected with HIV or not at risk of becoming infected with HIV is considered to be safe.

Risk-reducing sexual activities decrease the risk of contact with HIV through the use of barriers. Barriers should be used when engaging in insertive sexual activity (oral, vaginal, or anal) with a partner who is known to be HIV infected or with a partner whose HIV status is not known. The most commonly used bar-

NURSING DIAGNOSES

TABLE 14-10	HIV Infection

Acute pain
Anticipatory grieving
Anxiety
Caregiver role strain
Chronic low self-esteem
Decisional conflict
Diarrhea
Disturbed body image
Disturbed sleep pattern
Disturbed thought processes
Fatigue
Fear
Hyperthermia
Imbalanced nutrition: less than body requirements
Impaired oral mucous membrane
Ineffective coping
Ineffective denial
Ineffective therapeutic regimen management
Interrupted family processes
Noncompliance
Powerlessness
Relocation stress syndrome
Risk for disuse syndrome
Self-care deficit
Situational low self-esteem
Social isolation
Spiritual distress

TABLE 14-11 Nursing Interventions in HIV Disease		
LEVELS OF CARE/GOALS	**ASSESS**	**INTERVENTIONS**
Health Promotion 1. Prevent HIV infection 2. Detect HIV infection early	*Risk factors:* What behaviors or social, physical, emotional, pathologic, and immune factors place the patient at risk? Does the patient need to be tested for HIV?	Education, including knowledge, attitudes, and behaviors, with an emphasis on risk reduction to: • General population: cover general information • Pregnant women: general information and information specific to HIV infection and pregnancy • Individual patient: specific to assessed need Empower patients to take control of prevention measures. Provide HIV antibody testing with pretest and posttest counseling.
Acute Intervention 1. Promote health and limit disability 2. Manage problems caused by HIV infection	*Physical health:* Is patient experiencing problems? *Mental health status:* How is the patient coping? *Resources:* Does the patient have family/social support? Is patient accessing community services? Is money/insurance a problem? Does the patient have access to spiritual support?	Provide case management. Educate regarding HIV, the spectrum of infection, options for care, signs and symptoms to watch for, treatment options, immune enhancement, harm reduction, and ways to adhere to treatment regimens. Refer to needed resources. Establish long-term, trusting relationship with patient, family, and significant others. Provide emotional and spiritual support. Provide care during acute exacerbations: recognition of life-threatening developments, life support, rapid intervention with treatments and drugs, patient and family emotional support during crisis, comfort, and hygiene needs. Develop resources for legal needs: discrimination prevention, wills and powers of attorney, child care wishes. Empower patient to identify needs, direct care, seek services.
Ambulatory and Home Care 1. Maximize quality of life 2. Resolve life and death issues	*Physical health:* Are new symptoms developing? Is the patient experiencing drug side effects or interactions? *Mental health:* How is the patient coping? What adjustments have been made? *Finances:* Can the patient maintain health care and basic standards of living? *Family/social/community supports:* Are these available? Is the patient using supports in an effective manner? Do family/significant others need education, encouragement, or stress relief? *Spirituality issues:* Does the patient desire support from a religious organization? Are spirituality issues private and personal? What assistance does the patient need?	Continue case management. Educate about changing treatment options and continued adherence. Empower patient to continue to direct care and to make desires known to family members and significant others. Continue physical care for chronic disease process: treatments, drugs, comfort, and hygiene needs. Support patient and family/significant others in a trusting relationship. Refer to resources that will assist in meeting identified needs. Promote health maintenance measures. Assist with end-of-life issues: resuscitation orders, comfort measures, funeral plans, estate planning, child care continuation, etc.

rier is the male condom (Fig. 14-6). Male condoms have been shown to be up to 100% effective in preventing the transmission of HIV when used correctly and consistently.[36] Major points for the correct use of male condoms are discussed in Table 14-12. Female condoms are also available (Fig. 14-7). Use can be complicated, so careful instruction and practice are required

(Table 14-13). In addition, squares of latex (known as dental dams) or plastic food wrap can be used to cover the external female genitalia during oral sexual activity.[30]

Decreasing risks related to drug use. Illicit drug use is harmful. It can cause immune suppression and malnutrition, as well as a host of psychosocial problems. However, drug use in and of it-

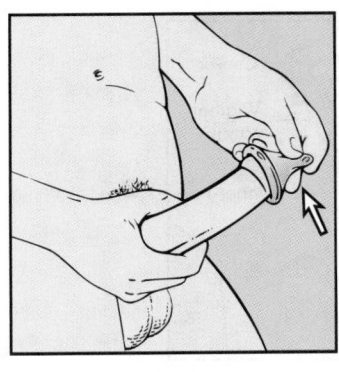 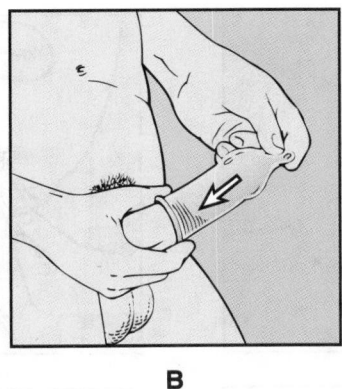 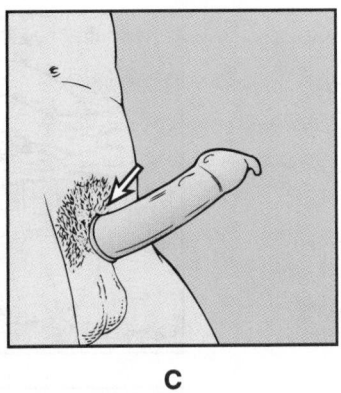

A   **B**   **C**

FIG. 14-6   Proper placement of the male condom. **A,** The condom is placed over the glans of the erect penis, being careful to squeeze air out of the reservoir. **B** and **C,** The condom is then rolled down the shaft of the penis to the hairline.

self does not cause HIV infection. The major risk for HIV infection is related to sharing injecting equipment and/or having unsafe sexual experiences while under the influence of drugs. The basic rules are as follows: (1) do not use drugs; (2) if you use drugs, do not share equipment; and (3) do not have sexual intercourse when under the influence of any drug (including alcohol) that impairs decision-making ability.[29]

The safest mechanism is to abstain from drugs. Although this is the best option for those who do not currently use drugs, it may not be a viable alternative for users who are not prepared to quit or for those who have no access to drug treatment services. The risk of HIV for these individuals can be eliminated if they use alternatives to injecting, such as smoking, snorting, or ingesting the drug. Risk for HIV can also be eliminated if users do not share injecting equipment. Injecting equipment (works) includes needles, syringes, cookers (spoons or bottle caps used to mix the drug), cotton, and rinse water. None of this equipment should be shared.[30] Another safe tactic is for the user to have access to sterile equipment. This can be accomplished through community needle and syringe exchange programs (NSEPs) that provide sterile equipment to users in exchange for used equipment. Opposition to these programs is supported by the fear that ready access to injecting supplies will increase drug use. However, studies have shown that in communities where exchange programs have been established, drug use does not increase, rates of HIV infection are controlled, and an overall cost benefit results.[37]

Cleaning equipment before use is a risk-reducing activity. It decreases the risk for those who share equipment (Table 14-14). This process takes time and may be difficult for a person in drug withdrawal.[29]

Decreasing risks of perinatal transmission. The best way to prevent HIV infection in infants is to prevent HIV infection in women. Women who are already infected with HIV should be asked about their reproductive desires. Women who choose not to have children need to have birth control methods discussed in detail. Should they become pregnant, abortion may be desired and should be discussed in conjunction with other options.[30]

If HIV-infected pregnant women are treated with zidovudine (ZDV, AZT, Retrovir), the rate of perinatal transmission is decreased. This treatment has minimal side effects for the baby. Combination ART as appropriate for the mother's HIV infection

TABLE 14-12	*Patient & Family Teaching Guide* **Proper Use of the Male Condom**

- Use only condoms (rubbers) that are made out of latex or polyurethane. "Natural skin" condoms have pores that are large enough for HIV to penetrate.
- Store condoms in a cool, dry place and protect them from trauma. The friction caused by carrying them in a back pocket, for instance, can wear down the latex.
- Do not use a condom if the expiration date has passed or if the package looks worn or punctured.
- Lubricants used in conjunction with condoms must be water soluble. Oil-based lubricants can weaken latex and increase the risk of tearing or breaking.
- Nonlubricated, flavored, or unflavored condoms can provide protection during oral intercourse.
- The condom must be placed on the erect penis before any contact is made with the partner's mouth, vagina, or rectum to prevent exposure to preejaculatory secretions that may contain HIV.
- See Fig. 14-6 for proper steps in male condom placement.
- Remove the penis and condom from the partner's body immediately after ejaculation and before the erection is lost. Hold the condom at the base of the penis and remove both at the same time. This keeps semen from leaking around the condom as the penis becomes flaccid.
- Remove the condom after use, wrap in tissue, and discard. Do not flush down the toilet, because this can cause plumbing problems.
- Condoms are not reusable! A new condom must be used for every act of intercourse.

can further decrease the risk of perinatal transmission to less than 2%. The current standard of care is that all women who are pregnant or contemplating pregnancy should be counseled about HIV infection, informed of their choices, routinely offered access to voluntary HIV antibody testing, and if infected, provided with optimal ART as desired. This area of HIV prevention is evolving

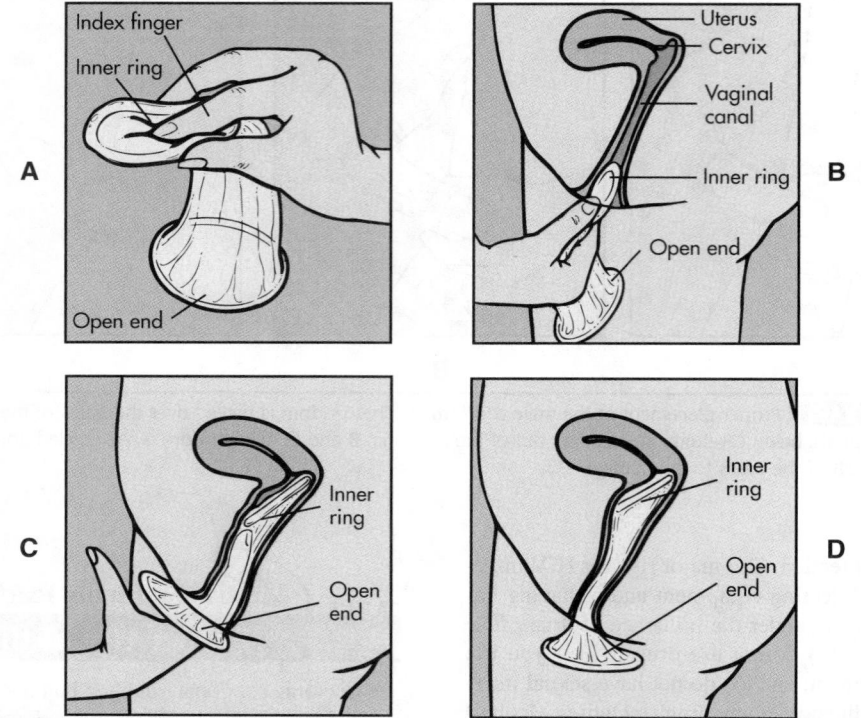

FIG. 14-7 Proper placement of the female condom. **A,** Inner ring is squeezed for insertion. **B,** Sheath is inserted similarly to a diaphragm. **C,** Inner ring is pushed up as far as it can go with the index finger. **D,** Proper placement of female condom.

TABLE 14-13

Patient & Family Teaching Guide
Proper Use of the Female Condom

- Female condoms consist of a polyurethane sheath with two spring-form rings.
  The smaller ring is inserted into the vagina and holds the condom in place internally. This ring can be removed if the condom is to be used for anal intercourse. It should not be removed if the condom is to be used for vaginal intercourse.
  The larger ring surrounds the opening to the condom. It functions to keep the condom in place while protecting the external genitalia.
- Use only water-soluble lubricants with female condoms.
  Female condoms come prelubricated and with a tube of additional lubricant.
  Lubrication is needed to protect the condom from tearing during sexual intercourse and can also decrease the noise that results from friction of the penis against the condom.
- Some men have reported that the female condom feels better than the male condom. Other men like male condoms better.

- The only way to find out which type of condom works best is to try them both.
- Practice inserting the female condom. The steps for proper insertion are shown in Fig. 14-7. Lubrication makes the condom slippery, but do not get discouraged, just keep trying.
- During sexual intercourse, ensure that the penis is inserted into the female condom through the outer ring. It is possible for the penis to miss the opening, thus making contact with the vagina and defeating the purpose of the condom.
- Do not use a male condom at the same time as a female condom.
- After intercourse, remove the condom before standing up.
- Twist the outer ring to keep the semen inside, gently pull the condom out of the vagina, and discard.
- Do not flush down the toilet, because this can cause plumbing problems.
- Do not reuse a female condom.

---

rapidly, and care should be taken to assess the latest treatment guidelines.[38,39]

Decreasing risks at work. The risk of infection from occupational exposure to HIV is small but real. The CDC and the Occupational Safety and Health Administration (OSHA) require employers to protect workers from exposure to blood and other potentially infectious materials. Precautions and safety devices decrease the risk of direct contact with blood and body fluids. Precautions for the prevention of occupational exposure to blood-borne diseases are discussed in Chapter 12. Should exposure to HIV-infected fluids occur, **postexposure prophylaxis** (PEP) with combination ART based on the type of exposure, the

TABLE 14-14 Patient & Family Teaching Guide
Proper Use of Injection Equipment

- When injecting drugs, it is always preferable to use new, sterile syringes, needles, cookers, and cotton (works).
- Find out if there is a needle and syringe exchange program in your community. If there is, take used equipment in and you will be provided with new works.
- Reusing your own equipment is acceptable. Just ensure that no one else uses your equipment.
- If you must share your equipment, it is very important to clean the works thoroughly before use.
- First, rinse the used needle and syringe twice with tap water.
- Then, fill the syringe with full strength household bleach, shake for 30 seconds, and squirt the bleach out.
- Repeat the bleaching process a second time, being sure to shake the bleach-filled syringe for 30 seconds.
- Finally, rinse equipment twice with tap water.
- Do not share your bleach or rinse water.
- Do not share your cooker. If you must share your cooker, clean it with bleach and water before using it again.

volume of the exposure, and the status of the source patient has been shown to significantly decrease the risk of infection. The possibility of treatment makes reporting of all blood exposures even more critical.[40]

HIV testing and counseling. Testing is the only sure way to determine if a person has HIV infection. Any individual who is at risk for HIV infection should be encouraged to be tested. When negative, testing can relieve anxieties about past behaviors and provide opportunities for prevention education. When positive, testing provides the needed impetus to seek treatment and to protect sexual and drug-using partners. All testing for HIV should be accompanied by pretest and posttest counseling (Table 14-15).[18,21,41]

Acute Intervention

Early intervention. Early intervention after detection of HIV infection can promote health and limit or delay disability. Because the course of HIV is variable, assessment is very important. Nursing interventions are based on and tailored to patient needs noted during assessment. The nursing assessment in HIV disease should focus on early detection of symptoms, opportunistic diseases, and psychosocial problems (see Table 14-9).[30]

Initial response to a diagnosis of HIV. Reactions to a positive HIV-antibody test are similar to the reactions of people who are

TABLE 14-15 Pretest and Posttest Counseling Associated with HIV–Antibody Testing

General Guidelines
People who are being tested for HIV are frequently fearful about the test results.
- Establish rapport with the patient.
- Assess patient's ability to understand HIV counseling.
- Determine the patient's ability to access support systems.

Explain the benefits of testing.
- Testing provides an opportunity for education that can decrease the risk of new infections.
- Infected individuals can be referred for early intervention and support programs.

Discuss negative aspects of testing.
- Confidentiality issues: breeches of confidentiality have led to discrimination.
- A positive test affects all aspects of the patient's life (personal, social, economic, etc.) and can raise difficult emotions (anger, anxiety, guilt, and thoughts of suicide).

Pretest Counseling
Determine the patient's risk factors and when the last risk occurred. Counseling should be individualized according to these parameters.
Provide education to decrease future risk of exposure.
Provide education that will help the patient protect sexual and drug-sharing partners.
Discuss problems related to the delay between infection and an accurate test. Testing will need to be repeated at intervals for up to 6 months after each possible exposure. Discuss the need to abstain from further risky behaviors. Discuss the need to protect partners during that interval.
Discuss the possibility of false-negative tests, which are most likely to occur during the window period.
Explain that a positive test shows HIV infection and not AIDS.
Assess support systems. Provide telephone numbers and resources as needed.

Discuss patient's personally anticipated responses to test results (positive and negative).
Outline assistance that will be offered if the test is positive.

Posttest Counseling
If the test is negative, reinforce pretest counseling and prevention education. Remind patient that test needs to be repeated at intervals for up to 6 months after the most recent exposure risk.
If the test is positive, understand that the patient may be in shock and not hear much of what you say.
Provide resources for medical and emotional support and help the patient get immediate assistance.
- Evaluate suicide risk and follow up as needed.
- Determine need to test others who have had risky contact with the patient.
- Discuss retesting to verify results. This tactic supports hope for the patient, but more important, it keeps the patient in the system. While waiting for the second test result, the patient has time to think about and adjust to the possibility of being HIV infected.
- Encourage optimism.
  - Remind patient that effective treatments are available.
  - Review health habits that can improve the immune system.
  - Arrange for patient to speak to HIV-infected people who are willing to share and assist newly diagnosed patients during the transition period.
  - Reinforce that a positive HIV test means that the patient is infected, but does not necessarily mean that the patient has AIDS.
- Educate to prevent new infections. HIV-infected people should be instructed to avoid donating blood, organs, or semen; to avoid sharing razors, toothbrushes, or other household items that may contain blood or other body fluids; and to protect sexual and needle-sharing partners.

Adapted from Bradley-Springer L, Fendrick R: *HIV instant instructor cards,* El Paso, Tex, 1994, Skidmore-Roth.

diagnosed with any life-threatening, debilitating, or chronic illness. They include anxiety, panic, fear, depression, denial, hopelessness, thoughts of suicide, anger, and guilt.[41] Many of these reactions are also seen in the patient's family members, friends, and caregivers. As time passes, patients and their loved ones must confront common issues associated with a life-threatening ill-

TABLE
14-16

Patient & Family Teaching Guide
Use of Antiretroviral Drugs

Resistance to antiretroviral drugs is a major problem in treating HIV infection. To decrease the risk of developing resistance:

1. Take at least three different antiretroviral drugs at a time; discuss other options with your health care provider.
2. Know what you are taking and how to take them (some have to be taken with food, some must be taken on an empty stomach, some cannot be taken together). If you do not understand, ask. Get your nurse to write the instructions clearly for you.
3. Take the full dose prescribed and take it on schedule. If you cannot take the drug because of side effects or other problems, report it to your health care provider.
4. Take all of the drugs prescribed. Do not quit taking one drug while continuing the others. If you cannot tolerate one of your drugs, your health care provider will recommend a completely new set of drugs.
5. Many of the antiretroviral drugs interact with other drugs, including a number of common drugs you can buy without a prescription. Be sure your health care provider and pharmacist know all of the drugs that you are taking, and do not take any new drugs without checking for possible interactions.
6. The goal of antiretroviral therapy is to decrease the amount of virus in your blood. This is called your *viral load*. Viral load can be determined by tests such as the PCR or bDNA. The results are reported in absolute numbers. The goal is to get your viral load to an undetectable level. Most health care providers will check this number on a regular basis whether you are taking antiretroviral agents or not.
7. Two to four weeks after you start on drug therapy (or change your therapy), your health care provider will test your viral load to find out if the drugs are working. These results are reported in absolute numbers or in logs (a mathematical concept). All you have to know is that you want to see the viral load drop. If reports are in logs, you want to see a drop of at least 1 log, which means that 90% of your viral load has been eliminated. If your viral load drops by 2 logs, your viral load will have decreased by 95%. If your viral load drops by 3 logs, your viral load will have decreased by 99%.
8. An undetectable viral load means that the amount of virus is extremely low and viruses cannot be found in the blood using the current technology. It does *not* mean that the virus is gone because much of the virus will be in lymph nodes and organs that the tests cannot detect. It also does *not* mean that you are no longer able to transmit HIV to others; you will need to continue protecting all of your sexual and drug-using partners.

PCR, Polymerase chain reaction.

ness. These include difficult treatment decisions; feelings of loss, anger, powerlessness, depression, and grief; social isolation imposed by self or others; altered concepts of the physical, social, emotional, and creative self; thoughts of suicide; and the possibility of death.[42-46] The nurse can help the patient gain control. Empowerment is particularly important because the individual with HIV infection often experiences multiple losses, including an overwhelming feeling of loss of control. Empowerment is facilitated by education and honest discussions about the patient's health status and treatment options.[30,44]

Antiretroviral therapy. Multidrug-therapy protocols have been shown to significantly reduce viral loads and reverse clinical progression of HIV.[13,20] However, nurses must be aware that the protocols are complex, the drugs have side effects and interactions, and they do not work for everyone. All of these factors contribute to problems with adherence to treatment, a dangerous situation because of the risk of developing drug resistance. Frequently, nurses are the health care providers who work most closely with patients who are trying to cope with these issues. Interventions include education about (1) the advantages and disadvantages of new treatments, (2) the dangers of nonadherence to therapeutic regimens, (3) how and when to take each drug, (4) drug interactions to avoid, and (5) side effects that must be reported to the primary care provider.[30] Table 14-16 provides guidance for patient teaching in these areas.

When to start antiretroviral therapy. ART has been in a state of continuous change since the first antiretroviral drug was released in 1987. When new drugs were developed, health care providers had the ability to combine and substitute drugs. However, as new treatments improve the quality and quantity of patients' lives, problems emerge. For a while, the preferred treatment strategy was known as "hit it early, hit it hard." This was thought to be appropriate because decreasing the viral load provides for better health outcomes. However, side effects and lack of adherence caused many patients to question their abilities to maintain ART for long periods of time. For this reason, new federal guidelines suggest that treatment can be delayed until higher levels of immune suppression are observed.[20] Despite the new guidelines, many health care providers and their patients prefer to start ART as soon as possible, and there is considerable debate on the optimum time to start treatment.[47] An important consideration is the patient's readiness to initiate ART. Nurses can provide in-depth education and counseling for patients as they struggle to make this decision.

Adherence. Adherence to drug regimens is a critical component of drug therapy for people with HIV infection and an area where nurses are uniquely well prepared to provide assistance. Taking drugs as ordered (right dose and time) every day is important for all drug therapy. The difference with HIV is that missing a dose can lead to viral mutations that allow HIV to become resistant to the drug.[20,48] It is now clear that adherence rates of better than 95% are required to prevent disease progression, opportunistic disease, and viral drug resistance. This is an amazing goal when one considers that adherence rates of 80% are thought to be acceptable for many other chronic diseases.[49,50]

The difficulty of adhering consistently is clear to anyone who has tried to take a 10-day course of antibiotics. Patients with HIV infection have to take anywhere from 3 to 20 pills a day, at precise times during the day. This process must be repeated every day for the rest of their lives even though they often suffer uncomfortable side effects.[50] Nurses have learned that helping people adhere to difficult treatment regimens requires a number of things. The most important is to remember that each patient is a unique individual who will have different ways of coping and of learning. Patients can be helped with technologies such as electronic reminders, beepers, or timers on pillboxes. Group support and individual counseling can also help, but the best assistance may be learning about the patient's life and assisting with problem solving within the confines of that life.[49-51]

Health promotion. HIV disease progression may also be delayed by promoting a healthy immune system whether the patient chooses to use ART or not. Useful interventions for HIV-infected patients include (1) nutritional support to maintain lean body mass and ensure appropriate levels of vitamins and micronutrients; (2) moderation or elimination of alcohol intake, smoking, and drug use; (3) adequate rest and exercise; (4) stress reduction; (5) avoidance of exposure to new infectious agents; (6) mental health counseling; and (7) involvement in support groups and community activities.

Patients should be taught to recognize symptoms that may indicate disease progression and/or drug side effects so that prompt medical care can be initiated. Table 14-17 provides an overview of symptoms that patients should report. In general, patients should have as much information as needed to make informed decisions about health care. These decisions then dictate the appropriate interventions.

Acute exacerbations. Chronic diseases are characterized by acute exacerbations of recurring problems.[32] This is especially true in HIV disease where infections, cancers, debility, and psychosocial/economic issues may interact to overwhelm the patient's ability to cope. Nursing care becomes more complex if the patient's immune system deteriorates and new problems arise to compound existing difficulties. When opportunistic diseases or difficult side effects of treatment develop, symptom management, education, and emotional support are necessary.

Nursing care assumes primary importance in helping patients prevent the many opportunistic diseases associated with HIV infection. The best prevention of opportunistic disease is adequate treatment of the underlying HIV infection. The following discussion gives additional information about some of these diseases.

Pneumocystis carinii *pneumonia.* *Pneumocystis carinii* pneumonia (PCP) is caused by a fungus so common that most people have been exposed to it by age 3 (Fig 14-8). A healthy immune system keeps *P. carinii* from causing disease, but an HIV-infected patient is at risk for PCP when the CD4$^+$ T cell count is less than $200/\mu l$. PCP can be prevented through the use of antibiotics (see Table 14-8), and most health care providers follow prevention protocols to help the patient avoid this opportunistic infection. The most common manifestations of PCP include shortness of breath, fever, night sweats, fatigue, and weight loss. It is frequently accompanied by oropharyngeal candidal infection and a nonproductive cough that may progress to a productive cough. Acute cases of PCP require intensive nursing intervention. Nursing care includes monitoring respiratory status, assessing fever and fever symptoms, administering drugs and oxygen, positioning to facilitate breathing, guiding relaxation exercises to decrease anxiety, promoting nutritional support and fluid replacement, and conserving energy to decrease oxygen demand.[13,52]

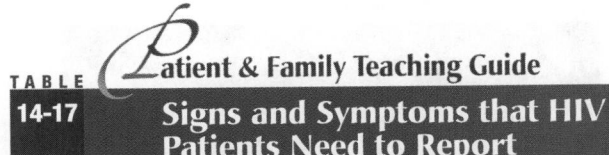

TABLE 14-17	*P*atient & Family Teaching Guide **Signs and Symptoms that HIV Patients Need to Report**

Report the Following Signs and Symptoms Immediately to Health Care Provider

- Any change in level of consciousness: lethargy, hard to arouse, unable to arouse, unresponsive, unconscious
- Headache accompanied by nausea and vomiting, changes in vision, changes in ability to perform coordinated activities, or after any head trauma
- Vision changes: blurry or black areas in vision field, new floaters
- Persistent shortness of breath related to activity and not relieved by a short rest period
- Nausea and vomiting accompanied by abdominal pain
- Dehydration: unable to eat or drink because of nausea, diarrhea, or mouth lesions; severe diarrhea or vomiting; dizziness when standing
- Yellow discoloration of the skin
- Any bleeding from the rectum that is not related to hemorrhoids
- Pain in the flank with fever and unable to urinate for more than 6 hours
- New onset of weakness in any part of the body, new onset of numbness that is not obviously related to pressure, new onset of difficulty speaking
- Chest pain not obviously related to cough
- Seizures
- New rash accompanied by fever
- New oral lesions accompanied by fever
- Severe depression, anxiety, hallucinations, delusions, or possible danger to self or others

Report the Following Signs and Symptoms within 24 Hours

- New or different headache; constant headache not relieved by aspirin or acetaminophen
- Headache accompanied by fever, nasal congestion, or cough
- Burning, itching, or discharge from the eyes
- New or productive cough
- Vomiting 2-3 times a day
- Vomiting accompanied by fever
- New, significant, or watery diarrhea (more than 6 times a day)
- Painful urination, bloody urine, urethral discharge
- New, significant rash (widespread, painful, itchy, or following a path down the leg or arm, around the chest, or on the face)
- Difficulty eating because of mouth lesions
- Vaginal discharge, pain, or itching

Cryptococcal meningitis. *Cryptococcus neoformans* is a yeast that causes disease in 6% to 10% of all HIV-infected patients. When it causes meningitis, the symptoms tend to be vague, including a prolonged waxing and waning period of fever, headache, and malaise, followed by nausea and vomiting, altered mental status, stiff neck, visual disturbances, papilledema, ataxia, seizures, aphasia, and sensitivity to light. Nursing care includes

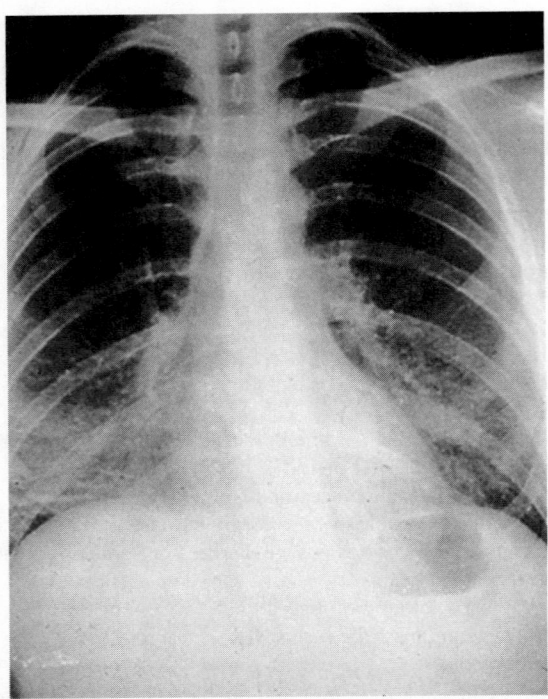

FIG. 14-8 Chest x-ray showing interstitial infiltrates as the result of *Pneumocystis carinii* pneumonia.

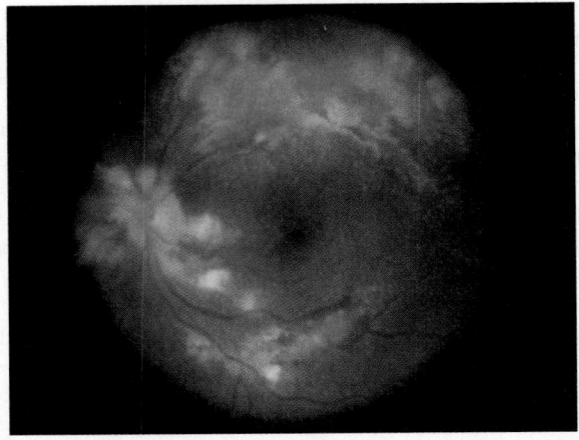

FIG. 14-9 The retina with "cottage cheese and ketchup" findings caused by cytomegalovirus (CMV) retinitis.

providing drugs for acute episodes and ensuring that patients understand the need to continue maintenance therapy after the acute episodes have resolved. Without this, 50% to 75% of patients with a history of cryptococcal meningitis will relapse within a year. Nursing care requirements include frequent neurologic assessments to detect subtle changes that can affect adherence to treatment regimens.[13,53]

Cytomegalovirus retinitis. Cytomegalovirus (CMV) is a common organism that can cause esophagitis, colitis, pneumonia, and several neurologic problems, including retinitis. Ocular disease generally will not appear until there is severe immune suppression (Fig. 14-9). Common symptoms of retinal disease include decreased vision, complaints of *floaters* (spots that appear to drift in front of the eye caused by vitreous humor debris), and one-sided visual field loss. Left untreated, CMV retinitis leads to blindness. Because symptoms occur relatively late in the progression of HIV infection, periodic eye examinations are recommended for early identification and treatment. Nursing care focuses on teaching the patient and caregiver about drug therapy (see Table 14-2) and follow-up care. The goal is to prevent vision loss, but there may be progression despite treatment. Nursing assistance can help patients cope with vision loss by altering activities of daily living, arranging referrals to agencies that provide services for vision-impaired patients, teaching about assistive devices, and providing support for loss-related grief.[13,54]

Mycobacterium avium *complex.* *Mycobacterium avium* complex (MAC) is a mycobacterial disease that frequently causes gastrointestinal (GI) tract problems for HIV-infected patients. It is also capable of causing widely disseminated infection, invading the blood, spleen, lymph nodes, bone marrow, and liver. The signs and symptoms of MAC infection include chronic diarrhea, abdominal pain, fever, malaise, weight loss, anemia, neutropenia, malabsorption syndrome, and obstructive jaundice. A major focus of nursing care for patients with MAC is to teach them about the complicated drug therapy (see Table 14-2). Nurses can also help patients deal with problems caused by diarrhea.[13,55]

Kaposi's sarcoma. **Kaposi's sarcoma (KS)** is a common neoplasm seen in HIV-infected patients, especially those who were infected as a result of unprotected male-to-male sexual intercourse. KS is thought to be caused by the human herpes virus 8 (HHV8), a sexually transmitted virus. KS can affect many organ systems, but lesions are most frequently seen on the skin and oral mucosa. The lesions can be flat or raised, of various shapes and sizes, and of various colors, and generally are not painful. Skin lesions are cosmetically disfiguring, but otherwise do not usually cause problems. However, KS lesions that occur in the GI tract or the lungs can cause bleeding and respiratory distress. Care once KS is diagnosed is generally considered to be palliative. Treatment with ART leading to immune reconstitution can resolve KS lesions without other treatments. Nurses can best help patients and their families by providing information about treatment options, assisting with the decision-making process, and providing caring support as the disease progresses.[13,56]

Ambulatory and Home Care

Ongoing care. HIV-infected patients share problems experienced by all individuals with chronic diseases, but these problems are exacerbated by social constructs surrounding HIV. Chronic diseases are characterized by negative social attitudes that label the patient as weak-willed or immoral for being sick. In HIV this stigma is compounded by several factors. HIV-infected people may be seen as lacking control over urges to have sex or use drugs. It is then easy to jump to the conclusion that they brought the disease on themselves and, therefore, somehow deserve to be sick. Behaviors associated with HIV infection may be viewed as immoral (e.g., homosexuality, having many sexual partners) and are sometimes illegal (e.g., injecting heroin, sex work). The fact that infected individuals can transmit the virus to others furthers the negative, stigmatizing social concept of HIV. Social stigmatization supports discrimination in all facets of life. For example, HIV-infected people have lost jobs, families, homes, and insurance because of such discrimination, even though many forms of discrimination are now illegal in the United States because of the Americans with Disabilities Act (ADA).[1,57]

The chronic nature of HIV infection can cause family stress, social isolation, dependence, frustration, lowered self-image, loss of control, and economic pressures. An interesting observation is that all of these variables may have contributed to the patient's infection in the first place. Low self-esteem, searching for social contact, frustration, and economic difficulties all contribute to drug use and risky sexual behaviors.

Disease and drug side effects. Physical problems related to HIV disease and/or the treatment of HIV can interrupt the patient's ability to maintain a desired lifestyle. HIV-infected patients frequently experience anxiety, fear, diarrhea, depression, peripheral neuropathy, pain, nausea and vomiting, and fatigue.[58] These are symptoms that nurses deal with routinely, and the interventions for them do not change significantly based on the primary diagnosis. Individual considerations will, of course, influence the way that the nurse approaches the patient. Nursing management of diarrhea, for instance, still includes helping patients collect specimens, recommending dietary changes, encouraging fluid and electrolyte replacement,[59] instructing the patient about skin care, and managing skin breakdown around the perianal area. Nursing approaches for fatigue in HIV include teaching patients to assess fatigue patterns, determine contributing factors, set activity priorities, conserve energy, schedule rest periods, exercise, and avoid substances such as caffeine, nicotine, alcohol, and other drugs that may disturb sleep.[60]

Over the past several years, a new set of metabolic disorders has emerged among HIV-infected patients, especially those who have been infected for a long time and who have been on ART. These disorders include a syndrome of changes in body shape (fat redistribution to the abdomen, upper back, and breasts along with wasting in the arms, legs, and face), hyperlipidemia (elevated triglycerides and decreases in high-density lipoproteins), insulin resistance and hyperglycemia, bone disease (osteoporosis, osteopenia, avascular necrosis), lactic acidosis, and cardiovascular disease.[61,62] It is still not clear why these disorders develop, but it is probably a combination of factors such as long-term survival after HIV diagnosis, ART side effects, genetic predisposition, and chronic stress.[61,62]

Management of metabolic disorders currently focuses on detecting problems early, dealing with the symptoms, and helping the patient cope with new problems and additional drugs. It is important to recognize and treat these problems early, especially since cardiovascular disease and lactic acidosis are potentially fatal complications. A frequent first intervention is to change ART because some drugs are more often associated with these problems (see Table 14-7). Lipid abnormalities are generally treated with lipid-lowering drugs (see Table 33-4), dietary changes, and exercise. Insulin resistance is treated with hypoglycemic drugs and weight loss. Bone disease may be improved with exercise, dietary changes, and calcium and vitamin D supplements.[63]

Body changes that combine fat accumulation and wasting are major problems for patients with this syndrome. Human growth hormone, testosterone, and anabolic steroids have been used to help resolve these changes, but the results are inconclusive. There is also little evidence that exercise or dietary changes make any difference.[63] Nursing interventions need to focus on helping the patient make treatment decisions and on dealing with negative changes in body image.

Terminal care. Dementia is an especially bothersome problem that can accompany the final stages of HIV disease. **AIDS-dementia complex (ADC),** also called *HIV-associated cognitive motor complex,* is caused by HIV infection in the brain, or HIV-related central nervous system problems caused by lymphoma,

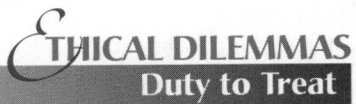

ETHICAL DILEMMAS
Duty to Treat

Situation

A nurse in a community clinic has just discovered that Maggie, a patient with respiratory problems, has HIV infection. The nurse is concerned about contact with Maggie and her bodily fluids. She requests that she not be assigned to Maggie's care. The nurse believes that she has the right to refuse to care for Maggie because she has her own family to support and protect.

Important Points for Consideration

- According to the American Nurses Association (ANA) Code of Ethics, the nurse must care for all patients regardless of background or medical condition.
- Health care providers have contact with patients every day who may have infectious blood or other body fluids.
- Infection precautions are instituted to protect health care workers from potentially infectious blood or other body fluids.
- There are two situations in which nurses can refuse to care for patients if employers are notified in advance: (1) when caring for a patient would conflict with a nurse's deeply held religious belief or (2) when there might be greater potential harm to the nurse than benefit to the patient (e.g., if the nurse were immunocompromised).
- The Rehabilitation Act and the Americans with Disabilities Act prohibit discrimination against the handicapped and disabled. People who are HIV infected are included under these acts.
- If a nurse's primary concern is personal safety, the nurse needs to reexamine her or his commitment to the nursing profession.

Critical Thinking Questions

1. How would you address this issue if this nurse was a colleague?
2. If nurses could select which patients they would care for, how would that affect their ability to care for patients in general?

toxoplasmosis, CMV, herpes virus, *Cryptococcus,* progressive multifocal leukoencephalopathy (PML), dehydration, or drug side effects. Dementia symptoms are sometimes reversible if a treatable cause is diagnosed. Treatable causes include dehydration, depression, opportunistic diseases, and drug side effects. Adequate ART has been instrumental in decreasing the rates of HIV dementia.[64]

The clinical manifestations of ADC include cognitive, behavioral, and motor abnormalities. Symptoms of ADC include decreased ability to concentrate, apathy, depression, inattention, forgetfulness, social withdrawal, personality change, insomnia, confusion, hallucinations, slowed response rates, clumsiness, and ataxia. ADC can progress from minor symptoms to global dementia, paraplegia, incontinence, and coma.[64] Nursing interventions focus on safety, including issues related to assistance devices, home environment, and smoking. Nurses need to encourage patients to continue self-care and to help caregivers support those activities, even as the patient loses the ability for total self-care. Preventing confusion and disorientation requires maintaining a meaningful environment, frequent reorientation, and stress reduction measures. A major emphasis also should be placed on providing support to family members and significant others who may have difficulty dealing with a patient's deteriorating mental and physical status.

Despite exciting new developments in the treatment of HIV infection, many patients will experience disease progression, disability, and death. Sometimes these occur because treatments do not work for the patient. This can be devastating because of the media hype related to "miracle" recoveries among those for whom the drugs work. In other cases, patients may make a calculated decision to forego further treatment, allowing the disease to progress toward death. This may be especially difficult for family members and loved ones to accept. Nursing care during the terminal phase of any disease needs to focus on keeping the patient comfortable, facilitating emotional and spiritual acceptance of the finite nature of life, and helping the patient's significant others deal with grief and loss. Nurses become pivotal care providers during the terminal phase of illness, especially in HIV disease where patients and families often choose terminal care at home. (End-of-life care is discussed in Chapter 10.)

■ Evaluation

The expected outcomes are that the patient at risk for HIV infection will

- analyze personal risk factors
- develop and implement a personal plan to decrease risks

The expected outcomes are that the patient with HIV infection will

- describe basic aspects of the effects of HIV on the immune system
- compare and contrast various treatment options for HIV disease
- work with a team of health care providers to achieve optimal health
- prevent transmission of HIV to others

CRITICAL THINKING EXERCISES

Case Study
At Risk for HIV Disease

Patient Profile. Emilio, a 20-year-old Hispanic male college student, comes to the student health center with pain on urination.

Subjective Data
- Describes pain as, "Just like it felt when I had the clap last year"
- Provides a history of sexual activity since age 15, reports lifetime sexual partners as six women and two men
- Denies injected drug use, tobacco use, or corticosteroid therapy
- Uses alcohol (mainly beer) at weekend parties and has smoked marijuana, but not recently
- Recent sexual activity has been on weekends during or after beer parties

Objective Data
Physical Examination
- 5 feet 11 inches tall, 168 pounds, temperature 100.4° F (38° C), purulent urethral discharge noted

Laboratory Studies
- Urine test for *Neisseria gonorrhoeae* is positive

Collaborative Care
- IM injection with 250 mg ceftriaxone (Rocephin)
- Doxycycline 100 mg PO bid for 7 days

CRITICAL THINKING QUESTIONS

1. Why should Emilio be encouraged to be tested for HIV?
2. How will you counsel Emilio about the testing process? How can you help him prepare for the test and the test results?
3. What further questions will you need to ask Emilio before you can determine his educational needs?
4. Ask a classmate to be "Emilio" and role-play HIV risk assessment, risk reduction counseling, and pretest and posttest counseling.
5. What are the main considerations to cover when teaching about barrier methods of protection? Are there components of Hispanic culture that may affect your approach to teaching about condoms?
6. How will you discuss the issue of partner notification with Emilio?
7. If Emilio's HIV test is positive, what nursing diagnoses most likely apply? If his HIV test is negative, what nursing diagnoses most likely apply?

Case Study
Symptomatic HIV Disease

Patient Profile. Janelle, a 35-year-old African American single mother, was admitted to the hospital with AIDS and CMV retinitis that were diagnosed 2 days ago.

Subjective Data
- Was initially seen by a doctor 6 years ago for pain behind the sternum and difficulty swallowing, diagnosed as esophageal candidiasis
- Had a positive HIV antibody test at that time
- Has consistently refused ART because "it's poison, I've seen how sick it makes other people, and besides, we can't afford it"
- Married to Jim, a former IV drug user, for 10 years until his recent death from AIDS-related complications
- Has two children, ages 8 and 11, who are both HIV-antibody negative
- Experiences fatigue and frequent oral and vaginal candidiasis outbreaks
- Expresses concern about welfare of children who are at home with her sister and says, "Maybe I should take better care of myself for them"

Objective Data
Physical Examination
5 feet 6 inches tall, 100 pounds, temperature 99.8° F (37.7° C)
Laboratory Studies
- CD4$^+$ T cell count 185/μl
- Viral load 25,328 (by bDNA)
- Hematocrit 30%

Collaborative Care
- Insertion of central venous catheter to be used for CMV treatment
- Trimethoprim-sulfamethoxazole
- Triple antiretroviral therapy: zidovudine + lamivudine (Combivir) and indinavir (Crixivan)

CRITICAL THINKING EXERCISES—cont'd

CRITICAL THINKING QUESTIONS

1. Why was Janelle's initial medical problem (esophageal candidiasis) unusual?
2. Why is Janelle taking trimethoprim-sulfamethoxazole, and what are its common side effects?
3. What drugs are used to treat CMV retinitis? What side effects do they have, and what problems are associated with their administration?
4. Is there a potential advantage to Janelle's refusal to take antiretroviral drugs in the past?
5. Women often put their children's welfare first. What problems could this cause for Janelle's treatment? How can these problems be solved?
6. What teaching needs to be done before Janelle is allowed to return home after this hospitalization? What referrals need to be made? How can Janelle be helped to adhere to her drug schedule?
7. What psychosocial and legal issues need to be assessed? What interventions might be appropriate?
8. What nursing interventions are immediately appropriate? What plans need to be made for continued nursing care after discharge?
9. Based on the assessment data presented, choose at least three appropriate nursing diagnoses. Are there any collaborative problems?

REVIEW QUESTIONS

The number of the question corresponds to the same-numbered objective at the beginning of the chapter.

1. Transmission of HIV from an infected individual to another occurs
   a. most commonly as a result of sexual contact.
   b. in all infants born to women with HIV infection.
   c. only when there is a large viral load in the blood.
   d. frequently in health care workers with needle-stick exposures.
2. Following infection with HIV
   a. the virus replicates mainly in B lymphocytes before spreading to CD4$^+$ T cells in lymph nodes.
   b. the immune system is impaired predominantly by infection and destruction of CD4$^+$ T cells.
   c. infection of monocytes may occur, but these cells are destroyed by antibodies produced by oligodendrocytes.
   d. within 2 to 3 days a long period develops during which the virus is not found in the blood and there is little viral replication.
3. Which of the following statements is false?
   a. Infection with HIV results in a chronic disease with acute exacerbations.
   b. Untreated HIV infection can remain in the early chronic stage for a decade or more.
   c. Late-stage infection is often called acquired immunodeficiency syndrome (AIDS).
   d. Opportunistic diseases occur more often when the CD4$^+$ T cell count is high and the viral load is low.
4. A diagnosis of AIDS is made when an HIV-infected patient has
   a. a CD4$^+$ T cell count below 200/μl.
   b. an increasing amount of HIV in the blood.
   c. a reversal of the CD4:CD8 ratio to less than 2:1.
   d. oral hairy leukoplakia, an infection caused by Epstein-Barr virus.
5. Screening for HIV infection generally involves
   a. laboratory analysis of blood to detect HIV antigen.
   b. electrophoretic analysis of HIV antigen in plasma.
   c. laboratory analysis of blood to detect HIV antibodies.
   d. analysis of lymph tissues for the presence of HIV RNA.
6. Antiretroviral drugs are used to
   a. cure acute HIV infection.
   b. treat opportunistic diseases.
   c. decrease viral RNA levels.
   d. supplement radiation and surgery.
7. Opportunistic diseases in HIV infection
   a. usually occur one at a time.
   b. are generally slow to develop and progress.
   c. occur in the presence of immunosuppression.
   d. are curable with appropriate pharmacologic intervention.
8. Which of the following statements about metabolic side effects of ART is false?
   a. These are an annoying set of symptoms that are ultimately harmless.
   b. Changes in body shape and size are often difficult for HIV-infected patients to accept.
   c. Lipid abnormalities include increases of triglycerides and decreases in high-density cholesterol.
   d. Insulin resistance and hyperlipidemia can be treated with drugs to control blood glucose and decrease cholesterol.
9. Which of the following eliminates the risk of transmission of HIV?
   a. using sterile equipment to inject drugs.
   b. cleaning equipment used to inject drugs.
   c. taking zidovudine (AZT, ZDV, Retrovir) during pregnancy.
   d. using latex barriers to cover genitals during sexual contact.
10. Of the following, which is the most appropriate nursing intervention to help an HIV-infected patient adhere to the treatment regimen?
    a. Give the patient a videotape and a brochure to view and read at home.
    b. Volunteer to "set up" a drug pillbox for a week at a time.
    c. Inform the patient that the side effects of the drugs are bad but that they go away after awhile.
    d. Assess the patient's lifestyle and find adherence cues that fit into the patient's lifestyle.

REFERENCES

1. Ungvarski P: The past 20 years of AIDS through the eyes of one nurse, *Am J Nurs* 101:26, 2001.
2. Centers for Disease Control and Prevention (CDC): US HIV and AIDS cases reported through December 2001, year-end edition, 13(2), 2001. Available at *www.cdc.gov/hiv/surveillance.htm* (accessed Nov. 25, 2002).
3. World Health Organization (WHO): Human immunodeficiency virus and acquired immune deficiency syndrome (HIV/AIDS), 2001. Available at *www.who.int/emc-documents/surveillance/docs/whocdscsrisr2001.html/hiv_aids/hiv_aids.htm* (accessed August 6, 2002).
4. World Health Organization (WHO): Global HIV/AIDS and STD surveillance, 2001. *Available at http://who.int/emc-hiv* (accessed August 6, 2002).
5. Miramontes HM: The global challenges of the HIV/AIDS pandemic, *J Assoc Nurses AIDS Care* 11:11, 2000.
6. Janes S et al: Sexually transmitted diseases and HIV/AIDS. In Lundy KS, Janes S, editors: *Community health nursing: caring for the public's health,* Boston, 2001, Jones & Bartlett.
7. Centers for Disease Control and Prevention (CDC): HIV and its transmission, 2001. Available at *www.cdc.gov/hiv/pubs/facts/transmission.htm* (accessed August 6, 2002).
8. Talotta D: Health care workers risk reduction in HIV/AIDS care. In Kirton CA, Talotta D, Zwolski K, editors: *Handbook of HIV/AIDS nursing,* St Louis, 2001, Mosby.
9. CDC National Prevention Information Network (NPIN): HIV/AIDS prevention, 2001. Available at *http://cdcnpin.org/hiv/* (accessed August 6, 2002).
10. Zwolski K: HIV immunopathogenesis. In Kirton CA, Talotta D, Zwolski K, editors: *Handbook of HIV/AIDS nursing,* St Louis, 2001, Mosby.
11. Centers for Disease Control and Prevention (CDC): Surveillance of health care workers with HIV/AIDS, 2002. Available at *www.cdc.gov/hiv/pubs/facts/hcwsurv.htm* (accessed August 6, 2002).
12. Anderson JR: HIV and reproduction. In Anderson JR, editor: *A guide to the clinical care of women with HIV, 2001 edition,* Rockville, Md, 2001, HRSA HIV/AIDS Bureau.
13. Bartlett JG, Gallant JE: *2001-2002 medical management of HIV infection,* Baltimore, 2001, Johns Hopkins University.
14. Greenblatt RM, Hessol NA: Epidemiology and natural history of HIV infection in women. In Anderson JR, editor: *A guide to the clinical care of women with HIV, 2001 edition,* Rockville, Md, 2001, HRSA HIV/AIDS Bureau.
15. Simon VA: HIV-1 drug resistance testing, *IAPAC Monthly* 7:235, 2001.
16. Stapranks SI, Feinberg MB: Natural history and immunopathogenesis of HIV-1 disease. In Sande MA, Volberding PA, editors: *The medical management of AIDS,* ed 5, Philadelphia, 1997, WB Saunders.
17. Sonza S, Crowe SM: Reservoirs for HIV infection and their persistence in the face of undetectable viral load, *AIDS Patient Care and STDs* 15:511, 2001.
18. Kirton CA: Risk assessment, identification, and HIV counseling. In Kirton CA, Talotta D, Zwolski K, editors: *Handbook of HIV/AIDS nursing,* St Louis, 2001, Mosby.
19. Centers for Disease Control and Prevention (CDC): Recommendations and reports: 1993 revised classification system for HIV infection and expanded surveillance case definition for AIDS among adolescents and adults, *MMWR* 41:1, 1992.
20. Centers for Disease Control and Prevention (CDC): Guidelines for the use of antiretroviral agents in HIV-infected adults and adolescents, 2002. Available at *www.hivatis.org/* (accessed August 6, 2002).
21. Kirton CA: Clinical application of immunological and virological markers. In Kirton CA, Talotta D, Zwolski K, editors: *Handbook of HIV/AIDS nursing,* St Louis, 2001, Mosby.
22. Kirton CA: Guidelines for the initiation of antiretroviral therapy. In Kirton CA, Talotta D, Zwolski K, editors: *Handbook of HIV/AIDS nursing,* St Louis, 2001, Mosby.
23. Wolbach J et al: *A pharmacist's guide to antiretroviral medications for HIV-infected adults and adolescents,* Denver, 2001, Mountain Plains AIDS Education and Training Center.
24. Project Inform: Drug interactions, 2002. Available at *www.projectInform.org* (accessed August 6, 2002).
25. Schackman BR et al: Cost-effectiveness of earlier initiation of antiretroviral therapy for uninsured HIV-infected adults, *Am J Public Health* 91:1456, 2001.

26. Centers for Disease Control and Prevention (CDC): USPHS/IDSA guidelines for the prevention of opportunistic infections in persons with human immunodeficiency virus, 2001. Available at *http://hivatis.org/trtgdlns.html* (accessed August 6, 2002).
27. National Institutes of Allergies and Infectious Disease, Division of AIDS: HIV vaccine development status report, 2000. Available at *www.niaid.nih.gov/daids/vaccine/whsummarystatus.htm* (accessed August 6, 2002).
28. Little K, Surjadi M: A scientific overview of the development of AIDS vaccines, *J Assoc Nurses AIDS Care* 11:19, 2000.
29. Bradley-Springer L: HIV prevention: What works? *Am J Nurs* 101:45, 2001.
30. Bradley-Springer L: *HIV/AIDS care plans,* ed 2, El Paso, Tex, 1999, Skidmore-Roth.
*31. Bova C: Adjustment to chronic illness among HIV-infected women, *J Nurs Scholarship* 33:217, 2001.
32. Paterson BL: The shifting perspectives model of chronic illness, *J Nurs Scholarship* 33:21, 2001.
33. Levi J: An HIV agenda for the new administration, *Am J Public Health* 91:1015, 2001.
*34. Tigges BB: Affiliative preferences, self-change, and adolescent condom use, *J Nurs Scholarship* 33:231, 2001.
35. Roberts JR: HIV prevention: Relentless pursuit of an elusive goal, 2001. Available at *http://nursing.medscape.com/Medscape/CNO/2001/anac/public/index-ANAC.html* (accessed August 6, 2002).
36. Centers for Disease Control and Prevention (CDC): How effective are latex condoms in preventing HIV? 1998. Available at *www.cdc.gov/hiv/pubs/faq/faq23.htm* (accessed August 6, 2002).
37. HIVdent: Public policy: evidence-based findings on the efficacy of syringe exchange programs: an analysis from the Assistant Secretary of Health and Surgeon General of the scientific research completed since April 1998, 2001. Available at *www.hivdent.org/publicp/ppebsotsr062000.htm* (accessed August 6, 2002).
38. Sherman D, Sherman N: HIV/AIDS and pregnancy. In Kirton CA, Talotta D, Zwolski K, editor: *Handbook of HIV/AIDS nursing,* St Louis, 2001, Mosby.
39. Centers for Disease Control and Prevention (CDC): Public Health Service Task Force recommendations for the use of antiretroviral drugs in pregnant HIV-1 infected women for maternal health and interventions to reduce perinatal HIV-1 transmission in the United States, 2001. Available at *http://hivatis.org/trtgdlns.html* (accessed August 6, 2002).
40. Centers for Disease Control and Prevention (CDC): Updated US Public Health Service guidelines for the management of occupational exposures to HBV, HCV, and HIV and recommendations for postexposure prophylaxis, 2001. Available at *http://hivatis.org/trtgdlns.html* (accessed August 6, 2002).
41. Centers for Disease Control and Prevention (CDC): Revised guidelines for HIV counseling, testing, and referral and revised recommendations for HIV screening of pregnant women, 2001. Available at *www.cdc.gov/hiv/testing.htm* (accessed August 6, 2002).
*42. Riley TA, Toth JM, Fava JL: The transtheoretical model and stress management practices in women at risk for, or infected with, HIV, *J Assoc Nurses AIDS Care* 11:67, 2000.
*43. Corless IB et al: Predictors of perception of cognitive functioning in HIV/AIDS, *J Assoc Nurses AIDS Care* 11:19, 2000.
*44. Inouye J, Flannelly L, Flannelly KJ: The effectiveness of self-management training for individuals with HIV/AIDS, *J Assoc Nurses AIDS Care* 12:73, 2001.
45. Kemppainen JK: Predictors of quality of life in AIDS patients, *J Assoc Nurses AIDS Care* 12:61, 2001.
*46. Hudson AL et al: Social interactions, perceived support, and level of distress in HIV-positive women, *J Assoc Nurses AIDS Care* 12:68, 2001.
47. Gulik RM: Evolving approaches to initial antiretroviral therapy: when to start and with what, *Top HIV Med* 9:4, 2001.
48. Esch JF, Frank SV: HIV drug resistance and nursing practice, *Am J Nurs* 101:30, 2001.
49. Williams AB: HIV adherence regimens: 10 vital lessons, *Am J Nurs* 101:37, 2001.

---

*Nursing research–based reference.

50. Jones SG: From pill fatigue to pill counts: medication adherence in HIV/AIDS, 2001. Available at *http://nursing.medscape.com/Medscape/CNO/2001/anac/public/index-ANAC.html* (accessed August 6, 2002).

*51. Holzemer WL et al: The client adherence profiling-intervention tailoring (CAP-IT) intervention for enhancing adherence to HIV/AIDS medications: a pilot study, *J Assoc Nurses AIDS Care* 11:36, 2000.

52. Winson G, Kirton CA, Zwolski K: Parasitic infections. In Kirton CA, Talotta D, Zwolski K, editors: *Handbook of HIV/AIDS nursing,* St Louis, 2001, Mosby.

53. Zwolski K: Fungal infections. In Kirton CA, Talotta D, Zwolski K, editors: *Handbook of HIV/AIDS nursing,* St Louis, 2001, Mosby.

54. Zwolski K: Viral infections. In Kirton CA, Talotta D, Zwolski K, editors: *Handbook of HIV/AIDS nursing,* St Louis, 2001, Mosby.

55. Zwolski K, Talotta D: Bacterial infections. In Kirton CA, Talotta D, Zwolski K, editors: *Handbook of HIV/AIDS nursing,* St Louis, 2001, Mosby.

56. Kirton CA: Oncologic conditions. In Kirton CA, Talotta D, Zwolski K, editors: *Handbook of HIV/AIDS nursing,* St Louis, 2001, Mosby.

57. The Americans with Disability Act, 42 U.S.C.s. 1201 et seq. (1992 and 1994).

58. Holzemer WL: The symptom experience, *Am J Nurs* 102:48, 2002.

59. Winson SKG: Management of HIV-associated diarrhea and wasting, *J Assoc Nurses AIDS Care* 12(suppl):55, 2001.

60. Adinolfi A: Assessment and treatment of HIV-related fatigue, *J Assoc Nurses AIDS Care* 12(suppl):29, 2001.

61. Lyon DE, Truban E: HIV-related lipodystrophy: a clinical syndrome with implications for nursing practice, *J Assoc Nurses AIDS Care* 11:36, 2000.

62. Currier JS, Havlir DV: Complications of HIV infection and its therapies, *Top HIV Med* 9:8, 2001.

63. Keithly JK: Management of antiretroviral-related nutritional problems: state of the science, *J Assoc Nurses AIDS Care* 12(suppl):67, 2001.

64. Zwolski K: Neurologic disorders in HIV/AIDS. In Kirton CA, Talotta D, Zwolski K, editors: *Handbook of HIV/AIDS nursing,* St Louis, 2001, Mosby.

RESOURCES

AIDS Action
www.aidsaction.org
AIDS Infonet
www.aidsinfonet.org
AIDS Education Global Information System (AEGIS)
www.aegis.com
AIDS Education and Training Centers (AETC) National Resource Center
www.aids-etc.org
American Foundation for AIDS Research (amfAR)
800-39-amfAR
www.amfar.org
Association of Nurses in AIDS Care (ANAC)
3538 Ridgewood Road
Akron, OH 44333
800-260-6780
Fax: 330-670-0109
E-mail: anac@anacnet.org
www.anacnet.org

Center for AIDS Prevention Studies (CAPS)
AIDS Research Institute
University of California, San Francisco
74 New Montgomery, Suite 600
San Francisco, CA 94105
415-597-9100
Fax: 415-597-9213
www.caps.ucsf.edu
HIV/AIDS Bureau (HAB)
Health Services and Resources Administration (HRSA)
Office of Communications
5600 Fishers Lane
Rockville, MD 20852
301-443-3376
http://hab.hrsa.gov
HIV/AIDS Clinical Treatment Information Service (ATIS)
800-HIV-0440 (800-448-0440)
E-mail: atis@hivatis.org
www.hivatis.org
Joint United Nations Programme on HIV/AIDS (UNAIDS)
E-mail: unaids@unaids.org
www.unaids.org
National Association of People with AIDS (NAPWA)
1413 K Street, NW
Washington, DC 20005
202-898-0414
Fax: 202-898-0435
E-mail: napwa@napwa.org
www.napwa.org
National HIV/AIDS Clinical Consultation Center
415-476-7070
Fax: 415-476-3454
800-933-3413 (telephone consultation service)
www.ucsf.edu/hivcntr/
National Institute for Allergy and Infectious Diseases (NIAID)
Building 31, Room 7A-50
31 Center Drive MSC 2520
Bethesda, MD 20892-2520
301-496-5717
www.niaid.nih.gov
National Minority AIDS Council (NMAC)
1931 13th Street, NW
Washington, DC 20009
202-483-6622
Fax: 202-483-1135
E-mail: info@nmac.org
www.nmac.org

For additional Internet resources, see the website for this book at *http://evolve.elsevier.com/Lewis/medsurg/.*

CHAPTER 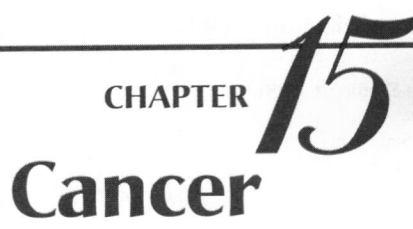 15

Cancer

Catherine M. Bender
Margaret Rosenzweig

LEARNING OBJECTIVES

1. Describe the prevalence, incidence, and death rates of cancer in the United States.
2. Describe the processes involved in the biology of cancer.
3. Differentiate the three phases of cancer development.
4. Describe the role of the immune system related to cancer.
5. Describe the use of the classification systems for cancer.
6. Explain the role of the nurse in the prevention and detection of cancer.
7. Explain the use of surgery, radiation therapy, chemotherapy, and biologic therapy in the treatment of cancer.
8. Differentiate between external beam radiation and brachytherapy.
9. Identify the classifications of chemotherapeutic agents and methods of administration.
10. Describe the effects of radiation therapy and chemotherapy on normal tissues.
11. Identify the types and effects of biologic therapy agents.
12. Describe the nursing management of the patient receiving radiation therapy, chemotherapy, and biologic therapy.
13. Describe the nutritional therapy for patients with cancer.
14. Describe the complications that can occur in advanced cancer.
15. Describe the appropriate psychologic support of the patient with cancer and the patient's family.

KEY WORDS

benign neoplasms, p. 292	metastasis, p. 295
biologic therapy, p. 318	nadir, p. 316
bone marrow transplantation, p. 321	oncogenes, p. 292
	protooncogenes, p. 292
brachytherapy, p. 304	radiation, p. 303
cancer, p. 290	sarcomas, p. 297
carcinogens, p. 293	staging, p. 298
carcinoma in situ, p. 299	tumor angiogenesis, p. 295
carcinomas, p. 297	tumor-associated antigens, p. 296
histologic grading, p. 298	
immunologic surveillance, p. 296	vesicants, p. 313
malignant neoplasms, p. 292	

Cancer is a group of more than 200 diseases characterized by uncontrolled and unregulated growth of cells. It can occur in persons of all ages and all ethnicities and is a major health problem. An estimated 30% of Americans now living will experience cancer at some point in their lives. An estimated 1,284,900 persons were diagnosed with cancer in 2002 (excluding nonmelanoma skin cancer and carcinoma in situ).[1] Some cancers, such as cancer of the stomach and uterus, have decreased in incidence in recent times whereas others, such as non-Hodgkins lymphoma, have increased in incidence.[2] The incidence of melanoma is rising faster than any other malignancy in the United States.[3] Differences are found in the incidence of certain cancers in men and women (Table 15-1).

Considerable progress has been made in controlling cancer for long periods. More than 8 million Americans alive today have a history of cancer, and the 5-year survival rate is now 62%. This statistic represents Americans living with cancer, including those who are disease free, in remission, or under treatment. However, these 5-year survival rates do not include the number of people who are "cured" of cancer.[4]

Cancer is the second most common cause of death in the United States (heart disease is the most common). One of every five deaths is caused by cancer, with one half of these deaths occurring before age 65. The death rate as a result of cancer is leveling off or decreasing except for an increasing rate of deaths from lung cancer in women (Table 15-2). In 2002 an estimated 555,500 Americans died from cancer—more than 1500 people per day. About 172,000 of these cancer deaths were caused by tobacco use, and it is estimated that one third of cancer deaths are attributable to nutritional factors such as high-fat, low-fiber diets.[1]

The cancer incidence and death rate are higher in African Americans than in whites. This rate is especially high among male African Americans. Most of the differences in cancer rates between African Americans and whites are attributed to environmental and social rather than biologic factors, such as diagnosis at a later stage of disease.[1]

Statistics cannot reveal the physiologic, psychologic, and sociologic impact of cancer. Cancer is known to be the most feared of all diseases, feared far more than heart disease. The word *cancer* is viewed as being synonymous with death, pain, and disfigurement. However, attitudes toward cancer do not fit today's status of the treatment and control of cancer. Education of health

Reviewed by Barbara I. Damron, RN, PhD, Educational Psychologist; President, Damron Oncology Consulting; and Oncology Clinical Nurse Specialist, St. Vincent Hospital, Santa Fe, N.M. and Erica Camarillo, RN, BSN, Pediatric Nurse, University Hospital, San Antonio, Tex.

TABLE 15-1	Cancer Incidence by Site and Sex in 2002*			
MALE			**FEMALE**	
TYPE	**%**		**TYPE**	**%**
Prostate	30		Breast	31
Lung	14		Lung	12
Colon/rectum	11		Colon/rectum	12
Urinary tract	7		Uterus	6
Melanoma (skin)	5		Melanoma	4

Source: *Cancer facts and figures*, Atlanta, 2002, American Cancer Society.
*Excluding basal and squamous cell skin cancers and carcinoma in situ.

care professionals and the public is essential if current attitudes about cancer and cancer treatment are to become more positive and realistic.

BIOLOGY OF CANCER

Cancer is a group of many diseases of multiple causes that can arise in any cell of the body capable of evading regulatory controls over proliferation and differentiation. Two major dysfunctions present in the process of cancer are defective cellular proliferation (growth) and defective cellular differentiation.

TABLE 15-2	Estimates of Cancer Deaths by Site and Sex in 2002		
MALE		**FEMALE**	
TYPE	**%**	**TYPE**	**%**
Lung and bronchus	31	Lung and bronchus	25
Prostate	11	Breast	15
Colon/rectum	10	Colon/rectum	11
Pancreas	5	Pancreas	6
Non-Hodgkin's lymphoma	5	Ovary	5

Source: *Cancer facts and figures,* Atlanta, 2002, American Cancer Society.

CULTURAL & ETHNIC CONSIDERATIONS
Cancer

- The death rate from the four most common cancers (lung, colorectal, breast, prostate) is higher among minorities (except Asian Americans) than in whites.
- Asian Americans have the lowest death rate from cancer of any ethnic group.
- However, cancer is the leading cause of death among Asian American women.
- At all stages of cancer diagnosis, African Americans with cancer have shorter survival times than whites.
- Although African American women are less likely than white women to develop breast cancer, they are more likely to die from the disease if they develop it.
- The death rate for African American women with breast cancer has increased 60%.
- African American men have almost twice the rate of prostate cancer than white men and are more than twice as likely to die from the disease.
- The death rate for African American men with colorectal cancer has increased 20%.
- The incidence rate of cervical cancer is five times higher in Vietnamese women than in white American women.
- Hispanic women have the highest incidence rate of invasive cervical cancer of any group other than Vietnamese, and twice the incidence rate of non-Hispanic white women.
- Native Americans and Alaska Natives have the highest death rate from "all cancers combined" compared with other ethnic groups.

Source: *Cancer facts and figures,* Atlanta, 2002, American Cancer Society.

Defect in Cellular Proliferation

Normally, most tissues of the human adult contain a population of predetermined, undifferentiated cells known as stem cells. *Predetermined* means that the stem cells of a particular tissue will ultimately differentiate and become mature, functioning cells of that tissue and only that tissue.

Cell proliferation originates in the stem cell and begins when the stem cell enters the cell cycle (Fig. 15-1). The time from when a cell enters the cell cycle to the time the cell divides into two identical cells is called the *generation time of the cell.* A mature cell continues to function until it degenerates and dies.

All cells of a tissue are controlled by an intracellular mechanism that determines when cellular proliferation is necessary. Under normal conditions, a state of dynamic equilibrium is constantly maintained (i.e., cellular proliferation equals cellular degeneration or death). Normally the process of cellular division and proliferation is activated only in the presence of cellular degeneration or death. Cellular proliferation will also occur if the body has a physiologic need for more cells. For example, a normal increase in white blood cell (WBC) count occurs in the presence of infection.

Another explanation for the phenomenon of proliferation control of normal cells is *contact inhibition.* Normal cells respect the boundaries and territory of the cells surrounding them. They will not invade a territory that is not their own. The neighboring cells are thought to inhibit cellular growth through the physical contact of the surrounding cell membranes. Cancer cells grown in tissue culture are characterized by loss of contact inhibition. These cells have no regard for cellular boundaries and will grow on top of one another and also on top of or between normal cells.

The rate of normal cellular proliferation (from the time of cellular birth to the time of cellular death) differs in each body tissue. In some tissues, such as bone marrow, hair follicles, and epithelial lining of the gastrointestinal (GI) tract, the rate of cellular proliferation is rapid. In other tissues, such as myocardium, neurons, and cartilage, cellular proliferation does not occur.

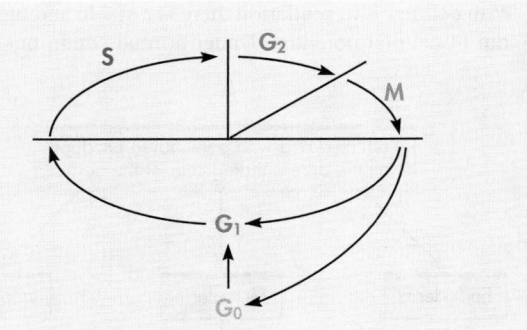

G_1 = relatively dormant with some RNA and protein synthesized
S = DNA is synthesized; RNA and protein synthesis continue
G_2 = some RNA synthesized
M = mitosis (cellular division)
G_0 = resting phase, cells are not in the process of cellular division

FIG. 15-1 Cell life cycle and metabolic activity. Generation time is the period from M phase to M phase. Cells not in the cycle but capable of division are in the resting phase (G_0).

Cancer cells usually proliferate in the manner and at the same rate of the normal cells of the tissue from which they arise. However, cancer cells respond differently than normal cells to the intracellular signals that regulate the state of dynamic equilibrium. Cancer cells divide indiscriminately and haphazardly. Sometimes they produce more than two cells at the time of mitosis.

The stem cell theory proposes that the loss of intracellular control of proliferation results from a mutation of the stem cells.[5] The stem cells are viewed as the target or the origin of cancer development. The deoxyribonucleic acid (DNA) of the stem cell is substituted or permanently rearranged. When this happens, the stem cell is mutated. Once the cell has mutated, one of three things can occur: (1) the cell can die, either from the damage resulting from the mutation or by initiating a programmed cellular suicide called *apoptosis;* (2) the cell can recognize the damage and repair itself; or (3) the mutated cell can survive and pass along the damage to its daughter cells.[6] Mutated cells that survive have the potential to become malignant (i.e., cells with invasive and metastatic potential). The stem cell theory of cancer development is not complete because malignant stem cells can differentiate to form normal tissue cells.[5]

A common misconception regarding the characteristics of cancer cells is that the rate of proliferation is more rapid than that of any normal body cell. In most situations, cancer cells proliferate at the same rate as the normal cells of the tissue from which they originate. The difference is that proliferation of the cancer cells is indiscriminate and continuous. In this way, with each cell division creating two or more offspring cells, there is continuous growth of a tumor mass: $1 \rightarrow 2 \rightarrow 4 \rightarrow 8 \rightarrow 16$ and so on. This is termed the *pyramid effect.* The time required for a tumor mass to double in size is known as its *doubling time.*

Defect in Cellular Differentiation

Cellular differentiation is normally an orderly process that progresses from a state of immaturity to a state of maturity. Because all body cells are derived from the fertilized ova, all cells have the potential to perform all body functions. As cells differentiate, this potential is repressed and the mature cell is capable of performing only specific functions (Fig. 15-2).

With cellular differentiation there is a stable and orderly phasing out of cellular potential. Under normal conditions the differentiated cell is stable and will not *dedifferentiate* (i.e., revert to a previous undifferentiated state).

The exact mechanism that controls cellular differentiation and proliferation is not completely understood. Two types of normal genes that can be affected by mutation are protooncogenes and tumor suppressor genes. **Protooncogenes** are normal cellular genes that are important regulators of normal cellular processes. Protooncogenes promote growth whereas tumor suppressor genes, such as p53, suppress growth. Mutations that alter the expression of protooncogenes can activate them to function as **oncogenes** (tumor-inducing genes). Mutations that alter *tumor suppressor genes* render them inactive, resulting in a loss of their tumor suppressor actions.[5]

The protooncogene has been described as the genetic lock that keeps the cell in its mature functioning state. When this lock is "unlocked," as may occur through exposure to *carcinogens* (agents that cause cancer) or oncogenic viruses, genetic alterations and mutations occur. The abilities and properties that the cell had in fetal development are again expressed. Oncogenes interfere with normal cell expression under some conditions, causing the cell to become malignant. This cell regains a fetal appearance and function. For example, some cancer cells produce new proteins, such as those characteristic of the embryonic and fetal periods of life. These proteins located on the cell membrane include carcinoembryonic antigen (CEA) and α-fetoprotein (AFP). They can be detected in human blood by laboratory studies (see Role of the Immune System later in this chapter). Other cancer cells, such as small (oat) cell carcinoma of the lung, produce hormones (see Complications Resulting from Cancer, later in this chapter) that are ordinarily produced by cells arising from the same embryonic cells as the tumor cells.

Tumors can be classified as benign or malignant. In general, **benign neoplasms** are well differentiated, and **malignant neoplasms** range from well differentiated to undifferentiated. The ability of malignant tumor cells to invade and metastasize is the major difference between benign and malignant neoplasms. Other differences between benign and malignant neoplasms are presented in Table 15-3.

Development of Cancer

The following is a theoretic model of the development of cancer. The cause and development of each type of cancer are likely to be multifactorial. It is not known how many tumors have a

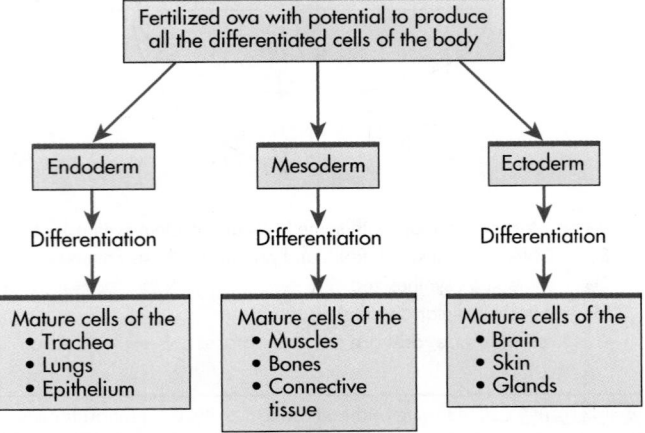

FIG. 15-2 Normal cellular differentiation.

TABLE 15-3	Comparison of Benign and Malignant Neoplasms	
CHARACTERISTIC	**MALIGNANT**	**BENIGN**
Encapsulated	Rarely	Usually
Differentiated	Poorly	Partially
Metastasis	Frequently present	Absent
Recurrence	Frequent	Rare
Vascularity	Moderate to marked	Slight
Mode of growth	Infiltrative and expansive	Expansive
Cell characteristics	Cells abnormal, become more unlike parent cells	Fairly normal; similar to parent cells

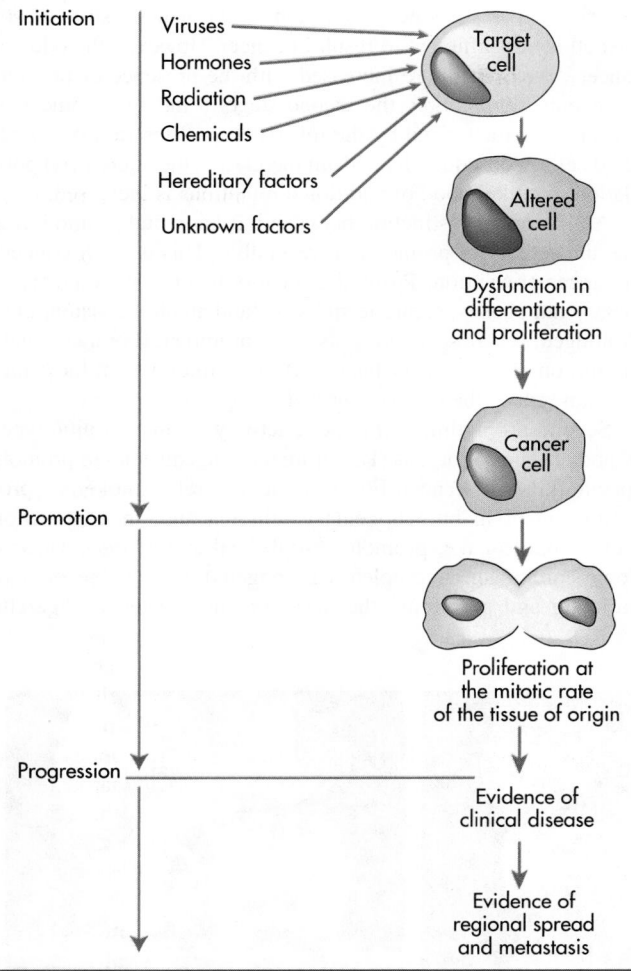

Initiation

Viruses
Hormones
Radiation
Chemicals
Hereditary factors
Unknown factors

Target
cell

Altered
cell

Dysfunction in
differentiation
and proliferation

Cancer
cell

Promotion

Proliferation at
the mitotic rate
of the tissue of origin

Progression

Evidence of
clinical disease

Evidence of
regional spread
and metastasis

FIG. 15-3   Process of cancer development.

chemical, environmental, genetic, immunologic, or viral origin. Cancers may arise spontaneously from causes that are thus far unexplained.

It is a common belief that the development of cancer is a rapid, haphazard event. However, the natural history of cancer is an orderly process comprising several stages and occurring over a period of time. These stages include initiation, promotion, and progression (Fig. 15-3).

Initiation. The first stage, *initiation,* is a mutation in the cell's genetic structure resulting from an inherited mutation, an error that occurs during DNA replication, or following exposure to a chemical, radiation, or viral agent. This altered cell has the potential for developing into a *clone* (group of identical cells) of neoplastic cells.[6]

Many **carcinogens** (cancer-causing agents capable of producing cellular alterations) are detoxified by protective enzymes and are harmlessly excreted. If this protective mechanism fails, carcinogens can enter the cell's nucleus and alter DNA. The cell may die or repair itself. However, if cell death or repair does not occur before cell division, the cell will replicate into daughter cells, each with the same genetic alteration.[7]

Carcinogens may be chemical, radiation, or viral in nature. In addition, some genetic anomalies increase the susceptibility of individuals to certain cancers. Common characteristics of car-

cinogens are that their effects in the stage of initiation are usually irreversible and additive.

Chemical carcinogens. Chemicals were identified as cancer-causing agents in the latter part of the eighteenth century when Percival Pott noted that chimney sweeps had a higher incidence of cancer of the scrotum associated with exposure to soot residues in chimneys. As the years passed, more chemical agents were identified as actual and potential carcinogens. Evidence indicated that persons exposed to certain chemicals over a period of time had a greater incidence of certain cancers than others. The long latency period from the time of exposure to the development of cancer makes it difficult to identify cancer-causing chemicals. Also, those chemicals that cause cancer in animals may or may not cause the same specific cancer in humans. Some chemicals are cancer causative in their environmental form, but others must first undergo certain changes to become carcinogenic.

Certain drugs have also been identified as carcinogens. Drugs that are capable of interacting with DNA (e.g., alkylating agents) and immunosuppressive agents have the potential to cause neoplasms in humans. The use of alkylating agents (e.g., cyclophosphamide [Cytoxan] and nitrogen mustard), either alone or in combination with radiation therapy, has been associated with an increased incidence of acute myelogenous leukemia in persons treated for Hodgkin's disease, non-Hodgkin's lymphomas, and multiple myeloma. These secondary leukemias are relatively refractory to induction of remission with combination chemotherapy. Secondary leukemia has also been observed in persons who have undergone transplant surgery and who have taken immunosuppressive drugs.

Radiation. Since the beginning of the twentieth century, it has been known that ionizing radiation can cause cancer in almost any human body tissue. Presently, the dose of radiation that causes cancer is not known, and there is considerable debate surrounding the effect of exposure to low-dose radiation over a period of time. When cells are exposed to a source of radiation, damage occurs to one or both strands of DNA. Certain malignancies have been correlated with radiation as a carcinogenic agent:

1. Leukemia, lymphoma, thyroid cancer, and other cancers increased in incidence in the general population of Hiroshima and Nagasaki after the atomic bomb explosions.
2. A higher incidence of bone cancer occurs in persons exposed to radiation in certain occupations, such as radiologists, radiation chemists, and uranium miners.
3. Thyroid cancer has a higher incidence in those persons who have received radiation to the head and neck area for treatment of a variety of disorders, such as acne, tonsillitis, sore throat, or enlarged thyroid gland.
4. A higher incidence of childhood cancer occurs in children exposed to radiation during fetal life.

Ultraviolet (UV) radiation has long been associated with melanoma and squamous and basal cell carcinoma of the skin. Skin cancer is the most common type of cancer among whites in the United States. Of great concern is the increase in the incidence of melanoma, a skin cancer that is poorly responsive to systemic treatment. Although the cause of melanoma is probably multifactorial, mounting evidence suggests that UV radiation secondary to sunlight exposure is linked to the development of melanoma.[5]

Viral carcinogens. Certain DNA and ribonucleic acid (RNA) viruses, termed *oncogenic,* can transform the cells they infect and induce malignant transformation. Viruses have been identified as causative agents of cancer in animals and humans. Burkitt's lymphoma has consistently shown evidence of the presence of the Epstein-Barr virus (EBV) in vitro.[4] This virus is also present in infectious mononucleosis, but the explanation of why an infectious disease develops in some persons and a lymphoma in others is not known. Persons with acquired immunodeficiency syndrome (AIDS), which is caused by a virus, have a high incidence of Kaposi's sarcoma (see Chapter 14). Other viruses that have been linked to the development of cancer include hepatitis B virus, which is associated with hepatocellular carcinoma, and human papillomavirus, which is believed to be capable of inducing lesions that progress to squamous cell carcinomas, such as cervical cancers.

Genetic susceptibility. Cancer-related genes have been identified that increase an individual's susceptibility to development of certain cancers. For example, a woman who carries the genes BRCA-1 or BRCA-2 has a 50% to 85% risk of developing breast cancer in her lifetime. However, in reality, 95% of women who develop breast cancer do not possess these genes. With our current knowledge, it is believed that only 10% of cancers have a strong genetic link.[4]

Promotion. A single alteration of the genetic structure of the cell is not sufficient to result in cancer. However, the odds of cancer development are increased with the presence of promoting agents.[2] *Promotion,* the second stage in the development of cancer, is characterized by the reversible proliferation of the altered cells. Consequently, with an increase in the altered cell population, the likelihood of additional mutations is increased.

An important distinction between initiation and promotion is that the activity of promoters is reversible. This is a key concept in cancer prevention. Promoting factors include such agents as dietary fat, obesity, cigarette smoking, and alcohol consumption. Prolonged, severe stress may also be a promoter. (For a complete discussion of stress, see Chapter 8.) The withdrawal of these factors can reduce the risk of cancer development.

Several promoting agents exert activity against specific types of body tissues or organs. Therefore these agents tend to promote specific kinds of cancer. For example, cigarette smoke is a promoting agent in bronchogenic carcinoma and, in conjunction with alcohol intake, promotes esophageal and bladder cancers. Some carcinogens (complete carcinogens) are capable of both initiating and promoting the development of cancer. Cigarette

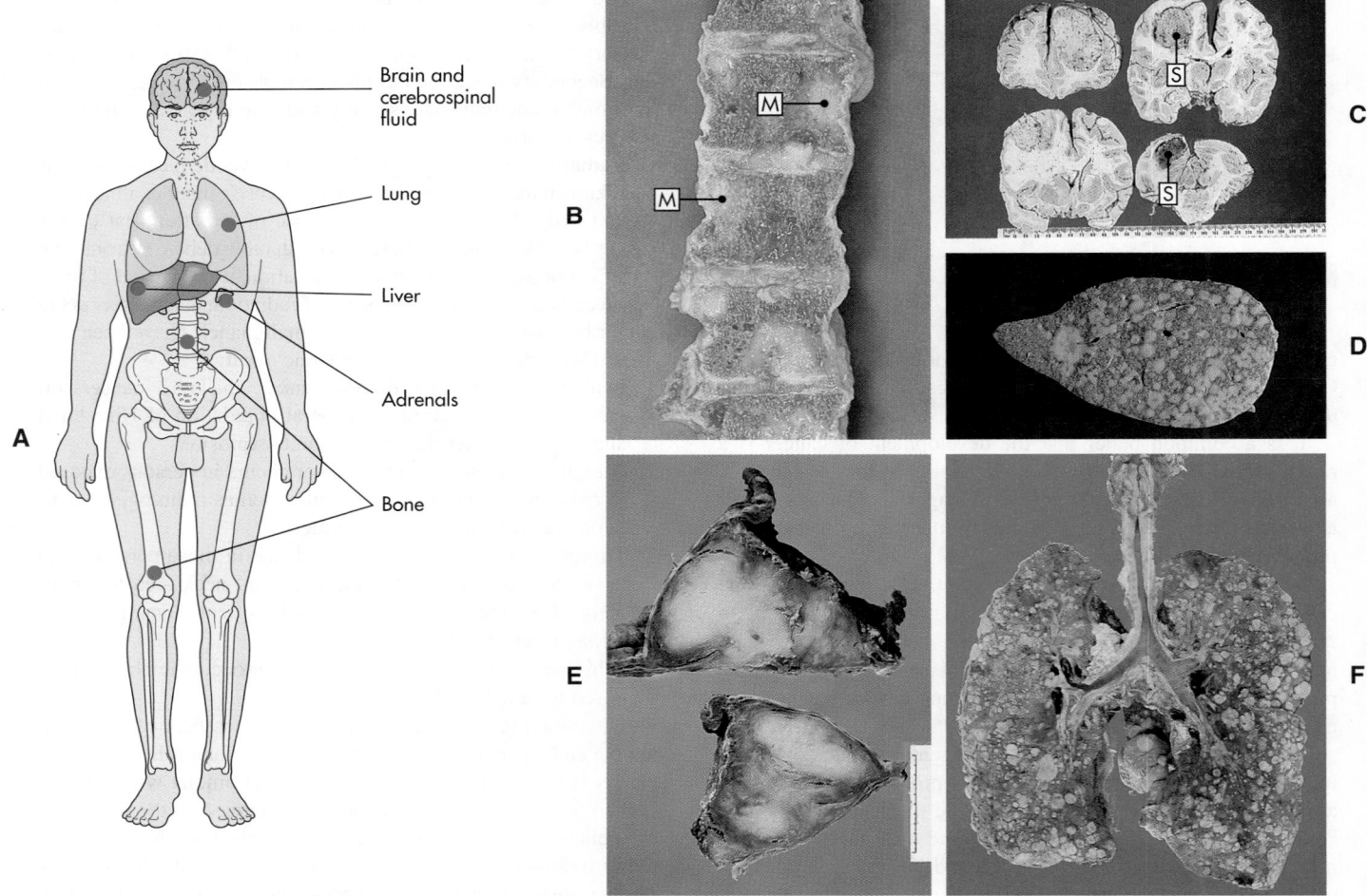

FIG. 15-4 Main sites of blood–borne metastasis. **A,** Sites of hematogenous metastasis. **B,** Metastasis in bone. **C,** Metastasis in brain. **D,** Metastasis in liver. **E,** Metastasis in adrenals. **F,** Metastasis in lungs. *M,* lesions in vertebrae; *S,* metastasis from neoplasm of the stomach. (From Stevens A, Lowe J: *Pathology: an illustrated review in color,* ed 2, London, 2000, Mosby.)

smoke is an example of a complete carcinogen capable of initiating and promoting cancer.

A period of time, ranging from 1 to 40 years, elapses between the initial genetic alteration and the actual clinical evidence of cancer. This period, called the *latent* period, is now theorized to comprise both the initiation and the promotion stages in the natural history of cancer.[2] The variation in the length of time that elapses before the cancer becomes clinically evident is associated with the mitotic rate of the tissue of origin and environmental factors. In most cancers, the process of developing cancer is years or even decades in length.

For the disease process to become clinically evident, the cells must reach a critical mass. A 1 cm tumor (the size usually detectable by palpation) contains 1 billion cancer cells. A 0.5 cm tumor is the smallest that can be detected by current diagnostic measures, such as magnetic resonance imaging (MRI).

Progression. *Progression* is the final stage in the natural history of a cancer. This stage is characterized by increased growth rate of the tumor, as well as by increased invasiveness and metastasis. **Metastasis** is the spread of the cancer from the initial or primary site to a distant site. Certain biochemical and mor-

phologic alterations take place during this stage, enabling the tumor to survive and thrive in its primary environment and throughout the process of metastasis.

Some cancers metastasize early in the process of development (e.g., premenopausal breast cancer), whereas others spread regionally and rarely metastasize (e.g., glioblastoma multiforme, basal cell carcinoma of the skin). Certain cancers seem to have an affinity for a particular tissue or organ as a site of metastasis; other cancers are unpredictable in their pattern of metastasis (e.g., melanoma). Certain cancers such as ovarian cancer ("seed") require a particular site for proliferation ("soil"). The most frequent sites of metastasis are the lungs, brain, bone, liver, and adrenals (Fig. 15-4). Most metastatic lesions are multiple and widely disseminated, but a few cancers, such as adenocarcinoma of the kidney, usually produce a single metastatic lesion.

Metastasis is a multistep process beginning with the rapid growth of the primary tumor (Fig. 15-5). As the tumor increases in size, development of its own blood supply is critical to its survival and growth. The process of the formation of blood vessels within the tumor itself is termed **tumor angiogenesis** and is facilitated by tumor angiogenesis factors produced by the cancer

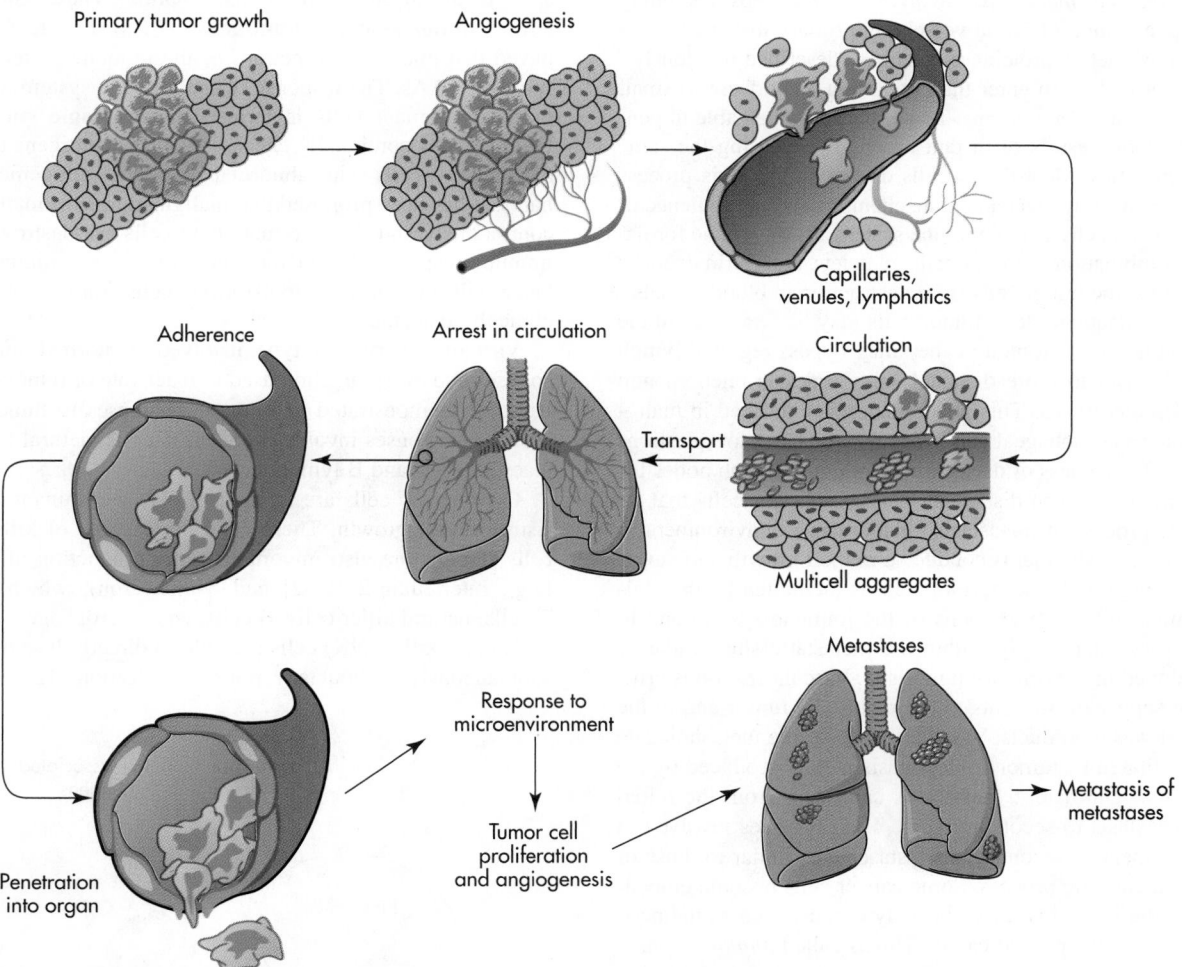

FIG. 15-5 The pathogenesis of cancer metastasis. To produce metastases, tumor cells must detach from the primary tumor and enter the circulation, survive in circulation, adhere to capillary basement membrane, gain entrance into the organ parenchyma, respond to growth factors, proliferate and induce angiogenesis, and evade host defenses.

cells. As the tumor grows, it can begin to mechanically invade surrounding tissues, growing into areas of least resistance.[6]

Certain subpopulations (segments) of tumor cells are able to detach from the primary tumor, invade the tissue surrounding the tumor, and penetrate the walls of lymph or vascular vessels for metastasis to a distant site. Unique capabilities of some tumor cells facilitate this process.[6] First, rapid proliferation of malignant cells causes mechanical pressure leading to penetration of surrounding tissues. Second, certain cells have decreased cell-to-cell adhesion in comparison with normal cells. This property equips these cancer cells with the mobility needed to move to the exterior of the primary tumor and to move within other vascular and organ structures. Some cancer cells produce metalloproteinase enzymes (a family of enzymes) that are capable of destroying the basement membrane (a tough barrier surrounding tissues and blood vessels) not only of the tumor itself, but also of lymph and blood vessels, muscles, nerves, and most epithelial boundaries. Once free from the primary tumor, metastatic tumor cells frequently travel to distant organ sites via lymphatic and hematogenous routes. These two routes of metastasis are interconnected. Thus it is theorized that tumor cells metastasize via both routes.

Hematogenous metastasis involves several steps beginning with the penetration of blood vessels by primary tumor cells via the release of metalloproteinase enzymes (described previously). These tumor cells then enter the circulation and adhere to small blood vessels of distant organs. Tumor cells are then able to penetrate the blood vessels of distant organs by releasing the same types of enzymes. Most tumor cells do not survive this process and are destroyed by mechanical mechanisms (e.g., turbulence of blood flow) and cells of the immune system. However, the formation of a combination of tumor cells, platelets, and fibrin deposits may protect some tumor cells from destruction in blood vessels.

In the lymphatic system, tumor cells may be "trapped" in the first lymph node confronted or they may bypass regional lymph nodes and travel to more distant lymph nodes, a phenomenon termed *skip metastasis*. This phenomenon is exhibited in malignancies such as esophageal cancers and is the basis for questions about the effectiveness of dissection of regional lymph nodes for the prevention of some distant metastases.[7] Tumor cells that do survive the process of metastasis must create an environment in the distant organ site that is conducive to their growth and development. This growth and development is facilitated by the ability of tumor cells to evade cells of the immune system and to produce a vascular supply within the metastatic site similar to that developed in the primary tumor site. Vascularization is critical to the supply of nutrients to the metastatic tumor and to the removal of waste products. Vascularization of the metastatic site is also facilitated by tumor angiogenesis factors produced by the cancer cells.[8] Ultimately, metastases can occur from the initial site of metastasis to secondary sites. The processes involved in the development of secondary metastases are similar to those of the initial metastatic process. Some cancer cells become embedded along the serosal surfaces of body organs, such as the peritoneal cavity or the pleural cavity. This is called *implantation.*

Cells of the primary tumor and metastatic site may develop from a single cell or a clone. However, as the primary and metastatic sites develop, the cells quickly become more heterogeneous. This change occurs as a result of spontaneous genetic mutations that take place in the tumor cells. The heterogeneous

nature of the cells in the primary and metastatic tumor makes it difficult to treat. Surgical removal of metastatic tumors is of value only if the tumor or tumors are small. Some cells of heterogeneous, primary, and metastatic tumors have the ability to become resistant to chemotherapy and radiation therapy.

Role of the Immune System

This section is limited to a discussion of the role of the immune system in the recognition and destruction of tumor cells. (For a detailed discussion of immune system function, see Chapter 13.)

The immune system has the potential to distinguish normal (self) from abnormal (nonself) cells. For example, cells of transplanted organs can be recognized by the immune system as *nonself* and thus elicit an immune response. This response can ultimately result in the rejection of the organ. Similarly, cancer cells can be perceived as nonself and elicit an immune response resulting in their rejection and destruction. However, unlike transplanted cells, cancer cells arise from normal, human cells and although they are mutated and thus different, the immune response that is mounted against cancer cells may be inadequate to reject or destroy the cancer cells.[9]

Some cancer cells have changes on their cell surface antigens as a result of malignant transformation. These antigens are termed **tumor-associated antigens** (TAAs) (Fig. 15-6). It is believed that one of the functions of the immune system is to respond to TAAs. The response of the immune system to antigens of the malignant cells is termed **immunologic surveillance.** Lymphocytes continually check cell surface antigens and detect and destroy cells with abnormal or altered antigenic determinants. It has been proposed that malignant transformation occurs continuously and that the malignant cells are destroyed by the immune response. Under most circumstances, immune surveillance will prevent these transformed cells from developing into clinically detectable tumors.[10]

Virtually every cell type involved in normal immune responses and every function used to inactivate or remove antigens has been demonstrated in immune responses to tumors. These immune responses involve cytotoxic T cells, natural killer cells, macrophages, and B lymphocytes.

Cytotoxic T cells are thought to play a dominant role in resisting tumor growth. These cells are capable of killing tumor cells. T cells are also important in the production of cytokines (e.g., interleukin-2 [IL-2] and γ-interferon), which stimulate T cells, natural killer cells, B cells, and macrophages.

Natural killer (NK) cells are able to directly lyse tumor cells spontaneously without any prior sensitization. These cells are

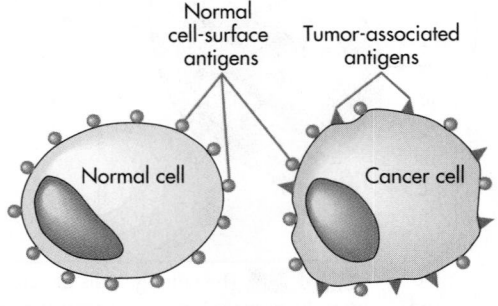

FIG. 15-6 Tumor-associated antigens appear on the cell surface of malignant cells.

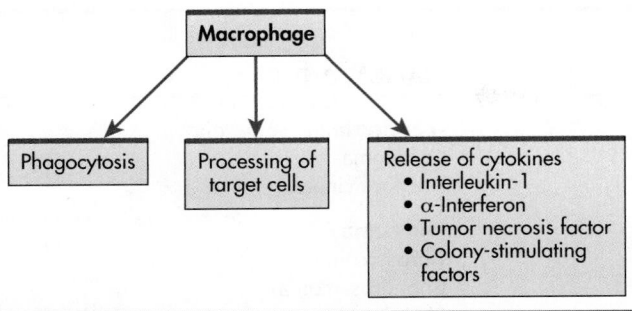

FIG. 15-7 Macrophage functioning in response to malignant target cells.

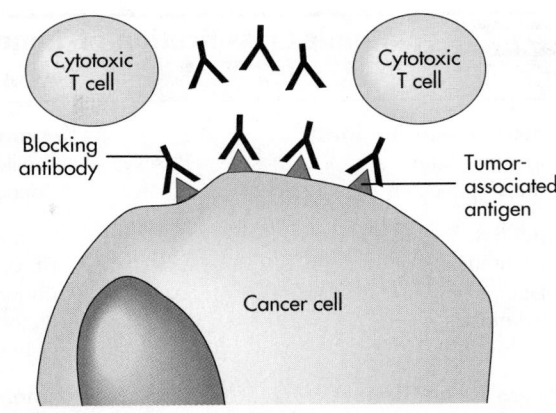

FIG. 15-8 Blocking antibodies prevent T cells from interacting with tumor-associated antigens and from destroying the malignant cell.

stimulated by γ-interferon and IL-2 (released from T cells), resulting in increased cytotoxic activity.

Monocytes and macrophages have several important roles in tumor immunity (Fig. 15-7). Macrophages can be activated by γ-interferon (produced by T cells) to become nonspecifically lytic for tumor cells. Macrophages also secrete cytokines, including IL-1, tumor necrosis factor (TNF), and colony-stimulating factors. The release of IL-1, coupled with the presentation of the processed antigen, stimulates T lymphocyte activation and production. α-Interferon augments the killing ability of NK cells. TNF causes hemorrhagic necrosis of tumors and exerts cytocidal or cytostatic actions against tumor cells. Colony-stimulating factors regulate the production of various blood cells in the bone marrow and stimulate the function of various WBCs.

B lymphocytes can produce specific antibodies that bind to tumor cells and can kill these cells by complement fixation and lysis (see Chapter 12). These antibodies are often detectable in the serum and saliva of the patient. In some persons, antibodies that are specific for both the person's own tumor and a similar tumor in other persons have been found.[10]

Escape Mechanisms from Immunologic Surveillance. The process by which cancer cells evade the immune system is termed *immunologic escape*.[9] Theorized mechanisms by which cancer cells can escape immunologic surveillance include (1) suppression of factors that stimulate T cells to react to cancer cells, (2) weak surface antigens allowing cancer cells to "sneak through" immunologic surveillance, (3) the development of tolerance of the immune system to some tumor antigens, (4) suppression of the immune response by products secreted by cancer cells, (5) the induction of suppressor T cells by the tumor, and (6) blocking antibodies that bind TAAs, thus preventing their recognition by T cells (Fig. 15-8).

Oncofetal Antigens. *Oncofetal antigens* are a type of tumor antigen. They are found on both the surfaces and the inside of cancer cells, as well as fetal cells. These antigens are an expression of the shift of cancerous cells to a more immature metabolic pathway, an expression usually associated with embryonic or fetal periods of life. The reappearance of fetal antigens in malignant disease is not well understood, but it is believed to occur as a result of the cell regaining its embryonic capability to differentiate into many different cell types.

Examples of oncofetal antigens are carcinoembryonic antigen (CEA) and α-fetoprotein (AFP). CEA is found on the surfaces of cancer cells derived from the GI tract and from normal cells from the fetal gut, liver, and pancreas. Normally, it disap-

pears during the last 3 months of fetal life. CEA was originally isolated from colon cancer cells. However, elevated CEA levels have also been found in nonmalignant conditions (e.g., cirrhosis of the liver, ulcerative colitis, and heavy smoking). Presently, the major value of CEA is its use as an indicator of the success of cancer treatment. For example, the persistence of elevated preoperative CEA titers after surgery indicates that the tumor is not completely removed. A rise in CEA levels after chemotherapy or radiation therapy may indicate recurrence or spread of the cancer.

AFP is produced by malignant liver cells, as well as fetal liver cells. AFP levels have also been found to be elevated in some cases of testicular carcinoma, viral hepatitis, and nonmalignant liver disorders. AFP has diagnostic value in primary cancer of the liver (hepatoma), but it is also produced when metastatic liver growth occurs. The detection of AFP is of value in tumor detection and determination of tumor progression.

Other examples of oncofetal antigens currently being studied are CA-125, found in ovarian carcinoma; CA-19-9, found in pancreatic, colon, and breast cancer; and prostate-specific antigen (PSA), found in prostate cancer.

CLASSIFICATION OF CANCER

Tumors can be classified according to anatomic site, histologic analysis (grading), and extent of disease (staging). Tumor classification systems are intended to provide a standardized way to (1) communicate the status of the cancer to all members of the health care team, (2) assist in determining the most effective treatment plan, (3) evaluate the treatment plan, (4) serve as a factor in determining the prognosis, and (5) compare like groups for statistical purposes.

Anatomic Site Classification

In the *anatomic classification* of tumors, the tumor is identified by the tissue of origin, the anatomic site, and the behavior of the tumor (i.e., benign or malignant) (Table 15-4). **Carcinomas** originate from embryonal *ectoderm* (skin and glands) and *endoderm* (mucous membrane linings of the respiratory tract, GI tract, and genitourinary [GU] tract). **Sarcomas** originate from embryonal *mesoderm* (connective tissue, muscle, bone, and fat). Lymphomas and leukemias originate from the hematopoietic system.

TABLE 15-4	Anatomic Classification of Tumors	
SITE	**BENIGN**	**MALIGNANT**
Epithelial Tissue Tumors*	**–oma**	**–carcinoma**
Surface epithelium	Papilloma	Carcinoma
Glandular epithelium	Adenoma	Adenocarcinoma
Connective Tissue Tumors†	**–oma**	**–sarcoma**
Fibrous tissue	Fibroma	Fibrosarcoma
Cartilage	Chondroma	Chondrosarcoma
Striated muscle	Rhabdomyoma	Rhabdomyosarcoma
Bone	Osteoma	Osteosarcoma
Nervous Tissue Tumors	**–oma**	**–oma**
Meninges	Meningioma	Meningeal sarcoma
Nerve cells	Ganglioneuroma	Neuroblastoma
Hematopoietic Tissue Tumors		
Lymphoid tissue		Hodgkin's disease, non-Hodgkin's lymphoma
Plasma cells		Multiple myeloma
Bone marrow		Lymphocytic and myelogenous leukemia

*Body surfaces, lining of body cavities, and glandular structures.
†Supporting tissue, fibrotic tissue, and blood vessels.

Histologic Analysis Classification

In **histologic grading** of tumors, the appearance of cells and the degree of differentiation are evaluated. For many tumor cells, four grades are used:

Grade I. Cells differ slightly from normal cells (mild dysplasia) and are well differentiated.

Grade II. Cells are more abnormal (moderate dysplasia) and moderately differentiated.

Grade III. Cells are very abnormal (severe dysplasia) and poorly differentiated.

Grade IV. Cells are immature and primitive (anaplasia) and undifferentiated; cell of origin is difficult to determine.

Extent of Disease Classification

Classifying the extent and spread of disease is termed **staging.** This classification system is based on a description of the extent of the disease rather than on cell appearance. Although there are similarities in the staging of cancers, there are many differences based on a thorough knowledge of the natural history of each specific type of cancer.

Clinical Staging. The clinical staging classification system determines the extent of the disease process of cancer by stages:

Stage 0: cancer in situ

Stage I: tumor limited to the tissue of origin; localized tumor growth

Stage II: limited local spread

Stage III: extensive local and regional spread

Stage IV: metastasis

This classification system has been used as a basis for staging in cancer of the cervix (see Chapter 52, Table 52-14) and Hodgkin's disease (see Chapter 30, Fig. 30-12).

TNM Classification System. The *TNM classification system* represents the standardization of the clinical staging of cancer by the International Union Against Cancer (UICC). This classification system (Table 15-5) is used to determine the extent of

TABLE 15-5	TNM Classification System
Primary Tumor (T)	
T_0	No evidence of primary tumor
T_{is}	Carcinoma in situ
T_{1-4}	Ascending degrees of increase in tumor size and involvement
Regional Lymph Nodes (N)	
N_0	No evidence of disease in lymph nodes
N_{1-4}	Ascending degrees of nodal involvement
N_x	Regional lymph nodes unable to be assessed clinically
Distant Metastases (M)	
M_0	No evidence of distant metastases
M_{1-4}	Ascending degrees of metastatic involvement of the host, including distant nodes

the disease process of cancer according to three parameters: tumor size (T), degree of regional spread to the lymph nodes (N), and metastasis (M). (An example of the TNM classification system can be found in Table 50-6.)

Staging of the disease can be done initially and at several intervals. Clinical diagnostic staging is done at the time of diagnosis to determine the most effective treatment plan. Examples of diagnostic studies that may be performed to assess for spread of disease include bone and liver scans, ultrasonography, computed tomography (CT), and MRI.

Surgical staging is used to describe the extent of the disease process after biopsy or surgical exploration. For example, a laparotomy and a splenectomy may be performed in staging of Hodgkin's disease. During a staging laparotomy, lymph node biopsies may be done and margins of any masses may be marked

TABLE 15-6	Karnofsky Performance Scale
100	Normal; no complaints; no evidence of disease
90	Ability to carry on normal activity; minor signs or symptoms of disease
80	Normal activity with effort; some signs or symptoms of disease
70	Ability to care for self; inability to carry on normal activity or do active work
60	Occasional assistance necessary but ability to care for most needs
50	Considerable assistance and frequent medical care necessary
40	Disabled; special care and assistance necessary
30	Severely disabled; indication for hospitalization although death not imminent
20	Very sick; hospitalization necessary; active supportive treatment necessary
10	Moribund; fatal processes progressing rapidly
0	Dead

with metal clips. These clips are used as markers when radiotherapy is used as a treatment modality.

After the extent of the disease is determined, the stage classification is not changed. The original description of the extent of the tumor remains part of the original record. If additional treatment is needed, or if treatment fails, re-treatment staging is done to determine the extent of the disease process at the time of re-treatment.

Carcinoma in situ is a commonly used term in classification of cancer. It is defined as a lesion with all the histologic features of cancer except invasion. If left untreated, carcinoma in situ will eventually become invasive.

In addition to tumor classification systems, there are also classification systems used to describe the status of the patient with cancer. The status of the patient is recorded at the time of diagnosis, treatment, and re-treatment and at each follow-up examination. The Karnofsky functional performance scale is an example of a method used to evaluate the performance status of the patient (Table 15-6).

PREVENTION AND DETECTION OF CANCER

The nurse plays a prominent role in the prevention and detection of cancer. Early detection and prompt treatment are directly responsible for increased survival rates in patients with cancer. One important aspect is to educate the public to do the following:

1. Reduce or avoid exposure to known or suspected carcinogens and cancer-promoting agents, including cigarette smoke and sun exposure.
2. Eat a balanced diet that includes vegetables (green, yellow, and orange), fresh fruits, whole grains, and adequate amounts of fiber, and reduce the amount of fat and preservatives, including smoked and salt-cured meats.
3. Participate in a regular exercise regimen.
4. Obtain adequate, consistent periods of rest (at least 6 to 8 hours per night).
5. Have a health examination on a regular basis that includes a health history, a physical examination, and specific diagnostic tests for common cancers in accordance with the guide-

lines published by the American Cancer Society (*www.cancer.org*) (Table 15-7).
6. Eliminate, reduce, or change the perceptions of stressors and enhance the ability to effectively cope with stressors (see Chapter 8).
7. Enjoy consistent periods of relaxation and leisure.
8. Know the seven warning signs of cancer (Table 15-8). (These actually detect fairly advanced disease.)
9. Learn and practice self-examination (e.g., breast self-examination, testicular self-examination).
10. Seek immediate medical care if you notice a change in what is normal for you and if cancer is suspected. Early detection of cancer has a positive impact on prognosis.

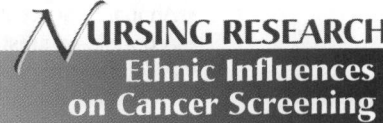

NURSING RESEARCH
Ethnic Influences on Cancer Screening

Citation
Foxall MJ, Barron CR, Houfek JF: Ethnic influences on body awareness, trait anxiety, perceived risk, and breast and gynecologic cancer screening practices, *Oncol Nurs Forum* 28:727, 2001.

Purpose
To examine ethnic influences on body awareness, trait anxiety, perceived risk, and breast and gynecologic cancer screening practices.

Methods
Two hundred twenty-three healthy women (59% white, 17% African American, 12% Hispanic, 12% American Indian) ages 18 and older responded to questionnaires that obtained information about their breast and gynecologic cancer screening practices, body awareness, anxiety, and perceived risk of breast and gynecologic cancer.

Results and Conclusions
Ethnicity predicted breast and gynecologic cancer screening practices, body awareness, trait anxiety, and perceived risk. Hispanic and American Indian women reported greater breast self-examination frequency than white and African American women. White and African American women reported more mammogram use than Hispanic and American Indian women. Increased body awareness was related to fewer gynecologic examinations for American Indian women. Women of different ethnic backgrounds respond differently to breast and gynecologic cancer screening practices. The influence of psychosocial variables on these practices varied with different groups.

Implications for Nursing Practice
The key to successful treatment of breast and gynecologic cancers is early detection. Chances of early detection of cancer are increased by participation in recommended screening procedures such as mammography and gynecologic examinations. Nursing interventions that are aimed at improving women's participation in cancer screening examinations must be ethnic specific so that they meet the needs of women of different ethnicities. These interventions must be also implemented in a way that is sensitive to the potential for anxiety about a cancer diagnosis because anxiety may prevent some women from participating in cancer screening practices.

TABLE 15-7 **Summary of American Cancer Society Recommendations for Early Detection of Cancer in Asymptomatic People**

SITE	RECOMMENDATION
Breast	Yearly mammograms starting at age 40 and continuing for as long as a woman is in good health. Clinical breast exams (CBE) should be part of periodic health exam, about every three years for women in their 20s and 30s and every year for women 40 and over. Women should report any breast change promptly to their health care providers. Women at increased risk (e.g., family history, genetic tendency, past breast cancer) should talk with their doctors about the benefits and limitations of starting mammography screening earlier, having additional tests (e.g., breast ultrasound, MRI), or having more frequent exams.
Colon and rectum	Beginning at age 50, men and women should follow one of the examination schedules below: • A fecal occult blood (FOBT) test every year, or • A flexible sigmoidoscopy (FSIG) every 5 years, or • Annual fecal occult blood test and flexible sigmoidoscopy every 5 years.* • A double-contrast barium enema every 5 to 10 years. • A colonoscopy every 10 years.
Prostate	The prostate-specific antigen (PSA) test and the digital rectal examination should be offered annually, beginning at age 50, to men who have a life expectancy of at least 10 years. Men at high risk (African American men and men with a strong family history of one or more first-degree relatives diagnosed with prostate cancer at an early age) should begin testing at age 45. Information should be provided to patients about what is known and what is uncertain about the benefits and limitations of early detection and treatment of prostate cancer, so that they can make an informed decision.
Uterus	*Cervix:* All women who are or have been sexually active or who are 18 and older should have an annual Pap test and pelvic examination. After three or more consecutive satisfactory examinations with normal findings, the Pap test may be performed less frequently. *Endometrium:* The American Cancer Society recommends that all women should be informed about the risks and symptoms of endometrial cancer, and strongly encouraged to report any unexpected bleeding or spotting to their health care providers. Annual screening for endometrial cancer with endometrial biopsy beginning at age 35 should be offered to women with or at risk for hereditary nonpolyposis colon cancer (HNPCC).
Cancer-related checkup	A cancer-related checkup is recommended every 3 years for people age 20 to 39 years and every year for people age 40 and older. This examination should include health counseling and, depending on a person's age, might include examinations for cancers of the thyroid, oral cavity, skin, lymph nodes, testes, and ovaries, as well as for some non-malignant diseases.

*Combined testing is preferred over either annual FOBT or FSIG every 5 years, alone. People who are at moderate or high risk for colorectal cancer should talk with a health care provider about a different testing schedule.
Source: *Cancer facts and figures,* Atlanta, 2002, American Cancer Society.

When the public is educated regarding the disease process of cancer, care should be taken to minimize the fear that surrounds the diagnosis of cancer. Tactics that increase fear should never be used. The facts should be taught in an accurate, low-key manner at the level of the learner. The goal of public education is to motivate the learner to change the pattern of behavior as necessary to achieve and maintain an optimal state of health. The nurse can play a significant role in meeting this goal. Although the general public must be taught, those who are at an increased risk of cancer are the target population for effective cancer control (see Table 15-7). The nurse can have a definite impact in convincing people that a change in lifestyle patterns will have a positive influence on health. If the nurse is to have a significant impact, the challenge must be recognized and strategies must be developed to teach cancer control effectively.

Diagnosis of Cancer

When a patient has a possible diagnosis of cancer, it is a stressful time for the patient and the family. The patient typically undergoes several days to weeks of diagnostic studies. During this time the fear of the unknown may be more stressful than ultimately being told of a positive diagnosis of cancer.

During the time the patient is waiting for the results of the diagnostic studies, the nurse should be available to actively listen to the patient's concerns. False reassurance that everything will be all right is inappropriate and may shut off further communication with the patient. During this time of high anxiety the patient may need repeated explanations regarding the diagnostic workup. Explanations should include as much information as needed by the patient and the family; the information should be given in clear, understandable terms and should be reinforced as

TABLE 15-8 **Seven Warning Signs of Cancer**

C	hange in bowel or bladder habits
A	sore that does not heal
U	nusual bleeding or discharge from any body orifice
T	hickening or a lump in the breast or elsewhere
I	ndigestion or difficulty in swallowing
O	bvious change in a wart or mole
N	agging cough or hoarseness

necessary. Written information is helpful for reinforcement of verbal information.

A diagnostic plan for the person in whom cancer is suspected includes health history, identification of risk factors, physical examination, and specific diagnostic studies. (The specifics of the health history and the screening physical examination are presented in Chapter 3.)

The health history includes particular emphasis on risk factors, such as family history of cancer, exposure to or use of known carcinogens (e.g., cigarette smoking, exposure to occupational pollutants or chemicals), diseases characterized by chronic inflammation (e.g., ulcerative colitis), and drug ingestion (e.g., hormone therapy). Other important information relates to dietary habits, ingestion of alcohol, lifestyle, and patterns and degree of coping with perceived stressors.

The physical examination should be thorough, and particular attention should be given to the respiratory system, the GI system (including colon, rectum, and liver), the lymphatic system (including the spleen), the breasts, the skin, the reproductive system (testes and prostate gland in men; cervix, uterus, and ovary in women), and the musculoskeletal and neurologic systems.

Diagnostic studies to be performed will depend on the suspected primary or metastatic site(s) of the cancer. (Specific procedures as they relate to each body system are discussed in the respective assessment chapters.) Examples of studies that may be included in the process of diagnosing cancer include the following:

1. Cytology studies (e.g., Papanicolaou [Pap] test)
2. Chest x-ray
3. Complete blood count
4. Sigmoidoscopy or colonoscopy examination (including guaiac for occult blood)
5. Liver function studies
6. Radiologic studies (e.g., mammography)
7. Radioisotope scans (e.g., bone, lung, liver, brain)
8. CT
9. MRI
10. Presence of oncofetal antigens such as CEA and AFP or genetic markers such as BRCA-1 and BRCA-2
11. Bone marrow examination (if a hematolymphoid malignancy is suspected)
12. Biopsy

Biopsy. The *biopsy* procedure is the definitive means of diagnosing cancer. It involves the histologic examination by a pathologist of a piece of tissue from the suspicious area. A biopsy is essential in planning a treatment regimen for the patient. A biopsy will determine whether the tissue is benign or malignant, the anatomic tissue from which the tumor arises, and the degree of cellular differentiation of the cancer cells present in the tumor.

The procedure may be a needle biopsy, an incisional biopsy, or an excisional biopsy. A *needle biopsy* specimen can be obtained by aspiration (e.g., bone marrow aspiration) or by the use of a large-bore needle. These needles are used in obtaining samples of prostate gland, breast, liver, and kidney tissues.

Incisional biopsy performed with a scalpel or dermal punch is a common technique used for obtaining a tissue sample for making a diagnosis of cancer. The premise that incisional biopsy may contribute to the spread of cancer has not been proven.

Excisional biopsy involves removal of the entire tumor. It is usually used for small tumors (smaller than 2 cm), skin le-

sions, intestinal polyps, and breast masses. This procedure can be considered therapeutic, as well as diagnostic. Often when a tumor is not easily accessible, a major surgical procedure (laparotomy, thoracotomy, craniotomy) is necessary to obtain a piece of the tumor tissue. Biopsy specimens of the GI, respiratory, and GU systems can usually be obtained by endoscopic procedures.

COLLABORATIVE CARE

Goals and Modalities

The goal of cancer treatment is cure, control, or palliation (Fig. 15-9). Factors that determine the treatment modality are the cell type of the cancer, the location and size of the tumor, and the extent of the disease. The physiologic and psychologic status and the expressed needs of the patient also have an important part in determining the treatment plan. These factors influence the modalities chosen for treatment and the length of time the treatment is administered.

When caring for the patient with cancer, the nurse should know the goals of the treatment plan to appropriately communicate with and support the patient. When *cure* is the goal, it is expected that after treatment the patient will be free of disease and will have a normal life span. Many kinds of cancer have the potential to go into permanent remission with an initial course of treatment or with treatment that extends for several weeks, months, or years. Basal cell carcinoma of the skin is usually cured by surgical removal of the lesion or by several weeks of radiation therapy. Acute lymphocytic leukemia (ALL) in children has the potential for cure. The treatment plan for ALL includes the administration of several chemotherapy drugs on a scheduled basis over a time span of 6 months to several years. Curative cancer therapy may involve surgery alone or extended periods of systemic therapy.

Until a few years ago, a 5-year disease-free period was thought to be indicative of a cancer cure. This is not true for all cancers. The patient with a tumor that has a rapid mitotic rate (e.g., testicular cancer) is considered in remission if cancer is not detected in a 2-year time span. The patient with a tumor that has slower mitotic rate (e.g., postmenopausal breast cancer) needs 20 or more disease-free years before she can be considered cured of cancer.

Control is the goal of the treatment plan for many cancers considered to be chronic. The patient undergoes the initial course of therapy and is continued on maintenance therapy for a period of time or is followed closely so that early signs and symptoms of recurrence can be detected. These cancers are usually not cured, but they are controlled by therapy for long periods of time. They are controlled in a manner similar to other chronic illnesses, such as diabetes mellitus, chronic lung disease, and congestive heart failure. An example of this type of cancer is chronic lymphocytic leukemia (see Chapter 30).

Palliation can also be a goal of the treatment plan. With this treatment goal, relief or control of symptoms and the maintenance of a satisfactory quality of life are the primary goals rather than cure or control of the disease process. Radiation therapy given to relieve the pain of bone metastasis is an example of treatment with a goal of palliation.

The goals of cure, control, and palliation are achieved through the use of four treatment modalities for cancer: surgery, radiation

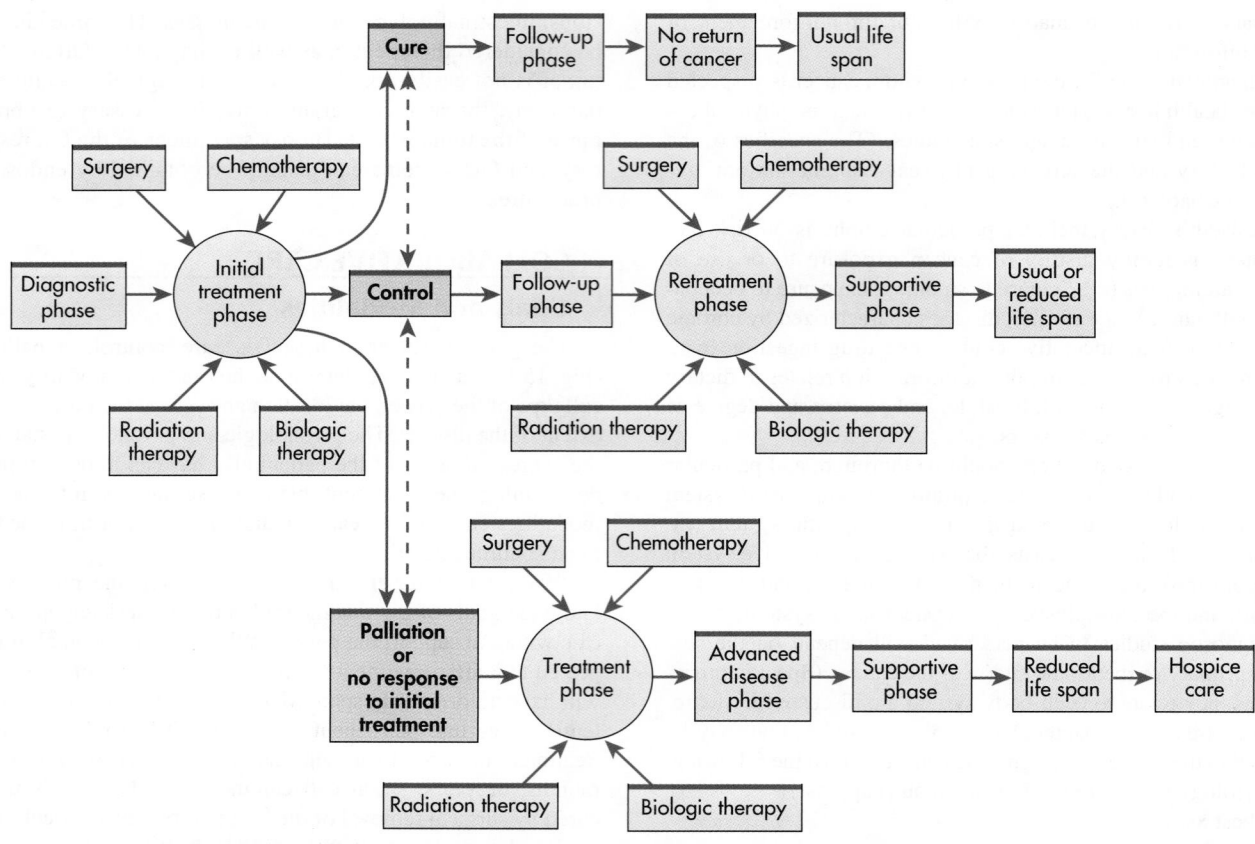

FIG. 15-9 Goals of cancer treatment.

therapy, chemotherapy, and biologic therapy. Surgery, radiation therapy, chemotherapy, and biologic therapy can be used alone or in any combination in the initial treatment phase, as well as in the re-treatment phase(s) of cancer. For many cancers, two or more of the treatment modalities are used to achieve the goal of cure or control for a long period of time.

Clinical Trials

A *clinical trial* is a research study conducted with patients and is usually designed with the intent of evaluating new treatments. The evaluation of treatments in cancer research begins in the laboratory and with animal studies. From these studies, those treatments determined to be most effective, with reasonable levels of toxicity, are further evaluated in a series of studies on patients with cancer. Progress in cancer care depends on clinical trials. New drugs or treatments, evaluated for the first time in human beings, usually go through three phases:

In *Phase I trials,* researchers test a new drug or treatment in a small group of people (20-80) for the first time to evaluate its safety, determine a safe dosage range, and identify side effects.

In *Phase II trials,* the study drug or treatment is given to a larger group of people (100-300) to see if it is effective and to further evaluate its safety.

In *Phase III trials,* the study drug or treatment is given to large groups of people (1,000-3,000) to confirm its effectiveness, monitor side effects, compare it to commonly used treatments, and collect information that will allow the drug or treatment to be used safely.

The rights of the patient who participates in clinical trials are closely guarded by institutional review boards (IRBs) in each agency conducting research. IRBs not only review clinical trials at their inception but also continue to review and monitor the study until its completion. Informed consent is a process in which information is fully disclosed to the patient by a physician and a nurse regarding the nature of the treatment being evaluated and the potential risks and benefits of entering the clinical trial. The patient must understand that she or he may elect to leave a clinical trial at any time.

The guidelines for the administration of a research protocol are included in the study's protocol. All the health care providers follow the protocol in order to ensure uniform treatment of patients in a clinical study.

SURGICAL THERAPY

Surgery is the oldest form of cancer treatment, and for many years it was the only effective method of cancer diagnosis and treatment. The treatment of choice for many years was to remove the cancer and as much of the surrounding normal tissue as possible.

Cure and Control

Several principles are applicable when surgery is used to cure or control the disease process of cancer (Fig. 15-10):

1. Cancer that arises from a tissue with a slow rate of cellular proliferation or replication is the most amenable to surgical treatment.

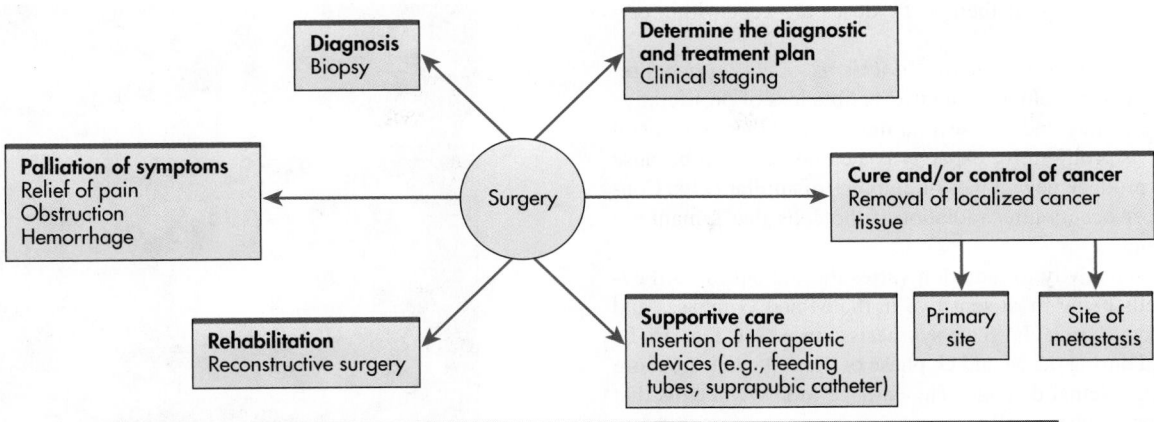

FIG. 15-10 Role of surgery in the treatment of cancer.

2. A margin of normal tissue must surround the tumor at the time of resection.
3. Only as much tissue as necessary is removed, and adjuvant therapy is used. The current trend among health care providers is toward less radical surgery. Adjuvant, or "additional," therapy is used after postoperative pathologic evaluation identifies the specific risk for metastatic disease. The risk for metastatic disease is tumor dependent. Each tumor has a designated staging system that allows treatment decisions to be made based on extent of disease. The decision regarding adjuvant therapy is customized to the patient's tumor type, stage, comorbidities, and preferences.
4. Preventive measures are used to reduce the surgical seeding of cancer cells.
5. The usual sites of regional spread may be surgically removed.
   Examples of surgical procedures used for cure or control of cancer include radical neck dissection, lumpectomy, mastectomy, pneumonectomy, orchiectomy, thyroidectomy, and bowel resection.

A *debulking* procedure may be used if the tumor cannot be completely removed (e.g., attached to a vital organ). When this occurs, as much tumor as possible is removed, and the patient may be given chemotherapy or radiation therapy. This type of surgical procedure makes chemotherapy or radiation therapy more effective.

Supportive Care

Surgical procedures can also be used to provide supportive care throughout the disease process of cancer. Examples of supportive surgical procedures include the following:
1. Insertion of feeding tubes in the stomach
2. Creation of a colostomy to allow healing of rectal abscess
3. Suprapubic cystostomy for the patient with advanced prostatic cancer

Palliation of Symptoms

When cure or control of cancer is no longer possible, the quality of life must be maintained at the highest possible level for the longest possible period of time. Examples of surgical procedures performed for palliative care include the following:
1. Debulking of tumor to relieve pain or pressure
2. Colostomy for the relief of a bowel obstruction (see Chapter 41)
3. Laminectomy for the relief of a spinal cord compression (see Chapter 59)

Rehabilitative Management

Cancer surgery can produce a change in body image. It is often difficult for the patient to cope with body image changes as well as a diagnosis of cancer while attempting to maintain usual lifestyle patterns. As the treatment for certain cancers becomes more effective, the length of time the patient must live with an alteration created by surgery will be increased. If quality of life is to be maintained, the body image must be one that the patient is able to accept and cope with on a daily basis. A greater emphasis has been placed on the rehabilitative role of surgery in cancer care to increase the quality of life. Breast reconstruction after a mastectomy is an example of a rehabilitative surgical procedure. The new appliances and the care of ostomies are other major focuses of rehabilitative management.

RADIATION THERAPY

Radiation therapy is a local treatment modality for cancer. It is one of the oldest methods of cancer treatment. Historically, workers exposed to radiation had a higher incidence of skin desquamation and developed carcinomas of the fingers. Marie and Pierre Curie both developed leukemia related to radiation exposure.[11]

The experience of radiation exposure causing tissue damage led scientists to explore the use of radiation to treat tumors. The hypothesized association was that if radiation resulted in the destruction of the highly mitotic skin cells of workers it could be used in a controlled way to prevent the continued growth of highly mitotic cancer cells. It was not until the 1960s that highly sophisticated equipment and treatment planning facilitated the delivery of adequate radiation doses to tumors and tolerable doses to normal tissues. It is estimated in current practice that up to 60% of all persons with cancer will receive radiation therapy at some point in the treatment of their disease.[12]

Effects of Radiation

Radiation is the emission and distribution of energy through space or a material medium. The energy produced by radiation, when absorbed into tissue, produces ionization and excitation. This local energy is sufficient to break chemical bonds in DNA, which leads to a biologic effect. Loss of proliferative capacity results in cellular death at the time of division. Therefore cancer cells are more likely to be permanently damaged by cumulative doses of radiation. Normal tissues are usually able to recover from radiation damage if therapeutic doses are kept within certain ranges.

Cellular Death and Tissue Reactions. *Cellular death* related to radiation is defined as an irreversible loss of proliferative capacity. Cells may undergo several mitoses and then die. A cell that retains its proliferative capacity is a clonogenic cell because it is able to produce new clones or colonies of similar cells. Control of cancer occurs after radiation if the cells that remain are nonclonogenic.

Cellular sensitivity to radiation varies throughout the cell cycle, with cells being most sensitive in the M and G_2 phases and least sensitive during the S or synthesis phase (see Fig. 15-1). Cells treated during the M and G_2 phase of the cell cycle are more likely to suffer lethal damage. The damage to DNA in cells that are not in the M phase will be expressed when division occurs.

The amount of time that is required for the manifestations of radiation damage is determined by the mitotic rate of the tissue. Sufficient cells within the tissue must be killed to establish a noticeable effect. This is true in both normal and cancer cells. Rapidly dividing cells in the gastrointestinal tract, oral mucosa, and bone marrow will die fast and exhibit early acute responses to radiation. Tissues with slowly proliferating cells such as cartilage, bone, and kidneys manifest late responses to radiation.

This differential rate of cellular death explains the timing of clinical manifestations related to radiation therapy. Normal cells within the radiation field will also be affected by treatment. For each normal cell type there is a maximally tolerated radiation dose. Administration of radiation above the maximally tolerated doses results in limited ability of normal cells to recover from damage and potentially irreversible side effects. Treatment planning and computerized dosimetry ensure that normal tissue tolerance is not exceeded.[13,14]

Table 15-9 describes the relative radiosensitivity of a variety of tumors. In responsive tumors, even a large tumor burden will be affected by therapy. In less responsive tumors, a large tumor burden may result in a slower and perhaps incomplete response.

Simulation and Treatment

Simulation is a part of radiation treatment planning used to determine the optimal treatment method. The patient lies on a table in the treatment position. Under fluoroscopy the critical normal structures that will be included in the treatment field or portal are identified. A film is taken to verify the field, and marks are placed on the skin so that the field can be reproduced on a daily basis. Fig. 15-11 illustrates the radiation simulator. Com-

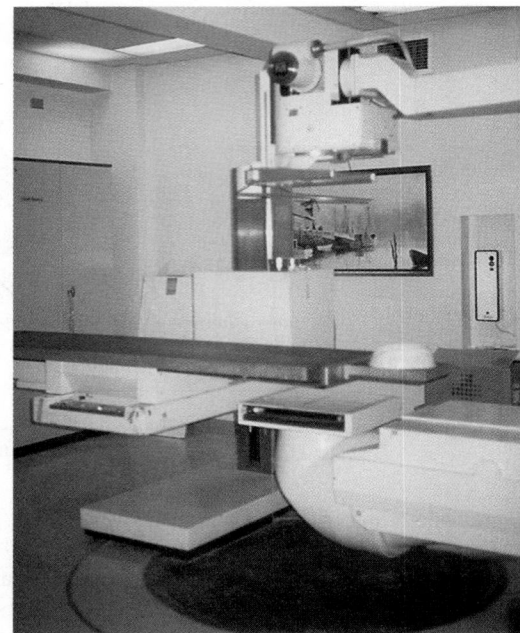

FIG. 15-11 Radiation simulator.

puterized dosimetry using CT scanning is used to produce a treatment plan that delivers the maximum amount of radiation to the tumor within the acceptable dose to normal tissue.[15]

External Radiation. Radiation treatment can be given by *external beam radiation therapy* (teletherapy), which is the most common form of treatment delivery. In this treatment the patient is exposed to radiation from the treatment machine (Fig. 15-12). The patient is never radioactive during this treatment.

Internal Radiation. Another radiation delivery system is **brachytherapy.** This means "close" treatment and consists of the implantation or insertion of radioactive materials directly into the tumor or in close proximity to the tumor. An implant may be temporary, with the source placed into a catheter or tube inserted into the tumor area and left in place for several days. This method is commonly used for tumors of the head and neck and gynecologic malignancies. Implants, such as prostate implants, may also be permanent, with insertion of radioactive seeds into tumors. Brachytherapy is used in the clinical situation where the tumor dose must be high to eradicate the tumor. However, this dose is too high for the tolerance of nearby normal tissues. The sources used in brachytherapy are not as energetic or penetrating as those

TABLE 15-9	Tumor Radiosensitivity		
HIGH RADIOSENSITIVITY	**MODERATE RADIOSENSITIVITY**	**MILD RADIOSENSITIVITY**	**POOR RADIOSENSITIVITY**
Ovarian dysgerminoma	Skin carcinoma	Soft tissue sarcomas (e.g., chondrosarcoma)	Osteosarcoma
Testicular seminoma	Oropharyngeal carcinoma	Gastric adenocarcinoma	Malignant melanoma
Hodgkin's disease	Esophageal carcinoma	Renal adenocarcinoma	Malignant gliomas
Non-Hodgkin's lymphoma	Breast adenocarcinoma	Colon adenocarcinoma	Testicular nonseminoma
Wilms' tumor	Uterine and cervical carcinoma		
Neuroblastoma	Prostate carcinoma		
	Bladder carcinoma		

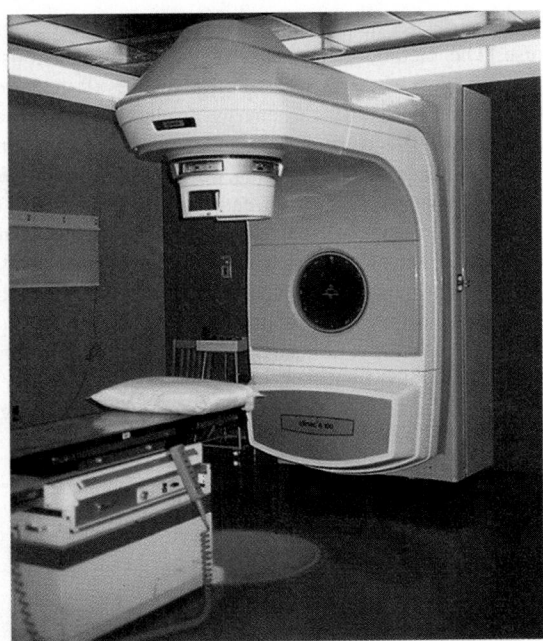

FIG. 15-12 Radiation treatment machine.

TABLE 15-10	Measurement of Radiation
UNIT	**DEFINITION**
Curie (Ci)	A measure of the number of atoms of a particular radioisotope that disintegrate in 1 sec
Roentgen (R)	A measure of the radiation required to produce a standard number of ions in air; a unit of exposure to radiation
Rad	Measurement of radiation dosage absorbed by the tissues
Rem	Measurement of the biologic effectiveness of various forms of radiation on the human cell (1 rem = 1 rad)
Gray (Gy)	100 rads = 1 Gy

used in the external beam machines and thus deliver most of the dose locally. Often external beam radiation and brachytherapy will be used in combination.

Caring for the person with a radiation implant requires that the nurse be aware that the patient is radioactive. If a patient has a temporary implant, the patient is radioactive during the time the source is in place. If the patient has a permanent implant, the radioactive exposure to the outside and others is low, and the patient may be discharged with precautions. The principles of time, distance, and shielding are used when caring for the person with an implant. Nursing care should be organized so that a limited amount of time is spent with the patient. The patient should be prepared for the implant before the procedure and be aware of time limitations. The radiation safety officer will indicate how much time at a specific distance can be spent with the patient. This is determined by the dose delivered by the implant. Because the source is nonpenetrating, small differences in distance are critical. Only care that must be delivered near the source, such as checking placement of the implant, is performed in close proximity. Shielding, if available, should be used, and no care should be delivered without wearing a film badge. This badge will indicate any radiation exposure. The film badge should not be shared, should not be worn other than at work, and should be returned according to the agency's protocol.

Measurement of Radiation

Several different units are used to measure radiation (Table 15-10). Grays and centigrays are the units currently used in clinical practice.

Goals of Radiation Therapy

The goals of radiation therapy are cure, control, or palliation. To accomplish these treatment goals, radiation therapy can be used alone or as an adjuvant treatment modality in combination with surgery, chemotherapy, and biologic therapy.

Cure is the goal when radiation therapy is used alone as a curative modality for treating patients with basal cell carcinoma of the skin, tumors confined to the vocal cords, and stage I or IIA Hodgkin's disease. Radiation therapy can be combined with surgery and chemotherapy to cure certain cancers, such as (1) stage IIB, IIIA, and IIIB Hodgkin's disease in combination with chemotherapy; (2) Ewing's sarcoma in combination with chemotherapy; (3) head and neck cancer in combination with surgery and chemotherapy; and (4) stage I and II breast cancer.

Control of the disease process of cancer for a period of time is considered to be a reasonable goal in some situations. Initial treatment is offered at the time of diagnosis, and additional treatment is instituted each time symptoms of disease recur. Most patients enjoy a satisfactory quality of life during the symptom-free period. Radiation therapy can be combined with surgery to further enhance the local control of cancer. It can be given preoperatively to reduce the size of the tumor so that it can be more easily resected, or it can be given postoperatively to destroy any remaining tumor cells. Intraoperative radiation therapy is now being given at some research centers. In this procedure, radiation is administered directly to the site of the tumor during surgery.

Inoperable tumors can be treated with radiation therapy. These tumors are large and have extended regionally. An example of an inoperable cancer treated for control with radiation therapy is small (oat) cell cancer of the lung.

Palliation is often the goal of radiation therapy. The patient can be treated to control the distressing symptoms that are occurring as a result of the disease process. Tumors can be reduced in size to relieve symptoms such as pain and obstruction. Examples of the use of radiation therapy for palliation include relief of the following:

1. Pain associated with bone metastasis
2. Pain and neurologic symptoms associated with brain metastasis
3. Spinal cord compression
4. Intestinal obstruction
5. Superior vena cava obstruction
6. Bronchial or tracheal obstruction
7. Bleeding (e.g., bladder and intrabronchial)

NURSING MANAGEMENT
RADIATION THERAPY

The nurse has an important role in helping the patient deal with the side effects of radiation therapy. Common side effects of radiation therapy are presented in Table 15-11. Fatigue, anorexia, bone marrow suppression, skin reactions, mucosal reactions, and pulmonary, GI, and reproductive effects are discussed in this section.

■ Nursing Implementation

Fatigue. Fatigue is a commonly reported side effect of radiation therapy. The pathophysiologic mechanisms that result in radiation-induced fatigue are unclear. Accumulation of metabolites from the destruction of cells during treatment is one probable cause. The metabolites include lactate, hydrogen ions, and other end products of cellular destruction and result in decreased muscle strength. Alterations in energy production in the patient with cancer may also result from cachexia, anorexia, fever, and infection. Fatigue generally begins during the third to fourth week of treatment, persists after treatment ends, and then gradually subsides. It is proposed that good symptom management can reduce fatigue. Factors such as weight loss, anemia, depression, nausea, and other symptoms exacerbate the sensation of fatigue.

The patient must recognize that fatigue is an expected side effect of radiation therapy. Otherwise the patient may interpret fatigue as a sign that the treatment is not effective and that the cancer must be spreading. A patient may report more energy on

TABLE 15-11 Nursing Management of Problems Caused by Radiation Therapy and Chemotherapy		
PROBLEM	**ETIOLOGY**	**NURSING MANAGEMENT**
Gastrointestinal System		
Stomatitis, mucositis, esophagitis	• Cells destroyed when located in radiation treatment field • Epithelial cells are destroyed by chemotherapy • Inflammation and ulceration occur due to rapid cell destruction	• Be aware that eating, swallowing, and talking are difficult • Encourage patient to use artificial saliva • Assess oral mucosa daily and teach patient to do this • Discourage use of irritants such as tobacco and alcohol • Apply topical anesthetics, such as viscous Xylocaine or oxethazaine
Nausea and vomiting	• Cellular breakdown stimulates vomiting center in brain • Drugs also stimulate vomiting center • GI lining destroyed with radiation and chemotherapy	• Teach to eat and drink when not nauseated • Administer antiemetics as needed • Use diversional activities (if appropriate)
Anorexia	• Release of TNF and IL-1 from macrophages have appetite-suppressant effect • General reaction to therapy	• Monitor weight • Provide small, frequent meals of high-protein, high-calorie foods • Gently encourage patient to eat, but avoid nagging • Serve food in pleasant environment
Diarrhea	• Denuding of epithelial lining of intestines	• Give antidiarrheal agents as needed
Constipation	• Autonomic nervous system dysfunction • Caused by neurotoxic effects of plant alkaloids (vincristine, vinblastine)	• Provide stool softeners as needed • Encourage to eat high-fiber foods
Hepatotoxicity	• Toxic effects from chemotherapy drugs	• Monitor liver function tests
Hematologic System		
Anemia	• Bone marrow depressed secondary to therapy • Malignant infiltration of bone marrow by cancer	• Monitor hemoglobin and hematocrit levels • Encourage intake of foods that promote RBC production (see Chapter 30, Table 30-5)
Leukopenia	• Depression of bone marrow secondary to chemotherapy or radiation therapy • Infection most frequent cause of morbidity and death in cancer patients • Respiratory and genitourinary system usual sites of infection	• Monitor WBC count, especially neutrophils • Teach to report temperature elevation and any other manifestations of infection • Teach to avoid large crowds and people with infections • Teach to use good hand-washing techniques
Thrombocytopenia	• Bone marrow depressed secondary to chemotherapy • Malignant infiltration of bone marrow • Spontaneous bleeding can occur with platelet counts ≤20,000/μl	• Observe for signs of bleeding (e.g., petechiae, ecchymosis) • Monitor hemoglobin and hematocrit and platelet counts • Teach to use soft-bristle toothbrush and use electric razor • Discuss impact of hair loss on self-image

BUN, Blood urea nitrogen; *ECG,* electrocardiogram; *GI,* gastrointestinal; *IL-1,* interleukin 1; *RBC,* red blood cell; *TNF,* tumor necrosis factor; *WBC,* white blood cell.

TABLE 15-11 Nursing Management of Problems Caused by Radiation Therapy and Chemotherapy—cont'd

PROBLEM	ETIOLOGY	NURSING MANAGEMENT
Integumentary System		
Alopecia	• Destruction of hair follicles by chemotherapy or radiation to scalp • Hair loss usually temporary with chemotherapy; usually permanent in response to radiation	• Suggest ways to cope with hair loss (e.g., hair pieces, scarves, wigs) • Cut long hair before therapy • Avoid excessive shampooing, brushing, and combing of hair • Avoid use of electric hair dryers, curlers, and curling rods
Skin reactions	• Extravasation of vesicant chemotherapeutic drugs • Radiation therapy damage to skin	• Protect skin from trauma • Lubricate dry skin with nonirritating creams • Avoid the use of harsh soaps
Genitourinary Tract		
Cystitis	• Cells lining bladder destroyed from chemotherapy • Side effect of radiation when located in treatment field	• Monitor manifestations such as urgency, frequency, and hematuria
Reproductive dysfunction	• Cells of testes or ova are damaged from therapy	• Discuss these changes with patients
Nephrotoxicity	• Accumulation of drugs in the kidney and tumor lysis causes necrosis of proximal renal tubules	• Monitor BUN and serum creatinine levels
Nervous System		
Increased intracranial pressure	• May result from radiation edema in central nervous system	• May be controlled with steroids and pain medication
Peripheral neuropathy	• Paresthesias, areflexia, skeletal muscle weakness, and smooth muscle dysfunction can occur as a side effect of plant alkaloids and cisplatin	• Monitor for these manifestations in patients on these drugs
Respiratory System		
Pneumonitis	• Radiation pneumonitis develops 2-3 mo after start of treatment • After 6-12 mo fibrosis occurs and is evident on x-ray • Side effect of some chemotherapy drugs	• Monitor for dry, hacking cough, fever, and exertional dyspnea
Cardiovascular System		
Pericarditis and myocarditis	• Inflammation secondary to radiation injury • Complication when chest wall is radiated; may occur up to 1 year after treatment • Side effect of some chemotherapy drugs	• Monitor for clinical manifestations of these disorders
Cardiotoxicity	• Some chemotherapy drugs (e.g., doxorubicin, daunorubicin) can cause ECG changes and rapidly progressive heart failure	• Monitor heart with ECG and cardiac ejection fractions • Drug therapy may need to be modified
Biochemical		
Hyperuricemia	• Increased uric acid levels due to cell destruction by chemotherapy • Can cause secondary gout and obstructive uropathy	• Monitor uric acid levels • Allopurinol (Zyloprim) may be given as a prophylactic measure • Encourage high fluid intake
Psychoemotional		
Fatigue	• Increased metabolic rate • Anabolic processes resulting in accumulation of metabolites from cell breakdown	• Tell patient that fatigue is an expected side effect of therapy • Encourage patient to rest when fatigued, to maintain usual lifestyle patterns as closely as possible, and to pace activities in accordance with energy level
Pain	• Compression or infiltration of tumor involving nerves • Inflammation, ulceration, or necrosis of tissues	• Use an analgesic ladder (see Fig. 15-20) to provide basis for pain medication administration • Teach use of imagery, relaxation therapy, etc. (see Chapters 7 and 8)

some days than on others. Encouraging the individual to identify days or times during the day when feeling better may allow the patient to remain more active. Resting before activity and having others assist with work or home management may be necessary. Ignoring the fatigue or overstressing the body when fatigue is tolerable may lead to an increase in symptoms. Maintaining nutritional status and managing other symptoms also helps reduce fatigue. Walking programs are a way of keeping the patient active. Most patients are able to participate in walking programs.[16] Fatigue is one symptom that shows improvement during walking programs.[17] Walking programs have also been found to lessen anxiety and improve sleep in women receiving radiation for breast cancer.[18] The ability to remain active has been shown to improve mood and avoid the debilitating cycle of fatigue-depression-fatigue that can occur.

Anorexia. Anorexia may develop as a general reaction to treatment. The mechanisms for anorexia are unclear, but several theories exist. Macrophages release tumor necrosis factor (TNF) and interleukin-1 (IL-1) in an attempt to fight the cancer. Both TNF and IL-1 have an appetite-suppressing (anorectic) effect. As tumors are destroyed by therapy, it is proposed that increased levels of these factors may be released into the system and cross the blood-brain barrier, exerting an influence on the satiety center. Large tumors produce more of these factors, thus resulting in the cachexia seen in advanced cancer. In addition, treatments to the head and neck and GI areas exacerbate eating difficulties. Anorexia peaks at about 4 weeks of treatment and seems to resolve more quickly than fatigue when treatment ends.

The patient with anorexia will need to be monitored carefully during treatment to ensure that weight loss does not become excessive. Body weight should be measured at least twice weekly. Small, frequent meals of high-protein, high-calorie foods are better tolerated than large meals. Nutritional supplements are indicated if anorexia is present or if other factors contribute to difficulty in eating.[19]

Bone Marrow Suppression. Bone marrow within the treatment field will be affected by radiation at a rate matching the cellular turnover rate. White blood cells (WBCs) are affected within 1 week, platelets in 2 to 3 weeks, and red blood cells (RBCs) in 2 to 3 months. In the adult about 40% of active marrow is in the pelvis, and 25% is in the thoracic and lumbar vertebrae. If the marrow is irradiated, destruction of blood cells occurs within the treatment field. As a consequence, the nonirradiated marrow becomes more active in an attempt to compensate.

The experience of immunosuppression is not clinically as significant a problem in radiation as it is in the patient receiving certain chemotherapeutic agents. Combination radiation and chemotherapy may cause drops in WBC, RBC, and platelet counts, as does radiation following chemotherapy when bone marrow reserves are limited. Blood counts (including WBC, RBC, and platelets) in these individuals must be closely monitored. Bleeding and infection as consequences of immunosuppression are rare when radiation therapy is delivered alone.

If anemia occurs and the hemoglobin level drops below 10 g/dl (100 g/L), the patient may require blood transfusions. Radiation therapy is more effective against well-oxygenated cells. Therefore there is a concern that a hemoglobin level below 10 g/dl (100 g/L) does not provide for adequate oxygenation of cells in the treatment field.

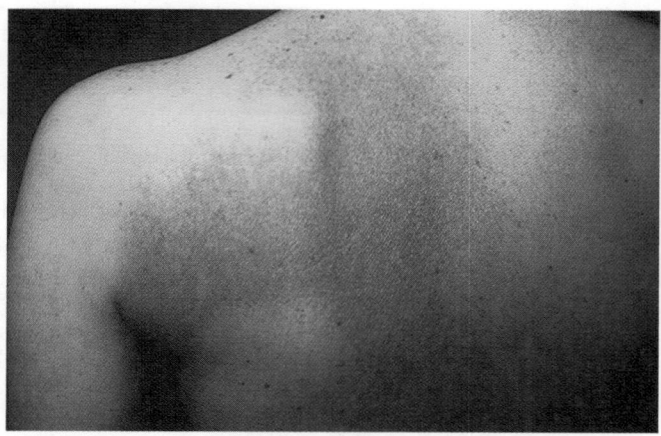

FIG. 15-13 Dry desquamation.

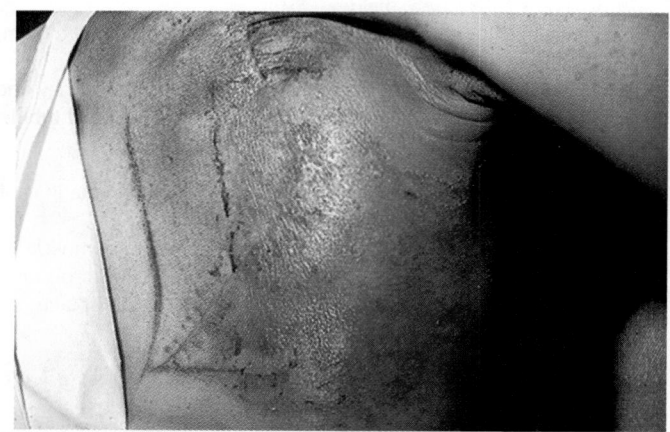

FIG. 15-14 Wet desquamation.

Skin Reactions. Both acute and chronic changes can occur in the skin within the radiation field. The skin-sparing property of modern radiation equipment limits the severity of these reactions. Although the skin reaction begins as early as the first treatment, it is initially transitory. Erythema may develop 1 to 24 hours after a single treatment. Erythema is an acute response followed by dry desquamation (Fig. 15-13). If the rate of cellular sloughing is faster than the ability of the new epidermal cells to replace dead cells, a wet desquamation occurs with exposure of the dermis and oozing of serum (Fig. 15-14). Skin reactions are particularly evident in areas subjected to pressure such as behind the ear and in gluteal folds, perineum, breast, collar line, and bony prominences.

Although there is a lack of consistency in protocols for the management of irradiated skin in terms of products used, there are basic principles of skin care.[19] Dry reactions are uncomfortable and result in pruritus. Wet reactions result in discomfort and drainage. Dry skin should be lubricated with a nonirritating lotion or solution that contains no metal, alcohol, perfume, or additives that irritate the skin. Wet reactions must be kept clean and protected from further damage. Prevention of infection and facilitation of wound healing are the therapeutic goals.

TABLE 15-12

Patient & Family Teaching Guide
Radiation Skin Reactions

1. Gently cleanse the skin in the treatment field using a mild soap (Ivory, Dove), tepid water, a soft cloth, and a gentle patting motion. Rinse thoroughly and pat dry.
2. Apply nonmedicated, nonperfumed, moisturizing lotion or creams, such as baby lotion, oil, aloe gel, or cream to alleviate dry skin. This substance must be gently cleansed from the treatment field before each treatment and reapplied. (NOTE: Care differs from institution to institution.) Dusting with cornstarch may reduce itching.
3. Rinse the area with saline solution. Expose the area to air as often as possible. If copious drainage is present, nonadhesive absorbent dressings are warranted, and they must be changed as soon as they become wet. Observe the area daily for signs of infection.
4. Instruct the patient to avoid wearing tight-fitting clothing such as brassieres, girdles, and belts over the treatment field.
5. Instruct the patient to avoid wearing harsh fabrics, such as wool and corduroy. A lightweight cotton garment is best. If possible, expose the treatment field to air.
6. Instruct the patient to use gentle detergents such as Dreft and Ivory Snow to wash clothing that will come in contact with the treatment field.
7. Instruct the patient to avoid direct exposure to the sun. If the treatment field is in an area that is exposed to the sun, protective clothing such as a wide-brimmed hat should be worn during exposure to the sun.
8. Avoid all sources of heat (hot water bottles, heating pads, and sun lamps) on the treatment field.
9. Avoid exposing the treatment field to cold temperatures (ice bags or cold weather).
10. Instruct the patient to avoid swimming in salt water or in chlorinated pools during the time of treatment.
11. Instruct the patient to avoid the use of all medication, deodorants, perfumes, powders, or cosmetics on the skin in the treatment field. Tape, dressings, and adhesive bandages should also be avoided unless permitted by the radiation therapist. Avoid shaving the hair in the treatment field.
12. Sensitive skin must continue to be protected after the treatment is completed. Teach the patient to do the following:
    a. Avoid direct exposure to the sun. A sunscreen agent and protective clothing must be worn if the potential of exposure to the sun is present.
    b. Use an electric razor if shaving is necessary in the treatment field.

Irradiated skin should be protected from extremes of temperature to prevent trauma. Heating pads, ice packs, and hot water bottles cannot be used in the treatment field. Constricting garments, rubbing, harsh chemicals, and deodorants may also traumatize the skin and should be avoided. The use of corticosteroids and hydrogen peroxide remains controversial because of their interference with wound healing. Because protocols vary widely, the guidelines presented in Table 15-12 should be clarified with the department of radiotherapy before being instituted.

Oral, Oropharynx, and Esophageal Reactions. The mucosal linings of the oral cavity, oropharynx, and esophagus are sensitive to the effects of radiation therapy. A decrease in salivary flow with resultant *xerostomia* (dry mouth) can occur during therapy. Food must be dissolved in saliva to be tasted. Thick saliva is less able to perform the functions of cleansing teeth and moistening food. Taste loss is progressive during therapy, and by the end of treatment patients often report that all food has lost its flavor.[20]

The oral cavity and esophageal effects of radiotherapy have the potential to compromise nutritional status. Oral assessment and meticulous intervention are essential to prevent infection and to facilitate nutritional intake. Difficulty swallowing, which characterizes esophageal reactions, further impedes eating. Patients report feeling that they have a "lump" as they swallow and that "foods get stuck."

The patient should be taught to examine the oral cavity. The mucous membranes, characteristics of saliva, and ability to swallow must be assessed. Oral care includes pretreatment evaluation by a dentist to perform all necessary dental work before the initiation of treatment. The patient should also be taught how to perform oral care. Compliance with this protocol significantly reduces the risk of radiation caries, which develop as a result of loss of saliva. These dental caries are extremely damaging to the teeth, resulting in the need for extraction. Saliva substitutes are available and may be offered to patients, although many patients find that drinking small amounts of water frequently has an equivalent effect. Oral care should be performed at least before and after each meal and at bedtime. A saline solution of 1 teaspoon of salt in 1 L of water is an effective cleansing agent. One teaspoon of sodium bicarbonate may be added to the oral care solution to decrease odor, alleviate pain, and dissolve mucin. Tooth brushing and flossing are critical unless contraindicated by decreased platelet counts.

Alleviation of mucositis or pain in the throat can be achieved by systemic analgesics and antibiotics, as well as coating agents, which include antacids and sucralfate suspension.[21] Combinations of coating and analgesic compounds may be used. Antacids, diphenhydramine (Benadryl), and viscous lidocaine (Xylocaine) have been mixed in equal proportions to use as a component of oral care. The solutions may be swallowed to alleviate esophagitis. Any coating solution must be cleansed and not allowed to build up on the mucosa where it could serve as a medium for infection. Infection, particularly *Candida albicans*, can occur in individuals receiving head and neck radiation. The incidence increases dramatically in protocols using concomitant chemotherapy. Antifungal agents may be prescribed to treat the infection.

Feedings of soft, nonirritating high-protein and high-caloric foods should be offered frequently throughout the day. Extremes of temperature, as well as tobacco and alcohol, should be avoided. Nutritional supplements (e.g., Ensure) as an adjunct to meals and fluid intake must be encouraged. The patient should be weighed at least twice each week to ensure that excessive amounts of weight have not been lost. Families are an integral part of the health care team. As taste loss increases, the family's role in assisting the patient to eat becomes increasingly critical. If family members are not available, alternative support such as volunteers and home aides are indicated.

Pulmonary Effects. The effects of radiation on the lung include both acute and late reactions. Radiation doses in the lung are magnified because there is no reduction of the dose through tissue. Pneumonitis can be an acute inflammatory reaction related to radiation. This reaction is often asymptomatic, although an increase in cough, fever, and night sweats may occur. Treatment with bronchodilators, expectorants, bed rest, and oxygen is preferable to treatment with corticosteroids.

The pulmonary effects of radiation are frightening to the patient because they may involve an exacerbation of the symptoms that precipitated the cancer diagnosis. Cough and dyspnea may increase. The cough becomes more productive as alveoli that had been blocked are opened as the tumor responds to treatment. As treatment continues, the cough can become dry as the mucosa begins to be altered by the radiation. Cough suppressants may be indicated at night.

Oxygen, if prescribed for symptomatic pneumonitis, must be used judiciously if the patient has chronic obstructive pulmonary disease (see Chapter 28). The patient may mistakenly believe that increasing oxygen flow is an appropriate response to treat increasing dyspnea. If the patient experiences dyspnea, anxiety may be pronounced. Lying flat on the radiation treatment table and being alone in the room may potentiate anxiety.

Gastrointestinal Effects. The mucosa of the GI tract is highly proliferative, with surface cells being replaced every 2 to 6 days. The intestinal mucosa is one of the most radiosensitive tissues. Radiation alters gastric secretion by direct injury to cells. The secretion of mucus, hydrochloric acid, and pepsin decreases with further treatment. Nausea, vomiting, and diarrhea result from irradiation of the GI tissue.

Nausea and vomiting are early reactions of GI tract irradiation, occurring as soon as immediately following the first treatment. The etiology of GI reactions may be related to the release of serotonin from the GI tract, which then stimulates the chemoreceptor trigger zone and the vomiting center in the brain. Further GI irritation is related to cellular death. Prophylactic administration of antiemetics 1 hour before treatment is recommended. The patient may find that eating a light meal of nonirritating food before treatment is also helpful. The development of *anticipatory nausea and vomiting* can occur in the patient receiving radiation. This conditioned response develops over time in the individual who has unrelieved nausea and vomiting. As the patient repeatedly experiences these symptoms, a framework of cues is created associated with nausea and vomiting to the point that encountering the cues even without receiving treatment may precipitate nausea and vomiting. This is called anticipatory nausea and vomiting. In some individuals this response persists after treatment ends. This type of reaction does not usually develop in the patient who does not experience posttreatment vomiting, which underscores the necessity for prophylactic treatment.

The patient experiencing nausea and vomiting must be assessed for signs and symptoms of dehydration and alkalosis. Fluid intake is recorded to ensure that an adequate volume is being consumed and retained. Nausea and vomiting can be successfully managed when conventional radiation doses and field sizes are used.

Diarrhea is a reaction of the bowel to radiation. The small bowel is extremely sensitive and does not tolerate significant radiation doses. Treating the patient with a full bladder may serve to move the small bowel out of the treatment field. Nonirritating diets and low-residue diets, as well as antidiarrheals and antispasmodics, are recommended. Lukewarm sitz baths may alleviate discomfort and cleanse the rectal area. The rectal area must be kept clean and dry to maintain mucosal integrity. The nurse should inspect the anal area. The number, volume, consistency, and character of stools per day should be noted. Adequate food and fluid intake promote healing and mucosal integrity. Meticulous perianal care is essential. Systemic analgesia is warranted for the painful skin irritations that may develop.

Reproductive Effects. The effects of radiation on the ovary and testes are determined by the dose delivered. The testes are highly sensitive to radiation, and protection of the testicles is achieved whenever possible. Doses of 15 to 30 cGy temporarily decrease the sperm count, with aspermia at 35 to 230 cGy. In some cases, 200 cGy may result in permanent aspermia. The patient receiving 300 to 600 cGy either recovers in 2 to 5 years or not at all. Pretreatment status may be a significant factor because a low sperm count and loss of motility are seen in individuals with testicular cancer and Hodgkin's disease before any therapy. Combined modality treatment or prior chemotherapy with alkylating agents enhances and prolongs the effects of radiation on the testes. When radiation is used alone with conventional doses and appropriate shielding, testicular recovery often occurs. Compromise of reproductive function in men may also result from erectile dysfunction following pelvic radiation and related vascular and neurologic effects.

The radiation dose necessary to induce ovarian failure changes with age. Permanent cessation of menses occurs in 95% of women less than 40 years of age at 500 to 1000 cGy and at 375 cGy in women more than 40 years of age. Unlike the testes, there is no avenue for repair of ovarian function. The ovaries are shielded whenever possible. Other factors that influence reproductive or sexual functioning in women include reactions in the cervix and endometrium. These tissues withstand a high radiation dose with minimal sequelae, accounting for the ability to treat endometrial and cervical cancer with high external and brachytherapy doses. Acute reactions such as tenderness, irritation, and loss of lubrication compromise sexual activity. Late effects of combined internal and external therapy include vaginal shortening related to fibrosis and loss of elasticity and lubrication.

The patient and her or his partner require information about the expected effects of treatment relative to reproductive and sexual issues. Potential infertility can be a significant consequence for the individual, and counseling may be indicated. Pretreatment harvesting of sperm or ova may be considered. Specific suggestions to manage side effects that have an impact on sexual functioning include using a water-soluble vaginal lubricant and a vaginal dilator after pelvic irradiation. The nurse must be able to encourage discussion of issues related to sexuality, offer specific suggestions, and make referrals for ongoing counseling when indicated.[22]

Coping with Radiation Therapy. Assisting the patient to cope with the anxieties of receiving radiation is an essential component of the nursing role. The necessity of coming for treatment five times per week for several weeks forces the individual to confront the cancer on an almost daily basis. In conjunction with the social worker, the nurse should assist with planning for transportation, nutrition, and emotional support with available resources such as the American Cancer Society, churches, and community resources.

Anxiety is usually present in the patient receiving therapy. The uncertainties regarding treatment and the fears of receiving radiation are most evident at the beginning of therapy. Anxiety continues to be a factor at the end of treatment when outcomes are still unknown. Anxiety may increase in some patients when treatment ends. The patient must realize that he or she will be followed and that support is ongoing. The impact of radiation on the quality of life of the patient undergoing therapy may be minimized with information and support. The nurse plays an important role in the management of the individual receiving radiation therapy. Patient teaching and symptom management allow the individual to cope with therapy while maintaining the highest possible quality of life.[22]

CHEMOTHERAPY

The use of chemicals as a systemic therapy for cancer has been evolving over the past several decades. In the 1940s chemotherapy was in its infancy. Nitrogen mustard, a chemical warfare agent used in World Wars I and II, was used in the treatment of acute leukemia, and a folic acid antimetabolite (5-FU) was found to have antitumor activity. In the 1970s chemotherapy was established as an effective treatment modality for cancer. Chemotherapy is now used in the treatment of many solid tumors and is the primary therapy for leukemias and some lymphomas. Chemotherapy as a treatment option has evolved from a palliative, "last-ditch effort" treatment modality to one that can offer cure for certain cancers, control other cancers for long periods of time, and offer palliative relief of symptoms when cure or control no longer is possible (Fig. 15-15). Although states vary in their practice laws, optimally nurses administering chemotherapy should be specifically trained in the drugs, administration, and possible side effects.[23]

Effect on Cells

The effect of chemotherapy is at the cellular level. All cells (cancer cells and normal cells) enter the cell cycle for replication and proliferation (see Fig. 15-1). The effects of the chemotherapeutic agents are described in relationship to the cell cycle. The two major categories of chemotherapeutic drugs are cell cycle–nonspecific and cell cycle phase–specific drugs.

Cell cycle–nonspecific chemotherapeutic drugs have their effect on the cells that are in the process of cellular replication and proliferation, as well as on the cells that are in the resting phase (G_0).

Cell cycle phase–specific chemotherapeutic drugs have their effect on cells that are in the process of cellular replication or proliferation (G_1, S_1, G_2, or M). These drugs exert their most significant effect during specific phases of the cell cycle. Cell cycle phase–specific and cell cycle–nonspecific agents are often administered in combination with one another. The aim of this approach is to promote a better response using agents that function by differing mechanisms.[24]

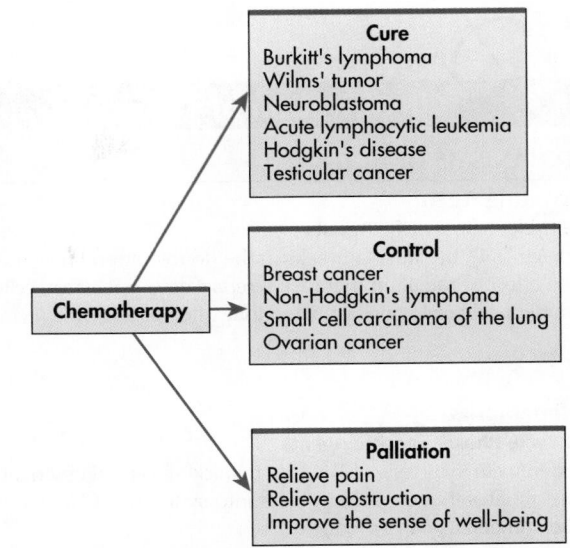

FIG. 15-15 Goals of chemotherapy.

The goal of chemotherapy is to reduce the number of cancer cells present in the primary tumor site(s) and metastatic tumor site(s). Several factors determine the response of cancer cells to chemotherapy:

1. *Mitotic rate of the tissue from which the tumor arises.* The more rapid the mitotic rate, the greater the response to chemotherapy. Chemotherapy is the treatment of choice for acute leukemia, Wilms' tumor (used in conjunction with surgery), and neuroblastoma. These cancer cells have a rapid rate of cellular proliferation.
2. *Size of the tumor.* The smaller the number of cancer cells, the greater the response to chemotherapy.
3. *Age of the tumor.* The younger the tumor, the greater the response to chemotherapy. Younger tumors have a greater percentage of proliferating cells.
4. *Location of the tumor.* Certain anatomic sites provide a protected environment from the effects of chemotherapy. For example, only a few drugs (nitrosoureas and bleomycin) cross the blood-brain barrier.
5. *Presence of resistant tumor cells.* Mutation of cancer cells within the tumor mass can result in variant cells that are resistant to chemotherapy. Resistance can also occur because of the biochemical inability of some cancer cells to convert the drug to its active form.

As cancer first begins to grow, most of the cells are actively dividing. As the tumor increases in size, more cells become inactive and convert to a resting state (G_0). Because most chemotherapeutic agents are most effective against dividing cells, cells can escape death by staying in the G_0 phase. The main problem in cancer chemotherapy is the presence of drug-resistant resting and noncycling cells.

Classification of Chemotherapeutic Drugs

Chemotherapeutic drugs are categorized or classified according to their structure and mechanisms of action (Table 15-13). Each drug in a particular classification has many similarities, but major differences in the drugs are also evident.

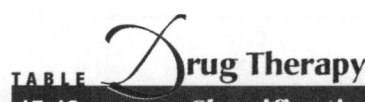

TABLE
15-13
Drug Therapy
Classification of Chemotherapy Drugs

MECHANISMS OF ACTION	EXAMPLES
Alkylating Agents **Cell Cycle–Nonspecific Agents** Damage DNA by causing breaks in the double-strand helix (similar to the effect of radiation therapy); if repair does not occur, cells will die immediately (cytocidal) or when they attempt to divide (cytostatic)	mechlorethamine (nitrogen mustard), cyclophosphamide (Cytoxan), chlorambucil (Leukeran), melphalan (Alkeran), busulfan (Myleran), dacarbazine (DTIC), lomustine (CCNU), oxaliplatin (Eloxatin), streptozocin (Zanosar), cisplatin (Platinol), carboplatin (Paraplatin)
Antimetabolites **Cell Cycle Phase–Specific Agents** Interfere with synthesis of DNA by mimicking certain essential cellular metabolites that cell incorporates into synthesis of DNA; cells will die immediately (cytocidal)	methotrexate, cytarabine (Ara-C, Cytosar), fluorouracil (5-FU), mercaptopurine (6-MP), thioguanine (6-TG), floxuridine (FUDR), pentostatin (Nipent), fludarabine (Fludara), hydroxyurea (Hydrea), gemcitabine (Gemzar), cladribine (Leustatin)
Antitumor Antibiotics **Cell Cycle–Nonspecific Agents** Modify function of DNA and interfere with transcription of RNA; cells will die immediately (cytocidal) or when they attempt to divide (cytostatic)	doxorubicin (Adriamycin), bleomycin (Blenoxane), mitomycin (Mutamycin), daunorubicin (Daunomycin), dactinomycin (Cosmegen), idarubicin (Idamycin), mithramycin (Mithracin), epirubicin (Ellence), mitoxantrone (Novantrone)
Plant Alkaloids (Mitotic Inhibitors) **Cell Cycle Phase–Specific Agents** Interrupt cellular replication in mitosis at metaphase; cells will die immediately (cytocidal)	vinblastine (Velban), vincristine (Oncovin), etoposide (VePesid), paclitaxel (Taxol), docetaxel (Taxotere), teniposide (Vumon)
Nitrosoureas **Cell Cycle–Nonspecific Agents** Have similar effect to alkylating agents and also block specific enzymes needed for the synthesis of purine; cells will die immediately (cytocidal) or when they attempt to divide (cytostatic)	carmustine (BCNU), lomustine (CCNU)
Corticosteroids **Cell Cycle–Nonspecific Agents** Disrupt the cell membrane and inhibit synthesis of protein; decrease circulating lymphocytes; inhibit mitosis; depress immune system; increase feeling of well-being	cortisone (Cortone), hydrocortisone (Cortef), methylprednisolone (Medrol), prednisone, dexamethasone (Decadron)
Hormone Therapy **Cell Cycle–Nonspecific Agents** Stimulate the process of cellular differentiation; metastatic lesions are less able to survive in unfavorable environment; decrease the process of cellular proliferation	androgens (testosterone), fluoxymesterone (Halotestin), estrogens, progestins
Aromatase Inhibitors Inhibit the enzyme aromatase, a p450 enzyme involved in estrogen synthesis	anastrozole (Arimidex), letrozole (Femara), vorozole (Rizivor), exemestane (Aromasin), aminoglutethimide (Cytadren)
Selective Estrogen Receptor Modulator (SERM) Selectively modulates estrogen receptors, thus acting as an estrogen antagonist	raloxifene (Evista)
Miscellaneous Destroys exogenous supply of L-asparagine, which is needed for cellular proliferation; normal cells can synthesize but cannot be synthesized by cancer cells	L-asparaginase (Elspar)
Antiestrogens used in breast cancer	tamoxifen (Nolvadex), toremifene (Fareston), fulvestrant (Faslodex)
Suppresses mitosis at interphase, appears to alter preformed DNA, RNA, and protein	procarbazine (Matulane, Natulan)

Preparation and Administration of Chemotherapy

It is very important to know the specific guidelines for administration of chemotherapeutic drugs. In addition, it is important to understand that drugs may be hazardous for health care professionals. A person preparing or giving chemotherapy may absorb the drug through inhalation of particles when reconstituting a powder in an open ampule and through skin contact. There may also be some risk in handling the vomitus and excreta of persons receiving chemotherapy. Guidelines for the safe handling of chemotherapeutic agents have been developed by the Occupational Safety and Health Administration (OSHA) and the Oncology Nursing Society (see the website at *www.ons.org*).

Methods of Administration

Chemotherapy can be administered by several routes (Table 15-14). The oral and intravenous (IV) routes are the most common. One of the major concerns with the IV administration of antineoplastic drugs is possible irritation of the vessel wall by the drug or, even worse, *extravasations* (infiltration of drugs into tissues surrounding the infusion site) causing local tissue damage. Many chemotherapeutic drugs are **vesicants,** agents that when accidentally infiltrated into the skin cause severe local tissue breakdown and necrosis.[24]

Pain is the cardinal symptom of extravasation, although extravasation has been known to occur without causing pain. Swelling, redness, and the presence of vesicles on the skin are other signs of extravasation. After a few days, the tissue may begin to ulcerate and necrose. The process has the potential to progress to a deep, wide crater that often warrants closure with skin grafts.

Chemotherapy can also be administered by means of a central vascular access device. Central vascular access devices are placed in large vessels (venous or arterial) and permit frequent, continuous, or intermittent administration of chemotherapy, biologic therapy, and other products, thus avoiding multiple punctures for vascular access. These devices are indicated in instances of limited vascular access, intensive chemotherapy, continuous infusion of vesicant agents, and projected long-term need for vascular access. In addition to their usefulness in administration of chemotherapeutic agents, vascular access devices can be used to administer additional fluids, such as blood products, parenteral nutrition, or other drugs, and for venous blood sampling.

The trends in cancer care toward combination therapies requiring venous access have necessitated the increased use of vascular access devices. The advantages of vascular access devices are that they provide for rapid dilution of chemotherapy, decreased incidence of extravasation, and reduced need for venipuncture. The disadvantages are that central catheters can be a source of systemic infection, particularly if the patient becomes immunosuppressed during therapy. Three major types of vascular access devices are Silastic right atrial catheters, implanted infusion ports, and infusion (external and implanted) pumps.

Silastic Right Atrial Catheters. Silastic right atrial catheters are single-, double-, or triple-lumen catheters approximately 90 cm in length with internal diameters ranging from 1 to 2 mm (Fig. 15-16). These catheters are inserted with the aid of local or general anesthesia through a central vein with the tip resting in the right atrium of the heart. The other end of the catheter is tunneled through subcutaneous tissue and exits through a separate incision on the chest or abdominal wall. A Dacron cuff on the catheter serves to stabilize the catheter and may decrease the incidence of infection. Accurate placement must be verified by chest x-ray before the catheter can be used. Care requirements include cap change, cleansing, heparin flush, and dressing change. The exact frequency and procedures for these requirements vary from institution to institution. Reported complications with these catheters include occlusion, sepsis, bleeding, venous thrombosis, technical problems, and local infection at the exit site.

The Groshong catheter is a distinct type of tunneled central venous catheter. The unique features of this catheter are the existence of a pressure-sensitive valve near the distal end, which precludes the need for heparin flushing and clamping, and its placement 2 to 3 cm above the right atrium in the superior vena cava.

Peripherally Inserted Central Venous Catheters and Midline Catheters. Peripherally inserted central venous catheters (PICCs) and midline catheters (MLCs) are single- or double-lumen, nontunneled, polymer catheters that are primarily

METHOD	EXAMPLES
Oral	cyclophosphamide
Intramuscular	bleomycin
Intravenous	doxorubicin, vincristine
Intracavitary (pleural, peritoneal)	radioisotopes, alkylating agents, methotrexate
Intrathecal	methotrexate, cytarabine
Intraarterial	DTIC, 5-FU, methotrexate, floxuridine
Perfusion	Alkylating agents
Continuous infusion	5-FU, methotrexate, cytarabine
Subcutaneous	cytarabine
Topical	5-FU cream

TABLE 15-14 Drug Therapy Methods of Chemotherapy Administration

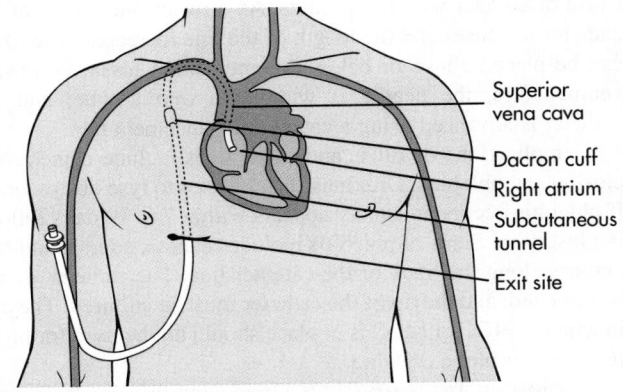

FIG. 15-16 Silastic right atrial catheter placement. Note tip of the catheter in the right atrium.

Superior vena cava

Dacron cuff

Right atrium

Subcutaneous tunnel

Exit site

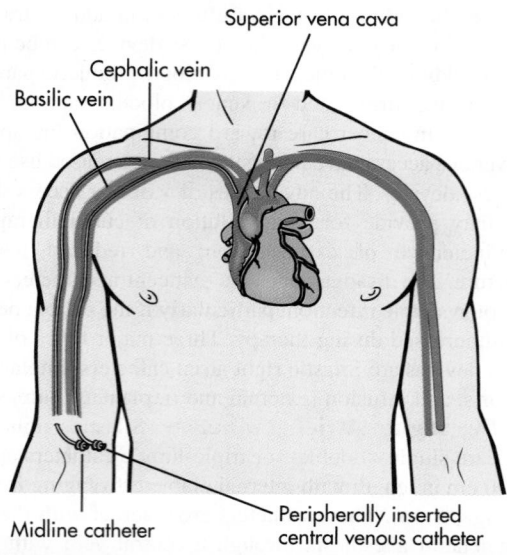

FIG. 15-17 Placement of peripherally inserted central venous catheters(PICC) and midline catheters (MLC).

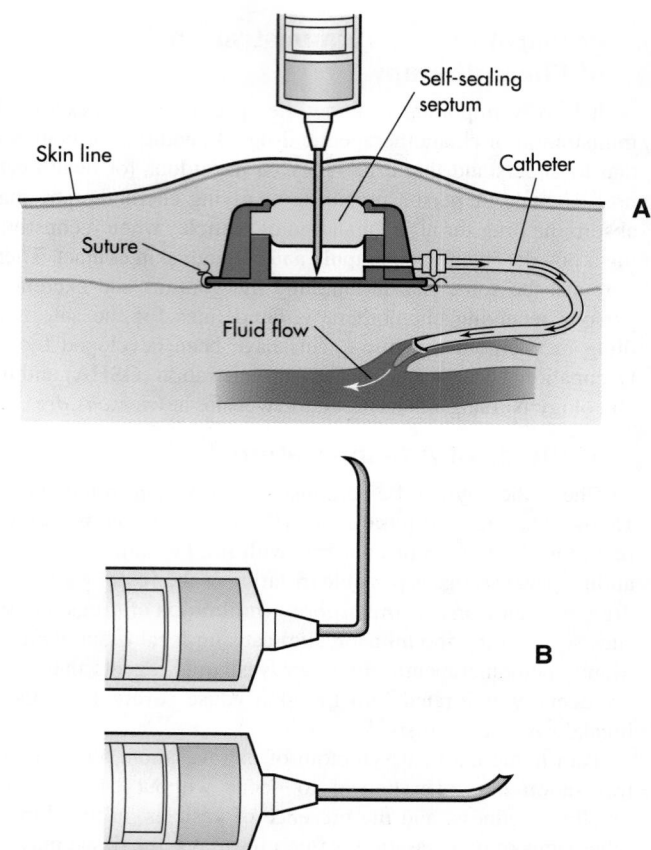

FIG. 15-18 A, Cross section of implantable port displaying access of the port with the Huber needle. Note the deflected point of the Huber needle, which prevents coring of the port's septum. B, Two Huber needles used to enter the implanted port. The 90-degree needle is used for top-entry ports for continuous infusion.

used in cancer care for immediate central venous access or when the need for infusion therapy is beyond the capacity of the patient's existing, long-term venous access device (Fig. 15-17). These catheters are used for short-term IV therapy, frequent administration of blood products, blood drawing, and intermittent or continuous drug infusions. A physician or a specially trained nurse places these catheters.

PICC lines are inserted at or just above the antecubital fossa and advanced to a position with the tip ending in the distal one third of the superior vena cava. These lines are up to 60 cm in length with gauges ranging from 24 to 16. They can be in place for up to 6 months. The technique for placement of a PICC line involves insertion of the catheter through a needle with the use of a guide wire or forceps to advance the line.

MLC lines are catheters that are placed between the antecubital fossa and the head of the clavicle. These catheters are shorter than PICC lines (15 to 20 cm) with the tip resting in the larger vessels of the upper arm. PICC lines can be used for this purpose. However, specific MLCs have been developed. MLCs are made of an elastomeric hydrogel that becomes approximately 50 times softer approximately 2 hours following insertion because of contact with body fluids. As a result, the gauge of the catheter increases and the length of the line increases. The MLC can be placed above or below the antecubital fossa. Following venipuncture, the needle is withdrawn into a tube, and the catheter is advanced using a catheter advancement tab.

Complications of PICC and MLC lines include catheter occlusion and phlebitis. Urokinase can be used to lyse obstructions. If phlebitis occurs, it usually appears within 7 to 10 days following insertion. Signs of phlebitis include redness, edema, and tenderness along the track of the catheter line. The catheter should be removed, and the tip of the catheter must be cultured. The arm in which a PICC or MLC is in place should not be used for blood pressures or blood drawing.

Implanted Infusion Ports. Implanted infusion ports consist of a central venous catheter connected to an implanted, single or double subcutaneous injection port (Fig. 15-18). The

catheter is placed into the desired vein and the other end is connected to a port that is sutured to the chest wall muscle and surgically implanted in a subcutaneous pocket on the chest wall. The port consists of a metal sheath with a self-sealing silicone septum. It is accessed via the septum by means of a special Huber-point needle that has a deflected tip to prevent coring of the septum. Huber-point needles are also available with the tip at a 90-degree angle for longer infusions. Care requirements include dressing change, cleansing, and flushing. Complications attributed to implanted infusion ports include clotting, catheter migration, infection, bleeding, thrombosis, air embolism, and infection at the exit site or in the pocket. Formation of "sludge" (accumulation of clotted blood and drug precipitate) may also occur within the port septum.

Infusion Pumps. Infusion pumps are used primarily for the continuous infusion of chemotherapy by IV, subcutaneous, intraarterial, and epidural routes. Infusion pumps can be worn externally or implanted surgically. The various types of external infusion pumps differ in terms of their mechanisms of action, components, and capabilities.

Implanted infusion pumps are used primarily for intraarterial administration of chemotherapy (Fig. 15-19). This approach permits continuous infusion of the chemotherapeutic agent directly to the

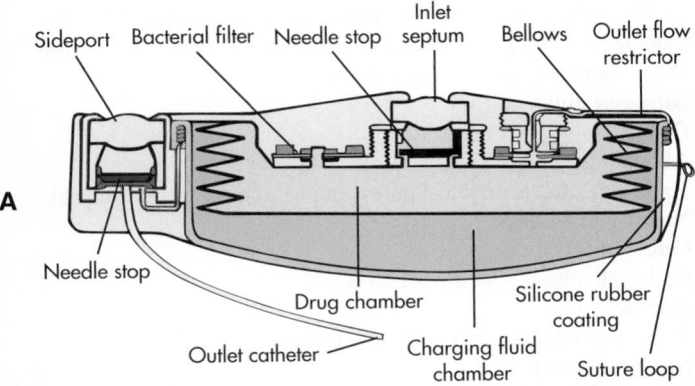

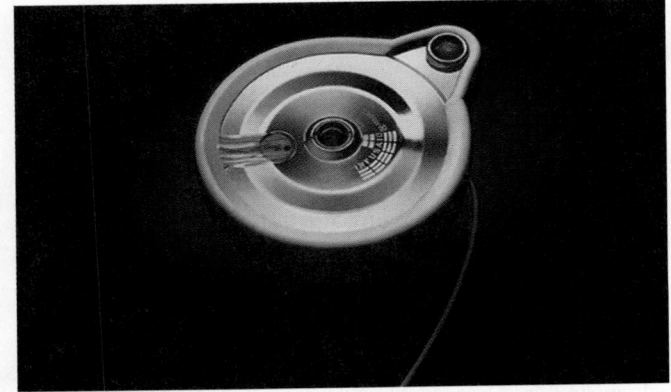

FIG. 15-19 A, Cross section of the implantable pump displaying its two chambers: the drug chamber (inner) and the charging fluid chamber (outer). As the drug chamber is filled, the bellows expand, compressing the charging fluid in the outer chamber. The resulting increased pressure in the outer chamber forces the drug through a membrane filter and preset flow restrictor, thus ensuring a nearly constant flow. B, Infusaid pump.

area of the tumor while sparing the patient the systemic effects of the drug. Some implanted pumps have two silicone septums. The second septum can be used for bolus medication administration. The most common use of this method of chemotherapy administration has been hepatic artery infusion in the treatment of liver metastasis, usually from primary colon cancer.

Implanted pumps also consist of a catheter that is threaded into the designated artery. The catheter is attached to a pump apparatus that consists of two chambers: an inner chamber that serves as the drug reservoir and an outer chamber that contains vapor pressure providing a source of power for the pump. The pump is implanted surgically in a subcutaneous pocket. Access to the pump is via a silicone septum with a Huber-point needle. Flow rate of the pump can be affected by drug concentration, the length and diameter of the Silastic catheter, and the patient's body temperature. Thus dose alterations may be required if the patient experiences a change in temperature or travels to higher altitudes. Complications that have been associated with implanted infusion pumps include infection, thrombosis, clotting of the catheter, and pump malfunction.

Other access devices used in the treatment of the person with cancer include the Tenckhoff catheter used in the administration of intraperitoneal chemotherapy and the Ommaya reservoir, which delivers agents directly to the central nervous system (CNS).

Regional Chemotherapy Administration

Regional treatment with chemotherapy involves the delivery of the drug directly to the tumor site. The advantage of administering chemotherapy by this method is that higher concentrations of the drug can be delivered to the tumor with reduced systemic toxicity. Several regional delivery methods have been developed, including intraarterial, intraperitoneal, intrathecal or intraventricular, and intravesical bladder chemotherapy.

Intraarterial Chemotherapy. Intraarterial chemotherapy delivers the drug to the tumor via the arterial vessel supplying the tumor. This method has been used for the treatment of osteogenic sarcoma; cancers of the head and neck, bladder, brain, and cervix; melanoma; primary liver cancer; and metastatic liver disease. One method of intraarterial drug delivery involves the surgical placement of a catheter that is subsequently connected to an external infusion pump or an implanted infusion pump for infusion of the chemotherapeutic agent. Generally, intraarterial chemotherapy results in reduced systemic toxicity. The type of toxicity experienced by the patient depends on the site of the tumor being treated.

Intraperitoneal Chemotherapy. Intraperitoneal chemotherapy involves the delivery of chemotherapy to the peritoneal cavity for treatment of peritoneal metastases from primary colorectal and ovarian cancers and malignant ascites. Temporary Silastic catheters (Tenckhoff, Hickman, and Groshong) are percutaneously or surgically placed into the peritoneal cavity for short-term administration of chemotherapy. Alternatively, an implanted port can be used to administer chemotherapy intraperitoneally. Chemotherapy is generally infused into the peritoneum in 1 to 2 L of fluid and allowed to "dwell" in the peritoneum for a period of 1 to 4 hours. Following the "dwell time," the fluid is usually drained from the peritoneum. Complications of peritoneal chemotherapy include abdominal pain; catheter occlusion, dislodgement, and migration; and infection.[25]

Intrathecal or Intraventricular Chemotherapy. Cancers that metastasize to the CNS, most commonly breast, lung, GI, leukemia, and lymphoma, are difficult to treat because the blood-brain barrier often prevents distribution of chemotherapy to this area. One method used to treat metastasis to the CNS is intrathecal chemotherapy. This method involves a lumbar puncture and injection of chemotherapy through the dura and arachnoid and into the subarachnoid space. However, this method has resulted in incomplete distribution of the drug in the CNS, particularly to the cisternal and ventricular areas.

To ensure more uniform distribution of chemotherapy to the cisternal and ventricular areas, an Ommaya reservoir is often inserted. An Ommaya reservoir is a Silastic, dome-shaped disk with an extension catheter that is surgically implanted through the cranium into a lateral ventricle. In addition to more consistent drug distribution, the Ommaya reservoir precludes the use of repeated, painful lumbar punctures. Complications of intrathecal or intraventricular chemotherapy include headache, nausea, vomiting, fever, and nuchal rigidity.[26]

Intravesical Bladder Chemotherapy. The patient with superficial transitional cell cancer of the bladder often has recurrent disease following traditional surgical therapy. Instillation of chemotherapy into the bladder promotes destruction of cancer cells and reduces the incidence of recurrent disease. Additional benefits of this therapy include reduced urinary and sexual dysfunction. The chemotherapeutic agent is instilled into the bladder via a urinary catheter and retained for 1 to 3 hours. Complications of this therapy include dysuria, urinary frequency, hematuria, and bladder spasms.

Effects of Chemotherapy on Normal Tissues

Chemotherapeutic agents cannot selectively distinguish between normal cells and cancer cells. When normal cells are destroyed, the patient experiences certain signs and symptoms that are the expected side effects or toxic effects of chemotherapy. Effects of chemotherapy are caused by specific drug toxicities and destruction of cells (Table 15-15). Response of the body to the products of cellular destruction in circulation may cause fatigue, anorexia, and taste alterations.

The adverse effects of these drugs can be classified as acute, delayed, or chronic. Acute toxicity includes vomiting, allergic reactions, and arrhythmias. Delayed effects include mucositis, alopecia, and bone marrow suppression. Mucositis can result in mouth sores, gastritis, and diarrhea. Chronic toxicities involve damage to organs such as the heart, liver, kidneys, and lungs.

Treatment Plan

When chemotherapy is used in the treatment of cancer, several drugs are usually given in combination. Today, single-drug chemotherapy is rarely chosen for a treatment plan. The drugs given are carefully selected to most effectively kill the cancer cells while allowing the normal cells to repair themselves and proliferate. The dose of each drug is carefully calculated according to the body weight or the body surface area of the patient being treated. The choice of the drugs selected to be given together to treat a particular cancer is based on the following principles of combination chemotherapy:

1. The drugs used in the treatment plan are effective against the cancer being treated.
2. When drugs are given in combination, a synergistic effect occurs.
3. The combination includes cell cycle phase–specific and cell cycle–nonspecific drugs and drugs that have different mechanisms of action.
4. The combination includes drugs that have different toxic side effects.
5. The combination includes drugs that cause nadirs occurring at different time intervals. The **nadir** is the lowest level of the peripheral blood cell counts (particularly WBC) that occurs secondary to bone marrow depression. The nadir following administration of most chemotherapy drugs occurs in 7 to 28 days.

TABLE 15-15	Cells with Rapid Rate of Proliferation
CELLS AND GENERATION TIME	**EFFECT OF CELL DESTRUCTION**
Bone marrow stem cell, 6-24 hr	Myelosuppression; infection, bleeding, anemia
Neutrophils, 12 hr	Leukopenia, infection
Epithelial cells lining the gastrointestinal tract, 12-24 hr	Anorexia, stomatitis, esophagitis, nausea and vomiting, diarrhea
Cells of the hair follicle, 24 hr	Alopecia
Ova or testes, 24-36 hr	Reproductive dysfunction

The MOPP protocol, the first combination protocol for the treatment of Hodgkin's disease, is an example of a combination chemotherapy treatment regimen:

Nitrogen mustard (M)
Cell cycle–nonspecific drug
Alkylating agent
Toxic side effects: myelosuppression, nausea, vomiting, alopecia
Nadir: 7 to 14 days
Oncovin (O)
Cell cycle phase–specific drug
Plant alkaloid
Toxic side effects: neurotoxicity, alopecia
Nadir: unknown
Procarbazine (P)
Cell cycle phase–specific drug
Monoamine oxidase (MAO) inhibitor
Toxic side effects: myelosuppression, nausea, vomiting
Nadir: 2 to 8 weeks
Prednisone (P)
Toxic side effects: corticosteroid effects
Nadir: unknown

The agents in this drug protocol differ in mechanisms of action, toxic side effects, and nadir, but the combination is synergistic in nature and effectively destroys the cancer cells present in the early stages of Hodgkin's disease.

The drugs are given according to a specific schedule that includes a time of drug administration and a time of rest from drug administration. The rest period is necessary to allow the normal cells to proliferate and repair the damaged tissue. The example in Table 15-16 describes a typical MOPP schedule. This drug schedule is repeated a specific number of times. The patient is evaluated before the administration of each course of chemotherapy to determine whether the normal cells have proliferated to a sufficient degree.

NURSING MANAGEMENT CHEMOTHERAPY

One of the most important responsibilities of the nurse is that of differentiating between toxic effects of the drug and progression of the malignant process. The nurse also must differentiate between tolerable side effects and acute toxic effects of chemotherapeutic agents. For example, nausea and vomiting are expected and controllable side effects of many drugs. However, if paresthesia occurs with the use of vincristine (Oncovin) or signs of heart failure appear with the use of doxorubicin (Adriamycin), these serious reactions must be reported to the physician so that drug dosages can be modified or discontinued. Some toxicities associated with chemotherapy may not be reversible. For example, ototoxicity may be an irreversible effect of cisplatin (Platinol) therapy, especially at higher doses. Periodic testing of hearing may be necessary to monitor for this toxicity. Specific nursing considerations related to problems caused by chemotherapy are presented in Table 15-11.

■ Nursing Implementation

Side Effects. Many side effects of chemotherapy are similar to those of radiation therapy. (Fatigue, anorexia, bone marrow suppression, mucositis, and nausea and vomiting are discussed on pp. 306-310.)

TABLE 15-16 Drug Therapy
MOPP Chemotherapeutic Drug Schedule

Drug	Days 1	2	3	4	5	6	7	8	9	10	11	12	13	14	15-28
Nitrogen mustard (intravenous administration)	↔							↔							
Oncovin (intravenous administration)	↔							↔							*
Procarbazine (oral administration)	←———————————————————————————→														
Prednisone (oral administration)	←———————————————————————————→														

*No drugs given.

Nausea and vomiting are the most commonly observed GI side effects. Vomiting may occur within 1 hour of administration and may last for 24 hours or more. Several antiemetic drugs are available (see Chapter 40 and Table 40-1). Metoclopramide (Reglan), ondansetron (Zofran), granisetron (Kytril), and dexamethasone (Decadron) have been used to decrease nausea and vomiting caused by chemotherapy. Aprepitant (Emend) is a new antinausea drug that is especially effective in treating delayed nausea and vomiting that patients experience after receiving chemotherapy.

Results of laboratory studies of the patient who is receiving chemotherapy should be monitored. Particular attention should be given to the WBC (especially neutrophil count), platelet, and RBC counts. If the WBC count falls to less than $2000/\mu l$ (2×10^9/L), the drug regimen may need to be modified or discontinued. Every possible measure should be taken to prevent infections in a patient with leukopenia (see nursing care plan on neutropenia [NCP 30-3]). If the platelet count falls to less than $50,000/\mu l$ (50×10^9/L), the patient must be assessed for signs of bleeding, and measures should be taken to prevent bleeding (see the nursing care plan on thrombocytopenia [NCP 30-2]). Platelet

transfusions may be necessary. RBC transfusions may also be indicated for treatment of symptomatic anemia.

Patient Teaching. Patient teaching is an extremely important part of the nurse's role related to chemotherapy. To decrease the fear and anxiety often associated with chemotherapy, the patient must be told what to expect during a course of treatment. The patient's attitude toward treatment should be explored so that any misconception or fear can be discussed. The patient must be told of the possible side effects of chemotherapy that may be experienced during treatment. Good nursing judgment is essential to determine the amount of information that the patient can assimilate. The patient must be reassured that this is a temporary situation and that she or he should be feeling better within a few weeks after chemotherapy is discontinued. The patient should also be informed that supportive care (e.g., antiemetics, antidiarrheals) will be provided as needed.

Management of Hair Loss. Many emotions are experienced and expressed when hair loss occurs, including anger, grief, embarrassment, and fear. For some persons, the loss of hair is one of the most stressful events experienced during the course of chemotherapy. Alopecia caused by the administration of chemotherapeutic agents is usually reversible. The degree and duration of hair loss depend on the type and dose of the chemotherapeutic agent, the duration of the treatment, and the nutritional status of the patient. Sometimes the hair grows back while the patient is still receiving chemotherapeutic agents, but generally the hair does not grow back until the agents are discontinued. Often the new hair has a different color and texture than the hair that was lost.

LATE EFFECTS OF RADIATION AND CHEMOTHERAPY

Cancer survivors are achieving long-term remission and survival rates because of advancements in treatment modalities. However, these forms of therapy (especially radiation and chemotherapy) may produce long-term sequelae termed *physiologic late effects* that occur months to years after cessation of therapy. Every body system can be affected to some extent by chemotherapy and radiation therapy. The effects of radiation on the body's tissues are caused by cellular hypoplasia of stem cells and alterations in the fine vasculature and fibroconnective tissues. In addition to the acute toxicities, chemotherapy can have long-term effects related to the loss of cells' proliferative reserve capacity. The additive effects of multiagent chemotherapy before, during, or after a course of radiotherapy can significantly increase the resulting physiologic late effects.

EVIDENCE-BASED PRACTICE
Anemia and Cancer

Clinical Problem
What is the effect of anemia on survival in patients with cancer?

Best Clinical Practice
- Anemia is associated with shorter survival times for patients with lung cancer, cervicouterine cancer, head and neck cancer, prostate cancer, lymphoma, and multiple myeloma.
- Anemia in cancer patients must be treated to decrease the risk of death from cancer.

Implications for Nursing Practice
- The patient should be frequently assessed during the treatment of cancer for clinical manifestations related to anemia and have hemoglobin and/or hemocrit levels done on a regular basis.
- The patient and family need to be taught about foods high in iron and other factors that will promote red blood cell production (see Chapter 30, Table 30-5).
- Drug therapy, including iron and erythropoietin, should be considered in the management of anemia in cancer patients.

Reference for Evidence
Caro J, Goss G: Anemia as an independent prognostic factor for survival in patients with cancer: a systematic, quantitative review, *Cancer* 91:2214, 2001.

The cancer survivor may also be at risk for leukemias and other secondary malignancies resulting from therapy for the primary cancer. However, the potential risk for developing a second malignancy does not contraindicate the use of cancer treatment. The overall risk of developing neoplastic complications is low, and the latency period may be long.

The cancer treatments most frequently implicated in causing secondary malignancy are the alkylating chemotherapeutic agents and high-dose radiation, which can induce cancers at the exposure site. The exact mechanism of oncogenesis secondary to radiation and chemotherapy remains unclear. It could be related to interactions between immunosuppressive factors, direct cellular damage, and carcinogenic effects along with other environmental carcinogens.

Acute leukemias occurring as secondary malignancies have been most widely reported after treatment for Hodgkin's disease, but they also occur in survivors of ovarian, lung, and breast cancers. Secondary malignancies other than leukemias include multiple myeloma after radiation therapy for breast cancer; non-Hodgkin's lymphoma after treatment for Hodgkin's disease; and cancers of the bladder, kidney, and ureters after the use of cyclophosphamide. Radiation therapy for breast, lung, ovarian, uterine, and thyroid cancers, non-Hodgkin's lymphoma, and Hodgkin's disease has been linked to secondary osteosarcoma of the rib, scapula, clavicle, humerus, sternum, ilium, and pelvis. Fibrosarcomas have been reported several years after radiation therapy for astrocytoma, glioblastoma, and pituitary adenoma. Unfortunately, secondary malignancies are usually resistant to therapy.

BIOLOGIC THERAPY

Biologic therapy is the fourth cancer treatment modality. **Biologic therapy** can be effective alone or in combination with surgery, radiotherapy, and chemotherapy. Biologic therapy, or biologic response modifier therapy, consists of agents that modify the relationship between the host and the tumor by altering the biologic response of the host to the tumor cells. Biologic agents may affect host-tumor response in three ways: (1) they have direct antitumor effects; (2) they restore, augment, or modulate host immune system mechanisms; and (3) they have other biologic effects, such as interfering with the cancer cells' ability to metastasize or differentiate.[27]

Interferons

Interferons are naturally occurring complex proteins of which there are three types: α-interferon, β-interferon, and γ-interferon. Interferons are cytokines that have antiviral, antiproliferative, and immunomodulatory properties (see Chapter 13, Tables 13-5 and 13-6). Interferons protect cells infected by viruses from attack by other viruses, and they inhibit replication of viral DNA (see Fig. 13-7). The antiproliferative effects of interferons are not completely understood. However, they have been shown to inhibit DNA and protein synthesis in tumor cells and to stimulate the expression of tumor-associated antigens on tumor cell surfaces, thus increasing the potential for an immune response against the tumor cell. Interferons modulate the immune response by their direct interaction with lymphocytes and monocytes or macrophages. They are also capable of mediating the function of other cytokines such as IL-2 and TNF. Interferons have also been shown to increase the cytotoxic activity and killing potential of NK cells.[27]

Because of the protein nature of interferons, they cannot be administered orally. Therefore they are administered intravenously, intramuscularly, subcutaneously, or intracavitarily. In addition, α-interferon is available as interferon alfa-2a (Roferon-A) and interferon alfa-2b (Intron-A). It is important to stress to the patient that these different brands of interferon are not interchangeable. If the patient begins to take one form of interferon, the brand of interferon being taken must not be changed unless recommended by the physician.

α-Interferon has been approved by the Food and Drug Administration (FDA) for the treatment of chronic myelogenous leukemia, hairy cell leukemia, Kaposi's sarcoma (KS), melanoma, genital warts (caused by papillomavirus), and hepatitis B and C. α-Interferons have also demonstrated effectiveness in the treatment of renal cell carcinoma, lymphomas, multiple myeloma, ovarian cancer, and carcinoid tumors. Clinical trials continue to investigate the use of interferons to treat malignancies.

The severity of side effects associated with interferons depends on the dose and route of administration. The most common side effects include flulike syndrome, which includes fever, chills, myalgias, and headaches. Additional side effects include fatigue, lethargy, depression, changes in cognitive function, anorexia, weight loss, bone marrow depression, and changes in liver function tests.

Interleukins

Many ILs have been identified (see Table 13-5), although not all are undergoing clinical investigation. The ILs are a family of biologic agents that perform a variety of functions. Most ILs induce a multitude of biologic activities resulting in the activation of the immune system or alteration in the functional capacity of cancer cells. Currently, many of the ILs are in the clinical or preclinical research phases of development for potential use in the treatment of cancer and other diseases. Aldesleukin (Proleukin), a recombinant form of IL-2, has been used in the treatment of metastatic renal cell carcinoma, advanced metastatic melanoma, acute myelogenous leukemia, and non-Hodgkin's lymphoma.[28]

IL-2 is a cytokine produced by T lymphocytes that can stimulate proliferation of T lymphocytes and activate NK cells. IL-2 also stimulates the release of other cytokines, including γ-interferon, TNF, IL-1, and IL-6. IL-2 can be administered by IV bolus, continuous infusion, subcutaneous injection, and peritoneal infusion. The agent can be administered alone and in combination with chemotherapeutic agents.

A major toxicity of IL-2 therapy is *capillary leak syndrome,* which occurs as a result of changes in capillary permeability and vascular tone. As a consequence of the increase in capillary permeability, fluids shift from intravascular to extravascular compartments. This causes intravascular fluid depletion. Manifestations of capillary leak syndrome can include hypotension, peripheral edema, ascites, interstitial pulmonary infiltrates, weight gain, and decreased systemic vascular resistance. Additional toxicities of IL-2 therapy include renal, cardiovascular, pulmonary, gastrointestinal, and integumentary toxicities; bone marrow suppression; and changes in cognitive function.

Monoclonal Antibodies

Monoclonal antibodies are antibodies or immunoglobulins produced by B lymphocytes that are capable of binding to specific target cells, including tumor cells. A large number of monoclonal antibodies (MoAbs) are currently being investigated for diagnostic and treatment capabilities. (Hybridoma technology for the production of MoAbs is described in Chapter 13.) The diagnostic use of MoAbs is primarily for the imaging of tumors to locate areas of metastatic disease and for laboratory studies.

MoAbs can be unconjugated or conjugated. Unconjugated MoAbs are used alone to directly attack tumor cells. Conjugated MoAbs are attached to agents such as radioisotopes, toxins, chemotherapeutic agents, and other biologic agents. The goal of this approach is for the antibody to deliver the MoAb directly to the targeted cancer cells for their ultimate destruction.

MoAbs have demonstrated limited effectiveness in treating lymphomas, acute and chronic lymphocytic leukemias, T cell leukemia, and ovarian, gastric, and colon cancers. Muromonab-CD3 (Orthoclone OKT-3) is a MoAb targeted to the CD3 receptor of human T cells and is used for the treatment of acute rejection in renal transplant patients. Satumomab pendetide (Onco Scint CR/OV) is used for the detection of colorectal and ovarian cancers. Rituximab (Rituxan) is a monoclonal antibody against the CD20 antigen on the surface of normal and malignant B lymphocytes and is used to treat non-Hodgkin's lymphoma.

The HER2/neu oncogene is overexpressed in certain cancers (especially breast cancers) and is associated with more aggressive disease and decreased survival. Trastuzumab (Herceptin) is a MoAb that binds to HER2 and inhibits the growth of breast cancer cells that overexpress the HER2 protein. Trastuzumab has been approved by the FDA for treatment of metastatic breast cancers that overexpress the HER2 oncogene.[29]

MoAbs are administered by the infusion method. Patients may experience infusion-related symptoms, which can include fever, chills, urticaria, mucosal congestion, nausea, diarrhea, and myalgias. There is also a risk, although rare, of anaphylaxis associated with the administration of MoAbs. This potential exists because most MoAbs are produced by mouse lymphocytes and thus represent a foreign protein to the human body. Onset of anaphylaxis can occur within 5 minutes of administration and can be a life-threatening event. Administration of the MoAb should be stopped immediately, an emergency code called, and 0.5 ml IV epinephrine 1:10,000 solution administered over 5 minutes. (See Chapter 13 for a discussion of nursing management of anaphylaxis.) Other toxicities of MoAbs can include capillary leak syndrome, hepatotoxicity, bone marrow depression, and central nervous system effects. Patients who receive traztuzumab may also experience cardiac dysfunction, especially when it is administered in higher doses or in combination with anthracycline antibiotics such as doxorubicin (Adriamycin).[29]

Hematopoietic Growth Factors

Colony-Stimulating Factors. Colony-stimulating factors (CSFs) are a family of glycoproteins produced by various cells. CSFs stimulate production, maturation, regulation, and activation of cells of the hematologic system. After release, CSFs attach to receptors on the cell surface of peripheral blood cells and hematopoietic precursors (precursors of mature blood cells). CSFs then stimulate production, maturation, release from the bone marrow, and functional ability of blood cells. The name of the CSF is based on the specific cell line it affects. These include granulocyte colony–stimulating factor (G-CSF), granulocyte-macrophage colony–stimulating factor (GM-CSF), macrophage colony–stimulating factor (M-CSF or CSF-1), and multicolony-stimulating factor (IL-3).

There are a number of potential clinical uses of CSFs. They may hasten recovery from bone marrow depression after stan-

dard and high-dose chemotherapy and bone marrow transplantation or decrease bone marrow suppression associated with chemotherapy administration. CSFs may also reestablish bone marrow function in aplastic anemia, myelodysplastic syndrome, and leukemia and may be effective in the management of sepsis.

G-CSF is available as filgrastim (Neupogen) for the treatment of neutropenia. Pegfilgrastim (Neulasta) is a longer-acting form of filgrastim. G-CSF stimulates the production and function of neutrophils. It can be administered subcutaneously or by IV infusion. The most commonly reported side effect of G-CSF therapy is medullary bone pain, which occurs most often in the lower back, pelvis, and sternum. This pain generally develops at the time the neutrophil count begins to recover and lasts for about 24 hours. The pain associated with G-CSF therapy is usually relieved with nonnarcotic analgesics.

GM-CSF is available as sargramostim (Leukine, Prokine) for the treatment of (1) neutropenia associated with bone marrow transplantation, (2) bone marrow transplant failure or delay in bone marrow engraftment, and (3) acute myelogenous leukemia after chemotherapy. GM-CSF stimulates the production and function of neutrophils, eosinophils, and monocytes. In addition, GM-CSF stimulates these cells to produce cytokines. GM-CSF can be administered either subcutaneously or by IV infusion. The most common side effects associated with GM-CSF administration include medullary bone pain (similar to the bone pain associated with G-CSF administration), leukocytosis, and eosinophilia.

IL-3 is a multipotential stimulator of hematopoietic stem cells. IL-3 has been shown to stimulate the growth of neutrophils, monocytes, eosinophils, basophils, and platelet cell lines. IL-3 is being investigated for the treatment of bone marrow failure and for its ability to enhance myeloid recovery after chemotherapy, radiotherapy, and bone marrow transplantation. M-CSF is also undergoing investigation for its potential role in cancer treatment.

Erythropoietin. Erythropoietin (EPO) is a CSF responsible for stimulating growth of the erythroid precursor cells that ultimately mature into red blood cells. EPO is normally made by the kidneys. EPO (Epogen) was initially approved by the FDA in 1987 for the management of chronic anemia associated with end-stage renal disease. In 1993 FDA approval was expanded to include the use of EPO (Procrit) for the management of chemotherapy-related anemia. Darbepoetin (Aranesp), a long-acting form of erythropoietin, is now available.

Oprelvekin. Oprelvekin (Neumega) is a platelet growth factor. It is indicated for the prevention of severe thrombocytopenia and the reduction of the need for platelet transfusions following myelosuppresive chemotherapy in patients with nonmyeloid malignancies who are at high risk for severe thrombocytopenia. Adverse effects are mild or moderate in severity, associated with fluid retention, and reversible after discontinuation of the drug. The most adverse events included peripheral edema, dyspnea, tachycardia, and conjunctiva redness. Papilledema and pulmonary edema have also been reported.

Toxic and Side Effects of Biologic Agents

The administration of one biologic agent usually induces the endogenous release of other biologic agents. The release and action of these biologic agents results in systemic immune and inflammatory responses. The toxicities and side effects of biologic agents are related to dose and schedule. Table 15-17 summarizes the potential side effects associated with specific biologic agents. Common side effects include constitutional flulike

TABLE 15-17 Side Effects of Biologic Therapy

INTERFERONS	INTERLEUKIN-2 (IL-2)	MONOCLONAL ANTIBODIES	GRANULOCYTE COLONY–STIMULATING FACTOR (G-CSF)	GRANULOCYTE-MACROPHAGE COLONY–STIMULATING FACTOR (GM-CSF)
		BIOLOGIC AGENT		
Flulike Syndrome Fever, chills, malaise, fatigue	Fever, chills, malaise, fatigue, myalgia	Fever, chills, fatigue, headache	Fever, chills, myalgias, headache	Fever, chills, myalgias, headache, fatigue
Central Nervous System Impaired concentration and memory, confusion, lethargy, somnolence, seizures	Disorientation, impaired concentration and memory, somnolence, severe anxiety and agitation			
Renal-Hepatic Proteinuria, increased transaminase levels	Oliguria; anuria; azotemia; increased BUN, serum creatinine, serum bilirubin, and liver enzymes; hypoalbuminemia, hepatomegaly			
Gastrointestinal Nausea, vomiting, diarrhea, anorexia	Nausea, vomiting, anorexia, diarrhea, stomatitis	Nausea		
Hematologic Leukopenia, thrombocytopenia, anemia	Anemia, thrombocytopenia, lymphopenia, eosinophilia			Leukocytosis, eosinophilia
Cardiovascular-Pulmonary Hypotension, tachycardia, arrhythmias, myocardial ischemia	Capillary leak syndrome, hypotension, tachycardia, arrhythmias, myocardial ischemia, rare myocardial infarction, pulmonary congestion	Cardiac dysfunction, pulmonary reactions (primarily with trastuzumab [Herceptin])		Dyspnea
Integumentary Alopecia, irritation at injection site	Diffuse, pruritic, erythematous rash, dry desquamation, inflammatory reaction at injection site		Generalized rash	Facial flushing, generalized rash, inflammation at injection site
Endocrine	Hypothyroidism; increased ACTH, cortisol, prolactin, growth hormone, and acute phase proteins		Generalized rash	
Miscellaneous Photophobia, impotence, decreased libido	Decreased libido, arthralgia	Allergic reactions, anaphylaxis	Bone pain	Bone pain, fluid retention

BUN, Blood urea nitrogen.

symptoms, including headache, fever, chills, myalgias, fatigue, malaise, weakness, photosensitivity, anorexia, and nausea. With interferons the flulike symptoms almost invariably appear. However, the severity of the flulike symptoms associated with interferon therapy generally decreases over time. Acetaminophen administered every 4 hours, as prescribed, often reduces the severity of the flulike syndrome. The patient is commonly premedicated with acetaminophen in an attempt to prevent or decrease the intensity of these symptoms. In addition, large amounts of fluids help decrease the symptoms.

Tachycardia and orthostatic hypotension are also commonly reported. IL-2 and monoclonal antibodies can cause capillary leak syndrome, which can result in pulmonary edema. Other toxic and side effects may involve the CNS, renal and hepatic systems, and cardiovascular system. These effects are found particularly with interferons and IL-2.

NURSING MANAGEMENT BIOLOGIC THERAPY

Some problems experienced by the patient receiving biologic therapy are different from those observed with more traditional forms of cancer therapy. For example, capillary leak syndrome and pulmonary edema are problems that require critical care nursing. These critical care requirements are new to many oncology nurses. Other problems, such as bone marrow depression and fatigue, are more familiar but exist at different levels of severity than those customarily associated with other forms of cancer therapy. Bone marrow depression occurring with biologic therapy administration is generally more transient and less severe than that observed with chemotherapy. Fatigue associated with biologic therapy can be so severe that it can constitute a dose-limiting toxicity.

Nursing interventions for flulike syndrome include the administration of acetaminophen before treatment and every 4 hours after treatment. Intravenous meperidine (Demerol) has been used to control the severe chills associated with some biologic agents. Other nursing measures include monitoring of vital signs and temperature, planning for periods of rest for the patient, and assisting with activities of daily living (ADLs).

A wide range of neurologic deficits have been observed with interferon and IL-2 therapy. The nature and extent of these problems have not been completely elucidated. However, these problems are understandably frightening to the patient and the family, who must be taught to observe for neurologic problems (e.g., confusion, memory loss, difficulty making decisions, insomnia), report their occurrence, and institute appropriate safety and support measures.

BONE MARROW AND STEM CELL TRANSPLANTATION

Bone marrow transplantation (BMT) has become an effective, lifesaving procedure for a number of malignant and nonmalignant diseases (Table 15-18). BMT allows for the safe use of very high doses of chemotherapy or radiation therapy to patients whose tumors have developed resistance or failed to respond to standard doses of chemotherapy and radiation. BMT offers hope to many patients with disease responsive to increased doses of systemic therapy.[30] BMT has become one of the most promising treatments for a number of cancers. In recent years there has been a dramatic increase in the number of BMT and transplant centers.

TABLE 15-18	Uses for Bone Marrow Transplantation	
MALIGNANT DISEASES	**NONMALIGNANT DISEASES**
Acute and chronic myelogenous leukemia	Sickle cell disease
Acute lymphocytic leukemia	Thalassemia
Myelodysplastic syndrome	Aplastic anemia
Hodgkin's disease	Immunodeficiency diseases
Non–Hodgkin's lymphoma	Severe autoimmune diseases
Multiple myeloma	
Breast cancer	
Testicular cancer	
Ovarian cancer	

Whether the diagnosis is a malignant or nonmalignant disease, the goal of BMT is cure. Cure rates are still low, but are steadily increasing. Even if there is no cure, most transplants result in a period of remission. BMT is an intensive procedure with many risks, and some patients die from complications of the BMT or from relapse of the original disease. Because it is a highly toxic therapy, the patient must weigh the significant risks of treatment-related death or treatment failure (relapse) with the hope of cure.

Types of Bone Marrow Transplants

Bone marrow transplants can be allogeneic, autologous, or syngeneic. In *allogeneic marrow transplantation* the infused bone marrow is acquired from a donor who has been determined to be human leukocyte antigen (HLA) matched to the recipient in terms of tissue typing. HLA typing involves testing WBCs to identify genetically inherited antigens common to both donor and recipient that are important in compatibility of transplanted tissue. (HLA tissue typing is discussed in Chapter 13.) Often this is a family member but may be an unrelated donor found through a bone marrow registry. The goal is to administer large doses of systemic therapy and then "rescue" the bone marrow through the engraftment and subsequent normal proliferation and differentiation of the donated marrow in the host. The most common indication for allogeneic transplant is leukemia.

In *autologous marrow transplantation* patients receive their own bone marrow. The aim of this approach is to enable patients to receive intensive chemotherapy or radiation while supporting them with their own bone marrow. In this type of BMT the patient's own marrow is removed, treated, stored, and reinfused. *Syngeneic marrow transplantation* involves obtaining stem cells from one identical twin and infusing them into the other. Identical twins have identical HLA types and are a perfect match.

Procedures

Harvest Procedures. Bone marrow can be "harvested" via a procedure conducted in the operating room using general or spinal anesthesia in which multiple bone marrow aspirations are carried out, usually from the iliac crest, but also from the sternum. The entire harvest procedure usually takes 1 to 2 hours, and the patient can be discharged following recovery. Following harvest the donor may experience pain at the collection site, which can be treated with mild analgesics. The donor's body will replace the bone marrow in a few weeks.

After harvest, autologous bone marrow may be treated (purged) to remove cancer cells. Many different pharmacologic, immunologic, physical, and chemical agents have been used for this purpose. The bone marrow is then frozen *(cryopreserved)* and stored until it is used for transplantation. In allogeneic transplants, the marrow can be harvested, processed, and infused into the recipient within a few hours of donation.

Preparative Regimens. In malignant diseases the goal of BMT is to rescue the marrow after the patient has received high doses of chemotherapy with or without radiation aimed at treating the underlying disease. Following harvesting of the marrow, the patient is given high-dose chemotherapy with or without radiation therapy. Total body radiation can be used for immunosuppression or to treat the disease.

After the therapy the marrow that was removed is thawed and given back to the patient through a needle in a vein to replace the destroyed marrow. The stem cells reconstitute, or "rescue," the recipient's hematopoietic system. Usually 2 to 4 weeks are required for the transplanted marrow to start producing hematopoietic blood cells. During this pancytopenic period it is critical for the patient to be in a protective isolation environment receiving supportive care. RBC and platelet transfusions usually are necessary to maintain circulating RBCs and platelets during this time.

Complications. Bacterial, viral, and fungal infections are common following BMT. Prophylactic antibiotic therapy may reduce their incidence. A potentially serious complication of allogeneic transplant is graft-versus-host disease. This occurs when the T lymphocytes from the donated marrow (graft) recognize the recipient (host) as foreign and begin to attack certain organs such as the skin, liver, and intestines. Graft-versus-host disease is discussed in Chapter 13.

Peripheral Stem Cell Transplantation

An alternative to the harvest procedure is *peripheral stem cell transplant* (PSCT). Peripheral or circulating stem cells are capable of repopulating the bone marrow. PSCT is a type of transplant that differs from BMT primarily in the stem cell collection method. Because there are fewer stem cells in the blood than in the bone marrow, mobilization of stem cells from the bone marrow into the peripheral blood can be done using chemotherapy or hematopoietic growth factors. Common growth factors that are used are GM-CSF and G-CSF. The donor's blood is collected via pheresis, in which the person is attached to a cell separator machine that removes peripheral stem cells and then returns the blood to the person. This procedure is called *leukapheresis* and usually takes 2 to 4 hours to complete. In autologous transplants the stem cells are purged to kill any cancer cells and then frozen and stored until used for transplantation. Although many of the same steps (harvesting, intensive chemotherapy, reinfusion) of BMT are used in PSCT, the hematologic recovery period in PSCT is shorter, and fewer, less severe complications are seen.[30]

Cord Blood Stem Cells

Umbilical cord blood is rich in hematopoietic stem cells, and successful allogeneic transplants have been performed using this source. Cord blood can be HLA typed and cryopreserved. A disadvantage of cord blood is the possibility of insufficient numbers of stem cells to permit transplant to adults.

GENE THERAPY

Gene therapy involves the transfer of exogenous genes (transgenes) into the cells of patients in an effort to correct the defective gene. The effect of gene therapy for cancer can be a temporary gene transfer with the additional goal of instigating an immune response to the transgene. The use of this new therapeutic approach for cancer is currently investigational. Several clinical trials are underway evaluating the safety, tolerability, and efficacy of gene therapy for malignancies such as melanoma, brain tumors, and mesothelioma.[31,32] (Gene therapy is discussed in Chapter 13.)

COMPLICATIONS RESULTING FROM CANCER

The patient may develop complications related to the continual growth of the malignancy or the side effects of treatment.

Nutritional Problems

Malnutrition. The patient with cancer often experiences protein and calorie malnutrition characterized by fat and muscle depletion. (Assessment of the degree of malnutrition is discussed in Chapter 39.) Foods suggested for increasing the protein intake to facilitate repair and regeneration of cells are presented in Table 15-19. High-caloric foods that provide energy and minimize weight loss are presented in Table 15-20. A sample high-caloric, high-protein diet is presented in Chapter 39, Table 39-14.

The nurse should suggest the need for a nutritional supplement to the health care provider as soon as a 5% weight loss is noted or if the patient has the potential for protein and caloric malnutrition. Albumin and prealbumin levels should be monitored. Once a 10 lb (4.5 kg) weight loss occurs, it is difficult to maintain the nutritional status. The patient can be taught to use nutritional supplements in place of milk when cooking or baking. Foods to which nutritional supplements can be easily added include scrambled eggs, pudding, custard, mashed potatoes, cereal, and cream sauces. Packages of instant breakfast can be used as indicated or sprinkled on cereals, desserts, and casseroles.[33]

If the malnutrition cannot be treated with dietary intake, it may be necessary to use enteral or parenteral nutrition as an adjunct nutritional measure.[34] (Enteral and parenteral nutrition are discussed in Chapter 39.)

Altered Taste Sensation. It is theorized that cancer cells release substances that resemble amino acids and stimulate the bitter taste buds. The patient may also experience an alteration in the sweet taste sensation, as well as in the sour and salty taste sensations. Meat may also taste bitter to the patient. At this time the physiologic basis of these varied taste alterations is unknown. The patient with an altered taste problem should be instructed to avoid foods that are disliked. Frequently the patient may feel compelled to eat certain foods because those foods are believed to be beneficial. The patient can be taught to experiment with spices and other seasoning agents in an attempt to mask the taste alterations that are occurring. Lemon juice, onion, mint, basil, and fruit juice marinades may improve the taste of certain meats and fish. Bacon bits, onion, and pieces of ham may enhance the taste of vegetables. An additional amount of a spice or seasoning agent is usually not an effective way to enhance the taste.

TABLE 15-19   Nutritional Therapy
Protein Foods with High Biologic Value

Milk

Whole milk (1 cup) = 9 g protein

Double-strength milk–1 quart of whole milk plus 1 cup of dried skim milk blended and chilled: 1 cup = 14 g protein

Milk shake–1 cup of ice cream plus 1 cup of milk = 15 g protein, 416 calories

Use evaporated milk, double-strength milk, or half-and-half to make casseroles, hot cereals, sauces, gravies, puddings, milk shakes, and soups

Yogurt (regular and frozen)–check labels and purchase brand with highest protein content: 1 cup = 10 g protein

Eggs

Egg = 6 g protein

Eggnog (1 cup) = 15.5 g protein

Add eggs to salads, casseroles, and sauces. Deviled eggs are especially well tolerated.

Desserts that contain eggs include angel food cake, sponge cake, custard, and cheesecake

Cheese

Cottage	½ cup	15 g protein
American	1 slice	3 g protein
Cheddar	1 slice	6 g protein
Cream	1 tbs	1 g protein

Use cheese in a sandwich or as a snack.

Add cheese to salads, casseroles, sauces, and baked potatoes.

Cheese spread with crackers is a wholesome snack that can be made and stored in the refrigerator for easy accessibility.

Meat, Poultry, Fish

Beef	3 oz	approx. 21 g protein
Pork	3 oz	approx. 19 g protein
Chicken	½ breast	approx. 26 g protein
Fish	3 oz	approx. 30 g protein
Tuna fish	6½ oz	approx. 44.5 g protein

Add meat, poultry, and fish to salads, casseroles, and sandwiches.

Add strained and junior baby meats to soups and casseroles.

Cocktail weiners or deviled ham on crackers are wholesome snacks. These snacks can be made and stored in the refrigerator for easy accessibility.

TABLE 15-20   Nutritional Therapy
High-Caloric Foods

Mayonnaise	1 tbs	=	101 cal
Butter or margarine	1 tsp	=	35 cal
Sour cream	1 tbs	=	72 cal
Peanut butter	1 tbs	=	94 cal
Whipped cream	1 tbs	=	53 cal
Corn oil	1 tbs	=	119 cal
Jelly	1 tbs	=	49 cal
Ice cream	1 cup	=	256 cal
Honey	1 tbs	=	64 cal

Infection

Infection can be a cause of death in the patient with cancer. The usual sites of infection include the lungs, GU system, mouth, rectum, peritoneal cavity, and blood (septicemia). Infection occurs as a result of the ulceration and necrosis caused by the tumor, compression of vital organs by the tumor, and neutropenia caused by the disease process or the treatment of cancer. Outpatients with risk for neutropenia should be instructed to call with a temperature of 100.5° F (38° C) or greater. Assessment most often includes signs and symptoms of fever, determination of possible etiology, and complete blood count.

Many patients are neutropenic when an infection develops. In these individuals, infection may cause significant morbidity and may be rapidly fatal if not treated promptly. The classic manifestations of infection are not often present in a patient with neutropenia and a depressed immune system. (Neutropenia is discussed in Chapter 30.)

Oncologic Emergencies

Oncologic emergencies are life-threatening emergencies that can occur as a result of cancer or cancer treatment. These emergencies can be obstructive, metabolic, or infiltrative.

Obstructive Emergencies. Obstructive emergencies are primarily caused by tumor obstruction of an organ or blood vessel. Obstructive emergencies include superior vena cava syndrome, spinal cord compression syndrome, third space syndrome, and intestinal obstruction.

Superior vena cava syndrome. *Superior vena cava syndrome* results from obstruction of the superior vena cava by a tumor. The clinical manifestations include facial edema, periorbital edema, distention of veins of the neck and chest, headache, and seizures. A mediastinal mass is often visible on chest x-ray. The most common causes are Hodgkin's disease, non-Hodgkin's lymphoma, and lung cancer. Superior vena cava syndrome is considered a serious medical problem, and management usually involves radiation therapy to the site of obstruction and treatment of the primary tumor. Chemotherapy may be administered concurrently with the radiation therapy.

Spinal cord compression. *Spinal cord compression* is the result of the presence of a malignant tumor in the epidural space of the spinal cord. The most common primary tumors that produce this problem are breast, lung, prostate, GI, melanoma, and renal tumors. Lymphomas also pose a risk if diseased lymph tissue invades the epidural space. The manifestations are back pain that is intense, localized, and persistent, accompanied by vertebral tenderness and aggravated by the Valsalva maneuver; motor weakness and dysfunction; sensory paresthesia and loss; and autonomic dysfunction. One of the clinical symptoms that reflect autonomic dysfunction is a reported change in bowel or bladder function. Radiation therapy is used for the patient with slowly progressive neurologic deficits and radiosensitive tumors. Surgery is usually recommended for the patient with rapidly progressive neurologic signs, especially if the tumors are relatively radioresistant. Activity limitations and pain management are important nursing interventions.

Third space syndrome. *Third space syndrome* involves a shifting of fluid from the vascular space to the interstitial space that primarily occurs secondary to extensive surgical procedures, biologic therapy, or septic shock. Initially patients exhibit signs of hypovolemia, including hypotension, tachycardia, low central venous pressure, and decreased urine output. Treatment includes fluid, electrolyte, and plasma protein replacement. During recovery hypervolemia can occur, resulting in hypertension, elevated central venous pressure, weight gain, and shortness of breath. Treatment generally involves reduction in fluid administration and fluid balance monitoring.

Intestinal obstruction. Chapter 41 contains a complete discussion of intestinal obstruction.

Metabolic Emergencies.
Metabolic emergencies are caused by the production of ectopic hormones directly from the tumor or secondary to cancer treatment. Ectopic hormones arise from tissues that do not normally produce these hormones. Cancer cells return to a more embryologic form, thus allowing the stored potential of the cells to become evident. Metabolic emergencies include syndrome of inappropriate antidiuretic hormone, hypercalcemia, tumor lysis syndrome, septic shock, and disseminated intravascular coagulation.

Syndrome of inappropriate antidiuretic hormone. Syndrome of inappropriate antidiuretic hormone (SIADH) results from abnormal or sustained production of antidiuretic hormone (ADH) (see Chapter 48). SIADH occurs most frequently in carcinoma of the lung but can also occur in cancer of the pancreas, duodenum, brain, esophagus, colon, ovary, prostate, bronchus, and nasopharynx; leukemia; mesothelioma; reticulum cell sarcoma; Hodgkin's disease; thymoma; and lymphosarcoma. Cancer cells in these tumors are actually able to manufacture, store, and release ADH. The chemotherapeutic agents vincristine and cyclophosphamide (Cytoxan) also stimulate the release of ADH from the pituitary or tumor cells. Symptoms of SIADH include weight gain, weakness, anorexia, nausea, vomiting, personality changes, seizures, and coma. Treatment of SIADH includes fluid restriction and, in severe cases, IV administration of 3% sodium chloride solution.[35]

Hypercalcemia. Hypercalcemia can occur in the presence of cancer that involves the bone such as in metastatic disease of the bone or multiple myeloma, or when a parathyroid hormone–like substance is secreted by cancer cells in the absence of bony metastasis. Hypercalcemia resulting from malignancies that have metastasized occurs most frequently in patients with lung, breast, kidney, colon, ovarian, or thyroid cancer. Hypercalcemia resulting from secretion of parathyroid hormone–like substance occurs most frequently in hypernephromas; squamous cell carcinoma of the lung; head and neck, cervical, and esophageal cancer; lymphomas; and leukemia. Immobility and dehydration can contribute to or exacerbate hypercalcemia.

The primary manifestations of hypercalcemia include apathy, depression, fatigue, muscle weakness, electrocardiogram changes, polyuria and nocturia, anorexia, nausea, and vomiting. Serum levels of calcium in excess of 12 mg/dl (3 mmol/L) can be life threatening. Chronic hypercalcemia can result in nephrocalcinosis and irreversible renal failure. The long-term treatment of hypercalcemia is aimed at the primary disease. Acute hypercalcemia is treated by hydration (3 L/day), diuretic (particularly loop diuretics) administration, and a bisphosphonate, a drug that inhibits the action of osteoclasts. Infusion of the bisphosphonate pamidronate (Aredia) is the treatment of choice.[35]

Tumor lysis syndrome. Acute *tumor lysis syndrome* (TLS) is a metabolic complication that occurs in some patients with cancer and is frequently triggered by chemotherapy. It results from the rapid destruction of a large number of tumor cells, which can cause fatal biochemical changes. TLS is often associated with tumors that have high growth rates and are sensitive to the effects of chemotherapy. If not identified and treated quickly, TLS can result in acute renal failure.

The four hallmark signs of TLS are hyperuricemia, hyperphosphatemia, hyperkalemia, and hypocalcemia. TLS usually occurs within the first 24 to 48 hours after the initiation of chemotherapy and may persist for approximately 5 to 7 days. The primary goal of TLS management is preventing renal failure and severe electrolyte imbalances. The primary treatment includes increasing urine production using hydration therapy and decreasing uric acid concentrations using allopurinol.[36]

Septic shock and disseminated intravascular coagulation. Septic shock is discussed in Chapter 65, and disseminated intravascular coagulation is discussed in Chapter 30.

Infiltrative Emergencies.
Infiltrative emergencies occur when malignant tumors infiltrate major organs or secondary to cancer therapy. The most common infiltrative emergencies are cardiac tamponade and carotid artery rupture.

Cardiac tamponade. Cardiac tamponade results from fluid accumulation in the pericardial sac, constriction of the pericardium by tumor, or pericarditis secondary to radiation therapy to the chest. Manifestations include a heavy feeling over the chest, shortness of breath, tachycardia, cough, dysphagia, hiccups, hoarseness, nausea, vomiting, excessive perspiration, decreased level of consciousness, pulsus paradoxus, distant or muted heart sounds, and extreme anxiety. Emergency management is aimed at reduction of fluid around the heart and includes surgical establishment of a pericardial window or an indwelling pericardial catheter. Supportive therapy includes administration of oxygen therapy, intravenous hydration, and vasopressor therapy.

Carotid artery rupture. Rupture of the carotid artery occurs most frequently in patients with cancer of the head and neck secondary to invasion of the arterial wall by tumor or erosion following surgery or radiation therapy. Bleeding can manifest as minor oozing or spurting of blood in the case of a "blowout" of the artery. In the presence of a blowout, pressure should be applied to the site with a finger. Intravenous fluid and blood products are administered in an attempt to stabilize the patient for surgery. Surgical management involves ligation of the carotid artery above and below the rupture site and reduction of local tumor.

MANAGEMENT OF CANCER PAIN

Patients with cancer commonly experience pain, which can be caused by both the disease and its treatment. Undertreatment of cancer pain is common.[37,38]

Data such as vital signs and patient behaviors are not reliable indicators of pain, especially long-standing, chronic pain. Therefore it is essential that every patient with cancer be assessed for

TABLE 15-21 **Cancer Pain Assessment**

Location	Where is the pain? (There may be more than one place.)
Intensity	How bad is the pain? (See Chapter 9 for rating scales.)
Quality	What does the pain feel like? (See Chapter 9 for descriptors.)
Pattern	Has the pain changed? What makes the pain better or worse?
Relief measures	What do you do to control your pain? Are medications used? Does the relief measures help much? How much?

Modified from Agency for Health Care Policy and Research: *Patient guide, clinical practice guideline, managing cancer pain*, Rockville, MD, 1994, US Department of Health and Human Services.

pain by first asking the question "Do you have pain?" If the patient's self-report is affirmative, further data are obtained and documented initially and at regular intervals on the location and intensity of the pain, what it feels like, and how it is relieved. Patterns of change also should be assessed. The patient report should always be believed and accepted as the primary source of assessment data. Table 15-21 presents assessment questions that may facilitate this data collection.

Drug therapy, including nonsteroidal antiinflammatory drugs, opioids, and adjuvant pain medications, should be used following the World Health Organization analgesic ladder (Fig. 15-20). Analgesic medications should be given on a regular schedule, around the clock, with additional doses as needed for breakthrough pain. Oral administration of the medication is preferred. It is important to remember that with opioid drugs such as morphine the appropriate dose is whatever is necessary to control the pain with the least side effects. Principles of patient-controlled analgesia should also be followed. Fear of addiction is not warranted but must be addressed as

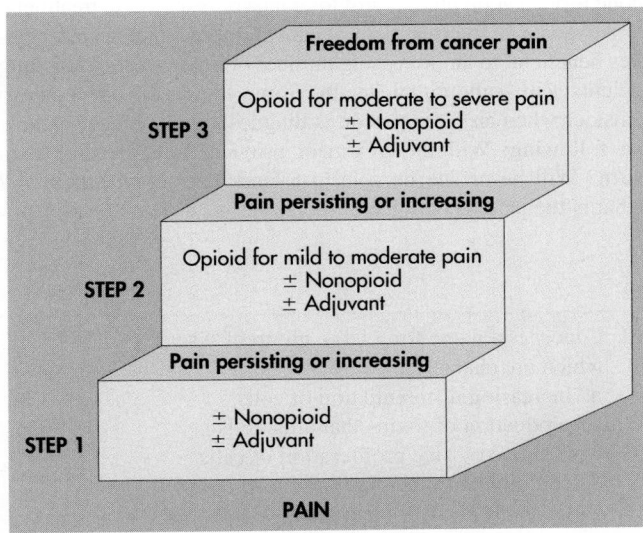

FIG. 15-20 The World Health Organization (WHO) three-step analgesic ladder.

part of patient teaching relevant to pain control, since it is a significant barrier for both the patient and the nurse to appropriate pain management.[39]

Nonpharmacologic interventions, including relaxation therapy and imagery, can be effectively used to manage pain (see Chapter 8). Additional strategies to relieve pain are discussed in Chapter 9.

PSYCHOLOGIC SUPPORT

Psychologic support of the patient is an important aspect of cancer care.[40] Because of the effectiveness of cancer treatment, many patients with cancer are cured or their disease is controlled for long periods. In light of this trend in cancer treatment, emphasis must be placed on maintaining an optimal quality of life after the diagnosis of cancer. A positive attitude of patient, family, and health care providers toward cancer and cancer treatment has a significant positive impact on the quality of life that the patient experiences. A positive attitude may also influence the prognosis of the patient with cancer.

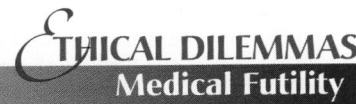

ETHICAL DILEMMAS
Medical Futility

Situation

A 65-year-old Jewish woman has breast cancer with metastasis to the liver and bone. The family asks the nurse why their mother is not receiving chemotherapy. In addition, they want to make certain that she will be resuscitated should her heart stop. They are aware of her diagnosis and that she may have less than 1 month to live. The nurse was told in morning rounds that the woman does not want any treatment that would prolong her life.

Important Points for Consideration

- If the patient is competent, the patient is legally and ethically the decision maker regarding his or her own care in consultation with the patient's family and the health care team as desired.
- Members of the health care team have no obligation to provide care that is medically futile. Care that is futile may be inappropriate, prolong dying, or provide little or no benefit to the patient.
- Palliative care is health care that would provide comfort, control pain, reduce symptoms, or improve the quality of her remaining life, as defined by the patient.
- Patients or families do not have a right to demand treatment that offers no clear benefit to the patient.
- The nurse should work in collaboration with other members of the health care team to have discussions with the family members, ease the acceptance of their mother's diagnosis, incorporate their mother's goals into the plan of care, discuss a do-not-resuscitate (DNR) order and a referral to hospice, and plan for her eventual death.

Critical Thinking Questions

1. How can the nurse help the patient communicate her wishes to her family?
2. How can the nurse and the health care team help the family plan end-of-life care that incorporates the wishes of their mother?

The diagnosis of cancer is viewed by most persons as a crisis. The most common fears experienced by the patient with cancer include disfigurement, dependency, pain, emaciation, financial depletion, abandonment, and death.

To cope with these fears, the patient with cancer will use and experience different behavioral patterns: shock, anger, denial, bargaining, depression, helplessness, hopelessness, rationalization, acceptance, and intellectualization. These behavioral patterns may occur at any time during the process of cancer. However, some patterns appear to occur more frequently or at a greater intensity at certain specific stages of the disease process. The following factors may determine how the patient will cope with the diagnosis of cancer:

1. *Ability to cope with stressful events in the past* (e.g., loss of job, major disappointment). By simply asking how the patient has coped with stressful events, the nurse can gain an understanding of the patient's coping patterns, the effectiveness of the usual coping patterns, and the usual coping time framework.

2. *Availability of significant others.* The patient who has effective support systems tends to cope more effectively than the patient who does not have a meaningful, available support system.

3. *Ability to express feelings and concerns.* The patient who is able to express feelings and needs and who seeks and asks for help appears to cope more effectively than the patient who internalizes feelings and needs.

4. *Age at the time of diagnosis.* Age determines the coping strategies to a great degree. For example, a young mother with cancer may have concerns that differ from those of a 70-year-old woman with cancer.

5. *Extent of disease.* Cure or control of the disease process is usually easier to cope with than the reality of terminal illness.

6. *Disruption of body image.* Disruption of the body image (e.g., radical neck dissection, alopecia, mastectomy) may intensify the psychologic impact of cancer.

7. *Presence of symptoms.* Symptoms such as fatigue, nausea, diarrhea, and pain may intensify the psychologic impact of cancer.

8. *Past experience with cancer.* If past experiences with cancer have been negative, the patient will probably view the present status as negative.

9. *Attitude associated with the cancer.* A patient who feels in control and has a positive attitude about cancer and cancer treatment is better able to cope with the diagnosis and treatment of cancer than the patient who feels hopeless, helpless, and out of control.

To facilitate the development of a hopeful attitude about cancer and to support the patient and the family during the various stages of the process of cancer, the nurse should do the following:

1. Be available and continue to be available, especially during difficult times.
2. Exhibit a caring attitude.
3. Listen actively to fears and concerns.
4. Provide relief from distressing symptoms.
5. Provide essential information regarding cancer and cancer care.
6. Maintain a relationship based on trust and confidence; be open, honest, and caring in the approach.
7. Use touch to exhibit caring. A squeeze of the hand or a hug may at times be more effective than words.
8. Assist the patient in setting realistic, reachable short-term and long-term goals.
9. Assist the patient in maintaining usual lifestyle patterns.
10. Maintain hope, which is the key to effective cancer care. Hope varies, depending on the status of the patient—hope that the symptoms are not serious, hope that the treatment is curative, hope for independence, hope for relief of pain, hope for a longer life, or hope for a peaceful death. Hope provides control over what is occurring and is the basis of a positive attitude toward cancer and cancer care.

Organizations and journals available as resources for the nurse are listed in the Resources section at the end of this chapter. In many cities, local units of the American Cancer Society provide a wide variety of services.

■ Gerontologic Considerations: Cancer

Cancer is a disease of aging. Most cancers occur in people over age 65. Cancer is the leading cause of death in people 65 to 74 years of age.[41] Clinical manifestations of cancer in older adults may be mistakenly attributed to age-related changes and ignored by the person.

Older adults are particularly vulnerable to the complications of both cancer and cancer therapy. This is due to their decline in physiologic functioning, social and emotional resources, and cognitive function.[42] The functional status of an older adult should be taken into consideration when selecting a treatment plan. Age alone is not a good predictor of tolerance or response to treatment.

Advances in the treatment of cancer are making cancer therapies beneficial to an increasing number of older adults, including patients with suboptimal health. Some important questions to consider when an older person is diagnosed with cancer include the following: Will the treatment provide more benefits than harm? Will he or she be able to tolerate the treatment safely? What is the patient's choice of therapy?[42] ■

REVIEW QUESTIONS

The number of the question corresponds to the same-numbered objective at the beginning of the chapter.

1. Trends in the incidence and death rates of cancer include the fact that
   a. lung cancer is the most common type of cancer in men.
   b. breast cancer is the leading cause of cancer deaths in women.
   c. a higher percentage of women than men have lung cancer.
   d. African Americans have a higher death rate from cancer than whites.

2. Cancer is a name for a large group of diseases, all of which are characterized by
   a. increasing differentiation of cells.
   b. production of toxins that alter cells.
   c. rapid, explosive proliferation of cells.
   d. cell growth that escapes normal control.

REVIEW QUESTIONS—cont'd

3. A characteristic of the stage of progression in the development of cancer is
   a. oncogenic viral transformation of target cells.
   b. a reversible steady growth facilitated by carcinogens.
   c. a period of latency before clinical detection of cancer.
   d. proliferation of cancer cells in spite of host control mechanisms.

4. The primary protective role of the immune system related to malignant cells is
   a. surveillance for cells with tumor-associated antigens.
   b. binding with free antigen released by malignant cells.
   c. production of blocking factors that immobilize cancer cells.
   d. responding to a new set of antigenic determinants on cancer cells.

5. The primary difference between benign and malignant neoplasms is the
   a. rate of cell proliferation.
   b. site of malignant tumor.
   c. requirements for cellular nutrients.
   d. characteristic of tissue invasiveness.

6. Important nursing roles related to prevention and detection of cancer include
   a. instructing people to eat low-fiber, refined-carbohydrate diets.
   b. instructing persons on ways to increase capacity to cope with stress.
   c. teaching people to have annual screening tests for all detectable cancer sites.
   d. using people's natural fear of cancer to motivate changes in unhealthy lifestyles.

7. The goals of cancer treatment are based on the principle that
   a. surgery is the single most effective treatment for cancer.
   b. initial treatment is always directed toward cure of the cancer.
   c. a combination of treatment modalities is effective for controlling many cancers.
   d. although cancer cure is rare, quality of life can be increased with treatment modalities.

8. The nurse explains to a patient undergoing brachytherapy of the cervix that she
   a. must undergo simulation to locate the treatment area.
   b. requires the use of radioactive precautions during nursing care.
   c. may experience desquamation of the skin on the abdomen and upper legs.
   d. requires shielding of the ovaries during treatment to prevent ovarian damage.

9. The most effective method of administering a chemotherapeutic agent that is a vesicant is to
   a. give it orally.
   b. give it intraarterially.
   c. use an Ommaya reservoir.
   d. use a central venous access device.

10. Stomatitis, a common side effect of chemotherapeutic agents, occurs because the
    a. site of the malignancy is near the oral cavity.
    b. general health of the patient with cancer is poor.
    c. chemotherapeutic drugs have an external, local, and irritating effect.
    d. rapidly dividing cells of the mucous membranes of the mouth are being destroyed.

11. The nurse teaches the patient receiving IL-2 about the drug based on the knowledge that this agent is administered primarily for the purpose of
    a. stimulating the immune system.
    b. inhibiting DNA and protein synthesis in tumor cells.
    c. decreasing the antigenic expression of antigens on tumor cell surfaces.
    d. preventing bone marrow suppression associated with chemotherapy administration.

12. The nurse counsels the patient receiving radiation therapy or chemotherapy that
    a. effective birth control methods should be used for the rest of the patient's life.
    b. if nausea and vomiting occur during treatment, the treatment plan will be modified.
    c. following successful treatment a return to the person's previous functional level can be expected.
    d. the cycle of fatigue-depression-fatigue that may occur during treatment can be reduced by restricting activity.

13. An inappropriate nursing intervention to promote nutrition in the patient with cancer is
    a. providing bland, pureed food because the person's taste sensation is altered.
    b. providing increased protein for normal cell recovery and immune system function.
    c. encouraging the patient to eat a high-calorie, high-protein snack every few hours to prevent weight loss.
    d. alerting the physician that nutritional supplements may be needed when the patient has a 10 lb weight loss.

14. Syndrome of inappropriate ADH (SIADH) that occurs in certain types of cancer is primarily due to
    a. autoimmune reaction.
    b. gram-negative septicemia.
    c. invasiveness of cancer cells.
    d. ectopic hormonal production.

15. A patient has recently been diagnosed with early stages of breast cancer. Which of the following is most appropriate for the nurse to focus on?
    a. maintaining patient's hope
    b. preparing a will and advance directives
    c. discussing replacement child care for patient's children
    d. discussing the patient's past experiences with her grandmother's cancer

REFERENCES

1. *Cancer facts and figures,* Atlanta, 2002, American Cancer Society.
2. DeVita VT, et al: *Cancer: principles and practice of oncology,* ed 6, Philadelphia, 2001, Lippincott-Raven.
3. Rigel DS: Malignant melanoma: prevention, early detection, and treatment in the 21st century, *CA Cancer J Clin* 50:4, 2000.
4. LeMarbre PJ, Groenwald SL: Biology of cancer. In Groenwald SL et al, editors: *Cancer nursing: principles and practice,* ed 4, Boston, 1997, Jones & Bartlett.
5. Abeloff MD: *Clinical oncology,* New York, 2000, Churchill Livingstone.
6. Ross DW: Cancer: the emerging molecular biology, *Hosp Pract* 35:63, 2000.
7. Loud JT et al: Applications of advances in molecular biology and genomics to clinical cancer care, *Cancer Nurs* 25:110, 2002.
8. Fidler I, Kerbel R, Ellis L: Biology of cancer: angiogenesis. In Devita V et al, editors: *Cancer principles and practice of oncology,* ed 6, Philadelphia, 2001, Lippincott-Raven.
9. Davis ID: An overview of cancer immunotherapy, *Immunol Cell Biol* 78:179, 2000.
10. Kobayashi A et al: Recent developments in understanding the immune response to human papilloma virus infection and cervical neoplasia, *Oncol Nurs Forum* 27:643, 2000.
11. Kaplan H: Historic milestones in radiobiology and radiation therapy, *Semin Oncol* 4:479, 1979.
12. Stein J: Some observations of the history of irradiation therapy, *Endocur Hyperthermia Oncology* 1:59, 1985.
13. Iwamoto R: Radiation therapy. In Otto S, editor: *Oncology nursing,* ed 4, St Louis, 2001, Mosby.
14. Hellman S: Principles of cancer management: radiation therapy. In DeVita V et al, editors: *Cancer principles and practice of oncology,* ed 6, Philadelphia, 2001, Raven.
15. Withers HR: Biologic basis of radiation therapy. In Perez C, Brady L, editors: *Principles and practice of radiation oncology,* ed 3, Philadelphia, 1998, Lippincott.
16. Buschel P, Barton-Burke M, Winningham M: Treatment: an overview. In Winningham M, Barton-Burke M, editors: *Fatigue in cancer,* Sudbury, 2000, Jones & Bartlett.
17. Winningham M: Walking program for people with cancer: getting started, *Cancer Nurs* 4:270, 1991.
18. Mock V et al: Effects of exercise on fatigue, physical functioning and emotional distress during radiation for breast cancer, *Oncol Nurs Forum* 24:991, 1997.
19. Rosenzweig M: Taste alterations. In Yasko J, editor: *Nursing management of symptoms associated with chemotherapy,* ed 5, West Conshohocken, Pa, Meniscus Limited, 2001.
20. Miller M: Oral care for patients with cancer: a review of the literature, *Cancer Nurs* 24: 241, 2001.
21. Worthington HV: Interventions for treating oral mucositis for patients with cancer receiving treatment, *Cochrane Library* 1, 2002.
22. Shell J: Impact of cancer on sexuality. In Otto S, editor: *Oncology nursing,* ed 4, St Louis, 2001, Mosby.
23. Fishman M, Mrozek-Orlowski M: *Cancer chemotherapy guidelines and recommendations for practice,* ed 2, Pittsburgh, 1999, Oncology Nursing Society, Oncology Nursing Press.
24. Bender CM: Nursing implications of antineoplastic therapy. In Itano J, Taoka K, editors: *The core curriculum for oncology nursing practice,* ed 3, Philadelphia, 1997, WB Saunders.
25. Otto S: Chemotherapy. In Otto S, editor: *Oncology nursing,* ed 4, St Louis, 2001, Mosby.
26. Kosier M, Minkler P: Nursing management of patients with an implanted Ommaya reservoir, *Clin J Oncol Nurs* 3:63, 1999.
27. Appel C: Biotherapy. In Otto S, editor: *Oncology nursing,* ed 4, St Louis, 2001, Mosby.
28. Moldawer N: The promise of recombinant interleukin-2, *Am J Nurs* 100:35, 2000.
29. Weiner L, Adams G, Von Mehren M: Therapeutic monoclonal antibodies: General principles. In DeVita V et al, editors: *Cancer principles and practice of oncology,* ed 6, Philadelphia, 2001, Lippincott-Raven.
30. Keller C: Bone marrow and stem cell transplantation. In Otto S, editor: *Oncology nursing,* ed 4, St Louis, 2001, Mosby.
31. Fibison WJ: Gene therapy, *Nurs Clin North Am* 35:757, 2000.
32. Amor D: Gene therapy: principles and potential applications, *Aust Fam Physician* 30: 953, 2001.
33. Brown J et al: Nutrition during and after cancer treatment: a guide for informed choices by cancer survivors, *CA Cancer J Clin* 51:15, 2001.
34. Whitman M: The starving patient: supportive care for people with cancer, *Clin J Oncol Nurs* 4:3, 1999.
35. Myers M: Oncologic complications in oncology nursing. In Otto S, editor: *Oncology nursing,* ed 4, St Louis, 2001, Mosby.
36. Ezzone SA: Tumor lysis syndrome, *Semin Oncol Nurs* 15:202, 1999.
37. Fortner BV: A survey of pain-related hospitalizations, emergency department visits, and physician office visits reported by cancer patients with and without history of breakthrough pain, *J Pain* 3:38, 2002.
38. de Wit R: Assessment of pain cognitions in cancer patient with chronic pain, *J Pain Symptom Manage* 22:911, 2001.
39. Cherny NI: The management of cancer pain, *CA Cancer J Clin* 50:70, 2000.
40. Shell J, Kirsch S: Psychosocial issues outcomes and quality of life. In Otto S, editor: *Oncology nursing,* ed 4, St Louis, 2001, Mosby.
41. Extermann M: Cancer in the older patient: a geriatric approach, *Ann Long-Term Care* 10:49, 2002.
42. Balducci L, Beghe C: Management of cancer in the older person, *Clin Geriatrics* 10:54, 2002.

RESOURCES

American Association for Cancer Education (AACE)
www.aaceonline.com/
American Cancer Society
1599 Clifton Road NE
Atlanta, GA 30329
800-ACS-2345 or 404-320-3333
www.cancer.org
American Institute for Cancer Research
1759 R Street NW
Washington, DC 20009
800-843-8114 or 202-328-7744
Fax: 202-328-7226
www.aicr.org
American Society of Clinical Oncology (ASCO)
1900 Duke Street, Suite 200
Alexandria, VA 22314
703-299-0150
Fax: 703-299-1044
www.asco.org/
Association of Community Cancer Centers (ACCC)
11600 Nebel Street, Suite 201
Rockville, MD 20852-2557
301-984-9496
Fax: 301-770-1949
www.accc-cancer.org/
Canadian Cancer Society
10 Alcorn Avenue, Suite 200
Toronto, Ontario M4V 3B1
Canada
416-961-7223
Cancer Care, Inc.
275 Seventh Avenue
New York, NY 10001
800-813-HOPE or 212-712-8080
Fax: 212-712-8495
www.cancercare.org/
Cancer Federation, Inc.
PO Box 1298
Banning, CA 92220
909-849-4325
www.cancerfed.com/
Cancer Guide
http://cancerguide.org/

Cancer Hotline
800-525-3777
800-638-6070 (Alaska)
800-636-5700 (District of Columbia)
808-524-1234 (Hawaii, call collect)

Cancer Information Service: 888-939-3333
Fax: 416-961-4189
www.cancer.ca

Cancer Information Service (CIS), a program of the National Cancer Institute
800-4-CANCER
http://cis.nci.nih.gov/

Cancer News on the Net
www.cancernews.com

International Society of Nurses in Cancer Care
ISNCC Secretariat
PO Box 297
Macclesfield
Cheshire SK11 7FZ
UK
44 (0) 1625-428-192
Fax: 44 (0) 1625-428-128
www.isncc.org/

International Union Against Cancer
3 rue du Conseil General
1205 Geneva
Switzerland
41-22-809-18-11
www.uicc.ch/

Memorial Sloan-Kettering Cancer Center
1275 York Avenue
New York, NY 10021
212-639-2000
www.mskcc.org/

National Cancer Institute
NCI Public Inquiries Office
Suite 3036A
6116 Executive Boulevard, MSC8322
Bethesda, MD 20892-8322
800-4-CANCER or 301-496-4907
Fax: 301-402-0212
www.nci.nih.gov/

National Coalition for Cancer Survivorship (NCCS)
1010 Wayne Avenue, Suite 770
Silver Spring, MD 20910
877-NCCS-YES or 301-650-9127
Fax: 301-565-9670
www.canceradvocacy.org/

National Foundation for Cancer Research
4600 East West Highway, Suite 525
Bethesda, MD 20814
800-321-CURE or 301-654-1250
Fax: 301-654-5824
www.researchforacure.com/

OncoLink (cancer information site)
www.oncolink.upenn.edu

Oncology Nursing Society
125 Enterprise Drive
Pittsburgh, PA 15275-1214
412-859-6100
Fax: 877-369-5497
www.ons.org

Society of Gynecologic Oncologists
401 North Michigan Avenue
Chicago, IL 60611
312-644-6610
www.sgo.org/

For additional Internet resources, see the website for this book at *http://evolve.elsevier.com/Lewis/medsurg/.*

CHAPTER *16*
Fluid, Electrolyte, and Acid–Base Imbalances

Lisa B. Malick

LEARNING OBJECTIVES

1. Describe the composition of the major body fluid compartments.
2. Define the following processes involved in the regulation of movement of water and electrolytes between the body fluid compartments: diffusion, osmosis, filtration, hydrostatic pressure, oncotic pressure, and osmotic pressure.
3. Describe the etiology, laboratory diagnostic findings, clinical manifestations, and nursing and collaborative management of the following disorders:
   a. Water excess and deficit
   b. Sodium and volume imbalances: hypernatremia and hyponatremia
   c. Potassium imbalance: hyperkalemia and hypokalemia

   d. Magnesium imbalance: hypermagnesemia and hypomagnesemia
   e. Calcium imbalance: hypercalcemia and hypocalcemia
   f. Phosphate imbalance: hyperphosphatemia and hypophosphatemia
4. Identify the processes of acid–base regulation.
5. Discuss the etiology, laboratory diagnostic findings, clinical manifestations, and nursing and collaborative management of the following acid–base imbalances: metabolic acidosis, metabolic alkalosis, respiratory acidosis, and respiratory alkalosis.
6. Describe the composition and indications of common intravenous fluid solutions.

KEY TERMS

acidosis, p. 350	hypertonic, p. 334
active transport, p. 333	hypotonic, p. 334
alkalosis, p. 350	ions, p. 331
anions, p. 331	isotonic, p. 334
buffers, p. 350	oncotic pressure, p. 334
cations, p. 331	osmolality, p. 334
diffusion, p. 333	osmolarity, p. 334
electrolytes, p. 331	osmosis, p. 333
facilitated diffusion, p. 333	osmotic pressure, p. 333
fluid spacing, p. 335	pH, p. 350
homeostasis, p. 330	tetany, p. 347
hydrostatic pressure, p. 334	valence, p. 331

HOMEOSTASIS

Body fluids and electrolytes play an important role in homeostasis. **Homeostasis** is the state of equilibrium in the internal environment of the body, naturally maintained by adaptive responses that promote healthy survival.[1] Maintenance of the composition and volume of body fluids within narrow limits of normal is necessary to maintain homeostasis.[2] During normal metabolism the body produces many acids. These acids alter the internal environment of the body, including fluid and electrolyte balances, and must also be regulated to maintain homeostasis. Many diseases and their treatments have the ability to affect fluid and electrolyte balance. For example, a patient with metastatic breast cancer may develop hypercalcemia. Chemotherapy prescribed to treat the cancer may result in nausea and vomiting and, subsequently, dehydration and acid-base imbalances. Correction

of the dehydration with intravenous fluids must be monitored closely to prevent fluid overload.

It is important for the nurse to anticipate the potential for alterations in fluid and electrolyte balance associated with certain disorders and medical therapies, to recognize the signs and symptoms of imbalances, and to intervene with the appropriate action. This chapter describes the normal control of fluids, electrolytes, and acid-base balance; etiologies that disrupt homeostasis and resultant manifestations; and actions that the health care provider can take to prevent or restore fluid, electrolyte, and acid-base balance.

WATER CONTENT OF THE BODY

Water is the primary component of the body, accounting for approximately 60% of the body weight in the adult. Water is the solvent in which body salts, nutrients, and wastes are dissolved and transported. The water content varies with gender, body mass, and age (Fig. 16-1). In men, the percentage of body weight that is composed of water is generally greater than in women because men tend to have more lean body mass than women. Fat cells contain less water than an equivalent volume of lean tissue.[2] In the older adult, body water content averages 45% to 55% of body weight. In the infant, water content is 70% to 80% of the body weight. Thus infants and the elderly are at a higher risk for fluid-related problems than young adults.

Body Fluid Compartments

The two major fluid compartments in the body are intracellular and extracellular (Fig. 16-2). Approximately two thirds of the body water is located within cells and is termed *intracellular fluid* (ICF); the ICF constitutes approximately 42% of body

---

Reviewed by Elizabeth Speakman, RN, EdD, Associate Professor of Nursing, Community College of Philadelphia, Philadelphia, Pa.

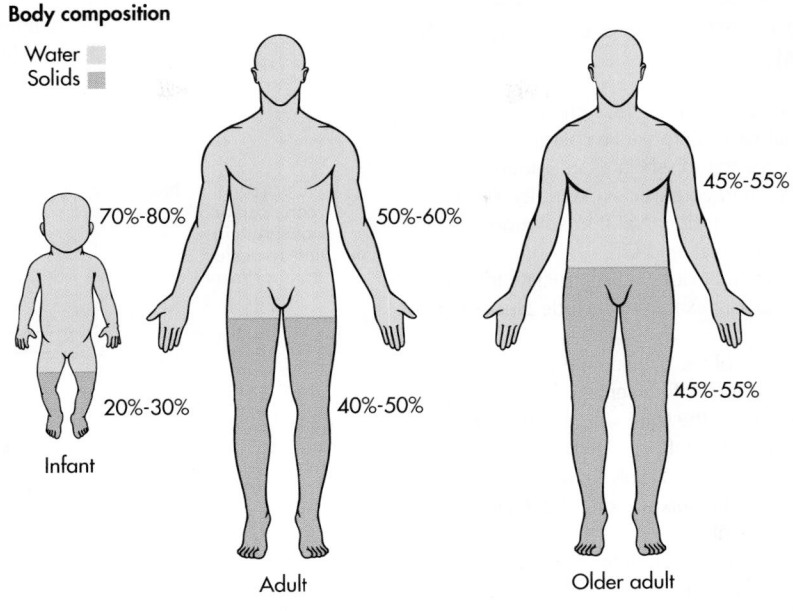

Body composition

Water
Solids

70%-80%

50%-60%

45%-55%

20%-30%

40%-50%

45%-55%

Infant

Adult

Older adult

FIG. 16-1   Changes in body water content with age.

weight. The body of a 70-kg man would contain approximately 42 L of water, of which 30 L would be located within cells. *Extracellular fluid* (ECF) consists of the fluid spaces between cells (interstitial fluid and lymph) and the plasma space. The ECF consists of one third of the body water, or about 17% of the total weight; this would amount to about 11 L in a 70-kg man. About one third of the ECF is in the plasma space (3 L in a 70-kg man), and two thirds is in the interstitial space (8 L in a 70-kg man).

A third small but important fluid compartment is the *transcellular space*. This usually consists of approximately 1 L. It includes fluid in the cerebrospinal space, gastrointestinal (GI) tract, and pleural, synovial, and peritoneal fluid spaces. If the transcellular fluid is not reabsorbed, but instead is lost (e.g., vomiting), the loss of the transcellular fluid can produce serious fluid and electrolyte imbalances.

Functions of Body Water

Body fluids are in constant motion transporting nutrients, electrolytes, and oxygen to cells and carrying waste products away from cells. Water is necessary in the regulation of body temperature. In addition, it lubricates joints and membranes and is a medium for food digestion.[2]

Calculation of Fluid Gain or Loss

One liter of water weighs 2.2 lb (1 kg). Body weight change, especially sudden change, is an excellent indicator of overall fluid volume loss or gain. For example, if a patient drinks 240 ml (8 oz) of fluid, weight gain will be 0.5 lb (0.24 kg). A patient receiving diuretic therapy who loses 4.4 lb (2 kg) in 24 hours has experienced a fluid loss of approximately 2 L. An adult patient who is fasting might lose approximately 1 to 2 lb per day. A weight loss exceeding this is likely due to loss of body fluid.

ELECTROLYTES

Electrolytes are substances whose molecules dissociate or split into ions when placed in water. **Ions** are electrically charged particles. **Cations** are positively charged ions. Examples include sodium (Na^+), potassium (K^+), calcium (Ca^{2+}), and magnesium (Mg^{2+}) ions. **Anions** are negatively charged ions. Examples include bicarbonate (HCO_3^-), chloride (Cl^-), and phosphate (PO_4^{3-}) ions. Most proteins bear a negative charge and are thus anions. The electrical charge of an ion is termed its **valence.** Cations and anions combine according to their valences. (Terminology related to body fluid chemistry is presented in Table 16-1.)

Measurement of Electrolytes

The measurement of electrolytes is important to the nurse in evaluating electrolyte balance, as well as determining the composition of electrolyte preparations. The concentration of electrolytes can be expressed in milligrams per deciliter (mg/dl), millimoles per liter (mmol/L), or milliequivalents per liter (mEq/L).

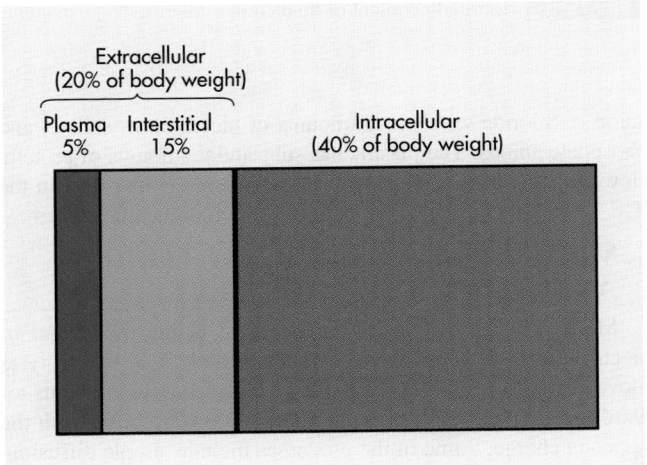

Extracellular
(20% of body weight)

Plasma Interstitial
5%   15%

Intracellular
(40% of body weight)

FIG. 16-2   Fluid compartments in the body.

TABLE 16-1	Terminology Related to Body Fluid Chemistry
Anion	Ion that carries a negative charge
Cation	Ion that carries a positive charge
Electrolyte	Substance that dissociates in solution into ions (charged particles); a molecule of sodium chloride (NaCl) in solution becomes Na⁺ and Cl⁻
Nonelectrolyte	Substance that does not dissociate into ions in solution; examples include glucose and urea
Osmolality	A measure of the total solute concentration per kilogram of solvent
Osmolarity	A measure of the total solute concentration per liter of solution
Solute	Substance that is dissolved in a solvent
Solution	Homogeneous mixture of solutes dissolved in a solvent
Solvent	Substance that is capable of dissolving a solute (liquid or gas)
Valence	The degree of combining power of an ion

The international standard for measuring electrolytes is mmol/L. One mole (mol) of a substance is the molecular (or atomic) weight of that substance in grams; hence a millimole (mmol) of a substance is the atomic weight in milligrams. Sodium's atomic weight is 23 mg; therefore 23 mg of sodium is 1 mmol of sodium. Sodium and chloride are monovalent elements that carry one electron and will match one to one. One mmol of sodium combines with one mmol of chloride.

An element with two electrons, such as calcium, will require two monovalent partners. To avoid keeping track of how to match millimoles, the milliequivalent is the favored unit of measure for electrolytes in the United States.[2,3] The following formula is used to convert millimoles to milliequivalents:

$$mEq = mmol/L \times valence$$

Electrolytes in body fluids are active chemicals that unite in varying combinations. Thus it is more practical to express their concentration as a measure of chemical activity (or milliequivalents) rather than as a measure of weight. Ions combine milliequivalent for milliequivalent; they match one to one. For example, 1 mEq (1 mmol) of sodium combines with 1 mEq (1 mmol) of chloride, and 1 mEq (0.5 mmol) of calcium combines with 1 mEq (1 mmol) of chloride. This combining power of electrolytes is important to maintain the balance of positively charged (cation) and negatively charged (anion) ions within body fluids.

Electrolyte Composition of Fluid Compartments

Electrolyte composition varies between the ECF and ICF. The overall concentration of the electrolytes is approximately the same in the two compartments. However, concentrations of specific ions differ greatly (Fig. 16-3). In the ICF the most prevalent cation is potassium with small amounts of magnesium and sodium. The prevalent anion is phosphate with some protein and a small amount of bicarbonate. In the ECF the main cation is sodium with small amounts of potassium, calcium, and magnesium. The primary ECF

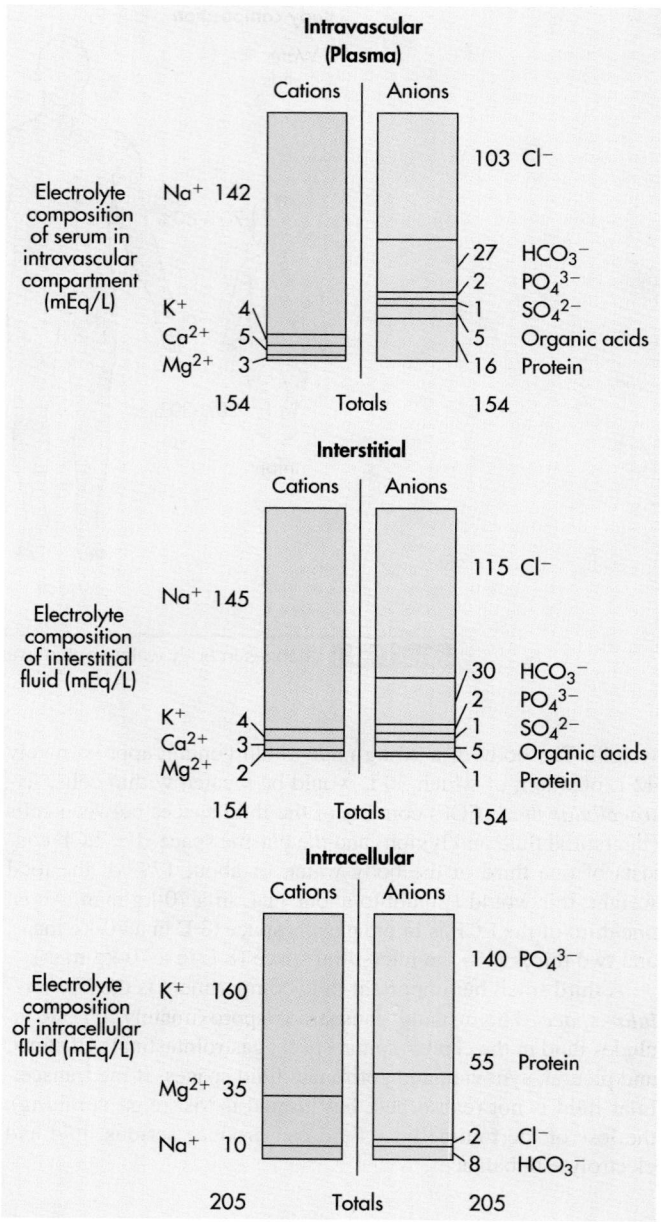

FIG. 16-3 Electrolyte content of fluid compartments.

anion is chloride with small amounts of bicarbonate, sulfate, and phosphate anions. The plasma has substantial amounts of protein. However, the amount of protein in the plasma is less than in the ICF. There is a very small amount of protein in the interstitium.

MECHANISMS CONTROLLING FLUID AND ELECTROLYTE MOVEMENT

Many different processes are involved in the movement of electrolytes and water between the ICF and ECF. Electrolytes move according to their concentration and electrical gradients toward the areas of lower concentration and toward areas with the opposite charge. Some of the processes include simple diffusion, facilitated diffusion, and active transport. Water moves as driven by two forces: hydrostatic pressure and osmotic pressure.

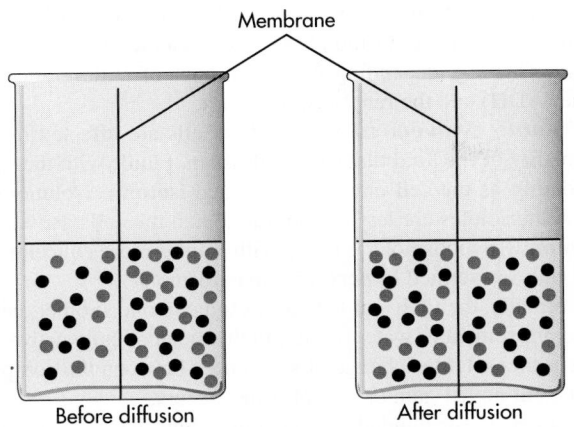

FIG. 16-4 Diffusion is the movement of molecules from an area of high concentration to an area of low concentration.

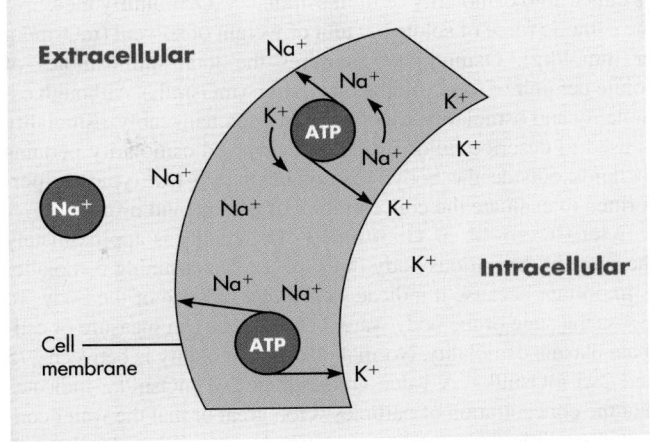

FIG. 16-5 Sodium-potassium pump. As sodium (Na^+) diffuses into the cell and potassium (K^+) diffuses out of the cell, an active transport system supplied with energy delivers Na^+ back to the extracellular compartment and K^+ to the intracellular compartment. *ATP*, adenosine triphosphate.

Diffusion

Diffusion is the movement of molecules from an area of high concentration to one of low concentration (Fig. 16-4). It occurs in liquids, gases, and solids. Net movement of molecules stops when the concentrations are equal in both areas. The membrane separating the two areas must be permeable to the diffusing substance for the process to occur. Simple diffusion requires no external energy. Gases (e.g., oxygen, nitrogen, carbon dioxide) and substances (e.g., urea) can permeate through cell membranes and are distributed throughout the body.

Facilitated Diffusion

Because of the composition of cellular membranes, some molecules diffuse slowly into the cell. However, when they are combined with a specific carrier molecule, the rate of diffusion accelerates. Like simple diffusion, **facilitated diffusion** moves molecules from an area of high concentration to one of low concentration. Facilitated diffusion is passive and requires no energy other than that of the concentration gradient. Glucose transport into the cell is an example of facilitated diffusion. There is a carrier molecule on most cells that increases or facilitates the rate of diffusion of glucose into these cells.

Active Transport

Active transport is a process in which molecules move against the concentration gradient. External energy is required for this process. The concentrations of sodium and potassium differ greatly intracellularly and extracellularly (see Fig. 16-3). By active transport, sodium moves out of the cell and potassium moves into the cell to maintain this concentration difference (Fig. 16-5). The energy source for the sodium-potassium pump is adenosine triphosphate (ATP), which is produced in the mitochondria.

Osmosis

Osmosis is the movement of water between two compartments separated by a membrane permeable to water but not to a solute. Water moves through the membrane from an area of low solute concentration to an area of high solute concentration (Fig. 16-6); that is, water moves from the more dilute compartment (has more water) to the side that is more concentrated (has

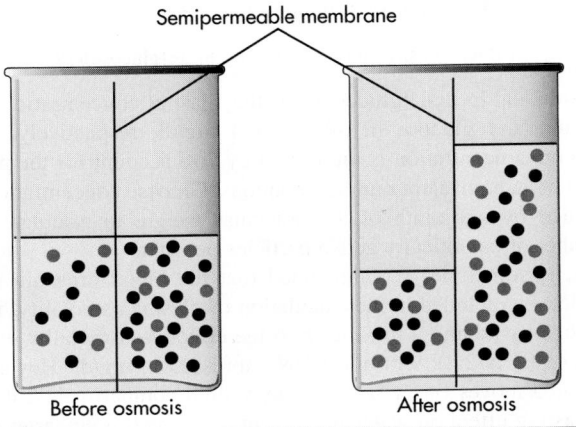

FIG. 16-6 Osmosis is the process of water movement through a semipermeable membrane from an area of low solute concentration to an area of high solute concentration.

less water). The semipermeable membrane prevents movement of solute particles. Osmosis requires no outside energy sources and stops when the concentration differences disappear or when hydrostatic pressure builds and is sufficient to oppose any further movement of water. Diffusion and osmosis are important in maintaining the fluid volume of body cells and the concentration of the solute.

Osmotic pressure is the amount of pressure required to stop the osmotic flow of water. Osmotic pressure can be understood in terms of imagining a chamber in which two compartments are separated by a membrane permeable to water and not to the solute (see Fig. 16-6). Water will move from the less concentrated side to the more concentrated side of the vessel. At some point the pressure generated by the height of the higher column of water will oppose the further movement of water.

Osmotic pressure is determined by the concentration of solutes in solution. It is measured in milliosmoles and may be expressed as either fluid osmolarity or fluid osmolality. **Osmolality** measures the osmotic force of solute per unit of weight of solvent (mOsm/kg or mmol/kg). **Osmolarity** measures the total milliosmoles of solute per unit of total volume of solution (mOsm/L). Although osmolality and osmolarity are often used interchangeably, osmolality is used to describe fluids inside the body and osmolarity pertains to fluids outside the body.[4] Osmolality is the test typically performed to evaluate the concentration of plasma and urine.

Measurement of Osmolality. Osmolality is approximately the same in the various body fluid spaces. Determining osmolality is important because it indicates the water balance of the body. To assess the state of the body water balance, one can measure or estimate plasma osmolality. Normal plasma osmolality is between 275 and 295 mOsm/kg. A value greater than 295 mOsm/kg indicates that the concentration of particles is too great or that the water content is too little. This condition is termed *water deficit*. A value less than 275 mOsm/kg indicates too little solute for the amount of water or too much water for the amount of solute. This condition is termed *water excess*. Both conditions are clinically significant.

Plasma and urine osmolality can be measured in most clinical laboratories. Because the major determinants of the plasma osmolality are sodium, glucose, and urea, one can calculate the effective plasma osmolality based on the concentrations of those compounds by using the following equation:

$$\text{Effective osmolality} = 2 \times [Na^+]p + [\text{glucose}]/18$$

where $[Na^+]p$ and [glucose] are the plasma concentrations of sodium and glucose in mEq/L and mg/dl, respectively. The sodium concentration is multiplied by 2 to account for the presence of an equivalent number of anions. Glucose concentration is divided by one tenth of its molecular weight to calculate the number of osmotically active particles per liter.

It is sometimes recommended that the blood urea nitrogen (BUN) be included in the calculation of plasma osmolality. This is done by adding a third term to the effective osmolality equation (+BUN/2.8), with the BUN expressed in mg/dl. However, the urea moves freely between body fluid compartments; it has no lasting effect on water movement across cell boundaries and is sometimes dubbed an "ineffective osmole." One can estimate the actual osmolality more accurately by including the BUN. However, the measure of the effective plasma osmolality without

consideration of the BUN term is the more physiologically meaningful estimate. Osmolality of urine can range from 100 to 1300 mOsm/kg, depending on the amount of antidiuretic hormone (ADH) and the renal response to it.

Osmotic Movement of Fluids. Cells are affected by the osmolality of the fluid that surrounds them. Fluids with the same osmolality as the cell interior are termed **isotonic.** Solutions in which the solutes are less concentrated than the cells are termed **hypotonic** (hypoosmolar). Those with solutes more concentrated than cells are termed **hypertonic** (hyperosmolar).

Normally, the ECF and ICF are isotonic to one another; hence no net movement of water occurs. In the metabolically active cell there is a constant exchange of substances between the compartments, but no net gain or loss of water occurs.

If a cell is surrounded by hypotonic fluid, water moves into the cell, causing it to swell and possibly to burst. If a cell is surrounded by hypertonic fluid, water leaves the cell to dilute the ECF; the cell shrinks and may eventually die (Fig. 16-7).

Hydrostatic Pressure

Hydrostatic pressure is the force within a fluid compartment. In the blood vessels hydrostatic pressure is the blood pressure generated by the contraction of the heart.[5] Hydrostatic pressure in the vascular system gradually decreases as the blood moves through the arteries until it is about 40 mm Hg at the arterial end of a capillary. Because of the size of the capillary bed and fluid movement into the interstitium, the pressure decreases to about 10 mm Hg at the venous end of the capillary. Hydrostatic pressure is the major force that pushes water out of the vascular system at the capillary level.

Oncotic Pressure

Oncotic pressure (colloidal osmotic pressure) is osmotic pressure exerted by colloids in solution. The major colloid in the vascular system contributing to the total osmotic pressure is protein. Protein molecules attract water, pulling fluid from the tissue space to the vascular space.[4] Unlike electrolytes, the large molecular size prevents proteins from leaving the vascular space through pores in capillary walls. Plasma oncotic pressure is approximately 25 mm Hg. Some proteins are found in the interstitial space; they exert an oncotic pressure of approximately 1 mm Hg.

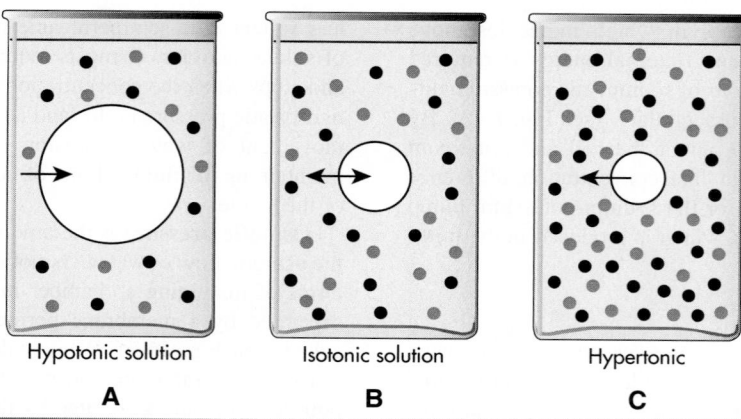

Hypotonic solution	Isotonic solution	Hypertonic
A	**B**	**C**

FIG. 16-7 Effects of water status on cell size. **A,** Hypotonic solution (H_2O excess) results in cellular swelling. **B,** Isotonic solution (normal H_2O balance) results in no change. **C,** Hypertonic solution (H_2O deficit) results in cellular shrinking.

FLUID MOVEMENT IN CAPILLARIES

There is normal movement of fluid between the capillary and the interstitium. The amount and direction of movement are determined by the interaction of (1) capillary hydrostatic pressure, (2) plasma oncotic pressure, (3) interstitial hydrostatic pressure, and (4) interstitial oncotic pressure.

Capillary hydrostatic pressure and interstitial oncotic pressure cause the movement of water out of the capillaries. Plasma oncotic pressure and interstitial hydrostatic pressure cause the movement of fluid into the capillary. At the arterial end of the capillary (Fig. 16-8), capillary hydrostatic pressure exceeds plasma oncotic pressure, and fluid is moved into the interstitium. At the venous end of the capillary, the capillary hydrostatic pressure is lower than plasma oncotic pressure, and fluid is drawn back into the capillary by the oncotic pressure created by plasma proteins.

Fluid Shifts

If capillary or interstitial pressures are altered, fluid may abnormally shift from one compartment to another, resulting in edema or dehydration.

Shifts of Plasma to Interstitial Fluid. Accumulation of fluid in the interstitium *(edema)* occurs if venous hydrostatic pressure rises, plasma oncotic pressure decreases, or interstitial oncotic pressure rises. Edema may also develop if there is an obstruction of lymphatic outflow that causes decreased removal of interstitial fluid.

Elevation of venous hydrostatic pressure. Increasing the pressure at the venous end of the capillary inhibits fluid movement back into the capillary. Causes of increased venous pressure include fluid overload, congestive heart failure, liver failure, obstruction of venous return to the heart (e.g., tourniquets, restrictive clothing, venous thrombosis), and venous insufficiency (e.g., varicose veins).

Decrease in plasma oncotic pressure. Fluid remains in the interstitium if the plasma oncotic pressure is too low to draw fluid back into the capillary. Decreased oncotic pressure is seen when the plasma protein content is low. This can result from excessive protein loss (renal disorders), deficient protein synthesis (liver disease), and deficient protein intake (malnutrition).

Elevation of interstitial oncotic pressure. Trauma, burns, and inflammation can damage capillary walls and allow plasma proteins to accumulate in the interstitium. The resultant increased interstitial oncotic pressure draws fluid into the interstitium and holds it there.

Shifts of Interstitial Fluid to Plasma. Fluid is drawn into the plasma space whenever there is an increase in the plasma osmotic or oncotic pressure. This could happen with administration of colloids, dextran, mannitol, or hypertonic solutions. Fluid is drawn from the interstitium. In turn, water is drawn from cells via osmosis, equilibrating the osmolality between ICF and ECF.

Increasing the tissue hydrostatic pressure is another way of causing a shift of fluid into plasma. The wearing of elastic compression gradient stockings or hose to decrease peripheral edema is a therapeutic application of this effect.

FLUID MOVEMENT BETWEEN EXTRACELLULAR FLUID AND INTRACELLULAR FLUID

Changes in the osmolality of the ECF alter the volume of cells. Increased ECF osmolality *(water deficit)* pulls water out of cells until the two compartments have a similar osmolality. Water deficit is associated with symptoms that result from cell shrinkage as water is pulled into the vascular system. For example, neurologic symptoms are caused by altered central nervous system (CNS) function as brain cells shrink. Decreased ECF osmolality (water excess) develops as the result of gain or retention of excess water. In this case, cells swell. Again, the primary symptoms are neurologic as a result of brain cell swelling as water shifts into the cells.

FLUID SPACING

Fluid spacing is a term sometimes used to describe the distribution of body water. *First spacing* describes the normal distribution of fluid in the ICF and ECF compartments. *Second spacing* refers to an abnormal accumulation of interstitial fluid (i.e., edema). *Third spacing* occurs when fluid accumulates in a portion of the body from which it is not easily exchanged with the rest of the ECF. Third-spaced fluid is trapped and essentially unavailable for functional use. Examples of third spacing are ascites, sequestration of fluid in the abdominal cavity with peritonitis, and edema associated with burns.

REGULATION OF WATER BALANCE

Hypothalamic Regulation

Water balance is maintained via the finely tuned balance of water intake and excretion. A body fluid deficit or increase in plasma osmolality is sensed by osmoreceptors in the hypothalamus, which in turn stimulates thirst and antidiuretic hormone (ADH) release. Thirst causes the patient to drink water. ADH, which is synthesized in the hypothalamus and stored in the posterior pituitary, acts in the renal distal and collecting tubules causing water reabsorption. Together these factors result in increased free water in the body and decreased plasma osmolality. If the

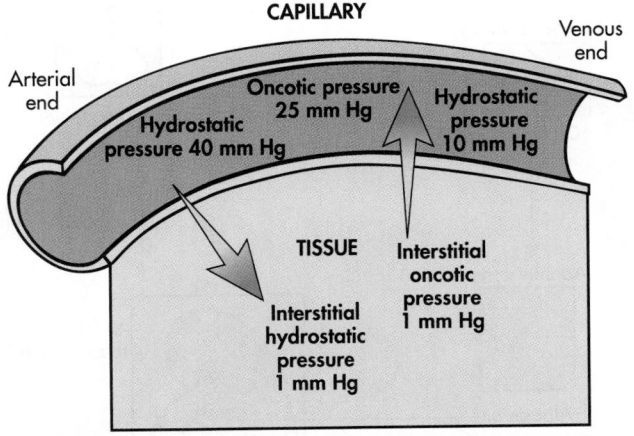

CAPILLARY

Arterial end — Venous end

Oncotic pressure 25 mm Hg

Hydrostatic pressure 40 mm Hg

Hydrostatic pressure 10 mm Hg

TISSUE

Interstitial oncotic pressure 1 mm Hg

Interstitial hydrostatic pressure 1 mm Hg

FIG. 16-8 Dynamics of fluid exchange between the capillary and the tissue. An equilibrium exists between forces filtering fluid out of the capillary and forces absorbing fluid back into the capillary. Note that the hydrostatic pressure is greater at the arterial end of the capillary than the venous end. The net effect of pressures at the arterial end of the capillary causes a movement of fluid into the tissue. At the venous end of the capillary there is net movement of fluid back into the capillary.

plasma osmolality is diminished or there is water excess, secretion of ADH is suppressed, resulting in urinary excretion of water.

An intact thirst mechanism is critical because it is the primary protection against the development of hyperosmolality. The patient who cannot recognize or act on the sensation of thirst is at risk for fluid deficit and hyperosmolality. The sensitivity of the thirst mechanism decreases in older adults.

The desire to consume fluids is also affected by social and psychologic factors not related to fluid balance. A dry mouth will cause the patient to drink, even when there is no measurable body water deficit. Water ingestion will equal water loss in the individual who has free access to water, a normal thirst and ADH mechanism, and normally functioning kidneys.

Pituitary Regulation

Under hypothalamic control, the posterior pituitary releases ADH, which regulates water retention by the kidneys. The distal tubules and collecting ducts in the kidneys respond to ADH by becoming more permeable to water so that water is reabsorbed from the tubular filtrate into the blood and not excreted in urine. An increase in plasma osmolality or a decrease in circulating volume will stimulate ADH secretion. Other factors that stimulate ADH release include stress, nausea, nicotine, and morphine. These factors usually result in shifts of osmolality within the range of normal values. It is common for the postoperative patient to have a lower serum osmolality after surgery, possibly because of the stress of surgery and narcotic analgesia.

A pathologic condition seen occasionally is *syndrome of inappropriate antidiuretic hormone* (SIADH) (see Chapter 48). Causes of SIADH include abnormal ADH production in CNS disorders (e.g., brain tumors, brain injury) and certain malignancies (e.g., small cell lung cancer). The inappropriate ADH causes water retention, which produces a decrease in plasma osmolality below the normal value and a relative increase in urine osmolality with a decrease in urine volume.

Reduction in the release or action of ADH produces diabetes insipidus (see Chapter 48). A copious amount of dilute urine is excreted because the renal tubules and collecting ducts do not appropriately reabsorb water. The patient with diabetes insipidus exhibits extreme polyuria and, if alert, *polydipsia* (excessive thirst). Symptoms of dehydration and hypernatremia develop if the water losses are not adequately replaced.

Adrenal Cortical Regulation

ECF volume is maintained by a combination of hormonal influences. ADH affects only water reabsorption. Hormones released by the adrenal cortex help regulate both water and electrolytes. Two groups of hormones secreted by the adrenal cortex are glucocorticoids and mineralocorticoids. The glucocorticoids (e.g., cortisol) primarily have an antiinflammatory effect and increase serum glucose levels, whereas the mineralocorticoids (e.g., aldosterone) enhance sodium retention and potassium excretion (Fig. 16-9). When sodium is reabsorbed, water follows as a result of osmotic changes.

Cortisol is the most common example of a naturally occurring glucocorticoid. In large doses, cortisol has both glucocorticoid (glucose-elevating and antiinflammatory) and mineralocorticoid (sodium-retention) properties. The adrenocortical hormone cortisol is secreted normally and whenever stress levels are increased. Many body systems, including fluid and electrolyte balance, are affected by stress (Fig. 16-10).

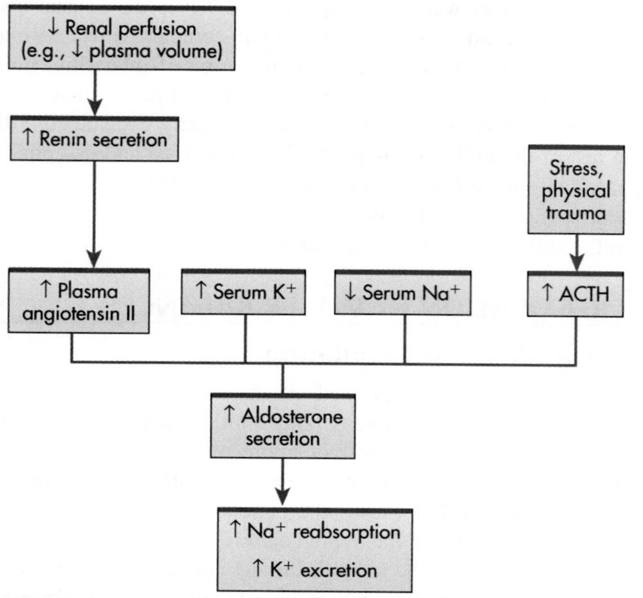

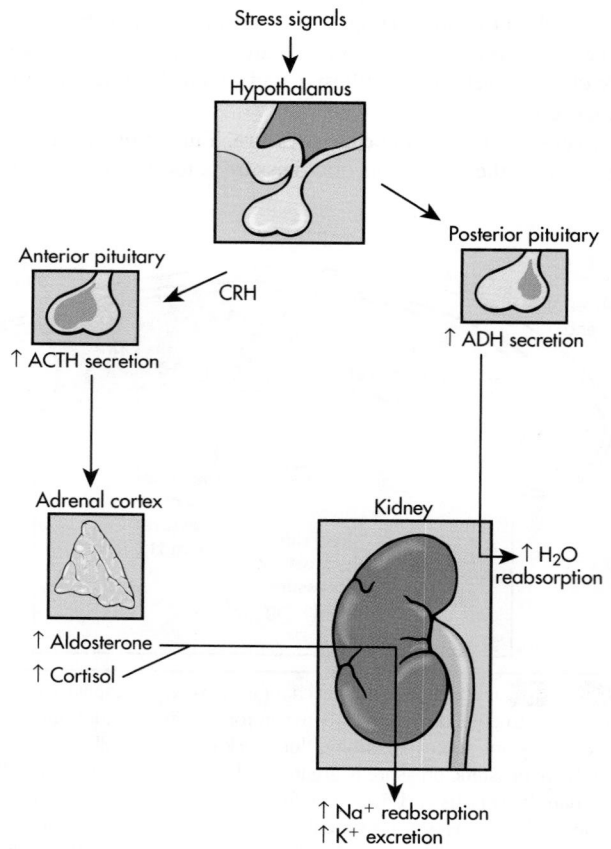

FIG. 16-9 Factors affecting aldosterone secretion.

FIG. 16-10 Effects of stress on fluid and electrolyte balance.

Aldosterone is the naturally occurring mineralocorticoid with potent sodium-retaining and potassium-excreting capability. The secretion of aldosterone may be stimulated by decreased renal perfusion or decreased sodium delivery to the distal portion of the renal tubule. The kidneys respond by secreting renin into the plasma. Angiotensinogen produced in the liver and normally found in blood is acted on by the renin to form angiotensin I, which converts to angiotensin II, which stimulates the adrenal cortex to secrete aldosterone. In addition to the renin-angiotensin mechanism, increased plasma potassium, decreased plasma sodium, and increased release of adrenocorticotropic hormone (ACTH) from the anterior pituitary all act directly on the adrenal cortex to stimulate the secretion of aldosterone (see Fig. 16-9).

Renal Regulation

The primary organs for regulating fluid and electrolyte balance are the kidneys (see Chapter 43). The kidneys regulate water balance through adjustments in urine volume. Similarly, urinary excretion of most electrolytes is adjusted so that a balance is maintained between overall intake and output. The total plasma volume is filtered by the kidneys many times each day. In the average adult the kidney reabsorbs 99% of this filtrate, producing approximately 1.5 L of urine per day. As the filtrate moves through the renal tubules, selective reabsorption of water and electrolytes and secretion of electrolytes result in the production of urine that is greatly different in composition and concentration than the plasma. This process helps maintain normal plasma osmolality, electrolyte balance, blood volume, and acid-base balance. The renal tubules are the site for the actions of ADH and aldosterone.

With severely impaired renal function, the kidneys cannot maintain fluid and electrolyte balance. This condition results in edema, potassium and phosphorus retention, acidosis, and other electrolyte imbalances (see Chapter 45). Renal function is typically decreased in the elderly person, placing the patient at increased risk for fluid and electrolyte imbalances. In particular, the ability to concentrate urine may be reduced in the older adult.

Cardiac Regulation

Atrial natriuretic factor (ANF) is a hormone released by the cardiac atria in response to increased atrial pressure (increased volume). The primary actions of ANF are vasodilation and increased urinary excretion of sodium and water, which decreases blood volume.[5]

Gastrointestinal Regulation

Daily water intake and output are between 2000 and 3000 ml (Table 16-2). The gastrointestinal (GI) tract accounts for most of the water intake. Water intake includes fluids, water from food metabolism, and water present in solid foods. Lean meat is approximately 70% water, whereas the water content of many fruits and vegetables approaches 100%.

Most of the body's water is excreted by the kidneys. A small amount of water is normally eliminated by the GI tract in feces, but diarrhea and vomiting can lead to significant fluid and electrolyte loss.

Insensible Water Loss

Insensible water loss, which is invisible vaporization from the lungs and skin, assists in regulating body temperature. Normally, about 900 ml per day is lost. The amount of water loss is increased by accelerated body metabolism, which occurs with increased body temperature and exercise.

Water loss through the skin should not be confused with the vaporization of water excreted by sweat glands. Only water is lost by insensible perspiration. Excessive sweating *(sensible perspiration)* caused by fever or high environmental temperatures may lead to large losses of water and electrolytes.

FLUID AND ELECTROLYTE IMBALANCES

Fluid and electrolyte imbalances occur to some degree in most patients with a major illness or injury because illness disrupts the normal homeostatic mechanism. Some fluid and electrolyte imbalances are directly caused by illness or disease (e.g., burns, congestive heart failure). At other times, therapeutic measures (e.g., intravenous fluid replacement, diuretics) cause or contribute to fluid and electrolyte imbalances.

The imbalances are commonly classified as *deficits* or *excesses.* Each imbalance is discussed separately. (For normal values, see Table 16-3.) In actual clinical situations, more than one imbalance occurring in the same patient is common. For example, a patient with prolonged nasogastric suction will lose Na^+, K^+, H^+, and Cl^-. These imbalances may result in a deficiency of both Na^+ and K^+, as well as metabolic alkalosis and fluid volume deficit.

TABLE 16-2	Normal Fluid Balance in the Adult	
Intake		
Fluids		1200 ml
Solid food		1000 ml
Water from oxidation		300 ml
		2500 ml
Output		
Insensible loss (skin and lungs)		900 ml
In feces		100 ml
Urine		1500 ml
		2500 ml

TABLE 16-3	Normal Serum Electrolyte Values	
ANIONS	**NORMAL VALUE**	
Bicarbonate (HCO_3^-)	20-30 mEq/L (20-30 mmol/L)	
Chloride (Cl^-)	96-106 mEq/L (96-106 mmol/L)	
Phosphate (PO_4^{3-})	2.8-4.5 mg/dl (0.90-1.45 mmol/L)	
Protein	6-8 g/dl (60-80 g/L)	
CATIONS	**NORMAL VALUE**	
Potassium (K^+)	3.5-5.5 mEq/L (3.5-5.5 mmol/L)	
Magnesium (Mg^{2+})	1.5-2.5 mEq/L (0.75-1.25 mmol/L)	
Sodium (Na^+)	135-145 mEq/L (135-145 mmol/L)	
Calcium (Ca^{2+}) (total)	9-11 mg/dl	
	4.5-5.5 mEq/L (2.25-2.75 mmol/L)	
Calcium (ionized)	4.5-5.5 mg/dl (1.13-1.38 mmol/L)	

SODIUM AND VOLUME IMBALANCES

Sodium plays a major role in maintaining the concentration and volume of the ECF. Sodium is the main cation of the ECF and the primary determinant of ECF osmolality. Sodium imbalances are typically associated with parallel changes in osmolality. Because of its impact on osmolality, sodium affects the water distribution between the ECF and the ICF. Sodium is also important in the generation and transmission of nerve impulses and the regulation of acid-base balance. Serum sodium is measured in milliequivalents per liter or millimoles per liter.

The GI tract absorbs sodium from foods. Typically, daily intake of sodium far exceeds the body's daily requirements. Sodium leaves the body through urine, sweat, and feces. The kidneys are the primary regulator of sodium balance. The kidneys regulate the ECF concentration of sodium by excreting or retaining water under the influence of ADH. Aldosterone also plays a part in sodium regulation by promoting sodium reabsorption from the renal tubules. The serum sodium level reflects the ratio of sodium to water, not necessarily the loss or gain of sodium. Thus changes in the serum sodium level may reflect either a primary water imbalance, a primary sodium imbalance, or a combination of the two. Sodium imbalances are typically associated with imbalances in ECF volume (Figs. 16-11 and 16-12).

HYPERNATREMIA

Common causes of hypernatremia are listed in Table 16-4. An elevated serum sodium may occur with water loss or sodium gain. Because sodium is the major determinant of the ECF osmolality, hypernatremia causes hyperosmolality. In turn, hyperosmolality causes a shift of water out of the cells, which leads to cellular dehydration.

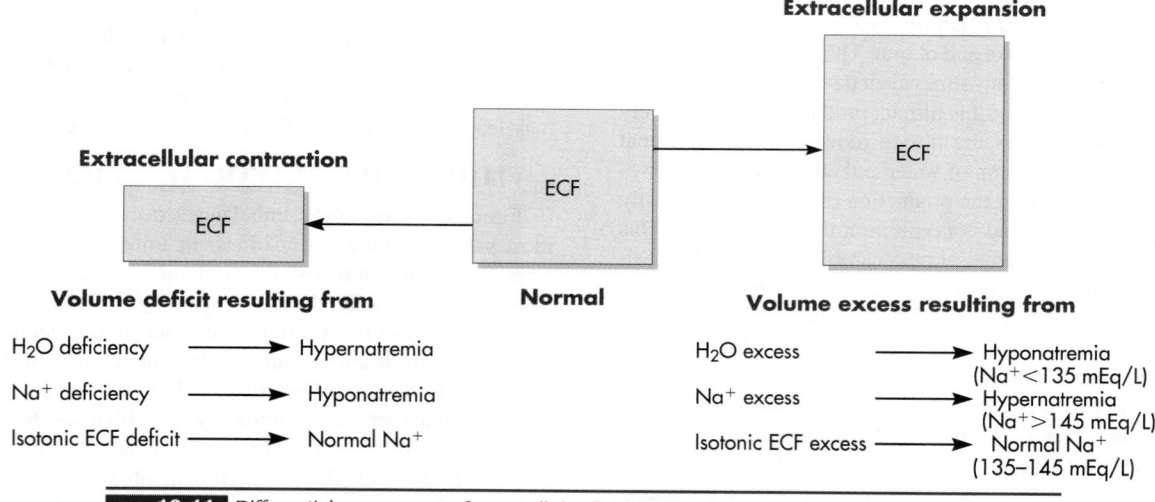

FIG. 16-11 Differential assessment of extracellular fluid (ECF) volume.

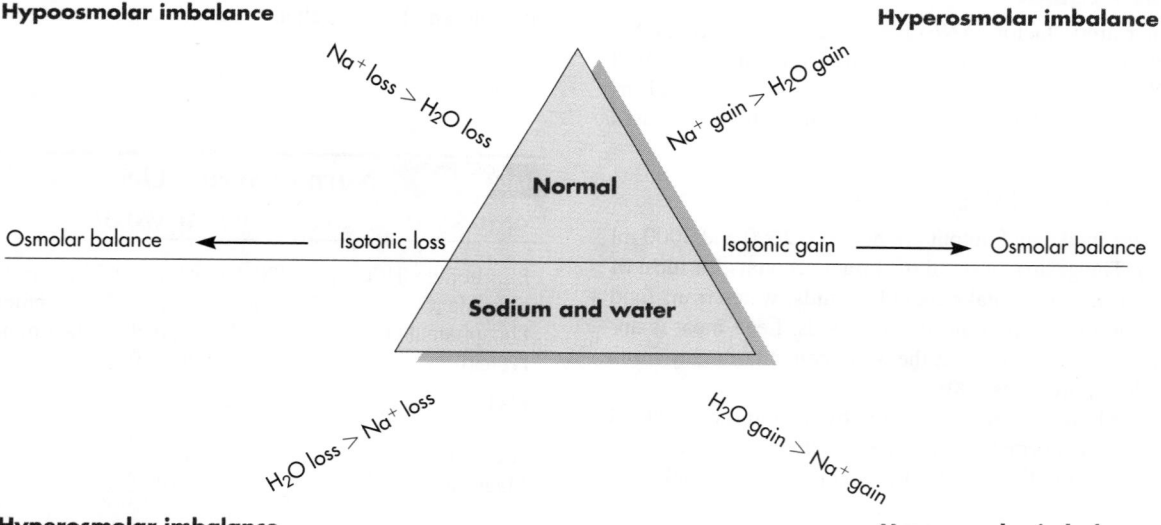

FIG. 16-12 Isotonic gains and losses affect mainly the extracellular fluid (ECF) compartment with little or no water movement into the cells. Hypertonic imbalances cause water to move from inside the cell into the ECF to dilute the concentrated sodium, causing cell shrinkage. Hypotonic imbalances cause water to move into the cell, causing cell swelling.

TABLE 16-4 Water and Sodium Imbalances: Causes and Clinical Manifestations	
WATER EXCESS/HYPONATREMIA (Na+ <135 mEq/L [mmol/L])	**WATER DEFICIT/HYPERNATREMIA** (Na+ >145 mEq/L [mmol/L])
Causes ***Sodium Loss*** GI losses: Diarrhea, vomiting, fistulas, NG suction Renal losses: Diuretics, adrenal insufficiency, Na+ wasting renal disease Skin losses: Burns, wound drainage ***Water Gain (Sodium Dilution)*** SIADH Congestive heart failure Excessive hypotonic IV fluids Primary polydipsia	***Water Loss (Sodium Concentration)*** ↑ Insensible water loss or perspiration (high fever, heatstroke) Diabetes insipidus Osmotic diuresis ***Sodium Gain*** IV hypertonic NaCl IV sodium bicarbonate IV excessive isotonic NaCl Primary hyperaldosteronism Saltwater near-drowning
Clinical Manifestations ***Decreased ECF Volume (Sodium Loss)*** Irritability, apprehension, confusion Postural hypotension Tachycardia Rapid, thready pulse ↓ CVP ↓ Jugular venous filling Nausea, vomiting Dry mucous membranes Weight loss Tremors, seizures, coma ***Normal or Increased ECF Volume (Water Gain)*** Headache, lassitude, apathy, weakness, confusion Nausea, vomiting Weight gain ↑ BP, ↑ CVP Muscle spasms, seizures, coma	***Decreased ECF Volume (Water Loss)*** Intense thirst, dry, swollen tongue Restlessness, agitation, twitching Seizures, coma Weakness Postural hypotension, ↓ CVP Weight loss ***Normal or Increased ECF Volume (Sodium Gain)*** Intense thirst Restlessness, agitation, twitching Seizures, coma Flushed skin Weight gain Peripheral and pulmonary edema ↑ BP, ↑ CVP

ECF, Extracellular fluid; *GI,* gastrointestinal; *IV,* intravenous; *NG,* nasogastric; *SIADH,* syndrome of inappropriate antidiuretic hormone.

As discussed earlier, the primary protection against the development of hyperosmolality is thirst. As the plasma osmolality increases, the thirst center in the hypothalamus is stimulated, and the individual seeks fluids.

Hypernatremia is not a problem in an alert person who has access to water, can sense thirst, and is able to swallow. Hypernatremia secondary to water deficiency is often the result of an impaired level of consciousness or an inability to obtain fluids. The unconscious patient or the cognitively impaired are at risk because of an inability to express thirst and act on it. The frail elderly, especially if ill, are at increased risk of free-water loss and subsequent development of hypernatremia secondary to impairment of the thirst mechanism and barriers to accessible fluids.[6]

Several clinical states can produce water loss and hypernatremia. A deficiency in the synthesis or a release of ADH from the posterior pituitary gland (central diabetes insipidus) or a decrease in kidney responsiveness to ADH (nephrogenic diabetes insipidus) can result in profound diuresis resulting in a water deficit and hypernatremia. Hyperosmolality can result from administration of concentrated hyperosmolar tube feedings and osmotic diuretics (mannitol), as well as hyperglycemia associated with uncontrolled diabetes mellitus. These situations result in osmotic diuresis. Dilute urine is lost, leaving behind a high solute load. Other causes of hypernatremia include excessive sweating and increased sensible losses from high fever.

Sodium intake in excess of water intake can also lead to hypernatremia. Examples of sodium gain include intravenous administration of hypertonic saline or sodium bicarbonate, use of sodium-containing drugs, excessive oral intake of sodium (ingestion of seawater), and *primary aldosteronism* (hypersecretion of aldosterone) caused by a tumor of the adrenal glands.

The clinical manifestations of hypernatremia are listed in Table 16-4. Symptoms are primarily the result of changes in the plasma osmolality that lead to changes in the volume of cellular water. Dehydration of neurons leads to neurologic manifestations such as intense thirst, lethargy, agitation, seizures, and even coma. Sodium excess also has a direct effect on the irritability and conduction of neurons, causing them to be more easily excited. Patients with hypernatremia will also exhibit the symptoms of any accompanying volume imbalance.

Collaborative Care. The goal of treatment in hypernatremia that is caused by either water loss or sodium gain is to treat the underlying cause. In primary water deficit the continued water loss must be prevented, and water replacement must be provided. If oral fluids cannot be ingested, intravenous solutions of 5% dextrose in water or hypotonic saline may be given initially. Serum sodium levels must be reduced gradually to prevent too rapid a shift of water back into the cells. Overly rapid correction of hypernatremia can result in cerebral edema. The risk is greatest in the patient who has developed hypernatremia over several days or longer.

The goal of treatment for sodium excess is to dilute the sodium concentration with salt-free intravenous (IV) fluids, such as 5% dextrose in water, and to promote excretion of the excess sodium by administering diuretics. Sodium intake will also be restricted. (See Chapter 48 for specific treatment of diabetes insipidus.) To prevent hypernatremia in the elderly or cognitively impaired patient, it is important to pay close attention to fluid intake and losses.[6] Regular administration of oral fluids must be incorporated into these patients' plan of care.[7]

HYPONATREMIA

Hyponatremia may result from loss of sodium-containing fluids or from water excess. Hyponatremia causes hypoosmolality with a shift of water into the cells.

Common causes of hyponatremia caused by water excess are inappropriate use of sodium-free or hypotonic IV fluids. This may occur in patients after surgery or major trauma, during administration of fluids in patients with renal failure, or in patients with psychiatric disorders associated with excessive water intake. SIADH will result in dilutional hyponatremia caused by abnormal retention of water. (See Chapter 48 for a discussion of the causes of SIADH.)

Losses of sodium-rich body fluids from the GI tract, kidney, or skin indirectly result in hyponatremia. Because these fluids are either isotonic or hypotonic, sodium is lost with an equal or greater proportion of water. However, hyponatremia develops as the body responds to the fluid volume deficit with activation of the thirst mechanism and by releasing ADH. The resultant retention of water lowers the sodium concentration.[3]

Symptoms of hyponatremia are related to cellular swelling and are first manifested in the CNS.[3] The excess water lowers plasma osmolality, shifting fluid into brain cells. The clinical manifestations of hyponatremia are listed in Table 16-4.

Collaborative Care. In hyponatremia that is caused by water excess, fluid restriction is often all that is needed to treat the problem. If severe symptoms (seizures) develop, small amounts of intravenous hypertonic saline solution (3% NaCl) are given to restore the serum sodium level while the body is returning to a normal water balance. Treatment of hyponatremia associated with abnormal fluid loss includes fluid replacement with sodium-containing solutions. Replacing losses with commercially available oral rehydration fluids containing electrolytes instead of pure water may help prevent the development of hyponatremia in the home setting.[6]

EXTRACELLULAR FLUID VOLUME IMBALANCES

ECF volume deficit (hypovolemia) and ECF volume excess (hypervolemia) are commonly occurring clinical conditions (Table 16-5). ECF volume imbalances are typically accompanied by one or more electrolyte imbalances. As previously discussed,

TABLE 16-5	Causes of ECF Volume Imbalances
ECF VOLUME DEFICIT	**ECF VOLUME EXCESS**
Increased Loss	**Increased Retention**
Vomiting	Congestive heart failure
Diarrhea	Cushing syndrome
Fistula drainage	Chronic liver disease with portal
GI tract suction	hypertension
Excessive sweating	Long-term use of corticosteroids
Third-space fluid shifts	Renal failure
(e.g., burns, intestinal	
obstruction)	
Overuse of diuretics	
Hemorrhage	
Decreased Intake	**Increased Intake**
Nausea	Rare with adequate renal function
Anorexia	Excessive IV administration of
Inability to drink	fluids
Inability to obtain water	

volume imbalances are often associated with changes in the serum sodium level. Fluid volume deficit can occur with abnormal loss of body fluids (e.g., diarrhea, fistula drainage, hemorrhage, polyuria), decreased intake, or a plasma-to-interstitial fluid shift. Fluid volume excess may result from excessive intake of fluids, abnormal retention of fluids (e.g., congestive heart failure, renal failure), or interstitial-to-plasma fluid shift. Although shifts in fluid between the plasma and interstitium do not alter the overall volume of the ECF, these shifts do result in changes in the clinically important intravascular volume.

Collaborative Care. The goal of treatment for fluid volume deficit is to correct the underlying cause and to replace both water and electrolytes. Balanced IV solutions, such as lactated Ringer's solution, are usually given. Isotonic sodium chloride is used when rapid volume replacement is indicated. Blood is administered when volume loss is due to blood loss.

The goal of treatment for fluid volume excess is removal of sodium and water without producing abnormal changes in the electrolyte composition or osmolality of ECF. The primary cause must be identified and treated. Intravenous therapy is usually not indicated for this type of fluid imbalance. Diuretics and fluid restriction are the primary forms of therapy. Restriction of sodium intake may also be indicated. If the fluid excess leads to ascites or pleural effusion, an abdominal paracentesis or thoracentesis may be necessary.

NURSING MANAGEMENT SODIUM AND VOLUME IMBALANCES

■ Nursing Diagnoses

Nursing diagnoses and collaborative problems for the patient with various fluid and sodium imbalances include, but are not limited to, the following.

Extracellular fluid volume excess:
- Excess fluid volume *related to* increased sodium and water retention
- Ineffective airway clearance *related to* sodium and water retention

- Risk for impaired skin integrity *related to* edema
- Disturbed body image *related to* altered body appearance secondary to edema
- Potential complications: pulmonary edema, ascites

Extracellular fluid volume deficit:

- Deficient fluid volume *related to* excessive ECF losses or decreased fluid intake
- Decreased cardiac output *related to* excessive ECF losses or decreased fluid intake
- Potential complication: hypovolemic shock

Hypernatremia:

- Risk for injury *related to* altered sensorium and seizures secondary to abnormal CNS function

Hyponatremia:

- Risk for injury *related to* altered sensorium and decreased level of consciousness secondary to abnormal CNS function

■ Nursing Implementation

Intake and Output. The use of 24-hour intake and output records gives valuable information regarding fluid and electrolyte problems. Sources of excessive intake or fluid losses can be identified on a properly recorded intake-and-output flowsheet. Intake should include oral, IV, and tube feedings and retained irrigants. Output includes urine, excess perspiration, wound or tube drainage, vomitus, and diarrhea. Fluid loss from wounds and perspiration should be estimated. Urine specific gravity measurements can be done. Readings of greater than 1.025 indicate a concentrated urine, whereas those of less than 1.010 indicate a dilute urine.

Cardiovascular Changes. Monitoring the patient for cardiovascular changes is necessary to prevent or detect complications from sodium and volume imbalances. Signs and symptoms of ECF volume excess and deficit are reflected in changes in blood pressure, pulse force, and jugular venous visibility. In fluid volume excess, the pulse is full and bounding. Because of the expanded intravascular volume, the pulse is not easily obliterated. Increased volume causes distended neck veins (jugular venous distention) and increased blood pressure.

In mild to moderate fluid volume deficit, compensatory mechanisms include sympathetic nervous system stimulation of the heart and peripheral vasoconstriction. Stimulation of the heart increases heart rate and, combined with vasoconstriction, maintains blood pressure within normal limits. A change in position from lying to sitting or standing may elicit a further increase in heart rate or a decrease in blood pressure (orthostatic hypotension). If vasoconstriction and tachycardia provide inadequate compensation, hypotension occurs when the patient is recumbent. Severe fluid volume deficit can cause a weak, thready pulse that is easily obliterated and flattened neck veins. Severe, untreated fluid deficit will result in shock.

Respiratory Changes. Both fluid excess and fluid deficit affect respiratory status. Fluid excess results in pulmonary congestion and pulmonary edema as increased hydrostatic pressure in the pulmonary vessels forces fluid into the alveoli. The patient will experience shortness of breath, irritative cough, and moist crackles on auscultation.[8] The patient with fluid deficit will demonstrate an increased respiratory rate due to decreased tissue perfusion and resultant hypoxia.

Neurologic Changes. Changes in neurologic function may occur with sodium and water imbalances. With increased water volume and hyponatremia, water moves by osmosis into the brain cells. Alternatively, decreased water volume and hypernatremia cause water to shift out of the brain cells with resultant shrinkage. In addition, profound volume depletion may cause an alteration in sensorium secondary to reduced cerebral tissue perfusion.

Assessment of neurologic function includes evaluation of (1) the level of consciousness, which includes responses to verbal and painful stimuli and the determination of a person's orientation to time, place, and person; (2) pupillary response to light and equality of pupil size; and (3) voluntary movement of the extremities, degree of muscle strength, and reflexes. Nursing care focuses on maintaining patient safety.

Daily Weights. Accurate daily weights provide the easiest measurement of volume status. An increase of 1 kg (2.2 lb) is equal to 1000 ml (1 L) fluid retention (provided the person has maintained usual dietary intake or has not been on nothing-by-mouth [NPO] status). However, weight changes can be relied on only if obtained under standardized conditions. An accurate weight requires the patient to be weighed at the same time every day, wearing the same garments, and on the same carefully calibrated scale. Excess bedding should be removed and all drainage bags should be emptied before the weighing. If bulky dressings or tubes are present, which may not necessarily be used every day, a notation regarding these variables should be recorded on the flowsheet or nursing notes.

Skin Assessment and Care. Clues to fluid volume deficit and excess can be detected by inspection of the skin. Skin should be examined for turgor and mobility. Normally a fold of skin, when pinched, will readily move and, on release, will rapidly return to its former position. Skin areas over the sternum, abdomen, and anterior forearm are the usual sites for evaluation of tissue turgor (Fig. 16-13). The preferred areas to assess for tissue turgor in the older person are areas where decreases in skin elasticity is less significant, such as the forehead or over the sternum.[2]

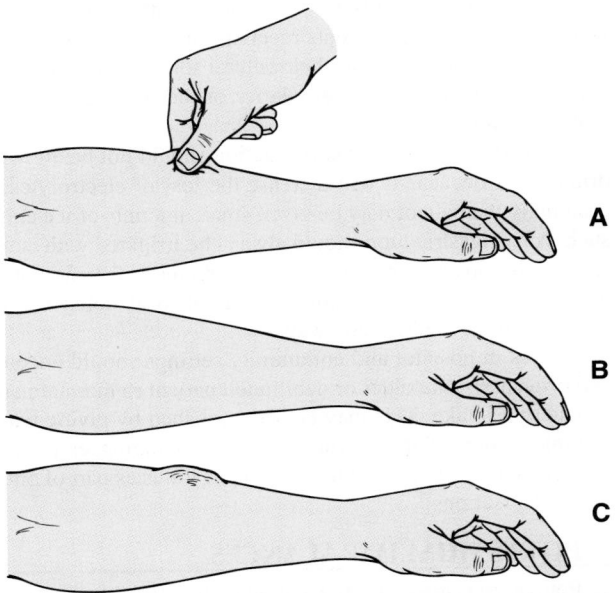

FIG. 16-13 Assessment of skin turgor. **A** and **B,** When normal skin is pinched, it resumes shape in seconds. **C,** If the skin remains wrinkled for 20 to 30 seconds, the patient has poor skin turgor.

In fluid volume deficit, skin turgor is diminished; there is a lag in the pinched skinfold's return to its original state (referred to as *tenting*). The skin may be cool and moist if there is vasoconstriction to compensate for the decreased fluid volume. Mild hypovolemia usually does not stimulate this compensatory response; consequently, the skin will be warm and dry. Volume deficit may also cause the skin to appear dry and wrinkled. These signs may be difficult to evaluate in the older adult because the patient's skin may be normally dry, wrinkled, and nonelastic. Oral mucous membranes will be dry, the tongue may be furrowed, and the individual often complains of thirst. Routine oral care is critical to the comfort of the dehydrated patient and the patient who is fluid restricted for management of fluid volume excess.

Skin that is edematous may feel cool because of fluid accumulation and a decrease in blood flow secondary to the pressure of the fluid. The fluid can also stretch the skin, causing it to feel taut and hard. Edema is assessed by pressing with a thumb or forefinger over the edematous area. A grading scale is used to standardize the description if an indentation (ranging from 1+ [slight, 2 mm indentation] to 4+ [pitting, 8 mm indentation]) remains when pressure is released. The areas to be evaluated for edema are those where soft tissues overlie a bone. Skin areas over the tibia, fibula, and sacrum are the preferred sites.

Good skin care for the person with fluid volume excess or deficit is important. Edematous tissues must be protected from extremes of heat and cold, prolonged pressure, and trauma. Frequent skin care and changes in position will protect the patient from skin breakdown. Elevation of edematous extremities helps promote venous return and fluid reabsorption. Dehydrated skin needs frequent care without the use of soap. The application of moisturizing creams or oils will increase moisture retention and stimulate circulation.

Other Nursing Measures. The rates of infusion of intravenous fluid solutions should be carefully monitored. Attempts to "catch up" should be approached with extreme caution, particularly when large volumes of fluid or certain electrolytes are involved. This is especially true in patients with cardiac, renal, or neurologic problems. Patients receiving tube feedings need supplementary water added to their enteral formula. The amount of water will depend on the osmolarity of the feeding and the patient's condition.

The patient with nasogastric suction should not be allowed to drink water because it will increase the loss of electrolytes. Occasionally the patient may be given small amounts of ice chips to suck. A nasogastric tube should always be irrigated with isotonic saline solution and not with water. Water causes diffusion of electrolytes into the gastric lumen from mucosal cells; the electrolytes are then suctioned away.

Nurses in hospital and community settings should encourage and often assist the older or debilitated patient to maintain an adequate oral intake. This may be accomplished by giving patients a drink as part of the morning care, encouraging extra sips of fluid with drugs, and including a drink of fluids as part of one-on-one conversations.[7]

POTASSIUM IMBALANCES

Potassium is the major ICF cation with 98% of the body potassium being intracellular. For example, potassium concentration within muscle cells is approximately 140 mEq/L; potassium concentration in the ECF is 3.5 to 5.5 mEq/L. The sodium-potassium pump in cell membranes maintains this concentration difference by pumping potassium into the cell and sodium out, a process fueled by the breakdown of ATP. The ratio of ECF potassium to ICF potassium is the major factor in the resting neuron's membrane potential. Many of the symptoms related to potassium imbalance are due to changes in the ratio of ECF to ICF potassium (increased or decreased ECF potassium).[5]

Potassium is critical for many cellular and metabolic functions. It is necessary for the transmission and conduction of nerve impulses, maintenance of normal cardiac rhythms, and skeletal and smooth muscle contraction. As the major intracellular cation, potassium regulates intracellular osmolality and promotes cellular growth. Potassium moves into cells during the formation of new tissues and leaves the cell during tissue breakdown.[5,9] Potassium also plays a role in acid-base balance that is discussed in acid-base regulation later in this chapter.

Diet is the source of potassium. The typical Western diet contains approximately 50 to 100 mEq of potassium daily, mainly from fruits, dried fruits, and vegetables. Many salt substitutes contain substantial potassium. Patients may receive potassium from parenteral sources, including IV fluids, stored transfused blood, and potassium-penicillin.

The kidneys are the primary route for potassium loss. About 90% of the daily potassium intake is eliminated by the kidneys; the remainder is lost in the stool and sweat. If kidney function is significantly impaired, toxic levels of potassium may be retained. There is an inverse relationship between sodium and potassium reabsorption in the kidneys. Factors that cause sodium retention (e.g., low blood volume, increased aldosterone level) cause potassium loss in the urine. Large urine volumes can be associated with excess loss of potassium in the urine. The ability of the kidneys to conserve potassium is weak even when body stores are depleted.[9]

Disruptions in the dynamic equilibrium between ICF and ECF potassium often cause clinical problems. Among the factors causing potassium to move from the ECF to the ICF are the following:

- Insulin
- Alkalosis
- β-adrenergic stimulation (catecholamine release in stress, coronary ischemia, delirium tremens, or administration of β-adrenergic agonist drugs)
- Rapid cell building (administration of folic acid or cobalamin [vitamin B_{12}] to patients with megaloblastic anemia resulting in marked production of red blood cells)

Factors that cause potassium to move from the ICF to the ECF include acidosis, trauma to cells (as in massive soft tissue damage or in tumor lysis), and exercise. Both digoxin-like drugs and β-adrenergic blocking drugs (e.g., propanolol [Inderal]) can impair entry of potassium into cells, resulting in the higher ECF potassium concentration. Causes of potassium imbalance are summarized in Table 16-6.

HYPERKALEMIA

Hyperkalemia (high serum potassium) may be caused by a massive intake of potassium, impaired renal excretion, shift of potassium from the ICF to the ECF, or a combination of these factors. The most common cause of hyperkalemia is renal failure. Hyperkalemia is also common in patients with massive cell destruction (e.g., burn or crush injury, tumor lysis), rapid transfusion of

TABLE 16-6   **Potassium Imbalances: Causes and Clinical Manifestations**

HYPOKALEMIA (K⁺ <3.5 mEq/L [mmol/L])	HYPERKALEMIA (K⁺ >5.5 mEq/L [mmol/L])
Causes ***Potassium Loss*** GI losses: Diarrhea, vomiting, fistulas, NG suction Renal losses: Diuretics, hyperaldosteronism, magnesium depletion Skin losses: Diaphoresis Dialysis ***Shift of Potassium into Cells*** Increased insulin (e.g., IV dextrose load) Alkalosis Tissue repair ↑ Epinephrine (e.g., stress) ***Lack of Potassium Intake*** Starvation Diet low in potassium Failure to include potassium in parenteral fluids if NPO	***Excess Potassium Intake*** Excessive or rapid parenteral administration Potassium-containing drugs (e.g., potassium-penicillin) Potassium-containing salt substitute ***Shift of Potassium Out of Cells*** Acidosis Tissue catabolism (e.g., fever, sepsis, burns) Crush injury Tumor lysis syndrome ***Failure to Eliminate Potassium*** Renal disease Potassium-sparing diuretics Adrenal insufficiency ACE inhibitors
Clinical Manifestations Fatigue Muscle weakness Leg cramps Nausea, vomiting, ileus Soft, flabby muscles Paresthesias, decreased reflexes Weak, irregular pulse Polyuria Hyperglycemia ***Electrocardiogram Changes*** ST segment depression Flattened T wave Presence of U wave Ventricular arrhythmias (e.g., PVCs) Bradycardia Enhanced digitalis effect	Irritability Anxiety Abdominal cramping, diarrhea Weakness of lower extremities Paresthesias Irregular pulse Cardiac standstill if hyperkalemia sudden or severe ***Electrocardiogram Changes*** Tall, peaked T wave Prolonged PR interval ST depression Loss of P wave Widening QRS Ventricular fibrillation Ventricular standstill

ACE, Angiotensin-converting enzyme; *NG,* nasogastric; *NPO,* nothing by mouth; *PVC,* premature ventricular contraction.

aged blood, and catabolic state (e.g., severe infections). Metabolic acidosis, particularly when the chloride is normal, is associated with a shift of potassium ion from the ICF to the ECF as hydrogen ions move into the cell. Adrenal insufficiency leads to retention of K⁺ in the serum because of aldosterone deficiency. Certain drugs, such as potassium-sparing diuretics (e.g., spironolactone [Aldactone], triamterene [Dyrenium]) and angiotensin-converting enzyme (ACE) inhibitors (e.g., enalapril [Vasotec], lisinopril [Prinivil]), may contribute to the development of hyperkalemia. Both of these types of drugs reduce the kidneys's ability to secrete and therefore excrete excess potassium (see Table 16-6).

Clinical Manifestations. Hyperkalemia causes membrane depolarization, altering cell excitability. Skeletal muscles become weak or paralyzed. The patient may experience cramping leg pain. Leg muscles are affected initially; respiratory muscles are spared. Disturbances in cardiac conduction occur as the potassium level rises.[2] Ventricular fibrillation or cardiac standstill may occur. Cardiac depolarization is impaired, leading to flatten-

ing of the P wave and widening of the QRS wave. Repolarization occurs more rapidly, resulting in shortening of the Q-T interval and causing the T wave to be narrower and more peaked. Fig. 16-14 illustrates the electrocardiographic (ECG) effects of hypokalemia and hyperkalemia. Abdominal cramping and diarrhea occur from hyperactivity of smooth muscles. Other clinical manifestations are listed in Table 16-6.

NURSING *and* COLLABORATIVE MANAGEMENT
HYPERKALEMIA

■ Nursing Diagnoses

Nursing diagnoses and collaborative problems for the patient with hyperkalemia include, but are not limited to, the following:
- Risk for injury *related to* lower extremity muscle weakness and seizures
- Potential complication: arrhythmias

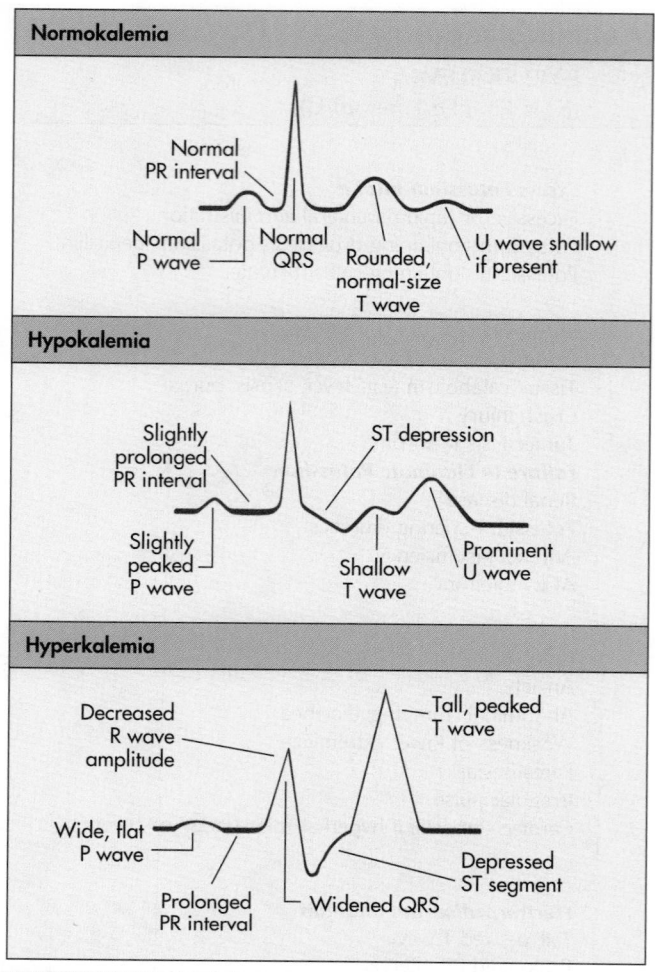

Normokalemia

Normal PR interval

Normal P wave

Normal QRS

Rounded, normal-size T wave

U wave shallow if present

Hypokalemia

Slightly prolonged PR interval

Slightly peaked P wave

ST depression

Shallow T wave

Prominent U wave

Hyperkalemia

Decreased R wave amplitude

Wide, flat P wave

Prolonged PR interval

Widened QRS

Tall, peaked T wave

Depressed ST segment

FIG. 16-14 Electrocardiogram changes associated with alterations in potassium status.

■ Nursing Implementation

Treatment of hyperkalemia consists of the following:

1. Eliminate oral and parenteral potassium intake (see Table 45-4).
2. Increase elimination of potassium. This is accomplished via diuretics, dialysis, and use of ion-exchange resins such as sodium polystyrene sulfonate (Kayexalate). Increased fluid intake can enhance renal potassium elimination.
3. Force potassium from the ECF to the ICF. This is accomplished by administration of intravenous insulin (along with glucose so the patient does not become hypoglycemic) or via administration of IV sodium bicarbonate in the correction of acidosis. Rarely, a β-adrenergic agonist (e.g., epinephrine) is administered.
4. Reverse the membrane effects of the elevated ECF potassium by administering calcium gluconate intravenously. Calcium ion can immediately reverse the effect of the depolarization on cell excitability.

In cases where the elevation of potassium is mild and the kidneys are functioning, it may be sufficient to withhold potassium from the diet and intravenous sources and increase renal elimination by administering fluids and possibly diuretics. Kayexalate, which is administered via the GI tract, binds potassium in exchange for sodium, and the resin is excreted in feces (see Chapter 45). All

patients with clinically significant hyperkalemia should be monitored electrocardiographically to detect arrhythmias and to monitor the effects of therapy. Patients with moderate hyperkalemia should additionally receive one of the treatments to force potassium into cells, usually IV insulin and glucose. The patient experiencing dangerous cardiac arrhythmias should receive IV calcium gluconate immediately to protect the patient while the potassium is being eliminated and forced into cells. Hemodialysis is an effective means of removing potassium from the body in the patient with renal failure.

HYPOKALEMIA

Hypokalemia (low serum potassium) can result from abnormal losses of potassium from a shift of potassium from ECF to ICF, or rarely from deficient dietary potassium intake. The most common causes of hypokalemia are abnormal losses, either via the kidneys or GI tract. Abnormal losses occur when the patient is diuresing, particularly in the patient with an elevated aldosterone level. Aldosterone is released when the circulating blood volume is low; it causes sodium retention in the kidneys but loss of potassium in the urine. Magnesium deficiency may contribute to the development of potassium depletion. Low plasma magnesium stimulates renin release and subsequent increased aldosterone levels, which results in potassium excretion.[5] GI tract losses of potassium secondary to diarrhea, laxative abuse, vomiting, and ileostomy drainage can cause hypokalemia.

Metabolic alkalosis can cause a shift of potassium into cells in exchange for hydrogen, thus lowering the potassium in the ECF and causing symptomatic hypokalemia. Hypokalemia is sometimes associated with the treatment of diabetic ketoacidosis because of a combination of factors, including an increased urinary potassium loss and a shift of potassium into cells with the administration of insulin and correction of acidosis. A less common cause of hypokalemia is the sudden initiation of cell formation; for example, the formation of red blood cells (RBCs) as in treatment of anemia with cobalamin, folic acid, or erythropoietin.

Clinical Manifestations. Hypokalemia alters resting membrane potential. It most commonly is associated with hyperpolarization, or increased negative charge within the cell. This causes excitability problems in many types of tissue. The most serious clinical problems are cardiac. The incidence of potentially lethal ventricular arrhythmias is increased in hypokalemia. Patients should be monitored with ECG for signs of hypokalemia. These changes include impaired repolarization, resulting in a flattening of the T wave and eventually in emergence of a U wave. The P wave amplitude may increase and may become peaked (see Fig. 16-14). Patients taking digoxin experience increased digoxin toxicity if their serum potassium is low. Skeletal muscle weakness and paralysis may occur with hypokalemia. As with hyperkalemia, symptoms are most often observed in the legs. Respiratory muscles and those innervated by cranial nerves are not involved. Muscle cramping and muscle cell breakdown (known as rhabdomyolysis) can be caused by hypokalemia. This can lead to myoglobin in the plasma and urine, which can, in turn, lead to renal failure.

Smooth muscle function is altered by hypokalemia. The patient may experience decreased GI motility (e.g., paralytic ileus), altered airway responsiveness, and impaired regulation of arteriolar blood flow, possibly contributing to muscle cell breakdown. Finally, hypokalemia can impair function in nonmuscle tissue. With prolonged hypokalemia, the kidneys are unable to concentrate urine and diuresis occurs.[9] Release of insulin is impaired, often causing hyperglycemia. Clinical manifestations of hypokalemia are presented in Table 16-6.

NURSING *and* COLLABORATIVE MANAGEMENT
HYPOKALEMIA

■ Nursing Diagnoses

Nursing diagnoses and collaborative problems for the patient with hypokalemia include, but are not limited to, the following:
▪ Risk for injury *related to* muscle weakness and hyporeflexia
▪ Potential complication: arrhythmias

■ Nursing Implementation

Hypokalemia is treated by giving potassium chloride supplements and increasing dietary intake of potassium. Potassium chloride (KCl) supplements can be given orally or intravenously. Except in severe deficiencies, KCl is never given unless there is urine output of at least 0.5 ml/kg of body weight per hour. KCl supplements added to IV solutions should never exceed 60 mEq/L. The preferred level is 40 mEq/L. The rate of IV administration of KCl should not exceed 10 to 20 mEq per hour to prevent hyperkalemia and cardiac arrest. When given intravenously, potassium may cause pain in the area of the vein where it is entering. Central IV lines should be used when rapid correction of hypokalemia is necessary. Potassium may also be replaced with potassium phosphate. Patients should be taught methods to prevent hypokalemia depending on their individual situations. Patients at risk should obtain regular serum potassium levels to monitor for hypokalemia (Table 16-7).

TABLE 16-7

*P*atient & Family Teaching Guide
Prevention of Hypokalemia

1. Teach the patient and family the signs and symptoms of hypokalemia and to report them to the health care provider.
2. For patient taking diuretics:
   ▪ Explain the importance of increasing dietary potassium intake, especially if on a thiazide or loop diuretic (see Chapter 32, Table 32-7).
   ▪ Teach patient which foods are high in potassium (see Chapter 45, Table 45-4).
   ▪ Explain that salt substitutes contain approximately 50 to 60 mEq of potassium per teaspoon and help raise potassium if taking a potassium-losing diuretic. Salt substitutes should be avoided if taking a potassium-sparing diuretic (see Chapter 32, Table 32-7).
3. For patient taking oral potassium supplements:
   ▪ Instruct the patient to take the medication as prescribed to prevent overdosage and to take the supplement with a full glass of water to help it dissolve in the GI tract.
4. For patient taking digitalis preparations and others at risk for hypokalemia:
   ▪ Explain the importance of having serum potassium levels regularly monitored because low potassium enhances the action of digitalis.

CALCIUM IMBALANCES

Calcium is obtained from ingested foods. However, only about 30% is absorbed in the GI tract. More than 99% of the body's calcium is combined with phosphorus and concentrated in the skeletal system. Bones serve as a readily available store of calcium. Thus wide variations in serum calcium levels are avoided by regulating the movement of calcium into or out of the bone. Usually the amount of calcium and phosphorus found in the serum has an inverse relationship; that is, as one increases, the other decreases.[9] The functions of calcium include transmission of nerve impulses, myocardial contractions, blood clotting, formation of teeth and bone, and muscle contractions.

Calcium is present in the serum in three forms: free or ionized; bound to protein (primarily albumin); and complexed with phosphate, citrate, or carbonate. The ionized form is the biologically active form. Approximately one half of the total serum calcium is ionized.

Calcium is typically measured in milligrams per deciliter (mg/dl). As usually reported, serum calcium levels reflect the total calcium level (all three forms), although ionized calcium levels may be reported separately. The levels listed in Table 16-8 reflect total calcium levels. Changes in serum pH will alter the level of ionized calcium without altering the total calcium level. Acidosis decreases calcium binding to albumin, leading to more ionized calcium, and alkalosis increases calcium binding, leading to decreased ionized calcium. Alterations in serum albumin levels affect interpretation of total calcium levels. Low albumin levels result in a drop in the total calcium level, although the level of ionized calcium does not change as much.

Calcium balance is controlled by parathyroid hormone (PTH), calcitonin, and vitamin D.[9] PTH is produced by the parathyroid gland. Its production and release are stimulated by low serum calcium levels. PTH increases bone resorption (movement of calcium out of bones), increases GI absorption of calcium, and increases renal tubule reabsorption of calcium.

Calcitonin is produced by the thyroid gland and is stimulated by high serum calcium levels. It opposes the action of PTH and thus lowers the serum calcium level by decreasing GI absorption, increasing calcium deposition into bone, and promoting renal excretion.

Vitamin D is formed through the action of ultraviolet (UV) rays on a precursor found in the skin or is ingested in the diet. Vitamin D is important for absorption of calcium from the gastrointestinal tract. Causes of calcium imbalances are listed in Table 16-8.

HYPERCALCEMIA

About two thirds of hypercalcemia cases are caused by hyperparathyroidism and one third are caused by malignancy, especially from breast cancer, lung cancer, and multiple myeloma.[10] Malignancies lead to hypercalcemia through bone destruction from tumor invasion or through tumor secretion of a parathyroid-related protein, which stimulates calcium release from bones. Hypercalcemia is also associated with vitamin D overdose. Prolonged immobilization results in bone mineral loss and increased calcium concentration. Hypercalcemia rarely occurs from increased calcium intake (e.g., ingestion of antacids containing calcium, excessive administration during cardiac arrest).

TABLE 16-8   Calcium Imbalances: Causes and Clinical Manifestations

HYPOCALCEMIA (Ca²⁺ <9 mg/dl [2.25 mmol/L])	HYPERCALCEMIA (Ca²⁺ >11 mg/dl [2.75 mmol/L])
Causes	
Decreased Total Calcium	***Increased Total Calcium***
Chronic renal failure	Multiple myeloma
Elevated phosphorus	Other malignancy
Primary hypoparathyroidism	Prolonged immobilization
Vitamin D deficiency	Hyperparathyroidism
Magnesium deficiency	Vitamin D overdose
Acute pancreatitis	Thiazide diuretics
Loop diuretics	Milk-alkali syndrome
Chronic alcoholism	
Diarrhea	
↓ Serum albumin (patient is usually asymptomatic due to normal ionized calcium level)	
Decreased Ionized Calcium	***Increased Ionized Calcium***
Alkalosis	Acidosis
Excess administration of citrated blood	
Clinical Manifestations	
Easy fatigability	
Depression, anxiety, confusion	Lethargy, weakness
Numbness and tingling in extremities and region around mouth	Depressed reflexes
Hyperreflexia, muscle cramps	Decreased memory
Chvostek's sign	Confusion, personality changes, psychosis
Trousseau's sign	Anorexia, nausea, vomiting
Laryngeal spasm	Bone pain, fractures
Tetany, seizures	Polyuria, dehydration
	Nephrolithiasis
	Stupor, coma
Electrocardiogram Changes	***Electrocardiogram Changes***
Elongation of ST segment	Shortened ST segment
Prolonged QT interval	Shortened QT interval
Ventricular tachycardia	Ventricular arrhythmias
	Increased digitalis effect

Excess calcium blocks the effect of sodium in skeletal muscles, which leads to reduced excitability of both muscles and nerves.[9] Manifestations of hypercalcemia include decreased memory, confusion, disorientation, fatigue, muscle weakness, constipation, cardiac arrhythmias, and renal calculi (see Table 16-8).

NURSING *and* COLLABORATIVE MANAGEMENT HYPERCALCEMIA

■ Nursing Diagnoses

Nursing diagnoses and collaborative problems for the patient with hypercalcemia include, but are not limited to, the following:
- Risk for injury *related to* neuromuscular and sensorium changes
- Potential complication: arrhythmias

■ Nursing Implementation

The basic treatment of hypercalcemia is promotion of excretion of calcium in urine by administration of a loop diuretic (e.g., furosemide [Lasix], ethacrynic acid [Edecrin]) and hydration of the patient with isotonic saline infusions. In hypercalcemia the patient must drink 3000 to 4000 ml of fluid daily to promote the renal excretion of calcium and to decrease the possibility of renal calculi formation.

Synthetic calcitonin can also be administered to lower serum calcium levels. A diet low in calcium may be prescribed. Mobilization with weight-bearing activity is encouraged to enhance bone mineralization. Plicamycin (Mithracin), a cytotoxic antibiotic, inhibits bone resorption and thus lowers the serum calcium level. In hypercalcemia associated with malignancy, the drug of choice is pamidronate (Aredia), which inhibits the activity of osteoclasts. Pamidronate is preferred over plicamycin because it does not have cytotoxic side effects and it inhibits bone resorption without inhibiting bone formation and mineralization.

HYPOCALCEMIA

Any condition that causes a decrease in the production of PTH may result in the development of hypocalcemia. This may occur with surgical removal of a portion of or injury to the parathyroid glands during thyroid or neck surgery. Acute pancreatitis is another potential cause of hypocalcemia. Lipolysis, a consequence of pancreatitis, produces fatty acids that combine with calcium ions, decreasing serum calcium levels.[2] The patient who receives multiple blood transfusions can become hypocalcemic because the citrate used to anticoagulate the blood binds with the calcium. Sudden alkalosis may also result in symptomatic hypocalcemia despite a normal total serum calcium level. The high pH increases calcium binding to protein, decreasing the amount of ionized calcium. Hypocalcemia can occur if the diet is low in calcium or if there is increased loss of calcium with laxative abuse and malabsorption syndromes. (See Table 16-8 for the clinical manifestations and etiologies of hypocalcemia.)

Low calcium levels allow sodium to move into excitable cells, increasing depolarization. This results in increased nerve excitability and sustained muscle contraction that is referred to as **tetany.** Clinical signs of tetany include the Trousseau's sign and Chvostek's sign. *Trousseau's sign* refers to carpal spasms induced by inflating a blood pressure cuff on the arm (Fig. 16-15). The blood pressure cuff is inflated above the systolic pressure. Carpal spasms become evident within 3 minutes if hypocalcemia is present. *Chvostek's sign* is contraction of facial muscles in response to a tap over the facial nerve in front of the ear (see Fig. 16-15), and it also indicates hypocalcemia with latent tetany. Other manifestations of tetany are laryngeal stridor, dysphagia, and numbness and tingling around the mouth or in the extremities.

Because calcium is necessary for cardiac contractions, hypocalcemia results in decreased cardiac contractility and ECG change. Clinical manifestations of hypocalcemia are listed in Table 16-8.

NURSING and COLLABORATIVE MANAGEMENT HYPOCALCEMIA

■ Nursing Diagnoses

Nursing diagnoses and collaborative problems for the patient with hypocalcemia include, but are not limited to, the following:
- Risk for injury *related to* tetany and seizures
- Potential complications: fracture, respiratory arrest

■ Nursing Implementation

The primary goal in treatment of hypocalcemia is aimed at treating the cause. Hypocalcemia can be treated with oral or IV calcium supplements. Calcium is not given intramuscularly (IM) because it will precipitate in the muscle. Intravenous preparations of calcium, such as calcium gluconate, are administered when severe symptoms of hypocalcemia are impending or present. A diet high in calcium-rich foods is usually ordered along with vitamin D supplements for the patient with hypocalcemia. Oral calcium supplements, such as calcium carbonate, may be used when patients are unable to consume enough calcium in the diet, such as those who do not tolerate dairy products. Pain and anxiety must be adequately treated in the patient with suspected hypocalcemia because hyperventilation-induced respiratory alkalosis can precipitate hypocalcemic symptoms. Any patient who has had thyroid or neck surgery must be observed closely in the immediate postoperative period for manifestations of hypocalcemia because of the proximity of the surgery to the parathyroid glands.

PHOSPHATE IMBALANCES

Phosphorus is a primary anion in the ICF and is essential to the function of muscle, red blood cells, and the nervous system. It is deposited with calcium for bone and tooth structure. It is also involved in the acid-base buffering system, in the mitochondrial energy production of ATP, in cellular uptake and use of glucose, and as an intermediary in the metabolism of carbohydrates, proteins, and fats.

Maintenance of normal phosphate balance requires adequate renal functioning because the kidneys are the major route of phosphate excretion. A small amount is lost in the feces. A reciprocal relationship exists between phosphorus and calcium in that a high serum phosphate level tends to cause a low calcium concentration in the serum.

HYPERPHOSPHATEMIA

The major condition that can lead to hyperphosphatemia is acute or chronic renal failure that results in an altered ability of the kidneys to excrete phosphate. Other causes include chemotherapy for certain malignancies (lymphomas), excessive ingestion of milk or phosphate-containing laxatives, and large intakes of vitamin D that increase GI absorption of phosphorus (Table 16-9).

Clinical manifestations of hyperphosphatemia (presented in Table 16-9) primarily relate to metastatic calcium-phosphate

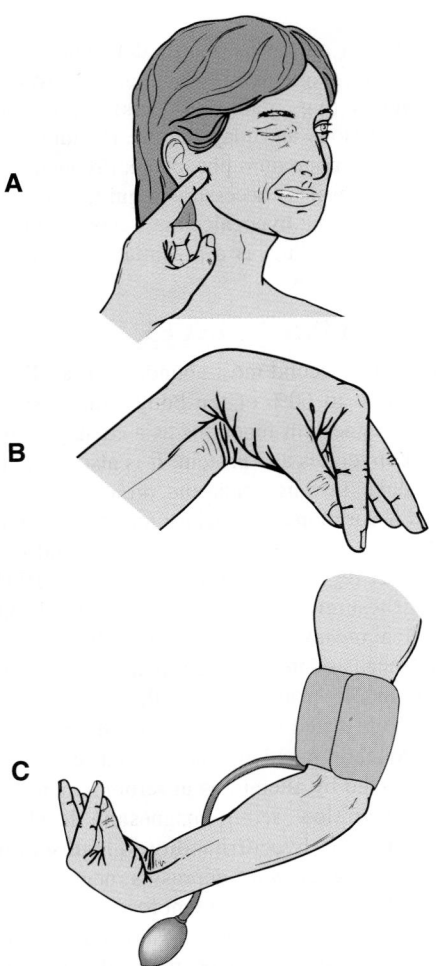

FIG. 16-15 Tests for hypocalcemia. **A,** Chvostek's sign is contraction of facial muscles in response to a light tap over the facial nerve in front of the ear. **B,** Trousseau's sign is a carpal spasm induced by **C,** inflating a blood pressure cuff above the systolic pressure for a few minutes.

TABLE 16-9	Phosphate Imbalances: Causes and Clinical Manifestations
HYPOPHOSPHATEMIA (PO$_4^{3-}$ <2.8 mg/dl [0.9 mmol/L])	**HYPERPHOSPHATEMIA (PO$_4^{3-}$ >4.5 mg/dl [1.45 mmol/L])**
Causes	
Malabsorption syndrome	Renal failure
Nutritional recovery syndrome	Chemotherapeutic agents
Glucose administration	Enemas containing phosphorus (e.g., Fleet Enema)
Total parenteral nutrition	Excessive ingestion (e.g., milk, phosphate-containing laxatives)
Alcohol withdrawal	Large vitamin D intake
Phosphate-binding antacids	Hypoparathyroidism
Recovery from diabetic ketoacidosis	
Respiratory alkalosis	
Clinical Manifestations	
Central nervous system dysfunction (confusion, coma)	Hypocalcemia
Rhabdomyolysis	Muscle problems; tetany
Renal tubular wasting of Mg^{2+}, Ca^{2+}, HCO$_3^-$	Deposition of calcium-phosphate precipitates in skin, soft tissue,
Cardiac problems (arrhythmias, decreased stroke volume)	cornea, viscera, blood vessels
Muscle weakness, including respiratory muscle weakness and difficulty weaning	
Osteomalacia	

precipitates. Ordinarily, calcium and phosphate are deposited only in bone. However, an increased serum phosphate concentration along with calcium precipitates readily, and calcified deposits can occur in soft tissue such as joints, arteries, skin, kidneys, and cornea (see Chapter 45). Other manifestations of hyperphosphatemia are neuromuscular irritability and tetany, which are related to the low serum calcium levels often associated with high serum phosphate levels.

Management of hyperphosphatemia is aimed at identifying and treating the underlying cause. Ingestion of foods and fluids high in phosphorus (e.g., dairy products) should be restricted. Adequate hydration and correction of hypocalcemic conditions can enhance the renal excretion of phosphate. For the patient with renal failure, measures to reduce serum phosphate levels include calcium supplements, phosphate-binding agents or gels, and dietary phosphate restrictions (see Chapter 45). Sevelamer (Renagel), an example of a binding agent, binds and removes dietary phosphorous in the GI tract.[11]

HYPOPHOSPHATEMIA

Hypophosphatemia (low serum phosphate) is seen in the patient who is malnourished or has malabsorption syndromes. Other causes include alcohol withdrawal and use of phosphate-binding antacids. Hypophosphatemia may also occur during parenteral nutrition with inadequate phosphorus replacement. Table 16-9 lists causes of phosphorus imbalances.

Most clinical manifestations of hypophosphatemia (presented in Table 16-9) relate to a deficiency of ATP or 2,3-diphosphoglycerate (2,3-DPG), an enzyme in RBCs. Both conditions result in impaired cellular energy resources and oxygen delivery to tissues. Hemolytic anemia may occur because of the fragility of the RBCs. Acute manifestations include CNS depression, confusion, and other mental changes. Other manifestations include muscle weakness and pain, arrhythmias, and cardiomyopathy.

Management of a mild phosphorus deficiency may involve oral supplementation (e.g., Neutra-Phos) and ingestion of foods high in phosphorus (e.g., dairy products). Severe hypophosphatemia can be serious and may require IV administration of sodium phosphate or potassium phosphate. Frequent monitoring of serum phosphate levels is necessary to guide intravenous therapy. Sudden symptomatic hypocalcemia, secondary to increased calcium phosphorus binding, is a potential complication of IV phosphorus administration.

MAGNESIUM IMBALANCES

Magnesium is the second most abundant intracellular cation. Approximately 50% to 60% of the body's magnesium is contained in bone. Magnesium functions as a coenzyme in the metabolism of carbohydrates and protein. It is also involved in metabolism of cellular nucleic acids and proteins. Magnesium is regulated by GI absorption and renal excretion.[12] The kidneys are able to conserve magnesium in times of need and excrete excesses. Factors that regulate calcium balance (e.g., PTH) appear to influence magnesium balance. Manifestations of magnesium balance are often mistaken for calcium imbalances. Because magnesium balance is related to calcium and potassium balance, all three cations should be assessed together.[12] Causes of magnesium imbalances are listed in Table 16-10. Magnesium acts directly on the myoneural junction, and neuromuscular excitability is profoundly affected by alterations in serum magnesium.

Hypomagnesemia (low serum magnesium level) produces neuromuscular and CNS hyperirritability. A high serum magnesium level *(hypermagnesemia)* depresses neuromuscular and CNS functions. Magnesium is important for normal cardiac function. There is an association between hypomagnesemia and cardiovascular problems, such as myocardial infarction, hypertension, and congestive heart failure.[12] Decreased intracellular magnesium may be a factor in the pathophysiologic consequences of diabetes mellitus, such as microangiopathies and

TABLE 16-10	Causes of Magnesium Imbalances
HYPOMAGNESEMIA	**HYPERMAGNESEMIA**
Diarrhea	Renal failure (especially if patient
Vomiting	is given magnesium products)
Chronic alcoholism	Excessive administration of
Impaired GI absorption	magnesium for treatment of
Malabsorption syndrome	eclampsia
Prolonged malnutrition	Adrenal insufficiency
Large urine output	
NG suction	
Poorly controlled diabetes	
mellitus	
Hyperaldosteronism	

macroangiopathies, and may contribute to insulin resistance common in diabetes.[12] However, it is not clear how hypomagnesemia and insulin resistance are related.[2]

HYPERMAGNESEMIA

Hypermagnesemia usually occurs only with an increase in magnesium intake accompanied by renal insufficiency or failure. A patient with chronic renal failure who ingests products containing magnesium (e.g., Maalox, milk of magnesia) will have a problem with excess magnesium. Magnesium excess could develop in the pregnant woman who receives magnesium sulfate for the management of eclampsia.

Initial clinical manifestations of a mildly elevated serum magnesium concentration include lethargy, drowsiness, and nausea and vomiting. As the levels of serum magnesium increase, deep tendon reflexes are lost, followed by somnolence; then respiratory and, ultimately, cardiac arrest can occur.

Management of hypermagnesemia should focus on prevention. Persons with renal failure should not take magnesium-containing drugs and must be cautioned to review all over-the-counter drug labels for magnesium content. The emergency treatment of hypermagnesemia is IV administration of calcium chloride or calcium gluconate to physiologically oppose the effects of the magnesium on cardiac muscle. Promoting urinary excretion with fluid will decrease serum magnesium levels. The patient with impaired renal function will require dialysis because the kidneys are the major route of excretion for magnesium.

HYPOMAGNESEMIA

A major cause of magnesium deficiency is prolonged fasting or starvation. Chronic alcoholism commonly causes hypomagnesemia as a result of insufficient intake and alcohol-related diuresis.[12] Fluid loss from the GI tract interferes with magnesium absorption. Prolonged parenteral nutrition without magnesium supplementation is another potential cause of hypomagnesemia. Diuretics increase the risk of magnesium loss through renal excretion.[13] In addition, osmotic diuresis caused by high glucose levels in uncontrolled diabetes mellitus increases renal excretion of magnesium. The significant clinical manifestations include confusion, hyperactive deep tendon reflexes, tremors, and seizures. Magnesium deficiency also predisposes to cardiac ar-

rhythmias. Clinically, hypomagnesemia resembles hypocalcemia and may contribute to the development of hypocalcemia. Hypomagnesemia may also be associated with hypokalemia that does not respond well to potassium replacement. This occurs because intracellular magnesium is critical to normal function of the sodium-potassium pump.

Mild magnesium deficiencies can be treated with oral supplements and increased dietary intake of foods high in magnesium (e.g., green vegetables, nuts, bananas, oranges, peanut butter, chocolate). If the condition is severe, parenteral IV or IM magnesium (e.g., magnesium sulfate) should be administered. Too rapid administration of magnesium can lead to cardiac or respiratory arrest.

PROTEIN IMBALANCES

Plasma proteins, particularly albumin, are a significant determinant of plasma volume. Because of their large molecular size, they remain in the vascular space and contribute to the colloidal oncotic pressure. Causes of protein imbalances are listed in Table 16-11. Hypoproteinemia can occur over time. Causes related to intake are anorexia, malnutrition, starvation, fad dieting, and poorly balanced vegetarian diets. Poor absorption of protein can occur in certain GI malabsorptive diseases, such as pancreatic insufficiency and inflammatory bowel disease. Protein can shift out of the intravascular space with inflammation. Increased breakdown of proteins occurs with elevated basal metabolic rates and catabolic states, such as fever, infection, and certain malignancies. Increased use of protein occurs with cell growth and repair after surgical wounds or burns. Hemorrhage with loss of red blood cells can be a cause of protein deficit. Impaired synthesis of albumin occurs in liver failure. The kidneys can lose large amounts of protein, especially albumin, in nephrotic syndrome (see Chapter 44).

Clinical manifestations of protein deficit include edema (from decreased oncotic pressure), slow healing, anorexia, fatigue, anemia, and muscle loss that results from the breakdown of body tissue to meet the body's need for protein. Intravascular fluid readily accumulates in the peritoneal cavity, producing ascites, when the vascular oncotic pressure is decreased in hypoproteinemia.

Management of protein deficit includes providing a high-carbohydrate, high-protein diet and dietary protein supplements. If the patient cannot meet the needs for protein orally, enteral nutrition or total parenteral nutrition may be used. (Protein-calorie malnutrition is discussed in Chapter 39.)

Hyperproteinemia is rare, but it can occur with dehydration-induced hemoconcentration.

TABLE 16-11	Causes of Protein Imbalances
HYPOPROTEINEMIA	**HYPERPROTEINEMIA**
Decreased food intake	Dehydration
Starvation	Hemoconcentration
Diseased liver	
Massive burns	
Loss of albumin in renal disease	
Major infection	

ACID-BASE IMBALANCES

The body normally maintains a steady balance between acids produced during metabolism and bases that neutralize and promote the excretion of the acids. Many health problems may lead to acid-base imbalances in addition to fluid and electrolyte imbalances. Patients with diabetes mellitus, chronic obstructive pulmonary disease, and kidney disease frequently develop acid-base imbalances. Vomiting and diarrhea may cause loss of acids and bases in addition to fluids and electrolytes. The kidneys are an essential buffer system for acids, and in the older adult, the kidneys are less able to compensate for an acid load. The older adult also has decreased respiratory function, leading to impaired compensation for acid-base imbalances. In addition, tissue hypoxia from any cause may alter acid-base balance. The nurse must always consider the possibility of acid-base imbalance in patients with serious illnesses.

pH and Hydrogen Ion Concentration

The acidity or alkalinity of a solution depends on its hydrogen ion (H^+) concentration. An increase in H^+ concentration leads to acidity; a decrease leads to alkalinity. (Definitions related to acid-base balance are presented in Table 16-12.)

Despite the fact that acids are produced by the body daily, the hydrogen ion concentration of body fluids is small (0.0004 mEq/L). This tiny amount is maintained within a narrow range to ensure optimal cellular function. Hydrogen ion concentration is usually expressed as a negative logarithm (symbolized as **pH**) rather than in milliequivalents. The use of the negative logarithm means that the lower the pH, the higher the hydrogen ion concentration. In contrast to a pH of 7, a pH of 8 represents a tenfold decrease in hydrogen ion concentration.

The pH of a chemical solution may range from 1 to 14. A solution with a pH of 7 is considered neutral. An acid solution has a pH less than 7, and an alkaline solution has a pH greater than 7. Blood is slightly alkaline (pH 7.35 to 7.45); yet if it drops be-

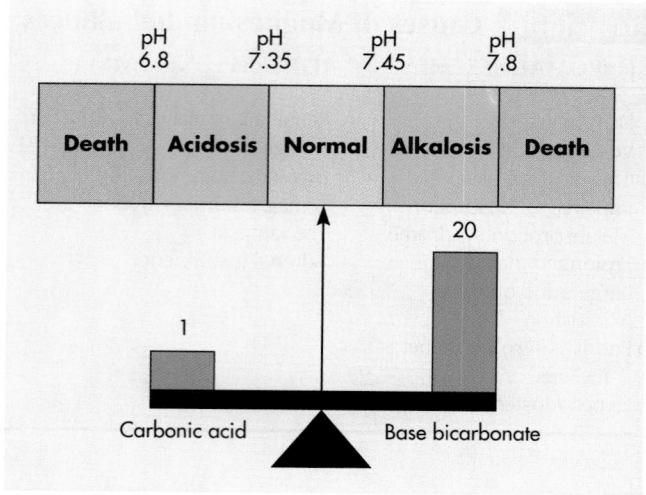

FIG. 16-16 The normal range of plasma pH is 7.35 to 7.45. A normal pH is maintained by a ratio of 1 part carbonic acid to 20 parts bicarbonate.

low 7.35, the person has **acidosis,** even though the blood may never become truly acidic. If the blood pH is greater than 7.45, the person has **alkalosis** (Fig. 16-16).

Acid-Base Regulation

The body's metabolic processes constantly produce acids. These acids must be neutralized and excreted to maintain acid-base balance. Normally the body has three mechanisms by which it regulates acid-base balance to maintain the arterial pH between 7.35 and 7.45. These mechanisms are the buffer systems, the respiratory system, and the renal system.

The regulatory mechanisms react at different speeds. Buffers react immediately; the respiratory system responds in minutes and reaches maximum effectiveness in hours; the renal response takes 2 to 3 days to respond maximally, but the kidneys can maintain balance for a long period of time.

Buffer System. The buffer system is the fastest-acting system and the primary regulator of acid-base balance. **Buffers** act chemically to change strong acids into weaker acids or to bind acids to neutralize their effect. The buffers in the body include carbonic acid–bicarbonate, monohydrogen-dihydrogen phosphate, intracellular and plasma protein, and hemoglobin buffers.

A buffer consists of a weakly ionized acid or a base and its salt. Buffers function to minimize the effect of acids on blood pH until they can be excreted from the body. The carbonic acid (H_2CO_3)-bicarbonate (HCO_3^-) buffer system neutralizes hydrochloric acid (HCl) in the following manner:

$$HCl \quad + \quad NaH_2CO_3 \quad \rightarrow \quad NaCl \quad + \quad H_2CO_3$$
strong acid   strong base   salt   weak acid

In this way, HCl is prevented from making a large change in the solution's pH, and more H_2CO_3 is formed. The carbonic acid, in turn, is broken down to H_2O and CO_2. The CO_2 is excreted by the lungs. In this process the buffer system maintains the 20:1 ratio between bicarbonate and carbonic acid and the normal pH.

The phosphate buffer system is composed of sodium and other cations in combination with HPO_4^{2-} and $H_2PO_4^-$. This buffer system acts in the same manner as the bicarbonate system.

TABLE 16-12	Terms in Acid-Base Physiology
Acid	Donor of hydrogen ion (H^+); separation of an acid into H^+ and its accompanying anion in solution
Acidemia	Signifying an arterial blood pH of less than 7.35
Acidosis	Process that adds acid or eliminates base from body fluids
Alkalemia	Signifying an arterial blood pH of more than 7.45
Alkalosis	Process that adds base or eliminates acid from body fluids
Anion gap	Reflection of normally unmeasured anions in the plasma; helpful in differential diagnosis of acidosis
Base	Acceptor of hydrogen ions; chemical combining of acid and base when hydrogen ions are added to a solution containing a base; bicarbonate (HCO_3^-) most abundant base in body fluids
Buffer	Substance that reacts with an acid or base to prevent a large change in pH
pH	Negative logarithm of the H^+ concentration

Strong acids are neutralized to form a weak acid of sodium biphosphate, which can be excreted in the urine, and sodium chloride: $Na_2HPO_4 + HCl \rightarrow NaCl + NaH_2PO_4$. When a strong base is added to the system, it is neutralized to form a weak base and H_2O:

$$NaOH + NaH_2PO_4 \rightarrow Na_2HPO_4 + H_2O$$

Intracellular and extracellular proteins are an effective buffering system throughout the body. The protein buffering system acts like the bicarbonate system. Some of the amino acids of proteins contain free acid radicals, —COOH, which can dissociate into CO_2 and H^+. Other amino acids have basic radicals, —NH_3OH, which can dissociate into NH_3^+ and OH^-; the OH^- can combine with an H^+ to form H_2O.

Using the "chloride shift" mechanism, hemoglobin regulates pH by shifting chloride in and out of RBCs in exchange for bicarbonate. This shift is regulated by the level of oxygen in blood.

The cell can also act as a buffer by shifting hydrogen in and out of the cell. With an accumulation of H^+ in the ECF, the intracellular compartment can accept hydrogen in exchange for another cation (e.g., Na^+).

The body buffers an acid load better than it neutralizes base excess. Buffers cannot maintain pH without the adequate functioning of the respiratory and renal systems.

Respiratory System. The lungs help maintain a normal pH by excreting carbon dioxide and water, which are by-products of cellular metabolism. When released into circulation, CO_2 enters RBCs and combines with H_2O to form H_2CO_3. The carbonic acid dissociates into hydrogen ions and bicarbonate. The free hydrogen is buffered by hemoglobin molecules, and the bicarbonate diffuses into the plasma. In the pulmonary capillaries, this process is reversed, and CO_2 is formed and excreted by the lungs. The overall reversible reaction is expressed as the following:

$$CO_2 + H_2O \rightleftarrows H_2CO_3 \rightleftarrows H^+ + HCO_3^-$$

The amount of CO_2 in the blood directly relates to carbonic acid concentration and subsequently to hydrogen ion concentration. With increased respirations, less CO_2 remains in the blood. This leads to less carbonic acid and fewer H^+ ions. With decreased respirations, more CO_2 remains in the blood. This leads to increased carbonic acid and more hydrogen ions.

The rate of excretion of CO_2 is controlled by the respiratory center in the medulla in the brainstem. If increased amounts of CO_2 or hydrogen ions are present, the respiratory center stimulates an increased rate and depth of breathing. Respirations are inhibited if the center senses low H^+ or CO_2 levels.

As a compensatory mechanism the respiratory system acts on the $CO_2 + H_2O$ side of the reaction by altering the rate and depth of breathing to "blow off" (through hyperventilation) or "retain" (through hypoventilation) CO_2. If a respiratory problem is the cause of an acid-base imbalance (e.g., respiratory failure), the respiratory system loses its ability to correct a pH alteration.

Renal System. Under normal conditions the kidneys reabsorb and conserve all of the bicarbonate they filter. The kidneys can generate additional bicarbonate and eliminate excess hydrogen ions as compensation for acidosis. The three mechanisms of acid elimination include (1) secretion of small amounts of free hydrogen into the renal tubule, (2) combination of hydrogen ions with ammonia (NH_3) to form ammonium (NH_4^+), and (3) excretion of weak acids.

The body depends on the kidneys to excrete a portion of the acid produced by cellular metabolism. Thus the kidneys normally excrete an acidic urine (average pH equals 6). As a compensatory mechanism, the pH of the urine can decrease to 4 and increase to 8. If the renal system is the cause of an acid-base imbalance (e.g., renal failure), it loses its ability to correct a pH alteration.

Alterations in Acid-Base Balance

An acid-base imbalance is produced when the ratio of 1:20 between acid and base content is altered (Table 16-13). A primary disease or process may alter one side of the ratio (e.g., CO_2 retention in pulmonary disease). The compensatory process attempts to maintain the other side of the ratio (e.g., increased renal bicarbonate reabsorption). When the compensatory mechanism fails, an acid-base imbalance results. The compensatory process may be inadequate because either the pathophysiologic process is overwhelming or there is insufficient time for the compensatory process to function.

Acid-base imbalances are classified as respiratory or metabolic. *Respiratory imbalances* affect carbonic acid concentrations; *metabolic imbalances* affect the base bicarbonate. Therefore acidosis can be caused by an increase in carbonic acid (respiratory acidosis) or a decrease in bicarbonate (metabolic acidosis). Alkalosis can be caused by a decrease in carbonic acid (respiratory alkalosis) or an increase in bicarbonate (metabolic alkalosis). Imbalances may be further classified as acute or chronic. Chronic imbalances allow greater time for compensatory changes.

Respiratory Acidosis. *Respiratory acidosis* (carbonic acid excess) occurs whenever there is hypoventilation (see Table 16-13). Hypoventilation results in a buildup of CO_2; subsequently, carbonic acid accumulates in the blood. Carbonic acid dissociates, liberating H^+, and there is a decrease in pH. If carbon dioxide is not eliminated from the blood, acidosis results from the accumulation of carbonic acid (Fig. 16-17, *A*).

To compensate, the kidneys conserve bicarbonate and secrete increased concentrations of hydrogen ion into the urine. In acute respiratory acidosis the renal compensatory mechanisms begin to operate within 24 hours. Therefore a normal serum bicarbonate level usually can be found until the kidneys have compensated for the imbalance.

Respiratory Alkalosis. *Respiratory alkalosis* (carbonic acid deficit) occurs with hyperventilation (see Table 16-13). Anxiety, CNS disorders, sepsis, and mechanical overventilation all increase ventilation and decrease the PCO_2 level. This leads to decreased carbonic acid and alkalosis (see Fig. 16-17, *A*).

Compensated respiratory alkalosis is uncommon unless the patient has been maintained on a ventilator or has a CNS problem. A decreased bicarbonate level differentiates compensated respiratory alkalosis from acute or uncompensated respiratory alkalosis.

Metabolic Acidosis. *Metabolic acidosis* (base bicarbonate deficit) occurs when an acid other than carbonic acid accumulates in the body or when bicarbonate is lost from body fluids (see Table 16-13 and Fig. 16-17, *B*). In both cases a bicarbonate deficit results. Ketoacid accumulation in diabetic ketoacidosis and lactic acid accumulation with shock are examples of accumulation of acids. Severe diarrhea results in loss of bicarbonate. In renal disease the kidneys lose their ability to reabsorb bicarbonate and secrete hydrogen ions.

The compensatory response to metabolic acidosis is to increase CO_2 excretion by the lungs. The patient often develops

TABLE 16-13 **Acid-Base Imbalances**

COMMON CAUSES	PATHOPHYSIOLOGY	LABORATORY FINDINGS
Respiratory Acidosis		
Chronic obstructive pulmonary disease	CO_2 retention from hypoventilation	Plasma pH ↓
Barbiturate or sedative overdose	Compensatory response to HCO_3^- retention by kidney	PCO_2 ↑
Chest wall abnormality (e.g., obesity)		HCO_3^- normal (uncompensated)
Severe pneumonia		HCO_3^- ↑ (compensated)
Atelectasis		Urine pH <6 (compensated)
Respiratory muscle weakness (e.g., Guillain-Barré syndrome)		
Mechanical hypoventilation		
Respiratory Alkalosis		
Hyperventilation (caused by hypoxia, pulmonary emboli, anxiety, fear, pain, exercise, fever)	Increased CO_2 excretion from hyperventilation	Plasma pH ↑
	Compensatory response of HCO_3^- excretion by kidney	PCO_2 ↓
Stimulated respiratory center caused by septicemia, encephalitis, brain injury, salicylate poisoning		HCO_3^- normal (uncompensated)
		HCO_3^- ↓ (compensated)
Mechanical hyperventilation		Urine pH >6 (compensated)
Metabolic Acidosis		
Diabetic ketoacidosis	Gain of fixed acid, inability to excrete acid or loss of base	Plasma pH ↓
Lactic acidosis	Compensatory response of CO_2 excretion by lungs	PCO_2 normal (uncompensated)
Starvation		PCO_2 ↓ (compensated)
Severe diarrhea		HCO_3^- ↓
Renal tubular acidosis		Urine pH <6 (compensated)
Renal failure		
Gastrointestinal fistulas		
Shock		
Metabolic Alkalosis		
Severe vomiting	Loss of strong acid or gain of base	Plasma pH ↑
Excess gastric suctioning	Compensatory response of CO_2 retention by lungs	PCO_2 normal (uncompensated)
Diuretic therapy		PCO_2 ↑ (compensated)
Potassium deficit		HCO_3^- ↑
Excess $NaHCO_3$ intake		Urine pH >6 (compensated)
Excessive mineralocorticoids		

Kussmaul respiration (deep, rapid breathing). In addition, the kidneys attempt to excrete additional acid.

Metabolic Alkalosis. *Metabolic alkalosis* (base bicarbonate excess) occurs when a loss of acid (prolonged vomiting or gastric suction) or a gain in bicarbonate (ingestion of baking soda) occurs (see Table 16-13 and Fig. 16-17, *B*). The compensatory mechanism is a decreased respiratory rate to increase plasma CO_2. Renal excretion of bicarbonate also occurs.

Mixed Acid-Base Disorders. A mixed acid-base disorder occurs when two or more simple disorders are present at the same time. The pH will depend on the type, severity, and acuity of each of the simple disorders involved. Respiratory acidosis combined with metabolic alkalosis (e.g., chronic obstructive lung disease treated with diuretic therapy) may result in a near-normal pH, while respiratory acidosis combined with metabolic acidosis will cause a greater decrease in pH than either disorder alone. An example of a mixed acidosis appears in a patient in cardiopulmonary arrest. Hypoventilation elevates the CO_2 level, and anaerobic metabolism produces lactic acid. An example of a mixed alkalosis is the case of a patient who is hyperventilating because of postoperative pain and is also losing acid secondary to nasogastric suctioning.

Clinical Manifestations

Clinical manifestations of acidosis and alkalosis are summarized in Tables 16-14 and 16-15. Because a normal pH is vital to all cellular reactions, the clinical manifestations of acid-base imbalances are generalized and nonspecific. The actual compensatory mechanisms also produce some clinical manifestations. For example, the deep, rapid respirations of a patient with metabolic acidosis are an example of respiratory compensation. In alkalosis, hypocalcemia may concurrently be found and accounts for many of the clinical manifestations.

Blood Gas Values. Arterial blood gas (ABG) values provide valuable information about a patient's acid-base status; the origin of the imbalance; an idea of the body's ability to regulate pH; and a reflection of the patient's overall oxygen status.[14] Diagnosis of acid-base disturbances and identification of compensatory processes are done by performing the following five steps:

1. Determine whether the pH is acidotic or alkalotic. Use 7.4 as the starting point. Label values less than 7.4 as acidotic and values greater than 7.4 as alkalotic.
2. Analyze the PCO_2 to determine if the patient has respiratory acidosis or alkalosis. CO_2 is controlled by the lungs and is thus con-

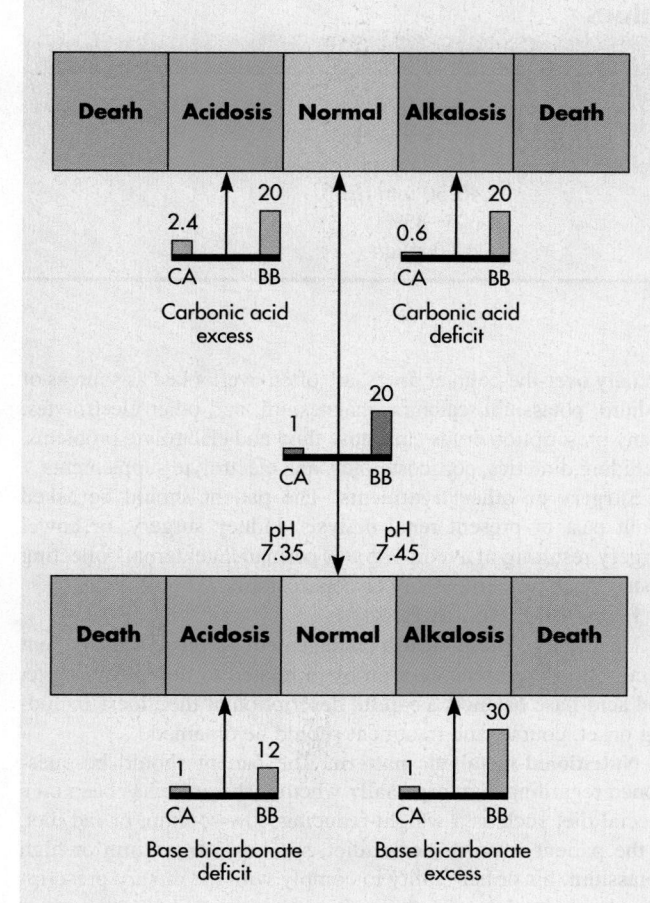

FIG. 16-17 Kinds of acid-base imbalances. **A,** Respiratory imbalances caused by carbonic acid *(CA)* excess and carbonic acid deficit. **B,** Metabolic imbalances caused by base bicarbonate *(BB)* deficit and base bicarbonate excess.

sidered the respiratory component of the ABG. Because CO_2 forms carbonic acid when dissolved in blood, high CO_2 levels indicate acidosis and low CO_2 levels indicate alkalosis.

3. Analyze the HCO_3^- to determine if the patient has metabolic acidosis or alkalosis. HCO_3^-, the metabolic component of the ABG, is controlled primarily by the kidneys. Because HCO_3^- is a base, high levels of HCO_3^- result in alkalosis and low levels result in acidosis.

4. Determine if the CO_2 or the HCO_3^- matches the acid or base alteration of the pH. For example, if the pH is acidotic and the CO_2 is high (respiratory acidosis), but the HCO_3^- is high (metabolic alkalosis), the CO_2 is the parameter that matches the pH derangement. The patient's acid-base imbalance would be diagnosed as respiratory acidosis.

5. Decide if the body is attempting to compensate for the pH change. If the parameter that does not match the pH is moving in the opposite direction, the body is attempting to compensate. In step 4, the HCO_3^- is alkalotic; this is in the opposite direction of respiratory acidosis and considered compensation. If compensatory mechanisms are functioning, the pH will return toward 7.40. When the pH is back to normal, the patient has *full compensation*. The body will not overcompensate for pH changes.

TABLE 16-14   Clinical Manifestations of Acidosis

RESPIRATORY ($\uparrow PCO_2$)	METABOLIC ($\downarrow HCO_3^-$)
Neurologic	
Drowsiness	Drowsiness
Disorientation	Confusion
Dizziness	Headache
Headache	Coma
Coma	
Cardiovascular	
↓ Blood pressure	↓ Blood pressure
Ventricular fibrillation (related to hyperkalemia from compensation)	Arrhythmias (related to hyperkalemia from compensation)
Warm, flushed skin (related to peripheral vasodilation)	Warm, flushed skin (related to peripheral vasodilation)
Gastrointestinal	
No significant findings	Nausea, vomiting, diarrhea, abdominal pain
Neuromuscular	
Seizures	No significant findings
Respiratory	
Hypoventilation with hypoxia (lungs are unable to compensate when there is a respiratory problem)	Deep, rapid respirations (compensatory action by the lungs)

TABLE 16-15   Clinical Manifestations of Alkalosis

RESPIRATORY ($\downarrow PCO_2$)	METABOLIC ($\uparrow HCO_3^-$)
Neurologic	
Lethargy	Dizziness
Light-headedness	Irritability
Confusion	Nervousness
	Confusion
Cardiovascular	
Tachycardia	Tachycardia
Arrhythmias (related to hypokalemia from compensation)	Arrhythmias (related to hypokalemia from compensation)
Gastrointestinal	
Nausea	Anorexia
Vomiting	Nausea
Epigastric pain	Vomiting
Neuromuscular*	
Tetany	Tremors
Numbness	Hypertonic muscles
Tingling of extremities	Muscle cramps
Hyperreflexia	Tetany
Seizures	Tingling of fingers and toes
	Seizures
Respiratory	
Hyperventilation (lungs are unable to compensate when there is a respiratory problem)	Hypoventilation (compensatory action by the lungs)

*Alkalosis decreases calcium binding to protein.

TABLE 16-16	Normal Arterial and Venous Blood Gas Values		
PARAMETER		**ARTERIAL**	**VENOUS**
pH		7.35–7.45	7.35–7.45
PCO_2		35–45 mm Hg	40–45 mm Hg
Bicarbonate (HCO_3^-)		22–26 mEq/L (mmol/L)	22–26 mEq/L (mmol/L)
PO_2*		80–100 mm Hg	40–50 mm Hg
Oxygen saturation		96%–100%	60%–85%
Base excess		±2.0 mEq/L	±2.0 mEq/L

*Decreases above sea level and with increasing age.

TABLE 16-17	Arterial Blood Gas (ABG) Analysis
ABG VALUES	**ANALYSIS**
pH 7.30 PCO_2 25 mm Hg HCO_3^- 16 mEq/L	1. pH < 7.4 indicates acidosis. 2. PCO_2 is low, indicating respiratory alkalosis. 3. HCO_3^- is low, indicating metabolic acidosis. 4. Metabolic acidosis matches the pH. 5. The CO_2 does not match, but is moving in the opposite direction, which indicates the lungs are attempting to compensate for the metabolic acidosis.

Interpretation
This ABG is interpreted as metabolic acidosis with partial compensation. If the pH returns to the normal range, the patient is said to have full compensation.

Table 16-16 lists normal blood gas values and Table 16-17 provides a sample ABG with interpretation. (Refer to the laboratory findings section of Table 16-13 for the ABG findings of the four major acid-base disturbances.) Knowledge of the patient's clinical situation and the physiologic extent of renal and respiratory compensation enables the clinician to identify mixed acid-base disorders.

Blood gas analysis will also show the PO_2 and oxygen saturation. These values are used to identify hypoxemia. Arterial blood gases are usually obtained. The values of blood gases differ slightly between arterial and venous samples (see Table 16-16). (Blood gases are discussed further in Chapter 25.)

ASSESSMENT OF FLUID, ELECTROLYTE, AND ACID–BASE IMBALANCES

Subjective Data

Important Health Information

Past health history. The patient should be questioned about any past health history of problems involving the kidneys, heart, GI system, or lungs that could affect the present fluid, electrolyte, and acid-base balance. Information about specific diseases such as diabetes mellitus, diabetes insipidus, chronic obstructive pulmonary disease, ulcerative colitis, and Crohn's disease should be obtained from the patient. The patient should also be questioned about the incidence of a prior fluid, electrolyte, or acid-base disorders.

Medications. An assessment of the patient's current and past use of medications is important. The ingredients in many drugs, es-

pecially over-the-counter drugs, are often overlooked as sources of sodium, potassium, calcium, magnesium, and other electrolytes. Many prescription drugs can cause fluid and electrolyte problems, including diuretics, corticosteroids, and electrolyte supplements.

Surgery or other treatments. The patient should be asked about past or present renal dialysis, kidney surgery, or bowel surgery resulting in a temporary or permanent external collecting system such as a colostomy or nephrostomy.

Functional Health Patterns

Health perception–health management pattern. If the patient is currently experiencing a problem related to fluid, electrolyte, and acid-base balance, a careful description of the illness including onset, course, and treatment should be obtained.

Nutritional-metabolic pattern. The patient should be questioned regarding diet, especially whether she or he has been on a special diet such as a weight-reducing, low-sodium, or fad diet. If the patient is on a special diet, such as low sodium or high potassium, his or her ability to comply with the dietary prescription should be determined.

Elimination pattern. Note should be made of the patient's usual bowel and bladder habits. Any deviations from the expected elimination pattern such as diarrhea, nocturia, or polyuria should be carefully documented.

Activity-exercise pattern. The patient's exercise pattern is important to determine because excessive perspiration secondary to exercise could result in a fluid and electrolyte problem. Also, the patient's exposure to extremely high temperatures as a result of leisure or work activity should be determined. The patient should be asked what practices are followed to replace fluid and electrolytes lost through excessive perspiration.

Cognitive-perceptual pattern. The patient should be queried about any changes in sensations such as numbness, tingling, *fasciculations* (uncoordinated twitching of a single muscle group), or muscle weakness that could indicate a fluid and electrolyte problem. Additionally, both the patient and the family should be asked if any changes in mentation or alertness have been noted such as confusion, memory impairment, or lethargy.

Objective Data

Physical Examination

There is no specific physical examination to assess fluid, electrolyte, and acid-base balance. Common abnormal assessment findings of major body systems offer clues to possible imbalances (Table 16-18).

Laboratory Values

Assessment of serum electrolyte values is a good starting point for identifying fluid and electrolyte imbalance (see Table 16-3). However, serum electrolyte values often provide only cursory in-

TABLE 16-18	Common Assessment Abnormalities — Fluid and Electrolyte Imbalances	
FINDING	**POSSIBLE CAUSE**
Skin	
Poor skin turgor	Fluid volume deficit
Cold, clammy skin	Na^+ deficit, shift of plasma to interstitial fluid
Pitting edema	Fluid volume excess
Flushed, dry skin	Na^+ excess
Pulse	
Bounding pulse	Fluid volume excess, shift of interstitial fluid to plasma
Rapid, weak, thready pulse	Shift of plasma to interstitial fluid, Na^+ deficit, fluid volume deficit
Weak, irregular, rapid pulse	Severe K^+ deficit
Weak, irregular, slow pulse	Severe K^+ excess
Blood Pressure	
Hypotension	Fluid volume deficit, shift of plasma to interstitial fluid, Na^+ deficit
Hypertension	Fluid volume excess, shift of interstitial fluid to plasma
Respirations	
Deep, rapid breathing	Compensation for metabolic acidosis
Shallow, slow, irregular breathing	Compensation for metabolic alkalosis
Shortness of breath	Fluid volume excess
Moist crackles	Fluid volume excess, shift of interstitial fluid to plasma
Skeletal Muscles	
Cramping of exercised muscle	Ca^{+2} deficit, Mg^+ deficit, alkalosis
Carpal spasm (Trousseau's sign)	Ca^{+2} deficit, Mg^+ deficit, alkalosis
Flabby muscles	K^+ deficit
Positive Chvostek's sign	Ca^{+2} deficit, Mg^+ deficit, alkalosis
Behavior or Mental State	
Picking at bedclothes	K^+ deficit, Mg^+ deficit
Indifference	Fluid volume deficit, Na^+ deficit
Apprehension	Shift of plasma to interstitial fluid
Extreme restlessness	K^+ excess, fluid volume deficit
Confusion and irritability	K^+ deficit, fluid volume excess, Ca^{+2} excess, magnesium excess, H_2O excess
Decreased level of consciousness	H_2O excess

formation. They reflect the concentration of that electrolyte in the ECF but do not necessarily provide information concerning the concentration of the electrolyte in the ICF. For example, the majority of the potassium in the body is found intracellularly. Changes in serum potassium values may be the result of a true deficit or excess of potassium or may reflect the movement of potassium into or out of the cell during acid-base imbalances.

An abnormal serum sodium level may reflect a sodium problem or, more likely, a water problem. A reduced hematocrit value could indicate anemia, or it could be caused by fluid volume excess.

Other laboratory tests that are helpful in evaluating the presence of or risk for fluid, electrolyte, and acid-base imbalances include serum and urine osmolality, serum glucose, BUN, serum creatinine, urine specific gravity, and urine electrolytes.

In addition to arterial and venous blood gases, serum electrolytes can provide important information concerning a patient's acid-base balance. Changes in the serum bicarbonate (often reported as total CO_2 or CO_2 content on an electrolyte panel) will indicate the presence of metabolic acidosis (low bicarbonate level) or alkalosis (high bicarbonate level). Calculation of the *anion gap* (serum sodium level minus chloride and bicarbonate levels) can help determine the source of metabolic acidosis. The anion gap is increased in metabolic acidosis associated with acid gain (e.g., lactic acidosis, diabetic ketoacidosis) but remains normal (10 to 14 mmol/L) in metabolic acidosis caused by bicarbonate loss (e.g., diarrhea).

ORAL FLUID AND ELECTROLYTE REPLACEMENT

In all cases of fluid, electrolyte, and acid-base imbalances the treatment is directed toward correction of the underlying cause. The specific diseases or disorders that cause these imbalances are discussed in various chapters throughout this text. Mild fluid and electrolyte deficits can be corrected using oral rehydration solutions containing water, electrolytes, and glucose. Glucose not only provides calories but also promotes sodium absorption in the small intestine. Commercial oral rehydration solutions are now available in markets and pharmacies for home use.

INTRAVENOUS FLUID AND ELECTROLYTE REPLACEMENT

IV fluid and electrolyte therapy are commonly used to treat many different fluid and electrolyte imbalances. Many patients need maintenance IV fluid therapy only while they cannot take oral fluids (e.g., during and after surgery). Other patients need corrective or replacement therapy for losses that have already occurred. The amount and type of solution are determined by the normal daily maintenance requirements and by imbalances identified by laboratory results. Table 16-19 provides a list of commonly prescribed IV solutions. The available selections have remained fairly constant over the years.

Solutions

Hypotonic. A hypotonic solution provides more water than electrolytes, diluting the ECF. Osmosis then produces a movement of water from the ECF to the ICF. After osmotic equilibrium has been achieved, the ICF and the ECF have the same osmolality, and both compartments have been expanded. Examples of hypotonic fluids are given in Table 16-19. Maintenance fluids are usually hy-

potonic solutions (e.g., 0.45% NaCl) because normal daily losses are hypotonic. Additional electrolytes (e.g., KCl) may be added to maintain normal levels. Hypotonic solutions have the potential to cause cellular swelling, and patients should be monitored for changes in mentation that may indicate cerebral edema.[4,15]

Although 5% dextrose in water is considered an isotonic solution, the dextrose is quickly metabolized, and the net result is the administration of free water (hypotonic) with proportionately equal expansion of the ECF and ICF. One liter of a 5% dextrose solution provides 50 g of dextrose, or 170 calories. Although this amount of dextrose is not enough to meet caloric requirements, it helps prevent ketosis associated with starvation. Pure water cannot be administered intravenously because it would cause hemolysis of red blood cells.

TABLE 16-19 Composition and Use of Commonly Prescribed Crystalloid Solutions

SOLUTION	TONICITY	mOsm/kg	GLUCOSE (g/L)	INDICATIONS AND CONSIDERATIONS
Dextrose in Water				
5%	Isotonic	278	50	• Provides free water necessary for renal excretion of solutes • Used to replace water losses and treat hypernatremia • Provides 170 calories/L • Does not provide any electrolytes
10%	Hypertonic	556	100	• Provides free water only, no electrolytes • Provides 340 calories/L
Saline				
0.45%	Hypotonic	154	0	• Provides free water in addition to Na+ and Cl− • Used to replace hypotonic fluid losses • Used as maintenance solution although it does not replace daily losses of other electrolytes • Provides no calories
0.9%	Isotonic	308	0	• Used to expand intravascular volume and replace extracellular fluid losses • Only solution that may be administered with blood products • Contains Na+ and Cl− in excess of plasma levels • Does not provide free water, calories, other electrolytes • May cause intravascular overload or hyperchloremic acidosis
3.0%	Hypertonic	1026	0	• Used to treat symptomatic hyponatremia • Must be administered slowly and with extreme caution because it may cause dangerous intravascular volume overload and pulmonary edema
Dextrose in Saline				
5% in 0.225%	Isotonic	355	50	• Provides Na+, Cl−, and free water • Used to replace hypotonic losses and treat hypernatremia • Provides 170 calories/L
5% in 0.45%	Hypertonic	432	50	• Same as 0.45% NaCl except provides 170 calories/L
5% in 0.9%	Hypertonic	586	50	• Same as 0.9% NaCl except provides 170 calories/L
Multiple Electrolyte Solutions				
Ringer's solution	Isotonic	309	0	• Similar in composition to plasma except that it has excess Cl−, no Mg2+, and no HCO3− • Does not provide free water or calories • Used to expand the intravascular volume and replace extracellular fluid losses
Lactated Ringer's (Hartmann's) solution	Isotonic	274	0	• Similar in composition to normal plasma except does not contain Mg2+ • Used to treat losses from burns and lower GI • May be used to treat mild metabolic acidosis but should not be used to treat lactic acidosis • Does not provide free water or calories

Modified from Heitz UE, Horne MM: *Pocket guide to fluid, electrolyte, and acid-base balance*, ed 4, St Louis, 2001, Mosby.

Isotonic. Administration of an isotonic solution expands only the ECF. There is no net loss or gain from the ICF. An isotonic solution is the ideal fluid replacement for a patient with an ECF volume deficit. Examples of isotonic solutions include lactated Ringer's solution and 0.9% NaCl. Lactated Ringer's solution contains sodium, potassium, chloride, calcium, and lactate (the precursor of bicarbonate) in about the same concentrations as those of the ECF. It is contraindicated in the presence of lactic acidosis because of the body's decreased ability to convert lactate to bicarbonate.

Isotonic saline (0.9% NaCl) has a sodium concentration (154 mEq/L) somewhat higher than plasma (135 to 145 mEq/L) and a chloride concentration (154 mEq/L) significantly higher than the plasma chloride level (96 to 106 mEq/L). Thus excessive administration of isotonic NaCl can result in elevated sodium and chloride levels. Isotonic saline may be used when a patient has experienced both fluid and sodium losses or as vascular fluid replacement in hypovolemic shock.

Hypertonic. A hypertonic solution initially raises the osmolality of ECF and expands it. It is useful in treatment of hypovolemia and hyponatremia. Examples are listed in Table 16-19. In addition, the higher osmotic pressure draws water out of the cells into the ECF. Hypertonic solutions (e.g., 3% NaCl) require frequent monitoring of blood pressure, lung sounds, and serum sodium levels and should be used with caution because of the risk for intravascular fluid volume excess, as well as intracellular dehydration.[15]

Although concentrated dextrose and water solutions (10% dextrose or greater) are hypertonic solutions, once the dextrose is metabolized, the net result is the administration of water. The free water provided by these solutions will ultimately expand both the ECF and ICF. The primary use of these solutions is in the provision of calories. Concentrated dextrose solutions may be combined with amino acid solutions, electrolytes, vitamins, and trace elements to provide total parenteral nutrition (see Chapter 39). Solutions containing 10% dextrose or less may be administered through a peripheral IV line. Solutions with greater concentrations of dextrose must be administered through a central line so that there is adequate dilution to prevent shrinkage of red blood cells.

Intravenous Additives. In addition to the basic solutions that provide water and a minimum amount of calories and electrolytes, there are additives to replace specific losses. These additives are mentioned previously during the discussion of the particular electrolyte deficiencies. KCl, CaCl, $MgSO_4$, and HCO_3^- are common additives to the basic IV solutions.

Recommendations for giving potassium vary, but in general no more than 10 to 20 mEq per hour is considered safe for routine administration. Potassium can be safely diluted as 40 mEq/L of solution with a maximum of 60 mEq/L. It must never be administered IV push or undiluted because it can cause fatal cardiac reactions.

Plasma Expanders. Plasma expanders stay in the vascular space and increase the osmotic pressure. Plasma expanders include colloids, dextran, and hetastarch. Colloids are protein solutions such as plasma, albumin, and commercial plasmas (e.g., Plasmanate). Albumin is available in 5% and 25% solutions. The 5% solution has an albumin concentration similar to plasma and will expand the intravascular fluid milliliter for milliliter. In contrast, the 25% albumin solution is hypertonic and will draw additional fluid from the interstitium. Dextran is a complex synthetic sugar. Because dextran is metabolized slowly, it remains in the vascular system for a prolonged period but not as long as the colloids. It pulls additional fluid into the intravascular space. Hetastarch (Hespan) is a synthetic colloid that works similarly to dextran. (Indications for plasma volume expanders are discussed in Chapter 65.)

If the patient has lost blood, whole blood or packed red blood cells are necessary. Packed red blood cells have the advantage of giving the patient primarily red blood cells; the blood bank can use the plasma for blood components. Whole blood, with its additional fluid volume, may cause circulatory overload. Although packed cells have a decreased plasma volume, they will increase the oncotic pressure and pull fluid into the intravascular space. Loop diuretics may be administered with blood to prevent symptoms of fluid volume excess in anemic patients who are not volume depleted. (Administration of blood is discussed in Chapter 30.)

CRITICAL THINKING EXERCISES

Case Study
Fluid and Electrolyte Imbalance

Patient Profile. Sarah Smith, a 73-year-old white woman with lung cancer, has been receiving chemotherapy on an outpatient basis. She completed her third treatment 5 days ago and has been experiencing nausea and vomiting for 2 days even though she has been taking prochlorperazine (Compazine) as directed. Ms. Smith's daughter brings her to the hospital, where she is admitted to the medical unit. The admitting nurse performs a thorough assessment.

Subjective Data
- Complains of lethargy, weakness, and a dry mouth
- States she has been too nauseous to eat or drink anything for 2 days

Objective Data
- Heart rate 110, pulse thready
- Blood pressure 100/65
- Weight loss of 5 pounds since she received her chemotherapy treatment 5 days ago
- Dry oral mucous membranes

CRITICAL THINKING QUESTIONS

1. Based on her clinical manifestations, what fluid imbalance does Ms. Smith have?
2. What additional assessment data should the nurse obtain?
3. What are the patient's risk factors for fluid and electrolyte imbalances?
4. The nurse draws blood for a serum chemistry evaluation. What electrolyte imbalances are likely and why?
5. The physician orders dextrose 5% in 0.45% saline to infuse at 100 ml/hr. What type of solution is this and how will it help Ms. Smith's fluid imbalance?
6. Because of the nature of her disease process, Ms. Smith is at risk for the development of SIADH. How would the nurse recognize this complication and what is the anticipated treatment?

REVIEW QUESTIONS

The number of the question corresponds to the same-numbered objective at the beginning of the chapter.

1. The majority of the body's water is contained in which of the following fluid compartments?
   a. interstitial
   b. intracellular
   c. extracellular
   d. intravascular

2. If the blood plasma has a higher osmolality than the fluid within a red blood cell, the mechanism involved in equalizing the fluid concentration is
   a. osmosis.
   b. diffusion.
   c. active transport.
   d. facilitated diffusion.

3a. An elderly woman was admitted to the medical unit with dehydration. A clinical indication of this problem is
   a. weight loss.
   b. full bounding pulse.
   c. engorged neck veins.
   d. Kussmaul respiration.

3b. Implementation of nursing care for the patient with hyponatremia includes
   a. fluid restriction.
   b. administration of hypotonic IV fluids.
   c. administration of a cation exchange resin.
   d. increased water intake for patients on nasogastric suction.

3c. A patient is receiving a loop diuretic. The nurse should be alert to which of the following symptoms?
   a. restlessness and agitation
   b. paresthesias and irritability
   c. weak, irregular pulse and poor muscle tone
   d. increased blood pressure and muscle spasms

3d. Which of the following patients would be at greatest risk for the potential development of hypermagnesemia?
   a. 83-year-old man with lung cancer and hypertension
   b. 65-year-old woman with hypertension taking β-adrenergic blockers
   c. 42-year-old woman with systemic lupus erythematosus and renal failure
   d. 50-year-old man with benign prostatic hyperplasia and a urinary tract infection

3e. It is especially important for the nurse to assess for which of the following in a patient who has just undergone a total thyroidectomy?
   a. weight gain
   b. depressed reflexes
   c. positive Chvostek's sign
   d. confusion and personality changes

3f. The nurse anticipates that the patient with hyperphosphatemia secondary to renal failure will require
   a. calcium supplements.
   b. potassium supplements.
   c. magnesium supplements.
   d. fluid replacement therapy.

4. The lungs act as an acid-base buffer by
   a. increasing respiratory rate and depth when CO_2 levels in the blood are high, reducing acid load.
   b. increasing respiratory rate and depth when CO_2 levels in the blood are low, reducing base load.
   c. decreasing respiratory rate and depth when CO_2 levels in the blood are high, reducing acid load.
   d. decreasing respiratory rate and depth when CO_2 levels in the blood are low, increasing acid load.

5. A patient has the following arterial blood gas results: pH 7.52; $PaCO_2$ 30 mm Hg; HCO_3^- 24 mEq/L. The nurse determines that these results indicate
   a. metabolic acidosis.
   b. metabolic alkalosis.
   c. respiratory acidosis.
   d. respiratory alkalosis.

6. The typical fluid replacement for the patient with an ICF fluid volume deficit is
   a. isotonic.
   b. hypotonic.
   c. hypertonic.
   d. a plasma expander.

REFERENCES

1. Anderson DM: *Mosby's medical, nursing, and allied health dictionary,* ed 6, St Louis, 2002, Mosby.
2. Metheny NM: *Fluid and electrolyte balance: nursing considerations,* ed 4, Philadelphia, 2000, Lippincott.
3. Pestana C: *Fluids and electrolytes in the surgical patient,* ed 5, Philadelphia, 2000, Lippincott Williams & Wilkins.
4. Porth CM: *Pathophysiology: concepts of altered health states,* ed 5, Philadelphia, 1998, Lippincott.
5. McCance KL, Huether SE: *Pathophysiology: the biologic basis for disease in adults and children,* ed 4, St Louis, 2002, Mosby.
6. Kugler JP, Hustead T: Hyponatremia and hypernatremia in the elderly, *Am Fam Physician* 61:12, 2000.
7. Kobriger AM: Dehydration—stopping a "sentinel event," *Nurs Homes* 48:10, 1999.
8. Schmidt TC, Williams-Evans SA: How to recognize hypokalemia, *Nursing* 30:2, 2000.
9. Bullock BA, Henze RL: *Focus on pathophysiology,* Philadelphia, 2000, Lippincott.
10. Camp-Sorrell D: Hypercalcemia, *Clin J Oncol Nurs* 2:2 1998.
11. Ramsdell R: Renagel—a new and different phosphate binder, *ANNA J* 26:3, 1999.
12. Innerarity S: Hypomagnesemia in acute and chronic illness, *Crit Care Nurs Q* 23:2, 2000.
13. Kee JL, Hayes ER: *Pharmacology: a nursing process approach,* ed 4, Philadelphia, 2003, WB Saunders.
14. Coleman NJ: Evaluating arterial blood gas results, *Aust Nurs J* 6:11, 1999.
15. Cooper A: IV fluid therapy—part 2: IV fluid selection, *Aust Nurs J* 7:6, 2000.

RESOURCE

Infusion Nurses Society
220 Norwood Park South
Norwood, MA 02062
781-440-9408
Fax: 781-440-9409
www.ins1.org

For additional Internet resources, see the website for this book at *http://evolve.elsevier.com/Lewis/medsurg/.*

Perioperative Care

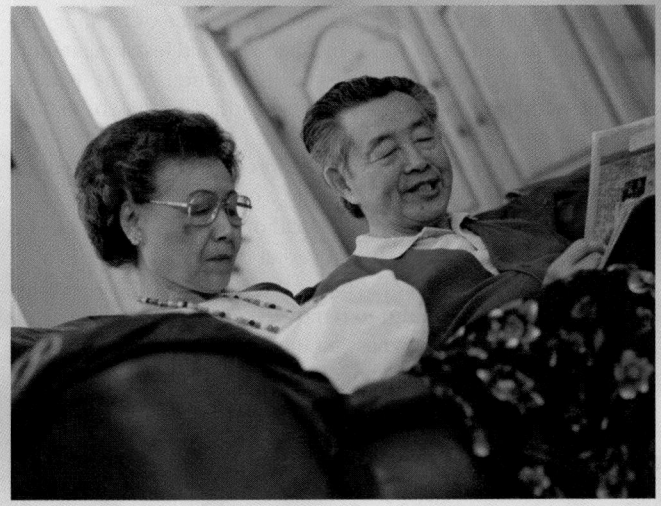

CHAPTER 17
NURSING MANAGEMENT
Preoperative Care

Nancy J. Girard

LEARNING OBJECTIVES

1. Identify the common purposes and settings of surgery.
2. Describe the purpose and components of a preoperative nursing assessment.
3. Interpret the significance of data related to the preoperative patient's health status and operative risk.
4. Explain the components and purpose of informed consent for surgery.
5. Describe the nursing role in the physical, psychologic, and educational preparation of the surgical patient.
6. Discuss the day-of-surgery preparation for the surgical patient.
7. Identify the purposes and types of preoperative medications.
8. Identify the special considerations of preoperative preparation for the older adult surgical patient.

KEY TERMS

ambulatory surgery, p. 360	informed consent, p. 370
elective surgery, p. 360	same-day admission, p. 360
emergency surgery, p. 360	surgery, p. 360

Surgery can be defined as the art and science of treating diseases, injuries, and deformities by operation and instrumentation. The surgical procedure involves the interaction of the patient, surgeon, and nurse. Surgery may be performed for any of the following purposes:

1. *Diagnosis:* determination of the presence and/or extent of pathology (e.g., lymph node biopsy or bronchoscopy)
2. *Cure:* elimination or repair of pathology (e.g., removal of a ruptured appendix or benign ovarian cyst)
3. *Palliation:* alleviation of symptoms without cure (e.g., cutting a nerve root [rhizotomy] to remove symptoms of pain, or creating a colostomy to bypass an inoperable bowel obstruction)
4. *Prevention:* examples include removal of a mole before it becomes malignant or removal of the colon in a patient with familial polyposis to prevent cancer
5. *Exploration:* surgical examination to determine the nature or extent of a disease (e.g., laparotomy)
6. *Cosmetic improvement:* examples include repairing a burn scar or changing breast shape

Specific suffixes are commonly used in combination with identifying a body part or organ in naming surgical procedures (Table 17-1).

SURGICAL SETTINGS

Surgery may be a carefully planned event **(elective surgery)** or may arise with unexpected urgency **(emergency surgery).** Both elective and emergency surgery may be performed in a variety of settings. The setting in which a surgical procedure may be safely and effectively performed is influenced by the complexity of the surgery, the potential complications, and the general health status of the patient. Changes in fiscal conditions, sur-

gical techniques, and technology have led to surgical patients most often admitted to the hospital on the day of surgery for inpatient surgery **(same-day admission).** Today the usual situation is that only those patients who are already hospitalized because of their medical conditions are in the hospital before surgery.

A large number and type of surgical procedures are being performed as **ambulatory surgery** (also called *same-day* or *outpatient surgery*). Many of these surgeries involve the use of endoscopic techniques and are described in chapters throughout the text that discuss surgical intervention for specific medical problems. Ambulatory surgery is conducted in emergency departments, endoscopy clinics, doctors' offices, freestanding surgical clinics, and outpatient surgery units in hospitals. These procedures can be performed with the use of a general, regional, or local anesthetic; usually take less than 2 hours; require less than a 3- to 4-hour stay in the postanesthesia care unit (PACU); and do not require an overnight hospital stay. In some cases, the patient will stay in the hospital overnight after surgery, but for less than a day. This is known as a "23-hour" stay. Ambulatory surgery is generally preferred by patients, physicians, and third-party payers when possible. Patients like the convenience, physicians prefer the flexibility in scheduling and availability of operating rooms, and the cost is usually less for both the patient and the insurer. Ambulatory surgery generally involves fewer laboratory tests, fewer preoperative and postoperative medications, less psychologic stress (especially for older adults), and less susceptibility to hospital-acquired infections. In some cases it is mandated by third-party payers, such as private insurance companies, government insurers (Medicare and Medicaid), and health maintenance organizations (HMOs).

Regardless of where the surgery is performed, the nurse is vital in preparing the patient for surgery, caring for the patient during surgery, and facilitating the patient's recovery following surgery. To perform these functions effectively, the nurse must have certain basic information. First, the nurse must have knowledge of the nature of the disorder requiring surgery and any coexisting disease processes. Second, the nurse must identify the individual patient's response to the stress of surgery. Third, the nurse must assess the results of appropriate preoperative diagnostic tests. Finally, the nurse must consider the bodily alterations and

Reviewed by Patricia A. Loflin, RN, MSN, FNP, Nursing Faculty, TVI Community College, Albuquerque, N.M.

TABLE 17-1	Suffixes Describing Surgical Procedures	
SUFFIX	**MEANING**	**EXAMPLE**
-ectomy	Excision or removal of	Appendectomy
-lysis	Destruction of	Electrolysis
-orrhaphy	Repair or suture of	Herniorrhaphy
-oscopy	Looking into	Endoscopy
-ostomy	Creation of opening into	Colostomy
-otomy	Cutting into or incision of	Tracheotomy
-plasty	Repair or reconstruction of	Mammoplasty

potential risks and complications associated with the surgical procedure and any coexisting medical problems. The nurse caring for the patient preoperatively is likely to be different from the nurse in the operating room (OR), PACU, surgical intensive care unit (SICU), or surgical unit. Thus communication and documentation of important preoperative assessment findings are essential.

The preoperative nursing measures included in this chapter are those that are applicable to the preparation of any surgical patient. Specific measures in preparation for specific surgical procedures (e.g., abdominal, thoracic, or orthopedic surgery) are covered in appropriate chapters of this text.

PATIENT INTERVIEW

The patient may be seen multiple times by multiple people before surgery. To prevent the patient from having to repeat the same information over and over, the nurse should check the documentation for information before asking common questions. Regardless of the source of information, one of the most important nursing actions is the preoperative interview. The interview may be done by the nurse who works in the physician's office, a preoperative admission clinic, the ambulatory surgery center, or the hospital preoperative area. The site of the interview and the time before surgery will dictate the depth and completeness of the interview. Important findings must be documented and communicated to others so that continuity and a continuum of care will be maintained.

The preoperative interview may occur in advance or on the day of surgery. The primary purposes of the patient interview are to (1) obtain patient health information, (2) determine the patient's expectations about surgery and anesthesia, (3) provide and clarify information about the surgical experience, and (4) assess the patient's emotional state and readiness for surgery. The nurse may also ensure that the patient's consent form for surgery is signed appropriately.

The interview also provides an opportunity for the patient and family to ask questions about surgery, anesthesia, and postoperative care. Often patients will ask about taking their routine medications, such as insulin or heart medications, or if they will experience pain. The nurse who is aware of a patient's and family's needs and perception of stressors can provide or arrange for the support needed during the perioperative period.

NURSING ASSESSMENT OF THE PREOPERATIVE PATIENT

Although nursing assessment and interventions are discussed separately here, both are done simultaneously in practice. The overall goal of the preoperative assessment is to gather data in or-

der to identify risk factors and plan care to ensure patient safety throughout the surgical experience. Goals of the assessment are to

1. Determine the psychologic status of the patient in order to reinforce coping strategies to undergo the proposed surgery.
2. Determine physiologic factors related and unrelated to the surgical procedure that may contribute to operative risk factors.
3. Establish baseline data for comparison in the intraoperative and postoperative period.
4. Identify prescription medications and over-the-counter drugs and herbs that have been taken by the patient that may affect the surgical outcome.
5. Identify if the results of all preoperative laboratory and diagnostic tests are documented and communicated to appropriate personnel.
6. Identify cultural and ethnic factors that may affect the surgical experience.
7. Determine if the patient has received adequate information from the surgeon to make an informed decision to have surgery and that the consent form is signed.

Subjective Data

Psychosocial Assessment. Surgery is a frightening event, even when the procedure is considered relatively minor. The psychologic and physiologic reactions to the surgery elicit the body's stress response.[1] The stress response is a desirable mechanism that enables the body to cope, adapt, and heal in the postoperative period. If stressors or the response to the stressors are excessive, the stress response can be magnified and recovery can be affected. Many factors influence the patient's susceptibility to stress, including age, past experiences, current health, and socioeconomic status. The nurse who is aware of a patient's perceived or actual stressors can provide support and the needed information during the preoperative period so that stress will not become distress. (See Chapter 8 for a discussion of stress.)

Emotional reactions to impending surgery and hospitalization often intensify in the older adult. Hospitalization may represent to the patient a physical decline and loss of health, mobility, and independence. The older adult may view the hospital as a place to die or as a stepping-stone to nursing home placement. The nurse can be instrumental in allaying anxieties and fears and maintaining and restoring the self-esteem of the older adult during the surgical experience (see the section on gerontologic considerations at the end of the chapter).

The nurse must use common language and avoid medical jargon. If the patient and family do not speak English, it is essential that the services of a competent translator are obtained. Hospitals are now required to provide translators for common languages other than English. Words and language that are familiar to the patient should be used to increase the patient's understanding of surgical consent and the surgical process. This also will decrease the anxiety level preoperatively.

The nurse's role in psychologically preparing the patient for surgery is to assess the patient for potential stressors that could negatively affect surgery (Table 17-2). The nurse may not be the health care provider who intervenes, but she or he should be able to communicate all concerns to the appropriate surgical team member. Because the patient may be admitted directly into the preoperative area from the community or home, the nurse must be skilled in assessing vital psychologic factors in a very short time. The most common psychologic factors are anxiety, fear, and hope.

TABLE 17-2 Psychosocial Assessment of the Preoperative Patient

Situational Changes
- Determine support systems, including family, significant others, group and institutional structure, and religious and spiritual orientation.
- Define current degree of personal control, decision making, and independence.
- Consider the impact of surgery and hospitalization and the possible effects on lifestyle.
- Identify the presence of hope and anticipation of positive results.

Concerns with the Unknown
- Identify specific areas and depth of anxiety and fears.
- Identify expectations of surgery, changes in current health status, and effects on daily living.

Concerns with Body Image
- Identify current roles or relationships and view of self.
- Determine perceived or potential changes in role or relationships and their impact on body image.

Past Experiences
- Review previous surgical experiences, hospitalizations, and treatments.
- Determine responses to those experiences (positive and negative).
- Identify current perceptions of surgical procedure in relation to the above and information from others (e.g., a neighbor's view of a personal surgical experience).

Knowledge Deficit
- Identify what amount and type of preoperative information this specific patient wants to know.
- Identify what this patient must know preoperatively.
- Assess understanding of the surgical procedure, including preparation, care, interventions, preoperative activities, restrictions, and expected outcomes.
- Identify the accuracy of information the patient has received from others, including health care team, family, friends, and the media.

Anxiety. Everyone is anxious when facing surgery because of the unknown. This is normal and is an inherent survival mechanism. However, if the anxiety level is extremely high, cognition, decision making, and coping abilities are diminished. Anxiety can arise from lack of knowledge, which may range from not knowing what to expect during the surgical experience to uncertainty about the outcome of surgery. The potential of the unknown often contributes to anxiety when the surgery is for diagnostic purposes. The patient may have totally unrealistic expectations of what surgery will be like, or what it will accomplish. This may be a result of past experiences or the vicarious experiences provided by friends' stories and the mass media, especially television. The nurse can decrease some anxiety for the patient by providing information about what can be expected.[2] The surgeon should be informed if the patient requires any additional information or if anxiety seems excessive.

The patient may experience anxiety when surgical interventions are in conflict with his or her religious and cultural beliefs.

In particular, the nurse should identify the patient's religious and cultural beliefs about the possibility of blood transfusions.[3] The need for blood replacement should have been discussed with the physician before admission, but may not have been communicated to all the perioperative staff.

Common fears. There are many reasons patients fear surgery. The most prevalent is the potential for death or permanent disability resulting from surgery. Sometimes the fear arises after hearing or reading about the risks during the informed consent process. Other fears can be pain, change in body image, or results of a diagnostic procedure.

Fear of death can be extremely detrimental. If the nurse identifies a strong death fear, this concern must be communicated to the physician immediately. A strong fear of impending death may prompt the physician to postpone the surgery if the patient is convinced that it will lead to death. Attitude and emotional state influence the stress response, and thus the surgical outcome.

Fear of pain and discomfort during and after surgery is universal. If the fear appears extreme, the nurse should notify the anesthesia care provider (ACP) so that an appropriate preoperative medication can be given. The nurse can encourage the patient to talk with the ACP for clarification. The patient should be reassured that drugs are available to eliminate pain during surgery. Drugs will be given that provide an amnesic effect so that the patient will not remember what occurs during the surgical episode. These medications can cause temporary cognitive deficits following surgery, and the patient should be told preoperatively that this is common. Some patients, particularly older adults, fear that they have had a stroke during surgery if they are not aware of temporary postoperative cognition problems. The nurse should stress that the patient should ask for medications following surgery if pain is present, and that taking these medications will not contribute to an addiction.

Fear of mutilation or alteration in body image can occur whether the surgery is radical, such as amputation, or minor, such as a bunion repair. The presence of even a small scar on the body can be repulsive to some, and others fear keloid development (overgrowth of a scar). The nurse must listen to and assess the patient's concern about this aspect of surgery with an open, nonjudgmental attitude.

Fear of anesthesia may arise from the unknown, from tales of others' bad experiences, or from personal past experience. These concerns can result from a prior unpleasant induction of anesthesia or information about hazards or complications (e.g., brain damage, paralysis). Many patients fear losing control while under the influence of anesthesia. If these fears are identified, the nurse should inform the ACP immediately so that he or she can talk further with the patient. Some patients will ask the nurse if it is safer to have general or spinal anesthesia. The nurse should not recommend one or the other, but should reassure the patient that both methods are equally safe and suggest they talk further with the ACP. The patient should also be reassured that a nurse and the ACP will be present at all times during surgery.

Fear of disruption of life functioning or patterns may be present in varying degrees. It can range from fear of permanent disability and loss of life to concern about not being able to play golf for a few weeks. Concerns about separation from family and about how spouse or children are managing are common. Financial concerns may be related either to an anticipated loss of income or to the costs of surgery.

If the nurse identifies any of these fears, consultation with a social worker, a spiritual or cultural advisor, a psychologist, or family members may prove valuable in providing assistance to the patient.

Hope. Most psychologic factors related to surgery seem to be negative, but hope stands out as a positive attribute.[4] Hope may be the patient's strongest method of coping, and to deny or minimize hope may negate the positive mental attitude necessary for a quick and full recovery. Some surgeries are hopefully anticipated. These can be the surgeries that repair (e.g., plastic surgery for burn scars), rebuild (e.g., total joint replacement to minimize pain and improve function), or save and extend life (e.g., repair of aneurysm, coronary artery bypass surgery). The nurse should assess and support the presence of hope and anticipation of positive results that the patient is expecting.

Past Health History. The nurse should ask about diagnosed medical conditions in the patient's past, as well as current health problems. A guideline for preoperative review of the patient's past health history and other subjective data will assist in asking the patient about specific problems. An organized approach elicits better information than just asking if the patient has had any medical problems. Initially the nurse should determine if the patient understands the reason for surgery. For example, the patient scheduled for a total knee replacement may indicate that the reason for the surgery is increasing problems with pain and mobility. Past hospitalizations should be documented, including what the hospitalizations were for. Any previous surgeries and dates of the surgeries should also be documented. Any problems with previous surgeries should be identified. For example, the patient may have experienced a bad wound infection or a reaction to an analgesic following a prior surgery.

Women should be asked about their menstrual and obstetric history. This includes obtaining the date of the patient's last menstrual period and the number of pregnancies. If the patient states that she might be pregnant, information should be immediately given to the surgeon to avoid maternal and subsequent fetal exposure to anesthetics during the first trimester. Questioning regarding reproductive functioning may be embarrassing for a teenager in the presence of parents or guardians. The nurse may elect to ask these questions with parents or guardians out of the room.

Possible inherited conditions may be identified by asking about the patient's family health history. A family history of cardiac and endocrine disease should be recorded. For example, if a patient reports a mother or father with hypertension, sudden cardiac death, myocardial infarction, or coronary artery disease, the nurse should be alerted to the possibility that the patient may also have a similar predisposition or condition. A family history of diabetes should also be investigated because of the familial predisposition to both type 1 and type 2 diabetes mellitus. Tendencies toward these conditions may be exacerbated during surgery and affect physiologic function during and after surgery. Racially inherited traits may contribute to the surgical outcome and need to be considered in the family histories.[5] For example, Native Americans have a high incidence of diabetes mellitus.

Information should also be obtained about the patient's family history of adverse reactions to or problems with anesthesia. Anesthesia care providers first became aware of a condition, later to be known as malignant hyperthermia, when a young man in Australia reported that 10 of his family members had died while undergoing anesthesia. The genetic predisposition for malignant hyperthermia is now well documented, and plans of care include minimizing complications associated with this condition. (For further information on malignant hyperthermia, see Chapter 18.)

Medications. Current medication use, including the use of over-the-counter drugs and herbal products, should be documented. In many ambulatory surgery centers, the patients are asked to bring their bottles of medications with them when reporting for surgery. This will enable the nurse to more accurately chart the names and dosage of drugs because patients frequently cannot remember specific details if they use a large number of drugs. For example, it is important to investigate if the patient is taking the drug as ordered, or has stopped taking the drug because of cost, side effects, or the feeling that ongoing therapy is no longer needed.

Drugs and herbal products may interact with anesthetics, often increasing or decreasing potency and effectiveness, or they may be needed during surgery to maintain physiologic function. It is especially important to consider the effects of drugs used for heart disease, hypertension, immunosuppression, seizure control, anticoagulation, and endocrine replacement. For example, tranquilizers potentiate the effect of narcotics and barbiturates, which are agents that can be used for anesthesia. Antihypertensive drugs may predispose the patient to shock from the combined effect of the drug and the vasodilator effect of some anesthetic agents. Insulin or oral hypoglycemic agents may require dose or agent adjustments during the perioperative period because of increased body metabolism, decreased caloric intake, stress, and anesthesia. Aspirin use is common in many people, but it inhibits platelet aggregation and may contribute to postoperative bleeding complications. Surgeons often require that patients not take any aspirin for at least 2 weeks before surgery.

The use of herbal therapy and dietary supplements is prevalent today. Many patients do not consider herbs and dietary supplements drugs, so they do not report them when asked what medications they are taking.[6] Therefore it is essential to specifically ask about the use of herbs and dietary supplements (see box in Chapter 3 on p. 34). One study that examined the frequency of herbal use by surgical patients showed that of 500 patients surveyed, 51% took herbs, vitamins, dietary supplements, or homeopathic medicine. These ranged from 1 to 22 products per person.[7]

Excessive use of vitamins and herbs can cause detrimental effects in surgery patients.[8] Complications from herbal products can include effects on blood pressure, increased sedation, cardiac effects, electrolyte alterations, and inhibition of platelet aggregation. In patients taking anticoagulants or platelet aggregation inhibitors, the additional use of herbal products can produce extensive postoperative bleeding that may necessitate a return to the operating room.[9] Some effects of specific herbs that can be of concern during the perioperative period are identified in the Complementary and Alternative Therapies box on p. 364.

The nurse must also ask the patient about possible recreational drug use, abuse, and addiction. The substances most likely to be abused include tobacco, alcohol, opioids, marijuana, and cocaine. Questions should be asked matter-of-factly, and the nurse should stress that recreational drug use may affect the type and amount of anesthesia that will be needed. When patients become aware of the potential interactions of these drugs with anesthetics, most patients will respond honestly about their drug use.

Chronic alcohol use will place the surgical patient at risk because of lung, gastrointestinal, or liver damage. When liver function is decreased, metabolism of anesthetic agents is prolonged, nutritional status is altered, and the potential for postoperative complications is increased. Alcohol withdrawal can also occur during

COMPLEMENTARY & ALTERNATIVE THERAPIES

Herbal Use of Concern during the Perioperative Period

HERB	PERIOPERATIVE CONSIDERATIONS
Dong quai	Increases the risk of bleeding.
Echinacea	Has immunostimulatory effect and should be avoided in patients who require preoperative immunosuppression; prolonged use may suppress the immune system.
Ephedra (Ma Huang)	Can interact with anesthetics to cause dangerous elevations in blood pressure and heart rate that can lead to arrhythmias, stroke, myocardial infarction, and cardiac arrest.
Feverfew	Increases the risk of bleeding.
Garlic	Inhibits platelet aggregation and increases the risk of bleeding and/or can result in an excessive response to anticoagulants.
Ginger	Increases the risk of bleeding.
Ginkgo biloba	Increases the risk of bleeding, especially in patients taking anticoagulants.
Ginseng	May cause rapid heart rate and increase in blood pressure; may decrease effect of certain anticholinergic drugs; may cause hypoglycemia; inhibits platelet aggregation.
Goldenseal	May cause or increase high blood pressure. Has anticoagulant effects.
Kava	May cause central nervous system depression and prolong the effects of anesthetic agents. Possible liver toxicity, especially with high doses.
St. John's wort	Prolongs the effects of certain anesthetics; has mild MAO inhibitor effects.
Valerian	May prolong the effects of anesthetic agents.

Recommendations: The American Society of Anesthesiologists recommends that all herbal products be stopped at least 2 to 3 weeks before surgery to avoid potential complications of herb use. If this is not possible, the herbal product in its original container should be brought to the surgery site so that the anesthesia care provider knows exactly what the patient is taking.

Sources: American Society of Anesthesiologists: What you should know about herbal use and anesthesia. Available at *www.asahp.org/PublicEducation/insidherb.html*; Mayo Clinic: Herbs and surgery. Available at *www.mayoclinic.com/invoke.cfm?id=SA00040.*
MAO, Monoamine oxidase.

lengthy surgery or in the postoperative period. This can be a life-threatening event, but it can be avoided with appropriate planning and management (see Chapter 11).

When assessing drugs, drug intolerance and drug allergies should be considered. Drug intolerance usually results in side effects that are uncomfortable or unpleasant for the patient but are not life threatening. These effects can include nausea, constipation, diarrhea, or idiosyncratic (opposite than expected) reactions. A true drug allergy produces hives and/or an anaphylactic reaction, causing cardiopulmonary compromise, including hypotension, tachycardia, bronchospasm, and possibly pulmonary edema. By being aware of drug intolerance and drug allergies, it will be possible to maintain patient comfort, safety, and stability. For example, some anesthetic agents contain sulfur, so the ACP should be notified if a history of allergy to sulfur is given. If a drug intolerance or drug allergy is noted, it must be documented, and an allergy wristband should be put on the patient on the day of surgery.

All findings of the medication history should be documented and communicated to the intraoperative and postoperative personnel. Although the ACP will determine the appropriate schedule and dose of the patient's routine medications before and after surgery based on the medication history, the nurse must ensure that all of the patient's medications are identified, implement the alterations in medication administration, and monitor the patient for potential interactions and complications.

Allergies. The nurse should inquire about nondrug allergies, including allergies to foods, chemicals, and pollen. The patient with a history of any allergic responsiveness has a greater potential for demonstrating hypersensitivity reactions to drugs administered during anesthesia.

Patients should also be screened for possible latex allergies[10] (see Chapter 13). The American College of Allergy, Asthma, and Immunology (ACAAI) recommends that patients be screened in the following five areas:
1. Risk factors
2. Contact dermatitis
3. Contact urticaria (e.g., hives)
4. Aerosol reactions
5. History of reactions that suggest an allergy to latex

Risk factors include long-term, multiple exposures to latex products, such as those experienced by health care personnel and rubber industry workers. Additional risk factors include a history of hay fever, asthma, and allergies to certain foods, such as avocados, kiwi, bananas, chestnuts, potatoes, peaches, and apricots.

Review of Systems. The last component of the patient history is the body systems review. Specific questions should be asked to confirm the presence or absence of disease. Past medical problems can alert the nurse to areas that should be more closely examined in the preoperative physical examination. If the patient is being evaluated before the day of surgery, the review of systems, combined with patient history data, will suggest the need for preoperative laboratory tests.

Cardiovascular system. The purpose of evaluating cardiovascular function is to determine the presence of preexisting disease or existing problems (e.g., mitral valve prolapse, valve replacements) so that the patient can be efficiently monitored during the surgical and recovery periods. In the review of systems the nurse may find that there is a history of cardiac problems, including hypertension, angina, arrhythmias, congestive heart failure, and/or myocardial infarction. The nurse should also inquire whether the patient has seen a cardiologist, who the cardiologist is, and if the patient is using any cardiac drugs. If the patient has had a recent myocardial infarction or has a pacemaker, a cardiologist should be consulted before surgery.

The patient's heart will be monitored continuously during surgery and, if indicated, postoperatively. The vital signs recorded preoperatively will be the baseline for the perioperative period. If pertinent, clotting and bleeding times should be present on the chart before surgery, as well as other laboratory reports. For example, the patient who receives digitalis therapy will have serum potassium levels drawn preoperatively and results should be available. If the patient has a history of hypertension, the ACP will maintain adequate blood flow with drugs during the surgery. If the patient has a history of congenital, rheumatic, or valvular heart disease, antibiotic prophylaxis before surgery may be given to decrease the risk of bacterial endocarditis (see Chapter 36).

Respiratory system. The patient should be asked about any recent or chronic upper respiratory infections. The presence of an upper airway infection normally results in the cancellation or postponement of elective surgery because the patient is at an increased risk of bronchospasm, laryngospasm, decreased oxygen saturation, and problems with respiratory secretions. If the patient has a history of dyspnea at rest or with exertion (e.g., breathing hard when carrying groceries), coughing (dry or productive), or hemoptysis (coughing blood), it should be brought to the attention of the perioperative team.

If a patient has a history of asthma, the nurse should inquire about the patient's use of inhaled or oral corticosteroids and bronchodilators and the frequency and triggers of asthma attacks. The patient with a history of chronic obstructive pulmonary disease (COPD) and asthma is at high risk for postoperative pulmonary complications, including hypoxemia and atelectasis.

The patient who smokes should be encouraged to stop at least 6 weeks preoperatively to decrease the risk of intraoperative and postoperative respiratory complications, but may find this difficult during such a stressful time. The greater the patient's pack-years of smoking (packs smoked per day times years), the greater the patient's potential for pulmonary complications during or after surgery. Any additional condition likely to influence or compromise respiratory function should also be noted. These include obesity and spinal, chest, and airway deformities. Depending on the patient's history and physical examination, baseline pulmonary function tests and arterial blood gases (ABGs) may be ordered preoperatively.

Nervous system. Preoperative evaluation of neurologic functioning includes assessing the patient's ability to respond to questions, follow commands, and maintain orderly thought patterns. Alterations in the patient's hearing and vision may affect responses and ability to follow directions and should also be evaluated. The ability to pay attention, concentrate, and respond appropriately must be documented to use as the baseline for postoperative comparison.

Cognitive function is particularly important for the patient who is expected to prepare for surgery and to complete preoperative preparation on an outpatient basis. If deficits are noted, careful assessment should determine their extent and if the problem can be corrected before surgery. If the problem cannot be corrected, it is important to determine whether there are appropriate resources and support to assist the patient.

Assessment of cognitive function is a major assessment area in older patients.[11] The older adult may have intact mental abilities preoperatively, but the stress of surgery, dehydration, hypothermia, and drugs affect older adults more than younger adults. These factors may contribute to the development of postoperative delirium, a condition that may be falsely labeled as senility or dementia. Thus preoperative findings are extremely important for postoperative comparison.

In the review of the nervous system it is also important to inquire about any presence of strokes, transient ischemic attacks, or spinal cord injury. The nurse should inquire about diseases of the nervous system, such as cerebral palsy, myasthenia gravis, Parkinson's disease, and multiple sclerosis, and drugs used for the conditions.

Urinary system. The preoperative patient should be asked about a history of renal or urinary diseases, such as glomerulonephritis, chronic renal insufficiency, or repeated urinary tract infections. The present status should be noted and documented. Renal dysfunction is associated with a number of alterations, including fluid and electrolyte imbalances, coagulopathies, increased risk for infection, and impaired wound healing. Another important consideration is the recognition that many drugs are metabolized and excreted by the kidneys. A decrease in renal function may contribute to an altered response to drugs and unpredictable drug elimination. Renal function tests, such as serum creatinine and blood urea nitrogen, are commonly ordered preoperatively, and results should be available on the chart before surgery.

If the patient has any problems voiding, it should be noted. Male patients may have physical alterations, such as an enlarged prostate, which would hinder the insertion of a urinary catheter during surgery. An enlarged prostate may also impair voiding in the postoperative period. This information is documented and shared with the perioperative team.

Hepatic system. The liver is involved in glucose homeostasis, fat metabolism, protein synthesis, drug and hormone metabolism, and bilirubin formation and excretion. The liver detoxifies many anesthetics and adjunctive drugs. The patient with hepatic dysfunction may have problems with glucose control, clotting abnormalities, and response to drug effects, all of which may increase perioperative risk. The nurse should consider the presence of liver disease if there is a history of jaundice, hepatitis, or alcohol abuse.

Integumentary system. The nurse should ask about a history of skin and musculoskeletal problems, especially in the older adult. A history of skin rashes, boils, ulcers, or other dermatologic conditions should be noted. A history of pressure ulcers may require extra padding during surgery, and skin problems may affect postoperative healing.

Musculoskeletal system. Mobility problems should also be noted. If the patient has arthritis, all affected joints should be identified. Mobility restrictions may influence intraoperative and postoperative positioning and postoperative ambulation. Spinal anesthesia may be difficult if the patient cannot flex his or her lumbar spine adequately to allow easy needle insertion. If the neck is affected, intubation and airway management may be difficult. Any mobility aids such as a cane, walker, or crutches should be brought with the patient on the day of surgery. Frequently, postoperative pain is due to chronic musculoskeletal pain and positioning during surgery, rather than the acute pain of the surgical procedure.

Endocrine system. Diabetes mellitus is a risk factor for both anesthesia and surgery. The diabetic patient is at risk for the development of hypoglycemia, hyperglycemia, ketosis, cardiovascular alterations, delayed wound healing, and infection. Preoperative capillary blood glucose (CBG) tests should be done to determine baseline levels. It is important to clarify with the patient's surgeon or ACP whether the patient should take the usual dose of insulin on the day of surgery. Some practitioners prefer that the patient take only half of the usual dose; others ask that the patient take either the usual dose or take no insulin at all. Regardless of the preoperative insulin orders, the patient's CBG will be determined periodically and managed, if necessary, with regular (short-acting, rapid-onset) insulin.

It should also be determined if the patient has a history of thyroid dysfunction. Either hyperthyroidism or hypothyroidism can place the patient at surgical risk because of alterations in metabolic rate. If the patient takes a thyroid replacement drug, the nurse should check with the ACP about administration of the drug the day of surgery. If the patient has a history of thyroid dysfunction, laboratory tests may be ordered to determine current levels of thyroid function.

Immune system. If the patient has a history of a compromised immune system or takes immunosuppressive drugs, it must be documented. Impairment of the immune system can lead to delayed wound healing and increased risk for postoperative infections. If the patient has an acute infection (e.g., active skin rash, acute sinusitis, flu), elective surgery is frequently cancelled. Patients with active chronic infections such as hepatitis, acquired immunodeficiency syndrome (AIDS), and tuberculosis may still have surgery. When preparing the patient for surgery, it should be remembered that infection control precautions must be taken with every patient. (Infection control guidelines are discussed in Chapter 12.)

Fluid and electrolyte status. The patient should be questioned about the recent presence of conditions that increase the risk for fluid and electrolyte imbalances, such as vomiting, diarrhea, or difficulty swallowing. For example, surgery may be planned for a patient with cholecystitis who has been vomiting for several days. Drugs that the patient takes that alter fluid and electrolyte status, such as diuretics, should also be identified. Serum electrolyte levels are often evaluated before surgery. Some patients may have restricted fluids for some time before surgery, and if the surgery is delayed, they could develop dehydration. A patient with or at risk for dehydration may require additional fluids and electrolytes before or during surgery. Although a preoperative fluid balance history should be completed for all patients, it is especially critical for the older adult because the reduced adaptive capacity leaves a narrow margin of safety between overhydration and underhydration.

Nutritional status. Nutritional deficits include overnutrition and undernutrition, both of which require considerable time to correct. However, knowing that a patient is at either end of the nutritional scale can help the team provide safer care. For example, with the very obese patient, timely notification can allow the perioperative nurse time to obtain a large operating bed or a large cart on which surgery can be performed where the patient does not have to be moved. Longer instruments can also be prepared, especially for abdominal surgery. These interventions can only happen if the information is communicated at least a day before surgery.

Obesity stresses both the cardiac and pulmonary system and makes access to the surgical site and anesthesia administration more difficult.[12] It predisposes the patient to wound dehiscence, wound infection, and incisional herniation postoperatively. Adipose tissue is less vascular than other types of tissue.[13] In addition, the patient may be slower to recovery from anesthesia because the inhalation anesthetic is absorbed and stored by adipose tissue, thus leaving the body more slowly.

Nutritional deficiencies of protein and vitamins A, C, and B complex are particularly significant because these substances are essential for wound healing.[14] Supplemental intravenous and oral nutrients can be administered during the perioperative period to promote adequate healing ability if the patient is malnourished. The older adult is often at risk for malnutrition and fluid volume deficits. If the patient is very thin, the perioperative team should be notified in order to provide more padding than usual (pressure points on all patients are protected routinely) on the operating bed. This is necessary to prevent pressure ulcers, especially during a lengthy procedure. Nutritional deficiencies impair the ability to recover from surgery. It is important to remember that the obese patient can also be protein and vitamin deficient. If the nutritional problem is severe, the surgery may be postponed until the patient loses or gains weight and nutritional deficiencies are corrected.

Dietary habits may affect postoperative recovery and should be identified if the patient will remain in the hospital postoperatively. For example, patients who consume large quantities of coffee or soft drinks containing high caffeine levels should be identified. In many cases, the withholding of caffeinated beverages preoperatively, as well as for a considerable length of time postoperatively, can lead to severe withdrawal headaches. Caffeine withdrawal headaches could be confused with spinal headaches if the preoperative data are not documented. Caffeinated beverages given postoperatively to the patient, when possible, will prevent caffeine withdrawal headaches.

Functional Health Patterns. The review of each functional health pattern of the patient provides valuable subjective data about the patient's physical and psychologic status, as well as cultural values and beliefs related to his or her health care. Questions to ask a preoperative patient are listed in Table 17-3.

Objective Data

Physical Examination. The Joint Commission on Accreditation of Healthcare Organizations (JCAHO)[15] requires that all patients admitted to the operating room have a documented physical examination (PE) in the chart. This examination may be done in advance of surgery or on the day of surgery. The PE may be performed by any number of qualified people, including nurses, nurse practitioners, physicians, physician assistants, or ACPs.

Findings from the patient's history and PE will enable the ACP to assign the patient a physical status rating for anesthesia administration (Table 17-4). This rating is an indicator of the patient's perioperative risk and overall outcome.

Many physiologic stressors may put the patient at risk for surgical complications, whether the surgery is an elective or an emergency procedure. A physiologic assessment of the preoperative patient is presented in Table 17-5. If the PE is done immediately before surgery, it will be focused because of the impending procedures that need to be completed before surgery. The nurse should review the documentation already present on the patient's chart, including the review of systems and the physician's PE report, to better proceed with the examination in a relevant way. All findings must be documented, with any relevant findings immediately communicated to members of the perioperative team.

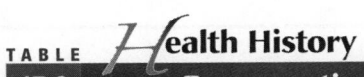

TABLE
17-3

Health History
Preoperative Patient

Health Perception–Health Management Pattern
- What has the doctor explained to you about your surgery?
- Have you had surgery before?*
- Have you or any family members ever experienced any problems with anesthesia?*
- Do you smoke?* If yes, how many packs daily? For how many years?
- Do you have any chronic illnesses?*
- Are you taking any medications?* Are you allergic to any medication?*
- What is your usual use of alcohol?

Nutritional-Metabolic Pattern
- What is your usual or present height and weight?
- Have you had a recent weight gain or loss?*
- Do you have any food preferences or dislikes?*
- Do you have any difficulty chewing or swallowing?*
- Do you take vitamins?*
- Do you have any problems healing?*
- Do you have a history of liver problems?*

Elimination Pattern
- Do you experience any problems with constipation?*
- Do you experience any problems with urinary elimination?*

Activity-Exercise Pattern
- Do you have a history of high blood pressure or cardiac disease?*
- Do you have any history of dyspnea, coughing, hemoptysis, COPD, or asthma?*
- Do you presently have an upper respiratory infection?*
- Do you have any musculoskeletal problems that might affect positioning during surgery or activity level after surgery?*
- Do you have any limitation in mobility of your neck?*
- Do you require any special equipment for ambulation?*

Sleep-Rest Pattern
- Describe any problems you have with sleeping.
- Do you use sleeping pills?*

Cognitive-Perceptual Pattern
- Do you wear glasses, contact lenses, or hearing aid?*
- How would you describe your pain tolerance?
- What methods have you found effective for pain relief?

Self-Perception–Self-Concept Pattern
- How do you feel about having this surgery?
- Have you experienced any changes in the way you feel about yourself or your body?*

Role-Relationship Pattern
- Will this surgery create any problems in your usual roles or relationships?*
- Will you have the support you feel you need following discharge?

Sexuality-Reproductive Pattern
- Do you expect this surgery to have any impact on your usual sexual activity?*

Coping–Stress Tolerance Pattern
- How do you feel about this surgery?
- Do you feel you will be able to cope following this surgery?

Value-Belief Pattern
- Do you have a conflict between your planned surgery and your value or belief system?*

*If yes, describe.
COPD, Chronic obstructive pulmonary disease.

TABLE 17-4	Preoperative Rating of Patient's Physical Status
RATING	**EXAMPLES**
I. Healthy patient with no systemic disease	Patient with no significant past or present health problems
II. Mild systemic disease without functional limitations	Patient with a history of asthma controlled with β-adrenergic agonist inhaler
III. Severe systemic disease associated with definite functional limitations	Patient with history of chronic asthma controlled with β-adrenergic agonist inhaler and inhaled corticosteroids; not wheezing
IV. Severe systemic disease that is an ongoing threat to life	Patient with history of asthma, poorly controlled with β-adrenergic agonists and corticosteroids; PaO$_2$ of 50 mm Hg; wheezing; chest x-ray changes
V. Patient unlikely to survive for more than 24 hr with or without surgery	Patient in status asthmaticus, intubated and on ventilator, receiving IV corticosteroids and IV aminophylline

Laboratory and Diagnostic Testing. The nurse should obtain and evaluate the results of laboratory and diagnostic tests ordered preoperatively. For example, if the patient is taking an anticoagulant (including aspirin), a coagulation profile may be done; a patient on diuretic therapy may need to have a potassium level obtained; a patient taking medications for arrhythmias will probably have a preoperative electrocardiogram (ECG). Blood glucose monitoring should be done for patients with diabetes.

The nurse can do a CBG if low or high glucose is suspected during the preoperative assessment if there are institutional policies in place to do so. Findings may require dose or agent adjustments during the perioperative period because of increased body metabolism, decreased caloric intake, stress, and anesthesia. Regulation of the stability of the blood glucose levels during surgery will promote a more positive outcome. Commonly ordered preoperative laboratory tests can be found in Table 17-6.

TABLE 17-5   Physiologic Assessment of the Preoperative Patient*

Cardiovascular System
- Identify acute or chronic problems; focus on the presence of angina, hypertension, congestive heart failure, and recent history of myocardial infarction.
- Auscultate and palpate baseline pulses: apical, radial, and pedal for rate and characteristics (compare one side to the other).
- Inspect and palpate for presence of edema (including dependent areas), noting location and severity.
- Inspect and palpate neck veins for distention.
- Take baseline blood pressure.
- Identify any drug or herbal product that may affect coagulation (e.g., aspirin, ginkgo, ginger).
- Review laboratory and diagnostic tests for cardiovascular function.

Respiratory System
- Identify acute or chronic problems; note the presence of infection or chronic obstructive pulmonary disease (COPD).
- Assess history of smoking, including the time interval since the last cigarette and the number of pack-years. (Remember that although smoking should be discouraged preoperatively, it may be difficult for patients to stop during this time of anxiety.)
- Auscultate lungs for breath sounds for normal and adventitious sounds.
- Determine baseline respiratory rate and rhythm, and regularity of pattern.
- Observe for cough, dyspnea, and use of accessory muscles of respiration.

Neurologic System
- Determine orientation to time, place, and person.
- Identify presence of confusion, disorderly thinking, or inability to follow commands.
- Identify past history of strokes, transient ischemic attacks, or diseases of the central nervous system such as Parkinson's disease or multiple sclerosis.

Urinary System
- Identify any preexisting disease.
- Determine ability of the patient to void. Prostate enlargement may affect catheterization during surgery and ability to void postoperatively.
- If necessary, note color, amount, and characteristics of urine.
- Review laboratory and diagnostic tests for renal function.

Hepatic System
- Inspect skin color and sclera of eyes for any signs of jaundice.
- Review past history of substance abuse, especially alcohol and IV drug use.
- Review laboratory and diagnostic tests for liver function.

Integumentary System
- Assess mucous membranes for dryness and intactness.
- Determine skin status; note drying, bruising, or breaks in integrity of surface.
- Inspect skin for rashes, boils, or infection, especially around the planned surgical site.
- Assess skin moisture and temperature.
- Inspect the mucous membranes and skin turgor for presence of dehydration.

Musculoskeletal System
- Examine skin/bone pressure points.
- Assess for presence of any pressure ulcers.
- Assess for limitations in joint range of motion and muscle weakness.
- Assess mobility, gait, and balance.
- Assess for presence of joint pain.

Nutritional System
- Determine food and fluid intake patterns and any recent weight loss.
- Weigh and measure patient.
- Assess for the presence of dentures and bridges (loose dentures or teeth may be dislodged during intubation).

*See related body system chapters for more specific assessments and related laboratory studies.

TABLE 17-6   Common Preoperative Laboratory Tests

TEST	AREA ASSESSED
Urinalysis	Renal status, hydration, urinary tract infection and disease
Chest x-ray	Pulmonary disorders, cardiac enlargement
Blood studies: RBC, Hb, Hct, WBC, WBC differential	Anemia, immune status, infection
Electrolytes	Metabolic status, renal function, diuretic side effects
ABGs, oximetry	Pulmonary and metabolic function
Prothrombin (INR) or partial thromboplastin time	Bleeding tendencies
Blood glucose	Metabolic status, diabetes mellitus
Creatinine	Renal function
Blood urea nitrogen	Renal function
Electrocardiogram	Cardiac disease, electrolyte abnormalities
Pulmonary function studies	Pulmonary status
Liver function tests	Liver function
Type and crossmatch	Blood availability for replacement (elective surgery patients may have own blood available)
Pregnancy	Reproductive status

ABGs, Arterial blood gases; *Hb,* hemoglobin; *Hct,* hematocrit; *INR,* international normalized ratio; *RBC,* red blood cells; *WBC,* white blood cells.

Ideally, preoperative laboratory tests should be ordered on the basis of the individual patient history and physical examination. However, many facilities or third-party reimbursement agencies have a written protocol or standards for preoperative laboratory tests, which may or may not include all the identified need areas. In addition, offices and preadmission clinics may do the preoperative tests days before surgery, and they will not be physically located near the surgical institution. Thus the nurse must ensure that all laboratory reports have arrived at the place of surgery at the right time and are on the chart. Lack of these reports may result in a delay or cancellation of the surgery.

NURSING MANAGEMENT PREOPERATIVE PATIENT

Preoperative nursing interventions are derived from the nursing assessment and must reflect each individual patient's specific needs. Physical preparations will be determined by the pending surgery and the routines of the surgery setting. Psychologic preparations should be tailored to each patient's needs. Preoperative teaching may be minimal or extensive. General information for surgery should be given.

■ Preoperative Teaching

The patient has a right to know what to expect and how to participate effectively during the surgical experience. Preoperative teaching increases patient satisfaction. It can reduce postoperative vomiting, pain, fear, anxiety, and stress.[16] It can also decrease complications, the duration of hospitalization, and the recovery time following discharge. However, the time to do effective teaching can be minimal.

In most surgical settings, patients often arrive only a short time before surgery is scheduled, even when the surgery is performed in a hospital and they will be hospitalized postoperatively. After ambulatory surgery, patients usually go home several hours after recovery. This means that patient teaching must be efficient and address needs of the highest priority. This may require teaching that is "just-in-time survival information." That is, what does the patient want to know, or need to know, right now, versus what would be nice to know for the whole surgical experience. If there is no time to allow for repetition, reinforcement, and verification of the patient's understanding, the family should be included to provide these actions. Written materials should also be provided for patients and families to use for review and reinforcement.

In preparing the patient for surgery, the nurse must strike a balance between telling so little that the patient is unprepared, and explaining so much that the patient is overwhelmed. The nurse who observes carefully and listens sensitively to the patient can usually determine how much information is enough in each instance, remembering that anxiety and fear may decrease learning ability. The nurse must also assess what the patient wants to know right away and give priority to his or her concerns.

Generally, preoperative teaching concerns three types of information: sensory, process, and procedural.[17] Different patients, with varying cultures, backgrounds, and experience, may want different types of information. With *sensory information,* patients want to know what they will see, hear, smell, and feel during the surgery. For example, the nurse may tell them that the OR will be cold, but they can ask the OR nurse for a warm blanket; the lights in the OR are very bright; or there will be lots of sounds that are unfamiliar

and there may be specific smells present. Patients wanting *process information* may not want specific details but desire the general flow of what is going to happen. For example, they can be told that they will be in a holding area and the nurse and anesthesia care provider will visit them. They will go to the OR; then, when they wake up, they will be in the PACU; and as soon as they are awake, their family can come in to visit them. With *procedural information,* desired details are more specific; for example, an intravenous line will be started while patients are in the holding area, and in the OR patients will be asked to move onto the narrow bed and a safety strap will be put over their thighs.

Preoperative patient teaching must be communicated to the postoperative care nurses so that learning can be evaluated from past teaching and duplication of teaching can be prevented. Because no nurse has unlimited time for teaching, the team approach is usually used. Nurses in offices, home, or clinics start the teaching; the perioperative nurses continue it; and the discharge nurse reinforces and supplements it. It may be important that community nurses also be aware if the patient has continuing learning needs, because they may be the ones who visit the patient at home, in the community, or in extended care facilities after surgery.

All teaching should be documented in the patient's medical record. A patient and family teaching guide for preoperative preparation is presented in Table 17-7. Additional information related to patient teaching may be found in Chapter 4.

General Surgery Information. Preoperative teaching includes essential information that the patient desires and needs to know during the surgical experience.[18] This information must be tailored to each individual patient and reflect the specific surgery. The nurse should determine what will best serve this patient rather than routinely giving information that may or may not be relevant. All patients should receive instruction about deep breathing, coughing, and moving postoperatively. This is essential because patients may not want to do these activities postoperatively unless they are taught the rationale for them and practice them preoperatively. Patients and families should be told if there will be tubes, drains, monitoring devices, or special equipment after surgery, and that these devices enable the nurse to safely care for the patient.

Examples of individualized teaching may include how to use incentive spirometers or postoperative patient-controlled analgesia pumps. The patient could also receive surgery-specific information, such as a patient with a total joint replacement having an immobilizer, a patient getting an epidural catheter for postoperative pain control, or the patient requiring extensive surgery being told about waking up in the intensive care unit.

Ambulatory Surgery Information. The ambulatory surgery patient or the patient admitted to the hospital the day of surgery will need to receive information before admission. The teaching is generally done in the surgeon's office or preadmission surgical clinic and reinforced on the day of surgery. Some ambulatory surgical centers have the staff telephone the patients the evening before surgery to answer last-minute questions and to reinforce teaching. Each surgical center has policies and procedures that direct and enable this communication in a timely manner. The nurse should identify this process for the institution in which he or she will be working.

Information for the patient includes the time to arrive at the surgery center and the time of surgery. Arrival time is usually 1 to 2 hours before the scheduled time of surgery to allow for the

TABLE 17-7   Patient & Family Teaching Guide
Preoperative Preparation

Sensory Information
- Holding area is often noisy.
- Drugs and cleaning solutions may be smelled.
- Operating room can be cold; warm blankets are available.
- Talking may be heard in the OR but will be distorted because of masks. Questions should be asked if something is not understood.
- OR bed will be narrow. A safety strap will be applied over the knees.
- Lights in the OR can be very bright.
- Machines (ticking and pinging noises) may be heard when awake. Their purpose is to monitor and ensure safety.

Procedural Information
- What to bring and what type of clothing to wear to the ambulatory surgery center.
- Any changes in time of surgery.
- Fluid and food restrictions.
- Physical preparation required (e.g., bowel or skin preparation).
- Purpose of frequent vital signs assessment.
- Pain control and other comfort measures.

- Why turning, coughing, and deep breathing postoperatively is important; practice sessions need to be done preoperatively.
- Insertion of intravenous lines.
- Procedure for anesthesia administration.

Process Information
Information about General Flow of Surgery
- Admission area.
- Preoperative holding area, OR, and recovery area.
- Families can usually stay in holding area until surgery.
- Families may be able to enter recovery area as soon as patient is awake.
- Identification of any technology that may be present on awakening, such as monitors and central lines.
Where Families Can Wait during Surgery
- Patient and family members need to be encouraged to verbalize concerns.
- OR staff will notify family when surgery is completed.
- Surgeon will usually talk with family following surgery.

---

completion of the preoperative assessment and paperwork preparation. Information can also include the day-of-surgery events such as patient registration, parking, what to wear, what to bring, and the need to have a responsible adult present for transportation home after surgery.

Preoperative preadmission information can include the need for a preoperative shower, an enema, and food and fluid restrictions. Historically, patients having elective surgery were usually instructed to have nothing by mouth (NPO) starting at midnight on the night before surgery. The American Society of Anesthesiologists has published guidelines that are much less stringent (Table 17-8). Providing the patient with the rationale for adhering to NPO orders can significantly increase the patient's perception of their importance.[19] Protocols may vary if the patient is having local anesthesia or the surgery is scheduled for late in the day. The NPO protocol of each surgical facility should be followed because varying NPO protocols exist. Restriction of fluids and food is designed to minimize the potential risk of aspiration and to decrease the risk of postoperative nausea and vomiting. The patient who has not followed this instruction may have surgery delayed or cancelled, so it is vital that the surgical patient understands and adheres to these restrictions.

■ Legal Preparation for Surgery

Legal preparation for surgery consists of checking that all required forms have been correctly signed and are present on the chart, and that the patient and family clearly understand what is going to happen. The most important of these forms is the signed consent form for the surgical procedure and blood transfusion. Other forms can include those that have been completed for advance directives, living wills, and power of attorney (see Chapter 10).

Consent for Surgery. Before nonemergency surgery can be legally performed, the patient must sign a voluntary and in-

TABLE 17-8   Preoperative Fasting Recommendations* of the American Society of Anesthesiologists

LIQUID AND FOOD INTAKE	MINIMUM FASTING PERIOD (HR)
Clear liquids (e.g., water, clear tea, black coffee, carbonated beverages, and fruit juice without pulp)	2
Breast milk	4
Nonhuman milk, including infant formula	6
Light meal (e.g., toast and clear liquids)	6
Regular or heavy meal (may include fried or fatty food, meat)	8

Source: Practice guidelines for preoperative fasting and the use of pharmacologic agents to reduce the risk of pulmonary aspiration: application to healthy patients undergoing elective procedures: a report by the American Society of Anesthesiologists Task Force on Preoperative Fasting, *Anesthesiology* 90:896, 1999.
*For healthy patients of all ages undergoing elective surgery (excluding women in labor).

formed consent in the presence of a witness. **Informed consent** is an active, shared decision-making process between the provider and the recipient of care. This process protects the patient, the surgeon, and the hospital and its employees. Every surgical facility has its own required informed consent form, and the nurse should become familiar with both the form and the process of obtaining consent in that institution.

Three conditions must be met for consent to be valid. First, there must be *adequate disclosure* of the diagnosis; the nature

EVIDENCE-BASED PRACTICE
Preoperative Fasting

Clinical Problem

Should patients be NPO after midnight before elective
surgery?

Best Clinical Practice

- Prolonged preoperative fasting is a time-honored tradition.
  The typical order of NPO after midnight (or no food or
  liquid after 12:00 AM on the day of surgery) has been challenged in recent years.
- Pulmonary aspiration is a rare complication of modern
  anesthesia.
- Based on extensive evidence, the American Society of Anesthesiologists (ASA) revised its practice guidelines for preoperative fasting in healthy patients undergoing elective
  procedures (see Table 17-8).
- The guidelines allow clear liquids up to 2 hours before elective surgery, a light breakfast (e.g., tea and toast) up to
  6 hours before, and a heavier meal up to 8 hours before.

Implications for Nursing Practice

More collaboration between nurses and surgeons is needed
to ensure that fasting instructions are according to ASA
guidelines and that patients understand them.

References for Evidence

Crenshaw JT, Winslow EH: Preoperative fasting: old habits die hard, *Am J
Nurs* 102:36, 2002.
www.asahq.org/practice/npo/npoguide.html.

ETHICAL DILEMMAS
Informed Consent

Situation

The nurse discusses a patient's impending surgery in the preoperative holding area. It becomes obvious that this competent adult patient was not fully informed of the alternatives
to this surgery. She has signed the consent form but clearly
was not fully informed about her treatment options.

Important Points for Consideration

- Informed consent requires that patients have complete
  information about the proposed treatment and its possible
  consequences, as well as alternative treatments and possible
  consequences.
- Risks and benefits of each treatment option must also be
  explained in order for patients to weigh treatment options.
- An opportunity to have questions answered about the
  various treatment options and their possible outcomes is
  also an important element of informed consent.
- Paternalism results when health care providers do not provide
  complete information for patients to make fully informed
  decisions or when they decide what is best for patients.

Critical Thinking Questions

1. What should the nurse do?
2. What is the nurse's role as patient advocate in the informed
   consent process?

and purpose of the proposed treatment; the risks and consequences of the proposed treatment; the probability of a successful outcome; the availability, benefits, and risks of alternative
treatments; and the prognosis if treatment is not instituted. Second, the patient must demonstrate clear *understanding* and *comprehension* of the information being provided. Because preoperative drugs may cloud a patient's comprehension, the operative
consent must be signed before any preoperative medication is
given. Third, the recipient of care must *give consent voluntarily.*
The patient must not be persuaded or coerced in any way to undergo the procedure.[20]

Although the physician is ultimately responsible for obtaining
the consent, the nurse may be responsible for obtaining and wit-
nessing the patient's signature on the consent form. At this time
the nurse can be a patient advocate, verifying that the patient (or
family member) understands the consent form and its implications and that consent for surgery is truly voluntary. The nurse
will contact the surgeon and explain the need for additional information if the patient is unclear about operative plans. The patient needs to be informed that permission may be withdrawn at
any time, including after the permit has been signed.

If the patient is a minor, is unconscious, or is mentally incompetent to sign the permit, the written permission may be
given by a legally appointed representative or responsible family
member.[21] Local hospital policies should be checked for further
clarification.

A true medical emergency may override the need to obtain
consent. When immediate medical treatment is needed to preserve life or to prevent serious impairment to life and the individual patient is incapable of giving consent, the next of kin may
give consent. If reaching the next of kin is not possible, the physician may institute treatment without written consent. A note is

written in the chart documenting the medical necessity of the
procedure.

Procedures for obtaining consent vary among states and institutions. The nurse should be aware of the state's nurse practice
act and the institutional or agency policies that apply to an individual situation.

■ Day-of-Surgery Preparation

Nursing Role. Day-of-surgery preparation will vary a great
deal depending on whether the patient is an inpatient or an outpatient. The nursing responsibility immediately before surgery
includes final preoperative teaching, assessment and communication of pertinent findings, and ensuring that all preoperative
preparation orders have been completed and that records and reports are present and complete to accompany the patient to the
OR. It is especially important to verify the presence of a signed
operative consent, laboratory data, a history and physical examination report, a record of any consultations, baseline vital signs,
and nurses' notes complete to that point.

If the patient is an inpatient, it will be the responsibility of the
hospital nurse to ensure that the patient is ready and appropriately prepared for surgery. If the patient is an outpatient, the patient or family member will share the responsibility for preoperative preparation.

Most institutions require that a patient wear a hospital gown
with no underclothes. Some surgery centers allow the patient
to wear underwear, depending on the surgical procedure to be
performed. The patient should wear no cosmetics because observation of skin color will be important. Nail polish should be removed because the pulse oximeter, used to monitor oxygenation,
will be placed on the patient's fingertip and cannot distinguish
blood oxygen through colored nail polish. An identification band

is put on the patient and, if applicable, an allergy band. All patient valuables are returned to a family member or locked up according to institutional protocol. If the patient prefers not to remove a wedding ring, the ring can be taped securely to the finger to prevent loss. All prostheses, including dentures, contact lenses, and glasses, are generally removed to prevent loss or damage to them. Hearing aids are usually left in place to allow the patient to better follow instructions. Glasses and hearing aids must be returned to the patient as soon as possible following surgery.

The patient must void shortly before surgery. Urination before surgery prevents involuntary elimination under anesthesia and reduces the possibility of urinary retention during early postoperative recovery. This should be done before the administration of any preoperative medication. Many preoperative medications can interfere with balance and could result in a fall when the patient is in the bathroom.

The nurse should determine that all preoperative preparations have been completed and that the signed consent for surgery is present before giving any preoperative medications. The use of a preoperative checklist (Fig. 17-1) ensures that no detail has been omitted.

Preoperative Medications. Preoperative medications are used for a variety of reasons (Table 17-9). A patient may receive a single drug or a combination of drugs (Table 17-10). Benzodiazepines and barbiturates are used for their sedative and amnestic properties. Anticholinergics are given to reduce secretions.

St. Joseph Hospital, Inc.
Albuquerque, New Mexico
☐ St. Joseph Hospital
☐ St. Joseph West Mesa Hospital

ADDRESSOGRAPH

PREOPERATIVE CHECKLIST

Name of procedure ______
Date of surgery ______

	INITIALS O.R.	UNIT
1. Operative permit signed and on chart: (initial if completed)		
2. History and physical in chart: (initial if present)		
3. New progress and doctor's order sheet on chart: (initial if present)		
4. Consultation: ______ NA ______		
5. Laboratory results: Hct: ______ Hgb: ______ K+ ______		
6. Miscellaneous pre-op lab studies: SMAC ______ Chest x-ray ______ ECG ______ Type & cross match ______ # of units ______		
7. Allergies: ______ NKA ______ Front of chart labelled ______ NPO ______		
8. Prosthetic removed: Contact lenses ______ Glasses ______ Limb ______ Eyes ______ Hearing aid ______ Dentures ______ Removable bridgework ______ Capped teeth present ______ Location ______ Etc. ______		
9. Old chart to O.R. with patient: ______ Not requested ______ No old chart ______		
10. Preoperative medication given: ______ TIME: ______ None ordered ______		
11. Vital Signs: (time taken) ______ B.P. ______ P ______ R ______ T ______		

12. Skin prep on unit: ______ wash ______ scrub ______ shower ______
13. Wearing hospital gown: ______ other: ______
14. Hairpins and/or wig removed: ______ NA ______
15. Make-up, false eyelashes and nail polish removed: ______ NA ______
16. Disposition of valuables: (money, credit cards)
To business office ______ family ______ none ______
To O.R. with patient: Rings (taped) ______ Religious articles ______ None ______
17. Antiembolism stockings/bandages: Applied ______ with patient ______ NA ______
18. Urinary status: Voided ______ Catheterized ______ Indwelling cath ______
19. Medications to O.R. with patient: ______ none ______
20. Addressograph on chart ______
21. Chart and transport slip checked ______
Chart signed off ______

Signature and title	initials	Signature and title	initials

FIG. 17-1 Preoperative checklist.

Narcotics may be given to decrease intraoperative anesthetic requirements and to decrease pain. Antiemetics may be given to decrease nausea and vomiting.

Other medications that may be administered preoperatively include antibiotics, eyedrops, and routine prescription drugs. Antibiotics may be administered throughout the perioperative period for a patient with a history of congenital or valvular heart disease to prevent the development of infective endocarditis. They may also be ordered for the patient undergoing surgery where wound contamination is either a potential risk (e.g., gastrointestinal surgery) or where wound infection could have serious postoperative consequences (e.g., cardiac and joint replacement surgery). Antibiotics are most commonly administered intravenously (IV) and may be started either preoperatively or in the OR.

Eyedrops are commonly ordered and administered preoperatively for the patient undergoing cataract and other eye surgery. Many times the patient will require multiple sets of eyedrops administered at 5-minute intervals. It is important to administer these drugs as ordered and on time to adequately prepare the eye for surgery.

A standard protocol for what routine medications are always given on the day of surgery and those that are never given on the day of surgery does not exist. In order to facilitate patient teaching and eliminate confusion about the medications, it is very important to carefully check written preoperative orders and to clarify which medications should and should not be taken on the day of surgery. If there is any question, the nurse should clarify the orders with the ACP. Most patients will be advised to take routine cardiac, antihypertensive, and asthma medications on the day of surgery. In the case of insulin it is important to clarify the time and amount of the last dose before surgery.

Premedications may be administered orally (PO), IV, subcutaneously (SC), or intramuscularly (IM). Oral medications should be given 60 to 90 minutes before the patient goes to the OR. Because patients are fluid restricted before surgery, the patient should swallow these medications with a minimal amount of water. IM and SC injections should be given 30 to 60 minutes before arrival at the OR (minimally 20 minutes). IV medications are usually administered to the patient after arrival in the preoperative holding area or operating room. The drug administration must be charted immediately. The patient should be told the effects of the medications, such as relaxation, drowsiness, and dryness of the mouth.

■ Transportation to the Operating Room

If the patient is an inpatient, the OR staff sends transport personnel to the patient's room with a cart to transport the patient to surgery. The nurse assists the patient in transferring from the hospital bed to the OR cart, and the side rails of the cart are raised and secured. The nurse should ensure that the completed chart goes with the patient, as well as any ordered preoperative equipment, such as antiembolism devices or the patient's inhaler. In many institutions the family may accompany the patient to the holding area.

If the patient is an outpatient, the patient may be transported to the OR by cart or wheelchair or, in the absence of premedication, may even walk accompanied to the OR. In all cases it is important for the nurse to ensure patient safety during transport. The method of transportation and who transported the patient should be documented by the nurse responsible for the transfer.

The family should be instructed where to wait for the patient during surgery. Many hospitals have a surgical waiting room where OR personnel communicate the status of the patient to the family. It is in this waiting room that the surgeon can locate the family after surgery and where families can be notified that the surgery is

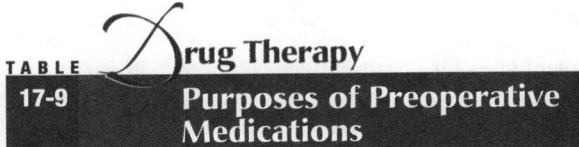

TABLE 17-9	Drug Therapy — Purposes of Preoperative Medications

- Provide analgesia
- Prevent nausea and vomiting
- Promote sedation and amnesia
- Decrease anesthetic requirements
- Facilitate induction of anesthesia
- Relieve apprehension and anxiety
- Prevent autonomic reflex response
- Decrease respiratory and gastrointestinal secretions

TABLE 17-10	Drug Therapy — Frequently Used Preoperative Medications

CLASS	DRUG	PURPOSE AND EFFECTS
Benzodiazepines	midazolam (Versed)	Reduce anxiety
	diazepam (Valium)	Induce sedation
	lorazepam (Ativan)	Induce amnesia
Narcotics	morphine	Relieve discomfort during preoperative procedures
	meperidine (Demerol)	
	fentanyl (Sublimaze)	
Histamine H$_2$-receptor antagonists	cimetidine (Tagamet)	Increase gastric pH
	famotidine (Pepcid)	Decrease gastric volume
	ranitidine (Zantac)	
Antacids	sodium citrate	Increase gastric pH
Antiemetics	metoclopramide (Reglan)	Increase gastric emptying
	droperidol (Inapsine)	Decrease nausea and vomiting
Anticholinergics	atropine	Decrease oral and respiratory secretions
	glycopyrrolate	Prevent bradycardia
	scopolamine	

complete. Some hospitals provide pagers to waiting family members so that they may eat or do errands during the surgery.

While the patient is in surgery the inpatient nurse can prepare the patient's room in consideration of the patient's needs after surgery. The bed is remade, and, if necessary, disposable pads are placed for any anticipated drainage. Any additional necessary equipment, including IV poles, oxygen, suction, and additional pillows for positioning, should also be placed in the room. The room should be organized to facilitate entry of the transport cart. By having these items readily available and the room ready, patient transfer from the PACU or the OR will be smooth.

Culturally Competent Care: Preoperative Patient

The nurse should include cultural and ethnic considerations when assessing and implementing care for the preoperative needs of a patient. For example, culture, not necessarily related to ethnicity, might determine one's expression of pain coping strategies, family expectations, and ability to verbally express needs.[22] Some studies have shown that there may be racial and ethnic differences in the types of surgical procedures and treatments chosen for individuals.[23] Cultural considerations may require including the

family in any decision-making. For example, many older Hispanic women may defer to their family for the decision to have or not to have surgery. These decisions must be respected and valued. (Culturally competent care is discussed in Chapter 2.) ■

Gerontologic Considerations: Preoperative Patient

Many surgical procedures are performed on patients older than 65 years of age, and surgery can even be safely performed on those in their nineties. Frequently performed procedures in the older adult are cataract extraction, coronary and vascular procedures, prostate surgery, herniorrhaphy, cholecystectomy, and hip repair.

The nurse must be particularly alert when assessing and caring for the older adult surgical patient. An event that has little effect on a younger patient may be overwhelming to the older patient. The risks associated with anesthesia and surgery increase in the older patient.[24] In general, the older the patient the greater the risk of complications after surgery. It is important to consider the physiologic status or condition of the patient in planning care and not simply the chronologic age. The patient's biologic age rather than the chronologic age is important to

CRITICAL THINKING EXERCISES

Case Study
Preoperative Patient

Patient Profile. Mrs. Frances Delarosa, an 82-year-old Hispanic retired librarian, is admitted to the hospital with compromised circulation of the right lower leg and a necrotic right foot. She is a diabetic and takes insulin to maintain appropriate blood glucose levels. She has not had anything to eat since last night at 8:00 PM. It is now 1:00 PM in the afternoon of the next day (surgery day).

Subjective Data
- History of type 2 diabetes mellitus for 40 years
- History of renal problems
- History of vision problems
- Surgical history that includes a cesarean section at age 30 and a cholecystectomy at age 65; did not heal well following the last surgery
- Blood glucose has not been well controlled
- Social security checks barely cover the cost of living and medications
- Lives alone but has family that wants her to move in with them following surgery
- Uses herbs to control diabetes and frequently refuses to take insulin

Objective Data
Physical Examination
- Alert, cognitively intact, anxious, obese, elderly woman with complaints of numbness and lack of feeling in right leg
- Weight 235 pounds, height 5 feet 3 inches
- Wears glasses
- Has macular degeneration in right eye

Diagnostic Studies
- Admission laboratory blood glucose level was 537 mg/dl (29.8 mmol/L)
- Morning finger-stick blood glucose level was 97 mg/dl (5.39 mmol/L)

- Doppler pulses for lower right leg very weak; absent in right foot
- Doppler pulses in left leg present, weak in left foot
- Serum creatinine 2.5 mg/dl (221 mmol/L)

Collaborative Care
- Scheduled for a below-the-knee amputation of the right leg as the last case of the day

CRITICAL THINKING QUESTIONS

1. What factors may influence Mrs. Delarosa's response to hospitalization and surgery?
2. Given Mrs. Delarosa's history, what preoperative nursing assessments would you want to complete and why?
3. What potential perioperative complications might you expect for Mrs. Delarosa?
4. What topics would you include in Mrs. Delarosa's preoperative teaching plan?
5. Based on the assessment data presented, identify one or more appropriate nursing diagnoses. What would be your plans and interventions for those diagnoses?

NURSING RESEARCH ISSUES

1. Can a patient assessment effectively predict the need for specific preoperative laboratory tests as opposed to using a predetermined list of required preoperative laboratory tests?
2. How can blood glucose levels best be monitored and controlled during the preoperative period?
3. What are the most pertinent interview data to obtain for planning preoperative instruction?
4. Is there a difference in the accuracy of preoperative assessment data collected by a patient-completed form as compared with a nurse-completed questionnaire?

consider in planning surgery and assessing risks. For example, a 75-year-old woman may be biologically healthy and be more like a 60-year-old in physiologic responses. Conversely, a 55-year-old may biologically be more like a 75-year-old if he or she has multiple chronic health problems. The surgical risk in the older adult relates to normal physiologic aging and changes that compromise organ function, reduce reserve capacity, and limit the body's ability to adapt to stress. This decreased ability to cope with stress, frequently compounded by the additional burden of one or more chronic illnesses, and the surgery itself increases the risk of complications.

When preparing the older adult for surgery, it is important to obtain a detailed history and complete physical examination. Preoperative laboratory tests, an ECG, and a chest x-ray can be important in planning the choice and technique of anesthesia. The patient's primary physician is usually not the surgeon, and frequently several physicians are involved in the patient's care. It is important for the nurse to help coordinate the care and the physicians' orders for the patient.

Consideration of family support is important with the older adult. With the increase in outpatient surgical procedures and shorter postoperative hospitalization, family support is an important consideration in the continuity of care for the older patient.

The nurse must remember that many older adults have sensory deficits. Vision and hearing may be diminished, and bright lights may bother those with eye problems. Thought processes and cognitive abilities may be slowed or impaired. This does not mean that every elderly person has cognitive deficits. Sensory function and cognition must be assessed and documented.[25] Physical reactions are often slowed as a result of mobility and balance problems. All of these changes may require more time for the older adult to complete preoperative testing, and understand preoperative instructions.

Some older adults live in extended care centers or nursing homes. Transportation from these agencies must be coordinated so that timely arrival allows for surgery preparation. If a long-term care patient is cognitively impaired, close attention must be given so that the patient does not inadvertently get out of bed and fall. A legal representative of the patient must be present to provide consent for surgery if the patient cannot sign for himself or herself.

Adding to the stress of the surgical procedure, even minimally invasive ones, the perceived situational change and loss may be overwhelming to the older adult. The threat to independence, lifestyle, and self-esteem may result in ineffective coping. The nurse must be particularly supportive and help the older adult cope with the surgical experience. ■

REVIEW QUESTIONS

The number of the question corresponds to the same-numbered objective at the beginning of the chapter.

1. Which of the following surgical procedures involves removal of a body organ?
   a. colostomy
   b. laparotomy
   c. mammoplasty
   d. cholecystectomy

2. One of the most important goals of the preoperative assessment by the nurse is to
   a. determine if the patient's psychologic stress is too high to undergo surgery.
   b. identify what information the patient needs to make a voluntary, informed consent for surgery.
   c. establish baseline data for comparison of the patient's status in the intraoperative and postoperative period.
   d. determine whether the patient's surgery should be done as an inpatient, an outpatient, or a same-day admission.

3. A patient who is scheduled for a hysterectomy reports using ginkgo biloba to improve her memory. Which of the following questions is the most important for the perioperative nurse to ask the patient?
   a. "How long have you used ginkgo biloba?"
   b. "How have you been able to tell if this herb is effective?"
   c. "Have you been taking this herb during the last several weeks?"
   d. "Have you experienced any side effects of taking this herbal product?"

4. The nurse's role in informed consent for surgery may include
   a. obtaining the patient's signature on the consent form.
   b. asking the patient for consent for the planned procedure.
   c. explaining the risks and consequences of the proposed surgery.
   d. informing the patient of the prognosis if the surgical procedure is refused.

5. A nursing intervention to assist a preoperative patient in coping with fear of pain would be to
   a. describe the degree of pain expected.
   b. explain the availability of pain medication.
   c. divert the patient when talking about pain.
   d. inform the patient of the frequency of pain medication.

6. The nursing measure that should be performed last on the morning of surgery is to
   a. ask patient to void in the bathroom.
   b. check chart for signed consent form.
   c. administer preanesthetic medications.
   d. lock up the patient's jewelry and money.

7. The nurse administering preoperative medications recognizes that
   a. preoperative medications may help reduce anesthetic requirements.
   b. intravenous medications can be administered only by an anesthesiologist on the day of surgery.
   c. a preoperative diazepam (Valium) tablet should be administered within 15 minutes of scheduled surgery.
   d. an intramuscular injection of secobarbital (Seconal) should be administered 2 hours before the scheduled surgery.

8. A primary consideration in the instruction of the older preoperative patient is
   a. using large-print material.
   b. teaching early in the morning.
   c. standing very close to aid communication.
   d. recognizing that cognitive function may be decreased.

REFERENCES

1. Garbee DD, Gentry JA: Case commentary: coping with the stress of surgery, *AORN J* 73:946, 2001.

*2. Morrell G: Effect of structured preoperative teaching on anxiety levels of patients scheduled for cataract surgery, *Insight* 26:4, 2001.

3. Podesta A, Carmagnini E: Erythropoietin in Jehovah's Witness heart surgery, *Minerva Cardioangiol* 47:261, 1999.

4. Snyder CR et al: Hope theory: updating a common process for psychological change. In Snyder CR, Ingram RE, editors: *Handbook of psychological change: psychotherapy processes and practices for the 21st century,* New York, 2000, Wiley.

5. Davila Y: Cultural considerations in perioperative nursing, *Semin Perioper Nurs* 8:128, 1999.

6. Murphy JM: Preoperative considerations with herbal medicines, *AORN J* 69:173, 1999.

7. Norred CL, Zamudio S, Palmer SK: Use of complementary and alternative medicines by surgical patients, *AANA J* 68:13, 2000.

8. Larkin M: Surgery patients are at risk for herb-anesthesia interactions, *Lancet* 354:1362, 1999.

9. Norred CL, Finlayson CA: Hemorrhage after the preoperative use of complementary and alternative medicines, *AANA J* 68:217, 2000.

10. Buhr V: Screening patients for latex allergies (published erratum), *J Am Acad Nurse Pract* 12:466, 2000.

11. Girard N: Care of the geriatric patient. In Phippen ML, Wells MP, editors: *Patient care during operative and invasive procedures,* Philadelphia, 2000, WB Saunders.

12. Keller C: The obese patient as surgical risk, *Semin Perioper Nurs* 8:109, 1999.

13. Armstrong M: Obesity as an intrinsic factor affecting wound healing, *J Wound Care* 7:220, 1998.

14. Ayello EA, Thomas DR, Litchford MA: Wound care 1999: nutritional aspects of wound healing, *Home Healthc Nurse* 17:719, 1999.

15. Joint Commission on Accreditation of Healthcare Organizations: *Comprehensive accreditation manual for hospitals: the official handbook,* Oakbrook Terrace, IL, 2001, The Commission.

16. Incorporating guided imagery into surgery areas: audiotapes provide self-direction for easing stress, *Patient Education Management* 7:90, 2000.

17. Krupat E, Fancey M, Cleary PD: Information and its impact on satisfaction among surgical patients, *Soc Sci Med* 51:1817, 2000.

18. Matiti M, Sharman J: Dignity: a study of preoperative patients, *Nurs Stand* 14:32, 1999.

19. Kramer FM: Patient perceptions of the importance of maintaining preoperative NPO status, *AANA J* 68:321, 2000.

20. Murphy EK: OR nursing law: continuing developments in informed consent, *AORN J* 72:717, 2000.

21. Kuther TL: Competency to provide informed consent in older adulthood, *Gerontol Geriatr Educ* 20:15, 1999.

22. Ernst G: The myth of the "Mediterranean syndrome": do immigrants feel different pain? *Ethn Health* 5:212, 2000. Available at *http://taylorandfrancis.metapress.com/app/home/contribution.asp?wasp=23* (accessed Feb 25, 2002).

23. Ford E, Newman J, Deosaransingh K: Racial and ethnic differences in the use of cardiovascular procedures: findings from the California cooperative cardiovascular project, *Am J Public Health* 90:1128, 2000.

24. Polanczyk CA et al: Impact of age on perioperative complications and length of stay in patients undergoing noncardiac surgery, *Ann Intern Med* 134:637, 2001.

25. Girard N: Gerontological nursing in acute care settings. In McConnell ES, Linton A, editors: *Gerontological nursing,* ed 3, Philadelphia, 2002, WB Saunders.

RESOURCES

Resources for this chapter are listed in Chapter 19 on pages 413-414.

---

*Nursing research–based references.

CHAPTER 18

NURSING MANAGEMENT
Intraoperative Care

Anita Shoup

LEARNING OBJECTIVES

1. Describe the three different areas of the surgery department and the proper attire for each area.
2. Describe the physical environment of the operating room and the holding area.
3. Describe the functions of the members of the surgical team.
4. Identify needs experienced by the patient undergoing surgical procedures.
5. Discuss the role of the perioperative nurse when managing the care of the patient undergoing surgery.
6. Describe basic principles of aseptic technique used in the operating room.
7. Discuss the importance of safety in the positioning of patients.
8. Differentiate between general and regional or local anesthesia, including advantages, disadvantages, and rationale for choice of the anesthetic technique.
9. Identify the basic techniques used to induce and maintain general anesthesia.
10. Discuss techniques for administering local and regional anesthesia.

KEY TERMS

anesthesia care provider, p. 380	malignant hyperthermia, p. 390
anesthesiologist, p. 380	nurse anesthetist, p. 381
conscious sedation, p. 385	operating room (OR) , p. 378
epidural block, p. 389	perioperative nurse, p. 379
function of circulating, p. 379	regional anesthesia, p. 385
function of scrubbing, p. 379	spinal anesthesia, p. 389
general anesthesia, p. 384	surgeon, p. 380
holding area, p. 378	surgical suite, p. 377
local anesthesia, p. 385	

Nursing care of the surgical patient requires an understanding of surgery and surgical interventions. This knowledge allows the nurse to monitor the patient's response to the stressors related to the surgical experience. Use of the nursing process during the operative phase of care is necessary as a framework for the delivery of care. The needs of the patient determine the type of nursing care delivered. These needs are based on the current health status of the patient and the type of surgical intervention anticipated.

Historically, surgical interventions have taken place in the traditional environment of the hospital operating room (OR) suite. Advancements in surgical technology, improvements in the administration of anesthesia, and changes in the health care environment have altered where and how surgery is performed.[1] The number of surgical procedures being performed in the ambulatory surgery setting has doubled in the last decade, thereby lowering the number of cases being performed in the hospital environment.[2] According to the SMG Marketing Group, hospitals are predicting a decrease of in-house surgical procedures and an increase in outpatient procedures in hospitals, surgery centers, and physician offices (Table 18-1). Although all surgical specialties are represented in the ambulatory surgery setting, ophthalmology, gynecology, plastic surgery, otorhinolaryngology, orthopedic, and general are the specialties with the highest patient loads.[1]

The perioperative nurse must remember that the surgical procedure has the same seriousness and potential for complications regardless of where it is performed. The patient and family members still have the same needs and fears. The nurse must still maintain asepsis in the surgical environment, keep current on new technologies, and continue to be a strong advocate for safe patient care.

Differences that are noted in the ambulatory surgery setting as compared with the traditional in-hospital surgery setting include healthier patient populations, shorter procedures, quicker turnovers, and less time available for perioperative teaching of the patient and family.

PHYSICAL ENVIRONMENT

Department Layout

The **surgical suite** is a controlled environment designed to minimize the spread of infectious organisms and allow a smooth flow of patients, personnel, and the instruments and equipment needed to provide safe patient care. The suite is divided into three distinct areas: the unrestricted, semirestricted, and restricted areas. The *unrestricted* area is where personnel in street clothes can interact with those in scrub clothing. These areas typically include the points of entry for patients (e.g., holding area), staff (e.g., locker rooms), and information (e.g., nursing station or control desk). The *semirestricted* area includes the peripheral support areas and corridors. Only authorized personnel are allowed access to the semirestricted areas. All personnel in the semirestricted area must wear surgical attire and cover all head and facial hair. In the restricted area masks are required to supplement surgical attire. The *restricted* area can include the operating rooms, scrub sink areas, and clean core.

In addition, the physical layout is designed to reduce cross-contamination. The flow of clean and sterile supplies and equipment should be separated from contaminated supplies, equip-

Reviewed by Virginia Printz-Feddersen, RN, CNS, MSN, RNC, CNRN, CNOR, Clinical Nurse Specialist, Lovelace Health System, Albuquerque, N.M. and Maureen P. Reilly, RN, PhD, CRNA, Staff Anesthetist, Audie L. Murphy Division, South Texas Veterans Health Care System, San Antonio, Tex.

TABLE 18-1	Inpatient vs. Outpatient Surgery Trends			
	HOSPITAL INPATIENT OPERATIONS (× 1000)	HOSPITAL OUTPATIENT OPERATIONS (× 1000)	FREESTANDING OUTPATIENT SURGERY CENTER OPERATIONS (× 1000)	PHYSICIAN'S OFFICE OPERATIONS (× 1000)
1990	10,903	11,020	2,318	2,256
1992	10,766	12,129	2,871	3,745
1994	10,326	12,691	3,641	5,254
1996	9,985	13,897	4,824	6,514
1998	9,755	15,905	5,784	7,896
2000	9,506	17,314	6,703	8,587
2002	9,255	18,791	7,449	9,196

Source: SMG Marketing Group Inc., Chicago, IL, Oct 2001.

ment, and waste by space, time, and traffic patterns.[3] Personnel move supplies from clean areas, such as the clean core, through the operating room for surgery, and on to peripheral areas, such as the instrument decontamination area.[3]

Holding Area

The **holding area,** frequently called the *preoperative holding area,* is a special waiting area inside or adjacent to the surgical suite. The size varies according to hospital design and can range from a centralized area to accommodate numerous patients to a small designated area immediately outside the actual room scheduled for the surgical procedure. In the holding area the perioperative nurse makes the final identification and assessment before the patient is transferred into the operating room for surgery. Many minor procedures can also be performed in the holding area, such as inserting intravenous (IV) catheters and arterial lines, removing casts, and drug administration.

In some settings another area for holding is identified as the admission, observation, and discharge (AOD) area. This area is designed to allow early-morning admissions for outpatient surgery, same-day admission, and inpatient holding before surgery. In this holding area the nurse can assess the patient for preoperative data, observe the patient both before and after surgery, and allow recovery for a sufficient length of time before discharge to either the home or an inpatient room. The AOD area significantly affects the patient's stay throughout outpatient surgery and prevents unnecessary overnight stays in the inpatient setting.

Separation from loved ones just before surgery can produce anxiety. Some institutions permit the family or a friend to wait with the patient until it is time to be transferred to the operating room. Allowing them to stay with the patient helps relieve anxiety.

Operating Room

The traditional surgical environment, or **operating room (OR),** is a unique acute care setting removed from other hospital clinical units. It is controlled geographically, environmentally, and bacteriologically, and it is restricted in terms of the inflow and outflow of personnel (Fig. 18-1). It is preferable to have the physical location of the OR adjacent to the *postanesthesia care unit* (PACU) and the surgical intensive care unit for quick transportation of the surgical postoperative patient and close proximity to anesthesia personnel if complications arise. This allows for close collaboration for postanesthesia recovery and intensive care follow-up. Careful consideration of the design, location, and control of the physical environment assists with the preven-

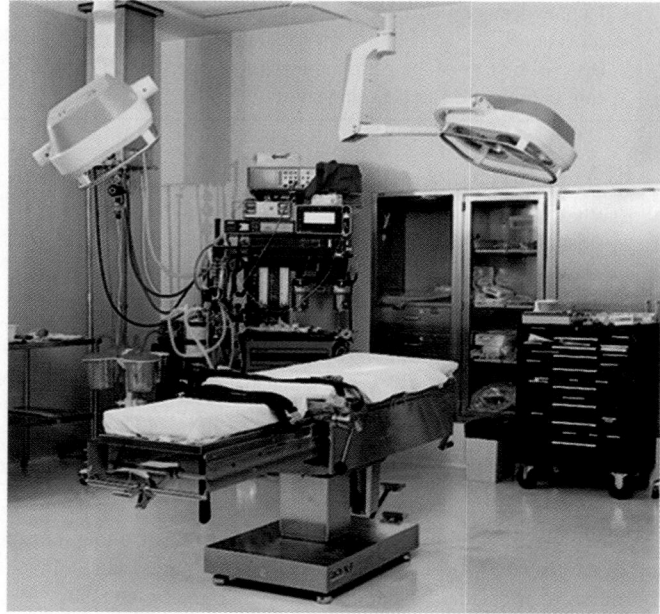

FIG. 18-1 Traditional operating room.

tion of infection and provides physical safety and comfort for the patient.

Several methods are used to prevent the transmission of infection. Filters and controlled airflow in the ventilating systems provide dust control. Positive air pressure in the rooms prevents air from entering the OR from the halls and corridors. Dust-collecting surfaces such as open shelves, windows, and ledges are omitted. Materials that are resistant to the corroding effects of strong disinfectants are used. The functional design facilitates the practice of aseptic technique by the OR team.

Physical safety and comfort are aided by the use of OR furniture that is adjustable, easy to clean, and easy to move. All equipment is checked frequently to ensure electrical safety. The lighting is designed to provide a low- to high-intensity range for a precise view of the surgical site. A communication system provides a means for the delivery of routine and emergency messages.[4-6]

The temperature is controlled from 68° F to 73° F (20° C to 24° C), and the humidity is regulated between 30% and 60% to facilitate patient comfort under the surgical drapes, team comfort during the procedure, and an environment that is unfavorable to bacterial incubation and growth.[6]

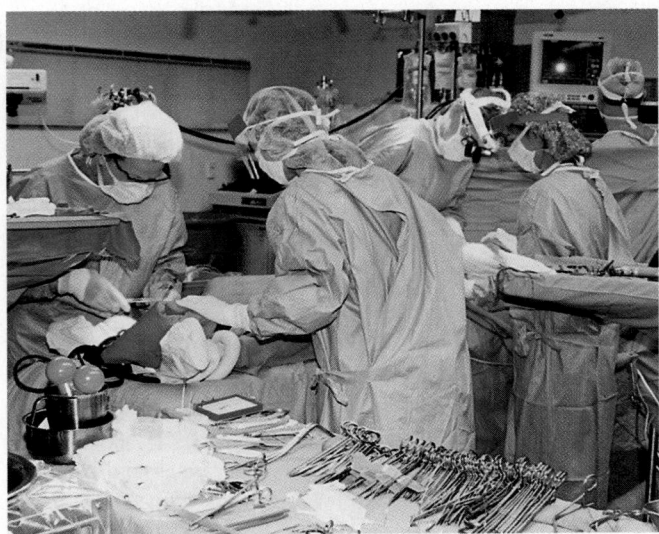

FIG. 18-2 The complexity of the operative procedure does not allow for the influx of extra personnel or visitors.

The privacy of the patient is achieved by restricting the influx of hospital personnel and visitors. The complexity of an ongoing operative procedure does not allow for the presence of extraneous personnel and visitors (Fig. 18-2).

SURGICAL TEAM

Registered Nurse

The **perioperative nurse** is a registered nurse who implements patient care based on the nursing process. Before the patient's arrival in the OR, the nurse, through close collaboration with the other members of the surgical team, prepares the OR for the patient. When the patient arrives from home or is transported from the acute care inpatient area to the holding area, the nurse is usually the first member of the surgical team encountered. The nurse is the patient's advocate throughout the intraoperative experience. Therefore the nurse assesses the patient to determine any additional needs or tasks to complete before surgery to meet the patient's individual plan of care. The nurse provides preoperative education regarding the upcoming experience and physical comfort measures. In addition, she or he helps reduce the patient's anxiety through communication and touch.

Different functions may be assumed by the perioperative nurse that involve either sterile or unsterile activities. If the nurse is not scrubbed, gowned, and gloved and remains in the unsterile field, the **function of circulating** is implemented. If the nurse follows the designated scrub procedure, is gowned and gloved in sterile attire, and remains in the sterile field, the **function of scrubbing** is implemented. Some specific intraoperative activities of each function are outlined in Table 18-2.

The perioperative nurse is not limited to task-oriented duties and actively implements nursing care throughout the patient's surgical experience. The majority of behaviors of perioperative nurses reflect critical thinking regarding safe patient care.[7] The nurse must anticipate the needs of not only the patient, but other members of the team as well. Ongoing assessment of the patient is essential because the patient's condition may change quickly. The perioperative nurse responds to these changes and revises the plan of care as needed. Examples of nursing activities that characterize each phase surrounding the surgical experience are presented in Table 18-3.

The nurse in the circulating role documents the nursing care of the patient. Documentation may be written or electronic. The Association of periOperative Registered Nurses (AORN) published the Perioperative Nursing Data Set (PNDS). The PNDS relates to the delivery of nursing care in the perioperative setting at

---

TABLE 18-2   Intraoperative Activities of the Perioperative Nurse

Circulating/Nonsterile Activities

- Reviews anatomy, physiology, and the surgical procedure.
- Assists with preparing the room:
  Practices aseptic technique.
  Monitors the activities of others.
  Ensures that needed items are available and sterile (if required).
  Checks mechanical and electrical equipment and environmental factors.
  Arranges the furniture in workable order.
- Identifies and assesses the patient. Then plans and coordinates the intraoperative nursing care.
- Checks the chart and relates pertinent data.
- Admits the patient to the operating room suite.
- Assists with transferring the patient to the operating room bed.
- Participates in insertion and application of monitoring devices.
- Protects the patient during induction of anesthesia.
- Positions the patient.
- Monitors the draping procedure and all activities requiring asepsis.
- Documents intraoperative care.
- Records, labels, and sends to proper locations tissue specimens and cultures.
- Measures blood and fluid loss.
- Records amount of drugs used during local anesthesia.

- Coordinates all activities in the room with team members and other health-related personnel and departments.
- Counts sponges, needles, and instruments.
- Monitors practices of aseptic technique in self and others.
- Accompanies the patient to the postanesthesia recovery area.
- Reports pertinent information to the recovery area nurses.

Scrubbed/Sterile Activities

- Reviews anatomy, physiology, and the surgical procedure.
- Assists with preparation of the room.
- Scrubs, gowns, and gloves self and other members of the surgical team.
- Prepares the instrument table and organizes sterile equipment for functional use.
- Assists with the draping procedure.
- Passes instruments to the surgeon and assistants by anticipating their needs.
- Counts sponges, needles, and instruments.
- Monitors practices of aseptic technique in self and others.
- Keeps track of irrigation solutions used for calculation of blood loss.
- Reports amounts of local anesthesia and epinephrine solutions used by anesthetist.

TABLE 18-3	Examples of Nursing Activities Surrounding the Surgical Experience	
BEFORE	**DURING**	**AFTER**
Assessment	**Implementation**	**Evaluation**
Home/Clinic/Holding Area	*Maintenance of Safety*	*Postanesthesia/Discharge Area*
Initiates preoperative assessment	Ensures the integrity of the sterile field	Determines patient's immediate response to surgical intervention
Plans teaching methods appropriate to patient's needs	Ensures that the sponge, needle, and instrument counts are correct	Monitors vital signs
Involves family in interview	Positions the patient to ensure correct alignment, exposure of surgical site, and prevention of injury	Safely administers appropriate medications
Surgical Unit		*Surgical Unit*
Completes preoperative assessment	Prevents chemical injury from prepping solutions, pharmaceuticals, etc.	Evaluates effectiveness of nursing care in the OR using patient outcome criteria
Coordinates patient teaching with other nursing staff	Ensures safe use of electrical equipment, lasers, and radiation	Determines patient's level of satisfaction with care given during perioperative period
Develops a plan of care	Safely administers appropriate medications	
Surgical Suite	*Monitoring of Physical Status*	Evaluates products used on patient in the OR
Identifies patient	Monitors and reports changes in patient's vital signs	Determines patient's psychologic status
Verifies surgical site	Monitors blood loss	
Assesses patient's level of consciousness, skin integrity, mobility, emotional status, and functional limitations	Monitors urine output as applicable	Assists with discharge planning
	Monitoring of Psychologic Status	*Home/Clinic*
Reviews chart	Provides emotional support to patient	Seeks patient's perception of surgery in terms of the effects of anesthetic agents, impact on body image, immobilization
Planning	Stands near or touches patient during procedures and induction	Determines family's perceptions of surgery
Determines a plan of care that incorporates and respects the patient's value system, lifestyle, ethnicity, and culture; care plan reflects the patient's level of function and ability during the perioperative period	Ensures the patient's right to privacy is maintained	
Ensures all supplies and equipment needed for surgery are available, functioning properly, and sterile, if appropriate	Communicates patient's emotional status to other appropriate members of the health care team	

OR, Operating room.

any point in time and is appropriate for use in any surgical setting. Documentation of the assessment and identification of clinical problems, diagnoses, and intervention differentiates the perioperative nurse's role from other members of the surgical team.[8,9]

Licensed Practical Nurse and Surgical Technician

In many institutions a trained OR surgical technician or a licensed practical nurse performs the scrubbed function. The scrubbed, or assistive, person assists the surgeon by passing instruments and implementing other technical functions during the surgical procedure. This role is supervised by and can also be assumed by a registered nurse.

Surgeon and Assistant

The **surgeon** is the physician who performs the surgical procedure. The surgeon may be the patient's primary physician or one who was selected by the patient's physician or the patient. The surgeon is primarily responsible for the following:

1. Preoperative medical history and physical assessment, including need for surgical intervention, choice of surgical procedure, and management of preoperative workup
2. Patient safety and management in the OR
3. Postoperative management of the patient

The surgeon's assistant can be a physician who functions in an assisting role during the surgical procedure. The assistant usu-

ally holds retractors to expose surgical areas and assists with hemostasis and suturing. In some instances, especially in educational settings, the assistant may perform some portions of the operative procedure under the direct supervision of the surgeon.

In some institutions the surgeon's assistant is a registered nurse or a nonphysician who functions in the role of the assistant under the direct supervision of the physician. Hospital policies define this role and physician responsibility when a nonphysician fills the assistant's position.

Registered Nurse First Assistant

Nursing roles in the perioperative setting change and evolve as technology and health care change. One of these changes is the use of the *registered nurse first assistant* (RNFA). The RNFA works in collaboration with the surgeon to produce an optimal surgical outcome for the patient. The AORN revised position statement of RNFAs states that this perioperative nurse must have formal education for this role and works collaboratively with the surgeon, patient, and surgical team by handling tissue, using instruments, providing exposure to the surgical site, assisting with hemostasis, and suturing.[6,10]

Anesthesia Care Provider

The term **anesthesia care provider** (ACP) is one who administers anesthesia and can be an anesthesiologist or a nurse anesthetist. An **anesthesiologist** is a medical doctor who has completed a residency in the field of anesthesia and is credentialed by the American Board of Anesthesiology. A **nurse anesthetist** is a registered nurse who has graduated from an accredited nurse anesthesia program and successfully completed a national certification examination to become a certified registered nurse anesthetist (CRNA). Both the anesthesiologist and the CRNA are qualified to administer anesthetics to the patient and assume responsibility for the maintenance of physiologic homeostasis throughout the intraoperative period. Anesthesia may be provided by the anesthesiologist or CRNA, working alone or in combination.

The ACP generally accepts the following responsibilities:

1. Assess the patient preoperatively to determine the safest anesthetic for the particular patient's needs and anticipated operative procedure.
2. Prescribe preoperative and adjunctive medications.
3. Monitor patient's cardiac and respiratory status.
4. Monitor patient's vital signs throughout the procedure.
5. Administer the anesthetic during the surgical procedure, and inform the surgeon if difficulties arise during the patient's anesthetic course.
6. Administer fluids and electrolytes, medications, and blood products throughout the surgical procedure.
7. Supervise the postanesthesia recovery of the patient in the PACU, and document the patient's postanesthetic recovery in the first 24 hours.

In preparation for and carrying out the surgical procedure, all members of the surgical team (circulating nurse, scrub assistant, surgeon, assistant, and ACP) collaborate to ensure that the patient is receiving the best possible care.

NURSING MANAGEMENT
PATIENT BEFORE SURGERY

The preoperative assessment of the surgical patient establishes baseline data for intraoperative and postanesthesia care. Assessment data that are provided by the patient and family in the holding area and data from the inpatient nursing units are verified and are important to ensure that a plan of care can be developed.

■ Psychosocial Assessment

The perioperative nurse who cares for the patient in the OR is knowledgeable about the ongoing activities that occur when a patient is transferred into the surgical suite. This knowledge allows for informative and reassuring explanations, especially to the anxious patient. General questions regarding surgery or anesthesia can usually be answered by the perioperative nurse. Examples of these questions include, "When will I go to sleep?" "Who will be in the room?" "When will my doctor arrive?" "How much of my body will be exposed and to whom?" "Will I be cold?" "When will I wake up?" Specific questions relating to details of the surgical procedure and anesthesia may be referred to the surgeon or ACP.

It is especially important that the perioperative nurse has knowledge of the patient's spiritual and cultural habits and beliefs. For example, members of the Jehovah's Witness community may refuse blood transfusions.[11] For Islamics, the left hand is considered unclean, so the nurse should use the right hand to administer forms, drugs, and treatments.[12] Some Native American patients may request that surgically removed body tissue be preserved so that it may be ritually buried. Care must be taken to ensure that cultural practices are identified and respected.

■ Physical Assessment

A thorough physical assessment should be made during the preoperative preparation of the patient (see Chapter 17). Physical assessment data that are specifically important to intraoperative nursing care include baseline data such as vital signs, height, weight, and age; allergic reactions to food, drugs, and latex; condition and cleanliness of skin; skeletal and muscle impairments; perceptual difficulties; level of consciousness; nothing-by-mouth (NPO) status; and any sources of pain or discomfort.[13] Vital signs are important as baseline data to evaluate the effects of intraoperative medications and body positioning. Height and weight of the patient guide the nurse regarding the width and length of the operating bed. The need for extra warmth is indicated by the patient's age, metabolic problems, and planned surgical procedures. Some allergic reactions may be avoided with such simple measures as a change in "prepping" solutions or the type of tape used with dressings. Catastrophic reactions can possibly be avoided if latex sensitivity is determined before the procedure begins. (See the discussion of latex allergies in Chapter 13.) The condition and cleanliness of the skin determine the amount and type of intraoperative skin preparation solutions and will alert the team to the potential for infection as a result of open or closed skin lesions. Knowledge of skeletal and muscle impairments helps prevent injury during positioning. Perceptual difficulty, such as a vision or hearing impairment, will guide the nurse in adapting communication techniques to individual needs. An altered level of consciousness necessitates increased safety and protection techniques. Communicating identified sources of pain to other health team members prevents subjecting the patient to unnecessary discomfort.

The increased use of herbs and dietary supplements has increased the risk of complications for patients undergoing surgery. Herbs can potentially inhibit coagulation, alter blood pressure, cause sedation, have cardiac effects, or alter electrolyte levels.[14-17] (See Complementary and Alternative Therapies box in Chapter 17 on p. 364.)

■ Chart Review

Required chart data vary with hospital policy, patient condition, and specific surgical procedures. Because ambulatory surgery facilities tend to have a healthier population, fewer tests may be required. Examples of data that are obtained during the preoperative assessment include the following:

1. History and physical examination
2. Urinalysis
3. Complete blood cell count
4. Serum electrolyte values
5. Chest x-ray
6. Electrocardiogram
7. Other diagnostic tests (e.g., computed tomography [CT] scan)
8. Pregnancy testing (if applicable)
9. Surgical and blood transfusion consent
10. Allergies
11. Blood type and crossmatch if applicable

Knowledge of these chart data contribute to an understanding of past and present history, cardiopulmonary status, and potential for infection.[13]

■ Admitting the Patient

Hospital policy designates the exact procedure that should be followed when admitting the patient to the holding area and OR suite. A general routine includes initial greeting, extension of human contact and warmth, and proper identification. The identification process includes asking the patient to state her or his name, the surgeon's name, and the operative procedure and location. In addition, the hospital identification numbers are compared with the patient's own identification band and chart. The patient may be further identified by the surgeon before anesthesia induction. In some institutions identification may take place in the holding area and, in others, in the OR itself.

Complementary and alternative therapies such as therapeutic touch, aroma and music therapy, guided imagery, and humor are some of the integrative caring-healing therapies that are being used for surgical patients. These therapies may decrease anxiety, promote relaxation, reduce pain, and accelerate the healing process.[18-22] In some facilities these are initiated before the patient's admission to the OR. In others, such as ambulatory settings, they may be started after the patient's arrival in the holding area.

The admitting procedure is continued with reassessment of the patient and with time allowed for last-minute questions.

The nurse completes the review of the chart for the previously mentioned data and notes any abnormalities or changes. The patient is questioned concerning valuables, prostheses, and last intake of food and fluid. Validation is made that the correct preoperative medication was given, if ordered. A warm blanket, pillow, or position adjustment is provided if the patient is uncomfortable. Most hospitals require the patient's hair to be covered just before transfer to the OR suite to reduce potential shedding.

NURSING MANAGEMENT
PATIENT DURING SURGERY

■ Room Preparation

Before transferring the patient into the scheduled OR, the nurse spends significant time preparing the room to ensure privacy, safety, and prevention of infection. Surgical attire (pants and shirts, masks, protective eyewear, and caps or hoods) is worn by all persons entering the OR suite (Fig. 18-3). All electrical and mechanical equipment is checked for proper functioning. Aseptic technique is practiced as each surgical item is opened and placed systematically on the instrument table.[23] Sponges, needles, and instruments are counted to ensure accurate retrieval at the close of the procedure.[24]

During this time and during the procedure the functions of the team members are delineated. The scrub person will scrub hands and arms, don sterile gown and gloves, and touch only those items in the sterile field. The circulating nurse remains in the unsterile field and implements those activities that permit touching all unsterile items and the patient. Every person on the surgical team must share the responsibility for monitoring aseptic practice and initiating corrective action when a sterile field is compromised.[6]

COMPLEMENTARY & ALTERNATIVE THERAPIES
Music Therapy

Clinical Uses

Music can be used to (1) decrease stress, anxiety, and pain; (2) improve cognitive functioning; (3) alter mood states; (4) promote relaxation and sleep; and (5) enhance alertness. Music can be used in many different clinical settings, including occupational and physical therapy, elder care facilities, operating or procedure rooms, and hospices. Playing music in the background, while a person is seemingly unaware of the music itself, can reduce stress.

Preoperatively music can be used to decrease anxiety. Before and during surgery music can be used to distract attention of patients from their discomfort and the sounds of the equipment and staff. Surgical patients exposed to music have diminished analgesic and hypnotic requirements during conscious sedation. Postoperatively, music can decrease pain and the need for analgesics.

Effects

Music can have many different physiologic effects. Listening to calming music can result in slower, deeper breathing and a decrease in heart rate and blood pressure—an indication of relaxation. Music with a faster pace can energize a person and promote mental alertness.

Nursing Implications

To be effective, music selection needs to be appropriate for the situation. There is not a single type of music that is good for everyone. People have different tastes. It is important that the patient likes the music being played. There are no known side effects of this low-cost intervention. It is also well suited as a self-care technique. Combining music with relaxation therapy is more effective than doing relaxation therapy alone. Additional information can be found at *www.musictherapy.org*.

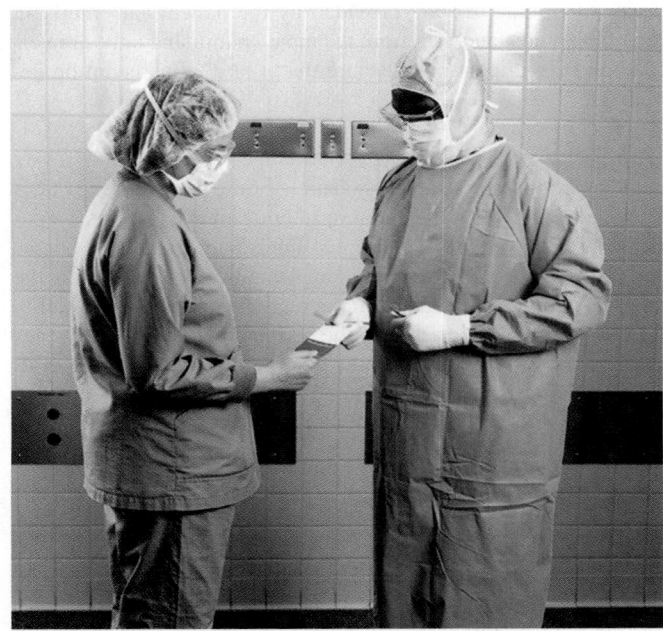

FIG. 18-3 Surgical attire is worn by all persons entering the operating room suite.

■ Transferring the Patient

Once the patient has been properly identified and the OR has been adequately prepared, the patient is transported into the room for the surgery. Each time a patient is transferred from one bed to another, the wheels of the stretcher should be locked, and a sufficient number of personnel should be available to lift, guide, and prevent accidental falling. Once the patient is on the operating bed, safety straps should be snugly placed across the patient's thighs. At this time the monitor leads (e.g., electrocardiograph leads) are usually applied and an IV catheter is inserted if it was not in place when the patient arrived from the holding area.

■ Scrubbing, Gowning, and Gloving

All sterile members of the surgical team (scrub assistant, surgeon, and assistant) are required to cleanse their hands and arms by scrubbing with a brush and detergent before entering the sterile field. This is done to eliminate dirt and skin oil and to decrease the microbial count as much as possible. The surgical scrub helps prevent the growth of microbes beneath the surgical gloves and gown. The detergent used should be an effective antimicrobial agent. The procedure should be standardized for all personnel. During the actual procedure of scrubbing, the team members' fingers and hands should be scrubbed first with progression to the forearms and elbows. The hands should be held away from surgical attire and higher than the elbows at all times to prevent contamination from clothing or detergent suds and water from draining from the unclean area above the elbows to the clean and previously scrubbed areas of the hands and fingers.[4,6,25] Waterless, alcohol-based agents are beginning to replace traditional soap and water in some facilities.[26]

Once the scrub procedure is completed, the team members enter the room to put on the surgical gowns and gloves. Because the gowns and gloves are sterile, it is permissible for the scrubbed people to manipulate and organize all sterile items for use during the procedure.

■ Basic Aseptic Technique

To prevent infections, aseptic technique is practiced in the OR. This is implemented through the creation and maintenance of a sterile field (Fig. 18-4). The center of the sterile field is the site of the surgical incision. Inanimate items in the sterile field include surgical items and equipment that have been sterilized by appropriate sterilization methods.

There are specific principles that the team members should understand to practice aseptic technique. Unless these principles are followed, the safety of the patient is compromised, and the potential for postoperative infection is increased. Table 18-4 presents basic principles of aseptic technique.[4,6,23]

In addition to following the principles of aseptic technique, the surgical team is responsible for following the guidelines established by the U.S. Occupational Safety and Health Administration (OSHA) and the Association of PeriOperative Registered Nurses to protect the patient and the team from exposure to blood-borne pathogens.[27] These guidelines emphasize standard and transmission-based precautions (see Table 12-19), engineering and work practice controls, and the use of personal protective equipment such as gloves, gowns, aprons, caps, face shields, masks, and protective eyewear (see Table 12-18 and Fig. 18-3). This is especially important in the OR environment because of the high potential for exposure to blood-borne pathogens.

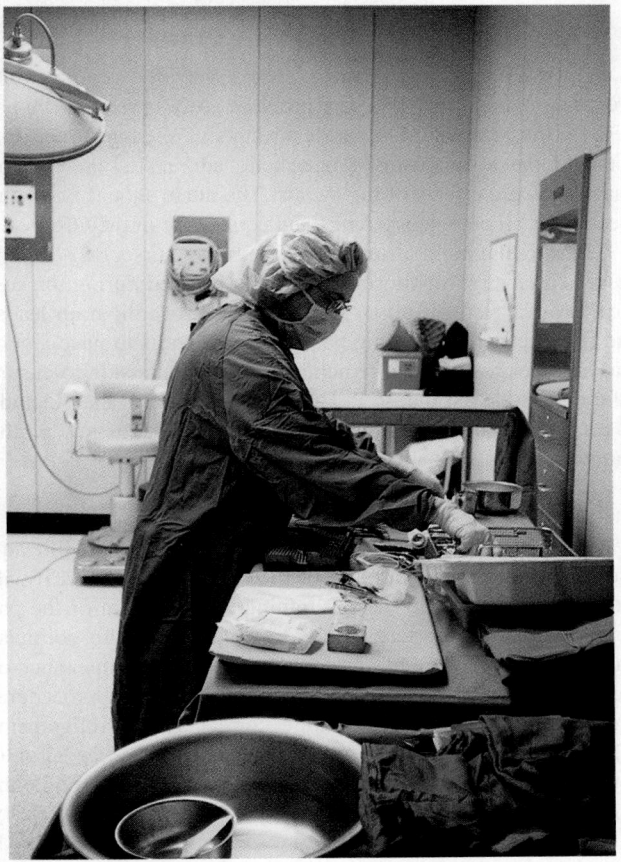

FIG. 18-4 A sterile field is created before surgery.

TABLE 18-4	Principles of Basic Aseptic Technique in the Operating Room

1. All materials that enter the sterile field must be sterile.
2. If a sterile item comes in contact with an unsterile item, it is contaminated.
3. Contaminated items should be removed immediately from the sterile field.
4. Sterile team members must wear only sterile gowns and gloves; once dressed for the procedure, they should recognize that the only parts of the gown considered sterile are the front from chest to table level and the sleeves to 2 inches above the elbow.
5. A wide margin of safety must be maintained between the sterile and unsterile field.
6. Tables are considered sterile only at tabletop level; items extending beneath this level are considered contaminated.
7. The edges of a sterile package are considered contaminated once the package has been opened.
8. Bacteria travel on airborne particles and will enter the sterile field with excessive air movements and currents.
9. Bacteria travel by capillary action through moist fabrics and contamination occurs.
10. Bacteria harbor on the patient's and the team members' hair, skin, and respiratory tracts and must be confined by appropriate attire.

■ Assisting the Anesthesia Care Provider

While the perioperative nurse checks the OR to complete its preparation, the anesthesia care provider (ACP) prepares the patient for the administration of the anesthetic. The nurse must understand the mechanism of anesthetic administration and the pharmacologic effects of the agents. The nurse should know the location of all emergency drugs and equipment in the OR area.

The circulating nonsterile perioperative nurse may be involved in placing monitoring devices to be used during the surgical procedure (e.g., urinary catheter, electrocardiogram leads) and the electrical grounding pad. If the patient is to have a general anesthetic, the nurse remains at the patient's side to ensure safety and to assist the ACP. These responsibilities may include obtaining blood pressure measurements and assisting in the maintenance of the patient's airway.

■ Positioning the Patient

Positioning the patient is a critical part of every procedure and usually follows administration of the anesthetic. The ACP will indicate when to begin the positioning. The position of the patient should allow for accessibility to the operative site, administration and monitoring of anesthetic agents, and maintenance of the patient's airway. When positioning for the surgical procedure, care must be used to (1) provide correct skeletal alignment; (2) prevent undue pressure on nerves, skin over bony prominences, and eyes; (3) provide for adequate thoracic excursion; (4) prevent occlusion of arteries and veins; (5) provide modesty in exposure; and (6) recognize and respect individual needs such as previously assessed aches, pains, or deformities. It is a nursing responsibility to secure the extremities, provide adequate padding and support, and obtain sufficient physical or mechanical help to avoid unnecessary straining of self or patient.[28]

Various positions in which the patient may be placed include supine, prone, Trendelenburg, lateral, kidney, lithotomy, jackknife, and sitting. The supine is the most common position used. It is suited for surgery involving the abdomen, heart, and breast. The prone position allows easy access for back surgeries (e.g., laminectomies). The lithotomy position is used for some types of pelvic organ surgery (e.g., vaginal hysterectomy).

Whatever position is required for the procedure, great care is taken to prevent injury to the patient. Because anesthesia has blocked the nerve impulses, the patient will not feel pain or discomfort, or stress being placed on the nerves, muscles, bones, and skin. Improper positioning could potentially result in muscle strain, joint damage, pressure ulcers, nerve damage, and other untoward effects.

General anesthesia causes peripheral vessels to dilate. Position changes affect where the pooling of blood occurs. If the head of the OR bed is raised, the lower torso will have increased blood volume and the upper torso may become compromised. Hypovolemia and cardiovascular disease can further compromise the patient's status. Consequently the perioperative nurse, working with the entire surgical team, carefully plans and implements the patient's positioning, and then closely monitors the patient throughout the surgical procedure.[6]

■ Preparing the Surgical Site

The purpose of skin preparation, or "prepping," is to reduce the number of organisms available to migrate to the surgical wound. The task of prepping is usually the responsibility of the circulating nurse.

The skin is prepared by mechanically scrubbing or cleansing around the surgical site with antimicrobial agents identified as being nonallergenic to the patient. If the patient is very hairy or if the hair will interfere with the surgical procedure, the nurse removes it using clippers. The area is then scrubbed in a circular motion. The principle of scrubbing from the clean area (site of the incision) to the dirty area (periphery) is observed at all times. A liberal area is cleansed to allow for added protection and unexpected occurrences during the procedure.[29]

After preparation of the skin, the sterile members of the surgical team drape the area. Only the site to be incised is left exposed.

■ Safety Considerations

All surgical procedures, regardless of where they take place, can put the patient at risk for injury. These injuries can be infections, physical injury from positioning or equipment used, or the surgery itself. Lasers and electrosurgical units can cause injury to the patient and surgical staff. The perioperative nurse must be familiar with fire safety issues to protect the patient and staff against burns. Airborne contaminants produced during laser procedures may contain trace hydrocarbons, including acetone, isopropanol, toluene, formaldehyde, and cyanide. Smoke can cause respiratory irritation and has mutagenic and carcinogenic potential.[30] Smoke evacuators are used in the OR.

Patient After Surgery

Through constant observation of the surgical progress, the ACP anticipates the end of the surgical procedure and uses appropriate types and doses of anesthetic agents so that their effects will be minimal at the end of the surgical procedure. This also allows greater physiologic control of the patient during the transfer to the postanesthesia care unit (PACU).

The ACP and the perioperative nurse or another member of the surgical team accompany the patient to the PACU. A report of the patient's status and the procedure is communicated. The OR nurse evaluates the patient's response to nursing care based on outcome criteria established when the plan of care was developed[8,31] (Table 18-5).

CLASSIFICATION OF ANESTHESIA

The anesthetic technique and agents are selected by the ACP in collaboration with the surgeon and the patient. Factors contributing to the decision include the patient's current health status and history, emotional stability, and factors relating to the operative procedure (e.g., length, position, site). The ACP validates this information during the preoperative assessment, obtains anesthesia consent, writes orders for the preoperative medication, and assigns the patient an anesthesia classification. The anesthesia classification, an independent guideline for the ACP, is based on the physiologic status of the patient with no regard to the surgical procedure to be performed. A scale of 1 to 5 is used, with 1 being a healthy patient and 5 being a moribund patient having surgery as a last resort or resuscitative effort. An intraoperative complication is more likely to develop with a higher classification number[6] (see Chapter 17, Table 17-4).

Anesthesia is classified according to the effect that it has on the patient's sensorium (central nervous system) and pain perception. **General anesthesia** is the loss of sensation with loss of consciousness, skeletal muscle relaxation, analgesia, and elimination of the somatic, autonomic, and endocrine responses, including coughing, gagging, vomiting, and sympathetic nervous

TABLE 18-5 Perioperative Nursing Data Set: Outcome Statements

Code: Outcome Statement
Domain: Perioperative Safety
- The patient is free from signs and symptoms of injury caused by extraneous objects.
- The patient is free from signs and symptoms of chemical injury.
- The patient is free from signs and symptoms of electrical injury.
- The patient is free from signs and symptoms of injury related to positioning.
- The patient is free from signs and symptoms of laser injury.
- The patient is free from signs and symptoms of radiation injury.
- The patient is free from signs and symptoms of injury related to transfer/transport.
- The patient receives appropriate medication(s), safely administered during the perioperative period.

Domain: Physiologic Responses
- The patient is free from signs and symptoms of infection.
- The patient has wound/tissue perfusion consistent with or improved from baseline levels established preoperatively.
- The patient is at or returning to normothermia at the conclusion of the immediate postoperative period.
- The patient's fluid, electrolyte, and acid–base balances are consistent with or improved from baseline levels established preoperatively.
- The patient's respiratory function is consistent with or improved from baseline levels established preoperatively.
- The patient's cardiovascular function is consistent with or improved from baseline levels established preoperatively.

- The patient demonstrates and/or reports adequate pain control throughout the perioperative period.
- The patient's neurologic function is consistent with or improved from baseline levels established preoperatively.

Domain: Behavioral Responses—Patient and Family
- The patient demonstrates knowledge of expected responses to the operative or invasive procedure.
- The patient demonstrates knowledge of nutritional requirements related to the operative or other invasive procedure.
- The patient demonstrates knowledge of medication management.
- The patient demonstrates knowledge of pain management.
- The patient participates in the rehabilitation process.
- The patient demonstrates knowledge of wound healing.
- The patient participates in decisions affecting his or her perioperative plan of care.
- The patient's care is consistent with the perioperative plan of care.
- The patient's right to privacy is maintained.
- The patient is the recipient of competent and ethical care within legal standards of practice.
- The patient receives consistent and comparable care regardless of the setting.
- The patient's value system, lifestyle, ethnicity, and culture are considered, respected, and incorporated in the perioperative plan of care.

Reprinted with permission from *AORN perioperative nursing data set*, ed 2, 2002, and *Standards, recommended practices and guidelines*, 2002. Copyright © 2002, AORN, Inc., 2170 South Parker Road, Suite 300, Denver, CO 80231.

system responsiveness. **Local anesthesia** is the loss of sensation without loss of consciousness. Local anesthesia may be induced topically or via infiltration intracutaneously or subcutaneously. **Conscious sedation** ("twilight sleep") is a minimally depressed level of consciousness with maintenance of the patient's protective airway reflexes. The primary goal of conscious sedation is to reduce the patient's anxiety and discomfort and to facilitate cooperation. Often a combination of sedative-hypnotic and opioid drugs is used.[32] Conscious sedation retains the patient's ability to maintain her or his own airway and respond appropriately to verbal commands, yet achieves a level of emotional and physical acceptance of a painful procedure (e.g., colonoscopy). **Regional anesthesia** is the loss of sensation to a region of the body without loss of consciousness when a specific nerve or group of nerves is blocked with the administration of a local anesthetic (e.g., spinal, epidural, or peripheral nerve block).

General Anesthesia

General anesthesia is usually the technique of choice for patients who (1) are having surgical procedures that require significant skeletal muscle relaxation, last for long periods of time, require awkward positions because of the location of the incision site, or require control of respiration; (2) are extremely anxious; (3) refuse or have contraindications for local or regional anesthetic techniques; and (4) are uncooperative because of their emotional status, lack of maturity, intoxication, head injury, or pathophysiologic processes that do not permit them to remain immobile for any length of time. Phases of general anesthesia are presented in Table 18-6.

General anesthesia may be administered intravenously, by inhalation, or rectally. A *balanced technique* (use of drugs from different classes) is the most common method used for general anesthesia. Table 18-7 presents common anesthetic drugs with advantages, disadvantages, and nursing interventions that are indicated for patients receiving the agents.

Intravenous Induction Agents. Virtually all routine adult general anesthetics begin with an IV induction agent. These agents induce a pleasant sleep, with a rapid onset of action that patients find desirable. A single dose lasts only a few minutes, which is long enough for an endotracheal tube to be placed and an inhalation agent to be started.

Inhalation Agents. Inhalation agents are the foundation of general anesthesia. The inhalation agents used for general anesthesia may be volatile liquids (liquid at room temperature) or gases (gas at room temperature). Volatile liquids are administered through a specially designed vaporizer after being mixed with oxygen as a carrier gas.

Inhalation agents enter the body through the alveoli in the lungs. They may be administered through a mask, an endotracheal tube, a laryngeal mask airway, or a tracheostomy. Ease of administration and rapid excretion by ventilation make them desirable agents. One undesirable characteristic is the irritating effect of inhalation agents on the respiratory tract. Complications that may arise are coughing, *laryngospasm* (muscular constriction of the larynx), bronchospasm, increased secretions, and respiratory depression.[33]

Inhalation agents are most commonly administered via an endotracheal tube placed into the trachea once the patient has been

TABLE 18-6	**Phases of General Anesthesia**		
PHASES	**INDUCTION**	**MAINTENANCE**	**EMERGENCE**
Definition	Time period starting with preoperative medication, initiation of appropriate IV/arterial access, application of monitors, initiation of sequence of medications that render the patient unconscious, securing the airway.	Time period during which the surgical procedure is performed; patient remains in an unconscious state with appropriate measures to ensure safety of the airway	Time period during which the surgical procedure is completed; patient is prepared for return to consciousness and removal of airway assist devices
ACP role	• Preanesthetic assessment • Determination of final anesthetic care plan • Application and monitoring of IV/arterial access • Administration of appropriate drugs • Securing the airway	• Monitor physiologic status of patient • Administer incremental medications as appropriate	• Reversal of residual neuromuscular blocking agents • Assessment for return of adequate respiratory reflexes and function • Removal of airway assist devices
Role of perioperative nurse related to anesthesia	• Preoperative assessment is completed • Assist with application of monitors (noninvasive and invasive) • Assist with airway management	• Adjust patient position as necessary • Monitor patient safety	• Assist in placement of dressing • Prepare the patient for movement to PACU

Anticipated classes of drugs to be used	Benzodiazepines
	Narcotics
	Hypnotics
	Volatile gases
		Benzodiazepines
		Narcotics
		Hypnotics
		Volatile gases
			Reversal agents:
			  Anticholinergics
			  Sympathomimetics
			  Narcotic antagonists (prn)
			  Benzodiazepine antagonists or supplemental narcotics (prn)

induced with an intravenous agent. The endotracheal tube permits control of ventilation and airway protection, both for patency and to prevent aspiration. Complications of endotracheal intubation include those primarily associated with its insertion and removal. These include damage to teeth and lips, laryngospasm, laryngeal edema, postoperative sore throat, and hoarseness caused by injury or irritation of the vocal cords or surrounding tissues.

Adjuncts to General Anesthesia. The administration of general anesthesia is rarely limited to one agent. Drugs added to an inhalation anesthetic (other than an IV induction agent) are termed *adjuncts*. These agents are added to the anesthetic regimen specifically to achieve unconsciousness, analgesia, amnesia, muscle relaxation, or autonomic nervous system control. Adjuncts include opioids (narcotics), benzodiazepines, neuromuscular blocking agents (muscle relaxants), and antiemetics. See Table 18-8 for commonly used adjunct agents, their uses during anesthesia, adverse effects, and nursing interventions.

Opioids. Opioids are used preoperatively for sedation and analgesia, intraoperatively for induction and maintenance of anesthesia, and postoperatively for pain management. Opioids alter the perception of pain and the response to painful stimuli. When administered before the end of a surgical procedure, the residual analgesia often carries over into the PACU, allowing the patient to awaken relatively pain free.

All opioids produce dose-related respiratory depression.[34] Respiratory depression may be difficult to detect in the OR and therefore requires close observation and pulse oximetry monitoring. Respiratory depression can be reversed with naloxone (Narcan). However, its use is often associated with a reversal of the analgesic effects of the narcotics as well.

Benzodiazepines. Sedative-hypnotic benzodiazepines are widely used for premedication before surgery for their amnestic effects, as agents for the induction and maintenance of anesthesia, for conscious sedation, as supplemental intravenous sedation during local and regional anesthesia, and for postoperative anxiety and agitation. Because of its excellent amnestic property, shorter duration of action, and absence of pain on injection, midazolam (Versed) is presently the most frequently used benzodiazepine. The other agents are limited in their usefulness because of their long duration of action. In both ambulatory surgery settings and in conscious sedation, midazolam is the most common anesthesia adjunct used. It is commonly administered intravenously or via intramuscular injection. Flumazenil (Romazicon) is a specific benzodiazepine antagonist that may be used to reverse marked benzodiazepine-induced respiratory depression.[35]

Neuromuscular blocking agents. Neuromuscular blocking agents (muscle relaxants) are used as adjuncts to general anesthesia to facilitate endotracheal intubation and to optimize surgical working conditions by providing relaxation (paralysis) of skeletal muscles. Neuromuscular blocking agents interrupt the transmission of nerve impulses at the neuromuscular junction. Based on their mechanisms of action, neuromuscular blocking agents are classified as either depolarizing or nondepolarizing muscle relaxants. The effects of nondepolarizing muscle relaxants are frequently reversed toward the end of the surgery by the administration of anticholinesterase agents (e.g., neostigmine [Prostigmin], pyridostigmine [Mestinon], edrophonium [Tensilon]).[6,36]

Disadvantages of the use of muscle relaxants are of special concern to the ACP and postanesthesia nurse. The duration of their action may be longer than the surgical procedure, or rever-

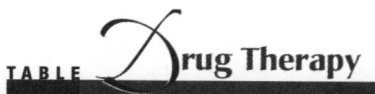

TABLE
18-7

rug Therapy
General Anesthesia

DRUGS	ADVANTAGES	DISADVANTAGES	NURSING INTERVENTIONS
Intravenous Agents			
Barbiturates			
thiopental (Pentothal) methohexital (Brevital)	Rapid induction, small dosage, duration of action less than 5 min	Higher doses: cardiac alterations, hypotension, tachycardia, and respiratory depression	Minimal postoperative effects due to extremely short effects
Nonbarbiturate Hypnotics			
etomidate (Amidate)	Produces little change in cardiovascular dynamics; useful for hemodynamically unstable patients	Associated with adverse effects of myoclonia, nausea and vomiting, hiccoughs, and adrenocortical inhibition	Observe for transient skeletal muscle movements (myoclonia), nausea and vomiting, hiccoughs, hypotension, and hypoglycemia
propofol (Diprivan)	Ideal for short outpatient procedures because of rapid onset of action and elimination; may be used for maintenance of anesthesia as well as induction	May cause bradycardia and other arrhythmias, hypotension; apnea, phlebitis, nausea and vomiting, hiccoughs	Short action leads to minimal postoperative effects; monitor injection site for phlebitis; cardiac monitoring if unstable
Inhalation Agents			
Volatile Liquids			
halothane (Fluothane) enflurane (Ethrane) isoflurane (Forane) desflurane (Suprane) sevoflurane (Ultane)	All volatile liquids: muscle relaxation, low incidence of nausea and vomiting Halothane: bronchodilation Isoflurane: less cardiac depression, devoid of toxicity to body organs Desflurane: rapid induction and emergence, most widely used volatile agent Sevoflurane: predictable effects on cardiovascular and respiratory systems, rapid acting, nonirritating to respiratory system	All volatile liquids: myocardial depression, early onset of pain because of rapid elimination Halothane: hypotension and possible hepatotoxicity Enflurane: increased intracranial pressure, seizures, unpredictable duration of action	Assess and treat pain during early anesthesia recovery; assess for adverse reactions such as cardiopulmonary depression with hypotension and prolonged respiratory depression; confusion, nausea and vomiting
Gaseous Agents			
Nitrous oxide	Potentiates volatile agents, allowing a reduction in their dosage and their negative side effects and increases the rate of induction	Weak anesthetic, rarely used alone; must be administered with oxygen to prevent hypoxemia	Produces little or no toxicity; monitor for effects of volatile liquids when nitrous oxide used as an adjunct
Dissociative Anesthetics			
ketamine (Ketalar)	Can be administered IV or IM; potent analgesic and amnestic	May cause hallucinations and nightmares, increased intracranial and intraocular pressure, increased heart rate, hypertension	Rarely used; anticipate administration of a benzodiazepine if agitation and hallucinations occur

IV, Intravenous; *IM,* intramuscular.

sal agents may not be effective in completely eliminating the residual effects. The patient should be carefully observed for airway patency and adequacy of respiratory muscle movement. Lack of movement or poor return of reflexes and strength may indicate the need for an artificial airway and ventilator. If the patient is intubated, the endotracheal tube should not be removed without careful assessment of return of muscular strength, level of consciousness, and the minute volume (respiratory rate times tidal volume [amount of air inhaled and exhaled during a normal ventilation]).

Antiemetics. Antiemetics are used preoperatively, intraoperatively, and postoperatively to prevent and treat nausea and vomiting associated with the administration of anesthesia. Antiemetics listed in Table 18-8 are most frequently used preoperatively or postoperatively.

Dissociative Anesthesia. *Dissociative anesthesia* interrupts associative brain pathways while blocking sensory pathways. The patient appears catatonic, is amnestic, and experiences profound analgesia that lasts into the postoperative period. This type of anesthetic is used for diagnostic or therapeutic procedures

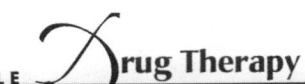

TABLE 18-8   Adjuncts to General Anesthesia

AGENTS	USES DURING ANESTHESIA	ADVERSE EFFECTS	NURSING INTERVENTIONS
Opioids fentanyl (Sublimaze) sufentanil (Sufenta) morphine sulfate meperidine (Demerol) alfentanil (Alfenta) remifentanil (Ultiva) methadone (Dolophine)	Induce and maintain anesthesia, reduce stimuli from sensory nerve endings, provide analgesia during anesthetic recovery	Respiratory depression, stimulation of vomiting center, possible bradycardia and peripheral vasodilation (when combined with anesthetics)	Assess respiratory status, monitor pulse oximetry, protect airway in anticipation of vomiting
Benzodiazepines midazolam (Versed) diazepam (Valium) lorazepam (Ativan)	Induce and maintain anesthesia, provide conscious sedation or sedation during local and regional anesthesia	Potentiation of the effects of opioids, increasing the potential for respiratory depression; hypotension and tachycardia	Monitor cardiopulmonary status, level of consciousness
Neuromuscular Blocking Agents Depolarizing agents: succinylcholine (Anectine) Nondepolarizing agents: vecuronium (Norcuron) atracurium (Tracrium) pancuronium (Pavulon) tubocurarine (Tubarine) pipecuronium (Arduan) doxacurium (Nuromax) rocuronium (Zemuron) mivacurium (Mivacron)	Facilitate endotracheal intubation, promote skeletal muscle relaxation (paralysis) to enhance access to surgical sites; effects of nondepolarizing agents are usually reversed toward the end of surgery by the administration of anticholinesterase agents (e.g., neostigmine, pyridostigmine, edrophonium)	Apnea related to paralysis of respiratory muscles, prolonged muscle relaxation due to longer action of nondepolarizing agents than reversal agents, cardiac alterations	Monitor respiratory rate and pattern until patient able to cough and return to previous levels of muscle strength; maintain patent airway for the patient; ensure availability of nondepolarizing reversal agents and respiratory support equipment
Antiemetics droperidol (Inapsine) ondansetron (Zofran) metoclopramide (Reglan) prochlorperazine (Compazine) promethazine (Phenergan)	Prevention of vomiting with aspiration during surgery, counteract the emetic effects of inhalation agents and opioids; droperidol most often used during surgery, others used postoperatively	Droperidol: arrhythmias, laryngospasm, bronchospasm, tachycardia, hypotension, central nervous system alterations	Monitor cardiopulmonary status, level of consciousness, and ability to move limbs Droperidol: administer with caution in patients with heart disease

that do not require muscle relaxation yet require profound analgesia and amnesia (e.g., burn scrubs and dressing changes).

Ketamine (Ketalar) is the agent most commonly administered as a dissociative anesthetic. It is particularly advantageous because ketamine can be administered intravenously or intramuscularly; it is a potent analgesic and amnestic. It is used in asthmatic patients undergoing surgery because it promotes bronchodilation and in trauma patients requiring surgery because it increases heart rate and helps maintain cardiac output. Because ketamine is a phencyclidine (PCP) derivative, the drug may cause hallucinations and nightmares, particularly in adult patients, greatly limiting its usefulness.[33]

Local Anesthesia

Local anesthetics block the initiation and transmission of electrical impulses along nerve fibers. With progressive increases in local anesthetic concentration, the transmission of autonomic, then somatic sensory, and finally somatic motor impulses is blocked. This produces autonomic nervous system blockade, anesthesia, and skeletal muscle paralysis in the area of the affected nerve.

Local anesthesia allows an operative procedure to be performed on a particular part of the body without loss of consciousness or sedation. Because there is little systemic absorption of the drug, recovery is rapid with little residual drug "hangover." The duration of action of the local anesthetic frequently carries over into the postoperative period, providing continued analgesia.[37] In addition, the use of a local anesthetic in a regional technique provides an alternative to a general anesthetic in a physiologically compromised patient.

The disadvantages of local anesthetics include the technical difficulty and discomfort that may be associated with injections, inadvertent intravenous administration producing hypotension and potential seizures, and the inability to precisely match the

TABLE 18-9	Methods for Administering Local Anesthesia

Topical application
Local infiltration
Regional injection
   Peripheral nerve block
   Intravenous regional block (Bier block)
   Spinal anesthesia (block)
   Epidural anesthesia (block)

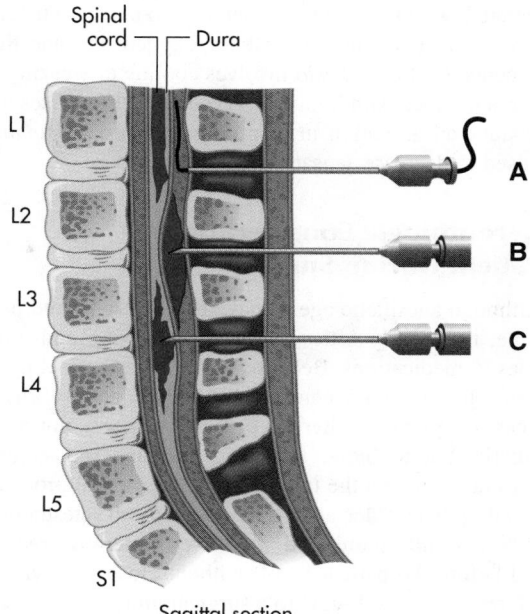

FIG. 18-5 Location of needle point and injected anesthetic relative to dura. **A,** Epidural catheter. **B,** Single-injection epidural. **C,** Spinal anesthesia. (Interspaces most commonly used are L4-5, L3-4, and L2-3.)

duration of action of the agents administered to the duration of the surgical procedure.

Methods of Administration. There are a variety of methods for administering local anesthetics (Table 18-9). *Topical application* is application of the agent directly to the skin, mucous membranes, or open surface. Eutectic mixture of local anesthetics (EMLA cream), a combination of lidocaine and prilocaine, can be applied to the skin to produce localized dermal anesthesia (see Chapter 9). EMLA should be applied to the site 30 to 60 minutes before painful procedures. *Local infiltration* is the injection of the agent into the tissues through which the surgical incision will pass.

Regional (peripheral) nerve block is achieved by the injection of a local anesthetic into or around a specific nerve or group of nerves. Nerve blocks may be used to provide intraoperative anesthesia and postoperative analgesia and for the diagnosis and treatment of chronic pain. Examples of common regional nerve blocks include brachial plexus, intercostal, and retrobulbar blocks. Intravenous regional nerve block (Bier block) is the intravenous injection of a local anesthetic into an extremity following mechanical exsanguination using a compression bandage and a tourniquet. This type of block provides not only analgesia, but the ability to work in a bloodless field.

Spinal and epidural anesthesia. Spinal and epidural anesthesia are also types of regional anesthesia. **Spinal anesthesia** involves the injection of a local anesthetic into the cerebrospinal fluid found in the subarachnoid space, usually below the level of L2. The local anesthetic mixes with cerebrospinal fluid, and, depending on the extent of its spread, various levels of anesthesia are achieved. Because the local anesthetic is administered directly into the cerebrospinal fluid, a spinal anesthetic produces an autonomic, sensory, and motor blockade. Patients experience vasodilation and may become hypotensive as a result of the autonomic block, feel no pain as a result of the sensory block, and are unable to move as a result of the motor block. The duration of action of the spinal anesthetic depends on the agent selected and the dose administered. A spinal anesthetic may be used for procedures involving the lower abdomen, groin, perineum, or lower extremity.[38]

An **epidural block** involves injection of a local anesthetic into the epidural (extradural) space via either a thoracic or lumbar approach. The anesthetic agent does not enter the cerebrospinal fluid, but works by binding to nerve roots as they enter and exit the spinal cord. By using a low concentration of local anesthetic, sensory pathways are blocked, but motor fibers remain intact. In higher doses, both sensory and motor fibers are blocked (Fig. 18-5). Epidural anesthesia may be used as the sole

anesthetic for a surgical procedure, or a catheter may be placed to allow for intraoperative use with continued use into the postoperative period for analgesia, using lower doses of epidurally administered local anesthetic, usually in combination with an opioid.[37] Epidural anesthesia is commonly used for vascular procedures involving the lower extremity and hip and knee replacement surgeries.

During the surgical procedure when spinal or epidural anesthesia is used, the patient can remain fully conscious or sedation can be achieved intravenously. The onset of spinal anesthesia is faster than that seen with an epidural, but the end results with either approach are usually similar. The patient must be closely observed for signs of autonomic nervous system blockade, including hypotension, bradycardia, nausea, and vomiting. There is less autonomic nervous system blockade with epidural anesthesia as compared with spinal anesthesia. Should "too high" a block be achieved, the patient may experience inadequate respiratory excursion and apnea.[38]

One advantage of epidural (extradural) injection over spinal (subarachnoid) injection is a decreased incidence of headache. A headache may be experienced after spinal anesthesia following leakage of spinal fluid at the site of injection. The incidence of headache is decreasing with the common use of smaller-gauge spinal needles (25 to 27 gauge) and the use of noncutting, "pencil-point" spinal needles. A headache following an epidural may occur when a 17- to 18-gauge needle is advanced too far and the dura is punctured, resulting in the leakage of cerebrospinal fluid.[38]

Additional Anesthetic Considerations

Controlled hypotension is a technique used to decrease the amount of expected blood loss by lowering the blood pressure during the administration of anesthesia. *Hypothermia* is the deliberate lowering of body temperature to decrease metabolism, thus reducing both the demand for oxygen and anesthetic requirements. *Cryoanesthesia* involves cooling or freezing a localized area to block pain impulses. *Hypnoanesthesia* uses hypnosis to produce an alteration in pain consciousness. *Acupuncture* is also used to decrease sensation[39] (see Chapter 7).

■ Gerontologic Considerations: Patient During Surgery

Although anesthetic agents have become safer and more predictable, the elderly often demonstrate varying and unique responses to medications. Because of this, anesthetic drugs should be carefully titrated when given to older adults. Physiologic changes in aging may alter the patient's response not only to the anesthetic, but to blood and fluid loss and replacement, hypothermia, pain, and the tolerance of the surgical procedure and positioning. The older adult's response to all anesthetic agents must be carefully monitored and the postoperative recovery assessed before the patient is left without close supervision (e.g., transferred from the PACU to a surgical unit).

Many older adults experience a decrease in their ability to communicate and follow directions as a result of alterations in vision or hearing. These factors pose a special need for clear and concise communication in the OR, especially when preoperative sedation is superimposed on the existing sensory deficit. Skin elasticity in the older adult is decreased because of loss of collagen. As a result, the skin is sensitive to injury from tape, electrodes, warming and cooling blankets, and certain types of dressing. In addition, the older adult often has osteoporosis and osteoarthritis. These factors reinforce the need for careful transferring, lifting, and positioning techniques. ■

CATASTROPHIC EVENTS IN THE OPERATING ROOM

Unanticipated intraoperative events occasionally occur. Although some might be anticipated (e.g., cardiac arrest in an unstable patient, massive blood loss during trauma surgery), others may occur without warning, demanding immediate intervention by all members of the OR team. Two such events are anaphylactic reactions and malignant hyperthermia.

Anaphylactic Reactions

Anaphylaxis is the most severe form of an allergic reaction, manifesting with life-threatening pulmonary and circulatory complications. The initial clinical manifestations of anaphylaxis may be masked by anesthesia. ACPs administer an array of drugs to patients, such as anesthetics, antibiotics, blood products, and plasma expanders, and because any parenterally administered material can theoretically produce an allergic response, vigilance and rapid intervention are essential. An anaphylactic reaction causes hypotension, tachycardia, bronchospasm, and possibly pulmonary edema. Antibiotics and latex are responsible for many perioperative allergic reactions.[39,40] (Anaphylaxis is discussed in Chapter 13.)

Latex allergy has become a particular concern in the perioperative setting, given the use of gloves, catheters, and many other devices containing natural rubber latex (NRL). Reactions to NRL have ranged from urticaria to anaphylaxis with symptoms appearing immediately or at some time during the surgical proce-

dure. Latex allergy protocols should be set up in each institution so that a latex-safe environment can be provided in susceptible individuals.[40,41] (Latex allergies are discussed in Chapter 13.)

Malignant Hyperthermia

Malignant hyperthermia (MH) is a rare metabolic disease characterized by hyperthermia with rigidity of skeletal muscles that can result in death. It occurs in affected people exposed to certain anesthetic agents. Succinylcholine (Anectine), especially in conjunction with the volatile inhalation agents, appears to be the primary trigger of the disorder, although other factors, such as stress, trauma, and heat, have been implicated. When it does occur, it is usually during general anesthesia, but it may manifest in the recovery period as well. It is autosomal dominant in inheritance but is variable in its genetic penetrance, so predictions based on family history are important but inconsistent. (Autosomal dominant disorders are discussed in Chapter 13.) The fundamental defect is hypermetabolism of skeletal muscle resulting from altered control of intracellular calcium, leading to muscle contracture, hyperthermia, hypoxemia, lactic acidosis, and hemodynamic and cardiac alterations.

Tachycardia, tachypnea, hypercarbia, and ventricular arrhythmias are generally seen but are nonspecific to MH. MH is generally diagnosed after all other causes of the hypermetabolism are ruled out. The rise in body temperature is not an early sign of MH. Unless promptly detected with rapid initiation of appropriate intervention, MH can result in cardiac arrest and death. The definitive treatment of MH is prompt administration of dantrolene (Dantrium), which slows metabolism, along with symptomatic support to correct hemodynamic instability, acidosis, hypoxemia, and elevated temperature. A treatment protocol is available from the Malignant Hyperthermia Association of the United States (*www.mhaus.com*) and is usually displayed in the OR.

To prevent MH it is important for the nurse to obtain a careful family history and be alert to its development perioperatively. The patient known or suspected to be at risk for this disorder can be anesthetized with minimal risks if appropriate precautions are taken. Patients with MH should be informed of the condition so that family members may be genetically tested.[42,43]

NEW AND FUTURE CONSIDERATIONS

Changes in technology and new developments in science provide new and better treatment modalities for the patient undergoing surgery. Historically, patients having surgery were instructed to be NPO starting at midnight the night before their surgery. The American Society of Anesthesiologists (ASA) published new practice guidelines that are much less stringent (see Table 17-8). Investigators have determined that ingestion of water, apple juice, black tea and coffee, pulp-free orange juice, and carbonated beverages 2 to 3 hours before surgery has no detrimental effect on the risk factors of gastric aspiration in healthy nonobese adults.[44,45]

"Bloodless surgery" is becoming more of a reality.[46] Various techniques can minimize blood loss during and after surgery, and others allow the surgical team to manage blood loss without the need for a blood transfusion. These include drug therapy and techniques for managing low hematocrit, hemostatic agents to enhance clotting and control bleeding, surgical devices and techniques to locate and stop internal bleeding, and surgical and anesthetic techniques to limit blood loss. There are also new alternatives to blood transfusions such as erythropoietin, deliberate hypotension, and normovolemic hemodilution.[47] Research is also continuing on the development of a synthetic, oxygen-carrying blood alternative.

After years of development and implementation in other fields, robotics is now a technology of the operating room and robots are being used to assist in surgery.[48] Although the first surgical systems were passive robotic aides, today most robotic aides have active mechanisms with a degree of autonomy. Surgical intervention using robotics, combined with advances in computer technology and communication systems, will vastly change and broaden the scope of practice for the perioperative nurse. These technologic developments have made telesurgery a reality. The first transatlantic operation was performed in September 2001 with the patient in Strasbourg, France, and the surgeon in New York City.[49] Telesurgery will reduce the need for seriously ill patients to travel long distances for care, allow surgeons to perform procedures in locations in which their expertise is not readily available, and permit surgeons to perform procedures on patients in hazardous environments such as battlefields.[48,50]

REVIEW QUESTIONS

The number of the question corresponds to the same-numbered objective at the beginning of the chapter.

1. Proper attire for the semirestricted area of the surgery department is
   a. street clothing.
   b. surgical attire and head cover.
   c. surgical attire, head cover, and mask.
   d. street clothing with the addition of shoe covers.
2. The characteristic of the operating room environment that facilitates the prevention of infection in the surgical patient is
   a. adjustable lighting.
   b. conductive furniture.
   c. filters in the ventilating system.
   d. explosion-proof electrical plugs.
3. An activity that is carried out by nurses performing both sterile and nonsterile activities in the operating room is
   a. checking electrical equipment.
   b. passing instruments to the surgeon and assistants.
   c. coordinating activities occurring in the operating room.
   d. assisting ACP with monitoring of patient during surgery.
4. Assessment of a patient with a musculoskeletal impairment on arrival to the operating room enables the nurse to meet the patient's needs during
   a. preparation of the skin.
   b. induction of anesthesia.
   c. positioning on the operating room bed.
   d. explanations about the surgical activities.
5. The perioperative nurse's primary responsibility for the care of the patient undergoing surgery is
   a. developing an individualized plan of nursing care for the patient.
   b. carrying out specific tasks related to surgical policies and procedures.
   c. ensuring that the patient has been assessed for safe administration of anesthesia.
   d. performing a preoperative history and physical assessment to identify patient needs.
6. When scrubbing at the scrub sink, the surgical team members should
   a. scrub from elbows to hands.
   b. scrub without mechanical friction.
   c. scrub for a minimum of 10 minutes.
   d. hold the hands higher than the elbows.
7. Which of the following is *not* a concern when positioning the surgical patient?
   a. provision of modesty for the patient
   b. avoiding compression of nerve tissue
   c. provision of correct skeletal alignment
   d. ensuring that students in the room can see the operative site
8. Mrs. Jones is scheduled for an abdominal hysterectomy. She is extremely anxious and has a tendency to hyperventilate when upset. The type of anesthetic that would probably be most appropriate for Mrs. Jones is
   a. a spinal block.
   b. an epidural block.
   c. a general anesthethic.
   d. a dissociative anesthethic.
9. Intravenous induction for general anesthesia is the method of choice for most patients because
   a. the patient is not intubated.
   b. the agents are nonexplosive.
   c. induction is rapid and pleasant.
   d. the odor of the agent is not offensive.
10. The injection of the local anesthetic into the tissues through which the surgical incision will pass is the technique of
    a. nerve block.
    b. local infiltration.
    c. topical application.
    d. regional application.

REFERENCES

1. Pandit SK: Ambulatory anesthesia and surgery in America: a historical background and recent innovations, *J Perianesth Nurs* 14:5, 1999.
2. Outpatient surgery doubles, *OR Manager* 17:1, 2001.
3. Association of periOperative Registered Nurses: Recommended practice for traffic patterns in the perioperative practice setting. In *Standards, recommended practices and guidelines,* Denver, 2001, Association of periOperative Registered Nurses.
4. Fortunato NH: *Berry and Kohn's operating room technique,* ed 9, St Louis, 2000, Mosby.
5. Groah L: *Operating room nursing,* ed 2, San Mateo, CA, 1995, Appleton & Lange.
6. Meeker MH, Rothrock JC: *Alexander's care of the patient in surgery,* ed 11, St Louis, 1999, Mosby.
*7. Reavis CW, Sandidge J, Bauer K: Critical thinking's role in perioperative patient safety outcomes, *AORN J* 68:5, 1998.
*8. Association of periOperative Registered Nurses: *Perioperative nursing data set: the perioperative nursing vocabulary,* Denver, 2000, Association of periOperative Registered Nurses.
9. Beyea SC: The ideal state for perioperative nursing, *AORN J* 73:5, 2001.
10. Association of periOperative Registered Nurses: *Revised AORN official statement on RN first assistants,* Denver, 2001, Association of periOperative Registered Nurses.
11. Trovarelli T, Kahn B, Vernon S: Transfusion-free surgery is a treatment plan for all patients, *AORN J* 68:5, 1998.
12. McKennis AT: Caring for the Islamic patient, *AORN J* 69:6, 1999.
13. Dunn D: Preoperative assessment criteria and patient teaching for ambulatory surgery patients, *J Perianesth Nurs* 13:5, 1998.
14. Flanagan K: Preoperative assessment: safety considerations for patients taking herbal products, *J Perianesth Nurs* 16:1, 2001.
*15. Norred CL, Zamudio S, Palmer SK: Use of complementary and alternative medicines by surgical patients, *AANA J* 68:1, 2000.
16. Murphy JM: Preoperative consideration with herbal medicines, *AORN J* 69:1, 1999.
17. Brumley C: Herbs and the perioperative patient, *AORN J* 72:5, 2000.
*18. Taylor LK et al: The effect of music in the postanesthesia care unit in women who have had abdominal hysterectomies, *J Perianesth Nurs* 13:2, 1998.
19. Norred CL; Minimizing preoperative anxiety with alternative caring-healing therapies, *AORN J* 72:5, 2000.
20. Touch, imagery help ready patients for their surgery, *OR Manager* 16:11, 2000.
21. Ramnaruine-Singh S: The surgical significance of therapeutic touch, *AORN J* 69:2, 1999.
22. Buckle J: Aromatherapy in perianesthesia nursing, *J Perianesth Nurs* 14:6, 1999.
23. Association of periOperative Registered Nurses: Recommended practice for sterile field—maintaining. In *Standards, recommended practices and guidelines,* Denver, 2001, Association of periOperative Registered Nurses.
24. Association of periOperative Registered Nurses: Recommended practice for counts—sponge, sharp and instrument. In *Standards, recommended practices and guidelines,* Denver, 2001, Association of periOperative Registered Nurses.
25. Association of periOperative Registered Nurses: Recommended practice for surgical hand scrubs. In *Standards, recommended practices and guidelines,* Denver, 2001, Association of periOperative Registered Nurses.
26. Williamson JE: CDC draft recommends alcohol rubs over traditional surgical scrub, *OR Today* 1:2, 2001.
27. Association of periOperative Registered Nurses: Recommended practice for standard and transmission-based precautions. In *Standards, recommended practice and guidelines,* Denver, 2001, Association of periOperative Registered Nurses.
28. Association of periOperative Registered Nurses: Recommended practice for positioning the patient in the perioperative practice setting. In *Standards, recommended practices and guidelines,* Denver, 2001, Association of periOperative Registered Nurses.
29. Association of periOperative Registered Nurses: Recommended practice for skin preparation of patients. In *Standards, recommended practices and guidelines,* Denver, 2001, Association of periOperative Registered Nurses.
30. Association of periOperative Registered Nurses: Recommended practice for electrosurgery. In *Standards, recommended practice and guidelines,* Denver, 2001, Association of periOperative Registered Nurses.
31. Association of periOperative Registered Nurses: Patient outcomes: standards of perioperative care. In *Standards, recommended practices and guidelines,* Denver, 2001, Association of periOperative Registered Nurses.
32. Association of periOperative Registered Nurses: Recommended practice for conscious sedation/analgesia: managing the patient. In *Standards, recommended practice and guidelines,* Denver, 2001, Association of periOperative Registered Nurses Association.
33. Berg M: An introduction to anesthesia-related medications, *J Perianesth Nurs* 13:4, 1998.
34. Bennett J, Wren KR, Haas R: Opioid use during the perianesthesia period: nursing implications, *J Perianesth Nurs* 16:4, 2001.
35. Borchardt M: Review of the clinical pharmacology and use of the benzodiazepines, *J Perianesth Nurs* 14:2, 1999.
36. Walker JR: Neuromuscular relaxation and reversal: an update, *J Perianesth Nurs* 12:264, 1997.
37. Pasero CL: Preemptive analgesia: it starts before surgery, *Am J Nurs* 96:12, 1996.
38. Kreger C: Spinal anesthesia and analgesia, *Nursing* 31:6, 2001.
39. Reilly MP: Clinical applications of acupuncture in anesthesia practice, *CRNA* 11:173, 2000.
40. Zaglaniczny K: Latex allergy: are you at risk? *AANA J* 69: 413, 2001.
41. Association of periOperative Registered Nurses: AORN latex guideline. In *Standards, recommended practices and guidelines,* Denver, 2001, Association of periOperative Registered Nurses.
42. Redmond MC: Malignant hyperthermia: perianesthesia recognition, treatment, and care, *J Perianesth Nurs* 16:4, 2001.
43. Rosenberg H: Malignant hyperthermia slide show. Available at *www.mhaus.org* (accessed 9/3/02).
44. American Society of Anesthesiologists: Practice guidelines for preoperative fasting and use of pharmacologic agents to reduce the risk of pulmonary aspiration: application to healthy patients undergoing elective procedures, *Anesthesiology* 90:3, 1999.
45. Pandit UA, Pandit SK: Fasting before and after ambulatory surgery, *J Perianesth Nurs* 12:3, 1997.
46. Maness CP et al: Bloodless medicine and surgery, *AORN J* 67:1, 1998.
47. Trovarelli T, Kahn B, Vernon S: Transfusion-free surgery is a treatment plan for all patients, *AORN J* 68:5, 1998.
48. Mathias JM: Robots assist in bypass surgery, *OR Manager* 15:12, 1999.
49. Larkin M: Transatlantic, robotic-assisted telesurgery deemed a success, *Lancet* 358(9287):1074, 2001.
50. Eckberg E: The future of robotics can be ours, *AORN J* 67:5, 1998.

RESOURCES

Resources for this chapter are listed in Chapter 19 on pages 413-414.

---

*Nursing research–based references.

CHAPTER *19*

NURSING MANAGEMENT
Postoperative Care

Debra J. Smith

LEARNING OBJECTIVES

1. Identify the components of an initial postanesthesia assessment.
2. Identify the nursing responsibilities in admitting patients to the postanesthesia care unit (PACU).
3. Explain the etiology and nursing assessment and management of potential problems of patients in the PACU.
4. Describe the initial nursing assessment and management after transfer from the PACU to the general care unit.

5. Explain the etiology and nursing assessment and management of potential problems during the postoperative period.
6. Identify the information needed by the postoperative patient in preparation for discharge.

KEY TERMS

airway obstruction, p. 395	hypothermia, p. 399
atelectasis, p. 395	hypoventilation, p. 397
bronchospasm, p. 397	hypoxemia, p. 395
delayed awakening, p. 399	patient-controlled analgesia (PCA), p. 409
emergence delirium, p. 399	
epidural analgesia, p. 409	syncope, p. 405
fast tracking, p. 393	wound dehiscence, p. 408
hiccoughs, p. 407	

The postoperative period begins immediately after surgery and continues until the patient is discharged from medical care. This chapter focuses on the common features of postoperative nursing care for the patient undergoing surgery. The problems and nursing care related to specific surgical procedures are discussed in the appropriate chapters of this text.

POSTOPERATIVE CARE IN THE POSTANESTHESIA CARE UNIT

The patient's immediate recovery period is supervised by a postanesthesia care nurse, an educated specialist working in a *postanesthesia care unit* (PACU). It is located adjacent to the operating room (OR) to minimize transportation of the patient immediately after surgery and to provide ready access to anesthesia and surgical personnel. There may be two patient areas designated to patient recovery. Patients who have undergone general anesthesia are admitted to the phase I area. Patients who have had local or regional anesthetic or conscious sedation and who will be discharged home from the PACU recover from surgery in phase II. These patients are considered the ambulatory surgery patients.

Postanesthesia Care Unit Admission

The initial admission of the patient to the PACU is a joint effort between the anesthesia care provider (ACP) and the PACU nurse. This collaborative effort fosters a smooth transfer of care

to the PACU and helps designate the area to which the patient is assigned.

Fast Tracking. Some PACUs use **fast tracking** in which patients are admitted to phase I or phase II recovery areas depending on the type of anesthesia and surgery experienced and expected discharge from the unit. *PACU phase I bypass* is the direct admission of patients from the OR to phase II recovery. This type of bypass is only appropriate for ambulatory surgery patients who are going to be discharged home. Inpatients must go to phase I recovery and then be transferred to the inpatient unit.

Rapid PACU progression is a type of fast tracking that applies to both inpatient and ambulatory surgery patients. Rapid progression is based on the patient's achievement of discharge criteria. All patients who received general anesthesia are admitted to phase I recovery but are transferred to phase II, the inpatient unit, and/or home as soon as discharge criteria are met. Technologic advances and shorter-acting anesthetic agents have been the reasons for instituting these changes. Fast tracking has been shown to result in cost savings and increased patient satisfaction.[1] Studies involving ambulatory surgery patients have shown that cost savings can occur without compromising patient safety.[2]

The American Society of PeriAnesthesia Nurses (ASPAN) recommends that before fast tracking is instituted, a collaborative team should address the following issues: (1) appropriate patient selection, (2) preoperative education, (3) anesthetic agents to be used, (4) assessment of readiness at end of surgery, (5) discharge criteria, and (6) patient outcomes.[3]

Initial Assessment. On admission of the patient to the PACU, the ACP gives a verbal report to the admitting PACU nurse. Table 19-1 summarizes the components of a complete anesthesia report. While the patient is in the PACU, priority care includes monitoring and management of respiratory and circulatory function, pain, temperature, and surgical site.[3]

Assessment should begin with an evaluation of the airway, breathing, and circulation (ABC) status of the patient. Assessment of the patient's airway patency and rate and quality of respirations is made. Breath sounds should be auscultated throughout all lung fields.

Oxygen therapy will be used if the patient has had general anesthesia and/or the ACP orders it. Oxygen therapy is given via nasal

Reviewed by Ann L. Lambeth, RN, MSN, Nursing Instructor, Mesa State College, Grand Junction, Colo.

TABLE 19-1	Postanesthesia Admission Report

General Information
- Patient name
- Age
- Anesthesia care provider
- Surgeon
- Surgical procedure

Patient History
- Indication for surgery
- Medical history, medications, allergies

Intraoperative Management
- Anesthetic medications
- Other medications received preoperatively or intraoperatively
- Blood loss
- Fluid replacement totals, including blood transfusions
- Urine output

Intraoperative Course
- Unexpected anesthetic events or reactions
- Unexpected surgical events
- Vital signs and monitoring trends
- Results of intraoperative laboratory tests

Postanesthesia Care Unit Plan
- Potential and expected problems (with plan for intervention)
- Suggested PACU course
- Acceptable parameters for laboratory test results
- PACU discharge plan

PACU, Postanesthesia care unit.

TABLE 19-2	Clinical Manifestations of Inadequate Oxygenation

Central Nervous System
- Restlessness
- Agitation
- Muscle twitching
- Seizures
- Coma

Cardiovascular System
- Hypertension
- Hypotension
- Tachycardia
- Bradycardia
- Arrhythmias

Integumentary System
- Cyanosis
- Prolonged capillary refill
- Flushed and moist skin

Respiratory System
- Increased to absent respiratory effort
- Use of accessory muscles
- Abnormal breath sounds
- Abnormal arterial blood gases

Renal System
- Urine output <0.5 ml/kg/hr

cannula or face mask. The use of oxygen aids in the elimination of anesthetic gases and helps meet the increased demand for oxygen needed due to decreased blood volume or increased cellular metabolism. If the patient requires postoperative ventilation, a ventilator will be provided. Pulse oximetry monitoring is initiated because it provides a noninvasive means of assessing the adequacy of oxygenation. (Pulse oximetry is discussed in Chapter 25.)

During the initial assessment, signs of inadequate oxygenation and ventilation should be identified (Table 19-2). Any evidence of respiratory compromise requires prompt intervention. Commonly occurring respiratory problems for patients in the PACU are discussed in the following sections (see pp. 395-397).

Electrocardiographic (ECG) monitoring is initiated to determine cardiac rate and rhythm. Deviations from preoperative findings should be noted and evaluated. Blood pressure should be measured and compared with baseline readings. Invasive monitoring (e.g., arterial blood pressure monitoring) will be initiated if needed. Body temperature and skin color and condition should also be assessed. Any evidence of inadequate circulatory status requires prompt intervention. Commonly occurring cardiovascular problems for patients in the PACU are discussed in the following sections (see p. 398.)

The initial neurologic assessment focuses on level of consciousness; orientation; sensory and motor status; and size, equality, and reactivity of the pupils. The patient may be awake, drowsy but arousable, or asleep. Occasionally the patient may wake up agitated in what is referred to as *emergence delirium.* If the patient has had a regional anesthetic (e.g., spinal or epidural), sensory and motor blockade may still be present.

The assessment of the urinary system focuses on intake and output and fluid balance. Intraoperative fluid totals are communicated as part of the anesthesia report. The PACU nurse should note the presence of all intravenous (IV) lines, irrigation solutions and infusions, and all output devices, including catheters and wound drains. Intravenous infusions are regulated according to postoperative orders.

The PACU nurse should also assess the surgical site, noting the condition of any dressings and the type and amount of any drainage. Postoperative orders related to site care are instituted. All data obtained in the admission assessment are documented on a PACU record, a form specific to postanesthesia and postsurgical care.

Even the patient who has been told what to expect after surgery may be frightened or confused on awakening in the strange environment. Because hearing is the first sense to return in the unconscious patient, the nurse should explain all activities from the moment of admission to the PACU. Orientation includes explaining to the patient that the surgery is completed, that the patient is in the recovery room, and that the family or significant other has been notified. The nurse also explains who is caring for the patient, what is being done, and what time it is.

After the initial assessment is completed, the PACU nurse continues to apply the skills of ongoing assessment, diagnosis, and intervention. The patient's response to intervention is also noted. The goal of PACU care is to identify actual and potential patient problems that may occur as a result of anesthetic administration and surgical intervention and to intervene appropriately. In 2000 ASPAN published *Standards of Perianesthesia Nursing Practice* to guide PACU care of adult, pediatric, and geriatric patients.[3]

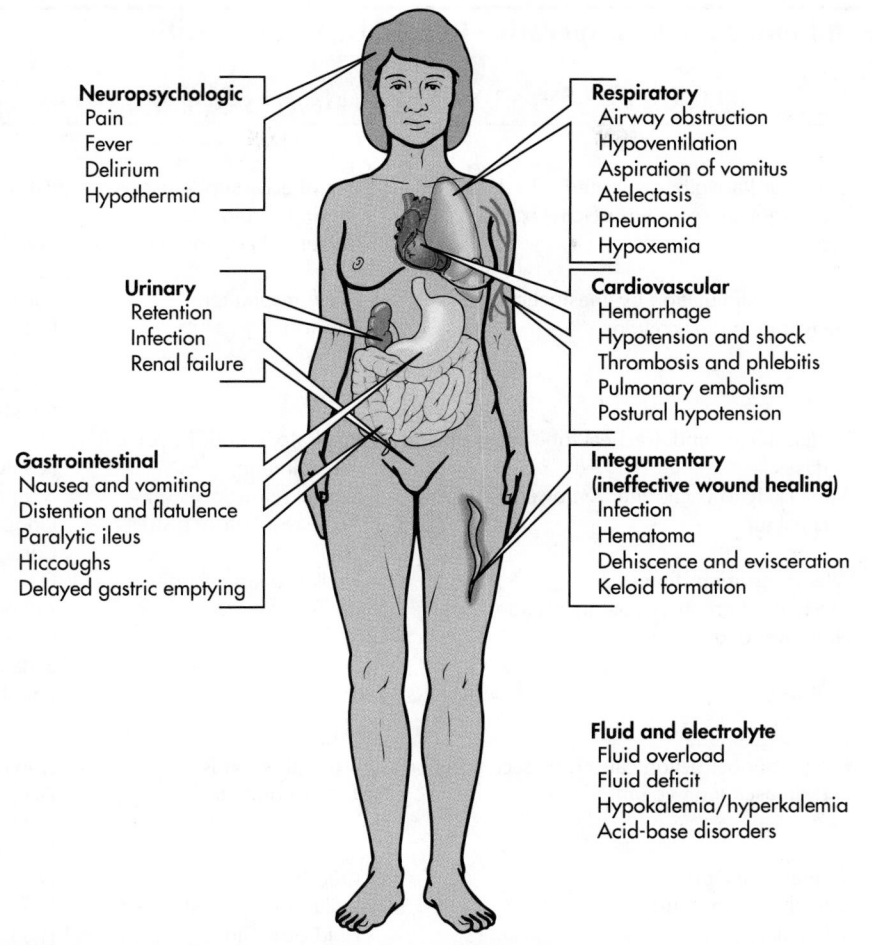

FIG. 19-1 Potential problems in the postoperative period.

Labels in figure:

Neuropsychologic
Pain
Fever
Delirium
Hypothermia

Urinary
Retention
Infection
Renal failure

Gastrointestinal
Nausea and vomiting
Distention and flatulence
Paralytic ileus
Hiccoughs
Delayed gastric emptying

Respiratory
Airway obstruction
Hypoventilation
Aspiration of vomitus
Atelectasis
Pneumonia
Hypoxemia

Cardiovascular
Hemorrhage
Hypotension and shock
Thrombosis and phlebitis
Pulmonary embolism
Postural hypotension

**Integumentary
(ineffective wound healing)**
Infection
Hematoma
Dehiscence and evisceration
Keloid formation

Fluid and electrolyte
Fluid overload
Fluid deficit
Hypokalemia/hyperkalemia
Acid-base disorders

Common postoperative problems the nurse should anticipate include airway compromise (obstruction), respiratory insufficiency (hypoxemia and hypercarbia), cardiac compromise (hypotension, hypertension, and arrhythmias), neurologic compromise (emergence delirium and delayed awakening), hypothermia, pain, and nausea and vomiting (Fig. 19-1). Each of these problems and appropriate nursing interventions are discussed in this chapter.

POTENTIAL ALTERATIONS IN RESPIRATORY FUNCTION

Etiology. In the immediate postanesthetic period the most common causes of airway compromise include obstruction, hypoxemia, and hypoventilation (Table 19-3). Patients at particular risk include those who have had general anesthesia, are older, smoke heavily, have lung disease, are obese, or have undergone airway, thoracic, or abdominal surgery. However, respiratory complications may occur with any patient who has been anesthetized.

Airway obstruction is most commonly caused by blockage of the airway by the patient's tongue (Fig. 19-2). The base of the tongue falls backward against the soft palate and occludes the pharynx. It is most pronounced in the supine position and in the patient who is extremely sleepy after surgery. Less common causes of airway obstruction include laryngospasm, retained secretions, and laryngeal edema.

Hypoxemia, specifically a PaO_2 of less than 60 mm Hg, is characterized by a variety of nonspecific clinical signs and symptoms, ranging from agitation to somnolence, hypertension to hypotension, and tachycardia to bradycardia. Pulse oximetry will indicate a low oxygen saturation (less than 90% to 92%). Arterial blood gas analysis should be used to confirm hypoxemia if the pulse oximetry indicates a low O_2 saturation.

The most common cause of postoperative hypoxemia is atelectasis. **Atelectasis** (alveolar collapse) may be the result of bronchial obstruction caused by retained secretions or decreased respiratory excursion. Hypotension and low cardiac output states can also contribute to the development of atelectasis. Other causes of hypoxemia that may occur in the PACU include pulmonary edema, aspiration, and bronchospasm.

Pulmonary edema is caused by an accumulation of fluid in the alveoli and may be the result of fluid overload; left ventricular failure; or prolonged airway obstruction, sepsis, or aspiration. Pulmonary edema is characterized by hypoxemia, crackles on auscultation, decreased pulmonary compliance, and the presence of infiltrates on chest x-ray.

Aspiration of gastric contents into the lungs is a potentially serious airway emergency. Symptoms include bronchospasm, hypoxemia, atelectasis, interstitial edema, alveolar hemorrhage, and respiratory failure. Gastric aspiration may also cause laryngospasm, infection, and pulmonary edema. Because of the serious

TABLE 19-3	Common Immediate Postoperative Respiratory Complications		
COMPLICATIONS AND CAUSES	**MECHANISMS**	**MANIFESTATIONS**	**INTERVENTIONS**
Airway Obstruction			
Tongue falling back	Muscular flaccidity associated with decreased consciousness and muscle relaxants	Use of accessory muscles Snoring respirations Decreased air movement	Patient stimulation Jaw thrust Chin lift Artificial airway
Retained thick secretions	Secretion stimulation by anesthetic agents Dehydration of secretions	Noisy respirations Rhonchi	Suctioning Deep breathing and coughing IV hydration IPPB with mucolytic agent Chest physical therapy
Laryngospasm	Irritation from endotracheal tube or anesthetic gases Most likely to occur after removal of endotracheal tube	Inspiratory stridor (crowing respiration) Sternal retraction Acute respiratory distress	O_2 Positive pressure ventilation IV muscle relaxant Lidocaine Corticosteroids
Laryngeal edema	Allergic drug reaction Mechanical irritation from intubation Fluid overload	Similar to laryngospasm	O_2 Antihistamines Corticosteroids Sedatives Possible intubation
Hypoxemia			
Atelectasis	Bronchial obstruction caused by secretions or decreased lung volumes	↓ Breath sounds ↓ O_2 saturation	Humidified O_2 Deep breathing Incentive spirometry Early mobilization
Pulmonary edema	↑ Hydrostatic pressure ↓ Interstitial pressure ↑ Capillary permeability	Crackles Infiltrates on chest x-ray Fluid overload ↓ O_2 saturation	O_2 therapy Diuretics Fluid restriction
Pulmonary embolism	Thrombus dislodged from peripheral venous system; lodged in pulmonary arterial system	Acute tachypnea Dyspnea Tachycardia Hypotension ↓ O_2 saturation	O_2 therapy Cardiopulmonary support Anticoagulant therapy
Aspiration	Inhalation of gastric contents	Bronchospasm Atelectasis Crackles Respiratory distress ↓ O_2 saturation	O_2 therapy Cardiac support Antibiotics
Bronchospasm	Increased smooth muscle tone with closure of small airways	Wheezing Dyspnea Tachypnea ↓ O_2 saturation	O_2 therapy Bronchodilators
Hypoventilation			
Depression of central respiratory drive	Medullary depression from anesthetics/narcotics/sedatives	Shallow respirations ↓ Respiratory rate/apnea ↓ PaO_2 ↑ $PaCO_2$	Stimulation Reversal of narcotics/ benzodiazepines Mechanical ventilation
Poor respiratory muscle tone	Neuromuscular blockade Neuromuscular disease	As above	Reversal of paralysis Mechanical ventilation
Mechanical restriction	Tight casts, dressings, positioning, and obesity prevent lung expansion	As above	Elevate head of bed Repositioning Loosen dressings
Pain	Shallow breathing to prevent incisional pain	As above Complaints of pain Guarding behavior	Narcotic analgesic therapy in reduced dose

IPPB, Intermittent positive pressure breathing.

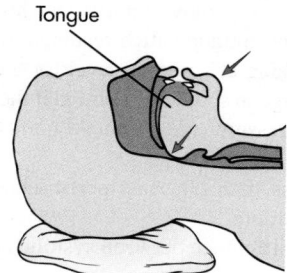

Tongue

Tongue occluding airway

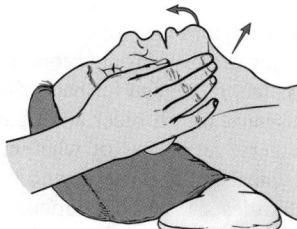

Manual elevation of
mandible to clear airway

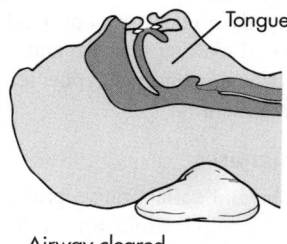

Tongue

Airway cleared

FIG. 19-2 Etiology and relief of airway obstruction caused by patient's tongue.

consequences of gastric aspiration, prevention, as opposed to treatment, is the goal. Patients identified as being at risk (obese, pregnant, history of hiatal hernia, gastroesophageal reflux disease [GERD], peptic ulcer, or trauma) may be premedicated with a histamine H_2-receptor antagonist (e.g., famotidine [Pepcid]) before induction of anesthesia. The ACP will take special precautions to protect the airway during induction of and emergence from anesthesia.

Bronchospasm is the result of an increase in bronchial smooth muscle tone with resultant closure of small airways. Airway edema develops, causing secretions to build up in the airway. The patient will have wheezing, dyspnea, use of accessory muscles, hypoxemia, and tachypnea. Bronchospasm may be due to aspiration, endotracheal intubation, suctioning, or chemical mediator release as a result of an allergic response. (Allergic responses are discussed in Chapter 13.) Bronchospasm is seen more frequently in patients with asthma and chronic obstructive pulmonary disease (COPD).

Hypoventilation, a common complication in the PACU, is characterized by a decreased respiratory rate or effort, hypoxemia, and an increasing $PaCO_2$ (hypercapnia). Hypoventilation may occur as a result of depression of the central respiratory drive (secondary to anesthesia or pain medication), poor respiratory muscle tone (secondary to neuromuscular blockade or disease), or a combination of both.

NURSING MANAGEMENT
RESPIRATORY COMPLICATIONS

■ Nursing Assessment

For an adequate respiratory assessment, the nurse must evaluate airway patency; chest symmetry; and the depth, rate, and character of respirations. The nurse can place a cupped hand over the patient's nose and mouth to evaluate the forcefulness of exhaled air.

The chest wall should be observed for symmetry of movement with a hand placed lightly over the xiphoid process. Impaired ventilation may initially be detected by the observation of slowed breathing or diminished chest and abdominal movement during the respiratory cycle. It should also be determined whether abdominal or accessory muscles are being used for breathing. Observable use of these muscles may indicate respiratory distress.

Breath sounds should be auscultated anteriorly, laterally, and posteriorly. Decreased or absent breath sounds will be detected when airflow is diminished or obstructed. The presence of crackles or wheezes requires notification of the ACP.

Regular monitoring of vital signs and use of pulse oximetry in conjunction with thorough respiratory assessment permit the nurse to recognize early signs of respiratory complications. The presence of hypoxemia from any cause may be reflected by rapid breathing, gasping, apprehension, restlessness, and a rapid or thready pulse.

The characteristics of sputum or mucus should be noted and recorded. Mucus from the trachea and throat is colorless and thin in consistency. Sputum from the lungs and bronchi is thick with a slight yellow tinge.

■ Nursing Diagnoses

Nursing diagnoses and collaborative problems related to potential respiratory complications for the patient in the PACU include, but are not limited to, the following:
■ Ineffective airway clearance
■ Ineffective breathing pattern
■ Impaired gas exchange
■ Risk for aspiration
■ Potential complication: hypoxemia

■ Nursing Implementation

In the PACU, nursing interventions are designed to both prevent and treat respiratory problems. Proper positioning of the patient to facilitate respirations and protect the airway is essential. Unless contraindicated by the surgical procedure, the unconscious patient is positioned in a lateral "recovery" position (Fig. 19-3). This recovery position keeps the airway open and reduces the risk of aspiration if vomiting occurs.[4] Once conscious, the patient is usually returned to a supine position with the head of the bed elevated. This position maximizes expansion of the thorax by decreasing the pressure of the abdominal contents on the diaphragm.

Deep breathing is encouraged to facilitate gas exchange and to promote the return to consciousness. The patient should be taught to take in slow, deep breaths, ideally through the nose, to hold the breath, and to then slowly exhale. This type of breathing is also useful as a relaxation strategy when the patient is anxious or in pain. Other nursing interventions appropriate for specific respiratory complications are detailed in Table 19-3.

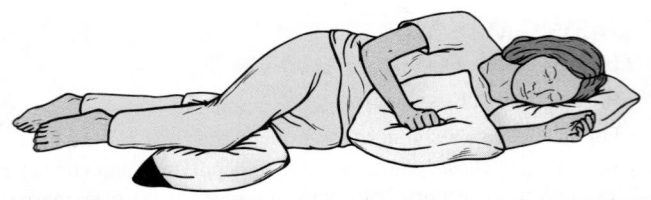

FIG. 19-3 Position of patient during recovery from general anesthesia.

POTENTIAL ALTERATIONS IN CARDIOVASCULAR FUNCTION

Etiology. In the immediate postanesthetic period the most common cardiovascular complications include hypotension, hypertension, and arrhythmias. Patients at greatest risk for alterations in cardiovascular function include those with alterations in respiratory function, those with a cardiac history, the elderly, the debilitated, and the critically ill.

Hypotension is evidenced by signs of hypoperfusion to the vital organs, especially the brain, heart, and kidneys. Clinical signs of disorientation, loss of consciousness, chest pain, oliguria, and anuria reflect hypoxemia and the loss of physiologic compensation. Intervention must be timely to prevent the devastating complications of cardiac ischemia or infarction, cerebral ischemia, renal ischemia, and bowel infarction.

The most common cause of hypotension in the PACU is unreplaced fluid and blood loss. As a result, treatment will be directed toward restoring circulating volume. If there is no response to fluid administration, cardiac dysfunction should be considered to be the cause of hypotension.

Primary cardiac dysfunction, as may occur in the case of myocardial infarction, cardiac tamponade, or pulmonary embolism, results in an acute fall in cardiac output. Secondary myocardial dysfunction occurs as a result of the negative chronotrope (rate) and negative inotrope (force) effects of drugs, such as β-adrenergic blockers, digoxin, or narcotics. Other causes of hypotension include decreased low systemic vascular resistance, arrhythmias, and measurement errors that may occur if a blood pressure cuff is incorrectly sized.

Hypertension, a common finding in the PACU, is most frequently the result of sympathetic nervous stimulation that may be the result of pain, anxiety, bladder distention, or respiratory compromise. Hypertension may also be the result of hypothermia and preexisting hypertension. It may be seen after vascular and cardiac surgery as a result of revascularization.

Arrhythmias are often the result of an identifiable cause as opposed to myocardial injury. The leading causes include hypokalemia, hypoxemia, hypercarbia, alterations in acid-base status, circulatory instability, and preexisting heart disease. Hypothermia, pain, surgical stress, and many anesthetic agents are also capable of causing arrhythmias.

NURSING MANAGEMENT CARDIOVASCULAR COMPLICATIONS

■ Nursing Assessment

The most important aspect of the cardiovascular assessment is frequent monitoring of vital signs. They are usually monitored every 15 minutes, or more often until stabilized, and then at less frequent intervals. Postoperative vital signs should be compared with preoperative and intraoperative readings to determine when the signs are stabilizing at a normal level for the patient's condition. The ACP or surgeon should be notified if the following occur:

1. Systolic blood pressure is less than 90 mm Hg or greater than 160 mm Hg.
2. Pulse rate is less than 60 beats per minute or greater than 120 beats per minute.
3. Pulse pressure (difference between systolic and diastolic pressures) narrows.
4. Blood pressure gradually decreases during several consecutive readings.
5. An irregular cardiac rhythm develops.
6. There is a significant variation from preoperative readings.

Cardiac monitoring is recommended for patients who have a history of cardiac disease and for all older adult patients who have undergone major surgery, regardless of whether they have cardiac problems. The apical-radial pulse should be assessed carefully, and any irregularities should be reported.

Assessment of skin color, temperature, and moisture provides valuable information in detecting cardiovascular problems. Hypotension accompanied by a normal pulse and warm, dry, pink skin usually represents the residual vasodilating effects of anesthesia and suggests only a need for continued observation. Hypotension accompanied by a rapid pulse and cold, clammy, pale skin may be caused by impending hypovolemic shock and requires immediate treatment.

■ Nursing Diagnoses

Nursing diagnoses and collaborative problems related to potential cardiovascular complications for the patient in the PACU include, but are not limited to, the following:

- Decreased cardiac output
- Deficient fluid volume
- Excess fluid volume
- Ineffective tissue perfusion
- Potential complication: hypovolemic shock

■ Nursing Implementation

Nursing interventions in the PACU are designed to prevent and treat cardiovascular complications. Treatment of hypotension should always begin with oxygen therapy to promote oxygenation of hypoperfused organs. Volume status should be assessed as described, and errors of blood pressure measurement should be ruled out. Because the most common cause of hypotension is fluid loss, IV fluid boluses will be given to normalize blood pressure. Primary cardiac dysfunction may require drug intervention. Peripheral vasodilation and hypotension may require vasoconstrictive agents to normalize systemic vascular resistance.

Treatment of hypertension will center on addressing the cause of sympathetic nervous system stimulation and eliminating the precipitating cause. Treatment may include the use of analgesics, assistance in voiding, and correction of respiratory problems. Rewarming will correct hypothermia-induced hypertension. If the patient has preexisting hypertension or has undergone cardiac or vascular surgery, drug therapy designed to reduce blood pressure will usually be required.

Because the majority of arrhythmias seen in the PACU have identifiable causes, treatment is directed toward eliminating the cause. Correction of these physiologic alterations will, in most instances, correct the arrhythmias. In the event of life-threatening arrhythmias, protocols of advanced cardiac life support will be applied (see Chapter 35).

POTENTIAL ALTERATIONS IN NEUROLOGIC FUNCTION

Etiology. Postoperatively, emergence delirium remains the neurologic alteration that causes the most concern to the practitioner. **Emergence delirium,** or *violent emergence,* can include behaviors such as restlessness, agitation, disorientation, thrashing, and shouting. This condition may be caused by anesthetic agents, hypoxia, bladder distention, pain, electrolyte abnormalities, or the patient's state of anxiety preoperatively. Nurses may be able to affect the patient's recovery by using interventions to decrease anxiety.[5]

Delayed awakening may also be a problem postoperatively. Fortunately, the most common cause of delayed awakening is prolonged drug action, particularly of narcotics, sedatives, and inhalational anesthetics, as opposed to neurologic injury. Normal awakening can be predicted by the ACP based on the drugs used in surgery.

NURSING MANAGEMENT
NEUROLOGIC COMPLICATIONS

■ Nursing Assessment

The patient's level of consciousness, orientation, and ability to follow commands should be assessed. The size, reactivity, and equality of the pupils should be determined. The patient's sensory and motor status should also be assessed. If the neurologic status is altered, possible causes should be determined.

■ Nursing Diagnoses

Nursing diagnoses related to potential neurologic complications for the patient in the PACU include, but are not limited to, the following:
- Disturbed sensory perception
- Risk for injury
- Disturbed thought processes
- Impaired verbal communication

■ Nursing Implementation

The most common cause of postoperative agitation is hypoxemia. As a result, attention must be addressed toward evaluation of respiratory function. Once hypoxemia has been ruled out as the cause of postoperative delirium and all potentially known causes have been addressed, sedation may prove beneficial in controlling the agitation and providing for patient and staff safety. Emergence delirium is usually time limited and will resolve before the patient is discharged from the PACU. Because the most common cause of delayed awakening is prolonged drug action, delays in awakening usually spontaneously resolve with time. If necessary, benzodiazepines and narcotics may be pharmacologically reversed with antagonists.

Until the patient is awake and able to communicate effectively, it will be the responsibility of the PACU nurse to act as a patient advocate and to maintain patient safety at all times. This includes having the side rails up, securing IV lines and artificial airways, verifying the presence of identification and allergy bands, and monitoring physiologic status.

PAIN AND DISCOMFORT

Etiology. Despite the availability of analgesic drugs and pain-relieving techniques, pain remains a common problem and a significant fear for the patient in the PACU and during the postoperative period. Pain may be the result of surgical manipulation, positioning, or the presence of internal devices such as an endotracheal tube or catheter, or it may occur as the patient begins to mobilize postoperatively. Pain is a common reason of a prolonged stay in the PACU.[6]

NURSING MANAGEMENT
PAIN

■ Nursing Assessment

The patient should be observed for indications of pain (e.g., restlessness) and questioned about the degree and characteristics of the pain. Identifying the location of the pain is important. Incisional pain is to be expected, but other causes of pain, such as a full bladder, may be present. In addition, the 1999-2000 Joint Commission on Accreditation of Healthcare Organizations (JCAHO) standards of practice include measurement of the patient's pain both before and after it is treated.[7]

■ Nursing Diagnoses

Nursing diagnoses for the patient experiencing pain and discomfort include, but are not limited to, the following:
- Acute pain
- Anxiety

■ Nursing Implementation

The most effective interventions for pain include both pharmacologic and nonpharmacologic approaches.[6] Intravenous narcotics provide the most rapid relief. Drugs are administered slowly and titrated to allow for optimal pain management with minimal to no adverse drug side effects. More sustained relief may be obtained through the use of epidural catheters, patient-controlled analgesia, or regional anesthetic blockade. Comfort measures, including touch, reuniting the patient and family, and rewarming, also contribute to patient comfort.

Pain management is most likely to be successful if the treatment plan is initiated with involvement of the patient, the ACP, and the PACU nurse. The goals should be to determine the most effective therapy, drug, and dose and to determine the best response to therapy. Once discharged from the PACU to an inpatient unit, the nurse will replace the PACU nurse as a member of the pain management team. For more information on nursing assessment and management of patients in pain, see Chapter 9.

HYPOTHERMIA

Etiology. Hypothermia, a core temperature of less than 96.8° F (36° C), occurs when heat loss exceeds heat production.[8] Hypothermia may be the result of loss of heat from a warm body to a cold OR or loss of heat from exposed body organs to the air.[9]

Although all patients are at risk for hypothermia, the older, debilitated, or intoxicated patient is at an increased risk. Long surgical procedures and prolonged anesthetic administration lead to redistribution of body heat from the core to the periphery. This places the patient at an increased risk for hypothermia.

Complications from hypothermia may include compromised immune function, postoperative pain, bleeding, myocardial ischemia, and delayed drug metabolism resulting in a prolonged PACU stay.[8-11]

NURSING MANAGEMENT
HYPOTHERMIA

■ Nursing Assessment

Vital signs, including temperature, should be determined. Temperature may be taken orally or via the tympanic membrane or axilla. Use of rectal temperature monitoring is rare; use of skin temperature monitoring is unreliable. The color and temperature of the skin should also be assessed.

■ Nursing Diagnoses

Nursing diagnoses for the patient with hypothermia include, but are not limited to, the following:
- Hypothermia
- Risk for imbalanced body temperature

■ Nursing Implementation

Passive rewarming (i.e., shivering) raises basal heat metabolism. *Active rewarming* requires the application of external warming devices and may include warm blankets, heated aerosols, radiant warmers, forced air warmers, or heated water mattresses. When using any external warming device, body temperature should be monitored at 15-minute intervals, and care should be taken to prevent skin injuries. In addition, oxygen therapy via nasal prongs or mask is used to treat the increased demand for oxygen accompanying the increase in body temperature. See Chapter 67 for additional management of hypothermia.

NAUSEA AND VOMITING

Etiology. Nausea and vomiting are significant problems in the immediate postoperative period. These problems are responsible for unanticipated hospital admission of day-surgery patients, increased patient discomfort, delays in discharge, and patient dissatisfaction with the surgical experience.[2] Numerous factors have been identified as contributing to the development of nausea and vomiting, including anesthetic agents and techniques, gender (female), length and type of surgery (eye, ear, abdominal, and gynecologic), and a history of nausea and vomiting after surgery or motion sickness.[12]

NURSING MANAGEMENT
NAUSEA AND VOMITING

■ Nursing Assessment

The patient should be questioned about feelings of nausea. If vomiting occurs, it is important to determine the quantity, characteristics, and color of the vomitus.

■ Nursing Diagnoses

Nursing diagnoses for the patient experiencing nausea and vomiting include, but are not limited to, the following:
- Nausea
- Risk for aspiration
- Risk for deficient fluid volume

■ Nursing Implementation

Intervention for nausea and vomiting is primarily the use of antiemetic or prokinetic drugs (see Chapter 40). In the PACU, oral fluids should be given only as indicated and tolerated. Intravenous fluids will provide hydration until the patient is able to tolerate oral fluids. Care should also be taken to prevent aspiration if the patient vomits while still sleepy from anesthesia. Having suction equipment readily available at the bedside and turning the patient's head to the side will help protect the patient from aspiration. Other nursing interventions that may be effective include placing the patient in the upright position; slow, deep breathing; mouth care; cool washcloth to the forehead; and emotional support.[13]

Surgical-Specific Care of the Patient in the Postanesthesia Care Unit

In addition to meeting the postanesthesia needs of the patient in the PACU, the PACU nurse will also attend to the surgery-specific (e.g., abdominal, thoracic) needs of the patient. The nursing assessment and management of the patient having a specific surgical procedure are discussed in the appropriate chapters of this text.

Discharge from the Postanesthesia Care Unit

The patient leaving the PACU may be discharged to an intensive care unit, an inpatient unit, an ambulatory care unit, or home. The choice of discharge site is based on patient acuity, access to follow-up care, and the potential for postoperative complications.

The decision to discharge the patient from the PACU is based on written discharge criteria. Discharge from an ambulatory care PACU requires that the patient meet additional criteria. Examples of discharge criteria are provided in Table 19-4.

Ambulatory Surgery Discharge. Ambulatory surgery patients include outpatients, same-day surgery patients, and short-stay patients. Because these patients are in the health care setting for such a short amount of time, it is difficult to do all the

TABLE 19-4	**Postanesthesia and Ambulatory Surgery Discharge Criteria**

Postanesthesia Discharge Criteria
- Patient awake (or baseline)
- Vital signs stable
- No excess bleeding or drainage
- No respiratory depression
- Oxygen saturation >90%
- Report given

Ambulatory Surgery Discharge Criteria
- All PACU discharge criteria met
- No IV narcotics for last 30 minutes
- Minimal nausea and vomiting
- Voided (if appropriate to surgical procedure/orders)
- Able to ambulate if age appropriate and not contraindicated
- Responsible adult present to accompany patient
- Discharge instructions given and understood

PACU, Postanesthesia care unit.

required teaching. Optimally, the patient and any caregivers should be contacted 1 or more days before surgery to collect assessment data and to provide teaching that will be needed postoperatively. The patient's anxiety level is lower at this time and learning may be enhanced.[14]

The patient leaving an ambulatory surgery setting must be mobile and alert to provide a degree of self-care when discharged to home. Postoperative pain and nausea and vomiting must be controlled. Overall, the patient must be stable and near the level of preoperative functioning for discharge from the unit. On discharge, instructions specific to the type of anesthesia received and the surgery are given to the patient verbally and reinforced with written directions. The type of information included in teaching is detailed later in this chapter (see pp. 410-411). The patient may not drive and must be accompanied by a responsible adult at the time of discharge. A follow-up evaluation of the patient's status is made by telephone, and any specific questions and concerns are addressed.

Although ambulatory surgical procedures are minimally invasive, the nurse must carefully determine not only readiness for discharge, but home care needs of the individual. It is important to determine availability of assistive personnel (e.g., family, friends), access to a pharmacy for prescriptions, access to a phone in the event of an emergency, and access to follow-up care.

CARE OF THE POSTOPERATIVE PATIENT ON THE CLINICAL UNIT

Before discharging the patient from the PACU to the clinical unit, the PACU nurse provides a verbal report about the patient to the receiving nurse. The report summarizes the operative and postanesthetic period.

The nurse who receives the patient on the clinical unit assists PACU transport personnel in transferring the patient from the PACU cart onto the bed. Care must be taken to protect IV lines, wound drains, dressings, and traction devices. The use of a draw sheet or transfer board and sufficient personnel facilitates transfer of the patient.

Vital signs should be obtained, and patient status should be compared with the report provided by the PACU. Documentation of the transfer is then completed, followed by a more in-depth assessment (Table 19-5). Postoperative orders and appropriate nursing care are then initiated.

Although many of the potential problems that may occur in the PACU are time limited to the immediate postoperative period, a number of potential complications may occur during the extended postoperative recovery period on the clinical unit. Nursing assessment and management are based on awareness of the potential complications of surgery in general, as well as complications specific to the surgical procedure. A general nursing care plan for the postoperative patient is presented in NCP 19-1.

Early ambulation is the most significant general nursing measure to prevent postoperative complications. Since it was first advocated nearly 40 years ago, the value of early ambulation has been obvious. The exercise associated with walking (1) increases muscle tone; (2) improves gastrointestinal (GI) and urinary tract function; (3) stimulates circulation, which prevents venous stasis and speeds wound healing; and (4) increases vital capacity and maintains normal respiratory function.[15]

POTENTIAL ALTERATIONS IN RESPIRATORY FUNCTION

Etiology. Atelectasis and pneumonia can occur in the postoperative surgical patient and are particularly common after abdominal and thoracic surgery. Atelectasis occurs when mucus blocks bronchioles or when the amount of alveolar surfactant (the substance that holds the alveoli open) is reduced (Fig. 19-4). As air becomes trapped beyond the plug and is eventually absorbed, the alveoli collapse. Atelectasis may affect a portion or an entire lobe of the lungs.

The postoperative development of mucous plugs and decreased surfactant production are directly related to hypoventilation, constant recumbent position, ineffective coughing, and smoking. Increased bronchial secretions occur when the respiratory passages are irritated by heavy smoking, acute or chronic pulmonary infection or disease, and the drying of mucous membranes that occurs with intubation, inhalation anesthesia, and dehydration. Without intervention, atelectasis can progress to pneumonia when microorganisms grow in the stagnant mucus and an infection develops.

TABLE 19-5 Nursing Assessment and Care of Patient on Admission to Clinical Unit	
Record time of patient's return to unit	Note last dose and type of pain control
Take baseline vital signs	Note current pain intensity
Assess airway and breath sounds	Position for airway maintenance, comfort, safety (bed in low
Assess neurologic status, including level of consciousness	position, side rails up)
and movement of extremities	Check IV infusion
Assess wound, dressing, drainage tubes	Note type of solution
Note type and amount of drainage	Note amount of fluid remaining
Connect tubing to gravity or suction drainage	Note flow rate
Assess color and appearance of skin	Check integrity of insertion site and size of catheter
Assess urinary status	Attach call light within reach and orient patient to use of call light
Note time of voiding	Ensure that emesis basin and tissues are available
Note presence of catheter and total output	Determine emotional condition and support
Check for bladder distention or urge to void	Check for presence of family member or significant other
Note catheter patency	Orient patient and family to immediate environment
Assess pain and discomfort	Check and carry out postoperative orders

NURSING CARE PLAN 19-1

Postoperative Patient*

EXPECTED PATIENT OUTCOMES	NURSING INTERVENTIONS and *RATIONALES*
NURSING DIAGNOSIS	**Acute pain** *related to* surgical incision and reflex muscle spasm *as manifested by* complaints of pain, tense and guarded body posture, facial grimacing, restlessness, irritability, moaning, diaphoresis, tachycardia.
• Satisfaction with pain relief • No interference with postoperative recovery	• Assess pain for character, location, and effectiveness of relief measures *to plan appropriate interventions.* • Teach and assess patient's correct use of patient-controlled analgesia *to ensure effectiveness.* • Use nonpharmacologic interventions to relieve pain such as distraction, massage, relaxation, and imagery *to enhance pharmacologic effects.*
NURSING DIAGNOSIS	**Nausea** *related to* gastrointestinal distention and medication or anesthesia effects *as manifested by* complaints of nausea, refusal to take fluids or solids, observed or reported vomiting.
• Reduced or no episodes of nausea and vomiting • No interference with postoperative recovery	• Assess precipitating factors and eliminate when possible (e.g., unpleasant smells, sights, pain) *to prevent initiating episode of nausea or vomiting.* • Maintain patency of nasogastric tube if present *to prevent accumulation of gastric secretions and subsequent vomiting.* • Assess bowel sounds *to determine presence, frequency, and characteristics of bowel sounds.* • Advance diet only as tolerated *to prevent gastrointestinal distention.* • Monitor gastrointestinal effects of medications, especially narcotics, *to determine if this is a possible source of the nausea.* • Administer antiemetics as indicated.
NURSING DIAGNOSIS	**Risk for infection** *related to* surgical incision, inadequate nutrition and fluid intake, presence of environmental pathogens, invasive catheters, and immobility.
• No evidence of infection such as fever, pain or swelling at operative site, or purulent wound drainage	• Monitor for and report the following *to determine possible presence of infection:* elevated body temperature; red, swollen, warm area surrounding incision, invasive lines, or indwelling catheters; elevated white blood cell count; elevated pulse and respiratory rate; purulent drainage from wound. • Use strict aseptic technique in providing wound care, including hand washing and sterile dressing technique and emptying drainage devices, *to prevent wound contamination.* • Administer antibiotics if ordered. • Ensure a minimum of 2000 calories and 2500 ml fluid per day (greater if metabolic demands are increased) *to ensure adequate calories for tissue repair.* • Help patient turn, cough, and breathe deeply every 1 to 2 hours while awake *to prevent respiratory infection.*
NURSING DIAGNOSIS	**Ineffective airway clearance** *related to* inability to clear tenacious secretions *as manifested by* abnormal breath sounds, shallow respirations, nonproductive cough, or low O₂ saturation.
• Clear breath sounds • Effective cough	• Provide for pain relief before having the patient cough and breathe deeply *to encourage cooperation and pain-free performance.* • Provide a minimum of 2500 ml fluids per day unless contraindicated *to liquefy secretions for easier removal.* • Assist patient with turning, coughing, and deep breathing every 1 to 2 hours while awake *to aid in removal of secretions and prevent formation of mucous plugs.* • Monitor use of incentive spirometer *to expand the lungs fully.* • Suction if necessary *to remove secretions the patient is unable to remove unaided.* • Monitor breath sounds and temperature *to detect early signs of infection.* • Assist with early mobility *to increase respiratory excursion.*

*This is a general nursing care plan for the postoperative patient. It should be used in conjunction with a nursing care plan specific to the type of surgery performed.

NURSING CARE PLAN 19–1

Postoperative Patient—cont'd

COLLABORATIVE PROBLEMS

NURSING GOALS	NURSING INTERVENTIONS and *RATIONALES*
POTENTIAL COMPLICATION • Monitor operative site for signs of hemorrhage • Report deviations from acceptable parameters • Carry out appropriate medical and nursing interventions	**Hemorrhage** *related to* ineffective vascular closure or alterations in coagulation. • Observe surgical site and dressings regularly, including dependent sites (q hr for 4 hr, then q4hr) *to detect signs of bleeding.* • Monitor vital signs regularly from q15min to q2-4hr as indicated *to detect signs of hypovolemia.* • Report abnormalities such as decreasing blood pressure; rapid pulse and respirations; cool, clammy skin; pallor; bright red blood on dressing. • Monitor for changes in mental status, such as restlessness and sense of impending doom, *as indicators of inadequate cerebral perfusion.* • Monitor hematocrit and hemoglobin levels *because decreases may indicate hemorrhage.* • Monitor platelet levels and coagulation function tests *because alterations indicate bleeding tendencies.*
POTENTIAL COMPLICATION • Monitor for signs of thromboembolism • Report deviations from acceptable parameters • Carry out appropriate medical and nursing interventions	**Thromboembolism** *related to* dehydration, immobility, vascular manipulation, or injury. • Assess for signs of thromboembolism, such as redness, swelling, pain; increased warmth along path of vein; edema or pain in extremity; chest pain; hemoptysis; tachypnea; dyspnea; restlessness. • Administer anticoagulants (e.g., heparin, enoxaprin [Lovenox]) as ordered *to decrease clot formation.* • Teach or perform range of motion to lower extremities and encourage early ambulation *to maintain muscle contractions and adequate vascular flow.* • Avoid pressure under knees from bed or pillows *to avoid pressure on veins, constriction of circulation, or pooling and stasis of blood.* • Apply antiembolism stockings and sequential compression device, if ordered. Remove for 1 hr every 8 to 10 hr *to allow for skin assessment.*
POTENTIAL COMPLICATION • Monitor for signs of urinary retention • Report deviation from acceptable parameters • Carry out appropriate medical and nursing interventions	**Urinary retention** *related to* horizontal positioning, pain, fear, analgesic and anesthetic medications, or surgical procedure. • Assess for bladder pain and distention, decreased or absent urinary output *to determine if a problem is present.* • Monitor intake and output *to determine fluid balance.* • Percuss bladder routinely for 48 hr postoperatively *to assess for distention.* • Notify physician if no urine output within 6 hr after surgery. • Position patient in as normal position as possible for voiding. • Use appropriate pain measures and provide privacy *to reduce anxiety so voiding will be easier.*
POTENTIAL COMPLICATION • Monitor for signs of paralytic ileus • Report deviation from acceptable parameters • Carry out appropriate medical and nursing interventions	**Paralytic ileus** *related to* bowel manipulation, immobility, pain medication, and anesthetics. • Assess for abdominal distention, presence of flatus or stool, bowel sounds, or nausea and vomiting *to determine if paralytic ileus is present.* • Maintain NPO status until peristalsis returns and ensure patency of nasogastric tube *to prevent vomiting with abdominal surgeries.* • Provide frequent oral hygiene *for patient comfort.*

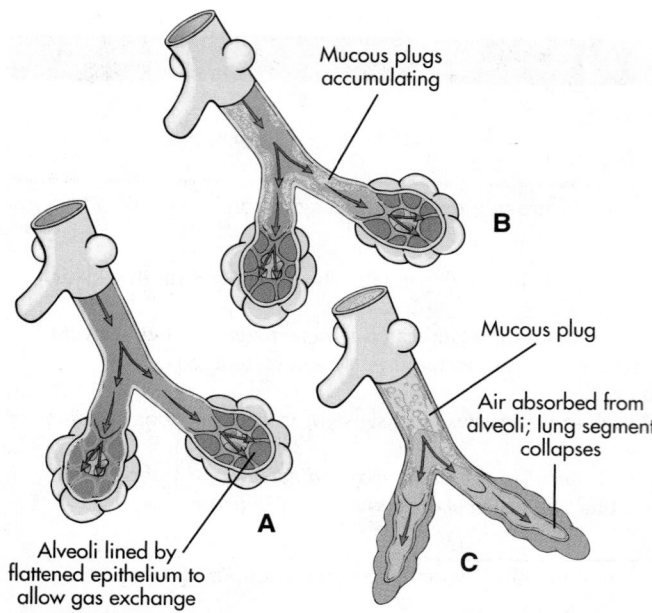

Mucous plugs accumulating

B

Mucous plug

Air absorbed from alveoli; lung segment collapses

A

C

Alveoli lined by flattened epithelium to allow gas exchange

FIG. 19-4 Postoperative atelectasis. A, Normal bronchiole and alveoli. B, Mucous plug in bronchiole. C, Collapse of alveoli due to atelectasis following absorption of air.

NURSING MANAGEMENT
RESPIRATORY COMPLICATIONS

■ Nursing Assessment

Nursing assessment of the patient's respiratory rate, patterns, and breath sounds is essential to identify potential respiratory problems.

■ Nursing Diagnoses

Nursing diagnoses and collaborative problems related to potential respiratory complications for the postoperative patient include, but are not limited to, the following:
- Ineffective airway clearance
- Ineffective breathing pattern
- Impaired gas exchange
- Potential complication: pneumonia
- Potential complication: atelectasis

■ Nursing Implementation

Deep-breathing and coughing techniques help the patient prevent alveolar collapse and move respiratory secretions to larger airway passages for expectoration. The patient should be assisted to breathe deeply 10 times every hour while awake. The use of an incentive spirometer is helpful in providing visual feedback of respiratory effort. Diaphragmatic or abdominal breathing is accomplished by inhaling slowly and deeply through the nose, holding the breath for a few seconds, and then exhaling slowly and completely through the mouth. The patient's hands should be placed lightly over the lower ribs and upper abdomen. This allows the patient to feel the abdomen rise during inspiration and fall during expiration.

Effective coughing is essential in mobilizing secretions (see Chapter 28). If secretions are present in the respiratory passages, deep breathing often will move them up to stimulate the cough

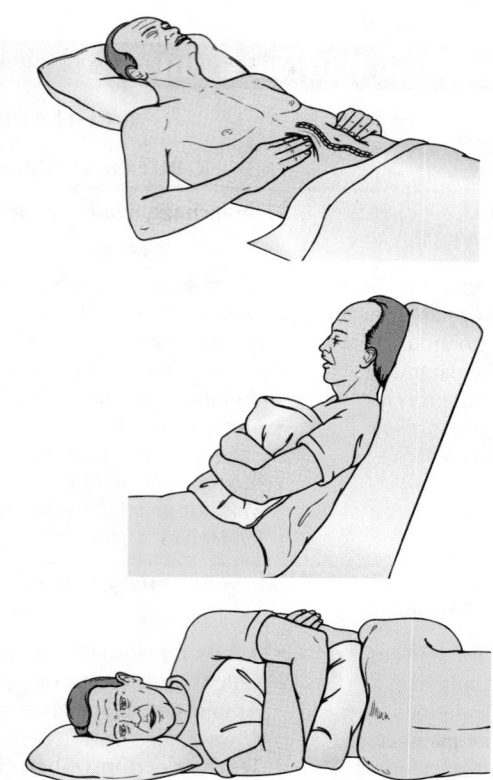

FIG. 19-5 Techniques for splinting wound when coughing.

reflex without any voluntary effort by the patient, and then they can be expectorated. Splinting an abdominal incision with a pillow or a rolled blanket provides support to the incision and aids in coughing and expectoration of secretions (Fig. 19-5).

The patient's position should be changed every 1 to 2 hours to allow full chest expansion and increase perfusion of both lungs. Ambulation, not just sitting in a chair, should be aggressively carried out as soon as physician approval is given. Adequate and regular analgesic medication should be provided because incisional pain often is the greatest deterrent to patient participation in effective ventilation and ambulation. The patient should also be reassured that these activities will not cause the incision to separate. Adequate hydration, either parenteral or oral, is essential to maintain the integrity of mucous membranes and to keep secretions thin and loose for easy expectoration.

POTENTIAL ALTERATIONS
IN CARDIOVASCULAR FUNCTION

Etiology. Postoperative fluid and electrolyte imbalances are contributing factors to alterations in cardiovascular function. They may develop as a result of a combination of the body's normal response to the stress of surgery, excessive fluid losses, and improper IV fluid replacement. The body's fluid status directly affects cardiac output. Fluid retention during the first 2 to 5 postoperative days can be the result of the stress response (see Chapter 8). This body response serves to maintain both blood volume and blood pressure (see Chapter 8, Fig. 8-6). Fluid retention results from the secretion and release of two hormones by the pituitary—antidiuretic hormone (ADH) and adrenocorticotropic hormone (ACTH)—and activation of the renin-angiotensin-aldosterone system. ADH release leads to increased H_2O reabsorption and decreased urinary output, increasing blood volume. ACTH stimulates the adrenal cortex to secrete aldosterone. Fluid losses resulting from surgery decrease kidney perfusion, stimulating the renin-angiotension-aldolsterone system and causing marked release of aldosterone (see Chapter 16). Both of the mechanisms that increase aldosterone lead to significant sodium and fluid retention, which also increase blood volume.

Fluid overload may occur during this period of fluid retention when IV fluids are administered too rapidly, when chronic (e.g., cardiac or renal) disease exists, or when the patient is an older adult. Conversely, fluid deficit may be related to slow or inadequate fluid replacement, which leads to decreases in cardiac output and tissue perfusion. Untreated preoperative dehydration or intraoperative or postoperative losses from vomiting, bleeding, wound drainage, or suctioning may be contributing factors to fluid deficits.

Hypokalemia can be a consequence of urinary and GI tract losses, and it results when potassium is not replaced in IV fluids. Low serum potassium levels directly affect the contractility of the heart and thus may also contribute to decreased cardiac output and overall body tissue perfusion. Adequate replacement of potassium is usually 40 mEq per day. However, it should not be given until adequate renal function has been established. A urine output of at least 0.5 ml/kg per hour is generally considered indicative of adequate renal function.

Cardiovascular status is also affected by the state of tissue perfusion or blood flow. The stress response contributes to an increase in clotting tendencies in the postoperative patient by increasing platelet production. Deep vein thrombosis (DVT) may form in leg veins as a result of inactivity, body position, and pressure, all of which lead to venous stasis and decreased perfusion. DVT, especially common in the older adult, obese individual, and immobilized patient, is a potentially life-threatening complication because it may lead to pulmonary embolism. Patients with a history of DVT have a greater risk for pulmonary embolism. Pulmonary embolism should be suspected in any patient complaining of tachypnea, dyspnea, and tachycardia, particularly when the patient is already receiving oxygen therapy. Manifestations may include chest pain, hypotension, hemoptysis, arrhythmias, and heart failure. Definitive diagnosis requires pulmonary angiography. Superficial thrombophlebitis is an uncomfortable but less ominous complication that may develop in a leg vein as a result of venous stasis or in the arm veins as a result of irritation from IV catheters or solutions. If a piece of a clot becomes dislodged and travels to the lung, it can cause a pulmonary infarction of a size proportionate to the vessel in which it lodges.

Syncope (fainting) is another factor that reflects the cardiovascular status. It may indicate decreased cardiac output, fluid deficits, or defects in cerebral perfusion. Syncope frequently occurs as a result of postural hypotension when the patient ambulates. It is more common in the older adult or in the patient who has been immobile for long periods of time. Normally when the patient quickly moves to a standing position, the arterial presoreceptors respond to the accompanying fall in blood pressure with sympathetic nervous stimulation, which produces vasoconstriction. This sympathetic nervous system response causes an increase in, and therefore maintains, blood pressure. These sympathetic and vasomotor functions may be diminished in the older adult and the immobile or postanesthetic patient.

NURSING MANAGEMENT
CARDIOVASCULAR COMPLICATIONS

■ Nursing Assessment

Specific assessment of cardiovascular function includes the regular monitoring of the patient's blood pressure, heart rate, pulse, and skin temperature and color. Results should be compared with preoperative status and the immediate postoperative and intraoperative findings.

■ Nursing Diagnoses

Nursing diagnoses and collaborative problems related to potential cardiovascular complications for the postoperative patient include, but are not limited to, the following:
- Decreased cardiac output
- Deficient fluid volume
- Excess fluid volume
- Ineffective tissue perfusion
- Activity intolerance
- Potential complication: thromboembolism

■ Nursing Implementation

An accurate intake and output record should be kept during the postoperative period, and laboratory findings (e.g., electrolytes, hematocrit) should be monitored. Nursing responsibilities relating to IV management are critical during this period. In particular the nurse should be alert for symptoms of too slow or too rapid a rate of fluid replacement. Assessment should also be made of the infusion site for discomfort and the hazards associated with the IV administration of potassium, such as cardiac arrest and pain in the area of the vein where it is entering. Thirst is one of the most annoying discomforts of postoperative patients. This may be related to the drying effects of anticholinergic drugs, anesthetic gases, and fluid deficits. Adequate and regular mouth care is helpful while the patient cannot ingest food or drink by mouth.

Leg exercises (Fig. 19-6) should be encouraged 10 to 12 times every 1 to 2 hours while awake. The muscular contraction produced by these exercises and by ambulation facilitates venous return from the lower extremities. The ambulating patient should pick up the feet rather than shuffling them so that muscular contraction is maximized. When confined to bed, the patient should alternately flex and extend the legs. When the patient is sitting in a chair or lying in bed, there should be no pressure to impede venous flow through the popliteal space. Crossed legs, pillows behind the knees, and extreme elevation of the knee gatch must be avoided.

Some surgeons routinely prescribe elastic stockings or mechanical aids such as sequential compressive devices to stimulate and enhance the massaging and milking actions that are transmitted to the veins when leg muscles contract. The nurse must remember that these aids are useless if the legs are not exercised and may actually impair circulation if the legs remain inactive or if the devices are sized or applied improperly. When in use, elastic stockings must be removed and reapplied at least twice daily for skin care and inspection. The skin of the heels and posttibial areas is particularly susceptible to increased pressure and breakdown.

The use of unfractionated heparin (UH) or low-molecular-weight heparin (LMWH) is a prophylactic measure for venous thrombosis and pulmonary embolism. Advantages of LMWH

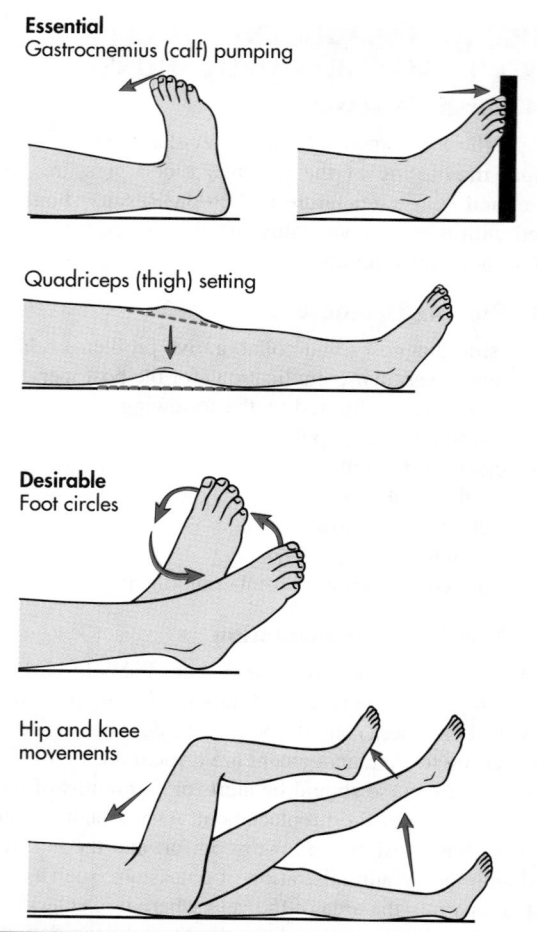

Essential
Gastrocnemius (calf) pumping

Quadriceps (thigh) setting

Desirable
Foot circles

Hip and knee
movements

FIG. 19-6 Postoperative leg exercises.

over UH include (1) less major bleeding, (2) decreased incidence of thrombocytopenia, (3) better absorption, (4) longer duration of action, (5) as effective or more effective, and (6) no laboratory monitoring required.[16] The nurse may prevent syncope by making changes slowly in the patient's position. Progression to ambulation can be achieved by first raising the head of the patient's bed for 1 to 2 minutes and then by assisting the patient to sit on the side of the bed while monitoring the radial pulse for rate and quality. If no changes or complaints are noted, ambulation can be started. If faintness occurs, the nurse can help the patient sit on the edge of the bed while continuing to monitor the pulse. If changes occur or if the patient complains of feeling faint during ambulation, the nurse should provide assistance to a nearby chair or ease the patient to the floor. The patient should remain in either location until recovery is evidenced by blood pressure stability, and then be helped back to the bed. If faintness occurs, it is often frightening for the patient and for the unprepared nurse, but syncope poses no real physiologic danger, although injury can result from a fall.

POTENTIAL ALTERATIONS IN URINARY FUNCTION

Etiology. Low urine output (800 to 1500 ml) in the first 24 hours may be expected, regardless of fluid intake. This low output is caused by increased aldosterone and ADH secretion resulting from the stress of surgery, fluid restriction before surgery, and loss of fluids during surgery, drainage, and diaphoresis. By the second or third day, the patient will begin to have increasing urinary output after fluid has been mobilized and the immediate stress reaction subsides.

Acute urinary retention can occur in the postoperative period for a variety of reasons. Anesthesia depresses the nervous system, including the micturition reflex arc and the higher centers that influence it. This allows the bladder to fill more completely than normal before the urge to void is felt. Anesthesia also impedes voluntary micturition. Anticholinergic and narcotic drugs may also interfere with the ability to initiate voiding or to empty the bladder completely.

Retention is more likely to occur after lower abdominal or pelvic surgery because spasms or guarding of the abdominal and pelvic muscles interferes with their normal function in micturition. Pain may alter perception and interfere with the patient's awareness of the less intense sensation arising as the bladder fills. Voiding ability is probably impaired to the greatest extent by immobility and the recumbent position in bed. Lack of skeletal muscle activity decreases smooth muscle (bladder detrusor) tone, and the supine position reduces the ability to relax the perineal muscles and external sphincter.

Oliguria, the diminished output of urine, can be a manifestation of acute renal failure and is a less common although more serious problem after surgery. It may result from renal ischemia caused by inadequate renal perfusion or altered cardiovascular function.

NURSING MANAGEMENT URINARY COMPLICATIONS

■ Nursing Assessment

The urine of the postoperative patient should be examined for both quantity and quality. The color, amount, consistency, and odor of the urine should be noted. Indwelling catheters should be assessed for patency, and urine output should be at least 0.5 ml/kg per hour. If a catheter is not present, the patient should be able to void approximately 200 ml of urine following surgery. Most people urinate within 6 to 8 hours after surgery. If no voiding occurs, the abdominal contour should be inspected and the bladder palpated and percussed for distention.

■ Nursing Diagnoses

Nursing diagnoses and collaborative problems related to potential urinary complications for the postoperative patient include, but are not limited to, the following:
- Impaired urinary elimination
- Potential complication: acute urinary retention

■ Nursing Implementation

The nurse may facilitate voiding by normal positioning of the patient—sitting for women and standing for men. Providing reassurance to the patient regarding the ability to void and the use of techniques such as running water, drinking water, or pouring warm water over the perineum may also be of assistance. Ambulation, preferably to the bathroom, and the use of a bedside commode are additional helpful measures to assist in voiding.

The surgeon often leaves an order to catheterize the patient in 8 to 12 hours if voiding has not occurred. Because of the possibility of infection associated with catheterization, the nurse should first try other measures to induce voiding and validate that the bladder is actually full. In assessing the need for catheterization, the nurse should consider fluid intake during and after surgery and determine bladder fullness (e.g., palpable fullness above the symphysis pubis, discomfort when pressure is applied over the bladder, or the presence of the urge to void). Straight catheterization is preferred because of the possibility of infection associated with an indwelling catheter.

POTENTIAL ALTERATIONS IN GASTROINTESTINAL FUNCTION

Etiology. Slowed GI motility and altered patterns of food intake may lead to the development of several distressing postoperative symptoms that are most pronounced after abdominal surgery. Nausea and vomiting may be caused by the action of anesthetics or narcotics, delayed gastric emptying, slowed peristalsis resulting from the handling of the bowel during surgery, and resumption of oral intake too soon after surgery.

Abdominal distention is another common problem caused by decreased peristalsis as a result of handling of the intestine during surgery and limited dietary intake before and after surgery. Following abdominal surgery, motility of the large intestine may be reduced for 3 to 5 days, although motility in the small intestine resumes within 24 hours. Swallowed air and GI secretions may accumulate in the colon, producing distention and gas pains.

Hiccoughs (singultus) are intermittent spasms of the diaphragm caused by irritation of the phrenic nerve, which innervates the diaphragm. Postoperative sources of direct irritation of the phrenic nerve may be gastric distention, intestinal obstruction, intraabdominal bleeding, and a subphrenic abscess. Indirect irritation of the phrenic nerve may be produced by acid-base and electrolyte imbalances. Reflex irritation may come from drinking hot or cold liquids or from the presence of a nasogastric tube. Hiccoughs usually last a short time and subside spontaneously; occasionally they may be persistent but are rarely debilitating.

NURSING MANAGEMENT GASTROINTESTINAL COMPLICATIONS

■ Nursing Assessment

The abdomen should be auscultated in all four quadrants to determine the presence, frequency, and characteristics of the bowel sounds. Bowel sounds are frequently absent or diminished in the immediate postoperative period when peristalsis is decreased. The return of normal bowel motility is usually accompanied by the passage of flatus in addition to normal bowel sounds. If vomiting occurs, the emesis should be evaluated for color, consistency, and amount.

■ Nursing Diagnoses

Nursing diagnoses and collaborative problems related to potential GI complications for the postoperative patient may include, but are not limited to, the following:

- Nausea
- Imbalanced nutrition: less than body requirements
- Potential complication: paralytic ileus
- Potential complication: hiccoughs

■ Nursing Implementation

Depending on the nature of the surgery, the patient may resume oral intake as soon as the gag reflex returns. The patient who had abdominal surgery is usually allowed nothing by mouth (NPO) until the presence of bowel sounds indicates the return of peristalsis. When the patient is NPO, IV infusions are given to maintain fluid and electrolyte balance. A nasogastric tube may be used to decompress the stomach to prevent nausea, vomiting, and abdominal distention. When oral intake is allowed, clear liquids are started and the IV infusion is continued, usually at a reduced rate. If oral intake is well tolerated by the patient, the IV is discontinued, and the diet is advanced until a regular diet is tolerated.

When the patient is on NPO status, regular mouth care is essential for comfort and stimulation of salivary glands. Nausea and vomiting may be prevented or relieved by the administration of an antiemetic drug given IV, intramuscularly, or by rectal suppository. In some instances a nasogastric tube is inserted if symptoms persist.

Abdominal distention may be prevented or minimized by early and frequent ambulation, which stimulates intestinal motility. The nurse should assess the patient regularly to detect the resumption of normal intestinal peristalsis as evidenced by the return of bowel sounds and the passage of flatus. The nasogastric tube must be clamped or suction turned off when the abdomen is auscultated. Resumption of a normal diet after bowel sounds have returned will also enhance the return of normal peristalsis.

The patient may need to be encouraged to expel flatus and assured that expulsion is necessary and desirable. Gas pains, which tend to become pronounced on the second or third postoperative day, may be relieved by ambulation and frequent repositioning. Positioning the patient on the right side permits gas to rise along the transverse colon and facilitates its release. Bisacodyl (Dulcolax) suppositories may be ordered to stimulate colonic peristalsis and expulsion of flatus and feces.

The postoperative patient who is hiccoughing should first be assessed in an attempt to determine the cause. In many instances simple irrigation of the nasogastric tube to restore patency will solve the problem.

POTENTIAL ALTERATIONS OF THE INTEGUMENT

Etiology. Surgery generally involves an incision through the skin and underlying tissues. An incision disrupts the protective skin barrier. Therefore wound healing is one of the major concerns during the postoperative period.

An adequate nutritional state is essential for wound healing. Amino acids are readily available for the healing process because of the catabolic effects of the stress-related hormones (e.g., cortisol). The patient who was well nourished preoperatively can tolerate the postoperative delay in nutritional intake for several days. However, the patient with preexisting nutritional deficits that occur with chronic diseases (e.g., diabetes, ulcerative colitis, alcoholism), is more prone to problems of wound healing. Wound healing is also a concern for the older adult and is affected by multiple factors. The patient who is unable to meet nutritional needs postoperatively may be provided with total parenteral nutrition to promote healing.

Wound infection may result from contamination of the wound from three major sources: (1) exogenous flora present in the environment and on the skin, (2) oral flora, and (3) intestinal flora. The incidence of wound sepsis is higher in patients who are malnourished, immunosuppressed, or older, or who have had a prolonged hospital stay or a lengthy surgical procedure (lasting more than 3 hours). Patients undergoing bowel surgery, particularly following a traumatic injury, are at a particularly high risk. Infection may involve the entire incision and may extend downward through the deeper tissue layers. An abscess may form locally, or the infection may penetrate entire body cavities, as in peritonitis. Evidence of wound infection usually does not become apparent before the third to the fifth postoperative day. The manifestations include local manifestations of redness, swelling, and increasing pain and tenderness at the site. Systemic manifestations are fever and leukocytosis.

An accumulation of fluid in a wound may create pressure, impair circulation and wound healing, and predispose to infection. Because of these reasons the surgeon may place a drain in the incision or make a stab wound adjacent to the incision to allow for drainage. These drains may be made of soft rubber and drain into a dressing, or they may be firm catheters attached to a Hemovac or other source of gentle suction. Wound healing and complications are discussed in Chapter 12.

NURSING MANAGEMENT
SURGICAL WOUNDS

■ Nursing Assessment

Nursing assessment of the wound and dressing requires knowledge of the type of wound, drains inserted, and expected drainage related to the specific type of surgery. A small amount of serous drainage is common from any type of wound. If a drain is in place, a moderate to large amount of drainage may be expected. For example, an abdominal incision with accompanying drain is expected to have a moderate amount of serosanguineous drainage in the first 24 hours. In contrast, an inguinal herniorrhaphy should have only minimal serous drainage during the postoperative period.

In general, drainage is expected to change from sanguineous (red) to serosanguineous (pink) to serous (clear yellow). The drainage output should decrease over hours or days, depending on the type of surgery.[17] Wound infection may be accompanied by purulent drainage. **Wound dehiscence** (separation and disruption of previously joined wound edges) may be preceded by a sudden discharge of brown, pink, or clear drainage.

■ Nursing Diagnoses

Nursing diagnoses related to surgical wounds of the postoperative patient include, but are not limited to, the following:
- Risk for infection
- Potential complication: impaired wound healing

■ Nursing Implementation

When drainage occurs on the dressing, the type, amount, color, consistency, and odor of drainage should be noted and recorded. Expected drainage from tubes is outlined in Table 19-6. The effect of position changes on drainage should also be assessed. The surgeon should be notified of any excessive or abnormal drainage and significant changes in vital signs.

The incision may be initially covered with a dressing immediately after surgery. If there is no drainage after 24 to 48 hours, the incision may be opened to the air. Agency policy determines whether the nurse may change the initial operative dressing or simply reinforce it if the dressing is saturated.

When a dressing is changed, the number and type of drains present should be noted. Care should be taken to avoid dislodging drains during dressing removal. When the dressing is changed, the incision site should be examined carefully. The area around the sutures may be slightly reddened and swollen, which is an expected inflammatory response. However, the skin around the incision should be normal color and temperature. Clinical manifestations of infection include redness, swelling, pain, fever, and increased white blood cell count.[17] The nurse should wear clean gloves when removing a dressing. Sterile technique should be used when any new dressing is applied. If healing is by primary intention, little or no drainage is present, and no drains are in place, a single-layer dressing or no dressing is sufficient. When drains are in place, when moderate to heavy drainage is occurring, or when healing occurs other than by primary intention, a multiple-layer dressing is needed. Wound healing and care are discussed in Chapter 12.

TABLE 19-6	**Expected Drainage from Tubes and Catheters**				
SUBSTANCE	**DAILY AMOUNT**	**COLOR**	**ODOR**	**CONSISTENCY**
Indwelling Catheter				
Urine	500-700 ml, 1-2 days postoperative; 1500-2500 ml thereafter	Clear, yellow	Ammonia	Watery
Nasogastric Tube/Gastrostomy Tube				
Gastric contents	Up to 1500 ml/day	Pale, yellow-green Bloody following gastrointestinal surgery	Sour	Watery
Hemovac				
Wound drainage	Variable with procedure	Variable with procedure Usually serosanguineous	Same as wound dressing	Variable
T-Tube				
Bile	500 ml	Bright yellow to dark green	Acid	Thick

PAIN AND DISCOMFORT

Etiology. The assessment and management of the patient in pain are discussed in Chapter 9. Postoperative pain is caused by the interaction of a number of physiologic and psychologic factors. The skin and underlying tissues have been traumatized by the incision and retraction during surgery. In addition, there may be reflex muscle spasms around the incision. Anxiety and fear, sometimes related to the anticipation of pain, create tension and further increase muscle tone and spasm. The effort and movement associated with deep breathing, coughing, and changing position may aggravate pain by creating tension or pull on the incisional area.

When the internal viscera is cut, no pain is felt. However, pressure in the internal viscera elicits pain. Therefore deep visceral pain may signal the presence of a complication such as intestinal distention, bleeding, or abscess formation.

Postoperative pain is usually most severe within the first 48 hours and subsides thereafter. Variation is considerable, according to the procedure performed and the patient's individual pain tolerance or perception.

NURSING MANAGEMENT
PAIN

■ Nursing Assessment

Research has shown that many patients are undermedicated for pain.[18] Pain assessment may be difficult in the early postoperative period. The patient may not be able to verbalize the presence or severity of pain. The nurse should observe for behavioral clues of pain such as a wrinkling face or brow, a clenched fist, moaning, diaphoresis, and an increased pulse rate.

■ Nursing Diagnoses

Nursing diagnoses related to pain for the postoperative patient may include, but are not limited to, the following:

- Acute pain
- Disturbed sensory perception

■ Nursing Implementation

Postoperative pain relief is a nursing responsibility because the surgeon's orders for analgesic medication and other comfort measures are usually written on an as-needed basis. During the first 48 hours or longer, narcotic analgesics (e.g., morphine) are required to relieve moderate-to-severe pain. After that time, nonnarcotic analgesics, such as nonsteroidal anti-inflammatory agents, may be sufficient as pain intensity decreases.

Effective pain management will promote optimal healing, prevent complications, and allow patients to participate in necessary activities.[3] The Agency for Healthcare Research and Quality has established practice guidelines for acute pain management in the perioperative setting.[19]

Analgesic administration should be timed to ensure that it is in effect during activities that may be painful for the patient, such as ambulating. Although narcotic analgesics are often essential for the postoperative patient's comfort, there are undesirable side effects. Side effects such as constipation, nausea and vomiting, respiratory and cough depression, and hypotension are most common with the opioids. Before administering any analgesic, the nurse should first assess the nature of the patient's pain, including location, quality, and intensity. If it is incisional pain, analgesic administration is appropriate. If it is chest or leg pain, medication may simply mask a complication that must be reported and documented. If it is gas pain, narcotic medication can aggravate it. The nurse should notify the physician and request a change in the order if the analgesic either fails to relieve the pain or makes the patient excessively lethargic or somnolent.

Patient-controlled analgesia (PCA) and epidural analgesia are two alternative approaches for pain control. The goals of PCA are to provide immediate analgesia and to maintain a constant, steady blood level of the analgesic agent. PCA involves self-administration of predetermined doses of analgesia by the patient. The route of delivery may be IV, oral, or epidural. (PCA is discussed in Chapter 9.)

Epidural analgesia is the infusion of pain-relieving medications through a catheter placed into the epidural space surrounding the spinal cord. The goal of epidural analgesia is delivery of medication directly to opiate receptors in the spinal cord. The administration may be intermittent or constant and is monitored by the nurse. The overall effectiveness and the technique of administration result in a constant circulating level and a total reduced dose of medication.

POTENTIAL ALTERATIONS IN TEMPERATURE

Etiology. Temperature variation in the postoperative period provides valuable information about the patient's status. Hypothermia may be present in the immediate postoperative period while the patient is recovering from the effects of anesthesia and body heat loss during surgery. Fever may occur at any time during the postoperative period (Table 19-7). A mild elevation (up to 100.4° F [38° C]) during the first 48 hours usually reflects the

TABLE 19-7	Significance of Postoperative Temperature Changes	
TIME AFTER SURGERY	**TEMPERATURE**	**POSSIBLE CAUSES**
Up to 12 hr	Hypothermia to 96.8° F (36° C)	Effects of anesthesia Body heat loss in surgical exposure
First 24-48 hr	Elevation to 100.4° F (38° C) Above 100.4° F (38° C)	Inflammatory response to surgical stress Lung congestion, atelectasis
Third day and later	Elevation above 100° F (37.7° C)	Wound infection Urinary infection Respiratory infection Phlebitis

surgical stress response. A moderate elevation (higher than 100.4° F [38° C]) is caused more frequently by respiratory congestion or atelectasis and less frequently by dehydration. After the first 48 hours a moderate to marked elevation (higher than 99.9° F [37.7° C]) is usually caused by infection.

Wound infection, particularly from aerobic organisms, is often accompanied by a fever that spikes in the afternoon or evening and returns to near-normal levels in the morning. The respiratory tract may be infected secondary to stasis of secretions in areas of atelectasis. The urinary tract may be infected secondary to catheterization. Superficial thrombophlebitis may occur at the IV site or in the leg veins. The latter may produce a temperature elevation between 7 and 10 days after surgery.

Nosocomial infectious diarrhea caused by *Clostridium difficile* may be signaled by fever, diarrhea, and abdominal pain. Surgical patients who receive antibiotics for a period of time are at risk.

Intermittent high fever accompanied by shaking chills and diaphoresis suggests septicemia. This may occur at any time during the postoperative period because microorganisms may have been introduced into the bloodstream during surgery, especially in GI or genitourinary (GU) procedures, or picked up later from the site of a wound or a urinary or vein infection.

NURSING MANAGEMENT
ALTERED TEMPERATURE

■ Nursing Assessment

Frequent assessment of the patient's temperature is important to detect patterns of hypothermia and/or fever that may be present in the postoperative period. The nurse should observe the patient for early signs of inflammation and infection so that any complications that arise may be treated in a timely manner.

■ Nursing Diagnoses

Nursing diagnoses related to potential temperature complications for the postoperative patient may include, but are not limited to, the following:
- Risk for imbalanced body temperature
- Hyperthermia
- Hypothermia

■ Nursing Implementation

The nurse's role with respect to postoperative fever may be preventive, diagnostic, and therapeutic. The patient's temperature is usually measured every 4 hours for the first 48 hours postoperatively and then less frequently if no problems develop. Meticulous asepsis is maintained with regard to the wound and IV site and airway clearance is encouraged. If fever develops, chest x-rays may be taken, and, depending on the suspected cause, cultures of the wound, urine, or blood are obtained. If infection is the source of the fever, antibiotics are started as soon as cultures have been obtained. If the fever rises above 103° F (39.4° C), antipyretic drugs and body-cooling measures may be employed.

POTENTIAL ALTERATIONS IN PSYCHOLOGIC FUNCTION

Etiology. Anxiety and depression may occur in the postoperative patient. These states may be more pronounced in the patient who has had radical surgery (e.g., colostomy) or amputation or whose findings suggest a poor prognosis (e.g., inoperable tumor).

A history of a neurotic or psychotic disorder should alert the nurse to the possibility of postoperative anxiety and depression. However, these responses may develop in any patient as part of the grief response to loss of a body organ or disturbance in body image and may be exacerbated by a lowered response to stress.

The patient who lives alone or requires rehabilitation after surgery may also develop anxiety and depression when faced with the need for assistance postoperatively until strength and independence can be regained. A lack of knowledge about Medicare or insurance payments for rehabilitation and the type of services needed often impair the patient's ability to make a decision regarding continuing care.

Confusion or delirium may arise from a variety of psychologic and physiologic sources, including fluid and electrolyte imbalances, hypoxemia, drug effects, sleep deprivation, and sensory alteration, deprivation, or overload. *Delirium tremens* may also occur as a result of alcohol withdrawal in a postoperative patient. Delirium tremens is a reaction characterized by restlessness, insomnia and nightmares, tachycardia, apprehension, confusion and disorientation, irritability, and auditory or visual hallucinations. Management of delirium tremens is discussed in Chapter 11.

NURSING MANAGEMENT
PSYCHOLOGIC FUNCTION

■ Nursing Diagnoses

Nursing diagnoses related to potential alterations in psychologic function in the postoperative patient include, but are not limited to, the following:
- Anxiety
- Ineffective coping
- Disturbed body image
- Decisional conflict

■ Nursing Implementation

The nurse attempts to prevent psychologic problems in the postoperative period by providing adequate support for the patient. Supportive measures include taking time to listen and talk with the patient, offering explanations and genuine reassurance, and encouraging the presence and assistance of significant others. The nurse must observe and evaluate the patient's behavior to distinguish a normal reaction to the stress situation from one that is becoming abnormal or excessive.

The nurse should discuss the patient's expectation of activity and assistance needed following discharge. The older patient may be particularly distressed that an immediate return to home is not feasible. The patient must be included in discharge planning and should be provided with the information and support to make informed decisions about continuing care.

The recognition of the alcohol withdrawal syndrome in a patient not previously known to be an alcoholic presents a particular challenge. Any unusual or disturbed behavior should be reported immediately so that diagnosis and treatment may be instituted.

Planning for Discharge and Follow-up Care

Preparation for the patient's discharge should be an ongoing process throughout the surgical experience that begins during the preoperative period. The informed patient is therefore prepared

NURSING RESEARCH
Educational Needs of Patients after Discharge

Citation
Jacobs V: Informational needs of surgical patients following discharge, *Appl Nurs Res* 13:12, 2000.

Purpose
To explore patient perceptions of information needed to manage care following early discharge, patient reports of information given, and satisfaction with the information given.

Method
A descriptive design was used. A self-administered questionnaire, the Patient Learning Needs Scale, was used to determine what information patients perceived they needed in order to manage their care at home.

Results and Conclusions
Forty-seven questionnaires were analyzed. Patients related that "activities of living" and "treatment and complications" were information areas that they considered to be the most important. Specifically, they wanted information about physical limitations, caring for wounds, and recognizing complications. Most of the patients reported that they received information about some of the identified topics. Less than 60% of the patients perceived that they were given recommendations for physical exercise, potential complications, or possible problems with elimination. Patients were satisfied with the information they did receive.

Implications for Nursing Practice
Patients in this study were very specific about what information they wanted to receive before being discharged. Guidelines for educational content should be established based on identified needs. Instructions should be individualized to patients, given in writing, and reviewed, and a follow-up contact should be made.

as events unfold and gradually assumes greater responsibility for self-care during the postoperative period. As the day of discharge approaches, the nurse should be certain that the patient and any caregivers have the following information:

1. Care of wound site and any dressings, including bathing recommendations
2. Action and possible side effects of any drugs; when and how to take them
3. Activities allowed and prohibited; when various physical activities can be resumed safely (e.g., driving a car, returning to work, sexual intercourse, leisure activities)
4. Dietary restrictions or modifications
5. Symptoms to be reported (e.g., development of incisional tenderness or increased drainage, discomfort in other parts of the body)
6. Where and when to return for follow-up care
7. Answers to any individual questions or concerns

If the physician has not provided information about particular diet or activity prescriptions or restrictions, the nurse should either obtain this information or encourage the patient to do so. Attention to complete discharge instruction may prevent needless distress for the patient. Written instructions are important for reinforcing verbal information. The nurse should specifically document in the record the discharge instructions provided to the patient and family. For the patient, the postoperative phase of care continues and extends into the recuperative period. Assessment and evaluation of the patient after discharge may be accomplished by a follow-up call or by a visit from a nurse (e.g., home health nurse).

Increasingly, patients are being discharged from the hospital with many medical or surgical needs. They may be transferred to transitional care facilities, to long-term care facilities, or directly to their homes (see Chapter 6). When discharged directly to home, it is expected that the patient, with assistance from family, friends, or home health care, will continue self-care in the home. This may include dressing changes, wound care, catheter or drain care, home antibiotics, or continued physical therapy. Working through the discharge planner for the hospital unit, or the case manager, the nurse can facilitate the transition of care from hospital-based to community-based and home care, without jeopardizing the quality of care.

■ Gerontologic Considerations: Postoperative Patient

The older postoperative patient deserves special consideration. The older adult has a decrease in respiratory function, including decreased ability to cough, decreased thoracic compliance, and decreased lung tissue. These alterations in pulmonary status lead to an increase in the work of ventilation and a decreased ability to readily eliminate pharmacologic agents. Reactions to anesthetic agents must be carefully monitored and their postoperative elimination assessed before the patient is left without close supervision. Pneumonia is a common postoperative complication in the elderly.[20]

Vascular function in the older adult is altered because of atherosclerosis and decreased elasticity in the blood vessels. Cardiac function is often compromised, and compensatory responses to changes in blood pressure and volume are limited. Circulating blood volume is decreased, and hypertension is common. Cardiovascular parameters must be closely monitored throughout surgery and the postoperative period.

Drug toxicity is a potential problem in the older adult. Renal perfusion in the older adult normally decreases with a reduction in the ability to eliminate drugs that are excreted by the kidney. Decreased liver function in the older adult also leads to decreased drug metabolism and increased drug activity. Renal and liver function must be carefully assessed in the postoperative phase of the patient's care to prevent drug overdosage and toxicity.

Observing for changes in mental status is an important part of postoperative care in older adults. Postoperative delirium is common in the elderly in the postoperative period. Factors such as age, alcohol abuse, low baseline cognition, severe metabolic derangement, hypoxia, hypotension, and type of surgery appear to contribute to postoperative delirium. Anesthetics, notably anticholinergic drugs and benzodiazepines, increase the risk for delirium. Despite knowledge of risk factors, postoperative delirium in the elderly is poorly understood.[21] One way that the nurse can differentiate delirium from dementia is to observe for alterations in the level of consciousness, because they may indicate a diagnosis of delirium rather than dementia.[20] In patients with an acute change in mental status, a potentially reversible cause should be considered, such as an infection or a side effect of analgesic medication. (Dementia and delirium are discussed in Chapter 58.)

Pain is a multidimensional experience that should include assessment of how pain affects function, mood, activities, and quality of life.[22] Older patients may be hesitant to request pain medication. They may believe that pain is an inevitable consequence of surgery and they need to just tolerate it. Nurses may not appropriately assess pain in patients who do not report their pain. Some older patients are hesitant to learn how to use PCA machines. The nurse should know that the surgery will usually result in pain, and if untreated, pain could have a negative effect on recovery. The nurse should emphasize this to the patient and family. ■

CRITICAL THINKING EXERCISES

Case Study
Postoperative Patient

Patient Profile. Edward Gray, 74-year-old African American retired college professor, has just undergone surgery for a fractured hip. He fell off of a ladder while painting his house. The surgery, performed while the patient was under general anesthesia, was uneventful.

Subjective Data
- Was in excellent health before fall
- Played tennis three times each week
- Walked 20 to 30 miles per week
- Always had problems sleeping
- Difficulty hearing, wears hearing aid
- Upset with injury and its impact on activity
- Has no relatives or friends to assist with care

Objective Data
- Admitted to PACU with abduction pillow between his legs, two peripheral IV catheters, a self-suction drain from the hip dressing, and an indwelling urinary catheter

Collaborative Care

Postoperative Orders
- Vital signs per PACU routine
- Dextrose 5% in 0.45 normal saline at 100 ml/hr
- Morphine via patient-controlled analgesia 1 mg q6min (30 mg max in 4 hr) for pain
- Advance diet as tolerated
- Triflow spirometry qhr × 10

CRITICAL THINKING QUESTIONS

1. What are the potential postanesthetic problems that the nurse might expect with Mr. Gray?
2. What nursing interventions would be appropriate to prevent these complications from occurring?

3. What factors may predispose Mr. Gray to the following problems: atelectasis, infection, pulmonary embolism, nausea and vomiting?
4. How should it be determined when Mr. Gray is sufficiently recovered from general anesthesia to be discharged to the clinical unit?
5. What potential postoperative problems might the nurse on the clinical unit expect?
6. Based on the assessment data presented, write one or more appropriate nursing diagnoses. Are there any collaborative problems?

Nursing Research Issues

1. Does early mobilization of specific patient groups prevent the development of postoperative respiratory complications?
2. What are the unique differences in discharging a patient to home as opposed to a clinical unit?
3. Does the use of written discharge criteria accurately predict patient readiness for discharge?
4. Is patient-controlled intravenous delivery of narcotics more effective in controlling postoperative pain than intramuscular injections of narcotics?
5. Does an early phone call from a nurse during the first week of postoperative discharge reduce the occurrence of hospital readmission and postoperative complications?
6. Do antiembolism/compression stockings assist in the prevention of deep vein thromboses?

REVIEW QUESTIONS

The number of the question corresponds to the same-numbered objective at the beginning of the chapter.

1. As soon as the patient enters the PACU, the priority assessment by the nurse is
   a. urinary output.
   b. ECG monitoring.
   c. level of consciousness.
   d. airway patency and respiratory status.

2. Nursing interventions indicated during the patient's recovery from general anesthesia in the PACU include
   a. placing the patient in a prone position.
   b. encouraging deep breathing and coughing.
   c. restraining patients during episodes of emergence delirium.
   d. withholding analgesics until the patient is discharged from PACU.

REVIEW QUESTIONS—cont'd

3. Postoperative nausea and vomiting presents the greatest risk for
   a. a 14-year-old, 40 kg boy following an orchiopexy under general anesthesia.
   b. an 81-year-old, 55 kg woman following a cystoscopy under local anesthesia.
   c. a 45-year-old, 70 kg man following an arthroscopy under epidural anesthesia.
   d. a 23-year-old, 125 kg woman following a diagnostic laparoscopy under general anesthesia.

4. Following admission of the postoperative patient to the clinical unit, which of the following assessment data requires the most immediate attention?
   a. oxygen saturation of 80%
   b. respiratory rate of 13/min
   c. blood pressure of 90/60 mm Hg
   d. temperature of 94.3° F (34.6° C)

5. A urine output averaging 20 ml/hr for the first postoperative day in a 154-pound patient
   a. is a normal, expected finding.
   b. requires a return to the operating room.
   c. requires an evaluation of the patient's fluid status.
   d. is normal if the patient had genitourinary surgery.

6. In preparation for discharge after surgery, the nurse should advise the patient regarding
   a. a time frame for when various physical activities can be resumed.
   b. the rationale for abstinence from sexual intercourse for 4 to 6 weeks.
   c. the need to call hospital clinical unit to report any abnormal signs or symptoms.
   d. the necessity of a referral to nutritional center for management of dietary restrictions.

REFERENCES

1. Mamaril M: Fast-tracking the postanesthesia patient: the pros and cons, *J Perianesth Nurs* 15:89, 2000.
*2. Apfelbaum J, Grasela T, Walawander C: Bypassing the PACU—a new paradigm in ambulatory surgery, *Anesthesiology* 87:32A, 1997.
3. American Society of PeriAnesthesia Nurses: *Standards of perianesthesia nursing practice,* New Jersey, 2000, The Society.
4. Cummins R: *ACLS provider manual,* Dallas, 2001, American Heart Assn.
5. Haynes C: Emergence delirium: a literature review, *Br J Theatre Nurs* 9:502, 1999.
*6. Shertzer K, Keck J: Music and the PACU environment, *J Perianesth Nurs* 16:90, 2001.
7. Summers S: Evidence-based practice part 2: reliability and validity of selected acute pain instruments, *J Perianesth Nurs* 16:35, 2001.
8. Connor E, Wren K: Detrimental effects of hypothermia: a systems analysis, *J Perianesth Nurs* 15:151, 2000.
*9. Defina J, Lincoln J: Prevalence of inadvertent hypothermia during the perioperative period: a quality assurance and performance improvement study, *J Perianesth Nurs* 13:229, 1998.
10. Burns S: Postanesthesia care revisiting hypothermia: a critical concept, *Crit Care Nurse* 21:83, 2001.
*11. Cory M et al: Constant temperature monitoring: a study of temperature patterns in the postanesthesia care unit, *J Perianesth Nurs* 13:292, 1998.
*12. Gunta K, Lewis C, Nuccio S: Prevention and management of postoperative nausea and vomiting, *Orthop Nurs* 19:39, 2000.
13. Brenner Z: Preventing postoperative complications: what's old, what's new, what's tried-and-true, *Nursing* 29:34, 1999.
14. Dunn D: Preoperative assessment criteria and patient teaching for ambulatory surgery patients, *J Perianesth Nurs* 13:274, 1998.
15. Verhaeghe R, Verstraete M: Prophylaxis of venous thromboembolism in surgery, *ACTA Chir Belg* 97:106, 1997.
*16. Merli G: Low-molecular-weight heparins versus unfractionated heparin in the treatment of deep vein thrombosis and pulmonary embolism, *Am J Phys Med Rehabil* 79(5 suppl):S9, 2000.
17. Ennis D: Reducing the risk of surgical site infection, *Nursing* 29:32hn1, 1999.
18. Summers S: Evidence-based practice part 1: pain definitions, pathophysiologic mechanisms, and theories, *J Perianesth Nurs* 15:357, 2000.
19. Agency for Healthcare Research and Quality: *Practice guidelines for acute pain management in the perioperative setting,* Washington, DC, 2001, US Department of Health and Human Services.
20. Nusbaum NJ: How do geriatric patients recover from surgery? *South Med J* 89:950, 1996.
21. Parikh SS, Chung F: Postoperative delirium in the elderly, *Anesth Analg* 80:1223, 1995.
22. Ferrill B, Stein W, Beck J: The geriatric pain measure: validity, reliability and factor analysis, *J Am Geriatr Soc* 48:1669, 2000.

RESOURCES

American Association of Nurse Anesthetists (AANA)
  222 South Prospect Avenue
  Park Ridge, IL 60068
  847-692-7050
  Fax: 847-692-6968
  www.aana.com/

American College of Surgeons
  633 North St. Clair Street
  Chicago, IL 60611-3211
  312-202-5000
  Fax: 312-202-5001
  www.facs.org/

American Society of Anesthesiologists
  520 North Northwest Highway
  Park Ridge, IL 60068-2573
  847-825-5586
  Fax: 847-825-1692
  www.asahq.org/

American Society of PeriAnesthesia Nurses (ASPAN)
  10 Melrose Avenue, Suite 110
  Cherry Hill, NJ 08003-3696
  877-737-9696
  Fax: 856-616-9601
  www.aspan.org/

Association of periOperative Registered Nurses (AORN)
  2170 South Parker Road, Suite 300
  Denver, CO 80231-5711
  303-755-6300
  800-755-2676
  www.aorn.org

*Nursing research–based references.

Association of Surgical Technologists
7108-C South Alton Way
Englewood, CO 80112
303-694-9130
Fax: 303-694-9169
www.ast.org/

Canadian Anesthetists' Society
1 Eglinton Avenue East, Suite 208
Toronto, ON
M4P 3A1 Canada
416-480-0602
Fax: 416-480-0320
www.cas.ca/

Centers for Disease Control and Prevention; Division of Healthcare Quality Promotion
1600 Clifton Road
Atlanta, GA 30333
404-639-3311
www.cdc.gov/ncidod/hip

National Latex Allergy Network: Latex Allergy Links
http://latexallergylinks.tripod.com

Malignant Hyperthermia Association of the United States
39 East State Street
PO Box 1069
Sherburne, NY 13460-1069
607-674-7901
Fax: 607-674-7910
www.mhaus.org

Operating Room Nurses Association of Canada
www.ornac.ca/

For additional Internet resources, see the website for this book at *http://evolve.elsevier.com/Lewis/medsurg/*.

Problems Related to Altered Sensory Input

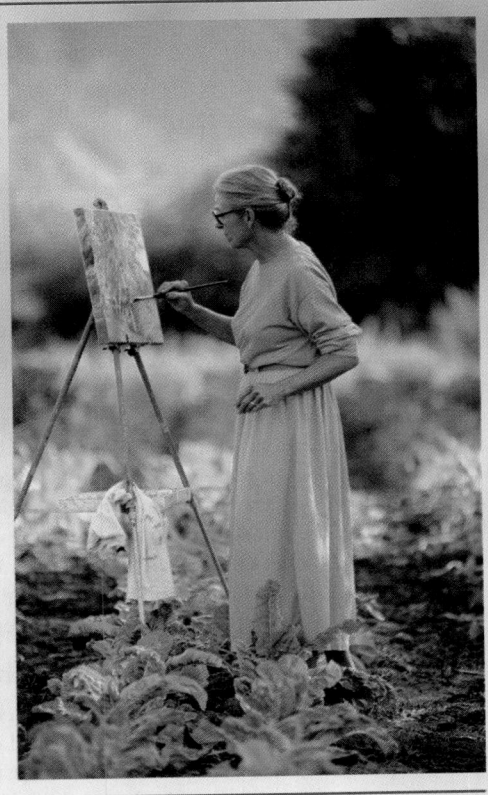

SECTION OUTLINE

CHAPTER *20*

NURSING ASSESSMENT
Visual and Auditory Systems

Sarah C. Smith
Mary E. Wilbur

LEARNING OBJECTIVES

1. Describe the structures and functions of the visual and auditory systems.
2. Describe the physiologic processes involved in normal vision and hearing.
3. Identify the significant subjective and objective assessment data related to the visual and auditory systems that should be obtained from the patient.
4. Describe the appropriate techniques used in the physical assessment of the visual and auditory systems.

5. Differentiate normal from common abnormal findings of a physical assessment of the visual and auditory systems.
6. Describe age-related changes in the visual and auditory systems and differences in assessment findings.
7. Describe the purpose, significance of results, and nursing responsibilities related to diagnostic studies of the visual and auditory systems.

KEY TERMS

aqueous humor, p. 416	presbycusis, p. 431
astigmatism, p. 417	presbyopia, p. 417
conjunctiva, p. 418	refraction, p. 417
hyperopia, p. 417	retina, p. 420
lens, p. 419	sclera, p. 418
myopia, p. 417	tinnitus, p. 431
nystagmus, p. 437	

STRUCTURES AND FUNCTIONS OF THE VISUAL SYSTEM

The visual system consists of the internal and external structures of the eyeball, the refractive media, and the visual pathway. The internal structures are the iris, lens, ciliary body, choroid, and retina. The external structures are the eyebrows, eyelids, eyelashes, lacrimal system, conjunctiva, cornea, sclera, and extraocular muscles. The entire visual system is important for visual function. Light reflected from an object in the field of vision passes through the transparent structures of the eye and, in doing so, is *refracted* (bent) so that a clear image can fall on the retina. From the retina, the visual stimuli travel through the visual pathway to the occipital cortex, where they are perceived as an image.

Structures and Functions of Vision

Eyeball. The eyeball, or globe, is composed of three layers (Fig. 20-1). The tough outer layer is composed of the sclera and the transparent cornea. The middle layer consists of the uveal tract (iris, choroid, and ciliary body), and the innermost layer is the retina. The anterior chamber lies between the iris and the posterior surface of the cornea, whereas the posterior chamber lies

between the anterior surface of the lens and the posterior surface of the iris. These chambers are filled with aqueous humor secreted by the ciliary body (Fig. 20-2). The anatomic space between the posterior lens surface and the retina is filled with the vitreous gel.

Refractive Media. For light to reach the retina, it must pass through a number of structures: the cornea, aqueous humor, lens, and vitreous. Each structure has a different density and plays a role in helping the image fall focused on the retina. All of these structures must remain clear for light to reach the retina and stimulate the photoreceptor cells. The transparent cornea is the first structure through which light passes. It is responsible for the majority of light refraction necessary for clear vision.[1]

Aqueous humor, a clear watery fluid, fills the anterior and posterior chambers of the anterior cavity of the eye. Aqueous humor is produced by the ciliary process and passes through the pupil from the posterior chamber into the anterior chamber (see Fig. 20-2). It drains through the trabecular meshwork located in the angle formed by the cornea and iris and into the canal of Schlemm. This circular canal conveys fluid into scleral veins, which enter the circulation of the body. The aqueous humor bathes and nourishes the lens and the endothelium of the cornea. Excess production or decreased outflow can elevate intraocular pressure above the normal 10 to 21 mm Hg, a condition termed *glaucoma.*

The lens is a biconvex structure located behind the iris and supported in place by small fibers called *zonules.* The primary function of the lens is to bend light rays, allowing the rays to fall onto the retina. The lens shape is modified by action of the ciliary zonules as part of *accommodation,* a process that allows the patient to focus on near objects, such as in reading. Anything altering the clarity of the lens affects light transmission.

Vitreous humor is located in the posterior cavity, the large area behind the lens and in front of the retina (see Fig. 20-1). Light passing through the vitreous may be blocked by any nontransparent substance within the vitreous. The effect on vision varies,

Reviewed by Mary Merchant, RN, MSN, FNP, Care Manager, Medical University of South Carolina Hospital, Department of Outcomes Management and Research, Charleston, S.C.

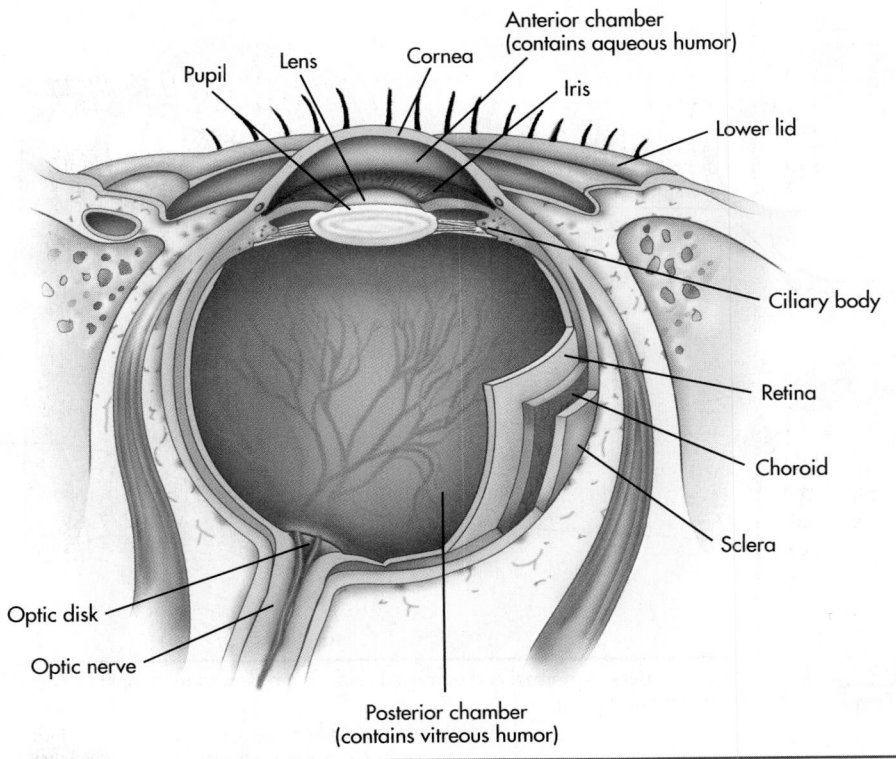

The human eye.

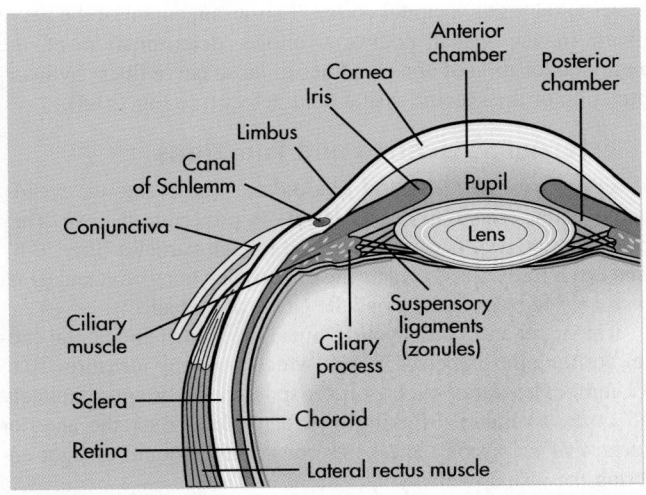

FIG. 20-2 Close-up view of ciliary body, zonules, lens, and anterior and posterior chambers. The aqueous humor flows from the ciliary process, over the anterior lens, and into the anterior chamber through the pupil, where it drains through the canal of Schlemm.

depending on the amount, type, and location of the substance blocking the light. For example, in the case of hemorrhage into the vitreous, little light will reach the retina, and vision will be severely compromised. However, cellular debris that accumulates from normal cell metabolism will cause only a relatively small shadow on the retina ("floater"). The vitreous becomes more liquid with aging.[2]

Refractive Errors. **Refraction** is the ability of the eye to bend light rays so that they fall on the retina. In the normal eye,

parallel light rays are focused through the lens into a sharp image on the retina. This condition is termed *emmetropia* and means that light is focused exactly on the retina, not in front of it or behind it. When the light does not focus properly, it is called a *refractive error.*

The individual with **myopia** can see near objects clearly (nearsightedness), but objects in the distance are blurred. This condition occurs when an image is focused in front of the retina, either because the eye is too long or because there is excessive refracting power (Fig. 20-3, *A*). A concave lens is used to correct the light refraction so that objects seen in the distance are focused clearly on the retina (Fig. 20-3, *B*).

The individual with **hyperopia** can see distant objects clearly (farsightedness), but close objects are blurred. This condition occurs when an image is focused behind the retina, either because the eye is too short or because there is inadequate refracting power (Fig. 20-3, *C*). A convex lens is used to correct the refraction (Fig. 20-3, *D*).

Astigmatism is caused by an unevenness in the corneal or lenticular curvature, causing horizontal and vertical rays to be focused at two different points on the retina, which results in visual distortion. It can be myopic or hyperopic in nature in relation to where the image falls.

Presbyopia is a form of hyperopia, or farsightedness, that occurs as a normal process of aging, usually around age 40. As the lens ages and becomes less elastic, it loses refractive power, and the eye can no longer accommodate for near vision. As with hyperopia, convex lenses are used to correct the light refraction so that the presbyopic individual can see clearly to read and accomplish other near-vision tasks.

Visual Pathways. Once the image travels through the refractive media, it is focused on the retina, inverted, and reversed

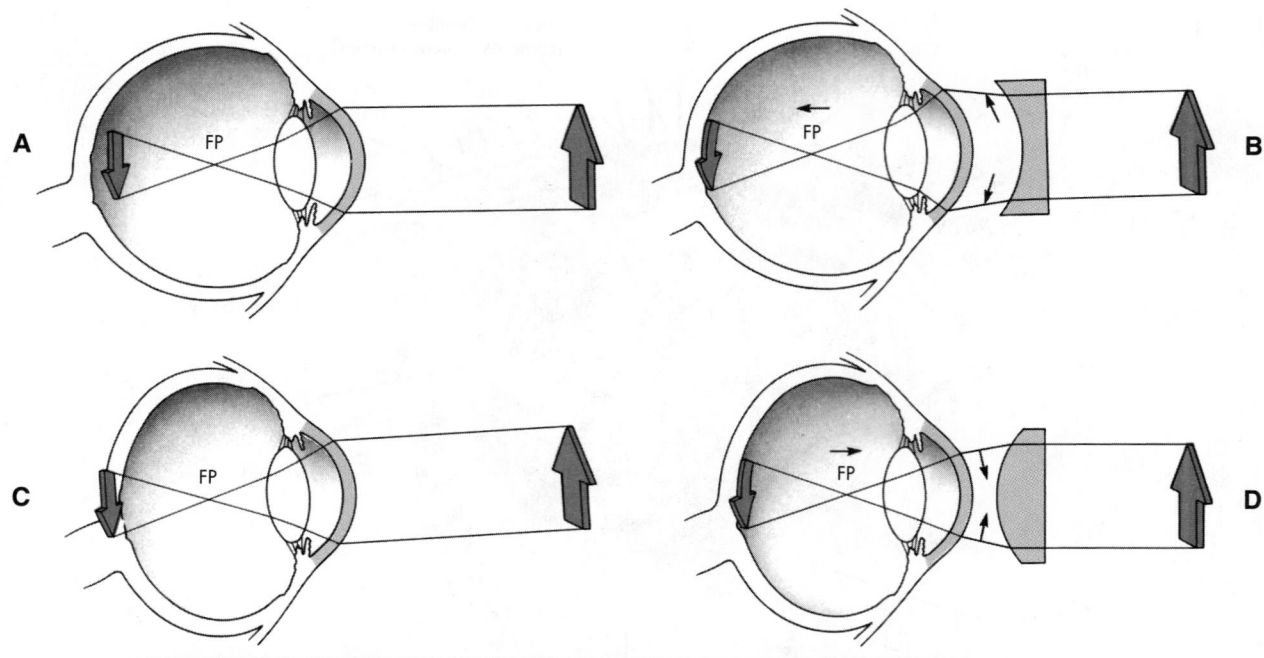

FIG. 20-3   Refraction disorders. Abnormal and corrected refraction observed in myopia (**A** and **B**) and hyperopia (**C** and **D**). *FP,* Focal point.

left to right (Fig. 20-4). For example, if the visualized object is in the upper part of the left temporal visual field, it will be focused in the lower part of the nasal retina, upside down, and as a mirror image. From the retina, the impulses travel through the optic nerve to the optic chiasm where the nasal fibers of each eye cross over to the other side. Fibers from the left field of both eyes form the left optic tract and travel to the left occipital cortex. The fibers from the right field of both eyes form the right optic tract and travel to the right occipital cortex. This arrangement of the nerve fibers in the visual pathways allows determination of the anatomic location of abnormalities in those nerve fibers by interpretation of the specific visual field defect (see Fig. 20-4).

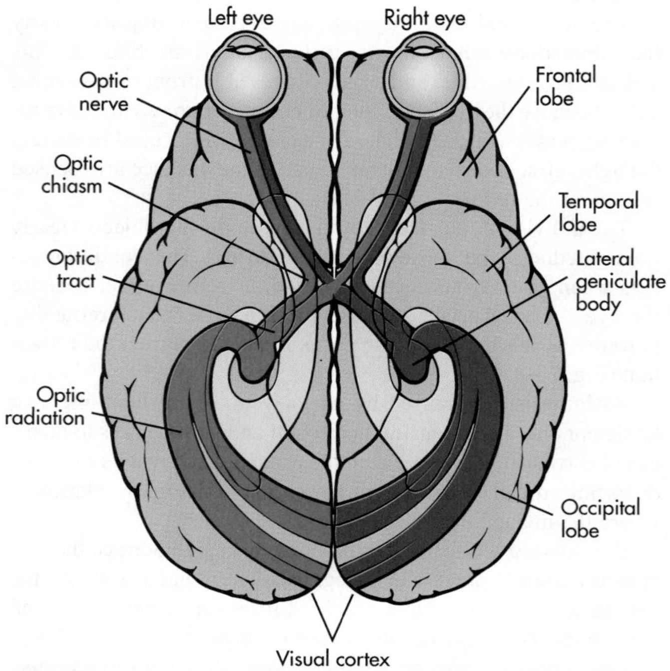

External Structures and Functions

Eyebrows, Eyelids, and Eyelashes. The eyebrows, eyelids, and eyelashes serve an important role in protecting the eye. They provide a physical barrier to dust and foreign particles (Fig. 20-5). The eye is further protected by the surrounding bony orbit and by fat pads located below and behind the globe, or eyeball.

The upper and lower eyelids join at the medial and lateral canthi, forming the palpebral fissure, which normally measures 10 to 12 mm.[3] The upper eyelid blinks spontaneously approximately 15 times a minute. Blinking distributes tears over the anterior surface of the eyeball and helps control the amount of light entering the visual pathway.

The eyelids open and close through the action of muscles innervated by cranial nerve (CN) VII, which is the facial nerve. Muscular action also helps hold the eyelids against the eyeball. Sebaceous glands, located in the eyelids, help form the lipid layer of the tear film.

Conjunctiva. The **conjunctiva** is a transparent mucous membrane that covers the inner surfaces of the eyelids (the palpebral conjunctiva) and also extends over the sclera (bulbar conjunctiva), forming a "pocket" under each eyelid. This structure takes on the pink color of the underlying tissue. The bulbar conjunctiva terminates at the corneal-scleral limbus and contains tiny blood vessels, most visible in the periphery. Glands in the conjunctiva secrete mucus and tears.

Sclera. The **sclera** is composed of collagen fibers meshed together to form an opaque structure commonly referred to as the

FIG. 20-4   The visual pathway. Fibers from the nasal portion of each retina cross over to the opposite side of the optic chiasm, terminating in the lateral geniculate body of the opposite side. Location of a lesion in the visual pathway determines the resulting visual defect.

Labels for Fig. 20-4:
Left eye
Right eye
Optic nerve
Frontal lobe
Optic chiasm
Temporal lobe
Optic tract
Lateral geniculate body
Optic radiation
Occipital lobe
Visual cortex

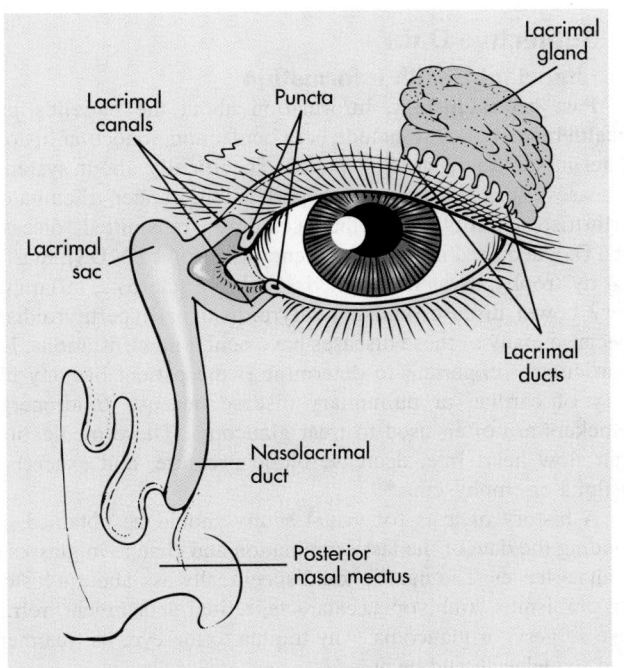

FIG. 20-5 External eye and lacrimal apparatus. Tears produced in the lacrimal gland pass over the surface of the eye and enter the lacrimal canal. From there the tears are carried through the naso-lacrimal duct to the nasal cavity.

"white" of the eye. It makes up the posterior five sixths of the external eye and encircles the globe to join the cornea at the limbus. The sclera forms a tough shell that helps protect the intraocular structures.

Cornea. The transparent and avascular cornea makes up the anterior one sixth of the globe and allows light to enter the eye (see Fig. 20-1). The curved cornea refracts (bends) incoming light rays to help focus them on the retina. It is innervated by the trigeminal nerve (CN V).

The cornea consists of five layers: the epithelium, Bowman's layer, the stroma, Descemet's membrane, and the endothelium. The epithelium consists of a layer of cells that helps protect the eye by serving as a barrier to fluid loss and to the entry of pathogens. The stroma consists of collagen fibrils separated by

the ground substance, which has a unique ability to hold water. The stroma is relatively water free to maintain transparency.

The avascular cornea obtains oxygen primarily through absorption from the tear film layer that bathes the epithelium. A small amount of oxygen is obtained from the aqueous humor through the endothelial layer, which is also responsible for transporting other nutrients into the corneal tissues.

Lacrimal Apparatus. The lacrimal system consists of the lacrimal gland and ducts, lacrimal canals and puncta, lacrimal sac, and nasolacrimal duct. In addition to the lacrimal gland, other glands provide secretions to make up the mucous, aqueous, and lipid layers of the tear film that covers the anterior surface of the globe. The tear film moistens the eye and provides oxygen to the cornea. Lid and globe movements are both involved in spreading tears over the anterior surface of the eye. The tears are drained from the eye through the upper and lower puncta, then through the lacrimal sac, and finally through the nasolacrimal duct into the nose (see Fig. 20-5).

Extraocular Muscles. Each eye is moved by three pairs of extraocular muscles: the superior and inferior rectus muscles, the medial and lateral rectus muscles, and the superior and inferior oblique muscles (Fig. 20-6). Neuromuscular coordination produces simultaneous movement of the eyes in the same direction (conjugate movement).

Internal Structures and Functions

Iris. The iris provides the color of the eye. This structure has a small round opening in its center, the *pupil,* which allows light to enter the eye. The pupil constricts via action of the iris sphincter muscle (innervated by CN III) and dilates via action of the iris dilator muscle (innervated by CN V) to control the amount of light that enters the eye. The constrictor muscle of the iris is stimulated by light falling on the retina and by accommodation. The autonomic nervous system also affects pupil size. Sympathetic stimulation results in contraction of the radial muscle and dilation of the pupil. Parasympathetic stimulation results in contraction of the circular muscle and constriction of the pupil.

Crystalline Lens. The crystalline **lens** is a biconvex, avascular, transparent structure located behind the iris. It is supported by the anterior and posterior ciliary zonules. The lens is composed of thick gelatinous material enclosed in a clear capsule. The primary function of the lens is to bend light rays so that they fall onto the retina. Accommodation occurs when the eye focuses

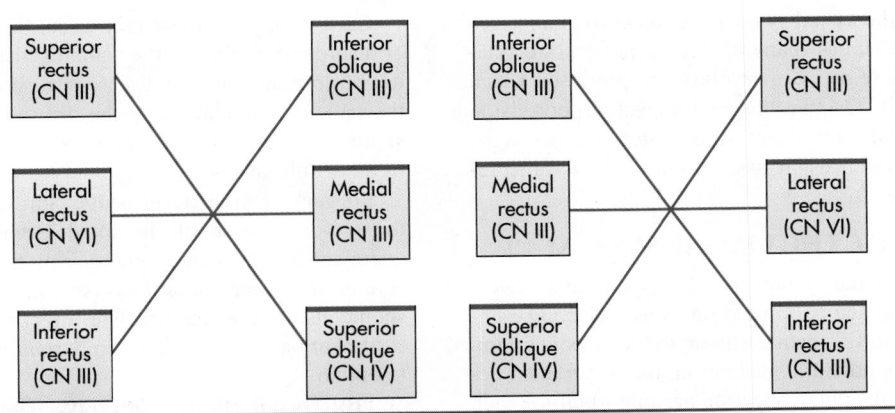

FIG. 20-6 Cardinal fields of gaze with corresponding muscles and nerves.

on a near object and is facilitated by contraction of the ciliary body, which changes the shape of the lens.

Ciliary Body. The ciliary body consists of the ciliary muscles, which surround the lens and lie parallel to the sclera; the ciliary zonules, which attach to the lens capsule; and the ciliary processes, which constitute the terminal portion of the ciliary body. The ciliary processes lie behind the peripheral part of the iris and secrete aqueous humor.

Choroid. The *choroid* is a highly vascular structure that serves to nourish the ciliary body, the iris, and the outer portion of the retina. It lies inside and parallel to the sclera and extends from the area where the optic nerve enters the eye to the ciliary body (see Fig. 20-1).

Retina. The **retina** is the innermost layer of the eye that extends and forms the optic nerve. Neurons make up the major portion of the retina. Therefore retinal cells are unable to regenerate if destroyed. The retina lines the inside of the eyeball, extending from the area of optic nerve to the ciliary body (see Fig. 20-1). It is responsible for converting images into a form the brain can understand and process as vision. The retina is composed of two types of photoreceptor cells: rods and cones. Rods are stimulated in dim or darkened environments, and cones are receptive to colors in bright environments. There are approximately 130 million photoreceptors in each human retina, with rods outnumbering cones by approximately 13:1.[4] The center of the retina is the *fovea centralis,* a pinpoint depression composed only of densely packed cones. This area of the retina provides the sharpest visual acuity. Surrounding the fovea is the *macula,* an area less than 1 square millimeter, which has a high concentration of cones and is relatively free of blood vessels.[5] Nourishment to the macula comes from two sources: the choroid and the underlying pigment epithelium, which is the deepest layer of the retina.

With the exception of the macula, the retina is nourished by retinal arterioles and veins. This blood supply enters the eye through the optic disk, located nasally from the macula. The optic disk is the area where the optic nerve (CN II) exits the eyeball. Within the disk is the physiologic cup, a depression that can be visualized through the pupil with an ophthalmoscope. The retinal veins and arteries can also be visualized in this way and can provide information about the vascular system in general.

■ Gerontologic Considerations: Effects of Aging on the Visual System

Every structure of the visual system is subject to changes as the individual ages. Whereas many of these changes are relatively benign, others may result in severely compromised visual acuity in the older adult. The psychosocial impact of poor vision or blindness can be highly significant. Age-related changes in the visual system and differences in assessment findings are presented in Table 20-1. ■

ASSESSMENT OF THE VISUAL SYSTEM

Assessment of the visual system may be as simple as determining a patient's visual acuity or as complex as collecting complete subjective and objective data pertinent to the visual system. To do an appropriate ophthalmic evaluation, the nurse must determine which parts of the data collection are important for each patient.

Subjective Data
Important Health Information

Past health history. Information about the patient's past health history should include both ocular and nonocular history. The nurse should ask the patient specifically about systemic diseases, such as diabetes, hypertension, cancer, rheumatoid arthritis, syphilis and other sexually transmitted diseases (STDs), acquired immunodeficiency syndrome (AIDS), muscular dystrophy, myasthenia gravis, multiple sclerosis, inflammatory bowel disease, and hypothyroidism or hyperthyroidism, because many of these diseases have ocular manifestations. It is particularly important to determine if the patient has any history of cardiac or pulmonary disease because β-adrenergic blockers are often used to treat glaucoma. These medications can slow heart rate, decrease blood pressure, and exacerbate asthma or emphysema.[6]

A history of tests for visual acuity should be obtained, including the date of the last examination and change in glasses or contact lenses. The nurse should specifically ask about a history of strabismus, amblyopia, cataracts, retinal detachment, refractive surgery, or glaucoma. Any trauma to the eye, its treatment, and sequelae should be noted.

The patient's nonocular history can be significant in assessing or treating the ophthalmic condition. Specifically, the nurse should ask the patient about previous surgeries or treatments related to the head, as well as about previous trauma to the head.

Medications. If the patient takes medication, the nurse should obtain a complete list, including over-the-counter (OTC) medicines, eyedrops, and herbal or "natural" supplements or substances. Many patients do not think OTC drugs, eyedrops, or herbal agents are "real" drugs and may not mention their use unless specifically questioned. However, many of these drugs have ocular effects. For example, many cold preparations contain a form of epinephrine that can dilate the pupil. The nurse should also note the use of any antihistamines or decongestants, because these drugs can cause ocular dryness. The nurse should specifically ask whether the patient uses any prescription drugs such as corticosteroids, thyroid medications, or agents such as oral hypoglycemics and insulin to lower blood glucose levels. Corticosteroid preparations can contribute to the development of glaucoma or cataracts. It is especially important to indicate whether the patient is taking any β-adrenergic blockers, because these can be potentiated by the β-adrenergic blockers used to treat glaucoma.

Each drug the patient uses should correspond with a disease or disorder described in the patient's history. If a medication cannot be correlated with a disease or disorder, the nurse should ask the patient to explain why the drug is used. Finally, the nurse should determine whether the patient has allergies to medications or other substances.

Surgery or other treatments. Surgical procedures related to the eye or brain should be noted. Brain surgery and the subsequent swelling can cause pressure on the optic nerve or tract, resulting in visual alterations. Any laser procedures to the eye should also be documented. The effect of any eye surgery or laser treatment on visual acuity is important information for the nurse to obtain.

Functional Health Patterns. The ophthalmic patient may seek health care for a specific problem or for regular ophthalmic

TABLE 20-1	Gerontologic Differences in Assessment — Visual System	
CHANGES	**DIFFERENCES IN ASSESSMENT FINDINGS**
Eyebrows and Eyelashes	
Loss of pigment in the hair	Graying of eyebrows, eyelashes
Eyelids	
Loss of orbital fat, decreased muscle tone	Entropion, ectropion, mild ptosis
Tissue atrophy, prolapse of fat into eyelid tissue	Blepharodermachalasis (excessive upper lid skin)
Conjunctiva	
Tissue damage related to chronic exposure to ultraviolet light or to other chronic environmental exposure	Pinguecula (small yellowish spot usually on the medial aspect of the conjunctiva)
Sclera	
Lipid deposition	Scleral color yellowish as opposed to bluish
Cornea	
Cholesterol deposits in peripheral cornea	Arcus senilis (milky or yellow ring encircling periphery of cornea)
Tissue damage related to chronic exposure	Pterygium (thickened, triangular bit of pale tissue that extends from the inner canthus of eye to the nasal border of the cornea)
Decrease in water content, atrophy of nerve fibers	Decreased corneal sensitivity
Epithelial changes	Loss of corneal luster
Accumulation of lipid deposits	Blurring of vision
Lacrimal Apparatus	
Decreased tear secretion	Dryness
Malposition of the eyelid resulting in tears overflowing the lid margins instead of draining through the puncta	Tearing, irritated eyes
Iris	
Increased rigidity of iris	Decreased pupil size
Dilator muscle atrophy or weakness	Slower recovery of pupil size after light stimulation
Loss of pigment	Change of iris color
Ciliary muscle becomes smaller, stiffer	Decrease in near vision and accommodation
Lens	
Biochemical changes in lens proteins, oxidative damage, chronic exposure to ultraviolet light	Cataracts
Increased rigidity of lens	Presbyopia
Opacities in the lens (may also be related to opacities in the cornea and vitreous)	Complaints of glare
Accumulation of yellow substances	Yellow color of lens
Retina	
Retinal vascular changes related to atherosclerosis and hypertension	Narrowed, pale, straighter arterioles; acute branching
Decrease in cones	Changes in color perception, especially blue and violet
Loss of photoreceptor cells, retinal pigment, epithelial cells, and melanin	Decreased visual acuity
Age-related macular degeneration as a result of vascular changes	Loss of central vision
Vitreous	
Liquefaction and detachment of the vitreous	Increased complaints of "floaters"

care. When the patient needs routine ophthalmic care, the nurse will focus the assessment of functional patterns on issues related to health promotion. When the patient has a recognized problem, the nurse will direct the assessment to identify those issues related to the patient's specific problem.

Ocular problems do not always affect the patient's visual acuity. For example, patients with blepharitis or diabetic retinopathy may not have any visual deficit. The nurse should be aware that many conditions can cause vision loss. The focus of the functional health pattern assessment depends on the presence or absence of vision loss and whether the loss is permanent or temporary. Table 20-2 lists suggested health history questions to obtain data relating to the functional health patterns.

TABLE 20-2	*H*ealth History **Visual System**

Health Perception–Health Management Pattern ▪ Describe the change in your vision. Describe how this affects your daily life. ▪ Do you wear protective eyewear (sunglasses or safety goggles)?* ▪ Do you wear contact lenses? If so, how do you take care of them? ▪ If you use eyedrops, how do you instill them? ▪ Do you have any allergies that cause eye symptoms? ▪ Do you have a family history of cataracts, glaucoma, or macular degeneration? **Nutritional-Metabolic Pattern** ▪ Do you take any nutritional supplements? ▪ Does your visual problem affect your ability to obtain and prepare food?* **Elimination Pattern** ▪ Do you have to strain to void or defecate?* **Activity-Exercise Pattern** ▪ Are your activities limited in any way by your eye problem?* ▪ Do you participate in any leisure activities that have the potential for eye injury?* **Sleep-Rest Pattern** ▪ Is your vision affected by the amount of sleep you get?*	**Cognitive-Perceptual Pattern** ▪ Does your eye problem affect your ability to read?* ▪ Do you have any eye pain?* Do you have any eye itching, burning, or foreign body sensation?* **Self-Perception–Self-Concept Pattern** ▪ How does your eye problem make you feel about yourself? **Role-Relationship Pattern** ▪ Do you have any problems at work or home because of your eyes?* ▪ Have you made any changes in your social activities because of your eyes? **Sexuality-Reproductive Pattern** ▪ Has your eye problem caused a change in your sex life?* ▪ For women—Are you pregnant? Do you use birth control pills?* **Coping–Stress Tolerance Pattern** ▪ Do you feel able to cope with your eye problem?* ▪ Are you able to acknowledge the effects of your eye problem on your life?* **Value-Belief Pattern** ▪ Do you have any conflicts about the treatment of your eye problem?*

*If yes, describe.

Health perception–health management pattern. The patient's age is pertinent in considering cataracts, macular problems, glaucoma, and other ophthalmic conditions. Men are more likely than women to have color blindness.[7] African Americans and older individuals are at higher risk of damage to the optic nerve from glaucoma.[8]

The ophthalmic patient in a clinic or office setting is often seeking routine eye care or a change in the prescription of eyewear. However, there can be some underlying concern that the patient may not mention or even recognize. The nurse should ask the patient, "Why are you here today?"

The patient's visual health can affect activities at home or at work. It is important to know how the patient perceives the current health problem. As outlined in Table 20-2, the nurse can guide the patient in defining the current problem and how it affects the patient's normal activities. The nurse should also assess the patient's ability to accomplish all necessary self-care, especially any eye care related to the patient's ophthalmic problem.

The nurse should assess the patient's ocular health care activities. The patient may not recognize the importance of eye safety practices such as wearing protective eyewear during potentially hazardous activities or avoiding noxious fumes and other eye irritants. Information about the use of sunglasses in bright light should be obtained. Prolonged exposure to ultraviolet (UV) light can affect the retina. Night driving habits and any problems encountered should be noted. Today, millions of people wear contact lenses, but many do not care for them properly.[9] The type of contact lenses used and the patient's wearing and care habits may provide information for teaching.

Information about allergies should be obtained. Allergies often cause eye symptoms such as itching, burning, watering, drainage, and blurred vision.

Many hereditary systemic diseases (e.g., sickle cell anemia) can significantly affect ocular health. In addition, many refractive errors and other eye problems are hereditary. For these reasons the nurse should obtain a careful family history of both ocular and nonocular diseases. Specifically, the nurse should ask if the patient has a family history of diseases such as atherosclerosis, diabetes, thyroid disease, hypertension, arthritis, or cancer. The nurse should also determine whether the patient has a family history of ocular problems such as cataracts, tumors, glaucoma, refractive errors (especially myopia and hyperopia), or retinal degenerative conditions (e.g., macular degeneration, retinal detachment, retinitis pigmentosa).

Nutritional-metabolic pattern. The patient's intake of antioxidants (vitamins C and E) and trace minerals can be important to ocular health. Adequate intake of vitamins C and E may be beneficial in preventing or delaying retinal damage, and zinc deficiency is linked to erythematous scales in the periorbital area.[10,11]

Elimination pattern. Straining to defecate (Valsalva maneuver) can raise the intraocular pressure. Although there is some evidence that elevating the intraocular pressure by normal activities is not detrimental to the surgical incision made during eye surgery, many surgeons do not want the patient to strain. The nurse should assess the patient's usual pattern of elimination and determine whether there is the potential for constipation in the patient who has had ophthalmic surgical procedures.

Activity-exercise pattern. The patient's usual level of activity or exercise may be affected by reduced vision, by symptoms accompanying an ocular problem, or by activity restrictions following a surgical procedure. For example, a patient with *hyphema* (intraocular bleeding) may be on bed rest or have severely restricted activity. The diabetic patient with lower limb prostheses will have additional ambulation difficulties if diabetic retinopathy with vision loss is present.

The nurse should also inquire about leisure activities during which the patient may incur an ocular injury. For example, gardening, woodworking, and other craft activities can result in corneal or conjunctival foreign bodies or even penetrating injuries of the globe. Injuries to the globe or bony orbit can also occur after blows to the head or eye during sports activities such as racquetball, baseball, and tennis. Cross-country skiers may develop corneal fungal ulcers after an abrasion caused by low-hanging tree limbs. Other leisure activities such as needlepoint, fly tying, or birdwatching may have high-level visual demands and produce eye strain.

Sleep-rest pattern. In the otherwise healthy person, lack of sleep may cause ocular irritation, especially in the patient who wears contact lenses. Normal sleep patterns may be disrupted in the patient with painful eye problems such as corneal abrasions. The patient with alkali burns of the eye requires continuous irrigation of the ocular surface until the pH of the conjunctival sac returns to normal levels.[12] Normal sleep will be disrupted during this time.

Cognitive-perceptual pattern. The entire assessment of the ophthalmic patient focuses on the sense of sight, but it is important not to overlook other cognitive or perceptual problems. For example, the functional ability of a patient with a visual deficit will be further compromised if the patient also has hearing problems. The patient who cannot see to read has increased difficulty in following postoperative instructions if there is also trouble hearing or remembering verbal instructions. The patient who does not understand or read English may require written or verbal instructions and information in the native language.

Eye pain is always an important symptom to assess. Corneal abrasions, iritis, and acute glaucoma manifest with pain and are serious eye problems. Infections and foreign bodies can also cause less severe eye discomfort and are also potentially serious. If eye pain is present, the patient should be questioned about treatment and response.

Self-perception–self-concept pattern. The loss of independence that can follow a partial or complete loss of vision, even if the condition is temporary, can have devastating effects on the patient's self-concept. The nurse should carefully evaluate the potential effect of vision loss on the patient's self-image. For instance, disabling glare from a cataract may prevent nighttime driving or even limit daytime driving, resulting in a diminished self-image. In today's highly mobile society, loss of ability to drive can represent a significant loss of independence and self-esteem. The patient with severe ptosis or other disfiguring ophthalmic conditions may be embarrassed by her or his appearance and suffer from a poor self-image.

Role-relationship pattern. The patient's ability to maintain the necessary or desired roles and responsibilities in the home, work, and social environments can be negatively affected by ocular problems. For example, macular degeneration may decrease the patient's visual acuity to a level inadequate to function at work. Many occupations place workers in conditions in which eye injury may occur. For example, factory workers may be at risk from flying metal debris. Information should be obtained about eye-safety practices, such as the use of goggles or safety glasses. Workers can also be exposed to eye strain in the office from video display terminals, poor lighting, and glare.

The patient with diabetes mellitus may not be able to see well enough to self-administer insulin. This patient may resent the dependence on a family member who takes over this function. The patient with exophthalmos (marked protrusion of eyeballs) may be embarrassed by his or her appearance and avoid usual social activities. The nurse should sensitively inquire if the patient's preferred roles and responsibilities have been affected by the ocular problem.

Sexuality-reproductive pattern. The inactivity that may be associated with low vision, blindness, and certain eye problems and surgeries can negatively affect a patient's sexuality. The patient with severe vision loss may develop such a poor self-image that the ability to be sexually intimate is lost. The nurse can assure the patient that low vision or blindness does not affect a person's ability to be sexually expressive. For many sexually expressive acts, touch is more important than vision.

If a patient with low vision or blindness has a family, assistance with child-rearing tasks may be necessary. The nurse should determine the need and availability of help if this situation is present.

Coping–stress tolerance pattern. The patient with temporary or permanent visual problems will experience emotional stress. The nurse should assess the patient's coping level, coping mechanisms, and availability of social and personal support systems.

The patient with permanent visual loss experiences the usual stages of grief after the loss. The nurse should assess the potential need for psychosocial counseling and eventual vocational rehabilitation.

Value-belief pattern. The nurse must be sensitive to the individual values and spiritual beliefs of each patient, because the patient makes decisions regarding ophthalmic care based on those values and beliefs. It can be difficult to understand why a patient refuses treatment that has potential benefit or wants treatment that may have limited potential benefit. The nurse should assess the patient's value-belief pattern that serves as the basis for making those decisions.

Objective Data

Physical Examination. Physical examination of the visual system includes inspecting the ocular structures and determining the status of their respective functions. Physiologic functional assessment includes determining the patient's visual acuity, determining the patient's ability to judge closeness and distance, assessing extraocular muscle function, evaluating the visual fields, observing pupil function, and measuring the intraocular pressure. Assessment of ocular structures should include examining the ocular adnexa, external eye, and internal structures. Some structures, such as the retina and blood vessels, must be visualized with the aid of ophthalmic observation equipment, such as the ophthalmoscope.

Assessment of the visual system may include all of the following components, or it may be as brief as measuring the patient's visual acuity. The nurse will assess what is appropriate and necessary for the specific patient. All of the following assessments are in the nurse's scope of practice, but some require special training. Normal physical assessment of the visual system is outlined in Table 20-3. Age-related visual changes and differences in assessment findings are listed in Table 20-1. Assessment techniques related to vision are summarized in Table 20-4, and common assessment abnormalities are listed in Table 20-5.

TABLE 20-3	Normal Physical Assessment of the Visual System

Visual acuity 20/20 OU; no diplopia
External eye structures symmetric without lesions or deformities
Lacrimal apparatus nontender without drainage
Conjunctiva clear; sclera white
PERRLA
Lens clear
EOMI
Disk margins sharp
Retinal vessels normal with no hemorrhages or spots

EOMI, Extraocular movements intact; *OU,* both eyes; *PERRLA,* pupils equal, round, reactive to light and accommodation.

Initial observation. The initial observation of the patient can provide information that will help the nurse focus the assessment. When first encountering the patient, the nurse may observe that the patient is dressed in clothing with unusual color combinations. This may indicate a color-vision deficit. The nurse may also note an unusual head position. The patient with diplopia may hold the head in a skewed position in an attempt to see a single image. The patient with a corneal abrasion or photophobia will cover the eyes with the hands to try to block out room light. The nurse can make a crude estimate of depth perception by extending a hand for the patient to shake.

During the initial observation, the nurse should also observe the overall facial and ophthalmic appearance of the patient. The eyes should be symmetric and normally placed on the face. The globes should not have a bulging or sunken appearance.

Assessing functional status

Visual acuity. The nurse should always record the patient's visual acuity for medical and legal reasons. The nurse must document the patient's visual acuity before the patient receives any care.

The patient sits or stands 20 feet (6 meters) from the Snellen chart with the usual correction (glasses or contact lenses) left in place unless they are used solely for reading. The nurse asks the patient to cover the left eye and read the smallest line that the patient can read comfortably. If the patient reads that line with two or fewer errors, the examiner instructs the patient to read the next

TABLE 20-4	Assessment Techniques: Visual System	
TECHNIQUE	**DESCRIPTION**	**PURPOSE**
• Visual acuity testing	Patient reads from Snellen chart at 20 ft (distance vision test) or Jaeger's chart at 14 in (near vision test); examiner notes smallest print patient can read on each chart.	To determine patient's distance and near visual acuity
• Extraocular muscle function testing	Examiner has patient follow a light source or other fixation object through a complete field of gaze; in the cover–uncover test, examiner covers patient's eye and then uncovers it to see if eye has deviated under the cover.	To determine if patient's extraocular muscles are functioning in a normal manner
• Confrontation visual field test	Patient faces examiner, covers one eye, fixates on examiner's face, and counts number of fingers that the examiner brings into patient's field of vision.	To determine if patient has a full field of vision, without obvious scotomas
• Pupil function testing	Examiner shines light into patient's pupil and observes pupillary response; each pupil is examined independently; examiner also checks for consensual and accommodative response.	To determine if patient has normal pupillary response
• Tono-pen tonometry	Covered end of probe is gently touched several times to the anesthesized corneal surface; examiner records several readings to obtain a mean intraocular pressure.	To measure intraocular pressure (normal pressure is 10-22 mm Hg)
• Slit lamp microscopy	Patient is seated with chin placed in chin rest; slit beam illuminates ocular structures; examiner looks through magnifying lens to assess various structures.	To provide magnified view of the conjunctiva, sclera, cornea, anterior chamber, iris, lens, and vitreous
• Ophthalmoscopy	Examiner holds ophthalmoscope close to patient's eye, shining light into back of eye and looking through aperture on ophthalmoscope; examiner adjusts dial to select one of the lenses in ophthalmoscope that produces the desired amount of magnification to inspect ocular fundus.	To provide magnified view of retina and optic nerve head
• Color vision testing	Patient identifies numbers or paths formed by pattern of dots in series of color plates.	To determine patient's ability to distinguish colors
• Stereopsis testing	From a series of plates, patient identifies geometric pattern or figure that appears closer to patient when viewed through special spectacles that provide a three-dimensional view.	To determine patient's ability to see objects in three dimensions; to test depth perception
• Keratometry	Examiner aligns the projection and notes the readings of corneal curvature.	To measure the corneal curvature; often done before fitting contact lenses, before doing refractive surgery, or after corneal transplantation

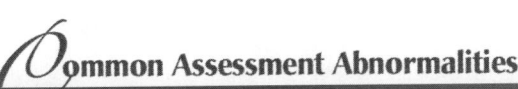

TABLE 20-5 **Common Assessment Abnormalities**

Visual System

FINDING	DESCRIPTION	POSSIBLE ETIOLOGY AND SIGNIFICANCE
Subjective Data		
▪ Pain	Foreign body sensation	Superficial corneal erosion or abrasion; can result from contact lens wear or trauma; conjunctival or corneal foreign body; usually lessened with lid closure
	Severe, deep, throbbing	Anterior uveitis, acute glaucoma, infection; acute glaucoma also associated with nausea, vomiting
▪ Photophobia	Persistent abnormal intolerance to light	Inflammation or infection of cornea or anterior uveal tract (iris and ciliary body)
▪ Blurred vision	Gradual or sudden inability to see clearly	Refractive errors, corneal opacities, cataracts, migraine aura, retinal changes (detachment, macular degeneration), optic neuritis or atrophy, central retinal vein or artery thrombosis, refractive changes related to fluctuations in serum glucose
▪ Scotoma	Blind or partially blind area in the visual field	Disorders of the optic chiasm, glaucoma, central serous chorioretinopathy, age-related macular degeneration, injury, migraine headache
▪ Spots, floaters	Patient describes seeing spots, "spider webs," "curtain," or floaters within the field of vision	Most common cause is vitreous liquefaction (benign phenomenon); other possible causes include hemorrhage into the vitreous humor, retinal holes or tears, impending retinal detachment, vitreous detachment, intraocular hemorrhage, chorioretinitis
▪ Dryness	Discomfort, sandy, gritty, irritation, or burning	Decreased tear formation or changes in tear composition because of aging or various systemic diseases
▪ Halo around lights	Presence of a halo around lights	Refractive changes, corneal edema as a result of a sudden rise in intraocular pressure in angle-closure glaucoma or secondary glaucoma
▪ Glare	Headache, ocular discomfort, reduced visual acuity	Related to corneal inflammation or to opacities in the cornea, lens, or vitreous that scatter the incoming light; can also result from light scatter around edges of an intraocular lens; worse at night when pupil dilated
▪ Diplopia	Double vision	Abnormalities of extraocular muscle action related to muscle or cranial nerve pathology
Objective Data		
Eyelids		
▪ Allergic reactions	Redness, excessive tearing, and itching of lid margins	Many possible allergens; associated eye trauma can occur from rubbing itchy eyelids
▪ Hordeolum (sty)	Small, superficial white nodule along lid margin	Infection of a sebaceous gland of eyelid; causative organism is usually bacterial (most commonly *Staphylococcus aureus*)
▪ Chalazion	Reddened, swollen area on eyelid; involves deeper tissues than hordeolum; can be inflamed and tender	Granuloma formed around a sebaceous gland; occurs as a foreign body reaction to sebum in the tissue; can develop from a hordeolum or from rupture of a sebaceous gland with resulting sebum in the tissue
▪ Blepharitis	Redness, swelling, and crusting along lid margins	Bacterial invasion of lid margins; often chronic
▪ Dacryocystitis	Redness, swelling, and tenderness of medial area of lower lid (in region of lacrimal sac)	Blockage of nasolacrimal duct and subsequent infection
▪ Xanthelasma	Raised, yellowish plaques on eyelids usually on nasal portion	Lipid disorders; may be normal finding
▪ Ptosis	Dropping of upper lid margin, unilateral or bilateral	Mechanical causes as a result of eyelid tumors or excess skin; myogenic causes attributable to condition involving the levator muscle or myoneural junction, such as myasthenia gravis; neurogenic causes affecting third cranial nerve that innervates the levator muscle
▪ Entropion	Inward turning of upper or lower lid margin, unilateral or bilateral	Congenital causes resulting in development abnormalities; involution entropion related to horizontal eyelid laxity; can cause irritation and tearing

Continued

TABLE 20-5   *C*ommon Assessment Abnormalities
Visual System—cont'd

FINDING	DESCRIPTION	POSSIBLE ETIOLOGY AND SIGNIFICANCE
Objective Data—cont'd		
Eyelids—cont'd		
• Ectropion	Outward turning of lower lid margin	Mechanical causes as a result of eyelid tumors, herniated orbital fat, or extravasation of fluid; paralytic ectropion occurs when orbicularis muscle function is disturbed as with Bell's palsy
• Lid lag	Slower or absent closing of one lid	Possible involvement of CN VII
• Blepharospasm	Increased blink rate; when severe spasms occur, inability to open eyelids	Inflammation; involvement of CNs V and VII; can occur as a response to bright lights
• Decreased blink	Decreased rate of eyelid closure	Decreased corneal sensation; possible involvement of CN VII; dry eye and corneal damage may result if blink rate significantly decreased
Conjunctiva		
• Conjunctivitis	Redness, swelling of conjunctiva; may be itchy	Bacterial or viral infection; may be allergic response or inflammatory response to chemical exposure
• Subconjunctival hemorrhage	Appearance of blood spot on sclera; may be small or can affect entire sclera	Conjunctival blood vessels rupture, leaking blood into the subconjunctival space; caused by coughing, sneezing, eye rubbing, or minor trauma; generally requires no treatment
• Pinguecula	Raised area (growth) on conjunctiva; horizontally oriented in medial area of bulbar conjunctiva	Degenerative lesion related to chronic ultraviolet light or other environmental exposure
• Jaundice	Yellowish color of entire sclera	Jaundice related to liver dysfunction; yellow color normal after diagnostic study requiring intravenous fluorescein injection
Cornea		
• Corneal abrasion	Localized painful disruption of the epithelial layer of cornea, can be visualized with fluorescein dye	Trauma; overwear or improper fit of contact lenses
• Corneal opacity	Whitish area of normally transplant cornea; may involve entire cornea	Scar tissue formation related to inflammation; infection, trauma; degree of visual acuity deficit depends on location and size of opacity
• Pterygium	Triangular, horizontally oriented thickening of bulbar conjunctiva that extends past cornea-scleral border onto cornea	Commonly thought to be an extension of a pinguecula; degenerative lesion related to chronic ultraviolet light or other environmental exposure; surgical removal necessary if progression to central cornea
Globe		
• Exophthalmos	Protrusion of globe beyond its normal position within bony orbit; sclera often visible above iris when eyelids are open	Intraocular or periorbital tumors; hyperthyroidism; swelling or tumors of the frontal sinus; dry eye and corneal damage may occur as a result of inability to close eyelid normally
Pupil		
• Mydriasis	Pupil is larger than normal (dilated)	Emotional influences, trauma, acute glaucoma (fixed, mid-dilated), systemic or local drugs, head injury
• Miosis	Pupil is smaller than normal	Iritis, morphine and similar drugs, glaucoma treated with miotic agents
• Anisocoria	Pupils are unequal (constricted)	Central nervous system disorders; slight difference in pupil size is normal in a small percentage of the population
• Dyscoria	Pupil is irregularly shaped	Congenital causes (e.g., iris coloboma); acquired causes (e.g., trauma, iris-fixated intraocular lens implant, posterior synechiae surgery on iris)
• Abnormal response to light or accommodation	Pupils respond asymmetrically or abnormally to light stimulus or accommodation	Central nervous system disorders, general anesthesia, Horner's syndrome (oculosympathetic paralysis)
Iris		
• Heterochromia	Irides are different colors	Congenital causes (Horner's syndrome); acquired causes (chronic iritis, metastatic carcinoma, diffuse iris nevus or melanoma)

CN, Cranial nerve.

TABLE 20-5	*C*ommon Assessment Abnormalities		
	Visual System—cont'd		

FINDING	DESCRIPTION	POSSIBLE ETIOLOGY AND SIGNIFICANCE
Objective Data—cont'd		
Iris—cont'd		
▪ Iridokinesis	Iris appears to shake on movement of eye	Aphakia
Extraocular Muscles		
▪ Strabismus	Deviation of eye position in one or more directions	Overaction or underaction of one or more extraocular muscles; can be congenital or acquired; neuromuscular involvement; CN III, IV, or VI involved
Visual Field Defect		
▪ Peripheral	Partial or complete loss of peripheral vision	Glaucoma; complete or partial interruption of visual pathway; migraine headache
▪ Central	Loss of central vision	Macular disease
Lens		
▪ Cataract	Opacification of lens, pupil can appear cloudy or white when opacity is visible behind pupil opening	Aging, trauma, electrical shock, diabetes, long–term systemic corticosteroid therapy, congenital
▪ Subluxation or dislocation	Edge of lens may be seen through pupil; "setting sun" sign	Trauma, systemic disease (e.g., Marfan syndrome)

lower line. The nurse notes the smallest line the patient can read with two or fewer errors, and records the standard of 20 feet (6 meters) and then the distance in feet on the line of the Snellen chart the patient read successfully. The nurse records the visual acuities using the ophthalmic abbreviations for right eye (*oculus dexter* [OD]), left eye (*oculus sinister* [OS]), and both eyes (*oculus uterque* [OU]). For example, for the patient who reads to the 30-foot (9-meter) line with the right eye, the nurse records the acuity as 20/30 OD. A visual acuity of 20/30 means that from 20 feet (6 meters) away, the patient can read the same letters that the person with normal vision can read from 30 feet (9 meters) away. *Legal blindness* is defined as the best-corrected vision in the better eye of 20/200 or less.[13] The nurse then asks the patient to cover the right eye, and the process is repeated.

If the patient cannot read letters, the examiner can use an eye chart with pictures or numbers. A second option is an eye chart that presents the letter E in four different directions. The examiner asks the patient to point in the direction the E faces.

To evaluate visual acuity when the patient is unable to see the 20/400 letter, the nurse holds up a number of fingers 3 to 5 feet (0.9 to 1.5 meters) in front of the patient and asks the patient to count them. If the patient is unable to count the fingers, the nurse holds up a different number of fingers at successively closer distances up to 1 foot and again asks the patient to count them. The examiner tests the opposite eye in the same manner and records the acuities of each eye. If the patient can count the number of fingers at 2 feet (0.6 meters), the nurse records the acuity as FC or CF ("finger counting" or "counts fingers") at 2 feet (0.6 meters). If the patient cannot count fingers, the nurse asks the patient to indicate if moving the hand is seen in front of the face. This level of visual acuity is HM ("hand motion"). LP ("light projection") is the term for a patient's visual acuity if only light can be seen.

If the patient has a complaint of visual problems with near vision, and for all patients 40 years of age or older, the nurse tests the near visual acuity. The patient is instructed to hold a Jaeger chart 14 inches (35.6 cm) from the eyes. The nurse covers the patient's left eye with the occluder, asks the patient to read successively smaller lines of print from the chart, and records the visual acuity that corresponds to the smallest line of print the patient can read comfortably. The procedure is repeated while covering the right eye. A near acuity of $Jaeger_1$ (J_1) indicates that the patient can read 4-point type at 14 inches (35.6 cm) and is considered normal. A near acuity of J_{10} indicates that the smallest print the patient can read at 14 inches (35.6 cm) is 14-point type and is moderately impaired. Normal newspaper print is 8-point type.

If the nurse must assess visual acuity without access to an eye chart, an accurate assessment is still possible. Examples of other stimuli acceptable for use include newsprint or the label on a container. The examiner records the acuity as "reads newspaper headline at ___ inches."

Extraocular muscle functions. The nurse observes the corneal light reflex to evaluate for weakness or imbalance of the extraocular muscles. In a darkened room, the nurse asks the patient to look straight ahead while a penlight is shone directly on the cornea. The light reflection should be located in the center of both corneas as the patient faces the light source.

Pupil function. Pupil function is determined by inspecting the pupils and their reactions to light. The pupils should be equal in size, round, and react briskly to light. In a small percentage of the population the pupils are unequal in size (anisocoria). The pupils should react to light directly (the pupil constricts when a light shines into the same eye) and consensually (the pupil constricts when a light shines into the opposite eye). The nurse should also check the accommodative response by having the patient fixate on an object held 2 to 3 feet (0.6 to 0.9 meters) away and then bringing the object closer to the patient until the patient is fixating on the object at 6 to 8 inches (15 to 20 cm) away. The pupils should constrict when the patient tries to focus on the near object.

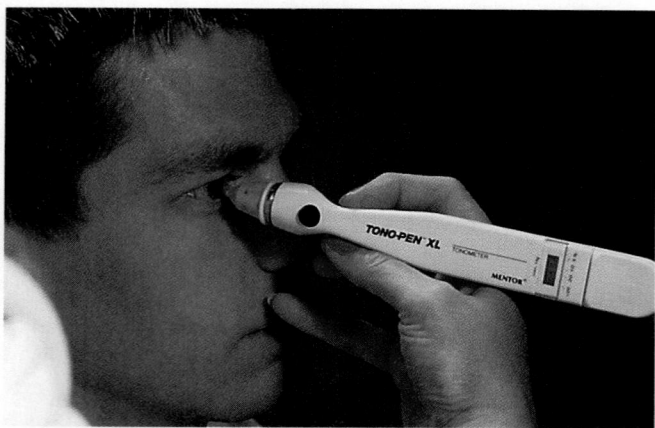

FIG. 20-7 Tono-pen tonometry.

Intraocular pressure. Intraocular pressure can be measured by a variety of methods, including the Tono-pen (Fig. 20-7). The Tono-pen is commonly used because it is simple to use and very accurate. The surface of the anesthetized cornea is touched lightly several times with the covered end of the probe. The instrument records several readings and provides a mean measurement on a digital light-emitting diode (LED) screen located on the front surface. Normal intraocular pressure ranges from 10 to 22 mm Hg.

Assessing structures. The structures that constitute the visual system are assessed primarily by inspection. The visual system is unique because the nurse can directly inspect not only the external structures but also many of the internal structures. The iris, lens, vitreous, retina, and optic nerve can all be visualized directly through the clear cornea and pupil opening.

This direct inspection requires the examiner to use special observation equipment such as the slit lamp microscope and the ophthalmoscope. This equipment permits examination of the conjunctiva, sclera, cornea, anterior chamber, iris, lens, vitreous, and retina under magnification. With the slit lamp microscope, a narrow beam or slit of light is directed onto the eye to brightly illuminate a small section. The patient's chin is positioned in a chin rest to stabilize the head. The *ophthalmoscope* is a handheld instrument with a light source and magnifying lenses that is held close to the patient's eye to visualize the posterior part of the eye. No pain or discomfort is associated with these examinations.

As with other skills, using this equipment requires some special training and practice. However, special equipment provides the means for a thorough ophthalmic assessment that gives the nurse information not only about the ocular structures themselves but also about the patient's systemic condition.

Eyebrows, eyelashes, and eyelids. All structures should be present and symmetric, and without deformities, redness, or swelling. Eyelashes extend outward from the lid margins. The eyelids are positioned symmetrically with the upper and lower eyelids approximately at the corneal-scleral limbus and the lid margins against the globe. In normal closing, the upper and lower eyelid margins just touch. The lacrimal puncta should be open and positioned properly against the globe, with no swelling or redness around the lower puncta indicating lacrimal sac inflammation. If the sac is inflamed, pressure over the lacrimal sac may cause purulent material to ooze from the puncta.

Conjunctiva and sclera. The nurse can easily examine the conjunctiva and sclera at the same time. The examiner evaluates the color, smoothness, and presence of lesions. To examine the palpebral conjunctiva, the examiner places a forefinger over the cheekbone and gently pulls down. This maneuver exposes the palpebral conjunctiva of the lower lid for the nurse to assess color (normally pale pink), texture (normally smooth), and the presence of lesions or foreign bodies. The bulbar conjunctiva covering the sclera is normally clear, with fine blood vessels visible. These blood vessels are more common in the periphery.

The sclera is normally white, but it may take on a yellowish hue in the older individual because of lipid deposition. A pale blue cast caused by scleral thinning can also be normal in the older adult and in the infant (who have naturally thinner scleras). The blue cast is actually the vascular choroid showing through. A slight yellow cast may also be found in some dark-pigmented persons, such as African Americans and Native Americans.

Cornea. The cornea should be clear, transparent, and shiny. The nurse can use either a handheld oblique light or the slit lamp microscope to inspect the anterior chamber. The iris should appear flat and not bulging toward the cornea. The area between the cornea and the iris should be clear with no blood or purulent material visible in the anterior chamber. Because blood and purulent material have a viscosity greater than aqueous humor, they will settle to the lower portion of the chamber, if present.

Iris. Both irides should be of similar color and shape. However, a color difference between the irides occurs normally in a small portion of the population. The iris should be inspected with the upper lid raised. Any area of missing iris will be evident, because the absence of the colored iris tissue leaves what appears to be a dark, abnormally shaped "pupil." Round or notched areas of missing iris tissue are often the result of cataract or glaucoma surgery. The nurse should determine the cause of these areas and document the findings.

Retina and optic nerve. To assess these structures, the nurse uses an ophthalmoscope to magnify the ocular structures and bring them into crisp focus. Blood vessels in the vascular choroid are visible through the retinal tissues, as is the optic disc (where the optic nerve enters the back of the eye). The ability to directly view arteries, veins, and the optic nerve in this manner is unique.

When using the ophthalmoscope, the nurse directs the beam of light obliquely into the patient's pupil. The *red reflex* should be visible. This reflex results from the light reflecting off the pink color of the retina. Any dense areas in the lens, such as a cataract, will decrease the red reflex. The reflex is followed inward until the *fundus,* or back of the eye, comes into view. Both arterioles and veins can be seen. Arterioles are smaller, thinner, and lighter red and reflect light better than veins. The nurse should examine the areas where arterioles and veins cross for nicking or narrowing. These changes are associated with diabetes mellitus and hypertension.

The examiner follows a blood vessel toward the optic nerve. The optic nerve or disk is examined for size, color, and abnormalities. The disk is creamy yellow with distinct margins. A slight blurring of the nasal margin is common.

A central depression in the disk, called the *physiologic cup,* may be seen. This area is the exit site for the optic nerve. The cup should be less than one half the diameter of the disc. The nurse should document the presence of any unusual rings or crescents surrounding the disk.

Normally, no hemorrhages or exudates are present in the fundus (retinal background). Careful inspection of the fundus can reveal the presence of retinal holes, tears, detachments, or lesions. Small hemorrhages can be associated with diabetes or hypertension and can appear in various shapes, such as dots or flames. Finally, the nurse examines the macula for shape and appearance. This area of high reflectivity is devoid of any blood vessels.

The nurse can obtain important information about the vascular system and the central nervous system (CNS) through direct visualization with an ophthalmoscope. Skilled use of this instrument requires practice, and it is not unusual for the nurse to be frustrated initially.

Special Assessment Techniques

Color vision. Testing the patient's ability to distinguish colors can be an important part of the overall assessment because some occupations may require accurate color discrimination. The Ishihara color test determines the patient's ability to distinguish a pattern of color in a series of color plates. In individuals of European ancestry, approximately 6% of males and 0.3% of females have a congenital color vision defect. The incidence of congenital color vision defects in individuals of non-European ancestry is lower.[7] Older adults have a loss of color discrimination at the blue end of the color spectrum and loss of sensitivity throughout the entire spectrum.

Stereopsis. *Stereoscopic vision* allows a patient to see objects in three dimensions. Any event that causes a patient to have monocular vision (e.g., enucleation, patching) results in the loss of stereoscopic vision. When stereopsis is not present, the individual's ability to judge distances is impaired. This disability can have serious consequences if the patient trips over a step when walking or follows too closely behind another vehicle when driving.

DIAGNOSTIC STUDIES OF THE VISUAL SYSTEM

Diagnostic studies provide important information to the nurse in monitoring the patient's condition and planning appropriate interventions. These studies are considered objective data. Table 20-6 presents the most common basic diagnostic studies of the visual system.

TABLE 20-6 Diagnostic Studies / Visual System

STUDY	DESCRIPTION AND PURPOSE	NURSING RESPONSIBILITIES*
• Retinoscopy	Objective (though inexact) measure of refractive error; handheld retinoscopy directs focused light into the eye, refractive error distorts the light, distortion is neutralized to determine refractive error; useful for patient unable to cooperate during process of subjective refraction (e.g., confused patients).	Procedure is painless; may need to help patient hold head still. Pupil dilation will make it difficult to focus on near objects; dilation may last from 3-4 hr.
• Refractometry	Subjective measure of refractive error; multiple lenses are mounted on rotating wheels; patient sits looking through apertures at Snellen acuity chart, lenses are changed; patient chooses lenses that make acuity sharpest; cycloplegic drugs used to paralyze accommodation during refraction process.	Same as retinoscopy.
• Visual field perimetry	Detailed mapping of the visual field; study uses semicircular, bowl-like instrument that presents patient with a light stimulus in various parts of the bowl; specific pattern of visual field loss used to diagnose glaucoma and certain neurologic deficits.	Procedure is painless but may be fatiguing; elderly or debilitated patient may need rest periods; patient must fixate on center target for accurate testing.
• Ultrasonography	A-scan probe is applanated against patient's anesthetized cornea; used primarily for axial length measurement for calculating power of intraocular lens implanted after cataract extraction; B-scan probe is applied to patient's closed lid; used more often than A-scan for diagnosis of ocular pathology such as intraocular foreign bodies or tumors, vitreous opacities, retinal detachments.	Procedure is painless (cornea is anesthetized for A-scan).
• Indirect ophthalmoscopy	Indirect ophthalmoscope is worn on examiner's head; light is projected through a handheld lens into patient's eye; stereoscopic view is larger and provides a better view of peripheral retina; always used when some retinal abnormality is suspected.	Light source is bright; patient may be uncomfortably photophobic, especially because pupil is dilated.
• Fluorescein angiography	Fluorescein (a nonradioactive, noniodine dye) is intravenously injected into antecubital or other peripheral vein, followed by serial photographs (over 10 min period) of the retina through dilated pupils; provides diagnostic information about flow of blood through pigment epithelial and retinal vessels; often used in diabetic patients to accurately locate areas of diabetic retinopathy before laser destruction of neovascularization.	If extravasation occurs, fluorescein is toxic to tissue; systemic allergic reactions are rare, but nurse should be familiar with emergency equipment and procedures; tell patient that dye can sometimes cause transient nausea or vomiting; yellow discoloration of urine and skin is normal and transient.

*Patient education regarding the purpose and method of testing is a nursing responsibility for all diagnostic procedures.

Continued

TABLE 20-6   **Diagnostic Studies**   **Visual System—cont'd**

STUDY	DESCRIPTION AND PURPOSE	NURSING RESPONSIBILITIES*
• Amsler grid test	Test is self-administered using a handheld card printed with a grid of lines (similar to graph paper); patient fixates on center dot and records any abnormalities of the grid lines, such as wavy, missing, or distorted areas; used to monitor macular problems.	Regular testing is necessary to identify any changes in macular function.
• Schirmer tear test	Study measures tear volume produced throughout fixed time period; one end of a strip of filter paper is placed in lower lid cul-de-sac; area of tear saturation is measured after 5 min; useful in diagnosing keratoconjunctivitis sicca.	Test may be done with closed or open eyes.

STRUCTURES AND FUNCTIONS OF THE AUDITORY SYSTEM

The auditory system is composed of the peripheral auditory system and the central auditory system. The peripheral system includes the structures of the ear itself: the external, middle, and inner ear (Fig. 20-8). This system is concerned with the reception and perception of sound. The inner ear functions in hearing and balance. The central system (the brain and its pathways) integrates and assigns meaning to what is heard.

External Ear

The external ear consists of the *auricle,* or pinna, and the external auditory canal. The auricle is composed of cartilage and connective tissue covered with epithelium, which also lines the external auditory canal (see Fig. 20-8). The external auditory canal is a slightly S-shaped tube about 1 inch (2.5 cm) in length in the adult. The skin that lines the canal contains fine hairs and sebaceous (oil) glands and ceruminous (wax) glands. The oil and wax lubricate the ear canal and keep it free from debris and kill bacteria.[14]

Hair is present in the outer half of the canal. The inner half of the ear canal is highly sensitive. The function of the external ear and canal is to collect and transmit sound waves to the *tympanic membrane* (eardrum). This shiny, translucent, pearl-gray membrane is composed of skin, connective tissue, and mucous membrane. It serves as a partition between the external auditory canal and the middle ear.

Middle Ear

Mucous membrane lines the middle ear and is continuous from the nasal pharynx via the eustachian tube. The middle ear cavity is an air space located in the temporal bone. It contains three tiny bones: *malleus, incus,* and *stapes* (called the ossicular chain). Vibrations of the tympanic membrane cause the ossicles to move and transmit sound waves to the oval window. This oval window vibration causes the fluid in the inner ear to move and stimulates the receptors of hearing. The round window covered with mucous membrane also opens into the inner ear and allows for dissipation of the fluid disturbances (round window reflex). The superior part of the middle ear is called the *epitympanum,* or the attic, and also communicates with air cells within the mastoid bone. The air cells are lined with the same mucous membrane as the middle ear.

The middle ear cavity is filled with air. Equalization of atmospheric air pressure is accomplished by the eustachian tube opening during yawning or swallowing. Blockage of the tube can occur with allergies, nasopharyngeal infections, and enlarged adenoids. The facial nerve (CN VII) traverses above the oval window of the middle ear. The thin, bony covering of the facial nerve can become damaged by chronic ear infection, skull fracture, or trauma during ear surgery. Problems may result related to voluntary facial movements, eyelid closure, and taste discrimination.

The external and middle portions of the ear function to conduct and amplify sound waves from the environment. This portion of sound conduction is termed *air conduction.* Problems in these two parts of the ear may cause conductive hearing loss, resulting in an alteration in the patient's perception or sensitivity to sounds.

Inner Ear

The middle ear interfaces with the inner ear where the stapes meets the oval window. The inner ear is composed of the bony labyrinth and the membranous labyrinth and contains the functional organs for hearing and balance. The receptor organ for hearing is the *cochlea,* a coiled structure. It contains the *organ of Corti,* whose tiny hair cells respond to stimulation of selected portions of the basilar membrane according to pitch. This mechanical stimulus is converted into an electrochemical impulse and then transmitted by the acoustic portion of the vestibulocochlear nerve (CN VIII) to the brain to process and interpret sound.

Three semicircular canals and two sacs, the utricle and saccule, make up the organ of balance. These structures make up the membranous labyrinth, which is housed in a bony labyrinth. The membranous labyrinth is filled with endolymphatic fluid, and the bony labyrinth is filled with perilymphatic fluid. The perilymphatic fluid cushions these two sensitive organs and communicates with the brain and the subarachnoid spaces of the brain. The nervous stimuli are communicated by the vestibular portion of CN VIII.

Pathology of the inner ear or along the nerve pathway from the inner ear to the brain can result in *sensorineural hearing loss.* This may result in an alteration of the patient's perception or sensitivity to high-pitched tones. These may be experienced as a decrease in intensity, muffling of the intensity (increased sensitivity to loud sounds), or decrease in ability to understand spoken words (distortion). Problems within the central auditory system from the cochlear nuclei to the cortex cause *central hearing loss.* This type of hearing loss causes difficulty in understanding the meaning of the words heard. (Types of hearing loss are discussed in Chapter 21.)

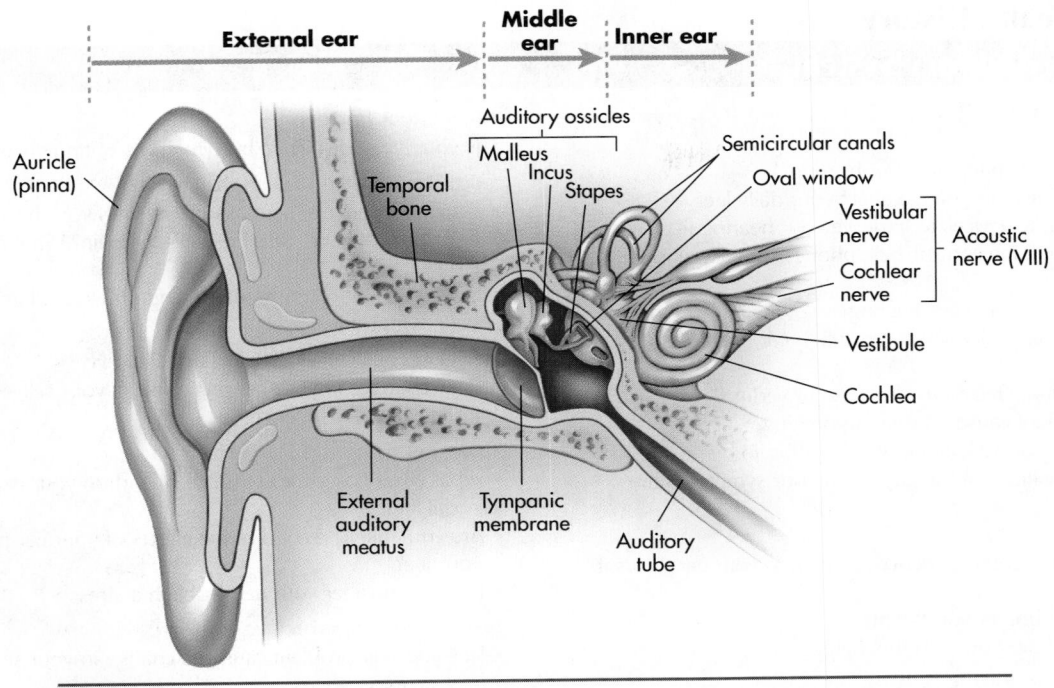

FIG. 20-8   External, middle, and inner ear.

Transmission of Sound. Sound waves are conducted by air and picked up by the auricles and auditory canal. The tympanic membrane is struck by the sound waves, causing it to vibrate. The central area of the tympanic membrane is connected to the malleus, which also starts to vibrate, transmitting the vibration to the incus and then the stapes. As the stapes moves back and forth, it pushes the membrane of the oval window in and out. Movement of the oval window produces waves in the perilymph.

Once sound has been transmitted to the liquid medium of the inner ear, the vibration is picked up by the tiny sensory hair cells of the cochlea, which initiate nerve impulses. These impulses are carried by nerve fibers to the main branch of the acoustic portion of CN VIII and then to the brain.[15]

■ Gerontologic Considerations: Effects of Aging on the Auditory System

Age-related changes of the auditory system can result in impaired hearing. **Presbycusis,** or hearing loss due to aging, has no clear-cut cause; however, several different variables in addition to aging are thought to be involved. The auditory system may encounter insults from a variety of sources, including noise exposure, vascular or systemic diseases, nutrition, ototoxic drugs, and pollution during the life span. **Tinnitus,** or ringing in the ears, may accompany the hearing loss that results from the aging process. Hearing loss, especially in the older adult, can have serious implications for the quality of life, including progressive physical and psychosocial dysfunction.[16] As the average life span increases, the number of people with hearing loss will also increase. Early identification of problems will ensure a more active and healthy patient population in their seventh and eighth decades.

Age-related changes in the auditory system and differences in assessment findings are presented in Table 20-7. ■

TABLE 20-7   *Gerontologic Differences in Assessment*   **Auditory System**

CHANGES	DIFFERENCES IN ASSESSMENT FINDINGS
External Ear	
Increased production of and drier cerumen	Impacted cerumen; potential hearing loss
Increased hair growth	Visible hair
Loss of elasticity in cartilage	Collapsed ear canal
Middle Ear	
Atrophic changes of tympanic membrane	Conductive hearing loss
Inner Ear	
Hair cell degeneration, neuron degeneration in auditory nerve and central pathways, reduced blood supply to cochlea	Presbycusis, diminished sensitivity to high-pitched sounds, impaired speech reception, tinnitus
Less effective vestibular apparatus in semicircular canals	Alterations in balance and body orientation

ASSESSMENT OF THE AUDITORY SYSTEM

Assessment of the auditory system includes assessment of the *vestibular* (balance) system because the auditory and vestibular systems are so closely related. It is often difficult to separate symptoms from the two systems. The nurse must help the patient describe symptoms and problems in order to differentiate the source of the problems. Health history questions to ask a patient with an auditory problem are listed in Table 20-8.

TABLE 20-8   Health History

Auditory System

Health Perception–Health Management Pattern

Hearing
- Have you had a change in your hearing?*
- If yes, how does this change affect your daily life?
- Do you use any devices to improve your hearing (e.g., hearing aid, special volume control, headphones for television or stereo)?*
- How do you protect your hearing?
- Do you have any allergies that result in ear problems?*

Balance
- Is your walking affected by dizziness or vertigo?*
- Does movement cause nausea or vomiting?
- Can you drive or walk alone? If no, elaborate.
- Are there any times of the day when your symptoms are worse?*

Tinnitus
- How long have you experienced ringing in your ears? Has it changed?
- When does it bother you the most?
- What things have you tried that help?

Nutritional-Metabolic Pattern
- Do you have any food allergies that affect your ears?*
- Do you notice any differences in symptoms with changes in diet?*

Elimination Pattern
- Does straining during a bowel movement cause you ear pain?*
- Does your ear problem cause nausea that interferes with your food intake?*
- Does chewing or swallowing cause you any ear discomfort?

Activity-Exercise Pattern
- Does your ear problem result in any change in your usual activity or exercise?*
- Do you need help with certain activities (lifting, bending, climbing stairs, driving, speaking) because of symptoms?*
- Do you have any limitations in activities of daily living because of your symptoms?*

Sleep-Rest Pattern
- Is your sleep disturbed by symptoms of tinnitus or dizziness?*

Cognitive-Perceptual Pattern
- Do you experience pain associated with your hearing or balance problem?* What relieves the pain? What makes it worse?
- Is your ability to communicate and understand affected by your symptoms?*

Self-Perception–Self-Concept Pattern
- Have changes in your hearing affected your self-esteem or feeling of independence?*

Role-Relationship Pattern
- What effect has your ear problem had on your work, family, or social life?
- Are you able to recognize the effects of your ear problems on your life?*
- Do you consider your ear problem a stressor?*

Sexuality-Reproductive Pattern
- Has your ear problem caused a change in your sex life?*

Coping–Stress Tolerance Pattern
- What coping mechanism do you use during time of exacerbation of symptoms?
- Do you feel able to cope with your hearing or balance problem? If no, describe.

Value-Belief Pattern
- Do you have a conflict between your planned treatment and your value-belief system?*

*If yes, describe.

Initially the nurse should try to categorize symptoms related to dizziness and vertigo and separate them from symptoms related to hearing loss or tinnitus. The symptoms can be combined later in the assessment to help make the diagnosis and plan for the patient.

Subjective Data

Important Health Information

Past health history. Many problems related to the ear are sequelae of childhood illnesses or result from problems of adjacent organs. Consequently a careful assessment of past health problems is important.

The patient should be questioned about previous problems regarding the ears, especially problems experienced during childhood. The frequency of acute middle ear infections (otitis media); surgical procedures (e.g., myringotomy); perforations of the eardrum; drainage; complications; and history of mumps, measles, or scarlet fever should be recorded. Congenital hearing loss can result from infectious diseases (rubella, influenza, or syphilis), teratogenic

medications, or hypoxia in the first trimester of pregnancy. Since a safe and effective rubella vaccine was developed in 1969, reported cases of deafness due to rubella have dropped to 1%.[17]

Symptoms such as dizziness, tinnitus, and hearing loss are recorded in the patient's words. It may be difficult for the patient to describe the dizziness. However, it is important that the patient describe the dizziness in detail using her or his own words. This careful description could help differentiate the cause.

Medications. Information about present or past medications that are *ototoxic* (cause damage to CN VIII) and can produce hearing loss, tinnitus, and vertigo should be obtained. The amount and frequency of aspirin use are important because tinnitus can result from high aspirin intake. Aminoglycosides, other antibiotics, salicylates, antimalarial agents, chemotherapeutic drugs, diuretics, and nonsteroidal antiinflammatory drugs (NSAIDs) are groups of drugs that are potentially ototoxic.[18] Careful monitoring is essential. Many drugs produce hearing loss that may be reversible if treatment is stopped.

Surgery or other treatments. Information regarding previous hospitalizations for ear surgery, as well as for tonsillectomy and adenoidectomy, should be obtained. History of a head injury should also be documented because a head injury may result in hearing loss. Use of and satisfaction with a hearing aid should be documented. Problems with impacted cerumen should also be noted.

Functional Health Patterns. Hearing and balance problems can affect all aspects of a person's life. To assess the impact of hearing loss, health history questions can be asked based on a functional health pattern approach (see Table 20-8).

Health perception–health management pattern. The nurse should note the onset of hearing loss, whether sudden or gradual. It should be recorded who noted the onset, whether it be the patient, family, or significant others. Gradual hearing losses are most often noted by those who communicate with the patient. Sudden losses and those exacerbated by some other condition are most often reported by the patient.

Information about allergies is important because they can cause the eustachian tube to become edematous and prevent aeration of the middle ear. Information regarding family members with hearing loss and type of hearing loss is important. Some congenital hearing loss is hereditary. The age of onset of presbycusis also follows a familial pattern.

The patient should be questioned about personal practices used to preserve hearing. The use of protective ear covers or earplugs is good practice for persons in high-noise environments. If the patient is a swimmer, the frequency and duration of swimming and use of ear protection should be documented. It is also important to note the type of water (pool, lake, or ocean) in which the swimming takes place.

Nutritional-metabolic pattern. Both alcohol and sodium affect the amount of endolymph in the inner ear system. Patients with Meniere's disease generally notice some improvement in their symptoms with alcohol restriction and a low-sodium diet. Improvements and exacerbations associated with food intake should be noted. The patient should also be questioned about any ear pain or discomfort associated with chewing or swallowing that might decrease nutritional intake. This situation is often associated with a problem in the middle ear.

Elimination pattern. Elimination patterns and their association with ear problems are mainly of interest in the patient with perilymph fistula or the patient who is immediately postoperative. If the patient experiences frequent constipation or straining with bowel or bladder elimination, this may interfere with healing of a perilymph fistula or its repair. The post-stapedectomy patient especially needs to prevent the increased intracranial (and consequent inner ear) pressure associated with straining during bowel movements. Stool softeners may be ordered postoperatively for the patient who reports chronic problems with constipation.

Activity-exercise pattern. Activity-exercise review is most important when assessing the patient with vestibular problems. The patient should be questioned specifically about activities that relieve or exacerbate symptoms of dizziness or cause nausea or vomiting. If dizziness is a problem, the patient should be questioned about the onset, duration, frequency, and precipitating factors of this symptom. The patient with chronic vertigo syndrome (benign paroxysmal positional vertigo [BPPV]) notes that the symptoms improve throughout the day as adjustment to the visual and positional input from the environment occurs.

In contrast, patients with Ménière syndrome demonstrate increasing inability to compensate for environmental input as the day progresses. Symptoms are experienced particularly in the evening. The nurse and the patient should identify a list of activities and exercises that affect dizziness and vertigo. The patient may use habituation exercises to help control the symptoms. Habituation exercises involve frequent repetition of an activity that causes symptoms until the body adjusts and the activity is no longer a problem.

Sleep-rest pattern. The patient with chronic tinnitus should be questioned about sleep problems. Tinnitus can disturb sleep and activities conducted in a quiet environment. If a sleep problem is associated with tinnitus, the patient should be asked if any masking devices or techniques are used or have been tried to drown out the tinnitus.

Cognitive-perceptual pattern. Pain is associated with some ear problems, particularly those involving the middle ear. If pain is present, the patient should be asked to describe the pain and the treatments used for relief. The effect on the pain level when the ear is moved should be noted.

Hearing loss is associated with many middle and inner ear problems. The nurse or family may report the patient's decreased hearing, or the patient may express concern about perceived hearing loss. If decreased hearing is noted, the patient and family should be questioned about the duration, severity, and circumstances associated with the decreased hearing.

Self-perception–self-concept pattern. The patient should be asked to describe how the ear problem has affected personal life and feelings about himself or herself. Hearing loss and chronic vertigo are particularly distressing for the patient. Hearing loss can result in embarrassing social situations that cause the patient to have a diminished self-concept. The nurse should sensitively question the patient about the occurrence of such situations.

The patient with chronic vertigo may at times be accused of alcohol intoxication. The patient should be asked if this has happened and how the situation was handled.

Role-relationship pattern. The patient should be questioned about the effect the ear problem has had on family life, work responsibilities, and social relationships. Hearing loss can result in strained family relations and misunderstandings. Failure to acknowledge hearing loss and failure to seek treatment can further hinder family relationships.

The patient should be questioned regarding employment or contact with environments that have excessive noise levels, such as work with jet engines and machinery, contact with the firing of firearms, and electronically amplified music. The use of preventive devices worn in noisy environments is important to document.

Many jobs rely on the ability to hear accurately and respond appropriately. If a hearing loss is present, the nurse should gather detailed information of the effect this has on the patient's job. The patient should be assisted to realistically evaluate the job situation.

Hearing loss often leaves the patient feeling isolated from valued social relationships. The nurse should gather information about social activities such as playing cards, going to movies, and attending church from before and since the hearing loss occurred. Comparison of the frequency and enjoyment of the events can indicate if a problem is present.

The unpredictability of vertigo attacks can have devastating effects on all aspects of a patient's life. Ordinary activities such as driving, child care, housework, climbing stairs, and cooking all have an element of danger. The patient should be asked to describe the effect of the vertigo on the many roles and responsibilities of life. Compensatory practices to avoid the development of dangerous situations should also be noted.

Sexuality-reproductive pattern. It should be determined if hearing loss or deafness has interfered with the establishment of a satisfactory sex life. Although intimacy does not depend on the ability to hear, it could interfere with establishing a relationship that could develop into a sexual relationship or maintaining a current relationship.

Coping–stress tolerance pattern. The patient should be asked to report the usual coping style, tolerance for stress, stress-reducing behaviors, and available support. This information enables the nurse to determine if the patient's resources are adequate to meet the demands imposed by the ear problem. If the nurse concludes that the patient seems unable to manage the situation, outside intervention may be required. Denial is a common response to a hearing problem and should be assessed.

Value-belief pattern. The patient should be questioned about any conflicts produced by the problem or treatment related to values or beliefs. Every effort should be made to resolve the problem so the patient does not experience additional stress.

Objective Data

Physical Examination. The nurse can collect valuable objective data regarding the patient's ability to hear during the health-history interview. Clues such as posturing of the head and appropriateness of responses should be noted. Does the patient ask to have certain words repeated? Does the patient intently watch the examiner but miss comments when not looking at the examiner? Such observations are significant and should be recorded. This is also important because the patient is often unaware of hearing loss or does not admit to changes in hearing until moderate losses have occurred. A normal assessment of the ear is listed in Table 20-9. Age-related changes of the auditory system and differences in assessment findings are listed in Table 20-7.

External ear. The external ear is inspected and palpated before examination of the external canal and tympanum. The auricle, preauricular area, and mastoid area are observed for symmetry of both ears, color of skin, nodules, swelling, redness, and lesions. The auricle and mastoid areas are then palpated for tenderness and nodules. Grasping the auricle may elicit pain, especially if inflammation of the external ear or canal is present.

External auditory canal and tympanum. Before inserting an otoscope, the nurse should inspect the canal opening for patency,

palpate the tragus, and move the ear about to check for discomfort. After inspecting the canal opening for patency, an otoscopic examination is performed. A speculum slightly smaller than the size of the ear canal is selected. The patient's head is tipped to the opposite shoulder. The top of the auricle is grasped and gently pulled up and back in adults and horizontally backward in children to straighten the canal. The otoscope, held in the examiner's hand and stabilized on the patient's head by the fingers, is inserted slowly (Fig. 20-9). The canal is observed for size and shape and the color, amount, and type of cerumen. If a large amount of cerumen is present, the tympanum may not be visible. The tympanum is observed for color, landmarks, contour, and intactness (Fig. 20-10).

The tympanic membrane separates the external ear from the middle ear. It is pearl gray, white, or pink; shiny; and translu-

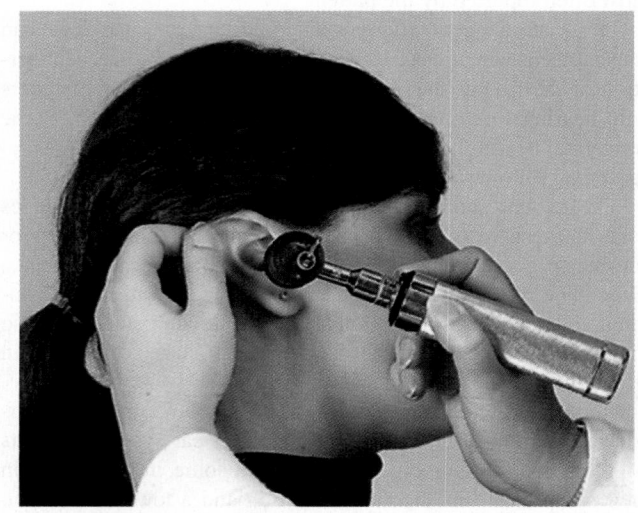

FIG. 20-9 Otoscopic examination of the adult ear. Auricle is pulled up and back. The hand holding the otoscope is braced against the face for stabilization.

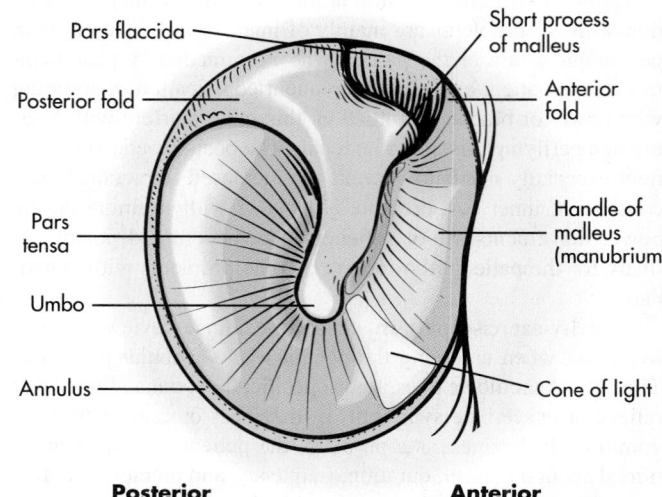

FIG. 20-10 Normal landmarks of the right tympanic membrane as seen through an otoscope.

TABLE 20-9	**Normal Physical Assessment of the Auditory System**

Ears symmetric in location and shape
Auricles and tragus nontender, without lesions
Canal clear, tympanic membrane intact, landmarks and light
   reflex intact
Able to hear low whisper at 30 cm; Rinne test results AC > BC;
   Weber's test results, no lateralization

AC, Air conduction; *BC,* bone conduction.

TABLE 20-10	Common Assessment Abnormalities — Auditory System	
FINDING	**DESCRIPTION**	**POSSIBLE ETIOLOGY AND SIGNIFICANCE**
External Ear and Canal		
• Sebaceous cyst behind ear	Usually within skin, possible presence of black dot (opening to sebaceous gland)	Removal or incision and drainage if painful
• Tophi	Hard nodules in the helix or antihelix consisting of uric acid crystals	Associated with gout, metabolic disorder; further diagnosis needed
• Impacted cerumen	Wax that has not normally been excreted from the ear; no visualization of eardrum	Decreased hearing possible, sensation of fullness in auditory canal, removal necessary before otoscopic examination
• Discharge in canal	Infection of external ear, usually painful	Swimmer's ear, infection of external ear; possibly caused by ruptured eardrum and otitis media
• Swelling of pinna, pain	Infection of glands of skin, hematoma caused by trauma	Aspiration (for hematoma)
• Scaling or lesions	Change in usual appearance of skin	Seborrheic dermatitis, squamous cell carcinoma, atrophic dermatitis
• Exostosis	Bony growth extending into canal causing narrowing of canal	Possible interference with visualization of tympanum, usually asymptomatic
Tympanum		
• Retracted eardrum	Appearance of shorter, more horizontal malleus; absent or bent cone of light	Vacuum in middle ear, blockage of eustachian tube, negative pressure in middle ear
• Hairline fluid level, yellow-amber bubbles above fluid level	Caused by transudate of blood and serum, meniscus of fluid producing hairline appearance	Serous otitis media
• Bulging red or blue eardrum, lack of landmarks	Fluid-filled middle ear, pus, blood	Acute otitis media, perforation possible
• Perforation of eardrum (central or marginal)	Previous perforations of the eardrum that have failed to heal; thin, transparent layer of epithelium surrounding eardrum	Chronic otitis media
• Recruitment	Disproportionate loudness of sound from malfunction of inner ear	Hearing aid difficult to use

cent. The anteroinferior quadrant is situated obliquely in the ear canal and is farthest from the examiner. The major landmarks are formed by the short process of the malleus superiorly; the handle, or *manubrium;* and the *umbo,* the most depressed point of the concave tympanum. From the innermost part of the tympanum a light reflex or cone of light is formed with the point directed toward the umbo. The circumference of the tympanum is thickened into a dense, whitish, fibrous ring, or annulus, except in the superior area. The tympanum within the annulus is taut and is called the *pars tensa.* Above the short process of the malleus is the *pars flaccida,* the flaccid part of the tympanum. The malleolar folds are anterior and posterior to the short process of the malleus. The middle and inner ear cannot be examined with the otoscope because of the tympanic membrane. Table 20-10 summarizes common assessment abnormalities of the auditory system.

DIAGNOSTIC STUDIES OF THE AUDITORY SYSTEM

Table 20-11 describes diagnostic studies commonly used to assess the auditory system.

Tests for Hearing Acuity

Tests involving the whispered and spoken voice can provide gross screening information about the patient's ability to hear. Audiometric testing provides more detailed information that can be used for diagnosis and treatment.

In the whispered test the examiner stands 12 to 24 inches (30 to 61 cm) to the side of the patient and, after exhaling, speaks using a low whisper. A louder whisper is used if the patient does not respond correctly. Spoken voice, increasing in loudness, is similarly used. The patient is asked to repeat numbers or words or answer questions. Each ear is tested. The ear not being tested is masked with the patient occluding the ear or with the examiner moving a finger rapidly, close to the ear canal.

In another test a ticking watch is placed 0.5 to 2 inches (1.3 to 5 cm) from the ear being tested, and the opposite ear is masked. The patient with normal hearing should be able to hear the ticking. However, with the popularity of quartz movement watches, ticking watches are harder to find and the variation among watches makes this test a difficult one for assessing hearing acuity. The patient with sensorineural loss may not be able to hear the high-pitched tones of a ticking watch.

TABLE 20-11 **Diagnostic Studies**
Auditory System

STUDY	DESCRIPTION AND PURPOSE	NURSING RESPONSIBILITIES
Auditory		
• Pure-tone audiometry	Sounds are presented through earphones in soundproof room. Patient responds nonverbally when sound is heard. Response is recorded on an audiogram. Purpose is to determine hearing range of patient in terms of dB and Hz for diagnosing conductive and sensorineural hearing loss. Tinnitus can cause inconsistent results.	Nurse does not usually participate in examination.
• Bone conduction	Tuning fork is placed on mastoid process, and hearing by bone conduction is recorded. Diagnoses conductive hearing loss.	
• One-syllable and two-syllable word lists	Words are presented and recorded at comfortable level of hearing to determine percentage correct and word understanding.	
• Auditory evoked potential (AEP)	Procedure is similar to electroencephalogram (see Chapter 54 and Table 54-8). Electrodes are attached to patient in a darkened room. Electrodes are placed typically at the vertex, mastoid process, or earlobes and forehead. A computer is used to isolate the auditory from other electrical activity of the brain.	Explain procedure to patient. Do not leave patient alone in the darkened room.
• Electrocochleography	Test is useful for uncooperative patient or patient who cannot volunteer useful information. Test records electrical activity in the cochlea and auditory nerve.	
• Auditory brainstem response (ABR)	Study measures electrical peaks along auditory pathway of inner ear to brain and provides diagnostic information related to acoustical neuromas, brainstem problems, and stroke.	
Vestibular		
• Caloric test stimulus	Endolymph of the semicircular canals is stimulated by irrigation of cold (68° F [20° C]) or warm (97° F [36° C]) solution into ear. Patient is seated or in supine position. Observation of type of nystagmus, nausea and vomiting, falling, or vertigo produced is helpful in diagnosing disease of labyrinth. Decreased function is indicated by decreased response and indicates disease of vestibular system. Other ear is tested similarly and results are compared.	Observe patient for vomiting, assist if necessary. Ensure patient safety.
• Electronystagmography (ENG)	Electrodes are placed near patient's eyes and movement of eyes (nystagmus) is recorded on graph during specific eye movements and when ear is irrigated. Study diagnoses diseases of vestibular system.	
• Posturography	Balance test that can isolate one semicircular canal from others to determine site of lesion.	Inform patient that test is time consuming and uncomfortable; test can be discontinued at any time at patient's request.
• Rotary chair testing	The patient is seated in a chair driven by a motor under computer control. Evaluates peripheral vestibular system.	

Tuning-Fork Tests. Tuning-fork tests aid in differentiating between conductive and sensorineural hearing loss. Tuning forks of 250, 500, and 1000 Hz are generally used for this examination. Both skill and experience are required to ensure accurate results. If a problem is suspected, further evaluation by pure-tone audiometry is essential. The most common tuning-fork tests are the Rinne test and Weber's test.

For the Rinne test the base of an activated tuning fork is held first against the mastoid bone and then in front of the ear canal (0.5 to 2 inches). The patient reports whether the sound is louder behind the ear (on the mastoid bone) or next to the ear canal.

When the sound is no longer perceived behind the ear, the fork is moved next to the ear canal until the patient indicates that the sound is no longer heard. The Rinne test is positive when the patient reports that air conduction (AC) is heard longer than bone conduction (BC). This can indicate normal hearing or a sensorineural loss. If the patient hears the tuning fork better by bone conduction, the Rinne test is negative and indicates that a conductive hearing loss is present.

For Weber's test an activated tuning fork is placed on the midline of the skull, the forehead, or the teeth. The patient is asked to indicate where the sound is heard best. In normal auditory function the patient perceives a midline tone. If a patient has a conductive hearing loss in one ear, sound is heard louder (lateralizes) in that ear. If a sensorineural loss is present, sound is louder (lateralizes) in the unaffected ear.

Results of tuning fork tests are subjective. The patient with inconsistent test results or questionable results should be referred for more objective audiometric evaluation.

Audiometry. *Audiometry* is beneficial as a screening test for hearing acuity and as a diagnostic test for determining the degree and type of hearing loss. The audiometer produces pure tones at varying intensities to which the patient can respond. Sound is characterized by the number of vibrations or cycles that occur each second. *Hertz* (Hz) is the unit of measurement used to classify the frequency of a tone; the higher the frequency, the higher the pitch. Hearing loss can affect certain sound frequencies. The specific pattern produced on the audiogram by these losses can assist in the diagnosis of the type of hearing loss. The intensity or strength of a sound wave is expressed in terms of decibels (dB), ranging from 0 to 140 dB. The intensity of a sound required to make any frequency barely audible to the average normal ear is 0 dB. Threshold refers to the signal level at which pure tones are detected (pure tone thresholds) or the signal level at which the patient correctly hears 50% of the signals (speech detection thresholds).

Normal speech is approximately 40 to 65 dB; a soft whisper is 20 dB. Normally, a child and a young adult can hear frequencies from about 16 to 20,000 Hz, but hearing is most sensitive between 500 and 4000 Hz. This is similar to the frequencies contained in speech. A 40 to 45 dB loss in these frequencies causes moderate difficulty in hearing normal speech. A hearing aid may be helpful because it amplifies sound. A patient with a loss primarily in the higher frequencies, such as 4000 through 8000 Hz, has difficulty distinguishing the high-pitched consonants. Words such as cat, hat, and fat may not be perceived accurately because the important information conveyed by the consonant is not heard. A hearing aid makes sound information louder but not clearer and so may not be helpful to the patient who has problems with discrimination of sounds or sound information because the consonants are still not heard enough to make speech understandable.

Screening audiometry. Screening audiometry is the testing of large numbers of persons with a fast, simple test to detect possible hearing problems. A pass-fail criterion is used to screen persons who will or will not be given additional diagnostic testing. Persons who fail the screening should be referred for threshold audiometry.

In screening audiometry, the audiometer is usually set at a hearing level of 10 to 20 dB. The patient wears earphones as the tester sweeps across the available signal frequencies. The patient is directed to raise a hand when a sound is heard. Responses to air-conducted tones are checked at each frequency setting.

Pure-tone audiometry. A pure-tone audiometer produces pure tones at varied frequencies and intensities. Threshold audiometry generally determines thresholds for seven frequencies from 250 to 8000 Hz. The intensity is plotted against the frequency on an audiogram.

In a quiet setting a tone loud enough to be clearly heard by the patient is presented. The threshold level for frequency is then determined. A person with thresholds at 25 dB or higher will demonstrate problems in everyday communication. A 26 dB hearing loss is used as a guideline for further action. A hearing aid or surgery is rarely recommended for a hearing loss of less than 25 to 30 dB.[19]

Specialized Tests

The more specialized tests of the auditory system are most often performed in an outpatient setting by an audiologist. An audiologist can perform many additional tests with the use of audiometers and computers that record electrical activity from the middle ear, inner ear, and brain (see Table 20-11). The most common test performed by the audiologist is pure-tone audiometry. The audiologist can also test bone conduction to aid in differentiating sensorineural from conductive hearing losses. The nursing responsibilities include (1) explaining the examination in general terms, (2) informing the patient if there are any dietary restrictions such as caffeine or other stimulants, and (3) advising the patient if sedation will be used.

More sophisticated tests are available to determine the origin of certain hearing losses. These include evoked potential studies (also called auditory brainstem response) and electrocochleography. Computed tomography (CT) and magnetic resonance imaging (MRI) scans are used to diagnose the site of a lesion, such as a tumor of the auditory nerve.

Test for Vestibular Function

Nystagmus, an abnormal involuntary repetitive movement of the eyes, can be caused by disturbances in the endolymph fluid. The movement of the endolymph fluid stimulates receptor cells and causes nystagmus. Lesions in the CNS (e.g., multiple sclerosis) and drug toxicity can also cause nystagmus. In a test for nystagmus the patient looks straight ahead and then follows the examiner's finger to an extreme lateral gaze. Quick jerking movements along the way, except on extreme lateral gaze, are considered abnormal. Caloric testing and electronystagmography are specific tests to evaluate the function of the vestibular system.

The caloric test is done to assess the function of the vestibular system. The ear canal is irrigated with cold or warm water, which causes disturbances in the endolymph. The patient's reaction is observed for nystagmus. This observation may be made subjectively by the examiner or objectively by placing electrodes around the eyes. A normal individual will have nystagmus when water is instilled in the ear, with cold water producing nystagmus on the opposite side of instillation. Peripheral or brain lesions are suspected in the patient with no nystagmus elicited by caloric testing. Drugs that may alter the test results include alcohol, CNS depressants, and barbiturates. The patient's use of these substances should be known before testing.

Posturography. Platform posturography and rotational chair tests isolate one semicircular canal from the other to determine the site of a lesion causing vestibular disturbance. They can also provide data concerning the degree of disability caused by the disorder. These tests are time consuming, and in the vestibularly compromised patient they can cause distress and discomfort, particularly nausea and vomiting. The patient will require pretest instructions regarding intake of substances that can affect test results. In addition, the patient should be reassured that the test can be discontinued if stimulation to the vestibular system cannot be tolerated.

REVIEW QUESTIONS

The number of the question corresponds to the same-numbered objective at the beginning of the chapter.

1. In a patient who has a hemorrhage in the posterior chamber of the eye, the nurse knows that blood is accumulating
   a. in the aqueous humor.
   b. between the cornea and the lens.
   c. between the lens and the retina.
   d. in the space between the iris and the lens.

2. Increased intraocular pressure may occur as a result of
   a. edema of the corneal stroma.
   b. dilation of the retinal arterioles.
   c. blockage of the lacrimal canals and ducts.
   d. increased production of aqueous humor by the ciliary process.

3. The nurse should specifically question patients using eyedrops to treat glaucoma about
   a. use of corrective lenses.
   b. their usual sleep pattern.
   c. a history of heart or lung disease.
   d. sensitivity to narcotics or depressants.

4. The nurse should always assess the patient with an ophthalmic problem for
   a. visual acuity.
   b. pupillary reactions.
   c. intraocular pressure.
   d. confrontation visual fields.

5. During assessment of hearing the nurse would expect to find
   a. absent cone of light.
   b. pearl-gray tympanic membrane.
   c. lateralization with Weber's test.
   d. bone conduction (BC) greater than air conduction (AC).

6. Arcus senilis is due to
   a. tissue atrophy.
   b. decreased pupil size.
   c. opacities in the lens.
   d. cholesterol deposits in the cornea.

7. Before injecting fluorescein for angiography, the nurse should
   a. obtain an emesis basin.
   b. ask if the patient is fatigued.
   c. administer topical anesthesia.
   d. determine whether the patient has a peripheral scotoma.

REFERENCES

1. Talamo JH, Steinert RF: Keratorefractive surgery. In Albert DM, Jakobiec FA, editors: *Principles and practice of ophthalmology: clinical practice,* ed 2, Philadelphia, 1999, WB Saunders.
2. Sahel JA, Brini A, Albert DM: Pathology of the retina and vitreous. In Albert DM, Jakobiec FA, editors: *Principles and practice of ophthalmology: clinical practice,* ed 2, Philadelphia, 1999, WB Saunders.
3. Maus M: Basic eyelid anatomy. In Albert DM, Jakobiec FA, editors: *Principles and practice of ophthalmology: clinical practice,* ed 2, Philadelphia, 1999, WB Saunders.
4. Berson EL: Hereditary retinal diseases: an overview. In Albert DM, Jakobiec FA, editors: *Principles and practice of ophthalmology: clinical practice,* ed 2, Philadelphia, 1999, WB Saunders.
5. Ogden T, Hinton D: Retina. In Ryan SJ et al, editors: *Basic science and inherited retinal disease,* ed 2, St Louis, 2001, Mosby.
6. *Physicians' desk reference of ophthalmology,* ed 25, Montvale, NJ, 2000, Medical Economics Data Production Company.
7. Reichel E: Hereditary cone dysfunction syndromes. In Albert DM, Jakobiec FA, editors: *Principles and practice of ophthalmology: clinical practice,* ed 2, Philadelphia, 1999, WB Saunders.
8. Jarvis C: *Physical examination and health assessment,* ed 3, Philadelphia, 2000, WB Saunders.
9. Bennett ES, Henry VA, editors: *Clinical manual of contact lenses,* ed 2, Philadelphia, 1999, Lippincott Williams & Wilkins.
10. De La Paz MA, D'Amico DJ: Photic retinopathy. In Albert DM, Jakobiec FA, editors: *Principles and practice of ophthalmology: clinical practice,* ed 2, Philadelphia, 1999, WB Saunders.
11. Bajart AM: Lid inflammations. In Albert DM, Jakobiec FA, editors: *Principles and practice of ophthalmology: clinical practice,* ed 2, Philadelphia, 1999, WB Saunders.
12. Mead MD: Evaluation and initial management of patients with ocular and adnexal trauma. In Albert DM, Jakobiec FA, editors: *Principles and practice of ophthalmology: clinical practice,* ed 2, Philadelphia, 1999, WB Saunders.
13. Riordan-Eva P, Vaughan D: Eye. In Tierney L, McPhee S, Papakadis M, editors: *Current medical diagnosis and treatment 2001,* ed 40, New York, 2001, McGraw-Hill.
14. Sinnatamby CS: *Last's anatomy, regional and applied,* Edinburgh, 1999, Churchill Livingstone.
15. Gelfand SA: *Hearing,* New York, 1998, Marcel Dekker.
16. McCarthy PA, Sapp JV: Rehabilitative needs of the aging population. In Alpiner JG, McCarthy PA, editors: *Rehabilitative audiology: children and adults,* Philadelphia, 2000, Lippincott Williams & Wilkins.
17. Brookhauser PE: Diseases of the cochlea and labyrinth. In Wetmore RF, Muntz HR, McGill TS, editors: *Pediatric otolaryngology: principles and practice pathways,* New York, 2000, Thieme.
18. Wackym PA, Storper IS, Newman AN: Cochlear and vestibular ototoxicity. In Canalis RF, Lambert PR, editors: *The ear: comprehensive otology,* Philadelphia, 2000, Lippincott Williams & Wilkins.
19. DeChicchis AR, Bess FH: Hearing aids and assistive listening devices. In Bailey BJ, Calhoun KH, editors: *Head and neck surgery—otolarylgology,* Philadelphia, 1998, Lippincott-Raven.

RESOURCES

Resources for this chapter are listed after Chapter 21 on page 474.

CHAPTER *21*

NURSING MANAGEMENT
Visual and Auditory Problems

Sarah C. Smith
Mary E. Wilbur

LEARNING OBJECTIVES

1. Describe the types of refractive errors and appropriate corrections.
2. Describe the etiology and collaborative care of extraocular disorders.
3. Explain the pathophysiology, clinical manifestations, and nursing management and collaborative care of the patient with selected intraocular disorders.
4. Describe the nursing measures that promote the health of the eyes and ears.
5. Explain the general preoperative and postoperative care of the patient undergoing surgery of the eye or ear.
6. Describe the action and uses of drug therapy used in treating problems of the eyes and ears.
7. Explain the pathophysiology, clinical manifestations, and nursing management and collaborative care of common ear problems.
8. Compare the causes, management, and rehabilitative potential of conductive and sensorineural hearing loss.
9. Explain the use, care, and patient teaching related to assistive devices for eye and ear problems.
10. Describe the common causes and assistive measures for un-correctable visual impairment and deafness.
11. Describe the measures used to assist the patient in adapting psychologically to decreased vision and hearing.

KEY TERMS

acoustic neuroma, p. 468	intraocular lens, p. 443
amblyopia, p. 439	keratitis, p. 447
aphakia, p. 441	keratoconus, p. 448
astigmatism, p. 441	labyrinthitis, p. 467
blepharitis, p. 446	laser photocoagulation, p. 454
cataract, p. 449	Ménière's disease, p. 466
chalazion, p. 446	myopia, p. 441
cholesteatoma, p. 464	otosclerosis, p. 466
conjunctivitis, p. 446	presbycusis, p. 471
enucleation, p. 461	presbyopia, p. 441
external otitis, p. 462	refractive error, p. 439
glaucoma, p. 456	retinal detachment, p. 453
hordeolum, p. 446	strabismus, p. 448
hyperopia, p. 441	

Visual Problems

CORRECTABLE REFRACTIVE ERRORS

The most common visual problem is **refractive error.**[1] This defect prevents light rays from converging into a single focus on the retina. Defects are a result of irregularities of the corneal curvature, the focusing power of the lens, or the length of the eye. The major symptom is blurred vision. In some cases the patient may also complain of ocular discomfort, eyestrain, or headaches. The patient with refractive errors needs to use corrective lenses to improve the focus of light rays on the retina (Fig. 21-1).

Myopia (nearsightedness) is the most common refractive error, with approximately 25% of Americans exhibiting this disorder. The prevalence of *hyperopia* (farsightedness) and *presbyopia* (farsightedness resulting from a decrease in the accommodative ability of the eye as a result of aging) is less common. However, approximately 80 million Americans have some type of correction for refractive errors, approximately 25 million wear contact lenses, and several hundred thousand more have had keratorefractive surgery to correct refractive errors.[2] Table 21-1 summarizes the types of refractive errors and the appropriate corrections. Contrary to common belief, uncorrected refractive errors do not worsen the error, nor do they cause further pathology. However, refractive errors in young children should be corrected because children may develop **amblyopia** (reduced vision in the affected eye) if their refractive error is uncorrected.[2]

CULTURAL & ETHNIC CONSIDERATIONS
Hearing and Visual Problems

- Whites have a higher incidence of hearing impairment than African Americans or Asian Americans.
- Incidence and severity of glaucoma are greater among African Americans than among whites.
- Hispanic Americans have an increased incidence of diabetic retinopathy.
- Native Americans have an increased incidence of otitis media when compared with whites.
- Whites have a higher incidence of macular degeneration than Hispanic Americans, African Americans, and Asian Americans.

Reviewed by Mary Merchant, RN, MSN, FNP, Care Manager, Medical University of South Carolina, Charleston, S.C.

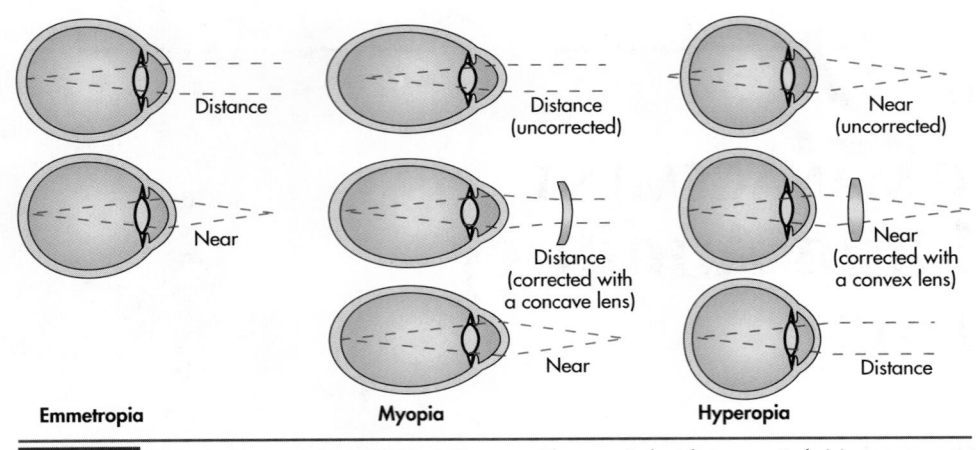

FIG. 21-1 Emmetropic, myopic, and hyperopic eyes with corrected and uncorrected vision.

TABLE 21-1 **Correction of Refractive Errors**

DESCRIPTION	SYMPTOMS	TYPE OF SPECTACLES	TYPE OF CONTACT LENSES*
Emmetropia Normal vision; light focuses on retina without accommodation for distance vision and with accommodation for near vision	None; vision is normal	Not indicated	Not indicated; some emmetropic patients wear tinted lenses for cosmetic reasons
Myopia Nearsightedness; light focuses in front of retina because eyeball is too long or because cornea or lens have excessive refractive power; light focuses on retina with accommodation for near vision	Blurred distance vision; patient may squint in an attempt to improve focus	Concave (minus); lens bends light rays outward	Rigid or soft; daily wear or extended wear; laser refractive or Intac procedures
Hyperopia Farsightedness; light focuses behind retina because eyeball is too short or because cornea or lens have inadequate refractive power; light focuses on retina for distance vision	Blurred near vision; ocular fatigue from accommodative effort	Convex (plus); lens bends light rays inward	Rigid or soft; daily wear or extended wear; laser refractive surgery
Astigmatism Light focuses as no clear point on the retina because corneal surface is irregularly curved; can occur with any of the above refractive errors	Blurred vision; ocular fatigue	Cylinder; lens bends light rays in different directions to align in a focused point	Rigid or soft toric; daily wear or extended wear; laser refractive surgery
Presbyopia Light does not focus on retina for near vision because the aging crystalline lens can no longer accommodate	Blurred near vision; patient may attempt to obtain clear vision by holding objects further from the eyes	Convex for near vision; can be reading glasses or bifocals with reading correction in lower part of lens	Bifocal rigid or soft; monovision (one eye corrected for distance, one for near)
Aphakia Crystalline lens is absent because of congenital defect, trauma, or surgery (cataract extraction); eye loses approximately 30% of its refractive power	No near vision; if one eye is involved, the retinal image is one third larger than in the normal eye	Thick, convex; almost never used after cataract extraction today because of visual distortion, discomfort from heavy glasses, poor appearance, and superiority of IOL implant for aphakic correction	Rigid, soft; daily wear or extended wear; not used after cataract extraction in most cases today because of difficulty in handling lenses, complications related to wear, and superiority of IOL implant as aphakic correction

*See Table 21-2 for explanation of contact lens types.
IOL, Intraocular lens.

Myopia

Myopia (nearsightedness) causes light rays to be focused in front of the retina. Myopia may occur because of excessive light refraction by the cornea or lens or because of an abnormally long eye. Myopia may also occur because of lens swelling that occurs when blood glucose levels are elevated, as in uncontrolled diabetes. This type of myopia is transient and variable and fluctuates with the blood glucose level.[3]

Hyperopia

Hyperopia (farsightedness) causes the light rays to focus behind the retina and requires the patient to use accommodation to focus the light rays on the retina for near and far objects. This type of refractive error occurs when the cornea or lens does not have adequate focusing power or when the eyeball is too short.

Presbyopia

Presbyopia is the loss of accommodation associated with age. This condition generally appears at about age 45 years. As the eye ages, the crystalline lens becomes larger, firmer, and less elastic. These changes, which progress with aging, decrease the eye's accommodative ability. People with presbyopia have difficulty focusing on near objects without some visual aid.[4]

Astigmatism

Astigmatism is caused by an irregular corneal curvature. This irregularity causes the incoming light rays to be bent unequally. Consequently, the light rays do not come to a single point of focus on the retina.

Aphakia

Aphakia is defined as the absence of the crystalline lens. The lens may be absent congenitally, or it may be removed during cataract surgery. A lens that is traumatically dislocated results in functional aphakia, although the lens remains in the eye. Because it accounts for approximately 30% of ocular refractive power, the absence of the lens results in a significant refractive error.[5] Without the focusing ability of the lens, images are projected behind the retina.

Nonsurgical Corrections

Corrective Glasses. Myopia, hyperopia, presbyopia, astigmatism, and aphakia can be modified by using the appropriate corrective lens (see Table 21-1). Myopia requires a minus corrective lens *(concave),* whereas hyperopia, presbyopia, and aphakia all require a plus corrective lens *(convex).* Glasses for presbyopia are often called "reading glasses" because they are usually worn for close work only. The presbyopic correction may also be combined with a correction for another refractive error, such as myopia or astigmatism. In these combined glasses the presbyopic correction is in the lower portion of bifocal or trifocal glasses. A newer type of correction for presbyopia, the "no-line" bifocal, is actually a multifocal lens that allows the patient to see clearly at any distance.

Aphakic glasses are very thick, making them heavy and unattractive to wear. The high degree of correction also causes images to be magnified about 25%. With the modern surgical procedures prevalent today, patients seldom wear aphakic glasses for correction because of the associated visual problems. Astigmatism can occur in conjunction with any of the other refractive errors.

Contact Lenses. Contact lenses are another way to correct refractive errors. Contact lenses generally provide better vision than glasses because the patient has more normal peripheral vision without the distortion and obstruction of the glasses and their frames. Aphakic contact lenses magnify objects only approximately 7% and are visually superior to aphakic glasses.[6] However, many older patients have difficulty handling and caring for contact lenses. Table 21-2 describes the various types of contact lenses and the advantages and disadvantages of each.

Lenses may be either rigid or flexible (soft lenses). Rigid contact lenses ride on the tear film layer of the cornea and are held in place by surface tension. Blinking causes the tear film to move under and over the contact lens, providing oxygen for the cornea. If the oxygen supply to the cornea is decreased, it becomes swollen, visual acuity decreases, and the patient experiences severe discomfort.

Because soft contact lenses do not ride on the corneal tear film layer, the cornea cannot receive oxygen from the tear film. Instead, the cornea receives oxygen through the soft contact lens, which is permeable to oxygen. Gas-permeable rigid contact lenses also allow oxygen to reach the cornea through the lens itself.

Altered or decreased tear formation can make wearing contact lenses difficult. Tear production can be decreased by antihistamines, decongestants, diuretics, birth control pills, and the hormones produced during pregnancy. Allergic conjunctivitis with itching, tearing, and redness can also affect contact lens wear.

In general, the nurse must know whether the patient wears contact lenses, the pattern of wear (daily versus extended), and care practices. The nurse must be able to identify whether contact lenses are present and should know how to remove them in an emergency situation. Shining a light obliquely on the eyeball can help the nurse visualize a contact lens. The nurse can remove a hard contact lens with a small suction cup designed for that purpose.

The patient should know the signs and symptoms of contact lens problems that must be managed by the eye care professional. The patient may remember these symptoms better if the nurse uses the mnemonic device RSVP:

Redness
Sensitivity
Vision problems
Pain

The nurse must stress the importance of removing contact lenses immediately if any of these problems occur.

Surgical Therapy

Refractive Surgery. Keratorefractive surgery (surgery to alter the corneal curvature) includes a variety of procedures, including those in which the surgeon either uses a laser and/or a special microsurgical knife to open and replace a flap of corneal tissue with the laser, or implants tiny semicircular pieces of plastic. Myopia is the refractive error most commonly corrected by refractive surgery. However, hyperopia, presbyopia, and various degrees of astigmatism correction are also now available.

Photorefractive keratectomy (PRK) is a procedure that uses a laser to reshape the central corneal surface. It is used for myopia, hyperopia, and astigmatism. *Laser-in-situ-keratomileusis* (LASIK) is a procedure in which first a corneal flap is folded back, and then a laser removes some of the internal layers of the cornea. Afterward, the flap is returned to normal position and allowed to heal in

TABLE 21-2	**Types of Contact Lenses**			
TYPE	**DESCRIPTION**	**ADVANTAGES**	**DISADVANTAGES**	**WEARING SCHEDULE**
Rigid Lenses				
• Standard	Rigid plastic; smaller than cornea	Can be tinted for easier visibility out of the eye; longer lasting, least expensive to purchase; corrects all types of refractive errors	Requires separate care solutions for cleaning, storing, wetting; new patients (or those resuming wear after a period of nonwear) must gradually increase wearing time; initially uncomfortable, requires adaptation to obtain adequate comfort level	Daily wear; sleeping in lenses (either inadvertently or purposely) can cause corneal edema or severe pain from lack of oxygen to cornea
• Gas permeable	Similar to standard rigid lenses, but plastic allows oxygen to pass through to cornea	Longer lasting than soft lenses; corrects all types of refractive errors; more comfortable initially than standard hard lenses; less adaptation time and fewer problems with corneal edema than standard hard lenses; flexible wearing schedule	Requires separate care solutions for cleaning, storing, wetting; more expensive to purchase then rigid standard contact lens	Daily wear
Soft Lenses				
• Standard	Soft, flexible plastic; covers entire cornea and a small rim of sclera	Fits snugly on eye, allowing less invasion of foreign particles under the lens; initially more comfortable and less adaptation time than rigid lenses; can be worn intermittently	Less durable and more expensive than rigid lenses (cost may be similar to gas-permeable rigid lenses); more susceptible to surface protein deposition that causes discomfort and vision problems; requires cleaning, sterilizing, and enzymatic removal of protein deposition, cannot correct for higher degrees of astigmatism	Daily wear only; sleeping in these lenses causes similar problems as sleeping in standard rigid lenses
• High water content	Similar to standard soft lenses, but with a higher water content	Similar to standard soft lenses; allows more oxygen through lens so lens can be worn up to a week at a time without removal	Similar to standard soft lenses (with the exception that these can be extended wear); greater risk of complications related to contact lens wear than with standard soft lenses	Daily wear or extended wear
• Toric	Similar to other standard soft lenses; special design to correct astigmatism	Similar to other soft lenses; can be custom ordered to correct patient's individual type of astigmatism	Similar to other soft lenses; more expensive than other types of lenses; can be more difficult to fit than nontoric soft lenses	Daily wear or extended wear
• Disposable	Similar to other soft lenses but thinner	Similar to other soft lenses; frequent replacement decreases risk of complications related to contact lens wear	Similar to other soft lenses; cost may be greater (can be similar, depending on prevalent charges for replacement lenses)	Daily wear or extended wear; each lens can be worn as long as 2 weeks before disposal
• Daily disposable	Similar to disposable	Similar to other soft lenses; daily disposal decreases risk of complications; no cleaning or disinfection necessary; commonly dispensed for new users, teenagers, and frequent travelers	Greater expense	Daily wear only; each lens is worn for 1 day and then discarded

place. Evidence supports claims that LASIK creates earlier visual stability in patients with a high degree of myopia than does PRK.[7]

Intacs, which are corneal ring segments, are the newest innovation in refractive procedures. Intacs are two tiny half rings of plastic. The Intac rings are placed between the layers of the cornea, around the pupil, after the surgeon makes a tunnel-like pathway with a specially designed surgical knife. They can also be removed if necessary, and the effects on refractive error are completely reversed.

Intraocular Lens Implantation. The most common reason for aphakia is surgical removal of the lens during cataract extraction. In the past, the aphakic patient had to use either aphakic glasses or, more recently, contact lenses for aphakic correction. However, the most common method of correction today is the surgical implantation of an **intraocular lens** (IOL), usually at the time of the initial cataract extraction. The IOL is a small plastic lens that can be implanted either in the anterior or posterior chamber; it provides very little optical distortion, especially compared with aphakic spectacles or even aphakic contact lenses. The type of IOL implanted depends on the cataract extraction technique and the surgeon's preference, but currently most IOLs are placed in the posterior chamber.

UNCORRECTABLE VISUAL IMPAIRMENT

The patient with correctable errors of vision is not functionally impaired. When no correction is possible, the patient's visual impairment may be moderate or profound. Approximately 4.8 million people in the United States have *severe visual impairment,* which is defined as the inability to read newsprint even with glasses. Of those individuals, only 9% have no useful vision, and the remaining 91% are considered partially sighted. The partially sighted individual may have significant visual abilities. It is important in working with the visually impaired patient to understand that a person classified as blind may have useful vision. Appropriate responses and interventions depend on the nurse's understanding of each patient's visual abilities.

Levels of Visual Impairment

The patient may be categorized by the level of visual loss.[8] *Total blindness* is defined as no light perception and no usable vision. *Functional blindness* is present when the patient has some light perception but no usable vision. The patient with either total or functional blindness is considered legally blind and may use vision substitutes such as guide dogs and canes for ambulation and Braille for reading. Vision enhancement techniques are not helpful.

The *legally blind individual* meets the criteria developed by the federal government to determine eligibility for federal and state assistance and income tax benefits (Table 21-3). The legally blind individual has some usable vision. The *partially sighted individual* who is not legally blind has a corrected visual acuity greater than 20/200 in the better eye and greater than 20 degrees

TABLE 21-3	Definition of Legal Blindness in the United States

- Central visual acuity for distance of 20/200 or worse in the better eye (with correction)
- Visual field no greater than 20 degrees in its widest diameter or in the better eye

of visual field, but the visual acuity is 20/50 or worse in the better eye. The patient who is partially sighted or legally blind can benefit greatly from vision enhancement techniques.

NURSING MANAGEMENT VISUAL IMPAIRMENT

■ Nursing Assessment

It is important to determine how long the patient has had a visual impairment because recent loss of vision has different implications for nursing care. The nurse should determine how the patient's visual impairment affects normal functioning. This may be done by questioning the patient about the level of difficulty encountered when doing certain tasks. For example, the nurse may ask how much difficulty the patient has when reading a newspaper, writing a check, moving from one room to the next, or viewing television. Other questions can help the nurse determine the personal meaning that the patient attaches to the visual impairment. The nurse can ask how the vision loss has affected specific aspects of the patient's life, whether the patient has lost a job, or what activities the patient does not engage in because of the visual impairment. The patient may attach many negative meanings to the impairment because of societal views of blindness. For example, the patient may view the impairment as punishment or view himself or herself as useless and burdensome. It is also important to determine the patient's primary coping strategies, the patient's emotional reactions, and the availability and strength of the patient's support systems.

■ Nursing Diagnoses

Nursing diagnoses depend on the degree of visual impairment and how long it has been present. Nursing diagnoses for the visually impaired patient include, but are not limited to, the following:

- Disturbed sensory perception *related to* visual deficit
- Risk for injury *related to* visual impairment and inability to see potential dangers
- Self-care deficits *related to* visual impairment
- Fear *related to* inability to see potential danger or accurately interpret environment
- Anticipatory grieving *related to* loss of functional vision

■ Planning

The overall goals are that the patient with recently impaired vision or the patient with impaired adjustment to long-standing visual impairment will (1) make a successful adjustment to the impairment, (2) verbalize feelings related to the loss, (3) identify personal strengths and external support systems, and (4) use appropriate coping strategies. If the patient has been functioning at an appropriate or acceptable level, the goal of the patient is to maintain the current level of function.

■ Nursing Implementation

Health Promotion. The nurse should encourage the partially sighted patient with preventable causes for further visual impairment to seek appropriate health care. For example, the patient with vision loss from glaucoma may prevent further visual impairment by complying with prescribed therapies and suggested ophthalmic evaluations.

Acute Intervention. The nurse provides emotional support and direct care to the patient with recent visual impairment. Active listening and grief work facilitation are important components of nursing care for the recently visually impaired patient. The nurse should allow the patient to express anger and grief and should help the patient to identify fears and successful coping strategies. The family is intimately involved in the experiences that follow vision loss. With the patient's knowledge and permission, the nurse should include family members in discussions and encourage members to express their concerns.

Many people are uncomfortable around a blind or partially sighted individual because they are not sure what behaviors are appropriate. Sensitivity to the patient's feelings without being overly solicitous or stifling the patient's independence is vital in creating a therapeutic nursing presence. The nurse should always communicate in a normal conversational tone and manner with the patient, and the nurse should address the patient, not a family member or friend that may be with the patient. Common courtesy dictates introducing oneself and any other persons who approach the blind or partially sighted patient and saying good-bye on leaving. Making eye contact with the partially sighted patient accomplishes several objectives. It ensures that the nurse speaks while facing the patient so the patient has no difficulty hearing the nurse. The nurse's head position validates that the nurse is attentive to the patient. Also, establishing eye contact ensures that the nurse can observe the patient's facial expressions and reactions.

The nurse should explain any activities or noises occurring in the patient's immediate surroundings. Orientation to the environment lessens the patient's anxiety or discomfort and facilitates independence. In orienting the partially sighted or blind patient to a new area, the nurse should identify one object as the focal point and describe the location of other objects in relation to it. For example, the nurse may say, "The bed is straight ahead, approximately 10 steps. The chair is to the left, and the nightstand is to the right, near the head of the bed. The bathroom is to the left of the foot of the bed."

The nurse should assist the patient to each major object in the area, using the sighted-guide technique. When using this technique, the nurse stands slightly in front and to one side of the patient and offers an elbow for the patient to hold. The nurse serves as the sighted guide, walking slightly ahead of the patient with the patient holding the back of the nurse's arm (Fig. 21-2). When using this technique in any situation, the nurse should describe the environment to help orient the patient. For example, the nurse may say, "We're going through an open doorway and approaching two steps down. There is an obstacle on the left." To assist the patient to sit, place one of his or her hands on the back of the chair.

Ambulatory and Home Care. Rehabilitation after partial or total loss of vision can foster independence, self-esteem, and productivity. The nurse should know what services and devices are available for the partially sighted or blind patient and should be prepared to make appropriate referrals for those services and devices. For the legally blind patient, the primary resource for services is the state agency for rehabilitation of the blind.[9] A list of agencies that serve the partially sighted or blind patient is available from the American Foundation for the Blind, 11 Penn Plaza, Suite 300, New York, NY 10001 (212-502-7600). Many of these agencies are listed in the resources section at the end of the chapter.

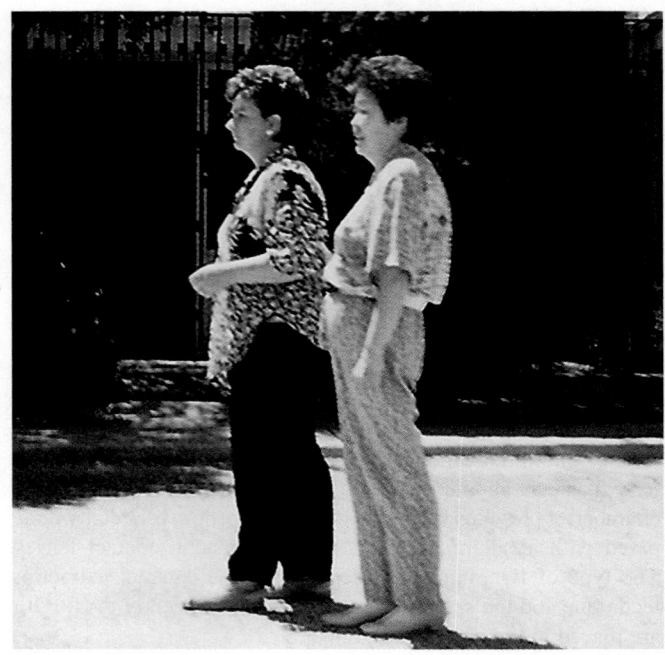

FIG. 21-2   Sighted-guide technique. The nurse serves as the sighted guide, walking slightly ahead of the patient with the patient holding the back of the nurse's arm.

Braille or audio books for reading and a cane or guide dog for ambulation are examples of vision substitution techniques. These are usually most appropriate for the patient with no functional vision. For most patients who have some remaining vision, vision enhancement techniques can provide enough help for many patients to learn to ambulate, read printed material, and accomplish activities of daily living (ADLs).

Optical devices for vision enhancement. Telescopic lenses for near or far vision and magnifiers of various types can often enhance the patient's remaining vision enough to allow the performance of many previously impossible tasks and activities. Most of these devices require some training and practice for successful use. Closed circuit television can provide magnification up to 60 times, allowing some patients to read, write, use computers, and do crafts. Although these systems are expensive and have limited portability, they are available in some public or university libraries.

Nonoptical methods for vision enhancement. *Approach magnification* is a simple but sometimes overlooked technique for enhancing the patient's residual vision. The nurse can recommend that the patient sit closer to the television or hold books closer to the eyes, which the patient may be reluctant to do unless encouraged. Contrast enhancement techniques include watching television in black and white, placing dark objects against a light background (e.g., a white plate on a black place mat), using a black felt-tip marker, and using contrasting colors (e.g., a red stripe at the edge of steps or curbs). Increased lighting can be provided by halogen lamps, direct sunlight, or gooseneck lamps that can be aimed directly at the reading material or other near objects. Large type is often helpful, especially in conjunction with other optical or nonoptical vision enhancements.

■ Evaluation

The overall expected outcomes are that the patient with severe visual impairment will

- have no further progressive loss of vision
- be able to express adaptive coping strategies
- not experience a decrease in self-esteem or social interactions
- function safely within her or his own environment

■ Gerontologic Considerations: Visual Impairment

The elderly patient is at an increased risk for vision loss because cataracts, glaucoma, diabetic retinopathy, macular degeneration, and other potential causes of visual impairment are more common in the older patient. The older patient may have other deficits, such as cognitive impairment or limited mobility, that further affect the ability to function in usual ways. Societal devaluation of the elderly may compound the self-esteem or isolation issues associated with the older patient's visual impairment. Financial resources may meet normal needs but can be inadequate in meeting increased demands of vision services or devices.

The older patient may become confused or disoriented when visually compromised. The combination of decreased vision and confusion increases the risk of falls, which have potentially serious consequences for the older adult. Decreased vision may compromise the older patient's ability to function, causing concerns about maintaining independence and causing a decreased self-image. Decreased manual dexterity may make the instillation of prescribed eyedrops difficult for some older adults. ■

EYE TRAUMA

Although the eyes are well protected by the bony orbit and by fat pads, everyday activities can result in ocular trauma. Ocular injuries can involve the ocular adnexa, the superficial structures, or the deeper ocular structures. In the United States an estimated 1.3 million eye injuries occur each year. Of these injuries, 40,000 result in permanent visual impairment. Table 21-4 outlines emergency management of the patient with an eye injury. Types of ocular trauma include blunt injuries, penetrating injuries, and chemical exposure injuries. Causes of ocular injuries include automobile accidents, falls, sports and leisure activity injuries, assaults, and work-related situations. Trauma is often a

---

TABLE 21-4 Emergency Management — Eye Injury

ETIOLOGY	ASSESSMENT FINDINGS	INTERVENTION
Blunt Injury Fist Other blunt objects **Penetrating Injury** Fragments such as glass, metal, wood Knife, stick, or other large object **Chemical Injury** Alkaline Acid **Thermal Injury** Direct burn from curling iron or other hot surface Indirect burn from UV light (e.g., welding torch, sun lamp) **Foreign Bodies** Glass Metal Wood **Trauma** Blunt Penetrating/perforating **Burns** Chemical Thermal	- Pain - Photophobia - Redness—diffuse or localized - Swelling - Ecchymosis - Tearing - Blood in the anterior chamber - Absent eye movements - Fluid drainage from eye (e.g., blood, CSF, aqueous humor) - Abnormal or decreased vision - Visible foreign body - Prolapsed globe - Abnormal intraocular pressure	**Initial** - Determine mechanism of injury. - Ensure airway, breathing, circulation. - Assess for other injuries. - Assess visual acuity after irrigation for chemical exposure. - Begin ocular irrigation *immediately* for chemical exposure. Use sterile saline or water if saline is unavailable. - Do not put pressure on the eye. - Instruct patient not to blow nose. - Begin ocular irrigation *immediately* in case of chemical exposure; do not stop until emergency personnel arrive to continue irrigation; sterile, pH-balanced, physiologic solution is best; if unavailable, use any nontoxic liquid. - Do not attempt to treat the injury (except as noted above for chemical exposure). - Stabilize foreign objects. - Cover the eye(s) with dry, sterile patches and a protective shield. - Do not give the patient food or fluids. - Elevate head of bed 45 degrees. - Do not put medication or solutions in the eye unless ordered by physician. - Administer analgesia as appropriate. **Ongoing Monitoring** - Reassure the patient. - Monitor pain. - Anticipate surgical repair for penetrating injury, globe rupture, or globe avulsion.

CSF, Cerebrospinal fluid; *UV*, ultraviolet.

preventable cause of visual impairment. Almost 90% of all sports-related eye injuries could be prevented by wearing protective eyewear during potentially hazardous work, hobbies, or sports activities.[10] The nurse's role in individual and community education is extremely important in reducing the incidence of ocular trauma.

Extraocular Disorders

INFLAMMATION AND INFECTION

One of the most common conditions encountered by the ophthalmologist is inflammation or infection of the external eye. Many external irritants or microorganisms affect the lids and conjunctiva and can involve the avascular cornea. It is a nursing responsibility to teach the patient appropriate interventions related to the specific disorder.

Hordeolum

A **hordeolum** (commonly called a *sty*) is an infection of the sebaceous glands in the lid margin. The most common bacterial infective agent is *Staphylococcus aureus*.[11] A red, swollen, circumscribed, and acutely tender area develops rapidly. The nurse should instruct the patient to apply warm, moist compresses at least four times a day until it improves. This may be the only treatment necessary. If there is a tendency for recurrence, the patient should perform lid scrubs daily. In addition, appropriate antibiotic ointments or drops may be indicated.

Chalazion

A **chalazion** is an inflammation of a sebaceous gland in the lids. It may evolve from a hordeolum. It may also occur as a response to the material released into the lid when a blocked gland ruptures. The chalazion appears as a swollen, nonpainful, reddened area, usually on the upper lid. Initial treatment is similar to that for a hordeolum. If warm, moist compresses are ineffective in causing spontaneous drainage, the ophthalmologist may surgically remove the chronic lesion (this is normally an office procedure), or the ophthalmologist may inject the chronic lesion with corticosteroids.

Blepharitis

Blepharitis is a common chronic bilateral inflammation of the lid margins. The lids are red rimmed with many scales or crusts on the lid margins and lashes. The patient may primarily complain of itching but may also experience burning, irritation, and photophobia. Conjunctivitis may occur simultaneously.

If the blepharitis is caused by a staphylococcal infection, collaborative care includes the use of an appropriate ophthalmic antibiotic ointment. Seborrheic blepharitis, related to seborrhea of the scalp and eyebrows, is treated with an antiseborrheic shampoo for the scalp and eyebrows. Often blepharitis is caused by both staphylococcal and seborrheal microorganisms, and the treatment must be more vigorous to avoid hordeolum, keratitis (inflammation of the cornea), and other eye infections. Conscientious hygienic practices involving skin and scalp must be emphasized. Gentle cleansing of the lid margins with baby shampoo can effectively soften and remove crusting.

Conjunctivitis

Conjunctivitis is an infection or inflammation of the conjunctiva. Conjunctival infections may be caused by bacterial or viral microorganisms. Conjunctival inflammation may result from exposure to allergens or chemical irritants (including cigarette smoke). The tarsal conjunctiva (lining the interior surface of the lids) may become inflamed as a result of a chronic foreign body in the eye, such as a contact lens or an ocular prosthesis.

Bacterial Infections. Acute bacterial conjunctivitis (pinkeye) is a common infection. Although it occurs in every agegroup, epidemics commonly occur in children because of their poor hygienic habits. In adults and children the most common causative microorganism is *S. aureus*. *Streptococcus pneumoniae* and *Haemophilus influenzae* are other common causative agents, but they are seen more often in children than adults. The patient with bacterial conjunctivitis may complain of irritation, tearing, redness, and a mucopurulent drainage. Although this typically occurs initially in one eye, it spreads rapidly to the unaffected eye. It is usually self-limiting, but treatment with antibiotic drops shortens the course of the disorder. Careful hand washing and using individual or disposable towels helps prevent spreading the condition.

Viral Infections. Conjunctival infections may be caused by many different viruses. The patient with viral conjunctivitis may complain of tearing, foreign body sensation, redness, and mild photophobia. Unless other ocular structures become involved, this condition is usually mild and self-limiting. However, it can be severe with increased discomfort and subconjunctival hemorrhaging. Adenovirus conjunctivitis may be contracted in contaminated swimming pools and through direct contact with an infected patient.[12] Good hygiene practices decrease spread of the virus. Treatment is usually palliative. If the patient is severely symptomatic, topical corticosteroids provide temporary relief but have no benefit in the final outcome. Antiviral drops are ineffective and therefore not indicated.

Chlamydial Infections. Adult inclusion conjunctivitis (AIC) is caused by the oculogenital type of *Chlamydia trachomatis*. AIC is becoming more prevalent in the United States because of the increase in sexually transmitted chlamydial disease. The patient complains of a mucopurulent ocular discharge, irritation, redness, and lid swelling. Systemic symptoms may be present as well. For unknown reasons, AIC does not carry the long-term consequences of trachoma (a sight-threatening keratoconjunctivitis caused by a different type of the *C. trachomatis* bacteria). AIC also differs from trachoma in that it is common in economically developed countries, whereas trachoma is rarely seen except in underdeveloped countries.[13]

Although topical treatment may be successful in the adult with chlamydial conjunctivitis, these patients have a high risk of concurrent chlamydial genital infection, as well as other sexually transmitted diseases. Consequently, all patients should be referred for further evaluation and systemic antibiotic therapy. The nurse's responsibility with the patient with chlamydial conjunctivitis includes education about the ocular condition, as well as the sexual implications of the condition.

Allergic Conjunctivitis. Conjunctivitis caused by exposure to some allergen can be mild and transitory, or it can be severe enough to cause significant swelling, sometimes ballooning the conjunctiva beyond the eyelids. The defining symptom of allergic conjunctivitis is itching. The patient may also complain of burning, redness, and tearing. Acutely, the patient may also have white or clear exudate. If the condition is chronic, the exudate is thicker and becomes mucopurulent. In addition to pollens, the patient may develop allergic conjunctivitis in response to animal dander, ocular solutions and medications, or even contact lenses. The nurse should instruct the patient to avoid the allergen if it is known. Artificial tears can be effective in diluting the allergen and washing it from the eye. Effective topical medications include antihistamines and corticosteroids.

Keratitis

Keratitis is an inflammation or infection of the cornea that can be caused by a variety of microorganisms or by other factors. The condition may involve the conjunctiva and/or the cornea. When it involves both, the disorder is termed *keratoconjunctivitis.*

Bacterial Infections. The intact cornea provides an effective defense against infection. However, when the epithelial layer is disrupted, the cornea can become infected by a variety of bacteria. Topical antibiotics are generally effective, but eradicating the infection may require subconjunctival antibiotic injection or, in severe cases, intravenous (IV) antibiotics. Risk factors include mechanical or chemical corneal epithelial damage, contact lens wear, debilitation, nutritional deficiencies, immunosuppressed states, and contaminated products (e.g., lens care solutions and cases, topical medications, cosmetics).[14]

Viral Infections. Herpes simplex virus (HSV) keratitis is the most frequently occurring infectious cause of corneal blindness in the Western hemisphere.[12] It is a growing problem, especially with immunosuppressed patients. It may be caused by HSV-1 or HSV-2 (genital herpes), although HSV-2 ocular infection is much less common. The resulting corneal ulcer has a characteristic dendritic (tree-branching) appearance, and it is often, although not always, preceded by infection of the conjunctiva or eyelids. Pain and photophobia are common. Up to 40% of patients with herpetic keratitis heal spontaneously. The spontaneous healing rate increases to 70% if the cornea is debrided to remove infected cells. Collaborative therapy includes corneal debridement followed by topical therapy with vidarabine (Vira-A) or trifluridine (Viroptic) used for 2 to 3 weeks. Corticosteroids are contraindicated because they contribute to a longer course, possible deeper ulceration of the cornea, and systemic complications. Drug therapy may also include acyclovir (Zovirax).

The varicella-zoster virus (VZV) causes both chickenpox and herpes zoster ophthalmicus (HZO). HZO may occur by reactivation of an endogenous infection that has persisted in latent form after an earlier attack of varicella or by direct or indirect contact with a patient with chickenpox or herpes zoster. It occurs most frequently in the older adult and in the immunosuppressed patient. Collaborative care of the patient with acute HZO may include narcotic or nonnarcotic analgesics for the pain, topical corticosteroids to reduce inflammation, antiviral agents such as acyclovir (Zovirax) to reduce viral replication, mydriatic agents to dilate the pupil and relieve pain, and topical antibiotics to combat secondary infection. The patient may apply warm compresses and povidone-iodine gel to the affected skin (gel should not be applied near the eye).

Epidemic keratoconjunctivitis (EKC) is the most serious ocular adenoviral disease. EKC is spread by direct contact, including sexual activity. In the medical setting, contaminated hands and in-struments can be the source of spread. The patient may complain of tearing, redness, photophobia, and foreign body sensation. In most patients, the disease involves only one eye. Treatment is primarily palliative and includes ice packs and dark glasses. In severe cases, therapy can include mild topical corticosteroids to temporarily relieve symptoms and topical antibiotic ointment.[12] The nurse's most important role is to teach the patient and family members regarding good hygienic practices to avoid spreading the disease.

Other Causes of Keratitis. Keratitis may also be caused by fungi (most commonly by the *Aspergillus, Candida,* and *Fusarium* species), especially in the case of ocular trauma in an outdoor setting where fungi are prevalent in the soil and moist organic matter. *Acanthamoeba* keratitis is caused by a parasite that is associated with contact lens wear, probably as a result of contaminated lens care solutions or cases. Homemade saline solution is particularly vulnerable to *Acanthamoeba* contamination. The nurse should instruct the patient who wears contact lenses about good lens care practices. Medical treatment of fungal and *Acanthamoeba* keratitis is difficult. Only one antifungal eyedrop (natamycin [Natacyn]) is approved by the Food and Drug Administration (FDA), and the *Acanthamoeba* organism is resistant to most drugs. If antimicrobial therapy fails, the patient may require a corneal transplant.

Exposure keratitis occurs when the patient cannot adequately close the eyelids. The patient with exophthalmos (protruding eyeball) from thyroid eye disease or masses posterior to the globe is susceptible to exposure keratitis.

Corneal Ulcer. Tissue loss due to infection of the cornea produces a *corneal ulcer* (infectious keratitis). The infection can be due to bacteria, viruses, or fungi. Corneal ulcers are often very painful, and patients may feel as if there is a foreign body in their eye. Other symptoms can include tearing, purulent or watery discharge, redness, and photophobia. Treatment is generally aggressive to avoid permanent loss of vision. Antibiotic, antiviral, or antifungal eyedrops may be prescribed as frequently as every hour night and day for the first 24 hours. An untreated corneal ulcer can result in corneal scarring and perforation (hole in the cornea). A corneal transplant may then be indicated.

NURSING MANAGEMENT
INFLAMMATION AND INFECTION

■ Nursing Assessment

The nurse should assess ocular changes, such as edema, redness, decreasing visual acuity, feeling as if a foreign body is present, or discomfort, and document the findings in the patient's record. The nurse's assessment should also consider the psychosocial aspects of the patient's condition, especially when the patient has visual impairment associated with the condition.

■ Nursing Diagnoses

Nursing diagnoses for the patient with inflammation or infection of the external eye include, but are not limited to, the following:

- Acute pain *related to* irritation or infection of the external eye
- Anxiety *related to* uncertainty of cause of disease and outcome of treatment
- Disturbed sensory perception (visual) *related to* diminished or absent vision

■ **Planning**

The overall goals are that the patient with inflammation or infection of the external eye will (1) avoid spread of infection, (2) maintain an acceptable level of comfort and functioning during the course of the specific ocular problem, (3) maintain or improve visual acuity, (4) comply with the prescribed therapy, and (5) promote appropriate health-seeking behaviors.

■ **Nursing Implementation**

Health Promotion. Careful asepsis and frequent, thorough hand washing are essential to prevent spreading organisms from one eye to the other, to other patients, to family members, and to the nurse. The nurse should dispose of any contaminated dressings in a proper waste container. The patient and family need information about avoiding sources of ocular irritation or infection and responding appropriately if an ocular problem occurs. The patient with infective disorders that may have a sexual mode of transmission or an associated sexually transmitted disease (STD) needs specific information about those disorders. The patient needs information about appropriate use and care of lenses and lens care products. The nurse should encourage the patient to follow the recommended regimens.

Acute Intervention. The nurse may apply warm or cool compresses if indicated for the patient's condition. Darkening the room and providing an appropriate analgesic are other comfort measures. If the patient's visual acuity is decreased, the nurse may need to modify the patient's environment or activities for safety.

The patient may require eyedrops as frequently as every hour. If the patient receives two or more different drops, the nurse should stagger the eyedrops to promote maximum absorption. For example, if two different eyedrops are ordered hourly, the nurse should administer one drop on the hour and one drop on the half hour unless otherwise prescribed. This staggered schedule promotes maximum absorption. The patient who needs frequent eyedrop administration may experience sleep deprivation.

Ambulatory and Home Care. The patient's primary need in the home environment is for information about required care and how to accomplish that care. The nurse should provide the patient and family with information about proper hygiene techniques to prevent contamination or limit the spread of infectious disorders. The patient and family also need information about proper techniques for medication administration. If the patient's vision is compromised, the nurse should provide suggestions for alternative ways to accomplish necessary daily activities and self-care. The patient who wears contact lenses and develops infections should discard all opened or used lens care products and cosmetics to decrease the risk of reinfection from contaminated products (a common problem and a probable source of infection for many patients).

■ **Evaluation**

The overall expected outcomes are that the patient with inflammation or infection of the external eye will
- cooperate with the treatment plan
- experience relief of ocular discomfort
- effectively cope with functional changes if decreased visual acuity is present
- obtain specific information to prevent recurrent disease

DRY EYE DISORDERS

Complaints of dry eye are caused by a variety of ocular disorders characterized by decreased tear secretion or increased tear film evaporation. *Keratoconjunctivitis sicca* is caused by lacrimal gland dysfunction from an autoimmune mechanism. If the patient with keratoconjunctivitis sicca has associated dry mouth, the patient may have primary Sjögren's syndrome (see Chapter 63). If the patient has associated rheumatoid arthritis, scleroderma, or systemic lupus erythematosus, the patient has secondary Sjögren's syndrome. The patient complains of a sandy or gritty sensation that typically worsens during the day and is better in the morning after eye closure with sleep. Treatment is directed at the underlying cause. With meibomian gland dysfunction, hot compresses and lid margin massage may be used. With decreased tear secretion, the patient may use artificial tears or ointments. They should be used sparingly because preservatives in the drops or overuse can cause further ocular irritation. In severe cases the ophthalmologist may temporarily or permanently surgically occlude the puncta, effectively providing the ocular surface with more available tears.

STRABISMUS

Strabismus is a condition in which the patient cannot consistently focus two eyes simultaneously on the same object. One eye may deviate in *(esotropia),* out *(exotropia),* up *(hypertropia),* or down *(hypotropia).* Strabismus in the adult may be caused by thyroid disease, neuromuscular problems of the eye muscles, entrapment of the extraocular muscles in orbital floor fractures, retinal detachment repair, or cerebral lesions. In the adult, the primary complaint with strabismus is double vision.

CORNEAL DISORDERS

Corneal Scars and Opacities

The cornea is an optically transparent tissue that allows light rays to enter the eye and focus on the retina, thus producing a visual image. Any wound causes the cornea to become abnormally hydrated and decreases the normal transparency. A rigid contact lens can be effective in correcting the irregular astigmatism that results from corneal scars. In other situations the treatment for corneal scars or opacities is *penetrating keratoplasty* (corneal transplant). In penetrating keratoplasty the ophthalmic surgeon removes the full thickness of the patient's cornea and replaces it with a donor cornea or "button" that is sutured into place.[15] Although corneal problems leading to blindness are uncommon, a corneal transplant can restore vision that otherwise would be lost. Approximately 40,000 corneal transplants are performed in the United States each year.

The time between the donor's death and the removal of the tissue should be as short as possible. Most surgeons prefer this interval to be 4 hours or less.[16] The eye banks test donors for human immunodeficiency virus (HIV) and hepatitis B and C. The tissue is preserved in a special nutritive solution, and it can be kept for up to 5 days in the storage media, if used for transplantation. Improved methods of tissue procurement and preservation, refined surgical techniques, postoperative topical corticosteroids, and careful follow-up have decreased graft rejection.

Keratoconus

Keratoconus is a noninflammatory, usually bilateral disease that is familial but has no exclusive inheritance pattern. It can be associated with Down syndrome, atopic dermatitis, Marfan syndrome, aniridia (congenital absence of the iris), and retinitis pigmentosa (hereditary disease characterized by bilateral primary degeneration of the retina beginning in childhood and progressing to blindness by middle age).

The anterior cornea thins and protrudes forward, taking on a cone shape. Keratoconus usually appears during adolescence and slowly progresses between ages 20 and 60 years. The only symptom is blurred vision caused by the variable astigmatism associated with the altered corneal shape. The astigmatism may be corrected with glasses or rigid contact lenses. The cornea can perforate as central corneal thinning progresses. Penetrating keratoplasty is indicated before perforation in advanced cases.

Intraocular Disorders

CATARACT

A **cataract** is an opacity within the crystalline lens. The patient may have a cataract in one or both eyes. If present in both eyes, one cataract may affect the patient's vision more than the other. Cataracts are the third leading cause of preventable blindness and the most common cause of self-declared visual disability in the United States. Approximately 50% of Americans between ages 65 and 74 years have some degree of cataract formation, and for those older than 75 years, the incidence increases to approximately 70%. Cataract removal is the most common surgical procedure for Americans older than 65 years. Congenital cataracts are relatively common, occurring in 1 of every 250 newborns (0.4%).[17]

Etiology and Pathophysiology

Although most cataracts are age related (*senile cataracts*), they can be associated with other factors. These include blunt or penetrating trauma, congenital factors such as maternal rubella, radiation or ultraviolet (UV) light exposure, certain drugs such as systemic corticosteroids or long-term topical corticosteroids, and ocular inflammation. The patient with diabetes mellitus tends to develop cataracts at a younger age than does the patient without diabetes.

Cataract development is mediated by a number of factors. In senile cataract formation, it appears that altered metabolic processes within the lens cause an accumulation of water and alterations in the lens fiber structure. These changes affect lens transparency, causing vision changes.[18]

COMPLEMENTARY & ALTERNATIVE THERAPIES
Bilberry

Clinical Uses
Cataracts, myopia, glaucoma, macular degeneration, night blindness, retinopathy, varicose veins.

Effects
May improve microcirculation in eyes. Has mild antiinflammatory effect. Anthocyanins in the herb act to prevent capillary fragility and inhibit platelet aggregation. May cause hypoglycemia.

Nursing Implications
Because it may increase the action of anticoagulants or antiplatelet agents, it should be used with caution if drugs such as aspirin, warfarin (Coumadin), or ticlopidine (Ticlid) are being used. Bilberry should not be used in large doses over a long period of time.

Clinical Manifestations

The patient with cataracts may complain of a decrease in vision, abnormal color perception, and glare. Glare is due to light scatter caused by the lens opacities, and it may be significantly worse at night when the pupil dilates. The visual decline is gradual, but the rate of cataract development varies from patient to patient. Some patients may complain of a sudden loss of vision because they inadvertently cover their unaffected eye, and the decreased acuity of the eye with cataracts becomes "suddenly" apparent. Secondary glaucoma can also occur if the enlarging lens causes increased intraocular pressure (IOP).

Diagnostic Studies

Diagnosis is based on decreased visual acuity or other complaints of visual dysfunction. The opacity is directly observable by ophthalmoscopic or slit lamp microscopic examination. As noted earlier, a totally opaque lens creates the appearance of a white pupil. Table 21-5 outlines other diagnostic studies that may be helpful in evaluating the visual impact of a cataract.

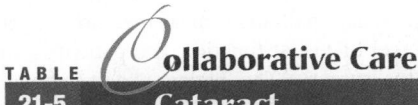

TABLE 21-5	Collaborative Care Cataract

Diagnostic
History and physical examination
Visual acuity measurement
Ophthalmoscopy (direct and indirect)
Slit lamp microscopy
Glare testing, potential acuity testing in selected patients
Keratometry and A-scan ultrasound (if surgery is planned)
Other tests (e.g., visual field perimetry) may be indicated to differentiate visual loss of cataract from visual loss of other causes

Collaborative Therapy
Nonsurgical
Change prescription of glasses
Strong reading glasses or magnifiers
Increased lighting
Lifestyle adjustment
Reassurance
Acute Care: Surgical Therapy
Preoperative
Mydriatic, cycloplegic agents
Nonsteroidal antiinflammatory drugs
Topical antibiotics
Antianxiety medications
Surgery
Removal of lens
   Phacoemulsification
   Extracapsular extraction
Correction of surgical aphakia
Intraocular lens implantation (most frequent type of correction)
Contact lens
Postoperative
Topical antibiotic
Topical corticosteroid or other antiinflammatory agent
Mild analgesia if necessary
Eye shield and activity as preferred by patient's surgeon

Collaborative Care

The presence of a cataract does not necessarily indicate a need for surgery. For many patients the diagnosis is made long before they actually decide to have surgery. Nonsurgical therapy may postpone the need for surgery. Collaborative care for cataracts is presented in Table 21-5.

Nonsurgical Therapy. Currently, there is no available treatment to "cure" cataracts other than surgical removal. If the cataract is not removed, the patient's vision will continue to deteriorate. However, palliative measures alone may help the patient. Often, changing the patient's eyewear prescription can improve the level of visual acuity, at least temporarily. Other visual aids, such as strong reading glasses or magnifiers of some type, may help the patient with close vision. Increasing the amount of light to read or accomplish other near-vision tasks is another useful measure. The patient may be willing to adjust his or her lifestyle to accommodate for visual decline. For example, if glare makes it difficult to drive at night, a patient may elect to drive only during daylight hours or to have a family member drive at night. Sometimes informing and reassuring the patient about the disease process makes the patient comfortable about choosing nonsurgical measures, at least temporarily.

Surgical Therapy. When palliative measures no longer provide an acceptable level of visual function, the patient is an appropriate candidate for surgery. The patient's occupational needs and lifestyle changes are also factors affecting the decision to have surgery. In some instances, factors other than the patient's visual needs may influence the need for surgery. Lens-induced problems such as increased IOP may require lens removal. Opacities may prevent the ophthalmologist from obtaining a clear view of the retina in the patient with diabetic retinopathy or other sight-threatening pathology. In those cases the cataract may be removed to allow visualization of the retina and adequate management of the problem.

Preoperative phase. The patient's preoperative preparation should include an appropriate history and physical examination. Because almost all patients have local anesthesia, many physicians and surgical facilities do not require an extensive preoperative physical assessment. However, most cataract patients are older adults and may have several medical problems that should be evaluated and controlled before surgery. The surgeon may order preoperative antibiotic eyedrops. The patient should not have food or fluids for approximately 6 to 8 hours before surgery. Almost all cataract patients are admitted to a surgical facility on an outpatient basis. The patient is normally admitted several hours before surgery to allow adequate time for necessary preoperative procedures.

The nurse will instill dilating drops and a nonsteroidal antiinflammatory eyedrop to reduce inflammation and to help maintain pupil dilation. One type of drug used for dilation is a *mydriatic,* an α-adrenergic agonist that produces pupillary dilation by contraction of the iris dilator muscle. Another type of drug is a *cycloplegic,* an anticholinergic agent that produces paralysis of accommodation (cycloplegia) by blocking the effect of acetylcholine on the ciliary body muscles. Cycloplegics produce pupillary dilation (mydriasis) by blocking the effect of acetylcholine on the iris sphincter muscle. Examples of mydriatics and cycloplegics are listed in Table 21-6, and nursing considerations are discussed on p. 452. The patient often receives preoperative antianxiety medication before the local anesthesia injection.

Intraoperative phase. Cataract extraction is an intraocular procedure. Rarely, intracapsular extraction is performed, in which the entire lens is removed with the capsule intact (this procedure may be necessary in instances of trauma). More commonly, extracapsular extraction is done, in which the anterior capsule is opened and the lens nucleus and cortex are removed, leaving the remaining capsular bag intact. In extracapsular ex-

TABLE 21-6

Drug Therapy

Topical Medications for Pupil Dilation

EXAMPLES	ONSET	DURATION	COMMENTS
Mydriatics			
phenylephrine HCl (Neo-Synephrine, Mydfrin)	45-60 min	4-6 hr	May cause tachycardia and elevated blood pressure, especially in elderly patient; can cause a reflexive decrease in heart rate when blood pressure rises; use punctal occlusion to limit systemic absorption
Cycloplegics			
tropicamide (Mydriacyl, Tropicacyl)	20-40 min	4-6 hr	1% solution used in cycloplegic refraction; 0.5% solution used in fundus examination
cyclopentolate HCl (AK-Pentolate, Cyclogyl, Ocu-Pentolate, Pentolair)	30-75 min	6-24 hr	Has been associated with psychotic reactions and behavioral disturbances, usually in children (especially in stronger concentrations); used in cycloplegic refraction, fundus examination, and uveitis
homatropine hydrobromide (AK-Homatropine, Isopto Homatropine)	30-60 min	1-3 days	Used in cycloplegic refraction, uveitis; may be used for pupil dilation to allow patient to see around a central lens opacity
scopolamine (Isopto Hyoscine)			
atropine (Atropisol, Atropair, Bufopto, Atropine, Isopto Atropine, Ocu-Tropine)	20-60 min 30-180 min	3-7 days 6-12 days	Used in cycloplegic refraction, uveitis Used in cycloplegic refraction, uveitis

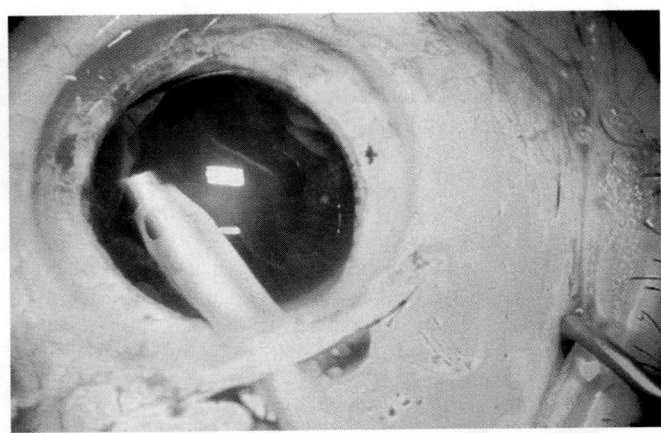

FIG. 21-3 Phacoemulsification of a cataractous lens through a self-sealing, scleral-tunnel incision. Note the circular opening in the anterior lens capsule.

traction, the surgeon can remove the lens nucleus by "scooping" it out with a lens loop, or by *phacoemulsification,* in which the nucleus is fragmented by ultrasonic vibration and aspirated from inside the capsular bag (Fig. 21-3). In either case, the remaining cortex is aspirated with an irrigation and aspiration instrument. The placement and type of incision vary among surgeons. Corneoscleral incisions require closure with sutures, whereas scleral tunnel incisions are self-sealing and require no closing suture. The incision required for phacoemulsification is considerably smaller than that required with intracapsular or standard extracapsular surgery.

Almost all patients now have an intraocular lens implanted at the time of cataract extraction surgery. Because most patients have an extracapsular procedure, the lens of choice is a posterior chamber lens that is implanted in the capsular bag behind the iris. At the end of the procedure, the patient receives injections of subconjunctival corticosteroid and antibiotic medications. Then an antibiotic and corticosteroid ointment is applied, and the patient's eye is covered with a patch and protective shield. The patch is usually worn overnight and removed during the first postoperative visit.

Postoperative phase. Unless complications occur, the patient is usually ready to go home within a few hours after the surgery as soon as the effects of sedative agents have dissipated. Postoperative medications usually include antibiotic and corticosteroid drops to prevent infection and decrease the postoperative inflammatory response. There is some evidence that postoperative activity restrictions and nighttime eye shielding are unnecessary. However, many ophthalmologists still prefer that the patient avoid activities that increase the IOP, such as bending or stooping, coughing, or lifting. Ophthalmologists may also recommend using an eye shield over the operative eye at night for protection.

The ophthalmologist will usually see the patient four to five times at increasing intervals throughout the 6 to 8 weeks following surgery. During each postoperative examination the surgeon will measure the patient's visual acuity, check anterior chamber depth, assess corneal clarity, and measure IOP. A flat anterior chamber may cause adhesions of the iris and cornea. The cornea may become hazy or cloudy from intraoperative trauma to the endothelium. Even on the first postoperative day the patient's un-

corrected visual acuity in the operative eye may be good. However, it is not unusual or indicative of any problem if the patient's visual acuity is reduced immediately after surgery. The postoperative eyedrops will be gradually reduced in frequency and finally discontinued when the eye has healed. When the eye is fully recovered, the patient will receive a final glasses prescription. Although the majority of the postoperative refractive error is corrected with the intraocular lens, the patient will still need corrective eyewear for near vision and for any residual refractive error.

NURSING MANAGEMENT
CATARACTS

■ Nursing Assessment

The nurse should assess the patient's distance and near visual acuity. If the patient is going to have surgery, the nurse should especially note the visual acuity in the patient's unoperated eye. With this information the nurse can determine how visually compromised the patient may be while the operative eye is patched and healing. In addition, the nurse should assess the psychosocial impact of the patient's visual disability and the patient's level of knowledge regarding the disease process and therapeutic options. Postoperatively it is important to assess the patient's level of comfort and ability to follow the postoperative regimen.

■ Nursing Diagnoses

Nursing diagnoses for the patient with a cataract include, but are not limited to, the following:
- Self-care deficits *related to* visual deficit
- Anxiety *related to* lack of knowledge about the surgical and postoperative experience

■ Planning

Preoperatively the overall goals are that the patient with a cataract will (1) make informed decisions regarding therapeutic options and (2) experience minimal anxiety. Postoperatively the overall goals are that the patient with a cataract will (1) understand and comply with postoperative therapy, (2) maintain an acceptable level of physical and emotional comfort, and (3) remain free of infection and other complications.

■ Nursing Implementation

Health Promotion. There are no proven measures to prevent cataract development. However, it is probably wise (and certainly does no harm) to suggest that the patient wear sunglasses, avoid extraneous or unnecessary radiation, and maintain appropriate intake of antioxidant vitamins (e.g., vitamins C and E) and good nutrition. The nurse can also provide information about vision enhancement techniques for the patient who chooses not to have surgery.

Acute Intervention. Preoperatively the patient with cataracts needs accurate information about the disease process and the treatment options, especially because cataract surgery is considered an elective procedure. For the patient who wants or needs to see better than is possible with medical interventions only, cataract surgery may not seem elective. However, in most cases there is no harm in not having surgery except that the patient has some degree of visual disability. The nurse should be available to

NURSING RESEARCH

Effect of Handholding on Anxiety in Cataract Surgery Patients

Citation

Moon J, Cho K: The effects of handholding on anxiety in cataract surgery patients under local anesthesia, *J Adv Nurs* 35:3, 2001.

Purpose

To determine the effectiveness of handholding on the anxiety of patients undergoing cataract surgery under local anesthesia.

Methods

A pretest and posttest design with 62 patients was used. Subjects were randomly assigned to a handholding during surgery group and an untreated control group. Handholding was provided by the researcher during the operation. The outcome variables measured were anxiety level; pulse rate and blood pressure; and concentrations of epinephrine, norepinephrine, cortisol, neutrophils, lymphocytes, and natural killer cells.

Results and Conclusions

A comparison of the two groups revealed a significant decrease in anxiety and epinephrine levels in the handholding group. The remaining physiologic parameters were not significantly different between the two groups. Anxiety levels were higher for both groups during the preoperative period than during the postoperative period.

Implications for Nursing Practice

Handholding during cataract surgery can lead to increased psychologic comfort and thus contribute to patient satisfaction with the surgery. During the preoperative period, when anxiety is reported as the highest, the patient's family (if allowed) could help reduce the patient's anxiety by handholding. Other types of therapeutic touch such as massage may be equally effective in reducing anxiety related to surgical procedures.

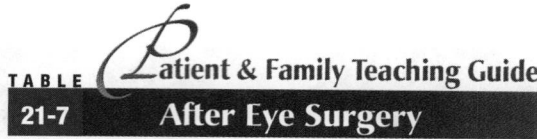

TABLE 21-7 Patient & Family Teaching Guide
After Eye Surgery

1. Teach patient and family proper hygiene and eye care techniques to ensure that medications, dressings, and/or surgical wound are not contaminated during necessary eye care.
2. Teach patient and family about signs and symptoms of infection and when and how to report those to allow early recognition and treatment of possible infection.
3. Instruct patient to comply with postoperative restrictions on head positioning, bending, coughing, and Valsalva maneuver to optimize visual outcomes and prevent increased intraocular pressure.
4. Instruct patient to instill eye medications using aseptic techniques and to comply with prescribed eye medication routine to prevent infection.
5. Instruct patient to monitor pain and take prescribed medication for pain as directed and to report pain not relieved by prescribed medications.
6. Instruct patient of the importance of continued follow-up as recommended to maximize potential visual outcomes.

Source: American Society of Ophthalmic Registered Nurses: *Core curriculum for ophthalmic nursing*, ed 2, Dubuque, Iowa, 2002, Kendall/Hunt Publishing.

give the patient and the family information to help them make an informed decision about appropriate treatment.

For the patient who elects to have surgery, the nurse is able to provide information, support, and reassurance about the surgical and postoperative experience that can reduce or alleviate the patient's anxiety.

When administering topical medications for pupil dilation before surgery (see Table 21-6 for examples), note that patients with dark irides may need a larger dose. Photophobia is common. Therefore using dark glasses is helpful. These medications produce transient stinging and burning and are contraindicated in patients with narrow-angle glaucoma because angle-closure glaucoma may be produced. Mydriatic agents can produce significant cardiovascular effects. When administering mydriatics, use punctal occlusion, especially in older and susceptible patients. When using cycloplegic agents for inflammatory disorders such as uveitis or iritis, the desired effect is to place the iris and ciliary body at rest, thus increasing patient comfort.

Table 21-7 outlines patient and family teaching following eye surgery. The nurse should inform all patients that they will not have depth perception until their patch is removed (usually within 24 hours). This necessitates special considerations to avoid possible falls or other injuries. The patient with significant visual impairment in the unoperated eye requires more assistance while the operative eye is patched. Once the patch is removed (usually within 24 hours), most patients with visual impairment in the unoperated eye will have adequate vision for necessary activities because the implanted IOL provides immediate visual rehabilitation in the operated eye. Occasionally the patient may require 1 or 2 weeks for the visual acuity in the operated eye to reach an adequate level for most visual needs. This patient will also need some special assistance until the vision improves. The postoperative cataract patient usually experiences little or no pain. There may be some scratchiness in the operative eye. Mild analgesics are usually sufficient to relieve these problems. If the pain is intense, the patient should notify the surgeon because this may indicate hemorrhage, infection, or increased IOP. The nurse should also instruct the patient to notify the surgeon if there is increased or purulent drainage, increased redness, or any decrease in visual acuity.

Ambulatory and Home Care. For the patient with cataracts who has not had surgery, the nurse can suggest ways in which the patient may modify activities or lifestyle to accommodate the visual deficit caused by the cataract. The nurse should also provide the patient with accurate information about appropriate long-term eye care.

Patients with cataracts who have surgery remain in the surgical facility for only a few hours. This shift in practice patterns has dramatically affected how the nurse provides the patient with postoperative care and teaching. The patient and the family are now responsible for almost all postoperative care. It is essential that the nurse give them written and verbal instructions before discharge. These teachings should include information about postoperative eye care, activity restrictions, medications, follow-up visit schedule, and signs and symptoms of possible complications. The patient's family should be included in the instruction because some patients may have difficulty with self-care activities, especially if the vision in the unoperated eye is poor. The nurse should provide an opportunity for the patient and family to perform return demonstrations of any necessary self-care activities.

Most patients experience little visual impairment following surgery. IOL implants provide immediate visual rehabilitation, and many patients achieve a usable level of visual acuity within a few days following surgery. Also, the patient's eye remains patched for only 24 hours, and many patients have good vision in their unoperated eye. A few patients may experience significant visual impairment postoperatively. These include patients who do not have an IOL implanted at the time of surgery, those who require several weeks to achieve a usable level of visual acuity following surgery, or those with poor vision in their unoperated eye. For those patients the time between surgery and receiving aphakic glasses or contacts can be a period of significant visual disability. The nurse can suggest ways in which the patient and the family can modify activities and the environment to maintain an adequate level of safe functioning. Suggestions may include getting assistance with steps, removing area rugs and other potential obstacles, preparing meals for freezing before surgery, or obtaining audio books for diversion until visual acuity improves.

■ Evaluation

The overall expected outcomes are that the patient following cataract surgery will
- have improved vision
- be able to take care of self
- have minimal to no pain
- have hopeful attitude about expected outcomes

■ Gerontologic Considerations: Cataracts

Most patients with cataracts are elderly. When the older patient is visually impaired, even temporarily, the patient may experience a loss of independence, lack of control over her or his life, and a significant change in self-perception. Societal devaluation of the older individual complicates these experiences. The older patient often needs emotional support and encouragement, as well as specific suggestions to allow a maximum level of independent function. The nurse can assure the older patient that cataract surgery can be accomplished safely and comfortably with minimal sedation. The use of outpatient surgery for cataract surgery is particularly beneficial for the older patient who may become confused or disoriented during hospitalization. ■

RETINAL DETACHMENT

A **retinal detachment** is a separation of the sensory retina and the underlying pigment epithelium, with fluid accumulation between the two layers. The incidence of nontraumatic retinal detachment is approximately 1 out of every 10,000 individuals each year. This number increases when aphakic individuals are included because retinal detachment is more likely to occur in aphakic patients. If traumatic retinal detachments are included,

the incidence is only slightly increased. In the patient with no other risk factors who has had a retinal detachment in one eye, the risk of detachment in the second eye is 2% to 25%. Almost all patients with untreated, symptomatic retinal detachment become blind in the involved eye.

Etiology and Pathophysiology

There are many causes of retinal detachment. The most common cause is a retinal break. *Retinal breaks* are an interruption in the full thickness of the retinal tissue, and they can be classified as tears or holes. *Retinal holes* are atrophic retinal breaks that occur spontaneously. *Retinal tears* can occur as the vitreous humor shrinks during aging and pulls on the retina. The retina tears when the traction force exceeds the strength of the retina. Once there is a break in the retina, liquid vitreous can enter the subretinal space between the sensory layer and the retinal pigment epithelium layer, causing a *rhegmatogenous* retinal detachment. Less frequently, retinal detachment can occur when abnormal membranes mechanically pull on the retina. These are called *tractional* detachments. A third type of retinal detachment is the *secondary* or *exudative* detachment that occurs with conditions that allow fluid to accumulate in the subretinal space (e.g., choroidal tumors, intraocular inflammation). Risk factors for retinal detachment are listed in Table 21-8.

Clinical Manifestations

Patients with a detaching retina describe symptoms that include *photopsia* (light flashes), floaters, and a "cobweb," "hairnet," or ring in the field of vision. Once the retina has detached, the patient describes a painless loss of peripheral or central vision, "like a curtain" coming across the field of vision. The area of visual loss corresponds to the area of detachment. If the detachment is in the superior nasal retina, the visual field loss will be in the inferior temporal area. If the detachment is small or develops slowly in the periphery, the patient may not be aware of a visual problem.

TABLE 21-8   Risk Factors for Retinal Detachment

High Myopia
Premature, accelerated rate of vitreous detachment; increased incidence of lattice degeneration

Aphakia
Retinal tears that presumably occur because of surgical disturbance of the vitreous

Proliferative Diabetic Retinopathy
Vitreous remains attached to areas of neovascularization as normal process of vitreal contraction occurs

Retinal Lattice Degeneration
Retinal holes common in lattice degeneration; vitreous remains attached to area of degeneration as the normal process of vitreal contraction occurs

Ocular Trauma
Retinal breaks after blunt or penetrating trauma allow fluid to accumulate in the subretinal space

Diagnostic Studies

Visual acuity measurements should be the first diagnostic procedure with any complaint of vision loss (Table 21-9). The retinal detachment can be directly visualized using direct and indirect ophthalmoscopy or slit lamp microscopy in conjunction with a special lens to view the far periphery of the retina. Ultrasound may be useful to identify a retinal detachment if the retina cannot be directly visualized (e.g., when the cornea, lens, or vitreous is hazy or opaque).

Collaborative Care

The ophthalmologist will carefully evaluate the patient with retinal breaks to determine if prophylactic laser photocoagulation or cryopexy is necessary to avoid possible retinal detachment. Some retinal breaks are not likely to progress to detachment, and the ophthalmologist will simply watch the patient, giving precise information about the warning signs and symptoms of impending detachment and instructing the patient to seek immediate evaluation if any of those signs or symptoms are recognized. The general ophthalmologist will usually refer the patient with retinal detachments to a retinal specialist. Treatment of retinal detachment has two objectives. The first is to seal any retinal breaks, and the second is to relieve inward traction on the retina. Several techniques are used to accomplish these objectives.

Surgical Therapy

Laser photocoagulation and cryopexy. These techniques seal retinal breaks by creating an inflammatory reaction that causes a chorioretinal adhesion or scar. **Laser photocoagulation** involves using an intense, precisely focused light beam, such as the argon laser, to create an inflammatory reaction. The light is directed at the area of the retinal break. This produces a scar that seals the edges of the hole or tear and prevents fluid from collecting in the subretinal space and causing a detachment. The ophthalmologist may use photocoagulation alone if there is a single small tear with little or no detachment in the periphery and minimal subretinal fluid. For retinal breaks accompanied by significant detachment, the retinal surgeon may use photocoagulation intraoperatively in conjunction with scleral buckling. Tears or holes without accompanying retinal detachment may be treated prophylactically with laser photocoagulation if the ophthalmologist judges them to be at high risk of progressing to retinal detachment. When used alone, laser therapy is an outpatient procedure that usually requires only topical anesthesia, and the patient usually experiences minimal adverse symptoms during or following the procedure.

An alternative method used to seal retinal breaks is *cryopexy*. This procedure involves using extreme cold to create the inflammatory reaction that produces the sealing scar. The ophthalmologist applies the cryoprobe instrument to the external globe in the area over the tear. This is usually done on an outpatient basis and under local anesthesia. As with photocoagulation, cryotherapy may be used alone or during scleral buckling surgery. The patient may experience significant discomfort and eye pain following cryopexy. The nurse should encourage the patient to take the prescribed pain medication following the procedure.

Scleral buckling. *Scleral buckling* is an extraocular surgical procedure that involves indenting the globe so that the pigment epithelium, choroid, and sclera move toward the detached retina. This not only helps seal retinal breaks, but also helps relieve inward traction on the retina. The retinal surgeon sutures a silicone implant against the sclera, causing the sclera to buckle inward. The surgeon may place an encircling band over the implant if there are multiple retinal breaks, if the surgeon cannot locate suspected breaks, or if there is widespread inward traction on the retina (Fig. 21-4). If present, subretinal fluid may be drained by inserting a small-gauge needle to facilitate contact between the retina and the buckled sclera. Scleral buckling is usually accomplished under local anesthesia, and the patient may be discharged on the first postoperative day. Many surgeons now perform scleral buckling surgery as an outpatient procedure.

Intraocular procedures. In addition to the extraocular procedures described, retinal surgeons may use one or more intraocular procedures in treating some retinal detachments. *Pneumatic retinopexy* is the intravitreal injection of a gas to form a temporary bubble in the vitreous that closes retinal breaks and provides apposition of the separated retinal layers. Because the intravitreal bubble is temporary, this technique is combined with laser photocoagulation or cryotherapy. The patient with an intravitreal bubble must position the head so that the bubble is in contact with the retinal break. It may be necessary for the patient to maintain this position as much as possible for up to several weeks.[19]

Vitrectomy (surgical removal of the vitreous) may be used to relieve traction on the retina, especially when the traction results from proliferative diabetic retinopathy. Vitrectomy may be combined with scleral buckling to provide a dual effect in relieving traction. In *proliferative vitreoretinopathy* (PVR), membranes develop in the vitreous cavity and on the retinal surface, exerting traction that causes folds in the retina. Vitrectomy may be combined with membrane peeling to relieve traction in those cases.

TABLE 21-9	Collaborative Care
	Retinal Detachment

Diagnostic
History and physical examination
Visual acuity measurement
Ophthalmoscopy (direct and indirect)
Slit lamp microscopy
Ultrasound if cornea, lens, or vitreous are hazy or opaque

Collaborative Therapy
Preoperative
Mydriatic, cycloplegic
Photocoagulation of retinal break that has not progressed to detachment
Surgery to Seal Retinal Breaks and Relieve Traction on Retina
Laser photocoagulation
Cryoretinopexy
Scleral buckling procedure
Draining of subretinal fluid
Vitrectomy
Intravitreal bubble
Postoperative
Topical antibiotic
Topical corticosteroid
Analgesia
Mydriatics
Positioning and activity as preferred by patient's surgeon

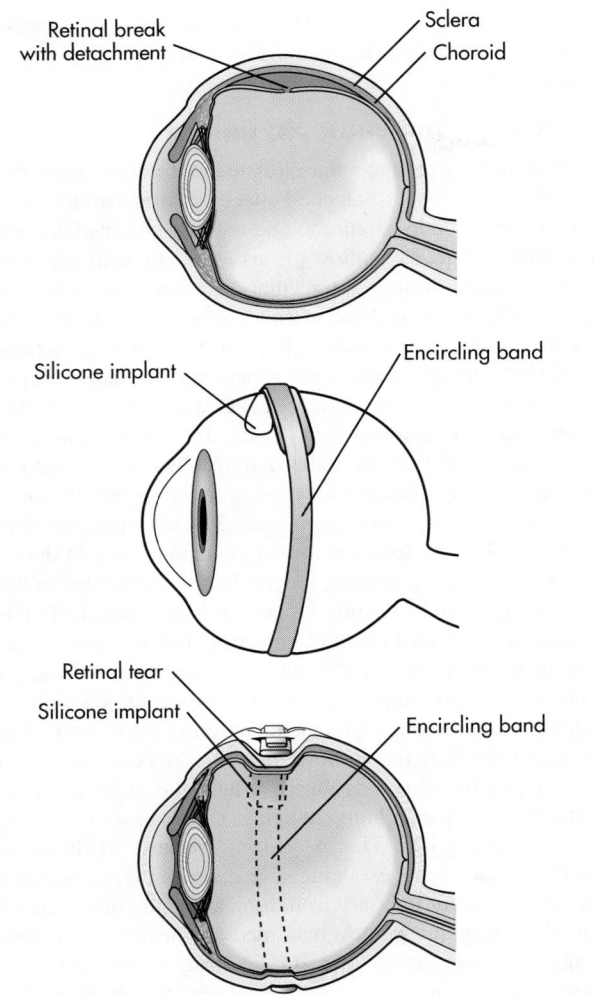

Retinal break with detachment

Sclera
Choroid

Silicone implant

Encircling band

Retinal tear
Silicone implant

Encircling band

FIG. 21-4 Retinal break with detachment: surgical repair by scleral buckling technique.

Postoperative considerations in scleral buckling and intraocular procedures. Reattachment is successful in 90% of retinal detachments. Visual prognosis varies, depending on the extent, length, and area of detachment. Postoperatively, the patient may be on bed rest and may require special positioning to maintain proper position of an intravitreal bubble. Overnight hospitalization varies according to physician preference and third-party payer guidelines. The patient may need multiple topical medications, including antibiotics, antiinflammatory agents, or dilating agents. Activity recommendations vary according to physician preference, extent of the detachment, and the particular repair procedure.

The nurse should teach the patient at risk for retinal detachment the signs and symptoms of retinal detachment. The nurse can also promote use of proper protective eyewear to help avoid retinal detachments related to trauma.

In most cases retinal detachment is an urgent situation, and the patient is confronted suddenly with the need for surgery. The patient needs emotional support, especially during the immediate preoperative period when preparations for surgery produce additional anxiety. When the patient experiences postoperative pain, the nurse should administer prescribed pain medications and teach the patient to take the medication as necessary after being discharged. The patient may go home within a few hours of surgery or may remain in the hospital for several days, depending on the surgeon and the type of repair. Discharge planning and teaching is important, and the nurse should begin this process as early as possible because the patient may not remain hospitalized long. Patient and family teaching following eye surgery is discussed in Table 21-7.

The level of activity restriction following retinal detachment surgeries varies greatly. The nurse should verify the prescribed level of activity with each patient's surgeon and help the patient plan for any necessary assistance related to activity restrictions. The nurse should teach the patient the signs and symptoms of retinal detachment because of the risk of retinal detachment in the other eye.

AGE-RELATED MACULAR DEGENERATION

Age-related macular degeneration (ARMD) is divided into two classic forms: dry (atrophic) and wet (exudative). ARMD is the most common cause of vision loss in persons over 55. People with dry ARMD notice that reading and other close-vision tasks become more difficult. In this form, the macular cells have wasted or atrophied and simply do not function as well as previously. Patients report that "sometimes I see the image and sometimes it sort of blinks at me, like I have a short circuit." ARMD is slowly progressive, and usually can result in a final visual outcome of 20/200. Many patients retain reading and other abilities with low-vision assistive devices, and many can retain a license to drive during daylight or at reduced speeds.

Wet (exudative) ARMD is characterized by the development of abnormal blood vessels in or near the macula. This results in a distinct area of blurred, darkened, and/or distorted vision. The process can occur rapidly over days or weeks. Only 10% to 15% of patients with dry ARMD go on to develop the wet form.

Etiology and Pathophysiology

Clearly, ARMD is related to retinal aging. In addition, studies support that heredity, environmental exposure to UV light, dietary intake, and use of carotenoids may alter the onset and course of the disease. The pathophysiologic mechanism is thought to be abnormal accumulation of waste material in the retinal pigment epithelium. Cigarette smokers have a significantly higher risk of developing ARMD.[20]

Clinical Manifestations

The hallmark sign of ARMD is the appearance of *drusen* in the fundus found on ophthalmoscopic evaluation. Drusen appear as yellowish exudates beneath the retinal pigment epithelium and represent localized or diffuse deposits of extracellular debris. The patient may complain of blurred vision, the presence of *scotomas* (blind spots in the visual field), or *metamorphopsia* (distortion of vision).

Diagnostic Studies

In addition to visual acuity measurement, the primary diagnostic procedure is ophthalmoscopy. The examiner looks for drusen and other fundus changes associated with ARMD. The Amsler grid test (see Chapter 20, Table 20-6) may help define the involved area, and it provides a baseline for future comparison. Fundus photography and IV angiography with fluorescein and/or indocyanine green dyes may be helpful in further defining the extent and type of degenerative disease.

Collaborative Care

Laser photocoagulation of the abnormal blood vessels when visual acuity is already compromised extensively has been the therapy of choice until recently. Patients undergoing macular photocoagulation may benefit from destroying the blood vessels, preventing additional central vision loss. However, the laser beam also destroys the retinal pigment epithelium and photoreceptor cells where it is applied, leaving a blind spot from the scarred area.

A new therapy available for patients with wet ARMD called *photodynamic therapy* (PDT) uses verteporfin (Visudyne) intravenously and a "cold" laser to excite the dye. This procedure destroys the abnormal blood vessels without permanent damage to the retinal pigment epithelium and photoreceptor cells. Current criteria for its use are very specific, and only about 10% of patients with wet ARMD are eligible at this time. Verteporfin is a photosensitizing drug that becomes active when exposed to the low-level laser light wave. Until the drug is completely excreted by the body, it can be activated by exposure to sunlight or other high-intensity light such as halogen. Therefore patients are cautioned to avoid direct exposure to sunlight and other intense forms of light for 5 days after treatment. Patients leave the clinic completely covered because any exposure to skin by sunlight could activate the drug in that area, resulting in a thermal burn.

The role of high-dose vitamin therapy, especially vitamins C and E and β-carotene, in slowing the progression of vision loss is currently under investigation.

The permanent loss of central vision associated with ARMD has significant psychosocial implications for nursing care. Nursing management of the patient with uncorrectable visual impairment is discussed on p. 443 and is appropriate for the patient with ARMD. It is especially important when caring for the patient to avoid giving the impression that "nothing can be done" about the problem. Although it is true that therapy will not recover lost vision, much can be done to augment the remaining vision. Just knowing that the health care provider has not abandoned them can give these patients a more positive outlook.

GLAUCOMA

Glaucoma is not one disease but rather a group of disorders characterized by (1) increased IOP and the consequences of elevated pressure, (2) optic nerve atrophy, and (3) peripheral visual field loss.

Glaucoma may occur congenitally, as a primary disease, or secondary to other ocular or systemic conditions. Intraocular pressure is regulated by the formation and reabsorption of aqueous humor. The presence of glaucoma is directly related to the balance or imbalance of this fluid. If elevated IOP is not recognized and treated, glaucomatous damage to the optic nerve and retinal cells results in atrophy and permanent vision loss. Glaucoma is the second leading cause of permanent blindness in the United States and the leading cause of blindness among African Americans. At least 2 million persons have glaucoma, and, of these, more than 50% are unaware of their condition. Another 5 to 10 million persons have elevated IOP, placing them at increased risk of developing the disease. The incidence of glaucoma increases with age. One in 50 whites is affected. However,

1 in 10 African Americans develops glaucoma. Blindness from glaucoma is largely preventable with early detection and appropriate treatment.

Etiology and Pathophysiology

The etiology of glaucoma is related to the consequences of elevated IOP. A proper balance between the rate of aqueous production (referred to as inflow) and the rate of aqueous reabsorption (referred to as outflow) is essential to maintain the IOP within normal limits. Intraocular pressures between 10 and 21 mm Hg are considered normal. When the rate of inflow is greater than the rate of outflow, IOP can rise above the normal limits. If IOP remains elevated, permanent visual damage may occur.

Primary open-angle glaucoma (POAG) represents 90% of the cases of primary glaucoma. In POAG, the outflow of aqueous humor is decreased in the trabecular meshwork. In essence, the drainage channels become clogged, like a clogged kitchen sink.[21]

Primary angle-closure glaucoma (PACG) represents approximately 10% of the total number of glaucoma cases in the United States. As the name implies, the mechanism reducing the outflow of aqueous is angle closure. Usually, this is caused from the lens bulging forward as a result of an age-related process. Angle closure may also occur as a result of pupil dilation in the patient with anatomically narrow angles. Dilation causes peripheral iris bulging with the same outcome of covering the trabecular meshwork and blocking the outflow channels. An acute attack may be precipitated by situations during which the pupil remains in a partially dilated state long enough to cause an acute and significant rise in the IOP. This may occur because of drug-induced mydriasis, emotional excitement, or darkness. Drug-induced mydriasis may occur not only from topical ophthalmic preparations but also from many systemic medications (both prescription drugs and over-the-counter [OTC] drugs). The nurse should check drug documentation before administering medications to the patient with angle-closure glaucoma and should instruct the patient not to take any mydriatic-producing medications.

In *secondary glaucoma,* increased IOP results from other ocular or systemic conditions that may block the outflow channels in some way. Secondary glaucoma may be associated with various inflammatory processes that block the outflow channels. Inflammatory processes may also damage the trabecular meshwork. Trauma, intraocular or periorbital neoplasms, iris neovascularization (new blood vessel growth), and other ocular or systemic disorders may also be associated with secondary glaucoma.

Clinical Manifestations

POAG develops slowly and without symptoms. The patient with POAG reports no symptoms of pain or pressure. The patient usually does not notice the gradual visual field loss until peripheral vision has been severely compromised. Eventually the patient with untreated glaucoma has "tunnel vision" in which only a small center field can be seen, and all peripheral vision is absent.

Acute angle-closure glaucoma causes definite symptoms, including sudden, excruciating pain in or around the eye. This is often accompanied by nausea and vomiting. Visual symptoms include seeing colored halos around lights, blurred vision, and ocular redness. The acute rise in IOP may also cause corneal edema, giving the cornea a frosted appearance.

Manifestations of subacute or chronic angle-closure glaucoma appear more gradually. The patient who has had a previous, unrecognized episode of subacute angle-closure glaucoma may report a history of blurred vision, seeing colored halos around lights, ocular redness, or eye or brow pain.

Diagnostic Studies

IOP is usually elevated in glaucoma. Normal IOP by applanation tonometry is 10 to 21 mm Hg. In the patient with elevated pressures, the ophthalmologist will usually repeat the measurements over a period of time to verify the elevation. In open-angle glaucoma, IOP is usually between 22 and 32 mm Hg. In acute angle-closure glaucoma, IOP may be 50 mm Hg or higher.

In open-angle glaucoma, slit lamp microscopy reveals a normal angle. In angle-closure glaucoma, the examiner may note a markedly narrow or flat anterior chamber angle, an edematous cornea, a fixed and moderately dilated pupil, and ciliary injection. Gonioscopy allows better visualization of the anterior chamber angle.

Measures of peripheral and central vision provide other diagnostic information. Whereas central acuity may remain 20/20 even in the presence of severe peripheral visual field loss, visual field perimetry may reveal subtle changes in the peripheral retina early in the disease process, long before actual scotomas develop. When visual field defects begin to appear, the initial scotoma is a small, football-shaped defect that gradually progresses to a nasal and superior field defect in chronic open-angle glaucoma. In acute angle-closure glaucoma, central visual acuity will be reduced if the patient has corneal edema, and the visual fields may be markedly decreased.

As glaucoma progresses, *optic disc cupping* occurs. This is visible with direct or indirect ophthalmoscopy (Fig. 21-5). The optic disc becomes wider, deeper, and paler (light gray or white). Optic disc cupping may be one of the first signs of chronic open-angle glaucoma. Optic disc photographs are useful for comparison over time to demonstrate an increase in the cup-to-disc ratio and progressive blanching.

Collaborative Care

The primary focus of glaucoma therapy is to keep the IOP low enough to prevent the patient from developing optic nerve damage. This damage is manifested by increasing visual field loss and progressive optic disc cupping. Specific therapies vary with the type of glaucoma. The diagnostic and collaborative care of glaucoma is summarized in Table 21-10.

Chronic Open-Angle Glaucoma. Initial treatment in chronic open-angle glaucoma is with drugs (Table 21-11). With all drug therapy, the patient must understand that continued treatment and supervision are necessary because the drugs control, but do not cure, the disease.

Argon laser trabeculoplasty (ALT) is a therapeutic option to lower IOP when medications are not successful or when the patient either cannot or will not use the drug therapy as recommended. ALT is an outpatient procedure that requires only topical

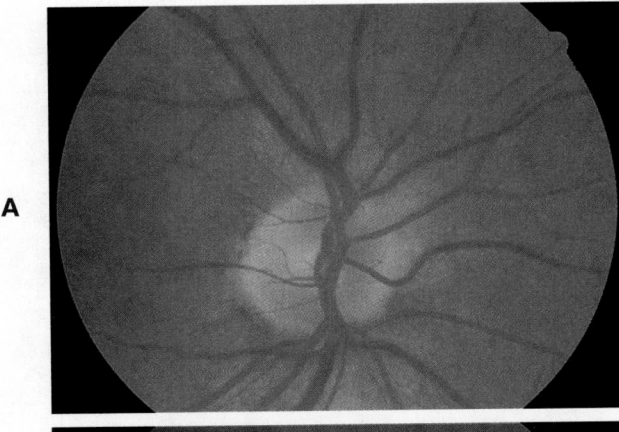

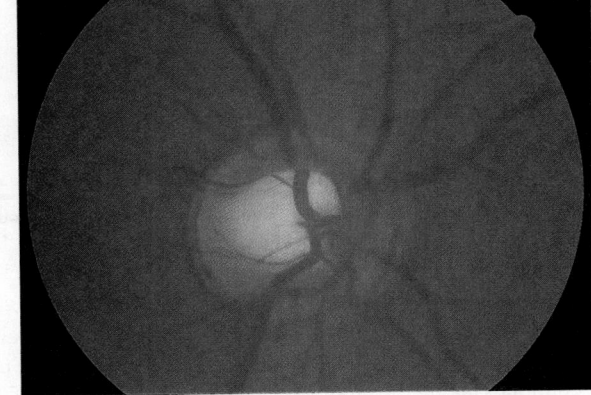

FIG. 21-5 **A,** In the normal eye, the optic cup is pink with little cupping. **B,** In the glaucomatous eye, the optic disc is bleached and optic cupping is present. (Note the appearance of the retinal vessels, which travel over the edge of the optic cup and appear to dip into it.)

TABLE 21-10 Collaborative Care

Glaucoma

Diagnostic
History and physical examination
Visual acuity measurement
Tonometry
Ophthalmoscopy (direct and indirect)
Slit lamp microscopy
Gonioscopy
Visual field perimetry
Fundus photography

Collaborative Therapy
Ambulatory/Home Care for Open-Angle Glaucoma
Drug therapy
  β-adrenergic blockers
  α-adrenergic agonists
  Cholinergic agents (miotics)
  Carbonic anhydrase inhibitors
Surgical therapy
  Argon laser trabeculoplasty (ALT)
  Trabeculectomy, with or without filtering implant
  Cyclocryotherapy destruction of ciliary body
Acute Care Angle-Closure Glaucoma
Topical cholinergic agent
Hyperosmotic agent
Laser peripheral iridotomy
Surgical iridectomy

TABLE 21-11   Drug Therapy
Acute and Chronic Glaucoma

DRUG	ACTION	SIDE EFFECTS	NURSING CONSIDERATIONS
β-Adrenergic Blockers			
betaxolol (Betoptic)	β_1 cardioselective blocker; probably decreases aqueous humor production	Transient discomfort; systemic reactions rarely reported but include bradycardia, heart block, pulmonary distress, headache, depression	Topical drugs; minimal effect on pulmonary and cardiovascular parameters; contraindicated in patient with bradycardia, cardiogenic shock, or overt cardiac failure; systemic absorption can have additive effect with systemic β-blocking agents
carteolol (Ocupress) levobunolol (Betagan) metipranolol (Optipranolol) timolol maleate (Timoptic)	β_1 and β_2 noncardioselective blockers; probably decrease aqueous humor production	Transient ocular discomfort, blurred vision, photophobia, blepharoconjunctivitis, bradycardia, decreased blood pressure, bronchospasm, headache, depression	Topical drops; same as betaxolol; these noncardioselective β-blockers are also contraindicated in patients with asthma or severe COPD
α-Adrenergic Agonists			
dipivefrin (Propine)	α- and β-adrenergic agonist; converted to epinephrine inside the eye; decreases aqueous humor production, enhances outflow facility	Ocular discomfort and redness, tachycardia, hypertension	Topical drops; contraindicated in patient with narrow-angle glaucoma; teach punctal occlusion to patient at risk of systemic reactions
epinephrine (Epifrin, Eppy, Gaucon, Epitrate, Epinal, Eppy/N)	Same as dipivefrin	Same as dipivefrin, but can be more pronounced	Topical drops; same as dipivefrin
apraclonidine (Lopidine) brimonidine (Alphagan)	α-Adrenergic agonist; probably decrease aqueous humor production	Ocular redness; irregular heart rate	Topical drops; used to control or prevent acute postlaser IOP rise (used 1 hr before, and immediately after ALT and iridotomy, Nd:YAG laser capsulotomy); teach patient at risk of systemic reactions to occlude puncta
latanoprost (Xalatan)	Prostaglandin F-analog	Increased brown iris pigmentation, ocular discomfort and redness, dryness, itching, and foreign body sensation	Topical drops; teach patient to not exceed 1 drop per evening; have patient remove contact lens 15 min before instilling
Cholinergic Agents (Miotics)			
carbachol (Isopto Carbachol)	Parasympathomimetic; stimulates iris sphincter contraction, causing miosis and opening of trabecular meshwork, facilitating aqueous outflow; also partially inhibits cholinesterase	Transient ocular discomfort, headache, browache, blurred vision, decreased dark adaptation, syncope, salivation, arrhythmias, vomiting, diarrhea, hypotension, retinal detachment in susceptible individual (rare)	Topical drops; caution patient about decreased visual acuity caused by miosis, particularly in dim light

ALT, Argon laser trabeculoplasty; *CHF,* congestive heart failure; *COPD,* chronic obstructive pulmonary disease; *GI,* gastrointestinal; *IOP,* intraocular pressure; *IV,* intravenous.

anesthetic. The topical drops anesthetize the cornea before the gonioscopy lens is applied, allowing visualization of the treatment area. Approximately 50 laser "spots" are evenly spaced around the superior or inferior 180 degrees of the trabecular meshwork. The laser stimulates scarring and contraction of the trabecular meshwork, opening the outflow channels. ALT reduces IOP approximately 75% of the time.[22] A second 180-degree area may be treated in a subsequent procedure. The patient uses

topical corticosteroids for approximately 3 to 5 days following surgery. The most common complication is an acute postoperative IOP rise. Because the decrease in pressure is gradual, the patient continues taking the preoperative glaucoma medication. The ophthalmologist examines the patient 1 week after the procedure and again 4 to 6 weeks following surgery.

A *filtering procedure,* such as trabeculectomy, may be indicated if medical management and laser therapy are not success-

TABLE 21-11	Drug Therapy — Acute and Chronic Glaucoma—cont'd		
DRUG	**ACTION**	**SIDE EFFECTS**	**NURSING CONSIDERATIONS**
Cholinergic Agents (Miotics)—cont'd			
pilocarpine (Akarpine; Isopto Carpine, Pilocar, Pilopine, Piloptic, Pilostat)	Parasympathomimetic; stimulates iris sphincter contraction, causing miosis and opening of tabecular meshwork, facilitating aqueous humor outflow	Same as carbachol	Topical drops; same as carbachol
Carbonic Anhydrase Inhibitors			
Systemic acetazolamide (Diamox) dichlorphenamide (Daranide) methazolamide (Neptazane)	Decreases aqueous humor production	Paresthesias, especially "tingling" in extremities; hearing dysfunction or tinnitus; loss of appetite; taste alteration; GI disturbances; drowsiness; confusion	Oral nonbacteriostatic sulfonamides; anaphylaxis and other sulfa-type allergic reactions may occur in patient allergic to sulfa; diuretic effect can lower electrolyte levels; ask patient about aspirin use; drug should not be given to patient on high-dose aspirin therapy
Topical brinzolamide (Azopt) dorzolamide (Trusopt)		Transient stinging, blurred vision, redness	Same as above
Combination Therapy timolol maleate and dorzolamide (Cosopt)	Combination of two drugs	See individual drugs for side effects	
Hyperosmolar Agents glycerin liquid (Ophthalgan, Osmoglyn Oral)	Increases extracellular osmolarity so intracellular water moves to the extracellular and vascular spaces, reducing IOP	Nausea, vomiting, headache, confusion, disorientation, arrhythmia, severe dehydration	Oral liquid; used in acute glaucoma attacks or preoperatively when decreased IOP is desired; assess patient for susceptibility to pulmonary edema and CHF before administering hyperosmolar agents
isosorbide solution (Ismotic)	Same as glycerin	Nausea, vomiting, headache, confusion, disorientation, syncope, lethargy, irritability	Oral liquid; same as glycerin
mannitol solution (Osmitrol)	Same as glycerin	Nausea, vomiting, diarrhea, thrombophlebitis, hypertension, hypotension, tachycardia	IV solution; same as glycerin

ful. In this procedure the surgeon makes conjunctival and scleral flaps, removes part of the iris and trabecular meshwork, and closes the scleral flap loosely. Aqueous humor may now "percolate" out through the area of missing iris where it is trapped under the repaired conjunctiva and absorbed into the systemic circulation. The success rate of this filtering surgery is 75% to 85%. The subconjunctival application of mitomycin (Mutamycin) or 5-fluorouracil (5-FU) may increase the success rate by preventing scarring and subsequent closure of the opening created during surgery.

Cyclocryotherapy is another procedure that reduces IOP. The cryoprobe is touched to the sclera outside of the ciliary body. This freezes parts of the ciliary body, causing local destruction of the ciliary tissue and decreasing production of aqueous humor. The procedure may be repeated and can also be used in treating acute glaucoma.

An implant is another surgical option, usually reserved for the patient in whom filtration surgery has failed. It involves surgical placement of a small tube and reservoir to shunt aqueous humor from the anterior chamber to the implanted reservoir.

Acute Angle-Closure Glaucoma. Acute angle-closure glaucoma is an ocular emergency that requires immediate intervention. Miotics and oral or IV hyperosmotic agents are usually successful in immediately lowering the IOP (see Table 21-10). A laser peripheral iridotomy or surgical iridectomy is necessary for long-term treatment and prevention of subsequent episodes. These procedures allow the aqueous humor to flow through a newly created opening in the iris and into normal outflow channels. One of these procedures may also be performed on the other eye as a precaution because many patients often experience an acute attack in the other eye.

Secondary Glaucoma. Secondary glaucoma is managed by treating the underlying problem and by using antiglaucoma drugs. If treatment fails, glaucoma can progress to absolute glaucoma, resulting in a hard, sightless, and usually painful eye requiring enucleation (surgical removal of the eye).

NURSING MANAGEMENT
GLAUCOMA

■ Nursing Assessment

Because glaucoma is a chronic condition requiring long-term management, the nurse must carefully assess the patient's ability to understand and comply with the rationale and regimen of the prescribed therapy. In addition, the nurse should assess the patient's psychologic reaction to the diagnosis of a potentially sight-threatening chronic disorder. The nurse must include the patient's family in the assessment process because the chronic nature of this disorder affects the family in many ways. Some families may become the primary providers of necessary care, such as eyedrop administration or insulin injections, if the patient is unwilling or unable to accomplish these self-care activities. The nurse also assesses visual acuity, visual fields, IOP, and fundus changes when appropriate.

■ Nursing Diagnoses

Nursing diagnoses for the patient with glaucoma include, but are not limited to, the following:

- Noncompliance *related to* the inconvenience and side effects of glaucoma medications
- Risk for injury *related to* visual acuity deficits
- Self-care deficits *related to* visual acuity deficits
- Acute pain *related to* pathophysiologic process and surgical correction

■ Planning

The overall goals are that the patient with glaucoma will (1) have no progression of visual impairment, (2) understand the disease process and rationale for therapy, (3) comply with all aspects of therapy (including medication administration and follow-up care), and (4) have no postoperative complications.

■ Nursing Implementation

Health Promotion. Glaucoma is a preventable problem. The nurse has an important role in teaching the patient and family about the risk of glaucoma. In addition, the nurse should stress the importance of early detection and treatment in preventing visual impairment. This knowledge should encourage the patient to seek appropriate ophthalmic health care. The patient should know that the incidence of glaucoma increases with age and that a comprehensive ophthalmic examination is invaluable in identifying persons with glaucoma or those at risk of developing glaucoma. The current recommendation is for an ophthalmologic examination every 2 to 4 years for persons between ages 40 and 64 years, and every 1 to 2 years for persons age 65 years or older. African Americans in every age category should have examinations more often because of the increased incidence and more aggressive course of glaucoma in these individuals.

Acute Intervention. Acute nursing interventions are directed primarily toward the patient with acute angle-closure glaucoma and the surgical patient. The patient with acute angle-closure glaucoma requires immediate medication to lower the IOP, which the nurse must administer in a timely and appropriate manner according to the ophthalmologist's prescription. This patient may also be uncomfortable, and appropriate nursing comfort interventions may include darkening the environment, applying cool compresses to the patient's forehead, and providing a quiet and private space for the patient. Most surgical procedures for glaucoma are outpatient procedures. Acutely, the patient needs postoperative instructions and may require nursing comfort measures to relieve discomfort related to the procedure. Patient and family teaching following eye surgery is discussed in Table 21-7.

Ambulatory and Home Care. Because of the chronic nature of glaucoma, the patient needs encouragement to follow the therapeutic regimen and follow-up recommendations prescribed by the ophthalmologist. The patient needs accurate information about the disease process and treatment options, including the rationale underlying each option. In addition, the patient needs information about the purpose, frequency, and technique for administration of prescribed antiglaucoma agents. In addition to verbal instructions, all patients should receive written instructions that contain the same information. This should be sufficiently detailed to provide all the necessary information without being so extensive that the patient becomes overwhelmed. The patient may be encouraged to comply with the medication regimen if the nurse promotes consideration of the sight-saving nature of the drops. The nurse can further encourage compliance by helping the patient identify the most convenient and appropriate times for medication administration or advocating a change in therapy if the patient reports unacceptable side effects.

■ Evaluation

The overall expected outcomes are that the patient with glaucoma will

- have no further loss of vision
- comply with recommended therapy
- safely function within own environment
- obtain relief from pain associated with the disease and surgery

■ Gerontologic Considerations: Glaucoma

Many older patients with glaucoma have systemic illnesses or take systemic medications that may affect their therapy. In particular, the patient using a β-adrenergic blocking glaucoma agent may experience an additive effect if a systemic β-adrenergic blocking drug is also being taken. All β-adrenergic blocking glaucoma agents are contraindicated in the patient with bradycardia, greater than first-degree heart block, cardiogenic shock, and overt cardiac failure. The noncardioselective β-adrenergic blocker glaucoma agents are also contraindicated in the patient with severe chronic obstructive pulmonary disease (COPD) or asthma. The hyperosmolar agents may precipitate congestive heart failure (CHF) or pulmonary edema in the susceptible patient. The older patient on high-dose aspirin therapy for rheumatoid arthritis should not take carbonic anhydrase inhibitors. The α-adrenergic agonists can cause tachycardia or hypertension, which may have serious consequences in the older patient. The nurse should teach the older patient to occlude the puncta to limit the systemic absorption of glaucoma medications. ■

INTRAOCULAR INFLAMMATION AND INFECTION

The term *uveitis* is used to describe inflammation of the uveal tract, the retina, the vitreous body, or the optic nerve. This inflammation may be caused by bacteria, viruses, fungi, or parasites. *Cytomegalovirus retinitis* (CMV retinitis) is an opportunistic infection that occurs in patients with acquired immunodeficiency syndrome (AIDS) and in other immunosuppressed patients. The etiology of sterile intraocular inflammation includes autoimmune disorders, AIDS, malignancies, or those associated with systemic diseases such as juvenile rheumatoid arthritis and inflammatory bowel disease. Pain and photophobia are common symptoms.

Endophthalmitis is an extensive intraocular inflammation of the vitreous cavity. Bacteria, viruses, fungi, or parasites can all induce this serious inflammatory response. The mechanism of infection may be endogenous, in which the infecting agent arrives at the eye through the bloodstream, or exogenous, in which the infecting agent is introduced through a surgical wound or a penetrating injury. Although rare, most cases of endophthalmitis are a devastating complication of intraocular surgery or penetrating ocular injury and can lead to irreversible blindness within hours or days. Manifestations include ocular pain, photophobia, decreased visual acuity, headaches, upper lid edema, reddened and swollen conjunctiva, and corneal edema.

When all the layers of the eye (vitreous, retina, choroid, and sclera) are involved in the inflammatory response, the patient has *panophthalmitis*. In the final stages of extensive cases, the scleral coat may undergo bacterial or inflammatory dissolution. Subsequent rupture of the globe spreads the infection into the orbit or eyelids.

Treatment of intraocular inflammation depends on the underlying cause. Intraocular infections require antimicrobial agents, which may be delivered topically, subconjunctivally, intravitreally, systemically, or in some combination. Sterile inflammatory responses require antiinflammatory agents such as corticosteroids. The site and the severity of the sterile inflammatory response determine whether topical, subconjunctival, or systemic corticosteroids are necessary.

The patient with intraocular inflammation is usually uncomfortable and may be noticeably anxious and frightened. The patient may fear sudden and total loss of vision. In some cases this fear is realistic, and the nurse should provide accurate information and emotional support to the patient and the family. In severe cases enucleation may be necessary. When the patient has lost visual function or even the entire eye, the patient will grieve the loss. The nurse's role includes helping the patient through the grieving process.

ENUCLEATION

Enucleation is the removal of the eye. The primary indication for enucleation is a blind, painful eye. This may result from absolute glaucoma, infection, or trauma. Enucleation may also be indicated in ocular malignancies, although many malignancies can be managed with cryotherapy, radiation, and chemotherapy. An extremely rare indication is *sympathetic ophthalmia,* in which the untraumatized eye develops an inflammatory response following the primary eye trauma. In this situation the traumatized eye is enucleated. The surgical procedure includes severing the extraocular muscles close to their insertion on the globe, inserting an implant to maintain the intraorbital anatomy, and suturing the ends of the extraocular muscles over the implant. The conjunctiva covers the joined muscles, and a clear conformer is placed over the conjunctiva until the permanent prosthesis is fitted. A pressure dressing helps prevent postoperative bleeding.

Postoperatively the nurse observes the patient for signs of complications, including excessive bleeding or swelling, increased pain, displacement of the implant, or temperature elevation. Patient teaching should include the instillation of topical ointments or drops and wound cleansing. The nurse should also instruct the patient in the method of inserting the conformer into the socket in case it falls out. The patient is often devastated by the loss of an eye, even when enucleation occurs following a lengthy period of painful blindness. The nurse should recognize and validate the patient's emotional response and provide support to the patient and the family.

Approximately 6 weeks following surgery the wound is sufficiently healed for the permanent prosthesis. The prosthesis is fitted by an ocularist and designed to match the remaining eye. The patient should learn how to remove, cleanse, and insert the prosthesis. Special polishing is required periodically to remove dried protein secretions.

OCULAR MANIFESTATIONS OF SYSTEMIC DISEASES

Many systemic diseases have significant ocular manifestations. Although it is not the purpose of this discussion to provide a full description of these disorders, it is important for the nurse to recognize that many systemic diseases have ocular symptoms. Conversely, ocular signs and symptoms may be the first finding or complaint in the patient with a systemic disease. One example is the patient with undiagnosed diabetes who seeks ophthalmic care for blurred vision. A careful history and examination of the patient can reveal that the underlying cause of the blurred vision is lens swelling caused by hyperglycemia. Another example is the patient who seeks care for a conjunctival lesion. The ophthalmologist may be the first health care professional to make the diagnosis of AIDS based on the presence of a conjunctival Kaposi's sarcoma (KS). Table 21-12 lists some systemic diseases and disorders and the associated ophthalmic manifestations.

TABLE 21-12   Ocular Manifestations of Systemic Diseases or Disorders

SYSTEMIC ENTITY	OCULAR MANIFESTATIONS
• AIDS	Herpes zoster ophthalmicus, keratitis (bacterial and viral), CMV retinitis, endophthalmitis (bacterial and fungal), cotton-wool spots and microvasculopathy of the retina, KS of eyelids or conjunctiva
• Albinism	Decreased visual acuity, photophobia, nystagmus, strabismus
• Diabetes mellitus	Fluctuating refractive errors, diabetic retinopathy, macular edema, premature cataract development, increased incidence of glaucoma
• Down syndrome	Myopia, cataracts, nystagmus, strabismus, keratoconus, upward and outward slant of palpebral fissures
• Hypertension	Cotton-wool spots and hemorrhage of the retina, retinal lipid deposits
• Systemic lupus erythematosus	Dry eye, retinal changes, uveitis, scleritis
• Marfan syndrome	Lens dislocation, severe myopia, keratoconus, retinal detachment
• Rheumatoid arthritis	Dry eye, keratitis, scleritis
• Infections	
Botulism	Blurred vision, ptosis, diplopia, fixed, dilated pupil
Endocarditis	Subconjunctival or retinal petechiae
Tuberculosis	Conjunctivitis, keratitis, uveitis
Leprosy	Conjunctivitis, keratitis, uveitis, ptosis
Genital herpes	Herpes simplex keratitis
CMV infection	CMV retinitis
Measles	Conjunctivitis, keratitis, retinopathy
Congenital rubella	Cataracts, glaucoma
Histoplasmosis	Chorioretinal lesions, subretinal neovascularization
Toxoplasmosis	Necrotic retinal lesions, vitreal inflammation, retinochoroiditis
Lyme disease	Conjunctivitis, keratitis, episcleritis, panophthalmitis, retinal detachment, diplopia
Syphilis	Conjunctivitis, keratitis, uveitis, retinal detachment, macular edema, lens dislocation, glaucoma (congenital syphilis)
• Temporal arteritis	Vision loss; palsies of CN III, IV, and VI; nystagmus; ptosis
• Thyroid disease	Lid retraction, lid lag, exophthalmos, abnormal eye movement, increased IOP
• Vitamin deficiencies	
A	Night blindness, corneal ulceration
B	Optic neuropathy, corneal changes, retinal hemorrhage, nystagmus
C	Hemorrhage in anterior chamber, retina, conjunctiva
D	Exophthalmos

AIDS, Acquired immunodeficiency syndrome; *CMV,* cytomegalovirus; *CN,* cranial nerve; *IOP,* intraocular pressure, *KS,* Kaposi's sarcoma.

Hearing Problems

EXTERNAL EAR AND CANAL

TRAUMA

Trauma to the external ear can cause injury to the subcutaneous tissue that may result in a hematoma. If the hematoma is not aspirated, inflammation of the membranes of the ear cartilage (perichondritis) can result. Antibiotics are given to prevent infection. Blows to the ear can also cause a conductive hearing loss if there is damage to the ossicles in the middle ear or if a perforation of the tympanic membrane results. It is important to obtain a careful history of the accident and to assess the hearing of a patient who has had a blow to the ear or side of the head.

EXTERNAL OTITIS

The skin of the external ear and canal is subject to the same problems as skin anywhere on the body. **External otitis** involves inflammation or infection of the epithelium of the auricle and ear canal. Frequent swimming may alter the flora of the external canal, resulting in an infection often referred to as "swimmer's ear." Trauma caused by picking the ear or the use of sharp ob-

jects, such as hairpins, frequently causes the initial break in the skin.

Etiology

Infections, dermatitis, or both may cause external otitis. Bacteria or fungi may be the cause. The bacteria most commonly cultured are *Pseudomonas aeruginosa* followed by *Klebsiella, Proteus, Escherichia coli,* and *S. aureus.* The most common fungi are *Candida albicans* and *Aspergillus* organisms.[23] Fungi are often the causative agents of external otitis, especially in warm, moist climates. The warm, dark environment of the ear canal provides a good medium for the growth of microorganisms.

Clinical Manifestations and Complications

Pain *(otalgia)* is one of the first signs of external otitis. Even in mild cases, the patient may experience pain that is disproportionate to the infection. Pain is caused by the swelling of the bony ear canal as a result of the inflammatory process. Pain is especially noted on movement of the auricle or on application of pressure to the tragus (directly in front of the ear). Drainage from the ear may be serosanguineous or purulent. If it is the result of an infection caused by *Pseudomonas,* the drainage will be green and have a musty smell. Temperature elevations occur when there is extensive involvement of the tissue. The swelling of the ear canal can block hearing and cause dizziness.

NURSING MANAGEMENT
EXTERNAL OTITIS

Diagnosis of external otitis is made by observation with the otoscope light using the largest speculum that the ear will accommodate without causing the patient unnecessary discomfort. The eardrum may be normal if it can be seen. Culture and sensitivity studies of the drainage may be done. Mild analgesics will usually control the pain. After the ear canal is cleansed, a wick of cotton is placed in the canal to help deliver the antibiotic eardrops. Cotton wicks should be used with caution in young patients and confused or psychotic patients, who may push them farther into the ear. Topical antibiotics include polymyxin B and neomycin (Neosporin) and chloramphenicol (Chloromycetin). Nystatin (Mycostatin) is used for fungal infections. Corticosteroids may also be used to decrease inflammation unless the infection is fungal, in which case they are contraindicated. If the surrounding tissue is involved, systemic antibiotics are prescribed. Warm, moist compresses or heat may be applied. Improvement should occur in 48 hours, but 7 to 14 days are required for complete resolution.

Careful handling and disposal of material saturated with drainage are important. Otic drops (eardrops) should be administered at room temperature because cold drops can cause dizziness in the patient due to stimulation of the semicircular canals. The tip of the dropper should not touch the ear during administration to prevent contamination of the entire bottle of drops. The ear is positioned so that the drops can run down the canal. This position should be maintained for 2 minutes after eardrop administration to allow dispersion of drops. Collaborative care of external otitis is shown in Table 21-13.

CERUMEN AND FOREIGN BODIES IN THE EXTERNAL EAR CANAL

Impacted cerumen can cause discomfort and decreased hearing, which is often described as a hollow sensation. In the older person, the earwax becomes dense and drier. Hair becomes thicker and coarser, entrapping the hard dry cerumen in the canal. Water that enters the canal during a shower or swimming may cause swelling of

TABLE 21-13	Collaborative Care External Otitis

Diagnostic
History and physical examination
Otoscopic examination
Culture and sensitivity

Collaborative Therapy
Analgesics (depending on severity)
Warm compresses
Cleansing of canal
Ear wick
Antibiotic otic drops
Systemic antibiotics

TABLE 21-14	Manifestations of Cerumen Impaction

Hearing loss
Otalgia
Tinnitus
Vertigo
Cough
Cardiac depression (vagal stimulation)

the cerumen, resulting in complete blockage of the canal. Symptoms of cerumen impaction are outlined in Table 21-14. Management involves irrigation of the canal with body-temperature solutions. Special syringes can be used and vary from the simple bulb syringe to special irrigating equipment used in the health care provider's office or clinic. The patient is placed in a sitting position with an emesis basin under the ear. The auricle is pulled up and back, and the flow of solution is directed to the top of the canal. It is important that the ear canal not be completely occluded with the syringe tip. If irrigation does not remove the wax, a cerumen spoon can be used. Mild lubricant drops may be used (sometimes overnight) to soften the earwax, and irrigation may then be effective in removing the impacted cerumen. It may need to be removed by a physician using an operating microscope, suction, and microsurgical instruments.

The list of objects removed from the ear is extensive and includes animate, inanimate, vegetable, and mineral objects. Attempts to remove the object occasionally result in pushing it further into the canal. An otolaryngologist should remove the object. Vegetable matter tends to swell and may create a secondary inflammation, making removal more difficult.

Animate objects must be immobilized before removal. Mineral oil or lidocaine can be used to drown an insect. The organism can then be removed with microscope guidance. The use of general anesthesia or conscious sedation may be necessary depending on the level of patient cooperation. Rarely, it may be necessary to make a canal incision to remove the foreign body.[24]

The patient should be instructed to keep objects out of the ear. Ears should be cleaned only with a washcloth and finger. Bobby pins and cotton-tipped applicators should especially be avoided. Penetration of the middle ear by a cotton-tipped applicator can cause serious injury to the tympanic membrane and ossicles and may result in facial paralysis as a result of nerve damage. The use of cotton-tipped applicators can also impact cerumen against the tympanic membrane and impair hearing.

MALIGNANCY OF THE EXTERNAL EAR

Malignancies of the external ear (other than skin cancers) and canal are uncommon. The predominant signs include a chronic ulcer of the auricle and persistent drainage from the canal much like that seen with otitis externa. This drainage may be tinged with blood and does not diminish with treatment. Collaborative care includes biopsy and other diagnostic studies such as a computed tomography (CT) scan to determine invasion of underlying tissue and bone. Treatment usually involves surgery. If the malignancy involves the ear canal and temporal bone, radical surgery of the middle and inner ear with resection of the facial nerve (CN VII), auditory nerve (CN VIII), and part of the temporal bone may be necessary.

Because of long-term sun exposure, the ears are at increased risk for development of cancer. The most common malignant neoplasms of the auricle are basal cell and squamous cell cancers.[25] These skin cancers can be excised surgically, or they may be serially excised using a special technique to microscopically examine the tissue to ensure that all residual cancer cells are resected. This procedure is known as Mohs' micrographic technique (described in Chapter 23). These skin cancers are usually not life threatening, and the cure rate after resection is greater than 90% in most cases. Melanoma occurs rarely on the external ear. Cancer of the ear often results in cosmetic deformities that are difficult to reconstruct.

MIDDLE EAR AND MASTOID
ACUTE OTITIS MEDIA

The most common problem of the middle ear is *acute otitis media,* usually a childhood disease associated with colds, allergies, sore throats, and blockage of the eustachian tube. The earlier the first episode, the greater the risk of subsequent episodes occurring. Risk factors include young age, congenital abnormalities, immune deficiencies, exposure to cigarette smoke, family history of otitis media, recent upper respiratory infections, male gender, and allergy.[26] Although most patients have mixed infections, bacteria are the predominant etiologic agents. Pain, fever, malaise, headache, and reduced hearing are signs and symptoms of acute otitis media.

Collaborative care involves the use of antibiotics to eradicate the causative organism. Amoxicillin for 10 days is the current therapy of choice in the United States. Surgical intervention is generally reserved for the patient who does not respond to medical treatment. A *myringotomy* involves an incision in the tympanum to release the increased pressure and exudate from the middle ear. A tympanostomy tube may be placed for short- or long-term use. Prompt treatment of an episode of acute otitis media generally prevents spontaneous perforation of the tympanic membrane. In the adult patient for whom allergy may be a causative factor, antihistamines may also be prescribed. Since the advent of treatment with antibiotics, the incidence of severe and prolonged infections of the middle ear and mastoid has been greatly reduced.

CHRONIC OTITIS MEDIA
AND MASTOIDITIS

Etiology and Pathophysiology

Untreated or repeated attacks of acute otitis media may lead to a chronic condition. Chronic infection of the middle ear is more common in persons who experience episodes of acute otitis media in early childhood. Organisms involved in chronic otitis media include *S. aureus, Streptococcus, Proteus mirabilis, P. aeruginosa,* and *E. coli.* Because the mucous membrane is continuous, both the middle ear and the air cells of the mastoid can be involved in the chronic infectious process.

Clinical Manifestations

Chronic otitis media is characterized by a purulent, mucoid, or serous discharge accompanied by hearing loss and occasionally by ear pain, nausea, and episodes of dizziness. The patient may complain of hearing loss that may be a result of destruction

of the ossicles, a tympanic membrane perforation, or the accumulation of fluid in the middle ear space. Occasionally a facial palsy or an attack of vertigo may alert the patient to this condition. Chronic otitis media is usually painless, but if pain is present, it indicates that fluid has accumulated.

Complications

Untreated conditions can result in perforation of the tympanic membrane and the formation of a **cholesteatoma** (an accumulation of keratinizing squamous epithelium in the middle ear). Its enlarging tumor-like behavior may destroy the adjacent bones, including the ossicles. Unless removed surgically, a cholesteatoma can cause extensive damage to the structures of the middle ear, can erode the bony protection of the facial nerve, may create a labyrinthine fistula, or can even invade the dura, threatening the brain. In addition to cholesteatoma, other complications of chronic otitis media include sensorineural hearing loss, facial paralysis, lateral sinus thrombosis, brain or subdural abscess, mastoiditis, labyrinthitis, and meningitis.[27]

Diagnostic Studies

Otoscopic examination may reveal a marginal or central perforation of the tympanic membrane (Fig. 21-6). Some tympanic membranes may be healed but have an area that is more flaccid and thinner, indicating a previous perforation. Culture and sensitivity tests are necessary to identify the organisms involved so that the appropriate antibiotic therapy can be prescribed. The audiogram may demonstrate no loss in hearing or a loss as great as 50 to 60 dB if the ossicles have been partially destroyed or disarticulated (separated). Sinus x-rays, magnetic resonance imaging (MRI), or a CT scan of the temporal bone may demonstrate bone destruction, absence of ossicles, or the presence of a mass, most likely a cholesteatoma.

Collaborative Care

The aim of treatment is to clear the middle ear of infection (Table 21-15). Systemic antibiotic therapy is initiated based on the culture and sensitivity results. In addition, the patient may need to undergo frequent evacuation of drainage and debris in an outpatient setting. Antibiotic eardrops and 2% acetic acid drops are also used to reduce infection. If there is a recurrence, the patient may need to be treated with parenteral antibiotics. In many cases of chronic otitis media, additional antibiotic

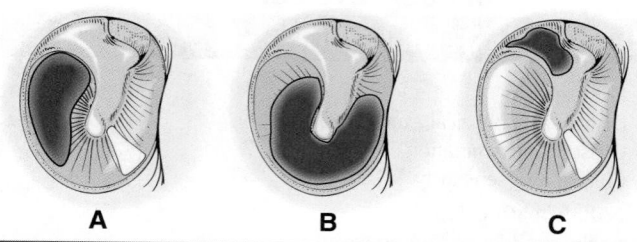

A **B** **C**

FIG. 21-6 Three common tympanic perforations. **A,** Small central perforation (hearing is usually good). **B,** Large central perforation around the handle of the malleus (hearing is usually poor). **C,** Marginal perforation of Shrapnell's membrane (hearing is usually good). Cholesteatomas commonly occur in patients with a marginal perforation and are always present with attic perforation.

TABLE 21-15	*C*ollaborative Care Chronic Otitis Media

Diagnostic
History and physical examination
Otoscopic examination
Culture and sensitivity of middle ear drainage
Mastoid x-ray

Collaborative Therapy
Ear irrigations
Acetic acid (equal amounts of white vinegar and warm water)
Otic drops, powders
Analgesics
Antiemetics
Systemic antibiotics
Surgery
  Tympanoplasty*
  Mastoidectomy

*See Table 21-17.

therapy loses its effectiveness as the number of treatments increases.

Surgical Therapy. Often chronic tympanic membrane perforations will not heal with conservative treatment, and surgery is necessary. Surgery involving reconstruction of the tympanic membrane and/or the ossicular chain is called a *tympanoplasty* (Table 21-16). Diseased tissue is removed, and the ossicles are examined and evaluated in reconstructing the conductive mechanism. This may be done with the use of partial or total ossicular prostheses in combination with a fascia graft to repair the perforation of the tympanic membrane. The incision may be endaural (within the ear canal) or postauricular (behind the auricle or ear), depending on the amount of involvement.

A *mastoidectomy* is often performed with a tympanoplasty to remove diseased tissue and the source of infection. A modified mastoidectomy attempts to preserve functioning by removing as little tissue as possible. Removal of tissue stops at the middle ear structures that appear capable of functioning in the conduction of sound.

TABLE 21-16	Surgical Therapy for Chronic Ear Infection

Myringoplasty
Surgical reconstruction limited to repair of a tympanic membrane perforation

Tympanoplasty without Mastoidectomy
An operation to eradicate disease in the middle ear and to reconstruct the hearing mechanism without mastoid surgery; with or without tympanic membrane grafting

Tympanoplasty with Mastoidectomy
An operation to eradicate disease in both the middle ear and the mastoid process and to reconstruct the middle ear conduction mechanism; with or without tympanic membrane grafting

NURSING MANAGEMENT
ACUTE OTITIS MEDIA

■ Following Tympanoplasty

Routine preoperative care is provided before tympanoplasty and includes teaching postoperative expectations. Postoperative concerns are the avoidance of complications such as disruption of the repair during the healing phase, facial nerve paralysis (rare), and increased pressure in the middle ear. The patient is instructed to avoid blowing the nose because this causes increased pressure in the eustachian tube and the middle ear cavity and could dislodge the tympanum graft. Coughing and sneezing can cause similar disruption and are to be avoided if possible. If the patient must cough or sneeze, leaving the mouth open will reduce the pressure. It is essential that the patient be helped when getting up the first time; because of dizziness and a loss of balance, a fall may occur.

A cotton ball dressing is used for an endaural incision. If a postauricular incision is used and a drain is in place, a mastoid dressing is used. A 4 × 4–inch dressing is cut to fit behind the ear, and fluffs are applied over the ear to prevent the outer circular head dressing from placing pressure on the auricle. It is necessary to monitor the tightness of the dressing (to prevent tissue necrosis) and the amount and type of drainage postoperatively.

CHRONIC OTITIS MEDIA WITH EFFUSION

Chronic otitis media with effusion is an inflammation of the middle ear in which a collection of fluid is present in the middle ear space. The fluid may be thin, mucoid, or purulent. This condition is commonly called *serous otitis media,* "glue ear," and *secretory otitis media.* It may occur at any age but is more frequent in children. The fluid usually collects because of a malfunction of the eustachian tube, which commonly follows upper respiratory and/or chronic sinus infections, barotrauma (caused by pressure change), or otitis media. If the eustachian tube does not open and allow equalization of atmospheric pressure, negative pressure within the middle ear causes fluid transudation from the tissues. Allergic reaction of the mucosa creating edema can also cause blockage of the eustachian tube and cause fluid within the ear. Overgrowth of nasopharyngeal lymphoid tissue and chronic sinusitis are also factors that may contribute to middle ear effusion.

Complaints include a feeling of fullness of the ear, "plugged" feeling or popping, and decreased hearing. The patient does not experience pain, fever, or discharge from the ear. Otoscopic examination may reveal a normal tympanic membrane or minimal dullness and retraction. Tympanometry and pneumatoscopy may demonstrate limited tympanic membrane motion consistent with decreased hearing acuity.

Decongestants, antihistamines, corticosteroids, and antibiotics have been used in the treatment of middle ear effusions. Exercises such as swallowing and gum chewing are used to open the eustachian tube. In addition, the patient may be taught the Valsalva maneuver, which forces air into the middle ear through the eustachian tube. If the effusion is not relieved after a period of time, a myringotomy is performed, usually under local or topical anesthesia with an operating microscope. A ventilating tube is frequently used for the person who has recurrent otitis media with effusion or dysfunction of the eustachian tube. The patient who has a ventilating tube in the tympanic membrane must be instructed not to swim or get water in the ear. Despite efforts to correct inadequate middle ear aeration, eustachian tube dysfunction may persist, causing collapse of the eardrum, conductive hearing loss, and formation of a cholesteatoma. Adenoidectomy may also be done in conjunction with myringotomy to correct the underlying problem of middle ear aeration.

OTOSCLEROSIS

Otosclerosis, an autosomal dominant disease, is the fixation of the footplate of the stapes in the oval window. It is a common cause of conductive hearing loss in young adults, especially women, and may accelerate during pregnancy. Otosclerosis is bilateral in about 80% of patients. Spongy bone develops from the bony labyrinth, causing immobilization of the footplate of the stapes, which reduces the transmission of vibrations to the inner ear fluids. Although hearing loss is typically bilateral, one ear may show greater hearing loss progression. The patient is often unaware of the problem until the loss becomes so severe that communication is difficult. Loss of hearing usually becomes increasingly severe.

Otoscopic examination may reveal a reddish blush of the tympanum (Schwartz's sign) caused by the vascular and bony changes within the middle ear. Tuning fork tests help identify the conductive component of the hearing loss. On the Rinne test, bone conduction will be better than air conduction if hearing loss is greater that 25 dB. Weber's test lateralizes to the ear with the greater conductive hearing loss. An audiogram demonstrates good hearing by bone conduction, but air conduction or an air-bone gap audiogram demonstrates poor hearing. Usually at least a difference of 20 to 25 dB between air-conduction and bone-conduction levels of hearing is seen in otosclerosis.

Collaborative Care

Stapedectomy is the surgical treatment for otosclerosis and is usually performed under local anesthesia with sedation. The ear with poorer hearing is repaired first, and the other ear may be operated on 6 months to a year later. (Collaborative care of otosclerosis is shown in Table 21-17.)

In stapedectomy an endaural incision is made using the operating microscope for visualization. Generally the stapes super-

TABLE 21-17   Collaborative Care   Otosclerosis

Diagnostic
History and physical examination
Otoscopic examination
Rinne test (512 Hz tuning fork)
Weber test
Audiometry
Tympanometry

Collaborative Therapy
Hearing aid
Surgery (stapedectomy)
Drug therapy
    Sodium fluoride
    Vitamin D
    Calcium carbonate

structure is removed, and a small hole is made in the footplate with a drill or laser. A prosthesis made of stainless steel, Teflon, or other synthetic material completes the ossicular chain. Sound is then conducted with the prosthesis. The tympanum is rolled back into normal position, and Gelfoam is placed on the flap. A cotton ball is placed in the ear canal and a Band-Aid dressing is used to cover the ear. During surgery the patient will often report an immediate improvement in hearing in the operative ear. Because of the accumulation of blood and fluid in the middle ear, the hearing level decreases postoperatively but does return to near-normal levels. After stapedectomy, 90% of patients experience an improvement in hearing, in many instances near normal. The hearing loss associated with otosclerosis may be stabilized by the use of sodium fluoride with vitamin D and calcium carbonate to retard bone resorption and encourage calcification of bony lesions.[28]

NURSING MANAGEMENT
OTOSCLEROSIS

Nursing management of the patient undergoing a stapedectomy is similar to that for the patient who has undergone a tympanoplasty. Postoperatively, the patient may experience dizziness, nausea, and vomiting as a result of stimulation of the labyrinth intraoperatively. Some patients demonstrate nystagmus on lateral gaze because of disturbance of the perilymph. Care should be taken to decrease sudden movements by the patient that may bring on or exacerbate dizziness. Actions such as coughing, sneezing, lifting, bending, and straining during bowel movements should also be minimized.

INNER EAR PROBLEMS

Three symptoms that indicate disease of the inner ear are vertigo, sensorineural hearing loss, and tinnitus. Symptoms of vertigo arise from the vestibular labyrinth, whereas hearing loss and tinnitus arise from the auditory labyrinth. There is an overlap between manifestations of inner ear problems and central nervous system (CNS) disorders.

MÉNIÈRE'S DISEASE

Ménière's disease is characterized by symptoms caused by inner ear disease, including episodic vertigo, tinnitus, fluctuating sensorineural hearing loss, and aural fullness. This disease causes significant disability for the patient because of sudden, severe attacks of vertigo with nausea and vomiting. Symptoms usually begin between 30 and 60 years of age. In 40% of patients with Ménière's disease, bilateral involvement is found.

The cause of the disease is unknown, but it results in an excessive accumulation of endolymph in the membranous labyrinth. The volume of endolymph increases until the membranous labyrinth ruptures, mixing high-potassium endolymph with low-potassium perilymph. Attacks of vertigo are sudden, with little or no warning. Attacks may be preceded by a sense of fullness in the ear, increasing tinnitus, and a decrease in hearing acuity. The patient may experience the feeling of being pulled to the ground ("drop attacks"). However, only 7% of patients with Ménière's disease report this symptom. Some patients report that they feel as if they are whirling in space. The duration of attacks may be hours or days, and attacks may occur several times a year. Autonomic symptoms include pallor, sweating, nausea, and vomiting.

The clinical course of the disease is highly variable. Low-pitched tinnitus may be present continuously in the affected ear or it may be intensified during an attack. It is often described as a "roar," or "like the ocean." Hearing loss fluctuates, and with continued attacks, hearing recovery is often less complete with each episode, eventually leading to progressive permanent hearing loss.

NURSING and COLLABORATIVE MANAGEMENT MÉNIÈRE'S DISEASE

Collaborative care of Ménière's disease (Table 21-18) includes diagnostic tests to rule out CNS disease. The audiogram demonstrates a mild low-frequency sensorineural hearing loss. Vestibular tests indicate decreased function.

A glycerol test may aid in the diagnosis of Ménière's disease. An oral dose of glycerol is given, followed by serial audiograms over 3 hours. Improvement in hearing or speech discrimination supports a diagnosis of Ménière's disease. The improvement is attributed to the osmotic effect of glycerol that pulls fluid from the inner ear. Although a positive test is diagnostic of Ménière's disease, a negative test does not rule out the condition.

During the acute attack, antihistamines, anticholinergics, and benzodiazepines can be used to decrease the abnormal sensation and lessen symptoms such as nausea and vomiting. Acute vertigo is treated symptomatically with bed rest, sedation, and antiemetics or drugs for motion sickness administered orally, rectally, or intravenously. The patient requires reassurance and counseling that the condition is not life threatening. Management between attacks may include vasodilation, diuretics, antihistamines, a low-sodium diet, and avoidance of caffeine and nicotine. Diazepam (Valium) and meclizine (Antivert [Bonamine plus nicotinic acid]) are commonly used to reduce the dizziness. Over a period of time, most patients respond to the prescribed medications but must learn to live with the unpredictability of the attacks. Approximately 75% to 85% of patients experience improvement with medical management and supportive therapy. The remainder of patients may, in time, require surgical intervention.[29]

Frequent and incapacitating attacks, reduced quality of life, and threatened unemployment are indications for surgical intervention. Surgical decompression of the endolymphatic sac is performed to reduce the pressure on the cochlear hair cells and to prevent further damage and hearing loss. If relief is not achieved with endolymphatic shunt surgery and hearing remains good, vestibular nerve resection may be performed to alleviate vertigo and preserve hearing. When involvement is unilateral, surgical ablation of the labyrinth, resulting in loss of the vestibular and hearing cochlear function, is performed. Careful management can decrease the possibility of progressive sensorineural loss in many patients.

Nursing interventions are planned to minimize vertigo and provide for patient safety. During an acute attack the patient is kept in a quiet, darkened room in a comfortable position. The patient needs to be taught to avoid sudden head movements or position changes. Fluorescent or flickering lights or watching television may exacerbate symptoms and should be avoided. An emesis basin should be available because vomiting is common. To minimize the risk of falling, the nurse should keep the side rails up and the bed low in position when the patient is in bed. The patient should be instructed to call for assistance when getting out of bed. Medications and fluids are administered parenterally, and intake and output are monitored. When the attack subsides, the patient should be assisted with ambulation because unsteadiness may remain. Similar nursing care is provided after surgical ablation of the labyrinth. The patient will have severe tinnitus and vertigo, which decrease during a period of days or weeks as the brain adjusts to loss of vestibular input and postural stability is regained.

LABYRINTHITIS

Labyrinthitis is an inflammation of the inner ear affecting the cochlear and/or vestibular portion of the labyrinth. Infection can enter from the meninges, the middle ear, or the bloodstream. Symptoms include vertigo, tinnitus, and sensorineural hearing loss on the affected side. This condition is rare since the advent of antibiotics. *Nystagmus,* an abnormal rhythmic, jerking movement of the eyes, accompanies the vertigo and has a horizontal beat.

Suppurative labyrinthitis from infection causes severe vertigo with nausea and vomiting similar to that of an attack of Ménière's disease. Complete destruction of the cochlea and labyrinth may occur, causing permanent deafness. Loss of vestibular input causes extreme unsteadiness in the patient. The patient requires physical therapy to recondition the brain to interpret vestibular input.

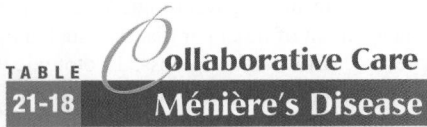

TABLE 21-18	**Collaborative Care**
	Ménière's Disease

Diagnostic
History and physical examination
Audiometric studies, including speech discrimination, tone decay
Vestibular tests, including caloric test, positional test
Electronystagmography
Neurologic examination
Glycerol test

Collaborative Therapy
Acute Care (one or more)
Sedative (diazepam [Valium])
Anticholinergic (atropine)
Vasodilators
Antihistamine (diphenhydramine [Benadryl])
Surgical Therapy
Conservative Surgical Intervention
Endolymphatic shunt
Vestibular nerve section
Destructive Surgical Intervention
Labyrinthotomy
Labyrinthectomy
Ambulatory/Home Care (one or more)
Diuretics
Antihistamines
Vasodilators
Antiseizure drugs
Vitamins
diazepam (Valium)
Low-salt diet
Restriction of caffeine, nicotine, and alcohol intake

Vestibular neuronitis causes vertigo, nausea, vomiting, and nystagmus. A viral infection may be the cause. The patient recovers after 7 to 10 days. Tinnitus is not present, and hearing loss does not occur. Toxic or serous labyrinthitis is associated with acute otitis media. It is caused by bacterial toxins diffusing through the round window membrane. High-frequency hearing loss and mild to moderate vertigo may occur.

ACOUSTIC NEUROMA

An **acoustic neuroma** (or *vestibular schwannoma*) is a benign tumor that occurs where the acoustic nerve (CN VIII) enters the internal auditory canal or the temporal bone from the brain. It is important that an early diagnosis be made because the tumor can compress the facial nerve and arteries within the internal auditory canal. Once the tumor has expanded and become an intracranial neoplasm, more extensive surgery is necessary, reducing the chances of preserving hearing and normal facial nerve function. It can expand into the cerebellopontine angle and involve other cranial nerves and the brain by compression.

Early symptoms are associated with CN VIII compression and destruction. They include unilateral, progressive, sensorineural hearing loss; unilateral tinnitus; and mild, intermittent vertigo. One of the earliest symptoms of an acoustic neuroma is reduced touch sensation in the posterior ear canal. Diagnostic tests include neurologic, audiometric, and vestibular tests and CT scans and MRI with gadolinium enhancement.

Surgery to remove small tumors is performed through the middle cranial fossa or retrolabyrinthine approach, which preserves hearing and vestibular function. A translabyrinthine approach is usually used for medium-sized tumors and when hearing is minimal. Although hearing is destroyed by this approach, advantages include good access to the tumor and preservation of the facial nerve. Retrosigmoid (suboccipital) or transotic approaches are used for large tumors (larger than 3 cm). It is almost impossible to preserve hearing when the tumor is larger than 2 cm.

HEARING LOSS AND DEAFNESS

Hearing disorders are the primary handicapping disability in the United States. Twenty-eight million persons in the United States have impaired hearing in one or both ears. The majority of persons lose their hearing as adults. Hearing impairment is common among older adults. Nearly half of the persons who need assistance with hearing disorders are 65 years of age or older. With the aging of the population, hearing loss is increasing. At age 50, one of every eight persons is hearing impaired.[30]

Types of Hearing Loss

Conductive Hearing Loss. *Conductive hearing loss* occurs in the outer and middle ear and impairs the sound being conducted from the outer to the inner ear. It is caused by conditions interfering with air conduction, such as impacted cerumen and foreign bodies, middle ear disease, otosclerosis, and stenosis of the external auditory canal. The audiogram demonstrates an air-bone gap of at least 15 dB. The most common cause of conductive hearing loss is otitis media with effusion.

An air-bone gap occurs when hearing sensitivity by bone conduction is significantly better than by air conduction. The patient may speak softly because he or she hears his or her voice, which is conducted by bone, as being loud. This patient hears better in a noisy environment. A hearing aid is helpful for a patient with a 40 to 50 dB loss or more, although the device often is not necessary because of the excellent results of treatment of the underlying problem.

Sensorineural Hearing Loss. *Sensorineural hearing loss* is caused by impairment of function of the inner ear or its central connections. Congenital and hereditary factors, noise trauma during a period of time, aging (presbycusis), Ménière's disease, and ototoxicity can cause sensorineural hearing loss. Systemic diseases, such as tuberculosis, syphilis, Lyme disease, cytomegalovirus, HIV, and Paget's disease of the bone, can also cause sensorineural deafness. Immune diseases, diabetes mellitus, bacterial meningitis, and trauma are also causes of this type of hearing loss.

The two main problems associated with sensorineural loss are the ability to hear sound but not to understand speech, and the lack of understanding of the problem by others. The ability to hear high-pitched sounds diminishes with a sensorineural hearing loss. Consonants are high-pitched sounds that give intelligibility to speech. Words become difficult to distinguish, and sound becomes muffled. An audiogram demonstrates a loss in dB levels of the 4000 Hz range, which can progress to the 2000 Hz range. A hearing aid may help the patient who has a 30 dB loss or more by reducing the strain of trying to hear, but the sounds will still be muffled. *Presbycusis,* degenerative change of the inner ear, is a major cause of sensorineural hearing loss in the older adult. It is a progressive problem that results in many psychologic and communication issues. The management of inner ear diseases such as Ménière's disease can prevent further hearing loss. If ototoxic drugs are used, hearing should be monitored frequently during treatment. Causes of hearing loss are shown in Fig. 21-7.

Mixed Hearing Loss. Mixed hearing loss is caused by a combination of conductive and sensorineural losses. Careful evaluation is needed before corrective surgery for conductive loss is planned because the sensorineural component of the hearing loss will still remain.

Central and Functional Hearing Loss. Central hearing loss is caused by problems in the CNS from the auditory nucleus to the cortex. The patient is unable to understand or to put mean-

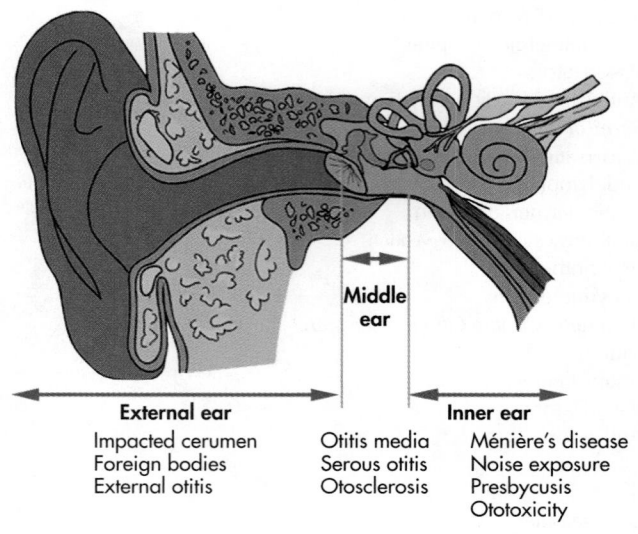

External ear	Middle ear	Inner ear
Impacted cerumen	Otitis media	Ménière's disease
Foreign bodies	Serous otitis	Noise exposure
External otitis	Otosclerosis	Presbycusis
		Ototoxicity

FIG. 21-7   Causes of hearing loss.

ing to the incoming sound. Functional hearing loss may be caused by an emotional or a psychologic factor. The patient does not seem to hear or respond to pure-tone subjective hearing tests, but no organic cause can be identified. A careful history is helpful because there is usually a reference to deafness within the family. Psychologic counseling may help. Referral to qualified hearing and speech services is indicated.

Classification of Hearing Loss. Hearing loss can also be classified by the decibel (dB) level or loss as recorded on the audiogram. Normal hearing is in the 0 to 15 dB range. Slight hearing loss is in the 16 to 25 dB range. A mild impairment is present at the 26 to 40 dB hearing level. A moderate impairment is in the 41 to 55 dB range. A moderately severe impairment is in the 56 to 70 dB range. The severely impaired have a loss in the 71 to 90 dB range. The profoundly deaf have a loss greater than 91 dB. Many persons in this last group are congenitally deaf.

Clinical Manifestations

Manifestations that indicate hearing loss include asking others to speak up, answering questions inappropriately, not responding when not looking at the speaker, straining to hear, cupping hand around ear, showing irritability with others who do not speak up, and increasing sensitivity to slight increases in noise level. Often the patient is unaware of minimal hearing loss or may compensate by using these mannerisms. Family and friends who get tired of repeating or talking loudly are often first to notice hearing loss.

Deafness is often called the "unseen handicap" because it is not until conversation is initiated with a deaf adult that the difficulty in communication is realized. It is important that the health professional be aware of the need for thorough validation of the deaf person's understanding of health teaching. Descriptive visual aids can be helpful.

Interference in communication and interaction with others can be the source of many problems for the patient and family. Often the patient refuses to admit or may be unaware of impaired hearing. Irritability is common because of the concentration with which the patient must listen to understand speech. The loss of clarity of speech in the patient with sensorineural hearing loss is most frustrating. The patient may hear what is said but not understand it. Withdrawal, suspicion, loss of self-esteem, and insecurity are commonly associated with advancing hearing loss.

NURSING *and* COLLABORATIVE MANAGEMENT HEARING LOSS AND DEAFNESS

■ Health Promotion

Environmental Noise Control. Hearing loss can be caused by acute loud noise (acoustic trauma) or by the chronic exposure to loud noise (noise-induced hearing loss). Acoustic trauma causes hearing loss from mechanical destruction of parts of the organ of Corti. Some recovery of function may occur in the first weeks after injury, but the remaining loss is permanent. Noise-induced hearing loss is probably caused by high-intensity stimulation of the cochlea resulting in mechanical damage of the hair cells and supporting cells in the organ of Corti.

Sensorineural hearing loss as a result of increased and prolonged environmental noise, such as amplified sound, is occurring in young adults at an increasing rate. Health teaching re-

TABLE 21-19	Range of Sounds Audible to Human Ear
TYPICAL	**EXAMPLE**
Decibel	
0	Lowest sound audible to the human ear.
30	Quiet library, soft whisper.
40	Living room, quiet office, bedroom away from traffic.
50	Light traffic at a distance, refrigerator, gentle breeze.
60	Air conditioner at 20 ft, conversation, sewing machine.
70	Busy traffic, noisy restaurant. At this decibel level, noise may begin to affect hearing if exposure is constant.
Hazardous Zone for Hearing Loss	
80	Subway, heavy city traffic, alarm clock at 2 ft, factory noise. These noises are dangerous if exposure to them lasts for more than 8 hr.
90	Truck traffic, noisy home appliances, shop tools, lawn mower. As loudness increases, the "safe" time exposure decreases; damage can occur in less than 8 hr.
100	Chain saw, stereo headphones, pneumatic drill. Even 2 hr of exposure can be dangerous at this decibel level; with each 5 dB increase the safe time is cut in half.
120	Rock band concert in front of speakers, sandblasting, thunderclap. The danger is immediate; exposure of 120 dB can injure ears.
140	Gunshot blast, jet plane. Any length of exposure time is dangerous; noise at this level may cause actual pain in the ear.
180	Rocket launching pad. Without ear protection, noise at this level causes irreversible damage; hearing loss is inevitable.

From American Academy of Otolaryngology, 1993.

garding avoidance of continued exposure to noise levels greater than 85 to 95 decibels (dB) is essential. Table 21-19 describes the range of sounds audible to humans.

In work environments known to have high noise levels (greater than 85 dB), ear protection should be worn. Occupational Safety and Health Administration (OSHA) standards require ear protection for workers in environments where the noise levels exceed 85 dB consistently. A variety of protectors are available that are worn over the ears or in the ears to prevent hearing loss. Periodic audiometric screening should be part of the health maintenance policies of industry. This provides baseline data on hearing to measure subsequent hearing loss.

The nurse should participate in hearing conservation programs in work environments. A hearing conservation program should include noise exposure analysis, provision for control of noise exposure (hearing protectors), measurements of hearing, and employee-employer notification and education. Often a multidisciplinary team including an industrial hygienist, engineer, nurse, and audiometric technician is responsible for such a program.

Ear protection should be worn during skeet shooting and other recreational pursuits with high noise levels. Young adults should be encouraged to keep amplified music at a reasonable level and limit their exposure time. Hearing loss caused by noise is not reversible.

Immunizations. Childhood and adult immunizations, including the measles, mumps, and rubella (MMR) immunization, should be promoted. Various viruses can cause deafness as a result of fetal damage and malformations affecting the ear. The period of greatest risk for birth defects due to rubella infection is during the first trimester. If infection occurs early in the second trimester, the result is often permanent hearing impairment.[31] Women of childbearing age should be tested for immunity. A rubella antibody titer of 1:8 or greater shows that the individual has immunity to rubella. If the titer is less, immunization with live vaccine should be given. The woman should avoid pregnancy for at least 3 months after being immunized. Immunization must be delayed if the woman is pregnant. Women who are susceptible to rubella can be vaccinated safely during the postpartum period.[32]

Ototoxic Drugs. The patient's reaction to drugs that are known to cause ototoxicity should be monitored. Ototoxic drugs are capable of damaging one or both branches of the auditory nerve (cranial nerve [CN] VIII) and the inner ear. Drugs commonly associated with ototoxicity include salicylates, antimalarial drugs, diuretics, antineoplastic drugs, and antibiotics. The patient who is receiving these drugs should be assessed for signs and symptoms associated with ototoxicity. The most common symptoms of drug-induced ototoxicity are tinnitus, sensorineural hearing loss, and vestibular dysfunction.[33] If these symptoms develop, immediate withdrawal of the drug may prevent further damage and may cause the symptoms to disappear.

■ Assistive Devices and Techniques

Hearing Aids. It is important that the patient with a suspected hearing loss have a hearing assessment by a qualified audiologist, including examination and audiometric testing. If a hearing aid is indicated, it should be fitted by an audiologist or a speech and hearing specialist. Many types of hearing aids are available, each with advantages and disadvantages: behind-the-ear, in-the-ear, in-the-canal, completely-in-the-ear (Fig. 21-8), and implantable hearing aids. The conventional hearing aid serves as a simple am-

plifier. For the patient with bilateral hearing impairment, binaural hearing aids provide the best sound lateralization and speech discrimination. Patients who are motivated and optimistic about using a hearing aid will be more successful users. The nurse must be prepared to give careful instruction on its use and maintenance and to assist the patient during the period of adjustment.

Initially, use of the hearing aid should be restricted to quiet situations in the home. The patient must first adjust to voices (including the patient's own) and household sounds. The patient should also experiment by increasing and decreasing the volume, as situations require. As adjustment to the increase in sounds and background noise occurs, the patient will be ready to try a different listening environment, such as a small party where several people will be talking simultaneously. Next the environment can be expanded to the outdoors. After adapting to controlled situations, the patient will be ready to encounter environments such as the shopping mall or grocery store. Adjustment to different environments occurs gradually, depending on the individual patient.

When the hearing aid is not being worn, it should be placed in a dry, cool area where it will not be inadvertently damaged or lost. The battery should be disconnected or removed. Battery life averages 1 week, and patients should be advised to purchase only a month's supply at a time. Earmolds should be cleaned weekly or as needed. Toothpicks or pipe cleaners may be used to clear a clogged ear tip.

Speech Reading. Speech reading, commonly called lip reading, can be helpful in increasing communication. It allows for approximately 40% understanding of the spoken word. The patient is able to use visual cues associated with speech, such as gestures and facial expression, to help clarify the spoken message. In speech reading, many words will look alike to the patient (e.g., rabbit, woman). If the patient wears glasses, the glasses should be used to facilitate speech reading. The nurse can help the patient by using and teaching verbal and nonverbal communication techniques as described in Table 21-20. If a hearing aid is used, it should be readily available to the patient.

TABLE 21-20 Communication with the Hearing-Impaired Patient

Nonverbal Aids
Draw attention with hand movements.
Have speaker's face in good light.
Avoid covering mouth or face with hands.
Avoid chewing, eating, smoking while talking.
Maintain eye contact.
Avoid distracting environments.
Avoid careless expression that the patient may misinterpret.
Use touch.
Move close to better ear.
Avoid light behind speaker.

Verbal Aids
Speak normally and slowly.
Do not overexaggerate facial expressions.
Do not overenunciate.
Use simple sentences.
Rephrase sentence; use different words.
Write name or difficult words.
Avoid shouting.
Speak in normal voice directly into better ear.

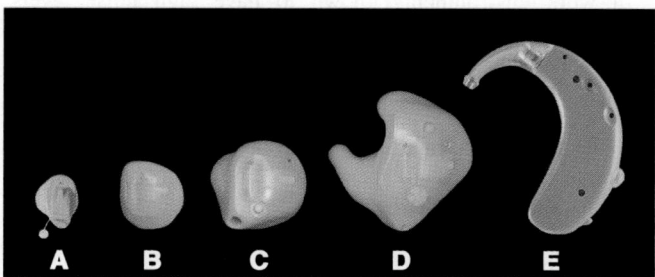

FIG. 21-8 Hearing aids are classified into five basic types. **A,** TRIANO Micro CIC (completely-in-the-canal) hearing aid. **B,** TRIANO ITC (in-the-canal) hearing aid. **C,** TRIANO HS (half shell) hearing aid. **D,** TRIANO ITE (in-the-ear) hearing aid. **E,** TRIANO 3 BTE (behind-the-ear) hearing aid. The TRIANO product family, its fitting philosophy, and its range of accessories were intended to satisfy individuals of all ages, from infants through senior citizens, who have hearing loss. (Image courtesy of Siemens Hearing Solutions.)

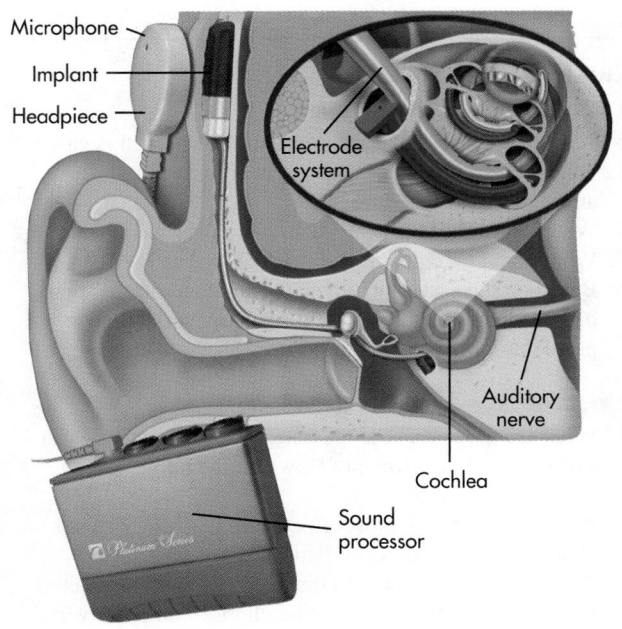

Microphone
Implant
Headpiece
Electrode system
Auditory nerve
Cochlea
Sound processor

FIG. 21-9 Cochlear implant.

Cochlear Implant. The *cochlear implant* is used as a hearing device for the profoundly deaf. The system consists of a surgically implanted induction coil beneath the skin behind the ear and an electrode wire placed in the cochlea (Fig. 21-9). The implanted parts interface with an externally worn speech processor. The system stimulates auditory nerve fibers by an electric current so that signals reach the brainstem's auditory nuclei and ultimately the auditory cortex. The implant is intended for the patient whose sensorineural hearing loss is either congenital or acquired. The ideal candidate is one who has become deaf after acquiring speech and language. The adult who was born deaf or became deaf before learning to speak may be considered a candidate for a cochlear implant if she or he has followed an aural/oral educational approach.[34]

The implant offers the profoundly deaf the ability to hear environmental sounds, including speech, at comfortable loudness levels. Multichannel cochlear implants also serve as aids to speech production. Extensive training and rehabilitation are essential to receive maximum benefit from these implants. The positive aspects of a cochlear implant include providing sound to the person who heard none, improving lip reading, monitoring the loudness of the person's own speech, improving the sense of security, and decreasing feelings of isolation. With continued research the cochlear implant may offer the possibility of aural rehabilitation for a wider range of hearing-impaired individuals.

Assisted Listening Devices. Numerous devices are now available to assist the hearing-impaired person. Direct amplification devices, amplified telephone receivers, alerting systems that flash when activated by sound, an infrared system for amplifying the sound of the television, and a combination FM receiver and hearing aid are all aids that can be explored by the nurse based on patient needs.

■ Gerontologic Considerations: Hearing Loss

Presbycusis, hearing loss associated with aging, includes the loss of peripheral auditory sensitivity, a decline in word recognition ability, and associated psychologic and communication issues. Because consonants (high-frequency sounds) are the letters by which spoken words are recognized, the ability of the older person with presbycusis to understand the spoken word is greatly affected. Vowels are heard, but some consonants fall into the high-frequency range and cannot be differentiated. This may lead to confusion and embarrassment because of the difference in what was said and what was heard.

The cause of presbycusis is related to degenerative changes in the inner ear such as loss of hair cells, reduction of blood supply, diminution of endolymph production, decreased basilar membrane flexibility, and loss of neurons in the cochlear nuclei. Noise exposure is thought to be a common factor related to presbycusis. Table 21-21 describes the classification of specific causes and associated hearing changes of presbycusis. Often, more than one type of presbycusis may be present in the same person. The prognosis for hearing depends on the cause of the loss. Sound amplification with the appropriate device is often helpful in improving the understanding of speech. In other situations an audiologic rehabilitation program can be valuable.

The older adult is often reluctant to use a hearing aid for sound amplification. Reasons cited most often include cost, appearance, insufficient knowledge about hearing aids, amplification of competing noise, and unrealistic expectations. Most hearing aids and batteries are small, and neuromuscular changes such as stiff fingers, enlarged joints, and decreased sensory perception often make the care and handling of a hearing aid a difficult and frustrating experience for an older person. Some elderly persons may also tend to accept their losses as part of getting older and believe there is no need for improvement. ■

TABLE 21-21	**Classification of Presbycusis**	
TYPE	**CAUSE**	**HEARING CHANGE AND PROGNOSIS**
• Sensory	Atrophy of auditory nerve; loss of sensory hair cells	Loss of high-pitched sounds, little effect on speech understanding; good response to sound amplification
• Neural	Degenerative changes in cochlea and spinal ganglion	Loss of speech discrimination; amplification alone not sufficient
• Metabolic	Atrophy of blood vessels in wall of cochlea with interruption of essential nutrient supply	Uniform loss for all frequencies accompanied by recruitment*; good response to hearing aid
• Cochlear	Stiffening of basilar membrane, which interferes with sound transmission in the cochlea	Hearing loss increases from low to high frequencies; speech discrimination affected with higher frequency losses; helped by appropriate forms of amplification

*Abnormally rapid increase in loudness as sound intensity increases.

CRITICAL THINKING EXERCISES

Case Study

Argon Laser Trabeculoplasty

Patient Profile. Anne Richards, a 70-year-old African American woman with rheumatoid arthritis, returns to the clinic for follow-up care of primary open-angle glaucoma (POAG). Her current medical regimen includes topical timolol maleate (Timoptic) 0.5% bid OU and latanoprost (Xalatan) 0.005% q hs OU. Her intraocular pressures are stable on this regimen.

Subjective Data
- Reports stable vision
- States she is not always successful in getting the eyedrops instilled because her hands are gnarled and painful from rheumatoid arthritis

Objective Data
- Distant and near visual acuity is stable at 20/40 OU.
- Goldmann visual field testing reveals a new scotoma in the right eye.

Collaborative Care

- Brimonidine (Alphagen) 0.2% OD 15 minutes before procedure
- Argon laser trabeculoplasty (ALT) in the right eye
- Postoperative, check intraocular pressure 1 hour after ALT
- Discharge medication 1% Pred Forte (topical corticosteroid) tid OD
- Continue previous antiglaucoma drug regimen
- Follow-up in 2 weeks for possible ALT in the left eye

CRITICAL THINKING QUESTIONS

1. Explain the etiology of Anne's new scotoma.
2. Why might ALT be an appropriate therapy in this case?
3. What is the purpose of the topical corticosteroid drops after the laser procedure?
4. What topics should the nurse discuss in discharge teaching?
5. What is the therapeutic goal of ALT?
6. Based on the assessment data, write one or more appropriate nursing diagnoses. Are there any collaborative problems?

Nursing Research Issues

1. What are the main coping strategies of the patient with severe visual impairment? How can the nurse best support these strategies?
2. What strategies are most effective in teaching patients about avoiding sources of ocular irritation?
3. What factors contribute to the decision-making process for a patient with cataracts who chooses surgery over continued palliative therapy?
4. Are there significant differences in outcomes for elderly patients when postoperative care following eye surgery includes visits by a home health care nurse?
5. Does family support significantly influence patient usage and adjustment to a hearing aid?
6. What motivates a patient following a tympanoplasty to comply with the therapeutic regimen?

REVIEW QUESTIONS

The number of the question corresponds to the same-numbered objective at the beginning of the chapter.

1. Presbyopia occurs in older individuals because
   a. the retina degenerates.
   b. the crystalline lens becomes inflexible.
   c. the corneal curvature becomes irregular.
   d. it is associated with cataract development.
2. The most important nursing intervention in patients with epidemic keratoconjunctivitis is
   a. applying patches to the affected eyes.
   b. accurately measuring intraocular pressure.
   c. monitoring near visual acuity every 4 hours.
   d. teaching patient and family members good hygiene techniques.
3. Patients with an eye inflammation or infection should be taught
   a. to wear dark glasses to prevent irritation from UV light.
   b. that acute conditions commonly lead to chronic problems.
   c. to apply a cold washcloth with pressure to the inflamed area frequently.
   d. that regular careful hand washing may prevent the infection from spreading.

4. Rubella can cause hearing problems if
   a. exposure is after 20 weeks of gestation.
   b. exposure is before 16 weeks of gestation.
   c. the mother had rubella before age 18 years.
   d. the mother is vaccinated during the postpartum.
5. In preparing patients for retinal detachment surgery, the nurse should
   a. begin explaining how to care for an ocular prosthesis.
   b. assure patients that they can expect 20/20 vision following surgery.
   c. teach the family how to recognize when the patient is hallucinating.
   d. assess the patient's level of knowledge about retinal detachment and provide information appropriate to the situation.
6. The nurse should instruct patients with glaucoma that
   a. they should see their family practitioner or internist every 2 months.
   b. punctal occlusion will lessen systemic absorption of glaucoma eyedrops.
   c. if they use their drops properly, they can expect full resolution of the glaucoma.
   d. the frequent pain caused by the increased intraocular pressure can be controlled with analgesics.

REVIEW QUESTIONS—cont'd

7. The nurse would suspect otosclerosis from assessment findings of hearing loss in
   a. a 26-year-old woman who has three biologic children under 5 years of age.
   b. a 52-year-old man whose hearing loss is accompanied by vertigo and tinnitus.
   c. a 42-year-old African American woman who has a history of serous otitis media.
   d. a 63-year-old man who can hear high-pitched sounds more effectively than low-pitched sounds.

8. The patient who has a sensorineural hearing loss
   a. has difficulty understanding speech.
   b. experiences clearer sounds with the use of a hearing aid.
   c. may have a reversal of damage caused by ototoxic drugs.
   d. hears low-pitched sounds better than high-pitched sounds.

9. The nurse teaches the patient with extended-wear contact lenses that
   a. the lenses may be moistened with saliva if necessary.
   b. the lenses may be worn for up to 1 week without removal.
   c. any saline solution may be used for moistening as long as it is hypertonic.
   d. the person may continue lens wear if he or she experiences only mild to moderate irritation or redness.

10. A nursing measure that is helpful in communicating with a hearing-impaired patient is to
    a. use simple sentences.
    b. overenunciate speech.
    c. raise the voice to a higher pitch.
    d. write out all questions and responses.

11. Patients with permanent visual impairment
    a. feel most comfortable with other visually impaired persons.
    b. may feel threatened when others make eye contact during a conversation.
    c. usually need others to speak louder so they can communicate appropriately.
    d. may experience the same grieving process that is associated with other losses.

REFERENCES

1. Thompson JM et al, editors: *Mosby's clinical nursing,* ed 5, St Louis, 2002, Mosby.
2. Lehmann OJ, Verity DH, Coombes AGA: *Clinical optics and refraction,* Oxford, England, 1998, Butterworth-Heineman.
3. Harkness GA, Dincher JJ, editors: *Medical-surgical nursing: total patient care,* ed 10, St Louis, 1999, Mosby.
4. Herlihy B, Maebius NK, editors: *The human body in health and illness,* Philadelphia, 2000, WB Saunders.
5. Mead MD, Sieck EA, Steinert RF: Optical rehabilitation of aphakia. In Albert DM, Jakobiec FA, editors: *Principles and practice of ophthalmology: clinical practice,* vol 2, Philadelphia, 1999, WB Saunders.
6. Tortora CM, Hersh PS, Blaker JW: Optics of intraocular lenses. In Albert DM, Jakobiec FA, editors: *Principles and practice of ophthalmology: clinical practice,* ed 2, vol 5, Philadelphia, 1999, WB Saunders.
7. Gimbel HW, Anderson-Penno EE: *Refractive surgery: a manual of principles and practice,* Thorofare, NJ, 2000, Slack.
8. Kraut JA, McCabe CP: The problem of low vision: definition and common problems. In Albert DM, Jakobiec FA, editors: *Principles and practice of ophthalmology: clinical practice,* ed 2, vol 5, Philadelphia, 1999, WB Saunders.
9. Brandt JT, Nason FE: Community resources for the ophthalmic practice. In Albert DM, Jakobiec FA, editors: *Principles and practice of ophthalmology: clinical practice,* ed 2, vol 5, Philadelphia, 1999, WB Saunders.
10. Hecimovich MD: Eyewear protection, *Journal of Sports Chiropractic and Rehabilitation* 14:24, 2000.
11. Bajart AM: Lid inflammations. In Albert DM, Jakobiec FA, editors: *Principles and practice of ophthalmology: clinical practice,* ed 2, vol 5, Philadelphia, 1999, WB Saunders.
12. Pavan-Langston D: Viral disease of the cornea and external eye. In Albert DM, Jakobiec FA, editors: *Principles and practice of ophthalmology: clinical practice,* ed 2, vol 5, Philadelphia, 1999, WB Saunders.
13. Adamis AP, Schein OD: *Chlamydia* and *Acanthamoeba* infections of the eye. In Albert DM, Jakobiec FA, editors: *Principles and practice of ophthalmology: clinical practice,* ed 2, vol 5, Philadelphia, 1999, WB Saunders.
14. Foulks GN: Bacterial infections of the conjunctiva and cornea. In Albert DM, Jakobiec FA, editors: *Principles and practice of ophthalmology: clinical practice,* ed 2, vol 5, Philadelphia, 1999, WB Saunders.
15. Talamo JH, Steinert RF: Keratorefractive surgery. In Albert DM, Jakobiec FA, editors: *Principles and practice of ophthalmology: clinical practice,* ed 2, vol 5, Philadelphia, 1999, WB Saunders.
16. Boruchoff SA: Penetrating keratoplasty. In Albert DM, Jakobiec FA, editors: *Principles and practice of ophthalmology: clinical practice,* ed 2, vol 5, Philadelphia, 1999, WB Saunders.
17. Streeten BW: Pathology of the lens. In Albert DM, Jakobiec FA, editors: *Principles and practice of ophthalmology: clinical practice,* ed 2, vol 5, Philadelphia, 1999, WB Saunders.
18. Watson G: Low vision in the geriatric population: rehabilitation and management, *J Am Geriatr Soc* 49:317, 2001.
19. Haynie GD, D'Amico DJ: Scleral buckling surgery. In Albert DM, Jakobiec FA, editors: *Principles and practice of ophthalmology: clinical practice,* ed 2, vol 5, Philadelphia, 1999, WB Saunders.
20. Delcourt C et al: Smoking and age-related macular degeneration, *Arch Ophthalmol* 116:1031, 1998.
21. Thomas JV: Primary open-angle glaucoma. In Albert DM, Jakobiec FA, editors: *Principles and practice of ophthalmology: clinical practice,* ed 2, vol 5, Philadelphia, 1999, WB Saunders.
22. Richter CU: Laser therapy of open-angle glaucoma. In Albert DM, Jakobiec FA, editors: *Principles and practice of ophthalmology: clinical practice,* ed 2, vol 5, Philadelphia, 1999, WB Saunders.
23. Williams MA: Diseases of the external ear. In Dershewitz RA, editor: *Ambulatory pediatric care,* Philadelphia, 1999, Lippincott-Raven.
24. Kryzer TC, Lambert PR: Diseases of the external auditory canal. In Canalis RF, Lambert PR, editors: *The ear: comprehensive otology,* Philadelphia, 2000, Lippincott Williams & Wilkins.
25. May JS, Fisch U: Neoplasms of the ear and lateral skull base. In Bailey BJ, Calhoun KH, editors: *Head and neck surgery—otolaryngology,* Philadelphia, 1998, Lippincott-Raven.
26. Kenna MA: Diagnosis and management of acute otitis media with effusion. In Wetmore RF, Muntz HR, McGill TJ, editors: *Pediatric otolaryngology: principles and practice pathways,* New York, 2000, Thieme.

27. Hashisaki GT: Complications of chronic otitis media. In Canalis RF, Lambert PR, editors: *The ear: comprehensive otology,* Philadelphia, 2000, Lippincott Williams & Wilkins.

28. Roland PS, Meyerhoff WL: Otosclerosis. In Bailey BJ, Calhoun KH, editors: *Head and neck surgery—otolaryngology,* Philadelphia, 1998, Lippincott-Raven.

29. Schessel DA, Minor LB, Nedzelski J: Meniere's disease and other peripheral vestibular disorders. In Cummings CW et al, editors: *Otolaryngology head and neck surgery,* St Louis, 1998, Mosby.

30. Alpiner JG, Hansen EM, Kaufman KJ: Transition rehabilitative audiology into the new millennium. In Alpiner JG, McCarthy PA, editors: *Rehabilitative audiology,* Philadelphia, 2000, Lippincott Williams & Wilkins.

31. Olds SB, London ML, Ladewig PA: *Maternal newborn nursing,* Upper Saddle River, NJ, 2000, Prentice Hall Health.

32. Novak JC, Broom BL: *Ingalls and Salernos' maternal and child health nursing,* ed 9, St Louis, 2000, Mosby.

33. Wackym PA, Storper IS, Newman AN: Cochlear and vestibular toxicity. In Canalis RF, Lambert PR, editors: *The ear: comprehensive otology,* Philadelphia, 2000, Lippincott Williams & Wilkins.

34. Miyamoto RT, Kirk KI: Cochlear implants. In Bailey BJ, Calhoun KH, editors: *Head and neck surgery—otolaryngology,* Philadelphia, 1998, Lippincott-Raven.

RESOURCES

Acoustic Neuroma Association
600 Peachtree Parkway, Suite 108
Cumming, GA 30041-6899
770-205-8211
Fax: 770-205-0239
E-mail: ANAusa@aol.com
http://anausa.org/

ADARA: Professionals Networking for Excellence in Service Delivery with Individuals Who Are Deaf or Hard of Hearing
ADARA National Office
PO Box 727
Lusby, MD 20657
E-mail: ADARAorgn@aol.com
www.adara.org/

Alexander Graham Bell Association for the Deaf and Hard of Hearing
3417 Volta Place, NW
Washington, DC 20007
202-337-5221 (voice/TTY)
Fax: 202-337-8314
www.agbell.org/

American Academy of Ophthalmology
PO Box 7424
San Francisco, CA 94120-7424
415-561-8500
Fax: 415-561-8533
http://206.14.84.20/aao/

American Academy of Otolaryngology—Head and Neck Surgery
One Prince Street
Alexandria, VA 22314-3357
703-836-4444
www.entnet.org/

American Foundation for the Blind
11 Penn Plaza, Suite 300
New York, NY 10001
212-502-7600
800-AFB-LINE
Fax: 212-502-7777
E-mail: afbinfo@afb.net
www.afb.org/

American Society of Cataract and Refractive Surgery
ASCRS-ASOA
4000 Legato Road, Suite 850
Fairfax, VA 22033
703-591-2220
Fax: 703-591-0614
E-mail: ascrs@ascrs.org
www.ascrs.org/

American Society of Ophthalmic Registered Nurses, Inc.
PO Box 193030
San Francisco, CA 94119
415-561-8513
Fax: 415-561-8531
www.asorn.org

American Speech-Language-Hearing Association
10801 Rockville Pike
Rockville, MD 20852
301-897-5700
800-498-2071 (professionals/students)
800-638-8255 (public)
www.asha.org/

Associated Services for the Blind
919 Walnut Street
Philadelphia, PA 19107
215-627-0600
Fax: 215-922-0692
E-mail:asbinfo@asb.org
www.asb.org/

Association for Education and Rehabilitation of the Blind and Visually Impaired
4600 Duke Street, Suite 430
PO Box 22397
Alexandria, VA 22304
703-823-9690
Fax: 703-823-9695
www.aerbvi.org/

Association for Research in Vision and Ophthalmology
12300 Twinbrook Parkway, Suite 250
Rockville, MD 20852-1606
240-221-2900
Fax: 240-221-0370
www.arvo.org/

Better Hearing Institute
515 King Street, Suite 420
Alexandria, VA 22314
703-684-3391
E-mail: mail@betterhearing.org
www.betterhearing.org/

Canadian Hard of Hearing Association
2435 Holly Lane, Suite 205
Ottawa, ON K1V 7P2
Canada
800-263-8068
613-526-1584
613-526-2692 (TTY)
Fax: 613-526-4718

Canadian National Institute for the Blind
1929 Bayview Avenue
Toronto, ON, Canada M4G 3E8
416-486-2500
Fax: 416-480-7677
www.cnib.ca/

Ear Foundation
1817 Patterson Street
Nashville, TN 37203
615-284-7807
800-545-HEAR
Fax: 615-284-7935
E-mail: earfound@earfoundation.org
www.theearfound.com/

Eye Bank Association of America
1015 Eighteenth Street NW, Suite 1010
Washington, DC 20036
202-775-4999
Fax: 202-429-6036
www.restoresight.org

Fight for Sight
381 Park Avenue South, Suite 809
New York, NY 10016
212-679-6060
Fax: 212-679-4466
E-mail: info@fightforsight.com
http://fightforsight.com/

Glaucoma Research Foundation
490 Post Street, Suite 830
San Francisco, CA 94102-9950
415-986-3162
Fax: 415-986-3763
www.glaucoma.org/

Guide Dogs for the Blind, Inc.
PO Box 151200
San Rafael, CA 94915-1200
415-499-4000
800-295-4050
Fax: 415-499-4035
www.guidedogs.com/

Guide Dog Users, Inc.
14311 Astrodome Drive
Silver Spring, MD 20906
301-598-5771
888-858-1008
Fax: 301-871-7591
www.gdui.org/

Guiding Eyes for the Blind
611 Granite Springs Road
Yorktown Heights, NY 10598
800-942-0149
Fax: 914-245-1609
www.guiding-eyes.org/

International Hearing Dog, Inc.
5901 East 89th Avenue
Henderson, CO 80640-8315
303-287-3277
Fax: 303-287-3425
http://hometown.aol.com/IHDI/IHDI.html

International Hearing Society
16880 Middlebelt Road
Livonia, MI 48154
734-522-7200
www.ihsinfo.org/

National Association for Visually Handicapped
NAVH New York
22 West 21st Street
New York, NY 10010
212-255-2804
Fax: 212-727-2931
www.navh.org/

National Association of the Deaf
814 Thayer Avenue
Silver Spring, MD 20910-4500
301-587-1788
301-587-1789 (TTY)
Fax: 301-587-1791
www.nad.org/

National Braille Association
3 Townline Circle
Rochester, NY 14623-2513
585-427-8620
Fax: 585-427-0263
www.nationalbraille.org/

National Federation of the Blind
1800 Johnson Street
Baltimore, MD 21230
410-659-9314
www.nfb.org/

National Institute on Deafness and Other Communication Disorders
National Institutes of Health
31 Center Drive, MSC 2320
Bethesda, MD 20892-2320
www.nidcd.nih.gov/

National Library Service for the Blind and Physically Handicapped
Library of Congress
202-707-5100 (voice)
202-707-0744 (TDD)
Fax: 202-707-0712
E-mail: nls@loc.gov
www.loc.gov/nls/

Prevent Blindness America
800-331-2020
www.preventblindness.org

Prevention of Blindness Society
1775 Church Street NW
Washington, DC 20036
202-234-1010
www.youreyes.org/

Recording for the Blind and Dyslexic
20 Roszel Road
Princeton, NJ 08540
609-452-0606
www.rfbd.org/

Self-Help for Hard of Hearing People (SHHH)
7910 Woodmont Avenue, Suite 1200
Bethesda, MD 20814
301-657-2248
301-657-2249 (TTY)
Fax: 301-913-9413
www.shhh.org/

Telecommunications for the Deaf
8630 Fenton Street, Suite 604
Silver Spring, MD 20910-3803
301-589-3006 (TTY)
301-589-3786 (voice)
Fax: 301-589-3797
www.tdi-online.org/

Vestibular Disorders Association
PO Box 4467
Portland, OR 97208-4467
503-229-7705
Fax: 503-229-8064
E-mail: veda@vestibular.org
www.vestibular.org/

For additional Internet resources, see the website for this book at
http://evolve.elsevier.com/Lewis/medsurg/.

CHAPTER 22

NURSING ASSESSMENT
Integumentary System

Shannon Ruff Dirksen

LEARNING OBJECTIVES

1. Describe the structures and functions of the integumentary system.
2. Describe age-related changes in the integumentary system and differences in assessment findings.
3. Identify the significant subjective and objective data related to the integumentary system that should be obtained from a patient.
4. Describe specific assessments to be made during the physical examination of the skin and appendages.
5. Explain the critical components for describing a lesion.

6. Describe the appropriate techniques used in the physical assessment of the integumentary system.
7. Explain the structural and assessment differences in dark skin color.
8. Differentiate normal from common abnormal findings in a physical assessment of the integumentary system.
9. Describe the purpose, significance of results, and nursing responsibilities related to diagnostic studies of the integumentary system.

KEY TERMS

alopecia, p. 480	keloids, p. 483
apocrine sweat glands, p. 477	keratinocytes, p. 476
dermis, p. 476	melanocytes, p. 476
eccrine sweat glands, p. 478	mongolian spots, p. 483
epidermis, p. 476	pseudofolliculitis, p. 483
intertriginous, p. 482	sebaceous glands, p. 477

The integumentary system is the largest body organ and is composed of the skin, hair, nails, and glands. The skin is further divided into three layers: epidermis, dermis, and subcutaneous tissue (Fig. 22-1).

STRUCTURES AND FUNCTIONS OF THE SKIN AND APPENDAGES

Structures

The epidermis is the outermost layer of the skin. The dermis, the second skin layer, contains a framework of highly vascular connective tissue. The subcutaneous layer is composed primarily of fat and loose connective tissue.

Epidermis. The **epidermis,** the thin avascular superficial layer of the skin, is made up of an outer dead cornified portion that serves as a protective barrier and a deeper, living portion that folds into the dermis. Together these layers measure 0.05 to 0.1 mm in thickness. The epidermis is nourished by blood vessels in the dermis. The epidermis is replaced with new cells every 30 days. The two types of epidermal cells are the melanocytes (5%) and the keratinocytes (95%).

Melanocytes are contained in the deep, basal layer (stratum germinativum) of the epidermis. They secrete melanin, a pigment that gives color to the skin and hair and protects the body from

damaging ultraviolet (UV) sunlight. Sunlight and hormones stimulate melanin production. The wide range of skin and hair colors is caused by the amount of melanin produced; more melanin results in darker skin color.[1]

Keratinocytes are synthesized from epidermal cells in the basal layer. Initially these cells are undifferentiated. As they mature (keratinize) they move to the surface where they flatten and die to form the outer skin layer (stratum corneum). Keratinocytes produce a specialized protein, keratin, which is vital to the protective barrier function of the skin. The upward movement of keratinocytes from the basement membrane to the stratum corneum takes approximately 4 weeks. If dead cells slough off too rapidly, the skin will appear thin and eroded. If new cells form faster than old cells are shed, the skin becomes scaly and thickened. Changes in this cell cycle account for many skin problems.

Dermis. The **dermis** is the connective tissue below the epidermis. Dermal thickness varies from 1 to 4 mm. The dermis is highly vascular and assists in body temperature and blood pressure regulation. It is divided into two layers, an upper thin papillary layer and a deeper, thicker reticular layer. The papillary layer is folded into ridges, or papillae, which extend into the upper epidermal layer. These exposed surface ridges form congenital patterns called fingerprints and footprints. The reticular layer contains collagen and elastic and reticular fibers.

Collagen forms the greatest part of the dermis and is responsible for the mechanical strength of the skin. Elastin fibers, nerves, lymphatic vessels, hair follicles, and sebaceous and sweat glands are also found in the dermis. The primary cell type in the dermis is the *fibroblast.* Fibroblasts produce collagen and elastin and are important in wound healing.

Subcutaneous Tissue. The subcutaneous tissue is below the dermis and is not part of the skin. The subcutaneous tissue is typically discussed with the skin because it attaches the skin to underlying tissues such as the muscle and bone. In addition, loose connective tissue and fat cells provide insulation. The anatomic distribution of subcutaneous tissue varies according to

---

Reviewed by Beverly Gay, RN, MSN, CCRN, Nurse Educator, Medical College of Virginia Hospitals at the Virginia Commonwealth University Health Systems, Richmond, Va.

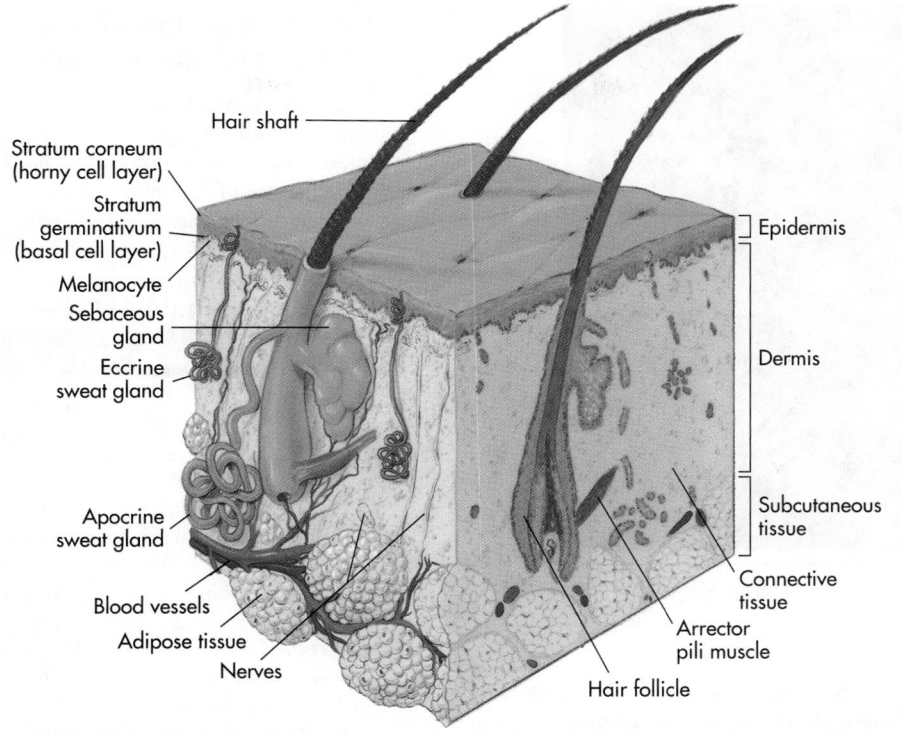

FIG. 22-1 Microscopic view of the skin in longitudinal section.

sex, heredity, age, and nutritional status. This layer also stores lipids, regulates temperature, and provides shock absorption.

Skin Appendages. Appendages of the skin include the hair, nails, and glands (sebaceous, apocrine, and eccrine). These structures develop from the epidermal layer and receive nutrients, electrolytes, and fluids from the dermis. Hair and nails form from specialized keratin that becomes hardened.

Hair grows on most of the body except for the lips, the palms of the hands, and the soles of the feet. The color of the hair is a result of heredity and is determined by the type and amount of melanin in the hair shaft. Hair grows approximately 1 cm per month. On average 100 hairs are lost each day; the rate of growth is not affected by cutting.[2] Baldness results when lost hair is not replaced. This absence of hair may be disease or treatment related or due to heredity, particularly in men.

Nails grow from under the *lunula,* which is the white crescent-shaped area nearest the nail root (Fig. 22-2). The cuticle is the part of the stratum corneum, which covers the nail root. The viable part of a nail is called the nail body. Nails grow at a rate of 0.5 mm per week, with toenail growth somewhat slower. Nails can be injured by direct trauma. A lost fingernail usually regenerates in 3 to 6 months, whereas a lost toenail may require 12 months or more for regeneration. Nail growth may vary according to the person's age and health. Nail color ranges from pink to yellow or brown depending on skin color. Pigmented bands may commonly occur in the nail bed in approximately 90% or more of all people with dark skin (Fig. 22-3).

Two major types of glands are associated with the skin: sebaceous and sweat (apocrine and eccrine) glands. The **sebaceous glands** secrete *sebum,* which is emptied into the hair follicles. Sebum prevents the skin and hair from becoming dry. Sebum is somewhat bacteriostatic and consists mainly of lipids. These

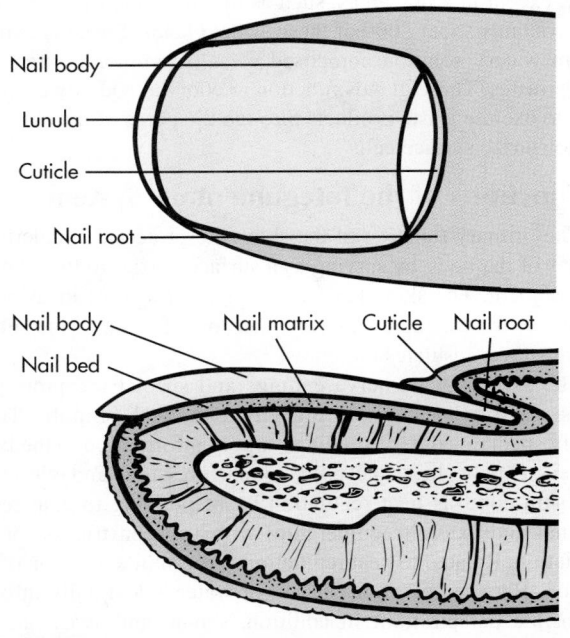

FIG. 22-2 Structure of a nail.

glands depend on sex hormones, particularly testosterone, to regulate sebum secretion and production. Sebum secretion varies across the life span according to sex hormone levels. Sebaceous glands are present on all areas of the skin except the palms and soles and are most abundant on the face, scalp, upper chest, and back.

The **apocrine sweat glands** are located mainly in the axillae, breast areolae, and anogenital area. These sweat glands secrete a

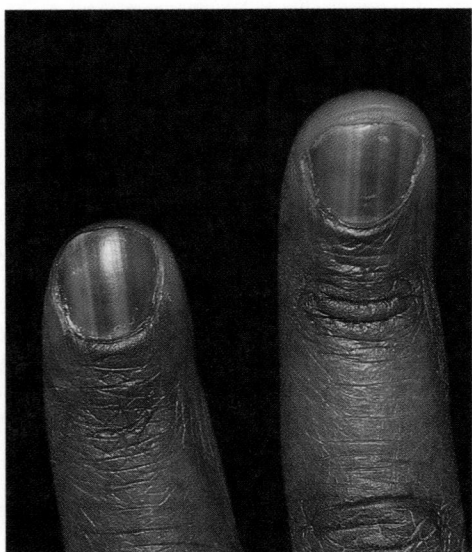

FIG. 22-3 Pigmented nail bed normally seen with dark skin color.

thick milky substance that becomes odoriferous when altered by skin surface bacteria. These glands enlarge and become active at puberty due to reproductive hormones.

The **eccrine sweat glands** are widely distributed over the body, except in a few areas, such as the lips. One square inch of skin contains about 3000 of these sweat glands. Sweat is a transparent watery solution composed of salts, ammonia, urea, and other wastes. These glands function to cool the body by evaporation, to excrete waste products through the pores of the skin, and to moisturize surface cells.

Functions of the Integumentary System

The primary function of the skin is to protect the underlying tissues of the body by serving as a surface barrier to the external environment. The skin also acts as a barrier against invasion by bacteria, viruses, and excessive water loss. The fat of the subcutaneous layer insulates the body.

The skin with its nerve endings and special receptors provides sensory perception for environmental stimuli. These highly specialized nerve endings supply information to the brain related to pain, heat and cold, touch, pressure, and vibration. The skin controls heat regulation by responding to changes in internal and external temperature with vasoconstriction or vasodilation. Related to heat regulation is the skin's function of excretion. Between 600 and 900 ml of water is lost daily through insensible perspiration. In addition, sebum and sweat are secreted by the skin and lubricate the skin surface. Endogenous synthesis of vitamin D, which is critical to calcium and phosphorus balance, occurs in the epidermis. Vitamin D is synthesized by the action of UV light on vitamin D precursors in epidermal cells.

The aesthetic functions of the skin include the mirroring of various emotions such as anger or embarrassment, as well as displaying the individual identity of a person. The role of absorption at the cutaneous level is a subject of ongoing research, and an increasing number of drugs are effectively delivered via patches applied directly to the skin.

Gerontologic Considerations: Effects of Aging on the Integumentary System

There are many changes in the skin of the aging person. Although many changes are not serious except for their cosmetic effect, others are more serious and need careful evaluation. Age-related changes of the integumentary system and differences in assessment findings are listed in Table 22-1.

TABLE 22-1   Gerontologic Differences in Assessment — Integumentary System

CHANGES	DIFFERENCES IN ASSESSMENT FINDINGS
Skin	
• Decreased subcutaneous fat, muscle laxity, degeneration of elastic fibers, collagen stiffening	Increased wrinkling, sagging breasts and abdomen, redundant flesh around eyes, slowness of skin to flatten when pinched together (tenting)
• Decreased extracellular water, surface lipids, and sebaceous gland activity	Dry, flaking skin with possible signs of excoriation caused by scratching
• Decreased activity of apocrine and sebaceous glands	Dry skin with minimal to no perspiration
• Increased capillary fragility and permeability	Evidence of bruising
• Increased melanocytes in basal layer with pigment accumulation	Senile lentigines on face and back of hands
• Diminished blood supply	Decrease in rosy appearance of skin and mucous membranes; skin is cool to touch; diminished awareness of pain, touch, temperature, and peripheral vibration
• Decreased proliferative capacity	Diminished rate of wound healing
• Decreased immunocompetence	Increase in neoplasms
Hair	
• Decreased melanin and melanocytes	Graying hair
• Decreased oil	Dry, coarse hair; scaly scalp
• Decreased density of hair follicles	Thinning and loss of hair; loss of hair in outer half or outer third of eyebrow and back of legs
• Cumulative androgen effect; decreasing estrogen levels	Facial hirsutism; baldness
Nails	
• Decreased peripheral blood supply	Thick, brittle nails with diminished growth
• Increased keratin	Ridging
• Decreased circulation	Prolonged return of blood to nails on blanching

The rate of age-related skin changes is influenced by heredity and a personal history of sun exposure, hygiene practices, nutrition, and general state of health. Skin changes that are related to aging include decreased firmness and flexibility, dryness, roughness, wrinkling, and benign neoplasms.

The junction between the dermis and the epidermis becomes flattened and the epidermis contains fewer melanocytes. In addition, the dermis loses volume and has fewer blood vessels. Scalp, pubic, and axillary hair becomes depigmented and thinner. A loss of melanin results in gray or white hair. The nail body thins and nails become brittle, thicker, and more prone to splitting and yellowing.

Chronic exposure to UV rays is the major contributor to the wrinkling of skin. Sun damage to the skin is cumulative.[3] The wrinkling of sun-exposed areas such as the face is more marked than in sun-shielded areas such as the buttocks. Poor nutrition contributes to aging of the skin resulting from a decreased intake of protein, calories, and vitamins. With aging, collagen fibers stiffen, elastic fibers degenerate, and the amount of subcutaneous tissue decreases. These changes, with the added effects of gravity, lead to wrinkling (Fig. 22-4).

Benign neoplasms related to the aging process can occur on the skin. These growths include seborrheic keratoses, cherry angiomas, and skin tags. A common premalignant lesion is an *actinic keratosis*, which appears on areas of chronic sun exposure, especially in the person who has a fair complexion and light eyes (blue, green, or hazel). These cutaneous lesions place an individual at increased risk for squamous cell and basal cell carcinomas. The aging person is more susceptible to skin cancers because there is a decline in the capacity to repair cellular (especially DNA) damage caused by sun exposure.

Decreased subcutaneous fat leads to an increased risk of trauma injury, hypothermia, and skin shearing, which may lead to pressure ulcers. With aging, the eccrine and apocrine sweat glands atrophy, causing dry skin and decreased body odor. The growth rate of the hair and nails decreases as a result of atrophy of the involved structures. Vitamin deficiencies can cause dry, thin hair that has a tendency to fall out.

The visible effects of aging on the skin and hair may have a profound psychologic effect on many people. A youthful look may be tied to a person's self-image. Although wrinkling skin, thinning hair, and brittle nails are normal changes with aging, they may result in an altered self-image.[4] ■

ASSESSMENT OF THE INTEGUMENTARY SYSTEM

Assessment of the skin begins at the initial contact with the patient and continues throughout the examination. Specific areas of the skin are examined during examination of other areas of the body unless the chief complaint is that of a dermatologic nature. A general statement about the physical condition of the skin should be recorded (Table 22-2), and specific problems should be noted under the appropriate system. In addition, health history questions presented in Table 22-3 should be asked when a skin problem is noted.

Subjective Data

Important Health Information

Past health history. Past health history will indicate previous trauma, surgery, or prior disease that involves the skin. The nurse should determine if the patient has noticed any dermatologic manifestations of systemic problems such as jaundice (liver disease), delayed wound healing (diabetes mellitus), cyanosis (respiratory disorder), and pallor (anemia). Table 23-13 lists diseases with dermatologic manifestations. Specific information related to food, pet, and drug allergies and skin reactions to insect bites and stings should also be obtained. A history of chronic or unprotected exposure to UV light, as well as radiation treatments, should be noted.

Medications. The patient should be questioned about skin-related problems that occurred as a result of taking prescription or over-the-counter (OTC) medications. A thorough medication history is important, especially in relation to vitamins, corticosteroids, hormones, antibiotics, and antimetabolites, because these medications may often cause side effects that are manifested in the skin.

The nurse should document the use of prescription or OTC medications used specifically to treat a primary skin problem such as acne or a secondary skin problem such as itching. If a preparation is used, the name, length of use, method of application, and effectiveness of the medication should be recorded.

Surgery or other treatments. It is important to determine if any surgical procedures, including cosmetic surgery, were performed on the skin. If a biopsy was done, the result should be

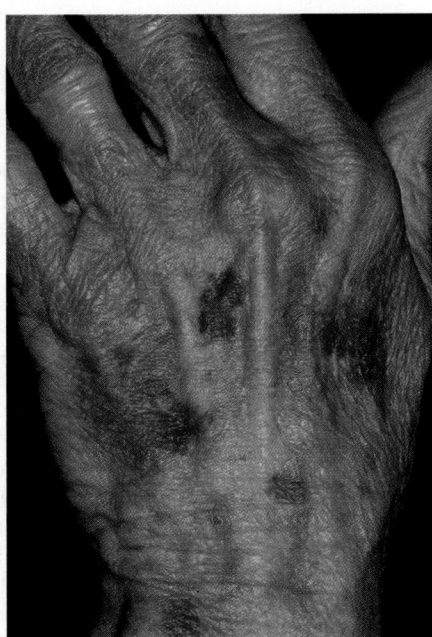

FIG. 22-4 Photoaging. Bleeding occurs with minor injury to the sun-damaged surfaces of the hands.

TABLE 22-2	**Normal Physical Assessment of the Integumentary System**

Skin: even-toned and warm; good turgor; no petechiae, purpura, lesions, or excoriations.
Nails: pink, round, and mobile with 160-degree angle.
Hair: shiny and full; amount and distribution appropriate for age and sex; no flaking of scalp, forehead, or pinna.

TABLE 22-3   Health History — Integumentary System

Health Perception–Health Management Pattern
- Describe your daily hygiene practices.
- What skin products are you currently using?
- Describe any current skin condition, including onset, course, and treatment (if any).
- Do you have any pets?

Nutritional-Metabolic Pattern
- Describe any changes in the condition of your skin, hair, nails, and mucous membranes.
- Are the conditions related to changes in your diet, including supplemental vitamins and minerals?*
- Have you noticed any changes in the way sores or lesions heal?*

Elimination Pattern
- Have you noticed changes in your skin related to excessive sweating, dryness, or swelling?

Activity-Exercise Pattern
- Do your leisure activities involve the use of any chemicals that are potentially toxic to the skin?*
- What is your sun protection program?

Sleep-Rest Pattern
- Does your skin condition keep you awake or awaken you after you have fallen asleep?

Cognitive-Perceptual Pattern
- Do you have any unusual sensations of heat, cold, or touch?*
- Do you have any pain associated with your skin condition?*
- Do you have any joint pain?*

Self-Perception–Self-Concept Pattern
- How does your skin condition make you feel about yourself?

Role-Relationship Pattern
- Has your skin condition changed your relationships with others?*
- Have you changed your lifestyle because of your skin condition?*
- Are there any environmental skin irritants at your current or previous work place or home?*

Sexuality-Reproductive Pattern
- Has your skin condition changed your intimate relationships with others?*
- Has your birth control method, if used, caused a skin problem?*

Coping–Stress Tolerance Pattern
- Are you aware of any situation or stressor that changes your skin condition?*
- Do you feel that stress plays a role in your skin condition?*
- How do you handle stress?

Value-Belief Pattern
- Are there any cultural beliefs that influence your thinking or feelings about your skin condition?*
- Are there any treatment options that you would be opposed to using?*

*If yes, describe.

---

recorded. Any treatments specific for a skin problem such as phototherapy or for a health problem such as radiation therapy should be noted. In addition, treatments undergone for primarily cosmetic purposes, such as tanning booth use or cosmetic "peels," should also be documented.

Functional Health Patterns

Health perception–health management pattern. The nurse should ask about the patient's health practices related to the integumentary system, such as the usual self-care habits related to daily hygiene. The frequency of use and sun protection factor (SPF) number of sun screen products should be documented. Assessment of the use of personal care products (e.g., shampoos, moisturizing agents, cosmetic products), including brand name, quantity, and frequency, should be noted. A description of any current skin problem including onset, symptoms, course, and treatment should be recorded. Medications used for treating hair loss also must be noted.

Information should be obtained about family history of any skin diseases, including congenital and familial diseases (e.g., **alopecia** [partial or incomplete lack of hair] and psoriasis) and systemic diseases with dermatologic manifestations (e.g., diabetes, thyroid disease, cardiovascular diseases, immune disorders). In addition, a family and personal history of skin cancer, particularly melanoma, should be noted.

Nutritional-metabolic pattern. The nurse should question the patient about any changes in the condition of skin, hair, nails, and mucous membranes and whether they are related to dietary changes. A diet history reveals the adequacy of nutrients essential to healthy skin such as vitamins A, D, E, and C; dietary fat; and protein. Food allergies that cause a skin reaction should also be noted. Obese patients should be asked if they have areas of chafing or maceration where moisture accumulates in overlapping skin areas. Amount and frequency of sweating should be noted. Changes in the time for wound healing to occur should also be questioned and recorded.[5]

Elimination pattern. The patient should be questioned about conditions of the skin such as dehydration, edema, and pruritus, which can indicate alterations in fluid balance. If urinary or fecal incontinence is a problem, the condition of the skin in the anal and perineal areas should be determined.

Activity-exercise pattern. Information should be obtained about environmental hazards in relation to hobbies and recreation activities, including exposure to known carcinogens, chemical irritants, and allergens. The patient should be asked if any changes occur in the skin during exercise or other activities.

Sleep-rest pattern. The patient should be questioned about disturbances in sleep patterns caused by a skin condition. For example, pruritus can be distressing and cause major alterations in normal sleep patterns. Also, poor sleep and resulting tiredness is often reflected in a patient's face by dark circles under the eyes and a decreased firmness in the facial skin.

Cognitive-perceptual pattern. The nurse should ascertain the patient's perception of the sensations of heat, cold, pain, and touch. Discomfort associated with a skin condition should be noted, especially when observed in intact skin. Joint pain related to the patient's skin condition should also be recorded.

Self-perception–self-concept pattern. Assessment should be made of the feelings related to sadness, anxiety, or despair in relation to the patient's skin condition. The patient should be observed for signs of decreased self-esteem and a poor or altered body image.

Role-relationship pattern. It is important to determine how the patient's skin condition affects relationships with family members, peers, and work associates. Assessment should be made of the changes in lifestyle that have occurred relative to the skin condition.

The patient should be questioned regarding the effect of environmental factors on the skin such as occupational exposure to irritants, sun, and unusually cold or unhygienic conditions. Contact dermatitis caused by allergies and irritants is a common skin problem associated with occupation.

Sexuality-reproductive pattern. The nurse should tactfully question and assess the effect of the patient's skin condition on sexual activity. The nurse should also make note of the reproductive status of the female patient relative to possible therapeutic interventions. For example, isotretinoin (Accutane), which is used to treat acne, is a teratogenic drug that may cause abnormal fetal development and, consequently, should not be used by a woman who could become pregnant.

Coping–stress tolerance pattern. It is important for the nurse to assess and question the patient about the role stress may play in creating or exacerbating the skin condition. The patient should be questioned as to what coping strategies are used to manage the skin condition.

Value-belief pattern. The patient should be questioned about cultural or religious beliefs that could influence the perception of self-image as related to the skin condition. Assessment should also be made of values and beliefs that might influence or limit the choice of treatment options.

Objective Data

Physical Examination. Primary skin lesions develop on previously unaltered skin. The common characteristics of primary skin lesions are shown in Table 22-4. Secondary skin lesions are lesions that change with time or because of a factor such as scratching or infection. Secondary skin lesions are shown in Table 22-5. General principles when conducting an assessment of the skin are as follows:

1. Have a private examination room of moderate temperature with good lighting; a room with exposure to daylight is preferred.
2. Ensure that the patient is comfortable and in a dressing gown that allows easy access to all skin areas.
3. Be systematic and proceed from head to toe.
4. Compare symmetric parts.
5. Perform a general inspection and then a lesion-specific examination.
6. Use the metric system when taking measurements.
7. Use appropriate terminology and nomenclature when reporting or documenting.

Photographs are useful when accurate findings are needed.

Inspection. The skin is inspected for general color and pigmentation, vascularity or bruising, and the presence of lesions or discolorations. The critical factor in assessment of skin color is change. A skin color that is normal for a particular patient can be

TABLE 22-4 Primary Skin Lesions	
LESION	**DESCRIPTION**
Macule 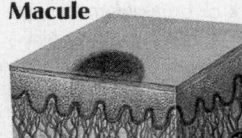	Circumscribed, flat area with a change in skin color; less than 1 cm in diameter *Examples:* freckles, petechiae, measles, flat mole (nevus)
Papule 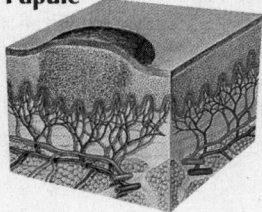	Elevated, solid lesion; less than 1 cm in diameter *Examples:* wart (verruca), elevated moles
Vesicle 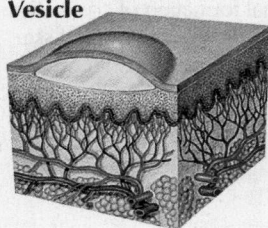	Circumscribed, superficial collection of serous fluid; less than 1 cm in diameter *Examples:* varicella (chicken pox), herpes zoster (shingles), second-degree burn
Plaque 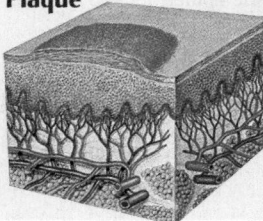	Circumscribed, elevated superficial, solid lesion; greater than 1 cm in diameter *Examples:* psoriasis, seborrheic and active keratoses
Wheal 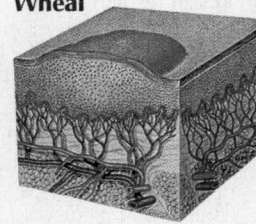	Firm, edematous, irregularly shaped area; diameter variable *Examples:* insect bite, urticaria
Pustule 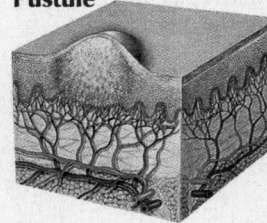	Elevated, superficial lesion filled with purulent fluid *Examples:* acne, impetigo

a sign of a pathologic condition in another patient. The color of the skin depends on the amount of melanin (brown), carotene (yellow), oxyhemoglobin (red), and reduced hemoglobin (bluish-red) present at a particular time. The most reliable areas in which to assess color are the areas of least pigmentation, such as the

TABLE 22-5 Secondary Skin Lesions

LESION	DESCRIPTION
Fissure 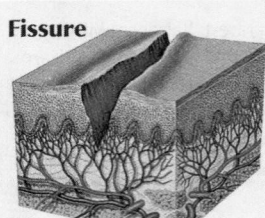	Linear crack or break from the epidermis to dermis; dry or moist *Examples:* athlete's foot, cracks at corner of the mouth
Scale 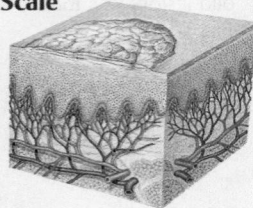	Excess, dead epidermal cells produced by abnormal keratinization and shedding *Examples:* flaking of skin after a drug reaction or scarlet fever
Scar 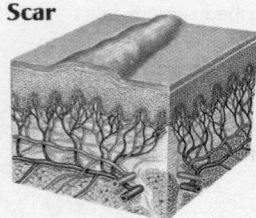	Abnormal formation of connective tissue that replaces normal skin *Examples:* surgical incision or healed wound
Ulcer 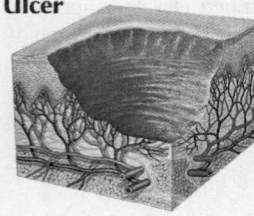	Loss of the epidermis and dermis; crater-like; irregular shape *Examples:* pressure ulcer, chancre
Atrophy 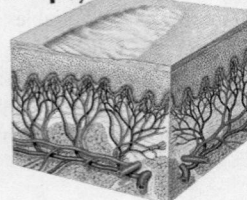	Depression in skin resulting from thinning of the epidermis or dermis *Examples:* aged skin, striae
Excoriation 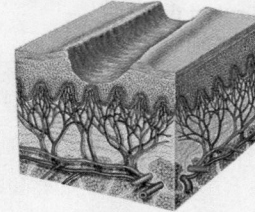	Area in which epidermis is missing, exposing the dermis *Examples:* scabies, abrasion, or scratch

sclera, conjunctiva, nail beds, lips, and buccal mucosa. Activity, emotions, cigarette smoking, and edema, as well as respiratory, renal, cardiovascular, and hepatic disorders, can all directly affect the color of the skin. Table 22-6 describes assessment variations in light- and dark-skinned individuals.

The skin is examined for possible problems related to vascularity, such as areas of bruising, and vascular and purpuric lesions, such as *angioma* (benign tumor of blood or lymph vessels), *petechiae* (tiny purple spots on skin), or *purpura* (bleeding disorder causing ecchymosis or petechiae). Reaction to direct pressure should be noted. If a lesion blanches on direct pressure and then refills, the redness is due to dilated blood vessels. If the discoloration remains, it is the result of subcutaneous or intradermal bleeding. Any pattern of bruising, for example, in the shape of the hand or fingers or bruises at different stages of resolution should be noted. These may be indications of other health problems or abuse and should be further investigated.

If lesions are found on the skin, the color, size, distribution, location, and shape should be recorded. Skin lesions are usually described in terms related to the lesions' configuration (pattern in relation to other lesions, Table 22-7) and distribution (arrangement of lesions over an area of skin, Table 22-8).

During systematic inspection it is important to note any unusual odors. Colonized lesions and overgrowth of yeast in calluses or **intertriginous** (overlapping) areas are often associated with distinctive odors. Tattoos and needle-track marks should be examined and noted for location and the characteristics of the surrounding skin area.

Inspection of the hair should include an examination of all body hair. Note the distribution, texture, and quantity of hair. Changes in the normal distribution of body hair and growth may indicate an endocrine disorder. Inspection of the nails should include a careful examination of nail shape, thickness, curvature, and surface. Any grooves, pitting, or ridges should be noted. Changes in nail smoothness or thickness can occur with anemia, psoriasis, thyroid problems, and decreased vascular circulation.

Palpation. The skin is palpated to provide information about temperature, turgor and mobility, moisture, and texture. Temperature of the skin is best assessed by using the backs of the hands. The skin should be warm without being hot. The temperature of the skin increases when blood flow to the dermis is increased. There will be a localized temperature increase with burns and local inflammation. A generalized increase in temperature will result from fever. A decreased body temperature may occur when shock, chilling, or emotional distress is present.

Turgor and mobility refer to the elasticity of the skin. The nurse assesses turgor by gently pinching an area of skin under the clavicle. Skin with good turgor should move easily when lifted and should immediately return to its original position when released. There is a loss of turgor with dehydration and aging that often causes tenting (Table 22-9).

Moisture of the skin is the dampness or dryness of the skin. Moisture increases in intertriginous areas and with high humidity. The amount of moisture on the skin varies with environmental temperature, muscular activity, body weight, and body temperature. The skin should be intact with no flaking, scaling, or cracking. Skin generally becomes drier with increasing age.

Texture refers to the fineness or coarseness of the skin. The skin should feel smooth and firm with the surface evenly thin in most areas. Thickened callus areas are normal on the soles and palms and relate to weight bearing. Increased thickness is often work related and as a result of excessive pressure.

TABLE 22-6   Assessment Variations in Light- and Dark-Skinned Individuals

CLINICAL SIGN	LIGHT SKIN	DARK SKIN
Cyanosis	Grayish-blue tone, especially in nail beds, ear lobes, lips, mucous membranes, and palms and soles of feet	Ashen or gray color most easily seen in the conjunctiva of the eye, mucous membranes, and nail beds
Ecchymosis	Dark red, purple, yellow, or green color, depending on age of bruise	Purple to brownish-black; difficult to see unless occurring in an area of light pigmentation
Erythema	Reddish tone, possibly accompanied by increased skin temperature secondary to localized inflammation	Deeper brown or purple skin tone with evidence of increased skin temperature secondary to inflammation
Jaundice	Yellowish color of skin, sclera, fingernails, palms of hands, and oral mucosa	Yellowish-green color most obviously seen in sclera of eye (do not confuse with yellow eye pigmentation, which may be evident in dark-skinned patients), palms of hands, and soles of feet
Pallor	Pale skin color that may appear white or ashen, also evident on lips, nail beds, and mucous membranes	Underlying red tone in brown or black skin is absent. Light-skinned African Americans may have yellowish brown skin; dark-skinned African Americans may appear ashen or gray
Petechiae	Lesions appear as small, reddish-purple pinpoints, best observed on abdomen and buttocks	Difficult to see; may be evident in the buccal mucosa of the mouth or conjunctiva of the eye
Rash	May be visualized as well as felt with light palpation	Not easily visualized, but may be felt with light palpation
Scar	Generally heals, showing narrow scar line	Higher incidence of keloid development, resulting in a thickened, raised scar

TABLE 22-7   Lesion Configuration Terminology

NAME	APPEARANCE
Annular	Ring-shaped
Gyrate	Ring-spiral–shaped
Iris lesions	Concentric rings or "bull's eyes"
Linear	In a line
Nummular, discoid	Coinlike
Polymorphous	Occurring in several forms
Punctuate	Marked by points or dots
Serpiginous	Snakelike

TABLE 22-8   Lesion Distribution Terminology

TERM	DESCRIPTION
Asymmetric	Unilateral distribution
Confluent	Merging together
Diffuse	Wide distribution
Discrete	Separate from other lesions
Generalized	Diffuse distribution
Grouped	Cluster of lesions
Localized	Limited areas of involvement that are clearly defined
Satellite	Single lesion in close proximity to a large grouping
Solitary	A single lesion
Symmetric	Bilateral distribution
Zosteriform	Bandlike distribution along a dermatome area

Common assessment abnormalities of the skin are described in Table 22-9.

Assessment of Dark Skin Color

A normal range of differences exists in the physical examination of skin, hair, and nails. Genetic factors determine the skin color of the individual and can vary from white to dark brown with overtones of yellow, olive, and red. The darker skin tones result from the reflection of light as it strikes the underlying skin pigment. An increased amount of melanin pigment produced by the melanocytes results in the darker skin color. This increased melanin forms a natural sun shield for dark skin and results in a decreased incidence of skin cancer in these individuals.

The structures of dark skin are no different than those of lighter skin, but they are often more difficult to assess (see Table 22-6). Assessment of color is more easily made in areas where the epidermis is thin and pigmentation is lighter, such as the lips, mucous membranes, palms, and nail beds. Rashes are often difficult to observe and may need to be palpated. Light-skinned individuals wrinkle earlier than dark-skinned individuals due to sun exposure.[6]

Individuals with dark skin are predisposed to certain skin conditions, including **pseudofolliculitis** (bacterial disorder caused by *Staphylococcus aureus* characterized by erythematous papules), **keloids** (overgrowth of collagenous tissue at site of skin injury), and **mongolian spots** (benign bluish-black macules). Because of the darkness of the skin of some individuals, color often cannot be used as an indicator of systemic conditions (e.g., flushed skin with fever). Cyanosis may be difficult to determine because a normal bluish hue occurs in dark-skinned persons.

TABLE 22-9

Common Assessment Abnormalities
Integumentary System

FINDING	DESCRIPTION	POSSIBLE ETIOLOGY AND SIGNIFICANCE
Alopecia	Loss of hair (localized or general)	Heredity, friction, rubbing, traction, trauma, stress, infection, inflammation, chemotherapy, pregnancy, emotional shock, tinea capitis, immunologic factors
Angioma	Tumor consisting of blood or lymph vessels	Normal increase with aging, liver disease, pregnancy, varicose veins
Carotenemia (carotenosis)	Yellow discoloration of skin, no yellowing of sclerae, most noticeable on palms and soles	Vegetables containing carotene (e.g., carrots, squash), hypothyroidism
Comedo (blackheads and whiteheads)	Keratin, sebum microorganism, and epithelial debris within a dilated follicular opening	Acne vulgaris
Cyanosis	Slightly bluish-gray or dark purple discoloration of the skin and mucous membranes caused by presence of excessive amounts of reduced hemoglobin in capillaries	Cardiorespiratory problems; vasoconstriction, asphyxiation, anemia, leukemia, and malignancies
Cyst	Sac containing fluid or semisolid material	Obstruction of a duct or gland, parasitic infection
Depigmentation (vitiligo)	Congenital or acquired loss of melanin resulting in white, depigmented areas	Genetic, chemical and pharmacologic agents, nutritional and endocrine factors, burns and trauma, inflammation and infection
Ecchymosis	Large, bruiselike lesion caused by collection of extravascular blood in dermis and subcutaneous tissue	Trauma, bleeding disorders
Erythema	Redness occurring in patches of variable size and shape	Heat, certain drugs, alcohol, ultraviolet rays, any problem that causes dilation of blood vessels to the skin
Hematoma	Extravasation of blood of sufficient size to cause visible swelling	Trauma, bleeding disorders
Hirsutism	Male distribution of hair in women	Abnormality of ovaries or adrenal glands, decrease in estrogen level, familial trait
Intertrigo	Dermatitis of overlying surfaces of the skin	Moisture, obesity, *Monilia* infection
Jaundice	Yellow (in whites) or yellowish-brown (in African Americans) discoloration of the skin, best observed in the sclera secondary to increased bilirubin in the blood	Liver disease, red blood cell hemolysis; pancreatic cancer, common bile duct obstruction
Keloid	Hypertrophied scar beyond margin of incision or trauma	Predisposition more common in African Americans
Lichenification	Thickening of the skin with accentuated skin markings	Repeated scratching, rubbing, and irritation
Mole (nevus)	Benign overgrowth of melanocytes	Defects of development; excessive numbers and large, irregular moles; often familial
Petechiae	Pinpoint, discrete deposit of blood less than 1 to 2 mm in the extravascular tissues and visible through the skin or mucous membrane	Inflammation, marked dilation, blood vessel trauma, blood dyscrasia that results in bleeding tendencies (e.g., thrombocytopenia)
Telangiectasia	Visibly dilated, superficial, cutaneous small blood vessels, commonly found on face and thighs	Aging, acne, sun exposure, alcohol, liver failure, corticosteroids, radiation, certain systemic diseases, skin tumors; normal variant
Tenting	Failure of skin to return immediately to normal position after gentle pinching	Aging, dehydration, cachexia
Varicosity	Increased prominence of superficial veins	Interruption of venous return (e.g., from tumor, incompetent valves, inflammation)

DIAGNOSTIC STUDIES OF THE INTEGUMENTARY SYSTEM

Diagnostic studies provide important information to the nurse in monitoring the patient's condition and planning appropriate interventions. These studies are considered to be objective data.

Table 22-10 contains diagnostic studies common to the integumentary system.

The main diagnostic techniques related to skin problems are inspection of an individual lesion and a careful history related to the problem. If a definitive diagnosis cannot be made by these techniques, additional tests may be indicated.

TABLE 22-10   Diagnostic Studies   Integumentary System

STUDY	DESCRIPTION AND PURPOSE	NURSING RESPONSIBILITY
Biopsy		
• Punch	Special punch biopsy instrument of appropriate size used. Instrument rotated to appropriate level to include dermis and some fat. Suturing may or may not be done.	Verify that consent form is signed (if needed). Assist with preparation of site, anesthesia, procedure, and hemostasis. Apply dressing, and give postprocedure instructions to patient. Properly identify specimen.
• Excisional	Useful when good cosmetic results and entire removal desired. Skin closed with subcutaneous and skin sutures.	Same as above.
• Incisional	Elliptical incision made in lesion too large to excise. Adequate specimen obtained without causing an extensive cosmetic defect.	Same as above.
• Shave	Single-edged razor blade used to shave off lesions. Performed on superficial lesions. Provides full-thickness specimen of stratum corneum.	Same as above.
Microscopic Tests		
• Potassium hydroxide (KOH)	Hair, scales, or nails examined for superficial fungal infection. Specimen is put on a glass slide and 10% to 20% concentration of potassium hydroxide added.	Instruct patient regarding purpose of test. Prepare slide.
• Tzanck test (Wright's and Giemsa's stain)	Fluid and cells from vesicles examined. Used to diagnose herpes infections. Specimen put on slide, stained, and examined microscopically.	Inform patient of purpose of test. Use sterile technique for collection of fluid.
• Culture	The test identifies fungal, bacterial, and viral organisms. For fungi, scraping performed if the fungus is systemic involving the skin. For bacteria, material obtained from intact pustules, bullae, or abscesses. For viruses, bullae scraped and exudate taken from center of lesion.	Instruct patient regarding purpose and procedure. Properly identify specimen. Follow instructions for storage of specimen if not immediately sent to laboratory.
• Mineral oil slides	To check for infestations, scrapings are placed on slide with mineral oil.	Instruct patient about purpose of test. Prepare slide.
• Immunofluorescent studies	Some cutaneous diseases have specific, abnormal antibody proteins that can be identified by fluorescent studies. Both skin and serum can be examined.	Inform patient about purpose of test. Assist in obtaining specimen.
Miscellaneous		
• Wood's lamp (black light)	Examination of skin with long-wave ultraviolet light causes specific substances to fluoresce (e.g., *Pseudomonas* organisms, fungal infections, vitiligo).	Explain purpose of examination. Inform patient it is not painful.
• Patch test	Used to determine whether patient is allergic to any testing material. Small amount of potentially allergenic material applied under occlusion, usually to skin on back.	Explain purpose and procedure to patient. Instruct patient to return in 48 hr for removal of allergens and evaluation. Inform patient if reevaluation is needed at 96 hr.

Biopsy is one of the most common diagnostic tests used in the evaluation of a skin lesion. A biopsy is indicated in all conditions in which a malignancy is suspected or a specific diagnosis is questionable. Techniques include punch, incisional, excisional, and shave biopsies. The method used is related to factors such as the site of the biopsy, cosmetic result desired, and the type of tissue to be obtained.

Other diagnostic procedures used include stains and cultures for fungal, bacterial, and viral infections. Immunofluorescence is a special technique used on biopsy specimens and may be indicated in certain conditions such as bullous diseases and systemic lupus erythematosus. Patch testing and photopatch testing may be used in the evaluation of allergic contact dermatitis and photoallergic reactions.[7]

REVIEW QUESTIONS

The number of the question corresponds to the same-numbered objective at the beginning of the chapter.

1. The primary function of the skin is
   a. insulation.
   b. protection.
   c. sensation.
   d. absorption.

2. Age-related changes in the skin include
   a. oily scalp.
   b. a loss of collagen.
   c. thinner, flexible nails.
   d. improved blood supply.

3. When assessing the sleep-rest pattern in relation to the skin, the nurse questions the patient regarding
   a. the presence of dry, flaky skin.
   b. occupational exposure to irritants.
   c. self-care habits related to daily hygiene.
   d. the presence of dark circles under the eyes.

4. During the physical examination of a patient's skin, the nurse would
   a. use a flashlight if the room is poorly lit.
   b. note cool, moist skin as a normal finding.
   c. pinch up a fold of skin to assess for turgor.
   d. perform a lesion-specific examination first and then a general inspection.

5. Skin lesions found by the nurse and described as firm, edematous, and irregularly shaped areas of varying diameter are called
   a. pustules.
   b. macules.
   c. vesicles.
   d. wheals.

6. To assess the skin for temperature and moisture, the most appropriate technique is
   a. auscultation.
   b. inspection.
   c. palpation.
   d. percussion.

7. Individuals with dark skin are more likely to develop
   a. sunburn.
   b. skin rashes.
   c. skin cancer.
   d. keloids.

8. On inspection of the patient's skin, the nurse notes the complete absence of melanin pigment in patchy areas on the patient's hands. This condition is called
   a. vitiligo.
   b. hirsutism.
   c. lichenification.
   d. telangiectasia.

9. Diagnostic testing is recommended for skin lesions when
   a. a health history cannot be obtained.
   b. a more definitive diagnosis is needed.
   c. percussion reveals an abnormal finding.
   d. treatment with prescribed medication has failed.

REFERENCES

1. Thibodeau GA, Patton KT: *Human body in health and disease,* ed 3, St Louis, 2002, Mosby.
2. Goldstein BG, Goldstein AO: *Practical dermatology,* ed 2, St Louis, 1997, Mosby.
3. Marks R: *Skin diseases in old age,* ed 2, Malden, MA, 1999, Blackwell Science Publications.
4. Jarvis C: *Physical examination and health assessment,* ed 3, Philadelphia, 2000, WB Saunders.
5. Morison M et al: *A color guide to the nursing management of chronic wounds,* ed 2, St Louis, 1999, Mosby.
6. Wilson S, Giddens J: *Health assessment for nursing practice,* ed 2, St Louis, 2001, Mosby.
7. Hooper BJ, Goldman MP: *Primary dermatologic care,* St Louis, 1999, Mosby.

23

NURSING MANAGEMENT
Integumentary Problems

Shannon Ruff Dirksen
Marcia J. Hill

LEARNING OBJECTIVES

1. Describe health promotion practices related to the integumentary system.
2. Explain the etiology, clinical manifestations, and nursing and collaborative care of common acute dermatologic problems.
3. Describe the psychologic and pathophysiologic effects of chronic dermatologic conditions.
4. Explain the etiology, clinical manifestations, and collaborative care of malignant dermatologic disorders.
5. Explain the etiology, clinical manifestations, and collaborative care of bacterial, viral, and fungal infections of the integument.
6. Explain the etiology, clinical manifestations, and collaborative care of infestations and insect bites.
7. Explain the etiology, clinical manifestations, and collaborative care of dermatologic disorders related to allergies.
8. Explain the etiology, clinical manifestations, and collaborative care related to benign dermatologic disorders.
9. Describe the dermatologic manifestations of common systemic diseases.
10. Explain the indications and nursing management related to plastic surgery and skin grafts..

KEY TERMS

actinic keratosis, p. 490
basal cell carcinoma, p. 490
cryosurgery, p. 502
curettage, p. 502
dermabrasion, p. 509
dysplastic nevus syndrome, p. 493

lichenification, p. 504
malignant melanoma, p. 492
pruritus, p. 503
squamous cell carcinoma, p. 490
sun protection factor (SPF), p. 487

HEALTH PROMOTION

Health promotion practices related to the skin often parallel practices appropriate for general good health. The skin reflects both physical and psychologic well-being. Specific health promotion activities appropriate to good skin health include avoidance of environmental hazards, adequate rest and exercise, proper hygiene and nutrition, and cautious use of self-treatment.

Environmental Hazards

Sun Exposure. Many people are unaware that the effects of years of exposure to the sun are cumulative and damaging. The ultraviolet (UV) rays of the sun cause degenerative changes in the dermis, resulting in premature aging (i.e., loss of elasticity, thinning, wrinkling, drying of the skin). Prolonged and repeated sun exposure is a major factor in precancerous and cancerous lesions.[1] Actinic keratoses, basal cell carcinoma, squamous cell carcinoma, and malignant melanoma are dermatologic problems associated directly or indirectly with sun exposure. These skin disorders are discussed in this chapter.

Nurses should be strong advocates of safe sun practices. Specific wavelengths of the sun (Table 23-1) have different effects on the skin. Ultraviolet B (UVB) appears to be the major factor in the development of skin cancer, and ultraviolet A (UVA) aug-

ments the carcinogenic effects of UVB. Tanning is the skin's response to injury by the sun and is caused by increased production of melanin. When sun exposure is excessive, the turnover time of the skin is shortened and results in peeling. Fair-skinned persons should be especially cautious about excessive sun exposure, because they have smaller amounts of the natural protection afforded by melanin.

Sunscreens can filter UVA and UVB wavelengths. There are two types of topical sunscreen—chemical and physical. *Chemical sunscreens* are light creams or lotions designed to absorb or filter UV light, resulting in diminished UV light penetration into the epidermis. *Physical sunscreens* are thick, opaque, heavy creams that reflect UV radiation. They block all UVA and UVB radiation, as well as all visible light.

The Food and Drug Administration (FDA) has rated popular sunscreen products according to their **sun protection factor (SPF).** This is a method of measuring the effectiveness of a sunscreen in filtering and absorbing UVB radiation. There is no similar rating of products to screen UVA. Patients should be taught to look for the term "broad spectrum" on the packaging, indicating a wide range of absorbance, particularly for UVB wavelengths.

TABLE 23-1	Wavelengths of the Sun and Effects on Skin
WAVELENGTH	**EFFECT**
Short (UVC)	Does not reach earth; blocked by atmosphere
Middle (UVB)	Causes sunburn and cumulative effect of sun damage; major factor in development of skin cancer
Long (UVA)	Can produce elastic tissue damage and actinic skin damage; contributes to formation of skin cancer

Reviewed by Beverly Gay, RN, MSN, CCRN, Nurse Educator, Medical College of Virginia Hospitals at the Virginia Commonwealth University Health Systems, Richmond, Va.

Consumers need to select the sunscreen most appropriate for their needs. PABA and PABA esters, cinnamates, salicylates, and methyl anthranilate block UVB rays. Para-aminobenzoic acid (PABA) has been removed from many sunscreen products because it stains clothing and can cause allergic reactions, including contact dermatitis.[2] Parsol (avobenzone) blocks UVA rays and has been added to most sunscreens. The benzophenones block both UVA and UVB rays (Table 23-2). Waterproof sunscreens should be used by swimmers and persons who perspire profusely. Directions accompanying specific products should be followed because application time before exposure varies according to the product.

The general recommendation is that everyone should use a sunscreen with a minimum SPF of 15 daily. Sunscreens with an SPF of 15 or more filter 92% of the UVB responsible for erythema and make sunburn unlikely in most individuals when applied appropriately.

The nurse can also inform the patient about other means of protection from the damaging effects of the sun, such as wearing a large-brimmed hat, sunglasses, and a long-sleeved shirt of a lightly woven fabric or carrying an umbrella.[3] Patients need to know that the rays of the sun are most dangerous between 10 AM and 2 PM standard time or 11 AM and 3 PM daylight saving time,

regardless of the latitude. Even on overcast days serious sunburn can occur, because up to 80% of UV rays can penetrate through the clouds. Other factors that increase the possibility of sunburn include being at high altitudes; being in snow, which reflects 85% of the sun's rays; or being in or near water. People should be warned of the dangers of tanning booths and sun lamps, which are predominantly UVA.[4] No presently available sunscreen blocks all UVA.

Certain topical and systemic medications potentiate the effect of the sun, even with brief exposure. Categories of drug therapy that may contain common photosensitizing medications are listed in Table 23-3. The nurse should be aware that many drugs are included in these categories, and the photosensitivity of each individual drug should be examined. The chemicals in these medications absorb light and release energy that harms cells and tissues. The clinical manifestations of drug-induced photosensitivity are similar to those of exaggerated sunburn, with swelling; erythema; papular, plaque-like lesions; and vesicles. Skin that is at risk for photosensitivity reactions can be protected by the use of sunscreen products. Nurses have a role in educating patients who are taking these drugs about their photosensitizing effect.

Irritants and Allergens. Patients can seek treatment for irritant or allergic dermatitis, two types of contact dermatitis. *Irritant contact dermatitis* is produced by direct chemical injury to the skin.[5] *Allergic contact dermatitis* is an agent-specific, type IV delayed hypersensitivity response. This response requires sensitization and occurs only in individuals who are predisposed to react to a particular antigen (see Chapter 13).

The nurse should counsel patients to avoid known irritants (e.g., ammonia, harsh detergents). Skin patch testing (application of allergens) is necessary to determine the most likely sensitizing agent. Usually the nurse is the first health care provider to detect a contact allergy to various tapes, gloves (latex), and adhesives. The nurse must also be aware that prescribed and over-the-counter (OTC) topical and systemic drugs used to treat a variety of conditions may cause dermatologic reactions.[6]

Radiation. Although most radiology departments are extremely cautious in protecting both themselves and their patients from the effects of excessive radiation, the nurse should help the patient make decisions about radiologic procedures. X-rays can be invaluable in both diagnosis and therapy, but indiscriminate use can cause serious side effects to the skin, as well as other body processes. In the past (30 years ago), cystic acne was treated with radiation. This information is important because the patients who have been treated in the past by this method have an increased incidence of basal cell carcinoma.[7]

Rest and Sleep

Rest and sleep are important health-promotion considerations in relation to the skin. Although the exact effects of sleep are not known, it is thought to be restorative. Rest reduces the threshold of itching and the potential skin damage from the resultant scratching.

Exercise

Exercise increases circulation and dilates the blood vessels. In addition to the healthy glow produced by exercise, the psychologic effects can also improve one's appearance and mental outlook. However, caution must be used to avoid or protect the

CULTURAL & ETHNIC CONSIDERATIONS
Integumentary Problems

- African Americans and Native Americans have a lower incidence of skin cancer than whites.
- Whites, especially those living in sunny climates, have a high incidence of skin cancer.
- Skin assessment may be difficult in individuals with darker skin. The oral mucous membranes and conjunctiva are areas where pallor, cyanosis, and jaundice are more readily detected. The palms of the hands and soles of the feet can also be used for assessment of the skin of darker individuals.
- When darker skin heals following injury or inflammation, it tends to be hypopigmented or hyperpigmented.

TABLE 23-2	Sunscreen Ingredients and Ultraviolet Light Protection
SUNSCREEN INGREDIENTS	**ULTRAVIOLET LIGHT (UVL) PROTECTION**
Chemical	
Benzophenones	UVA and UVB
PABA and PABA esters	UVB
Cinnametes	UVB
Salicylates	UVB
Miscellaneous	
Methyl anthranilate	UVB
Parsol (avobenzone)	UVA
Physical Sunscreens	
Titanium dioxide	UVA and UVB
Zinc oxide	UVA and UVB

UVA, Long wavelength of UVL; *UVB,* middle wavelength of UVL.

TABLE 23-3 Drug Therapy
Categories of Drugs That May Cause Photosensitivity

CATEGORIES	EXAMPLES
Anticancer drugs	methotrexate, vinorelbine (Navelbine)
Antidepressants	amitriptyline (Elavil), clomipramine (Anafranil), doxepin (Sinequan)
Antiarrhythmics	quinidine, amiodarone (Cordarone)
Antihistamines	diphenhydramine (Benadryl), chlorpheniramine, clemastine (Tavist)
Antimicrobials	tetracycline, sulfamethoxazole, azithromycin (Zithromax), ciprofloxacin (Cipro)
Antifungals	griseofulvin, ketoconazole (Nizoral)
Antipsychotics	chlorpromazine (Thorazine), haloperidol (Haldol)
Diuretics	furosemide (Lasix), hydrochlorothiazide (HydroDiuril)
Hypoglycemics	tolbutamide (Orinase), glipizide (Glucotrol), chlorpropamide (Diabinese)
Nonsteroidal antiinflammatory drugs	diclofenac (Voltaren), piroxicam (Feldene), sulindac (Clinoril)

exerciser from overexposure to heat, cold, and sun during outdoor exercise.

Hygiene

Hygienic practices should match the skin type, lifestyle, and culture of the patient. The person with oily skin should cleanse the skin with a drying agent more often than the person with dry skin. Dry skin might benefit from superfatted soaps and measures to increase moisture, such as the application of moisturizers to the skin.

The normal acidity of the skin (pH 4.2 to 5.6) and perspiration protect against bacterial overgrowth. Most soaps are alkaline and cause a neutralization of the skin surface and loss of protection. The use of more mild soaps such as Ivory, as well as avoiding hot water and vigorous rubbing, can noticeably decrease local irritation and inflammation.

In general, the skin and hair should be washed often enough to remove excess oil and excretions and to prevent odor. Older persons should avoid the use of harsh soaps and shampoos because of the increasing dryness of their skin and scalp. Moisturizers should be used after bath or shower while the skin is still damp to seal in this moisture.

Nutrition

A well-balanced diet adequate in all food groups can produce healthy skin, hair, and nails. Certain elements are particularly essential to good skin health. These elements include the following:

1. *Vitamin A*—essential for maintenance of normal cell structure, specifically epithelial cells. It is necessary for normal wound healing. The absence of vitamin A causes dryness of the conjuctiva and poor wound healing.
2. *Vitamin B complex*—essential for complex metabolic functions. Deficiencies of niacin and pyridoxine (B_6) manifest as dermatologic symptoms such as erythema, bullae, and seborrhea-like lesions.
3. *Vitamin C (ascorbic acid)*—essential for connective tissue formation and normal wound healing. Absence of vitamin C causes symptoms of scurvy, including petechiae, bleeding gums, and purpura.
4. *Vitamin K deficiency*—interferes with normal prothrombin synthesis in the liver and can lead to bruising.
5. *Protein*—necessary in amounts adequate for cell growth and maintenance. It is also necessary for normal wound healing.
6. *Unsaturated fatty acids*—necessary to maintain the function and integrity of cellular and subcellular membranes in tissue metabolism, especially linoleic and arachidonic acids.

Obesity has an adverse effect on the skin. The increase in subcutaneous fat can lead to stretching and overheating. Overheating secondary to the greater insulation provided by fat causes an increase in sweating, which has an adverse effect on inflamed skin. Obesity also has an influence on the development of type 2 diabetes mellitus with its concomitant skin complications (see Chapter 47).

Self-Treatment

The nurse needs to increase the patient's awareness of the dangers of self-diagnosis and treatment. The wide variety of OTC skin preparations can confuse the consumer. General instructions that the nurse can discuss with the patient would stress the duration of the treatment and the need to follow package directions closely. Skin problems are generally slow to produce symptoms and slow to resolve. If the package insert of an OTC drug says its use should not exceed 7 days, this warning should be heeded. If the directions say to apply twice daily, the urge to increase the dose and hasten the cure must be avoided. If any systemic signs of inflammation or extension of the skin problem (e.g., an increased number of lesions or increased erythema or swelling) develop, self-care should be stopped and the help of a professional should be enlisted.

Malignant Skin Neoplasms

Cancer of the skin is the most common cancer. Malignant neoplasms of the skin exhibit similar characteristics to other malignant conditions (see Chapter 15). However, skin malignancies generally grow slowly. The presence of a persistent lesion that does not heal is highly suspicious of a malignancy and should be biopsied. Adequate and early treatment can often lead to a highly favorable prognosis.[8] The fact that skin lesions are so visible increases the likelihood of early detection and diagnosis. Patients should be taught to self-examine their skin regularly.

Risk Factors

Risk factors for skin malignancies include having a fair skin type (blonde or red hair and blue or green eyes), history of chronic sun exposure, family history of skin cancer, and exposure to tar and systemic arsenicals. Environmental factors that increase the risk of skin malignancies include living near the equator, working outdoors, and frequent outdoor recreational activities.[9] Dark-skinned persons are less susceptible to skin cancer because of the naturally occurring increased melanin, an effective sunscreen. However, although dark skin lowers the risk of melanoma, people with dark skin do develop melanoma.

NONMELANOMA SKIN CANCERS

Nonmelanoma skin cancers, either basal cell carcinoma or squamous cell carcinoma, are the most common form of skin cancer.[10] Globally, there are more than 1 million new cases yearly.[11] Nonmelanoma skin cancers do not develop from melanocytes, the skin cells that make melanin, as melanoma skin cancers do. Instead, they are a neoplasm of the epidermis. The most common sites for development of nonmelanoma skin cancer are in sun-exposed areas and include the face, head, neck, back of the hands, and arms.

Although the number of deaths attributable to nonmelanoma skin cancer is small, the tumors have an inherent potential for severe local destruction, permanent disfigurement, and disability. The most common etiologic factor, chronic sun exposure, should be consciously avoided by the use of sunscreens and protective clothing.[12]

Actinic Keratosis

Actinic keratosis, also known as *solar keratosis,* consists of hyperkeratotic papules and plaques occurring on sun-exposed areas. Actinic keratosis is a premalignant form of squamous cell carcinoma that affects nearly all of the older white population. It is the most common of all precancerous skin lesions. The clinical appearance of actinic keratosis can be highly varied. The typical lesion is an irregularly shaped, flat, slightly erythematous macule or papule with indistinct borders and an overly-

ing hard keratotic scale or horn (Table 23-4). Many forms of treatment are used, including cryosurgery, fluorouracil (5-FU), surgical removal, tretinoin (Retin-A), and chemical peeling agents. Any lesion that persists should be evaluated for possible biopsy.

Basal Cell Carcinoma

Basal cell carcinoma (BCC) is a locally invasive malignancy arising from epidermal basal cells. It is the most common type of skin cancer and also the least deadly. BCC usually occurs in middle-aged to older adults. The clinical manifestations are described in Table 23-4. The cancerous cells of BCC almost never spread beyond the skin (Fig. 23-1). However, if left untreated, massive tissue destruction may result. Some basal cell carcinomas are pigmented with curled borders and an opaque appearance and may be misinterpreted as a melanoma. Therefore a tissue biopsy is needed to confirm the diagnosis.

Multiple treatment modalities are used depending on the tumor location and histologic type, history of recurrence, and patient characteristics.[12] Treatment modalities include electrodesiccation and curettage, excision, cryosurgery, radiation therapy, Mohs' micrographic surgery, topical chemotherapy (5-FU), and intralesional α-interferon. (These treatments are discussed later in this chapter.) Electrodesiccation, curettage, cryosurgery, and scalpel incision all have a cure rate of greater than 90% when used correctly on primary lesions.

Squamous Cell Carcinoma

Squamous cell carcinoma (SCC) is a malignant neoplasm of keratinizing epidermal cells (Fig. 23-2). It frequently occurs on sun-exposed skin. SCC is less common than BCC. SCC can be very aggressive, has the potential to metastasize, and may lead to death if not treated early and correctly. Pipe, cigar, and cigarette smoking contributes to the formation of SCC. Therefore lesions are commonly seen on the mouth and lips.

The clinical manifestations of SCC are described in Table 23-4. A biopsy should always be performed when a lesion is suspected to be SCC. Treatment consists of electrodesiccation and curettage, excision, radiation therapy, intralesional injection of 5-FU or

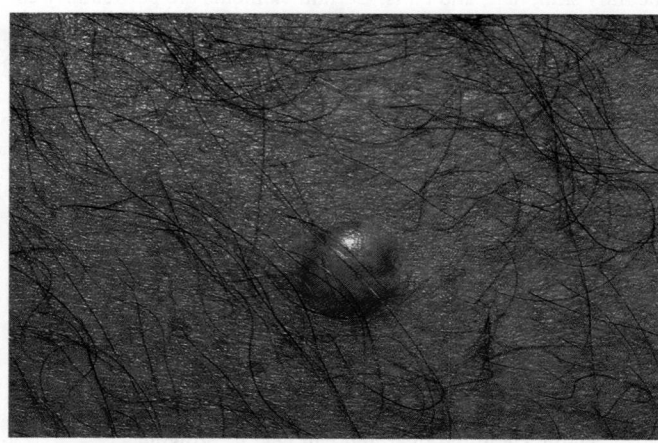

FIG. 23-1 Basal cell carcinoma. Pearly papule with slight erythema.

TABLE 23-4 Premalignant and Malignant Conditions of the Skin		
ETIOLOGY AND PATHOPHYSIOLOGY	CLINICAL MANIFESTATIONS	TREATMENT AND PROGNOSIS
Actinic Keratoses Actinic (sun) damage (precursor of squamous cell carcinoma)	Flat or slightly elevated, dry, hyperkeratotic scaly papule; possibly flat, rough, or verrucous; adherent scale, which returns when removed; often multiple; rough scale on red base; often on erythematous sun-exposed areas; increase in number with age	Curettage, electrosurgery, cryosurgery, chemical caustics, topical application of 5-FU over entire area for 14-21 days; no effect on healthy skin and other lesions; recurrence possible even with adequate treatment; untreated lesions possibly leading to squamous cell carcinoma (1% incidence)
Dysplastic Nevus Syndrome Morphologically between common acquired nevi and melanoma; histogenetic precursor of cutaneous malignant melanoma	Often larger than 5 mm; irregular border, possibly notched; variegated color mixture of tan, brown, black, red, and pink with single mole; presence of at least one flat portion, often at edge of mole; frequently multiple; uncommon before puberty; most common site on back, but possible in uncommon mole sites such as scalp or buttocks	Marker of increased risk for melanoma; careful monitoring of persons suspected of familial tendency to melanoma or dysplastic nevus syndrome necessary to increase likelihood of early diagnosis of melanoma; indication for excisional biopsy for suspicious lesions
Basal Cell Carcinoma Change in basal cells; no maturation or normal keratinization; continuing division of basal cells and formation of enlarging mass; related to excessive sun exposure, genetic skin type, x-ray radiation, scars, and some types of nevi; basal cells possibly pigmented but absent in nevi	**Nodular and Ulcerative** Small, slowly enlarging papule; borders semitranslucent or "pearly," with overlying telangiectasia; erosion, ulceration, and depression of center; normal skin markings lost (see Fig. 23-1) **Superficial** Erythematous, sharply defined, barely elevated multinodular plaques with varying scaling and crusting; similar to eczema but not pruritic	Excisional surgery, chemosurgery, electrosurgery, cryosurgery; 95% cure rate; slow-growing tumor that invades local tissue; metastasis rare
Squamous Cell Carcinoma Frequent occurrence on previously damaged skin (e.g., from sun, radiation, scar); malignant tumor of squamous (prickle) cell of epidermis; invasion of dermis, surrounding skin; metastasis possible	**Early** Firm nodules with indistinct borders with scaling and ulceration; opaque **Late** Covering of lesion with scale or horn from keratinization; most common on sun-exposed areas such as face and hands (see Fig. 23-2)	Surgical removal, cryosurgery, radiation therapy, chemosurgery, Mohs' procedure or microscopically controlled excision, electrodesiccation, and curettage; untreated lesion possibly metastasizes to regional lymph nodes; high cure rate with early detection and treatment
Cutaneous T Cell Lymphoma (mycosis fungoides) Origination in skin; chronic, slowly progressing disease, possible etiologies of environmental toxins and chemical exposure	Prevalence is twice as high in men as compared to women in United States; classic presentation involving three stages—patch, plaque, and tumor; history of persistent macular eruption followed by gradual appearance of indurated plaques	Topical nitrogen mustard, radiation therapy, systemic chemotherapy, PUVA, extracorporeal photopheresis, denileukin diftitox (Ontak); 5 yr life expectancy with only skin manifestations and no treatment; greatly decreased survival rate with generalized erythroderma with exfoliation and abnormal cells in bloodstream (Sézary syndrome)

HIV, Human immunodeficiency virus; *PUVA*, psoralen ultraviolet A.

Continued

TABLE 23-4	Premalignant and Malignant Conditions of the Skin—cont'd	
ETIOLOGY AND PATHOPHYSIOLOGY	**CLINICAL MANIFESTATIONS**	**TREATMENT AND PROGNOSIS**
Malignant Melanoma		
Neoplastic growth of melanocytes anywhere on skin, eyes, or mucous membranes; classification according to major histologic mode of spread; potential invasion and widespread metastases	Irregular color, irregular surface, irregular border; variegated color including red, white, blue, black, gray, brown; flat or elevated, eroded or ulcerated; often under 1 cm in size; most common sites in males and females on back; in females on chest and lower legs (see Fig. 23-3)	Wide excision, full-thickness surgical removal; correlation of survival rate with depth of invasion; poor prognosis unless diagnosis and treatment early; spreading by local extension, regional lymphatic vessels, and bloodstream; adjuvant therapy after surgery may be necessary if lesion greater than 1.5 mm in depth
Kaposi's Sarcoma*		
Multicentric neoplasms that occur most commonly in HIV-infected individuals; multiple vascular nodules appearing in the skin, mucous membranes, and viscera; severity ranges from minor to fulminant with extensive cutaneous and visceral involvement	Wide range of presentation; initially, small reddish, purple nodules on skin; lesions range in size from a few mm to several cm, can cause lymphedema and disfigurement particularly when confluent; systemic involvement has symptoms associated with organ (e.g., lungs and shortness of breath)	Diagnosis based upon biopsy of suspicious lesion; treatment dependent on severity of lesions and patient's immune status; attempt to avoid treatments to further suppress immune system; possible treatments include localized radiation, α-interferon, chemotherapy, cryotherapy

*Refer to Chapter 14 for more information.

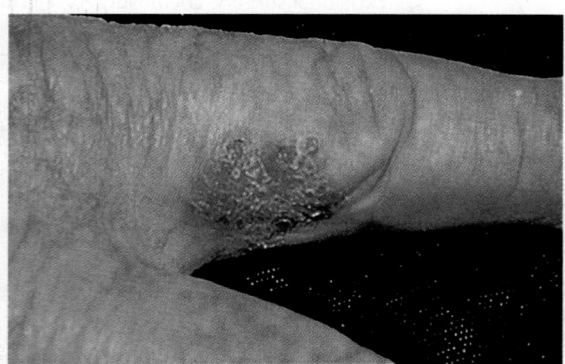

FIG. 23-2 Squamous cell carcinoma of the finger.

methotrexate, and Mohs' surgery. There is a high cure rate with early detection and treatment.

MALIGNANT MELANOMA

Malignant melanoma is a tumor arising in cells producing melanin, usually the melanocytes of the skin. Melanoma has the ability to metastasize to any organ, including the brain and heart. This is the most deadly skin cancer, and its incidence is increasing faster than any other cancer. It accounts for 40,000 deaths a year worldwide. Currently it accounts for 11% of all skin cancers.[11]

Melanoma is one of the most common cancers in Americans between ages 25 and 29.[13] The precise cause of melanoma is unknown, but risk factors include UV radiation; skin sensitivity; genetic, hormonal, and immunologic factors; and recreational lifestyle changes that lead to greater sun exposure. A sponta-

neous mutation in a gene (B-RAF) has been identified that is responsible for 70% of the cases of melanoma.

Types of Melanoma

The four types of cutaneous melanoma are superficial spreading melanoma (SSM), lentigo maligna melanoma (LMM), acral-lentiginous melanoma (ALM), and nodular melanoma (NM). SSM is the most common type, the most curable, and often occurs on chronically sun-exposed areas such as the legs and upper back. It frequently arises from a preexisting mole. LMM is commonly located on the face and is often found in elderly patients. Lesions appear as flat, brown, irregular patches. These patches increase in size for many years before the development of cancer occurs. ALM appears on the soles, palms, mucous membranes, and terminal phalanges. ALM is more common in Asian people and people with dark skin. NM occurs more often in men and can be located anywhere on the body. It is the most frequently misdiagnosed melanoma because it resembles a blood blister or polyp. It is believed to be a more aggressive type of melanoma that can develop and invade rapidly.[14]

Clinical Manifestations

About one third of melanomas occur in existing nevi or moles. Melanoma frequently occurs on the lower legs in women and on the trunk, head, and neck in men. Because most melanoma cells continue to produce melanin, melanoma tumors are often brown or black. Individuals should consult their health care provider immediately if their moles or lesions show any of the clinical signs (ABCDs) of melanoma (Fig. 23-3). Any sudden or progressive increase in the size, color, or shape of a mole should be checked. When melanoma begins in the skin it is called *cutaneous melanoma*. Melanoma can also occur in the eyes, meninges, lymph nodes, digestive tract, and anywhere else in the body where melanocytes are found.

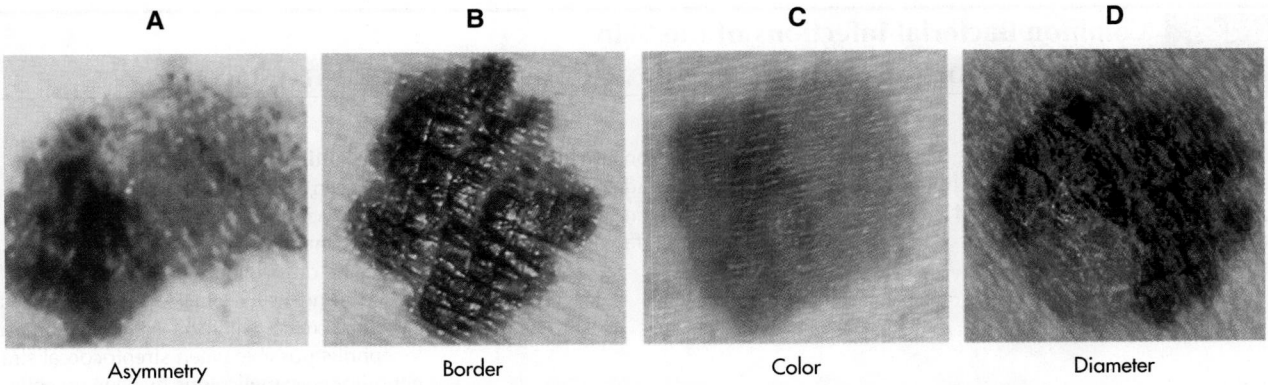

A   **B**   **C**   **D**

Asymmetry   Border   Color   Diameter

FIG. 23-3 The ABCDs of melanoma. **A,** Asymmetry: one half unlike the other half. **B,** Border irregularity: edges are ragged, notched, or blurred. **C,** Color: varied pigmentation; shades of tan, brown, and black. **D,** Diameter: larger than 6 mm (diameter of a pencil eraser).

Collaborative Care

Treatment depends on the site of the original tumor, stage of the cancer, and patient's age and general health. The initial treatment of malignant melanoma is surgery. Melanoma that has spread to the lymph nodes or nearby sites usually requires additional therapy such as chemotherapy, biologic therapy (e.g., α-interferon, interleukin-2), and/or radiation therapy. The type of therapy depends on the stage of the disease.[15] Examples of chemotherapy agents that are used include dacarbazine (DTIC), temozolomide (TMZ), procarbazine (Matulane), carmustine (BCNU), and lomustine (CCNU). Gene therapy is currently being examined as another treatment option (see Chapter 15 for discussion of these therapies). Any pigmented lesions believed to be melanoma should never be shave-biopsied, shave-excised, or electrocauterized.

Cutaneous melanoma is nearly 100% curable by excision if diagnosed early when the malignant cells are restricted to the epidermis. The most important prognostic factor is tumor thickness at the time of presentation. If spread to regional lymph nodes occurs, the patient has a 50% chance of 5-year survival. If metastasis to other organs occurs, treatment is largely palliative.

Dysplastic Nevus Syndrome

An abnormal mole pattern called **dysplastic nevus syndrome** (DNS) places a person at increased risk of melanoma. Approximately 30% of the population has moles classified as dysplastic nevi. Dysplastic nevi, or atypical moles, are moles that are larger than usual (greater than 5 mm across) with irregular borders and various shades of color. The earliest clinically detectable abnormality associated with this syndrome is an increase in the number of morphologically normal-looking nevi at around age 2 to 6 years. Another proliferation occurs around adolescence, and new nevi appear throughout life. Obtaining a detailed family history related to melanoma and DNS is an important responsibility of the health care provider. The risk of developing melanoma doubles with the presence of one dysplastic nevus, and having 10 or more increases the chance by twelvefold.[16]

SKIN INFECTIONS AND INFESTATIONS

Bacterial Infections

The skin is covered with numerous microorganisms, especially bacteria. *Staphylococcus epidermidis* and diphtheroids are the most common bacteria present on the skin. The skin provides an ideal environment for bacterial growth with an abundant supply of warmth, nutrients, and water.

Bacterial infection occurs when the balance between the host and the microorganisms is altered. This can occur as a primary infection following a break in the skin. It can also occur as a secondary infection to already damaged skin or as a sign of a systemic disease (Table 23-5).

Healthy persons can develop bacterial skin infections. Predisposing factors such as moisture, obesity, skin disease, systemic corticosteroids and antibiotics, chronic disease, and diabetes mellitus all increase the likelihood of infection. Good hygiene practices and general good health inhibit bacterial infections. If an infection is present, the resulting drainage is infectious. Meticulous skin hygiene and infection control practices are necessary to prevent spread of the infection.

Trauma is a common predisposing factor to skin infection. Table 23-6 outlines the emergency care of a patient with a surface skin wound.

Viral Infections

Viral infections of the skin are as difficult to treat as viral infections anywhere in the body. When a cell is infected by a virus, a lesion can result (Fig. 23-4). Lesions can also result from an inflammatory response to the viral infections. Herpes simplex, herpes zoster (Fig. 23-5), and warts are the most common viral infections affecting the skin (Table 23-7).

Fungal Infections

Because of the large number of identified fungi, it is almost impossible to avoid exposure to some pathologic varieties. However, some fungi can cause serious infections, including tinea corporis and candidiasis (Figs. 23-6 and 23-7). Common fungal infections of the skin are presented in Table 23-8.

Text continued on page 498

TABLE 23-5	Common Bacterial Infections of the Skin	
ETIOLOGY AND PATHOPHYSIOLOGY	**CLINICAL MANIFESTATIONS**	**TREATMENT AND PROGNOSIS**
Impetigo		
Group A β-hemolytic streptococci, staphylococci, or combination of both; associated with poor hygiene and low socioeconomic status; primary or secondary infection; contagious	Vesiculopustular lesions that develop thick, honey-colored crust surrounded by erythema; pruritic; most common on face	**Systemic Antibiotics** Oral penicillin, benzathine penicillin IM, erythromycin **Local Treatment** Warm saline or aluminum acetate soaks followed by soap-and-water removal of crusts; topical antibiotic cream; with no treatment, glomerulonephritis possible when streptococcal strain nephritogenic; meticulous hygiene essential
Folliculitis		
Usually staphylococci; present in areas subjected to friction, moisture, rubbing, or oil; increased incidence in patients who have diabetes mellitus	Small pustule at hair follicle opening with minimal erythema; development of crusting; most common on scalp, beard, extremities in men; tender to touch	Soap (e.g., Hibiclens) and water cleansing; topical antibiotics (e.g., Bactroban); warm compresses of water or aluminum acetate solution; healing usually without scarring; if lesions extensive and deep, possible scarring and loss of involved hair follicles
Furuncle		
Deep infection with staphylococci around hair follicle, often associated with severe acne or seborrheic dermatitis	Tender erythematous area around hair follicle; draining of pus and core of necrotic debris on rupture; most common on face, back of neck, axillae, breasts, buttocks, perineum, thighs; painful	Incision and drainage, occasionally antibiotics, meticulous care of involved skin, frequent application of warm, moist compresses
Furunculosis		
Increased incidence in patients who are obese, chronically ill, or regularly exposed to moisture, pressure, or irritation or who have diabetes mellitus	Lesions as above; malaise, regional adenopathy, elevated temperature	Warm compresses; systemic antibiotic after culture and sensitivity study of drainage (usually semisynthetic, penicillinase-resistant, oral penicillin such as cloxacillin and oxacillin); measures to reduce surface staphylococci include antimicrobial cream to nares, armpits, and groin and antiseptic to entire skin; often recurrent with scarring; incision and drainage of soft lesions; prevention or correction of predisposing factors; meticulous personal hygiene
Carbuncle		
Multiple, interconnecting furuncles	Many pustules appearing in erythematous area, most common at nape of neck	Treatment same as furuncles; often recurrent despite production of antibodies; healing slow with scar formation
Cellulitis		
Inflammation of subcutaneous tissues; possibly secondary complication or primary infection; often following break in skin; *S. aureus* and streptococci usual causative agents; deep inflammation of subcutaneous tissue from enzymes produced by bacteria	Hot, tender, erythematous, and edematous area with diffuse borders; malaise and fever	Moist heat, immobilization and elevation, systemic antibiotic therapy, hospitalization if severe; progression to gangrene possible if untreated
Erysipelas		
Superficial cellulitis primarily involving the dermis; group A β-hemolytic streptococci	Red, hot, sharply demarcated plaque that is indurated and painful; bacteremia possible; most common on face and extremities; toxic signs, such as fever, ↑ white blood cell count, headache, malaise	Systemic antibiotics—usually penicillin; hospitalization often required

IM, Intramuscular.

TABLE 23-6	Emergency Management Surface Skin Wound	

ETIOLOGY	ASSESSMENT FINDINGS	INTERVENTIONS
Blunt Direct blow to skin (e.g., fist, baseball bat, rock) Indirect blow to skin (e.g., blast wave from gunshot) **Penetrating** Puncture or cutting of skin surface (e.g., knife, stick, glass)	• Contusion • Laceration • Avulsion • Abrasion • Bleeding • Pain • Neurovascular compromise	**Initial** • Ensure airway, breathing, and circulation before management of surface injury. • Identify and treat other more serious injuries. • Control bleeding with direct pressure or pressure dressing. • Assess for impaled objects, pieces of glass, or debris. • Do not remove *impaled* object. Stabilize for removal under controlled environment. • Cleanse wounds carefully with isotonic solution. Cover with moist saline gauze until wound is closed. • Shave or clip as small an area as possible with scalp wound. • Never shave eyebrows. • Fold avulsed skin flap into normal position, then control bleeding. Apply bulky sterile dressing to area and immobilize injured part. • Determine tetanus immunization status. • Use sticky side of a wide piece of tape to remove surface slivers of glass. **Ongoing** • Monitor vital signs. • Check neurovascular status of injured extremity.

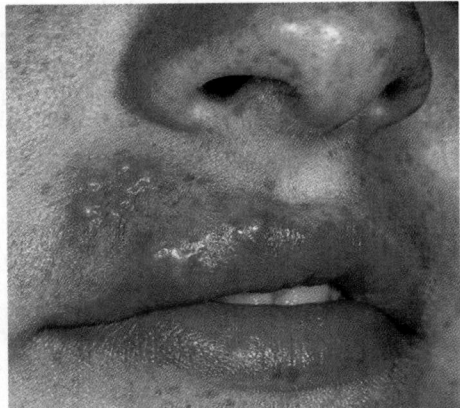

FIG. 23-4 Herpes viral infection on the lips. Typical presentation with vesicles on the lips and extending on to the skin.

FIG. 23-5 Herpes zoster with bullae and vesicles on the anterior chest.

TABLE 23-7	**Common Viral Infections of the Skin**	
ETIOLOGY AND PATHOPHYSIOLOGY	**CLINICAL MANIFESTATIONS**	**TREATMENT AND PROGNOSIS**
Herpes Simplex Virus Type 1* Generally oral infections; virus remaining in nerve root ganglion and possibly returning to skin to produce recurrence when exacerbated by sunlight, trauma, menses, stress, and systemic infection; contagious to those not previously infected; increase in severity with age, transmission by respiratory droplets or virus-containing fluid, such as saliva or cervical secretions; no protection against subsequent infection in other areas with episodes of infection in one area	**First Episode** Symptoms occurring 3-7 days or more after contact; painful local reaction; grouped vesicles on erythematous base; systemic symptoms, such as fever and malaise possible or asymptomatic presentation possible (see Fig. 23-4) **Recurrent** Small; recurrence in similar spot; characteristic grouped vesicles on erythematous base	Symptomatic medication; soothing, moist compresses; petrolatum to lesions; scarring not usual result; antiviral agents such as acyclovir (Zovirax), famciclovir (Famvir), and valacyclovir (Valtrex)
Herpes Simplex Virus Type 2 Generally genital infections; recurrence more frequent than oral-labial infections	Same as for herpes simplex virus type 1	Same as for herpes simplex virus type 1
Herpes Varicella Virus Highly contagious, primary infection characterized by successive crops of pruritic vesicles that evolve to pustules, crusts, and in some instances scars	Exanthem, vesicular lesions in successive crops ("dewdrop on a rose petal") seen on face/scalp, then spreading to trunk and extremities	Self-limiting in children, pneumonia and encephalitis may develop in adults; immunization now available; oral acyclovir, valcyclovir, or famciclovir for systemic treatment; symptomatic treatment and control of risk of secondary infection
Herpes Zoster Activation of the varicella-zoster virus; frequent occurrence in immunosuppressed patients; potentially contagious to anyone who has not had varicella or who is immunosuppressed	Linear patches along dermatome of grouped vesicles on erythematous base; usually unilateral and on trunk; burning, pain, and neuralgia preceding outbreak; mild to severe pain during outbreak (see Fig. 23-5)	Symptomatic; antiviral agents such as acyclovir, famciclovir, and valacyclovir; wet compresses, white petrolatum to lesions; analgesia; mild sedation at bedtime; systemic corticosteroids to shorten course and decrease likelihood of postherpetic neuralgia (controversial); usual healing without complications but scarring possible; postherpetic neuralgia possible
Verruca Vulgaris Caused by human papillomavirus; spontaneous disappearance in 1-2 yr possible; mildly contagious by autoinoculation; specific response dependent on body part affected	Circumscribed, hypertrophic, flesh-colored papule limited to epidermis; painful on lateral compression	Multiple treatments, including surgery—scoop removal with scissors and currette; liquid nitrogen therapy; blistering agents—cantharidin; keratolytic agents—salicylic acid; CO_2 laser therapy, treatment can result in scarring
Plantar Warts Caused by human papillomavirus (HPV)	Wart on bottom surface of foot, growing inward because of pressure of walking or standing; painful when pressure applied; interrupted skin markings; cone-shaped with black dots (thrombosed vessels) when pared	Usual treatment is liquid nitrogen or frequent paring followed by application of patches of impregnated chemicals to decrease regrowth; overaggressive destruction possibly resulting in painful, hypertrophic scar

*Herpes simplex is also discussed in Chapter 51.

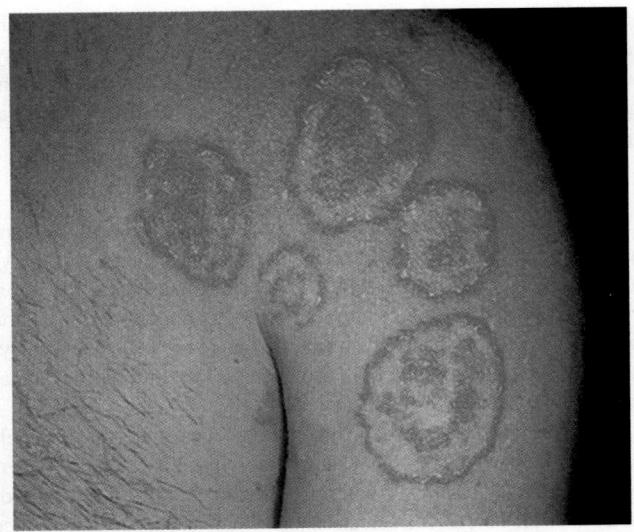

FIG. 23-6 Tinea corporis (ringworm). Typical presentation with an advancing red scaly border. Designation of "ring worm" is obvious.

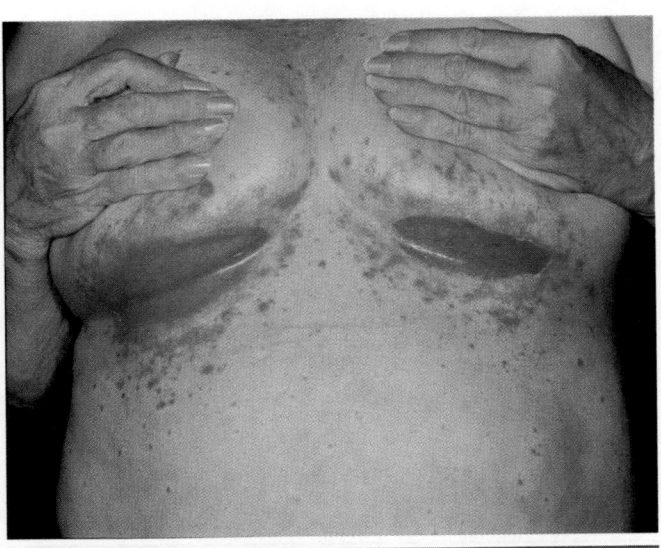

FIG. 23-7 Candidiasis in intertriginous (submammary) folds.

TABLE 23-8 Common Fungal Infections of the Skin and Mucous Membranes

ETIOLOGY AND PATHOPHYSIOLOGY	CLINICAL MANIFESTATIONS	TREATMENT AND PROGNOSIS
Candidiasis Caused by *Candida albicans*; also known as moniliasis; 50% of adults symptom-free carriers; presenting in warm, moist areas such as crural area, oral mucosa, and submammary folds; HIV infection, chemotherapy, radiation, and organ transplantation related to depression of cell-mediated immunity that allow yeast to become pathogenic; production of symptoms by imbalance between host and normal inhabitant of gastrointestinal tract, mouth, and vagina	**Mouth** White, cheesy plaque, resembles milk curds **Vagina** Vaginitis, with red, edematous, painful vaginal wall, white patches; vaginal discharge; pruritus; pain on urination and intercourse **Skin** Diffuse papular erythematous rash with pinpoint satellite lesions around edges of affected area (see Fig. 23-7)	Microscopic examination and culture; nystatin or other specific medication as vaginal suppository or oral lozenge; abstinence or use of condom; eradication of infection with appropriate medication; skin hygiene to keep it clean and dry; mycostatin powder effective on skin lesions
Tinea Corporis Various dermatophytes, commonly referred to as ringworm (see Fig. 23-6)	Typical annular appearance, well-defined margins; erythematous	Cool compresses; topical antifungals for isolated patches; creams or solutions of miconazole (Monistat), clotrimazole (Lotrimin), and butenafine (Mentax)
Tinea Cruris Various dermatophytes, commonly referred to as jock itch	Well-defined border in groin area	Topical antifungal cream or solution
Tinea Unguium Various dermatophytes	Only few nails on one hand affected; nails on toes possibly affected; fungal scale close to outer margin of lesion; brittle, thickened, broken nails with white or yellow discoloration	Topical antifungal cream or solution; griseofulvin moderately successful on fingernails; poor response on toenails; debridement of toenails to normal contour if problematic
Tinea Pedis Various dermatophytes, commonly referred to as athlete's foot	Interdigital scaling and maceration; erythema and blistering; pruritus; painful	Topical antifungal cream or solution

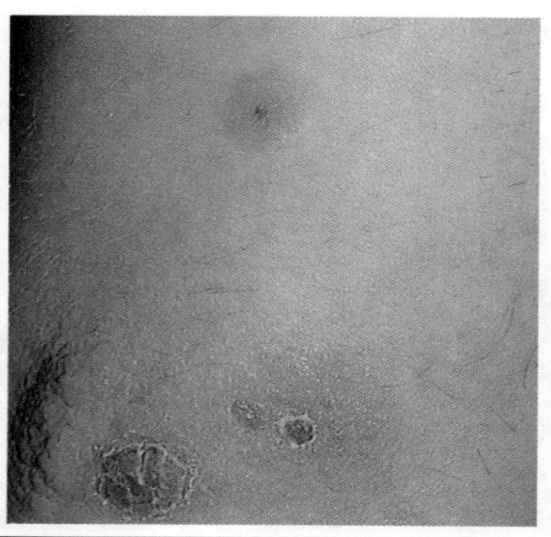

FIG. 23-8 Insect bites with characteristic purpuric spots in center of papule.

Microscopic examination of the scraping of suspicious skin lesions in 10% to 20% potassium hydroxide (KOH) is an easy, inexpensive diagnostic measure to determine the presence of fungus. The appearance of *hyphae* (threadlike structures) is indicative of a fungal infection.

Infestations and Insect Bites

The possibilities for exposure to insect bites and infestations are numerous. In many instances, an allergy to the venom plays a major role in the reaction (Fig. 23-8). In other cases, the clinical manifestations are a reaction to the eggs, feces, or body parts of the invading organism. Certain persons react with a severe hypersensitivity *(anaphylaxis)*, which can be life threatening. (Anaphylaxis is discussed in Chapter 13.)

Prevention of insect bites by avoidance or by the use of repellents is somewhat effective. Meticulous hygiene related to personal articles, clothing, bedding, and examination and care of pets, as well as careful selection of sexual partners, can reduce the incidence of infestations. Routine inspection is necessary where there is a risk of tick bites and Lyme disease (Table 23-9).

TABLE 23-9	**Common Infestations and Insect Bites**		
NAME	**ETIOLOGY AND PATHOPHYSIOLOGY**	**CLINICAL MANIFESTATIONS**	**TREATMENT AND PROGNOSIS**
Bees and Wasps	*Hymenoptera*	Intense, burning, local pain; swelling and itching; severe hypersensitivity possibly leading to anaphylaxis	Cool compresses; local application of antipruritic lotion; antihistamines if indicated; usually uneventful recovery
Bedbugs	*Cimicidae*; feeding periodic, usually at night; present in furniture, walls during day	Wheal surrounded by vivid flare; firm urticaria transforming into persistent lesion; severe pruritus; often grouped in threes appearing on noncovered parts of body	Bedbug controlled by chlorocyclohexane; lesions usually requiring no treatment; severe itching possibly requiring use of antihistamines or topical corticosteroids
Pediculosis Head lice Body lice Pubic lice	*Pediculus humanus* var. *capitis*; *Pediculus humanus* var. *corporis*; *Phthirius pubis*; obligate parasites that suck blood, leave excrement and eggs on skin, live in seams of clothing (if body lice) and in hair as nits; transmission of pubic lice often by sexual contact	Minute, red, noninflammatory; points flush with skin; progression to papular wheal-like lesions; pruritus; secondary excoriation, especially parallel linear excoriations in intrascapular region; firmly attached to hair shaft in head and body lice	γ-Benzene hexachloride or pyrethrins to treat various parts of body; application as directed; contact screening with bed partners, playmates, shared head gear
Scabies	*Sarcoptes scabiei*; penetration of stratum corneum; depositing of eggs; allergic reaction resulting from presence of eggs, feces, mite parts; transmission by direct physical contact, only occasionally by shared personal items	Severe itching, especially at night, usually not on face; presence of burrows, especially in interdigital webs, flexor surface of wrists, and anterior axillary folds; redness, swelling, vesiculation	10% crotamiton, γ-benzene hexachloride, benzyl benzoate 12-25%; complete eradication possible; recurrence possible; treatment of sexual partner in positively diagnosed scabies; antibiotics if dermatitis and secondary infections present
Ticks	*Borrelia burgdorferi* (spirochete transmitted by ticks in certain areas) causes Lyme disease; endemic areas that include Northeast, Mid-Atlantic states, parts of Midwest and West (see Chapter 63)	Spreading, ringlike rash 3-4 wk after bite; commonly in groin, buttocks, axillae, trunk, and upper arms and legs; warm, itchy, or painful rash; flulike symptoms; cardiac, arthritic, and neurologic manifestations possible; unreliable laboratory test; no acquired immunity	Oral antibiotics, such as doxycycline, tetracycline; intravenous antibiotics for arthritic, neurologic, and cardiac symptoms; rest and healthy diet; most patients recover

ALLERGIC DERMATOLOGIC PROBLEMS

Dermatologic problems associated with allergies and hypersensitivity reactions may present a challenge to the clinician (Table 23-10). The pathophysiology related to allergic and contact dermatitis is discussed in Chapter 13. A careful family history and discussion of exposure to possible offending agents provide valuable data. Patch testing involves the application of allergens to the patient's skin (usually on the back) for 48 hours, after which the test sites are examined for erythema, papules, vesicles, or all of these. Patch testing is used to determine possible causative agents. The best treatment of allergic dermatitis is avoidance of the causative agent. The extreme pruritus of contact dermatitis and its potential for chronicity make it a frustrating problem for the patient, nurse, and dermatologist.

GENERAL MEASURES TO TREAT ACUTE DERMATOLOGIC PROBLEMS

Diagnostic Studies

A careful history is of prime importance in the diagnosis of skin problems. The clinician must be skilled at detecting any evidence that could lead to the cause of the extraordinary number of skin problems. After a careful history and physical examination, individual lesions are inspected. On the basis of the history, physical examination, and appropriate diagnostic tests, either medical, surgical, or combination therapy is planned.

Collaborative Care

Many different treatment methods are used in dermatology. Advances in this field have brought relief to many previously chronic, untreatable conditions. Many of the specific therapeutic treatments require specialized equipment and are usually reserved for use by the dermatologist. Drug therapy is prescribed by many clinicians. The effectiveness of this therapy can often be related to the base (or vehicle) in which the medication is prepared. Table 23-11 summarizes the common agents used as bases for topical preparations and their therapeutic considerations.

Phototherapy. Two types of ultraviolet light (UVL), or a combination of the two types (UVA, UVB), are used to treat many dermatologic conditions. Ultraviolet wavelengths cause erythema, desquamation, and pigmentation and may cause a temporary suppression of basal cell mitosis followed by a rebound increase in cell turnover.

Psoralen plus UVA light (PUVA) is a form of phototherapy. The photosensitizing drug psoralen is given to patients 90 minutes before exposure to UVA to enhance the effect of UVL in the UVA spectrum. Usually a moisturizing agent or a tar preparation is applied to the affected area in a thin layer before exposure to UVB. Conditions that are responsive to effective wavelengths with or without drugs include atopic dermatitis, cutaneous T cell lymphoma, pruritus, psoriasis, and vitiligo.

UVL in the specific wavelengths can be produced artificially. Therapeutic doses of UVA and UVB can be measured and used to treat spectrum-specific diseases (Fig. 23-9). Frequent skin

---

TABLE 23-10 **Common Allergic Conditions of the Skin**		
ETIOLOGY AND PATHOPHYSIOLOGY	**CLINICAL MANIFESTATIONS**	**TREATMENT AND PROGNOSIS**
Contact Dermatitis Manifestation of delayed hypersensitivity, absorbed agent acting as antigen, sensitization after several exposures, appearance of lesions 2-7 days after contact with allergen	Red, hivelike papules and plaques; sharply circumscribed with occasional vesicles; exposed areas more common; usually pruritic; relation of area of dermatitis to causative agent (e.g., metal allergy and dermatitis on ring finger)	Topical corticosteroids, antihistamines; skin lubrication; elimination of contact allergen; avoidance of irritating affected area; systemic corticosteroids if sensitivity severe
Urticaria Usually allergic phenomena; presence of edema in upper dermis resulting from a local increase in permeability of capillaries, usually from histamine	Spontaneously occurring and rounded elevations, varying size, usually multiple	Removal of source, if known; antihistamine therapy; cool compresses
Drug Reaction Any drug that acts as antigen and causes hypersensitivity reaction is possible cause, certain drugs more prone to reactions (e.g., penicillin) mediated by circulating antibodies	Rash of any morphology; often red, macular and papular, semiconfluent, generalized rash with abrupt onset; appearance as late as 14 days after cessation of drug; possibly pruritic	Withdrawal of drug if possible; antihistamines, local or systemic corticosteroids possibly necessary
Atopic Dermatitis Exact cause unknown, often beginning in infancy and decreasing in incidence with age, association with allergic conditions, elevation of IgE levels common, genetically determined, often family history; decreased itch threshold, stress, and increased water contact (e.g., frequent hand washing) possible contributing factors	Scaly, red to red-brown, circumscribed lesions; accentuation of skin markings; pruritic; symmetric eruptions common in antecubital and popliteal space in adults	Topical corticosteroids, phototherapy, coal tar therapy, intralesional corticosteroids, lubrication of dry skin, systemic corticosteroids if severe, reduction of stress, antibiotics for secondary infection

IgE, Immunoglobin E.

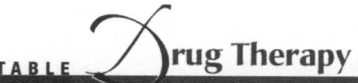

AGENT	THERAPEUTIC CONSIDERATIONS
Powder	Promotion of dryness, increase in evaporation, absorbing of moisture possible, common base for antifungal preparations
Lotion	Suspension of insoluble powders in water; cooling and drying, with residual powder film after evaporation of water; useful in subacute pruritic eruptions
Cream	Emulsions of oil and water, most common base for topical medications, lubrication, and protection
Ointment	Oil with differing amounts of water added in suspension, lubrication and prevention of dehydration, petrolatum most common
Paste	Mixture of powder and ointment, used when drying effect necessary because moisture is absorbed

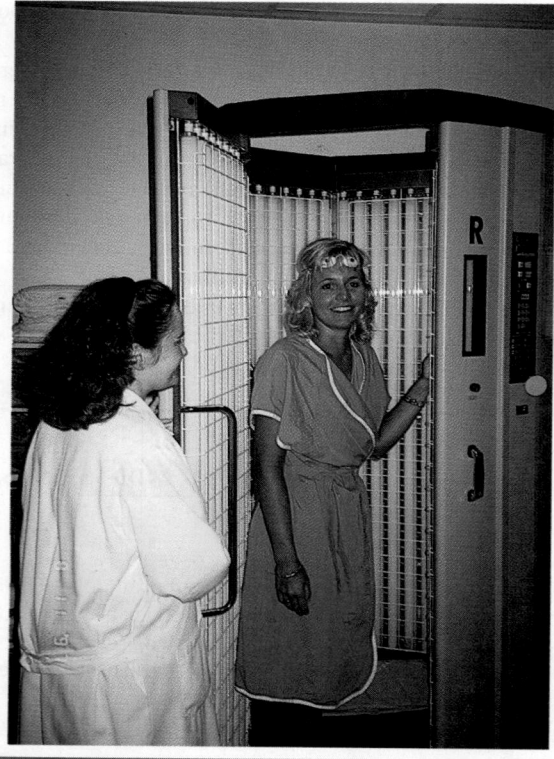

FIG. 23-9 Phototherapy is a method for treating spectrum-specific diseases. The patient's eyes must be protected during the phototherapy session. PUVA unit is illustrated in photo.

assessments must be performed on all patients receiving phototherapy. Inappropriate exposure to UVL can result in basal or squamous cell carcinoma, as well as severe erythema or burn to the skin. Patients should be cautioned about the potential hazards of using photosensitizing chemicals and further exposure to UV rays from sunlight or artificial UVL during the course of phototherapy. Protective eyewear that blocks 100% of UVL is prescribed for patients receiving PUVA, because psoralen is absorbed by the lens of the eye. The eyewear is used to prevent cataract formation. Patients are instructed to use the eyewear for 24 hours after taking the medication when outdoors or near a bright window because UVA penetrates glass. The immunosuppressive effects related to the use of PUVA require careful ongoing monitoring of these patients.

Radiation Therapy. The use of radiation for the treatment of cutaneous malignancies varies greatly according to local practice and availability. Even if radiation therapy is planned, a biopsy must first be performed to obtain a pathologic diagnosis.

Radiation to malignant cutaneous lesions is a painless treatment that is similar in cost to surgery. It produces minimal damage to surrounding tissue. It is a particularly effective treatment for the older adult or debilitated patient who cannot tolerate even a minor surgical procedure and for such areas as the nose, eyelids, and canthal areas, where preservation of the surrounding tissue is of prime consideration. Careful shielding is necessary to prevent ocular lens damage if the irradiated area is around the eyes.

Radiation therapy usually requires multiple visits to a radiology department. It is most effective on lesions above the neck. However, it produces permanent hair loss (*alopecia*) of the irradiated areas. Other adverse effects include telangiectasia, atrophy, hyperpigmentation, depigmentation, ulceration, chronic radiodermatitis, basal cell carcinoma, and squamous cell carcinoma. (Radiation therapy is discussed in Chapter 15.)

Total-body skin irradiation (body is bombarded with high-energy electrons) may be the treatment of choice or adjunctive therapy for cutaneous T cell lymphoma. Treatment follows a lengthy course. Patients experience varying degrees of hair loss and radiation dermatitis with transient loss of sweat gland function. This treatment causes premature aging of the skin.

Laser Technology. Laser treatment is expanding rapidly as an efficient surgical tool for many types of dermatologic problems. Lasers are able to produce measurable, repeatable, consistent zones of tissue damage. They can cut, coagulate, and vaporize tissue to some degree. The wavelength determines the type of delivery system used and the intensity of the energy delivered.

The surgical use of laser energy requires a focusing device to produce a small, high-density spot of energy that can be carefully focused on the surgical site and controllably directed to the operative site. Written policies and procedures should cover laser safety and be reviewed by all personnel working with laser equipment. Laser light does not accumulate in body cells and cannot cause cumulative cellular changes or damage.

Several types of lasers are available in most offices and hospitals. The CO_2 laser is the most common treatment. This laser has numerous applications as a vaporizing and cutting tool for most tissues. The argon laser emits light that is primarily absorbed by hemoglobin and helps in the treatment of vascular and other pigmented lesions. Other, less common lasers include the use of copper and gold vapors, tunable dye, and neodymium:

yttrium-aluminum-garnet (Nd:YAG). Dermatologic uses of the various lasers include coagulation of vascular lesions, skin resurfacing, removal of birthmarks, and the treatment of basal cell carcinoma, condylomas, plantar warts, and keloids.

Drug Therapy

Antibiotics. Antibiotics are used both topically and systemically to treat dermatologic problems, and they are often used in combination. If used, topical antibiotics should be applied to clean skin lightly. Common OTC topical antibiotics include bacitracin and polymyxin B. Prescription topical antibiotics include mupirocin (used for *Staphylococcus*), gentamicin (used for *Staphylococcus* and most gram-negative organisms), and erythromycin (used for gram-positive cocci [staphylococci and streptococci] and gram-negative cocci and bacilli). Topical erythromycin and clindamycin (Cleocin) (solutions or gels) are used in the treatment of acne vulgaris. Many of the more popular systemic antibiotics are not used topically because of the danger of allergic contact dermatitis.

If there are signs of systemic infection, a systemic antibiotic should be used. Systemic antibiotics are useful in the treatment of bacterial infections and acne vulgaris. The most frequently used are synthetic penicillin, erythromycin, and tetracycline. These drugs are particularly useful for erysipelas, cellulitis, carbuncles, and severe, infected eczema. Culture and sensitivity of the lesion can guide the choice of antibiotic. Patients require drug-specific instructions on the proper technique of taking or applying antibiotics. For instance, oral tetracycline must be taken on an empty stomach and should never be taken with a dairy product, which would interfere with absorption.

Corticosteroids. Corticosteroids are particularly effective in treating a wide variety of dermatologic conditions and can be used topically, intralesionally, or systemically. Topical corticosteroids are used for their local antiinflammatory action, as well as for their antipruritic effects.[17] Attempts to diagnose a lesion should be made before a corticosteroid preparation is applied, because corticosteroids will mask the clinical manifestations. Once a sufficient amount of medication is dispensed, limits should be set on the duration and frequency of application. The potency of a particular preparation is related to the concentration of active drug in the preparation. With prolonged use, the more potent corticosteroid formulations can cause adrenal suppression, especially if occlusive dressings are used. High-potency corticosteroids may produce side effects when their use is prolonged, including atrophy of the skin resulting from impaired cell mitosis and capillary fragility and susceptibility to bruising. In general, dermal and epidermal atrophy does not occur until a corticosteroid has been used for 2 to 3 weeks. If drug use is discontinued at the first sign of atrophy, recovery usually occurs in several weeks. Rosacea eruptions, severe exacerbations of acne vulgaris, and dermatophyte infections may also occur. Rebound dermatitis is not uncommon when therapy is stopped, and this can be reduced by tapering the use of high-potency topical corticosteroids when patient improvement is noted.

Low-potency corticosteroids such as hydrocortisone act more slowly but can be used for a longer period of time without producing serious side effects. Low-potency corticosteroids are safe to use on the face and intertriginous (opposing skin surfaces) areas, such as the axillae. The potency of a particular preparation is related to the concentration of active drug in the preparation. The ointment form represents the most efficient delivery system.

Creams and ointments should be applied in thin layers and slowly massaged into the site one to three times a day as prescribed. Accurate and adequate topical therapy is often the key to a successful outcome.

Intralesional corticosteroids are injected directly into or just beneath the lesion. This method provides a reservoir of medication with an effect lasting several weeks to months. Intralesional injection is commonly used in the treatment of psoriasis, *alopecia areata* (patchy hair loss), cystic acne, hypertrophic scars, and keloids. Triamcinolone acetonide (Kenalog) is the most common drug used for intralesional injection.

Systemic corticosteroids can have remarkable results in the treatment of dermatologic conditions. However, they often have undesirable systemic effects (see Chapter 48). Corticosteroids can be administered as short-term therapy for acute conditions such as contact dermatitis caused by poison ivy. Long-term corticosteroid therapy for dermatologic conditions is reserved for chronic bullous diseases, for severe systemic effects of collagen and immunologic responses, and as a last resort when other therapies have failed.

Antihistamines. Oral antihistamines are used to treat conditions that exhibit urticaria; angioedema; pruritus associated with many dermatologic problems such as atopic dermatitis, psoriasis, and contact dermatitis; and other allergic cutaneous reactions. Antihistamines compete with histamine for the receptor site, thus preventing its effect. Antihistamines may have anticholinergic and/or sedative effects. Several different antihistamines may have to be tried before the satisfactory therapeutic effect is achieved. Sedating antihistamines are often preferred, because the tranquilizing and sedative effects offer symptomatic relief. The patient should be warned about sedative effects, a particular problem when driving or operating heavy machinery. A newer generation of antihistamines such as loratidine (Claritin) and fexofenadine (Allegra) bind to peripheral histamine receptors, providing antihistamine action without sedation. Antihistamines should be used with particular caution in older adults because of their long half-life and their anticholinergic effects.

Topical fluorouracil. Fluorouracil (5-FU) is a topical cytotoxic agent with selective toxicity for sun-damaged cells. 5-FU is available in three strengths (1%, 2%, and 5%) and is used for the treatment of premalignant skin disease, especially actinic keratosis. Because systemic absorption of the drug is minimal, systemic side effects are virtually nonexistent. When a diagnosis of skin cancer has been established, 5-FU is generally not used.

Patient compliance is the major problem with the use of 5-FU. The medication produces painful, eroded areas over the damaged skin within 4 days. Treatment must continue with applications one to two times a day for 2 to 4 weeks. Healing may take up to 3 weeks after medication is stopped. Because 5-FU is a photosensitizing drug, the patient must be instructed to avoid sunlight during treatment. Patients should be educated about the effect of the medication and should be warned that they will look worse before they look better. After effective treatment, treated skin is smooth and free of actinic keratoses, although sometimes a second course is necessary due to recurrence.

Diagnostic and Surgical Therapy

Skin Scraping. Scraping is done with a scalpel blade to obtain a sample of surface cells for microscopic inspection and diagnosis.

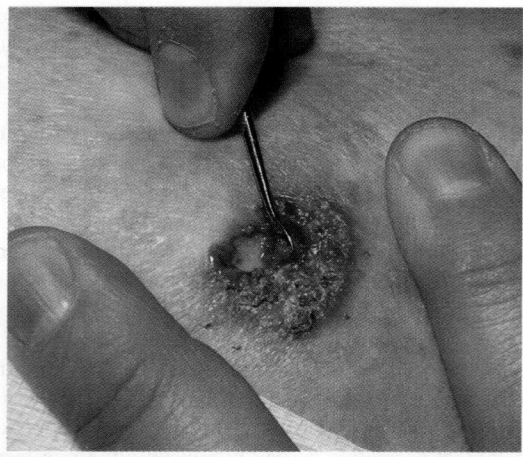

FIG. 23-10 Curettage of an inflamed seborrheic keratosis.

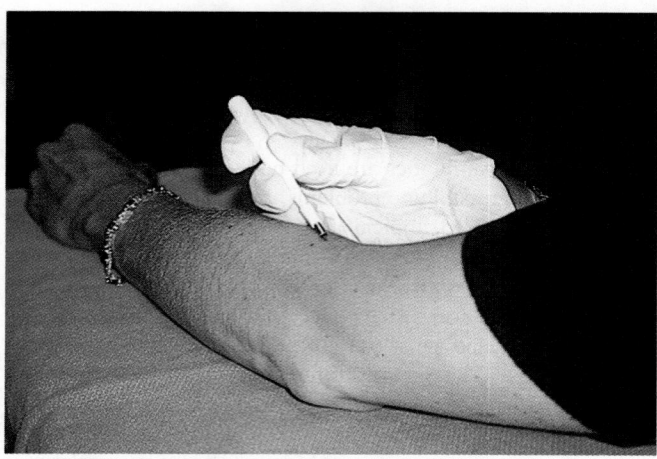

FIG. 23-11 Punch biopsy used to obtain tissue sample.

Electrodesiccation and Electrocoagulation. Electrical energy can be converted to heat by the tip of an electrode. This results in tissue being destroyed by burning. The major uses of this type of therapy are point coagulation of bleeding vessels to obtain hemostasis and destruction of small telangiectasias. *Electrodesiccation* usually involves more superficial destruction, and a monopolar electrode is used. *Electrocoagulation* has a deeper effect, with better hemostasis and an increased possibility of scarring. A dipolar electrode is used for electrocoagulation.

Curettage. **Curettage** is the removal of tissue using an instrument with a circular cutting edge attached to a handle (Fig. 23-10). The tissue is scooped away. Although the curette is not usually strong enough to cut normal skin, it is useful for removing many types of small skin tumors, such as warts, seborrheic keratoses, and small basal and squamous cell cancers. The area to be curetted is anesthetized before the procedure. Hemostasis is obtained by use of one of several methods: electrocoagulation, ferric subsulfate (Monsel's solution), gelatin foam, aluminum chloride, or a gauze pressure dressing. A small scar may form. The specimen may be sent for biopsy.

Punch Biopsy. Punch biopsy is a common dermatologic procedure used to obtain a tissue sample for histologic study or to remove small lesions (Fig. 23-11). Its use is generally reserved for lesions smaller than 0.5 cm. Before local anesthesia is used, the biopsy area is outlined so that landmarks will not be obscured by the anesthetizing agent. The biopsy punch cores out a small cylinder of skin when its sharp edge is twirled between the fingers. The core of skin is snipped from the subcutaneous fat and appropriately preserved for examination. Hemostasis is achieved by using methods as with curettage, but sites of 3 mm or larger are often closed with sutures. Other types of biopsies are discussed in Table 22-10 and Chapter 22.

Cryosurgery. **Cryosurgery** is the use of subfreezing temperatures to perform surgery. Cryosurgery is a useful treatment for common and genital warts, cutaneous tags, seborrheic keratoses, actinic keratoses, and many other less common skin conditions. Topical liquid nitrogen is the agent most commonly used for cryosurgery. Although the exact mechanism is not clearly un-

derstood, the use of liquid nitrogen causes death or destruction of the treated skin.

Liquid nitrogen can be applied topically (directly onto the benign or precancerous lesion) with a cotton swab or with the appropriate container (Cry-AC) for several freeze-and-thaw cycles. Patients are informed that they will feel a cold sensation. The lesion will first become swollen and red, and it may blister. Next, a scab will form and fall off in 1 to 3 weeks. The skin lesion will be sloughed along with the scab. Growth of new skin follows.

Cryosurgery is inexpensive, rapid, and leaves minimal scarring. The major disadvantages of this treatment are lack of a tissue specimen and potential for destruction of adjacent healthy tissue.

Excision. Excision should be considered if the lesion involves the dermis. Complete closure of the excised area usually results in a good cosmetic result.

A specific type of excision is the *Mohs' micrographic surgery,* which is a microscopically controlled removal of a cutaneous malignancy.[18] This procedure sections the surgical specimen horizontally, so that 100% of the surgical margin can be examined. Tissue is removed in thin layers, and all margins of the specimen are mapped to determine whether tumor remains. Any residual tumor not removed by the first surgical excision can be removed in serial excisions performed the same day. The benefit of this treatment is preservation of normal tissue, producing the smallest possible wound. The procedure is done on an outpatient basis with the patient receiving a local anesthetic.

NURSING MANAGEMENT
DERMATOLOGIC PROBLEMS

■ Ambulatory and Home Care

Dermatologic conditions are not common reasons for hospitalization. Although it may not be the primary reason for hospitalization, many hospitalized patients will exhibit concurrent skin problems that warrant nursing intervention and patient education.

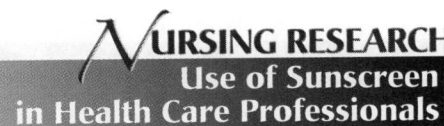

NURSING RESEARCH
Use of Sunscreen in Health Care Professionals

Citation

Grubbs L, Tabano L: Use of sunscreen in health care professionals: the health belief model, *Cancer Nurs* 23:164, 2000.

Purpose

To explore the relationship among health care providers' perceived susceptibility, actual risk of skin cancer, and use of sunscreen.

Methods

A descriptive design used a convenience sample of 90 health care providers in the southeastern United States. The sample included nurses, physicians, and pharmacists. Subjects completed two questionnaires related to skin cancer risk assessment and perceived susceptibility to skin cancer. Four percent of the sample had a personal and/or family history of skin cancer.

Results and Conclusions

Participants at actual low risk or high risk reported appropriate perceived susceptibility scores. However, those with an average risk of getting skin cancer perceived their risk as low. The relationship between use of sunscreen and perceived susceptibility was not significant. Older subjects were found to have a higher level of perceived susceptibility to skin cancer. Persons at high risk reported using sunscreen 75% of the time.

Implications for Nursing Practice

Health care providers have the ability to teach persons to use sunscreen with all sun exposure activities. An accurate perception of the providers' own susceptibility to skin cancer is important in influencing good sunscreen behavior. Skin cancer susceptibility and prevention education targeting young adults, who may be more unaware of safe sun exposure than older persons, is especially important.

If the patient is in an acute care setting, the nurse will both administer and teach the appropriate treatments. If the patient is in an outpatient setting, the nursing focus is on patient teaching, with opportunities provided for demonstration and repeated demonstration. Subsequent visits provide the opportunity to evaluate patient understanding and treatment effectiveness.

Nursing interventions related to dermatologic conditions fall into broad categories. They are applicable to many skin problems in both inpatient and outpatient settings. The nursing care for a patient with chronic skin lesions is presented in NCP 23-1.

Wet Dressings. Wet dressings are commonly used when the skin is weepy from infection and/or inflammation. The best drying agent for this type of skin condition is water. These dressings are also used to relieve itching, suppress inflammation, and debride a wound. In addition, wet dressings increase penetration of topical medications, promote sleep by relieving discomfort, and enhance removal of scales, crusts, and exudate. Such materials as thin sheeting, gauze sponges, thermal underwear, or tube socks can be used for dressings. Ingenuity is sometimes required when odd-shaped parts of the body must be covered.

The prescribed dressing is put into fresh solution, squeezed until it is no longer dripping, and then applied to the affected area, avoiding normal skin tissue. The dressing should be left in place 10 to 30 minutes. This treatment is generally done two to four times a day. If the skin appears macerated (softened), the dressings should be discontinued for 2 to 3 hours. The patient should be protected from discomfort and chilling by using linens and bedclothes with pads or plastic.

Wet dressings do not need to be sterile. They should be cool when an antiinflammatory effect is desired and tepid when the purpose is to debride an infected, crusted lesion. These treatments are excellent ways to remove the scabs left by the collection of debris at a wound site.

Tap water at room temperature is the most common solution where water quality is adequate. Filtered or sterile water may be indicated in some locations. Potassium permanganate must be completely dissolved before use, because the crystals that do not dissolve may burn the skin. This solution must be freshly prepared to maintain its oxidative properties. If potassium permanganate solution turns brown, it should be discarded and fresh solution made. Boric acid is not recommended as a wet dressing solution because of potential systemic toxicity as a result of percutaneous absorption, especially on open skin.

Baths. Baths are appropriate when large body areas need to be treated. They also have sedative and antipruritic effects. Some medications, such as oilated oatmeal (Aveeno), potassium permanganate, and sodium bicarbonate, can be added directly to the bath water. One cup of the mixture can be added to 2 cups of water and then added to the bath water. The tub should be full enough to cover affected areas. Both the bath water and the prescribed solution should be at a temperature that is comfortable for the patient. The patient can soak for 15 to 20 minutes three to four times a day, depending on the severity of the dermatitis and the patient's discomfort. It is important to stress to the patient that the skin not be rubbed dry with a towel but gently patted to prevent increasing irritation and inflammation. The addition of oils makes the bathtub extremely slippery and should be avoided. If oils are used in the tub, the utmost caution must be used in transferring patients to prevent accidents. To sustain the hydrating effect, sealing moisturizers or medications should be applied to the skin directly after the bath. This helps retain the moisture in the hydrated cells.

Topical Medications. A thin layer of ointment, cream, or lotion should be applied to clean skin and spread evenly in a downward motion. An alternative method is to apply the medication directly onto the dressings. Pastes are designed to protect the affected area. They should be applied thickly with a tongue blade or a gloved hand. Draining lesions and lesions with greasy medication can be covered with a light dressing to prevent soiling clothes. Patients need specific directions on proper application technique of prescribed topical medications.

Control of Pruritus. **Pruritus** (itching) can be caused by almost any physical or chemical stimulus to the skin, such as drugs, insects, and dry skin. The itch sensation is carried by the same nonmyelinated nerve fibers as pain. If the epidermis is damaged or absent, the sensation will be felt as pain rather than an itch.

NURSING CARE PLAN 23-1

Patient with Chronic Skin Lesions

EXPECTED PATIENT OUTCOMES	NURSING INTERVENTIONS and *RATIONALES*
NURSING DIAGNOSIS	**Risk for infection** *related to* open lesion, presence of environmental pathogens.
• No evidence of secondary infection such as redness, edema, or exudate	• Monitor for open draining lesions; redness, swelling, and pain at lesion sites; lymphadenopathy and fever; indications of scratching *to detect presence of infection.* • Practice and teach careful hand washing and bathing. Use proper disposal of dressings and contaminated linens *to prevent secondary infections.* • Keep patient's nails trimmed short *to prevent skin excoriation from scratching.*
NURSING DIAGNOSIS	**Impaired skin integrity** *related to* scratching, dehydration, frequent wetting and drying of skin, dryness from treatment medications *as manifested by* destruction of skin layers.
• Moist, well-lubricated, intact skin	• Decrease environmental irritants (e.g., heat, scratchy coverings) *to reduce vasodilation and sensory stimulation.* • Provide adequate fluid intake (2000 to 3000 ml/day) *to maintain normal hydration status.* • Avoid frequent wetting and drying of skin without proper use of topical lubricants. • Encourage use of superfatted soap *to prevent drying of skin and encourage moisture retention.* • Apply skin lotion/cream/ointments immediately after bathing *to trap moisture and reduce water loss.* • Provide diversional activities *to distract patient from discomfort or pruritus.*
NURSING DIAGNOSIS	**Situational low self-esteem** *related to* presence of unsightly lesions *as manifested by* verbalization of self-disgust and despair over appearance of lesions, isolation, reluctance to look at lesions or participate in self-care.
• Realistic hope for resolution of open lesions • Maintenance of normal social relationships	• Discuss situation with patient in open, accepting manner *to assist patient to express feelings.* • Do not show shock or disgust at the sight of lesions *to prevent further decrease in self-esteem.* • Provide counseling, if indicated, *to assist patient in accepting situation.*
NURSING DIAGNOSIS	**Ineffective health maintenance** *related to* lack of knowledge of disease process, management plan, prevention of scarring, and use of over-the-counter (OTC) medications *as manifested by* questions about self-care.
• Confidence in ability to care for self and explore surgical options • Understanding of disease process and management plan	• Answer questions completely *to foster knowledge base of pertinent issues.* • Teach patient about disease process, management plan, care of lesions *to foster independence and boost confidence in ability to manage self-care.* • Discuss possible cosmetic surgery options *so patient can make informed decisions.* • Advise patient to carefully follow guidelines for OTC medications *to prevent misuse or worsening of condition.*
NURSING DIAGNOSIS	**Social isolation** *related to* decreased activities secondary to poor self-image, fear of rejection, and lack of knowledge related to cover-up techniques *as manifested by* lack of social activities, verbalization of dissatisfaction with social life.
• Satisfaction with social life	• Encourage socialization in patient's interest areas *to reduce sense of isolation and worthlessness.* • Teach skillful use of cosmetics, cover-up agents, and clothing *to maximize personal appearance and encourage socialization.*

The itch-scratch cycle must be broken to prevent excoriation. Control of pruritus is also important because it is difficult to diagnose a lesion that is excoriated and inflamed. Certain circumstances make itching worse. Anything that causes vasodilation, such as heat or rubbing, should be avoided. Dryness of the skin lowers the itch threshold and increases the itch sensation.

Lichenification is a thickening of skin as a result of the proliferation of keratinocytes with accentuation of the normal markings of the skin. Lichenification is caused by scratching or rubbing of the skin and is often associated with atopic dermatoses and pruritic conditions. Although any area of the body may be af-

fected, the hands and forearms are common sites. Treatment of the cause of the itching is the key to prevention of lichenification. Excoriations are often evident in the thickened skin as a result of the pruritus.

The nurse can use or teach the patient various methods to break the itch cycle. A cool environment may cause vasoconstriction and decrease itching. The use of topical corticosteroids reduces inflammation and promotes vasoconstriction, but should be reserved for use with appropriate dermatologic problems. Menthol, camphor, or phenol can be used to numb the itch receptors. Systemic antihistamines can be used if necessary to provide relief to a patient while the underlying cause of the pruritus is diagnosed and treated. The principle side effect of most antihistamines is sedation. This may, in fact, be desirable, because pruritus is often worse at night and interferes with sleep.

Wet dressings can be used effectively to relieve pruritus. Thin, cotton sheets or thermal underwear is placed in warm water, wrung out, and placed over the pruritic area. After 10 to 15 minutes the dressing is removed and the skin is patted dry and a lubricant or medication applied. This procedure can be repeated as necessary for comfort.

Prevention of Spread. Although most skin problems are not contagious, infection precautions indicate the need for gloves with open or bleeding wounds. Procedures should be explained to the patient in order to avoid demoralizing an already sensitive patient. However, if in doubt, the nurse should wear gloves until a definite diagnosis has been established. The most common contagious lesions that the nurse should be cautious with include impetigo, staphylococcus, pyoderma, primary chancre and secondary syphilis lesions, scabies, and pediculosis. Careful hand washing and safe disposal of soiled dressings are the best means of preventing spread of skin problems.

Prevention of Secondary Infections. Open lesions on the skin are susceptible to invasion by other viral, bacterial, or fungal organisms. Meticulous hygiene, hand washing, and dressing changes are important to prevent secondary infections. Also, the patient should be warned about scratching lesions, which can cause excoriations and create a portal of entry for pathogens. The patient's nails should be trimmed short to minimize trauma from scratching.

Specific Skin Care. Nurses are often in a position to advise patients regarding care of the skin following simple dermatologic surgical procedures, such as skin biopsy, excision, and cryosurgery. Patient follow-up should be individualized. In general, instructions include dressing changes, use of topical antibiotics, and the signs and symptoms of infection. After a dermatologic procedure any oozing wound should be regularly cleansed with a saline solution. An antibiotic ointment may then be applied with a dressing that is both absorbent and nonadherent.

Wounds that are kept moist and covered heal more rapidly and with less scarring. Initially, a scab should be left alone to be a protective coating for the damaged skin beneath it. Scabs can be covered during the day for cosmetic purposes and should be protected at night from premature removal through rubbing against sheets. Scabs will separate naturally from healed epidermis.

A wound that required stitches can be covered with a variety of different dressings. Stitches will generally be removed in 4 to 10 days. Sometimes every other stitch is removed after the third day. Incision lines may require daily cleansing, usually with plain tap water. If necessary, a topical antibiotic is applied and the wound is either covered with a dry sterile dressing or left open to air. The patient may experience some swelling and discomfort in the first 24 hours. Mild analgesics such as acetaminophen should control the discomfort. The patient needs to know the manifestations of inflammation such as redness, fever, or increased pain or swelling and signs of infection, such as purulent drainage. If these manifestations occur, they should be reported to the health care provider.

Psychologic Effects of Chronic Dermatologic Problems. Emotional stress can occur for persons who suffer from chronic skin problems such as psoriasis, atopic dermatitis, or severe acne.

The sequelae of chronic skin problems could result in employment problems with subsequent financial implications, a poor self-image, problems with sexuality, and increasing and progressive frustration. The usual lack of systemic overt illness coupled with the visibility of the skin lesions often presents a real problem to the patient.

The nurse must continue to be optimistic and help the patient comply with the prescribed regimen. The patient must be allowed to verbalize the "Why me?" question, even though there is no ready answer. Reinforcement of the prescribed hygiene and treatment measures is an important part of the nursing management. Dermatology patient support groups are listed with the American Academy of Dermatology (*www.aad.org*). These groups are extremely useful for accurate patient support and education materials.

Many lesions can be camouflaged with the skillful use of cosmetics. Individual sensitivity to product ingredients must always be considered in the selection of a cosmetic product. Oil-free, hypoallergenic cosmetics are available and could be beneficial to the allergic patient. Rehabilitative cosmetics are available to help camouflage and deemphasize such lesions as *vitiligo* (loss of pigmentation), *melasma* (tan to brown patches on the face), or healed postoperative wound sites. These commercially available products are opaque, smudge resistant, and water resistant.

In addition to specific skin conditions that tend to chronicity, other factors affecting the outcome of long-term dermatologic problems include skin type, history of previous exacerbations, family history, complications, intolerance to therapy, environmental factors, lack of adherence to the prescribed regimen, endocrine factors, and psychologic factors. Lesions that follow a chronic pattern often are associated with lichenification and scarring.

Pathophysiologic Effects of Chronic Dermatologic Problems. Scarring and lichenification are the result of chronic dermatologic problems. Scars occur when ulceration takes place and reflect the pattern of healing in the area. Scars are pink and vascular at first. As they age they become avascular and white with increasing strength. Different parts of the body scar differently, such as the face and neck, which heal fairly well because of a good blood supply. Scar formation is described in Chapter 12.

The location of the scar is the determining factor with respect to its cosmetic implications. Facial scars are the most damaging psychologically, because they are so visible. Creative use of cosmetics can do much to mask the scarring of chronic skin conditions. The best treatment is prevention of scarring by control of the problem in the acute phase.

BENIGN DERMATOLOGIC PROBLEMS

Although the list of benign dermatoses is extensive, some of the most commonly seen and distressing problems are summarized in Table 23-12. Psoriasis is one common benign disorder that may occur with skin irritation or injury (Fig. 23-12).

DISEASES WITH DERMATOLOGIC MANIFESTATIONS

Dermatologic manifestations of various diseases are listed in Table 23-13. The health care provider should always consider the possibility that a particular dermatosis is a clue to an internal, less obvious problem.

TABLE 23-12 Common Benign Conditions of the Skin

ETIOLOGY AND PATHOPHYSIOLOGY	CLINICAL MANIFESTATIONS	TREATMENT AND PROGNOSIS
Acne		
Inflammatory disorder of sebaceous glands; more common in teenagers but possible development and persistence in adulthood; can occur related to menstrual cycle; secondary result of iodides, bromides, corticosteroids, androgen–dominant birth control pills	Noninflammatory lesions, including comedones (blackheads) and closed comedones (whiteheads); inflammatory lesions, including papules and pustules; most common on face, neck, and upper back	Mechanical removal of multiple lesions with comedo extractor after comedo opened with fine needle or blade; topical application of benzoyl peroxide as antibacterial and peeling agent; use of peeling and irritating agents such as retinoic acid; long-term antibiotic therapy—topical or systemic; phototherapy; aim of treatment to suppress new lesions; spontaneous remission possible; often improvement with exposure to sun. Use of isotretinoin (Accutane) for severe cystic acne to possibly provide lasting remission; contraindicated in pregnant women or women intending to become pregnant while on drug; monitoring of liver function and pregnancy tests, cholesterol, and triglycerides essential
Moles		
Grouping of normal cells derived from melanocyte–like precursor cells; hereditary predisposition possible	Hyperpigmented areas that vary in form and color; flat, slightly elevated, haloid, verrucoid, polypoid, dome-shaped, sessile, or papillomatous; preservation of normal skin markings; hair growth possible	No treatment necessary except for cosmetic reasons; skin biopsy for diagnosis
Psoriasis		
Chronic dermatitis, which involves excessively rapid turnover of epidermal cells; family predisposition	Sharply demarcated scaling plaques of the scalp, elbows, and knees; palms, soles, and fingernails possibly affected; localized or general, intermittent or continuous (see Fig. 23-12)	Aim of retarding growth of epidermal cells; difficult to medicate; usually topical corticosteroids, tar, anthralin; intralesional injection of corticosteroids for chronic plaques; sunlight; ultraviolet light, alone or with topical or systemic potentiation; alefacept (Amevive), an injectable medication, for plaque psoriasis; no cure; control possible; antimetabolites (especially methotrexate) or systemic retinoids for difficult cases
Seborrheic Keratoses		
Benign, genetically determined growths; found in increasing number with age; no association with sun exposure	Irregularly round or oval, flat-topped papules or plaques; surface often warty; appearance of being stuck on; increase in pigmentation with age of lesion; usually multiple and possibly itchy	Removal by curettage or cryosurgery for cosmetic reasons or to eliminate source of irritation; minimal scarring
Skin Tags		
Common after midlife; appearance on neck, axillae, and upper trunk	Small, skin-colored, soft, pedunculated papules	No treatment unless for cosmetic reasons or because of repeated trauma; surgical removal possible (if requested); usually just "clipping off" without anesthesia
Lipoma		
Benign tumor of adipose tissue, often encapsulated, most common in 40- to 60-year-old age group	Rubbery, compressible, round mass of adipose tissue; single or multiple; variable in size, possibly extremely large; most common on trunk, back of neck, and forearms	Usually no treatment, biopsy to differentiate from liposarcoma, excision usual treatment (when indicated)

TABLE 23-12   Common Benign Conditions of the Skin—cont'd

ETIOLOGY AND PATHOPHYSIOLOGY	CLINICAL MANIFESTATIONS	TREATMENT AND PROGNOSIS
Vitiligo Unknown cause; genetically influenced, most noticeable in dark-skinned persons and those with a tan; complete absence of melanocytes; noncontagious	Focal amelanosis (complete loss of pigment); macular; variation in size and location; usually symmetric and permanent	Attempts at repigmentation with exposure to UVA and psoralens; depigmentation of pigmented skin with extensive disease (>50% of body involved); cosmetics and stains for camouflage and to deemphasize vitiliginous areas
Lentigo Increased number of normal melanocytes in basal layer of epidermis; senile lentigos ("liver spots") related to aging and sun exposure	Hyperpigmented, brown to black, flat lesion; usually on sun-exposed areas	Treatment only for cosmetic purposes, liquid nitrogen; possible recurrence in 1-2 yr

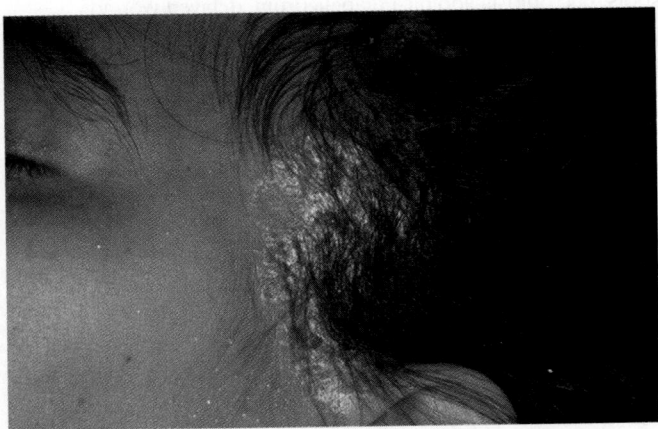

FIG. 23-12   Psoriasis on the scalp.

Certain life changes have recognized associated dermatoses. At puberty, male- or female-pattern hair growth will be evident as a secondary sex characteristic. Increased apocrine gland activity can lead to body odor. The increased sebaceous gland activity stimulated by androgens can result in seborrhea and acne.

PLASTIC SURGERY

Elective Cosmetic Surgery

The possible cosmetic changes that can be made surgically are almost limitless. Cosmetic surgery includes such techniques as breast enlargement; breast reduction; chemical, mechanical, and surgical face-lift; eyelid lift; hair transplant; nose corrections; removal of double chin; correction of receding or prominent chin; abdomen or thigh lift; buttocks reduction; correction of elephant ears; and liposuction of many body areas.

The reasons for the surgery are as varied as the techniques. The most common reason that people suffer the discomfort and financial expense (most are not covered by insurance) of cos-

metic surgery is to improve their body image. People project their personal image of themselves; if they feel better about themselves as a result of cosmetic surgery, they will often act more confident and self-assured. Often social position and economic considerations are part of the decision. Increased longevity provides a larger population to whom cosmetic surgery is especially appealing.

Regardless of the reason that the patient elects to have cosmetic surgery, the nurse should maintain a supportive, nonjudgmental attitude. If the patient wishes to change a body feature perceived as unattractive, it is a personal decision to undergo cosmetic surgery and the nurse should support this decision.

Chemical Face-Lift or Peel. A chemical face peel uses a cauterant to the skin to cause a controlled burn. This results in superficial destruction of the upper layers of the skin and a tightening of the deep layers. The most common indications for a chemical peel include pigmentation problems, skin damage as a result of radiation, freckles, superficial acne scarring, and actinic and seborrheic keratoses.

A solution (buffered phenol, trichloroacetic acid, or other exfoliation acids) is applied to the skin with care taken to avoid the eyes. Posttreatment care is prescribed specifically by the health care provider. It may include refraining from activities, talking, and chewing, and it may involve the application of compresses and topical ointments. There may be moderate swelling and crusting for 1 week. Within 7 to 8 days new skin appears, and healing is complete by 10 days. Redness will persist for 6 to 8 weeks. A pink tone will be apparent for several months. Once healing is complete, the skin will have a more youthful appearance because of a new superficial layer of skin.

Because there is a reduction of melanin as a result of this procedure, the patient must be instructed to absolutely avoid the sun for 6 months to prevent hyperpigmentation. Chemical peeling is accepted as a treatment for wrinkles and certain types of hyperpigmentation.

Topical Tretinoin. Topical application of tretinoin (Retin-A) provides some reversal of photodamaged skin and normal aging changes by influencing epithelial cell growth and differentiation.

TABLE 23-13 Diseases with Dermatologic Manifestations*

SYSTEMIC PROBLEM	DERMATOLOGIC MANIFESTATIONS
Endocrine	
Hyperthyroidism	Increased sweating, warm skin with persistent flush, thin nails, vitiligo and alopecia, fine, soft hair
Hypothyroidism	Cold, dry, pale to yellow skin; slightly hyperkeratotic epidermis with follicular plugging; generalized nonpitting edema; dry, coarse, brittle hair; brittle, slow-growing nails
Glucocorticoid excess (Cushing's syndrome), induced endogenously or exogenously	Atrophy; striae; epidermal thinning; telangiectasia; acne, decreased subcutaneous fat over extremities; thin, loose dermis; impaired wound healing; increased vascular fragility; mild hirsutism; excessive collection of fat over clavicles, back of neck, abdomen, and face; increased incidence of pyodermas (purulent bacterial dermatitis)
Addison's disease	Loss of body hair (especially axillary), generalized hyperpigmentation (especially in folds)
Androgen excess	Enlarged facial pores, male sex characteristics, acne, acceleration of coarse hair growth
Androgen deficiency–postpuberty	Development of sparse hair; marked reduction in sebum production
Hypoparathyroidism	Opaque, brittle nails with transverse ridges; coarse, sparse hair with patchy alopecia; eczematous and exfoliative dermatitis; hyperkeratotic and maculopapular eruptions
Hyperpituitarism (acromegaly)	Coarsened skin, deepened lines; increased oiliness and sweating; acne; increased number of nevi, hyperpigmentation; hypertrichosis (excess hair growth)
Hypopituitarism (Froëlich's syndrome)	Smooth skin; scant hair growth; obesity; small, thin fingernails
Diabetes mellitus	Increased xanthomas, shin spots, necrobiosis lipoidica diabeticorum, delayed wound healing
Gastrointestinal	
Ulcerative colitis, Crohn's disease	Pyoderma gangrenosum, mouth ulcers
Liver disease and biliary tract obstruction	Jaundice, itching, pigmentary abnormalities, alterations in nails and hair, spider angiomas, telangiectasia
Deficiency of essential fatty acids	Scaly skin
Malabsorption syndrome	Acquired ichthyosis (dry, scaly skin)
Cystic fibrosis	Abnormal sweat gland function resulting in failure to conserve sodium
Musculoskeletal and Connective Tissue	
Systemic lupus erythematosus	Maculopapular semiconfluent rash (butterfly rash)
Scleroderma	Leathery hardening and stiffness of skin
Dermatomyositis	Edema; purplish-red upper eyelids; butterfly rash; scaly, macular erythema over knuckles; linear telangiectasia of posterior nail fold
Metabolic	
Lipidoses	Xanthomas
Vitamin A deficiency	Generalized dry hyperkeratoses
Hypervitaminosis A	Hair loss, dry skin
Vitamin B_1 (thiamine) deficiency	Edema, redness of soles of feet
Vitamin B_2 (riboflavin) deficiency	Red fissures at corner of mouth, glossitis
Nicotinic acid (niacin) deficiency	Pellagra; redness of exposed areas of hand or foot; face or neck; infected dermatitis
Vitamin C deficiency	Petechiae, purpura, bleeding gums
Immune	
Drug sensitivity	Rash of any morphology
Serum sickness	Pruritus
Cancer of breast, stomach, lung, uterus, kidney, ovary, colon, bladder	Metastasis to skin
Hodgkin's disease	Pruritus and nonspecific erythemas
Lymphomas	Papules, nodules, plaques, pruritus
Cardiovascular	
Rheumatic heart disease	Petechiae, urticaria, rheumatoid nodules, erythema nodosum and multiforme
Periarteritis nodosa	Periarteritis nodules
Thromboangiitis obliterans (Buerger's disease)	Superficial migrating thrombophlebitis, pallor or cyanosis, gangrene, ulceration
Peripheral vascular disease	Loss of hair on hands and feet; delayed capillary filling; dependent rubor (redness)
Venous stasis ulcers	Leathery, brownish skin on lower leg; concave lesion with edema; scar tissue with healing

*Refer to the systemic disease for specific information.

TABLE 23-13   Diseases with Dermatologic Manifestations—cont'd

SYSTEM PROBLEM	DERMATOLOGIC MANIFESTATIONS
Respiratory	
Inadequate oxygenation secondary to respiratory disease	Cyanosis
Hematologic	
Anemia	Pallor, hyperpigmentation, pale mucous membranes, hair loss, nail dystrophy
Clotting disorders	Purpura, petechiae, ecchymosis
Renal	
Chronic kidney disease	Dry skin, pruritus, uremic frost, pallor, dry skin, bruises
Reproductive	
Primary syphilis	Chancre
Secondary syphilis	Generalized skin lesions
Late benign syphilis	Gummas
Paget's disease	Eczematous patch of nipple and areola
Neurologic	
Syringomyelia Chronic sensory polyneuropathies Spinal cord trauma	Trophic changes in skin resulting from sensory denervation, pressure ulcers, anesthesia, paresthesias

Fine and coarse wrinkling improves. There is a reduction in the number of *lentigines* (age spots) and in the color of freckles.[19] Actinic keratoses decrease in number. Deep wrinkles and expression lines are usually not affected by tretinoin. The main adverse effect is a cutaneous reaction characterized by erythema, swelling, and scaling, which generally improves when treated with emollients or when the frequency of tretinoin application is decreased to every other day or stopped altogether.

The response to tretinoin appears to be dose related. The usual dose is 0.025%, 0.05%, or 0.1% in a cream or gel base. Gradual introduction to tretinoin begins with application every other day, aiming for nightly application as tolerated. Treatment is not usually stopped when inflammation occurs unless the inflammation is severe. Maximum response occurs after 8 to 12 months of treatment. Thereafter application three to four times a week should maintain improvement. A sunscreen must be used in combination with tretinoin to prevent further sun damage and to protect against the greater photosensitivity that patients experience during tretinoin therapy.

α-Hydroxy Acids. Topical α-hydroxy acids are being used for similar indications as topical tretinoin. α-Hydroxy acids do not have many of the side effects associated with other peel products. On application, minimal stinging and redness may occur in some individuals.[20]

Dermabrasion. Dermabrasion is the removal of the epidermis and a portion of the superficial layer of the dermis with preservation of sufficient epidermal adnexa to allow for spontaneous reepithelialization of the abraded surface. Dermabrasion is used to treat acne scars, hypertrophic scars, and sun-damaged and wrinkled skin, and it is also used to correct pigmentary abnormalities, usually on the face.

In general, the instructions to patients who have dermabrasion are focused on prevention of drying. Emollients or antibiotic ointments and wet soaks are included in the instructions and are to be applied at varying times on particular postoperative days. Patients are instructed to use a heavy layer of emollient when not using wet soaks. Instructions for postoperative wound care vary widely among practitioners. Specific care should be well understood by the patient. Sunscreens (SPF 30) should be used if the patient is outdoors. The most common complications include hyperpigmentation, hypopigmentation, keloids, herpes simplex, milia, persistent erythema, telangiectasia, and infection.

Botulinum Toxin Injections. Botulinum toxin type A (BTX), a neurotoxin produced by *Clostridium botulinum,* temporarily interferes with neuromuscular transmission thereby paralyzing the affected muscle. Only the A serotype (Botox, Allergan, Irvine, Calif.) has been approved for clinical use in the United States.[21] Injections of BTX can be used safely and effectively for a variety of patient conditions, including migraine headaches; excess sweating of the axillae, palms, and soles; and strabismus. One currently popular use of BTX is to decrease wrinkles by paralyzing the small muscles involved in repetitive facial expressions. Treatment will not cause botulism because of the small dosages used. When used cosmetically, the mild and transitory side effects can include redness, pain, swelling, headaches, and double vision lasting for 1 to 2 weeks.[22] Injections can be expensive and must be repeated every 3 to 6 months to prevent the wrinkles from recurring.

Face-Lift. A face-lift *(rhytidectomy)* is the lifting and repositioning of the lower two thirds of the face and neck to improve appearance (Fig. 23-13). Indications for this procedure include the following:

1. Redundant soft tissue resulting from disease (e.g., acne scarring)
2. Asymmetric redundancy of soft tissues (e.g., facial palsy)
3. Redundant soft tissue resulting from trauma

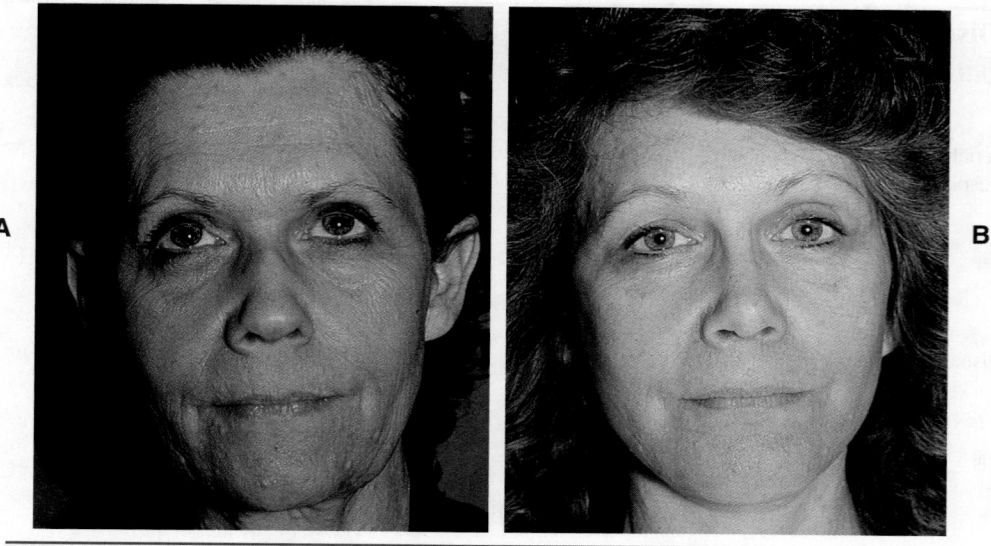

FIG. 23-13 Face-lift. **A,** Preoperative. **B,** Postoperative.

4. Preauricular lesions
5. Redundant soft tissues resulting from solar *elastosis* (sagging of the skin as a result of sun damage), changes in body weight, and the effects of gravity
6. Restoration of body image

The surgical approach and lines of incisions vary according to the nature of the deformity and the position of the hairline. Prevention of hematoma formation is the most important postoperative consideration. A pressure dressing is usually used the first 24 to 48 hours to reduce the possibility of hematoma formation. Complications can occur if the person smokes or is involved in vigorous exercise. Once the dressing is removed, there is little pain. The sutures are removed sometime from the fifth to the tenth postoperative day. Antibiotics are used at the discretion of the surgeon. Infection is not a common problem.

Liposuction. *Liposuction* is a technique for removing subcutaneous fat to improve facial and body contours. Although not a substitute for diet and exercise, it can be successful in removing areas of fat from virtually any body area that is resistant to other techniques (Fig. 23-14).

Although relatively free of complications, possible contraindications for the procedure include use of anticoagulants, uncontrolled hypertension, diabetes mellitus, and poor cardiovascular status. Persons under 40 years of age with good skin elasticity are the best candidates. However, patients ranging in age from 16 to 70 years can be treated successfully.

The procedure is usually performed on an outpatient basis with the aid of local anesthesia. One or more sessions may be necessary, depending on the size of the area to be treated. A blunt-tipped cannula is inserted through a 0.5-inch incision and pushed into the fat to break it loose from the fibrous stroma. Multiple repeated thrusts disrupt the fat and create tunnels. The loosened fat is removed with a powerful suction. The area is taped because firm bandaging helps contour the skin and reduce the chance of postoperative bleeding and fluid accumulation. It may take several months for the final results to be evident.

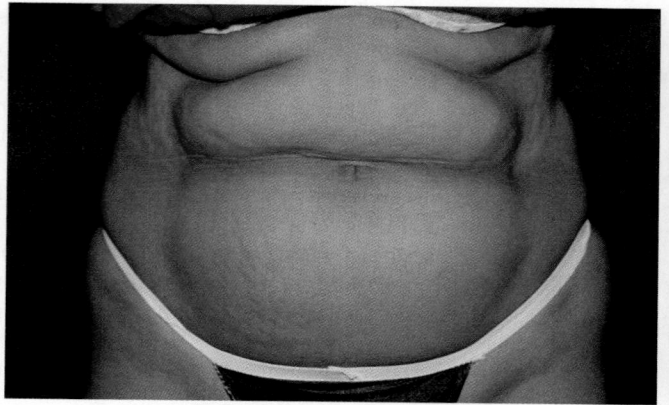
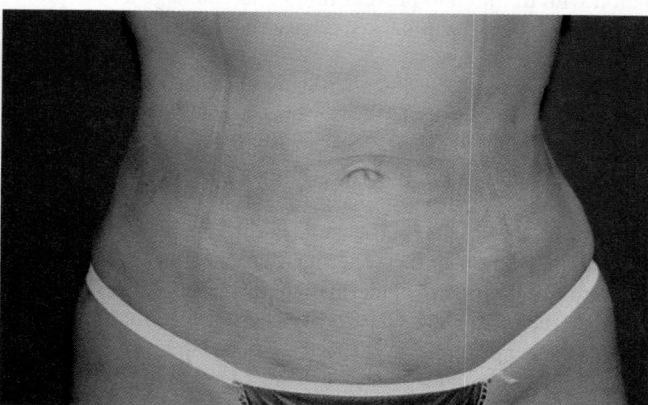

FIG. 23-14 Liposuction. **A,** Preoperative. **B,** Postoperative.

NURSING MANAGEMENT
COSMETIC SURGERY

Many cosmetic surgical procedures are performed in well-equipped day surgery units or in plastic surgeons' office surgery suites. Several nursing interventions are appropriate for the patient who has had cosmetic surgery, regardless of where the surgery was done.

■ Preoperative Management

A major consideration relates to informed consent and realistic expectations of what cosmetic surgery can accomplish. Although this information is usually provided by the surgeon, the nurse can and should reinforce this information and answer questions and concerns. For instance, a face-lift has little or no effect on deep wrinkling of the forehead and temples, deep nasolabial grooves, or vertical lip wrinkles. Before and after treatment photographs of similar cases are often useful in helping the patient to set realistic expectations.

The patient also needs to understand the time frame for healing. Complete results may not be evident until 1 year after the procedure. The oozing, crusting stage of the abrasive procedure must be explained so the patient can plan time off from work if this seems necessary. The final results of the cosmetic procedure are affected by the patient's age, general state of health, and skin type. If a health problem is present, efforts should be made to correct or control the problem before the procedure is performed.

■ Postoperative Mangement

Most of the cosmetic procedures are not extremely painful. Usually mild analgesics are sufficient to keep the patient comfortable.

Although infection is not a common problem after cosmetic surgery, the nurse should assess the surgical sites for signs of infection. The patient should be aware of signs of infection and told to report any such signs and symptoms immediately so that appropriate antibiotic intervention can be started.

If the surgery involved alteration in the circulation to the skin, such as the undermining done in a face-lift, a careful monitoring of adequate circulation is necessary. Warm, pink skin that blanches on pressure indicates that adequate circulation is present in the surgical area.

SKIN GRAFTS

Uses

Skin grafts may be necessary to provide protection to underlying structures or to reconstruct areas for cosmetic or functional purposes. Ideally, wounds heal by primary intention. However, large, surgically created wounds, trauma, and chronic wounds can cause extensive tissue destruction, making primary intention healing impossible. In these cases, skin grafting may be necessary. Improved surgical techniques make it possible to graft skin, bone, cartilage, fat, fascia, muscles, and nerves. For cosmetically pleasing results, the color, thickness, texture, and hair-growing nature of skin used for grafting must be chosen to match the recipient site. (Skin grafting is discussed in Chapter 24.)

Types

The two types of skin grafts are free grafts and skin flaps. *Free grafts* are further classified according to the method of providing a blood supply to the grafted skin. One method is to transfer the graft (epidermis and part or all of the dermis) to the recipient site from the donor site. If the graft is an *autograft* (from the patient's own body) or an *isograft* (from an identical twin), it will revascularize and become fixed to the new site. Chapter 24 discusses full and split skin grafts in detail. Another method of free skin grafting is by reconstructive microsurgery. With the use of an operating microscope, circulation is immediately established in the free flap by anastomosis of the blood vessels from the skin flap to the vessels in the recipient site.

Skin flaps involve moving a section of skin and subcutaneous tissue from one part of the body to another without terminating the vascular attachment. The vascular attachment is called a *pedicle*. Skin flaps are used to cover wounds with a poor vascular bed, when padding is needed, and to cover wounds over cartilage and bone. There may be a need for intermediate flap placement if the recipient site is far removed from the donor site. For instance, a skin flap from the thigh to the head would require an intermediate graft. The flap is advanced to the recipient site when circulation is well established at the intermediate site. The type of flap and the route of transfer are determined according to the needs of the patient and the nature of the defect to be repaired.

Soft tissue expansion is a technique for providing skin for resurfacing a defect, such as a burn scar, for removing a disfiguring mark, such as a tattoo, or as a preliminary step in breast reconstruction. A subcutaneous tissue expander of an appropriate size and shape is placed under the skin, usually as an outpatient procedure. Weekly expansion with saline solution can be done in a health care setting or by the patient at home. This expansion procedure is repeated until the skin reaches the size needed for the repair. This may take from several weeks to 3 to 4 months. Once sufficient skin is available, the old incision is opened, the expander is removed, and the soft tissue is ready to be used as an advancement flap. The tissue expander next to a defect retains the primary tissue characteristics such as color and texture.

CRITICAL THINKING EXERCISES

Case Study

Herpes Varicella Zoster Virus

Patient Profile. Jo Hill, 43, comes to the clinic for evaluation of the presence of generalized vesicular lesions in various stages of development.

Subjective Data

- States she had headache, general aches, severe backache, and malaise approximately 2 weeks before appearance of "rash"
- Explains that lesions began on face and spread to trunk—"They just keep popping up"
- Complains of severe pruritus
- Takes care of an elderly parent who has recently had shingles
- Did not have chickenpox as a child and has not had the vaccine

Objective Data

Physical Examination

- Has crops of lesions in various stages of evolution, vesicles on erythematous base (dewdrop on a rose petal), and excoriated crusted lesions

Diagnostic Studies

- Tzanck smear

CRITICAL THINKING QUESTIONS

1. What factors placed the patient at risk for this diagnosis?
2. What are the usual manifestations associated with varicella infection?
3. What treatment options are available for this patient?
4. What are some of the sequelae that Mrs. Hill might experience?
5. How long can the patient expect to have lesions/symptoms?
6. What would you include in a patient teaching plan for this individual?
7. Based on the assessment data presented, write one or more appropriate nursing diagnoses. Are there any collaborative problems?

Nursing Research Issues

1. What strategies are the most effective in educating patients regarding the source of infection and the risk of contagion? How might these strategies vary based on the patient's age?
2. What factors influence the decision to undergo cosmetic surgery? Is there a significant improvement in quality of life after this surgery?
3. Do adult patients with childhood dermatologic disorders significantly differ in their care needs as compared with adult patients who developed problems as an adult?
4. Is there a significant decrease in sun exposure after a diagnosis of actinic keratoses?

REVIEW QUESTIONS

The number of the question corresponds to the same-numbered objective at the beginning of the chapter.

1. The nurse advises a patient with photosensitivity to use a sunscreen that contains
   a. cinnamates.
   b. benzophenones.
   c. methyl anthranilate.
   d. PABA (para-aminobenzoic acid).
2. In teaching a patient who is using topical corticosteroids to treat an acute dermatitis, the nurse should tell the patient that
   a. the cream form is the most efficient system of delivery.
   b. topical corticosteroids usually do not cause systemic side effects.
   c. creams and ointments should be applied with a glove in small amounts to prevent further infection.
   d. abruptly discontinuing the use of topical corticosteroids will cause a reappearance of the dermatitis.
3. A patient with psoriasis tells the nurse that she has quit her job as a receptionist because she feels her appearance is disgusting to customers. The nursing diagnosis that best describes this patient response is
   a. ineffective coping related to lack of social support.
   b. impaired skin integrity related to presence of lesions.
   c. anxiety related to lack of knowledge of the disease process.
   d. social isolation related to decreased activities secondary to fear of rejection.
4. In teaching a patient with malignant melanoma about this disorder, the nurse recognizes that the prognosis of the patient is most dependent on
   a. the thickness of the lesion.
   b. the degree of color change in the lesion.
   c. how much superficial spread the lesion has.
   d. the amount of ulceration present in the lesion.

REVIEW QUESTIONS—cont'd

5. The nurse identifies that a patient with a diagnosis of which of the following disorders is most at risk for spreading the disease?
   a. tinea pedis
   b. impetigo on the face
   c. candidiasis of the nails
   d. psoriasis on the palms and soles

6. A mother and her two children have been diagnosed with pediculosis corporis at a health center. An appropriate measure in treating this condition is
   a. washing the body with pyrethrins.
   b. topical application of griseofulvin.
   c. moist compresses applied frequently.
   d. administration of systemic antibiotics.

7. A common site for the lesions associated with atopic dermatitis is the
   a. buttocks.
   b. temporal area.
   c. antecubital space.
   d. palmar surface of the feet.

8. During assessment of a patient the nurse notes an area of red, sharply defined plaques covered with silvery scales that are mildly itchy on the patient's knee and elbow. The nurse recognizes this finding as
   a. lentigo.
   b. psoriasis.
   c. actinic keratoses.
   d. seborrheic keratoses.

9. A dermatologic manifestations of Cushing's syndrome would include
   a. telangiectasia.
   b. thickened skin.
   c. increased sweating.
   d. generalized hyperpigmentation.

10. Important patient teaching after a chemical peel includes
    a. avoidance of sun exposure.
    b. application of firm bandages.
    c. limitation of vigorous exercise.
    d. use of mild heat to prevent drying.

REFERENCES

1. Berger T: Skin, hair, and nails. In Tierney L et al, editors: *Current medical diagnosis and treatment 2001,* ed 40, New York, 2001, McGraw-Hill.
2. Mackie B, Mackie L: The PABA story, *Aust J Dermatol* 40:51, 1999.
3. Benson L: Malignant melanoma. In Miaskowski C, Buchsel P, editors: *Oncology nursing: assessment and clinical care,* St Louis, 1999, Mosby.
4. Hill MJ: *Dermatology nursing essentials: a core curriculum,* New Jersey, 1998, Dermatology Nurses Association.
5. Herlihy B, Maebius NK: *The human body in health and illness,* Philadelphia, 2000, WB Saunders.
6. Jarvis C: *Physical examination and health assessment,* ed 3, Philadelphia, 2000, WB Saunders.
7. Lichter MD et al: Therapeutic ionizing radiation and the incidence of basal cell carcinoma and squamous cell carcinoma. The New Hampshire study group, *Arch Dermatol* 136:1007, 2000.
8. Rigel DS, Carrucci JA: Malignant melanoma: prevention, early detection and treatment in the 21st century, *CA Cancer J Clin* 50:215, 2000.
9. Espinosa A et al: Cutaneous malignant melanoma and sun exposure in Spain, *Melanoma Research* 9:199, 1999.
10. Hill L, Ferrini R: Skin cancer prevention and screening: summary of the American College of Preventative Medicine's practice policy statements, *CA Cancer J Clin* 48:232, 1998.
11. American Cancer Society: *Cancer facts and figures 2002,* Atlanta, 2002, American Cancer Society.
12. Burton R: Malignant melanoma in the year 2000, *CA Cancer J Clin* 50:209, 2000.
13. Epstein F: The pathogenesis of melanoma induced by ultraviolet radiation, *N Engl J Med* 340:1341, 1999.
14. Lamb L, Hwu W: Overview of cutaneous melanoma, *Oncol Nurs Updates* 8:1, 2001.
15. Oldhoffer I, Bolognia J: What's new in the treatment of cutaneous melanoma? *Semin Cutan Med Surg* 17:96, 1998.
16. Titus-Ernsthoff L: An overview of the epidemiology of cutaneous melanoma, *Clin Plast Surg* 27:305, 2000.
17. Pogue S, Mayhew MS: Skin, otic, mouth and vaginal agents. In Edmunds MW, Mayhew MS, editors: *Pharmacology for the primary care provider,* St Louis, 2000, Mosby.
18. Decker G: Nonmelanoma skin cancers. In Miaskowski C, Buchsel P, editors: *Oncology nursing: assessment and clinical care,* St Louis, 1999, Mosby.
19. Hooper BJ, Goldman MP: *Primary dermatologic care,* St Louis, 1999, Mosby.
20. Fortunato N, McCullough SM: *Plastic and reconstructive surgery,* St Louis, 1998, Mosby.
21. Blitzer A, Binder W: Current practices in the use of botulinum toxin A in the management of facial lines and wrinkles, *Facial Plast Surg Clin North Am* 9:395, 2001.
22. University of California, Berkeley: *Wellness Letter* 18:7, 2002, School of Public Health. Available at *www.WellnessLetter.com.* Hard copy available.

RESOURCES

AcneNet
 www.derm-infonet.com/acnenet/index.html
American Academy of Dermatology
 930 North Meacham Road
 Schaumburg, IL 60173
 847-330-0230
 Fax: 847-330-0050
 www.aad.org/
American Academy of Facial Plastic and Reconstructive Surgery
 310 South Henry Street
 Alexandria, VA 22314
 703-299-9291
 Fax: 703-299-8898
 www.facial-plastic-surgery.org/index.asp

American Social Health Association
PO Box 13827
Research Triangle Park, NC 27709
919-361-8400
Fax: 919-361-8425
www.ashastd.org

American Society of Plastic and Reconstructive Surgical Nurses
East Holly Avenue, Box 56
Pitman, NJ 08071-0056
609-256-2340
Fax: 609-589-7463

Dermatology Foundation
1560 Sherman Avenue, Suite 870
Evanston, IL 60201-4808
www.dermfnd.org/

National Arthritis and Musculoskeletal and Skin Diseases Information Clearinghouse
National Institutes of Health
1 AMS Circle
Bethesda, MD 20892-3675
301-495-4484
877-22-NIAMS
Fax: 301-718-6366
www.niams.nih.gov/

National Eczema Association for Science and Education
6600 SW 92nd Avenue, Suite 230
Portland, OR 97223-7195
503-228-4430
800-818-7546
Fax: 503-224-3363
www.nationaleczema.org/

National Pediculosis Association
50 Kearney Road
Needham, MA 02494
781-449-NITS
Fax: 781-449-8129
www.headlice.org/

National Psoriasis Foundation
6600 SW 92nd Avenue, Suite 300
Portland, OR 97223-7195
503-244-7404
800-723-9166
Fax: 503-245-0626
www.psoriasis.org/

Skin Cancer Foundation
245 5th Avenue Suite #1403
New York, NY 10016
800-SKIN-490
Fax: 212-725-5751
E-mail: info@skincancer.org
www.skincancer.org/

For additional Internet resources, see the website for this book at *http://evolve.elsevier.com/Lewis/medsurg/*.

CHAPTER 24

NURSING MANAGEMENT
Burns

Cynthia J. Knipe

LEARNING OBJECTIVES

1. Describe the causes and prevention of burn injuries.
2. Describe the burn injury classification system.
3. Describe the relationship between the involved structures and the clinical appearance of partial- and full-thickness burns.
4. Identify the parameters used to determine the severity of burns.
5. Describe the pathophysiology, clinical manifestations, complications, and nursing and collaborative management of the three burn phases.
6. Explain fluid and electrolyte shifts during the emergent and acute burn phases.
7. Describe the nutritional therapy of the burn patient during the three burn phases.
8. Describe the interventions that the nurse may use in the management of pain in the burn patient.
9. Explain the physiologic and psychosocial aspects of burn rehabilitation.
10. Describe the nursing management of the emotional needs of the burn patient and family.
11. Discuss the issues involved and rationale for preparing the burn patient to return home.

KEY TERMS

artificial skin, p. 534
burn, p. 515
chemical burns, p. 515
contracture, p. 536
cultured epithelial autograft, p. 533
debridement, p. 528
electrical burns, p. 517
enzymatic debridement, p. 532

escharotomy, p. 523
excision and grafting, p. 533
full-thickness burn, p. 518
hypermetabolic state, p. 530
partial-thickness burn, p. 518
smoke and inhalation injuries, p. 516
thermal burns, p. 515

A **burn** occurs when there is injury to the tissues of the body caused by heat, chemicals, electrical current, or radiation. The resulting effects are influenced by the intensity of the energy, duration of exposure, and type of tissue injured.

An estimated 2.5 million Americans seek medical care each year for burns.[1] Approximately 100,000 are hospitalized, and 70,000 require intensive care services. An estimated 12,000 of these people die annually as a direct result of their burns. Approximately 1 million sustain substantial or permanent disabilities resulting from their burn injury. The highest fatality rates occur in children (especially preschool-age children) and older adults.[2]

The major cause of fires in the home is carelessness with cigarettes. Other causes of burns include hot water from water heaters set above 140° F (60° C), cooking accidents, space heaters, combustibles such as gasoline and charcoal lighter fluid, steam from radiators, and chemicals.

Most burn injuries can be prevented. The nurse as a citizen and health care provider is in a good position to conduct home safety assessments and to teach people about burn injuries before accidents occur. Home safety measures include the use of smoke alarms, carbon monoxide detectors, and fire extinguishers. Families should have fire drills, and each family member should know where to go and what to do in case of a fire. Local fire departments can inform the public of regional fire codes and perform home safety checks.

Knowledge of potential sources for burn injury allows problem solving for burn prevention (Tables 24-1 and 24-2). Teaching people proper use of appliances (e.g., space heaters), electrical cords, wiring, outlets, outdoor grills, and hot water heaters can prevent burn injury. The nurse can be instrumental in teaching home care of minor burns to the public. The nurse should teach burn prevention in the industrial work setting.

TYPES OF BURN INJURY

Thermal Burns

Thermal burns, which can be caused by flame, flash, scald, or contact with hot objects, are the most common type of burn (Table 24-2 and Fig. 24-1).

Chemical Burns

Chemical burns are the result of tissue injury and destruction from necrotizing substances. Chemical burns are most commonly caused by acids. However, alkali burns also occur, and they are more difficult to manage than acid burns. Alkaline substances are not neutralized by tissue fluids as readily as acid substances. Alkalis adhere to tissue, causing protein hydrolysis and liquefaction. This damage continues even when the alkali is neutralized. Examples of alkalis that cause burn injury are cleaning agents, drain cleaners, and lyes.

Chemicals can cause respiratory problems and other systemic manifestations, as well as skin or eye injuries. When chlorine gas is inhaled, it produces respiratory distress. By-products of burning substances (e.g., carbon) are toxic to the sensitive respiratory mucosa.

With chemical injuries, it is important to remove the person from the burning agent, or vice versa. The latter is accomplished

Reviewed by Judy A. Knighton, RN, MScN, Clinical Nurse Specialist—Burns, Sunnybrook and Women's College Health Sciences Center, Sharon, Ontario, Canada.

| TABLE 24-1 | Common Places and Causes of Burn Injury |

Occupational Hazards

Steam pipes	Electricity from power lines
Chemicals	Combustible fuels
Hot metals	Fertilizers/pesticides
Tar	

Home and Recreational Hazards

Hot water heaters set higher than 140° F (60° C)	Improper use of outdoor grills
Multiple extension cords per outlet	Improper use of flammables (e.g., starter fluid, gasoline, kerosene)
Frayed or defective wiring	Hot grease or liquids from cooking
Pressure cookers	
Microwaved food	Excessive exposure to sunlight
Radiators	Electrical storms
Open space heaters	
Carelessness with cigarettes or matches	

| TABLE 24-2 | Causes of Burn Injury |

CAUSE	EXAMPLES
Flame	Clothing ignited with fire
Flash	Flame burn associated with explosion (combustible fuels)
Scald	Hot bath water
	Spilled hot beverages
	Hot grease or liquids from cooking
	Steam burns (pressure cookers, microwaved food, automobile radiators)
Contact	Hot metal (outdoor grill)
	Hot, sticky tar

by lavaging the affected area with copious amounts of water. Any clothing containing the chemical should be removed, because the burning process will continue as long as the chemical is in contact with the skin. Tissue destruction may continue for up to 72 hours after a chemical injury.

Smoke and Inhalation Injury

Smoke and inhalation injuries result from the inhalation of hot air or noxious chemicals and can cause damage to the tissues of the respiratory tract. Although damage to the respiratory mucosa can occur, it seldom happens because the vocal cords and glottis close as a protective mechanism. Redness and airway edema may result. However, gases are cooled to body temperature before they reach the lung tissue. Smoke inhalation injuries are an important determinant of mortality in fire victims.[3]

There are three types of smoke and inhalation injuries:

1. *Carbon monoxide poisoning.* Carbon monoxide (CO) poisoning and asphyxiation account for the majority of deaths at the fire scene. CO is produced by the incomplete combustion of burning materials. It is subsequently inhaled and displaces oxygen (O$_2$) on the hemoglobin molecule, caus-

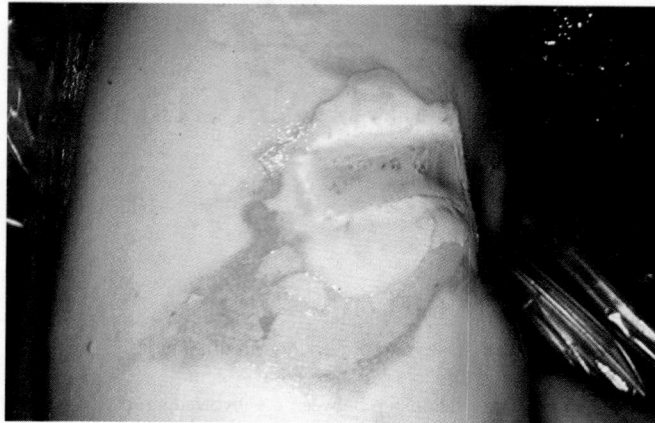

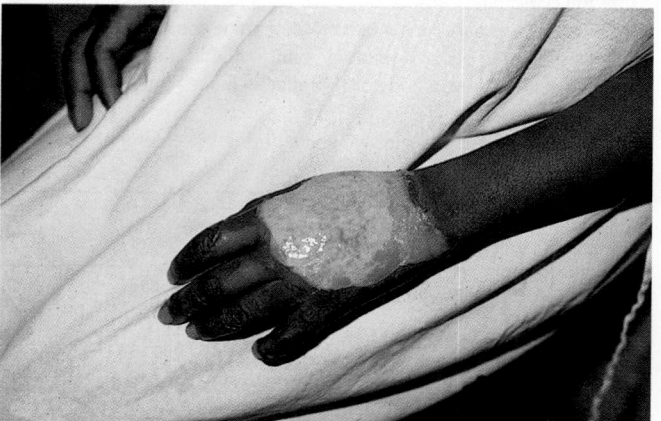

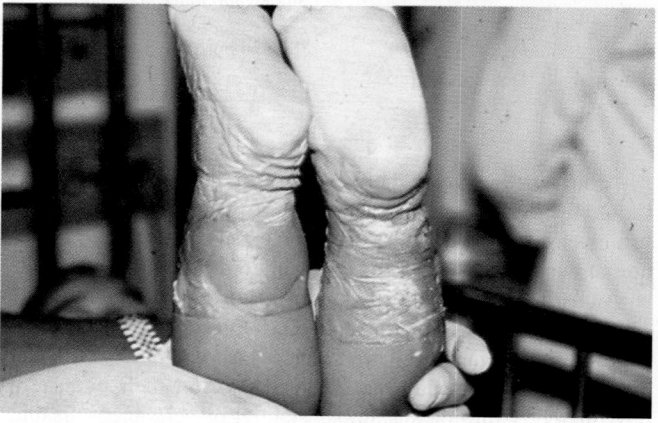

FIG. 24-1 Types of burn injury. **A,** Patient with full-thickness thermal burn. **B,** Parital-thickness burn to the hand. **C,** Partial-thickness burns secondary to immersion in hot water.

ing hypoxia, carboxyhemoglobinemia, and ultimately death when the CO levels are high. Often the victims of fires, especially those who have been trapped in a closed space, will have elevated carboxyhemoglobin levels. If CO intoxication is suspected, the patient should be quickly treated with 100% humidified O$_2$ and the carboxyhemoglobin level should be measured when feasible. Skin color is often described as "cherry red" in appearance with CO poisoning. CO poisoning may occur in the absence of burn injury to the skin.

2. *Inhalation injury above the glottis.* A general principle to remember is that inhalation injury above the glottis is ther-

mally produced, and below the glottis it is usually chemically produced. This injury may be caused by the inhalation of hot air, steam, or smoke. Mucosal burns of the oropharynx and larynx are manifested by redness, blistering, and edema. Mechanical obstruction can occur quickly, presenting a true medical emergency. Often a reliable clue that this injury is likely is the presence of facial burns, singed nasal hair, hoarseness, painful swallowing, and darkened oral and nasal membranes.

3. *Inhalation injury below the glottis.* The tissue injury to the lower respiratory tract is related to the length of exposure to smoke or toxic fumes. Clinical manifestations such as pulmonary edema may not appear until 12 to 24 hours after the burn, and then they may manifest as acute respiratory distress syndrome (see Chapter 66).

These patients must be observed closely for signs of respiratory distress or compromise and must be treated quickly and efficiently if they are to survive. Respiratory tract complications from burn injury are discussed in detail later in this chapter.

Electrical Burns

Electrical burns result from coagulation necrosis that is caused by intense heat generated from an electrical current (Fig. 24-2). It can also result from direct damage to nerves and vessels causing tissue anoxia and death. The severity of the electrical injury depends on the amount of voltage, tissue resistance, current pathways, and surface area in contact with the current and on the length of time the current flow was sustained. Tissue densities offer various amounts of resistance to electrical current. For example, fat and bone offer the most resistance, whereas nerves and blood vessels offer the least resistance. Current that passes through vital organs (e.g., brain, heart, kidneys) will produce more damage than current that passes through other tissue. In addition, electrical sparks may ignite the patient's clothing, causing a combination of thermal and electrical injury.

Nursing assessment of the patient with electrical injury should be thorough. Often the wounds of electrical current entry and exit are all that are visible, masking the possibility of extensive, underlying tissue damage. Noting the patient's position when the injury was sustained in conjunction with identifying the entry and exit wounds can help the nurse assess which underlying organ structures may have been affected. Contact with electrical current can cause muscle contractions strong enough to fracture the long bones and vertebrae. Another reason to suspect long bone or spinal fractures is a fall. Most electrical injuries occur when the victim is elevated above the ground (e.g., during the work of a utility pole lineperson) and comes in contact with a current source. For this reason, all patients with electrical burns should be considered at risk for a potential cervical spine injury. Cervical spine immobilization should be used during transport and subsequent spinal x-rays taken to rule out any injury.

Electrical injury puts the patient at risk for cardiac arrest or arrhythmias, severe metabolic acidosis, and myoglobinuria, which can lead to acute renal tubular necrosis (ATN). The electrical shock event can cause immediate cardiac standstill or fibrillation. If this occurs, cardiopulmonary resuscitation (CPR) should be initiated immediately. Delayed cardiac arrhythmias or arrest may also occur without warning during the first 24 to 48 hours after injury; therefore the patient should be monitored continuously. Because of extensive tissue destruction and cell rupture, severe

metabolic acidosis develops within minutes after the injury, even in the absence of cardiac arrest. Arterial blood gas (ABG) analysis should be performed to assess the acid-base balance. Sodium bicarbonate may be administered in amounts sufficient to maintain the serum pH at near-normal levels.

Myoglobin is released from muscle tissue and hemoglobin from damaged red blood cells (RBCs) into the circulation whenever massive muscle and blood vessel damage occurs. The released myoglobin pigments are then transported to the kidneys where they can mechanically block the renal tubules because of their large size. This process can result in ATN and eventual acute renal failure if not appropriately treated (see Chapter 45). Treatment consists of infusing Ringer's lactate solution at a rate sufficient to maintain urinary output at 75 to 100 ml per hour until the urine sample analyses indicate that the myoglobin and hemoglobin have been flushed from the circulatory system. In addition, an osmotic diuretic (e.g., mannitol)

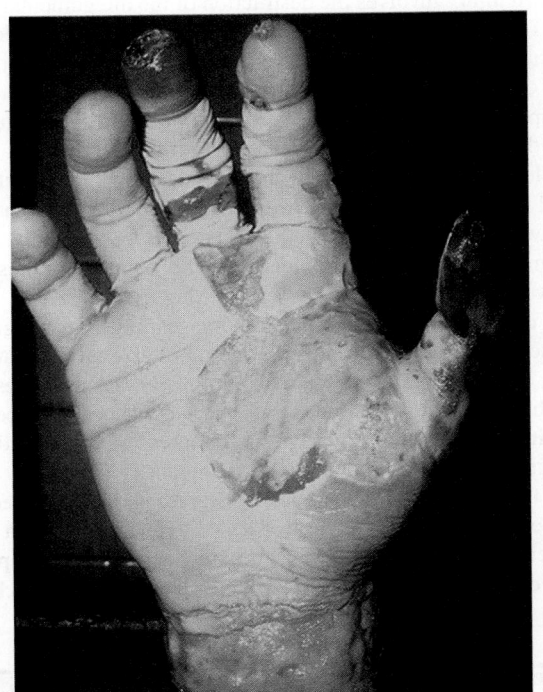

A

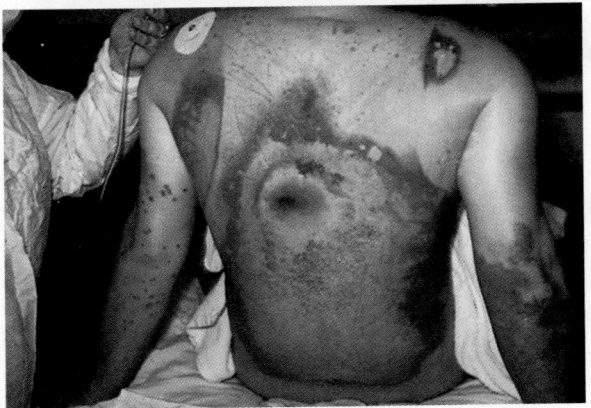

B

FIG. 24-2 Electrical injury produces heat coagulation of blood supply and contact area as electrical current passes through the skin. A, Hand. B, Back.

may be given to maintain urine output, along with sodium bicarbonate to alkalinize the urine.

Cold Thermal Injury

Cold thermal injury, or frostbite, is discussed in Chapter 67.

CLASSIFICATION OF BURN INJURY

The treatment of burns is related to the severity of the injury. Severity is determined by (1) depth of burn, (2) extent of burn calculated in percent of total body surface area (TBSA), (3) location of burn, and (4) patient risk factors.[4] The American Burn Association (ABA) classifies burn injuries into major, moderate uncomplicated, and minor (Table 24-3). The ABA recommends that major burn injuries be treated at burn centers or burn units that have optimal facilities and personnel for handling such severe trauma.

Depth of Burn

Burn injury involves the destruction of the integumentary system. The skin is divided into three layers: the epidermis, dermis, and subcutaneous tissue (Fig. 24-3). The *epidermis,* or nonvascular outer layer of the skin, is approximately as thick as a sheet of paper. It is composed of many layers of nonliving epithelial cells that provide a protective barrier to the skin, hold in fluids and electrolytes, regulate heat, and keep harmful agents in the external environment from injuring or invading the body. The *dermis,* which lies below the epidermis, is approximately 30 to 45 times thicker than the epidermis. The dermis contains connective tissues with blood vessels and highly specialized structures consisting of hair follicles, nerve endings, sweat glands, and sebaceous glands. Under the dermis lies the subcutaneous tissue, which contains major vascular networks, fat, nerves, and lymphatics. The *subcutaneous tissue* acts as a shock absorber and heat insulator for the underlying structures, which include the muscles, tendons, bones, and internal organs.

In the past, burns were defined by degrees: first-degree, second-degree, and third-degree burns. The ABA now advocates a more explicit definition categorizing the burn according to depth of skin destruction: **partial-thickness burn** and **full-thickness**

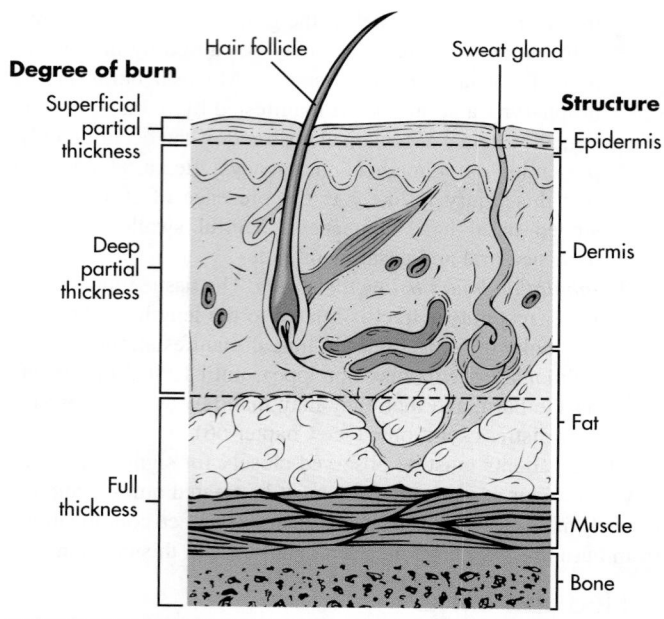

FIG. 24-3 Cross section of skin indicating the degree of burn and structures involved.

burn (see Fig. 24-3). Table 24-4 shows the comparison of the depth of injury.

Extent of Burn

Two commonly used guides for determining the *total body surface area* affected or the extent of a burn wound are the Lund-Browder chart (Fig. 24-4, *A*) and the *rule of nines* (Fig. 24-4, *B*). (Only partial-thickness and full-thickness burns are included when calculating TBSA.) The Lund-Browder chart is considered more accurate because the patient's age, in proportion to relative body-area size, is taken into account. The rule of nines, which is easy to remember, is considered adequate for initial assessment of an adult burn patient. For irregular- or odd-shaped burns, the palmar surface of the patient's hand is considered to

TABLE 24-3	American Burn Association Adult Burn Classification		
MAGNITUDE OF BURN INJURY	**PARTIAL-THICKNESS* (SECOND-DEGREE) BURN**	**FULL-THICKNESS* (THIRD-DEGREE) BURN**	**OTHER FACTORS**
Minor	<15%	<2%	Does not involve special care areas (eyes, ears, face, hands, feet, perineum); excludes electrical injury, inhalation injury, complicated injury (fractures), all high-risk patients (extremes of age, concomitant disease)
Moderate uncomplicated	15%-25%	<10%	Excludes electrical injury, inhalation injury, complicated injury, all high-risk patients; does not involve special care areas
Major	>25%	>10%	Includes all burns involving hands, face, eyes, ears, feet, or perineum; includes inhalation injury, electrical injury, complicated burn injury, and all high-risk patients; patient should be transferred to a burn unit

*Figures indicate percentage of total body surface area involved.

TABLE 24-4	Classification of Burn Injury Depth		
CLASSIFICATION	**CLINICAL APPEARANCE**	**CAUSE**	**STRUCTURE**
Partial-thickness skin destruction			
• Superficial (first-degree)	Erythema, blanching on pressure, pain and mild swelling, no vesicles or blisters (although after 24 hr skin may blister and peel)	Superficial sunburn Quick heat flash	Only superficial devitalization with hyperemia is present. Tactile and pain sensation intact.
• Deep (second-degree)	Fluid-filled vesicles that are red, shiny, wet (if vesicles have ruptured); severe pain caused by nerve injury; mild-to-moderate edema	Flame Flash Scald Contact burns Chemical tar	Epidermis and dermis involved to varying depth. Some skin elements, from which epithelial regeneration can occur, remain viable.
Full-thickness skin destruction			
• (Third- and fourth-degree)	Dry, waxy white, leathery, or hard skin; visible thrombosed vessels; insensitivity to pain and pressure because of nerve destruction; possible involvement of muscles, tendons, and bones	Flame Scald Chemical Tar Electric current	All skin elements and nerve endings destroyed. Coagulation necrosis present. Surgical intervention for wound closure.

be approximately 1% of the TBSA. The extent of a burn is often revised after edema has subsided and demarcation of zones of injury has occurred.

Location of Burn

The location of the burn wound is related to the severity of the burn injury. Burns to the face and neck and circumferential burns of the chest may inhibit respiratory function by virtue of mechanical obstruction secondary to edema or eschar formation. These injuries may also indicate the possibility of inhalation injury and respiratory mucosal damage.

Burns of the hands, feet, joints, and eyes are of concern because they make self-care very difficult and may jeopardize future function. Hands and feet are difficult to manage medically because of superficial vascular and nerve-supply systems.

The ears and nose, composed mainly of cartilage, are susceptible to infection because of poor blood supply to the cartilage. Burns of the buttocks or genitalia are highly susceptible to infection. Circumferential burns of the extremities can cause circulatory compromise distal to the burn with subsequent neurologic impairment of the affected extremity. Patients may also develop compartment syndrome (see Chapter 61) from direct heat damage to the muscles, multiple intravenous access attempts, or preburn vascular problems.

Patient Risk Factors

The older adult heals more slowly and may experience more difficulty with rehabilitation than a younger adult. Any patient with preexisting cardiovascular, respiratory, or renal disease has a poorer prognosis for recovery because of the tremendous demands placed on the body by a burn injury. The patient with diabetes mellitus or peripheral vascular disease is at high risk for poor healing and gangrene, especially with foot and leg burns. General physical debilitation from any chronic disease, including alcoholism, drug abuse, and malnutrition, renders the patient less

Head	7
Neck	2
Ant. trunk	13
Post. trunk	13
R. buttock	2½
L. buttock	2½
Genitalia	1
R.U. arm	4
L.U. arm	4
R.L. arm	3
L.L. arm	3
R. hand	2½
L. hand	2½
R. thigh	9½
L. thigh	9½
R. leg	7
L. leg	7
R. foot	3½
L. foot	3½
TOTAL	100%

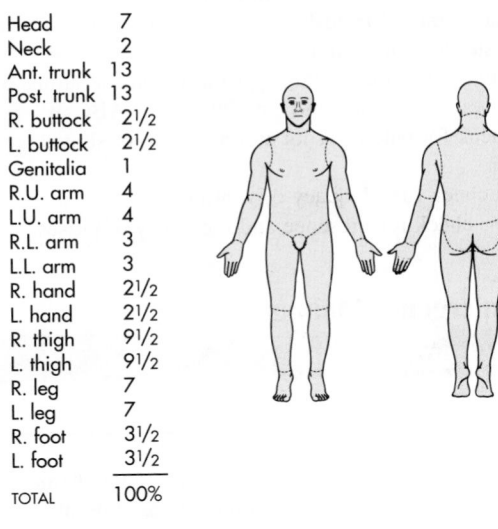

Head & neck	9%
Arms	9%
Ant. trunk	18%
Post. trunk	18%
Legs	18%
Perineum	1%
TOTAL	100%

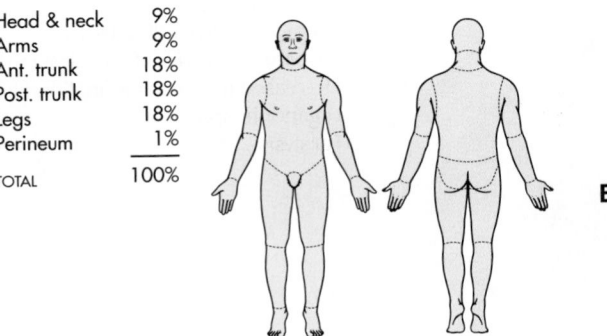

FIG. 24-4 A, Lund-Browder chart. By convention, areas of partial-thickness injury are colored in blue and areas of full-thickness injury in red. Superficial partial-thickness burns are not calculated. **B,** Rule of nines chart.

physiologically competent to deal with a burn injury. In addition, the patient who concurrently sustained fractures, head injuries, or other trauma has a poorer prognosis for recovery from the burn injury.

Phases of Burn Management

Burn management can be divided into three phases: emergent (resuscitative), acute, and rehabilitative. Prehospital care is also briefly discussed.

PREHOSPITAL CARE

The initial consideration in aiding the burn patient is to remove the person from the source of the burn and stop the burning process.[5] The caregiver must be protected from becoming part of the incident. In the case of electrical injuries, initial management involves removal of the patient from contact with the source of current by a trained individual. Most chemical burns are best treated by brushing solid particles off the skin, followed by thorough lavage with water. (For handling specific agents, refer to a hazardous materials text.) Small thermal burns (10% or less TBSA) may be covered with a clean, cool, tap water–dampened towel for the patient's comfort and protection until definitive medical care is instituted. The cooling of the injured area (if small) within 1 minute helps minimize the depth of the injury. Tap water is acceptable for flushing. Time should not be wasted trying to find sterile water, saline solution, or antidotes.

If the thermal burn area is large, primary considerations are focused on airway, breathing, and circulation (the ABCs):

Airway: check for patency, soot around nares, or singed nasal hair.
Breathing: check for adequacy of ventilation.
Circulation: check for presence and regularity of pulses.

If the burn is large, it is not advisable to immerse the burned body part in cool water because doing so would lead to extensive heat loss. The burn should never be packed in ice because this could cause frostbite. As much burned clothing as possible should be removed to prevent further tissue damage. The patient should be wrapped in a dry, clean sheet or blanket to prevent further contamination of the wound and to provide warmth.

The burn patient may also have sustained other injuries that take priority over the burn wound. It is important for the individual involved in the prehospital phase of burn care to adequately communicate the circumstances of the injury to the receiving hospital. This is especially important when the injury involves entrapment in a closed space, hazardous chemicals, or possible trauma.

Prehospital emergency care of the patient with various types of burns is presented in tables that describe chemical burns (Table 24-5), inhalation injury (Table 24-6), electrical burns (Table 24-7), and thermal burns (Table 24-8).

EMERGENT PHASE

The *emergent (resuscitative) phase* is the period of time required to resolve the immediate problems resulting from burn injury. This phase may last from burn onset to 5 or more days, but it usually lasts 24 to 48 hours. This phase begins with fluid loss and edema formation and continues until fluid mobilization and diuresis begin.

Pathophysiology

Fluid and Electrolyte Shifts. The greatest initial threat to a patient with a major burn is hypovolemic shock.[6] It is caused by a massive shift of fluids out of blood vessels as a result of increased capillary permeability. As the capillary walls become more permeable, water, sodium, and later plasma proteins (espe-

TABLE 24-5	**Emergency Management — Chemical Burns**	
ETIOLOGY	**ASSESSMENT FINDINGS**	**INTERVENTIONS**
Acids Alkalis Corrosives Organophosphates	• Burning • Redness, swelling of injured tissue • Degeneration of exposed tissue • Discoloration of injured skin • Localized pain • Edema of surrounding tissue • Respiratory distress if chemical inhaled • Decreased muscle coordination (if organophosphate) • Paralysis	**Initial** • Ensure patent airway. • Assess airway, breathing, and circulation before decontamination procedures. • Brush dry chemical from skin before irrigation. • Flush chemical from wound and surrounding area with saline solution or water. • Remove clothing, including shoes, watches, jewelry, and contact lenses if face exposed. • Establish IV access with large-bore catheter needle if greater than 15% TBSA burn. • Begin fluid replacement. • Blot skin dry with clean towels. Do *not* rub dry. • Cover burned areas with dry, sterile dressing or clean, dry sheet. • Anticipate intubation if significant inhalation injury present. • Contact poison control center for assistance. • Caregiver should protect self from potential exposure. **Ongoing Monitoring** • Monitor airway if airway exposed to chemicals.

TBSA, Total body surface area.

TABLE 24-6 Emergency Management — Inhalation Injury

ETIOLOGY	ASSESSMENT FINDINGS	INTERVENTIONS
Exposure of respiratory tract to intense heat or flames Inhalation of noxious chemicals, smoke, or carbon monoxide	• Rapid, shallow respirations • Increasing hoarseness • Coughing • Singled nasal or facial hair • Smoky breath • Carbonaceous sputum • Productive cough with black, gray, or bloody sputum • Irritation of upper airways or burning pain in throat or chest • Difficulty swallowing • Restlessness, anxiety • Altered mental status, including confusion, coma • Decreased oxygen saturation • Arrhythmias	**Initial** • Ensure patent airway. • Administer high-flow oxygen by non-rebreather mask. • Remove patient's clothing. • Establish IV access with large-bore catheter needle. • Begin fluid replacement. • Place in high Fowler's position unless spinal injury suspected. • Assess for facial/neck burns or other trauma. • Obtain arterial blood gas, carboxyhemoglobin levels, and chest x-ray. • Anticipate need for fiberoptic bronchoscopy or intubation. **Ongoing Monitoring** • Monitor vital signs, level of consciousness, oxygen saturation, respiratory status, and cardiac rhythm.

TABLE 24-7 Emergency Management — Electrical Burns

ETIOLOGY	ASSESSMENT FINDINGS	INTERVENTIONS
Alternating Current Electric wires Utility wires **Direct Current** Lightning Defibrillator	• Leathery, white, or charred skin • Burn odor • Impaired touch sensation • Minimal or absent pain • Arrhythmias • Cardiac arrest • Entrance and exit wounds • Diminished peripheral circulation in injured extremity • Thermal burns if clothing ignites • Fractures or dislocations from force of current • Head or neck injury if fall occurred • Depth and extent of wound difficult to visualize; assume injury greater than what is seen	**Initial** • Removal from current source must be done by trained personnel with special equipment to prevent injury to rescuer. • Assess and treat patient *after* removal from source of current. • Ensure patent airway. • Stabilize cervical spine. • Administer high-flow oxygen by non-rebreather mask. • Establish IV access with large-bore catheter needle. • Begin fluid replacement. • Remove patient's clothing. • Check pulses distal to burns. • Cover burn sites with dry dressing. • Assess for any other injuries (e.g., fractures, head injury). **Ongoing Monitoring** • Monitor cardiac rhythm, vital signs, level of consciousness, oxygen saturation, neurovascular status in injured limbs. • Monitor urine output to ensure adequate volume replacement. • Monitor urine for development of myoglobinuria secondary to muscle breakdown. • Anticipate administration of mannitol and $NaHCO_3$ for myoglobinuria and hemoglobinuria.

cially albumin) move into the interstitial spaces and other surrounding tissue (Fig. 24-5). The colloidal osmotic pressure decreases with progressive loss of protein from the vascular space. This results in more fluid shifting out of the vascular space into the interstitial spaces. (Fluid accumulation in the interstitium is termed *second spacing*.) Fluid also moves to areas that normally have minimal to no fluid, a phenomenon termed *third spacing*. Examples of third spacing in burn injury are exudate and blister formation.

The net result of the fluid shift is intravascular volume depletion. Edema, decreased blood pressure (BP), increased pulse, and other manifestations of hypovolemic shock are clinically detectable signs (see Chapter 65). If not corrected, these events can lead to irreversible shock and death.

Another source of fluid loss is insensible loss by evaporation from large, denuded body surfaces. The normal insensible loss of 30 to 50 ml per hour may increase to as much as 200 to 400 ml per hour in the severely burned patient.

TABLE 24-8   Emergency Management
Thermal Burns

ETIOLOGY	ASSESSMENT FINDINGS	INTERVENTIONS
Hot liquids or solids Flash flame Open flame Steam Hot surface Ultraviolet rays	**Partial-Thickness (Superficial)** • Redness • Pain • Moderate to severe tenderness • Minimal edema • Blanching with pressure **Partial-Thickness (Deep)** • Moist blebs, blisters • Mottled white, pink to cherry red • Hypersensitive to touch or air • Moderate to severe pain • Blanching with pressure **Full-Thickness** • Dry, leathery eschar • White, waxy, dark brown, or charred appearance • Strong burn odor • Impaired sensation when touched • Absence of pain with severe pain in surrounding tissues • Lack of blanching with pressure	**Initial** • Ensure patent airway. • Stop the burning process. • Inspect face and neck for singed nasal hair, hoarseness of voice, stridor, soot in the sputum. • Administer high-flow oxygen by non-rebreather mask. • Anticipate intubation with significant inhalation injury. • Establish IV access with large-bore catheter. • Begin fluid replacement. • Remove clothing and jewelry. • Identify and treat associated injuries (e.g., fractured ribs, pneumothorax). • Determine depth, extent, and severity of burn. • Administer IV analgesia. • Cover large burns with dry dressing. • Apply cool compresses or immerse in cool water for minor injuries only (less than 10% TBSA burn). • Insert urinary catheter for severe burns. • Prevent loss of body heat. • Transport as soon as possible to a burn center. • Do not debride burns or apply topical agents before transfer to a burn center. • Administer tetanus prophylaxis as appropriate. **Ongoing Monitoring** • Monitor vital signs, level of consciousness, oxygen saturation, cardiac rhythm, urine output. • Monitor temperature. • Monitor pain and medicate as needed based on patient response.

TBSA, Total body surface area.

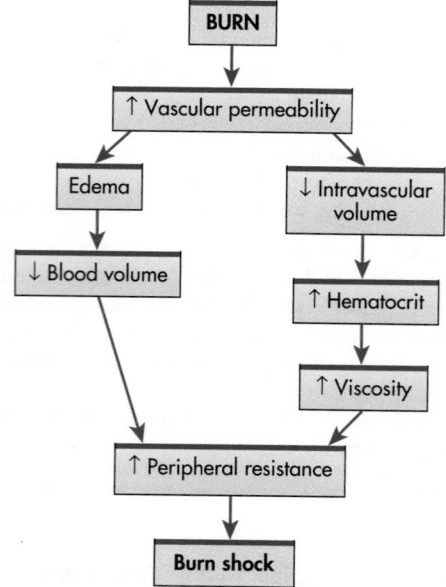

FIG. 24-5 At the time of major burn injury, there is increased capillary permeability. All fluid components of the blood begin to leak into the interstitium, causing edema and a decreased blood volume. The red blood cells and white blood cells do not leak. Therefore the hematocrit increases and the blood becomes more viscous. The combination of decreased blood volume and increased viscosity produces increased peripheral resistance. Burn shock, a type of hypovolemic shock, rapidly ensues and continues for about 24 hours.

The circulatory status is also impaired because of hemolysis of RBCs. The RBCs are hemolyzed by a circulating factor released at the time of the burn, as well as by the direct insult of the burn injury. Thrombosis in the capillaries of burned tissue causes an additional loss of circulating RBCs. An elevated hematocrit is commonly caused by hemoconcentration resulting from fluid loss. After fluid balance has been restored, lowered hematocrit levels are found secondary to dilution, and an anemic state is more readily detectable.

Sodium and potassium are involved in electrolyte shifts. Sodium rapidly shifts to the interstitial spaces and remains there until edema formation ceases (Fig. 24-6). A potassium shift develops initially because injured cells and hemolyzed RBCs release potassium into the extracellular spaces.

Toward the end of the emergent phase, if fluid replacement is adequate, capillary membrane permeability will be restored. Fluid loss and edema formation cease. Interstitial fluid gradually returns to the vascular space (see Fig. 24-6). Clinically, diuresis is noted with low urine specific gravities. Serum potassium levels may be markedly elevated initially as fluid mobilization brings potassium from the interstitium to the vascular space. Hypokalemia may occur later as a result of the loss of potassium from diuresis and potassium movement back into cells. Serum sodium levels increase as sodium returns from the interstitial space to the vascular space. Normal serum sodium values occur later with loss of sodium in urine.

Inflammation and Healing. Burn injury causes coagulation necrosis whereby tissues and vessels are damaged or de-

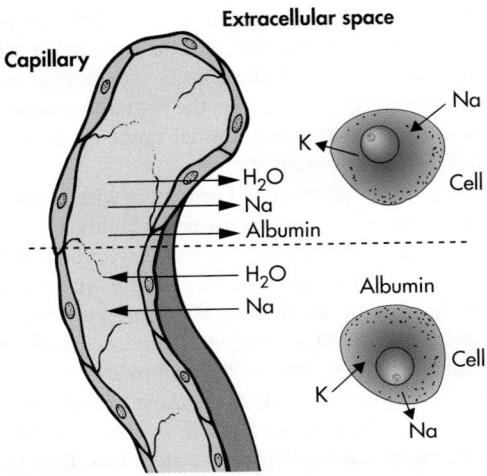

Extracellular space

Capillary

FIG. 24-6 The effects of burn shock during the first 24 hours are shown above the dotted line. As the capillary seal is lost, the interstitial edema fluid is formed. The cellular integrity is also altered, with sodium (Na) moving into the cell in abnormal amounts and potassium (K) leaving the cell. The shifts after the first 24 hours are shown below the dotted line. The water and sodium move back into the circulating volume through the capillary. The albumin remains in the interstitium. Potassium is transported into the cell and sodium is transported out as the cellular integrity returns.

stroyed. Neutrophils and monocytes accumulate at the site of injury. Fibroblasts and newly formed collagen fibrils appear and begin wound repair within the first 6 to 12 hours after injury. (The inflammatory response is discussed in Chapter 12.)

Immunologic Changes. Burn injury causes widespread impairment of the immune system. The skin barrier to invading organisms is destroyed, circulating levels of immunoglobulins are decreased, and many changes in white blood cells (WBCs), both quantitative and qualitative, occur. Depression of neutrophil chemotactic, phagocytic, and bactericidal activity is found after burn injury. Burn size–related alterations of lymphocyte populations include decreased T helper cells and increased T suppressor cells. In addition, decreased levels of interleukin-1 (produced by macrophages) and interleukin-2 (produced by lymphocytes) are also found in some patients with burn injury. Increases in interleukin-6 correlate with the severity of the injury.[7] All of these changes in the immune system can make the burn patient more susceptible to infection.

Clinical Manifestations

The burn patient may be in shock from pain and hypovolemia. Frequently, areas of full-thickness and deep partial-thickness burns are initially anesthetic because the nerve endings are destroyed. Superficial to moderate partial-thickness burns are painful. Blisters filled with fluid and protein may occur in partial-thickness burns. Fluid is not actually lost from the body as much as it is sequestered in the interstitial spaces and third spaces. It is hard to visualize severe dehydration in someone who is so obviously edematous. The patient may have signs of adynamic ileus such as absent or decreased bowel sounds as a result of the body's response to massive trauma and potassium shifts. Shivering may occur as a result of chilling that is caused by heat loss, anxiety, or pain.

The patient may have difficulty recalling the sequence of events that preceded the burn injury. Unconsciousness or altered mental status in a burn patient, however, is usually not a result of the burn. The most common reason is hypoxia associated with smoke inhalation. Other possibilities include head trauma or excessive amounts of sedative or pain medication.

Complications

The three major organ systems most susceptible to complications during the emergent phase of burn injury are the cardiovascular, respiratory, and urinary systems.

Cardiovascular System. Cardiovascular system complications include arrhythmias and hypovolemic shock, which may progress to irreversible shock. Circulation to the extremities can be severely impaired by circumferential burns and subsequent edema formation. These processes occlude the blood supply, causing ischemia, paresthesias, necrosis, and eventually gangrene. An **escharotomy** (a scalpel incision through the full-thickness eschar) is frequently performed to restore circulation to compromised extremities (Fig. 24-7).

Initially there is an increase in blood viscosity with burn injuries because of the fluid loss that occurs in the emergent period. Microcirculation is impaired because of the damage to skin structures that contain small capillary systems. These two events result in a phenomenon termed *sludging*. Sludging can be corrected by adequate fluid replacement.

Respiratory System. The respiratory system is especially vulnerable to two types of injury: (1) upper airway burns that cause edema formation and obstruction of the airway and (2) inhalation injury (Table 24-9). Upper airway distress may occur with or without smoke inhalation, and airway injury at either level may occur in the absence of burn injury to the skin.

Upper respiratory tract injury. Upper respiratory tract injury results from direct heat injury or edema formation and can lead to mechanical airway obstruction and asphyxia. The edema associated with an upper respiratory tract burn injury can be massive and the onset insidious, and it occurs in most patients with major thermal burn injuries. Mechanical obstruction of the airway is not

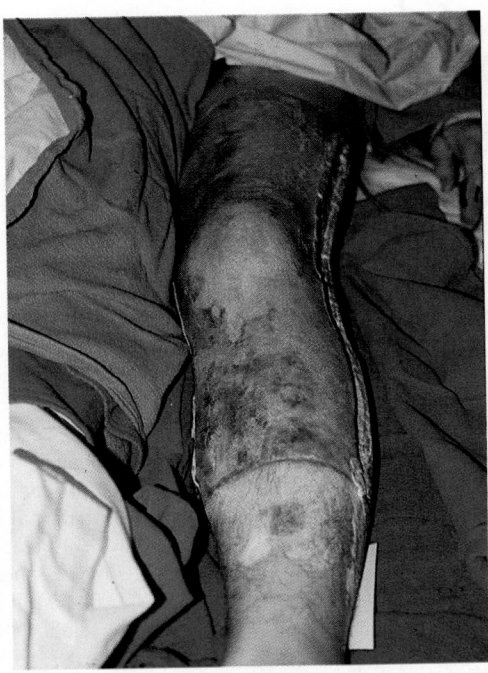

FIG. 24-7 Escharotomy of the lower extremity.

TABLE 24-9	Manifestations of Respiratory Injury Associated with Burns

Upper Respiratory Tract Injury
Edema, hoarseness, difficulty swallowing, copious secretions, stridor, substernal and intercostal retractions, total airway obstruction

Inhalation Injury
Initial absence of manifestations possible; high degree of suspicion if patient was trapped in fire and has facial burns, singed nasal or facial hair; dyspnea, carbonaceous sputum, wheezing, hoarseness, altered mental status

limited to the patient with flame burns to the upper airway. Swelling that accompanies scald burns to the face and neck can be lethal, as can pressure from the accumulated edema compressing the airway externally.[8] Flame burns to the neck and chest may contribute to respiratory difficulty because the inelastic eschar becomes tight and constricting due to the underlying edema.

Inhalation injury. Inhalation injury refers to a direct insult at the alveolar level secondary to the inhalation of chemical fumes or smoke. The result is interstitial edema that prevents the diffusion of oxygen from the alveoli into the circulatory system. The patient with smoke inhalation may not exhibit physical manifestations of injury during the first 24 hours after sustaining a major burn. Fiberoptic bronchoscopy can be used as an early diagnostic tool for suspected inhalation injury. Another diagnostic indicator may be a history of prolonged exposure to smoke or fumes; therefore the nurse must be especially sensitive to signs of respiratory distress such as increased agitation or change in the rate or character of respirations. Sputum that contains carbon may be present. Generally there is no correlation between the extent of

TBSA burn and severity of inhalation injury because inhalation injury is a factor of time exposure plus the type and density of the material inhaled. The initial chest x-ray may appear normal on admission, with changes noted over the next 24 to 48 hours. ABG values may also be within the normal range on admission and may change during hospitalization.

Other respiratory problems. The patient with preexisting respiratory problems (e.g., chronic obstructive pulmonary disease) is more predisposed to developing a respiratory infection. Pneumonia is a common complication of major burns (especially in the older adult) because of debilitation, abundant microbial flora, and the relative immobility of the patient. If fluid replacement is vigorous, the older adult patient can develop pulmonary edema.

Urinary System. The most common complication of the urinary system in the emergent phase is acute tubular necrosis (ATN). Because of the hypovolemic state, blood flow to the kidneys is decreased, causing renal ischemia. If this continues, acute renal failure may develop.

With full-thickness and electrical burns, myoglobin (from muscle cell breakdown) and hemoglobin (from RBC breakdown) are released into the bloodstream and occlude renal tubules. Adequate fluid replacement and diuretics can counteract myoglobin and hemoglobin obstruction of the tubules.

NURSING and COLLABORATIVE MANAGEMENT EMERGENT PHASE

In the emergent phase, patient survival depends on quick and thorough assessment and intervention.[9] It may be the nurse who makes the initial assessment of depth, degree, and percent of burn and coordinates the actions of the multidisciplinary burn team. From the onset of the burn event until the patient is stabilized, nursing and collaborative management predominantly consists of airway management, fluid therapy, and wound care (Table 24-10). See the accompanying nursing care plan (NCP 24-1).

TABLE 24-10	Collaborative Care	Patient with Burns

EMERGENT PHASE	ACUTE PHASE	REHABILITATION PHASE
Fluid therapy Assess fluid needs.* Begin IV fluid replacement. Insert indwelling urinary catheter. Monitor urine output. **Wound care** Start hydrotherapy or cleansing. Debride as necessary. Assess extent and depth of burns. Initiate topical antibiotic therapy. Administer tetanus toxoid or tetanus antitoxin. **Pain and anxiety** Assess and manage pain and anxiety.	**Fluid therapy** Replace fluids, depending on individual patient needs. **Wound care** Assess wound daily. Observe for complications. Continue hydrotherapy, cleansing. Continue debridement (if necessary). Continue assessing for and treating pain and anxiety. **Early excision and grafting** Provide homografts. Provide autografts. Care for donor site. **Nutritional therapy** Provide adequate diet to support wound healing. **Physical therapy** Begin physical therapy for maintenance and rehabilitation of motion.	Counsel and teach patient and family. Encourage and assist patient in resuming self-care. Prevent or minimize contractures and scarring (surgery, physical therapy, or splinting). Discuss possible cosmetic or reconstructive surgery.

*See Tables 24-11 and 24-12.
IV, Intravenous; *RBCs*, red blood cells.

NURSING CARE PLAN 24-1

Burn Patient

EXPECTED PATIENT OUTCOMES	NURSING INTERVENTIONS and *RATIONALES*		
	EMERGENCY PHASE	ACUTE PHASE	REHABILITATIVE PHASE
NURSING DIAGNOSIS	**Risk for deficient fluid volume** *related to* evaporative loss, plasma loss, and shift of fluid into interstitium secondary to burn injury.		
▪ Output >30 to 50 ml/hr ▪ Stable vital signs ▪ Clear sensorium ▪ Sodium and potassium levels within acceptable range ▪ Systolic blood pressure >90 mm Hg	▪ Assess every 1-2 hr: pulses, blood pressure, circulation, and sensation to all extremities; mental status; intake and output; pulmonary function *to determine status of major body systems.* ▪ Monitor weight daily *to evaluate fluid/nutritional status.* ▪ Monitor serial laboratory tests *to determine fluid and electrolyte status.* ▪ Give fluids according to patient needs.	▪ Use emergent phase interventions as necessary. ▪ Monitor electrolyte levels regularly. ▪ Provide oral fluids if patient is able to drink *to increase fluid intake and patient comfort.*	▪ No intervention is required.
NURSING DIAGNOSIS	**Acute pain** *related to* burn injury and treatments *as manifested by* demonstration of discomfort and pain.		
▪ Satisfaction with level of pain control	▪ Administer IV analgesia as needed *to manage pain.* ▪ Administer medication for pain 30 min before interventions. ▪ Administer antianxiety medications as needed *to manage anxiety and agitation.* ▪ Evaluate effectiveness of medication. ▪ Provide emotional support. ▪ Reposition patient carefully using lifting sheet as necessary *to avoid further trauma to skin.*	▪ Plan adequate rest periods *to facilitate coping.* ▪ Administer medication before interventions. ▪ Teach relaxation techniques, guided imagery, distraction *to augment other pain relief measures.* ▪ Plan diversional activities *to distract patient from present situation.*	▪ Be aware that patient's pain may be replaced by itchiness. ▪ Keep skin lubricated with water-based moisturizers *to prevent drying.* ▪ Caution patient to avoid injury to new, fragile skin.
NURSING DIAGNOSIS	**Bathing/hygiene, dressing/grooming, feeding, or toileting self-care deficit** *related to* pain, immobility, and perceived helplessness *as manifested by* inability or unwillingness to participate in self-care.		
▪ Optimal performance of self-care	▪ Assess patient's ability to perform self-care activities. ▪ Assist or intervene as appropriate.	▪ Increase patient's self-care activities as appropriate. ▪ Ensure that patient participates in planning care as able *to increase sense of control.*	▪ Assess and arrange for needed adaptations in living arrangements and lifestyle *to accommodate optimal self-care.*
NURSING DIAGNOSIS	**Imbalanced nutrition: less than body requirements** *related to* increased caloric demands and inability to ingest increased requirements *as manifested by* weight loss and negative nitrogen balance.		
▪ Positive nitrogen balance ▪ Weight loss not >10% of body weight	▪ Maintain patient NPO with NG tube to low intermittent suction *to allow for decompression of the stomach.* ▪ Insert feeding tube past pylorus to begin enteral feeding. ▪ Assess return of bowel sounds *to determine when oral intake can be resumed.* ▪ Institute progressive diet *to meet nutritional needs when bowel sounds return.* ▪ Chart caloric intake *to monitor adequacy of diet.*	▪ Continue to monitor peristalsis. ▪ Offer high-protein, high-carbohydrate diet *to meet increased nutritional needs.* ▪ Assess patient food preferences and offer favorite foods when patient is able to eat. ▪ Continue enteral feedings to meet needs until oral intake is adequate.	▪ Continue to meet nutritional needs. ▪ Once skin coverage is achieved, reduce calories *to prevent excess weight gain* (if necessary).

bid, Twice a day; *IV,* intravenous; *NG,* nasogastric; *NPO,* nothing by mouth; *ROM,* range of motion; *WBC,* white blood cell.

Continued

NURSING CARE PLAN 24-1

Burn Patient—cont'd

EXPECTED PATIENT OUTCOMES	NURSING INTERVENTIONS and *RATIONALES*		
	EMERGENCY PHASE	ACUTE PHASE	REHABILITATIVE PHASE

NURSING DIAGNOSIS   **Risk for infection** *related to* impaired skin integrity, endogenous flora, suppressed immune response.

• Wound free of debris and loose necrotic tissue • Absence of wound infections	• Use good hand-washing technique. • Use sterile technique during application of topical ointments and dressing changes *to prevent contaminating burn area.* • Shave appropriate areas *to reduce possibility of contamination.* • Remove devitalized tissue *to eliminate medium for bacterial growth.* • Apply topical antibiotic and sterile dressings as indicated *to decrease probability of infection.* • Give tetanus vaccine if necessary. • Observe wound daily for separation of eschar; check wound margins for cellulitis. • Monitor vital signs and temperature. • Blister should be left intact unless restricting ROM.	• Monitor burn wound bid *to detect signs of infection* such as purulent drainage, edema, redness. • Note any change in behavior or sensorium. • Perform hydrotherapy and debridement carefully *to remove wound debris and effectively cleanse wound.* • Monitor body temperature, WBC counts, and urine output *to detect signs of sepsis.* • Monitor donor sites *to detect possible infection.*	• Instruct patient and family about signs and symptoms of infection *so early treatment can be initiated.* • Teach family how to perform dressing changes *to ensure proper technique and increase their sense of control.*

NURSING DIAGNOSIS   **Anxiety** *related to* pain, guilt associated with injury, lack of knowledge about treatment and outcome, financial needs, and appearance *as manifested by* questions about treatment and prognosis, withdrawn or overtly angry behavior, expression of concerns about scarring.

• Reduction of anxiety • Body language indicating rest and comfort • Able to talk about changes in self-image	• Administer and evaluate effectiveness of pain medication. • Encourage family visits and participation in care *to increase feelings of support.* • Be open to patient's expressions of feelings about burn event *so patient has opportunity to express emotions.* • Describe burn process and clinical progress to patient and family. • Explain therapeutic interventions, precautionary measures (e.g., gowning, hand washing) *to elicit cooperation and decrease anxiety.* • Provide emotional support for patient and family.	• Assist patient and family in setting realistic expectations for patient's progress. • Consider psychiatric evaluation for patients and families who exhibit symptoms of posttraumatic stress disorder.	• Provide ways for patient and family to maintain contact with hospital personnel after discharge *to promote continuity of care and minimize anxiety.* • Consider referral to support group. • Plan counseling if needed.

NURSING DIAGNOSIS   **Disturbed body image** *related to* disfigurement secondary to burn *as manifested by* verbalized negative comments about appearance, unwillingness to look at self or participate in self-care.

• Realistic goals regarding future lifestyle • Acceptance of altered body image	• Reassure patient and family that swelling will subside in 2-4 days *so patient realizes that it is not permanent.*	• Plan for family interaction *to foster feeling of support and reduce sense of isolation.* • Explain expected appearance during treatments *to decrease misconceptions.* • Be realistic and positive during interventions. • Set goals within limitations *so patient can feel a sense of accomplishment.*	• Assess need for and provide means of professional counseling (psychologic and vocational) if appropriate *to reduce impact of the burn event on the patient's life.* • Reassure patient that appearance of burn wounds will continue to improve even after healing has taken place.

■ Airway Management

Airway management involves early nasotracheal or endotracheal intubation before the airway is actually compromised. Early intubation eliminates the necessity for emergency tracheostomy after respiratory problems have become apparent. In general the patient with major injuries involving burns to the face and neck requires intubation within 1 to 2 hours after burn injury. (Nasotracheal and endotracheal intubations are discussed in Chapter 64.) After intubation, the patient may be placed on ventilatory assistance, and the delivered oxygen concentration is determined by assessing ABG values. Extubation may be indicated when the edema resolves, usually 3 to 6 days after burn injury, unless severe inhalation injury is involved. Escharotomies of the chest wall may be needed to relieve respiratory distress secondary to circumferential, full-thickness burns of the neck and trunk.

Within 6 to 12 hours after injury in which smoke inhalation is probable, a fiberoptic bronchoscopy is performed to assess the lower respiratory tract. Significant findings include the appearance of carbonaceous material, mucosal edema, vesicles, erythema, hemorrhage, and ulceration.

Treatment of inhalation injury includes administration of humidified air and 100% oxygen as required. The patient should be placed in a high Fowler's position (unless contraindicated by a possible spinal injury), encouraged to cough and deep breathe every hour, repositioned every 1 to 2 hours, given chest physiotherapy, and suctioned as necessary. If respiratory failure is impending, nasotracheal or endotracheal intubation should be performed and the patient should be supported with mechanical ventilation. Positive end-expiratory pressure (PEEP) may be used to prevent collapse of the alveoli and progressive respiratory failure (see Chapter 64). Bronchodilators may be administered intravenously to treat severe bronchospasm. CO poisoning is treated by administering 100% O_2 until the carboxyhemoglobin levels return to normal. Hyperbaric oxygen therapy is contraindicated.

■ Fluid Therapy

As soon as the patient arrives at a health care facility, at least one (and usually two) large-bore intravenous (IV) replacement line is secured, preferably by percutaneous puncture. If this is not feasible, a jugular, subclavian, or femoral line is inserted through unburned or even burned tissue. A cutdown is a final measure but is rarely used because of the high incidence of infection and sepsis. It is critical to establish IV access that can accommodate large volumes of fluid.

The extent of an adult's burn wound should be assessed using the rule of nines (see Fig. 24-4). This universal standard will allow for the accurate estimation of fluid resuscitation requirements.

IV fluid therapy is usually instituted in the patient with burns greater than 15% TBSA. The type of fluid replacement is determined by size and depth of burn, age of the patient, and individual considerations such as dehydration in the preburn state or preexisting chronic illness. Each burn center has a preference for a replacement regimen. Fluid replacement is accomplished with crystalloid solutions (physiologic saline, lactated Ringer's, or 5% dextrose and saline), colloids (albumin, dextran, or other commercially prepared solutions), or a combination of the two.

Of the formulas that are used for fluid replacement, the Brooke and Parkland (Baxter) formulas are the most commonly used (Tables 24-11 and 24-12). It is important to remember that all formulas are estimates and must be titrated based on the patient's physical response. The Parkland formula is widely used in the United States because it is easy to calculate and monitor using the patient's weight, and it provides a reliable method of fluid replacement for most patients.[10]

Colloidal solutions (e.g., Hespan, albumin) are also routinely given. The amount is calculated based on the patient's body weight, which predicts the replacement volume (e.g., 0.3 to 0.5 ml/kg/% burn). Colloid administration is beneficial when capillary permeability returns to normal or near normal. After this time, the plasma remains in the vascular space and expands the circulating volume.

TABLE 24-12   Fluid Resuscitation with the Parkland (Baxter) Formula*

Formula

4 ml lactated Ringer's solution
per
kg body weight
per
% TBSA burn
= total fluid requirements for first 24 hr after burn

Application

½ of total in first 8 hr
¼ of total in second 8 hr
¼ of total in third 8 hr

Example

For a 70 kg patient with a 50% TBSA burn:

4 ml × 70 kg × 50% TBSA burn = 14,000 ml
= 14 L in 24 hr

½ of total in first 8 hr	= 7000 ml (875 ml/hr)
¼ of total in second 8 hr	= 3500 ml (436 ml/hr)
¼ of total in third 8 hr	= 3500 ml (436 ml/hr)

*Formulas are guidelines. Fluid is administered at a rate to produce 30 to 50 ml of urine output per hour.
TBSA, Total body surface area.

TABLE 24-11   Formulas for Estimating Fluid Replacement of an Adult Burn Patient

FORMULA	FIRST 24 HOURS CRYSTALLOIDS	SECOND 24 HOURS COLLOIDS	GLUCOSE IN WATER
Brooke (modified)	Lactated Ringer's solution: 2.0 ml/kg/% burn; ½ given during first 8 hr; ½ given during next 16 hr	0.3 to 0.5 ml/kg/% burn	Amount to replace estimated evaporative losses
Parkland (Baxter)	Lactated Ringer's solution: 4 ml/kg/% burn; ½ given first 8 hr; ¼ given each next 8 hr	20%-60% of calculated plasma volume	Amount to replace estimated evaporative losses

Assessment of the adequacy of fluid replacement is best made by use of more than one parameter. Urinary output is the most commonly used parameter. Assessment parameters include the following:

1. Urine output: 30 to 50 ml/hr in an adult; 75 to 100 ml/hr for electrical burn in an adult.
2. Cardiopulmonary factors: BP (systolic greater than 90 to 100 mm Hg), pulse rate (less than 120), respiration (16 to 20 breaths per minute). BP is most appropriately measured by an arterial line. Peripheral measurement is often invalid because of vasoconstriction and edema.
3. Sensorium: alert and oriented to time, place, and person.

■ Wound Care

Wound care should be delayed until a patent airway, adequate circulation, and adequate fluid replacement have been established. Full-thickness wounds will be dry and waxy white to dark brown/black and will have little to no sensation because nerve endings have been destroyed. Partial-thickness wounds are pink to cherry-red and wet and shiny with serous exudate. These wounds may or may not have intact blisters and are painful when touched or exposed to air.

Cleansing and debridement can be done in a hydrotherapy tub, cart shower (Fig. 24-8), shower, or bed. **Debridement** may need to be done in the operating room (OR) (Fig. 24-9). During these procedures, loose, necrotic skin is removed. Care should be taken to accomplish this procedure as quickly and effectively as possible. Patients may find the procedure to be both psychologically and physically demanding. Immersion in a tank for longer than 20 to 30 minutes can cause electrolyte loss from open burned areas. Prolonged immersion can lead to chilling after the bath and cross-contamination of wounds from one area of the body to another. Because of these factors, some institutions do

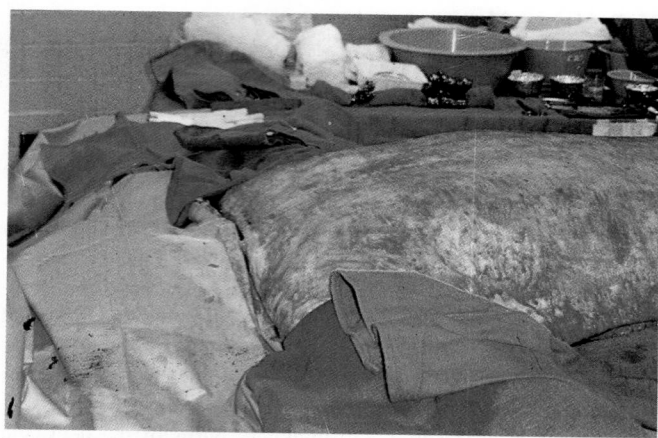

FIG. 24-9 Operative debridement of full-thickness burns is necessary to prepare the wound for grafting.

not submerge the patient. Instead the patient can be showered. The water does not need to be sterile, and tap water not exceeding 104° F (40° C) is acceptable. Because pathogenic organisms are present on the burn wound, a surgical detergent, disinfectant, or cleansing agent may be used. The patient may be bathed two times daily to limit the amount of bacterial growth. However, that degree of frequency may be too painful and psychologically demanding for many patients. A once-daily bath or shower followed by a dressing change in the patient's room is a popular alternative in many burn centers.

Infection is the most serious threat to further tissue injury and possible sepsis.[11] Survival is directly related to prevention of wound contamination. The source of infection in burn wounds is the patient's own flora, predominantly from the skin, respiratory tract, and gastrointestinal (GI) tract. The prevention of cross-contamination from one patient to another is a priority for nursing care.

Two types of wound treatment used to control infection are the open method and the use of multiple dressing changes. In the *open method* the patient's burn is covered with a topical antibiotic and has no dressing over the wound. In the *multiple dressing changes* method sterile gauze dressings are impregnated with or laid over a topical antibiotic. These dressings may be changed two to three times every 24 hours to once every three days.

When the patient's wounds are exposed, the staff must wear disposable hats, masks, gowns, and gloves. When removing dressings and washing the wound, the nurse should use nonsterile, disposable gloves. Sterile gloves are used when applying ointments and sterile dressings. In addition, the room must be kept warm (approximately 85° F [29.4° C]). All attire is changed before the nurse treats another patient. Careful hand washing is also required to prevent cross-contamination. After the patient has been treated in the tub, cart shower, or shower, the equipment is disinfected with a chemical preparation.

Coverage is the primary goal for burn wounds.[12] Because there is rarely enough unburned skin in the major burn patient for immediate skin grafting, other temporary wound closure methods are used. *Allograft* or *homograft skin* (usually from cadavers) is commonly used (Table 24-13). However, rejection eventually occurs because the patient's immune system reacts against the foreign substance.

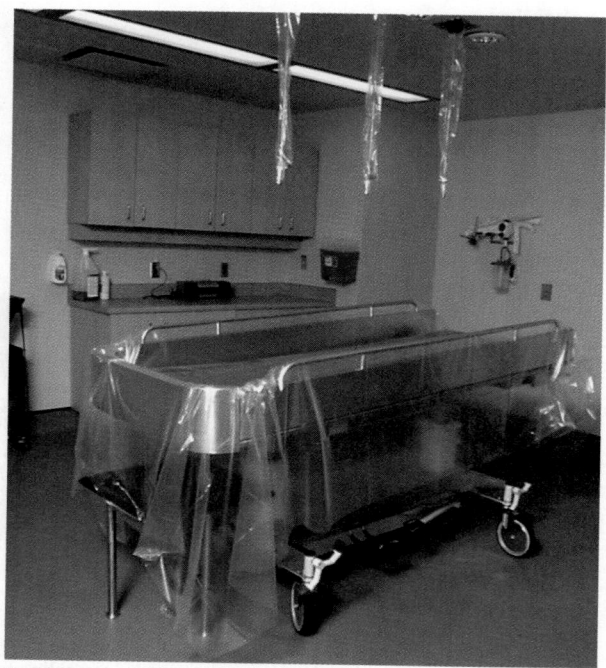

FIG. 24-8 Hydrotherapy cart shower. Bathing presents an opportunity for physical therapy as well as wound care.

TABLE 24-13 Sources of Grafts

SOURCE	GRAFT NAME	COVERAGE
Porcine skin	Heterograft or xenograft (different species)	Temporary (3 days to 2 wk)
Cadaveric skin	Homograft or allograft (same species)	Temporary (3 days to 2 wk)
Patient's own skin	Autograft	Permanent
Patient's own skin and cell culture	Cultured epithelial autograft (CEA)	Permanent

■ Other Care Measures

Care of special areas is initiated by the nurse. The face is highly vascular and subject to a greater amount of edema. Facial care is performed by the open method because facial dressings cause disorientation and confusion. Eye care for corneal burns or edema is done with slightly warmed physiologic saline rinses as often as every hour. An ophthalmology examination should occur soon after admission for all patients with facial burns.[13] Periorbital edema can prevent opening of the eyes. This can be frightening to the patient. The nurse must provide assurance that the swelling is not permanent and that vision will soon be restored. Instillation of methylcellulose drops or artificial tears into the eyes for moisture provides additional comfort and prevents corneal abrasions.

Hands and arms should be extended and elevated on pillows or in slings to minimize edema. Splints may need to be applied to burned hands and feet to maintain them in functional positions.

Ears should be kept free of pressure because of their poor vascularization and predisposition to infection. The patient with ear burns should not use pillows because of the danger of the burned ear sticking to the pillowcase, thereby causing bleeding, pain, or infection of the ear cartilage. The patient's head can be elevated using a donut roll, being careful to avoid pressure necrosis. The patient with neck burns cannot use pillows but should be hyperextended to prevent wound contraction.

The perineum must be kept as clean and dry as possible. In addition to providing hourly urine outputs, an indwelling catheter prevents urine contamination of the bowel and perineal area. Frequent perineal and catheter care in the presence or absence of a perineal burn wound is essential.

Routine laboratory tests are performed initially and serially to monitor electrolyte balance. Blood for measurement of ABGs may be drawn to determine adequacy of ventilation and perfusion.

Physical therapy is begun immediately, sometimes during hydrotherapy. Early range-of-motion (ROM) exercises are necessary to facilitate mobilization of the extravasated fluid back into the vascular bed. Exercise of body parts also maintains function, prevents contracture, and reassures the patient that movement is still possible.

■ Drug Therapy

Analgesics and Sedatives. Analgesics are ordered to promote patient comfort. Early in the postburn period, IV pain medications should be given because (1) GI function is slowed or impaired because of shock or paralytic ileus, and (2) intramuscular (IM) injections will not be absorbed adequately in burned or edematous areas, causing pooling of medications in the tissues. When fluid mobilization begins, the patient could be inadvertently overdosed from the interstitial accumulation of previous IM medications.

Common narcotics used for pain control are listed in Table 24-14. The need for analgesia must be evaluated. The drug of choice for pain control is morphine, but meperidine and methadone may also be used. When given appropriately, these drugs provide adequate pain control and a sedative effect. The patient may be in great pain

TABLE 24-14 Drug Therapy: Drugs Commonly Used in Burn Treatment

TYPES AND NAMES OF DRUGS	PURPOSE
Nutritional Support	
Vitamins A, C, E, and multivitamins	Promotes wound healing
Minerals: zinc, folate, iron (ferrous sulfate, ferrous gluconate)	Promotes cellular integrity and hemoglobin formation
Analgesia and Sedative	
morphine	Diminishes pain perception
meperidine (Demerol)	Diminishes pain perception
fentanyl (Sublimaze)	Diminishes pain perception
buprenorphine (Buprenex)	Diminishes pain perception
haloperidol (Haldol)	Produces antipsychotic and sedative effects, promotes sleep
lorazepam (Ativan)	Diminishes anxiety
midazolam (Versed)	Has short-acting amnestic properties
Gastrointestinal Support	
ranitidine (Zantac)	Decreases incidence of Curling's ulcer
nystatin (Mycostatin)	Prevents overgrowth of *Candida albicans* in oral mucosa
Mylanta, Maalox	Neutralizes stomach acid

with large burns (especially burns that are predominantly partial-thickness burns).

Tetanus Immunization. Tetanus toxoid is given routinely to all burn patients because of the likelihood of anaerobic burn-wound contamination. In the absence of active immunization within 10 years before the burn injury, tetanus immunoglobulin should be administered.

Antimicrobial Agents. After the wound is cleansed, topical agents are applied (Fig. 24-10) and may be covered with a light dressing or left open to air. Systemic antibiotics are not usually used in controlling burn wound flora, especially after 48 hours, because there is little or no blood supply to the burn eschar and consequently there is little delivery of the antibiotic to the wound. Topical burn agents penetrate the eschar, thereby inhibiting bacterial invasion of the wound (Table 24-15). Silver sulfadiazine (Silvadene) is commonly used because it is effective, and unlike mafenide acetate (Sulfamylon), it is painless. Silver-impregnated

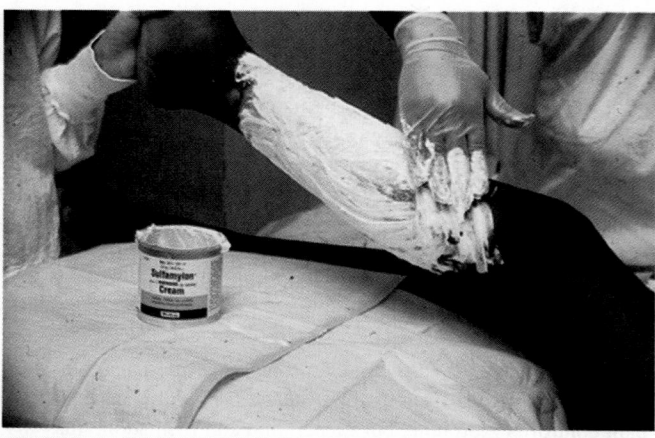

FIG. 24-10 Patient being treated with mafenide (Sulfamylon).

dressings that can be left on for up to 3 days are used in some burn units. They are effective against many organisms. Systemic sepsis remains a leading cause of death in the patient with major burns because resistant organisms develop with exposure of bacteria to topical agents over time. Most burn centers use one topical agent almost exclusively and change to another at the first sign of microbial resistance. Systemic antibiotic therapy is initiated when the clinical diagnosis of invasive burn wound sepsis is made or when some other source of sepsis is identified (e.g., pneumonia).

Frequently superinfections develop in the patient's mucous membranes (mouth and genitalia) as a result of antibiotic therapy and low resistance in the host. The offending organism is usually *Candida albicans.* Oral infection is treated with nystatin (Mycostatin) mouthwash. When a normal diet is resumed, yogurt or *Lactobacillus* (Lactinex) may be given by mouth to reintroduce the normal intestinal flora that have been destroyed by antibiotic therapy.

■ Nutritional Therapy

Fluid replacement takes priority over nutritional needs in the initial emergent phase. The patient with large burns frequently develops paralytic ileus within a few hours as a result of the body's response to major trauma. A nasogastric tube is inserted and connected to low intermittent suction for decompression. When bowel sounds return at 48 to 72 hours after injury, oral intake can be initiated beginning with clear liquids and progressing to a diet high in protein and calories.

A **hypermetabolic state** proportional to the size of the wound is observed. Resting metabolic expenditure may be increased by 50% to 100% above normal in patients with major burns. Core temperature is elevated. Plasma catecholamines, which stimulate heat production, are increased. Massive catabolism can occur and is characterized by protein breakdown and increased gluconeogenesis. Caloric needs are often in the 5000 kcal per day range. Failure to supply adequate calories and protein leads to malnutrition and delayed healing. The patient is not freely given water

TABLE 24-15	Drug Therapy — Topical Antibiotic Therapy		
TOPICAL	**INDICATIONS**	**ADVANTAGES**	**DISADVANTAGES**
silver sulfadiazine (Silvadene)	Gram-positive and gram-negative organisms, *Candida albicans*	Wide-spectrum antibacterial action No limit to motion Can use light or no dressings Fast, painless, easy to apply	Possible depression of granulocyte formation Possible allergic reaction to sulfa
mafenide acetate (Sulfamylon)	Gram-positive and gram-negative organisms Most anaerobes Ear burns Electrical burns	Wide-spectrum antibacterial action Most effective topical antibiotic Penetrates eschar, cartilage Open treatment possible	Possible pain on application Acid-base disturbance because it is a carbonic anhydrase inhibitor Possible allergic reaction to sulfa
bacitracin	Superficial burns Staphylococcal organisms Facial burns	Can be safely used on autografts and homografts Nonpainful Inexpensive Requires only 1-time daily application	May cause itching, rash
mupirocin (Bactroban)	Effective against many organisms resistant to silver sulfadiazine Use based on sensitivity results	Painless Safe for use on CEA Inhibits bacterial and protein synthesis	Possible itching, burning, rash Potential renal toxicity if used over large area

CEA, Cultured epithelial autograft.

to drink. Rather, calorie-containing liquids are given because of the great need for calories.

Major advances have been made in the area of liquid nutritional supplementation (see Chapter 39). A thin latex feeding tube can be advanced by fluoroscopic guidance into the duodenum, bypassing the stomach. This allows for quicker absorption of nutrients and a decrease in the nausea and vomiting associated with high-volume tube feedings into the stomach. The patient can be maintained on a more continuous feeding schedule, which does not have to be interrupted by surgical interventions (e.g., debridement, grafting). Because the liquid goes past the pyloric sphincter, the patient does not have to remain without food or water for extended periods as is required when the tube is in the stomach. Early and continuous enteral feeding promotes optimal conditions for wound healing and immunocompetence. Because of their direct effect on morbidity and mortality, early, continuous enteral feedings are recommended after burn injury.

Supplemental vitamins and iron may be given as early as the emergent phase. However, the need for these supplements usually does not occur until the acute phase.

ACUTE PHASE

The *acute phase* begins with the mobilization of extracellular fluid and subsequent diuresis. The acute phase is concluded when the burned area is completely covered by skin grafts or when the wounds are healed. This may take weeks or many months.

Pathophysiology

Burn injury involves pathophysiologic changes in many body systems. Diuresis from fluid mobilization occurs, and the patient is no longer grossly edematous. Areas that are full- or partial-thickness burns are more evident than in the emergent phase. Bowel sounds return. The patient is now aware of the enormity of body changes. Healing begins when WBCs have surrounded the burn wound and phagocytosis occurs. Necrotic tissue begins to slough. Fibroblasts lay down matrices of the collagen precursors that eventually form granulation tissue. Kept free from infection, a partial-thickness burn wound will heal from the edges and from below. However, full-thickness burn wounds, unless extremely small, must be covered by skin grafts. Often, healing time and length of hospitalization are decreased by early excision and grafting.[14]

Clinical Manifestations

Partial-thickness wounds form eschar that begins separating fairly soon after injury. Once the partial-thickness eschar is removed, epithelialization begins at the wound margins and appears as red or pink scar tissue. The epithelial buds eventually close in the wound, and the wound heals spontaneously without surgical intervention. This is expected to occur in 10 to 14 days.

Margins of full-thickness eschar take longer to separate than partial-thickness eschar, allowing for debridement of the wound. Full-thickness wounds require surgical debridement and skin grafting to speed the healing process.

Laboratory Values

Because the body is attempting to reestablish fluid and electrolyte homeostasis in the initial acute phase, it is important to follow serum electrolyte levels closely.

Sodium. *Hyponatremia* can occur if hydrotherapy is too lengthy (usually longer than 20 to 30 minutes), because the hypo-

tonicity of the bath water pulls sodium from the open burn areas. Other causes of hyponatremia include excessive GI drainage, diarrhea, and excessive water intake. Manifestations of hyponatremia include weakness, dizziness, muscle cramps, fatigue, headache, tachycardia, and confusion. The burn patient may also develop a dilutional hyponatremia called *water intoxication.* To avoid this condition, the patient should drink fluids other than water, such as juice, soft drinks, or nutritional supplements.

Hypernatremia may be seen following successful fluid replacement if copious amounts of hypertonic solutions were required. Other causes of hypernatremia include improper tube feeding therapy or inappropriate fluid administration. Manifestations of hypernatremia include thirst; dried, furry tongue; lethargy; confusion; and possibly seizures.

Potassium. *Hyperkalemia* is noted if the patient has renal failure, adrenocortical insufficiency, or massive deep muscle injury with large amounts of potassium released from damaged cells. Cardiac arrhythmias and ventricular failure can occur with excessive elevations. Muscle weakness and electrocardiographic changes are observed clinically (see Chapter 16).

Hypokalemia can be observed with lengthy hydrotherapy. Other causes of this deficit include vomiting, diarrhea, prolonged GI suction, and prolonged IV therapy without potassium supplementation. Constant potassium losses occur through the burn wound.

Complications

Infection. The body's first line of defense, the skin, has been destroyed by burn injury. Pathogens often proliferate before phagocytosis has adequately begun. If the bacterial density at the junction of the eschar with underlying viable tissue rises to greater than 10^5/g of tissue, the patient has a wound infection. In the presence of an infection, localized inflammation, induration, and suppuration can be seen at the burn wound margins. Partial-thickness burns can become full-thickness wounds in the presence of infection. A histologic examination of a burn-wound biopsy is the most reliable means of differentiating colonization of nonviable tissue from invasive infection of viable tissue. Invasive wound infections may be treated with systemic or topical antibiotics based on the culture results.

Wound infection may progress to transient bacteremia from wound manipulation (e.g., after debridement and hydrotherapy). The patient may develop sepsis. Manifestations of sepsis include an elevated temperature, increased pulse and respiratory rate, decreased BP, and decreased urine output. There may be mild confusion, chills, malaise, and loss of appetite. The WBC count will usually be between 10,000/μl (10 × 10^9/L) and 20,000/μl (20 × 10^9/L). There are functional defects in the WBCs, and the patient remains immunosuppressed for a period after the burn injury. The causative organisms of sepsis are usually gram-negative bacteria (e.g., *Pseudomonas, Proteus* organisms), putting the patient at further risk for septic shock.

When sepsis is suspected, cultures should be obtained immediately from all possible sources: urine, oropharynx, sputum, IV site, and wound. However, treatment should not be delayed pending results of the culture and sensitivity studies. Therapy will begin with antibiotics appropriate for the usual residual flora of the particular burn center. The topical antibiotic that is used may be continued or may be changed to another agent. At this stage, the patient's condition is critical, requiring close monitoring of vital signs.

Cardiovascular and Respiratory Systems. The same cardiovascular and respiratory system complications can be present in the emergent phase and may continue into the acute phase of care.

Neurologic System. Neurologically, the patient usually has no physically based problems unless severe hypoxia from respiratory injuries or complications from electrical injuries occur. However, some patients may demonstrate certain behaviors that are not completely understood. The patient can become extremely disoriented, may withdraw or become combative, and may have hallucinations and frequent nightmare-like episodes. Delirium is more acute at night and occurs more often in the older patient. This is a transient state lasting from a day or two to several weeks. Various causes have been considered, including electrolyte imbalance, stress, cerebral edema, sepsis, intensive care unit (ICU) psychosis syndrome, and the use of analgesics and antianxiety drugs.

Musculoskeletal System. The musculoskeletal system is especially watched for complications during the acute phase. As the burns begin to heal and scar tissue forms, the skin is less supple and pliant. ROM may be limited, and contractures can occur. Because of pain, the patient will prefer to assume a flexed position for comfort. Splinting can be beneficial to prevent contracture formation.

Gastrointestinal System. The GI system also exhibits complications during this phase. Adynamic ileus results from sepsis. However, diarrhea is more commonly present than ileus and can be caused by the use of supplemental feedings or antibiotics. Constipation can occur as a side effect of narcotic analgesics, decreased mobility, and a low-fiber diet. *Curling's ulcer,* a type of gastroduodenal ulcer characterized by diffuse superficial lesions, including mucosal erosion, is caused by a generalized stress response resulting in decreased production of mucus and increased gastric acid secretion. This condition is also due to the decreased blood flow to the GI tract during the hypovolemic shock phase. The best treatment of Curling's ulcer is prevention. The prophylactic use of antacids and H_2-histamine blockers (e.g., ranitidine [Zantac], cimetidine [Tagamet]) inhibits histamine and stimulation of hydrochloric acid (HCl) secretion. Many patients with major burns also have occult blood in their stools during the acute phase.

Endocrine System. An increase in blood glucose levels may be seen transiently because of stress-mediated cortisol and catecholamine release resulting in increased mobilization of glycogen stores, gluconeogenesis, and subsequent production of glucose. There is also an increase in insulin production and release. However, insulin's effectiveness is decreased because of relative insulin insensitivity, leading to an elevated blood glucose level. Later, hyperglycemia can be caused by the increased caloric intake necessary to meet some patients' metabolic requirements. When this occurs, the treatment is supplemental insulin, not decreased feeding. Serum glucose is checked frequently and an appropriate amount of insulin is given if hyperglycemia is present. Glucometers may be used to assess blood glucose; serum glucose samples are more accurate than capillary blood analysis by glucometer. As the patient's metabolic demands are met and less stress is placed on the entire system, this stress-induced condition is reversed.

NURSING and COLLABORATIVE MANAGEMENT ACUTE PHASE

The predominant therapeutic interventions in the acute phase are (1) wound care, (2) excision and grafting, (3) pain management, (4) physical and occupational therapy, (5) nutritional therapy, and (6) psychosocial care.

■ Wound Care

Goals of wound care are to (1) cleanse and debride the area of necrotic tissue and debris that would promote bacterial growth, (2) minimize further destruction of viable skin, (3) promote wound reepithelialization and/or success of skin grafting, and (4) promote patient comfort.

Wound care consists of daily observation, assessment, cleansing, and debridement. Wound care begun in the emergent phase continues during the acute phase. Debridement, dressing changes, topical antibiotic therapy, graft care, and donor site care may be performed from two to three times daily or once every few days. Enzymatic debriders may be used for the **enzymatic debridement** of burn wounds (Table 24-16). Appropriate coverage of the

TABLE 24-16 Drug Therapy

Enzymatic Debriders Used in Burn Therapy

TOPICAL	INDICATIONS	ADVANTAGES	DISADVANTAGES
collagenase (Santyl)	Aggressive debridement of necrotic tissue on deep partial-thickness wound	Does not harm healthy tissue Digests denatured collagen in devitalized tissue	Limited antimicrobial coverage Rare allergic sensitivity Expensive Effective only in narrow pH range of 6-8 Wound bed must be neutralized with Polysporin powder
fibrinolysin/ desoxyribonuclease (Elase)	Debridement of devitalized tissue in partial-thickness wound	Attacks denatured DNA and fibrin in necrotic wounds Can be applied one time daily Compatible with other topicals	Possible burning Can harm healthy tissue Expensive
Accuzyme	Debridement of necrotic tissue on partial-thickness wound Liquefaction of purulent drainage	Derived from papaya—digests nonviable protein matter Will not harm healthy tissue Compatible with other topicals	Burning Stinging sensation Expensive

graft (if it is not kept open to air) should include fine-mesh gauze next to the graft followed by middle and outer dressings. Fine-mesh, absorbent gauze dressings have a greasy base that keeps the gauze from adhering to graft sites.

Sheet skin grafts must be kept free of *blebs* (collections of serous fluid). Blebs prevent the graft from interfacing and growing to the wound itself. Evacuation of blebs is done by aspiration with a tuberculin syringe or by pricking or cutting the peripheral margin of the bleb and rolling (with a sterile swab) the fluid from the center of the bleb to the exit site. The bleb should never be rolled to the edge of the graft. This serves only to separate the adherent graft from the wound. The rolling of blebs may need to be done frequently as ordered by the health care provider.

Donor site care has been controversial throughout the years. The goals of care are to promote rapid healing, decrease pain at the donor site, and prevent infection. Many new methods are being evaluated. The average healing time for a donor site is 10 to 14 days. Several of the newer methods potentially can decrease this healing time, which would facilitate earlier reharvesting of skin at the site. There are many options for donor site dressings. Some centers use a transparent dressing (e.g., Opsite, Tegaderm, Biobrane) that adheres to the periphery of the donor site. This permits an occlusive yet visible wound. Pigskin (xenograft), silver sulfadiazene (Silvadene), and calcium alginate dressings are also used, with varying degrees of success. Another type of dressing is Acticoat, which releases silver; silver has an antimicrobial effect. Each donor site dressing has specific nursing care aspects, and use varies among centers. (Dressings are discussed in Chapter 12 and Table 12-17.)

■ Excision and Grafting

Current therapeutic management of burn wounds involves early removal of the necrotic tissue followed by application of split-thickness autograft skin. This therapy has changed the management and mortality rate of burn patients. In the past, patients with major burns had low rates of survival because healing and wound coverage took so long that the patient usually died of infection or malnutrition. Now, mortality rates have been greatly reduced and morbidity decreased by early intervention.[15] Candidates for early excision and grafting are those with a stable cardiovascular system after initial fluid resuscitation.

During the procedure of **excision and grafting,** eschar is removed down to the subcutaneous tissue or fascia, depending on the degree of injury. A graft is then placed on clean, viable tissue to achieve good adherence. Hemostasis is achieved by pressure and application of topical thrombin or epinephrine, after which the wound is covered with *autograft* (person's own) skin (see Table 24-13). With early excision, function is restored and scar tissue formation is minimized. Because the dead tissue is planed off until viable tissue is reached, extensive bleeding is expected to occur, which may pose a problem when grafting is performed. Clots between the graft and the wound keep the graft from adhering to the wound. Appropriate nursing interventions can help identify and manage excessive postoperative bleeding.

Donor skin is taken from the patient for grafting by means of a dermatome, which removes a thin layer (split-thickness) of skin from an unburned site (Fig. 24-11). The donor skin can be meshed to allow for greater wound coverage, or it may be applied as a sheet graft for a better cosmetic result when grafting the face, neck, and hands.

Cultured Epithelial Autografts. In the patient with large body surface area burns, limited unburned skin may be available as a donor site for grafting, and available skin may also be unsuitable for harvesting. **Cultured epithelial autograft** (CEA) is one method to obtain skin tissue from a person with limited available

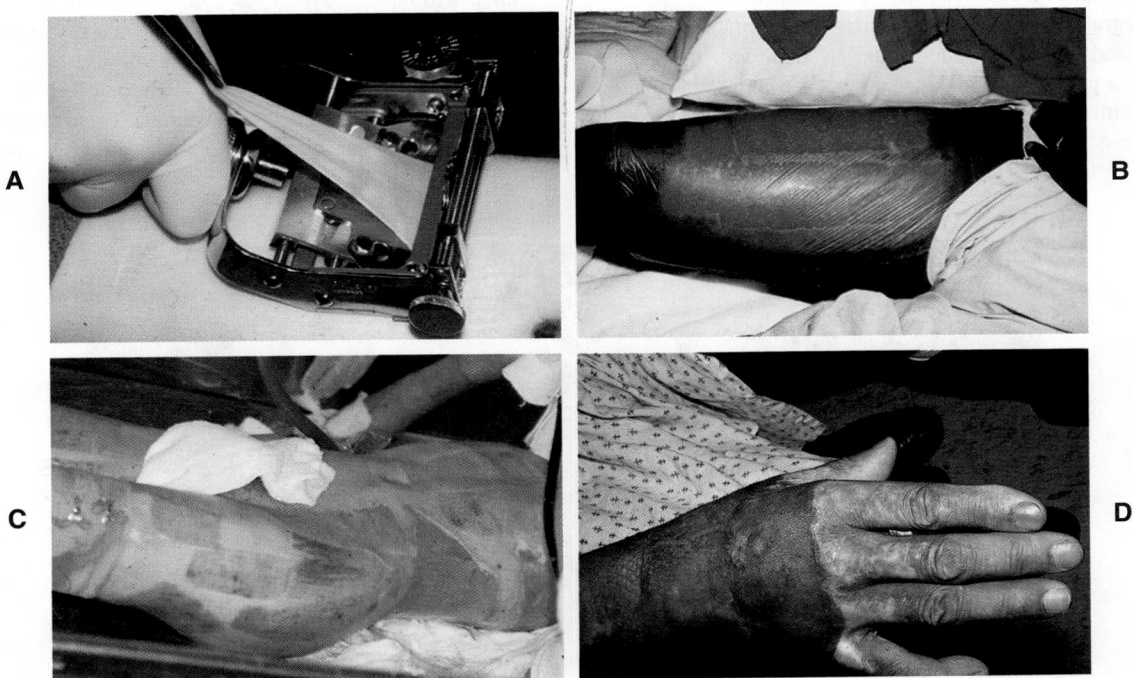

FIG. 24-11 A, The surgeon harvests skin from a patient's thigh using a dermatome. B, Appearance of donor site after harvesting split-thickness skin graft. Donor site is covered with a transparent occlusive dressing. C, Healed donor sites. D, Healed split-thickness skin graft to the hand.

skin for harvesting.[16] CEA is grown from biopsies obtained from the patient's own skin. The initial step in this process involves taking one or two small (2 to 3 cm long by 1 cm wide) biopsy specimens from unburned skin (usually the groin or axilla).

This procedure is performed as soon as possible after the patient has been identified as a candidate for this type of grafting. It can usually be done at the bedside using local anesthesia. The specimen is sent to a commercial laboratory where the skin biopsy specimens are disaggregated into single cells and are subsequently cultivated in a culture medium that contains epidermal growth factor. During the following 18 to 25 days, the originally cultivated keratinocytes expand up to 10,000 times until they form confluent sheets that can be used as skin grafts. The cultured skin is returned to the burn center where it is placed on the patient's excised burn wounds. Because CEA grafts are only epidermal cells, meticulous care is required to prevent shearing injury or infection.

CEA grafts generate permanent skin coverage because they originate from the patient's own cells. CEA is applied surgically using the same procedure as with split-thickness autografts. CEA grafts generally form a seamless, smooth replacement skin tissue (Fig. 24-12). This type of skin graft has played an important role in the survival of the patient with major burns with limited skin for donor harvesting. In 24 days enough CEA can be generated to cover the entire body surface. Problems related to CEA include thin, friable skin (resulting from lack of dermal cells) and contracture development.

Artificial Skin. It has been recognized that any successful **artificial skin** must replace all functions of the skin and consist of both a dermal and an epidermal portion. The Integra artificial skin dermal regeneration template is an example of one of the newest skin replacement systems available in burn care. It is indicated for use in postexcisional treatment of life-threatening full-thickness or deep partial-thickness burn wounds where conventional autograft is not available or advisable. It has also been used for reconstructive burn surgery procedures.

The Integra artificial skin has a bilayer membrane composed of dermis and silicone.[16] The wound is debrided, the bilayer membrane is placed dermal layer down first, and the wound is wrapped with dressings. The dermal layer functions as a biodegradable template that induces organized regeneration of new dermis by the body. The silicone layer remains intact as the dermal layer degrades. Final closure of the burn wound takes place several weeks later when thin epidermal autografts become available. The silicone is removed during surgery and replaced by the epidermal autografts.

Several other products are currently being investigated and evaluated in burn centers throughout North America, including Alloderm, a nonimmunogenic dermal transplant, and LifeSkin, a cultured composite autograft. Further evaluation must take place to determine the use and effectiveness of these products in burn wound management.

■ Pain Management

One of the most critical functions a nurse performs is individualized and consistent pain assessment and management. Almost every intervention that is performed for the patient causes pain. However, patients may experience moments of relative comfort if they receive adequate analgesia. The nurse must understand the physiologic and psychologic bases of pain in order to intervene with actions that may be helpful (see Chapter 9). Encouraging the patient to ventilate feelings of anger, hostility, and frustration can be a useful strategy. It is important to assess each patient's pain individually and consistently.

The nurse may use several interventions to help patients cope with their pain. These interventions can also help the nurse cope with interventions that cause pain. First, it is helpful to get an order for a dosage range of an opioid (e.g., morphine sulfate 5 to 10 mg IV) every 1 to 3 hours for pain. When the order is written this way, it allows the nurse some freedom to medicate the patient according to his or her response to the drug. That is, the nurse may find that giving morphine 5 mg every hour works better than giving 10 mg every 3 hours. Any strategy should include the patient's input if alert because it gives the patient a sense of control over the pain. If the patient is unable to participate, the nurse will have to assess response to pain medication by physiologic parameters (i.e., heart rate, BP, and respiratory rate).

The second intervention involves the use of several drugs in combination such as morphine with haloperidol (Haldol), lorazepam (Ativan), diazepam (Valium), or midazolam (Versed). The effect of midazolam is short-term amnesia, so if it is given

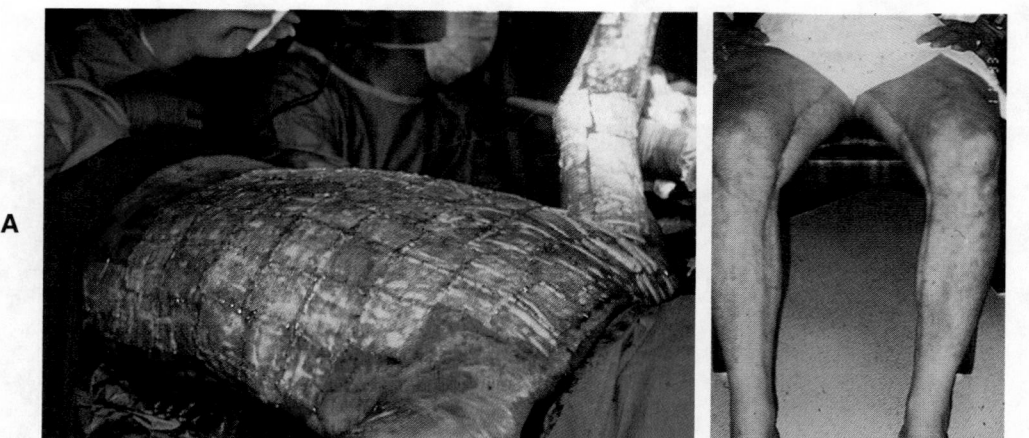

FIG. 24-12 Patient with cultured epithelial autograft (CEA). **A,** Intraoperative application of cultured epithelial autograft. **B,** Appearance of healed cultured epithelial autograft.

15 to 20 minutes before a dressing change, the patient will not necessarily recall the event. Midazolam lasts about 30 to 60 minutes after it is administered. Buprenorphine (Buprenex) is another drug that is useful to treat pain. The mechanism of action is not entirely understood, but it is proposed that it exerts its analgesic effect via high-affinity binding to opiate receptors in the central nervous system. It is an opioid antagonist so it cannot be used in combination with other opioid analgesics. Buprenorphine may work well for the patient who does not obtain relief even with high doses of opioids.

A third method of managing pain involves nonpharmacologic strategies such as the use of relaxation tapes, visualization, guided imagery, biofeedback, and meditation (see Chapters 7 and 8). These techniques are used as adjuncts to traditional pharmacologic treatments of pain. They are not meant to be used exclusively to control pain in the burn patient.

Visualization and guided imagery can be helpful to the nurse as well as the patient. These two techniques can take several forms, but the easiest method is for the nurse to ask the patient questions about a favorite hobby or recent vacation. The nurse can then explore these areas further by asking questions that make the patient visualize and describe a favorite hobby or recent vacation. When using this method, both the nurse and the patient must focus on things besides the task at hand (e.g., a dressing change) to keep the conversation flowing. Relaxation tapes can also be helpful, especially when played at night to help the patient fall asleep. The use of these techniques promotes a close nurse-patient relationship and can leave both with a sense of accomplishment.

The most important point to remember about pain management is that the more control the patient has in managing pain, the more successful the chosen strategies. There has been a recent trend toward the use of patient-controlled analgesia (PCA) pumps. An IV solution is made up to contain a certain dose of a narcotic per milliliter (e.g., morphine 2 mg/ml). The patient has a control that can be operated to deliver a preset dose of the IV narcotic. The machine is locked into this dose, so there is no possibility of the patient getting more than what is prescribed. (PCA is discussed in Chapters 9 and 19.)

■ Physical and Occupational Therapy

Rigorous physical therapy in partnership with the physical therapist is imperative to maintain optimal joint function. A good time for exercise is during and after hydrotherapy when the skin is softer and bulky dressings are removed. Passive and active ROM should be performed on all joints. The patient with neck burns should sleep without pillows or with the head hanging slightly over the top of the mattress to encourage hyperextension. Splints should be custom-fitted by the occupational therapist and used to keep joints in functional positions and reexamined frequently to ensure an optimal fit.

■ Nutritional Therapy

The goals of nutritional therapy of the burn patient during the acute phase are to minimize energy expenditure and provide adequate calories and protein to promote healing. The burn patient is in a hypermetabolic and highly catabolic state as a result of the burn injury.[14] Decreasing catecholamine release by minimizing pain, fear, anxiety, and cold can maximize patient comfort and conserve energy. Infection also increases the metabolic rate or expenditure.

Meeting daily caloric requirements is crucial. Estimated caloric needs for 24 hours for the adult can be calculated by the dietitian using one of a number of formulas currently recommended for burn patients.

By the end of the first 72 hours after burn injury, the patient's caloric and nutritional requirements should be met. The alert patient should be encouraged to eat high-protein, high-carbohydrate foods to meet increased caloric needs. Ideally, weight loss should not be more than 10% of preburn weight. Caloric requirements should be recalculated by the dietitian at least biweekly to prevent overfeeding and subsequent weight gain.

Optimally the patient should take a normal diet by mouth as soon as bowel function returns. If this is not possible, a feeding tube can be placed and a complete liquid diet administered. Diet supplements can be given by mouth or IV in the form of total parenteral nutrition if all other options are not effective (see Chapter 39).

If family members wish to bring in the patient's favorite foods, this should be encouraged. Appetite is usually diminished, and constant encouragement may be necessary to achieve adequate intake. The nurse should record the patient's caloric intake daily using calorie count sheets. Patients should also be weighed on a regular basis to monitor progress.

■ Psychosocial Care

The patient and family have many needs for psychosocial support during the often lengthy, unpredictable, and complex course of care. The social worker and nursing staff have important support and counseling roles. Pastoral care may be helpful when requested by patients and their families. (Patient and family emotional needs are discussed on p. 537.)

REHABILITATION PHASE

The *rehabilitation phase* is defined as beginning when the patient's burn wounds are covered with skin or healed and the patient is able to resume a level of self-care activity. This can occur as early as 2 weeks or as long as 2 or 3 months after the burn injury. Goals for this period are to assist the patient in resuming a functional role in society and to accomplish functional and cosmetic reconstruction.

Pathophysiologic Changes and Clinical Manifestations

The burn wound heals either by primary intention or by grafting. Layers of epithelialization begin rebuilding the tissue structure destroyed by the burn injury. Collagen fibers present in the new scar tissue help healing and add strength to weakened areas. After healing, the new skin appears flat and pink. In approximately 4 to 6 weeks the area becomes raised and hyperemic. If adequate ROM is not instituted, the new tissue will shorten, causing a contracture.[17] Mature healing is reached in 6 months to 2 years when suppleness has returned and the pink or red color has faded to a slightly lighter hue than the surrounding unburned tissue. It takes longer for more heavily pigmented skin to regain its dark color because many of the melanocytes are destroyed. Often skin never completely regains its original color. Cosmetics can help even out unequal skin tones.

Scarring has two components: discoloration and contour. The discoloration of scars will fade with time. However, scar tissue tends to develop altered contours; that is, it is no longer flat or slightly raised but becomes elevated and enlarged above the original burn injury area. Pressure can help keep a scar flat. Gentle pressure is maintained on the healed burn with pressure garments.

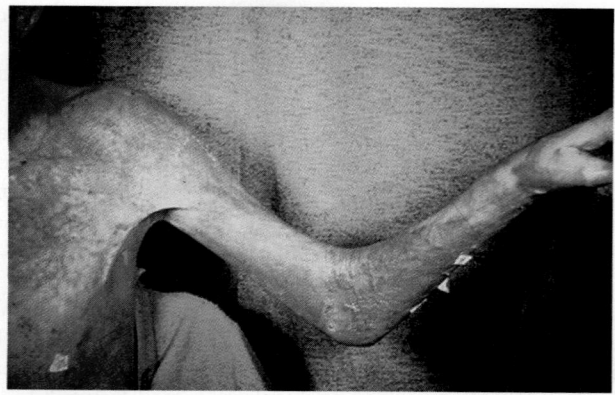

FIG. 24-13 Contracture of the axilla.

These garments are worn up to 24 hours a day for as long as 1 to 2 years after burn injury. They may be removed for short periods while bathing.

The patient may experience discomfort from itching where healing is occurring. Frequent applications of water-based moisturizers and diphenhydramine (Benadryl) help reduce the itching. As "old" epithelium is replaced by new cells, flaking will occur. The newly formed skin is extremely sensitive to trauma. Blisters are likely to form from slight pressure or friction. Additionally, these newly healed areas can be hypersensitive or hyposensitive to cold, heat, and touch. Grafted areas are more likely to be hyposensitive until peripheral nerve regeneration occurs. Healed burn areas must be protected from direct sunlight for 1 year to prevent hyperpigmentation and sunburn injury.

Complications

The most common complications during the rehabilitative phase are skin and joint contractures and hypertrophic scarring (Fig. 24-13). A **contracture** (an abnormal condition of a joint characterized by flexion and fixation) develops as a result of the shortening of scar tissue in the flexor tissues of a joint.[18] Areas that are most susceptible to contracture formation include the anterior and lateral neck areas, axillae, antecubital fossae, fingers, groin areas, popliteal fossae, and ankles. These areas encompass major joints. Not only does the skin over these areas develop contractures, but the underlying tissues such as the ligaments and tendons also have a tendency to shorten in the healing process.

Because of pain, the patient will prefer to assume a flexed position for comfort. This position predisposes the wounds to contracture formation. Positioning, splinting, and exercise should be instituted to minimize this complication. These procedures should be continued until the skin matures. Therapy is aimed at extension of body parts because the flexors are stronger than the extensors. Legs should be wrapped before ambulation after grafting and donor site healing. This pressure prevents blister formation and promotes venous return. Once the skin is completely healed, pressure garments can replace leg wraps to grafted areas.

NURSING *and* COLLABORATIVE MANAGEMENT REHABILITATION PHASE

During the rehabilitation phase, both patient and family are actively learning how to care for the healing wounds. Because the patient may go home with unhealed open areas, instruction will be needed in dressing changes and wound care. An emollient water-based cream (e.g., Vaseline Intensive Care lotion for sensitive skin) should be used routinely on healed areas to keep the skin supple and well moisturized and to decrease itching and flaking. Oral diphenhydramine may be used if itching persists. Cosmetic or reconstructive surgery is often needed following major burns. It is important for the patient to understand the need for or possibility of reconstructive surgery before leaving the hospital.

The role of exercise and appropriate physical therapy cannot be overemphasized. The progression from hydrotherapy to passive ROM, active ROM, stretching, ambulation, and ultimately restoration of function is a lengthy and painful process that lasts for at least 1 year after burn injury. Constant encouragement and reassurance are necessary to maintain a patient's morale. The patient must regard physical and occupational therapy as integral and ongoing parts of treatment and recovery.

Because of the severe psychologic impact of burn injury, health care providers must be sensitive and attuned to the patient's feelings. They play a key role in assisting patients to adjust emotionally by encouraging them to ventilate their fears regarding loss of function, deformity, disfigurement, return to

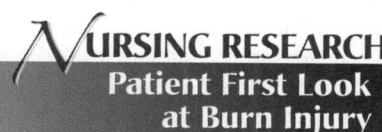

NURSING RESEARCH
Patient First Look at Burn Injury

Citation
Birdsall C, Weinberg K: Adult patients looking at their burn injuries for the first time, *J Burn Care Rehabil* 22:360, 2001.

Purpose
To describe how and when patients look at their burn injury for the first time and to identify qualitative themes that influence this patient response.

Methods
Nurses working in adult burn centers (*n* = 222) in North America completed a questionnaire focusing on how and when patients first see their burn injury, nursing behavior that may or may not influence the patient viewing his or her injury, and qualitative information on the nurse-patient interaction.

Results and Conclusions
The patient is most frequently with a nurse when the injury is first seen. This event is usually not planned or documented. Qualitative data revealed that nurses use verbal and nonverbal cues from patients to determine when they are ready to look at the injury. These cues include a curiosity and interest to see the injury despite some fears. The initial look "just happens," with the timing up to the patient. Family members are often not present at this event. There were no differences in patient response to the injury based on burn location or size of injury.

Implications for Nursing Practice
The approval and ongoing support of nurses can contribute to the patient's feelings of self-worth during the initial viewing of the burn injury. The nurse should be positive, hopeful, and honest in helping the patient through the experience. This event can also become an opportunity for nurses to teach patients about wound care, scar formation, and long-term outcomes.

work, and financial burdens. Care should also be taken to address individual spiritual and cultural needs. Having expressed these fears, patients can then be assisted in a realistic and positive appraisal of the particular situations, emphasizing what they can do, instead of what cannot be done.

An individual's self-esteem is usually adversely affected by a burn injury. In some individuals an overwhelming fear may be the loss of relationships because of perceived or actual physical disfigurement. In a society that values physical beauty, alterations in body image commonly result in psychologic distress. Encouraging appropriate independence, a return to preburn activities, and interactions with other burn survivors will involve the patient in activities that may help restore self-esteem. Counseling should be available after the patient goes home. Patients need reassurance that their feelings during this period of adjustment are normal and that frustration is to be expected as they attempt to resume normal lifestyles.

During this final phase of the patient's recovery, the negative nitrogen balance should have been corrected. However, it is still important to maintain a high-calorie, high-protein diet. The problem with anorexia decreases at this time. As the oral intake increases, tube feedings are gradually tapered and discontinued. The patient with functional limitations associated with eating, such as burn injury to the hands, may need assistance from occupational therapy to obtain devices to correct or lessen the problem. Often all that is necessary is padding the handle of a fork or spoon with several layers of gauze so that a better grip is established.

■ Gerontologic Considerations: Burns

The older patient presents many challenges for the burn team. Normal aging puts the patient at risk for injury because of the possibility of an unsteady gait, failing eyesight, and diminished hearing. Once injured, the older adult has more complications in the emergent and acute phases of burn resuscitation because of preexisting medical conditions that may be present. For example, older patients with diabetes, congestive heart failure, or chronic obstructive pulmonary disease will have morbidity and mortality rates exceeding those of healthy younger patients. In older patients, pneumonia is a frequent complication, wounds take longer to heal, and surgical procedures are less well tolerated. Because of these problems, strategies to prevent burn injuries in this population are particularly important. ■

EMOTIONAL NEEDS OF THE PATIENT AND FAMILY

Because the nurse has prolonged contact with the patient and family, she or he is seen as an important and continual source of emotional support. The nurse is a valuable person in assisting the patient to maintain a sense of personal worth and reestablish a satisfactory body image. Often the health care provider is the target for anger and hostility from the patient who has no other way of expressing these feelings.

Working with the family can be challenging for the nurse. Family members need to understand and appreciate the importance of reestablishing the patient's independence. They may be confused by all the changes they see in the various phases of care and can benefit from repeated explanations of what to expect as the patient recovers. It may be helpful for some family members to view the burn wounds frequently so that they can see the

progress of healing. The nurse should encourage the family to participate as team members during the patient's hospitalization.

The stress of the burn injury occasionally precipitates a time-limited psychiatric crisis. Treatment by a psychiatrist who can prescribe psychotropic drugs and begin ongoing dialogue with the patient is indicated when this occurs. Early psychiatric intervention is also crucial if the patient has been previously treated for a psychiatric disorder or if the burn injury was the result of a suicide attempt. The diagnosis of posttraumatic stress disorder is being made with increasing frequency in the burn patient population.[19] Early intervention by health care providers can be an important aspect of recovery.

Because of the suddenness and severity of burn trauma, the patient and family are plunged into physical and emotional crises. The health care provider must be prepared to assess psychoemotional cues and provide appropriate intervention throughout the course of recovery.

The patient may experience thoughts and feelings that are frightening and disturbing, such as guilt about the burn accident, reliving the experience, fear of death, and concern about future therapy and the concomitant pain. Families may share any or all of these feelings. At times, they may feel helpless when trying to assist their loved one. During this period of adjustment, the nurse should provide time for the patient and the family to be alone. Family members may also be encouraged to assist with position changes and eating.

For the nurse to adequately manage the enormous range of emotional responses that the burn patient may exhibit, it is important to have an understanding of the circumstances of the burn, past family interactions, and past coping experiences with stressful stimuli. At any time the various emotional responses of fear, anxiety, anger, guilt, and depression may be experienced (Table 24-17).

A common emotional response is regression. The patient will revert to behavior that helped in coping with stressful situations in the past. Major emotional tasks confront patients and families.

TABLE 24-17	Emotional Responses of Burn Patients
EMOTION	**POSSIBLE VERBAL EXPRESSION**
Fear	Will I die?
	What will happen next?
	Will I be disfigured?
	Will my spouse or friends still love me?
Anxiety	I feel out of control.
	What's happening to me?
	When will it end?
Anger	Why did this happen to me?
	Those nurses enjoy hurting me.
Guilt	If only I'd been more careful.
	I was punished because I was bad.
Depression	It's no use going on like this.
	I don't care what happens to me.
	I wish people would leave me alone.

As more and more independence is expected from the patient, new fears must be confronted: "Can I do it?" "Am I a desirable partner, parent?" Open communication among the patient, family members, friends, and burn team members is essential.

Therapeutic intervention for the patient can be provided by nurses, physicians, social workers, or anyone else who has a rapport with the patient and a good understanding of responses in such situations. The patient can best convey some of these negative but normal emotions to a health care provider with whom he or she can communicate. Acknowledgment that the feelings are real and valid can do much to help the patient. The nurse should be firm and consistent in guiding the patient toward positive coping responses.

The difficult issue of sexuality must be met with honesty. Physical appearance will be altered in the patient who has sustained a major burn. Acceptance of any changes is difficult at first for the patient and significant other. The nature of skin injury in itself causes modifications in processing sexual stimuli. Touch is an important part of sexuality, and immature scar tissue may make the sensation of touch unpleasant or may dull it. This is usually transient, but the patient and family need to know that it is normal and receive anticipatory guidance from health care personnel to avoid undue emotional strain.

Family and patient support groups may be beneficial in meeting the patient's and family's emotional needs at any phase of the recovery process. Speaking with others who have experienced burn trauma can be beneficial, both in terms of reaffirming that what the patient is feeling is normal and in allowing for the sharing of helpful advice.

SPECIAL NEEDS OF THE NURSING STAFF

The nurse cares for patients who, at times, may be unpleasant, hostile, apprehensive, and frustrated. The nurse will sometimes see many hours of patient care suddenly lost to sepsis and death. Because of long hospitalizations and intense contact, relationships between the caregiver and the care receiver can result in strong bonds that can be healthy and healing, or destructive and draining. The burn patient may demonstrate demanding or punitive behaviors, which may cause the nurse to be reluctant to provide care. The nurse and patient can also develop warm, trusting, mutually satisfying relationships not only during hospitalization but also during long-term rehabilitation. Sometimes the bond can be so strong that the patient has difficulty separating from the hospital and staff. The frequency and intensity of family contact can also be rewarding as well as draining to the nurse. Nurses new to burn nursing often find it difficult to cope with not only the deformities caused by burn injury but also the odor, the unpleasant sight of the wound, and the reality of the pain that accompanies the burn.

Many nurses believe that the care they provide makes a critical difference in helping patients not only to survive, but to cope with and triumph over a severe and multifaceted injury. It is this belief that keeps nurses caring for burn patients and their families.

Ongoing support services for the burn nurse or critical incident stress debriefings led by a psychiatrist, psychologist, psychiatric clinical nurse specialist, or social worker can be helpful.[20] Peer support groups can serve a similar purpose by helping nursing staff to cope with difficult feelings they may experience when caring for burn patients. A therapeutic communication process can support the nurse in delivering effective nursing care.

CRITICAL THINKING EXERCISES

Case Study
Severe Burn Patient

Patient Profile. Sylvia, a 44-year-old Amish woman, was brought to the emergency department with extensive full-thickness burns to her upper body. Her stove exploded while she was manually lighting the oven with firewood and kerosene. Her 10 children remain at home and her husband is in the fields, unable to be reached.

Subjective Data
- Complains of feeling very cold
- Cannot remember the accident
- Is hoarse and has difficulty talking
- Expresses a great deal of fear

Objective Data

Physical Examination
- Is awake and oriented but in obvious distress
- Has dark brown, leathery burns involving the head, neck, chest, and upper extremities
- Has hair and eyebrows that are singed
- Nurse is unable to palpate peripheral pulses; apical pulse: 140

CRITICAL THINKING QUESTIONS

1. What are the first priorities in the prehospital environment? How should her airway be managed?
2. Why would Sylvia be considered at high risk for an inhalation injury? What interventions can be anticipated?
3. What intervention should the nurse anticipate in a patient with full-thickness circumferential burns to the extremities?
4. Describe the rationale for Sylvia's lack of pain and her complaints of being cold. What drugs might be considered to promote her comfort?
5. What fluid and electrolyte disturbances would be expected in the first 48 hours of Sylvia's hospitalization? Explain the physiologic bases for these changes.
6. What measures should be taken to support Sylvia's family?
7. Based on the assessment data presented, write one or more appropriate nursing diagnoses. Are there any collaborative problems?

Nursing Research Issues

1. What nursing interventions are most effective in preparing patients, families, and community nurses for the early discharge and posthospitalization phase of burn care?
2. What pharmacologic and nonpharmacologic nursing interventions are most effective in the management of burn pain?
3. What nutritional supplements are best tolerated in the emergent and acute phases of burn recovery?
4. What are some expected psychologic or cultural issues that may occur with burn patients?

REVIEW QUESTIONS

The number of the question corresponds to the same-numbered objective at the beginning of the chapter.

1. In presenting a program on fire and burn prevention for parents, the nurse focuses on the most common cause of household fires as
   a. unattended cooking.
   b. frayed or defective wiring.
   c. carelessness with cigarettes.
   d. improper use of inflammables.

2. The injury that is least likely to result in a full-thickness burn is
   a. sunburn.
   b. scald injury.
   c. chemical burn.
   d. electrical injury.

3. When assessing a partial-thickness burn, the nurse would expect to find
   a. exposed fascia.
   b. dry, waxy appearance.
   c. red, shiny, wet appearance.
   d. absence of blanching with pressure.

4. The extent of burns is assessed by
   a. rating the location of burns at specific body sites.
   b. determining the presence of preexisting risk factors.
   c. estimating the ratio of full-thickness to partial-thickness burns.
   d. using guides to indicate burn location relative to total body surface.

5. An 82 kg patient has a 45% TBSA burn. Using 4 ml/kg/% TBSA during the first 12 hours after a burn injury, the nurse would anticipate a fluid replacement of
   a. 3690 ml.
   b. 7380 ml.
   c. 9225 ml.
   d. 14,760 ml.

6. Fluid and electrolyte shifts that occur during the early emergent phase include
   a. adherence of albumin to vascular walls.
   b. movement of potassium into the vascular space.
   c. sequestering of sodium and water in interstitial fluid.
   d. hemolysis of red blood cells from large volumes of rapidly administered fluid.

7. To maintain a positive nitrogen balance in a major burn, the patient must
   a. eat a high-protein, low-fat, low-carbohydrate diet.
   b. increase normal adult caloric intake by about 3 times.
   c. eat at least 1500 calories per day in small frequent meals.
   d. eat rice and whole wheat for the chemical effect on nitrogen balance.

8. Pain management for the burn patient is most effective when
   a. the nurse administers narcotics on a set schedule around the clock.
   b. the patient has as much control over the management of the pain as possible.
   c. the nurse has total freedom to administer narcotics within a dosage and frequency range.
   d. painful dressing changes and repositioning are delayed until the patient's pain is totally relieved.

9. A therapeutic measure used to prevent hypertrophic scarring during the rehabilitative phase of burn recovery is
   a. applying pressure garments.
   b. repositioning the patient every 2 hours.
   c. performing active ROM at least every 4 hours.
   d. massaging the new tissue with water-based moisturizers.

10. It is important for the burn patient and family to
    a. see the burn wound three times per day.
    b. talk frequently with the nurse about the patient's progress.
    c. allow nurses to do total care for the patient to prevent infection.
    d. avoid discussion of the patient's progress to minimize false hope.

11. Discharge planning for the burn patient begins
    a. after grafting.
    b. on admission.
    c. after the emergent phase.
    d. at least 1 week before discharge.

REFERENCES

1. Nortrade Medical: *Burnfacts. Burnfree,* 2001. Available at *www.burn-free.com/burnfact.html* (accessed March 14, 2002).
2. National Center for Injury Prevention and Control: *Fire and burn injuries fact sheet,* Centers for Disease Control and Prevention. Available at *www.cdc.gov/ncipc/duip/burn.htm* (accessed March 14, 2002).
3. Fultz J, Wells S, Welsh D: Acute burn injury. In Kidd P, Wagner K, editors: *High acuity nursing,* ed 3, Saddle Ridge, NJ, 2001, Prentice-Hall.
4. Kagan RJ, Smith SC: Evaluation and treatment of thermal injuries, *Dermatol Nurs* 12:335, 2000.
5. Jordan BS, Barillo BJ: Prehospital care and transport. In Carrougher GJ: *Burn care and therapy,* St Louis, 1998, Mosby.
6. Baldwin K, Morris S: Shock, multiple organ dysfunction syndrome, and burns in adults. In McCance KL, Huether SE, editors: *Pathophysiology: the biologic basis for disease in adults and children,* ed 4, St Louis, 2002, Mosby.
7. Nishiura T et al: Gene expression and cytokine and enzyme activation in the liver after a burn injury, *J Burn Care Rehabil* 21:35, 2000.
8. Gordon MD, Winfree JH: Fluid resuscitation after a major burn. In Carrougher GJ: *Burn care and therapy,* St Louis, 1998, Mosby.
9. Oman KS, Reilly EL: Initial assessment and care in the emergency department. In Carrougher GJ: *Burn care and therapy,* St Louis, 1998, Mosby.
10. Milner SM, Mottar S, Smith C: The burn wheel, *Am J Nurs* 101:35, 2001.
11. Cohen R, Moelleken B: Disorders due to physical agents. In Tierney L, McPhee S, Papadakis M, editors: *Medical diagnosis and treatment 2001,* ed 40, New York, 2001, McGraw-Hill.
12. Carrougher GJ: Burn wound assessment and topical treatment. In Carrougher GJ: *Burn care and therapy,* St Louis, 1998, Mosby.
13. Ho W, Leung T, Ying S: Corneal perforation with extrusion of lens in a burn patient, *Burns* 27:81, 2001.
14. Dhanaraj P: Changing trends in burn therapy, *Burns* 26:64, 2000.

15. Tang H et al: The experience in the treatment of patients with extensive full-thickness burns, *Burns* 25:757, 1999.

16. Sheridan R, Tompkins R: Skin substitutes in burns, *Burns* 25:97, 1999.

17. Dains J: Integumentary system. In Thompson JM et al, editors: *Mosby's clinical nursing,* ed 5, St Louis, 2002, Mosby.

18. Crowther C, Mourad L: Alterations of musculoskeletal function. In McCance KL, Huether SE, editors: *Pathophysiology: the biologic basis for disease in adults and children,* ed 4, St Louis, 2002, Mosby.

19. Taal LA, Faber AW: Posttraumatic stress and maladjustment among adult survivors 1-2 years postburn, *Burns* 24:285, 1998.

20. Badjer J: Burns: the psychological aspects, *Am J Nurs* 101:38, 2001.

RESOURCES

American Academy of Facial Plastic and Reconstructive Surgery
310 South Henry Street
Alexandria, VA 22314
703-299-9291
Fax: 703-299-8898
www.aafprs.org/

American Burn Association
ABA Central Office—Chicago
625 North Michigan Avenue, Suite 1530
Chicago, IL 60611
312-642-9260
Fax: 312-642-9130
www.ameriburn.org/

American Society of Plastic and Reconstructive Surgical Nurses
East Holly Avenue, Box 56
Pitman, NJ 08071
609-256-2340
Fax: 609-589-7463

Burn Foundation
1201 Chestnut Street, Suite 801
Philadelphia, PA 19107
215-988-9882
Fax: 215-988-9883
www.burnfoundation.org/

Canadian Association of Burn Nurses
The Wellesley Hospital
160 Wellesley Street East
Toronto, Ontario M4Y 1J3
Canada

International Society for Burn Injuries
Dr. Keith Judkins, ISBI Secretary-Treasurer–elect
Medical Director for Burn Care, Pinderfields Hospital, Aberford Road
Wakefield
WF1 4DG
England
44-1924-212331
Fax: 44-1924-814938
www.worldburn.org/

Phoenix Society for Burn Survivors, Inc.
2153 Wealthy Street SE, #215
East Grand Rapids, MI 49506
616-458-2773
800-888-2876
Fax: 616-458-2831
www.phoenix-society.org/

For additional Internet resources, see the website for this book at *http://evolve.elsevier.com/lewis/medsurg/.*

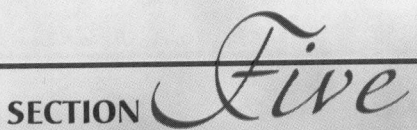
Problems of Oxygenation: Ventilation

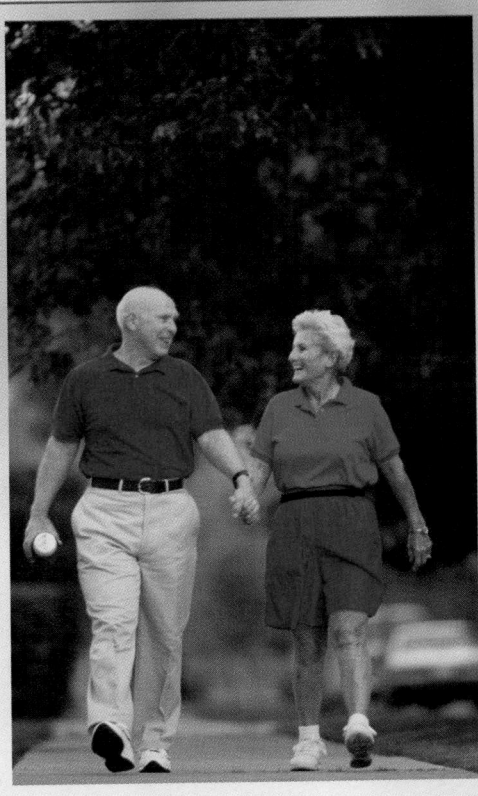

CHAPTER 25

NURSING ASSESSMENT
Respiratory System

Debra A. Hagler

LEARNING OBJECTIVES

1. Describe the structures and functions of the upper respiratory tract, the lower respiratory tract, and the chest wall.
2. Describe the process that initiates and controls inspiration and expiration.
3. Describe the process of gas diffusion within the lungs.
4. Identify the respiratory defense mechanisms.
5. Describe the significance of arterial blood gas values and the oxyhemoglobin dissociation curve in relation to respiratory function.
6. Identify the signs and symptoms of inadequate oxygenation and the implications of these findings.
7. Describe age-related changes in the respiratory system and differences in assessment findings.
8. Identify the significant subjective and objective data related to the respiratory system that should be obtained from a patient.
9. Describe the techniques used in physical assessment of the respiratory system.
10. Differentiate normal from common abnormal findings in a physical assessment of the respiratory system.
11. Describe the purpose, significance of results, and nursing responsibilities related to diagnostic studies of the respiratory system.

KEY TERMS

adventitious sounds, p. 556	mechanical receptors, p. 548
chemoreceptor, p. 548	pleural friction rub, p. 556
compliance, p. 545	rhonchi, p. 556
crackles, p. 556	surfactant, p. 543
dyspnea, p. 550	tidal volume, p. 543
elastic recoil, p. 545	ventilation, p. 545
fremitus, p. 555	wheezes, p. 556

STRUCTURES AND FUNCTIONS OF THE RESPIRATORY SYSTEM

The primary purpose of the respiratory system is gas exchange, which involves the transfer of oxygen and carbon dioxide between the atmosphere and the blood. The respiratory system is divided into two parts: the upper respiratory tract and the lower respiratory tract (Fig. 25-1). The upper respiratory tract includes the nose, pharynx, adenoids, tonsils, epiglottis, larynx, and trachea. The lower respiratory tract consists of the bronchi, bronchioles, alveolar ducts, and alveoli. With the exception of the right and left main-stem bronchi, all lower airway structures are contained within the lungs. The right lung is divided into three lobes (upper, middle, and lower) and the left lung into two lobes (upper and lower) (Fig. 25-2). The structures of the chest wall (ribs, pleura, muscles of respiration) are also essential to respiration.

Upper Respiratory Tract

The nose, made of bone and cartilage, is divided into two nares by the nasal septum. The interior of the nose is shaped into rolling projections called *turbinates* that increase the surface area for warming and moistening air. The internal nose opens directly into the sinuses. The nasal cavity connects with the pharynx, a tubular passageway that is subdivided from above downward into three parts: the nasopharynx, the oropharynx, and the laryngopharynx.

Breathing through the narrow nasal passages (rather than mouth breathing) provides protection for the lower airway. The nose is lined with mucous membrane and small hairs. Air entering the nose is warmed to near body temperature, humidified to nearly 100% water saturation, and filtered of particles larger than 10 μm (e.g., dust, bacteria).

The olfactory nerve endings (receptors for the sense of smell) are located in the roof of the nose. The adenoids and tonsils, which are small masses of lymphatic tissue, are found in the nasopharynx and the oropharynx, respectively.

The epiglottis is a small flap of tissue at the base of the tongue. During swallowing, the epiglottis covers the larynx, preventing solids and liquids from entering the lungs. A condition such as a stroke that alters the swallowing ability may impair the function of the epiglottis, thus predisposing to aspiration.

After passing through the oropharynx, air moves through the laryngopharynx and the larynx, where the vocal cords are located, and then down into the trachea. The trachea is a cylindric tube about 5 inches (10 to 12 cm) long and 1 inch (1.5 to 2.5 cm) in diameter. The support of U-shaped cartilages keeps the trachea open but allows the adjacent esophagus to expand for swallowing. The trachea bifurcates into the right and left main-stem bronchi at a point called the *carina*. The carina is located at the level of the manubriosternal junction, also called the *angle of Louis*. The carina is highly sensitive, and touching it during suctioning causes vigorous coughing.[1-3]

Lower Respiratory Tract

Once air passes the carina, it is in the lower respiratory tract. The main-stem bronchi, pulmonary vessels, and nerves enter the lungs through a slit called the *hilus*. The right main-stem bronchus is shorter, wider, and straighter than the left main-stem bronchus. For this reason, aspiration is more likely in the right lung than in the left lung.

Reviewed by Jane A. Madden, RN, MSN, Assistant Professor, Deaconess College of Nursing, St Louis, Mo.

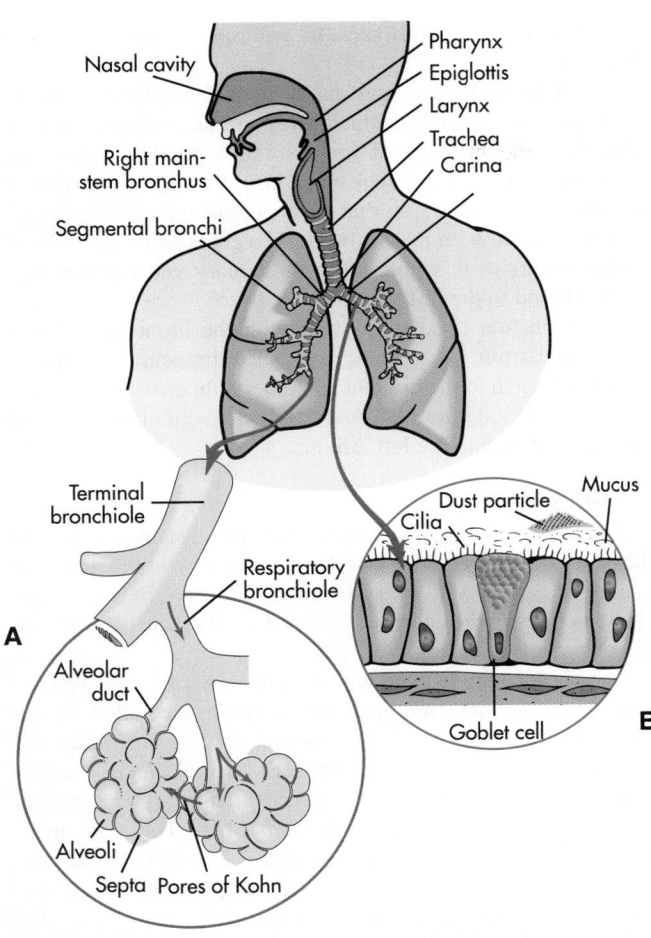

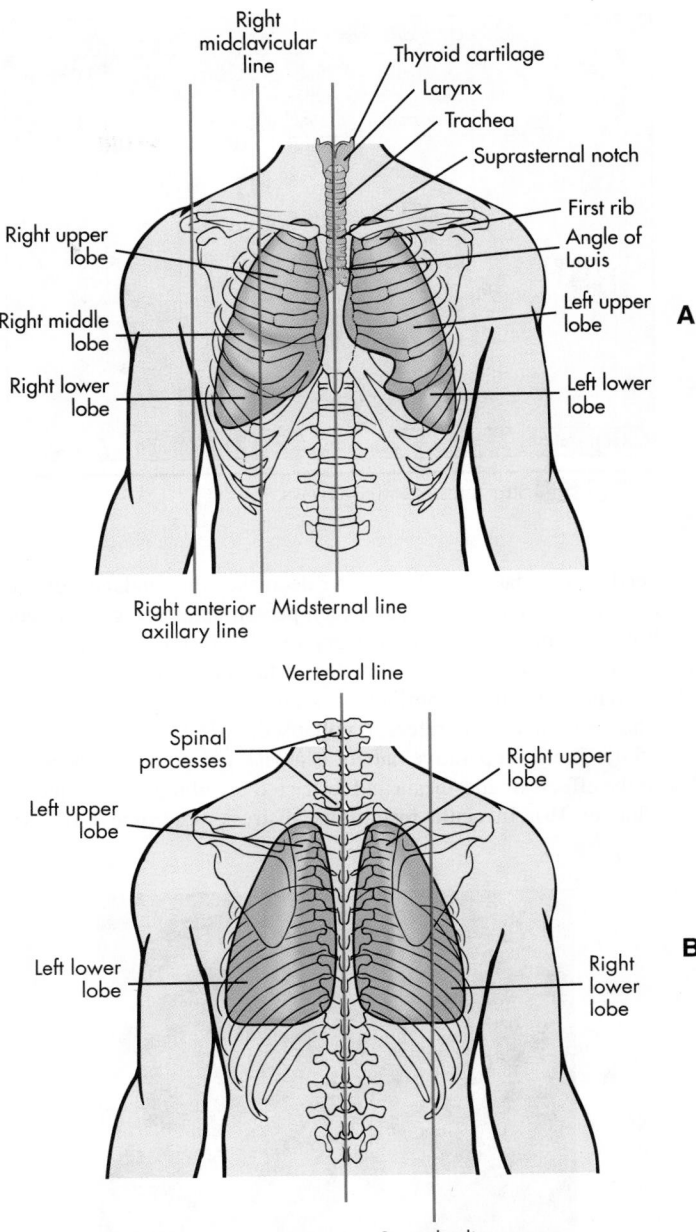

FIG. 25-1 Structures of the respiratory tract. **A,** Pulmonary functional unit. **B,** Ciliated mucous membrane.

FIG. 25-2 Landmarks and structures of the chest wall. **A,** Anterior view. **B,** Posterior view.

The main-stem bronchi subdivide several times to form the lobar, segmental, and subsegmental bronchi. Further divisions form the bronchioles. The most distant bronchioles are called the respiratory bronchioles. Beyond these lie the alveolar ducts and alveolar sacs (Fig. 25-3). The bronchioles are encircled by smooth muscles that constrict and dilate in response to various stimuli. The terms *bronchoconstriction* and *bronchodilation* are used to refer to a decrease or increase in the diameter of the airways caused by contraction or relaxation of these muscles.

No exchange of oxygen or carbon dioxide takes place until air enters the respiratory bronchioles. The area of the respiratory tract from the nose to the respiratory bronchioles serves only as a conducting pathway and is therefore termed the *anatomic dead space* (VD). This space must be filled with every breath, but the air that fills it is not available for gas exchange. In adults, a normal **tidal volume** (VT), or volume of air exchanged with each breath, is about 500 ml. Of each 500 ml inhaled, about 150 ml is VD.

After moving through the conducting zone, air reaches the respiratory bronchioles and alveoli (Fig. 25-4). *Alveoli* are small sacs that form the functional unit of the lungs. The alveoli are interconnected by pores of Kohn, which allow movement of air from alveolus to alveolus (see Fig. 25-1). Bacteria can also move through these pores, resulting in an extension of respiratory infection to previously noninfected areas. The 300 million alveoli

in the adult have a total volume of about 2500 ml and a surface area for gas exchange that is about the size of a tennis court. The alveolar-capillary membrane (Fig. 25-5) is very thin (less than $\frac{1}{5000}$ of an inch, or 5 μm) and is the site of gas exchange. In conditions such as pulmonary edema, excess fluid fills the interstitial space and alveoli, markedly impairing gas exchange.[3,4]

Surfactant. The lung can be conceptualized as a collection of 300 million bubbles (alveoli), each 0.3 mm in diameter.[1] Such a structure is inherently unstable and, as a consequence, the alveoli have a natural tendency to collapse. The alveolar surface is composed of cells that provide structure and cells that secrete surfactant (see Fig. 25-5). **Surfactant,** a lipoprotein that lowers the surface tension in the alveoli, reduces the amount of pressure

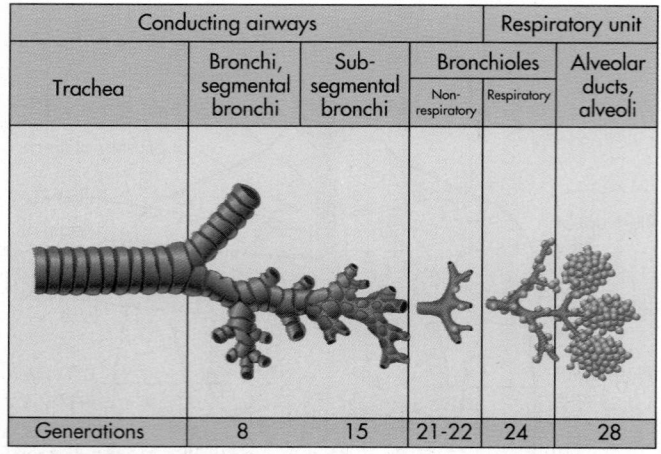

Conducting airways					Respiratory unit
Trachea	Bronchi, segmental bronchi	Sub-segmental bronchi	Bronchioles		Alveolar ducts, alveoli
			Non-respiratory	Respiratory	
Generations	8	15	21-22	24	28

FIG. 25-3   Structures of lower airways.

needed to inflate the alveoli and decreases the tendency of the alveoli to collapse. Normally, each person takes a slightly larger breath, termed a *sigh*, after every five to six breaths. This sigh stretches the alveoli and promotes surfactant secretion.

When insufficient surfactant is present, the alveoli collapse. The term *atelectasis* refers to collapsed, airless alveoli (see Fig. 25-4). The postoperative patient is at risk for atelectasis because of the effects of anesthesia and restricted breathing with pain (see Chapter 19). In acute respiratory distress syndrome (ARDS),

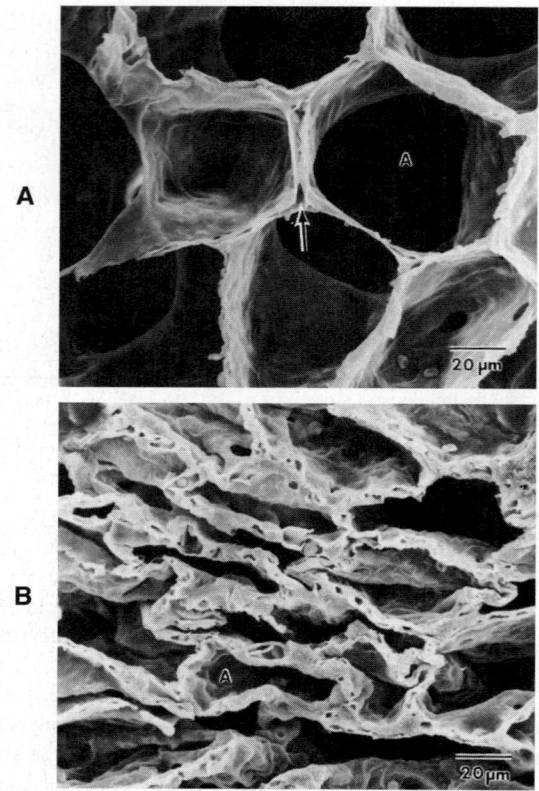

FIG. 25-4   Scanning electron micrograph of lung parenchyma. A, Alveoli (*A*) and alveolar capillary (*arrow*). B, Effects of atelectasis. Alveoli (*A*) are partially or totally collapsed.

lack of surfactant contributes to widespread atelectasis (see Chapter 66).[5,6]

Blood Supply. The lungs have two different types of circulation: pulmonary and bronchial. The pulmonary circulation provides the lungs with blood for gas exchange. The pulmonary artery receives deoxygenated blood from the right ventricle of the heart and branches so that each pulmonary capillary is directly connected with many alveoli. Oxygen–carbon dioxide exchange occurs at this point. The pulmonary veins return oxygenated blood to the left atrium of the heart.

The bronchial circulation starts with the bronchial arteries, which arise from the thoracic aorta. The bronchial circulation provides oxygen to the bronchi and other pulmonary tissues. Deoxygenated blood returns from the bronchial circulation through the azygos vein into the left atrium.

Chest Wall

The chest wall is shaped, supported, and protected by 24 ribs (12 on each side). The ribs and the sternum protect the lungs and heart from injury and are sometimes called the *thoracic cage.* The structures of the chest wall include the thoracic cage, pleura, and respiratory muscles.

The chest cavity is lined with a membrane called the *parietal pleura,* and the lungs are lined with a membrane called the *visceral pleura.* The parietal and visceral pleurae are joined and form a closed, double-walled sac. The visceral pleura does not have any afferent pain fibers or nerve endings. The parietal pleura, however, does have afferent pain fibers. Therefore, irritation of the parietal pleura causes severe pain with each breath.

The space between the pleural layers, termed the *intrapleural space,* is a potential space. In the normal adult, this space is filled with a thin film of fluid, which serves two purposes: it provides lubrication, allowing the layers of pleura to slide over each other

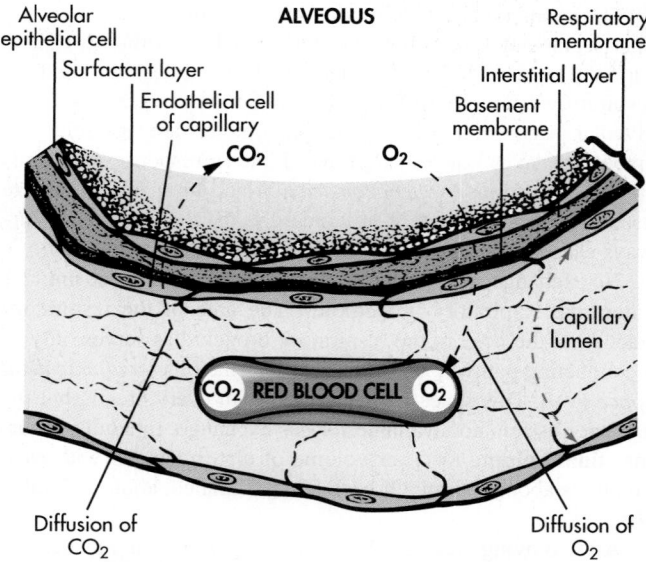

FIG. 25-5   A small portion of the respiratory membrane greatly magnified. An extremely thin interstitial layer of tissue separates the endothelial cell and basement membrane on the capillary side from the epithelial cell and surfactant layer on the alveolar side of the respiratory membrane. The total thickness of the respiratory membrane is less than $\frac{1}{5000}$ of an inch.

during breathing; and it increases cohesion between the pleural layers, thereby facilitating expansion of the pleura and lung during inspiration.

Normally, the pleural space contains 20 to 25 ml of fluid. Fluid is drained from the pleural space by the lymphatic circulation. Several pathologic conditions may cause the accumulation of greater amounts of fluid, termed a *pleural effusion.* Pleural fluid may accumulate because malignant cells block lymphatic drainage or because there is an imbalance between intravascular and oncotic fluid pressures, such as occurs in congestive heart failure. Purulent pleural fluid with bacterial infection is called *empyema.*

The diaphragm is the major muscle of respiration. During inspiration, the diaphragm contracts, pushing the abdominal contents downward. At the same time, the external intercostal muscles and scalene muscles contract, increasing the lateral and anteroposterior dimension of the chest. This causes the size of the thoracic cavity to increase (Fig. 25-6) and intrathoracic pressure to decrease, so air enters the lungs.

The diaphragm is made up of two hemidiaphragms, each innervated by the right and left phrenic nerves. The phrenic nerves arise from the spinal cord between C3 and C5, the third and fifth cervical vertebrae. Injury to the phrenic nerve results in hemidiaphragm paralysis on the side of the injury. Complete spinal cord injuries above the level of C3 result in total diaphragm paralysis and mechanical ventilator dependence.[7]

Physiology of Respiration

Ventilation. **Ventilation** involves *inspiration* (movement of air into the lungs) and *expiration* (movement of air out of the lungs). Air moves in and out of the lungs because intrathoracic pressure changes in relation to pressure at the airway opening. Contraction of the diaphragm and intercostal and scalene muscles increases chest dimensions, thereby decreasing intrathoracic pressure. Gas flows from an area of higher pressure (atmospheric) to one of lower pressure (intrathoracic) (see Fig. 25-6). When inspiration is difficult, neck and shoulder muscles can as-

sist the effort. Some conditions (e.g., phrenic nerve paralysis, rib fractures, neuromuscular disease) may limit diaphragm or chest wall movement and cause the patient to breathe with smaller tidal volumes. As a result, the lungs do not fully inflate, and gas exchange is impaired.

In contrast to inspiration, expiration is passive. The elastic recoil of the chest wall and lungs allows the chest to passively return to its normal position. Intrathoracic pressure rises, causing air to move out of the lungs. Exacerbations of asthma or emphysema cause expiration to become an active, labored process (see Chapter 28). Abdominal and intercostal muscles assist in expelling air during labored breathing.

Elastic Recoil and Compliance. **Elastic recoil** is the tendency for the lungs to recoil after being stretched or expanded. The elasticity of lung tissue is due to the elastin fibers found in the alveolar walls and surrounding the bronchioles and capillaries.

Compliance (distensibility) is a measure of the elasticity of the lungs and thorax. When compliance is decreased, the lungs are more difficult to inflate. Examples include conditions that increase fluid in the lungs (e.g., pulmonary edema, ARDS); conditions that make lung tissue less elastic (e.g., pulmonary fibrosis, sarcoidosis); and conditions that restrict lung movement (e.g., pleural effusion). Compliance is increased when there is destruction of alveolar walls and loss of tissue elasticity, as in emphysema.

Diffusion. Oxygen and carbon dioxide move back and forth across the alveolar capillary membrane by diffusion. The overall direction of movement is from the area of higher concentration to the area of lower concentration. Thus oxygen moves from alveolar gas (atmospheric air) into the arterial blood and carbon dioxide from the arterial blood into the alveolar gas. Diffusion continues until equilibrium is reached (see Fig. 25-5).

The ability of the lungs to oxygenate arterial blood adequately is determined by examination of the arterial oxygen tension (PaO_2) and arterial oxygen saturation (SaO_2). Oxygen is carried in the blood in two forms: dissolved oxygen and hemoglobin-bound oxygen. The PaO_2 represents the amount of oxygen dissolved in the plasma and is expressed in millimeters of mercury (mm Hg). The SaO_2 is the amount of oxygen bound to hemoglobin in comparison with the amount of oxygen the hemoglobin can carry. The SaO_2 is expressed as a percentage. For example, if the SaO_2 is 90%, this means that 90% of the hemoglobin attachments for oxygen have oxygen bound to them.

Oxygen-hemoglobin dissociation curve. The affinity of hemoglobin for oxygen is described by the *oxygen-hemoglobin dissociation curve* (Fig. 25-7). Oxygen delivery to the tissues depends on the amount of oxygen transported to the tissues and the ease with which hemoglobin gives up oxygen once it reaches the tissues. In the upper flat portion of the curve, fairly large changes in the PaO_2 cause small changes in hemoglobin saturation. For this reason, if the PaO_2 drops from 100 to 60 mm Hg, the saturation of hemoglobin changes only 7% (from the normal 97% to 90%). Thus the hemoglobin remains 90% saturated despite a 40 mm Hg drop in the PaO_2. This portion of the curve also explains the reason the patient is considered adequately oxygenated when the PaO_2 is greater than 60 mm Hg. Increasing the PaO_2 above this level does little to improve hemoglobin saturation.

The lower portion of the oxyhemoglobin dissociation curve indicates a different type of phenomenon. As hemoglobin is desaturated, larger amounts of oxygen are released for tissue use.

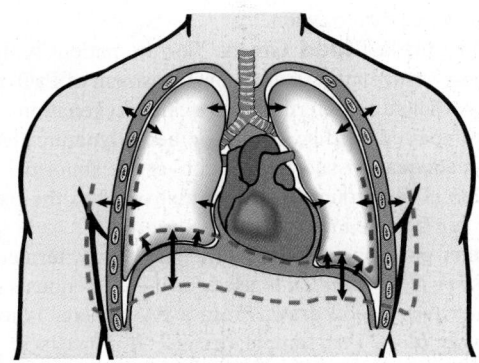

FIG. 25-6 Frontal section of chest showing movement of the lungs and chest wall during inspiration and expiration. During inspiration, the inspiratory muscles contract and the chest expands. Alveolar pressure becomes subatmospheric with respect to pressure at the airway opening and air flows into the lungs. During expiration, the inspiratory muscles relax. Recoil of the lung causes alveolar pressure to exceed pressure at the airway opening and air to flow out of the lungs. *Single arrows* show excursion of the lungs and chest wall. *Double arrows* show movement of the lung bases.

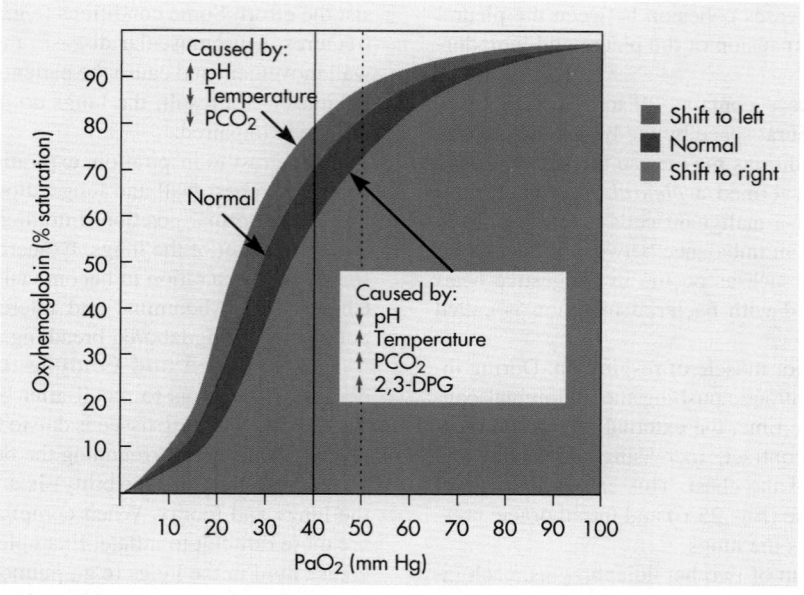

FIG. 25-7 Oxygen-hemoglobin dissociation curve. The effects of acidity and temperature changes are shown.

This is an important method of maintaining the pressure gradient between the blood and the tissues. It also ensures an adequate oxygen supply to peripheral tissues, even if oxygen delivery is compromised.

Many factors alter the affinity of hemoglobin for oxygen. When the oxygen dissociation curve shifts to the left, blood picks up oxygen more readily in the lungs but delivers oxygen less readily to the tissues. This is seen in alkalosis, in hypothermia, and with a decrease in arterial carbon dioxide tension ($PaCO_2$) (see Fig. 25-7). The patient with a condition that causes a leftward shift of the curve, such as with hypothermia that follows open heart surgery, may be given higher concentrations of oxygen until the body temperature normalizes. This helps compensate for decreased oxygen unloading in the tissues. When the curve shifts to the right, the opposite occurs. Blood picks up oxygen less rapidly in the lungs but delivers oxygen more readily to the tissues. This is seen in acidosis, in hyperthermia, and when the $PaCO_2$ is increased.

Two methods are used to assess the efficiency of gas transfer in the lung: analysis of *arterial blood gases* (ABGs) and oximetry. These measures are usually adequate if the patient is stable and not critically ill. The critically ill patient often has a condition that impairs tissue oxygen delivery. In this patient, cardiac output, oxygen consumption (VO_2), mixed venous oxygen tension (PvO_2), and venous oxygen saturation (SvO_2) may also be assessed[8] (see Chapter 64).

Arterial Blood Gases. ABGs are measured to determine oxygenation status and acid-base balance. ABG analysis includes measurement of the PaO_2, $PaCO_2$, acidity (pH), and bicarbonate (HCO_3^-) in arterial blood. The SaO_2 is either calculated or measured during this analysis.

Blood for ABG analysis can be obtained by arterial puncture or from an arterial catheter in the radial or femoral artery. Both techniques are invasive and allow only intermittent analysis. Continuous intraarterial blood gas monitoring is also possible via a fiberoptic sensor or an oxygen electrode inserted into an arter-

ial catheter. An arterial catheter permits ABG sampling without repeated arterial punctures.

Normal values for ABGs are given in Table 25-1. The normal PaO_2 decreases with advancing age. The normal PaO_2 also varies in relation to the distance above sea level. At higher altitudes, the barometric pressure is lower, resulting in a lower inspired oxygen pressure and a lower PaO_2 (see Table 25-1). Most airplanes are pressurized to approximate an altitude of 8000 feet above sea level. A normal person can expect a 16 to 32 mm Hg fall in PaO_2 at this altitude.[9] The patient who is already receiving oxygen therapy or the patient with a PaO_2 less than 72 mm Hg while breathing room air needs a careful evaluation before air travel. Supplemental oxygen or a change in liter flow may be required during the flight. If oxygen is required, the airline should be contacted several weeks in advance to determine the procedures regarding air travel with oxygen.

Mixed Venous Blood Gases. For the patient with a normal or near-normal cardiac status, an assessment of PaO_2 or SaO_2 is usually sufficient to determine adequate oxygenation. The patient with impaired cardiac output or hemodynamic instability may have inadequate tissue oxygen delivery or abnormal oxygen consumption. The amount of oxygen delivered to the tissues or consumed can be calculated.

A catheter positioned in the pulmonary artery, termed a *pulmonary artery (PA) catheter,* is used for mixed venous sampling (see Chapter 64). Blood drawn from a PA catheter is termed a *mixed venous blood gas* sample because it consists of venous blood that has returned to the heart from all tissue beds and "mixed" in the right ventricle. Normal mixed venous values are given in Table 25-1. When tissue oxygen delivery is inadequate or when inadequate oxygen is transported to the tissues by the hemoglobin, the PvO_2 and SvO_2 fall.

Oximetry. ABG values provide accurate information about oxygenation and acid-base balance. However, they are invasive, require laboratory analysis, and expose the patient to the risk of bleeding from an arterial puncture. Arterial oxygen saturation

TABLE 25-1	Normal Arterial and Venous Blood Gas Values*				
	ARTERIAL BLOOD GASES			**VENOUS BLOOD GASES**	
LABORATORY VALUE	**SEA LEVEL BP 760 mm Hg**	**1 MILE ABOVE SEA LEVEL (5280 ft) BP 629 mm Hg**		**MIXED VENOUS BLOOD GASES**	
pH	7.35-7.45	7.35-7.45	pH		7.34-7.37
PaO_2	80-100 mm Hg	65-75 mm Hg	PvO_2		38-42 mm Hg
SaO_2	>95%†	>95%†	SvO_2		60%-80%†
$PaCO_2$	35-45 mm Hg	35-45 mm Hg	$PvCO_2$		44-46 mm Hg
HCO_3^-	22-26 mEq/L	22-26 mEq/L	HCO_3^-		24-30 mEq/L

*Assumes patient is ≤60 years of age and breathing room air.
†The same normal values apply when SpO_2 and SvO_2 are obtained by oximetry.
BP, Barometric pressure; HCO_3^-, bicarbonate; $PvCO_2$, partial pressure of CO_2 in venous blood; PvO_2, partial pressure of oxygen in venous blood; SvO_2, venous oxygen saturation.

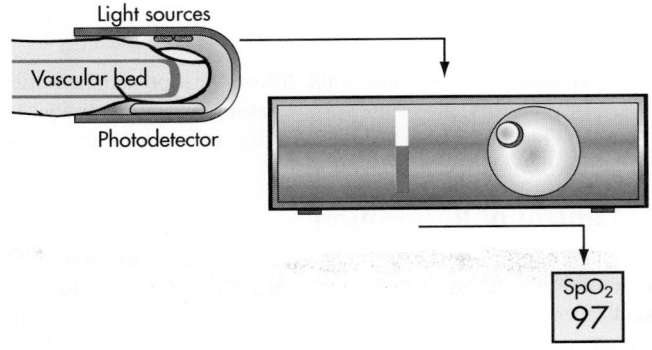

A

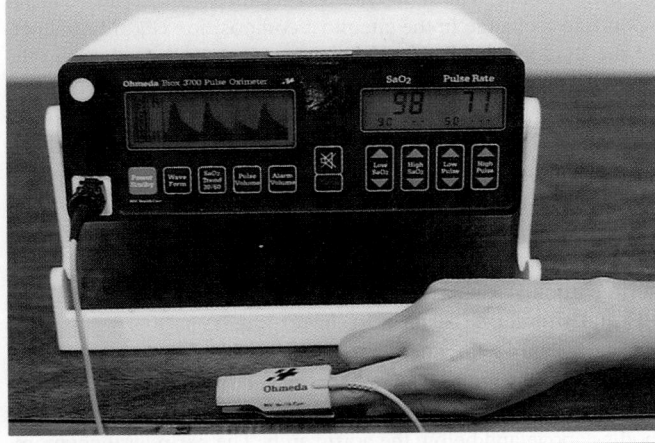

B

FIG. 25-8 **A,** A pulse oximeter passes light from a light–emitting diode through a vascular bed to a photodetector. The oximeter compares the amount of light emitted and absorbed and calculates the SpO_2. The oximeter displays SpO_2 as a digital reading. **B,** Portable pulse oximeter displays oxygen saturation and pulse rate.

TABLE 25-2	Signs and Symptoms of Inadequate Oxygenation	
SIGNS AND SYMPTOMS		**ONSET**
Central Nervous System		
Unexplained apprehension		Early
Unexplained restlessness or irritability		Early
Unexplained confusion or lethargy		Early or late
Combativeness		Late
Coma		Late
Respiratory		
Tachypnea		Early
Dyspnea on exertion		Early
Dyspnea at rest		Late
Use of accessory muscles		Late
Retraction of interspaces on inspiration		Late
Pause for breath between sentences, words		Late
Cardiovascular		
Tachycardia		Early
Mild hypertension		Early
Arrhythmias (e.g., premature ventricular contractions)		Early or late
Hypotension		Late
Cyanosis		Late
Cool, clammy skin		Late
Other		
Diaphoresis		Early or late
Decreased urinary output		Early or late
Unexplained fatigue		Early or late

can be monitored continuously using a *pulse oximetry* probe on the finger, toe, ear, forehead, or bridge of the nose (Fig. 25-8).

A pulse oximeter emits two wavelengths of light, one red and one infrared, which pass from a light-emitting diode (positioned on one side of the probe) to a photodetector (positioned on the opposite side). Well-oxygenated blood absorbs light differently than deoxygenated blood does. The oximeter determines the amount of light absorbed by the vascular bed and calculates the

saturation. SpO_2 is used to indicate the oxygen saturation value obtained by pulse oximetry. SpO_2 and heart rate are displayed on the monitor as digital readings (Fig. 25-8, *B*). The normal SpO_2 is greater than 95%.

Pulse oximetry is particularly valuable in intensive care and perioperative areas where sedation or decreased consciousness might mask hypoxia (Table 25-2). SpO_2 is assessed with each routine vital signs check in many inpatient areas. Changes in

TABLE 25-3	Critical Values for PaO_2 and SpO_2*	
PaO_2 (%)	SpO_2 (%)	CONSIDERATIONS
≥70	≥94	Adequate unless patient is hemodynamically unstable or has O_2-unloading problem. With a low cardiac output, arrhythmias, a leftward shift of the oxyhemoglobin dissociation curve, or carbon monoxide inhalation, higher values may be desired. Benefits of a higher blood O_2 value need to be balanced against the risk of O_2 toxicity.
60	90	Adequate in almost all patients. Values are at steep part of O_2-hemoglobin dissociation curve. Provides adequate oxygenation but with less margin of error than above.
55	88	Adequate for patients with chronic hypoxemia if no cardiac problems occur. These values are also used as criteria for prescription of continuous O_2 therapy.
40	75	Inadequate but may be acceptable on a short-term basis if the patient also has CO_2 retention. In this situation, respirations may be stimulated by a low PaO_2. Thus the PaO_2 cannot be raised rapidly. O_2 therapy at a low concentration (24%-28%) will gradually increase the PaO_2. Monitoring for arrhythmias is necessary.
<40	<75	Inadequate. Tissue hypoxia and cardiac arrhythmias can be expected.

*The same critical values apply for SpO_2 and SaO_2. Values pertain to rest or exertion.

SpO_2 can be detected quickly and treated (Table 25-3). Oximetry is also used during exercise testing and when adjusting flow rates during long-term oxygen therapy. Pulse oximetry alone does not provide information about ventilation status and acid-base balance. Therefore ABGs are also needed periodically.

Values obtained by pulse oximetry are less accurate if the SpO_2 is less than 70%. At this level, the oximeter may display a value that is 64% of the actual value. For example, if the SpO_2 reading is 70%, the actual value can range from 66% to 74%. Pulse oximetry is also inaccurate if hemoglobin variants (e.g., carboxyhemoglobin, methemoglobin) are present. Other factors that can alter the accuracy of pulse oximetry include motion, low perfusion, anemia, bright fluorescent lights, intravascular dyes, thick acrylic nails, and dark skin color. If there is doubt about the accuracy of the SpO_2 reading, an ABG analysis should be obtained to verify accuracy.

Oximetry can also be used to monitor SvO_2 via a PA catheter. A decrease in SvO_2 suggests that less oxygen is being delivered to the tissues or that more oxygen is being consumed. Changes in SvO_2 provide an early warning of a change in cardiac output or tissue oxygen delivery. Normal SvO_2 is 60% to 80%.

Oxygen Delivery. Information from ABGs or oximetry is used to assess adequacy of oxygenation. Several questions must be asked to determine if oxygenation is adequate:

1. What is the patient's SpO_2 or PaO_2 compared with expected normal values? (Normal values are given in Table 25-1.)
2. What is the degree of hypoxemia and what is the trend? Has there been a rapid decline in SpO_2 or PaO_2? A sudden drop in blood oxygen level can be life threatening. A gradual decline is tolerated with fewer symptoms. Critical values for SpO_2 and PaO_2 are given in Table 25-3.
3. Are there signs or symptoms of inadequate oxygenation? Changes in central nervous system, respiratory, cardiovascular, and renal function are seen when tissue oxygen delivery is inadequate (see Table 25-2). Because the brain is highly sensitive to a decrease in tissue oxygen delivery, the first evidence of hypoxemia may be apprehension, restlessness, or irritability. If these signs or symptoms are observed, a change in the management plan is needed.
4. What is the oxygenation status with activity or exercise? Pulse oximetry is used to monitor SpO_2 levels during a standardized 6-minute walk distance test or with activities of daily living to assess for desaturation with activity. An SpO_2 value of 88% or less during exertion indicates the need for supplemental oxygen.[9]

Control of Respiration

The respiratory center in the brainstem medulla responds to chemical and mechanical signals from the body. Impulses are sent from the medulla to the respiratory muscles through the spinal cord and phrenic nerves.

Chemoreceptors. A **chemoreceptor** is a receptor that responds to a change in the chemical composition ($PaCO_2$ and pH) of the fluid around it. Central chemoreceptors are located in the medulla and respond to changes in the hydrogen ion (H^+) concentration. An increase in the H^+ concentration (*acidosis*) causes the medulla to increase the respiratory rate and tidal volume (V_T). A decrease in H^+ concentration (*alkalosis*) has the opposite effect. Changes in $PaCO_2$ regulate ventilation primarily by their effect on the pH of the cerebrospinal fluid. When the $PaCO_2$ level is increased, more CO_2 is available to combine with H_2O and form carbonic acid (H_2CO_3). This lowers the cerebrospinal fluid pH and stimulates an increase in respiratory rate. The opposite process occurs with a decrease in $PaCO_2$ level.

Peripheral chemoreceptors are located in the carotid bodies at the bifurcation of the common carotid arteries and in the aortic bodies above and below the aortic arch. The peripheral chemoreceptors respond to decreases in PaO_2 and pH and to increases in $PaCO_2$. These changes also cause stimulation of the respiratory center.

In a healthy person an increase in $PaCO_2$ or a decrease in pH causes an immediate increase in the respiratory rate. The process is extremely precise. The $PaCO_2$ does not vary more than about 3 mm Hg if lung function is normal. Conditions such as chronic obstructive pulmonary disease (COPD) alter lung function and may result in chronically elevated $PaCO_2$ levels. In these instances, the patient will be relatively insensitive to further increases in $PaCO_2$ as a stimulus to breathe and may be maintaining ventilation largely because of a hypoxic drive from the peripheral chemoreceptors (see Chapter 28).

Mechanical Receptors. **Mechanical receptors** (juxtacapillary and irritant) are located in the lungs, upper airways, chest wall, and diaphragm. They are stimulated by a variety of physiologic factors, such as irritants, muscle stretching, and alveolar wall distortion. Signals from the stretch receptors aid in the control of respiration. As the lungs inflate, pulmonary stretch receptors activate the inspiratory center to inhibit further lung expansion. This is termed the *Hering-Breuer reflex* and it prevents overdistention of the lungs. Impulses from the mechanical sensors are sent through the vagus nerve to the brain. Juxtacapillary (J) receptors are believed to cause the rapid respiration (tachypnea) seen in pulmonary edema. These receptors are stimulated by fluid entering the pulmonary interstitial space.

Respiratory Defense Mechanisms

Respiratory defense mechanisms are efficient in protecting the lungs from inhaled particles, microorganisms, and toxic gases. The defense mechanisms include filtration of air, the mucociliary clearance system, the cough reflex, reflex bronchoconstriction, and alveolar macrophages.

Filtration of Air. Nasal hairs filter the inspired air. In addition, the abrupt changes in direction of airflow that occur as air moves through the nasopharynx and larynx increase air turbulence. This causes particles and bacteria to contact the mucosa lining these structures. Most large particles (greater than 5 μm in diameter) are removed in this manner.

The velocity of airflow slows greatly after it passes the larynx, facilitating the deposition of smaller particles (1 to 5 μm in size). They settle out similar to sand in a river, a process termed *sedimentation*. Particles less than 1 μm in size are too small to settle in this manner and are deposited in the alveoli. One example of small particles that can build up is coal dust, which can lead to pneumoconiosis (see Chapter 27). Particle size is important. Particles greater than 5 μm in size are less dangerous because they are removed in the nasopharynx or bronchi and do not reach the alveoli.

Mucociliary Clearance System. Below the larynx, movement of mucus is accomplished by the mucociliary clearance system, commonly referred to as the *mucociliary escalator.* This term is used to indicate the interrelationship between the secretion of mucus and the ciliary activity. Mucus is continually secreted at a rate of about 100 ml per day by goblet cells and submucosal glands. It forms a mucous blanket that contains the impacted particles and debris from distal lung areas (see Fig. 25-1). The small amount of mucus normally secreted is swallowed without being noticed. Secretory immunoglobulin A (IgA) in the mucus contributes to protection against bacteria and viruses.[10]

Cilia cover the airways from the level of the trachea to the respiratory bronchioles (see Fig. 25-1). Each ciliated cell contains approximately 200 cilia, which beat rhythmically about 1000 times per minute in the large airways, moving mucus toward the mouth. The ciliary beat is slower further down the tracheobronchial tree. As a consequence, particles that penetrate more deeply into the airways are removed less rapidly. Ciliary action is impaired by dehydration, smoking, inhalation of high oxygen concentrations, infection, and ingestion of drugs such as atropine, anesthetics, alcohol, cocaine, or crack. Patients with chronic bronchitis and cystic fibrosis have repeated upper respiratory infections. Cilia are often destroyed during these infections, resulting in impaired secretion clearance, a chronic productive cough, and frequent respiratory infections.

Cough Reflex. The cough is a protective reflex action that clears the airway by a high-pressure, high-velocity flow of air. It is a backup for mucociliary clearance, especially when this clearance mechanism is overwhelmed or ineffective. Coughing is only effective in removing secretions above the subsegmental level (large or main airways). Secretions below this level must be moved upward by the mucociliary mechanism or by interventions such as postural drainage before they can be removed by coughing.

Reflex Bronchoconstriction. Another defense mechanism is reflex bronchoconstriction. In response to the inhalation of large amounts of irritating substances (e.g., dusts, aerosols), the bronchi constrict in an effort to prevent entry of the irritants. A person with hyperreactive airways, such as a person with asthma, experiences bronchoconstriction after inhalation of cold air, perfume, or other strong odors.

Alveolar Macrophages. Because ciliated cells are not found below the level of the respiratory bronchioles, the primary defense mechanism at the alveolar level is alveolar macrophages. *Alveolar macrophages* rapidly phagocytize inhaled foreign particles such as bacteria. The debris is moved to the level of the bronchioles for removal by the cilia or removed from the lungs by the lymphatic system. Particles (e.g., coal dust, silica) that cannot be adequately phagocytized tend to remain in the lungs for indefinite periods and can stimulate inflammatory responses (see Chapter 27). Because alveolar macrophage activity is impaired by cigarette smoke, the smoker who is employed in an occupation with heavy dust exposure (e.g., mining, foundries) is at an especially high risk for lung disease.

■ Gerontologic Considerations: Effects of Aging on the Respiratory System

Age-related changes in the respiratory system can be divided into alterations in structure, defense mechanisms, and respiratory control. Structural alterations include a decrease in elastic recoil of the lung and a decrease in chest wall compliance. The anteroposterior diameter of the thoracic cage increases. Within the lung there is a decrease in the number of functional alveoli. Small airways in the lung bases close earlier in expiration. As a consequence, more inspired air is distributed to the lung apices and ventilation is less well matched to perfusion, causing a lowering of the PaO_2. The PaO_2 associated with a given age can be calculated by means of the following equation:

$$PaO_2 \text{ (mm Hg)} = 103.5 - 0.42 \times \text{Age in years}$$

For example, the normal PaO_2 for a patient 80 years of age is 70 mm Hg [$103.5 - (0.42 \times 80) = 70$ mm Hg] as compared with a PaO_2 of 93 mm Hg for a 25-year-old person [$103.5 - (0.42 \times 25) = 93$ mm Hg].

Respiratory defense mechanisms are less effective because of a decline in cell-mediated immunity and formation of antibodies. The alveolar macrophages are less effective at phagocytosis. An elderly patient has a less forceful cough and fewer and less functional cilia. Formation of secretory IgA, an important mechanism in neutralizing the effect of viruses, is diminished.

Respiratory control is altered, resulting in a more gradual response to changes in blood oxygen or carbon dioxide level. The PaO_2 drops to a lower level and the $PaCO_2$ rises to a higher level before the respiratory rate changes.

TABLE 25-4 *Gerontologic Differences in Assessment*
Respiratory System

CHANGES	DIFFERENCES IN ASSESSMENT FINDINGS
Structure ↓ Elastic recoil ↓ Chest wall compliance ↑ Anteroposterior diameter ↓ Functioning alveoli	Barrel chest appearance; ↓ chest wall movement; ↓ respiratory excursion; ↓ vital capacity; ↑ functional residual capacity; diminished breath sounds particularly at lung bases; ↓ PaO_2 and SaO_2; normal pH and $PaCO_2$.
Defense Mechanisms ↓ Cell-mediated immunity ↓ Specific antibodies ↓ Cilia function ↓ Cough force ↓ Alveolar macrophage function	↓ Cough effectiveness; ↓ secretion clearance; ↑ risk of upper respiratory infection, influenza, pneumonia. Respiratory infections may be more severe and last longer.
Respiratory Control ↓ Response to hypoxemia ↓ Response to hypercapnia	Greater ↓ in PaO_2 and ↑ in $PaCO_2$ before respiratory rate changes. Significant hypoxemia or hypercapnia may develop from relatively small incidents. Retained secretions, excessive sedation, or positioning that impairs chest expansion may substantially alter PaO_2 or SpO_2 values.

There is much variability in the extent of these changes in persons of the same age. The elderly patient who has a significant smoking history, is obese, and is diagnosed with a chronic illness is at greatest risk of adverse outcomes.[11]

Age-related changes in the respiratory system and differences in assessment findings are presented in Table 25-4. ■

ASSESSMENT OF THE RESPIRATORY SYSTEM

Correct diagnosis depends on an accurate health history and a thorough physical examination. A respiratory assessment can be done as part of a comprehensive physical examination or as an examination in itself. Judgment must be used in determining whether all or part of the history and physical examination will be completed based on problems presented by the patient and the degree of respiratory distress. If respiratory distress is severe, only pertinent information should be obtained and a thorough assessment should be deferred until the patient's condition stabilizes.

Subjective Data

Important Health Information

Past health history. The nurse should determine the frequency of upper respiratory problems (e.g., colds, sore throats, sinus problems, allergies) and if weather changes affect these problems. The patient with allergies should be questioned about possible precipitating factors such as medications, pollen, smoke, or pet exposure. Characteristics of the allergic reaction, such as runny nose, wheezing, scratchy throat, or tightness in the chest, and severity should be documented. The frequency of asthma exacerbations and cause, if known, should also be determined. Prior use of a peak expiratory flow rate (PEFR) meter and personal best values can be helpful information in determining the patient's current asthma status.

A history of lower respiratory problems, such as asthma, COPD, pneumonia, and tuberculosis, should also be elicited. Respiratory symptoms are often manifestations of problems that involve other body systems. Therefore the patient should be asked if there is a history of other health problems in addition to those involving the respiratory system. For example, the patient with cardiac dysfunction may experience **dyspnea** (shortness of breath) as a consequence of congestive heart failure. The patient with human immunodeficiency virus (HIV) infection may experience frequent respiratory infections because immune function is compromised.

Medications. The patient should be questioned carefully about prescription and over-the-counter drugs used to manage respiratory problems, such as antihistamines, bronchodilators, corticosteroids, cough suppressants, and antibiotics. Information about the reason for taking the medication, its name, the dose and frequency, length of time taken, its effect, and any side effects should be obtained.

If the patient is using oxygen to ease a breathing problem, the amount, method of administration, and effectiveness of the therapy should be documented. Safety practices related to using oxygen should also be assessed.

Surgery or other treatments. The nurse should determine if the patient has been hospitalized for a respiratory problem. If so, the dates, therapy (including surgery), and current status of the problem should be recorded. The nurse should ask about the use and results of respiratory treatments such as nebulizer, humidifier, and airway clearance modalities, including a Flutter valve, high-frequency chest oscillation, postural drainage, and percussion.

Functional Health Patterns. Health history questions to ask a patient with a respiratory problem are presented in Table 25-5.

Health perception–health management pattern. The patient should be asked if there has been a perceived change in health status within the last several days, months, or years. In COPD, lung function declines slowly over many years. The patient may not notice this decline because activity is altered to accommodate reduced exercise tolerance. If an upper respiratory infection is superimposed on a chronic problem, dyspnea and decreased exer-

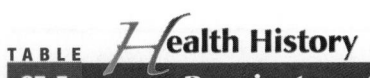

TABLE 25-5   Health History

Respiratory System

Health Perception–Health Management Pattern

- Describe your daily activities. Has there been a change in activities you can perform in the last several days? Months? Years? If changed, was this because of your health?
- How do your breathing problems affect your self-care abilities?
- Have you ever smoked? Do you smoke now? If yes, how many cigarettes each day and for how long? Did you stop or cut back on your smoking because of your health?*
- Have you had a Pneumovax vaccination? When was your last flu shot?
- What types of alcoholic beverages do you drink? How often? How much?
- Do you ever use drugs to get high?* How often?
- What equipment helps you manage your respiratory problems? How often do you use it? Does it help? Cause problems?

Nutritional-Metabolic Pattern

- Have you recently lost weight because of difficulty eating secondary to a respiratory problem? How much? Voluntarily?
- Do any particular foods affect your sputum production or breathing?*

Elimination Pattern

- Does your respiratory problem make it difficult for you to get to the toilet?*
- Are you inactive because of dyspnea to the point where it causes constipation?

Activity-Exercise Pattern

- Are you ever short of breath during exercise?* At rest?*
- Do you get too short of breath to do the things you want to do?*
- Is your home one story? Two stories? How many steps from the street to your door?
- Are you able to maintain your typical activity pattern? If not, explain.
- What do you do when you get short of breath?

Sleep-Rest Pattern

- Do breathing problems cause you to awaken during the night?*
- Can you lie flat at night? If not, how many pillows do you use? Do you need to sleep upright in a chair?
- Are you or your sleep partner aware of any snoring?

Cognitive-Perceptual Pattern

- Do you have any pain associated with breathing?*
- Do you ever feel restless, irritable, or confused without a reason?*
- Do you have difficulty remembering things?*

Self-Perception–Self-Concept Pattern

- Describe how your respiratory problems have changed your life.
- Do you ever go out without using your oxygen? When and why?

Role-Relationship Pattern

- Has your respiratory problem caused any difficulties in your work, family, or social relationships?*

Sexuality-Reproductive Pattern

- Has your respiratory problem caused a change in your sexual activity?*
- Do you want to discuss ways to decrease dyspnea during sexual activity?

Coping–Stress Tolerance Pattern

- How often do you leave your home?
- Would you want to join a support group? Pulmonary rehabilitation program?
- Does stress have an effect on your breathing?*
- What effect does your respiratory problem have on your emotions?

Value-Belief Pattern

- What do you believe causes your respiratory problems?
- Do you think the things you have been told to do for your respiratory problems really help? If not, why?

*If yes, describe.

---

cise tolerance may occur very quickly. In asthma, symptoms may occur or worsen in the presence of exercise, animals, or change in temperature, causing the patient to avoid these activities.

Common cues that should alert the nurse to the possibility of respiratory problems should be explored and documented (Table 25-6). The course of the patient's illness, including when it began, the type of symptoms, and factors that alleviate or aggravate these symptoms, should be described. Because of the chronic nature of respiratory problems, the patient may relate a change in symptoms rather than the onset of new symptoms when describing the present illness. Such changes should be carefully documented because they often suggest the cause of illness. For example, a change in the volume, tenacity (thickness), or color of sputum may suggest the onset of a lower respiratory tract infection in a patient with COPD.

If dyspnea is present, the nurse should determine if it occurs at rest or with physical exertion. The nurse should explore if the patient has difficulty breathing in a certain position, or if relief of dyspnea can be obtained by assuming a different position. To de-

termine the intensity of dyspnea, the use of a Borg scale or visual analog scale (VAS) may be helpful[12] (Fig. 25-9).

If a cough is present, the nurse should evaluate the quality of the cough. For example, a loose-sounding cough indicates the presence of secretions; a dry, hacking cough indicates airway irritation or obstruction; a harsh, barky cough suggests upper airway obstruction from inhibited vocal cord movement related to subglottic edema. The nurse should assess whether the cough is weak or strong and whether it is productive or unproductive of secretions. Determining the onset and chronicity of a cough is helpful in the differential diagnosis process. The pattern of the cough is determined by asking questions such as the following: What has been the pattern of coughing? Has it been regular, paroxysmal, related to a time of day or weather, certain activities, talking, deep breaths? Any change over time? What efforts have been tried to alleviate the coughing? Were any prescription or over-the-counter drugs tried?

If the patient has a productive cough, the following characteristics of sputum should be evaluated: amount, color, consistency,

TABLE 25-6   Cues to Respiratory Problems

MANIFESTATION	DESCRIPTION
Shortness of breath (dyspnea)	Distressful sensation of uncomfortable breathing. Most common complaint of people with respiratory problems. Person may become accustomed to sensation and not recognize its presence. Difficult to evaluate because it is a subjective experience.
Wheezing	May or may not be heard by patient. May be described as chest tightness.
Pleuritic chest pain	Described on a continuum from discomfort during inspiration to intense, sharp pain at the end of inspiration. Pain is usually aggravated by deep breathing and coughing.
Cough	Characteristics of cough are important diagnostic cues.
Sputum production	Material coughed up from lungs. Contains mucus, cellular debris, or microorganisms, and may contain blood or pus. Amount, color, and constituents of sputum are important diagnostic information.
Hemoptysis	Coughing up of blood; either gross, frankly bloody sputum, or blood-tinged sputum. Precipitating events should be investigated.
Voice change	Hoarseness, stridor (whistling sound during inspiration), muffling, or a barking cough may indicate abnormalities of upper airway, vocal cord dysfunction, or gastroesophageal reflux disease (GERD).
Fatigue	Sense of overwhelming tiredness not completely relieved by sleep or rest.

Breathlessness

0	Nothing at all
0.5	Very, very slight
1	Very slight
2	Slight
3	Moderate
4	Somewhat severe
5	Severe
6	
7	Very severe
8	
9	Very, very severe (almost maximal)
10	Maximal

FIG. 25-9 Borg category-ratio scale. Using this scale from 0 to 10, how much shortness of breath do you have right now?

and odor. The amount should be quantified in teaspoons, tablespoons, or cups per day. The nurse should note any recent increases or decreases in the amount. The normal color is clear or slightly whitish. If a patient is a cigarette smoker, the sputum is usually clear to gray with occasional specks of brown. The patient with COPD may exhibit clear, whitish, or slightly yellow sputum, especially in the morning on rising. If the patient reports any change from baseline to yellow, pink, red, brown, or green sputum, pulmonary complications should be suspected. Changes in consistency of sputum to thick, thin, or frothy should be noted. These changes may indicate dehydration, postnasal drip or sinus drainage, or possible pulmonary edema. Normally sputum should be odorless. A foul odor suggests an infectious process.

The patient should be asked if the sputum was produced along with a position change (e.g., increased with lying down) or a change in activity.

The patient should be questioned about a family history of respiratory problems that may be genetic or familial tendencies, such as asthma, emphysema resulting from α_1-antitrypsin deficiency, or cystic fibrosis. A history of family exposure to tuberculosis bacilli should be noted.

The nurse should ask where the patient has lived and traveled. Risk factors for tuberculosis include prior residence in Asia, Africa, or Latin America. Risk factors for fungal infections of the lung include living or traveling in the Southwest (coccidioidomycosis) and the Mississippi River Valley (histoplasmosis).

The nurse should also ask about current and past smoking habits and quantify exposure in pack-years. This is done by multiplying the number of packs smoked per day by the number of years smoked. For example, a person who smoked 1 pack per day for 15 years has a 15 pack-year history. The risk of lung cancer rises in direct proportion to the number of cigarettes smoked. Smoking increases the risk of COPD and exacerbates symptoms of asthma and chronic bronchitis. In addition to asking about cigarette use, it is important to find out the use of any tobacco products, including cigars, pipes, chewing tobacco, and smokeless tobacco products. It is also important to know about exposure to secondhand smoke. The nurse should also ask if efforts have been made to quit the use of these tobacco products, including prescription, over-the-counter, and herbal remedies.

The nurse should ask if the patient received immunization for influenza (flu) and pneumococcal pneumonia (Pneumovax). Influenza vaccine should be administered yearly in the fall. Pneumovax is recommended for persons 65 years or older or those individuals with chronic cardiovascular disease, chronic pulmonary disease, or diabetes mellitus. Revaccination is currently advised only if the patient received the vaccine more than 5 years previously and was less than 65 years old at the time of vaccination. In immunocompromised persons (e.g., transplant recipient), an initial vaccine is recommended followed by revaccination every 5 years.

The patient should be asked about the use of equipment to manage respiratory symptoms (e.g., home oxygen therapy equipment, metered-dose inhaler [MDI] with spacer or nebulizer for medication administration, positive airway pressure device for relief of sleep apnea). The patient should be questioned about the type of equipment used, frequency of use, its effect, and any side effects. The patient should be asked to demonstrate use of the MDI. Many patients do not know how to correctly use MDI devices (see Chapter 28).

Nutritional-metabolic pattern. Weight loss is a symptom of many respiratory diseases. The nurse should determine if weight loss was intentional and, if not, if food intake is altered by anorexia (from medications), fatigue (from hypoxemia, increased work of breathing), early satiety (from lung hyperinflation), or social isolation. Anorexia and weight loss are common symptoms in patients with COPD, acquired immunodeficiency syndrome (AIDS), lung cancer, and tuberculosis. Fluid intake should also be noted. Dehydration can result in thickened mucus, which can cause airway obstruction.

Excessive weight interferes with normal ventilation and may cause sleep apnea (see Chapter 26). Rapid weight gain from fluid retention may decrease pulmonary gas exchange.

Elimination pattern. Healthy elimination habits depend on the ability to reach a toilet when necessary. Activity intolerance secondary to dyspnea could result in incontinence. Dyspnea can also be the cause of limited mobility, which can cause constipation. The patient with dyspnea should be questioned about both of these possibilities.

Activity-exercise pattern. The nurse should determine if the patient's activity is limited by dyspnea at rest or during exercise. The nurse should also note whether the patient's housing (e.g., number of steps, levels) poses a problem that increases social isolation.

The nurse should also inquire if the patient is able to carry out activities of daily living without dyspnea or other respiratory symptoms. If unable, the amount and type of care needed should be documented. Self-care strategies to minimize dyspnea should be reinforced. Immobility and sedentary habits can be risk factors for hypoventilation leading to atelectasis or pneumonia.

Sleep-rest pattern. The nurse should ask if the patient can sleep throughout the night. The patient with asthma or COPD may awaken at night with chest tightness, wheezing, or coughing. This suggests a need for a longer-acting bronchodilator or other medication change. The patient with cardiovascular disease (e.g., congestive heart failure) may sleep with the head elevated on several pillows. The patient with sleep apnea may have snoring, insomnia, and daytime drowsiness. Night sweats may be a manifestation of tuberculosis.

Cognitive-perceptual pattern. Because hypoxia can cause neurologic symptoms, the nurse should ask about apprehension, restlessness, and irritability, which can indicate inadequate cerebral oxygenation (see Table 25-2). Hypoxemia interferes with the ability to learn and retain information. For this reason, teaching may be more effective if another person is present during the teaching session to provide reinforcement at a later date.

The patient's cognitive ability to cooperate with treatment should be assessed. Failure to participate in needed therapy can result in exacerbation of respiratory problems.

The nurse should inquire about any discomfort or pain with breathing. A complaint of chest pain must be explored carefully to rule out cardiac involvement. Respiratory system problems such as pleurisy, fractured ribs, and costochondritis cause chest pain. Pleuritic pain is described as a sharp, stabbing pain associated with movement or deep breathing. Fractured ribs cause localized sharp pain associated with breathing. The pain of costochondritis is along the borders of the sternum and is associated with breathing.

Self-perception–self-concept pattern. Dyspnea limits activity, impairs ability to fulfill normal developmental role functions, and often alters self-esteem. Concern about a highly visible nasal cannula and the difficulty of managing equipment may cause the patient to resist using oxygen in public. The nurse should ask how the patient views his or her personal body image. Referral to a support group or pulmonary rehabilitation program may be beneficial in developing a support system and coping strategies.

Role-relationship pattern. Acute or chronic respiratory problems can seriously affect performance in work or other activities. The nurse should ask about the impact of medications, oxygen, and special routines (e.g., pulmonary hygiene for cystic fibrosis) on the patient's family, job, and social life.

The nurse should document the nature of the patient's work and the frequency and intensity of exposure to fumes, toxins, asbestos, coal, or silica. Patient-specific allergens such as dust or fumes, which could be present in the work environment, should be investigated. Hobbies such as woodworking (sawdust) or pottery (silica) and exposure to animals (allergies) may also cause respiratory problems. Because of hyperreactive airways, exposure to fumes, smoke, and other chemicals may trigger wheezing in the asthmatic patient.

Sexuality-reproductive pattern. Most patients can continue to have good sexual relationships despite marked physical limitations. In a tactful manner, the nurse should determine whether breathing difficulties have caused alterations in sexual activity. If so, teaching can be provided about positions that decrease dyspnea during sexual activity and alternative strategies for sexual fulfillment.

Coping–stress tolerance pattern. Dyspnea causes anxiety and anxiety exacerbates dyspnea. The result is a vicious cycle—the patient avoids activities that cause dyspnea, becoming more deconditioned and more dyspneic. The outcome is often physical and social isolation. The nurse should ask how often the patient leaves home and interacts with others. Referral to a support group or pulmonary rehabilitation program may be beneficial.

The chronic nature of many respiratory problems such as COPD and asthma can cause prolonged stress. Inquiry should be made into the patient's coping strategies to manage this stress.

Value-belief pattern. The nurse should determine the patient's adherence to the management regimen. Reasons for lack of adherence should be explored, including conflict with culturally specific beliefs, financial constraints (costs of prescriptions), failure to note benefit, or other reasons.[13]

Objective Data

Physical Examination. Vital signs, including temperature, pulse, respirations, and blood pressure, are important data to collect before examination of the respiratory system.

Nose. The nose is inspected for patency, inflammation, deformities, symmetry, and discharge. Each nare is checked for air patency with respiration while the other nare is briefly occluded. The nurse tilts the patient's head backward and pushes the tip of the nose upward gently. With a nasal speculum and a good light, the interior of the nose is inspected. The mucous membrane should be pink and moist, with no evidence of edema (bogginess), exudate, or bleeding. The nasal septum should be observed for deviation, perforations, and bleeding. Some nasal deviation is normal in an adult. The turbinates should be observed for polyps, which are abnormal, fingerlike projections of swollen nasal mucosa. Polyps may result from long-term irritation of the mucosa, as from allergies. Any discharge should be assessed for color and consistency. The presence of purulent and malodorous discharge could indicate the presence of a foreign body. Watery discharge could be secondary to allergies or from cerebrospinal fluid. Bloody discharge could be from trauma. Thick mucosal discharge could indicate the presence of infection.

Mouth and pharynx. Using a good light source, the nurse inspects the interior of the mouth for color, lesions, masses, gum retraction, bleeding, and poor dentition. The tongue is inspected for symmetry and presence of lesions. The nurse observes the pharynx by pressing a tongue blade against the middle of the back of the tongue. The pharynx should be smooth and moist, with no evidence of exudate, ulcerations, swelling, or postnasal drip. The color, symmetry, and any enlargement of the tonsils are noted. The nurse stimulates the gag reflex by placing a tongue blade along the side of the pharynx behind the tonsil. A normal response (gagging) indicates that the cranial nerves IX (glossopharyngeal) and X (vagus) are intact and that the airway is protected. Each side of the pharynx should be checked for the gag reflex.

Neck. The nurse inspects the neck for symmetry and presence of tender or swollen areas. The lymph nodes are palpated while the patient is sitting erect with the neck slightly flexed. Progression is from the nodes around the ears, to the nodes at the base of the skull, and then to those located under the angles of the mandible to the midline. The patient may have small, mobile, nontender nodes *(shotty nodes)*, which are not a sign of a pathologic condition. Tender, hard, or fixed nodes indicate disease. The location and characteristics of any palpable nodes are described.

Thorax and lungs. Imaginary lines can be pictured on the chest to help in identifying abnormalities (see Fig. 25-2). Abnormalities can be described in relation to their location relative to these lines (e.g., 2 cm from the right midclavicular line).

Chest examination is best performed in a well-lighted, warm room with measures taken to ensure the patient's privacy. Either the anterior or the posterior chest may be examined first.

Inspection. The patient's anterior chest should be exposed while sitting upright or with the head of the bed upright. The patient may need to lean forward to support himself or herself on the bedside table to facilitate breathing. First, the nurse observes the patient's appearance and notes any evidence of respiratory distress, such as tachypnea or use of accessory muscles. Next, the nurse determines the shape and symmetry of the chest. Chest movement should be equal on both sides, and the anteroposterior (AP) diameter should be equal to the side-to-side diameter. Normal AP is less than the transverse by a ratio of 1:2. An increase in AP diameter (e.g., barrel chest) may be a normal aging change or result from lung hyperinflation. The nurse observes for abnormalities in the sternum (e.g., *pectus carinatum* [a prominent protrusion of the sternum] and *pectus excavatum* [an indentation of the lower sternum above the xiphoid process]).

Next the respiratory rate, depth, and rhythm should be observed. The normal rate is 12 to 20 breaths per minute; in the elderly, it is 16 to 25 breaths per minute. Inspiration (I) should take half as long as expiration (E) (I:E = 1:2). The nurse should ob-

serve for abnormal breathing patterns, such as Kussmaul (rapid, deep breathing), Cheyne-Stokes (abnormal pattern of respiration characterized by alternating periods of apnea and deep, rapid breathing), or Biot's (irregular breathing with apnea every 4 to 5 cycles) respirations.[14]

Skin color provides clues to respiratory status. Cyanosis is best observed in a dark-skinned patient in the conjunctivae, lips, palms, and soles of the feet. Causes of cyanosis include hypoxemia or decreased cardiac output. The fingers should be inspected for evidence of *clubbing* (an increase in the angle between the base of the nail and the fingernail to 180 degrees or more, usually accompanied by an increase in the depth, bulk, and sponginess of the end of the finger).

When the nurse is inspecting the posterior chest, the patient should be asked to lean forward with arms folded. This position moves the scapula away from the spine, so there is more exposure of the area to be examined. The same sequence of observations that were done on the anterior part of the chest is performed on the posterior part. In addition, any spinal curvature is noted. Spinal curvatures that affect breathing include kyphosis, scoliosis, and kyphoscoliosis.

Palpation. The nurse determines tracheal position by gently placing the index fingers on either side of the trachea just above the suprasternal notch and gently pressing backward. Normal tracheal position is midline; deviation to the left or right is abnormal. Tracheal deviation occurs away from the side of a tension pneumothorax or a neck mass, but toward the side of a pneumonectomy or lobar atelectasis.[15]

The nurse determines symmetry of chest expansion and extent of movement at the level of the diaphragm. The nurse places the hands over the lower anterior chest wall along the costal margin and moves them inward until the thumbs meet at midline. The patient is asked to breathe deeply, and the nurse observes the movement of the thumbs away from each other. Normal expansion is 1 inch (2.5 cm). On the posterior side of the chest, the nurse places the hands at the level of the tenth rib and moves the thumbs until they meet over the spine (Fig. 25-10).

Normal chest movement is equal. Unequal expansion occurs when air entry is limited by conditions involving the lung (e.g., atelectasis, pneumothorax) or the chest wall (e.g., incisional

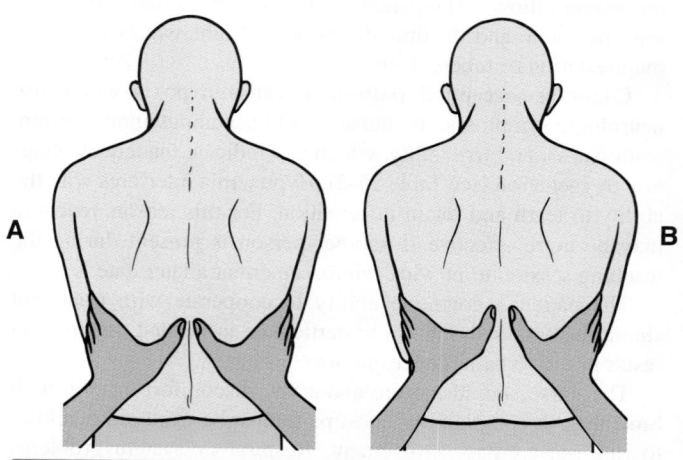

FIG. 25-10 Estimation of thoracic expansion. **A,** Exhalation. **B,** Maximal inhalation.

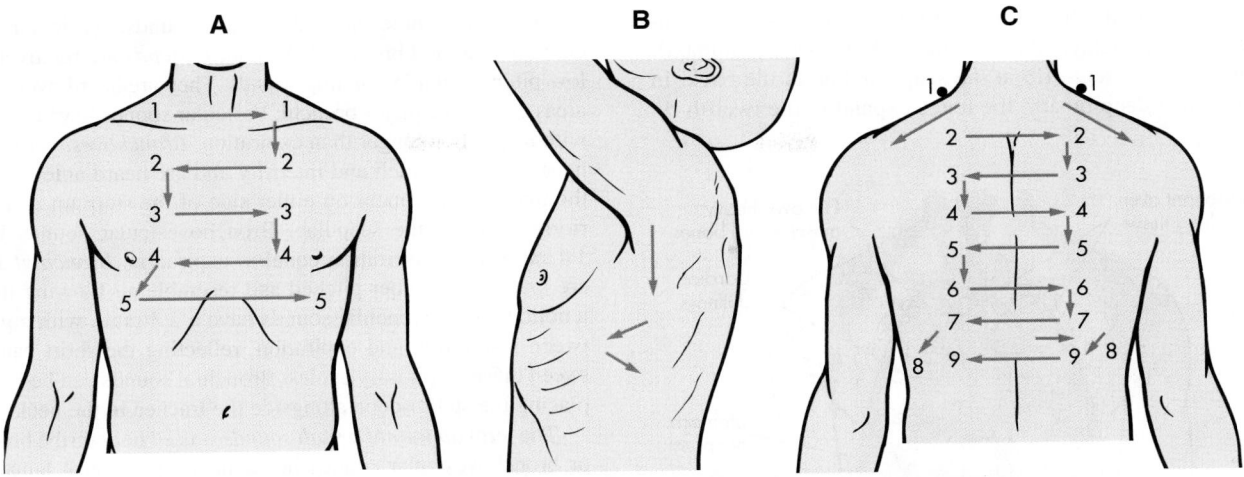

FIG. 25-11 Sequence for examination of the chest. **A,** Anterior sequence. **B,** Lateral sequence. **C,** Posterior sequence. For palpation, place the palms of the hands in the position designated as "1" on the right and left sides of the chest. Compare the intensity of vibrations. Continue for all positions in each sequence. For percussion, tap the chest at each designated position, moving downward from side to side, while comparing percussion notes. For auscultation, place the stethoscope at each position and listen to at least one complete inspiratory and expiratory cycle.

pain). Equal but diminished expansion occurs in conditions that produce a hyperinflated or barrel chest or in neuromuscular diseases (e.g., amyotrophic lateral sclerosis, spinal cord lesions). Movement may be absent or unequal over a pleural effusion, an atelectasis, or a pneumothorax.

Fremitus is vibration of the chest wall produced by vocalization. To elicit tactile fremitus, the nurse places the palms of the hands against the patient's chest and asks the patient to repeat a phrase such as "ninety-nine." The nurse moves the hands from side to side and from top to bottom on the patient's chest (Fig. 25-11). All areas of the chest should be palpated and vibrations compared from similar areas. Tactile fremitus is most intense in the first and second interspace lateral to the sternum and between the scapulae because these areas are closest to the major bronchi. Fremitus is less intense farther away from these areas.

Increase, decrease, or absence of fremitus should be noted. Increased fremitus occurs when the lung becomes filled with fluid or more dense. This is noted in pneumonia, in lung tumors, and above a pleural effusion (the lung is compressed upward). Fremitus is decreased if the hand is farther from the lung (e.g., pleural effusion) or the lung is hyperinflated (e.g., barrel chest). Absent fremitus may be noted with pneumothorax or atelectasis. The anterior of the chest is more difficult to palpate for fremitus because of the presence of large muscles and breast tissue.

Rhonchial fremitus is an abnormal palpable vibration caused by air traveling past thick bronchial mucus. It can be felt with the hand on the chest while the patient takes a deep inspiration, and may change or clear with coughing.

Percussion. Percussion is done to assess density or aeration of the lungs. Percussion sounds are described in Table 25-7. (The technique for percussion is described in Chapter 3.)

The anterior chest is usually percussed with the patient in a semisitting or supine position. Starting above the clavicles, the nurse percusses downward, interspace by interspace (see Fig. 25-11). The area over lung tissue should be resonant, with the exception of the area of cardiac dullness (Fig. 25-12). For

TABLE 25-7	Percussion Sounds
SOUND	**DESCRIPTION**
Resonance	Low-pitched sound heard over normal lungs
Hyperresonance	Loud, lower-pitched sound than normal resonance heard over hyperinflated lungs, such as in chronic obstructive lung disease and acute asthma
Tympany	Drumlike, loud, empty quality heard over gas-filled stomach or intestine, or pneumothorax
Dull	Medium-intensity pitch and duration heard over areas of "mixed" solid and lung tissue, such as over the top area of the liver, partially consolidated lung tissue (pneumonia), or fluid-filled pleural space
Flat	Soft, high-pitched sound of short duration heard over very dense tissue where air is not present

percussion of the posterior chest, the patient should sit leaning forward with arms folded. The posterior chest should be resonant over lung tissue to the level of the diaphragm (Fig. 25-13).

Auscultation. During chest auscultation, the patient is instructed to breathe slowly and deeply through the mouth. The nurse should proceed comparing opposite areas of the chest, from the lung apices to the bases (see Fig. 25-11). The stethoscope should be placed over lung tissue, not over bony prominences. At each placement of the stethoscope, the nurse should listen to at least one cycle of inspiration and expiration. Note the pitch (e.g., high, low), duration of sound, and presence of adventitious or abnormal sounds. The location of normal auscultatory sounds is more easily understood by visualization of a lung model (Fig. 25-14).

The lung sounds should be heard down to the sixth rib anteriorly at the midclavicular line, the eighth rib at the midaxillary line, and the tenth rib at the scapular line in the back. In addition, on a deep breath, the lungs expand to the twelfth rib posteriorly.

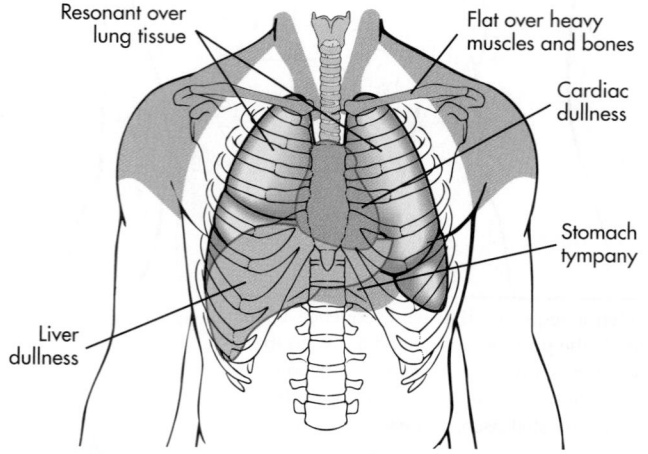

FIG. 25-12 Diagram of percussion areas and sounds in the anterior side of the chest.

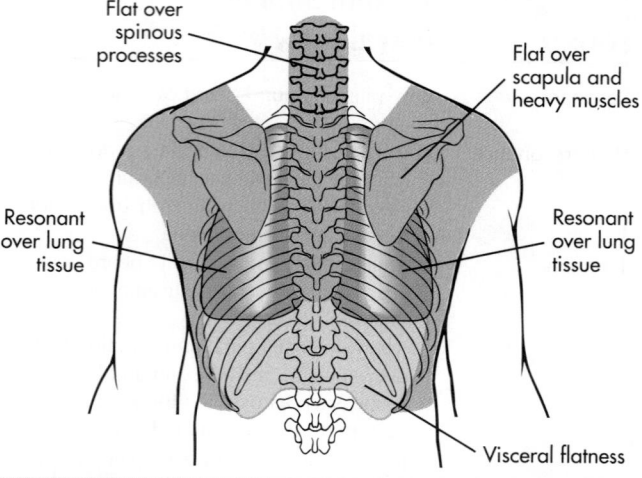

FIG. 25-13 Diagram of percussion areas and sounds in the posterior side of the chest. Percussion proceeds from the lung apices to the lung bases, comparing sounds in opposite areas of the chest.

There are three normal breath sounds: vesicular, bronchovesicular, and bronchial. *Vesicular sounds* are relatively soft, low-pitched, gentle, rustling sounds. They are heard over all lung areas except the major bronchi. Vesicular sounds have a 3:1 ratio, with inspiration longer than expiration. *Bronchovesicular sounds* have a medium pitch and intensity and are heard anteriorly over the main-stem bronchi on either side of the sternum and posteriorly between the scapulae. Bronchovesicular sounds have a 1:1 ratio, with inspiration equal to expiration. *Bronchial sounds* are louder and higher pitched and resemble air blowing through a hollow pipe. Bronchial sounds have a 2:3 ratio, with a gap between inspiration and expiration, reflecting the short pause between these respiratory cycles. Bronchial sounds can be heard by placing the stethoscope alongside the trachea in the neck.

The term *abnormal breath sounds* is used to describe bronchial or bronchovesicular sounds heard in the peripheral lung fields. **Adventitious sounds** are extra breath sounds that are abnormal. Adventitious breath sounds include **crackles, rhonchi, wheezes,** and **pleural friction rub** (described in Table 25-9).

A record of the normal physical assessment of the respiratory system is shown in Table 25-8. Common assessment abnormalities of the thorax and lungs are presented in Table 25-9. Chest examination findings in common pulmonary problems are presented in Table 25-10. Age-related changes in the respiratory system and assessment findings are presented in Table 25-4.

TABLE 25-8   Normal Physical Assessment of the Respiratory System

- Nose is symmetric with no deformities. Nasal mucosa is pink and moist with no edema, exudate, blood, or polyps. Nasal septum is straight, without perforations.
- Oral mucosa is light pink and moist, with no exudate or ulcerations.
- Tonsils are not inflamed or enlarged.
- Pharynx is smooth, moist, and pink.
- Neck is symmetric and trachea is in the midline. No nodes are palpable.
- Chest is oval and symmetric. Respirations are easy, at the rate of 14/min. Excursion is equal bilaterally, with no increase in tactile fremitus. Percussion is resonant throughout. Breath sounds are vesicular at periphery, without crackles, rhonchi, or wheezes. No axillary nodes are palpable.

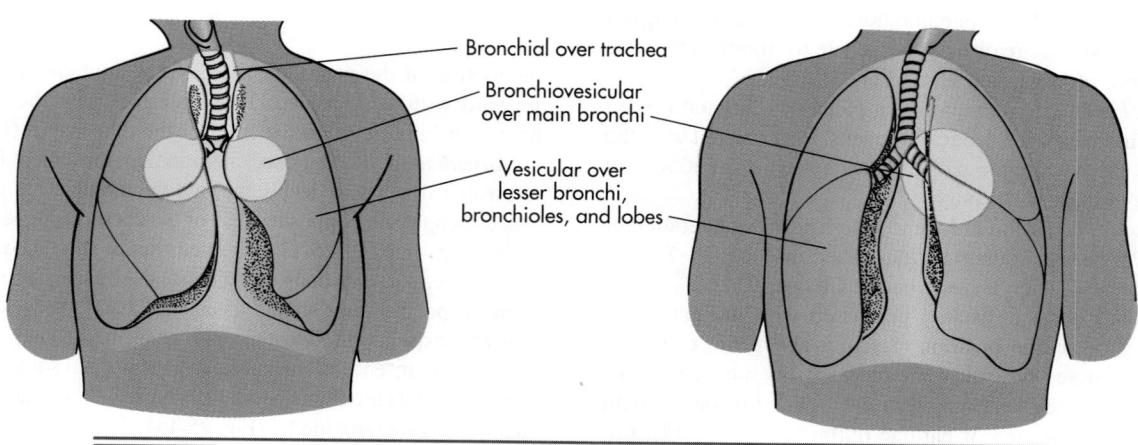

FIG. 25-14 Normal auscultatory sounds.

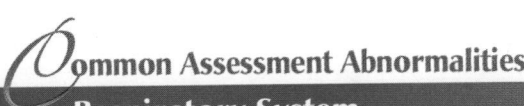

| TABLE 25-9 | Common Assessment Abnormalities | Respiratory System |

FINDING	DESCRIPTION	POSSIBLE ETIOLOGY AND SIGNIFICANCE*
Inspection		
▪ Pursed-lip breathing	Exhalation through mouth with lips pursed together to slow exhalation.	COPD, asthma. Suggests ↑ breathlessness. Strategy taught to slow expiration, ↓ dyspnea.
▪ Tripod position; inability to lie flat	Learning forward with arms and elbows supported on overbed table.	COPD, asthma in exacerbation, pulmonary edema. Indicates moderate to severe respiratory distress.
▪ Accessory muscle use; intercostal retractions	Neck and shoulder muscles used to assist breathing. Muscles between ribs pull in during inspiration.	COPD, asthma in exacerbation, secretion retention. Indicates severe respiratory distress, hypoxemia.
▪ Splinting	Voluntary ↓ in tidal volume to ↓ pain on chest expansion.	Thoracic or abdominal incision. Chest trauma, pleurisy.
▪ ↑ AP diameter	AP chest diameter equal to lateral. Slope of ribs more horizontal (90 degrees) to spine.	COPD, asthma, cystic fibrosis. Lung hyperinflation. Advanced age.
▪ Tachypnea	Rate >20 breaths/min; >25 breaths/min in elderly.	Fever, anxiety, hypoxemia, restrictive lung disease. Magnitude of ↑ above normal rate reflects increased work of breathing.
▪ Kussmaul's respirations	Regular, rapid, and deep respirations.	Metabolic acidosis; ↑ in rate aids body in ↑ CO_2 excretion.
▪ Cyanosis	Bluish color of skin best seen in earlobes, under the eyelids, or nail beds.	↓ Oxygen transfer in lungs, ↓ cardiac output. Nonspecific, unreliable indicator.
▪ Clubbing of fingers	↑ Depth, bulk, sponginess of distal digit of finger.	Chronic hypoxemia. Cystic fibrosis, lung cancer, bronchiectasis.
▪ Abdominal paradox	Inward (rather than normal outward) movement of abdomen during inspiration.	Inefficient and ineffective breathing pattern. Nonspecific indicator of severe respiratory distress.
Palpation		
▪ Tracheal deviation	Leftward or rightward movement of trachea from normal midline position.	Nonspecific indicator of change in position of mediastinal structures. Medical emergency if caused by tension pneumothorax.
▪ Altered tactile fremitus	Increase or decrease in vibrations.	↑ In pneumonia, pulmonary edema; ↓ in pleural effusion, lung hyperinflation; absent in pneumothorax, atelectasis.
▪ Altered chest movement	Unequal or equal but diminished movement of two sides of chest with inspiration.	Unequal movement caused by atelectasis, pneumothorax, pleural effusion, splinting; equal but diminished movement caused by barrel chest, restrictive disease, neuromuscular disease.
Percussion		
▪ Hyperresonance	Loud, lower-pitched sound over areas that normally produce a resonant sound.	Lung hyperinflation (COPD), lung collapse (pneumothorax), air trapping (asthma).
▪ Dullness	Medium-pitched sound over areas that normally produce a resonant sound.	↑ Density (pneumonia, large atelectasis), ↑ fluid pleural space (pleural effusion).
Auscultation		
▪ Fine crackles	Series of short, explosive, high-pitched sounds heard just before the end of inspiration; result of rapid equalization of gas pressure when collapsed alveoli or terminal bronchioles suddenly snap open; similar sound to that made by rolling hair between fingers just behind ear	Interstitial fibrosis (asbestosis), interstitial edema (early pulmonary edema), alveolar filling (pneumonia), loss of lung volume (atelectasis), early phase of congestive heart failure.
▪ Coarse crackles	Series of short, low-pitched sounds caused by air passing through airway intermittently occluded by mucus, unstable bronchial wall, or fold of mucosa; evident on inspiration and, at times, expiration; similar sound to blowing through straw under water; increase in bubbling quality with more fluid	Congestive heart failure, pulmonary edema, pneumonia with severe congestion COPD.

*Limited to common etiologic factors. (Further discussion of conditions listed may be found in Chapters 26 through 28.)
AP, Anteroposterior; COPD, chronic obstructive pulmonary disease.

Continued

TABLE
25-9

Common Assessment Abnormalities

Respiratory System—cont'd

FINDING	DESCRIPTION	POSSIBLE ETIOLOGY AND SIGNIFICANCE*
Auscultation—cont'd		
Rhonchi	Continuous rumbling, snoring, or rattling sounds from obstruction of large airways with secretions; most prominent on expiration; change often evident after coughing or suctioning	COPD, cystic fibrosis, pneumonia, bronchiectasis.
Wheezes	Continuous high-pitched squeaking sound caused by rapid vibration of bronchial walls; first evident on expiration but possibly evident on inspiration as obstruction of airway increases; possibly audible without stethoscope	Bronchospasm (caused by asthma), airway obstruction (caused by foreign body, tumor), COPD.
Stridor	Continuous musical sound of constant pitch; result of partial obstruction of larynx or trachea	Croup, epiglottitis, vocal cord edema after extubation, foreign body.
Absent breath sounds	No sound evident over entire lung or area of lung	Pleural effusion, main-stem bronchi obstruction, large atelectasis, pneumonectomy, lobectomy.
Pleural friction rub	Creaking or grating sound from roughened, inflamed surfaces of the pleura rubbing together; evident during inspiration, expiration, or both and no change with coughing; usually uncomfortable, especially on deep inspiration	Pleurisy, pneumonia, pulmonary infarct.
Bronchophony, whispered pectoriloquy	Spoken or whispered syllable more distinct than normal on auscultation	Pneumonia.
Egophony	Spoken "e" similar to "a" on auscultation because of altered transmission of voice sounds	Pneumonia, pleural effusion.

TABLE 25-10   Chest Examination Findings in Common Pulmonary Problems

PROBLEM	INSPECTION	PALPATION	PERCUSSION	AUSCULTATION
Chronic bronchitis	Barrel chest; cyanosis	↓ Movement ↑ Fremitus	Hyperresonant or dull if consolidation	Crackles; rhonchi; wheezes
Emphysema	Barrel chest; tripod position; use of accessory muscles	↓ Movement	Hyperresonant or dull if consolidation	Crackles; rhonchi; diminished if no exacerbation
Asthma In exacerbation	Prolonged expiration; tripod position; pursed lips	↓ Movement ↓ Fremitus if hyperinflation	Hyperresonance	Wheezes; ↓ breath sounds ominous sign if no improvement (severely diminished air movement)
Not in exacerbation	Normal	Normal	Normal	Normal
Pneumonia	Tachypnea; use of accessory muscles; duskiness or cyanosis	Unequal movement if lobar involvement; ↑ fremitus over affected area	Dull over affected areas	Early: Bronchial sounds Later: Crackles; rhonchi
Atelectasis	No change unless involves entire segment, lobe	If small, no change If large, ↓ movement; ↑ fremitus	Dull over affected areas	Crackles (may disappear with deep breaths); absent sounds if large
Pulmonary edema	Tachypnea; labored respirations; cyanosis	↓ Movement or normal movement	Dull or normal depending on amount of fluid	Fine or coarse crackles
Pleural effusion	Tachypnea; use of accessory muscles	↓ Movement ↑ Fremitus above effusion; absent fremitus over effusion	Dull	Diminished or absent over effusion; egophony over effusion
Pulmonary fibrosis	Tachypnea	↓ Movement	Normal	Crackles

DIAGNOSTIC STUDIES OF THE RESPIRATORY SYSTEM

Blood Studies

Common blood studies used to assess the respiratory system are the hemoglobin (Hb), hematocrit (Hct), and ABG determinations. Table 25-11 describes nursing responsibilities associated with these tests.

Oximetry

Oximetry is used to noninvasively monitor SpO_2 and SvO_2 (see Tables 25-1 and 25-2). Nursing care associated with oximetry is discussed in Table 25-11.

Sputum Studies

Sputum samples can be obtained by expectoration, tracheal suction, or bronchoscopy, a technique in which a flexible scope is inserted into the airways. The specimens may be examined for culture and sensitivity to identify an infecting organism (e.g., *Mycobacterium, Pneumocystis carinii*) or to confirm a diagnosis (e.g., malignant cells). Nursing responsibilities for specimen collection are given in Table 25-11. Regardless of whether specimen tests are ordered, it is important to observe the sputum for color, blood, volume, and viscosity.

Skin Tests

Skin tests may be performed to test for allergic reactions or exposure to tuberculous bacilli or fungi. Skin tests involve the intradermal injection of an antigen. A positive result indicates that the patient has been exposed to the antigen. It does not indicate that disease is currently present. A negative result indicates that there has been no exposure or there is depression of cell-mediated immunity such as occurs in HIV infection.

Nursing responsibilities are similar for all skin tests. First, to prevent a false-negative reaction, the nurse should be certain that the injection is intradermal and not subcutaneous. After the injection, the sites should be circled and the patient instructed not to remove the marks. When charting administration of the antigen, the nurse should draw a diagram of the forearm and hand and label the injection sites. The diagram is especially helpful when more than one test is administered.

When reading test results, the nurse should use a good light. If an induration is present, a marking pen should be brought in from the periphery on all four sides of the induration. As the pen touches the raised area, a mark should be made. The nurse then determines the diameter of the induration in millimeters. Reddened, flat areas are not measured. See Table 25-12 for a description of reactions that indicate a positive tuberculosis skin test.[16]

Radiologic Studies

Chest X-ray. A chest x-ray is the most commonly used test for assessment of the respiratory system. It is also used to assess progression of disease and response to treatment. The most common views used are the posteroanterior and lateral. (See Table 25-11 for nursing responsibilities related to chest x-rays.)

Computed Tomography. A computed tomography (CT) scan may be used to examine cross sections of the entire body. CT scans are used to evaluate areas that are difficult to assess by conventional x-ray, such as the mediastinum, hilum, and pleura. With the addition of a contrast-enhanced medium, high-resolution technique, or newer spiral CT scans, even pulmonary arteries can be inspected for emboli.

Magnetic Resonance Imaging. While in a strong magnetic field, the alignment of spinning nuclei can be changed with a superimposed radio frequency and the rate at which they return to alignment with the field can be measured. Magnetic resonance imaging (MRI) uses this technique to produce images of body structures. MRI has limited indications. It is most useful when evaluating images near the lung apex or spine and for distinguishing vascular from nonvascular structures.

Ventilation-Perfusion Scan. A ventilation-perfusion scan is used primarily to check for the presence of a pulmonary embolus. There is no specific preparation or aftercare. An intravenous (IV) radioisotope is given for the perfusion portion of the test, and the pulmonary vasculature is outlined and photographed. For the ventilation portion, the patient inhales a radioactive gas, which outlines the alveoli, and another photograph is taken. Normal scans show homogeneous radioactivity. Diminished or absent radioactivity suggests lack of perfusion or airflow.

Pulmonary Angiography. Pulmonary angiography is used to confirm the diagnosis of an embolus if findings of the lung scan are inconclusive. A series of x-rays is taken after radiopaque dye is injected into the pulmonary artery. This test also detects congenital and acquired lesions of the pulmonary vessels.

Positron Emission Tomography. Positron emission tomography (PET) scans involve the use of radionuclides with short half-lives. PET scans are used to distinguish benign and malignant solitary pulmonary nodules. Because malignant lung cells have an increased uptake of glucose, the PET scan, which uses an IV glucose preparation, can demonstrate increased uptake of glucose in malignant lung cells.

Endoscopic Examinations

Bronchoscopy. *Bronchoscopy* is a procedure in which the bronchi are visualized through a fiberoptic tube. Bronchoscopy may be used to obtain biopsy specimens, assess changes resulting from treatment, and remove mucous plugs or foreign bodies. Small amounts (30 ml) of sterile saline may be injected through the scope and withdrawn and examined for cells, a technique termed *bronchoalveolar lavage* (BAL). BAL is used to diagnose *Pneumocystis carinii* pneumonia (Fig. 25-15).

Bronchoscopy can be performed in an outpatient procedure room, in a surgical suite, or at the bedside in the intensive care unit or on a medical-surgical floor, with the patient lying down or seated. After the nasal pharynx and oral pharynx are anesthetized with local anesthetic, the bronchoscope is coated with lidocaine (Xylocaine) and inserted, usually through the nose, and threaded down into the airways. Bronchoscopy can be done on mechanically ventilated patients through the endotracheal tube. The nursing care for the patient undergoing this procedure is described in Table 25-11.

Mediastinoscopy. For *mediastinoscopy,* a scope is inserted through a small incision in the suprasternal notch and advanced into the mediastinum to inspect and biopsy lymph nodes. The test is used to diagnose carcinoma, granulomatous infections, and sarcoidosis. The procedure is performed in the operating room and the patient is given a general anesthetic.

TABLE 25-11

Diagnostic Studies
Respiratory System

STUDY	DESCRIPTION AND PURPOSE	NURSING RESPONSIBILITY
Blood Studies		
• Hemoglobin	Test reflects amount of hemoglobin available for combination with oxygen. Venous blood is used. *Normal level* for adult man is 13.5-18 g/dl (135-180 g/L); *normal level* for adult woman is 12-16 g/dl (120-160 g/L).	Explain procedure and its purpose.
• Hematocrit	Test reflects ratio of red blood cells to plasma. Increased hematocrit (polycythemia) found in chronic hypoxemia. Venous blood is used. *Normal* for adult man is 40%-54% (0.40-0.54); *normal* for adult woman is 38%-47% (0.38-0.47).	Explain procedure and its purpose.
• ABGs	Arterial blood is obtained through puncture of radial or femoral artery or through arterial catheter. ABGs are performed to assess acid-base balance, ventilation status, need for oxygen therapy, change in oxygen therapy, or change in ventilator settings.* Continuous ABG monitoring is also possible via a sensor or electrode inserted into the arterial catheter.	Indicate whether patient is using O_2 (percentage, L/min). Avoid change in oxygen therapy or interventions (e.g., suctioning, position change) for 20 min before obtaining sample. Assist with positioning (e.g., palm up, wrist slightly hyperextended if radial artery is used). Collect blood into heparinized syringe. To ensure accurate results, expel all air bubbles, and place sample in ice, unless it will be analyzed in less than 1 min. Apply pressure to artery for 5 min after specimen is obtained to prevent hematoma at the arterial puncture site.
• Oximetry	Test monitors arterial or venous oxygen saturation. Device attaches to the earlobe, finger, or nose for SpO_2 monitoring or is contained in a pulmonary artery catheter for SvO_2 monitoring. Oximetry is used for intermittent or continuous monitoring and exercise testing.†	Apply probe to finger, forehead, earlobe, or bridge of nose. When interpreting SpO_2 and SvO_2 values, first assess patient status and presence of factors that can alter accuracy of pulse oximeter reading. For SpO_2, these include motion, low perfusion, bright lights, use of intravascular dyes, acrylic nails, dark skin color. For SvO_2, these include change in O_2 delivery or O_2 consumption. For SpO_2, notify health care provider of $\pm 4\%$ change from baseline or $\downarrow$ to $<90\%$. For SvO_2, notify health care provider of $\pm 10\%$ change from baseline or $\downarrow$ to $<60\%$.
Sputum Studies		
• Culture and sensitivity	Single sputum specimen is collected in a sterile container. Purpose is to diagnose bacterial infection, select antibiotic, and evaluate treatment.	Instruct patient on how to produce a good specimen (see Gram stain). If patient cannot produce specimen, bronchoscopy may be used (see Fig. 25-15).
• Gram stain	Staining of sputum permits classification of bacteria into gram-negative and gram-positive types. Results guide therapy until culture and sensitivity results are obtained.	Instruct patient to expectorate sputum into the container after coughing deeply. Obtain sputum (mucoidlike), not saliva. Obtain specimen in early morning because secretions collect during night. If unsuccessful, try increasing oral fluid intake unless fluids are restricted. Collect sputum in sterile container (sputum trap) during suctioning or by aspirating secretions from the trachea. Send specimen to laboratory promptly.
• Acid-fast smear and culture	Test is performed to collect sputum for acid-fast bacilli (tuberculosis). A series of 3 early morning specimens is used.	Instruct patient on how to produce a good specimen (see Gram stain). Cover specimen and send to laboratory for analysis.
• Cytology	Single sputum specimen is collected in special container with fixative solution. Purpose is to determine presence of abnormal cells that may indicate malignant condition.	Send specimen to laboratory promptly. Instruct patient on how to produce a good specimen (see Gram stain). If patient cannot produce specimen, bronchoscopy may be used (see Fig. 25-15).

*For normal values, see Tables 25-1 and 25-2.
†For normal values see Table 25-12 and 25-13.
ABGs, Arterial blood gases; *ICUs,* intensive care units; *IV,* intravenous; *NPO,* nothing by mouth.

TABLE 25-11 ## *Diagnostic Studies*
Respiratory System—cont'd

STUDY	DESCRIPTION AND PURPOSE	NURSING RESPONSIBILITY
Radiology		
▪ Chest x-ray	Test is used to screen, diagnose, and evaluate change. Most common views are posteroanterior and lateral.	Instruct patient to undress to waist, put on gown, and remove any metal between neck and waist.
▪ Computed tomography (CT)	Test is performed for diagnosis of lesions difficult to assess by conventional x-ray studies, such as those in the hilum, mediastinum, and pleura. Images show structures in cross section.	Same as for chest x-ray.
▪ Magnetic resonance imaging (MRI)	Test is used for diagnosis of lesions difficult to assess by CT scan (e.g., lung apex near the spine).	Same as for chest x-ray. Instruct the patient to remove all metal (e.g., jewelry, watch) before test.
▪ Ventilation-perfusion (V̇/Q̇)	Test is used to identify areas of the lung not receiving airflow (ventilation) or blood flow (perfusion). It involves injection of radioisotope and inhalation of small amount of radioactive gas (xenon). A gamma-detecting device is used to record radioactivity. Ventilation without perfusion suggests pulmonary embolus.	Same as for chest x-ray. No precautions needed afterward because the gas and isotope transmit radioactivity for only a brief interval.
▪ Pulmonary angiogram	Study is used to visualize pulmonary vasculature and locate obstruction or pathologic conditions such as pulmonary embolus. Contrast medium is injected through a catheter into the pulmonary artery or right side of the heart.	Same as for chest x-ray. Know that contrast injection may cause flushing, warm sensation, and coughing. Check pressure dressing site after procedure. Monitor blood pressure, pulse, and circulation distal to injection site. Report and record significant changes.
▪ Positron emission tomography (PET)	Test is used to distinguish benign and malignant lung nodules. It involves IV injection of a radioisotope with short half-life.	Same as for chest x-ray study. No precautions needed afterward because isotope only transmits radioactivity for brief interval.
Endoscopic Examinations		
▪ Bronchoscopy	Study is typically performed in outpatient procedure room. Flexible fiberoptic scope is used for diagnosis, biopsy, specimen collection, or assessment of changes. It may also be done to suction mucous plugs or to remove foreign objects.	Instruct patient to be on NPO status for 6-12 hr. Obtain signed permit. Give sedative if ordered. After procedure, keep patient NPO until gag reflex returns and monitor for laryngeal edema; monitor for recovery from sedatives. If biopsy was done, monitor for hemorrhage and pneumothorax.
▪ Mediastinoscopy	Test is used for inspection and biopsy of lymph nodes in mediastinal area.	Prepare patient for surgical intervention. Obtain signed permit. Afterward, monitor as for bronchoscopy.
Biopsy		
▪ Lung biopsy	Specimens may be obtained by transbronchial or open-lung biopsy. This test is used to obtain specimens for laboratory analysis.	Same as bronchoscopy if procedure done with bronchoscope, and same as thoracotomy if open-lung biopsy done. Obtain signed permit.
Other		
▪ Thoracentesis	Test is used to obtain specimen of pleural fluid for diagnosis, to remove pleural fluid, or to instill medication. The physician inserts a large-bore needle through the chest wall into pleural space. Chest x-ray is always obtained after procedure to check for pneumothorax.	Explain procedure to patient and obtain signed permit before procedure. Position patient upright, instruct not to talk or cough, and assist during procedure. Observe for signs of hypoxia and verify breath sounds in all fields after procedure. Send labeled specimens to laboratory.
▪ Pulmonary function test	Test is used to evaluate lung function. It involves use of a spirometer to diagram air movement as patient performs prescribed respiratory maneuvers.[†]	Avoid scheduling immediately after mealtime. Avoid administration of inhaled bronchodilator for 6 hr before procedure. Explain procedure to patient. Provide rest after the procedure.

TABLE 25-12   Interpreting Skin Reactions to Tuberculosis Testing

TYPES OF RESPONSES	CONSIDER POSITIVE IN THE FOLLOWING GROUPS
5 mm or greater induration	Recent close contact with person diagnosed with infectious TB.
	Chest x-ray with fibrotic lesions likely to be healed TB.
	Known or suspected HIV infection.
	Patients with organ transplants and other immunosuppressed patients (e.g., patient receiving ≥15 mg/day of prednisone for 1 month or more).
10 mm or greater induration	Other medical risk factors known to substantially ↑ risk of TB once infection has occurred (e.g., diabetes mellitus, end-stage renal disease, cancer of oropharynx or upper GI tract).
	Recent immigrants (within the last 5 years) from high-prevalence countries.
	Medically underserved groups, homeless.
	Residents of long-term care facilities, prisons.
	IV drug users.
	Health care workers.
15 mm or greater induration	All other persons who are at low risk.

False-Negative Reactions

False-negative reactions may occur in persons who were infected with TB many years ago and persons with an active current infection; 10%-25% of persons with TB have a negative reaction if tested with tuberculin	Immunosuppression, overwhelming TB infection.
	Testing too soon after exposure to TB (up to 12 wk may be required to develop immune response).
	Aging (may result in decrease in delayed-type hypersensitivity).
	Long time since TB infection. Sensitivity to tuberculin may wane over the years, resulting in a negative reaction. However, the tuberculin test may stimulate (boost) ability to react to tuberculin, causing a positive reaction to future tests.
	Two-step testing is therefore recommended for individuals likely to be tested often (e.g., health care providers and individuals who may have decrease in delayed hypersensitivity).
	Interpret as follows:
	• First test positive, consider the person infected.
	• First test negative, repeat 1-3 wk later.
	• Second test positive, consider active or prior infection (depending on risk factors) and care for accordingly.
	• Second test negative, consider uninfected. Interpret future positive test as a new infection.

Source: American Thoracic Society, 2000.
GI, Gastrointestinal; *HIV,* human immunodeficiency virus; *TB,* tuberculosis.

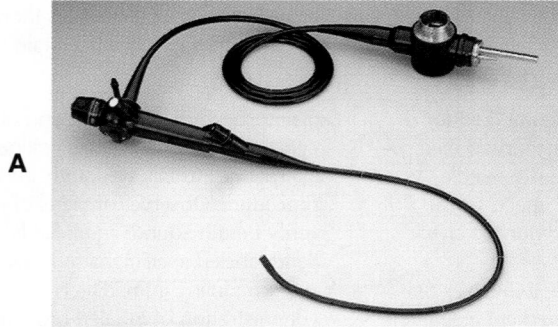
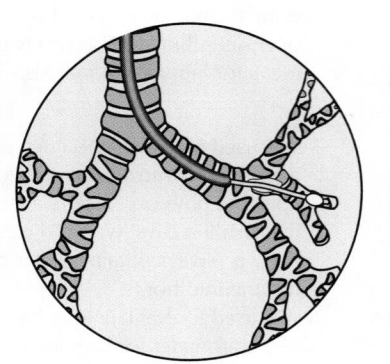

FIG. 25-15 Fiberoptic bronchoscope. **A,** The transbronchoscopic balloon-tipped catheter and the flexible fiberoptic bronchoscope. **B,** The catheter is introduced into a small airway and the balloon inflated with 1.5 to 2 ml air to occlude the airway. Bronchoalveolar lavage is performed by injecting and withdrawing 30 ml aliquots of sterile saline solution, gently aspirating after each instillation. Specimens are sent to the laboratory for analysis.

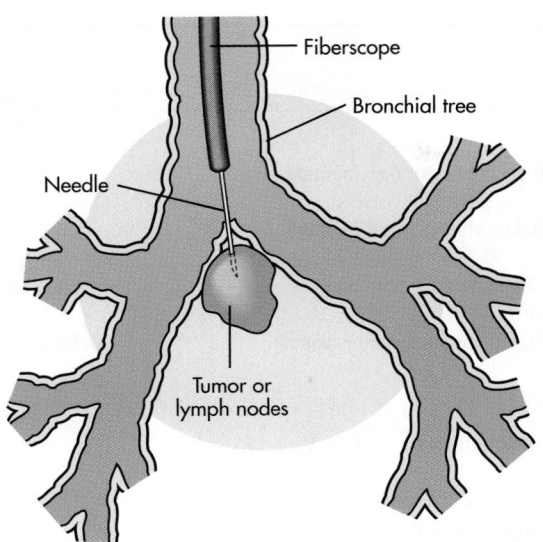

FIG. 25-16 Transbronchial needle biopsy. The diagram shows a transbronchial biopsy needle penetrating the bronchial wall and entering a mass of subcarinal lymph nodes or tumor.

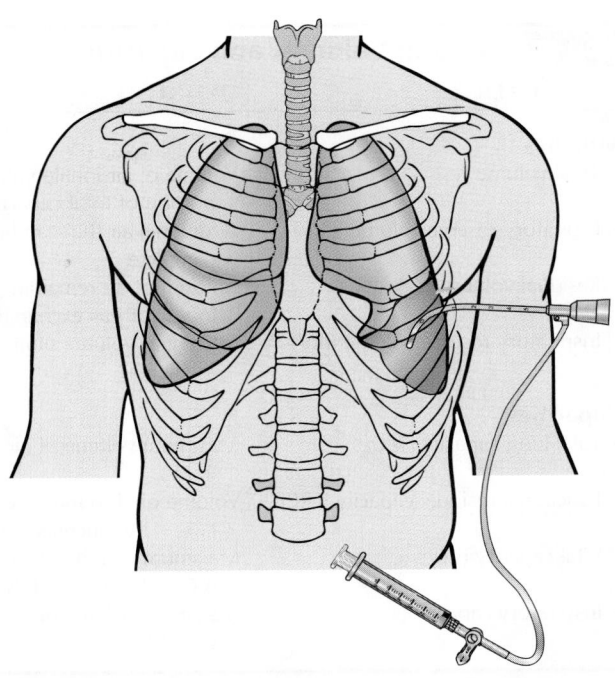

FIG. 25-17 Thoracentesis. A catheter is positioned in the pleural space to remove accumulated fluid.

Lung Biopsy

Lung biopsy may be done transbronchially or as an open-lung biopsy. The purpose is to obtain tissue, cells, or secretions for evaluation. Transbronchial lung biopsy involves passing a forceps or needle through the bronchoscope for a specimen (Fig. 25-16). Specimens can be cultured or examined for malignant cells. A combination of transbronchial lung biopsy and BAL is used to differentiate infection and rejection in lung transplant recipients. Nursing care is the same as for fiberoptic bronchoscopy. Open-lung biopsy is used when pulmonary disease cannot be diagnosed by other procedures. The patient is anesthetized, the chest is opened with a thoracotomy incision, and a biopsy specimen is obtained. Nursing care for the procedure is the same as after thoracotomy[17] (see Chapter 27).

Thoracentesis

Thoracentesis is the insertion of a needle through the chest wall into the pleural space to obtain specimens for diagnostic evaluation, remove pleural fluid, or instill medication into the pleural space (Fig. 25-17). The patient is positioned upright with elbows on an overbed table and feet supported. The skin is cleansed and a local anesthetic (Xylocaine) is instilled subcutaneously. A chest tube may be inserted to permit further drainage of fluid. Nursing care is described in Table 25-11.

Pulmonary Function Tests

Pulmonary function tests (PFTs) measure lung volumes and airflow. The results of PFTs are used to diagnose pulmonary disease, monitor disease progression, evaluate disability, and evaluate response to bronchodilators. PFTs are performed using a spirometer. The patient's age, sex, height, and weight are entered into the PFT computer to calculate predicted values. The patient inserts a mouthpiece, takes as deep a breath as possible, and exhales as hard, fast, and long as possible. Verbal coaching is given to ensure that the patient continues blowing out until exhalation is complete. The computer determines the actual value, predicted (normal) value, and percentage of the predicted value for each test. A normal value is 80% to 120% of the predicted value. Normal values for PFTs are shown in Tables 25-13 and 25-14 and Fig. 25-18.

Home spirometry may be used to monitor lung function in persons with asthma or cystic fibrosis, as well as before and after lung transplant. Spirometry changes at home can warn of early lung transplant rejection or infection. Feedback from a peak expiratory flow (PEF) meter can increase the sense of control when

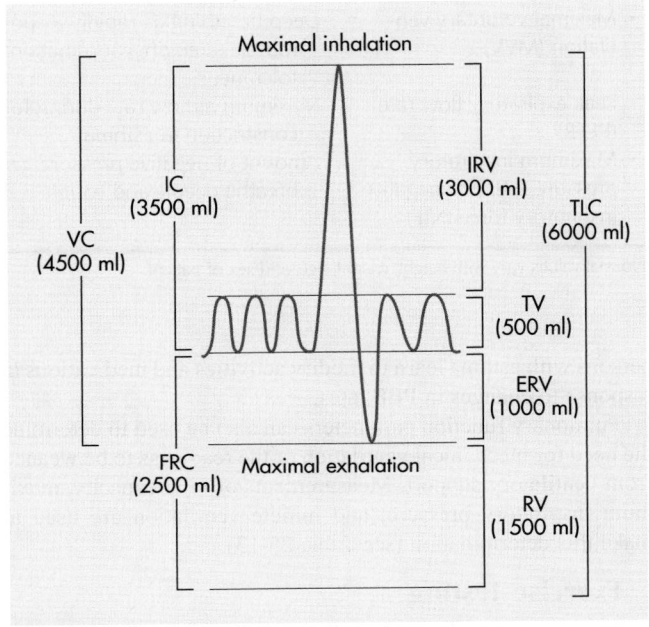

FIG. 25-18 Relationship of lung volumes and capacities.

TABLE 25-13   Lung Volumes and Capacities

PARAMETER	DEFINITION	NORMAL VALUES
Volumes		
▪ Tidal volume (V_T)	Volume of air inhaled and exhaled with each breath; only a small proportion of total capacity of lungs	0.5 L
▪ Expiratory reserve volume (ERV)	Additional air that can be forcefully exhaled after normal exhalation is complete	1.0 L
▪ Residual volume (RV)	Amount of air remaining in lungs after forced expiration; air available in lungs for gas exchange between breaths	1.5 L
▪ Inspiratory reserve volume (IRV)	Maximum volume of air that can be inhaled forcefully after normal inhalation	3.0 L
Capacities		
▪ Total lung capacity (TLC)	Maximum volume of air that lungs can contain (TLC = IRV + V_T + ERV + RV)	6.0 L
▪ Functional residual capacity (FRC)	Volume of air remaining in lungs at end of normal exhalation (FRC = ERV + RV); increase or decrease possible with lung disease	2.5 L
▪ Vital capacity (VC)	Maximum volume of air that can be exhaled after maximum inspiration (VC = IRV + V_T + ERV); higher VC for men (generally)	4.5 L
▪ Inspiratory capacity (IC)	Maximum volume of air that can be inhaled after normal expiration (IC = V_T + IRV)	3.5 L

TABLE 25-14   Common Measures of Pulmonary Function

MEASURE	DESCRIPTION	NORMAL VALUE*
▪ Forced vital capacity (FVC)	Amount of air that can be quickly and forcefully exhaled after maximum inspiration	Over 80% of predicted
▪ Forced expiratory volume in first second of expiration (FEV_1)	Amount of air exhaled in first second of FVC; valuable clue to severity of airway obstruction	Over 80% of predicted
▪ FEV_1/FVC	Dividing of value for FEV_1 by value for FVC; useful in differentiating obstructive and restrictive pulmonary dysfunction	Over 80% of predicted
▪ Forced midexpiratory flow rate ($FEF_{25\%-75\%}$)	Measurement of airflow rate in middle half of forced expiration; early indicator of disease of small airways	Over 80% of predicted
▪ Maximal voluntary ventilation (MVV)	Deep breathing as rapidly as possible for specified period; test for airflow, muscle strength, coordination, airway resistance; important factor in exercise tolerance	About 170 L/min
▪ Peak expiratory flow rate (PEFR)	Maximum airflow rate during forced expiration; aid in monitoring bronchoconstriction in asthma	Up to 600 L/min
▪ Maximum inspiratory pressure (MIP) or negative inspiratory force (NIF)	Amount of negative pressure generated on inspiration; indication of ability to breathe deeply and cough	<-80 cm H_2O

*Normal values vary with height, weight, age, and sex of patient.

persons with asthma learn to modify activities and medications in response to changes in PEF rates.

Pulmonary function parameters can also be used to determine the need for mechanical ventilation or the readiness to be weaned from ventilatory support. Measurements of vital capacity, maximum inspiratory pressure, and minute ventilation are used to make this determination (see Table 25-13).

Exercise Testing

Exercise testing is used in diagnosis, in determining exercise capacity, and for disability evaluation. A complete exercise test involves walking on a treadmill while expired oxygen and carbon dioxide, respiratory rate, heart rate, and rhythm are monitored. A modified test (desaturation test) may also be used. In this case, only SpO_2 is monitored. A desaturation test can also be used to determine the oxygen flow needed to maintain the SpO_2 at a safe level during activity or exercise in patients who use home oxygen therapy.

A timed walk can also be used to measure exercise capacity. The patient is instructed to walk as far as possible during a timed period (6 or 12 minutes), stopping when short of breath, and continuing when able. The distance walked is measured and used to monitor progression of disease or improvement after rehabilitation.

REVIEW QUESTIONS

The number of the question corresponds to the same-numbered objective at the beginning of the chapter.

1. The mechanism that stimulates the release of surfactant is
   a. fluid accumulation in the alveoli.
   b. alveolar collapse from atelectasis.
   c. alveolar stretch from deep breathing.
   d. air movement through the alveolar pores of Kohn.

2. During inspiration, air enters the thoracic cavity as a result of
   a. contraction of the accessory abdominal muscles.
   b. increased carbon dioxide and decreased oxygen in the blood.
   c. stimulation of the respiratory muscles by the chemoreceptors.
   d. decreased intrathoracic pressure relative to pressure at the airway.

3. The ability of the lungs to adequately oxygenate the arterial blood is determined by examination of the
   a. arterial oxygen tension.
   b. carboxyhemoglobin level.
   c. arterial carbon dioxide tension.
   d. venous carbon dioxide tension.

4. The most important respiratory defense mechanism distal to the respiratory bronchioles is the
   a. alveolar macrophage.
   b. impaction of particles.
   c. reflex bronchoconstriction.
   d. mucociliary clearance mechanism.

5. A rightward shift of the oxygen-hemoglobin dissociation curve
   a. is caused by metabolic alkalosis.
   b. is seen in postoperative hypothermia.
   c. facilitates release of oxygen at the tissue level.
   d. causes oxygen to have a greater affinity for hemoglobin.

6. Very early signs or symptoms of inadequate oxygenation include
   a. dyspnea and hypotension.
   b. apprehension and restlessness.
   c. cyanosis and cool, clammy skin.
   d. increased urine output and diaphoresis.

7. During the respiratory assessment of the older adult, the nurse would expect to find
   a. hypercapnia while at rest.
   b. increased breath sounds in the lung apices.
   c. decreased pH and increased $PaCO_2$ levels.
   d. increased anteroposterior chest diameter.

8. When assessing activity-exercise patterns related to respiratory health, the nurse inquires about
   a. dyspnea during rest or exercise.
   b. recent weight loss or weight gain.
   c. willingness to wear oxygen in public.
   d. ability to sleep through the entire night.

9. The vibration of tactile fremitus is best assessed using the nurse's
   a. palms.
   b. fingertips.
   c. stethoscope.
   d. index fingers.

10. Which of the following is an abnormal assessment finding of the respiratory system?
    a. presence of rhonchial fremitus
    b. inspiratory chest expansion of 1 inch
    c. percussion resonance over the lung bases
    d. symmetric chest expansion and contraction

11. A diagnostic procedure done to remove pleural fluid for analysis is
    a. thoracentesis.
    b. bronchoscopy.
    c. pulmonary angiography.
    d. sputum culture and sensitivity.

REFERENCES

1. Woodson GE: *Ear, nose and throat disorders in primary care,* Philadelphia, 2001, WB Saunders.
2. Altose MD, Kawakami Y: *Control of breathing in health and disease,* New York, 1999, Marcel Dekker.
3. Thibodeau GA, Patton KT: *The human body in health and disease,* ed 3, St Louis, 2002, Mosby.
4. Kidd PS, Wagner KD: *High acuity nursing,* ed 3, Upper Saddle River, NJ, 2001, Prentice-Hall.
5. Notter RH: *Lung surfactants: basic science and clinical applications,* New York, 2000, Marcel Dekker.
6. Roca J, Rodriguez-Roisin R, Wagner PD: *Pulmonary and peripheral gas exchange in health and disease,* New York, 2000, Marcel Dekker.
7. Herlihy B, Malbius NK: *The human body in health and illness,* Philadelphia, 2000, WB Saunders.
8. Cox CL, McGarth A: Respiratory assessment in critical care units, *Intensive Crit Care Nurs* 15:226, 1999.
9. McCance KL, Huether SE: *Pathophysiology: the biologic basis for disease in adults and children,* ed 4, St Louis, 2002, Mosby.
10. Ho JC et al: The effect of aging on nasal mucociliary clearance, beat frequency, and ultrastructure of respiratory cilia, *Am J Respir Crit Care Med* 163:983, 2001.
11. Bonder BR, Wagner MB: *Functional performance in older adults,* ed 2, Philadelphia, 2001, Davis.
12. Kedrick KR, Baxi SC, Smith RM: Usefulness of the modified 0-10 Borg scale in assessing the degree of dyspnea in patients with COPD and asthma, *Emerg Nurs* 26:216, 2000.
13. Jarvis C: *Physical examination and health assessment,* ed 3, Philadelphia, 2000, WB Saunders.
14. Seidel HM et al: *Mosby's guide to physical examination,* ed 5, St Louis, 2002, Mosby.
15. Wilson SF, Giddens JF: *Health assessment for nursing practice,* ed 2, St Louis, 2001, Mosby.
16. Reichman LB, Hershfield ES: *Tuberculosis: a comprehensive international approach,* ed 2, New York, 2000, Marcel Dekker.
17. Cagle PT: *Diagnostic pulmonary pathology,* New York, 2000, Marcel Dekker.

RESOURCES

Resources for this chapter are listed after Chapter 28 on page 686.

Debra A. Hagler

CHAPTER 26
NURSING MANAGEMENT
Upper Respiratory Problems

LEARNING OBJECTIVES

1. Describe the clinical manifestations and nursing management of problems of the nose.
2. Describe the clinical manifestations and nursing management of problems of the paranasal sinuses.
3. Describe the clinical manifestations and nursing management of problems of the pharynx and larynx.
4. Discuss the nursing management of the patient who requires a tracheostomy.
5. Identify the steps involved in performing tracheostomy care and suctioning an airway.
6. Describe the risk factors and warning symptoms associated with head and neck cancer.
7. Discuss the nursing management of the patient with a laryngectomy.
8. Describe the methods used in voice restoration for the patient with temporary or permanent loss of speech.

KEY TERMS

allergic rhinitis, p. 568
apnea, p. 574
deviated septum, p. 566
epistaxis, p. 567
esophageal speech, p. 589

nasal polyps p. 573
obstructive sleep apnea, p. 574
rhinoplasty, p. 566
tracheostomy, p. 575
tracheotomy, p. 575

Structural and Traumatic Disorders of the Nose

DEVIATED SEPTUM

Deviated septum is a deflection of the normally straight nasal septum. It is most commonly caused by trauma to the nose or congenital disproportion, a condition in which the size of the septum is not proportional to the size of the nose. On inspection, the septum is bent to one side, altering the air passage. Symptoms are variable. The patient may experience obstruction to nasal breathing, nasal edema, or dryness of the nasal mucosa with crusting and bleeding (epistaxis). A severely deviated septum may block drainage of mucus from the sinus cavities, resulting in infection (sinusitis).[1]

Medical management of deviated septum includes nasal allergy control as in allergic rhinitis (see p. 568). For patients with severe symptoms, a nasal septoplasty is performed to reconstruct and properly align the deviated septum.

NASAL FRACTURE

Nasal fracture is most often caused by trauma of substantial force to the middle of the face. Some cases of facial trauma can be prevented by using protective sports equipment and protecting against falls. Complications of the fracture include airway obstruction, epistaxis, meningeal tears, and cosmetic deformity.

Nasal fractures are classified as unilateral, bilateral, or complex. A unilateral fracture typically produces little or no displacement. Bilateral fractures, the most common fractures, give the nose a flattened look. Powerful frontal blows cause complex fractures, which may also shatter frontal bones. Diagnosis is based on the health history, direct observation, and x-ray findings.

On inspection, the nurse should assess the patient's ability to breathe through each side of the nose and note the presence of edema, bleeding, or hematoma. There may be ecchymosis under one or both eyes. Ecchymosis involving both eyes is often termed *raccoon eyes*. The nose is inspected internally for evidence of septal deviation, hemorrhage, or clear drainage, which suggests leakage of cerebrospinal fluid (CSF). If clear drainage is observed, a specimen may be sent to the laboratory to determine if it is CSF. Injury of sufficient force to fracture nasal bones results in considerable swelling of soft tissues. With extensive swelling, it may be difficult to verify the extent of deformity or to repair the fracture until several days later when the edema subsides.

The goals of nursing management are to reduce edema, prevent complications, and provide emotional support. Ice may be applied to the face and nose to reduce edema and bleeding. When a fracture is confirmed, the goal of management is to realign the fracture using closed or open reduction (septoplasty, rhinoplasty). These procedures reestablish cosmetic appearance and proper function of the nose and provide an adequate airway.[2,3]

RHINOPLASTY

Rhinoplasty, the surgical reconstruction of the nose, is performed for cosmetic reasons or to improve airway function when trauma or developmental deformities result in nasal obstruction. Assessment of the patient's expectations is a critical aspect of preparation for rhinoplasty. Any actual or perceived alteration in body image (e.g., a deformed or enlarged nose) can affect self-esteem and interactions with others. The patient's expectations concerning surgical results should be assessed with regard to the expected change. Computerized photographs made to life-size

Reviewed by Patricia Cryer, RN, MS, MSN, CENP, Instructor, Associate Degree Nursing, Tyler Junior College, Tyler, Tex.

measurements can be used to simulate appearance after the surgery and may help the patient decide whether to undergo rhinoplasty. Expected results of surgery should be explained frankly and truthfully to avoid disappointment.

Collaborative Care

Rhinoplasty is performed as an outpatient procedure using regional anesthesia. Nasal tissue may be added or removed, and the nose may be lengthened or shortened. Plastic implants are sometimes used to reshape the nose. After surgery, nasal packing may be inserted to apply pressure and prevent bleeding or septal hematoma formation. Nasal septal splints (small pieces of plastic or Silastic) may be inserted to help prevent scar tissue formation between the surgical site and lateral nasal wall. An external plastic splint is molded to the new shape of the nose and placed on the nose. Steri-Strips are placed to hold the skin against the septal cartilage. Typically, nasal packing is removed the day after surgery, and the splint is removed in 3 to 5 days.

NURSING MANAGEMENT
NASAL SURGERY

Examples of nasal surgery include rhinoplasty, septoplasty, and nasal fracture reductions. Before surgery, the patient should be instructed to not take aspirin-containing drugs or nonsteroidal antiinflammatory drugs (NSAIDs) for 2 weeks to reduce the risk of bleeding. Nursing interventions during the immediate postoperative period include assessment of respiratory status, pain management, and observation of the surgical site for hemorrhage and edema. Teaching is important because the patient must be able to detect early and late complications at home. There is an interim period while edema and ecchymosis resolve before the final cosmetic effect can be achieved.

EPISTAXIS

Epistaxis (nosebleed) occurs in all age-groups, especially in children and the elderly. Epistaxis may be caused by trauma, foreign bodies, nasal spray abuse, street drug use, anatomic malformation, allergic rhinitis, or tumors. Any condition that prolongs bleeding time or alters platelet counts will predispose the patient to epistaxis. Bleeding time may also be prolonged if the patient takes aspirin or nonsteroidal antiinflammatory drugs (NSAIDs). Conditions such as hypertension do not increase the risk of epistaxis. Elevated blood pressure, however, makes bleeding more difficult to control.

Children and young adults have a tendency to develop anterior nasal bleeding, whereas older adults more commonly have posterior nasal bleeding. Anterior bleeding usually stops spontaneously or can be self-treated; posterior bleeding may require medical treatment.[3]

NURSING *and* COLLABORATIVE MANAGEMENT
EPISTAXIS

Simple first aid measures should be used first to control epistaxis. The nurse should (1) keep the patient quiet; (2) place the patient in a sitting position, leaning forward, or if not possible, in a reclining position with head and shoulders elevated; (3) apply direct pressure by pinching the entire soft lower portion of the nose for 10 to 15 minutes; (4) apply ice compresses to the nose, and have the patient suck on ice; (5) partially insert a small gauze pad into the bleeding nostril, and apply digital pressure if bleeding continues; and (6) obtain medical assistance if bleeding does not stop.

If first aid is not effective, management involves localization of the bleeding site and application of a vasoconstrictive agent, cauterization, or anterior packing by a health care provider. Anterior packing may consist of ribbon gauze impregnated with antibiotic ointment that is wedged firmly in the desired location and remains in place for 48 to 72 hours. If posterior packing is required, the patient should be hospitalized. Inflatable balloons may be used as a nasal pack or gauze rolls may be inserted (Fig. 26-1). Strings attached to the packing are brought to the outside and taped to the cheek for ease of removal. A nasal sling (a folded 2 × 2–inch gauze pad) should be taped over the nares to absorb drainage.

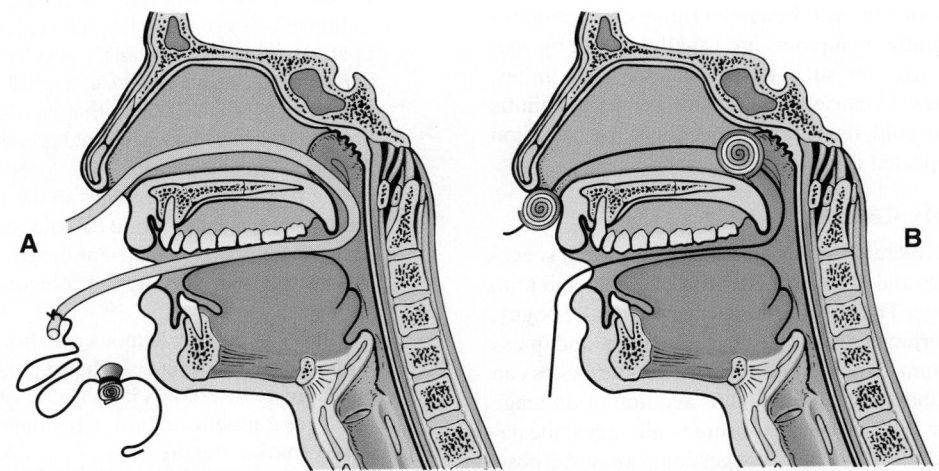

FIG. 26-1 Method for placing posterior nasal pack. **A,** Catheter is passed through the bleeding side of the nose and pulled out through the mouth with a hemostat. Strings are tied to the catheter and the pack is pulled up behind the soft palate and into the nasopharynx. **B,** Nasal pack in position in the posterior nasopharynx. Dental roll at the nose helps maintain correct position.

Posterior packing may alter respiratory status, especially in older adults. Some patients experience *hypoventilation* (increase in $PaCO_2$) and *hypoxemia* (decrease in PaO_2) sufficient to lead to cardiac arrhythmias or respiratory arrest. The nurse should closely monitor respiratory rate, heart rate and rhythm, oxygen saturation using pulse oximetry (SpO_2), and level of consciousness and observe for signs of aspiration. Because of the risk of complications, the patient may be admitted to a monitored unit to permit closer observation.

Packing is painful because sufficient pressure must be applied to stop the bleeding. Nasal packing predisposes to infection from bacteria (e.g., *Staphylococcus aureus*) present in the nasal cavity. The patient should receive a mild narcotic analgesic for pain (e.g., acetaminophen with codeine) and an antibiotic effective against staphylococci to protect against infection.

Posterior packs are left in place for a minimum of 3 days. Before removal, the patient should be medicated for pain, because this procedure is very uncomfortable. After removal, the nares may be gently cleaned and lubricated with petroleum jelly.

Failure of posterior packing to control epistaxis indicates the need for surgery or radiologic embolization of the affected artery. The most common surgical procedure involves ligation of the internal maxillary artery performed through a Caldwell-Luc incision under the upper lip to gain access to the artery.

The patient can be discharged after being taught about home care. The patient should be instructed to avoid vigorous nose blowing, strenuous activity, lifting, and straining for 4 to 6 weeks. The patient should be taught to sneeze with the mouth open and to avoid the use of aspirin-containing products or NSAIDs.

Inflammation and Infection of the Nose and Paranasal Sinuses

ALLERGIC RHINITIS

Allergic rhinitis is the reaction of the nasal mucosa to a specific allergen. Attacks of seasonal rhinitis usually occur in the spring and fall and are caused by allergy to pollens from trees, flowers, or grasses. The typical attack lasts for several weeks during times when pollen counts are high, disappears, and recurs at the same time the following year. Perennial rhinitis is present intermittently or constantly. Symptoms are usually caused by specific environmental triggers such as pet dander, dust mites, molds, or cockroaches. Because symptoms of perennial rhinitis resemble the common cold, the patient may believe the condition is a continuous or repeated cold.

Clinical Manifestations

Manifestations of allergic rhinitis are nasal congestion; sneezing; watery, itchy eyes and nose; altered sense of smell; and thin, watery nasal discharge. The nasal turbinates appear pale, boggy, and swollen. The turbinates may fill the air space and press against the nasal septum. The posterior ends of the turbinates can become so enlarged that they obstruct sinus aeration or drainage and result in sinusitis. With chronic exposure to allergens, the patient's responses include headache, congestion, pressure, postnasal drip, and nasal polyps. The patient may complain of cough, hoarseness, or the recurrent need to clear the throat. Congestion may cause snoring.[4]

NURSING *and* COLLABORATIVE MANAGEMENT ALLERGIC RHINITIS

Several steps are used in managing allergic rhinitis. The most important step involves identifying and avoiding triggers of allergic reactions (Table 26-1). The patient should be instructed to keep a diary of times when the allergic reaction occurs and the activities that precipitate the reaction. Steps can then be taken to avoid these triggers.

Drug therapy involves using nasal sprays, antihistamines, and decongestants to manage symptoms (Table 26-2). Intranasal corticosteroid or cromolyn sprays are effective for seasonal and perennial rhinitis. Nasal corticosteroid sprays are used to decrease inflammation locally with little absorption in the systemic circulation. Therefore systemic side effects are rare. Relief may require combining a nasal corticosteroid spray and an antihista-

TABLE 26-1 *Patient & Family Teaching Guide*

How to Reduce Symptoms of Allergic Rhinitis

1. **Avoidance is the best treatment.**
2. **Avoid house dust.** Use the approach "less is best." Focus on the bedroom. Remove carpeting. Limit furniture. Enclose the pillows, mattress, and springs in air-tight, vinyl encasements. Limit clothing in the bedroom to items used frequently. Place clothing in air-tight, zipper-sealed, vinyl clothes bags. Install an air filter. Close the air-conditioning vent into the room.
3. **Avoid house dust mites.** Wash bedding in hot water (130° F [54° C]) weekly. Wear a mask when vacuuming. Double-bag the vacuum cleaner. Install a filter on the outlet port of the vacuum cleaner. Avoid sleeping or lying on upholstered furniture. Remove carpets that are laid on concrete. If possible, have someone else clean the house.
4. **Avoid mold spores.** The three *Ds* that promote growth of mold spores are darkness, dampness, and drafts. Avoid places where humidity is high (e.g., basements, camps on the lake, clothes hampers, greenhouses, stables, barns). Dehumidifiers are rarely helpful. Ventilate closed rooms, open doors, and install fans. Consider adding windows to dark rooms. Consider keeping a small light on in closets. A basement light with a timer that provides light several hours a day may decrease mold growth.
5. **Avoid pollens.** Stay inside with closed doors and windows during high-pollen season. Avoid the use of fans. Install an air conditioner with a good air filter. Wash filters weekly during high pollen season. Put the car air conditioner on "recirculate" when driving. Get someone else to tend to your yard.
6. **Avoid pet allergens.** Remove pets from the interior of the home. Clean the living area thoroughly. Do not expect instant relief. Symptoms usually do not improve significantly for 2 months following pet removal.
7. **Avoid smoke.** The presence of a smoker will sabotage the best of all possible symptom reduction programs.

Adapted from Boggs P: *Sneezing your head off? How to live with your allergic nose,* 1994, Boggs, pp. 125-137.

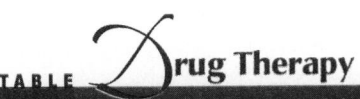

TABLE
26-2 **rug Therapy**

Allergic Rhinitis and Sinusitis

PREPARATION	MECHANISM OF ACTION	SIDE EFFECTS	NURSING ACTIONS
Corticosteroids **Nasal spray** beclomethasone (Vancenase) budesonide (Rhinocort) flunisolide (Nasalide) fluticasone (Flonase) triamcinolone (Nasacort)	Inhibits inflammatory response. At recommended dose, systemic side effects are unlikely because of low systemic absorption. Systemic effects may occur with greater than recommended doses.	Mild transient nasal burning and stinging. In rare instances, localized fungal infection with *Candida albicans*.	• Teach patient correct use (see Fig. 26-1). • Instruct patient to use on regular basis and not prn. • Reinforce that spray acts to decrease inflammation and effect is not immediate, as with decongestant sprays. • Discontinue use if nasal infection develops.
Mast Cell Stabilizer **Nasal spray** cromolyn spray (Nasalcrom)	Inhibits degranulation of sensitized mast cells which occurs after exposure to specific antigens.	Minimal side effects. Occasional burning or nasal irritation.	• Teach patient correct use (see Fig. 26-1). • Reinforce that spray prevents symptoms. • Begin 2 weeks before pollen season starts and use throughout pollen season. • If isolated allergy, such as cat, use prophylactically (i.e., 10-15 min before exposure to allergen).
Anticholinergic **Nasal spray** ipratropium bromide (Atrovent)	Blocks hypersecretory effects by competing for binding sites on the cell. Reduces rhinorrhea in the common cold, allergic and nonallergic rhinitis.	Dryness of the mouth and nose may occur. Does not cause systemic side effects.	• Teach patient correct use (see Fig. 26-1). • Reinforce that spray prevents symptoms with onset of action within 1 hr of use. • May reduce the need for other rhinitis medications.
Antihistamines *First-Generation Agents* **Ethanolamines** carbinoxamine (Clistin) clemastine (Tavist) diphenhydramine (Benadryl) **Ethylenediamines** tripelennamine (PBZ) **Alkylamines** brompheniramine (Dimetane) chlorpheniramine (Chlor-Trimeton) dexchlorpheniramine (Polaramine) triprolidine (Actidil) **Piperidine** azatadine (Optimine) **Phenothiazines** phenothiazine (Phenergan)	Bind with H_1 receptors on target cells, blocking histamine binding. Relieve acute symptoms of allergic response (itching, sneezing, excessive secretions, mild congestion).	**First-generation agents** cross blood-brain barrier, bind to H_1 receptors in brain, cause *sedation* (diminished alertness, slow reaction time, somnolence) and *stimulation* (restless, nervous, insomnia). Some drugs (e.g., ethanolamines) are more likely to cause sedation. Patients vary in their sensitivity to these side effects. The next most common side effects involve the GI system and include loss of appetite, epigastric distress, constipation, or diarrhea. May cause palpitations, tachycardia, urinary retention or frequency.	**First-generation agents:** • Warn patient that operating machinery and driving may be dangerous because of sedative effect. Drowsiness usually passes after 2 weeks of treatment. • Teach patient to report palpitations, change in heart rate, change in bowel, bladder habits. • Instruct patient not to use alcohol with antihistamines because of additive depressant effect. • Rapid onset of action, no drug tolerance with prolonged use.

Continued

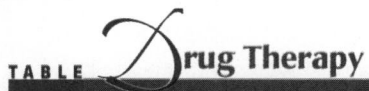

TABLE
26-2   Allergic Rhinitis and Sinusitis—cont'd

PREPARATION	MECHANISM OF ACTION	SIDE EFFECTS	NURSING ACTIONS
Antihistamines—cont'd *Second-Generation Agents* loratadine (Claritin) cetirizine (Zyrtec) fexofenadine (Allegra) desloratadine (Clarinex)		**Second-generation agents** have limited affinity for brain H₁ receptors. Cause minimal sedation, few effects on psychomotor activities, bladder function.	**Second-generation agents:** • Teach patient to expect few, if any, side effects. • More expensive than classic antihistamines. • Rapid onset of action, no drug tolerance with prolonged use. *General interactions:* • Do not take with alcohol or any form of tranquilizer or sedative. • Do not take with any monoamine oxidase inhibitor.
Decongestants *Oral* pseudoephedrine (Sudafed) phenylpropanolamine	Stimulate adrenergic receptors on blood vessels, promote vasoconstriction and reduce nasal edema and rhinorrhea.	CNS stimulation, causing insomnia, excitation, headache, irritability, increased blood and ocular pressure, dysuria, palpitations, tachycardia.	• Advise patient of adverse reactions. • Advise that some preparations are contraindicated for patients with cardiovascular disease, hypertension, diabetes, glaucoma, prostate hyperplasia, hepatic and renal disease.
Topical (Nasal Spray) oxymetazoline (Dristan) phenylephrine (Neo-Synephrine)	Same as above.	Same as above, plus rhinitis medicamentosa (rebound nasal congestion).	• Teach patient that these drugs should not be used for >3 days or more than 3-4 times a day. Longer use increases risk of rhinitis medicamentosa.
azelastine (Astelin)	Blocks action of histamine.	Headache, bitter taste, somnolence, nasal irritation.	

CNS, Central nervous system.

mine. The patient who is using first-generation antihistamines should be warned about sedative side effects. Second-generation (nonsedating) antihistamines eliminate or reduce drowsiness but are more costly. The patient using nasal inhalers needs careful instructions about proper use (Fig. 26-2). Nasal decongestant sprays can cause a rebound effect from prolonged use.

Omalizumab (Xolair) is a monoclonal antibody to immunoglobulin E (IgE) that is being investigated for use in the treatment of allergic rhinitis. By binding to IgE antibodies, it prevents IgE from attaching to mast cells and thus prevents the release of mediators such as histamine. It blocks the allergic cascade for multiple allergens. (The mechanisms involved in the allergic response and discussed in Chapter 13.)

Immunotherapy ("allergy shots") may be used if drugs are not tolerated, or are not effective, when a specific unavoidable allergen is identified. Immunotherapy involves controlled exposure to small amounts of a known allergen through frequent (at least weekly) injections with the goal to decrease sensitivity. (Immunotherapy is discussed in Chapter 13.)

ACUTE VIRAL RHINITIS

Acute viral rhinitis (common cold or acute coryza) is caused by viruses that invade the upper respiratory tract. It is the most prevalent infectious disease and is spread by airborne droplet

sprays emitted by the infected person while breathing, talking, sneezing, or coughing or by direct hand contact. Frequency increases in the winter months, when people stay indoors and overcrowding is more common. Other factors, such as chilling, fatigue, physical and emotional stress, and compromised immune status, may increase susceptibility. The patient with acute viral rhinitis typically first experiences tickling, irritation, sneezing, or dryness of the nose or nasopharynx, followed by copious nasal secretions, some nasal obstruction, watery eyes, elevated temperature, general malaise, and headache. After the early profuse secretions, the nose becomes more obstructed, and the discharge is thicker. Within a few days the general symptoms improve, nasal passages reopen, and normal breathing is established.

NURSING *and* COLLABORATIVE MANAGEMENT ACUTE VIRAL RHINITIS

Rest, fluids, proper diet, antipyretics, and analgesics are recommended. Complications of acute viral rhinitis include pharyngitis, sinusitis, otitis media, tonsillitis, and lung infections. Unless symptoms of complications are present, antibiotic therapy is not indicated. Antibiotics have no effect on viruses and, if taken injudiciously, may produce antibiotic-resistant bacteria.

COMPLEMENTARY & ALTERNATIVE THERAPIES
Echinacea

Clinical Uses
Common cold, upper respiratory tract infection, wound healing, urinary tract infections.

Effects
Stimulates immune system; has antibacterial and antiinflammatory activity.

Nursing Implications
Because it has immunomodulating actions, individuals with systemic lupus erythematous, tuberculosis, multiple sclerosis, leukemia, or acquired immunodeficiency syndrome (AIDS) should not use it. Long-term use may suppress the immune system. Should not be used in conjunction with corticosteroids or immunosupression therapy. May be used in conjunction with antibiotics.

Is considered safe when used in recommended doses. Therapy for 10 to 14 days is usually long enough. Should not be taken for more than 8 weeks.

Before using the inhaler, gently blow your nose, making sure your nostrils are clear.

Then follow these steps:

1. Remove the protective cap from the nasal inhaler.

2. Shake the canister well.

3. Hold the inhaler between the thumb and forefinger.

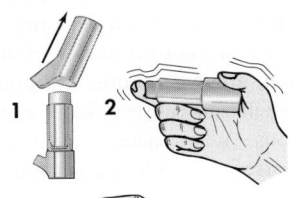

4. Tilt the head back slightly and insert the end of the inhaler into one nostril, pointing it slightly toward the outside nostril wall. Hold the other nostril closed with one finger.

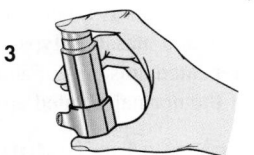

5. Press down on the canister to release one dose and, at the same time, inhale gently.

6. Hold your breath for a few seconds, then breathe out slowly through the mouth.

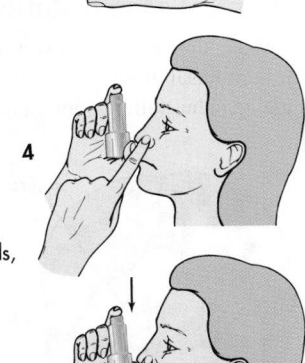

7. Withdraw the inhaler from the nostril and repeat the process for the other nostril. If more than one puff is prescribed per nostril, repeat steps 4-6. To avoid irritation, direct the spray at a different area of the mucosa for each puff.

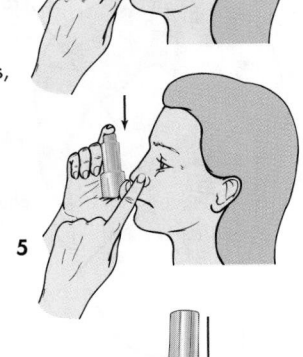

8. Replace the protective cap on the inhaler.

FIG. 26-2 Method for using an intranasal inhaler.

During the cold season, the patient with a chronic illness or a compromised immune status should be advised to avoid crowded, close situations and other persons who have obvious cold symptoms. Frequent hand washing and avoiding hand-to-face contact may help prevent direct spread.

Interventions are directed toward relieving annoying symptoms. The patient should be encouraged to drink increased amounts of fluids to liquefy secretions. Antihistamine or decongestant therapy reduces postnasal drip and significantly decreases severity of cough, nasal obstruction, and nasal discharge. The patient should also be taught to recognize the symptoms of secondary bacterial infection, such as a temperature higher than 100.4° F (38° C); purulent nasal exudate; tender, swollen glands; and a sore, red throat. In the patient with pulmonary disease, signs of infection include a change in consistency, color, or volume of the sputum. Because infection can progress rapidly, the patient with chronic respiratory disease may be taught to begin antibiotics for sputum changes.

INFLUENZA

Each year influenza (flu) causes significant morbidity and mortality rates. Influenza-related deaths average 20,000 per year in the United States. Most deaths occur in persons over 60 years of age with underlying heart or lung disease, but could be prevented with vaccination of high risk groups (Table 26-3).[5]

There are three groups of influenza viruses (A, B, and C, although influenza C has little pathogenic potential). Influenza viruses have a remarkable ability to change over time. This accounts for widespread disease and the need for annual vaccination against new strains. Fewer cases of influenza result when a minor change in the virus occurs because most persons have partial immunity.[6,7]

Clinical Manifestations

The onset of flu is typically abrupt with systemic symptoms of cough, fever, and myalgia often accompanied by a headache and sore throat. Milder symptoms, similar to the common cold, may also occur. Physical findings are usually minimal with normal assessment on chest auscultation. Dyspnea and diffuse

---

TABLE 26-3   Target Groups for Influenza Immunization

Groups at High Risk
- Anyone ≥50 years old
- Adults of any age with chronic cardiac or pulmonary disease
- Adults who had regular medical follow-up or were hospitalized during the preceding year
- Residents of long-term care facilities
- Immunocompromised adults
- Women who will be in second or third trimester of pregnancy during influenza season

Groups Who Can Transmit Influenza to High-Risk Persons
- Health care workers
- Providers of home care to high risk persons
- Household members of high risk persons

Modified from Centers for Disease Control and Prevention: Prevention and control of influenza. Recommendations of the Advisory Committee on Immunization Practices, *MMWR* 47(RR-6):1, 1998; Couch RB: Drug therapy: prevention and treatment of influenza, *N Engl J Med* 343:1778, 2000.

crackles are signs of pulmonary complications. In uncomplicated cases, symptoms subside within 7 days. Some patients, particularly older adults, experience weakness or lassitude that persists for weeks. The convalescent phase may be marked by hyperactive airways and a chronic cough. Important diagnostic factors include the patient's health history, clinical findings, and the presence of other cases of influenza in the community.

The most common complication of influenza is pneumonia. The patient who develops secondary bacterial pneumonia experiences gradual improvement of influenza symptoms, then worsening cough and purulent sputum. Treatment with antibiotics is usually effective if started early.

NURSING *and* COLLABORATIVE MANAGEMENT INFLUENZA

The nurse should advocate influenza vaccination in patients at high risk during routine office visits or, if hospitalized, at the time of discharge (see Table 26-3). The vaccine is 70% to 90% effective in preventing influenza in adults. To be effective, the vaccine must be given in the fall (mid-October) before exposure occurs. The present policy in the United States is for routine vaccination of persons over 50 years old.[5] High priority should also be given to groups that can transmit influenza to high risk persons, such as health care workers. By being vaccinated, the nurse can decrease the risk of transmitting influenza to those who have less ability to cope with the effects of this illness. Despite obvious benefits, many persons are reluctant to be vaccinated. Current vaccines are highly purified, and reactions are extremely uncommon. Soreness at the injection site is usually the only side effect. The only contraindication is hypersensitivity to eggs, because the vaccine is produced in eggs. FluMist, a nasally delivered influenza vaccine, is available for patients reluctant to get an injection. It should not be used for patients older than 49 or those with chronic medical disorders.

The primary goals in nursing management are supportive measures directed toward relief of symptoms and prevention of secondary infection. Unless at high risk or complications develop, the patient with influenza usually requires only symptomatic therapy.

COMPLEMENTARY &ALTERNATIVE THERAPIES
Goldenseal

Clinical Uses
Common cold, respiratory and gastrointestinal infections, wound healing, cirrhosis of the liver, gallbladder inflammation, peptic ulcers.

Effects
Has a wide variety of effects. Has antiinflammatory, antimicrobial, and immunostimulating actions. Can stimulate the flow of bile.

Nursing Implications
Has anticoagulant effects. Should not be used for longer than 2 weeks. Large doses may cause gastrointestinal distress (e.g., diarrhea, vomiting) and possible nervous system effects. Commonly combined with echinacea in preparations. May be used in conjunction with antibiotics. Should not be used concurrently with anticoagulants, antihypertensives, β-adrenergic blockers, or calcium channel blockers. Should not be used if person has heart or vascular disease, especially hypertension, heart failure, or arrhythmias.

Older adults and those with a chronic illness may require hospitalization. Drug therapy with oral rimantadine (Flumadine) or amantadine (Symmetrel) may be given to prevent or decrease symptoms of influenza A in high risk patients exposed to the flu but not vaccinated. Amantadine has a higher incidence of side effects (e.g., heartburn, hallucinations). These drugs are given orally.

Zanamivir (Relenza) and oseltamivir (Tamiflu) are relatively new drugs effective against both influenza A and B. These drugs are neuraminidase inhibitors that prevent the virus from budding and spreading to other cells. For maximum benefit they should be initiated as soon as possible and ideally within 2 days of the onset of symptoms. They shorten the course of influenza. Zanamivir is administered using an inhaler. Oseltamivir is available as an oral capsule. Both zanamavir and oseltamavir have been effectively shown to reduce symptom duration and severity of influenza. Both drugs can be used prophylactically for control of outbreaks of influenza.[7]

SINUSITIS

Sinusitis develops when the ostia (exit) from the sinuses is narrowed or blocked by inflammation or hypertrophy (swelling) of the mucosa (Fig. 26-3). The secretions that accumulate behind the obstruction provide a rich medium for growth of bacteria, viruses, and fungi, all of which may cause infection. Bacterial sinusitis is most commonly caused by *Streptococcus pneumoniae*, *Haemophilus influenzae*, or *Moraxella catarrhalis*.[8] Viral sinusitis follows an upper respiratory infection in which the virus penetrates the mucous membrane and decreases ciliary transport. Fungal sinusitis is uncommon and is usually found in patients who are debilitated or immunocompromised.

Acute sinusitis usually results from an upper respiratory infection, allergic rhinitis, swimming, or dental manipulation, all of which can cause inflammatory changes and retention of secretions. When acute sinusitis follows viral rhinitis, symptoms worsen after 5 to 7 days and are worse than the original rhinitis. *Chronic sinusitis* is a persistent infection usually associated with allergies and nasal polyps. Chronic sinusitis generally results from repeated episodes of acute sinusitis that result in irreversible loss of the normal ciliated epithelium lining the sinus cavity.

Clinical Manifestations

Acute sinusitis causes significant pain over the affected sinus, purulent nasal drainage, nasal obstruction, congestion, fever, and malaise. The patient looks and feels sick. Assessment involves

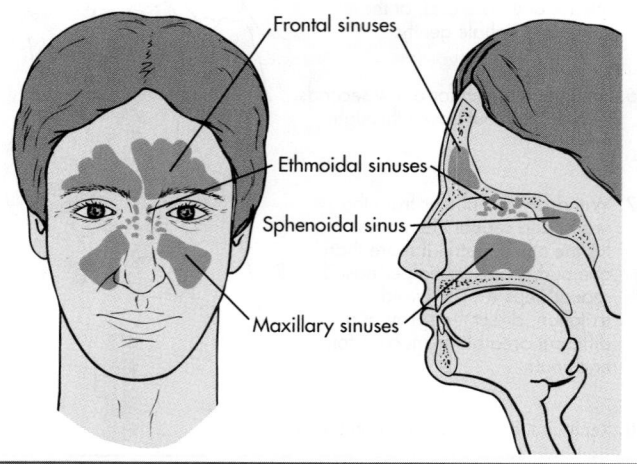

FIG. 26-3 Location of the sinuses.

inspection of the nasal mucosa and palpation of the sinus points for pain. Findings that indicate acute sinusitis include a hyperemic and edematous mucosa, enlarged turbinates, and tenderness over the involved sinuses. The patient may have recurrent headaches that change in intensity with position changes or when secretions drain.

Chronic sinusitis is difficult to diagnose because symptoms may be nonspecific. The patient is rarely febrile. Although there may be facial pain, nasal congestion, and increased drainage, severe pain and purulent drainage are often absent. Symptoms may mimic those seen with allergies. X-rays of the sinuses or a sinus computed tomography (CT) scan may be performed to confirm the diagnosis. CT scans may show the sinuses to be filled with fluid or the mucous membrane to be thickened. Nasal endoscopy with a flexible scope may be used to examine the sinuses, obtain drainage for culture, and restore normal drainage.

Many patients with asthma have sinusitis. The link between these diseases is unclear. Sinusitis may trigger asthma by stimulating reflex bronchospasm. Appropriate treatment of sinusitis often causes a reduction in asthma symptoms.[9]

NURSING and COLLABORATIVE MANAGEMENT SINUSITIS

If allergies are the precipitating cause of sinusitis, the patient needs to be instructed in ways to reduce sinus inflammation and infection, including environmental control of allergies and appropriate drug therapy (see section on allergic rhinitis, earlier in this chapter).

Treatment of acute sinusitis includes antibiotics to treat the infection, decongestants to promote drainage, nasal corticosteroids to decrease inflammation, and mucolytics to promote mucous flow (Table 26-4). Classic (first-generation) antihistamines increase the viscosity of mucus and promote continued symptoms, so they should be avoided. Nonsedating (second-generation) antihistamines do not cause this problem. Antibiotic therapy is usually continued for 10 to 14 days for acute sinusitis. If symptoms do not resolve, the antibiotic should be changed to a broader-spectrum agent. With chronic sinusitis, mixed bacterial flora are often present and infections are difficult to eliminate. Broad-spectrum antibiotics may be used for 4 to 6 weeks.

COMPLEMENTARY & ALTERNATIVE THERAPIES
Zinc

Clinical Uses
Common cold, upper respiratory tract infections, wound healing, dermatitis, acne, herpes simplex.

Effects
Prevents replication of viruses and stimulates the immune system. Severe zinc deficiency results in severely depressed immune function and frequent infections.

Nursing Implications
Zinc supplements are available as oral tablets and lozenges. Oral zinc should not be taken with foods that will reduce its absorption, such as coffee, bran, protein, or calcium. Long-term use of zinc supplements over 15 mg/day is not recommended without medical supervision.

TABLE 26-4 Patient & Family Teaching Guide
Acute or Chronic Sinusitis

1. Keep well hydrated by drinking six to eight glasses of water to liquefy secretions.
2. Take hot showers twice daily; use a steam inhaler (15-minute vaporization of boiled water), bedside humidifier, or nasal saline spray to promote secretion drainage.
3. Report temperature of 100.4° F (38° C), which may indicate infection.
4. Follow prescribed medication regimen:
   - Take analgesics to relieve pain.
   - Take decongestants/expectorants to relieve swelling and thin mucus.
   - Take antibiotics, as prescribed, for infection. Be sure to take entire prescription and report continued symptoms or a change in symptoms.
   - Administer nasal sprays correctly.
5. Do not smoke, and avoid exposure to smoke. Smoke is an irritant and may worsen symptoms.
6. If allergies predispose to sinusitis, follow instructions regarding environmental control, drug therapy, and immunotherapy to reduce the inflammation and prevent sinus infection.

The patient should be encouraged to increase fluid intake (six to eight glasses daily) and use nasal cleaning techniques. This many include taking a hot shower in the morning and evening followed by blowing the nose thoroughly. Other intervention to cleanse the nasal passages and promote drainage include irrigating the nose with salt water (¼ to ½ teaspoon per quart of water) or steam inhalations.

The patient with persistent or recurrent sinus complaints not alleviated by medical therapy may require nasal endoscopic surgery to relieve blockage caused by hypertrophy or septal deviation. This is an outpatient procedure usually performed under local anesthesia.

Obstruction of the Nose and Paranasal Sinuses

POLYPS

Nasal polyps are benign mucous membrane masses that form slowly in response to repeated inflammation of the sinus or nasal mucosa. Polyps, which appear as bluish, glossy projections in the nare, can exceed the size of a grape. The patient may be anxious, fearing they are malignant. Clinical manifestations include nasal obstruction, nasal discharge (usually clear mucus), and speech distortion. Nasal polyps can be removed with endoscopic or laser surgery, but recurrence is common. Topical or systemic corticosteroids may slow polyp growth.

FOREIGN BODIES

A variety of foreign bodies may lodge in the upper respiratory tract. Inorganic foreign bodies such as buttons and beads may cause no symptoms, lie undetected, and be accidentally discovered on routine examination. Organic foreign bodies such as wood, cotton, beans, peas, and paper produce a local inflammatory reaction and nasal discharge, which may become purulent and foul smelling. Foreign bodies should be removed from the nose through the route of entry. Sneezing with the opposite nostril closed may be effective in assisting the removal of foreign bodies. Irrigation of the nose or pushing the object backward should not be done, because either could cause aspiration and airway obstruction. If sneezing or blowing the nose does not remove the object, the patient should see a health care provider.

Problems Related to the Pharynx

ACUTE PHARYNGITIS

Acute pharyngitis is an acute inflammation of the pharyngeal walls. It may include the tonsils, palate, and uvula. It can be caused by a viral, bacterial, or fungal infection. Viral pharyngitis accounts for approximately 70% of cases. Acute follicular pharyngitis ("strep throat") results from β-hemolytic streptococcal invasion and accounts for an additional 15% to 20% of episodes.[3] Fungal pharyngitis, especially candidiasis, can develop with prolonged use of antibiotics or inhaled corticosteroids or in immunosuppressed patients, especially those with human immunodeficiency virus (HIV).

Clinical Manifestations

Symptoms of acute pharyngitis range in severity from complaints of a "scratchy throat" to pain so severe that swallowing is difficult. Both viral and strep infections appear as a red and edematous pharynx, with or without patchy yellow exudates. Appearance is not always diagnostic. Cultures or a rapid strep antigen test is done to establish the cause and direct appropriate management. Inadequate treatment of acute streptococcal pharyngitis can result in rheumatic heart disease or glomerulonephritis.

White, irregular patches suggest fungal infection with *Candida albicans*. In diphtheria, a gray-white false membrane, termed a *pseudomembrane,* is seen covering the oropharynx, nasopharynx, and laryngopharynx and sometimes extends to the trachea.

NURSING *and* COLLABORATIVE MANAGEMENT ACUTE PHARYNGITIS

The goals of nursing management are infection control, symptomatic relief, and prevention of secondary complications. The patient with documented strep throat is treated with antibiotics. *Candida* infections are treated with nystatin (Mycostatin), an antifungal antibiotic. The preparation should be swished in the mouth as long as possible before it is swallowed, and treatment should continue until symptoms are gone. The patient should be encouraged to increase fluid intake. Cool, bland liquids and gelatin will not irritate the pharynx; citrus juices can be irritating.

PERITONSILLAR ABSCESS

Peritonsillar abscess is a complication of acute pharyngitis or acute tonsillitis when bacterial infection invades one or both tonsils. The tonsils may enlarge sufficiently to threaten airway patency. The patient experiences a high fever, leukocytosis, and chills. Intravenous (IV) antibiotic therapy is given along with needle aspiration or incision and drainage of the abscess. An emergency tonsillectomy may be performed, or an elective tonsillectomy may be scheduled after the infection has subsided.

OBSTRUCTIVE SLEEP APNEA

Obstructive sleep apnea (OSA) is a condition characterized by partial or complete upper airway obstruction during sleep, causing apnea and hypopnea.[10] **Apnea** is the cessation of spontaneous respirations. *Hypopnea* is abnormally shallow and slow respirations. Airflow obstruction occurs when the tongue and the soft palate fall backward and partially or completely obstruct the pharynx (Fig. 26-4). The obstruction may last from 15 to 90 seconds. During the apneic period, the patient experiences severe *hypoxemia* (decreased PaO_2) and *hypercapnia* (increased $PaCO_2$). These changes are ventilatory stimulants and cause the patient to partially awaken. The patient has a generalized startle response, snorts, and gasps, which causes the tongue and soft palate to move forward and the airway to open. Apnea and arousal cycles occur repeatedly, as many as 200 to 400 times during 6 to 8 hours of sleep.[11,12]

Sleep apnea occurs in 2% to 10% of the population. The disorder is more common in men than women and more common after age 65.[12]

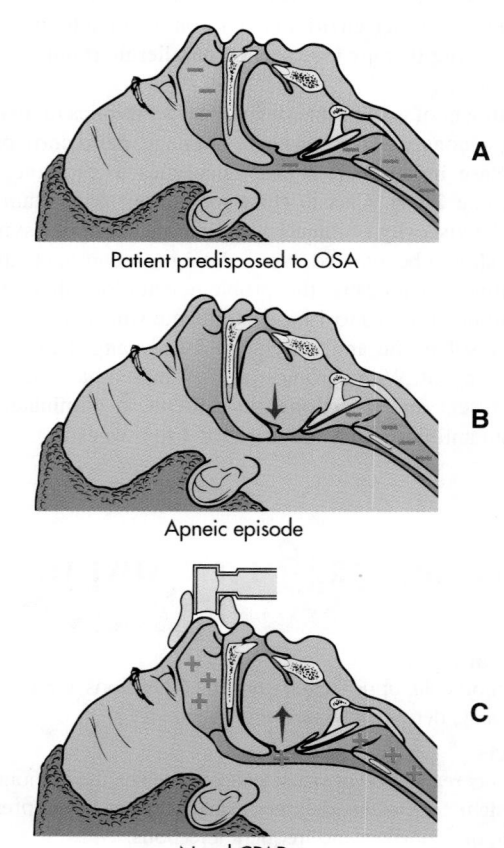

A

Patient predisposed to OSA

B

Apneic episode

C

Nasal CPAP

FIG. 26-4 How sleep apnea occurs. **A,** The patient predisposed to obstructive sleep apnea (OSA) has a small pharyngeal airway. **B,** During sleep, the pharyngeal muscles relax, allowing the airway to close. Lack of airflow results in repeated apneic episodes. **C,** With nasal CPAP, positive pressure splints the airway open, preventing airflow obstruction.

Clinical Manifestations and Diagnostic Studies

Clinical manifestations of sleep apnea include frequent awakening at night, insomnia, excessive daytime sleepiness, and witnessed apneic episodes. The patient's bed partner may complain about the patient's loud snoring. The snoring may be so loud that both persons cannot sleep in the same room. Other symptoms include morning headaches (from hypercapnia, which causes vasodilation of cerebral blood vessels), personality changes, and irritability. Systemic hypertension and cardiac arrhythmias are serious complications that may occur.

Symptoms of sleep apnea alter many aspects of the patient's lifestyle. Chronic sleep loss predisposes to diminished ability to concentrate, impaired memory, failure to accomplish daily tasks, and interpersonal difficulties. The male patient may experience impotence. Driving accidents are more common in habitually sleepy persons.[13] Family life and the patient's ability to maintain employment are also often compromised. As a result, the patient may experience severe depression. Appropriate referral should be made if problems are identified. Cessation of breathing reported by the bed partner is usually a source of great anxiety because of the fear that breathing may not resume.

Diagnosis of sleep apnea is made during sleep with the use of polysomnography. The patient's chest and abdominal movement, oral airflow, nasal airflow, SpO_2, ocular movement, and heart rate and rhythm are monitored, and time in each sleep stage is determined. A diagnosis of sleep apnea requires documentation of multiple episodes of apnea (no airflow with respiratory effort) or hypopnea (airflow diminished 30% to 50% with respiratory effort). Polysomnography may be carried out in a sleep laboratory, or the patient may be taught to attach monitoring leads for a home sleep study.

NURSING and COLLABORATIVE MANAGEMENT
SLEEP APNEA

Mild sleep apnea may respond to simple measures. The patient should be instructed to avoid sedatives and alcoholic beverages for 3 to 4 hours before sleep. Referral to a weight loss program may help, because excessive weight exacerbates symptoms. Symptoms resolve in half of the patients with OSA who use an oral appliance during sleep to prevent airflow obstruction. Oral appliances bring the mandible and tongue forward to enlarge the airway space, thereby preventing airway occlusion. Some individuals find a support group beneficial where concerns and feelings can be expressed and strategies discussed for resolving problems.

In patients with more severe symptoms, nasal continuous positive airway pressure (nCPAP) may be used.[14] With nCPAP, the patient applies a nasal mask that is attached to a high-flow blower (Fig. 26-5). The blower is adjusted to maintain sufficient positive pressure (5 to 15 cm H_2O) in the airway during inspiration and expiration to prevent airway collapse. Some patients cannot adjust to exhaling against the high pressure. A technologically more sophisticated therapy, bilevel positive airway pressure (BiPAP), capable of delivering a higher pressure during inspiration (when the airway is most likely to be occluded) and a lower pressure during expiration (when the airway is least likely to be occluded), may be helpful and is better tolerated. Although nCPAP is highly

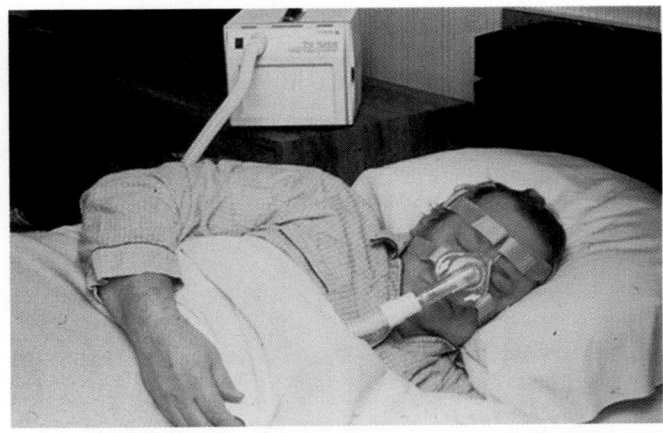

FIG. 26-5 Management of sleep apnea often involves sleeping with a nasal mask in place. The pressure supplied by air coming from the compressor opens the oropharynx and nasopharynx.

effective, compliance is poor even if symptoms of sleep apnea are relieved.[13]

If other measures fail, sleep apnea may be managed surgically. The two most common procedures are uvulopalatopharyngoplasty (UPPP or UP3) and genioglossal advancement and hyoid myotomy (GAHM). UPPP involves excision of the tonsillar pillars, uvula, and posterior soft palate with the goal of removing the obstructing tissue. GAHM involves advancing the attachment of the muscular part of the tongue on the mandible. When GAMH is performed, UPPP is generally done as well. Symptoms are relieved in up to 60% of patients.[10] Laser-assisted uvulopalatoplasty (LAUP) is a new surgical procedure than has been used to treat OSA.

Problems Related to the Trachea and Larynx

AIRWAY OBSTRUCTION

Airway obstruction may be complete or partial. Complete airway obstruction is a medical emergency. Partial airway obstruction may occur as a result of aspiration of food or a foreign body. In addition, partial airway obstruction may result from laryngeal edema following extubation, laryngeal or tracheal stenosis, CNS depression, and allergic reactions. Symptoms include stridor, use of accessory muscles, suprasternal and intercostal retractions, wheezing, restlessness, tachycardia, and cyanosis. Prompt assessment and treatment are essential because partial obstruction may quickly progress to complete obstruction. Interventions to reestablish a patent airway include the obstructed airway (Heimlich) maneuver (see Chapter 35), cricothyroidotomy, endotracheal intubation, and tracheostomy. Unexplained or recurrent symptoms indicate the need for additional tests, such as a chest x-ray, pulmonary function tests, and bronchoscopy.

TRACHEOSTOMY

A **tracheotomy** is a surgical incision into the trachea for the purpose of establishing an airway. A **tracheostomy** is the stoma (opening) that results from the tracheotomy. Indications for a tracheostomy are to (1) bypass an upper airway obstruction,

(2) facilitate removal of secretions, (3) permit long-term mechanical ventilation, and (4) permit oral intake and speech in the patient who requires long-term mechanical ventilation. Most patients who require mechanical ventilation are initially managed with an endotracheal tube, which can be quickly inserted in an emergency. (Care of the patient with an endotracheal tube is discussed in Chapter 64.) A tracheostomy requires surgical dissection and is therefore not typically an emergency procedure.

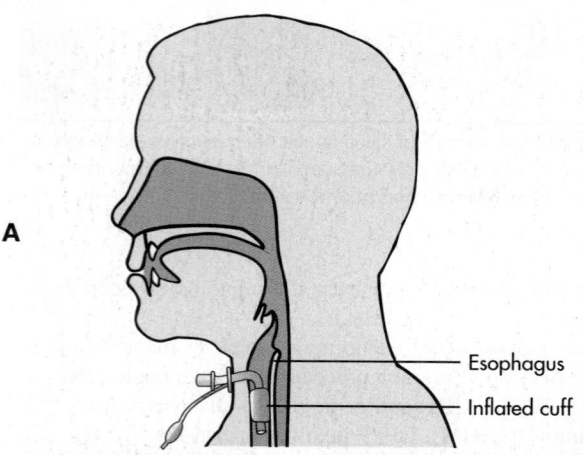

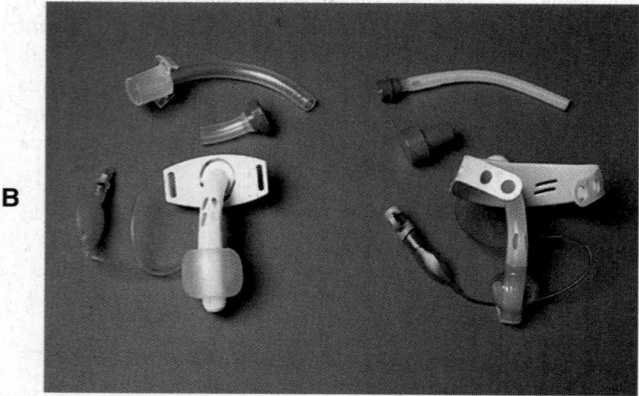

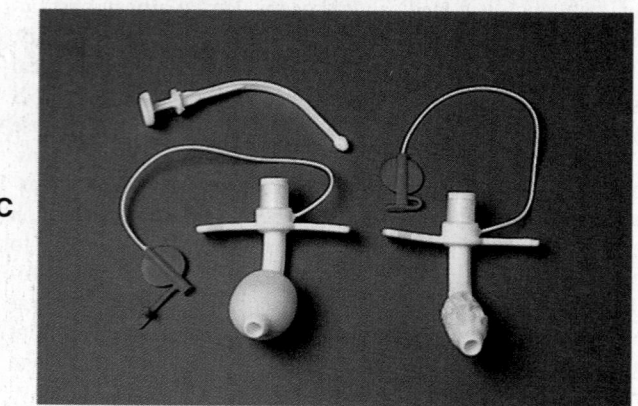

Esophagus

Inflated cuff

FIG. 26-6 Types of tracheostomy tubes. **A**, Tracheostomy tube inserted in airway with inflated cuff. **B**, Shiley and Portex fenestrated tracheostomy tube with cuff, inner cannula, decannulation plug, and pilot balloon. **C**, Bivona (Fome) tracheostomy tube with foam cuff and obturator (one cuff is deflated on tracheostomy tube). (See Table 26-5 and NCP 26-1 for related nursing management.)

Several advantages make a tracheostomy the better option for long-term care. With a tracheostomy, there is less risk of long-term damage to the airway. Patient comfort may be increased because no tube is present in the mouth. The patient can eat with a tracheostomy because the tube enters lower in the airway (Fig. 26-6). Because the tracheostomy tube is more secure, mobility may be increased.[15]

NURSING MANAGEMENT
TRACHEOSTOMY

■ Providing Tracheostomy Care

Before the tracheotomy procedure, the nurse should explain to the patient and the family the purpose of the procedure and inform them that the patient will not be able to speak while an inflated cuff is used.

A variety of tubes are available to meet individual patient needs (Table 26-5). All tracheostomy tubes contain a faceplate or flange, which rests on the neck between the clavicles and outer cannula. In addition, all tubes have an obturator, which is used when inserting the tube (see Fig. 26-6, *C*). During insertion of the tube, the obturator is placed inside the outer cannula with its rounded tip protruding from the end of the tube to ease insertion. After insertion, the obturator must be immediately removed so air can flow through the tube. The obturator should be kept in an easily accessible place at the bedside (e.g., taped to the wall) so that it can be used quickly in case of accidental decannulation.[16]

Some tracheostomy tubes also have an inner cannula, which can be removed for cleaning (see Fig. 26-6, *B*). The cleaning procedure removes mucus from the inside of the tube. If humidification is adequate, mucus may not accumulate and a tube without an inner cannula can be used. Care of the patient with a tracheostomy involves suctioning the airway to remove secretions[17] (Fig. 26-7 and Table 26-6) and cleaning around the stoma. In addition, tracheostomy care includes changing tracheostomy ties (Fig. 26-8 and Table 26-7). If a disposable or nondisposable inner cannula is used, tracheostomy care also involves inner cannula care[18] (see Table 26-7).

Both cuffed and uncuffed tracheostomy tubes are available. A tracheostomy tube with an inflated cuff is used if the patient is at risk of aspiration or needs mechanical ventilation. Because an inflated cuff exerts pressure on tracheal mucosa, it is important to inflate the cuff with the minimum volume of air required to obtain an airway seal. Cuff inflation pressure should not exceed 20 mm Hg or 25 cm H_2O because higher pressures may compress tracheal capillaries, limit blood flow, and predispose to tracheal necrosis. An alternative approach, termed the *minimal leak technique* (MLT), involves inflating the cuff with the minimum amount of air to obtain a seal and then withdrawing 0.1 ml of air. A disadvantage of MLT is risk of aspiration from secretions leaking around the cuff. MLT should not be used when the tracheostomy was placed to bypass an upper airway obstruction, such as with head and neck surgical patients.

In some patients, cuff deflation is performed to remove secretions that accumulate above the cuff. Before deflation, the patient should cough up secretions, if possible, and the tracheostomy tube and mouth should be suctioned (see Fig. 26-7 and Table 26-6). This step is important to prevent secretions from being aspirated during deflation. The cuff is deflated during exhalation because

TABLE 26-5	**Characteristics and Nursing Management of Tracheostomies**	
TUBE	**CHARACTERISTICS**	**NURSING MANAGEMENT**
Tracheostomy tube with cuff and pilot balloon (see Fig. 26-6, *A* and *B*)	When properly inflated, low-pressure, high-volume cuff distributes cuff pressure over large area, minimizing pressure on tracheal wall.	**Procedure for cuff inflation** - *Mechanically ventilated patient:* Inflate the cuff to *minimal occlusion pressure* by slowly injecting air into the cuff until no leak (sound) is heard at peak inspiratory pressure (end of ventilator inspiration) when a stethoscope is placed over the trachea. Use cuff pressure monitor to determine cuff inflation pressure. An alternative approach, termed *minimal leak technique* (MLT), involves inflating the cuff to minimal occlusion pressure and then withdrawing 0.1 ml of air. - *Spontaneously breathing patient:* Inflate cuff to minimal occlusion pressure by slowly injecting air into the cuff until no sound is heard after deep breath or during inhalation with manual resuscitation bag. If using MLT, remove 0.1 ml of air while maintaining seal. MLT should not be used if there is risk of aspiration. - *Immediately after cuff inflation (both groups):* Verify pressure is within accepted range ($\leq$20 mm Hg or $\leq$25 cm H_2O) with a manometer. Record cuff pressure and volume of air used for cuff inflation in chart. **Care of patients with an inflated cuff** - Monitor and record cuff pressure q8h. Cuff pressure should be $\leq$20 mm Hg or $\leq$25 cm H_2O to allow adequate tracheal capillary perfusion. If needed, remove or add air to the pilot tubing using a syringe and stopcock. Afterward, verify cuff pressure is within accepted range with manometer. - Report inability to keep the cuff inflated or need to use progressively larger volumes of air to keep cuff inflated. Potential causes include tracheal dilation at the cuff site or a crack or slow leak in the housing of the one-way inflation valve. If the leak is due to tracheal dilation, the physician may intubate the patient with a larger tube. Cracks in the inflation valve may be temporarily managed by clamping the small-bore tubing with a hemostat. The tube should be changed within 24 hours.
Fenestrated tracheostomy tube (Shiley, Portex) with cuff, inner cannula, and decannulation plug (see Fig. 26-6, *B*; Fig. 26-9, *A*)	When inner cannula is removed, cuff deflated, and decannulation plug inserted, air flows around tube, through fenestration in outer cannula, and up over vocal cords. Patient can then speak.	- Assess risk of aspiration before removing inner cannula. Deflate cuff. Note coughing. Have patient swallow a small amount of clear liquid (grape juice) or 30 ml of water with a few drops of blue food coloring. Observe secretions after patient coughs or when suctioned for presence of colored secretions. If no aspiration is noted, a fenestrated tube may be used. - **Never** insert decannulation plug in tracheostomy tube until cuff is deflated and inner cannula removed. Prior insertion will prevent patient from breathing (no air inflow). This may precipitate a respiratory arrest. - Assess for signs of respiratory distress when a fenestrated cannula is first used. If this occurs, the cap should be removed, the inner cannula replaced, and the cuff reinflated. - Cuff management as described above.
Speaking tracheostomy tube (Portex, National) with cuff, two external tubings (see Fig. 26-9, *B*)	Has two tubings, one leading to cuff and second to opening above the cuff. When port is connected to air source, air flows out of opening and up over the vocal cords, allowing speech with cuff inflated.	- Once tube is inserted, wait 2 days before use so that the stoma can close around the tube and prevent leaks. - When patient desires to speak, connect port to compressed air (or oxygen). Be certain to identify correct tubing. If gas enters the cuff, it will overinflate and rupture, requiring an emergency tube change. Use lowest flow (typically 4-6 L/min) that results in speech. High flows dehydrate mucosa. - Cover port adaptor. This will cause the air to flow upward. Instruct patient to speak in short sentences because voice becomes a whisper with long sentences. - Disconnect flow when patient does not want to speak to prevent mucosal dehydration. - Cuff management as described above.
Tracheostomy tube (Bivona Fome-Cuf) foam-filled cuff (see Fig. 26-6, *C*)	Cuff is filled with plastic foam. Before insertion, cuff is deflated. After insertion, cuff is allowed to fill passively with air. Pilot tubing is not capped, and no cuff pressure monitoring is required.	- Before insertion, withdraw all air from the cuff using a 20 ml syringe. Cap pilot balloon tubing to prevent reentry of air. After tracheostomy is inserted, remove cap from pilot tubing allowing cuff to passively reinflate. - Do not inject air into tubing or cap pilot balloon tubing while in patient. Air will flow in and out in response to pressure changes (head turning). Place tag on tubing alerting staff not to cap or inflate cuff. - Deflate cuff daily via pilot balloon to evaluate integrity of cuff. Also assess ability to easily deflate cuff. Difficulty deflating cuff indicates a need for tube change. If aspirate returns with air, the cuff is no longer intact. - Tube can be used for up to 1 month in patients on home mechanical ventilation. Good choice for patients who require inflated cuff at home since teaching about cuff pressure is simplified.

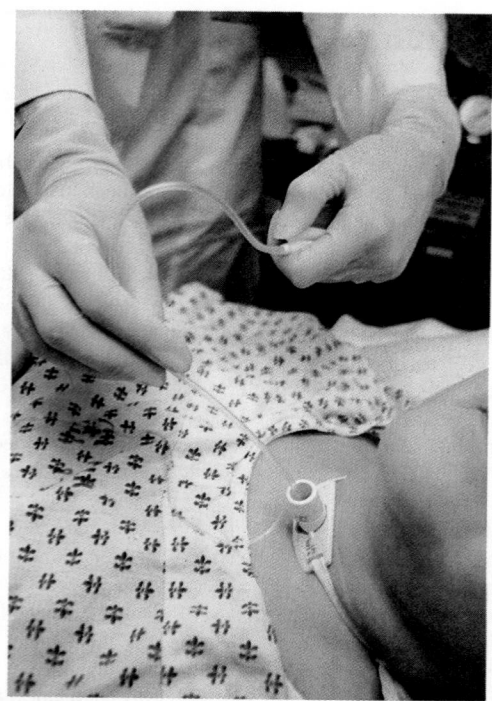

FIG. 26-7 Suctioning a tracheostomy. Using sterile technique, the suction catheter is being withdrawn from the airway while suction is applied. The pilot balloon tubing may be seen lying on the patient's chest.

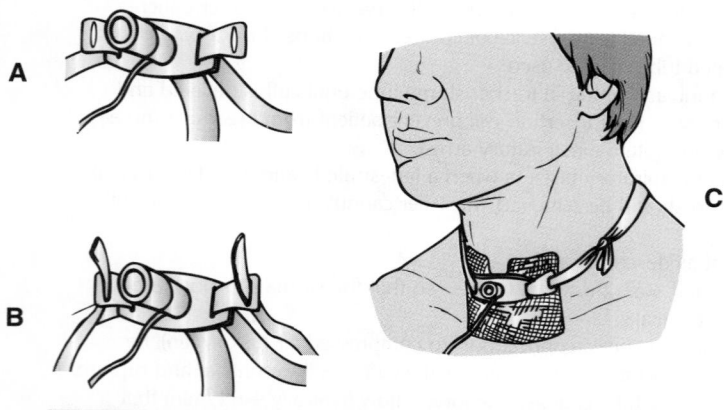

FIG. 26-8 Changing tracheostomy ties. **A,** A slit is cut about 1 inch (2.5 cm) from the end. The slit end is put into the opening of the cannula. **B,** A loop is made with the other end of the tape. **C,** The tapes are tied together with a double knot on the side of the neck.

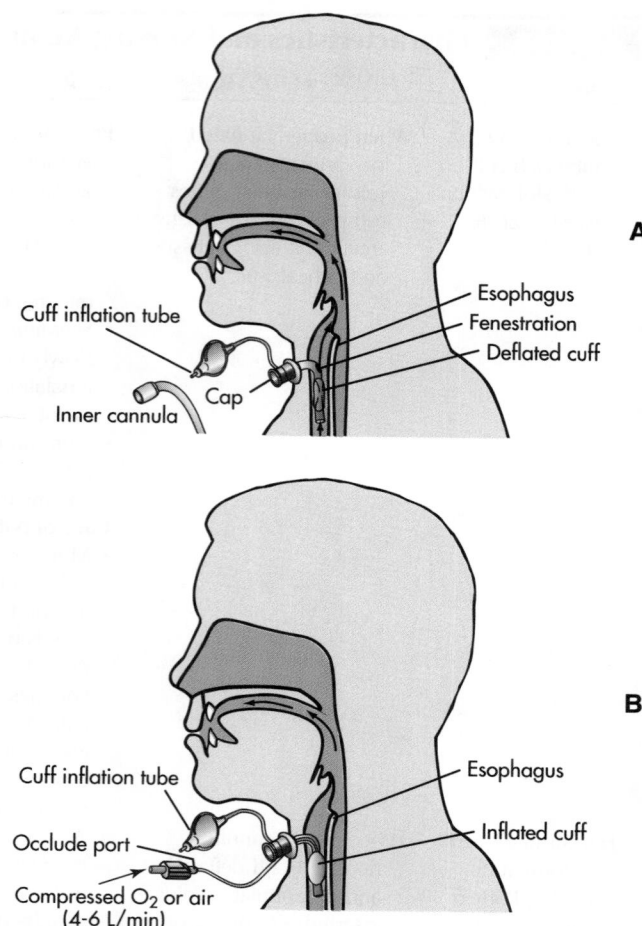

FIG. 26-9 Speaking tracheostomy tubes. **A,** Fenestrated tracheostomy tube with cuff deflated, inner cannula removed, and tracheostomy tube capped to allow air to pass over the vocal cords. **B,** Speaking tracheostomy tube. One tubing is used for cuff inflation. The second tubing is connected to a source of compressed air or oxygen. When the port on the second tubing is occluded, air flows up over the vocal cords, allowing speech with an inflated cuff. (See Table 26-5 and NCP 26-1 for related nursing management.)

the exhaled gas helps propel secretions into the mouth. The patient should also cough or be suctioned after cuff deflation. The cuff should be reinflated during inspiration. The volume of air required to inflate the cuff should be monitored daily because this volume may increase if there is tracheal dilation from cuff pressure. The nurse should assess the ability of the patient to protect the airway from aspiration and remain with the patient when the cuff is initially deflated unless the patient can protect the airway from aspiration and breathe without respiratory distress. When the patient can protect the airway from aspiration and does not require

mechanical ventilation, a cuffless tracheostomy tube should be used.

Retention sutures are often placed in the tracheal cartilage when the tracheostomy is performed. The free ends should be taped to the skin in a place and manner that leaves them accessible if the tube is dislodged. Care should be taken not to dislodge the tracheostomy tube during the first few days when the stoma is not mature (healed). Because tube replacement can be difficult, several precautions are required: (1) a replacement tube of equal or smaller size is kept at the bedside, readily available for emergency reinsertion; (2) tracheostomy tapes are not changed for at least 24 hours after the insertion procedure; and (3) the first tube change is performed by a physician usually no sooner than 7 days after the tracheostomy.

If the tube is accidentally dislodged, the nurse should immediately attempt to replace it. The retention sutures (if present) are grasped and the opening is spread. A hemostat can also be used to spread the opening to facilitate replacing the tube. The obtura-

TABLE 26-6   Procedure for Suctioning a Tracheostomy Tube

1. Assess the need for suctioning q2h. Indications include coarse crackles or rhonchi over large airways, moist cough, increase in peak inspiratory pressure on mechanical ventilator, and restlessness or agitation if accompanied by decrease in SpO_2 or PaO_2. Do not suction routinely or if patient is able to clear secretions with cough.
2. If suctioning is indicated, explain procedure to patient.
3. Collect necessary sterile equipment: suction catheter (no larger than half the lumen of the tracheostomy tube), gloves, water, cup, and drape. If a closed tracheal suction system is used, the catheter is enclosed in a plastic sleeve and reused. No additional equipment is needed.
4. Check suction source and regulator. Adjust suction pressure until the dial reads -120 to -150 mm Hg pressure with tubing occluded.
5. Wash hands. Put on goggles and gloves.
6. Use sterile technique to open package, fill cup with water, put on gloves, and connect catheter to suction. Designate one hand as contaminated for disconnecting, bagging, and operating the suction control. Suction water through the catheter to test the system.
7. Assess SpO_2, heart rate, and rhythm to provide baseline for detecting change during suctioning.
8. Provide preoxygenation by (1) adjusting ventilator to deliver 100% O_2; (2) using a reservoir-equipped manual resuscitation bag (MRB) connected to 100% oxygen; or (3) asking the patient to take 3-4 deep breaths while administering oxygen. The method chosen will depend on the patient's underlying disease and acuity of illness. The patient who has had a tracheostomy for an extended period of time and is not acutely ill may be able to tolerate suctioning without use of an MRB or the ventilator.
9. Gently insert catheter *without suction* to minimize the amount of oxygen removed from the lungs. Insert the catheter approximately 5-6 inches (13-15 cm). Stop if an obstruction is met.
10. Withdraw the catheter $1/2$-$3/4$ inch (1-2 cm) and apply suction intermittently, while withdrawing catheter in a rotating manner. If secretion volume is large, apply suction continuously.
11. *Limit suction time to 10 seconds.* Discontinue suctioning if heart rate decreases from baseline by 20 beats per minute, increases from baseline by 40 beats per minute, an arrhythmia occurs, or SpO_2 decreases to less than 90%.
12. After each suction pass, oxygenate with 3-4 breaths by ventilator, MRB, or deep breaths with oxygen.
13. Rinse catheter with sterile water (if in suction kit).
14. Repeat procedure until airway is clear. Limit insertions of suction catheter to as few as needed.
15. Return oxygen concentration to prior setting.
16. Rinse catheter and suction the oropharynx or use mouth suction.
17. Dispose of catheter by wrapping it around fingers of gloved hand and pulling glove over catheter. Discard equipment in proper waste container.
18. Auscultate to assess changes in lung sounds. Record time, amount, and character of secretions and response to suctioning.

TABLE 26-7   Tracheostomy Care

1. Explain procedure to patient.
2. Use tracheostomy care kit or collect necessary sterile equipment (e.g., suction catheter, gloves, water, basin, drape, tracheostomy ties, tube brush or pipe cleaners, 4 × 4s, hydrogen peroxide [3%], sterile water, and tracheostomy dressing [optional]). Note: Clean rather than sterile technique is used at home.
3. Position patient in semi-Fowler's position.
4. Assemble needed materials on bedside table next to patient.
5. Wash hands. Put on goggles and clean gloves.
6. Auscultate chest sounds. If rhonchi or coarse crackles are present, suction the patient if unable to cough up secretions (see Table 26-6). Remove soiled dressing and clean gloves.
7. Open sterile equipment, pour sterile H_2O and hydrogen peroxide in basins, and put on sterile gloves.
8. Unlock and remove inner cannula, if present. Many tracheostomy tubes do not have inner cannulas. Care for these tubes includes all steps except for inner cannula care.
9. If disposable inner cannula is used, replace with new cannula. If a nondisposable cannula is used:
   a. Immerse inner cannula in 3% hydrogen peroxide and clean inside and outside of cannula using tube brush or pipe cleaners.
   b. Drain hydrogen peroxide from cannula. Immerse cannula in sterile water. Remove from sterile water and shake to dry.
   c. Insert inner cannula into outer cannula with the curved part downward and lock in place.
10. Remove dried secretions from stoma using 4 × 4 soaked in hydrogen peroxide. Rinse with another 4 × 4 soaked in sterile water. Gently pat area around the stoma dry. Be sure to clean under the tracheostomy face plate, using cotton swabs to reach this area.
11. Maintain position of tracheal retention sutures, if present, by taping above and below the stoma.
12. Change tracheostomy ties. Secure new ties to flanges before removing the old ones. Tie tracheostomy ties securely with room for one finger between ties and skin (see Fig. 26-8). To prevent accidental tube removal, secure the tracheostomy tube by gently applying pressure to the flange of the tube during the tie changes. *Do not change tracheostomy ties for 24 hr after the tracheotomy procedure.*
13. As an alternative, some patients prefer tracheostomy ties made of Velcro, which are easier to adjust.
14. If drainage is excessive, place dressing around tube (see Fig. 26-8). A tracheostomy dressing or unlined gauze should be used. Do not cut the gauze because threads may be inhaled or wrap around the tracheostomy tube. Change the dressing frequently. Wet dressings promote infection and stoma irritation.
15. Repeat care three times a day and as needed.

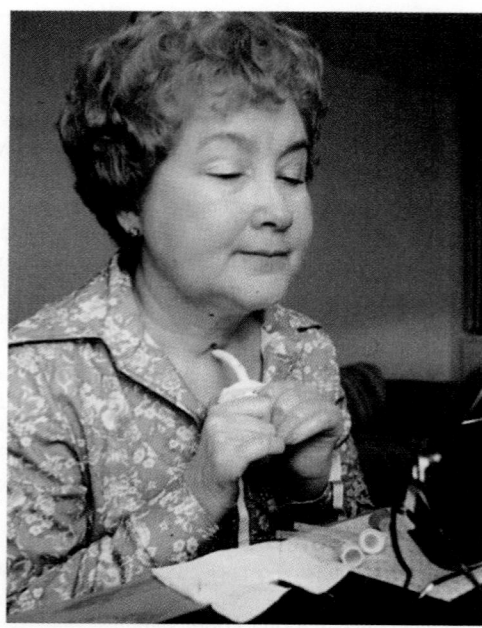

FIG. 26-10 Changing the tracheostomy tube at home. When a tracheostomy has been in place for several months, the tract will be well formed. The patient can then be taught to change the tube using a clean technique at home.

tor is inserted in the replacement tube, lubricated with saline poured over the tip, and the tube is inserted in the stoma at a 45-degree angle to the neck. If insertion is successful, the obturator is removed immediately so that air can flow through the tube. Another method is to insert a suction catheter to allow passage of air and to serve as a guide for insertion. The tracheostomy tube should be threaded over the catheter and the suction catheter removed. If the tube cannot be replaced, assess the level of respiratory distress. Minor dyspnea may be alleviated by use of semi-Fowler's position until assistance arrives. Severe dyspnea may progress to respiratory arrest. If this situation occurs, the stoma should be covered with a sterile dressing, and the patient should be ventilated with bag-mask ventilation until help arrives.

After the first tube change, the tube should be changed approximately once a month. When a tracheostomy has been in place for several months, the healed tract will be well formed. The patient can then be taught to change the tube using a clean technique at home (Fig. 26-10). Teaching will vary, depending on the illness of the patient and the device selected.

Nursing diagnoses for the patient with a tracheostomy include, but are not limited to, those presented in NCP 26-1.

■ Swallowing Dysfunction

The patient who cannot protect the airway from aspiration requires an inflated cuff. However, an inflated cuff may promote swallowing dysfunction because the cuff interferes with the normal function of muscles used to swallow. For this reason, it is important to evaluate the risk for aspiration with the cuff deflated. The patient may be able to swallow without aspirating when the cuff is deflated but not when it is inflated. The cuff may then be left deflated or a cuffless tube substituted (see Fig. 26-9).

To evaluate aspiration risk, the cuff is deflated and the patient is instructed to swallow a small amount of clear liquid such as grape juice or 30 ml of water that has blue food coloring added. Any coughing and secretions are noted. If needed, the trachea is suctioned to check for the presence of blue-colored secretions. If there is no indication of aspiration, the patient is judged to have adequate epiglottic function without risk for aspiration. A formal swallowing evaluation may be done by a speech therapist.

■ Speech with a Tracheostomy Tube

A number of techniques promote speech in the patient with a tracheostomy. The spontaneously breathing patient may be able to talk by deflating the cuff, which allows exhaled air to flow upward over the vocal cords. This can be enhanced by the patient occluding the tube. Frequently, a small cuffless tube is inserted so exhaled air can pass freely around the tube. If the patient is on mechanical ventilation, speech may be possible by allowing a constant air leak around the cuff. In addition, tracheostomy tubes and valves have been designed to facilitate speech. The nurse can be an advocate in promoting use of these specialized devices. Their use can provide great psychologic benefit and facilitate self-care for the patient with a tracheostomy.

A fenestrated tube has openings on the surface of the outer cannula that permit air from the lungs to flow over the vocal cords (see Fig. 26-6, *B*, and Fig. 26-9, *A*). A fenestrated tube allows the patient to breathe spontaneously through the larynx, speak, and cough up secretions while the tracheostomy tube remains in place. It can be used by the patient who can swallow without risk of aspiration but requires suctioning for secretion removal. It may also be used by the patient who requires mechanical ventilation for fewer than 24 hours a day (e.g., during sleep).

Before the fenestrated tube is used, the patient's ability to swallow without aspiration is determined (see Table 26-5 and NCP 26-1). If there is no aspiration, (1) the inner cannula is removed, (2) the cuff is deflated, and (3) the decannulation cap is placed in the tube (see Fig. 26-9, *A*). It is important to perform the steps in order because severe respiratory distress may result if the tube is capped before the inner cannula is removed and the cuff deflated. When a fenestrated cannula is first used, the nurse should frequently assess the patient for signs of respiratory distress. If the patient is not able to tolerate the procedure, the cap should be removed, the inner cannula replaced, and the cuff reinflated. A disadvantage of fenestrated tubes is the potential for development of tracheal polyps from tracheal tissue granulating into the fenestrated openings.[19]

A speaking tracheostomy tube has two pigtail tubings. One tubing connects to the cuff and is used for cuff inflation, and the second connects to an opening just above the cuff (see Fig. 26-9, *B*). When the second tubing is connected to a low-flow (4 to 6 L/min) air source, sufficient air moves up over the vocal cords to permit speech. The patient can then speak, although the cuff is inflated.

When a speaking tracheostomy valve is used, a cuffless tube must be in place or the cuff deflated to allow exhalation (Fig. 26-11). Ability to tolerate cuff deflation without aspiration or respiratory distress must also be evaluated in patients using this device. If there is no aspiration, the cuff is deflated and the valve is placed over the tracheostomy tube opening. The speaking valve contains a thin plastic diaphragm that opens on inspi-

NURSING CARE PLAN 26-1

Patient with a Tracheostomy

EXPECTED PATIENT OUTCOMES	NURSING INTERVENTIONS and *RATIONALES*
NURSING DIAGNOSIS	**Ineffective airway clearance** *related to* presence of tracheostomy tube and difficulty expectorating sputum *as manifested by* adventitious breath sounds, tenacious secretions, increase in restlessness, ineffective or absent cough.
• Maintenance of patent airway • Secretions expectorated without need to suction airway • Clear lung sounds • Normal SpO_2	• Assess for respiratory distress (e.g., abnormal breath sounds, dyspnea, SpO_2 less than 90%) *to determine need for interventions.* • Keep head of bed elevated 30 to 40 degrees *to allow a more forceful cough and to relieve dyspnea.* • Provide humidification and hydration *to liquefy secretions.* • Encourage coughing, deep breathing, and ambulation *to assist in mobilizing secretions.* • Clean and/or change inner cannula, if present, as needed *to minimize buildup of secretions on inside lumen of cannula.* • Maintain minimum cuff pressure while obtaining airway seal by measuring with manometer at no more than 25 cm H_2O pressure or with minimal leak technique (MLT) *to minimize pressure on trachea.* MLT cannot be used if tracheostomy is to bypass upper airway obstruction such as head and neck surgery. • If cuff is to be deflated, deflate during exhalation and reinflate during inhalation. Clear mouth and trachea before and after deflation by coughing or suctioning *to minimize aspiration.* • Keep tracheostomy tube tied securely, allowing room for one finger between ties and skin, *to secure tube from dislodging.*
NURSING DIAGNOSIS	**Impaired verbal communication** *related to* use of artificial airway and cuff *as manifested by* inability to speak and signs of frustration.
• Able to communicate needs	• If patient is alert, provide call bell within easy reach and respond immediately in person *to allay anxiety.* • Assess patient's ability to read and write; provide with magic slate, pad and pencil, communication board with illustrations of requests, electrolarynx (Cooper-Rand) *as alternative means of communication.* • Reassure patient that speech will return when tube can be removed (if total laryngectomy has not been performed) *to allay fear that situation is permanent.* • Suggest use of speaking tubes (small, cuffless tube, fenestrated tube, speaking valve, speaking tracheostomy tube) *to permit speech.* • Encourage gesturing *to communicate needs and desires.*
NURSING DIAGNOSIS	**Risk for infection** *related to* bypass of airway defense mechanisms and impaired skin integrity.
• Normal white blood cell count • Normal temperature • Clear mucus • No erythema or purulent secretions from stoma site	• Monitor and report elevated white blood cell count and temperature, change in color of secretions, purulent drainage or redness around the site *to identify signs of infection and permit early medical intervention.* • Use strict aseptic technique for suctioning and tracheostomy care during hospitalization *to reduce occurrence of infection.* • Change oxygen-delivery equipment per agency policy *to prevent contaminated tubing from being a source of infection.* • Keep stoma clean and dry with frequent tracheostomy care.
NURSING DIAGNOSIS	**Imbalanced nutrition: less than body requirements** *related to* decreased oral intake, altered taste sensation, and swallowing difficulty *as manifested by* inadequate caloric intake, weight loss.
• Usual appetite • Maintenance or progression toward normal body weight	• Provide ongoing assessment of oral intake and caloric count *to assess adequacy of diet.* • Monitor weight *to provide information for evaluation.* • Provide high-calorie, high-protein food and beverages *to maximize nutritional intake.* • Thicken foods and beverages if needed *to ease swallowing and minimize aspiration.* • Assess for swallowing dysfunction *to determine if presence of inflated cuff is predisposing to aspiration.* • Perform mouth care q8h and prn *to promote patient comfort and appetite.*

Continued

NURSING CARE PLAN 26-1

Patient with a Tracheostomy—cont'd

EXPECTED PATIENT OUTCOMES	NURSING INTERVENTIONS and *RATIONALES*
NURSING DIAGNOSIS	**Impaired swallowing** *related to* tracheostomy tube *as manifested by* inability to swallow without difficulty and/or without aspiration.
• Normal swallowing function • No aspiration	• Assess swallow and gag reflexes by deflating cuff; note coughing *because it is an indicator of aspiration.* • If patient tolerates cuff deflated, have patient swallow clear liquid (grape juice) or water with blue food coloring *to determine presence of aspiration.* If patient does not cough or no colored secretions are suctioned, the patient may tolerate eating with cuff deflated.
NURSING DIAGNOSIS	**Ineffective therapeutic regimen management** *related to* lack of knowledge about care of tracheostomy at home *as manifested by* questioning about care (patient and/or family), agitation, and restlessness when planning for discharge.
• Demonstration of techniques by patient and significant others for tracheostomy care • Able to verbalize expected outcomes and when to contact health care professionals if problems arise	• Assess ability of patient and significant other to provide care at home, including tracheostomy tube care, stoma care, airway care, and ability to respond appropriately to emergencies, *to determine if home care is feasible.* • Teach good hand-washing technique *to minimize risk for infection.* • Teach clean tracheostomy tube care and home preparation of sterile saline solution *so patient can care for self at home.* • Teach clean suctioning, if needed, *so patient can care for self at home.* • Teach patient and significant other the signs and symptoms to report to health care professionals such as changes in secretions (yellow, green, or blood tinged) and/or elevated temperature *because these may be early signs of respiratory infection.* • Make referral to home health nurse *to provide ongoing assistance and support.*

COLLABORATIVE PROBLEM

NURSING GOALS	NURSING INTERVENTIONS and *RATIONALES*
POTENTIAL COMPLICATION	**Hypoxemia** *related to* misplaced or improperly functioning tube, accumulated secretions.
• Monitor for signs of hypoxemia • Carry out appropriate medical and nursing interventions	• Assess patient for restlessness, agitation, confusion, tachycardia, bradycardia, arrhythmias; SpO_2 less than 90% *to detect presence of hypoxemia.* • Elevate head of bed if tolerated. • Auscultate chest *to determine need for suctioning.* If coarse crackles or rhonchi are present and patient cannot cough and clear secretions, suction airway. • If unable to pass suction catheter, tube is dislodged and emergency measures must be implemented. • Monitor tube and inner cannula for placement. • If tube is dislodged or misplaced, grasp the retention sutures (if present) or hemostat and spread opening. Lubricate tube and insert with obturator in place at 45-degree angle to neck. If successful, remove obturator immediately. • Another method is to insert a suction catheter to allow the passage of air and to serve as a guide for insertion. Thread the tracheostomy tube over catheter and remove the suction catheter. • If tube cannot be reinserted, assess the level of respiratory distress *to determine whether patient can breathe without tube for a short interval.* • Notify physician. If distress is severe, ventilate with bag-mask until assistance arrives *to ensure adequate ventilation.*

ration and closes on expiration. During inspiration, air flows in through the valve. During expiration, the diaphragm prevents exhalation and air flows upward over the vocal cords and into the mouth.

If speaking devices are not used, the patient should be provided with a paper and pencil or magic slate. A word (communication) board can usually be obtained from speech therapy or one can be devised with pictures of common needs and an alphabet for spelling words.

■ Decannulation

When the patient can adequately exchange air and expectorate secretions, the tracheostomy tube can be removed. The stoma is closed with tape strips and covered with an occlusive dressing. The dressing must be changed if it gets soiled or wet. The patient should be instructed to splint the stoma with the fingers when coughing, swallowing, or speaking.[20] Epithelial tissue begins to form in 24 to 48 hours, and the opening will close in several days. Surgical intervention to close the tracheostomy is not required.

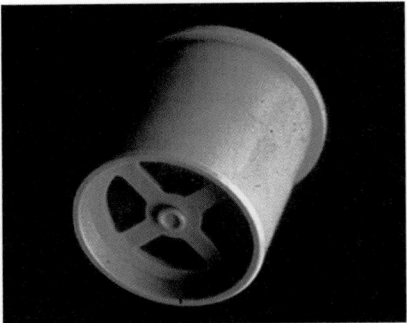

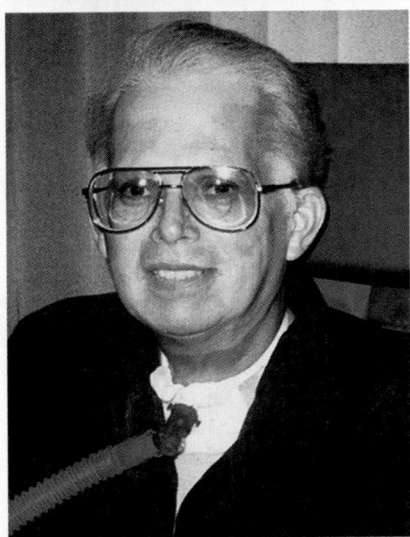

FIG. 26-11 Passy-Muir speaking tracheostomy valve. The valve is placed over the hub of the tracheostomy tube after the cuff is deflated. Two options are available: a white valve for nonventilated patients and an aqua valve (shown) for ventilated patients. The valve contains a one-way valve that allows air to enter the lungs during inspiration and redirects air upward over the vocal cords into the mouth during expiration.

LARYNGEAL POLYPS

Laryngeal polyps may develop on the vocal cords from vocal abuse (e.g., excessive talking, singing) or irritation (e.g., intubation, cigarette smoking). The most common symptom is hoarseness. Polyps may be treated conservatively with voice rest. Surgical removal may be indicated for large polyps, which may cause dyspnea and stridor. Polyps are usually benign but may be removed because they may later become malignant.

HEAD AND NECK CANCER

Head and neck cancer arises from mucosal surfaces and is typically squamous cell in origin. This category of tumors includes the paranasal sinuses, the oral cavity, and the nasopharynx, oropharynx, and larynx. (Cancer of the oral cavity is discussed in Chapter 40.) An estimated 30,100 new cases of oral and pharyngeal cancer were diagnosed in the United States in 2002, with nearly 7800 deaths. Although this type of cancer is not common, disability is great because of the potential loss of voice, disfigurement, and social consequences. Most (90%) head and neck cancers occur in individuals 50 years or older after prolonged use of tobacco and alcohol. The male-to-female ratio is 2:1.[21]

Clinical Manifestations

Early signs and symptoms of head and neck cancer vary with the tumor location. Cancer of the oral cavity may be a painless growth in the mouth, an ulcer that does not heal, or a change in fit of dentures. Pain is a late symptom that may be aggravated by acidic food. Cancers of the oropharynx, hypopharynx, and supraglottic larynx rarely produce early symptoms and are usually diagnosed in late stages. The patient may complain of persistent unilateral sore throat or otalgia (ear pain). Hoarseness may be a symptom of early laryngeal cancer. If a lump in the neck or hoarseness lasts longer than 2 weeks, a medical evaluation is indicated. Some patients experience what feels like a lump in the throat or a change in voice quality.

Late stages of head and neck cancers have easily detectable signs and symptoms, including pain, dysphagia, decreased mobility of the tongue, airway obstruction, and cranial nerve neuropathies. The nurse should thoroughly examine the oral cavity, including the area under the tongue and dentures. The floor of the mouth, tongue, and lymph nodes in the neck should be bimanually palpated. There may be thickening of the normally soft and pliable oral mucosa. *Leukoplakia* (white patch) or *erythroplakia* (red patch) may be seen and should be noted for later biopsy. Both leukoplakia and carcinoma in situ (localized to a defined area) may precede invasive carcinoma by many years.

Diagnostic Studies

If lesions are suspected, the upper airways may be examined using indirect laryngoscopy, which involves using a laryngeal mirror to visualize the laryngeal area, or a flexible nasopharyngoscope may be used. The larynx and vocal cords are visually inspected for lesions and tissue mobility. A CT scan or magnetic resonance imaging (MRI) may be performed to detect local and regional spread. Neoplastic tissue is identifiable because it contains tissue of greater density or because it distorts, displaces, or destroys normal anatomic structures. Typically, multiple biopsy specimens are obtained to determine the extent of the disease.

Collaborative Care

The stage of the disease will be determined based on tumor size (T), number and location of involved nodes (N), and extent of metastasis (M). TNM staging classifies disease as stage I to stage IV and guides treatment. Choice of treatment is based on medical history, extent of disease, cosmetic considerations, urgency of treatment, and patient choice. Approximately one third of patients with head and neck cancers have highly confined lesions that are stage I or II at diagnosis. Such patients can undergo radiation therapy or surgery with the goal of cure.

Radiation therapy may be effective in curing early vocal cord lesions. This therapy is usually successful in eliminating the tumor while preserving the quality of the voice. If radiation therapy is not successful or the lesion is too advanced for this therapy, surgery may be performed. A *cordectomy* (partial removal of one vocal cord) is used when there is a superficial tumor involving one cord (Fig. 26-12). A *hemilaryngectomy* involves removal of one vocal cord or part of a cord and requires a temporary tracheostomy. A *supraglottic laryngectomy* involves removing structures above the true cords—the false vocal cords and epiglottis. The patient is left at high risk of aspiration following surgery and requires a temporary tracheostomy. Both a hemilaryngectomy

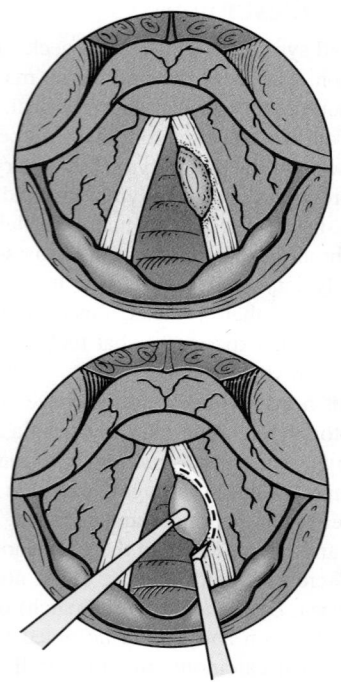

FIG. 26-12 Excision of laryngeal cancer. This cancer of the right vocal cord meets criteria for resection by transoral cordectomy. The cord is fully mobile and the lesion can be fully exposed. It does not approach or cross the anterior commissure.

and supraglottic laryngectomy allow the voice to be preserved, but quality is breathy and hoarse.

Advanced lesions are treated by a total laryngectomy in which the entire larynx and preepiglottic region is removed and a permanent tracheostomy performed. Airflow patterns before and after total laryngectomy are shown in Fig. 26-13. *Radical neck dissection* frequently accompanies total laryngectomy to decrease the risk of lymphatic spread. Depending on the extent of involvement, extensive dissection and reconstruction may be performed. This procedure involves wide excision of the lymph nodes and their lymphatic channels (Fig. 26-14). The following structures may also be removed or transected: sternocleidomastoid muscle and other closely associated muscles, internal jugular vein, mandible, submaxillary gland, part of the thyroid and parathyroid glands, and the spinal accessory nerve.

A *modified neck dissection* is performed whenever possible as an alternative to a radical neck dissection. The dissection is modified by sparing as many structures as possible to limit disfigurement and functional loss. A modified neck dissection usually involves dissection of the major cervical lymphatic vessels and lateral cervical space with preservation of nerves and vessels, including the sympathetic and vagus nerves, spinal accessory nerves, and internal jugular vein. Neck dissection with vocal cord cancer usually involves one side of the neck. However, if the lesion is midline, a bilateral neck dissection may be performed. When a bilateral neck dissection is performed, it is always modified on at least one side to minimize structural and functional deficits.

The patient may refuse surgical intervention for advanced lesions because of the extent of the procedure or may be judged to be at too great a medical risk to undergo the procedure. In this sit-

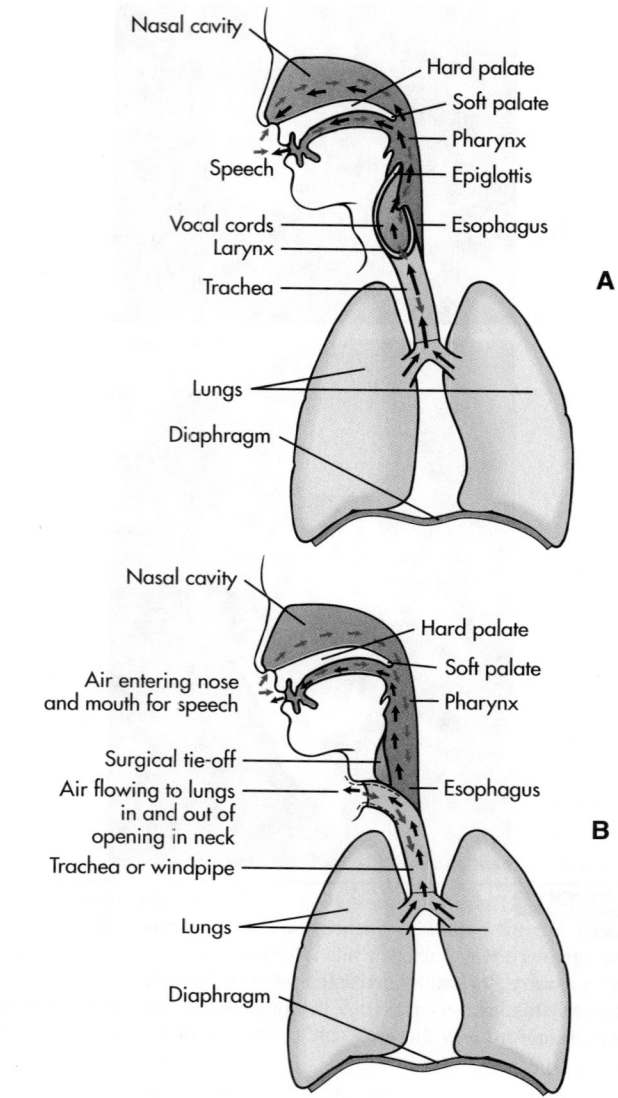

FIG. 26-13 A, Normal airflow in and out of the lungs. B, Airflow in and out of the lungs after total laryngectomy. Patients using esophageal speech trap air in the esophagus and release it to create sound.

uation, external radiation therapy may be used as the sole treatment or in combination with chemotherapy.

In addition, brachytherapy, a concentrated and localized method of delivering radiation that involves placing a radioactive source into or near the tumor, may be used to treat head and neck cancer. The goal is to deliver high doses of radiation to the target area while limiting exposure of surrounding tissues. Thin, hollow, plastic needles are inserted into the tumor area, and radioactive iridium seeds are placed in the needles. The seeds emit continuous radiation. Brachytherapy can be used alone or combined with external radiation or surgical intervention. (Radiation therapy and brachytherapy are discussed in Chapter 15.)

Nutritional Therapy. After radical neck surgery, the patient may be unable to take in nutrients through the normal route of ingestion because of swelling, the location of sutures, or difficulty with swallowing. Parenteral fluids will be given for the first 24 to 48 hours. Tube feedings are usually given via a nasogastric, nasointestinal, or gastrostomy tube that was placed during

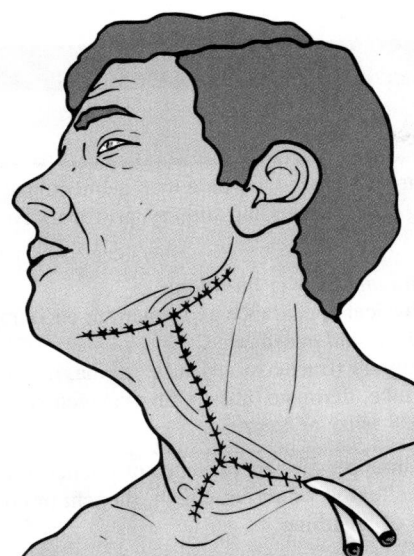

FIG. 26-14 Radical neck incision with suction tubing in place.

surgery. (Nasogastric and gastrostomy feedings are described in Chapter 39.) The nurse must observe for tolerance of the feedings and adjust the amount, time, and formula if nausea, vomiting, diarrhea, or distention occurs. The patient is instructed about the tube feedings. When the patient can swallow, small amounts of water are given. Close observation for choking is essential. Suctioning may be necessary to prevent aspiration.

Swallowing problems should be anticipated when the patient resumes eating. The type and degree of difficulty vary, depending on the procedure. When a supraglottic laryngectomy is performed, the surgeon excises the upper portion of the larynx, including the epiglottis and false vocal cords. The patient can speak because the true vocal cords remain intact. However, a new technique, the *supraglottic swallow*, must be learned to compensate for removal of the epiglottis and minimize risk of aspiration (Table 26-8). When learning this technique, it may be helpful to start with carbonated beverages because the effervescence provides cues about the liquid's position. With this exception, thin, watery fluids should be avoided because they are difficult to swallow and increase the risk of aspiration. A better choice is nonpourable pureed foods, which are thicker and allow more

control during swallowing. Swallowing can be enhanced by thickening liquids through the use of a commercially available thickening agent (Thick It).

Good nutrition is important during radiation therapy because calories and protein are needed for tissue repair. Antiemetics or analgesics may be given before meals to reduce nausea and mouth pain. Bland foods may be better tolerated. Caloric intake may be increased by adding dry milk to foods during preparation, selecting foods high in calories, and using oral supplements. It is helpful to add sauces and gravies to food, which adds calories and moistens food so it is more easily swallowed. If an adequate intake cannot be maintained, enteral feedings may be used. The patient should always be in a position with the head elevated.

NURSING MANAGEMENT HEAD AND NECK CANCER

■ Nursing Assessment

Subjective and objective data that should be obtained from a person with head and neck cancer are presented in Table 26-9.

■ Nursing Diagnoses

Nursing diagnoses for the patient with head and neck cancer include, but are not limited to, those presented in NCP 26-2.

TABLE 26-8	*Patient & Family Teaching Guide* **Steps for Performing the Supraglottic Swallow**

1. Take a deep breath to aerate lungs.
2. Perform Valsalva maneuver to approximate cords.
3. Place food in mouth and swallow. Some food will enter airway and remain on top of closed vocal cords.
4. Cough to remove food from top of vocal cords.
5. Swallow so food is moved from top of vocal cords.
6. Breathe after cough-swallow sequence to prevent aspiration of food collected on top of vocal cords.

TABLE 26-9	*Nursing Assessment* **Head and Neck Cancer**

Subjective Data
Important Health Information
Past health history: Positive family history; prolonged tobacco use (cigarettes, pipes, cigars, chewing tobacco, smokeless tobacco); prolonged, heavy alcohol use
Medications: Prolonged use of over-the-counter medication for sore throat, decongestants
Functional Health Patterns
Health perception–health management: Does not value preventive health measures, long history of alcohol and tobacco use
Nutritional-metabolic: Mouth ulcer that does not heal, change in fit of dentures, change in appetite, weight loss, swallowing difficulty (e.g., sensation of lump in throat, pain with swallowing, aspiration when swallowing)
Activity-exercise: Fatigue with minimal exertion
Cognitive-perceptual: Sore throat, pain on swallowing, referred ear pain

Objective Data
Respiratory
Hoarseness, change in voice quality, chronic laryngitis, nasal voice, palpable neck mass and lymph nodes (tender, hard, fixed), tracheal deviation; dyspnea, stridor (late sign)
Gastrointestinal
White (leukoplakia) or red (erythoplakia) patches inside mouth, ulceration of mucosa, asymmetric tongue, exudate in mouth or pharynx, mass or thickening of mucosa
Possible Findings
Mass on direct or indirect laryngoscopy; tumor on soft tissue x-ray, computed tomography (CT) scan, or magnetic resonance imaging (MRI); positive biopsy

NURSING CARE PLAN 26-2

Patient Having Total Laryngectomy and/or Radical Neck Surgery

EXPECTED PATIENT OUTCOMES	NURSING INTERVENTIONS and *RATIONALES*
NURSING DIAGNOSIS	**Anxiety** *related to* lack of knowledge regarding surgical procedure, pain management, and prevention of complications *as manifested by* questioning about impending surgery, postoperative care, agitation, and restlessness.
• Decrease in anxiety and a calm appearance • Verbalization of confidence regarding surgical therapy	• Assess knowledge desired by patient *to allay fears and answer questions.* • Facilitate discussion of expected alterations in physical appearance and function; encourage sharing of feelings and concerns *to begin adjustment and acceptance.* • Provide information about what to expect after surgery (tracheostomy tube, stoma, incisions, alternative communication methods, nasogastric tube, drainage tubes, pain management) *to reduce patient's sense of helplessness and increase sense of control.*
NURSING DIAGNOSIS	**Ineffective airway clearance** *related to* alteration in upper airway, presence of tracheostomy tube, difficulty expectorating sputum *as manifested by* ineffective or absent cough, rhonchi or coarse crackles on auscultation, abnormal rate and pattern of breathing.
• Patent airway • Normal respiratory rate and pattern	• Auscultate chest and monitor respiratory rate, pattern, SpO$_2$, and level of consciousness q4h for 24 hr postoperatively *to determine adequacy of respirations.* • Encourage coughing, deep breathing, and ambulation *to assist in mobilizing secretions.* • Suction tracheostomy tube/stoma as needed *to clear secretions.* • Administer humidified air or oxygen as prescribed into tracheostomy/stoma *to help keep secretions moist.* • Clean inner cannula of tracheostomy/laryngectomy tube three times daily and as needed *to prevent mucous crusting which may occlude the lumen.*
NURSING DIAGNOSIS	**Ineffective tissue perfusion** *related to* tissue edema and disruption of blood flow and lymphatic drainage *as manifested by* tissue swelling, serous drainage from wound drainage tubes.
• Decrease in tissue edema • Minimal to no drainage from tubes • Healing of incision lines	• Maintain head of bed at 30 to 40 degrees *to decrease tissue edema.* • Monitor heart rate, blood pressure, hemoglobin, and hematocrit *to detect excessive bleeding.* • Monitor patency of drainage tubes, amount, color of drainage *to determine if drainage is excessive.* • Clean incision as prescribed *to prevent infection.*
NURSING DIAGNOSIS	**Imbalanced nutrition: less than body requirements** *related to* surgical procedure, edema, and dysphagia *as manifested by* absence of or inadequate oral intake.
• Normal oral intake • Able to swallow • Maintenance of body weight	• Provide frequent oral hygiene with saline rinses or dilute hydrogen peroxide *to promote comfort and remove drainage.* • Administer tube feedings as ordered *to provide adequate nutrients while wound heals.* • When oral feedings begin, give clear liquids and advance as tolerated *to allow patient time to adjust to initiation of oral intake.* • Monitor caloric intake and weight *to evaluate response.*
NURSING DIAGNOSIS	**Impaired verbal communication** *related to* removal of vocal cords *as manifested by* inability to speak.
• Able to communicate clearly	• Evaluate the patient's ability to read and write. • Instruct in alternative methods of communication (magic slate, communication board, electrolarynx). • Encourage use of communication tools and allow adequate time for communication. • Consult with speech therapist *to learn use of voice prosthesis, electrolarynx, or esophageal speech.*

■ Planning

The overall goals are that the patient will have (1) a patent airway, (2) no spread of cancer, (3) no complications related to therapy, (4) adequate nutritional intake, (5) minimal to no pain, (6) the ability to communicate, and (7) an acceptable body image.

■ Nursing Implementation

Health Promotion. Development of head and neck cancer is closely related to personal habits, primarily tobacco use, including the use of cigarettes, cigars, chewing tobacco, and snuff. Snuff dipping, or the placement and retention of tobacco in the

NURSING CARE PLAN 26-2

Patient Having Total Laryngectomy and/or Radical Neck Surgery—cont'd

EXPECTED PATIENT OUTCOMES	NURSING INTERVENTIONS and *RATIONALES*
NURSING DIAGNOSIS	**Disturbed body image** *related to* disfiguring surgery and loss of speaking ability *as manifested by* withdrawal, depression, isolation, unwillingness to look at self or assist with care, and refusal to see visitors.
• Acknowledgement of changes in body image • Able to communicate feelings about surgical changes • Participation in self-care	• Assess patient's body image *to identify patients at high risk for impaired adjustment.* • Provide privacy *to respect patient's request while adjusting to change in body function and appearance.* • Encourage attention to personal hygiene *because improved appearance can boost self-esteem.* • Encourage socialization with family and friends *because acceptance by significant others is a critical factor in patient's own acceptance.* • Provide information about measures to help improve appearance such as wearing clothes with high collars and wearing accessories *to aid in successful adjustment.* • Answer questions honestly about changes in body image *to convey acceptance and to provide accurate information.* • Involve patient in self-care *because participation in self-care is a sign of successful adjustment.* • Assure patient of self-worth *to increase acceptance of altered physical appearance.*
NURSING DIAGNOSIS	**Acute pain** *related to* surgical procedure *as manifested by* report of discomfort; facial mask of pain; changes in blood pressure, pulse, and respiratory rate.
• Satisfactory pain control	• Assess patient's manifestations of pain (e.g., facial expression, reluctance to cough or move) *to plan appropriate interventions.* • Administer pain medication as prescribed and assess response *to determine if it is effective.* • Keep head of bed elevated 30 to 40 degrees *to prevent edema.*
NURSING DIAGNOSIS	**Ineffective therapeutic regimen management** *related to* lack of knowledge about home care after discharge *as manifested by* verbalized concern about ability to manage self-care at home.
• Demonstration of steps to be used in carrying out self-care	• Provide written instructions for patient and family *because an accurate reference reduces error.* • Teach patient and family about laryngectomy tube and stoma care, allowing them to perform care repeatedly in hospital, *to ensure correct performance of technique.* • Teach patient to cover stoma before performing activities such as shaving, application of makeup *to avoid inhalation of foreign materials.* • Teach patient to report changes, such as stoma narrowing, difficulty swallowing, lump in the throat, *to detect possible recurrence of tumor or tracheal stenosis.* • Teach patient to provide adequate humidity at home using a bedside humidifier or sitting in a steamy bathroom. • Teach patient to report changes in mucus production such as color changes (yellow or green) or blood-tinged secretions *because these may be signs of infection or tracheal irritation.* • Make referral for home health care visit *to evaluate self-care.*

cheek, is becoming more common among U.S. youth. Another popular fad is cigar smoking. Long-term snuff users and cigar smokers are at increased risk of oral cancer. Prolonged alcohol use has been implicated as a potentiating factor in head and neck cancer.

The nurse should include information about risk factors in health teaching. If cancer has been diagnosed, tobacco cessation is still important. The patient with head and neck cancer who continues to smoke during radiation therapy has a lower rate of response and survival than the patient who does not smoke during radiation therapy. Additionally, risk of a second primary cancer is significantly increased in patients who continue to smoke.

Acute Intervention. The patient and the family must be taught about the type of therapy to be performed and care re-

quired. Assessment of concerns is integral to the plan of care. The patient and family must deal with the psychologic impact of the diagnosis of cancer, alteration of physical appearance, and possible need for altered methods of communication. The care plan should include assessment of the patient's support system. The patient may not have someone to provide assistance after discharge, may not be employed, or may be employed in a job that cannot be continued.

Radiation therapy. The nurse can suggest interventions to reduce side effects of radiation therapy. Dry mouth (*xerostomia*), the most frequent and annoying problem, typically begins within a few weeks of treatment. The patient's saliva decreases in volume and becomes thick. The change may be temporary or permanent. Pilocarpine hydrochloride (Salagen) can be effective in increasing saliva production and should be started before the initiation of radiation therapy and continued for 90 days. Symptom relief can also be obtained by increasing fluid intake, chewing sugarless gum or sugarless candy, using nonalcoholic mouth rinses (baking soda or glycerin solutions), and using artificial saliva.

The patient may also complain of stomatitis, especially if the oral cavity is in the field of therapy. Irritation, ulceration, and pain are common complaints. Rinses of water and hydrogen peroxide (3:1 ratio) or baking soda and water (1 tsp baking soda to 8 oz water) can be used to clean and soothe irritated tissues. Commercial mouthwashes and hot or spicy foods should be avoided because they are irritating. If the problem is severe, a mixture of equal parts of antacid, diphenhydramine (Benadryl), and topical lidocaine can be used.

Skin over the irradiated area often becomes reddened and sensitive to touch. It is common for patients to require a break from their scheduled radiation program because of altered skin integrity. All exposure to the sun should be avoided to reduce discomfort.

Surgical therapy. Preoperative care for the patient who is to have a radical neck dissection involves consideration of the patient's physical and psychosocial needs. Physical preparation is the same as for any major surgery, with special emphasis on oral hygiene. Explanations and emotional support are of special significance and should include postoperative measures relating to communication and feeding. The surgical procedure should be explained to the patient and family, and the nurse should make sure that the information is understood.

Teaching must be tailored to the planned surgical procedure. For surgeries that involve a laryngectomy, teaching should include information about expected changes in speech. The nurse or speech pathologist should demonstrate means of communicating other than speaking that can be used temporarily or permanently. This may include some type of communication board.

After surgery, maintenance of a patent airway is essential. The inflammation in the surgical area may compress the trachea. A tracheostomy tube will be in place. The patient will be placed in a semi-Fowler's position to decrease edema and limit tension on the suture lines. Vital signs should be monitored frequently because of the risk of hemorrhage and respiratory compromise. Pressure dressings, packing, or drainage tubes (Hemovac, Jackson Pratt) may be used for wound management, depending on the type of surgical procedure. When a radical neck dissection is performed, wound suction using a portable system, such as a Hemovac, is usually used. If skin flaps are employed, dressings are typically not used. This allows better visualization of the incision and avoids excessive pressure on tissue (see Fig. 26-14). The drainage should be serosanguineous and gradually decrease in volume over 24 hours. Patency of drainage tubes should be monitored every 4 hours to ensure that they are properly removing serous drainage and for the amount and character of drainage. If the tubing becomes obstructed, fluid will accumulate under the skin flap and predispose to impaired wound healing and infection. After drainage tubes are removed, the area should be closely monitored to detect any swelling. If fluid continues to accumulate, aspiration may be necessary.

Immediately after surgery, the patient with a laryngectomy requires frequent suctioning via the laryngectomy tube. Secretions typically change in amount and consistency over time. The patient may initially have copious blood-tinged secretions that diminish and thicken. If the patient develops mucous plugs or thick secretions, a 3 to 5 ml bolus of normal saline may be instilled into the airway to loosen secretions enough to clear the airway either through coughing or suctioning. However, this practice is no longer recommended by many respiratory departments. The patient will benefit from the use of a humidifier while hospitalized and at home.

Following a neck dissection, an exercise program should be instituted to maintain strength and movement in the affected shoulder and neck. This is especially important when the spinal accessory nerve and sternocleidomastoid muscles are removed or damaged. Without exercise, the patient will be left with a "frozen" shoulder and limited range of neck motion. This exercise program should be continued following discharge to prevent future functional disabilities. The patient may need support of the neck to move the head after surgery.

Voice rehabilitation. A speech therapist should meet with the patient following a total laryngectomy to discuss voice restoration options. The International Association of Laryngectomees, an association of laryngectomy patients, focuses on assisting patients to reestablish speech. Local groups, called Lost Cord Clubs, often provide member volunteers to visit the patient, preferably preoperatively. Several options are available to restore speech. These include use of a voice prosthesis, esophageal speech, and an electrolarynx.

The most commonly used voice prosthesis is the Blom-Singer prosthesis (Fig. 26-15). This soft plastic device is inserted into a fistula made between the esophagus and the trachea. The puncture may be created at the time of surgery or afterward, depending on the preference of the surgeon. A red rubber catheter is placed in the tracheoesophageal puncture and must remain intact until a tract is formed. Once the tract is formed, the speech prosthesis is inserted. This prosthesis allows air from the lungs to en-

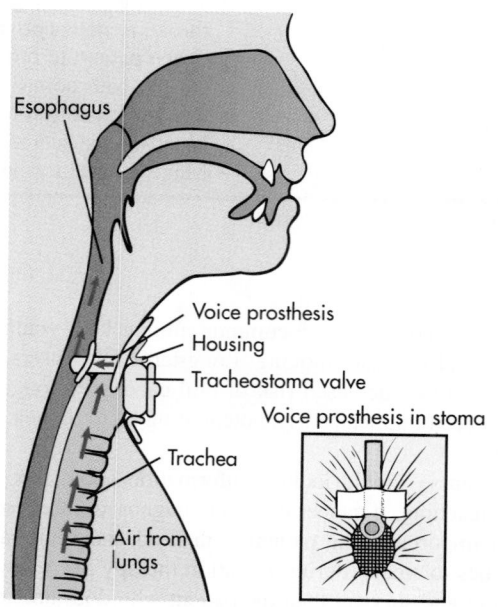

FIG. 26-15 Blom-Singer voice prosthesis and tracheostoma valve. With this prosthesis and valve, patients with a laryngectomy can speak normally. *Inset* shows laryngectomy stoma and voice prosthesis with tracheostoma valve removed.

ter the esophagus by way of the tracheal stoma. A one-way valve prevents aspiration of food or saliva from the esophagus into the tracheostomy. To speak, the patient manually blocks the stoma with the finger. Air moves from the lungs, through the prosthesis, into the esophagus, and out the mouth. Speech is produced by the air vibrating against the esophagus and is formed into words by moving the tongue and lips. A valve may also be used with this device. When the valve is in place, the stoma does not need to be closed with the finger to speak. The prosthesis must be cleaned regularly and replaced when it becomes blocked with mucus.

An electrolarynx is a handheld, battery-powered device that creates speech with the use of sound waves. One device, the Cooper-Rand, uses a plastic tube placed in the corner of the roof of the mouth to create vibrations. To create the most normal sound when using this device, the patient should (1) avoid trying to use the tongue to hold the tube in place; (2) compress the tone generator for short intervals and speak in phrases, rather than full sentences; (3) speak using large movements of the lips, tongue, and jaw, rather than keeping the mouth partially closed; (4) talk face-to-face with the listener; and (5) practice because development of skill takes time.

An artificial larynx is placed against the neck rather than in the mouth. This device is used after surgical healing is complete and there is no edema remaining (Fig. 26-16). With experience the patient can learn to move the lips in ways that create normal-sounding speech. With both devices, voice pitch is low, and the sound is mechanical.

Esophageal speech is a method of swallowing air, trapping it in the esophagus, and releasing it to create sound. The air causes vibration of the pharyngoesophageal segment and sound (which initially is similar to a belch). With practice 50% of patients develop some speech skills, but only 10% develop fluent speech.

Stoma care. Before discharge the patient should be instructed in the care of the laryngectomy stoma. The area around the stoma should be washed daily with a moist cloth. If a laryngectomy tube is in place, the entire tube must be removed at least daily and cleaned in the same manner as a tracheostomy tube. The inner cannula may need to be removed and cleaned more frequently. A scarf, a loose shirt, or a crocheted shield can be used to shield the stoma.

The patient should cover the stoma when coughing (because mucus may be expectorated) and during any activity (e.g., shaving, applying makeup) that might lead to inhalation of foreign materials. Because water can easily enter the stoma, the patient should wear a plastic collar when taking a shower. Swimming is contraindicated. Initially, humidification will be administered via a tracheostomy mask. After discharge, a bedside humidifier can be used. A high oral fluid intake must be maintained, especially in dry weather.

The patient should be told the importance of wearing a Medic Alert bracelet or other identification that alerts others in an emergency situation of the use of neck breathing (Fig. 26-17). Because the patient no longer breathes through the nose, the ability to smell smoke and food may be lost. Advise the patient to install smoke and carbon monoxide detectors in the home. It is important for food to be colorful, attractively prepared, and nutritious, because taste may also be diminished secondary to the loss of smell, as well as radiation therapy.

Depression. Depression is common in the patient who has had a radical neck dissection. The patient may not be able to speak because of the laryngectomy and cannot control saliva. The neck and shoulders may be numb because of the transected nerves. The facial appearance may be significantly altered, with swelling, edema, and deformities. The patient must understand that many of the physical changes are reversible as the edema subsides and the tracheostomy tube is removed. Depression may also be related to concern about the prognosis. The nurse can help the patient through the depression by allowing verbalization of feelings, conveying acceptance, and helping the patient regain an acceptable self-concept. Sometimes it is appropriate to obtain a psychiatric referral for the patient who is experiencing prolonged or severe depression.[22]

Sexuality. Surgery and the presence of foreign attachments such as tracheostomy and gastrostomy tubes may affect body

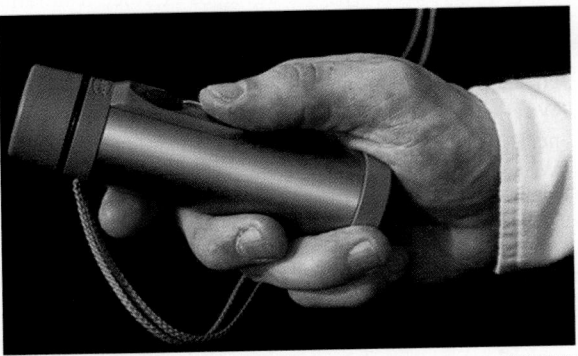

FIG. 26-16   Artificial larynx. Battery-powered electronic artificial larynx for patient who has total laryngectomy.

TOTAL NECK BREATHER

(Front of Card)   (Back of All Cards)

EMERGENCY!

I am a Total Neck Breather
(Laryngectomee–No Vocal Cords)

I breathe ONLY through an opening in my neck, NOT through my nose or mouth.

If I have stopped breathing:
1. Expose my entire neck.

2. Give me **mouth to neck breathing only.**

3. Keep my head straight—chin up.

4. Keep neck opening clear with clean CLOTH (not tissue).

5. Use oxygen supply to neck opening ONLY, when I start to breathe again.

BE PROMPT–SECONDS COUNT I NEED AIR NOW!

Medical Problems
☐ Epilepsy   ☐ Glaucoma
☐ Diabetes   ☐ Peptic Ulcer
☐ Other _____
Medicines Taken Regularly
☐ Anticoagulants ☐ Cortisone or
☐ Heart drugs   ACTH
(Name and dose)
☐ Other _____
Dangerous Allergies
☐ Drugs (Name)
☐ Penicillin
☐ Other _____
Other Information
☐ Hard of hearing
☐ Speaks No English (Other)
☐ Wearing Contact Lenses
☐ Other _____
NAME _____
ADDRESS _____
PLEASE NOTIFY:
NAME _____
PHONE _____
ADDRESS _____
CITY _____
OR
NAME _____
PHONE _____
ADDRESS _____
INTERNATIONAL ASSOCIATION OF LARYNGECTOMEES

FIG. 26-17   Emergency identification of a neck breather.

image dramatically. The patient may feel less desirable sexually. The nurse can assist the patient by allowing discussions regarding sexuality and encouraging the patient to discuss this problem with the sexual partner. It may be difficult for the patient to orally discuss sexual problems because of the alteration in communication. The nurse can allow the patient to plan how to communicate with the sexual partner and offer support and guidance to the sexual partner. Helping the patient see that sexuality involves much more than appearance may relieve some anxiety.[23]

Ambulatory and Home Care. The patient is often discharged with a tracheostomy and a nasogastric or gastrostomy feeding tube. Home health care may need to be provided initially to evaluate the family's or the patient's ability to perform self-care activities. The patient and the family must be taught how to manage tubes and who to call if there are problems.

The patient can resume exercise, recreation, and sexual activity when able. Most patients can return to work 1 to 2 months after surgery. However, many never return to full-time employment. The changes that follow a total laryngectomy can be upsetting. Loss of speech, loss of the ability to taste and smell, inability to produce audible sounds (including laughing and weeping), and the presence of a permanent tracheal stoma that produces undesirable mucus are often overwhelming to the patient. Although changes are discussed before surgery, the patient may not be prepared for the extent of these changes. If the patient has a significant other, the reaction of this person to the patient's altered appearance is important. Acceptance by another person can promote an improved self-image. Encouraging the patient to participate in self-care is another important part of rehabilitation.

Reconstructive surgery may be performed at the time of the initial surgery or soon after the tumor is removed. Various types of flaps and grafts are used. It may be necessary to rebuild the nose or the mandible or to close oral cutaneous openings. Prosthetic materials, such as Silastic and Plastigel (which is soft), are often used to reconstruct various deformities.

Despite the use of surgical interventions and radiation therapy, the cure rate is disappointingly low for advanced head and neck cancer. Metastatic cancer is often painful, leaving the affected person in a severely debilitated state. If pain is a problem, a pain control regimen should be identified to provide comfort, and referral should be made to a hospice if indicated.

■ Evaluation

Expected outcomes for the patient with head and neck cancer who is treated surgically are addressed in NCP 26-2.

CRITICAL THINKING EXERCISES

Case Study
Laryngeal Cancer
Patient Profile. Mr. Carlson, a 60-year-old white man, was admitted for evaluation of mild pain on swallowing and a persistent sore throat over the past year.

Subjective Data
- States that his symptoms worsened in the last 2 months
- Has used various cold remedies to relieve symptoms without relief
- Has lost weight because of decrease in appetite and difficulty swallowing
- Has smoked 3 packs of cigarettes a day for 40 years
- Consumes 6 cans of beer a day

Objective Data
Laryngoscopy
- Subglottic mass

Physical Examination
- Enlarged cervical nodes

Computed Tomography Scan
- Subglottic lesion with lymph node involvement

Collaborative Care
- Total laryngectomy with tracheostomy with inflated cuff
- Nasogastric tube

CRITICAL THINKING QUESTIONS
1. What information in the assessment suggests that Mr. Carlson might be at risk for cancer of the larynx?
2. What diagnostic tests are typically performed to evaluate the extent of this problem?
3. What teaching should the nurse plan for Mr. Carlson before and after laryngectomy?
4. Discuss methods used to restore speech after laryngectomy.
5. What teaching is required to assist this patient to assume self-care after his surgery? What precautions should the patient take because of his stoma?
6. Based on the assessment data presented, write one or more nursing diagnoses. Are there any collaborative problems?

Nursing Research Issues
1. What are the effects of sleep apnea on functional ability and overall quality of life?
2. After a laryngectomy, what methods of voice restoration provide the most satisfaction for the patient?
3. What are the most effective ways for a patient with a tracheostomy to communicate?
4. What is the quality of life of patients following a radical neck dissection?
5. What factors are most likely to promote compliance with CPAP therapy?

REVIEW QUESTIONS

The number of the question corresponds to the same-numbered objective at the beginning of the chapter.

1. A patient was seen in the clinic for an episode of epistaxis, which was controlled by placement of anterior nasal packing. During discharge teaching, the nurse instructs the patient to
   a. use aspirin for pain relief.
   b. remove the packing later that day.
   c. skip the next dose of antihypertensive medication.
   d. avoid vigorous nose blowing and strenuous activity.

2. A patient with allergic rhinitis reports severe nasal congestion, sneezing, and watery, itchy eyes and nose at various times of the year. To teach the patient to control these symptoms, the nurse advises the patient to
   a. avoid all intranasal sprays and oral antihistamines.
   b. limit the duration of use of nasal decongestant spray to 10 days.
   c. use oral decongestants at bedtime to prevent symptoms during the night.
   d. keep a diary of when the allergic reaction occurs and what precipitates it.

3. A patient with sleep apnea would like to avoid using a nasal CPAP device, if possible. To help him reach this goal the nurse suggests that he
   a. lose excess weight.
   b. take a nap during the day.
   c. eat a high-protein snack at bedtime.
   d. use mild sedatives or alcohol at bedtime.

4. A type of tracheostomy tube that prevents speech is
   a. a cuffless tracheostomy tube.
   b. a fenestrated tracheostomy tube.
   c. a tube with an inflated foam cuff.
   d. a cuffed tube with the cuff deflated.

5. To prevent excessive pressure on tracheal capillaries, pressure in the cuff on a tracheostomy tube should be
   a. monitored every 2 to 3 days.
   b. less than 20 mm Hg or 25 cm H_2O.
   c. less than 30 mm Hg or 35 cm H_2O.
   d. sufficient to fill the pilot balloon until it is tense.

6. Which of the following is not an early symptom of head and neck cancer?
   a. hoarseness
   b. change in fit of dentures
   c. mouth ulcers that do not heal
   d. decreased mobility of the tongue

7. Nursing management of the patient immediately after a total laryngectomy includes all of the following except
   a. changing the surgical dressing.
   b. monitoring function of the drainage tubes.
   c. ensuring that the nasogastric tube is patent.
   d. placing the patient in semi-Fowler's position.

8. When using a voice prosthesis, the patient
   a. places a vibrating device in the mouth.
   b. places a speaking valve over the stoma.
   c. blocks the stoma entrance with a finger.
   d. swallows air using Valsalva maneuver.

REFERENCES

1. Alvarez H et al: Sequelae after nasal septum injuries in children, *Auris Nasus Larynx* 27:339, 2000.
2. Rohrich RJ, Adams WP: Nasal fracture management: minimizing secondary nasal deformities, *Plast Reconstr Surg* 106:266, 2000.
3. Woodson GE: *Ear, nose and throat disorders in primary care,* Philadelphia, 2001, WB Saunders.
4. Lagnese MS, Kelsen SG: Allergic rhinitis: practical clues to diagnosis and treatment, *Hosp Med* 35:32, 1999.
5. Valley J, Blue CL: Influenza: overview and recommendations for control, *Topics in Advanced Practice Nursing eJournal* vol 2, 2002. Available at http://www.medscape.com/viewarticle/421478 (accessed 10/28/02).
6. Couch RB: Drug therapy: prevention and treatment of influenza, *N Engl J Med* 343:1778, 2000.
7. Fleming D: Influenza in the elderly, *Ann Long-Term Care* 10:23, 2002.
8. Klein L: Sinusitis: when to treat and how, *RN* 64:42, 2001.
9. Slavin RG: Sinusitis: answers to key questions, *Consultant* 37:745, 1997.
10. Attarian HP, Sabri AN: When to suspect obstructive sleep apnea syndrome, *Postgrad Med* 111:70, 2002.
11. Yantis MA: Obstructive sleep apnea syndrome, *Am J Nurs* 102:83, 2002.
12. Bradley TD, Flores JSL: *Sleep apnea implication in cardiovascular and cerebrovascular disease,* New York, 1999, Marcel Dekker.
13. Masa JF et al: Habitually sleepy drivers have a high frequency of automobile crashes associated with respiratory disorders during sleep, *Am J Respir Crit Care Med* 162:1407, 2000.
*14. Smith CE et al: Continuous positive airway pressure: patients' and caregivers' learning needs and barriers to use, *Heart Lung* 27:99, 1998.
15. Thelan LA et al: *Critical care nursing: diagnosis and management,* ed 4, St Louis, 2002, Mosby.
16. Seay SJ, Gray SL, Strauss M: Trachestomy emergencies, *Am J Nurs* 102:59, 2002.
17. McConnell EA: Suctioning a tracheostomy tube, *Nursing* 30:80, 2000.
18. McConnell EA: Providing tracheostomy care, *Nursing* 32:17, 2002.
19. Kidd PS, Wagner KD: *High acuity nursing,* ed 3, Upper Saddle River, NJ, 2001, Prentice-Hall.
20. Schreiber D: Trach care at home: a how-to guide, *RN* 64:43, 2001.
21. Forastiere A et al: Head and neck cancer, *N Engl J Med* 345:1890, 2001.
*22. Clarke C, Cooper C: Psychological rehabilitation after disfiguring injury or disease: investigating the training needs of specialist nurses, *J Adv Nurs* 34:18, 2001.
*23. Schneider SM et al: Outcome of patients treated with home enteral nutrition, *Journal of Parenteral and Enteral Nutrition* 25:203, 2001.

*Nursing research–based articles.

RESOURCES

American Academy of Sleep Medicine
One Westbrook Corporate Center, Suite 920
Westchester, IL 60154
708-492-0930
Fax: 708-492-0943
www.asda.org

American Sleep Apnea Association
www.sleepapnea.org

International Association of Laryngectomees
8900 Thornton Road, Box 99311
Stockton, CA 95209
866-IAL-FORU (425-3678)
Fax: 209 472-0516
www.larynxlink.com

National Sleep Foundation
1522 K Street NW, Suite 500
Washington, DC 20005
202-347-3471
Fax: 202-347-3472
www.sleepfoundation.org

For additional Internet resources, see the website for this book at *http://evolve.elsevier.com/Lewis/medsurg/.*

CHAPTER 27

NURSING MANAGEMENT
Lower Respiratory Problems

Janet T. Crimlisk

LEARNING OBJECTIVES

1. Describe the pathophysiology, types, clinical manifestations, and collaborative care of pneumonia.
2. Explain the nursing management of the patient with pneumonia.
3. Describe the pathogenesis, classification, clinical manifestations, complications, diagnostic abnormalities, and nursing and collaborative management of tuberculosis.
4. Identify the causes, clinical manifestations, and nursing and collaborative management of pulmonary fungal infections.
5. Explain the pathophysiology, clinical manifestations, and nursing and collaborative management of bronchiectasis and lung abscess.
6. Identify the causative factors, clinical features, and management of environmental lung diseases.
7. Describe the causes, risk factors, pathogenesis, clinical manifestations, and nursing and collaborative management of lung cancer.
8. Identify the mechanisms involved and the clinical manifestations of pneumothorax, fractured ribs, and flail chest.
9. Describe the purpose, methods, and nursing responsibilities related to chest tubes.
10. Explain the types of chest surgery and appropriate preoperative and postoperative care.
11. Compare and contrast extrapulmonary and intrapulmonary restrictive lung disorders in terms of causes, clinical manifestations, and collaborative management.
12. Describe the pathophysiology, clinical manifestations, and management of pulmonary hypertension and cor pulmonale.
13. Discuss the use of lung transplantation as a treatment for pulmonary disorders.

KEY TERMS

acute bronchitis, p. 592	pleural effusion, p. 627
atelectasis, p. 630	pleurisy (pleuritis), p. 629
bronchiectasis, p. 608	pneumoconiosis, p. 611
chylothorax, p. 621	pneumonia, p. 593
community-acquired pneumonia, p. 593	pneumothorax, p. 620
cor pulmonale, p. 632	pulmonary edema, p. 630
empiric therapy, p. 597	pulmonary embolism, p. 630
empyema, p. 628	pulmonary hypertension, p. 631
flail chest, p. 621	tension pneumothorax, p. 621
hemothorax, p. 621	thoracentesis, p. 628
hospital-acquired pneumonia, p. 594	thoracotomy, p. 626
lung abscess, p. 610	tuberculosis, p. 601

A wide variety of problems affect the lower respiratory system. Lung diseases that are characterized primarily by an obstructive disorder, such as asthma, emphysema, chronic bronchitis, and cystic fibrosis, are discussed in Chapter 28. All other lower respiratory problems are discussed in this chapter.

Respiratory tract infections are common. Lower respiratory tract infections are the most common cause of death in the world. Chronic lower respiratory disease is the fourth leading cause of death in the United States, and pneumonia ranks as the sixth leading cause of death despite the availability of antimicrobial agents.[1]

Tuberculosis, although potentially curable and preventable, is a worldwide public health threat of epidemic proportion.

ACUTE BRONCHITIS

Acute bronchitis is an inflammation of the bronchi in the lower respiratory tract usually due to infection. It is one of the most common conditions seen in primary care. It usually occurs as a sequela to an upper respiratory tract infection. A type of acute bronchitis is acute exacerbation of chronic bronchitis (AECB). AECB represents acute infection superimposed on chronic bronchitis. AECB is a potentially serious condition that may lead to respiratory failure. (Chronic bronchitis is discussed in Chapter 28.)

The cause of most cases of acute bronchitis is viral (rhinovirus, influenza). However, bacterial causes are also common both in smokers (e.g., *Streptococcus pneumoniae, Haemophilus influenzae*) and nonsmokers (e.g., *Mycoplasma pneumoniae, Chlamydia pneumoniae*).

In acute bronchitis, persistent cough following an acute upper airway infection (e.g., rhinitis, pharyngitis) is the most common symptom. Cough is often accompanied by production of clear, mucoid sputum, although some patients produce purulent sputum. Associated symptoms include fever, headache, malaise, and shortness of breath on exertion. Physical examination may reveal mildly elevated temperature, pulse, and respiratory rate with either normal breath sounds or rhonchi and expiratory wheezing. Chest x-rays can differentiate acute bronchitis from pneumonia because there is no evidence of consolidation or infiltrates on x-ray with bronchitis.

Acute bronchitis is usually self-limiting and the treatment is generally supportive, including fluids, rest, and antiinflammatory agents. Cough suppressants or bronchodilators may be prescribed for symptomatic treatment of nocturnal cough or wheezing.

Reviewed by Patricia Cryer, RN, MS, MSN, CENP, Instructor, Associate Degree Nursing Program, Tyler Junior College, Tyler, Tex.

Antibiotics are generally not prescribed unless the person has a prolonged infection associated with constitutional symptoms, or if the person is a smoker or has chronic obstructive pulmonary disease (COPD).[2,3]

The patient with AECB is usually treated empirically with broad-spectrum antibiotics. Often the patient with COPD is taught to recognize symptoms of acute bronchitis and to begin a course of antibiotics when symptoms occur. Many health care providers believe that a more severe infection often results if the patient delays taking antibiotics until after a clinical examination. Early initiation of antibiotic treatment in COPD patients has resulted in a decrease in relapses and a decrease in hospital admissions.[4]

PNEUMONIA

Pneumonia is an acute inflammation of the lung parenchyma caused by a microbial agent. Until 1936 pneumonia was the leading cause of death in the United States. The discovery of sulfa drugs and penicillin was pivotal in the treatment of pneumonia. Since that time there has been remarkable progress in the development of antibiotics to treat pneumonia. However, despite the new antimicrobial agents, pneumonia is still common and is associated with significant morbidity and mortality rates. Pneumonia is the leading cause of death from an infectious disease in the United States.[1]

Etiology

Normal Defense Mechanisms. Normally, the airway distal to the larynx is sterile because of protective defense mechanisms. These mechanisms include the following: filtration of air, warming and humidification of inspired air, epiglottis closure over the trachea, cough reflex, mucociliary escalator mechanism, secretion of immunoglobulin A, and alveolar macrophages (see Chapter 25).

Factors Predisposing to Pneumonia. Pneumonia is more likely to result when defense mechanisms become incompetent or are overwhelmed by the virulence or quantity of infectious agents. Decreased consciousness depresses the cough and epiglottal reflexes, which may allow aspiration of oropharyngeal contents into the lungs. Tracheal intubation interferes with the normal cough reflex and the mucociliary escalator mechanism. It also bypasses the upper airways in which filtration and humidification of air normally take place. The mucociliary escalator mechanism is impaired by air pollution, cigarette smoking, viral upper respiratory infections (URIs), and normal changes of aging. In cases of malnutrition the functions of lymphocytes and polymorphonuclear leukocytes are altered. Certain diseases such as leukemia, alcoholism, and diabetes mellitus are associated with an increased frequency of gram-negative bacilli in the oropharynx. (Gram-negative bacilli are not normal flora in the respiratory tract.) Altered oropharyngeal flora can also occur secondary to antibiotic therapy given for an infection elsewhere in the body. The factors predisposing to pneumonia are listed in Table 27-1.

Acquisition of Organisms. Organisms that cause pneumonia reach the lung by three methods:

1. *Aspiration* from the nasopharynx or oropharynx. Many of the organisms that cause pneumonia are normal inhabitants of the pharynx in healthy adults.
2. *Inhalation* of microbes present in the air. Examples include *Mycoplasma pneumoniae* and fungal pneumonias.
3. *Hematogenous spread* from a primary infection elsewhere in the body. An example is *Staphylococcus aureus*.

TABLE 27-1 Factors Predisposing to Pneumonia

- Aging
- Air pollution
- Altered consciousness: alcoholism, head injury, seizures, anesthesia, drug overdose, stroke
- Altered oropharyngeal flora
- Bed rest and prolonged immobility
- Chronic diseases: chronic lung disease, diabetes mellitus, heart disease, cancer, end-stage renal disease
- Debilitating illness
- Human immunodeficiency virus (HIV) infection
- Immunosuppressive drugs (corticosteroids, cancer chemotherapy, immunosuppressive therapy after organ transplant)
- Inhalation or aspiration of noxious substances
- Intestinal and gastric feedings
- Malnutrition
- Smoking
- Tracheal intubation (endotracheal intubation, tracheostomy)
- Upper respiratory tract infection

Types of Pneumonia

Pneumonia can be caused by bacteria, viruses, *Mycoplasma*, fungi, parasites, and chemicals. Although pneumonia can be classified according to the causative organism, a clinically effective way is to classify pneumonia as community-acquired or hospital-acquired pneumonia. Classifying pneumonia is important because of differences in the likely causative organisms and the selection of appropriate antibiotics (Table 27-2).

Community-Acquired Pneumonia. **Community-acquired pneumonia** (CAP) is defined as a lower respiratory tract infection of the lung parenchyma with onset in the community or during the first 2 days of hospitalization. The incidence in the United States is increasing; 6.5 million adults develop CAP annually, 1.5 million of whom are eventually hospitalized. Every year almost 90,000 people die because of pneumonia, making it the sixth leading cause of

TABLE 27-2 Organisms Associated with Pneumonia

COMMUNITY-ACQUIRED PNEUMONIA	HOSPITAL-ACQUIRED PNEUMONIA
*Streptococcus pneumoniae**	*Pseudomonas aeruginosa*
Mycoplasma pneumoniae	*Enterobacter*
Haemophilus influenzae	*Escherichia coli*
Respiratory viruses	*Proteus*
Chlamydia pneumoniae	*Klebsiella*
Legionella pneumophila	*Staphylococcus aureus*
Oral anaerobes	*Streptococcus pneumoniae*
Moraxella catarrhalis	Oral anaerobes
Staphylococcus aureus	
Nocardia	
Enteric aerobic gram-negative bacteria (e.g., *Klebsiella*)	
Fungi	
Mycobacterium tuberculosis	

*Most common cause of community-acquired pneumonia (CAP).

death in the United States.[5] The incidence of CAP is highest in the winter months. Smoking is an important risk factor. The causative organism in CAP is identified only 50% of the time. Organisms that are commonly implicated in CAP include *S. pneumoniae* and atypical organisms (e.g., *Legionella, Mycoplasma, Chlamydia,* viral) (see Table 27-2). The American Thoracic Society (ATS) guidelines classify patients with CAP into four categories based on place of therapy, presence of cardiopulmonary disease, and presence of modifying factors.

Category 1: Outpatients with no history of cardiopulmonary disease, no modifying factors

Category 2: Outpatients with cardiopulmonary disease and/or modifying factors

Category 3: Inpatients, not admitted to intensive care unit (ICU)

Category 4: ICU-admitted patients

Modifying risk factors include age greater than 65 years, alcoholism, multiple medical comorbidities, and immunosuppressive disease[6] (Table 27-3). The Infectious Diseases Society of America (IDSA) guidelines on CAP identify CAP classifications as outpatient versus hospitalized and identify empiric treatment of CAP; they also recommend medical management based on the isolated pathogen.[7]

Hospital-Acquired Pneumonia. **Hospital-acquired pneumonia** (HAP) is pneumonia occurring 48 hours or longer after hospital admission and not incubating at the time of hospitalization.[7] HAP is estimated to occur at a rate of 5 to 10 cases per 1000 hos-

TABLE 27-3   Drug Therapy

Patient Categories and Treatment for Community-Acquired Pneumonia

	SEVERITY OF ILLNESS			
	CATEGORY 1 **MILD TO MODERATE**	**CATEGORY 2** **MILD TO MODERATE**	**CATEGORY 3** **MODERATELY SEVERE**	**CATEGORY 4** **SEVERE**
Hospitalization	No	No	Yes, not ICU	ICU
Cardiopulmonary disease	No	Yes	Yes or no	
Modifying factors	No	Yes	Yes or no	
Risk for *Pseudomonas*				Yes and no
Antibiotic therapy	Advanced generation macrolide (azithromycin [Zithromax], clarithromycin [Biaxin]) *or* doxycycline	β-lactam* *plus* macrolide or doxycycline *or* antipseudomonal fluoroquinolone[†] (used alone)	*If cardiopulmonary disease and +/− modifying factors:* IV β-lactam[‡] *plus* IV or oral macrolide or doxycycline *or* IV antipseudomonal fluoroquinolone alone *If no cardiopulmonary disease, no modifying factors:* IV azithromycin alone *or* Monotherapy with antipseudomonal fluoroquinolone	*No risk for* P. aeruginosa: IV β-lactam (cefotaxime, ceftriaxone) *plus either* IV macrolide (azithromycin) *or* IV fluoroquinolone *Risk for* P. aeruginosa: IV antipseudomonal β-lactam[§] *plus* IV antipseudomonal fluoroquinolone (ciprofloxacin) *or* selected IV antipseudomonal β-lactam[§] *plus* IV aminoglycoside *plus either* IV macrolide (azithromycin) *or* IV nonpseudomonal fluoroquinolone

Source: American Thoracic Society (ATS), 2001.

*Oral cefpodoxime (Vantin), cefuroxime (Ceftin), high–dose amoxicillin, amoxicillin/clavulanate (Augmentin); or parenteral ceftriaxone (Rocephin) followed by oral cefpodoxime.

[†]Antipseudomonal fluoroquinolones include ciprofloxacin (Cipro), levofloxacin (Levaquin), sparfloxacin (Zagam), gatifloxacin (Tequin), moxifloxacin (Avelox).

[‡]Cefotaxime (Claforan), ceftriaxone, amoxicillin/sulbactam, high–dose ampicillin.

[§]Cefepime (Maxipime), imipenem (Primaxin), meropenem (Merrem), piperacillin/tazobactam (Zosyn).

ICU, Intensive care unit; *IV,* intravenous.

pital admissions, with the rate increasing by 6 to 20 times in patients requiring mechanical ventilation. Pneumonia has the highest morbidity and mortality rates of any nosocomial infection.[8] The microorganisms responsible for HAP are different from those organisms implicated in CAP (see Table 27-2). Bacteria are responsible for the majority of HAP infections, including *Pseudomonas, Enterobacter, S. aureus,* and *S. pneumoniae.* Many of the organisms causing HAP enter the lungs after aspiration of particles from the patient's own pharynx. Immunosuppressive therapy, general debility, and endotracheal intubation may be predisposing factors. Contaminated respiratory therapy equipment is another source of infection. Patients with HAP are classified into three groups based on (1) severity of the patient's illness, (2) whether specific host or therapeutic factors predisposing to specific pathogens are present, and (3) whether the pneumonia is of early (less than 5 days after admission) or late (more than 5 days after admission) onset.[8] The three groups are as follows (Table 27-4):

Group 1: Patients without unusual risk factors who have mild to moderate HAP with onset at any time during hospitalization or severe HAP of early onset

Group 2: Patients with specific risk factors who have mild to moderate HAP occurring any time during hospitalization

Group 3: Patients with severe HAP either of early onset with specific risk factors or of late onset

Fungal Pneumonia. Fungi may also be a cause of pneumonia (see section on pulmonary fungal infections).

Aspiration Pneumonia. *Aspiration pneumonia* refers to the sequelae occurring from abnormal entry of secretions or substances into the lower airway. It usually follows aspiration of material from the mouth or stomach into the trachea and subsequently the lungs. The person who has aspiration pneumonia usually has a history of loss of consciousness (e.g., as a result of seizure, anesthesia, head injury, stroke, alcohol intake). With loss of consciousness the gag and cough reflexes are depressed, and aspiration is more likely to occur. Another risk factor is tube

---

TABLE 27-4 Drug Therapy

Organisms Associated with Hospital-Acquired Pneumonia and Recommended Antibiotics

Group 1: Mild to moderate HAP, no unusual risk factors, onset at any time; or severe HAP with early onset

CORE ORGANISMS	CORE ANTIBIOTICS
▪ Enteric gram-negative bacilli (non-pseudomonal, e.g., *Enterobacter, Escherichia coli, Proteus, Klebsiella, Serratia marcescens, Haemophilus influenzae*) ▪ Methicillin-sensitive *Staphylococcus aureus* ▪ *Streptococcus pneumoniae*	Cephalosporin (second generation or nonantipseudomonal third generation) *or* β-lactam/β-lactamase inhibitor *or* If allergic to penicillin, a fluoroquinolone* or clindamycin + aztreonam

Group 2: Mild to moderate HAP with risk factors associated with additional specific organisms, onset at any time

RISK FACTORS	CORE *PLUS* SPECIFIC AT-RISK ORGANISMS	CORE ANTIBIOTICS *PLUS* ADDITIONAL SPECIFIC COVERAGE
Abdominal surgery, aspiration	▪ Anaerobes	Clindamycin or beta-lactam/beta-lactamase inhibitor
Coma, head trauma, diabetes mellitus, renal failure	▪ *S. aureus*	+/− vancomycin (until MRSA ruled out)
High-dose corticosteroids	▪ *Legionella*	Erythromycin +/− rifampin
Prolonged ICU stay, corticosteroids, antibiotics, lung disease	▪ *Pseudomonas aeruginosa*	Treat as severe HAP (group 3)

Group 3: Severe HAP with risk factors, early onset; or severe HAP, late onset

CORE ORGANISMS PLUS	ANTIBIOTICS
▪ *P. aeruginosa* ▪ *Acinetobacter* species	Aminoglycoside or ciprofloxacin, *plus* One of the following: antipseudomonal penicillin, β-lactam/β-lactamase inhibitor, ceftazidime or cefoperazone (Cefobid), imipenem (Primaxin), aztreonam (Azactam) *and*
▪ Consider MRSA	+/− vancomycin (if MRSA is a concern)

Adapted from American Thoracic Society: Hospital-acquired pneumonia in adults: diagnosis, assessment of severity, initial antimicrobial therapy: a consensus statement, *Am J Respir Crit Care Med* 153:1711, 1996.
*If *S. pneumoniae* not a concern.
HAP, Hospital-acquired pneumonia; *ICU,* intensive care unit; *MRSA,* methicillin-resistant *S. aureus.*

feedings. The dependent portions of the lung are most often affected, primarily the superior segments of the lower lobes and the posterior segments of the upper lobes, which are dependent in the supine position.

The aspirated material, food, water, vomitus, or toxic fluids, is the triggering mechanism for the pathology of this type of pneumonia. There are three distinct forms of aspiration pneumonia. If the aspirated material is an inert substance (e.g., barium), the initial manifestation is usually caused by mechanical obstruction of airways. When the aspirated materials contain toxic fluids such as gastric juices, there is chemical injury to the lung with infection as a secondary event, usually 48 to 72 hours later; this is identified as *chemical (noninfectious) pneumonitis.* The most important form of aspiration pneumonia is bacterial infection. The infecting organism is usually one of the normal oropharyngeal flora, and multiple organisms, including both aerobes and anaerobes, are isolated from the sputum of the patient with aspiration pneumonia. Antibiotic therapy is based on an assessment of the severity of illness, where the infection was acquired (community versus hospital), and type of organisms present.

Opportunistic Pneumonia. Certain patients with altered immune response are highly susceptible to respiratory infections. Individuals considered at risk include those who have severe protein-calorie malnutrition; those who have immune deficiencies; those who have received transplants and been treated with immunosuppressive drugs; and patients who are being treated with radiation therapy, chemotherapy drugs, and corticosteroids (especially for a prolonged period). The individual has a variety of altered conditions, including altered B and T lymphocyte function, depressed bone marrow function, and decreased levels or function of neutrophils and macrophages. In addition to the causative agents (especially gram-negative bacteria), other agents that cause pneumonia in the immunocompromised patient are *Pneumocystis carinii,* cytomegalovirus (CMV), and fungi.

Pneumocystis carinii is an opportunistic pathogen whose natural habitat is the lung. Although its classification has been historically considered to be protozoa, it is now considered a fungus. This organism rarely causes pneumonia in the healthy individual. *Pneumocystis carinii* pneumonia (PCP) affects 70% of human immunodeficiency virus (HIV)–infected individuals and is the most common opportunistic infection in patients with acquired immunodeficiency syndrome (AIDS). In this type of pneumonia the chest x-ray usually shows a diffuse bilateral alveolar pattern of infiltration. In widespread disease the lungs are massively consolidated.

Clinical manifestations are insidious and include fever, tachypnea, tachycardia, dyspnea, nonproductive cough, and hypoxemia. Pulmonary physical findings are minimal in proportion to the serious nature of the disease. Treatment consists of a course of trimethoprim-sulfamethoxazole (Bactrim) as the primary agent. An alternative medication for the Bactrim-intolerant patient is dapsone-trimethoprim. In populations at risk for development of *P. carinii* pneumonitis (e.g., patients with hematologic malignancies or AIDS), prophylaxis with trimethoprim-sulfamethoxazole may be advocated. Aerosolized pentamidine (Nebupent), although less commonly used, is an alternative for prophylaxis in Bactrim-intolerant patients. (PCP is discussed in Chapter 14.)

Cytomegalovirus (CMV) is a cause of viral pneumonia in the immunocompromised patient, particularly in transplant recipients. CMV, a type of herpes virus, gives rise to latent infections

and reactivation with shedding of infectious virus. This type of interstitial pneumonia can be a mild disease, or it can be fulminant and produce pulmonary insufficiency and death. Often, CMV coexists with other opportunistic bacterial or fungal agents in causing pneumonia. Ganciclovir (Cytovene) is recommended for treatment of CMV pneumonia.

Pathophysiology

Pneumococcal pneumonia is the most common cause of bacterial pneumonia, and the pathophysiology related to this type of pneumonia is discussed below. (The pathophysiology of other types of pneumonia is similar.) There are four characteristic stages of the disease process:

1. *Congestion.* After the pneumococcus organisms reach the alveoli via droplets or saliva, there is an outpouring of fluid into the alveoli. The organisms multiply in the serous fluid, and the infection is spread. The pneumococci damage the host by their overwhelming growth and interference with lung function.
2. *Red hepatization.* There is massive dilation of the capillaries, and alveoli are filled with organisms, neutrophils, red blood cells (RBCs), and fibrin (Fig. 27-1). The lung appears red and granular, similar to the liver, which is why the process is called hepatization.
3. *Gray hepatization.* Blood flow decreases, and leukocytes and fibrin consolidate in the affected part of the lung.
4. *Resolution.* Complete resolution and healing occur if there are no complications.

The exudate becomes lysed and is processed by the macrophages. The normal lung tissue is restored, and the person's gas-exchange ability returns to normal.

Clinical Manifestations

Patients with CAP usually have a constellation of symptoms including sudden onset of fever, chills, cough productive of purulent sputum, and pleuritic chest pain (in some cases). In the elderly or

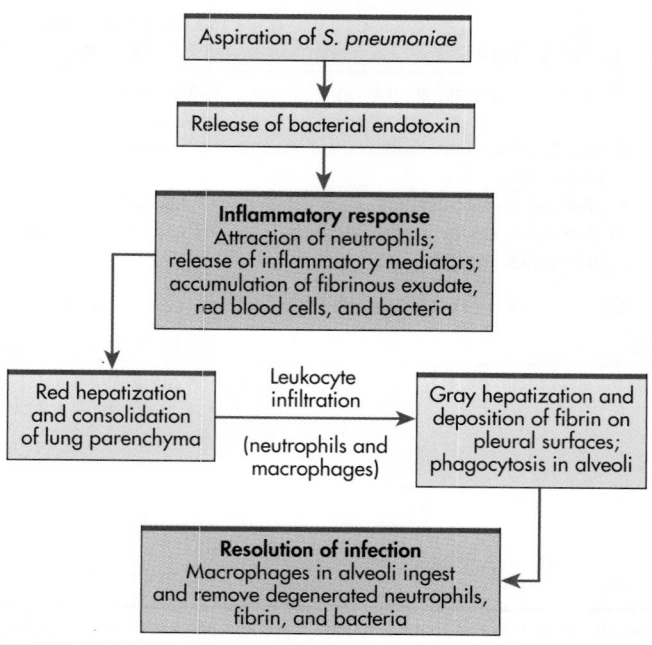

FIG. 27-1 Pathophysiologic course of pneumococcal pneumonia.

debilitated patient, confusion or stupor (possibly related to hypoxia) may be the predominant finding. On physical examination signs of pulmonary consolidation, such as dullness to percussion, increased fremitus, bronchial breath sounds, and crackles, may be found. The typical pneumonia syndrome is usually caused by the most common pathogen in CAP, which is *S. pneumoniae,* but can also be due to other bacterial pathogens, such as *H. influenzae.*

CAP may also manifest atypically with a more gradual onset, a dry cough, and extrapulmonary manifestations such as headache, myalgias, fatigue, sore throat, nausea, vomiting, and diarrhea. On physical examination crackles are often heard. This presentation of symptoms is classically produced by *M. pneumoniae* but can also be caused by *Legionella* and *C. pneumoniae.* Patients with hematogenous *S. aureus* pneumonia may have only dyspnea and fever. This necrotizing infection causes destruction of lung tissue, and these patients are usually very sick.

Although the initial manifestations of viral pneumonia are highly variable, viruses also cause pneumonia that is usually characterized by an atypical presentation with chills, fever, dry nonproductive cough, and extrapulmonary symptoms. Primary viral pneumonia can be caused by influenza virus infection. Viral pneumonia is also found in association with systemic viral diseases such as measles, varicella-zoster, and herpes simplex.

Complications

Most cases of pneumonia generally run an uncomplicated course. However, complications can occur, and they develop more frequently in individuals with underlying chronic diseases and other risk factors. Complications may include the following:

1. *Pleurisy* (inflammation of the pleura) is a relatively common accompanying problem of pneumonia.
2. *Pleural effusion* can occur, and usually the effusion is sterile and is reabsorbed in 1 to 2 weeks. Occasionally, it requires aspiration by means of thoracentesis.
3. *Atelectasis* (collapsed, airless alveoli) of one or part of one lobe may occur. These areas usually clear with effective coughing and deep breathing.
4. *Delayed resolution* results from persistent infection and is seen on x-ray as residual consolidation. Usually, the physical findings return to normal within 2 to 4 weeks. Delayed resolution occurs most frequently in the patient who is older, is malnourished, is alcoholic, or has COPD.
5. *Lung abscess* is not a common complication of pneumonia. It is seen with pneumonia caused by *S. aureus* and gram-negative pneumonias (see section on lung abscess later in this chapter).
6. *Empyema* (accumulation of purulent exudate in the pleural cavity) is relatively infrequent but requires antibiotic therapy and drainage of the exudate by a chest tube or open surgical drainage.
7. *Pericarditis* results from spread of the infecting organism from an infected pleura or via a hematogenous route to the pericardium (the fibroserous sac around the heart).
8. *Arthritis* results from systemic spread of the organism. The affected joints are swollen, red, and painful, and a purulent exudate can be aspirated.
9. *Meningitis* can be caused by *S. pneumoniae.* The patient with pneumonia who is disoriented, confused, or somnolent should have a lumbar puncture to evaluate the possibility of meningitis.

10. *Endocarditis* can develop when the organisms attack the endocardium and the valves of the heart. The clinical manifestations are similar to those of acute bacterial endocarditis (see Chapter 36).

Diagnostic Studies

The common diagnostic measures for pneumonia are presented in Table 27-5. History, physical examination, and chest x-ray often provide enough information to make management decisions without costly laboratory tests.

Chest x-ray often shows a typical pattern characteristic of the infecting organism and is an invaluable adjunct in the diagnosis of pneumonia. Lobar or segmental consolidation suggests a bacterial cause, usually *S. pneumoniae* or *Klebsiella.* Diffuse pulmonary infiltrates are most commonly caused by infection with viruses, *Legionella,* or pathogenic fungi. Cavitary shadows suggest the presence of a necrotizing infection with destruction of lung tissue commonly caused by *S. aureus,* gram-negative bacteria, and *Mycobacterium tuberculosis.* Pleural effusions, which can occur in up to 30% of patients with CAP, can also be seen on x-ray.

Sputum cultures are recommended if a drug-resistant pathogen or an organism that is not covered by the usual empiric therapy is suspected. (**Empiric therapy** is based on observation and experience without always knowing the exact cause.) A Gram stain of the sputum provides information on the predominant causative organism. A sputum culture should be collected before initiating antibiotic therapy. Because of the poor sensitivity and specificity of sputum cultures, any sputum culture results should be correlated with the predominant organisms found on Gram stain results. If a delay in the time from collecting the sputum to incubation exceeds 2 to 5 hours, results are less reliable. Before treatment, two blood cultures may be done for patients who are seriously ill. Although microbial studies are expected before treatment, initiation of antibiotics should not be delayed.[6]

Arterial blood gases (ABGs), if obtained, usually reveal hypoxemia. Leukocytosis is found in the majority of patients with

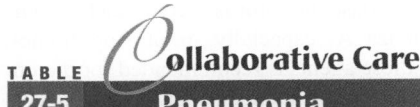

TABLE 27-5	Collaborative Care — Pneumonia

Diagnostic
History and physical examination
Chest x-ray
Gram stain of sputum
Sputum culture and sensitivity test (if drug-resistant pathogen or organism not covered by empiric therapy)
Pulse oximetry or ABGs (if indicated)
Complete blood count, differential, and routine blood chemistries (if indicated)
Blood cultures (if indicated)

Collaborative Therapy
Appropriate antibiotic therapy (see Tables 27-3 and 27-4)
Increased fluid intake (at least 3 L/day)
Limited activity and rest
Antipyretics
Analgesics
Oxygen therapy (if indicated)

ABGs, Arterial blood gases.

bacterial pneumonia, usually with a white blood cell (WBC) count greater than 15,000/μl (15 × 10^9/L) with the presence of bands (immature neutrophils).

Collaborative Care

Prompt treatment with the appropriate antibiotic almost always cures bacterial and mycoplasma pneumonia. In uncomplicated cases, the patient responds to drug therapy within 48 to 72 hours. Indications of improvement include decreased temperature, improved breathing, and reduced chest pain. Abnormal physical findings can last for more than 7 days.

In addition to antibiotic therapy, supportive measures may be used, including oxygen therapy to treat hypoxemia, analgesics to relieve the chest pain for patient comfort, and antipyretics such as aspirin or acetaminophen for significantly elevated temperature. During the acute febrile phase, the patient's activity should be restricted, and rest should be encouraged and planned.

Most individuals with mild to moderate illness who have no other underlying disease process can be treated on an outpatient basis. If there is a serious underlying disease or if the pneumonia is accompanied by severe dyspnea, hypoxemia, or other complications, the patient should be hospitalized. Guidelines for hospitalization for CAP are presented in Table 27-3.

Currently, there is no definitive treatment for viral pneumonia. Two antiviral drugs, amantadine (Symmetrel) and rimantadine (Flumadine), are approved for oral use in the treatment of influenza A virus. The new neuraminidase inhibitors, zanamivir (Relenza) and oseltamivir (Tamiflu), are active against both influenza A and B (see Chapter 26). An influenza vaccine is available. It is modified annually to reflect the anticipated strains in the upcoming season. Influenza vaccine is considered a mainstay of prevention and is recommended annually for use in the individual considered to be at risk. Individuals at risk for influenza include the elderly, nursing home residents, patients with COPD or diabetes mellitus, and health care workers. For elderly with signs and symptoms of influenza, including those who have received the influenza vaccine, empiric treatment with amantadine, rimantadine, or a neuraminidase inhibitor is recommended. During epidemics of influenza A, especially in nursing homes, chemoprophylaxis with these agents is recommended for the unvaccinated patients, immunodeficient patients, or those who have received the vaccine within the past 2 weeks.[9]

Pneumococcal Vaccine. Pneumococcal vaccine is indicated primarily for the individual considered at risk who (1) has chronic illnesses such as lung and heart disease and diabetes mellitus, (2) is recovering from a severe illness, (3) is 65 years of age or older, or (4) is in a long-term care facility. This is particularly important because the rate of drug-resistant *S. pneumoniae* infections is increasing. Pneumococcal vaccine can be given simultaneously with other vaccines such as the flu vaccine, but each should be administered in a separate site.[6]

The current recommendation is that pneumococcal vaccine is good for a person's lifetime. However, in the immunosuppressed individual at risk for development of fatal pneumococcal infection (e.g., asplenic patient; patient with nephrotic syndrome, renal failure, or AIDS; or transplant recipient), revaccination is recommended every 5 years.

Drug Therapy. The main problems with the use of antibiotics in pneumonia are the development of resistant strains of organisms and the patient's hypersensitivity or allergic reaction to certain antibiotics.

Most cases of CAP in otherwise healthy adults do not require hospitalization.[10] The oral antibiotic therapy administered is frequently empiric treatment with broad-spectrum antibiotics. Once the patient is categorized (see Table 27-3), empiric therapy can be based on the likely infecting organism. For example, in the category 1 patients these organisms include *S. pneumoniae, M. pneumoniae,* respiratory viruses, *C. pneumoniae,* and *H. influenzae.* Macrolides are the recommended therapy, including either azithromycin (Zithromax) or clarithromycin (Biaxin) because erythromycin is not active against *H. influenzae.* Doxycycline (Vibramycin) is recommended for the patient who is allergic to macrolides, but this antibiotic is not reliably active against pneumococcus organisms.[6]

For hospital-acquired pneumonia, the American Thoracic Society recommends that empiric antibiotic therapy be based on the likely pathogens in the various patient groups (see Table 27-4).[8] Even with extensive diagnostic testing an etiologic organism is often not identified.

When using empiric therapy, it is important to recognize the nonresponding patient. Therapy may require modification based on the patient's culture results or clinical response. Clinical response is evaluated by factors such as a change in fever, sputum purulence, leukocytosis, oxygenation, or x-ray patterns. Improvement is often not apparent for the first 48 to 72 hours, and empiric therapy need not be altered during this period unless deterioration is noted or culture results dictate that a different antibiotic should be used.[8]

Patients with ventilator-associated pneumonia may experience rapid deterioration. Patients who deteriorate or fail to respond to therapy will require aggressive evaluation to assess noninfectious etiologies, complications, other coexisting infectious processes, or pneumonia caused by a resistant pathogen. It may be necessary to broaden antimicrobial coverage while awaiting results of cultures and other studies, such as computed tomography (CT) scan, ultrasound, or lung scans.[9]

Nutritional Therapy. Fluid intake of at least 3 L per day is important in the supportive treatment of pneumonia. If the patient has heart failure, fluid intake must be individualized. If oral intake cannot be maintained, IV administration of fluids and electrolytes may be necessary for the acutely ill patient. An intake of at least 1500 calories per day should be maintained to provide energy for the increased metabolic processes in the patient. Small, frequent meals are better tolerated by the dyspneic patient.

NURSING MANAGEMENT
PNEUMONIA

■ Nursing Assessment

Subjective and objective data that should be obtained from a patient with pneumonia are presented in Table 27-6.

■ Nursing Diagnoses

Nursing diagnoses for the patient with pneumonia may include, but are not limited to, those presented in NCP 27-1.

■ Planning

The overall goals are that the patient with pneumonia will have (1) clear breath sounds, (2) normal breathing patterns, (3) no signs of hypoxia, (4) normal chest x-ray, and (5) no complications related to pneumonia.

TABLE 27-6	Nursing Assessment
	Pneumonia

Subjective Data

Important Health Information

Past health history: Lung cancer, COPD, diabetes mellitus, chronic debilitating disease, malnutrition, altered consciousness, AIDS, exposure to chemical toxins, dust, or allergens

Medications: Use of antibiotics; corticosteroids, chemotherapy, or any other immunosuppressants

Surgery or other treatments: Recent abdominal or thoracic surgery, splenectomy, endotracheal intubation, or any surgery with general anesthesia; tube feedings

Functional Health Patterns

Health perception–health management: Cigarette smoking, alcoholism; recent upper respiratory tract infection, malaise

Nutritional-metabolic: Anorexia, nausea, vomiting; chills

Activity-exercise: Prolonged bed rest or immobility; fatigue, weakness; dyspnea, cough (productive or nonproductive); nasal congestion

Cognitive-perceptual: Pain with breathing, chest pain, sore throat, headache, abdominal pain, muscle aches

Objective Data

General

Fever, restlessness or lethargy; splinting of affected area

Respiratory

Tachypnea; pharyngitis; asymmetric chest movements or retraction; decreased excursion; nasal flaring; use of accessory muscles (neck, abdomen); grunting; crackles, friction rub on auscultation; dullness on percussion over consolidated areas, increased tactile fremitus on palpation; pink, rusty, purulent, green, yellow, or white sputum (amount may be scant to copious)

Cardiovascular

Tachycardia

Neurologic

Changes in mental status, ranging from confusion to delirium

Possible Findings

Leukocytosis; abnormal ABGs with ↓ or normal PaO_2, ↓ $PaCO_2$, and ↑ pH initially, and later ↓ PaO_2, ↑ $PaCO_2$, and ↓ pH; positive sputum Gram stain and culture; patchy or diffuse infiltrates, abscesses, pleural effusion, or pneumothorax on chest x-ray.

ABGs, Arterial blood gases; *AIDS,* acquired immunodeficiency syndrome; *COPD,* chronic obstructive pulmonary disease.

■ **Nursing Implementation**

Health Promotion. There are many nursing interventions to help prevent the occurrence of, as well as the morbidity associated with, pneumonia. Teaching the individual to practice good health habits, such as proper diet and hygiene, adequate rest, and regular exercise, can maintain the natural resistance to infecting organisms. If possible, exposure to URIs should be avoided. If a URI occurs, it should be treated promptly with supportive measures (e.g., rest, fluids). If symptoms persist for more than 7 days, the person should obtain medical care. The individual at risk for pneumonia (e.g., the chronically ill, older adult) should be encouraged to obtain both influenza and pneumococcal vaccines.[10]

In the hospital, the nursing role involves identifying the patient at risk (see Table 27-1) and taking measures to prevent the development of pneumonia. The patient with altered consciousness should be placed in positions (e.g., side-lying, upright) that will prevent or minimize the risk of aspiration. The patient should be turned and repositioned at least every 2 hours to facilitate adequate lung expansion and to discourage pooling of secretions.

The patient who has a feeding tube generally requires attention to measures to prevent aspiration (see Chapter 39). Although the feeding tube is small, an interruption in the integrity of the lower esophageal sphincter still exists, which can allow reflux of gastric and intestinal contents.

The patient who has difficulty swallowing (e.g., stroke patient) needs assistance in eating, drinking, and taking medication to prevent aspiration. The patient who has recently had surgery and others who are immobile need assistance with turning and deep-breathing measures at frequent intervals (see Chapter 19). The nurse must be careful to avoid overmedication with narcotics or sedatives, which can cause a depressed cough reflex and accumulation of fluid in the lungs. The gag reflex should be present in the individual who has had local anesthesia to the throat before the administration of fluids or food.

Strict medical asepsis and adherence to infection control guidelines should be practiced by the nurse to reduce the incidence of nosocomial infections.[11] Poor hand-washing practices allow spread of pathogens via the hands of the health care worker. Staff should wash their hands each time before they provide care to a patient. Respiratory devices can harbor microorganisms and have been associated with outbreaks of pneumonia. Strict sterile aseptic technique should be used when suctioning the trachea of a patient.

Acute Intervention. Although many patients with pneumonia are treated on an outpatient basis, the nursing care plan for a patient with pneumonia (see NCP 27-1) is applicable to both these individuals and in-hospital patients. It is important for the nurse to remember that pneumonia is an acute, infectious disease. Although most cases of pneumonia are potentially completely curable, complications can result. The nurse must be aware of these complications and their manifestations. The infection control nurse can be a valuable resource in assisting with the care of patients with pneumonia.

Ambulatory and Home Care. The patient needs to be reassured that complete recovery from pneumonia is possible. It is extremely important to emphasize the need to take all of the prescribed drug and to return for follow-up medical care and evaluation. The patient needs to be taught about the drug-drug and the food-drug interactions for the prescribed antibiotic. Adequate rest is needed to maintain progress toward recovery and to prevent a relapse. The patient should be told that it may be weeks before the usual vigor and sense of well-being are felt. A prolonged period of convalescence may be necessary for the older adult or chronically ill patient.

The patient considered to be at risk for pneumonia should be told about available vaccines and should discuss them with the health care provider. Deep-breathing exercises should be practiced for 6 to 8 weeks after the patient is discharged from the hospital.

■ **Evaluation**

The expected outcomes for the patient with pneumonia are presented in NCP 27-1.

NURSING CARE PLAN 27-1

Patient with Pneumonia

NURSING DIAGNOSIS   **Ineffective breathing pattern** *related to* inflammation and pain *as manifested by* rapid respirations, dyspnea, tachypnea, nasal flaring, altered chest excursion.

OUTCOMES—NOC	INTERVENTIONS—NIC and *RATIONALES*
Respiratory Status: Gas Exchange (0402) • Ease of breathing _____ • Dyspnea at rest not present _____ • SpO$_2$ WNL _____ _____ **Outcome Scale** 1 = Extremely compromised 2 = Substantially compromised 3 = Moderately compromised 4 = Mildly compromised 5 = Not compromised	*Ventilation Assistance (3390)* • Monitor respiratory and oxygenation status *to provide baseline assessment.* • Auscultate breath sounds, noting areas of decreased or absent ventilation, and presence of adventitious sounds. • Position to minimize respiratory efforts *to reduce oxygen needs.* • Monitor effects of position change on oxygenation (SpO$_2$) *to assess appropriate position.* • Initiate and maintain supplemental oxygen as prescribed *to improve respiratory status.* • Administer drugs (e.g., bronchodilators) *that promote airway patency and gas exchange.*

NURSING DIAGNOSIS   **Ineffective airway clearance** *related to* thick secretions *as manifested by* ineffective cough or thick, tenacious sputum; abnormal breath sounds; dyspnea.

OUTCOMES—NOC	INTERVENTIONS—NIC and *RATIONALES*
Respiratory Status: Airway Patency (0410) • Respiratory rate IER _____ • Free of adventitious breath sounds _____ • Moves sputum out of airway _____ _____ **Outcome Scale** 1 = Extremely compromised 2 = Substantially compromised 3 = Moderately compromised 4 = Mildly compromised 5 = Not compromised	*Cough Enhancement (3250) and Respiratory Monitoring (3350)* • Monitor rate, rhythm, depth, and effort of respirations *to provide baseline assessment.* • Auscultate breath sounds, noting areas of decreased or absent ventilation, and presence of adventitious sounds *to obtain ongoing data on patient's response to therapy.* • Assist patient to a sitting position with head slightly flexed, shoulders relaxed, and knees flexed *to improve respiratory status.* • Encourage use of incentive spirometry as appropriate *to aid in lung expansion and prevent atelectasis.* • Promote systemic fluid hydration as appropriate *to help liquefy secretions.*

NURSING DIAGNOSIS   **Acute pain** *related to* inflammation and ineffective pain management and/or comfort measures *as manifested by* pleuritic chest pain, pleural friction rub, shallow respirations, decreased breath sounds.

OUTCOMES—NOC	INTERVENTIONS—NIC and *RATIONALES*
Pain Control (1605) • Reports pain controlled _____ • Recognizes causal factors _____ • Uses nonanalgesic relief measures _____ • Uses analgesics appropriately _____ _____ **Outcome Scale** 1 = Never demonstrated 2 = Rarely demonstrated 3 = Sometimes demonstrated 4 = Often demonstrated 5 = Consistently demonstrated	*Pain Management (1400)* • Perform a comprehensive assessment of pain to include location, characteristics, onset/duration, frequency, quality, intensity or severity of pain, and precipitating factors *to create baseline status of pain.* • Consider cultural influences related to pain response. • Encourage patient to monitor own pain and to intervene appropriately *to allow independence and prepare for discharge.* • Teach the use of nonpharmacologic techniques (e.g., biofeedback, hypnosis, relaxation, guided imagery, music therapy, distraction, massage) before, after, and, if possible, during painful activities; before pain occurs or increases; and along with other pain relief measures *to relieve pain and reduce the need for analgesia.* • Use pain control measures before pain becomes severe *because mild to moderate pain is controlled more quickly.* • Medicate before an activity to increase participation, but evaluate the hazard of sedation *to help minimize pain that will be experienced.*

IER, In expected range; *WNL,* within normal limits.

NURSING CARE PLAN 27-1

Patient with Pneumonia—cont'd

NURSING DIAGNOSIS **Imbalanced nutrition: less than body requirements** *related to* increased metabolism, fatigue, and anorexia *as manifested by* weight loss and patient's statement of foul taste in mouth.

OUTCOMES—NOC

Nutritional Status: Food and Fluid Intake (1008)
- Oral food intake _____
- Fluid intake _____
- Weight gain _____

_____

Outcome Scale
1 = Extremely compromised
2 = Substantially compromised
3 = Moderately compromised
4 = Mildly compromised
5 = Not compromised

INTERVENTIONS—NIC and *RATIONALES*

Nutritional Monitoring (1160) and Nutrition Therapy (1120)
- Weigh patient at specified intervals *to assess status of weight.*
- Schedule treatment and procedures at times other than feeding times *to conserve energy for breathing.*
- Monitor food/fluid ingested and calculate daily caloric intake *to assess if meeting patient's needs.*
- Determine food preferences with consideration of cultural and religious preferences *to provide appropriate intake.*
- Provide oxygen therapy via nasal cannula if needed during meals *to maintain oxygen status.*
- Position patient in high Fowler's position at meal times *to help relieve dyspnea.*
- Provide patient with high-protein, high-caloric, nutritious finger foods and drinks that can be readily consumed, as appropriate, *to provide nutritional needs.*

NURSING DIAGNOSIS **Activity intolerance** *related to* interrupted sleep/wake cycle, hypoxia, and weakness *as manifested by* fatigue, unwillingness or inability to exert self, dyspnea, increased pulse and respiration, dizziness on exertion.

OUTCOMES—NOC

Activity Tolerance (0005)
- Oxygen saturation IER in response to activity _____
- Heart rate IER in response to activity _____
- Reported activities of daily living performance _____

_____

Outcome Scale
1 = Extremely compromised
2 = Substantially compromised
3 = Moderately compromised
4 = Mildly compromised
5 = Not compromised

INTERVENTIONS—NIC and *RATIONALES*

Energy Management (0185)
- Determine patient's physical limitations *to establish patient's needs and capabilities.*
- Monitor cardiorespiratory and oxygen response to activity (e.g., tachycardia, other arrhythmias, dyspnea, diaphoresis, pallor, hemodynamic pressures, respiratory rate, and pulse oximetry) *to help establish obtainable goals and create appropriate interventions.*
- Plan activities for periods when patient has the most energy and alternate rest and activity periods *to provide activity based on patient's response and promote increased feeling of accomplishment.*
- Encourage afternoon nap, if appropriate, *to reduce stress and promote rest.*

TUBERCULOSIS

Tuberculosis (TB) is an infectious disease caused by *Mycobacterium tuberculosis.* It usually involves the lungs, but it also occurs in the larynx, kidneys, bones, adrenal glands, lymph nodes, and meninges and can be disseminated throughout the body. TB kills more people worldwide than any other infectious disease. It is estimated that between 19% and 43% of the world's population is infected with *M. tuberculosis.* The World Health Organization (WHO) estimates that more than 8 million new cases of TB occur each year, and approximately 3 million people die from the disease.[12]

With the introduction of chemotherapeutic agents (streptomycin, isoniazid [INH]) in the late 1940s and early 1950s, there was a dramatic decrease in the prevalence of TB. However, between 1985 and 1992, there was a significant increase in TB cases. The trend has been decreasing since 1993 because of improvements in TB control programs, with the United States seeing an all-time low of 5.8 cases per 100,000 reported in 2000.[13] Today in the United States, it is estimated that 15 million people

are infected with the tubercle bacillus. These statistics indicate that TB, despite being potentially curable and preventable, is still a major public health problem in the United States. HIV infection and immigration of persons from areas of high incidence have resulted in increases in the number of cases.[12]

The major factors that have contributed to the resurgence of TB have been (1) epidemic proportions of TB among patients with HIV infection and (2) the emergence of multidrug-resistant (MDR) strains of *M. tuberculosis.* During the past three decades, the prevalence of MDR strains of TB in the United States has steadily increased from 2% to 9%.[14] MDR strains of TB have developed because of poor compliance with drug therapy leading to treatment failure and development of resistant strains. Patients were lost to follow-up treatment or placed on drug regimens to which their infections were no longer susceptible. In general there has been decreased vigilance in treating patients diagnosed with TB.

TB is seen disproportionately in the poor, the underserved, and minorities. Individuals at risk for TB include homeless persons, residents of inner-city neighborhoods, foreign-born persons, older adults, those in institutions (long-term care facilities, prisons), injection drug users, the socioeconomically disadvantaged, and medically underserved of all races. Immunosuppression from any etiology (e.g., HIV infection, malignancy) increases the risk of TB infection. The prevalence of TB is high in a few areas of the United States where there is a large population of Native Americans, such as Arizona and New Mexico, and in counties near the Mexican border. Health care workers with increased exposure to TB are also at high risk.

Etiology and Pathophysiology

M. tuberculosis, a gram-positive, acid-fast bacillus, is usually spread from person to person via airborne droplets, which are produced when the infected individual with pulmonary or laryngeal TB coughs, sneezes, speaks, or sings. Once released into a room, the organisms are dispersed and can be inhaled. Brief exposure to a few tubercle bacilli rarely causes an infection. Rather, it is more commonly spread to the individual who has had repeated close contact with an infected person. TB is not highly infectious, and transmission usually requires close, frequent, or prolonged exposure. The disease cannot be spread by hands, books, glasses, dishes, or other fomites.

When the bacilli are inhaled, they pass down the bronchial system and implant themselves on the respiratory bronchioles or alveoli. The lower parts of the lungs are usually the site of initial bacterial implantation. After implantation, the bacilli multiply with no initial resistance from the host. The organisms are engulfed by phagocytes (initially neutrophils and later macrophages) and may continue to multiply within the phagocytes.

While a cellular immune response is being activated, the bacilli can be spread through the lymphatic channels to regional lymph nodes and via the thoracic duct to the circulating blood. Thus organisms may be spread throughout the body before sufficient activation of the cell-mediated immune response is available to bring the infection under control. The organisms find favorable environments for growth primarily in the upper lobes of the lungs, kidneys, epiphyses of the bone, cerebral cortex, and adrenal glands.

Eventually the cellular immunity limits further multiplication and spread of the infection. A characteristic tissue reaction called

an *epithelioid cell granuloma* results after the cellular immune system is activated. This granuloma is a result of fusion of the infiltrating macrophages. The granuloma is surrounded by lymphocytes. This reaction usually takes 10 to 20 days. The central portion of the lesion (called a Ghon tubercle) undergoes necrosis characterized by a cheesy appearance and hence is named *caseous necrosis.* The lesion may also undergo liquefactive necrosis in which the liquid drains into connecting bronchi and produces a cavity. Tubercular material may enter the tracheobronchial system, allowing airborne transmission of infectious particles.

Healing of the primary lesion usually takes place by resolution, fibrosis, and calcification. The granulation tissue surrounding the lesion may become more fibrous and form a collagenous scar around the tubercle. A *Ghon complex* is formed, consisting of the Ghon tubercle and regional lymph nodes. Calcified Ghon complexes may be seen on chest x-ray.

When a tuberculosis lesion regresses and heals, the infection enters a latent period in which it may persist without producing a clinical illness. The infection may develop into clinical disease if the persisting organisms begin to multiply rapidly, or it may remain dormant.

If the initial immune response is not adequate, control of the organisms is not maintained and clinical disease results. Certain individuals are at a higher risk for clinical disease, including those who are immunosuppressed for any reason (e.g., patients with HIV infection, those receiving cancer chemotherapy or long-term corticosteroid therapy) or have diabetes mellitus.

Dormant but viable organisms persist for years. Reactivation of TB can occur if the host's defense mechanisms become impaired. The reasons for reactivation are not well understood, but they are related to decreased resistance found in older adults, individuals with concomitant diseases, and those who receive immunosuppressive therapy.

Classification

The American Thoracic Association and American Lung Association adopted a classification system that covers the entire population (Table 27-7).

Clinical Manifestations

In the early stages of TB the person is usually free of symptoms. Many cases are found incidentally when routine chest x-rays are taken, especially in older adults.

Systemic manifestations may initially consist of fatigue, malaise, anorexia, weight loss, low-grade fevers, and night sweats. The weight loss may not be excessive until late in the disease and is often attributed to overwork or other factors.

A characteristic pulmonary manifestation is a cough that becomes frequent and produces mucoid or mucopurulent sputum. Dyspnea is unusual. Chest pain characterized as dull or tight may be present. Hemoptysis is not a common finding and is usually associated with more advanced cases. Sometimes TB has more acute, sudden manifestations; the patient has high fever, chills, generalized flulike symptoms, pleuritic pain, and a productive cough.

The HIV-infected patient with TB often has atypical physical examination and chest x-ray findings. Classic signs such as fever, cough, and weight loss may be attributed to *Pneumocystis carinii* pneumonia (PCP) or other HIV-associated opportunistic diseases. Clinical manifestations of respiratory problems in patients with HIV must be carefully investigated to determine the cause.

TABLE 27-7	Classification of Tuberculosis (TB)	
Class 0	No TB exposure	No TB exposure, not infected (no history of exposure, negative tuberculin skin test)
Class 1	TB exposure, no infection	TB exposure, no evidence of infection (history of exposure, negative tuberculin skin test)
Class 2	Latent TB infection, no disease	TB infection without disease (significant reaction to tuberculin skin test, negative bacteriologic studies, no x-ray findings compatible with TB, no clinical evidence of TB)
Class 3	TB clinically active	TB infection with clinically active disease (positive bacteriologic studies or both a significant reaction to tuberculin skin test and clinical or x-ray evidence of current disease)
Class 4	TB, but not clinically active	No current disease (history of previous episode of TB or abnormal, stable x-ray findings in a person with a significant reaction to tuberculin skin test; negative bacteriologic studies if done; no clinical or x-ray evidence of current disease)
Class 5	TB suspect	TB suspect (diagnosis pending); person should not be in this classification for more than 3 months

Source: American Thoracic Society, 2000.

Complications

Miliary TB. If a necrotic Ghon complex erodes through a blood vessel, large numbers of organisms invade the bloodstream and spread to all body organs. This is called *miliary* or *hematogenous* TB. The patient may be either acutely ill with fever, dyspnea, and cyanosis or chronically ill with systemic manifestations of weight loss, fever, and gastrointestinal (GI) disturbance. Hepatomegaly, splenomegaly, and generalized lymphadenopathy may be present.

Pleural Effusion and Empyema. A pleural effusion is caused by the release of caseous material into the pleural space. The bacteria-containing material triggers an inflammatory reaction and a pleural exudate of protein-rich fluid. A form of pleurisy called dry pleurisy may result from a superficial tuberculosis lesion involving the pleura. It appears as localized pleuritic pain on deep inspiration. Empyema is less common than effusion but may occur from large numbers of organisms spilling into the pleural space, usually from rupture of a cavity.

Tuberculosis Pneumonia. Acute pneumonia may result when large amounts of tubercle bacilli are discharged from the liquefied necrotic lesion into the lung or lymph nodes. The clinical manifestations are similar to those of bacterial pneumonia, including chills, fever, productive cough, pleuritic pain, and leukocytosis.

Other Organ Involvement. Although the lungs are the primary site of TB, other body organs may also be involved. The meninges may become infected. Bone and joint tissue may be involved in the infectious disease process. The kidneys, adrenal glands, lymph nodes, and both female and male genital tracts may also be infected.

Diagnostic Studies

Tuberculin Skin Testing. The body's immune response can be demonstrated by hypersensitivity to a tuberculin skin test. A positive reaction occurs 2 to 12 weeks after the initial infection, corresponding to the time needed to mount an immune response.

Purified protein derivative (PPD) of tuberculin is used primarily to detect the delayed hypersensitivity response. (The procedure for performing the tuberculin skin test is described in Chapter 25.) Once acquired, sensitivity to tuberculin tends to persist throughout life. A positive reaction indicates the presence of a tuberculosis infection, but it does not show whether the infection is dormant or active, causing a clinical illness.

Because the response to TB skin testing may be decreased in the immunocompromised patient, induration reactions equal to or greater than 5 mm are considered positive. Two-step testing is recommended for initial testing for health care workers who get repeated testing and for those who have a decreased response to allergens. For these people a second PPD test later may cause an accelerated response ("booster effect") misinterpreted as a new PPD conversion.[12] See Chapter 25, Table 25-12, for guidelines in interpreting TB skin tests. Recent guidelines for targeted tuberculin testing emphasize targeting only high risk groups and discourage testing low risk individuals.[15]

Chest X-ray. Although the findings on chest x-ray examination are important, it is not possible to make a diagnosis of TB solely on the basis of this examination. This is because other diseases can mimic the x-ray appearance of TB. The abnormality most commonly found in TB is multinodular lymph node involvement with cavitation in the upper lobes of the lungs. Calcification of the lung lesions generally occurs within several years of the infection.

Bacteriologic Studies. The demonstration of tubercle bacilli bacteriologically is essential for establishing a diagnosis. Microscopic examination of stained sputum smears for acid-fast bacilli is usually the first bacteriologic evidence of the presence of tubercle bacilli. This is a quick, easy examination that provides valuable information. Three consecutive sputum specimens collected on different days are obtained and sent for smear and culture. In addition to sputum, material for examination can be obtained from gastric washings, cerebrospinal fluid (CSF), or pus from an abscess.

The most accurate means of diagnosis is a culture technique. The major disadvantage of this method is that it may take 6 to 8 weeks for the mycobacterium to grow. The advantage is that it can detect small quantities (as few as 10 bacteria per milliliter of specimen).

A new test for TB, a nucleic acid amplification (NAA), is a rapid diagnostic test for TB. Test results are available in a few hours. This does not replace routine sputum smears and cultures, but it offers a health care provider increased confidence in the diagnosis.[16]

Collaborative Care

Hospitalization for initial treatment of TB is not necessary in most patients. Most patients are treated on an outpatient basis (Table 27-8), and many can continue to work and maintain their lifestyles with few changes. Hospitalization may be used for diagnostic evaluation, for the severely ill or debilitated, and for those who experience adverse drug reactions or treatment failures.

The mainstay of TB treatment is drug therapy. Drug therapy is used to treat an individual with clinical disease and to prevent disease in an infected person.

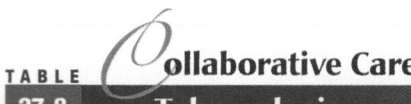

TABLE 27-8	Collaborative Care — Tuberculosis

Diagnostic
History and physical examination
Tuberculin skin test
Chest x-ray
Bacteriologic studies
  Sputum smear
  Sputum culture

Collaborative Therapy
Long-term treatment with antimicrobial drugs (see Tables 27-9 and 27-10)
Follow-up bacteriologic studies and chest x-rays

Drug Therapy

Active disease. In view of the growing prevalence of multidrug-resistant TB, the patient with active TB should be managed aggressively. Multidrug-resistant TB occurs when resistance develops to two or more anti-TB drugs. Standard therapy has been revised because of the increase in prevalence of drug-resistant TB. Treatment of TB usually consists of a combination of at least four drugs. The reason for combination therapy is to increase the therapeutic effectiveness and decrease the development of resistant strains of *M. tuberculosis.* It has been shown that single-drug therapy can result in rapid development of resistant strains.

The five primary drugs used are isoniazid (INH), rifampin (Rifamate), pyrazinamide, streptomycin, and ethambutol (Myambutol) (Table 27-9). Fixed-dose combination antituberculous drugs may enhance adherence to treatment recommendations. Combinations of isoniazid and rifampin (Rifamate) and of isoniazid, ri-

TABLE 27-9	Drug Therapy — Tuberculosis (TB)

DRUG	MECHANISMS OF ACTION	SIDE EFFECTS	COMMENTS
First-Line Drugs			
• isoniazid (INH)	Interferes with DNA metabolism of tubercle bacillus	Peripheral neuritis, hepatotoxicity, hypersensitivity (skin rash, arthralgia, fever), optic neuritis, vitamin B_6 neuritis	Metabolism primarily by liver and excretion by kidneys, pyridoxine (vitamin B_6) administration during high-dose therapy as prophylactic measure; use as single prophylactic agent for active TB in individuals whose PPD converts to positive; ability to cross blood-brain barrier
• rifampin (Rifadin)	Has broad-spectrum effects, inhibits RNA polymerase of tubercle bacillus	Hepatitis, febrile reaction, GI disturbance, peripheral neuropathy, hypersensitivity	Most common use with isoniazid; low incidence of side effects; suppression of effect of birth control pills; possible orange urine
• ethambutol (Myambutol)	Inhibits RNA synthesis and is bacteriostatic for the tubercle bacillus	Skin rash, GI disturbance, malaise, peripheral neuritis, optic neuritis	Side effects uncommon and reversible with discontinuation of drug; most common use as substitute drug when toxicity occurs with isoniazid or rifampin
• streptomycin	Inhibits protein synthesis and is bactericidal	Ototoxicity (eighth cranial nerve), nephrotoxicity, hypersensitivity	Cautious use in older adults, those with renal disease, and pregnant women; must be given parenterally
• pyrazinamide	Bactercidal effect (exact mechanism is unknown)	Fever, skin rash, hyperuricemia, jaundice (rare)	High rate of effectiveness when used with streptomycin or capreomycin
Second-Line Drugs			
• ethionamide (Trecator)	Inhibits protein synthesis	GI disturbance, hepatotoxicity, hypersensitivity	Valuable for treatment of resistant organisms; contraindicated in pregnancy
• capreomycin (Capastat)	Inhibits protein synthesis and is bactericidal	Ototoxicity, nephrotoxicity	Cautious use in older adults
• kanamycin (Kantrex) and amikacin	Interferes with protein synthesis	Ototoxicity, nephrotoxicity	Use in selected cases for treatment of resistant strains
• para-aminosalicylic acid (PAS)	Interferes with metabolism of tubercle bacillus	GI disturbance (frequent), hypersensitivity, hepatotoxicity	Interference with absorption of rifampin; infrequent use
• cycloserine (Seromycin)	Inhibits cell-wall synthesis	Personality changes, psychosis, rash	Contraindicated in individuals with a history of psychosis; use in treatment of resistant strains

DNA, Deoxyribonucleic acid; *GI,* gastrointestinal; *PPD,* purified protein derivative; *RNA,* ribonucleic acid.

fampin, and pyrazinamide (Rifater) are available to simplify therapy. Patients on antiretroviral drugs for HIV cannot take rifampin because it can impair the effectiveness of the antiretroviral drugs. Other drugs are primarily used for treatment of resistant strains or if the patient develops toxicity to the primary drugs. Many second-line drugs carry a greater risk of toxicity and require closer monitoring. Newer drugs for the treatment of TB that have not been placed in categories of first- or second-line drugs include the quinolones, especially ciprofloxacin (Cipro), ofloxacin (Floxin), and sparfloxacin (Zagam). Rifapentine (Priftin), a new drug to treat TB, can be used in combination with other TB drugs.

A problem with therapy for TB has been the length of time medication must be taken. Shorter courses of therapy (6 to 9 months) have now been shown to be effective. Three options for a treatment regimen are available (Table 27-10). The Centers for Disease Control and Prevention (CDC) recently reported that the 2-month rifampin and pyrazinamide regimen was associated with severe liver disease. The CDC recommends that this 2-month

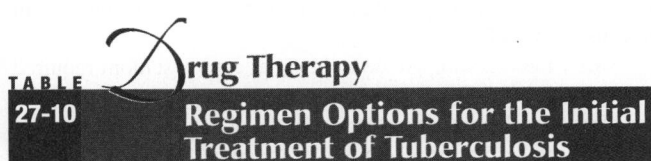

TABLE 27-10	**Drug Therapy** **Regimen Options for the Initial Treatment of Tuberculosis**

TB without HIV Infection: Four-Drug Therapy

Option 1   Four-drug regimen consisting of isoniazid (INH), rifampin (Rifadin), pyrazinamide, and either ethambutol (Myambutol) or streptomycin. Therapy may be given daily or 2-3 times weekly if DOT. Ethambutol or streptomycin may be discontinued if susceptibility to isoniazid or rifampin is documented. Pyrazinamide should be discontinued after 8 weeks. The total duration of therapy should be at least 6 months and at least 3 months after sputum cultures convert to negative. Fixed-dose combinations of rifampin and isoniazid (Rifamate) and rifampin, isoniazid, and pyrazinamide (Rifater) are available to simplify therapy.

Option 2   Daily isoniazid, rifampin, pyrazinamide, and streptomycin or ethambutol for 2 weeks, followed by DOT twice-weekly administration of the same drugs for 6 weeks, followed by DOT twice-weekly administrations of isoniazid and rifampin for 16 weeks.

Option 3   DOT 3 times/week administration of isoniazid, rifampin, pyrazinamide, and ethambutol or streptomycin for 6 months.

TB with HIV Infection

Option 1, 2, or 3 can be used, but treatment regimens should continue for a total of 9 months and at least 6 months beyond culture conversion.

Source: Centers for Disease Control and Prevention (CDC).
NOTE: The CDC advises consultation with a TB medical expert if the patient is symptomatic or smear or culture is positive after 3 months.
DOT, Directly observed therapy; *HIV*, human immunodeficiency virus; *TB*, tuberculosis.

treatment regimen be used with caution in patients with liver disease and alcoholism.[17]

Treatment in geographic areas where drug resistance is known to be a problem may consist of initial addition of drugs not in the resistance pattern for that area. Drug regimens should be adapted to the resistance pattern evident from sputum culture. In follow-up care for patients on long-term therapy, it is important to monitor the effectiveness of drugs and the development of toxic side effects. Usually sputum specimens are initially obtained weekly and then monthly to assess the effectiveness of the medication. The regimen is considered to be effective if the patient converts to a negative TB sputum status.

Although TB tends to have a rapidly progressive course in the patient co-infected with HIV, it responds well to standard medication. The co-infected patient should receive treatment for TB for at least 6 months beyond the conversion of sputum cultures to negative status.

An important reason for follow-up care in the patient with TB is to ensure adherence to the treatment regimen. Noncompliance is a major factor in the emergence of multidrug resistance and treatment failures. Many individuals do not adhere to the treatment program in spite of understanding the disease process and the value of treatment. Directly observed therapy (DOT) is recommended for patients known to be at risk for noncompliance with therapy. DOT is an expensive but essential public health issue. DOT involves observing the ingestion of every dose of medication for the TB patient's entire course of treatment. Completing therapy is important because of the danger of reactivation of TB and multidrug-resistant TB seen in patients who do not complete the full course of therapy. In many areas the public health nurse administers DOT at a clinic site. The patient needs to have follow-up visits for 12 months after completion of therapy to check for the presence of resistant strains.

Teaching patients about the side effects of these drugs and when to seek prompt medical attention is critical. The major side effect of isoniazid, rifampin, and pyrazinamide is hepatitis.[15] Liver function tests should be monitored.[15] Baseline liver function tests are done at the start of treatment, and routine monitoring of liver function tests is done if baseline tests are abnormal.

Latent tuberculosis infection. *Latent TB infection* (LTBI) occurs when an individual becomes infected with *M. tuberculosis* but does not become acutely ill. Drug therapy can be used to prevent a TB infection from developing into a clinical disease. Previously used terms such as "preventive therapy" and "chemoprophylaxis" were confusing. Therefore LTBI is the preferred terminology.[15] The indications for treatment of LTBI are presented in Table 27-11.

The drug generally used in treatment of LTBI is isoniazid (INH). It is effective and inexpensive and can be administered orally. Isoniazid is usually administered once daily for 6 to 9 months. INH can be given daily or twice weekly. The 9-month regimen is more effective, but compliance issues may make the 6-month regimen preferable. For HIV patients and those with fibrotic lesions on chest x-ray, INH is given for 9 months.

Vaccine. Immunization with bacille Calmette-Guérin (BCG) vaccine to prevent tuberculosis is currently in use in many parts of the world. Although millions of people have been vaccinated with BCG, the efficacy of the vaccine is not clear. BCG vaccination can result in a positive PPD reaction. The BCG vaccine reaction will wane over time, and the mean reaction size among persons who

TABLE 27-11 Indications for Treatment of Latent Tuberculosis Infection

- Newly infected patient at high risk
- Person with known or suspected HIV infection and positive skin test
- Exposure of household members and other close associates to newly diagnosed patient
- Significant tuberculin skin test reactors with abnormal chest x-ray
- Significant tuberculin skin test reactors in special clinical situations (immunosuppression therapy, use of corticosteroids, diabetes mellitus, silicosis, gastrectomy, end-stage renal disease, head and neck cancer)
- Other significant tuberculin skin test converters (10 mm increase within a 2-yr period regardless of age)
- Other significant tuberculin skin test reactors (persons born outside of the United States from high-prevalence countries; medically underserved low-income populations including high risk racial or ethnic populations [e.g., Asian/Pacific Islanders, American Indian/Alaskan Native, African Americans, Hispanics], residents in long-term care facilities, health care workers, mycobacteriology laboratory technicians)

Source: American Thoracic Society, 2000.
HIV, Human immunodeficiency virus.

received BCG is less than 10 mm. Because it may be difficult to determine the relevance of increases in individuals who have undergone BCG vaccination, the American Thoracic Society recommends a conversion to "positive" defined as an increase in induration by 10 mm from a previous PPD test. Persons who receive BCG are from high-prevalence areas of the world, and it is important that a positive skin reaction be evaluated for TB.

NURSING MANAGEMENT
TUBERCULOSIS

■ Nursing Assessment

It is important to determine whether the patient was ever exposed to a person with TB. The patient should be assessed for productive cough, night sweats, afternoon temperature elevation, weight loss, pleuritic chest pain, and crackles over the apices of the lungs. If the patient has a productive cough, an early-morning sputum specimen will be required for an acid-fast bacillus (AFB) smear to detect the presence of mycobacteria.

■ Nursing Diagnoses

Nursing diagnoses for the patient with TB may include, but are not limited to, the following:

- Ineffective breathing pattern *related to* decreased lung capacity
- Imbalanced nutrition: less than body requirements *related to* chronic poor appetite, fatigue, and productive cough
- Noncompliance *related to* lack of knowledge of disease process, lack of motivation, and long-term nature of treatment
- Ineffective health maintenance *related to* lack of knowledge about the disease process and therapeutic regimen
- Activity intolerance *related to* fatigue, decreased nutritional status, and chronic febrile episodes

■ Planning

The overall goals are that the patient with TB will (1) comply with therapeutic regimen, (2) have no recurrence of disease, (3) have normal pulmonary function, and (4) take appropriate measures to prevent the spread of the disease.

■ Nursing Implementation

Health Promotion. The ultimate goal related to TB in the United States is eradication. Selective screening programs in known risk groups are of value in detecting individuals with TB. The person with a positive tuberculin skin test should have a chest x-ray to assess for the presence of TB. Another important measure is to identify the contacts of the individual who has TB. These contacts should be assessed for the possibility of infection and the need for chemoprophylactic treatment.

When an individual has respiratory symptoms such as cough, dyspnea, or sputum production, especially if accompanied by a history of night sweats or unexplained weight loss, the nurse should assess for exposure to persons with TB. Even if the suspected respiratory problem is something else, such as emphysema, pneumonia, or lung cancer, it is possible that the patient may also have TB.

Acute Intervention. Acute in-hospital care is seldom required for the patient with TB. If hospitalization is needed, it is usually for a brief period. Patients strongly suspected of having TB should (1) be placed on respiratory isolation; (2) receive four-drug therapy; and (3) receive an immediate medical workup, including chest x-ray, sputum smear, and culture. Respiratory isolation is indicated for the patient with pulmonary or laryngeal TB until the patient is considered to be noninfectious (effective drug therapy, improving clinically, three negative AFB smears).[18] A negative pressure isolation room that offers six or more exchanges per hour may be used. Ultraviolet radiation of the air in the upper part of the room is another approach to reduce airborne TB organisms. Ultraviolet lights are commonly seen in clinics and homeless shelters. Masks are needed to filter out droplet nuclei. High-efficiency particulate air (HEPA) masks are indicated because they can remove almost 100% of particles greater than 3 mm in diameter.[19] The mask must be molded to fit tightly around the nose and mouth.

The patient should be taught to cover the nose and mouth with paper tissue every time he or she coughs, sneezes, or produces sputum. The tissues should be thrown into a paper bag and disposed of with the trash, burned, or flushed down the toilet. The patient should also be taught careful hand-washing techniques after handling sputum and soiled tissues. Special precautions should be taken during high risk procedures such as sputum induction, aerosolized pentamidine (NebuPent) treatments, intubation, bronchoscopy, or endoscopy.

Ambulatory and Home Care. Patients who have responded clinically are discharged home despite positive smears if their household contacts have already been exposed and the patient is not posing a risk to susceptible persons. Determination of absolute noninfectiousness requires negative cultures. Most treatment failures occur because the patient neglects to take the drug, discontinues it prematurely, or takes it irregularly. On discharge, the physician may order Rifater or Rifamate, a fixed-dose combination drug, to increase compliance and ensure that all drugs are being taken, reducing the risk of drug resistance.

It is important for the nurse to develop a therapeutic, consistent relationship with each patient. The nurse must understand

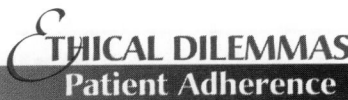

ETHICAL DILEMMAS
Patient Adherence

Situation

The health clinic for the homeless discovers that a Native American man with tuberculosis (TB) has not been complying with taking his medication. He tells the nurse that it is hard for him to get to the clinic to obtain the medication, much less to keep on a schedule. The nurse is concerned not only about this patient, but also about the risks for the other people at the shelter, in the park, and at the meal sites.

Important Points for Consideration

- Adherence is a complex issue involving a person's culture and values, perceived risk of disease, availability of resources, access to treatment, and perceived consequences of available choices.
- Nurses in the community are concerned not only with providing benefits and supporting decision making for individual patients, but also the health and well-being of the entire community.
- Greater harm may result for the community when more virulent drug-resistant strains of microorganisms develop as a consequence of partial treatment or inability of the patient to complete a course of therapy.
- Advocacy for the patient and the community obliges the nurse to involve other members of the health care team, such as social services, to assist in obtaining the necessary resources or support to facilitate completing the course of treatment by the patient.
- If the patient is unable to comply with the treatment program even with necessary supports in place, concern for the public's health would take priority and necessitate placing him in a supervised living situation until his treatment is completed.

Critical Thinking Questions

1. Under what circumstances are health care providers justified in overriding a patient's autonomy or decision making?
2. How would you determine if there were cultural beliefs interfering with this man's ability to understand the importance of completing the treatment? What would you do about it?

the patient's lifestyle and provide flexibility in planning a program that facilitates the patient's participation in and completion of therapy. The nurse should teach the patient so that the need for dedication to the prescribed regimen is fully understood by the patient. Ongoing reassurance helps the patient understand that adherence can mean cure. If the patient cannot or will not adhere to a self-administered medication regimen, medication may have to be given by a responsible person on a daily or intermittent basis. Notification of the public health department is essential if drug compliance is questionable so that follow-up of close contacts can be accomplished. In some cases the public health nurse will be responsible for DOT. In other situations, a spouse, grown child, other relative living with the patient, or co-worker may be asked to supervise drug taking.

Some patients may feel that there is a social stigma attached to TB. These feelings should be discussed, and the patient should be reassured that an individual with TB can be cured if the prescribed regimen is followed. Many people still remember when TB patients were sent away to TB sanitariums and isolated from society. The American Lung Association provides excellent literature for teaching about the disease, as well as providing emotional support to the patient and family.

When the chemotherapy regimen has been completed and there is evidence of negative cultures, the patient is improving clinically, and there is radiologic evidence of improvement, most individuals can be considered adequately treated. Follow-up care may be indicated during the subsequent 12 months, including bacteriologic studies and chest x-ray. Because approximately 5% of individuals experience relapses, the patient should be taught to recognize the symptoms that indicate recurrence of TB. If these symptoms occur, immediate medical attention should be sought.

The patient needs to be instructed about certain factors that could reactivate TB, such as immunosuppressive therapy, malignancy, and prolonged debilitating illness. If the patient experiences any of these events, the health care provider must to be told so that reactivation of TB can be closely monitored. In some situations it may be necessary to put the patient on anti-TB therapy.

■ Evaluation

The expected outcomes are that the patient with TB will have
- complete resolution of the disease
- normal pulmonary function
- absence of any complications
- no transmission of TB

ATYPICAL MYCOBACTERIA

Pulmonary disease that closely resembles TB may be caused by atypical acid-fast mycobacteria. This type of pulmonary disease is indistinguishable from TB clinically and radiologically but can be differentiated by bacteriologic culture. These organisms are not believed to be airborne and thus are not transmitted by droplet nuclei.

Atypical mycobacteria that affect the lung include *M. kansasii, M. scrofulaceum, M. intracellulare,* and *M. xenopi.* These bacteria (especially *M. avium-intracellulare* and *M. scrofulaceum*) may also invade the cervical lymph nodes, causing lymphadenitis. This type of pulmonary disease typically occurs in white men with a history of COPD, cystic fibrosis, or silicosis. *Mycobacterium avium-intracellulare* is a common cause of opportunistic infections in the patient with HIV infection (see Chapter 14).

Treatment depends on identification of the causative agent and determination of drug sensitivity. Many of the drugs used in treating TB are used in combating infections from atypical mycobacteria.

PULMONARY FUNGAL INFECTIONS

Pulmonary fungal infections are increasing in incidence. They are found most frequently in seriously ill patients being treated with corticosteroids, antineoplastic and immunosuppressive drugs, or multiple antibiotics. They are also found in patients with AIDS and cystic fibrosis. Types of fungal infections are presented in Table 27-12. These infections are not transmitted from person to person, and the patient does not have to be placed in isolation. The clinical manifestations are similar to those of bacterial pneumonia. Skin and serology tests are available to assist in identifying the infecting organism. However, identification of

TABLE 27-12   **Fungal Infections of the Lung**

ORGANISM	CHARACTERISTICS
Histoplasmosis *Histoplasma capsulatum*	Indigenous to soil of North American river valleys, inhalation of mycelia into lungs, infected individual often free of symptoms, generally self-limiting, chronic disease similar to TB
Coccidioidomycosis *Coccidioides immitis*	Indigenous to semiarid regions of southwestern United States, inhalation of arthrospores into lungs, suppurative and granulomatous reaction in lungs, symptomatic infection in one third of individuals
Blastomycosis *Blastomyces dermatitidis*	Indigenous to southeastern and midwestern United States, inhalation of fungus into lungs, progression of disease often insidious, possible involvement of skin
Cryptococcosis *Cryptococcus neoformans*	True yeast, indigenous worldwide in soil and pigeon excreta, inhalation of fungus into lungs, possible meningitis
Aspergillosis *Aspergillus niger or* *Aspergillus fumigatus*	True mold inhabiting mouth, widely distributed, invasion of lung tissue resulting in possible necrotizing pneumonia; in individual with asthma, allergic bronchopulmonary aspergillosis may require corticosteroid therapy
Candidiasis *Candida albicans*	Leading cause of mycotic infections in hospitalized and immunocompromised hosts, ubiquitous and frequent colonization of upper respiratory and GI tracts, infections often following broad-spectrum antibiotic therapy (systemic or inhaled), possible development of localized pulmonary infiltrate to widespread bilateral consolidation with hypoxemia
Actinomycosis *Actinomyces israeli*	Not a true fungus, pseudohyphae present; anaerobic; gram-positive, higher bacteria with branching hyphae; presence of necrotizing pneumonia after aspiration; pneumonitis, commonly in lower lobes with abscess or empyema formation
Nocardiosis *Nocardia asteroides*	Not a true fungus; aerobic, higher bacteria with branching hyphae; soil saprophyte widely distributed in nature; acquisition of infection from nature; rarely present in sputum without accompanying disease

the organism in a sputum specimen or in other body fluids is the best diagnostic indicator.

Collaborative Care

Amphotericin B is the drug most widely used in treating serious systemic fungal infections. It must be given intravenously to achieve adequate blood and tissue levels because it is poorly absorbed from the GI tract. Amphotericin B is considered a toxic drug with many possible side effects, including hypersensitivity reactions, fever, chills, malaise, nausea and vomiting, thrombophlebitis at the injection site, and abnormal renal function. Many of the side effects during infusion can be avoided by premedicating with an antiinflammatory or diphenhydramine (Benadryl) 1 hour before the infusion. Inclusion of a small amount of hydrocortisone in the infusion helps decrease the irritation of the veins. Monitoring of renal function and ensuring adequate hydration is essential while a person is receiving this drug. Renal changes are at least partially reversible. Amphotericin infusions are incompatible with most other drugs. Amphotericin is frequently administered every other day after an initial period of several weeks of daily therapy. Total treatment with the drug may range from 4 to 12 weeks.

Oral imidazole and triazole compounds with antifungal activity such as ketoconazole (Nizoral), fluconazole (Diflucan), or itraconazole (Sporanox) have been successful in the treatment of fungal infections. Their effectiveness in treatment allows an alternative to the use of amphotericin B in many cases. Effectiveness of therapy can be monitored with fungal serology titers.

Flucytosine (Ancobon) has also been used in selected types of pulmonary fungal infections. It is given orally. Common adverse reactions include nausea, vomiting, diarrhea, and abdominal discomfort. Antiemetics may be helpful. Hepatotoxicity and bone marrow suppression may occur. Frequent blood monitoring, including complete blood count (CBC), potassium levels, and renal and hepatic function, is done.

BRONCHIECTASIS

Etiology and Pathophysiology

Bronchiectasis is characterized by permanent, abnormal dilation of one or more large bronchi.[20] The pathophysiologic change that results in dilation is destruction of the elastic and muscular structures of the bronchial wall. There are two pathologic types of bronchiectasis: saccular and cylindric (Fig. 27-2). *Saccular*

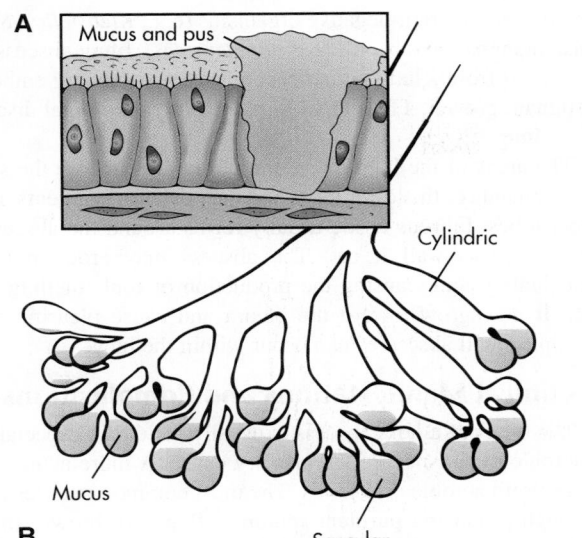

FIG. 27-2 Pathologic changes in bronchiectasis. A, Longitudinal section of bronchial wall where chronic infection has caused damage. B, Collection of purulent material in dilated bronchioles, leading to persistent infection.

bronchiectasis occurs mainly in large bronchi and is characterized by cavity-like dilations. The affected bronchi end in large sacs. *Cylindric bronchiectasis* involves medium-sized bronchi that are mildly to moderately dilated.

Almost all forms of bronchiectasis are associated with bacterial infections. A wide variety of infectious agents can initiate bronchiectasis, including adenovirus, influenza virus, *S. aureus, Klebsiella,* and anaerobes. Infections cause the bronchial walls to weaken, and pockets of infection begin to form. When the walls of the bronchial system are injured, the mucociliary mechanism is damaged, allowing bacteria and mucus to accumulate within the pockets. The infection becomes worse and results in bronchiectasis.

The incidence of bronchiectasis has shown a decline in recent years. The emergence of atypical mycobacteria, especially *M. avium-intracellulare* (MAI), presents a new threat because MAI can progress to bronchiectasis. MAI is an opportunistic infection found in patients with HIV.

Clinical Manifestations

The hallmark of bronchiectasis is persistent or recurrent cough with production of greater than 20 ml of purulent sputum per day. The cough is paroxysmal and is often stimulated with position changes. Other manifestations include exertional dyspnea, fatigue, weight loss, anorexia, and fetid breath. On auscultation of the lungs, any combination of crackles, rhonchi, and wheezing may be heard. Sinusitis frequently accompanies diffuse bronchiectasis. The manifestations of advanced, widespread bronchiectasis are generalized wheezing, digital clubbing, and cor pulmonale.

Diagnostic Studies

An individual with a chronic productive cough with copious purulent sputum (which may be blood streaked) should be suspected of having bronchiectasis. Chest x-rays are usually done and may show streaky infiltrates or may be normal. With the

availability of CT scanning, detecting bronchiectasis has improved. High-resolution CT scan of the chest has excellent sensitivity for detecting bronchiectasis. Bronchoscopy can also be useful in identifying the source of secretions, in identifying sites of hemoptysis, or for collecting microbiologic samples.

Sputum may provide additional information regarding the severity of impairment and the presence of active infection. Pulmonary function studies may be abnormal in advanced bronchiectasis, showing a decrease in vital capacity, expiratory flow, and maximum voluntary ventilation. CBC may be normal or show evidence of leukocytosis or anemia from chronic infection.

Collaborative Care

Bronchiectasis is difficult to treat. Therapy is aimed at treating acute flare-ups and preventing decline in lung function. Antibiotics are the mainstay of treatment and are given on the basis of sputum culture results. Long-term suppressive therapy with antibiotics is occasionally used but is fraught with risks of antibiotic resistance. A form of treatment gaining popularity is the use of nebulized antibiotics. Studies indicate that it is safe and may reduce the number of flare-ups and hospitalizations in bronchiectatic patients.[20] Antipseudomonal antibiotics, such as tobramycin (Nebcin), are commonly used. Concurrent bronchodilator therapy is given to prevent bronchospasm. Other forms of drug therapy may include mucolytic agents and expectorants. Maintaining good hydration is important to liquefy secretions. Chest physical therapy and other airway clearance techniques are important to facilitate expectoration of sputum. (These techniques are discussed in Chapter 28.) The individual should reduce exposure to excessive air pollutants and irritants, avoid cigarette smoking, and obtain pneumococcal and influenza vaccinations.

Surgical resection of parts of the lungs, although not used as often as previously, may be done if more conservative treatment is not effective. Surgical resection of an affected lobe or segment may be indicated for the patient with repeated bouts of pneumonia, hemoptysis, and disabling complications. Surgery is not advisable when there is diffuse or widespread involvement. For selected patients who are disabled in spite of maximal therapy, lung transplantation is an option. (Lung transplantation is discussed later in this chapter.)

NURSING MANAGEMENT
BRONCHIECTASIS

The early detection and treatment of lower respiratory tract infections will help prevent complications such as bronchiectasis. Any obstructing lesion or foreign body should be removed promptly. Other measures to decrease the occurrence or progression of bronchiectasis include avoiding cigarette smoking and decreasing exposure to pollution and irritants.

An important nursing goal is to promote drainage and removal of bronchial mucus. Various airway clearance techniques can be effectively used to facilitate secretion removal. The patient should be taught effective deep-breathing exercises and effective ways to cough (see Chapter 28, Table 28-21). Chest physical therapy with postural drainage should be done on affected parts of the lung (see Chapter 28, Fig. 28-16). Some individuals require elevation of the foot of the bed by 4 to 6 inches to facilitate drainage. Pillows may be used in the hospital and at home to help the patient assume postural drainage positions. A Flutter mucus clearance device is a handheld device that provides airway vibration during the expiratory phase of breathing (see Chapter 28, Fig. 28-17). Two to four 15-minute sessions daily by a patient who has been properly trained can provide satisfactory mucus clearance. Positive expiratory pressure (PEP) therapy is a breathing maneuver against an expiratory resistance often used in conjunction with nebulized medications. (Respiratory therapy procedures are explained in Chapter 28.)

Administration of the prescribed antibiotics, bronchodilators, or expectorants is important. The patient needs to understand the importance of taking the prescribed regimen of drugs to obtain maximum effectiveness. The patient should be aware of possible side effects or adverse effects that must be reported to the physician.

Rest is important to prevent overexertion. Bed rest may be indicated during the acute phase of the illness. Chilling and excess fatigue should be avoided.

Good nutrition is important and may be difficult to maintain because the patient is often anorexic. Oral hygiene to cleanse the mouth and remove dried sputum crusts may improve the patient's appetite. Offering foods that are appealing may also increase the desire to eat. Adequate hydration to help liquefy secretions and thus make it easier to remove them is extremely important. Unless there are contraindications such as concomitant congestive heart failure or renal disease, the patient should be instructed to drink at least 3 L of fluid daily. To accomplish this, the patient should be advised to increase fluid consumption from the baseline by increasing intake by one glass per day until the goal is reached. Generally the patient should be counseled to use low-sodium fluids to avoid systemic fluid retention.

Direct hydration of the respiratory system may also prove beneficial in the expectoration of secretions. Usually a bland aerosol with normal saline solution delivered by a jet-type nebulizer is used. The patient with bronchiectasis should avoid ultrasonic nebulizers because they often induce bronchospasm. At home a steamy shower can prove effective; expensive equipment that requires frequent cleaning is usually unnecessary. It is important that the patient medicate with an inhaled bronchodilator 10 to 15 minutes before using a bland aerosol to prevent bronchoconstriction.

The patient and family should be taught to recognize significant clinical manifestations to be reported to the health care provider. These manifestations include increased sputum production, grossly bloody sputum, increasing dyspnea, fever, chills, and chest pain.

LUNG ABSCESS

Etiology and Pathophysiology

Lung abscess is a pus-containing lesion of the lung parenchyma that gives rise to a cavity. The cavity is formed by necrosis of the lung tissue. In many cases the causes and pathogenesis of lung abscess are similar to those of pneumonia. Most lung abscesses are caused by aspiration of material from the oral cavity (the gingival crevices) into the lungs. Risk factors for aspiration include alcoholism, seizure disorders, neuromuscular diseases, drug overdose, general anesthesia, and stroke. Infectious agents generally cause lung abscesses. The organisms involved cause infection and necrosis of the lung tissue. Examples

include enteric gram-negative organisms (e.g., *Klebsiella*), *S. aureus,* and anaerobic bacilli (e.g., *Bacteroides*). Lung abscess can also result from a lung infarct secondary to pulmonary embolus, malignant growth, TB, and various parasitic and fungal diseases of the lung.

The areas of the lung most commonly affected are the superior segments of the lower lobes and the posterior segments of the upper lobes. Fibrous tissue usually forms around the abscess in an attempt to wall it off. The abscess may erode into the bronchial system, causing the production of foul-smelling sputum. It may grow toward the pleura and cause pleuritic pain. Multiple small abscesses can occur within the lung.

Clinical Manifestations and Complications

The onset of a lung abscess is usually insidious, especially if anaerobic organisms are the primary cause. A more acute onset occurs with aerobic organisms. The most common manifestation is cough-producing purulent sputum (often dark brown) that is foul smelling and foul tasting. Hemoptysis is common, especially at the time that an abscess ruptures into a bronchus. Other common manifestations are fever, chills, prostration, pleuritic pain, dyspnea, cough, and weight loss.

Physical examination of the lungs indicates dullness to percussion and decreased breath sounds on auscultation over the segment of lung involved. There may be transmission of bronchial breath sounds to the periphery if the communicating bronchus becomes patent and drainage of the segment begins. Crackles may also be present in the later stages as the abscess drains. Oral examination often reveals dental caries, gingivitis, and periodontal infection.

Complications that can occur include chronic pulmonary abscess, bronchiectasis, and brain abscess as a result of the hematogenous spread of infection, bronchopleural fistula, and empyema from abscess perforation into the pleural cavity.

Diagnostic Studies

A chest x-ray will reveal a solitary cavitary lesion with fluid.[21] CT scanning is used if there is a question of cavitation not clearly seen. Lung abscess, in contrast to other types of abscesses, does not require assisted drainage, as long as there is drainage via the bronchus. Routine sputum cultures can be collected, but contaminants can confuse the results and it is difficult to isolate anaerobic bacteria. Pleural fluid and blood cultures may be obtained. Bronchoscopy may be used in cases of abscess in which drainage is delayed or in which there are factors that suggest an underlying malignancy.

NURSING *and* COLLABORATIVE MANAGEMENT LUNG ABSCESS

Antibiotics given for a prolonged period (up to 2 to 4 months) are usually the primary method of treatment. Penicillin has historically been the drug of choice because of the frequent presence of anaerobic organisms. However, recent studies suggest that there is β-lactamase production by the anaerobic bacteria involved in abscesses of the lung and they are resistant to penicillin. Clindamycin (Cleocin) has been shown to be superior to penicillin and is the standard treatment for an anaerobic lung infection. Patients with putrid lung abscesses usually show clinical improvement with decreased fever within 3 to 4 days of beginning antibiotics.

Because of the need for prolonged antibiotic therapy, the patient must be aware of the importance of continuing the medication for the prescribed period. The patient needs to know about untoward side effects to be reported to the health care provider. Sometimes the patient is asked to return periodically during the course of antibiotic therapy for repeat cultures and sensitivity tests to ensure that the infecting organism is not becoming resistant to the antibiotic. When antibiotic therapy is completed, the patient is reevaluated.

The patient should be taught how to cough effectively (see Chapter 28, Table 28-21). Chest physiotherapy and postural drainage are sometimes used to drain abscesses located in the lower or posterior portions of the lung. Postural drainage according to the lung area involved will aid the removal of secretions (see Chapter 28, Fig. 28-16). Frequent (every 2 to 3 hours) mouth care is needed to relieve the foul-smelling odor and taste from the sputum. Diluted hydrogen peroxide and mouthwash are often effective.

Rest, good nutrition, and adequate fluid intake are all supportive measures to facilitate recovery. If dentition is poor and dental hygiene is not adequate, the patient should be encouraged to obtain dental care.

Surgery is rarely indicated but occasionally may be necessary when reinfection of a large cavitary lesion occurs or to establish a diagnosis when there is evidence of an underlying neoplasm or chronic associated disease. The usual procedure in such cases is a lobectomy or pneumonectomy. An alternative to surgery is percutaneous drainage, but this has a high risk of contamination of the pleural space.

ENVIRONMENTAL LUNG DISEASES

Environmental or occupational lung diseases result from inhaled dust or chemicals. The duration of exposure and the amount of inhalant have a major influence on whether the exposed individual will have lung damage. Another factor is the susceptibility of the host.

Pneumoconiosis is a general term for lung diseases caused by inhalation and retention of dust particles. The literal meaning of *pneumoconiosis* is "dust in the lungs." Examples of this condition are silicosis, asbestosis, and berylliosis. The classic response to the inhaled substance is diffuse parenchymal infiltration with phagocytic cells. This eventually results in diffuse pulmonary fibrosis (excess connective tissue). Fibrosis is the result of tissue repair after inflammation. Pneumoconiosis and other environmental lung diseases are presented in Table 27-13. Hantavirus, a potentially fatal disease with outbreaks reported in the United States and Canada, is transmitted by inhalation of aerosolized rodent excreta.[22]

Chemical pneumonitis results from exposures to toxic chemical fumes. Acutely there is diffuse lung injury characterized as pulmonary edema. Chronically the clinical picture is that of bronchiolitis obliterans, which is usually associated with a normal chest x-ray or one that shows hyperinflation. An example is silo filler's disease.

Hypersensitivity pneumonitis or extrinsic allergic alveolitis is the response seen when antigens are inhaled to which an individual is allergic. Examples include bird fancier's lung and farmer's lung.

Lung cancer, either squamous cell carcinoma or adenocarcinoma, is the most frequent cancer associated with asbestos exposure. People with more exposure are at a greater risk of disease. There is a minimum lapse of 15 to 19 years between first exposure and development of lung cancer. Mesotheliomas, both pleural and peritoneal, are also associated with asbestos exposure.

Clinical Manifestations

Acute symptoms of pulmonary edema may be seen following early exposures to chemical fumes. However, symptoms of many environmental lung diseases may not occur until at least 10 to 15 years after the initial exposure to the inhaled irritant. Dyspnea and cough are often the earliest manifestations. Chest pain and cough with sputum production usually occur later. Complications that often result are pneumonia, chronic bronchitis, emphysema, and lung cancer. Cor pulmonale is a late complication, especially in conditions characterized by diffuse pulmonary fibrosis. Manifestations of these complications can be the reason the patient seeks health care.

Pulmonary function studies often show reduced vital capacity. A chest x-ray will often reveal lung involvement specific to the primary problem. CT scans have been shown to be useful in detecting early lung involvement.

Occupational asthma refers to the development of symptoms of shortness of breath, wheezing, cough, and chest tightness as a result of exposure to fumes or dust that trigger an allergic response. The obstruction may initially be reversible or intermittent, but continued exposure results in permanent obstructive changes. The best-known causative agent in occupational asthma is toluene diisocyanate (TDI), which is used in the production of rigid polyurethane foam.

Collaborative Care

The best approach to management is to try to prevent or decrease environmental and occupational risks. Well-designed, effective ventilation systems can reduce exposure to irritants. Wearing masks is appropriate in some occupations. Periodic inspections and monitoring of workplaces by agencies such as the Occupational Safety and Health Administration (OSHA) and the National Institute for Occupational Safety and Health (NIOSH) reinforce the obligations of employers to provide a safe work environment.

Cigarette smoking adds increased insult to the lungs, and the person at risk for occupational lung disease should not smoke. Additionally, secondhand smoke is an important source of occupational exposure with increased risk for development of lung cancer. This has led to regulations requiring a smoke-free workspace for all employees.

Early diagnosis is essential if the disease process is to be halted. Some places of employment, where there is a known risk of lung disease, may require periodic chest x-rays and pulmonary function studies for exposed employees. These measures can detect pulmonary changes before symptoms develop.

There is no specific treatment for most environmental lung diseases. The best treatment is to decrease or stop exposure to the harmful agent. Strategies are directed toward providing symptomatic relief. If there are coexisting problems, such as pneumonia, chronic bronchitis, emphysema, or asthma, they are treated.

TABLE 27-13 **Environmental Lung Diseases**

DISEASE	AGENTS/INDUSTRIES	DESCRIPTION	COMPLICATIONS
• Asbestosis	Asbestos fibers present in insulation, construction material (roof tiling, cement products), shipyards, textiles (for fireproofing), automobile clutch and brake linings	Disease appears 15-35 yr after first exposure. Interstitial fibrosis develops. Pleural plaques, which are calcified lesions, develop on pleura. Dyspnea, basal crackles, and decreased vital capacity are early manifestations.	Diffuse interstitial pulmonary fibrosis; lung cancer, especially in cigarette smokers; mesothelioma (rare type of cancer affecting pleura and peritoneal membrane)
• Berylliosis	Beryllium dust present in aircraft manufacturing, metallurgy, rocket fuels	Formation of noncaseating granulomas. Acute pneumonitis occurs after heavy exposure. Interstitial fibrosis can also occur.	Progress of disease possible after removal of stimulating inhalant
• Bird fancier's, breeder's, or handler's lung	Bird droppings or feathers	Hypersensitivity pneumonitis is present.	Progressive fibrosis of lung
• Byssinosis	Cotton, flax, and hemp dust (textile industry)	Airway obstruction is caused by contraction of smooth muscles. Chronic disease results from severe airway obstruction and decreased elastic recoil.	Progression of chronic disease after cessation of dust exposure
• Coalworker's pneumoconiosis (black lung)	Coal dust	Incidence is high (20-30%) in coal workers. Deposits of carbon dust cause lesions to develop along respiratory bronchioles. Bronchioles dilate because of loss of wall structure. Chronic airway obstruction and bronchitis develop. Dyspnea and cough are common early symptoms.	Progressive, massive lung fibrosis; increased risk of chronic bronchitis and emphysema with smoking
• Farmer's lung	Inhalation of airborne material from moldy hay or similar matter	Hypersensitivity pneumonitis occurs. *Acute* form is similar to pneumonia, with manifestations of chills, fever, and malaise. *Chronic*, insidious form is type of pulmonary fibrosis.	Progressive fibrosis of lung
• Hantavirus pulmonary syndrome (HPS)	Rodent droppings inhaled while in rodent-infested areas	Acute hemorrhagic fever associated with severe pulmonary and cardiovascular collapse and death. Incubation period is 1-4 wk with prodrome (3-5 days) of flulike symptoms. No cure or specific treatment exists.	CDC recommends rapid transfer to ICU with careful monitoring of fluid and electrolyte balance and blood pressure; supportive therapy and early intervention vital; research on this virus is done in high-level biocontainment facilities
• Siderosis	Iron oxide present in welding materials, foundries, iron ore mining	Dust deposits are found in lung.	
• Silicosis	Silica dust present in quartz rock in mining of gold, copper, tin, coal, lead; also present in sandblasting, foundries, quarries, pottery making, masonry	In *chronic disease*, dust is engulfed by macrophages and may be destroyed, resulting in fibrotic nodules. *Acute disease* results from intense exposure in short time period. Within 5 yr, it progresses to severe disability from lung fibrosis.	Increased susceptibility to tuberculosis; progressive, massive fibrosis; high incidence of chronic bronchitis
• Silo filler's disease	Nitrogen oxides from fermentation of vegetation in freshly filled silo	Chemical pneumonitis occurs.	Progressive bronchiolitis obliterans

CDC, Centers for Disease Control and Prevention; *ICU,* intensive care unit.

LUNG CANCER

Lung cancer is the leading cause of cancer-related deaths in men and women in the United States. In 2002 an estimated 157,400 deaths were expected.[21] Beginning in 1987, deaths from lung cancer in women exceeded deaths from all other cancers. The Surgeon General's report, *Women and Smoking: A Report of the Surgeon General—2001,* identified a 600% increase in women's death rates from lung cancer and attributes this to smoking. Lung cancer in women is now considered to be an epidemic.[23] In 2002, 25% of all female deaths were estimated to be due to lung cancer. In addition, a total of 36.5% of teenagers, male and female, smoke. The overall 5-year survival rate from lung cancer is 14%. California, with an aggressive antismoking campaign, has seen a decline in rates, whereas the rest of the nation's rates continue to escalate.

Lung cancer most commonly occurs in individuals more than 50 years of age who have a long history of cigarette smoking. The disease is found most frequently in persons 40 to 75 years of age, with peak incidence between 55 and 65 years of age.

Etiology

Cigarette smoking is the most important risk factor in the development of lung cancer. Smoking is responsible for approximately 80% to 90% of all lung cancers. Tobacco smoke contains 60 carcinogens in addition to substances (carbon monoxide, nicotine) that interfere with normal cell development. Cigarette smoking, a lower airway irritant, causes a change in the bronchial epithelium, which usually returns to normal when smoking is discontinued. The risk of lung cancer is gradually lowered when smoking ceases and continues to decline with time. After 10 years following cessation of smoking, lung cancer mortality risk is reduced 30% to 50%.[21]

The risk of developing lung cancer is directly related to total exposure to cigarette smoke measured by total number of cigarettes smoked in a lifetime, earlier age of smoking onset, depth of inhalation, tar and nicotine content, and the use of unfiltered cigarettes. Sidestream smoke contains the same carcinogens found in mainstream smoke. This environmental tobacco smoke (ETS) inhaled by nonsmokers poses a 35% increased risk of the development of lung cancer in nonsmokers.[24] This exposure can occur early in life for children of smokers. Children are more vulnerable to ETS than adults because their respiratory and immune systems are not fully developed. Recent data suggest that childhood exposure to ETS is associated with increased prevalence of asthma among adults and that children exposed to ETS are more likely to become smokers.[25]

CULTURAL & ETHNIC CONSIDERATIONS
Lung Cancer

- Lung cancer occurs more frequently and has a higher mortality rate among African Americans than among whites.
- The mortality rate of lung cancer for white women surpasses that for African American women.
- Cigarette consumption has decreased dramatically in developed countries such as the United States and Canada; however, it is increasing in developing countries (e.g., nations in Africa, Asia, Latin America).

Those who smoke pipes and cigars have also been shown to have an increased risk of developing lung cancer, which is slightly higher than that of nonsmokers. Cigar smokers are at higher rate for lung cancer than are pipe smokers. However, heavy smoking of cigars and inhalation of smoke from small cigars have been shown to correlate with the rates of lung cancer observed in cigarette smokers.

Another major risk factor for lung cancer is inhaled carcinogens. These include asbestos, radon, nickel, iron and iron oxides, uranium, polycyclic aromatic hydrocarbons, chromates, arsenic, and air pollution. Exposure to these substances is common for employees of industries involved in mining, smelting, or chemical or petroleum manufacturing. The cigarette smoker who is also exposed to one or more of these chemicals or to high amounts of air pollution is at significantly higher risk for lung cancer.

There are marked variations in a person's propensity to develop lung cancer. To date no genetic abnormality has conclusively been defined for lung cancer. It is known that the carcinogens in cigarette smoke directly damage DNA. One theory is that people have different genetic carcinogen-metabolizing pathways.

Pathophysiology

The pathogenesis of primary lung cancer is not well understood. More than 90% of cancers originate from the epithelium of the bronchus (bronchogenic). They grow slowly, and it takes 8 to 10 years for a tumor to reach 1 cm in size, which is the smallest detectable lesion on an x-ray. Lung cancers occur primarily in the segmental bronchi or beyond and have a preference for the upper lobes of the lungs (Fig. 27-3). Pathologic changes in the bronchial system show nonspecific inflammatory changes with hypersecretion of mucus, desquamation of cells, reactive hyperplasia of the basal cells, and metaplasia of normal respiratory epithelium to stratified squamous cells. (Pathologic types of lung cancer are presented in Fig. 27-4.)

Primary lung cancers are often categorized into two broad subtypes (Table 27-14), non–small cell lung cancer (75%) and small cell lung cancer (25%). Lung cancers metastasize primar-

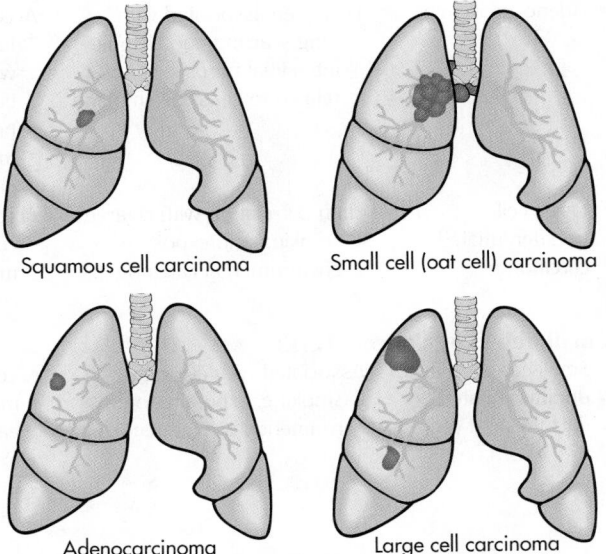

Squamous cell carcinoma   Small cell (oat cell) carcinoma

Adenocarcinoma   Large cell carcinoma

FIG. 27-3 Predominant sites of types of lung cancer.

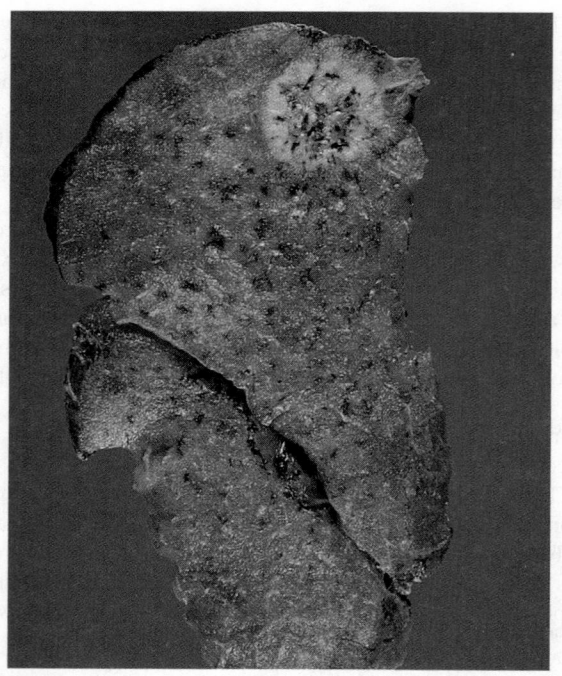

FIG. 27-4 | Lung cancer. Peripheral adenocarcinoma. The tumor shows prominent black pigmentation, suggestive of having evolved in an anthracotic scar.

ily by direct extension and via the blood circulation and the lymph system. The common sites for metastatic growth are the liver, brain, bones, scalene lymph nodes, and adrenal glands.

Paraneoplastic Syndrome. Certain lung cancers cause the *paraneoplastic syndrome,* which is characterized by various systemic manifestations caused by factors (e.g., hormones, enzymes, antigens) produced by the tumor cells. Small cell lung cancers (SCLCs) are most commonly associated with the paraneoplastic syndrome. The systemic manifestations seen are hormonal, dermatologic, neuromuscular, vascular, hematologic, and connective tissue syndromes. These syndromes can respond temporarily to symptomatic treatment, but they are impossible to control without successful treatment of the underlying lung cancer.

Clinical Manifestations

Lung cancer is clinically silent for most individuals for the majority of its course. The clinical manifestations of lung cancer are usually nonspecific and appear late in the disease process. Manifestations depend on the type of primary lung cancer, its location, and metastatic spread. Often there is extensive metastasis before symptoms become apparent. Persistent pneumonitis that is a result of obstructed bronchi may be one of the earliest manifestations, causing fever, chills, and cough.

One of the most significant symptoms, and often the one reported first, is a persistent cough that may be productive of sputum. Blood-tinged sputum may be produced because of bleeding

TABLE 27-14 | **Comparison of the Types of Primary Lung Cancer**

CELL TYPE	RISK FACTORS	CHARACTERISTICS	RESPONSE TO THERAPY
Non–Small Cell Lung Cancer (NSCLC)			
• Squamous cell (epidermoid) carcinoma	Almost always associated with cigarette smoking; is associated with exposure to environmental carcinogens (e.g., uranium, asbestos)	Accounts for 30%–35% of lung cancers; is more common in men; arises from the bronchial epithelium, produces earlier symptoms because of bronchial obstructive characteristics; does not have a strong tendency to metastasize, metastasizes locally by direct extension, causes cavitating pulmonary lesions	Surgical resection is often attempted; life expectancy is better than for small cell lung cancer
• Adenocarcinoma	Has been associated with lung scarring and chronic interstitial fibrosis; is not related to cigarette smoking	Accounts for approximately 35%–45% of lung cancers; is more common in women; often has no clinical manifestations until widespread metastasis is present; metastasizes via bloodstream; is most commonly located in peripheral portions of lungs*	Surgical resection is often attempted; cancer does not respond well to chemotherapy
• Large cell undifferentiated carcinoma	High correlation with cigarette smoking and exposure to environmental carcinogens	Accounts for 5%–10% of lung cancers; commonly causes cavitation; is highly metastatic via lymphatics and blood; commonly peripheral rather than central	Surgery is not usually attempted because of high rate of metastases; tumor may be radiosensitive but often recurs
Small Cell Lung Cancer (SCLC)			
• Small cell anaplastic undifferentiated (includes oat cell)	Associated with cigarette smoking, exposure to environmental carcinogens	Accounts for 15%–25% of lung cancers; is most malignant form; tends to spread early via lymphatics and bloodstream; is frequently associated with endocrine disturbances; predominantly central and can cause bronchial obstruction and pneumonia	Cancer has poorest prognosis; however, chemotherapy advances have been substantial; radiation is used as adjuvant therapy, as well as palliative measure; average median survival is 12-18 mo

*See Fig. 27-3.

caused by malignancy, but hemoptysis is not a common early symptom. Chest pain may be present and localized or unilateral, ranging from mild to severe. Dyspnea and an auscultatory wheeze may be present if there is bronchial obstruction.

Later manifestations may include nonspecific systemic symptoms such as anorexia, fatigue, weight loss, and nausea and vomiting. Hoarseness may be present as a result of involvement of the recurrent laryngeal nerve. Unilateral paralysis of the diaphragm, dysphagia, and superior vena cava obstruction may occur because of intrathoracic spread of the malignancy. There may be palpable lymph nodes in the neck or axilla. Mediastinal involvement may lead to pericardial effusion, cardiac tamponade, and arrhythmias.

Diagnostic Studies

Chest x-rays are widely used in the diagnosis of lung cancer. The findings may show the presence of the tumor or abnormalities related to the obstructive features of the tumor such as atelectasis and pneumonitis. The x-ray can also show evidence of metastasis to the ribs or vertebrae and the presence of pleural effusion.

CT scanning is the single most effective noninvasive technique for evaluating lung cancer. CT scans of the brain and bone scans complete the evaluation for metastatic disease. With CT scans, the location and extent of masses in the chest can be identified, as well as any mediastinal involvement or lymph node enlargement. Magnetic resonance imaging (MRI) may be used in combination with or instead of CT scans. Positron emission tomography (PET) promises to be a useful diagnostic tool in early clinical staging. PET allows measurement of differential metabolic activity in normal and diseased tissues.

A definitive diagnosis of lung cancer is made by identifying malignant cells. Sputum specimens are usually obtained for cytologic studies. An early-morning specimen that has been obtained by having the patient cough deeply provides the most accurate results. However, malignant cells may not be obtained even in the presence of a lung cancer.

The use of the fiberoptic bronchoscope is important in the diagnosis of lung cancer, particularly when the lesions are endobronchial or are in close proximity to an airway. It provides direct visualization and allows biopsy specimens to be obtained. A biopsy is usually the best method for establishing the presence of a malignant tumor.

Mediastinoscopy involves the insertion of a scope via a small anterior chest incision into the mediastinum. This is done to examine for metastasis in the anterior mediastinum or hilum or in the chest extrapleurally. It is also used to determine the stage of the lung cancer, which is important in determining the treatment plan. Video-assisted thoracoscopy (VATS) involving a scope into a small thoracic incision may be used to explore areas inaccessible by mediastinoscopy.

Pulmonary angiography and lung scans may be performed to assess overall pulmonary status. Fine-needle aspiration (FNA) may be used to obtain a tissue sample to determine tumor histology. FNA is most useful in cases involving a peripheral lesion near the chest wall, and it is usually attempted in an effort to avoid a thoracotomy. If a thoracentesis is performed to relieve a pleural effusion, the fluid should be analyzed for malignant cells. (Table 27-15 summarizes the diagnostic management of lung cancer.)

Staging. Staging of non–small cell lung cancer (NSCLC) is performed according to the TNM staging system in a manner

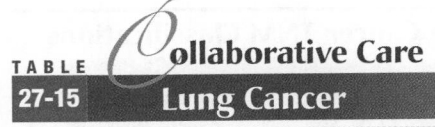

TABLE 27-15	Collaborative Care Lung Cancer

Diagnostic
History and physical examination
Chest x-ray
Sputum for cytologic study
Bronchoscopy
CT scan
MRI
Positron emission tomography (PET)
Spirometry (preoperative)
Mediastinoscopy
Video-assisted thoracoscopy (VAT)
Pulmonary angiography
Lung scan
Fine-needle aspiration

Collaborative Therapy
Surgery
Radiation therapy
Chemotherapy
Biologic therapy
Bronchoscopic laser therapy
Phototherapy
Airway stenting
Cryotherapy

CT, Computed tomography; *MRI,* magnetic resonance imaging.

similar to that for other tumors (Table 27-16). Assessment criteria are T, which denotes tumor size, location, and degree of invasion; N, which indicates regional lymph node involvement; and M, which represents the presence or absence of distant metastases. Depending on the TNM designation, the tumor is then staged, which assists in estimating prognosis and determining the appropriate therapy.

Staging of small cell lung cancer (SCLC) has not been useful because the cancer has usually metastasized by the time a diagnosis is made. Instead, SCLC is determined to be limited (confined to one hemothorax and to regional lymph nodes) or extensive (any disease exceeding those boundaries).

Screening for Lung Cancer. Early screening for lung cancer is controversial. No current recommendations exist in the United States because previous lung cancer screening studies indicated no significant difference in lung cancer deaths between those who were screened and those who were not. High-resolution CT and/or sputum cytology reduces morbidity and mortality rates in high risk patients. In Japan, the standard of care for lung cancer screening includes chest x-ray and sputum cytology with an increase seen in 5-year survival rates. Physicians in the United States and Canada may begin to screen their highest risk patients (i.e., smokers more than 40 years old with spirometry changes, patients with strong family history of lung cancer).[26]

Collaborative Care

Surgical Therapy. Surgical resection is usually the only hope for cure in lung cancer. Unfortunately, detection is often so late that the tumor is no longer localized and is not amenable to resection. Resectability of the tumor is a major consideration in

TABLE 27-16 Lung Cancer TNM Classifications

Tumor Descriptor

T_x	Tumor proved by cytologic studies but not visualized by x-ray or bronchoscope
T_0	No evidence of tumor
T_{is}	Carcinoma in situ
T_1	Tumor 3 cm or less in greatest dimension
T_2	Tumor greater than 3 cm in diameter
T_3	Tumor with extension to pleura, chest wall, or pericardium
T_4	Tumor invading mediastinum or carina or with malignant pleural effusion

Nodal Involvement

N_0	No nodal metastasis
N_1	Metastasis to peribronchial or ipsilateral hilar lymph nodes
N_2	Metastasis to ipsilateral mediastinal or subcarinal lymph nodes
N_3	Metastasis to contralateral mediastinal or hilar lymph nodes or any scalene or supraclavicular node

Distant Metastasis

M_0	No known metastasis
M_1	Presence of distant metastasis

Stage Grouping

Occult carcinoma	T_x	N_0	M_0
Stage 0	T_{is}	Carcinoma in situ	M_0
Stage IA	T_1	N_0	M_0
Stage IB	T_2	N_0	M_0
Stage IIA	T_1	N_1	M_0
Stage IIB	T_2	N_1	M_0
	T_3	N_0	M_0
Stage IIIA	T_3	N_1	M_0
	T_{1-3}	N_2	M_0
Stage IIIB	Any T	N_3	M_0
	T_4	Any N	M_0
Stage IV	Any T	Any N	M_1

Source: Revised international system for staging lung cancer, 1997.
TNM, Tumor node metastasis.

planning the surgical intervention. Small cell carcinomas usually have widespread metastasis at the time of diagnosis. Therefore surgery is usually contraindicated. In contrast, squamous cell carcinomas are more likely to be treated with surgery because they remain localized, or if they metastasize they primarily do so by local spread.

When the tumor is considered operable with a potential for cure, the patient's cardiopulmonary status must be evaluated to determine the ability to withstand surgery. This is done by clinical studies of pulmonary function, arterial blood gases (ABGs), and others, as indicated by the individual's status. Contraindications for thoracotomy include hypercapnia, pulmonary hypertension, cor pulmonale, and markedly reduced lung function. Coexisting conditions such as cardiac, renal, and liver disease may also be contraindications for surgery.

A tumor may be considered inoperable. If operable, the type of surgery performed is usually a *lobectomy* (removal of one or more lobes of the lung) and less often a *pneumonectomy* (removal of one entire lung).

Radiation Therapy. Radiation therapy is used as a curative approach in the individual who has a resectable tumor but who is considered a poor surgical risk. There has been improved survival when radiation therapy is used in combination with surgery and chemotherapy.[21] Adenocarcinomas are the most radioresistant type of cancer cell. Although SCLC are radiosensitive, radiation (even when used in combination with chemotherapy) does not significantly improve the mortality rate because of the early metastases of this type of cancer.

Radiation therapy is also done as a palliative procedure to reduce distressing symptoms such as cough, hemoptysis, bronchial obstruction, and superior vena cava syndrome. It can be used to treat pain that is caused by metastatic bone lesions or cerebral metastasis. Radiation used as a preoperative or postoperative adjuvant measure has not been found to significantly increase survival in the patient with lung cancer.

Chemotherapy. Chemotherapy may be used in the treatment of nonresectable tumors or as adjuvant therapy to surgery in NSCLC with distant metastases. A variety of chemotherapy drugs and multidrug regimens (i.e., protocols) including combination chemotherapy have been used. These drugs include etoposide (VePesid), carboplatin (Paraplatin), cisplatin (Platinol), paclitaxel (Taxol), vinorelbine (Navelbine), cyclophosphamide (Cytoxan), ifosfamide (Ifex), docetaxel (Taxotere), gemcitabine (Gemzar), topotecan (Hycamtin), irinotecan (Camptosar), and gefitinib (Iressa).[21]

Chemotherapy has improved survival in patients with advanced NSCLC and is now considered standard treatment. Chemotherapy in SCLC has a strong response rate, but the majority (80%) of patients still die from the disease.

Biologic Therapy. Biologic therapy as adjuvant therapy has been used in individuals with cancer, including malignant lung tumors. (Biologic therapy is discussed in Chapter 15.)

Other Therapies

Prophylactic cranial radiation. Brain metastasis is a common complication of SCLS. Most chemotherapy drugs do not adequately penetrate the blood-brain barrier. Prophylactic cranial radiation may be used as a potential way to improve the prognosis of patients, especially those who have a complete response to chemotherapy. Toxicity of this therapy may include scalp erythema, fatigue, and alopecia.

Bronchoscopic laser therapy. Bronchoscopic laser therapy makes it possible to remove obstructing bronchial lesions. The neodymium:yttrium-aluminum-garnet (Nd:YAG) is most commonly used for laser resection. The thermal energy of the laser is transmitted to the target tissue. It is a complicated procedure that often requires general anesthesia to control the patient's cough reflex. Relief of the symptoms from airway obstruction as a result of thermal necrosis and shrinkage of the tumor can be dramatic. However, it is not a curative therapy for cancer.

Phototherapy. Photodynamic therapy is a safe, nonsurgical therapy for lung cancer. Porfimer (Photofrin) is injected intravenously and selectively concentrates in tumor cells. After a set time period (usually 48 hours) the tumor is exposed to laser light, producing a toxic form of oxygen that destroys tumor cells. Necrotic tissue is removed through a bronchoscope.

Airway stenting. Stents can be used alone or in combination with other techniques for palliation of dyspnea, cough, or respiratory insufficiency. The advantage of an airway stent is that it supports the airway wall against collapse or external compression and can impede extension of tumor into the airway lumen.

Cryotherapy. Cryotherapy is a technique in which tissue is destroyed as a result of freezing. Bronchoscopic cryotherapy is used to ablate (destroy) bronchogenic carcinomas, especially polypoid lesions. A repeat bronchoscope is performed 8 to 10 days after the first session. The second examination enables assessment of cryodestruction, removal of any slough, and repeat cryotherapy if required for the treatment of large lesions.

The American Society of Clinical Oncology (*www.asco.org*) and Cancer Care Ontario, *Lung Cancer Clinical Practice Guidelines* (*http://hiru.mcmaster.ca/ccOpgi/*), have both published clinical practice guidelines for lung cancer that present evidence-based recommendations.

NURSING MANAGEMENT
LUNG CANCER

■ Nursing Assessment

It is important to determine the understanding of the patient and the family concerning the diagnostic tests (those completed as well as those planned), the diagnosis or potential diagnosis, the treatment options, and the prognosis. At the same time the nurse can assess the level of anxiety experienced by the patient and the support provided and needed by the patient's significant others. Subjective and objective data that should be obtained from a patient with lung cancer are presented in Table 27-17.

■ Nursing Diagnoses

Nursing diagnoses for the patient with lung cancer may include, but are not limited to, the following:

- Ineffective airway clearance *related to* increased tracheobronchial secretions and presence of tumor
- Anxiety *related to* lack of knowledge of diagnosis or unknown prognosis and treatments
- Acute pain *related to* pressure of tumor on surrounding structures and erosion of tissues
- Imbalanced nutrition: less than body requirements *related to* increased metabolic demands, increased secretions, weakness, and anorexia
- Ineffective health maintenance *related to* lack of knowledge about the disease process and therapeutic regimen
- Ineffective breathing pattern *related to* decreased lung capacity

■ Planning

The overall goals are that the patient with lung cancer will have (1) effective breathing patterns, (2) adequate airway clearance, (3) adequate oxygenation of tissues, (4) minimal to no pain, and (5) a realistic attitude toward treatment and prognosis.

■ Nursing Implementation

Health Promotion. The best way to halt the epidemic of lung cancer is for people to stop smoking. Important nursing activities to assist in the progress toward this goal include promoting smoking cessation programs and actively supporting education and policy changes related to smoking. Important changes have occurred as the result of the recognition that sidestream smoke is a health hazard; laws require designation of nonsmoking areas in most public places or prohibiting smoking and a ban on smoking on airline flights. Other actions aimed at controlling tobacco use include restrictions on tobacco advertising on television and warning label requirements for cigarette packaging.

TABLE 27-17	Nursing Assessment Lung Cancer

Subjective Data
Important Health Information
Past health history: Exposure to secondhand smoke; airborne carcinogens (e.g., asbestos, uranium, chromates, hydrocarbons, arsenic) or other pollutants; urban living environment; chronic lung disease, including TB, COPD, bronchiectasis
Medications: Use of cough medicines or other respiratory medications
Functional Health Patterns
Health perception–health management: Smoking history; family history of lung cancer; frequent respiratory infections
Nutritional-metabolic: Anorexia, nausea, vomiting, dysphagia (late); weight loss; chills
Activity-exercise: Fatigue; persistent cough (productive or nonproductive); dyspnea, hemoptysis (late symptom)
Cognitive-perceptual: Chest pain or tightness, shoulder and arm pain, headache, bone pain (late symptom)

Objective Data
General
Fever, neck and axillary lymphadenopathy, paraneoplastic syndromes (e.g., syndrome of inappropriate ADH; ACTH secretion)
Integumentary
Jaundice (liver metastasis); edema of neck and face (superior vena cava syndrome), digital clubbing
Respiratory
Wheezing, hoarseness, stridor, unilateral diaphragm paralysis, pleural effusions (late signs)
Cardiovascular
Pericardial effusion, cardiac tamponade, arrhythmias (late signs)
Neurologic
Unsteady gait (brain metastasis)
Musculoskeletal
Pathologic fractures, muscle wasting (late)
Possible Findings
Observance of lesion on chest x-ray, CT scan, or lung scan; positive sputum or bronchial washings for cytologic studies; positive fiberoptic bronchoscopy and biopsy findings; low serum sodium and hypercalcemia (paraneoplastic syndrome)

ACTH, Adrenocorticotropic hormone; *ADH,* antidiuretic hormone; *COPD,* chronic obstructive pulmonary disease; *CT,* computed tomography; *TB,* tuberculosis.

These are examples of beginning steps toward the goal of a smokeless society. Despite the small advances being made, tobacco-producing states and tobacco companies still have strong political influences.

For the individual who does have a smoking habit, efforts should be made to assist the smoker to stop smoking. The updated evidence-based guideline, *A Clinical Practice Guideline for Treating Tobacco Use and Dependence, 2000,* describes a framework (the five *As*) for approaching patients who are willing to attempt to quit smoking.[24] The five *As* stand for the five strategies: ask, advice, assess, assist, and arrange (see Chapter 11, Table 11-13). The four stages of change identified in smokers attempting to quit include precontemplation ("I want"), contemplation ("I might"), preparation ("I will"), and action ("I am").[27]

(The stages of change in relationship to patient teaching are discussed in Chapter 4, Table 4-3.) Each stage requires specific actions to progress to the next stage. Nurses working with patients at their individual stage of change will help them progress to the next stage. For patients unwilling to quit, motivational interviewing is recommended (discussed in Chapter 11 on p. 197).

The evidence-based guideline also offers the five Rs strategy for motivating smokers to quit: relevance, risk, reward, roadblocks, and repetition (see Chapter 11, Table 11-13). Because some patients relapse months or years after having stopped smoking, nurses need to continually provide interactions to prevent relapse. (Tobacco use and dependence and strategies to assist patients stop smoking are discussed in Chapter 11 and Tables 11-13 and 11-14.)

Nicotine's addictive properties make quitting a difficult task that requires much support. Nicotine replacement significantly lessens the urge to smoke and increases the percentage of smokers who successfully quit smoking. There is no evidence that one product has better results than another, so the choice of agent is dependent on the health care provider and patient preferences.[28] Stop-smoking aids are presented in Chapter 11, Table 11-14.

Research into smoking behaviors and successful strategies to promote smoking cessation is ongoing. A combination of both behavioral and nicotine replacement products is the most effective strategy to help smokers quit.[24] Therefore all patients should be offered some form of nicotine replacement.

The advice and motivation of health care professionals can be a powerful force in smoking cessation. (See the Evidence-Based Practice box in Chapter 11 on p. 194.) Nurses are in a unique position to promote smoking cessation because they see large numbers of smokers who may be reluctant to seek help. Support for the smoker includes education that smoking a few cigarettes during a cessation attempt (a slip) is much different than resuming the full smoking habit (a relapse). Despite the slip, smokers should be encouraged to continue the attempt at cessation without viewing the effort as a failure. Measures to assist an individual in quitting should be directed toward the meaning that smoking has to that individual. The nurse needs to be aware of resources in the community to assist the individual who is interested in quitting.

Acute Intervention. Care of the patient with lung cancer will initially involve support and reassurance during the diagnostic evaluation. (Specific nursing measures related to the diagnostic studies are outlined in Chapter 25.)

Another major responsibility of the nurse is to help the patient and their family deal with the diagnosis of lung cancer. The patient may feel guilty about cigarette smoking having caused the cancer and need to discuss this feeling with someone who has a nonjudgmental attitude. Questions regarding each patient's condition should be answered honestly. Additional counseling from a social worker, psychologist, or member of the clergy may be needed. Nursing research focused on the nutritional assessment, intervention, and evaluation of weight loss in patients with lung cancer indicated that although assessments were routinely completed, interventions were initiated only 60% of the time.[29] Nurses can make a great impact on the care of the patient with lung cancer by focusing not only on assessment but on implementing the appropriate interventions more frequently.

Specific care of the patient will depend on the treatment plan. Postoperative care for the patient having surgery is discussed later in this chapter. Care of the patient undergoing radiation therapy and chemotherapy is discussed in Chapter 15. The nurse has a major role in providing patient comfort, teaching methods to reduce pain, and assessing indications for hospitalization.

Ambulatory and Home Care. The patient who has had a surgical resection with intent to cure should be followed up carefully for manifestations of metastasis. The patient and family should be told to contact the physician if symptoms such as hemoptysis, dysphagia, chest pain, and hoarseness develop.

For many individuals who have lung cancer, little can be done to significantly prolong their lives. Radiation therapy and chemotherapy can be used to provide palliative relief from distressing symptoms. Constant pain becomes a major problem. (Measures used to relieve pain are discussed in Chapter 9. Care of the patient with cancer is discussed in Chapter 15.)

■ Evaluation

The expected outcomes are that the patient with lung cancer will have
- adequate breathing patterns
- minimal to no pain
- realistic attitude about prognosis

OTHER TYPES OF LUNG TUMORS

Other types of primary lung tumors include sarcomas, lymphomas, and bronchial adenomas. Bronchial adenomas are small tumors that arise from the lower trachea or major bronchi and are considered malignant because they are locally invasive and frequently metastasize. Clinical manifestations of bronchial adenomas include hemoptysis, persistent cough, localized obstructive wheezing, and pneumonia. Bronchial adenomas can usually be treated successfully with surgical resection.

The lungs are a common site for secondary metastases and are more often affected by metastatic growth than by primary lung tumors. The pulmonary capillaries, with their extensive network, are ideal sites for tumor emboli. In addition, the lungs have an extensive lymphatic network. The primary malignancies that spread to the lungs often originate in the gastrointestinal (GI) or genitourinary (GU) tracts and in the breast. General symptoms of lung metastases are chest pain and nonproductive cough.

Benign tumors of the lung are generally classified as *mesenchymal*. Their occurrence is rare, and they have the potential to become malignant. The most common mesenchymal tumors are *chondromas,* which arise in the bronchial cartilage, and *leiomyomas,* which are myomas of smooth, nonstriated muscle fibers.

Hamartomas of the lung are the most common benign tumor. These tumors, composed of fibrous tissue, fat, and blood vessels, are congenital malformations of the connective tissue of the bronchiolar walls. Hamartomas are slow-growing tumors.

Chest Trauma and Thoracic Injuries

Traumatic injuries fall into two major categories: (1) blunt trauma and (2) penetrating trauma. *Blunt trauma* occurs when the body is struck by a blunt object, such as a steering wheel. The external injury may appear minor, but the impact may cause severe, life-threatening internal injuries, such as a ruptured spleen. *Contrecoup trauma,* a type of blunt trauma, is caused by the impact of parts of the body against other objects. This type of injury differs from blunt trauma primarily in the velocity of the impact. Internal organs are rapidly forced back and forth within the bony structures that surround them so that internal injury is sustained not only on the side of the impact but also on the opposite side, where the organ or organs hit bony structures. If the velocity of impact is great enough, organs and blood vessels can literally be torn from their points of origin. Many head injuries are caused by contrecoup trauma.

Penetrating trauma occurs when a foreign body impales or passes through the body tissues (e.g., gunshot wounds, stab-bings). Table 27-18 describes selective traumatic injuries as they relate to the categories of trauma and the mechanism of injury. Emergency care of the patient with a chest injury is presented in Table 27-19.

Thoracic injuries range from simple rib fractures to life-threatening tears of the aorta, vena cava, and other major vessels. The most common thoracic emergencies and their management are described in Table 27-20.

TABLE 27-18 **Common Traumatic Chest Injuries and Mechanisms of Injury**

MECHANISM OF INJURY	COMMON RELATED INJURY
Blunt Trauma	
Blunt steering–wheel injury to chest	Rib fractures, flail chest, pneumothorax, hemopneumothorax, cardiac contusion, pulmonary contusion, cardiac tamponade, great vessel tears
Shoulder-harness seat belt injury	Fractured clavicle, dislocated shoulder, rib fractures, pulmonary contusion, pericardial contusion, cardiac tamponade
Crush injury (e.g., heavy equipment, crushing thorax)	Pneumothorax and hemopneumothorax, flail chest, great vessel tears and rupture, decreased blood return to heart with decreased cardiac output
Penetrating Trauma	
Gunshot or stab wound to chest	Open pneumothorax, tension pneumothorax, hemopneumothorax, cardiac tamponade, esophageal damage, tracheal tear, great vessel tears

---

TABLE 27-19 **Emergency Management** **Chest Trauma**

ETIOLOGY	ASSESSMENT FINDINGS	INTERVENTIONS
Blunt Motor vehicle accident Pedestrian accident Fall Assault with blunt object Crush injury Explosion **Penetrating** Knife Gunshot Stick Arrow Other missiles	**Respiratory** • Dyspnea, respiratory distress • Cough with or without hemoptysis • Cyanosis of mouth, face, nail beds, mucous membranes • Tracheal deviation • Audible air escaping from chest wound • Decreased breath sounds on side of injury • Decreased O_2 saturation • Frothy secretions **Cardiovascular** • Rapid, thready pulse • Decreased blood pressure • Narrowed pulse pressure • Asymmetric blood pressure values in arms • Distended neck veins • Muffled heart sounds • Chest pain • Crunching sound synchronous with heart sounds • Arrhythmias **Surface Findings** • Bruising • Abrasions • Open chest wound • Asymmetric chest movement • Subcutaneous emphysema	**Initial** • Ensure patent airway. • Administer high-flow O_2 with non-rebreather mask. • Establish IV access with two large-bore catheters. Begin fluid resuscitation as appropriate. • Remove clothing to assess injury. • Cover sucking chest wound with nonporous dressing taped on three sides. • Stabilize impaled objects with bulky dressings. *Do not remove.* • Assess for other significant injuries and treat appropriately. • Stabilize flail rib segment with hand followed by application of large pieces of tape horizontal across the flail segment. • Place patient in a semi-Fowler's position or position patient on the injured side if breathing is easier *after* cervical spine injury has been ruled out. **Ongoing Monitoring** • Monitor vital signs, level of consciousness, oxygen saturation, cardiac rhythm, respiratory status, and urinary output. • Anticipate intubation for respiratory distress. • Release dressing if tension pneumothorax develops after sucking chest wound is covered.

TABLE 27-20 Emergency Management — Thoracic Injuries

INJURY	DEFINITION	CLINICAL MANIFESTATIONS	EMERGENCY MANAGEMENT
Pneumothorax	Air in pleural space (see Fig. 27-5).	Dyspnea, decreased movement of involved chest wall, diminished or absent breath sounds on the affected side, hyperresonance to percussion	Chest tube insertion with chest drainage system
Hemothorax	Blood in the pleural space, usually occurs in conjunction with pneumothorax.	Dyspnea, diminished or absent breath sounds, dullness to percussion, shock	Chest tube insertion with chest drainage system; autotransfusion of collected blood, treatment of hypovolemia as necessary
Tension pneumothorax	Air in pleural space that does not escape. Continued increase in amount of air shifts intrathoracic organs and increases intrathoracic pressure (see Fig. 27-6).	Cyanosis, air hunger, violent agitation, tracheal deviation away from affected side, subcutaneous emphysema, neck vein distention, hyperresonance to percussion	Medical emergency: needle decompression followed by chest tube insertion with chest drainage system
Flail chest	Fracture of two or more adjacent ribs in two or more places with loss of chest wall stability (see Fig. 27-7).	Paradoxic movement of chest wall, respiratory distress, associated hemothorax, pneumothorax, pulmonary contusion	Stabilize flail segment with intubation in some patients; taping in others; oxygen therapy; treat associated injuries; analgesia
Cardiac tamponade	Blood rapidly collects in pericardial sac, compresses myocardium because the pericardium does not stretch, and prevents heart from pumping effectively.	Muffled, distant heart sounds, hypotension, neck vein distention, increased central venous pressure	Medical emergency: pericardiocentesis with surgical repair as appropriate

PNEUMOTHORAX

A **pneumothorax** is air in the pleural space. There is a resultant complete or partial collapse of a lung due to the accumulation of air in the pleural space. This condition should be suspected after any blunt trauma to the chest wall. Pneumothorax may be closed or open. Pneumothorax associated with trauma may be accompanied by hemothorax, a condition called *hemopneumothorax*.

Types of Pneumothorax

Closed Pneumothorax. *Closed pneumothorax* has no associated external wound. The most common form is a spontaneous pneumothorax, which is accumulation of air in the pleural space without an apparent antecedent event. It is caused by rupture of small blebs on the visceral pleural space. The cause of the blebs is unknown. This condition occurs most commonly in underweight male cigarette smokers between 20 and 40 years of age. There is a tendency for this condition to recur.

Other causes of closed pneumothorax include the following:
1. Injury to the lungs from mechanical ventilation
2. Injury to the lungs from insertion of a subclavian catheter
3. Perforation of the esophagus
4. Injury to the lungs from broken ribs
5. Ruptured blebs or bullae in a patient with COPD

Open Pneumothorax. *Open pneumothorax* occurs when air enters the pleural space through an opening in the chest wall (Fig. 27-5, *B*). Examples include stab or gunshot wounds and surgical thoracotomies. A penetrating chest wound is often referred to as a sucking chest wound.

An open pneumothorax should be covered with a vented dressing. (A vented dressing is one secured on three sides with

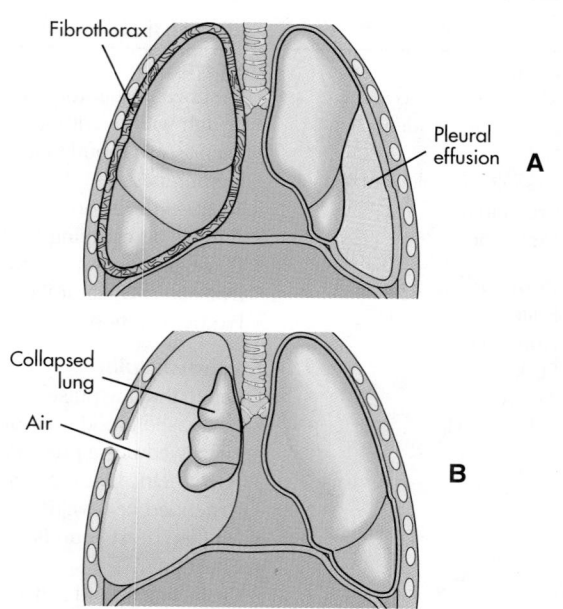

FIG. 27-5 Disorders of the pleura. **A,** Fibrothorax resulting from an organization of inflammatory exudate and pleural effusion. **B,** Open pneumothorax resulting from collapse of lung due to disruption of chest wall and outside air entering.

the fourth side left untaped.) This allows air to escape from the vent and decreases the likelihood of tension pneumothorax developing. If the object that caused the open chest wound is still in place, it should not be removed until a physician is present. The impaled object should be stabilized with a bulky dressing.

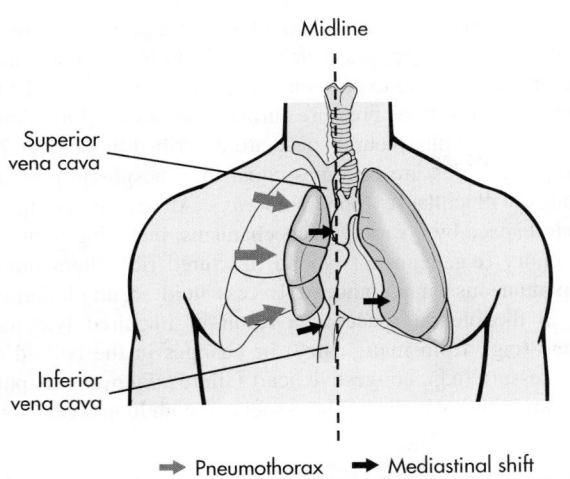

Midline

Superior
vena cava

Inferior
vena cava

➡ Pneumothorax   ➡ Mediastinal shift

FIG. 27-6 Tension pneumothorax. As pleural pressure on the affected side increases, mediastinal displacement ensues with resultant respiratory and cardiovascular compromise.

Tension Pneumothorax. Tension pneumothorax is a pneumothorax with rapid accumulation of air in the pleural space causing severely high intrapleural pressures with resultant tension on the heart and great vessels. It may result from either an open or a closed pneumothorax (Fig. 27-6). In an open chest wound, a flap may act as a one-way valve; thus air can enter on inspiration but cannot escape. The intrathoracic pressure increases, the lung collapses, and the mediastinum shifts toward the unaffected side, which is subsequently compressed. As the pressure increases, cardiac output is altered because of decreased venous return and compression of the vena cava and aorta. Tension pneumothorax can occur with mechanical ventilation and resuscitative efforts. It can also occur if chest tubes are clamped or become blocked in a patient with a pneumothorax. Unclamping the tube or relief of the obstruction will remedy this situation.

Tension pneumothorax is a medical emergency with both the respiratory and circulatory systems affected. If the tension in the pleural space is not relieved, the patient is likely to die from inadequate cardiac output or marked hypoxemia. Nurses and paramedics are now being trained to insert large-bore needles and chest tubes into the chest wall to release the trapped air.

Hemothorax. Hemothorax is an accumulation of blood in the intrapleural space. It is frequently found in association with open pneumothorax and is then called a *hemopneumothorax*. Causes of hemothorax include chest trauma, lung malignancy, complications of anticoagulant therapy, pulmonary embolus, and tearing of pleural adhesions.

Chylothorax. Chylothorax is lymphatic fluid in the pleural space due to a leak in the thoracic duct. Causes include trauma, surgical procedures, and malignancy. The thoracic duct is disrupted and the chylous fluid, milky white with high lipid content, fills the pleural space. Total lymphatic flow through the thoracic duct is 1500 to 2400 ml/day. Fifty percent will heal with conservative treatment (chest drainage, bowel rest, and total parenteral nutrition [TPN]). Surgery and pleurodesis are options if conservative therapy fails. *Pleurodesis* is the artificial production of adhesions between the parietal and visceral pleura, usually done with a chemical sclerosing agent.

Clinical Manifestations

If the pneumothorax is small, mild tachycardia and dyspnea may be the only manifestations. If the pneumothorax is large, respiratory distress may be present, including shallow, rapid respirations, dyspnea, and air hunger. Chest pain and a cough with or without hemoptysis may be present. On auscultation there are no breath sounds over the affected area, and hyperresonance may be present. A chest x-ray shows the presence of pneumothorax.

If a tension pneumothorax develops, severe respiratory distress, tachycardia, and hypotension occur. Mediastinal displacement occurs, and the trachea shifts to the unaffected side.

Collaborative Care

Treatment depends on the severity of the pneumothorax and the nature of the underlying disease. If the patient is stable, and the amount of air and fluid accumulated in the intrapleural space is minimal, no treatment may be needed as the pneumothorax resolves spontaneously. If the amount of air or fluid is minimal, the pleural space can be aspirated with a large-bore needle. As a lifesaving measure, needle venting (using a large-bore needle) of the pleural space may be used. A Heimlich valve may also be used to evacuate air from the pleural space. The most definitive and common form of treatment of pneumothorax and hemothorax is to insert a chest tube and connect it to water-seal drainage. Repeated spontaneous pneumothorax may need to be treated surgically by a partial pleurectomy, stapling, or pleurodesis to promote adherence of the pleurae to one another.

FRACTURED RIBS

Rib fractures are the most common type of chest injury resulting from trauma. Ribs 5 through 10 are most commonly fractured because they are least protected by chest muscles. If the fractured rib is splintered or displaced, it may damage the pleura and lungs.

Clinical manifestations of fractured ribs include pain (especially on inspiration) at the site of injury. The individual splints the affected area and takes shallow breaths to try to decrease the pain. Because the individual is reluctant to take deep breaths, atelectasis may develop because of decreased ventilation.

The main goal in treatment is to decrease pain so that the patient can breathe adequately to promote good chest expansion. Intercostal nerve blocks with local anesthesia may be used to provide pain relief. The effect of the anesthesia lasts for a period of hours to days. It must be repeated as necessary to provide pain relief. Strapping the chest with tape or using a binder is not common practice. Most physicians believe that these measures should be avoided because they reduce lung expansion and predispose the individual to atelectasis. Narcotic drug therapy must be individualized and used with caution because these drugs can depress respirations.

FLAIL CHEST

Flail chest results from multiple rib fractures, causing instability of the chest wall (Fig. 27-7). The chest wall cannot provide the bony structure necessary to maintain bellows action and ventilation. The affected (flail) area will move paradoxically to the intact portion of the chest during respiration. During inspiration the affected portion is sucked in, and during expiration it bulges out. This paradoxic chest movement prevents adequate ventilation of the lung in the injured area. The underlying lung may or may not have a serious injury. Associated pain and any lung in-

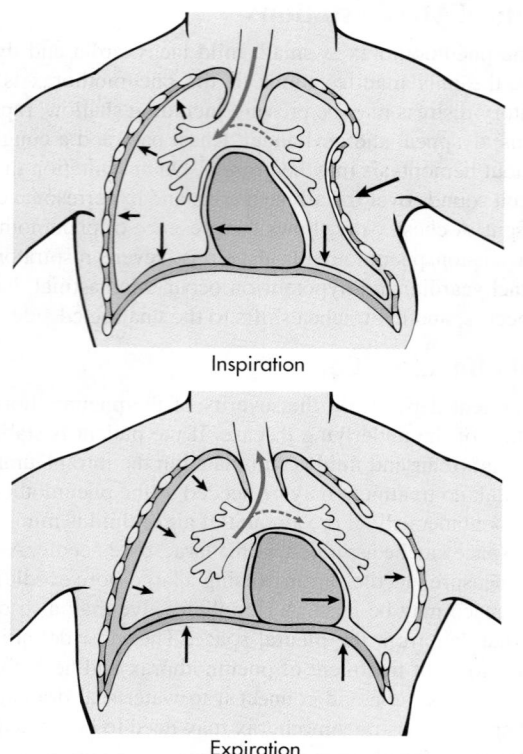

Inspiration

Expiration

FIG. 27-7 Flail chest produces paradoxic respiration. On inspiration the flail section sinks in with the mediastinal shift to the uninjured side. On expiration the flail section bulges outward with the mediastinal shift to the injured side.

jury, giving rise to loss of compliance, will contribute to an alteration in breathing patterns and lead to hypoxemia.

A flail chest is usually apparent on visual examination of the unconscious patient. The patient manifests rapid, shallow respirations and tachycardia. A flail chest may not be initially apparent in the conscious patient as a result of splinting of the chest wall. The patient moves air poorly, and movement of the thorax is asymmetric and uncoordinated. Palpation of abnormal respiratory movements, crepitus of the rib, chest x-ray, and ABGs assist in the diagnosis.

Initial therapy consists of adequate ventilation, humidified O_2, and careful administration of crystalloid IV solutions. The definitive therapy is to reexpand the lung and ensure adequate oxygenation. Although many patients can be managed without the use of mechanical ventilation, a short period of intubation and ventilation may be necessary until the diagnosis of the lung injury is complete.

Positive end-expiratory pressure (PEEP) used with mechanical ventilation to improve oxygenation will maintain positive pressure in the lungs throughout the respiratory cycle. Mechanical ventilation is discussed in Chapter 66. The lung parenchyma and fractured ribs will heal with time.

CHEST TUBES AND PLEURAL DRAINAGE

The purpose of chest tubes and pleural drainage is to remove the air and fluid from the pleural space and to restore normal intrapleural pressure so that the lungs can reexpand. Small accumulations of air or fluid in the pleural space may not require removal by thoracentesis or chest-tube insertion. Instead the air and fluid may be reabsorbed over time.

Under normal conditions, intrapleural pressure is below atmospheric pressure (approximately 4 to 5 cm H_2O below atmospheric pressure during expiration and approximately 8 to 10 cm H_2O below atmospheric pressure during inspiration). (Intrapleural pressure and the intrapleural space are described in Chapter 25.) If intrapleural pressure becomes equal to atmospheric pressure, the lungs will collapse (pneumothorax). Air can enter the intrapleural space by a variety of mechanisms, including traumatic chest injury (e.g., gunshot wound, fractured rib), thoracotomy, and spontaneous pneumothorax. Excess fluid accumulation can occur in the pleural space as a result of impaired lymphatic drainage (e.g., from malignancy) or changes in the colloid osmotic pressure (e.g., congestive heart failure). *Empyema* is purulent pleural fluid, which may be associated with lung abscesses or pneumonia.

Chest Tube Insertion

Chest tubes can be inserted in the emergency department (ED), at the patient's bedside, or in the operating room (OR), depending on the situation. In the OR the chest tube is inserted via the thoracotomy incision. In the ED or at the bedside the patient is placed in a sitting position or is lying down with the affected side elevated. The area is prepared with antiseptic solution, and the site is infiltrated with a local anesthetic agent. After a small incision is made, one or two chest tubes are inserted into the pleural space. One catheter is placed anteriorly through the second intercostal space to remove air (Fig. 27-8). The other is placed posteriorly through the eighth or ninth intercostal space to drain fluid and

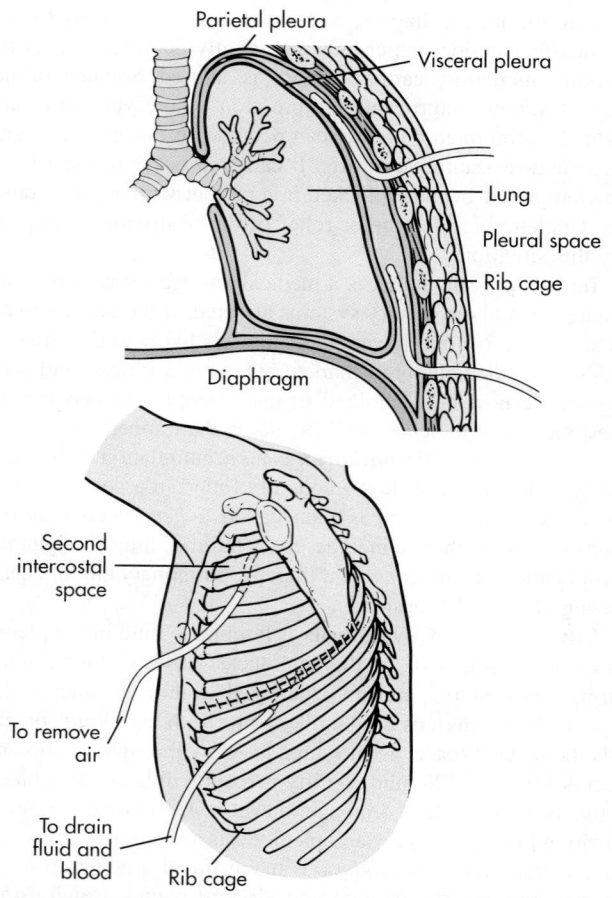

FIG. 27-8 Placement of chest tubes.

blood. The tubes are sutured to the chest wall, and the puncture wound is covered with an airtight dressing. During insertion, the tubes are kept clamped. After the tubes are in place in the pleural space, they are connected to drainage tubing and pleural drainage and the clamp is removed. Each tube may be connected to a separate drainage system and suction. More commonly, a Y-connector is used to attach both chest tubes to the same drainage system.

Pleural Drainage

Most pleural drainage systems have three basic compartments, each with its own separate function. The three compartments were bottles in early drainage systems and were known as the three-bottle system (Fig. 27-9). Modern products incorporate these same basic concepts in their disposable plastic chest drainage systems.

The *first compartment,* or collection chamber, receives fluid and air from the chest cavity. The fluid stays in this chamber while the air vents to the second compartment. The *second compartment,* called the water-seal chamber, contains 2 cm of water, which acts as a one-way valve. The incoming air enters from the collection chamber and bubbles up through the water. (The water acts as a one-way valve to prevent backflow of air into the patient from the system.) The air then exits the water seal and enters the suction chamber. Initial bubbling of air is seen in this chamber when a pneumothorax is evacuated. Intermittent bubbling can also be seen during exhalation, coughing, or sneezing due to an increase in the patient's intrathoracic pressure. In this chamber fluctuations, or "tidaling," will be seen that reflect the pressures in the pleural space. If tidaling is not seen, either the lungs have reexpanded or there is a kink or obstruction in the tubing.

A *third compartment,* the suction control chamber, applies controlled suction to the chest drainage system. The classic suction control chamber uses tubing with one end submerged in a column of water and the other end vented to the atmosphere (see Fig. 27-9). It is typically filled with 20 cm of water. When the negative pressure generated by the suction source exceeds 20 cm, the air from the atmosphere enters the chamber through a vent

and begins bubbling up through the water. As a result, excess pressure is relieved. The amount of suction applied is regulated by the depth of the suction control tube in the water and not by the amount of suction applied to the system. An increase in suction does not result in an increase in negative pressure to the system because any excess suction merely draws in air through the vented tubing. The suction pressure is usually ordered to be -20 cm H_2O.[30]

Two types of suction control chambers are available on the market: wet and dry. The wet suction control chamber system is the classic system outlined previously. Bubbling is one way to tell that suction is functioning. To start the suction, the vacuum source is turned up until gentle bubbling appears. Turning the vacuum source higher just makes the bubbling more vigorous and makes the water evaporate faster.[31] Even at gentle bubbling, water evaporates in this chamber, and water must be added periodically. The dry suction control chamber system contains no water. It uses either a restrictive device or a regulator to dial the desired negative pressure; this is internal in the chest drainage system. The dry system has a visual alert that indicates if the suction is working, so bubbling is not seen in a third chamber. To increase the suction pressures, the dial is turned on the drainage system. Increasing the vacuum suction source will not increase the pressure.

A variety of commercial disposable plastic chest drainage systems are available. One popular system is the Pleur-evac shown in Fig. 27-10. (Note the correspondence of the chambers to the bottles shown in the three-bottle system in Fig. 27-9.) The manufacturer's suggestions for use are included with the equipment. The plastic units allow the patient mobility and decrease the risk of breaking or spilling the drainage system.

Heimlich Valves. Another device that may be used to evacuate air from the pleural space is the Heimlich valve. This device

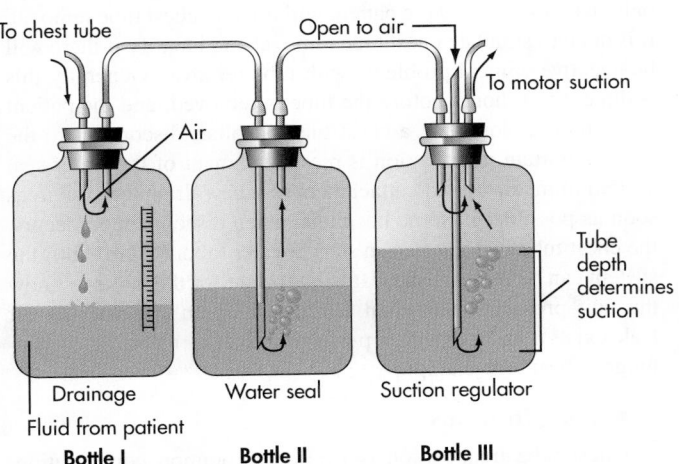

FIG. 27-9 Three-bottle water-seal suction. *Bottle I* is the drainage bottle. A vertical piece of tape should be applied to the outer surface of the drainage bottle. The time and the fluid level should be marked hourly on the tape. *Bottle II* is the water-seal bottle. *Bottle III* is the suction control bottle. The length of tube below the water surface determines the amount of suction.

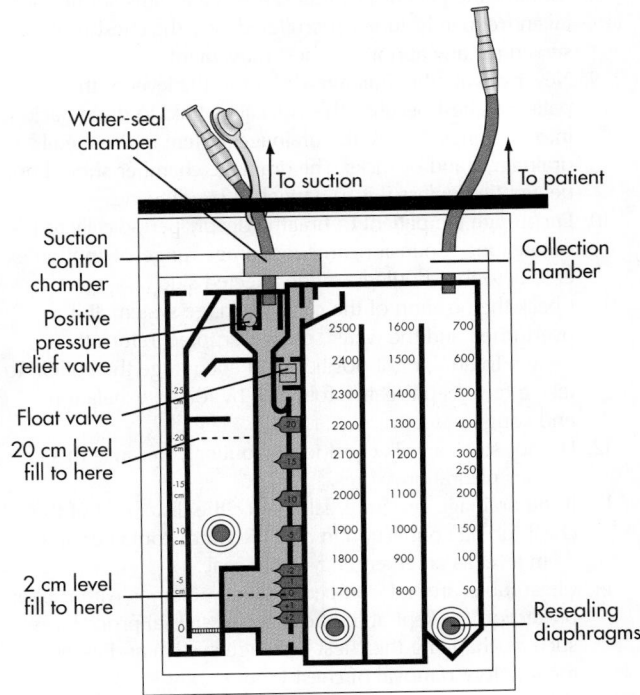

FIG. 27-10 Pleur-evac disposable chest suction system (displaying the wet suction control system).

TABLE 27-21	**Guidelines for Care of Patient with Chest Tubes and Water-Seal Drainage**

1. Keep all tubing as straight as possible and coiled loosely below chest level. Do not let the patient lie on it.
2. Keep all connections between chest tubes, drainage tubing, and the drainage collector tight and tape at connections.
3. Keep the water seal and suction control chamber at the appropriate water levels by adding sterile water as needed because water loss by evaporation may occur.
4. Mark the time of measurement and the fluid level on the drainage chamber according to the prescribed orders. Marking intervals may range from once per hour to every 8 hours. Any change in the quantity or characteristics of drainage (e.g., clear yellow to bloody) should be reported to the physician and recorded.
5. Monitor the fluid drainage and evacuate no more than 1000 to 1200 ml of pleural fluid from the pleural space at one time to prevent rebound hypotension or reexpansion pulmonary edema.
6. Observe for air bubbling in the water-seal chamber and fluctuations (tidaling). If no tidaling is observed (rising with inspiration and falling with expiration in the spontaneously breathing patient; the opposite occurs during positive-pressure mechanical ventilation), the drainage system is blocked or the lungs are reexpanded. If bubbling increases, there may be an air leak.
7. Bubbling in the water seal may occur intermittently. When bubbling is continuous and constant, the source of the air leak may be determined by momentarily clamping the tubing at successively distal points away from the patient until the bubbling ceases. Retaping tubing connections or replacing the drainage apparatus may be necessary to correct the air leak.
8. Monitor the patient's clinical status. Vital signs should be taken frequently, lungs auscultated, and the chest wall observed for any abnormal chest movements.
9. Never elevate the drainage system to the level of the patient's chest because this will cause fluid to drain back into the lungs. Secure the drainage system to the metal drainage stand or racks. The drainage chamber should not be emptied unless it is in danger of overflowing.
10. Encourage the patient to breathe deeply periodically to facilitate lung expansion, and encourage range-of-motion exercises to the shoulder on the affected side.
11. Check the position of the chest drainage system. If it is overturned and the water seal is disrupted, return the system to an upright position and encourage the patient to take a few deep breaths, followed by forced exhalations and cough maneuvers.
12. Do not strip or milk chest tubes routinely because this increases pleural pressures.
13. If the drainage system breaks, place the distal end of the chest tubing connection in a sterile water container at a 2 cm level as an emergency water seal.
14. Chest tubes are not clamped routinely. Clamps with rubber protection are kept at the bedside for special procedures such as changing the chest drainage system and assessment before removal of chest tubes.

consists of a rubber flutter one-way valve within a rigid plastic tube. It is attached to the external end of the chest tube. The valve opens whenever the pressure is greater than atmospheric pressure and closes when the reverse occurs. The Heimlich valve functions like a water seal and is usually used for emergency transport or in special home care situations.

Small Chest Tubes. Small chest tubes ("pigtail catheters") are used in selected patients because they are less traumatic. They drain air and fluid equally as well as large-bore chest tubes.[32] The drains may be straight catheters or "pigtail" catheters (curled at the distal end to look like a pig's tail). Curled catheters are considered to be less traumatic than straight catheters. These catheters, if occluded, can be irrigated by the physician using sterile water. Clinical pleurodesis can also be performed through this catheter. This system is not suitable for trauma or for drainage of blood.

NURSING MANAGEMENT
CHEST DRAINAGE

Some general guidelines for nursing care of the patient with chest tubes and water-seal drainage systems are presented in Table 27-21. The traditional practice of routine milking and/or stripping of chest tubes to maintain patency is no longer necessary. Drainage and blood are not likely to clot inside chest tubes because the tube is defibrinogenated. Additionally, the newer chest tubes are made with coating that makes them nonthrombogenic.[1] Clinical unit protocol and physician preferences should be ascertained before initiation of stripping or milking. The nurse should remember that these procedures can cause the patient to experience pain and that dislodgment of the tube may occur if the tube is not stabilized above the area being stripped.

Clamping of chest tubes during transport or when the tube is accidentally disconnected is no longer advocated. The danger of rapid accumulation of air in the pleural space causing tension pneumothorax is far greater than that of a small amount of atmospheric air entering the pleural space. Chest tubes may be momentarily clamped to change the drainage apparatus or to check for air leaks. Clamping for more than a few moments is indicated only in assessing how the patient will tolerate chest tube removal. It is done to simulate chest tube removal and identify if there will be negative clinical problems with tube removal. Generally this is done 4 to 6 hours before the tube is removed, and the patient is monitored closely. If a chest tube becomes disconnected, the most important intervention is reestablishment of the water-seal system immediately and attachment of a new drainage system as soon as possible. In some hospitals, when disconnection occurs, the chest tube is immersed in sterile water (about 2 cm) until the system can be reestablished. It is important for the nurse to know the unit protocol, individual clinical situation (whether an air leak exists), and physician preference before resorting to prolonged chest tube clamping.

■ Complications

Chest tube malposition is the most common complication. Routine monitoring is done by the nurse to evaluate if the chest drainage is successful by observing for tidaling in the water-seal chamber, listening for breath sounds over the lung fields, and measuring the amount of fluid drainage. Reexpansion pulmonary edema can occur after rapid expansion of a collapsed lung in patients with a pneumothorax or evacuation of large volumes of pleural fluid (greater than 1 to 1.5 L). A vasovagal response with symptomatic hypotension can occur from too rapid removal of fluid.

Infection at the skin site is also a concern. Meticulous sterile technique during dressing changes can reduce the incidence of infected sites. Other complications include (1) pneumonia from not taking deep breaths, from not using incentive spirometers, and by splinting on the affected side and (2) shoulder disuse ("frozen shoulder") from lack of range-of-motion exercises. Poor patient compliance or lack of patient teaching can contribute to these complications. Nurses can make a tremendous impact on preventing these complications.[33]

■ Chest Tube Removal

The patient with chest tubes may have chest x-rays to follow the course of lung expansion. The chest tubes are removed when the lungs are reexpanded and fluid drainage has ceased. Generally suction is discontinued and the patient is placed on gravity drainage for a period of time before the tubes are removed. The tube is removed by cutting the sutures; applying a sterile petroleum jelly gauze dressing; having the patient take a deep breath, exhale, and bear down (Valsalva maneuver); and then removing the tube. Pain medication is generally given before chest tube removal. The site is covered with an airtight dressing, the pleura seals itself off, and the wound is healed in several days. A chest x-ray is done after chest tube removal to evaluate for pneumothorax and/or reaccumulation of fluid. The wound should be observed for drainage and should be reinforced if necessary. The patient should be observed for respiratory distress, which may signify a recurrent or new pneumothorax.

CHEST SURGERY

Chest surgery is performed for a variety of reasons, some of which are unrelated to primary lung problems. For example, a thoracotomy is performed for heart and esophageal surgery. The types of chest surgery are compared in Table 27-22.

Preoperative Care

Before chest surgery, baseline data are obtained on the respiratory and cardiovascular systems. Diagnostic studies performed are pulmonary function studies, chest x-rays, electrocardiogram (ECG), ABGs, blood urea nitrogen (BUN), serum creatinine, blood glucose, serum electrolytes, and complete blood count. Additional studies of cardiac function such as cardiac catheterization may be done for the patient who is to un-

---

TABLE 27-22   Chest Surgeries

TYPE AND DESCRIPTION	INDICATION	COMMENTS
Lobectomy Removal of one lobe of lung	Lung cancer, bronchiectasis, TB, emphysematous bullae, benign lung tumors, fungal infections	Most common lung surgery; postoperative insertion of chest tubes; expansion of remaining lung tissue to fill up space
Pneumonectomy Removal of entire lung	Lung cancer (most common), extensive TB, bronchiectasis, lung abscess	Done only when lobectomy or segmental resection will not remove all diseased lung; no drainage tubes (generally), fluid gradually filling space where lung has been removed; position patient on operative side to facilitate expansion of remaining lung
Segmental resection Removal of one or more lung segments	Bronchiectasis, TB	Technically difficult; done to remove lung segment, insertion of chest tubes, expansion of remaining lung tissue to fill space
Wedge resection Removal of small, localized lesion that occupies only part of a segment	Lung biopsy, excision of small nodules	Need for chest tubes postoperatively
Decortication Removal of stripping of thick, fibrous membrane from visceral pleura	Empyema	Use of chest tubes and drainage postoperatively
Exploratory thoracotomy Incision into thorax to look for injured or bleeding tissues	Chest trauma	Use of chest tubes and drainage postoperatively
Thoracotomy not involving lungs* Incision into thorax for surgery on other organs	Hiatal hernia repair, open heart surgery, esophageal surgery, tracheal resection, aortic aneurysm repair	—
Thorascopy (endoscopic thoracotomy) One to four 1-in incisions through which a special fiberoptic camera is introduced as well as other instruments and suction	Patient without prior thoracotomy; peripheral or mediastinal lesions; lung function must be sufficient to undergo conventional thoracotomy	Possible complications include heavy bleeding, diaphragmatic perforation, air emboli, tension pneumothorax; chest tube is inserted through one of the incisions; incisions may be sutured or closed with adhesive wound-approximating strips

*For comments on thoracotomy not involving the lungs, see discussion of individual diseases in text.
TB, Tuberculosis.

dergo a pneumonectomy. A careful physical assessment of the lungs, including percussion and auscultation, should be done. This will allow the nurse to compare preoperative and postoperative findings.

The patient should be encouraged to stop smoking before surgery to decrease secretions and increase O_2 saturation. In the anxious period before surgery this is not an easy thing for the habitual smoker to do. Chest physiotherapy may be indicated to help drain the lungs of accumulated secretions. This is especially indicated for the patient with a lung abscess or bronchiectasis.

Preoperative teaching should include exercises for effective deep breathing and incentive spirometry. If the patient practices these techniques before surgery, the techniques will be easier to perform postoperatively. The patient should be told that adequate medication will be given to reduce the pain, and the patient is helped to splint the incision with a pillow to facilitate deep breathing.

For most types of chest surgery, chest tubes are inserted and connected to water-sealed drainage systems. The purpose of these tubes should be explained to the patient. In addition, O_2 is frequently given the first 24 hours after surgery. Range-of-motion exercises on the surgical side similar to those for the mastectomy patient should be taught (see Chapter 50).

The thought of losing part of a vital organ is frequently frightening. The patient should be reassured that the lungs have a large degree of functional reserve. Even after the removal of one lung there is enough lung tissue to maintain adequate oxygenation.

The nurse should be available to deal with the questions asked by the patient and the family. Questions should be answered honestly. The nurse should try to facilitate the expression of concerns, feelings, and questions. (General preoperative care and teaching are discussed in Chapter 17.)

Surgical Therapy

Thoracotomy (surgical opening into the thoracic cavity) surgery is considered major surgery because the incision is large, cutting into bone, muscle, and cartilage. The two types of thoracic incisions are median sternotomy, performed by splitting the sternum, and lateral thoracotomy. The median sternotomy is primarily used for surgery involving the heart. The two types of lateral thoracotomy are posterolateral and anterolateral. The posterolateral thoracotomy is used for most surgeries involving the lung. The incision is made from the anterior axillary line below the nipple level posteriorly at the fourth, fifth, or sixth intercostal space. It is rarely necessary to remove the ribs. Strong mechanical retractors are used to gain access to the lung. The anterolateral incision is made in the fourth or fifth intercostal space from the sternal border to the midaxillary line. This procedure is commonly used for surgery or trauma victims, mediastinal operations, and wedge resections of the upper and middle lobes of the lung.

The extensiveness of the thoracotomy incision often results in severe pain for the patient after surgery. Because muscles have been severed, the patient is reluctant to move the shoulder and arm on the surgical side. Chest tubes are placed in the pleural space except in pneumonectomy surgery. In a pneumonectomy the space from which the lung was removed gradually fills with serosanguineous fluid.

Thoracopic Surgery. *Thorascopic surgery* (endoscopic thoracotomy) is a procedure that in many cases can avoid the impact of a full thoracotomy. The procedure involves three to four 1-inch incisions made on the chest that allow the thorascope (a special fiberoptic camera) and instruments to be inserted and manipulated. Video-assisted thorascopes improve visualization because the surgeon can view the thoracic cavity from the video monitor. The thorascope is equipped with a camera that magnifies the image on the monitor. Thorascopy can be used to diagnose and treat a variety of conditions of the lung, pleura, and mediastinum.

The candidate for this type of procedure should not have a prior history of conventional thoracic surgery because the probability of adhesion formation would make access more difficult. The patient whose lesions are in the lung periphery or the mediastinum is a better candidate because of better accessibility. The patient considered for thorascopic surgery should have sufficient pulmonary function preoperatively to allow the surgeon to perform conventional thoracotomy if complications occur. Complications that may occur are bleeding, diaphragmatic perforation, air emboli, persistent pleural air leaks, and tension pneumothorax.

There are many benefits of thorascopic surgery when compared with a conventional thoracotomy procedure. These include less adhesion formation, minimal blood loss, less time under anesthesia, shorter hospitalization, faster recovery, less pain, and no need for postoperative rehabilitation therapy because of minimal disruption of thoracic structures.

Chest tubes are placed at the end of the procedure through one of the incisions. The incisions are closed with sutures or a wound-approximating adhesive bandage. Nursing assessment and care postoperatively include monitoring respiratory status and lung reexpansion with the chest tubes and checking the incisions for drainage or dehiscence. The most common complication is prolonged air leak. A return to prior activities should be encouraged as quickly as possible. The hospital stay averages from 1 to 5 days, depending on the type of surgery.

Postoperative Care

Specific measures related to the care after a thoracotomy are presented in NCP 27-2. The specific follow-up care depends on the type of surgical procedure. General postoperative care is discussed in Chapter 19.

Restrictive Respiratory Disorders

Restrictive respiratory disorders are characterized by decreased compliance of the lungs or chest wall or both. This is in contrast to obstructive disorders, which are characterized by increased resistance to airflow. Pulmonary function tests are the best means to use in differentiating between restrictive and obstructive respiratory disorders (Table 27-23). Mixed obstructive and restrictive disorders are often manifested. For example, a patient may have both chronic bronchitis (an obstructive problem) and pulmonary fibrosis (a restrictive problem).

Restrictive problems are generally categorized into extrapulmonary and intrapulmonary disorders. Extrapulmonary causes of restrictive lung disease include disorders involving the central nervous system (CNS), neuromuscular system, and chest wall (Table 27-24). In these disorders the lung tissue is normal. Intrapulmonary causes of restrictive lung disease involve the pleura or the lung tissue (Table 27-25).

NURSING CARE PLAN 27-2

Patient After Thoracotomy

EXPECTED PATIENT OUTCOMES	NURSING INTERVENTIONS and *RATIONALES*
NURSING DIAGNOSIS	**Impaired gas exchange** *related to* air and fluid collection in lungs and pleural space *as manifested by* chest tube or tubes with drainage, decreased breath sounds, abnormal pulse oximetry.
▪ Full expansion of lungs ▪ Normal breath sounds bilaterally ▪ Normal pulse oximetry	▪ Monitor chest drainage system (see text) *to ensure adequate ventilation and to detect hemorrhage.* ▪ Monitor respiratory rate and pattern and manifestations of hypoxia *to allow early recognition of significant changes in respiratory function.* ▪ Administer low-flow oxygen (1-2 L /min) via nasal prongs or cannula *to treat hypoxemia.* ▪ Assist with position changes *to increase patient's comfort and facilitate aeration of the lungs.*
NURSING DIAGNOSIS	**Ineffective breathing pattern** *related to* pain, position, and possible complication on affected side *as manifested by* shortness of breath, shallow respirations, use of accessory muscles.
▪ Respiratory rate 12-18 breaths/min ▪ Ease of respiration	▪ Auscultate lungs every 2-3 hr *to evaluate the rate, quality, and depth of patient's respirations and the need for tracheal suctioning.* ▪ Observe for manifestations of complications such as pneumothorax or hemothorax with symptoms of acute shortness of breath, shallow rapid respirations, dyspnea, cough, abnormal pulse oximetry, and air hunger. ▪ Assess patency of and drainage from chest tubes *to validate proper functioning.* ▪ Assist patient with deep breathing *to provide encouragement and improve results.* ▪ Position patient for comfort and ease of breathing *to increase compliance with respiratory treatments.* ▪ Encourage use of incentive spirometer every 2-3 hr *to provide visual feedback to the patient on effectiveness of respirations.*
NURSING DIAGNOSIS	**Anxiety** *related to* feelings of dyspnea and pain *as manifested by* anxious facial expression, inability to cooperate with instructions to breathe slowly.
▪ Relief from anxiety or able to manage level of anxiety	▪ Stay with patient during procedures *to provide encouragement and explanations.* ▪ Provide feedback about effective breathing *to provide encouragement and reduce anxiety.* ▪ Administer pain medication as ordered or implement nonpharmacologic measures such as distraction and relaxation *because pain increases anxiety and decreases compliance with necessary treatments.*

TABLE 27-23   Relationship of Lung Volumes to Type of Ventilatory Disorder

LUNG VOLUMES	RESTRICTIVE	OBSTRUCTIVE	RESTRICTIVE AND OBSTRUCTIVE
Vital capacity (VC)	↓	Normal or ↓	↓
Total lung capacity (TLC)	↓	↑	Variable
Residual volume (RV)	Normal or ↓	↑	Variable
Forced expiratory volume in 1 second (FEV_1)	Normal or ↓	↓	↓
FEV_1/Functional vital capacity (FVC)	Normal or ↑	↓	↓

PLEURAL EFFUSION

Types

The pleural space lies between the lung and chest wall and normally contains a very thin layer of fluid. **Pleural effusion** is a collection of fluid in the pleural space (see Fig. 27-5, *A*). It is not a disease but rather a sign of a serious disease. Pleural effusion is frequently classified as transudative or exudative according to whether the protein content of the effusion is low or high, respectively.[34] A *transudate* occurs primarily in noninflammatory conditions and is an accumulation of protein-poor, cell-poor fluid. Transudative pleural effusions (also called *hydrothorax*) are caused by

(1) increased hydrostatic pressure found in congestive heart failure (CHF), which is the most common cause of pleural effusion, or (2) decreased oncotic pressure (from hypoalbuminemia) found in chronic liver or renal disease. In these situations, fluid movement is facilitated out of the capillaries and into the pleural space.

An *exudative effusion* is an accumulation of fluid and cells in an area of inflammation. An exudative pleural effusion results from increased capillary permeability characteristic of the inflammatory reaction. This type of effusion occurs secondary to conditions such as pulmonary malignancies, pulmonary infections, pulmonary embolization, and GI disease (e.g., pancreatic disease, esophageal perforation).

TABLE 27-24 Extrapulmonary Causes of Restrictive Lung Disease

DISEASE OR ALTERATION	DESCRIPTION	COMMENTS
Central Nervous System		
▪ Head injury, CNS lesion (e.g., tumor, stroke)	Injury to or impingement on respiratory center, causing hypoventilation or hyperventilation; relationship of manifestations to increased intracranial pressure (see Chapters 55 and 56)	Management is directed toward treating the underlying cause, maintaining the airway, using mechanical ventilation for supportive care, and assessing for manifestations of increased intracranial pressure.
▪ Narcotic and barbiturate use	Depression of respiratory center, respiratory rate of <12 breaths/min	Respiratory depression is caused by drug overdose or inadvertent administration of drugs to a person with respiratory difficulty. These drugs should not be administered to a person with a respiratory rate of <12 breaths/min.
Neuromuscular System		
▪ Guillain-Barré syndrome	Acute inflammation of peripheral nerves and ganglia; paralysis of intercostal nerves leading to diaphragmatic breathing; paralysis of vagal preganglionic and postganglionic fibers leading to reduced ability of bronchioles to constrict, dilate, and respond to irritants	Patient often has to be put on mechanical ventilation for supportive care (see Chapter 59).
▪ Amyotrophic lateral sclerosis	Progressive degenerative disorder of the motor neurons in the spinal cord, brain stem, and motor cortex; respiratory system involvement as a result of interruption of nerve transmission to respiratory muscles, especially diaphragm	See Chapter 57 for clinical manifestations and management.
▪ Myasthenia gravis	Defect in neuromuscular junction, respiratory system involvement as a result of interruption of nerve transmission to respiratory muscles	See Chapter 57 for clinical manifestations and management.
▪ Muscular dystrophy	Hereditary disease; eventual involvement of all skeletal muscles; paralysis of respiratory muscles, including intercostals, diaphragm, and accessory muscles	Pulmonary problems develop late in disease process.
Chest Wall		
▪ Chest-wall trauma (e.g., flail chest, fractured rib)	Rib fracture causing inspiratory pain; voluntary splinting of chest, resulting in shallow, rapid breathing; impaired ventilatory ability caused by paradoxical breathing	Strapping the chest wall to stabilize the fractures is not recommended because this increases the restrictive defect.
▪ Pickwickian syndrome (extreme obesity)	Excess adipose tissue interfering with chest-wall and diaphragmatic excursion, somnolence from hypoxemia and CO_2 retention, polycythemia from chronic hypoxia	Weight loss generally causes reversal of symptoms. Prevention and prompt treatment of respiratory infections are important. Condition is worsened in supine position.
▪ Kyphoscoliosis	Posterior and lateral angulation of the spine; restriction of ventilation as a result of alteration in thoracic excursion; increase in work of breathing; pattern of rapid, shallow breathing; reduction of lung volume; compression of alveoli and blood vessels	Only small number of persons with condition develop severe respiratory problems. Atelectasis and pneumonia are common complications.

The type of pleural effusion can be determined by a sample of pleural fluid obtained via **thoracentesis** (a procedure done to remove fluid from the pleural space). Exudates have a high protein content, and the fluid is generally dark yellow or amber. Transudates have a low protein content or contain no protein, and the fluid is clear or pale yellow.[35] The fluid can also be analyzed for red and white blood cells, malignant cells, bacteria, and glucose.

An **empyema** is a pleural effusion that contains pus. It is caused by conditions such as pneumonia, TB, lung abscess, and infection of surgical wounds of the chest. A complication of empyema is *fibrothorax,* in which there is fibrous fusion of the visceral and parietal pleurae (see Fig. 27-5, *A*).

Clinical Manifestations

Common clinical manifestations of pleural effusion are progressive dyspnea and decreased movement of the chest wall on the affected side. There may be pleuritic pain from the underlying disease. Physical examination of the chest will indicate dull-

TABLE 27-25	Intrapulmonary Causes of Restrictive Lung Disease
DISEASE OR ALTERATION	**DESCRIPTION**
Pleural Disorders	
▪ Pleural effusion	Accumulation of fluid in pleural space secondary to altered hydrostatic or oncotic pressure; fluid collection >250 ml, showing up on chest x-ray
▪ Pleurisy (pleuritis)	Inflammation of pleura; classification as fibrinous (dry) or serofibrinous (wet); wet pleurisy accompanied by an increase in pleural fluid and possibly resulting in pleural effusion
▪ Pneumothorax	Accumulation of air in pleural space with accompanying lung collapse
Parenchymal Disorders	
▪ Atelectasis	Condition of lung characterized by collapsed, airless alveoli; possibly acute (e.g., in postoperative patient) or chronic (e.g., in patient with malignant tumor)
▪ Pneumonia	Acute inflammation of lung tissue caused by bacteria, viruses, fungi, chemicals, dusts, and other factors
▪ Interstitial lung diseases (ILDs)	General term that includes a variety of chronic lung disorders characterized by some type of injury, inflammation, and scarring (or fibrosis); this process occurs in the interstitium (tissue between the alveoli) and the lung becomes stiff (fibrotic); can be caused by occupational and environmental exposures (see Table 27-13), infections (e.g., TB), and connective tissue disorders (e.g., rheumatoid arthritis); when all known causes of ILDs are ruled out, the condition is termed idiopathic pulmonary fibrosis (IPF)
▪ ARDS*	Atelectasis, pulmonary edema, congestion, and hyaline membrane lining the alveolar wall; result of variety of conditions, including shock lung, O_2 toxicity, gram-negative sepsis, cardiopulmonary bypass, and aspiration pneumonia

*See Chapter 66 for clinical manifestations and management.
ARDS, Acute respiratory distress syndrome.

ness to percussion and absent or decreased breath sounds over the affected area. The chest x-ray will indicate an abnormality if the effusion is greater than 250 ml. Manifestations of empyema include the manifestations of pleural effusion, as well as fever, night sweats, cough, and weight loss. A thoracentesis reveals an exudate containing thick, purulent material.

Thoracentesis

If the cause of the pleural effusion is not known, a diagnostic thoracentesis is needed to obtain pleural fluid for analysis (see Chapter 25, Fig. 25-17). If the degree of pleural effusion is severe enough to impair breathing, a therapeutic thoracentesis is done to remove fluid for analysis.

A thoracentesis is performed by having the patient sit on the edge of a bed and lean forward over a bedside table. The puncture site is determined by chest x-ray, and percussion of the chest is used to assess the maximum degree of dullness. The skin is cleaned with an antiseptic solution and anesthetized locally. The thoracentesis needle is inserted into the intercostal space. Fluid can be aspirated with a syringe, or tubing can be connected to allow fluid to drain into a sterile collecting bottle. After the fluid is removed, the needle is withdrawn, and a bandage is applied over the insertion site.

Usually only 1000 to 1200 ml of pleural fluid is removed at one time. Because high volumes are removed, rapid removal can result in hypotension, hypoxemia, or pulmonary edema.[36] A follow-up chest x-ray should be done to detect a possible pneumothorax that could have been induced by perforation of the visceral pleura. During and after the procedure the patient should be observed for any manifestations of respiratory distress.

Collaborative Care

The main goal of management of pleural effusions is to treat the underlying cause. For example, adequate treatment of CHF with diuretics and sodium restriction will result in decreased pleural effu-

sions. The treatment of pleural effusions secondary to malignant disease represents a more difficult problem. These types of pleural effusions are frequently recurrent and accumulate quickly after thoracentesis. Chemical pleurodesis may be used to sclerose the pleural space and prevent reaccumulation of effusion fluid. Although doxycycline (Vibramycin) and bleomycin (Blenoxane) have been used for sclerosing with good results, talc appears to be the most effective agent for pleurodesis. Thoracoscopy can be used to perform talc pleurodesis after inspection of the pleural space. After instillation of the sclerosing agent, patients are usually instructed to rotate their positions to spread the agent uniformly throughout the pleural space. Chest tubes are left in place after pleurodesis until fluid drainage is greater than 150 ml/day and no air leaks are noted.

Treatment of empyema is directed at drainage of the pleural space via thoracentesis or a closed thoracotomy tube. Appropriate antibiotic therapy is also needed to eradicate the causative organism. If a fibrothorax results from the empyema and causes severe pulmonary restriction, a decortication surgical procedure is done in which the pleural membranes are separated.

PLEURISY

Pleurisy (pleuritis) is an inflammation of the pleura. The most common causes are pneumonia, TB, chest trauma, pulmonary infarctions, and neoplasms. The inflammation usually subsides with adequate treatment of the primary disease. Pleurisy can be classified as fibrinous (dry) with fibrinous deposits on the pleural surface or serofibrinous (wet) with increased production of pleural fluid that may result in pleural effusion.

The pain of pleurisy is typically abrupt and sharp in onset and is aggravated by inspiration. The patient's breathing is shallow and rapid to avoid unnecessary movement of the pleura and chest wall. A pleural friction rub may occur, which is the sound over areas where inflamed visceral pleura and parietal pleura rub over one another during inspiration. This sound is usually loudest at peak inspiration but can be heard during exhalation as well.

Treatment of pleurisy is aimed at treating the underlying disease and providing pain relief. Taking analgesics and lying on or splinting the affected side may provide some relief. The patient should be taught to splint the rib cage when coughing. Intercostal nerve blocks may be done if the pain is severe.

ATELECTASIS

Atelectasis is a condition of the lungs characterized by collapsed, airless alveoli. The most common cause of atelectasis is airway obstruction that results from retained exudates and secretions. This is frequently observed in the postoperative patient. Normally the pores of Kohn (see Chapter 25, Fig. 25-1) provide for collateral passage of air from one alveolus to another. Deep inspiration is necessary to open the pores effectively. For this reason, deep-breathing exercises are important in preventing atelectasis in the high risk patient (e.g., postoperative, immobilized patient). Pulmonary fibrosis can occur as a complication of chronic atelectasis. (The prevention and treatment of atelectasis are discussed in Chapter 19.)

Interstitial Lung Disease

Many acute and chronic lung disorders with variable degrees of pulmonary inflammation and fibrosis are collectively referred to as *interstitial lung diseases* (ILDs). ILDs have been difficult to classify because more than 200 known disease have diffuse lung involvement, either as the primary condition or as a significant part of a multiorgan process, as may occur in connective tissue disorders (e.g., systemic lupus erythematosus, rheumatoid arthritis).

Among the ILDs of known cause, the largest group comprises occupational and environmental exposures, especially the inhalation of dusts and various fumes or gases. The most common ILDs of unknown etiology are idiopathic pulmonary fibrosis and sarcoidosis.

IDIOPATHIC PULMONARY FIBROSIS

Idiopathic pulmonary fibrosis (IPF) is characterized by scar tissue in the connective tissue of the lungs as a sequela to inflammation or irritation. A common risk factor for IPF is environmental or occupational inhalation of organic and inorganic substances (see section earlier in this chapter). Other risk factors include cigarette smoking and history of chronic aspiration. There also may be genetic risk factor.

Clinical manifestations of IPF include exertional dyspnea, nonproductive cough, and inspirational crackles with or without clubbing. Chest x-ray shows changes characteristic of IPF. Pulmonary function tests show a typical pattern characteristic of restrictive lung disease (see Table 27-23).

The clinical course is variable, with a 5-year survival rate of 30% to 50% after diagnosis. Treatment includes corticosteroids, cytotoxic agents (azathioprine [Imuran], cyclophosphamide [Cytoxan]), and antifibrotic agents (colchicine). However, there is no good evidence that any of these treatments improves survival or quality of life. Lung transplantation is an option that should be considered for those who meet the criteria. (Lung transplantation is discussed later in this chapter.)

SARCOIDOSIS

Sarcoidosis is a chronic, multisystem granulomatous disease of unknown cause that primarily affects the lungs. The disease may also involve the skin, eyes, liver, kidney, heart, and lymph nodes. The disease is often acute or subacute and self-limiting, but in many individuals it is chronic with remissions and exacerbations. Marked pulmonary fibrosis can be present with severe restrictive lung disease. Cor pulmonale can develop in the advanced stages. There is no specific treatment for sarcoidosis. Often the disease is self-limiting, and the patient gets well without treatment. Corticosteroids have been used to relieve symptoms and suppress the acute inflammation.

Vascular Lung Disorders

PULMONARY EDEMA

Pulmonary edema is an abnormal accumulation of fluid in the alveoli and interstitial spaces of the lungs. It is a complication of various heart and lung diseases (Table 27-26). It is considered a medical emergency and may be life threatening.

Normally, there is a balance between the hydrostatic and oncotic pressures in the pulmonary capillaries. If the hydrostatic pressure increases or the colloid oncotic pressure decreases, the net effect will be fluid leaving the pulmonary capillaries and entering the interstitial space. This stage is referred to as *interstitial edema*. At this stage the lymphatics can usually drain away the excess fluid. If fluid continues to leak from the pulmonary capillaries it will enter the alveoli. This stage is referred to as *alveolar edema*. Pulmonary edema interferes with gas exchange by causing an alteration in the diffusing pathway between the alveoli and the pulmonary capillaries.

The most common cause of pulmonary edema is left-sided CHF. (The clinical manifestations and management of pulmonary edema are described in Chapter 34.) Chronic forms of pulmonary edema are not common. This condition can be asymptomatic for a long period of time while changes occur resulting in pulmonary fibrosis. An early manifestation of this condition may be paroxysmal nocturnal dyspnea as a result of increased hydrostatic pressure in the lungs in the recumbent position.

PULMONARY EMBOLISM

A **pulmonary embolism** arises from thrombi in the venous circulation or right side of the heart (thromboembolism) and from other sources, such as amniotic fluid, air, fat, bone marrow, and foreign intravenous material. The most common source of the thrombus is the deep veins of the legs. The thrombus breaks loose and travels as an embolus until it lodges in the pulmonary vasculature.

The result of the thromboembolic occlusion is complete or partial occlusion of the pulmonary arterial blood flow to parts of

---

TABLE 27-26 | **Causes of Pulmonary Edema**

Congestive heart failure
Overhydration with intravenous fluids
Hypoalbuminemia: nephrotic syndrome, hepatic disease, nutritional disorders
Altered capillary permeability of lungs: inhaled toxins, inflammation (e.g., pneumonia), severe hypoxia, near-drowning
Malignancies of the lymph system
Respiratory distress syndrome (e.g., O_2 toxicity)
Unknown causes: neurogenic condition, narcotic overdose, high altitude

the lung. Thus the lung tissue distal to the embolus is ventilated but not perfused. As the pressure increases in the pulmonary vasculature, pulmonary hypertension may result. (Pulmonary embolism is described in detail in Chapter 37.)

Pulmonary Hypertension

Pulmonary hypertension comprises a variety of disorders occurring as a primary disease (primary pulmonary hypertension) or as a complication of a large number of respiratory and cardiac disorders (secondary pulmonary hypertension). Pulmonary hypertension is elevated pulmonary pressure resulting from an increase in pulmonary vascular resistance to blood flow through small arteries and arterioles. A 60% to 70% reduction in the pulmonary vascular bed is required before pulmonary hypertension develops.

PRIMARY PULMONARY HYPERTENSION

Primary pulmonary hypertension (PPH) is a rare disease whose exact cause in unknown. PPH is characterized by mean pulmonary arterial pressure greater than 25 mm Hg at rest or greater than 30 mm Hg with exercise, in the absence of a demonstrable cause. PPH is associated with a poor prognosis because there is no definitive therapy.

Etiology and Pathophysiology

The exact etiology of PPH is unknown. PPH has been linked to the use of fenfluramine in the drug Fen-Phen, which was used as an appetite suppressant to treat obesity. The drug was withdrawn from the market in 1996. PPH affects more women than men. It may have a genetic component; the incidence is higher in families.

Normally the pulmonary circulation is characterized by low resistance and low pressure. In pulmonary hypertension the pulmonary pressures are elevated. Until recently the pathophysiology of PPH was poorly understood. Recently it was discovered that a key mechanism involved in PPH is a deficient release of vasodilator mediators from the pulmonary epithelium with a resultant cascade of injury (Fig. 27-11).

Clinical Manifestations

Classic symptoms of pulmonary hypertension are dyspnea on exertion and fatigue. Exertional chest pain, dizziness, and exertional syncope are other symptoms. These symptoms are related to the inability of cardiac output to increase in response to increased oxygen demand. Eventually as the disease progresses, dyspnea occurs at rest. Pulmonary hypertension increases the workload of the right ventricle and causes right ventricular hypertrophy (a condition called *cor pulmonale*) and eventually heart failure. A chest x-ray generally shows enlarged central pulmonary arteries and clear lung fields. An enlarged right heart may be seen. Echocardiogram usually reveals right ventricular hypertrophy.

Collaborative Care

Diagnostic evaluation includes ECG, chest x-ray, and echocardiogram. If the diagnosis is still in doubt, right cardiac catheterization to measure pulmonary artery pressures is recommended.[37] Additional tests may be done to exclude secondary factors. Early recognition of pulmonary hypertension is essential

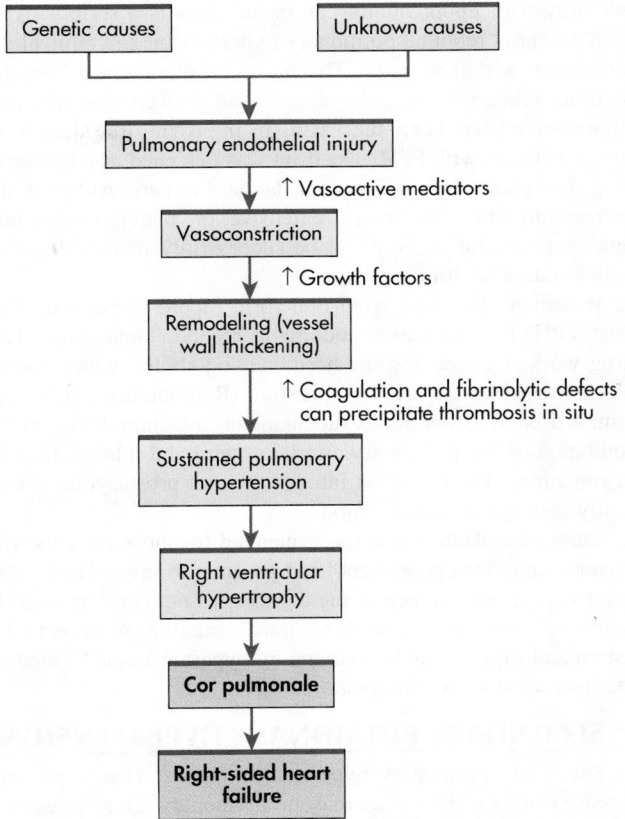

FIG. 27-11 Pathogenesis of pulmonary hypertension and cor pulmonale.

to interrupt the self-perpetuation cycle responsible for the progression of this problem (see Fig. 27-11).

Although there is no cure for PPH, treatment can relieve symptoms, increase quality of life, and prolong life. Diuretic therapy relieves dyspnea and peripheral edema and may be useful in reducing right ventricular volume overload. Anticoagulation therapy is recommended for patients with severe pulmonary hypertension to prevent in situ thrombus formation and venous thrombosis.

Vasodilator therapy is used to reduce right ventricular overload by dilating pulmonary vessels and reversing remodeling. Many patients with pulmonary hypertension can be effectively managed with calcium channel blocker therapy, such as nifedipine (Adalat) and diltiazem (Cardizem).

Epoprostenol (Flolan), a prostacyclin that promotes pulmonary vasodilation and reduces pulmonary vascular resistance, has revolutionized the management of PPH. Continuous epoprostenol has been shown to have significant improvement in clinical symptoms and long-term survival.[38] It is now the treatment of choice for selected patients unresponsive to calcium channel blockers. Its administration requires the placement of an indwelling central line catheter and continuous infusion pump. The patient and family must be trained to use the portable intravenous infusion pump, mix medications, manage the central line, and monitor for complications. The half-life of the drug is less than 6 minutes. If the central line is disrupted, stopped, or dislodged for any reason, clinical deterioration from abrupt withdrawal of epoprostenol can occur. This is a serious event with potential rebound pulmonary hypertension and clinical deterioration within minutes. The major problems have been infections related to vascular access and broken central lines. Epoprostenol has been successful in improving the quality of life of patients with PPH. The drug was designed as a bridge to lung transplantation but is now a standard of care. Although the patient and family teaching is extensive, the patient on continuous epoprostenol therapy can be successfully managed with a collaborative health care team.

Bosentan (Tracleer) is an oral form of prostacyclin used to treat PPH. It is an active endothelin receptor antagonist. This drug works by blocking the hormone endothelin, which causes blood vessels to constrict. Treprostinil (Remodulin), a prostacyclin, is used as a continuous subcutaneous injection. It causes vasodilation of the pulmonary arterial system and inhibits platelet aggregation. The use of an inhaled form of prostacyclin is currently undergoing investigation.

Lung transplantation is recommended for those patients who do not respond to epoprostenol and progress to severe right-sided heart failure. Recurrence of the disease has not been reported in individuals who have undergone transplantation. A patient education and support site for pulmonary hypertension is located on the Internet at *www.phassociation.org*.

SECONDARY PULMONARY HYPERTENSION

Secondary pulmonary hypertension occurs when a primary disease causes a chronic increase in pulmonary artery pressures. The specific primary disease pathology may result in anatomic or vascular changes causing the pulmonary hypertension. Anatomic changes causing increased vascular resistance include (1) loss of capillaries as a result of alveolar wall damage (e.g., COPD), (2) stiffening of the pulmonary vasculature (e.g., pulmonary fibrosis connective tissue disorders), and (3) obstruction of blood flow (chronic emboli).

Vasomotor increases in pulmonary vascular resistance are found in conditions characterized by alveolar hypoxia. Hypoxia causes localized vasoconstriction and shunting of blood away from poorly ventilated alveoli. Alveolar hypoxia can be caused by a wide variety of conditions (e.g., pickwickian syndrome, kyphoscoliosis, neuromuscular disease).

It is possible to have a combination of anatomic restriction and vasomotor constriction. This is found in the patient with long-standing chronic bronchitis who has chronic hypoxia in addition to loss of lung tissue.

Treatment of pulmonary hypertension caused primarily by pulmonary or cardiac disorders consists mainly of treating the underlying disorder, such as COPD or pulmonary emboli.

COR PULMONALE

Cor pulmonale is enlargement of the right ventricle secondary to diseases of the lung, thorax, or pulmonary circulation. Pulmonary hypertension is usually a preexisting condition in the individual with cor pulmonale. Cor pulmonale may be present with or without overt cardiac failure. The most common cause of cor pulmonale is COPD. Almost any disorder that affects the respiratory system can cause cor pulmonale. The etiology and pathogenesis of pulmonary hypertension and cor pulmonale are outlined in Fig. 27-11.

Clinical Manifestations

Clinical manifestations of cor pulmonale include dyspnea, chronic productive cough, wheezing respirations, retrosternal or substernal pain, and fatigue. Chronic hypoxemia leads to polycythemia and increased total blood volume and viscosity of the blood. (Polycythemia is often present in cor pulmonale secondary to COPD.) Compensatory mechanisms that are secondary to hypoxemia can aggravate the pulmonary hypertension. Episodes of cor pulmonale in a person with underlying chronic respiratory problems are frequently triggered by an acute respiratory tract infection.

If heart failure accompanies cor pulmonale, additional manifestations such as peripheral edema; weight gain; distended neck veins; full, bounding pulse; and enlarged liver will also be found. (Heart failure is discussed in Chapter 34.) A chest x-ray will show an enlarged right ventricle and pulmonary artery.

Collaborative Care

The primary management of cor pulmonale is directed at treating the underlying pulmonary problem that precipitated the heart problem (Table 27-27). Long-term low-flow O_2 therapy is used to correct the hypoxemia and reduce vasoconstriction in chronic states of respiratory disorders. If fluid, electrolyte, and acid-base imbalances are present, they must be corrected. Diuretics and a low-sodium diet will help decrease the plasma volume and the load on the heart. Bronchodilator therapy is indicated if the underlying respiratory problem is due to an obstructive disorder. Digitalis may be used if there is left-sided heart failure. Other treatments include those for pulmonary hypertension and include vasodilator therapy, calcium channel blockers, and anticoagulants. Theophylline and terbutaline may help reduce dyspnea, possibly due to myocardial contractility and acute decompensation of cor pulmonale. Phlebotomy may be needed in the patient with severe polycythemia (hematocrit above 55%) because a reduction in volume is associated with a resultant decrease in pulmonary pres-

TABLE 27-27	Collaborative Care Cor Pulmonale
Diagnostic	
History and physical examination	
ABGs	
Serum and urine electrolytes	
Monitoring with ECG	
Chest x-ray	
Collaborative Therapy	
O_2 therapy	
Bronchodilators	
Diuretics	
Low-sodium diet	
Fluid restriction	
Antibiotics (if indicated)	
Digitalis (if left-sided heart failure)	
Vasodilators (if indicated)	
Calcium channel blockers (if indicated)	

ABGs, Arterial blood gases; *ECG,* electrocardiogram.

sures. When medical treatment fails, lung transplantation is an option for some patients.

Chronic management of cor pulmonale resulting from COPD is similar to that described for COPD (see Chapter 28). Continuous low-flow O_2 during sleep; exercise; and small, frequent meals may allow the patient to feel better and be more active.

Lung Transplantation

Lung transplantation has evolved as a viable therapy for patients with end-stage lung disease. Improved selection criteria, technical advances, and better methods of immunosuppression have resulted in improved survival rates. A variety of pulmonary disorders are potentially treatable with some type of lung transplantation (Table 27-28). Various transplant options are available, including single lung transplant, bilateral lung transplant, and heart-lung transplant.

Patients being considered for a lung transplant need to undergo extensive evaluation. The candidate for lung transplantation should not have a malignancy or recent history of malignancy (within the last 2 years), renal or liver insufficiency, or HIV. The current wait for a lung transplant is greater than 1 year. The candidate and the family undergo psychologic screening to determine the ability to cope with a postoperative regimen that requires strict adherence to immunosuppressive therapy, continuous monitoring for early signs of infection, and prompt reporting of manifestations of infection for medical evaluation.

Postoperatively, infection is the leading cause of morbidity and mortality. Viral infection with CMV and herpes simplex occur frequently. CMV is a leading cause of mortality, usually seen 4 to 8 weeks postoperatively. Bacterial pathogens and fungal infections are seen. Empiric antibiotic regimen is routine perioperatively for potential pathogens isolated from donor or recipient. Pulmonary clearance measures, including aerosolized bronchodilators, chest physiotherapy, and deep-breathing and coughing techniques, are mandatory to minimize potential complications. Maintenance of fluid balance is vital in the postoperative phase.

Immunosuppressive therapy usually includes a triple-drug regimen of cyclosporine, azathioprine (Imuran), and prednisone. Immunosuppressive drugs are discussed in Chapter 13 and Table 13-17.

Acute rejection can be seen as soon as 5 to 7 days after surgery. It is characterized by low-grade fever, fatigue, and oxygen desaturation with exercise. Accurate diagnosis is by transtracheal biopsy. Treatment is bolus corticosteroids, which results in complete remission of symptoms.

TABLE 27-28 Indications for Lung Transplant

- α_1-Antitrypsin deficiency
- Bronchiectasis
- Cystic fibrosis
- Emphysema
- Idiopathic pulmonary fibrosis
- Interstitial lung disease
- Pulmonary fibrosis secondary to other diseases (e.g., sarcoidosis)
- Pulmonary hypertension

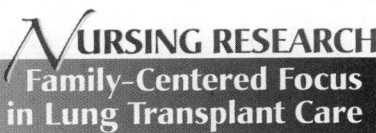

NURSING RESEARCH
Family-Centered Focus in Lung Transplant Care

Citation
Kurz JM: Experiences of well spouses after lung transplantation, *J Adv Nurs* 34:493, 2001.

Purpose
To explore what life is like for well spouses after their partners' lung transplantation.

Methods
A convenience sample of 12 well spouses of lung transplant recipients from eight states participated in this study, which was posted on an Internet listserve. Spouses completed a demographic form, the Family Inventory of Life Events (FILE), and the Center for Epidemiologic Studies Depression Scale (CES-D). In addition, a taped telephone interview was done in which the spouses shared details of their lives after their partners' lung transplant.

Results and Conclusions
The core theme was a "roller coaster ride" characterized by a series of ups and downs. Major themes expressed included coping, giving drugs, knowing the donor, making comparisons (life before transplant versus life after transplant), and caring for themselves. Most spouses thought that their knowledge of drugs and side effects was deficient, with the frequent refrain, "I was not prepared." Five stages of life for well spouses after lung transplant were identified: (1) the transplant event, (2) cocooning (community reintegration), (3) normalizing, (4) branching out, and (5) settling down. Spousal adjustment was associated with patient recovery.

Implications for Nursing Practice
This study supports the premise that nurses should use a family-centered focus for transplant patients, as opposed to a patient-centered focus, and should specifically address the needs of the family members. Family teaching is seen as vital. By incorporating the information of the five stages in family-patient teaching materials, the nurse can initiate discussions around changes in roles, stressors, and activities over time. The nurse can apply information from this study to help spouses anticipate changes at each stage and develop effective coping strategies.

Bronchiolitis obliterans (an obstructive airways disease causing progressive occlusion) is considered to represent chronic rejection in lung transplant patients. The onset is often subacute, with gradual onset of progressive obstructive airflow defect, including cough, dyspnea, and recurrent lower respiratory tract infection. Treatment involves optimum maintenance immunosuppression.

Discharge planning begins in the preoperative phase. Patients are placed in an outpatient rehabilitation program to improve physical endurance. The use of home spirometry has been useful in monitoring trends in lung function. Patients are taught to keep logs of medications, laboratory results, and spirometry. Over the past decade, lung transplantation has become an increasingly important mode of therapy for patients with a variety of end-stage lung diseases.

CRITICAL THINKING EXERCISES

Case Study
Aspiration Pneumonia

Patient Profile. Sam, a 27-year-old African American man, was admitted to the hospital because of an uncontrollable fever. He was transferred from a long-term care facility. He has a history of a gunshot wound to his left chest. Following a cardiac arrest after the accident he developed hypoxic encephalopathy. He has a tracheostomy and gastrostomy tube. He has a history of methicillin-resistant *Staphylococcus aureus* (MRSA) in his sputum.

Subjective Data
- Family says that they visit him regularly and are very devoted to him.

Objective Data

Physical Examination
- Thin, cachectic African American man in moderate respiratory distress
- Unresponsive to voice, touch, or painful stimuli
- Vital signs: temperature 104° F (40° C), heart rate 120, respiratory rate 30, O_2 saturation 90%
- Chest auscultation revealed crackles and scattered rhonchi in the left upper lobe

Diagnostic Studies
- Serum albumin 2.8 g/dl (28 g/L)
- White blood cell (WBC) count 18,000/μl (18 × 10⁹/L)
- Sputum specimen: thick, green colored, foul smelling; cultures pending
- Arterial blood gases: pH 7.29, PaO_2 80 mm Hg, $PaCO_2$ 40 mm Hg, bicarbonate 16 mEq/L
- Stool culture positive for *Clostridium difficile*
- Chest x-ray: infiltrate in left upper lobe; no pleural effusions noted

CRITICAL THINKING QUESTIONS

1. What types of infectious disease precautions should be taken related to Sam's hospitalization?
2. What clinical manifestations of aspiration pneumonia did Sam exhibit? Explain their pathophysiologic bases.
3. What antibiotic medication is likely to be prescribed?
4. What is his oxygenation status and metabolic state?
5. What other clinical issues must be addressed in his plan of care?
6. What family interventions would you initiate?
7. Based on the assessment data presented, write one or more appropriate nursing diagnoses. Are there any collaborative problems?

Nursing Research Issues

1. What are effective measures that a nurse can institute to increase patient compliance with long-term antituberculosis medication?
2. Indicate which strategy to use when helping a patient who is unwilling to quit smoking.
3. What position should a patient assume following lung surgery for comfort and maximum oxygenation?
4. Is there a significant impact on the quality of life and survival of pulmonary hypertension patients on epoprostenol therapy?
5. Does a patient-focused approach for the lung transplant patient meet the family's needs?

REVIEW QUESTIONS

The number of the question corresponds to the same-numbered objective at the beginning of the chapter.

1. In assessing a patient with pneumococcal pneumonia, the nurse recognizes that clinical manifestations of this condition include
   a. fever, chills, and a productive cough with rust-colored sputum.
   b. a nonproductive cough and night sweats that are usually self-limiting.
   c. a gradual onset of nasal stuffiness, sore throat, and purulent productive cough.
   d. an abrupt onset of fever, nonproductive cough, and formation of lung abscesses.

2. An appropriate nursing intervention for a patient with pneumonia with the nursing diagnosis of ineffective airway clearance related to thick secretions and fatigue would be to
   a. perform postural drainage every hour.
   b. provide analgesics as ordered to promote patient comfort.
   c. administer oxygen as prescribed to maintain optimal oxygen levels.
   d. teach the patient how to cough effectively to bring secretions to the mouth.

3. A patient with TB has a nursing diagnosis of noncompliance. The nurse recognizes that the most common etiologic factor for this diagnosis in patients with TB is
   a. fatigue and lack of energy to manage self-care.
   b. lack of knowledge about how the disease is transmitted.
   c. little or no motivation to adhere to a long-term drug regimen.
   d. feelings of shame and the response to the social stigma associated with TB.

4. A patient has been receiving high-dose corticosteroids and broad-spectrum antibiotics for treatment of serious trauma and infection. The nurse plans care for the patient knowing that the patient is most susceptible to
   a. candidiasis.
   b. aspergillosis.
   c. histoplasmosis.
   d. coccidioidomycosis.

5. A primary goal for the patient with bronchiectasis is that the patient will
   a. have no recurrence of disease.
   b. have normal pulmonary function.
   c. maintain removal of bronchial secretions.
   d. avoid environmental agents that precipitate inflammation.

REVIEW QUESTIONS—cont'd

6. A common pathophysiologic characteristic of many types of pneumoconiosis is
   a. liquefactive necrosis.
   b. benign tumor growth.
   c. diffuse airway obstruction.
   d. diffuse pulmonary fibrosis.

7. The type of lung cancer generally associated with the best prognosis because it is potentially surgically resectable is
   a. adenocarcinoma.
   b. small cell carcinoma.
   c. squamous cell carcinoma.
   d. undifferentiated large cell carcinoma.

8. The nurse identifies a flail chest in a trauma patient when
   a. multiple rib fractures are determined by x-ray.
   b. a tracheal deviation to the unaffected side is present.
   c. paradoxic chest movement occurs during respiration.
   d. there is decreased movement of the involved chest wall.

9. The nurse notes tidaling of the water level in the tube submerged in the water-seal chamber in a patient with closed chest-tube drainage. The nurse should
   a. continue to monitor this normal finding.
   b. check all connections for a leak in the system.
   c. lower the drainage collector further from the chest.
   d. clamp the tubing at progressively distal points away from the patient until the tidaling stops.

10. A nursing measure that should be instituted after a pneumonectomy is
    a. monitoring chest-tube drainage and functioning.
    b. positioning the patient on the unaffected side or back.
    c. range-of-motion exercises on the affected upper extremity.
    d. auscultating frequently for lung sounds on the affected side.

11. Guillain-Barré syndrome causes respiratory problems primarily by
    a. depressing the CNS.
    b. deforming chest-wall muscles.
    c. paralyzing the diaphragm secondary to trauma.
    d. interrupting nerve transmission to respiratory muscles.

12. A patient with COPD asks why the heart is affected by the respiratory disease. The nurse's response to the patient is based on the knowledge that cor pulmonale is characterized by
    a. pulmonary congestion secondary to left ventricular failure.
    b. excess serous fluid collection in the alveoli caused by retained respiratory secretions.
    c. right ventricular hypertrophy secondary to increased pulmonary vascular resistance.
    d. right ventricular failure secondary to compression of the heart by hyperinflated lungs.

13. In responding to a patient with emphysema who asks about the possibility of a lung transplant, the nurse knows that lung transplantation is contraindicated in patients
    a. with cor pulmonale.
    b. who currently smoke.
    c. older than 50 years of age.
    d. with end-stage lung disease.

REFERENCES

1. Centers for Disease Control and Prevention: National Center for Health Statistics. Available at *www.cdc.gov/nchs/fastats* (accessed 10/28/02).
2. Bartlett JG: Acute and chronic cough syndromes. In Bartlett JG: *Management of respiratory tract infections,* Philadelphia, 2001, Lippincott Williams & Wilkins.
3. Poole MD: Appropriate antibiotic use in treating respiratory tract infections, *American Journal of Managed Care* 7(suppl):S178, 2001.
4. Niederman MS: Antibiotic therapy of acute exacerbations of chronic bronchitis, *Semin Respir Infect* 15:59, 2000.
5. Kim MK et al: Guidelines for treatment of community-acquired pneumonia, *Conn Med* 65:473, 2001.
6. American Thoracic Society: Guidelines for the management of adults with community-acquired pneumonia: diagnosis, assessment of severity, antimicrobial therapy and prevention, *Am J Respir Crit Care Med* 163:1730, 2000.
7. Bartlett JG et al: Practice guidelines for the management of community-acquired pneumonia in adults, *Clin Infect Dis* 31:347, 2000.
8. American Thoracic Society: Hospital-acquired pneumonia in adults: diagnosis, assessment of severity, initial microbial therapy, and preventative strategies, *Am J Respir Crit Care Med* 153:1711, 1996.
9. Boldt MD, Kiresuk T: Community-acquired pneumonia in adults, *Nurse Pract* 26:14, 2001.
10. Chan ED, Fernandez E: The challenge of pneumonia in the elderly: part 2, *J Respir Dis* 22:236, 2001.
11. Harris JR, Miller TH: Preventing nosocomial pneumonia: evidence-based practice, *Crit Care Nurse* 20:51, 2000.
12. American Thoracic Society: Diagnostic standards and classification of tuberculosis in adults and children, *Am J Respir Crit Care Med* 161:1376, 2000.
13. Centers for Disease Control and Prevention: Press release: US TB cases decline seven percent in 2000, reaching all-time low. Available at *www.cdc.gov/nchstp/tb* (accessed 10/22/02).
14. Mahmoudi A, Iseman MD: Pitfalls in the care of patients with tuberculosis: common errors and their association with the acquisition of drug resistance, *JAMA* 270:65, 1993.
15. American Thoracic Society: Targeted tuberculin testing and treatment of latent TB infection, *Am J Respir Crit Care Med* 16:5221, 2000.
16. Catanzaro A: Assessing the indications for rapid diagnostic tests for tuberculosis, *J Respir Dis* 22:202, 2001.
17. Centers for Disease Control and Prevention: Fatal and severe liver injuries associated with rifampin and pyrazinamide for latent tuberculosis infection, revisions in the American Thoracic Society/CDC recommendations—United States, 2001, *MMWR* 50:34, 2001.
18. Horsburg CR, Feldman S, Ridzon R: Guidelines from the Infectious Disease Society of America: practice guidelines for the treatment of tuberculosis, *Clin Infect Dis* 31:633, 2000.
19. Boutotte JM: Keeping TB in check, *Nursing* 29:34, 1999.
20. Ahya V, Tino G: Bronchiectasis: new perspectives, *J Respir Dis* 22:252, 2001.

21. Joyce M, Houlihan N: Current strategies in the diagnosis and treatment of lung cancer, *Oncology Nursing* 8:1, 2001.
22. Myers F: Hunting down hantavirus, *Nursing* 32:56, 2002.
23. Women and smoking: a report of the Surgeon General—2001. Available at *www.cdc.gov/tobacco/sgr/sgr_forwomen/ataglance.htm* (accessed 10/28/02).
24. Fiore MC: Clinical practice guideline: treating tobacco use and dependence. Available at *www.surgeongeneral.gov/tobacco* (accessed 10/28/02).
25. Larsson ML et al: Environmental tobacco smoke exposure during childhood is associated with increased prevalence of asthma in adults, *Chest* 120:711, 2001.
26. Petty TL: Screening strategies for early detection of lung cancer: the time is now, *JAMA* 284: 1977, 2000.
*27. Spoljoric D: How to implement an effective smoking cessation plan, *Patient Care for the Nurse Practitioner* 3:59, 2000.
*28. Goolsby MJ: Treating tobacco use and dependence, *J Am Acad Nurse Pract* 13:101, 2001.
29. Smoking tools for quitting. One third of American smokers try to quit each year, but few take advantage of effective smoking-cessation aids, *Health News* 8:3, 2002.
30. Lazzara D: Eliminate the air of mystery from chest tubes, *Nursing* 32:36, 2002.
31. Carroll P: Exploring chest drain options, *RN* 63:50, 2000.
32. Charnock Y, Evans D: Nursing management of chest drains: a systematic review, *Aust Crit Care* 14:156, 2001.
33. Lancey RA, Gaca C, Vander Salm TJ: The use of smaller, more flexible chest drains following open heart surgery: an initial evaluation, *Chest* 119:19, 2001.
34. Hayes DD: Stemming the tide of pleural effusions, *Nursing* 31:49, 2001.
35. Clinical update: managing malignant pleural effusions, *J Respir Dis* 22:248, 2001.
36. Russo-Magno PM, Hill NR: New approaches to pulmonary hypertension, *Hosp Pract* 36:29, 2001.
37. Adiutori DM: Primary pulmonary hypertension: a review for advanced practice nurses, *Medsurg Nurs* 9:255, 2000.
*38. Crimlisk JT et al: An epoprostenol therapy program in an inner city hospital, *Am J Crit Care Med* 163 (suppl):A114, 2001.

RESOURCES

American Cancer Society
800-ACS-2345
www.cancer.org/

American Lung Association
1740 Broadway
New York, NY 10019
212-315-8700
800-586-4872
www.lungusa.org

*Nursing research–based reference.

American Society of Clinical Oncology
1900 Duke Street, Suite 200
Alexandria, VA 22314
703-299-0150
Fax: 703-299-1044
www.asco.org/

Cancer Care Ontario
Lung Cancer Clinical Practice Guidelines
www.ccopebc.ca/lungcpg.html

Cancer Information Service
NCI Public Inquiries Office
6116 Executive Boulevard, MSC8322, Suite 3036A
Bethesda, MD 20892-8322
800-422-6237
www.nci.nih.gov/

Centers for Disease Control and Prevention, National Center for Health Statistics
Division of Data Services
Hyattsville, MD 20782-2003
301-458-4636
www.cdc.gov/nchs/fastats/

Centers for Disease Control and Prevention, Office on Smoking and Health Publications
Surgeon General's Report: Women and Smoking 2001
Mail Stop K-50
4770 Buford Highway, NE
Atlanta, GA 30341-3717
770-488-5705
www.cdc.gov/tobacco/sgr/sgr_forwomen/ataglance.htm

Pulmonary Hypertension Association (PHA)
850 Sligo Ave Suite #800
Silver Spring, MD 20910
www.phassociation.org/

Smoking Cessation Consumer Tool Kit
Agency for Healthcare Research and Quality (AHRQ)
2101 East Jefferson Street, Suite 501
Rockville, MD 20852
301-594-1364
www.ahrq.gov/

Tobacco Information and Prevention Source (TIPS)
National Center for Chronic Disease Prevention and Health Promotion
800-CDC-1311
www.cdc.gov/tobacco/

Try To Stop
Massachusetts Department of Public Health
800-TRY-TO-STOP (800-879-8678)
www.trytostop.org/

For additional Internet resources, see the website for this book at *http://evolve.elsevier.com/Lewis/medsurg/*.

CHAPTER *28*

NURSING MANAGEMENT
Obstructive Pulmonary Diseases

Maria A. Connolly

LEARNING OBJECTIVES

1. Describe the etiology, pathophysiology, clinical manifestations, and collaborative care of asthma.
2. Describe the nursing management of the patient with asthma.
3. Differentiate between the etiology, pathophysiology, clinical manifestations, and collaborative care of the patient with chronic bronchitis and emphysema.
4. Describe the effects of cigarette smoking on the lungs.
5. Explain the nursing management of the patient with chronic bronchitis and emphysema.
6. Identify the indications for O_2 therapy, methods of delivery, and complications of O_2 administration.
7. Describe the pathophysiology, clinical manifestations, collaborative care, and nursing management of the patient with cystic fibrosis.

KEY TERMS

absorption atelectasis, p. 669	cor pulmonale, p. 663
α_1-antitrypsin (AAT) deficiency, p. 660	cystic fibrosis, p. 681
asthma, p. 637	emphysema, p. 659
chest physiotherapy, p. 672	O_2 toxicity, p. 669
chronic bronchitis, p. 659	postural drainage, p. 672
chronic obstructive pulmonary disease, p. 659	pursed-lip breathing, p. 672
	status asthmaticus, p. 641

"When you can't breathe, nothing else matters," is the mantra of the American Lung Association. More than 30 million Americans are living with chronic lung disease.[1] Obstructive pulmonary diseases, the most common chronic lung diseases, include diseases characterized by increased resistance to airflow as a result of airway obstruction or airway narrowing. Airway obstruction may result from accumulated secretions, edema, and swelling of the inner lumen of airways, bronchospasm, or destruction of lung tissue. *Asthma,* a reactive airway disease, is a chronic inflammatory lung disease that results in airflow obstruction, but is reversible in the early stages of disease. *Emphysema* and *chronic bronchitis* are also forms of *chronic obstructive pulmonary disease* (COPD), and most often are irreversible in nature. The patient with asthma has variations in airflow over time, whereas the limitation in expiratory airflow in the patient with emphysema or chronic bronchitis is generally more constant. The patient with a diagnosis of obstructive pulmonary disease may have distinguishing features of two or all three of these diseases.[2] *Cystic fibrosis,* another form of obstructive pulmonary disease, is a genetic disorder that produces airway obstruction because of changes in glandular secretions.

ASTHMA

Asthma is a chronic inflammatory disorder of the airways in which inflammation causes varying degrees of obstruction in the airways.[3] This inflammation causes recurrent episodes of wheezing, breathlessness, chest tightness, and cough, particularly at night and in the early morning, and is associated with an increase in existing hyperresponsiveness to a variety of stimuli. The airway obstruction may reverse spontaneously or with treatment. The hyperresponsiveness of the airways is variable, producing spontaneous fluctuations in the severity of obstruction. The clinical course of asthma is unpredictable, ranging from paroxysms of dyspnea and wheezing to unremitting symptoms.

Asthma affects an estimated 1 in 20 Americans, with 14 to 15 million people affected. The incidence of asthma has increased 60% since the 1980s.[3] It is not known why the incidence has increased. The morbidity associated with asthma is dramatic. It accounts for 5000 deaths per year. It affects school attendance (10 million absences per year), occupational choices, physical activity, and many other aspects of life. Asthma hospitalization rates have markedly increased. The highest hospitalization rates are among African Americans.[4] Death rates for asthma are consistently highest among African Americans ages 15 to 24 years. Underdiagnosis and inappropriate therapy are the major contrib-

CULTURAL & ETHNIC CONSIDERATIONS
Obstructive Pulmonary Diseases

- African Americans have a higher hospitalization rate and mortality rate from asthma than whites.
- Whites have the highest incidence of cystic fibrosis.
- Cystic fibrosis is uncommon among African Americans and Asian Americans.

Reviewed by Jean K. Berry, RN, PhD, CS, Clinical Assistant Professor and Adult Nurse Practitioner, Medical Surgical Nursing, University of Illinois at Chicago; and Barbara Velsor-Friedrich, RN, PhD, Associate Professor, Department of Maternal Child Health, Niehoff School of Nursing, Loyola University, Chicago, Ill.

utors to asthma morbidity and mortality. The high morbidity rates related to asthma may be attributed to limited access to health care, an inaccurate assessment of disease severity, a delay in seeking help, inadequate medical treatment, nonadherence to prescribed therapy, and an increase in allergens in the environment.[3]

Triggers of Asthma Attacks

Although the exact mechanisms that cause asthma remain unknown, triggers are involved (Table 28-1 and Fig. 28-1). These triggers are discussed in this section.

Allergens. In some persons with asthma, an exaggerated immunoglobulin E (IgE) response to certain allergens (e.g., dust, pollen, grasses, mites, roaches, molds, animal danders, latex) occurs.[5] These allergens attach to IgE receptors on mast cells (Fig. 28-2) (see Chapter 13, Fig. 13-9). The IgE–mast cell complexes remain for a long time so that a second exposure to the allergen triggers mast cell degranulation even years after the initial exposure to the allergen. (Allergic reactions are discussed in Chapter 13.)

Exercise. Asthma that is induced or exacerbated during physical exertion is called *exercise-induced asthma* (EIA). Typically, EIA occurs after several minutes of vigorous exercise (e.g., jogging, aerobics, walking briskly, climbing stairs) and is characterized by bronchospasm, shortness of breath, cough, and wheezing. Cromolyn (Intal), nedocromil (Tilade), and β_2-adrenergic ago-

nists have successfully maintained bronchodilation during exercise when they were inhaled 10 to 20 minutes before exercise. Long-acting β_2-adrenergic agonists (e.g., salmeterol [Serevent]) may also be of value. The patient should perform a brief warm-up of stretching for 2 to 3 minutes before exercise. When exercising in cold or dry climate conditions, breathing through a scarf or mask may decrease the likelihood of symptoms, because cold air or airway temperature changes are thought to trigger this response.

Respiratory Infections. Respiratory infections (especially viral infections) are one of the most common precipitating factors of an acute asthma attack. Bacterial respiratory infections, with the exception of sinusitis, often play a major role in exacerbations of asthma. Infections cause inflammatory changes in the tracheobronchial system and alter the mucociliary mechanism. Therefore they increase the hyperresponsiveness of the bronchial system. Increased airway responsiveness can last from 2 to 8 weeks after the infection in both normal and asthmatic persons. The patient with asthma should avoid people with colds or flu, get yearly influenza vaccinations, and avoid taking over-the-counter (OTC) cold remedies unless approved by the health care

---

TABLE 28-1   Triggers of Acute Asthma Attacks

Allergen inhalation
- Animal danders
- House dust mite
- Cockroaches
- Pollens
- Molds

Air pollutants
- Exhaust fumes
- Perfumes
- Oxidants
- Sulfur dioxides
- Cigarette smoke
- Aerosol sprays

Viral upper respiratory infection
Sinusitis
Exercise and cold, dry air
Stress
Drugs
- Aspirin
- Nonsteroidal antiinflammatory drugs
- β-adrenergic blockers

Occupational exposure
- Metal salts
- Wood and vegetable dusts
- Industrial chemicals and plastics
- Pharmaceutical agents

Food additives
- Sulfites (bisulfites and metabisulfites)
- Beer, wine, dried fruit, shrimp, processed potatoes
- Monosodium glutamate
- Tartrazine

Hormones/menses
Gastroesophageal reflux disease (GERD)

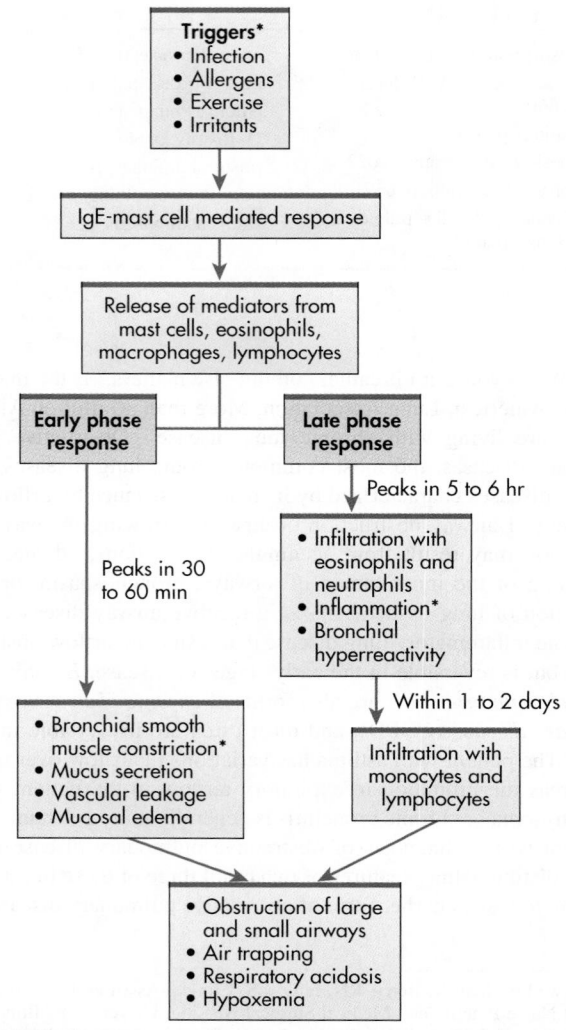

FIG. 28-1 Early- and late–phase responses of asthma. Items with an *asterisk (*)* are primary processes.

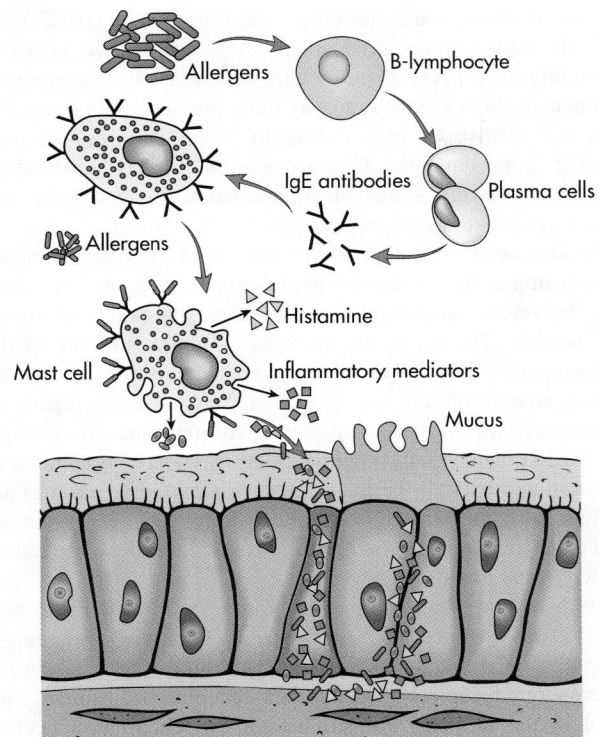

FIG. 28-2 The early-phase response in asthma is triggered when an allergen or irritant cross-links IgE receptors on mast cells, which are then activated to release histamine and other inflammatory mediators.

found in fruits, beer, and wine and used extensively in salad bars to protect vegetables from oxidation).

These drugs and food additives are thought to interfere with prostaglandin metabolic pathways, leading to enhanced production of leukotrienes, some of which are potent bronchoconstrictors. The onset of a typical reaction occurs 15 minutes to 3 hours after ingestion and is marked by profuse rhinorrhea, often accompanied by nausea, vomiting, intestinal cramps, and diarrhea. Acute asthma begins after the nasal symptoms appear. Pretreatment with corticosteroids or cromolyn does not prevent the reaction. Epinephrine, given shortly after the onset, usually controls the symptoms.

Although sensitivity to salicylates persists for many years, the nature and severity of the reaction can change over time. Dietary restrictions of tartrazine (if applicable) and avoidance of aspirin and NSAIDs are required.

Food allergies may cause asthma symptoms. Avoidance diets may be needed to prevent asthma. However, food allergies triggering asthma in adults are rare but are more common in children.

Gastroesophageal Reflux Disease. The exact mechanism by which gastroesophageal reflux disease (GERD) triggers asthma is unknown. It is postulated that reflux of stomach acid into the esophagus can be aspirated into the lungs, causing reflex vagal stimulation and bronchoconstriction. Although GERD is primarily involved in nocturnal asthma, it can trigger daytime asthma as well. Patients with hiatal hernia, excessive stress, and a prior history of reflux or ulcer disease may have acid reflux as an asthma trigger. Monitoring esophageal pH simultaneously with peak expiratory flow rate (PEFR) can determine if this is the cause of the asthma. (GERD is discussed in Chapter 40.)

Emotional Stress. Another factor often discussed in relationship to the etiology of asthma is psychologic or emotional stress. Asthma is not a psychosomatic disease, although some people still believe this to be true. However, psychologic factors can interact with the asthmatic response to worsen or ameliorate the disease process. An asthma attack caused by any trigger can produce panic and anxiety, which are not unexpected emotions during this experience. The extent to which psychologic factors contribute to the induction and continuation of any given acute exacerbation is unknown, but it probably varies from patient to patient and in the same patient from episode to episode.

Pathophysiology

The hallmarks of asthma are *airway inflammation* and *nonspecific hyperirritability* or *hyperresponsiveness* of the tracheobronchial tree. The airway hyperresponsiveness seen in asthma is caused by bronchoconstriction in response to physical, chemical, and pharmacologic agents. Traditionally asthma has been considered a disease characterized by bronchospasm. However, the pathophysiologic changes associated with asthma are also primarily due to inflammation in the airways.[7]

The *early-phase response* in asthma is characterized by bronchospasm, which induces the inflammatory sequelae of the late-phase response (see Fig. 28-1). The early-phase response is triggered when an allergen or irritant cross-links IgE receptors on mast cells found beneath the basement membrane of the bronchial wall (see Fig. 28-2). The mast cells become activated, with subsequent release of granules and disruption of the phospholipid cell membrane. Both processes result in the release of inflammatory mediators, including histamine, bradykinin, leukotrienes, prostaglandins,

provider. Influenza vaccines are safe for children and adults with asthma, regardless of the severity of their asthma.[6]

Nose and Sinus Problems. Some patients with asthma have chronic sinus problems and more have nasal problems. Nasal problems include allergic rhinitis, which can be seasonal or perennial, and nasal polyps. Sinus problems are usually related to inflammation of the mucous membranes, most commonly from noninfectious causes such as allergies. However, bacterial sinusitis may also occur. Sinusitis must be treated and large nasal polyps removed for the asthma patient to have good control. (Sinusitis is discussed in Chapter 26.)

Drugs and Food Additives. Sensitivity to specific drugs may occur in some asthmatic persons, especially those with nasal polyps. Some people with asthma have what is termed the *asthma triad*—nasal polyps, asthma, and sensitivity to aspirin and nonsteroidal antiinflammatory drugs (NSAIDs). Salicylic acid can be found in many OTC drugs and some foods, beverages, and flavorings. In some asthmatics who ingest aspirin or NSAIDs (e.g., ibuprofen [Motrin], indomethacin [Indocin]), wheezing will develop in approximately 2 hours. Some patients are also sensitive to salicylates, which are found in many foods, beverages, and flavorings. β-Adrenergic blockers (e.g., propranolol [Inderal], timolol [Timoptic]) may trigger asthma because they inhibit adrenergic stimulation of the bronchioles and thus prevent bronchodilation. Angiotensin-converting enzyme (ACE) inhibitors may produce cough in susceptible individuals, thus making asthma symptoms worse. Other agents that may precipitate asthma in the susceptible patient are tartrazine (yellow dye no. 5 found in many foods), vitamins, and sodium metabisulfite (a food preservative commonly

platelet-activating factor, chemotactic factors, and cytokines (e.g., interleukins-4 and -5).[8] (A similar process can occur in a susceptible patient after exercise.) These mediators cause intense inflammation associated with the classic immediate reaction of asthma, which consists of bronchial smooth muscle constriction, increased vasodilation and permeability, and epithelial damage. Clinically the effects are bronchospasm, increased mucus secretion, edema formation, and increased amounts of tenacious sputum (see Fig. 28-1). This immediate response peaks within 30 to 60 minutes of exposure to the trigger (e.g., allergen, irritant) and subsides in another 30 to 90 minutes. Clinically the patient has wheezing, chest tightness, dyspnea, and cough.

The *late-phase response* in asthma peaks 5 to 6 hours after exposure and may last for several hours or days. It is characterized primarily by inflammation. Eosinophils and neutrophils infiltrate the airways. These cells can subsequently release mediators that cause mast cells to release histamine and other mediators that eventually set up a self-sustaining cycle. In addition, lymphocytes and monocytes influx into the area.

These events, which define the late-phase response, increase airway reactivity, which may worsen the symptoms of future asthma attacks. The person becomes hyperresponsive to specific allergens and nonspecific stimuli such as air pollution, cold air, and dust. Identifying the original trigger may be difficult at this point, and less stimulation is required to produce a reaction. The airway hyperreactivity may be related to the exposure of sensory nerve endings as a result of epithelial injury caused by the repeated late-phase responses. Increased airway resistance leads to air trapping in the alveoli and hyperinflation of the lungs.

In summary, the prominent pathophysiologic features of asthma are a reduction in airway diameter and an increase in airway resistance related to mucosal inflammation, constriction of bronchial smooth muscle, and excess production of mucus (Fig. 28-3). Accompanying these changes are bronchial smooth muscle hypertrophy, basement membrane thickening, mucous gland hypertrophy, thick and tenacious sputum, hyperinflation, and air trapping in the alveoli leading to an increased work of breathing. As a consequence of these events, alterations in respiratory muscle function, abnormal distribution of both ventilation and perfusion, and altered arterial blood gases (ABGs) occur. Although asthma is considered a disease of the airways, eventually all aspects of pulmonary function are compromised during an asthma attack. If airway inflammation is not treated or does not resolve, it may eventually cause progressive, irreversible lung damage. This irreversible airway obstruction thought to be the result of inflammation-induced structural changes is called *airway remodeling*.[7]

In addition to the inflammatory aspects of asthma, alterations in the neural control of the airways have been postulated. It is possible, however, that these defects are secondary to the inflammatory process. The autonomic nervous system, consisting of the parasympathetic and sympathetic systems, innervates the bronchi. Airway smooth muscle tone is regulated by the parasympathetic nervous system via the vagus nerve. Afferent and efferent impulses are conducted through the vagus nerve to the medulla in the brain and back to the lungs. When airway nerve endings are stimulated by mechanical or chemical stimuli (e.g., air pollution, cold air, dust, allergens), increased release of acetylcholine causes bronchoconstriction.

Both α- and β-adrenergic receptors of the sympathetic nervous system are located in the bronchi. When the α-adrenergic receptors are stimulated, bronchoconstriction occurs. When the β-adrenergic receptors (β_2-adrenergic receptors are primarily located in the bronchi) are stimulated, bronchodilation occurs. Epinephrine acts on α-, β_1-, and β_2-adrenergic receptors. β_2-Adrenergic drugs act primarily on β-adrenergic receptors.

Clinical Manifestations

Asthma is characterized by an unpredictable and variable course. It causes recurrent episodes of wheezing, breathlessness, chest tightness, and cough, particularly at night and in the early morning. An attack of asthma may have an abrupt onset or may be more gradual. Attacks often occur at night and may last for a few minutes to several hours. Between attacks the patient may be asymptomatic with normal or near-normal pulmonary function, depending on severity of disease. However, in some persons, compromised pulmonary function may result in a state of continuous asthma and chronic debilitation characterized by irreversible airway disease.

The characteristic clinical manifestations of asthma are wheezing, cough, dyspnea, and chest tightness after exposure to a precipitating factor or trigger. Expiration may be prolonged. Instead of a normal inspiratory-expiratory ratio of 1:2, it may be prolonged to 1:3 or 1:4. Normally the bronchioles constrict during expiration. However, as a result of bronchospasm, edema, and mucus in the bronchioles, the airways become narrower than usual. Thus it takes longer for the air to move out of the bronchioles. This produces the characteristic wheezing, air trapping, and hyperinflation.

Wheezing is an unreliable sign to gauge the severity of an attack. Many patients with minor attacks wheeze loudly, whereas others with severe attacks do not wheeze. The patient with severe asthmatic attacks may have no audible wheezing because of the marked reduction in airflow. For wheezing to occur, the patient must be able to move enough air to produce the sound. Wheezing usually occurs first on exhalation. As asthma progresses the patient may wheeze during inspiration and expiration. Severely diminished breath sounds, often referred to as the "silent chest," is an ominous sign, indicating severe obstruction and impending respiratory failure.

In some patients with asthma, cough is the only symptom. The bronchospasm may not be severe enough to cause airflow

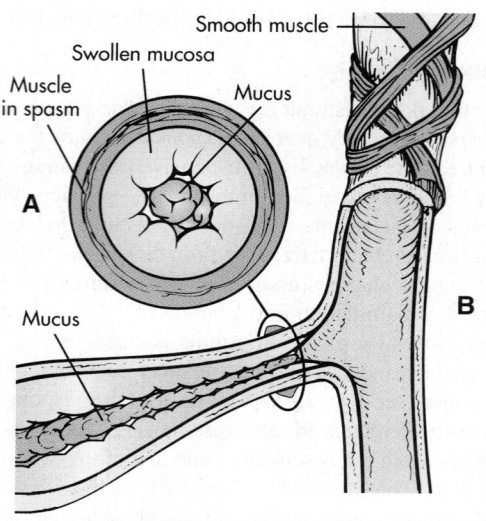

FIG. 28-3 Factors causing airway obstruction in asthma. **A,** Cross section of a bronchiole occluded by muscle spasm, swollen mucosa, and mucus in the lumen. **B,** Longitudinal section of a bronchiole.

(Figure labels: Smooth muscle; Swollen mucosa; Muscle in spasm; Mucus; Mucus; A; B)

obstruction, but it can increase bronchial tone and cause irritation and stimulation of the cough receptors. The cough may be non-productive. Mobilizing secretions may be difficult. Secretions may be thick, tenacious, white, gelatinous mucus.

The person with asthma has difficulty with air movement in and out of the lungs, which creates a feeling of suffocation. Therefore during an acute attack, the person with asthma usually sits upright or slightly bent forward using the accessory muscles of respiration to try to get enough air. The more difficult the breathing becomes, the more anxious the patient feels.

Examination of the patient during an acute attack usually reveals signs of hypoxemia, which may include restlessness, increased anxiety, inappropriate behavior, increased pulse and blood pressure, and *pulsus paradoxus* (a drop in systolic pressure during the inspiratory cycle greater than 10 mm Hg). The respiratory rate is significantly increased (usually greater than 30 breaths per minute) with the use of accessory muscles. Percussion of the lungs indicates hyperresonance, and auscultation indicates the presence of inspiratory or expiratory wheezing. Diminished or absent breath sounds may indicate a significant decrease in air movement resulting from exhaustion and an inability to generate enough muscle force to ventilate. Diminished or absent breath sounds may also indicate atelectasis or pneumothorax.

Classification of Asthma

Asthma can be classified as mild intermittent, mild persistent, moderate persistent, or severe persistent[9] (Table 28-2). Patients may progress up or down in the level of asthma severity over the course of their disease. Good asthma control correlates with minimal symptoms, ability to sleep through the night, and ability to participate in sports, exercise, and strenuous activity.

Complications

Severe acute asthma can result in complications such as rib fractures, pneumothorax, pneumomediastinum, atelectasis, pneumonia, and status asthmaticus.

Status Asthmaticus. **Status asthmaticus** is a severe, life-threatening asthma attack that is refractory to usual treatment and places the patient at risk for developing respiratory failure. An axiom describes status asthmaticus: "The longer it lasts, the worse it gets, and the worse it gets, the longer it lasts." Acute asthmatic attacks account for nearly 1 million emergency department (ED) visits a year in the United States, with hundreds of thousands of hospital admissions each year. Of the persons with asthma admitted to the hospital, approximately 10% require intensive care unit (ICU) monitoring or ventilatory assistance for status asthmaticus.[3]

TABLE 28-2	Classification of Asthma Severity: Clinical Features Before Treatment		
CATEGORY	**SYMPTOMS**	**NOCTURNAL SYMPTOMS**	**PULMONARY FUNCTION***
Step 4 **Severe persistent**	Continual symptoms Limited physical activity Frequent exacerbations	Frequent	FEV_1/PEFR is no greater than 60% of predicted. PEFR variability exceeds 30%.
Step 3 **Moderate persistent**	Daily symptoms Daily use of inhaled short–acting β_2-agonist Exacerbations affect activity Exacerbations at least twice weekly and may last for days	More frequent than once weekly	FEV_1/PEFR exceeds 60% but is less than 80% of predicted. PEFR variability exceeds 30%.
Step 2 **Mild persistent**	Symptoms more frequent than twice weekly but less than once a day Exacerbations may affect activity	More frequent than twice monthly	FEV_1/PEFR is at least 80% of predicted. PEFR variability is between 20% and 30%.
Step 1 **Mild intermittent**	Symptoms no more frequent than twice weekly Asymptomatic and with normal PEFR between exacerbations Exacerbations brief (hours to days) Intensity of exacerbations varies	No more frequent than twice monthly	FEV_1/PEFR is at least 80% of predicted. PEFR variability is less than 20%.

Source: *Practical guide for the diagnosis and management of asthma, based on Expert Panel Report 2: guidelines for the diagnosis and management of asthma,* Washington, DC, 1997, National Institutes of Health.
*Percent predicted values for forced expiratory volume in 1 second (FEV_1) and percent of personal best for peak expiratory flow rate (PEFR).
NOTES:
- Patients should be assigned to the most severe step in which *any* feature occurs. Clinical features for individual patients may overlap across steps.
- An individual's classification may change over time.
- Patients at any level of severity of chronic asthma can have mild, moderate, or severe exacerbations of asthma. Some patients with intermittent asthma experience severe and life-threatening exacerbations separated by long periods of normal lung function and no symptoms.
- Patients with two or more asthma exacerbations per week (i.e., progressively worsening symptoms that may last hours or days) tend to have moderate to severe persistent asthma.

Causes of status asthmaticus include viral illnesses, ingestion of aspirin or other NSAIDs, emotional stress, increases in environmental pollutants or other allergen exposure, abrupt discontinuation of drug therapy (especially corticosteroids), abuse of aerosol medication, and ingestion of β-adrenergic blockers. Usually the patient reports a history of poorly controlled asthma progressing over days or weeks.

The clinical manifestations of status asthmaticus result from increased airway resistance as a consequence of edema, mucous plugging, and bronchospasm with subsequent air trapping and hyperinflation. The patient has clinical manifestations similar to those of asthma, but they are more severe and more prolonged. Extreme anxiety, fear of suffocation, severely increased work of breathing, and diaphoresis are common. Absence of diaphoresis may indicate significant dehydration. Sternocleidomastoid, intercostal, and supraclavicular muscle retractions reflect increased work of breathing. If obtainable, the PEFR is usually less than 100 to 150 L per minute.

Although wheezing is often audible without a stethoscope, auscultation may not always be reliable because the airflow obstruction may be so severe in some patients that audible wheezing or other abnormal lung sounds may not be produced because of insufficient airflow. Absence of a wheeze (i.e., silent chest) is a life-threatening situation that may require mechanical ventilation. The chest appears fixed in a hyperinflated position and is often described as "tight," indicating severely decreased movement of air through the constricted bronchial airways.

Forced exhalation with the use of the abdominal musculature can result in increased intrathoracic pressure transmitted to the great vessels and heart. Neck vein distention and a pulsus paradoxus of 40 mm Hg or higher may result. Usually it is difficult to auscultate pulsus paradoxus secondary to a noisy chest or increased work of breathing. (Pulsus paradoxus is described in Chapter 36 and Table 36-10.) Hypertension, sinus tachycardia, and ventricular arrhythmias may occur. These three conditions are related to hypoxemia, catecholamines due to an endogenous response to hypoxia, and underlying coronary artery disease in the older adult population. Electrocardiogram (ECG) results may show sinus tachycardia or signs of strain on the right side of the heart secondary to pulmonary vasoconstriction, which may be seen as P pulmonale and a right axis deviation.

Hypoxemia with hypocapnia usually occurs initially as the patient attempts to hyperventilate and maintain adequate oxygenation and ventilation. As the severity of the attack increases, the work of breathing increases, making it more difficult for the patient to overcome the increased resistance to breathing. The patient becomes fatigued, causing more CO_2 retention. ABGs initially show hypocapnia due to increased respiratory rate. Ultimately, they deteriorate to hypercapnia and hypoxemia (Table 28-3). A moderate elevation in $PaCO_2$ may be tolerated without intubation and mechanical ventilation if the patient remains alert and cooperative and continues to improve during the first 2 to 3 hours of treatment.

Complications of status asthmaticus include pneumothorax, pneumomediastinum, acute cor pulmonale with right ventricular failure, and severe respiratory muscle fatigue leading to respiratory arrest. Death from status asthmaticus is usually the result of respiratory arrest or cardiac failure.

Diagnostic Studies

Wheezing and respiratory distress characterize a variety of disorders, including asthma, chronic bronchitis, emphysema, cystic fibrosis, pulmonary edema, upper airway and bronchial obstruction, tracheobronchitis, bronchiolitis, aspiration, and pulmonary embolism. Therefore certain diagnostic studies must be performed to determine whether these symptoms are caused primarily by asthma (Table 28-4). The severity of the clinical manifestations of asthma determines the appropriate diagnostic studies.

In the patient who is not in distress, a detailed history may indicate previous attacks of a similar nature, often precipitated by a known cause. Seasonal attacks may indicate pollen triggers. Attacks that occur at night may be caused by sleeping with a cat, sleep apnea, GERD, or mattress dust mites. It is important to determine whether the patient can sleep through the night or participate in an aerobic exercise program. This information helps identify some of the asthma triggers.

Pulmonary function tests are usually within normal limits between attacks if the patient has no other underlying pulmonary disease. Pulmonary function tests are frequently used to diagnose and manage asthma and are an essential objective measurement of airflow obstruction. The patient with asthma usually has a decrease in forced expiratory volume in 1 second (FEV_1), PEFR, FEV_1 to forced vital capacity (FVC) ratio (FEV_1/FVC), and forced expiratory flow rate measured during the middle of FVC ($FEF_{25\%-75\%}$), with the degree of obstruction depending on the values obtained. (The normal values for pulmonary function tests are discussed in

TABLE 28-3				Arterial Blood Gas Results Correlated with Clinical Manifestations during an Acute Asthmatic Attack	
TIME FRAME	**pH**	**$PaCO_2$**	**PaO_2**	**PHYSIOLOGIC EVENT**	**CLINICAL MANIFESTATIONS**
Early in attack	↑	↓	↓	Alveolar hyperventilation → hypocarbia Hypoxemia secondary to ventilation-perfusion mismatch Adequate alveolar ventilation	Use of all accessory muscles of ventilation to overcome increased airway resistance Increased heart rate, diaphoresis, chest tightness, cough, wheezing
Progressive attack	N	N	↓	CO_2 not being eliminated as well Decrease in effective alveolar ventilation	Tiring of patient and difficulty with increased work of breathing
Prolonged attack, status asthmaticus	↓	↑	↓	Hypercarbia indicating that ventilation is no longer adequate Alveolar hypoventilation → respiratory acidosis Worsening hypoxemia as result of hypoventilation and ventilation-perfusion mismatch	Exhaustion, diminished breath sounds, intubation and mechanical ventilation necessary

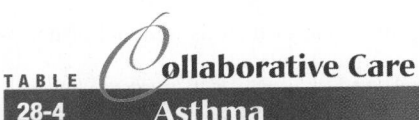

TABLE	Collaborative Care
28-4	**Asthma**

Diagnostic
History and physical examination
Pulmonary function studies including response to bronchodilator therapy
Peak expiratory flow monitoring
Chest x-ray
Measurement of ABGs or oximetry
Allergy skin testing (if indicated)
Blood level of eosinophils and IgE (if indicated)

Collaborative Therapy
Mild Intermittent or Persistent Asthma
Identification and avoidance/elimination of triggers
Desensitization (immunotherapy) if indicated
Patient and family teaching
Drug therapy (see Tables 28-5 and 28-6)
Asthma management plan (see Table 28-11)
Status Asthmaticus
Inhaled β_2-adrenergic drugs or anticholinergic agents
IV aminophylline (if indicated)
O_2 by mask or nasal prongs
IV corticosteroids
IV fluids
IV magnesium
Intubation and assisted ventilation (if indicated)
Heliox therapy

ABGs, Arterial blood gases; *IgE,* immunoglobulin E.

Chapter 25.) PEFR correlates with FEV_1 and is a helpful tool for the health care provider to diagnose and manage asthma.

These parameters decrease from their baseline levels during an exacerbation, and some patients may be within normal limits during a remission. Rarely do health care providers require confirmation of the diagnosis by inducing bronchospasm during pulmonary function testing with bronchial provocation testing with known quantities of bronchial irritants such as histamine and methacholine. An increase of 12% to 15% or more in the FEV_1 in response to a bronchodilator when the patient is not experiencing an exacerbation is another diagnostic indicator of asthma.

Eosinophils in the sputum and serum eosinophilia (greater than or equal to 5% of the total white blood cell [WBC] count) and elevated serum IgE levels are highly suggestive of asthma in a symptomatic patient. A chest x-ray in an asymptomatic patient with asthma is usually normal. A chest x-ray obtained during an acute attack usually shows hyperinflation and may reveal other complications of asthma such as mucoid impaction, pneumothorax, atelectasis, or pneumomediastinum.

In a mild asthma attack, ABGs (if obtained) would indicate respiratory alkalosis with an arterial O_2 pressure (PaO_2) near normal. Hypercapnia and respiratory and metabolic acidosis indicate severe disease. In mild asthma pulse oximetry monitoring is sufficient to determine oxygenation status.

Allergy skin testing may be of some value to determine sensitivity to specific allergens (antigens). However, a positive skin test does not necessarily mean that the allergen (antigen) is causing the asthma attack. On the other hand, a negative allergy test does not mean that the asthma is not allergy related. A radioallergosorbent test (RAST) is sometimes used to identify allergic

causes in certain patients who show negative skin tests and in those who should not be tested (e.g., patients with severe eczema). (Allergy testing is discussed in Chapter 13.)

If the patient has wheezing and acute distress, it is not feasible to obtain a detailed health history (although a family member may supply some pertinent information). During an acute attack of asthma, bedside spirometry (specifically FEV_1 or FVC, but usually PEFR) may be used to monitor obstruction. Pulmonary function test results, serial spirometric parameters, oximetry, and measurement of ABGs help provide information about the severity of the attack and the response to therapy. A complete blood cell count (CBC) and serum electrolytes are also obtained to help monitor the course of therapy.

A sputum specimen for culture and sensitivity may be obtained to rule out the presence of bacterial infection, especially if the patient has purulent sputum, a history of upper respiratory tract infection, a fever, or an elevated WBC count.

Collaborative Care

To help health care professionals bridge the gap between current knowledge and practice, the National Asthma Education and Prevention Program (NAEPP) of the National Heart, Lung, and Blood Institute (NHLBI) has convened two expert panels to prepare guidelines for the diagnosis and management of asthma. The charge of the first panel was to develop a report that would provide a general approach to diagnosing and managing asthma based on current science.[3] The second expert panel report (EPR-2) critically reviewed and expanded on the first. The goal of the expert panel is to serve as a comprehensive guide to diagnosing and managing asthma. Implementation of EPR-2 recommendations is likely to increase some costs of asthma care by increasing the initial care and use of medications, but asthma diagnosis and management are expected to improve, which should reduce the numbers of lost school and work days, hospitalizations, ED visits, and deaths caused by asthma.[3,9]

Education for an active partnership with patients remains the cornerstone of asthma management and should be carried out by health care providers delivering asthma care (see the Evidence-Based Practice box on p. 644). Education should start at the time of asthma diagnosis and be integrated into every step of clinical asthma care. Asthma self-management should be tailored to the needs of each patient, maintaining a sensitivity to cultural beliefs and practices. Emphasis should be placed on evaluating outcomes in terms of the patient's perceptions of improvement, especiallyquality of life and the ability to engage in usual activities. A description of asthma education programs for adults can be accessed through the American Lung Association website at *www.lungusa.org.*

Mild Intermittent and Persistent Asthma. The patient who has persistent airflow obstruction and frequent attacks of asthma should be taught to avoid triggers of acute attacks and to premedicate before exercising. The choice of drug therapy depends on the severity of symptoms (Table 28-5). The patient with mild intermittent asthma or EIA should use inhaled β_2-adrenergic agonists, cromolyn (Intal), or nedocromil (Tilade) before exercising or when anticipating exposure to allergens known to cause asthma. Moderate persistent asthma requires regular or maintenance use of inhaled antiinflammatory medication. These include inhaled corticosteroids (used at lowest possible dose to manage symptoms), cromolyn (Intal), and nedocromil (Tilade). In mild persistent asthma cromolyn and nedocromil can be used in place

EVIDENCE-BASED PRACTICE
Asthma Education for Self-Management

Clinical Problem

Do asthma education, education in self-management, and regular review by health care providers improve health outcomes for adults with asthma?

Best Clinical Practice

- Moderately strong evidence suggests that asthma self-management training that includes self-monitoring by either peak expiratory flow or symptoms together with regular medical review and a written action plan improves health outcomes for adults with asthma.
- These patients have a low incidence of hospital admissions, unscheduled doctor visits, days off work, and nocturnal asthma.
- Reductions are greater when self-management education includes a written care plan.
- Limited asthma education (information only) does not improve health outcomes in adults.

Implications for Nursing Practice

- A key component of asthma management is patient education with regular, ongoing reviews.

References for Evidence

Gibson PG et al: Self-management education and regular practitioner review for adults with asthma, *The Cochrane Library.* Issue 1, 2002.

Gibson PG et al: Limited (information only) patient education programs for adults with asthma, *The Cochrane Library.* Issue 1, 2002.

of inhaled corticosteroids. For severe persistent asthma, inhaled or oral corticosteroids, inhaled or oral β_2-adrenergic agonists, and theophylline may be used to alleviate symptoms. Some persons require continuous oral corticosteroids, which should be maintained at as low a dosage as possible and administered on alternate days (if possible) to reduce systemic side effects.

Acute Asthma Episode. A patient frequently comes to the ED or a health care provider's office in acute respiratory distress. The choice of treatment of acute asthma depends on the severity of the attack and response to initial therapy. Severity can be measured objectively by measuring FEV_1 or PEFR. Assessing the degree or amount of change from the patient's personal best PEFR (if known) and the patient's baseline pulse oximetry results can help determine the severity of the attack. O_2 therapy should be started immediately, and its administration should be monitored by pulse oximetry and in more severe cases by measurement of ABGs. Initial therapy should include inhaled β_2-adrenergic agonists administered by metered-dose inhaler (MDI) using spacer devices or nebulizer. Generally, aerosolized medications by nebulizer therapy or by MDI used correctly with a spacer are given every 20 minutes to 4 hours as necessary.[3]

Corticosteroids are indicated if the initial response is insufficient (e.g., no response within 30 to 60 minutes), if the patient has had several recent asthma attacks, or if the patient is receiving oral corticosteroid therapy. The choice of oral or IV administration of corticosteroids depends on the severity of the attack. Therapy should be continued until the patient is breathing comfortably, wheezing has disappeared, and pulmonary function study results are near baseline values. Although the value of administering aminophylline in the treatment of acute asthma has been questioned, intravenous (IV) aminophylline may be considered if the asthma attack is severe or there is minimal or no response to inhaled β_2-adrenergic agonists.[2]

Status Asthmaticus. Management of the patient with status asthmaticus focuses on correcting hypoxemia and improving ventilation. Most of the therapeutic measures are the same as for acute asthma. It may be necessary, however, to increase the frequency and dose of inhaled bronchodilators. When an MDI is used, the typical dose is two to six puffs every 5 to 20 minutes, depending on the medication selected. Continuous β-adrenergic agonist nebulizer therapy may be given. Therapy with inhaled agents is usually initiated despite prior home use, because drug delivery at home may have been submaximal and higher doses given under supervision may be beneficial.

Continuous monitoring of the patient is critical. Obtaining a PEFR during a severe asthma attack is usually not possible. IV aminophylline administration may be added to the treatment regimen if the patient does not respond to β-adrenergic agonists. IV corticosteroids (methylprednisolone) are administered every 4 to 6 hours, although their peak effect is not apparent for 6 to 12 hours. Sometimes IV magnesium sulfate is given to act as a bronchodilator. Although it is no longer listed in the guidelines for asthma management, subcutaneous epinephrine is occasionally administered. If administered, patients need their blood pressure (BP) and ECG monitored closely.

Supplemental O_2 is given by mask or nasal prongs to achieve a PaO_2 of at least 60 mm Hg or an O_2 saturation of 90% or greater. An arterial catheter may be inserted to facilitate frequent ABG monitoring. Because the patient's insensible loss of fluids is increased and the metabolic rate is increased, IV fluids are given to provide optimal hydration. Sodium bicarbonate administration is usually limited to treatment of severe metabolic or respiratory acidosis (pH less than 7.29) in the mechanically ventilated patient because effective bronchodilation by β-adrenergic agonists is not possible if the patient has extreme acidosis. Bronchoscopy, although rarely performed during an acute attack, may be necessary to remove thick mucous plugs.

Occasionally, asthma attacks are so severe that the patient requires mechanical ventilation if there is no response to treatment. Indications for mechanical ventilation are persistent or progressive CO_2 retention and respiratory acidosis, clinical deterioration indicated by fatigue, hypersomnolence, metabolic acidosis, and cardiopulmonary arrest. In status asthmaticus, the goals of initiating mechanical ventilation are to achieve a PaO_2 greater than or equal to 60 mm Hg, an O_2 saturation greater than or equal to 90%, and a normal pH. Heliox therapy, which is a mixture of O_2 and helium, has been used with limited success during mechanical ventilation or with continuous nebulization to decrease airway resistance and improve ventilation.[10]

Louder wheezing may actually occur in the airways that are responding to the therapy as airflow in the airways increases. As improvement continues and airflow increases, breath sounds increase and wheezing decreases. As the patient begins to respond to therapy and symptoms begin to subside, it is important to remember that despite the disappearance of most of the bronchospasm, the edema and cellular infiltration of the airway mucosa and the viscous mucous plugs may take several days to improve. Thus intensive therapy must be continued even after clinical improvement has occurred.

IV corticosteroids are usually tapered rapidly, and the patient is placed on oral corticosteroids, which are tapered over several weeks. Inhaled corticosteroids are usually added when the oral dose is tapered. IV aminophylline (if used), frequent airway care

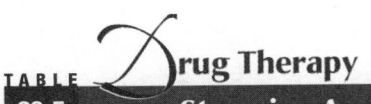

TABLE 28-5   Drug Therapy

Stepwise Approach for Managing Asthma in Adults

CLASSIFY SEVERITY: CLINICAL FEATURES BEFORE TREATMENT OR ADEQUATE CONTROL			MEDICATIONS REQUIRED TO MAINTAIN LONG-TERM CONTROL
	SYMPTOMS/DAY SYMPTOMS/NIGHT	PEF OR FEV$_1$ PEF VARIABILITY	DAILY MEDICATIONS
Step 4 **Severe Persistent**	Continual Frequent	≤60% >30%	• Preferred treatment High-dose inhaled corticosteroids *and* Long-acting inhaled β_2-agonists *and, if needed,* Corticosteroids
Step 3 **Moderate Persistent**	Daily >1 night/week	>60% but <80% >30%	• Preferred treatment Low-to-medium dose inhaled corticosteroids and long-acting inhaled β_2-agonists. • Alternative treatment (listed alphabetically) Increase inhaled corticosteroids within medium-dose range *or* Low-to-medium dose inhaled corticosteroids and either leukotriene modifier or theophylline. If needed (particularly in patients with recurring severe exacerbations): • Preferred treatment Increase inhaled corticosteroids within medium-dose range and add long-acting inhaled β_2-agonists. • Alternative treatment Increase inhaled corticosteroids within medium-dose range and add either leukotriene modifier or theophylline.
Step 2 **Mild Persistent**	>2/week but <1×/day >2 nights/month	≥80% 20%-30%	• Preferred treatment Low-dose inhaled corticosteroids. • Alternative treatment (listed alphabetically): cromolyn, leukotriene modifier, nedocromil, *or* sustained release theophylline.
Step 2 **Mild Intermittent**	≤2 days/week ≤2 nights/month	≥80% <20%	• No daily medication needed. • Severe exacerbations may occur, separated by long periods of normal lung function and no symptoms. A course of systemic corticosteroids is recommended.

Quick Relief
All Patients
Short-acting bronchodilator: 2-4 puffs short-acting inhaled β_2-agonists as needed for symptoms.
Intensity of treatment will depend on severity of exacerbation; up to three treatments at 20-minute intervals or a single nebulizer treatment as needed. Course of systemic corticosteroids may be needed.
Use of short-acting β_2-agonists >2 times a week in intermittent asthma (daily, or increasing use in persistent asthma) may indicate the need to initiate (increase) long-term control therapy.
Step down Review treatment every 1 to 6 months; a gradual stepwise reduction in treatment may be possible.
Step up If control is not maintained, consider step up. First, review patient medication technique, adherence, and environmental control.

Source: Quick Reference of the National Asthma Education and Prevention Program (NAEPP) Expert Panel Report: *Guidelines for the Diagnosis and Management of Asthma—Update on Selected Topics 2002.* http://www.nhlbi.nih.gov/guidelines/asthma/asthsumm.htm.

with aerosolized medications, and chest physiotherapy (if indicated) are continued for several days after clinical improvement is noted. The patient's cough often becomes productive of mucous plugs, and breath sounds improve. If the patient is asked to perform a forced expiratory maneuver, a faint wheeze may still be heard. Finally, the patient can be switched to oral bronchodilators and can use a β-adrenergic MDI before discharge.

Drug Therapy

The NAEPP recommends a stepwise approach to drug therapy, with the type and amount of medication dictated by asthma severity (see Table 28-5). The NAEPP emphasizes that persistent asthma requires daily long-term therapy in addition to appropriate medications to manage acute asthma exacerbations.[9] To clarify this concept, the NAEPP now categorizes medications into two general classifications: (1) long-term–control medications to achieve and maintain control of persistent asthma and (2) quick-relief medications to treat symptoms and exacerbations.[3] Because inflammation is considered an early and persistent component of asthma, drug therapy for persistent asthma must be directed toward long-term suppression of the inflammation (Table 28-6).

TABLE 28-6 Drug Therapy — Asthma and Chronic Obstructive Pulmonary Disease

DRUG	ROUTE OF ADMINISTRATION	MECHANISMS OF ACTION	SIDE EFFECTS	COMMENTS
β-Adrenergic Agonists				
metaproterenol (Alupent, Metaprel)	Nebulizer, oral tablets, elixir, MDI	Stimulates β-adrenergic receptors, producing bronchodilation. Increases mucociliary clearance.	Tachycardia, BP changes, nervousness, palpitations, muscle tremors, nausea, vomiting, vertigo, insomnia, dry mouth, headache, hypokalemia.	Should not be used in patient with angina or other cardiac disorders. Has fairly rapid onset of action (5–10 min). Duration of action is 3–4 hr. Oral lasts up to 8 hr.
albuterol (Proventil, Ventolin, Proventil HFA)	Nebulizer, MDI, oral tablets, rotahaler	Selectively stimulates β₂ receptors, producing bronchodilation.	Same as above but cardiac effects are less.	Has rapid onset of action (1–3 min). Duration of action is 4–8 hr.
levalbuterol (Xopenex)	Nebulizer	Same as above.	Tachycardia, nervousness, tremor.	Too frequent use can result in loss of effectiveness.
pirbuterol (Maxair)	MDI	Same as above.	Same as metaproterenol but cardiac effects are less.	Has slow onset of action (except nebulized and subcutaneous route). Duration of action is 4–6 hr.
terbutaline (Bricanyl, Brethine, Brethair)	Oral tablets, nebulizer, subcutaneous, MDI	Same as above.	Same as above.	Duration of action is 4–8 hr.
bitolterol (Tornalate)	MDI, nebulizer	Same as above.	Same as above.	Not to exceed 2 puffs every 12 hours. Not to be used for acute exacerbations.
salmeterol (Serevent)	MDI, DPI	Long acting.	Headache, throat dryness, tremor, dizziness, pharyngitis.	Can affect blood glucose levels. Should be used with caution in patients with diabetes.
formoterol (Foradil)	DPI in aerolizer inhaler	Same as above.	Angina, tachycardia, nervousness, headache, tremor, dizziness.	Used primarily to treat severe bronchial asthma attacks. Should not be used in patient with arrhythmias or hypertension.
epinephrine (Adrenalin)	Subcutaneous	Long acting. Stimulates α, β₁, and β₂ receptors, producing bronchodilation.	Headache, dizziness, palpitations, tremors, restlessness, hypertension, arrhythmias, tachycardia.	
Antiinflammatory Agents				
hydrocortisone (Solu-Cortef)	IV	Have antiinflammatory and immunosuppressive effects. Decrease edema in bronchial airways. Act synergistically with β₂-agonists. Decrease mucus secretion. Effective in late-phase reaction of asthma.	Cushingoid appearance, skin changes (acne, striae, bruising), osteoporosis, increased appetite, obesity; peptic ulcer, hypertension, hypokalemia, cataracts, menstrual irregularities, muscle weakness, immunosuppression, catabolism, dysphonia, growth retardation.	Alternate-day therapy minimizes side effects. Oral dose should be taken in morning with food or milk. When given in high doses, patient must be observed for epigastric distress. Histamine H₂ blockers (ranitidine, cimetidine) and antacids may help minimize GI effects. The patient taking long-term corticosteroids may be given vitamin D and calcium to prevent osteoporosis. Should never be abruptly discontinued but tapered gradually over time to prevent adrenal insufficiency. If during tapering patient has recurrence of symptoms, health care provider should be notified. May be used concomitantly with bronchodilator.
methylprednisolone (Medrol) (Solu-Medrol)	Oral IV			
prednisone	Oral			

Drug	Route	Action	Side Effects	Nursing Considerations
beclomethasone (Vanceril, Beclovent, Vanceril DS, Qvar)	MDI, nasal spray	Same as above. Acts locally in respiratory tract with relatively little systemic absorption.	Oral thrush infections, hoarseness, irritated throat, dry mouth, cough, few systemic effects.	Not recommended for acute asthma attack. Rinse mouth with water or mouthwash after use to prevent oral fungal infections. Use of space device with MDI may decrease incidence of thrush. Use after MDI bronchodilator. MDI steroids may be discontinued during acute asthma attack. Nasal spray is used for allergic rhinitis.
triamcinolone (Azmacort)	MDI	Same as above.	Same as above.	Same as above. Advantage is that it has a built-in spacer device.
flunisolide (AeroBid, AeroBid-M)	MDI	Same as above.	Same as above.	AeroBid-M contains menthol.
fluticasone (Flovent)	MDI, DPI	Same as above but with higher potency.	High incidence of yeast infections.	Same as beclomethasone.
budesonide (Pulmicort)	MDI, DPI Nebulizer	Same as above.	Same as above.	
cromolyn (Intal)	MDI	Inhibits release of histamine and SRS-A by acting directly on mast cell. May act by interference with calcium ion influx across cell membrane. Exact mechanism unknown.	Irritation of throat, relatively nontoxic effects, bronchospasm.	Used for asthma (e.g., before exercise) prophylactically if allergen is causative agent. Instruct patient in correct use of inhaler. May follow treatment with glass of water to reduce pharyngeal irritation. May take 4-6 wk before clinical response occurs. Nasal spray (Nasalcrom) used for allergic rhinitis.
nedocromil (Tilade)	MDI	Similar to cromolyn but with broad-spectrum effects.	Same as above. Transient unpleasant taste, rhinitis.	
Anticholinergics				
ipratropium (Atrovent)	Nebulizer, MDI	Blocks action of acetylcholine, resulting in bronchodilation.	Drying of oral mucosa, cough, flushing of skin, bad taste.	Alternating schedules of β-adrenergic agonists and atropine administration may be helpful in some patients. Temporary blurred vision will occur if sprayed in eyes.
ipratropium and albuterol (Combivent)	MDI	Combination of anticholinergic and β-agonist		Patients must be careful not to overuse and take as prescribed.
ipratropium and albuterol (DuoNeb)	Nebulizer	Same as above.	Chest pain, pharyngitis, diarrhea, nausea.	Should be used cautiously in patients with seizure disorders, hyperthyroidism, diabetes mellitus.

Continued

BP, Blood pressure; *CNS,* central nervous system; *DPI,* dry powder inhaler; *GI,* gastrointestinal; *IV,* intravenous; *MDI,* metered-dose inhaler; *SRS-A,* slow-reacting substance of anaphylaxis.

Drug Therapy

TABLE 28-6	Asthma and Chronic Obstructive Pulmonary Disease—cont'd			
DRUG	**ROUTE OF ADMINISTRATION**	**MECHANISMS OF ACTION**	**SIDE EFFECTS**	**COMMENTS**
Methylxanthine Derivatives				
IV agent: aminophylline Oral: Aerolate Choledyl SA Elixophyllin Quibron Slo-Bid Slo-Phyllin Theo-Dur Theolair Theo 24 Uni-Dur Uniphyl	Oral tablets, IV, elixir, sustained release tablets	Major effects are relaxation of bronchial smooth muscles and improved contractility of fatigued diaphragm. Other effects are mild diuresis, increased gastric acid secretion, stimulation of mucociliary clearance, stimulation of CNS and respiration, pulmonary vasodilation, improved exercise tolerance.	Tachycardia, BP changes, arrhythmias, anorexia, nausea, vomiting, nervousness, irritability, headache, muscle twitching, flushing, epigastric pain, diarrhea, insomnia, palpitations.	Wide variety of response to drug metabolism exists. Half-life is decreased by smoking and is increased by heart failure and liver disease. Cimetidine, ciprofloxacin, erythromycin, and several other drugs may rapidly increase theophylline levels. Gastrointestinal side effects may be alleviated by taking drug with food or antacids. Patient should be instructed to lie down if dizziness is experienced. Patient must be encouraged to take drugs even when feeling well. Extra doses should not be taken when symptoms are present unless prescribed. Side effects should be reported but medication not stopped unless symptoms are severe.
Mucolytics				
acetylcysteine (Mucomyst) (10% and 20%)	Nebulizer	Enzyme breaks down mucoproteins. Decreases viscosity of mucus and enhances mobilization of secretions.	Bronchospasm, hemoptysis, nausea, vomiting.	After administration of mucolytics, secretions may become profuse. Use of mucolytic agents may not be necessary if patient is kept well hydrated and humidified. Usually combined with bronchodilator when administered.
guaifenesin (Humibid)	Oral tablets	Expectorant that helps loosen phlegm.	No serious side effects.	
Leukotriene Modifiers				
Leukotriene Receptor Antagonist				
zafirlukast (Accolate) montelukast (Singulair)	Oral tablets, chewable tablets	Blocks the action of leukotrienes once they are formed. Has both bronchodilator and antiinflammatory effects.	Headache, dizziness; nausea, vomiting diarrhea, fatigue, abdominal pain.	Take at least 1 hour before or 2 hours after meals. Affects metabolism of erythromycin and theophylline. Not to be used to treat acute asthma episodes.
Leukotriene Inhibitors				
zileuton (Zyflo)	Oral tablets	Inhibits the synthesis of leukotrienes. Has both bronchodilator and antiinflammatory effects.	Elevated liver enzymes; dizziness, insomnia, dyspepsia, abdominal pain.	Monitor liver enzymes. May interfere with metabolism of warfarin (Coumadin) and theophylline. Not to be used to treat acute asthma episodes.

Antiinflammatory Drugs

Corticosteroids. Because chronic inflammation is a primary component of asthma, corticosteroids, which suppress the inflammatory response, are the most potent and effective antiinflammatory medication currently available. The inhaled form is used in the long-term control of asthma. Systemic corticosteroids are used to gain prompt control of asthma in exacerbations and also to manage severe persistent asthma that is not controlled with maximal inhaled therapy.[3] Corticosteroids are remarkably effective in suppressing the inflammation induced by asthma, but are still greatly underused.[11]

Corticosteroids do not block the classic immediate response to irritants, allergens, or exercise, but they do block the late-phase response and subsequent bronchial hyperresponsiveness. The onset of action of corticosteroids occurs approximately 3 to 6 hours after oral administration. They act by inhibiting the release of mediators from macrophages and eosinophils, reducing the microvascular leakage in the airways, inhibiting the influx of inflammatory cells into the reactive site, and decreasing peripheral blood eosinophilia.

Usually inhaled corticosteroids must be administered for at least 4 to 5 days before a therapeutic effect can be seen. Newer inhaled corticosteroids (e.g., fluticasone [Flovent], budesonide [Pulmicort]) begin to have a therapeutic effect in 48 to 72 hours. Corticosteroids given by inhalation are active topically and can usually control the disease without systemic side effects. When administered in the aerosol form as MDIs, little systemic absorption occurs, thus eliminating the side effects that result from adrenal suppression seen with oral or IV corticosteroids.

Oropharyngeal candidiasis, hoarseness, and dry cough are local adverse effects caused by inhalation of corticosteroids. These problems can be reduced or prevented by using a spacer (Fig. 28-4) with the MDI and by gargling the mouth with water after each use. Using a spacer or holding device for inhalation of inhaled corticosteroids can be helpful in getting more medication into the lungs and less into the gastrointestinal tract, thus decreasing systemic side effects.

Short courses of orally administered corticosteroids are indicated for acute exacerbations of asthma. Side effects associated

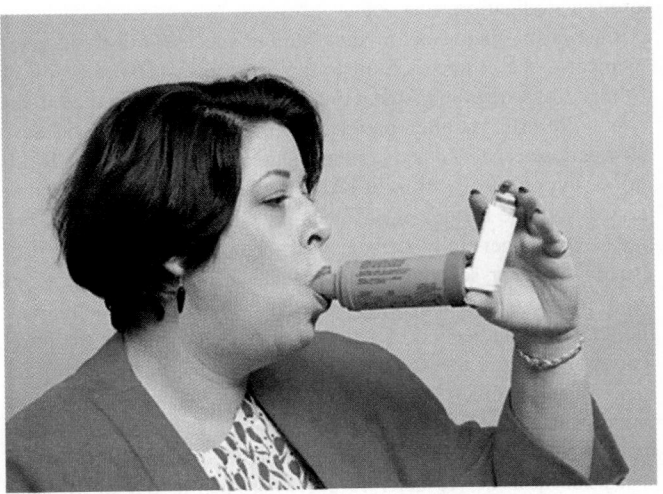

FIG. 28-4 Example of an AeroChamber spacer used with a metered-dose inhaler.

with short-term therapy include insomnia, heartburn, mood swings, blurry vision, headache, increased appetite, and weight gain. Maintenance doses of oral corticosteroids may be necessary to control asthma in a minority of patients with severe chronic asthma when long-term therapy is required. A single dose in the morning to coincide with endogenous cortisol production and alternate-day dosing are associated with fewer side effects. Side effects of long-term corticosteroid therapy are discussed in Chapter 48.

Women, especially postmenopausal women, who have asthma and who use corticosteroids should take adequate amounts of calcium and vitamin D and participate in regular weight-bearing exercise. (Osteoporosis is discussed in Chapter 62.)

Cromolyn and nedocromil. Cromolyn (Intal) and nedocromil (Tilade) are often classified as mast cell stabilizers. However, their exact mechanism of action is unknown. They inhibit the immediate response from exercise and allergens and prevent the late-phase response. Long-term administration can reduce bronchial hyperreactivity and prevent the increased bronchial hyperreactivity associated with pollens in susceptible asthmatics. They can be used successfully for seasonal asthma. They are particularly effective in exercise-induced asthma when used 10 to 20 minutes before exercise. Patient teaching should emphasize the rationale for use and the correct method of administration of these drugs.

Leukotriene modifiers. Leukotriene modifiers include leukotriene receptor antagonists (zafirlukast [Accolate], montelukast [Singulair]) and leukotriene synthesis inhibitors (zileuton [Zyflo]). These types of drugs interfere with the synthesis or block the action of leukotrienes.[12,13] Leukotrienes are produced from arachidonic acid metabolism (see Chapter 12, Fig. 12-7). Leukotrienes are potent bronchoconstrictors, and some also cause airway edema and inflammation, thus contributing to the symptoms of asthma. A broad range of patients, from those with mild symptoms to those with more severe asthma, can benefit from taking leukotriene modifiers. They are not indicated for use in the reversal of bronchospasm in acute asthma attacks. It is also recommended that these drugs not be used as the only therapy for treatment of persistent asthma. A major advantage of these drugs is that they have both bronchodilator and antiinflammatory effects.

Bronchodilators. Three classes of bronchodilator drugs currently used in asthma therapy are β-adrenergic agonists, methylxanthine derivatives, and anticholinergics.

β-Adrenergic agonist drugs. Inhaled β_2-adrenergic agonists such as albuterol (Proventil, Proventil HFA, and Ventolin), metaproterenol (Alupent), bitolterol (Tornalate), and pirbuterol (Maxair) have an onset of action within minutes and are effective for 4 to 8 hours. Inhaled β_2-adrenergic agonists are indicated for the short-term relief of bronchoconstriction and are the treatment of choice for acute exacerbations of asthma.[14] β_2-Adrenergic agonists are also useful in preventing bronchospasm precipitated by exercise and other stimuli because they prevent mediator release from mast cells. They do not inhibit the late-phase response. If used frequently, inhaled β_2-adrenergic agonists may produce tremors, anxiety, tachycardia, palpitations, and nausea. Overuse of β_2-adrenergic agonists may cause rebound bronchospasm, especially common with albuterol. Too frequent use of β_2-adrenergic agonists indicates poor asthma control, may mask asthma severity, and may lead to reduced drug effectiveness.

Longer-acting (8 to 12 hours or 24 hours) inhaled β_2-adrenergic agonists include salmeterol (Serevent). These drugs are useful for nocturnal asthma. Patient teaching should stress that these drugs are used only once every 12 hours and are not used to obtain quick relief from bronchospasm.

The most common side effects of inhaled β_2-adrenergic agonists are tremor, tachycardia, and palpitations. Some of these side effects can be decreased by teaching the patient to avoid contact between the medication and the tongue. Because the tongue has many blood vessels, rapid absorption of these drugs can occur. Excessive use of β_2-adrenergic agonists may cause hypokalemia. Therefore their use should be monitored carefully in patients on long-term diuretic or corticosteroid therapy.

Combination therapy using an inhaled corticosteroid (fluticasone) and an inhaled long-acting β_2-adrenergic agonist (salmeterol) is one of the outlined treatment options in the NHLBI asthma guidelines.[3] Adding an inhaled corticosteroid to an inhaled long-acting β_2-adrenergic agonist results in greater improvement in lung function and overall asthma control compared with higher-dose inhaled corticosteroids.[3] Advair Diskus is an example of a combination-therapy dry powder inhaler (DPI).

Methylxanthines. Methylxanthine (theophylline) preparations are less effective bronchodilators than inhaled β_2-adrenergic agonists.[9] The trend is now toward introducing theophylline as an additional bronchodilator later in the therapeutic regimen. Theophylline may have a synergistic effect with β_2-adrenergic agonists. It is not effective as an inhalant and must be given orally or intravenously as aminophylline. Sustained-release theophylline preparations are preferable for maintenance therapy.

Although the exact mechanism of action is unknown, the main therapeutic action of methylxanthine derivatives is bronchodilation, which is useful in the early-phase response. Only minimal bronchodilation occurs at therapeutic theophylline concentrations.

Theophylline alleviates the early phase of asthma attacks and the bronchoconstrictive portion of the late-phase asthmatic response. However, it has no effect on bronchial hyperresponsiveness. Long-acting theophylline products administered at bedtime may be used to treat the patient with nocturnal asthma. The main problem with theophylline is the relatively high incidence of side effects, which include nausea, headache, insomnia, gastrointestinal distress, tachycardia, arrhythmias, and seizures.

Anticholinergic drugs. Airway diameter is predominantly controlled by the parasympathetic division of the autonomic nervous system. The effects of acetylcholine on the airways are increased mucus secretion and smooth muscle contraction, resulting in bronchoconstriction. Anticholinergic agents (e.g., ipratropium [Atrovent]) inhibit only the component of bronchoconstriction related to the parasympathetic nervous system. Thus these drugs are less effective than β_2-adrenergic agonists and are usually used in combination with other bronchodilators. Anticholinergic agents produce most of their bronchodilation in larger airways, in contrast to β_2-adrenergic agonists, which act primarily in smaller airways. Anticholinergics are not useful in routine asthma management but may be used as alternative bronchodilators for patients with severe adverse effects from β_2-adrenergic agonist inhalers. They may also provide additive effects used in combination with β_2-adrenergic agonists (e.g., ipratropium and albuterol [Combivent]).

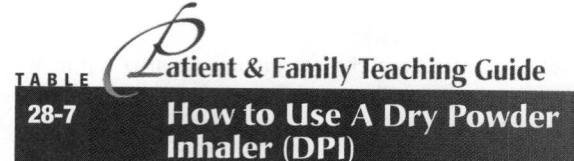

TABLE 28-7 Patient & Family Teaching Guide

How to Use A Dry Powder Inhaler (DPI)

1. Remove mouthpiece cap. Check for dust or dirt.
2. Load the medicine into the inhaler. Some DPIs should be held upright while loading. Others should be held sideways or in a horizontal position.
3. Do not shake your medicine.
4. Tilt your head back slightly and breathe out, getting as much air out of your lungs as you can (see Fig. 28-5). Do not breathe into your inhaler because this could affect the dose.
5. Close your lips tightly around the mouthpiece of the inhaler.
6. Breathe in deeply and quickly. This will ensure that the medicine moves down deeply into your lungs. You may not taste or sense the medicine going into your lungs.
7. Hold your breathe for 10 seconds or as long as you can to disperse the medicine into your lungs.
8. If you need to take another draw of medicine, follow the directions for your inhaler to reload another dose of medicine.

Source: Reinke LF, Hoffman L: Asthma education: creating a partnership, *Heart Lung* 29:225, 2000.

The onset of action of anticholinergics is slower than β_2-adrenergic agonists, peaking at 1 hour and lasting longer, usually up to 4 to 6 hours. Systemic side effects of inhaled anticholinergics are uncommon because they are poorly absorbed.

Monoclonal antibody to IgE. Omalizumab (Xolair) is a monoclonal antibody to IgE that decreases circulating free IgE levels. Omalizumab prevents IgE from attaching to mast cells, thus preventing the release of chemical mediators. It is used to treat patients who have been inadequately controlled with inhaled corticosteroids.[15]

Patient Teaching Related to Drug Therapy. Information about medications should include the name, dosage, method of administration, and schedule, taking into consideration meal times and other activities of daily living (ADLs), purpose, side effects, appropriate action if side effects occur, consequences of improper use, and the importance of refilling the prescription before the medication runs out.

One of the major factors determining success in asthma management is the correct administration of drugs.[16] The majority of asthma drugs are administered only or preferably by inhalation. Inhalation of drugs is often preferred to oral administration because a lower dose is needed and systemic side effects are reduced. In addition, the onset of action of bronchodilators is faster. Inhalation devices include nebulizers, MDIs, and DPIs (Table 28-7). Nebulizers, which generally deliver a larger dose of medication, are usually used for severe asthma. MDIs are usually effective, but some persons, particularly older adults, may have problems with the coordination needed to activate the MDI and inhale the medication. Poor coordination can be solved by the use of spacer devices (Aerochamber, Inspirease) (see Fig. 28-4) or the use of a breath-activated MDI (Maxair Autoinhaler). If the patient is still unable to receive adequate medication, a nebulizer may be used.

In addition, newer delivery systems, such as dry powder inhalers (DPIs), are now available and are simpler to use (Advair

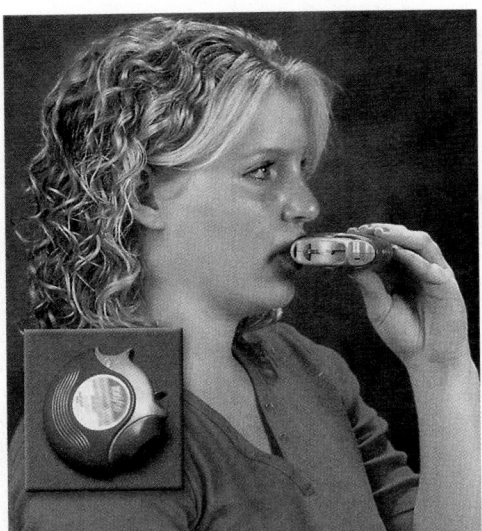

FIG. 28-5   Example of a dry powder inhaler (DPI).

TABLE 28-8   **Problems Encountered with Metered-Dose Inhaler (MDI) Use**

1. Failing to coordinate activation with inspiration
2. Activating MDI in the mouth while breathing through nose
3. Inspiring too rapidly
4. Not holding the breath for 10 sec (or as close to 10 sec as possible)
5. Holding MDI upside down or sideways
6. Inhaling more than 1 puff with each inspiration
7. Not shaking MDI before use
8. Not waiting a sufficient amount of time between each puff
9. Not opening mouth wide enough, causing medication to bounce off teeth, tongue, or palate
10. Not having adequate strength to activate MDI
11. Unable to understand and incorporate directions

Diskus) (Fig. 28-5). The DPI contains dry, powdered medication and is breath activated. No propellant is used; instead an aerosol is created when the patient inhales through a reservoir containing a dose of powder. This convenient-to-carry diskus has several advantages over MDIs: (1) less manual dexterity is needed; (2) the patient does not need to coordinate device puffs with inhalation; (3) an easily visible color or number system indicates the number of doses left in the diskus; and (4) its use does not require a spacer. Disadvantages are that commonly prescribed drugs are not yet available in DPIs and the medication may clump if exposed to humidity.[17]

The inhaler should be cleaned by removing the dust cap and rinsing it in warm water (Fig. 28-6). The patient who needs to use several MDIs is often unclear about the order in which to take the medications. As a general rule, β_2-adrenergic agonists should be used first to open the airway if needed at that time. Corticosteroid inhalers should be used last because they require gargling after use to prevent oral candidiasis. Numbering the inhalers in order of use and marking the number of puffs in large, indelible markers on the inhaler has proved valuable for some patients.

One of the major problems with metered-dose drugs is the potential for overuse (i.e., using them much more frequently than prescribed rather than seeking needed medical care), especially β_2-adrenergic agonist MDIs (Table 28-8). As a patient develops additional asthmatic symptoms, she or he may use the β_2-adrenergic agonist MDI repeatedly. β_2-Adrenergic agonists help by relieving bronchospasm; they do not treat the inflammatory response. Therefore the patient must receive explicit instructions in the correct therapeutic use of these drugs.

Poor adherence with asthma therapy is a major challenge in the long-term management of chronic asthma. The patient will use β_2-adrenergic agonist inhalers because they provide immediate relief of symptoms. The patient, however, often does not take the long-term therapy (inhaled corticosteroids or cromolyn) regularly because no immediate benefit is seen. It is important to explain to the patient the importance and purpose of taking the long-term therapy regularly, emphasizing that maximum improvement may take more than 1 week. It is important to emphasize that without regular use the swelling in the airways may progress and the asthma will likely worsen over time.

Nonprescription Combination Drugs. Several nonprescription combination drugs are available over the counter (OTC). They are usually combinations of a bronchodilator, an expectorant, and a sedative (Table 28-9). These agents are advertised as drugs to relieve bronchospasm. In general they should be avoided. Many persons consider these drugs safe because they can be obtained without a prescription. Some of the dangers of these drugs are as follows:

1. Epinephrine, found in Primatene spray, acts only for a short time and may increase the patient's heart rate and blood pressure. This drug is not recommended for use.
2. Theophylline, taken with other xanthines including caffeine, has an additive effect. Side effects include central nervous system (CNS) and cardiovascular effects, vomiting, nausea, and anorexia.
3. A combination of ephedrine (found in many OTC decongestants) and theophylline causes synergistic stimulation of the central nervous and cardiovascular systems. Side effects include nervousness, heart palpitations and arrhythmias, tremors, insomnia, and increases in blood pressure.

An important teaching responsibility is to warn the patient about the dangers associated with nonprescription combination drugs. These drugs are especially dangerous to a patient with underlying cardiac problems. The patient who persists in taking one of these medications should be cautioned to read and follow the accompanying directions on the label. Another way of discouraging the use of these drugs is to carefully monitor and reevaluate the effectiveness of the prescribed drug therapy. The drug regimen may have to be adjusted to help the patient obtain maximum relief from bronchospasm. An attitude of understanding and caring will often reassure the patient that the health care professional is concerned. This may prevent the patient from attempting to find relief at the local drugstore.

Using an inhaler seems simple, but most patients do not use it the right way. When you use your inhaler the wrong way, less medicine gets to your lungs. (Your doctor may give you other types of inhalers.)

For the next 2 weeks, read these steps aloud as you do them or ask someone to read them to you. Ask your doctor or nurse to check how well you are using your inhaler.

Use your inhaler in one of the three ways pictured below (**A** or **B** are best, but **C** can be used if you have trouble with **A** and **B**).

Steps for Using Your Inhaler

Getting ready
1. Take off the cap and shake the inhaler.
2. Breathe out all the way.
3. Hold your inhaler the way your doctor said (**A**, **B**, or **C** below).

Breathe in slowly
4. As you start breathing in **slowly** through your mouth, press down on the inhaler **one** time. (If you use a holding chamber, first press down on the inhaler. Within 5 sec, begin to breathe in slowly.)
5. Keep breathing in **slowly**, as deeply as you can.

Hold your breath
6. Hold your breath as you count to 10 slowly, if you can.
7. For inhaled quick-relief medicine (β_2-agonists), wait about 1 min between puffs. There is no need to wait between puffs for other medicines.

A. Hold inhaler 1 to 2 in in front of your mouth (about the width of two fingers).

B. Use a spacer/holding chamber. These come in many shapes and can be useful to any patient.

C. Put the inhaler in your mouth. Do not use for steroids.

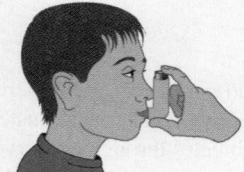

Clean Your Inhaler as Needed

Look at the hole where the medicine sprays out from your inhaler. If you see "powder" in or around the hole, clean the inhaler. Remove the metal canister from the L-shaped plastic mouthpiece. Rinse only the mouthpiece and cap in warm water. Let them dry overnight. In the morning, put the canister back inside. Put the cap on.

Know When to Replace Your Inhaler

For medicines you take each day (an example):
Say your new canister has 200 puffs (number of puffs is listed on canister) and you are told to take 8 puffs per day.

$$8 \text{ puffs per day} \overline{)\begin{array}{c} 25 \text{ days} \\ 200 \text{ puffs} \\ \text{in canister} \end{array}}$$

So this canister will last 25 days. If you started using this inhaler on May 1, replace it on or before May 25.
You can write the date on your canister.

For quick-relief medicine take as needed and count each puff.

Do not put your canister in water to see if it is empty. This does not work.

FIG. 28-6 How to use your metered-dose inhaler correctly.

TABLE 28-9   Nonprescription Combination Asthma Drugs

DRUG PRODUCT	INGREDIENTS		
	SYMPATHOMIMETIC	XANTHINE	OTHER
Amodrine	Ephedrine	Aminophylline	Phenobarbital
Asthma Nefrin inhalant	Epinephrine	—	Chlorobutanol
Bronkaid tablets	Ephedrine	Theophylline	Guaifenesin
Bronkaid Mist	Epinephrine	—	Ascorbic acid, alcohol
Bronkotabs	Ephedrine	Theophylline	Guaifenesin, phenobarbital
Primatene M tablets	Ephedrine	Theophylline	Pyrilamine
Primatene P tablets	Ephedrine	Theophylline	Phenobarbital
Primatene Mist	Epinephrine	—	Ascorbic acid, alcohol
Tedral	Ephedrine	Theophylline	Phenobarbital
Vaponefrin inhalant	Epinephrine	—	Chlorobutanol

NURSING MANAGEMENT
ASTHMA

■ Nursing Assessment

If a patient can speak and is not in acute distress, a detailed health history, including identification of any precipitating factors and what has helped alleviate attacks in the past, can be taken. Subjective and objective data that should be obtained from a patient with asthma are presented in Table 28-10.

■ Nursing Diagnoses

Nursing diagnoses for the patient with asthma may include, but are not limited to, those presented in NCP 28-1.

■ Planning

The overall goals are that the patient with asthma will have (1) normal or near-normal pulmonary function, (2) normal activity levels (including exercise and other physical activity), (3) no recurrent exacerbations of asthma or decreased incidence of asthma attacks, and (4) adequate knowledge to participate in and carry out management.

■ Nursing Implementation

Health Promotion. The nursing role in preventing asthma attacks or decreasing their severity focuses primarily on teaching the patient and family. The patient should be taught to identify and avoid known personal triggers for asthma (e.g., cigarette smoke, pet dander) and irritants (e.g., cold air, aspirin, foods, cats, indoor air pollution) (see Table 28-1). Use of dust covers on mattresses can significantly reduce exposure to dust mites. If cold air cannot be avoided, dressing properly with scarves or using a mask helps reduce the risk of an asthma attack. Aspirin and

NURSING RESEARCH
Ethnic Differences between African American and White Asthma Patients

Citation
Hardie GE et al: Ethnic differences: word descriptors used by African Americans and white asthma patients during induced bronchoconstriction, *Chest* 117: 935, 2000.

Purpose
To determine if African American and white patients with asthma (1) differ in the words they use to describe their breathlessness and (2) differ in their perception of breathlessness.

Methods
The study was conducted in an ethnically and economically diverse area. A total of 32 subjects (16 per group) completed the study. All had a provocation concentration of methacholine causing a 30% fall in FEV_1. Serial pulmonary function testing was performed. Breathlessness was measured using the Borg scale* and the visual analog scale. Word descriptors were measured by an open-ended word descriptor questionnaire.

Results and Conclusions
There were significant ethnic differences in the words used to describe the sensation of breathlessness. African Americans used upper airway word descriptors: tight throat, scared-agitated, voice tight, itchy throat, and tough breath. Whites used lower airway or chest-wall symptom descriptors: deep breath, light-headed, out of air, aware of breathing, and it hurts to breathe. The African Americans required a significantly smaller dose of methacholine to achieve breathlessness.

Implications for Nursing Practice
This study provides nurses with valuable new information about ethnicity and the words used to describe breathlessness during airflow obstruction. African Americans used different words than whites to describe breathlessness. If nurses are to be effective in asthma symptom monitoring, it requires asking the correct questions and being aware that ethnic differences may exist.

*The Borg scale is shown in Chapter 25, Fig. 25-9.
FEV_1, Forced expiratory volume in 1 second.

TABLE 28-10   Nursing Assessment
Asthma

Subjective Data

Important Health Information

Past health history: Allergic rhinitis or sinusitis; previous asthma attack; exposure to pollen, danders, feathers, mold, dust, inhaled irritants, weather changes, exercise, smoke; sinus infections; gastroesophageal reflux

Medications: Use of and compliance with corticosteroids, bronchodilators, cromolyn sodium, anticholinergics, antibiotics; medications that may precipitate an attack in susceptible asthmatics such as aspirin, nonsteroidal antiinflammatory drugs, β-adrenergic blockers

Functional Health Patterns

Health perception–health management: Family history of allergies or asthma; recent upper respiratory infection or sinus infection

Activity-exercise: Fatigue, decreased or absent exercise tolerance; dyspnea, cough, productive cough with yellow or green sputum; chest tightness, feelings of suffocation, air hunger

Sleep-rest: Interrupted sleep, insomnia

Coping–stress tolerance: Fear, anxiety, emotional distress, stress in work environment or in the home

Objective Data

General

Restlessness or exhaustion, confusion, upright or forward-leaning body position

Integumentary

Diaphoresis, cyanosis (circumoral, nailbed)

Respiratory

Wheezing, crackles, diminished or absent breath sounds, and rhonchi on auscultation; hyperresonance on percussion; sputum (thick, white, tenacious), ↑ work of breathing with use of accessory muscles; intercostal and supraclavicular retractions; tachypnea with hyperventilation; prolonged expiration

Cardiovascular

Tachycardia, pulsus paradoxus, jugular venous distention, hypertension or hypotension, premature ventricular contractions

Possible Findings

Abnormal ABGs during attacks, ↓ O_2 saturation, serum and sputum eosinophilia, ↑ serum IgE, positive skin tests for allergens, chest x-ray demonstrating hyperinflation with attacks, abnormal pulmonary function tests showing ↓ flow rates; FVC, FEV_1, PEFR, and FEV_1/FVC ratio that improve between attacks and with bronchodilators

FEV_1, Forced expiratory volume at 1 second; *FVC,* forced vital capacity, *PEFR,* peak expiratory flow rate.

NURSING CARE PLAN 28-1

Patient with Asthma

NURSING DIAGNOSIS **Ineffective airway clearance** *related to* bronchospasm, ineffective cough, excessive mucus production, tenacious secretions, and fatigue *as manifested by* ineffective cough, inability to raise secretions, adventitious breath sounds.

OUTCOMES—NOC

Respiratory Status: Airway Patency (0410)
- Respiratory rate IER ____
- Respiratory rhythm IER ____
- Moves sputum out of airway ____
- Free of adventitious breath sounds ____

Outcome Scale
1 = Extremely compromised
2 = Substantially compromised
3 = Moderately compromised
4 = Mildly compromised
5 = Not compromised

INTERVENTIONS—NIC and *RATIONALES*

Cough Enhancement (3250)
- Assist patient to a sitting position with head slightly flexed, shoulders relaxed, and knees flexed *to allow for adequate chest expansion.*
- Encourage patient to take a deep breath, hold for 2 seconds, and cough two or three times in succession *to prepare for exhalation and distribution of the inhaled air.*

Airway Management (3140)
- Monitor respiratory and oxygenation status *to determine need for intervention or note improvement.*
- Instruct how to use prescribed inhalers (see Tables 28-7 and 28-8 and Fig. 28-6).
- Regulate fluid intake *to optimize fluid balance and liquefy secretions to facilitate removal.*
- Administer drug therapy (e.g., bronchodilators, corticosteroids) *to improve respiratory function.*
- Auscultate lung sounds after treatments *to note results.*

NURSING DIAGNOSIS **Anxiety** *related to* difficulty breathing, perceived or actual loss of control, and fear of suffocation *as manifested by* restlessness; elevated pulse, respiratory rate, and blood pressure.

OUTCOMES—NOC

Anxiety Control (1402)
- Monitors intensity of anxiety ____
- Plans coping strategies for stressful situations ____
- Uses relaxation techniques to reduce anxiety ____

Outcome Scale
1 = Never demonstrated
2 = Rarely demonstrated
3 = Sometimes demonstrated
4 = Often demonstrated
5 = Consistently demonstrated

INTERVENTIONS—NIC and *RATIONALES*

Anxiety Reduction (5820)
- Identify level of anxiety and when it changes *to assess possible precipitating factors.*
- Use calm, reassuring approach *to provide reassurance.*
- Stay with patient *to promote safety and reduce fear.*
- Encourage verbalization of feelings, perceptions, and fears *to identify problem areas so concentrated planning can take place.*
- Instruct patient on the use of relaxation techniques *to relieve muscle tension and to promote ease of respirations.*

NURSING DIAGNOSIS **Ineffective therapeutic regimen management** *related to* lack of information about asthma and its treatment *as manifested by* frequent questioning regarding all aspects of long-term management.

OUTCOMES—NOC

Asthma Control (0704)
- Demonstrates appropriate use of inhalers, spacers, and nebulizers ____
- Initiates action to manage personal triggers ____
- Seeks early treatment of infections ____

Outcome Scale
1 = Never demonstrated
2 = Rarely demonstrated
3 = Sometimes demonstrated
4 = Often demonstrated
5 = Consistently demonstrated

INTERVENTIONS—NIC and *RATIONALES*

Teaching: Disease Process (5602)*
- Appraise the patient's current level of knowledge related to specific disease process *to define level of knowledge.*
- Instruct the patient on measures to prevent/minimize side effects of treatment for the disease *to plan for future problems.*

Teaching: Prescribed Medication (5616)*
- Evaluate the patient's ability to self-administer medications *to assess competence and correct usage.*
- Instruct the patient on the purpose, action, dosage, and duration of each medication *to promote understanding of effects.*
- Instruct the patient on the proper administration of each medication (e.g., inhalers, spacers) *to ensure proper use.*
- Include the family and significant other as appropriate *to ensure knowledgeable help when the patient is in need.*

*Refer to Patient and Family Teaching Guides (Tables 28-7, 28-12, and 28-13).
IER, In expected range.

NSAIDs should be avoided if they are known to precipitate an attack. Many OTC drugs contain aspirin, and the patient should be instructed to read the labels carefully. β-Adrenergic receptor blockers (e.g., propranolol [Inderal]) are contraindicated because they inhibit bronchodilation. Desensitization (immunotherapy) may be partially effective in decreasing the patient's sensitivity to known allergens (see Chapter 13).

Prompt diagnosis and treatment of upper respiratory tract infections and sinusitis may prevent an exacerbation of asthma. If occupational irritants are involved as etiologic factors, the patient may need to consider changing jobs. The patient should be encouraged to maintain a fluid intake of 2 to 3 L per day, good nutrition, and adequate rest. If exercise is planned, administering a β$_2$-adrenergic agonist, cromolyn, or nedocromil 10 to 20 minutes before the activity should prevent bronchospasm.

Acute Intervention. During an acute attack of asthma, it is important to monitor the patient's respiratory and cardiovascular systems. This includes auscultating lung sounds; taking the pulse rate, respiratory rate, and BP; and monitoring ABGs, pulse oximetry, and FEV$_1$ and PEFR. The patient's work of breathing (i.e., use of accessory muscles, degree of fatigue) and response to therapy should also be evaluated. If the patient's condition deteriorates, the health care provider must be notified immediately to initiate prompt medical intervention. Nursing interventions include administering O$_2$, bronchodilators, chest physiotherapy, and medications (as ordered) and ongoing patient monitoring, including the effectiveness of these interventions.

An important nursing goal during an acute attack is to decrease the patient's sense of panic. A calm, quiet, reassuring attitude may help the patient relax. The patient should be positioned comfortably (usually sitting) to maximize chest expansion. Staying with the patient and being available provide additional comfort. Encouraging slow breathing using pursed lips for prolonged exhalation can be helpful.

When the acute attack subsides, the nurse should provide rest and a quiet, calm environment for the patient. When the patient has recovered from exhaustion, the nurse should attempt to obtain information about the patient's health history and pattern of asthma. If family members are present, they may be able to provide information about the patient's health history. A thorough physical assessment should be completed (see Table 28-10). This information is important in planning an individualized nursing care plan for the patient. Well-thought-out written plans involving the patient and significant others increase the patient's knowledge and control of the situation and may help improve confidence and compliance.

Ambulatory and Home Care. It is important to remember that asthma is potentially controllable and that every effort should be made to keep the patient free of symptoms. The patient with asthma usually takes several medications with different routes of administration and time frames for dosage (e.g., tapering corticosteroid schedules, using several different inhalers with different indications). The drug regimen itself can be confusing and complex. The patient with asthma must learn about the numerous medications and develop self-management strategies. The patient and the health professional need to monitor the patient's responsiveness to medication. It is easy to undermedicate or overmedicate a patient with asthma unless careful monitoring is ongoing. Some patients may benefit from keeping a diary to record medication use, the presence of wheezing or coughing,

PEFR, the drug's side effects, and the activity level. This information will be valuable in helping the health care provider adjust the medication. The patient must understand the importance of continuing the medication even when symptoms are not present. If worsening bronchospasm or severe side effects of the drugs occur, the patient should seek medical attention. (Additional information related to patient teaching related to drug therapy is discussed on pp. 650-651.)

Good nutrition is important. Physical exercise (e.g., swimming, walking, stationary cycling) within the patient's limit of tolerance is also beneficial. If dyspnea occurs on exertion, it can often be prevented with the use of a β$_2$-adrenergic agonist MDI, cromolyn, or nedocromil. Sleep that is uninterrupted by asthma symptoms is important.

A written asthma management plan (Table 28-11) should be developed together with the patient and family. Most plans are developed based on the patient's asthma symptoms and peak flow readings. A management plan can be established when the patient's best peak flow is established and the patient has good asthma control (e.g., not waking up at night with asthma symptoms, able to perform some type of aerobic exercise or strenuous activity, not having frequent daily symptoms).

To follow the management plan, the patient must measure his or her peak flow at least daily. Patients with asthma frequently do not perceive changes in their breathing. Therefore peak flow monitoring when done correctly can be a good objective measurement of asthma (Table 28-12). Using PEFR is similar to using BP monitoring in a person with hypertension.

If a patient's PEFR is within the green zone (usually 80% to 100% of the person's personal best), the patient should remain on her or his usual medications. If the PEFR is within the yellow zone (usually 50% to 80% of personal best), it indicates caution. Something is triggering the patient's asthma. Patients who get a cold or sinus infection, which may trigger asthma, can usually increase the dose of the corticosteroid inhaler one third to one half, depending on the asthma management plan. The dose can be decreased once the cold subsides. Different strategies may be employed by the patient based on the asthma management plan. For example, the patient could use the β$_2$-adrenergic agonist inhaler more frequently.

If the PEFR is in the red zone (50% or less of personal best), it indicates a serious problem. Definitive action must be taken. In addition to increasing the use of β$_2$-adrenergic agonist inhalers, oral corticosteroids may be indicated. The patient needs to contact or be seen by the health care provider.

It is important to emphasize to the patient the need to monitor PEFR daily because asthma tends to worsen gradually over time. Although it may occur, it is unusual for a patient's PEFR to drop from the green zone to the red zone quickly. Usually the patient has time to make changes in medications, avoid triggers, and notify the health care provider.

When developing a management plan, it is important to involve the patient's family. Often the family member feels frustrated and does not know how to help. The family member or significant other should be taught what can be done to help the patient during an asthmatic attack. This person should know where the patient's inhalers, oral medications, and emergency phone numbers are located. The significant other can also be instructed on how to decrease the patient's anxiety if an asthma attack occurs. When the patient is stabilized or controlled, the significant other can gently remind the patient about doing daily

TABLE 28-11 Asthma Management Plan

NAME	PERSONAL BEST PEAK FLOW	DATE

Green—GO
- Breathing is good
- No coughing, wheezing, chest tightness, or shortness of breath
- No problems talking or walking

> **Peak Flow Number:**
> _____ to _____
> (80%–100% of Best)

PLAN A: Continue regular medicines. Use **preventer** medicines all the time.
Bronchodilator Inhaler (**Quick Reliever**): _____
Steroid Inhaler (**Preventer/Controller**): _____
Other Inhaler/Nebs: _____
Additional Instructions:
- At the first sign of a cold, you may double the dose of the steroid inhaler *until the cold subsides.* Then resume usual dose.
- Monitor your peak flows daily. When exposed to triggers or when you have a cold, monitor your peak flows at least 2 times/day or more.
- Use quick reliever medicine 10 minutes before exercise if you have exercise-induced asthma.

Yellow—CAUTION
- Mild to moderate symptoms
- Coughing, wheezing, chest tightness, or shortness of breath
- No problems talking or walking but may feel anxious
- Unable to sleep because of asthma symptoms

> **Peak Flow Number:**
> _____ to _____
> (50%–80% of Best)

PLAN B: Continue Plan A and add quick reliever medicine.
❶ Immediately take 2-4 puffs or quick reliever _____ or by nebulizer treatment.
❷ Wait 20 minutes.
- If peak flow returns to Green Zone or asthma symptoms subside, follow Green Zone plan.
- If peak flow remains in the Yellow Zone and/or symptoms do not improve, repeat ❶ and ❷. You may repeat this a third time if still not improved.
❸ If still in the Yellow Zone after _____ hours and/or symptoms do not improve, _____ or begin prednisone (Deltasone) or Medrol on the following schedule: _____

WARNING: If at any time you progress to the Red Zone, proceed to Plan C.

Red—STOP—Danger
Severe Symptoms
- Continuous coughing, wheezing, chest tightness, or shortness of breath
- Able to speak in short sentences only but feel very anxious
- Lips and nails still pink color

> **Peak Flow Number:**
> _____ to _____
> (0%–50% of Best)

PLAN C: This is the **DANGER ZONE!** Act immediately.
❶ Immediately take 2-6 puffs of quick reliever or nebulizer treatment _____
❷ If you are still in the Red Zone in 10-20 minutes, begin prednisone (Deltasone) or Medrol in the following schedule, if instructed to do so: _____
_____
❸ Repeat ❶ and ❷ for a total of three times in 1 hour if asthma symptoms persist.
❹ Call your health care provider if you do not have instructions to begin prednisone (Deltasone) or Medrol or if your symptoms do not improve.

Very Severe Symptoms →
- Severe chest tightness, struggling to breathe, hunching over, chest pulled or sucked in with each breath
- Having trouble walking and talking
- Must stop activity you are doing and cannot start again
- Lips and nails may be blue

STOP

PLAN D: Call 911 immediately to be taken to the emergency room.
- Take 6 puffs of beta bronchodilator (quick reliever) inhaler every 5-10 minutes OR take a continuous nebulizer treatment while waiting or in route.
- If you have prednisone, take 40 mg immediately.

Any time you are having an asthma episode, **STAY CALM.** Breathe out slowly through pursed lips. If possible, identify the specific trigger for this episode and try to avoid it. If you need help, call your health care provider.

_____   _____
Provider Signature   *Patient Signature*

Source: Lovelace Health Systems Adult Asthma Program, Albuquerque, N.M.

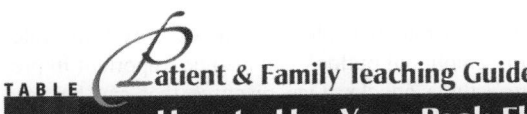

TABLE 28-12

TABLE
28-12

Patient & Family Teaching Guide

How to Use Your Peak Flow Meter

A peak flow meter helps you check how well your asthma is controlled. Peak flow meters are most helpful for people with moderate or severe asthma.

This guide will tell you (1) how to find your personal best peak flow number, (2) how to use your personal best number to set your peak flow zones, (3) how to take your peak flow, and (4) when to take your peak flow to check your asthma each day.

Starting Out: Find Your Personal Best Peak Flow Number

To find your personal best peak flow number, take your peak flow each day for 2 to 3 weeks. Your asthma should be under good control during this time. Take your peak flow as close to the times listed below as you can. (These times for taking your peak flow are *only* for finding your personal best peak flow. To check your asthma each day, you will take your peak flow in the morning.)

- Between noon and 2:00 PM each day.
- Each time you take your quick-relief medicine to relieve symptoms. (Measure your peak flow *after* you take your medicine.)
- Any other time your doctor suggests.

Write down the number you get for each peak flow reading. The highest peak flow number you had during the 2 to 3 weeks is your personal best.

Your personal best can change over time. Ask your doctor when to check for a new personal best.

Your Peak Flow Zones

Your peak flow zones are based on your personal best peak flow number. The zones will help you check your asthma and take the right actions to keep it controlled. The colors used with each zone come from the traffic light.

Green Zone (80%-100% of your personal best) signals **good control.** Take your usual daily long-term–control medicines, if you take any. Keep taking these medicines even when you are in the yellow or red zones.

Yellow Zone (50%-79% of your personal best) signals **caution: your asthma is getting worse.** Add quick-relief medicines. You might need to increase other asthma medicines as directed by your doctor.

Red Zone (below 50% of your personal best) signals **medical alert!** Add or increase quick-relief medicines and call your doctor ***now.***

Ask your doctor to write an action plan for you that tells you:

- The peak flow numbers for *your* green, yellow, and red zones. Mark the zones on your peak flow meter with colored tape or a marker.
- The medicines you should take while in each peak flow zone.

How to Take Your Peak Flow

1. Move the marker to the bottom of the numbered scale.
2. Stand up or sit up straight.
3. Take a deep breath. Fill your lungs all the way.
4. Hold your breath while you place the mouthpiece in your mouth, between your teeth. Close your lips around it. Do **not** put your tongue inside the hole.
5. Blow out as hard and fast as you can. Your peak flow meter will measure how fast you can blow out air.
6. Write down the number you get. But if you cough or make a mistake, do not write down the number. Do it over again.
7. Repeat steps 1 through 6 two more times. Write down the highest of the three numbers. This is your peak flow number.
8. Check to see which peak flow *zone* your peak flow number is in. Do the actions your doctor told you to do while in that zone.

Your doctor may ask you to write down your peak flow numbers each day. You can do this on a calendar or other paper. This will help you and your doctor see how your asthma is doing over time.

Checking Your Asthma: When to Use Your Peak Flow Meter

- **Every morning** when you wake up, *before* you take medicine. Make this part of your daily routine.
- **When you are having asthma symptoms or an attack.** And after taking medicine for the attack. This can tell you how bad your asthma attack is and whether your medicine is working.
- Any other time your doctor suggests.

If you use more than one peak flow meter (such as at home and at school), be sure that both meters are the same brand.

Bring to Each of Your Doctor's Visits

- Your peak flow meter.
- Your peak flow numbers if you have written them down each day.

Also, ask your doctor or nurse to check how you use your peak flow meter—just to be sure you are doing it right.

Source: *Practical guide for the diagnosis and management of asthma, based on Expert Panel Report 2: guidelines for the diagnosis and management of asthma,* Washington, DC, 1997, National Institutes of Health.

PEFR by asking questions such as, "What zone are you in? How's your peak flow today?"

Counseling may be indicated to help the patient and the family resolve personal, family, social, and occupational problems that have resulted from asthma. Relaxation therapies (e.g., yoga, meditation, relaxation techniques, breathing techniques) may be of value in helping a patient relax respiratory muscles and de-crease the respiratory rate. (Chapter 8 discusses relaxation strategies.) A healthy emotional outlook can also be important in preventing future asthma attacks. One resource that can be used when teaching the patient about asthma is the American Lung Association, which has educational materials about asthma, including *The Asthma Handbook*. Table 28-13 is a patient and family teaching guide for the patient with asthma.

TABLE 28-13 *Patient & Family Teaching Guide*

Asthma

Goal: To assist patient in improving quality of life through education, increased understanding, and promotion of lifestyle practices that support successful living with asthma.

TEACHING TOPIC	RESOURCES
What Is Asthma? • Basic anatomy and physiology of lung • Pathophysiology of asthma • Relationship of pathophysiology to signs and symptoms • Measurement and correlation of pulmonary function tests and peak expiratory flow rate	*Teach Your Patient about Asthma: A Clinician's Guide* (Publication 92-2737, National Institutes of Health) *The Asthma Handbook* (American Lung Association)
What Is Good Asthma Control?	Discussion with patient on personal ideas of good control. Videotape—*Essence of Life* (Glaxo—sponsored by Allen and Hansbury's Respiratory Institute)
Hindrances to Asthma Treatment and Control • Intermittent nature of symptoms • Role of denial • Poor perception of asthma severity by patient	Discussion with patient and family about possible hindrances
Environmental/Trigger Control • Identifications of possible triggers and possible preventive measures • Avoidance of allergens and other triggers • Need to maintain good hydration	Trigger diary kept by patient Handouts from National Asthma Education and Prevention Program (NIH Publication 97-4053)
Medications • Types (include mechanism of action) β_2-agonists cromolyn/nedocromil Corticosteroids Methylxanthines Leukotriene modifiers • Establishing medication schedule • Use of preventive/maintenance agents (e.g., antiinflammatory agents) • Regular use	*Understanding Lung Medications: How They Work—How to Use Them* (American Lung Association) Asthma Management Plan (see Table 28-11) Write out medication list and schedule
Correct Use of Meter-Dose Inhaler, Spacer, and Nebulizer	Videotape—*Managing Your Asthma* (Glaxo) (see Fig. 28-6)
Breathing Techniques • Pursed-lip breathing • Diaphragmatic breathing	Demonstration–return demonstration
Correct Use of Peak Flow Meter	See Table 28-12 Videotape—*Managing Your Asthma* (Glaxo) *Facts about Peak Flow Meters* (American Lung Association)
Asthma Management Plan • Peak flow zones • Individualize plan • Early recognition of infection	See Table 28-11 Living with Asthma and the Asthma Handbook (American Lung Association) Patient completes plan and discusses it with health care provider

■ Evaluation

The expected outcomes for the patient with asthma are presented in NCP 28-1.

EMPHYSEMA AND CHRONIC BRONCHITIS

Chronic obstructive pulmonary disease (COPD) is a disease state characterized by the presence of airflow obstruction caused by chronic bronchitis or emphysema. The airflow obstruction is generally progressive, may be accompanied by airway hyperreactivity, and may be partially reversible. In the past, asthma was generally defined along with COPD. Now, inflammation is considered the distinguishing feature of asthma, and therefore asthma has now been defined separately. Patients with COPD may have asthma, and some patients with asthma may go on to develop fixed or irreversible airflow obstruction. **Chronic bronchitis** is the presence of chronic productive cough for 3 months in each of 2 successive years in a patient in whom other causes of chronic cough have been excluded. **Emphysema** is an abnormal permanent enlargement of the airspaces distal to the terminal bronchioles, accompanied by destruction of their walls and without obvious fibrosis. There is usually some overlap between chronic bronchitis and emphysema.[2,18]

More than 15 million persons in the United States suffer from emphysema and chronic bronchitis. The estimated number of those with COPD has doubled in the last 25 years. The number of women with COPD is on the rise because of the increased number of women smoking cigarettes. COPD is the fourth-leading cause of death in the United States. More than one half of COPD patients die within 10 years of diagnosis. The decrease in cigarette smoking in the United States should lead to a decrease in COPD mortality rates in the future. However, there has been a marked increase in cigarette smoking in developing countries, which will increase COPD mortality rates worldwide.[19]

Etiology

Exposure to tobacco smoke is the primary cause of COPD in the United States.

Cigarette Smoking. The major risk factor for developing COPD is cigarette smoking. Although the prevalence of cigarette smoking in the United States has decreased since 1964, it is still a major public health concern among young people. Nearly all first use of tobacco occurs before high school graduation, and each day 3000 teenagers start to smoke.[20]

Clinically significant airway obstruction develops in 15% of smokers, and 80% to 90% of COPD deaths in the United States are related to tobacco smoking. For most Americans who die of lung diseases related to cigarette smoking, death is preceded by a long period of debilitation characterized by frequent hospitalizations and loss of many years of productivity. Cigarette smoking is extremely costly to both the individual and society. More than one out of every five deaths in the United States is the result of smoking. Cigarette smoking remains the most preventable cause of premature death in the United States. In addition to being linked with emphysema, chronic bronchitis, and lung cancer, cigarette smoking has also been implicated as a factor in cancers of the mouth, pharynx, larynx, esophagus, pancreas, kidney, stomach, cervix, and bladder.

When cigarettes are smoked, approximately 4000 chemicals and gases are inhaled into the lungs. Many carcinogens have been isolated from cigarette smoke; 3,4-benzpyrene is the most dangerous. At least 43 other components have been identified as carcinogens, co-carcinogens, tumor promoters, tumor initiators, and mutagens. Nicotine is probably not a carcinogen, but it has other deleterious effects. It acts by stimulating the sympathetic nervous system, resulting in increased heart rate, increased peripheral vasoconstriction, increased BP, and increased cardiac workload. These effects of nicotine compound the problems in a person with coronary artery disease. (The effects of nicotine are discussed in Chapter 11.)

Cigarette smoke has several direct effects on the respiratory tract (Table 28-14). The irritating effect of the smoke causes hyperplasia of cells, including goblet cells, which subsequently results in increased production of mucus. Hyperplasia reduces airway diameter and increases the difficulty in clearing secretions. Smoking reduces the ciliary activity and may cause actual loss of ciliated cells. Smoking also produces abnormal dilation of the distal air space with destruction of alveolar walls. Many cells develop large, atypical nuclei, which is considered a precancerous condition.

After only 1 year of smoking, changes in small airway function can develop. In the early stages these changes are mostly inflammatory with mucosal edema and an influx of inflammatory cells. In later stages, however, peribronchiolar fibrosis is present. These inflammatory changes in small airways can be reversed with smoking cessation, at least in the younger person.

Carbon monoxide (CO), a component of tobacco smoke, is also present in similar concentrations in automobile exhaust. CO

TABLE 28-14   Effects of Tobacco Smoke on the Respiratory System

AREA OF DEFECT	ACUTE EFFECTS	LONG-TERM EFFECTS
Respiratory mucosa		
Nasopharyngeal	↓ Sense of smell	Cancer
Tongue	↓ Sense of taste	Cancer
Vocal cords	Hoarseness	Chronic cough, cancer
Bronchus and bronchioles	Bronchospasm, cough	Chronic bronchitis, asthma, cancer
Cilia	Paralysis, sputum accumulation, cough	Chronic bronchitis, cancer
Mucous glands	↑ Secretions, ↑ cough	Hyperplasia and hypertrophy of glands, chronic bronchitis
		↑ Incidence of infection
Alveolar macrophages	↓ Function	
Elastin and collagen fibers	↑ Destruction by proteases, ↓ function of antiproteases (α_1-antitrypsin), ↓ synthesis and repair of elastin	Emphysema

has a high affinity for hemoglobin and combines with it more readily than does O_2, thereby reducing the smoker's O_2-carrying capacity. The smoker inhales a lower percentage of O_2 than normal, resulting in less O_2 available at the alveolar level. The heart's need for O_2 is increased because of the stimulatory effect of nicotine on the sympathetic nervous system. Because the blood's O_2-carrying capacity is reduced, the heart must pump more rapidly to adequately supply tissues with O_2. CO also seems to impair psychomotor performance and judgment.

Passive smoking is the exposure of nonsmokers to cigarette smoke, also known as *environmental tobacco smoke* (ETS) or secondhand smoke. In adults, involuntary smoke exposure is associated with decreased pulmonary function, increased risk for lung cancer, and increased mortality rates from ischemic heart disease.[2]

Infection. Recurring respiratory tract infections are a major contributing factor to the aggravation and progression of COPD. Recurring infections impair normal defense mechanisms, making the bronchioles and alveoli more susceptible to injury. In addition, the person with COPD is more prone to respiratory infections, which subsequently intensify the pathologic destruction of lung tissue and the progression of COPD. The most common causative organisms are *Haemophilus influenzae, Streptococcus pneumoniae,* and *Moraxella catarrhalis.* Retained secretions provide a good medium for their proliferation.

Heredity. α_1-Antitrypsin (AAT) deficiency is the only known genetic abnormality that leads to COPD[21] (see the Genetics in Clinical Practice box). AAT deficiency accounts for less than 1% of COPD in the United States. Also known as α_1-protease inhibitor, AAT is a serum protein produced by the liver and normally found in the lungs. Severe AAT deficiency leads to premature emphysema, often with chronic bronchitis and occasionally with bronchiectasis. Emphysema results when lysis of lung tissues by proteolytic enzymes from neutrophils and macrophages occurs because of the AAT deficiency. Normally AAT inhibits the action of these enzymes. Therefore lower levels of AAT result in insufficient inactivation and subsequent destruction of lung tissue. Smoking greatly exacerbates the disease process in these patients.

The level of AAT is controlled by a pair of autosomal codominant genes. Low levels of AAT are related to homozygosity for the deficiency gene (ZZ), intermediate levels to heterozygosity (MZ), and normal values to homozygosity for the normal gene (MM). In the recessive gene homozygous group, onset of symptoms often occurs by age 40, and the disease is found as frequently in women as in men. The people with this type of emphysema are primarily of northern European origin.[21,22]

IV or nebulizer-administered AAT (Prolastin) augmentation therapy has recently been approved for persons with AAT deficiency. The infusions are administered weekly.[21,22] Its effectiveness in slowing the progression of the disease continues to be evaluated.

Aging. Some degree of emphysema is common in the lungs of the older person, even a nonsmoker. Aging results in changes in the lung structure, the thoracic cage, and the respiratory muscles. Clinically significant emphysema, however, is usually not caused by aging alone.

As people age there is gradual loss of the elastic recoil of the lung. The lungs become more rounded and smaller. The number of functional alveoli decreases as a result of the loss of the alveolar supporting structures and loss of the intraalveolar septum. These changes are similar to those seen in the patient with emphysema. Thinner alveolar walls contribute to loss of alveolar septal tissue and alveolar capillaries. With fewer capillaries available for gas exchange, arterial O_2 levels decrease. The PaO_2 falls at a rate of 4 mm Hg for each decade of life, beginning after 20 years of age. The surface area available for gas exchange decreases from 80 m[2] at 20 years of age to 65 to 70 m[2] by 70 years of age.[23]

Thoracic cage changes result from osteoporosis and calcification of the costal cartilages. The thoracic cage becomes stiff and rigid, and the ribs are less mobile. The shape of the rib cage gradually changes because of the increased functional residual capacity (FRC), causing it to expand and become rounded. These changes result in a decreased compliance of the chest wall and an increase in the work of breathing.

Pathophysiology

It is common clinically to find a combination of emphysema and chronic bronchitis in the same person, often with one condition predominating (Fig. 28-7).

Emphysema. Structural changes in emphysema include (1) hyperinflation of alveoli; (2) destruction of alveolar walls; (3) destruction of alveolar capillary walls; (4) narrowed, tortuous, small airways; and (5) loss of lung elasticity.

There are two major types of emphysema: centrilobular and panlobular (Fig. 28-8). In centrilobular emphysema the primary area of involvement is the central part of the lobule. Respiratory bronchioles enlarge, the walls are destroyed, and the bronchioles become confluent. Chronic bronchitis is often associated with centrilobular emphysema, which is more common than panlobular emphysema.

In contrast, panlobular emphysema involves distention and destruction of the whole lobule. Respiratory bronchioles, alveolar ducts and sacs, and alveoli are all affected. There is progressive loss of lung tissue and a decreased alveolar-capillary surface area. Severe panlobular emphysema is usually found in persons with AAT deficiency. In some patients with emphysema, *bullae*

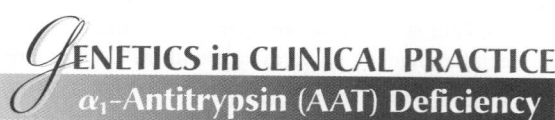

GENETICS in CLINICAL PRACTICE
α_1-Antitrypsin (AAT) Deficiency

Genetic Basis
- Autosomal codominant disorder
- Gene for AAT is located on chromosome 14
- Several allelic variants of AAT gene

Incidence
- 1 in 1700 to 3500 live births in the United States
- Persons of Northern European decent most affected
- Found equally in males and females

Genetic Testing
- DNA testing available
- Serum assay available to measure the amount of α_1-antitrypsin

Clinical Implications
- Only genetic disorder that is linked specifically to chronic obstructive pulmonary disease (COPD)
- Treatment includes α_1-antitrypsin replacement (Prolastin)
- Predisposes to early-onset emphysema

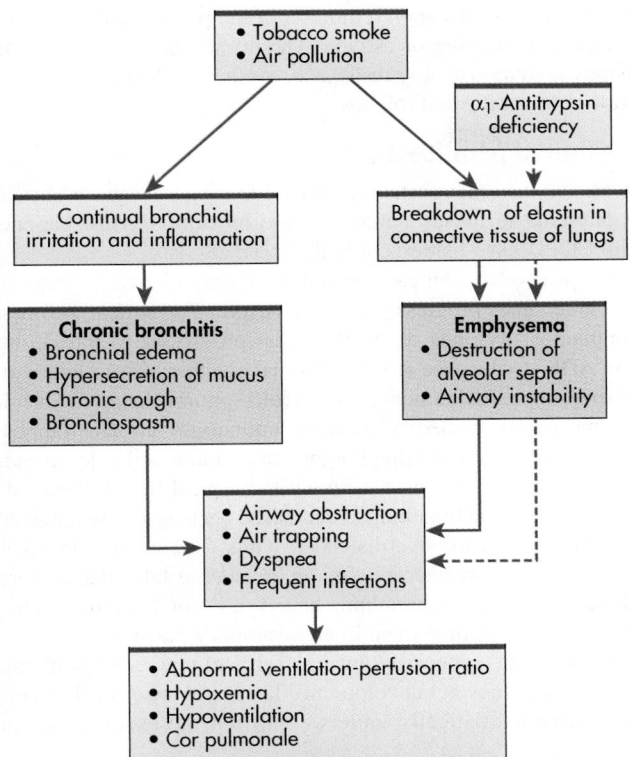

FIG. 28-7 Pathophysiology of chronic bronchitis and emphysema. *Dashed arrows*, role of α₁-antitrypsin deficiency, if present.

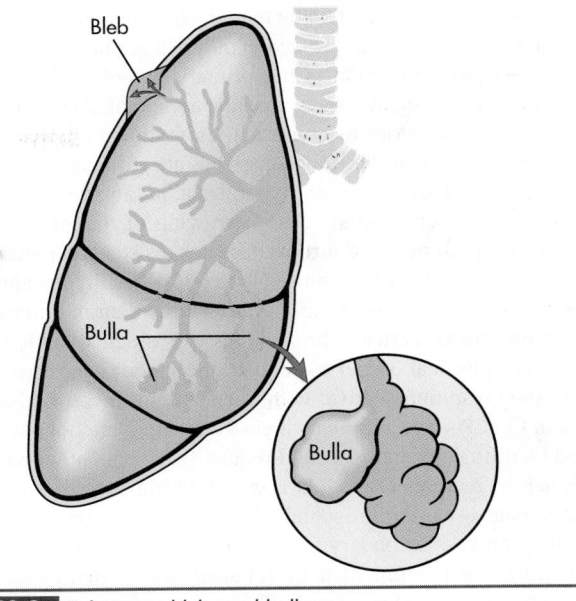

FIG. 28-9 Pulmonary blebs and bullae.

(large cystic areas) develop. When emphysema is severe, it is difficult to distinguish the two types, which may coexist in the same lung.

The pathophysiologic mechanisms involved in emphysema are not totally understood. Small bronchioles become obstructed as a result of mucus, smooth muscle spasm, the inflammatory process, and collapse of bronchiolar walls. Recurrent infectious processes lead to increased production and stimulation of neutrophils and macrophages. These cells release proteolytic enzymes that can destroy alveolar tissue. This process results in more inflammation, more edema, and exudate formation.

In a healthy person there is a balance between elastases and proteases and antiproteases in the lungs. In smokers the numbers of neutrophils and macrophages are increased. Release of their elastases and proteases may overwhelm the normal antiprotease defense. In addition, smoking inactivates AAT. In AAT-related emphysema, AAT activity is greatly diminished and may be overwhelmed by normal protease activity.

In emphysema, elastin and collagen, the supporting structures of the lung, are destroyed. As a result there is no pull or traction on the walls of the bronchioles. Like air being blown into a paper bag, air goes into the lungs easily but is unable to come out on its own and remains in the lung. Thus the bronchioles tend to collapse (especially on expiration) and air is trapped in the distal alveoli, resulting in hyperinflation and overdistention of the alveoli. This trapped air in the lungs gives the patient the typical barrel-chested appearance. In emphysema the lungs can be inflated easily but can deflate only partially. As more alveoli are destroyed and alveoli coalesce, larger air spaces called *blebs* (in the visceral pleura) and *bullae* (in the lung parenchyma) may develop (Fig. 28-9).

Because of the loss of alveolar walls and the capillaries surrounding them, the amount of surface area that is available for diffusion of O_2 in the blood decreases. The patient with emphysema compensates for this problem by increasing the respiratory rate to increase alveolar ventilation. Typically the patient with pure emphysema does not have difficulty with hypoxemia at rest until late in the disease. However, hypoxemia may develop during exercise, and the patient may benefit from supplemental O_2. Hypercapnia and respiratory acidosis do not develop until late in the disease process.

Chronic Bronchitis. *Chronic bronchitis* is excessive production of mucus in the bronchi accompanied by a recurrent cough that persists for at least 3 months of the year during at least 2 successive years. Pathologic changes in the lung consist of (1) hyperplasia of mucous-secreting glands in the trachea and bronchi, (2) increase in goblet cells, (3) disappearance of cilia, (4) chronic inflammatory changes and narrowing of small airways, and (5) altered function of alveolar macrophages, leading to increased bronchial infections. Frequently the airways are colonized with microorganisms. Infections can occur when the organisms increase. Excess amounts of mucus are found in the airways and sometimes may occlude small bronchioles. Eventually,

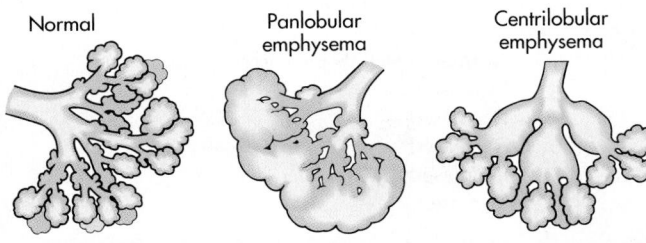

FIG. 28-8 Morphologic types of emphysema. In panlobular emphysema, the entire primary lobule is involved, with destruction and distention distal to the respiratory bronchioles. In centrilobular emphysema, destruction is central, involving primarily the respiratory bronchioles.

scarring of the bronchial walls may occur. In contrast to emphysema, the alveolar structure and capillaries are normal.

Chronic inflammation is the primary pathologic mechanism involved in causing the changes characteristic of chronic bronchitis. The inflammatory response causes vasodilation, congestion, and mucosal edema. The mucous glands are stimulated to become hyperplastic. These changes (hyperplasia, inflammatory swelling, and excess, thick mucus) cause narrowing of the airway lumen and result in diminished airflow. Greater resistance to airflow increases the work of breathing. Hypoxemia and hypercapnia develop more frequently in chronic bronchitis than in emphysema. Because the constricted bronchioles are clogged with mucus, there is a physical barrier to ventilation. In addition, there is a diminished respiratory drive, with a tendency to hypoventilate and retain CO_2. As a result, many areas of the lung are not ventilated, and O_2 diffusion cannot occur. Frequently the patient with chronic bronchitis requires O_2 both at rest and during exercise as the disease progresses. Peribronchial fibrosis may also result from the healing process secondary to inflammatory changes.

Coughing is stimulated by retained mucus that cannot adequately be removed as a result of decreased cilia and mucociliary activity. The cough is often ineffective to remove secretions adequately because the person cannot inspire deeply enough to cause air to flow distal to retained secretions. Frequently, bronchospasm develops in the patient with chronic bronchitis. Bronchospasm is usually more common in the patient with a history of cigarette smoking or asthma. The bronchospasm adds to the already increased airway resistance, resulting in further increased work of breathing and impaired gas exchange.

Clinical Manifestations

The clinical manifestations of COPD vary from those of pure emphysema to those of pure chronic bronchitis. Most patients with COPD have features of both (Table 28-15).

Emphysema. An early symptom of emphysema is dyspnea, which becomes progressively more severe. The patient will first complain of dyspnea on exertion that progresses to interfering with ADLs to dyspnea at rest. Minimal coughing is present, with no sputum or small amounts of mucoid sputum. As more alveoli become overdistended, increasing amounts of air are trapped. This causes a flattened diaphragm and an increased anteroposterior diameter of the chest, forming the typical barrel chest. Effective abdominal breathing is decreased because of the flattened diaphragm from the overdistended lungs. The person becomes more of a chest breather, relying on the intercostal and accessory muscles. This type of breathing, however, is not that effective because the ribs become fixed in an inspiratory position.

Hypoxemia (especially during exercise) may be present, but hypercapnia does not develop until late in the disease. The person is characteristically underweight, but the exact cause for

---

TABLE 28-15   **Comparison of Emphysema and Chronic Bronchitis***

	EMPHYSEMA	CHRONIC BRONCHITIS
Clinical Features		
Age	30-40 yr (onset) 60-70 yr (disabling)	20-30 yr (onset) 40-50 yr (disabling)
Body build	Thin	Tendency toward obesity
Health history	Generally healthy, occasional insidious dyspnea, smoking	Recurrent respiratory tract infections, smoking
Weight loss	Often marked	Absent or slight
Dyspnea	Slowly progressive and eventually disabling	Variable, relatively late
Sputum	Scanty, mucoid	Copious, mucopurulent
Cough	Negligible	Considerable
Chest examination	Marked increase in AP diameter, quiet or diminished breath sounds, limited diaphragmatic excursion	Slight to marked increase in AP diameter, scattered crackles, rhonchi, wheezing
Cor pulmonale	Rare except terminally	Frequent with many episodes
Diagnostic Study Results		
ABGs	Near-normal, mild ↓ PaO_2, normal or ↓ $PaCO_2$	↓ PaO_2, ↑ $PaCO_2$
Chest x-ray	Hyperinflation, flat diaphragm, attenuated peripheral vessels, small or normal heart, widened intercostal margins	Cardiac enlargement, normal or flattened diaphragm, evidence of chronic inflammation, congested lung fields
Lung volumes		
Total lung capacity	Increased	Normal or slightly increased
Residual volume	Increased	Increased
Vital capacity	Decreased	Decreased
FEV_1	Decreased	Decreased
FEV_1/FVC	Decreased (<70%)	Decreased (<70%)
Hematocrit and hemoglobin	Normal until late in disease	Increased
Pathology	Panlobular emphysema	Centrilobular emphysema

*Most persons with COPD have features of both pulmonary emphysema and chronic bronchitis.
ABGs, Arterial blood gases; *AP,* anteroposterior; *FEV₁,* forced expiratory volume in 1 second; *FVC,* forced vital capacity.

this is not well understood. One possibility is that the patient is in a hypermetabolic state with increased energy requirements that are partly due to the increased work of breathing. However, even when the patient has adequate calorie intake, weight loss is still experienced. The patient with emphysema often has protein-calorie malnutrition with loss of lean muscle mass and subcutaneous fat.[24] (Malnutrition is discussed in Chapter 39.) Later in the course of the disease, secondary chronic bronchitis may develop. Other characteristics are presented in Table 28-15.

Chronic Bronchitis. The earliest symptom in chronic bronchitis is usually a frequent, productive cough during most winter months. It is often exacerbated by respiratory irritants and cold, damp air. Bronchospasm can occur at the end of paroxysms of coughing. Frequent respiratory infections are another common manifestation. Somewhat later, dyspnea on exertion may develop. A history of cigarette smoking for many years is almost always present. Unfortunately, a patient often attributes chronic cough to smoking rather than lung disease, thus delaying initiation of treatment. In addition, the patient may not be aware of the cough because she or he becomes accustomed to it. A person with chronic bronchitis is usually of normal weight or heavyset, with a ruddy appearance.

Hypoxemia and hypercapnia result from hypoventilation caused by increased airway resistance in addition to problems with alveolar gas exchange. The bluish-red color of the skin results from polycythemia and cyanosis. Polycythemia develops as a result of increased production of red blood cells secondary to the body's attempt to compensate for chronic hypoxemia. Hemo-globin concentrations may reach 20 g/dl (200 g/L) or more. Cyanosis develops when there is at least 5 g/dl (50 g/L) or more of circulating unoxygenated hemoglobin.

Complications

Cor Pulmonale. **Cor pulmonale** is hypertrophy of the right side of the heart, with or without heart failure, resulting from pulmonary hypertension. In COPD, pulmonary hypertension is caused primarily by constriction of the pulmonary vessels in response to alveolar hypoxia, with acidosis further potentiating the vasoconstriction (Fig. 28-10). Chronic alveolar hypoxia causes pulmonary arteriolar muscle hypertrophy. Chronic hypoxia also stimulates erythropoiesis, which causes polycythemia and increases the viscosity of the blood.

Normally the right ventricle and pulmonary circulatory system are low-pressure systems compared with the left ventricle and systemic circulation. When pulmonary hypertension develops, the pressures on the right side of the heart must increase to push blood into the lungs. Eventually, right-sided heart failure develops.

The clinical manifestations of cor pulmonale are related to dilation and failure of the right ventricle with subsequent intravascular volume expansion and systemic venous congestion. Heart sound changes include accentuation of the pulmonic component of the second heart sound, right-sided ventricular diastolic S_3 gallop, and early systolic ejection click along the left sternal border. ECG changes include increased P wave amplitude (P pulmonale), a tendency for right axis deviation, and incomplete right bundle branch block. Overt manifestations of right-sided heart

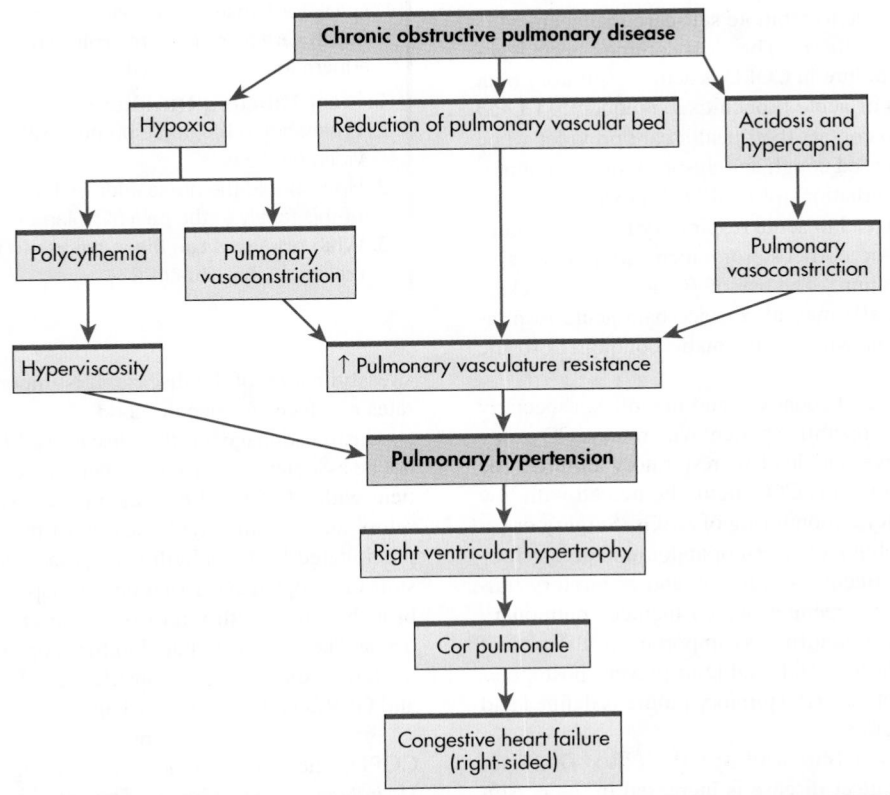

FIG. 28-10 Mechanisms involved in the pathophysiology of cor pulmonale secondary to chronic obstructive pulmonary disease.

failure may develop, which include distended neck veins (jugular venous distention), hepatomegaly with right upper quadrant tenderness, ascites, epigastric distress, peripheral edema, and weight gain.

Management of cor pulmonale includes continuous low-flow O_2. Long-term O_2 therapy can slow but not reverse the progression of pulmonary hypertension in the patient with COPD. Although use of digitalis is not indicated for right-sided heart failure, it is used when a left-sided heart failure is present. Dietary salt restriction is sometimes recommended, especially if overt congestive heart failure (CHF) is present. Although diuretics are generally used, they are prescribed with caution because of their tendency to deplete potassium and chloride and reduce intravascular volume and cardiac output. (Cor pulmonale is discussed further in Chapter 27.)

Acute Exacerbations of Chronic Bronchitis. The airways of patients with stable chronic COPD are colonized with *Streptococcus pneumoniae* and *Haemophilus influenzae,* which are relatively nonpathogenic in these patients. Factors that impair the normal function of the mucociliary system and thus slow or prevent the removal of particulate matter may result in the potential for acute infection. The most common organisms causing acute bronchitis are *H. influenzae, M. catarrhalis,* and *S. pneumoniae.* As COPD becomes more severe, *Pseudomonas, Klebsiella pneumoniae,* and *E. coli* are frequent causes of infection.[25]

Clinical manifestations of an acute exacerbation include worsened cough, hemoptysis, wheezing, increased shortness of breath, and changes in the amount, color, consistency, or viscosity of the sputum. Patients are treated with antibiotics, increases in bronchodilator usage, possibly corticosteroids, humidification, and postural drainage. Teaching the patients and families regarding these treatments is done to promote self-care management.

Acute Respiratory Failure. The most common event leading to acute respiratory failure in COPD is acute respiratory tract infection (usually viral) or acute bronchitis.[26] Frequently COPD patients wait too long to contact their health care provider when they develop fever, increased cough and dyspnea, or other symptoms suggestive of exacerbations of COPD. An exacerbation of cor pulmonale may also lead to acute respiratory failure. Discontinuing bronchodilator or corticosteroid medication may also precipitate respiratory failure. The use of β-adrenergic blockers (e.g., propranolol [Inderal]) may also exacerbate acute respiratory failure in the patient with an asthmatic component to the COPD.

The indiscriminate use of sedatives and narcotics, especially in the preoperative or postoperative patient who retains CO_2, may suppress ventilatory drive and lead to respiratory failure. The person with COPD who retains CO_2 should be treated with low flow rates of O_2 with careful monitoring of ABGs. Surgery or severe, painful illness involving the chest or abdominal organs may lead to splinting and ineffective ventilation and respiratory failure. Careful preoperative screening, which includes pulmonary function tests and ABG monitoring, is important in the patient with a heavy smoking history and COPD to prevent postoperative pulmonary complications. (Respiratory failure is defined and discussed in Chapter 66.)

Peptic Ulcer and Gastroesophageal Reflux Disease. The incidence of peptic ulcer disease is increased in the person with COPD. The reason for this occurrence is not known. It may be because of side effects from the long-term use of bronchodilator or corticosteroid drugs. Another factor may be the

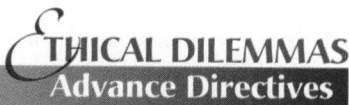

ETHICAL DILEMMAS
Advance Directives

Situation

A 79-year-old man with emphysema is admitted to the hospital in respiratory failure. He is placed on a ventilator and responds occasionally by opening his eyes. His living will was executed 5 years ago, and a copy was given to his wife and health care provider at that time. The wife brings the document to the intensive care unit and tells the nurse that the hospital must stop treating her husband and allow him to die as he requested. However, the oldest son is threatening the hospital with a lawsuit if the staff does not provide full care to his father.

Important Points for Consideration

- A living will is one type of an advance directive provided for under the Patient Self-Determination Act of 1991.
- A living will is prepared by the person in advance, indicating the person's treatment wishes should he or she become terminally ill or in a situation where there is no hope of recovery.
- Durable power of attorney for health care is another form of advance directive in which a person names another to make health care decisions in the event that the person is no longer able to do so.
- An advance directive respects the patient's autonomy, that is, the right to self-determination regarding health care at the end of life.
- A legally executed living will is legally binding in most states.
- Health care providers are obligated to follow the patient's advance directive when the patient is no longer able to speak for himself or herself.
- Health care providers are protected from liability when they adhere to advance directives.

Critical Thinking Questions

1. What should the nurse do next with the information provided by the wife?
2. How should the nurse address the needs of each member of this family in the patient's plan of care?
3. What resources can the nurse use to facilitate decision making in this situation?

stressful nature of the disease. It is important to test gastric aspirates and feces for occult blood.

Gastroesophageal reflux disease (GERD), which may or may not be associated with a hiatal hernia, occurs frequently in the patient with COPD and may aggravate respiratory symptoms. The reflux and accompanying heartburn may be aggravated or even precipitated by theophylline or β_2-adrenergic agonists. As a result of esophageal irritation or aspiration into the tracheobronchial tree, reflux airway constriction and obstruction may occur. The presence of acid in the esophagus can cause a vagally mediated reflex bronchoconstriction. (Treatment of hiatal hernia and GERD is discussed in Chapter 40.)

Pneumonia. Pneumonia is a frequent complication of COPD. The most common causative agents are *S. pneumoniae, H. influenzae,* and viruses. The most common manifestation is purulent sputum. Systemic manifestations such as fever, chills, and leukocytosis may not be present. (Treatment of pneumonia is discussed in Chapter 27.)

Diagnostic Studies

An important goal of the diagnostic workup is to determine the major disease component of COPD, the severity of the disease, and the impact of disease on the patient's quality of life. These factors enable the health care provider to design an individualized treatment plan. Chest x-rays taken early in the disease may not show abnormalities. Later in the disease the findings presented in Table 28-15 may be present.

A history and physical examination are extremely important in a diagnostic workup of the patient.[27] Pulmonary function studies are useful in diagnosing and assessing the severity of COPD. Usually spirometry before and after bronchodilation is ordered. The most significant findings are related to increased resistance to expiratory airflow. Typical findings include the following:

- Reduced FEV_1, $FEF_{25\%-75\%}$, maximum voluntary ventilation (MVV), vital capacity (VC), FEV_1/FVC ratio, diffusing capacity for carbon monoxide
- Increased residual volume, total lung capacity, FRC

When the FEV_1/FVC ratio is less than 70%, it suggests the presence of obstructive lung disease. The value of FEV_1 in milliliters can provide a rough guideline to determine the severity of the patient's lung disease and the degree of disease progression (Table 28-16).

ABGs are usually monitored. In the later stages of COPD, typical findings are low PaO_2, elevated $PaCO_2$, decreased pH, and increased bicarbonate levels. In the early stages there may be a normal or only slightly decreased PaO_2 and a normal $PaCO_2$. An exercise test to determine O_2 saturation in the blood with pulse oximetry may be performed to evaluate how much desaturation of O_2 occurs with exercise. An ECG may be normal or show signs indicative of right ventricular failure (e.g., low voltage, right-axis deviation, P pulmonale). An echocardiogram or gated pool nuclear blood studies (see Chapter 31) can be used to evaluate right-sided ventricular as well as left ventricular function.

Collaborative Care

In general, COPD is an irreversible process. The reversible components are airway size and secretions. Most patients with COPD have emphysema that may be described as fixed airway disease; that is, there is little or no reversibility. Collaborative care guidelines are presented in Table 28-17. The primary goals of care for the COPD patient are to (1) improve ventilation, (2) promote secretion removal, (3) prevent complications and progression of symptoms, (4) promote patient comfort and participation in care, and (5) improve quality of life as much as possible. The majority of these patients are treated as outpatients. They are hospitalized for acute exacerbations and complications such as respiratory failure, pneumonia, and CHF.

TABLE 28-16	Correlation of FEV_1 with Probable Clinical Manifestations
APPROXIMATE FEV_1 (ml)	**PROBABLE CLINICAL MANIFESTATION**
1500	Shortness of breath just beginning to be noticed
1000	Shortness of breath with activity
500	Shortness of breath at rest

TABLE 28-17   Collaborative Care: Chronic Obstructive Pulmonary Disease

Diagnostic
History and physical examination
Chest x-ray
Pulmonary function tests
Sputum specimen for Gram stain and culture (if indicated)
ABGs
ECG
Exercise testing with oximetry (if indicated)
Echocardiogram or cardiac nuclear scans (if indicated)

Collaborative Therapy
Treatment of respiratory infections
Bronchodilator therapy (see Table 28-6)
   β_2-adrenergic agonists
   Anticholinergic agents
   Long-acting theophylline preparations
Corticosteroids
PEFR monitoring (if indicated)
Chest physiotherapy and postural drainage (if indicated)
Breathing exercises and retraining
Hydration of 3 L/day (if not contraindicated)
Cessation of cigarette smoking
Appropriate rest periods
Patient and family teaching
Influenza immunization yearly
Pneumovax immunization
Low flow rate O_2 (if indicated)
Progressive plan of exercise
Pulmonary rehabilitation program

ABGs, Arterial blood gases; *ECG,* electrocardiogram; *PEFR,* peak expiratory flow rate.

Environmental or occupational irritants should be evaluated for their possible negative effect, and ways to control or avoid them should be determined. For example, aerosol hair sprays and smoke-filled rooms should be avoided. The patient with COPD should have a vaccination with influenza virus vaccine yearly and with pneumococcal vaccine. Pneumococcal revaccination is recommended every 5 years for the patient with COPD. The patient with COPD is extremely susceptible to pulmonary infections.

Respiratory infections should be treated as soon as possible. Often the best indication of the presence of a respiratory infection is the increasing quantity, viscosity, or purulence of sputum. Some patients are given a 7- to 10-day supply of antibiotics and are instructed to begin taking them at the first signs of change in sputum. The most common antibiotics given are amoxicillin, amoxicillin with clavulanate (Augmentin), ciprofloxacin (Cipro), erythromycin, and trimethoprim-sulfamethoxazole (Bactrim, Septra).[26]

Smoking Cessation. Cessation of cigarette smoking in the early stages is probably the most significant factor in slowing the progression of the disease. After discontinuation of smoking, the accelerated decline in pulmonary function slows and pulmonary function usually improves. Thus the sooner the smoker stops, the less pulmonary function is lost and the sooner the symptoms decrease, particularly cough and sputum production. (Smoking cessation techniques are discussed in Chapter 11 and in Tables 11-13, 11-14, and 11-17.)

Drug Therapy. Bronchodilator drug therapy decreases airway resistance and dynamic hyperinflation of the lungs, which results in reducing the degree of breathlessness.[27] Although patients with COPD do not respond as dramatically as those with asthma to bronchodilator therapy, a reduction in dyspnea and an increase in FEV_1 are usually achieved. Bronchodilator therapy is best given as maintenance therapy rather than as a treatment for acute symptoms. However, the routine use of bronchodilator therapy in all patients with COPD is controversial, especially in people with pure emphysema.

β_2-Adrenergic agonists are routinely used as bronchodilators in the treatment of COPD.[28] The preferred route of administration is by MDI or nebulizer. Anticholinergic agents, especially ipratropium (Atrovent) by inhaler, are even more effective bronchodilators than β_2-adrenergic agonists in the patient with emphysematous COPD. Inhaled anticholinergics are the preferred route of delivery, and they have minimal side effects. These medications are also available in combination (albuterol and ipratropium [Combivent]) via MDI and aerosol therapy. These drugs are best taken on a regular basis. The use of long-acting theophylline in the treatment of COPD is controversial. Although it has some action as a mild bronchodilator in the patient with partial reversibility of airflow obstruction, its main value may be to improve contractility of the diaphragm and decrease diaphragmatic fatigue. (Bronchodilator drugs are discussed in Table 28-6.)

The use of corticosteroid therapy in COPD is controversial.[29] The person most likely to benefit from these drugs has a history of childhood asthma, has bronchospasm, has a relatively short duration of disease, or has frequent exacerbations that do not respond to therapy with β_2-adrenergic agonists and theophylline.[2]

O_2 Therapy. O_2 therapy is frequently used in the treatment of COPD and other problems associated with hypoxemia. O_2 is a colorless, odorless, tasteless gas that constitutes 20.95% of the atmosphere. Administering supplemental O_2 raises the partial pressure of O_2 (PO_2) in inspired air. Used clinically it is considered a drug, but for reimbursement purposes, it is considered durable medical equipment.

Indications for use. O_2 is usually administered to treat hypoxemia caused by (1) respiratory disorders such as COPD, cor pulmonale, pneumonia, atelectasis, lung cancer, and pulmonary emboli; (2) cardiovascular disorders such as myocardial infarction, arrhythmias, angina pectoris, and cardiogenic shock; and (3) CNS disorders such as overdose of narcotics, head injury, and disordered sleep (sleep apnea).

Methods of administration. The goal of O_2 administration is to supply the patient with adequate O_2 to maximize the O_2-carrying ability of the blood. There are various methods of O_2 administration (Table 28-18 and Figs. 28-11 and 28-12). The method selected depends on factors such as the fraction of inspired O_2 (FIO_2) and mobility of the patient, humidification required, patient cooperation, comfort, cost, and available financial resources.

O_2 delivery systems are classified as low- or high-flow systems. Most methods of O_2 administration are low-flow devices that deliver O_2 in concentrations that vary with the person's respiratory pattern. In contrast, the Venturi mask is a high-flow de-

---

TABLE 28-18 **Methods of Oxygen Administration**

ADVANTAGES	DISADVANTAGES	NURSING INTERVENTIONS
Low-Flow Delivery Devices		
Nasal Cannula		
Cannula may be used by a restless patient. It is a safe and simple method that is relatively comfortable and acceptable. It is useful for a patient requiring low O_2 concentrations (e.g., those with chronic CO_2 retention). It allows patient to move about in bed. Patient can eat, talk, or cough while wearing device (Fig. 28-11, *F*).	Cannula is difficult to maintain in position and can be easily dislodged. Patient must be alert and cooperative to keep cannula in proper place. High flow rates (>5 L/min) dry nasal membranes and may cause pain in frontal sinuses.	Nasal cannula should be stabilized when caring for a restless patient. A flow rate of 2 L/min gives an O_2 concentration of approximately 28%. Amount of O_2 inhaled depends on room air and patient's breathing pattern. Most patients with COPD can tolerate 2 L/min via cannula.
Simple Face Mask		
O_2 can be given quickly for short periods. O_2 concentrations of 35%–50% can be achieved with flow rates of 6-12 L/min. Mask provides adequate humidification of inspired air (Fig. 28-11, *A*).	Lack of patient tolerance results in inadequate therapy. Mask may be uncomfortable because tight seal must be maintained between face and mask. Mask may produce pressure necrosis of the skin and confines heat radiating from the face about nose and mouth. It must be removed to eat or drink.	Wash and dry under mask q2hr. Mask must fit snugly. Nasal cannula may be provided while patient is eating. Watch for pressure necrosis at the top of ears from elastic straps. (Gauze or other padding may be used to alleviate this problem.) Method requires at least 5 L/min flow to prevent accumulation of expired air in the mask.
Nasal Catheter		
Catheter allows continuous uninterrupted O_2 therapy. Patient receives O_2 even if a mouth breather. Catheter does not interfere with patient care. It is rarely used except for short-term procedures (e.g., bronchoscopy).	Catheter must be inserted into nasopharynx through a nostril and can produce excoriation of the nares. High flow rates (>6 L/min) can cause drying of nasal membranes. Inadvertent gas flow distends the stomach. Cannula does not permit a high degree of humidification and must be taped to patient's face.	Catheter should be changed q8hr, alternating the nostrils. Distance that catheter is to be inserted is measured from distance between tip of nose and earlobe. A flow rate of 5-6 L/min gives an O_2 concentration of approximately 30%. Method is best used for short-term therapy.

ABGs, Arterial blood gases; *COPD,* chronic obstructive pulmonary disease.

TABLE 28-18	Methods of Oxygen Administration—cont'd	
ADVANTAGES	**DISADVANTAGES**	**NURSING INTERVENTIONS**

Low-Flow Delivery Devices—cont'd

Partial Rebreathing Mask

Mask is lightweight and easy to use. Reservoir bag conserves O_2. Concentrations of 40%-60% can be achieved using flow rates of 6-10 L/min.	Mask cannot be used with a high degree of humidity.	Method is useful when blood O_2 concentrations must be raised. It is not recommended for patient with COPD and should never be used with a nebulizer. Bag should not be allowed to deflate during inspiration.

Non-Rebreathing Mask

High concentrations of O_2 can be delivered accurately. O_2 flows into bag and mask during inhalation. Valve prevents expired air from flowing back into bag. Concentrations of 60%-90% can be achieved.	Mask cannot be used with a high degree of humidity.	Mask should fit snugly. Flow rate must be sufficient to keep bag from collapsing during inspiration. Bag should not be allowed to deflate during inspiration.

Oxygen-Conserving Cannula

Cannula has a built-in reservoir that increases O_2 concentration delivered and allows patient to use lower flow, usually 30%-50%, which increases comfort and lowers cost. It is reportedly more comfortable than standard cannulas (Fig. 28-13).	Cannula cannot be cleaned: manufacturer recommends changing cannula every week. It is more expensive than standard cannulas and requires evaluation with ABGs and oximetry to determine correct flow for patient. Cannula is highly visible. Cannula heavy on ears.	Method is generally indicated for patient requiring long-term O_2 therapy at home versus during hospitalization. It may be "moustache" or "pendant" type. May cause necroses over the tops of the ears; can be padded.

Transtracheal Catheter

Catheter is less visible. Flow requirement may be reduced 60%-80%, which greatly increases amount of time available from portable source of O_2. Less nasal irritation occurs (Fig. 28-12).	Patient and family must learn entire program of care for tracheostoma and how to replace catheter. Procedure is invasive. Procedure and replacement adds costs to O_2 therapy.	Method may not be appropriate for patient with excessive mucus production from mucous plugging.

Face Tent

Tent is ideal for providing moderate-to-high-density aerosol. O_2 concentration administered varies with O_2 flow rate (Fig. 28-11, *E*).	Face tent is less reliable than face mask for maintaining high inspiration of O_2 concentration.	Open plastic mask fits under chin. Temperature of aerosol must be checked to maintain at or near body temperature. It is rarely used.

Tracheostomy Collar

Collar can deliver high humidity and O_2 via tracheostomy.	Condensed fluid in tubing may drain into tracheostomy. Water traps are usually put in. Secretions collect inside collar and around tracheostomy. O_2 concentration is lost into atmosphere because collar does not fit tightly.	Collar attaches to neck with elastic strap and should be removed and cleaned at least q4hr to prevent aspiration of fluid and infection.

Tracheostomy T Bar

Tight fit allows better O_2 and humidity delivery than tracheostomy collar.	Condensed fluid in tubing may drain into tracheostomy. Water traps are usually put in.	T bar must be removed for suctioning. Mörch swivel may be used to eliminate the need for removal. It should be emptied as necessary.

Tent or Incubator

Tent or incubator has ability to control temperature and humidity.	Tent or incubator has limited usefulness. It is difficult to maintain adequate concentrations of O_2. Method isolates patient from environment.	Tent should be flushed with O_2 every time it is opened. Nurse should assess for leaks around canopy.

High-Flow Delivery Devices

Venturi Mask

Mask can deliver precise, high flow rates of O_2. Lightweight plastic, cone-shaped device is fitted to face. Masks are available for delivery of 24%, 28%, 31%, 35%, 40%, and 50% O_2. Adaptors can be applied to increase humidification (Fig. 28-11, *C*).	Mask is uncomfortable and must be removed when patient eats. Patient can talk but voice may be muffled. Other disadvantages are the same as those discussed for the simple face mask.	Entrainment device on mask must be changed to deliver higher concentrations of O_2. Method is especially helpful for administering low, constant O_2 concentrations to patients with COPD. Air entrainment ports must not be occluded.

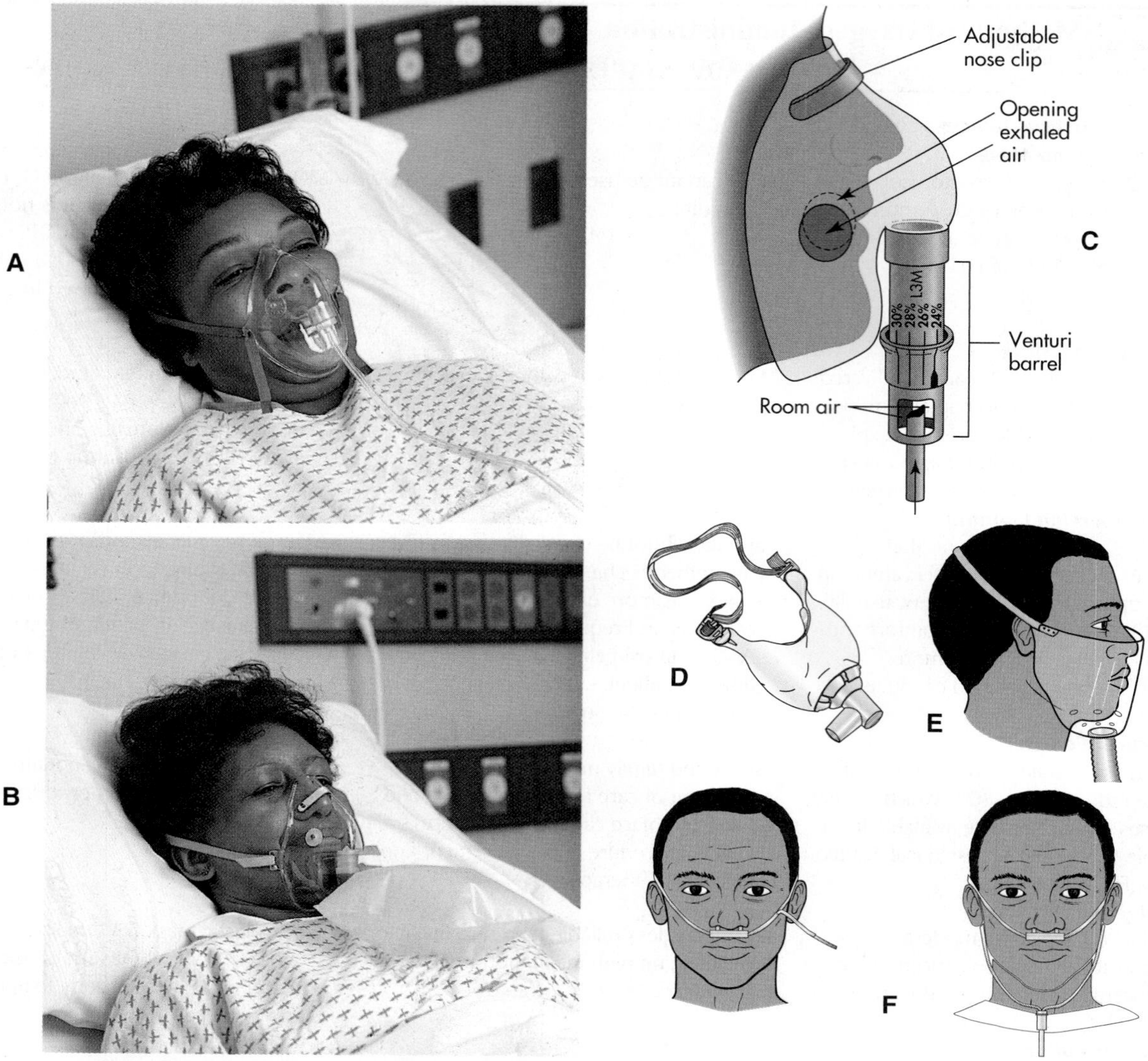

FIG. 28-11 Methods of oxygen administration. **A,** Simple face mask. **B,** Plastic face mask with reservoir bag. **C,** Venturi mask. **D,** Tracheostomy mask. **E,** Face tent. **F,** Standard nasal cannulas.

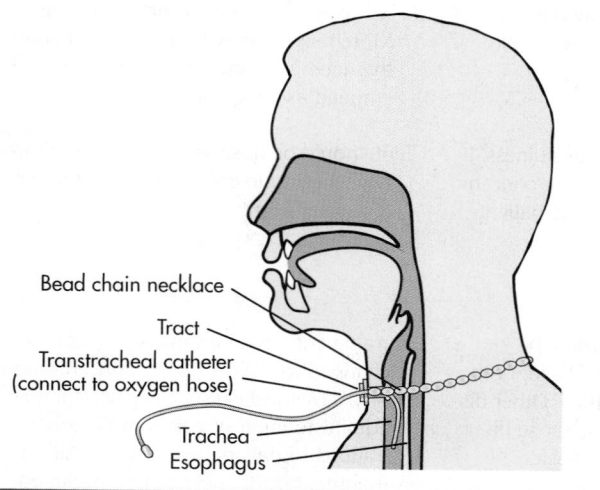

FIG. 28-12 Transtracheal catheter for oxygen pulmonation.

vice that delivers fixed concentrations of O_2 independent of the patient's respiratory pattern. With the Venturi mask, O_2 is delivered to a small jet (Venturi device) in the center of a wide-based cone (see Fig. 28-11, *C*). Air is entrained (pulled through) openings in the cone as O_2 flows through the small jet. The mask has large vents through which exhaled air can escape. The degree of restriction or narrowness of the jet determines the amount of entrainment and dilution of pure O_2 with room air and thus the concentration of O_2. Mechanical ventilators are another example of a high-flow O_2 delivery system.

Humidification and nebulizers. O_2 obtained from cylinders or wall systems is dry. Dry O_2 has an irritating effect on mucous membranes and dries secretions. Therefore it is important that O_2 be humidified when administered, either by humidification or nebulization. A common device used for humidification when the patient has a catheter, cannula, or low-flow mask is a bubble-through humidifier. It is a small plastic jar filled with sterile distilled water that is attached to the O_2 source by means of a flowmeter. O_2 passes into the jar, bubbles through the water, and then goes through tubing to the patient's catheter, cannula, or mask. The purpose of the bubble-through humidifier is to restore the humidity conditions of room air. However, the need for bubble-through humidifiers at flow rates between 1 and 4 L per minute is controversial when humidity in the environment is adequate.

Another means of administering humidified O_2 is via a nebulizer. It delivers particulate water mist (aerosols) with nearly 100% humidity. The humidity can be raised by heating the water, which increases the ability of the gas to hold moisture. Heated (98.6° F [37° C]) and humidified (100%) gas is required when the upper airway is bypassed in acute care. However, patients with established tracheotomies do not always require 100% humidity. When nebulizers are used, large-size tubing should be employed to connect the device to a face mask or T bar. If small-size tubing is used, condensation can occlude the flow of O_2.

Vapotherm can deliver high flows (15 to 20 L/min) of warm humidified air (either sterile air or O_2) to the patient through a nasal cannula or transtracheal cannula using technology to warm and saturate the gas stream. Preliminary findings in COPD patients in pulmonary rehabilitation suggest increases in exercise tolerance with Vapotherm high-flow therapy.[30]

Complications

Combustion. O_2 supports combustion and increases the rate of burning. This is why it is important that smoking be prohibited in the area in which O_2 is being used. A "No Smoking" sign should be prominently displayed on the patient's door. The patient should also be cautioned against smoking cigarettes with O_2 prongs or a catheter in place.

CO_2 narcosis. The two chemoreceptors in the respiratory center that control the drive to breathe are CO_2 and O_2. Normally, CO_2 accumulation is the major stimulant of the respiratory center. Over time COPD patients develop a tolerance for high CO_2 levels (the respiratory center loses its sensitivity to the elevated CO_2 levels). Theoretically, for these individuals the "O_2 drive" to breathe is hypoxemia. Thus there has been concern regarding the dangers of administering O_2 to COPD patients and wiping out their drive to breathe. This has been a pervasive myth but is not regarded as a serious threat. In fact, not providing adequate O_2 to these patients is much more detrimental. Although O_2 administration should be titrated to the lowest effective dose, many patients who have end-stage chronic obstructive disease require high flow rates and higher concentrations for survival. They may, in fact, exhibit higher than normal levels of CO_2 in their blood, but this is of little concern. What is important is careful, ongoing assessment when providing O_2 to these patients.

It is critical to start O_2 at low flow rates until ABGs can be obtained. ABGs are used as a guide to determine what FIO_2 level is sufficient and can be tolerated. The patient's mental status and vital signs should be assessed before starting O_2 therapy and frequently thereafter.

O_2 toxicity. Pulmonary **O_2 toxicity** may result from prolonged exposure to a high level of O_2 (PaO_2). The development of O_2 toxicity is determined by patient tolerance, exposure time, and effective dose. It is believed that high concentrations of O_2 may inactivate pulmonary surfactant and lead to the development of acute respiratory distress syndrome (ARDS).

Early manifestations of O_2 toxicity are reduced vital capacity, cough, substernal chest pain, nausea and vomiting, paresthesia, nasal stuffiness, sore throat, and malaise. The later stages of O_2 toxicity affect the alveolar-capillary gas exchange unit, causing edema and production of copious sputum. The end stage of O_2 toxicity is progressive fibrosis of the lungs. Prevention of O_2 toxicity is important for the patient who is receiving O_2. The amount of O_2 administered should be just enough to maintain the PaO_2 within a normal or acceptable range for the patient. ABGs should be monitored frequently to evaluate the effectiveness of therapy and to guide the tapering of supplemental O_2. A safe limit of O_2 concentrations has not yet been established. All levels above 50% and used for longer than 24 hours should be considered potentially toxic. Levels of 40% and below may be regarded as relatively nontoxic and may not result in development of significant O_2 toxicity if the exposure period is short.

Absorption atelectasis. Normally nitrogen, which constitutes 79% of the air that is breathed, is not absorbed into the bloodstream. This prevents alveolar collapse. When high concentrations of O_2 are given, nitrogen is washed out of the alveoli and replaced with O_2. If airway obstruction occurs, the O_2 is absorbed into the bloodstream and the alveoli collapse. This process is called **absorption atelectasis.**

Infection. Infection can be a major hazard of O_2 administration. Heated nebulizers present the highest risk. The constant use of humidity supports bacterial growth, with the most common infecting organism being *Pseudomonas aeruginosa.* Disposable equipment that operates as a closed system should be used. There should be a hospital policy stating the required frequency of equipment changes based on the type of equipment used at that particular institution. Both equipment and respiratory secretions should be stained using Gram stain and cultured frequently.

Chronic O_2 therapy at home. Improved prognosis and enhanced quality of life have been noted in patients with COPD who receive nocturnal or continuous O_2 to treat hypoxemia. The improved prognosis results from preventing progression of the disease and subsequent cor pulmonale. The benefits of long-term continuous O_2 therapy include improved neuropsychologic function, increased exercise tolerance, decreased hematocrit, and reduced pulmonary hypertension. It also improves sleep, may reduce nocturnal arrhythmias, and may extend life.[31]

The potential benefit of long-term O_2 therapy (LTOT) should be evaluated when the patient's condition has stabilized. There should be an accurate, current diagnosis and an optimal medical regimen prescribed by a health care provider knowledgeable in the treatment of respiratory disease. Short-term home O_2 therapy (1 to 30 days) may be indicated for the patient in whom hypoxemia persists after discharge from the hospital. For example, the patient with underlying COPD who develops a serious respiratory infection may continue to have clearing of the infection after completion of antibiotic therapy and discharge from the hospital. This patient may demonstrate continued hypoxemia for 4 to 6 weeks after discharge. It is important to measure the patient's oygenation status by pulse oximetry 2 to 3 months after an acute episode to determine if the O_2 is still warranted.[31]

Patients whose disease is stable with a PaO_2 of 55 mm Hg or less (corresponding to an SaO_2 of 88% or less) should receive LTOT. A patient whose PaO_2 is between 55 and 59 mm Hg (SaO_2 89%) and who exhibits signs of tissue hypoxia, such as cor pulmonale, erythrocytosis, peripheral edema from right-sided heart failure, or impaired mental status, should also receive long-term O_2 therapy. Desaturation only during exercise or sleep suggests consideration of O_2 therapy specifically under those conditions.

Patients may receive O_2 only during exercise or sleep or at both times. The need for O_2 during these periods should be evaluated with oximetry. (Pulse oximetry is discussed in Chapter 25.)

Periodic reevaluations are necessary for the patient who is using chronic supplemental O_2. Generally the recommendation is that the patient should be reevaluated every 30 to 90 days during the first year of therapy and annually after that, as long as the patient remains stable.

Nasal cannulas, either regular or the O_2-conserving type (see Table 28-18 and Figs. 28-11 and 28-13) are usually used to de-

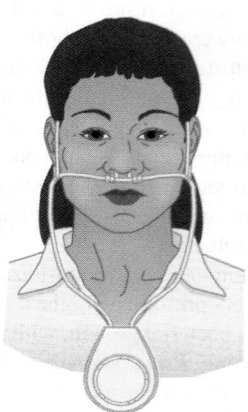

FIG. 28-13 Pendant-type oxygen-conserving cannula.

liver O_2 from a central source in the home. The source may be a liquid O_2 storage system, compressed O_2 in tanks, or an O_2 concentrator or extractor, depending on the patient's home environment, insurance coverage, activity level, and proximity to an O_2 supply company (Table 28-19). The patient can use extension tubing (up to 50 feet) without adversely affecting the O_2 flow delivery to increase mobility in the home, provided that the flowmeter is the back pressure–compensated type. Small portable systems, such as liquid O_2, may be provided for the patient who remains active outside the home (Fig. 28-14).

Reservoir cannulas operate on the principle of storing O_2 in a small reservoir during exhalation. The O_2 is then delivered to the patient during the subsequent inhalation, similar to a bolus effect. The reservoir cannulas can reduce flow requirements by approximately 50%. There is a pendant type (see Fig. 28-13). Another type that fits onto the frame of eyeglasses is also available and is less visible on the face.

Other delivery devices for chronic O_2 therapy include transtracheal O_2 delivery and intermittent-demand O_2 delivery systems. Transtracheal O_2 delivery requires a surgical procedure to insert the small O_2 catheter into the patient's trachea (see Fig. 28-12). Nursing care involves teaching the patient and family how to care for the stoma and the transtracheal catheter. The transtracheal catheter is less visible than nasal cannulas and there is no nasal irritation. It also reduces the O_2 flow requirement by 30% to 50%.

Intermittent-demand delivery systems are mechanically complex devices. They deliver "pulses" of O_2 to the patient, usually dur-

---

TABLE 28-19 Home Oxygen Delivery Systems

SYSTEM	ADVANTAGES	DISADVANTAGES	COMMENTS
• Liquid oxygen	Portable unit* can be refilled by patient from reservoir. Portable unit holds 6-8 hr supply at 2 L/min; reservoir will last approximately 7-10 days at 2 L/min continuously.	Liquid system slightly more expensive, depending on location; not available everywhere; generally limited to urban areas.	As liquid warms to gas, some is vented from the system. In summer, evaporation is accelerated and may decrease reservoir duration to <1 wk.
• Compressed tank O_2 (H or J tank/E or A cylinder)	Good availability in most areas. Portability possible with cart. Aluminum E or A cylinders available that are markedly lighter than steel and easier to maneuver.	Duration of H or J tank at 2 L/min flow about 50 hr; storage of 4-5 large cylinders in the home necessary to have 1 wk to 10-day supply; portable cylinder on cart is cumbersome and heavy. Duration of E cylinder at 2 L/min approximately 4-5 hr; a cylinder at 2 L/min will last approximately 8-10 hr.	Some smaller tanks (D or M) may be used; these can be refilled from large cylinders and weigh about 10 lb. Tank can be carried on shoulder strap, backpack, or fanny pack or placed on portable cart.
• Concentrator or extractor (E or A cylinder)	On wheels, movable from room to room; weekly delivery of supply not necessary, because unit delivers oxygen continuously; compact, excellent system for rural or homebound patient.	Older models can be noisy; increase in electricity bill by $20-$30 a month (not reimbursable by insurance); >3 L flow resulting in significant decrease in concentration. Patient will need backup O_2 tank in case electricity fails.	Concentrator should be kept in room other than bedroom; extension tubing should be used if noise disturbs sleep.
• Pulse or demand delivery system	Simple to use; delivery rate changes with respiratory rate, (i.e., the faster the patient's rate, the higher the rate of delivery).	Mechanically complex; only safe use with portable system when patient is awake unless there is an alarm to detect disconnection of patient. Oxygenation possibly less efficient with exertion.	System may be a separate unit that can be used with liquid or cylinder, or can be "built in" to portable liquid oxygen unit. Less drying, rarely needs humidification.

*Portable usually refers to units weighing more than 10 lb (4.5 kg) and ambulatory units weigh less than 10 lb.

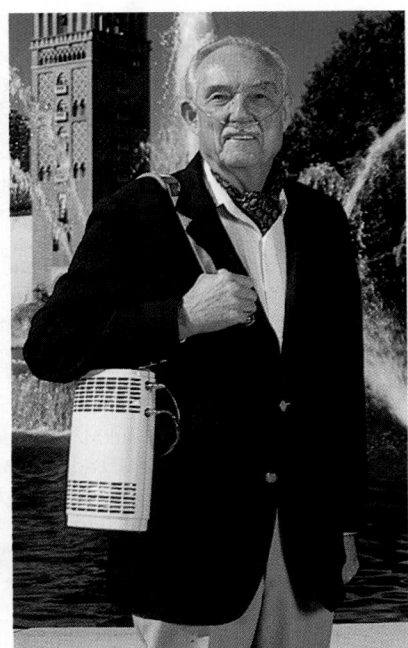

FIG. 28-14 Ambulatory liquid oxygen system.

TABLE
28-20

Patient & Family Teaching Guide

Home Oxygen Use

Mask/Cannula
- Ensure that the straps are not too tight
- Remove 2-3 times/day to wash and dry skin where straps are and stimulate skin
- Pad any pressure points
- Observe tops of ears for skin breakdown from pressure points

Oral and Nasal Mucous Membranes
- Assess oral and nasal mucous membranes 2-3 times/day
- Use water-based gel on lips and nasal mucosa
- Provide frequent oral hygiene
- Provide humidification via humidifier or nebulizing device

Decreasing Risk for Infection
- Remove mask or collar and cleanse with water 2-3 times/day
- Cleanse skin carefully at this time and observe for cuts, scratches, and bruises
- Change disposable equipment frequently
- Remove secretions that are coughed out

Decreasing Risk of Fire Injuries
- Post "No Smoking" warning signs in home where they can be seen
- Do not use electric razors, portable radios, open flames, wool blankets, or mineral oils in the area where oxygen is in use
- Do not allow smoking in the home

NOTE: A good resource for patients is *About Oxygen Therapy at Home,* a booklet published by the American Lung Association.

ing inspiration, and thus eliminate wasted flow during exhalation as is experienced during continuous flow. There are intermittent-demand units that operate independently of a particular system and units that are built into the delivery device itself.

Home O_2 systems are usually rented from a company that sends a respiratory therapist or pulmonary nurse specialist to the patient's home. The therapist teaches the patient how to use the O_2 system, how to care for it, and how to recognize when the supply is running low and needs to be reordered. A patient and family teaching guide for the use of O_2 at home is presented in Table 28-20.

The patient who uses home O_2 should be encouraged to remain active and to travel normally. If travel is by automobile, arrangements can be made for O_2 to be available at the destination point. O_2 supply companies can often assist in these arrangements. If a patient wishes to travel by bus, train, or airplane, these parties require notification when reservations are made of the need for O_2 during the travel. A high-altitude simulation test (HAST) may be performed in a hospital pulmonary function laboratory to determine the O_2 prescription required for the altitude at which the patient will be flying. Because airplane cabins are pressurized to an elevation of 7000 or 8000 feet, the patient who uses supplemental O_2 should have O_2 provided during flight. The plane's O_2 system must be used. Patients may not use their own O_2 system during flight because it is not properly pressurized. Airlines allow patients to bring their O_2 system to be carried in the baggage compartment for use at the point of destination, but the reservoirs (liquid or tank) must be empty and the valves left open. Some patients may need to avoid prolonged exposure to high elevations during travel unless they are instructed by their health care provider regarding adjustments in their O_2 flow to attempt to compensate for altitude.

Surgical Therapy for COPD. Two different surgical procedures have been used in severe COPD. One type of surgery is *lung volume reduction surgery* (LVRS).[32] The rationale for this type of surgery is that by reducing the size of the hyperinflated emphysematous lungs, there is decreased airway obstruction and increased room for the remaining normal alveoli to function. The procedure reduces lung volume and improves lung and chest wall mechanics. There are different types of LVRS. In one approach a median sternotomy is performed and parts of each lung are removed and tissue reattached using a stapling device. Another approach is a video-assisted thoracoscopy that can be performed unilaterally or bilaterally. In this approach either a stapling or laser procedure can be done, or they can be done together. The most common postoperative complication is pneumonia.[33]

The second surgical procedure is *lung transplantation.* COPD patients are the largest group of patients on waiting lists for lung transplantation. Although single-lung transplant is the most commonly used technique, bilateral transplantation can be performed. In appropriately selected patients with COPD, lung transplantation prolongs life, improves functional capacity, and enhances quality of life. However, rejection and effects of immunosuppressive therapy remain an obstacle. (Lung transplantation is discussed in Chapter 27.)

Respiratory Therapy. Respiratory therapy and pulmonary rehabilitation are usually a collaborative effort involving respiratory therapists and nurses. Respiratory care includes breathing retraining, effective cough techniques, chest physiotherapy, and aerosol-nebulization therapy.[34] Pulmonary nurses are responsible for the management of many pulmonary rehabilitation centers. Along with exercise and pulmonary conditioning, smoking cessation strategies, and COPD support groups, a large part of the nurse's role is to teach COPD patients in self-management of their disease.

Breathing retraining. The patient with COPD develops an increased respiratory rate with a prolonged expiration to compensate for obstruction to airflow resulting in dyspnea. In addition, the accessory muscles of breathing in the neck and upper part of the chest are used excessively to promote chest wall movement. These muscles are not designed for long-term use and as a result the patient experiences increased fatigue. Breathing exercises can assist the patient during rest and activity (e.g., lifting, walking, stair climbing). The main types of breathing exercises are (1) pursed-lip breathing and (2) diaphragmatic breathing.

The purpose of using **pursed-lip breathing** is to prolong exhalation and thereby prevent bronchiolar collapse and air trapping. The patient is taught to inhale slowly through the nose and then to exhale slowly through pursed lips, almost as if whistling. Exhalation should be at least three times as long as inhalation. It is helpful to have the nurse demonstrate the breathing exercises so the patient can imitate the action. The following techniques can be used to teach pursed-lip breathing:

1. Blow through a straw in a glass of water with the intent of forming small bubbles.
2. Blow at a lit candle enough to bend the flame without blowing it out.
3. Steadily blow a table-tennis ball across a table.

Diaphragmatic (abdominal) breathing focuses on using the diaphragm instead of the accessory muscles to achieve maximum inhalation and to slow the respiratory rate. The patient should be made aware of the difference between chest breathing and abdominal breathing. This can be achieved by having the patient lie down or assume a semi-Fowler position and by placing one hand on the chest and the other on the abdomen. The patient should observe which hand moves during inspiration. The abdomen should protrude on inhalation with diaphragmatic breathing and contract on exhalation as the diaphragm pushes the air out of the lungs. The nurse should emphasize the value of diaphragmatic movement in increasing lung expansion.

To practice diaphragmatic breathing, the patient should keep the hand on the abdomen and concentrate on filling up the abdomen by inhaling slowly through the nose. Another technique is to wrap a towel gently around the abdomen and to pull it tight during exhalation. The patient then attempts to stretch the towel with slow inhalation by diaphragmatic breathing. On exhalation the patient uses pursed-lip breathing and draws the towel tighter to promote effective expiration.

Another technique to assist in diaphragmatic breathing is to place a small pillow, magazine, book, or small bag of beans on the abdomen. This approach provides tactile stimulation and visual feedback. If the object rises on inspiration, the patient is given positive feedback that diaphragmatic breathing is taking place.

Pursed-lip breathing and diaphragmatic breathing should be practiced together for 8 to 10 repetitions three or four times a day. These techniques give the patient more control over breathing, especially during exercise and periods of dyspnea.

In the setting of extreme acute dyspnea when the patient is hospitalized for infection or heart failure, it is more important to focus on helping the patient slow the respiratory rate by using the

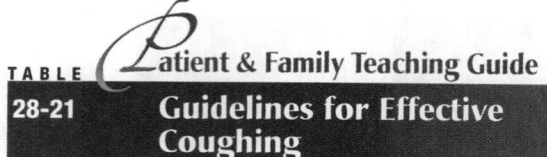

TABLE 28-21

Patient & Family Teaching Guide

Guidelines for Effective Coughing

1. Patient assumes a sitting position with head slightly flexed, shoulders relaxed, knees flexed, and forearms supported by pillow, and if possible, with feet on the floor.
2. Patient then drops head and bends forward while using slow, pursed-lip breathing to exhale.
3. Sitting up again, patient uses diaphragmatic breathing to inhale slowly and deeply.
4. Patient repeats steps 2 and 3 three to four times to facilitate mobilization of secretions.
5. Before initiating a cough, patient should take a deep abdominal breath, bend slightly forward, and then huff cough (cough three to four times on exhalation). Patient may need to support or splint thorax or abdomen to achieve a maximum cough.

principles of pursed-lip breathing. Diaphragmatic (abdominal) breathing requires more energy and thus should be taught only when the patient has achieved a stable rehabilitative state such as before discharge or in a home care rehabilitation program.

Effective coughing. Many patients with COPD have developed ineffective coughing patterns that do not adequately clear their airways of sputum. In addition, they fear they may develop spastic coughing, resulting in increased dyspnea. Guidelines for effective coughing are presented in Table 28-21. *Huff coughing* is an effective technique that the patient can be easily taught. The main goals of effective coughing are to conserve energy, reduce fatigue, and facilitate removal of secretions.

Chest physiotherapy. Chest physiotherapy (CPT) is indicated in the patient with (1) excessive bronchial secretions who has difficulty clearing secretions with expectorated sputum production greater than 25 to 30 ml per day, (2) evidence or suggestion of retained secretions in the presence of an artificial airway, or (3) lobar atelectasis caused by or suspected of being caused by mucous plugging.

Chest physiotherapy consists of percussion, vibration, and postural drainage (Table 28-22). Percussion and vibration are manual or mechanical techniques used to augment postural drainage. **Postural drainage** uses the principle of gravity to assist in bronchial drainage. Percussion and vibration are used after the patient has assumed a postural drainage position to assist in loosening the mobilized secretions. Percussion, vibration, and postural drainage may assist in bringing secretions into larger, more central airways. Effective coughing is then necessary to help raise these secretions. After each drainage position change, the patient should be given time to cough and deep breathe. These techniques are individualized based on the patient's pulmonary condition and response to the initial treatment. Sometimes it takes several hours after CPT for secretions to be expectorated. It is important to evaluate CPT for both its effectiveness and relief of the patient's symptoms. CPT should be performed by an individual who has been properly trained. Complications associated with improperly performed CPT include fractured ribs, bruising, hypoxemia, and discomfort to the patient. CPT may not be beneficial and may be stressful for some patients.

TABLE 28-22 **Steps in Chest Physiotherapy**

1. Perform procedure 1 hr before meals or 1-3 hr after meals.
2. Administer bronchodilator (if nebulized or MDI is ordered) approximately 15 min before procedure.
3. Collect needed equipment such as tissues, emesis basin, paper bag, and pillows.
4. Help patient assume correct position for postural drainage based on findings from x-ray, auscultation, palpation, and percussion of chest. Position should be maintained for 5-15 min to mobilize secretions via gravity.
5. Observe patient during treatment to assess tolerance. Particularly observe breathing and color changes, especially duskiness in face.
6. Have patient take several deep abdominal breaths.
7. Percuss appropriate area for 1-2 min.
8. Vibrate the same area while the patient exhales 4-5 deep breaths.*
9. Assist patient to cough while assuming same position. Splinting with towel or hands may be necessary to aid in effective coughing. Patient may have to assume sitting position to generate enough airflow to expel secretions. (Coughing productively may be a long waiting process that may occur 30 min after procedure.) Suction may be necessary if coughing is not effective.
10. Repeat percussion, vibration, and coughing until patient no longer expectorates mucus.
11. Repeat same procedure in all necessary positions.
12. After procedure, help patient assume a comfortable position, assist with oral hygiene, and discard used tissues.
13. Monitor for hypoxemia if patient having any respiratory difficulty during the procedure.
14. Evaluate and chart effectiveness of treatment by amount of sputum produced and the results of auscultation. Also chart patient tolerance.

*If using an electronic vibrator, use for periods of 5-20 min in each position according to the patient's tolerance.
MDI, Metered dose inhaler.

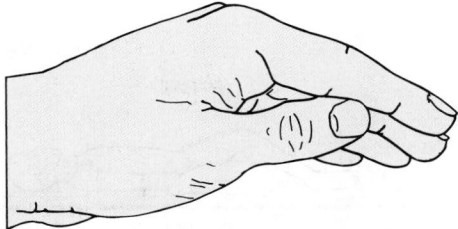

FIG. 28-15 Cupped-hand position for percussion. The hand should be cupped as though scooping up water.

Some patients may develop hypoxemia and bronchospasms with CPT.

Percussion. Percussion is performed in the appropriate postural drainage position with the hands in a cuplike position (Fig. 28-15). The hands are cupped, and the fingers and thumbs are closed. The cupped hand should create an air pocket between the patient's chest and the hand. Both hands are cupped and used in an alternating rhythmic fashion. Percussion is accomplished with flexion and extension of the wrists. If it is performed correctly, a hollow sound should be heard. The air-cushion impact facilitates the movement of thick mucus. A thin towel should be placed over the area to be percussed, or the patient may choose to wear a T-shirt or hospital gown. Percussion should not be performed over the kidneys, sternum, spinal cord, or any tender or painful area. Other contraindications to percussion include hemoptysis, carcinoma, and induced bronchospasm.

Vibration. Vibration is accomplished by tensing the hand and arm muscles repeatedly and pressing mildly with the flat of the hand on the affected area while the patient slowly exhales a deep breath. The vibrations facilitate movement of secretions to larger airways. Mild vibration is tolerated better than percussion and can be used in situations where percussion may be contraindicated. Commercial vibrators are available for hospital and home use.

Postural drainage. The lungs are divided into five lobes, with three on the right side and two on the left side. There are 18 segments in the lungs, which can be drained by 18 positions. Fig. 28-16 shows the modified postural drainage positions most often used in clinical practice. The purpose of various positions in postural drainage is to drain each segment toward the larger airways. The postural drainage positions are determined by the areas of involved lung, which are assessed by chest x-rays, percussion, palpation, and auscultation. Aerosolized bronchodilators and hydration therapy are frequently administered before postural drainage. The chosen postural drainage position is maintained for 5 to 15 minutes. The degree of slope can be obtained with pillows, blocks, books, or a tilt board.

The frequency and choice of postural drainage positions depend on the location of retained secretions and patient tolerance to dependent positions. A common order is two to four times a day. In acute situations, postural drainage may be performed as frequently as every 1 to 2 hours. The procedure should be planned to occur and be completed at least 1 hour before meals or 3 hours after meals.

If a patient has difficulty in assuming various positions, adaptations will need to be made by reducing the angle or length of time of the procedure. A side-lying position can be used for the patient who cannot tolerate a head-down position. Some positions for postural drainage (e.g., Trendelenburg) should not be performed on the patient with chest trauma, hemoptysis, heart disease, or head injury, and in other situations where the patient's condition is not stable.

Flutter mucus clearance device. The Flutter mucus clearance device is a handheld device that provides positive expiratory pressure (PEP) treatment for patients with mucus-producing conditions (Fig. 28-17). The Flutter valve works by (1) vibrating the airways, which loosens mucus from airway walls; (2) intermittently increasing the endobronchial pressure, which helps maintain the patency of the airway; and (3) accelerating expiratory airflow. It helps move mucus up through the airways to the mouth where the mucus can be expectorated.

The Flutter valve has been used in place of CPT in some patients in whom chest physiotherapy cannot be used (e.g., patients with pneumothorax or right-sided heart failure). Although the Flutter valve is mostly used in patients with cystic fibrosis, it has been effectively used in patients with chronic bronchitis and bronchiectasis.

Aerosol-nebulization therapy. Medications for COPD patients are most often delivered via metered-dose inhalers. This is the preferred delivery route, although devices that deliver a sus-

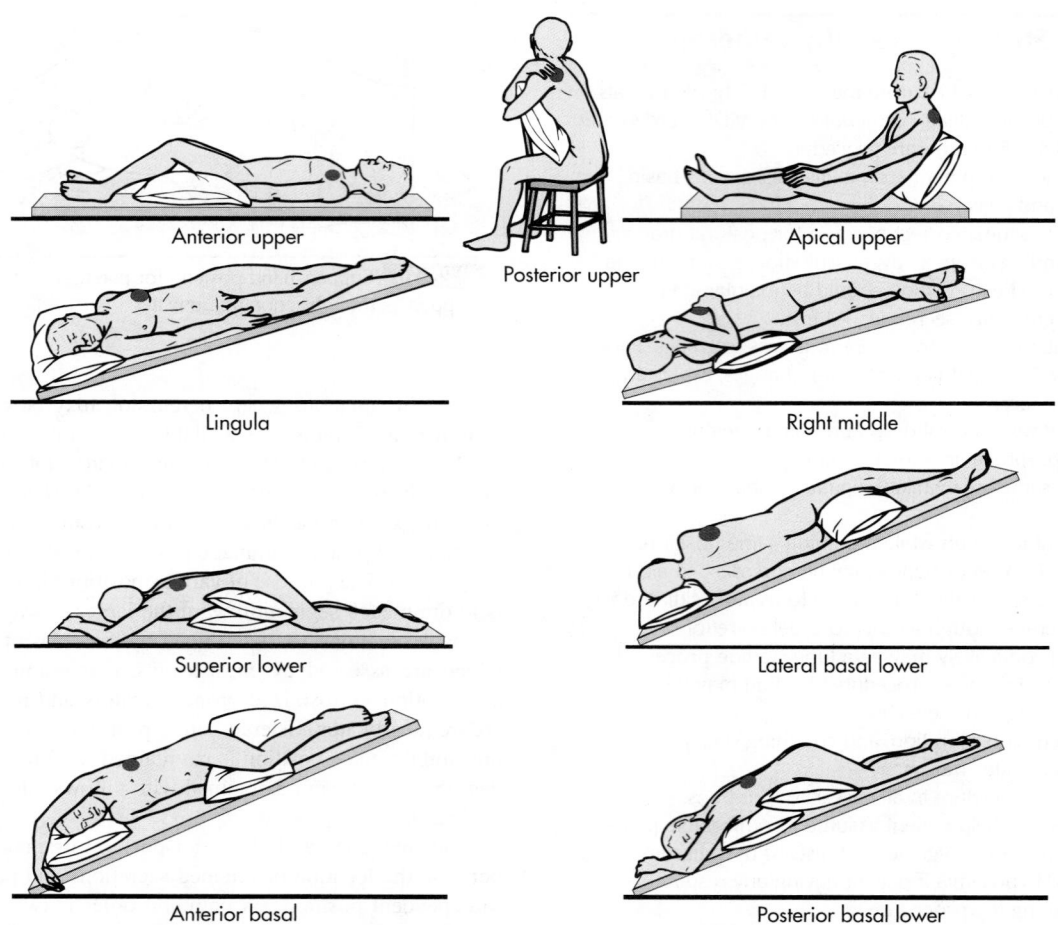

FIG. 28-16 Representative positions for postural drainage. *Shaded areas* in each drawing indicate the segment of the lung in which drainage is promoted.

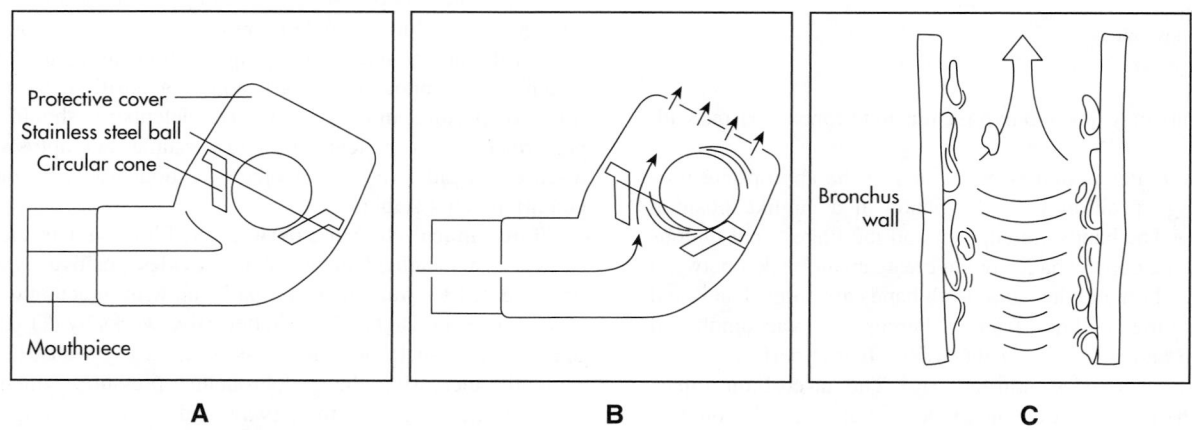

FIG. 28-17 Flutter mucus clearance device is a small handheld device that provides positive expiratory pressure (PEP) therapy. It is used to facilitate removal of mucus from the lungs. **A,** It consists of a hard plastic mouthpiece, a plastic perforated cover, and a high-density stainless steel ball resting in a circular cone. **B,** The Flutter effects occurs during expiration. Before exhalation, the steel ball blocks the conical canal of the Flutter. During exhalation, the position of the steel ball is the result of an equilibrium between the pressure of the exhaled air, the force of gravity on the ball, and the angle of the cone where the contact with the ball occurs. As the steel ball rolls and moves up and down, it creates an opening and closing cycle that repeats itself many times throughout each exhalation. The net result is that vibrations occur in the airways, resulting in the "fluttering" sensation. **C,** These vibrations loosen mucus from the airway walls and facilitate its movement up the airways.

pension of fine particles of liquid in a gas may also be used to deliver medications to the COPD patient. Nebulizers are usually powered by a compressed air or O_2 generator. At home the patient may have an air-powered compressor; in the hospital, wall O_2 or compressed air is used to power the nebulizer.

Aerosolized medication orders must include the medication, dose, diluent, and whether it is to be nebulized with O_2 or compressed air. Medication is nebulized or reduced to a fine spray, and depending on several factors, including droplet size, it can be inhaled into the patient's tracheobronchial tree. The advantage to aerosol-nebulization therapy is that it is easy to use. Medications that are routinely nebulized include albuterol and ipratropium. Other medications infrequently used that can be administered by nebulization include antibiotics, pentamidine (Nebupent), and DNase (Pulmozyme).

The patient is placed in an upright position that allows for most efficient breathing to ensure adequate penetration and deposition of the aerosolized medication. The patient must breathe slowly and deeply through the mouth and hold inspiration for 2 to 3 seconds. Deep diaphragmatic breathing helps ensure deposition of the medication. The patient is instructed to do normal breathing in between these larger forced vital capacity breaths to prevent alveolar hypoventilation and dizziness. After the treatment the patient should be instructed to cough effectively. Postural drainage and CPT are ideally administered after bronchodilator medications are given.

A disadvantage of nebulizer equipment use is the possibility that the nebulizer unit will be a source of respiratory infection. Because home nebulization is used for the patient with COPD, it is important for the health care professional in the hospital and home care setting to review cleaning procedures for home respiratory equipment with the patient. A frequently used, effective home-cleaning method is to wash the nebulizer daily in soap and water, rinse it with water, and soak it for 20 to 30 minutes in a 1:1 white vinegar–water solution followed by a water rinse and air drying. Commercial respiratory cleaning agents may also be used if directions are followed carefully. Cleaning the nebulizer in the top shelf of an automatic dishwasher saves time, and the hot water destroys most organisms.

Nutritional Therapy. The patient with COPD should try to keep body weight for height in standard range. Weight loss and malnutrition are commonly seen in the patient with severe emphysema. The cause of this weight loss is unknown. Eating becomes an effort, especially in the later stages of COPD. A full stomach presses up on the flattened diaphragm, causing increased dyspnea and discomfort. It is difficult for some patients to eat and breathe at the same time; therefore inadequate amounts of food are eaten. Other proposed reasons for malnutrition include loss of appetite related to a decreased sense of taste and smell and gastrointestinal disturbances.[24]

To decrease dyspnea and conserve energy, the patient should rest for at least 30 minutes before eating, use the bronchodilator before meals, and select foods that can be prepared in advance. The patient should eat five to six small, frequent meals to avoid feelings of bloating and early satiety when eating. A full stomach puts pressure on the diaphragm and decreases lung movement. Liquid, blenderized, or commercial diets may be helpful (see the Evidence-Based Practice box). Foods that require a great deal of chewing should be avoided or served in another manner (e.g., grated, pureed). Cold foods

$\mathcal{E}$VIDENCE-BASED PRACTICE

Enteral Feeding for Patients with Chronic Obstructive Pulmonary Disease

Clinical Problem

Is enteral feeding better than a blenderized diet in patients with stable chronic obstructive pulmonary disease?

Best Clinical Practice

- Comparison of the effectiveness of a formula diet with a blenderized diet on nutritional and respiratory function was made.
- There was a slight increase in weight and in pulmonary function in both groups, but these results did not differ significantly.
- In the overall assessment, health care providers and patients rated both formulas as comparable.

Implications for Nursing Practice

- Either enteral feeding or blenderized diet is acceptable to keep body weight in the standard range.
- The convenience and palatability for an individual patient should guide the decision for the type of diet chosen.

Reference for Evidence

Tanchoco C: Enteral feeding in stable chronic obstructive pulmonary disease patients, *Respirology* 6:43, 2001.

may give less of a sense of fullness than hot foods. Exercises and treatments should be avoided for at least 1 hour before and after eating. The exertion involved in the preparation and eating of food is often fatiguing. The use of frozen foods and a microwave oven may help conserve patient energy in food preparation.

Many patients with COPD have feelings of bloating and early satiety when eating. This sensation can be attributed to swallowing air while eating, side effects of medication (especially corticosteroids and theophylline), and the abnormal position of the diaphragm relative to the stomach in association with hyperinflation. Intestinal gas–forming foods should be avoided, such as cabbage, brussels sprouts, and beans.

The patient with emphysema has a greater than normal nutritional requirement for protein and calories. A high-calorie, high-protein diet is recommended and can be divided into five to six small meals a day. High-protein, high-calorie nutritional supplements can be offered between meals. Ice cream added to these supplements can help increase calories. (Nutritional supplements are discussed in Chapter 39.) A high-carbohydrate diet may need to be avoided in the patient who retains CO_2 because carbohydrates metabolize into CO_2 and increase the CO_2 load of the patient. However, research is currently being done in this area, and it remains controversial. In most cases just getting the patients to eat adequate amounts of any foods can be difficult. If the patient has O_2 prescribed, use of supplemental O_2 by nasal prongs while eating may also be beneficial, because eating expends energy. Fluid intake should be at least 3 L per day unless contraindicated for other medical conditions, such as heart failure. Fluids should be taken between meals (rather than with them) to prevent excess stomach distention and to decrease pressure on the diaphragm. Sodium restriction may be indicated if there is accompanying heart failure.

NURSING MANAGEMENT
EMPHYSEMA AND CHRONIC BRONCHITIS

■ Nursing Assessment

Subjective and objective data that should be obtained from a person with emphysema or chronic bronchitis are presented in Table 28-23.

■ Nursing Diagnoses

The nursing diagnoses for the patient with emphysema and chronic bronchitis may include, but are not limited to, those presented in NCP 28-2.

■ Planning

The overall goals are that the patient with COPD will have (1) return of baseline respiratory function, (2) ability to perform ADLs, (3) relief from dyspnea, (4) no complications related to COPD, (5) knowledge and ability to implement a long-term treatment regimen, and (6) overall improved quality of life.

■ Nursing Implementation

Health Promotion. The incidence of COPD would decrease if more people would not begin smoking or would stop smoking. (Techniques to help patients stop smoking are discussed in Chapter 11 and Tables 11-14, 11-15, and 11-17.) Avoiding or controlling exposure to occupational and environmental pollutants and irritants is another preventive measure to maintain healthy lungs. (These factors are discussed in the section on nursing management of lung cancer in Chapter 27.)

Early detection of small-airway disease is important. The person who has smoked for only a few years may have early evidence of obstructive airway disease on spirometry testing. These changes often cannot be detected from pulmonary function studies until extensive damage is present. It is extremely important for the person to stop smoking and avoid inhaling irritants while the disease is still reversible. Failure to follow this advice will inevitably lead to irreversible COPD.

As health care professionals, nurses who smoke should reevaluate their own smoking behavior and its relationship to their health. Nurses, health care providers, and respiratory therapists who smoke and smell of cigarette smoke should be aware that the odor of their clothes can be offensive to patients.

Early diagnosis and treatment of respiratory tract infections are other ways to decrease the incidence of COPD. Avoiding exposure to large crowds in the peak periods for influenza may be necessary, especially for the older adult and the person with a history of respiratory problems. Influenza and pneumococcal pneumonia vaccines are recommended for the patient with COPD.

Families with a history of COPD, as well as AAT deficiency, should be aware of the genetic nature of the disease. Genetic counseling may be appropriate for the patient with ATT deficiency who is planning to have children.

Acute Intervention. The patient with COPD will require acute intervention for complications such as pneumonia, cor pulmonale, and acute respiratory failure. (The nursing care for these conditions is discussed in Chapters 27 and 66.) Once the crisis in these situations has been resolved, the nurse can assess the degree and severity of the underlying respiratory problem. The information obtained will help plan the nursing care.

TABLE 28-23	Nursing Assessment Emphysema or Chronic Bronchitis

Subjective Data

Important Health Information

Past health history: Long-term exposure to chemical pollution, respiratory irritants, occupational fumes, dust; recurrent respiratory infections; previous hospitalizations

Medications: Use and duration of O_2 use, bronchodilators, corticosteroids, antibiotics, anticholinergics, OTC drugs, herbs

Functional Health Patterns

Health perception–health management: Smoking (pack-years, including passive smoking); family history of respiratory disease

Nutritional-metabolic: Anorexia, weight loss or gain

Activity-exercise: Fatigue, inability to perform ADLs; palpitations, swelling of feet; progressive dyspnea, especially on exertion; wheezing; recurrent cough; sputum production with changes in color, odor, viscosity, amount; orthopnea

Elimination: Constipation, gas, bloating

Sleep-rest: Insomnia; sitting up position for sleeping, paroxysmal nocturnal dyspnea

Cognitive-perceptual: Chest and abdominal soreness, headache

Objective Data

General

Debilitation, anxiety, depression, restlessness, assumption of upright position

Integumentary

Cyanosis (bronchitis), pallor or ruddy color, poor skin turgor, thin skin, digital clubbing, easy bruising; peripheral edema (cor pulmonale)

Respiratory

Rapid, shallow breathing; inability to speak; prolonged expiratory phase; pursed-lip breathing; wheezing; rhonchi, crackles, diminished or bronchial breath sounds; ↓ chest excursion and diaphragm movement; use of accessory muscles; hyperresonant or dull chest sounds on percussion

Cardiovascular

Tachycardia; arrhythmias, jugular vein distention, distant heart tones, right-sided S_3 (cor pulmonale), edema (especially in feet)

Gastrointestinal

Ascites, hepatomegaly (cor pulmonale)

Musculoskeletal

Muscle atrophy, ↑ anteroposterior diameter (barrel-chest)

Possible Findings

Abnormal ABGs, polycythemia, pulmonary function tests showing expiratory airflow obstruction (e.g., low FEV_1, low FEV_1/VC, large RV, low PEFR compared with baseline, ↓ expiratory flow rate), chest x-ray showing flattened diaphragm and hyperinflation or infiltrates, ECG showing arrhythmias

ABGs, Arterial blood gases; *ADLs,* activities of daily living; *OTC,* over-the-counter; *RV,* residual volume; *VC,* vital capacity.

NURSING CARE PLAN 28-2

Patient with Chronic Obstructive Pulmonary Disease (COPD)

EXPECTED PATIENT OUTCOMES	NURSING INTERVENTIONS and *RATIONALES*

NURSING DIAGNOSIS

Ineffective airway clearance *related to* expiratory airflow obstruction, ineffective cough, decreased airway humidity, and infection in airways *as manifested by* ineffective or absent cough, presence of abnormal breath sounds, or absence of breath sounds.

- Normal breath sounds for patient
- Effective coughing

- Facilitate deep breathing by elevating head or sitting patient up *to maximize ventilation and prolong expiratory phase.*
- Position in semi-Fowler position *to facilitate cough and prevent aspiration.*
- Ensure hydration (oral intake approximately 2-3 L/day, humidified ambient air) *to liquefy secretions for easier expectoration.*
- Teach effective cough techniques *to minimize airway collapse and aid in proper coughing.*
- Provide chest physiotherapy (positioning, percussion, and vibration) when indicated *to use effect of gravity in removing secretions.*
- Coordinate inhaled bronchodilator administration *to facilitate clearance of retained secretions.*

NURSING DIAGNOSIS

Impaired gas exchange *related to* alveolar hypoventilation *as manifested by* headache on awakening, $PaCO_2 \geq 45$ mm Hg and abnormal for patient's baseline, $PaO_2 <60$ mm Hg, or $SaO_2 <90\%$ at rest.

- $PaCO_2$ of 35-45 mm Hg or usual compensated baseline value
- Return of PaO_2 to normal range for patient
- Improved mental status

- Teach pursed-lip breathing *to prolong expiratory phase and slow rate.*
- Assist patient to assume position of comfort (e.g., tripod position, elevated backrest, supported upper extremities to fix shoulder girdle) *to maximize respiratory excursion.*
- Administer and teach appropriate use of bronchodilators *to open the airways.*
- Teach signs, symptoms, and consequences of hypercapnia (e.g., confusion, somnolence, headache, irritability, decrease in mental acuity, increase in respiration, facial flush, diaphoresis) *so problem can be recognized early and treatment initiated.*
- Teach avoidance of central nervous system depressants *because they further depress respirations.*
- Administer O_2 if appropriate *to increase O_2 saturation.*
- Select O_2 supply systems and devices (e.g., nasal cannula, mask) that are appropriate to patient's activities of daily living (rest, sleep, exercise) *to minimize impact on preferred lifestyle.*

NURSING DIAGNOSIS

Imbalanced nutrition: less than body requirements *related to* poor appetite, lowered energy level, shortness of breath, gastric distention, sputum production, and depression *as manifested by* weight loss > 10% of ideal body weight, serum albumin level below normal laboratory values, lack of interest in food.

- Maintenance of body weight within normal range for height and age
- Normal serum protein and albumin levels

- Monitor caloric intake, weight, and serum albumin *to determine adequacy of intake.*
- Provide menu suggestions for high-protein, high-calorie foods.
- Give patient high-protein, high-calorie liquid supplements if necessary *to provide adequate calories and protein to prevent weight loss and muscle wasting.*
- Plan periods of rest after food intake *to compensate for blood flow diversion to the gastrointestinal tract for digestion.*
- Refer to agency for financial or nutritional assistance as necessary (e.g., meals-on-wheels, food stamps) *to ensure nutritional adequacy after discharge.*
- Be aware that patient may benefit from six small meals throughout the day *because this reduces bloating.*

NURSING DIAGNOSIS

Disturbed sleep pattern *related to* anxiety, dyspnea, depression, hypoxemia and/or hypercapnia, and shortness of breath *as manifested by* insomnia, lethargy, fatigue, restlessness, irritability; orthopnea, paroxysmal nocturnal dyspnea.

- Feeling of being rested
- Improvement in sleep pattern
- Rested feeling on awakening

- Identify usual sleep habits *to provide baseline data.*
- Ask patient why he or she is having difficulty sleeping, and identify causes of discomfort and wakefulness.
- Observe for signs and symptoms of sleep apnea such as frequent awakening at night, insomnia, and excessive daytime sleepiness *so appropriate interventions can be initiated.*
- Identify patient-specific methods of relaxation and teach patient relaxation methods *to foster sleep.*
- Encourage exercise and activity during daylight hours *because this will improve sleep at night.*
- Instruct patient in maintaining an environment conducive to rest (e.g., clothing, temperature, position, noise level).
- Teach avoidance of alcoholic beverages, caffeine products, or other stimulants before bedtime *to reduce interference with sleep.*

Continued

NURSING CARE PLAN 28-2

Patient with Chronic Obstructive Pulmonary Disease (COPD)—cont'd

EXPECTED PATIENT OUTCOMES	NURSING INTERVENTIONS and *RATIONALES*
NURSING DIAGNOSIS	**Risk for infection** *related to* decreased pulmonary function, possible corticosteroid therapy, ineffective airway clearance, and lack of knowledge regarding signs and symptoms of infection and preventive measures.
• Use of behaviors designed to minimize risk of infection • Aware of need to seek medical attention for appropriate treatment • No infection	• Assess for change in color, quantity, odor, and viscosity of sputum; difficulty in mobilizing secretions; foul oral odor; increase in cough; increase in dyspnea; fever; chills; diaphoresis; increase in respiratory rate; abnormal breath sounds (gurgles, wheezing); hypoxemia and/or hypercapnia; excessive fatigue *to determine if an infection is present.* • Teach patient to use good hand-washing techniques and avoid contact (whenever possible) with persons with respiratory infections *to minimize source of infection.* • Encourage patient to obtain vaccines for influenza and pneumococcal pneumonia *to decrease occurrence or severity of influenza or pneumonia.* • Teach proper care and cleaning of home respiratory equipment *to eliminate this source of infection.* • Instruct patient to seek medical attention for manifestations of early infection *so treatment can be started promptly.* • Teach patient to initiate plan of care previously discussed with physician when infections occur (e.g., increase fluid intake, begin antibiotics, increase corticosteroid dosage) *so appropriate self-care is initiated promptly.*

Ambulatory and Home Care. By far the most important aspect in the long-term care of the patient with COPD is teaching (Table 28-24). (Patient teaching is discussed in Chapter 4.)

Pulmonary rehabilitation. Pulmonary rehabilitation should be recommended for all patients with symptomatic COPD. According to the American Thoracic Society, the objectives of pulmonary rehabilitation are to (1) control and alleviate as much as possible the symptoms and pathophysiologic complications of respiratory impairment and (2) teach the patient how to achieve optimal capability for carrying out ADLs. The overall goal is to increase the quality of life. The components of pulmonary rehabilitation include physical therapy (e.g., bronchial hygiene, exercise conditioning, breathing retraining, energy conservation), nutrition, and education and other topics such as smoking cessation, environmental factors, health promotion, psychologic counseling, and vocational rehabilitation. Although much of this intervention should be routinely included in the comprehensive approach to the patient with COPD, the referral of the patient to a structured pulmonary rehabilitation program should also be a goal for the patient with moderate to severe COPD.[35]

Activity considerations. Energy conservation is another important component in COPD rehabilitation. This patient is typically an upper thoracic and neck breather who uses accessory muscles rather than the diaphragm. Thus the patient has difficulty performing upper-extremity activities, particularly those activities that require arm elevation above the head. Exercise training of the upper extremities may improve function and reduce dyspnea. Frequently the patient has already adapted alternative energy-saving practices for ADLs. Alternative methods of hair care, shaving, showering, and reaching may need to be explored. An occupational therapist may help with ideas in these areas. Assuming a tripod posture (elbows supported on a table, chest in fixed position) and a mirror placed on the table during use of an electric razor or hair dryer conserves much more energy than when the patient stands in front of a mirror to shave or blow-dry hair. If the patient uses home O_2 therapy, it is essential that the

ETHICAL DILEMMAS
Durable Power of Attorney

Situation

A 50-year-old woman is being treated for complications of COPD. She is currently on a ventilator and not coherent because of the drugs she is receiving. Her life partner, another woman, has been with her throughout this hospitalization. The patient had executed a valid durable power of attorney for health care decisions before this admission and had named her partner as her primary agent. However, the patient's parents and siblings have arrived and demand to be in charge of her treatment decisions. They do not accept the partner or the patient's appointment of this woman to make decisions for her.

Important Points for Consideration

• Durable power of attorney for health care is one type of advance directive in which persons, when they are competent, identify someone else to make decisions for them, should they lose their decision-making ability in the future.
• The surrogate decision maker, who is named as durable power of attorney for health care, is often selected because the person believes that personal values, beliefs, and wishes will be respected when making treatment decisions for him or her.
• Advance directives are legal documents. However, it is often difficult for health care providers when family members or designated surrogates do not agree.
• State laws may differ regarding surrogate decision makers, so it is imperative to be familiar with the statutes in the state in which one practices.

Critical Thinking Questions

1. How would you handle a situation in which the family and surrogate decision maker disagree?
2. What resources would you consult or seek assistance from under these circumstances?

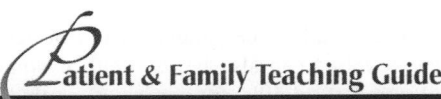

TABLE

28-24

Patient & Family Teaching Guide

Chronic Obstructive Pulmonary Disease

Goal: To assist a patient and family in improving quality of life through education and promotion of lifestyle practices that support successful living with chronic obstructive pulmonary disease (COPD).

TEACHING TOPIC	RESOURCES
What Is COPD? • Basic anatomy and physiology of lung • Basic pathophysiology of COPD • Signs and symptoms of COPD, respiratory infection, heart failure	*Help Yourself to Better Breathing* (American Lung Association) Videos (American Lung Association)
Breathing Retraining • Pursed-lip breathing • Abdominal (diaphragm) breathing	Demonstration and return demonstration
Energy Conservation Techniques • Pacing and pursing (pacing activity and using pursed-lip breathing with activities)	*Around the Clock with COPD: Helpful Hints for Respiratory Patients* (American Lung Association)

Medications
• Types (include mechanism of action)
  Methylxanthines
  β_2-adrenergic agonists
  Corticosteroids
  Anticholinergics
  Antibiotics
• Establishing medication schedule
	Understanding Lung Medications: How They Work—How to Use Them (American Lung Association)
	Write out medication list and schedule

Correct Use of Metered-Dose Inhaler, Spacer, and Nebulizer	See Fig. 28-6
Home Oxygen • Explanation of rationale for use • Guide for home O_2 use	*About Oxygen Therapy at Home* (American Lung Association) See Table 28-20

Psychosocial Emotional Issues
• Concerns about interpersonal relationships
  Dependency
  Intimacy
• Problems with emotions
  Depression
  Anxiety
  Panic
• Effects of medications
• Support and rehabilitation groups
	Intimacy and Lung Disease (American Lung Association)
	Open discussion (sharing with patient, significant other, and family)

COPD Management Plan • Focusing on self-management • Knowing usual signs/symptoms • Need to report changes • Cause of flare-ups • Recognition of signs and symptoms of respiration infection, heart failure • Yearly follow-up	Nurse and patient develop and write up COPD management plan that meets individual needs
Healthy Nutrition • Strategies to lose weight (if overweight) • Strategies to gain weight (if underweight)	Consultation with dietitian

patient use the O_2 during activities of hygiene, because these are energy consuming. The patient should be encouraged to make a schedule and plan daily and weekly activities so as to leave plenty of time for rest periods. The patient should also try to sit as much as possible when performing activities. Another energy-saving tip is to exhale when pushing, pulling, or exerting effort during an activity and inhale during rest.

Walking is by far the best physical exercise for the COPD patient. Coordinated walking with slow, pursed-lip breathing without breath holding is a difficult task that requires conscious effort and frequent reinforcement. During coordinated walking and breathing, the patient is taught to breathe in through the nose while taking one step, then to breathe out through pursed lips while taking two to four steps (the number depends on the patient's tolerance). Walking should occur at a slow pace with rest periods when necessary so the patient can sit or lean against an object such as a tree or post. The patient may need to ambulate using O_2. Once the patient is able to successfully perform coordinated walking with pursed-lip breathing, diaphragmatic breathing may also be incorporated if the patient has practiced and mastered this technique at rest. The nurse should walk with the patient, giving verbal reminders when necessary regarding breathing (inhalation and exhalation) and steps. Walking with the patient helps decrease anxiety and helps maintain a slow pace. It also enables the nurse to observe the patient's actions and physiologic responses to the activity. Many patients with moderate or severe COPD are anxious and fearful of walking or performing exercise. These patients and their families require much support while they build the confidence they need to walk or to perform daily exercises.

The patient should be encouraged to walk 15 to 20 minutes a day with gradual increases. Severely disabled patients can begin at a slow pace by walking for 2 to 5 minutes three times a day and slowly building up to 20 minutes a day, if possible. Adequate rest periods should be allowed. Some patients benefit from using their β_2-adrenergic agonist MDI approximately 10 minutes before exercise. Parameters that may be monitored in the patient with mild COPD are resting pulse and pulse rate after walking. Pulse rate after walking should not exceed 75% to 80% of the maximum heart rate (maximum heart rate is age in years subtracted from 220). In the patient with other than mild COPD and without significant heart disease, it is usually dyspnea and the limitation in breathing rather than increased heart rate that limits the exercise. Thus it is better to use the patient's perceived sense of dyspnea as an indication of exercise tolerance. The Borg scale (see Chapter 25, Fig. 25-9) can be used to have the patient determine the intensity of dyspnea.

The patient should be told that shortness of breath will probably increase during exercise (as it does for a healthy individual) but that the activity is not being overdone if this increased shortness of breath returns to baseline within 5 minutes after the cessation of exercise. The patient should be told to wait 5 minutes after completion of exercise before using the β_2-adrenergic agonist MDI to allow a chance to recover. During this time, slow, pursed-lip breathing should be used. If it takes longer than 5 minutes to return to baseline, the patient most likely has overdone it and should proceed at a slower pace during the next exercise period. The patient may benefit from keeping a diary or log of the exercise program. The diary can help provide a realistic evaluation of the patient's progress. In addition, the diary can help mo-

tivate the patient and add to the patient's sense of accomplishment. Stationary cycling can also be used either alone or with walking. Cycles and treadmills are particularly valuable when weather prevents walking outside.

Sexual activity. Modifying but not abstaining from sexual activity can also contribute to a healthy psychologic well-being. Using an inhaled bronchodilator before sexual activity can help ventilation. The patient with COPD will also use less energy if these guidelines are followed: (1) plan sexual activity during the part of the day when breathing is best, (2) use slow pursed-lip breathing, (3) refrain from sexual activity after eating or other strenuous activity, (4) do not assume a dominant position, and (5) do not prolong foreplay. These aspects of sexual activity require open communication between partners regarding their needs and expectations.

Sleep. Adequate sleep is extremely important. Getting adequate amounts of sleep can be difficult for the COPD patient. Medications may cause restlessness and insomnia. Many patients with COPD have postnasal drip or nasal congestion that may cause coughing and wheezing at night. Nasal saline sprays before sleep and in the morning may help. The health care provider may also prescribe a nasal decongestant or nasal steroid inhaler that may be used at bedtime. Long-acting theophylline preparations frequently aid in promoting sleep by decreasing bronchospasm and airway obstruction. If the patient is a restless sleeper, snores, stops breathing while asleep, and has a tendency to fall asleep during the day, the patient may need to be tested for sleep apnea (see Chapter 26).

Psychosocial considerations. Healthy coping is often the most difficult task for a patient with COPD to accomplish. People with COPD frequently have to deal with many lifestyle changes that may involve decreased ability to care for themselves, decreased energy for social activities, and loss of a job.

When a patient with COPD is first diagnosed or when a patient has complications that require hospitalization, the nurse should expect a variety of emotional responses. Emotions frequently encountered include guilt, depression, anxiety, social isolation, denial, and dependence. Guilt may result from the knowledge that the disease was caused largely by cigarette smoking. Depression may be experienced as the severity and chronicity of the disease are realized. The nurse should convey a sense of understanding and caring to the patient.

The patient with COPD may benefit from several relaxation techniques. One is the use of a progressive relaxation technique in which the patient listens either to a tape or to the patient's own or another voice and gradually begins to tighten and relax muscle groups. Self-hypnosis, biofeedback, meditation, and massage (self-massage or massage from others) are other alternative relaxation therapies (see Chapters 7 and 8). Support groups at local American Lung Associations, hospitals, and clinics can also be helpful.

Patients frequently ask whether moving to a warmer or drier climate will help. In general, such a move is not significantly beneficial. Moving to places with an elevation of 4000 feet or more should be discouraged because of the lower partial pressure of O_2 found in the air at higher elevations. A disadvantage of moving may be that a person leaves an occupation, friends, and familiar environment, which could be psychologically stressful. Any advantage gained from a different climate may be outweighed by the psychologic effects of the move.

■ Evaluation

The expected outcomes for the patient with COPD are presented in NCP 28-2.

CYSTIC FIBROSIS

Cystic fibrosis (CF) is an autosomal recessive, multisystem disease characterized by altered function of the exocrine glands involving primarily the lungs, pancreas, and sweat glands. (Autosomal recessive disorders are discussed in Chapter 13.) Abnormally thick, abundant secretions from mucous glands can lead to a chronic, diffuse, obstructive pulmonary disorder in almost all patients. Exocrine pancreatic insufficiency is associated with most cases of CF. Sweat glands excrete increased amounts of sodium and chloride.

Cystic fibrosis affects approximately 30,000 persons in the United States. The disease occurs primarily in Whites, with a frequency of 1 in 2000 births among Whites and 1 in 17,000 births among African Americans.[36] Both sexes are equally affected. Approximately 4% to 5% (1 in 20 to 25) of the general population are carriers of the gene transmitting CF, with 20% of these being young adults. The first signs and symptoms typically occur in children, but some patients are not diagnosed until they are adults.

The severity and progression of the disease vary from person to person. In the last decade, it has been shown that with early diagnosis and improvements in therapy, the prognosis has been significantly improved. Approximately 34% of patients reach adulthood, and nearly 10% live past age 30. The average life span is 28 years.[37]

Etiology and Pathophysiology

CF results from mutations in a gene located on chromosome 7. The most common mutation in the CF gene is known as the CF transmembrane regulator (CFTR). The primary defect in CF is abnormally regulated chloride channel activity. This defect alters ionic transport of sodium and chloride across epithelial surfaces. The high concentrations of sodium and chloride in the sweat of the patient with CF result from decreased chloride reabsorption in the sweat duct. The basic pathophysiologic mechanism is obstruction of the ducts of exocrine gland with thick, viscous secretions that adhere to the lumen of the ducts. The glands distal to the duct eventually undergo fibrosis.

In the respiratory system, both upper and lower respiratory tracts can be affected. Upper respiratory tract manifestations may be present and include chronic sinusitis and nasal polyposis. The hallmark of respiratory involvement in CF is its effect on the airways. The disease progresses from being a disease of the small airways (chronic bronchiolitis) to an entity that eventually involves the larger airways and finally causes destruction of lung tissue. Thick secretions obstruct bronchioles and lead to air trapping and hyperinflation of the lungs. The stasis of mucus provides an excellent growth medium for bacteria. CF is characterized by chronic airway infection. The most common organisms cultured from the sputum of a patient with CF are *S. aureus,* *H. influenzae,* and *P. aeruginosa.*[38]

Lung disorders that can result include pneumonia, bronchiolitis, bronchitis, bronchiectasis, atelectasis, and emphysema. There is progressive loss of lung tissue from inflammation and scarring, and the resultant chronic hypoxia leads to pulmonary hyperten-

GENETICS in CLINICAL PRACTICE
Cystic Fibrosis (CF)

Genetic Basis
- Autosomal recessive disorder
- Gene location on chromosome 7
- Many different mutations of the gene have been identified

Incidence
- 1 in 2000 whites
- Uncommon in other ethnic populations
- 1 in 20 to 25 are carriers of the gene
- If both parents carry the affected gene, there is a 25% chance each offspring will have the disease (see Chapter 13, Fig. 13-3)

Genetic Testing
- DNA testing available
- Testing usually done if parents have an affected child
- In parents who are known carriers, amniocentesis or chorionic villus sampling in pregnant women may be useful for prenatal testing

Clinical Implications
- Most common autosomal recessive disease in whites
- Wide range of clinical expression of disease
- Requires long-term medical management
- Advances in medical care have improved life expectancy
- Current recommendations are that CF screening be offered to individuals with a family history of CF and reproductive partners of individuals who have CF

sion and cor pulmonale. Blebs and large cysts in the lung are also severe manifestations of lung destruction. Other pulmonary complications include hemoptysis, which can sometimes be fatal, and pneumothorax. Hemoptysis may range from scant streaking to major bleeding.

Initially, CF is an obstructive lung disease caused by the overall obstruction of the airways with mucus. Later, CF also progresses to a restrictive lung disease because of the fibrosis, lung destruction, and thoracic wall changes. Death usually results from loss of pulmonary function. Cor pulmonale is a common late complication caused by extensive loss of lung tissue and chronic hypoxia.

Pancreatic insufficiency is caused primarily by mucous plugging of the pancreatic duct and its branches, which results in fibrosis of the acinar glands of the pancreas. The exocrine function of the pancreas is altered and may be lost completely. Pancreatic enzymes such as trypsinogen, lipase, and amylase do not reach the intestine to digest ingested nutrients. There is malabsorption of fat, protein, and fat-soluble vitamins (vitamins A, D, E, and K). Fat malabsorption results in steatorrhea, and protein malabsorption results in failure to grow and gain weight. In advanced pancreatic insufficiency, endocrine function may also be affected.[39]

Diabetes mellitus may occur if the islets of Langerhans become fibrotic. Cystic fibrosis–related diabetes mellitus affects approximately 15% of all patients with CF. It differs from type 1 diabetes in that some insulin is secreted, it is nonketotic, and it is slow in onset. It differs from type 2 diabetes in that individuals are underweight (as opposed to being obese), the onset is in a younger age population, and the individual is hypoinsulinemic.

Routine screening is indicated to follow serum glucose levels. Insulin may be required for treatment of CF-related diabetes.

The sweat glands of the CF patient secrete normal volumes of sweat but are unable to absorb sodium chloride from sweat as it moves through the sweat duct. Therefore they excrete four times the normal amount of sodium and chloride in sweat. This abnormality does not seem to affect the general health of the person, but it is useful as a diagnostic indicator.

Individuals with CF often have gastrointestinal problems. Intestinal obstruction resulting in meconium ileus is seen in the newborn. However, GERD, distal intestinal obstructive syndrome (DIOS), and constipation are common. GERD is a major problem in individuals with CF, particularly in those with pulmonary disease. The relationship between reflux and exacerbation of respiratory disease is not known, but it is known that these two entities enhance each other.

DIOS is a syndrome that results from intermittent obstruction in the ileal-cecal area in patients with pancreatic insufficiency. The degree to which the bowel is obstructed may vary with each episode, and a partial obstruction may progress to a complete obstruction. Complete obstruction requires gastric decompression and a surgical consultation; partial and uncomplicated episodes of DIOS are treated with ingestion of a balanced polyethylene glycol electrolyte solution. Constipation develops in the sigmoid colon and progresses proximally, whereas DIOS develops in the ileal-cecal area and progresses distally. Careful monitoring of bowel habits and patterns is essential.

The liver may become involved. Biliary cirrhosis may not be recognized until late in the disease. Hepatobiliary disease is common in the older patient. Chronic cholestasis, inflammation, fibrosis, and portal hypertension can occur.[40]

Clinical Manifestations

The clinical manifestations of CF vary depending on the severity of the disease. An initial finding of meconium ileus in the newborn infant is present in 10% to 15% of persons with CF. Early manifestations in childhood are failure to grow, clubbing, persistent cough with mucus production, tachypnea, and large, frequent bowel movements. A large, protuberant abdomen may develop with an emaciated appearance of the extremities.

The first symptom of CF in the adult is frequently cough. With time the cough becomes persistent and produces viscous, purulent, often greenish-colored sputum. Other respiratory problems that may be indicative of CF are recurring lung infections such as bronchiolitis, bronchitis, and pneumonia. As the disease progresses, periods of clinical stability are interrupted by exacerbations characterized by increased cough, weight loss, increased sputum, and decreases in pulmonary function. Over time the exacerbations become more frequent and the recovery of lost lung function less complete, ultimately leading to respiratory failure.

Distal intestinal obstruction causes right lower quadrant pain, loss of appetite, emesis, and often a palpable mass. Insufficient pancreatic enzyme release causes the typical pattern of protein and fat malabsorption with frequent, bulky, foul-smelling stools.

The function of the reproductive system is altered. This finding is important because more persons with CF are living to adulthood. The male adult is usually sterile (although not impotent) as a result of structural changes in the vas deferens, seminal vesicles, and epididymis. The female adult usually has delayed menarche. During exacerbations, menstrual irregularities and secondary amenorrhea are fairly common. The woman may be unable to become pregnant because of the increased viscosity of the cervical mucus. Women with CF do become pregnant, but the fertility rate is lower than in healthy women. The baby is heterozygous (and hence a carrier) for CF if the father is not a carrier. If the father is a carrier, there is a 50% chance that the baby will have CF. (See Chapter 13, Fig. 13-3, for explanation of genetic transmission of CF.)

Complications

Pneumothorax is common (greater than 10% of patients) in patients with cystic fibrosis. The presence of small amounts of blood in sputum is common in the CF patient with lung infection. Massive hemoptysis is life threatening. With advanced lung disease, digital clubbing becomes evident in almost all patients with CF. Respiratory failure and cor pulmonale are late complications of CF.

Diagnostic Studies

The main diagnostic test for CF is the sweat chloride test with the pilocarpine iontophoresis method. Pilocarpine carried by a small electric current is used to stimulate sweat production. The sweat is collected on filter paper or gauze and then analyzed for sodium and chloride concentrations. The test takes approximately 40 minutes. Values greater than 65 mEq/L for both sodium and chloride are suggestive of CF, especially in a person who has other clinical features of the disease. The degree of sodium and chloride elevation does not necessarily correlate with the severity of the disease. Other diagnostic studies include chest x-ray, pulmonary function tests, fecal analysis for fat, and duodenoscopy for quantitative determination of pancreatic enzymes.

Because of the large number of CF mutations, DNA analysis is not used for the primary diagnostic test. DNA analysis may be performed in CF patients to corroborate the diagnosis. Fetal diagnosis can be done from samples obtained by amniocentesis or chorionic villus sampling.

Collaborative Care

The major objectives of therapy in CF are to (1) promote clearance of secretions, (2) control infection in the lungs, and (3) provide adequate nutrition. Management of pulmonary problems in CF aims at relieving airway obstruction and controlling infection. Drainage of thick bronchial mucus is assisted by aerosol and nebulization treatments of medications used to liquefy mucus and to facilitate coughing. The abnormal viscoelastic properties of CF secretions are primarily caused by mucus glycoproteins and DNA from degenerated neutrophils. Agents that degrade the high concentrations of DNA in CF sputum (e.g., DNase [Pulmozyme]) decrease sputum viscosity and increase airflow. Bronchodilators (e.g., β_2-adrenergic agonists, theophylline) and mucolytics may be used.

Airway clearance techniques are critical in reducing mucus. These techniques include CPT, postural drainage, and PEP breathing. Flutter mucus clearance devices are also effective in promoting mucus removal (see Fig. 28-17). Individuals with CF may have a preference for a certain technique that works well for them in a daily routine. (These airway clearance techniques are discussed in the section on respiratory therapy for COPD earlier in this chapter.)

Aerobic exercise seems to be effective in clearing the airways. Important needs to consider when planning an aerobic exercise program for the patient with CF are (1) frequent rest periods interspersed throughout the exercise regimen, (2) meeting increased nutritional demands of exercise, (3) observing for manifestations of hyperthermia, and (4) drinking large amounts of fluid and replacing salt losses.

Most CF patients die of complications resulting from lung infection. Antimicrobial treatment is initiated for the treatment of infection. The use of antibiotics should be carefully guided by sputum culture results. Early intervention with antibiotics is useful, and long courses of antibiotics are the usual treatment.[41] Prolonged high-dose therapy may be necessary because many drugs are abnormally metabolized and rapidly excreted in the patient with CF. Pharmacokinetic and kidney function studies therefore should be monitored closely. Oral agents commonly used are trimethoprim-sulfamethoxazole, tetracycline, chloramphenicol, cephalosporins, antistaphylococcal penicillins, and oral quinolones, especially ciprofloxacin (Cipro).

Although oral and aerosolized antimicrobial therapy is usually adequate, some patients require a 2- to 4-week course of IV antimicrobial therapy. If home facilities are adequate, the CF patient and the family may choose to continue parenteral therapy at home. The usual treatment for acute infectious exacerbation is an aminoglycoside combined with penicillin, or a third-generation cephalosporin. Aerosolized bronchodilators and antiinflammatory agents (e.g., cromolyn) are used in selected patients, particularly before CPT (see Table 28-22). The patient with cor pulmonale or hypoxemia may require home O_2 therapy. (O_2 therapy is discussed earlier in this chapter.) Sclerosing of the pleural space or partial pleural stripping and pleural abrasion performed surgically are usually indicated for recurrent episodes of pneumothorax.

CF has become a leading indication for either heart-lung or lung transplantation. (Lung transplants are discussed in Chapter 27.) Lung transplantations for the patient with CF have resulted in significant improvement of pulmonary function and prolonging life.

The management of pancreatic insufficiency includes pancreatic enzyme replacement of lipase, protease, and amylase (e.g., Cotazym, Creon, Ultrase, Viokase, Zymase) administered before each meal and snack. A high-calorie, high-protein diet and multivitamins are recommended. Fat restriction usually is not necessary. Fat-soluble vitamins (vitamins A, D, E, and K) must be supplemented. Use of caloric supplements improves nutritional status. Added dietary salt is indicated whenever sweating is excessive, such as during hot weather, in the presence of fever, or from intense physical activity.

Gene therapy has been used as an experimental therapy for treating CF.[42] (Gene therapy is discussed in Chapter 13.)

NURSING MANAGEMENT
CYSTIC FIBROSIS

■ Nursing Assessment

Subjective and objective data that should be obtained from the patient with cystic fibrosis are presented in Table 28-25.

■ Nursing Diagnoses

Nursing diagnoses for the patient with CF may include, but are not limited to, the following:
- Ineffective airway clearance *related to* abundant, thick bronchial mucus, weakness, and fatigue

TABLE 28-25	Nursing Assessment Cystic Fibrosis

Subjective Data
Important Health Information
Past health history: Recurrent respiratory and sinus infections, persistent cough with excessive sputum production
Medications: Use of and compliance with corticosteroids, bronchodilators, antibiotics, herbs
Functional Health Patterns
Health perception–health maintenance: Family history of cystic fibrosis; diagnosis of cystic fibrosis in childhood
Nutritional-metabolic: Dietary intolerances, voracious appetite, weight loss
Elimination: Intestinal gas; large, frequent bowel movements
Activity-rest: Fatigue, ↓ exercise tolerance; dyspnea, cough, excessive mucus or sputum production
Cognitive-perception: Abdominal pain
Sexuality-reproductive: Delayed menarche, menstrual irregularities, and secondary amenorrhea; ↓ fertility in men and women

Objective Data
General
Anxiety, depression, restlessness; failure to thrive
Integumentary
Cyanosis (circumoral, nailbed), digital clubbing; salty skin
Respiratory
Persistent runny nose, diminished breath sounds, sputum (thick, white, tenacious), hemoptysis, ↑ work of breathing, use of accessory muscles of respiration, barrel chest
Cardiovascular
Tachycardia
Gastrointestinal
Protuberant abdomen; abdominal distention; foul, fatty stools
Possible Findings
Abnormal ABGs and pulmonary function tests; abnormal sweat chloride test, chest x-ray, fecal fat analysis

- Ineffective breathing pattern *related to* bronchoconstriction, anxiety, and airway obstruction
- Impaired gas exchange *related to* recurring lung infections
- Imbalanced nutrition: less than body requirements *related to* dietary intolerances, intestinal gas, and altered pancreatic enzyme production

■ Planning

The overall goals are that the patient with CF will have (1) adequate airway clearance, (2) reduced risk factors associated with respiratory infections, (3) ability to perform ADLs, (4) no complications related to CF, and (5) active participation in planning and implementing a therapeutic regimen.

■ Nursing Implementation

The nurse and other health professionals can assist young adults to gain independence by helping them assume responsibility for their care and for their vocational or school goals. An important issue that should be discussed is sexuality. Delayed or irregular menstruation is not uncommon. There may be delayed development of secondary sex characteristics such as breasts in girls. The person may use the illness to avoid certain events or relationships. The healthy person may hesitate to make friends with someone who is sick. Other crises and life transitions that must be dealt with in the young adult include building confidence and self-respect on the basis of achievements, persevering with employment goals, developing motivation to achieve, learning to cope with the treatment program, and adjusting to the need for dependence if health fails.

The issue of marrying and having children is difficult. Genetic counseling may be an appropriate suggestion for the couple considering having children. Many men with CF are sterile. Women with the disease may have difficulty becoming pregnant. In addition, any children produced will either be a carrier of CF or have the disease. Another concern is the shortened life span of the parent with CF, and the parent's ability to care for the child must be taken into consideration.

Acute intervention for the patient with CF includes relief of bronchoconstriction, airway obstruction, and airflow limitation. Interventions include aggressive CPT, antibiotics, O_2 therapy, and corticosteroids in severe disease. Good nutrition is important to support the immune system. Advances in long-term vascular access (e.g., implanted ports) have made IV access and administration of medication much easier. This has also eased the transition for IV treatment at home.

CPT is the mainstay of intervention for ineffective airway clearance for these patients. Home management of cystic fibrosis includes an aggressive plan of postural drainage with percussion and vibration, aerosol-nebulization therapy, and breathing retraining. The patient is taught controlled coughing techniques, deep-breathing exercises, and progressive exercise conditioning such as a bicycling program.

The family and the person with CF have a great financial and emotional burden. The cost of drugs, special equipment, and health care is often a financial hardship. Because many CF patients live to childbearing age, family planning and genetic counseling are important. The burden of living with a chronic disease at a young age can be emotionally overwhelming. Community resources are often available to help the family. In addition, the Cystic Fibrosis Foundation can be of assistance. As the person continues toward and into adulthood, the nurse and other skilled health professionals should be available to help the patient and family cope with complications resulting from the disease.

CRITICAL THINKING EXERCISES

Case Study
Asthma
Patient Profile. Mrs. S., a 30-year-old African American mother of two preschoolers, comes to the emergency department (ED) with severe wheezing, dyspnea, and anxiety. She was in the ED only 6 hours ago with an acute asthma attack.

Subjective Data
- Treated in the ED previously with nebulized albuterol and responded quickly
- Can speak only one- to three-word sentences
- Is allergic to cigarette smoke
- Began to experience increased shortness of breath and tightness in her chest when she returned home
- Used albuterol MDI (without a spacer) repeatedly at home with no relief

Objective Data
Physical Examination
- Uses accessory muscles to breathe
- Has audible wheezing
- Respiratory rate 34/min
- Auscultation reveals no air movement in lower lobes
- Heart rate 126 beats/min

Diagnostic Studies
- ABGs: PaO_2 80 mm Hg, $PaCO_2$ 35 mm Hg, pH 7.46
- PEFR: 150 L/min (personal best: 400 L/min)

CRITICAL THINKING QUESTIONS
1. Why did Mrs. S. return to the ED? Explain the pathophysiology of this exacerbation of asthma.
2. What are the nursing care priorities for Mrs. S.?
3. What are the complications that the nurse must be ready for based on her assessment of Mrs. S.?
4. What should be included in her discharge plan of care?
5. Based on the assessment data presented, write one or more nursing diagnoses. Are there any collaborative problems?

Nursing Research Issues
1. What effect does a planned exercise program have on respiratory function in the patient with COPD?
2. Can the use of relaxation techniques reduce dyspnea in the patient with asthma or COPD?
3. What types of breathing retraining techniques result in the greatest improvement in oxygenation?
4. What are the most common patient care problems with an adult who has CF?
5. What are the most effective measures to improve upper arm strength and endurance and reduce dyspnea in the patient with COPD?

REVIEW QUESTIONS

The number of the question corresponds to the same-numbered objective at the beginning of the chapter.

1. Asthma is best characterized as
   a. an inflammatory disease.
   b. a steady progression of bronchoconstriction.
   c. an obstructive disease with loss of alveolar walls.
   d. a chronic obstructive disorder characterized by mucus production.

2. In evaluating the asthmatic patient's knowledge of self-care, the nurse recognizes that additional instruction is needed when the patient says,
   a. "I use my corticosteroid inhaler when I feel short of breath."
   b. "I get a flu shot every year and see my health care provider if I have an upper respiratory infection."
   c. "I use my bronchodilator inhaler before I visit my aunt who has a cat, but I only visit for a few minutes because of my allergies."
   d. "I walk 30 minutes every day but sometimes I have to use my bronchodilator inhaler before walking to prevent me from getting short of breath."

3. A plan of care for the patient with COPD would include
   a. chronic corticosteroid therapy.
   b. reduction of risk factors for infection.
   c. high flow rate O_2 administration.
   d. lung exercises that involve inhaling longer than exhaling.

4. The effects of cigarette smoking on the respiratory system include
   a. increased proliferation of ciliated cells.
   b. hypertrophy of the alveolar membrane.
   c. destruction of all alveolar macrophages.
   d. hyperplasia of goblet cells and increased production of mucus.

5. One of the most important things that a nurse can teach a patient with emphysema is to
   a. move to a hot, dry climate.
   b. perform chest physiotherapy.
   c. obtain adequate rest in the supine position.
   d. know the early signs of respiratory infection.

6. The major advantage of a Venturi mask is that it can
   a. deliver up to 80% O_2.
   b. provide continuous 100% humidity.
   c. deliver a precise concentration of O_2.
   d. be used while a patient eats and sleeps.

7. Diagnostic studies that the nurse would expect to be abnormal in a person with CF are
   a. insulin tolerance and blood glucose.
   b. pancreatic enzymes and hormones.
   c. sweat test and vitamin B tolerance test.
   d. pulmonary function test and sweat test.

REFERENCES

1. American Lung Association: Data and statistics: prevalence on Revised National Health Interview Survey (on line), 2001. Available at *www.lungusa.org/data* (accessed Mar 20, 2001).
2. American Thoracic Society: Standards for the diagnosis and care of patients with chronic obstructive pulmonary disease, *Am J Respir Crit Care Med* (Suppl) 152:5, 1995.
3. National Institutes of Health: *Highlights of the Expert Panel Report 2: guidelines for the diagnosis and management of asthma,* pub no 97-4051A, 1997, US Department of Health and Human Services.
4. Krishnaswamy G: Treatment strategies for bronchial asthma: an update, *Hosp Pract* 35: 25, 2001.
5. Custovic A et al: Controlling indoor allergens, *Ann Allergy Asthma Immunol* 88:432, 2002.
6. Einarsson O, Wirth JA: Sinopulmonary syndromes, *Clin Pulm Med* 3:199, 1996.
7. Busse W, Lemanske RF: Asthma, *N Engl J Med* 344:350, 2001.
8. Smurthwaite L, Durham SR: Local IgE synthesis in allergic rhinitis and asthma, *Curr Allergy Asthma Rep* 2:231, 2002.
9. Richman E: Asthma diagnosis and management: new severity classifications and therapy alternatives, *Clin Rev* 7:76, 1997.
10. Rodrigo G et al: Heliox for treatment of exacerbations of chronic obstructive pulmonary disease, *Cochrane Database of Systematic Reviews,* 2002.
11. Singer R, Wood-Baker R: Review of the effect of the dosing interval for inhaled corticosteroids in asthma control, *Intern Med J* 32:72, 2002.
12. Janson S, Lazarus SC: Where do leukotriene modifiers fit in asthma management? *Nurse Pract* 27:19, 2002.
13. Milanese M et al: Role of leukotriene receptor antagonists in the management of mild to moderate asthma, *Monaldi Arch Chest Dis* 56:508, 2001.
14. Rodrigo GJ, Rodrigo C: Continuous vs intermittent beta-agonists in the treatment of acute adult asthma: a systematic review with meta-analysis, *Chest* 122:160, 2002.
15. Johansson SG, Haahtela T, O'Byrne PM: Omalizumab and the immune system: an overview of preclinical and clinical data, *Ann Allergy Asthma Immunol* 89:132, 2002.
16. Pope B: Asthma, *Nursing* 32:44, 2002.
17. Togger D, Brenner P: Metered dose inhalers, *Am J Nurs* 101:26, 2001.
18. Barnes PJ: Chronic obstructive pulmonary disease, *Medical Progress* 343:269, 2000.
19. Petty TL: COPD in perspective, *Chest* 121:116S, 2002.
20. Rennard SI: Overview of causes of COPD, *Postgrad Med* 111:28, 2002.
21. Banasik J: Diagnosing alpha₁-antitrypsin deficiency, *Nurse Pract* 26:58, 2001.
*22. Scharnweber K: Alpha₁-antitrypsin deficiency and the impact of nursing interventions and treatment with intravenous therapy, *J Intravenous Nurs* 22:258, 1999.
23. Hall CS, Fein AM: The management of chronic obstructive pulmonary disease in the elderly, *Clin Geriatr* 40:21, 2002.
24. Berry JK, Baum CL:Malnutrition in chronic obstructive pulmonary disease: Adding insult to injury, *AACN Clinical Issues: Advanced Practice in Acute and Critical Care* 12:210, 2001.
25. Stoller JK: Acute exacerbation of chronic obstructive pulmonary disease, *N Engl J Med* 346:998, 2002.
26. Blanchard AR: Treatment of COPD exacerbations: pharmacologic options and modification of risk factors, *Postgrad Med* 111:65, 2002.
27. Doherty DE: Early detection and management of COPD: what you can do to reduce the impact of this disabling disease, *Postgrad Med* 111:51, 2002.
28. Chitkara RK, Sarinas PS: Recent advances in diagnosis and management of chronic bronchitis and emphysema, *Curr Opin Pulmonary Med* 8:126, 2002.
29. Sahn S: Pharmacologic management of patients with COPD, *J COPD Manage* 2:4, 2001.

*Nursing research–based reference.

30. Baroody OS, Mehta KD, Cortez F: Effects of breathing warm humidified air on pulmonary function in asthmatic patients with chronic rhinitis, *Chest* 216:291S, 1999.

31. Petty TL, Casaburi R: Recommendations of the Fifth O_2 Consensus Conference, *Respir Care* 45:957, 2000.

32. Schedel E, Connolly M: Lung volume reduction surgery: a new hope for emphysema patients, *DCCN* 18:28, 1999.

33. National Emphysema Treatment Trial Research Group: Patients at high risk of death after lung-volume-reduction surgery, *N Engl J Med* 345:1075, 2001.

34. Goodfellow LT, Jones M: Bronchial hygiene therapy: from traditional hands-on techniques to modern technological approaches, *Am J Nurs* 102:37, 2002.

*35. McBride S et al: The therapeutic use of music for dyspnea and anxiety in patients with COPD who live at home, *Journal of Holistic Nursing* 17: 229, 1999.

36. Sigmon HD, Grady PA: Increasing nursing research in cystic fibrosis, *Heart Lung* 31:81, 2002.

37. Jaffe A, Bush A: Cystic fibrosis: a review of the decade, *Monaldi Arch Chest Dis* 56:240, 2001.

38. Yu H, Head NE: Persistent infections and immunity in cystic fibrosis, *Frontiers in Bioscience* 7:d442, 2002.

39. Modolell I, Guarner L, Malagelada JR: Digestive system involvement in cystic fibrosis, *Pancreatology* 2:12, 2002.

40. Tombazzi CR, Riely CA: Liver disease in cystic fibrosis, *Revista Medica de Chile* 129:1071, 2001.

41. Smyth A, Walter S: Prophylactic antibiotics for cystic fibrosis, *Cochrane Database of Systematic Reviews* 2, 2000.

42. Griesenbach U, Alton EW: Recent progress in gene therapy for cystic fibrosis, *Current Opinion in Molecular Therapeutics* 3:385, 2001.

---

*Nursing research–based reference.

RESOURCES

Alpha-1 Association
815 Connecticut Avenue NW, Suite 1200
Washington, DC 20006-4004
800-521-3025 or 202-887-1900
Fax: 202-887-1964
www.alpha1.org

American Lung Association
61 Broadway, 6th Floor
New York, NY 10006
212-315-8700
www.lungusa.org

American Thoracic Society
1740 Broadway
New York, NY 10019
212-315-8700
Fax: 212-315-6498
www.thoracic.org

Cystic Fibrosis Foundation
2785 East Desert Inn Road, Suite 240
Las Vegas, NV 89121
702-383-8500
www.cff.org

Global Initiative for Asthma (GINA)
www.ginasthma.com

Global Initiative for Chronic Obstructive Lung Disease (GOLD)
www.goldcopd.com

National Heart, Lung, and Blood Institute (NHLBI)
National Institutes of Health
4733 Bethesda Avenue, Suite 530
Bethesda, MD 20814
301-951-3260
www.nhlbi.nih.gov/index.htm

NHLBI Asthma Management Model System
www.nhlbisupport.com/asthma/index.html

NHLBI Clinical Guidelines
www.nhlbi.nih.gov/guidelines/index.htm

For additional Internet resources, see the website for this book at *http://evolve.elsevier.com/Lewis/medsurg.*

Problems of Oxygenation: Transport

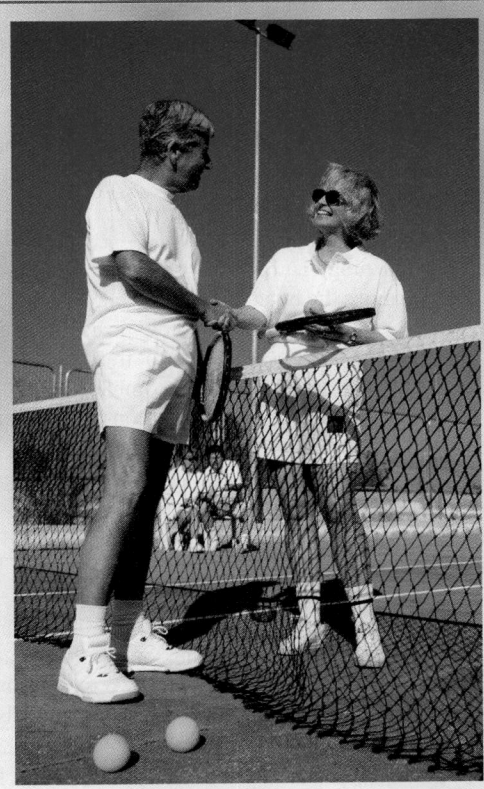

CHAPTER 29

NURSING ASSESSMENT
Hematologic System

Jean Foret Giddens

LEARNING OBJECTIVES

1. Describe the structures and functions of the hematologic system.
2. Differentiate among the different types of blood cells and their functions.
3. Explain the process of hemostasis.
4. Describe the age-related changes in the hematologic system and differences in hematologic studies.
5. Describe the significant subjective and objective assessment data related to the hematologic system that should be obtained from a patient.
6. Describe the appropriate techniques used in the physical assessment of the hematologic system.
7. Differentiate normal from common abnormal findings of a physical assessment of the hematologic system.
8. Describe the purpose, significance of results, and nursing responsibilities related to diagnostic studies of the hematologic system.

KEY TERMS

bone marrow, p. 688
erythrocytes, p. 688
erythropoiesis, p. 689
fibrinolysis, p. 691
hematemesis, p. 695
hematology , p. 688
hematopoiesis, p. 688
hemoglobin, p. 688
hemolysis, p. 690
hemostasis, p. 691

leukocytes, p. 688
leukopenia, p. 700
neutropenia, p. 700
pancytopenia, p. 697
phagocytosis, p. 690
reticulocyte, p. 690
stem cell, p. 688
thrombocytes, p. 688
thrombocytopenia, p. 700

Hematology is the study of blood and blood-forming tissues. This includes the bone marrow, blood, spleen, and lymph system. A basic knowledge of hematology is useful in clinical settings to evaluate the patient's ability to transport oxygen and carbon dioxide, coagulate blood, and combat infections. Assessment of the hematologic system is based on the patient's health history, physical examination, and results of diagnostic studies.

STRUCTURES AND FUNCTIONS OF THE HEMATOLOGIC SYSTEM

Bone Marrow

Blood cell production (**hematopoiesis**) occurs within the bone marrow. **Bone marrow** is the soft material that fills the central core of bones. Although there are two types of bone marrow (yellow and red), it is the red marrow that actively produces blood cells. In the adult, the red marrow is found primarily in the flat and irregular bones, such as the ends of long bones, pelvic bones, vertebrae, sacrum, sternum, ribs, flat cranial bones, and scapulae.

All three types of blood cells (red blood cells [RBCs], white blood cells [WBCs], and platelets) develop from a common hematopoieitic stem cell within the bone marrow. The **stem cell**

is best described as a nondifferentiated immature blood cell found in the bone marrow. As the cells mature and differentiate, several different types of blood cells are formed (Fig. 29-1). The marrow is able to respond to increased demands for various types of blood cells by increasing production.

Blood

Blood is a type of connective tissue that performs three major functions: transportation, regulation, and protection (Table 29-1). The blood is responsible for the *transportation* of oxygen, nutrients, hormones, and waste products around the body. Blood also plays a role in the *regulation* of fluid, electrolyte, and acid-base balance. Finally, the blood has a *protective role* in its ability to coagulate (or clot) and combat infections. There are two major components to blood: plasma and blood cells.

Plasma. Approximately 55% of blood is plasma (Fig. 29-2). Plasma is composed primarily of water, but it also contains proteins, electrolytes, gases, nutrients, and waste. The term *serum* refers to plasma minus its clotting factors.[1] Plasma proteins include albumin, globulin, and fibrinogen.

Blood Cells. About 45% of the blood (see Fig. 29-2) is composed of formed elements, or blood cells. There are three types of blood cells: **erythrocytes** (RBCs), **leukocytes** (WBCs), and **thrombocytes** (platelets). The primary function of erythrocytes is oxygen transportation, whereas the leukocytes are involved in protection of the body from infection. Platelets mainly function to promote blood coagulation.

Erythrocytes. The primary functions of erythrocytes include transport of gases (both oxygen and carbon dioxide) and assistance in maintaining acid-base balance. The composition and features of an erythrocyte are ideal for its gas transportation role. It is a flexible cell with a unique biconcave shape (Fig. 29-3). Flexibility enables the cell to alter its shape so that it can easily pass through tiny capillaries. The cell membrane is very thin to facilitate the diffusion of gases. Erythrocytes are primarily composed of a large molecule called hemoglobin. **Hemoglobin,** a complex protein-iron compound composed of heme (an iron compound) and globin (a simple protein), functions to bind with oxygen and

---

Reviewed by Sandra Rome, RN, MN, OCN, Hematology/Oncology Clinical Nurse Specialist, Cedars-Sinai Medical Center, Torrance, Calif.

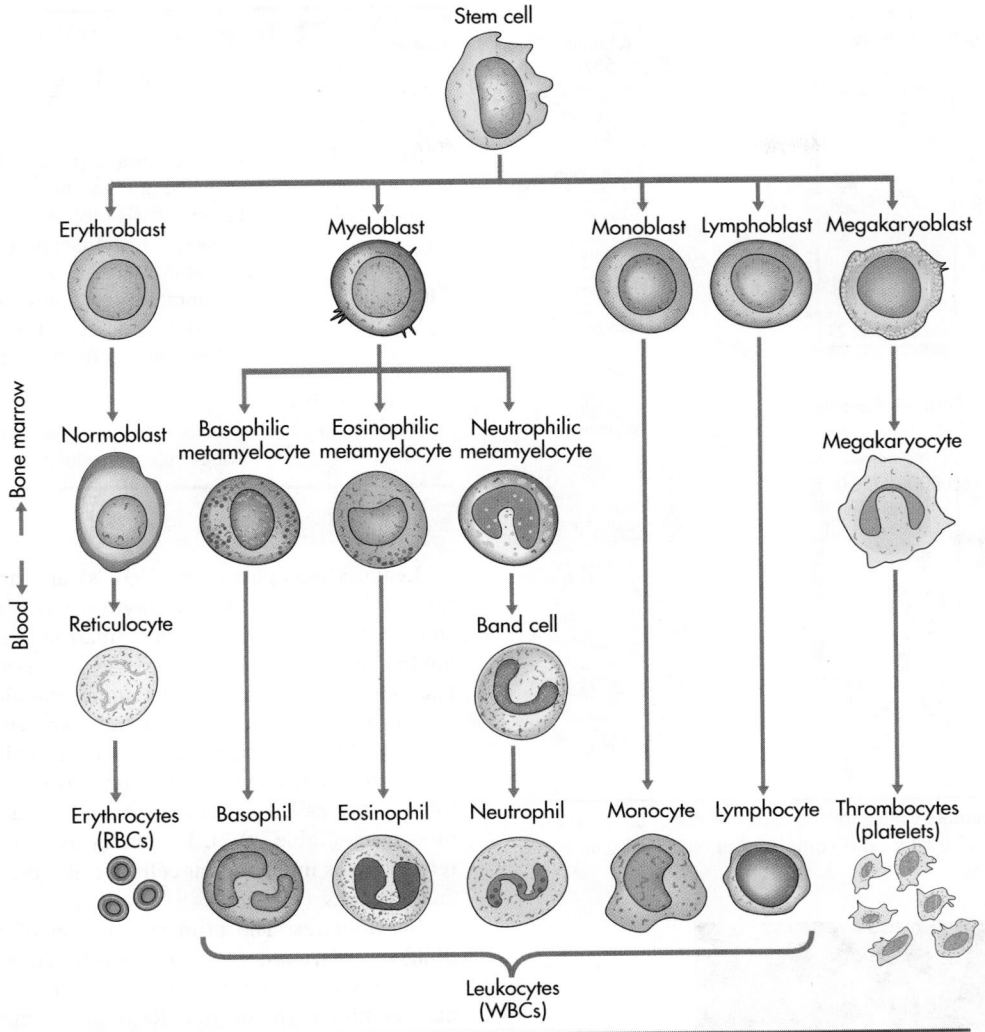

Bone marrow ← → Blood

Stem cell

Erythroblast   **Myeloblast**   **Monoblast** **Lymphoblast** **Megakaryoblast**

Normoblast   **Basophilic** **Eosinophilic** **Neutrophilic**   **Megakaryocyte**
metamyelocyte metamyelocyte metamyelocyte

Reticulocyte   **Band cell**

Erythrocytes **Basophil** **Eosinophil** **Neutrophil** **Monocyte** **Lymphocyte** **Thrombocytes**
(RBCs)   (platelets)

Leukocytes
(WBCs)

FIG. 29-1   Development of blood cells. *RBCs,* Red blood cells; *WBCs,* white blood cells.

carbon dioxide. As erythrocytes circulate through the capillaries surrounding alveoli within the lung, oxygen attaches to the iron on the hemoglobin. The oxygen-bound hemoglobin is referred to as *oxyhemoglobin* and is responsible for giving arterial blood its bright red appearance. As erythrocytes flow to body tissues, oxygen detaches from the hemoglobin and diffuses from the capillary into tissue cells. Carbon dioxide diffuses from tissue cells into the capillary, attaches to the globin portion of hemoglobin, and is transported to the lungs for removal. Hemoglobin also acts as a buffer and plays a role in maintaining acid-base balance. This buffering function is described further in Chapter 16.

Erythropoiesis (the process of RBC production) is regulated by cellular oxygen requirements and general metabolic activity. Erythropoiesis is stimulated by hypoxia and controlled by *erythropoietin,* a hormone synthesized and released by the kidney. Erythropoietin stimulates the bone marrow to increase erythrocyte production. Erythropoiesis is also influenced by the availability of nutrients. Many essential nutrients are necessary for erythropoiesis, including protein, iron, folate (folic acid), cobalamin (vitamin B_{12}), riboflavin (vitamin B_2), and pyridoxine (vitamin B_6).[2]

TABLE 29-1	**Functions of Blood**
FUNCTION	**EXAMPLES**
Transportation	▪ Oxygen from lungs to cells
	▪ Nutrients from gastrointestinal tract to cells
	▪ Hormones from endocrine glands to tissues and cells
	▪ Metabolic waste products (e.g., CO_2, NH_3, urea) from cells to lungs, liver, and kidneys
Protection	▪ Combating invasion of pathogens and other foreign substances
	▪ Maintaining homeostasis of blood coagulation
Regulation	▪ Fluid and electrolyte balance
	▪ Acid-base balance
	▪ Body temperature

Plasma
(percentage by weight)

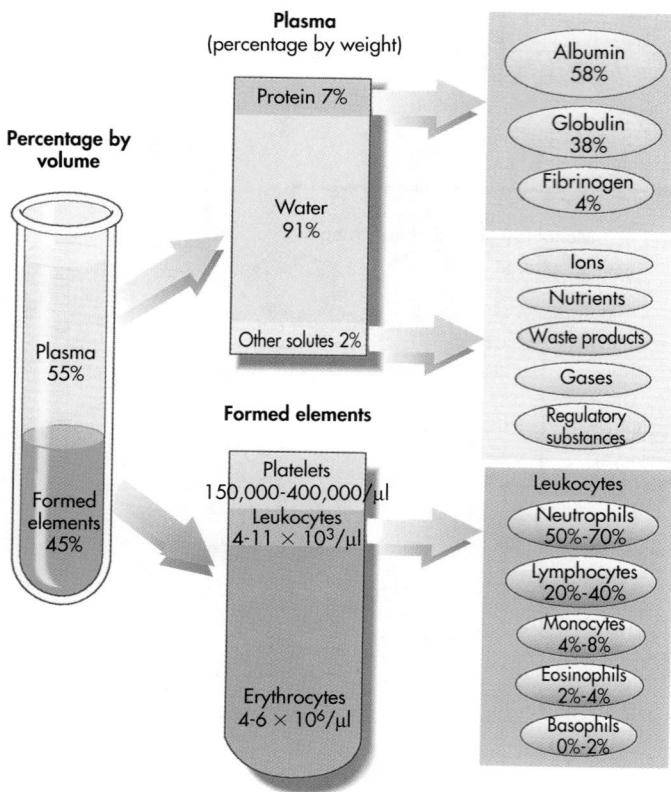

Percentage by volume

Plasma 55%

Formed elements 45%

Protein 7%

Water 91%

Other solutes 2%

Formed elements

Platelets
150,000-400,000/μl

Leukocytes
4-11 × 10³/μl

Erythrocytes
4-6 × 10⁶/μl

Albumin 58%

Globulin 38%

Fibrinogen 4%

Ions

Nutrients

Waste products

Gases

Regulatory substances

Leukocytes

Neutrophils 50%-70%

Lymphocytes 20%-40%

Monocytes 4%-8%

Eosinophils 2%-4%

Basophils 0%-2%

FIG. 29-2 Approximate values for the components of blood in the adult. Normally, 45% of the blood is composed of blood cells, and 55% is composed of plasma.

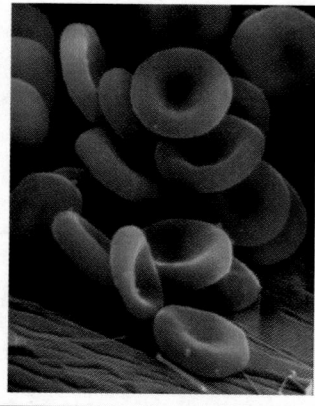

FIG. 29-3 Mature erythrocytes.

Several distinct cell types evolve during erythrocyte maturation (see Fig. 29-1). The **reticulocyte** is an immature erythrocyte. The reticulocyte count measures the rate at which new RBCs appear in the circulation. Reticulocytes can develop into mature erythrocytes within 48 hours of release into circulation. Therefore assessing the number of reticulocytes is a useful means of evaluating the rate and adequacy of erythrocyte production.

Hemolysis (destruction of erythrocytes) by monocytes and macrophages removes abnormal, defective, damaged, and old RBCs from circulation. Hemolysis occurs in the bone marrow, liver, and spleen and results in increased bilirubin. The normal life span of an erythrocyte is 120 days.

TABLE 29-2	**Types and Functions of Leukocytes**
TYPE	**CELL FUNCTION**
Granulocytes	
Neutrophil	Phagocytosis, especially during the early phase of inflammation
Eosinophil	Phagocytosis (not as effective as neutrophil); allergic response; protection from parasitic infections
Basophil	Inflammatory response and allergic response; release of bradykinin, heparin, histamine, serotonin; limited phagocytosis
Agranuloctyes	
Lymphocyte	Cellular and humoral immune response
Monocyte	Phagocytosis; cellular immune response

Leukocytes. Leukocytes (WBCs) appear white when separated from blood. Like the erythrocytes, leukocytes originate from stem cells within the bone marrow (see Fig. 29-1). There are five different types of leukocytes, each of which has a different function. Leukocytes containing granules within the cytoplasm are called *granulocytes* (also known as polymorphonuclear leukocytes) and include neutrophils, basophils, and eosinophils. Leukocytes that do not have granules within the cytoplasm are called *agranulocytes* and include lymphocytes and monocytes (Table 29-2). Lymphocytes and monocytes are also referred to as mononuclear cells because they have only one discrete nucleus.

Granulocytes. The primary function of the granulocytes is **phagocytosis,** a process by which WBCs ingest or engulf any unwanted organism and then digest and kill it. The *neutrophil* is the most common type of granulocyte, accounting for 50% to 70% of all WBCs. Neutrophils are the primary phagocytic cells involved in acute inflammatory responses. A mature neutrophil is called a *segmented neutrophil* or "seg" because the nucleus is segmented into two to five lobes connected by strands. An immature neutrophil is called a *band* (for the band appearance of the nucleus). Although band cells are sometimes found in the peripheral circulation of normal persons and are capable of phagocytosis, the mature neutrophil is much more effective.

Eosinophils account for only 2% to 4% of all WBCs. They have a similar but reduced ability for phagocytosis. One of their primary functions is to engulf antigen-antibody complexes formed during an allergic response. They also are able to defend against parasitic infections. *Basophils* make up less than 2% of all leukocytes. They have a limited role in phagocytosis. These cells have cytoplasmic granules that contain heparin, serotonin, and histamine. If a basophil is stimulated by an antigen or by tissue injury, it will respond by releasing substances within the granules. This is part of the response seen in allergic and inflammatory reactions.

Lymphocytes. Lymphocytes, one of the agranular leukocytes, constitute 20% to 40% of the WBCs. The main function of lymphocytes is related to the immune response (see Chapter 13). Lymphocytes originate from stem cells in the bone marrow and form the basis of the cellular and humoral immune responses. Two lymphocyte subtypes are B cells and T cells. Although T-cell precursors originate in the bone marrow, these cells migrate to the thymus gland for further differentiation into T cells. (Details of lymphocyte function are presented in Chapter 13.)

Monocytes. Monocytes are the other type of agranular leukocytes. These cells account for approximately 4% to 8% of the total WBCs. Monocytes are potent phagocytic cells. They can ingest small or large masses of matter, such as bacteria, dead cells, tissue debris, and old or defective RBCs. Monocytes are the second type of WBCs to arrive at the scene of an injury. These cells are only present in the blood for a short time before they migrate into the tissues and become macrophages.

In addition to macrophages that have differentiated from monocytes, resident macrophages can also be found in tissues. These resident macrophages are given special names (e.g., Kupffer cells in the liver, osteoclasts in the bone, alveolar macrophages in the lung) (see Table 12-5). These macrophages protect the body from pathogens at these entry points and are more phagocytic than monocytes. Macrophages also interact with lymphocytes to facilitate the humoral and cellular immune responses.

Thrombocytes. The primary function of thrombocytes, or *platelets,* is to aid in blood clotting. Platelets must be available in sufficient numbers and must be structurally and metabolically sound for blood clotting to occur. Platelets are also involved in hemostasis. They maintain capillary integrity by working as "plugs" to close any openings in the capillary wall. At the site of any capillary damage, platelet activation is initiated. Increasing numbers of platelets accumulate to form a platelet plug. Platelets are also important in the process of clot shrinkage and retraction.

Platelets, like other blood cells, originate from stem cells within the bone marrow (see Fig. 29-1). The stem cell undergoes differentiation by transforming into a *megakaryocyte,* which produces platelets. Technically, platelets are not actually cells but rather are fragments of megakaryocytes.[3] Platelet production is partly regulated by *thrombopoietin,* a growth factor acting on bone marrow to stimulate platelet production. Typically, platelets only have a life span of 5 to 9 days.

Normal Clotting Mechanisms

Hemostasis is a term used to describe the blood clotting process. This process is important in minimizing blood loss when various body structures are injured. Three components contribute to normal clotting: vascular response, platelet response, and plasma clotting factors.

Vascular Response. When a blood vessel is injured, an immediate local vasoconstrictive response occurs. Vasoconstriction reduces the leakage of blood from the vessel not only by restricting the vessel size but also by pressing the endothelial surfaces together. The latter reaction enhances vessel wall stickiness and maintains closure of the vessel even after the vasoconstriction subsides. Vascular spasm may last for 20 to 30 minutes, allowing time for the platelet response and plasma clotting factors to be activated.

Platelet Response. Platelets are activated when they are exposed to interstitial collagen from an injured blood vessel. Platelets stick to one another and form clumps. The stickiness is termed *adhesiveness,* and the formation of clumps is termed *aggregation* or *agglutination.* When a blood vessel is injured, the circulating platelets are exposed to the collagen from the inner lining of the vessel. This interaction causes the platelets to release substances such as platelet factor 3 and serotonin, which facilitate coagulation. At the same time, platelets release adenosine diphosphate, which increases platelet adhesiveness and aggregation, thereby enhancing the formation of a platelet plug.

In addition to their independent contribution to clotting, platelets also facilitate the reactions of the plasma clotting factors. As Fig. 29-4 shows, platelet lipoproteins stimulate necessary conversions in the clotting process.

Plasma Clotting Factors. The plasma clotting factors are labeled with both names and Roman numerals (Table 29-3). Plasma proteins circulate in inactive forms until stimulated to initiate clotting through one of two pathways, intrinsic or extrinsic. The intrinsic pathway is activated by collagen exposure from endothelial injury when the blood vessel is damaged. The extrinsic pathway is initiated when tissue thromboplastin is released extravascularly from injured tissues.

Regardless of whether clotting is initiated by substances internal or external to the blood vessel, coagulation ultimately follows the same final common pathway of the clotting cascade. Thrombin, in the common pathway, is the most powerful enzyme in the coagulation process (Fig. 29-5). It converts fibrinogen to fibrin, which is an essential component of a blood clot.

Anticoagulants. Just as some blood elements foster coagulation (*procoagulants*), others interfere with clotting (*anticoagulants*). This countermechanism to blood clotting serves to keep blood in its fluid state. Anticoagulation may be achieved by two means, antithrombins and fibrinolysis. As the name implies, antithrombins keep blood fluid by antagonizing thrombin, a powerful coagulant. Endogenous heparin is an example of an anticoagulant.

The second means of maintaining blood in its fluid form is **fibrinolysis,** a process resulting in the dissolution of fibrin. The fibrinolytic system is initiated when plasminogen is activated to plasmin (see Fig. 29-5). Thrombin is one of the substances that can activate the conversion of plasminogen to plasmin, thereby propagating fibrinolysis. The plasmin attacks either fibrin or fibrinogen by splitting the molecules into smaller elements known as *fibrin split products* (FSPs) or *fibrin degradation products* (FDPs). (More information about FSPs can be found in Table 29-9 later in this chapter and in the discussion of disseminated intravascular coagulation in Chapter 30.)

If fibrinolysis is excessive, the patient will be predisposed to bleeding. In such a situation, bleeding results from the destruction of fibrin in platelet plugs or from the anticoagulation effects of increased FSPs. Increased FSPs lead to impaired platelet aggregation, reduced prothrombin, and an inability to stabilize fibrin.

Spleen

Another component of the hematologic system is the spleen, which is located in the upper left quadrant of the abdomen. The functions of the spleen can be classified into the following four general groups:

1. *Hematopoietic function.* The spleen produces RBCs during fetal development.
2. *Filter function.* The splenic structure provides an ideal filter mechanism. For example, the spleen removes old and defective erythrocytes from the circulation by the mononuclear phagocyte system. Another example of filtering involves the reuse of iron. The spleen is able to catabolize hemoglobin released by hemolysis and return the iron component of the hemoglobin to the bone marrow for reuse.
3. *Immune function.* The spleen contains a rich supply of lymphocytes and monocytes.
4. *Storage function.* Approximately 30% of the platelet mass is stored in the spleen.

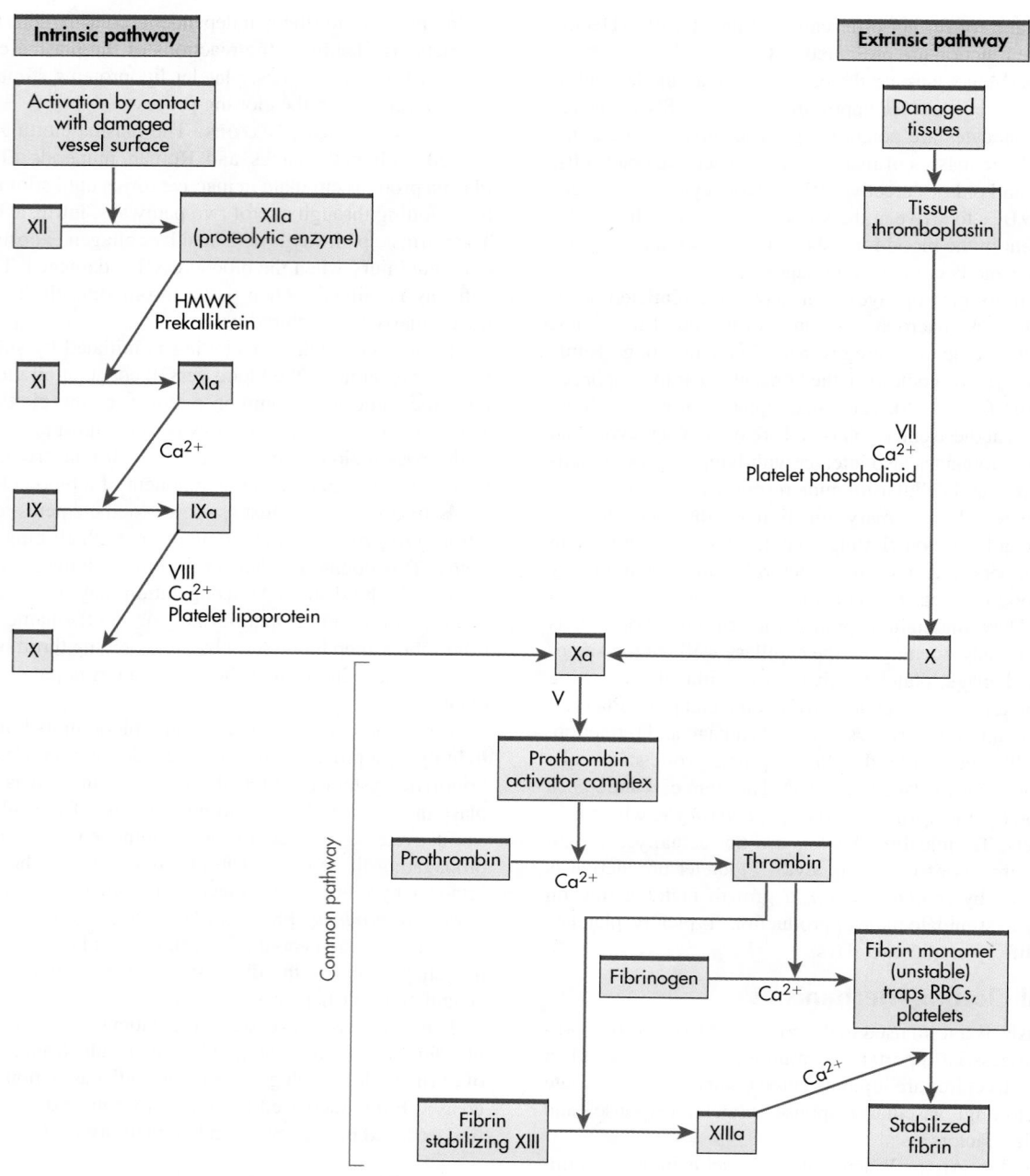

FIG. 29-4 Coagulation mechanism showing steps in the intrinsic pathway and extrinsic pathway as it would occur in the test tube. *HMWK,* High-molecular-weight kininogen; *RBCs,* red blood cells.

Lymph System

The lymph system, consisting of lymph fluid, lymphatic capillaries, ducts, and lymph nodes, carries fluid from the interstitial spaces to the blood. It is by means of the lymph that proteins and fat from the gastrointestinal (GI) tract and certain hormones are able to return to the circulatory system. The lymph system also returns excess interstitial fluid to the blood, which is important in preventing the development of edema.

Lymph fluid is pale yellow interstitial fluid that has diffused through lymphatic capillary walls. It circulates through a special vasculature, much as blood moves through blood vessels. The formation of lymph fluid increases when interstitial fluid increases, thereby forcing more fluid into the lymph system.

When too much interstitial fluid develops or when something interferes with the reabsorption of lymph, lymphedema develops. The lymphedema that may occur as a complication of mastectomy or lumpectomy with dissection of axillary nodes is often caused by the obstruction of lymph flow from the removal of lymph nodes.

The lymphatic capillaries are thin-walled vessels that have an irregular diameter. They are somewhat larger than blood capillaries and do not contain valves. Lymphatic capillaries unite to form lymphatic vessels that carry all lymph fluid to either the right lymphatic duct or the thoracic duct. These large lymphatic ducts drain into subclavian veins in the neck (Fig. 29-6).

TABLE 29-3   Coagulation Factors

COAGULATION FACTOR	NAMES
I	Fibrinogen
II	Prothrombin
III	Thromboplastin
	Thrombokinase
	Tissue factor
IV	Calcium
V	Proaccelerin
	Labile factor
	Ac globulin
VI	Not in use (now obsolete)
VII	Prothrombin conversion accelerator
VIII	Antihemophilic globulin
	Antihemophilic factor
IX	Plasma thromboplastin component
	Antihemophilic factor B
X	Stuart factor
XI	Plasma thromboplastin antecedent
	Antihemophilic factor C
XII	Hageman factor
XIII	Fibrin-stabilizing factor

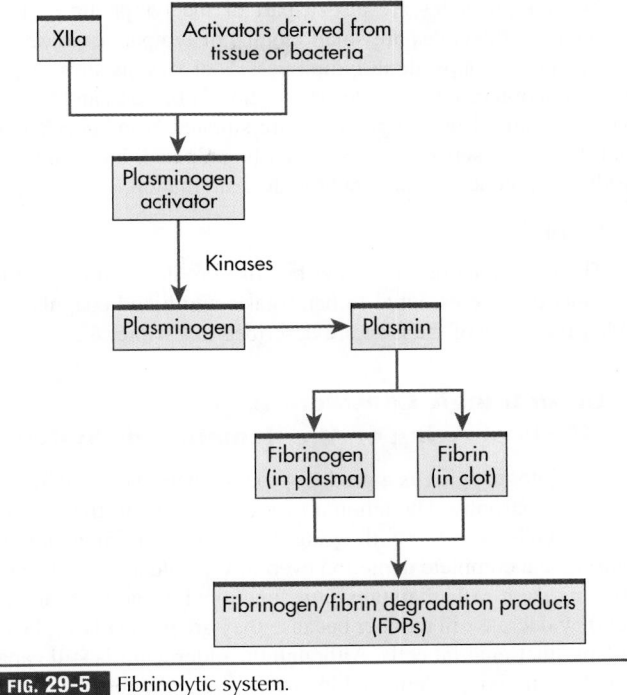

FIG. 29-5 Fibrinolytic system.

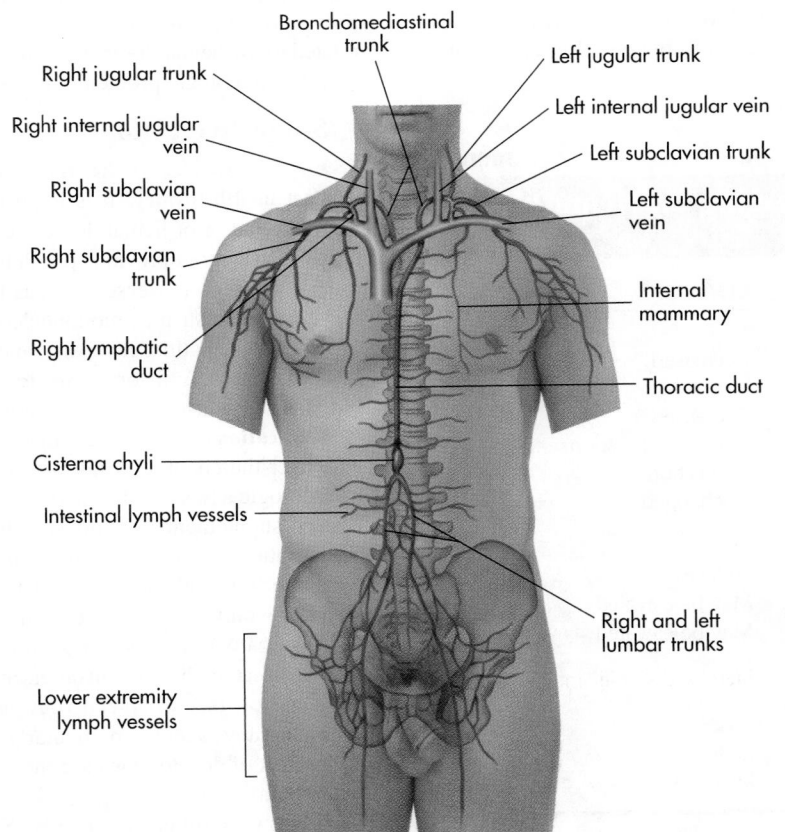

FIG. 29-6 Lymphatic drainage. Lymph fluid drains from tiny lymph vessels. Lymph vessels drain into large lymph ducts. Lymph ducts merge into the venous system at the subclavian veins.

The lymph nodes are also a part of the lymphatic system. Structurally the nodes are small clumps of lymphatic tissue and are found in groups along lymph vessels at various sites. A primary function of lymph nodes is filtration of bacteria and foreign particles carried by lymph. They are situated both superficially and deep. The superficial nodes can be palpated, but evaluation of the deep nodes requires radiologic examination.

Liver

The liver functions as a filter but also produces all the procoagulants that are essential to hemostasis and blood coagulation. Other functions of the liver are described in Chapter 42.

■ Gerontologic Considerations: Effects of Aging on the Hematologic System

Physiologic aging is a gradual process that involves cell loss and organ atrophy. The amount of red marrow and the number of stem cells decrease with aging. However, there does not appear to be a complete depletion even in very old adults.[4] The remaining stem cells maintain their functional capacity to divide, but they decrease in number because they are gradually replaced by nonfunctional fat cells. Although the older adult is still capable of maintaining adequate blood cell levels, the reserve capacity leaves the older adult more vulnerable to possible problems with clotting, oxygen transport, and fighting infection, especially during periods of increased demand. This results in a diminished ability of an older adult to compensate for an acute or chronic illness.[4]

Hemoglobin levels begin to decrease in both men and women after middle age, with the lowest levels seen in older people. Estimates of the prevalence of anemia in the elderly range from a low of 2% among the upper socioeconomic class of independently living elderly to a high of 40% among institutionalized elderly.[5] Although iron deficiency is usually responsible for the low hemoglobin levels, the cause of anemia in many older patients is unknown. Iron absorption is not impaired in the older patient, but adequate nutritional intake of iron may be decreased. It is essential to assess for signs of disease processes such as GI bleeding before concluding that decreased hemoglobin levels are caused solely by aging.

The osmotic fragility of RBCs is increased in the older person, and this may account for the increased mean corpuscular volume (MVC) and the decreased mean corpuscular hemoglobin concentration (MCHC) of RBCs of the older person.

The total WBC count and differential are generally not affected by aging.[4] Leukocyte function is also well preserved. However, during an infection, the older adult may have only a minimal elevation in the total WBC count. These laboratory findings suggest a diminished bone marrow reserve of granulocytes in older adults. Platelets are unaffected by the aging process. However, changes in vascular integrity from aging can manifest as easy bruising.

The effects of aging on hematologic studies are presented in Table 29-4. Immune changes related to aging are presented in Chapter 13. ■

ASSESSMENT OF THE HEMATOLOGIC SYSTEM

Much of the evaluation of the hematologic system is based on a thorough health history. Consequently, the nurse must be knowledgeable about what to include in the health history so that questions may be phrased in a manner eliciting the most information related to the hematologic problem. Key questions to ask a patient with a hematologic problem are presented in Table 29-5.

Subjective Data

Important Health Information

Past health history. It is important to learn whether the patient has had prior hematologic problems. Specifically the nurse needs to ask about previous problems with anemia, bleeding disorders, and blood diseases such as leukemia. Other related medical conditions such as mononucleosis, malabsorption, liver disorders (e.g., hepatitis, cirrhosis), and spleen disorders should also be documented. A history of recurrent infection or problems with blood clotting also important to note.

Medications. A complete medication history of prescription and over-the-counter drugs is an important component of a hematologic assessment. The use of vitamins, herbal products, or dietary supplements should specifically be addressed because many patients may not consider these to be drugs. Many drugs may interfere with normal hematologic function (Table 29-6). Herbal therapy can interfere with clotting (see Complementary and Alternative Therapies box on p. 934). Antineoplastic agents used to treat malignant disorders may cause depression of the bone marrow (see Chapter 15). A patient previously treated with chemotherapy agents, particularly alkylating agents, is at a higher risk of developing a secondary malignancy of leukemia or lymphoma.

Surgery or other treatments. Specific past surgical procedures to ask the patient about include splenectomy, tumor removal, prosthetic heart valve placement, surgical excision of the

TABLE 29-4	*Gerontologic Differences in Assessment* Effects of Aging on Hematologic Studies	
STUDY	**CHANGES**
CBC Studies	
Hb	Decreased
MCV	Increased
MCHC	Decreased
WBC count	Diminished response to infection
Platelets	Unchanged
Clotting Studies	
Partial thromboplastin time	Reduced
Fibrinogen	May be elevated
Factors V, VII, VIII, IX	May be elevated
ESR	Increased significantly
Iron Studies	
Serum iron	Reduced
Total iron–binding capacity	Reduced

CBC, Complete blood count; *ESR,* erythrocyte sedimentation rate; *Hb,* hemoglobin; *MCHC,* mean corpuscular hemoglobin concentration; *MCV,* mean corpuscular volume; *WBC,* white blood cell.

TABLE 29-5 *Health History* **Hematologic System**

Health Perception–Health Management Pattern
- Do you have any difficulty performing daily activities because of a lack of energy?*
- Do you smoke or drink alcohol?*
- Have you ever received a blood transfusion?*
- Is there any family history of anemia, cancer, bleeding, or clotting problems?*
- List the medications you are taking.

Nutritional-Metabolic Pattern
- Do you have any difficulties with eating, chewing, or swallowing?*
- How has your appetite been?
- Do you take any vitamins, nutritional supplements, or iron?*
- Is nausea and vomiting a problem for you?*
- Have you had any unusual bleeding or bruising?*
- Have there been recent changes in the condition of your skin?*
- Have you experienced night sweats or cold intolerance?*
- Have you noticed any swelling in your armpits, neck, or groin?*

Elimination Pattern
- Have you had black or tarry stools?*
- Have you noticed any blood in your urine?*
- Have you had any decrease in urinary output?*
- Do you ever have diarrhea?*

Activity-Exercise Pattern
- Have you experienced excessive fatigue recently?*
- Do you have any shortness of breath at rest? With activity?*
- Do you have any limitations in joint motion?*
- Do you have a problem with unsteady gait?*
- After activity do you ever notice bleeding or bruising?*

Sleep-Rest Pattern
- Do you feel fatigued? Are you more fatigued than usual?*
- Do you feel rested on awakening? If no, explain.

Cognitive-Perceptual Pattern
- Have you experienced any numbness or tingling?*
- Have you had any problems with your vision, hearing, or taste?*
- Have you noticed any changes in your mental functions?*
- Do you have any pain, such as bone, joint, or abdominal pain, or abdominal fullness?*
- Do you have pain when moving your joints?*
- Have your muscles been sore or achy recently?*

Self-Perception–Self-Concept Pattern
- Does your health problem make you feel differently about yourself?*
- Do you have any physical changes that cause you distress?*

Role-Relationship Pattern
- Does your occupation bring you into contact with hazardous substances?*
- Has your present illness caused a change in your roles and relationships?*

Sexuality-Reproductive Pattern
- Has your hematologic problem caused any sexual problems that concern you?*
- Women: When was your last menses? Do you consider your cycle normal? How long does your bleeding usually last? Have you had any increase in cramping or clotting?*
- Men: Do you experience impotence?*

Coping–Stress Tolerance Pattern
- Do you have a support system to assist you when needed?
- What coping strategies do you use during exacerbation of symptoms?

Value-Belief Pattern
- How do you feel about blood transfusions?
- Do you have any conflicts between your planned therapy and your value-belief system?*

*If yes, describe.

---

duodenum (where iron absorption occurs), partial or total gastrectomy (which removes parietal cells, thus reducing intrinsic factor needed for the absorption of cobalamin [vitamin B_{12}]) and ileal resection (where cobalamin absorption takes place). The nurse should also ascertain how wound healing progressed postoperatively and if and when any bleeding problems occurred in relation to the surgery. Wound healing and bleeding should be discussed as responses to past injuries (including minor trauma) and to dental extractions. The number of previous blood transfusions and possible complications during administration should also be determined.

Functional Health Patterns

Health perception–health management pattern. The nurse should ask the patient to describe the usual and present state of health. To assist the patient in maintaining optimal health, it is important to identify the health perceptions, health practices, and preventive practices.

Complete biographic data are needed, including age, sex, race, and ethnic background. There is a known genetic influence in certain hematologic conditions, as well as in other blood diseases that follow familial patterns. For example, sickle cell dis-

ease occurs primarily in African Americans, and pernicious anemia occurs most commonly in persons of Northern European descent. When a family health history is taken, the following health problems should be explored: jaundice, anemia, malignancies, RBC disorders such as sickle cell disease, and bleeding disorders such as hemophilia. The number of previous blood transfusions and possible complications during administration should be determined.

Risk factors such as alcohol and cigarette use that might disrupt the hematologic system must be assessed. Alcohol use must be explored tactfully. Alcohol is a caustic agent to GI mucosa, and damage to the GI tract secondary to alcohol can cause GI bleeding. **Hematemesis** (bright red, brown, or black vomitus) can be a symptom of this problem and should be investigated. Chronic alcohol abusers frequently have vitamin deficiencies. Alcohol also exerts a damaging effect on platelet function and the liver, where clotting factors are produced. Consequently, bleeding problems can develop and should be anticipated in cases of known alcohol abuse.

Nutritional-metabolic pattern. During the patient interview and assessment, the nurse should obtain the patient's weight and

TABLE 29-6 **Drugs Affecting Hematologic Function and Laboratory Values***

DRUG	CLINICAL USE	HEMATOLOGIC EFFECT
aminosalicyclic acid (Pamisyl, PAS)	Antituberculin	Leukocytosis secondary to hypersensitivity
amphotericin B (Fungizone)	Antifungal	Anemia
acetylsalicyclic acid (aspirin) and aspirin-containing compounds (e.g., Empirin, Percodan)	Analgesic, antipyretic, antiinflammatory	Reduced platelet aggregation, prolonged bleeding time
azathioprine (Imuran)	Immunosuppression	Anemia, leukopenia
carbamazepine (Tegretol)	Antiseizure agent	Anemia, leukopenia, thrombocytopenia
chloramphenicol (Chloromycetin)	Antibiotic	Anemia, neutropenia, thrombocytopenia
chlorothiazide (Diuril)	Diuretic	Thrombocytopenia (occasional)
Oral contraceptives and diethylstilbestrol	Birth control, menopausal symptoms, functional uterine bleeding, cancer of prostate	Increase in factors II, V, VII, VIII, IX, X; increase in fibrinogen; increase in thrombin; decrease in prothrombin and partial thromboplastin times; increase in coagulation and thromboemboli formation (overall)
phenytoin (Dilantin)	Antiseizure agent, antiarrhythmic	Anemia
epinephrine (Adrenalin)	Sympathomimetic	Leukocytosis
prednisone	Antiinflammatory	Lymphopenia, neutrophilia
isoniazid (INH)	Antituberculin	Neutropenia
methyldopa (Aldomet)	Antihypertensive	Hemolytic anemia
phenacetin (APC, Empirin compound)	Analgesic, antipyretic	Anemia
phenylbutazone (Butazolidin)	Antiinflammatory	Anemia, leukopenia, neutropenia, thrombocytopenia
procainamide (Pronestyl)	Antiarrhythmic	Agranulocytosis
quinidine sulfate	Antiarrhythmic	Agranulocytosis, anemia, thrombocytopenia
trimethoprim-sulfamethoxazole (Bactrim, Septra)	Antibacterial	Anemia, leukopenia, neutropenia, thrombocytopenia
Antineoplastic agents	Immunosuppression, malignances	Anemia, leukopenia, thrombocytopenia
Nonsteroidal antiinflammatory drugs	Antiinflammatory, analgesic, antipyretic	Inhibition of platelet aggregation

*This represents only a partial listing of drugs affecting the hematologic system.

determine if the patient has experienced any anorexia, nausea, vomiting, or oral discomfort. A dietary history may provide clues about the cause of anemia. Iron, cobalamin, and folic acid are necessary for the development of RBCs. Iron and folic acid deficiencies are associated with inadequate intake of foods such as liver, meat, eggs, whole-grain and enriched breads and cereals, potatoes, leafy green vegetables, dried fruits, legumes, and citrus fruits. Folic acid deficiencies may be offset by a diet including foods that are also high in iron.[6]

Any changes in the skin's texture or color should be explored. The patient should be asked about any bleeding of gum tissue. Any *petechiae* or *ecchymotic* areas on the skin should be noted. If present, the frequency, size, and cause should be documented. The location of petechiae can indicate an accumulation of blood in the skin or mucous membranes. Small vessels leak under pressure, and the platelet numbers are insufficient to stop the bleeding. Petechiae are more likely to occur where clothing constricts the circulation.

The patient should also be questioned about any lumps or swelling in the neck, armpits, or groin. Specifically the patient needs to be asked what the lumps feel like (i.e., hard or soft, tender or nontender) and if they are mobile or fixed. Primary lymph tumors are usually not painful. A nontender swollen lymph node may be a sign of Hodgkin's disease or non-Hodgkin's lymphoma. Lymph nodes that are enlarged and tender are usually as-

sociated with an acute infection.[7] Any incidents of fever should be explored thoroughly. It should be determined if the patient currently has a fever, recurring fevers, chills, or night sweats.

Elimination pattern. The patient should be asked if blood has been noted in the urine or stool or if black, tarry stools have occurred. Also, any decrease in urinary output or diarrhea should be documented.

Activity-exercise pattern. Because fatigue is a prominent symptom in many hematologic disorders, the patient should be asked about feelings of tiredness. Weakness and complaints of heavy extremities should also be determined. Symptoms of apathy, malaise, dyspnea, or palpitations should be documented. Any change in the patient's ability to perform activities of daily living (ADLs) should be noted.

Sleep-rest pattern. The patient's feeling of being rested after a night's sleep should be determined. Fatigue secondary to a hematologic problem often will not be resolved following sleep.

Cognitive-perceptual pattern. *Arthralgia* (joint pain) may be caused by a hematologic problem and should be assessed. Pain in the joint may indicate an autoimmune disorder or may be caused by gout secondary to increased uric acid production as a result of a hematologic malignancy or hemolytic anemia. Aching bones may result from pressure of expanding bone marrow with diseases such as leukemia. *Hemarthrosis* (blood in a joint) occurs in the patient with bleeding disorders and can be painful.

Paresthesias, numbness, and tingling may be related to a hematologic disorder and should be noted. Any changes in vision, hearing, taste, or mental status should also be assessed carefully.

Self-perception–self-concept pattern. The effect of the health problem on the patient's perception of self and personal abilities should be determined. The effect of certain problems, such as bruising, petechiae, and lymph node swelling, on the patient's personal appearance should also be assessed.

Role-relationship pattern. The patient should be questioned about any past or present occupational or household exposures to radiation or chemicals. If such exposure has occurred, the type, amount, and duration of the exposure should be determined.

It is known that a person who has been exposed to radiation, as a treatment modality or by accident, has a higher incidence of certain hematologic problems. The same is true of a person who has been exposed to chemicals (e.g., benzene, lead, naphthalene, phenylbutazone). These chemicals are commonly used by potters, dry cleaners, or individuals involved with occupations that use adhesives. The patient should also be questioned about a history in the military. Many Vietnam War veterans were exposed to dioxin-containing defoliant (Agent Orange), which has been linked with leukemia and lymphoma. The nurse also should assess the effect of the present illness on the patient's usual roles and responsibilities.

Sexuality-reproductive pattern. A careful menstrual history should be obtained from women, including the age at which menarche and menopause began, duration and amount of bleeding, incidence of clotting and cramping, and any associated problems. Any intrapartum or postpartum bleeding problems should also be documented. Men should be asked if they have any problems related to impotence because this is not uncommon in men with hematologic problems. The patient should also be questioned about sexual behavior because human immunodeficiency virus (HIV) infection is potentially a concern, particularly among high-risk groups.[8]

Coping–stress tolerance pattern. The patient with a hematologic problem often needs assistance with ADLs. The patient should be asked if adequate support is available to meet daily needs. The patient's usual methods of handling stress should also be determined. In the patient with platelet disorders or hemophilia, the potential for hemorrhage can be so frightening that usual life patterns may be drastically curtailed, affecting the person's quality of life. The nurse should explore the accuracy of the patient's understanding of the problem.

Value-belief pattern. Some hematologic problems are treated with blood transfusions or a bone marrow transplant. The nurse should determine if these types of treatments cause any conflicts with the patient's value-belief system. The nurse should be aware of a patient's cultural and religious beliefs related to blood and blood transfusions.

Objective Data

Physical Examination. A complete physical examination is necessary to accurately examine all systems that affect or are affected by the hematologic system (see Chapter 3). The nurse must be aware that disorders of the hematologic system can manifest in various ways; thus a patient's presenting symptoms may not immediately point to a hematologic problem[8] (Table 29-7). For example, increasing abdominal girth may be related to an en-

larged spleen, an enlarged liver, or abdominal bleeding. This finding warrants the need for a complete GI examination as part of the physical examination.

Although a full examination should be performed on patients suspected of a hematologic disorder, certain aspects of the physical examination are specifically relevant. These include the skin, lymph nodes, spleen, and liver. Examination of the skin is discussed in Chapter 22; spleen and liver examination is found in Chapter 38.

Lymph nodes are distributed throughout the body. Superficial lymph nodes can be evaluated by light palpation (Fig. 29-7). Deep lymph nodes cannot be palpated and are best evaluated by radiologic examination. Lymph nodes should be assessed symmetrically with regard to location, size (in centimeters), degree of fixation (e.g., movable, fixed), tenderness, and texture. To assess superficial lymph nodes, the examiner should lightly palpate the nodes using the pads of the fingers. The examiner should gently roll the skin over the area and concentrate on feeling for possible lymph node enlargement. Ordinarily, lymph nodes are not palpable in adults. If a node is palpable, it should be small (0.5 to 1 cm), mobile, firm, and nontender to be considered a normal finding. Abnormal findings, warranting further investigation, include any of the following: tender, hard, fixed, or enlarged (regardless if they are tender or not). Tender nodes are usually a result of inflammation, whereas hard or fixed nodes suggest malignancy.[7]

It is important to develop a sequence when examining the lymph nodes. A convenient sequence for examination is to start at the head and neck. First the preauricular, posterior auricular, occipital, tonsillar, submaxillary, submental, superficial cervical, posterior cervical chain, deep cervical chain, and supraclavicular nodes are palpated. Next the axillary lymph nodes and pectoral, subscapular, and lateral groups of nodes are palpated. The epitrochlear nodes, located in the antecubital fossa between the biceps and triceps muscles, are then examined. The inguinal lymph nodes, found in the groin, are palpated last.

DIAGNOSTIC STUDIES OF THE HEMATOLOGIC SYSTEM

The most direct means of evaluating the hematologic system is through laboratory analysis and other diagnostic studies. Repeated acquisition of blood specimens may be distressing for the patient. Some patients may become concerned that the amount of blood withdrawn for tests could lead to adverse effects. Although multiple blood studies may be uncomfortable, it is only in rare situations that diagnostic blood withdrawal predisposes the patient to significant loss of blood. For patients requiring frequent blood studies for several months, a central venous catheter may be recommended for venous access.

Laboratory Studies

Complete Blood Count. The complete blood count (CBC) involves several laboratory tests (Table 29-8), each of which serves to assess the three major blood cells formed in the bone marrow. Although the status of each cell type is important, the entire system may be disrupted by diseases, as well as by treatment of diseases. When the entire CBC is suppressed, a condition termed **pancytopenia** (marked decrease in the number of RBCs, WBCs, and platelets) exists. In such cases the patient needs care directed toward the management of anemia, infection, and hem-

TABLE 29-7 *Common Assessment Abnormalities*

Hematologic System

FINDING	DESCRIPTION	POSSIBLE ETIOLOGY AND SIGNIFICANCE
Skin		
Pallor of skin or nail beds	Paleness; decreased or absence of skin coloration	Low hemoglobin level (anemia)
Flushing	Transient, episodic redness of skin (usually around face and neck)	Increase in hemoglobin (polycythemia), congestion of capillaries
Jaundice	Yellow appearance of skin and mucous membranes	Accumulation of bile pigment caused by rapid or excessive hemolysis or liver damage
Cyanosis	Bluish discoloration of skin and mucous membranes	Reduced hemoglobin, excessive concentration of deoxyhemoglobin in blood
Excoriation	Scratch or abrasion of skin	Scratching from intense pruritus
Pruritus	Unpleasant cutaneous sensation that provokes the desire to rub or scratch the skin	Hodgkin's disease, increased bilirubin
Leg ulcers	Prominent on the malleoli on the ankles	Sickle cell disease
Angioma	Benign tumor consisting of blood or lymph vessels	Most are congenital; some may disappear spontaneously
Telangiectasis	Small angioma with tendency to bleed; focal red lesions, coarse or fine red lines	Dilation of small vessels
Spider nevus	Form of telangiectasis characterized by a round red central portion and branching radiations resembling the profile of a spider; usually develop on face, neck, or chest	Elevated estrogen levels as in pregnancy or liver disease
Purpura	Any of a small group of conditions characterized by ecchymosis or other small hemorrhages in skin and mucous membranes	Decreased platelets or clotting factors resulting in hemorrhage into the skin; vascular abnormalities; break in blood vessel walls resulting from trauma
Petechiae	Pinpoint, nonraised, perfectly round area >2 mm; purple, dark red, or brown	Same as above
Ecchymosis (bruise)	Small hemorrhagic spot, larger than petechiae; nonelevated; round or irregular	Same as above
Hematoma	A localized collection of blood, usually clotted	Same as above
Eyes		
Jaundiced sclera	Yellow appearance of the sclera	Accumulation of bile pigment resulting from rapid or excessive hemolysis or liver disease
Conjunctival pallor	Paleness; decreased or absence of coloration in the conjunctiva	Low hemoglobin level (anemia)
Mouth		
Gingival and mucous membrane changes	Pallor	Low hemoglobin level (anemia)
	Gingival/mucosal ulceration, swelling, or bleeding	Neutropenia; inability of impaired leukocytes to combat oral infections; thrombocytopenia
Smooth tongue	Tongue surface is smooth and shiny; mucosa is thin and red from decreased papillae	Pernicious anemia, iron-deficiency anemia
Lymph Nodes		
Lymphadenopathy	Lymph nodes are enlarged (>1 cm); may be tender to the touch	Infection, foreign infiltrations, or systemic disease such as leukemia, lymphoma, Hodgkin's disease, and metastatic cancer
Heart and Chest		
Tachycardia	Heart rate >100 beats/min	Compensatory mechanism in anemia to increase cardiac output
Sternal tenderness	Abnormal sensitivity to touch or pressure on sternum	Leukemia resulting from increased bone marrow cellularity, causing increase in pressure and bone erosion; multiple myeloma as a result of stretching of periosteum

TABLE 29-7	Common Assessment Abnormalities Hematologic System—cont'd		
FINDING	**DESCRIPTION**		**POSSIBLE ETIOLOGY AND SIGNIFICANCE**
Abdomen			
Hepatomegaly	Palpable liver		Leukemia, cirrhosis, or fibrosis secondary to iron overload from sickle cell disease or thalassemia
Splenomegaly	Palpable spleen		Anemia, thrombocytopenia, leukemia, lymphomas, leukopenia, mononucleosis, malaria, cirrhosis, trauma, portal hypertension
Nervous System			
Paresthesias of feet and hands; ataxia	Numbness sensation and extreme sensitivity experienced in central and peripheral nerves; impaired muscle movement		Cobalamin (vitamin B_{12}) deficiency
Weakness	Lacking physical strength or energy		Low hemoglobin level (anemia)
Musculoskeletal System			
Bone pain	Pain in pelvis, ribs, spine, sternum		Multiple myeloma related to enlarged tumors that stretch periosteum; bone invasion by leukemia cells; bone demineralization resulting from various malignancies; sickle cell disease
Arthralgia	Joint pain		Sickle cell disease from hemarthrosis

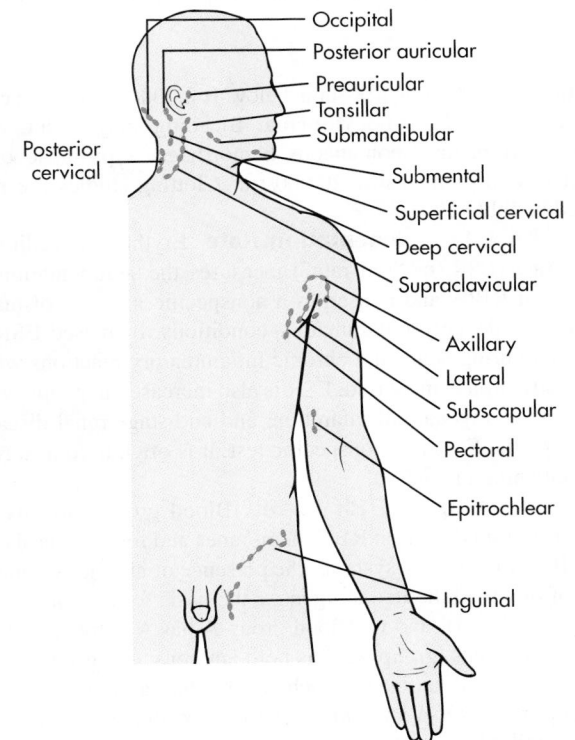

- Occipital
- Posterior auricular
- Preauricular
- Tonsillar
- Submandibular
- Posterior cervical
- Submental
- Superficial cervical
- Deep cervical
- Supraclavicular
- Axillary
- Lateral
- Subscapular
- Pectoral
- Epitrochlear
- Inguinal

FIG. 29-7 Palpable superficial lymph nodes.

orrhage (see Chapter 30). The effects of aging on hematologic studies are presented in Table 29-4.

Red blood cells. Normal values of some RBC tests are reported separately for men and for women because normal values are based on body mass and men usually have a larger body mass than women.

The *hemoglobin (Hb) value* is reduced in cases of anemia, hemorrhage, and states of hemodilution, such as those that occur when the fluid volume is excessive. Increases in hemoglobin are found in polycythemia or in states of hemoconcentration, which can develop from volume depletion (dehydration).

The *hematocrit (Hct) value* is determined by spinning blood in a centrifuge, which causes erythrocytes and plasma to separate. The erythrocytes, being the heavier elements, settle to the bottom. The hematocrit value represents the percentage of RBC compared with the total blood volume. Reductions and elevations of hematocrit value are seen in the same conditions that raise and lower the hemoglobin value. The hematocrit value generally is 3 times the hemoglobin value.

The total RBC count is reported as RBC $\times 10^6/\mu l$. However, total RBC count is not always reliable in determining the adequacy of RBC function. Consequently, other data, such as hemoglobin, hematocrit, and RBC indices, must also be evaluated. The RBC count is altered by the same conditions that raise and lower the hemoglobin and hematocrit values.

RBC indices are special indicators that reflect RBC volume, color, and hemoglobin saturation (see Table 29-8). These parameters may provide insight into the cause of anemia. (The significance of these parameters is discussed further in Chapter 30.)

White blood cells. The WBC count provides two different sets of information. The first is a total count of WBCs in 1 μl of peripheral blood. Elevations in WBC count over 11,000/μl are

TABLE 29-8   Complete Blood Count Studies

STUDY	DESCRIPTION AND PURPOSE	NORMAL VALUES
Hb	Measurement of gas-carrying capacity of RBC	Women: 12-16 g/dl (120-160 g/L) Men: 13.5-18 g/dl (135-180 g/L)
Hct	Measure of packed cell volume of RBC expressed as a percentage of the total blood volume	Women: 38%-47% (0.38-0.47) Men: 40%-54% (0.40-0.54)
Total RBC count	Count of number of circulating RBCs	Women: $4-5 \times 10^6/\mu l$ ($4-5 \times 10^{12}/L$) Men: $4.5-6 \times 10^6/\mu l$ ($4.5-6 \times 10^{12}/L$)
Red cell indices $MCV = \dfrac{Hct \times 10}{RBC \times 10^6}$	Determination of relative size of RBC; low MCV reflection of microcytosis, high MCV reflection of macrocytosis	82-98 fl
$MCH = \dfrac{Hb \times 10}{RBC \times 10^6}$	Measurement of average weight of Hb/RBC; low MCH indication of microcytosis or hypochromia, high MCHC indication of macrocytosis	27-33 pg
$MCHC = \dfrac{Hb}{Hct} \times 100$	Evaluation of RBC saturation with Hb; low MCHC indication of hypochromia, high MCHC evident in spherocytosis	32%-36% (0.32-0.36)
WBC count	Measurement of total number of leukocytes	$4000-11,000/\mu l$ ($4-11 \times 10^9/L$)
WBC differential	Determination of whether each kind of WBC is present in proper proportion, determination of absolute value by multiplying percentage of cell type by total WBC count and dividing by 100	Neutrophils: 50%-70% (0.50-0.70) Eosinophils: 2%-4% (0.02-0.04) Basophils: 0%-2% (0-0.02) Lymphocytes: 20%-40% (0.20-0.40) Monocytes: 4%-8% (0.04-0.08)
Platelet count	Measurement of number of platelets available to maintain platelet clotting functions (not measurement of quality of platelet function)	$150,000-400,000/\mu l$ ($150-400 \times 10^9/L$)

Hb, Hemoglobin; *Hct,* hematocrit; *MCH,* mean corpuscular hemoglobin; *MCHC,* mean corpuscular hemoglobin concentration; *MCV,* mean corpuscular volume; *RBC,* red blood cell; *WBC,* white blood cell.

associated with infection, inflammation, tissue injury or death, and malignancies (e.g., leukemia, lymphoma). A total WBC count less than $4000/\mu l$ (**leukopenia**) is associated with bone marrow depression or some types of leukemia.

The second aspect of the WBC count, the differential count, measures the percentage of each type of leukocyte. The information from the WBC differential provides valuable clues in determining the cause of illness. An important concept related to neutrophil counts is the *shift to the left.* When infections are severe, more granulocytes are released from the bone marrow as a compensatory mechanism. To meet the increased demand, many young, immature polymorphonuclear neutrophils (bands) are released into circulation. The usual laboratory procedure is to report the WBCs in order of maturity, with the less mature forms on the left side of the written report. Consequently, the existence of many immature cells is termed a "shift to the left."

The WBC differential is of considerable significance because it is possible for the total WBC count to remain essentially normal despite a marked change in one type of leukocyte. For example, a patient may have a normal WBC count of $8800/\mu l$ while the differential count may show a relative proportion of lymphocytes to be reduced to 10%. This is an abnormal finding that warrants further investigation.

When the bone marrow does not produce enough neutrophils, neutropenia occurs. **Neutropenia** is a condition associated with a neutrophil count less than 1000 cells/μl; severe neutropenia is associated with a neutrophil count less than 500 cells/μl. Neutropenia results from a number of disease processes, such as leukemia, or from bone marrow depression (see Chapter 30).

Platelet count. The platelet count is the number of platelets per microliter of blood. Normal platelet counts are between 150,000 and $400,000/\mu l$; counts below $100,000/\mu l$ signify a condition termed **thrombocytopenia.** Bleeding may occur with thrombocytopenia. Spontaneous hemorrhage is probable once platelet counts fall below $20,000/\mu l$.[9] Clotting studies are presented in Table 29-9.

Erythrocyte Sedimentation Rate. Erythrocyte sedimentation rate (ESR, or "sed rate") measures the sedimentation or settling of RBCs and is used as a nonspecific measure of many diseases, especially inflammatory conditions. Increased ESR is common during acute and chronic inflammatory reactions when cell destruction is increased. ESR is also increased in people with malignancy, myocardial infarction, and end-stage renal disease. Although the ESR is a nonspecific test, it is often used as a routine screening procedure.

Blood Typing and Rh Factor. Blood group antigens (A and B) are found only on RBC membranes and form the basis for the ABO blood typing system. The presence or absence of one or both of the two inherited antigens is the basis for the four blood groups: A, B, AB, and O. Blood group A has A antigens, group B has B antigens, group AB has both antigens, and group O has neither A nor B antigens. Each person has antibodies in the serum termed *anti-A* and *anti-B* that react with A or B antigens. These antibodies are found when the corresponding antigen is absent from the RBC surface. For example, B antibodies are found in the serum of persons with blood group A (Table 29-10).

Blood reactions based on ABO incompatibilities result from intravascular hemolysis of the RBCs.[9] Erythrocytes *agglutinate* (or clump) when a serum antibody is present to react with the antigens on the RBC membrane. For example, agglutination would occur in the blood of a person with type A blood when blood is transfused from a person with B antigens (i.e., type B or

TABLE 29-9	Clotting Studies	
STUDY	**DESCRIPTION AND PURPOSE**	**NORMAL VALUES**
Platelet count	Count of number of circulating platelets	150,000–400,000/μl
Prothrombin time (PT)	Assessment of extrinsic coagulation by measurement of factors I, II, V, VII, X	12–15 sec
International normalized ratio (INR)	Standardized system of reporting PT based on a reference calibration model and calculated by comparing the patient's PT with a control value	2–3*
Activated partial thrombo-plastin time (APTT)	Assessment of intrinsic coagulation by measuring factors I, II, V, VIII, IX, X, XI, XII; longer with use of heparin	30–45 sec
Automated coagulation time (ACT)	Evaluation of intrinsic coagulation status; more accurate than APTT; used during dialysis, coronary artery bypass procedure, arteriograms	150–180
Thromboplastin generation test (TGT)	Reflection of generation of thromboplastin; if abnormal, second stage done to identify missing coagulation factor	<12 sec (100%)
Bleeding time	Measurement of timed small skin incision bleeds; reflection of ability of small blood vessels to constrict	1–6 min
Thrombin time	Reflection of adequacy of thrombin; prolonged thrombin time indicates that coagulation is inadequate secondary to decreased thrombin activity	8–12 sec
Fibrinogen	Reflection of level of fibrinogen; increase in fibrinogen possible indication of enhancement of fibrin formation, making patient hypercoagulable; decrease in fibrinogen indicates that patient possibly predisposed to bleeding	200–400 mg/dl (2–4 g/L)
Fibrin split products[†]	Reflection of degree of fibrinolysis; reflection of excessive fibrinolysis and pre-disposition to bleed (if present); possible indication of disseminated intravascular coagulation	<10 mg/L
Clot retraction	Reflection of clot shrinkage or retraction from sides of test tube after 24 hours; used to confirm a platelet problem	50%–100% in 24 hr
Capillary fragility test (tourniquet test, Rumpel-Leede test)	Reflection of capillary integrity when positive or negative pressure is applied to various areas of the body; positive test indication of thrombocytopenia, toxic vascular reactions	No petechiae or negative
Protamine sulfate tests	Reflection of presence of fibrin monomer (portion of fibrin remaining after elements that polymerize and stabilize clot detach); positive test indication of predisposition to bleed and possible presence of disseminated intravas-cular coagulation	Negative

*Desired level for anticoagulation regimens.
[†]Also called fibrin degradation products (FDPs).

TABLE 29-10	ABO Blood Group Names and Compatibilities*			
BLOOD GROUP	**RED BLOOD CELL AGGLUTINOGEN(S)**	**SERUM AGGLUTININ(S)**	**COMPATIBLE DONOR BLOOD GROUPS**	**INCOMPATIBLE DONOR BLOOD GROUPS**
A	A	Anti-B	A and O	B and AB
B	B	Anti-A	B and O	A and AB
AB	A and B	Neither	A, B, AB, and O	None
O	Neither (universal donor)	Anti-A and anti-B	O	A, B, and AB

*ABO blood groups are named for the antigen found on the RBCs. Compatibility is based on the antibodies present in the serum.

AB) into the person with type A blood. The anti-B antibodies in the type A blood would react with the B antigens, thus initiating the process that results in RBC hemolysis.

The Rh system is based on a third antigen, D, which is also found on the RBC membrane. Rh-positive persons have the D antigen, whereas Rh-negative persons do not. As a result of transfusion therapy or during childbirth, an Rh-negative person may be exposed to Rh-positive blood. Such exposure results in formation of an antibody, anti-D, which acts against Rh antigens.

(Rh-positive persons normally have no anti-D.) The person is then sensitized to Rh-positive blood, and a second exposure to Rh-positive blood will cause a severe hemolytic reaction. A Coombs test can be used to evaluate the person's Rh status (Table 29-11).

Radiologic Studies

Radiologic studies for the hematology system involve primarily the use of computed tomography (CT) or magnetic resonance imaging (MRI) for evaluating the spleen, liver, and lymph nodes.

TABLE 29-11   Miscellaneous Laboratory Blood Studies

STUDY	DESCRIPTION AND PURPOSE	NORMAL VALUES
ESR	Measurement of sedimentation or settling of RBCs in 1 hr; inflammatory processes cause an alteration in plasma proteins, resulting in aggregation of RBCs and making them heavier; the faster the sedimentation rate, the higher the ESR	Women: 1-20 mm in 1 hr Men: 1-15 mm in 1 hr
Reticulocyte count	Measurement of immature RBCs; reflection of bone marrow activity in producing RBCs	0.5%-1.5% of RBC count (0.005-0.015 of RBC count)
Bilirubin	Measurement of degree of RBC hemolysis or liver's inability to excrete normal quantities of bilirubin; increase in indirect bilirubin with hemolytic problems	Total: 0.2-1.3 mg/dl (3.4-22 μmol/L) Direct: 0.1-0.3 mg/dl (1.7-5.1 μmol/L) Indirect: 0.1-1 mg/dl (1.7-17 μmol/L)
Iron	Reflection of amount of iron combined with proteins in serum; accurate indication of status of iron storage and use	
Serum iron		50-150 μg/dl (9-26.9 μmol/L)
Total iron-binding capacity	Measurement of percentage of saturation of transferrin, a protein that binds iron; evaluation of amount of extra iron that can be carried	250-410 μg/dl (45-73 μmol/L)
Coombs test	Differentiation among types of hemolytic anemias; detection of immune antibodies; detection of Rh factor	
Direct	Detection of antibodies that are attached to RBCs	Negative
Indirect	Detection of antibodies in serum	Negative

ESR, Erythrocyte sedimentation rate.

In the past, lymphangiography with the use of contrast dye was a common procedure used to evaluate deep lymph nodes. CT is now the preferred method to evaluate lymph nodes. Nursing responsibilities related to these studies are presented in Table 29-12.

Biopsies

Biopsy procedures specific to hematologic assessment are bone marrow examination and lymph node biopsy. In general, these procedures are done when a diagnosis cannot be established from a peripheral blood smear or when more information about the possible hematologic problem is needed.

Bone Marrow Examination. Bone marrow examination is important in the evaluation of many hematologic disorders. The examination of the marrow may involve aspiration only or aspiration with biopsy. The benefit gained from bone marrow examination is a full evaluation of hematopoiesis.

The preferred site for both aspiration and biopsy of bone marrow is the posterior iliac crest.[10] In adults, the anterior iliac crest and sternum are alternative sites; however, the sternum is usually used only for aspiration.

Bone marrow aspiration and biopsy are performed by a physician or specially credentialed nurse. Conscious sedation is often used to minimize anxiety and pain that the patient may experience. For bone marrow aspiration, the skin over the puncture site is cleansed with a bactericidal agent. The skin, subcutaneous tissue, and periosteum are infiltrated with a local anesthetic agent. The patient may be uncomfortable when the periosteum is penetrated. Once the area is anesthetized, a bone marrow needle is inserted through the cortex of the bone. The stylet of the needle is then removed, the hub is attached to a 10-ml syringe, and 0.2 to 0.5 ml of the fluid marrow is aspirated (Fig. 29-8). The patient experiences pain with aspiration. Although it lasts for only a few seconds, the pain may be quite uncomfortable. After the marrow aspiration, the needle is removed. Pressure is applied over the aspiration site to ensure hemostasis. If the patient is thrombocytopenic, pressure may be required for 5 to 10 minutes or longer.

If a bone biopsy is required, the preparatory procedure remains the same, but a different needle is used. The needle has a cutting blade that allows a specimen of the bone to be removed. When either a marrow aspirate or a biopsy specimen is acquired, a glass slide is carefully prepared with a thin film of the marrow.

Although complications of bone marrow aspiration are minimal, there is a possibility of penetrating the bone and damaging underlying structures. This hazard is greatest in aspiration procedures involving the sternum.[10] Other complications include hemorrhage (particularly if the patient is thrombocytopenic) and infection (particularly if the patient is leukopenic).[9]

Lymph Node Biopsy. Lymph node biopsy involves obtaining lymph tissue for histologic examination to determine the diagnosis and therapy. This may be accomplished by either an open biopsy or a closed (needle) biopsy. In the *open biopsy procedure*, an incision is made, and the lymph node and surrounding tissue are dissected whenever possible. Care must be taken because neoplastic cells can be disseminated during the biopsy procedure if the scalpel passes through tissues containing cancerous cells. An open biopsy is performed in the operating room using either local or general anesthesia.

A *closed (needle) biopsy* may also be performed to analyze lymph tissue. This procedure is performed by a physician at the bedside or in an outpatient area. Sterile technique is essential throughout the procedure. Nursing personnel must recognize the possibility of insidious bleeding, and direct pressure should be applied to the area after the biopsy procedure to achieve hemostasis. Frequent observations of the site for bleeding and monitoring of vital signs should be done, especially if the platelet count is low. The sterile dressing should be changed as ordered, and the wound should be inspected for healing and infection. It is important to recognize that if the results from a needle biopsy are negative, it may only indicate that the cancer cells were not part of the tissue in the biopsy specimen. However, a positive finding is sufficient evidence for confirming a diagnosis.

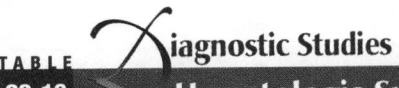

TABLE 29-12   Diagnostic Studies
Hematologic System

STUDY	DESCRIPTION AND PURPOSE	NURSING RESPONSIBILITY
Urine Studies		
• Bence Jones protein	An electrophoretic measurement is used to detect the presence of the Bence Jones protein, which is found in most cases of multiple myeloma. Negative finding is considered normal.	Acquire random urine specimen.
Radioisotope Studies		
• Liver/spleen scan	Radioactive isotope is injected intravenously. Images from the radioactive emissions are used to evaluate the structure of the spleen and liver. Patient is not a source of radioactivity.	No specific nursing responsibilities.
• Bone scan	Same procedure as for the spleen scan except used for evaluating the structure of the bones.	No specific nursing responsibilities.
Radiologic Studies		
• Computed tomography (CT)	Noninvasive radiologic examination using computer-assisted x-ray evaluates the lymph nodes. Contrast medium often is used in abdominal studies of the liver or spleen.	Investigate iodine sensitivity if contrast medium used.
• Magnetic resonance imaging (MRI)	Noninvasive procedure produces sensitive images of soft tissue without using contrast dyes. No ionizing radiation is required. Technique is used to evaluate spleen, liver, and lymph nodes.	Instruct patient to remove all metal objects and ask about any history of surgical insertion of staples, plates, or other metal appliances. Inform patient of need to lie still in small chamber.
Biopsies		
• Bone marrow	Technique involves removal of bone marrow through a locally anesthetized site to evaluate the status of the blood-forming tissue. It is used to diagnose multiple myeloma, all types of leukemia, and some lymphomas and to stage some solid tumors (e.g., breast cancer). It is also done to assess efficacy of leukemic therapy.*	Explain procedure to patient. Obtain signed consent form. Consider preprocedure analgesic administration to enhance patient comfort and cooperation. Apply pressure dressing after procedure. Assess biopsy site for bleeding.
• Lymph node biopsy	Purpose is to obtain lymph tissue for histologic examination to determine diagnosis and therapy.	Explain procedure to patient. Obtain signed consent form. Use sterile technique in dressing changes after procedure. Carefully evaluate wound for healing. Assess patient for complications, especially bleeding and edema.
Open	Test is performed in operating room with direct visualization of the area.	
Closed (needle)	Test is performed at bedside or in office.	
Blood Studies†		

*See Chapter 30.
†See Tables 29-8, 29-9, and 29-11.

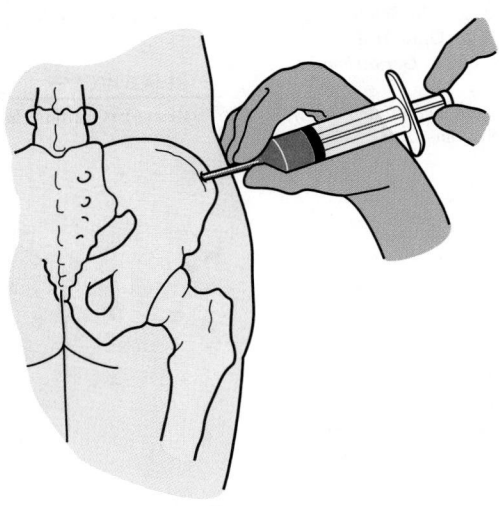

FIG. 29-8   Bone marrow aspiration from the posterior iliac crest.

REVIEW QUESTIONS

The number of the question corresponds to the same-numbered objective at the beginning of the chapter.

1. An individual who lives at a high altitude may normally have an increased RBC count because
   a. high altitudes cause vascular fluid loss, leading to hemoconcentration.
   b. hypoxia caused by decreased atmospheric oxygen stimulates erythropoiesis.
   c. the function of the spleen in removing old erythrocytes is impaired at high altitudes.
   d. impaired production of leukocytes and platelets leads to proportionally higher red cell counts.

2. Disorders such as myeloblastic leukemia that arise from myeloblast cells in the bone marrow will have the primary effect of causing
   a. increased incidence of cancer.
   b. decreased production of antibodies.
   c. decreased phagocytosis of bacteria.
   d. increased allergic and inflammatory reactions.

3. An anticoagulant such as warfarin (Coumadin) that interferes with the production of prothrombin will alter the clotting mechanism during
   a. platelet aggregation.
   b. activation of thrombin.
   c. the release of tissue thromboplastin.
   d. stimulation of factor activation complex.

4. When reviewing laboratory results of an 83-year-old patient with an infection, the nurse would expect to find
   a. minimal leukocytosis.
   b. decreased platelet count.
   c. increased hemoglobin and hematocrit levels.
   d. decreased erythrocyte sedimentation rate (ESR).

5. Significant information obtained from the patient's health history that relates to the hematologic system includes
   a. jaundice.
   b. bladder surgery.
   c. early menopause.
   d. multiple pregnancies.

6. While assessing the lymph nodes, the nurse
   a. applies gentle, firm pressure to deep lymph nodes.
   b. palpates the deep cervical and supraclavicular nodes last.
   c. lightly palpates superficial lymph nodes with the pads of the fingers.
   d. uses the tips of the second, third, and fourth fingers to apply deep palpation.

7. If a lymph node is palpated, which of the following is a normal finding?
   a. firm, mobile nodes.
   b. hard, fixed nodes.
   c. enlarged, tender nodes.
   d. hard, nontender nodes.

8. Immediately following a bone marrow biopsy and aspiration, the nurse should instruct the patient to
   a. expect to receive a blood transfusion.
   b. lie still with a sterile pressure dressing intact.
   c. lie with knees slightly bent and head elevated.
   d. cleanse the site immediately with povidone-iodine.

REFERENCES

1. Thibodeau GA, Patton KT: *The human body in health and disease,* ed 3, St Louis, 2002, Mosby.
2. McCance KL, Huether SE, editors: *Pathophysiology: the biologic basis for disease in adults and children,* ed 4, St Louis, 2002, Mosby.
3. Herlihy B, Maebius NK: *The human body in health and illness,* Philadelphia, 2000, WB Saunders.
4. Lichtman MA, Williams WJ: Hematology in the aged. In Beutler E, editor: *Williams hematology,* ed 6, New York, 2001, McGraw-Hill.
5. Walsh JR: Hematologic problems. In Cassel CK, editor: *Geriatric medicine,* ed 3, New York, 1997, Springer.
6. Grodner M, Anderson SL, DeYoung S: *Foundations and clinical applications of nutrition: a nursing approach,* ed 2, St Louis, 2000, Mosby.
7. Wilson SF, Giddens JF: *Health assessment for nursing practice,* ed 2, St Louis, 2001, Mosby.
8. Beutler E et al: Approach to the patient. In Beutler E, editor: *Williams hematology,* ed 6, New York, 2001, McGraw-Hill.
9. Pagana KD, Pagana TJ: *Mosby's diagnostic and laboratory test reference,* ed 5, 2001, Mosby.
10. Ryan DH: Examination of the marrow. In Beutler E, editor: *Williams hematology,* ed 6, New York, 2001, McGraw-Hill.

RESOURCES

Resources for this chapter are listed in Chapter 30 on pp. 753-754.

CHAPTER 30

NURSING MANAGEMENT
Hematologic Problems

Kathleen J. Jones

LEARNING OBJECTIVES

1. Describe the general clinical manifestations and complications of anemia.
2. Describe the etiologies, clinical manifestations, diagnostic findings, and nursing and collaborative management of iron-deficiency, megaloblastic, and aplastic anemias and anemia of chronic disease.
3. Explain the nursing management of anemia secondary to blood loss.
4. Describe the pathophysiology, clinical manifestations, and nursing and collaborative management of anemia caused by increased erythrocyte destruction, including sickle cell disease and acquired hemolytic anemias.
5. Describe the pathophysiology and nursing and collaborative management of polycythemia.
6. Explain the pathophysiology, clinical manifestations, and nursing and collaborative management of various types of thrombocytopenia.
7. Describe the types, clinical manifestations, diagnostic findings, and nursing and collaborative management of hemophilia and von Willebrand's disease.

8. Explain the pathophysiology, diagnostic findings, and nursing and collaborative management of disseminated intravascular coagulation.
9. Describe the etiology, clinical manifestations, and nursing and collaborative management of neutropenia.
10. Describe the pathophysiology, clinical manifestations, and nursing and collaborative management of myelodysplastic syndrome.
11. Compare and contrast the major types of leukemia regarding distinguishing clinical and laboratory findings.
12. Explain the nursing and collaborative management of acute and chronic leukemias.
13. Compare Hodgkin's disease and non-Hodgkin's lymphomas in terms of clinical manifestations, staging, and nursing and collaborative management.
14. Describe the pathophysiology, clinical manifestations, and nursing and collaborative management of multiple myeloma.
15. Describe the spleen disorders and related collaborative care.
16. Describe the nursing management of the patient receiving transfusions of blood and blood components.

KEY TERMS

anemia, p. 705
aplastic anemia, p. 714
disseminated intravascular coagulation, p. 729
hemochromatosis, p. 719
hemolytic anemia, p. 716
hemophilia, p. 726
Hodgkin's disease, p. 741
iron-deficiency anemia, p. 709
leukemia, p. 735
lymphomas, p. 741
megaloblastic anemias, p. 712

multiple myeloma, p. 744
myelodysplastic syndrome, p. 735
neutropenia, p. 732
non-Hodgkin's lymphomas, p. 742
pernicious anemia, p. 712
polycythemia, p. 720
sickle cell disease, p. 716
thalassemia, p. 711
thrombocytopenia, p. 721

Anemia

Definition and Classification

Anemia is a deficiency in the number of erythrocytes (red blood cells [RBCs]), the quantity of hemoglobin, and/or the volume of packed RBCs (hematocrit). It is a prevalent condition with many diverse causes such as blood loss, impaired production of erythrocytes, or increased destruction of erythrocytes. Because RBCs transport oxygen (O_2), erythrocyte disorders can lead to tissue hypoxia. This hypoxia accounts for many of the signs and symptoms of anemia. Anemia is not a specific disease; it is a manifestation of a pathologic process. Anemia is identified and classified by laboratory diagnosis. Once anemia is identified, further investigation is done to determine its cause.[1]

Anemia can result from primary hematologic problems or can develop as a secondary consequence of defects in other body systems. The various types of anemia can be grouped according to either a *morphologic* (cellular characteristic) or an *etiologic* (underlying cause) classification. Morphologic classification is based on descriptive, objective laboratory information about erythrocyte size and color. (The terms used in this classification system are explained in Chapter 29.) Etiologic classification is related to the clinical conditions causing the anemia, such as decreased erythrocyte

CULTURAL & ETHNIC CONSIDERATIONS
Hematologic Problems

- Sickle cell disease has a high incidence among African Americans.
- Thalassemia has a high incidence among African Americans and people of Mediterranean origin.
- Tay-Sachs disease has the highest incidence in families of Eastern European Jewish origin, especially the Ashkenazi Jews.
- Pernicious anemia has a high incidence among Scandinavians and African Americans.

Reviewed by Sandra Rome, RN, MN, OCN, Hematology/Oncology Clinical Nurse Specialist, Cedars-Sinai Medical Center, Torrance, Calif.

TABLE 30-1	Etiologic Classification of Anemia

Decreased Erythrocyte Production
Decreased Hemoglobin Synthesis
  Iron deficiency
  Thalassemias (decreased globin synthesis)
  Sideroblastic anemia (decreased porphyrin)
Defective DNA Synthesis
  Cobalamin (vitamin B$_{12}$) deficiency
  Folic acid deficiency
Decreased Number of Erythrocyte Precursors
  Aplastic anemia
  Anemia of leukemia and myelodysplasia
  Chronic diseases or disorders
Chemotherapy

Blood Loss
Acute
  Trauma
  Blood vessel rupture
Chronic
  Gastritis
  Menstrual flow
  Hemorrhoids

Increased Erythrocyte Destruction*
Intrinsic
  Abnormal hemoglobin (HbS—sickle cell anemia)
  Enzyme deficiency (G6PD)
  Membrane abnormalities (paroxysmal nocturnal
    hemoglobinuria)
Extrinsic
  Physical trauma (prosthetic heart valves, extracorporeal
    circulation)
  Antibodies (isoimmune and autoimmune)
  Infectious agents and toxins (malaria)

*Hemolytic anemias.
DNA, Deoxyribonucleic acid; *G6PD,* glucose-6-phosphate dehydrogenase;
HbS, hemoglobin S.

TABLE 30-2	Relationship of Morphologic Classification and Etiologies of Anemia

MORPHOLOGY	ETIOLOGY
Normocytic, normochromic (normal size and color)	Acute blood loss, hemolysis, chronic renal disease, chronic disease, cancers, sideroblastic anemia, refractory anemia, diseases of endocrine dysfunction, aplastic anemia, pregnancy
Macrocytic, normochromic (large size, normal color)	Cobalamin (vitamin B$_{12}$) deficiency, folic acid deficiency, liver disease (including effects of alcohol abuse), postsplenectomy
Microcytic, hypochromic (small size, pale color)	Iron-deficiency anemia, thalassemia, lead poisoning

production, blood loss, or increased erythrocyte destruction (Table 30-1). Although the morphologic system is the most accurate means of classifying anemias, it is easier to discuss patient care by focusing on the cause or etiology of the anemia. Table 30-2 relates morphologic classifications to various etiologies.

Clinical Manifestations

The clinical manifestations of anemia are caused by the body's response to tissue hypoxia. Specific manifestations vary depending on the severity of the anemia and the presence of co-existing disease. Hemoglobin (Hb) levels are often used to determine the severity of anemia. Mild states of anemia (Hb 10 to 14 g/dl [100 to 140 g/L]) may exist without causing symptoms. If symptoms develop, it is because the patient has an underlying disease or is experiencing a compensatory response to heavy exercise. Symptoms include palpitations, dyspnea, and diaphoresis. In cases of moderate anemia (Hb 6 to10 g/dl [60 to 100 g/L]), the cardiopulmonary symptoms are increased and the patient may experience them while resting as well as with activity. The patient with severe anemia (Hb less than 6 g/dl [60 g/L]) displays many clinical manifestations involving multiple body systems (Table 30-3).

Integumentary Changes. Integumentary changes include pallor, jaundice, and pruritus. Pallor results from reduced amounts of hemoglobin and reduced blood flow to the skin. Jaundice occurs when hemolysis of RBCs results in an increased concentration of serum bilirubin. Pruritus occurs because of increased serum and skin bile salt concentrations. In addition to the skin, the sclera of the eyes and mucous membranes should be evaluated for jaundice because they reflect the integumentary changes more accurately, especially in a dark-skinned individual.

Cardiopulmonary Manifestations. Cardiopulmonary manifestations of severe anemia result from additional attempts by the heart and lungs to provide adequate amounts of oxygen to the tissues. Cardiac output is maintained by increasing the heart rate and stroke volume. The low viscosity of the blood contributes to the development of systolic murmurs and bruits. In extreme cases or when concomitant heart disease is present, angina pectoris and myocardial infarction (MI) may occur if myocardial O_2 needs cannot be met. Congestive heart failure (CHF), cardiomegaly, pulmonary and systemic congestion, ascites, and peripheral edema may develop if the heart is overworked for an extended period of time.

NURSING MANAGEMENT
ANEMIA

This section discusses general nursing management of anemia. Specific care related to various types of anemia is discussed later in this chapter.

■ Nursing Assessment

Subjective and objective data that should be obtained from a patient with anemia are presented in Table 30-4.

■ Nursing Diagnoses

Nursing diagnoses for the patient with anemia include, but are not limited to, those presented in NCP 30-1.

■ Planning

The overall goals are that the patient with anemia will (1) assume normal activities of daily living, (2) maintain adequate nutrition, and (3) develop no complications related to anemia.

TABLE 30-3   Clinical Manifestations of Anemia

	SEVERITY OF ANEMIA		
BODY SYSTEM	**MILD** (Hb 10-14 g/dl [100-140 g/L])	**MODERATE** (Hb 6-10 g/dl [60-100 g/L])	**SEVERE** (Hb <6 g/dl [<60 g/L])
Integument	None	None	Pallor, jaundice,* pruritus*
Eyes	None	None	Icteric conjunctiva and sclera,* retinal hemorrhage, blurred vision
Mouth	None	None	Glossitis, smooth tongue
Cardiovascular	Palpitations	Increased palpitations	Tachycardia, increased pulse pressure, systolic murmurs, intermittent claudication, angina, CHF, MI
Pulmonary	Exertional dyspnea	Dyspnea	Tachypnea, orthopnea, dyspnea at rest
Neurologic	None	None	Headache, vertigo, irritability, depression, impaired thought processes
Gastrointestinal	None	None	Anorexia, hepatomegaly, splenomegaly, difficulty swallowing, sore mouth
Musculoskeletal	None	None	Bone pain
General	None	Fatigue	Sensitivity to cold, weight loss, lethargy

*Caused by hemolysis.
CHF, Congestive heart failure; *Hb,* hemoglobin; *MI,* myocardial infarction.

TABLE 30-4   Nursing Assessment
Anemia

Subjective Data
Important Health Information
Past health history: Recent blood loss or trauma; chronic liver, endocrine, or renal disease (including dialysis); GI disease (malabsorption syndrome, ulcers, gastritis, or hemorrhoids); inflammatory disorders (especially Crohn's disease); exposure to radiation or chemical toxins (arsenic, lead, benzenes, copper)
Medications: Use of vitamin and iron supplements; aspirin, anticoagulants, oral contraceptives, phenobarbital, penicillins, nonsteroidal antiinflammatory drugs, phenacetin, quinine, quinidine, phenytoin (Dilantin), methyldopa (Aldomet), sulfonamides
Surgery or other treatments: Recent surgery, small bowel resection, gastrectomy, prosthetic heart valves, chemotherapy, radiation therapy.

Functional Health Patterns
Health perception–health management: Family history of anemia; malaise
Nutritional-metabolic: Nausea, vomiting, anorexia, weight loss; dysphagia, dyspepsia, heartburn, night sweats, cold intolerance
Elimination: Hematuria, decreased urinary output; diarrhea, constipation, flatulence, tarry stools, bloody stools
Activity-exercise: Fatigue, muscle weakness and decreased strength; dyspnea, orthopnea, cough, hemoptysis; palpitations; shortness of breath with activity
Cognitive-perceptual: Headache; abdominal, chest, and bone pain; painful tongue; paresthesias of feet and hands; pruritus; disturbances in vision, taste, or hearing; vertigo; hypersensitivity to cold

Sexuality-reproductive: Menorrhagia, metrorrhagia; recent or current pregnancy; male impotence

Objective Data
General
Lethargy, apathy, general lymphadenopathy, fever
Integumentary
Pale skin and mucous membranes; blue, pale white, or icteric sclera; cheilitis; poor skin turgor; brittle, spoon-shaped fingernails; jaundice; petechiae; ecchymoses; nose or gingival bleeding; poor healing; dry, brittle, thinning hair
Respiratory
Tachypnea
Cardiovascular
Tachycardia, systolic murmur, arrhythmias; postural hypotension, widened pulse pressure, bruits (especially carotid); intermittent claudication, ankle edema
Gastrointestinal
Hepatosplenomegaly; glossitis; beefy, red tongue; stomatitis; abdominal distention; anorexic
Neurologic
Confusion, impaired judgment, irritability, ataxia, unsteady gait, paralysis
Possible Findings
↓ RBCs; ↓ Hb; ↓ Hct; ↓ serum iron, ferritin, folate, or cobalamin (vitamin B$_{12}$); heme (guaiac)–positive stools; ↓ serum erythropoietin level

GI, Gastrointestinal; *Hb,* hemoglobin; *Hct,* hematocrit; *RBCs,* red blood cells.

NURSING CARE PLAN 30-1

Patient with Anemia

EXPECTED PATIENT OUTCOMES	NURSING INTERVENTIONS and *RATIONALES*
NURSING DIAGNOSIS	**Activity intolerance** *related to* weakness and malaise *as manifested by* difficulty in tolerating increased activity (e.g., increased pulse, respiration).
• Participation in activities of daily living (e.g., bathing, dressing, grooming, feeding) to greatest extent possible • Vital signs within acceptable range	• Plan care to alternate periods of rest and activity *to provide activity without tiring the patient.* • Strive for a 1:3 rest/activity ratio; assist patient with activities of daily living as needed. • Limit visitors, phone calls, noise, and interruptions by hospital staff *to reduce demands placed on patient.* • Monitor vital signs *to evaluate activity tolerance.* • Monitor hematocrit and hemoglobin *as a guide to planning activities.*
NURSING DIAGNOSIS	**Imbalanced nutrition: less than body requirements** *related to* poor nutritional intake, anorexia, and treatment *as manifested by* weight loss, low serum albumin, decreased iron levels, vitamin deficiencies, below usual body weight.
• Maintenance of body weight, then gradual increase to within range of ideal body weight • Hematocrit, hemoglobin, and serum albumin within normal ranges	• Teach patient about foods high in protein, iron, calories, and other nutrients *to increase intake of essential nutrients needed for hematopoiesis* (see Table 30-5). • With input from patient, establish range of optimal weight outcomes and dietary plan *to involve patient and increase compliance.* • Teach and monitor use of a food diary *to increase patient's awareness of actual intake and increase intake.* • Suggest eating small, frequent meals with snacks throughout the day.
NURSING DIAGNOSIS	**Ineffective therapeutic regimen management** *related to* lack of knowledge about appropriate nutrition and medication regimen *as manifested by* questioning about lifestyle adjustments, diet, medication prescriptions.
• Knowledge about lifestyle changes, nutrition, and medication regimens	• Review and teach patient about nutrition and medication information *to promote compliance.* • Teach about and monitor response to supplemental drugs that aid in red blood cell production *because it is often difficult to correct anemia by diet alone.* • Suggest follow-up resources *to help patient maintain gains and adjustments throughout recovery.*

COLLABORATIVE PROBLEM

NURSING GOALS	NURSING INTERVENTIONS and *RATIONALES*
POTENTIAL COMPLICATION	**Hypoxemia** *related to* decreased hemoglobin.
• Monitor for signs of hypoxemia • Report deviations from acceptable parameter • Carry out appropriate medical and nursing interventions	• Assess for manifestations of hypoxemia such as dyspnea, decrease in O_2 saturation, increase in $PaCO_2$, cyanosis *to initiate early intervention.* • Administer O_2 as ordered *to saturate all available hemoglobin.* • Transfuse with blood products as ordered *to increase red blood cells.* • Monitor hemoglobin *to determine severity of anemia and response to treatment.* • Teach effective breathing exercises and relaxation techniques *to relieve dyspnea and to promote maximum thoracic excursion.*

■ Nursing Implementation

The numerous causes of anemia necessitate different nursing interventions specific to the needs of the patient. Nevertheless, there are certain general components of care for all patients with anemia that are presented in NCP 30-1.

Dietary and lifestyle changes (described with specific types of anemia) can reverse some anemias so that the patient can return to the former state of health. Acute interventions include blood or blood product transfusions, drug therapy (e.g., erythropoietin, vitamin supplements), and oxygen therapy. However, correcting the cause of the anemia is ultimately the goal of therapy. Ongoing assessment of the patient's knowledge regarding adequate

nutritional intake and compliance with drug therapies should be included in the plan of care.[2]

■ Gerontologic Considerations: Anemia

Anemia is common in older adults. The most common form of anemia in older adults is that of chronic disease. Nutritional deficiencies rank second. Physical debilitation and depression among older adults can interfere with their ability to maintain adequate nutrition (Table 30-5).[3] Signs and symptoms of anemia may go unrecognized in the older adult because they may be mis-

TABLE 30-5 Nutritional Therapy

Nutrients Needed for Erythropoiesis

Nutrient	Role in Erythropoiesis	Food Sources
Cobalamin (vitamin B$_{12}$)	RBC maturation	Red meats, especially liver
Folic acid	RBC maturation	Green leafy vegetables, liver, meat, fish, legumes, whole grains
Iron	Hemoglobin synthesis	Liver and muscle meats, eggs, dried fruits, legumes, dark green leafy vegetables, whole-grain and enriched bread and cereals, potatoes
Vitamin B$_6$	Hemoglobin synthesis	Meats (especially pork and liver), wheat germ, legumes, potatoes, cornmeal, bananas
Amino acids	Synthesis of nucleoproteins	Eggs, meat, milk and milk products (cheese, ice cream), poultry, fish, legumes, nuts
Vitamin C	Conversion of folic acid to its active forms, aids in iron absorption	Citrus fruits, leafy green vegetables, strawberries, cantaloupe

RBC, Red blood cell.

taken for normal aging changes. These symptoms include pallor, confusion, ataxia, fatigue, worsening angina, and CHF. Multiple comorbid conditions in older adults increase the likelihood of occurrence of many types of anemia. The nurse plays a major role in providing appropriate health assessment and related interventions for the older adult.[4] ■

Anemia Caused by Decreased Erythrocyte Production

Normally RBC production (termed *erythropoiesis*) is in equilibrium with RBC destruction and loss. This balance ensures that an adequate number of erythrocytes are available at all times. The normal life span of an RBC is 120 days. Three alterations in erythropoiesis may occur that decrease RBC production: (1) decreased hemoglobin synthesis may lead to iron-deficiency anemia, thalassemia, and sideroblastic anemia; (2) defective DNA synthesis in RBCs (e.g., cobalamin [vitamin B$_{12}$] deficiency, folic acid deficiency) may lead to megaloblastic anemias; and (3) diminished availability of erythrocyte precursors may result in aplastic anemia and anemia of chronic disease (see Table 30-1).

IRON-DEFICIENCY ANEMIA

Iron-deficiency anemia, one of the most common chronic hematologic disorders, is found in 30% of the world's population. In the United States, those most susceptible to iron-deficiency anemia are the very young, those on poor diets, and women in their reproductive years.[5]

Iron is present in all RBCs as heme in hemoglobin and in a stored form. The heme in hemoglobin accounts for two thirds of the body's iron. The other one third of iron is stored as ferritin and hemosiderin in the bone marrow, spleen, liver, and macrophages. Normally, 1 mg of iron is lost daily through feces, sweat, and urine. When the stored iron is not replaced, hemoglobin production is reduced.

Etiology

Iron deficiency may develop from inadequate dietary intake, malabsorption, blood loss, or hemolysis. Iron is obtained from food and dietary supplements. Approximately 1 mg of every 10 to 20 mg of iron ingested is absorbed in the duodenum. Therefore only 5% to 10% of ingested iron is absorbed. This amount of dietary iron is adequate to meet the needs of men and older women, but it may be inadequate for those individuals who have higher iron needs (e.g., menstruating or pregnant women). Table 30-5 lists nutrients needed for erythropoiesis.

Malabsorption of iron may occur after certain types of gastrointestinal (GI) surgery and in malabsorption syndromes. Iron absorption occurs in the duodenum. Surgical procedures may involve removal or bypass of the duodenum (see Chapter 40). Malabsorption syndromes may involve disease of the duodenum in which the absorption surface is altered or destroyed.

Blood loss is a major cause of iron deficiency in adults. Two milliliters of whole blood contain 1 mg of iron. The major sources of chronic blood loss are from the GI and genitourinary (GU) systems. GI bleeding is often not apparent and therefore may exist for a considerable time before the problem is identified. Loss of 50 to 75 ml of blood from the upper GI tract is required for stools to appear black (*melena*). The black color results from the iron in the RBCs. Common causes of GI blood loss are peptic ulcer, gastritis, esophagitis, diverticuli, hemorrhoids, and neoplasia. GU blood loss occurs primarily from menstrual bleeding. The average monthly menstrual blood loss is about 45 ml and causes the loss of about 22 mg of iron. Postmenopausal bleeding can contribute to anemia in a susceptible older woman.

Pregnancy contributes to iron deficiency because of the diversion of iron to the fetus for erythropoiesis, blood loss at delivery, and lactation. In addition to anemia of chronic renal failure, dialysis treatment may induce iron-deficiency anemia because of the blood lost in the dialysis equipment and frequent blood sampling.

Clinical Manifestations

In the early course of iron-deficiency anemia, the patient may be free of symptoms. As the disease becomes chronic, any of the general manifestations of anemia may develop (see Table 30-3). In addition, specific clinical symptoms may occur related to iron-deficiency anemia. Pallor is the most common finding, and *glossitis* (inflammation of the tongue) is the second most common; another finding is *cheilitis* (inflammation of the lips). In addition, the patient may report headache, paresthesias, and a burning sensation of the tongue, all of which are caused by lack of iron in the tissues.

Diagnostic Studies

Laboratory abnormalities characteristic of iron-deficiency anemia are presented in Table 30-6. Other diagnostic studies are done to determine the cause of the iron deficiency (e.g., stool

TABLE 30-6   Laboratory Study Findings in Anemias

	IRON DEFICIENCY	THALASSEMIA MAJOR	COBALAMIN (VITAMIN B₁₂) DEFICIENCY	FOLIC ACID DEFICIENCY	APLASTIC ANEMIA	CHRONIC DISEASE	ACUTE BLOOD LOSS	CHRONIC BLOOD LOSS	SICKLE CELL ANEMIA	HEMOLYTIC ANEMIA
Hb/Hct	↓	↓	↓	↓	↓	↓	↓	↓	↓	↓
MCV	↓	N	↑	↑	N	N	N	↓	N	N
MCH	↓	N	N or slight ↓	N or slight ↓	N	N	N	↓	N	N
MCHC	↓	N	↑	↑	N	N	N	↓	N	N
Reticulocytes	N or ↓	↑	↓	N	↓	↓	N	N or ↑	↑	↑
Serum iron	↓	↑	N	N	±N	↓	N	↓	N to ↑	↑
TIBC	↑	↑	N	N	±N	±N	N	N to ↓	N to ↓	↓
Bilirubin	N to ↓	↑	N	N	N	↑	N	N to ↑	↑	N to ↑
Platelets	N or ↑	—	↓	—	↓	—	—	—	—	—
Other findings	—	—	↓ Cobalamin, positive Schilling test, achlorhydria	↓ Folate	↓ WBC	—	—	—	—	—

MCH, Mean corpuscular hemoglobin; MCHC, mean corpuscular hemoglobin concentration; MCV, mean corpuscular volume; N, normal; TIBC, total iron-binding capacity; WBC, white blood cell.

guaiac test). Endoscopy and colonoscopy may be used to detect GI bleeding.

Collaborative Care

The main goal of collaborative care of iron-deficiency anemia is to treat the underlying disease that is causing reduced intake (e.g., malnutrition, alcoholism) or absorption of iron. In addition, efforts are directed toward replacing iron (Table 30-7). This may be done through increasing the intake of iron. The patient should be taught which foods are good sources of iron (see Table 30-5). If nutrition is already adequate, increasing iron intake by dietary means may not be practical. Consequently, oral or occasionally parenteral iron supplements are used. If the iron deficiency is from acute blood loss, the patient may require a transfusion of packed RBCs.

Drug Therapy. Oral iron should be used whenever possible because it is inexpensive and convenient. Many iron preparations are available. The following five factors should be considered in the administration of iron:

1. Iron is absorbed best from the duodenum and proximal jejunum. Therefore enteric coated or sustained release capsules, which release iron farther down in the GI tract, are counterproductive and expensive.
2. The daily dosage should provide 150 to 200 mg of elemental iron. This can be ingested in three or four daily doses, with each tablet or capsule of the iron preparation containing between 50 and 100 mg of iron (e.g., a 300 mg tablet of ferrous sulfate contains 60 mg of elemental iron).
3. Iron is best absorbed as ferrous sulfate (Fe^{2+}) in an acidic environment. For this reason and to avoid binding the iron with food, iron should be taken about an hour before meals, when the duodenal mucosa is most acidic. Taking iron with vitamin C (ascorbic acid) or orange juice, which contains ascorbic acid, also enhances iron absorption. Gastric side effects, however, may necessitate ingesting iron with meals.
4. Undiluted liquid iron may stain the patient's teeth; therefore it should be diluted and ingested through a straw.

5. GI side effects of iron administration may occur, including heartburn, constipation, and diarrhea. If side effects develop, the dose and type of iron supplement may be adjusted. For example, many individuals who need supplemental iron cannot tolerate ferrous sulfate because of the effects of the sulfate base. However, ferrous gluconate may be an acceptable substitute. All patients should know that the use of iron preparations will cause their stools to become black because the GI tract excretes excess iron. Constipation is common, and the patient should be started on stool softeners and laxatives when started on iron.

In some situations, it may be necessary to administer iron parenterally. Parenteral use of iron is indicated for malabsorption, intolerance of oral iron, a need for iron beyond oral limits, or poor patient compliance in taking the oral preparations of iron. Parenteral iron can be given intramuscularly (IM) or intravenously (IV). The most generally available parenteral iron preparation in the United States is an iron-dextran complex (Infed), which contains 50 mg/ml of elemental iron in 2 ml.

Because IM iron solutions may stain the skin, separate needles should be used for withdrawing the solution and for injecting the medication. Approximately 0.5 ml of air should be left in the syringe to clear the iron completely from the syringe. Iron should be given deep IM in the upper outer quadrant of the buttocks, with a 2- to 3-inch, 19- to 20-gauge needle. Preferably, no more than 2 ml of iron is given in a single injection. A Z-track technique should be used for injection to prevent leakage of the iron solution to the subcutaneous (SQ) tissue. The site should not be massaged after the injection is given. IV administration of iron dextran should not be mixed with other medications or added to parenteral nutrition solutions. It should be given undiluted and at a rate of no more than 1 ml/min. The IV line should be flushed with normal saline.

NURSING MANAGEMENT
IRON-DEFICIENCY ANEMIA

It is important to recognize groups of individuals who are at an increased risk for the development of iron-deficiency anemia. These include premenopausal and pregnant women, persons from low socioeconomic backgrounds, older adults, and individuals experiencing blood loss. Diet teaching, with an emphasis on foods high in iron, is important for these groups. Supplemental iron is especially important for the pregnant woman. Appropriate nursing measures are presented in NCP 30-1. It is important to discuss with the patient the need for diagnostic studies to identify the cause. The hemoglobin and RBC counts are reassessed to evaluate the response to therapy. Compliance with dietary and drug therapy is emphasized. To replenish the body's iron stores, the patient needs to continue to take iron therapy for 2 to 3 months after the hemoglobin level returns to normal. Patients who require lifelong iron supplementation should be monitored for potential liver problems related to the iron storage.

THALASSEMIA

Etiology

Another cause of decreased erythrocyte production is thalassemia. **Thalassemia** is an autosomal recessive genetic disorder of inadequate production of normal hemoglobin. Hemolysis also

TABLE	Collaborative Care
30-7	**Iron-Deficiency Anemia**

Diagnostic
History and physical examination
Hct and Hb levels
RBC count, including morphology
Reticulocyte count
Serum iron
Serum ferritin
Total iron-binding capacity
Stool examination for occult blood

Collaborative Therapy
Identification and treatment of underlying cause
Ferrous sulfate or ferrous gluconate
Iron dextran IM or IV
Diet rich in foods containing iron
Nutritional therapy (see Table 30-5)
Transfusion of packed RBCs (symptomatic patient only)

Hb, Hemoglobin; *Hct,* hematocrit; *IM,* intramuscular; *IV,* intravenous; *RBC,* red blood cell.

occurs in thalassemia, but insufficient production of normal Hb is the predominant problem. In contrast to iron-deficiency anemia, in which heme synthesis is the problem, thalassemia involves a problem with the globulin protein. Therefore the basic defect of thalassemia is abnormal Hb synthesis.

Thalassemia is commonly found in members of ethnic groups whose origins are near the Mediterranean Sea and equatorial or near-equatorial regions of Asia and Africa. An individual with thalassemia may have a heterozygous or homozygous form of the disease. A person who is heterozygous has one thalassemic gene and one normal gene and is said to have *thalassemia minor* (or thalassemic trait), which is a mild form of the disease. A homozygous person has two thalassemic genes, causing a severe condition known as *thalassemia major.*

Clinical Manifestations

The patient with thalassemia minor is frequently asymptomatic. The patient has mild to moderate anemia with *microcytosis* (small cells) and *hypochromia* (pale cells). Occasionally, splenomegaly may develop in this patient, and mild jaundice may occur if malformed erythrocytes are rapidly hemolyzed. Thalassemia major is a life-threatening disease in which growth, both physical and mental, is often retarded. The person who has thalassemia major is pale and displays other general symptoms of anemia (see Table 30-3). The symptoms develop in childhood and can cause growth and development deficits. In addition, the person has pronounced splenomegaly and hepatomegaly. Jaundice from RBC hemolysis is prominent. Chronic bone marrow hyperplasia leads to expansion of the marrow space. This may cause thickening of the cranium and maxillary cavity, leading to an appearance resembling Down syndrome.

Collaborative Care

The laboratory abnormalities of thalassemia major are summarized in Table 30-6. No specific drug or diet therapies are effective in treating thalassemia. Thalassemia minor requires no treatment because the body adapts to the reduction of normal hemoglobin. The symptoms of thalassemia major are managed with blood transfusions in conjunction with IV deferoxamine (Desferal) (a chelating agent that binds to iron) to reduce the iron overloading that sometimes occurs with chronic transfusion therapy. Transfusions are administered to keep the Hb level at approximately 10 g/dl (100 g/L). This level is low enough to foster the patient's own erythropoiesis without enlarging the spleen. Because RBCs are sequestered in the enlarged spleen, thalassemia may be treated by splenectomy. However, even with therapy, the person with thalassemia major will experience growth failure, hemochromatosis, and cardiac failure that is often fatal.[6]

MEGALOBLASTIC ANEMIAS

Megaloblastic anemias are a group of disorders caused by impaired DNA synthesis and characterized by the presence of large RBCs. When DNA synthesis is impaired, defective RBC maturation results. The RBCs are large (macrocytic) and abnormal and are referred to as *megaloblasts*. Macrocytic RBCs are easily destroyed because they have fragile cell membranes. Although the overwhelming majority of megaloblastic anemias result from cobalamin (vitamin B$_{12}$) and folic acid deficiencies, this type of RBC deformity can also occur from suppression of DNA synthesis by drugs, from inborn errors of cobalamin and folic

TABLE 30-8	Classification of Megaloblastic Anemias

Cobalamin (Vitamin B$_{12}$) Deficiency
Dietary deficiency
Deficiency of gastric intrinsic factor
   Pernicious anemia
   Gastrectomy
Intestinal malabsorption
Increased requirement

Folic Acid Deficiency
Dietary deficiency
Impaired absorption
Increased requirement

Drug-Induced Suppression of DNA Synthesis
Folate antagonists
Metabolic inhibitors
Alkylating agents

Inborn Errors
Defective folate metabolism
Defective transport of cobalamin

Erythroleukemia

acid metabolism, and from *erythroleukemia* (malignant blood disorder characterized by a proliferation of erythropoietic cells in bone marrow). Two common forms of megaloblastic anemia are cobalamin deficiency and folic acid deficiency (Table 30-8).

COBALAMIN DEFICIENCY

Normally, a protein termed *intrinsic factor* (IF) is secreted by the parietal cells of the gastric mucosa. IF is required for cobalamin (extrinsic factor) absorption. Therefore if IF is not secreted, cobalamin will not be absorbed. (Cobalamin is normally absorbed in the distal ileum.) There are many causes of cobalamin deficiency. The most common cause is pernicious anemia. The term **pernicious anemia** has been used incorrectly to describe any cobalamin deficiency. However, it is actually only one cause of cobalamin deficiency. The term should only be used to describe situations in which the gastric mucosa is not secreting IF. Other causes of cobalamin deficiency include nutritional deficiency and hereditary enzymatic defects of cobalamin utilization (see Table 30-8).

Pernicious anemia is a disease of insidious onset that begins in middle age or later (usually after age 40) with 60 years being the most common age at diagnosis. Pernicious anemia occurs frequently in persons of Northern European ancestry (particularly Scandinavians) and African Americans. In African Americans, the disease tends to begin early, occurs with higher frequency in women, and is often severe.

Etiology

Pernicious anemia is caused by an absence of IF, from either gastric mucosal atrophy or autoimmune destruction of parietal cells. This results in a decrease of hydrochloric acid secretion by the stomach. An acid environment in the stomach is required for the secretion of IF.

Cobalamin deficiency can occur in patients who have had GI surgery such as gastrectomy; patients who have had a small bowel resection involving the ileum; and patients with Crohn's disease, ileitis, diverticuli of the small intestine, and/or chronic atrophic gastritis. In these cases, cobalamin deficiency results from the loss of IF-secreting gastric mucosal cells or impaired absorption of cobalamin in the distal ileum. Cobalamin deficiency is also found in long-term users of H_2-histamine receptor blockers.

Clinical Manifestations

General symptoms of anemia related to cobalamin deficiency develop because of tissue hypoxia (see Table 30-3). GI manifestations include a sore tongue, anorexia, nausea, vomiting, and abdominal pain. Typical neuromuscular manifestations include weakness, paresthesias of the feet and hands, reduced vibratory and position senses, ataxia, muscle weakness, and impaired thought processes ranging from confusion to dementia. Because cobalamin deficiency–related anemia has an insidious onset, it may take several months for these manifestations to develop.

Diagnostic Studies

Laboratory data reflective of cobalamin deficiency anemia are presented in Table 30-6. The RBCs appear large (macrocytic) and have abnormal shapes. This structure contributes to erythrocyte destruction because the cell membrane is fragile. Serum cobalamin levels are reduced. Serum folate levels are also obtained. If they are normal and cobalamin levels are low, it suggests that megaloblastic anemia is due to a cobalamin deficiency. Because the potential for gastric cancer is increased in patients with pernicious anemia, a gastroscopy and biopsy of the gastric mucosa may also be done.

Another means of assessing parietal cell function is by a Schilling test. After radioactive cobalamin is administered to the patient, the amount of cobalamin excreted in the urine is measured. An individual who cannot absorb cobalamin excretes only a small amount of this radioactive form. The same procedure may be followed with the parenteral administration of IF. Absorption of cobalamin when IF is added is diagnostic of pernicious anemia.

Collaborative Care

Regardless of how much is ingested, the patient is not able to absorb cobalamin if intrinsic factor is lacking or if there is impaired absorption in the ileum. For this reason, increasing dietary cobalamin does not correct the anemia. However, the patient should be instructed on adequate dietary intake to maintain good nutrition (see Table 30-6). Parenteral administration of cobalamin (cyanocobalamin or hydroxocobalamin) is the treatment of choice. Without cobalamin administration, these individuals will die in 1 to 3 years. The efficacy of cobalamin injections in altering the otherwise fatal course cannot be overemphasized. The dosage and frequency of cobalamin administration may vary. A typical treatment schedule consists of 1000 mg of cobalamin IM daily for 2 weeks and then weekly until the hematocrit is normal, then monthly for life. An intranasal form of cyanocobalamin (Nascobal) is now available. It is a nasal gel that is self-administered once weekly. High-dose oral cobalamin and sublingual cobalamin are also available. As long as supplemental cobalamin is used, the anemia can be reversed. However, if the person has had long-standing neuromuscular complications, they may not be reversible.

NURSING MANAGEMENT
COBALAMIN DEFICIENCY ANEMIA

Because there is a familial predisposition for pernicious anemia, the most common type of cobalamin deficiency, patients who have a positive family history of pernicious anemia should be evaluated for symptoms. Although disease development cannot be prevented, early detection and treatment can lead to reversal of symptoms.

The nursing measures presented in the nursing care plan for the patient with anemia (see NCP 30-1) are appropriate for the patient with cobalamin deficiency anemia. In addition to these measures, the nurse should ensure that injuries are not sustained because of the diminished sensations to heat and pain resulting from the neurologic impairment. The patient must be protected from burns and trauma. If heat therapy is required, the patient's skin must be evaluated at frequent intervals to detect redness.

Ongoing care is focused on ensuring good patient compliance with treatment. There must also be careful follow-up to assess for neurologic difficulties that were not fully corrected by adequate cobalamin replacement therapy. Because the potential for gastric carcinoma is increased in patients with atrophic gastritis-related pernicious anemia, the patient should have frequent and careful evaluation of this problem.

FOLIC ACID DEFICIENCY

Folic acid deficiency also causes megaloblastic anemia. Folic acid is required for DNA synthesis leading to RBC formation and maturation. Common causes of folic acid deficiency include the following:

1. Poor nutrition, especially a lack of leafy green vegetables, liver, citrus fruits, yeast, dried beans, nuts, and grains
2. Malabsorption syndromes, particularly small bowel disorders
3. Drugs that impede the absorption and use of folic acid (e.g., methotrexate, oral contraceptives), as well as anti-seizure drugs (e.g., phenobarbital, diphenylhydantoin [Dilantin])
4. Alcohol abuse and anorexia
5. Hemodialysis patients because folic acid is lost during dialysis

The clinical manifestations of folic acid deficiency are similar to those of cobalamin deficiency. The disease develops insidiously, and the patient's symptoms may be attributed to other coexisting problems such as cirrhosis or esophageal varices. GI disturbances include dyspepsia and a smooth, beefy red tongue. The absence of neurologic problems is an important diagnostic finding. This lack of neurologic involvement differentiates folic acid deficiency from cobalamin deficiency.

The diagnostic findings for folic acid deficiency are presented in Table 30-6. In addition, the serum folate level is low (normal is 3 to 25 mg/ml [7 to 57 mol/L]), the serum cobalamin level is normal, and the gastric analysis is positive for hydrochloric acid.

Folic acid deficiency is treated by replacement therapy. The usual dose is 1 mg per day by mouth. In malabsorption states, up to 5 mg per day may be required. The duration of treatment depends on the reason for the deficiency. The patient should be encouraged to eat foods containing large amounts of folic acid (see Table 30-5).

ANEMIA OF CHRONIC DISEASE

Diverse systemic illnesses may cause anemias with similar features. The anemia of chronic disease is associated with an underproduction of RBCs and mild shortening of RBC survival. The RBCs are usually normocytic, normochromic, and hypoproliferative. The anemia is usually mild, but it can be more severe. One cause is end-stage renal disease. There is a relationship between the degree of anemia and the severity of uremia. Although several mechanisms may be involved in the development of anemia with renal disease, the primary factor is decreased erythropoietin, a hormone made in the kidneys that is necessary for erythropoiesis. With impaired renal function, decreased levels of erythropoietin are produced (see Chapter 45).

Other chronic, inflammatory, infectious, or malignant diseases can lead to the anemia of chronic disease. Chronic liver disease may also contribute to the development of anemia. Anemia may result from the folic acid deficiencies caused by inadequate nutrition in abusers of alcohol or from blood loss caused by chronic gastritis. The use of alcohol itself may reduce erythropoiesis. Anemia may also result from splenomegaly, which is commonly found in advanced stages of cirrhosis. Anemia can also result from hepatitis (see Chapter 42).

Chronic inflammation and malignant tumors are other conditions in which anemia may be present. The mechanisms involved include increased RBC destruction accompanied by a failure to augment erythropoiesis to compensate for the rise in destruction. Many chemotherapy agents cause myelosuppression and thus some degree of anemia. Human immunodeficiency virus (HIV) and its treatments are other causes of anemia.

Chronic endocrine diseases may also lead to anemia. Hypopituitary and hypothyroid states both lead to reduced tissue metabolism; therefore tissue oxygen needs are diminished, leading to a reduced production of erythropoietin by the kidneys. Adrenal dysfunction caused by either adrenalectomy or Addison's disease also results in anemia.

Anemia of chronic disease must first be recognized and differentiated from anemias of other etiologies. Findings of elevated serum ferritin and increased iron stores distinguish it from iron-deficiency anemia; normal folate and cobalamin blood levels distinguish it from those types of anemias. The best treatment of anemia of chronic disease is correction of the underlying disorder. Unless the anemia is severe, blood transfusions are rarely indicated. Erythropoietin therapy (Epogen, Procrit) is used for anemia related to renal disease or anemia related to cancer therapies (see Chapter 45).[7] Darbepoetin (Aranesp) is a newer formulation of erythropoietin. It has a longer duration of action than erythropoietin.

APLASTIC ANEMIA

Aplastic anemia is a disease in which the patient has peripheral blood *pancytopenia* (decrease of all blood cell types—RBCs, white blood cells [WBCs], and platelets) and hypocellular bone marrow. The signs and symptoms can range from a chronic condition managed with erythropoietin or blood transfusions to a critical condition with hemorrhage and sepsis.

Etiology

The incidence of aplastic anemia is low, affecting approximately 4 of every 1 million persons. There are various etiologic classifications for aplastic anemia, but they can be divided into two major groups: congenital or acquired (Table 30-9).

TABLE 30-9   Causes of Aplastic Anemia

Congenital
- Fanconi syndrome

Acquired
- Chemical agents and toxins
- Drugs
- Idiopathic
- Pregnancy
- Radiation
- Viral and bacterial infections

1. *Congenital origin* is caused by chromosomal alterations. Approximately 30% of the aplastic anemias that appear in childhood are inherited.
2. *Acquired aplastic anemia* results from exposure to ionizing radiation, chemical agents (e.g., benzene, insecticides, arsenic, alcohol), viral and bacterial infections (e.g., hepatitis, parvovirus, biliary tuberculosis), and prescribed medications (e.g., alkylating agents, antiseizure agents, antimetabolites, antimicrobials, gold). Approximately 70% of the acquired aplastic anemias are idiopathic.[8]

Clinical Manifestations

Aplastic anemia usually develops gradually. Clinically the patient may have symptoms caused by suppression of any or all bone marrow elements. General manifestations of anemia such as fatigue and dyspnea, as well as cardiovascular and cerebral responses, may be seen (see Table 30-3). The patient with neutropenia (low neutrophil count) is susceptible to infection and may be febrile. Thrombocytopenia is manifested by a predisposition to bleeding (e.g., petechiae, ecchymosis, epistaxis).

Diagnostic Studies

The diagnosis is confirmed by laboratory studies. Because all marrow elements are affected, hemoglobin, WBC, and platelet values are often decreased in aplastic anemia. Other RBC indices are normal (see Table 30-6). The condition is therefore classified as a normocytic, normochromic anemia. The reticulocyte count is low. Bleeding time is prolonged.

Aplastic anemia can be further evaluated by assessing various iron studies. The serum iron and total iron-binding capacity (TIBC) are elevated as initial signs of erythropoiesis suppression. Bone marrow biopsy, aspiration, and pathologic examination may be done for any anemic state. However, the findings are especially important in aplastic anemia because the marrow is hypocellular, with increased yellow marrow (fat content), a finding sometimes referred to as a "dry tap."

NURSING *and* COLLABORATIVE MANAGEMENT
APLASTIC ANEMIA

Management of aplastic anemia is based on identifying and removing the causative agent (when possible) and providing supportive care until the pancytopenia reverses. Nursing interventions appropriate for the patient with pancytopenia from aplastic anemia are presented in the nursing care plan for the patient with anemia (NCP 30-1) earlier in this chapter and the nursing care plans for thrombocytopenia (NCP 30-2) and neutropenia (NCP 30-3) later in this chapter. Nursing actions are directed at preventing complications from infection and hemorrhage.

The prognosis of untreated aplastic anemia is poor (approximately 75% fatal). However, advances in medical management, including bone marrow transplantation and immunosuppressive therapy with antithymocyte globulin (ATG) and cyclosporine, have improved outcomes significantly. ATG is a horse serum that contains polyclonal antibodies against human T cells. The rationale for this therapy is that aplastic anemia is an immune-mediated disease.[8] (ATG and cyclosporine are discussed in Chapter 13.)

The treatment of choice for adults less than 45 years of age who have a human leukocyte antigen (HLA)–matched donor is bone marrow transplantation. The best results occur in a younger patient who has not had previous blood transfusions. Prior transfusions increase the risk of graft rejection. (Bone marrow transplants are discussed in Chapter 15).

For the older adult or the patient without an HLA-matched donor, the treatment of choice is immunosuppression with ATG or cyclosporine. Although this therapy may be only partially beneficial, transfusions usually can be avoided.

Anemia Caused by Blood Loss

Anemia resulting from blood loss may be caused by either acute or chronic problems.

ACUTE BLOOD LOSS

Acute blood loss occurs as a result of sudden hemorrhage. Causes of acute blood loss include trauma, complications of surgery, and conditions or diseases that disrupt vascular integrity. There are two clinical concerns in such situations. First, there is a sudden reduction in the total blood volume that can lead to hypovolemic shock. Second, if the acute loss is more gradual, the body maintains its blood volume by slowly increasing the plasma volume. Although the circulating fluid volume is preserved, the number of RBCs available to carry oxygen is significantly diminished.

Clinical Manifestations

The clinical manifestations of anemia from acute blood loss are caused by the body's attempts to maintain an adequate blood volume and meet oxygen requirements. Table 30-10 summarizes the clinical manifestations of patients with varying degrees of blood volume loss. It is essential to understand that the clinical signs and symptoms the patient is experiencing are more important than the laboratory values. The nurse should be alert to the patient's expression of pain. Internal hemorrhage may cause pain because of tissue distention, organ displacement, and nerve compression. Pain may be localized or referred. In the case of retroperitoneal bleeding, the patient may not experience abdominal pain. Instead, the patient may have numbness and pain in a lower extremity secondary to compression of the lateral cutaneous nerve, which is located in the region of the first to third lumbar vertebrae. The major complication of acute blood loss is shock (see Chapter 65).

Diagnostic Studies

When blood volume loss is sudden, plasma volume has not yet had a chance to increase, the loss of RBCs is not reflected in laboratory data, and values may seem normal or high for 2 to 3 days. However, once the plasma is replaced by endogenous and exogenous

TABLE 30-10	Clinical Manifestations of Acute Blood Loss	
VOLUME LOST (%)	**CLINICAL MANIFESTATIONS**
10	None
20	No detectable signs of symptoms at rest, tachycardia with exercise and slight postural hypotension
30	Normal supine blood pressure and pulse at rest, postural hypotension and tachycardia with exercise
40	Blood pressure, central venous pressure, and cardiac output below normal at rest; rapid, thready pulse and cold, clammy skin
50	Shock and potential death

means, the RBC mass is less concentrated. At this time, RBC, hemoglobin, and hematocrit levels are low and reflect the blood loss.

Collaborative Care

Collaborative care is initially concerned with (1) replacing blood volume to prevent shock and (2) identifying the source of the hemorrhage and stopping the blood loss. IV fluids used in emergencies include dextran, Hetastarch, albumin, or crystalloid electrolyte solutions such as lactated Ringer's. The amount of infusion varies with the solution used. (Management of shock is discussed in Chapter 65.)

Once volume replacement is established, attention can be directed to correcting RBC loss. The body needs 2 to 5 days to manufacture more RBCs in response to increased erythropoietin. Consequently, blood transfusions (packed RBCs) may be needed if the blood loss is significant.

The patient may also need supplemental iron because the availability of iron affects the marrow production of erythrocytes. When anemia exists after acute blood loss, dietary sources of iron will probably not be adequate to maintain iron stores. Therefore oral or parenteral iron preparations are administered.

NURSING MANAGEMENT ACUTE BLOOD LOSS

In the case of trauma, it may be impossible to prevent the situation leading to the blood loss. For the postoperative patient, the nurse carefully monitors the blood loss from various drainage tubes and dressings and implements appropriate actions. The nursing care plan for the patient with anemia resulting from acute blood loss will most likely include administration of blood products (described at the end of this chapter).

Once the source of hemorrhage is identified, blood loss is controlled, and fluid and blood volumes are replaced, the anemia should begin to correct itself. There should be no need for long-term treatment of this type of anemia.

CHRONIC BLOOD LOSS

The sources of chronic blood loss are similar to those of iron-deficiency anemia (e.g., bleeding ulcer, hemorrhoids, menstrual and postmenopausal blood loss). The effects of chronic blood loss are usually related to the depletion of iron stores and are usually considered as iron-deficiency anemia. Management of chronic blood loss anemia involves identifying the source and stopping the bleeding. Supplemental iron may be required. The nursing measures presented in NCP 30-1 are relevant to anemia of chronic blood loss.

Anemia Caused by Increased Erythrocyte Destruction

The third major cause of anemia is termed **hemolytic anemia,** a condition caused by the destruction or hemolysis of RBCs at a rate that exceeds production. Hemolysis can occur because of problems intrinsic or extrinsic to the RBCs. *Intrinsic hemolytic anemias* result from defects in the RBCs themselves caused by abnormal hemoglobin (e.g., sickle cells), enzyme deficiencies that alter glycolysis (glucose-6-phosphate dehydrogenase [G6PD] deficiency), or RBC membrane abnormalities. Intrinsic hemolytic anemias are usually hereditary. More common are the *extrinsic hemolytic anemias,* which are acquired. In this type of anemia the patient's RBCs are normal, but damage is caused by external factors such as trapping of cells within the sinuses of the liver or spleen, antibody-mediated destruction, toxins, or mechanical injury (e.g., prosthetic heart valves).

The two sites of hemolysis are classified as intravascular or extravascular. *Intravascular* destruction occurs within the circulation; *extravascular* hemolysis takes place in the macrophages of the spleen, liver, and bone marrow. The spleen is the primary site of the destruction of RBCs that are old, defective, or moderately damaged. Fig. 30-1 indicates the sequence of events involved in extravascular hemolysis.

The patient with hemolytic anemia manifests the general symptoms of anemia and clinical manifestations specific to this type of anemia (see Table 30-3). Jaundice is likely because the increased destruction of RBCs causes an elevation in bilirubin levels. The spleen and liver may enlarge because of their hyper-

activity, which is related to macrophage phagocytosis of the defective erythrocytes.

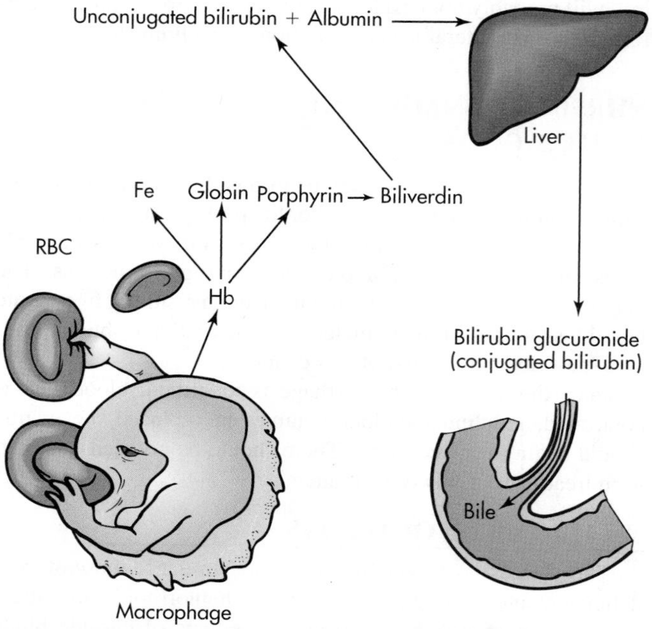

In all causes of hemolysis a major focus of treatment is to maintain renal function. When an RBC is hemolyzed, the hemoglobin molecule is released and filtered by the kidneys. The accumulation of hemoglobin molecules can obstruct the renal tubules and lead to acute tubular necrosis (see Chapter 45).

SICKLE CELL DISEASE

Sickle cell disease (SCD) is a group of inherited, autosomal recessive disorders characterized by the presence of an abnormal form of hemoglobin in the erythrocyte. (Autosomal recessive genetic disorders are discussed in Chapter 13.) This abnormal hemoglobin, *hemoglobin S* (HbS), causes the erythrocyte to stiffen and elongate taking on a sickle shape in response to low oxygen levels. Hemoglogin S results from substitution of valine for glutamic acid on the β-globin chain of hemoglobin. Because this is a genetic disorder, SCD is usually identified during infancy or early childhood. It is an incurable disease that is often fatal by middle age from renal and pulmonary failure.[9]

SCD affects more than 50,000 Americans and is predominant in African Americans, occurring in an estimated prevalence of 1 in 350 to 500 live births. It can also affect people of Mediterranean, Caribbean, South and Central American, Arabian, or East Indian ancestry.

Etiology and Pathophysiology

Types of Sickle Cell Disease. Types of SCD disorders include sickle cell anemia, sickle cell–thalassemia, sickle cell HbC disease, and sickle cell trait. *Sickle cell anemia* is the most severe

FIG. 30-1 Sequence of events in extravascular hemolysis.

GENETICS in CLINICAL PRACTICE
Sickle Cell Disease

Genetic Basis
- Autosomal recessive disorder
- Mutation in β–globin gene; sickle hemoglobin (HbS) on chromosome 11
- HbS variant involves substitution of valine for glutamic acid in the β–globin gene

Incidence
- 1 in 350 to 500 African Americans
- Also affects people of Mediterranean, Caribbean, South and Central American, Arab, and East Indian descent

Genetic Testing
- DNA testing available but costly
- Electrophoresis of hemoglobin and sickling screening test are more commonly used

Clinical Implications
- Requires ongoing continuity of care and extensive patient education.
- Sickle cell trait is the carrier state for sickle cell disease and represents a mild type of sickle cell disease. One in 10 to 12 African Americans has sickle cell trait.
- Management of sickle cell disease should focus on the prevention of sickle cell crisis.
- Genetic counseling is recommended for individuals with a family history of sickle cell disease. Individuals should understand the risks of transmitting the genetic mutation.

of the SCD syndromes. This occurs when a person is homozygous for hemoglobin S (HbSS); the person has inherited HbS from both parents. *Sickle cell–thalassemia* and *sickle cell HbC* occur when a person inherits HbS from one parent and another type of abnormal hemoglobin (such as thalassemia or hemoglobin C) from the other parent. Both of these forms of SCD are less common and less severe than sickle cell anemia. *Sickle cell trait* occurs when a person is heterozygous for hemoglobin S (HbAS); the person has inherited hemoglobin S from one parent and normal hemoglobin (hemoglobin A) from the other parent. Sickle cell trait is typically a very mild to asymptomatic condition.

Sickling Episodes. The major pathophysiologic event of SCD is the sickling of RBCs. Sickling episodes are most commonly triggered by low oxygen tension in the blood. Hypoxia or deoxygenation of the RBCs can be caused by viral or bacterial infection, high altitude, emotional or physical stress, surgery, and blood loss. Infection is the most common precipitating factor.[9] Other events that can trigger or sustain a sickling episode include dehydration, increased hydrogen ion concentration (acidosis), increased plasma osmolality, decreased plasma volume, and low body temperature. A sickling episode can also occur without an obvious cause.

Sickled RBCs become rigid and take on an elongated, crescent shape (Fig. 30-2). Sickled cells cannot easily pass through capillaries or other small vessels and can cause vascular occlusion, leading to acute or chronic tissue injury. The resulting hemostasis promotes a self-perpetuating cycle of local hypoxia, deoxygenation of more erythrocytes, and more sickling. Circulating sickled cells are hemolyzed by the spleen, leading to anemia. Initially the sickling of cells is reversible with reoxygenation, but it eventually becomes irreversible due to cell membrane damage from recurrent sickling.

Sickle cell crisis is a severe, painful, acute exacerbation of RBC sickling causing a vasoocclusive crisis. As blood flow is impaired by sickled cells, vasospasm occurs, further restricting blood flow. Severe capillary hypoxia causes changes in membrane permeability, leading to plasma loss, hemoconcentration, the development of thrombi, and further circulatory stagnation. Tissue ischemia, infarction, and necrosis eventually occurs from lack of oxygen. Shock is a possible life-threatening consequence of sickle cell crisis due to severe oxygen depletion of the tissues and a reduction of the circulating fluid volume. Sickle cell crisis can begin suddenly and persist for days to weeks.

The frequency, extent, and severity of sickling episodes is highly variable and unpredictable, but is largely dependent on the percentage of HbS present. Individuals with sickle cell anemia have the most severe form because the erythrocytes contain a high percentage of HbS.

Clinical Manifestations

The effects of sickle cell disease vary greatly from person to person. Many people with sickle cell anemia are in reasonably good health the majority of the time. The typical patient is anemic but asymptomatic except during sickling episodes. Clinical manifestations of chronic anemia include pallor of mucous membranes, fatigue, and decreased exercise tolerance. Because most individuals with sickle cell anemia have dark skin, pallor is more readily detected by examining the mucous membranes. The skin may have a grayish cast. Because of the hemolysis, jaundice is common and patients are prone to gallstones (cholelithiasis).

The primary symptom associated with sickling is pain. During sickle cell crisis the pain is severe due to ischemia of tissue. Aching in the joints, especially those of the hands and feet, is a common complaint. The painful bone infarction of the *hand-foot syndrome* (painful swelling of hands and feet) is often the first symptom of SCD. The pain associated with these attacks is often described as deep gnawing and throbbing.[10] *Priapism* (persistent penile erection) may occur if penile veins become occluded.

Complications

With repeated episodes of sickling there is gradual involvement of all body systems, especially the spleen, lungs, kidneys, and brain. Organs that have a high need for oxygen are most often affected and form the basis for many of the complications of sickle cell disease (Fig. 30-3). The heart may become ischemic and enlarged, leading to congestive heart failure. *Acute chest syndrome* is characterized by fever, chest pain, cough, pulmonary infiltrates, and dyspnea. Pulmonary infarctions may cause pulmonary hypertension, MI, heart failure, and ultimately cor pulmonale. Retinal vessel obstruction may result in hemorrhage, scarring, retinal detachment, and blindness. The kidneys may be injured from the increased blood viscosity and the lack of oxygen and can lead to renal failure. The spleen becomes small because of repeated scarring, a phenomenon termed *autosplenectomy.* Stroke can result from thrombosis and infarction of cerebral blood vessels. Bone changes may include osteoporosis and osteosclerosis after infarction. Chronic leg ulcers can result from the hypoxia and are especially prevalent around the ankles. The patient with SCD is particularly prone to infection. One reason for this is the failure of the spleen to phagocytize foreign substances. Pneumonia is the most common infection and often is of pneumococcal origin.

Diagnostic Studies

A peripheral blood smear may reveal sickled cells. The presence of sickle hemoglobin can be diagnosed by the sickling test, which uses RBCs (in vitro) and exposes them to a deoxygenation agent. Electrophoresis of hemoglobin readily identifies the presence of abnormal hemoglobin. DNA testing can be done, but is costly.

As a result of the accelerated RBC breakdown, the patient has characteristic clinical findings of hemolysis (jaundice, elevated serum bilirubin levels) and abnormal laboratory test results (see Table 30-6). Skeletal x-rays will demonstrate bone and joint deformities and flattening. Magnetic resonance imaging may be used to diagnose a stroke caused by blocked cerebral vessels from sickled cells.

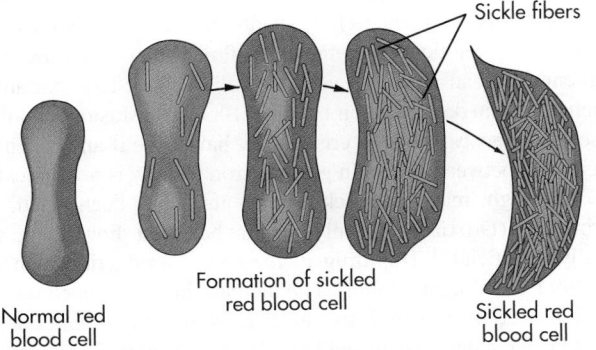

FIG. 30-2   Sickle cell hemoglobin aggregates into long chains and alters the shape of the RBC.

Sickle fibers

Normal red blood cell

Formation of sickled red blood cell

Sickled red blood cell

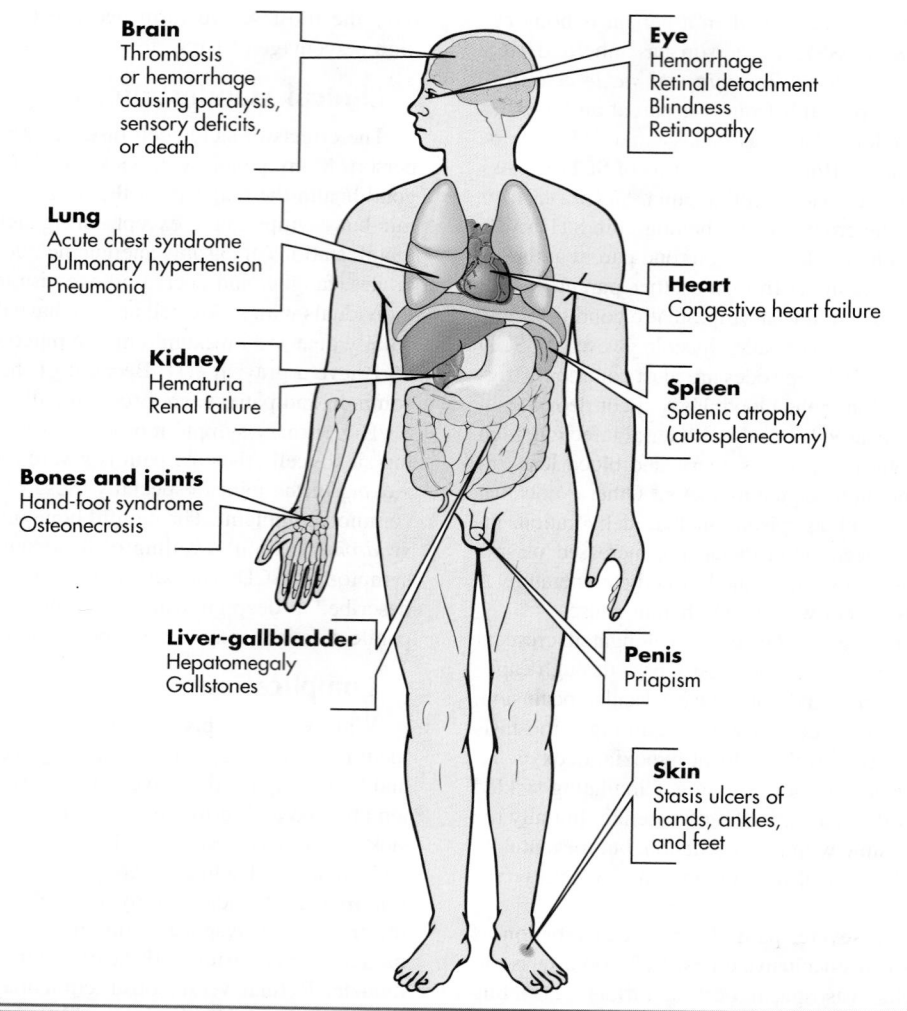

Brain
Thrombosis
or hemorrhage
causing paralysis,
sensory deficits,
or death

Eye
Hemorrhage
Retinal detachment
Blindness
Retinopathy

Lung
Acute chest syndrome
Pulmonary hypertension
Pneumonia

Heart
Congestive heart failure

Kidney
Hematuria
Renal failure

Spleen
Splenic atrophy
(autosplenectomy)

Bones and joints
Hand-foot syndrome
Osteonecrosis

Liver-gallbladder
Hepatomegaly
Gallstones

Penis
Priapism

Skin
Stasis ulcers of
hands, ankles,
and feet

FIG. 30-3 Clinical manifestations and complications of sickle cell disease.

NURSING *and* COLLABORATIVE MANAGEMENT
SICKLE CELL DISEASE

Collaborative care for a patient with SCD is directed toward alleviating the symptoms from the complications of the disease and minimizing end target-organ damage. There is no specific treatment for the disease. Patients with SCD should be taught to avoid high altitudes, maintain adequate fluid intake, and treat infections promptly. Pneumovax, *Haemophilus influenzae,* influenza, and hepatitis immunizations should be administered. Chronic leg ulcers may be treated with bed rest, antibiotics, warm saline soaks, mechanical or enzyme debridement, and grafting if necessary. Priapism is managed with pain medication and nifedipine (Procardia).

Sickle cell crises may require hospitalization. Oxygen may be administered to treat hypoxia and control sickling. Rest is instituted to reduce metabolic requirements, and fluids and electrolytes are administered to reduce blood viscosity and maintain renal function. Transfusion therapy is indicated when an aplastic crisis occurs. These patients, like those with thalassemia major, may require chelation therapy to reduce transfusion-produced iron overload.

Pain management poses a number of challenges to the health care provider. Undertreatment of sickle cell pain is a major prob-

lem.[10] Large doses of continuous (rather than as-needed [prn]) narcotic analgesics are the mainstay of pain management during the acute phase. Patient-controlled analgesia (PCA) may be used during an acute crisis. (PCA is discussed in Chapter 9.) After discharge patients will often continue on oral narcotic analgesics. Health care personnel must overcome their fears of narcotic addiction to treat pain optimally and to avoid prolonging the duration of pain.

Infection is a frequent complication and must be treated. Pain is the most common symptom of patients with SCD seeking medical care. Patients with acute chest syndrome are treated with broad-spectrum antibiotics, O_2 therapy, and fluid therapy. Because these patients have an increased need for folic acid, it is important for them to obtain daily supplementation. Blood transfusions should be used judiciously to treat a crisis. They have little if any role in the treatment between crises. In general, iron therapy is not indicated.

Although many antisickling agents have been tried, hydroxyurea (Droxia) is the only one that has been shown to be clinically beneficial.[11] This drug increases the production of hemoglobin F (fetal hemoglobin). The increase in HbF is accompanied by a reduction in hemolysis, an increase in hemoglobin concentration, and a decrease in sickled cells. Erythropoietin can be used in patients not responding to hydroxyurea.

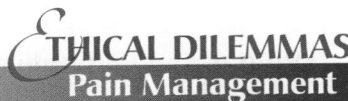
ETHICAL DILEMMAS
Pain Management

Situation

A 21-year-old African American man is admitted to the emergency department in sickle cell crisis with complaints of excruciating pain. He is known to several of the nurses and physicians in the department. One of the nurses remarks to you that it must be time for his "fix" of narcotics. Pain management is a major concern for both the patient and the health care team.

Important Points for Consideration

- The experience of pain is subjective, and experts in pain management agree that "pain is what the patient says it is."
- Acute or chronic pain can have serious and debilitating physical and psychologic effects for patients.
- The nurse's duty to prevent harm and provide benefit to patients is undermined when a patient's complaints of unrelieved pain are attributed to attention-seeking or drug-seeking behavior.
- The nurse's obligation to provide holistic individualized care to patients is compromised when stereotypes or myths interfere with the ability to accurately assess a patient's problems.

Critical Thinking Questions

1. How would you respond to the nurse's negative remark?
2. What important factors would need to be included in your assessment of this patient?

Bone marrow transplantation is the only available treatment that can cure some patients with SCD. The selection of appropriate recipients, scarcity of appropriate donors, risk, and cost-effectiveness limit the use of bone marrow transplant for SCD. (Bone marrow transplants are discussed in Chapter 15.) Recent advances in gene therapy technology provide some promise for the future treatment of SCD. (Gene therapy is discussed in Chapter 13.)

Patient teaching is important in the long-term care of the patient. The patient and family must understand the basis of the disease and the reasons for supportive care. The patient must be taught ways to avoid crises, which include taking steps to reduce the chance of developing hypoxia, such as avoiding high altitudes and seeking medical attention quickly to counteract problems such as upper respiratory tract infections. Education on pain control is also needed because the pain during a crisis may be severe and often requires considerable analgesia.

ACQUIRED HEMOLYTIC ANEMIA

Extrinsic causes of hemolysis can be separated into three categories: (1) physical factors, (2) immune reactions, and (3) infectious agents and toxins. Physical destruction of RBCs results from the exertion of extreme force on the cells. Traumatic events causing disruption of the RBC membrane include hemodialysis, extracorporeal circulation used in cardiopulmonary bypass, and prosthetic heart valves. In addition, the force needed to push blood through abnormal vessels, such as those that have been burned or affected by angiopathic disease (e.g., diabetes mellitus), may also physically damage RBCs.

Antibodies may destroy RBCs by the mechanisms involved in antigen-antibody reactions. The reactions may be of an isoim-

mune or autoimmune type. *Isoimmune reactions* occur when antibodies develop against antigens from another person of the same species. Blood transfusion reactions typify this response, when the recipient's antibodies hemolyze donor cells.

Autoimmune reactions result when individuals develop antibodies against their own RBCs. Autoimmune hemolytic reactions may be idiopathic, developing with no prior hemolytic history as a result of the immunoglobulin IgG covering the RBCs, or secondary to other autoimmune diseases (e.g., systemic lupus erythematosus), leukemia, lymphoma, or drugs (penicillin, indomethacin [Indocin], phenylbutazone [Butazolidin], phenacetin, quinidine, quinine, and methyldopa [Aldomet]).

Infectious agents and toxins cause the third category of acquired hemolytic disorders. Infectious agents foster hemolysis in four ways: (1) by invading the RBC and destroying its contents (e.g., parasites such as in malaria); (2) by releasing hemolytic substances (e.g., *Clostridium perfringens*); (3) by generating an antigen-antibody reaction; and (4) by contributing to splenomegaly as a means of increasing removal of damaged RBCs from the circulation. Various agents may be toxic to RBCs and cause hemolysis. These hemolytic toxins involve chemicals such as oxidative drugs, arsenic, lead, copper, and snake venom.

Laboratory findings in hemolytic anemia are presented in Table 30-6. Treatment and management of acquired hemolytic anemias involve general supportive care until the causative agent can be eliminated or at least rendered less injurious to the RBCs. Because a hemolytic crisis is a potential consequence, the nurse needs to be ready to institute appropriate emergent therapy. Supportive care may include administering corticosteroids and blood products or removing the spleen.

HEMOCHROMATOSIS

Hemochromatosis is an autosomal recessive disease characterized by increased intestinal iron absorption and, as a result, increased tissue iron deposition (see the Genetics in Clinical Practice box). It is the most common genetic disorder among whites, with an incidence of 1 in 100 to 500 whites of European ancestry. The normal range for total body iron is 2 to 6 g. Individuals with hemochromatosis accumulate iron at a rate of 0.5 to 1.0 g each year and may exceed total iron concentrations of 50 g. Symptoms of hemochromatosis usually develop between 40 and 60 years of age. In addition to the primary genetic defect, hemochromatosis occurs secondary to diseases such as thalassemia and sideroblastosis. It may also be caused by multiple blood transfusions.[12]

Initially the excess iron accumulates in the liver and causes liver enlargement and eventually cirrhosis. Then other organs become affected, resulting in diabetes mellitus, skin pigment changes (bronzing), cardiac changes (e.g., cardiomyopathy), arthritis, and testicular atrophy. Physical examination reveals an enlarged liver and spleen and pigmentation changes in the skin. Laboratory values demonstrate an elevated serum iron, TIBC, and serum ferritin. A liver biopsy can quantify the amount of iron and is the definitive way to establish the diagnosis.

The goal of treatment is to remove excess iron from the body and minimize any symptoms the patient may have. Iron removal is achieved by removing 500 ml of blood each week for 2 to 3 years until the iron stores in the body are depleted. Then less frequent removal of blood is needed to maintain iron levels within normal limits. Management of organ involvement (e.g., diabetes mellitus, heart failure) is the same as conventional treat-

GENETICS in CLINICAL PRACTICE
Hemochromatosis

Genetic Basis
- Autosomal recessive trait
- Most common mutations: C282Y and H63D
- Genetic defect located in close proximity to the major histo-compatibility complex on chromosome 6

Incidence
- Most common genetic disease in people of European ancestry
- Affects 1 in 100 to 500 whites of European ancestry
- Very low prevalence in other ethnic populations

Genetic Testing
- Genetic testing is recommended for all first-degree relatives of people with disease.
- American Hemochromatosis Society recommends genetic testing regardless of family history.
- Useful diagnostic tests include serum iron concentration, total iron-binding capacity, and transferrin saturation.
- Liver biopsy, once considered the gold standard diagnostic test, is primarily used to quantify iron deposition and esti-mate the prognosis and extent of disease.

Clinical Implications
- Early treatment can prevent serious complications.
- Clinical expression is variable depending on dietary iron, blood loss, and other modifying factors.
- If untreated, progressive iron deposits can lead to multiple organ failure.

ment for these problems. The most common causes of death are cirrhosis, liver failure, hepatic carcinoma, and cardiac failure. With early diagnosis and treatment, life expectancy is normal. However, many cases go undetected and untreated.

POLYCYTHEMIA

Polycythemia is the production and presence of increased numbers of RBCs. The increase in RBCs can be so great that blood circulation is impaired as a result of the increased blood viscosity (hyperviscosity) and volume (hypervolemia).

Etiology and Pathophysiology

The two types of polycythemia are primary polycythemia, or polycythemia vera, and secondary polycythemia (Fig. 30-4). Their etiologies and pathogenesis differ, although their compli-cations and clinical manifestations are similar. *Polycythemia vera* is considered a myeloproliferative disorder arising from a chro-mosomal mutation in a single pluripotent stem cell. Therefore not only are RBCs involved but also granulocytes and platelets, leading to increased production of each of these blood cells. The disease develops insidiously and follows a chronic, vacillating course. It usually develops in patients more than 50 years of age. With this myeloproliferative disorder the patient has enhanced blood viscosity and blood volume and congestion of organs and tissues with blood. Splenomegaly is common.

Chronic hypoxia causes *secondary polycythemia*. Hypoxia stimulates erythropoietin production in the kidney, which in turn stimulates erythrocyte production. The need for O_2 may be due to high altitude, pulmonary disease, cardiovascular disease, alveolar hypoventilation, defective O_2 transport, or tissue hypoxia. Conse-quently, secondary polycythemia is a physiologic response in which the body tries to compensate for a problem rather than a pathologic response. (Secondary polycythemia is discussed in the section on chronic obstructive pulmonary disease in Chapter 28.)

Clinical Manifestations and Complications

Circulatory manifestations of polycythemia vera occur be-cause of the hypertension caused by hypervolemia and hypervis-cosity. They are often the first symptoms and include subjective complaints of headache, vertigo, dizziness, tinnitus, and visual disturbances. In addition, the patient may experience angina, congestive heart failure, intermittent claudication, and throm-bophlebitis, which may be complicated by embolization. These manifestations are caused by blood vessel distention, impaired blood flow, circulatory stasis, thrombosis, and tissue hypoxia caused by the hypervolemia and hyperviscosity. The most com-mon serious complication is stroke secondary to thrombosis. Generalized pruritus may be a striking symptom and is related to histamine release from an increased number of basophils.

Hemorrhagic phenomena caused by either vessel rupture from overdistention or inadequate platelet function may result in pe-

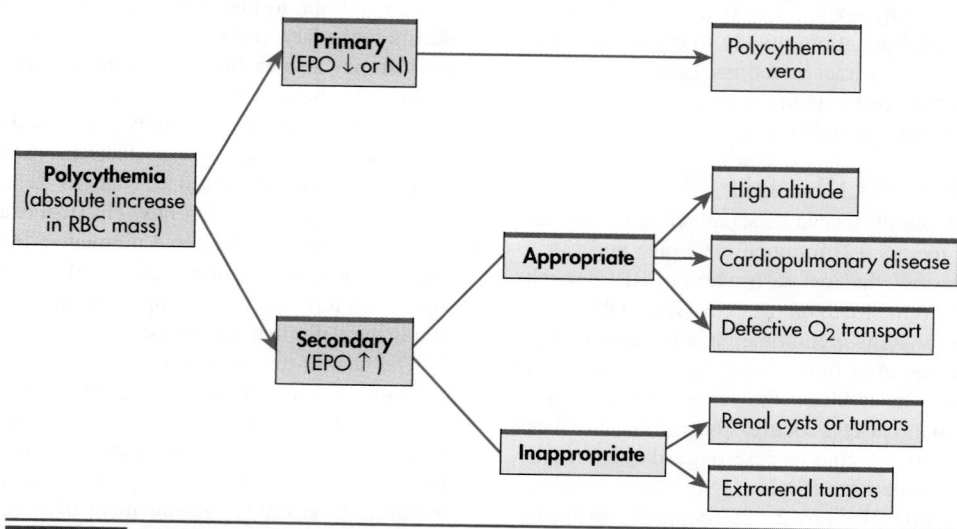

FIG. 30-4 Differentiating between primary and secondary polycythemia. *EPO*, Erythropoietin; *N*, normal.

techiae, ecchymoses, epistaxis, or GI bleeding. Hemorrhage can be acute and catastrophic. Hepatomegaly and splenomegaly from organ engorgement may contribute to patient complaints of satiety and fullness. The patient may also experience pain from peptic ulcer caused by either increased gastric secretions or liver and spleen engorgement. *Plethora* (ruddy complexion) may also be present. Hyperuricemia is caused by the increase in RBC destruction that accompanies excessive RBC production. Uric acid is one of the products of cell destruction. As RBC destruction increases, uric acid production also increases, thus leading to hyperuricemia. This problem may cause a form of gout.

Diagnostic Studies

The following laboratory manifestations are seen in a patient with polycythemia vera: (1) elevated hemoglobin and RBC count; (2) elevated WBC count with basophilia; (3) elevated platelets (thrombocytosis) and platelet dysfunction; (4) elevated leukocyte alkaline phosphatase, uric acid, and cobalamin levels; and (5) elevated histamine levels. Bone marrow examination in polycythemia vera shows hypercellularity of RBCs, WBCs, and platelets. Splenomegaly is found in 90% of patients with primary polycythemia but does not accompany secondary polycythemia.

Collaborative Care

Once the diagnosis of polycythemia vera is made, treatment is directed toward reducing blood volume and viscosity and bone marrow activity. Phlebotomy may be done to diminish blood volume until the desired hematocrit level is achieved. The aim of phlebotomy is to reduce the hematocrit and keep it less than 45% to 48%. Generally, at the time of diagnosis 300 to 500 ml of blood may be removed every other day until the hematocrit is reduced to normal levels. An individual managed with repeated phlebotomies eventually becomes deficient in iron, although this effect is rarely symptomatic. Iron supplementation should be avoided. Hydration therapy is used to reduce the blood's viscosity. Myelosuppressive agents such as busulfan (Myleran), hydroxyurea (Hydrea), melphalan (Alkeran), and radioactive phosphorus may be given to inhibit bone marrow activity. Allopurinol may reduce the number of acute gouty attacks. Antiplatelet agents, such as aspirin and dipyridamole (Persantine), used to prevent thrombotic complications are controversial because of increased irritation of the gastric mucosa resulting in GI problems, including bleeding.

NURSING MANAGEMENT
POLYCYTHEMIA VERA

Primary polycythemia vera is not preventable. However, because secondary polycythemia is generated by any source of hypoxia, maintaining adequate oxygenation may prevent problems. Therefore controlling chronic pulmonary disease, stopping smoking, and avoiding high altitudes may be important.

When acute exacerbations of polycythemia vera develop, the nurse has several responsibilities. Depending on the institution's policies, the nurse may either assist with or perform the phlebotomy. Fluid intake and output must be evaluated during hydration therapy to avoid fluid overload (which further complicates the circulatory congestion) and underhydration (which can cause the blood to become even more viscous). If myelosuppressive agents are used, the nurse must administer the drugs as ordered, observe the patient, and teach the patient about medication side effects.

Assessment of the patient's nutritional status in collaboration with the dietitian may be necessary to offset the inadequate food intake that can result from GI symptoms of fullness, pain, and dyspepsia. Activities must be instituted to decrease thrombus formation. The relative immobility normally imposed by hospitalization puts the patient at risk for thrombus formation. Active or passive leg exercises and ambulation when possible should be initiated.

Because of its chronic nature, polycythemia vera requires ongoing evaluation. Phlebotomy may need to be done every 2 to 3 months, reducing the blood volume by about 500 ml each time. The nurse must evaluate the patient for the development of complications.

Although the incidence is low, leukemia and lymphomas develop in some patients with polycythemia vera. These occurrences may be caused by the chemotherapeutic drugs used to treat the disease, or they may be secondary to a disorder in the stem cells that progresses to erythroleukemia. The major cause of morbidity and mortality from polycythemia vera is related to thrombosis (e.g., stroke).

Problems of Hemostasis

The homeostatic process involves the vascular endothelium, platelets, and coagulation factors, which normally function together to arrest hemorrhage and repair vascular injury. (These mechanisms are described in Chapter 29.) Disruption in any of these components may result in bleeding or thrombotic disorders.

Three major disorders of hemostasis discussed in this section are (1) thrombocytopenia (low platelet count), (2) hemophilia and von Willebrand's disease (inherited disorders of specific clotting factors), and (3) disseminated intravascular coagulation (DIC).

THROMBOCYTOPENIA

Etiology and Pathophysiology

Thrombocytopenia is a reduction of platelets below $150,000/\mu l$ $(150 \times 10^9/L)$. Acute, severe, or prolonged decreases from this normal range can result in abnormal hemostasis that manifests as prolonged bleeding from minor trauma to spontaneous bleeding without injury.

Platelet disorders can be inherited (e.g., Wiskott-Aldrich syndrome), but the vast majority are acquired. Acquired disorders occur because of decreased platelet production or increased platelet destruction (Table 30-11). Many of these abnormalities of platelet number occur following ingestion of some foods, herbs, or drugs (Table 30-12). Aspirin doses as low as 81 mg (a baby aspirin) can alter the function of circulating platelets. Normal function is restored with the generation of newly formed platelets. It is important for the nurse to be aware of the numerous conditions that may affect platelet production and destruction.[13]

Immune Thrombocytopenic Purpura. The most common acquired thrombocytopenia is a syndrome of abnormal destruction of circulating platelets termed *immune thrombocytopenic purpura* (ITP). It was originally termed *idiopathic thrombocytopenic purpura* because its cause was unknown. However, it is now known that ITP is an autoimmune disease. In ITP, platelets are coated with antibodies. Although these platelets function normally, when they reach the spleen, the antibody-coated platelets are recognized as foreign and are destroyed by macrophages.[14,15]

TABLE 30-11   Causes of Thrombocytopenia

Decreased Platelet Production
Inherited
 Fanconi syndrome (pancytopenia)
 Hereditary thrombocytopenia
Acquired
 Aplastic anemia
 Hematologic malignant disorders
 Myelosuppressive drugs
 Chronic alcoholism
 Exposure to ionizing radiation
 Viral infections
 Deficiencies of cobalamin, folic acid

Increased Platelet Destruction
Nonimmune
 Thrombotic thrombocytopenic purpura
 Pregnancy
 Infection
 Severe burns
Immune
 Immune thrombocytopenic purpura
 Human immunodeficiency virus infection
Splenomegaly
Drug Induced
 (Heparin, quinidine, valproic acid
 [Depakene], interferons, sulfonamides)

TABLE 30-12   Causes of Abnormal Platelet Function

Suppression of Platelet Production
• Thiazide diuretics, alcohol, estrogen, chemotherapeutic drugs

Abnormal Platelet Aggregation
• Nonsteroidal antiinflammatory drugs: ibuprofen (Advil, Motrin), indomethacin (Indocin), naproxen (Naprosyn, Aleve)
• Antibiotics: penicillins, cephalosporins
• Analgesics: aspirin and aspirin-containing drugs
• Spices: ginger, cumin, turmeric, cloves
• Vitamins: vitamin C, vitamin E
• Heparin
• Herbs: angelica, bilberry, evening primrose, feverfew, garlic, ginger, ginkgo biloba, ginseng, goldenseal

Platelets normally survive 8 to 10 days. However, in ITP survival of platelets is only 1 to 3 days. Chronic ITP occurs most commonly in women between 20 and 40 years of age. Chronic ITP has a gradual onset, and transient remissions occur.

Thrombotic Thrombocytopenic Purpura. *Thrombotic thrombocytopenic purpura* (TTP) is an uncommon syndrome characterized by hemolytic anemia, thrombocytopenia, neurologic abnormalities, fever (in the absence of infection), and renal abnormalities. The disease is associated with enhanced agglutination of platelets, which form microthrombi that deposit in arterioles and capillaries. The cause of the platelet agglutination is unknown. TTP is seen primarily in adults between 20 and 50 years of age, with a slight female predominance. The syn-drome is occasionally precipitated by the use of estrogen or by pregnancy. TTP is a medical emergency because bleeding and clotting occur simultaneously.

Heparin-Induced Thrombocytopenia and Thrombosis Syndrome. One of the risks associated with the broad and increasing use of heparin is the development of the life-threatening condition called *heparin-induced thrombocytopenia and thrombosis syndrome* (HITTS), also called white clot syndrome.

Platelet destruction and vascular endothelial injury are the two major responses to what is believed to be an immune-mediated response to heparin. The immune response promotes platelet aggregation, leading to decreased circulating platelets and ultimately thrombocytopenia. In addition, platelet-fibrin thrombi are formed. Platelet aggregation also induces heparin to be neutralized. Thus more heparin is required to maintain therapeutic activated partial thromboplastin times. HITTS can be mild (type I) or severe (type II), and estimates vary from 5% to as high as 25% incidence rate in patients on heparin therapy. A lower incidence is seen in patients receiving porcine preparations of heparin as compared with other types.

Clinical Manifestations

Many patients with thrombocytopenia are asymptomatic. The most common symptom is bleeding, usually mucosal or cutaneous. Mucosal bleeding may be manifest as epistaxis and gingival bleeding, and large bullous hemorrhages may appear on the buccal mucosa due to the lack of vessel protection afforded by the submucosal tissue. Bleeding into the skin is manifested as petechiae or superficial ecchymoses. *Petechiae* are small, flat, pinpoint red or reddish brown microhemorrhages. When the platelet count is low, RBCs may leak out of the blood vessels and into the skin to cause petechiae. When petechiae are numerous, the resulting reddish skin bruise is called *purpura*. Larger purplish lesions caused by hemorrhage are termed *ecchymoses* (Fig. 30-5). Ecchymoses may be flat or raised; pain and tenderness sometimes are present.

Prolonged bleeding after routine procedures such as venipuncture or IM injection may also indicate thrombocytopenia. Because the bleeding may be internal, the nurse must also be aware of manifestations that reflect this type of blood loss, including weakness, fainting, dizziness, tachycardia, abdominal pain, and hypotension.

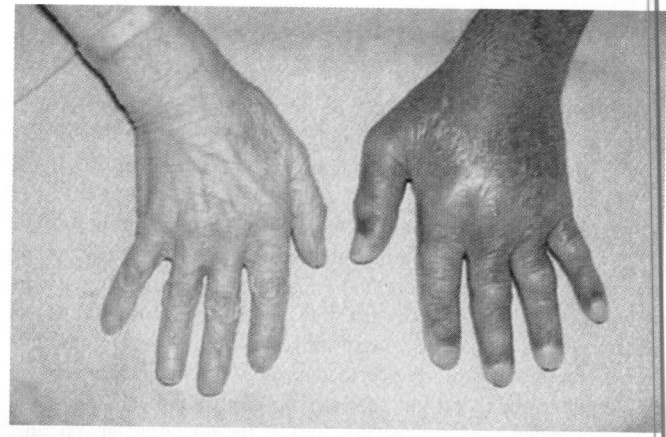

FIG. 30-5   Severe ecchymosis of the left hand.

The major complication of thrombocytopenia is hemorrhage. The hemorrhage may be insidious or acute and internal or external. It may occur in any area of the body, including the joints, retina, and brain.

Cerebral hemorrhage may be fatal in persons with ITP. Insidious hemorrhage may first be detected by discovering the anemia that accompanies blood loss.

Diagnostic Studies

The platelet count is decreased in cases of thrombocytopenia. Any reduction below 150,000/μl (150 $\times$ 10^9/L) may be termed thrombocytopenia. However, prolonged bleeding from trauma or injury does not usually occur until platelet counts are less than 50,000/μl (50 $\times$ 10^9/L). When the count drops below 20,000/μl (20 $\times$ 10^9/L), spontaneous, life-threatening hemorrhages (e.g., intracranial bleeding) can occur. Platelet transfusions are generally not recommended until the count is below 20,000/μl (20 $\times$ 10^9/L) unless the patient is actively bleeding.

Laboratory tests that assess secondary hemostasis or coagulation, such as the prothrombin time (PT) and activated partial thromboplastin time (APTT), can be normal even in severe thrombocytopenia. Bone marrow examination is done to rule out production problems as the cause of thrombocytopenia (e.g., leukemia, aplastic anemia, other myeloproliferative disorders). When destruction of circulating platelets is the etiology, bone marrow analysis shows *megakaryocytes* (precursors of platelets) to be normal or increased, even though circulating platelets are reduced. The absence or decreased numbers of megakaryocytes on bone marrow biopsy is consistent with thrombocytopenia due to decreased bone marrow production (e.g., aplastic anemia). Special blood analyses using flow cytometry and other techniques can detect antiplatelet antibodies as the source of destruction.

The nurse needs to monitor the patient's hemoglobin and hematocrit levels and observe the patient for cardiopulmonary distress and other manifestations of anemia. When thrombocytopenia occurs with anemia characterized by altered RBC morphology, including *spherocytes* (small globular, completely hemoglobinated erythrocytes), fragmented cells (schistocytes), and pronounced reticulocytosis, a diagnosis of TTP should be suspected. These findings are partially as a result of intravascular fibrin deposition causing a "slicing" of RBCs. In TTP, thrombocytopenia may be severe, but coagulation studies are normal.

Collaborative Care

Collaborative care of thrombocytopenia differs based on the etiology of the thrombocytopenia. Discussion of management strategies for these different etiologies follows (Table 30-13).

Immune Thrombocytopenic Purpura. Multiple therapies are used to manage the patient with ITP. Corticosteroids (e.g., prednisone) are used to treat ITP because of their ability to suppress the phagocytic response of splenic macrophages. This alters the spleen's recognition of platelets and increases the life span of the platelets. In addition, corticosteroids depress antibody formation. Corticosteroids also reduce capillary fragility and bleeding time. The mechanism of action for this response is poorly understood. If these are neurologic manifestations related to intracranial bleeding, high-dose methylprednisolone (Solu-Medrol) can be administered IV. Methylprednisolone has also been used when patients are resistant to prednisone.

TABLE 30-13	Collaborative Care Thrombocytopenia

Diagnostic
History and physical examination
Bone marrow aspiration and biopsy
CBC including platelet count

Collaborative Therapy
Immune Thrombocytopenic Purpura
Corticosteroids
Platelet transfusions
Intravenous immunoglobulin
Danazol
Immunosuppressives (cyclophosphamide [Cytoxan], azathioprine [Imuran])
Splenectomy
Thrombotic Thrombocytopenic Purpura
Plasmapheresis (plasma exchange)
High-dose prednisone
Splenectomy
Decreased Production Problem
Identification and treatment of cause
Corticosteroids
Platelet transfusions
Thrombopoietin (investigational)

CBC, Complete blood count.

Treatment may also include high doses of IV immunoglobulin (IVIG) and a component of IVIG, anti-Rh(D) (anti-D, WinRho), in the patient who is unresponsive to corticosteroids or splenectomy. These agents work by competing with the antiplatelet antibodies for macrophage receptors. They effectively raise the platelet count, but the beneficial effects are temporary.[16]

Danazol, an androgen, has been used with success in some patients. Immunosuppressive therapy used in refractory cases includes vincristine (Oncovin), vinblastine (Velban), azathioprine (Imuran), cyclophosphamide (Cytoxan), and cyclosporine.[17]

Splenectomy is indicated if the patient does not respond to prednisone initially or requires unacceptably high doses to maintain an adequate platelet count. Approximately 80% of patients benefit from splenectomy, resulting in a complete or partial remission. The effectiveness of splenectomy is based on four factors. First, the spleen contains an abundance of the macrophages that sequester and destroy platelets. Second, structural features of the spleen enhance antibody-coated platelets and macrophage interaction. Third, some antibody synthesis occurs in the spleen; thus antiplatelet antibodies decrease after splenectomy. Fourth, the spleen normally sequesters approximately one third of the platelets, so its removal increases the number of platelets in circulation.

Platelet transfusions may be used to increase platelet counts in cases of life-threatening hemorrhage.[18] Platelets should not be administered prophylactically because of the possibility of antibody formation. ABO compatibility is not a necessary prerequisite for platelet transfusions. However, after multiple platelet transfusions, a patient may develop anti-HLA antibodies to the transfused platelets.

By using lymphocyte typing to match HLA types of the donor and the recipient, multiple platelet transfusions can be given with fewer complications. In addition, the patient may be premedicated with an antihistamine (e.g., diphenhydramine [Benadryl]) and hydrocortisone to decrease the possibility of reacting to platelet transfusions. Aspirin and aspirin-containing compounds should be avoided in the patient with thrombocytopenia.

Thrombotic Thrombocytopenic Purpura. TTP may be treated in a variety of ways. Corticosteroids are used initially. Plasma exchange or plasmapheresis (see Chapter 13) may be needed to aggressively reverse the process. Treatment should be continued daily until the patient is in complete remission. Splenectomy, corticosteroids, dextran (antiplatelet agent), and vincristine (Oncovin) or vinblastine (Velban) have also been used with success.[19]

TABLE 30-14	Nursing Assessment Thrombocytopenia

Subjective Data

Important Health Information

Past health history: Recent hemorrhage, excessive bleeding, or viral illness; HIV infection; cancer (especially leukemia or lymphoma); aplastic anemia; systemic lupus erythematosus; cirrhosis; exposure to radiation or toxic chemicals; disseminated intravascular coagulation

Medications: Use of thiazide diuretics, furosemide (Lasix), aspirin, acetaminophen, estrogens, gold salts, nonsteroidal antiinflammatory drugs, phenylbutazone (Butazolidin), penicillins, cephalothin, streptomycin, sulfonamides, quinidine, quinine, phenobarbital, methyldopa (Aldomet), phenytoin (Dilantin), chlorpropamide (Diabinese), meprobamate (Equanil), chemotherapy drugs, others listed in Table 30-12.

Functional Health Patterns

Health perception–health management: Family history of bleeding problems; malaise

Nutritional-metabolic: Bleeding gingiva; coffee-ground or bloody vomitus; easy bruising

Elimination: Hematuria, dark or bloody stools

Activity-exercise: Fatigue, weakness, fainting; epistaxis, hemoptysis; dyspnea

Cognitive-perceptual: Pain and tenderness in bleeding areas (e.g., abdomen, head, extremities); headache

Sexuality-reproductive: Menorrhagia, metrorrhagia

Objective Data

General

Fever, lethargy

Integumentary

Petechiae, ecchymoses, purpura

Gastrointestinal

Splenomegaly, abdominal distention; guaiac-positive stools

Possible Findings

Platelet count <150,000/μl (150 × 10^9/L), prolonged bleeding time, ↓ hemoglobin and hematocrit; normal or ↑ megakaryocytes in bone marrow examination

HIV, Human immunodeficiency virus.

Heparin-Induced Thrombocytopenia and Thrombosis Syndrome. Heparin must be discontinued when HITTS is first recognized.[13] The most commonly used treatment modalities are plasmapheresis to clear the platelet-aggregating IgG from the blood, protamine sulfate to interrupt the circulating heparin, thrombolytic agents to treat the thromboembolic events, and surgery to remove clots. Lepirudin (Refludan), an inhibitor of thrombin, may also be used to treat HITTS. It is important to note that platelet transfusions are not effective because they may enhance thromboembolic events.

Acquired Thrombocytopenia from Decreased Platelet Production. The management of acquired thrombocytopenia is based on identifying the cause and treating the disease or removing the causative agent. If the precipitating factor is unknown, the patient may receive corticosteroids. Platelet transfusions are given if life-threatening hemorrhage develops. Splenectomy is not used because the spleen is not contributing to this type of thrombocytopenia.

Often, acquired thrombocytopenia is caused by another underlying condition (e.g., aplastic anemia, leukemia) or therapy used to treat another problem. For example, in acute leukemia all blood cell types may be depressed. Additionally, the patient may receive chemotherapeutic drugs that cause bone marrow suppression. If the patient can be adequately supported throughout the course of chemotherapy-induced thrombocytopenia, the thrombocytopenia will also resolve.

Oprelvekin (Neumega), a platelet growth factor that is a recombinant form of interleukin-11, stimulates the bone marrow to produce platelets.[20] It may be used to treat chemotherapy-induced thrombocytopenia. (Oprelvekin is discussed in Chapter 15.)

Since thrombopoietin (a hematopoeitic growth factor that stimulates the bone marrow to make platelets) was discovered in 1994, there has been much progress in the development of recombinant thrombopoietin. However, no thrombopoietin products have yet been approved for clinical use.

NURSING MANAGEMENT THROMBOCYTOPENIA

■ Nursing Assessment

Subjective and objective data that should be obtained from a patient with thrombocytopenia are presented in Table 30-14.

■ Nursing Diagnoses

Nursing diagnoses for the patient with thrombocytopenia may include, but are not limited to, those presented in NCP 30-2.

■ Planning

The overall goals are that the patient with thrombocytopenia will (1) have no gross or occult bleeding, (2) maintain vascular integrity, and (3) manage home care to prevent any complications related to an increased risk for bleeding.

■ Nursing Implementation

Health Promotion. It is important for the nurse to discourage excessive use of over-the-counter (OTC) medications known to be possible causes of acquired thrombocytopenia. Many medica-

NURSING CARE PLAN 30-2

Patient with Thrombocytopenia

EXPECTED PATIENT OUTCOMES	NURSING INTERVENTIONS and *RATIONALES*
NURSING DIAGNOSIS	**Impaired oral mucous membrane** *related to* low platelet counts, treatment, disease *as manifested by* bleeding and blood-filled bullae.
• Pink, moist, lesion-free oral mucosa, tongue, and lips	• Assess oral mucosa daily for presence of blood-filled bullae in mouth; bleeding; tender gingivae and lips *to provide information for planning interventions.* • Remove dentures daily (if present) and assess oral cavity *to assess underlying gums and mouth for bullae or bleeding areas.* • Provide oral hygiene with minimal friction: use soft-bristle toothbrush, cotton swabs, mild mouthwash, or irrigating syringe *to gently cleanse mouth without trauma.* • Evaluate integrity of nares, especially if nasogastric tube, endotracheal tube, or nasal O_2 is in use *to determine need for prophylactic or treatment interventions.*
NURSING DIAGNOSIS	**Risk for injury** *related to* low platelet counts and treatments.
• Maintenance of tissue integrity • No evidence of petechiae, ecchymoses, purpura, hematoma	• Initiate IV therapy judiciously; consider use of alternative venous access devices *to reduce number of venipunctures.* • Avoid IM and SQ injections; if used, apply local pressure with dry, sterile 2 × 2–inch gauze for 5-10 min after needle is removed *to prevent bleeding into tissue surrounding puncture site.* • Teach patient to use electric razor for shaving *to reduce potential for skin nicks.* • Pad rails and other firm surfaces, especially if patient is combative or at risk for seizures; be very gentle when turning patient or changing dressings *to reduce tissue trauma and subsequent bleeding into tissue.*
NURSING DIAGNOSIS	**Ineffective therapeutic regimen management** *related to* lack of knowledge of disease process, activity, and medication *as manifested by* frequent questioning about disease management, anxiety, restlessness.
• Verbalization and/or demonstration by patient and/or family of required knowledge and skills to manage home care	• Assess learning needs related to disease management *to plan appropriate interventions.* • Teach patient about disease process, medication, and activity recommendations *to decrease anxiety and prevent complications.* • Discuss (1) complications and signs that should be reported such as trauma prevention, (2) need for high fluid intake, (3) medication management, and (4) need for periods of rest and exercise *so patient will be knowledgeable and able to manage own care or direct others in care.* • Provide opportunities for patient to verbalize concerns *because discussing these with a supportive other decreases anxiety.*

COLLABORATIVE PROBLEM

NURSING GOALS	NURSING INTERVENTIONS and *RATIONALES*
POTENTIAL COMPLICATION	**Acute blood loss** *related to* decreased platelets, use of antiplatelet aggregating drugs.
• Monitor for signs of hemorrhage • Report deviations from acceptable parameter • Carry out appropriate medical and nursing interventions	• Evaluate mucous membranes and skin *to detect presence of epistaxis, petechiae, ecchymoses, hematomas.* • Test emesis, sputum, feces, urine, nasogastric secretions, and wound secretions regularly for occult blood and observe for blood *to detect potential presence of bleeding.* • Assess CBC and platelet count daily or more often if warranted *to monitor for bleeding.* • Do not administer and tell patient not to use aspirin or aspirin-containing products *because of their effects on platelet adhesiveness.* • Use ice, packing, or direct pressure *to control active bleeding.* • Teach patient to avoid Valsalva maneuver (e.g., straining at stool); administer stool softeners as ordered; avoid rectal temperatures, suppositories, and enemas; teach patient to cough, sneeze, and blow nose gently; administer medications to suppress vomiting and coughing *to avoid activities that could cause hemorrhage.* • Administer platelets or other blood components as ordered *to treat bleeding or replace blood loss due to hemorrhage.*

CBC, Complete blood count; *IM,* intramuscular; *IV,* intravenous; *SQ,* subcutaneous.

tions contain aspirin as an ingredient. Aspirin reduces platelet adhesiveness, thus contributing to bleeding.

It is also important for the nurse to encourage persons to have a complete medical evaluation if manifestations of bleeding tendencies (e.g., prolonged epistaxis, petechiae) develop. In addition, the nurse must observe for early signs of thrombocytopenia in the patient receiving cancer chemotherapy drugs.

Acute Intervention. The goal during acute episodes of thrombocytopenia is to prevent or control hemorrhage (see NCP 30-2). In the patient with thrombocytopenia, bleeding is usually from superficial sites; deep bleeding (into muscles, joints, and abdomen) usually occurs only when clotting factors are diminished. It is important to emphasize that a seemingly minor nosebleed or new petechiae may indicate potential hemorrhage and the physician should be notified. Bleeding from the posterior nasopharynx may be difficult to detect because the blood may be swallowed. If an IM or SQ injection is unavoidable, the use of a small-gauge needle and application of direct pressure for at least 5 to 10 minutes after injection is indicated or application of an ice pack may be helpful.

In a woman with thrombocytopenia, menstrual blood loss may exceed the usual amount and duration. Counting sanitary napkins used during menses is another important intervention to detect excess blood loss. Fifty milliliters of blood will completely soak a sanitary napkin. Suppression of menses with hormonal agents may be indicated during predictable periods of thrombocytopenia to reduce blood loss from menses (e.g., during chemotherapy and bone marrow transplantation).

The proper administration of platelet transfusions is an important nursing responsibility. Platelet concentrates, derived from fresh whole blood, can increase the platelet level effectively. Centrifuging 500 ml of whole blood derives 1 unit of platelets, a yellow liquid that is usually 30 to 50 ml in volume. Platelet concentrates from multiple units of blood (usually from six to eight different donors) can be pooled together for a single administration. The degree of increase or increment from a pooled platelet product varies widely and is usually measured by performing a platelet count within 1 hour following the transfusion.

Platelet transfusions can also be prepared by pheresing or removing the platelets from a single donor. This may be indicated when HLA-matched platelets are needed, especially for patients requiring multiple platelet transfusions. In this procedure, blood is removed from the donor, the platelets are removed, and the rest of the blood is reinfused into the donor. This procedure results in 200 to 400 ml of platelets and plasma. Once acquired from a donor, platelets can be stored at room temperature for 1 to 5 days. Gentle agitation of the bag is useful to prevent the platelets from adhering to the plastic. In a severely immunocompromised patient, these products are also irradiated to further ensure WBC removal and prevent the complication of graft-versus-host disease (see Chapter 13).

Ambulatory and Home Care. The patient with ITP who is receiving corticosteroids should be monitored frequently for the response to therapy. If the ITP is reversed by splenectomy, there is usually no recurrence. The person with acquired thrombocytopenia must be taught to avoid causative agents when possible (see Table 30-12). If the causative agents cannot be avoided (e.g., chemotherapy), the patient should learn to avoid injury or trauma during these periods and to detect the clinical signs and symp-

toms of bleeding caused by thrombocytopenia. The patient with either ITP or acquired thrombocytopenia should have planned periodic medical evaluations to assess the patient's status and to intercede in situations in which exacerbations and bleeding are likely to occur.

■ Evaluation

The expected outcomes for the patient with thrombocytopenia are presented in NCP 30-2.

HEMOPHILIA AND VON WILLEBRAND'S DISEASE

Hemophilia is a sex-linked recessive genetic disorder caused by defective or deficient coagulation factor (see the Genetics in Clinical Practice box and Fig. 13-2). (Sex-linked genetic disorders are discussed in Chapter 13.) The two major forms of hemophilia, which can occur in mild to severe forms, are hemophilia A (classic hemophilia, factor VIII deficiency) and hemophilia B (Christmas disease, factor IX deficiency). Von Willebrand's disease is a related disorder involving a deficiency of the von Willebrand coagulation protein. Factor VIII is synthesized in the liver and circulates as a complex with von Willebrand factor (vWF).[21]

Hemophilia A is the most common form of hemophilia; it makes up approximately 80% of all cases. The incidence of hemophilia A is approximately 1 in 5000 to 20,000 males; hemophilia B is seen in 1 in 30,000 to 50,000 males. Von Willebrand's disease is considered the most common congenital bleeding disorder in humans, with estimates as high as 1 in 100. However, because this disease can exist in mild to severe forms, life-threatening hemorrhage in patients is rare (1 in 1 million).[22] The deficiency and inheritance patterns of these three forms of inherited coagulopathies are compared in Table 30-15.

𝒢ENETICS in CLINICAL PRACTICE
Hemophilia A and B

Genetic Basis
- X-linked recessive disorder
- Mutations in gene that encodes clotting factor VIII (hemophilia A) or IX (hemophilia B)

Incidence
- 1 in 5000 to 20,000 male births (hemophilia A)
- 1 in 30,000 to 50,000 male births (hemophilia B)

Genetic Testing
- Possible with DNA technology

Clinical Implications
- Female carriers will transmit the genetic defect to 50% of their sons, and 50% of their daughters will be carriers.
- Men with hemophilia will not transmit the genetic defect to their sons, but all of their daughters will be carriers.
- Female hemophilia can occur if a man with hemophilia mates with a female carrier.
- Clinical manifestations of hemophilia A and B are very similar.
- Replacement therapy is available for factors VIII and IX (see Table 30-17).

TABLE 30-15	Comparison of Types of Hemophilia	
DISORDER	**DEFICIENCY**	**INHERITANCE PATTERN**
Hemophilia A	Factor VIII	Recessive sex-linked (transmitted by female carriers, displayed almost exclusively in men)
Hemophilia B	Factor IX	Recessive sex-linked (transmitted by female carriers, displayed almost exclusively in men)
von Willebrand's disease	vWF and platelet dysfunction	Autosomal dominant, seen in both sexes Recessive (in severe forms of the disease)

vWF, von Willebrand factor.

Clinical Manifestations and Complications

Clinical manifestations and complications related to hemophilia include (1) slow, persistent, prolonged bleeding from minor trauma and small cuts (Fig. 30-6); (2) delayed bleeding after minor injuries (the delay may be several hours or days); (3) uncontrollable hemorrhage after dental extractions or irritation of the gingiva with a hard-bristle toothbrush; (4) epistaxis, especially after a blow to the face; (5) GI bleeding from ulcers and gastritis; (6) hematuria from GU trauma and splenic rupture resulting from falls or abdominal trauma; (7) ecchymoses and subcutaneous hematomas; (8) neurologic signs, such as pain, anesthesia, and paralysis, which may develop from nerve compression caused by hematoma formation; and (9) hemarthrosis (bleeding into the joints) (Fig. 30-7), which may lead to joint deformity severe enough to cause crippling (most commonly in the knees, elbows, shoulders, hips, and ankles).

In children these symptoms may lead to the diagnosis. In adults, these developments may be the first sign of a newly diagnosed mild form of the disease that escaped detection through a childhood free of major injuries, dental procedures, or surgeries. All clinical manifestations relate to bleeding, and any bleeding episode in persons with hemophilia may lead to a life-threatening hemorrhage.

Historically, hemophilia was a disease of childhood because of early death from complications. In the early 1900s the average life expectancy was 11 years. By the 1970s advances in treatment enabled persons with hemophilia to have an average life expectancy of 68 years. Unfortunately, the acquired immunodeficiency syndrome (AIDS) epidemic and the HIV contamination of blood products reduced average life expectancy to 49 years in the late 1980s. Presently, about 90% of older persons severely affected with hemophilia are seropositive for HIV, which was transmitted via replacement therapy. Longer-term survival is now being observed because of improved preparation of replacement products, improved screening of donor populations, and use of recombinant replacement factors.[23] The development of hepatitis C in hemophilia patients was also common for many years because of lack of an available test to detect it and the use of pooled blood products. Hepatitis C antibody screening is now routinely done on all donated blood and blood products.

Diagnostic Studies

Laboratory studies are used to determine the type of hemophilia present. Any factor deficiency within the intrinsic system (factors VIII, IX, XI, or XII or vWF) will yield the laboratory results presented in Table 30-16.

Collaborative Care

The goals of collaborative care are to prevent and treat bleeding. Collaborative care for persons with hemophilia or von Willebrand's disease requires the provision of preventive care, the use replacement therapy during acute bleeding episodes and as prophylaxis, and the treatment of the complications of the disease and its therapy.

Replacement of deficient clotting factors is the primary means of supporting a patient with hemophilia. In addition to treating acute crises, replacement therapy may be given before surgery and dental care as a prophylactic measure. Examples of replacement therapy are listed in Table 30-17. Fresh frozen plasma, once commonly used for replacement therapy, is rarely used today.

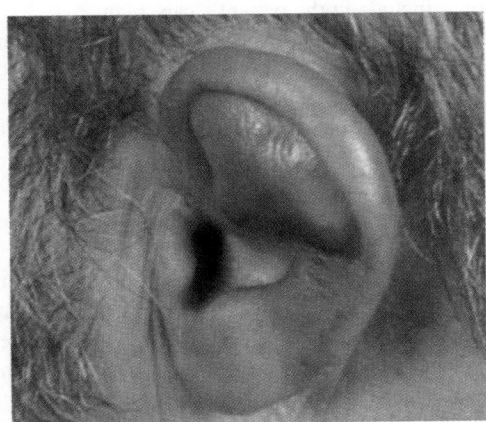

FIG. 30-6 Hematoma that developed in a person with hemophilia after trauma to the ear.

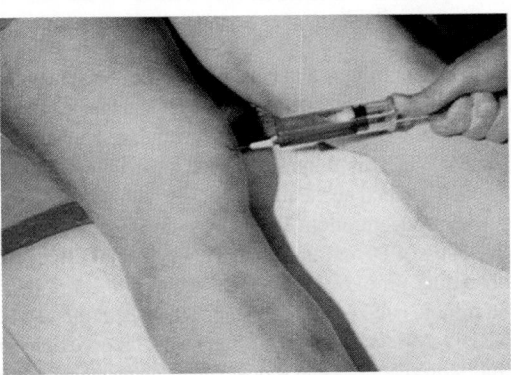

FIG. 30-7 Acute hemarthrosis of right knee in a patient with severe hemophilia. Blood from the synovial cavity is being aspirated with a needle and syringe.

TABLE 30-16	Laboratory Results in Hemophilia
TEST	**COMMENTS**
Prothrombin time	No involvement of extrinsic system
Thrombin time	No impairment of thrombin-fibrinogen reaction
Platelet count	Adequate platelet production
Partial thromboplastin time	Prolonged because of deficiency in any intrinsic clotting system factor
Bleeding time	Prolonged in von Willebrand's disease because of structurally defective platelets, normal in hemophilia A and B because platelets not affected
Factor assays	Reduction of factor VIII in hemophilia A, vWF in von Willebrand's disease, reduction of factor IX in hemophilia B

vWF, von Willebrand factor.

TABLE 30-17	_D_rug Therapy Replacement Factors Used in Treating Hemophilia

FACTOR VIII	FACTOR IX
Alphanate	Alphanine
Bicolate	Bebulin
Haemoctin SDH	Benefix
Helixate	Konyne
Hemofil	Mononine
Humate	Profilnine
Hyate	
Koate	
Kogenate	
Monoclate	
Melate	
Nybcen	
Omrixate	
Profilate	
Recombinate	
ReFacto	

For mild hemophilia A and certain subtypes of von Willebrand's disease, desmopressin acetate (also known as DDAVP), a synthetic analog of vasopressin, may be used to stimulate an increase in factor VIII and vWF. This drug acts on endothelial cells to cause the release of vWF, which subsequently binds with factor VIII, thus increasing their concentration. It can be administered intravenously, subcutaneously, or by intranasal spray. Beneficial effects (e.g., decreased bleeding time) of DDAVP, when administered IV, are seen within 30 minutes and can last for more than 12 hours. Because the effect of DDAVP is relatively short-lived, the patient must be closely monitored and repeated doses may be necessary. It is an appropriate therapy for minor bleeding episodes and dental procedures. The intranasal form may be indicated for home therapy for some patients with mild to moderate forms of the disease.[22]

Antifibrinolytic therapy (tranexamic acid [Cyklokapron] and epsilon aminocaproic acid [EACA]) inhibits fibrinolysis by inhibiting plasminogen activation in the fibrin clot, thereby enhancing clot stability. These agents are useful therapeutic adjuncts to stabilize clots in areas of increased fibrinolysis, such as the oral cavity, and in patients with difficult episodes of epistaxis and menorrhagia.

Complications of treatment of hemophilia include development of inhibitors to factors VIII or IX, transfusion-transmitted infectious disorders, allergic reactions, and thrombotic complications with the use of factor IX because it contains activated coagulation factors. Because of the improved viral-detecting processes and donor screening practices, the risk of HIV and hepatitis B and C transmission is greatly reduced.

The most common difficulties with acute management are starting factor replacement therapy too late and stopping it too soon. Generally, minor bleeding episodes should be treated for at least 72 hours. Surgery and traumatic injuries may need support for 10 to 14 days. Because of the short half-life of the factors, regular intermittent or continuous infusions have been used to manage bleeding episodes or expected traumatic procedures. Chronically, development of inhibitors to the factor products has occurred and requires individualized expert patient management by the health care team.

Designated treatment centers have been established in the United States and many other countries to provide multidisciplinary care of hemophilia and related disorders. The multidisciplinary team provides optimal chronic disease management.

Gene therapy has been used on an experimental basis to treat hemophilia. These clinical trials have involved (1) removing cells from the patient and genetically modifying them to secrete factor VIII or IX and (2) injecting vectors with the genes for factors VIII and IX.[24] (Gene therapy is discussed in Chapter 13.)

NURSING MANAGEMENT
HEMOPHILIA

■ Nursing Implementation

Health Promotion. Because of the hereditary nature of hemophilia, referral for genetic counseling is essential when considering preventive measures. This is especially important because many persons with hemophilia live into adulthood. Reproductive concerns and long-term effects are issues that the nurse should include in the patient's care plan.

Acute Intervention. Interventions are related primarily to controlling bleeding and include the following:

1. Stop the topical bleeding as quickly as possible by applying direct pressure or ice, packing the area with Gelfoam or fibrin foam, and applying topical hemostatic agents such as thrombin.
2. Administer the specific coagulation factor to raise the patient's level of the deficient coagulation factor.
3. When joint bleeding occurs, in addition to administering replacement factors, it is important to totally rest the involved joint to prevent crippling deformities from hemarthrosis. The joint may be packed in ice. Analgesics (e.g., acetaminophen, codeine) are given to reduce severe pain. However, aspirin and aspirin-containing compounds should never be used. As soon as bleeding ceases, it is important to encourage mobilization of the affected area

through range-of-motion exercises and physical therapy. Weight bearing is avoided until all swelling has resolved and muscle strength has returned.

4. Manage any life-threatening complication that may develop as a result of hemorrhage. Examples include nursing interventions to prevent or treat airway obstruction from hemorrhage into the neck and pharynx, as well as early assessment and treatment of intracranial bleeding.

Ambulatory and Home Care. Home management is a primary consideration for the patient with hemophilia because the disease follows a progressive, chronic course. The quality and the length of life may be significantly affected by the patient's knowledge of the illness and how to live with it. The patient and family can be referred to a local chapter of the National Hemophilia Society to encourage associations with other individuals who are dealing with the problems of hemophilia. The nurse must provide ongoing assessment of the patient's adaptation to the illness. Psychosocial support and assistance should be readily available as needed.

Most of the long-term care measures are related to patient teaching. The patient with hemophilia must be taught to recognize disease-related problems and to learn which problems can be resolved at home and which require hospitalization. Immediate medical attention is required for severe pain or swelling of a muscle or joint that restricts movement or inhibits sleep and for a head injury, a swelling in the neck or mouth, abdominal pain, hematuria, melena, and skin wounds in need of suturing.

Daily oral hygiene must be performed without causing trauma. Understanding how to prevent injuries is another consideration. This is no easy task; there are many potential sources of trauma. The patient can learn to participate in noncontact sports (e.g., golf) and wear gloves when doing household chores to prevent cuts or abrasions from knives, hammers, and other tools. The patient should wear a Medic Alert tag to ensure that health care providers know about the hemophilia in case of an accident.

The patient needs information about routine follow-up care, and the compliance with scheduled visits must be assessed. A reliable person can be taught to self-administer some of the factor replacement therapies at home.

■ Evaluation

The overall expected outcomes are similar to those for the patient with thrombocytopenia and are presented in NCP 30-2.

DISSEMINATED INTRAVASCULAR COAGULATION

Disseminated intravascular coagulation (DIC) is a serious bleeding disorder resulting from abnormally initiated and accelerated clotting. Subsequent decreases in clotting factors and platelets ensue, which may lead to uncontrollable hemorrhage. The term *disseminated intravascular coagulation* can be misleading because it suggests that blood is clotting. However, the paradox of this condition is characterized by the profuse bleeding that results from the depletion of platelets and clotting factors. An underlying disease or condition always causes DIC. The underlying disease must be treated for the DIC to resolve.

Etiology and Pathophysiology

DIC is not a disease; it is an abnormal response of the normal clotting cascade stimulated by a disease process or disorder. The diseases and disorders known to predispose a patient to DIC are

---

TABLE 30-18	**Predisposing Conditions to Development of Disseminated Intravascular Coagulation**

Acute DIC
Shock
  Hemorrhagic
  Cardiogenic
  Anaphylactic
Septicemia
Hemolytic processes
  Transfusion of mismatched blood
  Acute hemolysis from infection or immmunologic disorders
Obstetric conditions
  Abruptio placentae
  Amniotic fluid embolism
  Septic abortion
Tissue damage
  Extensive burns and trauma
  Heatstroke
  Severe head injury
  Transplant rejections
  Postoperative damage, especially after extracorporeal membrane oxygenation
  Fat and pulmonary emboli
  Snakebites
  Glomerulonephritis
  Acute anoxia (e.g., after cardiac arrest)
  Prosthetic devices

Subacute DIC
Malignant disease
  Acute leukemias
  Metastatic cancer
Obstetric
  Retained dead fetus

Chronic DIC
Liver disease
Systemic lupus erythematosus
Localized malignancy

DIC, Disseminated intravascular coagulation.

---

listed in Table 30-18. DIC can occur as an acute, catastrophic condition, or it may exist at a subacute or chronic level. Each condition may have one or multiple triggering mechanisms to start the clotting cascade. For example, tumors and traumatized or necrotic tissue release tissue factors into circulation. Endotoxin from gram-negative bacteria activates several steps in the coagulation cascade.

Initially in DIC, the normal coagulation mechanisms are enhanced. Abundant intravascular thrombin, the most powerful coagulant, is produced (Fig. 30-8). It catalyzes the conversion of fibrinogen to fibrin and enhances platelet aggregation. There is widespread fibrin and platelet deposition in capillaries and arterioles, resulting in thrombosis. This excessive clotting activates the fibrinolytic system, which in turn breaks down the newly formed clot, creating fibrin split (fibrin degradation) products. These products have anticoagulant properties and inhibit normal blood clotting. Ultimately with fibrin split products accumulating

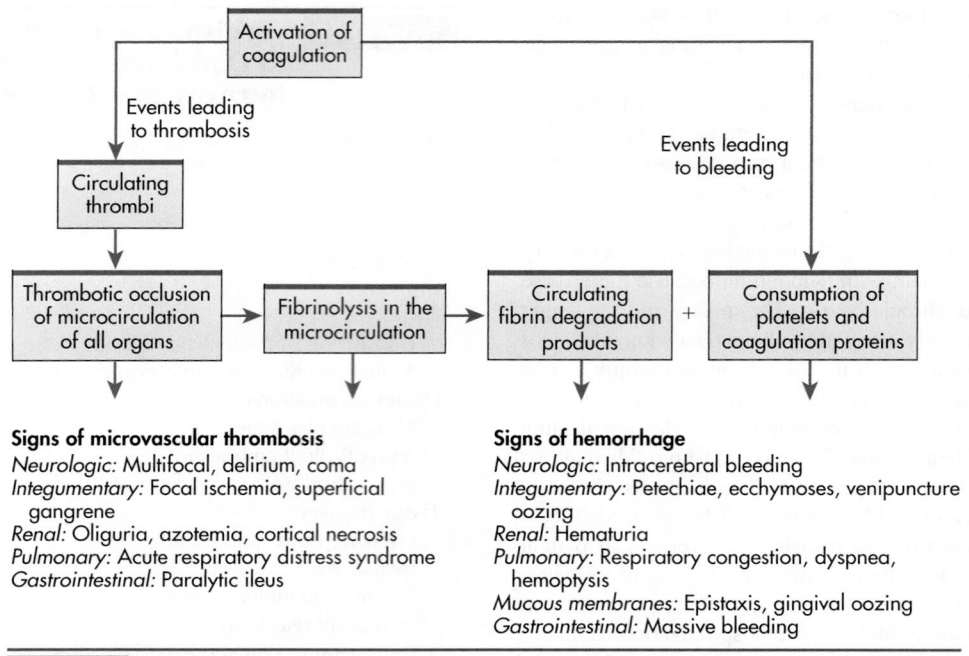

FIG. 30-8 The sequence of events that occur during disseminated intravascular coagulation (DIC).

and clotting factors being depleted, the blood loses its ability to clot. Therefore a stable clot cannot be formed at injury sites. This situation predisposes the patient to hemorrhage.

Chronic DIC is most commonly seen in patients with long-standing illnesses such as malignant disorders or autoimmune diseases. The incidence of DIC associated with malignancy ranges from 10% to 75%.[25] Occasionally these patients have sub-clinical disease manifested only by laboratory abnormalities. However, the clinical spectrum ranges from easy bruising to hemorrhage and from hypercoagulability to thrombosis.

Clinical Manifestations

There is no well-defined sequence of events in acute DIC. Bleeding in a person with no previous history or obvious cause should be questioned because it may be one of the first manifestations of acute DIC. Other nonspecific manifestations can include weakness, malaise, and fever.

There are both bleeding and thrombotic manifestations in DIC. Bleeding manifestations of DIC are multifactorial (see Fig. 30-8) and result from consumption and depletion of platelets and coagulation factors, as well as clot lysis and formation of fibrin split products that have anticoagulant properties.

Bleeding manifestations include integumentary manifestations, such as pallor, petechiae, oozing blood, venipuncture site bleeding, hematomas, and occult hemorrhage; respiratory manifestations such as tachypnea, hemoptysis, and orthopnea; cardiovascular manifestations, such as tachycardia and hypotension; GI manifestations, such as upper and lower GI bleeding, abdominal distention, and bloody stools; urinary manifestations, such as hematuria; neurologic changes, such as vision changes, dizziness, headache, changes in mental status, and irritability; and musculoskeletal complaints, such as bone and joint pain.

Thrombotic manifestations are a result of fibrin or platelet deposition in the microvasculature (see Fig. 30-8) and include integumentary changes, such as cyanosis, ischemic tissue necrosis (e.g., gangrene), and hemorrhagic necrosis; respiratory changes,

such as tachypnea, dyspnea, pulmonary emboli, and acute respiratory distress syndrome (ARDS); cardiovascular changes, such as electrocardiogram (ECG) changes and venous distention; GI changes, such as abdominal pain and paralytic ileus; and urinary changes, such as oliguria.

Diagnostic Studies

Tests used to diagnose acute DIC and their findings are listed in Table 30-19. As more clots are made in the body, more breakdown products from fibrinogen and fibrin are also formed. These are termed *fibrin split products* (FSPs) or *fibrin degradation products* (FDPs), and they work in three ways to interfere with blood coagulation. First, they coat the platelets and interfere with platelet function. Second, they interfere with thrombin and thereby disrupt coagulation. Third, the FSPs attach to fibrinogen, which interferes with the polymerization process necessary to form a stable clot. A much more specific test that is replacing measurement of FSP is the D-dimer assay. D-dimer, a specific polymer resulting from the breakdown of fibrin (and not fibrinogen), is a specific marker for the degree of fibrinolysis. In general, tests that measure raw materials needed for coagulation (e.g., platelets, fibrinogen) are reduced, and values that measure times to clot are prolonged. Fragmented erythrocytes (schistocytes), indicative of partial occlusion of small vessels by fibrin thrombi, may be found on blood smears.

Collaborative Care

It is important to diagnose DIC quickly, institute therapy that will resolve the underlying causative disease or problem, and provide supportive care for the manifestations resulting from the pathology of DIC itself. The treatment of DIC remains controversial and under investigation as researchers attempt to determine the most suitable means of managing this dangerous syndrome. Consequently it is imperative that the nurse maintain an ongoing awareness of current modes of therapy. Diagnosing and treating the primary disease process is essential to the resolution of DIC.

TABLE 30-19	Laboratory Abnormalities of Acute Disseminated Intravascular Coagulation
TEST	**FINDING (INCIDENCE)**
Screening Tests	
Prothrombin time	Prolonged (75%)
	Normal or shortened (25%)
Partial thromboplastin time	Prolonged (50%-60%)
Activated partial thromboplastin time	Prolonged
Thrombin time	Prolonged
Fibrinogen	Reduced
Platelets	Reduced to below 100,000/μl (100 × 10^9/L) to 5000/μl (5 × 10^9/L) in some patients
Special Tests	
Fibrin split products (FSP)*	Elevated (75%-100%)
Factor assays (for factors V, VII, VIII, X, XIII)	Reduced
D-dimers (cross-linked fibrin fragments)	Elevated (more reliable than FSP)
Antithrombin III	Reduced (90%)

*Fibrin degradation products (FDP).

Depending on its severity, a variety of different methods are used to provide supportive and symptomatic management of DIC (Fig. 30-9). First, if chronic DIC is diagnosed in a patient who is not bleeding, no therapy for DIC is necessary. Treatment of the underlying disease may be sufficient to reverse the DIC (e.g., an-

tineoplastic therapy when DIC is caused by malignancy). Second, when the patient with DIC is bleeding, therapy is directed toward providing support with necessary blood products while treating the primary disorder. The blood products are administered on the basis of specific component deficiencies. Platelets are given to correct thrombocytopenia, cryoprecipitate replaces factor VIII and fibrinogen, and fresh frozen plasma (FFP) replaces all clotting factors except platelets and provides a source of antithrombin.

A patient with manifestations of thrombosis is often treated by anticoagulation with heparin or low-molecular-weight heparin (LMWH). However, the use of heparin in the treatment of DIC remains controversial. Antithrombin III (AT III), a cofactor of heparin that becomes depleted during DIC, has been used alone or in conjunction with heparin when levels of this factor are low. Hirudin, a thrombin inhibitor and neutralizer, is also being studied as a blocker of the abnormal coagulation process.[25] Another treatment that has been used is epsilon aminocaproic acid (EACA, Amicar) because of its ability to inhibit fibrinolysis. The use of EACA is controversial because it can enhance thrombosis. Generally it is used only as adjunctive therapy to heparin.

Blood product support with platelets, cryoprecipitate, and FFP is usually reserved for a patient with life-threatening hemorrhage. The concern is that one is adding "fuel to the fire" of already activated coagulation. However, it may be the only method to avoid fatal hemorrhage in some patients. Therapy will stabilize a patient, prevent exsanguination or massive thrombosis, and permit institution of definitive therapy to treat the underlying cause.

Chronic DIC does not respond to oral anticoagulants, but it can be controlled with long-term use of heparin. Some patients with indolent (inactive and slowly developing) tumors and se-

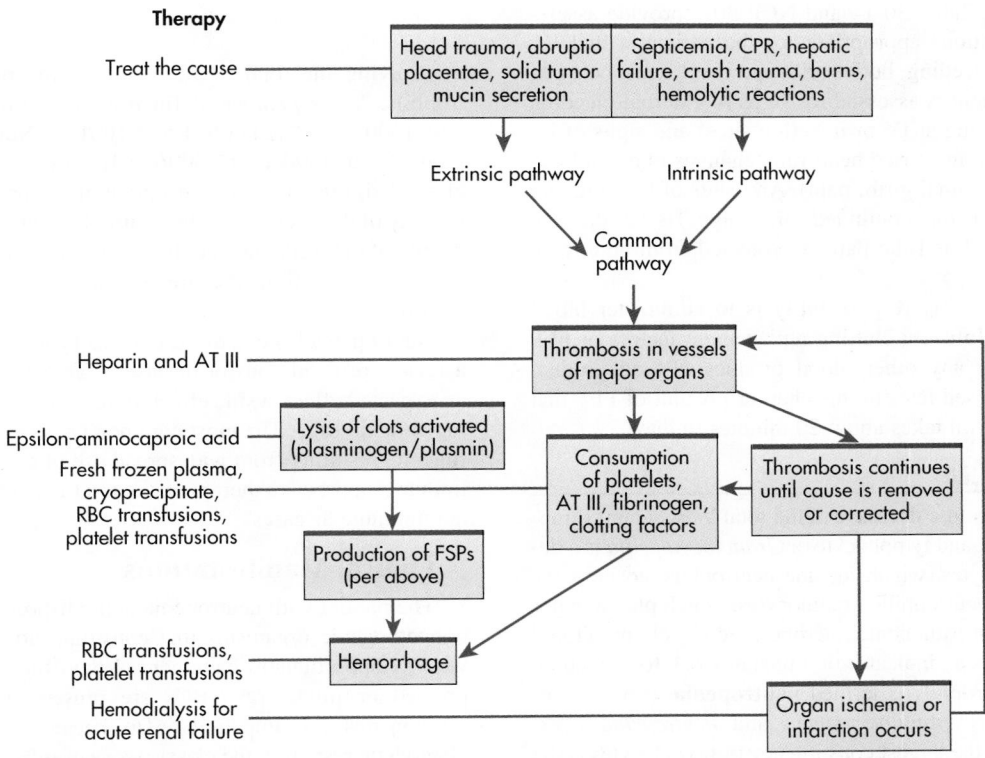

FIG. 30-9 Intended sites of action for therapies in disseminated intravascular coagulation. *AT III,* Antithrombin III; *CPR,* cardiopulmonary resuscitation; *FSPs,* fibrin split products.

vere, chronic DIC may need continuous infusion of heparin with portable pumps.

NURSING MANAGEMENT
DISSEMINATED INTRAVASCULAR COAGULATION

■ Nursing Diagnoses

Nursing diagnoses for the patient with DIC may include, but are not limited to, the following:
- Ineffective tissue perfusion (cerebral, cardiopulmonary, renal, GI, and peripheral) *related to* bleeding and sluggish or diminished blood flow secondary to thrombosis
- Acute pain *related to* bleeding into tissues and diagnostic procedures
- Decreased cardiac output *related to* fluid volume deficit and hypotension
- Anxiety *related to* fear of the unknown, disease process, diagnostic procedures, and therapy

■ Nursing Implementation

Nurses must be alert to the possible development of DIC and especially to the precipitating factors listed in Table 30-18. This may be difficult because the nurse is focusing on the complex care often required by the primary problem that precipitated the DIC. The nurse must also remember that because DIC is secondary to an underlying disease, appropriate care for managing the causative problem must be provided while providing supportive care related to the manifestations of DIC.

Appropriate nursing interventions are essential to the survival of a patient with acute DIC. Astute, ongoing assessment; active attention to manifestations of the syndrome; and institution of appropriate treatment measures are challenging and sometimes paradoxic nursing responsibilities (e.g., administering heparin to a bleeding patient). Table 30-14 and NCP 30-2 provide assessments and interventions appropriate for the patient with DIC. Early detection of bleeding, both occult and overt, must be a primary goal. The patient is assessed for signs of external bleeding (e.g., petechiae, oozing at IV or injection sites) and signs of internal bleeding (e.g., increased heart rate, changes in mental status, increasing abdominal girth, pain). Any sites of bleeding are carefully monitored for continued bleeding. Tissue damage should be minimized and the patient protected from additional foci of bleeding.

An additional nursing responsibility is to administer blood products correctly. Infusing clotting replacement factors or FFP is similar to giving any other blood product. (Blood product transfusion is discussed later in this chapter.) A unit of FFP that contains 200 to 280 ml takes about 20 minutes to thaw.

NEUTROPENIA

Leukopenia refers to a decrease in the total WBC count (granulocytes, monocytes, and lymphocytes). *Granulocytopenia* is a deficiency of granulocytes, which include neutrophils, eosinophils, and basophils. The neutrophilic granulocytes, which play a major role in phagocytizing pathogenic microbes, are closely monitored in clinical practice as an indicator of a patient's risk for infection. A reduction in neutrophils is termed **neutropenia.** (Some clinicians use the terms *granulocytopenia* and *neutropenia* interchangeably because the largest constituency of granulocytes is the neutrophils.) The absolute neutrophil count is determined by

TABLE 30-20	Causes of Neutropenia

Drug-Induced Causes
- Antitumor antibiotics (daunorubicin, doxorubicin)
- Alkylating agents (nitrogen mustards, busulfan)
- Antimetabolites (methotrexate, 6-mercaptopurine)
- Antiinflammatory drugs (phenylbutazone)
- Psychotropics and antidepressants (clozapine, imipramine)
- Miscellaneous (gold, penicillamine, mepacrine, amodiaquine)
- zidovudine (AZT)

Hematologic Disorders
- Idiopathic neutropenia
- Cyclic neutropenia
- Aplastic anemia
- Leukemia

Autoimmune Disorders
- Systemic lupus erythematosus
- Felty syndrome
- Rheumatoid arthritis

Infections
- Viral (e.g., hepatitis, influenza, HIV, measles)
- Fulminant bacterial infection (e.g., typhoid fever, miliary tuberculosis)

Miscellaneous
- Severe sepsis
- Bone marrow infiltration (e.g., carcinoma, tuberculosis, lymphoma)
- Hypersplenism (e.g., portal hypertension, Felty syndrome, storage diseases [e.g., Gaucher's disease])
- Nutritional deficiencies (cobalamin, folic acid)

HIV, Human immunodeficiency virus.

multiplying the total WBC count by the percentage of neutrophils. *Neutropenia* is defined as a neutrophil count of less than 1000 to 1500/μl (1 to 1.5 × 10^9/L).[26] Normally, neutrophils range from 4000 to 11,000/μl. However, in considering the clinical significance of neutropenia it is important to know the rapidity of the decrease in the neutrophil count (gradual or rapid), degree of neutropenia, and duration. The faster the drop and the longer the duration, the greater the likelihood of developing infection.

Neutropenia is not a disease; it is a syndrome that occurs with a variety of conditions or diseases (Table 30-20). It can also be an expected effect, a side effect, or an unintentional effect of taking certain drugs. The most common cause of neutropenia is iatrogenic, resulting from widespread use of chemotherapeutic and immunosuppressive therapy in the treatment of malignancies and autoimmune diseases.

Clinical Manifestations

The patient with neutropenia is predisposed to infection with nonpathogenic organisms that constitute normal body flora, as well as opportunistic pathogens. When the WBC count is depressed or immature WBCs are present, normal phagocytic mechanisms are impaired. Also because of the diminished phagocytic response, the classic signs of inflammation—redness, heat, and swelling—may not occur. WBCs are the major component of pus. Therefore in the patient with neutropenia, pus formation (e.g., as a visible skin lesion or as pulmonary infiltrates on a chest x-ray) is also absent. Because neutropenia masks some of the signs and symptoms of infection, the presence of even a low-grade fever is of great significance.[27]

When fever occurs in a neutropenic patient, it is assumed to be caused by infection and requires immediate attention. The immunocompromised, neutropenic patient has little or no ability to fight infection. Thus minor infections can lead rapidly to sepsis. The mucous membranes of the throat and mouth, the skin, the perianal area, and the pulmonary system are common entry points for pathogenic organisms in susceptible hosts. Clinical manifestations related to infection at these sites include complaints of sore throat and dysphagia, appearance of ulcerative lesions of the pharyngeal and buccal mucosa, diarrhea, rectal tenderness, vaginal itching or discharge, shortness of breath, and nonproductive cough. These seemingly minor complaints can progress to fever, chills, sepsis, and septic shock if not recognized and treated in early stages.

Systemic infections caused by bacterial, fungal, and viral organisms are common in patients with neutropenia. The patient's own flora (normally nonpathogenic) contributes significantly to life-threatening infections such as pneumonia. Organisms that are known to be common sources of infection include gram-positive *Staphylococcus aureus* and aerobic gram-negative organisms. Fungi that are involved include *Candida* (usually *C. albicans*) and *Aspergillus*. Viral infections caused by reactivation of herpes simplex and zoster are common following prolonged periods of neutropenia.[27]

Diagnostic Studies

The primary diagnostic tests for assessing neutropenia are the peripheral WBC count and bone marrow aspiration and biopsy (Table 30-21). A total WBC count of less than $4000/\mu l$ ($4 \times 10^9/L$) reflects leukopenia. However, only a differential count can confirm the presence of neutropenia (neutrophil count, 1000 to $1500/\mu l$ [1 to $1.5 \times 10^9/L$]). If the differential WBC count reflects an absolute neutropenia of 500 to $1000/\mu l$ (0.5 to $1.0 \times 10^9/L$), the patient is at moderate risk for a bacterial infection. An absolute neutropenia of less than $500/\mu l$ ($0.5 \times 10^9/L$) places the patient at severe risk.

A peripheral blood smear is used to assess for immature forms of WBCs. The hematocrit level, reticulocyte count, and platelet count are done to evaluate bone marrow function. If the cause of neutropenia is unknown, bone marrow aspirations and biopsies are done to examine cellularity and cell morphology. Additional studies may be done as indicated to assess spleen and liver function.

NURSING *and* COLLABORATIVE MANAGEMENT NEUTROPENIA

The factors involved in the nursing and collaborative care of neutropenia include (1) determining the cause of the neutropenia; (2) identifying the offending organisms if an infection has developed; (3) instituting prophylactic, empiric, or therapeutic antibiotic therapy; (4) administering hematopoietic growth factors (e.g., granulocyte colony–stimulating factor [G-CSF] and granulocyte-macrophage colony–stimulating factor [GM-CSF]); and (5) instituting protective isolation practices, such as strict hand washing, visitor restrictions, private room, high-efficiency particulate

TABLE 30-21 *C*ollaborative Care Neutropenia
Diagnostic
History and physical examination
WBC count with differential count
WBC morphology
Hct and Hb values
Reticulocyte and platelet count
Bone marrow aspiration or biopsy
Cultures of nose, throat, sputum, urine, stool, obvious lesions, blood (as indicated)
Chest x-ray
Collaborative Therapy
Identification and removal of cause of neutropenia (if possible)
Identification of site of infection (if present) and causative organism
Antibiotic therapy
Hematopoietic growth factors (G-CSF, GM-CSF)
Protective (reverse) isolation
High-efficiency particulate air (HEPA) filtration
Laminar airflow isolation

G-CSF, Granulocyte colony–stimulating factor; *GM-CSF*, granulocyte-macrophage colony–stimulating factor; *Hb*, hemoglobin; *Hct*, hematocrit; *WBC*, white blood cell.

air (HEPA) filtration, or laminar air flow (LAF) environment (see Table 30-21).

Occasionally the cause of the neutropenia can be easily treated (e.g., nutritional deficiencies). However, neutropenia can also be a side effect that must be tolerated as a necessary step in therapy (e.g., chemotherapy, radiation therapy). In some situations the neutropenia resolves when the primary disease is treated (e.g., tuberculosis).

The nurse needs to monitor the neutropenic patient for signs and symptoms of infection and early septic shock. Early identification of a potentially infective organism depends on acquiring cultures from various sites. Serial blood cultures (at least two) or one from a peripheral site and one from a venous access device and cultures of sputum, throat, lesions, wounds, urine, and feces are essential in the surveillance of the patient. It may also be necessary to do a tracheal aspiration, bronchoscopy with bronchial brushings, or lung biopsy to diagnose the cause of pneumonic infiltrates. Despite these many tests, the causative organism is identified only in approximately one half of neutropenic patients.[27]

When a febrile episode occurs in a neutropenic patient, antibiotic therapy is initiated immediately (within 1 hour) even before the determination of a specific causative organism by culture. Administration of broad-spectrum antibiotics is usually by the IV route because of the rapidly lethal effects of infection. However, some oral antibiotics are highly effective and routinely used for prophylaxis against infection in some neutropenic patients. Antibiotics are often used in combinations because of their synergistic effects. Combinations of antibiotics are also used in the event that multiple organisms are responsible for the infectious symptoms. Usually an aminoglycoside is used with an antipseudomonal penicillin or cephalosporin. Regardless of the combination, the nurse must observe for side effects of antimicrobial agents. Side effects common to aminoglycosides include nephrotoxicity and ototoxicity; side effects common to cephalosporins include rashes, fever, and pruritus.

The duration of the neutropenia also increases the infection risk of the patient. The longer the neutropenia, the greater the risk of a fungal infection. Antifungal therapy is initiated whenever a culture is positive, or in patients who do not become afebrile with broad-spectrum antibiotic coverage.

G-CSF (filgrastim [Neupogen] and pegfilgrastim [Neulasta]) and GM-CSF (sargramostim [Leukine, Prokine]) can be used to treat a neutropenic patient. G-CSF stimulates the production and function of neutrophils. GM-CSF stimulates the production and function of neutrophils and monocytes. These agents can be given IV or SQ. The nurse can teach the patient and family how to administer the SQ medication. These factors are especially beneficial in enhancing granulocyte recovery after chemotherapy and shorten the period of vulnerability to fatal infections. (G-CSF and GM-CSF are discussed in Chapter 15.)

An important consideration in the care of a neutropenic patient is the determination of the best means to protect the patient whose own defenses against infection are compromised. To accomplish this goal, the following principles must be kept in mind: (1) the patient's normal flora is the most common source of microbial colonization and infection; (2) transmission of organisms from humans most commonly occurs by direct contact with the hands; (3) air, food, water, and equipment provide additional opportunities for infection transmission; and (4) health care providers with transmittable illnesses and other patients with infections can also be sources of infection transmission under certain conditions.

Strict hand washing by all persons coming in contact with the compromised patient is the major method to prevent transmission of harmful pathogens. The Centers for Disease Control and Prevention (CDC) advocates hand washing before, during, and after care. This seemingly routine technique has a significant effect in reducing infection. It must be emphasized and enforced despite its seeming simplicity.

The CDC also encourages separating immunocompromised patients from those who are infected or who have conditions that increase the probability of transmitting infections (e.g., poor hygiene caused by lack of understanding or cognitive dysfunction). Private rooms are useful whenever possible. High-efficiency particulate air (HEPA) filtration is an air-handling method with a high-flow filtering system that can reduce or eliminate the number of aerosolized pathogens in the environment. Although it is expensive to install, it is often used for a patient with severe prolonged neutropenia (e.g., bone marrow transplant patients). Care routines in a HEPA environment are essentially the same as care in any other private room.

For severely immunocompromised patients (e.g., bone marrow transplants, high-dose chemotherapy) routine protective isolation techniques may be warranted. These include laminar airflow (LAF) rooms, prophylactic antibiotics, and avoidance of fresh fruit and vegetables. Although LAF rooms can reduce the incidence of hospital-acquired infections in severely neutropenic patients, it has not been shown to increase survival. Cost, lack of sufficient improvement in long-term survival, and the psychologic effects of being isolated in an LAF room have contributed to the declining construction of new LAF rooms.[28] The nursing measures presented in NCP 30-3 are important in the treatment of the patient with neutropenia.

The value of effective nursing care in reducing the development of infection or limiting its extent cannot be overempha-

---

NURSING CARE PLAN 30-3

Patient with Neutropenia

EXPECTED PATIENT OUTCOMES	NURSING INTERVENTIONS and *RATIONALES*
NURSING DIAGNOSIS	**Risk for infection** *related to* decreased neutrophils and altered response to microbial invasion and presence of environmental pathogens.
• Free from signs and symptoms of infection • Minimal exposure to environmental pathogens	• Monitor for fever and absolute neutrophil count *to identify signs of and potential for infection.* • Evaluate for presence of chills. Take vital signs q4hr *because fever may be the only indication of infection and septic shock.* • Report temperature elevations >100.4° F (38° C) to health care provider immediately *in order to promptly initiate antibiotic therapy due to the rapidly lethal effects of infection.* • Be aware of chills, complaints of being cold when environment is warm, sore throat, persistent cough, chest pain, burning on urination *because these may be signs of infection.* • Use proper skin preparation techniques for initiating and maintaining IV lines, caring for venous access devices, or obtaining blood culture specimens *to reduce the risk of introducing infection through the skin.* • Assess for superinfections *that may develop with extended use of antibiotics.* • Institute good hand-washing technique with antiseptic solution for all persons in contact with patient; place patient in private room; limit and/or screen visitors and hospital staff members with colds or potentially communicable illnesses *to prevent the transmission of harmful pathogens to patient.* • Teach patient necessary personal hygiene techniques (e.g., hand washing, oral care, skin hygiene, and pulmonary hygiene) and potential infection risks. • Avoid invasive procedures to the greatest extent possible (e.g., venipunctures, urinary catheters). • Administer hematopoietic growth factors as ordered (e.g., G-CSF, GM-CSF) *to increase patient's WBC count and reduce infection risk during periods of neutropenia.*

G-CSF, Granulocyte colony–stimulating factor; *GM-CSF,* granulocyte-monocyte colony–stimulating factor; *IV,* intravenous; *WBC,* white blood cell.

sized. Regular assessment and early detection of infectious sources are key roles for the nurse in reducing morbidity and mortality rates from infection.

MYELODYSPLASTIC SYNDROME

Myelodysplastic syndrome (MDS) is a group of related hematologic disorders characterized by a change in the quantity and quality of bone marrow elements. Other terms used to describe this hematologic syndrome include *preleukemia, hematopoietic dysplasia, refractory anemia with excessive myeloblasts, subacute myeloid leukemia, oligoplastic leukemia,* and *smoldering leukemia.*[29]

Etiology and Pathophysiology

The etiology of MDS is unknown. Its manifestations result from neoplastic transformation of the pluripotent hematopoietic stem cells within the bone marrow. Occasionally one type of MDS transforms into another. In some cases, MDS will progress to acute myelogenous leukemia.

MDS is referred to as a *clonal disorder* because some bone marrow stem cells continue to function normally whereas others (a specific clone) do not. The abnormal clone of the stem cells is usually found in the bone marrow but eventually may be found in circulation. In contrast to *acute myelogenous leukemia* (AML), in which the leukemic cells show little normal maturation, the clonal cells in MDS always display some degree of maturity. Disease progression is slower than in AML. However, eventually the abnormal cells replace the bone marrow. Typically, life-threatening anemia, thrombocytopenia, and neutropenia occur during the advanced stage of MDS.

Clinical Manifestations

MDS commonly manifests as infection and bleeding caused by inadequate numbers of ineffective functioning circulating granulocytes or platelets. MDS is often discovered in the elderly as a result of testing for the symptoms of anemia, thrombocytopenia, or neutropenia. It may also be diagnosed incidentally from a routine complete blood count (CBC).

Diagnostic Studies

Bone marrow biopsy with aspirate analysis is essential for both the diagnosis and the classification of the specific types of myelodysplasia. In MDS the bone marrow is normocellular, hypocellular, or hypercellular and the patient has peripheral cytopenia. MDS is staged according to clinical and laboratory findings. The relationship between the number of circulating blast cells and the number of blast cells in the bone marrow serves as the main indicator of prognosis in this disease.

NURSING *and* COLLABORATIVE MANAGEMENT
MYELODYSPLASTIC SYNDROME

Supportive treatment of MDS is based on the premise that the aggressiveness of treatment should match the aggressiveness of the disease. Supportive treatment consists of hematologic monitoring (serial bone marrow and peripheral blood examinations), antibiotic therapy, or transfusions with blood products. Side effects and toxicities from supportive treatment include anemia, thrombocytopenia, and blood transfusion reactions.

Drugs can be used to correct the defective maturation of the hematopoietic stem cell clone in the marrow in about 25% to

35% of patients. Some agents have been shown to transform nonfunctional immature blasts and promyelocytes into functional mature granulocytes.[29] These agents include retinoic acid (Tretinoin) and cytarabine (Ara-C, Cytosar). Side effects and toxicities from retinoic acid include dry skin, dry lips, myalgias, lethargy, and hypercalcemia. Bone marrow transplantation, biologic therapy, and colony-stimulating factors have also been used in an attempt to treat bone marrow dysfunction of MDS. However, because of the aggressiveness of these treatments, older patients do not often tolerate them.

Nursing care of a patient with MDS is similar to that of a patient with manifestations of anemia (see nursing care plan for the patient with anemia [NCP 30-1]), thrombocytopenia (see nursing care plan for the patient with thrombocytopenia [NCP 30-2]), and neutropenia (see nursing care plan for the patient with neutropenia [NCP 30-3]).

LEUKEMIA

Leukemia is the general term used to describe a group of malignant disorders affecting the blood and blood-forming tissues of the bone marrow, lymph system, and spleen. Leukemia occurs in all age-groups. It results in an accumulation of dysfunctional cells because of a loss of regulation in cell division. It follows a progressive course that is eventually fatal if untreated. An estimated 30,800 new cases are diagnosed each year. Although often thought of as a disease of children, the number of adults affected with leukemia is 10 times that of children.[30]

Etiology and Pathophysiology

Regardless of the specific type of leukemia, there is generally no single causative agent in the development of leukemia. Most leukemias result from a combination of factors, including genetic and environmental influences. Chromosomal changes, first recognized in chronic myelogenous leukemia, have led to discoveries of how normal genes, once transformed, can result in abnormal genes (oncogenes) capable of causing many types of cancers, including leukemias (see Chapter 15). Chemical agents (e.g., benzene), chemotherapeutic agents (e.g., alkylating agents), viruses, radiation, and immunologic deficiencies have all been associated with the development of leukemia in susceptible hosts. There is an increased incidence of leukemia in radiologists, persons who have lived near nuclear bomb test sites or nuclear reactor accidents (e.g., Chernobyl), survivors of the bombing of Nagasaki and Hiroshima, and persons previously treated with radiation therapy or chemotherapy. Although RNA retroviruses cause a number of leukemias in animals, a viral cause for a human leukemia has been established only for some patients with adult T cell leukemia. This form of leukemia is endemic in southwestern Japan and parts of the Caribbean and central Africa and is caused by the human T cell leukemia virus type 1 (HTLV-1).

Classification

Classification of leukemia can be done based on acute versus chronic and on the type of WBC involved. The terms *acute* and *chronic* refer to cell maturity and nature of disease onset. Acute leukemia is characterized by the clonal proliferation of immature hematopoietic cells. The leukemia develops following malignant transformation of a single type of immature hematopoietic cell, followed by cellular replication and expansion of that malignant

TABLE 30-22   Types of Leukemia

TYPE	AGE OF ONSET	CLINICAL MANIFESTATIONS	DIAGNOSTIC FINDINGS
Acute myelogenous leukemia (AML)	Increase in incidence with advancing age, peak incidence between 60-70 yr of age	Fatigue and weakness, headache, mouth sores, minimal hepatosplenomegaly and lymphadenopathy, anemia, bleeding, fever, infection, sternal tenderness	Low RBC count, Hb, Hct; low platelet count; low to high WBC count with myeloblasts; greatly hypercellular bone marrow with myeloblasts
Acute lymphocytic leukemia (ALL)	Before 14 yr of age, peak incidence between 2-9 yr of age and in older adults	Fever; pallor; bleeding; anorexia; fatigue and weakness; bone, joint, and abdominal pain; generalized lymphadenopathy; infections; weight loss; hepatosplenomegaly; headache; mouth sores; neurologic manifestations, including CNS involvement, increased intracranial pressure, secondary to meningeal infiltration	Low RBC count, Hb, Hct; low platelet count; low, normal, or high WBC count; transverse lines of rarefaction at ends of metaphysis of long bones on x-ray; hypercellular bone marrow with lymphoblasts; lymphoblasts also possible in cerebrospinal fluid
Chronic myelogenous leukemia (CML)	25-60 yr of age, peak incidence around 45 yr of age	No symptoms early in disease, fatigue and weakness, fever, sternal tenderness, weight loss, joint pain, bone pain, massive splenomegaly, increase in sweating	Low RBC count, Hb, Hct; high platelet count early, lower count later; increase in polymorphonuclear neutrophils, normal number of lymphocytes, and normal or low number of monocytes in WBC differential; low leukocyte alkaline phosphatase; presence of Philadelphia chromosome in 90% of patients
Chronic lymphocytic leukemia (CLL)	50-70 yr of age, rare below 30 yr of age, predominance in men	No symptoms frequently, detection of disease often during examination for unrelated condition, chronic fatigue, anorexia, splenomegaly and lymphadenopathy, hepatomegaly	Mild anemia and thrombocytopenia with disease progression; total WBC count >100,000/μl; increase in peripheral lymphocytes; increase in presence of lymphocytes in bone marrow

CNS, Central nervous system; *Hb,* hemoglobin; *Hct,* hematocrit; *RBC,* red blood cell; *WBC,* white blood cell.

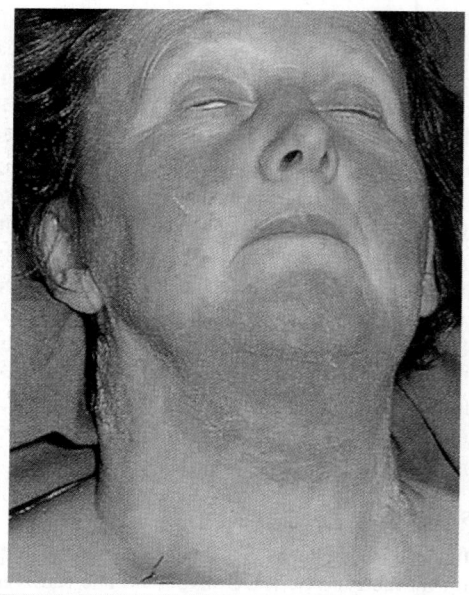

FIG. 30-10 Complications of acute leukemia. Spreading cellulitis of the neck and chin in this woman with acute myelogenous leukemia results from streptococcal and candidal infection. She was at risk because of previous chemotherapy and prolonged neutropenia.

clone. Chronic leukemias involve more mature forms of WBC, and the disease onset is more gradual.

Leukemia can also be classified by identifying the type of leukocyte involved, whether it is of myelogenous origin or of lymphocytic origin. By combining the acute and chronic categories with the cell type involved, specific types of leukemia can be identified. Four major types of leukemia are acute lymphocytic leukemia (ALL), acute myelogenous leukemia (AML) (also called acute nonlymphoblastic leukemia [ANLL]), chronic myelogenous (granulocytic) leukemia (CML), and chronic lymphocytic leukemia (CLL). Other defining features of these leukemic subtypes are presented in Table 30-22.

Acute Myelogenous Leukemia. AML (also referred to as ANLL) represents only one fourth of all leukemias, but it makes up approximately 85% of the acute leukemias in adults (Fig. 30-10). Its onset is often abrupt and dramatic. A patient may have serious infections and abnormal bleeding from the onset of the disease.[31,32]

AML is characterized by uncontrolled proliferation of myeloblasts, the precursors of granulocytes. There is hyperplasia of the bone marrow and spleen. The clinical manifestations are usually related to replacement of normal hematopoietic cells in the marrow by leukemic myeloblasts and, to a lesser extent, to infiltration of other organs (see Table 30-22).

Acute Lymphocytic Leukemia. ALL is the most common type of leukemia in children and accounts for about 15% of acute leukemia in adults. In ALL, immature lymphocytes proliferate in the bone marrow. Fever is present in the majority of patients at the time of diagnosis. Signs and symptoms may appear abruptly with bleeding or fever, or they may be insidious with progressive weakness, fatigue, and bleeding tendencies.

CNS manifestations are especially common in ALL and represent a serious problem. Leukemic meningitis caused by arachnoid infiltration occurs in many patients with ALL.

Chronic Myelogenous Leukemia. CML is also termed *chronic granulocytic leukemia* (CGL). CML is caused by excessive development of mature neoplastic granulocytes in the bone marrow. The excess neoplastic granulocytes move into the peripheral blood in massive numbers and ultimately infiltrate the liver and spleen. These cells contain a distinctive cytogenetic abnormality, the *Philadelphia chromosome,* which serves as a disease marker and results from translocation of genetic material between chromosomes 9 and 22.

The natural history of CML is a chronic stable phase, followed by the development of a more acute, aggressive phase referred to as the *blastic phase.* The chronic phase of CML can last for several years and can usually be well controlled with treatment. Even with treatment, the chronic phase of the disease will eventually progress to the accelerated phase, ending in a blastic phase. Once CML transforms to an acute or blastic phase, it is often refractory to therapy and the patient may live for only a few months.

Chronic Lymphocytic Leukemia. CLL is characterized by the production and accumulation of functionally inactive but long-lived, mature-appearing lymphocytes. The type of lymphocyte involved is usually the B cell. The lymphocytes infiltrate the bone marrow, spleen, and liver. Lymph node enlargement (lymphadenopathy) is present throughout the body, and there is an increased incidence of infection. B cell CLL is considered to be identical to the mature B cell small lymphocytic lymphoma, a type of non-Hodgkin's lymphoma. Complications from early-stage CLL are rare but may develop as the disease advances. Pressure on nerves from enlarged lymph nodes causes pain and even paralysis. Mediastinal node enlargement leads to pulmonary symptoms. Because CLL is usually a disease of older adults, treatment decisions must be made by considering the progression of the disease and the side effects of treatment. Many individuals in the early stages of CLL require no treatment.

Hairy Cell Leukemia. *Hairy cell leukemia* accounts for approximately 2% of all adult leukemias. Hairy cell leukemia is usually seen in male patients over 40 years of age. It is a chronic disease of lymphoproliferation predominantly involving B lymphocytes that infiltrate the bone marrow and spleen. Cells have a "hairy" appearance under the microscope. The spleen sequesters increasing numbers of normal hematopoietic cells, making splenomegaly a common finding.

A patient with hairy cell leukemia usually has symptoms from splenomegaly, pancytopenia, infection caused by impaired host defense, or vasculitis. Many asymptomatic patients are detected on routine CBC. α-Interferon, pentostatin (Nipent), and cladribine (Leustatin) are effective agents in the treatment of this type of leukemia.

Unclassified Leukemias. Occasionally the subtype of leukemia cannot be identified. The malignant leukemic cells may have lymphoid, myeloid, or mixed characteristics. Frequently these patients do not respond to treatment and have a poor prognosis.

Clinical Manifestations

The clinical manifestations of leukemia are varied (see Table 30-22). Essentially they relate to problems caused by bone marrow failure and the formation of leukemic infiltrates. Bone marrow failure results from (1) bone marrow overcrowding by abnormal cells and (2) inadequate production of normal marrow elements. The patient is predisposed to anemia, thrombocytopenia, and decreased number and function of WBCs.

As leukemia progresses, fewer normal blood cells are produced. The abnormal WBCs continue to accumulate because they do not go through the normal cell life cycle to death (*apoptosis*). The leukemic cells infiltrate the patient's organs, leading to problems such as splenomegaly, hepatomegaly, lymphadenopathy, bone pain, meningeal irritation, and oral lesions. Solid masses resulting from collections of leukemic cells called *chloromas* can also occur.

Diagnostic Studies

Peripheral blood evaluation and bone marrow examination are the primary methods of diagnosing and classifying the subtypes of leukemia. Morphologic, histochemical, immunologic, and cytogenetic methods are all used to identify cell subtypes and the stage of development of leukemic cell populations. This is important because different subtypes have different natural histories, prognoses, and chemotherapeutic regimens. Other studies such as lumbar puncture and computed tomography (CT) scan can determine the presence of leukemic cells outside of the blood and bone marrow.

The malignant cells in most patients with AML and ALL have chromosomal abnormalities. In some cases, specific cytogenetic abnormalities are associated with distinct subsets of the disease. In addition to establishing the type of AML or ALL, specific cytogenetic abnormalities have diagnostic, prognostic, and therapeutic importance. In CML, the finding of the Philadelphia chromosome has diagnostic value.

Collaborative Care

Once a diagnosis of leukemia has been made, collaborative care is focused on the initial goal of attaining remission. Because cytotoxic chemotherapy is the mainstay of the treatment, the nurse must understand the principles of cancer chemotherapy, including cellular kinetics, the use of multiple drugs rather than single agents, and the cell cycle. (See the section on chemotherapy in Chapter 15.)

Although not all forms of leukemia are considered curable at this time, attaining remission or disease control is a realistic option for the majority of patients. In *complete remission* there is no evidence of overt disease on physical examination, and the bone marrow and peripheral blood appear normal. A lesser state of control is known as partial remission. *Partial remission* is characterized by a lack of symptoms and a normal peripheral blood smear, but there is still evidence of disease in the bone marrow. The patient's prognosis is directly related to the ability to maintain a remission. The patient's prognosis becomes more unfavorable with each relapse. Each time there is a relapse, the succeeding remission may be more difficult to achieve and shorter in duration.

The chemotherapeutic treatment of acute leukemia is divided into stages. The first stage, *induction therapy,* is the attempt to induce or bring about a remission. Induction is aggressive treatment that seeks to destroy leukemic cells in the tissues, peripheral blood, and bone marrow. During induction therapy a patient may become critically ill because the bone marrow is severely depressed by the chemotherapeutic agents. Throughout the induction phase, nursing interventions focus on neutropenia, thrombocytopenia, and anemia, as well as providing psychosocial support to the patient and family. Common chemotherapy agents for induction of AML include cytarabine (Ara-C, Cytosar) and antitumor antibiotics (anthracyclines) such as daunorubicin, doxorubicin, idarubicin, amsacrine, or mitoxantrone. After one course of induction therapy, approximately 70% of newly diagnosed patients achieve complete remission.[33,34] It is generally assumed that leukemia cells persist undetected after induction therapy. This could lead to relapse within a few months if no further therapy is administered.

Terms used to describe postinduction or postremission chemotherapy include intensification, consolidation, and maintenance. *Intensification therapy,* or high-dose therapy, may be given immediately after induction therapy for several months. This therapy may use the same drugs as those used in induction but at higher dosages. Other drugs that target the cell in a different way than those administered during induction may also be added.

Consolidation therapy is started after a remission is achieved. It may consist of one or two additional courses of the same drugs given during induction or involve high-dose therapy (intensive consolidation). The purpose of consolidation therapy is to eliminate remaining leukemic cells that may not be clinically or pathologically evident.

Maintenance therapy is treatment with lower doses of the same drugs used in induction or other drugs given every 3 to 4 weeks for a prolonged period of time. Like consolidation or intensification, the goal is to keep the body free of leukemic cells. Each leukemia requires different maintenance therapy. In AML maintenance therapy is rarely effective and therefore rarely administered.[34]

In addition to chemotherapy, corticosteroids and radiation therapy can also have a role in the complex therapeutic plans for the patient with leukemia. Total body radiation may be used to prepare a patient for bone marrow transplantation, or it may be restricted to certain areas (fields) such as the liver and spleen or other organs affected by infiltrates. In ALL, prophylactic intrathecal methotrexate is given to decrease the chance of CNS involvement, which is common in this particular type of leukemia. When CNS leukemia does occur, cranial radiation may be given. Biologic therapy may be indicated for specific leukemias. (Biologic therapy is discussed in Chapter 15.)

Chemotherapy Regimens. The chemotherapeutic agents used to treat leukemia vary. Table 30-23 lists chemotherapeutic agents used to treat leukemia. Table 30-24 gives examples of treatment regimens used in various types of leukemia.

Combination chemotherapy is the mainstay of treatment for leukemia. The three purposes for using multiple drugs are to (1) decrease drug resistance, (2) minimize the drug toxicity to the patient by using multiple drugs with varying toxicities, and (3) interrupt cell growth at multiple points in the cell cycle.

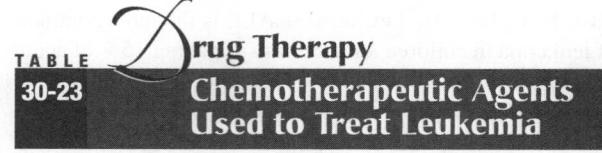

TABLE 30-23   Drug Therapy: Chemotherapeutic Agents Used to Treat Leukemia

DRUG CLASSIFICATION	DRUG NAME
Alkylating agents	busulfan (Myleran)
	chlorambucil (Leukeran)
	cyclophosphamide (Cytoxan)
Antitumor antibiotics (anthracyclines)	daunorubicin (Cerubidine)
	doxorubicin (Adriamycin)
	mitoxantrone (Novantrone)
	idarubicin (Idamycin)
Antimetabolites	cytarabine (Cytosar, Ara-C)
	6-mercaptopurine (Purinethol)
	methotrexate (Folex)
	6-thioguanine (6-TG)
	fludarabine (Fludara)
Corticosteroid	prednisone
Nitrosoureas	carmustine (BCNU)
Mitotic inhibitors	vincristine (Oncovin)
	vinblastine (Velban)
Monoclonal antibodies	rituximab (Rituxan)
	alemtuzumab (Campath)
Miscellaneous	L-asparaginase (Elspar)
	hydroxyurea (Hydrea)
	etoposide (VePesid)
	retinoic acid (tretinoin)
	arsenic trioxide (Trisenox)
	imatinib mesylate (Gleevec)

Acronyms made from the letters of the drugs used in combination chemotherapy are used to identify the regimen. For example, COAP stands for cyclophosphamide, Oncovin, arabinoside, and prednisone. This combination of drugs is used to treat ALL.

New chemotherapeutic drugs include arsenic trioxide (Trisenox) and imatinib mesylate (Gleevec). Arsenic trioxide is used in the treatment of acute promyelocytic leukemia. Its mechanism of action is not completely understood. It causes morphologic changes and DNA fragmentation. It inhibits proliferation. Imatinib mesylate represents a new class of drugs that specifically target an abnormal cell. It targets an abnormal version of a normal cell protein (the bcr-abl protein) that is present in nearly all patients with CML. This abnormal protein is probably the cause of the disease. The bcr-abl gene is located on the Philadelphia chromosome. Thus this drug kills only cancer cells, leaving healthy cells alone.

The use of monoclonal antibodies is an exciting new treatment modality in lymphoid malignancies. Rituximab (Rituxan) binds to the B cell antigen (CD 20) and has been used with CLL. Alemtuzumab (Campath) binds to CD52, a panlymphocyte antigen present on both T and B cells, and is used to treat CLL. After the monoclonal antibodies bind to the lymphocytes, the drug induces antibody-dependent lysis (killing). This causes the removal of malignant lymphocytes from the blood, bone marrow, and other affected organs.

Bone Marrow and Stem Cell Transplantation. Bone marrow transplantation (BMT) and stem cell transplantation are other therapies used to treat patients with different forms of

TABLE 30-24   Drug Therapy — Treatments Used in Leukemia

DRUG THERAPY	OTHER THERAPY
Acute Myelogenous Leukemia Daunorubicin, cytarabine, doxorubicin, idarubicin, 6-thioguanine, mitoxantrone, combination chemotherapy of antitumor antibiotic and cytosine arabinoside or antitumor antibiotic and cytosine arabinoside and thioguanine, arsenic trioxide (Trisenox)*	Bone marrow and stem cell transplant (see Chaper 15)
Acute Lymphocytic Leukemia Daunorubicin, doxorubicin, vincristine, prednisone, L-asparaginase, cyclophosphamide, methotrexate, 6-mercaptopurine, cytarabine, combination chemotherapy of cyclophosphamide and vincristine and prednisone and antitumor antibiotic and L-asparaginase, combination chemotherapy of daunorubicin and cytarabine and 6-mercaptopurine and vincristine and prednisone	Cranial radiation therapy, intrathecal methotrexate
Chronic Myelogenous Leukemia Hydroxyurea (Hydrea); combination chemotherapy including any of the following: cytarabine, thioguanine, daunorubicin, methotrexate, prednisone, vincristine, L-asparaginase, carmustine, 6-mercaptopurine, imatinib mesylate (Gleevec)	Radiation (total body or spleen), bone marrow and stem cell transplant, α-interferon, leukapheresis
Chronic Lymphocytic Leukemia Chorambucil (Leukeran), cyclophosphamide (Cytoxan), prednisone, (CVP protocol [cyclophosphamide, vincristine, and prednisone]), fludarabine, rituximab (Rituxan), alemtuzumab (Campath)	Radiation (total body, lymph nodes, or spleen), splenectomy, colony-stimulating factors, α-interferon

*Used for acute promyelocytic leukemia.

leukemia.[35] The goal of transplant is to totally eliminate leukemic cells from the body using combinations of chemotherapy with or without total body irradiation. This treatment also eradicates the patient's hematopoietic stem cells, which are then replaced with those of an HLA-matched sibling or volunteer donor (allogeneic), with those of an identical twin (syngeneic), or with the patient's own (autologous) stem cells that were removed (harvested) before the intensive therapy. (Bone marrow and peripheral stem cell transplantation is discussed in Chapter 15.)

The primary complications of patients with allogeneic BMT are graft-versus-host disease (GVHD), relapse of leukemia (especially ALL), and infection (especially interstitial pneumonia). GVHD is discussed in Chapter 13. Because transplantation has serious associated risks, the patient must weigh the significant risks of treatment-related death or treatment failure (relapse) with the hope of cure.[36,37]

NURSING MANAGEMENT
LEUKEMIA

■ Nursing Assessment

Subjective and objective data that should be obtained from a patient with leukemia are presented in Table 30-25.

■ Nursing Diagnoses

Nursing diagnoses for the patient with leukemia includes those appropriate for anemia, thrombocytopenia, and neutropenia (see the appropriate nursing care plans [NCPs 30-1, 30-2, and 30-3] in this chapter).

■ Planning

The overall goals are that the patient with leukemia will (1) understand and cooperate with the treatment plan, (2) experience minimal side effects and complications associated with both the disease and its treatment, and (3) feel hopeful and supported during the periods of treatment, relapse, or remission.

■ Nursing Implementation

Acute Intervention. The nursing role during acute phases of leukemia is extremely challenging because the patient has many physical and psychosocial needs. As with other forms of cancer, the diagnosis of leukemia can evoke great fear and be equated with death. It may be viewed as a hopeless, horrible disease with many painful and undesirable consequences. The nurse helps the patient realize that although the future may be uncertain, one can have a meaningful quality of life while in remission or with disease control. The family also needs help in adjusting to the stress of this abrupt onset of serious illness (e.g., dependence, withdrawal, changes in role responsibilities, alterations in body image) and the losses imposed by the sick role. The diagnosis of leukemia often brings with it the need to make difficult decisions at a time of profound stress for the patient and family.

The nurse is an important advocate in helping the patient and family understand the complexities of treatment decisions and manage the side effects and toxicities. A patient empowered by knowledge of the disease and treatment can have a more positive outlook and improved quality of life. A patient may require isolation or may need to temporarily relocate to an appropriate treatment center. These situations can lead a patient to feel deserted and isolated at a time when support is most needed. The nurse has contact with a patient 24 hours a day, and can help reverse feelings of abandonment and loneliness by balancing the demanding technical needs with a humanistic, caring approach. Nurses face special challenges when meeting the intense psychosocial needs of a patient with leukemia while

TABLE	**Nursing Assessment**
30-25	**Leukemia**

Subjective Data

Important Health Information

Past health history: Exposure to chemical toxins (e.g., benzene, arsenic), radiation, or viruses (Epstein–Barr, HTLV–1); chromosome abnormalities (Down syndrome, Klinefelter syndrome, Fanconi syndrome), immunologic deficiencies; organ transplantation; frequent infections; bleeding tendencies

Medications: Use of phenylbutazone (Butazolidin), chloramphenicol, chemotherapy

Surgery or other treatments: Radiation exposure; prior radiation and chemotherapy for cancer

Functional Health Patterns

Health perception–health management: Family history of leukemia; malaise

Nutritional-metabolic: Mouth sores, weight loss; chills, night sweats; nausea, vomiting, anorexia, dysphagia, early satiety; easy bruising

Elimination: Hematuria, decreased urine output; diarrhea, dark or bloody stools

Activity-exercise: Fatigue with progressive weakness; dyspnea, epistaxis, cough

Cognitive-perceptual: Headache; muscle cramps; sore throat; generalized sternal tenderness, bone, joint, abdominal pain; paresthesias, numbness, tingling, visual disturbances

Sexuality-reproductive: Prolonged menses, menorrhagia, impotence

Objective Data

General

Fever, generalized lymphadenopathy, lethargy

Integumentary

Pallor or jaundice; petechiae, ecchymoses, purpura, reddish-brown to purple cutaneous infiltrates, macules, and papules

Cardiovascular

Tachycardia, systolic murmurs

Gastrointestinal

Gingival bleeding and hyperplasia; oral ulcerations, herpes and *Candida* infections; perirectal irritation and infection; hepatosplenomegaly

Neurologic

Seizures, disorientation, confusion, decreased coordination, cranial nerve palsies, papilledema

Musculoskeletal

Muscle wasting

Possible Findings

Low, normal, or high WBC count with shift to the left (↑ blast cells); anemia, ↓ hematocrit and hemoglobin, thrombocytopenia, Philadelphia chromosome; hypercellular bone marrow aspirate or biopsy with myeloblasts, lymphoblasts, and markedly ↓ normal cells

HTLV-1, Human T cell leukemia virus, type 1; *WBC,* white blood cell.

---

continuing to offer the complex physical care that is required. The needs of the patient with leukemia are best met by a multidisciplinary team (e.g., psychiatric and oncology clinical nurse specialists, case managers, dietitians, chaplains and social workers).

From a physical care perspective, the nurse is challenged to make astute assessments and plan care to help the patient manage the severe side effects of chemotherapy. The life-threatening results of bone marrow suppression (neutropenia, thrombocytopenia, and anemia) require aggressive nursing interventions (see NCPs 30-1, 30-2, and 30-3). Additional complications of chemotherapy may affect the patient's GI tract, nutritional status, skin and mucosa, cardiopulmonary status, liver, kidneys, and neurologic system. (Nursing interventions related to chemotherapy are discussed in Chapter 15.)

The nurse must be knowledgeable about all drugs being administered. This includes the mechanism of action, purpose, routes of administration, usual doses, potential side effects, safe-handling considerations, and toxic effects of the drugs. In addition, the nurse must know how to assess laboratory data reflecting the effects of the drugs. Patient survival and comfort during aggressive chemotherapy are significantly affected by the quality of nursing care.

Ambulatory and Home Care. Ongoing care for the patient with leukemia is necessary to monitor for signs and symptoms of disease control or relapse. For a patient requiring long-term or maintenance chemotherapy, the fatigue of long-term chronic disease management can become arduous and discouraging. There-

fore a patient and the significant other must be taught to understand the importance of the continued diligence in disease management and the need for follow-up care. The patient and significant other must be taught about the drugs, self-care measures, and when to seek medical attention.

The goals of rehabilitation for long-term survivors of childhood and adult leukemia are to manage the physical, psychologic, social, and spiritual consequences and delayed effects from the disease and its treatment. (Delayed effects are discussed in Chapter 15.) Assistance may be needed to reestablish the various relationships that are a part of the patient's life. Friends and family may not know how to interact with the patient. The patient and family must learn to regain attitudes of health and life while facing the real fear of relapse of disease. Involving the patient in survivor networks, support groups, or services such as Can Surmount and Make Today Count may help the patient adapt to living after a life-threatening illness. Exploring resources in the community (e.g., American Cancer Society, Leukemia Society, Meals-on-Wheels, wheelchair taxis) may reduce the financial burden and the feelings of dependence. Spiritual support may give the patient inner strength and peace.

The patient will need support in adapting to any physical limitations or changes imposed by the illness. Vigilant follow-up care by providers who are aware of the unique needs of a cancer survivor is of the utmost importance for early recognition and treatment of long-term or delayed physical, psychologic, and social effects. The nurse may involve other health care providers in meeting the patient's needs. However, often these needs will require the initiation of a referral or consultation. For example, physical therapy personnel may be asked to develop an exercise program to prevent posttreatment deficits caused by drug-induced peripheral neuropathy. These needs can also include other concerns such as growth and development concerns for childhood survivors, vocational retraining, and reproductive concerns for a patient of childbearing age. The long-term recovery following treatment for leukemia affects the quality of the patient's life.

■ Evaluation

The expected outcomes are that the patient with leukemia will (1) cope effectively with diagnosis, treatment regimen, and prognosis; (2) attain and maintain adequate nutrition; (3) experience no complications related to the disease or its treatment; and (4) feel comfortable and supported throughout treatment.

Lymphomas

Lymphomas are malignant neoplasms originating in the bone marrow and lymphatic structures resulting in the proliferation of lymphocytes. Lymphomas are the fifth most common type of cancer in the United States.[38] Two major types of lymphoma—Hodgkin's disease and non-Hodgkin's lymphoma (NHL)—are discussed in this chapter. A comparison of these two types of lymphoma is presented in Table 30-26.

HODGKIN'S DISEASE

Hodgkin's disease, which makes up about 15% of all lymphomas, is a malignant condition characterized by proliferation of abnormal giant, multinucleated cells, called *Reed-Sternberg cells,* which are located in lymph nodes. The disease has a bimodal age-specific incidence, occurring most frequently in persons from 15 to 35 years of age and above 50 years of age. In adults, it is twice as prevalent in men as in women. Approximately 7200 new cases of Hodgkin's disease are diagnosed each year, and approximately 1300 deaths occur each year.[38]

Etiology and Pathophysiology

Although the cause of Hodgkin's disease remains unknown, several key factors are thought to play a role in its development. The main interacting factors include infection with Epstein-Barr virus (EBV), genetic predisposition, and exposure to occupational toxins.

Normally, the lymph nodes are composed of connective tissues that surround a fine mesh of reticular fibers and cells. In Hodgkin's disease the normal structure of lymph nodes is destroyed by hyperplasia of monocytes and macrophages. The main

diagnostic feature of Hodgkin's disease is the presence of Reed-Sternberg cells in lymph node biopsy specimens. The disease is believed to arise in a single location (it originates in lymph nodes in 90% of patients) and then spreads along adjacent lymphatics. It eventually infiltrates other organs, especially the lungs, spleen, and liver. In approximately two thirds of patients the cervical lymph nodes are the first to be affected. When the disease begins above the diaphragm, it remains confined to lymph nodes for a variable period of time. Disease originating below the diaphragm frequently spreads to extralymphoid sites such as the liver.

Clinical Manifestations

The onset of symptoms in Hodgkin's disease is usually insidious. The initial development is most often enlargement of cervical, axillary, or inguinal lymph nodes (Fig. 30-11). This lymphadenopathy affects discrete nodes that remain movable and nontender. The enlarged nodes are not painful unless they exert pressure on adjacent nerves.

The patient may notice weight loss, fatigue, weakness, fever, chills, tachycardia, or night sweats. A group of initial findings including fever, night sweats, and weight loss (termed *B symptoms*) correlates with a worse prognosis. After the ingestion of even small amounts of alcohol, individuals with Hodgkin's disease may complain of a rapid onset of pain at the site of disease. The cause for the alcohol-induced pain is unknown. Generalized pruritus without skin lesions may develop. Cough, dyspnea, stridor, and dysphagia may all reflect mediastinal node involvement.

In more advanced disease there is hepatomegaly and splenomegaly. Anemia results from increased destruction and decreased production of erythrocytes. Other physical signs vary de-

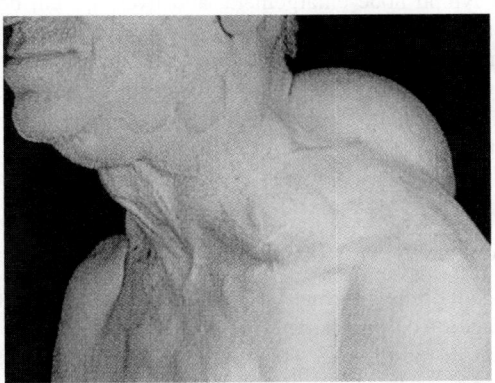

FIG. 30-11 Hodgkin's disease (stage IIA). This patient has enlargement of the cervical lymph nodes.

TABLE 30-26	Comparison of Hodgkin's Disease and Non-Hodgkin's Lymphoma	
	HODGKIN'S DISEASE	**NON-HODGKIN'S LYMPHOMA**
Cellular origin	B lymphocytes	B lymphocytes (90%)
		T lymphocytes (10%)
Extent of disease	Localized to regional	Disseminated
B symptoms*	Common	Uncommon
Extranodal involvement	Rare	Common
Histopathologic classification	Singular	Many different classifications

*B symptoms include fever, night sweats, and weight loss.

pending on where the disease is located. For example, intrathoracic involvement may lead to superior vena cava syndrome, enlarged retroperitoneal nodes may cause palpable abdominal masses or interfere with renal function, jaundice may occur from liver involvement, and spinal cord compression leading to paraplegia may occur with extradural involvement. Bone pain occurs as a result of bone involvement.

Diagnostic and Staging Studies

Peripheral blood analysis, lymph node biopsy, bone marrow examination, and radiologic evaluation are important means of evaluating Hodgkin's disease. Peripheral blood analysis often reveals a microcytic hypochromic anemia, neutrophilic leukocytosis (15,000 to 28,000/μl [15 to 28 × 10^9/L]), which may be associated with lymphopenia and an increased platelet count. Leukopenia and thrombocytopenia may develop, but they are usually a consequence of treatment, advanced disease, or superimposed hypersplenism. Other blood studies may show hypoferremia caused by excessive iron uptake by the liver and spleen, elevated leukocyte alkaline phosphatase from liver and bone involvement, hypercalcemia from bone involvement, and hypoalbuminemia from liver involvement.

Excisional lymph node biopsy offers a definitive means of diagnosis. The removed peripheral lymph node is examined for the presence of the diagnostic Reed-Sternberg cells. Bone marrow biopsy is performed as an important aspect of staging. Reed-Sternberg cells may also be found in the bone marrow of patients.

Radiologic evaluation can help define all sites and determine the clinical stage of the disease. Chest x-rays, radioisotope studies, and CT scans may show mediastinal lymphadenopathy, renal displacement caused by retroperitoneal node enlargement, abdominal lymph node enlargement, and liver, spleen, bone, and brain infiltration. Some clinicians also use lymphangiography, a radiographic dye study that uses blue dye injected into the lymphatic system to assess the lymph nodes and lymph vessels. This test can also visualize the sometimes difficult to see retroperitoneal structures.

NURSING *and* COLLABORATIVE MANAGEMENT HODGKIN'S DISEASE

Using all of the information from the various diagnostic studies, a stage of disease is determined (Fig. 30-12). The stage is the extent of the disease. This is important because Hodgkin's disease may be localized or diffuse (advanced). Treatment depends on the nature and extent of the disease. The nomenclature used in staging involves an A or B classification, depending on whether symptoms are present when the disease is found, and a Roman numeral (I to IV) that reflects the location and extent of the disease.

Once the stage of Hodgkin's disease is established, management focuses on selecting a treatment plan. The least amount of treatment is used to achieve cure yet minimize the short-term and long-term complications. Radiation therapy given to affected areas over 4 to 6 weeks can cure 95% of patients with stage I or stage II disease. Combination chemotherapy is used in some early stages in patients believed to have resistant disease or to be at high risk for relapse. Chemotherapy regimens include MOPP and ABVD. MOPP consists of mechlorethamine, vincristine (Oncovin), procarbazine, and prednisone. ABVD consists of doxorubicin (Adriamycin), bleomycin, vinblastine, and dacarbazine. Stage IIIA disease is treated with both radiation therapy and chemotherapy. The role of radiation as a supplement to chemotherapy in stages III and IV varies depending on sites of disease. Advances in treatment now enable some stage IIIB and stage IV diseases to be cured with high-dose chemotherapy and bone marrow or peripheral stem cell transplantation (see Chapter 15).

Intensive chemotherapy with or without the use of bone marrow and peripheral stem cell transplantation and hematopoietic growth factors is the treatment of choice for advanced Hodgkin's disease (stages IIIB and IV). Transplantation has allowed patients to receive higher, potentially curative doses of chemotherapy while reducing life-threatening leukopenia. Combination chemotherapy works well because, as in leukemia, drugs are used that have an additive antitumor effect without increasing side effects. As with leukemia, therapy must be aggressive; therefore potentially life-threatening problems are encountered in an attempt to achieve a remission.[38]

Maintenance chemotherapy does not contribute to increased survival once a complete remission is achieved. Occasionally, single drugs may be administered palliatively to patients who cannot tolerate intensive combination therapy. A serious consequence of the treatment for Hodgkin's disease is the later development of secondary malignancies (see Chapter 15). The estimated risk of a secondary cancer is approximately 18% at 15 years after treatment for Hodgkin's disease. The most common secondary malignancies are acute nonlymphoblastic leukemia, non-Hodgkin's lymphoma, and solid tumors.

The nursing care for Hodgkin's disease is largely based on managing pancytopenia and other side effects of therapy. Because the survival of patients with Hodgkin's disease depends on their response to treatment, supporting the patient through the immunosuppressive state is extremely important.

The patient undergoing radiation therapy has special nursing needs. The skin in the radiation field requires attention. Also, the nurse must understand the concepts related to administration of radiation therapy (see Chapter 15).

Psychosocial considerations are just as important as they are with leukemia. Although the prognosis for Hodgkin's disease is better than that for many forms of cancer or leukemia, attention to the physical, psychologic, social, and spiritual consequences of the patient's disease must be addressed. Fertility issues may be of particular concern because this disease is frequently seen in adolescents and young adults. In this light, the nurse must help ensure that these issues have been addressed soon after diagnosis. Evaluation of patients for long-term effects of therapy is important because delayed consequences of disease and treatment may not be apparent for many years. (Secondary malignancies and delayed effects are discussed in Chapter 15.)

NON-HODGKIN'S LYMPHOMA

Non-Hodgkin's lymphomas (NHLs) are a heterogeneous group of malignant neoplasms of the immune system affecting all ages. They are classified according to different cellular and lymph node characteristics. A variety of clinical presentations and courses are recognized, from indolent (slowly developing) to rapidly progressive disease. B cell lymphomas constitute about 90% of all NHLs. Common names for different types of NHLs include Burkitt's lymphoma, reticulum cell sarcoma, and lymphosarcoma. There is no hallmark feature in NHLs that parallels

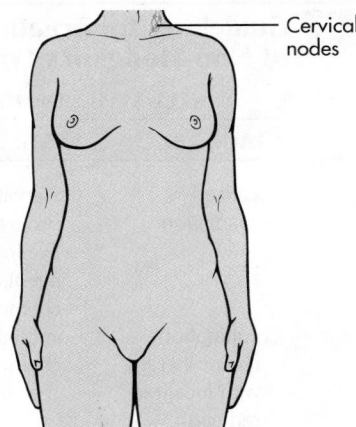

Stage I
Involvement of a single lymph node
or a single extranodal site

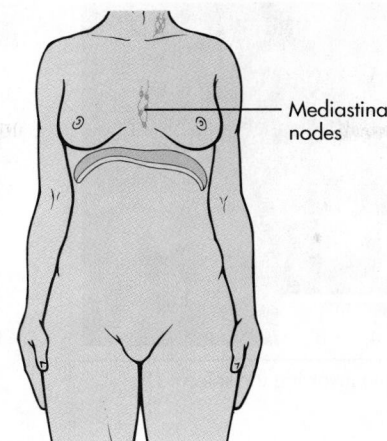

Stage II
Involvement of two or more lymph node regions
on the same side of the diaphragm or localized
involvement of an extranodal site and one or more
lymph node regions of the same side of diaphragm

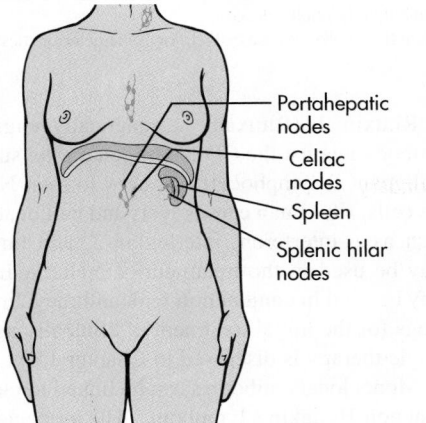

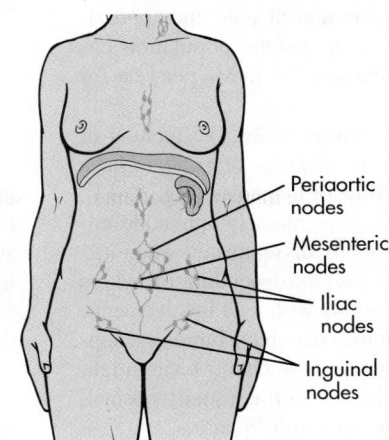

Stage III
Involvement of lymph node regions on both sides of the diaphragm. May include a single extranodal site, the spleen,
or both; now subdivided into lymphatic involvement of the upper abdomen in the spleen (splenic, celiac, and portal
nodes) (*Stage III₁*) and the lower abdominal nodes in the paraaortic, mesenteric, and iliac regions (*Stage III₂*)

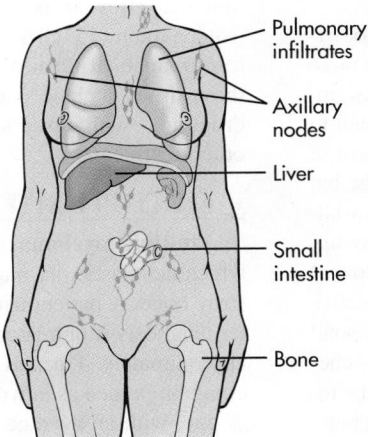

Stage IV
Diffuse or disseminated disease of one or more extralymphatic
organs or tissues with or without associated lymph node
involvement; the extranodal site is identified as *H*, hepatic;
L, lung; *P*, pleura; *M*, marrow; *D*, dermal; *O*, osseous

FIG. 30-12 Staging system for Hodgkin's disease and non–Hodgkin's lymphoma.

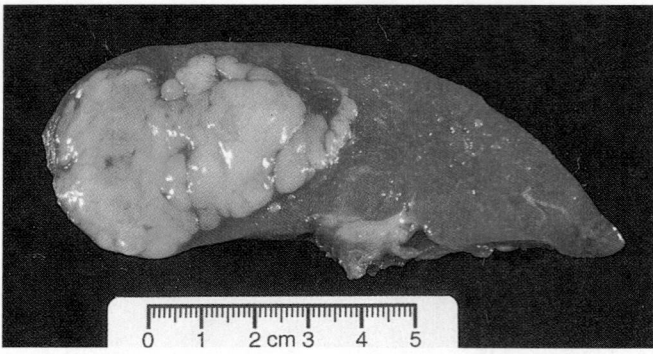

FIG. 30-13 Non-Hodgkin's lymphoma involving the spleen. The presence of an isolated mass is typical.

TABLE 30-27	Guidelines for Treatment of Non-Hodgkin's Lymphoma	
	RECOMMENDED THERAPY	
GRADE	**STAGE I, II₁***	**STAGES II₂,† III, IV**
Low	Localized irradiation	Observation until disease progression, then palliative irradiation or single-agent or combination chemotherapy
Intermediate	Combination chemotherapy with localized radiation	Combination chemotherapy
High	Combination chemotherapy (high dose) with localized radiation	Combination chemotherapy (high dose)

*Stage II₁ = nonbulky disease.
†Stage II₂ = bulky disease >10 cm or ⅓ diameter of chest.

the Reed-Sternberg cell of Hodgkin's disease. However, all NHLs involve lymphocytes arrested in various stages of development.

NHL is the most commonly occurring hematologic cancer and the fifth leading cause of cancer death. Approximately 54,000 new cases of NHL are diagnosed each year, and approximately 25,000 deaths occur each year. As the population has aged, the incidence of NHL has increased 2% to 3% per year for at least the past 30 years.[38]

NHLs can originate outside the lymph nodes, the method of spread can be unpredictable, and the majority of patients have widely disseminated disease at the time of diagnosis (Fig. 30-13). The primary clinical manifestation is painless lymph node enlargement. Because the disease is usually disseminated when it is diagnosed, other symptoms will be present depending on where the disease has spread (e.g., hepatomegaly with liver involvement).

Patients with high-grade lymphomas may have lymphadenopathy and constitutional ("B") symptoms such as fever, night sweats, and weight loss. The peripheral blood is usually normal, but some lymphomas manifest in a "leukemic" phase.

Diagnostic studies used for NHL resemble those used for Hodgkin's disease. Lymph node biopsy establishes the cell type and pattern. Staging, as described for Hodgkin's disease, is used to guide therapy (see Fig. 30-12). The prognosis for NHL is generally not as good as that for Hodgkin's disease.

Treatment for NHL involves radiation therapy and chemotherapy (Table 30-27). Ironically, more aggressive lymphomas are more responsive to treatment and more likely to be cured. In contrast, indolent lymphomas have a naturally long course but are difficult to effectively treat. Radiation alone may be effective for treatment of localized stage I or II disease. Patients who are asymptomatic but with advanced disease are usually followed with "watchful waiting" to assess the progress of the disease. Once the disease is symptomatic, chlorambucil (Leukeran) or cyclophosphamide (Cytoxan) with or without prednisone is a standard approach. Complete remissions are uncommon, but the majority of patients will respond with improvement in adenopathy and symptoms. Numerous chemotherapy combinations have been used to try to overcome the resistant nature of this disease. The most common chemotherapeutic regimen is CHOP (cyclophosphamide, doxorubicin [Adriamycin], vincristine [Oncovin], and prednisone). Other combination therapies include cyclophosphamide, vincristine, and prednisone (CVP) and cyclophosphamide, vincristine [Oncovin], procarbazine, and prednisone (COPP). Furthermore, high-dose chemotherapy with peripheral blood stem cell or BMT is used.

Rituximab (Rituxan), a genetically engineered monoclonal antibody against the CD20 antigen on the surface of normal and malignant B lymphocytes, is used to treat NHL. Once bound to the cells, rituximab causes lysis and cell death. Biologic therapy, such as α-interferon, interleukin-2, and tumor necrosis factor, may be used in the treatment of NHL. α-Interferon (Intron A) may be used in conjunction with anthracycline chemotherapeutic drugs for the initial treatment of clinically aggressive NHL. (Biologic therapy is discussed in Chapter 15.)

Monoclonal antibodies can be linked to radioactive isotopes to treat non-Hodgkin's lymphoma. The monoclonal antibody targets the CD 20 antigen which is on the surface of mature B cells and B cell tumors. This allows for the delivery of radiation directly to the malignant B cells. Ibritumomab tiuxetan (Zevalin) is a monoclonal antibody linked to radioactive isotope yttrium-90 and tositumomab (Bexxar) is a monoclonal antibody linked to radioactive isotope iodine 131. These drugs can be used in patients refractory to rituximab (Rituxam) or in conjunction with it. Side effects of these drugs include pancytopenia. Because of the risks, these drugs are usually used for patients who have failed to respond to other treatments.

MULTIPLE MYELOMA

Multiple myeloma, or *plasma cell myeloma,* is a condition in which neoplastic plasma cells infiltrate the bone marrow and destroy bone. A patient usually lives for approximately 2 years after diagnosis if untreated. The incidence of multiple myeloma is approximately 4 per 100,000 people. The disease is twice as common in men as in women and usually develops after 40 years of age, with an average age of 65 years. Multiple myeloma occurs in African Americans more commonly than in whites.[39]

Etiology and Pathophysiology

The cause of multiple myeloma is unknown. Exposure to radiation, organic chemicals (such as benzene), herbicides, and insecticides may play a role. Genetic factors and viral infection may also influence the risk of developing multiple myeloma.

The disease process involves excessive production of plasma cells. Plasma cells are activated B cells, which produce immunoglobulins (antibodies) that normally serve to protect the body. However, in multiple myeloma the malignant plasma cells infiltrate the bone marrow and produce abnormal and excessive amounts of immunoglobulin (usually IgG, IgA, IgD, or IgE). This abnormal immunoglobulin is termed a *myeloma protein.* Furthermore, plasma cell production of excessive and abnormal amounts of cytokines (interleukins [ILs]; IL-4, IL-5, and IL-6) also plays an important role in the pathologic process of bone destruction. As myeloma protein increases, normal plasma cells are reduced, which further compromises the body's normal immune response. In some patients, excessive production and secretion of free light-chain proteins (called *Bence Jones* proteins) is also seen and can be detected in the urine. Proliferation of malignant plasma cells and the overproduction of immunoglobulin and proteins result in the end-organ effects of myeloma to the bone marrow, bone, and kidneys and possibly the spleen, lymph nodes, liver, and even heart muscle.

Clinical Manifestations

Multiple myeloma develops slowly and insidiously. The patient often does not manifest symptoms until the disease is advanced, at which time skeletal pain is the major manifestation. Pain in the pelvis, spine, and ribs is particularly common. The pain is triggered by movement. Diffuse osteoporosis develops as the myeloma protein destroys bone. Osteolytic lesions are seen in the skull, vertebrae, and ribs (Fig. 30-14). Vertebral destruction can lead to collapse of vertebrae with ensuing compression of the spinal cord. Loss of bone integrity can lead to the development of pathologic fractures.

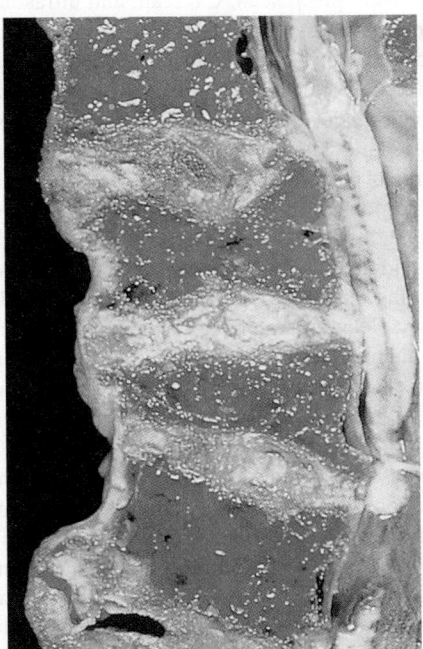

FIG. 30-14 Multiple myeloma. This segment of the lower thoracic spine has been sectioned to show the extensive replacement of the bone and marrow with red gelatinous tissue.

Bony degeneration also causes calcium to be lost from bones, eventually causing hypercalcemia. Hypercalcemia may cause renal, GI, or neurologic manifestations such as polyuria, anorexia, confusion, and ultimately seizures, coma, and cardiac problems. High protein levels caused by the presence of the myeloma protein can result in renal failure, from renal tubular obstruction by the myeloma protein, and interstitial nephritis. The patient may also display manifestations of anemia, thrombocytopenia, and granulocytopenia, all of which are related to the replacement of normal bone marrow with plasma cells.

Diagnostic Studies

Evaluating multiple myeloma involves laboratory, radiologic, and bone marrow examination. The presence of a monoclonal (M) antibody protein can be found in the blood and urine. Pancytopenia, hypercalcemia, the presence of Bence Jones protein in the urine, and an elevated serum creatinine are possible findings.

X-rays show distinct lytic areas of bone erosions, generalized thinning of the bones, and/or fractures, especially in the vertebrae, ribs, pelvis, and bones of the thigh and upper arms. Bone marrow analysis shows significantly increased numbers of plasma cells in the bone marrow. The simplest measure of prognosis in multiple myeloma is based on blood levels of two markers: β_2-microglobulin and albumin. In general, higher levels of β_2-microglobulin and lower levels of albumin are associated with a poorer prognosis.

Collaborative Care

Collaborative care involves managing both the disease and its symptoms. The current treatment options include watchful waiting (for early multiple myeloma), chemotherapy, biologic therapy, and stem cell transplantation. Multiple myeloma is seldom cured, but treatment can relieve symptoms, produce remission, and prolong life. Ambulation and adequate hydration are used to treat hypercalcemia, dehydration, and potential renal damage. Weight bearing helps the bones reabsorb some calcium, and fluids dilute calcium and prevent protein precipitates from causing renal tubular obstruction. Control of pain and prevention of pathologic fractures are other goals of management. Analgesics, orthopedic supports, and localized radiation help reduce the skeletal pain. Bisphosphonates, such as pamidronate (Aredia), zoledronic acid (Zometa), and etidronate (Didronel), inhibit bone breakdown and are used for the treatment of skeletal pain and hypercalcemia. They inhibit bone resorption without inhibiting bone formation and mineralization. They are given monthly by IV infusion.

Chemotherapy is usually the first treatment recommended for multiple myeloma. It is used to reduce the number of plasma cells. The agents most frequently used are the alkylating drugs, including melphalan (Alkeran), cyclophosphamide (Cytoxan), and carmustine (BCNU). Other drugs used include vincristine (Oncovin), doxorubicin (Adriamycin), and bortezomib (Velcade). Corticosteroids (prednisone, dexamethasone [Decadron]) may be added because they exert an antitumor effect in some patients. α-Interferon therapy has been used following chemotherapy. It works by altering the receptors for IL-6, which is a growth factor for myeloma cells.[40] Radiation therapy is another important component of treatment, primarily because of its effect on localized lesions.

Thalidomide (Thalomid) is an immune-modulating drug that may slow the growth of plasma cells and reduce their numbers. Thalidomide is currently considered experimental, but it may be given alone or with corticosteroids or chemotherapy drugs. The use of thalidomide is contraindicated in pregnant women because it is known to cause birth defects. Bone marrow and peripheral blood stem cell transplantation, when successful, prolongs life and can lead to remission.

Drugs may be used to treat complications of multiple myeloma. For example, allopurinol (Zyloprim) may be given to reduce hyperuricemia, and IV furosemide (Lasix) promotes renal excretion of calcium. Calcitonin can be used to decrease the risk of fractures and reduce bone pain.

NURSING MANAGEMENT
MULTIPLE MYELOMA

A major focus of care relates to the bone involvement and sequelae from bone breakdown. Maintaining adequate hydration is a primary nursing consideration to minimize problems from hypercalcemia. Fluids are administered to attain a urinary output of 1.5 to 2 L per day. This may require an intake of 3 to 4 L. In addition, weight bearing helps bones reabsorb some of the circulating calcium, and corticosteroids may augment the excretion of calcium. Once chemotherapy is initiated, the uric acid levels may rise because of the increased cell destruction. Hyperuricemia is treated by ensuring adequate hydration and using allopurinol to prevent any renal damage.

Because of the potential for pathologic fractures, the nurse must be careful when moving and ambulating the patient. A slight twist or strain in the wrong area (e.g., a weak area in the patient's bones) may be sufficient to cause a fracture.

Pain management requires innovative and knowledgeable nursing interventions. Analgesics, such as nonsteroidal antiinflammatory drugs, acetaminophen, or an acetaminophen/opioid combination, may be more effective than opioids alone in diminishing bone pain. Braces, especially for the spine, may also help control pain. As in any pain management situation, the nurse is responsible for assessing the patient and for implementing necessary measures to alleviate the pain. (Pain management is discussed in Chapter 9.)

The patient's psychosocial needs require sensitive, skilled management. It is important to help the patient and significant others adapt to changes fostered by chronic sickness, deal with reality, and adjust to the losses related to the disease process. The symptoms of multiple myeloma remit and exacerbate. Consequently acute care is needed at various times during the course of the illness. The final, acute phase is unresponsive to treatment and usually short in duration. The way in which patients and families deal with confronting death may be affected by the manner in which they learned to accept and live with the chronic nature of the disease.

DISORDERS OF THE SPLEEN

The spleen performs many functions and is affected by many illnesses. There are many different causes of *splenomegaly* (enlarged spleen) (Table 30-28). The term *hypersplenism* refers to the occurrence of splenomegaly and peripheral cytopenias (anemia, leukopenia, and thrombocytopenia). The degree of splenic enlargement varies with the disease. For example, massive splenic enlargement occurs with chronic myelogenous leukemia, hairy cell leukemia, and thalassemia major. Mild splenic enlargement occurs with congestive heart failure and systemic lupus erythematosus.

TABLE 30-28	Causes of Splenomegaly

Hereditary hemolytic anemias
  Sickle cell disease
  Thalassemia

Autoimmune cytopenias
  Acquired hemolytic anemia
  Immune thrombocytopenia

Infections and inflammations
  Bacterial endocarditis
  Infectious mononucleosis
  Systemic lupus erythematosus
  Sarcoidosis
  Human immunodeficiency virus infection
  Viral hepatitis

Infiltrative diseases
  Acute and chronic leukemia
  Lymphomas
  Polycythemia vera

Congestion
  Cirrhosis of the liver
  Congestive heart failure

When the spleen enlarges, its normal filtering and sequestering capacity increases. Consequently there is often a reduction in the number of circulating blood cells. A slight to moderate enlargement of the spleen is usually asymptomatic and found during a routine examination of the abdomen. Even massive splenomegaly can be well tolerated, but the patient may complain of abdominal discomfort and early satiety. In addition to physical examination, other techniques to assess the size of the spleen include ^{99}Tc-colloid liver-spleen scan, CT scan, and ultrasound scan.

Occasionally laparotomy and splenectomy are indicated in the evaluation or treatment of splenomegaly. Splenectomy can have a dramatic effect in increasing peripheral RBC, WBC, and platelet counts. Another major indication for splenectomy is splenic rupture. The spleen may rupture from trauma, inadvertent tearing during other surgical procedures, and diseases such as mononucleosis.

Nursing responsibilities for the patient with spleen disorders vary depending on the nature of the problem. Splenomegaly may be painful and may require analgesic administration; care in moving, turning, and positioning; and evaluation of lung expansion because spleen enlargement may impair diaphragmatic excursion. If anemia, thrombocytopenia, or leukopenia develops from splenic enlargement, nursing measures must be instituted to support the patient and prevent life-threatening complications. If splenectomy is performed, the nurse must provide the meticulous care warranted after any surgery. In addition, there must be special observation for hemorrhage, which could lead to shock, fever, and abdominal distention.

After splenectomy, immunologic deficiencies may develop. IgM levels are reduced, and IgG and IgA values remain within normal limits. Postsplenectomy patients have a lifelong risk for infection, especially from encapsulated organisms such as pneumococcus. This risk is reduced by immunization with pneumococcal vaccine (e.g., Pneumovax).

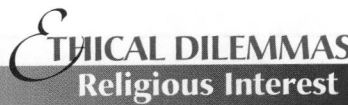

ETHICAL DILEMMAS
Religious Interest

Situation

An elderly woman is transferred from a nursing home because of gastrointestinal bleeding from an unknown cause. Some of her family members tell the nurse that she is a Jehovah's Witness and must not receive blood products. If she does not have exploratory surgery and transfusions, the surgeon believes that she will die.

Important Points for Consideration

- Competent adults have the right to make health care decisions based on their religious beliefs, including the right to refuse treatment.
- Health care professionals should make every effort to incorporate the patient's values and beliefs into the treatment plan. When the extent of the patient's beliefs is not clear, members of the health care team should consult other available resources, such as family, friends, or church officials, in an attempt to ascertain the patient's commitment to his or her faith.
- Jehovah's Witnesses believe that if they receive blood or blood products there are eternal consequences.
- When a clear determination of the patient's beliefs cannot be made, the patient is unable to communicate his or her wishes, or there are no advance directives, a decision by the health care team to perform the lifesaving surgery and transfusion would be acceptable.

Critical Thinking Questions

1. What resources do you have available to consult on religious practices?
2. How could you determine whether the family members were acting in the patient's best interest or their own?

BLOOD COMPONENT THERAPY

Blood component therapy is frequently used in managing hematologic diseases. Many therapeutic and surgical procedures depend on blood product support. However, blood component therapy only temporarily supports the patient until the underlying problem is resolved. Because transfusions are not free from hazards, they should be used only if necessary. Nurses must be careful to avoid developing a complacent attitude about this common but potentially dangerous therapy.[41]

Traditionally, the term *blood transfusion* meant the administration of whole blood. Blood transfusion now has a broader meaning because of the ability to administer specific components of blood such as platelets, packed red blood cells (PRBCs), or plasma (Table 30-29). (See Chapter 15 for discussion of stem cell and BMT infusions.)

Administration Procedure

Blood components can be administered safely through a 19-gauge or larger needle into a free-flowing IV line. Larger needles (e.g., 18 or 16 gauge) may be preferred if rapid transfusions are given. Smaller needles can be used for platelets, albumin, and clotting factor replacement. Most blood product administration tubing is of a "Y type" with a microaggregate filter (filters out particulate) with one Y for the isotonic saline solution and the other Y for the blood product. Dextrose solutions or lactated Ringer's should not be used because they induce RBC hemolysis. No other additives (including medications) should be given via the same tubing as the blood unless the tubing is cleared with saline solution.

When the blood or blood components have been obtained from the blood bank, positive identification of the donor blood and recipient must be made. Improper product-to-patient identification causes 90% of hemolytic transfusion reactions, thus placing a great responsibility on nursing personnel to carry out the identification procedure appropriately. The nurse must follow the policy and procedures at the place of employment. The blood bank is responsible for typing and crossmatching the donor's blood with the recipient's blood.

The blood should be administered as soon as it is brought to the patient. It should not be refrigerated on the nursing unit. If the blood is not used right away, it should be returned to the blood bank. During the first 15 minutes or 50 ml of blood infusion, the nurse should remain with the patient. If there are any untoward reactions, they are most likely to occur at this time. The rate of infusion during this period should be no more than 2 ml/min. PRBCs should not be infused quickly unless an emergency exists. Rapid infusion of cold blood may cause the patient to become chilled. If rapid replacement of large amounts of blood is necessary, a blood-warming device may be used. Other blood components, such as fresh frozen plasma and platelets, may be infused over 30 minutes.

After the first 15 minutes, the rate of infusion is governed by the clinical condition of the patient and the product being infused. Most patients not in danger of fluid overload can tolerate the infusion of 1 unit of PRBCs over 2 hours. The transfusion should not take more than 4 hours to administer. Blood unrefrigerated for 4 hours or longer should not be infused and should be returned to the blood bank.

Blood Transfusion Reactions

A *blood transfusion reaction* is an adverse reaction to blood transfusion therapy that can range in severity from mild symptoms to a life-threatening condition. Because complications of transfusion therapy may be significant, judicious evaluation of the patient is required. Blood transfusion reactions can be classified as acute or delayed (Tables 30-30 and 30-31).

If an acute transfusion reaction occurs, the following steps should be taken: (1) stop the transfusion; (2) maintain a patent IV line with saline solution; (3) notify the blood bank and the health care provider immediately; (4) recheck identifying tags and numbers; (5) monitor vital signs and urine output; (6) treat symptoms per physician order; (7) save the blood bag and tubing and send them to the blood bank for examination; (8) complete transfusion reaction reports; (9) collect required blood and urine specimens at intervals stipulated by hospital policy to evaluate for hemolysis; and (10) document on transfusion reaction form and patient chart. The blood bank and laboratory are responsible for identifying the type of reaction.

Acute Transfusion Reactions

Acute hemolytic reactions. The most common cause of hemolytic reactions is transfusion of ABO-incompatible blood (see Table 30-30). This is an example of a type II cytotoxic hypersensitivity reaction (see Chapter 13). Severe hemolytic reactions are

TABLE 30-29   Blood Products*

DESCRIPTION	SPECIAL CONSIDERATIONS	INDICATIONS FOR USE
Packed RBCs Packed RBCs are prepared from whole blood by sedimentation or centrifugation. One unit contains 250-350 ml.	Use of RBCs for treatment allows remaining components of blood (e.g., platelets, albumin, plasma) to be used for other purposes. There is less danger of fluid overload. Packed RBCs are preferred RBC source because they are more component specific.	Severe or symptomatic anemia, acute blood loss.
Frozen RBCs Frozen RBCs are prepared from RBCs using glycerol for protection and frozen. They can be stored for 3 yr at $-188.6°$ F (-87 C°).	They must be used within 24 hr of thawing. Successive washings with saline solution remove majority of WBCs and plasma proteins.	Autotransfusion, patient with previous febrile reactions to transfusions. Infrequently used because filters remove most WBCs.
Platelets Platelets are prepared from fresh whole blood within 4 hr after collection. One unit contains 30-60 ml of platelet concentrate.	Multiple units of platelets can be obtained from one donor by plateletpheresis. They can be kept at room temperature for 1-5 days depending on type of collection and storage bag used. Bag should be agitated periodically. Expected increase is 10,000/μl/U. Failure to have a rise may be due to fever, sepsis, splenomegaly, or DIC.	Bleeding caused by thrombocytopenia, platelet levels <10,000-20,000/μl (10-20 $\times$ 10^9/L).
Fresh Frozen Plasma Liquid portion of whole blood is separated from cells and frozen. One unit contains 200-250 ml. Plasma is rich in clotting factors but contains no platelets. It may be stored for 1 yr. It must be used within 2 hr after thawing.	Use of plasma in treating hypovolemic shock is being replaced by pure preparations such as albumin plasma expanders.	Bleeding caused by deficiency in clotting factors (e.g., DIC, hemorrhage, massive transfusion).
Albumin Albumin is prepared from plasma. It can be stored for 5 yr. It is available in 5% or 25% solution.	Albumin 25 g/100 ml is osmotically equal to 500 ml of plasma. Hyperosmolar solution acts by moving water from extravascular to intravascular space.	Hypovolemic shock, hypoalbuminemia.
Cryoprecipitates and Commercial Concentrates Cryoprecipitate is prepared from fresh frozen plasma, with 10-20 ml/bag. It can be stored for 1 yr. Once thawed, must be used.	See Table 30-17.	Replacement of clotting factors, especially factor VIII and fibrinogen.

*Component therapy has replaced the use of whole blood, which accounts for less than 10% of all transfusions.
DIC, Disseminated intravascular coagulation; RBCs, red blood cells; WBCs, white blood cells.

rare. Mislabeling specimens and administering blood to the wrong individual cause most acute hemolytic reactions.

When an acute hemolytic reaction occurs, antibodies in the recipient's serum react with antigens on the donor's RBCs. This results in agglutination of cells, which can obstruct capillaries and block blood flow. Hemolysis of the RBCs releases free hemoglobin into the plasma. The hemoglobin is filtered by the kidney and may be found in the urine (hemoglobinuria). Hemoglobin may obstruct the renal tubules, leading to acute renal failure (see Chapter 45).

The clinical manifestations of an acute hemolytic reaction may be mild or severe and usually develop within the first 15 minutes of transfusion. Free hemoglobin in blood and urine specimens obtained at the onset of the reaction will provide evidence of an acute hemolytic reaction. Delayed transfusion reactions occur 2 to 14 days after the administration of blood. (The clinical manifestations and nursing management for the patient with a hemolytic reaction are presented in Table 30-30.)

Febrile reactions. Febrile reactions are most commonly caused by leukocyte incompatibility. Many individuals who receive five or more transfusions develop circulating antibodies to the small amount of WBCs in the blood product. Febrile reactions can often be prevented by using additional filters in the tubing to leukocyte deplete RBCs and platelets. Leukocyte-poor

TABLE 30-30   Acute Transfusion Reactions

REACTION	CAUSE	CLINICAL MANIFESTATIONS	MANAGEMENT	PREVENTION
Acute hemolytic	Infusion of ABO-incompatible whole blood, RBCs or components containing 10 ml or more of RBCs. Antibodies in the recipient's plasma attach to antigens on transfused red blood cells causing RBC destruction.	Chills, fever, low back pain, flushing, tachycardia, tachypnea, hypotension, vascular collapse, hemoglobinuria, acute jaundice, dark urine, bleeding, acute renal failure, shock, cardiac arrest, death.	Treat shock if present. Draw blood samples for serologic testing slowly to avoid hemolysis from the procedure. Send urine specimen to the laboratory. Maintain BP with IV colloid solutions. Give diuretics as prescribed to maintain urine flow. Insert indwelling urinary catheter or measure voided amounts to monitor hourly urine output. Dialysis may be required if renal failure occurs. Do not transfuse additional RBC–containing components until blood bank has provided newly crossmatched units.	Meticulously verify and document patient identification from sample collection to component infusion.
Febrile, nonhemolytic (most common)	Sensitization to donor WBCs, platelets, or plasma proteins.	Sudden chills and fever (rise in temperature of >1° C), headache, flushing, anxiety, muscle pain.	Give antipyretics as prescribed—avoid aspirin in thrombocytopenic patients. *Do not restart transfusion* unless physician orders.	Consider leukocyte-poor blood products (filtered, washed, or frozen) for patients with a history of two or more such reactions. Treat prophylactically with antihistamines. Consider washed RBCs and platelets.
Mild allergic	Sensitivity to foreign plasma proteins.	Flushing, itching, urticaria (hives).	Give antihistamine as directed. If symptoms are mild and transient, transfusion may be restarted slowly. Do not restart transfusion if fever or pulmonary symptoms develop.	
Anaphylactic and severe allergic	Sensitivity to donor plasma proteins. Infusion of IgA proteins to IgA-deficient recipient who has developed IgA antibody.	Anxiety, urticaria, wheezing progressing to cyanosis, shock, and possible cardiac arrest.	Initiate CPR, if indicated. Have epinephrine ready for injection (0.4 ml of a 1:1000 solution SQ or 0.1 ml of 1:1000 solution diluted to 10 ml with saline for IV use). *Do not restart transfusion.*	Transfuse extensively washed RBC products, from which all plasma has been removed. Use blood from IgA-deficient donor. Use autologous components.
Circulatory overload	Fluid administered faster than the circulation can accommodate.	Cough, dyspnea, pulmonary congestion, headache, hypertension, tachycardia, distended neck veins.	Place patient upright with feet in dependent position. Administer prescribed diuretics, oxygen, morphine. Phlebotomy may be indicated.	Adjust transfusion volume and flow rate based on patient size and clinical status. Have blood bank divide unit into smaller aliquots for better spacing of fluid input.
Sepsis	Transfusion of bacterially infected blood components.	Rapid onset of chills, high fever, vomiting, diarrhea, marked hypotension, or shock.	Obtain culture of patient's blood and send bag with remaining blood and tubing to blood bank for further study. Treat septicemia as directed—antibiotics, IV fluids, vasopressors.	Collect, process, store, and transfuse blood products according to blood banking standards and infuse within 4 hr of starting time.

Modified from Transfusion Therapy Guidelines for Nurses, National Blood Resources Education Program, US Department Health and Human Services.
BP, Blood pressure; *CPR,* cardiopulmonary resuscitation; *IgA,* immunoglobulin A; *IV,* intravenous; *RBC,* red blood cell; *SQ,* subcutaneous; *WBC,* white blood cell.

TABLE 30-31 Delayed Transfusion Reactions

REACTION	CLINICAL MANIFESTATIONS
Delayed hemolytic	Fever, mild jaundice, decreased hematocrit. Occurs as early as 3 days or as late as several months, but usually 7-14 days posttransfusion as the result of destruction of transfused RBCs by alloantibodies not detected during crossmatch. Generally, no acute treatment is required, but hemolysis may be severe enough to warrant further transfusions.
Hepatitis B*	Elevated liver enzymes (AST and ALT), anorexia, malaise, nausea and vomiting, fever, dark urine, jaundice. Usually resolves spontaneously within 4-6 wk. Chronic carrier state can develop and can result in permanent liver damage. Treat symptomatically. (See Chapter 42.)
Hepatitis C*	Similar to hepatitis B, but symptoms are usually less severe. Chronic liver disease and cirrhosis may develop. Before introduction of anti-HCV test, accounted for 90%-95% of all posttransfusion hepatitis. Treat symptomatically. (See Chapter 42.)
Human immunodeficiency virus (HIV)	Can be asymptomatic for up to several years or may develop flulike symptoms within 2-4 wk. Later signs and symptoms include weight loss, diarrhea, fever, lymphadenopathy, thrush, *Pneumocystis* pneumonia.
Iron overload	Excess iron is deposited in the heart, liver, pancreas, and joints, causing dysfunction. Congestive heart failure, arrhythmias, impaired thyroid and gonadal function, diabetes, arthritis, cirrhosis. Commonly occurs in patients receiving >100 units for chronic anemia over a period of time. Treat symptomatically. Deferoxamine (Desferal), which chelates and removes accumulated iron via the kidneys, may be administered IV or SQ.
Graft-versus-host disease	Fever, rash, diarrhea, hepatitis. Result of replication of donor lymphocytes (graft) in the transfusion recipient (host). No effective therapy available. To prevent, irradiate blood products intended for immunocompromised patients. Some believe that irradiated blood products are indicated for first-degree family members' donations also. (See Chapter 13.)
Other	Other infectious diseases and agents may be transmitted via transfusion, including cytomegalovirus, HTLV-1, and those causing malaria.

Modified from Transfusion Therapy Guidelines for Nurses, National Blood Resources Education Program, US Department Health and Human Services.
*New cases of transfusion-related hepatitis B and C are not common.
ALT, Alanine aminotransferase; *AST,* aspartate aminotransferase; *HTLV-1,* human T cell leukemia virus, type 1; *IV,* intravenous; *RBCs,* red blood cells; *SQ,* subcutaneous.

blood products (filtered, washed, or frozen) can also be used to prevent febrile reactions.

Allergic reactions. Allergic reactions result from the recipient's sensitivity to plasma proteins of the donor's blood. These reactions are more common in an individual with a history of allergies. Antihistamines may be used to prevent allergic reactions. Epinephrine or corticosteroids may be used to treat a severe reaction.

Circulatory overload. An individual with cardiac or renal insufficiency is at risk for developing circulatory overload. This is especially true if a large quantity of blood is infused in a short period of time, particularly in an elderly patient. A fluid balance assessment, including baseline auscultation of the patient's lungs, is performed. Complaints of shortness of breath and the presence of adventitious breath sounds may indicate fluid overload in any patient.

Sepsis. Blood products can become infected from improper handling and storage. Bacterial contamination of blood products can result in bacteremia, sepsis, or septic shock.

Massive blood transfusion reaction. An acute complication of transfusing large volumes of blood products is termed *massive blood transfusion reaction.* Massive blood transfusion reactions can occur when replacement of RBCs or blood exceeds the total blood volume within 24 hours. In this situation, an imbalance of normal blood elements results because clotting factors, albumin, and platelets are not found in RBC transfusions.

Additional problems such as hypothermia, citrate toxicity, hypocalcemia, and hyperkalemia may occur when massive blood transfusions are given. Hypothermia and cardiac arrhythmias can result from rapid infusion of large quantities of cold blood. Blood-warming equipment prevents this problem. Citrate toxicity and hypocalcemia can occur from the use of large quantities of blood products, because citrate is part of the storage solution; calcium binds to the citrate. Citrate toxicity is likely to develop when blood is transfused at a rate of 1 unit in 10 minutes (or 8 to 10 units of RBCs within a few hours). Manifestations such as muscle tremors and ECG changes may be observed with hypocalcemia but can be prevented or reversed by the infusion of 10% calcium gluconate (10 ml with every liter of citrated blood).[42] Hyperkalemia results when potassium leaks from RBCs in stored blood. Mild to severe signs and symptoms can occur, including nausea, muscle weakness, diarrhea, paresthesias, flaccid paralysis of the cardiac or respiratory muscles, and cardiac arrest. Electrolyte monitoring is an important aspect of care of the patient receiving massive transfusions of blood products.

Delayed Transfusion Reactions. Delayed transfusion reactions include delayed hemolytic reactions (discussed previously), infections, iron overload, and graft-versus-host disease (see Table 30-31).

Infection. Infectious agents transmitted by blood transfusion include hepatitis B and C viruses, HIV, human herpesvirus type 6 (HSV-6), Epstein-Barr virus (EBV), human T cell leukemia (HTLV-1), cytomegalovirus (CMV), and malaria. Hepatitis is still the most common viral infection transmitted, although its incidence has been decreasing. Hepatitis B virus can be detected in the blood by the presence of hepatitis B surface antigen (HBsAg). A test for hepatitis C antibodies in donor blood is used to exclude the use of any donated blood testing positive for hepatitis C. Therefore the risk of transmission of hepatitis C has been reduced. Leukocyte-reduced blood products drastically reduce the risk of blood transfusion–associated viral infection.

In the past, HIV was transmitted by contaminated blood and blood products. This posed a serious problem for an individual who received infected transfusions. Patients with hemophilia who received antihemophilic factors, which had been prepared from pooled plasma of a large number of donors of which some donors were infected, have a high rate of HIV infection from transfusion sources. Presently, the use of recombinant antihemophilic factors (see Table 30-17), donor education, donor screening, and HIV-antibody testing has greatly reduced the transmission of HIV by blood transfusion or factor replacement therapy.

Autotransfusion

Autotranfusion, or autologous transfusion, consists of removing whole blood from a person and transfusing that blood back into the same person. The problems of incompatibility, allergic reactions, and transmission of disease can be avoided. Methods of autotransfusion include the following:

- *Autologous donation or elective phlebotomy* (predeposit transfusion). A person donates blood before a planned surgical procedure. The blood can be frozen and stored for up to 3 years. Usually the blood is stored without being frozen

and is given to the person within a few weeks of donation. This technique is especially beneficial to the patient with a rare blood type or for any patient who might be expected to require limited blood product support during a major surgical procedure (e.g., elective orthopedic surgery).

- *Autotransfusion.* A newer method for replacing blood volume involves safely and aseptically collecting, filtering, and returning the patient's own blood lost during a major surgical procedure or from a traumatic injury. This system was originally developed in response to patients' concerns about the safety of blood from blood products. However, today it provides an important way to safely replace volume and stabilize bleeding patients.[42] Collection devices can be attached to drains following chest or orthopedic procedures. Sometimes the collection device is a component of the drainage system. Some systems allow blood to be automatically and continuously reinfused; others require collection for a period of time (usually no longer than 2 to 4 hours) and then the blood is reinfused.

Drainage after the first 24 hours or drainage that is suspected to contain pathogens should not be reinfused. Anticoagulants may or may not be added before reinfusion. Development of clots after blood is filtered through the collection system can sometimes prevent reinfusion of the blood. Sometimes blood that has been collected has become depleted of its normal coagulation factors; therefore monitoring coagulation studies in the patient receiving an autotransfusion is important.

CRITICAL THINKING EXERCISES

Case Study
Leukemia

Patient Profile. JJ, a 35-year-old white man, went to the emergency department because of severe bruising caused by a fall while hiking.

Subjective Data
- Complains of oral pain and white patches covering his tongue
- Has had a 2-month history of fatigue, malaise, and flu symptoms
- Has taken numerous prescribed antibiotics and increased rest and sleep in the past 2 months without relief of symptoms

Objective Data
Physical Examination
- Has bruises and ecchymoses from fall
- Gingiva has petechiae and patchy white spots
- Temperature 102.2° F (39° C)
- Has splenomegaly

Laboratory Results
- Hematocrit 30%
- WBC count 120,000/μl (120 $\times$ 10^9/L)
- Platelet count 25,000/μl (25 $\times$ 10^9/L)

Bone Marrow Biopsy
- Multiple myeloblasts (greater than 50%)

CRITICAL THINKING QUESTIONS

1. What components of the laboratory test results suggest acute leukemia?
2. How is acute myelogenous leukemia treated?
3. What is the prognosis for JJ?
4. What are the main priorities for patient teaching with a newly diagnosed young adult with leukemia?
5. Based on the assessment data presented, write one or more nursing diagnoses. Are there any collaborative problems?

Nursing Research Issues

1. What nursing interventions can assist the patient to manage fatigue from anemia?
2. What is the quality of life for a patient following bone marrow transplantation?
3. What is the impact on the family when one of its members is receiving chemotherapy for leukemia?
4. What are the most effective ways to train a nurse to administer blood and blood products?
5. What strategies are effective for pain management in patients with sickle cell crises?

REVIEW QUESTIONS

The number of the question corresponds to the same-numbered
objective at the beginning of the chapter.

1. In a severely anemic patient, the nurse would expect to find
   a. dyspnea and tachycardia.
   b. cyanosis and pulmonary edema.
   c. cardiomegaly and pulmonary fibrosis.
   d. ventricular arrhythmias and wheezing.

2. When obtaining assessment data from a patient with a microcytic, normochromic anemia, the nurse would question the patient about
   a. folic acid intake.
   b. dietary intake of iron.
   c. a history of gastric surgery.
   d. a history of sickle cell anemia.

3. A nursing intervention for a patient with severe anemia of chronic kidney disease includes
   a. monitoring stools for guaiac.
   b. instructions in high-iron diet.
   c. monitoring urine intake and output.
   d. teaching self-injection of erythropoietin.

4. The nursing management of a patient in sickle cell crisis includes
   a. bed rest and heparin therapy.
   b. blood transfusions and iron replacement.
   c. aggressive analgesic and oxygen therapy.
   d. platelet administration and monitoring of CBC.

5. A complication of the hyperviscosity of polycythemia is
   a. thrombosis.
   b. cardiomyopathy.
   c. pulmonary edema.
   d. disseminated intravascular coagulation (DIC).

6. When providing care for a patient with thrombocytopenia, the nurse must avoid administering aspirin or aspirin-containing products because they
   a. interfere with platelet aggregation.
   b. may contribute to the destruction of thrombocytes.
   c. may mask the fever that occurs with thrombocytopenia.
   d. alter blood flow to the homeostatic mechanisms in the brain.

7. The nurse would anticipate that a patient with von Willebrand's disease undergoing surgery would be treated with administration of vWF and
   a. thrombin.
   b. factor VI.
   c. factor VII.
   d. factor VIII.

8. DIC is a disorder in which
   a. the coagulation pathway is genetically altered, leading to thrombus formation in all major blood vessels.
   b. an underlying disease depletes hemolytic factors in the blood, leading to diffuse thrombotic episodes and infarcts.
   c. a disease process stimulates coagulation processes with resultant depletion of clotting factors, leading to diffuse hemorrhage.
   d. an inherited predisposition causes a deficiency of clotting factors that leads to overstimulation of coagulation processes in the vasculature.

9. Appropriate nursing actions when caring for a hospitalized patient with severe neutropenia include
   a. perirectal care and platelet administration.
   b. oral care and red blood cell administration.
   c. monitoring lung sounds and invasive blood pressures.
   d. strict hand washing and frequent temperature assessment.

10. Because myelodysplastic syndrome arises from the pluripotent hematopoietic stem cell in the bone marrow, laboratory results the nurse would expect to find include
    a. an excess of T cells.
    b. an excess of platelets.
    c. a deficiency of granulocytes.
    d. a deficiency of all cellular blood components.

11. A type of leukemia that is common but rarely fatal in older adults is
    a. acute myelocytic leukemia.
    b. acute lymphocytic leukemia.
    c. chronic lymphocytic leukemia.
    d. chronic granulocytic leukemia.

12. Multiple drugs are primarily used in combinations to treat leukemia and lymphoma because
    a. there are fewer toxic and side effects.
    b. the chance that one drug will be effective is increased.
    c. they can interrupt cell growth at multiple points in the cell cycle.
    d. they are more effective without having exacerbating side effects.

13. The nurse is aware that a major difference between Hodgkin's disease and non-Hodgkin's lymphoma is that
    a. Hodgkin's disease occurs only in young adults.
    b. Hodgkin's disease is considered potentially curable.
    c. non-Hodgkin's lymphoma requires a staging laparotomy.
    d. non-Hodgkin's lymphoma is treated only with radiation therapy.

14. A patient with multiple myeloma becomes confused and lethargic. The nurse would expect that these clinical manifestations may be explained by diagnostic results that indicate
    a. hyperkalemia.
    b. hyperuricemia.
    c. hypercalcemia.
    d. CNS myeloma.

15. When reviewing the patient's hematologic laboratory values after a splenectomy, the nurse would expect to find
    a. leukopenia.
    b. RBC abnormalities.
    c. decreased hemoglobin.
    d. increased platelet count.

16. Complications of transfusions that can be decreased by the use of leukocyte reduction filters for red blood cells and platelets are
    a. chills and back pain.
    b. leukostasis and neutrophilia.
    c. fluid overload and pulmonary edema.
    d. transmission of cytomegalovirus and alloimmunization.

REFERENCES

1. Loney M, Chernecky C: Anemia, *Oncol Nurs Forum* 27:951, 2000.
2. Hoffman R et al: *Hematology: basic principles and practice,* New York, 2000, Harcourt Brace.
3. Worrall L, Tompkins C, Rust DM: Recognizing and managing anemia, *Clin J Oncol Nurs* 3:153, 1999.
4. Smith D: Management and treatment of anemia in the elderly, *Clin Geriatr* 10:47, 2002.
5. Blackwell S, Hendrix P: Common anemias: what lies beneath, *Clin Rev* 11:3, 2001.
6. Blackwell S, Hendrix P: Less common anemias: beyond iron deficiency, *Clin Rev* 11:57, 2001.
7. Glaspy J, Cavill I: Role of iron in optimizing responses of anemic cancer patients to erythropoietin, *Oncology* 13:461, 1999.
8. Huffstutler SY: Adult anemia, *Adv Nurse Pract* 8:89, 2000.
9. Mitchell R: Sickle cell anemia, *Am J Nurs* 99:36, 1999.
10. Gorman K: Sickle cell disease, *Am J Nurs* 99:38, 1999.
11. Day SE, Wynn LW: Sickle cell pain and hydroxyurea, *Am J Nurs* 100:34, 2000.
12. Press R: Hemochromatosis: a "simple" genetic trait, *Hosp Pract* 34:55, 1999.
13. Horrell CJ, Rothman J: Establishing the etiology of thrombocytopenias, *Nurse Pract* 25:68, 2000.
14. Cines DB, Blanchette VS: Immune thrombocytopenic purpura, *N Engl J Med* 346:995, 2002.
15. Portielje JE et al: Morbidity and mortality in adults with idiopathic thrombocytopenic purpura, *Blood* 97:2549, 2001.
16. Godeau B et al: Intravenous immunoglobulin or high-dose methylprednisolone, with or without oral prednisone, for adults with untreated severe autoimmune thrombocytopenic purpura: a randomized, multicentre trial, *Lancet* 359:23, 2002.
17. Kappers-Klunne MC, van'T Veer MB: Cyclosporin A for the treatment of patients with chronic idiopathic thrombocytopenic purpura refractory to corticosteroids or splenectomy, *Br J Haematol* 114:121, 2001.
18. Gobel BH: Bleeding. In Groenwald SL et al, editors: *Cancer nursing principles and practice,* ed 5, Boston, 2000, Jones & Bartlett.
19. Moake J: Thrombotic thrombocytopenic purpura today, *Hosp Pract* 34:53, 1999.
20. Rust DM: FDA approves first biologic drug to promote platelet production, *Oncol Nurs Forum* 25:603, 1998.
21. Mannucci PM, Tuddenham EG: The hemophilias—from royal genes to gene therapy, *N Engl J Med* 344:1773, 2001.
22. Kleinert D et al: von Willebrand's disease: a nursing perspective, *J Obstet Gynecol Neonatal Nurs* 26: 271, 1997.
23. Lozier JN, Kessler CM: Clinical aspects and therapy of hemophilia. In Hoffman R et al, editors: *Hematology basic principles and practice,* ed 3, New York, 2000, Harcourt Brace.
24. Pasi KJ: Gene therapy for haemophilia, *Br J Haematol* 115:744, 2001.
25. Maxson JH: Management of disseminated intravascular coagulation, *Crit Care Nurs Clin North Am* 12:341, 2000.
26. Freifeld AG, Walsh TJ, Pizzo DA: Clinical approaches to infections in the compromised host. In Hoffman R et al, editors: *Hematology basic principles and practice,* ed 3, New York, 2000, Harcourt Brace.
27. Noskin GA, Phair JP, Murphy RL: Diagnosis and management of infections in the immunocompromised host. In Shulman ST et al, editors: *The biologic and clinical basis of infectious disease,* ed 5, Philadelphia, 1997, WB Saunders.
28. Whedon MB, Roach M: Principles of bone marrow and hematopoietic cell transplantation. In Groenwald SL et al, editors: *Cancer nursing: principles and practice,* ed 5, Boston, 2000, Jones & Bartlett.
29. Utley SM: Myelodysplastic syndromes, *Semin Oncol Nurs* 12:51, 1996.
30. *Cancer facts and figures (www.cancer.org),* 2002, American Cancer Society.
31. Seiter K: Treatment of acute myelogenous leukemia in the elderly patient, *Clin Geriatr* 10:41, 2002.
32. Estey EH: Therapeutic options for acute myelogenous leukemia, *Cancer* 92:1059, 2001.
33. Wujcik D: Leukemia. In Groenwald SL et al, editors: *Cancer nursing: principles and practice,* ed 5, Boston, 2000, Jones & Bartlett.
34. Medoff E: Leukemia, *RN* 63:42, 2000.
35. Gorin NC et al: Feasibility and recent improvement of autologous stem cell transplantation for acute myelocytic leukemia in patients over 60 years of age: importance of the source of stem cells, *Br J Haematol* 110:887, 2000.
36. O'Connell SA, Schmit-Pokorny K: Blood and marrow stem cell transplantation: indications, procedure, process. In Whedon MB, Wvjcik D, editors: *Blood and marrow stem cell transplantation,* ed 2, Boston, 1997, Jones & Bartlett.
37. DeMeyer E, Whedon MB, Ferrell B: Quality of life after transplantation. In Whedon MB, Wvjcik D, editors: *Blood and marrow stem cell transplantation,* ed 2, Boston, 1997, Jones & Bartlett.
38. McFadden ME: Malignant lymphomas. In Groenwald SL et al, editors: *Cancer nursing: principles and practice,* ed 5, Boston, 2000, Jones & Bartlett.
39. Diagnosis and management of multiple myeloma, *Br J Haematol* 115:522, 2001.
40. Crowley J, Jacobson J, Alexanian R: Standard-dose therapy for multiple myeloma: the Southwest Oncology Group Experience, *Semin Hematol* 38:203, 2001.
41. Fitzpatrick L: When to administer modified blood products, *Nursing* 32:36, 2002.
42. Medes P: Transfusion medicine technology transfer: traps to avoid, *Transfus Med Rev* 16:25, 2002.

RESOURCES

American Cancer Society
1599 Clifton Road, NE
Atlanta, GA 30329
800-ACS-2345 or 404-320-3333
www.cancer.org/

American Sickle Cell Anemia Association
10300 Carnegie Avenue
Cleveland Clinic/East Office Building (EEb18)
Cleveland, OH 44106
216-229-8600
Fax: 216-229-4500
www.ascaa.org/

Cooley's Anemia Foundation
129-09 26th Avenue #203
Flushing, NY 11354
800-522-7222 or 718-321-CURE (2873)
Fax: 718-321-3340
www.thalassemia.org/

Hemochromatosis Foundation
PO Box 8569
Albany, NY 12208-0596
518-489-0972
Fax: 518-489-0227
www.hemochromatosis.org/

International Myeloma Foundation
12650 Riverside Drive, Suite 206
North Hollywood, CA 91607-3421
800-452-2873 or 818-487-7455
Fax: 818-487-7454
www.myeloma.org/

Leukemia and Lymphoma Society
1311 Mamaroneck Avenue
White Plains, NY 10605
914-949-5213
Fax: 914-949-6691
www.leukemia.org/

National Cancer Institute
Suite 3036A
6116 Executive Boulevard, MSC8322
Bethesda, MD 20892-8322
800-4-CANCER (422-6237) or 301-435-3848
www.nci.nih.gov

National Heart, Lung, and Blood Institute
National Institutes of Health
Building 31, Room 5A52
31 Center Drive MSC 2486
Bethesda, MD 20892
301-592-8573
Fax: 301-592 8563
www.nhlbi.nih.gov/

National Hemophilia Foundation
116 West 32nd Street, 11th Floor
New York, NY 10001
800-42-HANDI or 212-328-3700
Fax: 212-328-3777
www.hemophilia.org/

Sickle Cell Disease Association of America, Inc.
200 Corporate Point, Suite 495
Culver City, CA 90230-7633
800-421-8453 or 310-216-6363
Fax: 310-215-3722
www.sicklecelldisease.org/

For additional Internet resources, see the website for this book at
http://evolve.elsevier.com/Lewis/medsurg/.

Problems of Oxygenation: Perfusion

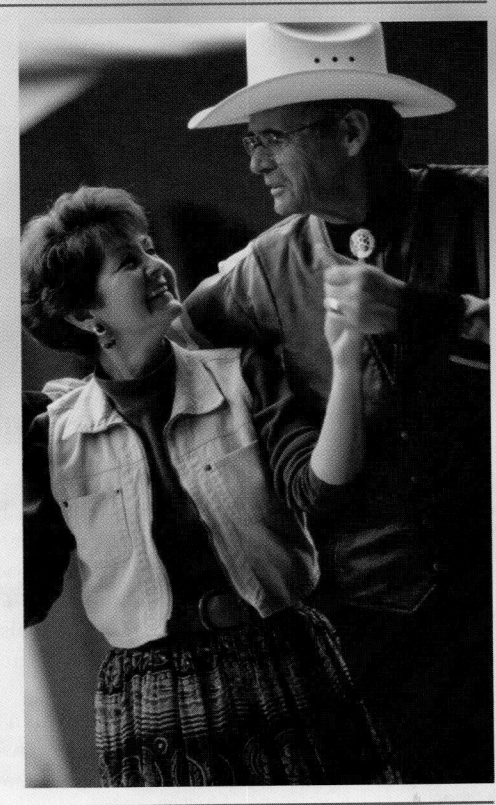

CHAPTER *31*
NURSING ASSESSMENT
Cardiovascular System

Anita Ralstin

LEARNING OBJECTIVES

1. Describe the anatomic location and function of the following cardiac structures: pericardial layers, atria, ventricles, semilunar valves, and atrioventricular valves.
2. Describe coronary circulation and the areas of heart muscle supplied by each blood vessel.
3. Explain the normal sequence of events involved in the conduction pathway of the heart.
4. Describe the structure and function of arteries, capillaries, and veins.
5. Define blood pressure and the mechanisms involved in its regulation.
6. Identify the significant subjective and objective assessment data related to the cardiovascular system that should be obtained from a patient.
7. Describe the appropriate techniques used in the physical assessment of the cardiovascular system.
8. Differentiate normal from common abnormal findings of a physical assessment of the cardiovascular system.
9. Describe the age-related changes of the cardiovascular system and differences in assessment findings.
10. Describe the purpose, significance of results, and nursing responsibilities of invasive and noninvasive diagnostic studies of the cardiovascular system.
11. Identify waveforms of a normal electrocardiogram and components of the normal sinus rhythm.

KEY TERMS

action potential, p. 758
afterload, p. 759
arterial blood pressure, p. 760
cardiac index, p. 758
cardiac output, p. 758
cardiac reserve, p. 759
diastole, p. 758
diastolic blood pressure, p. 760
heaves, p. 766

Korotkoff sounds, p. 760
mean arterial pressure, p. 760
murmurs, p. 767
point of maximal impulse, p. 756
preload, p. 759
pulse pressure, p. 760
systole, p. 758
systolic blood pressure, p. 760

STRUCTURES AND FUNCTIONS OF THE CARDIOVASCULAR SYSTEM

Heart

Structure. The heart is a four-chambered hollow muscular organ approximately the size of a fist. The heart lies within the thorax between the lungs in the mediastinal space. Its beating is often palpable at the fifth intercostal space approximately 2 inches left of the midline (Fig. 31-1). This pulsation, arising at the apex of the heart, is termed the **point of maximal impulse** (PMI).

The heart is composed of three layers: a thin inner lining, the *endocardium;* a layer of muscle, the *myocardium;* and a fibrous outer layer, the *epicardium.* The heart is surrounded by the pericardium. The inner (visceral) layer of the pericardium is in contact with the epicardium, and the outer (parietal) layer is in contact with the mediastinum. A small amount of pericardial fluid lubricates the space between the pericardial layers (*pericardial space*) and prevents friction between the surfaces as the heart beats.

The heart is divided vertically by the septum. This creates a right and left atrium and a right and left ventricle. The thickness of the wall of each chamber is different. The atrial myocardium is thinner than that of the ventricles, and the left ventricular wall is three times thicker than the right ventricular wall.[1] The thickness of the ventricle provides the force to pump the blood into the systemic circulation.

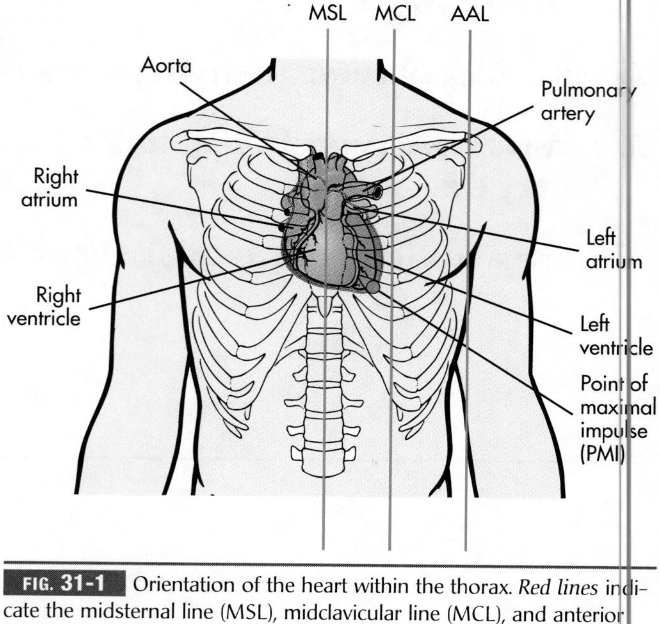

FIG. 31-1 Orientation of the heart within the thorax. *Red lines* indicate the midsternal line (MSL), midclavicular line (MCL), and anterior axillary line (AAL).

Reviewed by Elizabeth J. Bridges, RN, PhD, CCNS, Deputy Commander, 59th Clinical Research Squadron and Director of Nursing Research, Lackland Air Force Base, San Antonio, Tex.

Blood Flow Through the Heart. The right atrium receives venous blood from the inferior and superior venae cavae and the coronary sinus. The blood then passes through the tricuspid valve into the right ventricle. With each contraction, the right ventricle pumps blood through the pulmonic valve into the pulmonary artery.

Blood flows to the left atrium by way of the pulmonary veins. It then passes through the mitral valve and into the left ventricle. As the heart contracts, blood is ejected through the aortic valve into the aorta and thus enters the high-pressure systemic circulation (Fig. 31-2).

Cardiac valves. The four valves of the heart serve to keep blood flowing in a forward direction. The cusps of the mitral and tricuspid valves are attached to thin strands of fibrous tissue termed *chordae tendineae* (Fig. 31-3). Chordae are anchored in the papillary muscles of the ventricles. This support system prevents the eversion of the leaflets into the atria during ventricular contraction. The pulmonic and aortic valves (also known as *semilunar valves*) prevent blood from regurgitating into the ventricles at the end of each ventricular contraction.

Blood Supply to the Myocardium. The myocardium has its own blood supply, the *coronary circulation* (Fig. 31-4). Blood flow into the coronary arteries occurs primarily during diastole.

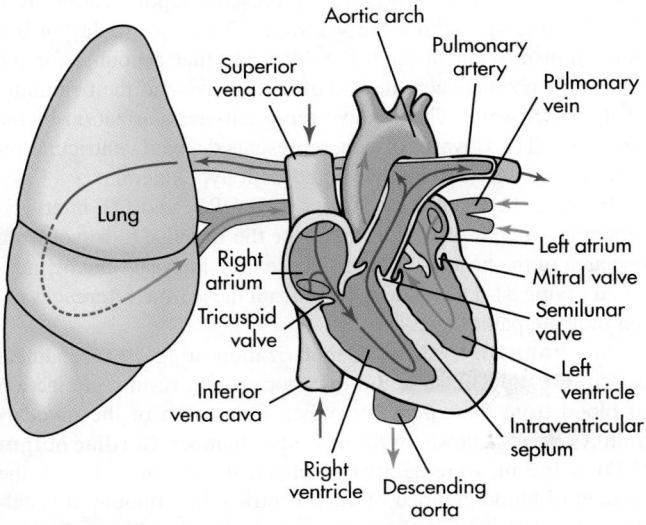

FIG. 31-2 Schematic representation of blood flow through the heart. *Arrows* indicate direction of flow.

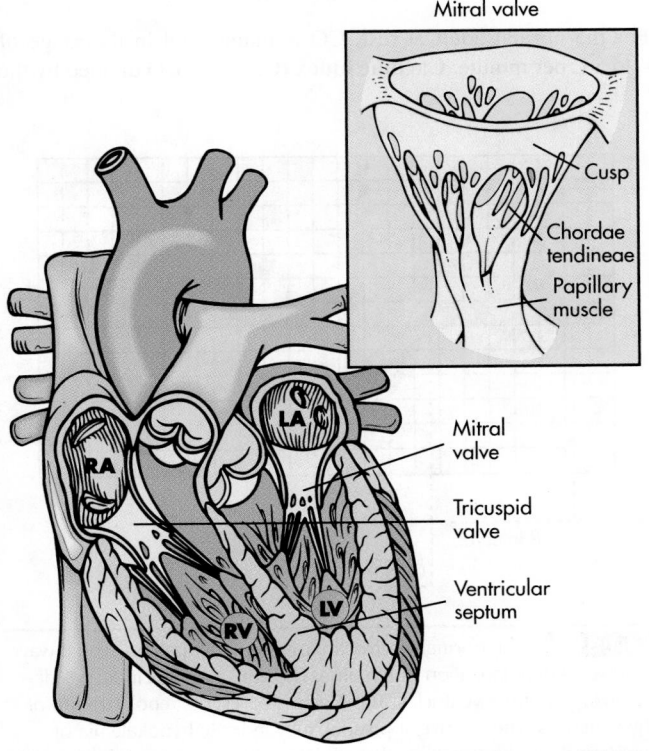

FIG. 31-3 Anatomic structures of the atrioventricular (AV) valves. *LA*, Left atrium; *LV*, left ventricle; *RA*, right atrium; *RV*, right ventricle.

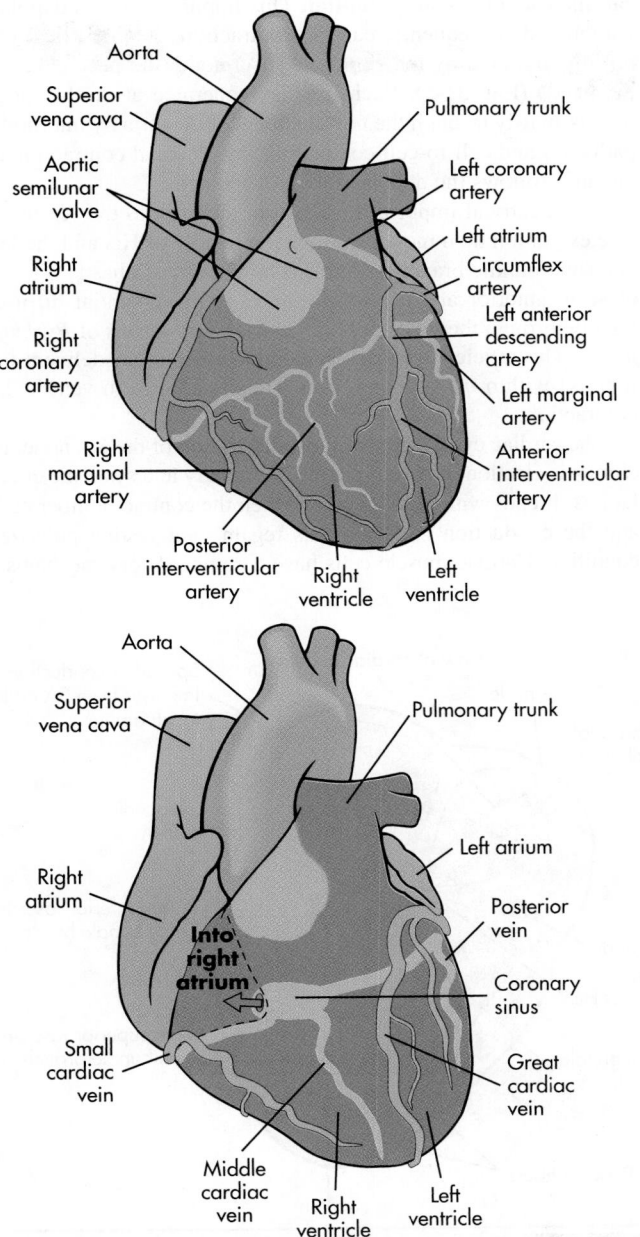

FIG. 31-4 Coronary arteries and veins.

The right coronary artery and its branches usually supply the right atrium, the right ventricle, and a portion of the posterior wall of the left ventricle. The left coronary artery and its branches (left anterior descending artery and left circumflex artery) supply the left atrium and the left ventricle. In 90% of people, the atrioventricular (AV) node and the bundle of His, part of the cardiac conduction system, receive blood supply from the right coronary artery. For this reason, obstruction of this artery often causes serious defects in cardiac conduction.

The divisions of coronary veins parallel the coronary arteries. Most of the blood from the coronary system drains into the coronary sinus, which empties into the right atrium near the entrance to the inferior vena cava (see Fig. 31-4).

Conduction System. The conduction system is specialized nerve tissue responsible for creating and transporting the electrical impulse, or **action potential.** This impulse initiates depolarization and subsequently cardiac contraction. The electrical impulse is initiated by the sinoatrial (SA) node (the pacemaker of the heart) (Fig. 31-5). Each impulse generated at the SA node travels swiftly through the muscle fibers of the atria by internodal pathways and cell-to-cell conduction. Mechanical contraction of the atria follows the depolarization of the cells.

The electrical impulse travels from the atria to the AV node. The excitation then moves through the bundle of His and the left and right bundle branches. The left bundle branch has two fascicles, an anterior and a posterior. The action potential diffuses widely through the walls of both ventricles by means of *Purkinje fibers.* The efficient ventricular conduction system delivers the impulse within 0.12 second. This triggers a uniform ventricular contraction.

The cardiac cycle starts with depolarization of the SA node. Its climax is ejection of blood into the pulmonary and systemic circulations. It ends with repolarization when the contractile fiber cells and the conduction pathway cells regain their resting polarized condition. Cardiac muscle cells have a compensatory mechanism that makes them unresponsive or refractory to restimulation during the action potential. During systole there is an *absolute refractory period* during which cardiac muscle does not respond to any stimuli. After this period, cardiac muscle gradually recovers its excitability and a *relative refractory period* occurs by early diastole.

Electrocardiogram. The electrical activity of the heart can be detected on the body surface and is recorded on an electrocardiogram (ECG). The letters P, QRS, T, and U are used to identify the separate waveforms (Fig. 31-6). The first wave, P, begins with the firing of the SA node and represents depolarization of the fibers of the atria. The QRS wave represents depolarization from the AV node throughout the ventricles. There is a delay of impulse transmission through the AV node that accounts for the time sequence between the end of the P wave and the beginning of the QRS wave. The T wave represents repolarization of the ventricles. The U wave, if seen, represents delayed ventricular repolarization and may be associated with hypokalemia.

Intervals between these waves (PR, QRS, and QT intervals) reflect the length of time it takes for the impulse to travel from one area of the heart to another. These time intervals can be measured (Table 31-1), and deviations from these time references often indicate pathology.

Mechanical System. Depolarization triggers mechanical activity. **Systole,** contraction of myocardium, results in ejection of blood from the cardiac chamber. Relaxation of the myocardium, **diastole,** allows for filling of the chamber. **Cardiac output** (CO) is the measurement of mechanical efficiency. CO is the amount of blood pumped by each ventricle in 1 minute. It is calculated by multiplying the amount of blood ejected from the ventricle with the heartbeat, the stroke volume (SV), by the heart rate (HR) per minute:

$$CO = SV \times HR$$

For the normal adult at rest, CO is maintained in the range of 4 to 8 L per minute. **Cardiac index** (CI) is the CO divided by the

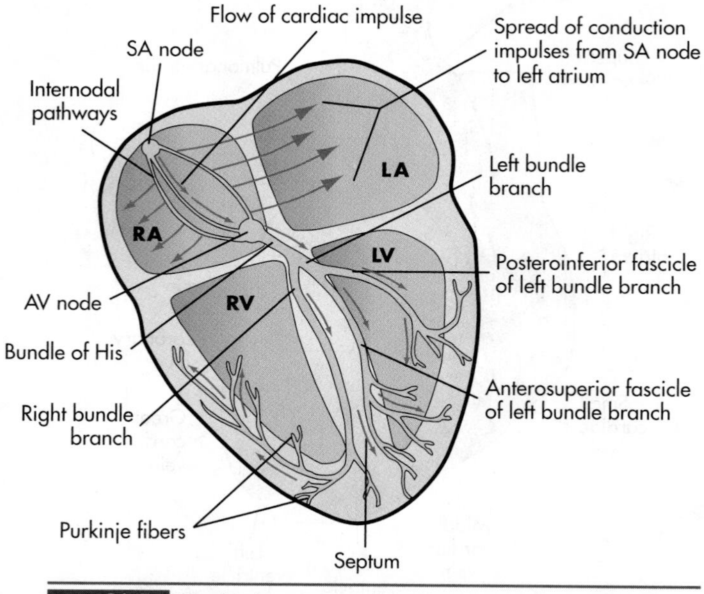

FIG. 31-5 Conduction system of the heart. *AV,* Atrioventricular; *LA,* left atrium; *LV,* left ventricle; *RA,* right atrium; *RV,* right ventricle; *SA,* sinoatrial.

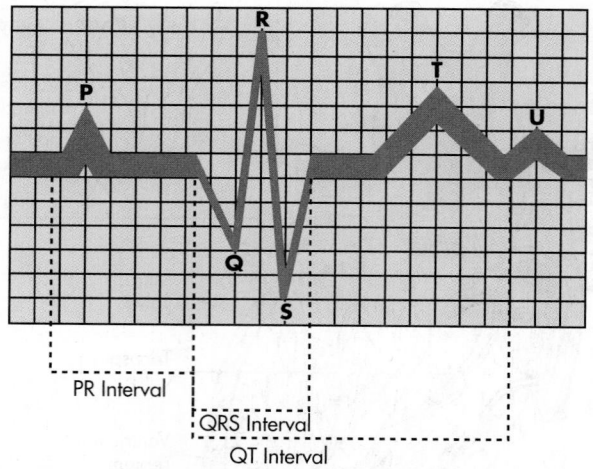

FIG. 31-6 The normal electrocardiogram (ECG) pattern. The P wave represents depolarization of the atria. The QRS complex indicates depolarization of the ventricles. The T wave represents repolarization of the ventricles. The U wave, if present, may indicate hypokalemia or repolarization abnormalities. The PR interval is a measure of the time required for the impulse to spread from the sinoatrial node to the ventricles.

TABLE 31-1 Electrocardiogram Waves		
NORMAL WAVEFORMS AND INTERVALS	**NORMAL TIMING**	**NORMAL SINUS RHYTHM***
P	0.06-0.12 sec	Precedes QRS-T waves
QRS	0.04-0.12 sec	Follows each P wave
T	0.16 sec	Follows each QRS wave
PR interval	0.12-0.20 sec	Should not vary from one complex to another
QT interval	Varies with pulse rate (0.31-0.38 sec at heart rate of 72 beats/min)	Should not vary from one complex to another. Should not be more than half the preceding RR interval
RR interval	Varies with pulse rate	Should be equidistant, with slight variations on respiration

*At 60-100 beats/min.

body mass index (BMI). The CI adjusts the CO to the body size. The normal CI is 2.8 to 4.2 L per minute per meter squared ($L/min/m^2$).

Factors affecting cardiac output. Numerous factors can affect either the HR or the SV and thus the CO. The HR is regulated primarily by the autonomic nervous system. The factors affecting the SV are preload, contractility, and afterload.[1] Increasing preload, contractility, and afterload increases the workload of the myocardium, resulting in increased oxygen demand.

Starling's law states that, to a point, the more the fibers are stretched, the greater their force of contraction. The volume of blood in the ventricles at the end of diastole, before the next contraction, is called **preload.** Preload determines the amount of stretch placed on myocardial fibers.

Contractility can be increased by norepinephrine released by the sympathetic nervous system, as well as by epinephrine. Increasing contractility raises the SV by increasing ventricular emptying.

Afterload is the peripheral resistance against which the left ventricle must pump. Afterload is affected by the size of the ventricle, wall tension, and arterial blood pressure. If the arterial blood pressure is elevated, the ventricles will meet increased resistance to ejection of blood, increasing the work demand. Eventually this results in *ventricular hypertrophy* (enlargement of the cardiac muscle tissue without an increase in the size of cavities).

Cardiac Reserve. The cardiovascular system must respond to numerous situations in health and illness (e.g., exercise, stress, hypovolemia). The ability to respond to these demands by altering CO threefold or fourfold is termed **cardiac reserve.**

The increase in CO results from an increase in HR or SV. The HR can increase to as high as 180 beats per minute for short periods without deleterious effects. The SV can be increased by increasing either preload or contractility.

Vascular System

Blood Vessels. The three major types of blood vessels in the vascular system are the arteries, veins, and capillaries. Arteries carry blood away from the heart and, except for the pulmonary artery, carry oxygenated blood. Veins carry blood toward the heart and, except for the pulmonary veins, carry deoxygenated blood. Small branches of arteries and veins are arterioles and venules, respectively. Blood circulates from the heart into arteries, arterioles, capillaries, venules, veins, and back to the heart.

Arteries and arterioles. The arterial system differs from the venous system by the amount and type of tissue that makes up arterial walls (Fig. 31-7). The large arteries have thick walls that are composed mainly of elastic tissue. This elastic property cushions the impact of the pressure created by ventricular contraction and provides recoil that propels blood forward into the circulation. Large arteries also contain some smooth muscle. Examples of large arteries are the aorta and the pulmonary artery.

Arterioles have relatively little elastic tissue and more smooth muscle. Arterioles serve as the major control of arterial blood pressure and distribution of blood flow. They respond readily to local conditions such as low O_2 and increasing levels of CO_2 by dilating or constricting.

Capillaries. The thin capillary wall is made up of endothelial cells, with no elastic or muscle tissue (see Fig. 31-7). There are many miles of capillaries in an adult. The exchange of cellular nutrients and metabolic end products takes place through these thin-walled vessels.

Veins and venules. Veins are large-diameter, thin-walled vessels that return blood to the right atrium (see Fig. 31-7). The venous system is a low-pressure, high-volume system. The larger veins contain semilunar valves at intervals to maintain the blood flow toward the heart and to prevent backward flow. The amount of blood in the venous system is affected by a number of factors, including arterial flow, compression of veins by skeletal muscles, alterations in thoracic and abdominal pressures, and right atrial pressure.

The largest veins are the *superior vena cava,* which returns blood to the heart from the head, neck, and arms, and the *inferior vena cava,* which returns blood to the heart from the lower part

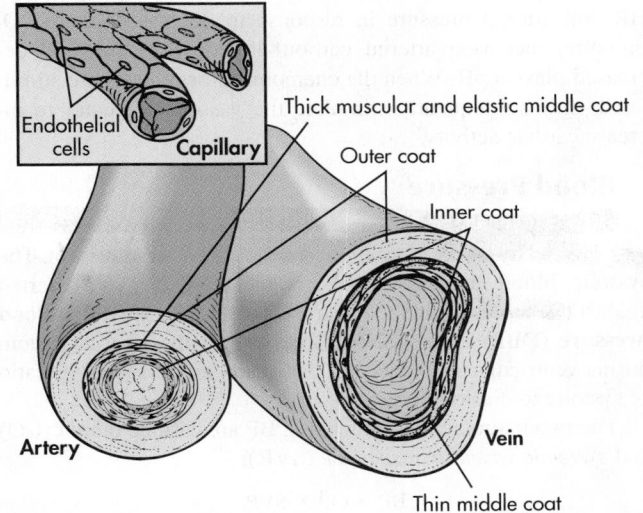

FIG. 31-7 Comparative thickness of layers of the artery, vein, and capillary.

of the body. These large-diameter vessels are affected by the pressure in the right side of the heart. Elevated right atrial pressure can cause distended neck veins or liver engorgement as a result of resistance to blood flow.

Venules are relatively small vessels made up of a small amount of muscle and connective tissue. Venules collect blood from various capillary beds and channel it to the larger veins.

Regulation of the Cardiovascular System

Autonomic Nervous System. The autonomic nervous system consists of the sympathetic nervous system and the parasympathetic nervous system.

Effect on the heart. Stimulation of the sympathetic nervous system increases the HR, the speed of impulse conduction through the AV node, and the force of atrial and ventricular contractions. This effect is mediated by specific sites in the heart called β-adrenergic receptors that are receptors for norepinephrine and epinephrine.

In contrast, stimulation of the parasympathetic system (mediated by the vagus nerve) causes a decrease in HR by the action on the SA node and slows conduction through the AV node.

Effect on the blood vessels. The source of neural control of blood vessels is the sympathetic nervous system. The α-adrenergic receptors are located in vascular smooth muscles. Stimulation of the α-adrenergic receptors results in vasoconstriction. Decreased stimulation to the α-adrenergic receptors causes vasodilation. (Sympathetic nervous system receptors that influence blood pressure are presented in Chapter 32, Table 32-1.)

The parasympathetic nerves have selective distribution in the blood vessels. Blood vessels in skeletal muscle do not receive parasympathetic input.

Baroreceptors. *Baroreceptors* in the aortic arch and carotid sinus (at the origin of the internal carotid artery) are sensitive to stretch or pressure within the arterial system. Stimulation of these receptors sends information to the vasomotor center in the brainstem. This results in temporary inhibition of the sympathetic nervous system and enhancement of the parasympathetic influence, causing a decreased HR and peripheral vasodilation. Decreased arterial pressure causes the opposite effect.

Chemoreceptors. *Chemoreceptors* are located in the aortic arch and carotid body. They are capable of initiating changes in HR and arterial pressure in response to decreased arterial O_2 pressure, increased arterial carbon dioxide pressure, and decreased plasma pH. When the chemoreceptor reflexes are stimulated, they subsequently stimulate the vasomotor center to increase cardiac activity.

Blood Pressure

The **arterial blood pressure** (BP) is a measure of the pressure exerted by blood against the walls of the arterial system. The **systolic blood pressure** (SBP) is the peak pressure exerted against the arteries when the heart contracts. The **diastolic blood pressure** (DBP) is the residual pressure of the arterial system during ventricular relaxation. BP is usually expressed as the ratio of systolic to diastolic pressure.

The two main factors influencing BP are cardiac output (CO) and *systemic vascular resistance* (SVR):

$$BP = CO \times SVR$$

SVR is the force opposing the movement of blood. This force is created primarily in small arteries and arterioles.

Measurement of Arterial Blood Pressure. BP can be measured by invasive and noninvasive techniques. The invasive technique consists of catheter insertion into an artery. The catheter is attached to a recording device, and the pressure is measured directly (see Chapter 64).

Noninvasive, indirect measurement of BP can be done with a sphygmomanometer and a stethoscope. The sphygmomanometer consists of an inflatable cuff and a pressure gauge. The BP is measured externally by listening for sounds of turbulent blood flow through a compressed artery (termed **Korotkoff sounds**). The brachial artery is the usual site for taking a BP.

After placing the appropriate size cuff on the extremity, the cuff is inflated to a pressure in excess of the systolic pressure. This causes blood flow in the artery to cease. As the pressure in the cuff is lowered, the artery is auscultated for Korotkoff sounds. There are five phases of Korotkoff sounds. The first phase is a tapping sound caused by the spurt of blood into the constricted artery as the pressure in the cuff is gradually deflated. This sound is considered the SBP. The fifth phase occurs when the sound disappears and is known as the DBP.[3] Clinically the BP is recorded as SBP/DBP (120/80). Occasionally an auscultatory gap is heard. An auscultatory gap is a loss of sound between the SBP and the DBP. The BP could be measured incorrectly if the cuff is not inflated to exceed the true SBP.

In addition to the manual technique, another noninvasive way to measure BP indirectly is to use automatic BP monitors (see Chapter 32).

Ambulatory BP monitoring may be used to diagnose hypertension more accurately in some patients (see Chapter 32). The monitor consists of a BP cuff and a lightweight microprocessing unit. This method records a patient's BP at preset intervals during routine activities over 24 to 48 hours.

Pulse Pressure and Mean Arterial Pressure. **Pulse pressure** is the difference between the SBP and DBP. It is normally about one third of the SBP. If the BP is 120/80, the pulse pressure is 40. An increased pulse pressure may occur during exercise or in individuals with atherosclerosis of the larger arteries due to increased SBP. A decreased pulse pressure may be found in cardiac failure or hypovolemia.

Another measurement related to BP is **mean arterial pressure** (MAP). It is not the average of the diastolic and systolic pressures because the duration of diastole exceeds that of systole at normal HRs. MAP is calculated by adding the diastolic pressure to one third of the pulse pressure:

$$MAP = DBP + \tfrac{1}{3} \text{ pulse pressure}$$

A person with a BP of 120/60 has a MAP of 80.

■ Gerontologic Considerations: Effects of Aging on the Cardiovascular System

Cardiovascular disease is the most common cause of hospitalization and death in older adults in North America. The most common cardiovascular problem is coronary artery disease (CAD) secondary to atherosclerosis. It is difficult to separate normal aging changes from the pathophysiologic changes of atherosclerosis. Current research suggests that some of the normal changes of aging promote atherosclerosis, hypertension, and cardiac failure.[4]

With increased age, the amount of collagen in the heart increases and elastin decreases. These changes affect the contractile and distensible properties of the myocardium. One of the major age-associated alterations in the cardiovascular response to exercise is a striking decrease in the cardiac response caused by decreased contractility and HR response to increased work. The resting HR is not markedly affected by aging.

Cardiac valves become thicker and stiffer from lipid accumulation, degeneration of collagen, and calcification. The aortic and mitral valves are most frequently affected. This can lead to valve incompetence or stenosis. The turbulent blood flow across the affected valve results in a *murmur*.

The number of pacemaker cells in the SA node decreases with age. An elderly person may have only 10% of the normal number of pacemaker cells.[5] This increases the likelihood of sinus node dysfunction causing sinus bradycardia. Fibrosis and increased microcalcification of the conduction system involving the left bundle branch in ventricular conduction may precipitate chronic heart block. A normal ECG of an aging patient may show small, inconspicuous increases in PR, QRS, and QT intervals.

The sympathetic nervous system control of the cardiovascular system decreases with aging. The number and function of β-adrenergic receptors in the heart decrease with age. Therefore the older adult has a decreased response to physical and emotional stress and is less sensitive to β-adrenergic agonist drugs.

Arterial blood vessels thicken and become less elastic with age. Arteries increase their sensitivity to vasopressin (antidiuretic hormone).[4] Both of these changes contribute to an increase in blood pressure with age. An increase in systolic pressure and a lower rate of increase in the diastolic pressure cause a widening of the pulse pressure. Despite the changes associated with aging, the heart is able to function adequately under normal circumstances, and hypertension is not considered a normal consequence of aging.

Age-related changes in the cardiovascular system and differences in assessment findings are presented in Table 31-2.

ASSESSMENT OF THE CARDIOVASCULAR SYSTEM

Subjective Data

A careful health history and physical examination should aid the nurse in differentiating symptoms that reflect a cardiovascular problem from problems of other body systems. For instance, it is important to determine if weight gain is because of overeating or a manifestation of fluid retention. Common chief cues that should alert the nurse to the possibility of underlying cardiovascular problems should be explored and documented (Table 31-3).

Important Health Information

Past health history. Many illnesses affect the cardiovascular system directly or indirectly. The patient should be questioned about a history of chest pain, shortness of breath, alcoholism or excessive drinking, anemia, rheumatic fever, streptococcal sore throat, congenital heart disease, stroke, syncope, hypertension, thrombophlebitis, intermittent claudication, varicosities, and edema.

Medications. An assessment of the patient's current and past use of medications should be made. This includes both over-the-counter (OTC) drugs and prescription drugs. For example, aspirin, which prolongs the blood clotting time, is contained in many drugs used to alleviate cold symptoms.

A medication assessment should list the name of the drug and the patient's understanding of its purpose and side effects. Drugs that may adversely affect the cardiovascular system also should be assessed. Some of these, and examples of their effect on the cardiovascular system, are as follows:

Tricyclic antidepressants—arrhythmias
Phenothiazines—arrhythmias and hypotension
Oral contraceptives—thrombophlebitis
Doxorubicin (Adriamycin)—cardiomyopathy
Lithium—arrhythmias
Corticosteroids—sodium and fluid retention
Theophylline preparations—tachycardia and arrhythmias
Recreational or abused drugs—tachycardia and arrhythmias

TABLE 31-2 *Gerontologic* Differences in Assessment — Cardiovascular System	
CHANGES	**DIFFERENCES IN ASSESSMENT FINDINGS**
Chest Wall	
Senile kyphosis	Altered chest landmarks for palpation, percussion, and auscultation; distant heart sounds
Heart	
Myocardial hypertrophy, ↑ collagen and scarring, ↓ elastin	↓ Cardiac reserve, slight ↓ HR
Downward displacement	Difficulty in isolating apical pulse
↓ CO, HR, SV in response to exercise or stress	Slowed, ↓ response to stress; slowed recovery from activity
Cellular aging changes and fibrosis of conduction system	↓ Amplitude of QRS complex and lengthening of PR, QRS, and QT intervals; left axis deviation; irregular cardiac rhythms
Valvular rigidity from calcification, sclerosis, or fibrosis, impeding complete closure of valves	Systolic murmur (aortic or mitral) possible without being indication of cardiovascular pathology
Blood Vessels	
Arterial stiffening caused by loss of elastin in arterial walls, thickening of intima of arteries and progressive fibrosis of media	Elevation in systolic and possibly diastolic BP (e.g., 160/90); possible widened pulse pressures; more pronounced arterial pulses; pedal pulses diminished

BP, Blood pressure; *CO,* cardiac output; *HR,* heart rate; *SV,* stroke volume.

TABLE 31-3　Cues to Cardiovascular Problems

MANIFESTATION	DESCRIPTION
Fatigue	No energy, need more rest than usual, normal activities result in tiring
Fluid retention	Weight gain, bloated feeling; swelling; tightening of clothing; shoes no longer fitting comfortably; marks or indentations left from constricting garments
Irregular heartbeat	Sensation of heart in throat or skipped beats, racing heart; dizziness
Dyspnea	Air hunger, especially after exertion; pillows or upright chair necessary for sleep
Pain	Indigestion, burning, numbness, tightness, or pressure in midchest; epigastric or substernal pain radiating to shoulder, neck, arms
Tenderness in calf of leg	Inability to bear weight; swelling of the involved extremity; inflamed, warm skin over vein
	Distended, discolored, tortuous veins in calves of legs; ache in lower extremities after standing for short periods
Dizzy, light-headed	Dizzy with change of position; woozy, unstable, weak
Altered neurologic function	Change in sensory or motor function, temporary or permanent
Leg pain	Tight squeezing pain in buttock, thigh, calf muscles with walking

Surgery or other treatments. The patient should also be asked about specific treatments, past surgeries, or hospital admissions related to cardiovascular problems. Any hospitalizations for diagnostic workups or cardiovascular symptoms should be explored. It should be noted whether an ECG or a chest x-ray was taken for baseline data.

Functional Health Patterns. The strong correlation between components of a patient's lifestyle and cardiovascular health supports the need to review each functional health pattern. Key questions to ask a person with a cardiovascular problem are listed in Table 31-4.

Health perception–health management pattern. The nurse should ask the patient about the presence of cardiovascular risk factors. Major risk factors include elevated serum lipids, hypertension, cigarette smoking, sedentary lifestyle, and obesity. Stressful lifestyle and diabetes mellitus should also be investigated.

If the patient smokes, the number of pack-years of smoking (number of packs smoked per day multiplied by the number of years the patient has smoked) should be estimated. The patient's attitude about smoking, as well as attempts to stop, should be documented. Alcohol use should also be recorded. This information should include type of beverage, amount, frequency, and any changes in the reaction to it. The use of habit-forming drugs, including recreational drugs, also should be noted. It is also important to obtain information on the patient's perception of how this illness may affect the future level of wellness and ability for self-care.

A question about the patient's allergies is appropriate. The nurse should determine whether a drug reaction or an allergic reaction was ever experienced. If the patient has been treated for allergies, understanding of this therapy should be ascertained. The patient should also be asked whether an anaphylactic reaction has ever been experienced.

Confirmed illnesses of blood relatives can highlight any hereditary or familial tendencies toward coronary artery disease, peripheral vascular disease, hypertension, bleeding, cardiac disorders, diabetes mellitus, atherosclerosis, and stroke. In addition, disorders affecting the vascular system, such as intermittent claudication and varicosities, may be familial. Finally, a family health history of noncardiac conditions such as asthma, renal disease, and obesity should be assessed because they can affect the cardiovascular system.

Nutritional-metabolic pattern. Being underweight or overweight may indicate potential cardiovascular problems. Thus it is important to assess the patient's weight history in relation to height and build. A typical day's diet should be examined for its adequacy in relation to the patient's lifestyle. The amount of salt, saturated fats, and triglycerides in the patient's diet should be determined. In addition to actual food habits, which may be influenced greatly by ethnicity, the patient's attitudes and plans in relation to diet should be investigated.

Elimination pattern. The patient on diuretics may report increased urinary elimination. Problems with constipation should be investigated and documented. Straining at stool (Valsalva maneuver) should be avoided in a patient with cardiovascular problems. Cardiovascular problems may impair the patient's ability to get to a toilet as quickly as necessary. The patient should be questioned about this if incontinence or constipation is problematic.

Activity-exercise pattern. The benefit of exercise to cardiovascular health is indisputable, with sustained aerobic exercise being most beneficial. The nurse should inquire about the types of exercise done, the duration and frequency of each, and the occurrence of any unwanted effects. The length of time the exercise program has been practiced should be recorded, along with participation in individual or group sports. Any symptoms indicative of cardiovascular problems such as light-headedness, chest pain, shortness of breath, or claudication during exercise should be noted.

The patient should also be questioned about any limitations in activities of daily living (ADLs) as a result of a cardiovascular problem. Such problems are often associated with fatigue and depression, which are symptoms of cardiac disease. The nurse should also gather information about the patient's leisure and recreational activities. Any decrease in previous abilities should be noted.

Sleep-rest pattern. Although there are many possible causes, cardiovascular problems are often the cause for interrupted sleep. *Paroxysmal nocturnal dyspnea* (attacks of shortness of breath especially at night that awaken the patient) are associated with advanced heart failure. Many patients with heart failure may need to sleep with their head elevated on pillows. The nurse should note the number of pillows needed for comfort. Nocturia, a common finding with cardiovascular patients, interrupts normal sleep patterns.

Cognitive-perceptual pattern. It is important that the nurse ask both the patient and significant others about cognitive-perceptual problems. Any pain associated with the cardiovascular system such as chest pain and claudication should be reported.

TABLE
31-4

Health History
Cardiovascular System

Health Perception–Health Management Pattern
- Have you noticed an increase in cardiovascular symptoms such as chest pain or dyspnea?*
- Do you practice any preventive measures to decrease cardiac risk factors?*
- Do you foresee any potential self-care problems because of your cardiovascular problem?*

Nutritional-Metabolic Pattern
- Describe your usual daily dietary intake, including fat, sodium, and fluid.
- What is your present weight? What was your weight one year ago? If different, explain.
- Does eating cause fatigue or shortness of breath?*

Elimination Pattern
- Do your feet or ankles ever swell?*
- Have you ever taken medication to help you get rid of excess fluid?*

Activity-Exercise Pattern
- Are your activities or exercise limited because of your cardio-vascular problem?*
- Are your activities of daily living restricted because of your cardiovascular problem?*
- Do you experience any discomfort or side effects as a result of exercise or activity?*

Sleep-Rest Pattern
- How many pillows do you sleep on at night?
- How many times a night do you awaken to urinate?
- Do you ever wake up suddenly and feel as if you cannot catch your breath?*

Cognitive-Perceptual Pattern
- Have you noticed any changes in your memory of level of awareness?*
- Do you ever experience dizziness?*
- Do you find it difficult to verbally express yourself?*
- Do you experience any pain (e.g., chest pain, leg pain with activity) as a result of your cardiovascular problem?*

Self-Perception–Self-Concept Pattern
- Have your perceptions of yourself changed since you were diagnosed with a cardiovascular disease?*
- How has your cardiovascular disease affected your life and your self-esteem?

Role-Relationship Pattern
- Describe how this illness has affected the roles that you play in your daily life.
- Describe how this illness has affected your relationships.
- How have your significant others been affected by your disease?

Sexuality-Reproductive Pattern
- Has your sexual behavior changed?*
- Do you experience any cardiac-related symptoms during intercourse?*
- Do any of your medications affect your ability to participate in sexual activities?*

Coping–Stress Tolerance Pattern
- Do you practice any stress reduction techniques?*
- Describe your normal coping mechanisms for stress.
- Who or where would you turn to during a time of stress? Are these people or services helping you now?*
- Do you feel capable of handling your present health situation? Explain.
- Do you experience any cardiovascular symptoms such as chest pain or palpitations during times of stress?*

Values-Belief Pattern
- What influence has your value-belief system had during your illness?
- Do you feel any conflicts between your value-belief system and your planned therapy?*
- Describe any cultural or religious beliefs that may influence the treatment of your cardiovascular problem.

*If yes, describe.

Cardiovascular problems such as arrhythmias, hypertension, and stroke may cause problems with vertigo, language, and memory.

Self-perception–self-concept pattern. If a cardiovascular event has been of acute origin, the patient's self-perception may be affected. Invasive diagnostic and palliative procedures often lead to body image concerns for the patient. When the cardiovascular disease is chronic in nature, the patient may not be able to identify the cause but can often describe the inability to "keep up" previous levels of activity or accomplishments. This too may affect the patient's self-esteem. Therefore it is essential to inquire about the effects of the illness on the patient.

Role-relationship pattern. The patient's sex, race, and age are all related to cardiovascular health and are therefore important basic information. In addition, discussing the patient's marital status, role in the household, number of children and their ages, living environment, and significant others assists the nurse in identifying strengths and support systems in the patient's life.

The nurse must assess the patient's level of satisfaction or dissatisfaction in each assigned role, which may alert the health care provider to possible areas of stress or conflict.

Sexuality-reproductive pattern. The patient should be asked about the effect of the cardiovascular problem on sexual patterns and satisfaction. It is common for the patient to have a fear of sudden death during sexual intercourse, causing a major alteration in sexual behavior. Fatigue or shortness of breath may also curtail sexual activity. Impotence may be a symptom of peripheral vascular disease and is a side effect of some medications used in treating cardiovascular problems (e.g., β-adrenergic blockers, diuretics).

Many medications used to treat cardiovascular problems, particularly those used to treat hypertension, can result in impotence (see Chapter 32, Table 32-8). This side effect may result in noncompliance with medical treatment. Counseling of both the patient and partner may be indicated.

Coping–stress tolerance pattern. The patient should be asked to identify areas that cause stress or anxiety. Potentially stressful areas include marital relationships, family, occupation, church, friends, finances, and housing. Although many persons enjoy certain activities, these activities can be stressful at the same time that they are rewarding. The usual methods of coping with stress should be investigated.

Behaviors such as explosive, rapid speech and emotions such as anger and hostility have been associated with a risk of cardiac disease. Further research has made a strong link between hostility and heart disease.[6] The patient and the family should be asked about the frequency of these types of behavior.

Information about support systems such as family, extended family and friends, psychologists, or religious groups may provide excellent resources for developing a plan of care.

Values-belief pattern. Individual values and beliefs, which are greatly affected by culture, may play a significant role in the level of conflict a patient faces when dealing with a diagnosis of cardiovascular disease. Some patients may attribute their illness to punishment from God; others may feel that a "higher power" may assist them. Information about a patient's values and beliefs will help the nurse intervene during periods of crisis. It is also important to determine if the proposed plan of care causes any conflict with the patient's value system.

Objective Data

Physical Examination

Vital signs. After the patient's general appearance has been observed, vital signs, including BP, heart and respiratory rate, and temperature, are taken. The BP should be measured while the patient is sitting, lying, and standing. An appropriate cuff size should be used for accurate readings. Normally there is a reduction of up to 15 mm Hg in the systolic BP and 3 to 5 mm Hg in the diastolic BP in the standing position. BP measurements should be taken in both arms. These readings may vary from 5 to 15 mm Hg. A greater variance indicates pathology. BP in the lower extremities is expected to be about 10 mm Hg higher than in the upper extremities.

Peripheral vascular system

Inspection. Inspection of the skin color, hair distribution, and venous blood flow provides information about arterial blood flow and venous return. The extremities should be inspected for conditions such as edema, thrombophlebitis, varicose veins, and lesions such as stasis ulcers. Edema in the extremities can be caused by gravity, interruption of venous return, or elevation of right atrial pressure.

A measure used for assessing arterial flow to the extremities is the *capillary filling time.* The patient's nail beds are squeezed to produce blanching and observed for the return of color. With normal arterial capillary perfusion, the color will return within 3 seconds.

The large veins in the neck (internal and external jugular) should be inspected while the patient is gradually elevated to an upright position. Distention and prominent pulsations of these neck veins can be caused by right atrial pressure elevation.

Palpation. Palpation of the pulses in the neck and extremities also provides information on arterial blood flow. The pulses should be palpated to assess the volume and pressure within each vessel. Characteristics of the arteries on the right and left sides of the body should be compared. It is important to palpate each

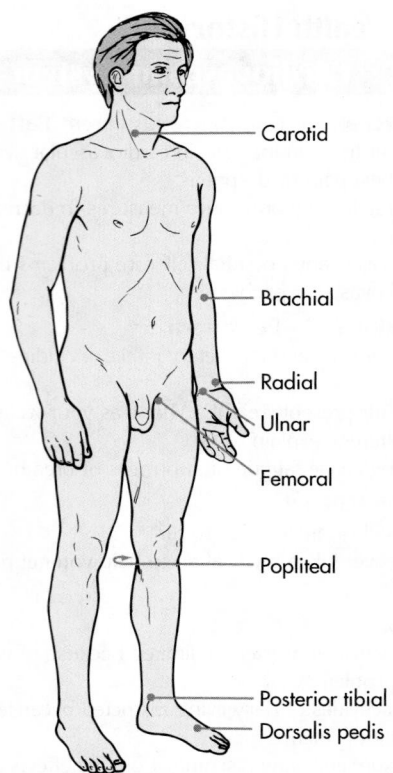

FIG. 31-8   Common sites for palpating arteries.

carotid pulse separately to avoid vagal stimulation and subsequent arrhythmias.

When palpating the arteries identified in Fig. 31-8, the assessor should note the pressure of the pulse wave, or how far the vessel wall distends when the pulse occurs. This judgment of the pulsation volume is recorded as normal, bounding, thready, or absent. A scale may be used to document pulse volume or amplitude:[3]

0	Absent
1+	Weak, thready
2+	Normal
3+	Full, bounding

The *rigidity* (hardness) of the vessel should also be noted. The normal pulse will feel like a tap, whereas a vessel wall that is narrowed or bulging will vibrate. A term ifor a palpable vibration is *thrill.*

Auscultation. An artery that has a narrowed or bulging wall may create turbulent blood flow. This abnormal flow can create a buzzing or humming termed a *bruit.* It can be heard with a stethoscope placed over the vessel. Auscultation of major arteries such as the carotid arteries, abdominal aorta, and femoral arteries should be part of the initial cardiovascular assessment. Abnormalities of the cardiovascular system are described in Table 31-5.

Thorax

Inspection and palpation. An overall inspection and palpation of the bony structures of the thorax is the initial step in the examination.

Next, inspect and palpate the areas where the cardiac valves project their sounds by identifying the intercostal spaces (ICSs). The raised notch, the *angle of Louis,* that is created where the manubrium and the body of the sternum are joined is readily pal-

TABLE 31-5

Common Assessment Abnormalities
Cardiovascular System

FINDINGS	DESCRIPTION	POSSIBLE ETIOLOGY AND SIGNIFICANCE
Pulse		
Pulse volume		
Bounding	Sharp, brisk, rapidly rising pulse	Bradycardia, anemia, aortic valve incompetence
Thready	Weak, slowly rising pulse	Blood loss, mitral valve stenosis
Absent	Lack of pulse	Atherosclerosis, thrombus, trauma, embolus
Thrill	Vibration of vessel or chest wall	Aneurysm, aortic regurgitation, arteriovenous fistula
Rigidity	Stiffness or inflexibility of vessel wall	Hardening or thickening of wall
Bruit	Humming heard through stethoscope placed over vessel	Narrowing of vessel, atherosclerosis, or aneurysm
Tachycardia	Heart rate greater than 100 beats/min	Exercise, anxiety, shock, need for increased cardiac output, hyperthyroidism
Bradycardia	Heart rate less than 60 beats/min	Rest, SA or AV node damage, athletic conditioning, side effect of drugs (e.g., β-adrenergic blockers), hypothyroidism
Arrhythmia	Irregular heart rate, skipped heart beats	Damage to cardiac conduction pathway, ischemia, side effect of drugs
Venous Abnormalities		
Distended neck veins	Vertical distance between intersection of angle of Louis and level of jugular distention greater than 3 cm with patient sitting at 45-degree angle	Elevated right atrial pressure
Pitting edema of lower extremities or sacral area	Visible finger indentation after application of firm pressure	Interruption of venous return to heart, fluid in tissues
Thrombophlebitis	Inflammation of vein associated with red, warm, tender, hard vein; edema, pain, tenderness of extremity	Venous stasis, damage to endothelial layer of vein, hypercoagulability of blood
Positive Homans' sign	Presence of calf pain during sharp dorsiflexion of foot	Thrombophlebitis
Skin		
Unusually warm hands or feet	Warmer than normal	Possible thyrotoxicosis and severe anemia
Cold hands or feet	Cold to touch, external covering necessary for comfort	Intermittent claudication, peripheral arterial obstruction, low cardiac output
Central cyanosis	Bluish or purplish tinge in central areas such as tongue, conjunctivae, inner surface of lips	Incomplete O_2 saturation of arterial blood due to pulmonary or cardiac disorders (e.g., congenital defects)
Peripheral cyanosis	Bluish or purplish tinge in extremities or in nose and ears	Reduced blood flow because of heart failure, vasoconstriction, cold environment
Color changes in extremities with postural change	Pallor, cyanosis, mottling of skin after limb elevation; glossy skin	Chronic decreased arterial perfusion
Stasis ulcers	Necrotic crater-like lesion of skin (usually lower leg); characterized by slow wound healing	Poor venous return, varicose veins, incompetent venous valves
Extremities		
Clubbing of nail beds	Obliteration of normal angle between base of nail and skin	Endocarditis, congenital defects, prolonged O_2 deficiency
Splinter hemorrhages	Small red to black streaks under fingernails	Infective endocarditis (infection of endocardium, usually in area of cardiac valves)
Abnormal capillary filling time	Blanching of nail bed for more than 3 sec after release of pressure	Reduced arterial capillary perfusion, anemia
Varicose veins	Visible dilated, tortuous vessels in lower extremities	Incompetent valves in vein
Asymmetry in limb circumference	Measurable swelling of involved limb	Thrombophlebitis, varicose veins
Arterial bruit	Turbulent flow sound in peripheral artery	Arterial obstruction or aneurysm

Continued

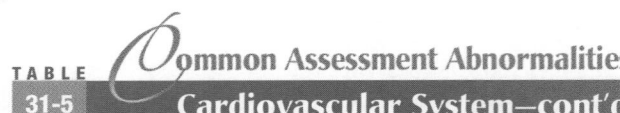

TABLE 31-5 Common Assessment Abnormalities

Cardiovascular System—cont'd

FINDINGS	DESCRIPTION	POSSIBLE ETIOLOGY AND SIGNIFICANCE
Cardiac Auscultatory Abnormalities		
Third heart sound (S₃)	Extra heart sound, low pitched, ending in early diastole, similar to sound of a gallop	Left ventricular failure; mitral valve regurgitation, volume overload, hypertension (possible)
Fourth heart sound (S₄)	Extra heart sound, low pitched, ending in late diastole, similar to sound of a gallop	Forceful atrial contraction from resistance to ventricular filling (e.g., in left ventricular hypertrophy, pulmonary stenosis, hypertension, coronary artery disease, aortic stenosis)
Cardiac murmurs	Turbulent sounds occurring between normal heart sounds; characterized by loudness, pitch, shape, quality, duration, timing	Cardiac valve disorder, abnormal blood flow patterns

AV, Atrioventricular; *SA,* sinoatrial.

pable in the midline of the sternum. The angle of Louis is at the level of the second rib and can therefore be used to count ICSs and locate specific auscultatory areas.

The following auscultatory areas can be located (Fig. 31-9): the aortic area in the second ICS to the right of the sternum, the pulmonic area in the second ICS to the left of the sternum, the tricuspid area in the fifth left ICS close to the sternum, and the mitral area in the left midclavicular line at the level of the fifth ICS. A fifth auscultatory area is *Erb's point,* located at the third left ICS near the sternum. Normally, no pulsations are felt in these areas unless the patient has a thin chest wall.

Valvular disorder may be suspected if abnormal pulsations or thrills are felt. Next, the epigastric area, which lies on either side of the midline just below the xyphoid process, is inspected and palpated. In a thin person the pulsation of the abdominal aorta may be visible and can normally be palpated here. Next, the precordium, which is located between the apex and the sternum, is inspected for heaves. **Heaves** are sustained lifts of the chest wall in the precordial area that can be seen or palpated. They may be caused by left ventricular enlargement. Normally no pulsations are seen or felt here.

When the patient is recumbent, the mitral valve area is inspected and palpated for the *point of maximal impulse* (PMI), which is due to the pulsation of the apex of the heart. This pulsation or ventricular thrust lies within the midclavicular line in the fifth ICS. If the PMI is palpable, its position is recorded in relation to the midclavicular line and ICSs. When the PMI is left of the midclavicular line, the heart may be enlarged.

Percussion. The borders of the right and left sides of the heart can be estimated by percussion. The nurse stands to the right of the recumbent patient and percusses along the curve of the rib in the fourth and fifth ICSs, starting at the midaxillary line. The percussion note over the heart is dull in comparison with the resonance over the lung and is recorded in relation to the midclavicular line.

Auscultation. The movement of the cardiac valves creates some turbulence in the blood flow resulting in normal heart sounds (Fig. 31-10). These sounds can be heard through a stethoscope placed on the chest wall. The first heart sound (S₁), which

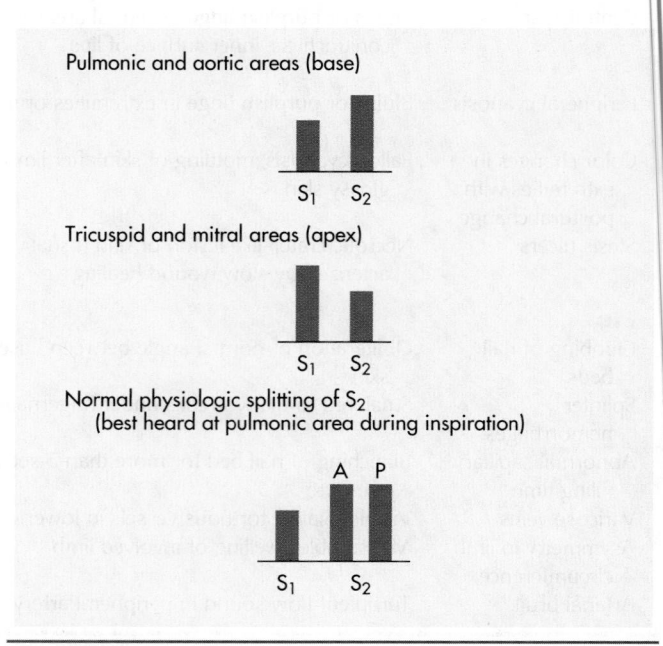

FIG. 31-9 Cardiac auscultatory areas.

FIG. 31-10 Heart sounds. *A,* Aortic; *P,* pulmonic.

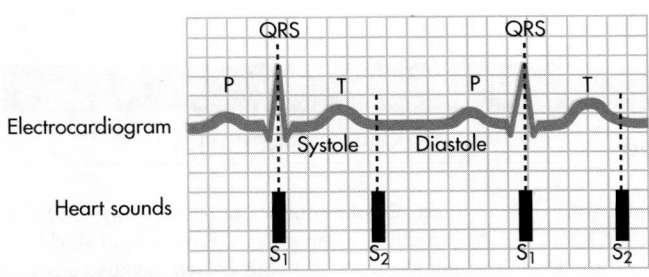

FIG. 31-11 Relationship of electrocardiogram, cardiac cycle, and heart sounds.

TABLE 31-6	Normal Physical Assessment of the Cardiovascular System
Inspection	Normal skin color with capillary refill <3 sec; thorax symmetric with no visible PMI; no JVD with patient at 45-degree angle
Palpation	PMI palpable in fifth ICS at MCL; no forceful pulsations, thrills, or heaves; slight palpable pulsations of abdominal aorta in epigastric area; carotid and extremity pulses 2+ and equal bilaterally; no evidence of impaired arterial flow or venous return in lower extremities
Percussion	Unable to distinguish right-sided heart border
Auscultation	S_1 and S_2 heard; HR 72 and regular; no murmurs or extra heart sounds

HR, Heart rate; *ICS,* intercostal space; *JVD,* jugular venous distention; *MCL,* mid-clavicular line; *PMI,* point of maximal impulse.

is associated with the closure of the tricuspid and mitral (AV) valves, has a soft *lubb* sound. The second heart sound (S_2), which is associated with the closure of the aortic and pulmonic (semilunar) valves, has a sharp *dupp* sound. S_1 signals the beginning of systole. S_2 signals the beginning of diastole (Fig. 31-11). The nurse should listen to the auscultatory areas in sequence with both the diaphragm and bell of the stethoscope.

The first and second heart sounds are heard best with the diaphragm of the stethoscope because they are high pitched. Extra heart sounds (S_3 or S_4), if present, are heard best with the bell of the stethoscope because they are low pitched. Having the patient leaning forward while sitting accentuates sounds from the second ICSs (aortic and pulmonic areas), whereas the left lateral decubitus position accentuates sounds produced at the mitral area.

The nurse listens at the apical area with the diaphragm of the stethoscope while simultaneously palpating the radial pulse. If fewer radial than apical pulses are counted, a *pulse deficit* is present. A judgment about the rhythm (regular or irregular) is also made when listening at the apex.

Palpating one carotid artery while auscultating it allows differentiation of S_1 from S_2 and systole from diastole. Because S_1 (lubb) occurs almost simultaneously with ventricular ejection, it is heard when the carotid pulse is felt.

Normally no sound is heard between S_1 and S_2 during the periods of systole and diastole. Sounds that are heard during these periods may represent abnormalities and should be described. An exception to this is a normal splitting of S_2, which is best heard at the pulmonic area during inspiration. Splitting of this heart sound can be abnormal if it is heard during expiration or if it is constant (fixed) during the respiratory cycle.

The S_3 heart sound is a low-intensity vibration of the ventricular walls usually associated with ventricular filling. An S_3 heart sound may occur in patients with left ventricular failure or mitral valve regurgitation. It is heard closely after S_2 and is known as a *ventricular gallop.* The S_4 heart sound is a low-frequency vibration caused by atrial contraction. It precedes S_1 of the next cycle and is known as an *atrial gallop.* An S_4 heart sound may occur in patients with coronary artery disease, left ventricular hypertrophy, or aortic stenosis.

Murmurs are sounds produced by turbulent blood flow through the heart or the walls of large arteries. Most murmurs are the result of cardiac abnormalities, but some occur in normal cardiac structures. Murmurs are graded on a six-point scale of loudness and recorded as a Roman numeral ratio; the numerator is the intensity of the murmur and the denominator is always VI, which indicates that the six-point scale is being used. An I/VI indicates

a soft, faint murmur; a VI/VI indicates a murmur that can be heard without a stethoscope.

If an abnormal sound is heard, it should be documented. This description should include the timing (during systole or diastole), location (the site on the chest where it is heard the loudest), pitch (heard best with the diaphragm or the bell of the stethoscope), position (heard best when patient is recumbent, sitting and leaning forward, or in the left lateral decubitus position), characteristic (harsh, musical, soft, short, long), and any other abnormal findings (irregular cardiac rhythms or palpable chest wall heaves) associated with the sound.

The most common abnormal sounds and abnormal assessment findings are described in Table 31-5. A method of recording data from the cardiovascular assessment is presented in Table 31-6.

DIAGNOSTIC STUDIES OF THE CARDIOVASCULAR SYSTEM

Numerous diagnostic procedures add to the information obtained from the history and physical examination of the cardiovascular system. These procedures are usually classified as noninvasive or invasive. If only needle insertion for withdrawal of blood or injection of contrast media is used, these studies are usually considered noninvasive. Catheter insertion for angiography is considered an invasive procedure. The most common studies used to assess the cardiovascular system are presented in Table 31-7.

Noninvasive Studies

Chest X-Ray. A radiographic picture can depict cardiac contours, heart size and configuration, and anatomic changes in individual chambers (Fig. 31-12). The radiographic image records any displacement or enlargement of the heart, presence of extra fluid around the heart (pericardial effusion), and pulmonary congestion.

Electrocardiogram. The basic P, QRS, and T waveforms (see Table 31-1) are used to assess cardiac function. Deviations from the normal sinus rhythm can indicate abnormalities in heart function. There are many types of electrocardiographic monitoring, including resting ECG, ambulatory monitoring, and exercise or stress testing.

TABLE 31-7 *Diagnostic Studies*
Cardiovascular System

STUDY	DESCRIPTION AND PURPOSE	NURSING RESPONSIBILITY
Noninvasive **Chest x-ray**	Patient is placed in two upright positions to examine the lung fields and size of the heart. The two common positions are posteroanterior (PA) and lateral. Normal heart size and contour for the individual's age, sex, and size are noted.	Inquire about frequency of recent x-rays and possibility of pregnancy. Provide lead shielding to areas not being viewed. Remove any jewelry or metal objects that may obstruct the view of the heart and lungs.
ECG	Electrodes are placed on the chest and extremities, allowing the ECG machine to record cardiac electrical activity from different views. Can detect rhythm of heart, activity of pacemaker, conduction abnormalities, position of heart, size of atria and ventricles, presence of injury, and history of myocardial infarction.	Inform patient that no discomfort is involved. Instruct to avoid moving to decrease motion artifact.
Ambulatory ECG **monitoring** ▪ Holter monitoring	Recording of ECG rhythm for 24-48 hr and then correlating rhythm changes with symptoms recorded in diary. Normal patient activity is encouraged to simulate conditions that produce symptoms. Electrodes are placed on chest and a recorder is used to store information until it is recalled, printed, and analyzed for any rhythm disturbance. It can be performed on an inpatient or outpatient basis.	Prepare skin and apply electrodes and leads. Explain importance of keeping an accurate diary of activities and symptoms. Tell patient that no bath or shower can be taken during monitoring. Skin irritation may develop from electrodes.
▪ Transtelephonic event recorder	It allows more freedom than a regular Holter monitor. It records rhythm disturbances that are not frequent enough to be recorded in one 24-hr period. Some units have electrodes that are attached to the chest and have a loop of memory that captures the onset and end of an event. Other types are placed directly on patient's wrist, chest, or fingers and have no loop of memory, but record the patient's ECG in real time. Recordings are transmitted over the phone to a receiving unit, and the recordings are printed out for review. Tracings can then be erased and the unit can be reused.	Instruct in the use of equipment for recording and transmitting of transient events. Teach patient about skin preparation for lead placement or steady skin contact for units not requiring electrodes. This will ensure the reception of optimal ECG tracings for analysis.
Exercise treadmill test	Various protocols are used to evaluate the effect of exercise tolerance on myocardial function. A common protocol uses 3 min stages at set speeds and elevation of the treadmill belt. Continual monitoring of vital signs and ECG rhythms for ischemic changes are important in the diagnosis of left ventricular function and coronary artery disease. An exercise bike may be used if the patient is unable to walk on the treadmill.	Instruct patient to wear comfortable clothes and shoes that can be used for walking and running. Instruct patient about procedure and application of lead placement. Monitor vital signs and obtain 12-lead ECG before exercise, during each stage of exercise, and after exercise until all vital signs and ECG changes have returned to normal. Monitor patient's symptoms throughout procedure.
Echocardiogram ▪ M-mode ▪ Two-dimensional ▪ Cardiac Doppler ▪ Color-flow imaging or color Doppler	Transducer that emits and receives ultrasound waves is placed in four positions on the chest above the heart. Transducer records sound waves that are bounced off the heart. Also records direction and flow of blood through the heart and transforms it to audio and graphic data that measure valvular abnormalities, congenital cardiac defects, wall motion, and cardiac function.	Place patient in a supine position on left side facing equipment. Instruct family and patient about procedure and sensations (pressure and mechanical movement from head of transducer). No contraindications to procedure exist.
▪ Stress echocardiogram	Combination of exercise treadmill test and echocardiogram. Resting images of the heart are taken with ultrasound and then the patient exercises. Postexercise images are taken immediately after exercise (within 1 min of stopping exercise). Differences in left ventricular wall motion and thickening before and after exercise are evaluated.	Instruct and prepare patient for exercise treadmill. Inform patient of importance of timely return to examination table for imaging after exercise. Contraindications include any patient unable to reach peak exercise.

ECG, Electrocardiogram.

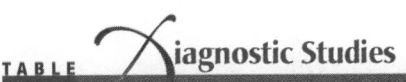

TABLE
31-7

Diagnostic Studies
Cardiovascular System—cont'd

STUDY	DESCRIPTION AND PURPOSE	NURSING RESPONSIBILITY
Noninvasive—cont'd		
▪ Dobutamine echocardiogram	Used as a substitute for the exercise stress test in individuals unable to exercise. Dobutamine (a positive inotropic agent) is infused IV and dosage is increased in 5 min intervals while echocardiogram is performed to detect wall motion abnormalities at each stage.	Start IV infusion. Administer dobutamine. Monitor vital signs before, during, and after test until baseline achieved. Monitor patient for signs and symptoms of distress during procedure.
▪ Transesophageal echocardiogram	A probe with an ultrasound transducer at the tip is swallowed. The physician controls angle and depth. As it passes down the esophagus, it sends back clear images of heart size, wall motion, valvular abnormalities, and possible source of thrombi without interference from lungs or chest ribs. A contrast medium may be injected IV for evaluating direction of blood flow if an atrial or ventricular septal defect is suspected. Doppler ultrasound and color flow imaging can also be used concurrently.	Instruct patient to be NPO for at least 6 hr before test. Remove dentures. A bite block is placed in the mouth. A sedative will be given and throat locally anesthetized, so if done as an outpatient, a designated driver is needed. Monitor vital signs and oxygen saturation levels and perform suctioning continually during procedure. Assist patient to relax. Patient may not eat or drink until gag reflex returns. Sore throat is temporary.
Nuclear cardiology	Study involves IV injection of radioactive isotopes. Radioactive uptake is counted over the heart by scintillation camera. It supplies information about myocardial contractility, myocardial perfusion, and acute cell injury.	Explain procedure to patient. Establish IV line for injection of isotopes. Explain that radioactive isotope used is a small, diagnostic amount and will lose most of its radioactivity in a few hours. Inform the patient that he or she will be lying still on back with arms extended overhead for 20 min. Repeat scans are performed within a few minutes to hours after the injection.
▪ Cardiolite scan	Cardiolite (technetium-99m sestamibi) is injected intravenously and used to evaluate blood flow in different parts of the heart. It is taken up in area of MI, producing hot spots. Images are taken at rest and after exercise. For stress testing, the injection of the technetium is given at maximum heart rate on bicycle or treadmill. Patient is then required to continue exercise for 3 min to circulate the radioactive isotope. Scanning is done 15-60 min after exercise. A resting scan is performed 60-90 min after initial infusion. A 3-4 hr interval between rest and stress studies is required. Follow-up scan may be done 24 hr later.	Explain procedure to patient. Instruct patient to eat only a light meal between scans. Certain medications may need to be held for 1-2 days before the scan.
▪ Dipyridamole Cardiolite scan	As with a Cardiolite exercise test, dipyridamole (Persantine) is injected. Dipyridamole acts as a powerful vasodilator and will increase blood flow to well-perfused coronary arteries. Scanning procedure is same as with Cardiolite scan.	Explain procedure to patient. Instruct patient to hold all caffeine products for 12 hr before procedure.
▪ Blood pool imaging	Technetium 99m pertechnetate is injected intravenously. Single injection allows sequential evaluation of heart for several hours. Study is indicated for patients with recent MI or congestive heart failure, especially if not recovering well. It can be used to measure effectiveness of various cardiac medications and can be done at patient's bedside.	Explain procedure to patient. Inform patient that procedure involves little or no risk.
▪ Positron emission tomography (PET)	Uses two radionuclides. Nitrogen-13-ammonia is injected intravenously first and scanned to evaluate myocardial perfusion. A second radioactive isotope, fluoro-18-deoxyglucose, is then injected and scanned to show myocardial metabolic function. In the normal heart, both scans will match, but in an ischemic or damaged heart, they will differ. The patient may or may not be stressed. A baseline resting scan is usually obtained for comparison.	Instruct patient on procedure. Explain that patient will be scanned by a machine and will need to stay still for a period of time. Patient's glucose level must be between 60 and 140 mg/dl (3.3-7.8 μmol/L) for accurate glucose metabolic activity. If exercise is included as part of testing, patient will need to be NPO and refrain from tobacco and caffeine for 24 hr before test.

MI, Myocardial infarction; *NPO,* nothing by mouth.

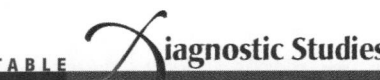

TABLE
31-7

Diagnostic Studies

Cardiovascular System—cont'd

STUDY	DESCRIPTION AND PURPOSE	NURSING RESPONSIBILITY
Noninvasive—cont'd		
Magnetic resonance imaging (MRI)	Noninvasive imaging technique obtains information about cardiac tissue integrity, aneurysms, ejection fractions, cardiac output, and patency of proximal coronary arteries. It does not involve ionizing radiation and is an extremely safe procedure. It provides images in multiple planes with uniformly good resolution. It cannot be used in persons with any implanted metallic devices.	Explain procedure to patient. Inform patient that the small diameter of the cylinder, along with loud noise of the procedure, may cause panic or anxiety. Antianxiety drugs and music may be recommended. Patient must lie still during MRI.
▪ Magnetic resonance angiography (MRA)	Same as MRI but with use of gadolinium as IV contrast medium to evaluate arterial disease.	
Blood studies		
▪ CK-MB	Immunochemical process using monoclonal antibodies that measures this cardiospecific enzyme. Concentrations >5% of total CK are highly indicative of MI. Serum levels increase within 3-12 hr after MI.	Serial sampling should be done in conjunction with ECG.
▪ Myoglobin	Low-molecular-weight protein that is 99%-100% sensitive for myocardial injury. Serum concentrations rise 1-2 hr after MI. *Normal:* <92 ng/ml (men) <76 ng/ml (women)	Cleared from the circulation rapidly and therefore must be measured within first 18 hr of onset of chest pain.
▪ Troponin	Contractile proteins that are released following an MI. Both troponin T and troponin I are highly specific to cardiac tissue. *Normal:* Troponin T (cTnT): <0.1 ng/ml Troponin I (cTnI): <0.1-3.1 ng/ml	Rapid bedside assays are available.
Serum lipids		
▪ Cholesterol	Cholesterol is a blood lipid. Elevated cholesterol is considered a risk factor for atherosclerotic heart disease. Level can be measured at any time of the day in a nonfasting state. *Normal:* 140-200 mg/dl (3.62-5.17 mmol/L) (varies with age and sex)	Explain procedure to patient. Cholesterol levels can be obtained in a nonfasting state, but for triglyceride levels and lipoproteins, fasting state for at least 12 hr (except for water) is necessary, and no alcohol intake is allowed for 24 hr before testing.
▪ Triglycerides	Triglycerides are mixtures of fatty acids. Elevations are associated with cardiovascular disease. *Normal:* 40-190 mg/dl (0.45-2.15 mmol/L) (varies with age)	
▪ Lipoproteins	Electrophoresis is done to separate lipoproteins into HDL, LDL, and VLDL and chylomicrons. There are marked day-to-day fluctuations in serum lipid levels. More than one determination is needed for accurate diagnosis and treatment. *Normal:* varies with age. Desirable LDL is <130 mg/dl (3.4 mmol/L). Desirable HDL is 37-70 mg/dl (0.97-1.83 mmol/L) for men; 40-88 mg/dl (1.05-2.30 mmol/L) for women.	Cardiac risk factors are assessed by dividing the total cholesterol level by the HDL level.
Invasive		
Cardiac catheterization	Study involves insertion of catheter into heart. Information can be obtained about O_2 saturation and pressure readings within chambers. Contrast medium is injected to assist in examining structure and motion of heart. Procedure is done by insertion of catheter into a vein (for right side of heart) or an artery (for left side of heart) (see text).	Before procedure, obtain written permission. Check for iodine sensitivity. Withhold food and fluids for 6-18 hr before procedure. Give sedative, if ordered. Inform patient about use of local anesthesia, insertion of catheter, and feeling of warmth and fluttering sensation of heart as catheter is passed. Note that patient may be instructed to cough or take a deep breath when catheter is inserted and that patient is monitored by ECG throughout procedure.

ECG, Electrocardiogram; *HDL,* high-density lipoproteins; *LDL,* low-density lipoproteins; *VLDL,* very low–density lipoproteins.

TABLE 31-7 Diagnostic Studies
Cardiovascular System—cont'd

STUDY	DESCRIPTION AND PURPOSE	NURSING RESPONSIBILITY
Invasive—cont'd **Cardiac catheterization—cont'd**		After procedure, assess circulation to extremity used for catheter insertion. Check peripheral pulses, color, and sensation of extremity every 15 min for 1 hr and then with decreasing frequency. Observe injection site for swelling and bleeding. Place sandbag over arterial site, if indicated. Monitor vital signs. Assess for abnormal HR, arrhythmias, and signs of pulmonary emboli (respiratory difficulty).
Coronary angiography	Study involves injection of radiopaque contrast medium directly into coronary arteries by same procedure as for cardiac catheterization. It is used to evaluate patency of coronary arteries and collateral circulation.	Same as for cardiac catheterization.
Intracoronary ultrasound (ICUS)	Invasive study used to provide ultrasound information about the coronary arteries. A very small ultrasound probe is introduced into the coronary artery, similar to coronary angiography. Information obtained is used to assess size and consistency of plaque, arterial walls, and effectiveness of intracoronary artery treatment.	Same as for cardiac catheterization.
Hemodynamic monitoring	Hemodynamic monitoring of arterial blood pressures, pulmonary artery pressure, pulmonary artery wedge pressure, and cardiac output are discussed in Chapter 64.	
Electrophysiology study (EPS)	Invasive study used to record intracardiac electrical activity using catheters (with multiple electrodes) inserted via the femoral vein into the right side of heart. The catheter electrodes record the electrical activity in different cardiac structures. In addition, arrhythmias can be induced.	Obtain written consent. Antiarrhythmic medications may be discontinued several days before study. Keep patient NPO 6-8 hr before test. Give premedication to promote relaxation and throughout the procedure if ordered. Place the patient on cardiac monitor after the procedure.
Peripheral arteriography and venography*	Study involves injection of radiopaque contrast medium into either arteries or veins. Serial x-rays taken to detect and visualize any atherosclerotic plaques, occlusion, aneurysms, or traumatic injury.	Carefully explain procedure to patient. Check for iodine allergy. Give mild sedative, if ordered. Check extremity with puncture site for pulsation, warmth, color, and motion after procedure. Inspect insertion site for bleeding or swelling. Observe patient for allergic reactions to dye.

*Additional peripheral vascular diagnostic studies are found in Table 37-8.
HR, heart rate.

A resting ECG helps identify at one point in time primary conduction abnormalities, cardiac arrhythmias, cardiac hypertrophy, pericarditis, myocardial ischemia, site and extent of myocardial infarction (MI), pacemaker performance, and effectiveness of drug therapy. It is also used to monitor recovery from an MI.

Electrocardiogram leads. Recording of an ECG involves the use of multiple electrodes. An electrode is placed on each of the four limbs. The right-leg electrode is used as an inactive ground electrode. Six electrodes are placed in specific locations on the chest wall (precordium). Electrical impulses generated by the heart are detected by the electrodes, magnified by an amplifier, and recorded on graph paper.

Each combination of electrodes used in standard electrocardiography is called a *lead*. Like a camera taking a picture from different angles, a 12-lead ECG records the electrical activity in the myocardium from 12 different views. The three limb leads are I, II, and III. Lead I records the direction of electric current and voltage detected between the right- and left-arm electrodes. Lead II is a right-arm and left-leg combination. Lead III records the electrical activity using the left-arm and left-leg electrodes. The unipolar augmented limb leads (aV$_R$, aV$_F$, and aV$_L$) measure electrical potential between one augmented limb lead and the electrical midpoint of the remaining two leads. The chest electrodes are placed in various locations, starting at the right sternal border in the fourth ICS (V$_1$) and moving across the chest (V$_1$ through V$_6$), as indicated in Fig. 31-13. These are known as chest or V leads.

Unfortunately, the 12-lead ECG has limitations, with some areas of the myocardium left completely invisible to "the camera's

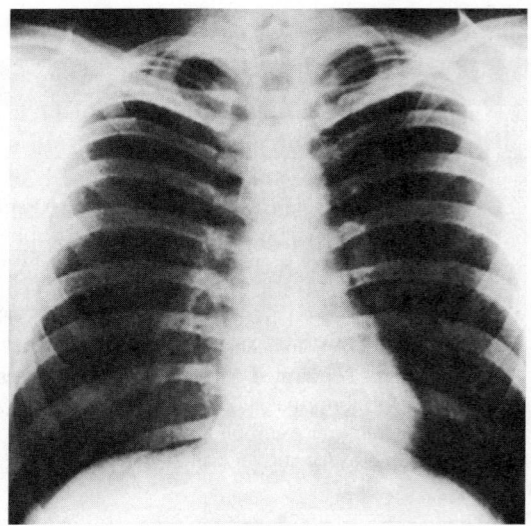

FIG. 31-12 Chest x-ray showing outline of the heart.

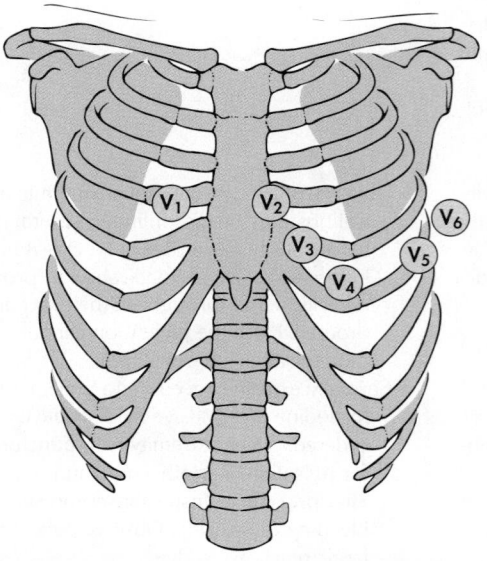

FIG. 31-13 Placement of chest leads (V leads) for a 12-lead electrocardiogram.

vision." Because of lead placement, invisible areas of the myocardium include portions of the right ventricle and the posterior wall of the left ventricle. If a more definitive diagnosis is needed for a posterior wall or right ventricular infarct, six V leads of the right chest may be obtained. Similar to the 12-lead ECG, the additional six leads are obtained by placing electrodes across the right side of the chest in the mirror image of the left chest leads.

Ambulatory electrocardiogram monitoring. Continuous ambulatory ECG can provide diagnostic information over a greater period of time than a standard resting ECG. In Holter monitoring a recorder is worn by the patient for 24 to 48 hours, and the resulting ECG information is then stored until it is played back for printing and evaluation. While the person performs usual activities, Holter monitoring gives the patient freedom to perform those activities that are associated with the cardiovascular symptoms while documenting any ECG changes associated with these

activities. The person maintains a record of activity and sleep to correlate with the ECG findings (see Table 31-7).

Transtelephonic event recorders. This type of recorder is helpful for monitoring less frequent ECG events. The monitor is a portable unit using electrodes to transmit a limited ECG over the phone to a receiving device. A disadvantage of this type of monitoring is that if the event occurs for only a short duration, the symptoms may be over before the patient puts on the device and calls the assigned number.

Exercise or stress testing. Cardiac symptoms frequently occur only with activity. Exercise testing is a method used to evaluate the cardiovascular response to physical stress. This is helpful in assessing cardiovascular disease and defining limits for exercise programs. Patient selection for exercise testing is appropriate for individuals who do not have limitations related to walking or using a bicycle and those without abnormal ECGs that limit diagnostic interpretation (e.g., pacemakers, left bundle branch block).

The placement of electrodes is similar to a regular 12-lead placement for chest leads V_1 through V_6. Limb leads are placed on upper and lower chest walls to alleviate muscle interference during exercise. Resting BP and ECGs are performed in the supine position, while standing, and after hyperventilation to provide a baseline for comparison of any changes during exercise.

As the patient exercises on a treadmill or stationary bicycle, the BP, ECG, and often the oxygen saturation level are measured and monitored. The patient exercises to either peak HR (calculated by subtracting the person's age from 220) or to peak exercise tolerance, at which time the test is terminated and the treadmill is slowed while the patient continues walking. The test is also terminated for moderate to severe chest discomfort or significant ST segment depression indicating ischemic changes associated with coronary artery disease. After the treadmill belt is stopped, the patient lies down to rest. The ECG is monitored after exercise for rhythm disturbances or, if ECG changes occurred with exercise, for return to baseline.

Echocardiogram. The echocardiogram uses ultrasound waves to record the movement of the structures of the heart. In the normal heart, ultrasonic sound waves directed at the heart are reflected back in typical configurations (Fig. 31-14). The echocardiogram provides information about abnormalities of (1) valvular

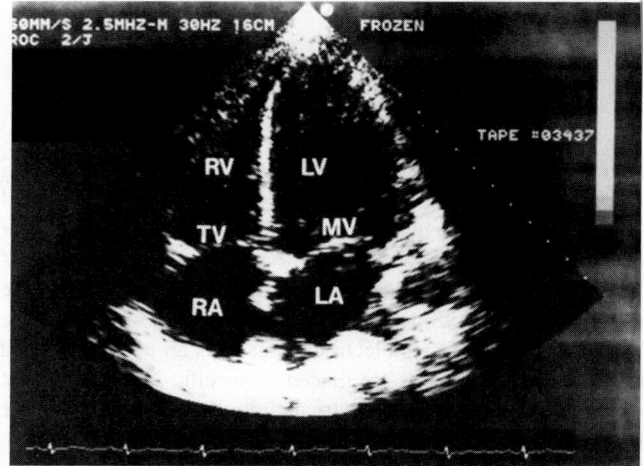

FIG. 31-14 Apical four-chamber two-dimensional echocardiographic view in a normal patient. *LA,* Left atrium; *LV,* left ventricle; *MV,* mitral valve; *RA,* right atrium; *RV,* right ventricle; *TV,* tricuspid valve.

structure and motion, (2) cardiac chamber size and contents, (3) ventricular muscle and septal motion and thickness, (4) the pericardial sac, and (5) the ascending aorta.

Two commonly used types are the *M-mode* (motion-mode) and the *two-dimensional* (2-D, real-time, cross-sectional) *echocardiogram.* In the M-mode, a single ultrasound beam is directed toward the heart, recording the motion of the intracardiac structures, as well as detecting wall thickness and chamber size. The 2-D echocardiogram sweeps the ultrasound beam through an arc, producing a cross-sectional view, and shows correct spatial relationships among the structures.

Doppler technology and color-flow imaging enhance echocardiogram studies. Doppler technology allows for sound evaluation of the flow or motion of the scanned object (heart valves, ventricular walls, blood flow). Color-flow imaging (duplex) is the combination of 2-D echocardiography and Doppler technology. It uses color changes to demonstrate the velocity and direction of blood flow. Pathologic conditions, such as valvular leaks and congenital defects, can be diagnosed more effectively.

Stress echocardiography, a combination of treadmill test and ultrasound images, evaluates segmental wall motion abnormalities.[7] By using a digital computer system to compare images before and after exercise, wall motion and segmental function can be clearly seen. This diagnostic test provides the information of an exercise stress test with the information gained from an echocardiogram. For those individuals unable to exercise, infusion of dobutamine causes a pharmacologic stress on the heart while the patient is resting. The same ultrasound technology is used.

Transesophageal echocardiography (TEE) is used to provide more precise echocardiography of the heart than surface 2-D echocardiography by eliminating interference from the chest wall and lungs. The TEE uses a modified, flexible endoscope probe with an ultrasound transducer in the tip for imaging of the heart and great vessels. The probe is introduced into the esophagus to the level of the heart, and M-mode, 2-D, pulsed Doppler, and color-flow imaging can be obtained.

TEE is used frequently in an outpatient setting. In addition, TEE has application in the operating room to assess presurgical and postsurgical cardiac function.

The risks of TEE are minimal. However, complications may include perforation of the esophagus, hemorrhage, arrhythmias, vasovagal reactions, and transient hypoxemia. TEE is contraindicated if the patient has a history of esophageal disorders, dysphagia, or radiation therapy to the chest wall.

New advances in echocardiography include real-time 3-D ultrasound and contrast echocardiography.[8,9] These methods are currently being researched and developed.

Nuclear Cardiology. Single photon emission computed tomography (SPECT) is used for the evaluation of the myocardium at risk of infarction and to determine infarction size. Small amounts of radioactive isotope are injected intravenously, and recordings are made of the radioactivity emitted over a specific area of the body. The total radiation exposure is minimal. The circulation of this tagged material can be used to detect coronary artery blood flow, intracardiac shunts, motion of ventricles, and size of the heart chambers. The most commonly used nuclear imaging tests include technetium-99m sestamibi (Cardiolite) scanning and blood pool imaging. Positron emission tomography (PET) scanning uses two isotopes (see Table 31-7). PET scans are highly sensitive in distinguishing between viable and nonviable myocardial tissue. Cost limits the widespread use of PET scanning.[10,11]

Perfusion imaging is also used with exercise testing to determine whether the coronary blood flow changes with increased activity. Stress exercising imaging may show an abnormality even when a resting image is normal. This procedure is indicated to diagnose coronary artery disease, determine the prognosis in already diagnosed coronary disease, assess the physiologic significance of a known coronary lesion, and assess the effectiveness of various therapeutic modalities such as bypass surgery or angioplasty.

If a patient is unable to tolerate exercise, an IV infusion of dipyridamole (Persantine) is given to dilate the coronary arteries and therefore simulate the effect of exercise. After the dipyridamole takes effect, the isotope is injected and the procedure proceeds. The patient is required to lie flat for 40 minutes while the pictures are taken. All caffeine and theophylline products must be held 12 hours before the study. Calcium channel blockers and β-adrenergic blockers should be held 24 hours before the use of dipyridamole.

Magnetic Resonance Imaging. Although not widely used because of equipment size and access, magnetic resonance imaging (MRI) allows detection and localization of MI areas. Further research is underway to determine if this imaging technique will become more commonly used in diagnosing cardiac problems.

Magnetic resonance angiography (MRA) is being used for imaging vascular occlusive disease and abdominal aortic aneurysms. The contrast material is non-iodine based and is injected through an intravenous line. The MRA images compare favorably to duplex ultrasound of arterial stenosis.[12]

Computed Tomography. Computed tomography (CT) with spiral technology is a noninvasive scan used to quantify calcium deposits in coronary arteries. Debate continues on the clinical relevance of coronary artery calcium scoring as a screening tool for coronary artery disease.[13]

Blood Studies. Numerous blood studies contribute information about the cardiovascular system. For example, studies of the blood itself reflect the O_2-carrying capacity (red blood cell count and hemoglobin) and coagulation properties (clotting times). (See Chapter 29 for hematology studies.)

Diagnostic tests for myocardial infarction. When cells are injured, they release their cell contents, including enzymes and other proteins, into the circulation. These biochemical markers are useful in the diagnosis of myocardial injury and necrosis. The enzymes characteristic of cardiac injury are creatine kinase (CK), lactic dehydrogenase (LDH), and serum aspartate aminotransferase (AST), formerly called serum glutamic-oxaloacetic transaminase (SGOT). Because these enzymes are found in a variety of body tissues, they can be elevated as a result of injury to the muscles, liver, brain, and other organs. LDH and AST levels are no longer typically used as markers of myocardial injury. CK is present in heart muscle, skeletal muscle, and brain tissue. CK-MM is found primarily in the skeletal muscle, and CK-BB is found in the brain and nervous tissue. CK-MB elevation is specific for myocardial tissue injury.

Troponin is a myocardial muscle protein released into circulation after injury. There are two subtypes, troponin T (cTnT) and troponin I (cTnI), and they are specific to myocardial tissue. Normally there is no circulating troponin, so a rise in its level is diagnostic of myocardial damage. Troponin T reaches peak levels within 12 hours and has a high specificity at 3 to 6 hours following the onset of symptoms.[14]

Myoglobin is a low-molecular-weight heme protein found in cardiac and skeletal muscle. Myoglobin elevation is a sensitive indicator of early myocardial injury, and serum elevations occur within 1 to 2 hours after injury but decline rapidly after 7 hours. Its clinical value is limited to the brief presence of myoglobin following infarction (24 hours).[15]

Correct interpretation of diagnostic tests requires consideration of the time frame from the onset of symptoms together with the time frame of the expected presence and elevated levels of the biomarkers. The adjunctive data (patient symptoms, history, and ECG changes) complete the diagnostic picture for the patient with a suspected MI.[15]

Blood lipids. Blood lipids consist of triglycerides, cholesterol, and phospholipids. They circulate in the blood bound to protein. Thus they are often referred to as *lipoproteins* (see Chapter 33, Fig. 33-6).

Triglycerides are the main storage form of lipids and constitute approximately 95% of fatty tissue. Cholesterol, a structural component of cell membranes and plasma lipoproteins, is a precursor of corticosteroids, sex hormones, and bile salts. In addition to being absorbed from food in the gastrointestinal tract, cholesterol can also be synthesized in the liver. Phospholipids contain glycerol, fatty acids, phosphates, and a nitrogenous compound. Although formed in most cells, phospholipids usually enter the circulation as lipoproteins synthesized by the liver. Apoproteins are water-soluble proteins that combine with most lipids to form lipoproteins.

Different classes of lipoproteins contain varying amounts of the naturally occurring lipids. These include the following:

1. *Chylomicrons:* primarily exogenous triglycerides from dietary fat
2. *Low-density lipoproteins (LDLs):* mostly cholesterol with moderate amounts of phospholipids
3. *High-density lipoproteins (HDLs):* about one-half protein and one-half phospholipids and cholesterol
4. *Very-low-density lipoproteins (VLDLs):* primarily endogenous triglycerides with moderate amounts of phospholipids and cholesterol

A lipid profile test usually consists of cholesterol, triglycerides, LDL, and HDL measurements. An elevation in LDL has a strong and direct association with coronary artery disease (CAD); an increased HDL has been associated with a decreased risk of CAD.[3] High levels of HDL serve a protective role by mobilizing cholesterol from tissues. Increased triglyceride levels are also linked to the progression of CAD.[16] Although the association between elevated serum cholesterol levels and CAD exists, determination of total cholesterol level is not sufficient for an assessment of coronary risk. A risk assessment for CAD is given by comparing the total cholesterol to HDL ratio.[17] An increase in the ratio indicates increased risk. This combination provides more information than either value alone. The patient must fast for 12 to 14 hours before the blood draw to eliminate the effects of a recent meal. A specimen should not be drawn if the patient is having acute stress.

Plasma levels of apolipoprotein A-1 (Apo A-1) (the major HDL protein) and apolipoprotein B (Apo B) (the major LDL protein) are better predictors of CAD than HDL or LDL. Measurements of these lipoproteins may replace cholesterol-lipoprotein determinations in assessing the risk of CAD.

Lipoprotein (a), or Lp(a), is being assessed for its role in CAD. Increased levels of Lp(a), especially with increased levels of LDH, are strongly associated with the progression of atherosclerosis. In addition, Lp(a) is found to have thrombogenic properties that increase the risk of clot formation at the site of intravascular lesions.[17]

Invasive Studies

Invasive studies are performed if definitive information is required. These include cardiac catheterization, coronary angiography, electrophysiology, and intracoronary ultrasound.

Cardiac Catheterization and Coronary Angiography. Cardiac catheterization is a common outpatient procedure. It provides a means of obtaining information about CAD, congenital heart disease, valvular heart disease, and ventricular function. Cardiac catheterization can be used to measure intracardiac pressures and O_2 levels in various parts of the heart, as well as CO. With injection of contrast media and fluoroscopy, the coronary arteries can be visualized, chambers of the heart can be outlined, and wall motion can be observed.

Cardiac catheterization is performed by insertion of a radiopaque catheter into the right or left side of the heart. For the right side of the heart, a catheter is inserted through an arm vein (basilic or cephalic) or a leg vein (femoral). The catheter is advanced into the vena cava, the right atrium, and the right ventricle. The catheter is further inserted into the pulmonary artery, and pressures are recorded. The catheter is then advanced until it is wedged or lodged in position. This position is called the *pulmonary artery wedge position.* The pulmonary artery wedge position (wedge pressure) obstructs the flow and pressure from the right side of the heart and looks forward through the pulmonary capillary bed to the pressure in the left side of the heart. The wedge pressure is used to determine the function of the left side of the heart.

The left heart catheterization is performed by insertion of a catheter into a femoral or brachial artery. The catheter is passed in a retrograde manner up the aorta, across the aortic valve, and into the left ventricle. Coronary angiography can be done with a left heart catherization.

Patients frequently feel a temporary hot and flushed sensation with contrast media injection. (See Table 31-7 for the nursing responsibilities related to cardiac catheterization.)

Complications of cardiac catheterization include looping, kinking, or breaking off of the catheter; blood loss; allergic reaction to the contrast media; infection; thrombus formation; air or blood embolism; arrhythmias; MI; stroke; puncture of the ventricles, cardiac septum, or lung tissue; and, rarely, death.

Electrophysiology Study. Electrophysiology study (EPS) is the direct study and manipulation of the electrical activity of the heart using electrodes placed inside the cardiac chambers. It provides information on SA node function, AV node conduction, and ventricular conduction. It is particularly helpful in diagnosing the source of arrhythmias. Patients with a history of symptomatic supraventricular or ventricular tachycardias may obtain an accurate diagnosis and treatment with this technique.[18]

Catheters are inserted in a similar method as for right and left heart catheterization. These catheters are placed at specific anatomic sites within the heart to record electrical activity. Nursing care for patients after EPS includes close ECG monitoring, puncture site assessment, vital signs, and other responsibilities related to care following a cardiac catheterization.

Intracoronary Ultrasound. Intracoronary ultrasound (ICUS), also known as intravascular ultrasound (IVUS), is an invasive procedure performed in the catheterization laboratory. The 2-D or 3-D ultrasound images provide a cross-sectional view of the arterial walls of the coronary arteries.

A miniature transducer attached to a small catheter is introduced through a peripheral artery and advanced to the artery to be studied. Once in the artery, ultrasound images are obtained. The health of the arterial layers is assessed, as is the composition, location, and thickness of plaque.

ICUS is currently used in conjunction with coronary angiography to diagnose severity of CAD. It may also evaluate the vessel response to treatments such as stent placement and atherectomy.

Because the patient will most often have ICUS in addition to angiography or an invasive treatment, nursing care of the patient following ICUS is similar to that following cardiac catheterization (see Table 31-7).

Blood Flow and Pressure Measurements

Peripheral vessel blood flow. Duplex imaging is useful in the diagnosis of occlusive disease in the peripheral blood vessels and for the diagnosis of thrombophlebitis. Peripheral vessel blood flow can be assessed by injection of contrast media into the appropriate arteries or veins (arteriography and venography). With these tests, arterial occlusions and venous abnormalities can be located. (Additional studies of peripheral blood vessels are discussed in Chapter 37 and Table 37-8.)

Hemodynamic monitoring. Bedside hemodynamic monitoring of pressures of the cardiovascular system is frequently used to assess cardiovascular status. Invasive hemodynamic monitoring using intraarterial and pulmonary artery catheters can be used to monitor arterial BP, intracardiac pressures, and CO (see Chapter 64). The central venous pressure (CVP) is a measurement of preload and can be used to monitor the pressure in the right atrium and right ventricle. The CVP reading is influenced by the function of the left side of the heart, pressures in the pulmonary vessels, venous return to the heart, and the position of the patient when the reading is taken. The last factor must be kept in mind to obtain an accurate reading. The CVP can be used as a guide in fluid volume management of overhydration or dehydration.

CVP can be measured with a pulmonary artery catheter (see Chapter 64) or a central venous line threaded through the jugular or subclavian vein into the superior vena cava. Two different methods to take CVP measurements include a mercury (mm Hg) system or a water (cm H_2O) manometer system. The end of the catheter is connected to a three-way stopcock, a fluid system, and a water manometer or to a pressure transducer. The normal CVP is 2 to 9 mm Hg (3 to 12 cm H_2O).

For an accurate reading, the base of the manometer should be at the level of the right atrium (the phlebostatic axis).

REVIEW QUESTIONS

The number of the question corresponds to the same-numbered objective at the beginning of the chapter.

1. A patient with a tricuspid valve disorder will have impaired blood flow between the
   a. vena cava and right atrium.
   b. left atrium and left ventricle.
   c. right atrium and right ventricle.
   d. right ventricle and pulmonary artery.

2. A patient with an MI of the anterior wall of the left ventricle most likely has an occlusion of the
   a. right marginal artery.
   b. left circumflex artery.
   c. left anterior descending artery.
   d. right anterior descending artery.

3. If the Purkinje system is damaged, conduction of the electrical impulse is impaired through the
   a. atria.
   b. AV node.
   c. ventricles.
   d. bundle of His.

4. Prolonged pressure on the skin causes reddened areas at the point of contact due to
   a. arterial vasodilation from smooth muscle relaxation.
   b. compression of veins resulting in venous engorgement.
   c. occlusion of major arteries causing infarction of the tissue.
   d. tissue damage and inflammation resulting from impaired capillary blood flow.

5. When a person's blood pressure rises, the homeostatic mechanism to compensate for an elevation involves stimulation of
   a. chemoreceptors that inhibit the sympathetic nervous system, causing vasodilation.
   b. baroreceptors that inhibit the parasympathetic nervous system, causing vasodilation.
   c. baroreceptors that inhibit the sympathetic nervous system, causing a decreased heart rate.
   d. chemoreceptors that stimulate the sympathetic nervous system, causing an increased heart rate.

6. When checking the capillary filling time of a patient, the color returns in 10 seconds. The nurse recognizes this finding as indicative of
   a. a normal response.
   b. thrombus formation in the veins.
   c. lymphatic obstruction of venous return.
   d. impaired arterial flow to the extremities.

7. The auscultatory area in the left midclavicular line at the level of the fifth ICS is the
   a. aortic area.
   b. mitral area.
   c. tricuspid area.
   d. pulmonic area.

8. When assessing the patient, the nurse notes a palpable precordial thrill. This finding may be caused by
   a. heart murmurs.
   b. gallop rhythms.
   c. pulmonary edema.
   d. right ventricular hypertrophy.

Continued

REVIEW QUESTIONS—cont'd

9. When assessing the cardiovascular system of a 79-year-old patient, the nurse expects to find
   a. a narrowed pulse pressure.
   b. diminished carotid artery pulses.
   c. difficulty in isolating the apical pulse.
   d. an increased heart rate in response to stress.

10. An important nursing responsibility for a patient having an invasive cardiovascular diagnostic study is
    a. checking the peripheral pulses and percutaneous site.
    b. instructing the patient about radioactive isotope injection.
    c. informing the patient that general anesthesia will be given.
    d. assisting the patient to do a surgical scrub of the insertion site.

11. A P wave on an ECG represents an impulse
    a. arising at the SA node and repolarizing the atria.
    b. arising at the SA node and depolarizing the atria.
    c. arising at the AV node and depolarizing the atria.
    d. arising at the AV node and spreading to the bundle of His.

REFERENCES

1. Berne RM, Levy MN: *Cardiovascular physiology,* ed 8, St Louis, 2000, Mosby.
2. Woods SL et al: *Cardiac nursing,* ed 4, Philadelphia, 1999, Lippincott.
3. Kinney MR, Packa DR: *Andreoli's comprehensive cardiac care,* ed 9, St Louis, 2000, Mosby.
4. Frolkis VV, Bezrukov VV, Kulchitshy OK: *The aging cardiovascular system: physiology and pathology,* New York, 1996, Springer.
5. Matteson MA: *Gerontological nursing: concepts and practice,* ed 2, Philadelphia, 1997, WB Saunders.
6. Delonas LR: Beyond type A: hostility and coronary artery disease—implication for research, *Rehabil Nurs* 21:4, 1996.
7. Gottdiener JS: Overview of stress echocardiography: uses, advantages, and limitations, *Prog Cardiovasc Dis* 43:315, 2001.
8. Arbeille P et al: Real-time 3-D ultrasound acquisition and display for cardiac volume and ejection fraction evaluation, *Ultrasound Med Biol* 26:273, 2000.
9. Binder T et al: NC100100, a new echo contrast agent for the assessment of myocardial perfusion: safety and comparison with technetium-99m sestamibi single photon emission computer tomography in a randomized multicenter study, *Clin Cardiol* 22:273, 1999.
10. Shaw LJ et al: Clinical and economic outcomes assessment in nuclear cardiology, *Q J Nucl Med* 4:138, 2000.
11. Beller GA, Zaret BL: Contributions of nuclear cardiology to diagnosis and prognosis of patients with coronary artery disease, *Circulation* 101:1465, 2000.
12. Botnar RM et al: Coronary magnetic resonance angiography, *Cardiol Rev* 9:77, 2001.
13. Higgins CB: Cardiac imaging, *Radiology* 217:4, 2000.
14. Jaffe AS: The World Health Organization. The European Society of Cardiology. The American College of Cardiology: New standard for the diagnosis of acute myocardial infarction, *Car Rev* 9:318, 2001.
15. Braunwald E et al: ACC/AHA guidelines for the management of patients with unstable angina and non-ST-segment elevation myocardial infarction. A report of the American College of Cardiology/American Heart Association Task Force on Practice Guidelines (Committee on the Management of Patients with Unstable Angina), *J Am Coll Cardiol* 36:970, 2000.
16. Assmann G, Schulte H, von Eckardstein A: Hypertriglyceridemia and elevated lipoprotein (a) are risk factors for major coronary events in middle-aged men, *Am J Cardiol* 77:1179, 1996.
17. Busby-Whitehead MJ, Blackman MC: Clinical implications of abnormal lipoprotein metabolism. In Barker LR et al, editors: *Principles of ambulatory medicine,* ed 5, Baltimore, 1999, Williams & Wilkins.
18. Josephson ME: *Clinical cardiac electrophysiology: techniques and interpretations,* Philadelphia, 2001, Lippincott.

RESOURCES

Resources for this chapter are listed in Chapter 33 on p. 837.

CHAPTER **32**

NURSING MANAGEMENT
Hypertension

New hypertension guidelines based on *The Seventh Report of the Joint National Committee on Prevention, Detection, Evaluation, and Treatment of High Blood Pressure (JNC-7)* are available on the Evolve site at http://evolve.elsevier.com/Lewis/medsurg/

Barbara S. Levine

LEARNING OBJECTIVES

1. Describe the mechanisms involved in the regulation of blood pressure.
2. Identify the pathophysiologic mechanisms associated with primary hypertension.
3. Describe the clinical manifestations and complications of hypertension.
4. Describe strategies for the prevention of primary hypertension.
5. Describe the collaborative care for hypertension, including drug and nutritional therapy.
6. Discuss the collaborative care of the older adult patient with hypertension.
7. Describe the nursing management of the patient with hypertension, emphasizing patient teaching.
8. Describe the clinical manifestations and collaborative care of hypertensive crisis.

KEY TERMS

baroreceptors, p. 778
blood pressure, p. 777
cardiac output, p. 777
hypertension, p. 779
hypertensive crisis, p. 796
isolated systolic hypertension, p. 795

orthostatic hypotension, p. 793
primary (essential) hypertension, p. 780
secondary hypertension, p. 780
systemic vascular resistance, p. 777

NORMAL REGULATION OF BLOOD PRESSURE

Blood pressure (BP) is the force exerted by the blood against the walls of the blood vessel and must be adequate to maintain tissue perfusion during activity and rest. The maintenance of normal BP and tissue perfusion requires the integration of both systemic factors and local peripheral vascular effects. Arterial BP is primarily a function of cardiac output and systemic vascular resistance. The relationship is summarized by the following equation:

$$\text{Arterial blood pressure} = \text{Cardiac output} \times \text{Systemic vascular resistance}$$

Cardiac output (CO) is the total blood flow through the systemic or pulmonary circulation per minute. CO can be described as the stroke volume (amount of blood pumped out of the left ventricle per beat [approximately 70 ml]) multiplied by the heart rate (HR) for 1 minute. **Systemic vascular resistance** (SVR) is the force opposing the movement of blood within the blood vessels. Radius of the small arteries and arterioles is the principal factor determining vascular resistance. A small change in the radius of the arterioles creates a major change in the SVR. If SVR is increased and CO remains constant or increases, arterial BP will increase.

The mechanisms that regulate BP can affect either CO or SVR, or both. Regulation of BP is a complex process involving

nervous, cardiovascular, renal, and endocrine functions (Fig. 32-1). BP is regulated by both short-term (seconds to hours) and long-term (days to weeks) mechanisms. Short-term mechanisms, including the sympathetic nervous system and vascular endothelium, are active within a few seconds. Long-term mechanisms include renal and hormonal processes that regulate arteriolar resistance and blood volume.

Sympathetic Nervous System

The nervous system, which reacts within seconds after a decrease in arterial pressure, increases BP primarily by activation of the sympathetic nervous system (SNS). Increased SNS activity increases HR and cardiac contractility, produces widespread vasoconstriction in the peripheral arterioles, and promotes the release of renin from the kidneys. The net effect of SNS activation is to increase arterial pressure by increasing both CO and SVR.

Changes in BP are sensed by specialized nerve cells called *baroreceptors* and transmitted to the vasomotor centers in the brainstem. Information received in the brainstem is relayed throughout the brain by complex networks of interneurons exciting or inhibiting efferent nerves, thereby influencing cardiovascular function. Sympathetic efferent nerves innervate cardiac and vascular smooth muscle cells. Under normal conditions, a low level of continuous sympathetic activity maintains tonic vasoconstriction. BP may be reduced by withdrawal of SNS activity or by stimulation of the parasympathetic nervous system, which decreases the HR (via the vagus nerve) and thereby decreases CO.

The neurotransmitter norepinephrine (NE) is released from sympathetic nerve endings. NE activates receptors located in the sinoatrial node, myocardium, and vascular smooth muscle. The response to NE depends on the type and density of receptors present. Sympathetic nervous system receptors are classified as α_1, α_2, β_1, and β_2 (Table 32-1). α-Adrenergic receptors located in peripheral vasculature cause vasoconstriction when stimulated by NE. β_1-Adrenergic receptors in the heart respond to NE with increased HR (*chronotropic*), increased force of contraction (*inotropic*), and increased speed of conduction. Diminished responsiveness of cardiovascular cells to sympathetic stimulation is one

Reviewed by Martha S. Tingen, RN, PhD, ANP, CS, Associate Professor, School of Nursing, Medical College of Georgia, Augusta, Ga.

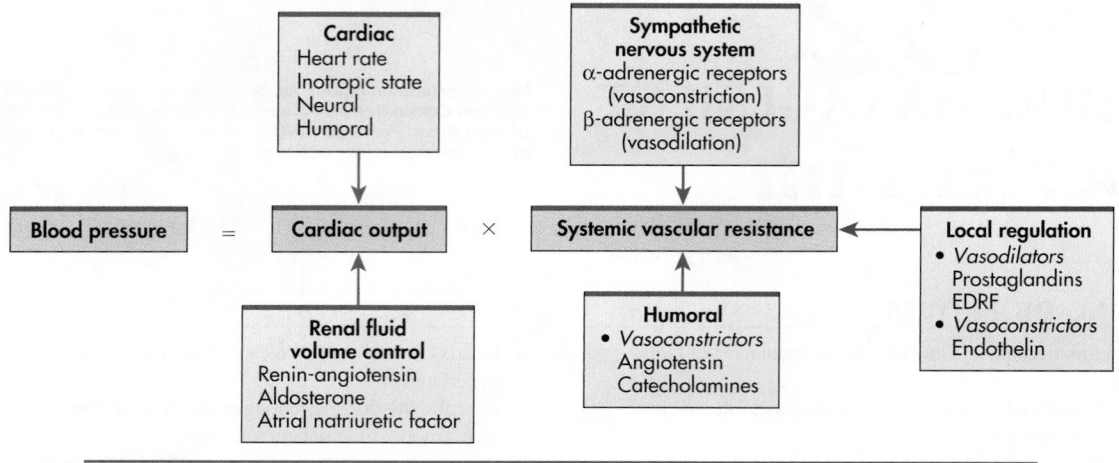

FIG. 32-1 Factors influencing blood pressure. *EDRF,* Endothelium-derived relaxing factor.

of the most significant cardiovascular effects of aging. The smooth muscle of the blood vessels has α_1-adrenergic and β_2-adrenergic receptors. β_2-Adrenergic receptors are activated primarily by epinephrine released from the adrenal medulla and cause vasodilation.

The sympathetic vasomotor center, located in the medulla, interacts with many areas of the brain to maintain normal BP under various conditions. During exercise the motor area of the cortex is stimulated, activating the vasomotor center and the SNS through neuronal connections. This causes an appropriate increase in BP to accommodate the increased oxygen demand of the exercising muscles. During postural change from lying to standing, there is a transient decrease in BP. The vasomotor center is stimulated and activates the SNS, causing peripheral vasoconstriction and increased venous return to the heart. If this response did not occur, there would be inadequate blood flow to the brain, resulting in dizziness. Cerebral cortical perceptions such as pain and stress activate the vasomotor centers through the neuronal connections.

Baroreceptors. Baroreceptors (pressoreceptors) are specialized nerve cells located in the carotid arteries and arch of the aorta. They are sensitive to stretching and, when stimulated by an increase in BP, send inhibitory impulses to the sympathetic vaso-

motor center in the brainstem. Inhibition of sympathetic activity results in decreased heart rate, decreased force of contraction, and vasodilation in peripheral arterioles. Increased parasympathetic activity (vagus nerve) reduces HR.

A fall in BP, sensed by the baroreceptors, leads to activation of the SNS. The result is constriction of the peripheral arterioles, increased HR, and increased contractility of the heart. The baroreceptors have an important role in the maintenance of BP stability during normal activities. In the presence of long-standing hypertension, the baroreceptors become adjusted to elevated levels of BP and recognize this level as "normal." The baroreceptor reflex is less responsive in some older adults.

Vascular Endothelium

The vascular endothelium is a single cell layer that lines the blood vessels. Previously considered inert, it has the ability to produce vasoactive substances and growth factors. Nitric oxide, an endothelium-derived relaxing factor (EDRF), helps maintain low arterial tone at rest, inhibits growth of the smooth muscle layer, and inhibits platelet aggregation. Other substances released by the vascular endothelium with local vasodilator effects include prostacyclin and endothelium-derived hyperpolarizing factor.

TABLE 32-1	**Sympathetic Nervous System Receptors Influencing Blood Pressure**	
RECEPTOR	**LOCATION**	**RESPONSE WHEN ACTIVATED**
α_1	Vascular smooth muscle	Vasoconstriction
	Heart	Increased contractility
α_2	Presynaptic membrane	Inhibition of norepinephrine release
	Vascular smooth muscle	Vasoconstriction
β_1	Heart	Increased contractility (positive inotropic effect)
		Increased heart rate (positive chronotropic effect)
		Increased conduction (positive dromotropic effect)
	Juxtaglomerular cells	Increased renin secretion
β_2	Smooth muscle of peripheral blood vessels in skeletal muscle and coronary arteries	Vasodilation
Dopaminergic receptors	Primarily renal and mesenteric blood vessels	Vasodilation

Endothelin (ET), produced by the endothelial cells, is an extremely potent vasoconstrictor. There are three subclasses of endothelins (ET-1, ET-2, and ET-3). ET-1 is the most potent endothelin in producing vasoconstriction. ET-1 also causes adhesion and aggregation of neutrophils and stimulates smooth muscle growth. Endothelial function and dysfunction is an area of ongoing investigation. There is some evidence that vascular endothelial dysfunction may contribute to atherosclerosis and primary hypertension. The prevention or reversal of endothelial dysfunction may become important for therapeutic interventions in the future.

Renal System

The kidneys contribute to BP regulation by controlling sodium excretion and extracellular fluid (ECF) volume (see Chapter 43). Sodium retention results in water retention, which causes an increased ECF volume. This increases the venous return to the heart, increasing the stroke volume, which elevates the BP through an increase in CO.

The renin-angiotensin-aldosterone system also plays an important role in BP regulation. In response to sympathetic stimulation, decreased blood flow through the kidneys, or decreased serum sodium concentration, renin is secreted from the juxtaglomerular apparatus in the kidney. Renin is an enzyme that converts angiotensinogen to angiotensin I. Angiotensin-converting enzyme (ACE) converts angiotensin I into angiotensin II (A-II), which can increase BP by two different mechanisms (see Chapter 43, Fig. 43-4). First, A-II is a potent vasoconstrictor and increases vascular resistance, resulting in an immediate increase in BP. Second, over a period of hours or days, A-II increases BP indirectly by stimulating the adrenal cortex to secrete aldosterone, which causes sodium and water retention by the kidneys resulting in increased blood volume and increased CO (Fig. 32-2).

Angiotensin II also functions at a local level within the heart and blood vessels. The local vasoactive effects of A-II (vasoconstriction and growth promotion) may contribute to atherosclerosis and primary hypertension.

Prostaglandins (PGE_2 and PGI_2) secreted by the renal medulla have a vasodilator effect on the systemic circulation. This results in decreased systemic vascular resistance and lowering of BP. (Prostaglandins are discussed in Chapter 12.)

Endocrine System

Stimulation of the SNS results in release of epinephrine along with a small fraction of norepinephrine by the adrenal medulla. Epinephrine increases CO by increasing HR and myocardial contractility. Epinephrine activates β_2-adrenergic receptors in peripheral arterioles of skeletal muscle, causing vasodilation. In peripheral arterioles with only α_1-adrenergic receptors (skin and kidneys), epinephrine causes vasoconstriction.

The adrenal cortex is stimulated by A-II to release aldosterone. (Release of aldosterone is also regulated by other factors, such as low sodium levels [see Chapters 46 and 48].) Aldosterone stimulates the kidneys to retain sodium and therefore water. This increases BP by increasing CO (see Fig. 32-2).

An increased blood sodium osmolarity level stimulates the release of antidiuretic hormone (ADH) from the posterior pituitary gland. ADH increases the ECF volume by promoting the reabsorption of water in the distal and collecting tubules of the kidneys. The resulting increase in blood volume can cause an elevation in BP.

In the healthy person, these regulatory mechanisms function in response to the demands of the body. When hypertension develops, one or more of the BP-regulating mechanisms are defective.

HYPERTENSION

Hypertension is sustained elevation of BP. In adults, hypertension exists when systolic blood pressure (SBP) is equal to or greater than 140 mm Hg or diastolic blood pressure (DBP) is equal to or greater than 90 mm Hg for extended periods of time[1] (Table 32-2). The diagnosis of hypertension requires that elevated readings be present on at least three occasions during several weeks.

TABLE 32-2	Classification of Blood Pressure for Adults Age 18 Years and Older*		
	BLOOD PRESSURE, MM HG		
CATEGORY	**SYSTOLIC**		**DIASTOLIC**
Optimal[†]	<120	and	<80
Normal	<130	and	<85
High normal	130-139	or	85-89
Hypertension[‡]			
Stage 1	140-159	or	90-99
Stage 2	160-179	or	100-109
Stage 3	≥180	or	≥110

From US Department of Health and Human Services: *The sixth report of the Joint National Committee on Detection, Evaluation, and Treatment of High Blood Pressure (JNC-VI)*, Washington, DC, 1997, National Institutes of Health.
*Not taking antihypertensive drugs and not acutely ill.
†Optimal blood pressure with respect to cardiovascular risk is less than 120/80 mm Hg. However, unusually low readings should be evaluated for clinical significance.
‡Based on the average of two or more readings taken at each of two or more visits after an initial screening. When systolic and diastolic blood pressures fall into different categories, the higher category should be selected to classify the individual's blood pressure status. For example, 160/92 should be classified as stage 2 hypertension, and 174/120 should be classified as stage 3 hypertension. Isolated systolic hypertension is defined as systolic blood pressure 140 mm Hg or greater and diastolic blood pressure less than 90 mm Hg and staged appropriately (e.g., 170/82 mm Hg is defined as stage 2 isolated systolic hypertension).
NOTE: In addition to classifying stages of hypertension based on average blood pressure levels, the clinician should specify presence or absence of target organ disease and additional risk factors. This specificity is important for risk classification and treatment.

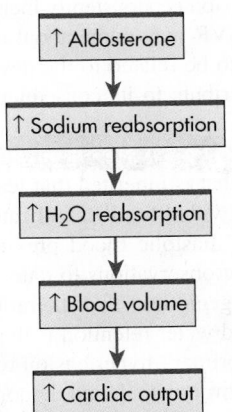

FIG. 32-2 Mechanism of action of aldosterone.

CULTURAL & ETHNIC CONSIDERATIONS
Hypertension

- African Americans, Puerto Ricans, Cubans, and Mexican Americans have a higher incidence of hypertension than whites.
- African Americans have the highest incidence of hypertension.
- African Americans develop hypertension at a younger age than whites.
- African American women have a particularly high incidence of hypertension.
- Hypertension is more aggressive in African Americans and results in more severe end-organ damage.
- African Americans have a higher mortality rate related to hypertension than whites.
- African Americans and whites living in the southeastern United States have a higher incidence of hypertension than similar ethnic groups living in other parts of the United States.
- African Americans produce less renin and do not respond as well to angiotensin inhibitors.

High BP means that the heart is working harder than normal, putting both the heart and the blood vessels under strain. High BP may contribute to myocardial infarction, stroke, renal failure, and atherosclerosis.

Hypertension is a worldwide epidemic with an estimated 690 million people having high BP. The prevalence of high BP among citizens of the United States and Canada is 20.4% and 22%, respectively. In the United States, 50 million people (one out of four adults) either have elevated BP (SBP of 140 mm Hg or greater or DBP of 90 mm Hg or greater) or are taking antihypertensive medication.[2] Only half of them have their BP under control. Many people with hypertension do not know they have it because it causes no symptoms.

The prevalence of hypertension increases with age and is higher in African Americans than in whites. In comparison to whites, African Americans develop high BP at an earlier age, and it is more severe at any decade. As a result, African Americans have a higher prevalence of stroke, heart disease, and end-stage renal disease when compared with whites. In addition, African Americans have a higher mortality rate at every level of BP elevation compared with whites. In both races, the prevalence is higher in less educated than in more educated people. Hypertension is more prevalent in men than in women until age 55; after age 55 it is more prevalent in women than men.[2]

The status of hypertension control has improved considerably over the past 20 years. Large-scale education programs provided by various organizations have increased awareness of hypertension. The percentage of patients with hypertension on medication who have their BP controlled has also improved substantially.

Classification of Hypertension

Table 32-2 describes the BP classification used in the United States for people 18 years of age and older. The Joint National Commission classifies hypertension according to stages (1 through 3) with the addition of a "high normal" category.[1] These experts consider the person with BP in the high normal category to be at higher risk for the development of definite hypertension and recommend more frequent monitoring than the person with lower BP. The risk of progression from high normal to definite hypertension is controversial.[1] The etiology of hypertension can be classified as either primary or secondary.

Primary Hypertension. Primary (essential) hypertension is elevated BP without an identified cause and accounts for 90% to 95% of all cases of hypertension.[3] Although the exact cause of primary hypertension is unknown, several contributing factors, including increased SNS activity, overproduction of sodium-retaining hormones and vasoconstrictors, increased sodium intake, greater than ideal body weight, diabetes mellitus, and excessive alcohol intake, have been identified. Primary hypertension is the focus of this chapter because of its prevalence in clinical practice.

Secondary Hypertension. Secondary hypertension is elevated BP with a specific cause that often can be identified and corrected. This type of hypertension accounts for 5% to 10% of hypertension in adults and more than 80% of hypertension in children. If a person below age 20 or over age 50 suddenly develops hypertension, especially if it is severe, a secondary cause should be suspected. Clinical findings that suggest secondary hypertension include unprovoked hypokalemia, abdominal bruit, variable pressures with history of tachycardia, sweating and tremor, or a family history of renal disease.

Causes of secondary hypertension include the following: (1) coarctation or congenital narrowing of the aorta; (2) renal disease such as renal artery stenosis and parenchymal disease (see Chapter 44); (3) endocrine disorders such as pheochromocytoma, Cushing syndrome, and hyperaldosteronism (see Chapter 48); (4) neurologic disorders such as brain tumors, quadriplegia, and head injury; (5) sleep apnea; (6) medications such as sympathetic stimulants (including cocaine), monoamine oxidase inhibitors taken with tyramine-containing foods, estrogen replacement therapy, oral contraceptive pills, and nonsteroidal antiinflammatory drugs (NSAIDs); and (7) pregnancy-induced hypertension. Treatment of secondary hypertension is directed at eliminating the underlying cause. Secondary hypertension is a contributing factor to hypertensive crisis (see section at end of this chapter).

Pathophysiology of Primary Hypertension

For arterial pressure to rise, there must be an increase in either CO or SVR. Increased CO is sometimes found in the early and borderline hypertensive person. Later in the course of hypertension, SVR rises and the CO returns to normal. The hemodynamic hallmark of hypertension is persistently increased SVR. This persistent elevation in SVR may come about in various ways. Factors that are known to be related to the development of primary hypertension or contribute to its consequences are presented in Table 32-3.

Heredity. The level of BP is strongly familial, although it is not known exactly what is inherited that leads to high BP. Studies of BP correlation within families indicate that the heritability of both systolic and diastolic blood pressure is approximately 20% to 40%. Genetic observations to date suggest that primary hypertension is polygenic and that alteration in renal function with resultant salt and water retention is the final common pathway. In most cases, primary hypertension results from the interaction of genetic, environmental, and demographic factors.[3]

Water and Sodium Retention. Excessive sodium intake is considered responsible for initiation of hypertension in some

TABLE 32-3	Risk Factors for Primary Hypertension
• Age	BP rises progressively with increasing age. Elevated BP is present in approximately 50% of people over 60 years of age.
• Alcohol	Excessive alcohol intake is strongly associated with hypertension. Patients with hypertension should limit their daily intake to 1 oz of alcohol.
• Cigarette smoking	Smoking greatly increases the risk of cardiovascular disease. People with hypertension who smoke are at even greater risk for cardiovascular disease.
• Diabetes mellitus	Hypertension is more common in diabetics. When hypertension and diabetes coexist, complications are more severe.
• Elevated serum lipids	Elevated levels of cholesterol and triglycerides are primary risk factors in atherosclerosis. Hyperlipidemia is more common in people with hypertension.
• Excess dietary sodium	High sodium intake can contribute to hypertension in some patients and can decrease the efficacy of certain antihypertensive medications.
• Gender	Hypertension is more prevalent in men in young adulthood and early middle age. After age 55, hypertension is more prevalent in women.
• Family history	Level of BP is strongly familial. Risk of hypertension increases for those with a close relative having hypertension.
• Obesity	Weight gain is associated with increased frequency of hypertension. The risk is greatest with central abdominal obesity.
• Ethnicity	Incidence of hypertension is twice as high in African Americans as in whites.
• Sedentary lifestyle	Regular physical activity can help control weight and reduce cardiovascular risk. Physical activity may decrease BP.
• Socioeconomic status	Hypertension is more prevalent in lower socioeconomic groups and among the less educated.
• Stress	People exposed to repeated stress may develop hypertension more frequently than others. People who become hypertensive may respond differently to stress than those who do not become hypertensive.

BP, Blood pressure.

people. Studies of populations with a low sodium intake (usually primitive hunter-gatherer societies) show little or no hypertension and no progressive increase in BP with age as is found in industrialized societies. In addition, when people from these societies adopt industrialized lifestyles, the prevalence of hypertension increases. When sodium is restricted in many hypertensive people, their BP falls. A high sodium intake may activate a number of pressor mechanisms and cause water retention. Although almost everyone in Western countries consumes a high-sodium diet, only about 20% develop hypertension. This indicates that some degree of sodium sensitivity must be present for high sodium intake to trigger the development of hypertension.

Altered Renin-Angiotensin Mechanism. High plasma renin activity (PRA) results in the increased conversion of angiotensinogen to angiotensin I (see Chapter 43, Fig. 43-4). Angiotensin II causes direct arteriolar constriction, promotes vascular hypertrophy, and induces aldosterone secretion. Thus altered renin-angiotensin mechanisms may contribute to the development and maintenance of hypertension. However, only about 20% of patients with primary hypertension have high PRA.[4]

Stress and Increased Sympathetic Nervous System Activity. It has long been recognized that arterial pressure is influenced by factors such as anger, fear, and pain. Physiologic responses to stress, which are normally protective, may persist to a pathologic degree, resulting in prolonged increase in SNS activity. Increased sympathetic stimulation produces increased vasoconstriction, increased HR, and increased renin release. Increased renin activates the angiotensin mechanism and increases aldosterone secretion, both leading to elevated BP. People exposed to high levels of repeated psychologic stress develop hypertension to a greater extent than those who do not experience as much stress.

Insulin Resistance and Hyperinsulinemia. Abnormalities of glucose, insulin, and lipoprotein metabolism are common in primary hypertension. They are not present in secondary hypertension and do not improve when hypertension is treated. Therefore insulin resistance is a risk factor for the development of hypertension and cardiovascular disease. High insulin concentration in the blood stimulates SNS activity and impairs nitric oxide–mediated vasodilation. Additional pressor effects of insulin include vascular hypertrophy and increased renal sodium reabsorption.

Endothelial Cell Dysfunction. Vascular endothelial cells are known to be the source of multiple vasoactive substances. Some hypertensive people have a reduced vasodilator response to nitric oxide. Endothelin produces pronounced and prolonged vasoconstriction. The role of endothelial dysfunction in the pathogenesis and treatment of hypertension is an area of ongoing investigation.

Clinical Manifestations

Hypertension is often called the "silent killer" because it is frequently asymptomatic until it becomes severe and target organ disease has occurred. A patient with severe hypertension may experience a variety of symptoms secondary to effects on blood vessels in the various organs and tissues or to the increased workload of the heart. These secondary symptoms include fatigue, reduced activity tolerance, dizziness, palpitations, angina, and dyspnea. In the past, symptoms of hypertension were thought to include headache, nosebleeds, and dizziness. However, unless BP is very high or low these symptoms are not more frequent in people with hypertension than in the general population.[5]

Complications

The most common complications of hypertension are *target organ diseases* (Table 32-4) occurring in the heart (hypertensive heart disease), brain (cerebrovascular disease), peripheral vasculature (peripheral vascular disease), kidney (nephrosclerosis), and eyes (retinal damage).

TABLE 32-4	Manifestations of Target Organ Disease
ORGAN	**MANIFESTATIONS**
Cardiac	Clinical, electrocardiographic, or radio-logic evidence of coronary artery disease
	Left ventricular hypertrophy or "strain" by electrocardiography or left ventricular hypertrophy by echocardiography
	Left ventricular dysfunction or cardiac failure
Cerebrovascular	Transient ischemic attack or stroke
Peripheral vascular	Absence of one or more major pulses in the extremities (except for dorsalis pedis) with or without intermittent claudication; aneurysm
Renal	Serum creatinine ≥1.5 mg/dl (130 μmol/L)
	Proteinuria (1+ or greater)
	Microalbuminuria
Retinopathy	Hemorrhages or exudates, with or without papilledema

From US Department of Health and Human Services: *The sixth report of the Joint National Committee on Detection, Evaluation, and Treatment of High Blood Pressure (JNC-VI)*, Washington, DC, 1997, National Institutes of Health.

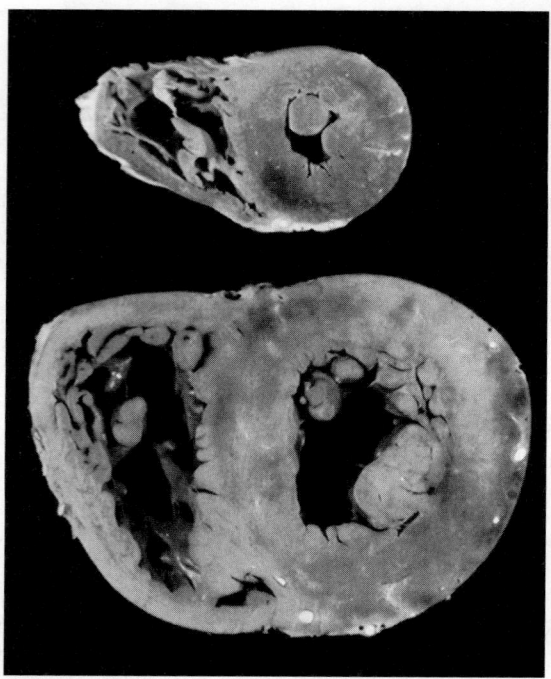

FIG. 32-3 Massively enlarged heart caused by hypertrophy of both ventricles. The normal heart weighs 325 g. The heart with biventricular hypertrophy weighs 1100 g. The patient had suffered from severe systemic hypertension.

Hypertensive Heart Disease

Coronary artery disease. Hypertension is a major risk factor for coronary artery disease. The mechanisms by which hypertension contributes to the development of atherosclerosis are not fully known. The "response-to-injury" hypothesis of atherogenesis suggests that hypertension disrupts the coronary artery endothelium, thus exposing the intimal layer to activated white blood cells and platelets. Growth factors released by the vascular endothelium and platelets may induce smooth muscle proliferation within the lesion. These arteriolar changes may account for a high incidence of coronary artery disease and the resulting problems of angina and myocardial infarction (MI).

Left ventricular hypertrophy. Sustained high BP increases the cardiac workload and produces left ventricular hypertrophy (LVH) (Fig. 32-3). Initially, LVH is an adaptive or compensatory mechanism that strengthens cardiac contraction and increases cardiac output. However, increased contractility increases myocardial work and oxygen consumption. When the heart can no longer meet the demands for myocardial oxygen, heart failure develops. Progressive LVH, especially in association with coronary artery disease, is associated with the development of heart failure.

Heart failure. Heart failure occurs when the heart's compensatory adaptations are overwhelmed and the heart can no longer pump enough blood to meet the metabolic needs of the body (see Chapter 34). Contractility is depressed, and stroke volume and cardiac output are decreased. The patient may complain of shortness of breath on exertion, paroxysmal nocturnal dyspnea, and fatigue. Signs of an enlarged heart may be present on x-ray, and an electrocardiogram (ECG) may show electrical changes indicative of LVH.

Cerebrovascular Disease. Atherosclerosis is the most common cause of cerebrovascular disease. Hypertension is a major risk factor for cerebral atherosclerosis and stroke. Even in mildly hypertensive people, the risk of stroke is four times higher than in normotensive people. Adequate control of BP effectively diminishes the risk of stroke.

Atherosclerotic plaques are commonly distributed at the bifurcation of the common carotid artery into the internal and external carotid arteries. Portions of the atherosclerotic plaque, or the blood clot that forms on the plaque, may break off and travel to intracerebral vessels, producing a thromboembolism. The patient may experience transient ischemic attacks or a stroke. (These conditions are discussed in Chapter 56.)

Hypertensive encephalopathy may occur after a marked rise in BP if the cerebral blood flow is not decreased by autoregulation. Autoregulation is a physiologic process that maintains constant cerebral blood flow despite fluctuations in arterial blood pressure. Normally as pressure in the cerebral blood vessels rises, the vessels constrict to maintain constant flow. When arterial blood pressure exceeds the body's ability to autoregulate, the cerebral vessels suddenly dilate and cerebral edema develops, producing a rise in intracranial pressure. If left untreated, patients die quickly from brain damage. (Cerebral blood flow and autoregulation are discussed in Chapter 55.)

Peripheral Vascular Disease. As it does with other vessels, hypertension speeds up the process of atherosclerosis in the peripheral blood vessels, leading to the development of aortic aneurysm, aortic dissection, and peripheral vascular disease (see Chapter 37). *Intermittent claudication* (ischemic muscle pain precipitated by activity and relieved with rest) is a classic symptom of peripheral vascular disease.

Nephrosclerosis. Hypertension is one of the leading causes of end-stage renal disease, especially among African Americans. Some degree of renal dysfunction is usually present in the hypertensive patient, even one with a minimally elevated BP. Renal dysfunction is the direct result of ischemia caused by the narrowed lumen of the intrarenal blood vessels. Gradual narrowing of the arteries and arterioles leads to atrophy of the tubules, destruction of the glomeruli, and eventual death of nephrons. Initially intact nephrons can compensate, but these changes may eventually lead to renal failure. Common laboratory indications of renal dysfunction are microalbuminuria, proteinuria, elevated blood urea nitrogen (BUN) and serum creatinine levels, and microscopic hematuria. The earliest manifestation of renal dysfunction is usually nocturia.

Retinal Damage. The appearance of the retina provides important information about the severity and duration of the hypertensive process. The retina is the only place in the body where the blood vessels can be directly visualized. Therefore damage to retinal vessels provides an indication of vessel damage in the heart, brain, and kidney. An ophthalmoscope is used to visualize the blood vessels of the eye. Manifestations of severe retinal damage include blurring of vision, retinal hemorrhage, and loss of vision.

Diagnostic Studies

The diagnosis of hypertension is not based on a single elevated reading (if lower than 180/110 mm Hg) but requires several elevated readings over several weeks. (Measurement of BP is discussed in Chapter 31 and on p. 760 and p. 794.)

There is some controversy as to how extensive a diagnostic workup should be performed in the initial evaluation of a person with hypertension.[5] Because most hypertension is classified as primary hypertension, testing for secondary causes is not routinely done. Basic laboratory studies are performed to evaluate target organ disease, determine overall cardiovascular risk, or establish baseline levels before initiating therapy.

Table 32-5 lists basic laboratory studies that are performed in a person with sustained hypertension. Routine urinalysis, BUN, and serum creatinine levels are used to screen for renal involvement and to provide baseline information about kidney function. *Creatinine clearance,* the rate at which creatinine is cleared from the circulation, reflects the glomerular filtration rate. Decreases in creatinine clearance indicate renal insufficiency. Creatinine clearance can be measured quantitatively in a timed urine collection. It can also be estimated from the serum creatinine level. (Serum creatinine and creatinine clearance are discussed in Chapters 43 and 45.)

Measurement of serum electrolytes, especially potassium levels, is important to detect hyperaldosteronism, a cause of secondary hypertension. Blood glucose levels should be assessed to assist in the diagnosis of diabetes mellitus. Serum cholesterol and triglyceride levels provide information about additional risk factors that predispose to atherosclerosis. Uric acid levels are determined to establish a baseline, because the levels often rise with diuretic therapy. An ECG provides baseline information about the cardiac status. It is helpful in identifying the presence of LVH and cardiac ischemia. Because of the prognostic importance of LVH, echocardiography is performed frequently. If the patient's age, history, physical examination findings, or severity of hypertension points to a secondary cause, further diagnostic tests may be indicated.

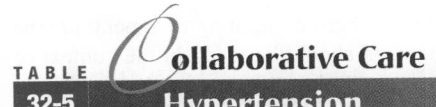

TABLE 32-5	Collaborative Care Hypertension

Diagnostic
History and physical examination
Routine urinalysis
Serum electrolytes and uric acid
BUN and serum creatinine
Blood glucose (fasting, if possible)
Complete blood count
Serum lipid profile, cholesterol, and triglycerides
Electrocardiogram (ECG)
Echocardiogram

Collaborative Therapy
Periodic monitoring of BP
• Every 3-6 months once BP is stabilized
Assignment of risk level (see Table 32-6)
Nutritional therapy (see Table 32-7)
• Restrict sodium
• Reduce weight (if indicated)
• Restrict cholesterol and saturated fats
• Maintain adequate intake of potassium
• Maintain adequate intake of calcium and magnesium
Physical activity
Cessation of smoking (see Chapter 11, Tables 11-13 and 11-14)
Modification of alcohol intake
Antihypertensive drugs (see Table 32-8)

BUN, Blood urea nitrogen.

Ambulatory Blood Pressure Monitoring. Some patients have elevated BP readings in a clinical setting and normal readings when BP is measured elsewhere. This phenomenon is referred to as "white coat" hypertension. When this type of hypertension is suspected, BP measurement at home or in the community may be helpful. Many fire stations and hospital auxiliaries provide BP measurement as a community service. Alternatively, a fully automated system that measures BP at preset intervals over a 24-hour period may be used. The equipment includes a BP cuff and a small microprocessing unit that fits into a pouch worn on a shoulder strap or belt. Patients are asked to maintain a diary of activities that may affect BP. This procedure may be helpful in patients with suspected white coat hypertension, apparent drug resistance, hypotensive symptoms with hypertensive medications, episodic hypertension, or autonomic nervous system dysfunction.

As with most physiologic phenomena, BP demonstrates diurnal variability expressed as sleep-wakefulness difference. For day-active people, BP is highest in the early morning, decreases during the day, and is lowest at night. Some patients with hypertension do not show a normal, nocturnal fall in BP. The absence of diurnal variability has been associated with more target organ damage. The presence or absence of diurnal variability can be determined by continuous ambulatory BP monitoring.

Collaborative Care

Clinical guidelines for the management of hypertension have been published.[1] Consensus among the guidelines exists in the following areas: (1) BP elevation should usually be assessed carefully over several months before initiating treatment; (2) the decision to treat hypertension should be made in the context of overall cardiovascular risk; (3) lifestyle modifications should provide the foundation for treatment; (4) primary and systolic hypertension should be treated in older adults up to 85 years; and (5) there are five categories of first-line drugs.

Risk Stratification. The risk of cardiovascular disease in people with hypertension is determined by the level of BP, the presence of target organ disease, and other risk factors. These factors independently modify the risk for cardiovascular disease. The Joint National Committee on Detection, Evaluation, and Treatment of High Blood Pressure (JNC-VI) guidelines (1997) for the management of hypertension assign patients to risk groups based on these factors.[1] Risk group A includes patients with high normal BP or stage 1, 2, or 3 hypertension who do not have clinical cardiovascular disease, target organ disease, or other risk factors. Risk group B includes patients with hypertension who do not have clinical cardiovascular disease or target organ disease, have one or more cardiovascular risk factors, but do not have diabetes. Risk group C includes patients with hypertension who have clinical cardiovascular disease, target organ damage, or diabetes.[1] The goal in treating a hypertensive patient is to reduce overall cardiovascular risk factors and to control BP by the least intrusive means possible. Treatment recommendations by risk group are summarized in Table 32-6.

Follow-up monitoring of the BP is very important. The frequency of monitoring varies initially with the level of BP. After the BP has stabilized, follow-up visits should be scheduled every 3 to 6 months to ensure continued control of BP, provide support for lifestyle changes, assess for target organ damage, and detect side or adverse effects of medications.

Lifestyle Modifications. Lifestyle modifications should be used in all hypertensive patients either as definitive or adjunctive therapy.[6] These modifications are directed toward reducing BP and overall cardiovascular risk factors. Modifications include (1) dietary changes, (2) limitation of alcohol intake, (3) regular physical activity, and (4) avoidance of tobacco use (smoking and chewing). Based on assigned risk group (see Table 32-6), lifestyle modifications are usually continued for up to 1 year before drug therapy is used (Fig. 32-4). Factors that may prompt a decision for early drug therapy include stage 2 or 3 hypertension, the presence of risk factors, target organ disease, clinical cardiovascular or cerebrovascular disease, and diabetes.

Nutritional therapy. Dietary management of hypertension consists of restriction of sodium; maintenance of dietary potassium, calcium, and magnesium intake; and calorie restriction if the patient is overweight. The American Heart Association recommends the DASH (Dietary Approaches to Stop Hypertension) diet. This diet involves eating several servings of fish each week, eating plenty of fruits and vegetables, increasing fiber intake, and drinking a lot of water[7] (see Table 32-7).

The average American adult's intake of salt totals 15 g per day. The American Heart Association and the JNC-VI recommend restricting salt intake to less than 6 g of salt (NaCl) or less than 2.3 g of sodium per day for healthy adults. This involves not adding salt in the preparation of foods or at meals and avoiding foods known to be high in sodium (see Chapter 34, Tables 34-9, 34-10, and 34-11).

The patient and family, especially the member who prepares the meals, should be taught about sodium-restricted diets. Instruction should include reading labels of over-the-counter drugs, packaged foods, and health products (e.g., baking soda–containing toothpaste) to identify hidden sources of sodium. It is helpful to review the patient's normal diet and to identify foods high in sodium. Analysis of a 3-day diet history will help identify foods high in sodium in the patient's usual diet.

Sodium restriction may be enough to control BP in some patients with stage 1 hypertension. If drug therapy is needed, a lower dose may be effective if the patient also restricts sodium intake. Furthermore, moderate sodium restriction lessens the risk of hypokalemia associated with diuretic therapy. However, people with hypertension respond differently to salt restriction. This heterogeneity of response has led to attempts to define subgroups of people with hypertension as "salt sensitive" or "salt resistant." Patients

---

TABLE 32-6   Risk Stratification and Treatment of Hypertension*

BLOOD PRESSURE STAGES (mm Hg)	RISK GROUP A (no risk factors; no TOD/CCD)	RISK GROUP B (at least one risk factor, not including diabetes; no TOD/CCD)	RISK GROUP C (TOD/CCD and/or diabetes with or without other risk factors)
High normal (130–135/85–89)	Lifestyle modifications	Lifestyle modifications	Drug therapy† Lifestyle modifications
Stage 1 (140–159/90–99)	Lifestyle modifications (up to 12 months)	Lifestyle modifications‡ (up to 6 months)	Drug therapy Lifestyle modifications
Stages 2 and 3 (≥160/≥100)	Drug therapy Lifestyle modifications	Drug therapy Lifestyle modifications	Drug therapy Lifestyle modifications

From US Department of Health and Human Services: *The sixth report of the Joint National Committee on Detection, Evaluation, and Treatment of High Blood Pressure (JNC-VI)*, Washington, DC, 1997, National Institutes of Health.
*For example, a patient with diabetes mellitus and BP of 142/94 mm Hg plus left ventricular hypertrophy (LVH) should be classified as having stage 1 hypertension with target organ disease (LVH) with another major risk factor (diabetes mellitus). This patient would be categorized as "stage 1, risk group C," and recommended for immediate initiation of drug therapy.
†For patients with multiple risk factors, health care providers should consider drugs as initial therapy plus lifestyle modifications.
‡For those with heart failure, renal insufficiency, or diabetes.
TOD/CCD, Target organ disease/clinical cardiovascular disease.

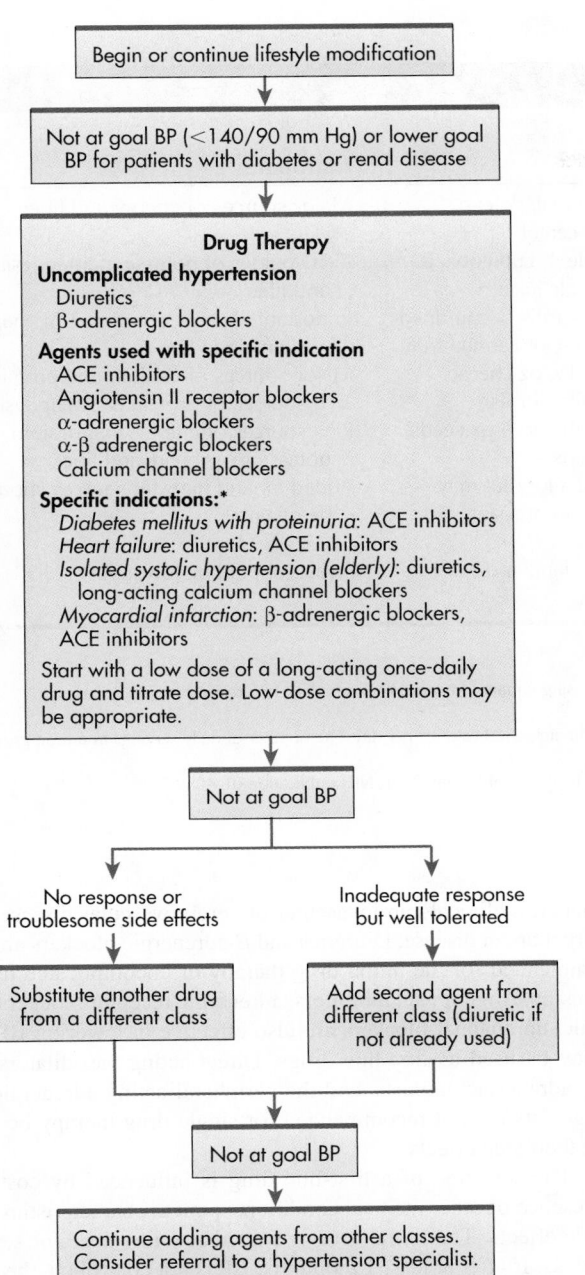

FIG. 32-4 Treatment algorithm for hypertension. *ACE,* Angiotensin-converting enzyme; *ISA,* intrinsic sympathetic activity.
*See reference 1 for further explanation.

with low renin activity, such as African Americans and older adults, are more likely to respond to salt restriction with a reduction in BP.

The significance of other dietary elements for the control of hypertension is not certain. There is evidence that greater levels of dietary potassium, calcium, and vitamin D are associated with lower BP in the general population and in those with hypertension. Based on available data, it is recommended that people with hypertension maintain adequate potassium and calcium intake from food sources. Although it is important to maintain an adequate intake of calcium for general health, calcium supplements are not recommended to lower BP. Caffeine may raise BP

acutely, but there is no long-term relationship between caffeine intake and elevated BP.

Overweight individuals have an increased incidence of hypertension and increased cardiovascular disease risk. Weight reduction has a significant effect on lowering BP in many people, and the effect is seen with even moderate weight loss. When a person decreases caloric intake, sodium and fat intake may also be reduced. Although reducing the fat content of the diet has not been shown to produce sustained benefits in BP control, it may slow the progress of atherosclerosis and reduce overall cardiovascular disease risk (see Chapter 33). Weight reduction through a combination of dietary calorie restriction and physical activity is recommended for overweight hypertensive patients.

Modification in alcohol consumption. Excessive alcohol consumption is strongly associated with hypertension. Consumption of three or more alcoholic drinks daily is a risk factor for heart disease and stroke. Hypertensive patients who drink alcohol should be advised to limit their alcohol intake to 1 oz per day (the amount of alcohol in 2 oz of 100-proof whiskey, 8 oz of wine, or 24 oz of beer). Because women absorb more ethanol than men and lighter-weight people are more susceptible to the effects of alcohol than heavier-weight people, women and lighter-weight men should further restrict alcohol to 0.5 oz per day. Excessive alcohol consumption is the most frequent cause of secondary hypertension in the United States.

Physical activity. To promote cardiovascular health, it is recommended that all adults have 30 minutes or more of moderate-intensity physical activity on most, or preferably all, days of the week. Moderately intense activity such as brisk walking, jogging, and swimming can lower BP, promote relaxation, and decrease or control body weight. Regular activity of this type can reduce SBP in the hypertensive patient by approximately 10 mm Hg. Sedentary people should be advised to increase activity levels gradually. People with heart disease or other serious health problems need a thorough examination, possibly including a stress test, before beginning an exercise program.

Avoidance of tobacco products. Nicotine contained in tobacco causes vasoconstriction and increases BP in hypertensive people. In addition, smoking tobacco is a major risk factor for cardiovascular disease. The cardiovascular benefits of discontinuing tobacco use can be seen within 1 year in all age groups. Everyone, especially a hypertensive patient, should be strongly advised to avoid tobacco use. The lower amounts of nicotine contained in smoking cessation aids usually will not raise BP and may be used as indicated. People who continue to use tobacco products should be advised to monitor their BP during use. (Tobacco use and smoking cessation are discussed in Chapter 11 and Tables 11-13 and 11-14.)

Stress management. Although stress can raise BP on a short-term basis and has been implicated in the development of hypertension, controversy exists as to the benefit of stress management in the prevention and treatment of hypertension.[1] Relaxation therapy, guided imagery, and biofeedback may be useful in helping patients manage stress, thus decreasing BP.

Drug Therapy. The general goals of drug therapy are to achieve BP less than 131/85 in young adults with mild hypertension. Treatment to lower levels, if tolerated, may be useful in people with diabetes, cardiovascular disease, and/or renal disease. In older adults with elevation of both systolic and diastolic BP, lowering BP to less than 140/90 mm Hg is desirable.

TABLE 32-7	Nutritional Therapy		
Hypertension			

Food Group	Daily Servings*	Serving Sizes	Rationale
Grains and grain products	8	1 slice bread, 1 oz dry cereal,[†] ½ cup cooked rice, pasta, or cereal	Major sources of energy and fiber
Vegetables	4.5	1 cup raw leafy vegetable, ½ cup cooked vegetable, 6 oz vegetable juice	Rich sources of potassium, magnesium, and fiber
Fruits	5	6 oz fruit juice, 1 medium fruit, ¼ cup dried fruit, ½ cup fresh, frozen, or canned fruit	Important sources of potassium, magnesium, and fiber
Low-fat or fat-free dairy foods	3	8 oz milk, 1 cup yogurt, 1½ oz cheese	Major sources of calcium and protein
Meat, poultry, and fish	2	3 oz cooked meats, poultry, or fish	Rich sources of protein and magnesium
Nuts, seeds, and dry beans	4-5/wk	⅓ cup or 1½ oz nuts, 2 tbs or ½ oz seeds, ½ cup cooked dry beans	Rich sources of energy, magnesium, potassium, protein, and fiber
Fats and oils[‡]	2-3	1 tsp soft margarine, 1 tbs low-fat mayonnaise, 2 tbs light salad dressing, 1 tsp vegetable oil	Added fat and high-fat sources should be minimal
Sweets	5/wk	1 tbs sugar, 1 tbs jelly or jam, ½ oz jelly beans, 8 oz lemonade	Sweets should be low in fat

*Except as noted.
[†]Equals ½-1¼ cup, depending on cereal type. Check the nutrition label on the product.
[‡]Fat content changes serving counts for fats and oils. For example, 1 tbs of regular salad dressing equals 1 serving; 1 tbs of a low-fat dressing equals ½ serving; 1 tbs of a fat-free dressing equals 0 servings.
DASH, Dietary Approaches to Stop Hypertension. The DASH eating plan is based on approximately 2100 calories per day. The number of daily servings in a food group may vary from those listed, depending on specific caloric needs.
Source: *The DASH diet.* National Heart, Lung, and Blood Institute. Washington, DC: National Institutes of Health, 2001; NIH publication 01-4082.

The drugs currently available for treating hypertension have two main actions: (1) they reduce SVR and (2) they decrease the volume of circulating blood (see Table 32-8). The drugs used in the treatment of hypertension include diuretics, adrenergic (sympathetic) inhibitors, direct vasodilators, angiotensin inhibitors, and calcium channel blockers. The various sites and methods of action are presented in Fig. 32-5.

Although the precise action of diuretics in the reduction of BP is unclear, it is known that they promote sodium and water excretion, reduce plasma volume, decrease sodium in the arteriolar walls, and reduce the vascular response to catecholamines. Adrenergic-inhibiting agents act by diminishing the sympathetic effects that increase BP. Adrenergic inhibitors include drugs that act centrally on the vasomotor center and peripherally to inhibit norepinephrine release or to block the adrenergic receptors on blood vessels. Direct vasodilators decrease the BP by relaxing vascular smooth muscle and reducing SVR. Calcium channel blockers increase sodium excretion and cause arteriolar vasodilation by preventing the movement of extracellular calcium into cells.

There are two types of angiotensin inhibitors. The first type is angiotensin-converting enzyme (ACE) inhibitors, which prevent the conversion of angiotensin I to angiotensin II and thus reduce angiotensin II (A-II)–mediated vasoconstriction and sodium and water retention. The second type is A-II receptor blockers (ARBs), which prevent angiotensin II from binding to its receptors in the walls of the blood vessels.

Drug therapy is recommended for all patients with stage 2 or 3 hypertension that is not controlled by lifestyle modifications. Because of the higher risk of hypertensive complications, drug therapy is also recommended for all hypertensive patients with diabetes, clinical cardiovascular or cerebrovascular disease, and target organ disease. Diuretics and β-adrenergic blockers are recommended for the initial drug therapy of uncomplicated hypertension. Angiotensin inhibitors, adrenergic receptor blockers, and calcium channel blockers are also effective in lowering BP and may be used as first-line drugs. Direct-acting vasodilators, the α_2-adrenergic agonists, and the peripheral-acting adrenergic antagonists are not recommended for single-drug therapy because of their side effects.

The selection of a first-line drug is influenced by cost, the presence of other medical conditions, patient characteristics, and side effects. The initial drug is started at a low dose for several weeks. If after at least 1 month the BP is not controlled, the dose of the first-line drug can be increased. A second drug from a different class can be substituted, or a second drug from a different class can be added if the initial drug was ineffective or there were adverse side effects to the initial drug. If the addition of the second drug controls the BP, the health care provider may try withdrawing the first drug. Many times, mild to moderate hypertension can be controlled with only one drug. Before proceeding with the addition or substitution of medication, consideration should be given to possible reasons for the lack of response to drug therapy (Table 32-9).

For stage 3 hypertension, the plan is essentially the same, but the interval between medication changes may be shortened, and therapy may need to be started with more than one drug. The addition of a third or fourth drug, including the centrally and peripherally acting adrenergic antagonists and direct vasodilators, may be necessary, but only after the maximum doses of the first and second drugs have been achieved.

Text continued on p. 792

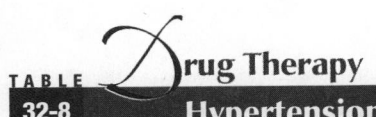

TABLE
32-8

Drug Therapy
Hypertension

DRUG	MECHANISM OF ACTION	SIDE EFFECTS AND ADVERSE EFFECTS	NURSING CONSIDERATIONS
Diuretics			
Thiazide and Related Diuretics			
bendroflumethiazide (Naturetin) benzthiazide (Aquatag, Exna) chlorothiazide (Diuril) chlorthalidone (Hygroton) hydrochlorothiazide (Esidrix, Hydrodiuril, Oretic) metolazone (Zaroxolyn) methyclothiazide (Enduron) trichlormethiazide (Metahydrin, Naqua)	Inhibit NaCl reabsorption in the distal convoluted tubule; increases excretion of Na^+ and Cl^-. Initial decrease in ECF; sustained decrease in SVR. Lower BP moderately in 2-4 wk.	Fluid and electrolyte imbalances (volume depletion, hypokalemia, hyponatremia, hypochloremia, hypomagnesemia, hypercalcemia, hyperuricemia, metabolic alkalosis); CNS effects (vertigo, headache, weakness); GI effects (anorexia, nausea, vomiting, diarrhea, constipation, pancreatitis); sexual problems (impotence and decreased libido); blood dyscrasias; and dermatologic (photosensitivity, skin rash) effects. Decreased glucose tolerance.	Monitor for orthostatic hypotension, hypokalemia, and alkalosis. Thiazides may potentiate cardiotoxicity of digoxin by producing hypokalemia. Dietary sodium restriction reduces the risk of hypokalemia. NSAIDs can decrease diuretic and antihypertensive effect of thiazide diuretics. Advise patient to supplement with potassium-rich foods. Current doses are lower than previously recommended.
Loop Diuretics			
bumetanide (Bumex) ethacrynic acid (Edecrin) furosemide (Lasix) torsemide (Demadex)	Inhibit NaCl reabsorption in the thick ascending limb of the loop of Henle. Increase excretion of Na^+ and Cl^-. More potent diuretic effect than thiazides, but shorter duration of action, less effective for hypertension.	Fluid electrolyte imbalance as with thiazides, except no hypercalcemia. Ototoxicity (hearing impairment, deafness, vertigo) that is usually reversible. Metabolic effects, including hyperuricemia, hyperglycemia, increased LDL cholesterol and triglycerides with decreased HDL cholesterol.	Monitor for orthostatic hypotension and electrolyte abnormalities. Loop diuretics remain effective despite renal insufficiency. Diuretic effect of drug increases at higher doses.
Potassium-Sparing Diuretics			
amiloride (Midamor) triamterene (Dyrenium)	Reduce K^+ and Na^+ exchange in the distal and collecting tubules. Reduces excretion of K^+, H^+, Ca^{2+}, and Mg^{2+}.	Hyperkalemia, nausea, vomiting, diarrhea, headache, leg cramps, and dizziness.	Monitor for orthostatic hypotension and hyperkalemia. Potassium-sparing diuretics are contraindicated in patients with renal failure and used with caution in patients on ACE inhibitors or angiotensin II blockers. Avoid potassium supplements.
spironolactone (Aldactone) eplerenone (Inspra)	Inhibit the Na^+ retaining and K^+ excreting effects of aldosterone in the distal and collecting tubules.	Same as amiloride and triamterene; may cause gynecomastia, impotence, decreased libido, and menstrual irregularities.	
Adrenergic Inhibitors			
Central-Acting Adrenergic Antagonists			
clonidine (Catapres)	Reduces sympathetic outflow from CNS. Reduces peripheral sympathetic tone, produces vasodilation; decreases SVR and BP.	Dry mouth, sedation, impotence, nausea, dizziness, sleep disturbance, nightmares, restlessness, and depression. Symptomatic bradycardia in patients with conduction disorder.	Sudden discontinuation may cause withdrawal syndrome including rebound hypertension, tachycardia, headache, tremors, apprehension, and sweating. Chewing gum or hard candy may relieve dry mouth. Alcohol and sedatives increase sedation. May be given transdermally with fewer side effects and better compliance.

BP, Blood pressure; *CNS*, central nervous system; *ECF*, extracellular fluid; *GI*, gastrointestinal; *HDL*, high density lipoproteins; *LDL*, low density lipoproteins; *NSAIDs*, nonsteroidal antiinflammatory drugs; *SVR*, systemic vascular resistance.

Continued

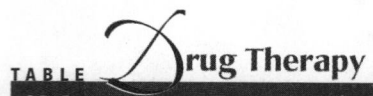

TABLE
32-8

Drug Therapy
Hypertension—cont'd

DRUG	MECHANISM OF ACTION	SIDE EFFECTS AND ADVERSE EFFECTS	NURSING CONSIDERATIONS
Adrenergic Inhibitors—cont'd			
Central-Acting Adrenergic Antagonists—cont'd			
guanabenz (Wytensin)	Same as clonidine.	Same as clonidine.	Same as clonidine, but not available in transdermal formulation.
guanfacine (Tenex)	Same as clonidine.	Same as clonidine.	Same as clonidine, but not available in transdermal formulation.
methyldopa (Aldomet)	Same as clonidine.	Sedation, fatigue, orthostatic hypotension, decreased libido, impotence, dry mouth, hemolytic anemia, hepatotoxicity, sodium and water retention, psychic depression.	Instruct patient about daytime sedation and avoidance of hazardous activities. Administration of a single daily dose at bedtime minimizes sedative effect.
Peripheral-Acting Adrenergic Antagonists			
guanethidine (Ismelin)	Prevents peripheral release of norepinephrine, resulting in vasodilation; lowers CO and reduces SBP more than DBP.	Marked orthostatic hypotension, diarrhea, cramps, bradycardia, retrograde or delayed ejaculation, sodium and water retention.	May cause severe postural hypotension; not recommended for use in patients with cerebrovascular or coronary insufficiency or in older adults; advise patient to rise slowly and wear support stockings. Hypotensive effect is delayed for 2-3 days and lasts 7-10 days after withdrawal. Once-daily dosing.
guanadrel sulfate (Hylorel)	Same as guanethidine.	Similar to guanethidine.	Must be given twice daily.
reserpine (Serpasil)	Depletes central and peripheral stores of norepinephrine; results in peripheral vasodilation (decreases SVR and BP).	Sedation and inability to concentrate; depression; nasal stuffiness.	Contraindicated in patients with history of depression. Monitor mood and mental status regularly. Advise patient to avoid barbiturates, alcohol, and narcotics.
α₁-Adrenergic Blockers			
doxazosin (Cardura) prazosin (Minipress) terazosin (Hytrin)	Block α₁-adrenergic effects producing peripheral vasodilation (decreases SVR and BP).	Variable amount of postural hypotension depending on the plasma volume. May see profound orthostatic hypotension with syncope within 90 minutes after initial dose. Retention of salt and water.	Reduced resistance to the outflow of urine in benign prostatic hyperplasia. Taking drug at bedtime reduces risks associated with orthostatic hypotension. Beneficial effects on lipid profile.
phentolamine (Regitine)	Blocks α₁-adrenergic receptors, resulting in peripheral vasodilation (decreases SVR and BP).	Acute, prolonged hypotension, cardiac arrhythmias, tachycardia, weakness, flushing. Abdominal pain, nausea, and exacerbation of peptic ulcer.	Used in short-term management of pheochromocytoma. Also used locally to prevent necrosis of skin and subcutaneous tissue after extravasation of an α-adrenergic drug. No oral formulation.

CO, Cardiac output; *DBP,* diastolic blood pressure; *SBP,* systolic blood pressure.

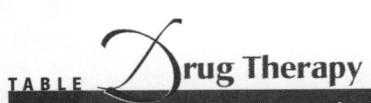

TABLE 32-8

Drug Therapy
Hypertension—cont'd

DRUG	MECHANISM OF ACTION	SIDE EFFECTS AND ADVERSE EFFECTS	NURSING CONSIDERATIONS
Adrenergic Inhibitors—cont'd			
β-Adrenergic Blockers			
acebutolol (Sectral) atenolol (Tenormin) betaxolol (Kerlone) bisoprolol (Zebeta) carteolol (Cartrol) carvedilol (Coreg) metoprolol (Lopressor) nadolol (Corgard) penbutolol (Levatol) pindolol (Visken) propranolol (Inderal) timolol (Blocadren)	Reduce BP by antagonizing β-adrenergic effects. Decrease CO and reduce sympathetic vasoconstrictor tone. Decrease renin secretion by kidney.	Bronchospasm, atrioventricular conduction block, impaired peripheral circulation. Nightmares, depression, weakness, reduced exercise capacity. May induce or exacerbate heart failure in susceptible patients. Sudden withdrawal of β-adrenergic blockers may cause rebound hypertension and exacerbate symptoms of ischemic heart disease.	β-Adrenergic blockers vary in lipid solubility, selectivity, and presence of partial sympathomimetic effect, which explains different therapeutic and side effect profiles of specific agents. Monitor pulse regularly. Caution in patients with diabetes mellitus because drug may mask signs of hypoglycemia.
esmolol (Brevibloc)	Reduces BP by antagonizing β₁-adrenergic effects.		IV administration; rapid onset and very short duration of action.
Combined α– and β-Adrenergic Blocker			
labetalol (Normodyne, Trandate)	α₁-, β₁-, and β₂-adrenergic blocking properties producing peripheral vasodilation and decreased heart rate. Reduces CO, SVR, and BP.	Dizziness, fatigue, nausea, vomiting, dyspepsia, paresthesia, nasal stuffiness, impotence, edema. Hepatic toxicity.	Same as β-adrenergic blockers. IV form available for hypertensive crisis in hospitalized patients. Patients must be kept supine during IV administration. Assess patient tolerance of upright position (severe postural hypotension) before allowing upright activities (e.g., commode).
Direct Vasodilators			
diazoxide (Hyperstat)	Reduces SVR and BP by direct arterial vasodilation.	Reflex sympathetic activation producing increased HR, CO, and salt and water retention. Hyperglycemia, especially in patients with type 2 diabetes.	IV use only for hypertensive crisis in hospitalized patients. Administer only into peripheral vein.
hydralazine (Apresoline)	Reduces SVR and BP by direct arterial vasodilation.	Headache, nausea, flushing, palpitation, tachycardia, dizziness, and angina. Hemolytic anemia, vasculitis, and rapidly progressive glomerulonephritis.	IV use for hypertensive crisis in hospitalized patients. Twice-daily oral dosage. Not used as monotherapy because of side effects. Contraindicated in patients with coronary artery disease; used with caution in patients over 40 years of age.
minoxidil (Loniten)	Reduces SVR and BP by direct arterial vasodilation.	Reflex tachycardia, marked sodium and fluid retention (may require loop diuretics for control), and hirsuitism. May cause ECG changes (flattened and inverted T waves) not related to ischemia.	Reserved for treatment of severe hypertension associated with renal failure and resistant to other therapy. Once- or twice-daily dosage.
nitroglycerin (Tridil)	Relaxes arterial and venous smooth muscle reducing preload and SVR. At low dose, venous dilation predominates; at higher dose arterial dilation is present.	Hypotension, headache, vomiting, flushing.	IV use for hypertensive crisis in hospitalized patients with myocardial ischemia. Administered by continuous IV infusion with pump or control device.

ECG, Electrocardiogram; *HDL,* high-density lipoproteins; *HR,* heart rate; *IV,* intravenous.

Continued

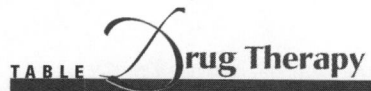

TABLE
32-8   Hypertension—cont'd

DRUG	MECHANISM OF ACTION	SIDE EFFECTS AND ADVERSE EFFECTS	NURSING CONSIDERATIONS
Direct Vasodilators—cont'd			
sodium nitroprusside (Nipride)	Direct arterial vasodilation reduces SVR and BP.	Acute hypotension, nausea, vomiting, muscle twitching. Signs of thiocyanate toxicity include anorexia, nausea, fatigue, and disorientation.	IV use for hypertensive crisis in hospitalized patients. Administered by continuous IV infusion with pump or control device. Use intraarterial monitoring of BP. Light-resistant bags, bottles, and administration sets must be used; stable for 24 hr. Monitor thiocyanate levels with prolonged (≥24 to 48 hr) use.
Ganglionic Blockers			
trimethaphan (Arfonad)	Interrupts adrenergic control of arteries, results in vasodilation, and reduces SVR and BP.	Visual disturbance, dilated pupils, dry mouth, urinary hesitancy, subjective chilliness.	IV use for initial control of BP in patient with dissecting aortic aneurysm. Administered by continuous IV infusion with pump or control device.
Angiotensin Inhibitors			
Angiotensin-Converting Enzyme Inhibitors			
benazepril (Lotensin) captopril (Capoten) enalapril (Vasotec) fosinopril (Monopril) lisinopril (Prinivil, Zestril) moexipril (Univasc) perindopril (Aceon) quinapril (Accupril) ramipril (Altace) trandolapril (Mavik) enalaprilat (Vasotec Injection)	Inhibit angiotensin-converting enzyme; reduce conversion of angiotensin I to angiotensin II (A-II); prevent A-II-mediated vasoconstriction. Inhibit angiotensin-converting enzyme when oral agents not appropriate.	Hypotension, loss of taste, cough, hyperkalemia, acute renal failure, skin rash, angioneurotic edema. Same as oral forms.	Aspirin and NSAIDs may reduce drug effectiveness. Addition of diuretic enhances drug effect. Should not be used with potassium-sparing diuretics. Can cause fetal morbidity or mortality. Captopril may be given orally for hypertensive crisis. Given IV over 5 minutes; may be given every 6 hr.
Angiotensin II Receptor Blockers			
candesartan (Atacand) eprosartan (Teveten) irbesartan (Avapro) losartan (Cozaar) olmesartan (Benicar) telmisartan (Micardis) tasosartan (Verdia) valsartan (Diovan)	Prevent action of angiotensin II and produce vasodilation and increased salt and water excretion.	Hyperkalemia, decreased renal function.	Full effect on BP may not be seen for 3-6 wk.
Calcium Channel Blockers			
amlodipine (Norvasc) diltiazem (Cardizem) felodipine (Plendil) isradipine (DynaCirc) mibefradil (Posicor) nicardipine (Cardene) nifedipine (Procardia) nisoldipine (Sular) verapamil (Isoptin)	Block movement of extracellular calcium into cells, causing vasodilation and decreased SVR.	Nausea, headache, dizziness, peripheral edema. Reflex tachycardia (with dihydropyridines). Reflex decrease HR (with diltiazem); constipation (with verapamil).	Use with caution in patients with heart failure. Contraindicated in patients with second- or third-degree heart block. IV nicardipine available for hypertensive crisis in hospitalized patients. Sustained-release formulations for some drugs. Avoid grapefruit when on nifedipine.

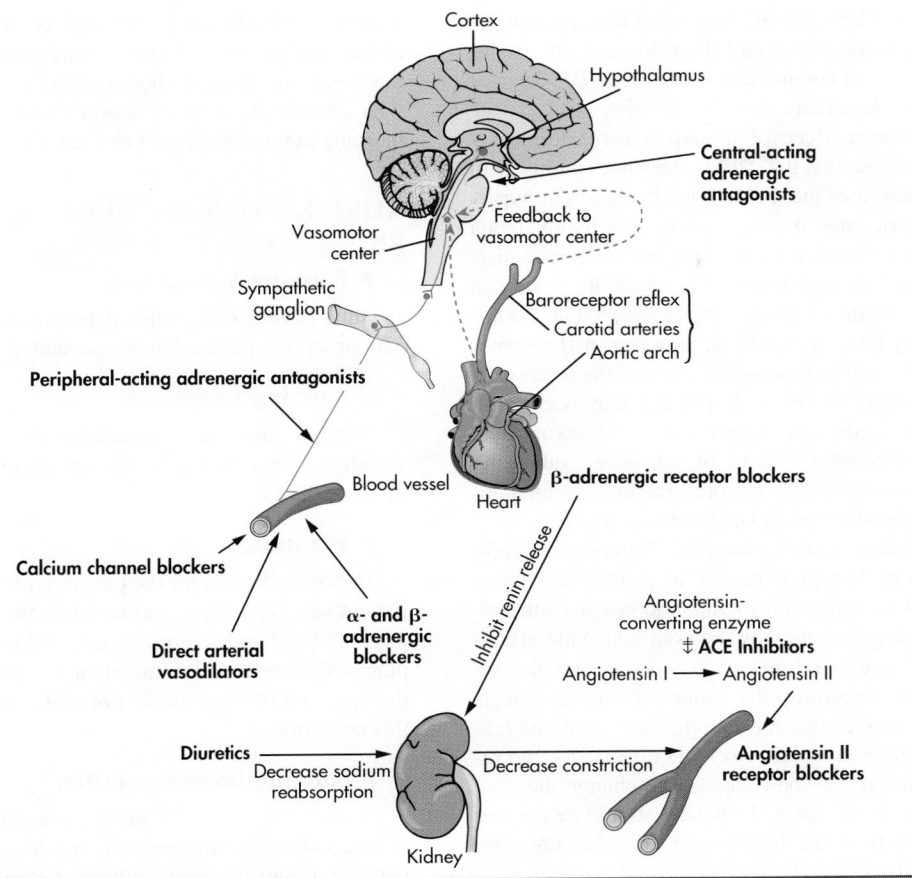

FIG. 32-5 Site and method of action of various antihypertensive drugs. *ACE,* Angiotensin-converting enzyme.

TABLE 32-9   Causes for Lack of Responsiveness to Therapy

Nonadherence to Therapy
- Cost of medication
- Instructions not clear or not given to the patient in writing
- Inadequate or no patient teaching
- Lack of involvement of the patient in the treatment plan
- Side effects of medication
- Dementia
- Inconvenient dosing

Drug-Related Causes
- Dosages too low
- Inappropriate combinations
- Rapid inactivation
- Drug interactions*
  Nonsteroidal antiinflammatory drugs
  Oral contraceptives
  Sympathomimetics
  Antidepressants
  Adrenal corticosteroids
  Nasal decongestants
  Licorice-containing substances (e.g., chewing tobacco)
  Cocaine
  Cyclosporine
  Erythropoietin

Associated Conditions
- Increasing obesity
- Alcohol intake more than 1 oz/day

Secondary Hypertension
- Renal insufficiency
- Renovascular hypertension
- Pheochromocytoma
- Primary aldosteronism

Volume Overload
- Inadequate diuretic therapy
- Excess sodium intake
- Fluid retention from reduction of blood pressure
- Progressive renal damage

Pseudohypertension

From US Department of Health and Human Services. *The sixth report of the Joint National Committee on Detection, Evaluation, and Treatment of High Blood Pressure (JNC-VI),* Washington, DC, 1997, National Institutes of Health.
*Especially in older adults.

After 1 year of good BP control, step-down therapy may be tried. The number of medications and their dosages are gradually decreased to the lowest amount that controls the BP. Regular follow-up is needed to detect any elevation of BP.

Side effects and adverse effects of antihypertensive drugs may be so severe or undesirable that the patient does not comply with therapy. Table 32-8 describes the major side effects of antihypertensive drugs. Hyperuricemia, hyperglycemia, and hypokalemia are common side effects with both thiazide and loop diuretics. ACE inhibitors can lead to high levels of bradykinin, which can cause coughing. An individual who develops a cough with the use of ACE inhibitors may be switched to an angiotensin II receptor blocker. Hyperkalemia can be a serious side effect of the potassium-sparing diuretics and ACE inhibitors. Impotence may occur with some of the diuretics. Orthostatic hypotension and sexual dysfunction are two undesirable effects of adrenergic-inhibiting agents. Tachycardia and orthostatic hypotension are potential adverse effects of both vasodilators and angiotensin inhibitors.

Patient teaching related to drug therapy. Patient and family teaching related to drug therapy is needed to identify and minimize side effects and to cope with therapeutic effects. Side effects of antihypertensive drug therapy are common. Side effects may be an initial response to a drug and may decrease with continued use of the drug. Informing the patient about side effects that lessen with time may enable the individual to continue taking the drug. The number or severity of side effects may be related to the dosage, and it may be necessary to change the drug or decrease the dosage. In this case, the patient should be advised to report the side effects to the health care provider who prescribed the medication.

A common side effect of several of these drugs is orthostatic hypotension. This condition is caused by an alteration of the autonomic nervous system's mechanisms for regulating pressure, which are required for position changes. Consequently, the patient may feel dizzy, weak, and faint when assuming an upright position after sitting or lying down. (Specific measures to control or decrease orthostatic hypotension are presented in Table 32-13.)

Sexual dysfunction may occur with many of the antihypertensive drugs (see Table 32-8) and can be a major reason that a patient does not adhere to the treatment plan. Rather than discussing a sexual problem with a health care professional, the patient may decide to discontinue using the drug. Often the nurse must approach the patient on this sensitive subject and encourage discussion of any sexual dysfunction that may be experienced. The sexual problems may be easier for the patient to discuss and handle once it has been explained that the drug may be the source of the problem and the side effects can be decreased or eliminated by changing to another antihypertensive drug. The patient should be encouraged to discuss side effects with the health care provider who prescribed the medication. If the patient is reluctant to do so, the nurse may offer to alert the health care provider to the sexual side effect that the patient is experiencing. There are so many options now in treating hypertension that a plan that is acceptable to the patient should be achievable.

Some unpleasant effects of drugs result from their therapeutic effect, but the impact can be minimized. For example, dry mouth and frequent voiding are unpleasant effects of diuretics. Sugarless gum or candy may relieve the dry mouth. The nurse can assist the patient to develop a medication schedule to minimize unpleasant effects. When frequent urination interrupts sleep, taking the diuretic earlier in the day may be beneficial. Side effects of va-

sodilators and adrenergic inhibitors decrease if the drugs are taken in the evening. It should be remembered that BP is lowest during the night and highest shortly after awakening. Therefore drugs with 24-hour duration of action should be taken as early in the morning as possible (e.g., 4 or 5 AM if the patient awakens to void).

NURSING MANAGEMENT PRIMARY HYPERTENSION

■ Nursing Assessment

Subjective and objective data that should be obtained from a patient with hypertension are presented in Table 32-10.

■ Nursing Diagnoses

Nursing diagnoses and collaborative problems for the patient with hypertension include, but are not limited to, those presented in Table 32-11.

■ Planning

The overall goals for the patient with hypertension are that the patient will (1) achieve and maintain the individually determined target BP; (2) understand, accept, and implement the therapeutic plan; (3) experience minimal or no unpleasant side effects of therapy; and (4) be confident of ability to manage and cope with this condition.

■ Nursing Implementation

Health Promotion. Primary prevention of hypertension provides an attractive alternative to the costly cycle of managing hypertension and its complications. Current recommendations for primary prevention are based on lifestyle modifications that have been shown to prevent or delay the expected rise in BP in susceptible people. A diet rich in fruits, vegetables, and low-fat dairy foods, with reduced saturated and total fats, significantly lowers BP (see Table 32-7). This diet has been recommended for primary prevention in the general population. Dietary modifications that do not require active participation of the individual, such as a reduction in the amount of salt added to processed foods, may be even more effective.

Individual patient evaluation. The majority of cases of hypertension are identified through routine screening procedures such as insurance, preemployment, and military physical examinations. The nurse in these settings, as well as in most other practice settings, is in an ideal position to assess for the presence of hypertension, identify the risk factors for hypertension and coronary artery disease, and teach the patient about these conditions. In addition to BP determination, a complete health assessment should include such factors as age, sex, and race; diet history (including sodium and alcohol intake); weight patterns; and family history of heart disease, stroke, renal disease, and diabetes mellitus. Medications taken, both prescribed and over-the-counter, should be noted. The patient should be asked about a previous history of high BP and the results of treatment (if any) (see Table 32-10).

Initially, the BP is taken two or three times, at least 2 minutes apart, with the average pressure recorded as the value for that visit. Waiting for at least 2 minutes between readings allows the venous blood to drain from the arm and prevents inaccurate readings. Size and placement of BP cuff are important considerations for accurate measurement. The width of the inflatable bladder should be 40% and length should be 80% of the upper arm cir-

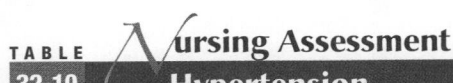

TABLE 32-10   Nursing Assessment
Hypertension

Subjective Data

Important Health Information

Past health history: Known duration and past workup of high BP; cardiovascular, cerebrovascular, renal, or thyroid disease; diabetes mellitus; pituitary disorders; obesity; dyslipidemia; menopause or hormone replacement status

Medications: Use of any prescription or over-the-counter, illicit, or herbal medications; previous use of antihypertensive drug therapy

Functional Health Patterns

Health perception–health management: Family history of hypertension or cardiovascular disease; smoking or other tobacco use, alcohol use; sedentary lifestyle

Nutritional-metabolic: Usual salt and fat intake; weight gain or loss

Elimination: Nocturia

Activity-exercise: Fatigue; dyspnea on exertion, palpitations on exertion, anginal chest pain; intermittent claudication, muscle cramps

Cognitive-perceptual: Dizziness; blurred vision, paresthesias

Sexual-reproductive: Impotence

Coping–stress tolerance: Stressful life events

Objective Data

Cardiovascular

BP consistently >140 mm Hg systolic or 90 mm Hg diastolic, orthostatic change in BP and pulse; retinal vessel changes, abnormal heart sounds; laterally displaced, sustained, forceful, apical pulse; diminished or absent peripheral pulses; carotid, renal, ischial, or femoral bruits; presence of edema

Musculoskeletal

Truncal obesity; abnormal waist-hip ratio

Neurologic

Mental status changes; localized edema

Possible Findings

Abnormal serum electrolytes (especially potassium); ↑ BUN, creatinine, glucose, cholesterol, and tryglyceride levels; proteinuria, microalbuminuria; evidence of ischemic heart disease and left ventricular hypertrophy on ECG; evidence of structural heart disease and left ventricular hypertrophy on echocardiogram

BP, Blood pressure; *BUN,* blood urea nitrogen; *ECG,* electrocardiogram; *MI,* myocardial infarction.

---

cumference. Use of a cuff that is too small or too large will result in readings that are falsely high or low, respectively.

BP measurements of both arms should be performed initially to detect any differences between arms. Atherosclerotic narrowing of the subclavian artery can cause a falsely low reading on the side where the narrowing occurs. Therefore the arm with the higher reading should be used for all subsequent BP measurements. The patient's arm is uncovered and placed at the level of the heart. The cuff should be inflated until no pulse is felt in the brachial artery located in the antecubital fossa of the arm being used. The cuff is then inflated an additional 10 to 20 mm Hg to ensure vascular occlusion. The pressure is released at 2 mm Hg per second. Releasing any slower or faster may create inaccurate readings. Both SBP and DBP should be recorded, with the DBP recorded as the disappearance of sound (Table 32-12).

The BP and pulse are initially measured with the patient in either the supine or the sitting position after at least 5 minutes of rest. BP and pulse should be measured again after 2 minutes in the standing position. Usually the SBP decreases on standing, whereas the DBP and pulse increase. A decrease of more than 10 mm Hg in SBP or any decrease in DBP when standing is abnormal and should prompt further investigation. Common causes of abnormal postural BP values include intravascular volume loss (e.g., with diuretic therapy or dehydration) and inadequate vasoconstrictor mechanisms related to disease or medications. Postural changes in BP and pulse should be measured in older adults, people taking antihypertensive drugs, and when **orthostatic hypotension** (abnormally low BP occurring when an individual assumes a standing position) is suspected.

Screening programs. Screening programs in the community are widely used to assess people's BP. At the time of the BP measurement, each person should be informed in writing of the nu-

NURSING DIAGNOSES & COLLABORATIVE PROBLEMS
TABLE 32-11   Hypertension

Nursing Diagnoses

Ineffective health maintenance *related to* lack of knowledge of pathology, complications, and management of hypertension

Anxiety *related to* complexity of management regimen, possible complications, and lifestyle changes associated with hypertension

Sexual dysfunction *related to* effects of antihypertensive medication

Ineffective therapeutic regimen management *related to*
- Lack of knowledge
- Unpleasant side effects of medication
- Return of blood pressure to normal while on medication
- High cost of some medications
- Inconvenient schedule for taking medications
- Lack of trusting relationship with health care provider

Disturbed body image *related to* diagnosis of hypertension

Ineffective tissue perfusion *related to* complications of hypertension (specify)
- Cerebral
- Cardiovascular
- Renal

Collaborative Problems

Potential complication: adverse effects from antihypertensive therapy

Potential complication: hypertensive crisis

Potential complication: stroke

TABLE 32-12	Appropriate Technique for Measuring Blood Pressure

1. Patient should be seated with the arm bared, supported, and positioned at heart level. The patient should not have smoked or ingested caffeine within 30 minutes before measurement.
2. Blood pressure should be taken in both arms initially.
3. Measurement should not begin until patient has had 5 minutes of quiet rest.
4. The appropriate cuff size must be used to ensure an accurate measurement. The rubber bladder should nearly (at least 80%) or completely encircle the arm. Cuff width should be at least 40% of the arm circumference. Several sizes of cuffs (e.g., child, adult, and large adult) should be available.
5. Measurements should be taken with a mercury sphygmomanometer, a recently calibrated aneroid manometer, or a calibrated electronic device.
6. Both systolic and diastolic pressures should be recorded. The disappearance of sound should be used for the diastolic reading.
7. Two or more readings (taken at least 2 minutes apart) should be averaged. If the first two readings differ by more than 5 mm Hg, additional readings should be obtained.
8. The patient should be informed of the reading and advised of the need for periodic remeasurement.

From US Department of Health and Human Services: *The sixth report of the Joint National Committee on Detection, Evaluation, and Treatment of High Blood Pressure (JNC-VI)*, Washington, DC, 1997, National Institutes of Health.

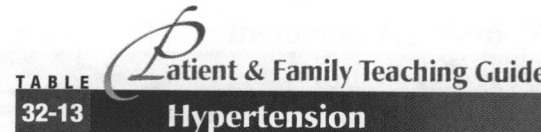

TABLE 32-13	Patient & Family Teaching Guide — Hypertension

When presenting information to the patient and/or family, the nurse should do the following:

1. Provide the numerical value of the patient's BP and explain what it means.
2. Inform the patient that hypertension is usually asymptomatic and symptoms do not reliably indicate BP levels.
3. Explain that hypertension means elevated blood pressure and does not relate to a "hyper" personality.
4. Explain that long-term follow-up and therapy are necessary to treat hypertension.
5. Explain that therapy will not cure, but should control hypertension.
6. Tell patient that controlled hypertension is usually compatible with an excellent prognosis and a normal lifestyle.
7. Explain the potential dangers of uncontrolled hypertension.
8. Be specific about the names, actions, dosages, and side effects of prescribed medications.
9. Tell the patient to plan regular and convenient times for taking medications.
10. Tell the patient not to discontinue drugs abruptly because withdrawal may cause a severe hypertensive reaction.
11. Tell the patient not to double up on doses when a dose is missed.
12. Inform the patient that if BP increases, the patient should not take an increased medication dosage before consulting with the health care provider.
13. Tell the patient not to take a medication belonging to someone else.
14. Inform the patient that side effects of medication often diminish with time.
15. Tell the patient to consult with the health care provider about changing drugs or dosages if impotence or other sexual problems develop.
16. Tell the patient to supplement diet with foods high in potassium (e.g., citrus fruits and green leafy vegetables) if taking potassium-losing diuretics.
17. Tell the patient to avoid hot baths, excessive amounts of alcohol, and strenuous exercise within 3 hr of taking medications that promote vasodilation.
18. Explain that to decrease orthostatic hypotension, the patient should arise slowly from bed, sit on the side of the bed for a few minutes, stand slowly, not stand still for prolonged periods of time, do leg exercises to increase venous return, sleep with the head of the bed raised or on pillows, and lie or sit down when dizziness occurs.
19. Caution about potentially high-risk over-the-counter medications, such as high-sodium antacids, appetite suppressants, and cold and sinus medications. Advise to read warning labels and to consult with pharmacist.

BP, Blood pressure.

meric value of the reading and, if necessary, why further evaluation is important. Effort and resources should be focused on controlling BP in the person already identified as having hypertension; identifying and controlling BP in high-risk groups such as African Americans, obese people, and blood relatives of people with hypertension; and screening those with limited access to the health care system.

Cardiovascular risk factor modification. Education regarding cardiovascular risk factors is appropriate for individual and targeted screening programs. Modifiable cardiovascular risk factors include hypertension, obesity, diabetes mellitus, elevated serum lipids, tobacco use, and physical inactivity. Risk factors can easily be identified and modification discussed with the patient. (Health-promoting behaviors for cardiovascular risk factors are discussed in Chapter 33, Table 33-3.)

Ambulatory and Home Care. The primary nursing responsibilities for long-term management of hypertension are to assist the patient in reducing BP and complying with the treatment plan. Nursing actions include patient and family teaching, detection and reporting of adverse treatment effects, compliance assessment and enhancement, and evaluation of therapeutic effectiveness (Table 32-13). Patient and family teaching includes the following: (1) nutritional therapy, (2) drug therapy, (3) physical activity, (4) home monitoring of BP (if appropriate), and (5) tobacco cessation (if applicable).

Physical activity. Physical activity is bodily movement produced by skeletal muscles that requires energy expenditure. Health benefits from physical activity can be achieved with moderate-intensity activities. The goal for all adults is to accumulate 30 minutes of moderate-intensity activity daily. Generally physi-

cal activity is more likely to be sustained if it is safe and enjoyable, fits easily into the daily schedule, and does not generate financial or social costs. Shopping malls in many communities are open early in the morning (before shopping hours) and provide a warm, safe, flat area for walking. In some communities, health clubs offer special "off-peak" rates to encourage physical activity among older adults. Cardiac rehabilitation programs offer supervised exercise with education about reduction of cardiovascular risk factors. Nurses can assist people with hypertension to increase their physical activity by identifying and communicating the need for increased activity, explaining the difference between physical activity and exercise, assisting in initiating activity, and following up appropriately.

Home blood pressure monitoring. Some patients benefit from regularly monitoring their BP at home. Home BP measurement may give a more valid indication of the BP because the patient is more relaxed. It is important to emphasize to the patient that a single reading is not as important as a series of readings over a period of time. The patient should be instructed to take BP readings weekly (unless otherwise instructed) once the BP has stabilized. A log of the BP measurements should be maintained by the patient and brought to office visits.

Home BP readings may help achieve patient compliance by reinforcing the need to remain on therapy. A patient may become excessively concerned with the BP readings when using home monitoring. Generally, however, this practice should reassure the patient that the treatment is effective.

Patient compliance. A major problem in the long-term management of the patient with hypertension is poor compliance with the prescribed treatment plan. The reasons are many and include inadequate patient teaching, unpleasant side effects of drugs, return of BP to normal range while on medication, lack of motivation, high cost of drugs, and lack of a trusting relationship between the patient and the health care provider. In addition to using BP determinations as an indicator of compliance, the nurse should also assess the patient's diet, activity level, and lifestyle.

Individual assessment to determine the reasons the patient is not complying with the treatment plan and the development of an individualized plan with the patient's assistance are essential. The plan should be compatible with the patient's personality, habits, and lifestyle. Active patient participation increases the likelihood of adherence to the treatment plan. Measures such as involving the patient in scheduling medication convenient to a daily routine, helping the patient link pill taking with another daily activity, and involving family members (if necessary) help increase patient compliance. Substituting combination tablets for multiple drugs once the BP is stabilized may also facilitate compliance, because the patient has to take fewer drugs each day and the cost may be less. It is important to help the patient and the family understand that hypertension is a chronic condition that cannot be cured but can be controlled with drug therapy, diet therapy, physical activity, periodic evaluation, and other relevant lifestyle changes.

■ Evaluation

The overall expected outcomes are that the patient with hypertension will
- achieve and maintain desired BP as defined for the individual
- understand, accept, and implement the therapeutic plan
- experience minimal or no unpleasant side effects of therapy

SPECIAL TYPES OF HYPERTENSION

Isolated Systolic Hypertension

Isolated systolic hypertension (ISH) is defined as a sustained elevation in SBP equal to or greater than 160 mm Hg with a DBP less than 90 mm Hg. (A one-time isolated reading of increased SBP is not classified as ISH.) SBP in the range of 140 to 159 mm Hg with DBP less than 90 mm Hg constitutes borderline ISH. Although ISH does occur in younger adults, it is much more common in older adults. Older adults often have ISH caused by loss of elasticity in large arteries from atherosclerosis.

In the past, ISH was not treated because of the belief that excessive lowering of the DBP would occur, leading to greater problems. Side effects of medication were also a concern. It is both safe and beneficial to treat ISH in the elderly, and doing so decreases the incidence of stroke and cardiovascular morbidity and mortality. For older adults with isolated systolic hypertension, the goal of treatment should be to achieve a systolic BP less than 140 mm Hg if tolerated.

Pseudohypertension

Pseudohypertension, or false hypertension, can occur with sclerosis of the large arteries. Sclerotic arteries do not collapse under the cuff, presenting much higher cuff pressures than are actually present within the vessels. Pseudohypertension is suspected if arteries feel rigid or when few retinal or cardiac signs are found relative to the pressures obtained by cuff. *Osler's sign* (a palpable radial artery after the blood pressure cuff is inflated above peak SBP) has a low sensitivity and specificity for pseudohypertension and is not recommended. The only way to accurately measure BP in pseudohypertension is through the use of an intraarterial catheter.

■ Gerontologic Considerations: Hypertension

Hypertension is common in people 60 years of age and older. It is found in 71% of older African Americans, 61% of older Hispanic Americans, and 60% of older whites.[5] In industrialized coun-

---

ℰVIDENCE-BASED PRACTICE
Hypertension

Clinical Problem
What is the effectiveness of various antihypertensive treatments in patients with hypertension and diabetes mellitus?

Best Clinical Practice
- Intensive blood-pressure control using drug therapy and monitoring reduces cardiovascular morbidity and mortality rates in patients with hypertension and diabetes mellitus.
- These findings were similar regardless of which of the four classes of antihypertensive drugs (diuretics, β-adrenergic blockers, angiotensin-converting enzyme [ACE] inhibitors, and calcium channel blockers) is used as first-line therapy.

Implications for Nursing Practice
- Monitor blood pressure and pulse frequently during initial dosage adjustment and periodically throughout the course of therapy.
- Notify health care provider of significant changes in blood pressure and pulse.
- Monitor frequency of prescription refills to determine compliance.

Reference for Evidence
EBM reviews: intensive blood-pressure control and drugs reduce morbidity and mortality in hypertension and diabetes mellitus, *ACP Journal Club* 134:48, 2001.

tries, SBP rises throughout the life span and DBP rises until age 55 or 60 years and then levels off. The following age-related physical changes play a role in the pathophysiology of hypertension in the older adult: (1) loss of tissue elasticity; (2) increased collagen content and stiffness of the myocardium; (3) increased peripheral vascular resistance; (4) decreased α-adrenergic receptor sensitivity; (5) blunting of baroreceptor reflexes; (6) decreased renal function; and (7) decreased renin response to sodium and water depletion.[5]

In the older adult taking antihypertensive medication, absorption of some drugs may be altered as a result of decreased splanchnic blood flow. Metabolism and excretion of drugs may also be prolonged.

Careful technique is important in assessing BP in older adults. In some older people, there is a wide gap between the first Korotkoff sound and subsequent beats. This is called the *auscultatory gap.* Failure to inflate the cuff high enough may result in seriously underestimating the SBP. This problem can be avoided by palpating the brachial or radial artery while inflating the cuff to a level above the disappearance of the pulse.

Older adults are sensitive to BP changes; therefore reducing SBP to less than 120 mm Hg in a person with long-standing hypertension could lead to inadequate cerebral blood flow. Older adults also produce less renin and are more resistant to the effects of ACE inhibitors and angiotenion II receptor blockers.[8]

Because of varying degrees of impaired baroreceptor reflex mechanisms, postural or orthostatic hypotension occurs often in older adults, especially in those with ISH. Postural hypotension in this age group is often associated with volume depletion or chronic disease states, such as decreased renal and hepatic function or electrolyte imbalance. To reduce the likelihood of postural hypotension, antihypertensive drugs should be started at low doses and increased cautiously. BP and pulse should be measured in the reclining and standing positions at every visit.[9]

HYPERTENSIVE CRISIS

Hypertensive crisis is a severe and abrupt elevation in BP, arbitrarily defined as a diastolic BP of above 120 to 130 mm Hg. The rate of rise of BP is more important than the absolute value in determining the need for emergency treatment. Patients with chronic hypertension can tolerate much higher BP than previously normotensive people.[10] Prompt recognition and management of hypertensive crisis is essential to decrease the threat to organ function and life.

Hypertensive crisis occurs most commonly in patients with a history of hypertension who have failed to comply with their prescribed medications or who have been undermedicated. In this setting, rising BP is thought to trigger endothelial damage and the release of vasoconstrictor substances. A vicious cycle of BP elevation ensues leading to life-threatening damage to target organs. Hypertensive crisis related to cocaine or crack use is becoming a more frequent problem. Other drugs such as amphetamines, phencyclidine (PCP), and lysergic acid diethylamide (LSD) may also precipitate hypertensive crisis that may be complicated by drug-induced seizures, stroke, myocardial infarction, or encephalopathy. Table 32-14 lists causes of hypertensive crisis.

Hypertensive crisis is classified by the degree of organ damage and the rapidity with which the BP must be lowered. *Hypertensive emergency,* which develops over hours to days, is a situation in which a patient's BP is severely elevated with evidence of acute target organ damage, especially damage to the central nervous system. Hypertensive emergencies include hypertensive encephalopathy,

TABLE 32-14	Causes of Hypertensive Crisis

Exacerbation of chronic hypertension
Renovascular hypertension
Preeclampsia, eclampsia
Pheochromocytoma
Drugs (cocaine, amphetamines)
Monoamine oxidase inhibitors taken with tyramine-containing foods
Rebound hypertension (from abrupt withdrawal of clonidine or β-adrenergic blockers)
Necrotizing vasculitis
Head injury
Acute aortic dissection

intracranial or subarachnoid hemorrhage, acute left ventricular failure with pulmonary edema, myocardial infarction, renal failure, and dissecting aortic aneurysm. *Hypertensive urgency,* which develops over days to weeks, is a situation in which a patient's BP is severely elevated but there is no clinical evidence of target organ damage.

Clinical Manifestations. A hypertensive emergency may be manifested as *hypertensive encephalopathy,* a syndrome in which a sudden rise in BP is associated with headache, nausea, vomiting, seizures, confusion, stupor, and coma. Other common manifestations are blurred vision and transient blindness. The manifestations of encephalopathy are probably the results of cerebral edema and spasms of cerebral vessels.

Renal insufficiency ranging from minor impairment to complete renal shutdown may occur. Rapid cardiac decompensation ranging from unstable angina to infarction and pulmonary edema is also possible with chest pain and dyspnea. Aortic dissection causes excruciating chest and back pain often accompanied by diaphoresis and the loss of pulses in an extremity.

Patient assessment is extremely important, especially monitoring for signs of neurologic dysfunction, retinal damage, heart failure, pulmonary edema, and renal failure. The neurologic manifestations are often similar to the presentation of a stroke. However, a hypertensive crisis does not show focal or lateralizing signs often seen with a stroke.

NURSING *and* COLLABORATIVE MANAGEMENT HYPERTENSIVE CRISIS

BP level alone is a poor indicator of the seriousness of the patient's condition and is not the major factor in deciding the treatment for a hypertensive crisis. The association between elevated BP and signs of new or progressive end-organ damage (e.g., cerebrovascular, cardiac, retinal, or renal involvement) determines the seriousness of the situation.

When treating hypertensive emergencies, the mean arterial pressure (MAP) is often used instead of systolic and diastolic readings to guide and evaluate therapy. MAP is calculated as DBP plus one third of the pulse pressure (SBP minus DBP):

$$MAP = DBP + \tfrac{1}{3} \text{ Pulse pressure}$$

Hypertensive emergencies require hospitalization, parenteral administration of antihypertensive drugs, and intensive care monitoring. Generally, the initial treatment goal is to decrease MAP 10% to 20% in the first 1 to 2 hours with further gradual reduction over the next 24 hours. Lowering the BP too far or too fast may decrease cerebral perfusion and could precipitate a stroke. A patient who has aortic dissection, unstable angina, or signs of myocardial infarction must have the SBP lowered to 100 to 120 mm Hg as quickly as possible.

The intravenous (IV) drugs used for hypertensive emergencies include vasodilators (e.g., sodium nitroprusside, nitroglycerin, diazoxide [Hyperstat], and hydralazine [Apresoline]), adrenergic inhibitors (e.g., phentolamine [Regitine], labetalol [Normodyne], and esmolol [Brevibloc]), and the ACE inhibitor enalaprilat (Vasotec). Sodium nitroprusside is the most effective parenteral drug for the treatment of hypertensive emergencies. Fenoldopam (Corlopam), an IV drug for the treatment of hypertensive emergencies, selectively activates dopamine receptors, resulting in renal and systemic vasodilation.[11] Oral agents may be administered in addition to the parenteral drugs to help make an earlier transition to long-term therapy. The mechanisms of action and the adverse effects of these drugs are presented in Table 32-7.

Administered intravenously the drugs have a rapid (within seconds to minutes) onset of action. The patient's BP and pulse should be taken every 2 to 3 minutes during the initial administration of these drugs. The use of an intraarterial line (see Chapter 64) or an automated BP monitoring machine (e.g., Dynamap) to monitor the BP is ideal. The rate of drug administration is titrated according to the level of BP. It is important to prevent hypotension and its effects in a person whose body has adjusted to hypertension. An excessive reduction in BP may cause stroke, MI, or visual changes. Continual ECG monitoring is frequently done to observe for cardiac arrhythmias. Extreme caution is needed in treating the patient with coronary artery disease or cerebrovascular insufficiency. Hourly urinary output should be measured to assess renal perfusion. Careful monitoring of vital signs and urinary output provides information regarding the effectiveness of these drugs and the patient's response to therapy. Patients receiving IV antihypertensive drugs may be restricted to bed; getting up (e.g., to use the commode) may cause severe cerebral ischemia and fainting.

Regular, ongoing assessment is essential to evaluate the patient with severe hypertension. Frequent neurologic checks, including level of consciousness, pupillary size and reaction, movement of extremities, and reactions to stimuli, help detect any changes in the patient's condition. Cardiac, pulmonary, and renal systems should be monitored for decompensation caused by the severe elevation in BP (e.g., pulmonary edema, CHF, angina, renal failure).

Hypertensive urgencies usually do not require IV medications but can be managed with oral agents. The patient with a hypertensive urgency may not need hospitalization, but requires frequent follow-up. The oral drugs most frequently used for hypertensive urgencies are captopril (Capoten) and clonidine (Catapres) (see Table 32-8). The disadvantage of oral medications is the inability to regulate the dosage moment to moment, as can be done with IV medications. If a patient with a hypertensive urgency is not hospitalized, outpatient follow-up should be arranged within 24 hours.

A patient with severe elevation of BP but without target organ damage may not require emergent drug therapy or hospitalization. Allowing the patient to sit for 20 or 30 minutes in a quiet environment may significantly reduce BP. Oral drugs may then be instituted or adjusted. Additional nursing interventions include encouraging the patient to verbalize fears, answering questions concerning the hypertension, and eliminating excess noise in the patient's environment.

Once the hypertensive crisis is resolved, it is important to determine the cause. The patient will need appropriate management and extensive education to avoid future crises.

CRITICAL THINKING EXERCISES

Case Study
Primary Hypertension

Patient Profile. Roger is a 45-year-old African American man with no previous history of hypertension. At a screening clinic, his BP was found to be 180/120 mm Hg.

Subjective Data
- Father died of stroke at age 60
- Mother is alive but has hypertension
- States that he feels fine and is not a "hyper" person
- Smokes one pack of cigarettes daily
- Drinks a six-pack of beer on Friday and Saturday nights
- Has been told that BP medication interferes with sexual relationships

Objective Data
Physical Examination
- Retinopathy
- Sustained apical impulse palpable in the fourth intercostal space just lateral to the midclavicular line

Diagnostic Studies
- ECG: left ventricular hypertrophy
- Urinalysis: protein 31 mg/dl (0.3 g/L)
- Serum creatinine level: 1.6 mg/dl (141 mmol/L)

Collaborative Care
- Low-sodium diet
- Hydrochlorothiazide 12.5 mg/day

CRITICAL THINKING QUESTIONS

1. What risk factors for hypertension does Roger have?
2. What evidence of target organ damage is present?
3. What misconceptions about hypertension should be corrected?
4. What areas would you focus on in teaching this patient about his illness?
5. Based on the assessment data presented, write one or more appropriate nursing diagnoses. Are there any collaborative problems?

Nursing Research Issues

1. Does a person believe that if the personal risk factors for hypertension are reduced, chances of developing hypertension will be reduced?
2. What are the perceptions and attitudes of the nurse toward the efficacy of hypertension screening?
3. Do the perceptions of daily stress in the hypertensive patient differ from the perceptions of daily stress in the normotensive patient?
4. Do the patient and family members who are taught BP measurement by videotaped instruction measure BP as accurately as those who are taught by personal instruction?
5. Does home monitoring of BP increase the patient's compliance with antihypertensive therapy?

REVIEW QUESTIONS

The number of the question corresponds to the same-numbered objective at the beginning of the chapter.

1. If a patient has decreased cardiac output caused by fluid volume deficit and marked vasodilation, the regulatory mechanism that will increase the blood pressure by improving both of these is
   a. release of antidiuretic hormone (ADH).
   b. secretion of prostaglandins PGE_2 and PGI_2.
   c. stimulation of the sympathetic nervous system.
   d. activation of the renin-angiotensin-aldosterone system.

2. While obtaining subjective assessment data from a patient with hypertension, the nurse recognizes that a modifiable risk factor for the development of hypertension is
   a. hyperlipidemia.
   b. excessive alcohol intake.
   c. a family history of hypertension.
   d. consumption of a high-carbohydrate, high-calcium diet.

3. Target organ damage that can occur from hypertension includes
   a. headache and dizziness.
   b. retinopathy and diabetes.
   c. hypercholesterolemia and renal dysfunction.
   d. renal dysfunction and left ventricular hypertrophy.

4. A high-risk population that should be targeted in the primary prevention of hypertension is
   a. smokers.
   b. African Americans.
   c. business executives.
   d. middle-aged women.

5. In teaching a patient with hypertension about controlling the condition, the nurse recognizes that
   a. all patients with elevated BP require medication.
   b. it is not necessary to limit salt in the diet if taking a diuretic.
   c. obese persons must achieve a normal weight in order to lower BP.
   d. lifestyle modifications are indicated for all persons with elevated BP.

6. A major consideration in the management of the older adult with hypertension is to
   a. prevent pseudohypertension from converting to true hypertension.
   b. recognize that the older adult is less likely to comply with the drug therapy than a younger adult.
   c. ensure that the patient receives larger initial doses of antihypertensive drugs because of impaired absorption.
   d. use careful technique in assessing the BP of the patient because of the possible presence of an auscultatory gap.

7. A patient with newly diagnosed hypertension has a blood pressure of 158/98 after 12 months of exercise and diet modifications. The nurse advises the patient that
   a. medication may be required because the BP is still not within the normal range.
   b. continued monitoring of the BP every 3 to 6 months is all that will be necessary for treatment.
   c. because lifestyle modifications were not effective they do not need to be continued and drugs will be used.
   d. he will have to make more vigorous changes in his lifestyle if he wants to stay off medication for his hypertension.

8. A patient is admitted to the hospital in hypertensive crisis. The nurse recognizes that the hypertensive urgency differs from hypertensive emergency in that
   a. the BP is always higher in a hypertensive emergency.
   b. hypertensive emergencies are associated with evidence of target organ damage.
   c. hypertensive urgency is treated with rest and tranquilizers to lower the BP.
   d. hypertensive emergencies require intraarterial catheter measurement of the BP.

REFERENCES

1. Sixth report of the Joint National Committee on Detection, Evaluation, and Treatment of High Blood Pressure (JNC-VI), *Arch Intern Med* 157:2413, 1997.
2. American Heart Association: *2001 heart stroke statistical update,* Dallas, 2000, American Heart Association.
3. Woods AD: Improving the odds against hypertension, *Nursing* 31:36, 2001.
4. Weir MR: Appropriate use of calcium antagonists in hypertension, *Hosp Pract* 36:47, 2001.
5. Vaitkevicius PV, Niranjan BS: Hypertension, *Clin Geriatr* 9:18, 2001.
6. Woods A: High blood pressure (hypertension), *Nursing* 32:52, 2002.
7. Moore TJ et al: DASH diet may be enough to control stage 1 isolated systolic hypertension, *Hypertension* 38:115, 2001.
8. Lee C: Chronic angiotensin-converting enzyme inhibitor therapy in the elderly, *Clin Geriatr* 10:61, 2002.
9. Dunn EC, Small RE: Economics of antihypertensive therapy in the elderly, *Drugs Aging* 18:515, 2001.
10. Miracle VA: Act fast during a hypertensive crisis, *Nursing* 31:50, 2001.
11. Wood AJ: Fenoldopam: a selective peripheral dopamine-receptor agonist for the treatment of severe hypertension, *N Engl J Med* 345:1548, 2001.

RESOURCES

American Heart Association
National Center
7272 Greenville Avenue
Dallas, TX 75231
800-AHA-USA-1 or 800-242-8721
www.americanheart.org/

American Society of Hypertension
515 Madison Avenue, Suite 1212
New York, NY 10022
212-644-0650
Fax: 212-644-0658
www.ash-us.org/

National High Blood Pressure Education Program
National Heart, Lung, and Blood Institute
4733 Bethesda Avenue, Suite 530
Bethesda, MD 20814
301-951-3260
www.nhlbi.nih.gov/hbp/index.html

For additional Internet resources, see the website for this book at *http://evolve.elsevier.com/Lewis/medsurg.*

CHAPTER **33**

NURSING MANAGEMENT
Coronary Artery Disease and Acute Coronary Syndrome

Linda Griego Martinez

LEARNING OBJECTIVES

1. Describe the etiology and pathophysiology of coronary artery disease.
2. Explain the nursing role in health promotion related to risk factors for coronary artery disease.
3. Describe the precipitating factors, types, clinical manifestations, collaborative care, and nursing management of angina pectoris.
4. Describe the clinical spectrum of acute coronary syndrome.
5. Describe the pathophysiology of myocardial infarction from the onset of injury through the healing process.

6. Describe the clinical manifestations, complications, diagnostic study results, and collaborative care of the patient with a myocardial infarction.
7. Identify commonly used drug therapy in treating patients with coronary artery disease and acute coronary syndrome.
8. Describe the nursing management of the patient following a myocardial infarction.
9. Describe the precipitating factors, types, clinical presentation, and collaborative care of the patient with or at risk for sudden cardiac death.

KEY TERMS

acute coronary syndrome, p. 810
angina pectoris, p. 811
atherosclerosis, p. 799
collateral circulation, p. 801
coronary artery disease, p. 799
Dressler syndrome, p. 815
metabolic equivalent (MET), p. 831
myocardial infarction, p. 810
myocardial revascularization, p. 822

percutaneous coronary intervention, p. 821
Prinzmetal's angina, p. 812
silent ischemia, p. 812
stable angina, p. 809
stents, p. 821
sudden cardiac death, p. 833
unstable angina, p. 812

CORONARY ARTERY DISEASE

Coronary artery disease (CAD) is a type of blood vessel disorder that is included in the general category of atherosclerosis. The term **atherosclerosis** is derived from two Greek words: *athere,* meaning "fatty mush," and *skleros,* meaning "hard." This word combination indicates that atherosclerosis begins as soft deposits of fat that harden with age. Atherosclerosis is often referred to as "hardening of the arteries." Although this condition can occur in any artery in the body, the *atheromas* (fatty deposits) have a preference for the coronary arteries. Arteriosclerotic heart disease (ASHD), cardiovascular heart disease (CVHD), ischemic heart disease (IHD), coronary heart disease (CHD), and CAD are synonymous terms used to describe this disease process.

Cardiovascular diseases are the major cause of death in the United States (Fig. 33-1). The American Heart Association (AHA) reports that an estimated 1.1 million Americans will have an acute myocardial infarction (MI) in 2003 and 460,000 will die, half of them before reaching a hospital. Although the death

rate decreased by 26.3% between 1988 and 1998, heart attacks are still the leading cause of all cardiovascular disease deaths and deaths in general. An estimated 60,800,000 persons have one or more types of cardiovascular disease.[1] The estimated prevalence of CAD by age is presented in Fig. 33-2.

Etiology and Pathophysiology

Atherosclerosis is the major cause of CAD. It is characterized by a focal deposit of cholesterol and lipids, primarily within the intimal wall of the artery. The genesis of plaque for-

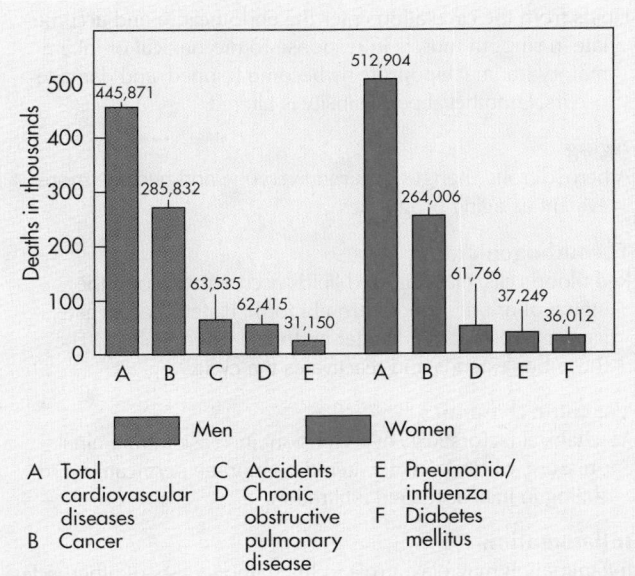

FIG. 33-1 Leading causes of death for men and women.

A Total cardiovascular diseases
B Cancer
C Accidents
D Chronic obstructive pulmonary disease
E Pneumonia/ influenza
F Diabetes mellitus

Reviewed by Janis L. Carelock, RN, MSN, CCRN, CNS, Clinical Instructor, School of Nursing, University of Texas at Austin, Austin, Tex.

mation is the result of complex interactions between the components of the blood and the elements forming the vascular wall.[2-4] Table 33-1 summarizes theories of atherogenesis, with endothelial injury being the leading theory for the cause of atherosclerotic disease.

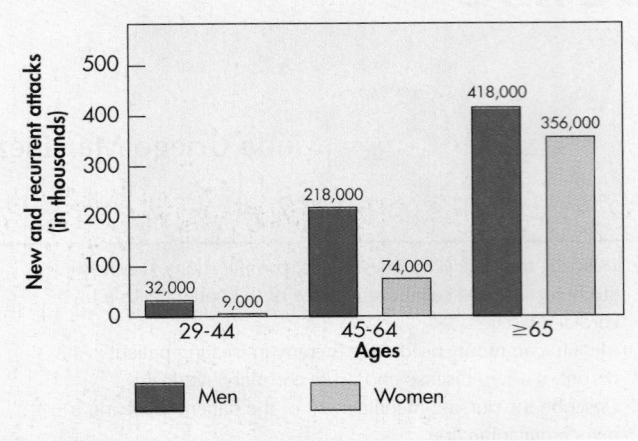

FIG. 33-2 Estimated annual number of Americans diagnosed with a heart attack by age and sex.

TABLE 33-1   Theories of Atherogenesis

Endothelial Injury
Endothelium is "injured" by hyperlipidemia, hypertension, or other chemical irritants. Factors are released into the subendothelium and induce the migration of smooth muscle cells into the intima. Smooth muscle cells initiate synthesis of collagen, elastic fiber proteins, and proteoglycans (a substance that tends to provide a nonthrombogenic surface). Intracellular and extracellular lipids begin to accumulate, as well as platelets and other clotting factors, and a lesion-associated superimposed thrombus is formed.

Lipid Infiltration
Lipids from the circulation enter the endothelium and accumulate in smooth muscle in response to mechanical or inflammatory trauma. Lipoproteins become trapped, and damage occurs. Endothelial permeability is altered.

Aging
Atherosclerotic changes occur in everyone and become more evident as aging progresses.

Thrombogenic
Red blood cells, platelets, and lipids accumulate along the intima of arteries. Microthrombi form. Platelets aggregate, releasing substances that alter endothelial permeability. The thrombus extends and reactivates the cycle.

Vascular Dynamics
Mechanical factors (e.g., hypertension) increase intraluminal pressure, which leads to altered membrane permeability, resulting in increased lipid infiltration.

Inflammation
Inflammation may play a role in the pathogenesis of atherosclerosis. The inflammatory reaction may be a consequence of infectious stimuli.

Intact normal endothelium is nonreactive to platelets and leukocytes, as well as coagulation, fibrinolytic, and complement factors. However, the endothelial lining can be altered as a result of chemical injuries, such as hyperlipidemia (nondenuding), or high-shear stress, such as hypertension (denuding). There is some evidence to suggest that certain systemic bacterial and viral infections play a role in damaging endothelium by causing a local inflammatory response, thus contributing to the development of atherosclerosis.[4] C-reactive protein (CRP), a nonspecific marker of inflammation, is increased in many patients with CAD. Chronic exposure to CRP triggers the rupture of plaques.[4]

With endothelial alteration, platelets are activated, and they release a growth factor that stimulates smooth muscle proliferation. The smooth muscle cell proliferation entraps lipids, which are calcified over time and form an irritant to the endothelium on which platelets adhere and aggregate. Thrombin is generated, and fibrin formation and thrombi occur (Fig. 33-3). Endothelial

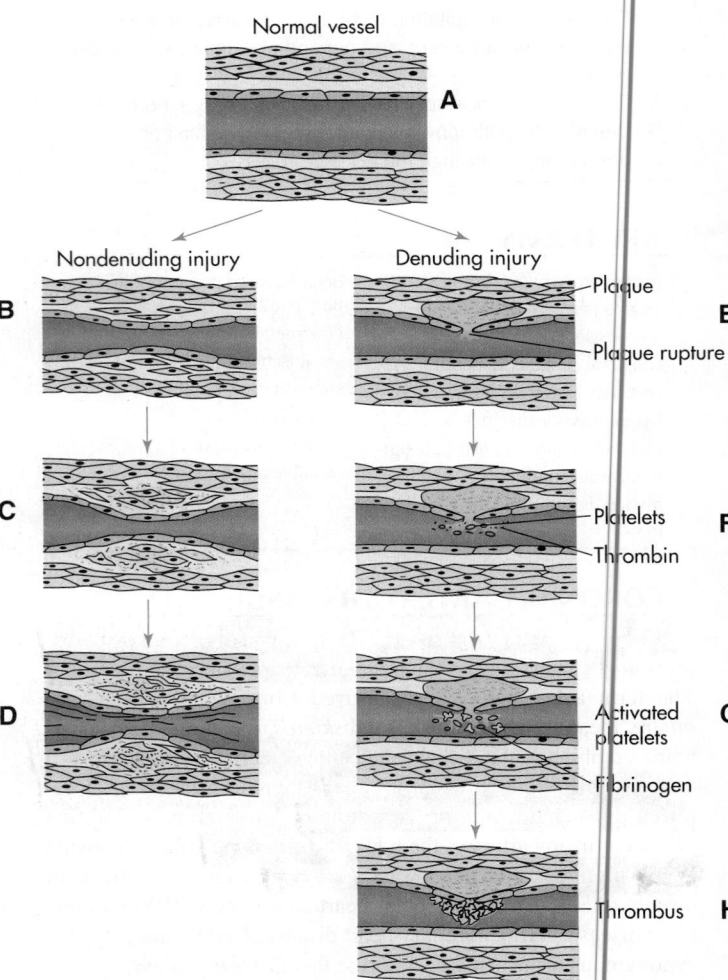

FIG. 33-3 Response to endothelial injury. **A,** Normal vessel, endothelium intact. **B,** Nondenuding injury (e.g., hyperlipidemia) with smooth muscle proliferation. **C,** Addition of collagen and fibroelastic tissues that narrow lumen. **D,** Narrowed lumen with calcification and irregular blood flow. **E,** Denuding injury with plaque rupture. **F,** As platelets adhere to the damaged area, they are activated. **G,** Activation of the exposed platelets causes expression of glycoprotein IIb/IIIa receptors that bind fibrinogen. **H,** Further platelet aggregation and adhesion eventually results in an enlarging thrombus.

replication is normally slow in adults, but in the presence of hypertension and hyperlipidemia, increased cell turnover leads to transient repeated denuding of the endothelium.

Developmental Stages. CAD takes many years to develop. When it becomes symptomatic, the disease process is usually well advanced. The stages of development in atherosclerosis are (1) fatty streak, (2) raised fibrous plaque resulting from smooth muscle cell proliferation, and (3) complicated lesion (Fig. 33-4).

Fatty streak. *Fatty streaks,* the earliest lesions of atherosclerosis, are characterized by lipid-filled smooth muscle cells.[2,3] As streaks of fat develop within the smooth muscle cells, a yellow tinge appears. Fatty streaks are usually observed in the coronary arteries by age 15 and involve an increasing amount of surface area as the patient ages. It is generally believed that they are reversible.

Raised fibrous plaque. The *raised fibrous plaque stage* is the beginning of progressive changes in the arterial wall. These changes appear in the coronary arteries by age 30 and increase with age. The arterial wall changes are initiated by chronic endothelial injury that results from many factors, including elevated blood pressure (BP), high blood cholesterol, heredity, carbon monoxide produced by smoking, immune reactions, and possibly toxic substances within the blood.

Normally the endothelium repairs itself immediately, but in the person with CAD the endothelium is not rapidly replaced, allowing low-density lipoproteins and growth factors from platelets to stimulate smooth muscle proliferation and thickening of the arterial wall. Once endothelial injury has occurred, lipoproteins (the carrier substances within the bloodstream) transport cholesterol and other lipids into the arterial intima (see Fig. 33-4). Lipids may cause smooth muscle damage and contribute to plaque thickening and instability.[2-4] As these lipids and other substances pass through the vessels, they adhere to the roughened, damaged wall,

thereby causing the lesion buildup or structural abnormality. Collagen tissue, elastic fibers, and smooth muscle cells filled with fat cover the lesion. The fibrous plaque appears grayish or whitish. These plaques can form on one portion of the artery or in a circular fashion involving the entire lumen. The borders can be smooth or irregular with rough, jagged edges.[2,5]

Platelets also play a part in the hypertrophy of smooth muscle cells. Once the artery's inner wall has become damaged, platelets may accumulate in large numbers, leading to a thrombus. The thrombus may adhere to the wall of the artery, leading to narrowing or total occlusion of the artery.

Activation of the exposed platelets causes expression of glycoprotein IIb/IIIa receptors that bind fibrinogen. This, in turn, leads to further platelet aggregation and adhesion, further enlarging the thrombus.

Complicated lesion. The final stage in the development of the atherosclerotic lesion is the most dangerous. The plaque consists of a core of lipid materials (mainly cholesterol) within an area of dead tissue. With the incorporation of lipids, thrombi, damaged tissue, and accumulation of calcium, the growing lesion becomes complex. As the lesion continues to grow and become complex, necrotic tissue that is hardened appears within the arteries, causing rigidity and hardening. This complicated lesion may totally or partially occlude the artery.

Collateral Circulation. Normally some arterial branching, termed **collateral circulation,** exists within the coronary circulation. The growth of collateral circulation is attributed to two factors: (1) the inherited predisposition to develop new blood vessels and (2) the presence of chronic ischemia. When an atherosclerotic plaque occludes the normal flow of blood through a coronary artery and ischemia is chronic, increased collateral circulation develops (Fig. 33-5). When occlusion of the coronary arteries occurs slowly over a long period, there is a greater chance of adequate collateral circulation developing, and the myocardium may still receive an adequate amount of oxygen. However, with rapid-onset CAD or coronary spasm, the time is inadequate for collateral development, and a diminished arterial flow results in a more severe ischemia or infarction. Clinically the younger person will have a more severe myocardial infarction as a result of inadequate collateral formation.

Risk Factors for Coronary Artery Disease

Risk factors are characteristics or conditions that are statistically associated with a high incidence of a disease. Many risk factors have been associated with CAD. Risk factors in differ-

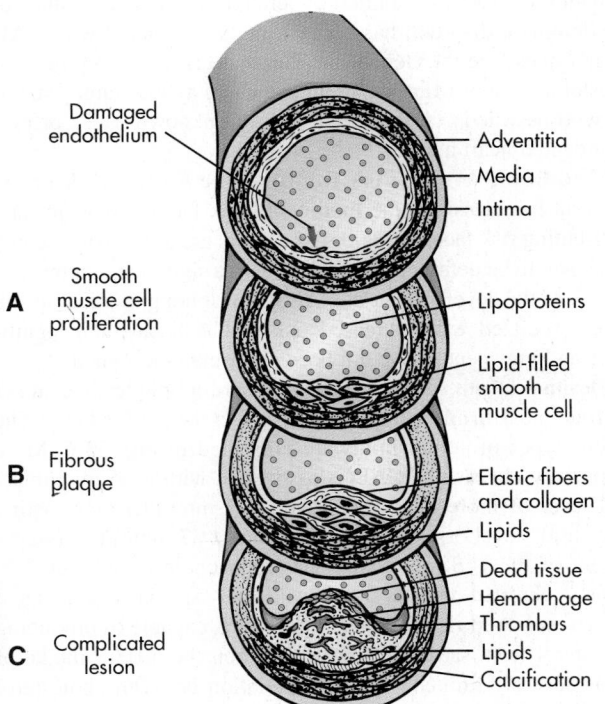

FIG. 33-4 The stages of development in the progression of atherosclerosis include **A,** smooth muscle cell proliferation, which creates **B,** a raised fibrous plaque and **C,** a complicated lesion.

Damaged endothelium
Adventitia
Media
Intima
A Smooth muscle cell proliferation
Lipoproteins
Lipid-filled smooth muscle cell
B Fibrous plaque
Elastic fibers and collagen
Lipids
Dead tissue
Hemorrhage
Thrombus
Lipids
C Complicated lesion
Calcification

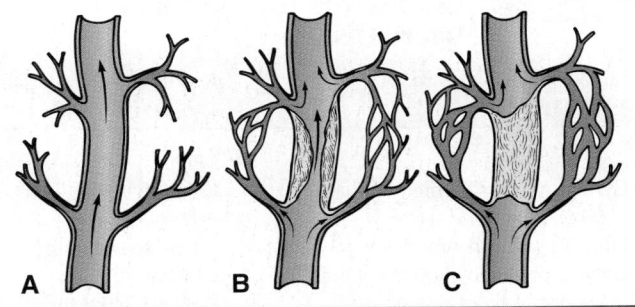

FIG. 33-5 Vessel occlusion with collateral circulation. **A,** Open, functioning coronary artery. **B,** Partial coronary artery closure with collateral circulation being established. **C,** Total coronary artery occlusion with collateral circulation bypassing the occlusion to supply the myocardium.

CULTURAL & ETHNIC CONSIDERATIONS
Coronary Artery Disease

- White, middle-aged men have the highest incidence of coronary artery disease.
- African Americans have an early age of onset of coronary artery disease.
- African American women have a higher incidence and death rate related to coronary artery disease than white women.
- African Americans have more severe coronary artery disease than whites.
- Native Americans less than 35 years of age have heart disease mortality rates twice as high as other Americans.
- Major modifiable cardiovascular risk factors for Native Americans are obesity and diabetes mellitus.
- Hispanics have lower death rates from heart disease than non-Hispanics.

GENETICS in CLINICAL PRACTICE
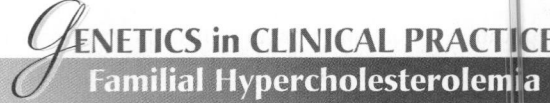
Familial Hypercholesterolemia

Genetic Basis
- Autosomal dominant disorder
- Mutation in gene coding for the low-density lipoprotein (LDL) receptor
- Multiple mutant alleles

Incidence
- Heterozygotes: 1 in 500
- Homozygotes: rare

Genetic Testing
- Disorder characterized by elevated serum LDL
- Serum lipid profile can be used to measure total cholesterol, triglycerides, LDLs, and high-density lipoproteins (HDLs)
- DNA testing available

Clinical Implications
- Common genetic disease
- Leading cause of coronary artery disease
- High cholesterol levels are a result of defective function of the LDL receptors
- Plasma levels of LDL elevated throughout life
- Develop severe atherosclerosis in early to middle years

ent populations may vary. For example, major risk factors for CAD in the United States, such as high serum cholesterol and hypertension, are less prevalent in Japanese and Puerto Rican populations.[2,3]

Risk factors can be categorized as unmodifiable and modifiable (Table 33-2). *Unmodifiable risk factors* are age, gender, ethnicity, and genetic inheritance. *Modifiable risk factors* include elevated serum lipids, hypertension, smoking, obesity, physical inactivity, and stress in daily living. Control of diabetes is highly recommended based on evidence that high glucose levels accelerate atherosclerosis.[6,7]

Data on risk factors have been obtained in several major studies. In the Framingham study (one of the most widely known), 5209 men and women were observed for 20 years. Over time, it was noted that elevated serum cholesterol (greater than 240 mg/dl), elevated systolic BP (greater than 160 mm Hg), and cigarette smoking (one or more packs a day) were positively correlated with an increased incidence of CAD. Other implicated risk factors and indicators included diabetes mellitus, physical inactivity, electrocardiogram (ECG) abnormalities, and reduced lung vital capacity.

Unmodifiable Risk Factors

Age and gender. The incidence of MI is highest among white, middle-aged men. After age 65, the incidence in men and women equalizes, although there is early evidence suggesting that more

women have CAD earlier because of increased stress, increased cigarette smoking, presence of hypertension, and use of birth control pills.

Family history and heredity. Genetic predisposition is an important factor in the occurrence of CAD, although the exact mechanism of inheritance is not fully understood. Some congenital defects in coronary artery walls predispose the person to the formation of plaques. Familial hypercholesterolemia, an autosomal dominant disorder, has been strongly associated with CAD at early ages (see the Genetics in Clinical Practice box). In most cases of angina or MI, the patient can name a close family member who has died either suddenly of an unknown cause or of a documented heart attack.

Modifiable Major Risk Factors. The American Heart Association has classified the modifiable risk factors as major and contributing risk factors. Major risk factors are those that research has shown to be definitely associated with a significant increase in the risk of the development of CAD. Contributing risk factors are those associated with increased risk of CAD, but their significance and prevalence have not been precisely determined.[3,8]

Elevated serum lipids. An elevated serum lipid level is one of the four most firmly established risk factors for CAD.[2,3,8] The various types of serum lipids are presented in Fig. 33-6. More specifically, the risk of CAD is associated with a serum cholesterol level of more than 200 mg/dl (5.2 mmol/L) or a fasting triglyceride level of more than 200 mg/dl (1.7 mmol/L). Twenty percent of the U.S. population has high cholesterol levels.[9] In women, elevated triglyceride levels are especially associated with an increased risk of CAD. The liver is capable of producing cholesterol from saturated fats, even when the dietary intake of fats is severely limited. A high correlation between cholesterol and triglyceride levels has been found. Elevated triglyceride and cholesterol levels are correlated with obesity, physical inactivity, high alcohol intake, and intake of trans fatty acids found in such snack foods as cookies, crackers, and french fries.

TABLE 33-2 **Risk Factors for Coronary Artery Disease**

UNMODIFIABLE RISK FACTORS	MODIFIABLE RISK FACTORS
Age	*Major*
Gender (men > women until 60 yr of age)	Elevated serum lipids
Ethnicity (African Americans <whites)	Hypertension
Genetic predisposition and family history of heart disease	Cigarette smoking
	Obesity
	Physical inactivity
	Contributing
	Diabetes mellitus*
	Stressful lifestyle

*A person may have a genetic predisposition to developing diabetes.

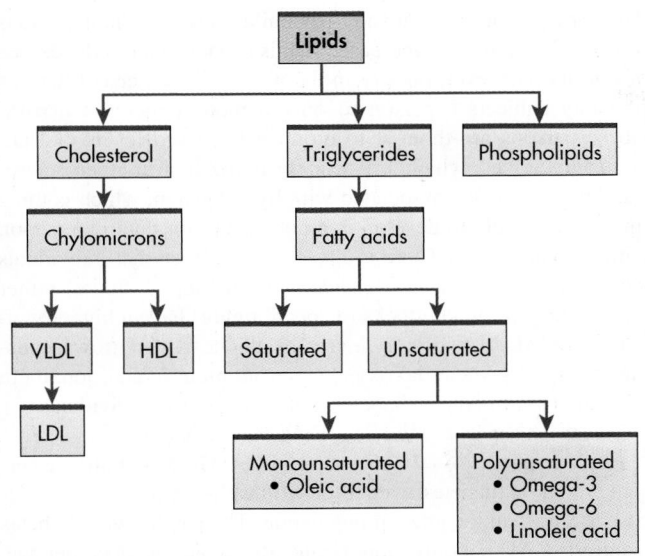

FIG. 33-6 Types of serum lipids. *HDL,* High-density lipoprotein; *LDL,* low-density lipoprotein; *VLDL,* very-low-density lipoprotein.

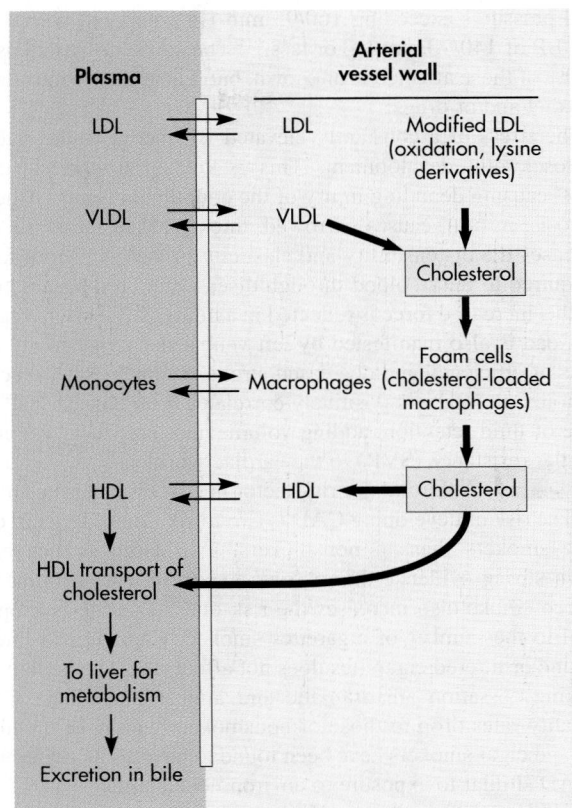

FIG. 33-7 Specific types of plasma lipoproteins (*LDL* and *VLDL*) deliver cholesterol to cells of the blood vessel wall, mostly to macrophages that become cholesterol foam cells. These are predominant early features of atherosclerotic lesions. *HDL* is an important cholesterol-transporting carrier, delivering cholesterol to the liver to be excreted in the bile.

For lipids to be used and transported by the body, they must become soluble in blood by combining with proteins. Lipids combine with protein to form *lipoproteins.* Lipoproteins are vehicles for fat mobilization and transport. The different types of lipoprotein vary in composition and are classified as high-density lipoproteins (HDLs), low-density lipoproteins (LDLs), and very-low-density lipoproteins (VLDLs) (see Fig. 33-6).

HDLs contain more protein by weight and less lipid than any other lipoprotein. HDLs carry lipids away from arteries and to the liver for metabolism (Fig. 33-7). Therefore high serum HDL levels are desirable. This process of HDL transport prevents lipid accumulation within the arterial walls. The higher the HDL levels in the blood, the lower the risk of CAD. HDL levels are generally higher in women than in men and are increased by physical activity. The person who has had an MI usually has lower concentrations of HDL than matched controls. In general, HDL levels are high in children and women, decrease with age, and are low in persons with CAD. Current research on drug and dietary therapy is concentrating on ways to increase HDL levels.[10-12]

HDLs are broken down into HDL_2 and HDL_3. HDL_2 helps clear out the fat load from the plasma. HDL_2 protects the arteries from developing atherosclerosis. Exercise can raise HDL_2, but more so in men than postmenopausal women and older adults. Premenopausal women have HDL_2 levels approximately three times greater than men. After menopause, their HDL_2 levels quickly approximate those of men.

LDLs contain more cholesterol than any of the other lipoproteins and have an affinity for arterial walls.[9-11] Elevated LDL levels correlate most closely with an increased incidence of atherosclerosis. Therefore low serum LDL levels are desirable.[11-13]

VLDLs contain most of the triglycerides. The direct correlation of VLDLs with heart disease is uncertain. High VLDL concentrations may increase the risk of premature atherosclerosis when associated with other factors such as diabetes, hypertension, and cigarette smoking.

Other lipoproteins of importance in CAD include apolipoprotein A-1 (Apo A-1), apolipoprotein B (Apo B), and lipoprotein (a), or Lp (a). Apo A-l is primarily found in the HDL particle. It

is a convenient marker for assessing cholesterol clearing capacity of the blood. It is associated with a lower risk for heart disease. Over 90% of LDL is composed of Apo B. It is a convenient marker of the cholesterol-depositing capacity of the blood. Apo B is associated with high levels of LDL and is an independent risk factor for CAD. Lp (a), which is genetically inherited, is bound to both HDL and LDL. It interferes with plasminogen, the enzyme that dissolves clots. Elevated Lp (a) levels contribute to blood clot formation and over a prolonged period of time can lead to significant damage to the coronary arteries.[13]

LDL levels below 130 mg/dl (3.36 mmol/L) are desirable. LDL levels of 130 to 159 mg/dl (3.36 to 4.12 mmol/L) place a person at a borderline high risk of cardiovascular disease. Levels above 160 mg/dl (4.14 mmol/L) place a person at high risk. People with HDL levels of 36 to 44 mg/dl (0.9 to 1.1 mmol/L) have a moderate risk of cardiovascular disease. HDL levels below 35 mg/dl (0.9 mmol/L) are a major risk factor. People with HDL levels between 45 and 59 mg/dl (1.2 and 1.5 mmol/L) carry an average risk for cardiovascular disease. HDL levels above 60 mg/dl (1.6 mmol/L) are a negative risk factor. Total cholesterol/HDL ratio represents the relationship between the total cholesterol and the HDL. It is useful in assessing a person's risk for developing CAD.

Hypertension. The second major risk factor in CAD is hypertension, which is defined as a BP greater than or equal to 140/90 mm Hg. In the Framingham study, a threefold increase in the incidence of CAD was reported for middle-aged men with arterial pressures exceeding 160/95 mm Hg compared with those with BP of 140/90 mm Hg or less.[8,11] The cause of hypertension in 90% of those affected is unknown, but it is usually controllable with diet and/or drugs.

The stress of a constantly elevated BP increases the rate of atherosclerotic development. This is related to the shearing stress, causing denuding injury of the endothelial lining. Atherosclerosis, in turn, causes narrowed, thickened arterial walls and decreases the distensibility and elasticity of vessels. More force is required to pump blood through diseased arterial vasculature, and this increased force is reflected in a higher BP. This increased workload is also manifested by left ventricular hypertrophy and a loss of efficiency and decreased stroke volume with each contraction. Salt intake is positively correlated with elevated BP because of fluid retention, adding volume and increasing systemic vascular resistance (SVR) to the cardiac workload.

Smoking. A third major risk factor in CAD is cigarette smoking. The risk of developing CAD is two to six times higher in cigarette smokers than in nonsmokers. Two large studies have shown strong evidence that chronic exposure to environmental tobacco smoke also increases the risk of CAD. Risk is proportional to the number of cigarettes smoked. Changing to lower-nicotine or filtered cigarettes does not affect risk. The benefits of smoking cessation are dramatic and almost immediate. CAD mortality rates drop to those of nonsmokers within 12 months.[8] Pipe and cigar smokers have been found to have an increased risk of CAD similar to exposure to environmental smoke.

Nicotine in cigarette smoke causes catecholamine (epinephrine, norepinephrine) release. These hormones cause an increased heart rate (HR), peripheral vasoconstriction, and increased BP. These changes increase the cardiac workload, necessitating greater myocardial oxygen consumption. Nicotine also increases platelet adhesion.[8]

Carbon monoxide, a by-product of combustion, affects the oxygen-carrying capacity of hemoglobin by reducing the sites available for oxygen transport. Thus the effects of an increased cardiac workload, combined with the oxygen-depleting effect of carbon monoxide from smoking, significantly decrease the oxygen available to the myocardium. There is also some indication that carbon monoxide may be a chemical irritant as well, thus causing nondenuding injury to the endothelium.[8]

Physical inactivity. Physical inactivity is a fourth major modifiable risk factor. Physical inactivity implies a lack of adequate physical exercise on a regular basis. Some practitioners define regular physical exercise as exercise that occurs at least three times a week for at least 30 minutes, causing perspiration and an increase in HR by 30 to 50 beats per minute.

The mechanism by which physical inactivity predisposes to CAD is still unknown. Physically active people have increased HDL levels and exercise enhances fibrinolytic activity, thus reducing the risk of clot formation. It is also believed that exercise encourages the development of collateral circulation.

Exercise training for those who are physically inactive decreases the risk of CAD through more efficient lipid metabolism, increased HDL_2 production, and more efficient oxygen extraction from the working muscle groups, thereby decreasing the cardiac workload. It may be observed that physically active persons are seldom obese, thus eliminating two risk factors in CAD.[11]

Obesity. The mortality rate from CAD is statistically higher in obese (defined as a weight 30% or more than that considered standard for a person's height and body build) persons than in persons of normal weight. The increased risk is proportional to the degree of obesity. However, obesity in the absence of other risk factors probably subjects a person to only a modest increase in risk. Obese persons are thought to produce increased levels of LDL and triglycerides, which are strongly implicated in atherosclerosis. Obesity is often associated with hypertension, which is three times more likely to develop in an obese person than in a person with normal weight. There is also some evidence that individuals who tend to store fat in the abdomen (an "apple" figure) rather than in the hips and buttocks (a "pear" figure) have a higher incidence of CAD.[11] As obesity increases, the heart size grows, causing increased myocardial oxygen consumption. In addition, there is an increase in type 2 diabetes mellitus in obese individuals.

Modifiable Contributing Risk Factors

Diabetes mellitus. The incidence of CAD is greater among persons who have diabetes, even those with well-controlled blood glucose levels, than the general population. The patient with diabetes manifests CAD not only more frequently but also at an earlier age. There is no age difference between male or female patients with diabetes in the onset of manifestations of CAD. Diabetes virtually eliminates the lower incidence of CAD in women. Latent diabetes is frequently diagnosed at the time of MI. Because the person with diabetes has an increased tendency toward connective tissue degeneration, it is thought that this condition may account for the tendency toward atheroma development seen in the patient with diabetes. Diabetic patients also have alterations in lipid metabolism and tend to have high cholesterol and triglyceride levels.[6,11]

Stress and behavior patterns. Several behavior patterns have been correlated with CAD. However, the study of these behaviors remains controversial and complex. The Framingham study provided evidence that certain behaviors and lifestyles are conducive to the development of CAD.[14,15] Type A and type B behaviors were described by Friedman and Rosenman in the 1960s and were further elaborated in the 1970s by Jenkins and Zyzanski.[8,15] Type A behaviors include perfectionism and a hardworking, driving personality. The type A person suppresses anger and hostility, has a sense of time urgency, is impatient, and creates stress and tension, often when a situation does not warrant it. This person is more prone to heart attacks than a type B person, who is more easygoing, takes upsets in stride, knows personal limitations, takes time to relax, is not an overachiever, and is able to keep priorities in perspective. Although not all characteristics are present in one person all the time, people tend to be either type A or type B. Meta-analysis of the type A personality studies has shown that the studies that demonstrated a positive correlation between type A personality and CAD were equal in number to the studies that failed to show a correlation with CAD.[14,15]

Studies now are focusing on specific components of the type A personality. Specifically, hostility and anger have both been linked with CAD, especially in men.[14] Continued research is needed in the field of personality, behavior, and risk for CAD.

Stress has also been correlated with the development of CAD. Sympathetic nervous system (SNS) stimulation and its effect on the heart are generally considered to be the physiologic mechanism by which stress predisposes to the development of CAD. SNS stimulation causes an increased release of epinephrine and norepinephrine. This stimulation influences the heart by increasing the HR and intensifying the force of myocardial contraction. Therefore the demand for oxygen greatly increases. Also, stress-induced mechanisms can cause elevated lipid levels and alterations in blood coagulation, which can lead to increased atherogenesis.[8]

Homocysteine. High blood levels of homocysteine have been linked to an increased risk for CAD and other cardiovascular diseases.[10,14] Homocysteine, a sulfur-containing amino acid, is produced by the breakdown of the essential amino acid methionine, which is found in dietary protein. High homocysteine levels possibly contribute to atherosclerosis by (1) damaging the inner lining of blood vessels, (2) promoting plaque buildup, and (3) altering the clotting mechanism to make clots more likely to occur.

Research is ongoing to determine if a decline in homocysteine can reduce the risk of heart disease. Generally, a screening test for homocysteine is not recommended, but limited to those suspected of having elevated levels such as older patients with pernicious anemia or people who develop CAD at an early age. B-complex vitamins (B_6, B_{12}, folic acid) have been shown to work together to lower blood levels of homocysteine.

Health Promotion. The appropriate management of risk factors in CAD may prevent, modify, or retard the progression of the disease. In the United States during the past 20 to 30 years there has been a gradual and persistent decline in coronary deaths. The decline can be attributed to the efforts of people to become generally healthier and individual initiatives to alter unhealthy and hazardous lifestyles. Emphasis on prevention and early treatment of heart disease must be ongoing.

Identification of high-risk persons. In both the acute care setting and the community, the nurse should identify the person at risk for CAD. Risk screening involves obtaining personal and family health histories. The patient should be questioned about a family history of heart disease in parents, grandparents, or siblings. The presence of any cardiovascular symptoms should be noted. Environmental factors, such as eating habits, type of diet, and level of exercise, are assessed to elicit lifestyle patterns. A psychosocial history is included to determine smoking habits, alcohol ingestion, type A behaviors, recent life-stressing events, sleeping habits, and the presence of anxiety or depression. The place of work and the type of work can provide important information on the kind of activity performed; exposure to pollutants, allergens, or noxious chemicals; and the degree of emotional stress associated with employment.

The nurse should identify the patient's attitudes and beliefs about health and illness. This information can give some indication of how disease and lifestyle changes may affect the patient and can reveal possible misconceptions about heart disease. Knowledge of the patient's educational background is frequently helpful in deciding at what level to begin teaching. If the patient is taking medications, it is important to know what they are, when they are taken, and what the patient's compliance and attitudes are regarding the taking of medications.

Management of high-risk persons. Once a high-risk person is identified, preventive measures can be taken. Risk factors such as age, gender, and genetic inheritance cannot be modified. However, the person with any of these risk factors can modify the risk of CAD by controlling or changing the additive effects of modifiable risk factors. For example, a young man with a family history of heart disease can decrease the risk of an MI by maintaining an ideal weight, getting adequate physical exercise, reducing intake of saturated fats, and not smoking.

The person who has modifiable risk factors should be encouraged and motivated to make changes in lifestyle to reduce the risk

of heart disease. The nurse can play a major role in teaching health-promoting behaviors to the person at risk for CAD (Table 33-3). For highly motivated persons, knowing how to reduce this risk may be the only information needed to get them to make changes.

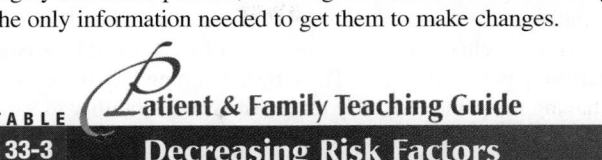

TABLE 33-3	Patient & Family Teaching Guide — Decreasing Risk Factors for Coronary Artery Disease	
RISK FACTOR	**HEALTH-PROMOTING BEHAVIORS**
Hypertension	• Have regular blood pressure (BP) checkups • Take prescribed medications for BP control • Reduce salt intake • Stop smoking • Control or reduce weight • Exercise regularly
Elevated Serum Lipids	• Reduce total fat intake • Reduce animal (saturated) fat intake • Adjust total caloric intake to achieve and maintain ideal body weight • Engage in regular exercise program • Increase amount of complex carbohydrates and vegetable proteins in diet
Smoking*	• Enroll in program to stop smoking • Change daily routines associated with smoking to reduce desire to smoke • Substitute other activities for smoking • Ask family members to support efforts to stop smoking
Physical Inactivity	• Develop and maintain routine for physical activity that is done at least three to four times a week • Increase activities to a fitness level
Stressful Lifestyle	• Increase awareness of behaviors that are detrimental to health • Alter patterns that are conducive to stress and rushing (e.g., get up 30 min earlier so breakfast is not eaten on way to work) • Set realistic goals for self • Reassess priorities in light of health needs • Learn effective coping strategies • Avoid excessive and prolonged stress • Take 20 min/day to meditate • Plan time for adequate rest and sleep
Obesity	• Change eating patterns and habits • Reduce caloric intake • Exercise regularly to increase caloric expenditure • Avoid fad and crash diets, which are not effective in the long run • Avoid large, heavy meals
Diabetes Mellitus†	• Follow the recommended diet • Reduce weight and control diet • Monitor blood glucose levels regularly

*Smoking cessation is discussed in Chapter 11 and Tables 11-13 and 11-14.
†See Chapter 47 for additional health-promoting behaviors.

For the person who is less motivated to assume responsibility for health, the idea of risk factor reduction may be so remote that the person is unable to perceive a threat of CAD in his or her life. Especially in the absence of symptoms, few persons desire to make lifestyle changes. The nurse should first assist this person in clarifying personal values. Then, by explaining the risk factors and having the person identify the personal vulnerability to various risks, the nurse may help the person recognize the susceptibility to CAD. The nurse may also help the person set realistic goals and allow the person to choose which risk factor to change first. Some persons are reluctant to change until they begin to manifest overt symptoms or actually suffer an MI. Others, having suffered an MI, may find the idea of changing lifelong habits totally unacceptable. The nurse must be able to identify such attitudes and respect them.

Physical fitness. In the past 30 years there has been a surge of interest in attaining and maintaining health. Physical fitness has become a field of major importance. Communities are developing exercise programs for persons of all ages and with all health needs, ranging from aerobic exercise classes to cardiac walking-jogging programs. Local YMCAs often sponsor exercise classes, jogging courses, bicycling courses, and related offerings. Many shopping malls open their doors in the early morning to allow people to walk indoors. The AHA takes pride in its annual "Heart Walk," as well as other events dramatizing the need for physical activity to promote health. Many large corporations provide gymnasiums where their employees can exercise. For many people, running may be inadvisable; these people should be encouraged to pursue walking, swimming, or whatever exercise will accommodate their individual physical abilities.

Health education in schools. The recent awareness of the body and physical health is also seen in school systems. The school nurse has an important role in teaching good health practices. Besides teaching physical fitness topics, the school nurse can inform students on how the body functions and responds to daily living. Lifestyle habits can be positively influenced at early ages to decrease the need for drastic changes later in life that confront the students' parents. The school nurse should take advantage of the social climate that promotes health and health practices and find innovative ways to present these values to a receptive, youthful audience before the habits of that audience become inflexible. The AHA has established school programs such as "Heart Power," which provides teaching materials for teachers to incorporate into their curriculum. Volunteers from the AHA are also available to help teachers educate children in their schools about healthy habits for better cardiac health.

Nutritional Therapy. The patient with elevated serum cholesterol and triglyceride levels should first achieve a normal weight if overweight. Then the patient should be maintained on a diet that emphasizes a decreased intake of saturated fat and cholesterol, such as the step 1 diet recommended by the AHA.[9-12] Red meats, eggs, and milk products are major sources of saturated fat and cholesterol. If the serum triglyceride level is elevated, alcohol intake and simple sugars should be reduced or eliminated. If within 6 months there is no trend toward lower blood cholesterol, the patient should be placed on the step 2 diet of the AHA, which further restricts intake of saturated fats and cholesterol[9-12] (Table 33-4).

The average reduction in total serum cholesterol levels with diet is 5% to 15%.[15] The highly motivated individual who adheres stringently to a low-fat diet may reduce total cholesterol more dramatically. Several studies have demonstrated regression in coronary atherosclerosis and reduction in coronary events by lifestyle changes, including a low-saturated-fat diet, smoking cessation, and increase in physical activity.[16,17] Many of these studies also included drug therapy as well.[9,11,17,18]

Drug Therapy. In the United States an estimated 65 million Americans have high cholesterol levels. A complete lipid profile is recommended every 5 years beginning when a person is 20 years old. The person with serum cholesterol levels greater than 200 mg/dl (5.2 mmol/L) is at high risk for CAD and should be treated. Treatment usually begins with dietary caloric restriction, decreased dietary fat content, lower cholesterol intake, and exercise instruction. The guidelines for treatment of high cholesterol focus on LDL levels (Table 33-5). Serum cholesterol levels are reassessed after 6 months of diet therapy. If they remain elevated, drug therapy may be started (see Table 33-5). Various drugs are available to treat hyperlipidemia[9,11,19-21] (Table 33-6).

Drugs that increase lipoprotein removal. The major route of elimination of cholesterol is via conversion to bile acids in the liver. Resins primarily lower LDL and also cause an increase in HDL. Resins are nonabsorbable compounds that interfere with the enterohepatic circulation of bile acids. Resins increase conversion of cholesterol to bile acids and decrease hepatic cholesterol content.

The resins are cholestyramine (Questran), colestipol (Colestid), and colesevelam (Welchol). A preparation of cholestyramine (Colybar) containing 4 g of cholestyramine in a bar form is also available. Administration of these drugs can be associated with complaints related to palatability and with a variety of upper and lower gastrointestinal (GI) symptoms, including constipation, abdominal pain, belching, heartburn, and nausea. The resins have been known to interfere with absorption of other drugs, such as warfarin, thiazides, thyroid hormones, and β-adrenergic block-

EVIDENCE-BASED PRACTICE
Fruits and Vegetables Protect Against Cardiovascular Disease

Clinical Problem
Do fruits and vegetables reduce the risk of cardiovascular disease (CVD)?

Best Clinical Practice
- Higher intake of fruit and vegetables may be protective against CVD.
- These data support current dietary guidelines to increase fruit and vegetable intake.

Implications for Nursing Practice
- Nutrition has a key role in preventing and reducing the risk of CVD.
- Patients and families need to be taught the value of including fruits and vegetables in their diet.

References for Evidence
Liu S et al: Fruit and vegetable intake and risk of cardiovascular disease: the Women's Health Study, *Am J Clin Nutr* 72:922, 2000.
Liu S et al: Intake of vegetables rich in carotenoids and risk of coronary heart disease in men: the Physicians' Health Study, *Int J Epidemiol* 30:130, 2001.

TABLE 33-4	**Nutritional Therapy**
	Coronary Artery Disease

Comparison of Step 1 Low-Fat Diet and Step 2 Low-Fat Diet

Principles of Step 1 Diet

8% to 10% of total calories come from saturated fat; ≤30% of total calories come from fat.

- Visible fat (e.g., butter, cream, margarine, salad dressing, cooking oil) is restricted to 1 tsp per meal.
- Unsaturated vegetable oils should be used.
- Only lean meats, skim milk or 1% milk, and no more than 3 egg yolks per week are used.
- Food high in fat content (e.g., avocados, fat, meat, olives, nuts) are avoided.
- Cooking methods such as steaming, baking, broiling, grilling, or stir-frying in small amounts of fat are recommended.

Principles of Step 2 Diet

<7% of total calories come from saturated fat; ≤30% of total calories come from fat.

- Only leanest cuts of meats are allowed.
- Organ meats and shrimp are restricted because they are high in cholesterol although low in total fat.
- Only 1 egg yolk per week is used because egg yolk is high in cholesterol. Egg whites or egg substitutes may be used as desired.
- Vegetable oils are used in cooking and food preparation. Coconut and palm oils are not allowed because of their high content of saturated fats. Choose margarine that contains 2 g or less of saturated fat per tablespoon.
- Skim milk is highly recommended. Low-fat yogurt and low-fat cheeses may be used. Low-fat ice milk or frozen yogurt or sherbet.

Sample Menus

	Step 1				Step 2		
Breakfast							
1 fruit	½ cup orange	1 banana	¼ cantaloupe	½ cup orange	1 banana	¼ cantaloupe	
1 starch	juice	½ cup oatmeal	½ cup corn meal	juice	½ cup oatmeal	½ cup corn meal	
3 eggs/wk	¾ cup dry	1 flour tortilla	mush	¾ cup dry cereal	1 corn tortilla	mush	
1 fat	cereal	1 cup skim milk	1 scrambled egg	Low-cholesterol	with 1 tsp	1 slice toast with	
1 skim milk	1 poached egg	Coffee with 1 tsp	1 slice toast with	egg	special	1 tsp special	
	1 slice toast with	cream	1 tsp butter or	1 slice toast with	vegetable oil	vegetable oil	
	1 tsp butter or		margarine	1 tsp special	margarine	margarine	
	margarine		1 cup skim milk	vegetable oil	1 cup skim milk	1 cup skim milk	
	1 cup skim milk		Coffee with	margarine	Coffee with	Coffee with	
	Coffee with		sugar	1 cup skim milk	sugar	sugar	
	sugar			Coffee with sugar			
Lunch							
2 meat	2 oz baked	3 oz lean	2 oz baked fish	3 oz baked chicken	¾ cup dry	4 oz baked fish	
2 starch	chicken	hamburger	Baked potato	(skinless)	cottage cheese	Fried potatoes	
1 vegetable	Mashed potato	Hamburger bun	Zucchini	Mashed potato with	with peach slices	(cooked with	
1 starch	Tossed salad with	Lettuce, tomato,	Bread with 1 tsp	1 tsp special	Saltine crackers	allowed oils)	
1 fat	vinegar, lemon	pickle, 1 tsp	butter or	vegetable oil	Cucumber and	Zucchini	
1 dessert	juice	mustard	margarine	margarine	tomato slices	Cornbread (made	
	Bread with	Sherbet	Gelatin dessert	Tossed salad with	1 tsp special	with allowed	
	1 tsp margarine	Carbonated	Lemonade	vinegar,	vegetable oil	oils)	
	or butter	beverage		vegetable oil	Sherbet	Gelatin dessert	
	Angel food cake			Angel food cake	Carbonated	Lemonade	
	Iced tea with sugar			Iced tea with sugar	beverage		
	and lemon			and lemon			
Dinner							
2 meat	2 oz lean roast	Green chili stew	2 oz lean pork	2 oz lean roast	Green chili stew	3 oz breaded	
2 starch	beef	(made with 2	chop	beef	(made with 2 oz	lean pork chop	
1 vegetable	Rice	oz lean beef	Corn on the cob	Rice with 1 tsp	lean beef cubes,	Corn on the cob	
1 fat	Green beans	cubes, potato	Okra	special	potato slices,	with 1 tsp	
1 fruit	Dinner roll with	slices, tomato,	Bread with	vegetable oil	tomato, chili)	special	
1 skim milk	1 tsp butter or	chili)	1 tsp margarine	margarine	1 corn tortilla with	vegetable oil	
	margarine	1 flour tortilla	or butter	Green beans	1 tsp special	margarine	
	Canned peach	Pudding (made	Watermelon	Dinner roll with	vegetable oil	Okra	
	1 cup skim milk	from skim milk	slice	1 tsp special	margarine	Biscuit (made	
		and egg	Buttermilk	vegetable oil	Pudding (made	with allowed	
		whites)		margarine	from skim milk	oils)	
		Fruit punch		Canned peach	and egg whites)	Watermelon slice	
				1 cup skim milk	Fruit punch	Buttermilk	

TABLE 33-5   **Treatment Decisions for High Blood Cholesterol Based on Low-Density Lipoprotein Levels**

| CATEGORY | LOW-DENSITY LIPOPROTEIN LEVELS | | |
	GOAL (mg/dl [mmol/L])	INITIATE LIFESTYLE CHANGES (mg/dl [mmol/L])	CONSIDER DRUG THERAPY (mg/dl [mmol/L])
CAD, CAD risk factors, or 10 yr risk of >20%	<100 (2.59)	≥100 (2.59)	≥130 (3.36); at 100-129 (2.59-3.34), drug therapy is optional
≥ 2 risk factors and 10 yr risk ≤ 20%	<130 (3.36)	≥130 (3.36)	≥130 (3.36) if 10 yr risk of 10%-20% >160 (4.14) if 10 yr risk of <10%
0-1 risk factor	<160 (4.14)	≥160 (4.14)	≥190 (4.91); at 160-189 (4.14-4.89), drug therapy is optional

Source: Executive Summary of the Third Report of the National Cholesterol Education Program (NCEP) Expert Panel on Detection, Evaluation, and Treatment of High Blood Cholesterol in Adults (Adult Treatment Panel III), *JAMA* 285:2486, 2001.
NOTE: Risk factors considered in the treatment of high LDL include age, family history of premature CAD, smoking, hypertension, and low HDL levels. At risk score refers to the probability of having a nonfatal MI or dying of a coronary event within 10 years.
CAD, Coronary artery disease; *HDL,* high-density lipoprotein; *LDL,* low-density lipoprotein.

TABLE 33-6   Drug Therapy   Hyperlipidemia

TYPE AND NAME	MECHANISM OF ACTION	SIDE EFFECTS	NURSING CONSIDERATIONS
Bile Acid Sequestrants cholestyramine (Questran, Colybar) colestipol (Colestid) colesevelam (Welchol)	Bind with bile acids in intestine, forming insoluble complex and excreted in feces Binding results in removal of LDL and cholesterol	Unpleasant gritty quality to taste GI disturbances (e.g., nausea, dyspepsia, constipation)	Effective and safe for long-term use; side effects diminish with time; interfere with absorption of digoxin, thiazides, β-adrenergic blockers, fat-soluble vitamins, folic acid, vancomycin (Vancocin)
Niacin nicotinic acid (niacin, Nicobid, Slo-Niacin, Niacor, Niaspan, Nicotinex)	Inhibits synthesis and secretion of VLDL and LDL Increases HDL levels	Hot flashes and pruritus in upper torso and face GI disturbances (e.g., nausea and vomiting, dyspepsia, diarrhea)	Most side effects subside with time; decreased liver function and arrhythmias may occur with high doses Taking aspirin 30 min-1 hr before drug may prevent flushing; take drug with food
Fibric Acid Derivatives clofibrate (Atromid) fenofibrate (Tricor) gemfibrozil (Lopid)	Reduce triglycerides by ↓ VLDL Decrease hepatic synthesis and secretion of VLDL ↑ HDL	Mild GI disturbances (e.g., nausea, diarrhea)	May ↑ effects of anticoagulants and hypoglycemics
HMG CoA Reductase Inhibitors (Statins) atorvastatin (Lipitor) fluvastatin (Lescol) lovastatin (Mevacor, Altocor) pravastatin (Pravachol) rosuvastatin (Crestor) simvastatin (Zocor)	Block synthesis of cholesterol ↓ LDL and triglycerides ↑ HDL	Rash, mild GI disturbances, insomnia, elevated liver enzymes, lens opacities, rhabdomyolysis (specifically lovastatin)	Well tolerated with few side effects Monitor patient with liver function tests and eye examinations
Cholesterol Absorption Inhibitor ezetimibe (Zetia)	Inhibits the intestinal absorption of cholesterol	Infrequent, but may include headache and mild GI distress	Can be used alone or with other antilipidemic drugs; should not be used by patients with active liver disease who are also taking statins

GI, Gastrointestinal; *HDL,* high-density lipoprotein; *LDL,* low-density lipoprotein; *VLDL,* very-low-density lipoprotein.

COMPLEMENTARY & ALTERNATIVE THERAPIES
Natural Lipid-Lowering Agents*

AGENT	COMMENTS
Niacin (nicotinic acid)	• Inhibits synthesis and secretion of low-density lipoproteins (LDLs) • Increases high-density lipoproteins (HDLs)
Garlic	See Complementary and Alternative Therapies box below
Omega-3 fatty acids	• Found in fish oil and flaxseed oil • Fish with high levels include cold-water ocean fish such as salmon, herring, mackerel, halibut, and sardines • ↓ Triglycerides and ↑ HDL levels
Milk thistle	• Silymarin, active part of milk thistle, has a cholesterol-lowering effect • ↑ HDL
Fiber	• Soluble fiber (e.g., pectin, oat bran, psyllium husk, fruits, beans) • ↓ Cholesterol and LDL levels by binding bile acids and slowing rate of lipid absorption
Phytosterols (plant sterols and stanols)	• Plant sterols are found in nuts, seeds, soybeans, and vegetable oils • Natural plant alcohols ↓ serum cholesterol
Soy	• ↓ Cholesterol, LDL, and triglyceride levels and ↑ HDL • Acts by ↓ absorption of cholesterol from GI tract
Coenzyme Q_{10} (ubiquinome)	• HMG CoA reductase inhibitors (e.g., lovastatin [Mevacor]) decrease plasma levels of coenzyme Q_{10}

*Cardiovascular disease is a serious health problem. Herbal or other natural therapy should not be initiated without consultation with a health care provider. This is especially important when conventional drug therapy for cardiovascular disease is also being used.

GI, Gastrointestinal; *HMG CoA*, hydroxy-methyl-glutaryl coenzyme A.

ers. Separating the time of administration of the resins from that of other drugs may decrease this adverse effect.

Drugs that restrict lipoprotein production. Nicotinic acid (niacin) is a B vitamin that has been used in conjunction with diet therapy. Nicotinic acid is highly effective in lowering cholesterol and triglyceride levels by interfering with their synthesis. Adverse effects of this drug may include severe flushing, pruritus, and GI distress. Aspirin taken 30 minutes to 1 hour before administration may eliminate flushing.

The fibric acid derivatives lower VLDL levels and triglycerides, and also increase HDL levels. These drugs include clofibrate (Atromid), fenofibrate (Tricor), and gemfibrozil (Lopid). Although most patients tolerate the drugs well, complaints may include GI irritability. Fenofibrate is particularly effective in treating patients with very high serum triglyceride levels. This drug should not be taken with statin medications.

The statin drugs reduce the synthesis of cholesterol in the liver by blocking hydroxy-methyl-glutaryl coenzyme A (HMG-CoA) reductase, a key enzyme in cholesterol synthesis, and increased activity of LDL receptors in liver cells. Lovastatin (Mevacor), pravastatin (Pravachol), simvastatin (Zocor), fluvastatin (Lescol), atorvastatin (Lipitor), and rosuvastatin (Crestor) are all competitive inhibitors of the biosynthesis of cholesterol. Adverse effects of these drugs include rash, gas, upper GI distress, elevated liver enzymes, nausea, constipation or diarrhea, headaches, opacities of eye lenses, and rarely rhabdomyolysis. Liver enzymes must be monitored during therapy.

Drugs that decrease cholesterol absorption. Ezetimibe (Zetia) selectively inhibits the absorption of dietary and biliary cholesterol across the intestinal wall (see Table 33-6).

Drug therapy for hyperlipidemia is likely to be prolonged, perhaps continuing for a lifetime. It is essential that diet modification be used to minimize the need for drug therapy. The patient must fully understand the rationale and goals of treatment, as well as the safety and side effects of drugs.[19-21] A new laboratory

COMPLEMENTARY & ALTERNATIVE THERAPIES
Garlic

Clinical Uses
High blood cholesterol and hypertension

Effects
Antihyperlipidemic, antihypertensive, antioxidant, antithrombotic, and hypoglycemic activity. Due to garlic's hypoglycemic effect, blood glucose levels should be monitored closely when used. Moderate garlic consumption has few adverse effects other than a peculiar odor on the breath and body.

Nursing Implications
Relatively safe herb, but may be contraindicated in persons with bleeding disorders, gastrointestinal infection, diabetes, and inflammation. Enhances the effects of warfarin and should not be used with anticoagulant or antiplatelet drugs. Odor-modified garlic preparations are just as effective as fresh garlic, but dried garlic has little to no effect.

test (Cholesterol 1, 2, 3) is available to measure the amount of cholesterol in skin using the palm of the hand. The test is intended for people suspected of having severe coronary artery disease and those with a history of an MI.

Clinical Manifestations of Coronary Artery Disease

The three major clinical manifestations of CAD are angina pectoris, acute coronary syndrome, and sudden cardiac death (discussed later in this chapter). They result from *ischemia* (lack of oxygen supply to the heart). When the lack of oxygen supply is temporary and reversible, **stable angina** pectoris results. When

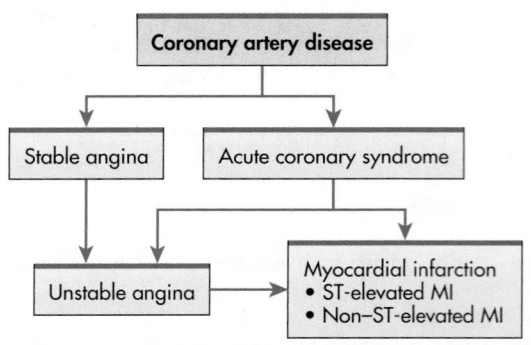

FIG. 33-8 Relationships among coronary artery disease, stable angina, unstable angina, and myocardial infarction.

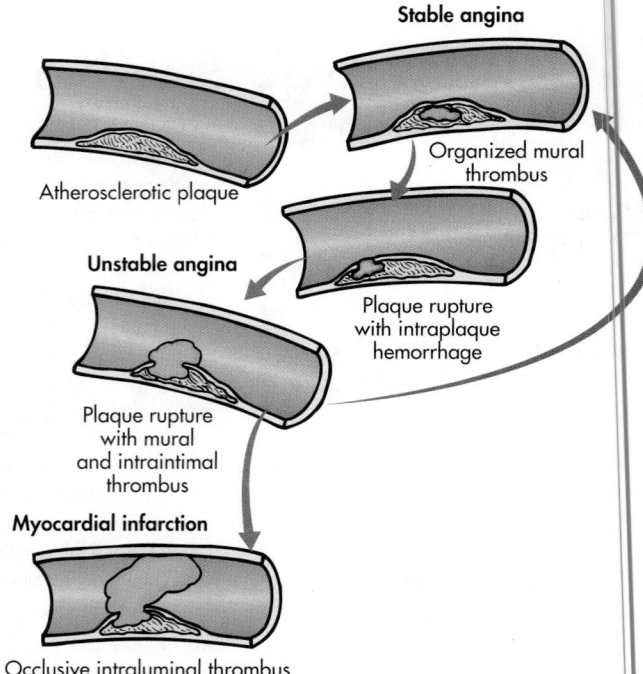

FIG. 33-9 Coronary thrombogenesis secondary to atherosclerotic plaque progression.

the oxygen supply is prolonged and not immediately reversible, **acute coronary syndrome** (ACS) develops. ACS encompasses the spectrum of unstable angina, non–ST-segment-elevation myocardial infarction (NSTEMI), and ST-segment-elevation STEMI (Fig. 33-8). Although each remains a distinct diagnosis, this shift in nomenclature reflects the relationships among the pathophysiology, diagnosis, prognosis, and therapy of these disorders.

Etiology and Pathophysiology

Myocardial ischemia develops when the demand for myocardial oxygen exceeds the ability of the coronary arteries to supply the heart with oxygen. Either an increased demand for oxygen or a decreased supply of oxygen can lead to myocardial ischemia (Table 33-7). The primary reason for insufficient blood flow is narrowing of coronary arteries by atherosclerosis. If myocardial oxygen needs are not met, coronary blood flow is increased through vasodilation and increased rate of flow.

In a person with CAD the coronary arteries are unable to dilate to meet increased metabolic needs because they are already chronically dilated beyond the obstructed area. For ischemia secondary to atherosclerosis to occur, the artery is usually 75% or

more stenosed. In addition, the diseased heart has difficulty increasing the rate of blood flow. This creates an oxygen deficit. In addition to atherosclerotic stenosis, oxygen deficit is caused by coronary artery spasm and coronary thrombosis. In *coronary artery spasm* the constriction is transient and reversible and causes either subtotal or total narrowing of the coronary artery. Although a coronary artery spasm is usually associated with an underlying atherosclerotic plaque (Fig. 33-9), spasms do occur in arteries without significant stenosis. The duration of the spasm determines whether the myocardium will sustain ischemia (not resulting in cell death) or actual infarction (resulting in cell death).

On the cellular level, the myocardium becomes cyanotic within the first 10 seconds of coronary occlusion, and ECG changes appear. With total occlusion of the coronary arteries, contractility ceases after several minutes, depriving the myocardial cells of glucose for aerobic metabolism. Anaerobic metabolism begins and lactic acid accumulates. Myocardial nerve fibers are irritated by the increased lactic acid and transmit a pain message to the cardiac nerves and upper thoracic posterior nerve roots. This is the reason for referred cardiac pain to the left shoulder and arm. In ischemic conditions, cardiac cells are viable for approximately 20 minutes. With restoration of blood flow, aerobic metabolism resumes and contractility is restored. Cellular repair also begins.

Angina is a result of ischemia caused by reversible cell injury. A **myocardial infarction** occurs as a result of sustained ischemia, causing irreversible cellular death (Fig. 33-10).

Cardiac cells can withstand ischemic conditions for approximately 20 minutes before cellular death (necrosis) begins. Contractile function of the heart stops in the areas of myocardial necrosis. The degree of altered function depends on the area of the heart involved and the size of the infarct. Most infarcts involve the left ventricle (LV). A transmural MI occurs when the

TABLE 33-7   Factors Determining Myocardial Oxygen Needs

DECREASED OXYGEN SUPPLY	INCREASED OXYGEN DEMAND OR CONSUMPTION
Noncardiac	
Anemia	Anxiety
Hypoxemia	Cocaine use
Pneumonia	Hypertension
Asthma	Hyperthermia
Chronic obstructive pulmonary	Hyperthyroidism
disease	Physical exertion
Low blood volume	
Cardiac	
Arrhythmias	Aortic stenosis
Congestive heart failure	Arrhythmias
Coronary artery spasm	Cardiomyopathy
Coronary artery thrombosis	Hypertension
Valve disorders	Tachycardia

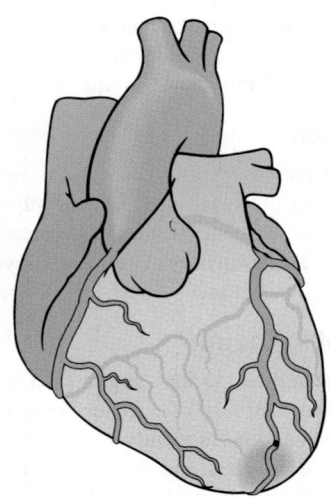

FIG. 33-10 Occlusion of coronary artery, resulting in a myocardial infarction.

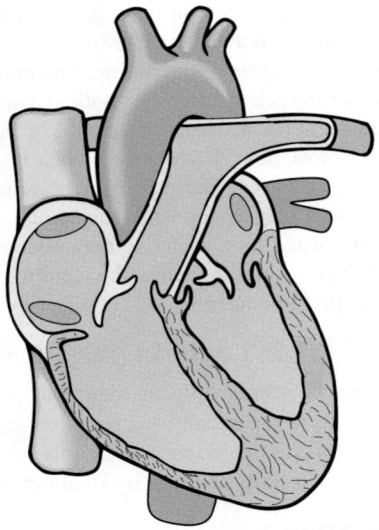

FIG. 33-11 Transmural myocardial infarction involving the thickness of the total wall.

entire thickness of the myocardium in a region is involved (Fig. 33-11). A subendocardial MI exists when the damage has not penetrated through the entire thickness of the myocardial wall.

Infarctions are described by the area of occurrence as anterior, inferior, lateral, or posterior wall infarctions. Common combinations of areas are the anterolateral or anteroseptal MI. An inferior MI is also called a diaphragmatic MI.

The location and area of the infarct correlate with the part of the coronary circulation involved. For example, inferior wall infarctions are usually the result of right coronary artery lesions. Anterior wall infarctions are usually caused by lesions in the left anterior descending artery. Lesions in the left circumflex artery usually cause lateral, posterior, or inferior wall MIs.

The degree of preestablished collateral circulation also determines the severity of infarction (see Fig. 33-5). In an individual with a history of heart disease, adequate collateral channels may

have been established that provide the area surrounding the infarction site with a blood supply and oxygen. This is one explanation why the younger person who has a severe MI is often more likely to have a more serious impairment than an older person with the same degree of occlusion.

Healing Process. The body's response to cell death is the inflammatory process (see Chapter 12). Within 24 hours, leukocytes infiltrate the area. Enzymes are released from the dead cardiac cells and are important diagnostic indicators of MI. (See section on serum cardiac markers later in this chapter.) The proteolytic enzymes of the neutrophils and macrophages remove all necrotic tissue by the second or third day. During this time, the necrotic muscle wall is thin. The development of collateral circulation improves areas of poor perfusion and may limit the zones of injury and infarction. Once infarction takes place, catecholamine-mediated lipolysis and glycogenolysis occur. These processes allow the increased plasma glucose and free fatty acids to be used by the oxygen-depleted myocardium for anaerobic metabolism. For this reason, serum glucose levels are frequently elevated after MI.

The necrotic zone is identifiable by ECG changes and by nuclear scanning after the onset of symptoms. At this point, the neutrophils and monocytes have cleared the necrotic debris from the injured area, and the collagen matrix that will eventually form scar tissue is laid down.

At 10 to 14 days after MI, the beginning scar tissue is still weak. The myocardium is considered to be especially vulnerable to increased stress because of the unstable state of the healing heart wall. (It is also at this time that the patient's activity level may be increasing, so special caution and assessment are necessary.) By 6 weeks after MI, scar tissue has replaced necrotic tissue. At this time, the injured area is said to be healed. The scarred area is often less compliant than the surrounding fibers. This condition may be manifested by uncoordinated wall motion, ventricular dysfunction, or pump failure.

These changes in the infarcted muscle also cause changes in the unaffected myocardium as well. In an attempt to compensate for the infarcted muscle, the normal myocardium will hypertrophy and dilate. This process is called *ventricular remodeling*. Remodeling of normal myocardium can lead to the development of late heart failure, especially in the individual with atherosclerosis of other coronary arteries and/or an anterior MI.

TYPES OF ANGINA

Stable Angina Pectoris

Angina pectoris is literally translated as pain *(angina)* in the chest *(pectoris)*. It refers to chest pain occurring intermittently over a long period with the same pattern of onset, duration, and intensity of symptoms. The pain usually lasts for only a few minutes (3 to 5 minutes) and commonly subsides when the precipitating factor (usually exertion) is relieved. (Precipitating factors are listed in Table 33-8.) Pain at rest is unusual. An ECG usually reveals ST segment depression, indicating subendocardial ischemia. The discomfort may be mild or severe and disabling, but it is usually infrequent.

Stable angina can be controlled with medications on an outpatient basis. Because stable angina is often predictable, medications can be timed to provide peak effects during the time of day when angina is likely to occur. For example, if angina occurs

TABLE 33-8	Precipitating Factors of Angina

Physical Exertion
- Increases HR, which decreases the time the heart spends in diastole (the time of greatest coronary blood flow).
- Walking outdoors is the most common form of exertion.
- Isometric exertion of the arms (e.g., raking, lifting heavy objects, or snow shoveling) also causes exertional angina.

Temperature Extremes
- Increase workload of the heart.
- Blood vessels constrict in response to a cold stimulus.
- Blood vessels dilate and blood pools in the skin in response to a hot stimulus.

Strong Emotions
- Stimulate the sympathetic nervous system.
- Increase the workload of the heart.

Consumption of Heavy Meal
- Can increase the workload of the heart.
- During the digestive process, blood is diverted to the GI system, causing a decreased flow rate in the coronary arteries.

Cigarette Smoking
- Nicotine stimulates catecholamine release.
- Causes vasoconstriction and an increased HR.
- Diminishes available oxygen by increasing the level of carbon monoxide.

Sexual Activity
- Increases the cardiac workload and sympathetic stimulation.
- In a person with severe CAD, the extra cardiac workload may precipitate angina.

Stimulants (e.g., cocaine, amphetamines)
- Cause increased HR and subsequent myocardial oxygen demand.

Circadian Rhythm Patterns
- Are related to the occurrence of stable angina, Prinzmetal's angina, MI, and sudden cardiac death.
- Manifestations of CAD tend to occur in the early morning after awakening.

CAD, Coronary artery disease; *GI,* gastrointestinal; *HR,* heart rate; *MI,* myocardial infarction.

when rising, the patient can take medication as soon as awakening and wait 30 minutes to 1 hour before engaging in activity. (The different types of angina are compared in Table 33-9.)

Silent Ischemia

Up to 80% of patients with myocardial ischemia are asymptomatic.[22] This type of ischemia is termed **silent ischemia.** Ischemia with pain or without pain has the same prognosis. Diabetes mellitus and hypertension are associated with an increased prevalence of silent ischemia.

Prinzmetal's Angina

Prinzmetal's angina (variant angina) often occurs at rest, usually in response to spasm of a major coronary artery. It is a rare form of angina and is frequently seen in patients with a history of migraine headaches and Raynaud's phenomenon. The spasm may occur in the absence of CAD, as well as with documented disease. Prinzmetal's angina is not usually precipitated by increased physical demand. Coronary spasm can be described as a strong contraction of smooth muscle in the coronary artery caused by an increase in intracellular calcium. Factors that may precipitate coronary artery spasm include increased myocardial oxygen demand and increased levels of a variety of substances (e.g., histamine, angiotensin, epinephrine, norepinephrine, prostaglandins). When spasm occurs, the patient experiences pain and marked, transient ST segment elevation. The pain may occur during rapid eye movement (REM) sleep when myocardial oxygen consumption increases. The pain may be relieved by some form of exercise or it may disappear spontaneously. Cyclic, short bursts of pain at a usual time each day may also occur with this type of angina. It is usually treated with calcium channel blockers or nitrates as first-line agents.

Nocturnal Angina and Angina Decubitus

Nocturnal angina occurs only at night but not necessarily when the person is in the recumbent position or during sleep. Angina decubitus is chest pain that occurs only while the person is lying down and is usually relieved by standing or sitting.

Unstable Angina

Angina that is new in onset, occurs at rest, or has a worsening pattern is called **unstable angina.** Unlike stable angina, unstable angina is unpredictable and is considered to be an acute coronary syndrome. The patient with stable angina may develop unstable angina, or unstable angina may be the first clinical manifestation

TABLE 33-9	Comparison of Types of Angina		
	STABLE ANGINA	**UNSTABLE ANGINA**	**PRINZMETAL'S ANGINA**
Etiology	Myocardial ischemia, usually secondary to atherosclerosis	Rupture of thickened plaque, exposing thrombogenic surface	Coronary vasospasm
Characteristics	• Episodic pain lasting 5-15 min • Provoked by exertion • Relieved by rest or nitroglycerin	• New-onset angina • Angina of increasing frequency, duration, or severity • Occurs at rest or minimal exertion • Pain refractory to nitroglycerin	• Occurs primarily at rest • Triggered by smoking • May occur in presence or absence of CAD

CAD, Coronary artery disease.

of CAD. The patient with previously diagnosed stable angina will describe a significant change in the pattern of angina if unstable angina develops. It will occur with increasing frequency and is easily provoked by minimal or no exertion, during sleep, or even at total rest. The patient without previously diagnosed angina will describe anginal pain that has progressed rapidly in the last few days or weeks, often culminating in pain at rest.[23]

Unstable angina is often associated with deterioration of a once stable atherosclerotic plaque (see Fig. 33-9). The once stable plaque ruptures, exposing the intima to blood and stimulating platelet aggregation and local vasoconstriction with thrombus formation. This unstable lesion is at increased risk of complete thrombosis of the lumen with progression to MI. This is why patients with unstable angina require immediate hospitalization with ECG monitoring and bed rest. The unstable lesion can progress to an MI, or it can return to a stable lesion (see Fig. 33-9). Aspirin and systemic anticoagulation with low-molecular-weight heparin given subcutaneously or intravenous (IV) heparin is the treatment of choice for unstable angina. IV antiplatelet agents may also be used if coronary angioplasty is anticipated. If the patient is not already on antianginal agents, nitrates or β-adrenergic blockers are the first line of treatment.[24,25] Calcium channel blockers or nitrates can be added if the patient is already on adequate doses of β-adrenergic blockers or if the patient cannot tolerate β-adrenergic blockers or has Prinzmetal's angina.[24,25]

CLINICAL MANIFESTATIONS

Angina

The most common initial manifestation of angina is chest pain or discomfort. The exact cause of the pain is unknown, but neurogenic pain at the site of ischemia is most likely. On direct questioning (Table 33-10), some patients may deny feeling pain but will refer to a vague sensation, a strange feeling, pressure, or ache in the chest. It is an unpleasant feeling, often described as a constrictive, squeezing, heavy, choking, or suffocating sensation. Angina is almost never sharp or stabbing, and it usually does not change with position or breathing. These characteristic features distinguish angina pain from pain associated with an MI. Many people with angina complain of severe indigestion or burning. Although most of the discomfort experienced by persons with angina appears substernally, the sensation may occur in the neck or radiate to various locations, including the jaw, shoulders, and down the arms (Fig. 33-12). Often people will complain of pain between the shoulder blades and dismiss it as not being heart pain.

Depending on the severity of the anginal attack, the person may remain motionless or may clench a fist over the sternal area. The person experiencing angina often refers to a feeling of anxiety and impending doom. Associated symptoms may include shortness of breath, cold sweat, weakness, or paresthesias of one or both arms. Relief of stable angina is usually obtained with rest or cessation of activity. Unstable angina is not relieved by rest. Prinzmetal's angina differs from stable or unstable angina in that it is longer in duration and may wake the patient from sleep.

Myocardial Infarction

Pain. Severe, immobilizing chest pain not relieved by rest, position change, or nitrate administration is the hallmark of an MI. Persistent and unlike any other pain, it is usually described as a heaviness, pressure, tightness, burning, constriction, or crushing. Common locations are substernal, retrosternal, or epigastric. The pain may radiate to the neck, jaw, and arms or to the back (see Fig. 33-12). It may occur while the patient is active or at rest, or asleep or awake. However, it commonly occurs in the early morning hours. It usually lasts for 20 minutes or more and is described as more severe than anginal pain. The pain may be located atypically in the epigastric area. The patient may have taken antacids without relief.

However, not everyone has classic symptoms. Some patients may not experience pain but may have "discomfort," weakness, or shortness of breath. Women may experience atypical discomfort, shortness of breath, or fatigue. Patients with diabetes mellitus are more likely to experience silent (asymptomatic) MIs. An older patient may experience shortness of breath, pulmonary edema, dizziness, altered mental status, or an arrhythmia.

Nausea and Vomiting. The patient may be nauseated and vomit. Nausea and vomiting can result from reflex stimulation of the vomiting center by the severe pain. These symptoms can also result from vasovagal reflexes initiated from the area of the infarcted myocardium.

Sympathetic Nervous System Stimulation. During the initial phases of MI, increased catecholamines (norepinephrine and epinephrine) are released. The increased sympathetic nervous system stimulation results in diaphoresis and vasoconstriction of peripheral blood vessels. On physical examination, the

	FACTOR	QUESTIONS TO ASK PATIENT
P	Precipitating events	What events or factors precipitated the pain or discomfort (e.g., activity, exercise, resting)?
Q	Quality of pain or discomfort	What does the pain or discomfort feel like (e.g., dull, aching, sharp, tight)?
R	Radiation of pain	Where is the pain located? Where does the pain radiate to (e.g., back, arms, jaw, teeth, shoulder, elbow)?
S	Severity of pain	On a scale of 0 to 10 with 10 being the most severe pain, how would you rate the pain or discomfort?
T	Timing	When did the pain or discomfort begin? Has the pain changed since that time? Have you had pain like this before?

TABLE 33-10 PQRST Assessment

The following can be used as a memory device to assist in obtaining information from the patient who has chest pain or discomfort.

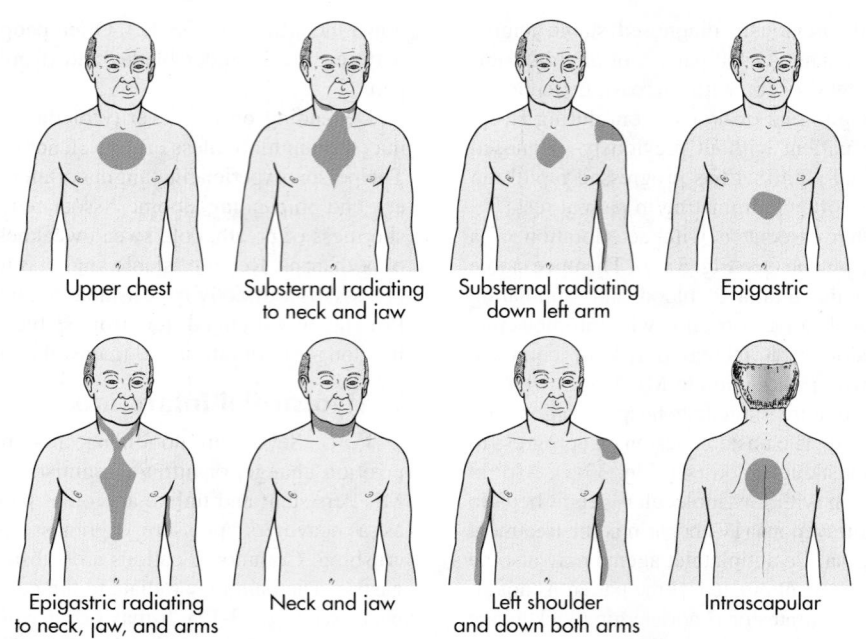

Upper chest

Substernal radiating to neck and jaw

Substernal radiating down left arm

Epigastric

Epigastric radiating to neck, jaw, and arms

Neck and jaw

Left shoulder and down both arms

Intrascapular

FIG. 33-12 Location of chest pain during angina or myocardial infarction.

patient's skin will be ashen, clammy, and cool. This condition is often referred to as a "cold sweat."

Fever. The temperature may increase within the first 24 hours up to 100.4° F (38° C) and occasionally to 102.2° F (39° C). The temperature elevation may last for as long as 1 week. This increase in temperature is a systemic manifestation of the inflammatory process caused by cell death in the infarcted myocardium.

Cardiovascular Manifestations. The BP and heart rate may be elevated initially. Later the BP may drop because of decreased cardiac output (CO). Urine output may be decreased. Crackles may be noted in the lungs, persisting for several hours to several days. Hepatic engorgement and peripheral edema may indicate overt cardiac failure. Jugular veins may be distended and may have obvious pulsations, indicating early right ventricular dysfunction and pulmonary congestion.

Cardiac examination may reveal abnormal precordial movements suggestive of ventricular aneurysm. Heart sounds may seem distant, but close auscultation may reveal splitting of heart sounds. Other abnormal sounds suggesting ventricular dysfunction are S₃ and S₄. In addition, a loud holosystolic apical murmur may develop and may indicate a septal defect or valve incompetency. Valve incompetency results from ischemia to papillary muscle and can lead to rupture or dysfunction of the muscle.

Complications of Myocardial Infarction

Arrhythmias. The most common complication after an MI is arrhythmias, which are present in 80% of MI patients. Arrhythmias are the most common cause of death in patients in the prehospital period. Arrhythmias are caused by any condition that affects the myocardial cell's sensitivity to nerve impulses, such as ischemia, electrolyte imbalances, and sympathetic nervous system stimulation. The intrinsic rhythm of the heartbeat is disrupted, causing a fast HR (tachycardia), a slow HR (bradycardia), or an irregular beat, all of which adversely affect the ischemic myocardium.

Life-threatening arrhythmias occur most often with anterior wall infarction, heart failure, and shock. Complete heart block is seen in massive infarction. Ventricular fibrillation, a common cause of sudden death, is a lethal arrhythmia that most often occurs within the first 4 hours after the onset of pain. Premature ventricular contractions (PVCs) may precede ventricular tachycardia and fibrillation. Life-threatening ventricular arrhythmias must be treated immediately. (See Chapter 35 for a detailed description of arrhythmias and their management.)

Congestive Heart Failure. *Congestive heart failure* (CHF) is a complication that occurs when the pumping power of the heart has diminished. Depending on the severity and extent of the injury, CHF occurs initially with subtle signs such as slight dyspnea, restlessness, agitation, or slight tachycardia. Jugular vein distention from right-sided heart failure, crackles heard in the lungs, distention of upper lobe veins on an upright chest x-ray, and the presence of an S₃ or S₄ heart sound may indicate the onset of heart failure. (The treatment of acute CHF is discussed in Chapter 34.)

Cardiogenic Shock. *Cardiogenic shock* occurs when inadequate oxygen and nutrients are supplied to the tissues because of severe left ventricular (LV) failure. Cardiogenic shock occurs less often since the advent of fibrinolytic therapy and percutaneous coronary intervention (PCI), but when it occurs, it has a high mortality rate. Cardiogenic shock often requires aggressive management, including control of arrhythmias, intraaortic balloon pump therapy, and support of contractility with the use of vasoactive drugs. The goal of therapy is to maximize oxygen delivery and prevent complications such as acute renal failure.[24] (Cardiogenic shock is discussed in Chapter 65.)

Papillary Muscle Dysfunction. *Papillary muscle dysfunction* may occur if the infarcted area includes or is adjacent to these structures. Papillary muscle dysfunction causes mitral valve regurgitation, which increases the volume of blood in the left atrium. This condition aggravates an already compromised

LV. Papillary muscle dysfunction is detected by a systolic murmur at the cardiac apex radiating toward the axilla. Papillary muscle rupture is a severe complication causing massive mitral valve regurgitation, which results in dyspnea, pulmonary edema, and decreased CO. There is rapid clinical deterioration of the patient. Treatment consists of rapid afterload reduction with nitroprusside or intraaortic balloon pumping and immediate open heart surgery with mitral valve replacement.[24]

Ventricular Aneurysm. *Ventricular aneurysm* results when the infarcted myocardial wall becomes thinned and bulges out during contraction. The patient with a ventricular aneurysm may experience intractable CHF, arrhythmias, and angina. Besides ventricular rupture, which is fatal, ventricular aneurysms harbor thrombi, cause arrhythmias, and promote LV dysfunction.

Pericarditis. Acute *pericarditis,* an inflammation of the visceral and/or parietal pericardium, may result in cardiac compression, decreased ventricular filling and emptying, and cardiac failure. It may occur 2 to 3 days after an acute MI as a common complication of the infarction. Chest pain, which may vary from mild to severe, is aggravated by inspiration, coughing, and movement of the upper body and usually accompanies acute pericarditis. The pain may be relieved by sitting in a forward position. The pain is usually different from pain associated with an MI.

Assessment of the patient with pericarditis may reveal a friction rub over the pericardium. The sound may be best heard with the diaphragm of the stethoscope at the mid to lower sternal border. It may be persistent or intermittent. Fever may also be present.

Diagnosis of pericarditis can be made with serial 12-lead ECGs. Characteristic ECG changes are persistent ST-T segment elevations that reflect the inflammation. Treatment may include pain relief by aspirin, corticosteroids, or nonsteroidal antiinflammatory drugs. (Pericarditis is discussed in Chapter 36.)

Dressler Syndrome. **Dressler syndrome** (post-MI syndrome) is characterized by pericarditis with effusion and fever that develops 1 to 4 weeks after MI. It may also occur after open heart surgery. It is thought to be caused by an antigen-antibody reaction to the necrotic myocardium. The patient experiences pericardial pain, fever, a friction rub, left pleural effusion, and arthralgia. Laboratory findings include an elevated white blood cell (WBC) count and an elevated sedimentation rate. Short-term corticosteroids are used to treat this condition.

Pulmonary Embolism. Pulmonary embolism may be seen in the patient with acute MI who has had CHF or arrhythmias or has been extremely immobile because of prolonged bed rest. The source of the thrombus may be the roughened endocardium or leg veins. Early detection of emboli is accomplished by observing for pallor or cyanosis, heart failure unresponsive to treatment, and an unexplained pleural effusion. Acute massive pulmonary embolism causes sudden, severe dyspnea and is usually fatal. (Pulmonary emboli are discussed in more detail in Chapter 36.)

DIAGNOSTIC STUDIES

Angina

When a patient has a history indicating CAD, the physician may order diagnostic studies (Fig. 33-13). After a detailed health history and physical examination, a chest x-ray is usually taken to look for cardiac enlargement, cardiac calcifications, and pulmonary congestion. An ECG is obtained and compared with an earlier tracing when possible. Laboratory tests may be done to

assess serum lipid levels, cardiac markers, and C-reactive protein (CRP). Serum lipid levels are assessed to screen for positive risk factors, and cardiac markers are determined to rule out the occurrence of an MI.

Treadmill exercise testing is an important diagnostic test done for the patient with stable angina. ST segment and T wave changes during exercise are an indirect assessment of coronary artery perfusion. Severely abnormal ECGs on exercise testing indicate a significant disease process, and may indicate the need for coronary angiography. Unfortunately, the ECG stress test is not always conclusive for CAD. A false-positive reaction may be found (especially in women), and a false-negative reaction may be seen if the patient is exercised submaximally or if only one coronary artery is involved. Ambulatory 24- to 48-hour ECG monitoring with patient-recorded activity may be effective in identifying silent ischemia. It is also helpful in differentiating Prinzmetal's angina because the incidence of spasm occurs more commonly in the early morning hours (5:00 to 6:00 AM). Perfusion imaging and dobutamine echocardiography can complement exercise testing, especially in people with inconclusive results on the exercise testing.

Nuclear imaging has become increasingly important in establishing the diagnosis of myocardial perfusion. It is considered an extremely sensitive indicator of myocardial damage. Myocardial nuclear scans, done by injecting IV radioactive isotopes, can help establish the diagnosis of acute MI when other data are inconclusive. After an IV injection of a radioisotope, the amount of radioisotope present in each myocardial region is determined by two factors: the amount of coronary blood flow to that region and the degree of viable myocardium. Ischemia or infarcted myocardial regions receiving little or no coronary blood flow accumulate little or no radioisotope. Such regions appear as "cold spots" on the scan and thus indicate an area of ischemia or infarct. However, this technique does not differentiate old from new infarcts.

Positron emission tomography (PET), a noninvasive technique, is also useful in identifying and quantifying ischemia and infarction (see Chapter 31 and Table 31-7).

Coronary angiography allows visualization of the coronary arteries and helps determine the treatment and prognosis. The patient with unstable angina may undergo coronary angiography to evaluate the extent of the disease and to determine the most appropriate therapeutic modality. Others may be treated with conservative medical management. It remains controversial which is the best management for unstable angina.[23] Coronary angiography is the only way to confirm the diagnosis of Prinzmetal's angina.

Other techniques for diagnosing coronary artery stenosis include the use of echocardiography with exercise. Stress echocardiograms may be used when a patient has an abnormal baseline ECG. The patient has a baseline echocardiogram before exercise stress testing and then proceeds with the treadmill exercise test. Immediately after the conclusion of the test, another echocardiogram is performed to detect any new regional abnormal wall motion. This increases the sensitivity of the treadmill test.

Another technique using an echocardiogram can be used for the patient who is unable to exercise. In this patient, a dobutamine (Dobutrex) stress echocardiogram can be performed. Echocardiography is done during a stepwise infusion of dobutamine, which causes a progressive increase in HR just as occurs with exercise; that is, the heart is being exercised chemically.

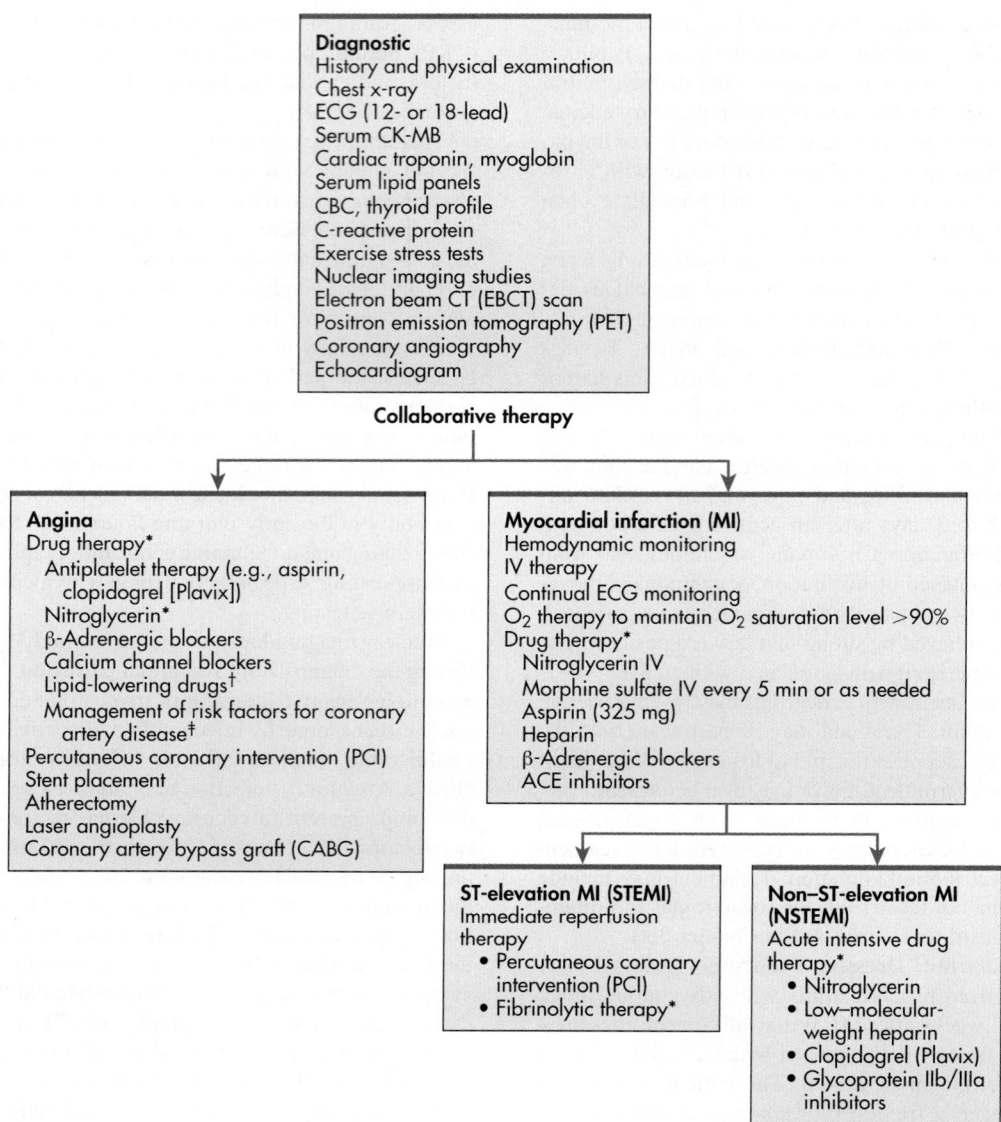

FIG. 33-13 Collaborative care: angina and myocardial infarction. *ASA*, Acetylsalicylic acid; *ACE*, angiotensin–converting enzyme; *CAD*, coronary artery disease; *CBC*, complete blood count; *CK*, creatine kinase.
*See Table 33-13.
†See Table 33-6.
‡See Table 33-3.

Again, abnormality of the regional wall motion is determined. The test is stopped if a wall motion abnormality or angina develops or the patient reaches the target HR or the peak dobutamine dose.

Electron beam computed tomography (EBCT) is a noninvasive procedure that can assess CAD in all stages but can also identify patients at risk before symptoms develop. EBCT creates a three-dimensional image of the heart and its arteries. EBCT images can reveal coronary artery plaque and other abnormalities in coronary structures and blood vessels. Individuals who benefit most from EBCT scanning are those who have a personal or family history of CAD, have risk factors for CAD, are symptomatic for CAD, or are on therapy for CAD.

Myocardial Infarction

Common diagnostic parameters used to determine whether a person has sustained an acute MI include (1) the patient's history of pain, risk factors, and health history; (2) ECG consistent with acute MI (ST segment elevations of greater than 1 mm or more in two contiguous leads); and (3) serial measurement of cardiac markers (see Fig. 33-13).

Electrocardiogram Findings. Serial ECGs are needed to rule out or confirm an MI. Changes in the QRS complex, ST segment, and T wave caused by ischemia and infarction can develop quickly after an MI. For diagnostic and treatment purposes, it is important to distinguish between ST-elevation MI (STEMI) (Fig. 33-14) and non–ST-elevation MI (NSTEMI). Patients with STEMI

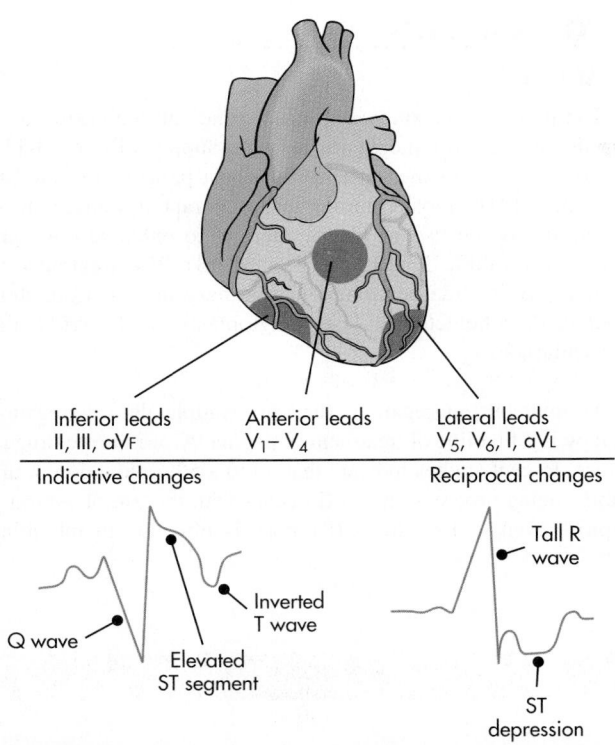

FIG. 33-14 Indicative changes occur in leads that examine the area of infarction. Reciprocal changes occur in leads opposite the area of infarction.

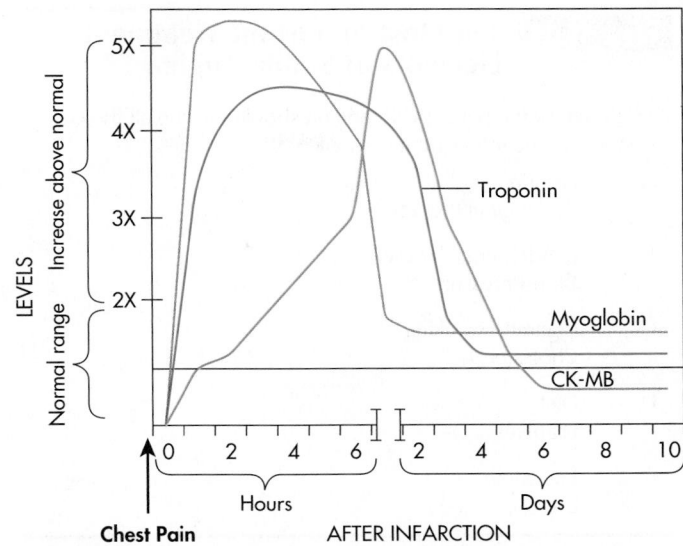

FIG. 33-15 Serum cardiac markers in the blood after myocardial infarction. *CK,* Creatine kinase.

tend to have a more extensive MI that is associated with prolonged and complete coronary thrombosis. Patients with NSTEMI usually have transient thrombosis or incomplete coronary artery occlusion. Areas of ischemia or infarction may be noted on the ECG. Because the acute infarction is a dynamic process that occurs with time, the ECG may reveal the time sequence of ischemia, injury, infarction, and resolution of the infarction.

The ECG may be normal when the patient comes to the emergency department (ED) with a complaint of pain typical of ischemic chest pain, but within a few hours it may have changed to show the infarction process. These changes take place when cellular damage has occurred, interrupting the normal electrical depolarization. Many patients with an acute MI have nondiagnostic ECGs on admission to an ED. Diagnosis will then depend on serial cardiac markers and repeat ECG in 6 to 8 hours.[25]

Figure 33-14 correlates the anatomy with areas of infarction and with changes that occur on the 12-lead ECG. Changes that are present in the leads that examine infarcted areas of the heart are called *indicative* changes (i.e., they are indicative of infarction). Changes in the leads opposite infarcted areas are called *reciprocal* changes.

Serum Cardiac Markers. Certain proteins, called *serum cardiac markers,* are released into the blood in large quantities from necrotic heart muscle after an MI. These markers, specifically cardiac serum enzymes and troponin, are important diagnostic criteria for an acute MI. The cardiac enzyme of primary importance is creatine kinase (CK). When cardiac cells die, their cellular enzymes are released into circulation. The increase in serum enzymes that occurs after cellular death can indicate whether cardiac damage is present and the approximate extent of the damage. CK and troponin are typically measured to diagnose

an MI. (Fig. 33-15 indicates the peak level and duration of these markers in the presence of MI.)

CK levels begin to rise approximately 3 to 12 hours after an acute MI, peak in 24 hours, and return to normal within 2 to 3 days. The CK enzymes may be fractionated into bands, including the MB band. The MB band is specific to the myocardial cell and may more specifically quantify myocardial damage. Depending on the individual laboratory, MB bands greater than 3% indicate MI.

Troponin is a myocardial muscle protein released into circulation after an injury. In the heart there are two subtypes: troponin T and troponin I. Cardiac-specific troponin T (cTnT) and cardiac-specific troponin I (cTnI) have different amino acid sequences than skeletal muscle forms of these proteins. Therefore these markers are highly specific indicators of MI and have greater sensitivity and specificity for myocardial injury than CK-MB.

Troponin rises as quickly as CK and remains elevated for 2 weeks. It is usually used for diagnostic purposes in conjunction with total CK and the MB fraction.[26] Serum levels of cTnI and cTnT increase 3 to 12 hours after the onset of MI, peak at 24 to 48 hours, and return to baseline over 5 to 14 days.

Myoglobin is released into circulation within a few hours after an MI. Although it is one of the first serum cardiac markers that increase after an MI, it lacks cardiac specificity. In addition, it is rapidly excreted in urine so that blood levels return to normal range within 24 hours after an MI.

Other Measures. A new blood test for evaluating a patient with an MI is the albumin cobalt-binding (ACB) test, which measures how much cobalt is bound to albumin. Changes in the structure of albumin occur in MI. The ACB test is used in conjunction with ECG and troponin testing.

For the assessment of cardiac size and pulmonary congestion, an initial chest x-ray is helpful but not diagnostic of an acute MI. The appearance of distended upper lobe veins may indicate early LV dysfunction. The WBC count may rise to 12,000 to 14,000/μl (12 to 14 × 10⁹/L) or higher. Increases in fasting blood glucose levels to 300 mg/dl (16.7 mmol/L) may also occur secondary to the body's stress response to injury.

TABLE 33-11	**Ten Most Important Treatment Elements of Stable Angina**

Treatment of the patient with angina should include all the elements in the following mnemonic:

A	Aspirin Antianginal therapy
B	β-Adrenergic blocker Blood pressure
C	Cigarette smoking Cholesterol
D	Diet Diabetes
E	Education Exercise

COLLABORATIVE CARE

Angina

The treatment of stable angina is aimed at decreasing oxygen demand and/or increasing oxygen supply (Table 33-11). Emergency care of the patient with chest pain is presented in Table 33-12. The most common initial therapeutic intervention for angina is the use of nitrate therapy to enhance coronary blood flow (Table 33-13; see Fig. 33-13). The treatment of angina may include percutaneous coronary intervention, stent placement, atherectomy, laser angioplasty, and myocardial revascularization.

Drug Therapy (see Table 33-13)

Antiplatelet aggregation therapy. Antiplatelet aggregation therapy is a first line of treatment of angina. Aspirin is the drug of choice. Recent studies indicate that up to a 50% reduction in unstable angina progression to MI occurs with the use of aspirin.[27] Aspirin, even in low doses (81 mg), is effective in inhibiting

TABLE 33-12	**Emergency Management** — **Chest Pain**

ETIOLOGY	ASSESSMENT FINDINGS	INTERVENTIONS
Cardiovascular • Angina • Myocardial infarction • Arrhythmia • Pericarditis • Aortic aneurysm • Aortic valve disease **Respiratory** • Costochondritis • Pleurisy • Pneumonia • Pneumothorax • Pulmonary edema • Pulmonary embolus **Chest Trauma** • Rib/sternal fracture • Flail chest • Cardiac tamponade • Pneumothorax • Pulmonary contusion • Great vessel injury **Gastrointestinal** • Esophagitis • GERD • Hiatal hernia • Peptic ulcer • Cholecystitis **Others** • Stress • Strenuous exercise • Drugs • Acute anxiety	• Pain in chest, neck, arm, or shoulder • Cold, clammy skin • Diaphoresis • Nausea and vomiting • Abdominal pain • Heartburn • Dyspnea • Weakness • Anxiety • Feeling of impending doom • Tachycardia • Irregular HR • Palpitations • Arrhythmias • Decreased BP • Narrowed pulse pressure • Unequal BP readings in upper extremities • Syncope, loss of consciousness • Decreased O₂ saturation • Decreased or absent breath sounds • Pericardial friction rub	**Initial** • Ensure patent airway. • Administer O₂ by nasal cannula or non-rebreather mask. • Insert two IV catheters. • Obtain 12-lead ECG. • Determine location of pain. Assess severity using pain scale (0-10). • Medicate for pain as ordered (e.g., morphine, nitroglycerin). • Identify underlying rhythm. • Obtain cardiac marker levels. • Obtain portable chest x-ray. • Assess for fibrinolytic therapy as appropriate. • Administer aspirin and β-adrenergic blockers for cardiac-related chest pain unless contraindicated. • Administer antiarrhythmic drugs as indicated. **Ongoing Monitoring** • Monitor vital signs, level of consciousness, cardiac rhythm, and O₂ saturation. • Monitor pain and remedicate as needed. • Reassure patient. • Anticipate need for intubation if respiratory distress is evident. • Prepare for CPR, defibrillation, transcutaneous pacing, or cardioversion.

BP, Blood pressure; *CPR*, cardiopulmonary resuscitation; *ECG*, electrocardiogram; *GERD*, gastroesophageal reflux disease; *HR*, heart rate.

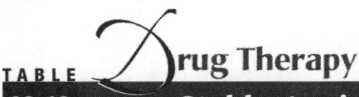
DRUG	MECHANISM OF ACTION AND COMMENTS
Antiplatelet Agents aspirin 325 mg (can be chewed)	• Inhibits cyclooxygenase, which in turn produces thromboxane A_2, a potent platelet activator • Should be administered as soon as ACS is suspected
β-Adrenergic Blockers metoprolol (Lopressor) propranolol (Inderal) esmolol (Brevibloc)	• Inhibit sympathetic nervous stimulation of the heart • Reduce both heart rate and contractility • Decrease afterload
Nitrates Sublingual nitroglycerin (Nitrostat, NitroQuick) Spray nitroglycerin (Nitrolingual, Translingual Spray) Nitroglycerin ointment (Nitro-Bid, Nitrol) Transdermal nitroglycerin (Transderm-Nitro, Minitran) IV nitroglycerin (Nitro-Bid, Tridil) Extended-release buccal tablets (Nitrogard) Extended-release capsules (Nitroglyn, Nitrospan) Long-acting formulations (isosorbide dinitrate [Isordil, Sorbitrate])	• Promote peripheral vasodilation, decreasing preload and afterload • Coronary artery vasodilation
Glycoprotein (GP) IIB/IIIA Inhibitors abciximab (ReoPro) eptifibatide (Integrilin) tirofiban (Aggrastat)	• Prevent the binding of fibrinogen to platelets, thereby blocking platelet aggregation • Standard antiplatelet therapy in combination with aspirin for patients at high risk for unstable angina
Low-Molecular-Weight Heparin dalteparin (Fragmin) enoxaparin (Lovenox)	• Bind to antithrombin III, enhancing its effect • Heparin–antithrombin III complex inactivates activated factor X and thrombin • Prevent conversion of fibrinogen to fibrin
Direct Thrombin Inhibitors bivalirudin (Angiomax) lepirudin (Refludan)	• Bind directly to the receptor for thrombin, thus preventing the binding of thrombin and subsequent clot formation
Adenosine Diphosphate (ADP) Receptor Antagonists ticlopidine (Ticlid) clopidogrel (Plavix)	• Inhibit platelet aggregation • Alternative for patient who cannot use aspirin
Fibrinolytic Therapy recombinant plasminogen activator (rPA, reteplase [Retavase]) streptokinase (Streptase) tissue plasminogen activator (tPA, alteplase [Activase]) TNK-tPA (Tenecteplase)	• Break up fibrin meshwork in clots • Used only in ST elevation MI
Calcium Channel Blockers verapamil (Calan, Isoptin) nifedipine (Procardia) nicardipine (Cardene) felodipine (Plendil) amlodipine (Norvasc) diltiazem (Cardizem)	• Prevent calcium entry into vascular smooth muscle cells and myocytes (cardiac cells) • Coronary and peripheral vasodilation • ↓ AV conduction • ↓ Myocardial contractility
Morphine	• Acts as an analgesic and sedative • Reduces preload and myocardial O_2 consumption
Angiotensin-Converting Enzyme Inhibitors* captopril (Capoten) enalapril (Vasotec)	• Prevent conversion of angiotensin I to angiotensin II • Decrease endothelial dysfunction • Useful with heart failure, tachycardia, MI, hypertension, and diabetes

*See Table 32-8.

ACS, Acute coronary syndrome; *AV,* atrioventricular; *IV,* intravenous; *MI,* myocardial infarction.

EVIDENCE-BASED PRACTICE
Aspirin Reduces Coronary Artery Disease

Clinical Problem

What is the effectiveness of aspirin in prevention of coronary artery disease (CAD) in those people at risk for CAD?

Best Clinical Practice

- In persons at risk, aspirin reduces the incidence of CAD.
- For patients at risk for CAD, treatment with aspirin for primary prevention was reported to be valuable and safe, with benefits likely to outweigh harms.
- People taking aspirin had an increased incidence of bleeding complications.

Implications for Nursing Practice

- It is important to identify people at risk for CAD.
- Those identified as at risk for CAD should be taught that low-dose aspirin (81 mg) taken on a daily basis can reduce their risk.
- Patients should be taught to assess for manifestations of bleeding, including bleeding gums, frequent nosebleeds, unusual bruising, tarry stools, and blood in urine.

Reference for Evidence

Review: aspirin reduces the incidence of coronary artery disease in persons at risk, *ACP Journal Club* 88, Nov/Dec 2001.

platelet aggregation. For patients unable to tolerate aspirin or in patients with recent gastrointestinal bleeding, ticlopidine (Ticlid) or clopidogrel (Plavix) may be given.[28]

Nitrates. Nitrates are first-line therapy for treatment of acute anginal symptoms (see Table 33-13). Nitrates produce their principal effects by the following:

1. *Dilating peripheral blood vessels.* This results in decreased SVR, venous pooling, and decreased venous blood return to the heart. Therefore myocardial oxygen demand is decreased because of the reduced cardiac workload.
2. *Dilating coronary arteries and collateral vessels.* This may increase blood flow to the ischemic areas of the heart. However, when the coronary arteries are severely atherosclerotic, coronary dilation is difficult to achieve.[28]

Sublingual nitroglycerin. Nitroglycerin given sublingually will usually relieve pain in approximately 3 minutes and has a duration of approximately 20 to 45 minutes. The usual recommended dose is one tablet taken sublingually, which can be followed at 5-minute intervals with two more doses. If nitroglycerin tablets have been necessary and relief from anginal pain has not been obtained after three tablets and 15 minutes, the patient should be instructed to seek immediate medical attention.

The patient must be instructed in the proper use of SL nitroglycerin. It should be easily accessible to the patient at all times. However, patients should be taught not to carry nitroglycerin in their pockets because heat from the body can cause loss of potency of the tablets. For protection from degradation, it should be kept in a tightly closed dark glass bottle. The patient should be instructed to place a nitroglycerin tablet beneath the tongue and allow it to dissolve. This may cause a fizzing or slightly warm feeling locally. The patient should be warned that HR may increase and a pounding headache, dizziness, or flushing may occur. The patient should be cautioned against quickly rising to a standing position because postural hypotension may occur after nitroglycerin ingestion.

Nitroglycerin can be used prophylactically before undertaking an activity that the patient knows may precipitate an anginal attack. In these instances the patient can take a tablet 5 to 10 minutes before beginning the activity. Any changes in the usual pattern of pain, especially increasing frequency or nocturnal angina, should be reported to the health care provider.

Nitroglycerin tablets are marketed in light-resistant bottles closed with metal caps. Because they tend to lose potency once a bottle has been opened, the patient should be advised to purchase a new supply every 6 months.

Nitroglycerin ointment. Nitroglycerin (Nitrol, Nitropaste) is a 2% nitroglycerin topical ointment dosed by the inch. It is placed on the skin, where it is absorbed, producing anginal prophylaxis for 3 to 6 hours. It has been found to be especially useful for nocturnal and unstable angina because it acts for a longer period of time than sublingual (SL) nitroglycerin. Its disadvantages include its messiness and its rapid absorption, necessitating repeated application.[29]

Transdermal controlled-release nitrates. Currently two systems are available for transdermal drug administration: reservoir and matrix. Transderm-Nitro is the reservoir system, in which the drug migrates to the absorption site through a rate-controlled permeable membrane. Nitro-Dur and Nitro-Disc are the matrix system, in which the drug is slowly dispersed through a polymer matrix to the skin absorption site. Both reservoir and matrix delivery systems offer the advantages of steady plasma levels within the therapeutic range during 24 hours, thus making only one application a day necessary. The reservoir system has the disadvantage of dose dumping if the reservoir seal is punctured or broken. An advantage of the matrix system is that there can be no dose dumping. Both systems achieve plasma drug level steady states by 2 hours.

Long-acting nitrates. Long-acting nitrates such as isosorbide dinitrate and isosorbide mononitrate (Isordil, Sorbitrate, Imdur) are longer acting than SL nitroglycerin and, when used in adequate doses, are effective in reducing the incidence of anginal attacks. The effects of oral isosorbide dinitrate may last for as long as 8 hours.

Because of the vasodilating properties of nitrates, the predominant side effect of all nitrate drugs is headache from the dilation of cerebral blood vessels. Sometimes the body can build up a tolerance to the drug so that the headaches abate but the principal antianginal effect is still present. Patients can be advised to take acetaminophen with their nitrate to relieve the headache. Another problem with nitrates is that the body has a tendency to develop a tolerance to the therapeutic effects of nitrates.[29] A strategy found effective to combat this tolerance is providing a nitrate-free period of at least 8 hours within each 24-hour period. This nitrate-free period should be at night unless the patient experiences nocturnal angina. Other complications of the vasodilator drugs are orthostatic hypotension (nitrate syncope) and an aggravation of cerebrovascular insufficiency.

Intravenous nitroglycerin. IV nitroglycerin (Nitrol IV, Nitrostat IV, Nitro-Bid IV, Tridil) has been used in treating the hospitalized patient with unstable angina. It has an immediate onset of action and can be titrated to prevent, treat, and stop acute attacks of angina. The goal of therapy is to reduce anginal pain.[25,30] IV nitroglycerin has also been used in treatment of MI. The rationale for use in MI is to increase the collateral blood flow to the ischemic area and reduce myocardial oxygen demand because of decreasing preload and afterload. Tolerance is a side effect of IV nitrate therapy. An effective strategy for this phenomenon is titrating down the dose at night during sleep and titrating the dose up during the day.

β-Adrenergic blockers. β-Adrenergic blockers decrease morbidity and mortality rates in patients with CAD, especially following acute MI. However, β-adrenergic blockers have many side effects and are sometimes poorly tolerated.[28] β-Adrenergic blockers available for the prophylaxis of angina are propranolol (Inderal), metoprolol (Lopressor), esmolol (Brevibloc), nadolol (Corgard), atenolol (Tenormin), oxyprendol (Trasicor), pindolol (Visken), and timolol (Blocadren). These drugs decrease myocardial contractility, HR, SVR, and BP, all of which reduce the myocardial oxygen demand. Side effects of β-adrenergic blockers may include bradycardia, hypotension, wheezing, and GI complaints. Many patients also complain of weight gain, depression, and sexual dysfunction. β-Adrenergic blockers should not be discontinued abruptly without medical supervision. β-Adrenergic blockers may mask the signs of hypoglycemia in diabetics.

Calcium channel blockers. Calcium channel blockers such as nifedipine (Procardia), verapamil (Calan, Isoptin), diltiazem (Cardizem), and nicardipine (Cardene) are the next step in the management of angina. However, calcium channel blockers are not used in the treatment of MI. Most of these agents have sustained-release versions for longer action with the hope of increased patient adherence. The three primary effects of calcium channel blockers are (1) systemic vasodilation with decreased SVR, (2) decreased myocardial contractility, and (3) coronary vasodilation. Each drug manifests these effects to a different degree.

Cardiac muscle and vascular smooth muscle cells are more dependent on extracellular calcium than skeletal muscles and are therefore more sensitive to calcium channel blocking agents. The effect of calcium channel blockers on smooth muscle of both coronary and systemic arteries is to cause relaxation and relative vasodilation, thus increasing blood flow. The long-acting nifedipine-like drugs primarily cause vasodilation. Verapamil and diltiazem also have antiarrhythmic properties (see Chapter 35). Myocardial perfusion is enhanced with calcium channel blockers by increased coronary blood flow through vasodilation and reduction in myocardial oxygen demand mediated through a decrease in HR and afterload. Calcium channel blockers have also been effective in controlling angina from either "fixed" atherosclerotic lesions or vasospasm. Verapamil, nifedipine, and diltiazem have also been shown to consistently decrease systemic BP in the hypertensive patient.

Calcium channel blockers potentiate the action of digoxin by increasing serum digoxin levels during the first week of therapy. Therefore serum digoxin levels should be closely monitored on institution of this therapy, and the patient should be taught the signs and symptoms of digoxin toxicity.

Percutaneous Coronary Intervention. A common intervention for angina is an elective **percutaneous coronary intervention** (PCI). (In a person with an MI, an emergent PCI may be done). In a catheterization laboratory a catheter equipped with an inflatable balloon tip is inserted into the appropriate coronary artery. When the lesion is located, the catheter is passed through and just past the lesion, the balloon is inflated, and the atherosclerotic plaque is compressed, resulting in vessel dilation. Bivalirudin (Angiomax), lepirudin (Refludan), and argatroban (Acova) are thrombin inhibitors used as anticoagulants in patients with unstable angina undergoing PCI.

The advantages of PCI are that (1) it provides an alternative to surgical intervention; (2) it is performed with local anesthesia; (3) the patient is ambulatory 24 hours after the procedure; (4) the length of hospital stay is approximately 1 to 3 days compared with the 4- to 6-day stay of someone having open heart surgery with a coronary artery bypass graft (CABG), thus reducing hospital costs; and (5) there is rapid return to work (approximately 5 to 7 days after PCI) instead of a 2- to 8-week convalescence after CABG.

Many advancements have been made in PCI during the last decade. Guide wires and catheters with greater flexibility have been developed, enabling cardiologists to maneuver the catheters to distal and proximal lesions. Today PCI is more frequently performed than CABG. Reduction of lesion size by greater than 50% occurs in 90% of patients.[23] New techniques have been developed to provide blood flow to the distal myocardium during balloon inflation, increasing the safety of the procedure. Dilation may also be done for stenotic grafts from a previous CABG, although these vessels usually require repeated dilation.

The most serious complication of PCI is dissection of the dilated artery. If the damage is extensive, the coronary artery could rupture, causing cardiac tamponade, ischemia and infarction, a fall in CO, and possible death. There is also danger from infarction should the lesion be calcified and a portion of the plaque dislodge and occlude the vessel distal to the catheter. Coronary spasm from the mechanical irritation of the catheter or balloon can occur, as well as chemical irritation from the contrast media injection used to visualize the artery. Abrupt closure is another complication that can occur in the first 24 hours after PCI. Restenosis after PCI can occur.

Stent Placement. Intracoronary stents are usually inserted during PCI. Stents are used to treat abrupt or threatened abrupt closure and restenosis following PCI. **Stents** are expandable meshlike structures designed to maintain vessel patency by compressing the arterial walls and resisting vasoconstriction (Fig. 33-16). Stents are carefully placed over the angioplasty site to hold the vessel open. Because stents are thrombogenic, the patient is usually treated with antiplatelet agents such as aspirin, ticlopidine (Ticlid), or clopidogrel (Plavix). An IV infusion of a glycoprotein IIb/IIIa inhibitor (e.g., abciximab [ReoPro], epifibatide [Integrilin], tirobifan [Aggrastat]), has been found to be beneficial for preventing abrupt closure of the stents (see Table 33-13). The primary complications

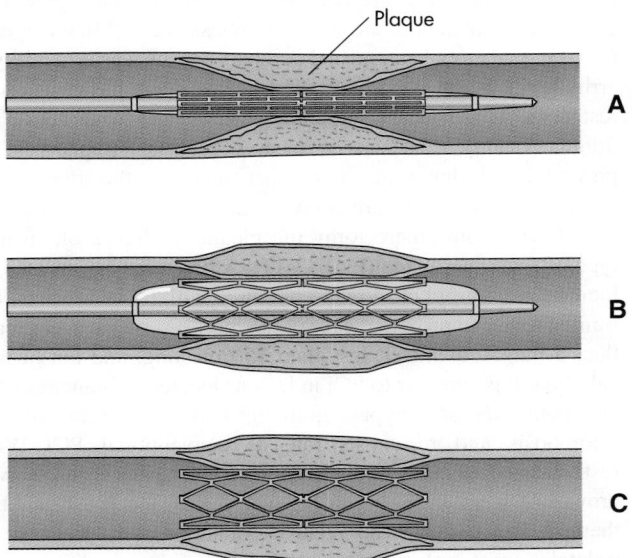

FIG. 33-16 Placement of a coronary artery stent. **A**, The stent is positioned at the site of the lesion. **B**, The balloon is inflated, expanding the stent. The balloon is then deflated and removed. **C**, The implanted stent is left in place.

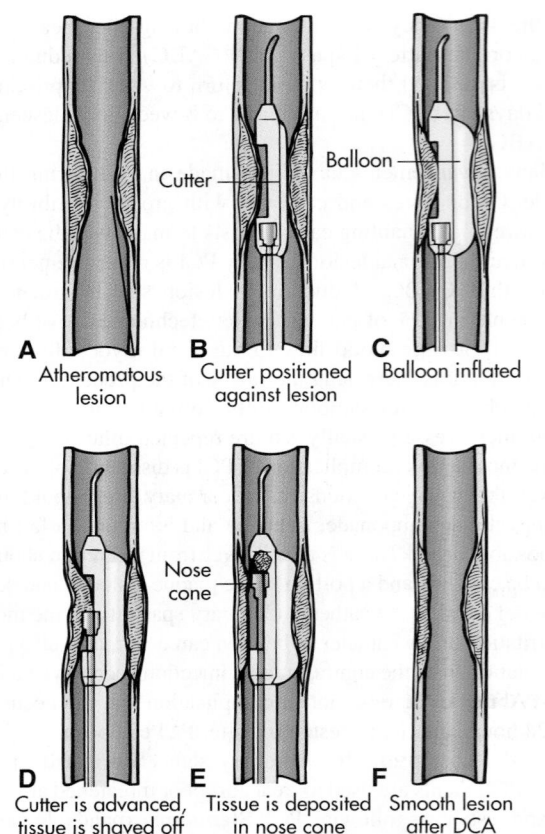

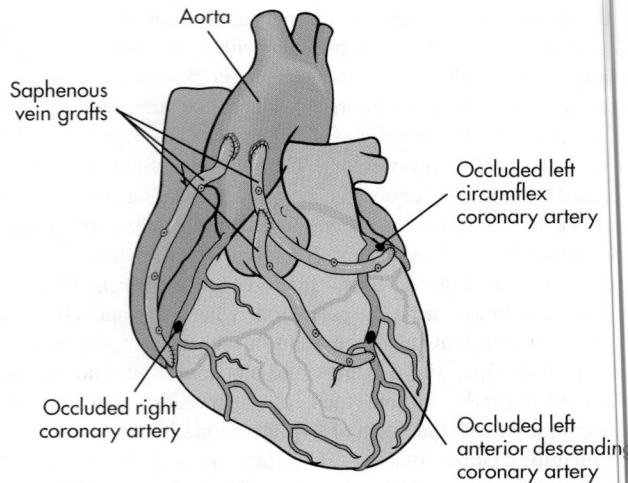

FIG. 33-18 Saphenous aortocoronary artery bypass or revascularization involves taking a piece of saphenous vein from the leg and creating a conduit for blood from the aorta to the area below the blockage in the coronary artery. A triple bypass is illustrated.

FIG. 33-17 Directional coronary atherectomy (DCA). A, Atheromatous lesion. B, DCA cutter is introduced over a guide wire into the coronary artery and positioned with the window against the lesion. C, Balloon is inflated to maintain cutting position against the lesion. D, As the rotating cutter is advanced across the lesion, atheromatous tissue is shaved off. E, Tissue is deposited in the nose cone. F, Smooth lesion after DCA.

from stent placement are hemorrhage and vascular injury. Less common complications are stent thrombosis, acute MI, emergency CABG, stent embolization, and coronary spasm. The possibility of arrhythmias is always present. The use of stents has reduced the restenosis rate of PCI. Drug-eluting stents can also be used. The drug-containing stent slowly releases sirolimus (rapamycin) to prevent the buildup of new tissue that can reclog the artery.

Atherectomy. *Atherectomy* is another technique used to treat CAD. With atherectomy the plaque is shaved off using a type of rotational blade (Fig. 33-17). Atherectomy decreases the incidence of abrupt closure as compared with PCI. However, it is limited to use in proximal and middle portions of a vessel greater than 3 mm in diameter, less than 15 mm long, and not heavily calcified. It is superior to PCI in lesions located in branches or attachment sites of a bypass graft but carries the same risk for thrombosis and restenosis rate as conventional PCI. When restenosis occurs in a stent site, it is usually caused by an overgrowth of scar tissue. It can be treated with localized radiation therapy. The patient who receives radiation will need an antiplatelet agent such as clopidogrel or ticlopidine for life because the stent will not endothelialize and will be prone to clotting.

Laser Angioplasty. Laser angioplasty, or excimer laser coronary angioplasty (ECLA), is performed with a catheter containing fibers that carry laser energy. The laser energy is used to precisely dissolve the blockage in the coronary artery. The excimer is a cool laser and does not generate the heat that a conventional laser does.

Myocardial Revascularization. **Myocardial revascularization,** or CABG, is the primary surgical treatment for CAD. The patient with CAD who has failed medical management or who has advanced disease is considered a candidate for surgical revascularization.

CABG procedure. The CABG operation consists of the construction of new conduits (vessels to transport blood) between the aorta, or other major arteries, beyond the obstructed coronary artery (or arteries) (Fig. 33-18). This procedure provides blood flow beyond the stenosis so that the myocardium distal to the obstruction continues to receive blood flow. The procedure requires the use of cardiopulmonary bypass.

This procedure usually involves a graft from the saphenous vein, the internal mammary artery (also called the internal thoracic artery), radial artery, gastroepiploic artery, or inferior epigastric artery. The saphenous vein from one or both of the legs of the patient is removed and is used as a free graft and anastomosed proximally to the ascending aorta and distally to one (or more) coronary artery. Saphenous veins used as grafts develop diffuse intimal hyperplasia, which contributes to ultimate stenosis and occlusions of the graft. Patency rates of these grafts are lower when the anastomosis is to a small coronary artery and to arteries supplying areas with scar tissue (infarction areas). The use of aspirin (81 to 325 mg orally daily) improves vein graft patency.

The internal mammary artery (IMA) is the most common artery used for bypass. Because the patency rate of the IMA is higher than that of saphenous veins, the IMA may prove to be a better conduit for improving long-term prognosis. The left IMA, which is left attached to its origin from the left subclavian artery, is mobilized from the chest wall and anastomosed to the coronary artery distal to the stenosis. The right IMA may also be used in a similar fashion. Use of both internal mammary arteries is not usually done because the major blood flow to the chest wall would be compromised.

If a patient has had previous CABG using saphenous vein grafts and/or IMA, and at the time of reoperation has no conduits to harvest (is not a candidate for radial artery harvest), the gastroepiploic artery or inferior epigastric artery may be used. These arteries are excellent conduits. However, use of these arteries creates the additional need for a laparotomy. This increases the length of surgery, and wound complications at the harvest site are not uncommon, especially in an obese or diabetic patient. Because of the number of patients requiring reoperation, the use of alternative arteries and veins will become increasingly more common.

CABG remains a palliative treatment for CAD and not a cure. It provides the patient with improved outcomes, quality of life, and survival. The results of coronary revascularization are less favorable for women than men. The severity of the clinical variables in women, including a more severe angina and the smaller mean diameter of the coronary vessels, are all considered possible causes of their higher mortality rates, which are often double that of men the same age.

Nursing care for the patient with a CABG involves caring for two surgical sites: the chest and the arm, leg, or abdomen. Care of the radial artery harvest site includes careful observation and monitoring of the skin site, as well as sensory and motor function of the distal thumb and fingers, and oximetry of the distal fingers. The patient with radial artery harvest should be on a calcium channel blocker for approximately 3 months to decrease the incidence of arterial spasm at the arm or anastomosis site. The care of the leg wound is similar to the postoperative care after the stripping of varicose veins (see Chapter 37). The management of the chest wound, which involves a sternotomy, is similar to that of other chest surgeries (see Chapter 27).

MIDCABG procedure. With recent efforts to reduce cost, length of hospital stay, and morbidity, a new approach to CABG surgery has been developed. *Minimally invasive direct coronary artery bypass grafting* (MIDCABG) has been used as an alternative to traditional CABG. This newer technique offers the patient with left anterior descending (LAD) or single-vessel disease, in whom medical management is not effective, an approach to surgical treatment other than sternotomy and the traditional CABG.

Several small incisions are made between the ribs. A thoracoscope is used to mobilize the left IMA (LIMA). The heart is slowed using an IV infusion of β-adrenergic or calcium channel blockers. The LIMA is then anastomosed to the distal LAD (and/or right coronary artery using the right IMA). (The radial artery and the saphenous vein may also be used.) Before closure, the IV infusion of β-adrenergic or calcium channel blockers is stopped. A chest tube is placed in the left lateral chest, and a mediastinal tube is also placed.

Postoperative nursing care of the patient with a MIDCABG procedure is similar to that for routine cardiac surgery patients. IV nitroglycerin is used to minimize ischemia and coronary artery spasm. Pain management in these patients is essential because a thoracotomy incision has a higher incidence of pain than a sternotomy. The recovery time is somewhat shorter, and patients may resume their routine activities in a shorter time than patients who have a standard CABG procedure.

MIDCABG is often performed without the use of cardiopulmonary bypass (CPB). The off-pump coronary artery bypass (OPCAB) procedure utilizes full or partial sternotomy to enable access to all coronary vessels. OPCAB is then performed on a beating heart without CPB. Vessel stabilizer devices and techniques allow the surgeon to suture the distal end of the bypass graft to the coronary artery without stopping or slowing the heart.

Transmyocardial laser revascularization. *Transmyocardial laser revascularization* (TMR) is an indirect revascularization procedure that uses a laser to create channels between the left ventric-

ular cavity and the coronary microcirculation (ventriculocoronary anastomoses). The channels allow blood to flow into ischemic areas. The procedure may be performed during cardiac catheterization as a percutaneous TMR or during surgery using a left anterior thoracotomy incision. A high-energy laser, triggered electrocardiographically, is focused through the wall of the ventricle, and usually as many as 40 transmural connections are established in the ischemic myocardium. The laser perforations are completed in 15 to 45 minutes. Currently treatment is limited to patients with advanced CAD who are not candidates for traditional bypass surgery and have failed maximum medical therapy.

Complications following TMR include ventricular arrhythmias, postoperative bleeding and cardiac tamponade, accidental perforation of the great vessels or epicardial coronary arteries, damage to the chordae tendineae, and low cardiac output. Although blood flow to the myocardium is improved immediately through the patent channels extending from the outside of the heart to the interior of the left ventricle, optimal results are not seen until the formation of new blood vessels arise from laser channels and begin to feed the myocardium. Optimal results are seen at about 3 to 6 months.

COLLABORATIVE CARE

Myocardial Infarction

It is extremely important that a patient with a suspected MI is rapidly diagnosed and treated to preserve cardiac muscle. Initial management of the patient with MI is best accomplished in an intensive care unit (ICU), where constant monitoring is available. Arrhythmias may be detected and appropriate treatment can be instituted. An IV route is established to provide an accessible means for emergency drug therapy. Morphine sulfate may be given intravenously for relief of pain. Oxygen is usually administered by nasal cannula at a rate of 2 to 4 L per minute. The collaborative care management of MI is presented in Fig. 33-13.

A continuous IV infusion of amiodarone may be given to the patient who has frequent PVCs, which may precede ventricular fibrillation. The use of prophylactic lidocaine is not recommended by the American College of Cardiology (ACC)/AHA practice guidelines for the treatment of acute MI. However, lidocaine may be a treatment option for the patient who has sustained ventricular tachycardia or ventricular fibrillation.[25,31]

Vital signs are taken frequently during the first few hours after admission and are monitored closely thereafter. Bed rest and limitation of activity are initially used for 12 to 24 hours, with a gradual increase in activity unless contraindicated.

A pulmonary artery (PA) catheter and an intraarterial line may be used to accurately monitor intracardiac, pulmonary artery, and systolic arterial pressures. In the presence of severe LV dysfunction, an intraaortic balloon pump (IABP) may be used to assist ventricular ejection and promote coronary artery perfusion. (Pulmonary artery catheters and IABP are discussed in Chapter 64.)

For a patient with STEMI, reperfusion therapy is used (see Fig. 33-13). *Reperfusion therapy* can include fibrinolytic (thrombolytic) therapy or PCI. The goal in the treatment of acute MI is to salvage as much myocardial muscle as possible. Historically, treatment of acute MI had been directed only at the patient's signs and symptoms (i.e., arrhythmia, CHF), and nothing was done for the acute process of infarction.

Fibrinolytic Therapy. Fibrinolytic therapy offers the advantages of availability and rapid administration. With the advent of fibrinolytic therapy, treatment has progressed to actually stopping the infarction process instead of just treating symptoms. Mortality rates have decreased 2.5% to 5% with fibrinolytic treatment.[25,31]

It is now known that 80% to 90% of all acute MIs are secondary to thrombus formation.[25] In this situation perfusion to the myocardium distal to the occlusion is halted, causing progressive ischemia, cell death, and necrosis. The acute MI process takes time. The earliest tissue to become ischemic is the subendocardium (the innermost layer of tissue in the cardiac muscle). Necrosis spreads toward the epicardium in a phenomenon termed the *wave front of necrosis.* Myocardial cells do not die instantly. It takes approximately 4 to 6 hours for the entire thickness of the muscle to become necrosed in the majority of patients; this is termed a *transmural infarction.*

Treatment of the acute MI is geared to quickly dissolve the thrombus in the coronary artery and reperfuse the myocardium before cellular death occurs. To be of most benefit, fibrinolytic therapy must be given as soon as possible, ideally within the first hour after onset of symptoms and preferably within the first 6 hours after the onset of symptoms. If reperfusion occurs within 6 hours, a 25% reduction in mortality rate has been shown.[31]

Indications and contraindications. The commonly used fibrinolytics (see Table 33-13) are given intravenously. The choice of a thrombolytic agent is guided by considerations of cost, efficacy, and ease of administration. Streptokinase is the least expensive. Although these drugs have different mechanisms of action and different pharmacokinetics, they all produce an open artery by lysis of the thrombus in the coronary artery.

Because all the fibrinolytics produce lysis of the pathologic clot, they may also lyse other clots (e.g., a postoperative site). Therefore patient selection is important because persons receiving fibrinolytic therapy may have a minor or major bleeding episode as a consequence of therapy. Not all patients who have an acute MI are candidates for fibrinolytic therapy (Table 33-14). Inclusion criteria to receive an IV thrombolytic agent are (1) chest pain typical of acute MI less than or equal to 6 hours in duration (some centers extend the time limit to 12 hours); (2) chest pain for more than 6 hours if intermittent with ongoing ischemia; (3) 12-lead ECG findings consistent with acute MI, irrespective of location; and (4) no condition that may cause a predisposition to hemorrhage.[31]

Procedure. Once the patient has been assessed for risk factors of possible side effects of the therapy and is considered a candidate, fibrinolytic therapy is begun. Each hospital has a protocol to follow for administration of thrombolytic agents. However, there are several common factors. Blood is drawn, two to three lines for IV therapy are started, and all other invasive procedures are done before the thrombolytic agent is given, reducing the possibility of bleeding in the patient.

The time at which therapy begins is noted, and the patient is monitored frequently during and after the period of time that the thrombolytic is administered. ECG, vital signs, and heart and lung assessments are completed as often as every 5 minutes to evaluate the patient's response to therapy. When reperfusion occurs (i.e., the coronary artery that was occluded is patent, and blood flow is reestablished to the myocardium), several clinical markers may occur. These include return of ST segment to baseline on the ECG; resolution of chest pain; the presence of reperfusion arrhythmias; and marked, rapid rise of the CK-MB enzyme within 3 hours of therapy, peaking within 12 hours. The CK-MB levels increase as the dead myocardial cells release

TABLE 33-14	Contraindications for the Use of Fibrinolytic Therapy

Absolute Contraindications
Active internal bleeding
Active inflammatory bowel disease
Active peptic ulcer disease
Acute pericarditis
Defective hemostasis
Gastrointestinal/genitourinary bleeding <6 months
History of hemorrhagic stroke
Known bleeding disorder
Neurosurgical procedure <2 months
Pregnancy
Recent surgery or trauma <3 months
Suspected aortic dissection
Uncontrolled hypertension
- Systolic BP >180 mm Hg
- Diastolic BP >110 mm Hg

Relative Contraindications
Bacterial endocarditis
Chronic warfarin therapy
Diabetic hemorrhagic retinopathy
Poorly controlled hypertension
Recent, brief CPR <10 minutes
Severe renal or liver disease
Stroke or TIA ≤12 months ago

BP, Blood pressure; *CPR,* cardiopulmonary resuscitation; *TIA,* transient ischemic attack.

CK-MB enzymes into the circulation after perfusion has been restored to the area.

The nurse must closely monitor the patient for signs of *reperfusion arrhythmias,* including an increase in premature ventricular contractions, ventricular tachycardia, and ventricular fibrillation, and accelerated idioventricular rhythm. Sometimes bradycardia, AV blocks, and asystole can occur, depending on the location of the infarction.

Another major concern with therapy is reocclusion of the artery. In this situation the patient seems to have a reperfused artery and is stable. However, because the area around the thrombus is unstable, another clot may form or spasm of the artery may occur. Because of this possibility, most physicians begin heparin therapy. An IV bolus is given, followed by a heparin drip to maintain the patient's partial thromboplastin time (PTT) at one to two times normal. This prevents another clot from forming in the coronary artery. If another clot develops, the patient will have similar complaints of chest pain, and ECG changes occur. The physician is notified and further action is taken to determine the cause of the reocclusion. The patient may go to the cardiac catheterization laboratory for further invasive diagnostic procedures or PCI. Sometimes the patient will again receive fibrinolytic therapy.

The major complication with fibrinolytic therapy is bleeding. Prevention of bleeding is essential. Ongoing nursing assessment is also essential. Minor bleeding is expected. If minor bleeding does occur (such as surface bleeding from IV sites or gingival bleeding), it can be controlled by pressure dressing or ice packs, and fibrinolytic therapy should not be stopped. If, however, there is a major bleeding episode, the physician should be notified and therapy should be stopped. The nurse must pay particular attention to signs and symptoms of bleeding such as a drop in BP, an increase in HR, blood in the nasogastric aspirate or stool, hematuria, a sudden decrease in the patient's level of consciousness, and oozing of blood from IV or catheter sites. If any of these manifestations develop, the physician should be notified and fibrinolytic therapy may be discontinued.

Cardiac Catheterization. Although the treatment for acute MI is to lyse the thrombus and reperfuse the myocardium, some patients may not be candidates for fibrinolytic therapy or may have a complicated course necessitating an emergent cardiac catheterization. The patient with an acute MI may have a catheterization early in the treatment phase to locate the exact lesion (or lesions) and to assess the severity, the presence of collateral circulation, and LV function. With actual visualization of the coronary artery system and LV function, the physician can prescribe a treatment modality most beneficial to the patient. Possible therapies include direct intracoronary thrombolytic therapy, PCI, IABP insertion, or CABG.

Percutaneous Coronary Intervention. PCI is a mechanical reperfusion of a thrombotic coronary occlusion. PCI is often performed as first-line treatment instead of fibrinolytic therapy, especially in institutions that have an interventional cardiologist, a cardiac catheterization laboratory, and cardiac surgery capability (PCI is discussed on p. 821).

Drug Therapy. Drug therapy for patients with MI is presented in Table 33-13 and Fig. 33-13 and discussed on pp. 818 to 821. Specific discussion of a few drugs is presented in this section.

IV nitroglycerin. IV nitroglycerin (Tridil) may be used in the initial therapeutic treatment of the patient with an acute MI. Nitroglycerin given intravenously may reduce pain and decrease preload and afterload while increasing the myocardial oxygen supply. Its action may also increase collateral circulation to the ischemic areas of the myocardium.

Antiarrhythmic drugs. Arrhythmias are the most common complications after an MI. In general, they are not treated aggressively, unless they are life threatening. (The drugs used in the treatment of arrhythmias are discussed in Chapter 35.)

Morphine. Morphine sulfate is given for acute chest pain relief because it reduces anxiety and fear and decreases the cardiac workload by lowering myocardial oxygen consumption, reducing contractility, lowering BP, and slowing the HR. Morphine can depress respirations, which may cause hypoxia, a condition to be avoided in myocardial ischemia and infarction.

β-Adrenergic blockers. β-Adrenergic blockers are used to decrease heart rate, myocardial contractility, and preload (see Table 33-13).

Angiotensin-converting enzyme inhibitors. Angiotensin-converting enzyme (ACE) inhibitors (e.g., captopril [Capoten], enalapril [Vasotec]) may be used following MIs. The use of ACE inhibitors can help prevent ventricular remodeling and prevent or slow the progression of heart failure. (See Chapter 32 and Table 32-8 for a discussion of ACE inhibitors.)

Stool softeners. After an MI the patient is predisposed to constipation as a result of bed rest and narcotic administration. Stool softeners such as docusate sodium (Colace) are given to facilitate and promote the comfort of bowel evacuation. This prevents straining and the resultant vagal stimulation from the Valsalva maneuver. Vagal stimulation produces bradycardia and can provoke arrhythmias. Another real danger of straining is that when the action is stopped, venous return to the heart is suddenly increased. This may result in overloading of a weakened heart.

Nutritional Therapy. Diet is restricted in saturated fats and cholesterol (see Table 33-4) and is sometimes low in sodium to prevent fluid retention. The patient may have a clear liquid diet the first day when there may still be nausea.

NURSING MANAGEMENT
ANGINA AND MYOCARDIAL INFARCTION

■ Nursing Assessment

Subjective and objective data that should be obtained from a patient with angina or an MI are presented in Table 33-15.

■ Nursing Diagnoses

Nursing diagnoses for the patient with angina or an MI may include, but are not limited to, those presented in NCP 33-1.

TABLE 33-15	Nursing Assessment
	Angina and Myocardial Infarction

Subjective Data

Important Health Information

Past health history: Previous history of MI, angina, aortic stenosis, or cardiomyopathy; hypertension, diabetes mellitus, anemia, lung disease; hyperlipidemia

Medications: Use of nitrates, calcium channel blockers, β-adrenergic blockers, antihypertensive drugs, antilipidemic agents

Functional Health Patterns

Health perception–health management: Family history of heart disease; sedentary lifestyle; smoking

Nutritional-metabolic: Indigestion, heartburn, nausea, belching, vomiting

Elimination: Desire to void, straining at stool

Activity-exercise: Palpitations; dyspnea; dizziness, weakness

Cognitive-perceptual: Substernal chest pain or pressure (squeezing, constricting, aching, sharp, tingling), possible radiation to jaw, neck, shoulders, back, or arms

Coping–stress tolerance: Stressful lifestyle; apprehension, anxiety; feeling of impending doom

Objective Data

General

Anxiety, fear, restlessness

Integumentary

Cool, clammy, pale skin

Cardiovascular

Tachycardia or bradycardia, pulsus alternans (alternating weak and strong heart beats), arrhythmias (especially ventricular), ventricular gallop, atrial gallop, ↑ or ↓ BP, murmur

Possible Findings

Negative or positive cardiac markers, ↑ serum lipids; ↑ WBC, positive exercise stress test and thallium scans; ST segment and T wave abnormalities on ECG; cardiac enlargement or calcifications, pulmonary congestion on chest x-ray; abnormal wall motion with stress echocardiogram; positive coronary angiography

BP, Blood pressure; *ECG,* electrocardiogram; *MI,* myocardial infarction; *WBC,* white blood cell.

NURSING CARE PLAN 33-1

Patient with Myocardial Infarction

NURSING DIAGNOSIS   **Acute pain** *related to* myocardial ischemia and decreased myocardial oxygen supply *as manifested by* severe chest pain and tightness, radiation of pain to the neck and arms.

OUTCOMES—NOC	INTERVENTIONS—NIC and *RATIONALES*
Pain Level (2102)	*Cardiac Care: Acute (4044)*
▪ Reported pain _____	▪ Evaluate chest pain noting intensity, location, radiation, duration, and precipitating and alleviating factors rating on a scale of 0 to 10 *to accurately evaluate, treat, and prevent further ischemia.*
	▪ Provide O_2 via nasal cannula and monitor the effectiveness of oxygen therapy *to increase oxygenation of myocardial tissue and prevent further ischemia.*
	▪ Administer morphine intravenously to relieve and prevent pain and ischemia as needed *to decrease anxiety and cardiac workload.*
Outcome Scale	▪ Obtain 12-lead ECG *during pain episode to help differentiate angina from extension of MI or pericarditis.*
1 = Never demonstrated	▪ Monitor cardiac rhythm, rate, and BP *to assess for hypotension and bradycardia, which may lead to hypoperfusion.*
2 = Rarely demonstrated	▪ Monitor peripheral pulses, capillary refill, and temperature and color of extremities *to assess for changes in systemic circulation.*
3 = Sometimes demonstrated	
4 = Often demonstrated	
5 = Consistently demonstrated	

NURSING DIAGNOSIS   **Ineffective tissue perfusion (cardiac)** *related to* myocardial injury and potential pulmonary congestion *as manifested by* decrease in BP, dyspnea, arrhythmias, peripheral edema, and oliguria.

OUTCOMES—NOC	INTERVENTIONS—NIC and *RATIONALES*
Cardiac Pump Effectiveness (0400)	*Cardiac Care (4040) and Hemodynamic Regulation (4150)*
▪ BP IER _____	▪ Monitor vital signs every hour and prn *to provide baseline and ongoing assessment.*
▪ Heart rate IER _____	▪ Monitor for cardiac arrhythmias, including disturbances of both rhythm and conduction through cardiac monitor, *to assess for any changes in rate or rhythm.*
▪ Peripheral edema not present _____	
▪ Pulmonary edema not present _____	▪ Provide rest periods *to avoid fatigue and decrease the oxygen demand on myocardium.*
▪ Arrhythmias not present _____	▪ Monitor respiratory status, including breath sounds and pulse oximetry, *to maintain appropriate levels of oxygenation and observe for signs of pulmonary edema.*
Outcome Scale	▪ Monitor fluid balance by measuring intake and output, assessing for peripheral edema, and daily weights *to assess renal perfusion and observe for fluid retention.*
1 = Extremely compromised	
2 = Substantially compromised	
3 = Moderately compromised	
4 = Mildly compromised	
5 = Not compromised	

NURSING DIAGNOSIS   **Anxiety** *related to* perceived or actual threat of death, pain, possible lifestyle changes *as manifested by* restlessness, agitation, and verbalization of concern over lifestyle changes and prognosis as evidenced by patient's statement, "What is going to happen when I die? Everyone relies on me."

OUTCOMES—NOC	INTERVENTIONS—NIC and *RATIONALES*
Anxiety Control (1402)	*Anxiety Reduction (5820) and Teaching: Disease Process (5602)*
▪ Monitors intensity of anxiety _____	▪ Assess for verbal and nonverbal signs of anxiety and when level of anxiety changes *because anxiety increases the need for oxygen.*
▪ Seeks information to reduce anxiety _____	▪ Use a calm, reassuring approach *so as not to increase patient's anxiety.*
▪ Controls anxiety response _____	▪ Instruct patient on the use of relaxation techniques such as guided imagery *to enhance self-control.*
▪ Uses relaxation techniques to reduce anxiety _____	▪ Encourage family to stay with patient as appropriate *to provide comfort.*
Outcome Scale	▪ Encourage verbalization of feelings, perceptions, and fears *to decrease anxiety and stress.*
1 = Never demonstrated	▪ If patient needs information, provide it clearly and simply *so it can be understood.*
2 = Rarely demonstrated	
3 = Sometimes demonstrated	
4 = Often demonstrated	
5 = Consistently demonstrated	

ADLs, Activities of daily living; *BP,* blood pressure; *ECG,* electrocardiogram; *IER,* in expected range; *MI,* myocardial infarction.

Patient with Myocardial Infarction—cont'd

NURSING DIAGNOSIS   **Activity intolerance** *related to* fatigue secondary to decreased cardiac output and poor lung and tissue perfusion *as manifested by* fatigue with minimal activity, and inability to care for self without dyspnea, and increased heart rate.

OUTCOMES—NOC

Energy Conservation (0002)
- Balances activity and rest _____
- Recognizes energy limitations _____
- Uses energy conservation techniques _____

_____

Outcome Scale
1 = Not at all
2 = To a slight extent
3 = To a moderate extent
4 = To a great extent
5 = To a very great extent

Activity Tolerance (1300)
- Oxygen saturation IER in response to activity _____
- Heart rate IER in response to activity _____
- Respiratory effort in response to activity _____

_____

Outcome Scale
1 = Extremely compromised
2 = Substantially compromised
3 = Moderately compromised
4 = Mildly compromised
5 = Not compromised

INTERVENTIONS—NIC and *RATIONALES*

Cardiac Care (4040) and Energy Management (01800)
- Monitor patient's response to antiarrhythmic medications *because these medications will affect BP and pulse before activity.*
- Assist patient to understand energy conservation principles, such as bed rest, *to conserve energy and promote independence.*
- Instruct patient and family on activity restrictions, such as bed rest and progressive activity, *so that the family can reinforce activities for the patient.*
- Arrange exercise and rest periods *to avoid fatigue and to increase activity tolerance without rapidly increasing cardiac workload.*
- Monitor patient's oxygen response (e.g., heart rate, cardiac rhythm, respiratory rate) to self-care or nursing activities *to monitor patient's response to activity and adjust as necessary.*
- Teach patient and significant other techniques in self-care that will minimize oxygen consumption, such as pacing self in ADLs, *to promote independence and minimize O_2 consumption.*

NURSING DIAGNOSIS   **Ineffective therapeutic regimen management** *related to* lack of knowledge of disease process, rehabilitation, home activities, and medications *as manifested by* frequent questioning about illness, management, and care after discharge.

OUTCOMES—NOC

Health Orientation (1705)
- Perception that health is a high priority in making lifestyle changes _____
- Perception that health behavior is relevant to self _____
- Focus on adjustments to life situations _____
- Focus on maintaining functional abilities _____

_____

Outcome Scale
1 = Very weak
2 = Weak
3 = Moderate
4 = Strong
5 = Very strong

Knowledge: Treatment Regimen (1813)
- Description of rationale for treatment regimen _____
- Description of expected effects of treatment _____

_____

Outcome Scale
1 = None
2 = Limited
3 = Moderate
4 = Substantial
5 = Extensive

INTERVENTIONS—NIC and *RATIONALES*

Self-Modification Assistance (4470)

Teaching: Disease Process (5602)

Teaching: Procedure/Treatment (5618)
- Appraise the patient's current level of knowledge related to specific disease process *to obtain information on patient's teaching needs.*
- Explain the pathophysiology of the disease and how it relates to the anatomy and physiology, as appropriate, *to individualize the information and to increase understanding.*
- Instruct the patient on the purpose, action, dose, route, and duration of each medication *so that the patient understands the reason for taking the medication and will be less likely to refuse to take medications.*
- Discuss lifestyle changes with patient and family that may be required to prevent further complications and/or control disease process *to get the cooperation of the patient's significant support system.*
- Assist the patient in identifying behaviors that need to change to achieve a desired goal *so that the patient has a clear understanding of how to change behaviors such as poor diet.*
- Assist the patient in identifying even small successes such as ambulating across the room *so that the patient has positive reinforcement at an early stage in recovery.*
- Refer the patient and family to local community agencies/support groups as appropriate *so that the patient and family have resources and support available.*
- Be specific when giving discharge instructions; write them down for patient to take home *to be available for reference.*

■ Planning

The overall goals are that the patient with angina and an MI will (1) experience relief of pain, (2) have no progression of MI, (3) receive immediate and appropriate treatment, (4) cope effectively with associated anxiety, (5) cooperate with the rehabilitation plan, and (6) modify or alter risk factors.

■ Nursing Implementation: Angina

Health Promotion. Behaviors to reduce risk factors for CAD are presented in Table 33-3 and discussed on p. 805.

Acute Intervention. If a nurse is present during an anginal attack, the following measures should be instituted: (1) administration of oxygen, (2) determination of vital signs, (3) ECG, (4) prompt pain relief first with a nitrate followed by a narcotic analgesic if needed, (5) auscultation of heart sounds, and (6) comfortable positioning of the patient. The patient will most likely appear distressed and have pale, cool, clammy skin. The BP and heart rate will probably be elevated, and an atrial gallop (S_4) sound may be heard. If a ventricular gallop (S_3) is heard, it may indicate LV decompensation. A murmur may be heard during an anginal attack secondary to ischemia of a papillary muscle. The murmur is likely to be transient and abates with the cessation of symptoms. Supportive and realistic assurance and a calm, soothing manner help reduce the patient's anxiety.

Ambulatory and Home Care. The patient with a history of angina should be reassured that a long, productive life is possible. Prevention of angina is preferable to its treatment, and this is where teaching is important. The patient should be taught regarding CAD and angina, precipitating factors, risk factors, and medications.

Patient teaching can be handled in a variety of ways. One-to-one contact between the nurse and the patient is often the most effective procedure. The time spent in providing daily care is often an ideal teaching period. Teaching tools, such as pamphlets, videotapes, a heart model, and especially written information, are necessary components of patient and family teaching (see Chapter 4).

The patient should be assisted in identifying factors that precipitate angina (see Table 33-8). The patient should be given instruction on how to avoid or control precipitating factors. For example, the patient should be cautioned to avoid exposures to extremes of weather and taught not to eat large, heavy meals. If a heavy meal is ingested, adequate rest should be planned for 1 to 2 hours after eating because blood is shunted to the GI tract to aid digestion and absorption.

The patient should be assisted in identifying personal risk factors in CAD. Once these risk factors are known, various methods of decreasing them should be discussed (see Table 33-3).

Teaching the patient and the family about diets that are low in sodium and reduced in saturated fats may be appropriate (see Table 33-4). Maintaining ideal body weight is important in controlling angina because weight above this level increases the myocardial workload and may cause pain.

Adhering to a regular, individualized exercise program that conditions the heart rather than overstresses the myocardium is important. Most patients can be advised to walk briskly on a flat surface 30 minutes a day at least 4 to 5 days a week.

It is important to teach the patient and the family in the proper use of nitroglycerin (see pp. 818-820). Nitroglycerin tablets or ointments may be used prophylactically before an emotionally stressful situation, sexual intercourse, or physical exertion (e.g., climbing a long flight of stairs).

Counseling should be provided to assess the psychologic adjustment of the patient and the family to the diagnosis of CAD and the resulting angina pectoris. Many patients feel a threat to their identity and self-esteem and are unable to fill their roles in society. These emotions are normal and real.

■ Nursing Implementation: Myocardial Infarction

Acute Intervention. Priorities for nursing interventions in the initial phase of MI include pain assessment and relief, physiologic monitoring, promotion of rest and comfort, alleviation of stress and anxiety, and understanding of the patient's emotional and behavioral reactions. Proper management of these priorities decreases the oxygen needs of a compromised myocardium. In addition, the nurse should institute measures to avoid the hazards of immobility while encouraging rest.

Pain. Morphine should be given as needed to eliminate or reduce chest pain. The nurse should instruct the patient to rate the pain on a scale of 0 to 10 to assist in the assessment and treatment of pain. Because a patient does not always verbalize pain, the nurse must be attuned to other manifestations of pain, such as restlessness, elevated heart rate or BP, clutching of the bedclothes, or other nonverbal cues. IV nitroglycerin, if given, should be titrated. Once pain is relieved, the nurse may have to deal with denial in a patient who interprets the absence of pain as an absence of cardiac damage. After the pain medication has been administered, the efficacy of the drug and the patient's response should be assessed and documented.

Monitoring. A patient has continuous ECG monitoring while in the emergency department and CCU and usually after transfer to a step-down or general unit. The nurse should be educated in ECG interpretation so that arrhythmias causing further deterioration of the cardiovascular status can be identified and treated. During the initial period after MI, ventricular fibrillation is the most common lethal arrhythmia. In many patients, this arrhythmia is preceded by PVCs or ventricular tachycardia (VT).

In addition to frequent vital signs, intake and output should be evaluated at least once a shift, and physical assessment should be carried out to detect deviations from the patient's baseline parameters. Included is an assessment of lung sounds and heart sounds and inspection for evidence of fluid retention (e.g., distended neck veins, hepatic engorgement, presacral or anterior tibial edema).

Assessment of the patient's oxygenation status is helpful, especially if the patient is receiving oxygen. Also, the nares should be checked for irritation or dryness, which can cause considerable discomfort if the nasal route is used for oxygen administration.

Rest and comfort. With a severe insult to the myocardium, as in the case of infarction, it is important for the nurse to promote rest and comfort. Bed rest may be ordered for the first few days in a severe MI. A patient with an uncomplicated MI may rest in a chair within 12 to 24 hours after the event. The use of a commode or bedpan is based on patient preference.

When sleeping or resting, the body requires less work from the heart than it does when active. It is important to plan nursing and therapeutic actions to ensure adequate rest periods free from interruption. Comfort measures that can promote rest are frequent oral care, adequate warmth, dim lighting, a quiet atmos-

TABLE 33-16	Phases of Rehabilitation Following a Myocardial Infarction

Phase I
Time when patient is in the hospital: Activity level depends on severity of MI; patient may initially rest in bed or chair and progress to ambulation in hallway; attention focuses on management of pain, anxiety, arrhythmias, and cardiogenic shock.

Phase II
Closely monitored exercise and classes at outpatient rehabilitation facility: Resumption of activities begins to the point of self-care at the time of discharge; information giving and teaching are appropriate at this time.

Phase III
Less closely monitored classes at outpatient rehabilitation facility: Patient and family examine and possibly restructure lifestyles and roles; exercise program begins, commonly a walking program, which progresses daily during first week and then weekly; patient undergoes exercise treadmill test at about 8 wk to determine workload of recovering myocardium.

Phase IV
Time of recovery and maintenance: Involvement with the community rehabilitation program for physical training and fitness continues.

MI, Myocardial infarction.

TABLE 33-17	Emotional and Behavioral Responses to Acute Myocardial Infarction

Denial
May have history of ignoring symptoms related to heart disease
Minimizes severity of medical condition
Ignores activity restrictions
Avoids discussing MI or its significance

Anger
Is commonly expressed as, "Why did this happen to me?"
May be directed at family, staff, or medical regimen

Anxiety and Fear
Fears death and long-term disability
Overtly manifests apprehension, restlessness, insomnia, tachycardia
Less overtly manifests increased verbalization, projection of feelings to others, hypochondriasis
Fears activity, recurrent heart attacks, and sudden death

Dependency
Is totally reliant on staff
Is unwilling to perform tasks or activities unless approved by health care provider
Wants to be monitored by ECG at all times
Is hesitant to leave ICU or hospital

Depression
Experiences mourning period concerning loss of health, altered body function, and changes in lifestyle
Realizes seriousness of situation
Begins to worry about future implications of health problem
Shows manifestations of withdrawal, crying, anorexia, apathy
May be more evident after discharge

Realistic Acceptance
Focuses on optimum rehabilitation
Plans changes compatible with altered cardiac function

ECG, Electrocardiogram; ICU, intensive care unit; MI, myocardial infarction.

phere, and assurance that personnel are nearby and responsive to the patient's needs.

It is important that the patient understand the reasons why activity is limited. However, in spite of this limitation the patient is not completely restricted. Gradually the cardiac workload is increased through more demanding physical tasks so that the patient can achieve a discharge activity level adequate for home care. Phases of rehabilitation are outlined in Table 33-16.

Anxiety. Anxiety is present in all patients with ACS to various degrees. The nurse's role is to identify the source of anxiety and assist the patient in reducing it. If the patient is afraid of being alone, a family member should be allowed to sit quietly by the bedside or to check in with the patient frequently. If a source of anxiety is fear of the unknown, the nurse should explore these concerns with the patient and help with appropriate reality testing.

If anxiety is caused by lack of information, the nurse should provide teaching appropriate to the patient's stated need and level. The nurse should answer the patient's questions with clear, simple explanations sufficient to reduce the patient's anxiety.

It is important to start teaching at the patient's level rather than to present a prepackaged protocol. Frequently the patient is not yet ready to hear about the pathogenesis of heart disease. The earliest questions usually relate to how the disease affects perceived control and independence. These questions include the following:

- When will I leave the intensive care unit?
- When can I be out of bed?
- When will I be discharged?
- When can I return to work?
- How much change will I have to make in my life?
- Will this happen again?

The nurse should advise that a more complete teaching program begins once the patient is feeling stronger. Frequently the patient may not be able to consciously examine the most pervasive concern of MI patients: Am I going to die? Even if a patient denies this concern, it is helpful for the nurse to initiate conversation by remarking that fear of dying is a common concern reported by most patients who have suffered an MI. This gives the patient "permission" to talk about an uncomfortable and fearful topic.

Emotional and behavioral reactions. The emotional and behavioral reactions of a patient are varied and frequently follow a predictable response pattern (Table 33-17). The role of the nurse in intervention is to understand what the patient is currently experiencing, to assist the patient in testing reality, and to support the use of constructive coping styles. Denial may be a positive coping style in the early phase of recovery from MI.

The nurse has an obligation to maximize and enhance the patient's social support systems. This entails assessing the support structure of the patient and family and allowing it to function. Often the patient is separated from the most significant support system at the time of hospitalization. The nurse's role can include talking with the family, informing them of the patient's progress, allowing the patient and the family to interact as necessary, and supporting the family members who will be able to provide the necessary support to the patient. Open visitation is helpful in decreasing anxiety and increasing support for the patient with an MI. Social isolation has been associated with negative outcomes following MI in both men and women.[15] It is important for the nurse to help the patient identify support systems that can help the patient after discharge.

Ambulatory and Home Care. Rehabilitation may be defined as the process of helping the patient adjust to a disability by teaching integration of all resources and concentrating more on existing abilities than on permanent disabilities. *Cardiac rehabilitation* is the restoration of a person to an optimal state of function in six areas: physiologic, psychologic, mental, spiritual, economic, and vocational. Many persons recover from an MI physically, yet they may never attain psychologic well-being because of misconceptions about the illness or a need to practice illness behaviors. Returning to work and resuming all activities have long been outcome measures of cardiac rehabilitation and are important in terms of the cost-effectiveness of cardiac care and rehabilitation.

In considering rehabilitation, the nurse and patient must recognize that CAD is a chronic disease. It will not be cured, nor will it disappear by itself. Therefore basic changes in lifestyle must be made to promote recovery and health. These changes must frequently be made at a time when a person is middle-aged. The patient must also realize that recovery takes time. Resumption of physical activity after MI is slow and gradual. However, with appropriate and adequate supportive care, recovery is more likely to occur.

Patient teaching. Once the acute stage of MI has passed, the patient is transferred to a step-down care or regular hospital unit. The goals of nursing care are ongoing. In addition, an important nursing goal is patient and family education. This teaching begins with the ED nurse and progresses through the staff nurse to the community health nurse. The purpose of teaching is to give the patient and family the tools they need to make informed decisions about attainment of health. For teaching to be meaningful, the patient must be aware of the need to learn. Careful assessment of the patient's learning needs helps the nurse set goals and objectives that are realistic.[32]

The timing of the teaching is important. When patients or families are in crisis (either physiologic or psychologic), they may not be very interested in patient teaching issues. It is important to remember that early questions should be answered initially in simple, brief terms, without detailed elaboration, and that the answers to these questions require repetition and follow-up (elaboration). When the shock and disbelief accompanying a crisis subside, the patient and family are better able to focus on new information.

In addition to teaching the patient and the family what they wish to know, several types of information are considered necessary in achieving optimal health. A teaching guide for the patient with MI is presented in Table 33-18.

When medical terminology is used, its meaning should be explained in lay terms. For example, it can be explained that the heart, a four-chambered pump, is a muscle that needs oxygen like all other muscles, and when vessels become narrowed by athero-

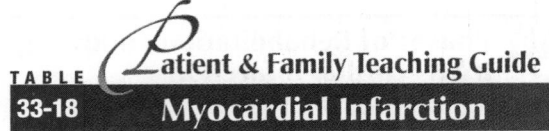

TABLE 33-18 Patient & Family Teaching Guide: Myocardial Infarction

The nurse needs to teach the following to the patient and the family:

- Anatomy and physiology of the heart and vessels
- Cause and effect of atherosclerosis
- Definition of terms (e.g., CAD, angina, MI, sudden cardiac death, CHF)
- Signs and symptoms of angina and MI and reasons they occur*
- Healing after infarction
- Identification of and decreasing risk factors (see Table 33-3)*
- Rationale for tests and treatments, including ECG, blood tests, and angiography, and monitoring, rest, diet, and medications*
- Appropriate expectations about recovery and rehabilitation (anticipatory guidance)
- Resumption of work, physical activity, sexual activity
- Measures to take to promote recovery and health
- Importance of the gradual, progressive resumption of activity*
- When to seek help (e.g., call 911)

*Identified by patients as most important to learn before discharge.
CAD, Coronary artery disease; *CHF*, congestive heart failure; *ECG*, electrocardiogram; *MI*, myocardial infarction.

sclerosis, the process is similar to a buildup of mineral deposits inside water pipes, which causes less water to flow through at a higher pressure. It is a good idea for the nurse to have a model of the heart or to use a pad and pencil to sketch what is being explained. Literature written for a nonmedical audience is available through the American Heart Association. Videotapes are also helpful tools that can be used to teach patients.

Anticipatory guidance involves preparing the patient and the family for what to expect in the course of recovery and rehabilitation. By learning what to expect during treatment and recovery, the patient gains a sense of control over life. This sense of perceived control allows the patient to consciously consider stressors and thus possibly to promote recovery.

The idea of perceived control is operationalized as the process by which the patient exercises choice and makes decisions by cutting back. Cutting back is one way of minimizing the psychologic and physiologic losses after MI (or any other life-changing event). The patient considers what must be cut back (changed), weighs this against what should be cut back, and finally determines what will be cut back. For example, a middle-aged man who smokes two packs of cigarettes a day, is 20 pounds overweight, and gets no physical exercise has a seemingly overwhelming task. He may decide that he can live with a weight-reduction diet and will get more exercise (although perhaps not daily) but that it is not possible for him to quit smoking. He reasons that because he is modifying two of the three risk factors, he will be safe if he cuts back on smoking. Ideally the smoking risk factors should be a priority for this patient, but if information regarding risks and effects of smoking is not accepted, the nurse must respect the patient's need for control.

Physical exercise. Exercise is an integral part of the rehabilitation program. It is necessary for optimal physiologic functioning and psychologic well-being. It has a direct, positive effect on maximal oxygen uptake, increasing CO, decreasing blood lipids, decreasing BP, increasing blood flow through the coronary arteries, increasing muscle mass and flexibility, improving the psychologic state, and assisting in weight loss and control. A regular schedule of moderate exercise, even after many years of sedentary living, is beneficial.

One method used to identify levels of physical activities is through **metabolic equivalent (MET)** units: 1 MET is the amount of oxygen needed by the body at rest—3.5 ml of oxygen per kilogram per minute or 1.4 cal/kg of body weight per minute. The MET is used to determine the energy costs of various exercises (Table 33-19).

In the hospital, the activity level is gradually increased so that by the time of discharge the patient can tolerate moderate-energy activities of 3 to 5 MET. Many patients with an uncomplicated MI are in the hospital for approximately 3 to 5 days. By day 3, the patient can ambulate in the hallway. Many physicians order low-level treadmill tests before discharge to assess readiness for discharge, accurate HR for an exercise prescription, and potential for reinfarction. If tests are positive (i.e., ischemia at a low level of energy expenditure), the patient is evaluated for cardiac catheterization before discharge and possible bypass grafting. If the test is negative, a catheterization may be suggested for 1 month after discharge. Because of the short hospitalization, it is critical to give the patient specific guidelines for activity and exercise so that overexertion will not occur. It is helpful to stress that when the patient "listens to what the body is saying"—the most important facet of recovery—uncomplicated recovery should proceed.

Teaching the patient to check the pulse rate is a nursing responsibility. The patient should be taught the parameters within which to exercise. The patient should be told the maximum HR that should be present at any point. If the HR exceeds this level or does not return to the rate of the resting pulse within a few minutes, the patient should stop. The patient should be instructed to stop exercising if pain or dyspnea occurs.

In a normal, healthy person the minimum threshold for improving cardiorespiratory fitness is 60% of the age-predicted maximum HR (which is calculated by subtracting the person's age from 220). The ideal training target HR is 80% of maximum HR. The patient who has been physically inactive and is just beginning an exercise program should do so under supervision whenever possible. The more important factor is the patient's response to exercise in terms of symptoms rather than absolute HR. This is a point that cannot be overstressed in teaching of the MI patient. In addition, a cardiac patient on medications (especially β-adrenergic blockers) may not be able to increase HR to any degree and should have a treadmill test to determine an individual target HR. Basic guidelines for cardiac conditioning are presented in Table 33-20.

The basic categories of exercise are static (isometric) and dynamic (isotonic). Most daily activities are a mixture of the two. *Static exercise* involves the development of tension during muscular contraction but produces little or no change in muscle length or joint movement. Lifting, carrying, and pushing heavy objects are primarily isometric activities. Because the HR and BP increase rapidly during isometric work, exercise programs involving isometric exercises should be limited.

Isotonic exercises involve changes in muscle length and joint movement with rhythmic contractions at relatively low muscular tension. Walking, jogging, swimming, bicycling, and jumping rope are examples of activities that are predominantly isotonic.

TABLE 33-19 Energy Expenditure in Metabolic Equivalents	
Low-Energy Activities (Less Than 3 METs or Less Than 3 cal/min)	**Calories Burned**
Activities in Hospital	
Resting supine	1.0
Sitting	1.2
Eating	1.4
Conversing	1.4
Washing hands, face	2.5
Activities Outside Hospital	
Sewing by hand	1.4
Sweeping floor	1.7
Painting, sitting	2.5
Driving car	2.8
Assembling radio	2.7
Sewing by machine	2.9
Moderate-Energy Activities (3-6 METs or 3-5 cal/min)	
Activities in Hospital	
Sitting on bedside commode	3.6
Walking at 2.5 mph	3.6
Showering	4.2
Using bedpan	4.7
Walking at 3.75 mph	5.6
Activities Outside Hospital	
Bricklaying	4.0
Tractor plowing	4.2
Ironing, standing	4.2
Mopping	4.2
Bowling	4.4
Cycling at 5.5 mph on level ground	4.5
Golfing	5.0
Dancing	5.5
High-Energy Activities (6-8 METs or 6-8 cal/min)	
Ambulating with braces and crutches	8.0
Performing carpentry	6.8
Mowing lawn by hand	7.7
Playing singles tennis	7.1
Riding on trotting horse	8.0
Walking at 5 mph	6.5
Ascending stairs	7.0
Very High–Energy Activities (8-10 METs or 8-10 cal/min)	
Skiing	9.9
Jogging at 5 mph	8.0
Shoveling snow	8.5
Ascending stairs with a 17 lb load	9.0
Extremely High–Energy Activities (more than 10 METs or more than 11 cal/min)	
Playing handball	
Cycling at 13 mph	
Ascending stairs with a 22 lb load	

MET, Metabolic equivalent unit.

Isotonic exercise can put a safe, steady load on the heart and lungs and may also improve the circulation in many organs.

Resumption of sexual activity. It is important to include sexual counseling for cardiac patients and their partners. This often-neglected area of discussion may be difficult for both patients

TABLE 33-20 *Patient & Family Teaching Guide* **Exercise Guidelines after Myocardial Infarction**

Type of Exercise
Exercise should be regular, rhythmic, and repetitive, using large muscles to build up endurance (e.g., walking, cycling, swimming, rowing).

Intensity
Exercise intensity should be determined by the patient's HR. If a treadmill test has not been performed, the person recovering from an MI should not exceed 20 beats per minute over the resting pulse rate.

Duration
Exercise can be from 20 to 30 minutes. It is important to begin slowly at personal tolerance (perhaps only 5 to 10 minutes) and build up to 30 minutes.

Frequency
The patient should exercise three to four times a week. If done at low duration (5 to 10 minutes), exercise can be done daily but is best done on nonconsecutive days.

Warm-up/Cool-down
Mild stretching for 3 to 5 minutes before the exercise activity and 5 minutes after the activity is important. Activity should not be started or stopped abruptly.

HR, Heart rate; *MI,* myocardial infarction.

TABLE 33-21 *Patient & Family Teaching Guide* **Sexual Activity after Myocardial Infarction**

- Planning of resumption of sexual activity should correspond to sexual activity before the heart attack.
- Physical training (exercise) seems to improve the physiologic response to coitus; therefore daily exercise during recovery should be encouraged.
- Consumption of food and alcohol should be reduced before intercourse is anticipated (e.g., waiting 3-4 hr after ingesting a large meal before engaging in sexual activity).
- Familiar surroundings and a familiar partner reduce anxiety.
- Masturbation may be a useful sexual outlet and may reassure the patient that sexual activity is still possible.
- Hot or cold showers should be avoided just before and just after intercourse.
- Foreplay is desirable because it allows a gradual increase in heart rate before orgasm.
- Positions during intercourse are a matter of individual choice.
- Orogenital sex places no undue strain on the heart.
- A relaxed atmosphere free of fatigue is optimal.
- Prophylactic use of nitrates is effective in decreasing angina during sexual activity.
- Anal intercourse may cause undue cardiac stress because of the possibility of inducing a vasovagal response.

and health care providers to approach. However, the patient's concern about resumption of sexual activity after MI often produces more stress than the physiologic act itself. About one third of men and women do not resume sexual activity or have a decrease in sexual activity after MI.[33] The majority of these patients changed their sexual behavior not because of physical problems, but because they were concerned about sexual inadequacy, death during coitus, and impotence. The misconceptions held by these persons could have been clarified with specific counseling by a concerned and knowledgeable health care provider.

Before the nurse provides guidelines on resumption of sexual activity, it is important to know the physiologic status of the patient, the physiologic effects of sexual activity, and the psychologic effects of having a heart attack. Sexual activity for middle-aged men with their usual partners is no more strenuous than climbing two flights of stairs.

Many nurses are unsure of how and when to begin counseling about resumption of sex. It is helpful to consider sex as a physical activity and to discuss or explore feelings in this area when other physical activities are discussed. One helpful approach is, "Many people who have had a heart attack wonder when they will be able to resume sexual activity. Has this been of concern to you?" Another is, "If this has been of concern to you, this information should be helpful." This type of nonthreatening statement brings up the topic, allows the patient to explore personal feelings, and gives the patient an opportunity to raise questions with the nurse or another health care provider. Common guidelines are presented in Table 33-21.

The patient needs to know that the inability to perform sexually after MI is common and that impotence usually disappears after several attempts. The nurse should reinforce the idea that patience and understanding usually solve the problem.

It is not uncommon for a patient who experiences chest pain on physical exertion to have some angina during sexual stimulation or intercourse. The patient should be instructed to take nitroglycerin prophylactically. It is also helpful to have the patient avoid sex soon after a heavy meal or after excessive ingestion of alcohol, when extremely tired or stressed, or with unfamiliar partners. Anal intercourse is to be avoided because of the likelihood of eliciting a vasovagal response.

The patient should be counseled that resumption of sex depends on the patient and his or her partner's emotional readiness and on the physician's assessment of the extent of recovery. It is now known that it is safe to resume sexual activity 7 to 10 days after an uncomplicated MI.[32] Some physicians believe that the patient should decide when he or she is ready to resume sex. Others say that a patient must be able to climb two flights of stairs briskly without dyspnea or angina before sexual activity can be resumed.

Reading material on resumption of sexual activity may be presented to the patient to facilitate discussion. The nurse should return to clarify and explain as necessary. Calmly and matter-of-factly introducing the subject of resumption of sexual activity during teaching about physical activity has positive effects of eliciting questions and concerns that might not have otherwise surfaced. For example, the nurse might begin, "Sexual activity is like other forms of activity and should be gradually resumed after MI. If your ability to perform sexually is concerning you, the energy expenditure has been found to be no more than walking briskly or climbing two flights of stairs." This forms a factual basis for the patient to begin to seek information and explore personal feelings about resuming sex.

Evaluation

The expected outcomes for the patient with an ACS are presented in NCP 33-1.

SUDDEN CARDIAC DEATH

Sudden cardiac death (SCD) is unexpected death from cardiac causes. In SCD there is a disruption in cardiac function, producing an abrupt loss of cerebral blood flow. Death usually occurs within 1 hour of the onset of acute symptoms. It occurs secondary to natural (not accidental or traumatic) causes. Sudden death from cardiac causes is estimated to account for about 50% of all deaths from cardiovascular causes. The affected person may or may not have a documented prior history of cardiovascular disease. In 25% of patients who die of CAD, sudden cardiac death may be the first sign of trouble.[1]

Sudden cardiac death accounts for approximately 400,000 deaths a year in the United States.[34] Only 20% of SCD survivors are discharged from the hospital without neurologic impairment. CAD is the most common cause of SCD, accounting for 80% of all SCDs. Fifty-six percent occur out of the hospital or in the ED. It is difficult to predict who is at risk for SCD. However, poor left ventricular function ejection fraction (less than 40%) has been found to be the strongest predictor.[34] Although increased sympathetic nervous system activity has been linked with the development of cardiac arrhythmias, continued research is needed.

Etiology and Pathophysiology

The majority of cases of SCD are caused by acute ventricular arrhythmias, often triggered by acute coronary events (e.g., acute myocardial ischemia). Victims of SCD usually have multivessel coronary artery disease. However, many of them have no known history of cardiovascular disease. Less commonly, SCD may occur as a result of a primary LV outflow obstruction. These obstructions may be secondary to such diseases as aortic stenosis, hypertrophic cardiomyopathy, and coarctation of the aorta.

Persons who experience SCD as a result of CAD fall into two groups: (1) those who had an acute MI and (2) those who did not have an acute MI. The latter group accounts for the majority of cases of SCD.[1] In this instance, victims usually have no warning signs or no known precedent symptoms. The patient is at risk for recurrent sudden death, probably because of continued electrical instability of the myocardium that caused the initial event to occur.

The second, smaller group of patients includes those who have had an acute MI and have suffered SCD. In these cases the patients usually do have prodromal symptoms, such as chest pain and dyspnea, and they have less chance of recurrent SCD than those who have not had MI.

Persons at increased risk for SCD include those with the following risk factors: (1) male gender (especially African American men), (2) family history of premature atherosclerosis, (3) cigarette smoking, (4) diabetes mellitus, (5) hypercholesterolemia, (6) hypertension, (7) cardiomegaly, (8) ejection fraction less than 40%, and (9) history of ventricular arrhythmias.

NURSING *and* COLLABORATIVE MANAGEMENT SUDDEN CARDIAC DEATH

Survivors of SCD generally require a diagnostic workup to determine whether they have had an acute MI. Thus serial analysis of cardiac markers and ECGs must be obtained, and the patient must be treated accordingly. (See section on collaborative care of MI.) In addition, because most persons with SCD have CAD secondary to multivessel coronary atherosclerosis, cardiac catheterization is indicated to determine the possible location and extent of coronary artery occlusion. PCI or CABG surgery may be indicated.

Most SCD patients have a lethal arrhythmia (usually ventricular arrhythmia) that is associated with a high incidence of recurrence. Thus it is useful to know when those persons are most likely to have a recurrence and what drug therapy is the most effective treatment. Assessment of arrhythmias in these patients includes 24-hour Holter monitoring, exercise stress testing, signal-averaged ECG, and electrophysiologic study (EPS).[35] EPS is performed under fluoroscopy; pacing electrodes are placed in selected intracardiac areas, and stimuli are selectively used to attempt to evoke arrhythmias. The patient's response to various antiarrhythmic medications can be determined and monitored in a controlled environment. (EPS is discussed in Chapters 31 and 35.)

The two most common approaches to preventing a recurrence are the use of antiarrhythmic drugs and the use of an implantable cardioverter-defibrillator (ICD). Commonly used drugs are sotalol (Betapace) and amiodarone (Cordarone). Current research is showing a trend toward improved survival with an ICD as compared with drug therapy alone.[36] (ICDs are discussed in Chapter 35.)

The nurse caring for a survivor of SCD should be attuned to the patient's psychosocial adaptation to this sudden "brush with death." Many of these patients develop a "time bomb" mentality. They fear the recurrence of cardiopulmonary arrest and may become anxious, angry, and depressed. Their families are likely to experience the same feelings. Wives of male survivors of SCD often experience a great deal of anxiety and fear of recurrence. The wives often feel responsible for the prevention of another event.[34] The grief response varies among persons and families. The nurse should be attuned to the specific needs of the patient and the family and teach them accordingly while providing appropriate emotional support.

■ Gerontologic Considerations: Coronary Artery Disease

The incidence of cardiac disease is greatly increased in older adults and is the leading cause of death in older persons. Angina can be disabling in this population, and affected persons increasingly rely on health care services to remain independent.[37]

The nurse caring for the older adult with CAD must be aware of the physiologic changes that occur in the cardiovascular system. Structural changes in the myocardium include increased collagen and fat deposition, myofibrillar degeneration, and endocardial thickening resulting in abnormalities in diastolic filling of the ventricles.[37] Calcification of the heart valves and degeneration of the conduction system can also occur. The majority of pacemakers are placed in persons over 65 years of age. In addition, resting HR decreases with age, and maximum HR with exercise decreases with age.

In the older adult, loss of elastic fibers and increased collagen in the arterial media diminish elasticity and distensibility of arteries. These changes cause an increased systolic BP and SVR, which can result in accelerated atherosclerosis.[37,38] These combined changes lead to a decrease in CO by 1% a year. This decrease in CO is probably secondary to decreased contractility of the myocardium and increased afterload caused by the increase in SVR. In addition, decreased arterial wall elasticity blunts the responsiveness to baroreceptors in the aortic arch and carotid arteries. Circulating norepinephrine levels also increase with age. However, β-adrenergic receptors may be less responsive to catecholamines.

The nurse must be aware of the changes in an older adult and must keep in mind the effect that nursing care may have on these patients. Because older adults have decreased responsiveness to catecholamines, their response to stress may be blunted; HR may not rise as quickly in response to pain or to declining CO. They often have atypical symptoms when experiencing an acute MI. Sudden shortness of breath may be more common than classic substernal chest pain. Associated diaphoresis may not be a predominant manifestation of an MI. The sudden occurrence of symptoms such as profound weakness and dyspnea should be investigated.

Many of the antianginal agents that cause postural hypotension and decrease preload may not be well tolerated in the older patient secondary to the decreased responsiveness of the baroreceptors and impaired diastolic filling of the ventricles.[37] The patient who has been on bed rest should sit for 3 to 5 minutes before ambulating. Also, antianginal agents that can slow HR must be used with caution in the patient who may have degeneration of the conduction system. The patient may be at increased risk of drug toxicity because of declining hepatic and renal function.

The older patient should be included in a cardiac rehabilitation program. Activity performance, endurance, and ability to tolerate stress can be improved in the older adult with physical training. Positive psychologic benefits can be derived from a planned exercise program and can include increased self-esteem and emotional well-being and improved body image.

When planning an exercise program for the older adult, the nurse should remember the following: (1) longer warm-up periods are needed, (2) longer periods of low-level activity or longer rest periods between sessions are advisable, and (3) heat intolerance may be caused by decreased ability to sweat efficiently. The patient should be taught to avoid exercising in extremes of temperature and to maintain a moderate pace. Target HR for an older adult is 60% to 75% of the maximum HR. The older adult should exercise a minimum of 30 to 40 minutes three or four times a week.

Aggressive treatment of hypertension and hyperlipidemia will stabilize plaques in the coronary arteries of older adults, and cessation of cigarette smoking helps decrease the risk of MI at any age.[37] Encouraging the older patient to adopt a healthy lifestyle may increase quality of life and reduce the risk of CAD.

Older adults have a greater incidence of unstable angina and more complications from an acute MI than younger patients.[36] Complications commonly found in an older patient with an acute MI include an increased incidence of atrial fibrillation, atrial flutter, complete heart block, CHF, myocardial rupture, and cardiogenic shock. Given this greater risk, aggressive management with

---

NURSING RESEARCH
Nursing Intervention for Survivors of Sudden Cardiac Arrest

Citation
Cowan MJ, Pike KC, Budzynski HK: Psychosocial nursing therapy following sudden cardiac arrest: impact of two-year survival, *Nurs Res* 50:68, 2001.

Purpose
Describe the effectiveness of psychosocial therapy on 2-year cardiovascular mortality rate in sudden cardiac arrest survivors.

Methods
Survivors of out-of-hospital ventricular fibrillation or asystole (N = 129) were randomized into a two-group, experimental, longitudinal design. The intervention consisted of 11 individual sessions implementing three components: relaxation with biofeedback training, cognitive-behavioral therapy, and cardiovascular health education. The primary outcome measure was cardiovascular mortality.

Results and Conclusions
Psychosocial therapy significantly reduced the risk of cardiovascular death in sudden cardiac arrest survivors. Risk of cardiovascular death was reduced 86% by psychosocial therapy. The risk of all-cause mortality was reduced by 62% in the therapy group.

Implications for Nursing Practice
It is important for nurses to focus on a multifaceted approach in managing survivors and those at risk for sudden cardiac arrest. This approach should include (1) relaxation therapy; (2) cognitive-behavioral therapy for coping with anger, depression, and anxiety; and (3) education about cardiac health.

---

thrombolytic therapy or direct PCI in the older adult patient with an acute MI is recommended.[38]

β-Adrenergic blocker therapy has also been shown to greatly benefit the older population, but side effects such as CHF and heart block are more common. PCI is another aggressive treatment used for controlling CAD in the older patient. However, in patients more than 70 years of age there is a significantly increased incidence of complications with this procedure.

Elective CABG is generally well tolerated in the older patient. However, the incidence of postoperative complications is high, including arrhythmias, stroke, and infection. The nurse caring for older adults must be aware that, although the benefits of treatment may outweigh risks in this population, complications are higher than in younger individuals. The nurse must be alert to early signs and symptoms of complications and aggressively try to prevent and treat them.

WOMEN AND CORONARY ARTERY DISEASE

Traditionally CAD has been viewed as an affliction of middle-aged men, when in fact CAD is the number one killer of American women. Approximately 500,000 deaths occur from cardiovascular disease in women per year. Heart disease kills almost 10 times more women than breast cancer. Cardiovascular disease causes more deaths in women than men.[39] Only recently has there been research focusing on the manifestations and course of CAD in women. Women tend to manifest CAD 10 years later in life than men, and most women have symptoms of angina rather than MI. The exercise treadmill test has a low sensitivity and specificity in women, and 30% to 40% of women have false-positive results. This may be because women have lower hematocrits, higher pulmonary and systolic BP responses to exercise, and ST segment depression from circulating estrogen. Exercise echocardiography is the most accurate test for the detection of CAD in women.[39]

Women also have a much higher mortality rate within 1 year following MI than men. Women are also more likely to have re-infarction within 1 year.[40] This increased mortality rate was thought to be a result of women developing CAD at a later age in life when they are more likely to have other illnesses such as diabetes, hypertension, and heart failure. However, even when these comorbidities have been taken into consideration, women still have a higher mortality rate following MI than men.

Women who have CABG surgery have a higher mortality rate and more complications after surgery than men. This is because women have smaller arteries, are older, and are referred more frequently for CABG with severe or unstable angina requiring urgent or emergent surgery.[39] Long-term survival rates are similar for men and women following CABG, but women report less relief from angina, poorer health, and more symptoms than men. Women also have higher rates of coronary artery dissection and hospital mortality than men following PCI, but men have a higher incidence of restenosis.[39,40] However, women have a decreased incidence of sudden cardiac death compared with men.

Although risk factors of CAD for men and women are similar, the significance of these risk factors may be different. Diabetes mellitus has been found to be the most single powerful predictor of CAD in women. Women with diabetes have five to seven times the risk for developing CAD than nondiabetic women.[39] Studies have shown that estrogen replacement in postmenopausal women does not reduce their risk for CAD even though estrogen replacement lowers LDL and raises HDL cholesterol.[41] Smoking, a major risk factor for both men and women, may also carry specific problems for women. Smoking has been linked to a decrease in estrogen levels and hence early menopause. Cigarette smoking has been identified as the most powerful contributor to CAD in women younger than age 50. Hypertension is a risk factor for CAD in women. In postmenopausal women, hypertension is associated with a higher incidence of CAD than men, and in premenopausal women, it increases the risk of death from CAD tenfold.[39]

Because CAD in women more often manifests with angina and women have a poorer prognosis following acute MI, aggressive teaching about the reduction of risk factors and counseling about lifestyle modification should be implemented after diagnosis of CAD in an attempt to prevent an acute MI. The nurse must recognize that women have significant post-MI and post-CABG morbidity and mortality rates. Women should be assessed for the presence of other diseases such as diabetes mellitus and hypertension that can affect their recovery after an MI. The nurse should closely assess for early complications following MI, PCI, and CABG.

Because women generally develop CAD at a later age than men, they often are widowed. The nurse should assess the patient's social support systems and refer to agencies that can assist in recovery where indicated. Cardiac rehabilitation programs are just as beneficial for women as men. Specific instruction should be given for activities that can be performed following recovery from MI or CABG. The American Heart Association website for women is *www.women.american-heart.org*.

CRITICAL THINKING EXERCISES

Case Study
Myocardial Infarction

Patient Profile. Matthew, a 46-year-old, white, successful businessman, was rushed to the hospital by a rescue squad after experiencing crushing substernal pain radiating down his left arm. He also complained of dizziness and nausea.

Subjective Data
- Has a history of angina pectoris and hypertension
- Is overweight but recently lost 10 pounds
- Rarely exercises
- Has three teenage children who are causing "problems"
- Recently experienced loss of best friend and business partner, who died from cancer

Objective Data
Physical Examination
- Diaphoretic, short of breath
- BP 165/100, pulse 120, respiratory rate 26/min

Diagnostic Studies
- CK-MB elevated
- Cholesterol 350 mg/dl (9.1 mmol/L)
- Myoglobin elevated
- ECG shows premature ventricular contractions and ST elevation in leads II, III, aVF, V_5, V_6
- Inferolateral wall MI

Collaborative Care
- reteplase (Retavase)
- Morphine 2 to 4 mg IV q5min prn for chest pain
- Nitroglycerin IV
- Oxygen 2 L/min
- ASA 325 mg per day
- Bed rest
- Vital signs every hour

CRITICAL THINKING QUESTIONS

1. Which coronary artery was most likely occluded in Matthew's coronary circulation?
2. Explain the pathogenesis of CAD. What risk factors may contribute to its development? What risk factors were present in Matthew's life?
3. What is angina pectoris? How does angina differ from MI?
4. List the clinical manifestations that Matthew exhibited and explain their pathophysiologic bases.
5. Explain the significance of the results of the laboratory tests and ECG findings.
6. For each treatment measure Matthew received, explain the physiologic reason for its use.
7. Based on the assessment data presented, write one or more appropriate nursing diagnoses. Are there any collaborative problems?

Continued

CRITICAL THINKING EXERCISES—con'td

Nursing Research Issues

1. Are patients with CABG more likely to make lifestyle changes than patients who are treated with PCI?
2. Do the activities that precipitate angina differ between those who are older than 75 years as compared with younger people?
3. Are there cultural differences in the presentation of CAD and how members of different cultural groups seek medical attention?
4. Are lipid-lowering agents as effective in women as in men?
5. Is a nurse-monitored rehabilitation program more effective than a self-monitored program?

REVIEW QUESTIONS

The number of the question corresponds to the same-numbered objective at the beginning of the chapter.

1. In teaching a patient about coronary artery disease, the nurse explains that the changes that occur in this disorder involve
   a. diffuse involvement of plaque formation in coronary veins.
   b. formation of fibrous tissue around coronary artery orifices.
   c. accumulation of lipid and fibrous tissue within the coronary arteries.
   d. chronic vasoconstriction of coronary arteries leading to permanent vasospasm.

2. After teaching about ways to decrease risk factors for CAD, the nurse recognizes that additional instruction is needed when the patient says,
   a. "I would like to add weight lifting to my exercise program."
   b. "I can't keep my blood pressure normal without medication."
   c. "I can change my diet to decrease my intake of saturated fats."
   d. "I will change my lifestyle to reduce activities that increase my stress."

3. A hospitalized patient with angina tells the nurse that she is having chest pain. The nurse bases her actions on the knowledge that anginal pain
   a. will be relieved by rest, nitroglycerin, or both.
   b. is less severe than pain of a myocardial infarction.
   c. indicates that irreversible cellular damage is occurring.
   d. is frequently associated with vomiting and extreme fatigue.

4. The clinical spectrum of acute coronary syndrome includes
   a. unstable angina and STEMI.
   b. unstable angina and NSTEMI.
   c. stable angina and sudden cardiac death.
   d. unstable angina, STEMI, and NSTEMI.

5. In planning activity for the patient recovering from an MI, the nurse recognizes that the healing heart wall is most vulnerable to stress
   a. 3 weeks after the infarction.
   b. 4 to 6 days after the infarction.
   c. 10 to 14 days after the infarction.
   d. when healing is complete at 6 to 8 weeks.

6. A patient is admitted to the CCU with chest pain of 24 hours' duration, ECG findings consistent with an acute MI, and occasional ventricular arrhythmias. The nurse plans care for the patient based on the expectation that the patient will be managed with
   a. endotracheal intubation.
   b. subcutaneous nitroglycerin.
   c. continuous ECG monitoring.
   d. thrombolytic therapy with tissue plasminogen activator.

7. A patient 5 days after MI is restless and apprehensive. The nurse can help by
   a. providing all care by doing everything for the patient.
   b. structuring the environment and routine so that the patient can rest.
   c. allowing the patient to participate in planning and carrying out activities.
   d. encouraging the family to provide for the patient's physical care and emotional support.

8. Three days after MI, a patient states that he does not understand what the alarm is about because his problem is just bad indigestion. His reaction is an example of
   a. anger.
   b. denial.
   c. projection.
   d. depression.

9. The most common pathologic finding in individuals with sudden cardiac death is
   a. cardiomyopathies.
   b. mitral valve disease.
   c. atherosclerotic heart disease.
   d. left ventricular hypertrophy.

REFERENCES

1. American Heart Association: *2002 heart and stroke facts statistics,* Dallas, 2002, American Heart Association.
2. Libby P: The vascular biology of atherosclerosis. In Braunwald E et al, editors: *Heart disease: a textbook of cardiovascular medicine,* ed 6, Philadelphia, 2001, WB Saunders.
3. American Heart Association: *A definition of initial, fatty streak, and intermediate lesions of atherosclerosis,* Dallas, 2002, American Heart Association.
4. Libby P, Ridker PM, Maseri A: Inflammation and atherosclerosis, *Circulation* 105:1135, 2002.
5. Schoenhagun P et al: The vulnerable coronary plaque, *J Cardiovasc Nurs* 15:1, 2000.
6. Vlassara H: Intervening in atherogenesis: lessons from diabetes, *Hosp Pract* 35:1, 2000.
7. Chyan D: Diabetes and coronary heart disease: a time for action, *Crit Care Nurse* 21:10, 2001.
8. Ridker PM, Genest J, Libby P: Risk factors for atherosclerotic disease. In Braunwald E et al, editors: *Heart disease: a textbook of cardiovascular medicine,* ed 6, Philadelphia, 2001, WB Saunders.

9. National Cholesterol Education Program (NCEP): Third report of the NCEP expert panel on detection, evaluation, and treatment of high cholesterol in adults, *JAMA* 285:2486, 2001.

10. Winston M, St Jeur S, Ashley J: Diet controversies in lipid therapy, *J Cardiovasc Nurs* 14:16, 2000.

11. Gualanick M, Cofer LA: Coronary risk factors: influences on the lipid profile, *J Cardiovasc Nurs* 14:16, 2000.

12. Holm K: Primary and secondary prevention using lipid lowering therapies, *J Cardiovasc Nurs* 14:1, 2000.

13. Futterman LG, Lemberg L: LP(a) lipoprotein—an independent risk factor for coronary heart disease after menopause, *Am J Crit Care* 10:63, 2001.

14. Futterman LG, Lemberg L: The Framingham heart study: a pivotal legacy of the last millennium, *Am J Crit Care* 9:147, 2000.

15. Barsky R: Psychiatric and behavioral aspects of cardiovascular disease. In Braunwald E et al, editors: *Heart disease: a textbook of cardiovascular medicine,* ed 6, Philadelphia, 2001, WB Saunders.

16. Ornish D et al: The Lifestyle Heart Trial: intensive lifestyle changes for reversal of coronary heart disease, *JAMA* 280:2001, 1998.

17. Barnard RJD, Lauro SC, Inkeles SB: Effects of intensive diet and exercise intervention in patients taking cholesterol lowering drugs, *Am J Cardiol* 79:1112, 1998.

18. Nutrition Screening Initiative of the American Academy of Family Physicians: Nutritional strategies efficacious in the prevention or treatment of coronary heart disease, *Geriatr Nurs* 22:47, 2001.

19. Kuncl N, Nelson KM: Getting the skinny on lipid lowering drugs, *Nursing* 30:52, 2000.

20. McCormick JJ, Deeg MA: Pharmacologic treatment of dyslipidemia, *Am J Nurs* 100:55, 2000.

21. Pradka LR: Lipids—how low do you go: plaque regression and passivation, *J Cardiovasc Nurs* 15:43, 2000.

22. Lewis L: Current thinking on silent ischemia, *Patient Care* 34:92, 2000.

23. Kong DF, Blazing MA, O'Connor CM: Advances in the approach to acute coronary syndromes, *Hosp Pract* 35:61, 2000.

24. Antman EM, Braunwald E: Acute myocardial infarction. In Braunwald E et al, editors: *Heart disease: a textbook of cardiovascular medicine,* ed 6, Philadelphia, 2001, WB Saunders.

25. Ryan TJ et al: ACC/AHA guidelines for the management of patients with acute myocardial infarction, *J Am Coll Cardiol* 34:890, 1999.

26. Murphy MJ, Berding CB: Use of measurements of myoglobin and cardiac troponins in the diagnosis of acute myocardial infarction, *Crit Care Nurse* 19:58, 1999.

27. ACC/AHA/ACP-ASIM guidelines for the management of chronic stable angina: executive summary and recommendations, *Circulation* 99:2829, 1999.

28. Palatnik AM: How cardiac drugs do what they do, *Nursing* 31:54, 2001.

29. McConnell EA: Applying nitroglycerin ointment, *Nursing* 31:17, 2001.

30. Casey K, Bedker DL, Roussel-McElmeel PC: Myocardial infarction: review of clinical trials and treatment strategies, *Crit Care Nurse* 18:39, 1998.

31. Furry B, House-Fancher MA: Reviewing the drug lineup against AMI, *Nursing* 30:32, 2000.

*32. Gentz CA: Perceived learning needs of the patient undergoing coronary angioplasty: an integrative review of the literature, *Heart Lung* 29:161, 2000.

33. Steinke EE: Sexual counseling after myocardial infarction, *Am J Nurs* 100:38, 2000.

34. Goldberger JJ: Treatment and prevention of sudden cardiac death, *Arch Intern Med* 159:1281, 1999.

*35. Tedesco C, Reigle J, Bergin J: Sudden cardiac death in heart failure, *J Cardiovasc Nurs* 14:38, 2000.

36. Josephson ME, Callans DJ, Buxton AE: The role of the implantable cardioverter-defibrillator for prevention of sudden cardiac death, *Ann Intern Med* 133:901, 2000.

37. Aronow WS: Treatment of older persons after myocardial infarction, *Ann Long-Term Care* 8:45, 2000.

38. Batchelor WB et al: Contemporary outcome trends in the elderly undergoing percutaneous coronary interventions: results in 7,472 octogen, *J Am Coll Cardiol* 36:723, 2000.

39. Halm MA, Penque S: Heart disease in women, *Am J Nurs* 99:26, 1999.

*40. King KB: Emotional and functional outcomes in women with coronary heart disease, *J Cardiovasc Nurs* 15:54, 2001.

41. Hulley S et al: Randomized trial of estrogen plus progestin for secondary prevention of coronary heart disease in postmenopausal women: Heart and Estrogen/progestin Replacement Study (HERS) research group, *JAMA* 280:605, 2000.

RESOURCES

American College of Cardiovascular Nursing (ACCN)
PO Box 3345
Riverview, FL 33568-3345
813-677-1116
Fax: 813-671-8912
www.accn.net/

American Heart Association
National Center
7272 Greenville Avenue
Dallas, TX 75231
800-AHA-USA-1 or 800-242-8721
www.americanheart.org/

Cardiovascular and Interventional Radiology Research and Education Foundation (CIRREF)
10201 Lee Highway, Suite 500
Fairfax, VA 22030
800-468-7284 or 703-691-1805
Fax: 703-691-1855
www.cirref.org/

Heartinfo.org
c/o Trigenesis Communications
26 Main Street
Chatham, NJ 07928
www.heartinfo.org/

International Society for Minimally Invasive Cardiac Surgery
13 Elm Street
Manchester, MA 01944
978-526-8330
www.ismics.org/

The Mended Hearts
7272 Greenville Avenue
Dallas, TX 75231-4596
888-HEART99 (888-432-7899) or 214-706-1442
Fax: 214-706-5245
www.mendedhearts.org/

National Cholesterol Education Program
National Heart, Lung, and Blood Institute
Building 31, Room 5A52
31 Center Drive MSC 2486
Bethesda, MD 20892
301-592-8573
Fax: 301-592-8563
www.nhlbi.nih.gov/chd/

National Heart Savers Association
http://heartsavers.org/

Nurse-Beat Cardiac Electronic Journal
www.nurse-beat.com/

Open the Door to a Healthy Heart
5775-G Peachtree-Dunwoody Rd., Suite 500
Atlanta, GA 30342
404-252-3663
www.healthyfridge.org/

Society for Cardiac Angiography and Interventions
9111 Old Georgetown Road
Bethesda, MD 20814
800-992-7224 or 301-581-3450
Fax: 301-581-3408
www.scai.org/

Society of Interventional Radiology
10201 Lee Highway, Suite 500
Fairfax, VA 22030
800-488-7284 or 703-691-1805
Fax: 703-691-1855
www.sirweb.org/

For additional Internet resources, see the website for this book at *http://evolve.elsevier.com/Lewis/medsurg/.*

---

*Nursing research–based references.

CHAPTER **34**

NURSING MANAGEMENT
Heart Failure and Cardiomyopathy

Mary Ann House-Fancher
Hatice Y. Foell

LEARNING OBJECTIVES

1. Compare the pathophysiology of systolic and diastolic ventricular failure.
2. Discuss the compensatory mechanisms involved in congestive heart failure.
3. Describe the nursing and collaborative management of the patient with acute congestive heart failure and pulmonary edema.
4. Describe the collaborative care and nursing management, including nutritional therapy, of the patient with chronic congestive heart failure.

5. Compare the pathophysiology, clinical manifestations, and nursing and collaborative management of different types of cardiomyopathy.
6. Describe the indications for cardiac transplantation and the nursing management of cardiac transplant recipients.

KEY TERMS

cardiac transplantation, p. 857
cardiomegaly, p. 854
cardiomyopathy, p. 853
congestive heart failure, p. 838
diastolic failure, p. 839
dilated cardiomyopathy, p. 854

hypertrophic cardiomyopathy, p. 855
paroxysmal nocturnal dyspnea, p. 842
pulmonary edema, p. 840
systolic failure, p. 839

CONGESTIVE HEART FAILURE

Congestive heart failure (CHF) is an abnormal condition involving impaired cardiac pumping. CHF is not a disease. It is associated with numerous types of heart disease, particularly with long-standing hypertension and coronary artery disease (CAD) (Table 34-1). CHF is characterized by ventricular dysfunction, reduced exercise tolerance, diminished quality of life, and shortened life expectancy.

Currently about 5 million people in the United States have CHF. It is the most rapidly increasing form of cardiovascular disease. The American Heart Association (AHA) estimates that 470,000 new cases are diagnosed each year. CHF dramatically increases with advancing age, and as the elderly population increases, CHF incidence and prevalence will increase. Approximately 1 in every 100 older adults has CHF. It is the most common reason for hospital admission in adults older than 65 years. The incidence of heart failure is similar in men and women.[1]

Heart failure is associated with high rates of morbidity, mortality, and economic costs.[1,2] Despite new advances in treatment, the number of deaths due to CHF has increased sixfold during the past 4 years. The annual health care cost of managing patients with CHF exceeds $57 billion.[1,2]

Etiology and Pathophysiology

Although CAD and advancing age are the primary risk factors for CHF, there are also other factors, including hypertension, diabetes, cigarette smoking, obesity, and high serum cholesterol. Hypertension is a major contributing factor, increasing the risk of CHF approximately threefold. The risk of CHF increases progressively with the severity of hypertension, and systolic and diastolic hypertension equally predict risk. Diabetes mellitus predisposes an individual to CHF regardless of the presence of concomitant CAD or hypertension. Diabetes is more likely to predispose women than men to CHF.[3]

TABLE 34-1	Common Causes of Congestive Heart Failure	
CHRONIC	**ACUTE**
Coronary artery disease	Acute myocardial infarction
Hypertensive heart disease	Arrhythmias
Rheumatic heart disease	Pulmonary emboli
Congenital heart disease	Thyrotoxicosis
Cor pulmonale	Hypertensive crisis
Cardiomyopathy	Rupture of papillary muscle
Anemia	Ventricular septal defect
Bacterial endocarditis	Myocarditis
Valvular disorders	

Reviewed by Linda Griego Martinez, RN, MSN, CS, CCRN, Clinical Nurse Specialist, Presbyterian Heart Group, Albuquerque, N.M.

CHF may be caused by any interference with the normal mechanisms regulating cardiac output (CO). CO depends on (1) preload, (2) afterload, (3) myocardial contractility, (4) heart rate (HR), and (5) metabolic state of the individual. (Preload and afterload are discussed in Chapter 31.) Any alteration in these factors can lead to decreased ventricular function and the resultant manifestations of CHF.[4] The major causes of CHF may be divided into two subgroups: (1) underlying diseases (see Table 34-1) and (2) precipitating causes (Table 34-2). Precipitating causes often increase the workload of the ventricles, causing a decompensated condition that leads to decreased myocardial function.

Pathology of Ventricular Failure. *Heart failure* can be described as systolic or diastolic.

Systolic failure. Systolic failure, the most common cause of CHF, results from an inability of the heart to pump blood. It is a defect in the ability of the ventricles to contract (pump). The left ventricle (LV) loses its ability to generate enough pressure to eject blood forward through the high-pressure aorta. The hallmark of systolic dysfunction is a decrease in the left ventricular *ejection fraction* (the fraction of total ventricular filling volume that is ejected during each ventricular contraction). Systolic failure is caused by impaired contractile function (e.g., myocardial infarction), increased afterload (e.g., hypertension), cardiomyopathy, and mechanical abnormalities (e.g., valvular heart disease).[5]

Diastolic failure. Diastolic failure is an impaired ability of the ventricles to fill during diastole. Decreased filling of the ventricles will result in decreased stroke volume. In diastolic failure there is normal systolic function. Diastolic failure is characterized by high filling pressures and the resultant venous engorgement in both the pulmonary and systemic vascular systems. The diagnosis of diastolic failure is made on the basis of the presence of pulmonary congestion and pulmonary hypertension with a normal ejection fraction.

Diastolic failure is usually the result of left ventricular hypertrophy from chronic systemic hypertension, aortic stenosis, or hypertrophic cardiomyopathy. Diastolic failure is commonly seen in older adults as a result of myocardial fibrosis and hypertension.[6]

Mixed systolic and diastolic failure. Systolic and diastolic failure of mixed origin is seen in disease states such as dilated cardiomyopathy (DCM), a condition in which poor systolic function (weakened muscle function) is further compromised by dilated left ventricular walls that are unable to relax. This patient often has extremely poor ejection fractions, high pulmonary pressures, and *biventricular failure* (both ventricles may be dilated and have poor filling and emptying capacity).

The patient with ventricular failure of any type has low systemic arterial blood pressure, low CO, and poor renal perfusion. Poor exercise tolerance and ventricular arrhythmias are also common. Whether a patient arrives at this point acutely from a myocardial infarction (MI) or chronically from worsening cardiomyopathy or hypertension, the body's response to this low CO is to mobilize its compensatory mechanisms to maintain CO and blood pressure (BP).

Compensatory Mechanisms. CHF can have an abrupt onset as with acute MI, or it can be an insidious process resulting from slow, progressive changes. The overloaded heart resorts to certain compensatory mechanisms to try to maintain adequate CO. The main compensatory mechanisms include (1) ventricular dilation, (2) ventricular hypertrophy, (3) increased sympathetic nervous system stimulation, and (4) neurohormonal responses.

Dilation. *Dilation* is an enlargement of the chambers of the heart. It occurs when pressure in the heart chambers (usually the left ventricle) is elevated over time. The muscle fibers of the heart stretch and thereby increase their contractile force. Initially this increased contraction leads to increased CO and maintenance of arterial blood pressure and perfusion. Therefore dilation is an adaptive mechanism to cope with increasing blood volume. Eventually this mechanism becomes inadequate because the elastic elements of the muscle fibers are overstretched and can no longer contract effectively, thereby decreasing the CO.

TABLE 34-2	Precipitating Causes of Congestive Heart Failure
CAUSE	**MECHANISM**
Anemia	↓ O₂-carrying capacity of the blood stimulating ↑ in CO to meet tissue demands
Infection	↑ O₂ demand of tissues, stimulating ↑ CO
Thyrotoxicosis	Changes the tissue metabolic rate, ↑ HR and workload of the heart
Hypothyroidism	Indirectly predisposes to ↑ atherosclerosis; severe hypothyroidism decreases myocardial contractility
Arrhythmias	May ↓ CO and ↑ workload and O₂ requirements of myocardial tissue
Bacterial endocarditis	*Infection:* ↑ metabolic demands and O₂ requirements
	Valvular dysfunction: causes stenosis and regurgitation
Pulmonary embolism	↑ Pulmonary pressure and exerts pressure on the RV, leading to RV hypertrophy and failure
Pulmonary disease	↑ Pulmonary pressure and exerts a pressure load on the RV, leading to RV hypertrophy and failure
Paget's disease	↑ Workload of the heart by ↑ vascular bed in the skeletal muscle
Nutritional deficiencies	May ↓ cardiac function by ↓ myocardial muscle mass and myocardial contractility
Hypervolemia	↑ Preload and causes volume load on the RV

CO, Cardiac output; *HR,* heart rate; *RV,* right ventricle.

Hypertrophy. In chronic CHF, *hypertrophy* is an increase in the muscle mass and cardiac wall thickness in response to overwork and strain. It occurs slowly because it takes time for this increased muscle tissue to develop. Hypertrophy generally follows persistent or chronic dilation and thus further increases the contractile power of the muscle fibers. This will lead to an increase in CO and maintenance of tissue perfusion. However, hypertrophic heart muscle has poor contractility.

Sympathetic nervous system activation. Sympathetic nervous system stimulation is often the first mechanism triggered in low-CO states. However, it is the least effective compensatory mechanism. Because there is inadequate stroke volume and CO, there is increased sympathetic nervous system activation, resulting in the increased release of epinephrine and norepinephrine. This results in an increased heart rate, myocardial contractility, and peripheral vascular constriction. Initially this increase in HR and contractility improves CO. However, over time these factors act in a detrimental fashion by increasing the myocardium's need for oxygen and the workload of the already failing heart. The vasoconstriction causes an immediate increase in preload, which may initially increase CO. However, an increase in venous return to the heart, which is already volume overloaded, actually worsens ventricular performance.

Neurohormonal response. As the CO falls, blood flow to the kidneys decreases, causing decreased glomerular blood flow. This is sensed by the juxtaglomerular apparatus in the kidney as decreased volume. In response, the kidneys release renin, which converts angiotensinogen to angiotensin I (see Chapter 43 and Fig. 43-4). The stimulation of renin and the resulting conversion of angiotensinogen to angiotensin I and II is known as the renin-angiotensin system. Angiotensin II causes (1) the adrenal cortex to release aldosterone, which causes sodium retention, and (2) increased peripheral vasoconstriction, which increases the arterial BP.

Low CO causes a decrease in cerebral perfusion pressure. The posterior pituitary then secretes antidiuretic hormone (ADH). ADH increases water reabsorption in the renal tubules, causing water retention and therefore increased blood volume. Therefore the blood volume is increased in a person who is already volume overloaded.

In addition to the sympathetic and renin-angiotensin systems, other factors also contribute to the development of CHF. *Endothelin* is produced by the endothelial cells primarily in the lining of blood vessels in response to sheer stress (stretch). Endothelin is a potent vasoconstrictor, which may contribute to hypertension. Circulating cytokines are also released in response to cardiac failure. The cytokines' tumor necrosis factor (TNF) and interleukin-1 (IL-1) depress cardiac function.[4]

The body's ability to try to maintain balance is demonstrated by several counterregulatory processes. Natriuretic peptides are hormones that promote vasodilation (thus reducing afterload and preload) and diuresis. In addition, they inhibit the development of cardiac hypertrophy. Atrial natriuretic peptide (ANP) is produced by the atrium, and brain natriuretic peptide (BNP) is produced by the ventricles. (The term *brain natriuretic peptide* is misleading. It was so named because it was first discovered in the porcine brain.) ANP is primarily triggered by increases in volume, whereas BNP is primarily triggered by increased pressure. Prolonged atrial distention (during heart failure) leads to a depletion of these factors.[7]

Stimulation of the sympathetic nervous system and renin-angiotensin system leads to elevated levels of norepinephrine, angiotensin II, aldosterone, and vasopressin. The effects of these mediators are vasoconstriction, increased blood volume, increased

HR, and increased contractility, all of which increase myocardial oxygen consumption.

Cardiac compensation occurs when compensatory mechanisms succeed in maintaining an adequate CO that is needed for tissue perfusion. *Cardiac decompensation* occurs when these mechanisms can no longer maintain adequate CO and inadequate tissue perfusion results.

Ventricular remodeling. The neurohormonal response discussed in the preceding paragraphs contributes to ventricular remodeling. This involves hypertrophy of the cardiac myocytes, resulting in large, abnormal cells. This eventually leads to increased ventricular mass, changes in ventricular shape, and impaired contractility. Although the ventricles become larger, they are a less effective pump.[4]

Types of Congestive Heart Failure

CHF is usually manifested by biventricular failure, although one ventricle may precede the other in dysfunction. Normally the pumping actions of the left and right sides of the heart complement each other, producing a continuous flow of blood. However, as a result of pathologic conditions, one side may fail while the other side continues to function normally for a period of time. Because of the prolonged strain, both sides of the heart will eventually fail, resulting in *biventricular failure*.

Left-Sided Failure. The most common form of initial heart failure is left-sided failure (Fig. 34-1). Left-sided failure results from LV dysfunction, which causes blood to back up through the left atrium and into the pulmonary veins. The increased pulmonary pressure causes fluid extravasation from the pulmonary capillary bed into the interstitium and then the alveoli, which is manifested as pulmonary congestion and edema.

Right-Sided Failure. Right-sided failure causes backward blood flow to the right atrium and venous circulation. Venous congestion in the systemic circulation results in peripheral edema, hepatomegaly, splenomegaly, vascular congestion of the gastrointestinal (GI) tract, and jugular venous distention. The primary cause of right-sided failure is left-sided failure. In this situation, left-sided failure results in pulmonary congestion and increased pressure in the blood vessels of the lung (pulmonary hypertension). Eventually, chronic pulmonary hypertension results in right-sided hypertrophy and failure. *Cor pulmonale* (right ventricular dilation and hypertrophy caused by pulmonary pathology) can also cause right-sided failure. (Cor pulmonale is discussed in Chapter 27.) Right ventricular infarction may also cause right ventricle (RV) failure.

Clinical Manifestations of Acute Congestive Heart Failure

Regardless of etiology, acute heart failure typically manifests as **pulmonary edema,** an acute, life-threatening situation in which the lung alveoli become filled with serosanguineous fluid (Fig. 34-2). The most common cause of pulmonary edema is acute LV failure secondary to CAD. (Other etiologic factors for pulmonary edema are listed in Chapter 27, Table 27-26.)

In most cases of acute heart failure, there is an increase in the pulmonary venous pressure caused by decreased efficiency of the LV. This results in engorgement of the pulmonary vascular system. As a result, the lungs become less compliant, and there is increased resistance in the small airways. In addition, the lymphatic system increases its flow to help maintain a constant volume of the pulmonary extravascular fluid. This early stage is

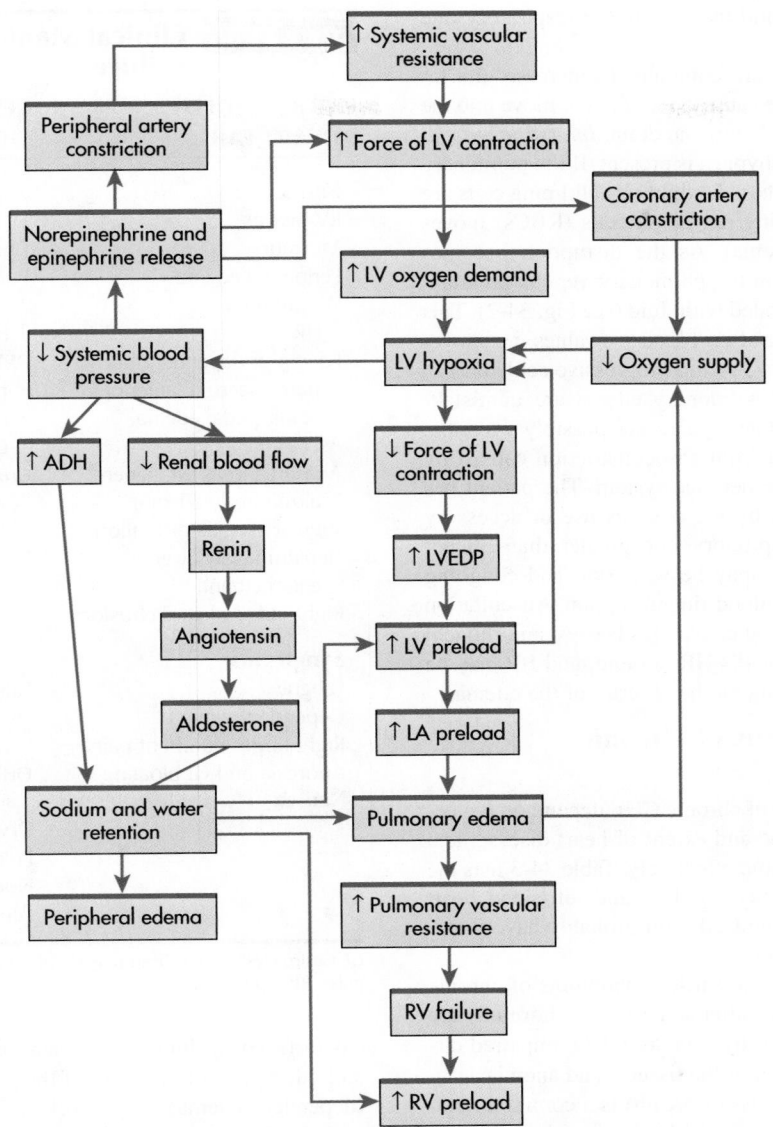

FIG. 34-1 Left-sided heart failure (congestive heart failure) from elevated systemic vascular resistance. Left-sided heart failure leads to right-sided heart failure. Systemic vascular resistance and preload are exacerbated by renal and adrenal mechanisms. *ADH,* Antidiuretic hormone; *LA,* left atrial; *LV,* left ventricle; *LVEDP,* left ventricular end–diastolic pressure; *RV,* right ventricle.

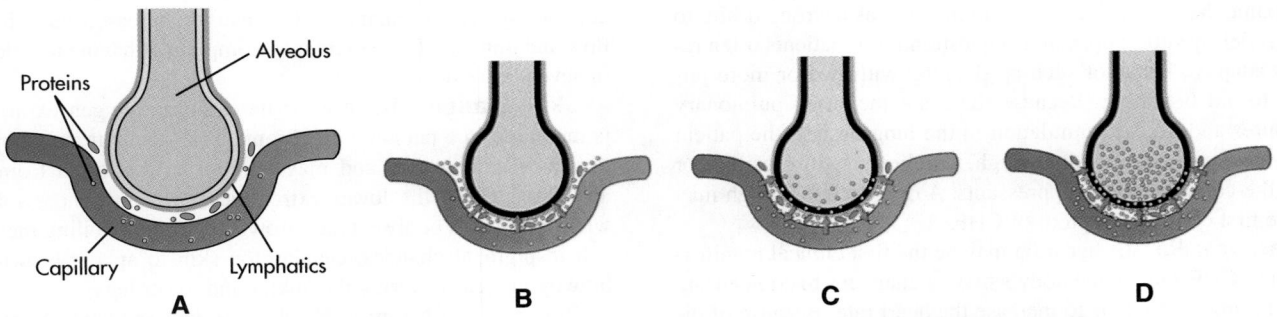

FIG. 34-2 As pulmonary edema progresses, it inhibits oxygen and carbon dioxide exchange at the alveolar capillary interface. **A,** Normal relationship. **B,** Increased pulmonary capillary hydrostatic pressure causes fluid to move from the vascular space into the pulmonary interstitial space. **C,** Lymphatic flow increases in an attempt to pull fluid back into the vascular or lymphatic space. **D,** Failure of lymphatic flow and worsening of left heart failure result in further movement of fluid into the interstitial space and into the alveoli.

clinically associated with a mild increase in the respiratory rate and a decrease in arterial PaO$_2$.

If pulmonary venous pressure continues to increase, the increase in intravascular pressure causes more fluid to move into the interstitial space than the lymphatics can drain. *Interstitial edema* occurs at this point. Severe tachypnea is present. If the pulmonary venous pressure increases further, the tight alveoli lining cells are disrupted and a fluid containing red blood cells (RBCs) moves into the alveoli (alveolar edema). As the disruption becomes worse from further increases in the pulmonary venous pressure, the alveoli and airways are flooded with fluid (see Fig. 34-2). This is accompanied by a worsening of the blood gas values (i.e., lower PaO$_2$ and possible increased PaCO$_2$ and progressive acidemia).

Clinical manifestations of pulmonary edema are unmistakable. The patient may be agitated, pale, and possibly cyanotic. The skin is clammy and cold from vasoconstriction caused by stimulation of the sympathetic nervous system. The patient has severe dyspnea, as evidenced by the obvious use of accessory muscles of respiration, a respiratory rate greater than 30 per minute, and orthopnea. There may be wheezing and coughing with the production of frothy, blood-tinged sputum. Auscultation of the lungs may reveal bubbling crackles, wheezes, and rhonchi throughout the lungs. The patient's HR is rapid, and BP may be elevated or decreased depending on the severity of the edema.

Clinical Manifestations of Chronic Congestive Heart Failure

The clinical manifestations of chronic CHF depend on the patient's age, the underlying type and extent of heart disease, and which ventricle is failing to pump effectively. Table 34-3 lists the manifestations of right-sided heart failure and left-sided heart failure. The patient with chronic CHF will probably have manifestations of biventricular failure.

Fatigue. Fatigue is one of the earliest symptoms of chronic CHF. The patient notices fatigue after activities that normally are not tiring. The fatigue is caused by decreased CO, impaired circulation, decreased oxygenation of the tissues, and anemia.

Dyspnea. *Dyspnea* (shortness of breath) is a common manifestation of chronic CHF. It is caused by increased pulmonary pressures secondary to interstitial and alveolar edema. Dyspnea can occur with mild exertion or at rest. *Orthopnea* is shortness of breath that occurs when the patient is in a recumbent position. **Paroxysmal nocturnal dyspnea** (PND) occurs when the patient is asleep. It is caused by the reabsorption of fluid from dependent body areas when the patient is recumbent. The patient awakens in a panic, has feelings of suffocation, and has a strong desire to seek relief by sitting up. Careful questioning of patients often reveals adaptive behavior such as sleeping with two or more pillows to aid breathing. Because there are increased pulmonary pressures and fluid accumulation in the lung tissues, the patient may have a persistent, dry cough, unrelieved with position or over-the-counter cough suppressants. A dry, hacking cough may be the first clinical symptom of CHF.

Tachycardia. Tachycardia may be the first clinical manifestation of CHF. One of the body's first mechanisms to compensate for a failing ventricle is to increase the heart rate. Because of diminished CO, there is increased sympathetic nervous system stimulation, which increases HR.

Edema. Edema is a common sign of CHF. It may occur in the legs (peripheral edema), liver (hepatomegaly), abdominal

TABLE 34-3 Clinical Manifestations of Heart Failure	
RIGHT-SIDED HEART FAILURE	**LEFT-SIDED HEART FAILURE**
Signs	
RV heaves	LV heaves
Murmurs	Cheyne-Stokes respirations
Peripheral edema	Pulsus alternans (alternating
Weight gain	pulses: strong, weak)
↑ HR	↑ HR
Edema of dependent body	PMI displaced inferiorly and
parts (sacrum, anterior	posteriorly (LV hypertrophy)
tibias, pedal edema)	↓ PaO$_2$, slight ↑ PaCO$_2$ (poor
Ascites	O$_2$ exchange)
Anasarca (massive gener-	Crackles (pulmonary edema)
alized body edema)	S$_3$ and S$_4$ heart sounds
Jugular venous distention	
Hepatomegaly (liver	
enlargement)	
Right-sided pleural effusion	
Symptoms	
Fatigue	Fatigue
Dependent edema	Dyspnea (shallow respirations
Right upper quadrant pain	up to 32-40/min)
Anorexia and GI bloating	Orthopnea (shortness of breath
Nausea	in recumbent position)
	Dry, hacking cough
	Pulmonary edema
	Nocturia
	Paroxysmal nocturnal dyspnea

GI, Gastrointestinal; *HR,* heart rate; *LV,* left ventricle; *PMI,* point of maximal impulse; *RV,* right ventricle.

cavity (ascites), lungs (pulmonary edema and pleural effusion), and other parts of the body. If the patient is in bed, sacral edema (dependent edema) may develop. Pressing the edematous skin with the finger may leave a transient indentation (pitting edema). The development of dependent edema or a sudden weight gain of 5 lb (2.3 kg) or more is often indicative of exacerbated CHF.

Nocturia. A person with chronic CHF who has decreased CO will also have impaired renal perfusion and decreased urinary output during the day. However, when the person lies down at night, fluid movement from interstitial spaces back into the circulatory system is enhanced. This causes increased renal blood flow and diuresis. The patient may complain of having to void six or seven times during the night.

Skin Changes. Because tissue capillary oxygen extraction is increased in a person with chronic CHF, the skin may appear dusky. It is also cool and may be cool to the touch from diaphoresis. Often the lower extremities are shiny and swollen, with diminished or absent hair growth. Chronic swelling may result in pigment changes, causing the skin to appear brown, or brawny in areas covering the ankles and lower legs.

Behavioral Changes. Cerebral circulation may be impaired with chronic CHF secondary to decreased CO. The patient or family may report unusual behavior, including restlessness, confusion, and decreased attention span or memory. This may also be secondary to poor gas exchange and worsening renal failure.

Chest Pain. CHF can precipitate chest pain because of decreased coronary perfusion from decreased CO and increased myocardial work. Anginal-type pain may accompany either acute or chronic CHF.

Weight Changes. Many factors contribute to weight changes. Initially there may be a progressive weight gain from fluid retention. However, over time the patient is often too sick to eat. Abdominal fullness from ascites and hepatomegaly frequently causes anorexia and nausea. Renal failure may also contribute to fluid retention. In many cases the muscle and fat loss is masked by the patient's edematous condition. The actual weight loss may not be apparent until after the edema subsides.

Complications of Congestive Heart Failure

Pleural Effusion. Pleural effusion results from increasing pressure in the pleural capillaries. A transudation of fluid occurs from these capillaries into the pleural space. (Pleural effusion is discussed in Chapter 27.)

Arrhythmias. Chronic CHF causes enlargement of the chambers of the heart. This enlargement (stretching of the atrial and ventricular tissues) may cause an alteration in the normal electrical pathway, and atrial fibrillation may result. When numerous sites in the atria fire spontaneously and rapidly, an organized spread of depolarization can no longer take place. Thus the atria cannot contract normally. This can promote thrombus formation within the atria, which may break loose and form emboli. Patients with atrial fibrillation require treatment with antiarrhythmics and anticoagulants. (Arrhythmias are discussed in Chapter 35.)

Patients with CHF have a high risk of fatal arrhythmias: nearly one half experience sudden cardiac death, usually because of ventricular tachyarrhythmias. (Sudden cardiac death is discussed in Chapter 33.)

Left Ventricular Thrombus. With acute or chronic CHF, the enlarged LV and decreased CO combine to increase the chance of thrombus formation in the LV. Current guidelines of the American College of Cardiology and AHA recommend anticoagulation in patients with CHF and atrial fibrillation or very poor LV function (e.g., ejection fraction less than 20%). Once a thrombus has formed, it may also decrease LV contractility, decrease CO, and further worsen the patient's perfusion. The development of emboli from the thrombus is also a possibility and can result in a stroke.

Hepatomegaly. CHF can lead to severe hepatomegaly, especially with RV failure. The liver lobules become congested with venous blood. The hepatic congestion leads to impaired liver function. Eventually liver cells die, fibrosis occurs, and cirrhosis can develop (see Chapter 42).

Classification of Congestive Heart Failure

The New York Heart Association has developed functional guidelines for classifying people with CHF. The classification is based on the person's tolerance to physical activity (Table 34-4).

Diagnostic Studies

The primary goal in diagnosis is to determine the underlying etiology of heart failure. Diagnostic measures to assess the cause and degree of heart failure include physical examination, chest x-ray, electrocardiogram (ECG), hemodynamic assessment, echocardiogram, stress testing, and cardiac catheterization. Ejection

TABLE 34-4	New York Heart Association Functional Classification of Persons with Cardiac Disease

Class 1
No limitation of physical activity. Ordinary physical activity does not cause fatigue, dyspnea, palpitations, or anginal pain.

Class 2
Slight limitation of physical activity. No symptoms at rest. Ordinary physical activity results in fatigue, dyspnea, palpitations, or anginal pain.

Class 3
Marked limitation of physical activity. Usually comfortable at rest. Ordinary physical activity causes fatigue, dyspnea, palpitations, or anginal pain.

Class 4
Inability to carry on any physical activity without discomfort. Symptoms of cardiac insufficiency or of angina may be present even at rest. If any physical activity is undertaken, discomfort is increased.

fraction (EF) can be measured using echocardiography and/or nuclear studies. EF can be used to differentiate between systolic and diastolic heart failure. (A normal EF is greater than 50%.) Diagnostic studies used for the patient with acute CHF are presented in Table 34-5, and those for the patient with chronic CHF are presented in Table 34-6. Plasma natriuretic peptide levels can

TABLE 34-5	*Collaborative Care* **Acute Congestive Heart Failure and Pulmonary Edema**

Diagnostic
History and physical examination
ABGs, serum chemistries, liver function tests
Chest x-ray
Hemodynamic monitoring
Twelve-lead ECG
Echocardiogram
Nuclear imaging studies
Cardiac catheterization

Collaborative Therapy
Treatment of underlying cause
High Fowler position
O₂ by mask or nasal catheter
Cardiac monitor and oximetry
Drug therapy: morphine IV; diuretics IV (furosemide [Lasix], bumetanide [Bumex], or torsemide [Demadex]); digitalis IV; nitroglycerin IV; nitroprusside IV; inotropic therapy (see Table 34-7); nesiritide (Natrecor)
BP, HR, RR, PAWP, urinary output at least q1hr
Daily weights
Possible cardioversion
Endotracheal intubation and mechanical ventilation

ABGs, Arterial blood gases; *BP,* blood pressure; *ECG,* electrocardiogram; *HR,* heart rate; *PAWP,* pulmonary artery wedge pressure; *RR,* respiratory rate.

TABLE 34-6 Collaborative Care: Chronic Congestive Heart Failure

Diagnostic
History and physical examination
Determination of underlying cause
Serum chemistries, liver function tests
Chest x-ray
Electrocardiogram
Echocardiography
Exercise-stress testing
Nuclear imaging studies
Hemodynamic monitoring
Cardiac catheterization

Collaborative Therapy
Treatment of underlying cause
Oxygen therapy at 2-6 L/min
Rest
Drug therapy (see Table 34-7)
Daily weights
Sodium-restricted diet
Intraaortic balloon pump
Ventricular assist device
Cardiac resynchronization therapy
Cardiac transplant

be used to assist in the diagnosis of CHF. In general, plasma levels correlate positively with the degree of LV dysfunction. Plasma BNP levels can be used in acute care settings to differentiate dyspnea caused by heart failure from dyspnea caused by pulmonary disease.

NURSING and COLLABORATIVE MANAGEMENT ACUTE CONGESTIVE HEART FAILURE AND PULMONARY EDEMA

The goal of therapy is to improve LV function by decreasing intravascular volume, decreasing venous return (preload), decreasing afterload, improving gas exchange and oxygenation, increasing CO, and reducing anxiety. Table 34-5 lists the major components of the therapeutic approach.

■ Decreasing Intravascular Volume

Decreasing intravascular volume with the use of diuretics improves LV function by reducing venous return. A loop diuretic (e.g., furosemide [Lasix], bumetanide [Bumex]) is the drug of choice for decreasing volume because it may be administered quickly by intravenous (IV) bolus and its action within the kidney occurs rapidly. By decreasing venous return to the LV and thereby reducing preload, the overfilled LV contracts more efficiently and CO improves. This increases LV function, decreases pulmonary vascular pressures, and improves gas exchange.

■ Decreasing Venous Return

Decreasing venous return *(preload)* reduces the amount of volume returned to the LV during diastole. This can be accomplished by placing the patient in a high Fowler position with the feet horizontal in the bed or dangling at the bedside. This position helps decrease venous return because of the pooling of blood in the extremities. This position also increases the thoracic capacity, allowing for improved ventilation. IV nitroglycerin is a vasodilator used in the treatment of acute and chronic CHF. It reduces circulating volume by decreasing preload and also increases coronary artery circulation by dilating the coronary arteries. Therefore nitroglycerin reduces preload, slightly reduces afterload (in high doses), and increases myocardial oxygen supply.[8]

■ Decreasing Afterload

Afterload is the amount of wall tension the LV must develop during systole to eject blood into the aorta; that is, it is the amount of work the LV has to produce to eject blood into the systemic circulation. Systemic vascular resistance (SVR) is a determinant of afterload, as is LV filling. If afterload is reduced, the CO of the LV improves and thereby decreases pulmonary congestion.

IV nitroprusside (Nipride) is a potent vasodilator that reduces preload and afterload. Because of its potent effects on the vascular system, it is the drug of choice for the patient with pulmonary edema. By reducing both preload and afterload (by arteriolar and venous dilation), myocardial contraction improves, increasing CO and reducing pulmonary congestion. Complications of IV nitroprusside include (1) hypotension, which may require the use of dobutamine (Dobutrex) IV to maintain a mean arterial BP greater than or equal to 60 mm Hg, and (2) thiocyanate toxicity, which can develop after 48 hours of use. Morphine also reduces preload and afterload. It dilates both the pulmonary and systemic blood vessels, a goal in decreasing pulmonary pressures and improving the exchange of gases. Morphine also reduces anxiety.

Nesiritide (Natrecor) is a recombinant form of brain natriuretic peptide (BNP). Nesiritide reduces both preload and afterload by venous and arterial dilation, increases cardiac output, and increases diuresis and sodium excretion. It causes a reduction in pulmonary artery wedge pressure (PAWP) and systemic arterial pressure. It is administered intravenously and is used in patients with acutely decompensated heart failure with dyspnea at rest or with minimal activity. Because it is a naturally occurring substance, it has few side effects.[9]

■ Improving Gas Exchange and Oxygenation

Gas exchange may be improved by several measures. IV morphine decreases oxygen demands, which may be raised as a result of anxiety and subsequent increased musculoskeletal and respiratory activity. Administration of oxygen helps increase the percentage of oxygen in inspired air. (Oxygen therapy is discussed in Chapter 28.) In severe pulmonary edema the patient may need to be intubated and placed on a mechanical ventilator.

■ Improving Cardiac Function

Digitalis improves LV function by its positive inotropic action. Digitalis increases contractility but also increases myocardial oxygen consumption. Newer inotropic drugs (e.g., dobutamine [Dobutrex], milrinone [Primacor]) that increase myocardial contractility without increasing oxygen consumption are also effective. Dobutamine and milrinone also cause increased peripheral vasodilation.

Hemodynamic monitoring may become necessary if rapid resolution of problems does not occur with diuretics, morphine, nitroprusside, and nitroglycerin or if the patient becomes hypotensive. (Hemodynamic monitoring is discussed in Chapter 64.) Once a pulmonary artery catheter is in position, accurate measurement of CO, pulmonary artery pressure (PAP), and PAWP may be made and effective therapy instituted to maximize CO. A PAWP of 14 to 18 mm Hg will generally achieve the goal of increasing CO. BP control can also be maintained with other drugs if needed (see Chapter 32).

■ Reducing Anxiety

Reduction of anxiety is facilitated by the sedative action of morphine administered intravenously. When morphine is used, the patient must be watched closely for respiratory depression. In addition, a calm approach in providing care helps reduce anxiety.

Once the patient is more stable, determination of the cause of pulmonary edema is important. Diagnosis of systolic or diastolic failure will then determine further management protocols. Aggressive drug therapy may continue with IV forms of inotropic drugs, vasodilators, and angiotensin-converting enzyme (ACE) inhibitors. Nursing care focuses on continual physical assessment, hemodynamic monitoring, and monitoring the patient's response to treatment.

Collaborative Care: Chronic Congestive Heart Failure

The main goal in the treatment of CHF is to treat the underlying cause and contributing factors, maximize CO, and provide treatment to alleviate symptoms (see Table 34-6). The management of arrhythmias is discussed in Chapter 35, hypertension in Chapter 32, valvular disorders in Chapter 36, and coronary artery disease in Chapter 33.

In a person with CHF, oxygen saturation of the blood is reduced because the blood is not adequately oxygenated in the lungs. Administration of oxygen improves saturation and assists greatly in meeting tissue oxygen needs. Thus oxygen therapy helps relieve dyspnea and fatigue. Optimally either arterial blood gases (ABGs) or pulse oximetry is used to monitor the effectiveness of oxygen therapy.

Physical and emotional rest allows the patient to conserve energy and decreases the need for additional oxygen. The degree of rest recommended depends on the severity of heart failure. A patient with severe CHF may be on bed rest with limited activity. A patient with mild to moderate CHF can be ambulatory with a restriction of strenuous activity. The patient should be instructed to participate in limited activities with adequate recovery periods.

Nonpharmacologic therapies are now being used in the management of CHF patients. One new technique is the utilization of biventricular pacing. Traditional pacemakers pace one or both chambers. *Cardiac resynchronization therapy* coordinates right and left ventricle contractility through biventricular pacing. The ability to have normal electrical conduction within the right and left ventricles increases LV performance and CO. This additional therapy allows patients to increase their exercise capacity and decrease their overall symptoms.[10] (Cardiac pacemakers are discussed in Chapter 35.)

Cardiac transplantation is often the treatment of choice. However, the lack of donor hearts and the challenges of care make it an option for only a small number of patients with CHF. Stringent criteria are necessary to select the few patients with advanced CHF who can even hope to receive a transplanted heart. (Heart transplants are discussed later in this chapter.)

Several mechanical options are available to sustain CHF patients with deteriorating conditions, especially those awaiting cardiac transplantation. The intraaortic balloon pump (IABP) is widely used as a short-term bridge to cardiac surgery, including transplantation. However, the limitations of bed rest, infection, and vascular complications preclude long-term use. (IABPs are discussed in Chapter 64.) Ventricular assist devices (VADs) provide highly effective long-term support for up to 2 years and have become standard care in many heart transplant centers. (VADs are discussed in Chapter 64.)

Drug Therapy: Chronic Congestive Heart Failure

General therapeutic objectives for drug management of chronic CHF include the following: (1) identification of the type of CHF and underlying causes, (2) correction of sodium and water retention and volume overload, (3) reduction of cardiac workload, (4) improvement of myocardial contractility, and (5) control of precipitating and complicating factors. The aims of treating CHF are to improve symptoms, minimize side effects of treatment, prevent morbidity, and prolong survival.[11] Current therapeutic approaches stress the role of ACE inhibitors, diuretics, inotropic agents, and vasodilator drugs[12] (Table 34-7).

Angiotensin-Converting Enzyme Inhibitors. The benefits of ACE inhibitors in the treatment of all stages of heart failure have been well documented.[13,14] ACE inhibitors are useful in both systolic and diastolic heart failure, and they are the first-line therapy in the treatment of CHF. Examples of ACE inhibitors include captopril (Capoten), benazepril (Lotensin), and enalapril (Vasotec). Other examples of ACE inhibitors are discussed in Chapter 32 and listed in Table 32-8.

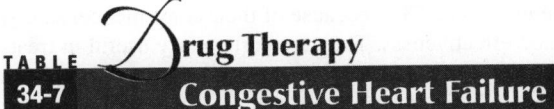

TABLE 34-7	**Drug Therapy** Congestive Heart Failure

ACE inhibitors (see Table 32-8)
Diuretics (see Table 32-8)
Inotropic drugs
   Digitalis preparations
      digoxin (Lanoxin)
   β-Adrenergic agonists
      dopamine (Intropin)
      dobutamine (Dobutrex)
   Phosphodiesterase inhibitors
      milrinone (Primacor)
   Calcium-sensitizing agent
      levosimendan (Simdax)*
Vasodilator drugs
   nitroprusside (Nipride)
   nitroglycerin
Antiarrhythmic drugs (see Table 35-8)
β-Adrenergic blockers
   carvedilol (Coreg)
   metoprolol (Toprol XL)
Human B-type natriuretic peptide
   nesiritide (Natrecor)

ACE, Angiotension-converting enzyme.
*FDA approval is pending.

The conversion of angiotensin I to the potent vasoconstrictor angiotensin II requires the presence of ACE (see Chapter 43, Fig. 43-4). ACE inhibitors exert their effects through blocking this enzyme, resulting in decreased levels of angiotensin II. As a result, plasma aldosterone levels are also reduced.

Because CO is dependent on afterload in chronic CHF, the reduction in SVR seen with the use of ACE inhibitors produces a significant increase in CO. Furthermore, with the use of ACE inhibitors, although BP may be decreased, tissue perfusion is maintained or is increased as a result of improvement of CO and redistribution of regional blood flow. Other hemodynamic changes include a reduction in (1) pulmonary artery pressure, (2) right arterial pressure, and (3) LV filling pressure.

Side effects of ACE inhibitors include symptomatic hypotension, chronic cough, and renal insufficiency (when ACE inhibitors are used in high doses). Aging and baseline renal insufficiency slow the metabolism of ACE inhibitors and may therefore lead to increased serum drug levels.[15,16] It is recommended that these drugs be started at the lowest dose and that BP and renal function be monitored at regular intervals. Overall, ACE inhibitors are well tolerated by patients.

In patients who are unable to tolerate the ACE inhibitors because of angioedema or cough, angiotensin II receptor blockers such as losartan (Cozaar) or valsartan (Diovan) may be used[17] (see Chapter 32, Table 32-8).

Diuretics. Diuretics are used in heart failure to mobilize edematous fluid, reduce pulmonary venous pressure, and reduce preload (see Chapter 32, Table 32-8). If excess extracellular fluid is excreted, blood volume returning to the heart can be reduced and cardiac function improved.

Diuretics act on the kidney by promoting excretion of sodium and water. Many varieties of diuretics are available, and some have specific indications for use. Thiazide diuretics may be the first choice in chronic CHF because of their convenience, safety, low cost, and effectiveness. They are particularly useful in treating edema secondary to CHF and in controlling hypertension. The thiazides inhibit sodium reabsorption in the distal tubule, thus promoting excretion of sodium and water.

Loop diuretics (e.g., furosemide [Lasix], bumetanide [Bumex], torsemide [Demadex]) are potent diuretics. These drugs act on the ascending loop of Henle to promote sodium, chloride, and water excretion. Furosemide is more commonly used in acute CHF and pulmonary edema because it is slightly more predictable in its response. Problems in using loop diuretics include reduction in serum potassium levels, ototoxicity, and possible allergic reaction in the patient who is sensitive to sulfa-type drugs.

Spironolactone (Aldactone) is a potassium-sparing diuretic that promotes sodium and water excretion but blocks potassium excretion by blocking the action of aldosterone. The drug is inexpensive and effective in patients with advanced heart failure.[17] Aldosterone receptor antagonism with spironolactone has been proven effective in the treatment of patients with CHF. Spironolactone appears to be additive to the benefits of ACE inhibitors, and is appropriate to use while renal function is adequate. A combination of diuretics may be administered for maximum effect.

Inotropic Drugs. The use of inotropic drugs in the patient with CHF is directed at improving cardiac contractility to increase CO, decrease LV diastolic pressure, and decrease systemic vascular resistance. Types of inotropic agents are listed in Table 34-7.

Digitalis preparations. Digitalis preparations (cardiac glycosides) have been the mainstay in the treatment of CHF and have been used for more than 200 years. However, the use of digitalis preparations has recently become controversial because they have never been shown to reduce mortality rates, but they do seem to offer some benefit in moderate to severe CHF by reducing hospitalizations and symptoms (see Evidence-Based Practice box). They are particularly useful in the treatment of CHF accompanied by atrial flutter and/or fibrillation with a rapid ventricular rate. Digitalis preparations increase the force or strength of cardiac contraction (inotropic action). They also decrease the conduction speed within the myocardium and slow the HR (chronotropic action). This action allows for more complete emptying of the ventricles, thus diminishing the volume remaining in the ventricles during diastole. CO increases because of an increased stroke volume from improved contractility.

An individual receiving digitalis preparations is subject to digitalis toxicity (Table 34-8). Some of the earliest symptoms of toxicity are anorexia, nausea, and vomiting. Visual disturbances, such as "yellow" vision, can occur with digitalis toxicity. Arrhythmias are a common indication of digitalis toxicity. Although almost any

EVIDENCE-BASED PRACTICE
Congestive Heart Failure and Digitalis

Clinical Problem
Is digitalis effective in treating congestive heart failure (CHF) in patients with normal sinus rhythm?

Best Clinical Practice
- Digitalis has a useful role in the treatment of patients with CHF who are in normal sinus rhythm.
- Digitalis therapy is associated with lower rates of hospitalization and clinical deterioration.

Implications for Nursing Practice
- If a patient with CHF is not taking digitalis therapy, the benefits of digitalis therapy should be discussed with the health care provider.
- The drugs being taken by a patient with CHF must be evaluated to assess for effectiveness and possible interactions.

Reference for Evidence
Hood WB et al: Digitalis for treatment of congestive heart failure in patients in sinus rhythm, *Cochrane Heart Group Cochrane Database of Systematic Reviews,* Issue 1, 2002.

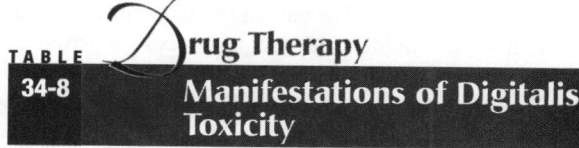

TABLE 34-8	**Drug Therapy** Manifestations of Digitalis Toxicity

Cardiovascular System
Bradycardia; tachycardia; pulse deficit; arrhythmias, including premature ventricular contractions, first-degree atrioventricular blocks, atrial fibrillation, junctional rhythms

Gastrointestinal System
Anorexia, nausea, vomiting, diarrhea, abdominal pain

Neurologic System
Headache, drowsiness, confusion, insomnia, muscle weakness

Visual System
Double vision, blurred vision, colored vision (usually green or yellow), visual halos

arrhythmia can occur, the types most frequently found are premature beats, atrial fibrillation, and first-degree heart block.

Hypokalemia is one of the most common causes of digitalis toxicity resulting in arrhythmias because low serum potassium levels enhance ectopic pacemaker activity. Monitoring the serum potassium levels of patients receiving both digitalis preparations and potassium-losing diuretics (e.g., thiazides, loop diuretics) is essential. Other electrolyte imbalances, such as hyperkalemia, hypercalcemia, and hypomagnesemia, can also precipitate toxicity.

Diseases of the kidney and liver increase the susceptibility to digitalis toxicity because most of the preparations are metabolized and eliminated by these organs. An older adult is especially prone to digitalis toxicity because digitalis accumulation occurs sooner with decreased liver and kidney function and slowed body metabolism, which occur with aging.

The usual treatment of toxicity consists of withholding the drug until the symptoms subside. In the case of life-threatening toxicity, digoxin immune Fab (ovine [Digibind]) is an antidote that can be given. The treatment of life-threatening arrhythmias is instituted as needed (see Chapter 35).

β-Adrenergic agonists. β-Adrenergic agonists include dopamine (Intropin), dobutamine (Dobutrex), epinephrine, and norepinephrine (Levophed). Stimulation of β-adrenergic receptors results in an increase in cyclic adenosine monophosphate (cAMP) within the myocardial cells and an increase in contractility (inotropic effect). The β-adrenergic agents are typically used as a short-term treatment of acute exacerbations of CHF in the intensive care unit (ICU). However, their role in long-term therapy of CHF is controversial. Potential problems related to long-term treatment with β-adrenergic agonists include tolerance, increased ventricular irritability, and increased need for oxygen by the myocardium.

Dopamine (Intropin) is an adrenergic agonist used for therapy of severe CHF and cardiogenic shock. In addition to increasing myocardial contractility, it also increases blood flow to the renal, mesenteric, coronary, and cerebrovascular beds. The action of dopamine is highly effective in the CHF patient because it increases CO (contractility), as well as urine output (decreases preload).

Phosphodiesterase inhibitors. Inhibition of phosphodiesterase increases cAMP, which enhances calcium entry into the cell and improves myocardial contractility. Phosphodiesterase inhibitors are also potent vasodilators. They increase CO and reduce arterial pressure (decrease afterload). These drugs are not currently available in oral form. Therefore they are limited to short-term use in the critical care setting.

Milrinone (Primacor) increases myocardial contraction, increases CO, promotes peripheral vasodilation, and decreases SVR, thus augmenting performance of the LV. Adverse reactions include arrhythmias, thrombocytopenia, and GI effects.

Calcium sensitizers. Levosimendan (Simdax)* is a positive inotropic drug. It binds to troponin C, a calcium-sensitive protein in heart muscle that plays an important role in regulating contractility. By binding to troponin C during the contraction phase of the cardiac cycle, levosimendan sensitizes heart muscle filaments to calcium, and thereby increases the pumping force of the heart. It is used in patients who need inotropic support who are also at risk for myocardial ischemia. It produces cardioprotective effects while simultaneously enhancing ventricular contractile function.

Vasodilator Drugs. Vasodilator drugs are a class of drugs clearly shown to improve survival in overt heart failure. The

goals of vasodilator therapy in the treatment of CHF include (1) increasing venous capacity, (2) improving ejection fraction through improved ventricular contraction, (3) slowing the process of ventricular dysfunction, (4) decreasing heart size, and (5) avoiding stimulation of the neurohormonal responses initiated by the compensatory mechanisms of CHF.

Sodium nitroprusside. Nitroprusside is the most commonly used IV vasodilator in the management of acute CHF and pulmonary edema (see earlier in this chapter).

Nitrates. Nitrates cause vasodilation by acting directly on the smooth muscle of the vessel wall. Their effects primarily involve increasing venous capacitance, dilating the pulmonary vasculature, and improving arterial compliance. Therefore the major hemodynamic effect of nitrates is to decrease preload. Nitrates are of particular benefit in the management of myocardial ischemia related to CHF because they promote vasodilation of the coronary arteries. One specific deterrent to the use of nitrates in CHF is nitrate tolerance.

β-Adrenergic Blockers. β-Adrenergic blockers are of increasing importance in the management of CHF. Marked improvement in patient survival occurs with the use of β-adrenergic blockers, specifically carvedilol (Coreg) and long-acting metoprolol (Toprol XL). β-Adrenergic blockers directly block the sympathetic nervous system's negative effects on the failing heart, such as increased heart rate. They are used in combination with ACE inhibitors, digitalis, and diuretics. β-Adrenergic blockers must be started gradually, increasing the dosage slowly every 2 weeks as tolerated by the patient. Patient teaching and close monitoring help identify side effects of β-adrenergic blockers, such as dizziness or edema.

Nutritional Therapy: Chronic Congestive Heart Failure

Diet education and weight management are critical to the patient's control of chronic CHF. The nurse or dietitian should obtain a detailed diet history, determining not only what foods the patient eats and when but also the sociocultural value of food. The nurse can use this database to assist the patient in solving problems and developing an individual diet plan. The patient should be taught what foods are low and high in sodium and ways to enhance food flavors without the use of salt (e.g., substituting lemon juice and various spices).

The edema of chronic CHF is often treated by dietary restriction of sodium. The degree of sodium restriction depends on the severity of the heart failure and the effectiveness of diuretic therapy. Diets that are severely restricted in sodium are rarely prescribed because they are unpalatable and patient compliance is poor. The Dietary Approach to Stop Hypertension (DASH) diet is effective as a first-line therapy for many individuals with isolated systolic hypertension (see Chapter 32, Table 32-7). This diet is now also widely used for the patient with CHF, with or without hypertension.[18]

The normal daily dietary intake of sodium ranges from 3 to 7 g. A commonly prescribed diet for a patient with mild CHF is a 2 g sodium diet (Table 34-9). All foods high in sodium should be eliminated (Tables 34-10 and 34-11). For more severe CHF, sodium intake is restricted to 500 to 1000 mg (see Table 34-9). On this diet, milk, cheese, bread, cereals, canned soups, and some canned vegetables must be eliminated. The patient and family must be instructed on how to read labels to look for sodium as an ingredient.

---

*FDA approval pending.

TABLE 34-9 — Nutritional Therapy: Low-Sodium Diets

General Principles

Do not add salt or seasonings containing sodium when preparing foods.
Do not use salt at the table.
Avoid high-sodium foods.
Limit milk products to 2 cups daily.

Sample Menu Plans for 2400 mg Sodium Diet

Breakfast	Sodium (mg)
⅔ cup bran cereal	161
(⅔ cup Shredded Wheat cereal)*	3
1 slice whole wheat bread	149
1 medium banana	1
6 oz fruit yogurt, fat free	85
1 cup fat-free milk	126
2 tbs jelly	5
Coffee, 8 oz	5

Lunch	
Chicken breast sandwich	
2 slices (3 oz) chicken breast, skinless	65
2 slices whole wheat bread	299
1 slice (¾ oz) American cheese	328
(1 slice ¾ oz Swiss cheese, natural)*	54
Large leaf romaine lettuce	1
2 slices tomato	90
1 tbs mayonnaise, low fat	90
1 medium peach	7

Dinner	
¾ cup vegetarian spaghetti sauce	459
(6 oz no–salt-added tomato paste)*	260
1 cup spaghetti	1
3 tbs Parmesan cheese	349
Spinach salad	
1 cup fresh spinach leaves	24
¼ cup fresh carrots (grated)	10
¼ cup fresh mushrooms (sliced)	1
2 tbs vinaigrette dressing	0
½ cup canned pears, juice pack	4
½ cup corn, cooked from frozen	4

Snack	
⅓ cup almonds	4
¼ cup dried apricots	3
6 oz fruit yogurt, fat free	85

Modifications for Other Low-Sodium Diets

500 mg Sodium Diet
Restrict milk products to 1 cup daily
Limit meat to 4 oz daily
Use salt-free butter, bread, vegetables, and starches

1000 mg Sodium Diet
Restrict milk products to 1 cup daily
Use salt-free butter and vegetables

4 g Sodium Diet
Allow cooking with small amounts of salt
Allow 3 cups milk products daily

*Substitutes to reduce to 1500 mg sodium diet.

TABLE 34-10 — Nutritional Therapy: Sodium Label Language

Phrase	What it Means
Sodium free or salt free	Less than 5 mg per serving
Very low sodium	35 mg or less of sodium per serving
Low sodium	140 mg or less of sodium per serving
Low-sodium meal	140 mg less of sodium per 3.5 oz
Reduced or less sodium	At least 25% less sodium than regular
Light in sodium	50% less sodium than regular
Unsalted or no salt added	No salt added to the product during process

Use caution with products advertised as no salt replacements—they may contain high potassium.

TABLE 34-11 — Nutritional Therapy: Sodium Content in Different Food Groups

Only a small amount of sodium occurs naturally in foods. Most sodium is added during processing. The following gives examples of varying amounts of sodium that occur in foods before and after processing.

Food Groups	Sodium (mg)
Grains and Grain Products	
Cooked cereal, rice, pasta, unsalted, ½ cup	0–5
Ready-to-eat cereal, 1 cup	100–360
Bread, 1 slice	110–175
Vegetables	
Fresh or frozen, cooked without salt, ½ cup	1–70
Canned or frozen with sauce, ½ cup	140–460
Tomato juice, canned, ¾ cup	820
Fruit	
Fresh, frozen, canned, ½ cup	0–5
Low-Fat or Fat-Free Dairy Foods	
Milk, 1 cup	120
Yogurt, 8 oz	160
Natural cheeses, 1½ oz	110–450
Processed cheeses, 1½ oz	600
Nuts, Seeds, and Dry Beans	
Peanuts, salted, ⅓ cup	120
Peanuts, unsalted, ⅓ cup	0–5
Beans, cooked from dried or frozen, without salt, ½ cup	400
Meats, Fish, and Poultry	
Fresh meat, fish, poultry, 3 oz	30–90
Tuna, canned, water pack, no salt added, 3 oz	34–45
Tuna, canned, water pack, 3 oz	250–350
Ham (lean) roasted, 3 oz	1020

Fluid restrictions are not commonly prescribed for the patient with mild to moderate CHF. Diuretic therapy and digitalis preparations act as effective diuretics to promote fluid excretion. However, in moderate to severe CHF and renal insufficiency, fluid restrictions are usually implemented.

Instructing patients to weigh themselves daily is important for monitoring fluid retention, as well as weight reduction. Patients should be instructed to weigh themselves at the same time each day, preferably before breakfast, while wearing the same type of clothing. This helps ensure valid comparisons from day to day and helps identify early signs of fluid retention. If a patient experiences a weight gain of 3 lb (1.4 kg) over 2 to 5 days, the primary care provider should be called.

NURSING MANAGEMENT
CHRONIC CONGESTIVE HEART FAILURE

■ Nursing Assessment

Subjective and objective data that should be obtained from a patient with CHF include those presented in Table 34-12.

■ Nursing Diagnoses

Nursing diagnoses for the patient with CHF include, but are not limited to, those presented in NCP 34-1.

■ Planning

The overall goals are that the patient with CHF will have (1) decreased peripheral edema, (2) decreased shortness of breath, (3) increased exercise tolerance, (4) compliance with drug regimen, and (5) no complications related to CHF.

■ Nursing Implementation

Health Promotion. An important measure used to prevent heart failure is the treatment or control of the underlying heart disease. For example, in valvular disease, valve replacement should be planned before lung congestion develops. Another important preventive measure concerns early and continued treatment of hypertension. Hyperlipidemic states in persons with CAD should be managed with diet, exercise, and medication. The use of antiarrhythmic agents or pacemakers is indicated for people with serious arrhythmias or conduction disturbances.

EVIDENCE-BASED PRACTICE
Telephone Interventions for Patients with Congestive Heart Failure

Clinical Problem

Is a nurse case-management telephone intervention effective in decreasing rehospitalization rates and other resource use in patients with congestive heart failure?

Best Clinical Practice

- Reduction in hospitalizations, costs, and other resources can be obtained with the use of a telephone case-management intervention.
- Patient satisfaction with care was higher in the telephone intervention group as compared with standard care.

Implications for Nursing Practice

- One role for nurses is case management.
- The nurse as a case manager can effectively promote continuity of care and decrease hospitalization rates in patients with congestive heart failure.
- Telephone interventions are effective in follow-up of patients.

Reference for Evidence

Riegel B et al: Effect of a standardized nurse case-management telephone intervention on resource use in patients with chronic heart failure, *Arch Intern Med* 162:705, 2002.

TABLE 34-12	Nursing Assessment Congestive Heart Failure

Subjective Data	Objective Data
Important Health Information	**Integumentary**
Past health history: CAD (including recent MI), hypertension, cardiomyopathy, valvular or congenital heart disease, diabetes mellitus, thyroid or lung disease, rapid or irregular heart rate	Cool, diaphoretic skin; cyanosis or pallor, peripheral edema (right-sided heart failure)
Medications: Use of and compliance with any cardiac medications; use of diuretics, estrogens, corticosteroids, phenylbutazone, nonsteroidal antiinflammatory drugs, over-the-counter drugs	**Respiratory**
	Tachypnea, crackles, rhonchi, wheezes; frothy, blood-tinged sputum
Functional Health Patterns	**Cardiovascular**
Health perception–health management: Fatigue, depression	Tachycardia, S_3, S_4, murmurs; pulsus alternans, PMI displaced inferiorly and posteriorly, jugular vein distention
Nutritional-metabolic: Usual sodium intake; nausea, vomiting, anorexia, stomach bloating; weight gain	**Gastrointestinal**
Elimination: Nocturia, decreased daytime urinary output, constipation	Abdominal distention, hepatosplenomegaly, ascites
Activity-exercise: Dyspnea, orthopnea, cough; palpitations; dizziness, fainting	**Neurologic**
Sleep-rest: Number of pillows used for sleeping; paroxysmal nocturnal dyspnea	Restlessness, confusion, decreased attention or memory
Cognitive-perceptual: Chest pain or heaviness; RUQ pain, abdominal discomfort; behavioral changes	**Possible Findings**
	Altered serum electrolytes (especially Na^+ and K^+), $\uparrow$ BUN, creatinine, or liver function tests; chest x-ray demonstrating cardiomegaly, pulmonary congestion, and interstitial pulmonary edema; echocardiogram showing increased chamber size and decreased wall motion; atrial and ventricular enlargement on ECG; $\downarrow$ O_2 saturation

BUN, Blood urea nitrogen; *CAD,* coronary artery disease; *ECG,* electrocardiogram; *MI,* myocardial infarction; *RUQ,* right upper quadrant.

NURSING CARE PLAN 34-1

Congestive Heart Failure

NURSING DIAGNOSIS   Activity intolerance *related to* fatigue secondary to cardiac insufficiency and pulmonary congestion *as manifested by* dyspnea, shortness of breath, weakness, increase in heart rate on exertion, and patient's statement, "I feel too weak to do anything."

OUTCOMES—NOC	INTERVENTIONS—NIC and *RATIONALES*
Activity Tolerance (0005)	*Energy Management (0180)*
▪ O$_2$ saturation IER in response to activity _____	▪ Encourage alternate rest and activity periods *to reduce cardiac workload.*
▪ Heart rate IER in response to activity _____	▪ Provide emotional and physical rest *to reduce O$_2$ consumption and to relieve dyspnea and fatigue.*
▪ Respiratory rate IER in response to activity _____	▪ Monitor cardiorespiratory response to activity *to determine level of activity that can be performed.*
▪ ECG WNL _____	
▪ Skin color WNL _____	▪ Teach patient and significant other the techniques of self-care *to minimize O$_2$ consumption.*
▪ Reported ADLs performance _____	
▪ Systolic BP IER in response to activity _____	*Activity Therapy (4310)*
▪ Diastolic BP IER in response to activity _____	▪ Assist to choose activities consistent with physical, psychologic, and social capabilities *to determine level of activity that can be performed.*
Outcome Scale	▪ Collaborate with occupational, physical, and/or recreational therapists *to plan and monitor activity program.*
1 = Extremely compromised	
2 = Substantially compromised	▪ Determine patient's commitment to ↑ frequency and/or range of activities *to provide patient with obtainable goals.*
3 = Moderately compromised	
4 = Mildly compromised	
5 = Not compromised	

NURSING DIAGNOSIS   Excess fluid volume *related to* cardiac failure *as manifested by* edema, dyspnea on exertion, increased weight gain, and patient's statement, "I'm short of breath and my ankles are so big and puffy!"

OUTCOMES—NOC	INTERVENTIONS—NIC and *RATIONALES*
Fluid Balance (0601)	*Fluid/Electrolyte Management (2080)*
▪ Peripheral pulses palpable _____	▪ Weigh daily and monitor trends *to monitor fluid retention and weight reduction.*
▪ Peripheral edema not present _____	▪ Monitor for serum electrolyte levels *to assess as a response to treatment.*
▪ Serum electrolytes WNL _____	
▪ Orthostatic hypotension not present _____	*Hypervolemia Management (4170)*
▪ BP IER _____	▪ Monitor respiratory pattern for symptoms of respiratory difficulty *for early recognition of pulmonary congestion.*
▪ Skin hydration _____	▪ Monitor hemodynamic status including CVP, MAP, PAWP, if available *because they help guide therapy.*
▪ Body weight stable _____	
Outcome Scale	▪ Monitor renal function and intake and output *to monitor fluid balance.*
1 = Extremely compromised	
2 = Substantially compromised	▪ Monitor for therapeutic effect of diuretic (↑ urine output, ↓ CVP, ↓ adventitious breath sounds) *to assess response to treatment.*
3 = Moderately compromised	
4 = Mildly compromised	
5 = Not compromised	

NURSING DIAGNOSIS   Disturbed sleep pattern *related to* nocturnal dyspnea, inability to assume favored sleep position, nocturia *as manifested by* inability to sleep through the night.

OUTCOMES—NOC	INTERVENTIONS—NIC and *RATIONALES*
Sleep (0004)	*Sleep Enhancement (1850)*
▪ Uninterrupted sleep _____	▪ Determine patient's sleep/activity pattern *to establish routine.*
▪ Hours of sleep _____	▪ Encourage patient to establish a bedtime routine to facilitate transition from wakefulness to sleep *in order to establish a pattern and decrease number of waking periods.*
▪ Feelings of rejuvenation after sleep _____	
▪ Vital signs IER _____	▪ Adjust environment *to promote sleep.*
Outcome Scale	▪ Regulate environmental stimuli to maintain normal day-night cycles *to help promote sleep cycle.*
1 = Extremely compromised	
2 = Substantially compromised	▪ Adjust medication administration schedule *to support patient's sleep cycle.*
3 = Moderately compromised	
4 = Mildly compromised	▪ Monitor patient's sleep pattern and number of sleep hours *to determine hours of sleep.*
5 = Not compromised	

ADLs, Activities of daily living; *CVP,* central venous pressure; *IER,* in expected range; *MAP,* mean arterial pressure; *PAWP,* pulmonary artery wedge pressure; *WNL,* within normal limits.

NURSING CARE PLAN 34-1

Congestive Heart Failure—cont'd

NURSING DIAGNOSIS   **Impaired gas exchange** *related to* increased preload, mechanical failure, or immobility *as manifested by* increased respiratory rate, shortness of breath, dyspnea on exertion, and patient's statement, "I just can't seem to catch my breath."

OUTCOMES—NOC

Respiratory Status: Gas Exchange (0402)
Vital Signs Status (0802)
- Ease of breathing _____
- Dyspnea with exertion not present _____
- O₂ saturation WNL _____
- Respiratory rate WNL _____

_____

Outcome Scale
1 = Extremely compromised
2 = Substantially compromised
3 = Moderately compromised
4 = Mildly compromised
5 = Not compromised

INTERVENTIONS—NIC and *RATIONALES*

Respiratory Monitoring (3350)
- Monitor rate, rhythm, depth, and effort of respirations.
- Auscultate breath sounds, noting areas of decreased/absent ventilation and presence of adventitious sounds, *to assess congestion.*
- Monitor for dyspnea and events that improve and worsen it *to detect events that can influence ADLs.*

Oxygen Therapy (3320)
- Administer supplemental O₂ as ordered *to maintain O₂ levels.*
- Change O₂ delivery device from mask to nasal prongs during meals as tolerated *to sustain O₂ levels while doing ADLs.*

Positioning (0840)
- Position to alleviate dyspnea (e.g., semi-Fowler position), as appropriate, *to improve ventilation by decreasing venous return to the heart and increasing thoracic capacity.*

Cardiac Care: Acute (4044)
- Monitor the effectiveness of O₂ therapy by measuring O₂ saturation *to identify hypoxemia and establish range of O₂ saturation.*

NURSING DIAGNOSIS   **Anxiety** *related to* dyspnea or perceived threat of death *as manifested by* restlessness, irritability, expression of feelings of life threat, and patient's statement, "Don't leave me alone, I'm afraid I might die."

OUTCOMES—NOC

Anxiety Control (1402)
- Uses effective coping strategies _____
- Reports decreased duration of episodes _____

_____

Outcome Scale
1 = Never demonstrated
2 = Rarely demonstrated
3 = Sometimes demonstrated
4 = Often demonstrated
5 = Consistently demonstrated

INTERVENTIONS—NIC and *RATIONALES*

Anxiety Reduction (5820)
- Use a calm, reassuring approach *to increase confidence in caregiver and relieve anxiety.*
- Explain all procedures, including sensations likely to be experienced during a procedure, *to promote sense of security.*
- Help patient identify situations that precipitate anxiety *to plan appropriate use of anxiety-reducing techniques.*
- Create an atmosphere to facilitate trust (e.g., answer call bell promptly and make frequent checks) *to promote sense of security.*
- Instruct patient on the use of relaxation techniques *to help alleviate anxiety.*

NURSING DIAGNOSIS   **Deficient knowledge** *related to* disease process *as manifested by* questions about the disease and patient's statement, "I don't know why I keep getting sick."

OUTCOMES—NOC

Knowledge: Disease Process (1803)
- Description of disease process _____
- Description of signs and symptoms of complications _____
- Descriptions of precautions to prevent complications _____

_____

Outcome Scale
1 = None
2 = Limited
3 = Moderate
4 = Substantial
5 = Extensive

INTERVENTIONS—NIC and *RATIONALES*

Teaching: Disease Process (5602)
- Assess the patient's current level of knowledge related to specific disease process *to assess needed areas of teaching.*
- Describe common signs and symptoms of the disease *so patient will know signs and symptoms of worsening CHF.*
- Instruct the patient on measures to prevent/minimize side effects of treatment for the disease *so patient may be able to decrease number of acute episodes of CHF.*
- Include family or significant others in teaching *to provide support for the patient.*

CHF, Congestive heart failure.

When a patient is diagnosed with CHF, preventive care should focus on slowing the progression of the disease. Knowledge of the importance of following the medication, diet, and exercise regimens and cardiac rehabilitation is essential. The in-hospital nurse may request home nursing care for the patient and family to provide for follow-up care and to monitor the patient's response to treatment. Early detection of signs and symptoms of worsening failure may help modify care and prevent an acute episode requiring further hospitalization.[19]

Acute Intervention. Successful CHF management depends on several important principles: (1) heart failure is a progressive disease, and treatment plans are established with quality-of-life goals; (2) symptom management is controlled by the patient with self-management tools (daily weights, drug regimens, exercise plans); (3) salt and water must be restricted; (4) exercise and energy must be conserved; and (5) support systems are essential to the success of the entire treatment plan.[20,21]

Many persons with CHF do not experience an acute episode. If they do, they are usually initially managed in an ICU and later transferred to a general unit when their condition has stabilized. The nursing care plan for the patient with CHF (see NCP 34-1) applies to the patient with stabilized acute or chronic CHF.

Ambulatory and Home Care. CHF is a chronic illness for most persons. Important nursing responsibilities are (1) teaching the patient about the physiologic changes that have occurred, (2) assisting the patient to adapt to both the physiologic and psychologic changes, and (3) integrating the patient and the patient's family or support system in the overall care plan.[22] It must be emphasized to the patient that it is possible to live productively with this health problem. Home health care can prevent future hospitalization. Home nursing care will follow up with ongoing clinical assessments, monitoring vital signs, and monitoring response to therapies. Managing these patients out of the hospital is a priority of care. A patient and family teaching guide for the patient with CHF is presented in Table 34-13.

Patients with CHF are usually required to take medication for the rest of their lives. This often becomes difficult because a patient may be asymptomatic when CHF is under control. It must be stressed that the disease is chronic and that medication must be continued to keep the heart failure under control.

The patient should evaluate the action of the prescribed drug and be taught to recognize the manifestations of drug toxicity. The patient should also be taught how to take her or his pulse rate and to know under what circumstances drugs, especially digitalis

---

TABLE 34-13

Patient & Family Teaching Guide
Congestive Heart Failure

Rest
1. Have a regular daily rest and activity program.
2. After exertion, such as exercise and ADLs, plan a rest period.
3. Shorten working hours or schedule rest period during working hours.
4. Avoid emotional upsets. Listen to concerns, fears, etc. and provide encouragement.

Drug Therapy
1. Take each drug as prescribed daily.
2. Develop a check-off system (e.g., daily chart) to ensure medications have been taken.
3. Take pulse rate each day before taking medications. Know the parameters that your health care provider wants for your heart rate.
4. Learn to take own BP at determined intervals. Know your acceptable BP limits.
5. Know signs and symptoms of orthostatic hypotension and how to prevent them.
6. Know signs and symptoms of internal bleeding; bleeding gums, increased bruises, blood in stool or urine, and what to do if on anticoagulants.
7. Know own INR if taking warfarin (Coumadin) and how often to have blood monitored.

Dietary Therapy
1. Consult the written diet plan and list of permitted and restricted foods.
2. Examine labels to determine sodium content. Also examine the labels of over-the-counter drugs such as laxatives, cough medicines, and antacids.
3. Avoid using salt.
4. Weigh yourself in the early morning after arising and emptying your bladder. Use the same scale and wear the same or similar clothes every day.
5. Report weight gain of more than 3 lb (0.4 kg) in 2 days.
6. Eat small, frequent meals.

Activity Program
1. Increase walking and other activities gradually, provided they do not cause fatigue and dyspnea.
2. Avoid extremes of heat and cold.
3. Keep regular appointments with health care provider.

Ongoing Monitoring
1. Know YOUR limit.
2. Know the signs and symptoms of recurring or progressing heart failure.
3. Recall the symptoms experienced when illness began; reappearance of previous symptoms may indicate a recurrence.
4. Report immediately to health care provider any of the following:
   - Difficulty breathing, especially with exertion or when lying flat
   - Waking up breathless at night
   - Frequent dry, hacking cough, especially when lying down
   - Fatigue, weakness
   - Swelling of ankles, feet, or abdomen
   - Nausea with abdominal swelling, pain, and tenderness
   - Dizziness or fainting
   - Weight gain of 3-5 lb
5. Join the local support group with your family members.

ADLs, Activities of daily living; *BP,* blood pressure; *INR,* international normalized ratio.

and β-adrenergic blockers, should be withheld and a health care provider consulted. The pulse rate should always be taken for 1 full minute. A pulse rate lower than 50 to 60 beats per minute may be a contraindication to taking a digitalis preparation unless specified otherwise by the health care provider. However, in the absence of primary heart block or the development of ventricular ectopy, a pulse rate of 60 beats per minute or less may not a contraindication to taking digitalis or β-adrenergic blockers. A pulse rate of 50 beats per minute (especially in a patient who is also taking β-adrenergic blockers) may be acceptable.

The patient should also be taught the symptoms of hypokalemia if diuretics that cause potassium excretion are being taken. (Manifestations of hypokalemia are discussed in Chapter 16.) Hypokalemia sensitizes the myocardium to digitalis. Consequently, toxicity may develop from an ordinary dose of digitalis. Frequently the patient who is taking thiazide or loop diuretics is given supplemental potassium.

The nurse, physical therapist, or occupational therapist can instruct the patient in energy-saving and energy-efficient behaviors after an evaluation of daily activities has been done. For example, once the nurse understands the patient's daily routine, suggestions can be made for simplification of work or modification of an activity. Frequently the patient needs a prescription for rest after an activity. Many hard-driving persons need the "permission" to not feel "lazy." Sometimes an activity that the patient enjoys may need to be eliminated. In such situations the patient should be helped to explore alternative activities that cause less physical and cardiac stress. The physical environment may require modification in situations in which there is an increased cardiac workload demand (e.g., frequent climbing of stairs). The nurse can help the patient identify areas where outside assistance can be obtained.

The home health nurse is essential in the care of the CHF patient and family. Frequent physical assessments, including vital signs and weight, are extremely important. Home health nurses frequently work within protocols set up with the patient's health care team. The protocols may enable the nurse and patient to identify problems, such as an increase in weight and HR as evidence of worsening failure, and institute interventions to prevent hospitalization. This may include altering medications and fluid restrictions. Home health nursing care of CHF patients is paramount in reducing the number of hospitalizations, increasing functional capacity, and increasing quality of life.[23]

■ Evaluation

The expected outcomes for the patient with CHF are presented in NCP 34-1.

Cardiomyopathy

Cardiomyopathy (CMP) is a term used to describe a group of heart muscle diseases that primarily affect the structural or functional ability of the myocardium. Diagnosis of CMP is made based on the patient's clinical manifestations and diagnostic noninvasive and invasive cardiac procedures.

CMPs can be classified as primary or secondary. Primary CMPs are those conditions in which the etiology of the heart disease is unknown. The heart muscle in this instance is the only portion of the heart involved, and other cardiac structures are unaffected. In secondary CMP the cause of the myocardial disease

is known and is secondary to another disease process. Common causes of secondary CMP are listed in Table 34-14.

The World Health Organization has classified CMP conditions into three general types: dilated (congestive), hypertrophic, and restrictive.[24] Each of these types has its own pathogenesis,

TABLE 34-14   Causes of Secondary Cardiomyopathy

DILATED	HYPERTROPHIC	RESTRICTIVE
Cardiotoxic agents— alcohol, cocaine, doxorubicin (Adriamycin) Genetic or familial Hypertension Idiopathic Ischemia (coronary artery disease) Metabolic disorders Muscular dystrophy Myocarditis Pregnancy Valvular disorder	Aortic stenosis Genetic Hypertension	Amyloidosis Endomyocardial fibrosis Idiopathic Neoplastic tumor Postradiation therapy Sarcoidosis Ventricular thrombus

TABLE 34-15   Characteristics of Cardiomyopathies

DILATED	HYPERTROPHIC	RESTRICTIVE
Major Manifestations		
Fatigue, weakness, palpitations, dyspnea, dry cough	Exertional dyspnea, fatigue, angina, syncope, palpitations	Dyspnea, fatigue, palpitations
Cardiomegaly		
Moderate to marked	Mild	Mild to moderate
Contractility		
Decreased	Increased or decreased	Normal or decreased
Valvular Incompetence		
Atrioventricular valves, particularly mitral	Mitral valve	Mitral valve
Arrhythmias		
Sinoatrial tachycardia, atrial and ventricular arrhythmias	Tachyarrhythmias	Atrial and ventricular arrhythmias
Cardiac Output		
Decreased	Decreased	Normal or decreased
Outflow Tract Obstruction		
None	Increased	None

clinical presentation, and treatment protocols (Table 34-15). All types of CMP can lead to cardiomegaly and CHF.

DILATED CARDIOMYOPATHY

Etiology and Pathophysiology

Dilated cardiomyopathy is the most common type of CMP, accounting for more than 90% of all cases, and is characterized by cardiomegaly with ventricular dilation, impairment of systolic function, atrial enlargement, and stasis of blood in the LV. **Cardiomegaly** (an enlargement of the heart) is the result of primarily ventricular dilation (Fig. 34-3). Although this disorder closely resembles CHF, the walls of the ventricles do not become hypertrophic as they do in CHF (Fig. 34-4).

Dilated CMP often follows an infectious myocarditis. Other common causes of dilated CMP are listed in Table 34-14. Regardless of the initial cause, dilated CMP is characterized by a diffuse inflammation and rapid degeneration of myocardial fibers that cause ventricular dilation and decreased contractile function.

Clinical Manifestations

The signs and symptoms of dilated CMP may develop acutely after an infectious process or insidiously over a period of time. Most people eventually develop CHF. Symptoms can include a change in exercise tolerance, fatigue, dry cough, dyspnea, paroxysmal nocturnal dyspnea, orthopnea, palpitations, and anorexia. Signs can include S_3, S_4, tachycardia, pulmonary crackles, edema, weak peripheral pulses, pallor, hepatomegaly, and jugular venous distention. The patient may also have arrhythmias. Because blood flows more slowly through an enlarged heart, blood clots easily form and may lead to systemic embolization.

Diagnostic Studies

The diagnosis of dilated CMP is made on the basis of the patient's history and by ruling out other conditions that cause CHF. The chest x-ray may show cardiomegaly with signs of pulmonary venous hypertension, as well as pleural effusion. The ECG may reveal tachycardia and arrhythmias with conduction disturbances. Echocardiography is useful in distinguishing dilated CMP from other structural abnormalities.

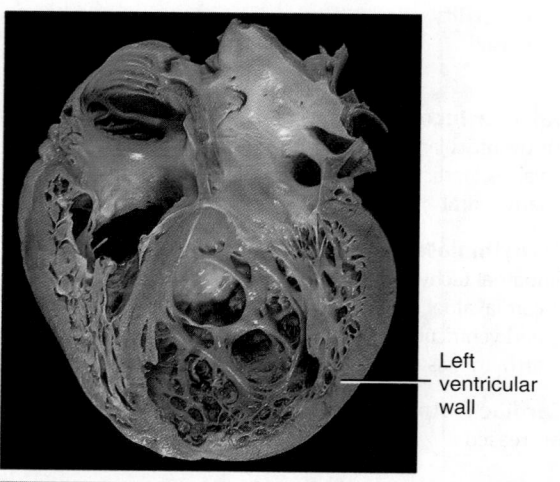

FIG. 34-3 Dilated cardiomyopathy. The dilated left ventricle has a thin wall.

Cardiac catheterization and coronary angiography are used in evaluating the manifestations of dilated CMP. The coronary arteries are usually normal. Left ventriculogram may reveal a thin-walled ventricle that is dilated. Endomyocardial biopsy may be done at the time of the right-sided heart catheterization to help make the diagnosis.

NURSING *and* COLLABORATIVE MANAGEMENT DILATED CARDIOMYOPATHY

Interventions focus on controlling CHF by enhancing myocardial contractility and decreasing afterload, similar to the treatment of chronic CHF (Table 34-16). Thus treatment is more palliative than curative. Digitalis is used to treat atrial fibrillation, diuretics are used to decrease preload, ACE inhibitors are used to reduce afterload, and β-adrenergic blockers and spironolactone are used to

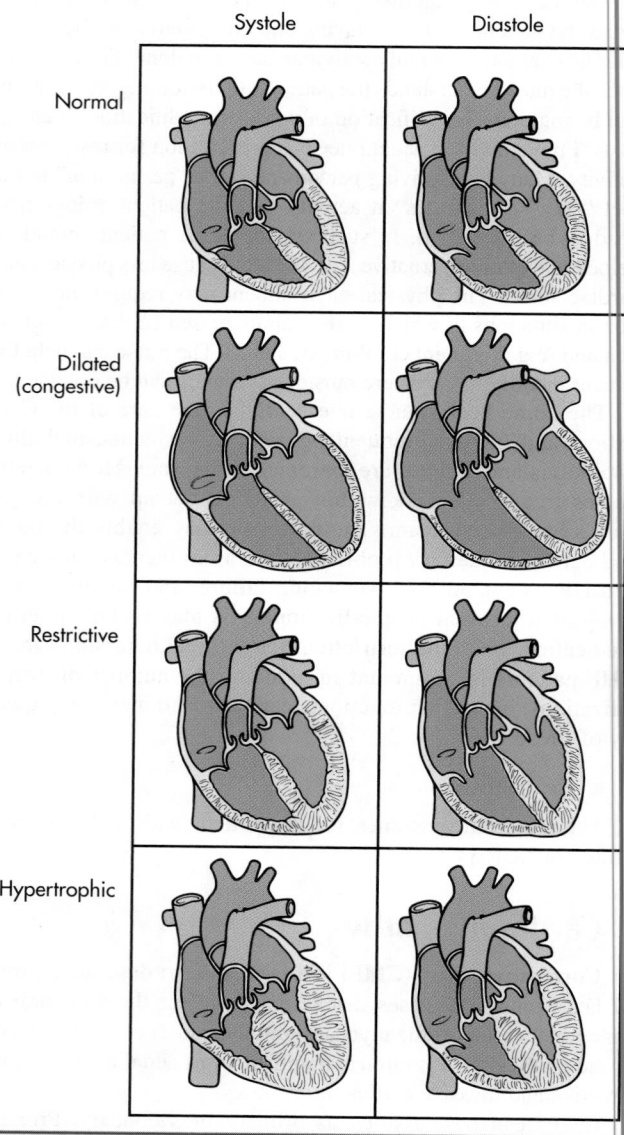

FIG. 34-4 Types of cardiomyopathies and the differences in ventricular diameter during systole and diastole, compared with a normal heart.

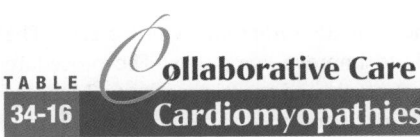

TABLE 34-16	**Collaborative Care** **Cardiomyopathies**

Diagnostic
History and physical examination
ECG, serum laboratory tests
Chest x-ray
Echocardiogram
Nuclear imaging studies
Cardiac catheterization
Endocardial biopsy

Collaborative Therapy
Treatment of underlying cause
Drug therapy
- ACE inhibitors (see Table 32-8)
- Diuretics (see Table 32-8)
- Digitalis (except in hypertrophic CMP in normal sinus rhythm)
- Anticoagulants (if indicated) (see Table 37-9)
- Antiarrhythmics (if indicated) (see Table 35-8)
- β-Adrenergic blockers (see Table 32-8)
Surgical correction
Cardiac transplant

ACE, Angiotensin-converting enzyme; *CMP,* cardiomyopathy; *ECG,* electrocardiogram.

control the neurohormonal system. Drug and nutritional therapy and cardiac rehabilitation may help alleviate symptoms of CHF and improve CO. A patient with secondary dilated CMP must be treated for the underlying disease process. For example, the patient with alcohol-induced dilated CMP must abstain from all alcohol intake.

Unfortunately, dilated CMP does not respond well to therapy. Intermittent dobutamine (Dobutrex) or milrinone (Primacor) infusions are used in the treatment of dilated cardiomyopathy. The patient is admitted to the hospital for a 72-hour infusion of dobutamine or milrinone followed by aggressive diuresis. Sometimes these infusions are done for an 8-hour period as an outpatient treatment or in the home. After infusion, many patients experience an improvement in symptoms that lasts several weeks after therapy.

The patient with terminal end-stage CMP may require cardiac transplantation. Currently approximately 50% of heart transplants are performed for treatment of cardiomyopathic conditions. Cardiac transplant recipients have a good prognosis for survival. However, donor hearts are difficult to obtain, and many patients with dilated CMP die while awaiting heart transplantation.

Patients with dilated cardiomyopathy are very ill people with a grave prognosis who need expert nursing care. The patient's family must learn cardiopulmonary resuscitation (CPR) and how to access emergency care in their neighborhood. The nurse should include family members and other support systems when planning a patient's care.

Home health care nursing can provide the patient and the family with the continuous assessments and therapeutic interventions that are required to maximize and maintain their functional status. Observing for signs and symptoms of worsening failure, arrhythmias, and embolic formation is paramount in this patient, as well as monitoring drug responsiveness. Because the goal of therapy is to keep the patient functional and out of the hospital,

home health nurses play a critical role in accomplishing these goals.

HYPERTROPHIC CARDIOMYOPATHY

Etiology and Pathophysiology

Hypertrophic cardiomyopathy (HCM) is asymmetric myocardial hypertrophy without ventricular dilation (Fig. 34-5). About one half of cases of HCM have a genetic basis. Other causes of HCM are listed in Table 34-14. HCM occurs less commonly than dilated CMP and is more common in men than in women.[25] HCM is the most common cause of sudden death in otherwise healthy young people. It is usually diagnosed in young adulthood and is often seen in active, athletic individuals. Another name for this disorder is *idiopathic hypertrophic subaortic stenosis* (IHSS). In one form of the disease, the septum between the two ventricles becomes enlarged and obstructs the blood flow from the left ventricle. It is termed *hypertrophic obstructive cardiomyopathy* (HOCM) or *asymmetric septal hypertrophy* (ASH).

The four main characteristics of HCM are (1) massive ventricular hypertrophy; (2) rapid, forceful contraction of the LV; (3) impaired relaxation; and (4) obstruction to aortic outflow (not present in all patients). Ventricular hypertrophy is associated with a thickened intraventricular septum and ventricular wall (see Fig. 34-4). The end result is impaired ventricular filling as the ventricle becomes noncompliant and unable to relax. The primary defect of HCM is diastolic dysfunction. Decreased ventricular filling and obstruction to outflow can result in decreased CO, especially during exertion, when increased CO is needed.[25]

Clinical Manifestations

Patients with HCM often are asymptomatic. Patient manifestations include exertional dyspnea, fatigue, angina, and syncope. The most common symptom is dyspnea, which is caused by an elevated left ventricular diastolic pressure. Fatigue occurs because of the resultant decrease in CO and in exercise-induced flow obstruction. Angina can occur and is most often caused by the increased LV muscle mass or compression of the small coronary arteries by the hypercontractile ventricular myocardium. The patient may also have syncope, especially during exertion.

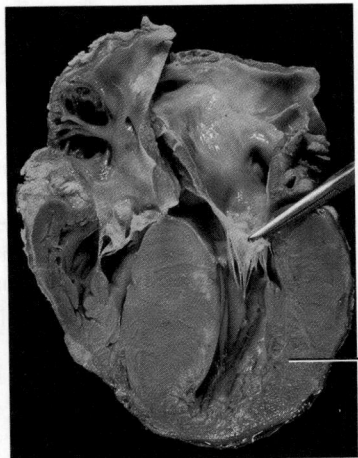

Left ventricular hypertrophy

FIG. 34-5 Hypertrophic cardiomyopathy. There is marked left ventricular hypertrophy.

Syncope in this population is most often caused by an increase in obstruction to aortic outflow during increased activity, resulting in decreased CO and cerebrovascular circulation. Syncope can also be caused by arrhythmias. Common arrhythmias include supraventricular tachycardia, atrial fibrillation, ventricular tachycardia, and ventricular fibrillation. Any of these arrhythmias may lead to loss of consciousness or sudden cardiac death of the patient, which is the most common cause of death in this population.

Diagnostic Studies

Clinical findings on examination may be unremarkable. However, there may be an abnormal arterial pulse by palpation; extra heart sounds, such as $S_3 S_4$; or a systolic murmur. The chest x-ray is usually normal except in a patient with severe disease causing an increased cardiac silhouette. Increased voltage and increased duration of the QRS complex are the most common abnormalities on the ECG. These findings usually indicate ventricular hypertrophy. Ventricular arrhythmias are also frequently seen, with ventricular tachycardia the most common.

The echocardiogram is the primary diagnostic tool revealing the classic feature of HCM, which is LV hypertrophy. The echocardiogram may also demonstrate wall motion abnormalities and diastolic dysfunction. Cardiac catheterization may also be helpful in the diagnosis of HCM.

NURSING *and* COLLABORATIVE MANAGEMENT
HYPERTROPHIC CARDIOMYOPATHY

Goals of intervention are to improve ventricular filling by reducing ventricular contractility and relieving LV outflow obstruction. These can be accomplished with the use of β-adrenergic blockers or calcium channel blockers. Digitalis preparations are contraindicated unless they are used to treat atrial fibrillation. CHF may also be present in varying degrees but is usually not present until later stages. Antiarrhythmics are also used to control arrhythmias. However, their use has not been proven to prevent sudden death. An alternative treatment for ventricular arrhythmias may be an implantable defibrillator (see Chapter 35). It has been found that ventricular or atrioventricular pacing can be beneficial for patients with HCM and outflow obstruction. By pacing the ventricles from the apex of the right ventricle, septal depolarization occurs first, allowing the septum to move away from the left ventricular wall and reducing the degree of obstruction of the outflow tract.

Some patients may be candidates for surgical treatment of their hypertrophied septum. The indications for surgery include severe symptoms refractory to therapy with marked obstruction to aortic outflow. The surgery is termed a *ventriculomyotomy and myectomy*. It involves incision of the hypertrophied septal muscle and resection of some of the hypertrophied muscle. Most patients have good symptomatic improvement after surgery and improved exercise tolerance.

Alcohol septal ablation or nonsurgical reduction of the hypertrophied septum is a new procedure that is performed in selected patients with HOCM. This procedure is performed in the cardiac catheterization laboratory and consists of administering absolute alcohol into the first septal artery branching off the left anterior descending artery. This causes ischemia and septal wall myocardial infarction. Ablation of the septal wall will decrease the obstruction to flow, and the patient's symptoms will decrease. The goal of this treatment is to improve symptoms. The procedure improves heart failure symptoms and exercise capacity 3 months after ablation. Mortality rates for the procedure are approximately 1% depending on the age and condition of the patient.[26]

Nursing interventions focus on relieving symptoms, observing for and preventing complications, and providing emotional and psychologic support. Teaching should focus on helping patients adjust their lifestyle to avoid strenuous activity and dehydration. Any activity or procedure that causes an increase in systemic vascular resistance (thus increasing the obstruction to forward flow) is dangerous and should be avoided.

RESTRICTIVE CARDIOMYOPATHY

Etiology and Pathophysiology

Restrictive cardiomyopathy is the least common of the cardiomyopathic conditions. It is a disease of the heart muscle that impairs diastolic filling and stretch (see Fig. 34-4). Systolic function remains unaffected. Although the specific etiology of restrictive CMP is unknown, a number of pathologic processes may be involved in its development. Myocardial fibrosis, hypertrophy, and infiltration produce stiffness of the ventricular wall with loss of ventricular compliance. Secondary causes of restrictive CMP include amyloidosis, endocardial fibrosis, glycogen deposition, hemochromatosis, sarcoidosis, fibrosis of different etiology, and radiation to the thorax. With restrictive cardiomyopathy, the ventricles are resistant to filling and therefore demand high diastolic filling pressures to maintain CO.

Clinical Manifestations

Angina, syncope, fatigue, and dyspnea on exertion are common signs. The most common symptom is that of exercise intolerance because the myocardium cannot increase CO by producing a tachycardia without further compromising the ventricular filling.

Signs and symptoms include those similar to CHF. The patient may have signs of both left-sided and right-sided heart failure, including dyspnea, peripheral edema, ascites, and hepatic dysfunction. Kussmaul's sign (bulging of the internal jugular neck veins on inspiration) may also be present.

Diagnostic Studies

The chest x-ray may be normal, or it may show cardiomegaly. Pleural effusions and pulmonary congestion may be evident in the patient with progression to CHF. The ECG may reveal a tachycardia at rest. The most common arrhythmias are atrial fibrillation and complex ventricular arrhythmias. Echocardiogram may reveal the thickened ventricular wall of restrictive CMP, small ventricular cavities, and dilated atria. Endomyocardial biopsy, computed tomography (CT) scan, and nuclear imaging may be helpful in a definitive diagnosis.

NURSING *and* COLLABORATIVE MANAGEMENT
RESTRICTIVE CARDIOMYOPATHY

Currently no specific treatment for restrictive CMP exists. Interventions are aimed at improving diastolic filling and the underlying disease process. Treatment includes conventional therapy for CHF and arrhythmias. Heart transplant may also be a consideration. Nursing care is similar to the care of a patient with CHF. As in the treatment of patients with HCM, the patient should be taught to avoid situations that impair ventricular filling, such as strenuous activity, dehydration, and increases in SVR.

CARDIAC TRANSPLANTATION

The first heart transplant was performed in 1967. Since that time, **cardiac transplantation** (transfer of a heart from one person to another) has become the treatment of choice for patients with end-stage heart disease. Patients with cardiomyopathy account for more than 50% of the cardiac transplant recipients. Inoperable CAD is the second most common indication for transplantation, accounting for 40% of candidates (Table 34-17).

Once an individual meets the criteria for cardiac transplantation, the goal of the evaluation process is to identify patients who would most benefit from a new heart. After a complete physical examination and diagnostic workup, the patient and family then undergo a comprehensive psychologic profile that includes assessing coping skills, family support systems, and motivation to follow the rigorous regimen that is essential to a successful transplantation. The complexity of the transplant process may be overwhelming to a patient with inadequate support systems and a poor understanding of the lifestyle changes required after transplant.

Once an individual is accepted as a transplant candidate (this may happen rapidly during an acute illness or over a longer period) he or she is placed on a transplant list. Patients may wait at home and receive ongoing medical care if their medical condition is stable. If their condition is not stable, they may require hospitalization for more intensive therapy. Unfortunately, the overall waiting period for a transplant is long, and many patients die while waiting for a transplant.

Donor and recipient matching is based on body and heart size and ABO type. Negative lymphocyte crossmatch (explained in Chapter 13) and avoidance of a transplantation from a cytomegalovirus (CMV)–positive donor to a CMV-negative recipient are important.

Most donor hearts are obtained at sites distant from the institution performing the transplant. The maximum acceptable ischemic time for cardiac transplant is 4 to 6 hours.

The recipient is prepared for surgery, and cardiopulmonary bypass is used. The usual surgical procedure involves removing the recipient's heart, except for the posterior right and left atrial walls and their venous connections. The recipient's heart is then

TABLE 34-17	Indications and Contraindications for Cardiac Transplantation

Indications: Transplant Center Specific

Suitable physiologic/chronologic age
End-stage heart disease refractory to medical therapy
Functional class III or IV status (NYHA)
Vigorous and healthy individual (except for end-stage cardiac disease) who would benefit from the procedure
Compliance with medical regimens
Demonstrated emotional stability and social support system
Financial resources available

Contraindications*

Systemic disease with poor prognosis
Active infection
Active or recent malignancy
Recent or unresolved pulmonary infarction
Severe pulmonary hypertension unrelieved with medication
Severe cerebrovascular or peripheral vascular disease
Irreversible renal or hepatic dysfunction
Active peptic ulcer disease
Severe osteoporosis
Severe obesity
History of drug or alcohol abuse or mental illness

NYHA, New York Heart Association.
*Contraindications may vary at different cardiac transplant centers.

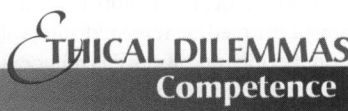

*E*THICAL DILEMMAS
Competence

Situation

An 83-year-old man has been a patient in intensive care for 1 month following cardiac surgery. During the surgery he suffered a stroke that left him paralyzed on his right side. He is only able to answer yes/no questions by shaking his head. He has required mechanical ventilation since surgery because of respiratory failure. For the past 2 weeks hemodialysis has been required because of renal failure. For the past several days when the nurses suction him, he tries to prevent the ventilator hose from being reconnected by turning his head or by pushing it away with his left hand. Although he does not have any advance directives, his wife and daughter state that on numerous occasions before his surgery, he expressed that he would not want to live if he lost his independence. His wife and daughter request to have the mechanical ventilator withdrawn.

Important Points for Consideration

- Informed consent related to treatment decisions entails four elements: (1) information provided about possible treatment options must be understandable to the patient; (2) possible outcomes of the various treatment options must be explained; (3) the patient must have the capacity to deliberate about the treatment choices and their consequences; and (4) the patient's treatment decision must be freely chosen or made without coercion.
- It may be difficult under certain circumstances, such as with impaired communication, to determine a patient's capacity to make an informed treatment decision.
- Health care providers cannot assume that a patient who does not have the capacity to make decisions in one area (e.g., hemodialysis) is incapable of making decisions related to other aspects of his or her care, such as continued mechanical ventilation.
- The wife, acting as the patient's surrogate decision maker, is using substituted judgment to indicate what the patient would want based on his previously expressed wishes.

Critical Thinking Questions

1. What would you do next given the patient's behavior and the information that you have obtained from the patient's wife?
2. What are your feelings about participating in the care of a patient in whom withdrawal of treatment will result in death?

replaced with the donor heart, which has been trimmed to match. Care is taken to preserve the integrity of the donor sinoatrial (SA) node so that a sinus rhythm may be achieved postoperatively.

Immunosuppressive therapy usually begins in the operating room. Regimens vary, but they usually include azathioprine (Imuran), corticosteroids, and cyclosporine. (The mechanisms of action and side effects of these and other immunosuppressants are discussed in Chapter 13 and Table 13-17.) Currently cyclosporine is used with corticosteroids for maintenance immunosuppression. Its use has resulted not only in reduced rejection, but also in slowing the rejection process so that early treatment can be instituted. Because of the use of immunosuppressants, infection is the primary complication following transplant.

Endomyocardial biopsies via the right internal jugular vein are performed at repeated intervals to detect rejection. In addition, peripheral blood T lymphocyte monitoring is done to assess the recipient's immune status.

Advances in surgical technique and postoperative care have improved early survival rates after cardiac transplantation. In the first year after transplantation, the major causes of death are acute rejection and infection. Later on, malignancy (especially lymphoma) and coronary artery vasculopathy are major causes of death. Nursing management throughout the posttransplant period focuses on promoting patient adaptation to the transplant process, monitoring, managing lifestyle changes, and ongoing teaching of the patient and family.

Artificial Heart

The lack of available transplant hearts and the increasing number of patients in need have triggered the movement to develop artificial hearts. A total artificial heart, which is fully implantable, has been developed. The internal thoracic unit weighs less than 2 lb and has two artificial ventricles with an electric motor driving the pumping system. It is made of titanium and a patented polyurethane designed to minimize coagulation. An electronic package in the abdomen monitors the system, including adjusting the speed of the heart based on the patient's activity. An external battery pack allows 6 to 8 hours of power, and it can be recharged by connecting it to an external stationary power source (often during sleep). The total artificial heart requires no immunosuppression. Further research is needed to improve the long-term usability of this device.

CRITICAL THINKING EXERCISES

Case Study
Congestive Heart Failure

Patient Profile. Mrs. E., a 70-year-old Hispanic woman, was admitted to the medical unit with complaints of increasing dyspnea on exertion.

Subjective Data
- Had a severe MI at 58 years of age
- Has experienced increasing dyspnea on exertion during the last 2 years
- Recently had a respiratory tract infection, frequent cough, and edema in legs 2 weeks ago
- Cannot walk two blocks without getting short of breath
- Has to sleep with head elevated on three pillows
- Does not always remember to take medication

Objective Data
Physical Examination
- In respiratory distress, use of accessory muscles, respiratory rate 36 breaths/min
- Heart murmur
- Moist crackles in both lungs
- Cyanotic lips and extremities
- Skin cool and diaphoretic

Diagnostic Studies
- Chest x-ray results: cardiomegaly with right and left ventricular hypertrophy; fluid in lower lung fields

Collaborative Care
- Digoxin 0.25 mg PO qd
- Furosemide (Lasix) 40 mg IV bid
- Potassium 40 mEq PO bid
- Enalapril (Vasotec) 5 mg PO qd

- 2 g sodium diet
- Oxygen 6 L/min
- Daily weights
- Daily 12-lead ECG, cardiac enzymes q8hr × 3

CRITICAL THINKING QUESTIONS
1. Explain the pathophysiology of Mrs. E.'s heart disease.
2. What clinical manifestations of heart failure did Mrs. E. exhibit?
3. What is the significance of the findings of the chest x-ray?
4. Explain the rationale for each of the medical orders prescribed for Mrs. E.
5. What are appropriate nursing interventions for Mrs. E.?
6. What teaching measures should be instituted to prevent recurrence of an acute episode of heart failure?
7. Based on the assessment data presented, write one or more appropriate nursing diagnoses. Are there any collaborative problems?

Nursing Research Issues
1. What nursing measures are most effective in relieving shortness of breath in a patient with CHF?
2. What are effective ways of promoting optimum sleep-rest patterns in a patient with end-stage CHF?
3. What are the psychoemotional needs of a spouse of an open heart surgical patient preoperatively and 2 months postoperatively?
4. What stressors are present for the family of a patient who is on a waiting list for a cardiac transplant?

REVIEW QUESTIONS

The number of the question corresponds to the same-numbered objective at the beginning of the chapter.

1. The nurse recognizes that primary manifestations of systolic ventricular failure include
   a. ↓ Afterload and ↓ LVEDP.
   b. ↓ Ejection fraction and ↑ PAWP.
   c. ↓ PAWP and ↑ left ventricular ejection fraction.
   d. ↑ Pulmonary hypertension associated with normal ejection fraction.

2. A compensatory mechanism involved in congestive heart failure that leads to inappropriate fluid retention and additional workload of the heart is
   a. ventricular dilation.
   b. ventricular hypertrophy.
   c. neurohormonal response.
   d. sympathetic nervous system activation.

3. The drug used in the management of a patient with acute pulmonary edema that will decrease both preload and afterload and provide relief of anxiety is
   a. morphine.
   b. amrinone.
   c. dobutamine.
   d. aminophylline.

4. A patient with chronic congestive heart failure and atrial fibrillation is treated with a digitalis preparation and a loop diuretic. To prevent possible complications of this combination of drugs, the nurse needs to
   a. monitor serum potassium levels.
   b. keep an accurate measure of intake and output.
   c. teach the patient about dietary restriction of potassium.
   d. withhold the digitalis and notify the health care provider if the heart rate is irregular.

5. The nurse plans care for the patient with dilated cardiomyopathy based on the knowledge that
   a. family members may be at risk because of the infectious nature of the disease.
   b. medical management of the disorder focuses on treatment of the underlying cause.
   c. the prognosis of the patient is poor, and emotional support is a high priority of care.
   d. the condition may be successfully treated with surgical ventriculomyotomy and myectomy.

6. The primary causes of death in patients with heart transplants in the first year include
   a. infection and rejection.
   b. rejection and arrhythmias.
   c. arrhythmias and infection.
   d. myocardial infarction and lymphoma.

REFERENCES

1. American Heart Association: *www.americanheart.org* (accessed Nov 29, 2002).
2. Gheorghiade M et al: Current medical therapy for advanced heart failure, *Heart Lung* 29:16, 2000.
3. Gomgerg-Maitland M, Baran DA, Fuster V: Treatment of congestive heart failure: guideline for the primary care physician and heart failure specialist, *Arch Intern Med* 161:342, 2001.
4. Carelock J, Clark AP: Heart failure: pathophysiologic mechanisms, *Am J Nurs* 101:26, 2001.
5. Pereira N, Cooper G: Systolic heart failure: practical implementation of standard guidelines, *Clin Cornerstone* 3:1, 2000.
6. Liew D, Krum H: Management of chronic heart failure in the elderly patient, *Clin Geriatr* 9:24, 2001.
7. Maisel AS: B-type natriuretic peptide (BNP) levels: diagnostic and therapeutic potential, *Rev Cardiovasc Med* 2:13, 2001.
8. Ammon S: Managing patients with heart failure, *Am J Nurs* 404:34, 2001.
9. Colucci WS et al: Intravenous nesiritide, a natriuretic peptide, in the treatment of decompensated congestive heart failure, *N Engl J Med* 343:246, 2000.
10. Cazeau S et al: Effect of multisite biventricular pacing in patients with heart failure and intraventricular conduction delay, *N Engl J Med* 344:873, 2001.
11. Pereira N, Cooper G: Systolic heart failure: practical guidelines, *Congestive Heart Failure* 6:12, 2001.
12. Heart Failure Society of America (HFSA) practice guidelines, *Congestive Heart Failure* 6:12, 2001.
13. Davis MK, Gibbs CR, Lip GY: Management: diuretics, ACE inhibitors, and nitrates, *BMJ* 320:428, 2000.
14. Kirk JK: Therapy with angiotensin receptor blockers, *Clin Geriatr* 9:35, 2001.
15. Torosoff M, Philbin E: Use of angiotensin-converting enzyme inhibitors for elderly patients with heart failure, *Clin Geriatr* 9:57, 2001.
16. Aronow WS: Therapy of older persons with congestive heart failure, *Annals of Long-Term Care* 9:21, 2001.
17. Bottorff M: Recent advances in the treatment of congestive heart failure, *Annals of Long-Term Care* 9:47, 2001.
18. US Department of Health and Human Resources: NIH pub no 01-4082, Washington, DC, 2001, USDHHR.
19. Whellan DJ et al: Cardiac rehabilitation and survival in patients with left ventricular systolic failure, *Am Heart J* 142:160, 2001.
*20. Deaton C: Outcome measurement, *J Cardiovasc Nurs* 14:116, 2000.
*21. Moser D, Worster PC: Effect of psychosocial factors on physiologic outcomes in patients with heart failure, *J Cardiovasc Nurs* 14:106, 2000.
22. Bither CJ, Apple S: Home management of the failing heart, *Am J Nurs* 101:41, 2001.
23. Fonarow GC: Medical management of heart failure in the elderly: clinical evidence and practical concerns, *Clin Geriatr* 10(suppl):1, 2002.
24. World Health Organization: *www.who.org* (accessed Nov 29, 2002).
25. Mohiddin S, Fananapazir L: Advances in understanding hypertrophic cardiomyopathy, *Hosp Pract* 36:23, 2001.
26. Oliver-McNeil S: Treating hypertrophic cardiomyopathy without surgery, *Nursing* 31:32CC1, 2001.

*Nursing research–based references.

RESOURCES

American Association of Cardiovascular and Pulmonary Rehabilitation (AACVPR)
401 North Michigan Avenue, Suite 2200
Chicago, IL 60611-4267
312-321-5146
Fax: 312-527-6635
www.aacvpr.org

American College of Cardiology
Heart House
9111 Old Georgetown Road
Bethesda, MD 20814-1699
800-253-4636, ext. 694 or 301-897-5400
Fax: 301-897-9745
www.acc.org

American Heart Association
7320 Greenville Avenue
Dallas, TX 75231
800-AHA-USA-1 (242-8721)
www.americanheart.org

Council on Cardiovascular Nursing
American Heart Association
7320 Greenville Avenue
Dallas, TX 75231
214-373-6300
http://216.185.112.5/presenter.jhtml?identifier=1148

The Mended Hearts, Inc.
7272 Greenville Avenue
Dallas, TX 75231-4596
888-HEART99 (432-7899) or 214-706-1442
Fax: 214-706-5245
www.mendedhearts.org

National Heart, Lung, and Blood Institute
National Institutes of Health
Building 31, Room 5A52
31 Center Drive MSC 2486
Bethesda, MD 20892
301-592-8573
Fax: 301-592-8563
www.nhlbi.nih.gov

National Heart Savers Association (NHSA)
9140 West Dodge Road
Omaha, NE 68114
402-398-1993
http://heartsavers.org

For additional Internet resources, see the website for this book at *http://evolve.elsevier.com/Lewis/medsurg/.*

CHAPTER 35
NURSING MANAGEMENT
Arrhythmias

Carolyn I. Johns

LEARNING OBJECTIVES

1. Identify the clinical characteristics and electrocardiographic patterns of common arrhythmias.
2. Describe the nursing and collaborative management of common arrhythmias.
3. Differentiate between defibrillation and cardioversion, identifying indications for use and physiologic effects.
4. Describe the management of patients with temporary and permanent pacemakers.
5. Describe the management of a patient with an implantable cardioverter-defibrillator.
6. Explain the management of a patient undergoing electrophysiologic testing and radiofrequency catheter ablation therapy.
7. Explain the essential elements of basic life support (BLS).
8. Explain the essential elements of advanced cardiac life support (ACLS).

KEY TERMS

advanced cardiac life support, p. 884
arrhythmias, p. 861
asystole, p. 874
atrial contraction, p. 865
atrial fibrillation, p. 870
atrial flutter, p. 869
automaticity, p. 865
basic life support, p. 879
cardiac arrest, p. 879
cardiac pacemaker, p. 876
cardiopulmonary resuscitation, p. 879

complete heart block, p. 872
electrocardiogram, p. 862
first-degree AV block, p. 871
premature atrial contraction, p. 869
premature ventricular contraction, p. 872
sudden cardiac death, p. 874
telemetry monitoring, p. 864
ventricular fibrillation, p. 873

ARRHYTHMIA IDENTIFICATION AND TREATMENT

The ability to recognize **arrhythmias,** which are abnormal cardiac rhythms, is an essential skill for the nurse. Cardiac monitoring is now used in a wide range of hospital, clinic, and home settings. Prompt assessment of an abnormal cardiac rhythm and the patient's response to the rhythm is critical. This chapter describes basic principles of common arrhythmias. For more information on arrhythmias, the reader should refer to detailed texts on electrocardiograph (ECG) interpretation.[1-3]

Conduction System

Four properties of cardiac tissue enable the conduction system to initiate an electrical impulse, which is transmitted through the cardiac tissue, stimulating muscle contraction (Table 35-1). The conduction system of the heart is made up of specialized neuromuscular tissue located throughout the heart (see Chapter 31,

Fig. 31-5). A normal cardiac impulse begins in the sinoatrial (SA) node in the upper right atrium. It is transmitted over the atrial myocardium via Bachmann's bundle and internodal pathways to the atrioventricular (AV) node. From the AV node, the impulse spreads through the bundle of His and down the left and right bundle branches, emerging in the Purkinje fibers, which transmit the impulse to the ventricles.

Conduction to the point just before the impulse leaves the Purkinje fibers takes place within the time of the PR interval of the ECG. When the impulse emerges from the Purkinje fibers, ventricular depolarization occurs, producing mechanical contraction of the ventricles and the QRS complex on the ECG. The electrical activity of the heart is illustrated in Chapter 31, Fig. 31-6.

Nervous Control of the Heart

The autonomic nervous system plays an important role in the rate of impulse formation, the speed of conduction, and the strength of cardiac contraction. The components of the autonomic nervous system that affect the heart are the right and left vagus nerve fibers of the parasympathetic nervous system and fibers of the sympathetic nervous system.

Stimulation of the vagus nerve causes a decreased rate of firing of the SA node, slowed impulse conduction of the AV node, and decreased force of cardiac muscle contraction. Stimulation of the sympathetic nerves that supply the heart has essentially the opposite effect on the heart.[1]

TABLE 35-1	Properties of Cardiac Tissue
Automaticity	Ability to initiate an impulse spontaneously and continuously
Contractility	Ability to respond mechanically to an impulse
Conductivity	Ability to transmit an impulse along a membrane in an orderly manner
Excitability	Ability to be electrically stimulated

Reviewed by Angela J. DiSabatino, RN, MS, Manager, Cardiovascular Research, Christiana Care Health Services, Newark, Del.; and Vanessa Briones, RN, BSN, Staff Nurse, Santa Rosa Hospital, San Antonio, Tex.

Electrocardiogram Monitoring

The **electrocardiogram** (ECG) is a graphic tracing of the electrical impulses produced in the heart. The wave forms on the ECG are produced by the movement of charged ions across the membranes of myocardial cells, representing depolarization and repolarization.

The membrane of a cardiac cell is semipermeable, allowing it to maintain a high concentration of potassium and a low concen-

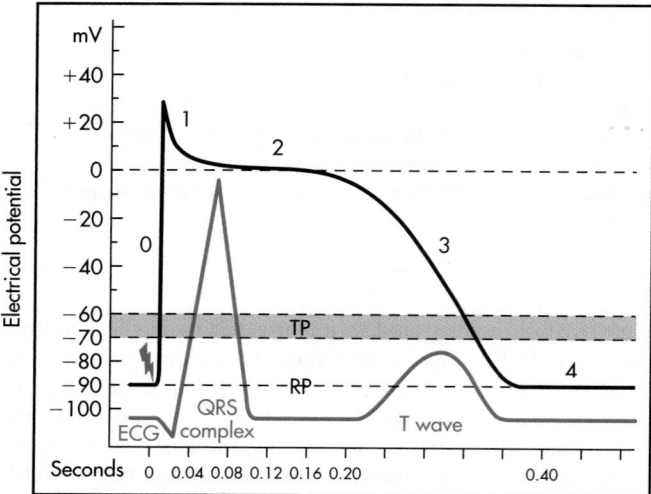

FIG. 35-1 Phases of the cardiac action potential. The electrical potential, measured in millivolts (mV), is indicated along the vertical axis of the graph. Time, measured in milliseconds (msec), is indicated along the horizontal axis. There are five phases of the action potential, labeled as phase 0 through phase 4. Each phase represents a particular electrical event or combination of electrical events. Phase 0 is the upstroke of rapid depolarization and corresponds with ventricular contraction. Phases 1, 2, and 3 represent repolarization. Phase 4 is known as complete repolarization (or the polarized state) and corresponds to diastole. *TP,* Threshold membrane potential; *RP,* resting membrane potential.

tration of sodium inside the cell. A high concentration of sodium and a low concentration of potassium are maintained outside the cell. The inside of the cell, when at rest, or in the polarized state, is negative compared with the outside. When a cell or groups of cells are stimulated, each cell membrane changes its permeability and allows sodium to migrate rapidly into the cell, making the inside of the cell positive compared with the outside (*depolarization*). A slower movement of ions across the membrane restores the cell to the polarized state, which is called *repolarization.* In Fig. 35-1 the phases are as follows: phase 4 is a polarized state; phase 0 is the upstroke of rapid depolarization; and phases 1, 2, and 3 represent repolarization.[2] Antiarrhythmic drugs have a direct effect on the action potential.[3] When antiarrhythmic drugs are used in a clinical setting, a nurse's understanding of the ionic shifts in the cardiac cell and the action potential mechanism is important.

Conventionally there are 12 recording leads in the ECG. Six of the 12 ECG leads measure electrical forces in the frontal plane (leads I, II, III, aVR, aVL, and aVF) (Fig. 35-2). The remaining six leads (V₁ through V₆) measure the electrical forces in the horizontal plane (precordial lead sites). The 12-lead ECG may show changes that are indicative of structural changes or damage such as ischemia, infarction, enlarged cardiac chambers, electrolyte imbalance, or drug toxicity.[2] Obtaining 12 views of the heart is also helpful in the assessment of arrhythmias. An example of a normal 12-lead ECG appears in Fig. 35-3.

When a patient's ECG is being continuously monitored, 1 to 12 ECG leads are used. The most common leads used are lead II and lead MCL₁ (which corresponds to V₁ in the standard 12-lead ECG) (Fig. 35-4). These leads most clearly demonstrate the P wave and QRS complexes.[4]

The ECG can be visualized continuously on a monitor oscilloscope. A recording of the ECG "strip" is done on ECG paper attached to the monitor. This provides documentation of the patient's rhythms. It is a way to thoroughly assess an arrhythmia and measure complexes and intervals.

It is essential to know how to measure time and voltage on the ECG paper to correctly interpret an ECG. ECG paper consists of

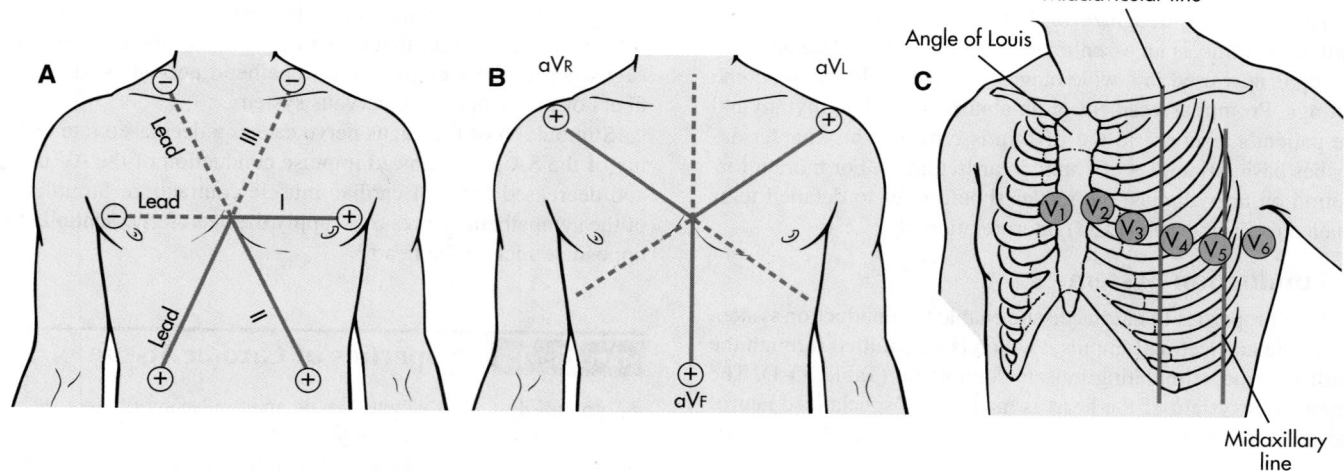

FIG. 35-2 **A,** Limb leads I, II, and III. Leads are located on the extremities. Illustrated are the angles from which these leads view the heart. **B,** Lead placement for limb leads aVR, aVL, and aVF. These unipolar leads use the calculated center of the heart as their negative electrode. **C,** Lead placement for the chest electrodes: V₁, fourth intercostal space at the right sternal border; V₂, fourth intercostal space at the left sternal border; V₃, equidistant between V₂ and V₄; V₄, fifth intercostal space at the left midclavicular line; V₅, anterior axillary line and same horizontal level as V₄; V₆, midaxillary line and same horizontal level as V₄.

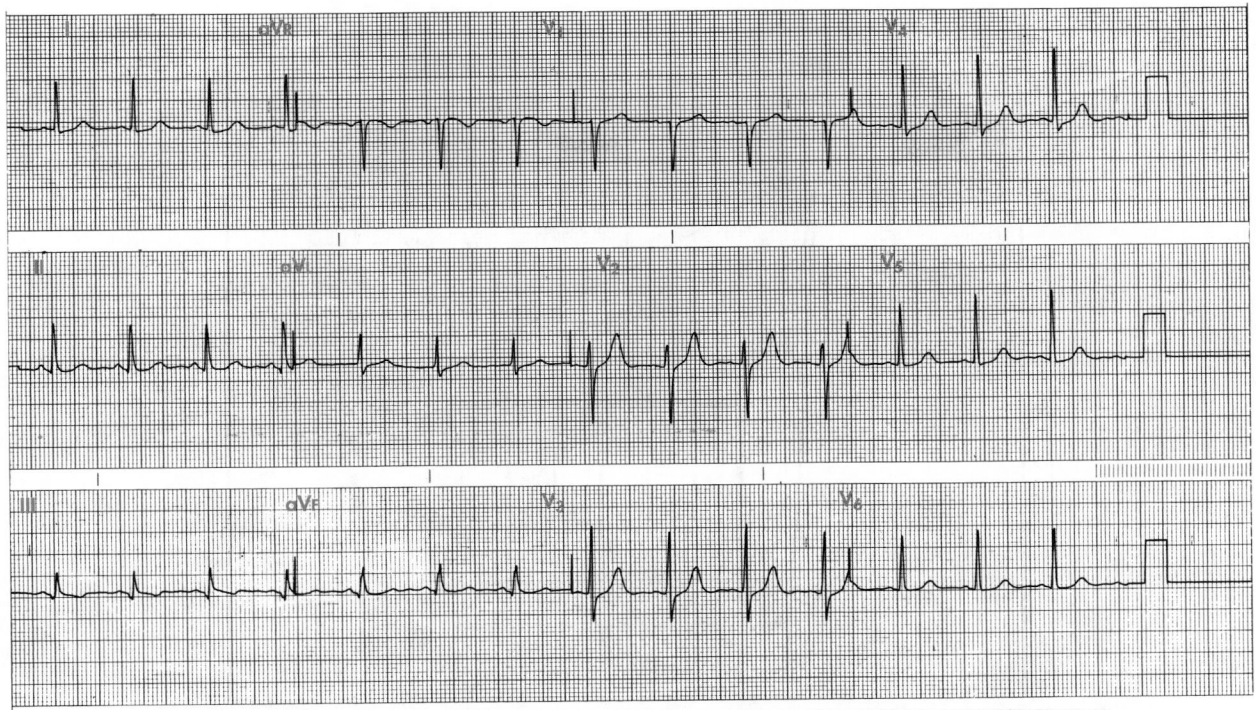

FIG. 35-3   Twelve-lead electrocardiogram showing a normal sinus rhythm.

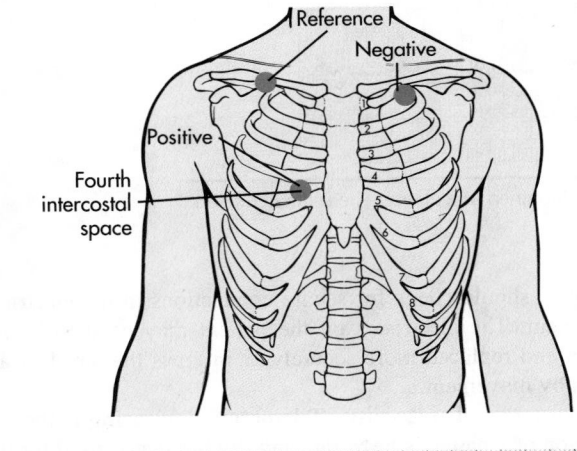

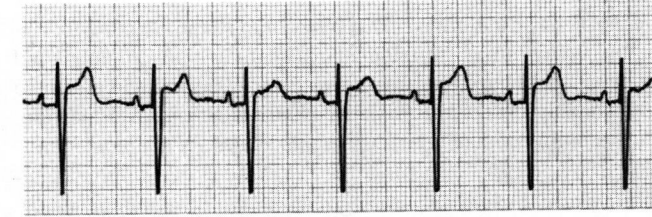

FIG. 35-4   A, Lead placement for MCL₁. B, Typical electrocardiogram tracing in lead MCL₁.

minute. Vertically, one large square is equal to 0.5 mV. These squares are used to calculate the heart rate (HR) and intervals between different ECG complexes.

A variety of methods can be used to calculate the HR from an ECG. Probably the most accurate way is to count the number of QRS complexes in 1 minute. However, this method is time consuming. If the rhythm is regular, a simpler process can be used. Every 3 seconds a marker appears on the ECG paper. The nurse can count the number of QRS complexes in 6 seconds and multiply that number by 10. This will yield the number of complexes or beats per minute (beats/min) (Fig. 35-6).

Another rapid method for calculating the HR when a regular rhythm is present is to count the number of small squares between two QRS complexes (R-R interval). An R wave is the first upward deflection of the QRS complex. The nurse divides 1500 by the number of small squares to get the precise HR. This method is accurate only if the rhythm is regular.

The nurse can also count the number of large squares between two R waves and divide into 300 (see Fig. 35-6). This method is accurate only if the rhythm is regular.

An additional way to measure distances on the ECG grid is to use calipers. Calipers are used for fine measurements, especially for points of a specific wave. Many times a P or R wave will not fall directly on a light or heavy line. The fine points of the calipers can be placed exactly on the components to be measured and then moved to another part of the grid for time measurement, which is accurate to 0.04 second.

ECG leads are attached to the patient's chest wall via an electrode pad fixed with electrical conductive paste. For best contact, hair on the chest wall should be shaved and skin should be prepared with acetone to remove excess oil and debris. In the case of a diaphoretic patient, benzoin may be applied to the skin

large (heavy lines) and small (light lines) squares (Fig. 35-5). Each large square incorporates 25 smaller squares (five horizontal and five vertical). Each small square represents 0.04 second horizontally and 0.1 mV vertically. This means that the large square equals 0.20 second and that 300 large squares equal 1.0

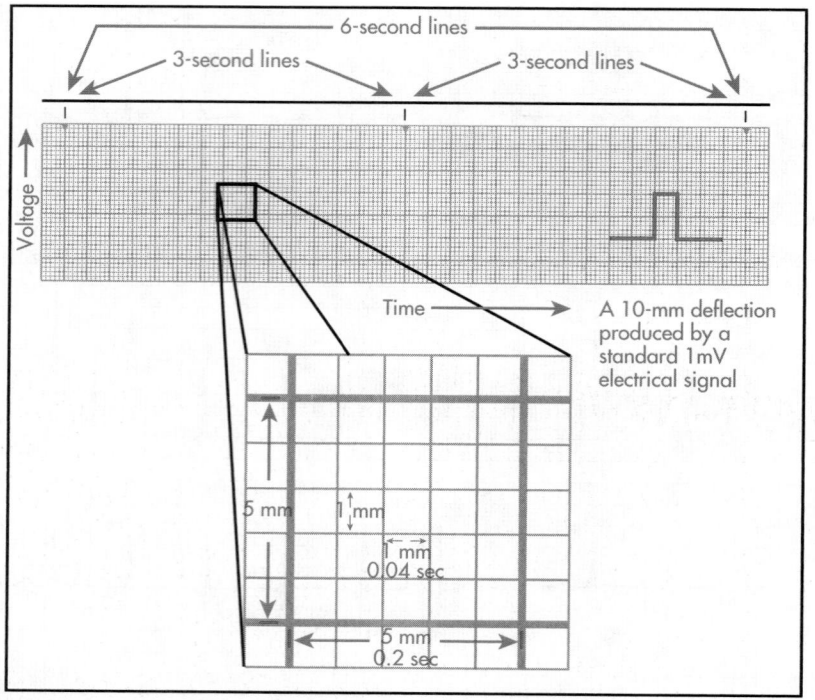

FIG. 35-5 Time and voltage on the electrocardiogram.

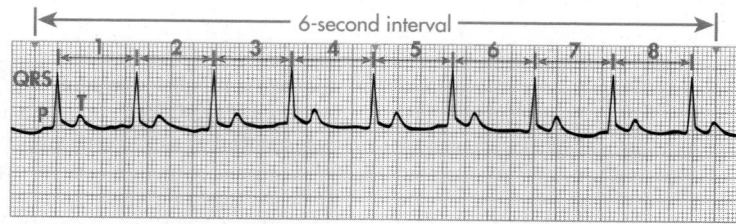

FIG. 35-6 When the rhythm is regular, heart rate can be determined at a glance. The estimated heart rate is 80. The actual heart rate is 86.

before electrode placement. If leads and electrodes are not firmly placed, or if there is muscle activity or electrical interference from an outside source, an artifact may be seen on the monitor. An artifact is a distortion of the baseline and waveforms seen on the ECG (Fig. 35-7). Accurate interpretation of cardiac rhythm is difficult when an artifact is present. If artifacts occur,

the nurse should check for secure connections in the electrical equipment. The electrodes on the patient may need to be removed and replaced more securely or in areas that are less affected by movement.[5]

Telemetry Monitoring. **Telemetry monitoring** is the observation of a patient's heart rate and rhythm that is used for the diagnosis of arrhythmias.[6] Two types of systems are used for detecting arrhythmias by telemetry. The first type, a centralized monitoring system, requires a nurse or telemetry technician to continuously observe all patients' rhythms at a central location. The second system of telemetry monitoring does not require constant nurse or technician surveillance. These systems have the capability of detecting and storing data on the type and frequency of arrhythmias. Sophisticated alarm systems provide different levels of detection of arrhythmias, depending on the severity of the arrhythmia. However, computerized monitoring systems are not fail-proof. Frequent nursing assessment is important when caring for monitored patients.

Assessment of Cardiac Rhythm

When assessing the cardiac rhythm, the nurse must make an accurate interpretation of an arrhythmia and immediately evaluate the consequences of that arrhythmia for the individual pa-

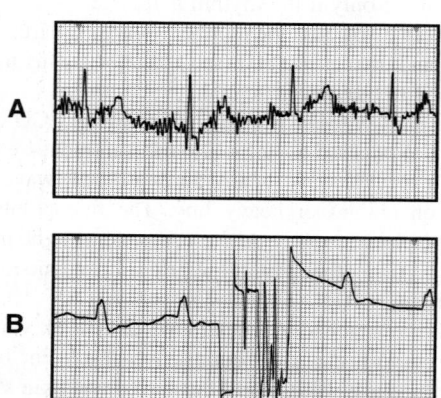

FIG. 35-7 A, Muscle tremor. B, Loose electrodes.

tient. Assessment of the patient's hemodynamic response to an arrhythmia provides guidance in therapeutic intervention. If possible, a determination of the cause of the arrhythmia should be made. Tachycardias may cause a decrease in cardiac output (CO) and possible hypotension. Certain arrhythmias may cause more life-threatening arrhythmias.[6] The patient, not just the arrhythmia, must be treated.

Normal sinus rhythm refers to the normal conduction pattern of the cardiac cycle, which originates in the SA node (Fig. 35-8). Fig. 35-9 shows the normal electrical pattern of the cardiac cycle. Table 35-2 provides a description of ECG intervals and the

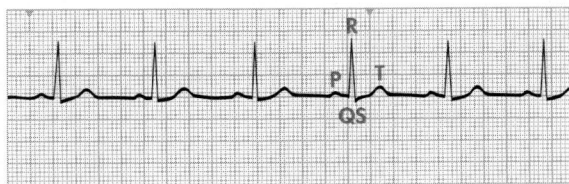

FIG. 35-8 Normal sinus rhythm in lead II.

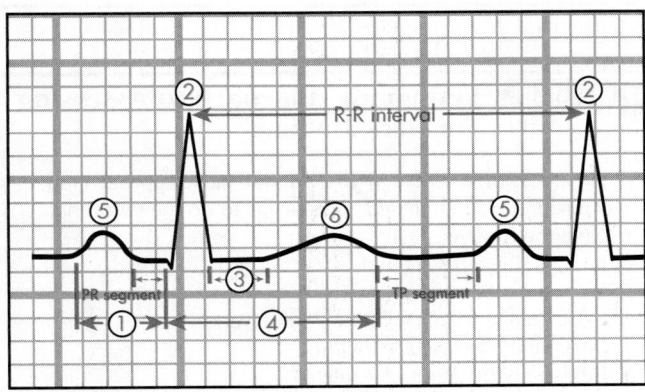

FIG. 35-9 The electrocardiogram complex as seen in a normal sinus rhythm. *1*, PR interval (normal is 0.12 to 0.20 sec); *2*, QRS complex (normal is 0.04 to 0.12 sec); *3*, ST segment (normal is 0.12 sec); *4*, QT interval (normal is 0.35 to 0.43 sec); *5*, P wave (normal is 0.06 to 0.12 sec); *6*, T wave (normal is 0.16 sec).

significance of disturbances. The P wave represents the depolarization of the atrium (passage of an electrical impulse through the atrial muscle), causing **atrial contraction.** The QRS complex represents depolarization of the ventricles, causing ventricular contraction. The T wave represents repolarization of the ventricles. The PR interval represents the period when the impulse spreads through the atria, AV node, bundle of His, and Purkinje fibers. The QRS interval represents the time it takes for depolarization of both ventricles. The QT interval represents the time it takes for complete depolarization and repolarization of the ventricles.

Electrophysiologic Mechanisms of Arrhythmias

Disorders of impulse formation can initiate arrhythmias. The heart has specialized cells found in the SA node, parts of the atria, the AV node, and the His-Purkinje system, which are able to discharge spontaneously. This is termed **automaticity.** Normally the main pacemaker of the heart is the SA node, which spontaneously discharges 60 to 100 times per minute (Table 35-3). A pacemaker from another site may be discharged in two ways. If the SA node discharges more slowly than a secondary pacemaker, the electrical discharges from the secondary pacemaker may passively "escape." The secondary pacemaker will then discharge automatically at its intrinsic rate. These secondary pacemakers may originate from the AV node or the His-Purkinje system at rates of 40 to 60 times per minute and 20 to 40 times per minute, respectively. Another way that secondary pacemakers can originate is when they discharge more rapidly than the normal pacemaker of the SA node. *Triggered beats* (early or late) may come from an *ectopic focus* in the atria, ventricles, or AV nodal area. This may begin a "run" of an arrhythmia, which replaces the normal sinus rhythm.

TABLE 35-3	Rates of the Conduction System
SA node	60-100 times/min
AV junction	40-60 times/min
Purkinje fibers	20-40 times/min

AV, Atrioventricular; *SA,* sinoatrial.

TABLE 35-2	Definition and Significance of Electrocardiogram Intervals*	
DESCRIPTION	**DURATION (SEC)**	**SIGNIFICANCE OF DISTURBANCE**
PR interval: From beginning of P wave to beginning of QRS complex; represents time taken for impulse to spread through the atria, AV node and bundle of His, the bundle branches, and Purkinje fibers, to a point immediately preceding ventricular activation	0.12-0.20	Disturbance in conduction usually in AV node, bundle of His, or bundle branches but can be in atria as well
QRS interval: From beginning to end of QRS complex; represents time taken for depolarization of both ventricles	0.04-0.12	Disturbance in conduction in bundle branches or in ventricles
QT interval: From beginning of QRS to end of T wave; represents time taken for entire electrical depolarization and repolarization of the ventricles	0.34-0.43	Disturbances usually affecting repolarization more than depolarization such as drug effects, electrolyte disturbances, and heart rate changes

*Heart rate influences the duration of these intervals, especially those of the PR and QT intervals.

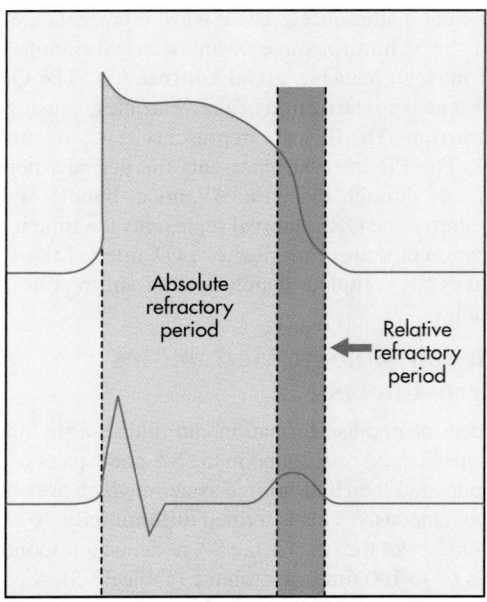

FIG. 35-10 Absolute and relative refractory periods correlated with the cardiac muscle's action potential and with an ECG tracing.

TABLE 35-4	**Common Causes of Arrhythmias**

Cardiac Conditions
Accessory pathways
Conduction defects
Congestive heart failure
Hypertrophy of cardiac muscle
Myocardial cell degeneration
Myocardial infarction

Other Conditions
Acid-base imbalances
Alcohol
Coffee, tea, tobacco
Connective tissue disorders
Drug effects or toxicity
Electric shock
Electrolyte imbalances
Emotional crisis
Hypoxia, shock
Metabolic conditions (e.g., thyroid dysfunction)
Near-drowning
Poisoning

TABLE 35-5	**Systematic Approach to Assessing Cardiac Rhythms**

When assessing a cardiac rhythm, a systematic approach must be used. A recommended approach is to do the following:
1. Note the P wave
2. Evaluate the atrial rhythm
3. Determine the atrial rate
4. Calculate the duration of the PR interval
5. Evaluate the ventricular rhythm
6. Determine the ventricular rate
7. Calculate the duration of the QRS complex
8. Calculate the duration of the QT interval
Questions to consider then include the following:
1. What is the dominant rhythm or arrhythmia?
2. What is the clinical significance of the arrhythmia?
3. What is the treatment for the particular arrhythmia?

The impulse started by a pacemaker focus must be conducted to the entire heart chamber. The property of myocardial tissue that allows it to be depolarized by a stimulus is called *excitability*. This is an important part of the transmission of the impulse from one fiber to another. The level of excitability is determined by the length of time after depolarization that the tissues can be restimulated. The recovery period after stimulation is called the *refractory phase* or period. The *absolute refractory phase* or period occurs when excitability is zero and heart tissue cannot be stimulated. The *relative refractory period* occurs slightly later in the cycle, and excitability is more likely. In states of *full excitability*, the heart is completely recovered. Fig. 35-10 shows the relationship between the refractory period and the ECG.

If conduction is depressed and if some areas of the heart are blocked, the unblocked areas are activated earlier than the blocked areas. When the block is unidirectional, this uneven conduction may allow the initial impulse to reenter areas that were previously not excitable but have recovered. The reentering impulse may be able to depolarize the atria and ventricles, causing a premature beat. If the reentrant excitation continues, tachycardia occurs.[3]

Evaluation of Arrhythmias

Arrhythmias occur as the result of various abnormalities and disease states.[2] The cause of an arrhythmia influences the treatment of the patient. Common causes of arrhythmias are presented in Table 35-4. Table 35-5 presents a systematic approach to assessing a cardiac rhythm.

Arrhythmias occurring in out-of-hospital settings present problems of management. Determination of the rhythm by cardiac monitoring is a high priority. Emergency care of the patient with an arrhythmia is outlined in Table 35-6. If indicated, the emergency medical system (EMS) is activated after the patient has been assessed.

In addition to continuous ECG monitoring during hospitalization, several other methods are used to evaluate cardiac arrhythmias and the effectiveness of antiarrhythmic drug therapy. An electrophysiology test (an invasive method) and Holter monitoring, event recorder monitoring, exercise treadmill testing, and signal-averaged ECG (all noninvasive methods) can be performed on both an inpatient and an outpatient basis.

Electrophysiology study (EPS) testing is performed to identify different mechanisms of tachyarrhythmias, as well as heart blocks, bradyarrhythmias, and arrhythmic causes of syncope. It can also be used to identify locations of accessory pathways and to determine the effectiveness of antiarrhythmic drugs. It involves introducing several electrode catheters transvenously to the right side of the heart with fluoroscopic guidance. Electrical stimulation to various areas of the atrium and ventricle is performed, and the inducibility of arrhythmias is determined. Serious arrhythmias can be provoked during the procedure, requiring immediate cardioversion or defibrillation; therefore the patient is

TABLE 35-6	**Emergency Management** Arrhythmias	
ETIOLOGY	**ASSESSMENT FINDINGS**	**INTERVENTIONS**
See Table 35-4	• Irregular rate and rhythm, palpitations • Chest, neck, shoulder, or arm pain • Dizziness, syncope • Dyspnea • Extreme restlessness • Decreased level of consciousness • Feeling of impending doom • Numbness, tingling of arms • Weakness and fatigue • Cold, clammy skin • Diaphoresis • Pallor • Nausea and vomiting • Decreased blood pressure • Decreased O_2 saturation	**Initial** • Ensure patent airway • Administer O_2 via nasal cannula or non-rebreather mask • Establish IV access • Apply cardiac monitoring electrodes • Identify underlying rhythm • Identify ectopic beats **Ongoing Monitoring** • Monitor vital signs, level of consciousness, O_2 saturation, and cardiac rhythm • Anticipate need for intubation if respiratory distress evident • Prepare to initiate CPR and/or defibrillation

CPR, Cardiopulmonary resuscitation; *IV,* intravenous.

sedated but conscious. Preprocedure anxiety is common for the patient undergoing EPS. Emotional support from the nurse is important. Nursing care before and after the procedure is similar to that for cardiac catheterization (see Chapter 31). (EPS testing is also discussed in Chapter 31.)

The Holter monitor is a device that records the ECG while the patient is ambulatory.[3] The device can record heart rhythm for 24 to 48 hours while the patient performs daily activities. The patient maintains a diary in which activities and any symptoms are recorded. Events in the diary can later be correlated with any arrhythmias observed on the recording. The monitor is generally a useful device for detecting significant arrhythmias and evaluating the effects of drugs during a patient's normal activities. It can also be used for detecting ischemia by analyzing ST segments. A limitation of the device is that the patient who has frequent ventricular arrhythmias, some of which may be lethal, may not have these arrhythmias during the monitored time. (Holter monitoring is also discussed in Chapter 31.)

Use of event monitors has greatly improved the evaluation of outpatient arrhythmias. Event monitors are recorders that are activated by the patient and can be used only at the time of the patient's symptoms related to the arrhythmia. The recorder is placed over the patient's chest during symptoms. The patient then transmits the rhythm to a central monitoring company via telephone. This is an easier method of documenting an arrhythmia than the 24-hour monitor, especially if symptoms are not occurring daily. (Ambulatory ECG monitoring is discussed in Chapter 31.)

The signal-averaged ECG (SAECG) is a high-resolution electrocardiogram used to identify the patient at risk for developing complex ventricular arrhythmias. A computerized program and ECG machine are used for the test. The identification of electrical activity called late potentials on the SAECG strongly suggests that the patient is at risk for developing serious ventricular arrhythmias.[3]

Exercise treadmill testing is used for evaluation of cardiac rhythm response to exercise. Exercise-induced arrhythmias can be reproduced and analyzed, and drug therapy can be eval-uated. These tests are performed with routine treadmill testing protocols.

Diagnostic procedures for assessment of the cardiovascular system are presented in Chapter 31, Table 31-7.

Types of Arrhythmias

Examples of the ECG tracings of common arrhythmias are presented in Figs. 35-11 through 35-19. Descriptive characteristics of common arrhythmias are presented in Table 35-7.

Sinus Bradycardia. In sinus bradycardia the conduction pathway is the same as that in sinus rhythm, but the sinus node discharges at a rate of less than 60 beats/min (Fig. 35-11, *A*).

Clinical associations. Sinus bradycardia is a normal sinus rhythm in aerobically trained athletes and in other individuals during sleep. It occurs in response to carotid sinus massage, Valsalva maneuver, hypothermia, increased intraocular pressure, increased vagal tone, and administration of parasympathomimetic drugs. Disease states associated with sinus bradycardia are hypothyroidism, increased intracranial pressure, obstructive jaundice, and inferior wall myocardial infarction (MI).

ECG characteristics. In sinus bradycardia, HR is less than 60 beats/min, and the rhythm is regular. The P wave precedes each QRS complex and has a normal contour and a fixed interval. The PR interval is normal, and the QRS complex has a normal contour and normal length.

Significance. The clinical significance of sinus bradycardia depends on how the patient tolerates it hemodynamically. Hypotension with decreased cardiac output (CO) may occur in some circumstances. An acute MI may predispose the heart to escape arrhythmias and premature beats.

Treatment. Treatment consists of administration of atropine (an anticholinergic drug) for the patient with symptoms. Pacemaker therapy may be required.

Sinus Tachycardia. The conduction pathway is the same in sinus tachycardia as that in normal sinus rhythm. The discharge rate from the sinus node is increased as a result of vagal inhibi-

TABLE 35-7   **Characteristics of Common Arrhythmias**

PATTERN	RATE AND RHYTHM	P WAVE	PR INTERVAL	QRS COMPLEX
NSR	60-100 beats/min and regular	Normal	Normal	Normal
Sinus bradycardia	<60 beats/min and regular	Normal	Normal	Normal
Sinus tachycardia	>100 beats/min and regular	Normal	Normal	Normal
PAC	Usually 60-100 beats/min and irregular	Abnormal shape	Normal or variable	Normal (usually)
PSVT	100-300 beats/min and regular	Abnormal shape, may be hidden	Variable	Normal (usually)
Atrial flutter	*Atrial:* 250-350 beats/min and regular *Ventricular:* >100 beats/min and irregular	Sawtooth	Variable	Normal (usually)
Atrial fibrillation	*Atrial:* 350-600 beats/min and irregular *Ventricular:* >100 beats/min and irregular or possibly any rate	Chaotic	Not measurable	Normal (usually)
Junctional rhythms	40-140 beats/min and regular	Abnormal (may be hidden)	Variable	Normal (usually)
First-degree AV heart block	Normal and regular	Normal	>0.20 sec	Normal
Second–degree AV heart block				
Type I (Mobitz I, Wenckebach)	*Atrial:* Normal and regular *Ventricular:* Slower and irregular	Normal	Progressively lengthened	Normal QRS width, with pattern of one nonconducted QRS
Type II (Mobitz II)	*Atrial:* Usually normal and regular or irregular *Ventricular:* Slower and regular or irregular	P wave occurs in multiples	Normal or prolonged	Widened QRS, preceded by two or more P waves
Third-degree AV heart block	Ventricular rate 20-40 beats/min and regular	Normal, but no connection with QRS complex	Variable	Normal or widened, no connection with P waves
PVC	60-100 beats/min and irregular	Not usually present	Not measurable	Wide and distorted
Ventricular tachycardia	100-250 beats/min and regular or irregular	Not usually present	Not measurable	Wide and distorted
Ventricular fibrillation	Not measurable and irregular	Absent	Not measurable	Not measurable

AV, Atrioventricular; *NSR,* normal sinus rhythm; *PAC,* premature atrial contraction; *PSVT,* paroxysmal supraventricular tachycardia; *PVC,* premature ventricular contraction.

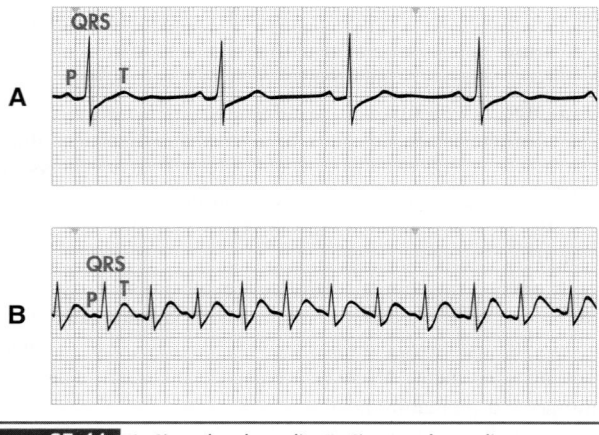

FIG. 35-11   A, Sinus bradycardia. B, Sinus tachycardia.

tion or sympathetic stimulation. The sinus rate is greater than 100 beats/min (see Fig. 35-11, *B*).

Clinical associations. Sinus tachycardia is associated with physiologic stressors such as exercise, fever, pain, hypotension, hypovolemia, anxiety, anemia, hypoxia, hypoglycemia, myocardial ischemia, congestive heart failure (CHF), and hyperthyroidism. It can also be an effect of drugs such as epinephrine, norepinephrine, caffeine, atropine, theophylline, nifedipine (Procardia), or hydralazine (Apresoline).

ECG characteristics. In sinus tachycardia, HR is greater than 100 beats/min, and the rhythm is regular. The P wave is normal, precedes each QRS complex, and has a normal contour and fixed interval. The PR interval is normal, and the QRS complex has a normal contour.

Significance. The clinical significance of sinus tachycardia depends on the patient's tolerance of the increased HR. The patient may have symptoms of dizziness, and hypotension may occur. Increased myocardial oxygen consumption is associated with an increased HR. Angina or an increase in infarct size may

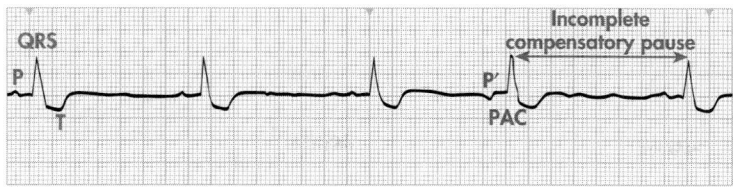

FIG. 35-12 Isolated premature atrial contraction (PAC).

accompany persistent sinus tachycardia in the patient with an acute MI.

Treatment. Treatment is determined by underlying causes. In certain settings, β-adrenergic blockers (e.g., metoprolol, atenolol) are used to reduce HR and decrease myocardial oxygen consumption.

Premature Atrial Contraction. A **premature atrial contraction** (PAC) is a contraction originating from an ectopic focus in the atrium in a location other than the sinus node. It originates in the left or right atrium and travels across the atria by an abnormal pathway, creating a distorted P wave (Fig. 35-12). At the AV node, it is stopped (nonconducted PAC), delayed (lengthened PR interval), or conducted normally. It moves through the AV node, and in most cases it is conducted normally through the ventricles.

Clinical associations. In a normal heart, a PAC can result from emotional stress or the use of caffeine, tobacco, or alcohol. A PAC can also result from disease states such as infection, inflammation, hyperthyroidism, chronic obstructive pulmonary disease (COPD), heart disease (including coronary artery disease), valvular disease, and other diseases. A PAC can also be caused by an enlarged atrium.

ECG characteristics. HR varies with the underlying rate and frequency of the PAC, and the rhythm is irregular. The P wave has a different contour from that of a normal P wave. It may be notched or have negative deflection, or it may be hidden in the preceding T wave. The PR interval may be shorter or longer than a normal PR interval originating from the sinus node, but it is within normal limits. The QRS complex is usually normal. If the QRS interval is 0.12 second or longer, abnormal conduction through the ventricles is present.

Significance. In persons with healthy hearts, isolated PACs are not significant. In persons with heart disease, frequent PACs may indicate enhanced automaticity of the atria, or a reentry mechanism. Such PACs may warn of or initiate supraventricular tachyarrhythmias.

Treatment. Treatment depends on the patient's symptoms. Withdrawal of sources of stimulation such as caffeine or sympathomimetic drugs may be warranted. β-Adrenergic blockers may be used to decrease PACs.

Paroxysmal Supraventricular Tachycardia. *Paroxysmal supraventricular tachycardia* (PSVT) is an arrhythmia originating in an ectopic focus anywhere above the bifurcation of the bundle of His (Fig. 35-13). Identification of the ectopic focus is sometimes difficult with a 12-lead ECG. It occurs with the reentrant phenomenon (reexcitation of the atria when there is a one-way block). A run of repeated premature beats is initiated and is usually heralded by a PAC. *Paroxysmal* refers to an abrupt onset and termination. Termination is sometimes followed by a brief period of asystole. Some degree of AV block may be present. PSVT can

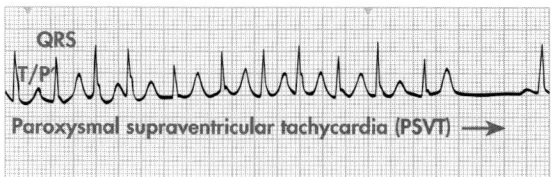

FIG. 35-13 Paroxysmal supraventricular tachycardia.

occur in the presence of Wolff-Parkinson-White (WPW) syndrome, or "preexcitation." In this syndrome, there are extra conduction pathways, or *accessory pathways*. The presence of accessory pathways is sometimes visible on the ECG with the presence of a widened QRS and delta wave at the beginning of the QRS.

Clinical associations. In the normal heart, PSVT is associated with overexertion, emotional stress, changes of position, deep inspiration, and stimulants such as caffeine and tobacco. PSVT is associated with rheumatic heart disease, digitalis toxicity, coronary artery disease (CAD), or cor pulmonale.

ECG characteristics. In PSVT, HR is 100 to 300 beats/min, and rhythm is regular. The P wave is often hidden in the preceding T wave and has an abnormal contour. The PR interval may be prolonged, shortened, or normal, and the QRS complex may have a normal or an abnormal contour.

Significance. The clinical significance of PSVT depends on symptoms and HR. A prolonged episode and HR greater than 180 beats/min may precipitate a decreased CO with hypotension and myocardial ischemia.

Treatment. Treatment includes vagal stimulation and drug therapy. Vagal stimulation induced by carotid massage or Valsalva maneuver may be used to treat PSVT. Adenosine (Adenocard) IV is most commonly used to convert PSVT to a normal sinus rhythm. This drug has a short half-life (10 seconds) and is well tolerated by most patients.[7,8] Intravenous diltiazem (Cardizem) or one of the following β-adrenergic blockers can be used: atenolol (Tenormin), metoprolol (Toprol XL), or esmolol (Brevibloc). Digitalis and amiodarone (Cordarone) can also be used. If the patient becomes hemodynamically unstable, DC cardioversion may be used. Note that digitalis and calcium channel blockers can cause hemodynamic collapse in WPW syndrome. Persistent, recurring PSVT in WPW may ultimately be treated with radiofrequency catheter ablation of the accessory pathway.[9] (Catheter ablation therapy is discussed on p. 878.)

Atrial Flutter. **Atrial flutter** is an atrial tachyarrhythmia identified by recurring, regular, sawtooth-shaped flutter waves (Fig. 35-14, *A*) and is best visualized in leads II, III, aVF, and V₁ on the 12-lead ECG. It is usually associated with a slower ventricular response.

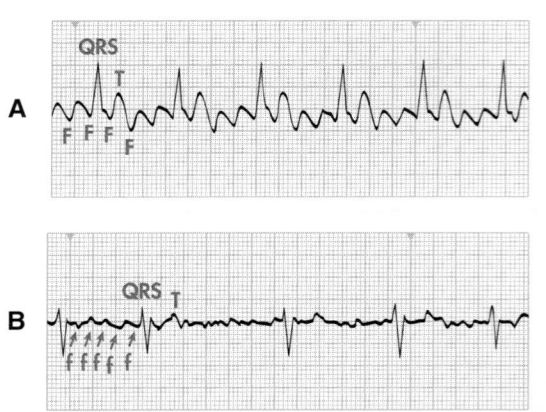

FIG. 35-14 **A,** Atrial flutter with a 4:1 conduction. **B,** Atrial fibrillation. Note the jagged, irregular baseline between the QRS complexes.

Clinical associations. Atrial flutter rarely occurs in a normal heart. In disease states, it is associated with CAD, hypertension, mitral valve disorders, pulmonary embolus, chronic lung disease, cor pulmonale, cardiomyopathy, hyperthyroidism, and the use of drugs such as digitalis, quinidine, and epinephrine.

ECG characteristics. Atrial rate is 250 to 350 beats/min. The ventricular rate varies according to the conduction ratio. In 2:1 conduction, the ventricular rate is typically found to be approximately 150 beats/min. Atrial rhythm is regular, and ventricular rhythm is usually regular. Atrial activity or "F" waves of a sawtooth appearance represents atrial depolarization followed by repolarization. The PR interval is variable. The QRS complex is normal unless bundle branch block or preexcitation is present. Because of the refractory characteristic of the AV node, there is usually some AV block in a fixed ratio of flutter waves to QRS complexes (e.g., 2:1, 3:1).

Significance. High ventricular rates and loss of atrial "kick" associated with atrial flutter can decrease CO and cause serious consequences such as heart failure, especially in the patient with underlying heart disease.[10] Patients with atrial flutter are at increased risk of stroke because of the risk of thrombus formation in the atria. Warfarin (Coumadin) is used to prevent stroke in patients with atrial flutter of greater than 48 hours duration.

Treatment. The primary goal in treatment of atrial flutter is to slow the ventricular response by increasing AV block. Electrical cardioversion may be used to convert the atrial flutter to sinus rhythm in an emergency situation. Drugs used to control ventricular rate include diltiazem, digoxin, and β-adrenergic blockers (atenolol, metoprolol, esmolol). Antiarrhythmic drugs used to convert atrial flutter to sinus rhythm or maintain sinus rhythm include amiodarone (Cordarone), propafenone (Rythmol), sotalol (Betapace), procainamide (Pronestyl), ibutilide (Corvert), and dofetilide (Tikosyn).[11,12] Radiofrequency catheter ablation is increasingly being used as curative therapy for atrial flutter.

Atrial Fibrillation. **Atrial fibrillation** is characterized by a total disorganization of atrial electrical activity without effective atrial contraction (Fig. 35-14, *B*). The arrhythmia may be chronic or intermittent. Atrial fibrillation is the most common arrhythmia in the United States and Canada. Its prevalence increases with age. As the elderly population increases, a 60% increase in this arrhythmia is predicted by 2020.[13]

Clinical associations. Atrial fibrillation usually occurs in the patient with underlying heart disease, such as CAD, rheumatic

heart disease, cardiomyopathy, hypertensive heart disease, CHF, and pericarditis. It is often acutely caused by factors such as thyrotoxicosis, alcohol intoxication, caffeine use, electrolyte disturbances, stress, and cardiac surgery. The term *lone atrial fibrillation* is used when no detectable cause is found for atrial fibrillation.[13]

ECG characteristics. During atrial fibrillation, atrial rate may be as high as 350 to 600 beats/min. Ventricular rate can vary from as low as 50 beats/min to as high as 180 beats/min. Atrial rhythm is chaotic, and ventricular rhythm is usually irregular. Ventricular rhythm may be regular if there is complete AV block (ventricular escape rhythm). The P wave shows fibrillatory waves, but no definite P wave can be observed. The PR interval is not measurable, and the QRS complex usually has a normal contour.

Significance. Atrial fibrillation can often result in a decrease in CO because of ineffective atrial contractions and a rapid ventricular response. Thrombi may form in the atria as a result of ineffective atrial contraction. An embolized clot may pass to the brain, causing a stroke. Risk of stroke increases fivefold with atrial fibrillation. Risk of stroke is even higher in patients with structural heart disease, with hypertension, and at an age over 65 years. Anticoagulation with warfarin (Coumadin) is used to prevent stroke in patients with atrial fibrillation[14] (see Evidence-Based Practice box below).

Treatment. The goals of treatment are a decrease in ventricular response and conversion to a sinus rhythm if possible. Drugs used for rate control include digoxin, β-adrenergic blockers (metoprolol, atenolol, esmolol), and calcium channel blockers (diltiazem [Cardizem], verapamil [Calan, Isoptin]). Antiarrhythmic drugs used for conversion to and maintenance of sinus rhythm include amiodarone (Cordarone), propafenone (Rythmol), sotalol (Betapace), flecainide (Tambocor), procainamide (Pronestyl), ibutilide (Corvert), and dofetilide (Tikosyn). Flecainide and propafenone should not be used in patients with CAD. DC cardioversion may be used to convert atrial fibrillation to a normal sinus rhythm. If

---

EVIDENCE-BASED PRACTICE
Atrial Fibrillation and Thrombosis

Clinical Problem

In patients with nonrheumatic atrial fibrillation, how effective are anticoagulants and antiplatelet drugs in preventing thromboembolic complications?

Best Clinical Practice

- In patients with nonrheumatic chronic atrial fibrillation, warfarin prevents stroke among those with average or higher risk and is more effective than antiplatelet drugs.
- Warfarin should be considered in all patients with chronic atrial fibrillation, and aspirin should be used only in patients with a contraindication to warfarin.

Implications for Nursing Practice

- Patients with atrial fibrillation are at an increased risk for thrombus formation and subsequent embolization to the brain.
- Anticoagulants are used to prevent thrombosis formation. They do not dissolve clots.
- Patients on anticoagulants need to be assessed for bleeding (see Chapter 37, Table 37-14).

Reference for Evidence

Warfarin prevents stroke in nonrheumatic atrial fibrillation but has a higher risk for hemorrhage than other agents, *ACP Journal Club* 135:59, 2001.

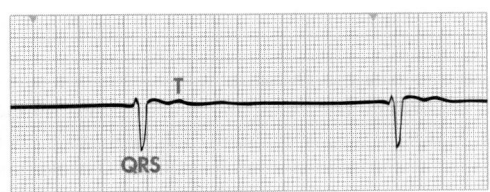

FIG. 35-15 Junctional escape rhythm.

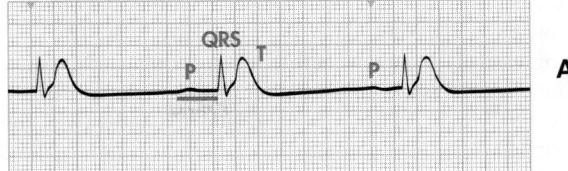

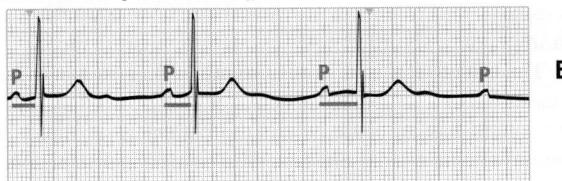

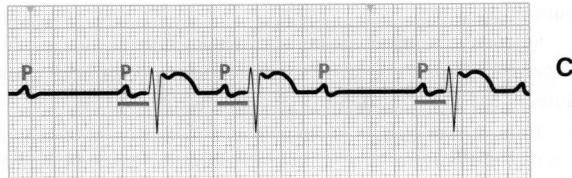

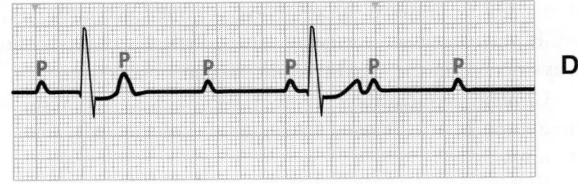

FIG. 35-16 Heart block. **A,** First-degree AV heart block. **B,** Second-degree AV heart block, type I (Wenckebach). **C,** Second-degree AV heart block, type II. **D,** Third-degree AV block (complete AV block).

a patient has been in atrial fibrillation for more than 48 hours, anticoagulation therapy with warfarin (Coumadin) is recommended for 3 to 4 weeks before any attempt at conversion to sinus rhythm.

Junctional Arrhythmia. *Junctional arrhythmia* refers to an arrhythmia that originates in the area of the AV node. The impulse may move in a retrograde fashion that produces an abnormal P wave occurring just before or after the QRS complex or that is hidden in the QRS complex. The impulse usually moves normally through the ventricles. Junctional premature beats may occur, and they are treated in a manner similar to that for PACs. Other junctional arrhythmias include junctional escape rhythm (Fig. 35-15), accelerated junctional rhythm, and junctional tachycardia. These arrhythmias are treated according to the patient's tolerance of the rhythm and the patient's clinical condition.

Clinical associations. Junctional escape rhythm is often associated with the aerobically trained individual who has sinus bradycardia. It may occur with acute MI, especially inferior MI, and dysfunction of the SA node. Accelerated junctional rhythm and junctional tachycardia are observed with acute inferior MI, digitalis toxicity, and acute rheumatic fever and during open heart surgery.

ECG characteristics. In junctional escape rhythm the HR is 40 to 60 beats/min, in accelerated junctional rhythm it is 60 to 100 beats/min, and in junctional tachycardia it is 100 to 140 beats/min. Rhythm is regular. The P wave is abnormal in contour and inverted, or it may be hidden in the QRS complex (see Fig. 35-15). The PR interval is less than 0.12 second when the P wave precedes the QRS complex. The QRS complex is usually normal.

Significance. Junctional escape rhythm serves as a safety mechanism occurring when the primary pacemaker has not been activated. Escape rhythms such as this should not be suppressed. Accelerated junctional rhythm and junctional tachycardia indicate a problem with the sinus node. If these rhythms are rapid, they may result in a reduction of CO and possible heart failure.

Treatment. Treatment varies according to the type of junctional arrhythmia. If a patient has symptoms with an escape junctional rhythm, atropine can be used. In accelerated junctional rhythm and junctional tachycardia caused by digoxin toxicity, the digoxin is withheld. In the absence of digitalis toxicity, β-adrenergic blockers, calcium channel blockers, and amiodarone are used. DC cardioversion should not be used.

First-Degree AV Block. **First-degree AV block** is a type of AV block in which every impulse is conducted to the ventricles but the duration of AV conduction is prolonged (Fig. 35-16). After the impulse moves through the AV node, it is usually conducted normally through the ventricles.

Clinical associations. First-degree AV block is associated with MI, chronic ischemic heart disease, rheumatic fever, hyperthyroidism, vagal stimulation, and drugs such as digitalis, β-adrenergic blockers, flecainide, and IV verapamil.

ECG characteristics. In first-degree AV block, HR is normal, and rhythm is regular. The P wave is normal, the PR interval is prolonged for more than 0.20 second, and the QRS complex usually has a normal contour.

Significance. First-degree AV block may be a precursor of higher degrees of AV block.

Treatment. There is no treatment for first-degree AV block.

Second-Degree AV Block, Type I. *Type I second-degree AV block (Wenckebach phenomenon)* includes a gradual lengthening of the PR interval, which occurs because of the AV conduction time that is prolonged until an atrial impulse is nonconducted and a QRS complex is dropped (see Fig. 35-16). Type I AV block most commonly occurs in the AV node, but it can also occur in the His-Purkinje system.

Clinical associations. Type I AV block may result from use of drugs such as digoxin or β-adrenergic blockers. It may also be associated with ischemic cardiac disease and other diseases that can slow AV conduction.

ECG characteristics. Atrial rate is normal, but ventricular rate may be slower as a result of dropped QRS complexes. Once a ventricular beat is dropped, the cycle repeats itself with progressive lengthening of the PR intervals until another QRS complex is dropped. The rhythm appears on the ECG in a pattern of grouped beats. Ventricular rhythm is irregular. The PR interval progressively lengthens before the nonconducted P wave occurs. The P wave has a normal contour. The PR interval lengthens progressively until a P wave is nonconducted and a QRS complex is dropped. The QRS complex has a normal contour. The duration of the QRS complex is normal or prolonged.

Significance. Type I AV block is usually a result of myocardial ischemia in an inferior MI. It is almost always transient and is usually well tolerated. However, it may be a warning signal of an impending significant AV conduction disturbance.

Treatment. If the patient is symptomatic, atropine is used to increase HR, or a temporary pacemaker may be needed, especially if the patient has an acute MI. If the patient is asymptomatic, the rhythm should be closely observed, with a transcutaneous pacemaker on standby. Bradycardia may become symptomatic when one or more of the following are present: (1) hypotension or shock, (2) congestive heart failure with pulmonary congestion, or (3) chest pain or dyspnea.

Second-Degree AV Heart Block, Type II. In *type II second-degree AV block* a P wave is nonconducted without progressive antecedent PR lengthening, and this almost always occurs when a bundle branch block is present (see Fig. 35-16). On conducted beats, the PR interval is constant. Second-degree heart block is a more serious type of block in which a certain number of impulses from the sinus node are not conducted to the ventricles. This occurs in ratios of 2:1, 3:1, and so on when there are two P waves to one QRS complex, three P waves to one QRS complex, and so on. It may occur with varying ratios. Type II AV block almost always occurs in the His-Purkinje system.

Clinical associations. Type II AV block is associated with rheumatic heart disease, CAD, acute anterior MI, and digitalis toxicity.

ECG characteristics. Atrial rate is usually normal. Ventricular rate depends on the intrinsic rate and the degree of AV block. Sinus rhythm is regular, but ventricular rhythm may be irregular. The P wave has a normal contour. The PR interval may be normal or prolonged but remains fixed on conducted beats. The QRS complex widens to more than 0.12 second because of bundle branch block.

Significance. Type II AV block often progresses to third-degree AV block and is associated with a poor prognosis. The reduced HR may result in decreased CO with subsequent hypotension and myocardial ischemia. Type II AV block is an indication for therapy with a permanent pacemaker.

Treatment. Temporary treatment before the insertion of a permanent pacemaker may involve the use of a temporary transvenous or transcutaneous pacemaker. Drugs such as atropine, epinephrine, isoproterenol, or dopamine can be tried as temporary measures to increase HR until pacemaker therapy is available.

Third-Degree AV Heart Block. Third-degree AV heart block, which is **complete heart block,** constitutes one form of AV dissociation in which no impulses from the atria are conducted to the ventricles (see Fig. 35-16). The atria are stimulated and contract independently of the ventricles. The ventricular rhythm is an escape rhythm, and the ectopic pacemaker may be above or below the bifurcation of the His bundle.

Clinical associations. Third-degree heart block is associated with fibrosis or calcification of the cardiac conduction system, CAD, MI, myocarditis, cardiomyopathy, open heart surgery, and

some systemic diseases such as amyloidosis and progressive systemic sclerosis (scleroderma).

ECG characteristics. The atrial rate is usually a sinus rate of 60 to 100 beats/min. The ventricular rate depends on the site of the block. If it is in the AV node, the rate is 40 to 60 beats/min, and if it is in the Purkinje system, it is 20 to 40 beats/min. Atrial and ventricular rhythms are regular but asynchronous. The P wave has a normal contour. The PR interval is variable, and there is no time relationship between the P wave and the QRS complex. The QRS complex is normal if escape rhythm is initiated in the bundle of His or above. It is widened if escape rhythm is initiated below the bundle of His.

Significance. Third-degree AV block almost always results in reduced CO with subsequent ischemia and heart failure. Syncope from third degree AV block may result from severe bradycardia or even periods of asystole.

Treatment. A temporary transvenous or transcutaneous pacemaker may be used on an emergency basis in a patient with acute MI. The use of drugs such as atropine, epinephrine, isoproterenol (Isuprel), and dopamine (Intropin) is a temporary treatment to increase HR and support blood pressure (BP) before pacemaker insertion.

Premature Ventricular Contractions. A **premature ventricular contraction** (PVC) is a contraction originating in an ectopic focus in the ventricles. It is the premature occurrence of a QRS complex, which is wide and distorted in shape, compared with a QRS complex initiated from the supraventricular tissue (Fig. 35-17). PVCs that are initiated from different foci appear different in contour from each other and are called *multifocal* PVCs. PVCs that appear to have the same contour are called *unifocal* PVCs. When every other beat is a PVC, it is called *ventricular bigeminy*. When every third beat is a PVC, it is called *ventricular trigeminy*. Two consecutive PVCs are called *couplets*. Three consecutive PVCs are called *triplets*. Ventricular tachycardia occurs when there are three or more consecutive PVCs. When a PVC falls on the T wave of a preceding beat, the *R on T phenomenon* occurs

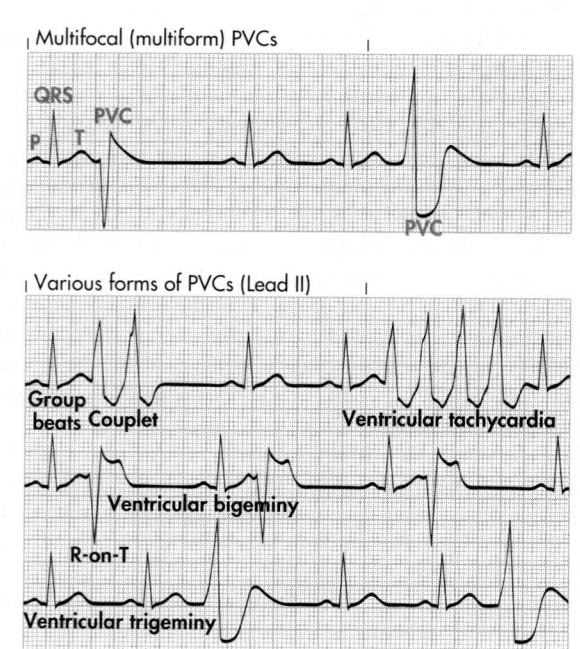

FIG. 35-17 Premature ventricular contractions (PVCs).

and is considered to be dangerous because it may precipitate ventricular tachycardia or ventricular fibrillation.

Clinical associations. PVCs are associated with stimulants such as caffeine, alcohol, aminophylline, epinephrine, isoproterenol (Isuprel), and digoxin. They are also associated with hypokalemia, hypoxia, fever, exercise, and emotional stress. Disease states associated with PVCs include MI, mitral valve prolapse (MVP), CHF, and CAD.

Electrocardiogram characteristics. HR varies according to intrinsic rate and number of PVCs. Rhythm is irregular because of premature beats. P wave is rarely visible and is usually lost in the QRS complex of PVC. Retrograde conduction may occur, and the P wave may be seen following the ectopic beat. The PR interval is not measurable. The QRS complex is wide and distorted in shape, more than 0.12 second. The T wave is generally large and opposite in direction to the major deflection of the QRS complex.

Significance. PVCs are usually a benign finding in the patient with a normal heart. In heart disease, depending on frequency, PVCs may reduce the CO and precipitate angina and heart failure. PVCs in ischemic heart disease or acute MI represent ventricular irritability. They may also occur as reperfusion arrhythmias after lysis of a coronary artery clot with thrombolytic therapy in acute MI, or following plaque reduction after percutaneous coronary intervention (PCI).

Treatment. Assessment of the patient's hemodynamic status is important to determine if treatment with drug therapy is indicated. Drugs that should be considered include β-adrenergic blockers, procainamide, amiodarone, or lidocaine.

Ventricular Tachycardia. The diagnosis of *ventricular tachycardia (VT)* is made when a run of three or more PVCs occurs. Different forms of ventricular tachycardia exist, depending on QRS configuration. Monomorphic VT (Fig. 35-18) has QRS complexes that are the same in shape, size, and direction. Polymorphic VT occurs when the QRS complexes gradually change back and forth from one shape, size, and direction to another over a series of beats. *Torsades de pointes* (French, "twisting around a point") is polymorphic VT associated with a prolonged QT interval of the underlying rhythm. Ventricular tachycardia may be sustained or nonsustained. Sustained VT lasts for greater than 30 seconds. Nonsustained VT lasts for 30 seconds or less. The appearance of ventricular tachycardia can be an ominous sign. It is considered to be a life-threatening arrhythmia because of decreased CO and the possibility of deterioration of ventricular tachycardia to ventricular fibrillation, which is a lethal arrhythmia.

Clinical associations. Ventricular tachycardia is associated with acute MI, CAD, significant electrolyte imbalances (e.g., potassium), cardiomyopathy, mitral valve prolapse, long QT syndrome, coronary reperfusion after thrombolytic therapy, digitalis toxicity, and central nervous system disorders. The arrhythmia has also been observed in patients who have no evidence of cardiac disease.

ECG characteristics. Ventricular rate is 100 to 250 beats/min. Rhythm may be regular or irregular. The P wave may be noted to "march through" the ventricular rhythm in AV dissociation, or it may occur after the QRS complex in a regular pattern of retrograde conduction. The PR interval is not measurable. The QRS complex is distorted in appearance, with a duration exceeding 0.12 second and with the ST-T direction pointing opposite to the major QRS deflection (see Fig. 35-18). It occurs when an ectopic focus or foci fire repetitively and the ventricle takes control as the pacemaker. The RR interval may be irregular or regular. AV dissociation may be present, with P waves occurring independently of the QRS complex. The atria may also be depolarized by the ventricles in a retrograde fashion.

Significance. Ventricular tachycardia may cause a severe decrease in CO as a result of decreased ventricular diastolic filling times and loss of atrial contraction. The result may be pulmonary edema, shock, and decreased blood flow to the brain. The arrhythmia must be treated quickly, even if it occurs only briefly and stops abruptly. Episodes may recur if prophylactic treatment is not begun. Ventricular fibrillation may also develop.

Treatment. If the VT is monomorphic and the patient is hemodynamically stable and has preserved left ventricular function, IV procainamide, amiodarone, or lidocaine is used. If the patient is unstable or has poor left ventricular function, amiodarone or lidocaine is given intravenously followed by synchronized cardioversion.

If VT is polymorphic with a normal baseline QT interval, any one of the following medications is used: β-adrenergic blockers, lidocaine, amiodarone, procainamide, or sotalol (Betapace). Synchronized cardioversion is used when drug therapy is ineffective.

If VT is polymorphic with a prolonged baseline QT interval, therapies include magnesium infusion, overdrive pacing, and possibly an IV β-adrenergic blocker. Drugs that prolong the QT interval should be discontinued. Unsynchronized cardioversion may be needed with the use sedation and/or anesthesia.

Ventricular tachycardia without a pulse is treated in the same manner as ventricular fibrillation. A rapid defibrillation attempt is performed.

Accelerated idioventricular rhythm (AIVR) is a "slow VT," originating in an ectopic pacemaker in the ventricles. The rate is between 40 and 100 beats/min. It is most commonly associated with acute MI and reperfusion of myocardium after thrombolytic therapy or angioplasty of coronary arteries. It can be an escape mechanism, appearing when the dominant pacemaker rate becomes less than that of the ventricular ectopic pacemaker. It can be seen with digitalis toxicity. In the setting of acute MI, AIVR is usually self-limited, well tolerated, and requires no treatment. If the patient becomes symptomatic, AIVR should be treated as one would treat VT.

Ventricular Fibrillation. **Ventricular fibrillation** is a severe derangement of the heart rhythm characterized on ECG by irregular undulations of varying contour and amplitude (Fig. 35-19). This represents the firing of multiple ectopic foci in the ventricle.

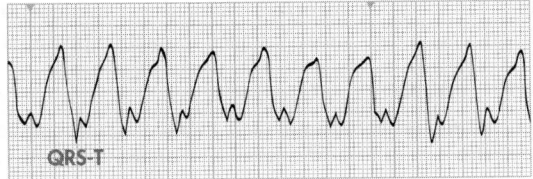

FIG. 35-18 Ventricular tachycardia.

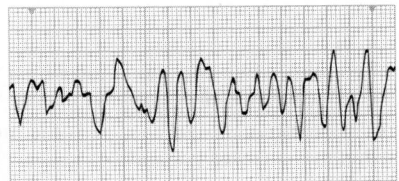

FIG. 35-19 Ventricular fibrillation.

Mechanically the ventricle is simply "quivering," and no effective contraction or CO occurs.

Clinical associations. Ventricular fibrillation occurs in acute MI and myocardial ischemia and in chronic diseases such as CAD and cardiomyopathy. It may occur during cardiac pacing or cardiac catheterization procedures as a result of catheter stimulation of the ventricle. It may also occur with coronary reperfusion after thrombolytic therapy. Other clinical associations are accidental electrical shock, hyperkalemia, hypoxemia, acidosis, and drug toxicity.

ECG characteristics. HR is not measurable. Rhythm is irregular and chaotic. The P wave is not visible, and the PR interval and the QRS interval are not measurable.

Significance. Ventricular fibrillation results in unconsciousness, absence of pulse, apnea, and seizures. If left untreated, the patient with this condition will die.

Treatment. Treatment consists of immediate initiation of cardiopulmonary resuscitation (CPR) and initiation of advanced cardiac life support (ACLS) measures with the use of defibrillation and definitive drug therapy. If a defibrillator is immediately available, there should be no delay in using it.[14]

Asystole. **Asystole** represents the total absence of ventricular electrical activity. Occasionally, P waves can be seen. No ventricular contraction occurs because depolarization does not occur. This is a lethal arrhythmia that requires immediate treatment. Ventricular fibrillation may masquerade as asystole; thus the rhythm should be assessed in more than one lead. The prognosis of a patient with asystole is poor.

Clinical associations. Asystole is usually a result of advanced cardiac disease, a severe cardiac conduction system disturbance, or end-stage CHF.

Significance. Generally the patient with asystole has end-stage cardiac function or has a prolonged arrest and cannot be resuscitated.

Treatment. Treatment consists of CPR with initiation of ACLS measures, which include intubation, transcutaneous pacing, and IV therapy with epinephrine and atropine.

Pulseless Electrical Activity. *Pulseless electrical activity* (PEA) describes a situation in which electrical activity can be observed on the ECG, but there is no mechanical activity of the ventricles and the patient has no pulse. Prognosis is poor unless the underlying cause can be identified and corrected. The most frequent causes of PEA include hypovolemia, hypoxia, acidosis, hyperkalemia or hypokalemia, hypothermia, drug overdose, cardiac tamponade, acute myocardial infarction, tension pneumothorax, and pulmonary embolus. Treatment begins with CPR followed by intubation and IV therapy with epinephrine. Atropine is also used if the ventricular rate is slow. Treatment is directed toward correction of the underlying cause.

Sudden Cardiac Death. The term **sudden cardiac death** (SCD), or *sudden death,* refers to cardiac death by an arrhythmia such as ventricular fibrillation. However, some electrophysiologists believe that the term can refer to death that is sudden by any cause. (SCD is discussed in Chapter 33.)

Proarrhythmia. Antiarrhythmic drugs may cause life-threatening arrhythmias similar to those for which they are administered. This concept is termed *proarrhythmia.* The patient who has severe left ventricular dysfunction is the most susceptible to a proarrhythmia. Class IA and IC drugs (Table 35-8), digoxin, and type III drugs can cause a proarrhythmic response. The first several days of drug therapy is the vulnerable period for

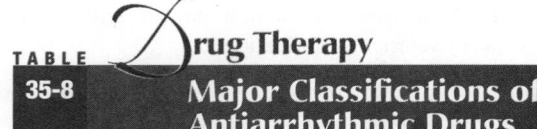

TABLE 35-8	**Drug Therapy** **Major Classifications of Antiarrhythmic Drugs**

Classification I: Drugs That Depress Upstroke of Action Potential
A. Prolong Repolarization
disopyramide (Norpace)
moricizine* (Ethmozine)
procainamide (Pronestyl)
quinidine
B. Accelerate Repolarization
lidocaine
mexiletine (Mexitil)
tocainide (Tonocard)
C. Have Little or No Effect on Repolarization
flecainide (Tambocor)
moricizine* (Ethmozine)
propafenone (Rythmol)

Classification II: β-Adrenergic Receptor Blockers
acebutolol (Sectral)
atenolol (Tenormin)
esmolol (Brevibloc)
labetalol (Normodyne)
metoprolol (Toprol XL)
nadolol (Corgard)
propranolol (Inderal)
sotalol† (Betapace)
timolol (Blocadren)

Classification III: Drugs That Prolong Repolarization
amiodarone (Cordarone)
dofetilide (Tikosyn)
ibutilide (Corvert)
sotalol† (Betapace)

Classification IV: Calcium Channel Blockers
diltiazem (Cardizem)
verapamil (Calan, Isoptin)

Potassium Channel Opener
adenosine (Adenocard)

Digitalis Preparations

*Moricizine has both class IA and IC properties.
†Sotalol has both class II and class III properties.

developing proarrhythmias. For this reason, the beginning of most oral antiarrhythmic drug regimens using these classes of drugs should be done in a monitored hospital setting.[15]

Antiarrhythmic Drugs

An increasing number of antiarrhythmic drugs have become available. Table 35-8 categorizes major drug classifications by primary effects on the cardiac intracellular action potential.

Defibrillation

Defibrillation is the most effective method of terminating ventricular fibrillation. It is most effective when the myocardial cells are not anoxic or acidotic. Therefore defibrillation should ideally be performed within 15 to 20 seconds of the onset of the ar-

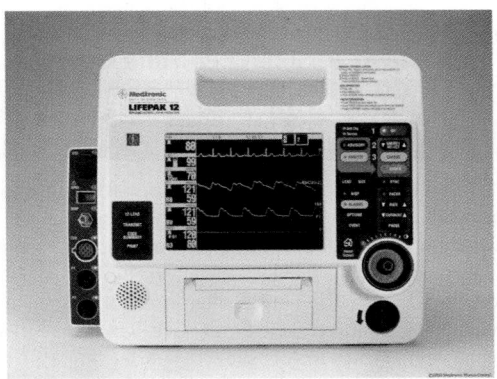

FIG. 35-20 LifePak: contains a monitor, defibrillator, and transcutaneous pacemaker.

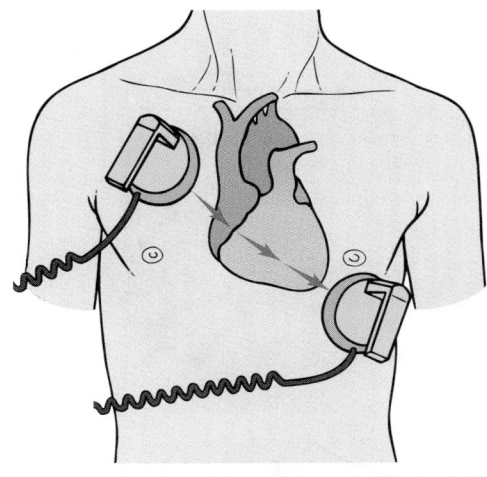

FIG. 35-21 Paddle placement and current flow in defibrillation.

rhythmia. Defibrillation is accomplished by the passage of a direct current (DC) electrical shock through the heart that is sufficient to depolarize the cells of the myocardium. The intent is that subsequent repolarization of myocardial cells will allow the SA node to resume the role of pacemaker.[16] The output of a defibrillator is quantified in joules, or watts per second. The recommended energy for initial shock in defibrillation is 200 joules with a second shock of 200 to 300 joules as needed and a third shock of 360 joules if defibrillation is unsuccessful. High doses of electricity during defibrillation have been found to cause myocardial damage; thus the lowest effective electrical output is the one with which to start.

A defibrillator is a standard item of emergency equipment (Fig. 35-20). There are many different models of defibrillators. The nurse should be familiar with the operation of the type of defibrillator that is used in the clinical setting. Proficiency verification in use of the defibrillator is recommended annually for nursing staff members who use it.

The following steps are to be taken for defibrillation: (1) CPR should be in progress if the defibrillator is not immediately available; (2) the defibrillator should be turned on, and the proper energy level should be selected; and (3) someone should make sure that the synchronizer switch is turned off. Conductive materials in the form of saline pads, electrode gel, or defibrillator gel pads are applied to the chest where defibrillator paddles will be placed. This decreases electrical impedance and helps prevent burns. The paddles are charged by a button on the defibrillator or a button on the paddles themselves. The paddles are placed on the chest wall (Fig. 35-21); one is placed to the right of the sternum just below the clavicle, and the other is placed to the left of the precordium. The operator applies 20 to 25 pounds of pressure to the paddles. The operator calls "all clear" to ensure that personnel are not touching the patient or the bed at the time of discharge. The defibrillator is then discharged by depressing buttons on both paddles simultaneously.

Cardioversion. *Electrical cardioversion* is the therapy of choice for the patient with hemodynamically unstable ventricular or supraventricular tachyarrhythmias. A synchronized circuit in the defibrillator is used to deliver a countershock that is programmed to occur during the QRS complex of the ECG.

The procedure for cardioversion is the same as for defibrillation with the following exceptions. If synchronized cardioversion is done on a nonemergency basis when the patient is awake and hemodynamically stable, the patient may be sedated with IV diazepam (Valium) or midazolam (Versed) before the procedure. Strict attention to maintenance of a patent airway is important in this situation. When a patient with supraventricular tachycardia or ventricular tachycardia is hemodynamically unstable, cardioversion is performed as quickly as possible.

Implantable Cardioverter-Defibrillator. The *implantable cardioverter-defibrillator* (ICD) has been developed as an acceptable treatment for the patient who has life-threatening ventricular arrhythmias. Indications for implantation of an ICD include cardiac arrest survivors, recurrent sustained VT, and prophylactically in patients who are at risk for SCD (e.g., history of MI and depressed heart function). Use of the ICD appears to significantly decrease cardiac mortality rates and has added a new dimension to the management of life-threatening arrhythmias and the prevention of SCD.[17,18]

The ICD consists of a lead system placed via a subclavian vein to the endocardium. A battery-powered pulse generator is implanted, usually subcutaneously, over the pectoral muscle. The pulse generator is similar to a pacemaker box but is somewhat larger. The newest systems are single-lead systems instead of previous multilead or patch systems (Fig. 35-22). The ICD sensing system monitors the HR and rhythm and identifies ventricular tachycardia or ventricular fibrillation. Approximately 25 seconds after the sensing system detects a lethal arrhythmia, the defibrillating mechanism delivers a 25-joule or less shock to the patient's heart muscle. If the first shock is unsuccessful, the generator recycles and can continue to deliver shocks.

In addition to defibrillation capabilities, the newest ICDs are equipped with antitachycardia and antibradycardia pacemakers. These sophisticated devices use arrhythmia algorithms that detect arrhythmias and determine the appropriate programmed response. These devices initiate overdrive pacing of supraventricular and ventricular tachycardias, sparing the patient painful shocks from the defibrillator device. They also provide backup pacing for bradyarrhythmias occurring after defibrillation discharges. Preprocedure and postprocedure nursing care of the patient undergoing ICD placement is similar to the care of a patient undergoing permanent pacemaker implantation (see p. 876).

Education of the patient who is receiving an ICD is of extreme importance. The patient experiences a variety of emotions, including fear of body image change, fear of recurrent arrhythmias,

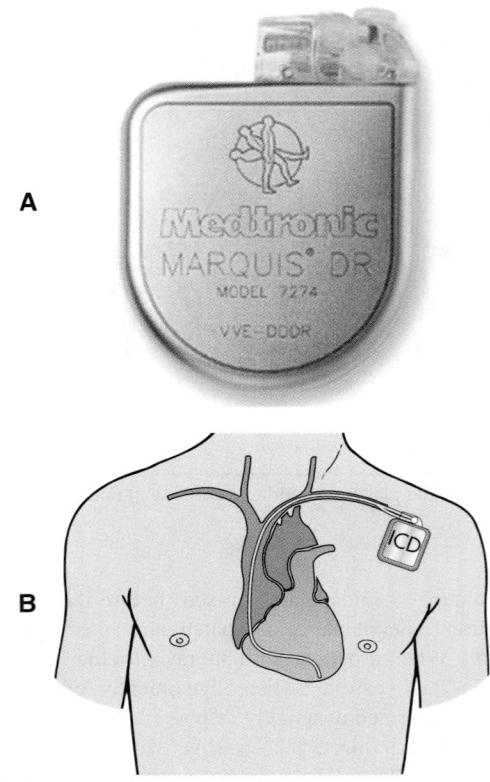

A

B

FIG. 35-22 **A,** The implantable cardioverter-defibrillator (ICD) pulse generator from Medtronic, Inc. **B,** The ICD is placed in a subcutaneous pocket over the pectoralis muscle. A single-lead system is placed transvenously from the pulse generator to the endocardium. The single lead detects arrhythmias and delivers an electrical shock to the heart muscle.

expectation of pain with ICD discharge (described as a feeling of a blow to the chest), and anxiety about going home. Table 35-9 describes the teaching guidelines for the patient with an ICD and the patient's family. Participation in an ICD support group should be encouraged.[18] Online resources for patients with an ICD include *www.implantable.com* and *www.casn.network.org* (Cardiac Arrest Survivor Network).

Pacemakers

The artificial **cardiac pacemaker** is an electronic device used in place of the SA node, the natural cardiac pacemaker of the heart. Implantable pacemakers were first developed in the 1950s. The artificial cardiac pacemaker is an electrical circuit in which the battery provides electricity that travels through a conducting wire to the myocardium, and the myocardium stimulates the heart to beat (i.e., it "captures" the heart).

Recent advances in technology have been applied extensively to pacemakers. This has resulted in sophisticated, noninvasive, programmable single- and dual-chambered pacemakers with specialized circuits that weigh only 40 to 50 g. Pacemakers have been developed that are more physiologically accurate, pacing both the atrium and the ventricle, as well as increasing HR when appropriate.[19] Pacemakers are primarily indicated for symptomatic bradyarrhythmias. However, there are multiple other indications for pacemakers. Atrial pacing is used for the prevention of atrial fibrillation. Pacemakers are indicated for neurocardiogenic syncope and long QT syndrome.

TABLE 35-9

Patient & Family Teaching Guide
Implantable Cardioverter–Defibrillator (ICD)

1. Maintain close follow-up with physician for testing of ICD function and for inspection of ICD insertion site.
2. Watch for signs of infection at incision site (e.g., redness, swelling, drainage).
3. Keep incision dry for 1 week after insertion.
4. Avoid lifting operative-side arm above shoulder for 1 week.
5. Avoid direct blows to ICD site.
6. When traveling, airport security should be informed of presence of ICD because it may set off the metal detector. If handheld screening wand is used, it should not be placed directly over the ICD.
7. When the ICD fires:
   - The patient should lie down.
   - If the patient loses consciousness or if there is repetitive firing, 911 should be called.
   - If the patient is feeling well and there is repetitive firing, contact the physician's office for ICD interrogation, including battery checks and safety and diagnostic checks.
8. Routine ICD check with interrogator/programmer device is needed every 2-3 months.
9. A Medic Alert bracelet should be worn at all times.
10. An information card about the ICD should be easily accessible in the patient's wallet.
11. Family members should learn CPR.
12. The nurse should assist the patient with the development of positive coping strategies to reduce stress.
13. Avoid large electromagnetic and vibratory forces because they may turn off the device.
14. Generally, patients should be told that they should not drive until they have been cleared by their physician. The release to drive is based on the presence of arrhythmias, the frequency of ICD firings, the patient's overall health, and state laws regarding drivers with ICDs.

Cardiac pacing is also used for the management of heart failure. More than 50% of heart failure patients have intraventricular conduction delays causing abnormal ventricular activation and contraction and subsequent dysynchrony between the right and left ventricles. This can result in reduced systolic function, pump inefficiency, and worsened heart failure. *Cardiac resynchronization therapy* (CRT) is a pacing technique that resynchronizes the cardiac cycle with both ventricles being paced, thus promoting improvement in ventricular function. This is an exciting development for improvement in left ventricular function for patients with heart failure. (Heart failure is discussed in Chapter 34.)

Permanent pacemakers are those that are implanted totally within the body (Fig. 35-23), and temporary pacemakers are those with the power source outside the body (Fig. 35-24). The permanent pacemaker power source is implanted subcutaneously in the chest (see Fig. 35-24) or abdomen and is attached to pacer electrodes, which are threaded transvenously to the right ventricle or the right atrium. Indications for insertion of permanent pacemakers are listed in Table 35-10.

Temporary pacemakers are usually used with a lead or wire threaded transvenously to the right ventricle and with a wire at-

Arrhythmias CHAPTER 35   877

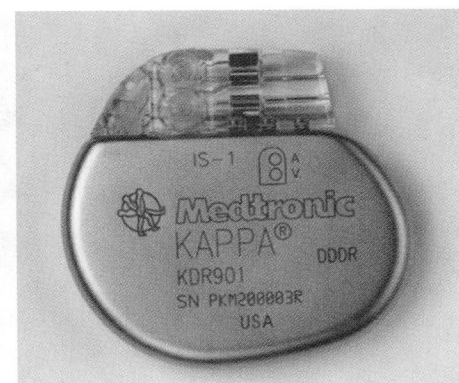

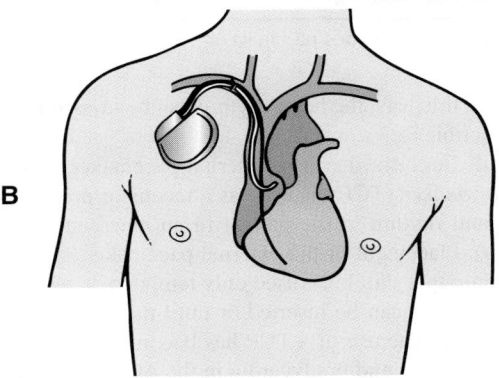

FIG. 35-23 **A,** A dual-chamber rate-responsive pacemaker from Medtronic, Inc., is designed to treat patients with chronic heart problems in which the heart beats too slowly to adequately support the body's circulation needs. **B,** Cardiac leads in both the atrium and ventricle enable a dual-chamber pacemaker to sense and pace in both heart chambers.

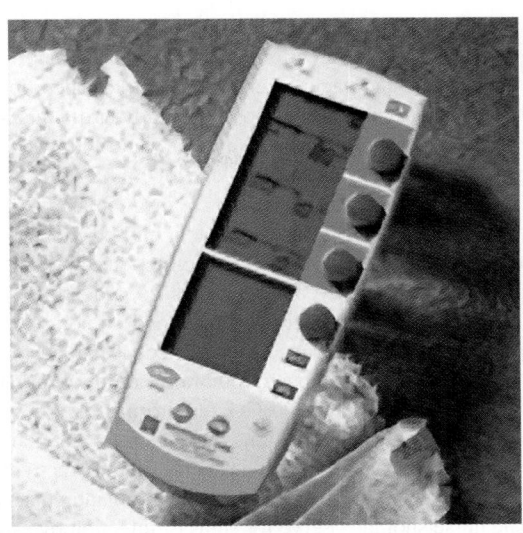

FIG. 35-24 Temporary external demand pacemaker.

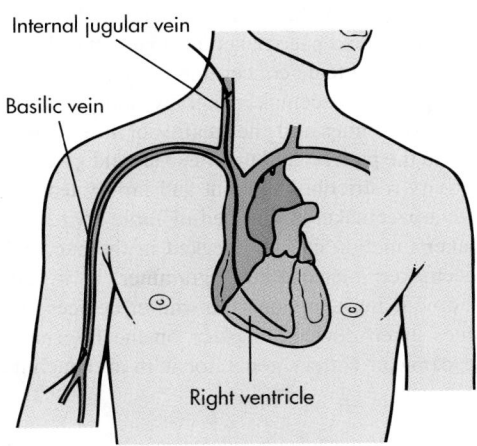

FIG. 35-25 Temporary pacemaker catheter insertion.

tached to a power source externally (Fig. 35-25). They are inserted in cardiac care units in emergency situations. Indications for temporary pacing are listed in Table 35-11.

Pacemaker malfunction is manifested by a failure to sense or a failure to capture. *Failure to sense* occurs when the pacemaker fails to recognize spontaneous atrial or ventricular activity, and it fires inappropriately. Failure to sense may be caused by pacer lead fracture, battery failure, or movement of electrode. *Failure to capture* occurs when the electrical charge to the myocardium is insufficient to produce atrial or ventricular contraction. Failure to capture may be caused by pacer lead fracture, battery failure, electrode movement, or fibrosis at the electrode tip.

TABLE 35-10 **Indications for Permanent Pacemaker Therapy**

- Chronic atrial fibrillation with slow ventricular response
- Fibrosis or sclerotic changes of cardiac conduction system
- Hypersensitive carotid sinus syndrome
- Sick sinus syndrome
- Sinus node dysfunction
- Tachyarrhythmias
- Third-degree AV block

AV, Atrioventricular.

TABLE 35-11 **Indications for Temporary Pacing**

- Maintenance of adequate HR and rhythm during special circumstances such as surgery and postoperative recovery, cardiac catheterization or coronary angioplasty, during drug therapy that may cause bradycardia, and before implantation of a permanent pacemaker
- As prophylaxis after open heart surgery
- Acute anterior MI with second-degree or third-degree AV block or bundle branch block
- Acute inferior MI with symptomatic bradycardia and AV block
- Termination of AV nodal reentry or reciprocating tachycardia associated with WPW syndrome, atrial flutter, or ventricular tachycardia
- Suppression of ectopic atrial or ventricular rhythm
- Electrophysiology studies to evaluate patient with bradyarrhythmias and tachyarrhythmias

AV, Atrioventricular; *HR,* heart rate; *MI,* myocardial infarction; *WPW,* Wolff-Parkinson-White.

Complications of invasive temporary or permanent pacemaker insertion include infection and hematoma formation at the site of insertion of the pacemaker power source, pneumothorax, failure to sense or capture with possible bradycardia and significant symptoms, perforation of the atrial or ventricular septum by the pacing wire, and appearance of "end-of-life" battery parameters on testing the pacemaker. A decrease in CO may also be seen when a ventricular demand–ventricular inhibited mode pacer is inserted because of loss of atrial contractions (atrial "kick").

Measures taken to prevent and assess complications include prophylactic IV antibiotic therapy before and after insertion, assessment of chest x-ray after insertion to check lead placement and to rule out the presence of a pneumothorax, careful observation of insertion site, and continuous ECG monitoring of the patient's rhythm. After pacemaker insertion, the patient is maintained on bed rest for 12 hours, and minimal arm and shoulder activity is allowed to prevent dislodgement of the newly implanted pacemaker leads. The nurse should observe for signs of infection by assessing the incision for redness, swelling, or discharge. Temperature elevation should also be noted. Careful monitoring of the patient's rhythm is used to detect problems with sensing or capturing.

The nurse must provide patient teaching in addition to observation for complications after pacemaker insertion. The patient with a newly implanted pacemaker has many questions about activity restrictions and fears concerning body image after the procedure. The goal of pacemaker therapy should be to enhance physiologic functioning and the quality of life. This should be emphasized to the patient, and the nurse should give concrete advice on activity restrictions. Patient and family teaching for the patient with a pacemaker is outlined in Table 35-12.

Pacemaker function can be checked in the pacemaker clinic by the pacemaker interrogator/programmer, or it can be done from the home using telephone transmitter devices. The patient is sometimes given devices to place on the fingers or directly over the pacemaker battery generator with an attachment to the

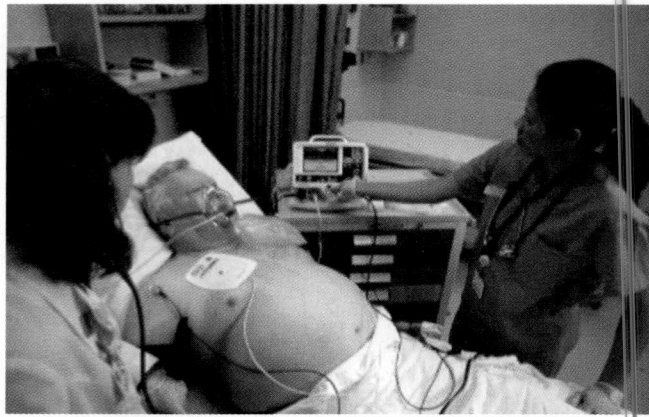
FIG. 35-26 Transcutaneous pacemaker.

telephone. In this way, the heart rhythm can be transmitted to the pacemaker clinic.[20]

External Pacemaker. The external pacemaker, or *transcutaneous pacemaker* (TCP), is used as a means of providing adequate HR and rhythm to the patient in an emergency situation (Fig. 35-26). Placement of the external pacemaker is a noninvasive procedure that should be used only temporarily until a transvenous pacemaker can be inserted or until more definitive therapy is available. The use of a TCP has become a cornerstone of therapy for asystole and bradycardia in the ACLS algorithms.

The external pacemaker consists of a power source and a rate- and voltage-control device that is attached to two large electrode pads. One pad is positioned on the anterior part of the chest, usually on the V_2 or V_5 lead position, and the other pad is placed on the back between the spine and the left scapula at the level of the heart.

Before initiating external pacemaker therapy, it is important to tell the patient what to expect. The uncomfortable muscle contractions that the pacemaker creates when the current passes through the chest wall should be explained. The patient should be reassured that the therapy is temporary and that every effort will be made to adjust the voltage settings of the pacemaker to improve comfort level. Mild analgesia may also be given.

Catheter Ablation Therapy

Catheter ablation therapy is a revolutionary development in the area of antiarrhythmic therapy. In 1981 transcatheter ablation of the AV node was introduced as a treatment for supraventricular arrhythmias. Radiofrequency energy (produced by high-frequency alternating current) has been most recently used to "burn" or ablate areas of the conduction system as definitive treatment of tachyarrhythmias.[21]

Ablation therapy is done after EPS has identified the source of the arrhythmia. An electrode-tipped ablation catheter is used to "burn" or ablate accessory pathways or ectopic sites in the atria, AV node, and ventricles. Catheter ablation is considered the nonpharmacologic treatment of choice for AV nodal reentrant tachycardia, for reentrant tachycardia related to accessory bypass tracts, and to control the ventricular response of certain tachyarrhythmias. The procedure is also used for atrial flutter. In some cases of uncontrolled ventricular response in atrial fibrillation or flutter that is unresponsive to medical therapy, complete ablation of the AV node or bundle of His is performed. Techniques for atrial flutter and atrial fibrillation circuit ablations are being used, and there is ongoing research in these techniques.

TABLE 35-12	*P*atient & Family Teaching Guide — Pacemaker

1. Maintain follow-up care with a physician to check the pacemaker site and begin regular pacemaker function checks with interrogator/programmer device.
2. Watch for signs of infection at incision site—redness, swelling, drainage.
3. Keep incision dry for 1 week after implantation.
4. Avoid lifting operative-side arm above shoulder level for 1 week.
5. Avoid direct blows to generator site.
6. Avoid close proximity to high-output electrical generators or to large magnets such as an MRI scanner. These devices can reprogram a pacemaker.
7. Microwave ovens are safe to use and do not threaten pacemaker function.
8. Travel without restrictions is allowed. The small metal case of an implanted pacemaker rarely sets off an airport security alarm.
9. The patient should be taught how to take the pulse.
10. Carry pacemaker information card at all times.

MRI, Magnetic resonance imaging.

The ablation procedure is a highly successful therapy with a low complication rate. Care of the patient following ablation therapy is similar to that of a patient undergoing cardiac catheterization (see Chapter 31).

SYNCOPE

Syncope (fainting or a brief lapse in consciousness) is a common diagnosis of patients coming into the emergency department and hospital. The most common cardiovascular causes of syncope include (1) neurocardiogenic syncope or "vasovagal" syncope (e.g., carotid sinus sensitivity) and (2) primary cardiac arrhythmias (e.g., tachycardias, bradycardias).[22,23]

A diagnostic workup for a patient with syncope from a cardiac standpoint begins with ruling out structural and/or ischemic heart disease. This is done with echocardiography and stress testing. In the older patient who is more likely to have ischemic and structural heart disease, electrophysiology study (EPS) is used to diagnose atrial and ventricular tachyarrhythmias, as well as conduction system disease causing bradycardias, all of which can cause syncope. These problems are treated with antiarrhythmic medical therapy, pacemakers, ICDs, or catheter ablation therapy.

In patients without structural heart disease or in whom EPS testing is not diagnostic, upright or head-up tilt table testing may be performed. This is a helpful test in identifying neurocardiogenic syncope. In this type of syncope, there is accentuated adrenergic activity in the upright position, with intense activation of cardiopulmonary mechanoreceptors resulting in bradycardia and hypotension.

In the tilt table test baseline ECG, blood pressure, and heart rate are recorded. The patient is placed on a table in the upright position, supported by a belt across the torso and feet. The upright position is maintained for 20 to 60 minutes at 60 to 80 degrees. In normal individuals in the upright position, there is central venous pooling, and this activates the renin-angiotensin system, which leads to compensatory mechanisms to increase cardiac output and maintain normal blood pressure. In patients with neurocardiogenic syncope, there is a marked decrease in blood pressure and heart rate. Neurocardiogenic syncope can be treated with β-adrenergic blockers, which promote maintenance of heart rate and blood pressure.

Other diagnostic tests for syncope include various recording devices. Holter monitors and event monitors are used, and are discussed in this chapter and Chapter 31. A newly developed implantable recording device is being increasingly used. The device can be interrogated after a syncopal event in order to determine the cardiac rhythm at the time to the event.

CARDIOPULMONARY RESUSCITATION

Cardiopulmonary resuscitation (CPR) is the process of externally supporting the circulation and respiration of a person who has a cardiac arrest. All health care professionals should be skilled in CPR because **cardiac arrest,** the sudden cessation of breathing and adequate circulation of blood by the heart, may occur at any time or in any setting. Resuscitation measures are divided into two components: *basic life support* (BLS) and *advanced cardiac life support* (ACLS). The American Heart Association (AHA) establishes the standards for CPR and is actively involved in teaching BLS and ACLS to health care professionals and laypeople.[6] The AHA recommends that nurses and physicians working with patients be certified in BLS and ACLS. Certification involves attending formal classes and passing cognitive and motor skill tests.

CPR alone is not enough to save lives in most cardiac arrests. It is a vital link in the chain of survival that supports the victim until more advanced help is available. The chain of survival is composed of the following sequence: early activation of the emergency medical services (EMS) system, early CPR, early defibrillation, and early advanced care.[24]

Basic Life Support

Basic life support (BLS) involves the external support of circulation and ventilation for a patient with cardiac or respiratory arrest through CPR.[24] *Artificial respiration* (mouth-to-mouth, mouth-to-mask, mouth-to-nose, mouth-to-stoma) and external *chest compression* substitute for spontaneous breathing and circulation. The major objective of performing CPR is to provide oxygen to the brain, heart, and other vital organs until appropriate therapeutic management and resuscitation efforts involving advanced life support methods can be initiated or until resuscitation efforts are ordered to be stopped.

Rapid intervention is the key to success and is critical in preventing biologic death or the death of brain cells. CPR must be initiated within 4 to 6 minutes of cardiac or pulmonary arrest. Brain cells begin to die (brain death) within 6 minutes of anoxia. It is critical that oxygenated blood be circulated during CPR. Unfortunately, even when CPR is performed with perfect technique, only 25% to 30% of the normal CO is achieved.[25] National standards for knowledge and technique must be met for personnel to be certified to deliver CPR. Assessment of the victim must be stressed in teaching CPR. Each of the broad areas—airway, breathing, and circulation (the ABCs of CPR)—should be reviewed.

The AHA now includes training in the use of automatic external defibrillators (AEDs) with instruction of health care personnel and laypersons in BLS. Shortening the time to defibrillation, along with CPR, improves survival from cardiac arrest. AEDs, which are simple to use with proper training, have become more available for use in out-of-hospital settings such as schools, shopping malls, sports arenas, airports, outpatient clinics, and commercial airliners.[6]

Airway. The first steps in administering BLS are to confirm the absence of breathing and to establish a patent airway. Fig. 35-27 demonstrates opening the airway and performing mouth-to-mouth ventilation. An adult's airway is opened by hyperextending the head. The *head tilt–chin lift maneuver* is used and involves tilting the head back with one hand and lifting the chin forward with the fingers of the other hand. If no respirations are detected, the rescuer attempts to ventilate the victim with mouth-to-mouth resuscitation.

Breathing. Breaths are given with the victim's nostrils pinched and the rescuer's mouth placed around the victim's mouth to make a tight seal. Mouth-to-barrier and bag-mask techniques can also be used. Two slow breaths are given by the rescuer (2 seconds per breath). The volume of air of each ventilation should be approximately 700 to 1000 ml, which can be determined by noting a rise of 1 to 2 inches in the victim's chest. Smaller volumes (400 to 600 ml) should be attempted during mouth-to-barrier and bag-mask ventilations. When the victim has a tracheostomy, ventilation should be given through the stoma.[6]

If airflow is obstructed, the rescuer should reposition the head and repeat the attempt to provide ventilation. If the victim cannot be ventilated after repositioning the head, the rescuer should proceed with maneuvers to remove foreign bodies that may be obstructing the airway (Table 35-13).

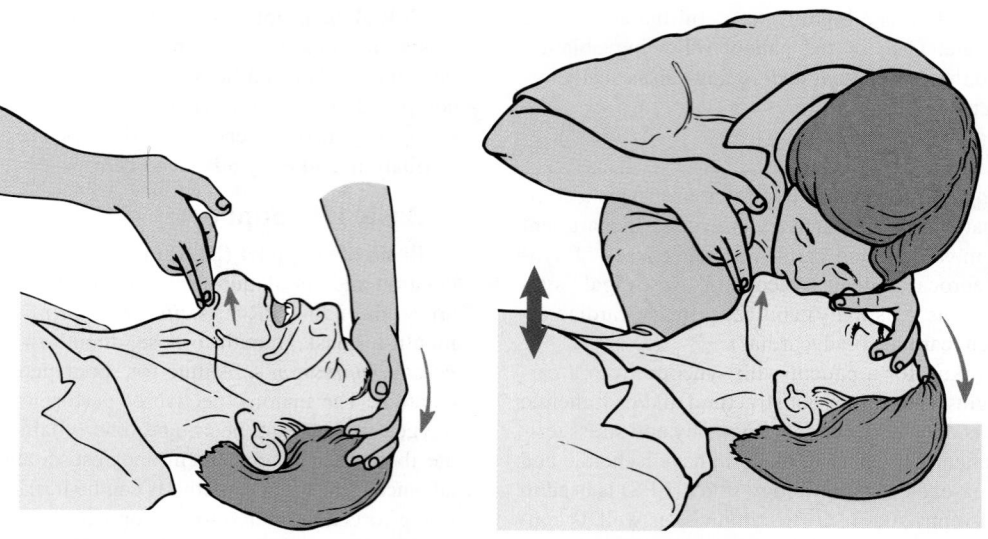

FIG. 35-27 The head tilt–chin lift maneuver is used to open the victim's airway to give mouth-to-mouth resuscitation. This procedure is carried out by placing one hand on the victim's forehead and applying firm, backward pressure with the palm to tilt the head back. The chin is lifted and brought forward with the fingers of the other hand.

TABLE 35-13   Management of Foreign Body Airway Obstruction (FBAO)

Conscious Adult Victim

Assess Victim for Airway Obstruction

Signs of airway obstruction:

- Universal choking sign (victim clutches neck with thumb and index finger)
- Inability to speak
  Ask the victim, "Are you choking?"
  Ask victim, "Can you speak?"
- Weak, ineffective cough
- High-pitched sound or no sound while inhaling
- Increased difficulty breathing
- Cyanosis

If the victim can cough forcefully and/or speak, the rescuer need not interfere. The rescuer simply stays with victim, monitors victim's condition, and, if partial obstruction persists, activates EMS

If the victim displays any of the above, severe or complete airway obstruction may be present and the rescuer must take action.

Heimlich Maneuver with Standing/Sitting Victim (Fig. 35-28)

1. Stand behind victim and wrap arms around waist.
2. Make fist with one hand.
3. Place thumb side of fist against victim's abdomen. Position fist midline, slightly above umbilicus and well below xiphoid process.
4. Grasp fist with other hand.
5. Press fist into victim's abdomen using quick upward thrusts. Each thrust should be a separate, distinct movement.
6. Repeat thrusts until object is expelled or victim becomes unresponsive.

Unconscious Adult Victim

Assessment

If rescuer sees victim collapse and knows that FBAO is the cause:

1. Activate the EMS system by calling 911.
2. Be sure victim is supine.

3. Perform tongue–jaw lift, then a finger sweep to remove object (Fig. 35-29).
4. Open airway and attempt to ventilate:
   - Give two rescue breaths.
   - If breaths are unsuccessful in making victim's chest rise:
     a. Reposition victim's head.
     b. Reopen airway.
     c. Reattempt to ventilate.
5. If efforts to ventilate are still unsuccessful, prepare to perform Heimlich maneuver.

Heimlich Maneuver with Unresponsive Victim

1. Place victim supine.
2. Kneel, straddling victim's thighs.
3. Place heel of one hand against victim's abdomen. Position fist midline, slightly above umbilicus and well below xiphoid process.
4. Place other hand directly over first hand.
5. Press both hands into victim's abdomen using quick upward thrusts.
6. Each thrust should be a separate, distinct movement.
7. After five abdominal thrusts open victim's airway using tongue–jaw lift.
8. Perform finger sweep to remove object.
9. Continue repeating this sequence until object is cleared or advanced procedures are available to establish a patent airway.
10. If obstruction is removed, assess breathing.
11. If victim is not breathing:
    - Provide two rescue breaths.
    - Assess for signs of circulation (breathing, coughing, movement, pulse).
12. If no signs of circulation are present, begin chest compressions.

Source: *2000 Handbook of emergency cardiovascular care for health care providers,* Dallas, 2000, American Heart Association.

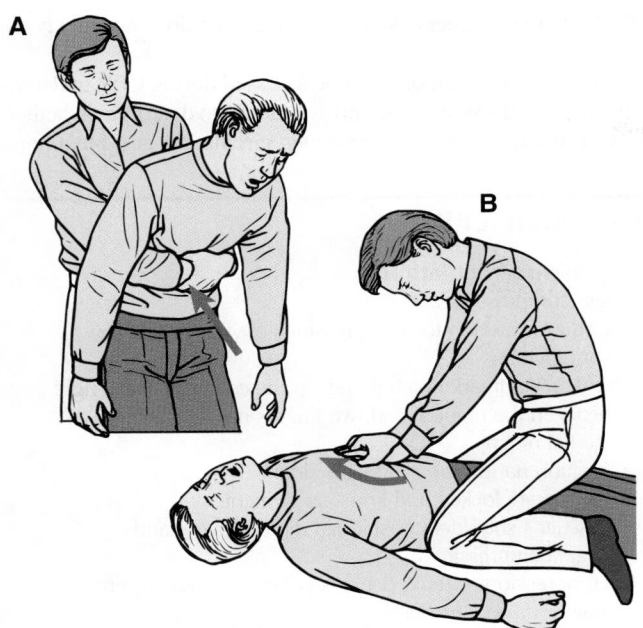

FIG. 35-28 **A**, Heimlich maneuver administered to a conscious (standing) victim of foreign body airway obstruction. **B**, Heimlich maneuver administered to an unconscious (lying) victim of foreign body airway obstruction—astride position.

In those rare instances when airway obstruction is not relieved by methods described in Table 35-13, additional procedures are necessary. These include transtracheal catheter ventilation and cricothyroidotomy, which should only be attempted by health care professionals experienced in these procedures.[11]

External Cardiac Compressions. Cardiac arrest is characterized by the absence of a pulse in the large arteries of an unconscious victim who is not breathing. The carotid artery is used to determine the absence of a pulse. After an airway has been established and two ventilations have been delivered, the rescuer checks the pulse. While maintaining the head-tilt position with one hand on the forehead, the rescuer locates the victim's trachea with two or three fingers of the other hand. The rescuer then slides these fingers into the groove between the trachea and the muscles of the side of the neck where the carotid pulse can be felt. The technique is more easily performed on the side nearest the rescuer. If no pulse is palpated, chest compressions should be initiated.[25]

The proper technique for administering chest compressions is shown in Fig. 35-30. External chest compression technique consists of serial, rhythmic applications of pressure on the lower half of the sternum. The victim must be in the horizontal supine position when the compressions are performed. The victim must be lying on a flat, hard surface, such as a CPR board (specially manufactured for use in CPR), a headboard from a cardiac care unit bed, or, if necessary, the floor. The rescuer should be positioned close to the side of the victim's chest.[6]

The guidelines for proper compression technique are presented in Tables 35-14 and 35-15 and Fig. 35-30, *C*. Rescue breathing and chest compressions are combined for an effective resuscitation effort of the victim of cardiopulmonary arrest. The compression-to-ventilation ratio for one- or two-person CPR is 15 compressions to 2 ventilations (see Tables 35-14 and 35-15). If the patient is intubated and airway is secure, a 5:2 compression-to-ventilation ratio is used in two-person CPR.

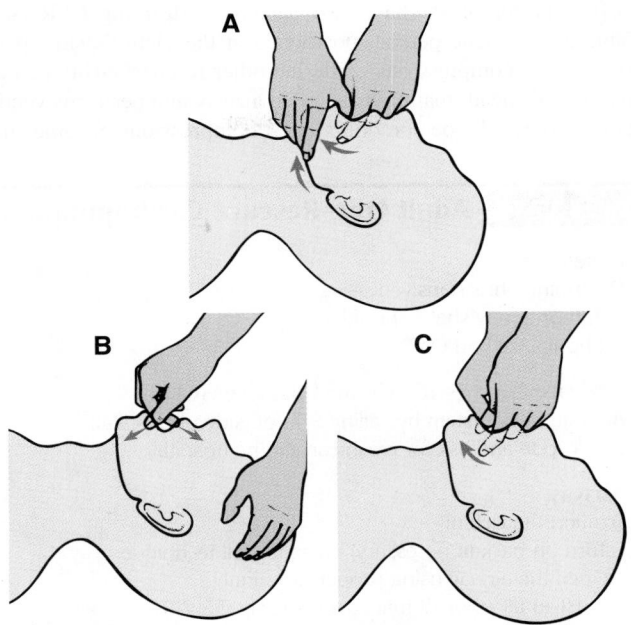

FIG. 35-29 **A**, Finger-sweep maneuver administered to an unconscious victim of foreign body airway obstruction. With the victim's head up, the rescuer opens the victim's mouth by grasping both the tongue and the lower jaw between the thumb and fingers and lifting (tongue-jaw lift). This action draws the tongue from the back of the throat and away from the foreign body. The obstruction may be partially relieved by this maneuver. **B**, Crossed-finger technique for opening the airway. If the rescuer is unable to open the mouth with the tongue-jaw lift, the crossed-finger technique may be used. The rescuer opens the mouth by crossing the index finger and thumb and pushing the teeth apart. **C**, The index finger of the rescuer's available hand is inserted along the inside of the cheek and deeply into the throat to the base of the tongue. A hooking motion is used to dislodge the foreign body and maneuver it into the mouth for removal.

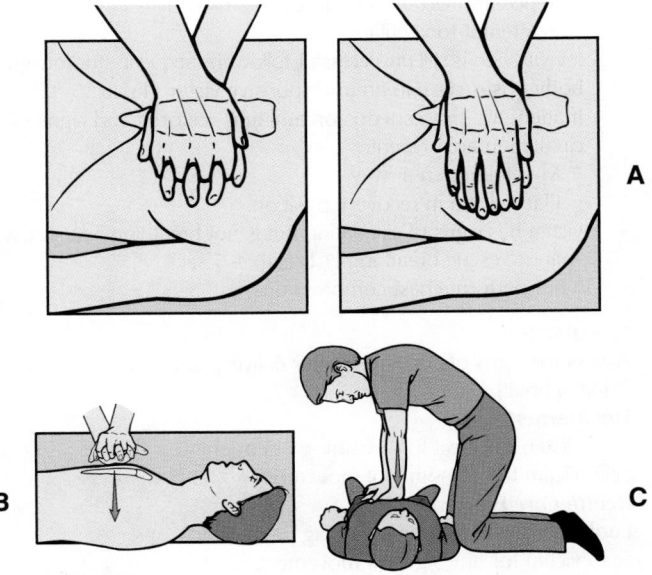

FIG. 35-30 Cardiopulmonary resuscitation (CPR). **A**, Position of the hands during application of external cardiac massage. **B**, When pressure is applied, the lower portion of the sternum is displaced posteriorly with the palm of the hand. **C**, To apply maximum downward pressure, the resuscitator leans forward so that both arms are at right angles to the patient's sternum and the elbows are locked.

It is preferable to have two persons performing CPR (see Table 35-15). One person, positioned at the victim's side, performs chest compressions while the other rescuer, positioned at the victim's head, maintains an open airway and performs ventilations. When the person doing chest compressions becomes fatigued, the two rescuers should exchange positions as quickly as possible.[6]

The victim's condition must be assessed during CPR to determine the effectiveness of compressions and to determine whether the victim has resumed spontaneous circulation and breathing.

TABLE 35-14   Adult One-Rescuer Cardiopulmonary Resuscitation (CPR)

Assess
Determine unresponsiveness:
  Tap or gently shake shoulder.
  Shout, "Are you OK?"

Activate Emergency Medical Services (EMS)*
Activate EMS system by calling 911 (outside of hospital).
Call a code and ask for crash cart (in the hospital).

Airway
Position the victim:
- Turn on back (if necessary) using logroll technique.
- Open the airway using proper technique:
    Head tilt–chin lift maneuver (see Fig. 35-27)
    Jaw-thrust maneuver (if cervical spine injury is suspected)

Breathing
1. Assess for cessation of breathing:
   - LOOK for chest rising and falling.
   - LISTEN for air escaping during exhalation.
   - FEEL for flow of air.
2. If victim is breathing adequately:
   - Continue to protect airway.
   - Place victim in recovery position.
3. If victim is unresponsive and not breathing:
   - Provide two slow breaths (2 sec/breath).
       Observe chest rise.
       Allow for complete exhalation between breaths.
   - If unable to give two effective breaths:
       Reposition victim to try to open airway.
       Reattempt to ventilate.
   - If ventilation is still unsuccessful, follow the sequence for foreign-body obstruction in an unresponsive victim (Table 35-13).
   - If adequate spontaneous breathing is restored and signs of circulation are present:
       Maintain open airway.
       Place victim in recovery position.
4. If victim has signs of circulation but is not breathing adequately:
   Continue rescue breathing (1 breath/4–5 sec).
   Do not perform chest compressions.

Circulation
Assess for signs of circulation after delivery of the two effective
  initial breaths.
Lay Rescuer†
Look, listen, and feel for breathing or coughing.
Scan victim for any signs of movement.
Health Care Professional
Look, listen, and feel for breathing or coughing.
Scan victim for any signs of movement.
Feel for carotid pulse.
If there are no signs of circulation, prepare to begin chest
  compressions.

Compression/Ventilation
1. Begin compressions:
   - Get into position for compressions at victim's side (by shoulders).
   - Locate landmark notch (hands in the center of chest, right between the nipples, and two fingers above the xiphoid-sternal notch).
   - Position hands, arms, and shoulders.
   - Elbows are locked and arms are straight.
   - Rescuer's shoulders positioned directly over hands.
   - Begin compressions.
   - Compressions should depress victim's sternum approximately 1½ to 2 inches.
   - Allow chest to rebound to normal position after each compression.
   - Perform compressions at the rate of 100 per minute.
   - Maintain correct position at all times.
2. Provide ventilation:
   - Open airway using proper technique.
   - Deliver two slow rescue breaths.
   - Return hands to chest.
   - Find proper landmark and hand position.
   - Restart compressions.
3. Compression-ventilation cycle:
   - Compression-ventilation ratio is 15:2.
   - Exhalation occurs between the two breaths and during the first chest compression of the next cycle.
   - Perform four complete cycles, then reassess for signs of breathing or circulation.

Reassessment
1. After four complete compression-ventilation cycles, reassess victim:
   - Assess for signs of breathing and circulation.
   - Take no more than 10 seconds to do this.
2. If signs of circulation are absent:
   - Resume CPR.
   - Start with chest compressions first.
3. If signs of circulation are present, assess for breathing.
   - If breathing is present:
       Place victim in recovery position.
       Monitor breathing and circulation.
   - If breathing is absent, provide rescue breathing:
       Provide one breath every 4 to 5 seconds.
       Monitor circulation closely.

Continuation of CPR
If CPR is continued:
- Reassess every few minutes.
- Do not interrupt CPR except in special circumstances.

Source: *2000 Handbook of emergency cardiovascular care for health care providers*, Dallas, 2000, American Heart Association.
*Rescuers should phone 911 for unresponsive adults before beginning CPR, except in the case of submersion, trauma, and drug intoxication/overdose.
†Lay rescuers are no longer taught a pulse check.

TABLE 35-15 Adult Two-Rescuer Cardiopulmonary Resuscitation (CPR)

Assess/Activate Emergency Medical Services (EMS)*

One Rescuer

Determine unresponsiveness:
  Tap or gently shake shoulder.
  Shout, "Are you OK?"

Other Rescuer

Activate EMS system by calling 911 (outside of hospital).
Call a code and ask for crash cart (in hospital).

Airway

Position the victim:

- Turn on back (if necessary) using logroll technique.
- Open the airway using proper technique:
    Head tilt–chin lift maneuver (Fig. 35-27).
    Jaw-thrust maneuver (if cervical spine injury is suspected).

Breathing

1. Assess for cessation of breathing:
    - LOOK for chest rising and falling.
    - LISTEN for air escaping during exhalation.
    - FEEL for flow of air.
2. If victim is breathing adequately:
    - Continue to protect airway.
    - Place victim in recovery position.
3. If victim has signs of circulation but is not breathing adequately:
    - Continue rescue breathing (1 breath/4-5 sec).
    - Do not perform chest compressions.
4. If victim is not breathing adequately:
    - Provide two slow breaths (2 sec/inflation).
        Observe chest rise.
        Allow for complete exhalation between breaths.
    - If unable to give two effective breaths:
        Reposition victim to try to open airway.
        Reattempt to ventilate.
    - If ventilation is still unsuccessful, follow the sequence for foreign-body obstruction in an unresponsive victim (Table 35-13).

Circulation

Assess for signs of circulation.

Lay Rescuer†

Look, listen, and feel for breathing or coughing.
Scan victim for any signs of movement.

Health Care Professional

Look, listen, and feel for breathing or coughing.
Scan victim for any signs of movement.
Feel for carotid pulse.
If no pulse is present:
- State assessment results:
    Say "No pulse."
- Prepare to perform compressions.

Compression/Ventilation

One Rescuer/Compressor

1. Get into position for compressions at victim's side.
2. Locate landmark notch (hands in the center of chest, right between the nipples, and two fingers above the xiphoid-sternal notch).

3. Position hands, arms, and shoulders:
    - Elbows are locked and arms are straight.
    - Rescuer's shoulders positioned directly over hands.
4. Begin compressions.
    - Compressions should depress victim's sternum approximately 1½ to 2 inches.
    - Allow chest to rebound to normal position after each compression.
    - Perform compressions at the rate of 100 per minute.
    - Maintain correct position at all times.

Other Rescuer/Ventilator

1. Get into position at victim's head.
2. Maintain an open airway.
3. Provide rescue breathing (two slow breaths of 2 seconds each).
4. Ensure that chest is rising with each ventilation.
5. Monitor carotid pulse to verify compression effectiveness.

Compression-Ventilation Cycle

Compression-ventilation ratio is 15:2.
Exhalation occurs between the two breaths and during the first chest compression of the next cycle.
Perform four complete cycles; then reassess for signs of breathing or circulation.

Switching

When the compressor becomes fatigued, the rescuer should call for a switch.
Rescuers should exchange positions simultaneously with minimal delay:
- Ventilator moves to chest.
- Compressor moves to head.

Reassessment

1. After four complete compression-ventilation cycles, reassess victim:
    - Assess for signs of breathing and circulation.
    - Take no more than 10 seconds to do this.
2. If signs of circulation are absent:
    - Resume CPR.
    - Start with chest compressions first.
3. If signs of circulation are present, assess for breathing.
    - If breathing is present:
        Place victim in recovery position.
        Monitor breathing and circulation.
    - If breathing is absent, provide rescue breathing:
        Provide one breath every 4 to 5 seconds.
        Monitor circulation closely.

Continuation of CPR

If CPR is continued:
- Reassess every few minutes.
- Do not interrupt CPR except in special circumstances.

Source: *2000 Handbook of emergency cardiovascular care for health care providers*, Dallas, 2000, American Heart Association.
*Rescuers should phone 911 for unresponsive adults before beginning CPR, except in the case of submersion, trauma, and drug intoxication/overdose.
†Lay rescuers are no longer taught a pulse check.

The pulse should be checked by the ventilating rescuer during the compressions to assess the effectiveness of compressions in two-rescuer CPR. Chest compressions are stopped for 5 seconds at the end of the first minute and every few minutes thereafter to determine whether the victim has resumed spontaneous breathing and circulation. The victim is also assessed for signs of coughing or spontaneous movements. The goal of CPR is the return of spontaneous breathing and circulation, but it is rarely achieved without more definitive therapy with ACLS.

Advanced Cardiac Life Support

Advanced cardiac life support (ACLS) involves a systematic approach to treatment of cardiac emergencies with knowledge and skills necessary to provide early treatment.[26] ACLS includes the primary survey and the secondary survey (see Chapter 67, Tables 67-3 and 67-5). In addition, the ACLS curriculum includes algorithms for the treatment of specific arrhythmia groups, as well as guidelines for clinical management of MI, acute myocardial ischemia, pulmonary edema, shock, stroke, drowning, hypothermia, and drug overdose.

The principle of early defibrillation has been emphasized in national emergency medical care organizations. With the invention of the AED, which is simple to use and available throughout communities, more trained rescuers are available to provide early defibrillation. The importance of early, effective BLS and defibrillation before entrance into the ACLS system cannot be overemphasized. Drugs used in ACLS are listed in Table 35-16.

Medical professionals trained in ACLS are taught treatment algorithms that are guidelines for treatment of specific cardiac emergencies. The algorithm can be adjusted to fit the needs of a particular patient or situation. Emphasis is placed on maintaining the basics of airway, breathing, and circulation and making judgments for effective treatment based on overall patient assessment.[26]

Nursing Role during a Code

There is potential for a "code," or cardiopulmonary arrest situation, in all health care settings. The nurse should be well prepared to participate in resuscitation of a patient. The nurse must

TABLE 35-16	**Drug Therapy** Drugs Used in Advanced Cardiac Life Support
CLASS	**DRUG**
Adrenergic agonist (sympathomimetic)	dobutamine (Dobutrex)
	dopamine (Intropin)
	epinephrine (Adrenalin)
	norepinephrine (Levophed)
Alkalizing agent	sodium bicarbonate
Antianginal, vasodilator	nitroglycerin
Antiarrhythmic	adenosine (Adenocard)
	amiodarone (Cordarone)
	ibutilide (Corvert)
	lidocaine
	procainamide (Pronestyl)
Anticholinergic	atropine sulfate
β-Adrenergic receptor blockers	atenolol (Tenormin)
	esmolol (Brevibloc)
	metoprolol (Toprol XL)
Calcium channel blocker	diltiazem (Cardizem)
Diuretic	furosemide (Lasix)
Electrolyte	magnesium sulfate
Cardiac glycoside	digoxin (Lanoxin)
Narcotic analgesic	morphine sulfate
Tranquilizer, amnesiac, sedative	diazepam (Valium)
	midazolam (Versed)
Vasoconstrictor	vasopressin (Pitressin)

be familiar with code protocols, be familiar with emergency equipment in the crash cart, and keep current with BLS and ACLS skills.

It is important for the nurse to be familiar with the crash cart location and contents. Most crash carts contain all necessary emergency supplies. Ideally, all crash carts in a health care setting are organized in the same fashion.

CRITICAL THINKING EXERCISES

Case Study
Arrhythmia

Patient Profile. J.M., a 68-year-old retired white postal worker, is admitted to the cardiac care unit following cardiac arrest. Defibrillation was performed by paramedics at his home. J.M. is awake and lethargic but responding appropriately.

Subjective Data
- Has had two MIs and a history of CHF
- Has shortness of breath, even in a sitting position

Objective Data

Physical Examination
- Appears anxious
- BP 92/60, pulse 98/min, respirations 28/min
- Lungs: bilateral coarse crackles
- Heart: S₃ gallop at apex

Diagnostic Studies
- ECG: frequent PVCs
- Echocardiogram: severe left ventricular dysfunction with ejection fraction of 20%
- Serum potassium 2.9 mEq/L (2.9 mmol/L)

Collaborative Care
- Amiodarone (Cordarone) infusion
- Scheduled for electrophysiology study (EPS)

CRITICAL THINKING QUESTIONS

1. Why is J.M. at risk for sudden cardiac death (ventricular fibrillation)?
2. Explain the rationale for using amiodarone after ventricular fibrillation.
3. What methods may be used to assess the effectiveness of an antiarrhythmic drug?
4. Would J.M. be a candidate for an ICD?
5. If J.M. had ventricular fibrillation again while on a amiodarone infusion, what other IV medications would be tried?
6. Explain the significance of the serum potassium value.
7. Based on the assessment data provided, write one or more appropriate nursing diagnoses. Are there any collaborative problems?

REVIEW QUESTIONS

The number of the question corresponds to the same-numbered objective at the beginning of the chapter.

1. A patient with a stable blood pressure and no symptoms has the following electrocardiogram characteristics: atrial rate—74 and regular; ventricular rate—62 and irregular; P wave—normal contour; PR interval—lengthens progressively until a P wave is not conducted; QRS—normal contour. The nurse would expect that treatment would involve
   a. epinephrine 1 mg IV push.
   b. isoproterenol IV continuous drip.
   c. immediate insertion of a temporary pacemaker.
   d. careful observation for symptoms of hypotension.

2. The cardiac monitor of a patient in the cardiac care unit following an acute MI indicates ventricular bigeminy. The nurse anticipates
   a. performing defibrillation.
   b. treatment with IV lidocaine.
   c. insertion of a temporary pacemaker.
   d. continuing monitoring without other treatment.

3. The nurse prepares a patient for electrical cardioversion knowing that cardioversion differs from defibrillation in that
   a. defibrillation requires a greater dose of electrical current.
   b. defibrillation is synchronized to countershock during the QRS complex.
   c. cardioversion is indicated only for treatment of atrial tachyarrhythmias.
   d. cardioversion may be done on a nonemergency basis with sedation of the patient.

4. When providing discharge instructions to a patient with a new permanent pacemaker, the nurse teaches the patient to
   a. take and record a daily pulse rate.
   b. request special hand scanning at airport and other security gates.
   c. immobilize the arm and shoulder on the side of the pacemaker insertion for 6 weeks.
   d. avoid microwave ovens because they emit radio waves that alter pacemaker function.

5. The nurse plans care for the patient with an implantable cardioverter-defibrillator based on the knowledge that
   a. antiarrhythmia drugs can be discontinued.
   b. all members of the patient's family should learn CPR.
   c. the patient should not drive until 1 month after the ICD has been implanted.
   d. the patient is usually relieved to have the device implanted to prevent arrhythmias.

6. Important teaching for the patient who will be undergoing electrophysiologic monitoring includes explaining that
   a. a catheter will be placed in each of the femoral arteries to allow double-catheter use.
   b. the patient will be given a general anesthetic to prevent the awareness of "near-death" experiences.
   c. ventricular tachycardia and ventricular fibrillation may be induced and treated during the procedure.
   d. the procedure is used to "burn" or ablate areas of the conduction system that are causing tachyarrhythmias.

7. The proper sequence for care of the obstructed airway victim who becomes unconscious is
   a. finger sweep into mouth; attempt rescue breathing; call 911; abdominal thrust if still obstructed.
   b. attempt rescue breathing; abdominal thrusts if still obstructed; finger sweep into mouth; call 911.
   c. abdominal thrusts; finger sweep into mouth; call for second rescuer; attempt rescue breathing.
   d. call 911; finger sweep into mouth; attempt rescue breathing; abdominal thrusts if still obstructed.

8. A procedure that is common to both BLS and ACLS is
   a. use of ECG monitoring.
   b. administration of emergency cardiac drugs.
   c. establishment and maintenance of IV access.
   d. establishment and maintenance of a patent airway.

REFERENCES

1. Podrid PJ, Kowey PR: *Cardiac arrhythmia: mechanisms, diagnosis, and management,* ed 2, Philadelphia, 2001, Lippincott Williams & Wilkins.
2. Huszar RJ: *Basic dysrhythmias: interpretation and management,* ed 3, St Louis, 2002, Mosby.
3. Wagner G: *Marriott's practical electrocardiography,* ed 10, Philadelphia, 2001, Lippincott Williams & Wilkins.
4. Third report of the American College of Cardiology/American Heart Association Task Force on Practice Guidelines, *J Am Coll Cardiol* 34:890, 1999.
5. Drew BJ: Celebrating the 100th birthday of the electrocardiogram: lessons learned from research in cardiac monitoring, *Am J Crit Care* 11:378, 2002.
6. *2000 handbook of emergency cardiovascular care for healthcare providers,* Dallas, 2000, American Heart Association.
7. Bubien RS: Atrial fibrillation treatment rationale, *AACN Clin Issues* 12:140, 2001.
8. Peters NS et al: Atrial fibrillation: strategies to control, combat, and cure, *Lancet* 359:593, 2002.
9. Lip GY, Hee FL: Paroxysmal atrial fibrillation, *QJM Monthly Journal of the Association of Physicians* 94:665, 2001.
10. Hiller G: Atrial fibrillation, soothing the savage beat, *Nursing 99* 30:27, 1999.
11. Saliba WI: Dofetilide (Tikosyn): a new drug to control atrial fibrillation, *Cleve Clin J Med* 68:353, 2001.
12. IV amiodarone, *DCCN* 19:29, 2000.
13. Greenbaum RA: Conversion of atrial fibrillation and maintenance of sinus rhythm by dofetilide. The EMERALD study, *Circulation* 27:98(suppl 1):1, 1998.
14. Ballew S: Medicines and management of ventricular dysrhythmias, *AACN Clin Issues* 12:140, 2001.
15. Roden DM: Mechanisms and management of proarrhythmia, *Am J Cardiol* 82:491, 1998.
16. Ellenbogen K, Kay G, Willicoff B, editors: *Clinical cardiac pacing and defibrillation,* ed 2, Philadelphia, 2000, WB Saunders.
17. Thomas F: Living with an implantable cardioverter-defibrillator, *AACN Clin Issues* 12:156, 2001.
18. Shaffer RS: ICD therapy: the patient's perspective, *Am J Nurs* 102:46, 2002.
19. What's the difference between a pacemaker and an implantable cardioverter defibrillator (ICD)? *Johns Hopkins Medical Letter, Health After 50* 13:8, 2001.
20. Boyle J, Rost MK: Present status of cardiac pacing: a nursing perspective, *Crit Care Nurs Q* 23:1, 2000.
21. Chen SA, Tai CT: Ablation of atrioventricular accessory pathways: current technique—state of the art, *Pacing Clinical Electrophysiology* 24:1795, 2001.
22. Kaufmann H: Treatment of patients with orthostatic hypotension and syncope, *Clin Neuropharmacol* 25:133, 2002.
23. Colgan J: Syncope: a fall from grace, *Prog Cardiovasc Nurs* 17:66, 2002.
24. Asselin M, Cullen HA: New BLS guidelines, *Nursing* 31:48, 2001.
25. Eisenberg MS, Mengert TS: Primary care: cardiac resuscitation, *N Engl J Med* 344:17, 2001.
26. Asselin M, Cullen HA: New ACLS guidelines, *Nursing* 31:48, 2001.

RESOURCES

Resources for this chaper are listed after Chapter 33 on page 837 and Chapter 34 on page 860.

CHAPTER 36

NURSING MANAGEMENT

Inflammatory and Valvular Heart Diseases

Nancy Stoetzner Kupper
De Ann F. Mitchell

LEARNING OBJECTIVES

1. Describe the etiology, pathophysiology, and clinical manifestations of infective endocarditis and pericarditis.
2. Discuss the collaborative care and nursing management of infective endocarditis and pericarditis.
3. Explain the importance of prophylactic antibiotic therapy in infective endocarditis.
4. Explain the etiology, clinical manifestations, collaborative care, and nursing management of myocarditis.
5. Describe the etiology, pathophysiology, and clinical manifestations of rheumatic fever and rheumatic heart disease.
6. Discuss the collaborative care and nursing management of the patient with rheumatic fever and rheumatic heart disease.
7. Identify the etiologies of congenital and acquired valvular heart diseases.
8. Discuss the pathophysiology, clinical manifestations, and diagnostic studies for the various types of valvular heart problems.
9. Describe the collaborative care and nursing management of the patient with valvular heart disease.
10. Describe surgical interventions used in management of the patient with valvular heart problems.

KEY TERMS

acute rheumatic fever, p. 897
aortic stenosis, p. 904
aortic valve regurgitation, p. 904
Aschoff's bodies, p. 897
cardiac tamponade, p. 893
chronic constrictive pericarditis, p. 895
endomyocardial biopsy, p. 896
infective endocarditis, p. 886
Janeway's lesions, p. 887
mitral valve prolapse, p. 903
myocarditis, p. 896

Osler's nodes, p. 887
pericardial effusion, p. 893
pericardial friction rub, p. 893
pericardiocentesis, p. 894
pericarditis, p. 892
regurgitation, p. 901
rheumatic fever, p. 897
rheumatic heart disease, p. 897
stenosis, p. 901
vegetation, p. 887

Inflammatory Disorders of the Heart

INFECTIVE ENDOCARDITIS

Infective endocarditis, previously known as *bacterial endocarditis,* is an infection of the endocardial surface of the heart.[1] The *endocardium,* the inner layer of the heart (Fig. 36-1), is contiguous with the valves of the heart. Therefore inflammation from infective endocarditis usually affects the cardiac valves.

Before the era of antibiotics, infective endocarditis was almost always fatal. The advent of penicillin therapy changed the prognosis dramatically, and mortality rates decreased appreciably. For example, the mortality rate of infective endocarditis from *Streptococcus viridans* is now less than 10%. In spite of the relatively uncommon nature of the disease, an estimated 5000 to 8000 new cases of infective endocarditis are diagnosed in the United States each year.[2]

Classification

Two forms of infective endocarditis, subacute and acute, have been described. The *subacute form* has a longer clinical course of more insidious onset and the causative organism is usually of low virulence (Table 36-1). In contrast, the *acute form* has a shorter clinical course with a more rapid onset and the organism is more virulent (see Table 36-1).[1] Although this classification system has been used historically and may be conceptually useful, clinicians prefer to classify infective endocarditis based on the etiologic agent or site of involvement such as prosthetic valve or native valve.

Etiology and Pathophysiology

The most common causative agents are bacterial, especially *Staphylococcus aureus, Streptococcus viridans, Streptococcus pyogenes* (a type of group A *Streptococcus*), and *Streptococcus*

FIG. 36-1 Layers of the heart.

Reviewed by Angela J. DiSabatino, RN, MS, Manager, Cardiovascular Research Program, Christiana Care Health Services, Newark, Del.

TABLE 36-1	**Etiologic Organisms Associated with Infective Endocarditis**

Organisms Usually Associated with Subacute Infection
Enterococci
Streptococcus bovis
Streptococcus viridans
Staphylococcus epidermidis
Coagulase-negative staphylococci
HACEK group *(Haemophilus, Actinobacillus, Cardiobacterium, Eikenella, Kingella)*

Organisms Usually Associated with Acute Infection
Streptococcus pneumoniae
Staphylococcus aureus
Streptococcus groups A, B, and C
Fungi

TABLE 36-2	**Predisposing Conditions for the Development of Infective Endocarditis**

Cardiac Conditions
Rheumatic heart disease
Aortic valve leaflet abnormalities
Mitral valve prolapse with murmur
Cyanotic congenital heart disease
Prosthetic valves
Degenerative valvular lesions
Prior endocarditis
Marfan syndrome
Asymmetric septal hypertrophy
Idiopathic hypertrophic subaortic stenosis

Noncardiac Diseases
Intravenous illicit drug use
Nosocomial bacteremia

Procedure-Associated Risks
Intravascular devices (leading to nosocomial bacteremia)
Procedures listed in Table 36-5

pneumoniae (see Table 36-1). Other possible pathogens include fungi, chlamydiae, rickettsiae, and viruses.

Infective endocarditis occurs when blood flow turbulence within the heart allows the causative organism to infect previously damaged valves or other endothelial surfaces. The damage may occur in individuals with underlying cardiac conditions (Table 36-2). A variety of invasive procedures (e.g., surgical interventions, intravenous injections, diagnostic procedures) can allow large numbers of organisms to enter the bloodstream and initiate the infectious process (see Tables 36-2 and 36-5).

Until recently rheumatic heart disease was the most common cause of infective endocarditis. Currently the main contributing factors include (1) aging (older people have more degenerative heart disease and undergo more invasive testing), (2) intravenous (IV) drug abuse, and (3) increased survival rate of children with congenital heart disease.[3] With the increasing use of valve replacement, the incidence of prosthetic valve endocarditis has continued to rise.[4] Left-sided endocarditis is more common in patients with bacterial infections and underlying heart disease. The primary cause of right-sided (tricuspid) lesions is IV drug abuse, especially cocaine abuse. Staphylococcal infections frequently occur in this patient population, although gram-negative bacilli or fungi may be the infecting organisms.

Vegetation, the primary lesions of infective endocarditis, consists of fibrin, leukocytes, platelets, and microbes that adhere to the valve surface or endocardium (Fig. 36-2). The loss of portions of these friable types of vegetation into the circulation results in *embolization.* Systemic embolization occurs from left-sided heart vegetation, progressing to organ (particularly the brain, kidneys, and spleen) and limb infarction. Right-sided heart lesions embolize to the lungs.

The infection may spread locally to cause damage to the valves or to their supporting structures. The resulting valvular incompetence and eventual invasion of the myocardium in the infectious disease result in congestive heart failure (CHF), generalized myocardial dysfunction, and sepsis (Fig. 36-3).

Clinical Manifestations

The findings in infective endocarditis are nonspecific and can involve multiple organ systems. Fever occurs in more than 90% of patients. Other nonspecific manifestations that may accom-

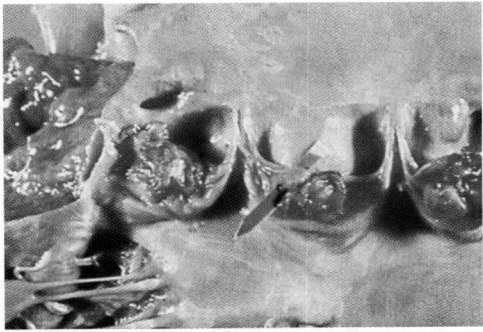

FIG. 36-2 Bacterial endocarditis of the mitral valve (caused by *Streptococcus viridans*).

pany fever include chills, weakness, malaise, fatigue, and anorexia. Arthralgias, myalgias, back pain, abdominal discomfort, weight loss, headache, and clubbing of fingers may occur in subacute forms of endocarditis.

Vascular manifestations of infective endocarditis include splinter hemorrhages (black longitudinal streaks) that may occur in the nail beds. Petechiae may occur as a result of fragmentation and microembolization of vegetative lesions and are common in the conjunctivae, the lips, the buccal mucosa, the palate, and over the ankles, the feet, and the antecubital and popliteal areas. **Osler's nodes** (painful, tender, red or purple, pea-size lesions) may be found on the fingertips or toes. **Janeway's lesions** (flat, painless, small, red spots) may be found on the palms and soles. Funduscopic examination may reveal hemorrhagic retinal lesions called *Roth's spots.*

The onset of a new murmur is noted in 80% of cases with infective endocarditis, with the aortic and mitral valves most commonly affected. The mitral murmur of endocarditis is generally a mid-to-late systolic regurgitant type. The aortic murmur may be early diastolic. Murmurs are often absent in tricuspid endocardi-

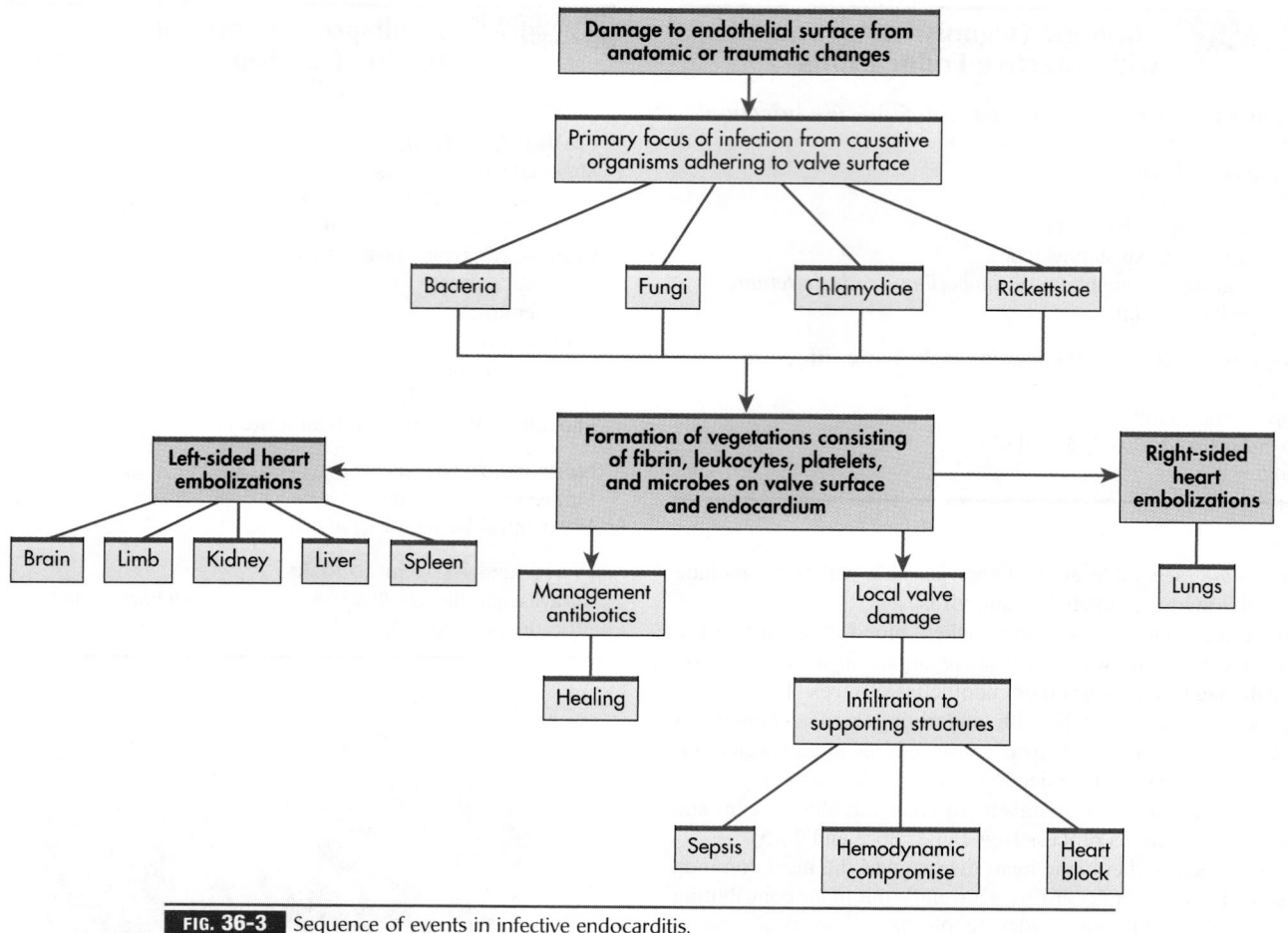

FIG. 36-3   Sequence of events in infective endocarditis.

tis because right-sided heart pressures are too low to be heard. CHF occurs in up to 80% of patients with aortic valve endocarditis and in approximately 50% of patients with mitral valve endocarditis.[5]

Clinical manifestations secondary to embolization in various body organs may also be present. Embolization to the spleen may result in sharp, left upper quadrant pain and splenomegaly. Local tenderness and abdominal rigidity may be present. Embolization to the kidneys may cause pain in the flank, hematuria, and azotemia. Emboli may lodge in small peripheral blood vessels of arms and legs and may cause gangrene. Embolization to the brain may cause neurologic problems such as hemiplegia, ataxia, aphasia, visual changes, and change in the level of consciousness. Pulmonary emboli may occur in right-sided endocarditis.

Diagnostic Studies

Obtaining the patient's recent health history is important in assessing infective endocarditis. Inquiry should be made regarding any recent (within the past 3 to 6 months) dental, urologic, surgical, or gynecologic procedures, including normal or abnormal obstetric delivery. Previous history of heart disease; recent cardiac catheterization; and skin, respiratory, or urinary tract infections should be documented.

Laboratory data, especially blood cultures, should also be assessed (Table 36-3). Blood cultures are the primary diagnostic tool for the evaluation of infective endocarditis. Positive blood cultures are found in 90% to 95% of patients with infective endocarditis. Two or three sets of blood cultures (a set consists of one aerobic and one anaerobic culture from one site) should be performed over a 24-hour period to assess for sustained bacteremia.[6] Negative cultures should be kept for 3 weeks if the clinical diagnosis remains endocarditis, because of the possibility of a slow-growing, causative organism. The blood cultures may be obtained at 20-minute intervals if immediate antibiotic therapy is deemed necessary. Blood-culture bottles containing a resin to bind the antibiotic should be used if the patient is already receiving antibiotics. Culture-negative endocarditis may occur in those patients who have had previous antibiotic therapy, in patients with causative organisms that cannot be grown from blood using routine media (e.g., *Mycobacterium tuberculosis*), or in patients with right-sided infection of the heart.

A mild leukocytosis occurs in acute endocarditis (uncommon in subacute) with average white blood cell (WBC) counts ranging from 10,000 to 11,000/μl (10 to 11 × 10^9/L). Erythrocyte sedimentation rates (ESRs) greater than 30 mm per hour are found in almost all cases. Proteinuria and positive rheumatoid factor may also be present in some patients with endocarditis.

Echocardiography is valuable in the diagnostic workup for a patient with infective endocarditis when the blood cultures are negative, or for the patient who is a surgical candidate and has an active infection. Transesophageal echocardiograms and digital

TABLE 36-3   Collaborative Care: Infective Endocarditis

Diagnostic
History and physical examination
Blood culture and sensitivity
WBC count with differential
Rheumatoid factor
Urinalysis
Chest x-ray
ECG
Echocardiography
Cardiac catheterization

Collaborative Therapy
Appropriate antibiotic therapy
Antipyretics
Rest
Repeat of blood cultures and sensitivity tests
Surgical valve repair or replacement (for severe valvular damage)

ECG, Electrocardiogram; *WBC,* white blood cell.

TABLE 36-4   Antibiotic Prophylaxis for Cardiac Conditions to Prevent Endocarditis*

High Risk Conditions
Prosthetic heart valve (including biosynthetic valve)
History of endocarditis
Surgically constructed systemic–pulmonary shunts

Moderate Risk Conditions
Organic heart murmur
Mitral valve prolapse with valvular regurgitation

Low Risk Conditions (No Prophylaxis)
"Functional," "physiologic," or "innocent" heart murmur
Mitral valve prolapse without valvular regurgitation
History of rheumatic fever without heart murmur

Source: American Heart Association.
*This table lists common conditions, but it is not all-inclusive.

TABLE 36-5   Procedures That Require Antibiotic Prophylaxis to Prevent Endocarditis*

Oropharyngeal
All dental procedures likely to produce gingival or mucosal bleeding (not simple adjustment of orthodontic appliances or shedding of deciduous teeth), including professional cleaning
Tonsillectomy or adenoidectomy

Respiratory
Surgical procedures or biopsy involving respiratory mucosa
Bronchoscopy, especially with a rigid bronchoscope

Gastrointestinal
Abdominal surgeries
Laparoscopy procedures
Esophageal dilation
Sclerotherapy of esophageal varices
Colonoscopy

Genitourinary
Cystoscopy
Laparoscopy procedures
Prostatic surgery
Urethral catheterization (in presence of infection)
Urinary tract surgery (in presence of infection)
Vaginal hysterectomy
Vaginal delivery in presence of infection

Cardiac
Placement of prosthetic heart valves
Surgically constructed systemic pulmonary shunts

*This table lists selected procedures and is not all-inclusive.

---

imaging using two-dimensional transthoracic echocardiograms can detect vegetation and abscesses on valves.[7]

A chest x-ray examination is done to detect the presence of an enlarged heart. An electrocardiogram (ECG) may show first- or second-degree AV block because the cardiac valves lie in proximity to cardiac conductive tissue, especially the atrioventricular (AV) node. Cardiac catheterization may be used to evaluate valve functioning when surgical intervention is being considered for patients with infective endocarditis.

Collaborative Care

Prophylactic Treatment. The principal risk factors for infective endocarditis are cardiac lesions, prosthetic valves, acquired valvular disease, mitral valve prolapse, prior endocarditis, and noncardiac diseases. Antibiotic prophylaxis is recommended for patients with specific cardiac conditions before they undergo certain dental or surgical procedures[8,9] (Table 36-4). Procedures that require endocarditis prophylaxis are summarized in Table 36-5. Specific antibiotic regimens are recommended for dental, respiratory tract, gastrointestinal (GI), and genitourinary (GU) procedures. Antibiotic prophylaxis should also be used for high risk patients who (1) are to undergo removal or drainage of infected tissue, (2) have indwelling cardiac pacemakers, (3) undergo renal dialysis, and (4) have ventriculoatrial shunts for management of hydrocephalus.[10]

Drug Therapy. When infective endocarditis has been diagnosed, accurate identification of the infecting organism is the key to successful treatment. The appropriate antibiotic (usually given intravenously) is chosen on the basis of sensitivity studies. The duration of therapy has to be sufficient to eradicate microorganisms growing within the valvular vegetations. Complete eradication of the organism generally takes weeks to achieve, and relapses are common. Traditionally this has meant a prolonged hospitalization for most patients with infective endocarditis. Currently, with the use of newer, more versatile antibiotics and in light of economic concerns, treatment of patients with infective endocarditis on an outpatient basis is becoming more common.[11] Table 36-6 outlines specific regimens for outpatient therapy of patients with endocarditis. Some patients require changes in antibiotics because of allergic reactions or other drug-related side effects.

The patient's antibiotic serum levels should be monitored periodically. Subsequent blood cultures may be performed to eval-

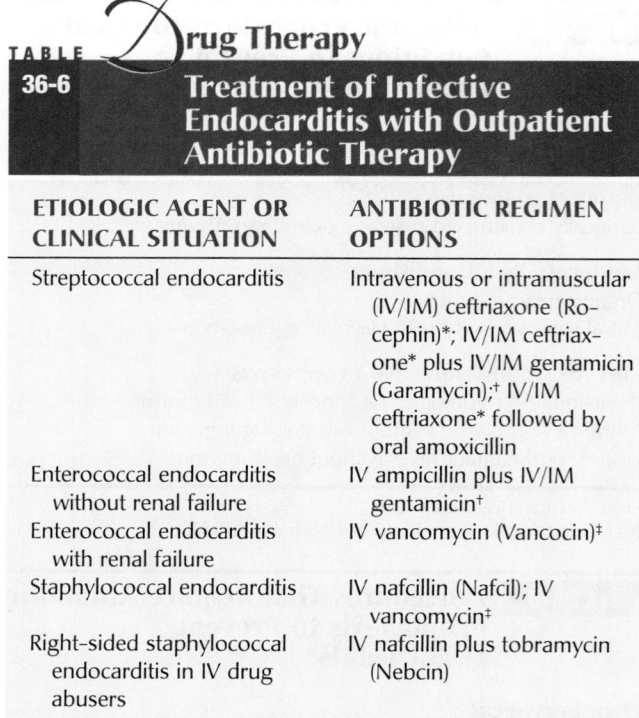

TABLE 36-6 Drug Therapy — Treatment of Infective Endocarditis with Outpatient Antibiotic Therapy

ETIOLOGIC AGENT OR CLINICAL SITUATION	ANTIBIOTIC REGIMEN OPTIONS
Streptococcal endocarditis	Intravenous or intramuscular (IV/IM) ceftriaxone (Rocephin)*; IV/IM ceftriaxone* plus IV/IM gentamicin (Garamycin);† IV/IM ceftriaxone* followed by oral amoxicillin
Enterococcal endocarditis without renal failure	IV ampicillin plus IV/IM gentamicin†
Enterococcal endocarditis with renal failure	IV vancomycin (Vancocin)‡
Staphylococcal endocarditis	IV nafcillin (Nafcil); IV vancomycin‡
Right-sided staphylococcal endocarditis in IV drug abusers	IV nafcillin plus tobramycin (Nebcin)

Source: Seto TB et al: Physicians' recommendations to patients for the use of antibiotic prophylaxis to prevent endocarditis, *JAMA* 284:68, 2000.
*Endocarditis is not a Food and Drug Administration (FDA)–approved indication for ceftriaxone therapy.
†Serum concentrations should be monitored.
‡Establish dose according to renal function and serum drug level.

uate the effectiveness of antibiotic therapy. Blood cultures that remain positive indicate inadequate or inappropriate antibiotic administration, aortic root or myocardial abscess, or the wrong diagnosis (e.g., an infection elsewhere). Fever may persist for several days after treatment has been started and can be treated with aspirin, acetaminophen, fluids, and rest. Complete bed rest is usually not indicated unless the temperature remains elevated or there are signs of heart failure.

The results of drug therapy alone are generally poor in patients with fungal endocarditis and prosthetic valve endocarditis. Early valve replacement followed by prolonged drug therapy is recommended in these situations. Valve replacement has become an important adjunct procedure in the management of endocarditis. It is used in more than 25% of cases. (Valve replacement is discussed later in this chapter.)

NURSING MANAGEMENT INFECTIVE ENDOCARDITIS

■ Nursing Assessment

Subjective and objective data that should be obtained from a patient with infective endocarditis are presented in Table 36-7. Heart sounds should be assessed together with vital signs to detect a change in the character of the cardiac murmur and the presence of extradiastolic sounds. *Arthralgia* is common and may involve multiple joints and may be accompanied by myalgias. The patient should be assessed for joint tenderness, decreased range of motion (ROM), and muscle tenderness. The

TABLE 36-7 Nursing Assessment — Infective Endocarditis

Subjective Data

Important Health Information

Past health history: Valvular, congenital, or syphilitic cardiac disease (including valve repair or replacement); previous endocarditis, childbirth, staphylococcal or streptococcal infections, nosocomial bacteremia

Medications: Immunosuppressive therapy

Surgery or other treatments: Recent obstetric or gynecologic procedures; invasive techniques including catheterization, cystoscopy, intravascular procedures; recent dental or surgical procedure

Functional Health Patterns

Health perception–health management: IV drug abuse, alcohol abuse; malaise

Nutritional-metabolic: Weight gain or loss; anorexia; chills, diaphoresis

Elimination: Bloody urine

Activity-exercise: Exercise intolerance, generalized weakness, fatigue; cough, dyspnea on exertion, orthopnea; palpitations

Sleep-rest: Night sweats

Cognitive-perceptual: Chest, back, or abdominal pain; headache; joint tenderness, muscle tenderness

Objective Data

General

Fever

Integumentary

Olser's nodes on extremities; splinter hemorrhages under nailbeds; Janeway's lesions on palms and soles; petechiae of skin, mucous membranes, or conjunctivae; purpura; peripheral edema, finger clubbing

Respiratory

Tachypnea, crackles

Cardiovascular

Arrhythmias, tachycardia, new or enhanced murmurs, S_3, S_4, retinal hemorrhages

Possible Findings

Leukocytosis, anemia, ↑ ESR and cardiac enzymes; positive blood cultures; microscopic hematuria; echocardiogram showing chamber enlargement, valvular dysfunction, and vegetations; chest x-ray showing cardiomegaly and pulmonary infiltrates; ECG demonstrating ischemia and conduction defects

ECG, Electrocardiogram; ESR, erythrocyte sedimentation rate.

oral mucosa, conjunctivae, upper chest, and lower extremities should be examined for petechiae. A general systems assessment should be completed to facilitate recognition of hemodynamic and embolic complications.

■ Nursing Diagnoses

Nursing diagnoses for the patient with infective endocarditis may include, but are not limited to, those presented in NCP 36-1.

■ Planning

The overall goals are that the patient with infective endocarditis will (1) have normal cardiac function, (2) have no residual cardiac damage, (3) perform activities of daily living (ADLs)

NURSING CARE PLAN 36-1

Patient with Infective Endocarditis

EXPECTED PATIENT OUTCOMES	NURSING INTERVENTIONS and *RATIONALES*

NURSING DIAGNOSIS   **Hyperthermia** *related to* infection of cardiac tissue *as manifested by* temperature elevation, diaphoresis, chills, headache, malaise, tachycardia, tachypnea.

• Normal temperature • Normal pulse (60-100 beats/min) • Normal respirations (12-20 breaths/min) • Absence of chills, diaphoresis, headache	• Monitor temperature *to determine effectiveness of therapy.* • Administer antipyretics and/or sedatives as ordered *to reduce fever and assist in sleep.* • Reduce physical activity *to decrease cardiac workload.* • Administer antibiotics *to treat the causative agent.* • Monitor blood cultures and WBC count *to evaluate patient's response to treatment.*

NURSING DIAGNOSIS   **Decreased cardiac output** *related to* valvular insufficiency and fluid overload *as manifested by* heart murmur, S_3, tachycardia, diminished peripheral pulses, adventitious breath sounds, decreased urine output, restlessness.

• Sufficient cardiac output to maintain mean arterial BP ≥60 mm Hg and urine output >0.5 ml/kg/hr	• Auscultate heart sounds, rate, and rhythm *to detect a change in the character of the cardiac murmur and the presence of extradiastolic sounds.* • Monitor for new onset of murmurs, *which could indicate infective endocarditis.* • Assess for peripheral and sacral edema *as indicators of ineffective circulation or fluid overload.* • Assess breath sounds *to identify pulmonary congestion and fluid overload.* • Provide O_2 therapy *to increase O_2 to the myocardium.* • Administer diuretics, inotropic therapy, and other medications as ordered *to promote diuresis and strengthen myocardial contractility.* • Assess urine output *to monitor renal function and evaluate fluid status.*

NURSING DIAGNOSIS   **Activity intolerance** *related to* generalized weakness and alteration in O_2 transport secondary to valvular dysfunction *as manifested by* fatigue, malaise, weakness, dyspnea, increased or decreased respiratory rate, and BP changes.

• Completion of activities of daily living with no to minimal fatigue or physiologic distress	• Monitor vital signs during activity *to evaluate cardiac response.* • Monitor for signs of activity intolerance (e.g., tachycardia, hypertension, diaphoresis, shortness of breath) *to plan or alter activities.* • Teach patient to check pulse rate and instruct patient to reduce activity if pulse increases >20 beats/min and to not increase activity if resting pulse >100 beats/per min *because these signs indicate excessive cardiac effort.* • Plan rest periods between activities *to reduce cardiac workload.*

NURSING DIAGNOSIS   **Ineffective health maintenance** *related to* lack of knowledge about disease and treatment process *as manifested by* nonperformance of desired prescribed health behaviors, verbalization of misconceptions about desired or prescribed health behaviors, requests for information.

Increased understanding of disease process and self-care management	• Assess patient's knowledge about disease and treatment process *to identify teaching needs.* • Discuss symptoms of recurrent infection (e.g., fatigue, malaise, chills, elevated temperature, anorexia) *so health care provider can be notified and treatment initiated promptly.* • Explain need to avoid persons with infections. • Encourage early treatment of common infections such as cold and flu *to reduce the risk of recurrent infective endocarditis.* • Explain need to report endocarditis history to the health care provider or dentist performing invasive procedures such as dental or gingival therapy, diagnostic tests, or medical and surgical procedures *so prophylactic antibiotic therapy can be initiated to prevent the possibility of infection.* • Discuss names of prescribed medications, dosages, times of administration, purpose, and side effects *to promote safe medication therapy.*

BP, Blood pressure; *WBC,* white blood cell.

without fatigue, and (4) understand the therapeutic regimen to prevent recurrence of endocarditis.

■ Nursing Implementation

Health Promotion. The incidence of infective endocarditis can be decreased by identifying individuals who are at risk for

the development of endocarditis (see Tables 36-2 and 36-4). Assessment of the patient's history and an understanding of the disease process are crucial for planning and implementing appropriate health promotion strategies.

Teaching the patient who is at risk or has had infective endocarditis helps reduce the incidence and recurrence of the disease.

Teaching is crucial for the patient's understanding of and adherence to the planned treatment regimen. The patient should understand the need to avoid persons with infection, especially upper respiratory infection, and to report cold, flu, and cough symptoms. The importance of avoiding excessive fatigue and the need to plan rest periods before and after activity should be carefully explained to the patient. Good oral hygiene, including daily care and regular dental visits, is also important. The patient must inform all health care providers performing dental, medical, or surgical procedures of the history of heart disease. The patient should understand the significance of the prescribed prophylactic antibiotic therapy before any invasive procedure.

Acute Intervention. A patient with infective endocarditis has many problems that require acute nursing management (see NCP 36-1). Infective endocarditis generally requires treatment with antibiotics for 4 to 6 weeks. The patient requires in-hospital treatment and then may be a candidate for outpatient parenteral antibiotic therapy.

Assessment findings are nonspecific (see Table 36-7) but can help confirm the diagnosis and assist with the treatment plan. Fever, chronic or intermittent, is a common early sign. Frequent assessment of body temperature is important because persistent, prolonged temperature elevations may mean that the drug therapy is ineffective.

The patient needs adequate periods of physical and emotional rest. Bed rest may be necessary when fever is present or when there are complications (e.g., heart damage). Otherwise the patient may ambulate and perform moderate activity.

Laboratory data should be monitored to determine the effectiveness of the long-term, high-dose antibiotic therapy. IV lines should be monitored for patency, and antibiotics should be given when scheduled. The patient should be monitored continuously for undesirable reactions to drugs. To prevent problems because of immobility, the patient should wear elastic compression gradient stockings, perform ROM exercises, and turn, cough, and deep breathe every 2 hours.

The patient may experience anxiety and fear associated with the illness. The nurse must recognize this problem and implement strategies to help reduce the patient's fears and anxieties.

Ambulatory and Home Care. Patients who receive outpatient antibiotics will require vigilant home nursing care. Patients with active endocarditis are at risk for life-threatening complications, such as cerebral emboli and pulmonary edema. The adequacy of the home environment in terms of in-home companions and hospital access must be determined for successful management. After therapy is completed in either the home or the hospital setting, management will focus on teaching the patient about the nature of the disease and on reducing the risk of reinfection. The patient should be instructed about symptoms that may indicate recurrent infection, such as fever, fatigue, malaise, and chills. If any of these symptoms occur, the patient should be aware of the importance of notifying the health care provider. The patient must be instructed about the need for prophylactic antibiotic therapy before any invasive procedure is performed (see Table 36-5). The nurse must explain to the patient the relationship of follow-up care, good nutrition, and early treatment of common infections (e.g., colds) to maintain good health.

■ Evaluation

Expected outcomes for the patient with infective endocarditis are presented in NCP 36-1.

ACUTE PERICARDITIS

Pericarditis is a condition caused by inflammation of the pericardial sac (the pericardium), which may occur on an acute basis. The pericardium is composed of the inner serous membrane (visceral pericardium) that closely adheres to the epicardial surface of the heart and the outer fibrous (parietal) layer (see Fig. 36-1). The pericardial space is the cavity between these two layers, and in the normal state it contains less than 50 ml of serous fluid. Although the pericardium may be congenitally absent or surgically removed, it serves a useful anchoring function, provides lubrication to decrease friction during systolic and diastolic heart movements, and assists in preventing excessive dilation of the heart during diastole.

Etiology and Pathophysiology

The common causes of acute pericarditis are listed in Table 36-8. Acute pericarditis most often is idiopathic, with a variety of suspected viral causes. The coxsackievirus B group is the most commonly identified virus. In addition to idiopathic or viral pericarditis, other causes of this syndrome include uremia, bacterial infection, acute myocardial infarction (MI), tuberculosis, neoplasm, and trauma.[12] Pericarditis in the acute MI patient may be described as two distinct syndromes. The first is *acute pericarditis*, which may occur within the initial 48 to 72 hours after an MI. The second is *Dressler syndrome* (late pericarditis), which appears 2 to 4 weeks after infarction (see Chapter 33).

TABLE 36-8	Etiologies of Pericarditis

Infectious

Viral: Coxsackievirus A and B, echovirus, adenovirus, mumps, Epstein-Barr, varicella zoster, hepatitis B, human immunodeficiency virus

Bacterial: Pneumococci, staphylococci, streptococci, *Neisseria gonorrhoeae*, *Legionella pneumophila*, septicemia from gram-negative organisms

Tuberculosis

Fungal: Histoplasma, *Candida* species

Infections: Toxoplasmosis, Lyme disease

Noninfectious

Uremia

Acute myocardial infarction

Neoplasms: Lung cancer, breast cancer, leukemia, Hodgkin's disease, lymphoma

Trauma: Thoracic surgery, pacemaker insertion, cardiac diagnostic procedures

Radiation

Dissecting aortic aneurysm

Myxedema

Hypersensitive or Autoimmune

Delayed post–myocardial-pericardial injury

Post–myocardial infarction (Dressler) syndrome

Postpericardiotomy syndrome

Rheumatic fever

Drug reactions (e.g., procainamide [Pronestyl], hydralazine [Apresoline])

Rheumatologic diseases: Rheumatoid arthritis, systemic lupus erythematosus, systemic sclerosis (scleroderma), ankylosing spondylitis

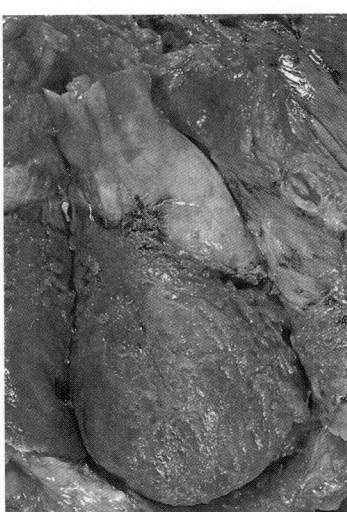

FIG. 36-4 Acute fibrinous pericarditis. There is a shaggy coat of fibrin covering the surface of the heart.

An inflammatory response is the characteristic pathologic finding in acute pericarditis. There is an influx of neutrophils, increased pericardial vascularity, and eventually fibrin deposition on the visceral pericardium (Fig. 36-4).

Clinical Manifestations

Characteristic clinical manifestations found in acute pericarditis include chest pain, dyspnea, and a pericardial friction rub. The intense, pleuritic chest pain is generally sharpest over the left precordium or retrosternally but may radiate to the trapezius ridge and neck (mimicking angina), or sometimes to the epigastrium or abdomen (mimicking abdominal or other noncardiac pathologic conditions). The pain is aggravated by lying supine, deep breathing, coughing, swallowing, and moving the trunk and is eased by sitting up and leaning forward. The dyspnea accompanying acute pericarditis is related to the patient's need to breathe in rapid, shallow breaths to avoid chest pain and may be aggravated by fever and anxiety.

The hallmark finding in acute pericarditis is the **pericardial friction rub.** The rub is a scratching, grating, high-pitched sound believed to arise from friction between the roughened pericardial and epicardial surfaces.[13] It is best heard with the stethoscope diaphragm firmly placed at the lower left sternal border of the chest. The pericardial friction rub does not radiate widely or vary in timing from the heartbeat, but it may require frequent auscultation to identify because it may be elusive and transient. Timing the pericardial friction rub with the pulse (and not respirations) will help distinguish it from pleural rub.

Complications

Two major complications that may result from acute pericarditis are pericardial effusion and cardiac tamponade. **Pericardial effusion** is an accumulation of excess fluid in the pericardium. It can occur rapidly (e.g., chest trauma) or slowly (e.g., tuberculous pericarditis). Large effusions may compress adjoining structures. Pulmonary tissue compression can cause cough, dyspnea, and tachypnea. Phrenic nerve compression can induce hiccups, and compression of the recurrent laryngeal nerve may

result in hoarseness. Heart sounds are generally distant and muffled, although blood pressure (BP) is usually maintained by compensatory mechanisms.

Cardiac tamponade develops as the pericardial effusion increases in size. It occurs because of an increase in intrapericardial pressure caused by fluid accumulation in the pericardial space. This results in compression of the heart. The speed of fluid accumulation affects the severity of clinical manifestations. Cardiac tamponade can occur acutely (e.g., rupture of heart, trauma) or subacutely (e.g., secondary to uremia, malignancy). The patient with cardiac tamponade is often confused, agitated, and restless and has tachycardia and tachypnea with a low-output state (Table 36-9). The neck veins are usually markedly distended because of jugular venous pressure elevation, and a significant pulsus paradoxus is present. *Pulsus paradoxus,* an inspiratory drop in systolic BP greater than 10 mm Hg, results because the normal inspiratory decline in systolic BP of less than 10 mm Hg is exaggerated in cardiac tamponade. (The technique for measurement of pulsus paradoxus is outlined in Table 36-10.) In a patient with a slow onset of a cardiac tamponade, dyspnea may be the only clinical manifestation.

TABLE 36-9	**Clinical Manifestations of Cardiac Tamponade**

Anxiety
Chest pain
Decrease in systolic blood pressure
Increase in venous pressure, distention of neck veins
Low-voltage electrocardiogram
Muffled heart sounds
Narrowing pulse pressure
Peripheral cyanosis
Possible friction rub
Pulsus paradoxus (>10 mm Hg)
Rapid enlargement of cardiac silhouette on chest x-ray
Tachycardia
Tachypnea

TABLE 36-10	**Measurement of Pulsus Paradoxus**

1. Make determination during quiet breathing with stable rhythm.
2. Determine systolic blood pressure.
3. Inflate blood pressure cuff until no sounds are heard with stethoscope.
4. Deflate cuff slowly until systolic sounds are heard on expiration, and note the pressure.
5. Deflate cuff until systolic sounds are heard throughout the respiratory cycle, and note the pressure.
6. Determine the difference between the measurements taken in steps 4 and 5. This will equal the amount of paradox:

Sounds heard in expiration at	110 mm Hg
Sounds heard throughout cycle at	82 mm Hg
Amount of paradox	28 mm Hg

The difference is usually less than 10 mm Hg. If the difference is greater than 10 mm Hg, cardiac tamponade may be present.

Diagnostic Studies

Electrocardiogram (ECG) changes in acute pericarditis are key diagnostic clues and evolve over a period of hours to days or weeks (Table 36-11). Four stages of ECG changes have been described: (1) initial diffuse ST segment elevations that concave upward and are present in all leads except aVR and V_1; (2) return of ST segments to baseline with T wave flattening several days later; (3) T wave inversion without the appearance of significant Q waves seen in acute MI; and (4) reversion of T wave changes to normal that may occur weeks or months later. PR segment depression may also be present in the early stages of ST segment changes. The changes are believed to be caused by superficial myocardial inflammation or epicardial injury. Arrhythmias can accompany these ECG changes but are generally rare occurrences. When encountered, there are usually atrial arrhythmias in patients who also have myocardial or valvular pathologic conditions.

The chest x-ray findings are generally normal or nonspecific in acute pericarditis unless the patient has a large pericardial effusion (Fig. 36-5). Echocardiographic findings are much more useful in determining the presence of a pericardial effusion or cardiac tamponade. Additional diagnostic studies such as radionuclide cardiac scans may be performed, although their sensitivity in diagnosing pericarditis has not yet been determined.

Laboratory testing focuses on the possible etiology of the pericarditis. For example, elevated blood urea nitrogen (BUN) levels and serum creatinine levels may indicate uremic pericarditis, or a positive tuberculin skin test may suggest tuberculous pericarditis. The fluid obtained during pericardiocentesis (Fig. 36-6) or the tissue from a pericardial biopsy may also be analyzed to determine the cause of the pericarditis.

Collaborative Care

Management of acute pericarditis is directed toward identification and treatment of the underlying problem (see Table 36-11). Antibiotics should be used to treat bacterial pericarditis. Corticosteroids are generally reserved for patients with pericarditis secondary to systemic lupus erythematosus, patients already taking corticosteroids for a rheumatologic or other immune system condition, or patients who do not respond to nonsteroidal antiinflammatory drugs (NSAIDs). When necessary, prednisone is usually given according to a tapering dosage schedule. Discriminate and careful administration of corticosteroids is advised because of their numerous side effects, such as upper GI bleeding, sodium retention, hyperglycemia, hypokalemia, and Cushing syndrome (see Chapter 48).

The pain and inflammation of acute pericarditis are usually treated with NSAIDs. High-dose salicylates (300 to 900 mg orally four times a day) or NSAIDs, such as indomethacin (Indocin), are commonly used.

Pericardiocentesis (see Fig. 36-6) is usually performed when acute cardiac tamponade has reduced the patient's systolic BP 30 mm Hg or more from baseline. Hemodynamic support for the patient being prepared for the pericardiocentesis may include ad-

TABLE 36-11	Collaborative Care
Acute Pericarditis	

Diagnostic
History and physical examination
Auscultation of chest
ECG
BUN, serum creatinine
TB test
Chest x-ray
Echocardiogram
Pericardiocentesis
Pericardial biopsy
CT scan
Cardiac nuclear scan

Collaborative Therapy
Treatment of underlying disease
Bed rest
Aspirin
Nonsteroidal antiinflammatory drugs
Corticosteroids
Pericardiocentesis (for large pericardial effusion or tamponade)

BUN, Blood urea nitrogen; *CT,* computed tomography; *ECG,* electrocardiogram; *TB,* tuberculosis.

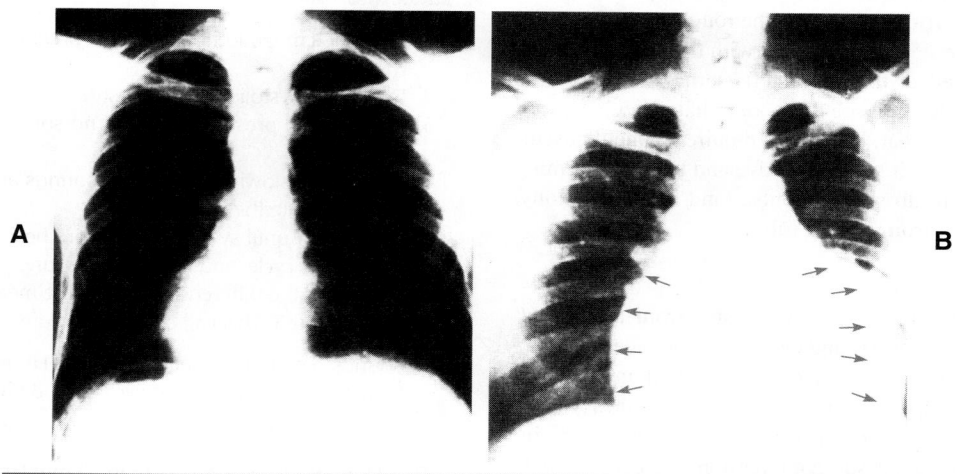

FIG. 36-5 **A,** X-ray of a normal chest. **B,** Pericardial effusion is present and the cardiac silhouette is enlarged with a globular shape *(arrows).*

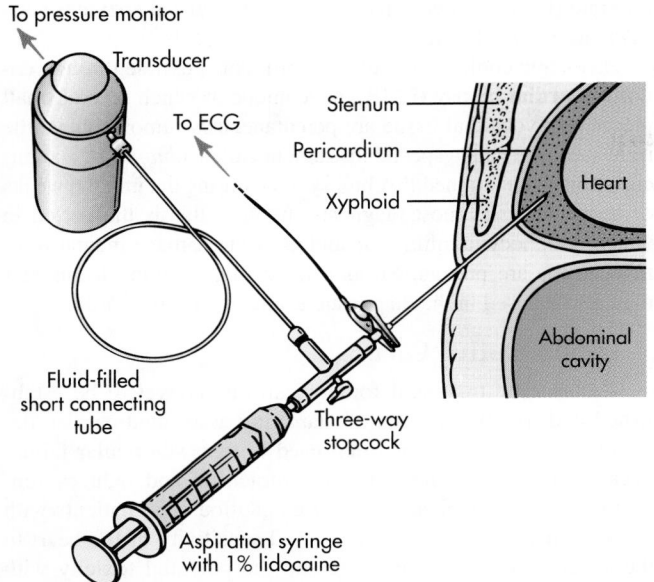

FIG. 36-6 Pericardiocentesis performed under sterile conditions in conjunction with electrocardiogram (ECG) and hemodynamic measurements.

ministration of volume expanders and inotropic agents (e.g., dopamine [Intropin]). The procedure is usually performed in the cardiac care unit or cardiac catheterization laboratory under sterile conditions and in conjunction with ECG, echocardiogram, and hemodynamic measurements. A 16- to 18-gauge needle is inserted into the pericardial space to remove fluid for analysis and to relieve cardiac pressure. Complications from pericardiocentesis include arrhythmias, pneumomediastinum, pneumothorax, myocardial laceration, cardiac tamponade, coronary artery laceration, and gastric fistula.

NURSING MANAGEMENT
ACUTE PERICARDITIS

The management of the patient's pain and anxiety during acute pericarditis is a primary nursing consideration. Assessment of the amount, quality, and location of the pain is important, particularly in distinguishing the pain of acute MI (or reinfarction) from the pain of pericarditis. Careful nursing observations should be made regarding ischemic chest pain, which is generally located retrosternal in the left shoulder and arm with a pressure-like, burning quality and is unaffected by posture. In contrast, pericarditic pain is usually located in the precordium, left trapezius ridge and has a sharp, pleuritic quality that changes with respirations. Relief from this pain is often obtained by leaning forward, and the pain is worsened by recumbency. The ECG also aids in distinguishing these types of pain because acute MI usually involves localized ST segment changes, as compared with the ST segment changes present in all ECG leads except aV$_R$ and V$_1$ during acute pericarditis.

Pain relief measures include maintaining the patient on bed rest with the head of the bed elevated to 45 degrees and providing a padded overbed table for the patient. Antiinflammatory medications help alleviate the patient's pain. However, because of the potential for upper GI bleeding with the use of high doses

of these medications, nursing interventions should be directed toward management of this potential problem. Specific interventions include the administration of these drugs with food or milk and instruction of the patient to avoid any alcoholic beverages while taking the medications.

Anxiety-reducing measures for the patient with acute pericarditis include providing simple, complete explanations of all procedures performed. These explanations are particularly important for the patient whose diagnosis of acute pericarditis is being established and for the patient who has already experienced an acute MI and has Dressler syndrome.

The real potential for decreased cardiac output (CO) also exists for the patient with acute pericarditis because of the possibility of cardiac tamponade. Monitoring for the signs and symptoms of tamponade (see Table 36-9) and making preparations for possible pericardiocentesis are important nursing responsibilities.

CHRONIC CONSTRICTIVE PERICARDITIS
Etiology and Pathophysiology

Chronic constrictive pericarditis results from scarring with consequent loss of elasticity of the pericardial sac. It usually begins with an initial episode of acute pericarditis (often secondary to neoplasia, radiation, previous surgery, or idiopathic causes) and is characterized by fibrin deposition with a clinically undetected pericardial effusion. Resorption of the effusion slowly follows with progression toward the chronic stage of fibrous scarring, thickening of the pericardium from calcium deposition, and eventual obliteration of the pericardial space. The fibrotic, thickened, and adherent pericardium encases the heart, thereby impairing the ability of the atria and ventricles to stretch adequately during diastolic filling.

Clinical Manifestations

Manifestations of chronic constrictive pericarditis occur over an extended time period and mimic those of CHF and cor pulmonale. Many of the clinical manifestations are related to decreased cardiac output. They include dyspnea on exertion, lower extremity edema, ascites, fatigue, anorexia, and weight loss. The most prominent finding at the physical examination is elevated jugular venous pressure. Unlike cardiac tamponade, the presence of significant pulsus paradoxus is uncommon. Auscultatory findings include a *pericardial knock,* which is a loud early diastolic sound often heard along the left sternal border.

Diagnostic Studies

ECG changes may be nonspecific in chronic constrictive pericarditis but usually consist of low QRS voltage, generalized T wave inversion or flattening, and either P mitrale or atrial fibrillation. The cardiac silhouette on the chest x-ray may be normal or enlarged depending on the degree of pericardial thickening and the presence of a coexisting pericardial effusion. Echocardiographic findings may reveal a thickened pericardium, but without the presence of a large pericardial effusion.

Cardiac catheterization pressure tracings are more specific diagnostic tools in constrictive pericarditis. Abnormalities include elevation of the right and left atrial pressures with equilibration of these pressures during diastole. Other valuable diagnostic tools used to evaluate this condition are computed tomography (CT) and magnetic resonance imaging (MRI).

NURSING *and* COLLABORATIVE MANAGEMENT
CHRONIC CONSTRICTIVE PERICARDITIS

Unless the patient is free of symptoms or the condition is inoperable, the treatment of choice for chronic constrictive pericarditis is a *pericardiectomy*. The pericardiectomy usually involves complete resection of the pericardium through a median sternotomy with the use of cardiopulmonary bypass. After surgery some patients show immediate improvement, but others may take weeks. The postoperative prognosis is improved when the surgery is performed before the development of severe clinical disability.

MYOCARDITIS

Etiology and Pathophysiology

Myocarditis is a focal or diffuse inflammation of the myocardium. Possible causes include viruses, bacteria, rickettsiae, fungi, parasites, radiation, and pharmacologic and chemical factors. Viruses are the most common etiologic agent in the United States and Canada, with a predominance of RNA viruses (coxsackievirus A and B, echovirus, influenza A and B, and mumps virus). Certain medical conditions such as metabolic disorders and collagen-vascular diseases (e.g., systemic lupus erythematosus) may also precipitate the development of myocarditis. Myocarditis may also occur when no causative agent or factor can be identified. Myocarditis is frequently associated with acute pericarditis, particularly when it is caused by coxsackievirus B strains or echoviruses.[14]

The pathophysiologic mechanisms of myocarditis are poorly understood because there is usually a period of several weeks after the initial infection before the development of manifestations of myocarditis. Immunologic mechanisms may play a role in the development of myocarditis. There is growing evidence that myocarditis and resulting cardiomyopathy are caused by progressive autoimmune disease of the myocardium.[15] The majority of infections are benign, self-limiting, and subclinical, although viral myocarditis in infants and pregnant women may be virulent.

Clinical Manifestations

The clinical features of myocarditis are variable, ranging from a benign course without any overt manifestations to severe heart involvement or sudden death. Fever, fatigue, malaise, myalgias, pharyngitis, dyspnea, lymphadenopathy, and nausea and vomiting are early systemic manifestations of the viral illness.

Early cardiac manifestations appear 7 to 10 days after viral infection and include pericardial chest pain with an associated friction rub because pericarditis often accompanies myocarditis. Cardiac signs (S_3, crackles, jugular venous distention, and peripheral edema) may progress to CHF, including pericardial effusion, syncope, and possibly ischemic pain.

Diagnostic Studies

The ECG changes for a patient with myocarditis are often nonspecific and reflect associated pericardial involvement, including diffuse ST segment abnormalities. Arrhythmias and conduction disturbances may be present. Laboratory findings are also often inconclusive, with the presence of mild to moderate leukocytosis and atypical lymphocytes, elevated viral titers (virus is generally only present in tissue and fluid samples during the initial 8 to 10 days of illness), increased erythrocyte sedimentation rate (ESR), and elevated levels of myocardial enzymes such as creatine kinase (CK).

Histologic confirmation of myocarditis is possible through **endomyocardial biopsy** (EMB), a technique in which several small pieces of myocardial tissue are percutaneously removed from the right ventricle with a special instrument called a *bioptome* and microscopically examined.[16] A biopsy done during the initial 6 weeks of acute illness is most diagnostic because this is the period in which lymphocytic infiltration and myocyte damage indicative of myocarditis are present. Special myocardial imaging techniques may also be used in the diagnostic evaluation of myocarditis.

Collaborative Care

The specific treatment for myocarditis has yet to be established and usually consists of managing associated cardiac decompensation. Digoxin is often used to treat ventricular failure because it improves myocardial contractility and reduces ventricular rate. Digoxin should be used cautiously in patients with myocarditis, because of the increased sensitivity of the heart to the adverse effects of this drug and the potential toxicity with minimal doses. Oxygen therapy, bed rest, restricted activity, and maintenance of standby emergency equipment are general supportive measures used for management of myocarditis.

Based on the infectious-immune theory of myocarditis, it has been thought that immunosuppressive therapy could be effective in the treatment of myocarditis. Immunosuppression with agents such as prednisone, azathioprine (Imuran), and cyclosporine has been used in a limited number of patients with myocarditis to reduce myocardial inflammation and to prevent irreversible myocardial damage. The actual effectiveness of immunosuppressive therapy has been difficult to evaluate because of the high rate of spontaneous recovery in patients with myocarditis. The use of corticosteroids for the treatment of myocarditis remains controversial because of the associated serious side effects and the lack of clear documentation of their efficacy.[17]

Intravenous immunoglobulin (IVIG) is being used on an experimental basis to treat myocarditis. It has been used for more than 20 years to treat immunopathologic disorders, despite its unknown mechanism of action.[18] Antiviral agents (e.g., ribavirin [Virazole], α-interferon) are undergoing clinical investigation for the treatment of acute viral myocarditis.

NURSING MANAGEMENT
MYOCARDITIS

Decreased cardiac output is an ongoing nursing diagnosis in the care of the patient with myocarditis. Interventions focus on assessment for the signs and symptoms of CHF and institution of measures to decrease cardiac workload, such as the use of semi-Fowler position, spacing of activity and rest periods, and provisions for a quiet environment. Prescribed medications that increase the heart's contractility and decrease the preload, afterload, or both are administered. Careful monitoring and evaluation of the patient taking these medications are necessary.

The patient may be anxious about the diagnosis of myocarditis, recovery from myocarditis, and therapy. Nursing measures include assessing the level of anxiety, instituting measures to decrease anxiety, and keeping the patient and family informed about therapeutic measures.

The patient who receives immunosuppressive therapy has additional problems of alterations in the immune response with the potential for infection and complications related to the therapy. Guidelines for care include monitoring for complications and providing the patient with a clean, safe environment by following proper infection control procedures.

The majority of individuals with myocarditis recover spontaneously. Occasionally, acute myocarditis progresses to chronic dilated cardiomyopathy (see Chapter 34).

RHEUMATIC FEVER AND HEART DISEASE

Rheumatic fever is an inflammatory disease of the heart potentially involving all layers (endocardium, myocardium, and pericardium). The resulting damage to the heart from rheumatic fever is termed **rheumatic heart disease,** a chronic condition characterized by scarring and deformity of the heart valves.

Acute rheumatic fever (ARF) is a complication of up to 3% of sporadic upper respiratory infections caused by group A β-hemolytic streptococci. The frequency of recurrence of rheumatic fever after streptococcal infection is greater in those patients with rheumatic heart disease than in those who have not had cardiac injury during previous attacks.[19] Recurrent attacks do occur in adulthood and are probably more common than previously believed. However, the sequelae of rheumatic heart disease are found primarily in young adults.

Etiology and Pathophysiology

Rheumatic fever occurs as a delayed sequela (usually after 2 to 3 weeks) of a group A β-hemolytic streptococcal infection of the upper respiratory system, usually a pharyngeal infection. Although all attacks of rheumatic fever follow a streptococcal infection, only a few streptococcal infections are followed by rheumatic fever.

In addition to the infecting organisms, socioeconomic factors, familial factors, and the presence of an altered immune response have a predisposing role in the development of rheumatic fever. The incidence of rheumatic fever is higher in low socioeconomic groups and remains a major public health problem in the poorer developing countries. Crowded living conditions may be the major factor contributing to this finding. There also seems to be a familial tendency toward rheumatic fever, which may be genetically determined, possibly leading to an altered immune response.

The correlation of streptococcal pharyngitis with rheumatic fever is conclusive, but the pathogenic mechanisms by which the streptococcal infection causes inflammation of the heart and other tissues are not well defined. The organism is not demonstrable in the lesions when rheumatic fever appears several days or weeks after the acute streptococcal infection. Normally, antibodies are produced in response to infections with streptococcal organisms. Episodes of primary and recurrent ARF have been associated with a greater antibody response than those found with uncomplicated streptococcal sore throats.[20]

Manifestations of ARF appear to be related (in susceptible individuals) to an abnormal immunologic response to an upper respiratory infection with group A β-hemolytic streptococci. ARF probably affects the heart, joints, central nervous system (CNS), and skin because of an abnormal humoral and cell-mediated immune response to group A β-hemolytic streptococcal cell membrane antigens. It is possible that these antigens cross-react with other tissues and bind to receptors on heart, muscle, joint, and brain cells, triggering immune and inflammatory responses.

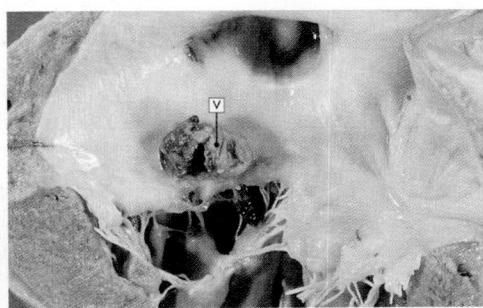

FIG. 36-7 Mitral stenosis and clumps of vegetation (V) containing platelets and fibrin. Mitral leaflets are thickened and fused and have clumps of vegetation containing platelets and fibrin.

Cardiac Lesions and Valvular Deformities. About 40% of ARF episodes are marked by carditis, and all layers of the heart (endocardium, myocardium, and pericardium) may be involved. This generalized involvement gives rise to the term *rheumatic pancarditis.*

Rheumatic endocarditis is found primarily in the valves, with swelling and erosion of the valve leaflets. Vegetations form from deposits of fibrin and blood cells in areas of erosion (Fig. 36-7). The lesions initially create fibrous thickening of the valve leaflets, fusion of commissures and chordae tendineae, and fibrosis of the papillary muscle. Valve leaflets may fuse and become thickened or even calcified, resulting in stenosis. Reduction in the mobility of valve leaflets may occur with failure of the leaflets to appose, resulting in regurgitation. The mitral and aortic valves are most commonly affected; less commonly involved are the tricuspid valve and, rarely, the pulmonic valve.

Myocardial involvement is characterized by **Aschoff's bodies,** which are nodules formed by a reaction to inflammation with accompanying swelling and fragmentation of collagen fibers. As the Aschoff's bodies age, they become more fibrous, and scar tissue is formed in the myocardium. In addition to Aschoff's bodies, a diffuse cellular infiltrate is present in interstitial tissues. This interstitial myocarditis may be more important than nodular Aschoff's bodies in producing heart failure.

Rheumatic pericarditis affects both layers of the pericardium, which become thickened and covered with a fibrinous exudate, and a serosanguineous pericardial fluid may be present. When healing occurs, fibrosis and adhesions develop that partially or completely obliterate the pericardial sac, but constrictive pericarditis does not occur.

These pathophysiologic changes in the heart may occur as a result of an initial attack of rheumatic fever. However, recurrent infections may cause further structural damage.

Extracardiac lesions. The lesions of rheumatic fever are systemic, especially involving the connective tissue. The joints (polyarthritis), skin (subcutaneous nodules), CNS (manifested as chorea), and lungs (fibrinous pleurisy and rheumatic pneumonitis) can be involved in rheumatic fever.

Clinical Manifestations

The diagnosis of ARF is suggested by a clustering of signs and symptoms as well as from laboratory findings. When not observed in its most severe form, the disease may be difficult to differentiate from many illnesses with similar clinical manifestations. Criteria were established by T.D. Jones in 1944, revised by

TABLE 36-12 Modified Jones Criteria for Acute Rheumatic Fever

MAJOR CRITERIA	MINOR CRITERIA
Carditis	Fever
Polyarthritis	Previous occurrence of rheumatic fever or rheumatic heart disease
Chorea	Arthralgia
Erythema marginatum	Prolonged PR interval
Subcutaneous nodules	Laboratory findings*

Source: American Heart Association.
*See Table 36-13.

TABLE 36-13 Laboratory Test Abnormalities in Acute Rheumatic Fever

LABORATORY TEST	ABNORMALITY
Antistreptolysin O titer	>250 IU/ml
Erythrocyte sedimentation rate	>15 mm/hr in men, >20 mm/hr in women
C-reactive protein	Positive
Throat culture	Positive for streptococci (usually negative)
WBC count	Elevated
Red blood cell parameters (Hct, Hb, RBCs)	Mild to moderate degree of normocytic, normochromic anemia

Hb, Hemoglobin; Hct, hematocrit; RBC, red blood cell; WBC, white blood cell.

the American Heart Association in 1965, and updated in 1992 to provide a logical basis for diagnosis (Table 36-12). The presence of two major criteria or one major and two minor criteria indicates a high probability of ARF. Either combination must have evidence of an existing streptococcal infection.

Major Criteria. Carditis is the most important manifestation of ARF (see Table 36-12), with three signs: (1) an organic heart murmur or murmurs of mitral or aortic regurgitation, or mitral stenosis; (2) cardiac enlargement and CHF occurring secondary to myocarditis; and (3) pericarditis resulting in distant heart sounds, chest pain, a pericardial friction rub, or signs of effusion. Large effusions are rare but can lead to cardiac tamponade.

Polyarthritis, which is not a cause of permanent disability, is the most common finding in rheumatic fever. The inflammatory process affects the synovial membranes of the joints, causing swelling, heat, redness, tenderness, and limitation of motion. The arthritis is migratory, affecting one joint and then moving to another. The larger joints are most frequently affected, particularly the knees, ankles, elbows, and wrists. The pain may prevent the patient from being able to walk.

Chorea (Sydenham's chorea) is the major CNS manifestation of ARF. It is characterized by weakness, ataxia, and choreic movement that is spontaneous, rapid, and purposeless, which tends to intensify with voluntary activity. When present in patients with ARF, it is often a delayed sign occurring 3 months or more after the initial infection.

Erythema marginatum lesions are a less common feature of ARF. The bright-pink maplike macular lesions occur mainly on the trunk or inner aspects of the upper arm and thigh but never on the face. The rash is nonpruritic and nonpainful and is neither indurated nor raised. It is usually transitory (lasting for a few hours), may recur intermittently for months, and is exacerbated by heat (e.g., warm bath).

Subcutaneous nodules are firm, small, hard, painless swellings found most commonly over bony prominences (e.g., knees, elbows, spine, scapulae). They frequently are not noticed by the person because the skin overlying the nodules moves freely and is not inflamed.

Minor Criteria. Minor clinical manifestations (see Table 36-12) are frequently present and are helpful in recognizing the disease. These criteria are too nonspecific to make a definitive diagnosis because they frequently occur in other diseases. The minor criteria are used as supplemental data to confirm the presence of rheumatic fever. Laboratory test abnormalities in rheumatic fever are presented in Table 36-13.

Complications

The course of rheumatic fever cannot be predicted at the onset of the disease, but generalizations can be made. Within a few months most symptoms disappear. Less than 5% of the symptoms last for more than 6 months.[19] Once all evidence of rheumatic inflammation has abated, rheumatic fever does not recur in the absence of a new streptococcal infection. If the initial episode is not associated with carditis, there is little likelihood of subsequent cardiac damage if repeated attacks do occur.

A complication that can result from ARF is *chronic rheumatic carditis.* It results from changes in valvular structure that may occur months to years after an episode of ARF. Rheumatic endocarditis can result in fibrous tissue growth in valve leaflets and chordae tendineae with scarring and contractures. The mitral valve is most frequently involved. Other valves that may be affected are the aortic and tricuspid valves.

Diagnostic Studies

No single diagnostic test exists for rheumatic fever, but the results of combinations of laboratory studies suggest the presence of the disease (see Table 36-13). Throat cultures are usually negative at the onset of the disease because of the relatively long latent period of 10 days to several weeks after the precipitating infection. The most specific diagnostic test to confirm a recent group A streptococcal infection is measurement of the antistreptolysin O (ASO) titer. The ESR and measurement of C-reactive protein (CRP) are nonspecific tests indicative of a systemic inflammatory response.

An echocardiogram may show valvular insufficiency and pericardial fluid or thickening. A chest x-ray may show an enlarged heart if CHF is present. The most consistent electrocardiographic change is delayed AV conduction as evidenced in prolongation of the PR interval. Other ECG changes are frequent but nondiagnostic.

Collaborative Care

No specific treatment will cure rheumatic fever. Treatment consists of drug therapy and supportive measures (Table 36-14). Antibiotic therapy does not modify the course of the acute disease or the development of carditis. Penicillin eliminates residual group A β-hemolytic streptococci remaining in the tonsils and pharynx and prevents the spread of organisms to close contacts.

TABLE 36-14	Collaborative Care Rheumatic Fever

Diagnostic
History and physical examination
ASO titer
Throat culture
ESR
C-reactive protein
WBC count
Chest x-ray
Echocardiogram
ECG

Collaborative Therapy
Bed rest (modified)
Benzathine penicillin (1.2 million units IM) or procaine penicillin (600,000 units IM) qd for 10 days
Acetylsalicylic acid
Corticosteroids

ASO, Antistreptolysin O; *ECG,* electrocardiogram; *ESR,* erythrocyte sedimentation rate; *WB,* white blood cell.

Salicylates and corticosteroids are the two antiinflammatory agents most widely used in the management of ARF. Both are effective in controlling the fever and joint manifestations. Salicylates are used when arthritis is the main manifestation, and corticosteroids are used if severe carditis is present.

NURSING MANAGEMENT
RHEUMATIC FEVER AND HEART DISEASE

■ Nursing Assessment

Subjective and objective data that should be obtained from a patient with rheumatic fever and heart disease are presented in Table 36-15. Rheumatic fever is five times more likely to occur in a person with a previous history of rheumatic fever than in the general population. A higher incidence of ARF occurs in lower socioeconomic groups and in crowded living conditions. This may be related to poor treatment of streptococcal infections.

The skin of the patient should be assessed for subcutaneous nodules and erythema marginatum. The procedure involves palpation for subcutaneous nodules over all bony surfaces and along extensor tendons of the hands and feet. The nodules range in size from 1 to 4 cm and are hard, painless, and freely movable. Erythema marginatum can occur on the trunk and inner aspects of the upper arm and thigh. The erythematous maplike macules do not itch and are not raised. The possible presence of these bright pink macules should be assessed in good light because the rash is difficult to observe.

■ Nursing Diagnoses

Nursing diagnoses for the patient with rheumatic fever and heart disease may include, but are not limited to, the following:

- Activity intolerance *related to* arthralgia secondary to joint pain and congestive heart failure.
- Ineffective therapeutic regimen management *related to* lack of knowledge concerning the need for long-term prophylactic antibiotic therapy and possible disease sequelae

TABLE 36-15	Nursing Assessment Rheumatic Fever

Subjective Data
Important Health Information
Past health history: Recent β-hemolytic streptococcal infection, previous rheumatic fever or rheumatic heart disease
Functional Health Patterns
Health perception–health management: Family history of rheumatic fever; malaise
Nutritional-metabolic: Anorexia, weight loss
Activity-exercise: Palpitations; generalized weakness, fatigue; ataxia
Cognitive-perceptual: Chest pain, abdominal pain; migratory joint pain and tenderness (especially large joints)

Objective Data
General
Low-grade fever
Integumentary
Subcutaneous nodules and erythema marginatum
Cardiovascular
Tachycardia, pericardial friction rub, distant heart sounds; gallop rhythm, diastolic and systolic murmurs, peripheral edema
Neurologic
Chorea (involuntary, purposeless, rapid motions; facial grimaces)
Musculoskeletal
Signs of polyarthritis including swelling, heat, redness, limitation of motion (especially of knees, ankles, elbows, shoulders, and wrists)
Possible Findings
Cardiomegaly on chest x-ray; delayed AV conduction on ECG; valve abnormalities, chamber dilation, and pericardial effusion on echocardiogram; ↑ ASO titer, ↑ ESR, positive C-reactive protein, leukocytosis, ↓ RBC, hemoglobin, and hematocrit

ASO, antistreptolysin O; *AV,* atrioventricular; *ECG,* electrocardiogram; *ESR,* erythrocyte sedimentation rate; *RBC,* red blood cell.

■ Planning

The overall goals are that the patient with rheumatic fever will (1) have no residual cardiac disease, (2) resume daily activities without joint pain, and (3) verbalize the ability to manage the disease.

■ Nursing Implementation

Health Promotion. Rheumatic fever is one of the cardiovascular diseases that is preventable. Prevention involves early detection and immediate treatment of group A β-hemolytic streptococcal pharyngitis. Adequate treatment of streptococcal pharyngitis prevents initial attacks of rheumatic fever. Treatment consists of intramuscular (IM) injection of 1.2 million units of benzathine penicillin G or oral penicillin V. If the patient is allergic to penicillin, erythromycin or azithromycin (Zithromax) may be substituted. Oral therapy requires faithful adherence to the full course of treatment. The nurse's role is to educate people in the community to seek medical attention for symptoms of streptococcal pharyngitis and to emphasize the need for adequate treatment of a streptococcal sore throat.

Acute Intervention. The primary goals of managing a patient with ARF are to control and eradicate the infecting organism; prevent cardiac complications; relieve joint pain, fever, and other symptoms; and support the patient psychologically and emotionally. The nurse should administer antibiotics as ordered to treat the streptococcal infection and teach the patient that oral antibiotic therapy requires faithful adherence to the full course of therapy. Precautions with respiratory secretions should be maintained for 24 hours after the initiation of antibiotic therapy. Antipyretics should be administered as prescribed. Oral fluids should be encouraged if the patient is able to swallow; IV fluids should be administered as prescribed.

Promotion of optimal rest is essential to reduce the cardiac workload and to diminish the metabolic needs of the body. After the acute symptoms have subsided, the patient without carditis should ambulate. The patient may resume normal activity after the antiinflammatory therapy is discontinued. If the patient has carditis with CHF, bed rest restrictions should be applied. Again, full activity should not be allowed until antiinflammatory therapy is discontinued. Nonstrenuous activities should be encouraged once recovery has begun.

Relief of joint pain is an important nursing goal. Painful joints should be positioned for comfort and proper alignment. Removal of covers from painful joints can be done with a bed cradle. Heat may be applied and salicylates may be administered to relieve joint pain.

Psychologic and emotional care can be more important than physical care, especially since the heart is often viewed as the center of life. Any alteration in cardiac function may be perceived as a threat to the person's body image.

Ambulatory and Home Care. Secondary prevention aims at preventing the recurrence of rheumatic fever. The patient with a previous history of rheumatic fever should be taught about the disease process, possible sequelae, and the continual need for prophylactic antibiotics. The patient must be made aware of the high risk of recurrence if a streptococcal infection develops and should be informed about the risk of exposure to individuals with streptococcal infections. Ongoing patient teaching should encourage good nutrition and hygienic practices and reinforce the importance of receiving adequate rest.

The patient should be instructed in the use of prophylactic antibiotic therapy. A person who has had rheumatic fever is more susceptible to a second attack after a streptococcal infection. The best prevention is monthly injections of penicillin. Alternative treatment is administration of oral penicillin or erythromycin one or two times a day. Prophylactic treatment should continue for life in individuals who had rheumatic heart disease. Rheumatic fever without carditis after age 18 may require only 5 years of prophylactic antibiotic therapy, or therapy may continue indefinitely in patients with frequent exposure to group A streptococcus.

The dosage of antibiotics used in maintenance prophylaxis of rheumatic fever is not adequate to prevent infective endocarditis when invasive procedures are performed. Additional prophylaxis is necessary if a patient with known rheumatic heart disease has dental or surgical procedures involving the upper respiratory, GI, or genitourinary (GU) tract. The nurse must explain the difference between these two prophylactic programs.

The patient should also be cautioned about the possibility of development of valvular heart disease. The nurse should teach the patient to seek medical attention if symptoms such as excessive fatigue, dizziness, palpitations, or exertional dyspnea develop.

■ Evaluation

The expected outcomes are that the patient with rheumatic fever and heart disease will

- be able to perform ADLs with minimal fatigue
- adhere to treatment regimen
- express confidence in managing disease

Valvular Heart Disease

The heart contains two atrioventricular valves, the mitral and the tricuspid, and two semilunar valves, the aortic and the pulmonic, which are located in four strategic locations to control unidirectional blood flow (Fig. 36-8). Types of valvular heart disease are defined according to the valve or valves affected and the two types of functional alterations, stenosis and regurgitation (Fig. 36-9).

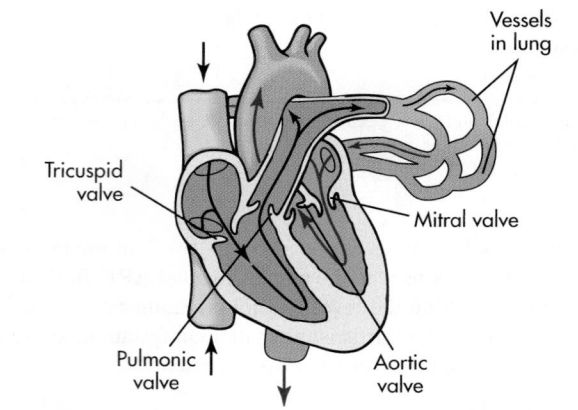

FIG. 36-8 Cross section of valves of the heart.

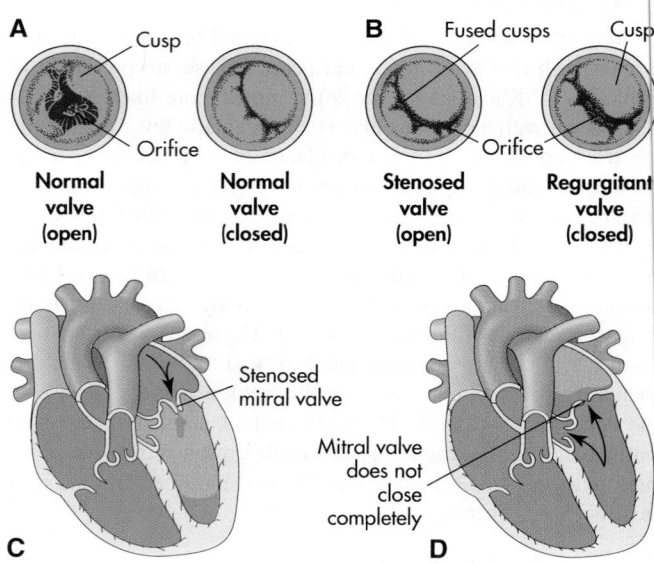

FIG. 36-9 Valvular stenosis and regurgitation. **A,** Normal position of the valve leaflets, or cusps, when the valve is open and closed. **B,** Open position of a stenosed valve *(left)* and position of closed regurgitant valve *(right).* **C,** Hemodynamic effect of mitral stenosis. The stenosed valve is unable to open sufficiently during left atrial systole, inhibiting left ventricular filling. **D,** Hemodynamic effect of mitral regurgitation. The mitral valve does not close completely during left ventricular systole, permitting blood to reenter the left atrium.

The pressure on either side of an open valve is normally equal. However, in a stenotic valve the valve orifice is restricted, impeding the forward flow of blood and creating a pressure gradient difference across an open valve. The degree of **stenosis** (constriction or narrowing) is reflected in the pressure gradient differences (i.e., the higher the gradient, the greater the stenosis). In **regurgitation** (also called *valvular incompetence* or *insufficiency*) incomplete closure of the valve leaflets results in the backward flow of blood.

Valvular disorders occur in children and adolescents primarily from congenital conditions such as tricuspid atresia, pulmonary stenosis, and aortic stenosis.[21] Valvular heart disease has remained prevalent because of an increase in the number of older adults, many of whom have degenerative heart disease. Aortic stenosis and mitral regurgitation are the most common valvular disorders in the elderly.[21] In the last 20 years, new types of cardiac valve disease have emerged. These include valvular disorders related to acquired immunodeficiency syndrome (AIDS) and anorectic drugs. Fenfluramine (Pondimin) and phentermine (Fastin, Adipex), used in combination to treat obesity, have been associated with valvular heart disease. The probability of developing valve disease is related to longer times of exposure and higher doses. Fenfluramine was withdrawn from the market in 1997.[19]

MITRAL VALVE STENOSIS

Etiology and Pathophysiology

The majority of adult cases of mitral valve stenosis result from rheumatic heart disease. Less common causes include congenital mitral stenosis, rheumatoid arthritis, and systemic lupus erythematosus. Rheumatic endocarditis causes scarring of the valve leaflets and the chordae tendineae. Contractures develop with adhesions between the commissures (the junctional areas) of the two leaflets (Fig. 36-10). The stenotic mitral valve assumes a funnel shape because of the thickening and shortening of the structures composing the mitral valve. Obstruction to flow through the mitral valve results from these structural deformities and creates a pressure gradient difference between the left atrium and the left ventricle during diastole. The flow obstruction increases left atrial pressure and volume, resulting in increased pressure in the pulmonary vasculature. Hypertrophy of the pulmonary vessels occurs in cases of chronic left atrial pressure elevations. In chronic mitral stenosis, pressure overload occurs on the left atrium, the pulmonary vasculature, and the right ventricle.

Clinical Manifestations

Dyspnea, sometimes accompanied by hemoptysis, is the primary symptom of mitral stenosis because of reduced lung compliance (Table 36-16). Palpitations from atrial fibrillation and fatigue may also be present. Auscultatory findings generally include a loud or accentuated first heart sound, an opening snap (best heard at the apex with the stethoscope diaphragm), and a low-pitched, rumbling diastolic murmur (best heard at the apex with the stethoscope bell). Less frequently, patients with mitral stenosis may have hoarseness (from atrial enlargement), chest pain (from decreased CO), seizures (from emboli), or a stroke (from emboli) (see Table 36-16). Emboli can arise from the stagnant blood in the left atrium.

MITRAL VALVE REGURGITATION

Etiology and Pathophysiology

Mitral valve patency depends on the integrity of the mitral leaflets, the mitral annulus, the chordae tendineae, the papillary muscles, the left atrium, and the left ventricle. An anatomic or functional abnormality of any of these structures can result in regurgitation. Causes of chronic and acute mitral regurgitation are numerous and may be inflammatory, degenerative, infective, structural, or congenital in nature. The majority of cases may be attributed to myocardial infarction, chronic rheumatic heart disease, isolated rupture of chordae tendineae, mitral valve prolapse, ischemic papillary muscle dysfunction, and infectious endocarditis. Myocardial infarction with resulting left ventricular failure places a patient at risk for rupture of the chordae tendineae. When this occurs, the patient experiences increased vascular resistance and pulmonary edema causing sudden acute mitral insufficiency.

The regurgitant mitral orifice is parallel with the aortic valve, so the burden imposed on the left ventricle and the left atrium is determined by the etiology, severity, and duration of the mitral regurgitation. In chronic mitral regurgitation, volume overload on the left ventricle, the left atrium, and the pulmonary bed is created by the backward flow of blood from the left ventricle into the left atrium during ventricular systole, resulting in varying degrees of left atrial enlargement and left ventricular dilation. Acute mitral regurgitation does not result in dilation of the left atrium or left ventricle. Without dilation to accommodate the regurgitant volume, pulmonary vascular pressures rise, ultimately causing pulmonary edema.

Clinical Manifestations

The clinical course of mitral regurgitation is determined by the nature of its onset (see Table 36-16). The left atrium is relatively noncompliant, and when the atrium is abruptly distended, as occurs in papillary muscle rupture following a myocardial infarction, the sudden increases of volume and pressure are transmitted directly to the pulmonary vasculature. The resultant clinical picture in acute mitral regurgitation is that of pulmonary edema and shock. Patients will have thready, peripheral pulses and cool, clammy extremities. Auscultatory findings of a new systolic murmur may be obscured by a low CO state. Rapid assessment is critical for a positive outcome.

Patients with chronic mitral regurgitation may remain asymptomatic for many years until the development of some degree of

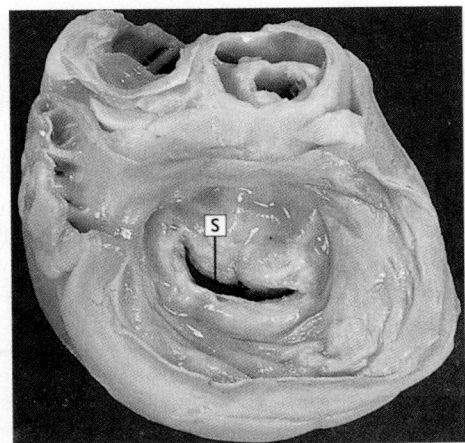

FIG. 36-10 Mitral stenosis with classic "fish mouth" orifice. *S,* Stenosis.

TABLE 36-16   Clinical Manifestations and Diagnostic Findings of Valvular Heart Diseases

	CLINICAL MANIFESTATIONS	ELECTRO-CARDIOGRAM	ECHOCARDIOGRAM	CARDIAC CATHETERIZATION
Mitral valve stenosis	Dyspnea, hemoptysis; fatigue; palpitations; loud, accentuated S_1; opening snap; low-pitched, rumbling diastolic murmur	Right axis deviation, left atrial enlargement, right ventricular hypertrophy, P mitrale (wide, M-shaped P wave), atrial flutter or fibrillation	Restricted movement of mitral valve leaflets; decreased size of orifice; diastolic turbulence	Left atrial pressure increased at end of diastole, reduction in CO
Mitral valve regurgitation	*Acute*—generally poorly tolerated with fulminating pulmonary edema and shock developing rapidly; systolic murmur	Left atrial enlargement, atrial fibrillation	Hyperdynamic left ventricular contraction in association with shock; regurgitant jets and flail chordae/leaflets	Contrast medium injection in left ventricle showing regurgitation of blood into left atrium
	Chronic—weakness, fatigue, exertional dyspnea, palpitations; an S_3 gallop, holosystolic or pansystolic murmur	P mitrale, left ventricular hypertrophy, atrial flutter or fibrillation	Left atrial enlargement; left ventricular hypertrophy; flail leaflets	Contrast medium injection in left ventricle showing regurgitation of blood into left atrium
Mitral valve prolapse	Palpitations, dyspnea, chest pain, activity intolerance, syncope; mobile midsystolic nonejection click and a late or holosystolic murmur	Usually normal; occasionally T wave inversion or biplasticity in leads II, III, and aVf are noted; PVCs and tachyarrhythmias possible	On the M-mode echo, late systolic posterior motion or holosystolic billowing of the mitral leaflets; on 2-D echo, systolic billowing of the mitral leaflets	Left ventricular angiogram reveals mitral leaflets with prominent scalloping as the leaflets billow into the left atrium during systole
Aortic valve stenosis	Angina pectoris, syncope, heart failure, normal or soft S_1, prominent S_4, crescendo-decrescendo murmur	Left ventricular hypertrophy, left bundle branch block, complete atrioventricular heart block	Restricted movement of aortic valve; diminished orifice; systolic turbulence	Left ventricular systolic pressure increased, reduction in CO
Aortic valve regurgitation	*Acute*—abrupt onset of profound dyspnea, transient chest pain, progression to shock	Left ventricular strain	Normal-sized left ventricle with hyperdynamic systolic contraction; aortic dissection can be seen, if cause of acute process	Significant elevation of left ventricular diastolic pressure
	Chronic—fatigue, exertional dyspnea; Corrigan's pulse; heaving precordial impulse; diastolic high-pitched soft decrescendo diastolic murmur, characteristic Austin Flint murmur at diastolic rumble, systolic ejection click	Left ventricular hypertrophy	Enlarged left ventricle and dilated aortic root	Increase in left ventricular diastolic pressure, aortic root contrast medium injection demonstrating regurgitation of blood into left ventricle
Tricuspid stenosis and regurgitation	Peripheral edema, ascites, hepatomegaly; diastolic low-pitched, decrescendo murmur with increased intensity during inspiration (stenosis), pansystolic murmur with increased intensity at inspiration (regurgitation)	Tall, peaked P waves; atrial fibrillation	Right ventricular dilation and paradoxic septal motion, usually poor visualization of tricuspid valve itself	Pressure gradient across tricuspid valve and increased right atrial pressure (stenosis), reflux of contrast medium into right atrium (regurgitation)

CO, Cardiac output; *PVCs*, premature ventricular contractions.

left ventricular failure. Initial symptoms include weakness, fatigue, and dyspnea that gradually progress to orthopnea, paroxysmal nocturnal dyspnea, and peripheral edema. Patients with chronic mitral regurgitation have brisk carotid pulses. Auscultatory findings reflect accentuated left ventricular filling leading to an audible third heart sound (S_3) even in the absence of left ventricular dysfunction. The murmur is a loud pansystolic or holosystolic murmur at the apex radiating to the left axilla.

MITRAL VALVE PROLAPSE

Etiology and Pathophysiology

Mitral valve prolapse (MVP) is a structural abnormality of the mitral valve leaflets and the papillary muscles or chordae that allows the leaflets to prolapse, or buckle, back into the left atrium during systole (Fig. 36-11).[22] The etiology of MVP is unknown but is related to diverse pathogenic mechanisms of the mitral valve apparatus. MVP can occur in the presence of redundant mitral valve leaflets, elongated chordae tendineae, enlarged mitral annulus, and abnormally contracting left ventricular wall segments. The use of the term *prolapse* is unfortunate because it is used even when the valve anomaly is functionally normal. MVP is the most common form of valvular heart disease in the United States.

MVP is usually benign, but serious complications can occur, including mitral regurgitation, infective endocarditis, sudden death, and cerebral ischemia. There is an increased familial incidence (autosomal dominant) in some patients with MVP resulting from a connective tissue defect affecting only the valve, or occurring as part of Marfan syndrome or other hereditary conditions that influence the structure of collagen in the body. In many patients the abnormality detected by echocardiography is not accompanied by any other clinical manifestations of cardiac disease, and the significance of the finding is uncertain.[22]

Clinical Manifestations

MVP encompasses a broad spectrum of severity. Most patients are asymptomatic and remain so for their entire lives. Although severe mitral regurgitation is an uncommon complication of MVP, the latter has become the most common cause of isolated severe mitral regurgitation. A characteristic of MVP is a murmur from insufficiency that gets more intense through systole. This could be a late or holosystolic murmur. Another major sign is one or more clicks usually heard in midsystole to late systole, between the first heart sound (S_1) and second heart sound (S_2), and less frequently in early systole. The clicks may be constant or vary from beat to beat. MVP does not alter S_1 or S_2. M-mode echocardiography confirms MVP by demonstrating late-systolic prolapse, and two-dimensional echocardiography reveals leaflet billowing into the left atrium.

Arrhythmias, most commonly ventricular premature contractions, paroxysmal supraventricular tachycardia, and ventricular tachycardia, may cause palpitations, light-headedness, and dizziness. Infective endocarditis may occur in patients with mitral regurgitation associated with MVP.

Patients may or may not have chest pain. Although the cause of the chest pain is not known, it may be due to abnormal tension on the papillary muscles. If episodes of chest pain occur, the episodes tend to occur in clusters, especially during periods of emotional stress. The chest pain may occasionally be accompanied by dyspnea, palpitations, and syncope. This chest pain does not respond to antianginal treatment (e.g., nitrates).

Patients with MVP generally have a benign, manageable course unless some severe problems associated with mitral regurgitation are present.[23] A teaching plan for patients with MVP is presented in Table 36-17.

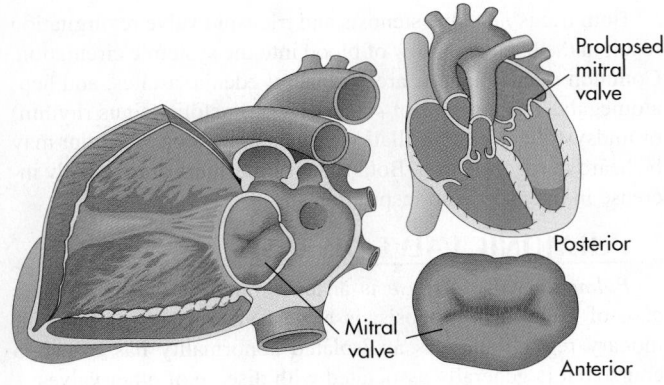

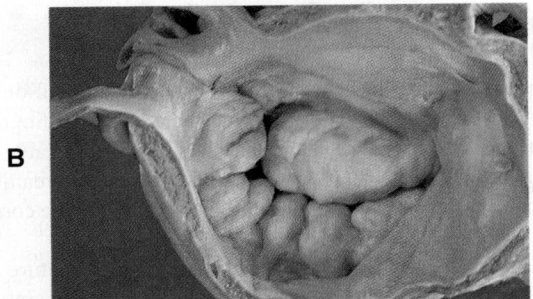

FIG. 36-11 Mitral valve prolapse. **A,** Normal mitral valve and prolapsed mitral valve *(upper right)*. Prolapse permits the valve leaflets to billow back into the atrium during left ventricular systole. The billowing causes the leaflets to part slightly, permitting regurgitation into the atrium. **B,** Looking down on the mitral valve, the ballooning of the leaflets is seen.

TABLE 36-17	*Patient & Family Teaching Guide* **Mitral Valve Prolapse (MVP)**

1. Recommend antibiotic prophylaxis for endocarditis before undergoing certain dental or surgical procedures if the patient has MVP with regurgitation (see Tables 36-4 and 36-6).
2. Monitor the patient treated with β-adrenergic blockers to control palpitations.
3. Advise the patient to adopt healthy eating patterns, such as avoiding caffeine because it is a stimulant and may exacerbate symptoms. Counsel the patient who uses diet pills containing stimulants that these preparations will exacerbate symptoms.
4. Instruct the patient to take over-the-counter drugs with caution and to check for common ingredients, including caffeine, ephedrine, and pseudoephedrine.
5. Develop a planned aerobic exercise program and help the patient implement it.

AORTIC VALVE STENOSIS

Etiology and Pathophysiology

Congenitally abnormal stenotic aortic valves are generally discovered in childhood, adolescence, or young adulthood. A patient seen later in life usually has **aortic stenosis** as a result of rheumatic fever or senile fibrocalcific degeneration of a normal valve. In rheumatic valvular disease, fusion of the commissures and secondary calcification cause the valve leaflets to stiffen and retract, resulting in regurgitation. If it does occur secondary to rheumatic heart disease, mitral valve disease accompanies aortic stenosis. In contrast to mitral stenosis, isolated aortic valve stenosis is almost always nonrheumatic in origin. Although the incidence of rheumatic aortic valvular disease has been decreasing, senile or degenerative stenosis is expected to increase as the population ages.

Aortic stenosis results in obstruction of flow from the left ventricle to the aorta during systole. The effect is left ventricular hypertrophy and increased myocardial oxygen consumption because of the increased myocardial mass. As the disease course progresses and compensatory mechanisms fail, reduced CO leads to pulmonary hypertension.

Clinical Manifestations

Symptoms of aortic stenosis (see Table 36-16) generally develop when the valve orifice becomes approximately one third its normal size and classically include angina pectoris, syncope, and heart failure. The prognosis is poor for a patient with symptoms and whose valve obstruction is not relieved. Nitroglycerin is contraindicated for the patient with significant aortic stenosis because it would reduce preload (the amount of blood returning to the heart). Preload is necessary with aortic stenosis to free the stiffened aortic valve so that it can open. Auscultatory findings of aortic stenosis typically reveal a normal or soft first heart sound (S_1); a diminished or absent second heart sound (S_2); a systolic, crescendo-decrescendo murmur that ends before the second heart sound (S_2); and a prominent fourth heart sound (S_4).

AORTIC VALVE REGURGITATION

Etiology and Pathophysiology

Aortic valve regurgitation may be the result of a primary disease of the aortic valve leaflets, the aortic root, or both. Acute aortic regurgitation is caused by bacterial endocarditis, trauma, or aortic dissection and constitutes a life-threatening emergency. Chronic aortic regurgitation is generally the result of rheumatic heart disease, a congenital bicuspid aortic valve, syphilis, or chronic rheumatic conditions such as ankylosing spondylitis or Reiter syndrome.

The basic physiologic consequence of aortic valve regurgitation is retrograde blood flow from the ascending aorta into the left ventricle resulting in volume overload. The left ventricle initially compensates for chronic aortic regurgitation by dilation and hypertrophy. Myocardial contractility eventually declines and blood volumes increase in the left atrium and pulmonary vasculature. Ultimately, pulmonary hypertension and right ventricular failure develop.

Clinical Manifestations

Patients with acute aortic valve regurgitation have sudden clinical manifestations of cardiovascular collapse (see Table 36-16). The left ventricle is exposed to aortic pressure during diastole. The patient develops weakness, severe dyspnea, and hypotension that generally constitutes a medical emergency. Patients with chronic, severe aortic regurgitation have pulses that are of the "water-hammer" or collapsing type with abrupt distention during systole and quick collapse during diastole (Corrigan's pulse). Auscultatory findings may include a soft or absent S_1, presence of S_3 or S_4, and a soft, decrescendo high-pitched diastolic murmur. A systolic ejection murmur may also be heard, and the *Austin-Flint murmur,* a low-frequency diastolic rumble similar to that of mitral stenosis, may be auscultated.

The patient with chronic aortic regurgitation generally remains asymptomatic for years and is seen with exertional dyspnea, orthopnea, and paroxysmal nocturnal dyspnea only after considerable myocardial dysfunction has occurred (see Table 36-16). Angina pectoris occurs less frequently in aortic regurgitation than in aortic stenosis. However, a nocturnal angina accompanied by diaphoresis and abdominal discomfort may be present.

TRICUSPID VALVE DISEASE

Etiology and Pathophysiology

Tricuspid valve stenosis is extremely uncommon and occurs almost exclusively in patients with rheumatic mitral stenosis. It is also seen in IV drug users. In tricuspid stenosis, right atrial outflow is obstructed, resulting in right atrial enlargement and elevated systemic venous pressures. Tricuspid regurgitation is usually the result of pulmonary hypertension or right ventricular dysfunction. Volume overload of the right atrium and ventricle occurs in tricuspid regurgitation.

Clinical Manifestations

Both tricuspid valve stenosis and tricuspid valve regurgitation result in the backward flow of blood into the systemic circulation. Common manifestations are peripheral edema, ascites, and hepatomegaly. The murmur of stenosis is presystolic (sinus rhythm) or midsystolic (atrial fibrillation), and a pansystolic murmur may be heard in regurgitation. Both types of murmurs dramatically increase in intensity with inspiration.

PULMONIC VALVE DISEASE

Pulmonic valve disease is an uncommon entity and, in the case of pulmonary stenosis, is almost always congenital. Pulmonary regurgitation as an isolated abnormality has a benign course but is generally associated with disease of other valves.

Diagnostic Studies for Valvular Heart Disease

Diagnosis of valvular heart disease is generally based on the results of a history, a physical examination, an echocardiogram, and a cardiac catheterization (if surgery is considered) (Table 36-18). Chest x-ray results, ECG findings, and the clinical manifestations exhibited by the patient also aid in establishing the correct diagnosis.

An echocardiogram provides information on the structure and function of the valves and on enlargement of the chambers. Transesophageal echocardiography and Doppler color-flow imaging are particularly valuable in diagnosing and monitoring the progression of valvular heart disease. Cardiac catheterization detects pressure changes in the cardiac chambers, as well as pressure gradients across the valves. It also quantifies the size of the valve area. An ECG shows variation in the heart rate and rhythm

TABLE	Collaborative Care
36-18	**Valvular Heart Disease**

Diagnostic
History and physical examination
Chest x-ray
ECG
Echocardiogram
Cardiac catheterization

Collaborative Therapy
Nonsurgical
Prophylactic antibiotic therapy
- Rheumatic fever
- Infective endocarditis*
Digitalis
Diuretics (see Table 32-8)
Sodium restriction
Anticoagulant agents
- warfarin (Coumadin)
- dipyridamole (Persantine)
- aspirin
Antiarrhythmic drugs (see Chapter 35, Table 35-8)
Oral nitrates†
β-Adrenergic blockers (see Chapter 32, Table 32-8)
Percutaneous transluminal balloon valvuloplasty

Surgical
Valvuloplasty
Closed commissurotomy (valvulotomy)
Open commissurotomy (valvulotomy)
Annuloplasty
Valve replacement

*See Tables 36–4 and 36–5.
†Sublingual nitroglycerin is contraindicated in aortic stenosis.
ECG, Electrocardiogram.

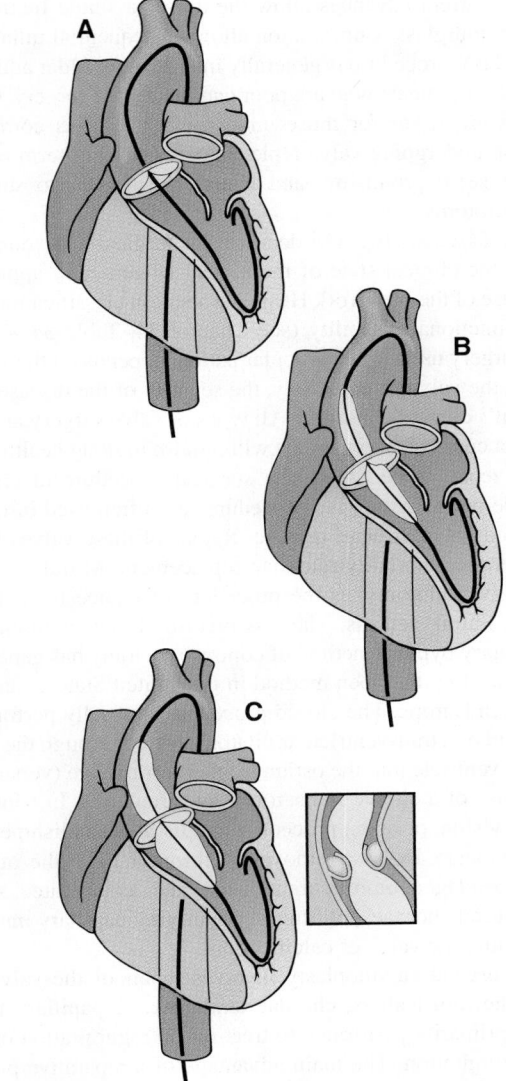

FIG. 36-12 Percutaneous transluminal balloon valvuloplasty procedure in a stenotic, calcific aortic valve. **A,** The loop of a guide wire, passed from the right femoral artery retrograde across the aortic valve, is seen nestling at the apex of the left ventricle. This positioning helps prevent perforation of the ventricular wall and minimizes ventricular ectopy. **B,** A 20 mm dilating balloon catheter, having been passed over the guide wire, is partially inflated; the indentation is caused by the stenosed valve. **C,** Full inflation of the balloon (*inset*) opens the aortic valve orifice.

and provides information about possible ischemia or chamber enlargement. Chest x-ray reveals the heart size, alterations in pulmonary circulation, and calcification of valves.

Collaborative Care of Valvular Heart Disease

Conservative Therapy. An important aspect of conservative management of valvular heart disease (see Table 36-18) is prevention of recurrent rheumatic fever and infective endocarditis. Treatment of valvular heart disease depends on the valve involved and the severity of the disease. It focuses on preventing exacerbations of heart failure, acute pulmonary edema, thromboembolism, and recurrent endocarditis. If manifestations of CHF develop, digitalis, diuretics, and a low-sodium diet are recommended (see Chapter 34). Anticoagulant therapy is used to prevent and treat systemic or pulmonary embolization, and it is also used as a prophylactic measure in patients with atrial fibrillation. Arrhythmias, especially atrial arrhythmias, are common with valvular heart disease and are treated with digitalis, antiarrhythmic drugs, or electrical cardioversion. β-Adrenergic blockers may be used to slow the ventricular rate in patients with atrial fibrillation. (Arrhythmias are discussed in Chapter 35.)

Percutaneous transluminal balloon valvuloplasty. An alternative treatment for some patients with valvular heart disease is the *percutaneous transluminal balloon valvuloplasty* (PTBV)

procedure, which splits open the fused commissures (Fig. 36-12). Balloon valvuloplasty has been used for pulmonic, aortic, and mitral stenosis.[24] The procedure, performed in the cardiac catheterization laboratory, involves threading a balloon-tipped catheter from the femoral artery or from the femoral vein with transatrial septal puncture to the stenotic valve so that the balloon may be inflated in an attempt to separate the valve leaflets. A single- or double-balloon technique may be used for the PTBV procedure. The double-balloon technique uses combinations of 10, 12, or 15 mm balloons inserted through each femoral artery to allow two balloons to be placed side by side into the valvular orifice, thus permitting a smaller arterial puncture and laceration.

However, current advances allow the use of a single Inoue balloon with hourglass configuration allowing sequential inflation.

The PTBV procedure is generally indicated for older adult patients and for patients who are poor candidates for surgery. Complications are fewer for those undergoing PTBV as compared with those undergoing valve replacement. The long-term results of PTBV seem promising, and results are similar to surgical commissurotomy.[24]

Surgical Therapy. The decision for surgical intervention is based on the clinical state of the patient as generally appraised through use of the New York Heart Association classification system for functional disability (see Chapter 34, Table 34-4). The type of surgery used for a particular patient depends on the valves involved, the valvular pathology, the severity of the disease, and the patient's clinical condition. All types of valve surgery are palliative, not curative, and patients will require lifelong health care.

Valve repair is becoming the surgical procedure of choice. Reparative or reconstructive procedures are often used in mitral or tricuspid valvular heart disease. Repair of these valves has a lower operative mortality rate than replacement. Mitral *commissurotomy* (valvulotomy) is the procedure of choice for patients with pure mitral stenosis. The less precise closed (without cardiopulmonary bypass) method of commissurotomy has generally been replaced by the open method in the United States, Canada, and Western Europe. The closed procedure is usually performed with the aid of a transventricular dilator inserted through the apex of the left ventricle into the ostium of the mitral valve (versus the previous use of a simple transatrial finger fracture). In contrast, the direct vision, or open, procedure entails the establishment of cardiopulmonary bypass; removal of thrombi from the atrium and its appendage; commissure incision; and, as indicated, separation of fused chordae, splitting of underlying papillary muscle, and debriding the valve of calcification.

Open surgical valvuloplasty involves repair of the valve by suturing the torn leaflets, chordae tendineae, or papillary muscles. It is primarily performed to treat mitral regurgitation or tricuspid regurgitation. The main advantage of a reparative procedure is that it avoids the risks associated with valve replacement. The disadvantage is that it may not be possible to establish total valve competence.

Further repair or reconstruction of the valve may be necessary and can be achieved by annuloplasty, a procedure also used in cases of mitral or tricuspid regurgitation. *Annuloplasty* entails reconstruction of the annulus, with or without the aid of prosthetic rings (e.g., a Carpentier ring).

Prosthetic valves. Valvular replacement may be required for mitral, aortic, tricuspid, and occasionally pulmonic valvular disease. The surgical treatment of choice for combined aortic stenosis and aortic regurgitation is valvular replacement (Fig. 36-13 and Table 36-19).

Prosthetic valves have improved since the first caged-ball valve was introduced in 1952. Early valves disintegrated, stuck, became incompetent, changed the structure of cardiac chambers, caused emboli, and traumatized blood cells. Newer valves and improved surgical techniques have made valve replacement safer and long-term valvular functioning more effective. A wide variety of valves have been introduced in an attempt to find the most sound, nonthrombogenic, durable valve, and one that creates the least amount of stenosis.

The two categories of prosthetic valves are mechanical and biologic (tissue) valves (see Table 36-19). *Mechanical valves* are manufactured from manmade materials and consist of combinations of metal alloys, pyrolite carbon, and Dacron. *Biologic valves* are constructed from bovine, porcine, and human cardiac tissue. Within the past few years, major innovations in freezing and thawing techniques have enabled human grafts to be preserved for extensive periods without losing viability. Mechanical prosthetic valves are more durable and last longer than biologic tissue valves but have an increased risk of thromboembolism, which necessitates the use of long-term anticoagulant therapy. Biologic valves offer the patient freedom from anticoagulant therapy as a result of their low thrombogenicity. However, their durability is limited by the tendency for early calcification, tissue degeneration, and stiffening of the leaflets. Other problems associated with prosthetic valves regardless of type include paravalvular leaks and endocarditis.

Long-term anticoagulation is recommended for all patients with mechanical prostheses and for patients with biologic tissue valves who are in atrial fibrillation. Some patients with biologic tissue valves or annuloplasty with prosthetic rings may require anticoagulation during the first few months after surgery.

The choice of a valvular prosthesis depends on many factors. For example, if a patient cannot take anticoagulant therapy (e.g., women of childbearing age), a biologic valve may be considered

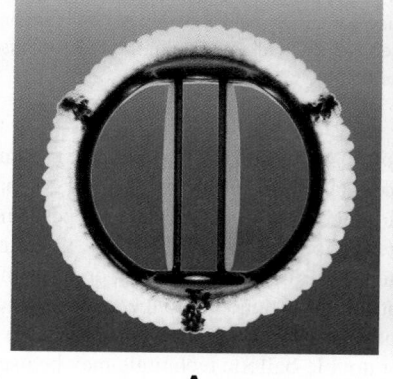 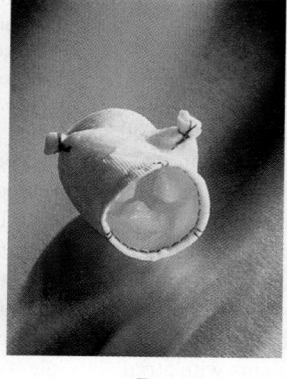 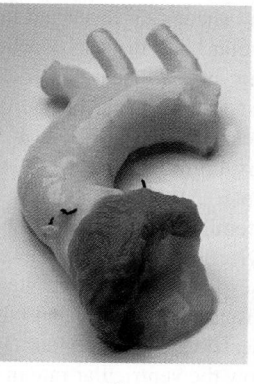

A   **B**   **C**

FIG. 36-13 Types of prosthetic and tissue valves. **A,** Bi-leaflet mechanical valve. **B,** Porcine heterograft. **C,** Carpentier-Edwards aortic pericardial valve.

TABLE 36-19 Types of Cardiac Prosthetic and Tissue Valves

TYPE	DESCRIPTION	ADVANTAGES	DISADVANTAGES
Mechanical			
Caged-Ball Valve Starr-Edwards Sutter Magovern-Cromie	Metal cage with several struts mounted on a circular ring; hollow metal or plastic ball (poppett) inside of cage	High durability (up to 20 yr)	Possibility of blood clots forming on or around valve (thrombogenic) with risk of embolism Need for long-term anticoagulation therapy Very large size
Tilting-Disk Valve Lillehei-Kaster Hall-Medtronic	Mobile, lens-shaped disk attached to a circular sewing ring by two offset transverse struts; pyrolytic carbon composition	Hemodynamic efficiency High durability Low thrombogenicity	Need for long-term anticoagulation therapy
Bi-leaflet Valve St. Jude Medical Duromedics CarboMedic	Two pivoting semicircular disks that open centrally, mounted directly onto a sewing ring	Compact size; successful use in children and patients with small aortic roots	Possibility of thrombogenicity and embolism Need for long-term anticoagulation therapy
Biologic			
Porcine **Heterograft** Hancock Carpentier-Edwards Medtronic	Harvested aortic valve of pig that is preserved in glutaraldehyde and mounted on specially designed sewing ring	Low thrombogenicity Need for anticoagulation therapy for only 3 mo after placement	Limited durability (failure rate increases sharply after 5-7 yr) Cumbersome structural design
Pericardial **Heterograft** Ionescu-Shiley Carpentier-Edwards	Three leaflets composed of pericardium from 16- to 18-month-old calves that are preserved in glutaraldehyde and mounted on a Dacron-covered frame	Low thrombogenicity Need for only short-term anticoagulation therapy Less resistance to blood flow; useful in patients with small aortic roots; outstanding durability	Limited durability Early valve failure secondary to calcification and degeneration
Homograft **Cadaver Valve**	Harvested aortic valve from human cadaver that is initially frozen until needed for valve replacement; then thawed, trimmed, and sewn into place with special mounting material	Excellent hemodynamics No hemolysis/low risk for embolism Only rare need for anticoagulation therapy	Limited durability Not useful for mitral or tricuspid valve replacement

A mechanical valve may be considered for a younger patient because it is more durable and lasts longer. For patients over age 65, durability is less important, but the risks of noncompliance or hemorrhage from anticoagulants may be greater.

NURSING MANAGEMENT VALVULAR DISORDERS

■ Nursing Assessment

Subjective and objective data should be obtained from an individual with valvular disease and are presented in Table 36-20.

■ Nursing Diagnoses

Nursing diagnoses for the patient with valvular disease may include, but are not limited to, those presented in NCP 36-2.

■ Planning

The overall goals are that the patient with valvular heart disease will have (1) normal cardiac function, (2) improved activity tolerance, and (3) an understanding of the disease process and preventive measures.

■ Nursing Implementation

Health Promotion. Prevention of acquired rheumatic valvular disease is achieved by diagnosing and treating streptococcal infection and providing prophylactic antibiotics for patients with a history of rheumatic fever. The patient at risk for endocarditis and any patient with valvular heart disease must also be treated with prophylactic antibiotics (see Tables 36-4 and 36-5).

The patient must adhere to recommended therapies. The individual with a history of rheumatic fever, endocarditis, and congenital heart disease should know the symptoms suggestive of valvular heart disease so that early medical treatment may be obtained.

Acute Intervention and Ambulatory and Home Care. A patient with progressive valvular heart disease may require hospitalization or outpatient care for management of CHF, endocarditis, embolic disease, or arrhythmias. CHF is the most common reason for ongoing medical care.

TABLE 36-20	Nursing Assessment Valvular Heart Disease

Subjective Data

Important Health Information

Past health history: Rheumatic fever, endocarditis, congenital defects, myocardial infarction, chest trauma, cardiomyopathy, syphilis, Marfan syndrome, staphylococcal or streptococcal infections

Functional Health Patterns

Health perception–health management: IV drug abuse; fatigue

Activity-exercise: Palpitations; generalized weakness, activity intolerance; dizziness, fainting; dyspnea on exertion, cough, hemoptysis, orthopnea

Sleep-rest: Paroxysmal nocturnal dyspnea

Cognitive-perceptual: Anginal or atypical chest pain

Objective Data

General

Fever

Integumentary

Diaphoresis, flushing, cyanosis, clubbing; peripheral edema

Respiratory

Crackles, wheezes, hoarseness

Cardiovascular

Abnormal heart sounds, including opening snaps, clicks, thrills, systolic and diastolic murmurs, S_3, and S_4; arrhythmias, including premature atrial contraction, atrial fibrillation; tachycardia; ↑ or ↓ in pulse pressure; hypotension, water-hammer or thready peripheral pulses, brisk carotid pulses

Gastrointestinal

Ascites, hepatomegaly

Possible Findings

Cardiomegaly, valve calcification, pulmonary congestion on chest x-ray; decrease in excursion, calcification or vegetation of leaflets or prolapse, chamber enlargement, turbulence on echocardiogram; abnormal chamber pressures and flow patterns on cardiac catheterization; atrial and ventricular hypertrophy, arrhythmias, conduction defects on ECG

ECG, Electrocardiogram; IV, intravenous; S_3 and S_4, third and fourth heart sounds.

ETHICAL DILEMMAS
Do Not Resuscitate

Situation

A 68-year-old man has been admitted for a second mitral valve surgery and possible coronary artery bypass. He did not adhere to the treatment plan following his original surgery 5 years ago. The nurse is concerned about his future compliance with medication to reduce blood clotting, appropriate diet, and exercise. His kidneys are failing and he is on dialysis, but not tolerating it well. Both the patient and family want complete therapeutic treatment and refuse to discuss do not resuscitate (DNR) orders.

Important Points for Consideration

- Nonadherence with the treatment plan in the past does not always indicate that the patient will not follow the plan of care in the future.
- A competent patient can decide if he or she wants continued treatment to be able to live. This is even more important when family members support the patient's decision.
- Health care providers have an obligation to respect the patient's request for treatment unless there is no clear benefit to continued treatment.
- DNR orders should reflect the patient's expressed wishes either through conversation, an advance directive, or a surrogate decision maker.
- DNR orders should be reevaluated periodically with the patient and family, especially before major diagnostic procedures or treatments.
- If a health care provider does not agree with a patient's treatment choice, a referral should be made to another provider.

Critical Thinking Questions

1. What measures or strategies would be beneficial to help the patient better adhere to the treatment plan?
2. What type of information should be provided to a patient and family in discussions about resuscitation? Who should provide this information?

The role of the nurse is to implement and evaluate the effectiveness of therapeutic management. Activity should be designed after considering the patient's limitations. An appropriate exercise plan can increase cardiac tolerance. However, activities that regularly produce fatigue and dyspnea should be restricted, and an explanation should be provided to the patient. Smoking should be discouraged. Strenuous physical exercise should be avoided because damaged valves may not be able to handle the required increase in CO. The patient should be assisted in planning the activities of daily living, with an emphasis on conserving energy, setting priorities, and taking planned rest periods. Referral to a vocational counselor may be necessary if the patient has a physically or emotionally demanding job.

Auscultatory assessment of the heart should be performed to monitor the effectiveness of digitalis, β-adrenergic blockers, and antiarrhythmic drugs. Patients should be instructed to wear a Medic Alert bracelet. The patient must understand the importance of prophylactic antibiotic therapy to prevent endocarditis (see Tables 36-4 and 36-5). If the valve disease was caused by rheumatic fever, prophylaxis to prevent recurrence is necessary.

The nurse should help the patient with a valvular disorder achieve and maintain an optimal level of health. Teaching regarding the actions and side effects of drugs is important to achieve compliance. When valvular heart disease can no longer be managed medically, surgical intervention is necessary. The patient who is on anticoagulation therapy after surgery for valve replacement must have the international normalized ratio (INR) checked regularly (usually monthly) to assess the adequacy of therapy. The INR is a standardized system of reporting prothrombin time.

NURSING CARE PLAN 36-2

Patient with Valvular Heart Disease

EXPECTED PATIENT OUTCOMES	NURSING INTERVENTIONS and *RATIONALES*
NURSING DIAGNOSIS	**Activity intolerance** *related to* insufficient oxygenation secondary to decreased cardiac output and pulmonary congestion *as manifested by* weakness, fatigue, shortness of breath, increase or decrease in pulse rate, BP changes.
▪ Demonstration of cardiac tolerance to increased activity (e.g., stable pulse, respirations, and BP)	▪ Assess and monitor patient responses to activity (e.g., pulse rate, respirations, BP) *to plan appropriate interventions.* ▪ Plan rest periods between activities *to conserve energy and decrease cardiac demands.* ▪ Organize care *to minimize unnecessary disturbance.* ▪ Progressively increase activity *to increase cardiac tolerance.*
NURSING DIAGNOSIS	**Excess fluid volume** *related to* cardiac failure secondary to incompetent valves *as manifested* by peripheral edema, weight gain, increased BP and pulse, adventitious breath sounds.
▪ Normal BP and pulse ▪ Normal breath sounds ▪ Peripheral edema not present	▪ Monitor for manifestations of hypervolemia such as peripheral edema; taut, shiny skin; adventitious breath sounds *to detect hypervolemia.* ▪ Assess vital signs, auscultate breath sounds, assess for jugular distention, measure intake and output, palpate for edema, and assess for weight gain (>2 lb [0.9 kg]/day or >5 lb [2.3 kg]/wk) *to monitor indicators of hypervolemia.* ▪ Restrict sodium as ordered *to prevent fluid retention.*
NURSING DIAGNOSIS	**Decreased cardiac output** *related to* valvular incompetence *as manifested by* heart murmurs, dyspnea, tachycardia, arrhythmias.
▪ No fatigue ▪ Normal heart rate and rhythm ▪ Normal breath sounds	▪ Monitor BP, apical pulse, respirations, breath and heart sounds *to assess for signs of decreased cardiac output* such as fatigue, malaise, shortness of breath, dyspnea on exertion, palpitations, angina, vertigo, heart murmur, widened pulse pressure. ▪ Maintain rest as ordered *to decrease cardiac workload and O_2 demands.* ▪ Elevate head of bed 30 to 40 degrees *to reduce venous return, reduce O_2 demand, and maximize chest excursion.* ▪ Administer O_2 as ordered *to improve O_2 saturation.* ▪ Monitor cardiac rhythm *to detect changes from baseline.* ▪ Administer inotropic medication as ordered *to increase myocardial contractility.*
NURSING DIAGNOSIS	**Ineffective therapeutic regimen management** *related to* lack of knowledge about disease process and prevention and treatment strategies *as manifested by* lack of compliance with therapeutic regimen.
▪ Knowledge of signs and symptoms that indicate a need to seek health care ▪ Knowledge of need and when to use prophylactic antibiotics ▪ Adherent to therapeutic regimen	▪ Explain nature and cause of disease process *to ensure patient has adequate knowledge base.* ▪ Teach signs and symptoms of heart failure and infective endocarditis *to ensure early reporting and treatment of complications.* ▪ Teach the need to avoid all invasive surgical or diagnostic procedures that may predispose to bacteremia until prophylactic antibiotics have been given. ▪ Explain the importance of notifying the dentist, urologist, gynecologist, and other health care providers of valvular disease *so prophylactic antibiotic treatment can be initiated.** ▪ Discourage smoking *to prevent an increased cardiac workload and the oxygen-depleting effect of carbon monoxide from decreasing the O_2 available to all tissues.* ▪ Discuss the name of prescribed medication, dosage, purpose, and side effects *to promote safe and accurate self-medication.* ▪ Instruct patient to wear a Medic Alert bracelet.

*See Tables 36-4 and 36-5.
BP, Blood pressure.

Teaching instructions related to anticoagulant therapy are listed in Chapter 37, Table 37-14. The patient must realize that valve surgery is not a cure, and that regular follow-up examinations by the health care provider will be required. The nurse also must teach the patient about when to seek medical care. Any manifestations of infection or congestive heart failure, any signs of bleeding, and any planned invasive or dental procedures require the patient to notify the health care provider.

■ Evaluation

The expected outcomes for a patient with valvular heart disease are addressed in NCP 36-2.

CRITICAL THINKING EXERCISES

Case Study

Valvular Heart Disease

Patient Profile. Mrs. S., a 54-year-old Hispanic woman, is admitted to the hospital for valvular heart disease.

Subjective Data
- Was told she had streptococcal throat infection as a child
- Was diagnosed 10 years ago with rheumatic heart disease
- Has shortness of breath at rest; cannot get out of bed without becoming dyspneic
- Takes digoxin (0.25 mg once a day)

Objective Data

Physical Examination
- Ankle edema
- Irregular pulse
- Crackles at lung bases
- Murmurs of mitral stenosis, mitral insufficiency, and aortic insufficiency

Diagnostic Studies
- Chest x-ray and ECG indicate enlarged left atrium

CRITICAL THINKING QUESTIONS

1. Explain the cause of Mrs. S.'s valvular heart disease. What valves are most likely to become involved with rheumatic heart disease?

2. Differentiate between the characteristics of mitral stenosis and mitral regurgitation.

3. What other conservative treatment measures might be initiated for this patient in addition to digoxin?

4. What are important nursing measures for Mrs. S.?

5. On the basis of the assessment data provided, write one or more nursing diagnoses. Are there any collaborative problems?

Nursing Research Issues

1. What are effective nursing measures to facilitate patient compliance with prophylactic antibiotic therapy for endocarditis?

2. How does the quality of life of a patient having valvular heart surgery differ preoperatively as compared with postoperatively?

3. Does a planned aerobic exercise program decrease symptoms associated with mitral valve prolapse?

4. What health problems are observed most frequently by the nurse caring for a patient with rheumatic heart disease?

REVIEW QUESTIONS

The number of the question corresponds to the same-numbered objective at the beginning of the chapter.

1. A patient with a history of IV cocaine use has acute infective endocarditis. The nurse closely assesses the patient for signs and symptoms of
   a. pulmonary emboli.
   b. increased cardiac output.
   c. streptococcal bacteremia.
   d. mitral valve regurgitation.

2. The nurse suspects cardiac tamponade in a patient with acute pericarditis based on the finding of
   a. chest pain.
   b. pulsus paradoxus.
   c. mitral valve murmur.
   d. pericardial friction rub.

3. Prophylactic antibiotics are indicated to prevent infective endocarditis for at-risk individuals who
   a. are undergoing any dental procedure.
   b. are entering the third trimester of pregnancy.
   c. have acquired a viral respiratory tract infection.
   d. are exposed to human immunodeficiency virus.

4. The most common cause of myocarditis is
   a. viruses.
   b. radiation.
   c. endocarditis.
   d. myocardial infarction.

5. Teaching the patient with rheumatic fever about the disease, the nurse explains that rheumatic fever is
   a. a *Streptococcus viridans* infection.
   b. a viral infection of endocardium and valves.
   c. a sequela of β-hemolytic streptococcal infection.
   d. frequently triggered by immunosuppressive therapy.

6. Penicillin therapy for the patient with rheumatic fever is indicated to
   a. prevent chronic rheumatic carditis.
   b. relieve arthralgia and inflamed joints.
   c. prevent reinfection and recurrent rheumatic fever.
   d. destroy the infective microorganism and cure the disease.

7. The most common cause of mitral valve stenosis is
   a. myocarditis.
   b. rheumatic heart disease.
   c. congenital heart disease.
   d. subacute infective endocarditis.

8. Which of the following findings is indicative of accentuated left ventricular filling in a patient with chronic mitral regurgitation?
   a. an audible third heart sound and a late diastolic murmur
   b. a midsystolic click followed by an early systolic murmur
   c. an audible third heart sound and a pansystolic or holosystolic murmur
   d. an audible third heart sound and a middiastolic click with a late diastolic murmur

REVIEW QUESTIONS—cont'd

9. A patient hospitalized with aortic stenosis has a nursing diagnosis of activity intolerance related to insufficient oxygen secondary to decreased cardiac output. An appropriate nursing intervention for this patient is to
   a. monitor ECG to assess cardiac output.
   b. maintain on bed rest to reduce tissue oxygen demands.
   c. progressively increase activity to increase cardiac tolerance.
   d. use a semi-Fowler position to decrease venous return and increase respiratory excursion.

10. The nurse caring for a patient scheduled for a percutaneous transluminal balloon valvuloplasty understands that this procedure
    a. is the treatment of choice for combined aortic stenosis and aortic regurgitation.
    b. involves the insertion of a transventricular dilator into the opening of the valve.
    c. is recommended for patients who are poor candidates for more extensive valvular surgery.
    d. is a last resort treatment when other valvular repair procedures have not been effective.

REFERENCES

1. Bridger A: Infective endocarditis: new strategies for diagnosis and prophylaxis, *J Am Acad Physician Assist* 14:35, 2001.
2. Mylonakis E, Calderwood SB: Infective endocarditis in adults, *N Engl J Med* 345:1318, 2001.
3. Dhawan VK: Infective endocarditis in elderly patients, *Clin Infect Dis* 34:806, 2002.
4. Mauri L, de Lemos JA, O'Gara PT: Infective endocarditis, *Curr Probl Cardiol* 26:562, 2001.
5. Thornton SE: Differential diagnosis of infective endocarditis, *J Am Acad Nurse Pract* 12:177, 2000.
6. Alestig K, Hogevik H, Olaison L: Infective endocarditis: a diagnostic and therapeutic challenge for the new millennium, *Scand J Infect Dis* 32:343, 2000.
7. Ryan EW, Bolger AF: Transesophageal echocardiography (TEE) in the evaluation of infective endocarditis, *Cardiol Clin* 18:773, 2000.
8. Press N, Montessori V: Prophylaxis for infective endocarditis. Who needs it? How effective is it? *Can Fam Physician* 46:2248, 2000.
9. Delahaye F et al: Treatment and prevention of infective endocarditis, *Expert Opinion on Pharmacotherapy* 3:131, 2002.
10. Seto TB et al: Physicians's recommendations to patients for use of antibiotic prophylaxis to prevent endocarditis, *JAMA* 284: 68, 2000.
11. Ellis-Pegler R et al: Prevention of infective endocarditis associated with dental treatment and other intervention, *N Z Med J* 113:289, 2000.
12. Maisch B, Ristic AD: The classification of pericardial disease in the age of modern medicine, *Current Cardiology Reports* 4:13, 2002.
13. Witte KK, Clark AL: The recognition and treatment of pericarditis, *Practitioner* 246:429, 2002.
14. Haas GJ: Etiology, evaluation, and management of acute myocarditis, *Cardiol Rev* 9:88, 2001.
15. Binah O: Immune effector mechanisms in myocardial pathologies, *International Journal of Molecular Medicine* 6:3, 2000.
16. Veinot JP: Diagnostic endomyocardial biopsy pathology: secondary myocardial diseases and other clinical indications—a review, *Can J Cardiol* 18:287, 2002.
17. D'Ambrosio A et al: The fate of acute myocarditis between spontaneous improvement and evolution to dilated cardiomyopathy: a review, *Heart* 85:449, 2001.
18. Tedeschi A et al: High-dose intravenous immunoglobulin in the treatment of acute myocarditis. A case report and review of the literature, *J Intern Med* 251:169, 2002.
19. Groves AM: Rheumatic fever and rheumatic heart disease: an overview, *Trop Doct* 29:129, 1999.
20. Guilherme L et al: Molecular evidence for antigen-driven immune responses in cardiac lesions of rheumatic heart disease patients, *Int Immunol* 12:1063, 2000.
21. Soler-Soler J, Galve E: Worldwide perspective valve disease, *Heart* 83:721, 2000.
22. Freed LA et al: Prevalence and outcome of mitral-valve prolapse, *N Engl J Med* 341:1, 1999.
23. Bouknight DP, O'Rourke RA: Current management of mitral valve prolapse, *Am Fam Physician* 61:3343, 2000.
24. Sutaria N, Elder AD, Shaw TRD: Long term outcome of percutaneous mitral balloon valvulotomy in patients aged 70 and older, *Heart* 83:433, 2000.

RESOURCES

Resources for this chapter are listed in Chapter 33 on page 837 and Chapter 34 on page 860.

CHAPTER 37

NURSING MANAGEMENT
Vascular Disorders

Deidre D. Wipke-Tevis
Kathleen Rich

LEARNING OBJECTIVES

1. Describe the etiology and pathophysiology of peripheral arterial disease.
2. Identify the major risk factors associated with peripheral arterial disease.
3. Describe the pathophysiology, clinical manifestations, and collaborative care of aortic aneurysms.
4. Discuss the perioperative nursing care of a patient having an aortic aneurysm repair.
5. Describe the pathophysiology, clinical manifestations, and collaborative care of aortic dissection.
6. Discuss the clinical manifestations, collaborative care, and surgical management of peripheral arterial disease of the lower extremities.
7. Discuss the nursing management of the patient with acute arterial insufficiency affecting the lower extremities.

8. Differentiate the pathophysiology, clinical manifestations, and collaborative care of thromboangiitis obliterans (Buerger's disease) and Raynaud's phenomenon.
9. Identify the risk factors predisposing to the development of superficial thrombophlebitis and deep vein thrombosis.
10. Differentiate between the clinical characteristics of superficial thrombophlebitis and deep vein thrombosis.
11. Describe the nursing management of the patient with deep vein thrombosis.
12. Explain the purpose and actions of commonly used anticoagulants and nursing management of the patients receiving them.
13. Discuss the pathophysiology, clinical manifestations, and collaborative and nursing management of venous leg ulcers.
14. Describe the pathophysiology, clinical manifestations, and collaborative and nursing management of pulmonary emboli.

KEY TERMS

aneurysms, p. 913	Raynaud's phenomenon, p. 927
aortic dissection, p. 918	thromboangiitis obliterans
atherosclerosis, p. 912	(Buerger's disease), p. 926
deep vein thrombosis, p. 928	thrombophlebitis, p. 927
intermittent claudication, p. 920	varicose veins, p. 935
peripheral arterial disease, p. 912	venous thrombosis, p. 927
pulmonary embolism, p. 938	Virchow's triad, p. 928

Problems of the vascular system include disorders of the arteries and veins. *Peripheral arterial disease* (PAD) is a term used to describe a wide variety of conditions affecting arteries in the neck, abdomen, and extremities. PAD can be subdivided into occlusive disease, aneurysmal disease, and vasospastic phenomenon. In contrast, venous diseases primarily affect the lower extremities and can be categorized into venous thrombosis and chronic venous insufficiency.

Peripheral Arterial Disease

Peripheral arterial disease (PAD) involves progressive narrowing and degeneration of the arteries of the neck, abdomen, and extremities. Regardless of the anatomic location, atherosclerosis is responsible for the majority of PAD, both occlusive and aneurysmal.[1] Although PAD typically appears in the sixth to

Reviewed by Anne M. Aquila, RN, MSN, CS, Advanced Practice Nurse and Vascular Program Coordinator, Hospital of Saint Raphael, New Haven, Conn.; and Karen R. Bruni, RN, MSN, NP, CVN, Nurse Practitioner, Vascular Surgery, The Institute for Vascular Health and Disease, Albany Medical Hospital, Albany, N.Y.

eighth decades of life, it occurs at an earlier age in persons with diabetes mellitus. Men in their sixties are almost twice as likely to have PAD as are women. However, as women age, the incidence of PAD is similar to or greater than that in men. After age 85, 30% to 50% of both men and women have PAD.[2,3] Thus as our population ages, PAD will become a major health care problem.

PAD is strongly related to other manifestations of cardiovascular disease and its risk factors. Specifically, those with PAD have a twofold to threefold risk of cardiovascular morbidity and mortality.[2] Therefore PAD must be thought of as a marker of advanced systemic atherosclerosis. If an individual has PAD, it is likely that she or he also has coronary artery disease and/or carotid artery disease.

Etiology and Pathophysiology

The leading cause of PAD is **atherosclerosis,** a gradual thickening of the intima and media of arteries, which leads to progressive narrowing of the vessel lumen. Although the exact cause (or causes) of atherosclerosis remains unknown, several theories exist (see Chapter 33). The pathologic changes that occur with atherosclerosis consist of migration and replication of smooth muscle cells, deposition of connective tissue, lymphocyte and macrophage infiltration, and accumulation of lipids.

The four most significant risk factors for PAD are cigarette smoking, hyperlipidemia, hypertension, and diabetes mellitus, with the most important being cigarette smoking. Other risk factors include obesity, hypertriglyceridemia, hyperuricemia, family history, sedentary lifestyle, and stress. Additional risk factors under investigation include elevated homocysteine and elevated ferritin levels.[4,5]

Although atherosclerosis is a diffuse process, certain segments of the arterial tree are more commonly involved, including the coronary arteries (see Chapter 33), carotid arteries (see Chap-

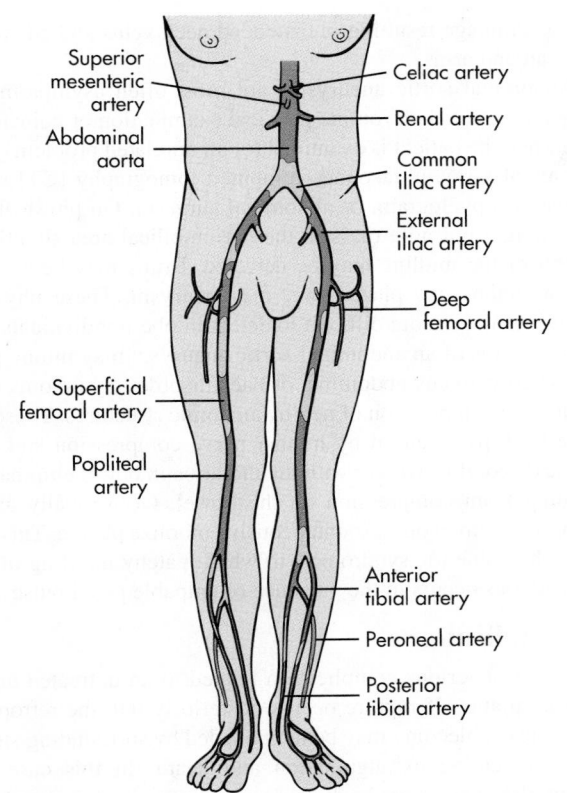

FIG. 37-1 Common anatomic locations of atherosclerotic lesions (shown in *yellow*) of the abdominal aorta and lower extremities.

Superior mesenteric artery
Abdominal aorta
Superficial femoral artery
Popliteal artery
Celiac artery
Renal artery
Common iliac artery
External iliac artery
Deep femoral artery
Anterior tibial artery
Peroneal artery
Posterior tibial artery

ter 56), aortic bifurcation, iliac and common femoral arteries, femoral profunda, superficial femoral artery, and distal popliteal artery (especially in diabetics) (Fig. 37-1).[1] The involvement is generally segmental, with normal segments interspersed between involved ones. Clinical manifestations occur when the vessel is between 60% and 75% occluded.

CAROTID ARTERY DISEASE

Atherosclerosis is the most common cause of carotid artery disease (cerebrovascular disease) in the United States. Over 80% of all strokes are ischemic in nature and result from an atherothrombotic event.[6] If carotid artery disease is identified early and treated, the risk of stroke decreases. Cerebrovascular disease and stroke are discussed in Chapter 56.

Disorders of the Aorta

The aorta is the largest artery and is responsible for supplying oxygenated blood to essentially all vital organs in the body. The most common vascular problems that affect the aorta are aneurysms, aortoiliac occlusive disease, and aortic dissection. Although the underlying etiology, pathophysiology, and clinical manifestations of these three aortic problems are slightly different, the diagnostic studies, surgical therapy, and nursing management are similar.

AORTIC ANEURYSMS

Aneurysms are outpouchings or dilations of the arterial wall and are common problems involving the aorta. Aneurysms of peripheral arteries can also occur but are far less common. An-

eurysms occur in men more often than in women, and their incidence increases with age. Abdominal aortic aneurysms occur in 5% to 7% of people over age 60 in the United States and account for about 16,000 deaths.[7] In Canada, abdominal aortic aneurysms are the tenth major cause of death in men over 65 years old.[8]

Etiology and Pathophysiology

Aortic aneurysms may involve the aortic arch, thoracic aorta, and/or abdominal aorta. Most aneurysms, however, are found in the abdominal aorta below the level of the renal arteries. The growth rate of aneurysms is unpredictable, but the larger the aneurysm, the greater the risk of rupture. The dilated aortic wall becomes lined with thrombi that can embolize, leading to acute ischemic symptoms to distal (downstream) branches. Three fourths of true aortic aneurysms occur in the abdomen (Fig. 37-2) and one fourth in the thoracic aorta. Popliteal artery aneurysms rank third in frequency. Patients may have an aneurysm in more than one location.

Although the exact cause of aneurysms remains unknown, several theories of pathogenesis exist. The most commonly accepted etiology of aneurysms is atherosclerosis.[9] It is known that atherosclerotic plaques deposit beneath the *intima* (the innermost layer of the arterial wall). This plaque formation is thought to cause degenerative changes in the *media* (middle layer of the arterial wall), leading to loss of elasticity, weakening, and eventual dilation of the aorta.

Several studies have shown a strong genetic predisposition in the development of abdominal aortic aneurysms. The familial tendency to develop aneurysms is related to either a specific defect in collagen (Ehlers-Danlos syndrome) or a premature degeneration of vascular elastic tissue (Marfan syndrome).[1] Less common causes of aneurysm formation include penetrating or blunt trauma, acute or chronic infections (e.g., *Salmonella*), and anastomotic disruptions.[9]

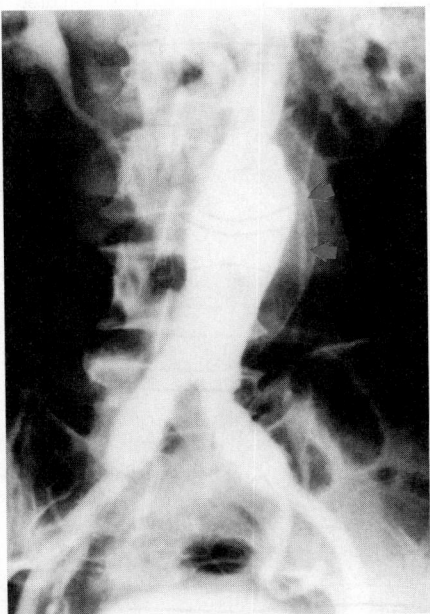

FIG. 37-2 Angiography demonstrating fusiform abdominal aortic aneurysm. Note calcification of the aortic wall *(arrows)* and extension of the aneurysm into the common iliac arteries.

Classification

Aneurysms are generally divided into two basic classifications: true and false aneurysms (Fig. 37-3). A *true aneurysm* is one in which the wall of the artery forms the aneurysm, with at least one vessel layer still intact. True aneurysms can be further subdivided into fusiform and saccular dilations. A *fusiform aneurysm* is circumferential and relatively uniform in shape. A *saccular aneurysm* is pouchlike with a narrow neck connecting the bulge to one side of the arterial wall.

A *false aneurysm,* or *pseudoaneurysm,* is not an aneurysm but a disruption of all layers of the arterial wall resulting in bleeding that is contained by surrounding structures. False aneurysms may result from trauma, from infection, or after peripheral artery bypass graft surgery at the site of the graft-to-artery anastomosis. They may also result from arterial leakage after removal of cannulae such as upper or lower extremity arterial catheters and intraaortic balloon pump devices.[10]

Clinical Manifestations

Thoracic aorta aneurysms are usually asymptomatic. When manifestations are present, they are varied. The most common manifestation is deep, diffuse chest pain. Aneurysms located in the ascending aorta and the aortic arch can produce hoarseness in the patient as a result of pressure on the recurrent laryngeal nerve. Pressure on the esophagus can cause dysphagia. If the aneurysm presses on the superior vena cava, it can cause decreased

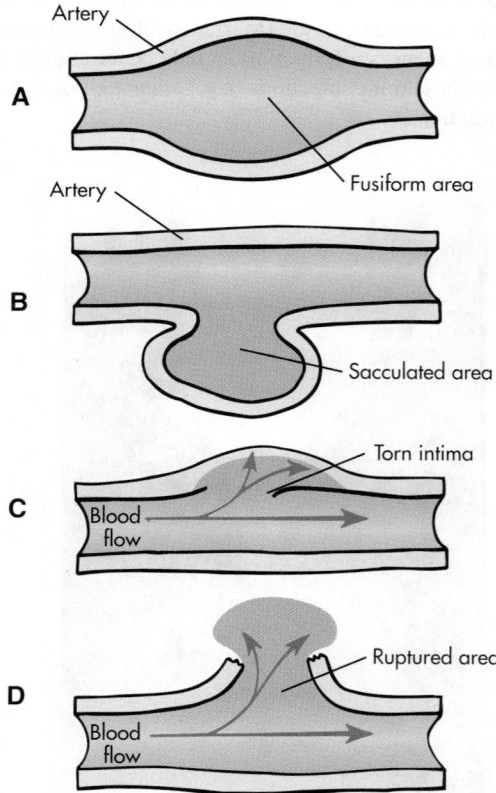

FIG. 37-3 A, True fusiform abdominal aortic aneurysm. B, True saccular aortic aneurysm. C, Aortic dissection. D, False aneurysm or pseudoaneurysm.

venous drainage resulting in distended neck veins and edema of the head and arms.

Abdominal aortic aneurysms are most often asymptomatic. They are detected on routine physical examination or coincidentally when the patient is examined for an unrelated problem (e.g., abdominal x-ray, ultrasound, computed tomography [CT] scan, intravenous pyelogram, or abdominal surgery). On physical examination, a pulsatile mass in the periumbilical area slightly to the left of the midline may be detected. Bruits may be audible with a stethoscope placed over the aneurysm. These physical findings may be more difficult to detect in obese individuals.

Symptoms of an abdominal aortic aneurysm may mimic pain associated with any abdominal or back disorder. Symptoms may result from compression of nearby anatomic structures. These include back pain caused by lumbar nerve compression and epigastric discomfort with or without alteration in bowel elimination resulting from compression on the bowel. Occasionally aneurysms, even small ones, spontaneously embolize plaque. This can cause the "blue toe syndrome," in which patchy mottling of the feet and toes occurs in the presence of palpable pedal pulses.

Complications

The most serious complication related to an untreated aneurysm is rupture. If rupture occurs posteriorly into the retroperitoneal space, bleeding may be tamponaded by surrounding structures, preventing exsanguination and death. In this case the patient often has severe back pain and may or may not have back or flank ecchymosis *(Grey Turner's sign).*

If rupture occurs anteriorly into the abdominal cavity, most patients do not survive long enough to get to the hospital; they die from massive hemorrhage. If the patient does reach the hospital, he or she is in hypovolemic shock with tachycardia, hypotension, pale clammy skin, decreased urine output, altered sensorium, and abdominal tenderness on palpation. (Shock is discussed in Chapter 65.) In this situation, simultaneous resuscitation and immediate surgical repair are necessary.

Diagnostic Studies

Most aneurysms are found on routine physical or x-ray examination. Chest x-rays are useful in demonstrating the mediastinal silhouette and any abnormal widening of the thoracic aorta. A plain x-ray of the abdomen may show calcification within the wall of an abdominal aortic aneurysm.

An electrocardiogram (ECG) may be performed to rule out evidence of myocardial infarction (MI) because some persons with thoracic aneurysms may have symptoms suggestive of angina. Echocardiography assists in the diagnosis of aortic insufficiency related to ascending aortic dilation. Ultrasonography is useful in screening for aneurysms, and in the case of a nonsurgical candidate it is used to serially monitor the aneurysm size. A CT scan is the most accurate test to determine the anterior-to-posterior length and cross-sectional diameter of the aneurysm and to identify the presence of thrombus in the aneurysm. Magnetic resonance imaging (MRI) may also be used to diagnose and assess the location and severity of aneurysms.

Angiography, anatomic mapping of the aortic system by contrast imaging, is not a reliable method of determining the diameter or length of an aneurysm. It may, however, be helpful in providing the surgeon with accurate information about the involvement of intestinal, renal, or distal vessels. It is also useful if a suprarenal or thoracoabdominal aneurysm is suspected. (Angiography is discussed in Chapter 31.)

Collaborative Care

The goal of management is to prevent rupture of the aneurysm. Therefore early detection and prompt treatment are imperative. Once an aneurysm is suspected, studies are performed to determine its exact size and location. A careful review of all body systems is necessary to identify any coexisting disorders, especially of the lungs, heart, or kidney, because they may influence the patient's risk for surgery. The carotid and coronary arteries should be assessed for atherosclerotic disease. If obstructions in these vessels are present, they may need to be corrected before the aneurysm is repaired. For individuals with small aneurysms (less than 4 cm), conservative therapy may be initiated, which consists of risk factor modification, decreasing blood pressure, and monitoring the size of the aneurysm every 6 months using ultrasound, MRI, or CT scan.[9] Generally, if coexisting medical problems are stable, surgical repair is the treatment of choice for aneurysms larger than 5 to 6 cm or if the aneurysm is expanding rapidly (0.5 cm or greater increase in diameter over a 6-month period) in a patient who is symptomatic. In individuals with stable, chronic comorbid conditions (e.g., chronic obstructive pulmonary disease, coronary artery disease, cerebrovascular disease) that meet specific anatomic criteria, endovascular repair of the aneurysm may be the treatment of choice.[11]

Surgical Therapy. Before surgery, the patient is hydrated and any abnormalities in electrolytes, coagulation, and hematocrit are corrected. The patient may receive preoperative antibiotics and showers with antiseptics before surgery to decrease risk of a postoperative infection. However, if the aneurysm has ruptured, immediate surgical intervention is required. Even with prompt care, the mortality rate is very high (over 50%) after rupture and increases with the age of the patient. Aneurysms repaired electively have a surgical risk of 1% to 5%.[12]

The surgical technique involves (1) incising the diseased segment of the aorta; (2) removing intraluminal thrombus or plaque; (3) inserting a synthetic graft (Dacron or polytetrafluoroethylene), which is sutured to the normal aorta proximal and distal to the aneurysm; and (4) suturing the native aortic wall around the graft so that it will act as a protective cover (Fig. 37-4). If the iliac arteries are also aneurysmal, the entire diseased segment is replaced with a bifurcation graft. With saccular aneurysms, it may be possible to excise only the bulbous lesion, repairing the artery by primary closure (suturing the artery together) or by application of an autogenous or synthetic patch graft over the arterial defect. Use of autotransfusion, which recycles the patient's own blood, has markedly reduced the need for blood transfusions in surgery. (Autotransfusion is discussed in Chapter 30.)

All aneurysm resections require cross-clamping of the aorta proximal and distal to the aneurysm. Most resections can be completed in 30 to 45 minutes, after which time the clamps are removed and blood flow to the lower extremities is restored. Fortunately, most abdominal aortic aneurysms originate below the origin of the renal arteries. However, if the aneurysm extends above the renal arteries or if the cross clamp must be applied above the renal arteries, adequate renal perfusion after removal of the clamp should be ascertained before closure of the abdominal incision. The risk of postoperative renal complications is significantly increased in patients who have surgical repair of aneurysms above the renal arteries.

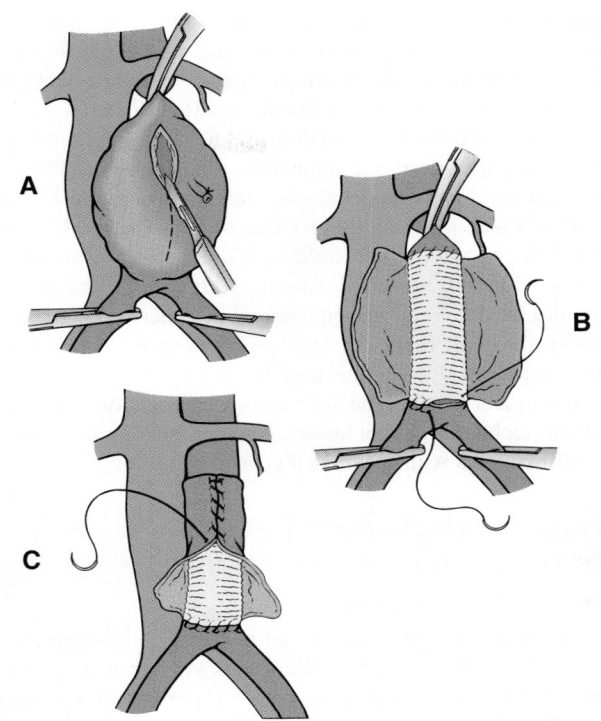

FIG. 37-4   Surgical repair of an abdominal aortic aneurysm. **A,** Incising the aneurysmal sac. **B,** Insertion of synthetic graft. **C,** Suturing native aortic wall over synthetic graft.

Endovascular graft procedure. The newest alternative to conventional surgical repair of an abdominal aortic aneurysm is the minimally invasive endovascular grafting technique.[11] The endovascular technique involves the placement of a sutureless aortic graft into the abdominal aorta inside the aneurysm through the femoral artery. The graft is constructed from a Dacron cylinder, and the surface of the graft is supported with multiple rings of extra flexible wire. After the compactly folded graft is delivered through the sheath to the predetermined point, the graft is deployed, pressed/implanted against the vessel wall by balloon inflation (creating a circumferential seal), and anchored to the vessel by a series of small hooks. The blood then flows through the endovascular graft, thus preventing further expansion of the aneurysm due to pressure. The aneurysmal wall will begin to shrink over time because the blood is now being diverted through the endograft. After the endovascular graft is in place, intravascular ultrasound (IVUS) may be used to assess how well the graft is seated in the aorta and the graft's proximity to the renal and/or hypogastric arteries.[13]

Patients must meet strict eligibility criteria to be a potential candidate for use of the endovascular devices. For example, patients are not considered suitable candidates if the aneurysm involves the renal arteries. Some of the devices are custom made for each patient using data from CT scans, angiography, and ultrasound. In other institutions, the surgeons use knitted Dacron grafts combined with balloon expandable stents.

The benefits of endovascular repair include decreased anesthesia and operative time, smaller operative blood loss, decreased morbidity and mortality rates, small bilateral groin incisions (as opposed to a large abdominal incision), more rapid resumption of physical activity, shortened length of hospital stay, quicker recovery, higher patient satisfaction, and reduction in overall costs.[11,14] Potential complications include perigraft leaks (endoleaks), aortic dissection, bleeding, graft dislocation and embolization, renal artery occlusion due to graft migration, graft thrombosis, incisional site hematoma, and incisional infection. The most commonly reported complication is perigraft leak (8% to 44%), which may require insertion of coils (beads) for hemostasis.[13] A perigraft leak (endoleak) is the seeping of blood from the new endograft back into the old aneurysm site. The perigraft leak may be due to an inadequate seal at either graft end, a tear through the graft fabric, or leakage between overlapping graft segments. Graft dysfunction may require conversion to a traditional surgical repair. The long-term complications associated with this technique are not known. Endovascular grafts cannot be used for patients with aortoiliac occlusive disease.

NURSING MANAGEMENT
AORTIC ANEURYSMS AND AORTOILIAC DISEASE

■ Nursing Assessment

A thorough nursing history and physical assessment should be performed. Because atherosclerosis is a systemic disease process, it is likely that the disease process is present throughout the body. Therefore it is important for the nurse to watch for signs of cardiac, pulmonary, cerebral, and lower extremity vascular problems. The patient should be monitored for indications of rupture of the aneurysm, such as diaphoresis; paleness; weakness; tachycardia; hypotension; abdominal, back, groin, or periumbilical pain; changes in sensorium; or a pulsating abdominal mass.

Establishing baseline data is important for later postoperative assessment and intervention. In addition to gathering data, the nurse should observe the patient closely for any abnormalities. Special attention should be paid to the character and quality of the peripheral pulses and the neurologic status. Pedal pulse sites (dorsalis pedis and posterial tibial) and skin lesions on the lower extremities should be marked and documented before surgery.

■ Planning

The overall goals for a patient undergoing aortic surgery include (1) normal tissue perfusion, (2) intact motor and sensory function, and (3) no complications related to surgical repair such as thrombosis or infection.

■ Nursing Implementation

Health Promotion. The nurse must be aware of cardiovascular disease risk factors and be alert for opportunities to teach health promotion measures to patients in the hospital and the community (see Chapter 33). Special attention should be given to the patient with a strong family history of aneurysm or any evidence of other cardiovascular disease.

The patient should be encouraged to reduce risk factors known to be associated with atherosclerosis (see Chapter 33, Table 33-3). These should include controlling hypertension, smoking cessation, and following a diet low in fats and cholesterol. These measures are also done to ensure continued graft patency following surgical repair.

Acute Intervention. The nursing role during the preoperative period includes patient and family teaching, providing support for the patient and family, and careful assessment of all body sys-

tems. Preoperative teaching should include a brief explanation of the disease process, the planned surgical procedure(s), preoperative routines, what to expect immediately after surgery (e.g., recovery room, tubes/drains), and usual postoperative timelines. Although specific preoperative routines often vary by institution and/or surgeon, in general, patients undergoing aortic surgery typically undergo some sort of bowel preparation (i.e., laxatives, enemas) and have a preoperative shower with an antimicrobial soap the day before surgery, receive nothing by mouth (NPO) after midnight the day before surgery, and often are given preoperative intravenous antibiotics immediately before surgery. If the patient will be going to the intensive care unit (ICU) after surgery, a tour of the ICU before surgery may be of interest to the patient and family.

Postoperatively patients undergoing aortic surgery typically go to an ICU where there are appropriate support services and equipment. When the patient arrives in the ICU, an endotracheal tube, an arterial line, a central venous pressure or pulmonary artery catheter, peripheral intravenous (IV) lines, an indwelling urinary catheter, and a nasogastric tube will likely be in place with continuous ECG and pulse oximetry monitoring. If the thorax is entered during surgery, chest tubes will also be in place. Pain medication may be administered via epidural catheter or patient-controlled analgesia.[9]

In addition to the usual goals associated with the care of a postoperative patient (e.g., maintaining adequate respiratory function, fluid and electrolyte balance, and pain control; see Chapter 19), the nurse must monitor graft patency and renal perfusion. The nurse can also assist in preventing arrhythmias, infections, and neurologic complications. Care of the patient with an aneurysm repair or other aortic surgery is described in NCP 37-1.

Graft patency. It is important to maintain adequate blood pressure to promote graft patency. Prolonged hypotension may result in graft thrombosis due to decreased blood flow. Administration of IV fluids and blood components (as indicated) is essential to maintaining adequate blood flow to the graft. Central venous pressure (CVP) readings or pulmonary artery (PA) pressures and urinary output should be monitored hourly in the immediate postoperative period to help assess the patient's state of hydration.

Severe hypertension may cause undue stress on the arterial anastomoses, resulting in leakage of blood or rupture at the suture lines. Drug therapy with diuretics or IV antihypertensive agents may be indicated if severe hypertension persists.

Cardiovascular status. In individuals with preexisting coronary artery disease, myocardial ischemia or infarction may occur in the perioperative period due to decreased oxygen supply to the heart or increased oxygen demands on the heart. Cardiac arrhythmias also may occur due to electrolyte imbalances, hypoxemia, hypothermia, or myocardial ischemia. Nursing interventions include continuous ECG monitoring, frequent electrolyte and arterial blood gas (ABG) determinations, administration of oxygen and IV antiarrhythmic medications as needed, replacement of electrolytes as indicated, adequate pain control, and resumption of preoperative cardiac medications.

Infection. The development of a prosthetic vascular graft infection is a relatively rare but possibly life-threatening complication. Nursing intervention to prevent infection should include ensuring that the patient receives a broad-spectrum antibiotic as prescribed. It is important to assess body temperature regularly

NURSING CARE PLAN 37-1

Patient after Surgical Repair of the Aorta

EXPECTED PATIENT OUTCOMES	NURSING INTERVENTIONS and *RATIONALES*
NURSING DIAGNOSIS	**Ineffective tissue perfusion (peripheral and/or renal)** *related to* graft thrombosis, embolism, prolonged aortic cross-clamping, hypotension, and blood loss *as manifested by* absent or diminished peripheral pulses, altered skin color, decreased urine output, altered ability to move extremities.
• Patent arterial graft with adequate distal perfusion • Urine output adequate	• Assess for diminished or absent peripheral pulses in the extremities; color or temperature changes in the extremities; altered sensation and movement of the extremities; increased pain level *because these are indicators of altered peripheral perfusion.* • Compare extremities for warmth, capillary refill, and color *because differences may indicate impaired blood flow.* • Administer IV fluids at prescribed rates *to ensure adequate hydration and renal perfusion.* • Maintain a warm environment *to prevent temperature-induced vasoconstriction.* • Administer anticoagulants and/or antiplatelet agents as prescribed *to prevent thrombus formation.* • Monitor urinary output daily weights, BUN, and serum creatinine *to detect signs of altered renal perfusion and renal failure.*
NURSING DIAGNOSIS	**Risk for infection** *related to* presence of a prosthetic vascular graft and invasive lines.
• Normal body temperature • No signs of infection • Wound is well approximated	• Monitor for signs of infection such as elevated body temperature, elevated WBC count, heart rate, and respiratory rate; decreased blood pressure; erythema and warmth along the incision line; persistent drainage from incisions, as well as sites of invasive lines; separation of wound edges. • Administer broad-spectrum antibiotic as ordered *to maintain adequate blood levels of the drug.* • Monitor WBC count *because a rising count may be the first sign of infection.* • Use aseptic technique in caring for incision and any indwelling IV line, tubing, or catheter *because these sites are potential portals of entry for infection.* • Ensure adequate nutrition, specifically a diet high in protein, vitamin C, vitamin A, and zinc, *to promote healing.*

BUN, Blood urea nitrogen; *IV,* intravenous; *WBC,* white blood cell.

and to report any elevations. Laboratory data should be monitored for elevated white blood cell (WBC) count, which may be the first indication of an infection. In addition, the nurse should ensure adequate nutrition and observe the surgical incision for any evidence of delayed healing, signs of infection, or prolonged drainage.

All IV, arterial, and central venous catheter insertion sites should be cared for carefully with the use of sterile technique because they are frequently a portal of entry for bacteria. Meticulous perineal care for the patient with an indwelling urinary catheter is also essential to minimize the risk of urinary tract infection. Surgical incisions should be kept clean and dry.

Gastrointestinal status. After abdominal aortic surgery, paralytic ileus may develop as a result of anesthesia and the manual manipulation and displacement of the bowel for long periods during surgery. The intestines may become swollen and bruised, and peristalsis ceases for variable intervals. A retroperitoneal surgical approach can be used to decrease the risk of bowel complications.

A nasogastric tube is inserted during surgery and connected to low, intermittent suction. This decompresses the stomach and duodenum, prevents aspiration of stomach contents, and decreases pressure on suture lines. The nasogastric tube should be irrigated with normal saline solution as needed, and the amount and character of the drainage should be recorded. The nurse should auscultate for the return of bowel sounds. The passing of flatus is a key sign of returning bowel function and should be noted. Early ambulation will assist with the resumption of bowel functioning. It is unusual for paralytic ileus to persist beyond the fourth postoperative day.

While the patient is NPO, meticulous mouth care should be given every few hours. In some situations ice chips or lozenges may be given to the patient to soothe an irritated throat.

If the blood supply to the bowel is disrupted during surgery, temporary ischemia or infarction (death) of intestinal tissue may result. This is evidenced by lack of bowel sounds, fever, abdominal distention, diarrhea, and bloody stools. When bowel infarction does occur as a result of mesenteric ischemia, reoperation is necessary as soon as possible to restore blood flow, with likely resection of the infarcted bowel. Fortunately, this serious complication is uncommon.

Neurologic status. Neurologic complications can occur after surgical procedures on the aorta. When the ascending aorta and aortic arch are involved, nursing interventions should include assessment of level of consciousness, pupil size and response to light, facial symmetry, tongue deviation, speech, ability to move upper extremities, and quality of hand grasps (see Chapter 55). When the descending aorta is involved, nursing assessment of the ability to move lower extremities is also important. These assessments should be recorded in detail with a careful description of the patient's response. Any alteration from the baseline assessment should be reported to the physician immediately.

Peripheral perfusion status. The anatomic location of the aneurysm indicates the areas of major concern related to peripheral perfusion. All peripheral pulses should be checked regularly and recorded. This should be done every hour for several hours, depending on the nursing policy, and routinely thereafter at frequent intervals. When the ascending aorta and aortic arch are involved, the carotid, radial, and temporal artery pulses should be assessed. After surgery involving the descending aorta, pulses to be assessed may include the femoral, popliteal, posterior tibial, and dorsalis pedis (see Chapter 31, Fig. 31-8).

When checking the pulses, the nurse should mark the locations lightly with a felt-tip pen so that others can locate them easily. An ultrasonic Doppler is useful in assessment of peripheral pulses. It is also important to note the skin temperature and color, capillary refill time, and sensation and movement of the extremities.

Occasionally pulses in the lower extremities may be absent for a short time following surgery. This is usually due to vasospasm and hypothermia. A decreased or absent pulse in conjunction with a cool, pale, mottled, or painful extremity may indicate embolization of aneurysmal thrombus or plaque or occlusion of the graft. Graft occlusion is treated with reoperation if identified early. In rare instances, thrombolytic therapy may also be considered. Therefore these findings should be reported to the surgeon immediately. In some patients the pulses may have been absent preoperatively because of coexistent peripheral arterial occlusive disease. Comparison with the preoperative status is essential to determine the etiology of a decreased or absent pulse and the proper treatment.

Renal perfusion status. One of the causes of decreased renal perfusion is embolization of a fragment of thrombus or plaque from the aorta that subsequently lodges in one or both of the renal arteries. This can cause ischemia of one or both kidneys. Hypotension, dehydration, prolonged aortic clamping, or blood loss can also lead to decreased renal perfusion.

The patient returns from surgery with an indwelling urinary catheter in place. In the immediate postoperative period, hourly urine outputs are recorded. An accurate record of fluid intake and urinary output should be kept until the patient resumes the preoperative diet. Daily weights also should be obtained. Central venous pressure readings and pulmonary artery pressures also provide important information regarding hydration status. Daily blood urea nitrogen (BUN) and serum creatinine studies are performed to evaluate renal function. (For signs and symptoms of acute renal failure, see Chapter 45.) Irreversible renal failure may occur after aortic surgery, particularly in high risk individuals (e.g., patients with diabetes).

Ambulatory and Home Care. The patient may be apprehensive about returning home after major surgery involving the aorta. The nurse should encourage the patient to express any concerns and reassure the patient that normal activities of daily living can be resumed. The patient should be instructed to gradually increase activities. Fatigue, poor appetite, and irregular bowel habits are to be expected. Heavy lifting is avoided for at least 4 to 6 weeks following surgery. Observation of incisions for signs and symptoms of infection is encouraged. Any redness, swelling, increased pain, drainage from incisions, or fever greater than 100° F (37.8° C) should be reported to the health care provider.

The patient should be taught to observe for changes in color or warmth of the extremities. Patients may be taught to palpate peripheral pulses and to assess changes in their quality. The patient who has received a synthetic graft should be aware that prophylactic antibiotics may be required before future invasive procedures, including any dental procedures.

Sexual dysfunction in male patients is not uncommon after aortic surgery. Sexual dysfunction may occur because the internal hypogastric artery is interrupted, leading to decreased arterial blood flow to the penis. In addition, the periaortic sympathetic plexus may be disrupted by the surgical procedure. Preoperatively, baseline sexual function should be documented and patient counseling is recommended. Postoperatively, a referral to a urologist may be considered if impotence is a problem.

There are situations in which operative repair is not performed. Examples of this are the presence of a very small aneurysm (less than 4 cm), a patient who is not a surgical candidate (e.g., severe lung or cardiac disease), or patient or family refusal to undergo repair. The patient who does not undergo surgical repair should be urged to receive regular routine physical examinations and should be reminded that any symptom, no matter how minor, must be investigated if it persists.

Evaluation

Expected outcomes for the patient who undergoes aortic surgery are addressed in NCP 37-1.

AORTIC DISSECTION

Aortic dissection, often misnamed "dissecting aneurysm," is not a type of aneurysm. **Aortic dissection,** occurring most commonly in the thoracic aorta, is the result of a tear in the intimal (innermost) lining of the arterial wall that allows blood to enter between the intima and media, thus creating a false lumen (Figs. 37-3 and 37-5). Aortic dissection affects men more often than women and occurs most frequently between the fourth and seventh decades of life. This process is usually acute and life threatening. However, it also may be self-limiting and result in a chronic and stable process for a period of time. If patients have an acute ascending aortic dissection and are not surgically treated, the mortality rate is 90%.[15]

Etiology and Pathophysiology

Aortic dissection results from a small tear in the intimal lining of the artery, allowing blood to "track" between the intima and media and creating a false lumen of blood flow. As the heart contracts, each systolic pulsation causes increased pressure on the damaged area, which further increases the dissection. As it

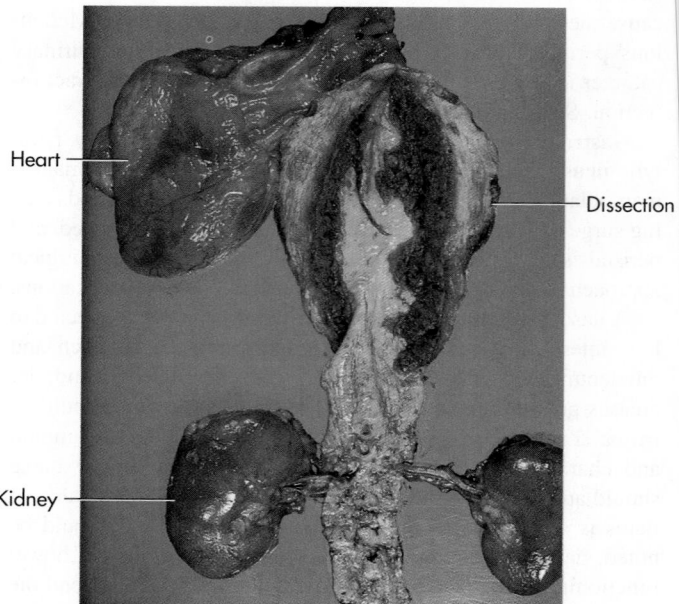

FIG. 37-5   Aortic dissection of the thoracic aorta.

extends proximally or distally, it may occlude major branches of the aorta, cutting off blood supply to areas such as the brain, abdominal organs, kidneys, spinal cord, and extremities. Occasionally a small tear develops distally and the blood flow reenters the true vessel lumen.

The exact cause of dissection is uncertain, although many authorities attribute the cause to the destruction of the medial layer elastic fibers. Most people with dissection problems are older and have chronic hypertension. Persons with Marfan syndrome (a premature degeneration of vascular elastic tissue) have a high incidence of aortic dissection. Pregnancy promotes increased vascular stress because of increased total blood volume, decreased peripheral vascular resistance, and increased aortic compliance.[16] Blunt trauma is also a precipitating factor associated with aortic dissection. Areas that undergo the greatest amount of stress and are thus most prone to dissection are the ascending aorta, the aortic arch, and the descending aorta beyond the origin of the left subclavian artery.

Clinical Manifestations

Clinical manifestations depend on the location of the intimal tear and the extent of the dissection. The typical patient with acute aortic dissection usually has sudden, severe pain in the anterior part of the chest or intrascapular pain radiating down the spine into the abdomen or legs.[17] The pain is described as "tearing" or "ripping." The severe pain may mimic that of a myocardial infarction. As the dissection progresses, pain may be located both above and below the diaphragm. Cardiovascular, neurologic, and respiratory signs may also be present.

If the arch of the aorta is involved, the patient may exhibit neurologic deficiencies, including an altered level of consciousness, dizziness, and weakened or absent carotid and temporal pulses. An ascending aortic dissection usually produces some degree of aortic valvular insufficiency, and a new high-pitched, diastolic cardiac murmur is audible on auscultation. Severe aortic valve insufficiency may produce left ventricular failure with the development of dyspnea and orthopnea caused by pulmonary edema. When either subclavian artery is involved, radial, ulnar, and brachial pulse quality and blood pressure (BP) readings may be significantly different between the left and right arms. As the dissection progresses down the aorta, the abdominal organs and lower extremities demonstrate evidence of altered tissue perfusion.

Complications

A severe and life-threatening complication of aortic dissection of the ascending aortic arch is *cardiac tamponade*, which occurs when blood escapes from the dissection into the pericardial sac. Clinical manifestations of cardiac tamponade include hypotension, narrowed pulse pressure, distended neck veins, muffled heart sounds, and pulsus paradoxus (see Chapter 36).

Because the aorta is weakened by the medial dissection, it may rupture. Hemorrhage may occur into the mediastinal, pleural, or abdominal cavities. Rupture of a dissected aorta typically results in exsanguination and death. Research indicates that 86% of deaths associated with aortic dissection are due to aortic rupture.[17]

Dissection can lead to occlusion of the arterial supply to many vital organs, such as the spinal cord, kidneys, and abdominal organs. Ischemia of the spinal cord produces symptoms varying from weakness and decreased pain sensation to complete paralysis of the lower extremities. Renal ischemia can lead to renal failure. Manifestations of abdominal ischemia include abdominal pain, decreased bowel sounds, and altered bowel elimination.

Diagnostic Studies

The diagnostic studies used to assess aortic dissection are similar to those performed for aortic aneurysms (Table 37-1). Left ventricular hypertrophy is a common finding on an echocardiogram and is possibly related to changes caused by systemic hypertension. A chest x-ray may show a widening of the mediastinal silhouette and left pleural effusion. A transesophageal echocardiogram (TEE) can identify dissections that are closest to the aortic root. A CT scan or MRI provides valuable information on the presence and severity of the dissection. After the patient's condition has stabilized, angiography may be necessary to assess the extent of the dissection.

Collaborative Care

The initial goal of therapy for aortic dissection without complications is to lower the BP and myocardial contractility to diminish the pulsatile forces within the aorta (see Table 37-1). IV trimethaphan (Arfonad) and nitroprusside (Nipride) rapidly reduce the systolic blood pressure. In addition, IV β-adrenergic blockers, such as propranolol (Inderal), decrease the force of myocardial contractility.

Conservative Therapy. The patient with aortic dissection without complications can be treated conservatively for a period. Supportive treatment is directed toward pain relief, blood transfusion (if required), and management of heart failure (if indicated). If the dissection is limited to the descending aorta, conservative therapy may be adequate to treat the problem. Success of the treatment is judged by relief of pain, which is an indication of stabilization of the dissection. However, if the dissection involves the ascending aorta, imminent surgery is usually indicated.

Surgical Therapy. Surgery is indicated when drug therapy is ineffective or when complications of aortic dissection (e.g., heart failure, leaking dissection, occlusion of an artery) are present.

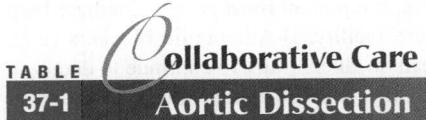

TABLE 37-1	***C*ollaborative Care **Aortic Dissection**

Diagnostic
Health history and physical examination
ECG
Chest x-ray
CT scan
Transesophageal echocardiogram (TEE)
Angiogram
Magnetic resonance imaging (MRI)

Collaborative Therapy
Bed rest
Pain relief with narcotics
Control of blood pressure
- trimethaphan (Arfonad)
- sodium nitroprusside (Nipride)
Control of myocardial contractility
- propranolol (Inderal)
- labetalol (Normodyne)
Aortic resection and repair

CT, Computed tomography; *ECG,* electrocardiogram.

The aorta is fragile following the dissection. Therefore surgery is delayed for as long as possible to allow time for edema in the area of the dissection to decrease, to permit clotting of the blood in the false lumen, and to allow the healing process to begin. Surgery for aortic dissection involves resection of the aortic segment containing the intimal tear and replacement with synthetic graft material. The extent of aortic replacement depends on the extent of the dissection.

NURSING MANAGEMENT AORTIC DISSECTION

Preoperatively, nursing management related to an aortic dissection includes keeping the patient in bed in a semi-Fowler position and maintaining a quiet environment. These measures assist in keeping the systolic BP at the lowest possible level that maintains vital organ perfusion (typically maintaining systolic BP between 110 and 120 mm Hg or mean arterial pressure between 70 and 80 mm Hg).[15] Narcotics and tranquilizers should be administered as ordered. Pain and anxiety must be managed for patient comfort, especially since they may cause elevations in the systolic BP.

Continuous IV administration of antihypertensive agents requires close nursing supervision. An ECG monitoring device is used, and an intraarterial pressure line is usually inserted (see Chapter 64). The nurse should observe for changes in the quality of peripheral pulses and for signs of increasing pain, restlessness, and anxiety. Vital signs are taken frequently, sometimes as often as every 2 to 3 minutes while obtaining control of the BP. If the blood vessels branching off the aortic arch are involved, decreased cerebral blood flow may alter the sensorium and level of consciousness. Postoperative care after surgery to correct the dissection is similar to that after aneurysmectomy (see section on nursing management of aneurysms earlier in this chapter and NCP 37-1).

In preparation for discharge, the nurse should focus on patient and family teaching. The therapeutic regimen includes antihypertensive drugs, which are usually taken orally. The patient needs to understand that these drugs must be taken to control BP. The nurse should instruct the patient that if the pain returns or other symptoms progress, the patient must seek immediate help at the nearest health care facility. β-Adrenergic blockers (e.g., propranolol [Inderal]) can be taken orally to continue to decrease myocardial contractility. It is important that the patient understand the drug regimen and potential side effects. The patient should be told to discuss any side effects with the health care provider before discontinuing the drug.

PERIPHERAL ARTERIAL DISEASE OF THE LOWER EXTREMITIES

Peripheral arterial disease (PAD) of the lower extremities may affect the aortoiliac, femoral, popliteal, tibial, or peroneal arteries, or any combination of these areas (see Fig. 37-1). The femoral-popliteal area is the site most commonly affected in nondiabetic patients. The patient with diabetes mellitus tends to develop disease in the arteries below the knee, especially the anterior tibial, posterior tibial, and peroneal arteries. In advanced stages, multiple levels of occlusions are found.

Clinical Manifestations

The severity of the clinical manifestations depends on the site and extent of the obstruction and the extent and amount of collateral circulation. The classic symptom of PAD of the lower ex-

tremities is **intermittent claudication,** ischemic muscle ache or pain that is precipitated by a consistent level of exercise, resolves within 10 minutes or less with rest, and is reproducible.[2] The ischemic pain is attributable to end products of anaerobic cellular metabolism, such as lactic acid accumulation. Once the patient stops exercising, the metabolites are cleared and the pain subsides. Disease involving the femoral or popliteal arteries causes claudication in the calf. PAD of the aortoiliac arteries produces claudication in the buttocks and the thighs. It should be noted, however, that sedentary patients with PAD of the lower extremities may never exert themselves sufficiently to experience claudication. If disease extends into the internal iliac (hypogastric) arteries, impotence often results. Sexual dysfunction occurs in as many as 30% to 50% of patients with aortoiliac occlusion.[18]

Paresthesia, manifested as numbness or tingling occurring in the toes or feet, may result from nerve tissue ischemia. True peripheral neuropathy occurs more commonly in patients with diabetes (see Chapter 47) and in those with progressive long-standing ischemia. The neuropathy produces excruciating shooting or burning pain in the extremity. It does not follow any particular nerve roots but may be present near ulcerated areas. Gradually diminishing perfusion to neurons produces loss of both pressure and deep pain sensations. Therefore injuries to the extremity often go unnoticed by the patient.

The physical appearance of the limb provides important information about the adequacy of blood flow. Trophic changes occur to the skin. The skin becomes thin, shiny, and taut, and there is a loss of hair on the lower legs. Diminished or absent pedal, popliteal, or femoral pulses may be noted. Pallor or blanching of the foot is noted in response to leg elevation *(elevation pallor)*. Conversely, *reactive hyperemia* (redness of the foot) is observed when the limb is hung in a dependent position *(dependent rubor)*.

However, as the disease process advances and involves multiple arterial segments, continuous pain develops at rest. *Rest pain* most often occurs in the forefoot or toes and is aggravated by limb elevation. Rest pain occurs when there is insufficient blood flow to maintain basic metabolic requirements of the tissues and nerves of the distal extremity. Rest pain occurs more often at night because cardiac output tends to drop during sleep and the limbs are at the level of the heart. At this severity of disease, patients will try to achieve partial pain relief by dangling the leg over the side of the bed to allow gravity to maximize arterial blood flow. Without revascularization, the limb may progress to ulceration and gangrene. Every attempt is made to save the limb, and surgery is usually indicated unless the patient is at high surgical risk and/or has numerous comorbid medical conditions.

Complications

Peripheral arterial disease of the lower extremities progresses slowly. Prolonged ischemia leads to atrophy of the skin and underlying muscles. Because of the decreased arterial blood flow to the lower extremities, even minor trauma to the feet (e.g., stubbing one's toe, blister from ill-fitting shoes) may result in delayed healing, wound infection, and tissue necrosis, especially in the diabetic patient. Arterial (ischemic) ulcers most commonly occur over bony prominences on the toes, feet, and lower leg (Table 37-2). Nonhealing arterial ulcers and gangrene are the most serious complications of end-stage PAD and may result in lower extremity amputation if blood flow is not adequately restored or if severe infection occurs. If atherosclerosis has been

TABLE 37-2	Comparison of Arterial and Venous Leg Ulcers	
CHARACTERISTIC	**ARTERIAL**	**VENOUS**
Peripheral pulses	Decreased or absent	Present; may be difficult to palpate with edema
Capillary refill	>3 sec	<3 sec
Ankle-brachial index	<0.75	>0.90
Edema	No edema	Lower leg edema
Hair	Loss of hair on legs, feet, toes	Hair may be present or absent
Ulcer location	Tips of toes, foot, or lateral malleolus	Near medial malleolus
Ulcer margin	Rounded, smooth, looks "punched out"	Irregularly shaped
Ulcer drainage	Minimal	Moderate to large amount
Pain	Intermittent claudication or rest pain in foot; ulcer may or may not be painful	Dull ache or heaviness in calf or thigh; ulcer often painful
Nails	Thickened; brittle	Normal or thickened
Skin color	Dependency rubor; elevation pallor	Bronze-brown pigmentation; varicose veins may be visible
Skin texture	Thin, shiny, friable, dry	Skin thick, hardened, and indurated
Skin temperature	Cool, temperature gradient down the leg	Warm, no temperature gradient
Dermatitis	Rarely occurs	Frequently occurs
Pruritus	Rarely occurs	Frequently occurs

present for an extended period, collateral circulation may prevent gangrene of the extremity.

Diagnostic Studies

Various tests have been developed to assess blood flow and to outline the vascular system (Table 37-3). Doppler ultrasound consists of a probe transducer containing a crystal that directs high-frequency sound waves toward the artery or vein being examined. The sound waves bounce off the blood cells at a rate that corresponds with the velocity (or speed) of blood flow through the vessel. This emits an audible signal. When palpation of a peripheral pulse is difficult because of severe PAD, the Doppler can be useful in determining the presence of blood flow. A palpable pulse and a dopplerable pulse are not equivalent, and these terms should not be used interchangeably. In addition, *segmental blood pressures* are also obtained (using a Doppler and sphygmomanometer) at the thigh, below the knee, and at ankle level while the patient is supine. A falloff in segmental pressure of more than 30 mm Hg indicates PAD.

The *ankle-brachial index* (ABI) is done using a handheld Doppler. The ABI is calculated by dividing the ankle systolic blood pressure (SBP) by the highest brachial SBP.[19] A normal ABI is 0.90 to 1.30. An ABI between 0.41 and 0.89 indicates mild to moderate PAD, and an index of 0 to 0.40 indicates severe PAD. The ABI technique is also used to follow patients postoperatively after revascularization to monitor patency of bypass grafts. This procedure has limited usefulness when arteries are calcified and noncompressible, as occurs in patients with diabetes mellitus. In these patients the ABI is frequently falsely elevated.

Duplex imaging, another noninvasive test, uses a bidirectional, color Doppler system to systematically map blood flow throughout the entire region of an artery. It provides anatomic and physiologic information about the blood vessels.

Angiography is used to further delineate the location and extent of the disease process. In addition, it provides information on inflow and outflow vessels to plan for surgery. Angiography is

TABLE 37-3	*Collaborative Care* **Peripheral Arterial Disease**

Diagnostic
Health history and physical examination, including palpation of peripheral pulses
Doppler ultrasound studies
Segmental blood pressures
Ankle-brachial index (ABI)
Duplex imaging
Angiogram
Magnetic resonance angiography (MRA)

Collaborative Therapy
Risk factor modification
- Smoking cessation
- Structured walking/exercise program
- Glucose control in diabetics
- Blood pressure control
- Treatment of high cholesterol

Antiplatelet agents
- aspirin
- ticlopidine (Ticlid)
- clopidogrel (Plavix)
- cilostazol (Pletal)
- pentoxifylline (Trental)

Nutritional therapy
Proper foot care (see Chapter 47, Table 47-21)
Percutaneous transluminal angioplasty with or without stent
Peripheral arterial bypass surgery
Patch graft angioplasty, often in conjunction with bypass surgery
Anticoagulation
Endarterectomy (for localized stenosis but rarely done)
Thrombolytic therapy
Amputation

useful when an intervention (i.e., surgery, angioplasty) is indicated. Magnetic resonance angiography (MRA) is sometimes used alternatively. (MRA is described in Chapter 54.)

Collaborative Care (see Table 37-3)

Risk Factor Modification. Regardless of the severity of symptoms, it is paramount that all patients with PAD undergo risk factor modification.[20,21] Smoking cessation is essential for slowing the progression of PAD to critical limb ischemia and reducing the risk of myocardial infarction and death.[20] Smoking cessation is a complex and difficult process with a high incidence of smoking relapse.[22] (Smoking cessation is discussed in Chapter 11 and Tables 11-14, 11-15, and 11-17.)

Aggressive treatment of hyperlipidemia (low-density lipoproteins [LDLs] less than 100 mg/dl and triglycerides less than 150 mg/dl) is another goal of therapy in PAD patients. Research has shown that treatment of PAD patients with a lipid-lowering agent such as a statin (e.g., simvastatin [Zocor]) lowers serum cholesterol levels, improves endothelial function, and stabilizes or reduces femoral atherosclerosis.[20] (Therapy to lower cholesterol is discussed in Chapter 33.)

Hypertension and diabetes mellitus are both important risk factors for PAD. However, data are not conclusive as to whether aggressive treatment will alter the progression of PAD.[20,21] Nonetheless, tight control of these two risk factors will likely decrease the risk of other cardiovascular-related morbidity and mortality (i.e., stroke, myocardial infarction). A glycosylated hemoglobin (A_{1C}) less than 7.0% is recommended for diabetics. Blood pressure should be maintained at less than 130/85 mm Hg.

Drug Therapy. Antiplatelet agents such as aspirin, ticlopidine (Ticlid), and clopidogrel (Plavix) are considered important for reducing the risks of myocardial infarction, ischemic stroke, and cardiovascular-related death in patients with PAD.[20] Aspirin, however, is not tolerated by some patients because of gastrointestinal distress. Ticlopidine and clopidogrel, both drugs that inhibit platelet activation, are also effective in reducing the risk of MI and stroke. Patients taking ticlopidine must be monitored carefully for thrombocytopenia, neutropenia, and thrombotic thrombocytopenic purpura, all of which necessitate stopping the drug. Clopidogrel is more effective than aspirin at reducing the risk of MI, stroke, and cardiovascular-related death in patients with PAD.[23]

Various drugs are prescribed to treat intermittent claudication. The most common drug therapy has been pentoxifylline (Trental), which increases erythrocyte flexibility and reduces blood viscosity, thus improving the supply of oxygenated blood to ischemic muscle. The use of heparin, low-molecular-weight heparin, and oral anticoagulants is not recommended for treating intermittent claudication.[24]

Cilostazol (Pletal) is the newest medication approved for the treatment of intermittent claudication. It is a phosphodiesterase inhibitor that promotes the effects of prostaglandin I_2, thus inhibiting platelet aggregation and increasing vasodilation. Cilostazol has been shown to significantly increase pain-free walking distance and maximal walking distance with minimal side effects.[24,25] The most common side effects are headache and transient diarrhea. Cilostazol should be used with caution in patients with New York Heart Association classification III and IV heart failure. (Heart failure is discussed in Chapter 34.)

Exercise Therapy. The primary nonpharmacologic treatment for claudication is a formal exercise-training program.[20] Al-though exercise training does not cause increased collateral blood flow to the legs, it does improve oxygen extraction in the legs and skeletal muscle metabolism.

Walking is the most effective exercise for individuals with claudication. Slow, progressive physical activity should be encouraged after a warm-up period. The patient should be instructed to walk to the point of discomfort, stop and rest, and then resume walking until the discomfort recurs. Walking should be done for a prescribed time, usually 30 to 40 minutes a day, in addition to normal activity. Patients in a formal rehabilitation program can exercise on other equipment (e.g., exercise bicycles, rowing machines) to improve whole body fitness and minimize boredom. An exercise therapy program should also be implemented in PAD patients after balloon angioplasty and/or peripheral arterial bypass surgery.

Nutritional Therapy. The patient with PAD should be taught how to alter his or her dietary intake. Overall caloric intake should be adjusted so that ideal body weight can be achieved and maintained. Within the diet, dietary cholesterol should be less than 200 mg per day and the saturated fat intake should be substantially reduced (see Chapter 33, Table 33-4). Soy protein products (e.g., tofu, miso) can be used in place of animal protein to help lower serum LDL cholesterol and triglycerides.[26] In addition, dietary sodium should be no more than 2 g per day (see Chapter 34, Tables 34-9, 34-10, and 34-11).

Complementary and Alternative Therapies. *Ginkgo biloba* is effective in increasing walking distance for patients with intermittent claudication.[27] Other nutritional supplements, which require additional randomized controlled trials, show promising results regarding the treatment of PAD. For example, folate, vitamin B_6, and cobalamin (vitamin B_{12}) appear to lower homocysteine levels.[28]

Care of the Leg with Critical Limb Ischemia. Conservative management goals of the patient with critical limb ischemia due to PAD include protecting the extremity from trauma, decreasing vasospasm, preventing and controlling infection, and maximizing arterial perfusion. Careful inspection, cleansing, and lubrication of both feet are advised to prevent cracking of the skin and infection. Although cleansing is important, soaking of the affected foot should be avoided to prevent skin maceration (or breakdown). If ulceration is present, the affected foot should be kept clean and dry. Covering the ulcer with a dry, sterile dressing helps maintain cleanliness and protects the limb. Ulcers with any significant depth may be treated with a variety of wound care products, but without restoration of blood flow healing is unlikely. Footwear should be soft, roomy, and protective. Chemicals, heat, and cold should be avoided. The patient's heels should be kept free of pressure. This can be accomplished by placing a pillow under the calves so that the heels do not touch the bed. There are also many commercially available devices that provide heel elevation.

Interventional Radiologic Procedures. Interventional radiologic procedures are indicated when (1) intermittent claudication symptoms become incapacitating, (2) the patient experiences pain at rest, or (3) ulceration or gangrene is severe enough to threaten the viability of the limb.

Similar to the angiography diagnostic procedure, *percutaneous transluminal balloon angioplasty* involves the insertion of a catheter through the femoral artery. However, the catheter is special and contains a cylindric balloon. The end of the catheter is advanced to the narrowed area of the artery, the balloon is inflated, and the balloon dilates the vessel by cracking the confining atherosclerotic intimal shell while also stretching the underlying media. This procedure is used selectively in certain patients who have localized, accessible lesions (less than 10 cm in length). Iliac and femoral artery lesions have responded most successfully to balloon angioplasty. It should be noted, however, that balloon angioplasty is not effective on arteries with diffuse or long segment lesions or in smaller vessels below the knee (tibial arteries).[29] Furthermore, there is a relatively high rate of restenosis after balloon angioplasty (up to 50% restenosis at 1 year). Successful angioplasty has been shown to improve health-related quality of life as much as arterial bypass surgery.[30]

Consequently, other adjunctive devices or techniques have been used in conjunction with balloon angioplasty in an attempt to improve patency rates. Atherectomy catheters and laser-tipped catheters have been used to either "shave" or "burn," respectively, the atherosclerotic plaque lining the arterial wall before balloon dilation. However, no significant improvement of patency has been obtained.[29]

In contrast, the placement of intravascular stents with balloon angioplasty helps relieve the problems of restenosis and arterial dissection. *Stents* are rigid or flexible metallic devices that are positioned within the artery immediately after the balloon angioplasty is performed. Antiplatelet agents are used after stenting procedures to reduce the risk of platelet aggregation and subsequent restenosis.

Surgical Therapy. Various surgical approaches can be used to improve arterial blood flow beyond a stenotic or occluded artery. The most common is a peripheral arterial bypass operation with autogenous vein or synthetic graft material to bypass or carry blood around the lesion (Fig. 37-6).

Other surgical options include *endarterectomy* (opening the artery and removing the obstructing plaque) and *patch graft angioplasty* (opening the artery, removing plaque, and sewing a patch to the opening to widen the lumen).[31] Antiplatelet agents are used often to prevent thrombosis after arterial bypass surgery. In addition, anticoagulation with heparin in the immediate postoperative period followed by long-term warfarin (Coumadin) therapy is sometimes used in the patient who has a tendency to occlude grafts secondary to a coagulopathy (clotting abnormality).

Amputation is the least desirable and is the end-stage surgical option, but it may be required if gangrene is extensive, infection is present in the bone (osteomyelitis), or all major arteries in the limb are occluded, precluding the possibility of successful peripheral arterial bypass surgery. Every effort is made to preserve as much of the limb as possible so that the potential for rehabilitation is optimized (see Chapter 61).

NURSING MANAGEMENT
LOWER EXTREMITY PERIPHERAL ARTERIAL DISEASE
■ Nursing Assessment

Subjective and objective data that should be obtained from a patient with PAD are presented in Table 37-4.

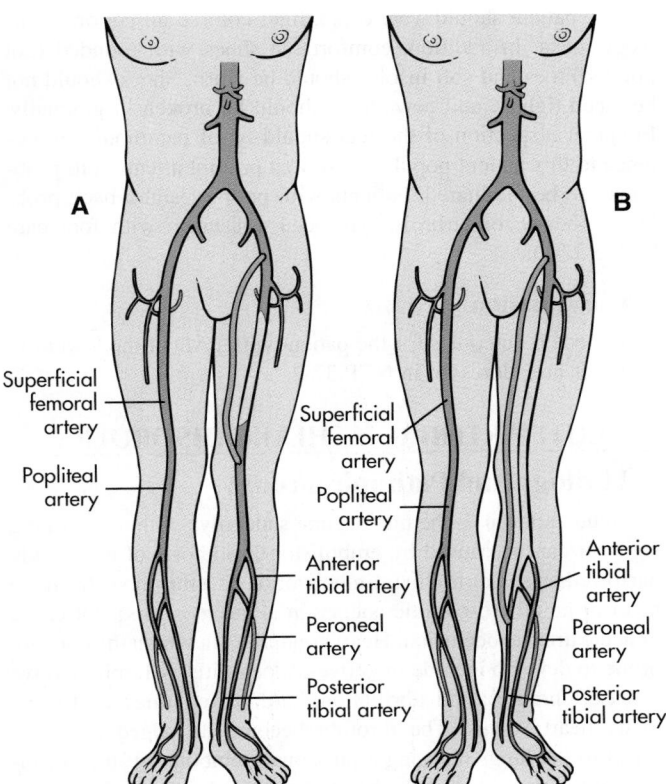

FIG. 37-6 A, Femoral-popliteal bypass graft around an occluded superficial femoral artery. B, Femoral-posterior tibial bypass graft around occluded superficial femoral, popliteal, and proximal tibial arteries.

TABLE 37-4	Nursing Assessment — Peripheral Arterial Disease

Subjective Data
Important Health Information
Past health history: Diabetes mellitus, smoking, hypertension, hyperlipidemia, hypertriglyceridemia, hyperuricemia, obesity, ↑ homocysteine or ferritin levels, positive family history, sedentary lifestyle, stress
Functional Health Patterns
Health perception–health management: Family history of vascular disease; smoking
Nutritional-metabolic: High saturated fat and cholesterol intake; elevated hemoglobin A1C
Activity-exercise: Exercise intolerance
Cognitive-perceptual: Buttock, thigh, or calf pain that is precipitated by exercise and that subsides with rest (intermittent claudication) or progresses to pain at rest; burning pain in forefeet and toes at rest; numbness, tingling, sensation of cold in legs or feet; progressive loss of sensation and deep pain in extremities
Sexuality-reproductive: Impotence

Objective Data
Integumentary
Loss of hair on legs and feet; thick toenails; pallor with elevation; dependent rubor; thin, cool, shiny skin with muscle atrophy; skin breakdown and arterial ulcers, especially over bony areas; gangrene
Cardiovascular
Decreased or absent peripheral pulses; feet cool to touch; bruits may be present at pulse sites
Neurologic
Mobility or sensation impairment
Possible Findings
Positive arterial duplex imaging, ↑ Doppler pressures, ↓ ankle-brachial index (ABI), angiography indicative of peripheral atherosclerosis

■ Nursing Diagnoses

Nursing diagnoses for the patient with PAD of the lower extremities (who has not undergone surgery) may include, but are not limited to, those presented in NCP 37-2.

■ Planning

The overall goals are that the patient with PAD of the lower extremities will have (1) adequate tissue perfusion; (2) relief of pain; (3) increased exercise tolerance; and (4) intact, healthy skin on extremities.

■ Nursing Implementation

Health Promotion. The patient should be assessed for risk factors and should be taught how to control them (see Chapter 33, Table 33-3). The nurse's role in the inpatient care facility includes identifying at-risk patients. The nurse should also be involved at the community level, such as in screening clinics for PAD, hyperlipidemia, hypertension, and diabetes. Young people and adults should be educated about the hazards of cigarette smoking. The nurse should also assist in teaching diet modification to reduce the intake of cholesterol, saturated fat, and refined sugars; proper care of the feet; and the avoidance of injury to the extremities. Patients with positive family histories of cardiac, diabetic, or vascular disease should be encouraged to obtain regular follow-up care.

Acute Intervention. After surgical or radiologic intervention the patient is placed in a recovery area for close observation. The operative extremity should be checked every 15 minutes initially and then hourly for skin color and temperature, capillary refill, presence of peripheral pulses distal to the operative site, and sensation and movement of the extremity. Loss of palpable pulses necessitates immediate notification of the surgeon and intervention. Ankle-brachial index (ABI) measurements may be ordered, and the indices should increase from the patient's preoperative baseline. They should remain constant if the bypass (or stent) remains patent. All of these findings should be compared with the patient's preoperative baseline and with findings in the opposite limb.[31]

After the patient leaves the recovery area, nursing care should focus on continued circulatory assessment and monitoring for the development of potential complications. These include bleeding, hematoma, thrombosis, embolization, and compartment syndrome. A dramatic increase in the level of pain, loss of a palpable pulse or pulses distal to the operative site, extremity pallor or cyanosis, decreasing ABIs, numbness or tingling, or a cold extremity temperature may indicate occlusion of the bypass graft and should be reported to the surgeon immediately.

Knee-flexed positions should be avoided except for exercise. The patient should be turned and positioned frequently with pillows to cushion the incision. By the first or second postoperative day, the patient should be out of bed several times daily. Sitting for long periods of time should be discouraged because leg dependency may cause significant edema, resulting in discomfort and stress to suture lines, and increases the risk of deep vein thrombosis. If significant swelling develops, a reclining position is preferred, with the edematous leg elevated above heart level. Occasionally elastic bandages (ACE) or elastic support stockings are used to help control edema of the limb. Walking even short distances is desirable. The use of a walker may be helpful initially, especially in the older patient. If no complications are present, discharge from the hospital can be anticipated 3 to 5 days postoperatively.

Ambulatory and Home Care. Atherosclerosis is a systemic disease process and not just localized to the lower extremities. Therefore the overall approach to the control of atherosclerotic occlusive disease involves management of risk factors (see Chapter 33, Table 33-3). Tobacco in any form is totally contraindicated, not only because of the vasoconstrictive effects of nicotine, but also because tobacco smoke impairs transport and cellular utilization of oxygen and increases blood viscosity. Continuance of cigarette smoking dramatically decreases the long-term patency rates of the bypass graft, as well as increases the risk of a myocardial infarction and stroke. (Smoking cessation is discussed in Chapter 11 and Tables 11-14, 11-15, and 11-17.)

All patients should be taught the importance of meticulous foot care to prevent injury. The patient should learn to inspect the legs and feet daily for skin color changes, mottling, alterations in the texture of the skin and subcutaneous fat, and reduction or absence of hair growth. Any ulceration or inflammation must be reported to the health care provider. Skin temperature should be noted, and capillary refill of the fingers and toes should be tested. In addition, selected patients may be taught to palpate pulses and report any changes to the health care provider. Thick or overgrown toenails and calluses are potentially serious lesions that require regular attention by a skilled health care provider (e.g., podiatrist). Emphasis on foot care is especially important in the diabetic patient with PAD because diabetic neuropathy (i.e., diminished peripheral sensation) increases the susceptibility to traumatic injury and results in delay in seeking treatment (see Chapter 47, Table 47-21).

The patient should wear clean, light-colored all-cotton or all-wool socks. In addition, comfortable shoes with rounded (not pointed) toes and soft insoles should be worn. Shoes should not be laced tightly, and new shoes should be broken in gradually. Frequent inspection of the feet should be of paramount importance to this patient population so that prompt attention to problems can be facilitated. Patients with poor eyesight, back problems, obesity, or arthritis may need assistance with foot care (Table 37-5).

■ Evaluation

Expected outcomes for the patient with PAD of the lower extremities are addressed in NCP 37-2.

ACUTE ARTERIAL ISCHEMIC DISORDERS

Etiology and Pathophysiology

Acute arterial ischemia occurs suddenly, without warning signs. It can be caused by embolism, thrombosis of an already narrowed artery, or trauma. Embolization of a thrombus from the heart or an atherosclerotic aneurysm is the most frequent cause of acute arterial occlusion. Heart conditions in which thrombi are prone to develop include infective endocarditis, MI, mitral valve disease, chronic atrial fibrillation, cardiomyopathies, and prosthetic heart valves. The thrombi become dislodged and may travel to the lungs (causing a pulmonary embolus) if they originate in the right side of the heart or to anywhere in the systemic circulation if they originate in the left side of the heart.

Arterial emboli tend to lodge at sites of arterial branching or in areas of atherosclerotic narrowing. An acute arterial occlusion

Patient with Peripheral Arterial Disease of the Lower Extremities

EXPECTED PATIENT OUTCOMES	NURSING INTERVENTIONS and *RATIONALES*

NURSING DIAGNOSIS | **Ineffective tissue perfusion (peripheral)** *related to* decreased arterial blood flow *as manifested by* intermittent claudication or rest pain; diminished or absent peripheral pulses; pallor or blanching on elevation of limb; hyperemia when limb is dependent.

- Able to identify activities that promote circulation
- Able to identify factors that impair circulation

- Assess for diminished or absent peripheral pulses in the extremities; color or temperature changes in the extremities; altered sensation and movement of the extremities; increased pain level *because these are indicators of worsening peripheral perfusion.*
- Compare extremities for warmth, capillary refill, and color *because differences may indicate impaired blood flow.*
- Encourage patient to participate in a structured walking program *to enhance O₂ utilization in the tissues.*
- Teach the patient to reduce risk factors for peripheral arterial disease by stopping smoking (see Chapter 11), lowering serum cholesterol and triglyceride levels, and controlling hypertension and diabetes mellitus *to prevent worsening of the atherosclerosis.*
- Teach patient to avoid tight girdles, garters, and socks, and avoid crossing legs, *because they impair peripheral circulation.*

NURSING DIAGNOSIS | **Impaired skin integrity** *related to* decreased peripheral circulation, altered sensation, and increased susceptibility to infection *as manifested by* ulcerations, nonhealing wounds, or gangrenous areas on lower extremities.

- Skin intact on lower extremities
- No evidence of wound or skin infection

- Teach patient to avoid trauma to lower extremities *because tissue is very fragile and wounds heal poorly due to poor circulation.*
- Teach patient to check temperature of bath water with fingers rather than toes to avoid burns *because sensation may be diminished.*
- Teach patient and significant other proper care and daily inspection of feet; the need to wear roomy, soft footwear and to obtain callus and toenail care by a health care professional *to avoid additional damage to the extremity.*
- Teach patient to apply a mild lotion daily to the lower extremities *to keep the skin moist and avoid cracking.*

NURSING DIAGNOSIS | **Acute pain** *related to* tissue ischemia secondary to decreased peripheral circulation *as manifested by* complaints of intermittent claudication or rest pain.

- Relief of pain

- Assess location, onset, degree, and duration of pain *so appropriate interventions are planned.*
- Encourage the patient to rest when pain occurs *so that tissue ischemia and pain are relieved or reduced,* and explain rationale to patient *to increase cooperation.*
- Teach patient relaxation techniques *because stress increases vasoconstriction and pain.*
- Teach patient to report rest pain *because this is an indication of worsening of the arterial blockages.*
- Teach patient the indications, benefits, and potential side effects of antiplatelet therapy (e.g., aspirin, ticlopidine [Ticlid]) *to prevent thrombosis* and pentoxyfylline (Trental) or cilostazol (Pletal) *because they help prevent pain and increase pain-free walking.*

NURSING DIAGNOSIS | **Activity intolerance** *related to* imbalance between oxygen supply and demand *as manifested by* intermittent claudication.

- Improved ability to ambulate without pain

- Assess the amount of exercise the patient can tolerate before the onset of pain *to provide a baseline for evaluation.*
- Instruct the patient to develop a structured exercise program that includes warm-up exercises, progressive walking, and cool-down exercises *to prevent injury during exercise.*
- Inform the patient that he or she should walk to point of pain, rest until pain subsides, and resume walking *so endurance can be increased and oxygen utilization in the tissues enhanced.*

NURSING DIAGNOSIS | **Ineffective therapeutic regimen management** *related to* lack of knowledge of disease and self-care measures *as manifested by* questions about disease process, wound, and treatment.

- Able to describe disease and treatment plan
- Able to demonstrate how to care for leg ulcers
- Able to identify risk factors for PAD and how to manage them

- Identify factors that influence learning such as perception of severity, available support systems, cognitive ability, and physical ability *so that teaching plan can be individualized.*
- Assess patient's knowledge of disease and its treatment *to determine extent of the problem and plan appropriate interventions.*
- Teach patient about the disease, treatment, activity restrictions, and ulcer care *so patient will be less anxious, be more cooperative with treatment plan, and make accurate adjustments in lifestyle.*
- Explain the importance of smoking cessation *so patient understands the effects of nicotine.*
- Emphasize the importance of meticulous foot care *to reduce the risk of infection and injury to feet.*

PAD, Peripheral arterial disease.

TABLE 37-5 Patient & Family Teaching Guide
Peripheral Artery Bypass Surgery

The nurse should include the following in a teaching plan:

1. Reduce your risk factors by stopping smoking and the use of tobacco products, controlling blood pressure and blood glucose levels (if diabetic), and lowering cholesterol and triglyceride levels.
2. Know reasons for and basic mechanism of action of medications such as antiplatelets, antihypertensives, anticholesterol therapy, and pain medication and how long anticipated therapy will last.
3. Eat healthy—it is essential to your recovery. You need to drink plenty of fluids, eat a well-balanced diet (including high-fiber foods and fresh fruits and vegetables), and eat less fried and high-fat foods.
4. Get a daily walk and/or participate in an exercise program. In the beginning, take several short walks a day and rest between activities. Gradually increase your walking to 30 to 40 minutes a day.
5. Care for your feet and legs. Inspect your feet and wash them daily. Wear clean cotton socks and well-fitting shoes. File toenails straight across. Avoid sitting with your legs crossed, extreme hot and cold temperatures, and prolonged standing.
6. Follow routine postoperative wound care that includes keeping incision clean and dry, not disturbing Steri-Strips, and eating a well-balanced diet that includes foods high in protein, vitamins C and A, and zinc.
7. Monitor for signs and symptoms of impaired healing and/or infection of the leg incision, and notify health care provider if any of the following occur:
   - Prolonged drainage or pus from the incision
   - Increased redness, warmth, pain, or hardness along incision
   - Separation of wound edges
   - Temperature greater than 100° F (37.8° C)
8. Keep all follow-up appointments with your health care provider.
9. Notify your physician immediately if you experience increased leg or foot pain or a change in the color or temperature of your foot and leg.

---

causes the blood supply distal to the embolus to acutely decrease. The degree and extent of symptoms depend on the size and location of the obstruction, the occurrence of clot fragmentation with embolism to smaller vessels, and the degree of PAD already present.

Sudden local thrombosis may occur at the location of an atherosclerotic plaque. Traumatic injury to the extremity itself may produce partial or total occlusion of a vessel from compression, shearing, or laceration. Acute arterial occlusion may also develop as a result of arterial dissection in the carotid artery or aorta or as a result of iatrogenic arterial injury (e.g., after angiography).

Clinical Manifestations

Signs and symptoms of an acute arterial ischemia usually have an abrupt onset. The exception is when a sudden occlusion is superimposed on preexisting PAD. In this case the symptoms may be insidious because collateral circulation is well developed.

Clinical manifestations of acute arterial ischemia include the "six Ps:" *pain, pallor, pulselessness, paresthesia, paralysis,* and *poikilothermia* (adaptation of the ischemic limb to its environmental temperature, most often cool). Without immediate intervention, ischemia may progress to tissue necrosis and gangrene within hours. It should be noted that paralysis is a very late sign of acute arterial ischemia and signals the death of nerves supplying the extremity. Because nerve tissue is extremely sensitive to hypoxia, limb paralysis or ischemic neuropathy may persist after revascularization and may be permanent.

Collaborative Care

With acute arterial ischemia due to occlusion, in the absence of adequate collateral circulation, early treatment is essential to keep the affected limb viable. Anticoagulant therapy is initiated immediately to prevent further enlargement of the thrombus and inhibit embolization. Continuous IV unfractionated heparin is the agent of choice. The thrombus should be removed as soon as possible by embolectomy or thrombectomy. Balloon catheters can be used and are passed distal and proximal to the site to remove the clot. Direct arteriotomy may be necessary to remove the clot.

If the ischemic limb is stable using heparin, recently formed emboli may be effectively treated with an intraarterial infusion of a thrombolytic agent (e.g., recombinant tissue plasminogen activator [tPA], streptokinase, or urokinase). A percutaneous catheter is inserted into the femoral artery and threaded to the site of the clot, and the drug is infused. Unlike anticoagulants, thrombolytic agents work by directly dissolving the clot over a period of 24 to 48 hours. (Thrombolytic therapy is discussed in Chapter 33.)

After the infusion of the thrombolytic agent, bed rest is maintained and periodic angiography is performed to monitor the dissolution of the clot. The most serious potential problem associated with this procedure can be life-threatening bleeding complications (e.g., cerebral hemorrhage). Therefore patients are carefully selected and monitored by experienced critical care providers.

If the patient remains at risk for further embolization from a persistent source such as chronic atrial fibrillation, treatment includes long-term oral anticoagulation to prevent further acute arterial ischemic episodes (see Table 37-9 later in this chapter).

THROMBOANGIITIS OBLITERANS

Thromboangiitis obliterans (Buerger's disease) is a somewhat rare nonatherosclerotic, segmental inflammatory disorder of the medium-sized arteries, veins, and nerves of the upper and lower extremities. The disorder occurs predominantly in younger men (25 to 40 years of age) and is more prevalent in the Middle and Far East than in North America and Europe.[32] A familial tendency has also been observed.

The underlying cause of Buerger's disease remains unknown. Unlike atherosclerosis, lipid accumulation does not occur in the vessel wall. Instead, a highly cellular and inflammatory thrombus forms inside the vessel, causing tissue ischemia. Buerger's disease typically begins with ischemia of the small, distal arteries and veins, progressing to more proximal arteries. Large arteries are rarely involved. The endothelial-dependent vasodilation of blood vessels is impaired in individuals with Buerger's disease.[32] There is a very strong relationship between Buerger's disease and tobacco use. It is thought that the disease occurs only in smokers, and when smoking is stopped, the disease improves.

The symptom complex of Buerger's disease is often confused with that of PAD and a variety of other inflammatory or autoimmune diseases.[33] Patients may have intermittent claudication of the feet, hands, or arms. As the disease progresses, rest pain and ischemic ulcerations develop. Other signs and symptoms may include color and temperature changes in the affected limb or limbs, paresthesia, superficial thrombophlebitis, and cold sensitivity. Up to 40% of patients with Buerger's disease also have Raynaud's phenomenon.[32] There are no laboratory or diagnostic tests specific to Buerger's disease. Diagnosis is made based on age of onset, history of tobacco usage, clinical symptoms, involvement of distal vessels, presence of ischemic ulcerations, and exclusion of diabetes mellitus, autoimmune disease, hypercoagulable states, and proximal source of emboli.[32]

Treatment includes complete cessation of tobacco usage in any form (including secondhand smoke). Nicotine-replacement products should not be used, and trauma to the extremity must be avoided. Patients are told that they have a choice between their cigarettes and their affected limbs; they cannot have both. Other than smoking cessation, no other therapies have proven success. Surgical revascularization is typically not an option because of the diffuse nature of the disease. Painful ulceration may necessitate finger or toe amputations. Amputation below the knee may be necessary in advanced cases.

RAYNAUD'S PHENOMENON

Raynaud's phenomenon is an episodic vasospastic disorder of small cutaneous arteries, most frequently involving the fingers and toes. The exact etiology of Raynaud's phenomenon remains unknown. One popular theory holds that the vasospasm occurs secondary to an exaggerated response to sympathetic nervous system stimulation. An alternative theory suggests that there are abnormalities in the endothelium and endothelium-derived vasoactive substances.[34] Other contributing factors include occupationally related trauma and pressure to the fingertips as noted in typists, pianists, and those who use handheld vibrating equipment. Exposure to heavy metals may also be a contributing etiologic factor. Raynaud's phenomenon occurs primarily in young women (typically between 15 and 40 years of age). It also is seen frequently in association with collagen diseases such as rheumatoid arthritis, scleroderma, and systemic lupus erythematosus.

Raynaud's phenomenon is characterized by vasospasm-induced color changes of the fingers, toes, ears, and nose (white, blue, and red) (Fig. 37-7). Decreased perfusion due to arteriole vasospasm

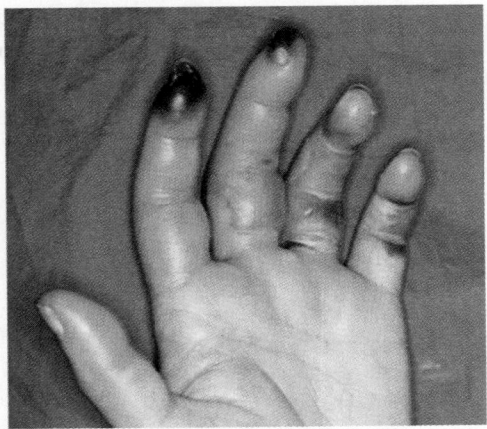

FIG. 37-7 Raynaud's phenomenon.

results in pallor (white). The digits then appear cyanotic (bluish-purple). These changes are subsequently followed by rubor, caused by the hyperemic response that occurs when perfusion is restored. The patient usually describes coldness and numbness in the vasoconstrictive phase followed by throbbing, aching pain; tingling; and swelling in the hyperemic phase. This type of episode usually lasts only minutes but in severe cases may persist for several hours. The symptoms are usually precipitated by exposure to cold, emotional upsets, caffeine, and tobacco use. After frequent, prolonged attacks the skin may become thickened and the nails brittle. Occasionally, in severe forms of the phenomenon, complications include punctuate (small hole) lesions of the fingertips and superficial gangrenous ulcers in advanced stages.

Similar to Buerger's disease, there is no simple diagnostic test for Raynaud's phenomenon. If the symptoms persist for at least 2 years in the absence of an associated underlying disorder, the diagnosis of *primary Raynaud's disease* is made. In contrast, if the symptoms exist in conjunction with a connective tissue or autoimmune disease, the diagnosis of *secondary Raynaud's phenomenon* is made.[33]

Patient teaching should be directed toward reassurance that no serious underlying disorder is present and that prevention of recurrent episodes is possible. Loose, warm clothing should be worn as protection from the cold, including gloves when the refrigerator-freezer is used or when cold objects are being handled. Temperature extremes should be avoided. The patient should stop using all tobacco products and avoid caffeine and other drugs with vasoconstrictive effects (amphetamines, cocaine, ergotamine, pseudoephedrine). If symptoms are exacerbated by stress, the patient needs to develop coping strategies for anxiety-producing situations. Biofeedback, relaxation training, and stress management are effective for some patients. Immersing hands in warm water often decreases the vasospasm.

When a patient's episodes are severe and other therapies are ineffective, drug therapy should be considered. Currently, calcium channel blockers are the first-line drug therapy.[34] Calcium channel blockers such as nifedipine (Procardia) and diltiazem (Cardizem) relax smooth muscles of the arterioles by blocking the influx of calcium into the cells, thus reducing the number of vasospastic attacks. Calcium channel blockers are effective for relieving symptoms in acute episodes. In addition, they can be used on a regular basis in treating patients with chronic Raynaud's phenomenon. Nifedipine is preferred over diltiazem because it has a stronger vasodilating effect and less effect on the calcium channels in the conduction system of the heart.[35] Adverse effects of calcium channel blockers include tachycardia, headache, flushing, dizziness, and peripheral edema. Sympathectomy is considered only in advanced cases. Patients with Raynaud's phenomenon should also receive routine follow-up to monitor possible connective tissue or autoimmune disease.

Disorders of the Veins

VENOUS THROMBOSIS

The most common disorder of the veins is **venous thrombosis,** the formation of a thrombus (clot) in association with inflammation of the vein. Venous thrombosis is classified as either superficial thrombophlebitis or deep vein thrombosis (Table 37-6). Superficial **thrombophlebitis** (inflammation of a vein), which

TABLE 37-6	Comparison of Superficial Thrombophlebitis and Deep Vein Thrombosis	
	SUPERFICIAL THROMBOPHLEBITIS	**DEEP VEIN THROMBOSIS**
Usual location	Superficial veins of arms and legs	Deep veins of arms (axillary, subclavian), legs (femoral), and pelvis (iliac, inferior or superior vena cava)
Clinical findings	Tenderness, redness, warmth, pain, inflammation and induration along the course of the superficial vein; vein appears as a palpable cord; edema rarely occurs	Tenderness over involved vein to pressure, induration of overlying muscle, venous distention; edema usually occurs; may have mild to moderate pain; deep reddish color to area due to venous congestion
Sequelae	Embolization rarely occurs	Embolization may occur; chronic venous insufficiency may develop

occurs in about 65% of all patients receiving IV therapy, is often of minor significance. **Deep vein thrombosis** (DVT) is a disorder involving a thrombus in a deep vein, most commonly the iliac and femoral veins. It occurs in at least 5% of all surgical patients. It is more serious than superficial thrombophlebitis because it can result in embolization of thrombi to the lungs. Pulmonary embolism (PE) is a life-threatening condition and, in the best case scenario, results in prolonged hospitalization.

Etiology

Three important factors (called **Virchow's triad**) in the etiology of venous thrombosis are (1) venous stasis, (2) damage of the endothelium (inner lining of the vein), and (3) hypercoagulability of the blood. The patient at risk for the development of venous thrombosis usually has predisposing conditions to these three disorders (Table 37-7).

Venous Stasis. Normal blood flow in the venous system depends on the action of muscles in the extremities and the functional adequacy of venous valves, which allow unidirectional flow. *Venous stasis* occurs when the valves are dysfunctional or

the muscles of the extremities are inactive. Venous stasis occurs more frequently in people who are obese, have congestive heart failure, have been on long trips without regular exercise, have a prolonged surgical procedure, or are immobile for long periods (e.g., with spinal cord injuries or fractured hips). Also at risk are pregnant women and women in the postpartum period.[36]

The patient with atrial fibrillation is also at high risk because of stagnation of blood in the atria and the eddying in blood flow caused by irregular ventricular contractions in response to the atrial fibrillation. Some medications (e.g., corticosteroids, quinine) predispose a patient to DVT formation.

Endothelial Damage. Damage to the endothelial surface of the vein may be caused by trauma or external pressure and occurs any time a venipuncture is performed. Damaged endothelium has decreased fibrinolytic properties, predisposing to thrombus development. Increased endothelial damage is sustained when patients on IV therapy are receiving caustic substances such as high-dose antibiotics, potassium, chemotherapeutic agents, or hypertonic solutions such as parenteral nutrition or contrast media.

TABLE 37-7	Risk Factors for Deep Vein Thrombosis	

Venous Stasis
Advanced age
Atrial fibrillation
Congestive heart failure
Obesity
Orthopedic surgery (especially lower extremity)
Postpartum period
Pregnancy
Prolonged immobility
- Bed rest
- Fractured leg or hip
- Long trip without adequate exercise
- Spinal cord injury
Stroke
Varicose veins

Endothelial Damage
Abdominal and pelvic surgery (e.g., gynecologic or urologic surgery)
Fractures of the pelvis, hip, or leg
History of previous deep vein thrombosis (DVT)
Indwelling femoral vein catheter
Intravenous drug abuse
Trauma

Hypercoagulability of Blood
Antithrombin III deficiency
Cigarette smoking
Dehydration or malnutrition
Factor V Leiden mutation
High-dose estrogen therapy
Malignancies (especially breast, brain, hepatic, pancreatic, and gastrointestinal)
Nephrotic syndrome
Oral contraceptives, especially in women older than 35 years who smoke cigarettes
Polycythemia vera
Protein C deficiency
Protein S deficiency
Sepsis
Severe anemias

Other factors predisposing to endothelial inflammation and damage include prolonged presence (longer than 48 hours) of an IV catheter in the same site, the use of contaminated IV equipment, a fracture that causes damage to the blood vessels, diabetes mellitus, blood pooling, burns, and any unusual physical exertion that results in muscle strain.

Hypercoagulability of Blood. Hypercoagulability of blood occurs in many hematologic disorders, particularly polycythemia, severe anemias, various malignancies (especially cancers of the breast, brain, pancreas, and gastrointestinal tract), antithrombin III deficiency, protein C deficiency, protein S deficiency, antiphospholipid antibodies, elevated homocysteine levels, and factor V Leiden mutation.[37] A patient with sepsis is predisposed to a hypercoagulable state in response to endotoxins that are released.

Women of childbearing age who take estrogen-based oral contraceptives or postmenopausal women who use hormone replacement therapy (HRT) are at increased risk for venous thromboembolism disease.[37] Women who use oral contraceptives and smoke double their risk because of the constricting effect of nicotine on the blood vessel wall. Smoking may also cause hypercoagulability. Women who smoke, use oral contraceptives, are over age 35, and have a family history of venous thrombosis are at an extremely high risk to develop a thrombotic event.

Pathophysiology

Red blood cells (RBCs), white blood cells (WBCs), platelets, and fibrin adhere to form a thrombus. A frequent site of thrombus formation is the valve cusps of veins, where venous stasis allows accumulation of blood products. As the thrombus enlarges, increased numbers of blood cells and fibrin collect behind it, producing a larger clot with a "tail" that eventually occludes the lumen of the vein.

If a thrombus only partially occludes the vein, the thrombus becomes covered by endothelial cells and the thrombotic process stops. If the thrombus does not become detached, it undergoes lysis or becomes firmly organized and adherent within 5 to 7 days. The organized thrombi may detach and result in emboli. Turbulence of blood flow is a major factor contributing to detachment of the thrombus from the vein wall. The thrombus can become an embolus that generally flows through the venous circulation to the heart and lodges in the pulmonary circulation. Thus it becomes a pulmonary embolus.

Superficial Thrombophlebitis

Clinical Manifestations. The patient with superficial thrombophlebitis may have a palpable, firm, subcutaneous cordlike vein (see Table 37-6). The area surrounding the vein may be tender to the touch, reddened, and warm. A mild systemic temperature elevation and leukocytosis may be present. Edema of the extremity may or may not occur. The most common cause of superficial thrombophlebitis in the upper extremities is trauma to the vein caused by IV therapy. Superficial thrombophlebitis in the lower extremities is usually related to trauma to the varicose veins. This type of superficial thrombophlebitis is more common in older patients with long-standing venous insufficiency and in women during pregnancy.[38] Superficial thrombophlebitis is typically diagnosed on the basis of physical examination alone.

Collaborative Care. The treatment of superficial thrombophlebitis includes elevation of the affected extremity to promote venous return and decrease the edema and the application of warm, moist heat. Heat is used to relieve the pain and treat the inflammation. If the superficial thrombophlebitis is associated with an IV catheter or solution, the IV catheter should be removed immediately. If the superficial thrombophlebitis has occurred in the lower extremity, elastic compression stockings are recommended once the acute thrombophlebitis has resolved.

Mild oral analgesics such as aspirin or acetaminophen with codeine may be used to relieve pain. Nonsteroidal antiinflammatory drugs (NSAIDs) such as ibuprofen (Motrin, Advil) have been used to treat the inflammatory process and accompanying pain. Anticoagulant therapy is usually not indicated unless the proximal greater saphenous vein or the saphenofemoral junction is involved. Antibiotics and/or corticosteroids are occasionally used in complicated situations where an infection or inflammation of the vein exists.[38]

Deep Vein Thrombosis

Clinical Manifestations. The patient with DVT may have no symptoms or have unilateral leg edema, extremity pain, warm skin, erythema (Fig. 37-8), and a systemic temperature greater than 100.4° F (38° C). If the calf is involved, tenderness may be present on palpation. A positive Homans' sign (pain on forced dorsiflexion of the foot when the leg is raised) is a classic but very unreliable sign (see Table 37-6). In fact, a positive Homans' sign appears in only 10% of DVT patients, and false positives are frequent.[39] If the inferior vena cava is involved, the lower extremities may be edematous and cyanotic. If the superior vena cava is involved, there may be symptoms of the upper extremities, neck, back, and face.

Complications. The most serious complications of DVT are pulmonary embolism, chronic venous insufficiency, and phlegmasia cerulea dolens. Pulmonary embolism is a life-threatening complication of DVT (see the section on pulmonary embolism later in this chapter).

Chronic venous insufficiency (CVI) results from valvular destruction, allowing retrograde flow of venous blood. Persistent edema, increased pigmentation, secondary varicosities, ulceration, and cyanosis of the limb when it is placed in a dependent position may develop in a person with CVI. Signs and symptoms of CVI often do not develop until several years following DVT.

Phlegmasia cerulea dolens (swollen, blue, painful leg), a very rare complication, may develop in a patient with severe lower extremity DVT(s). It causes sudden, massive swelling and intense cyanosis of the extremity. Gangrene occurs due to arterial occlusion secondary to venous obstruction.

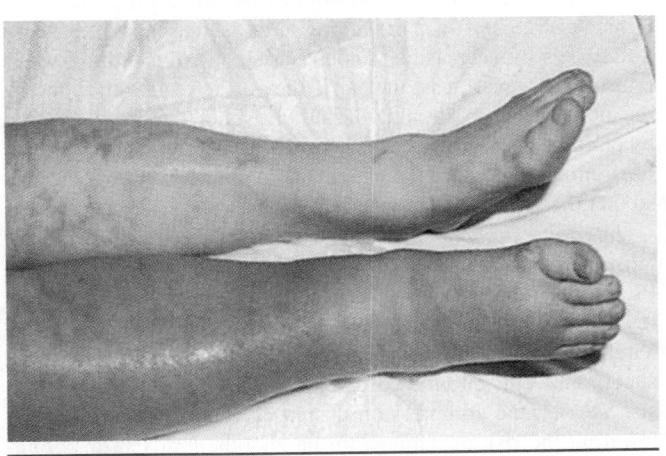

FIG. 37-8 Deep vein thrombosis (DVT).

TABLE 37-8 Diagnostic Studies

Deep Vein Thrombosis and Pulmonary Embolism

STUDY	DESCRIPTION AND ABNORMAL FINDINGS
Blood Laboratory Studies	
• Platelet count, bleeding time, INR, APTT	Elevation if patient has underlying blood dyscrasia; decrease possible if patient has polycythemia; alteration possible because of drug interaction
• D-dimer	Elevation suggestive but not diagnostic of pulmonary embolus
Noninvasive Venous Studies	
• Venous Doppler evaluation	Determination of venous flow in deep femoral, popliteal, and posterior tibial veins; normal finding of spontaneous flow with variation transmitted by respiration cycle; abnormal finding of absence of flow augmentation with distal compression and proximal release
• Duplex scanning	Combination of ultrasound imaging techniques and Doppler capabilities to determine location and extent of thrombus within veins (most widely used test to diagnose deep vein thrombosis)
Venogram (phlebogram)	X-ray determination of location and extent of clot using contrast media to outline filling defects; development of collateral circulation defined
Lung Scan (ventilation and perfusion)	Means of determining presence of pulmonary embolism and extent of resulting lung damage, abnormal finding of mismatch between ventilation and perfusion components; frequently inconclusive
Pulmonary Angiogram	X-ray determination (using contrast media) of location and size of pulmonary embolism
Spiral CT Scan	CT scan that obtains continuous slices allowing visualization of entire anatomic areas such as the lung; data can be computer reconstructed to allow for a 3-D picture

APTT, Activated partial thromboplastin time; *CT,* computed tomography; *INR,* international normalized ratio.

Diagnostic Studies. Various diagnostic studies are used to determine the site or location and extent of a deep vein thrombus or an embolism (Table 37-8).

Collaborative Care

Prevention and prophylaxis. In patients at risk for DVT, a variety of nonpharmacologic and pharmacologic interventions are used. Early mobilization is the easiest and most cost-effective method to decrease the risk of DVT. Patients on bed rest need to be instructed to change position, dorsiflex their feet, and rotate their ankles every 2 to 4 hours. Patients who are able to get out of bed need to be in the chair for all meals and ambulate at least three times per day.

Elastic compression stockings (e.g., TED hose) have long been part of DVT prevention. Studies show that these stockings (which exert about 18 mm Hg pressure) decrease distal calf vein thrombosis by decreasing venous stasis and augmenting venous return.[39] However, it is unclear if they are effective in reducing the incidence of proximal DVT and PE. Venous return is impeded by elastic stockings if the top elastic band is too tight.[39,40] Thus it is essential to measure the patient and obtain the appropriate size so that the stockings fit properly.

Intermittent compression devices (ICDs) are used for hospitalized patients at moderate, high, or very high risk for DVT and PE. These devices apply intermittent external pressure to the lower extremities, which, in effect, addresses all three aspects of Virchow's triad.[40] First, the compression pushes blood from the superficial veins into the deep veins, thus decreasing venous stasis. Second, the compression decreases venous distention, thus lowering the risk of damage to the endothelium. Third, the in-creased blood flow velocity enhances fibrinolysis (the body's natural anticoagulation factors). ICDs will not provide effective DVT prophylaxis if the device is not applied correctly or if the patient does not wear the device continuously except during bathing, skin assessment, and ambulation.[30,40] ICDs are not to be worn when a patient has an active DVT.

Preventive anticoagulation is used for patients at high or very high risk for DVT and PE and is addressed in the following drug therapy section. Anticoagulation may be used in combination with ICDs.

Nonpharmacologic therapy. The usual treatment of DVT in hospitalized patients involves bed rest, elevation of the extremity, and drug therapy. Typically, bed rest with elevation of the affected extremity above the level of the heart is indicated until the thrombus is stable and has adhered to the intraluminal wall, therapeutic levels of anticoagulation are achieved, and the edema is resolving. Warm compresses may also be applied to the affected area.

When the patient is allowed to resume ambulation, elastic compression stockings or 4-inch elastic bandages (e.g., Ace wrap) are recommended. Ideally, once the edema has resolved, the patient should be measured for specialized, custom-fit, graduated elastic compression stockings (e.g., Jobst stockings) that exert 30 to 40 mm Hg pressure at the ankle.[38] The use of elastic compression stockings (or sleeves in the case of an upper extremity) is recommended for several months (at least 3 to 6 months) to support the vein walls and valves and decrease swelling and pain on ambulation.

Drug therapy. Anticoagulants are routinely used for DVT. The goals of anticoagulation therapy in the treatment of DVT are to prevent propagation of the clot, development of any new thrombus, and embolization. Anticoagulant therapy does not dissolve the clot. Lysis of the clot begins spontaneously through the body's intrinsic fibrinolytic system (see Chapter 29).

The most commonly used anticoagulants are unfractionated heparin (UH), low-molecular-weight heparins (LMWHs), hirudin derivatives, and coumarin compounds (Table 37-9). Unfractionated heparin (heparin sodium, commonly known as heparin) acts directly on the intrinsic and common pathways of blood coagulation. Heparin inhibits thrombin-mediated conversion of fibrinogen to fibrin. It also potentiates the actions of antithrombin III, inhibits the activation of factor IX, and neutralizes activated factor X by activating factor X inhibitor. (Clotting factors and the clotting cascade are discussed in Chapter 29 and Fig. 29-4.)

LMWH is effective for the prevention and treatment of DVT. LMWHs are derived from heparin, but the molecule size is approximately one third that of heparin. Enoxaparin (Lovenox), dalteparin (Fragmin), and ardeparin (Normiflo) are examples of LMWHs. LMWH has a greater bioavailability, more predictable dose response, and longer half-life than heparin with less risk of bleeding complications. LMWH has the practical advantage that it does not require anticoagulant monitoring and dose adjustment.[41] LMWH is administered subcutaneously in fixed doses, once or twice daily. Duration of administration depends on the reason for use. Danaparoid (Orgaran), known as a heparinoid, does not contain heparin or heparin fragments. However, like heparin, it has antithrombotic action.

Hirudin was originally extracted from the salivary glands of the medicinal leech, *Hirudo medicinalis*. It is now manufactured through recombinant DNA technology. Hirudin binds with thrombin, thereby directly inhibiting its function without causing platelet reduction.[41] However, the hirudin/thrombin complex is not reversible, and there is no antidote if bleeding occurs. These drugs are indicated for use in patients experiencing heparin-induced thrombocytopenia who still require anticoagulation.[42] Hirudin derivatives such as lepirudin (Refludan), bivalirudin (Angiomax), and argatroban (Acova) are administered by continuous IV infusion.

Coumarin compounds, of which warfarin (Coumadin) is the most commonly used, exert their action indirectly on the coagulation pathway. Warfarin inhibits the hepatic synthesis of the vitamin K–dependent coagulation factors II, VII, IX, and X by competitively interfering with vitamin K. Vitamin K is normally required for the synthesis of these factors.

Oral anticoagulants are often administered concurrently with heparin. Warfarin requires 48 to 72 hours to influence prothrombin time (PT) and may take several days before maximum effect is achieved. Therefore an overlap of heparin and warfarin is re-

rug Therapy

TABLE 37-9   Anticoagulant Therapy

ANTICOAGULANT	DRUG	ROUTE OF ADMINISTRATION	COMMENTS
Unfractionated heparin (UH)	heparin sodium Liquaemin Hepalean Lipo-Hepin	Continuous IV Intermittent IV Subcutaneous	Therapeutic effects measured at regular intervals by the APTT or ACT. Monitor complete blood counts at regular intervals. If administering subcutaneously, inject deep subcutaneous preferably into the abdominal fatty tissue or above the iliac crest, inserting the entire length of the needle. Rotate sites. Do not aspirate. Do not inject IM. Hold skinfold during injection. Do not rub site after injection. Antidote is protamine sulfate.
Low-molecular-weight heparin (LMWH)	enoxaparin (Lovenox) ardeparin (Normiflo) tinzaparin (Innohep) dalteparin (Fragmin) danaparoid (Orgaran) nadroparin (Fraxiparine)* reviparin (Clivarine) certoparin (Sandoparin)	Subcutaneous	Routine coagulation tests typically not required. Monitor complete blood count at regular intervals. Do not expel air bubble before administering subcutaneously. Follow remaining administration guidelines as described above for unfractionated heparin. Extreme caution should be used in patients with a history of heparin-induced thrombocytopenia (risk versus benefit). Protamine sulfate partially reverses the effects of LMWH.
Hirudin derivatives	lepirudin (Refludan) bivalirudin (Angiomax) argatroban (Acova)	Continuous IV	Therapeutic effect measured by APTT ratio (1.5-2.5 times the control). Used in patients with heparin-induced thrombocytopenia when anticoagulation is still required. No antidote.
Coumarin derivatives	warfarin (Coumadin, Panwarfin, Sofarin, Warfilone) acenocoumarol (Sintrom) dicumarol (bishydroxycoumarin)	PO	INR is used rather than PT for monitoring therapeutic levels. Administer at the same time each day. Antidote is vitamin K.

*Available in Canada.
ACT, Activated clotting time; *APTT*, activated partial thromboplastin time; *IM*, intramuscular; *INR*, international normalized ratio; *IV*, intravenous; *PO*, oral (per os); *PT*, prothrombin time.

TABLE 37-10	Tests of Blood Coagulation		
TEST	**DRUG MONITORED**	**NORMAL VALUE**	**THERAPEUTIC VALUE**
International normalized ratio (INR)	Warfarin	0.75–1.25	2–3
Activated partial thromboplastin time (APTT)	Unfractionated heparin Hirudin derivatives	24–36 sec	46–70 sec
Activated clotting time (ACT)	Heparin	80–135 sec	3 min

quired for 3 to 5 days. The clotting status should be monitored by activated partial thromboplastin time (APTT) for heparin therapy and the international normalized ratio (INR) for coumarin derivatives. The INR is a standardized system of reporting PT based on a referenced calibration model and calculated by comparing the patient's PT with a control value. Other tests to monitor anticoagulation may be used (Table 37-10).

For DVT prophylaxis, low-dose unfractionated heparin, LMWH, or warfarin (Coumadin) can be prescribed depending on the patient's level of risk and weight.[39] Unfractionated heparin is typically taken subcutaneously (SQ) and prescribed at 5000 units q12hr SQ for low- and moderate-risk patients or 3500 to 5000 units q8hr SQ for high-risk patients. LMWH is usually dosed at 30 mg q12hr SQ or 40 mg qd SQ. LMWH is rapidly replacing heparin as the anticoagulant of choice to prevent DVT in high-risk patients. In fact, LMWH is considered the most effective form of prophylaxis in hip surgery, in knee surgery, and following major trauma.[43] Low-dose warfarin is usually reserved for patients with the highest DVT risk.

Patients with a very large DVT are usually hospitalized and receive an initial IV bolus of heparin followed by continuous IV heparin infusion for 5 to 7 days. Before discontinuing the IV heparin, oral anticoagulant therapy is started. The IV heparin is discontinued once the INR is at the desired level. Oral anticoagulants are prescribed for 3 to 6 months.

Fondaparinux (Arixta), a relatively new anticoagulant, selectively inhibits factor Xa. It is administered subcutaneously once daily. It has been used effectively for the prevention and treatment of DVT, especially in orthopedic surgery patients. Fondaparinux has no significant effect on APTT, bleeding time, or PT. Therefore these coagulation tests are not useful for monitoring.

Patients with a small, uncomplicated DVT (in the popliteal vein or a more proximal vein) can be managed on an outpatient basis with LMWH. Current guidelines recommend placing the patient on LMWH at a weight-based dose of 1 mg/kg administered q12hr SQ.[39] Warfarin is also prescribed and given concurrently with the LMWH until the warfarin is at a therapeutic level (INR 2.0 to 3.0). Warfarin is administered for 3 to 6 months after the DVT. Recurrent episodes of DVT require lifelong anticoagulation therapy unless contraindicated.

A careful history of pregnancy status and medications should be taken before initiating anticoagulation. Because coumarin compounds are contraindicated in pregnancy, pregnant patients requiring anticoagulation often receive subcutaneous heparin or LMWH. Antiplatelet agents (e.g., aspirin) are generally contraindicated while on anticoagulation. Other drugs that interact with coumarin compounds include nonsteroidal antiinflammatory drugs such as ibuprofen (Advil, Motrin), phenytoin (Dilan-

TABLE 37-11 Drug Therapy
Drugs That Interact with Oral Anticoagulants

INCREASE ANTICOAGULANT EFFECTS	DECREASE ANTICOAGULANT EFFECTS
alcohol (may increase or decrease)	barbiturates (e.g., secobarbitol, phenobarbital)
amiodarone (Cordarone)	carbamazepine (Tegretol)
anabolic steroids	chlordiazepoxide (Librium)
chloral hydrate	cholestyramine (Questran)
cimetidine (Tagamet)	ethchlorvynol (Placidyl)
clofibrate (Atromid)	griseofulvin (Grifulvin)
disulfiram (Antabuse)	rifampin (Rifadin)
erythromycin	
fluconazole (Diflucan)	
influenza (flu) vaccine	
isoniazid (INH)	
metronidazole (Flagyl)	
miconazole	
moxolactam (Moxam)	
neomycin	
nonsteroidal antiinflammatory drugs	
omeprazole (Prilosec)	
oxyphenbutazone (Tandearil)	
phenyramidol (Analexin)	
phenytoin (Dilantin)	
propafenone (Rythmol)	
quinidine	
salicylates	
sulfinpyrazone (Anturan, Antazone)	
sulfonamides	
tetracycline	

tin), and barbiturates (Table 37-11). Changes in diet can also interact with coumarin compounds. A diet high in vitamin K (e.g., green leafy vegetables) can make it difficult to maintain a patient within a therapeutic range. The patient should be instructed to follow a diet that includes foods containing vitamin K in moderate amounts but to avoid any additional supplements with vitamin K. In addition, the patient should be instructed to avoid excessive amounts of vitamin E and alcohol. While the patient is

TABLE 37-12   Nursing Interventions to Prevent Bleeding Complications in Patients Receiving Anticoagulants

Assessment
- Monitor vital signs as indicated.
- Examine appropriate laboratory coagulation tests for achieved therapeutic levels.
- Inspect skin frequently, especially under splinting devices.
- Perform assessments frequently to observe for signs and symptoms of bleeding and/or clotting.
- Evaluate lower extremity for ecchymosis/hematoma development if sequential compression hose used.
- Test urine and stool for occult blood as indicated.
- Notify the health care provider of any abnormalities in assessments, vital signs, or laboratory values.

Injections
- Minimize venipunctures.
- Do not give IM injections.
- Use small-gauge needles for venipunctures unless replacement therapy requires a larger gauge.
- Apply manual pressure for at least 10 minutes (or longer if needed) on venipuncture sites.

Patient Care
- Avoid restrictive clothing.
- Reposition the patient carefully at regular intervals.
- Use support pads, mattresses, bed cradles, and therapeutic beds as indicated.
- Avoid removing/disrupting established clots.
- Instruct patient not to forcefully blow nose.
- Administer stool softeners to avoid hard stools and constipation.
- Limit tape application—use paper tape as appropriate.
- Avoid restraints if possible—use only soft, padded restraints as needed.
- Perform care in a gentle manner.
- Use soft toothbrushes or foam swabs for oral care.
- Apply moisturizing lotion to skin.
- Do not use lemon-glycerin swabs.
- Humidify O_2 source.
- Utilize electric razors, not straight razors.
- Lubricate tubes adequately prior to insertion.
- Apply antiembolism stockings (e.g., TED hose) as ordered.

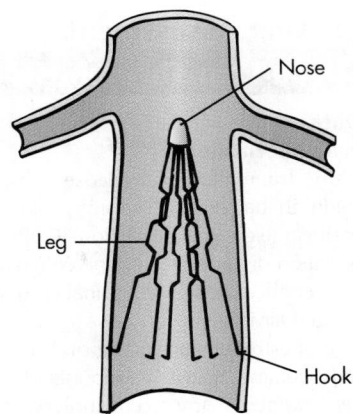

FIG. 37-9 Inferior vena caval interruption technique using Greenfield stainless steel filter to prevent pulmonary embolism.

perficial femoral or internal jugular veins. The filter device is opened and the spokes penetrate the vessel walls (see Fig. 37-9). These devices result in "sieve-type" obstruction, permitting filtration of clots without interruption of blood flow.

Complications after the insertion of the intravascular filter device are rare. They include air embolism, improper placement, and migration of the filter more distally into the venous system. Venous congestion is common and results from the accumulation of trapped clots at the filter site. Over time these clots may clog the filter and completely occlude the vena cava. Because this process is gradual, collateral vessels usually develop to maintain venous flow. However, these collateral venous pathways may also provide an alternate route for PE.

NURSING MANAGEMENT VENOUS THROMBOSIS

■ Nursing Assessment

Subjective and objective data that should be obtained from a patient with venous thrombosis are presented in Table 37-13.

■ Nursing Diagnoses

Nursing diagnoses and collaborative problems for the patient with venous thrombosis include, but are not limited to, the following:
- Acute pain *related to* venous congestion, impaired venous return, and inflammation
- Ineffective health maintenance *related to* lack of knowledge about disorder and its treatment
- Risk for impaired skin integrity *related to* altered peripheral tissue perfusion
- Potential complication: bleeding *related to* anticoagulant therapy
- Potential complication: pulmonary embolism *related to* embolization of thrombus, dehydration, and immobility

■ Planning

The overall goals are that the patient with venous thrombosis will have (1) relief of pain, (2) decreased edema, (3) no skin ulceration, (4) no complications from anticoagulant therapy, and (5) no evidence of pulmonary emboli.

hospitalized, nursing activities should be adjusted to monitor for and reduce the risk of bleeding that may occur with anticoagulant administration (Table 37-12).

Surgical Therapy. Although most patients are managed conservatively, small percentages require surgical intervention. The primary indication for surgery is to prevent PE. Surgical procedures include venous thrombectomy (rarely performed) and inferior vena cava interruption (Fig. 37-9). Venous thrombectomy involves the removal of a DVT through an incision in the vein. This procedure is done to prevent pulmonary embolism or to decrease the risk of the development of chronic venous insufficiency.

Vena cava interruption devices, such as the Greenfield or Simon-Nitinol filters, can be inserted percutaneously through su-

TABLE 37-13	Nursing Assessment
	Deep Vein Thrombosis

Subjective Data

Important Health Information

Past health history: Trauma to vein, varicose veins, pregnancy or recent childbirth, bacteremia, obesity, prolonged bed rest, irregular heartbeat (e.g., atrial fibrillation), COPD, CHF, cancer, coagulation disorders and hypercoagulable states, systemic lupus erythematosus, MI, spinal cord injury, stroke, prolonged air travel

Medications: Use of estrogens (including oral contraceptives), corticosteroids, quinine, excessive amounts of vitamin E

Surgery or other treatments: Any recent surgery, especially orthopedic, gynecologic, gastric, or urologic; previous surgery involving veins; central venous catheter

Functional Health Patterns

Health perception–health management: IV drug abuse, smoking, obesity

Activity-exercise: Inactivity

Cognitive-perceptual: Pain in area on palpation or ambulation

Objective Data

General

Fever, anxiety, pain

Integumentary

Increased size of extremity when compared with other side; taut, shiny warm skin, erythematous, tenderness to palpation

Cardiovascular

Distention and warmth of superficial veins; edema and cyanosis of extremities, neck, back, and face (superior vena cava involvement)

Possible Findings

Leukocytosis, abnormal coagulation, anemia or elevated hematocrit and RBC count, ↑ D-dimer level, positive venous duplex or Doppler studies, positive venogram

CHF, Congestive heart failure; *COPD,* chronic obstructive pulmonary disease; *MI,* myocardial infarction.

■ **Nursing Implementation**

Acute Intervention. Nursing care for the patient with venous thrombosis is directed toward the prevention of emboli formation and the reduction of inflammation. While the patient is receiving anticoagulation therapy, the nurse should closely observe for any indication of bleeding, including epistaxis and bleeding gingivae. Urine should be assessed for gross or microscopic hematuria. A smoky appearance to the urine is sometimes noted if blood is present. A specimen should be checked daily for hematuria. Particular attention should be paid to the protection of skin areas that may be traumatized. Surgical incisions should be closely observed for evidence of bleeding. Stools should be tested to determine the presence of occult blood from the gastrointestinal tract. Mental status changes, especially in the older patient, should be assessed as a possible indication of cerebral bleeding. Intramuscular injections should not be given.

The nurse should review with the patient any medications currently being taken that may interfere with anticoagulant therapy (see Table 37-11). In addition, the nurse should ask if the patient is taking any herbal products. Herbs can interfere with anticoag-

---

COMPLEMENTARY & ALTERNATIVE THERAPIES

Herbs That Affect Clotting

Many different herbs can interfere with clotting. These include garlic, ginger, ginkgo, ginseng, goldenseal, feverfew, chamomile, angelica, bilberry, and evening primrose.

Effects

Can interfere with clotting in various ways. One common mechanism is to inhibit platelet aggregation.

Nursing Implications

In general, these herbs should be used with caution or not at all in patients with bleeding or clotting disorders or those taking anticoagulant and antiplatelet drugs (e.g., warfarin [Coumadin], heparin, low-molecular-weight heparin, aspirin, ticlopidine [Ticlid], clopidogrel [Plavix]). Patients in these categories should consult with their health care provider before using any of these herbs. These herbs should be discontinued at least 2 to 3 weeks before surgery to avoid potential complications. If this is not possible, the herbal product in its original container should be brought to the health care provider or surgery site so that the anesthesia care provider knows exactly what the patient is taking.

ulant therapy[26] (see the Complementary and Alternative Therapies box). The nurse should monitor PTT, INR, hemoglobin, hematocrit, and platelet levels when a patient is receiving anticoagulant drugs. Platelet counts are monitored to assess for heparin-induced thrombocytopenia. Medication doses are titrated according to the results of clotting studies. The nurse should be cautious about administering either heparin or warfarin (Coumadin) without first checking the results of the clotting studies. The antidote for heparin is protamine sulfate, and the antidote for warfarin is vitamin K. These drugs must be immediately available if bleeding occurs. Fresh frozen plasma (FFP) may be administered for bleeding because it contains multiple clotting factors.

Ambulatory and Home Care. During all phases of care the nurse should evaluate the patient's psychologic response. Many patients are apprehensive that clots will move to the heart or lungs and cause sudden death. Every patient should be allowed to verbalize concerns, and an attempt should be made to clarify misconceptions. The patient hospitalized for an extended time requires diversional activities.

Discharge teaching should focus on elimination of modifiable risk factors for DVT, the importance of compression stockings and monitoring of laboratory values, medication instructions, and guidelines for follow-up. Modifiable risk factors for DVT include cigarette smoking, use of oral contraceptives, use of hormone replacement therapy, a sedentary lifestyle, and obesity. The patient should be taught to quit smoking and using nicotine products because nicotine increases the viscosity of the blood. Constrictive clothing, such as girdles or garters, should be avoided. Women with a history of DVT should be instructed to stop using oral contraceptives and hormone replacement therapy. Another important preventive measure is to avoid prolonged standing or sitting in a motionless, leg-dependent position. Frequent knee flexion, ankle rotation, and active walking should be done during long periods of sitting or standing, especially on long automobile or airplane trips. Dietary considerations for the overweight patient are aimed at limiting caloric intake to achieve and then maintain desired weight.

A balanced program of rest and exercise, along with proper posture and avoiding long periods of sitting, improves arterial filling and venous return. Exercise programs should be developed with an emphasis on walking, swimming, and wading. Exercises in water are particularly beneficial because of the gentle, even pressure of the water.

The patient and family should be taught about signs and symptoms of pulmonary embolism such as sudden onset of dyspnea, tachypnea, and pleuritic chest pain. (Pulmonary embolism is discussed later in this chapter.) They should be instructed to notify their health care provider immediately and/or go to the hospital.

If the patient is continuing on anticoagulant therapy, the patient and family need careful explanations of medication dosage, actions, and side effects, as well as the importance of routine blood tests and the need to report symptoms to the health care provider (Table 37-14). Home monitoring devices are now available for immediate testing of PT. Patients on LMWH will need to learn how to self-administer the drug or have a friend or family member administer it. The most common problems with LMWH are bruising at the injection site. Active or younger patients need to be instructed to avoid contact sports and other high-risk activities (e.g., in-line rollerblading). The older patient should be taught safety precautions to prevent injuries, such as falls. Should a bleeding episode occur, the patient and family should be instructed to apply pressure for 5 minutes. If the bleeding has not slowed significantly or completely resolved, they should call 911.

A well-balanced diet is important because calcium and vitamin E play active roles in the clotting mechanism. Proper hydration is required to prevent additional hypercoagulability of the blood, which may occur in the presence of deficient fluid intake.

■ **Evaluation**

The expected outcomes are that the patient with venous thrombosis will have
- minimal to no pain
- intact skin
- no signs of respiratory distress
- no signs of hemorrhage or occult bleeding

VARICOSE VEINS

Varicose veins, or *varicosities,* are dilated, tortuous subcutaneous veins most frequently found in the saphenous system. They may be small and innocuous or large and bulging. Primary varicosities are those in which the superficial veins are dilated and the valves may or may not be rendered incompetent. This condition tends to be familial, is characteristically found bilaterally, and is probably caused by congenital weakness of the veins. Secondary varicosities result from previous DVT of the deep femoral veins, with subsequent valvular incompetence. Secondary varicose veins may occur in the esophagus (esophageal varices), in the anorectal area (hemorrhoids), and as abnormal arteriovenous (AV) connections (AV fistulas and malformations).

Etiology and Pathophysiology

The etiology of varicose veins is unknown. Superficial veins in the lower extremities become dilated and tortuous, with increased venous pressure. This increased venous pressure may result from a congenital weakness of the vein structure, obesity, pregnancy, venous obstruction resulting from thrombosis or ex-

TABLE 37-14	**Patient & Family Teaching Guide** **Anticoagulant Therapy**

The nurse should include the following in a teaching plan:
1. Reasons for and basic mechanism of action of anticoagulant therapy and how long anticipated therapy will last.
2. Need to take medication at same time each day (preferably in afternoon or evening).
3. Requirement for frequent follow-up with blood tests to assess blood clotting and whether change in drug dosages is required.
4. Side effects and adverse effects of drug therapy requiring medical attention:
   - Any bleeding that does not stop after a reasonable amount of time (usually 10 to 15 minutes)
   - Blood in urine or stool, or black, tarry stools
   - Unusual bleeding from gums, throat, skin, or nose, or heavy menstrual bleeding
   - Severe headaches or stomach pains
   - Weakness, dizziness, mental status changes
   - Vomiting blood
   - Cold, blue, or painful feet
5. Avoid any trauma or injury that might cause bleeding (e.g., vigorous brushing of teeth, contact sports, in-line rollerblading).
6. Do not take aspirin-containing drugs or nonsteroidal anti-inflammatory drugs.
7. Limit alcohol intake to small to moderate amount.
8. Wear a Medic Alert bracelet or necklace indicating what anticoagulant is being taken.
9. Avoid marked changes in eating habits, such as dramatically increasing foods high in vitamin K (e.g., broccoli, spinach, kale, greens). Do not take supplemental vitamin K.
10. Consult with health care provider before beginning or discontinuing any medication.
11. Inform all health care providers, including dentist, of anticoagulant therapy.
12. Correct dosing is essential and supervision may be required (e.g., patients experiencing confusion).
13. Do not use herbal products that may alter coagulation (see Complementary and Alternative Therapies box on p. 934).
14. Physician should be notified immediately if chest pain, shortness of breath, a feeling of passing out, or palpitation (heart racing) is experienced.

trinsic pressure by tumors, or occupations that require prolonged standing.[38] As the veins enlarge, the valves are stretched and become incompetent, allowing venous blood flow to be reversed. As back pressure increases and the calf muscle pump (muscle movement that squeezes venous blood back toward the heart) fails, further venous distention results. The increased venous pressure is transmitted to the capillary bed, and edema develops.

Clinical Manifestations and Complications

Discomfort from varicose veins varies dramatically among people and tends to be worsened by superficial thrombophlebitis. In addition, many patients voice concern about cosmetic disfigurement (Fig. 37-10). The most common symptom of varicose veins is an ache or pain after prolonged standing, which is re-

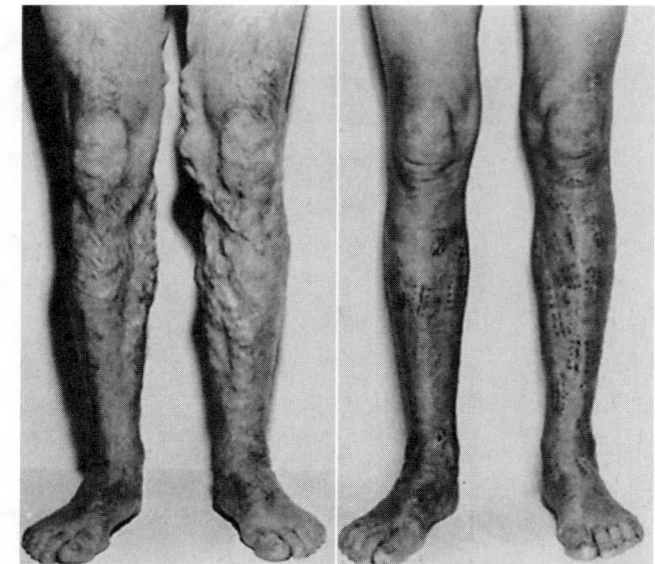

FIG. 37-10 Extensive varicosities (incompetency of the greater saphenous systems). **A,** Appearance preoperatively. **B,** Appearance 2 weeks postoperatively.

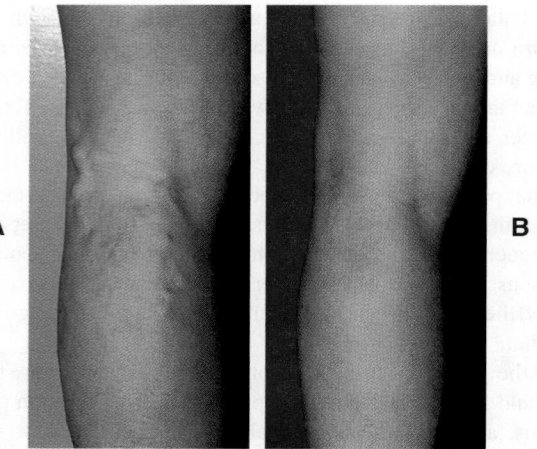

FIG. 37-11 Varicose veins and treatment with sclerotherapy. **A,** Before treatment. **B,** Clinical appearance 2½ years after treatment.

lieved by walking or by elevating the limb. Some patients feel pressure or a cramplike sensation. Swelling may accompany the discomfort. Nocturnal leg cramps in the calf may occur.

Superficial thrombophlebitis is the most frequent complication of varicose veins and may occur either spontaneously or after trauma, surgical procedures, or pregnancy. Rare complications include rupture of the varicose veins from weakening of the vessel wall and ulceration of the skin.

Diagnostic Studies and Collaborative Care

Superfical varicose veins can be diagnosed by appearance. A duplex ultrasound can detect obstruction and reflux in the venous system with considerable accuracy. It is the most widely used test to diagnose deep varicose veins.

Treatment is usually not indicated if varicose veins are only a cosmetic problem. If incompetency of the venous system develops, collaborative care involves rest with the affected limb elevated, compression stockings, and exercise, such as walking.

Sclerotherapy is a technique used in the treatment of unsightly superficial varicosities[44] (Fig. 37-11). Direct IV injection of a sclerosing agent such as sodium tetradecyl (Sotradecol) induces inflammation and results in eventual thrombosis of the vein. This procedure can be performed safely in an office setting and causes minimal discomfort. After injection the leg is wrapped with an elastic bandage for 24 to 72 hours to maintain pressure over the vein. Local tenderness subsides within 2 to 3 weeks, and eventually the thrombosed vein disappears. After sclerotherapy the patient should be advised to wear compression stockings to help prevent the development of further varicosities.

Surgical intervention for varicose veins involves ligation of the entire vein (usually the greater saphenous) and dissection and removal of its incompetent tributaries (see Fig. 37-11). Surgical intervention is indicated when chronic venous insufficiency cannot be controlled with conservative therapy. Recurrent thrombophlebitis in varicose veins is another indication for surgery. In selected patients, the use of lasers may be an option in the treatment of superficial varicosities instead of sclerotherapy or surgery.[45] Surgical treatment for varicose veins is typically done as an outpatient procedure.

NURSING MANAGEMENT
VARICOSE VEINS

Prevention is a key factor related to varicose veins. The nurse should instruct the patient to avoid sitting or standing for long periods of time, maintain ideal body weight, take precautions against injury to the extremities, avoid wearing constrictive clothing, and participate in a daily walking program.

After vein ligation surgery, the nurse should encourage deep breathing, which helps promote venous return to the right side of the heart. The extremities should be checked regularly for color, movement, sensation, temperature, presence of edema, and pedal pulses. Bruising and discoloration are considered normal. Postoperatively, the legs are elevated at a 15-degree angle to prevent edema. Compression stockings are applied and removed every 8 hours for short periods and reapplied.

Long-term management of varicose veins is directed toward improving circulation, relieving discomfort, improving cosmetic appearance, and avoiding complications, such as superficial thrombophlebitis and ulceration. Varicose veins can recur in other veins after vein ligation. The patient should be taught proper care of the lower extremities, including cleanliness and the use of individually fitted compression stockings. The patient should be taught to put on the stockings while still lying down just before rising in the morning. The importance of periodic positioning of the legs above the heart should be stressed. The overweight patient may need assistance with weight reduction. The patient whose occupation requires prolonged periods of standing or sitting needs to change position frequently.

CHRONIC VENOUS INSUFFICIENCY
AND VENOUS LEG ULCERS

Chronic venous insufficiency (CVI) is a common medical problem in the elderly. CVI, which often occurs as a result of previous episodes of DVT, can lead to *venous leg ulcers* (formerly called *venous stasis ulcers* or *varicose ulcers*). Venous ulcer prevalence on admission to nursing homes is 2.5% with an annual incidence in nursing home patients of 2.2%.[46] Although CVI and venous ulceration are not life-threatening diseases, they are painful, debilitating, and costly chronic conditions that can adversely affect the quality of patients' lives.

Etiology and Pathophysiology

The causes of CVI include vein incompetence, deep vein obstruction, congenital venous malformation, arteriovenous fistula, and calf muscle failure.[47] The basic dysfunction is incompetent valves of the deep veins. As a result, hydrostatic pressure in the veins increases and serous fluid and red blood cells (RBCs) leak from the capillaries and venules into the tissue, resulting in edema. Enzymes in the tissue eventually break down RBCs, causing the release of hemosiderin, which causes a brownish skin discoloration. Over time, the skin and subcutaneous tissue around the ankle are replaced by fibrous tissue, resulting in thick, hardened, contracted skin.

Although the causes of CVI are known, the exact pathophysiology of venous ulcers remains unknown. It is known that decreased fibrinolysis, pericapillary fibrin cuffs, and WBC trapping occur in venous ulcers.[47]

Clinical Manifestations and Complications

In individuals with CVI, the skin of the lower leg is leathery, with a characteristic brownish or "brawny" appearance from the hemosiderin deposition. Edema has usually been persistent for a prolonged period. Eczema, or "stasis dermatitis," is often present, and pruritus is a common complaint.

Venous ulcers classically are located above the medial malleolus. However, they can occur near the lateral malleolus (Fig. 37-12). The wound margins are irregularly shaped, and the tissue is typically a ruddy color (see Table 37-2). Venous ulcers are typically partial thick wounds that extend through the epidermis and portions of the dermis. Ulcer drainage may be extensive, especially when the leg is edematous. The ulcer is often quite painful, particularly when edema or infection is present.[48] Pain may be worse when the leg is in a dependent position. Ulcer pain adversely affects the patient's quality of life.[49]

If the venous ulcer is untreated, the lesion becomes more extensive, eroding wider and deeper, and increasing the likelihood

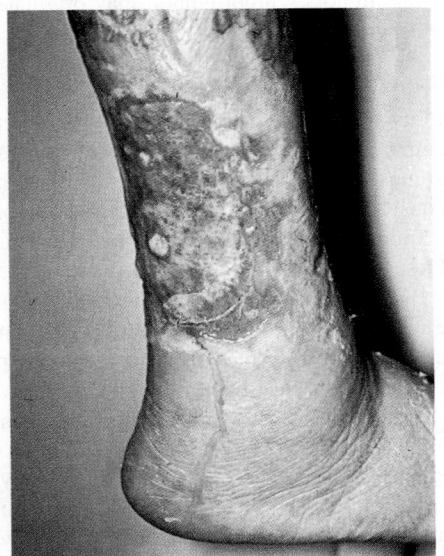

FIG. 37-12 Venous leg ulcer.

of wound infection and cellulitis. Recurrent episodes of cellulitis may lead to destruction of the superficial lymphatics, causing a secondary lymphedema to develop. On very rare occasions, severe CVI with long-standing nonhealing venous ulceration may result in the patient's need to have an amputation.

Collaborative Care

Compression is essential to the management of CVI, venous ulcer healing, and prevention of ulcer recurrence. A variety of options are available to achieve compression, including elastic wraps, custom-fitted compression stockings, elasticated tubular support bandages, a Velcro wrap (Circaid), sequential pneumatic compression devices, paste bandage (Unna's boot) with an elastic wrap, and multilayer (three or four) bandage regimens.[47] There are benefits to each type of compression therapy, and the nurse must evaluate each patient individually when choosing an extrinsic compression method. Before instituting compression therapy, assessment of the arterial status is necessary to make sure that coexistent arterial disease is not present. An ABI of 0.8 suggests that the patient also has PAD and should not have high levels of compression.

Moist environment dressings are the mainstay of wound care. A variety of dressings are available that provide a moist environment and include transparent film dressings, hydrocolloids, hydrogels, foams, calcium alginates, impregnated gauze, gauze moistened with saline, and combination dressings. When used in conjunction with extrinsic compression, moist environment dressings have proven to be more effective in hastening the healing of venous leg ulcers than dry dressings. (Hydrocolloid dressings and other dressings are discussed in Chapter 12 and Table 12-17.)

Nutritional status and intake should be evaluated in a patient with a venous leg ulcer.[50] A balanced diet with adequate protein, calories, and micronutrients is essential for healing. Nutrients most important for healing include protein, vitamins A and C, and zinc. Foods high in protein (e.g., meat, beans, cheese, tofu), vitamin A (green leafy vegetables), vitamin C (citrus fruits, tomatoes, cantaloupe), and zinc (meat, seafood) must be provided.[50] For patients with coexistent diabetes mellitus, maintaining normal blood glucose levels facilitates the healing process.[47] For overweight individuals with CVI and no active venous ulcer, a weight-reduction diet may be prescribed.

Routine prophylactic antibiotic therapy is not typically indicated. Clinical signs of infection in a venous ulcer include change in quantity, color, or odor of the drainage; presence of pus; erythema of the wound edges; change in sensation around the wound; warmth around the wound; increased local pain, edema, or both; dark-colored granulation tissue; induration around the wound; delayed healing; and cellulitis.[51] However, if signs of infection are present, a culture should be obtained and appropriate antibiotic therapy is then instituted. The usual treatment for infection is sharp debridement, wound excision, and systemic antibiotics. Moist-to-moist saline dressings are indicated until the infection clears, after which other moist environment dressings may be used.

If the ulcer fails to respond to conservative therapy, alternative treatments include use of a radiant heat bandage (Warm-Up Active Wound Therapy),[52] coverage with a split-thickness skin graft, cultured epithelial autografts, and allografts or bioengineered skin such as Apligraf. Typically when a split-thickness skin graft is used, the ulcer is debrided, varicosities in the area of the lesion are removed, and veins are ligated before the tissue from a donor site is applied. (Skin grafting is discussed in Chapter 24.)

NURSING MANAGEMENT
VENOUS LEG ULCERS

Long-term management of venous leg ulcers should focus on teaching the patient about self-care measures because the incidence of recurrence is high. This is particularly important because research indicates that patients with chronic venous disease lack understanding of appropriate treatments.[53] Patient and family teaching should include avoidance of trauma to the limbs, proper skin care measures, application of prescribed compression stockings, and appropriate activity and limb positioning.

Proper foot and leg care is essential to avoid additional trauma to the skin. In addition, because of the stasis dermatitis, patients

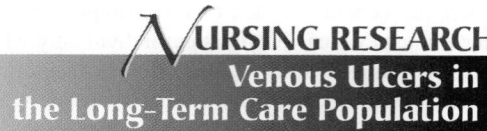

NURSING RESEARCH
Venous Ulcers in the Long-Term Care Population

Citation
Wipke-Tevis DD et al: Prevalence, incidence, management, and predictors of venous ulcers in the long-term-care population using the MDS, *Adv Skin Wound Care* 13:218, 2000.

Purpose
To describe the prevalence, incidence, management, and predictors of venous ulcers in residents of long-term care (LTC) facilities using the Minimum Data Set (MDS).

Methods
A retrospective study was performed using Missouri's MDS computerized database. The population consisted of all residents admitted to certified LTC facilities between January 1, 1996, and October 30, 1998, who had MDS assessments in the database (*n* = 32,221). Assessment items included selected measures from background information, disease diagnoses, physical functioning and structural problems, health conditions, oral/nutritional status, and skin condition.

Results and Conclusions
Venous ulcer prevalence on admission was 2.5%. The incidence of venous ulcer development for LTC residents admitted without an ulcer at 90, 180, 270, and 365 days after admission was 1.0%, 1.3%, 1.8%, and 2.2%, respectively. Venous ulcer prevalence and incidence are greater in the LTC population than in the general population. Residents with a venous ulcer are likely to have comorbid conditions such as diabetes mellitus, peripheral vascular disease, congestive heart failure, edema, wound infection, and pain. Factors associated with venous ulcer development within 1 year of admission were diabetes mellitus, peripheral vascular disease, and peripheral edema. The most frequent skin treatments were ulcer care, dressings, and ointments.

Implications for Nursing Practice
Risk factors such as history of leg ulcers, recent edema, diabetes mellitus, congestive heart failure, or peripheral vascular disease should prompt health care providers to carefully plan care that will decrease a person's risk for venous ulcer development. Teaching the patient, the patient's family, and the nursing staff about skin care, diet, and activity modifications will also reduce the incidence of ulcer development. In addition, patient sources of injury (e.g., scatter rugs) should be removed and passageways should be cleared for individuals at risk for venous ulcers.

---

with CVI have dry, flaky, itchy skin. Daily moisturizing of the skin decreases itching and prevents cracking. Creams or lotions with fragrance or lanolin should be avoided because of the potential for allergic reactions. The wound should be assessed for signs and symptoms of infection during each dressing change.

The patient with CVI with or without a venous ulcer is instructed to avoid standing or sitting with the feet dependent for long periods. Standing or sitting with the legs in a dependent position has been shown to decrease periulcer skin blood perfusion and oxygen levels.[54] Venous ulcer patients are also instructed to elevate their legs above the level of the heart. Once an ulcer is healed, a daily walking program is encouraged.

PULMONARY EMBOLISM

Etiology and Pathophysiology

Pulmonary embolism (PE) is the blockage of pulmonary arteries by thrombus, fat or air emboli, and tumor tissue. It is the most common pulmonary complication in hospitalized patients. Although the actual incidence of mortality and morbidity from PE is unknown, it is estimated that nearly 50,000 people die of PE each year in the United States and another 650,000 have nonfatal PEs.[55]

Most PEs arise from thrombi in the deep veins of the legs. Other sites of origin include the right side of the heart (especially with atrial fibrillation), upper extremities (rare), and the pelvic veins (especially after surgery or childbirth). Lethal PEs most commonly originate in the femoral or iliac veins. Emboli are mobile clots that generally do not stop moving until they lodge at a narrowed part of the circulatory system. The lungs are an ideal location for emboli to lodge because of their extensive arterial and capillary network. The lower lobes are most frequently affected because they have a higher blood flow than the other lobes. The presence of DVT is often unsuspected until a PE occurs.

Thrombi in the deep veins can dislodge spontaneously. However, a more common mechanism is jarring of the thrombus by mechanical forces, such as sudden standing, and changes in the rate of blood flow, such as those that occur with Valsalva maneuver.

In addition to dislodged thrombi, less common causes of PE include fat emboli (from fractured long bones), air emboli (from improperly administered IV therapy), bacterial vegetations, amniotic fluid, and tumors. Tumor emboli may originate from primary or metastatic malignancies.

Clinical Manifestations

The severity of clinical manifestations of PE depends on the size of the emboli and the size and number of blood vessels occluded. The most common manifestations of PE are anxiety and the sudden onset of unexplained dyspnea, tachypnea, or tachycardia. Other manifestations are cough, pleuritic chest pain, hemoptysis, crackles, fever, accentuation of the pulmonic heart sound, and sudden change in mental status as a result of hypoxemia.

Massive emboli may produce sudden collapse of the patient with shock, pallor, severe dyspnea, and crushing chest pain. However, some patients with massive PE do not have pain. The pulse is rapid and weak, the BP is low, and an ECG indicates right ventricular strain. When rapid obstruction of 50% or more of the pulmonary vascular bed occurs, acute cor pulmonale may result because the right ventricle can no longer pump blood into the lungs. Death occurs in more than 60% of patients with massive emboli.[5]

Medium-sized emboli often cause pleuritic chest pain, dyspnea, slight fever, and a productive cough with blood-streaked sputum. A physical examination may reveal tachycardia and a pleural friction rub.

Small emboli frequently are undetected or produce vague, transient symptoms. The exception to this is the patient with underlying cardiopulmonary disease, in whom even small or medium-sized emboli may result in severe cardiopulmonary compromise. However, repeated small emboli gradually cause a reduction in the capillary bed and eventual pulmonary hypertension. An ECG and chest x-ray may indicate right ventricular hypertrophy secondary to pulmonary hypertension.

Complications

Pulmonary infarction (death of lung tissue) is most likely when the following factors are present: (1) occlusion of a large- or medium-sized pulmonary vessel (greater than 2 mm in diameter), (2) insufficient collateral blood flow from the bronchial circulation, or (3) preexisting lung disease. Infarction results in alveolar necrosis and hemorrhage. Occasionally the infarcted tissue becomes infected and an abscess may develop. Concomitant pleural effusion is frequently found.

Pulmonary hypertension occurs when more than 50% of the area of the normal pulmonary bed is compromised. Pulmonary hypertension also results from hypoxemia. As a single event an embolus does not cause pulmonary hypertension unless it is massive. However, recurrent small- to medium-sized emboli may result in chronic pulmonary hypertension. Pulmonary hypertension eventually results in dilation and hypertrophy of the right ventricle. Depending on the degree of pulmonary hypertension and its rate of development, death may result rapidly or only mild or transient alterations may occur (see Chapter 27).

Diagnostic Studies

A lung scan (i.e., ventilation-perfusion scan) has traditionally been used in screening for initial (or recurrent) PE, assessing the natural history of the lesion, and evaluating the effectiveness of therapy. The lung scan has two components and is most accurate when both are performed:

1. Perfusion scanning involves IV injection of a radioisotope. A scanning device detects the adequacy of the pulmonary circulation.
2. Ventilation scanning involves inhalation of a radioactive gas such as xenon. Scanning reflects the distribution of gas through the lung. The ventilation component requires the cooperation of the patient and may be impossible to perform in the critically ill patient, particularly if the patient is intubated.

Alternatively, plasma D-dimer testing may be recommended when a PE is initially suspected. D-dimer is a degradation product of cross-linked fibrin generated by plasmin cleavage. When D-dimer levels are normal (less than 500 μg/L) it is highly unlikely that the patient has a PE.[56] Thus a normal or near-normal D-dimer level can rule out a PE. In the event that the D-dimer levels are elevated, a venous study (see Table 37-8) is indicated to look for a DVT as the likely source of a PE. If a DVT is located by venous ultrasound, the index of suspicion for PE is very high and anticoagulant treatment should be initiated immediately. Patients with an elevated D-dimer but normal venous ultrasound require a lung scan.

If the lung scan is inconclusive, pulmonary angiography is recommended. Pulmonary angiography is an invasive procedure that involves the insertion of a catheter through the antecubital or femoral vein, advancement to the pulmonary artery, and injection of contrast medium. This allows visualization of the pulmonary vascular system and location of the embolus.

A spiral (or helical) computed tomography (CT) scan, a relatively new noninvasive diagnostic test, may also be used to diagnose PE. Conventional CT scans rotate a frame 360 degrees in one direction, stop, make an image (called a slice), and then spin back in the opposite direction to make another slice after again stopping. The spiral CT scan is able to continuously rotate while obtaining slices and does not have to start and stop between each slice. This allows visualization of entire anatomic regions such as the lungs. The data can be computer reconstructed to allow for a three-dimensional picture of the area being imaged and assist in emboli visualization. In addition, multislice spiral CT scans are now becoming available that can collect even more data (by making more slices) than previous systems.

ABG analysis is important, but not diagnostic. The arterial oxygen partial pressure (PaO_2) is low because of inadequate oxygenation secondary to an occluded pulmonary vasculature. The arterial carbon dioxide partial pressure ($PaCO_2$) is usually low because of hyperventilation. The pH remains normal unless respiratory alkalosis develops as a result of prolonged hyperventilation or to compensate for lactic acidosis caused by shock. An ECG and chest x-ray are usually not diagnostic.

Collaborative Care

When the diagnosis of PE has been made, treatment should be instituted immediately (Table 37-15). The objectives of treatment are to (1) prevent further growth or multiplication of thrombi in the lower extremities, (2) prevent embolization from the upper or lower extremities to the pulmonary vascular system, and (3) provide cardiopulmonary support if indicated.

Conservative Therapy. Supportive therapy for the patient's cardiopulmonary status varies according to the severity of

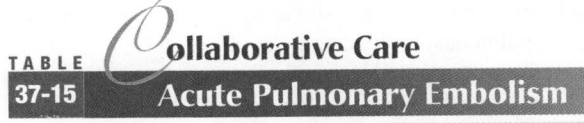

TABLE	*Collaborative Care*
37-15	**Acute Pulmonary Embolism**

Diagnostic
History and physical examination
Venous studies (see Table 37-8)
Chest x-ray
Continuous ECG monitoring
ABGs
CBC count with WBC differential
D-dimer level
Lung scan (ventilation and perfusion)
Pulmonary angiography
Spiral CT scan

Collaborative Therapy
O_2 by mask or cannula, may require intubation
Establishment of IV route for drugs and fluids
Continuous IV heparin for acute treatment
Warfarin (Coumadin) for long-term therapy
Bed rest
Narcotics for pain relief
Thrombolytic agents
Intracaval filter
Pulmonary embolectomy in life–threatening situation

ABGs, Arterial blood gases; *CBC,* complete blood count; *CT,* computed tomography; *ECG,* electrocardiogram; *IV,* intravenous; *WBC,* white blood cell.

the PE. The administration of O_2 by mask or cannula may be adequate for some patients. O_2 is given in a concentration determined by ABG analysis. In some situations, endotracheal intubation and mechanical ventilation may be needed to maintain adequate oxygenation. Respiratory measures such as turning, coughing, and deep breathing are necessary to prevent or treat atelectasis. If shock is present, vasopressor agents may be necessary to support systemic circulation (see Chapter 65). If heart failure is present, digitalis and diuretics are used (see Chapter 34). Pain resulting from pleural irritation or reduced coronary blood flow is treated with narcotics, usually morphine.

Drug Therapy. Properly managed anticoagulant therapy is effective in the treatment of many patients with PE. Heparin and warfarin (Coumadin) are the anticoagulant drugs of choice. Unless contraindicated, heparin should be started immediately and is continued while oral anticoagulants are initiated. The dosage of heparin is adjusted according to the PTT, and warfarin dose is determined by the INR.

Anticoagulant therapy for thromboembolic conditions may not be indicated if the patient has blood dyscrasias, hepatic dysfunction causing alteration in the clotting mechanism, injury to the intestine, overt bleeding, a history of hemorrhagic stroke, or neurologic conditions.

Thrombolytic agents, such as tPA, dissolve PE and the source of the thrombus in the pelvis or deep leg veins, thereby decreasing the likelihood of recurrent pulmonary emboli. (Thrombolytic therapy is discussed in Chapter 33.)

Surgical Therapy. If the degree of pulmonary arterial obstruction is severe (usually greater than 50%) and the patient does not respond to conservative therapy, an immediate embolectomy may be indicated. Pulmonary embolectomy, a rarely performed procedure, is possible with the use of temporary cardiopulmonary bypass. However, its role is limited because of a high mortality rate. Preoperative pulmonary angiography is necessary to identify and locate the site of the embolus. Fortunately, the need for pulmonary embolectomy is rare.

To prevent further pulmonary embolization, the surgical procedures appropriate for thrombophlebitis may be used (see the section on surgical interventions for venous thrombosis earlier in this chapter). These include the insertion of intracaval filter devices (see Fig. 37-9).

NURSING MANAGEMENT
PULMONARY EMBOLISM

■ Nursing Implementation

Health Promotion. Nursing measures aimed at prevention of pulmonary embolism parallel those for prophylaxis of deep vein thrombosis (see p. 930).

Acute Intervention. The prognosis of a patient with PE is good if therapy is promptly instituted. The patient should be kept on bed rest in a semi-Fowler position to facilitate breathing. An IV line should be maintained for medications and fluid therapy. The nurse should know the side effects of medications and observe for them. Oxygen therapy should be administered as ordered. Careful monitoring of vital signs, ECG, ABGs, and lung sounds is critical to assess the patient's status.

The patient is usually anxious because of pain, sense of doom, inability to breathe, and fear of death. The nurse should carefully explain the situation and provide emotional support and reassurance to help relieve the patient's anxiety. During the acute phase, someone should be with the patient as much as possible.

Ambulatory and Home Care. The patient affected by thromboembolic processes may require psychologic and emotional support. In addition to the thromboembolic problems, the patient may have an underlying chronic illness requiring long-term treatment. To provide supportive therapy, the nurse must understand and differentiate between the various problems caused by the underlying disease and those related to thromboembolic disease.

Long-term management is similar to that for the patient with deep vein thrombosis (see p. 930). Discharge planning is aimed at limiting progression of the condition and preventing complications and recurrence. The nurse must reinforce the need for the patient to return to the health care provider for regular follow-up examination.

Evaluation

The expected outcomes are that the patient who has a pulmonary embolism will have

- adequate tissue perfusion and respiratory function
- adequate cardiac output
- increased level of comfort
- no recurrence of PE

CRITICAL THINKING EXERCISES

Case Study
Peripheral Arterial Disease

Patient Profile. Mr. J., a 76-year-old African American man, was admitted to the hospital with rest pain and a nonhealing ulcer of the big toe on the right foot.

Subjective Data

- History of a myocardial infarction, stroke, hypertension, arthritis, and diabetes mellitus
- Underwent a left femoral-popliteal bypass 5 years ago
- Has a smoking history of 45 pack-years
- Has been using insulin for 30 years
- Complains of intense right foot pain for past 6 weeks
- Sleeps in recliner with right leg in dependent position

Objective Data
Physical Examination

- Has a diminished right femoral pulse with no palpable pulses below that level
- Has a small necrotic ulcer on the tip of the right big toe
- Has thickened toenails; has shiny, thin skin on the legs; and hair is absent on both feet

CRITICAL THINKING QUESTIONS

1. What are Mr. J.'s risk factors for peripheral arterial disease?
2. What additional information would you like to know about Mr. J.?

CRITICAL THINKING EXERCISES—cont'd

3. Are Mr. J.'s signs and symptoms evidence of an acute or a chronic peripheral arterial disease? Explain your answer.
4. What is the pathophysiology of rest pain?
5. What treatment modalities are possible for Mr. J.?
6. What are the primary nursing responsibilities in caring for Mr. J.?
7. Based on the assessment data presented, write one or more appropriate nursing diagnoses. Are there any collaborative problems?

Nursing Research Issues

1. What are the changes in quality of life that occur following vascular surgery (e.g., bypass surgery, aneurysm repair, or amputation)?

2. What are the outcomes of a structured versus an unstructured exercise program in the rehabilitation of vascular surgery patients?
3. Can complications of peripheral arterial disease be prevented in high-risk patients?
4. What are the most effective educational tools to teach emergency department nurses to promptly recognize a patient with aortic dissection and a ruptured abdominal aortic aneurysm?
5. What nursing interventions are most effective at preventing recurrence of venous leg ulcers?

REVIEW QUESTIONS

The number of the question corresponds to the same-numbered objective at the beginning of the chapter.

1. A 62-year-old woman weighs 92 kg and has a history of daily alcohol intake, smoking, high blood pressure, high sodium intake, and sedentary lifestyle. The nurse identifies the risk factors most highly related to peripheral arterial disease in this patient as
   a. sex and age.
   b. weight and alcohol intake.
   c. cigarette smoking and hypertension.
   d. sedentary lifestyle and high sodium intake.
2. Significant risk factors for peripheral arterial disease include
   a. sedentary lifestyle, stress, obesity.
   b. advanced age, female gender, familial tendency.
   c. cigarette smoking, hyperlipidemia, hypertension.
   d. protein S deficiency, protein C deficiency, factor V Leiden mutation.
3. A patient is being prepared for an abdominal aortic aneurysm repair. The nurse suspects rupture of the aneurysm when
   a. the patient becomes dizzy and short of breath.
   b. the patient complains of sudden, severe back pain.
   c. a bruit and thrill are present at the site of the aneurysm.
   d. the patient develops blue, patchy mottling of the feet and toes.
4. Important nursing measures after an abdominal aortic aneurysm repair are to
   a. elevate the legs and apply TED hose.
   b. assess cranial nerves and mental status.
   c. administer IV heparin and monitor APTT.
   d. monitor urine output, BUN, and creatinine.
5. Specific symptoms of aortic dissection vary depending on
   a. the medications that are administered.
   b. how elevated the blood pressure becomes.
   c. the aortic branches affected in the descent of the dissection.
   d. the respiratory status of the patient before dissection occurs.

6. Rest pain is a manifestation of peripheral arterial disease that occurs as a result of
   a. the beginning of a venous leg ulcer.
   b. inadequate blood flow to the nerves of the feet.
   c. inadequate blood flow to the muscles during exercise.
   d. inadequate blood flow to the skin after application of the heat.
7. A patient with infective endocarditis develops sudden left leg pain with pallor, paresthesia, and a loss of peripheral pulses. The nurse's initial action should be to
   a. notify the physician.
   b. elevate the leg to promote venous return.
   c. wrap the leg in a blanket to provide warmth.
   d. perform passive range of motion to stimulate circulation to the leg.
8. The usual medical treatment of Raynaud's phenomenon involves
   a. transluminal balloon angioplasty.
   b. amputation of the affected digits.
   c. peripheral arterial bypass surgery.
   d. prescribing calcium channel blockers.
9. The patient who is most likely to have the highest risk for deep vein thrombosis is a
   a. 25-year-old obese woman who is 3 days postpartum.
   b. 40-year-old woman who smokes and uses oral contraceptives.
   c. 62-year-old man who has had a stroke with left-sided hemiparesis.
   d. 72-year-old man who had a suprapubic prostatectomy for cancer of the prostate.
10. The nurse suspects the presence of a deep vein thrombosis based on the findings of
    a. paresthesia and coolness of the leg.
    b. pain in the calf that occurs with exercise.
    c. generalized edema of the involved extremity.
    d. pallor and cyanosis of the involved extremity.

Continued

REVIEW QUESTIONS—cont'd

11. Nursing interventions indicated in the plan of care for the patient with acute lower extremity deep vein thrombosis include
    a. applying elastic compression stockings.
    b. administering anticoagulants as ordered.
    c. positioning the leg dependently to promote arterial circulation.
    d. encouraging walking and leg exercises to promote venous return.

12. The nurse instructs the patient discharged on anticoagulant therapy to
    a. limit intake of vitamin C.
    b. report symptoms of nausea to the physician.
    c. have blood drawn routinely to check electrolytes.
    d. be aware of and report signs or symptoms of bleeding.

13. In planning care and patient teaching for the patient with venous leg ulcers, the nurse recognizes that the most important intervention in healing and control of this condition is
    a. application of antibiotic cream to the ulcers.
    b. debridement of the ulcers with skin grafting.
    c. elevation of the extremities to increase venous return.
    d. performance of leg exercises to increase collateral circulation.

14. A patient with a deep vein thrombosis suddenly develops dyspnea, tachypnea, and chest pain. Initially the most appropriate action by the nurse is to
    a. auscultate for abnormal lung sounds.
    b. administer oxygen and notify the physician.
    c. ask the patient to cough and deep breathe to clear the airways.
    d. elevate the head of the bed 30 to 45 degrees to facilitate breathing.

REFERENCES

1. Graham LM, Ford MB: Arterial disease. In Fahey VA, editor: *Vascular nursing,* ed 3, Philadelphia, 1999, WB Saunders.
2. Newman AB: Peripheral arterial disease: insights from population studies of older adults, *J Am Geriatr Soc* 48:1157, 2000.
3. Westendorp IC et al: Hormone replacement therapy and peripheral vascular disease: the Rotterdam study, *Arch Intern Med* 160:2498, 2000.
4. Langman LJ et al: Hyperhomocyst(e)inemia and the increased risk of venous thromboembolism, *Arch Intern Med* 160:961, 2000.
5. Howes PS et al: Role of stored iron in atherosclerosis, *J Vasc Nurs* 18:109, 2000.
6. Rosamond WD et al: Stroke incidence and survival among middle-aged adults: 9-year follow-up of the Atherosclerosis Risk in Communities (ARIC) cohort, *Stroke* 30:736, 1999.
7. American Heart Association: *2001 heart and stroke statistical update,* Dallas, 2000, American Heart Association.
8. Stokes J, Lindsay J: Major causes of death and hospitalization in Canadian seniors, *Chronic Diseases in Canada* 17:63, 1996.
9. Matsumura JS: Surgery of the aorta. In Fahey VA, editor: *Vascular nursing,* ed 3, Philadelphia, 1999, WB Saunders.
10. Gross KA: Ultrasonographic diagnosis and guided compression repair of femoral artery pseudoaneurysm: an update for the vascular nurse, *J Vasc Nurs* 17:59, 1999.
11. Jones MA, Hoffman LA, Makaroun MS: Endovascular grafting for repair of abdominal aortic aneurysm, *Crit Care Nurs* 20:38, 2000.
12. Phillips JK: Abdominal aortic aneurysm, *Nursing* 28:35, 1998.
13. Cox CC, Borgini LM: Intraoperative nursing care of the vascular patient. In Fahey VA, editor: *Vascular nursing,* ed 3, Philadelphia, 1999, WB Saunders.
*14. Kozon V, Fortner N, Holzenbein T: An empirical study of nursing in patients undergoing two different procedures for abdominal aortic aneurysm repair, *J Vasc Nurs* 16:1, 1998.
15. Karmy-Jones R, Aldea G, Boyle EM: The continuing evolution in the management of thoracic aortic dissection, *Chest* 5:1221, 2000.
16. Scott C et al: Acute ascending aortic dissection during pregnancy, *Am J Crit Care* 10: 6, 2001.
17. Meszaros I et al: Epidemiology and clinicopathology of aortic dissection, *Chest* 117: 1271, 2000.
18. Rice KL, Walsh ME: Peripheral arterial occlusive disease, part I: navigating a bottleneck, *Nursing* 28:33, 1998.

19. Sloan K, Wills EM: Ankle-brachial index: calculating your patient's vascular risks, *Nursing* 29:58, 1999.
20. Hiatt WR: Medical treatment of peripheral arterial disease and claudication, *N Engl J Med* 344:1608, 2001.
21. Ekers MA, Hirsch AT: Vascular medicine and vascular rehabilitation. In Fahey VA, editor: *Vascular nursing,* ed 3, Philadelphia, 1999, WB Saunders.
22. Cote MC: Vascular nurse as a smoking cessation specialist, *J Vasc Nurs* 18:47, 2000.
23. CAPRIE Steering Committee: A randomized, blinded trial of clopidogrel versus aspirin in patients at risk of ischaemic events (CAPRIE), *Lancet* 348:1329, 1996.
24. Beebe HG et al: A new pharmacological treatment for intermittent claudication: results of a randomized, multi-center trial, *Arch Intern Med* 159:2041, 1999.
25. Dawson DL et al: A comparison of cilostazol and pentoxifylline for treating intermittent claudication, *Am J Med* 109:523, 2000.
26. Keller KB, Lemberg L: Herbal or complementary medicine: fact or fiction? *Am J Crit Care* 10:438, 2001.
27. Pittler MH, Ernst E: Ginkgo biloba extract for the treatment of intermittent claudication: a meta-analysis of randomized trials, *Am J Med* 108:276, 2000.
28. Maxwell AJ, Anderson BE, Cooke JP: Nutritional therapy for peripheral vascular disease: a double blind, placebo-controlled, randomized trial of HeartBar, *Vasc Med* 5:11, 2000.
29. Vogelzang RL: Percutaneous vascular intervention and imaging techniques. In Fahey VA, editor: *Vascular nursing,* ed 3, Philadelphia, 1999, WB Saunders.
*30. Donaghue CC et al: Improved health-related quality of life 12 months after bypass or angioplasty for peripheral artery disease, *J Vasc Nurs* 18:75, 2000.
31. Fahey VA, McCarthy WJ: Arterial reconstruction of the lower extremity. In Fahey VA, editor: *Vascular nursing,* ed 3, Philadelphia, 1999, WB Saunders.
32. Olin JW: Thromboangiitis obliterans (Buerger's disease), *N Engl J Med* 343:864, 2000.
33. Frost-Rude JA, Nunnelee JD: Buerger's disease, *J Vasc Nurs* 18:128, 2000.
34. O'Connor CM: Raynaud's phenomenon, *J Vasc Nurs* 19:87, 2001.
35. Raynaud's Treatment Study Investigators: Comparison of sustained-released nifedipine and temperature feedback for treatment of primary Raynaud's phenomenon: results from a randomized clinical trial with 1-year follow-up, *Arch Intern Med* 160:1101, 2000.

*Nursing research–based reference.

*36. Olson HF, Nunnelee JD: Incidence of thrombosis in pregnancy and postpartum: a retrospective review in a large private hospital, *J Vasc Nurs* 16:84, 1998.

37. Page MJ: Factor V Leiden mutation: a nursing perspective, *J Vasc Nurs* 16:73, 1998.

38. Walsh EM, Rice KL: Venous thrombosis and pulmonary embolism. In Fahey VA, editor: *Vascular nursing*, ed 3, Philadelphia, 1999, WB Saunders.

39. Church V: Staying on guard for DVT and PE, *Nursing* 30:34, 2000.

40. Breen P: DVT: what every nurse should know, *RN* 63:58, 2000.

41. Weitz J, Hirsh J: New anticoagulant drugs, *Chest* 119:95S, 2001.

42. Becker R, Fintel D, Green D: *Antithrombotic therapy,* Caddo, Okla, 2000, Professional Communications.

43. Nazario R, Delorenzo LJ, Maguire AG: Treatment of venous thromboembolism, *Cardiol Rev* 10:249, 2002.

44. Green D: Sclerotherapy for the permanent eradication of varicose veins: theoretical and practical considerations, *J Am Acad Dermatol* 38:461, 1998.

45. Sadick NS: Long-term results with a multiple synchronized pulse 1064 nm Nd:YAG laser for the treatment of leg venulectasias and reticular veins, *Dermatol Surg* 27:365, 2001.

*46. Wipke-Tevis DD et al: Prevalence, incidence, management, and predictors of venous ulcers in the long-term-care population using the MDS, *Adv Skin Wound Care* 13:218, 2000.

47. Wipke-Tevis DD: Caring for vascular leg ulcers, *Home Healthc Nurs* 17:8, 1999.

48. Krasner D: Painful venous ulcers: themes and stories about living with the pain and suffering, *J WOCN* 25:158, 1998.

49. Krasner D: Painful venous ulcers: themes and stories about their impact on quality of life, *Ostomy Wound Manage* 44:38, 1998.

50. Wipke-Tevis DD, Stotts NA: Nutrition, tissue oxygenation, and healing of venous leg ulcers, *J Vasc Nurs* 16:48, 1998.

51. Wipke-Tevis DD: Vascular infections: medical and surgical therapies, *J Cardiovasc Nurs* 13:70, 1999.

52. Robinson C, Santilli SM: Warm-up Active Wound Therapy: a novel approach to the management of chronic venous ulcers, *J Vasc Nurs* 16:38, 1998.

53. Nunnelee JD, Spaner SD: Explanatory model of chronic venous disease in rural Midwest—a factor analysis, *J Vasc Nurs* 18:6, 2000.

54. Wipke-Tevis DD et al: Tissue oxygenation, perfusion, and position in patients with venous leg ulcers, *Nurs Res* 50:24, 2001.

55. Launius BK, Graham BD: Understanding and preventing deep vein thrombosis and pulmonary embolism, *AACN Clin Issues* 9:91, 1998.

56. Perrier A: Noninvasive diagnosis of pulmonary embolism, *Hosp Pract* 15:47, 1998.

RESOURCES

American Association of Cardiovascular and Pulmonary Rehabilitation (AACVPR)
401 North Michigan Avenue, Suite 2200
Chicago, IL 60611-4267
312-321-5146
Fax: 312-527-6635
www.aacvpr.org/

American College of Chest Physicians (ACCP)
3300 Dundee Road
Northbrook, IL 60062-2348
847-498-1400
Fax: 847-498-5460
www.chestnet.org/

American Venous Forum
13 Elm Street
Manchester, MA 01944
978-526-8330
www.venous-info.com/

Anticoagulation Forum
88 East Newton Street, E-113
Boston, MA 02118-2395
617-638-7265
Fax: 617-638-7267
www.acforum.org/

Canadian Cardiovascular Society (CCS)
222 rue Queen Street
Suite/Pièce 1403
Ottawa, ON K1P 5V9
613-569-3407
Fax: 613-569-6574
www.ccs.ca/

Council on Cardiovascular Nursing
American Heart Association
7320 Greenville Avenue
Dallas, TX 75231
214-373-6300
www.amhrt.org/Scientific/council/cvn/index.html

Heart and Stroke Foundation of Canada
222 Queen Street, Suite 1402
Ottawa, ON K1P 5V9
613-569-4361
Fax: 613-569-3278
http://www.heartandstroke.ca/

Mayo Clinic Heart and Blood Vessels Center
www.mayoclinic.com

National Heart, Lung, and Blood Institute
National Institutes of Health
4733 Bethesda Avenue, Suite 530
Bethesda, MD 20814
301-951-3260
www.nhlbi.nih.gov/

National Institute of Nursing Research
www.nih.gov/ninr/

National Lymphedema Network
Latham Square, 1611 Telegraph Avenue, Suite 1111
Oakland, CA 94612-2138
Hotline: 800-541-3259 or 510-208-320
Fax: 510-208-3110
www.lymphnet.org/

Peripheral Vascular Surgical Society
824 Munras Avenue, Suite C
Monterey, CA 93940
831-373-0508
Fax: 831-373-0460
www.pvss.org/

Society for Cardiovascular and Interventional Radiology
10201 Lee Highway, Suite 500
Fairfax, VA 22030
800-488-7284 or 703-691-1805
Fax: 703-691-1855
www.sirweb.org/

Society for Vascular Medicine and Biology
13 Elm Street
Manchester, MA 01944
978-526-8330
Fax: 978-526-4018
www.svmb.org/

Society for Vascular Nursing (SVN)
7794 Grow Drive
Pensacola, FL 32514
888-536-4786
Fax: 850-484-8762
www.svnnet.org/

Society for Vascular Surgery (SVS)
13 Elm Street
Manchester, MA 01944-1314
978-526-8330
Fax: 978-526-4018
http://svs.vascularweb.org/
Society of Vascular Technology
4601 Presidents Drive, Suite 260
Lanham, MD 20706
301-459-7550
Fax: 301-459-5651
www.svtnet.org/

Thrombosis Interest Group of Canada (TIGC)
www.tigc.org/
Vascular Disease Foundation
3333 South Wadsworth Boulevard #B104-37
Lakewood, CO 80227
866-PADINFO (723-4636) or 303-949-8337
Fax: 303-989-6522
www.vdf.org/
***www.dvt.org:* an Internet Resource on Venous Thromboembolism**
www.umassmed.edu/outcomes/dvt/

For additional Internet resources, see the website for this book at
http://evolve.elsevier.com/Lewis/medsurg/.

Problems of Ingestion, Digestion, Absorption, and Elimination

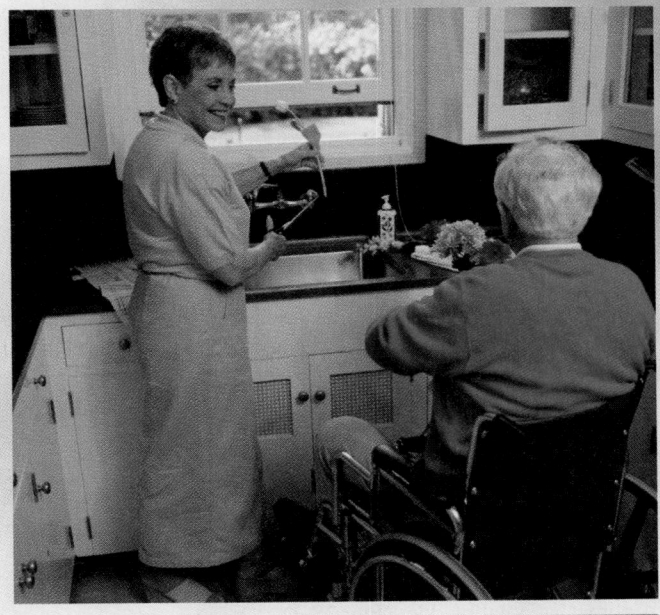

38

NURSING ASSESSMENT
Gastrointestinal System

Anne Croghan

LEARNING OBJECTIVES

1. Describe the structures and functions of the organs of the gastrointestinal tract.
2. Describe the structures and functions of the liver, gallbladder, biliary tract, and pancreas.
3. Explain the processes of ingestion, digestion, absorption, and elimination.
4. Explain the processes of biliary metabolism, bile production, and bile excretion.
5. Describe age-related changes in the gastrointestinal system and differences in assessment findings.
6. Identify the significant subjective and objective data related to the gastrointestinal system that should be obtained from a patient.
7. Describe the appropriate techniques used in the physical assessment of the gastrointestinal system.
8. Differentiate normal from common abnormal findings of a physical assessment of the gastrointestinal system.
9. Describe the purpose, significance of results, and nursing responsibilities related to diagnostic studies of the gastrointestinal system.

KEY TERMS

absorption, p. 948	ingestion, p. 947
bilirubin, p. 952	Kupffer cells, p. 951
borborygmi (Table 38-11), p. 960	melena (Table 38-11), p. 961
cheilosis (Table 38-11), p. 960	pyorrhea (Table 38-11), p. 960
defecation, p. 951	pyrosis (Table 38-11), p. 960
deglutition, p. 948	steatorrhea (Table 38-11), p. 961
digestion, p. 948	tenesmus (Table 38-11), p. 961
endoscopy, p. 965	Valsalva maneuver, p. 951
hematemesis (Table 38-11), p. 960	villi, p. 948
hepatocytes, p. 951	

The main function of the gastrointestinal (GI) system is to supply nutrients to body cells. This is accomplished through the processes of *ingestion* (taking in food), *digestion* (breakdown of food), and *absorption* (transfer of food products into circulation). *Elimination* is the process of excreting the waste products of digestion.

The GI system (also called the digestive system) consists of the GI tract and its associated organs and glands. Included in the GI tract are the mouth, esophagus, stomach, small intestine, large intestine, rectum, and anus. The associated organs are the liver, pancreas, and gallbladder (Fig. 38-1).

Factors outside the GI tract can influence its functioning. Both psychologic and emotional factors, such as stress and anxiety, influence GI functioning in many people. Stress may be manifested as anorexia, epigastric and abdominal pain, or diarrhea. However, GI problems should never be attributed solely to psychologic factors. Organic and psychologically based problems can exist independently or concurrently. Physical factors, such as dietary intake, ingestion of alcohol and caffeine-containing products, cigarette smoking, and fatigue, may also affect GI function. Some organic diseases of the GI system, such as peptic ulcer disease and ulcerative colitis, may be aggravated by stress.

STRUCTURES AND FUNCTIONS OF THE GASTROINTESTINAL SYSTEM

The GI tract is a tube approximately 30 feet (9 m) long extending from the mouth to the anus. The entire tract is composed of four common layers. From the inside to the outside, these layers are (1) mucosa, (2) submucosa, (3) muscle, and (4) serosa (Fig. 38-2). In the esophagus the outer coat is fibrous tissue rather than serosa. The muscular coat consists of two layers: the circular (inner) and the longitudinal (outer).

The GI tract is innervated by the parasympathetic and the sympathetic branches of the autonomic nervous system. The parasympathetic system is mainly excitatory, and the sympathetic system is mainly inhibitory. For example, peristalsis is increased by parasympathetic stimulation and decreased by sympathetic stimulation. Sensory information is relayed via both sympathetic and parasympathetic afferent fibers.

The GI tract also has its own nervous system: the enteric, or intrinsic, nervous system. The enteric nervous system is composed of two nerve layers that lie between the mucosa and the circular muscle layer and the circular and longitudinal muscle layers. These neurons contribute to the coordination of GI motor and secretory activities. The enteric nervous system is also known as the "gut brain." It contains numerous neurons (about as many as the spinal cord) and has the ability to control movement and secretion of the GI tract.

The GI tract and accessory organs receive approximately 25% to 30% of the cardiac output. Circulation in the GI system is unique in that venous blood draining the GI tract organs empties into the portal vein, which then perfuses the liver. The upper portion of the GI tract receives its blood supply from the splanchnic artery. The small intestine receives its blood supply from branches of the hepatic and superior mesenteric arteries. The large intestine receives its blood supply mainly from the superior and inferior

---

Reviewed by Phyllis Christiansen, RN, MN, ARNP, Adult and Geriatric Nurse Practitioner, University of Washington, Seattle, Wash.

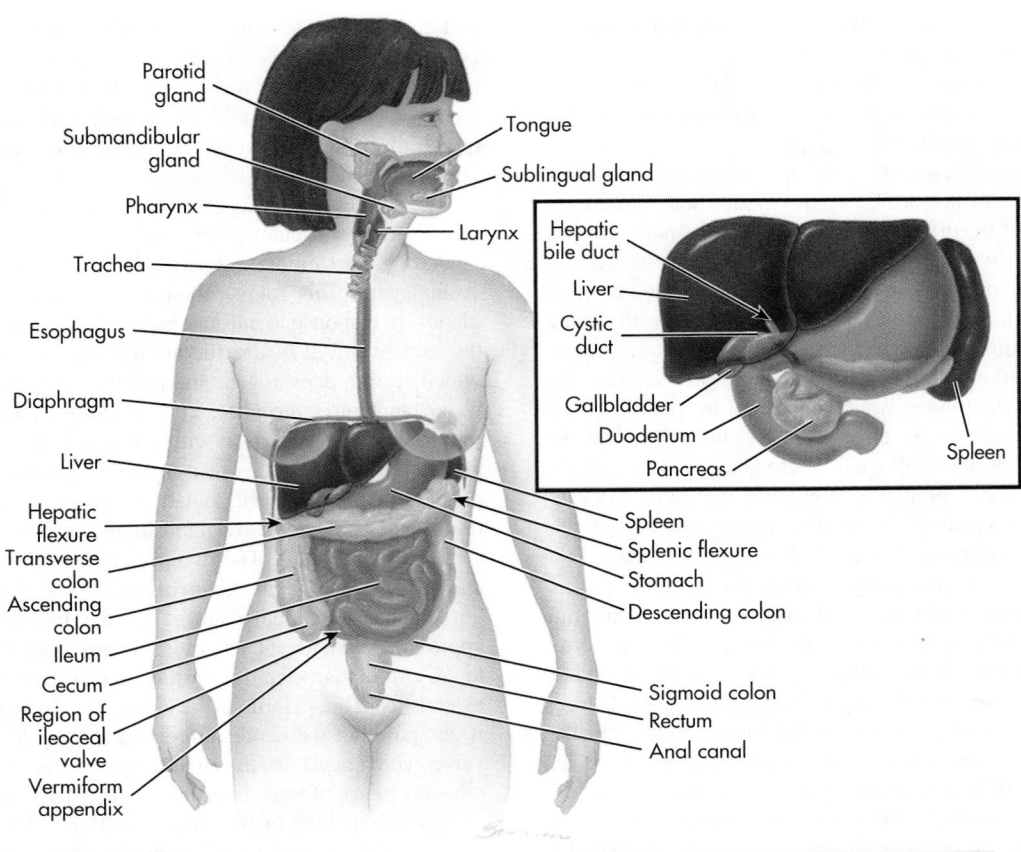

Parotid gland
Submandibular gland
Pharynx
Trachea
Esophagus
Diaphragm
Liver
Hepatic flexure
Transverse colon
Ascending colon
Ileum
Cecum
Region of ileoceal valve
Vermiform appendix

Tongue
Sublingual gland
Larynx

Hepatic bile duct
Liver
Cystic duct
Gallbladder
Duodenum
Pancreas
Spleen

Spleen
Splenic flexure
Stomach
Descending colon

Sigmoid colon
Rectum
Anal canal

FIG. 38-1 Location of organs of the gastrointestinal system.

mesenteric arteries. Because such a large percentage of the cardiac output perfuses these organs, the GI tract is a major source from which blood flow can be diverted during exercise or stress.

The two types of movement of the GI tract are mixing (segmentation) and propulsion (peristalsis). The secretions of the GI system consist of enzymes and hormones for digestion, mucus to provide protection and lubrication, and water and electrolytes.

The abdominal organs are almost completely covered by the peritoneum. The two layers of the peritoneum are the *parietal,* which lines the abdominal cavity wall, and the *visceral,* which covers the abdominal organs. The peritoneal cavity is the potential space between the parietal and visceral layers. The two folds of the peritoneum are the mesentery and omentum. The mesentery attaches the small intestine and part of the large intestine to the posterior abdominal wall and contains blood and lymph vessels. The lesser omentum goes from the lesser curvature of the stomach and upper duodenum to the liver, and the greater omentum hangs from the stomach over the intestines like an apron. The omentum contains fat and lymph nodes.

The primary functions of the GI system are (1) ingestion and propulsion (movement) of food, (2) digestion, (3) absorption, and (4) elimination. Each part of the GI system performs different activities to accomplish these functions.

Ingestion and Propulsion of Food

Ingestion is the intake of food. A person's appetite or desire to ingest food is a significant factor in how much food is eaten. Multiple factors are involved in the control of appetite. An ap-

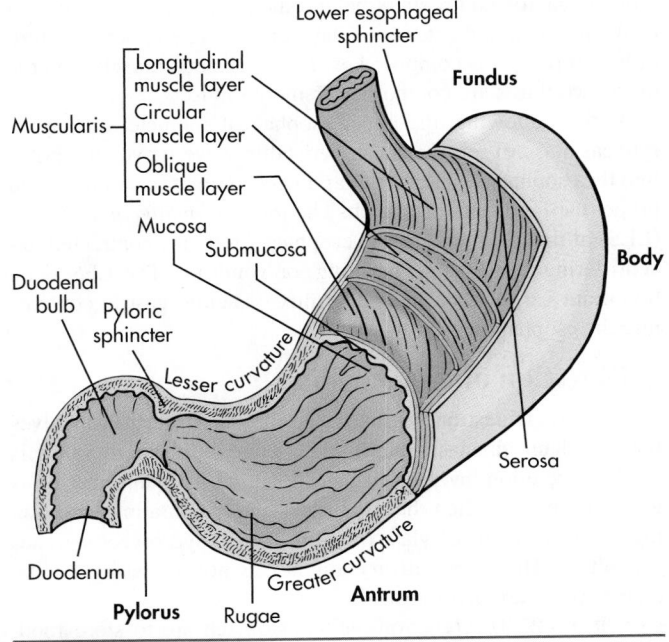

Lower esophageal sphincter
Longitudinal muscle layer
Circular muscle layer
Oblique muscle layer
Muscularis
Mucosa
Submucosa
Duodenal bulb
Pyloric sphincter
Lesser curvature
Duodenum
Pylorus
Rugae
Greater curvature
Fundus
Body
Serosa
Antrum

FIG. 38-2 Parts of the stomach.

petite center is located in the hypothalamus. It is directly or indirectly stimulated by hypoglycemia, an empty stomach, decrease in body temperature, and input from higher brain centers. The sight, smell, and taste of food frequently stimulate appetite. Appetite may be inhibited by stomach distention, illness (especially accompanied by fever), hyperglycemia, nausea and vomiting, and certain drugs (e.g., amphetamines).

Deglutition (swallowing) is the mechanical component of ingestion. The organs involved in the deglutition of food are the mouth, pharynx, and esophagus.

Mouth. The mouth consists of the lips and oral (buccal) cavity. The lips surround the orifice of the mouth and function in speech. The roof of the oral cavity is formed by the hard and soft palates. The oral cavity contains the teeth, used in mastication (chewing), and the tongue. The tongue is a solid muscle mass and assists in mastication by keeping food between the teeth during chewing and moving the food to the back of the throat for swallowing (deglutition). Taste receptors are found on the sides and tip of the tongue. The tongue is also important in speech.

Within the oral cavity are three pairs of salivary glands: the parotid, submaxillary, and sublingual. These glands produce saliva, which consists of water, protein, mucin, inorganic salts, and salivary amylase. Approximately 1 L of saliva is produced each day.

Pharynx. The pharynx is a musculomembranous tube that may be divided into the nasopharynx, oropharynx, and laryngeal pharynx. The mucous membrane of the pharynx is continuous with the nasal cavity, mouth, auditory tubes, and larynx. The oropharynx secretes mucus, which aids in swallowing. The epiglottis is a lid of fibrocartilage that closes over the larynx during swallowing. During ingestion the oropharynx provides a route for the food from the mouth to the esophagus. When receptors in the oropharynx are stimulated by food or liquid, the swallowing reflex is initiated.

Esophagus. The esophagus is a hollow, muscular tube that receives food from the pharynx and moves it to the stomach by peristaltic contractions. It is 9.2 to 10 inches (23 to 25 cm) long and 0.8 inch (2 cm) in diameter. The esophagus is located in the thoracic cavity, and it starts behind the trachea at the lower end of the pharynx and extends to the stomach. The upper one third of the esophagus is composed of striated skeletal muscle, and the distal two thirds are composed of smooth muscle.

With swallowing, the upper esophageal sphincter (cricopharyngeal muscle) relaxes and a peristaltic wave moves the bolus into the esophagus. The muscular layers contract (peristalsis) and propel the food to the stomach. The *lower esophageal sphincter* (LES) at the distal end of the esophagus remains contracted except during swallowing, belching, or vomiting. The LES is an important barrier that prevents reflux of acidic gastric contents into the esophagus.

Digestion and Absorption

Mouth. Digestion begins in the mouth. **Digestion** involves both mechanical (mastication) and chemical digestion. Saliva is the first secretion involved in digestion, and its main function is to lubricate and soften the food mass, thus facilitating swallowing. Saliva contains amylase (ptyalin), which hydrolyzes starches to maltose. However, salivary amylase is not necessary for the digestion of carbohydrates.

Stomach. The functions of the stomach are to store food, mix the food with gastric secretions, and empty contents into the small intestine at a rate at which digestion can occur. The stomach absorbs only small amounts of water, alcohol, electrolytes, and certain drugs.

The stomach lies obliquely in the epigastric, umbilical, and left hypochondriac regions of the abdomen (see Fig. 38-7 later in chapter). The shape and position of the stomach change based on the degree of gastric distention. It always contains gastric fluid

and mucus. The three main parts of the stomach are the fundus, body, and antrum (see Fig. 38-2). The pylorus is a small portion of the antrum that lies proximal to the pyloric sphincter. Sphincter muscles (the LES and the pyloric sphincter) guard the entrance to and exit from the stomach. The cardiac orifice is the opening between the esophagus and the stomach.

The serous (outer) layer of the stomach is formed by the peritoneum. The muscular layer consists of the longitudinal (outer) layer, circular (middle) layer, and oblique (inner) layer. The mucosal layer forms folds called *rugae* that contain many small glands. In response to nutrient intake, these glands secrete most of the gastric juice. In the fundus the glands contain chief cells, which secrete pepsinogen, and parietal cells, which secrete HCl, water, and intrinsic factor. The secretion of HCl makes gastric juice acidic in comparison with other body fluids. This acidic pH aids in the protection against ingested organisms. Intrinsic factor promotes cobalamin (vitamin B_{12}) absorption in the small intestine. Mucus is secreted by glands in the cardiac and pyloric areas.

Small Intestine. The two primary functions of the small intestine are digestion and **absorption** (uptake of nutrients from the gut lumen to the bloodstream). The small intestine is a coiled tube approximately 23 feet (7 m) in length and from 1 to 1.1 inches (2.5 to 2.8 cm) in diameter, diminishing in diameter at the lower end. It extends from the pylorus to the ileocecal valve. The small intestine is composed of the duodenum, jejunum, and ileum. The ileocecal valve, which separates the small intestine from the large intestine, prevents reflux of large intestine contents into the small intestine.

The serous coat of the small intestine is formed by the peritoneum. The mucosa is thick, vascular, and glandular. The circular folds in the mucous and submucous layers provide a greater surface area for digestion and absorption.

The functional units of the small intestine are villi. They are present in the entire small intestine. **Villi** are minute, fingerlike projections in the mucous membrane. They contain goblet cells that secrete mucus and epithelial cells that produce the intestinal digestive enzymes. The epithelial cells on the villi also have *microvilli,* which compose the brush border. Thus the presence of villi and microvilli greatly increases the surface area for absorption.

The digestive enzymes on the brush border of the microvilli chemically break down nutrients so that they can be absorbed. The villi are surrounded by the crypts of Lieberkühn, which contain the base columnar cells that are the stem cells for the other epithelial cell types. Brunner's glands in the submucosa of the duodenum secrete mucus.

Physiology of Digestion. *Digestion* is the physical and chemical breakdown of food into absorbable substances. Digestion in the GI tract is facilitated by the timely movement of food through the various organs and the secretion of specific enzymes. These enzymes break down foodstuffs to particles of appropriate size for absorption (Table 38-1).

The process of digestion begins in the mouth, where the food is chewed, mechanically broken down, and mixed with saliva. The saliva lubricates the food. In addition, salivary amylase begins the breakdown of starch. Salivary gland secretion is stimulated by chewing movements and the sight, smell, thought, and taste of food. The food is swallowed and passes into the esophagus, where peristaltic waves propel it to the stomach. No digestion or absorption occurs in the esophagus.

In the stomach the digestion of proteins begins with the release of pepsinogen from chief cells. The acidic environment of the stomach results in the conversion of pepsinogen to its active form, pepsin. Pepsin begins the initial breakdown of proteins. In the stomach there is minimal digestion of starches and fats. The food is mixed with gastric secretions, which are under neural and hormonal control (Tables 38-2 and 38-3). The stomach also serves as a reservoir for food, which is slowly expelled into the small intestine. The length of time that food remains in the stom-

ach depends on the composition of the food, but average meals remain from 3 to 4 hours.

Digestion is completed in the small intestine, where carbohydrates are hydrolyzed to monosaccharides, fats to glycerol and fatty acids, and proteins to amino acids. The physical presence of *chyme* (food mixed with gastric secretions), along with its chem-

TABLE 38-1 Gastrointestinal Secretions Related to Digestion

LOCATION	DAILY AMOUNT (ML)	SECRETIONS/ENZYMES	ACTION
Salivary glands	1000-1500	Salivary amylase (ptyalin)	Initiation of starch digestion
Stomach	2500	Pepsinogen	Protein digestion
		HCl	Protein digestion
		Lipase	Fat digestion
		Intrinsic factor	Essential for cobalamin absorption in ileum
Small intestine	3000	Enterokinase	Activation of trypsinogen to trypsin
		Amylase	Carbohydrate digestion
		Peptidases	Protein digestion
		Aminopeptidase	Protein digestion
		Maltase	Maltose to 2 glucose molecules
		Sucrase	Sucrose to glucose and fructose
		Lactase	Lactose to glucose and galactose
		Lipase	Fat digestion
Pancreas	700	Trypsinogen	Protein digestion
		Chymotrypsin	Protein digestion
		Amylase	Starch to disaccharides
		Lipase	Fat digestion
Liver and gallbladder	1000	Bile	Emulsification of fats and aid in absorption of fatty acids and fat-soluble vitamins (A, D, E, K)

TABLE 38-2 Phases of Gastric Secretion

PHASE	STIMULUS TO SECRETION	SECRETION
Cephalic (nervous)	Sight, smell, taste of food (before food enters stomach); initiated in the CNS and mediated by the vagus nerve	HCl, pepsinogen, mucus
Gastric (hormonal and nervous)	Food in antrum of stomach, vagal stimulation	Release of gastrin hormone from antrum into circulation to stimulate gastric secretions and motility
Intestinal (hormonal)	Presence of chyme in small intestine	Acidic chyme (pH <2): release of secretin, gastric inhibitory polypeptide, cholecystokinin into circulation to decrease acid secretion
Chyme (pH >3): release of duodenal gastrin to increase acid secretion

CNS, Central nervous system.

TABLE 38-3 Major Hormones Controlling Gastrointestinal Secretion and Motility

HORMONE	SOURCE	ACTIVATING STIMULI	FUNCTION
Gastrin	Gastric and duodenal mucosa	Stomach distention, partially digested proteins in pylorus	Gastric acid secretion, increased motility, maintenance of lower esophageal sphincter tone
Secretin	Duodenal mucosa	Acid entering small intestine	Inhibition of gastric motility and acid secretion, stimulation of pancreatic bicarbonate secretion
Cholecystokinin	Duodenal mucosa	Fatty acids and amino acids in small intestine	Contraction of gallbladder and relaxation of sphincter of Oddi, allowing increased flow of bile into duodenum; release of pancreatic digestive enzymes
Gastric inhibitory peptide	Duodenal mucosa	Fatty acids and lipids in the small intestine	Inhibition of gastric acid secretion and gastric motility

ical nature in the small intestine, stimulates motility and secretion. Secretions involved in digestion include enzymes from the pancreas, bile from the liver (see Table 38-1), and intestinal secretions from glands in the small intestine. Both secretion and motility are under neural and hormonal control.

When food enters the stomach and small intestine, hormones are released into the bloodstream (see Table 38-3). The hormone secretin stimulates the pancreas to secrete fluid with a high concentration of bicarbonate. This alkaline secretion enters the duodenum and neutralizes acid in the chyme. The duodenal mucosa also secretes mucus to protect against the HCl. In response to the presence of chyme, the hormone cholecystokinin (CCK), produced by the duodenal mucosa, enters the bloodstream and stimulates contraction of the gallbladder and relaxation of the sphincter of Oddi. These actions permit bile to flow from the common bile duct into the duodenum. Bile is necessary for the digestion of fats. CCK also stimulates the pancreas to synthesize and secrete enzymes for enzymatic digestion of carbohydrates, fats, and proteins.

Enzymes present on the brush border of the microvilli complete the digestion process. These enzymes hydrolyze disaccharides to monosaccharides and peptides to amino acids for absorption.

Absorption is the transfer of the end products of digestion across the intestinal wall to the circulation. Most absorption occurs in the small intestine. The surface area of the small intestine is greatly increased by its circular folds, villi, and microvilli. The movement of the villi enables the end products of digestion to come in contact with the absorbing membrane. Monosaccharides (from carbohydrates), fatty acids (from fats), amino acids (from proteins), water, electrolytes, and vitamins are absorbed.

Elimination

Large Intestine. The large intestine is a hollow, muscular tube approximately 5 to 6 feet (1.5 to 2 m) long and 2 inches (5 cm) in diameter. The four parts of the large intestine are (1) the cecum and appendix, a narrow tube at the end of the cecum; (2) the colon (ascending colon on the right side, transverse colon across the abdomen, descending colon on the left side, and the sigmoid colon); (3) the rectum; and (4) the anus, the terminal portion of the large intestine (Fig. 38-3).

The most important function of the large intestine is the absorption of water and electrolytes. It also forms feces and serves as a reservoir for the fecal mass until defecation occurs. Feces are composed of water (75%), bacteria, unabsorbed minerals, undigested foodstuffs, bile pigments, and desquamated epithelial cells. The large intestine secretes mucus, which acts as a lubricant and protects the mucosa.

Microorganisms in the colon are responsible for the breakdown of proteins not digested or absorbed in the small intestine. These amino acids are deaminated by the bacteria, leaving ammonia, which is carried to the liver and converted to urea. Bacteria in the colon also synthesize vitamin K and some of the B vitamins. Bacteria also play a part in the production of flatus.

The movements of the large intestine are usually slow. When the circular muscles contract, they produce a kneading action

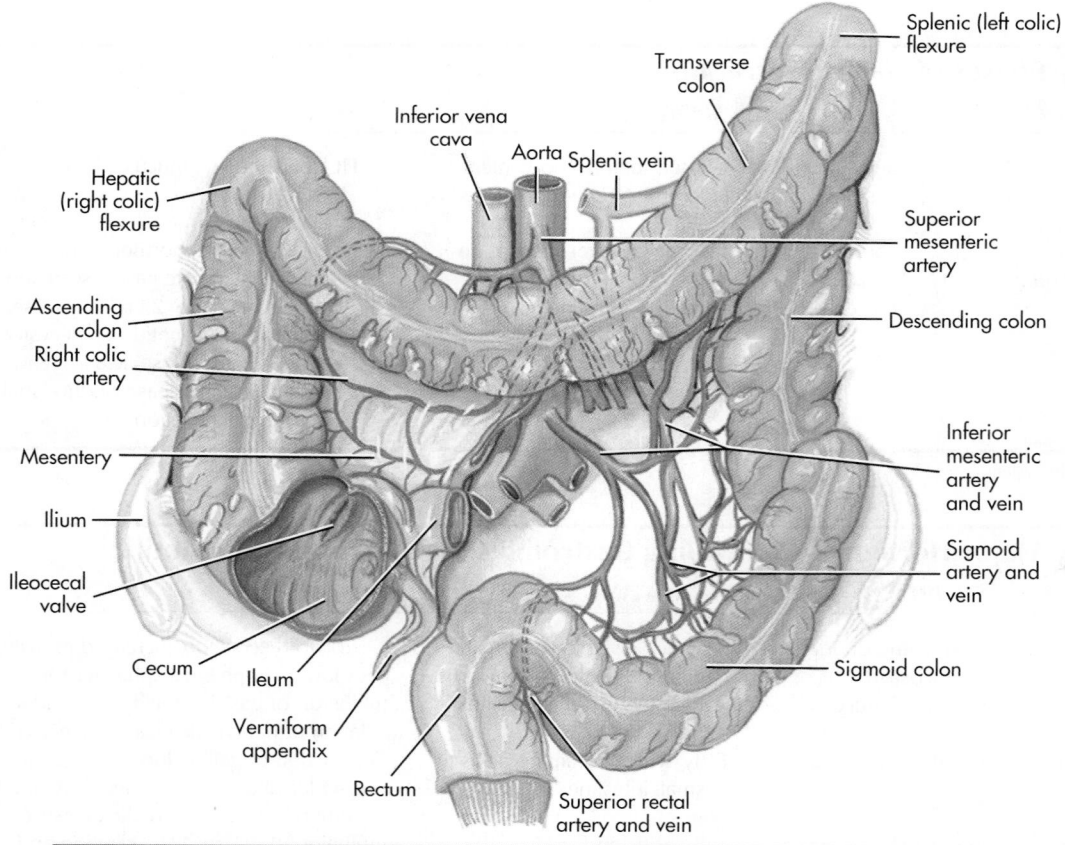

FIG. 38-3 Anatomic locations of the large intestine.

termed *haustral churning.* Propulsive (mass movements) peristalsis also occurs. When food enters the stomach and duodenum, the gastrocolic and duodenocolic reflexes are initiated, resulting in peristalsis in the colon. These reflexes are more active after the first daily meal and frequently result in bowel evacuation.

Defecation is a reflex action involving voluntary and involuntary control. Feces in the rectum stimulate sensory nerve endings that produce the desire to defecate. The reflex center for defecation is in the sacral portion of the spinal cord (parasympathetic nerve fibers). These fibers produce contraction of the rectum and relaxation of the internal anal sphincter. Defecation is controlled voluntarily by relaxing the external anal sphincter when the desire to defecate is felt. An acceptable environment for defecation is usually necessary or the urge to defecate will be ignored. If defecation is suppressed over long periods, problems can occur, such as constipation or stool impaction.

Defecation can be facilitated by the **Valsalva maneuver.** This maneuver involves contraction of the chest muscles on a closed glottis with simultaneous contraction of the abdominal muscles. These actions result in increased intraabdominal pressure. The Valsalva maneuver may be contraindicated in the patient with a head injury, eye surgery, cardiac problems, hemorrhoids, abdominal surgery, or liver cirrhosis with portal hypertension.

Constipation is common in the older adult and is due to many factors, including slower peristalsis, inactivity, decreased dietary fiber, decreased fluids, depression, constipating medications, and laxative abuse.[1] (Constipation is discussed in Chapter 41.)

Liver, Biliary Tract, and Pancreas

Liver. The liver is the largest internal organ in the body, weighing approximately 3 lb (1.37 kg) in the adult. It lies in the right hypochondriac and epigastric regions (see Fig. 38-7 later in chapter). Most of the liver is enclosed in peritoneum. It has a fibrous capsule that divides it into right and left lobes (Fig. 38-4).

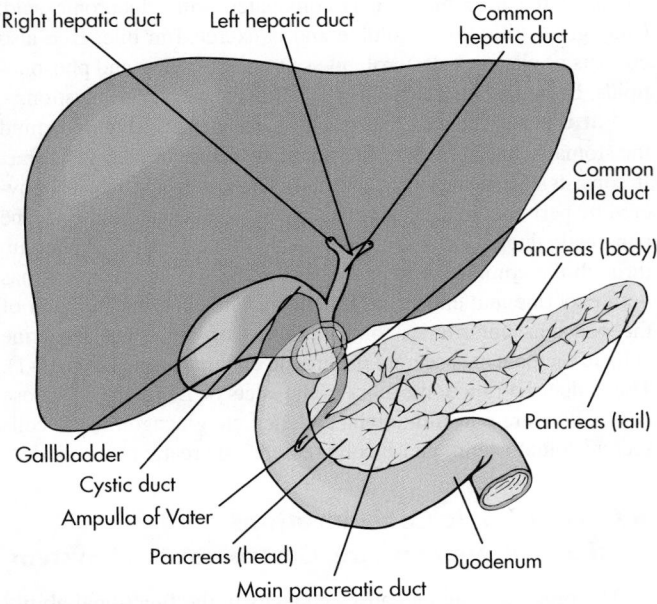

FIG. 38-4 Gross structure of the liver, gallbladder, and pancreas and the duct system.

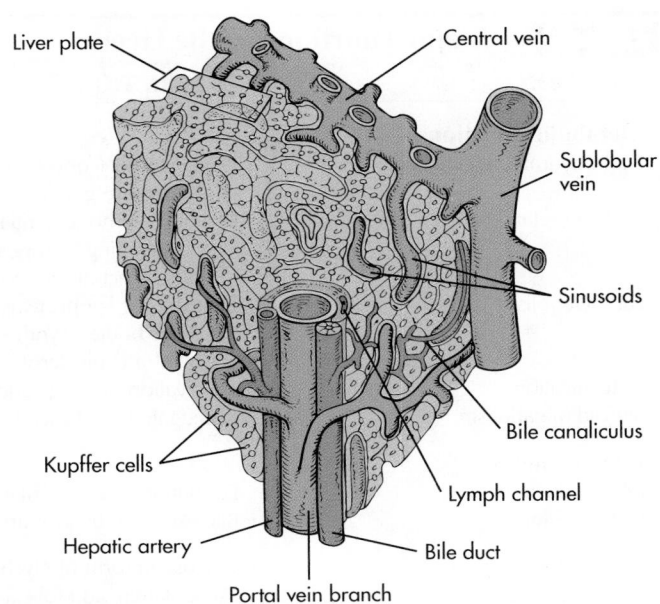

FIG. 38-5 Microscopic structure of liver lobule.

The functional units of the liver are lobules (Fig. 38-5). The lobule consists of rows of hepatic cells (**hepatocytes**) arranged around a central vein. The capillaries (sinusoids) are located between the rows of hepatocytes and are lined with **Kupffer cells,** which carry out phagocytic activity (removal of bacteria and toxins from the blood). Interlobular bile ducts form from bile capillaries (canaliculi). The hepatic cells secrete bile into the canaliculi.

The nerve supply to the liver is from the left vagus and sympathetic celiac plexus. About one third of the blood supply comes from the hepatic artery (branch of the celiac artery), and two thirds come from the portal vein.

The portal circulatory system (enterohepatic) brings blood to the liver from the stomach, intestines, spleen, and pancreas. This blood enters the liver through the portal vein. The portal vein carries absorbed products of digestion directly to the liver. In the liver the portal vein branches and comes in contact with each lobule. The blood in the sinusoids is a mixture of arterial and venous blood.

The liver is essential for life. It functions in the manufacture, storage, transformation, and excretion of a number of substances involved in metabolism. The functions of the liver are numerous but can be classified into four main areas, as identified in Table 38-4.

Biliary Tract. The biliary tract consists of the gallbladder and the duct system. The gallbladder is a pear-shaped sac located below the liver. The function of the gallbladder is to concentrate and store bile. It can hold approximately 45 ml of bile.

Bile is produced by the hepatic cells and secreted into the biliary canaliculi of the lobules. Bile then drains into the interlobular bile ducts, which unite into the two main left and right hepatic ducts. The hepatic ducts merge with the cystic duct from the gallbladder to form the common bile duct (see Fig. 38-4). Most bile is stored and concentrated in the gallbladder. It is then released into the cystic duct and moves down the common bile duct to enter the duodenum at the ampulla of Vater. In the intestines, most of the bilirubin is reduced to stercobilinogen and urobilinogen by bacterial action. Stercobilinogen accounts for the brown color of stool. A small amount of conjugated bilirubin is reabsorbed by the blood.

TABLE 38-4 **Major Functions of the Liver**

FUNCTION	DESCRIPTION
Metabolic Functions	
Carbohydrate metabolism	Glycogenesis (conversion of glucose to glycogen), glycogenolysis (process of breaking down glycogen to glucose), gluconeogenesis (formation of glucose from amino acids and fatty acids)
Protein metabolism	Synthesis of nonessential amino acids, synthesis of plasma proteins (except γ-globulin), synthesis of clotting factors, urea formation from NH_3 (NH_3 formed from deamination of amino acids by action of bacteria on proteins in colon)
Fat metabolism	Synthesis of lipoproteins, breakdown of triglycerides into fatty acids and glycerol, formation of ketone bodies, synthesis of fatty acids from amino acids and glucose, synthesis and breakdown of cholesterol
Detoxification	Inactivation of drugs and harmful substances and excretion of their breakdown products
Steroid metabolism	Conjugation and excretion of gonadal and adrenal steroid hormones
Bile Synthesis	
Bile production	Formation of bile, containing bile salts, bile pigments (mainly bilirubin), and cholesterol
Bile excretion	Bile excretion by liver about 1 L/day
Storage	Glucose in form of glycogen; vitamins, including fat soluble (A, D, E, K) and water soluble (B_1, B_2, cobalamin, and folic acid); fatty acids; minerals (iron and copper); amino acids in form of albumin and β-globulins
Mononuclear Phagocyte System	
Kupffer cells	Breakdown of old RBCs, WBCs, bacteria, and other particles; breakdown of hemoglobin from old RBCs to bilirubin and biliverdin

RBC, Red blood cell; *WBC,* white blood cell.

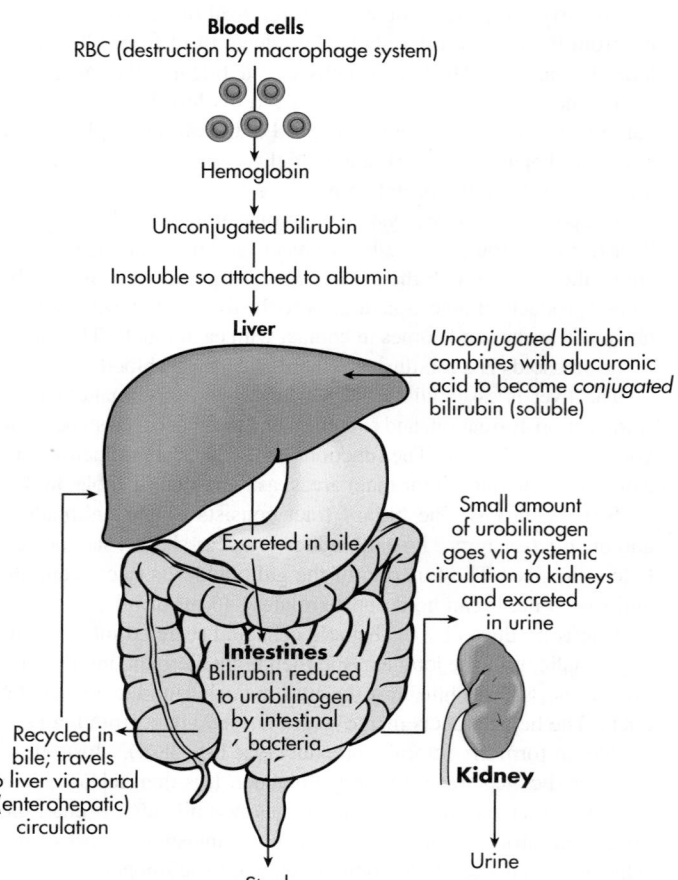

FIG. 38-6 Bilirubin metabolism and conjugation.

Some urobilinogen is reabsorbed by the blood and returned to the liver through the portal circulation (enterohepatic) and excreted in the bile. An insignificant amount of urobilinogen is excreted in the urine.[2] The sphincter of Oddi keeps the ampulla closed except when stimulated by the presence of food in the GI tract.

Bilirubin metabolism. Bilirubin, a pigment derived from the breakdown of hemoglobin, is constantly produced (Fig. 38-6). Because it is insoluble in water, it is bound to albumin for its transport to the liver. This form of bilirubin is referred to as unconjugated. In the liver bilirubin is conjugated with glucuronic acid. Conjugated bilirubin is soluble and is excreted in bile. Bile also consists of water, cholesterol, bile salts, electrolytes, and phospholipids. Bile salts are needed for fat emulsification and digestion.

Pancreas. The pancreas is a long, slender gland lying behind the stomach and in front of the first and second lumbar vertebrae. It consists of a head, body, and tail. The anterior surface is covered by peritoneum. The pancreas contains lobes and lobules. The pancreatic duct extends along the gland and enters the duodenum through the common bile duct (see Fig. 38-4). The pancreas has both exocrine and endocrine functions. The exocrine function of the pancreas contributes to the process of digestion. Exocrine cells in the pancreas secrete pancreatic enzymes (see Table 38-1). The endocrine function occurs in the islets of Langerhans, whose beta cells secrete insulin; alpha cells secrete glucagon; delta cells secrete somatostatin; and F cells secrete pancreatic polypeptide.

■ Gerontologic Considerations: Effects of Aging on the Gastrointestinal System

The process of aging causes changes in the functional ability of the GI system, although less than in other organ systems (Table 38-5). Tooth enamel and dentin wear down and make the

TABLE 38-5	*Gerontologic* Differences in Assessment **Gastrointestinal System**

CHANGES	DIFFERENCES IN ASSESSMENT FINDINGS
Mouth Loss of teeth Decreased taste buds, decreased sense of smell Decreased volume of saliva Atrophy of gingival tissue	Presence of dentures, difficulty chewing Diminished sense of taste (especially salty and sweet) Dry oral mucosa Poor-fitting dentures
Esophagus Decreased tone and motility	Complaints of pyrosis (heartburn), dysphagia, eructation
Abdominal Wall Thinner and less taut Decrease in number and sensitivity of sensory receptors	More visible peristalsis, easier palpation of organs Less sensitivity to surface pain
Stomach Decreased acid secretion, atrophy of gastric mucosa	Food intolerances, signs of anemia as result of cobalamin mal- absorption
Small Intestines Decreased secretion of most digestive enzymes, decreased motility	Complaints of indigestion
Liver Decreased size and lowered in position	Easier palpation
Large Intestine, Anus, Rectum Decreased anal sphincter tone and nerve supply to rectal area Decreased muscular tone, decreased motility Increase in transit time	Fecal incontinence Flatulence, abdominal distention, relaxed perineal musculature Constipation, fecal impaction

teeth susceptible to cavities. Periodontal disease can lead to the loss of teeth. Taste buds decrease, the sense of smell diminishes, and salivary secretions diminish, all of which can lead to a decrease in appetite and make eating less pleasurable.

Age-related changes in the esophagus include delayed emptying resulting from smooth muscle weakness and an incompetent lower esophageal sphincter.[1] Motility of the GI system decreases with age, but secretion and absorption are affected to a lesser extent. The elderly patient often experiences a decrease in HCl secretion (hypochlorhydria), delayed gastric emptying, and constipation. With chronic atrophic gastritis there is a decrease in the number of parietal cells and subsequent reduction in the amount of acid and intrinsic factor secreted.

The liver size decreases after 50 years of age, but results of liver function tests remain within normal ranges. Enzyme changes in the liver that are age-related decrease the ability of the liver to metabolize drugs and hormones. The size of the pancreas is unaffected by aging but does undergo structural changes such as fibrosis, fatty acid deposits, and atrophy. Aging does not cause changes in the structure and function of the gallbladder and bile ducts. However, with aging there is an increase in the incidence of gallstones.[3]

The economic inability to purchase food supplies may affect nutritional intake, especially in the older adult. Economic constraints may also reduce the number of fresh fruits and vegetables consumed and thus the amount of fiber. A reduction in dietary fiber, along with reduced fluid intake and decreased physical activity, contributes to constipation. Age-related changes in the GI system and differences in assessment findings are presented in Table 38-5.

ASSESSMENT OF THE GASTROINTESTINAL SYSTEM

Subjective Data

Important Health Information

Past health history. Information should be gathered from the patient about the history or existence of the following problems related to GI functioning: abdominal pain, nausea and vomiting, diarrhea, constipation, abdominal distention, jaundice, anemia, heartburn, dyspepsia, changes in appetite, hematemesis, food intolerance or allergies, indigestion, excessive gas, bloating, melena, hemorrhoids, or rectal bleeding. In addition, the patient should be asked about the history or existence of diseases such as gastritis, hepatitis, colitis, gallbladder disease, peptic ulcer, cancer, or hernias, especially hiatal hernias.

The patient should be questioned about weight history. Any unexplained or unplanned weight loss or weight gain within the past 12 months should be explored in detail. A history of chronic dieting and repeated weight loss and gain should be documented.

Medications. The health history should include an assessment of the patient's past and current use of medications. This is an important part of the assessment, particularly in relation to liver problems. It should include over-the-counter drugs, prescription drugs, and herbal products and nutritional supplements (see Complementary and Alternative Therapies box in Chapter 3 on p. 34). Many

TABLE 38-6	Potentially Hepatotoxic Chemicals and Drugs

acetaminophen
alcohol
anabolic steroids
arsenic
carbon tetrachloride
chloroform
gold compounds
halothane
isoniazid (INH)
6-mercaptopurine (6-MP)
mercury
methotrexate
phosphorus
propylthiouracil
sulfonamides
thiazide diuretics

TABLE 38-7	Surgeries of the Gastrointestinal System

SURGICAL PROCEDURE	DESCRIPTION
Antrectomy	Removal of antrum portion of stomach
Cecostomy	Opening into cecum
Cholecystectomy	Removal of gallbladder
Cholecystostomy	Opening into gallbladder
Choledochojejunostomy	Opening between common bile duct and jejunum
Choledocholithotomy	Opening into common bile duct for removal of stones
Colostomy	Opening into colon
Esophagoenterostomy	Removal of portion of esophagus with segment of colon attached to remaining portion
Esophagogastrostomy	Removal of esophagus and anastomosis of remaining portion to stomach
Gastrectomy	Removal of stomach
Gastrostomy	Opening into stomach
Glossectomy	Removal of tongue
Hemiglossectomy	Removal of half of tongue
Ileostomy	Opening into ileum
Mandibulectomy	Removal of mandible
Pyloroplasty	Enlargement and repair of pyloric sphincter area
Vagotomy	Resection of branch of vagus nerve

chemicals and drugs are potentially hepatotoxic (Table 38-6). Antibiotics can cause changes in the normal bacterial composition in the GI tract, resulting in diarrhea. The nurse should ask the patient if laxatives or antacids are taken, including the kind and frequency.

The nurse should assess the patient's use of over-the-counter pain medications. Chronic high doses of acetaminophen and nonsteroidal antiinflammatory drugs (NSAIDs) can be hepatotoxic. Chronic NSAID use can also predispose a person to upper GI bleeding.

The use of prescription or over-the-counter appetite suppressants should be noted. The names of drugs and frequency and duration of use are also important.

Surgery or other treatments. Information should be obtained about hospitalizations for any problems related to the GI system. Data should also be obtained related to any abdominal or rectal surgery, including the year, reason for surgery, postoperative course, and possible blood transfusions. Terms related to surgery of the GI system are presented in Table 38-7.

Functional Health Patterns. Key questions to ask a patient with a GI problem are presented in Table 38-8.

Health perception–health management pattern. The nurse should ask about the patient's health practices related to the GI system, such as maintenance of normal body weight, attention to proper dental care, maintenance of adequate nutrition, and effective elimination habits.

The patient should be asked about recent foreign travel with possible exposure to hepatitis, parasitic, or bacterial infestation. Past history of receiving hepatitis A and/or hepatitis B vaccination should be documented.

The patient should be assessed in relation to certain habits that directly affect GI functioning. The consumption of alcohol in large quantities has detrimental effects on the mucosa of the stomach and also increases the secretion of HCl and pepsinogen. Chronic alcohol exposure causes fatty infiltration of the liver and can cause damage leading to cirrhosis. The nurse should obtain a history of cigarette smoking. Nicotine is irritating to the entire GI tract mucosa. Cigarette smoking is related to various GI cancers (especially mouth and esophageal cancers), esophagitis, and ulcers. Smoking will also delay the healing of ulcers.

Nutritional-metabolic pattern. A thorough nutritional assessment is essential. A dietary history should be taken and compared with the food pyramid (see Fig. 39-1). The nurse should ask open-ended questions that will allow the patient to express beliefs and feelings about the diet. The nurse may need to ask the patient to do a 24-hour dietary recall to analyze the adequacy of the diet. The nurse should assist the patient in recalling the preceding day's food intake, including early morning and nighttime intake. The nurse should find out about the intake of snacks, liquids, and vitamin supplements. The nurse must then evaluate the diet in terms of the recommended groups and servings on the food pyramid and try to determine whether the 24-hour recall is typical of the patient's usual eating habits. If weekend eating habits vary greatly, the nurse should obtain a separate weekend diet history and assess the patient's intake for both quality and quantity of food.

The nurse should ask the patient about the use of sugar and salt substitutes, use of caffeine, and amount of fluid and fiber intake. The patient should be questioned about any changes in appetite, food tolerance, and weight. Anorexia and weight loss may indicate the presence of cancer. The nurse should ask the patient about allergies to any food and determine what GI symptoms such allergic responses cause. The patient should be asked about dietary intolerances including lactose and gluten.

Elimination pattern. A detailed account of the patient's bowel elimination pattern should be elicited. The frequency, time of day, and usual consistency of stool should be noted. The use

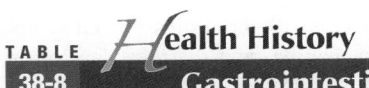

TABLE
38-8   Health History
Gastrointestinal System

Health Perception–Health Management Pattern
- Describe any measures used to treat GI symptoms such as diarrhea or vomiting.
- Do you smoke?* Do you drink alcohol?*
- Are you exposed to any chemicals on a regular basis?* Have you been exposed in the past?*
- Have you recently traveled outside the United States?*

Nutritional–Metabolic Pattern
- Describe your usual daily food and fluid intake.
- Do you take any supplemental vitamins or minerals?*
- Have you experienced any changes in appetite or food tolerance?*
- Has there been a weight change in the past?*
- Are you allergic to any foods?*

Elimination Pattern
- Describe the frequency and time of day you have bowel movements. What is the consistency of the bowel movement?
- Do you use laxatives or enemas?* If so, how often?
- Have there been any recent changes in your bowel pattern?*
- Describe any skin problems caused by GI problems.
- Do you need any assistive equipment, such as ostomy equipment?

Activity–Exercise Pattern
- Do you have limitations in mobility that make it difficult for you to procure and prepare food?*
- Are you able to feed yourself?
- Do you have any GI symptoms, such as vomiting or diarrhea, that affect your activity?*
- Do you have any difficulty accessing a toilet when needed?*
- Is a safe and comfortable environment for elimination available?

Sleep–Rest Pattern
- Do you experience any difficulty sleeping because of a GI problem?*
- Are you awakened by symptoms such as gas or esophageal burning?*

Cognitive–Perceptual Pattern
- Have you experienced any change in taste or smell that has affected your appetite?*
- Do you have any heat or cold sensitivity that affects eating?*
- Does pain interfere with food preparation, appetite, or chewing?*
- Do pain medications cause constipation or appetite suppression?*

Self-Perception–Self-Concept Pattern
- Describe any changes in your weight that have affected how you feel about yourself.
- Have you had any changes in normal elimination that have affected how you feel about yourself?*
- Have any symptoms of GI disease caused physical changes that are a problem for you?*

Role-Relationship Pattern
- Describe the impact of any GI problem on your usual roles and relationships.
- Have any changes in elimination affected your relationships?*
- Do you live alone? Describe how your family or others assist you with your GI problems.

Sexuality–Reproductive Pattern
- Describe the effect of your GI problem on your sexual activity.

Coping–Stress Tolerance Pattern
- Do you experience GI symptoms in response to stressful or emotional situations?
- Describe how you deal with any GI symptoms that result.

Value-Belief Pattern
- Describe any culturally specific health beliefs regarding food and food preparation that may influence the treatment of this GI problem.

*If yes, describe.

of laxatives and enemas, including type, frequency, and results, should be documented. Any recent change in bowel patterns should be investigated.

The amount and type of fluid and fiber intake should be determined because they have an important effect on the frequency and consistency of stools. Inadequate intake of fiber can be associated with constipation. Analysis of fluid intake and output could indicate the presence of a urinary problem and the possibility of fluid retention.

Food allergies can cause lesions, pruritus, and edema. Diarrhea can result in redness, irritation, and pain in the perianal area. External drainage systems such as an ileostomy or ileal conduit can cause local skin irritation. The possible association between a skin problem and a GI problem should be investigated.

Activity-exercise pattern. The patient's ambulatory status should be assessed to determine if the patient is capable of securing and preparing food. If the patient is unable to do these tasks, it should be determined if family or an outside agency is meeting this need. Any limitation in the patient's ability to feed self independently should be noted. Any difficulty accessing a safe environment of elimination should be assessed. Use of and access to elimination supplies should be assessed, such as a commode or ostomy supplies. Activity and exercise may affect GI motility. Immobility is a risk factor for constipation.

Sleep-rest pattern. Many food-related events can interrupt and interfere with the quality of sleep. Nausea, vomiting, diarrhea, indigestion, bloating, and hunger can produce sleep problems and should be investigated. The patient should be asked if GI symptoms affect sleep or rest. For example, a patient with a hiatal hernia may be awakened because of burning pain; sleep may be improved by elevating the head of the bed for this patient.

A patient often has a bedtime ritual that involves the use of a particular food or beverage. Milk is known to induce sleep through the effect of the serotonin precursor L-tryptophan. Herbal teas and melatonin are often sleep inducing. Individual routines should be noted and complied with whenever possible to avoid sleeplessness. Hunger can prevent sleep and should be relieved by a light, easily digested snack unless contraindicated.

Cognitive-perceptual pattern. Decreases in sensory adequacy can result in problems related to the acquisition, preparation, and ingestion of food. Changes in taste or smell can affect appetite and eating pleasure. Vertigo can make shopping and standing at a stove difficult and dangerous. Heat or cold sensitivity could make certain foods painful to eat. Problems in expressive communication could make it difficult and frustrating for the patient to make personal desires and preferences known. The nurse should assess the patient in this pattern to judge the effect of deficiencies on adequate nutritional intake. If the patient has been diagnosed as having a GI disorder, the nurse should ask questions to determine the patient's understanding of the illness and its treatment.

Pain is another area that requires careful assessment related to its effect on the GI system and nutrition. Relevant behaviors associated with chronic pain include avoidance of activity, fatigue, and disruption of eating patterns. The possible effects of narcotic pain medication related to constipation, nausea, sedation, and appetite suppression should be assessed.

Self-perception–self-concept pattern. Many GI and nutritional problems can have serious effects on the patient's self-perception. Overweight and underweight persons often have problems related to self-esteem and body image. Repeated attempts to achieve a personally acceptable weight can be discouraging and depressing for the patient. The manner in which a person recounts a weight history can alert the nurse to potential problems in this area.

Another potentially problematic area is the need for external devices to manage elimination, such as a colostomy or an ileostomy. The patient's willingness to engage in self-care and to discuss this situation should provide the nurse with valuable information related to body image and self-esteem.

The altered physical changes often associated with advanced liver disease can be problematic for the patient. Jaundice and ascites cause significant changes in external appearance. The patient's attitude toward these changes should be assessed.

Role-relationship pattern. Problems related to the GI system such as cirrhosis, alcoholism, hepatitis, ostomies, obesity, and carcinoma can have a major impact on the patient's ability to maintain usual roles and relationships. A chronic illness may necessitate leaving a job or reducing the number of hours worked. Changes in body image and self-esteem can affect relationships. The availability of and satisfaction with support should be determined. It is important that the nurse be aware of these possible consequences and assess for their presence.

Sexuality-reproductive pattern. Changes related to sexuality and reproductive status can result from problems of the GI system. For example, obesity, jaundice, anorexia, and ascites could decrease the acceptance of a potential sexual partner. The presence of an ostomy could affect the patient's confidence related to sexual activity. Chronic alcoholism could discourage a meaningful relationship that could develop into a sexual relationship. Sensitive questioning by the nurse could determine the presence of potential problems.

Anorexia can affect the reproductive status of a female patient. Alcoholism can affect the reproductive status of both men and women. A poor nutritional intake before and during pregnancy can result in a low-birth-weight infant.

Coping–stress tolerance pattern. The nurse should try to determine what is a stressor for the patient and what coping mechanisms the patient uses to function with these stressors. GI symptoms such as epigastric pain, nausea, and diarrhea develop in many people in response to stressful or emotional situations. Some GI problems such as peptic ulcers and irritable bowel syndrome are aggravated by stress.

Value-belief pattern. The patient's spiritual and cultural beliefs regarding food and food preparation should be assessed. Whenever possible, these preferences should be respected by the health care provider. In addition, it should be determined if any value or belief could interfere with planned interventions. For example, if the patient with anemia is a vegetarian, the prescription of a high-meat diet would be met with patient resistance. Thoughtful assessment and consideration of the patient's beliefs and values will usually increase patient compliance and satisfaction.

Objective Data

In addition to collecting subjective data related to a diet history and functional health patterns, objective data related to a nutritional assessment should be collected. Anthropometric measurements (height, weight, skinfold thickness) and blood studies such as serum protein, albumin, and hemoglobin are examples of important objective data related to the GI system. A physical examination also adds valuable information.

Physical Examination

Mouth

Inspection. The lips should be inspected for symmetry, color, and size. They should be observed for abnormalities such as pallor or cyanosis, cracking, ulcers, or fissures. The dorsum (top) of the tongue should have a thin white coating; the undersurface should be smooth. The nurse should observe for any lesions. Using a tongue blade, the nurse should inspect the buccal mucosa and note the color, any areas of pigmentation, and any lesions. Dark-skinned individuals normally have patchy areas of pigmentation. In assessing the teeth and gums, the nurse should look for caries; loose teeth; abnormal shape and position of teeth; and swelling, bleeding, discoloration, or inflammation of the gingivae. Any distinctive breath odor should be noted.

The pharynx is inspected by tilting the patient's head back and depressing the tongue with a tongue blade. The tonsils, uvula, soft palate, and anterior and posterior pillars should be observed. The nurse should have the patient say "ah." The uvula and soft palate should rise and remain in the midline.

Palpation. The nurse should palpate any suspicious areas in the mouth. Ulcers, nodules, indurations, and areas of tenderness should be palpated.

The mouth of the older adult requires careful assessment. Particular attention should be given to dentures (e.g., fit, condition), ability to swallow, the tongue, and lesions. The patient who has dentures must remove the dentures during an oral examination to allow for good visualization and palpation of the area.

Abdomen. Two systems are used to anatomically describe the surface of the abdomen. One system divides the abdomen into four quadrants by a perpendicular line from the sternum to the pubic bone and a horizontal line across the abdomen at the umbilicus (Fig. 38-7, *A*, and Table 38-9). The other system divides the abdomen into nine regions (Fig. 38-7, *B*), but only the epigastric, umbilical, and suprapubic or hypogastric regions are commonly addressed.

For the abdominal examination, good lighting should shine across the abdomen. The patient should be in the supine position

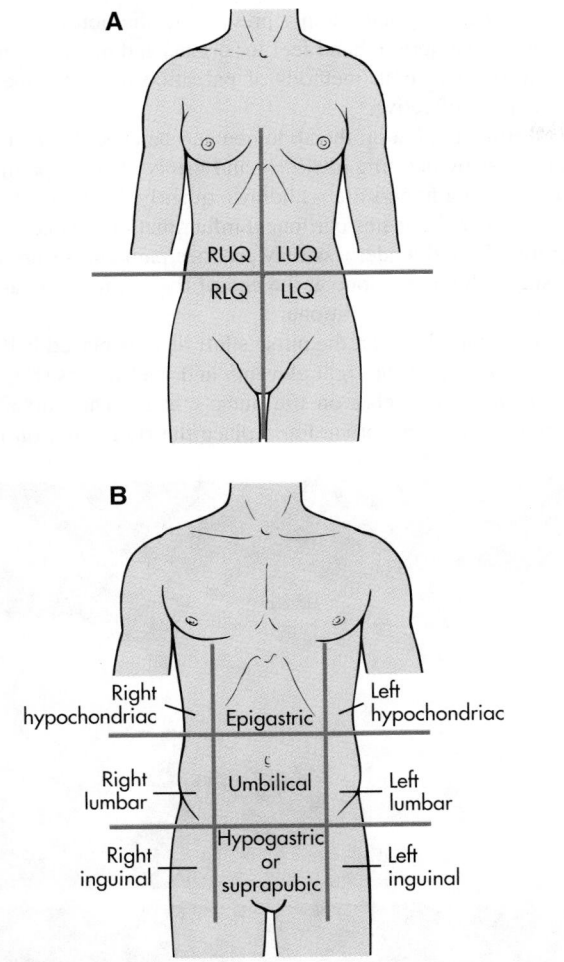

FIG. 38-7   A, Abdominal quadrants. B, Abdominal regions.

rounded [convex], concave, protuberant, distention), observable masses (hernias or other masses), and movement (pulsations and peristalsis). A normal aortic pulsation may be seen in the epigastric area. The nurse should look across the abdomen tangentially (across the abdomen in a line) for peristalsis. Peristalsis is not normally visible in an adult but may be visible in a thin person.

Auscultation. During examination of the abdomen, auscultation is done before percussion and palpation because these latter procedures may alter the bowel sounds. Auscultation of the abdomen includes listening for increased or decreased bowel sounds and vascular sounds. The diaphragm of the stethoscope is used to auscultate bowel sounds because they are relatively high pitched. The bell of the stethoscope is used to detect lower-pitched sounds. Normal bowel sounds occur 5 to 35 times per minute and sound like high-pitched clicks or gurgles.[4] Before auscultation, warming the stethoscope in the hands helps prevent abdominal muscle contraction. The nurse should listen in the epigastrium and in all four quadrants. The nurse should listen for bowel sounds for 2 to 5 minutes. Bowel sounds cannot be described as absent until no sound is heard for 5 minutes (in each quadrant).[5] The frequency and intensity of bowel sounds will vary, depending on the phase of digestion. Normally they will sound relatively high pitched and gurgling. Loud gurgles indicate hyperperistalsis and are termed *borborygmi* (stomach growling). The bowel sounds will be more high pitched (rushes and tinkling) when the intestines are under tension, such as in intestinal obstruction. The nurse should listen for decreased or absent bowel sounds. Terms used to describe bowel sounds include *present, absent, increased, decreased, high pitched, tinkling, gurgling,* and *rushing.* Normally no aortic bruits should be heard. A bruit, best heard with the bell of the stethoscope, is a swishing or buzzing sound and indicates turbulent blood flow.

Percussion. The purpose of percussion of the abdomen is to determine the presence of fluid, distention, and masses. Sound waves vary according to the density of underlying tissues; the presence of air produces a higher-pitched, hollow sound termed *tympany*; the presence of fluid or masses produces a short, high-pitched sound with little resonance termed *dullness.* The nurse should lightly percuss all four quadrants of the abdomen and assess the distribution of tympany and dullness. Tympany is the predominant percussion sound of the abdomen.

To percuss the liver, the nurse should start below the umbilicus in the right midclavicular line and percuss lightly upward until dullness is heard, thus determining the lower border of liver dullness. After the lower border of the liver has been determined, the nurse should start at the nipple line in the right midclavicular

and as relaxed as possible. To help relax the abdominal muscles, the patient should slightly flex the knees and the head of the bed should be raised slightly. The patient should have an empty bladder. The examiner should use warm hands when doing the abdominal examination to avoid eliciting muscle guarding. The patient should be asked to breathe slowly through the mouth.

Inspection. The nurse should assess the abdomen for skin changes (color, texture, scars, striae, dilated veins, rashes, and lesions), umbilicus (location and contour), symmetry, contour (flat,

TABLE 38-9	Abdominal Structures in Regions of the Abdomen		
RIGHT UPPER QUADRANT	**LEFT UPPER QUADRANT**	**RIGHT LOWER QUADRANT**	**LEFT LOWER QUADRANT**
Liver and gallbladder	Left lobe of liver	Lower pole of right kidney	Lower pole of left kidney
Pylorus	Spleen	Cecum and appendix	Sigmoid flexure
Duodenum	Stomach	Portion of ascending colon	Portion of descending colon
Head of pancreas	Body of pancreas	Bladder (if distended)	Bladder (if distended)
Right adrenal gland	Left adrenal gland	Right ovary and salpinx	Left ovary and salpinx
Portion of right kidney	Portion of left kidney	Uterus (if enlarged)	Uterus (if enlarged)
Hepatic flexure of colon	Splenic flexure of colon	Right spermatic cord	Left spermatic cord
Portion of ascending and transverse colon	Portion of transverse and descending colon	Right ureter	Left ureter

line and percuss downward between ribs to the area of dullness indicating the upper border of the liver. The height or vertical space between the two areas should be measured to determine the size of the liver. The normal range of liver height in the right midclavicular line is 2.4 to 5 inches (6 to 12 cm).

Palpation. *Light palpation* is used to detect tenderness or cutaneous hypersensitivity, muscular resistance, masses, and swelling. It also helps the patient to relax for deeper palpation. The nurse should keep fingers together and press gently with the pads of the fingertips, depressing the abdominal wall about 0.4 inch (1 cm). Smooth movements should be used and all quadrants palpated (Fig. 38-8, *A*).

Deep palpation is used to delineate abdominal organs and masses (Fig. 38-8, *B*). The palmar surfaces of the fingers should be used to press more deeply. Again, all quadrants should be palpated. When palpating masses, the nurse should note the location, size, shape, and presence of tenderness. The patient's facial expression should be observed during these maneuvers because it will provide nonverbal cues of discomfort or pain.

An alternative method for deep abdominal palpation is the two-hand method. One hand is placed on top of the other. The fingers of the top hand apply pressure to the bottom hand. The fingers of the bottom hand feel for organs and masses. The nurse should practice both methods of palpation to determine which one is most effective.[6]

A problem area on the abdomen can be checked for rebound tenderness by pressing in slowly and firmly over the painful site. The palpating fingers are withdrawn quickly. Pain on withdrawal of the fingers indicates peritoneal inflammation. Because assessing for rebound tenderness may produce pain and severe muscle spasm, it should be done at the end of the examination and only by an experienced practitioner.

To palpate the liver, the nurse's left hand is placed behind the patient to support the right eleventh and twelfth ribs (Fig. 38-9). The patient may relax on the nurse's hand. The nurse should press the left hand forward and place the right hand on the pa-

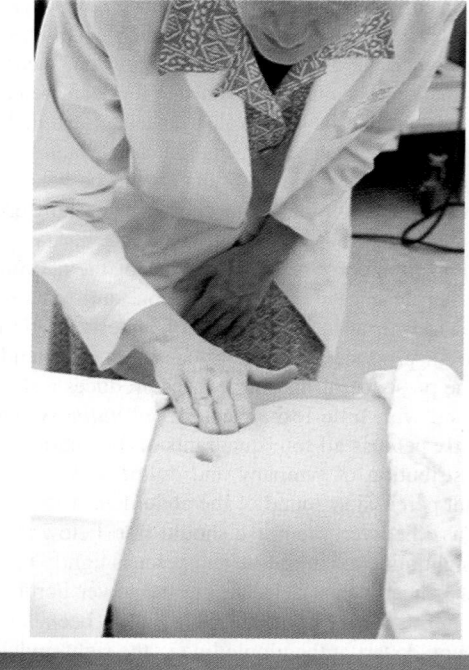

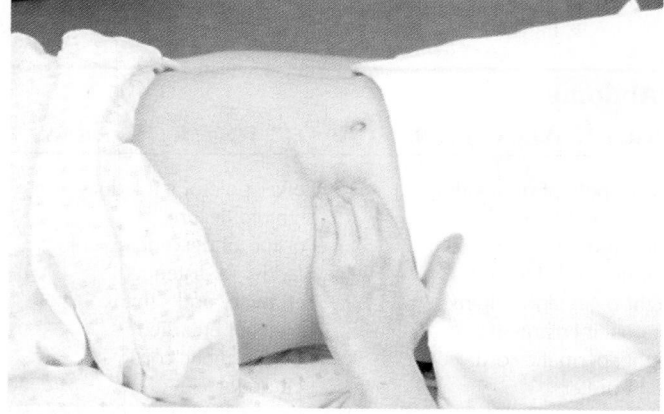

FIG. 38-8 **A,** Technique for light palpation of the abdomen. **B,** Technique for deep palpation.

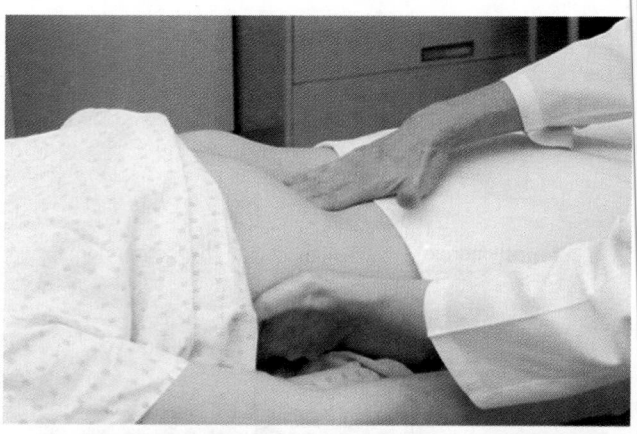

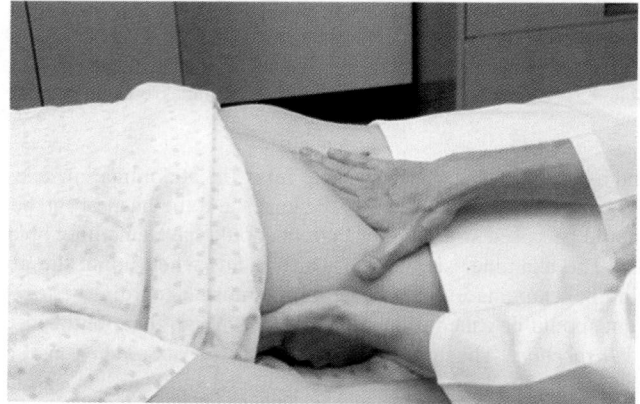

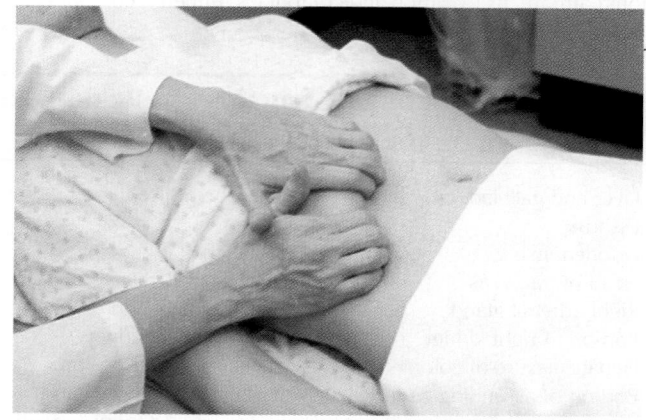

FIG. 38-9 **A,** Technique for liver palpation. **B,** Alternative technique. **C,** Palpation of liver with fingers hooked over the costal region.

tient's right abdomen lateral to the rectus muscle. The fingertips should be below the lower border of liver dullness and pointed toward the right costal margin. The nurse should gently press in and up. The patient should take a deep breath with the abdomen so that the liver drops and is in a better position to be palpated. The nurse should try to feel the liver edge as it comes down to the fingertips. During inspiration the liver edge should feel firm, sharp, and smooth. The surface and contour and any tenderness should be described.

To palpate the spleen, the nurse moves to the left side of the patient. The nurse places the right hand under the patient and supports and presses the patient's left lower rib cage forward. The left hand is placed below the left costal margin and presses it in toward the spleen. The nurse should ask the patient to breathe deeply. The tip or edge of an enlarged spleen will be felt by the fingertips. The spleen is normally not palpable. If it is palpable, the nurse should not continue because manual compression of an enlarged spleen may cause it to rupture.

The standard approach for examining the abdomen can be used on the older adult.[7] Palpation is important because it may reveal a tumor. The abdomen may be thinner and more lax unless the patient is obese. If the patient has chronic obstructive pulmonary disease, large lungs, or a low diaphragm, the liver may be palpated 0.4 to 0.8 inch (1 to 2 cm) below the right costal margin.

Rectum and anus. The perianal and anal area should be inspected for color, texture, lumps, rashes, scars, erythema, fissures, and external hemorrhoids. Any lumps or unusual areas should be palpated with a gloved hand.

For the digital examination of the rectum the gloved, lubricated index finger is placed against the anus while the patient strains (Valsalva maneuver). Then, as the sphincter relaxes, the finger is inserted. The finger is pointed toward the umbilicus. The nurse should try to get the patient to relax. The finger is inserted into the rectum as far as possible, and all surfaces are palpated. Nodules, tenderness, or any irregularities should be assessed. A sample of stool can be removed with the gloved finger and should be checked for occult blood.

Recording of the normal physical assessment of the GI system is found in Table 38-10. Gerontologic differences in the GI system and differences in assessment findings are described in Table 38-5. Common assessment abnormalities are presented in Table 38-11.

DIAGNOSTIC STUDIES OF THE GASTROINTESTINAL SYSTEM

Diagnostic studies provide important information to the nurse in monitoring the patient's condition and planning appropriate interventions. These studies are considered to be objective data. Table 38-12 presents diagnostic studies common to the GI system. For most diagnostic studies, nurses should make sure a signed consent form for the procedure has been completed and is in the medical record. It is the responsibility of the health care provider doing the procedure to explain the procedure and obtain the written consent. However, nurses play an important role in educating patients regarding the procedures. When preparing the patient it is important to ask about any known allergies to drugs or contrast medium.

Many of the diagnostic procedures of the GI system require measures to cleanse the GI tract, as well as the ingestion or injection of a contrast medium or a radiopaque tracer. Often the pa-

| TABLE 38-10 | Normal Physical Assessment of the Gastrointestinal System |

Mouth
Moist and pink lips
Pink and moist buccal mucosa and gingivae without plaques or lesions
Teeth in good repair
Protrusion of tongue in midline without deviation or fasciculations
Pink uvula in midline, soft palate, tonsils, and posterior pharynx
Swallows smoothly without coughing or gagging

Abdomen
Flat without masses or scars
No abdominal tenderness
No bruises
Bowel sounds in all quadrants
Nonpalpable liver and spleen
Liver 10 cm in right midclavicular line
Generalized tympany

Anus
Absence of lesions, fissures, and hemorrhoids
Good sphincter tone
Rectal walls smooth/soft
No masses
Stool soft, brown, and heme negative

tient has a series of GI diagnostic tests done. The nurse must monitor the patient closely to ensure adequate hydration and nutrition during the testing period. Some diagnostic studies of the GI system are especially difficult and uncomfortable for the older adult. It may be necessary to individualize and make adjustments. It is particularly important to prevent diarrhea from bowel-cleansing procedures and dehydration from prolonged fluid restriction.[8]

Many radiologic studies use either barium sulfate or meglumine diatrizoate (Gastrografin) as a contrast medium. Barium sulfate is more effective for visualizing mucosal detail. Gastrografin is water soluble and rapidly absorbed, so it is preferred when a perforation is suspected. Spillage of barium into the peritoneal cavity can result in peritonitis. Under other circumstances in a person at high risk for aspiration, water-soluble media are contraindicated and barium is preferred.

Radiologic Studies

Upper Gastrointestinal Series. A barium swallow allows examination of the esophagus after swallowing a thick barium solution. An upper GI series with small bowel follow-through provides visualization of the esophagus, stomach, and small intestine by means of fluoroscopy and x-ray examination. The procedure consists of the patient swallowing contrast medium (a thick barium solution) and then assuming different positions on the x-ray table. The movement of the contrast medium is observed with fluoroscopy, and several x-rays are taken (see Table 38-12). A barium swallow is used to identify esophageal, stomach, and small intestine disorders such as esophageal strictures, varices, polyps, tumors, hiatal hernia, foreign bodies, and peptic ulcers in the stomach or duodenum (Fig. 38-10).

Text continued on p. 965

TABLE
38-11

Common Assessment Abnormalities
Gastrointestinal System

FINDING	DESCRIPTION	POSSIBLE ETIOLOGY AND SIGNIFICANCE
Mouth		
Ulcer, plaque on lips or in mouth	Sore or lesion	Carcinoma, viral infections
Cheilosis	Softening, fissuring, and cracking of lips at angles of mouth	Riboflavin deficiency
Cheilitis	Inflammation of lips (usually lower) with fissuring, scaling, crusting	Often unknown
Geographic tongue	Scattered red, smooth (loss of papillae) areas on dorsum of tongue	Unknown
Smooth tongue	Red, slick appearance	Cobalamin deficiency
Leukoplakia	Thickened white patches	Premalignant lesion
Pyorrhea	Recessed gums, purulent pockets	Periodontitis
Herpes simplex	Benign vesicular lesion	Herpesvirus
Candidiasis	White, curdlike lesions surrounded by erythematous mucosa	*Candida albicans*
Glossitis	Reddened, ulcerated, swollen tongue	Exposure to streptococci, irritation, injury, vitamin B deficiencies, anemia
Acute marginal gingivitis	Friable, edematous, painful, bleeding gingivae	Irritation from ill-fitting dentures, calcium deposits on teeth, food impaction
Esophagus and Stomach		
Dysphagia	Difficulty in swallowing, sensation of food sticking in esophagus	Esophageal problems, cancer of esophagus
Hematemesis	Vomiting of blood	Esophageal varices, bleeding peptic ulcer
Pyrosis	Heartburn, burning in epigastric or substernal area	Hiatal hernia, esophagitis, incompetent lower esophageal sphincter
Dyspepsia	Burning or indigestion	Peptic ulcer, gallbladder disease
Odynophagia	Painful swallowing	Cancer of esophagus, esophagitis
Eructation	Belching	Gallbladder disease
Nausea and vomiting	Feeling of impending vomiting, expulsion of gastric contents through mouth	GI infections, common manifestation of many GI diseases; stress, fear, and pathologic conditions
Abdomen		
Distention	Excessive gas accumulation, enlarged abdomen; generalized tympany	Obstruction, paralytic ileus
Ascites	Accumulated fluid within abdominal cavity; eversion of umbilicus (usually)	Peritoneal inflammation, congestive heart failure, metastatic carcinoma, cirrhosis
Bruit	Humming or swishing sound heard through stethoscope over vessel	Partial arterial obstruction (narrowing of vessel), turbulent flow (aneurysm)
Hyperresonance	Loud, tinkling rushes	Intestinal obstruction
Borborygmi	Waves of loud, gurgling sounds	Hyperactive bowel as result of eating
Absent bowel sounds	No auscultation of bowel sounds	Peritonitis, paralytic ileus, obstruction
Absence of liver dullness	Tympany on percussion	Air from viscus (e.g., perforated ulcer)
Masses	Lump on palpation	Tumors, cysts
Rebound tenderness	Sudden pain when fingers withdrawn quickly	Peritoneal inflammation, appendicitis
Nodular liver	Enlarged, hard liver with irregular edge or surface	Cirrhosis, carcinoma
Hepatomegaly	Enlargement of liver, liver edge >1-2 cm below costal margin	Metastatic carcinoma, hepatitis, venous congestion
Splenomegaly	Enlargement of spleen	Chronic leukemia, hemolytic states, portal hypertension, some infections
Hernia	Bulge or nodule in abdomen, usually appearing on straining	Inguinal (in inguinal canal), femoral (in femoral canal), umbilical (herniation of umbilicus), or incisional (defect in muscles after surgery)

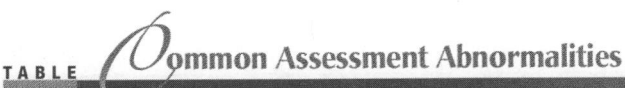

TABLE 38-11   Common Assessment Abnormalities
Gastrointestinal System—cont'd

FINDING	DESCRIPTION	POSSIBLE ETIOLOGY AND SIGNIFICANCE
Rectum and Anus		
Hemorrhoids	Thrombosed veins in rectum and anus (internal or external)	Portal hypertension, chronic constipation, prolonged sitting or standing, pregnancy
Mass	Firm, nodular edge	Tumor, carcinoma
Pilonidal cyst	Opening of sinus tract, cyst in midline just above coccyx	Probably congenital
Fissure	Ulceration in anal canal	Straining, irritation
Melena	Abnormal, black, tarry stool containing digested blood	Cancer, bleeding in upper GI tract from ulcers, varices
Tenesmus	Painful and ineffective straining at stool	Ulcerative colitis, diarrhea secondary to GI infection such as food poisoning
Steatorrhea	Fatty, frothy, foul-smelling stool	Chronic pancreatitis, biliary obstruction, malabsorption problems

TABLE 38-12   Diagnostic Studies
Gastrointestinal System

STUDY	DESCRIPTION AND PURPOSE	NURSING RESPONSIBILITY
Radiologic		
Upper Gastrointestinal (GI) or Barium Swallow	X-ray study with fluoroscopy with contrast medium. Study is used to diagnose structural abnormalities of the esophagus, stomach, and duodenal bulb.	Explain procedure to patient and that patient will need to drink contrast medium and assume various positions on x-ray table. Keep patient NPO for 8-12 hr before procedure. Tell patient to avoid smoking after midnight the night before the study. After x-ray, take measures to prevent contrast medium impaction (fluids, laxatives). Tell patient that stool may be white up to 72 hr after test.
Small Bowel Series	Contrast medium is ingested and films taken q20min until medium reaches terminal ileum.	Same as for upper GI.
Lower GI or Barium Enema	Fluoroscopic x-ray examination of colon uses contrast medium, which is administered rectally (enema). Double-contrast or air-contrast barium enema is test of choice. Air is infused after barium is evacuated.	Before the procedure, administer laxatives and enemas until colon is clear of stool evening before procedure. Administer clear liquid diet evening before procedure. Keep patient NPO for 8 hr before test. Instruct patient about being given barium by enema. Explain that cramping and urge to defecate may occur during procedure and that patient may be placed in various positions on tilt table. After the procedure, give fluids, laxatives, or suppositories to assist in expelling barium. Observe stool for passage of contrast medium.
Ultrasound	Noninvasive procedure uses high-frequency sound waves (ultrasound waves), which are passed into body structures and recorded as they are reflected (bounded). A conductive gel (lubricant jelly) is applied to the skin and a transducer is placed on the area.	
▪ Abdominal ultrasound	Study detects abdominal masses (tumors and cysts) and is also used to assess ascites.	Instruct patient to be NPO 8-12 hr before ultrasound. Air or gas can reduce quality of images. Food intake can cause gallbladder contraction, resulting in suboptimal study.

NPO, Nothing by mouth.

Continued

TABLE 38-12 — Diagnostic Studies Gastrointestinal System—cont'd

STUDY	DESCRIPTION AND PURPOSE	NURSING RESPONSIBILITY
Radiologic—cont'd **Ultrasound—cont'd**		
▪ Hepatobiliary ultrasound	Study detects subphrenic abscesses, cysts, tumors, and cirrhosis and is used to visualize biliary ducts.	Same as Abdominal ultrasound.
▪ Gallbladder (GB) ultrasound	Study detects gallstones (high degree of accuracy) and can be used for a patient with jaundice or allergic reaction to GB contrast media.	Same as Abdominal ultrasound.
Computed Tomography (CT)	Noninvasive radiologic examination combines special x-ray machine used for CT (exposures at different depths) with computer. Study detects mainly biliary tract, liver, and pancreatic disorders. Use of contrast medium accentuates density differences and helps detect biliary problems.	Explain procedures to patient. Determine sensitivity to iodine if contrast material used.
Magnetic Resonance Imaging (MRI)	Noninvasive procedure using radiofrequency waves and a magnetic field. Procedure is used to detect hepatic metastases and sources of GI bleeding and to stage colorectal cancer.	Keep patient NPO for 6 hr before procedure. Explain procedure to patient. Contraindicated in patient with metal implants (e.g., pacemaker) or who is pregnant.
Cholangiography		
▪ Percutaneous transhepatic cholangiogram (PTC)	After local anesthesia, liver is entered with long needle (under fluoroscopy), bile duct is entered, bile withdrawn, and radiopaque contrast medium injected. Fluoroscopy is used to determine filling of hepatic and biliary ducts.	Observe patient for signs of hemorrhage or bile leakage. Assess patient's medication for possible contraindications, precautions, or complications with the use of contrast medium.
▪ Surgical cholangiogram	Study is performed during surgery on biliary structures, such as GB. Contrast medium is injected into common bile duct.	Explain to patient that anesthetic will be used. Assess patient's medication for possible contraindications, precautions, or complications with the use of contrast medium.
▪ Magnetic resonance cholangiopancreatography (MRCP)	Noninvasive study uses MRI technology to obtain images of biliary and pancreatic ducts.	Same as MRI.
Nuclear Imaging Scans (Scintigraphy)	Purpose is to show size, shape, and position of organ. Functional disorders and structural defects may be identified. Radionuclide (radioactive isotope) is injected IV and a counter (scanning) device picks up radioactive emission, which is recorded on paper. Only tracer doses of radioactive isotopes are used.	Tell patient that substances contain only traces of radioactivity and pose little to no danger. Schedule no more than one radionuclide test on the same day. Explain to patient need to lie flat during scanning.
▪ Gastric emptying studies	Radionuclide study is used to assess ability of stomach to empty solids or liquids. In solid-emptying study, cooked egg white containing Tc-99m is eaten. In liquid-emptying study, orange juice with Tc-99m is drunk. Sequential images from gamma camera are recorded q2min for up to 60 min. Study is used in patients with emptying disorders from peptic ulcer, ulcer surgery, diabetes, or gastric malignancies.	Same as above.
▪ Hepatobiliary scintigraphy (HIDA)	Patient is given IV injection of Tc-99m and positioned under camera to record distribution of tracer in the liver, biliary tree, gallbladder, and proximal small bowel. Useful for identifying diffuse hepatic disease (such as cirrhosis or neoplasm), as well as to confirm acute cholecystitis.	Same as above.
▪ Scintigraphy of GI bleeding	Tc-99m–labeled sulfur colloid or Tc-99m labeling of the patient's own red blood cells (RBCs) can accurately determine the site of active GI blood loss. The sulfur colloid or the patient's RBCs are injected, and images of the abdomen are obtained at intermittent intervals.	Same as above.

IV, Intravenous.

TABLE
38-12

Diagnostic Studies
Gastrointestinal System—cont'd

STUDY	DESCRIPTION AND PURPOSE	NURSING RESPONSIBILITY
Endoscopic **Upper GI Endoscopy** ▪ Esophagogastroduodenoscopy (EGD)	Technique directly visualizes mucosal lining of esophagus, stomach, and duodenum with flexible, fiberoptic endoscope. Test may use video imaging to visualize stomach motility. Inflammations, ulcerations, tumors, or varices, or Mallory-Weiss tear may be detected.	Before the procedure, keep patient NPO for 8 hr. Make sure signed consent is on chart. Give preoperative medication if ordered (diazepam, midazolam, or meperidine). Explain to patient that local anesthetic may be sprayed on throat before insertion of scope and that patient will be sedated during the procedure. After the procedure, keep patient NPO until gag reflex returns. Gently tickle back of throat to determine reflex. Use warm saline gargles for relief of sore throat. Check temperature q15-30min for 1-2 hr (sudden temperature spike is sign of perforation).
Colonoscopy	Study directly visualizes entire colon up to ileocecal valve with flexible fiberoptic scope. Patient's position is changed frequently during procedure to assist with advancement of scope to cecum. Test is used to diagnose inflammatory bowel disease, detect tumors, and dilate strictures. Procedure allows for removal of colonic polyps without laparotomy.	Before the procedure, keep patient on clear liquids 1-3 days and NPO for 8 hr. Administer laxatives 1-3 days before and enemas night before. Explain to patient same information regarding insertion of scope as for sigmoidoscopy. Explain to patient that sedation will be given. Administer alternate preparation of 1 gal of Golytely or Colyte evening before (8-oz glass q10min). On morning of procedure, allow clear liquids. After the procedure, be aware that patient may experience abdominal cramps caused by stimulation of peristalsis because the patient's bowel is constantly inflated with air during procedure. Observe for rectal bleeding and signs of perforation (e.g., malaise, abdominal distention, tenesmus). Check vital signs.
Proctosigmoidoscopy	Study directly visualizes rectum and sigmoid colon with lighted endoscope. It is usually done with rigid metal scope but may be done with flexible endoscope. Sometimes special table is used to tilt patient into knee-chest position. Test may detect tumors, polyps, inflammatory and infectious diseases, fissures, hemorrhoids.	Administer enemas evening before and morning of procedure. Be aware that patient may have clear liquids day before or that no dietary restrictions may be necessary. Explain to patient knee-chest position (unless patient is older or very ill), need to take deep breaths during insertion of scope, and possible urge to defecate as scope is passed. Encourage patient to relax—let abdomen go limp. Observe for rectal bleeding after polypectomy or biopsy.
Endoscopic Retrograde Cholangiopancreatography (ERCP)	Fiberoptic endoscope (using fluoroscopy) is inserted through the oral cavity into descending duodenum, then common bile and pancreatic ducts are cannulated. Contrast medium is injected into ducts and allows for direct visualization of structures. Technique can also be used to retrieve a gallstone from distal common bile duct, dilate strictures, obtain biopsy of tumors, diagnose pseudocysts.	Before the procedure, explain procedure to patient, including patient role. Keep patient NPO 8 hr before procedure. Ensure consent form signed. Administer sedation immediately before and during procedure. Administer antibiotics if ordered. After the procedure, check vital signs. Check for signs of perforation or infection. Be aware that pancreatitis is most common complication. Check for return of gag reflex.
Endoscopic Ultrasound	Combined use of endoscopy and ultrasound using an ultrasound transducer attached to an endoscope. Enables visualization of the esophagus, stomach, intestine, liver, and pancreas.	Similar to upper GI endoscopy.

Continued

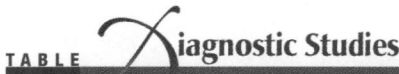

TABLE
38-12

Diagnostic Studies
Gastrointestinal System—cont'd

STUDY	DESCRIPTION AND PURPOSE	NURSING RESPONSIBILITY
Endoscopic—cont'd **Peritoneoscopy (Laparoscopy)**	Peritoneal cavity and contents are visualized with laparoscope. Biopsy specimen may also be taken. Done under general anesthesia in operating room. Double-puncture peritoneoscopy permits better visualization of abdominal cavity, especially liver. Technique can eliminate need for exploratory laparotomy in many patients.	Make sure signed permit is on chart. Keep patient NPO 8 hr before study. Administer preoperative sedative medication. Ensure that bladder and bowel are emptied. Instruct patient that local anesthetic is used before scope insertion. Observe for possible complications of bleeding and bowel perforation after the procedure.
Blood Chemistries • Serum amylase	Study measures secretion of amylase by pancreas and is important in diagnosing acute pancreatitis. Level of amylase peaks in 24 hr and then drops to normal in 48-72 hr. Depending on method, *normal finding* is 0-130 U/L (0-2.17 μkat/L).	Obtain blood sample in acute attack of pancreatitis. Explain procedure to patient.
• Serum lipase	Study measures secretion of lipase by pancreas. Level stays elevated longer than serum amylase. *Normal finding* is 0-160 U/L (0-2.66 μkat/L).	Explain procedure to patient.
Liver Biopsy	Percutaneous procedure uses needle inserted between sixth and seventh or eighth and ninth intercostal spaces on the right side to obtain specimen of hepatic tissue. Often done using ultrasound or CT guidance.	Before the procedure, check patient's coagulation status (prothrombin time, clotting or bleeding time). Ensure that patient's blood is typed and crossmatched. Take vital signs as baseline data. Explain holding of breath after expiration when needle is inserted. Ensure that informed consent has been signed. After the procedure, check vital signs to detect internal bleeding q15min × 2, q30min × 4, q1hr × 4. Keep patient lying on right side for minimum of 2 hr to splint puncture site. Keep patient in bed in flat position for 12-14 hr. Assess patient for complications such as bile peritonitis, shock, pneumothorax.
Miscellaneous Tests • Gastric analysis	Purpose is to analyze gastric contents for acidity and volume. NG tube is inserted, and gastric contents are aspirated. Contents are analyzed mainly for HCl, but pH, pepsin, and electrolytes may be determined. Histalog and pentagastrin may be used to stimulate HCl secretion. Exfoliative cytology may be done to determine whether malignant cells are present. With fasting, *normal acidity* is 2.5 mEq/L (2.5 mmol/L) and *normal volume* is 62 ml/hr; 30 min after Histalog or pentagastrin administration, *normal acidity* is 1.5 mEq/L (1.5 mmol/L) and *normal volume* is 110 ml/hr.	Keep patient NPO for 8-12 hr. Explain insertion of NG tube. Withhold drugs affecting gastric secretions 24-48 hr before test. Ensure no smoking morning of test (nicotine increases gastric secretion).
• Fecal analysis	Form, consistency, and color are noted. Specimen examined for mucus, blood, pus, parasites, and fat content. Tests for occult blood (guaiac test, Hemoccult, Hematest) are done.	Observe patient's stools. Collect stool specimens. Check stools for blood with Hemoccult or Hematest. Keep diet free of red meat for 24-48 hr before guaiac test.

NG, Nasogastric.

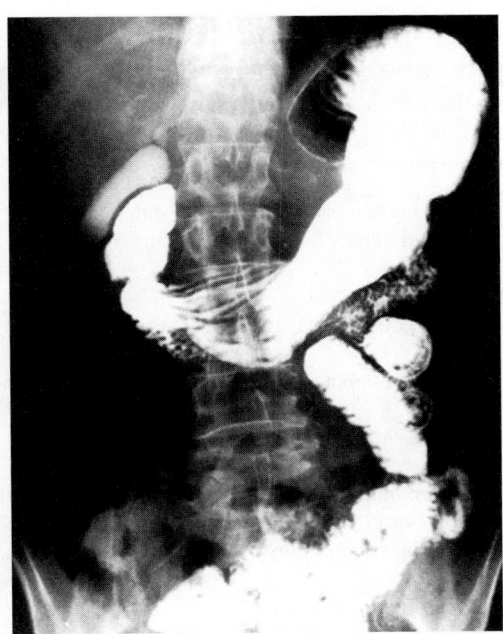

FIG. 38-10 Upper gastrointestinal tract x-ray.

Lower Gastrointestinal Series. The purpose of a lower GI series (barium enema) x-ray examination is to observe by means of fluoroscopy the filling of the colon with contrast medium and to observe by x-ray the filled colon. This procedure identifies polyps, tumors, and other lesions in the colon. It consists of administering an enema of contrast medium to the patient. The air-contrast barium enema provides better visualization of an inflammatory bowel disease, polyps, and tumors (Fig. 38-11). Because it requires the patient to retain the barium, it is not tolerated as well in an older or immobile patient.

Abdominal Ultrasound. Ultrasonography is used to show the size and configuration of organs. It is the diagnostic procedure of choice for detecting cholelithiasis (gallstones). Ultrasound is also used for detecting appendicitis, acute cholecystitis, and other changes in abdominal organs (see Table 38-12).

Endoscopy

Endoscopy refers to the direct visualization of a body structure through a lighted fiberoptic instrument (scope). The GI structures that can be examined by endoscopy include the esophagus, stomach, duodenum, colon, and, with the aid of fluoroscopy and x-rays, the pancreas and biliary tree. The pancreatic, hepatic, and common bile ducts can be visualized with side-viewing flexible endoscopes. This procedure is called *endoscopic retrograde cholangiopancreatography* (ERCP).[9]

The endoscope is an instrument channel through which biopsy forceps and cytology brushes may be passed. Cameras may be attached and video and still pictures taken. Endoscopy of the GI tract is often done in combination with biopsy and cytologic studies. The major complication of GI endoscopy is perforation through the structure being scoped. This complication is decreased with the use of the flexible fiberoptic scopes. All endoscopic procedures require informed, written consent. Specific endoscopy procedures are discussed in Table 38-12. In addition to diagnostic procedures, many invasive and therapeutic procedures may be done with endoscopes. These include procedures

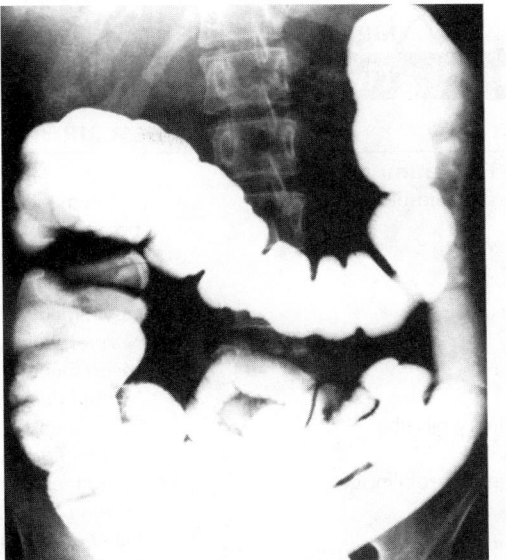
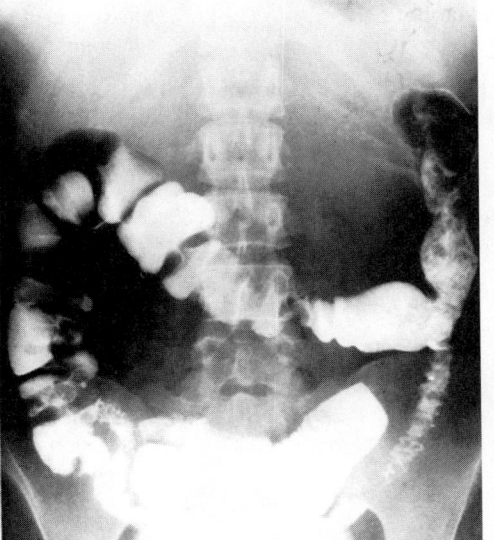
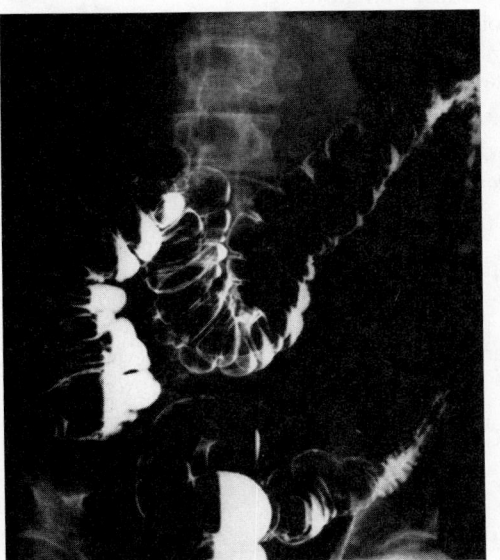

FIG. 38-11 Barium enema x-ray. **A,** Colon filled with barium. **B,** Colon after evacuation of barium. **C,** Air-contrast study of colon.

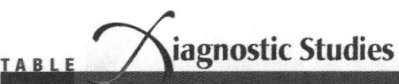

TABLE
38-13

Diagnostic Studies
Liver Function Tests

TEST	DESCRIPTION AND PURPOSE
Bile Formation and Excretion	
▪ Serum bilirubin	Measurement of ability of liver to conjugate and excrete bilirubin, allowing differentiation between unconjugated (indirect) and conjugated (direct) bilirubin in plasma
Total	Measurement of direct and indirect total bilirubin *Normal finding* of 0.2-1.3 mg/dl (3.4-22 μmol/L)
Direct	Measurement of conjugated bilirubin; elevation in obstructive jaundice *Normal finding* of 0.1-0.3 mg/dl (1.7-5.1 μmol/L)
Indirect	Measurement of unconjugated bilirubin; elevation in hepatocellular and hemolytic conditions *Normal finding* of 0.1-1 mg/dl (1.7-17 μmol/L)
▪ Urinary bilirubin	Measurement of urinary excretion of conjugated bilirubin *Normal finding* of 0
▪ Urinary urobilinogen	Measurement of urinary excretion of urobilinogen; maximum excretion midafternoon to early evening, collection of total urinary output for 2 hr in afternoon, sent to laboratory in dark container immediately because of oxidation of urobilinogen to urobilin on exposure to air *Normal finding* of 0.5-4 mg/day (0.8-6.8 μmol/day)
▪ Fecal urobilinogen	Measurement of fecal urobilinogen in stool specimen *Normal finding* of 30-220 mg/100 g stool (55-372 μmol/100 g of stool)
Dye Excretion Tests (Detoxification)	
▪ Indocyanine green	Determination of liver's ability to take up and excrete dye given IV, drawing of blood samples every 5 min for 20-30 min *Normal finding* of 500-800 ml/m² of body surface/min
Protein Metabolism	
▪ Serum protein levels	Measurement of serum proteins that are manufactured by the liver; measurement of albumin, *normal finding* of 3.5-5 g/dl (35-50 g/L); measurement of globulin, *normal finding* of 2-3.5 g/dl (20-35 g/L) *Normal total protein* of 6-8 g/dl (60-80 g/L) *Normal A/G ratio* of 1.5:1-2.5:1
▪ α-Fetoprotein	Indication of hepatic cancer *Normal finding* of <25 ng/ml (<25 μg/L)
▪ Blood ammonia levels	Conversion of ammonia to urea normally occurs in the liver; elevation can result in hepatic encephalopathy secondary to liver cirrhosis *Normal finding* of 30-70 μg/dl (17.6-41.1 μmol/L)
Hemostatic Functions	
▪ Prothrombin	Determination of prothrombin activity *Normal finding* of 12-15 sec
▪ Vitamin K production	Determination of response of liver to vitamin K, checking of prothrombin time necessary 24 hr after injection of vitamin K
Serum Enzyme Tests	
▪ Alkaline phosphatase (ALP)	Originating in bone and liver. Serum levels rise when excretion is impaired as a result of obstruction in the biliary tract. *Normal finding* of 30-120 U/L (0.5-2 μkat/L), depending on method and age
▪ Aspartate aminotransferase (AST)	Elevation in liver damage and inflammation *Normal finding* of 7-40 U/L (0.12-0.67 μkat/L)
▪ Alanine aminotransferase (ALT)	Elevation in liver damage and inflammation *Normal finding* of 5-36 U/L (0.08-0.6 μkat/L)
▪ γ-Glutamyl transpeptidase (GGT)	Present in biliary tract (not in skeletal muscle or cardiac), increase in hepatitis and alcoholic liver disease. More sensitive for liver dysfunction than ALP. *Normal finding* of 0-30 U/L (0-0.5 μkat/L)
Lipid Metabolism	
▪ Serum cholesterol	Synthesis and excretion by liver, increase in biliary obstruction, decrease in extensive liver disease and malnutrition *Normal finding* of 140-200 mg/dl (3.6-5.2 mmol/L), varying with age

such as polypectomy, sclerosis of varices, laser treatment, cauterization of bleeding sites, papillotomy, common bile duct stone removal, and balloon dilations. Many endoscopic procedures require intravenous short-acting sedation.

Endoscopic Ultrasound. Endoscopic ultrasound (EUS) is a relatively new endoscopic technique that provides highly accurate images of esophagus, GI tract, pancreas, and liver. EUS provides high-resolution imaging of the GI tract by its unique ability to differentiate the histologic layers of the GI tract wall. It is most often used for preoperative staging of esophageal, gastric, pancreatic, and colorectal cancers. It can also be used to detect gallstones.

Capsule Endoscopy. Capsule endoscopy is a new technique that uses a disposable video camera capsule swallowed by the patient. The image of the intestine is captured by the video camera and transmitted by radiofrequency. This procedure is particularly useful in visualization of the small bowel not within reach of standard upper and lower endoscopy. It allows more access to the small bowel for patients with an obscure source of GI bleeding. This technology may be particularly helpful in discovering the cause of GI bleeding when results of standard upper endoscopy and colonoscopy are negative.

Liver Biopsy

The purpose of a liver biopsy is to obtain hepatic tissue to be used in establishing a diagnosis such as fibrosis, cirrhosis, hepatitis, and neoplasms. It may also be useful for following the progress of liver disease.

The two types of liver biopsy are open and closed. The *open method* involves making an incision and removing a wedge of tissue. It is done in the operating room with the patient under general anesthesia, often concurrently with another surgical procedure. The *closed,* or *needle, biopsy* is a percutaneous procedure in which the site is infiltrated with a local anesthetic and a needle is inserted between the sixth and seventh or eighth and ninth intercostal spaces on the right side. The patient lies supine with the right arm over the head. The patient should be instructed to expire fully and not breathe while the needle is inserted (see Table 38-12). Nursing assessment before and after a liver biopsy is important.

Liver Function Studies

Liver function tests are usually described separately from other GI diagnostic studies. Liver function tests are laboratory (blood) studies that reflect hepatic disease. Table 38-13 describes some common liver function tests.

REVIEW QUESTIONS

The number of the question corresponds to the same-numbered objective at the beginning of the chapter.

1. A patient is admitted to the hospital with a diagnosis of diarrhea with dehydration. The nurse recognizes that increased peristalsis resulting in diarrhea can be related to
   a. sympathetic inhibition.
   b. mixing and propulsion.
   c. sympathetic stimulation.
   d. parasympathetic stimulation.

2. A patient has an elevated blood level of indirect (unconjugated) bilirubin. One cause of this finding is that
   a. the gallbladder is unable to contract to release stored bile.
   b. bilirubin is not being conjugated and excreted into the bile by the liver.
   c. the Kupffer cells in the liver are unable to remove bilirubin from the blood.
   d. there is an obstruction in the biliary tract preventing flow of bile into the small intestine.

3. As gastric contents move into the small intestine the bowel is normally protected from the acidity of gastric contents by the
   a. inhibition of secretin release.
   b. release of bicarbonate by the pancreas.
   c. release of pancreatic digestive enzymes.
   d. release of gastrin by the duodenal mucosa.

4. A patient is jaundiced and her stools are clay colored (gray). This is most likely related to
   a. decreased bile flow into the intestine.
   b. increased production of urobilinogen.
   c. increased production of cholecystokinin.
   d. increased bile and bilirubin in the blood.

5. An 80-year-old man states that although he adds a lot of salt to his food it still does not have much taste. The nurse's response is based on the knowledge that the older adult
   a. should not experience changes in taste.
   b. has a loss of taste buds, especially for sweet and salt.
   c. has some loss of taste but no difficulty chewing food.
   d. loses the sense of taste because the ability to smell is decreased.

6. When assessing the health promotion–health maintenance pattern as related to GI function, an appropriate question by the nurse is
   a. "What is your usual bowel elimination pattern?"
   b. "What percentage of your income is spent on food?"
   c. "Have you traveled to a foreign country in the last year?"
   d. "Do you have diarrhea when you are under a lot of stress?"

7. During an examination of the abdomen the nurse should
   a. position the patient in the supine position with the bed flat and knees straight.
   b. listen in the epigastrium and all four quadrants for 2 to 5 minutes for bowel sounds.
   c. use the following order of techniques: inspection, palpation, percussion, auscultation.
   d. describe bowel sounds as absent if no sound is heard in the lower right quadrant after 2 minutes.

8. A normal physical assessment finding of the GI system is
   a. tympany on percussion of the abdomen.
   b. liver edge 2 to 4 cm below the costal margin.
   c. finding of a firm, nodular edge on the rectal examination.
   d. easy palpation of the spleen edges with moderate pressure.

9. In preparing a patient for a colonoscopy the nurse explains that
   a. a signed permit is not necessary.
   b. sedation may be used during the procedure.
   c. only one cleansing enema is necessary for preparation.
   d. a light meal should be eaten the day before the procedure.

REFERENCES

1. Eliopoulos C: *Gerontological nursing*, ed 5, Philadelphia, 2000, Lippincott.
2. Porth CM: *Pathophysiology concepts of altered health states*, ed 6, Philadelphia, 2002, Lippincott.
3. Burke MM, Walsh MB: *Gerontologic nursing: wholistic care of the older adult*, ed 2, St Louis, 1997, Mosby.
4. Bickley LS et al: *Bates' guide to physical examination and history taking*, ed 7, Philadelphia, 1999, Lippincott.
5. Seidel HM et al: *Mosby's guide to physical examination*, ed 5, St Louis, 2003, Mosby.
6. Barkausus VH, Baumann LC, Darling-Fisher CS: *Health and physical assessment*, ed 3, St Louis, 2002, Mosby.
7. Ebersole P, Hess P: *Toward healthy aging*, ed 6, St Louis, 2001, Mosby.
8. Feldman M et al: *Sleisenger and Fordtran's gastrointestinal and liver disease: pathophysiology/diagnosis/management*, ed 6, Philadelphia, 1998, Saunders.
9. Domkowski, K: *Gastroenterology nursing: a core curriculum*, ed 2, St Louis, 1998, Mosby.

RESOURCES

Resources for this chapter are listed in Chapter 39 on page 1002, Chapter 40 on page 1051, Chapter 41 on page 1103, and Chapter 42 on page 1149.

CHAPTER 39

NURSING MANAGEMENT
Nutritional Problems

Peggi Guenter

LEARNING OBJECTIVES

1. Describe the essential components of a nutritionally sound diet and their importance to good health.
2. Describe possible adverse interactions between drugs and various foods.
3. Describe the common etiologic factors, clinical manifestations, and management of malnutrition.
4. Explain the indications for use, complications, and nursing management of tube feedings.
5. Describe the types of feeding tubes and related nursing management.
6. Define the indications, complications, and nursing management related to the use of parenteral nutrition.
7. Discuss the etiologies, complications, and collaborative care of obesity.
8. Describe the nursing management related to conservative and surgical therapies for obesity.
9. Compare the etiologic factors, clinical manifestations, and nursing management of eating disorders.

KEY TERMS

anorexia nervosa, p. 999
body mass index, p. 991
bulimia nervosa, p. 999
kwashiorkor, p. 973
lipectomy, p. 995
malabsorption syndrome, p. 973
malnutrition, p. 972
marasmus, p. 973
morbid obesity, p. 991

nutrition, p. 969
obesity, p. 991
overnutrition, p. 972
parenteral nutrition, p. 987
protein-calorie malnutrition, p. 972
total parenteral nutrition, p. 987
tube feeding, p. 982
undernutrition, p. 972

CULTURAL & ETHNIC CONSIDERATIONS
Nutritional Problems

- Incidence of obesity is higher among African American women compared with white women.
- Anorexia nervosa is most common among women from middle and upper-middle classes.
- Anorexia nervosa and bulimia have a higher incidence among whites than among African Americans and Asian Americans.
- Lactase deficiency has a higher incidence among African Americans and Asians than among whites.

This chapter focuses on problems related to nutrition. The primary nutritional problems discussed are malnutrition, obesity, and eating disorders.

NUTRITIONAL PROBLEMS

Nutritional problems can occur in all age groups, cultures, ethnic groups, and socioeconomic classes. Intelligence and wealth do not necessarily preclude the development of poor nutritional habits. The nurse in the roles of caregiver, teacher, and resource person can have a strong influence on the nutritional practices of patients and their families. Together with the physician, the registered dietitian, and the pharmacist, the nurse is in an excellent position to assess the dietary practices of the patient and provide important information, as well as provide nutritional resources within and outside the institutional setting.

The nutritional status of a person or a family may be influenced by many factors. Attitudes toward the importance of food and eating habits are established early. Cultural or religious preferences and requirements are frequently reflected in dietary intake. The financial status of a family or an individual can determine the type and amount of nutritionally sound food that can be

purchased. Findings support that generally the lower the socioeconomic status, the poorer the nutritional state.[1] The availability of food sources also contributes to the individual's nutritional status.

NORMAL NUTRITION

Nutrition is the process by which the body uses food for energy, growth, and maintenance and repair of body tissues. Good nutrition in the absence of any underlying disease process results from the ingestion of a balanced diet. The United States Department of Agriculture (USDA) has adopted the Food Guide Pyramid, which consists of food groups that are presented in proportions appropriate for a healthy diet. Fig. 39-1 and Table 39-1 show these food groups with the recommended daily requirements and examples of common sources. The essential components of the basic food groups are carbohydrates, fats, proteins, vitamins, and minerals.

Carbohydrates, the body's primary source of energy, yield approximately 4 kilocalories per gram. (Kilocalorie is the correct unit to designate caloric intake and expenditure. However, calorie is more commonly used.) Carbohydrates are either simple or complex. Simple carbohydrates come in two forms: *monosaccharides* (e.g., glucose and fructose), which are found in fruits and honey, and *disaccharides* (e.g., sucrose, maltose, and lac-

Reviewed by Karen Goff, RN, BSN, Case Manager, GI Services, Saint Joseph's Hospital of Atlanta, Atlanta, Ga.

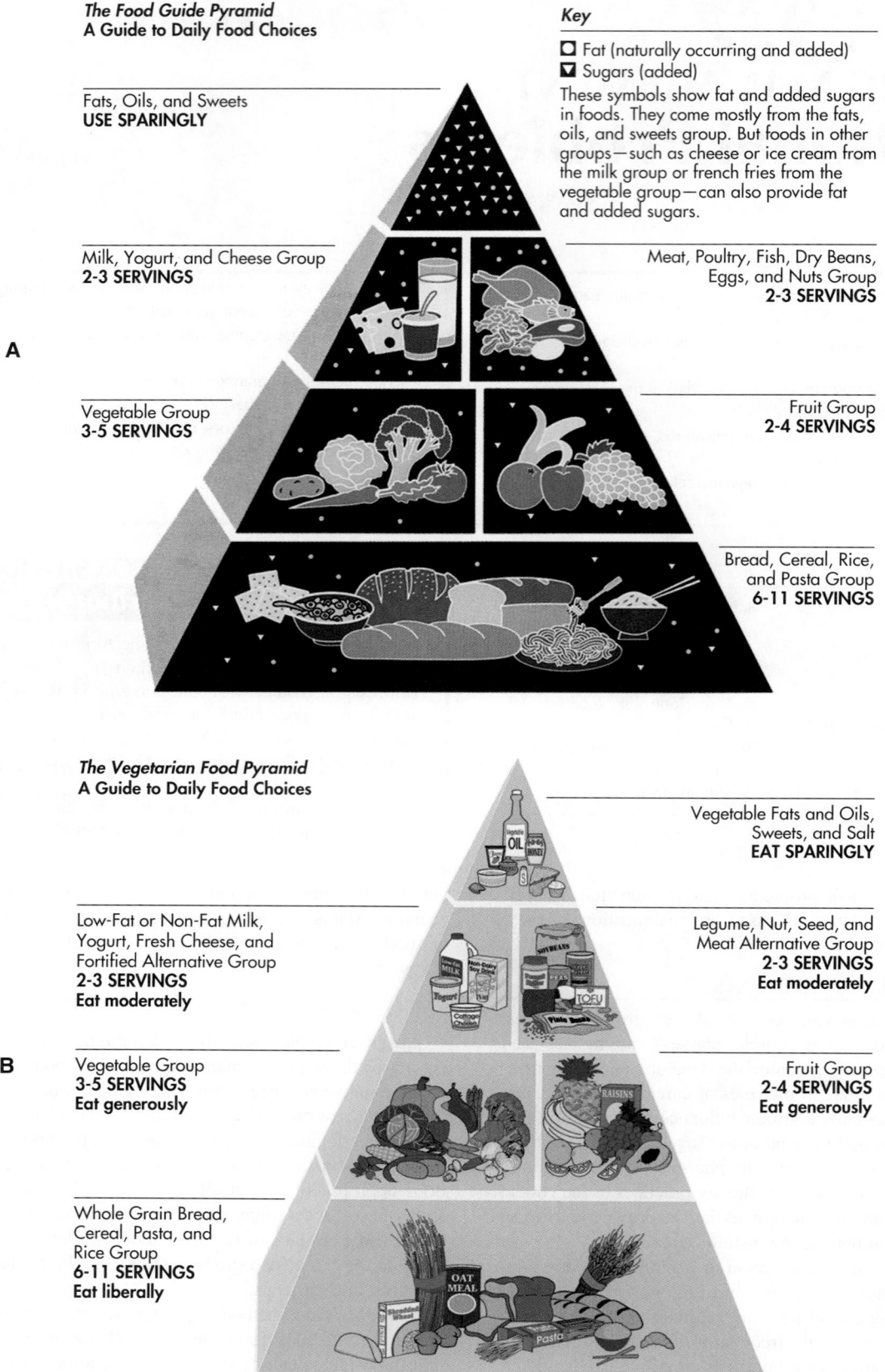

The Food Guide Pyramid
A Guide to Daily Food Choices

Fats, Oils, and Sweets
USE SPARINGLY

Key

☐ Fat (naturally occurring and added)
▼ Sugars (added)
These symbols show fat and added sugars in foods. They come mostly from the fats, oils, and sweets group. But foods in other groups—such as cheese or ice cream from the milk group or french fries from the vegetable group—can also provide fat and added sugars.

Milk, Yogurt, and Cheese Group
2-3 SERVINGS

Meat, Poultry, Fish, Dry Beans, Eggs, and Nuts Group
2-3 SERVINGS

Vegetable Group
3-5 SERVINGS

Fruit Group
2-4 SERVINGS

Bread, Cereal, Rice, and Pasta Group
6-11 SERVINGS

A

The Vegetarian Food Pyramid
A Guide to Daily Food Choices

Vegetable Fats and Oils, Sweets, and Salt
EAT SPARINGLY

Low-Fat or Non-Fat Milk, Yogurt, Fresh Cheese, and Fortified Alternative Group
2-3 SERVINGS
Eat moderately

Legume, Nut, Seed, and Meat Alternative Group
2-3 SERVINGS
Eat moderately

Vegetable Group
3-5 SERVINGS
Eat generously

Fruit Group
2-4 SERVINGS
Eat generously

Whole Grain Bread, Cereal, Pasta, and Rice Group
6-11 SERVINGS
Eat liberally

B

FIG. 39-1 **A,** Food guide pyramid: a guide to daily food choices and number of servings. **B,** Vegetarian food guide pyramid.

TABLE 39-1	Pyramid Food Groups and Recommended Number of Servings		
GROUP	**NUTRIENTS PROVIDED**	**NUMBER OF SERVINGS DAILY**	**SERVING SIZE**
• Bread, cereal, rice, pasta	Thiamine, niacin, iron, protein	6-11	1 slice of bread 1 oz ready-to-eat cereal ½ cup of cooked cereal, rice, or pasta
• Vegetable	Vitamins A and C, folic acid	3-5	1 cup of raw leafy vegetables ½ cup of other vegetables, cooked or raw ¾ cup of vegetable juice
• Fruit	Vitamins A and C	2-4	1 medium apple, banana, or orange ½ cup of chopped, cooked, or canned fruit ¾ cup of fruit juice
• Milk, yogurt, cheese	Calcium, protein, riboflavin, vitamin B₆, and cobalamin	2-3	1 cup of milk or yogurt 1½ oz of natural cheese 2 oz of processed cheese
• Meat, poultry, fish, dry beans, eggs, nuts	Protein, niacin, thiamine, iron, zinc, cobalamin, folic acid	2-3	2-3 oz of cooked lean meat, poultry, or fish ½ cup of cooked dry beans, 1 egg, or 2 tbs of peanut butter (count as 1 oz lean meat)

tose), which are found in such substances as table sugar, malted cereal, and milk, respectively. Complex carbohydrates or polysaccharides commonly appear in the diet as starches, such as cereal grains, potatoes, and legumes. Carbohydrates are the chief protein-sparing ingredient in a nutritionally sound diet and compose approximately 47% of the daily caloric needs of the body. The National Research Council recommends that at least half of the body's energy needs should come from carbohydrates, especially complex carbohydrates.[2]

Approximately 36% of the daily caloric intake in current American diets is derived from fat.[2] This level is considerably higher than that found in many other societies and is a cause for concern. The Food and Nutrition Board's Committee on Diet and Health recommends that people reduce their fat intake to 30% of their total daily caloric intake.[3] One gram of fat yields 9 calories. Fats are stored in adipose tissue and in the abdominal cavity. Besides being a major source of energy, fats act as insulation, which reduces loss of body heat in cold environments and provides padding and protection for vital organs. Fats also act as carriers of essential fatty acids and fat-soluble vitamins. Fats provide a feeling of satiety after eating, partly from the flavor added and partly from their slow rate of digestion, which delays hunger. The daily caloric requirements of a person are influenced by body build, age, gender, and physical activity. Adjustments in caloric intake are necessary depending on changes in health status and daily activity level. An average adult requires an estimated 20 to 35 calories per kilogram of body weight per day, leaning toward the higher end if the person is critically ill or very active and the lower end if the person is sedentary.[4]

Proteins, another essential component of a well-balanced diet, are obtained from both animal and plant sources. Ideally, proteins provide 15% to 20% of daily caloric needs.[3] The recommended daily protein intake is 0.8 to 1 g/kg of body weight. One gram of protein yields 4 calories. Proteins are complex nitrogenous organic compounds, of which amino acids are the fundamental units of structure. The 22 amino acids can be classified as essential and nonessential. The body is capable of synthesizing nonessential

TABLE 39-2	Good Sources of Protein
COMPLETE PROTEINS	**INCOMPLETE PROTEINS**
Milk and milk products (e.g., cheese) Eggs Fish Meats Poultry	Grains (e.g., corn) Legumes (e.g., navy beans, soybeans, peas) Nuts (e.g., peanuts) Seeds (e.g., sesame seeds, sunflower seeds)

amino acids if an adequate supply of protein is available. However, the nine essential amino acids cannot be synthesized, and their availability depends totally on dietary sources. Protein sources containing all the essential amino acids are called *complete proteins*. Proteins that lack one or more of the essential amino acids are called *incomplete proteins*. Table 39-2 lists good sources of protein. Proteins are essential for tissue growth, repair, and maintenance; body regulatory functions; and energy production.

Vitamins are organic compounds required in small amounts by the body for normal metabolism. Vitamins function primarily in enzyme reactions that facilitate the metabolism of amino acids, fats, and carbohydrates. The body must rely on a dietary source to meet requirements for some vitamins, such as cobalamin (vitamin B₁₂). Vitamins are divided into two categories: water-soluble vitamins (vitamin C and the B-complex vitamins) and fat-soluble vitamins (vitamins A, D, E, and K).

Mineral salts (e.g., magnesium, iron, calcium) make up approximately 4% of the total body weight. When minerals are present in minute amounts, they are referred to as trace elements. Minerals required in amounts greater than 100 mg per day are called major minerals. Table 39-3 lists the major minerals and trace elements. Minerals are necessary for the body to build tissues, regulate body fluids, and assist in various body functions. Some minerals are stored in a manner similar to that of the fat-

TABLE 39-3	Major Minerals and Trace Elements	
MAJOR MINERALS	**TRACE ELEMENTS**	
Calcium	Chromium	
Chloride	Copper	
Magnesium	Fluoride	
Phosphorus	Iodine	
Potassium	Iron	
Sodium	Manganese	
Sulfur	Molybdenum	
	Selenium	
	Zinc	

TABLE 39-4 Nutritional Therapy — Foods High in Iron*	
FOOD	**SELECTED SERVING SIZE**
Breads, Cereals, and Grain Products	
Farina, regular or quick cooked (enriched)	⅔ cup
Oatmeal, instant, fortified, prepared (enriched)	⅔ cup
Ready-to-eat cereals, fortified (enriched)	1 oz
Meat, Poultry, Fish, and Alternatives	
Beef liver, braised	3 oz
Pork liver, braised	3 oz
Chicken or turkey liver, braised	½ cup diced
Clams: steamed, boiled, or canned (drained)	3 oz
Oysters: baked, broiled, steamed, or canned (undrained)	3 oz
Soybeans, cooked	½ cup

*These foods provide 25% to 39% of the recommended dietary allowance (RDA) of iron.

soluble vitamins and can be toxic if taken in excess amounts. The amount of minerals needed in the daily diet varies greatly from a few micrograms of trace minerals to 1 g or more of the major minerals, such as calcium, phosphorus, and sodium. A well-balanced diet can usually meet the daily requirements of needed minerals. However, deficiency states can occur.

SPECIAL DIETS

Vegetarian Diet

The common element among all vegetarians is the exclusion of red meat from the diet. Vegetarians have a variety of reasons for following this dietary practice, including religious or cultural beliefs that it is a better way of attaining total health, respect for all living beings, ethical-ecologic ideals, and economics. Many vegetarians are *vegans,* who are pure or total vegetarians and eat only plant food, and *lacto-ovo-vegetarians,* who eat plant foods and sometimes dairy products and eggs.

Vegetarians can have vitamin or protein deficiencies unless their diets are well-planned. Plant protein, although of a lesser quality than that of animal origin, fulfills most of the protein requirements. Combinations of vegetable protein foods (e.g., cornmeal, kidney beans) can increase the nutritional value. Lacto-ovo-vegetarians obtain additional protein sources from dairy products and eggs. Milk made from soybeans is an excellent protein source, especially for the true vegan. The primary deficiency of a strict vegan is lack of cobalamin (vitamin B_{12}). This vitamin can be obtained only from animal protein, special supplements, or foods that have been fortified with the vitamin. Vegans not using cobalamin supplements are susceptible to the development of megaloblastic anemia and the neurologic signs of cobalamin deficiency. Strict vegetarians and lacto-ovo-vegetarians are also at risk for iron deficiency. Iron-enriched foods or iron supplements are prescribed during pregnancy, early childhood, and adolescence and after major blood loss. Table 39-4 lists examples of foods high in iron. Other deficiencies that may be present in a vegan diet include calcium, zinc, vitamins A and D, and protein.

MALNUTRITION

Malnutrition is an excess, deficit, or imbalance in the essential components of a balanced diet (Fig. 39-2). Terms such as undernutrition and overnutrition are also used to describe malnutrition. **Undernutrition** describes a state of poor nourishment as a result of inadequate diet or diseases that interfere with normal appetite and assimilation of ingested food. **Overnutrition** refers to the ingestion of more food than is required for body needs, as in obesity. An example of nutrient imbalance is a vitamin deficiency state such as *rickets,* a bone disorder caused by inadequate vitamin D. *Scurvy* is a condition characterized by weakness, anemia, and oral ulcerations that is associated with inadequate vitamin C intake.

Malnutrition is most prevalent in developing countries in which adequate food sources do not exist, the inhabitants are not well educated about their nutritional needs, and economic conditions often preclude the purchase of a balanced diet. Undernutrition does exist in the United States, and it is usually found in individuals or groups from the lower socioeconomic class or in individuals who have chronic or acute illnesses. Malnutrition is common in hospitalized patients, with an incidence of 30% to 55%.[5] The prevalence of elderly long-term care residents who can be found to have protein-calorie malnutrition ranges from 23% to 85%.[6]

Types of Malnutrition

Protein-Calorie Malnutrition. **Protein-calorie malnutrition** (PCM) is the most common form of undernutrition and can result from either primary or secondary factors. Primary PCM is present when nutritional needs are not met as a result of poor eat-

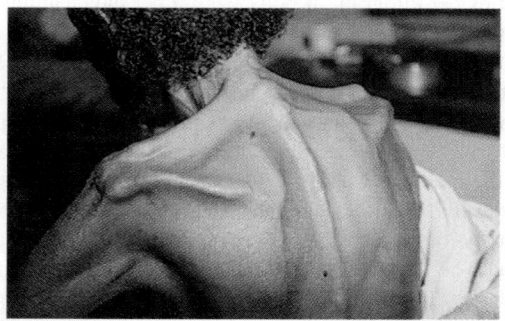

FIG. 39-2 Patient with malnutrition.

ing habits. Secondary PCM is the result of an alteration or defect in ingestion, digestion, absorption, or metabolism. In this type of malnutrition, tissue needs are not met even though the dietary intake would be satisfactory under normal conditions. Secondary malnutrition may occur as a result of gastrointestinal (GI) obstruction, surgical procedure, cancer, malabsorption syndromes, drugs, or infectious diseases.

PCM may also be due to the ingestion of foods deficient in protein. In addition to decreased quantities of protein, the diet is generally low in necessary vitamins and minerals. Most malnourished ill patients have this type of combined PCM.

Marasmus and Kwashiorkor. Marasmus is the result of a concomitant deficiency of both caloric and protein intake leading to generalized loss of body fat and muscle. Patients generally appear "wasted," or emaciated, but may have normal serum protein levels. **Kwashiorkor** is caused by a deficiency of protein intake that is superimposed on a catabolic stress event, such as a GI obstruction, a surgical procedure, cancer, a malabsorption syndrome, or an infectious disease. These patients may appear well nourished but have very low serum protein levels.

Etiology and Pathophysiology

Starvation Process. Knowledge of the phases of the starvation process is essential to better understand the physiologic changes that occur in PCM. Initially, the body selectively uses carbohydrates (glycogen) rather than fat and protein to meet metabolic needs. These carbohydrate stores, found in the liver and muscles, are minimal and may be totally depleted within 18 hours. During this early phase of starvation, the only use of protein is in its obligatory participation in cellular metabolism. However, once carbohydrate stores are depleted, protein begins to be converted to glucose for energy. Alanine and glutamine are the first amino acids to be used by the liver for the formation of glucose in a process termed *gluconeogenesis*. The resulting available plasma glucose allows the metabolic processes to continue. With these amino acids being used as energy sources, the person may be in negative nitrogen balance (greater nitrogen excretion). However, within 5 to 9 days, body fat is fully mobilized to supply much of the needed energy.

In prolonged starvation up to 97% of calories are provided by fat, and protein is conserved. Depletion of fat stores depends on the amount available, but fat stores are generally used up in 4 to 6 weeks. Once fat stores are used, body proteins, including those in internal organs and plasma, can no longer be spared and rapidly decrease because they are the only remaining body source of energy available.

If the malnourished patient has surgery, experiences bodily trauma, or has an infection, the stress response with concomitant increase in energy expenditure is superimposed on the starvation response. These body insults cause an increase in the metabolic rate, with a subsequent increase in energy requirements. Protein stores are no longer spared and are used with increasing frequency for body energy because of the increased metabolic energy needs.

As the protein depletion continues, liver function is impaired, and synthesis of proteins is diminished. The plasma oncotic pressure is decreased because of decreased protein synthesis. A major function of plasma proteins, primarily of albumin, is the maintenance of the osmotic pressure of the blood. Because of this decreased pressure, a shift in body fluids occurs from the vascular space into the interstitial compartment. As protein ingestion decreases and body stores are depleted, albumin eventu-

ally leaks into the interstitial space along with the fluid. Edema becomes clinically observable. Often the edema present in the face and legs of the patient masks the muscle wasting that occurs.

As the total blood volume is reduced, the skin appears dry and wrinkled. Along with the shift of fluids to the interstitial space, ions also move. Sodium (a predominant extracellular ion) is found in increased amounts within the cell, and potassium (a predominant intracellular ion) and magnesium are shifted to the extracellular space. The sodium-potassium exchange pump has high energy needs, using 20% to 50% of all calories ingested. When the diet is extremely deficient in calories and essential proteins, the pump will fail, leaving sodium inside the cell (along with water), and the cell will expand.

The liver is the body organ that loses the most mass during protein deprivation. It gradually becomes infiltrated with fat secondary to decreased synthesis of lipoproteins. Immediate restoration to a diet of protein and other necessary constituents must be instituted, or death will rapidly ensue.

Causes of Malnutrition. Many factors contribute to the development of malnutrition, including socioeconomic status, cultural influences, psychologic disorders, medical conditions, and medical treatments. Table 39-5 lists conditions that increase the risk of malnutrition. Because individuals and families from the lower socioeconomic class spend a greater percentage of their income on food, there is a tendency to seek out cheaper foods as the cost of food increases. These foods may not provide adequate or balanced nutrition. In contrast, some lower-income persons may prefer to select foods that are more expensive but only marginally nutritious because of their prestige value. The nurse and the registered dietitian can assist their patients in making food choices that meet nutritional requirements while staying within their limited resources.

Patients with physical illnesses. Regardless of the cause of the illness, the sick person has increased nutritional needs. Pathologic conditions are frequently aggravated by undernutrition, and an existing deficiency state is likely to become more severe during illness. Malnutrition is not an uncommon consequence of illness, surgery, injury, or hospitalization. Anorexia, nausea, vomiting, diarrhea, abdominal distention, and abdominal cramping may accompany diseases of the GI system. Any combination of these symptoms interferes with normal food consumption and metabolism. In addition, a patient may restrict the dietary intake to a few foods or fluids that may not be nutritionally sound out of fear of aggravating the already disturbed GI function.

Malabsorption syndrome is defined as the impaired absorption of nutrients from the GI tract. It may result from decreased amounts of necessary enzymes or a reduced bowel surface area

---

TABLE 39-5 Conditions That Increase the Risk for Malnutrition

- Chronic alcoholism
- Decreased mobility that limits access to food or its preparation
- Nutrient losses from malabsorption, dialysis, fistulas, or wounds
- Drugs with antinutrient or catabolic properties, such as corticosteroids and oral antibiotics
- Extreme need for nutrients because of hypermetabolism or stresses such as infection, burns, trauma, or fever
- No oral intake and/or receiving standard intravenous solutions (5% dextrose) for 10 days or for 5 days in older adults

and can quickly lead to a deficiency state. Many drugs may have undesirable GI side effects, as well as alter normal digestive and absorptive processes. For example, antibiotics change the normal flora of the intestines, decreasing the body's ability to synthesize biotin.

Fever accompanies many illnesses, injuries, and infections, with a concomitant increase in the body's basal metabolic rate (BMR). Each degree of temperature increase on the Fahrenheit scale raises the BMR by about 7%.[7] Without an increase in the amount of calories ingested in the diet, body protein stores will be used to supply calories, and protein depletion can become a problem.

The hospitalized patient, especially the older adult, is at risk of becoming malnourished. Prolonged illness, major surgery, sepsis, draining wounds, burns, hemorrhage, fractures, and immobilization can all contribute to malnutrition. The nurse must assume responsibility, along with the health care provider and the dietitian, for meeting the patient's nutritional needs. The nurse must also be knowledgeable of the requirements of a patient who is not overtly ill but who is undergoing diagnostic studies. This patient may be nutritionally fit on entering the hospital but can develop nutritional problems because of the dietary restrictions imposed by multiple diagnostic studies.

Incomplete diets. Vitamin deficiencies are rare in most of the developed countries of the world. When vitamin deficiencies are present, several vitamins are usually involved rather than a single vitamin deficiency. The recommended dietary allowances or Dietary Reference Intakes (DRIs) for essential vitamins and minerals can be obtained by eating a diet consisting of foods from the basic five food groups. DRIs from the Food and Nutrition Board have a safety margin because the levels exceed minimum daily requirements for most people.[8] When vitamin imbalances do occur, they are usually found among persons with a pattern of alcohol and drug abuse, persons who are chronically ill, and individuals who follow poor dietary practices. Followers of fad diets or poorly planned vegetarian diets are also subject to a potential deficiency state. Clinical manifestations of vitamin imbalances are most commonly exhibited as neurologic manifestations (Table 39-6). In the growing child, the central nervous system (CNS) is primarily involved, whereas the peripheral nervous system is most affected in the adult.

Food-drug interactions. When health conditions require drug therapy, drug and food interactions may not be explored before starting a prescription. Adverse interactions can include incompatibilities, altered drug effectiveness, and impaired nutritional status. Table 39-7 outlines examples of common drug

TABLE 39-6	Recommended Dietary Vitamin Allowances and Manifestations of Imbalance		
VITAMIN	**RDA**	**MANIFESTATIONS OF OVERDOSE**	**MANIFESTATIONS OF DEFICIENCIES**
Fat Soluble			
• A	Men: 1000 μg/retinol equivalents* Women: 800 μg/retinol equivalents	Hair loss, dry skin; headaches; dry mucous membranes; liver damage; bone and joint pain; blurred vision; nausea and vomiting	Dry, scaly skin; increased susceptibility to infection; night blindness; anorexia; eye irritation; xerosis (dry skin); keratinization of respiratory and GI mucosa; bladder stones; anemia; retarded growth
• D	Adults: 5-10 μg of cholecalciferol†	Deposits of calcium and phosphorus in soft tissue; kidney and heart damage; bone fragility; constipation; anorexia, nausea, vomiting; headache	Muscular weakness; excessive sweating; diarrhea and other GI disturbances; bone pain; active rickets; healed rickets; osteomalacia
• E	Men: 10 mg Women: 8 mg	Relatively nontoxic	Neurologic defects
• K	Men: 70-80 μg Women: 60-65 μg	Anemia	Defective blood coagulation
Water Soluble			
• B₁	Men: 1.2-1.5 mg Women: 1-1.1 mg	Not stored in body, therefore overdose does not occur	Loss of appetite; fatigue; nervous irritability; constipation; paresthesias; insomnia
• B₆	Men: 1.7-2 mg Women: 1.4-1.6 mg	Not stored in body, therefore overdose does not occur	Seizures; dermatitis; anemia; neuropathy with motor weakness; anorexia
• Cobalamin (B₁₂)	Adults: 2-10 μg	Not stored in body, therefore overdose does not occur	Megaloblastic anemia; inadequate myelin synthesis; anorexia; glossitis; sore mouth and tongue; pallor; neurologic problems such as depression and dizziness; weight loss; nausea; constipation
• C	Adults: 50-60 mg	Not stored in body, therefore overdose does not occur	Bleeding gums; loose teeth; easy bruising; poor wound healing; scurvy; dry, itchy skin
• Folic acid	Men: 200 μg Women: 180 μg	Not stored in body, therefore overdose does not occur	Impaired cell division and protein synthesis; megaloblastic anemia; anorexia; fatigue; sore tongue; diarrhea; forgetfulness

*1 Retinol equivalent = 10 IU vitamin A activity from β-carotene or 3.33 IU vitamin A activity from retinol.
†1 μg of cholecalciferol = 40 IU vitamin D.
GI, Gastrointestinal; *RDA,* recommended dietary allowance.

TABLE 39-7	Common Drug and Food/Nutrient Interactions	
DRUG CATEGORY/DRUG	**FOOD/NUTRIENT**	**DRUG-FOOD EFFECTS OR CAUTIONS**
Anticoagulants	Dietary vitamin K (e.g., green leafy vegetables, green tea, dairy products/meats)	Decrease or loss of anticoagulant effect
Antiseizure agents • phenytoin (Dilantin)	Folic acid	Long-term drug use may increase folic acid requirement
Antidepressants • trazodone (Desyrel) • Tricyclic antidepressants	Food Riboflavin	Food slows drug absorption Riboflavin requirements may increase with amitriptyline (Elavil) or imipramine (Tofranil)
Antidiabetic agents • glyburide (Micronase, DiaBeta)	High-fat diet	Drug should not be taken with high-fat diet
Antithyroid agents • methimazole (Tapazole)	Food	Foods may inconsistently alter bioavailability of methimazole
Barbiturates • phenobarbital • mephobarbital (Mebaral)	Folic acid	Drugs may increase folic acid requirements; long-term therapy may require vitamin D supplements for osteomalacia
β-Adrenergic blockers • labetalol (Normodyne) • metaproterenol (Alupent) • carteolol (Cartrol) • sotalol (Betapace)	Food	Bioavailability of these drugs may be enhanced when taken with food
Bronchodilators • theophylline • oxtriphylline (Choledyl) • dyphylline (Lufyllin)	High-carbohydrate, low-protein diets Caffeine-containing foods and fluids	↓ Drug elimination Caffeine may increase CNS stimulant effects of xanthine-derivative bronchodilators
cholestyramine (Questran)	Fat-soluble vitamins	Drug may interfere with their absorption
Corticosteroids (prolonged therapy)	Salt seasonings	May require decreased sodium and/or potassium supplementation intake
erythropoietin	Folic acid and/or cobalamin	Nutrient deficiencies may reduce/delay drug response
etidronate (Didronel)	Foods, fluids, or drugs high in calcium	May prevent drug absorption
furazolidone (Furoxone)	Food and fluids containing tyramine (e.g., aged cheese, smoked or pickled meats or poultry, fermented meat, overripe fruit, beer, wine, liqueurs)	MAO-inhibiting effects may last at least 2 wk after stopping drug. Dietary restrictions need to continue for at least 2 wk after MAO inhibitors discontinued if received large doses or prolonged therapy
isoniazid (INH)	Cheese (e.g., Swiss) or fish (e.g., tuna, skipjack)	Concurrent ingestion may lead to redness or itching, HR changes, sweating, chills or clammy feeling, headache or light-headedness; thought to be related to altered metabolism of tyramine in foods
Phenothiazines	Riboflavin	Drugs may increase riboflavin requirements
procarbazine (Matulane)	Food and fluids containing tyramine or other high-pressor amines (e.g., aged cheese, smoked or pickled meats or poultry, fermented meat, overripe fruit, beer, wine, liqueurs)	When used concurrently, may cause sudden and severe hypertensive reactions; dietary restrictions need to continue for at least 2 wk after MAO inhibitors discontinued
selegiline (Eldepryl)	Food and fluids containing tyramine (e.g., aged cheese, smoked or pickled meats or poultry, fermented meat, overripe fruit, beer, wine, liqueurs)	When used concurrently, may cause sudden and severe hypertensive reactions; dietary restrictions need to continue for at least 2 wk after MAO inhibitors discontinued
ticlopidine (Ticlid)	Food	Drug absorption increased when taken after a meal
zafirlukast (Accolate)	High-fat and high-protein meal	When taken concurrently, drug bioavailability reduced by about 40%
Zinc supplements	Foods	Many foods (e.g., fiber, milk casein) impair zinc absorption

CNS, Central nervous system; *HR,* heart rate; *MAO,* monoamine oxidase.

and food/nutrient interactions. As members of the health team, nurses have a responsibility for monitoring and preventing potential interactions for patients while in the hospital and at home.

Clinical Manifestations. The adult who is deprived of adequate protein and calories will have many of the clinical manifestations presented in Table 39-8. The most obvious clinical signs on physical examination are apparent in the skin, eyes, mouth, muscles, and CNS. The speed at which the protein deficiency develops depends on the quantity and quality of the protein intake, caloric value, illness, and the age of the person.

Clinical manifestations of malnutrition are the result of numerous interactions occurring at the cellular level. As protein intake is severely reduced, the muscles, which make up the largest reservoir of protein in the body, become wasted and flabby, leading to weakness, fatigability, and decreased endurance. There is decreased protein available for repair, and as a result, wound healing may be delayed. Malnutrition in the hospitalized patient may result in delayed recovery and prolonged hospitalization. The person is more susceptible to all types of infections. Both humoral and cell-mediated immunity are deficient in PCM. There is a decrease in leukocytes in the peripheral blood. Phagocytosis is altered as a result of the lack of energy (adenosine triphosphate [ATP]) necessary to drive the process. Most malnourished persons are anemic. Anemia resulting from PCM is usually caused by nutritional deficiencies in iron and folic acid, the necessary building blocks for red blood cells (RBCs).

The severity of complications from malnutrition ranges from mild to emaciation and death. Major complications center around

TABLE 39-8	Manifestations of Protein–Calorie Malnutrition	
BODY SYSTEM	**SUBCLINICAL MANIFESTATIONS**	**CLINICAL MANIFESTATIONS**
Integumentary	Slowed tissue turnover rate, surface temperature 1°–2° F cooler	Brittle nails, ↓ tone and elasticity of skin, xeroderma (dry skin), pigment changes (brown–gray), erythematous seborrheic dermatitis, scrotal dermatitis
Visual	Night blindness	Hair: easy loss of hair, color changes, lack of luster
		Blood vessel growth in cornea, Bitot's spots (gray keratinized epithelium on conjunctiva), dryness of conjunctiva and cornea, pale to red conjunctiva
Gastrointestinal		
Mouth and lips	Reduction in saliva production	Cheilosis (crusting and ulceration at angle of mouth)
Tongue	Mucosa more permeable to bacteria	Raw and beefy red, edematous and smooth, atrophy or hypertrophy of papillae
Teeth	Improper development, delayed eruption	Caries, loose teeth, discolored enamel
Gingivae		Periodontal disease, tendency to bleed easily, receding, pale, and soft
Stomach	↓ Gastric secretion, delayed gastric emptying	Constant hunger, ↑ incidence of ulcers
Intestines	↓ Motility and absorption, normal flora causing infection from ↑ permeability of mucosa	Diarrhea and flatulence, protruding abdomen, ↑ incidence of parasitic diseases
Liver–biliary	Fatty liver, ↓ absorption of fat-soluble vitamins	Hepatomegaly
Cardiovascular	↓ Cardiac output, ↓ hemoglobin, shift in heart position, ↑ risk of thrombophlebitis	↓ Blood pressure and pulse, slight cyanosis, anemia, body edema
Endocrine	↓ Insulin production	Thyroid enlargement, polydipsia, polyuria, ↑ sensitivity to cold
Immunologic	↓ Lymphocyte proliferation, ↓ albumin levels, ↓ antibody production, diminished febrile response to infection	↑ Number of infections, ↓ response to delayed hypersensitivity skin tests
Musculoskeletal	↓ Growth rate, ↓ body stature with chronic PCM, ↓ muscle mass	Prominence of bony structures such as face, clavicle, scapula, ribs, iliac crests, and spinal vertebrae due to subcutaneous tissue loss; weak and spindly arms and legs, flat buttocks, weak and flabby muscles; ↓ physical activity and ability to work; severe weight loss
Neurologic	Loss of ambition, feeling of being tired	Depression, confusion, ↓ reflexes in legs and ankles, ↓ position sense, ↓ vibratory sense, paresthesias of hands and feet, syncope, motor weakness
Renal	Negative nitrogen balance, ↓ BUN and creatinine levels	Nocturia, ↓ urinary output
Reproductive	↓ Gonadotropin levels	Amenorrhea, impotence, atrophied breasts
Respiratory	Pulmonary edema, ↓ strength of respiratory muscles	↑ Susceptibility to respiratory infection, ↓ respiratory rate, ↓ vital capacity

BUN, Blood urea nitrogen; *PCM,* protein–calorie malnutrition.

delayed wound healing and increased susceptibility to infection from decreased immune function.

Diagnostic Studies

History and physical examination. A diet history of foods eaten over the past week will reveal a great deal about the patient's dietary habits and knowledge of good nutrition. In addition to the height, weight, and vital signs, the patient's physical state should be thoroughly assessed and documented. Each body system should be assessed. Table 39-9 summarizes the assessment and findings of the patient with malnutrition.

The diagnosis of PCM can be determined by a variety of laboratory studies used in conjunction with the physical examination. Serum albumin is somewhat useful in the diagnosis of malnutrition. The degree of protein depletion can be identified with the use of the scale in Table 39-10. Serum albumin has a half-life of approximately 20 to 22 days. In the absence of marked fluid loss, such as from hemorrhage or burns, the serum albumin value lags behind actual protein changes by more than 2 weeks and

TABLE 39-10	Serum Albumin and Prealbumin Levels
Albumin	
Normal value	3.8-4.5 g/dl (38-45 g/L)
Mild depletion	3.0-3.7 g/dl (30-37 g/L)
Moderate depletion	2.5-2.9 g/dl (25-29 g/L)
Severe depletion	<2.5 g/dl (<25 g/L)
Prealbumin	
Normal value	20 mg/dl (200 mg/L)
Mild depletion	10-15 mg/dl (100-150 mg/L)
Moderate depletion	5-10 mg/dl (50-100 mg/L)
Severe depletion	<5 mg/dl (<50 mg/L)

TABLE 39-9   Nursing Assessment
Malnutrition

Subjective Data

Important Health Information

Past health history: Severe burns, major trauma, hemorrhage, draining wounds, bone fractures with prolonged immobility, chronic renal or liver disease, cancer, malabsorption syndrome, GI obstruction, infectious diseases (TB, AIDS)

Medications: Corticosteroids, chemotherapeutic agents, diet pills

Surgery or other treatments: Recent surgery, radiation

Functional Health Patterns

Health perception–health management: Alcohol or drug abuse; malaise, apathy

Nutritional-metabolic: Increase or decrease in weight, weight problems; increase or decrease in appetite, typical dietary intake; food preferences and aversions; food allergies or intolerance; ill-fitting or absent dentures; dry mouth, difficulty in chewing or swallowing; bloating or gas; ↑ sensitivity to cold; delayed wound healing

Elimination: Constipation, diarrhea, nocturia, decreased urinary output

Activity-exercise: Increase or decrease in activity patterns; weakness, fatigue, decreased endurance

Cognitive-perceptual: Pain in mouth; paresthesias; loss of position and vibratory sense

Role-relationship: Change in family (e.g., loss of a spouse); financial resources

Sexual-reproductive: Amenorrhea, impotence, decreased libido

Objective Data

General

Listless, cachectic; underweight for height

Integumentary

Dry, brittle, sparse hair with color changes and lack of luster, alopecia; dry, scaly lips, fever blisters, angular crusts and lesions at corners of mouth (cheilosis); brittle, ridged nails; decreased tone and elasticity of skin; cool, rough, dry, scaly skin with brown-gray pigment changes; reddened, scaly dermatitis, scrotal dermatitis; slight cyanosis; peripheral edema

Eyes

Pale or red conjunctivae, gray keratinized epithelium on conjunctiva (Bitot's spots); dryness and dull appearance of conjunctiva and cornea, soft cornea; blood vessel growth in cornea; redness and fissuring of eyelid corners

Respiratory

Decreased respiratory rate, ↓ vital capacity, crackles, weak cough

Cardiovascular

Increase or decrease in heart rate, ↓ BP, arrhythmias

Gastrointestinal

Swollen, smooth, raw, beefy red tongue (glossitis), hypertrophic or atrophic papillae; dental caries, absent or loose teeth, discolored tooth enamel; spongy, pale, receded gums with a tendency to bleed easily, periodontal disease; ulcerations, white patches or plaques, redness, swelling of oral mucosa; distended, tympanic abdomen; ascites, hepatomegaly, decreased bowel sounds; steatorrhea

Neurologic

Decreased or loss of reflexes, tremor; inattention, irritability, confusion, syncope

Musculoskeletal

Decreased muscle mass with poor tone, "wasted" appearance; bowlegs, knock-knees, beaded ribs, chest deformity, prominent bony structures

Possible Findings

↓ Hemoglobin and hematocrit; ↓ MCV, MCH, or MCHC (iron deficiency); ↑ MCV or MHC (folic acid or cobalamin deficiency); altered serum electrolyte levels, especially hyperkalemia; ↓ BUN and creatinine; ↓ serum albumin, transferrin, and prealbumin; ↓ lymphocytes; ↑ liver enzymes; ↓ serum vitamin levels

---

AIDS, Acquired immunodeficiency syndrome; *BUN,* blood urea nitrogen; *GI,* gastrointestinal; *MCH,* mean corpuscular hemoglobin; *MCHC,* mean corpuscular hemoglobin concentration; *MCV,* mean corpuscular volume; *TB,* tuberculosis.

therefore is not a good indicator of acute changes in nutritional status. Prealbumin, a protein synthesized by liver, has a half-life of 2 days and is a better indicator of recent or current nutritional status.[9] Serum transferrin level is another indicator of protein status. Transferrin, a protein synthesized by the liver and used to transport iron, decreases during states of protein deficiency.

Serum electrolyte levels reflect changes taking place between the intracellular and the extracellular spaces. The serum potassium level is often elevated. The RBC count and the hemoglobin level indicate the presence and degree of anemia. The total lymphocyte count decreases during malnutrition states. The total lymphocyte count is calculated by multiplying the percent of lymphocytes times the total white blood cell (WBC) count. Liver enzyme levels, a reflection of liver function, may be elevated during malnutrition. Serum levels of both fat-soluble and water-soluble vitamins are usually diminished in malnutrition. The lowered levels of the fat-soluble vitamins correlate with the clinical signs of *steatorrhea* (fatty stools).

Anthropometric measurements. Anthropometric measurements, which include gross measures of fat and muscle contents, may be ordered. These measurements tend to be most beneficial in evaluating long-term effects of malnutrition or responses to nutritional interventions. They consist of measures of skinfold thickness at various sites, which is an indicator of subcutaneous fat stores, and midarm muscle circumference, an indicator of protein stores. These measurements are then compared with standards for healthy persons of the same age and gender. Training and practice are required to perform these measurements accurately and reliably. To provide information on the patient's nutritional status in response to treatment, serial measurements are needed. Sites most reflective of body fat are those over the biceps and the triceps, below the scapula, above the iliac crest, and over the upper thigh. Both skinfold thickness and mid-arm muscle circumference measurements are decreased in chronic PCM and acute protein malnutrition. These measurements may also be influenced by shifts in hydration status. The exact relationship of the midarm circumference measure to body composition of functional protein, both muscle and nonmuscle, remains to be established.

NURSING MANAGEMENT
MALNUTRITION

■ Nursing Assessment

Across all settings of care delivery, the nurse must be aware of the nutritional status of the patient. The recording of the patient's height and weight is an important component of this assessment. The patient's current weight relative to usual body weight and ideal body weight, such as that listed in the Metropolitan Life Insurance tables (Table 39-11), is determined. The percent change in body weight over time provides information on the degree of weight loss. In addition, the nurse should get a record of the complete diet history from the patient or the family. The patient's nutritional state may not be the reason medical assistance was sought. However, it may well be a major factor in the outcome and perhaps the underlying reason for illness. The registered dietitian, pharmacist, and physician should also be involved in the assessment and planning of care. However, the nurse, as the first-line health care professional dealing with the patient, should take the initiative in determining the severity of any nutritional problems.

TABLE 39-11	Desirable Weights for Men and Women*		
	FRAME SIZE		
HEIGHT	**SMALL**	**MEDIUM**	**LARGE**
Men			
5'2"	128-134	131-141	138-150
5'3"	130-136	133-143	140-153
5'4"	132-138	135-145	142-156
5'5"	134-140	137-148	144-160
5'6"	136-142	139-151	146-164
5'7"	138-145	142-154	149-168
5'8"	140-148	145-157	152-172
5'9"	142-151	148-160	155-176
5'10"	144-154	151-163	158-180
5'11"	146-157	154-166	161-184
6'	149-160	157-170	164-188
6'1"	152-164	160-174	168-192
6'2"	155-168	164-178	172-197
6'3"	158-172	167-182	176-202
6'4"	162-176	171-187	181-207
Women			
4'10"	102-111	109-121	118-131
4'11"	103-113	111-123	120-134
5'	104-115	113-126	122-137
5'1"	106-118	115-129	125-140
5'2"	108-121	118-132	128-143
5'3"	111-124	121-135	131-147
5'4"	114-127	124-138	134-151
5'5"	117-130	127-141	137-155
5'6"	120-133	130-144	140-159
5'7"	123-136	133-147	143-163
5'8"	126-139	136-150	146-167
5'9"	129-142	139-153	149-170
5'10"	132-145	142-156	152-173
5'11"	135-148	145-159	155-176
6'	138-151	148-162	158-179

*From 1983 Metropolitan Life Insurance Company weight tables by height and size of frame for people aged 25 to 59, in 1-inch shoes and wearing 5 lb of indoor clothing for men or 3 lb for women.

In many institutions (acute and long-term care) and in home care, the nurse is responsible for nutritional screening. Nutritional screening identifies individuals who are malnourished or at risk for malnutrition. The purpose of the nutrition screening is to determine if a more detailed nutrition assessment is necessary.[9-12] Table 39-12 provides an example of a nursing nutrition screening tool.[11] In long-term care, the Minimum Data Set (MDS) form queries the health care team on a number of items related to nutritional status.[12] In home care, the Outcome and Assessment Information Set (OASIS) prompts the nurse to collect myriad information on diet, oral intake, dental health, swallowing difficulties, and any needs for meal assistance. If nutritional problems are identified, a referral to a dietitian is suggested.

If the nutrition screening identifies an individual at nutritional risk, a full nutrition assessment is most often warranted. A nutrition assessment is a comprehensive approach to defining nutrition status that uses medical, nutrition, and medication histories; physical examination; anthropometric measurements; and laboratory data.[9]

TABLE 39-12 Admission Nutrition Screening Tool

A. Diagnosis

If the patient has at least *one* of the following diagnoses, circle and proceed to section E to consider the patient AT NUTRITIONAL RISK and stop here.

- Anorexia nervosa/bulimia nervosa
- Malabsorption (celiac sprue, ulcerative colitis, Crohn's disease, short bowel syndrome)
- Multiple trauma (closed head injury, penetrating trauma, multiple fractures)
- Pressure ulcers
- Major gastrointestinal surgery within the past year
- Cachexia (temporal wasting, muscle wasting, cancer, cardiac)
- Coma
- Diabetes
- End-stage liver disease
- End-stage renal disease
- Nonhealing wounds

B. Nutrition Intake History

If the patient has at least *one* of the following symptoms, circle and proceed to section E to consider the patient AT NUTRITIONAL RISK and stop here.

- Diarrhea (>500 ml × 2 days)
- Vomiting (>5 days)
- Reduced intake (<½ normal intake for >5 days)

C. Ideal Body Weight Standards

Compare the patient's current weight for height to the ideal body weight chart.

If at <80% of ideal body weight, proceed to section E to consider the patient AT NUTRITIONAL RISK and stop here.

D. Weight History

Any recent unplanned weight loss? No ___ Yes ___
  Amount (lb or kg) _____
  If yes, within the past _____ weeks or _____ months
  Current weight (lb or kg) _____
  Usual weight (lb or kg) _____
  Height (ft, in, or cm) _____
Find percentage of weight loss:

$$\frac{\text{Usual wt} - \text{Current wt}}{\text{Usual wt}} \times 100 = \text{\_\_\_\_\_ \% wt loss}$$

Compare the % wt loss with the chart below and circle appropriate value

Length of Time	Significant (%)	Severe (%)
1 week	1–2	>2
2–3 weeks	2–3	>3
1 month	4–5	>5
3 months	7–8	>8
5+ months	10	>10

If the patient has experienced a significant or severe weight loss, proceed to section E and consider the patient AT NUTRITIONAL RISK

E. Nurse Assessment

Using the above criteria, what is this patient's nutritional risk? (circle one)

LOW NUTRITIONAL RISK   AT NUTRITIONAL RISK

Adapted from Kovacevich DS et al: Nutrition risk classification: a valid and reproducible tool for nurses, *Nutr Clin Practice* 12:20-25, 1997.

■ Nursing Diagnoses

Nursing diagnoses for the patient with malnutrition include, but are not limited to, the following:

- Imbalanced nutrition: less than body requirements *related to* decreased access, ingestion, digestion, or absorption of food or to anorexia
- Self-care deficit (feeding) *related to* decreased strength and endurance, fatigue, and apathy
- Constipation or diarrhea *related to* poor eating patterns, immobility, or medication effects
- Deficient fluid volume *related to* factors affecting access to or absorption of fluids
- Risk for impaired skin integrity *related to* poor nutritional state
- Noncompliance *related to* alteration in perception, lack of motivation, or incompatibility of regimen with lifestyle or resources
- Activity intolerance *related to* weakness, fatigue, and inadequate caloric intake or iron stores

■ Planning

The overall goals are that the patient with malnutrition will (1) achieve weight gain, (2) consume a specified number of calories per day (with a diet individualized for the patient), and (3) have no adverse consequences related to malnutrition or nutrition therapies.

■ Nursing Implementation

Health Promotion. The nurse is in a good position to teach and reinforce healthy eating habits with individuals and groups of persons throughout their life span. The gap between perceived importance of nutrition and care in selecting foods has widened. To assist in these efforts are the Food and Drug Administration (FDA)–mandated food labels that are now on all packaged foods. The Dietary Guidelines for Americans offers key recommendations for improving nutrition that are useful points for a teaching program (Table 39-13).[13]

Acute Intervention. The nurse must assess the patient's nutritional state, as well as focus on the other physical problems of the patient. The nurse must become more aware of who is at risk, why, and how to intervene appropriately. In states of increased stress, such as surgery, severe trauma, and sepsis, more calories and protein are needed. Wound healing requires increased protein synthesis. When fever is present, the metabolic rate is increased

TABLE 39-13 Patient & Family Teaching Guide — Good Nutrition

The following recommendations apply to most people:

- Eat a variety of foods
- Choose a diet moderate in sugars
- Choose a diet moderate in salt and sodium
- If you drink alcoholic beverages, do so in moderation
- Choose a diet low in fat, unsaturated fat, and cholesterol
- Choose a diet with plenty of grain products, vegetables, and fruits
- Balance the food you eat with physical activity to maintain or improve your weight

and nitrogen loss is accelerated. Despite the return of body temperature to normal, the rate of protein breakdown and resynthesis may be accelerated for several weeks. After major surgery, several weeks of increased protein and calorie intake are needed to promote healing and replenish body stores.

The nurse must have a thorough understanding of nutritional support and the rationale for recording the daily weight, intake, and output. Daily weights can give an ongoing record of body weight gain or loss. However, rapid gains and losses are usually the result of shifts in fluid balance. The body weight, in conjunction with accurate recording of food and fluid intake, provides a clearer picture of the patient's fluid and nutritional state. To obtain an accurate weight, the nurse should weigh the patient at the same time each day, on the same scale, with the same type or amount of clothing, and preferably with the bladder recently emptied.

The protein and calorie intake required in the malnourished patient depends on the cause of the malnutrition, the treatment being employed, and other stressors affecting the patient. If the patient is able to take food by mouth, a daily calorie count and diet diary can be obtained to give an accurate record of food intake. The nurse and the dietitian working with the patient and family can assist in the selection of high-calorie and high-protein foods (unless medically contraindicated). Preparation of foods preferred by the patient enhances the daily intake. Discussion with the patient and family about foods that should be eaten to provide high-protein, high-calorie content is important. The family can be encouraged to bring the patient's favorite foods from home while the patient is still hospitalized. Table 39-14 gives an example of a high-calorie, high-protein diet.

The undernourished patient usually needs to have between-meal supplements. These may consist of items prepared in the dietary department or commercially prepared products. Eating these items between meals increases the total daily intake and provides extra calories, proteins, fluids, and nutrients. In addition, multiple small feedings improve the tolerance for food intake by distributing the amount more evenly throughout the day. If the patient is unable to consume enough nutrition with a high-calorie, high-protein diet, nutrition supplements can be added.

TABLE 39-14	Nutritional Therapy
	High-Calorie, High-Protein Diet

General Principles

1. A normal diet is supplemented with larger portions to increase the protein and caloric content. It is used for patients with hypermetabolism, burns, excessive stress, and cancer.
2. It is important to eat regularly and not to skip meals or snacks.

MEAL	PROTEIN (G)	SAMPLE MENU PLAN 1	SAMPLE MENU PLAN 2	MENU PLAN 3
Breakfast				
Fruit	2	Large orange juice	Large apple juice	½ grapefruit
Starch, fat		1 toast with butter or jelly	Flour tortilla with butter	Biscuits and gravy
Starch, protein supplement	4	Cream of wheat with 2 tbs skim milk powder	Atole with 2 tbs skim milk powder	Grits with 2 tbs margarine
2 meat	14	2 poached eggs	2 fried eggs	Omelet with 2 eggs
Milk, protein supplement	10	High-protein milk shake (2 tbs skim milk powder added)	High-protein milk shake	High-protein milk shake
Lunch				
4 meat	28	Cheeseburger on bun with double meat patty, lettuce, tomato	2 burritos with extra cheese, meat	Split pea soup with ham hocks
4 starches	8			Grilled cheese sandwich
Vegetable	2		Lettuce and tomato salad with dressing	Watermelon wedge
4 fats		French fried potatoes	Biscochitos	Sugar cookies
Milk, protein supplement	10	High-protein milk shake	High-protein milk shake	High-protein milk shake
Dinner				
4 meat	28	Spaghetti with 4 oz meat sauce, Parmesan cheese	2 tamales with red chili sauce	4 oz fried chicken
3 starches	6			Sweet potato
Vegetable	2	Green beans with 2 tbs margarine	Spanish rice	Mustard greens with 2 tbs butter
			Peas with 2 tbs butter	
7 fats		Bread with butter	Custard	Biscuit
		Tapioca pudding		Vanilla ice cream
Milk, protein supplement	10	High-protein milk shake	High-protein milk shake	High-protein milk shake
Snack				
Milk	8	Fruit yogurt	Cottage cheese with fruit	½ sandwich with peanut butter
Fruit				Banana
TOTAL	132			

Elemental diets are liquid products (e.g., Peptamen) that can be used as dietary supplements or complete meal replacements. They contain glucose, peptides, essential fatty acids, vitamins, and minerals, and can be fed orally or enterally. They require minimal digestion and are easily absorbed in the small intestine.

If the patient is still unable to take in enough calories, tube feedings may be considered. Total parenteral nutrition (TPN) may be initiated if enteral feedings are not feasible.

Ambulatory and Home Care. With shortened hospital stays, many patients are discharged on a therapeutic diet. Discharge preparation for both the patient and the family is important. They must be carefully instructed on the cause of the undernourished state and ways to avoid the problem in the future. The patient must be made aware that undernourishment, whatever the cause, can recur and that adhering to a diet high in protein and calories for a few weeks cannot fully restore a normal nutritional state. Many months are needed to reach this goal. Diet instruction is usually carried out by the dietitian, but it is important for the nurse to assess the patient's understanding and reinforce the information whenever possible. The patient's ability to comply with the dietary instructions must be examined in light of past eating habits, religious and ethnic preferences, age, income, other resources, and state of health.

Unless the patient and the family can be convinced of the necessity for dietary change and have the resources to effect change, it is likely that no long-term benefits will be achieved. Ways should be found in which the patient can become actively involved in the recovery. The need for continuous follow-up care must be strongly emphasized if rehabilitation is to be accomplished and maintained.

The nurse is in an ideal position to determine the need for nutritious meals and snacks after discharge from the hospital. In addition, it is important to consider the availability and acceptability of community resources that provide meals. Such aspects can be integrated into discharge planning and follow-up home visits by the nurse.

Keeping a diet diary or a calorie count for 3 days at a time is one way to analyze and reinforce healthful eating patterns. These records are also helpful to the health care team in the follow-up care. Self-assessment of progress can be encouraged by having the patient weighed once or twice a week and keeping a weight record.

■ Evaluation

The expected outcomes are that the patient who is malnourished will

- achieve and maintain optimal body weight
- consume a well-balanced diet
- experience no adverse outcomes related to malnutrition

■ Gerontologic Considerations: Malnutrition

Older adults are at risk for malnutrition with many factors influencing their nutritional intake (Table 39-15). Many of these factors may occur at the same time, thus further increasing the risk of malnutrition. The unique nutritional requirements of an older adult are often overlooked. As a person grows older there are decreases in lean body mass (the metabolically active tissue), basal metabolic rate, and physical activity. Combined, these factors decrease the caloric needs for energy. The older person frequently reduces the consumption of needed protein, vitamins, and minerals and may take in "empty calories," such as candy and pastries. As a group,

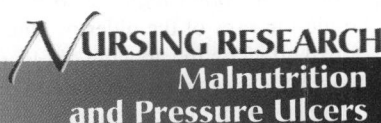

TABLE 39-15 Gerontologic Differences in Assessment
Factors Affecting Nutritional Intake in Older Adults

Physical Factors
Age
Anorexia
Decreased number of taste buds
Dental problems
Food intolerances
Health status
Physical disability
Prescribed diets
Prescribed or over-the-counter drugs

Psychosocial Factors
Importance of food in the past
Loneliness or loss
Mental awareness
Social isolation

Socioeconomic Factors
Available time for food preparation and eating
Availability of desired foods
Availability of transportation to food stores
Education level and nutritional knowledge
Food fads
Income level
Lack of food preparation equipment

∧ URSING RESEARCH
Malnutrition and Pressure Ulcers

Citation Guenter P et al: Survey of nutritional status in newly hospitalized patients with stage III or stage IV pressure ulcers, *Adv Skin Wound Care* 13:164, 2000.

Purpose To examine the relationship between nutritional status and pressure ulcers in patients newly admitted to an acute care facility.

Methods Newly admitted non-ICU patients (n = 120) with stage III or stage IV pressure ulcers were included in the study. Measures included demographic characteristics, weight, serum prealbumin and albumin levels, nutritional intake, and type of pressure ulcer.

Results and Conclusions The majority of patients were elderly; had a stage III sacral pressure ulcer, low prealbumin levels, and inadequate nutritional intake; and were below their usual weight. Patients admitted into acute care facilities with pressure ulcers are often malnourished, and aggressive nutritional therapy may be indicated.

Implications for Nursing Practice The nurse plays an important role in identifying patients at risk for malnutrition. The presence of pressure ulcers or delays in wound healing are important signs that nutritional intake may not be adequate. Older patients are particularly at risk for malnutrition and its adverse consequences.

ICU, Intensive care unit.

older adults may be less well informed about what constitutes a well-balanced diet.

When these factors are added to already existing medical problems, it is easy to see why poor dietary practices develop. In addition, poor dentition, ill-fitting dentures, anorexia, multiple losses affecting the social setting of meals, low income, and medical conditions involving the GI tract contribute to the type and amount of foods that are eaten. The nurse, working with the dietitian, must be aware of common medical and psychosocial factors in the older adult and should incorporate interventions for overcoming these problems in the plan of care.

Some of the physiologic changes associated with aging affect the nutritional status of older adults. The following changes are of particular interest:

1. Changes in the oral cavity (e.g., change in bite surfaces of the teeth, periodontal disease, drying of the mucous membrane of the mouth and tongue, poorly fitting dentures, decreased muscle strength for chewing, decreased number of taste buds, decreased saliva production)
2. Changes in digestion and motility (e.g., decreased absorption of cobalamin, vitamin A, and folic acid and decreased GI motility)
3. Changes in the endocrine system (e.g., decreased tolerance to glucose)
4. Changes in the musculoskeletal system (e.g., decreased bone density, degenerative joint changes)
5. Decrease in vision and hearing (e.g., procurement and preparation of food are more difficult)

Certain illnesses that are more prevalent in the older population are considered to be diet related. These include atherosclerosis, osteoporosis, diabetes mellitus, and diverticulosis. Multiple drugs are often required to treat these and other common chronic illnesses of the older patient. These drugs often have an adverse effect on the appetite of older adults, increasing the possibility of inadequate intake caused by anorexia.

To date, with the exception of calories, it has not been determined that older adults have different requirements for specific nutrients from those of middle-aged adults. Generally, caloric intake should decrease with age because of the progressive loss of lean body mass and a decrease in the basal metabolic rate. Therefore fewer calories are needed to meet metabolic needs. Unless caloric intake is decreased by careful attention to food intake, or energy expenditure is increased through greater physical activity and exercise, obesity will result.

Socioeconomic factors are important variables when assessing the nutritional status of an older adult. Because more than one third of older adults have incomes below the poverty level, obtaining adequate and nutritious food can be an ongoing problem. In many cases the older person cannot afford to purchase meat, fresh vegetables, and fruits that provide many necessary nutrients.

Lifestyle changes such as retirement or relocation to a nursing home can have a significant impact on the eating habits of the older adult. Other important considerations that should be assessed include the ethnic background, previous dietary practices, food preferences, knowledge of proper diet, availability and accessibility of food stores, transportation, and health status. Problems related to any or all of these areas can alert the nurse to the possibility of a nutritional problem.

Malnutrition can occur in an older person even though the caloric requirements decrease with age. If malnutrition is present, few malnourished older persons are able to ingest enough

food to correct the malnourished state. Special strategies, such as adaptive devices (e.g., large-handled eating utensils), often are helpful in increasing dietary intake. Some older persons may require nutritional support therapies until their strength and general health are improved.

Many community nutritional programs are available to the older person to make mealtime a pleasant, social event. Improving the social setting of a meal often improves the dietary intake. Home-delivered meals and meal sites in a central location are popular meal alternatives for many older adults. The use of food stamps is another alternative that allows low-income households, regardless of age, to buy more food of a greater variety.

TYPES OF SPECIALIZED NUTRITION SUPPORT

Oral Feeding

High-calorie oral supplements may be used in the patient whose nutritional intake is deficient. This may include milk shakes, puddings, or commercially available products (e.g., Ensure, Sustacal). Research suggests that ingestion of these beverages may have a role in improving the nutritional status of elderly patients.[14] These supplements should not be used as meal substitutes but between meals as snacks. In some long-term care facilities, these beverages are used instead of water with oral medication administration to increase caloric intake.

Tube Feeding

Tube feeding refers to the administration of a nutritionally balanced liquefied food or formula through a tube inserted into the stomach, duodenum, or jejunum. Tube feedings may be ordered for the patient who has a functioning GI tract but is unable to take any or enough oral nourishment. Specific indications for tube feeding include those persons with anorexia, orofacial fractures, head and neck cancer, neurologic or psychiatric conditions that prevent oral intake, and extensive burns and those who are receiving chemotherapy or radiation therapy. Tube feedings are considered to be easily administered, safer, more physiologically efficient, and definitely less expensive than parenteral nutrition. They are used to provide nutrients by way of the GI tract either alone or as a supplement to oral or parenteral nutrition.

Common delivery options are continuous infusion by pump, intermittent by gravity, intermittent bolus by syringe, and cyclic feedings by infusion pump. Continuous infusion is most often used with critically ill patients and feedings into the small intestine. Intermittent feeding may be preferred as the patient improves or is receiving such feedings at home.[15]

A nasogastric (NG) tube is most commonly used for short-term feeding problems. If the feedings are necessary for an extended time, other means of feeding may be used, such as an esophagostomy tube, a gastrostomy tube (placed surgically, endoscopically, or radiologically), or a jejunostomy tube that empties directly into the jejunum. Transpyloric (nasointestinal) tube placement or placement into the jejunum is used when physiologic conditions warrant feeding the patient below the pyloric sphincter. (Fig. 39-3 shows the locations of commonly used enteral feeding tubes.)

Nasogastric and Nasointestinal Tubes. Feeding tubes made of polyurethane or silicone materials have added to the comfort level of the patient over extended periods. These tubes are long, small in diameter, soft, and flexible, thereby decreasing the risk of mucosal damage from prolonged placement. The older

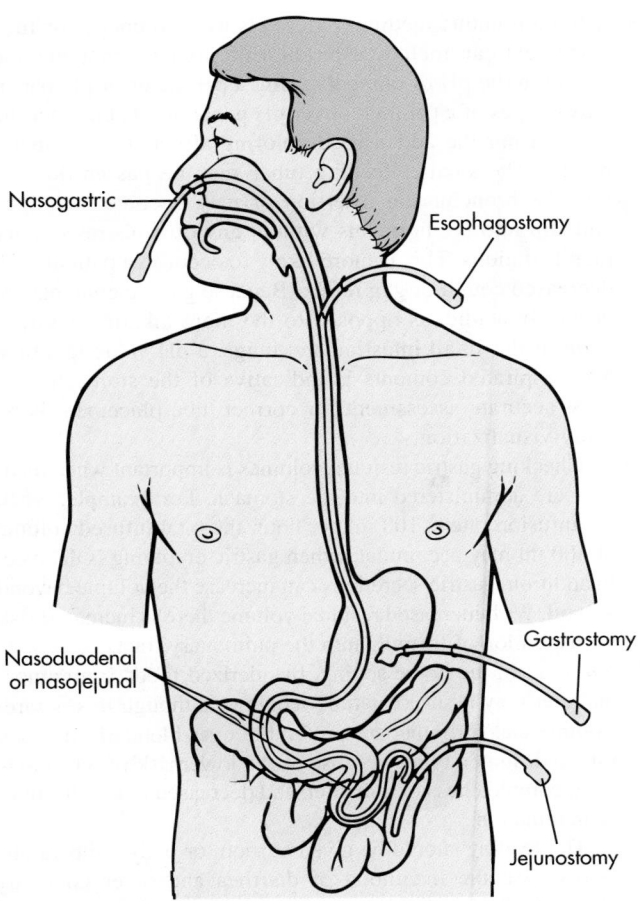

FIG. 39-3 Common enteral feeding tube placement locations.

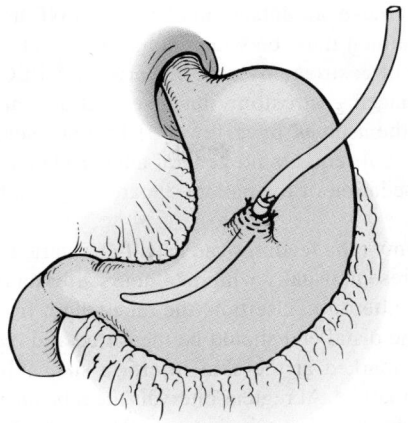

FIG. 39-4 Placement of a gastrostomy tube.

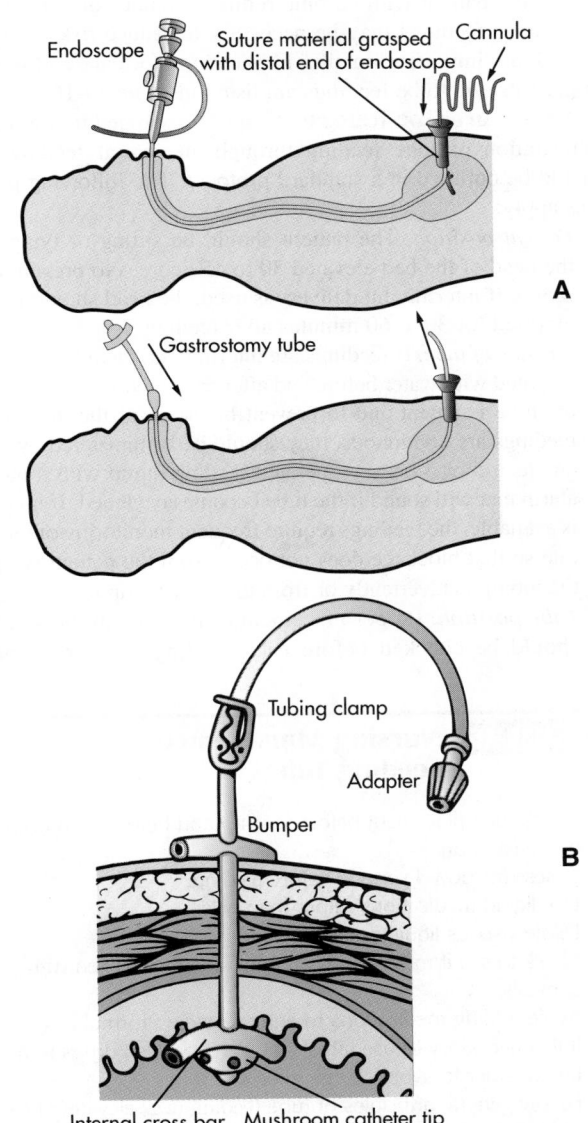

FIG. 39-5 Percutaneous endoscopic gastrostomy. **A,** Gastrostomy tube placement via percutaneous endoscopy. Using endoscopy, a gastrostomy tube is inserted through the esophagus into the stomach and then pulled through a stab wound made in the abdominal wall. **B,** A retention disk and bumper secure the tube.

tubes made of rubber or polyvinyl chloride tend to stiffen with time. Polyurethane and silicone tubes are radiopaque, making their position readily identified by x-ray. Many of these tubes also have weighted tips, allowing for easier passage of the tube through the pylorus into the duodenum. Placement into the intestine theoretically decreases the likelihood of regurgitation of contents into the esophagus and subsequent aspiration. With the use of a stylet, these tubes can be placed in a comatose patient because the ability to swallow is not essential during insertion.

Although the smaller feeding tubes have many advantages over wider-lumen tubes, such as the standard decompression NG tube, there are some disadvantages. Because of the small diameter, these tubes are more easily clogged when feedings are thick and are more difficult to use for checking residual volumes. They are particularly prone to obstruction when oral drugs have not been thoroughly crushed and dissolved in water before administration. They can become dislodged by vomiting or coughing and can also become knotted or kinked in the GI tract. Failure to flush the tubing after both drug administration and residual volume determinations can result in tube clogging. When the tube becomes clogged, it may necessitate removal and insertion of a new tube, adding to cost and patient discomfort.

Gastrostomy and Jejunostomy. A gastrostomy tube may be used for a patient who requires tube feedings over an extended time (Fig. 39-4). Gastrostomy tubes can be placed surgically, radiologically, or endoscopically. See Fig. 39-5 for the placement procedure of a percutaneous endoscopic gastrostomy (PEG). The patient must have an intact, unobstructed GI tract, and the esophageal lumen must be wide enough to pass the endoscope for this type of gastrostomy tube placement. A PEG and a radiologically placed gastrostomy have several advantages. These procedures themselves have fewer risks than surgical placement. Because it requires no general anesthesia and only minimum or no sedation of the patient, laparotomy can be done at a lower cost.

Gastrostomy tube feedings can usually be started when bowel sounds are present, usually within 24 hours after tube placement. Immediately after tube insertion, the tube length from the insertion site to the distal end should be measured and recorded. The tube is then marked at the skin insertion site, although many tubes are premarked. At regular intervals the tube insertion length should be rechecked. The tube is most often connected to a pump for continuous feeding. Water may be infused within 2 hours after placement.

For the patient with chronic reflux, a jejunostomy tube with continuous feedings may be necessary to reduce risk of aspiration. Some important nursing implications for care and feeding of patients with tube feedings are listed in Table 39-16.

Procedures for Tube Feedings. The procedure for the administration of tube feeding through an enteral feeding tube should be outlined in a standard protocol. The following principles apply:

1. *Patient position.* The patient should be sitting or lying with the head of the bed elevated 30 to 45 degrees to prevent aspiration. If intermittent delivery is used, the head should remain elevated for 30 to 60 minutes after feeding.

2. *Patency of tube.* If feedings are intermittent, the tube should be irrigated with water before and after each feeding to ensure that the tube is patent and to prevent blockage of the tube. If the feedings are continuous, they should be administered by using an electric or a battery-operated feeding pump with a built-in alarm that will sound if the tube becomes occluded. If no pump is available, the feedings require frequent monitoring of the drip rate so that blockage does not occur from the patient lying on the tubing inadvertently or from too slow a drip rate.

3. *Tube position.* Proper placement of the tube in the stomach should be checked before each feeding or every 8 hours

with continuous feedings. Methods used to check for tube placement can include aspiration of stomach contents and checking the pH of contents using a pH meter or pH paper. Advantages of a pH meter over pH paper are that neither the formula nor the added food coloring affects the pH meter results. The smaller feeding tubes may be passed directly into the bronchus on insertion or may become dislodged and slip into the bronchus without any obvious respiratory manifestations. This is more likely to occur in a patient with decreased cough or gag reflex. Because gastric contents are primarily acidic, as opposed to the more alkaline environment of the small intestine and lungs, a pH value less than 5 on aspirated contents is indicative of the stomach. The most accurate assessment for correct tube placement is by x-ray visualization.

Checking gastric residual volumes is important when feedings are administered into the stomach. For example, when the infusion rate is 100 ml per hour, the total infused volume of 400 ml may accumulate when gastric emptying is delayed. In addition, gastric secretions can increase the volume beyond 400 ml. With increased residual volume there is increased risk for aspiration of formula into the pulmonary tract.

4. *Formula.* In the home setting, blenderized foods from a normal diet may be used as tube feedings, although this is rare. Commercial formulas are preferable over blenderized foods for small-lumen tubes because of the lower risk of tube clogging, completeness of nutrition, and decreased risk of formula contamination.

The feeding should be given at room or body temperature to decrease the likelihood of diarrhea and other GI complaints. The pleasurable aspects of eating, such as smelling, seeing, tasting, and chewing the food, are frequently denied the tube-fed patient. If the clinical condition permits, the patient may be allowed to smell, taste, and even chew small amounts of food before the feeding, and then the chewed food must be spit out. The patient may hesitate to do this because it is not esthetic, but it stimulates salivary and gastric secretions and provides the pleasurable sensations associated with oral intake. Before initiating the feeding, the nurse should aspirate gastric contents and measure the amount. If the volume is greater than 200 ml and there are clinical signs of intolerance, including nausea or increase in abdominal girth, the next feeding is held for 1 hour and then the residual volume is rechecked. The aspirate should be reinstilled.[16]

5. *Administration of feeding.* Feedings are administered either by gravity drip method or by feeding pump. Applying pressure to force the feeding can damage the tube. The feeding rate or volume is increased gradually for 24 to 48 hours to minimize side effects, such as nausea or diarrhea. If intermittent feedings are ordered, the volume is usually 200 to 500 ml per feeding. It is important to remember that the patient still needs water, and this may be administered with flush water or as additional boluses of water as tolerated.

6. *General nursing considerations.* The patient should be weighed daily or several times a week, and accurate intake and output records should be maintained. These measures provide information on weight gain or loss, as well as tolerance of the feedings. Initially blood glucose checks to assess glucose tolerance are performed at the bedside. An older patient who has baseline glucose intolerance is particularly at risk for hyperglycemia.

TABLE 39-16   Nursing Management: Feeding Tubes

- Check tube placement before feeding and before each drug administration.
- Assess for bowel sounds before feeding.
- Use liquid medications rather than pills.
  Dilute viscous liquid medications.
  Check to see if medications are intended to be taken with meals.
  Avoid adding medications to enteral feeding formula.
- If it is necessary to use tablets, be sure to crush drugs to a fine powder to avoid clogging feeding tubes.
- Follow general principles of tube feeding (e.g., elevating head of bed, checking for residual volumes, and flushing tube with water).
- Assess regularly for complications (e.g., aspiration, diarrhea, abdominal distention, hyperglycemia, constipation, and fecal impaction).

Feedings that have been opened and not refrigerated or feedings that have been infusing longer than 8 hours should be discarded to prevent the administration of possible contaminated feedings. Feedings should be labeled with the date and time they are initially used. If a pump is used, pump tubing should be changed every 24 hours or per manufacturer's guidelines. See NCP 39-1 for care of the patient receiving enteral nutrition.

Complications Related to Tubes and Feedings. The types of problems encountered in patients receiving tube feedings and corrective measures are presented in Table 39-17. When commercial products are used, the concentration, flavor, osmolarity, and amounts of protein, sodium, and fat vary according to the manufacturer. Most commercial formulas are lactose free. The concentrations range from 1 to 2 kcal/ml, with most between 1 and 1.5 kcal/ml.

NURSING CARE PLAN 39-1

Patient Receiving Enteral Nutrition

EXPECTED PATIENT OUTCOMES	NURSING INTERVENTIONS and *RATIONALES*
NURSING DIAGNOSIS	**Imbalanced nutrition: less than body requirements** *related to* enteral feeding problems *as manifested by* body weight less than ideal, diarrhea, abdominal distention.
▪ Stable or gain in weight ▪ No diarrhea or abdominal distention	▪ Monitor weight and compare with baseline *to make adjustments as needed in calorie intake.* ▪ Progress the patient slowly from clear liquids to blenderized foods *to prevent gastric distention.* ▪ Gradually add high-calorie foods to patient's blenderized foods *to maintain body weight while preventing distention.*
NURSING DIAGNOSIS	**Impaired skin integrity** *related to* enzymatic action of gastric juices that may leak around tube *as manifested by* red, irritated tissue around the tube.*
▪ No skin breakdown around tube ▪ Daily inspections of skin performed and any problems reported	▪ Assess skin daily for signs of irritation *so that early treatment is provided.* ▪ Wash skin around the tube with soap and water daily; apply a protective skin barrier such as zinc oxide or petrolatum or a Stomahesive wafer *to maintain skin integrity.* ▪ Teach patient and family to assess and provide care *to ensure involvement in self-care and early detection of problems.*
NURSING DIAGNOSIS	**Disturbed body image** *related to* presence of feeding tube *as manifested by* refusal to participate in own feeding, verbalization of fear of rejection by family and friends, avoidance of social activities associated with food and eating.
▪ Participation in self-care related to feedings ▪ Verbalization of acceptance of enteral feeding	▪ Encourage patient to express feelings about the enteral feedings *to increase the patient's self-awareness.* ▪ Provide information about the tube, feedings, purpose, and patient progress *so that the patient makes decisions based on correct information.* ▪ Acknowledge the patient's fears *to establish a trusting nurse-patient relationship.*
NURSING DIAGNOSIS	**Risk for deficient fluid volume** *related to* diarrhea or inadequate fluid intake.
▪ No signs of fluid volume deficit ▪ Adequate fluid intake	▪ Monitor patient for poor skin turgor, decreased blood pressure, tachycardia, decreased urine output, and dry mucous membranes *to identify signs of fluid volume deficit.* ▪ Provide adequate fluid intake, including water, as determined by intake records. ▪ Monitor urine output for osmotic diuresis, *which may occur secondary to high glucose load of feedings or too rapid infusion.* ▪ Identify possible cause of diarrhea *so that appropriate treatment is started.*
NURSING DIAGNOSIS	**Ineffective therapeutic regimen management** *related to* care required for skin around tubing and tube feedings *as manifested by* questioning about self-care.
▪ Demonstration of skin care and tube feeding before discharge	▪ Assess the patient's home environment and lifestyle *to make teaching relevant to individual requirements.* ▪ Provide detailed information about how to prepare the formula and how to manage the tube feeding *to facilitate self-care.* ▪ Use return demonstration technique *to validate patient's and family's learning of the necessary skills.*
NURSING DIAGNOSIS	**Risk for aspiration** *related to* enteral tube with tube feedings.
▪ No aspiration Able to describe measures to prevent aspiration	▪ During feeding have the patient's head elevated at least 30 degrees; remain in this position 30 minutes after feeding *to prevent aspiration.* ▪ Aspirate gastric contents before feeding *to validate gastric emptying.* ▪ Reinstill the residual gastric contents *to prevent excessive fluid and electrolyte losses.*

*This applies to feeding tubes that have been inserted through the skin.

TABLE 39-17	Common Problems of Patients Receiving Tube Feedings
PROBLEMS AND POSSIBLE CAUSES	**CORRECTIVE MEASURES**

Vomiting and/or Aspiration

• Improper placement of tube	Replace tube in proper position. Check tube position before beginning feeding and every 8 hr if continuous feedings.
• Delayed gastric emptying, increased residual volume	Hold feeding 1 hr; then if residual volume is less than previous rate, resume feeding.
• Potential for aspiration	Keep head of bed elevated to 30- to 45-degree angle. Have patient sit up on side of bed or in chair. Encourage ambulation unless contraindicated.
• Contamination of formula	Refrigerate unused formula and record date opened. Discard outdated formula every 24 hr. Discard formula left standing for longer than manufacturer's guidelines: 8-12 hr for ready-to-feed formulas (cans) or 4 hr for reconstituted formula. Use closed system to prevent contamination.

Diarrhea

• Feeding too fast, hypertonic formula, or medications	Decrease rate of feeding. Change to continuous drip feedings. Check for drugs that may cause diarrhea (e.g., antibiotics).
• Lactose intolerance	Consult health care provider for change in formula to lactose-free solution.
• Contamination of formula or tubing	Change tubing every 24 hr. Hang 8-hr formula at a time. Do not exceed manufacturer's guidelines.
• Low-fiber formula	Change to formula with more fiber.
• Tube moving distally	Properly secure tube before beginning feeding. Check before each feeding or at least every 24 hr if continuous feedings.

Constipation

• Formula components	Consult health care provider for change in formula to one with more fiber content. Obtain laxative order.
• Poor fluid intake	Increase fluid intake if not contraindicated. Give free water, as well as formula. Give total fluid intake of 30 ml/kg body weight.
• Drugs	Check for drugs that may be constipating.
• Impaction	Perform rectal examinations to check and manually remove feces if present.

Dehydration

• Excessive diarrhea, vomiting	Decrease rate or change formula. Check drugs that patient is receiving, especially antibiotics. Take care to prevent bacterial contamination of formula and equipment.
• Poor fluid intake	Increase intake and check amount and number of feedings. Increase amount of intake if appropriate.
• High protein formula	Change formula.
• Hyperosmotic diuresis	Check blood glucose levels frequently. Change formula.

The osmolality of the solution is determined by the number and size of particles in solution. With regard to feeding formulas, the more hydrolyzed or broken down the nutrients, the greater the osmolality. Many tube feeding formulas are isotonic, although some are hypertonic. The more calorically dense the formula, the less water it contains. Protein content greater than 16% can lead to dehydration unless the patient is given supplemental fluids or is sufficiently alert to request additional fluids. The nurse must be aware of this potential problem and must provide extra fluids through the feeding tube or, if permitted, by mouth. Tube feedings with high sodium content are contraindicated in the patient with cardiovascular problems, such as congestive heart failure. High fat content is not advocated for a patient with short bowel syndrome or ileocecal resections because of impaired fat absorption.

The dietitian can be of considerable assistance to the nursing staff. When close consultation with the nursing staff occurs, existing problems with tube feedings can be quickly and efficiently addressed and resolved. Some institutions have nutrition support teams composed of a physician, nurse, dietitian, and pharmacist whose function is to oversee the nutrition support of select inpatients and outpatients.

In patients receiving gastrostomy or jejunostomy feeding, the nurse should be alert to two possible problems: (1) skin irritation and (2) pulling out of the tube. Skin care around the tube site is important because the action of the digestive juices is irritating to the skin. The skin around the feeding tube should be assessed daily for signs of redness and maceration. To keep the skin clean and dry, initially it should be rinsed with sterile water and dried. Once the site has healed, it can be washed with mild soap and water. A protective ointment (zinc oxide, petroleum gauze) or a skin barrier (Karaya, Stomahesive) may be used on the skin around the tube. A small dressing may be placed around the tube until the site is healed and must be changed promptly if it gets wet. Other types of drain or tube pouches may be used if there is a problem with skin irritation, and an enterostomal therapist can be of great assistance to the nurse if these issues arise. The patient and family members can be taught how to care for the feeding tube. Teaching should include skin care, care of the tube, and complete information about feeding administration and potential complications.[17]

■ Gerontologic Considerations: Enteral Nutrition

Enteral nutrition strategies, including NG, nasointestinal, and gastrostomy feedings, are often used in the older patient to improve nutritional status. Because of physiologic changes associated with aging, the older adult is more vulnerable to complications associated with these interventions, especially fluid and electrolyte imbalances. Complications such as diarrhea can leave the patient dehydrated. Decreased thirst perception or impaired cognitive function decreases the ability of the patient to seek additional fluids.

With aging there is decreased ability to handle glucose loads (glucose intolerance). As a result, the older patient may be more susceptible to problems of hyperglycemia in response to the high carbohydrate load of some enteral feeding formulas. If the older adult has compromised cardiovascular function (e.g., congestive heart failure), there will be a decreased ability to handle large volumes of formula. In this situation the use of more concentrated formulas may be warranted. The older adult also is at increased risk for aspiration caused by gastroesophageal reflux disease, hiatal hernia, or diminished gag reflex. Physical mobility, fine motor movement, and visual system changes associated with aging may contribute to difficulties in managing enteral nutrition equipment at home. In addition, age-related changes such as a decrease in lean muscle mass influence the reliability of measures used for nutritional assessment.

Total Parenteral Nutrition

When the GI tract cannot be used for the ingestion, digestion, and absorption of essential nutrients, TPN may be substituted. **Parenteral nutrition** refers to the administration of nutrients by a route (e.g., bloodstream) other than the GI tract. **Total parenteral nutrition** is the delivery of a nutritionally adequate hypertonic solution consisting of glucose, protein hydrolysates, minerals, and vitamins using an intravenous (IV) route. TPN has become a relatively safe and practical method of delivering total nutritional needs. The goal of using TPN is to meet the patient's nutritional needs and to allow growth of new body tissue. Regular IV solutions of 5% dextrose (5 g dextrose/100 ml) in water (D5W) or 5% dextrose in lactated Ringer's solution (D5LR) contain no protein and have approximately 170 calories per liter. The normal adult requires a minimum of 1200 to 1500 calories per day to carry out normal physiologic functions. Patients who sustain severe injury, surgery, or burns and those who are malnourished as a result of medical treatment or disease processes have greatly increased nutritional needs. The volume of regular dextrose solutions needed to meet these high caloric requirements could exceed the capacity of the cardiovascular system. Table 39-18 lists common indications for the use of TPN.

Composition. Commercially prepared TPN base solutions are available for both central and peripheral use. These base solutions contain dextrose and protein in the form of amino acids. The pharmacy adds the prescribed electrolytes (e.g., sodium, potassium, chloride, calcium, magnesium, and phosphate), vitamins, and trace elements (e.g., zinc, copper, chromium, and manganese) to customize the solution for the patient. A three-in-one

TABLE 39-18	Common Indications for Total Parenteral Nutrition

- Chronic diarrhea and vomiting
- Complicated surgery or trauma
- Gastrointestinal obstruction
- Gastrointestinal tract anomalies and fistulae
- Hypermetabolic states (sepsis, fractures)
- Intractable diarrhea
- Malnutrition
- Pancreatitis
- Severe anorexia nervosa
- Severe malabsorption
- Short bowel syndrome

or total nutrient admixture containing an IV fat emulsion, dextrose, and amino acids has become widely used, especially in the home setting.

Calories. Calories in TPN are supplied primarily by carbohydrates in the form of dextrose and by fat in the form of fat emulsion. The administration of between 100 and 150 g of dextrose (1 g provides approximately 3.4 calories, as opposed to oral carbohydrates, which provide 4 calories) daily has a protein-sparing effect. Adequate nonprotein calories in the form of glucose and lipids must be provided to allow metabolism of amino acids for wound healing and not as energy. However, overfeeding can lead to metabolic complications. To minimize these problems, an energy intake of 25 to 30 calories per kilogram per day in a nonobese patient is often recommended. Providing both lipid and carbohydrate components meets the energy requirement while minimizing problems of overfeeding. The FDA has approved the use of 10%, 20%, and 30% fat emulsion solutions. These lipid emulsions provide approximately 1 calorie per milliliter (10% solution) or 2 calories per milliliter (20% solution). The contents of fat emulsion are primarily soybean or safflower triglycerides with egg phospholipids added as an emulsifier. In practice, the conservative approach is IV-administered fat emulsions providing not more than 30% of the total energy to minimize possible immunosuppressive effects of linoleic acid. The maximum fat emulsion amount should not exceed a dose of 2.5 g/kg per day[18] and should be administered slowly over 12 to 24 hours. Nausea, vomiting, and elevated temperature have been reported, especially when lipids are infused quickly. The administration of fat emulsion is contraindicated in the patient with a disturbance in fat metabolism. It should also be used with caution in the patient who is in danger of fat embolism (e.g., fractured femur) and the patient with an allergy to eggs.

Protein. The normal healthy person of average body size needs approximately 45 to 65 g of protein daily. Protein should be provided at the rate of 1 to 1.5 g/kg per day depending on the patient's needs. In a nutritionally depleted patient under the stress of illness or surgery, requirements can exceed 150 g per day to ensure a positive nitrogen balance. In the most recent guidelines, protein intake levels of 1.5 to 2 g/kg per day are suggested for most patients with moderate to severe stress.[4]

Electrolytes. The assessment of individual requirements should take place daily at the beginning of therapy and then several times a week as the treatment progresses. The following are ranges for average daily electrolyte requirements for adult patients without renal or hepatic impairment:

Sodium: 1 to 2 mEq/kg
Potassium: 1 to 2 mEq/kg
Chloride: As needed to maintain acid-base balance
Magnesium: 8 to 20 mEq
Calcium: 10 to 15 mEq
Phosphate: 20 to 40 mmol

The exact amount needed depends on the patient's health problem and on electrolyte levels as determined by blood testing.

Trace elements. Zinc, copper, chromium, manganese, selenium, molybdenum, and iodine supplements may be added according to the patient's condition and needs. Levels of these elements are monitored in the patient receiving TPN. The health care provider may order additional amounts of these elements to be added to the solutions according to the patient's requirements.

Vitamins. The daily addition of a multivitamin preparation to the TPN generally meets the vitamin requirements. If multivitamin infusion is used, the cobalamin (vitamin B_{12}) requirement may be met without the need for supplemental injections. It may be necessary for the physician to order vitamin K separately because it is currently not included in the multivitamin preparation.

Methods of Administration. Parenteral nutrition may be administered by central or peripheral veins. *Central parenteral nutrition* is given through a catheter whose tip lies in the superior vena cava. The central venous catheter often originates at the subclavian or jugular vein. More recently, single- or double-lumen peripherally inserted central catheters (PICCs) are being placed, usually into the basilic or cephalic vein and then advanced into the central circulation. Such catheters are made of soft, flexible material (silicon, polymer) and are 20 to 24 inches long. Ease of placement, cost, and limited complications make this an attractive alternative to a subclavian vein catheter. Central TPN is indicated when long-term parenteral support is necessary or when the patient has high protein and caloric requirements.

Peripheral parenteral nutrition (PPN) is administered through a peripherally inserted catheter or vascular access device, which uses a large peripheral vein. PPN is used when (1) nutritional support is needed for only a short time, (2) protein and caloric requirements are not high, (3) the risk of a central catheter is too great, or (4) parenteral nutrition is used to supplement inadequate oral intake. Both central and peripheral parenteral nutrition are used in a patient who is not a candidate for enteral support.

Central and peripheral parenteral nutrition differ in tonicity, which is measured in milliosmoles (mOsm; the concentration of particles in a fluid). Blood is isotonic and measures approximately 280 mOsm/L. The standard IV solutions of D_5W and normal saline are essentially isotonic. Central TPN solutions are hypertonic, measuring at least 1600 mOsm/L. The high glucose content ranges from 20% to 50%. Central TPN must be infused in a large central vein so that rapid dilution can occur. The use of a peripheral vein for central TPN would cause irritation and thrombophlebitis. Nutrients can be infused using smaller volumes than PPN. PPN is hypertonic (using as much as 20% glucose), but less so than central TPN, and can be safely administered through a large peripheral vein, although phlebitis can occur. Another potential complication of PPN is fluid overload.

All TPN solutions should be prepared by a pharmacist or a trained technician using strict aseptic techniques under a laminar flow hood. Nothing should be added to parenteral nutrition solutions after they are prepared in the pharmacy. The danger of drug incompatibilities and contamination is high. The fewer the personnel involved in the preparation and administration of TPN, the lower the risk of infection for the patient. In most hospitals the health care provider must order the TPN solution daily. In this way the solution and additives can be adjusted to the patient's current needs. Each TPN solution label indicates the nutrient content, all additives, the time mixed, and the date and time of expiration. In general, solutions are good for 24 hours and must be refrigerated until a half hour before use.

Catheter Placement. The central placement of the catheter into a large main vein for TPN is performed by the physician or a specially trained advanced practice nurse. The vein most commonly used is the subclavian, although the innominate or the jugular vein may be used. The procedure is the same as for the insertion of a central venous pressure line and should be done under strict aseptic conditions.

A standard isotonic IV solution is infused through the central line until x-ray confirms proper placement of the catheter tip in the superior vena cava and not in the jugular vein. The catheter insertion site is covered with a sterile dressing. The date is marked on the dressing.

Placement of a PICC catheter is done under sterile conditions, often by a specially trained nurse. A baseline measurement of the upper arm circumference is recommended. A tourniquet is then placed around the upper arm near the axilla to allow examination of the antecubital fossa and selection of a vein. If possible, the patient should be supine with the arm straight and at a 90-degree angle. Preparation of the insertion site should be done according to institutional policy. The sterile catheter is cut to the predetermined length, depending on the vein selected.

A local anesthetic is usually used at the insertion site. This site should be cleaned, protected, and maintained according to institutional policy. As with the centrally placed line, a chest x-ray is needed to verify proper tip placement before administering any TPN solution. Proper placement of a catheter for central TPN is illustrated in Fig. 39-6. Complications frequently

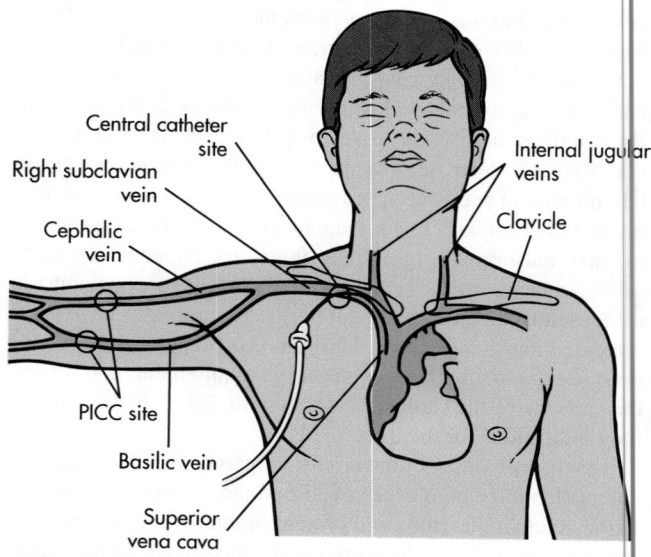

FIG. 39-6 Placement of a catheter for total parenteral nutrition using subclavian vein. Peripherally inserted central catheters (PICC) are inserted using the basilic or cephalic vein.

TABLE 39-19 **Complications of Total Parenteral Nutrition**

Infection
Fungus
Gram-positive bacteria
Gram-negative bacteria

Metabolic Problems
Hyperglycemia; hypoglycemia; and hyperosmolar, hyperglycemic state
Prerenal azotemia
Essential fatty acid deficiency
Electrolyte and vitamin excesses and deficiencies
Trace mineral deficiencies
Hyperlipidemia

Mechanical Problems
Insertion
    Air embolus
    Pneumothorax, hemothorax, and hydrothorax
    Hemorrhage
Dislodgement
Thrombosis of great vein
Phlebitis

associated with catheter placement are hemorrhage, hydrothorax and pneumothorax, hemothorax, air embolus, and venous thrombosis. Once established for TPN, a single-lumen central catheter should not be used for the administration of blood or antibiotics, the drawing of blood samples, or the monitoring of central venous pressure.

Administration of Solution. Because TPN solutions are excellent media for microbial growth, it is essential that proper aseptic techniques be followed. The FDA recommends that a 0.22-micron Millipore filter be placed on parenteral solutions not containing fat emulsion and a 1.2-micron filter placed on solutions containing fat emulsion.[18] Filters and IV tubing are changed every 24 hours. The tubing and the filter should be clearly labeled with the date and the time they are put into use. Complications of TPN can be divided into three categories: (1) infection, (2) metabolic, and (3) mechanical. The major complications of each category are presented in Table 39-19.

NURSING MANAGEMENT
TOTAL PARENTERAL NUTRITION

Vital signs should be monitored every 4 to 8 hours in the patient receiving TPN. Daily weights give an indication of the patient's hydration status as therapy progresses. Body weight is considered the sum of the changes in protein, fat, and water. On a daily basis, body water fluctuates more than protein or fat. Analysis must be made of whether gains or losses in weight are caused by fluid gained from edema, fluid lost through diuresis, or actual increase or decrease in tissue weight. Blood levels of glucose, electrolytes, and urea nitrogen; a complete blood count; and hepatic enzyme studies are followed 3 times per week until stable and then weekly as the patient's condition warrants. Assessment of these important values assists the nurse in evaluating the patient's tolerance of parenteral nutrition. A nursing care plan for the patient receiving parenteral nutrition is presented on page 990.

Dressings covering the catheter site are changed according to institutional protocol, ranging from every other day to once a week. Some institutions have specially trained nurses from the IV team or the nutritional support team who are responsible for these dressing changes, whereas others have the staff nurse do the dressing changes after special instruction. The procedure for changing the dressing is similar to that followed after catheter insertion. The institutional routine should be followed with respect to the appropriate use of solutions for the dressing change. The site is carefully observed for signs of inflammation and infection. Phlebitis can readily occur in the vein as a result of the hypertonic infusion, and the area can become infected. The patient receiving parenteral nutrition may be immunosuppressed and thus more susceptible to opportunistic infections. In this patient, signs of inflammation or infection can be subtle, if present at all. Many patients receiving TPN are receiving chemotherapy, corticosteroids, or antibiotics, which can mask signs of infection.

If sutures are used to anchor the catheter, they may become infected. If an infection is suspected during dressing change, a culture specimen of the site and drainage should be sent for analysis, and the health care provider should be notified immediately. The use of an occlusive dressing protects the wound from contamination.

Hyperglycemia is a metabolic complication of parenteral nutrition. At the beginning of TPN therapy, the solution is infused at a gradually increasing rate for 24 to 48 hours. This allows the pancreas to adapt to the increased amount of glucose in the circulation by producing more insulin. Blood glucose levels should be checked at the bedside every 4 to 6 hours with a glucose-testing meter (see Chapter 47). Some increase in the blood glucose level is expected during the first few days after TPN is started. A sliding scale dose of insulin may be ordered to keep the glucose level below 150 mg/dl (8.34 mmol/L).[19]

The nurse must be made aware that speeding or slowing the infusion rate is contraindicated. Speeding up the rate results in a large amount of glucose entering the circulation. Endogenous insulin levels often are not adequate to handle this increase in glucose, and a hyperglycemic state results. Conversely, slowing the rate may result in a hypoglycemic state because it takes time for the pancreatic islet cells to adjust to a reduced glucose level. Checking the amount infused and the rate every 30 minutes to 1 hour is recommended. An infusion pump must be used during administration of TPN so that the infusion rate can be maintained, and an alarm will sound if the tubing becomes obstructed. Even though an infusion pump is being used, the nurse should periodically check the volume infused because pump malfunctions can alter the rate.

Before setting up and administering TPN, the nurse must check the label and ingredients in the solution to see that they are what the health care provider ordered. Solutions must also be examined for signs of contamination, such as a cloudy appearance. If contamination is suspected, the solution should be returned promptly to the pharmacy for replacement. It is the nurse's responsibility to ensure that the TPN solution is discontinued and replaced with a new solution if the bag is not empty at the end of 24 hours. At room temperature, the solution is an excellent medium for microorganism growth.

NURSING CARE PLAN 39-2

Patient Receiving Total Parenteral Nutrition

EXPECTED PATIENT OUTCOMES	NURSING INTERVENTIONS and *RATIONALES*
NURSING DIAGNOSIS	**Risk for infection** *related to* placement of a central venous access catheter, inadequate aseptic practices, and decreased defense mechanisms.
▪ No manifestations of infection ▪ Normal body temperature	▪ Use protocols for infusion of solution and tubing and filter changes; change occlusive dressing over catheter site according to institutional policy *to minimize the possibility of infection.* ▪ Observe for signs of inflammation and infection; monitor vital signs q4hr *to ensure early detection of infection.*
NURSING DIAGNOSIS	**Anxiety** *related to* inability to ingest food and fluids; lack of knowledge regarding catheter position; benefits and management of TPN *as manifested by* restlessness and apprehension; frequent questioning regarding care of catheter and TPN line.
▪ Statement of rationale for and demonstration of care of TPN line	▪ Instruct patient on rationale and benefits of TPN and care of line *because knowledge and facts may reduce anxiety.* ▪ Illustrate catheter position by drawings and pictures *to increase patient understanding.*

COLLABORATIVE PROBLEMS

NURSING GOALS	NURSING INTERVENTIONS and *RATIONALES*
POTENTIAL COMPLICATIONS	**Hyperglycemia, hypoglycemia, and electrolyte imbalances.**
▪ Monitor blood glucose and serum electrolytes ▪ Report deviations from acceptable parameters ▪ Carry out medical and nursing interventions	▪ Monitor for signs of hyperglycemia such as thirst, polyuria, confusion, elevated blood glucose, blurred vision, dizziness, nausea and vomiting, and dehydration to plan appropriate treatment. ▪ Monitor for signs of hypoglycemia such as sweating, hunger, weakness, and tremors *to ensure early intervention.* ▪ Monitor serum electrolyte levels daily *to identify and treat complications early.* ▪ Check for symptoms of hyperkalemia (e.g., muscle weakness, flaccid paralysis, cardiac arrhythmias, abdominal cramps, diarrhea) and hypokalemia (e.g., general weakness, decreased muscle tone, weak or irregular pulse, low blood pressure, shallow respirations, abdominal distention, and ileus).* ▪ Maintain accurate infusion rate *to control the amount of glucose administered and prevent fluctuations in blood glucose levels.* ▪ Never increase or decrease flow rate by more than 10% *to prevent fluctuations in blood glucose levels.* ▪ Never stop TPN abruptly unless it is replaced by another glucose source *to prevent hypoglycemia.*

*Other manifestations of electrolyte imbalances are discussed in Chapter 16.

Sometimes fat emulsions are infused separately from the parenteral nutrition solution. The preferred delivery method is a continuous low volume, such as 20% lipids delivered over 12 hours, depending on patient needs. Adverse reactions that can occur are allergic manifestations, dyspnea, cyanosis, fever, flushing, phlebitis, chest and back pain, and pain at the IV site. A major benefit derived from IV fat administration is that a large number of calories can be provided in a relatively small amount of fluid. This is especially beneficial when the patient is at risk for fluid overload.

Catheter-related infection and septicemia can occur in patients receiving TPN through both peripherally and centrally placed lines. Local manifestations of infection include erythema, tenderness, and exudate at the catheter insertion site. Systemically the patient may have fever, chills, nausea, vomiting, and malaise. If no other causes can be identified, a catheter-related infection is suspected. Because of the risk of infection, catheters with antibiotic or antiseptic surfaces may be used. To diagnose the presence

of infection and to determine the causative organism, cultures are performed of the catheter tip if the catheter has been removed or of the blood in the catheter if still in place. Blood cultures are drawn simultaneously from the catheter and a peripheral vein. A chest x-ray is taken to detect changes in pulmonary status. The current TPN solution with tubing and filter should also be cultured and replaced with an entirely new setup. When the catheter tip is the source of infection, antibiotic therapy may not be necessary because removal of the catheter can eliminate the problem.[10] A new central line may be immediately established or replaced by a peripheral route. It is important that a glucose source be maintained to prevent rebound hypoglycemia.

The same precautions should be followed in weaning from TPN as when therapy is being initiated. The flow rate must be gradually decreased for 1 to 2 hours, while oral intake is increased. If an emergency situation precludes a slow weaning process, other dextrose- or glucose-containing nutrients should be administered. When the catheter is removed, the dressing should be changed daily until the wound heals. Oral nourishment should be encouraged, and a careful record of intake should be maintained. Recording of body weight and laboratory analysis of serum electrolyte and glucose levels may continue.

■ Home Nutrition Support

Home parenteral or enteral nutrition is an accepted mode of nutritional therapy for the person who does not require hospitalization but who benefits from continued nutritional support. Some patients have been successfully treated at home for many months and even years. It is important for the nurse to educate the patient or the family about catheter or tube care, proper technique in mixing and handling of the solutions and tubing, and side effects.

Home nutrition therapies are expensive. For patients to be reimbursed for expenses, there are specific criteria that must be met. The nurse should have the discharge planning personnel involved early in the admission to help plan for such issues. Home nutrition support may also be a burden on the patient and caregivers and may affect quality of life. The nurse should make the family aware of support groups such as the OLEY Foundation (see resources at end of chapter for information) who provide peer support and advocacy.[4]

OBESITY

Obesity is as an abnormal increase in the proportion of fat cells, mainly in the viscera and subcutaneous tissues of the body. Obesity has reached epidemic proportions in our society. In the United States obesity is the most common nutritional problem. Recent data document that over 50% of adults are overweight, 15% are obese, 5% are seriously obese, and 3% have clinically severe obesity.[21]

The calculated **body mass index** (BMI) is a common clinical index of obesity or altered body fat distribution. A well-accepted scale has been developed to calculate BMI by gender using weight-to-height ratios[22] (see Chapter 39, Fig. 39-6). Individuals with a BMI of 25 to 29.9 kg/m^2 are classified as being overweight, those with values of 30 kg/m^2 or more are classified as obese, and those with a BMI of more than 40 kg/m^2 have clinically severe obesity.

The waist-to-hip ratio is another way to define obesity. This ratio is a method of describing the distribution of both subcutaneous and intraabdominal adipose tissue. The waist measurement is divided by the hip measurement to calculate the ratio. A number greater than 1 in men and 0.8 in women indicates overweight. This ratio increases with age and excessive weight.[22] When body weight exceeds 100% of the ideal body weight, it is classified as **morbid obesity.**

In obese persons a variety of problems occur at a rate higher than the expected rate. These include hypertension, hyperlipidemia, type 2 diabetes mellitus, degenerative joint disease, gout, insulin resistance with hyperinsulinemia, respiratory problems, cardiovascular disease, gallbladder disease, non-alcoholic fatty liver disease, stroke, and some kinds of cancer (e.g., breast, colon).[23] Several of these conditions improve if weight loss occurs.

Etiology and Pathophysiology

Many factors have been investigated in an effort to identify the critical elements in the development and maintenance of obesity. Once obesity is present, the number of calories consumed must exceed the energy expended for the condition to continue. However, there is debate about processes leading to obesity.

When assessing the obese patient, the nurse should consider several different types of questions, such as the following:

1. What is the psychologic importance of food to the patient?
2. Is the patient's food intake influenced by hunger?
3. Do the taste and appearance of food or other physical factors in the environment stimulate the patient to eat?
4. Is an emotional problem stimulating the patient to eat?
5. Are any stressors influencing the patient's eating patterns?
6. Do members of the patient's family have a tendency to be overweight?

The nurse must recognize that environmental and genetic factors are important. The children of obese parents tend to be obese. Obesity tends to affect several persons within a family. One biologic component related to obesity is leptin. Leptin is a hormone that mediates the expression of a host of neuropeptides regulating energy intake and expenditure.[24,25] Much more research is needed in this area of biologic and genetic etiologies. Environmental factors play a role in the development of obesity. These include sedentary lifestyle, plentiful food in the household, and socioeconomic status.

The emotional component of the tendency to overeat is powerful. People use food for many reasons, including comfort and reward. Some people are triggered by specific foods to continue eating beyond satiety. The social component of eating develops early in life when food is associated with pleasure and fun at such events as birthday parties, Thanksgiving, and religious holidays. All of these factors must be included when considering the etiology of obesity.

Diagnostic Studies

The majority of obese persons have *primary obesity,* that is, excess calorie intake for the body's metabolic demands. Others have *secondary obesity,* which can result from various congenital anomalies, chromosomal anomalies, metabolic problems, or CNS lesions and disorders. The first step in the treatment process is to determine whether any physical conditions are present. A thorough history and physical examination are necessary and will reveal the extent and duration of the obese state.

The current approach to determining the presence of obesity is the BMI discussed earlier in this chapter. The BMI is not dependent on frame size. Because the BMI value rises with age, it has been suggested that age-specific guidelines for older adults be established. The way to determine BMI is to measure height without shoes and weight with minimal clothing. The weight (expressed in kilograms) is divided by the height squared (expressed in meters). Normal BMI is 20 to 24.9[26] (see Fig. 39-7).

More sophisticated measures of obesity use densitometry, dual photon absorption, magnetic resonance imaging, and ultrasonography. However, such measures are generally used only for research purposes.

Collaborative Conservative Care

The health care provider should explore genetic and endocrine factors such as hypothyroidism, hypothalamic tumors, Cushing syndrome, hypogonadism in men, or polycystic ovarian disease in women. Laboratory tests of liver function, fasting glucose level, triglyceride level, and low- and high-density lipoprotein cholesterol levels assist in evaluating the cause and effects of obesity.

When no organic cause can be found for obesity, it should be considered a chronic, complex illness. Any supervised plan of

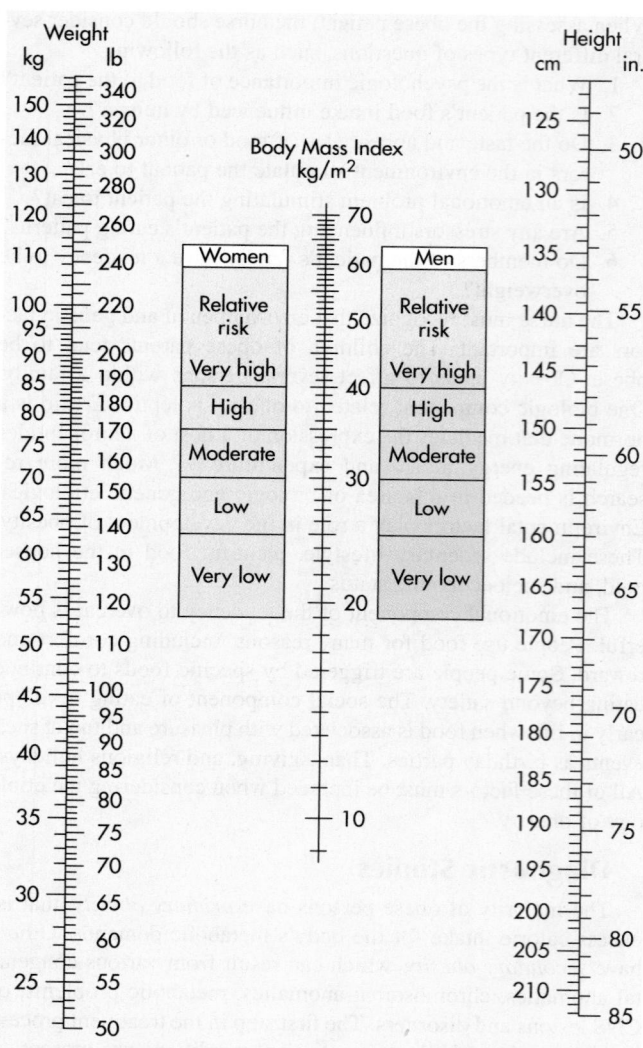

FIG. 39-7 Nomogram for determining body mass index (BMI). To use this nomogram, place a rule or other edge between the column for height and the column for weight connecting an individual's numbers for these two variables. Read the BMI in kg/m² where the straight line crosses the middle lines when the height and weight are connected. Overweight: BMI of 25 to 29.9 kg/m²; obesity: BMI of 30 kg/m² or more. Heights and weights are without shoes or clothes. Relative risk for health problems associated with obesity is shown.

care should be directed at (1) successful weight loss, requiring a short-term energy deficit, and (2) successful weight control, requiring long-term behavior changes. These are two different processes. A multipronged approach ought to be used with attention to multiple factors including dietary intake, physical activity, behavioral-cognitive modification, and perhaps drug therapy. Focusing on more than one aspect will likely give better balance to weight-loss and weight-control efforts.

Nutritional Therapy. Restricted food intake is a cornerstone for any weight loss or maintenance program. A good weight loss plan should contain foods from the basic food groups. Diets may be classified as low calorie (800 to 1200 calories per day) or very low calorie (less than 800 calories per day). Persons on low- and very low-calorie diets need frequent professional monitoring because the severe energy restriction places them at risk for mul-

EVIDENCE-BASED PRACTICE
Diet and Mortality Risk in Women

Clinical Problem
Is quality of diet associated with risk for mortality in women?

Best Clinical Practice
- Diet quality was assessed in 42,254 women over a 1–year period. Data were adjusted for age, race, education level, body mass index, smoking status, alcohol use, energy intake, hormone use, physical activity, and history of cancer, heart disease, or diabetes.
- Analyses showed an association between quality of diet (including fruits, vegetables, whole grains, low-fat dairy products, and lean meats) and risk of death from all causes, all types of cancer, coronary artery disease, and stroke.

Implications for Nursing Practice
Consumption of foods that are recommended in current dietary guidelines, including fruits, vegetables, whole grains, low-fat dairy products, and lean meats and poultry, can help decrease the risk for mortality in women.

Reference for Evidence
Kant AK et al: A prospective study of diet quality and mortality in women. *JAMA* 283:2109, 2000.

tiple nutrient deficiencies. A diet that includes adequate amounts of fruits and vegetables provides enough bulk to prevent constipation and meets daily vitamin A and vitamin C requirements. Lean meat, fish, and eggs provide sufficient protein, as well as the B-complex vitamins. Table 39-20 contains a sample 1200-calorie reducing diet.

The only effective method of treating primary obesity is to restrict dietary intake so that it is below energy requirements. It is rare to find an overweight person who has not at some time attempted to lose weight. Some have met with limited and temporary success, and others have met only with failure. It is likely that the majority of these persons attempted weight loss by trying out at least one of the many fad diets that offer the enticement to eat and get slim. In general, fad diets claim weight loss quickly, easily, and inexpensively. Although it is true that initially weight is lost, it is not fat but body water that is lost. The normal fat cell is composed of approximately 80% fat, 18% water, and 2% protein. It is also a storage area for small amounts of glycogen. Glycogen is known to bind with water. When reducing diets severely restrict carbohydrates, the body's glycogen stores become depleted within a few days. It is only when the glycogen pool is almost depleted that protein and adipose tissues are burned to release energy for bodily functions. An obese patient must understand that following a well-balanced, low-calorie diet is an essential part of weight loss.

The degree of success of any reducing diet depends in part on the amount of weight to be lost. A moderately obese person will obviously attain the goal more easily than will a massively obese person. Perhaps because men have a higher percentage of lean body mass, men are able to lose weight more quickly than women. Women have a higher percentage of body fat, which is metabolically less active than muscle tissue.

Motivation is an essential ingredient for successful achievement of weight loss. The obese patient must see the need for weight loss and weight control and the advantages that will oc-

TABLE	Nutritional Therapy
39-20	1200-Calorie-Restricted Weight-Reduction Diet*

General Principles
1. Eat regularly. Do not skip meals.
2. Measure foods to determine the correct portion size.
3. Avoid concentrated sweets, such as sugar, candy, honey, pies, cakes, cookies, and regular sodas.
4. Reduce fat intake by baking, broiling, or steaming foods.
5. Maintain a regular exercise program for successful weight loss.

MEAL	EXCHANGES	MEAL PLAN 1	MEAL PLAN 2	MEAL PLAN 3
Breakfast	1 meat	1 scrambled egg	1 hard-boiled egg	1 oz ham
	2 bread	1 slice toast	1 flour tortilla	2 griddle cakes with diet syrup
		¾ cup dry cereal (unsweetened)	½ cup Cream of Wheat	
	1 fruit	½ small banana	⅓ cup orange juice	⅓ cup pineapple juice
	1 fat	1 tsp margarine	1 slice bacon	1 tsp margarine
	1 dairy	1 cup low-fat milk	1 cup low-fat milk	1 cup low-fat milk
	Beverage	Coffee	Coffee	Coffee
Lunch	2 meat	1 slice bologna	Cheese enchiladas (made with 2 oz cheese, 2 corn tortillas, chili sauce)	2 oz baked breaded pork chop
		1 slice cheese		
	2 bread	2 slices bread		1 corn muffin
	Vegetable	Lettuce, pickles	Tomato wedges	Spinach
	1 fruit	Fresh grapes (12)	2 canned peach halves (packed in water)	Fresh orange
	Beverage	Diet soda	Artificially sweetened lemonade	Unsweetened iced tea
Dinner	2 meat	1 oz roast beef	Chili con carne (made with ½ cup ground beef, ½ cup pinto beans, and chili powder)	2 oz baked chicken
	1 bread	Baked potato with 1 tsp margarine†		Corn on the cob with 1 tsp margarine
	Vegetable	Cooked carrots	Tossed salad and 1 tbs salad dressing†	Okra
	1 fruit	¾ cup strawberries	Fresh apple	Fruit cocktail (packed in water)
	1 milk	1 cup low-fat milk	1 cup low-fat milk	1 cup low-fat milk

*For 1000 calories, omit 1 fruit exchange and change low-fat milk to skim milk. For 1500 calories, add 1 meat, 1 fruit, and 2 fat exchanges; change low-fat milk to whole milk. For 1800 calories, add 2 bread, 3 meat, 3 fat, and 1 fruit exchanges; change low-fat milk to whole milk.
†One extra fat exchange allowed for each cup of 2% low-fat milk; 2 extra fat exchanges allowed for each cup of skim milk.

cur. The nurse can assist by helping the patient track eating patterns by keeping a diet diary. A frank discussion of eating habits helps the patient realize that often eating is the result of bad habits picked up with time and not of hunger. The bad habits must be changed, or weight loss will be only temporary.

Setting a realistic goal, such as losing 1 to 2 pounds per week, must be mutually agreed on at the outset. Trying to lose too much too fast usually results in a sense of frustration and failure for the patient. The nurse can help the patient understand that losing large amounts of weight in a short period causes skin and underlying tissue to lose elasticity and tone and become unsightly folds of flabby tissue. Slower weight loss offers better cosmetic results. Inevitably, the patient reaches plateau periods during which no weight is lost. These plateaus may last from several days to several weeks. It is especially important for the patient to realize that these are normal occurrences during weight reduction, so that discouragement, frustration, and giving up of the prescribed dietary plan are prevented. A weekly check of body

weight is a good method of monitoring progress. Daily weighing is not recommended because of the frequent fluctuations resulting from retained water (including urine) and elimination of feces. The patient should be instructed to record the weight at the same time of the day, wearing the same type of clothing.

There is no firm agreement on the number of meals to be eaten when a person is on a diet. Some nutritionists advocate several small meals per day because the body's metabolic rate is temporarily increased immediately after eating. When several small meals a day are ingested, more calories are used. There seems to be general agreement that consumption of most of the daily caloric intake at a large evening meal results in less weight loss than when the calories are evenly distributed throughout the day.

When a person is first starting on a weight-reduction program, food portions should be weighed to stay within the dietary guidelines. After a time, weighing may not be necessary because the patient can make more accurate judgments of size and weight. A list of permitted foods serves as a good reference and permits an occasional meal to be eaten at a restaurant. The patient who carefully follows the prescribed diet may not need to take vitamin supplements. Appropriate fluid intake should be encouraged. Alcoholic beverages are usually not permitted on a reducing diet because they increase the caloric intake and are low in nutritional value.

Exercise. Exercise is an essential part of a weight-control program. There is no evidence that increased activity promotes an increase in appetite or leads to dietary excess. In fact, exercise frequently has the opposite effect. The addition of exercise produces more weight loss than does dieting alone. Exercise has a favorable effect on body fat distribution, with a reduction in waist-to-hip ratio with increased exercise. Exercise is especially important in maintaining weight loss in overweight persons. Overweight men and women who are active and fit have lower rates of morbidity and mortality than overweight persons who are sedentary and unfit. Therefore exercise is of benefit to overweight persons even if it does not make them lean.

Behavior-Cognitive Modification. For successful long-term weight loss management, behavior modification or cognitive therapy should be integrated into the management plan. Useful basic techniques include (1) self-monitoring, (2) stimulus control, and (3) rewards. Self-monitoring can focus on a record that shows what and when foods are eaten, as well as how the person was feeling when the foods were consumed. Stimulus control is aimed at separating events that trigger eating from the act of eating. Rewards may be used as incentive for weight loss. Short- and long-term goals are useful benchmarks for earning rewards. It is important that the reward for a specified weight loss not be associated with food, such as dinner out or a favorite treat. Reward items do not have to have a monetary component. For example, time for a hot bath or an hour of pleasure reading would be an enjoyable reward for many people. People may participate in group or individual sessions, or both, as they work toward their goals.

Drug Therapy. Drugs have been used in the treatment of obesity but only as adjuncts to a good diet and exercise program. Drugs approved for weight loss can be classified into two categories: (1) those that decrease food intake by reducing appetite or increasing satiety (sense of feeling full after eating) and (2) those that decrease nutrient absorption. Drugs that increase energy expenditure (e.g., ephedrine) are not FDA approved for weight loss in the United States at this time.

Appetite-suppressing drugs. Appetite suppressants reduce food intake through noradrenergic (drugs that mimic norepinephrine) or serotonergic mechanisms in the CNS. Noradrenergic agents include phentermine (Adipex-P, Fastin), diethylpropion (Tenuate, Tepanil), phendimetrazine (Bontril, Plegine), and benzphetamine (Didrex). Amphetamines are not recommended because of their abuse potential. Benzphetamine and phendimetrazine are also classified as Schedule III drugs by the Drug Enforcement Administration because of their potential for abuse. These drugs are recommended for short-term use (i.e., less than 12 weeks) in the management of obesity. Adverse effects of these drugs include palpitations, tachycardia, overstimulation, restlessness, dizziness, insomnia, weakness, and fatigue.[24,25]

Serotonergic drugs act to either increase the release of serotonin or decrease its uptake, thus reducing its metabolism. Fenfluramine (Pondimin) and dexfenfluramine (Redux) were the first drugs in this class. However, in 1997 these drugs were withdrawn from the market because of reported adverse effects (e.g., valvu-

lar heart disease, pulmonary hypertension). These drugs are mentioned to advise patients that their use is dangerous.[24]

Mixed noradrenergic-serotonergic agents are also used in weight management. Sibutramine (Meridia) inhibits both serotonin and norepinephrine uptake, thus increasing their levels in the CNS. Sibutramine along with a reduced-calorie diet has been shown to reduce body weight. Unlike fenfluramine it does not stimulate the release of serotonin, which is thought to be associated with adverse side effects.[25] Side effects include increased blood pressure and heart rate, dry mouth, headache, insomnia, and constipation. Other selective serotonin-reuptake inhibitors that are approved for the management of depression and other psychiatric conditions may have a short-term effect on weight loss, but the effect does not appear to last over time.[25]

Nutrient absorption–blocking drugs. Orlistat (Xenical), a drug that was developed for weight loss and maintenance, works by blocking fat breakdown and absorption in the intestine. It inhibits the action of intestinal lipases. The undigested fat is excreted in the feces. Though this drug has a high safety profile, some fat-soluble vitamin levels may drop and may need to be supplemented.[25,26] Side effects include increased intestinal gas (flatulence), fecal urgency, fecal incontinence, and steatorrhea.

Because drugs will not cure obesity without substantial changes in food intake and increased physical activity, weight gain will occur when short-term drug therapy is stopped. Supervised long-term drug therapy with safe compounds can contribute to weight management, as well as loss. As with any pharmacologic treatment, there are side effects. Careful evaluation for the presence of other medical conditions can help determine which drugs, if any, would be advisable for a given patient.

The role of the nurse in relation to drug therapy should center on teaching the patient about proper administration and side effects and how the drugs fit into the larger weight loss plan. The modification of dosage without consultation with the physician or the nurse can have detrimental effects. The nurse should reemphasize that the diet and exercise regimens are the cornerstones of permanent weight loss. Drugs may be helpful, but they do not help the patient change eating behavior. The purchase of over-the-counter diet aids should be discouraged.

Even with a comprehensive action plan, there is a high rate of weight regain among all age groups. For successful management of obesity, it helps if obesity is viewed as a chronic condition that necessitates day-to-day attention to maintain weight loss.

Collaborative Surgical Care

Many different types of surgical techniques have been described for treating obesity. These techniques can be classified as physical or mechanical (e.g., lipectomy) or nutrient intake limiting (e.g., gastric bypass, banding gastroplasty). For a patient to be selected for any of the operations for morbid obesity, the following criteria are considered:

1. Gross obesity for 5 years
2. Failure to reduce weight with other forms of therapy
3. Body weight 100% above the ideal for age, gender, and height
4. No serious endocrine problem causing the obesity
5. Absence of other medical conditions (liver disease, alcoholism, cardiovascular or pulmonary disease, inflammatory bowel disease, cancer)
6. Psychiatric and social stability and willingness to cooperate with long-term follow-up

7. Availability of a team of health care providers (nurses, physicians, dietitians) to provide immediate and long-term care
8. Presence of a high-risk condition (degenerative joint disease) that weight loss would ameliorate

Lipectomy. **Lipectomy** (adipectomy) is performed to remove unsightly flabby folds of adipose tissue. The patient who chooses lipectomy does so for cosmetic reasons. In some patients, up to 15% of the total fat cells can be removed from the breasts, abdomen, and lumbar and femoral areas. There is no evidence that a regeneration of adipose tissue occurs at the surgical sites. However, it must be emphasized to the patient that surgical removal does not prevent obesity from recurring, especially if lifetime eating habits remain the same. Although body image and self-esteem may be enhanced by such procedures, these operations are not without complications. The dangerous effects of anesthesia and the potential for poor wound healing in the obese patient cannot be overemphasized. It is more useful for the majority of patients contemplating a lipectomy to be instructed in preventive health measures, such as slow weight reduction to maintain and preserve tissue integrity, the value of exercise, and behavior-modification techniques.

Liposuction. Another surgical procedure is *liposuction,* or suction-assisted lipectomy. The current use is for cosmetic purposes and not for weight reduction. This surgical intervention helps improve facial appearance or body contours. A good candidate for this type of surgery is one who has achieved weight reduction but who has excess fat under the chin, along the jawline, in the nasolabial folds, over the abdomen, or around the waist and upper thighs. The procedure is relatively free of major complications. A long, hollow, stainless steel cannula is inserted through a small incision over the fatty tissue to be suctioned. The purpose of this type of surgery is to improve body appearance, thereby enhancing body image and self-concept. It is not usually recommended for the older person because the skin is less elastic and will not accommodate the new underlying shape.

Gastrointestinal Surgeries. Surgical approaches within the GI tract have been directed toward either limiting food intake or producing malabsorption. Many different types of GI surgery have been tried for severe obesity and rejected primarily because of complications or because they were not effective. However, two nutrient intake–limiting procedures currently used are vertical banded gastroplasty and Roux-en-Y gastric bypass[27] (Table 39-21 and Fig. 39-8).

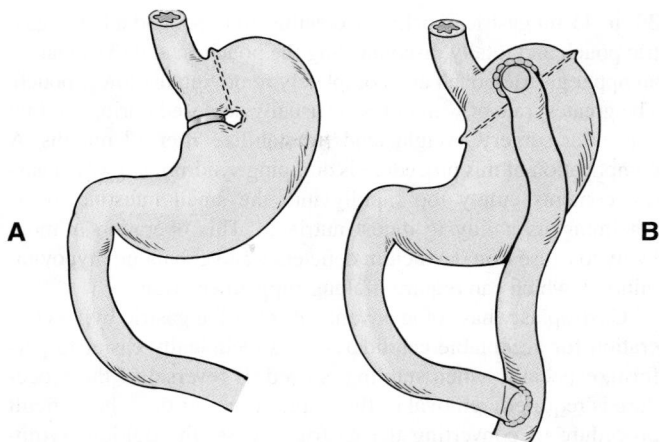

FIG. 39-8 Two gastrointestinal surgical procedures for limiting nutrient intake are currently being used in the treatment of morbid obesity. *A,* Vertical banded gastroplasty consists of constructing a small pouch with a restricted outlet along the lesser curvature of the stomach. This outlet may be externally reinforced to prevent disruption or dilation. *B,* Roux-en-Y gastric bypass procedure involves constructing a proximal gastric pouch whose outlet is a Y-shaped limb of small bowel.

Vertical banded gastroplasty. *Vertical banded gastroplasty* is the most frequently used procedure to produce weight loss in obese people. This approach leads to physical restriction of food intake. In vertical banded gastroplasty, the stomach is partitioned into a small (usually about 30 ml) upper portion along the lesser curvature of the stomach. This small pouch drastically limits capacity. In addition, the stoma opening to the rest of the stomach is banded to delay emptying of solid food from the proximal pouch. This procedure has achieved considerable success in management of weight loss. Problems associated with this gastric restriction operation include intractable vomiting from too rapid intake of solids, distention of the wall of the proximal pouch, rupture of the staple line, and erosion of the band into the stomach.

Gastric bypass. The Roux-en-Y surgical procedure is the most commonly used gastric bypass surgery. In this procedure, the stomach size is decreased with a gastric pouch anastomosis emptying directly into the jejunum. Variations of this procedure include (1) stapling the stomach without transection to create a small,

---

TABLE 39-21 **Surgical Interventions for Morbid Obesity**

PROCEDURE	METHOD OF WEIGHT LOSS	ANATOMIC CHANGES	ADVANTAGES	RISKS
• Roux-en-Y gastric bypass*	Reduced gastric capacity Some malabsorption	Gastric pouch and gastrojejunostomy	Large weight loss	Staple line dehiscence; iron, calcium, cobalamin deficiency; dumping syndrome with dietary intake of refined carbohydrates
• Vertical banded gastroplasty*	Reduced gastric capacity	Small gastric pouch along lesser stomach curvature	Easy to perform procedure (e.g., no anastomosis necessary); more normal anatomy and physiology maintained	Less weight loss than gastric bypass; disrupted staple line; dilated pouch; erosion at band into stomach (rare); potential for maladaptive eating (e.g., ingestion of calorically dense food)

*See Fig. 39-8.

30- to 45-ml gastric pouch; (2) creating an upper and a lower gastric pouch and totally disconnecting the pouches; and (3) creating an upper gastric pouch and completely removing the lower pouch. The greatest rate of weight loss is usually achieved during the first year after surgery. Weight tends to stabilize after 18 months. A complication of this procedure is dumping syndrome in which gastric contents empty too rapidly into the small intestine, overwhelming its ability to digest nutrients. This operation is more likely to cause iron or calcium deficiency and cobalamin hypovitaminosis, which can require lifelong supplementation.

Gastroplasty has some advantages over the gastric bypass operation for acceptable candidates. It is technically easier to perform, especially when stapling is used. If reversal of the procedure is required, removal of the staples is easier than the difficult procedure of converting the gastric bypass. In addition, symptoms of the dumping syndrome and malabsorption are eliminated. However, the weight loss record is often disappointing.[27]

An early surgery that led to malabsorption was the jejunoileal bypass. This procedure resulted in excellent weight loss. However, because of frequent serious health-related complications, including electrolyte imbalance, osteoporosis, bypass enteritis, and liver failure, this surgery is no longer performed. Many patients had surgical procedures done to reverse the bypass. A group of patients may still have a malabsorptive biliopancreatic diversion procedure performed. Weight loss is superior to the gastric bypass, but metabolic and nutritional disturbances remain with this technique.[27]

NURSING MANAGEMENT
OBESE PATIENT

■ Nursing Assessment

The nurse, working closely with the other members of the health care team, plays a major role in the planning and management of the obese patient. To be effective, the nurse must be aware of perceptions of and beliefs about obesity. If a health care provider associates this condition with lack of will power and gluttony, the patient can experience shame in a setting that claims to be a caring one. By being sensitive when asking specific and leading questions, the nurse can often obtain information that the patient may withhold out of embarrassment or shyness or because of being a poor historian. Information that can assist the nurse in understanding an obese patient and provide a basis for intervention is presented in Table 39-22. The nurse must provide acceptable reasons for such personally intrusive questions, respond to the patient's concerns about diagnostic tests, and interpret test outcomes. The patient's answers to questions must be treated with respect, understanding, and a nonjudgmental attitude.

Measurements used with the obese person may include skinfold thickness, height, weight, and BMI. *Android obesity,* in which fat is distributed over the abdomen and upper body (neck, arms, and shoulders), is associated with a greater cardiovascular risk of hypertension, type 2 diabetes mellitus, dyslipidemia, ischemic heart disease, stroke, and death. The nurse should emphasize the importance of vigorous treatment of this type of obesity. The patient should be informed that *gynecoid obesity* (fat distribution over hips) carries a better prognosis but may be more difficult to treat.

As part of the initial nursing physical assessment, each body system should be examined with particular attention to the organ system in which the patient has expressed a problem or concern. Providing specific documentation on these areas assists the physician with a more in-depth history and physical examination.

■ Nursing Diagnoses

Nursing diagnoses for the patient with obesity include, but are not limited to, the following:

1. Imbalanced nutrition: more than body requirements *related to* excessive intake in relation to metabolic need and decreased activity
2. Impaired physical mobility *related to* excessive body weight

TABLE 39-22	Nursing Assessment Obese Patient

Subjective Data	Role-relationship: Change in financial status or family; personal, social, and financial resources to support a reducing diet

Subjective Data

Important Health Information

Past health history: Time of obesity onset; diseases related to metabolism and obesity such as hypertension, cardiovascular problems, stroke, cancer, chronic joint pain, respiratory problems, diabetes mellitus, cholelithiasis

Medications: Thyroid preparations, use of diet pills

Surgery or other treatments: Weight-reduction procedures

Functional Health Patterns

Health perception–health management: Family history of obesity; perception of problem; methods of weight loss attempted

Nutritional-metabolic: Amount and frequency of eating; overeating in response to boredom, stress, specific times or activities

Elimination: Constipation

Activity-exercise: Typical physical activity; drowsiness, somnolence; dyspnea on exertion, orthopnea, paroxysmal nocturnal dyspnea

Sleep-rest: Sleep apnea

Cognitive-perceptual: Feelings of rejection, isolation, guilt, or shame; meaning or value of food; compliance with prescribed reducing diets, degree of long-term commitment to a weight-loss program

Role-relationship: Change in financial status or family; personal, social, and financial resources to support a reducing diet

Sexuality-reproductive: Menstrual irregularity, heavy menstrual flow in women, infertility; effect of obesity on sexual activity

Objective Data

General

Body mass index ≥30 kg/m²; waist-to-hip ratio greater than 0.8 (women) or 1 (men), body weight 20% above ideal for height and frame, triceps skinfold greater than 25 (women) or 15 (men)

Respiratory

Hypoventilation

Cardiovascular

Hypertension

Musculoskeletal

Decreased joint mobility

Possible Findings

Elevated serum glucose, cholesterol, triglycerides; polycythemia

3. Social isolation *related to* alterations in physical appearance and perceived unattractiveness
4. Impaired skin integrity *related to* alterations in nutritional state (obesity), immobility, excess moisture, and multiple skinfolds
5. Ineffective breathing pattern *related to* decreased lung expansion from obesity
6. Noncompliance *related to* alteration in perception or lack of motivation
7. Disturbed body image *related to* deviation from usual or expected body size and inability to lose or retain weight loss

■ Planning

The overall goals are that the obese patient will (1) achieve weight loss to a specified level, (2) maintain weight loss at a specified level, (3) modify eating levels, and (4) participate in a regular physical activity program.

■ Nursing Implementation

Health Promotion. In collaboration with the dietitian, the nurse is in a prime position to participate in formal and informal health and nutritional teaching activities. Targeting groups in the work setting is one way health promotion activities can be conducted and reinforced. Group competition within the work environment has been reported to offer moderate success for participants. Interrelated key factors are group support coupled with competition.

Acute Intervention. Special considerations are necessary in the care of the patient who is admitted to the hospital for surgical treatment of obesity, especially the morbidly obese. Most nursing units are not prepared to meet the needs of a patient who is often too large for a typical hospital or recovery room bed or who has arms that even a large-size blood pressure cuff will not fit. To eliminate embarrassment for the patient and frustration for the staff, plans for these special needs should be made before the patient's admission. Oversized blood pressure cuffs should be ready for use when the patient arrives. A private room may be necessary for privacy of the patient and to accommodate the bed and sitting arrangements. A strongly reinforced trapeze bar should be placed over the bed to facilitate movement and positioning. In some cases a specially constructed chair may have to be built and beds joined together to allow the patient to sit and sleep in comfort.

A care-planning conference should be a priority so that even simple nursing care measures do not become impossible tasks. Consideration should be given to questions such as how the patient will be weighed, how the patient will be transported throughout the hospital, and how simple physical assessment strategies may have to be adjusted to accommodate the morbidly obese patient. Anticipation of the need to use the hospital's meat or freight scales saves time and energy later for both the staff and the patient. Another need is a wheelchair with removable arms that is large enough to safely accommodate the patient and that will pass easily through doorways.

Strategies for bathing, turning, and ambulating the patient, including the number of extra people needed to carry out these measures, are invaluable when the actual need arises. Special gowns are also needed for the patient. Routine physical assessment strategies do not work well with a morbidly obese female patient who has numerous layers of skinfolds covering the chest and abdomen in addition to huge, pendulous breasts obscuring the area to be assessed. Without identifying alternatives or unique methods of dealing with this problem, assessment of respiratory status and bowel sounds or even wound inspection could be awkward for the nurse and embarrassing for the patient.

Wound infection is one of the most common complications after surgery. Because of the many layers of flabby skinfolds, especially in the abdominal area, preoperative skin preparation is important. Frequently the patient is instructed to take several showers a day for a few days before admission to the hospital. Careful cleansing with soap and warm water of the abdominal area from the breasts to below the waist is emphasized.

The patient must be instructed in the proper coughing technique, deep breathing, and methods of turning and positioning to prevent pulmonary complications after surgery. The use of a spirometer may be introduced before surgery. Because most obese patients breathe shallowly, use of the spirometer helps prevent and alleviate postoperative lung congestion. Practicing these strategies preoperatively can aid in performing them correctly postoperatively.

All patients admitted for major gastric surgery procedures have an NG tube inserted during surgery and attached to low suction after surgery. Allowing the patient to see a typical tube and explaining why it is necessary is a good method of involving the patient in the plan of care. The patient should know that oral nourishment will be impossible for a few days after the surgery and that IV fluids will be the main source of intake.

Early ambulation is essential for the obese patient. It is important that the patient know that it is usually necessary to get out of bed soon after surgery and with increasing frequency thereafter, generally 3 to 4 times each day. The dangers of thrombophlebitis and measures to counteract its development are a routine part of preoperative teaching. The patient should know that elastic stockings, elastic compression stockings, or elastic wraps will be applied to the legs and that active and passive range-of-motion exercises will be a frequent part of daily care. Low-dose heparin often will be ordered. (General preoperative nursing care is discussed in Chapter 17.)

The patient experiences considerable abdominal pain after surgery. Administration of pain medications should be given as frequently as necessary during the immediate postoperative period. If pain medication is not given by patient-controlled analgesia, the nurse must remember that intramuscular medications must be given with an extra-long needle, such as a spinal needle, so that the medication is administered into the muscle and not into the adipose or subcutaneous tissue, which will delay absorption. Keeping the head of the bed elevated at a 30-degree angle at all times facilitates ventilatory efforts. Encouraging and assisting the patient to turn, cough, and deep breathe at least every 1 to 2 hours minimizes the risk for atelectasis and pneumonia. Frequent mouth and nose care also helps breathing efforts because the NG tube is inserted through one nostril.

Position changes and range-of-motion exercises are instituted immediately after surgery and carried out every 1 to 2 hours. Ambulatory efforts generally are begun on the evening of surgery. For patient safety, the nurse should enlist the assistance of other staff members during these initial efforts, while encouraging the patient to help.

The abdominal wound requires frequent observation for the amount and type of drainage, condition of the sutures, and signs of infection. The incision must be protected against undue straining that accompanies turning and coughing. Wound dehiscence and wound healing are potential problems for all obese patients. Monitoring the vital signs assists in identifying problems such as infection.

It is important that the NG tube be kept patent and in the correct position. Vomiting is common following gastric procedures. If tube patency is blocked or the tube requires repositioning, the physician should be notified at once. The upper gastric pouch is small, and irrigating the tube with too much solution or manipulating tube position can lead to disruption of the anastomosis or staple line. In most cases the NG tube can be removed in approximately 48 hours, or when bowel sounds have resumed.

Skin care should be carried out several times each shift. Perspiration may be excessive at times. The many layers of skin should be kept clean and dry so that this source of irritation is eliminated. For the patient who has an indwelling catheter, perineal care is important so that a urinary tract infection can be prevented.

Clear liquids are given orally when tolerance is established. The amount offered at first is necessarily limited to approximately 1 ounce, which is to be sipped slowly. More solid types of food are given to the patient who has had gastric surgery as progress is made through the postoperative recovery period.

Ambulatory and Home Care. The patient who has undergone major surgical treatment for obesity has not, in the past, been successful in following or maintaining a prescribed diet. Now the patient is forced to reduce the oral intake as a result of the anatomic changes brought about by the operation. This patient finds that adherence to a reduced intake is necessary because of the concern for abdominal distention, cramping abdominal pain, and perhaps diarrhea.

Weight loss is considerable during the first 6 to 12 months. It is during this time that the patient must learn to adjust intake sufficiently to maintain a stable weight. Although behavior modification was not an intended outcome when these surgical procedures were devised, it becomes an unexpected secondary gain. The diet generally prescribed should be high in protein and low in carbohydrates, fat, and roughage and consist of six small feedings daily. Fluids should not be ingested with the meal, and in some cases, fluids should be restricted to less than 1000 ml per day. Fluids and foods high in carbohydrate tend to promote diarrhea and symptoms of the dumping syndrome. Generally, calorically dense foods (foods high in fat) should be avoided to permit more nutritionally sound food to be consumed.

Proper diet must be clearly understood by the patient. Late complications can be anticipated after gastric bypass or gastroplasty, including anemia, vitamin deficiencies, diarrhea, and psychiatric problems. Failure to lose weight or loss of too much weight may be caused by the surgical formation of too large a stomach pouch or of an outlet that is much too small, respectively. Peptic ulcer formation, dumping syndrome, and small bowel obstruction may be seen late in the recovery and rehabilitative stage.

Long-term follow-up care must be stressed, in part because of complications late in the recovery period. The patient must be encouraged to adhere strictly to the prescribed diet and to keep the care provider informed of any changes in physical or emotional condition. Some patients have been known to overeat when they return home and gain rather than lose weight.

The nurse must anticipate and recognize several potential psychologic problems after surgery. Some patients express guilt feelings concerning the fact that the only way they could lose weight was by surgical means rather than by the "sheer willpower" of reduced dietary intake. The nurse should be ready to provide support so that this patient does not dwell on negative feelings.

Many morbidly obese patients who blamed their feelings of social inferiority or inadequacies on their appearance before bypass surgery may suffer from episodes of depression. By 6 to 8 months after surgery, considerable weight loss has occurred, and they are able to see clearly how much their appearance has changed. Massive weight loss often leaves the patient with large quantities of flabby skin that can result in problems related to altered body image. Reconstructive surgery at least 1 full year after the initial surgery may alleviate this situation. Reduction of the breasts, upper arms, thighs, and excess abdominal skinfolds are possible solutions. Discussion of this possible outcome with the patient before surgery and again during the rehabilitation phase of recovery helps facilitate the patient's adjustment to a new body image and social reintegration.

Physical activity. Once a physical activity program has been outlined for the patient, the nurse can reinforce instruction and help individualize it to the patient's time schedule and physical limitations. The nurse should point out that engaging in weekend exercise only or in spurts of strenuous activity is not advantageous and can actually be dangerous. Joining a health club can be one mechanism of getting exercise. Walking, swimming, and cycling are sensible forms of exercise and have long-term benefits. The combination of a good reducing diet and an increased physical activity program can have profound effects on the patient's achievement of weight loss. When large muscles are involved in the exercise program, a primary benefit is cardiovascular conditioning.

Many psychologic benefits can be derived from an increased physical activity program. Reduction in tension and stress, better-quality sleep and rest, decreased desire to eat excessively, increased stamina and energy, improved self-concept and self-confidence, better attitudes toward work and play, and increased optimism about the future can be achieved.

Cognitive-behavior modification. The person who is on any type of restrictive dietary program is often encouraged to join a group of other obese persons who are receiving professional counseling to help them modify their eating habits. The assumption behind behavior modification is that obesity is a learned disorder caused by overeating and that the critical difference between an obese person and a nonobese person is in the cues that stimulate eating behavior. Therefore most behavior-modification programs de-emphasize the diet and focus on how and when the person eats. Participants often are taught to restrict their eating to designated meals and to increase the amount of physical activity in their lives. Persons who have undergone behavior therapy are more successful in maintaining their losses over an extended time than those who do not participate in such training.

Many self-help groups are available to the person who wants to learn more about successful dieting and who likes the support of others having the same problems and experiences. Take Off Pounds Sensibly (TOPS) is the oldest nonprofit organization of this type. Behavioral modification is an integral part of the program, along with nutrition education. Weight Watchers International, Inc., is probably the most successful commercial weight-reduction enterprise. Weight Watchers offers a food plan that is nutritionally balanced and practical to follow, and it has used behavior-modification techniques since 1974. There has been a proliferation of commercial weight-reduction centers across the nation. Many of these programs are staffed by nurses or dietitians, or both, and require an initial physical examination by a care provider before a candidate is accepted for weight reduction. These weight-reduction centers are costly and therefore are cost prohibitive for those with limited financial resources. Many of these programs also offer special prepackaged foods and supplements that must be purchased as part of the weight-reduction plan. Only these prescribed foods and drinks are to be consumed until an agreed-on amount of weight is lost. The patient is encouraged to buy the same type of foods for the maintenance phase of the program, lasting from 6 months to 1 year. Behavior-modification training is incorporated within these programs as well.

Regardless of the commercial products used, successful weight loss and control are limited and require individualized programs consisting of restricted caloric intake, behavior modification, and exercise. Although persons who follow this type of program are likely to lose weight, once they leave the program the weight is usually regained because they tend to resume previous eating behaviors and return to the foods previously eaten.

A new concept of influencing health behavior and better employee health has occurred recently. Programs on health teaching and maintenance have been started at places of employment. The rationale for such programs is that better health repays the cost of the programs through improved work performance, decreased absenteeism, and eventually less hospitalization. Weight-reduction and hypertension-reduction programs have been instituted and are popular with employees.

■ Evaluation

The expected outcomes are that the obese patient will
- experience long-term weight loss
- have improvement in obesity-related comorbidities
- integrate healthy practices into daily routines
- monitor for adverse side effects of surgical therapy
- have an improved self-image

EATING DISORDERS

Eating disorders are primarily psychiatric disorders. However, there are a number of nutritional problems associated with these disorders that require the nurse to implement a nutritional plan of care. According to the American Dietetic Association, over 5 million Americans suffer from eating disorders. It primarily affects young women. It is estimated that 6% of those with severe eating disorders will die, and only 50% report being cured.[28]

Anorexia Nervosa

Anorexia nervosa is characterized by a self-imposed weight loss, endocrine dysfunction, and a distorted psychopathologic attitude toward weight and eating.[29] Anorexia nervosa clinically manifests as abnormal weight loss, deliberate self-starvation, intense fear of gaining weight, *lanugo* (soft, downy hair covering the body except the palms and soles), refusal to eat, continuous dieting, hair loss, sensitivity to cold, compulsive exercise, absent or irregular menstruation, dry skin, and constipation. Diagnostic studies often show iron deficiency anemia and an elevated blood urea nitrogen level that is reflective of marked intravascular vol-

ume depletion and prerenal azotemia. Lack of potassium in the diet and loss of potassium in the urine lead to potassium deficiency. Manifestations of potassium deficiency include muscle weakness, cardiac arrhythmias, and renal failure. If the eating pattern is permitted to continue for a prolonged time, body wasting and signs of severe malnutrition are evident.

Multidisciplinary treatment must involve a combination of nutritional support and psychiatric care. Hospitalization may be necessary if there are severe physical complications that cannot be managed in an outpatient therapy program. Nutritional replenishment must be closely supervised to ensure consistent and ongoing weight gains. The use of tube or parenteral feedings may be necessary. Improved nutrition, however, is not a cure for anorexia nervosa. The underlying psychiatric problem must be addressed by identification of the disturbed patterns of individual and family interactions, followed by individual and family counseling.

Bulimia Nervosa

Bulimia nervosa is a disorder characterized by frequent binge eating and self-induced vomiting associated with loss of control over eating and a persistent concern with body image.[29] These individuals may have normal weight for height, or their weight may fluctuate with bingeing and purging. They may also abuse laxatives, diuretics, exercise, or diet drugs. They may have signs of frequent vomiting, such as macerated knuckles, swollen salivary glands, broken blood vessels in the eyes, and dental problems.

Bulimia is increasing in incidence and may be even more prevalent than anorexia nervosa. Female college students seem to be most susceptible to this syndrome. The cause remains unclear but is thought to be similar to that of anorexia nervosa. Substance abuse, anxiety, affective disorders, and personality disturbances have been reported among persons with bulimia.

The patient with bulimia, similar to the one with anorexia nervosa, goes to great lengths to conceal abnormal eating habits. As the behavior persists, many problems associated with the condition become increasingly hard to deal with effectively. As with anorexia, a treatment combination of psychologic counseling and diet therapy is essential. Education and emotional support for the patient and family are vital. Support groups such as the National Association of Anorexia Nervosa and Associated Disorders (see resources for information) are extremely helpful to those affected by these disorders.

■ Culturally Competent Care: Nutrition

People have unique cultural heritages that may affect eating customs and nutritional status. Culture along with personal preferences, socioeconomic status, and religious preferences can influence food choices. Each culture has its own beliefs and behaviors related to food and the role that food plays in the etiology and treatment of disease. In addition, culture can dictate what food is considered edible, as well as how it is prepared and when it is eaten. There are a wide array of cultural influences on diet ranging from what foods are selected to when meals are eaten and how and who prepares them. For example, some religions require periods of fasting.

The nurse should include cultural and ethnic considerations when assessing the patient's diet history and implementing interventions that require dietary changes. At the same time, the nurse needs to avoid *cultural stereotyping* by making assumptions or generalizations about diet based on the individual's cultural background. For example, not all Jewish patients eat only kosher foods.

It is important to know whether the patients eats "traditional foods" associated with the culture. If traditional foods are eaten, the nurse should assess for their impact on health. For example, "soul foods," which include traditional foods eaten by some African Americans, tend to be high in fat, cholesterol, and sodium. Traditional foods eaten by some Asian Americans may be high in fiber and low in fat and cholesterol but also low in calcium content because of the lack of milk products.

Consideration of cultural beliefs is very important when planning dietary changes and monitoring acceptance of dietary changes. For example, perception of body weight and size may also be influenced by culture. Thus the nurse needs to ask the patient or family about how culture affects dietary choices and weight maintenance. In some cultures an overweight person may be seen as a sign of success. Thus the nurse would have a challenging time trying to convince that person to lose weight. ■

Teaching related to dietary restrictions and recommended dietary changes should involve the patient's family. In many situations it is a family member who does the grocery shopping and cooking.

CRITICAL THINKING EXERCISES

Case Study
Obesity

Patient Profile. Mrs. Estella Rodriguez is a 60-year-old Hispanic woman who is 5 feet 4 inches tall and weighs 190 pounds.

Subjective Data
- Reports gradual weight gain during past 40 years
- Spends most of her free time watching television
- Reports health problems related to type 2 diabetes mellitus, shortness of breath, hypertension, chest pressure, and osteoarthritis
- Had knee replacement surgery at age 56 for osteoarthritis

Objective Data
Physical Examination
- Has obese, nontender, soft abdomen
- BP is 150/90

Laboratory Results
- Fasting blood glucose: 250 mg/dl (13.9 mmol/L)
- Total cholesterol: 205 mg/dl (5.3 mmol/L)
- Triglyceride: 298 mg/dl (3.36 mmol/L)
- HDL cholesterol: 31 mg/dl (0.8 mmol/L)

CRITICAL THINKING QUESTIONS

1. What are Mrs. Rodriguez's obesity risk factors?
2. What is her estimated BMI?
3. Of the possible complications of obesity, which ones does Mrs. Rodriguez have? What are contributing factors to her developing type 2 diabetes mellitus, cardiovascular disease manifestations, and osteoarthritis?
4. What would you, as the nurse, include in a successful weight loss and weight management program for Mrs. Rodriguez?
5. Is Mrs. Rodriguez a candidate for surgical intervention for obesity? If so, why? If not, why not?
6. Based on the assessment data presented, write one or more appropriate nursing diagnoses. Are there any collaborative problems?

Nursing Research Issues

1. What nursing interventions can be used to reduce diarrhea associated with tube feedings?
2. What happens to serum calcium and bone density in vegetarian patients over time?
3. What is the effect of surgical procedures for obesity on the quality of life or on functional abilities?
4. Does early enteral feeding reduce the risk of sepsis in critically ill patients?
5. Are there valid and reliable bedside methods for determining nasogastric (NG) and nasointestinal tube placement?
6. What are the ways to reduce the risk of catheter sepsis in a patient receiving TPN?

REVIEW QUESTIONS

The number of the question corresponds to the same-numbered objective at the beginning of the chapter.

1. The nurse identifies a need for dietary teaching for the patient whose daily intake of food groups consists of
   a. 2 to 4 servings of the fruit group.
   b. 2 to 3 servings of the milk, yogurt, and cheese group.
   c. 4 to 5 servings of the bread, cereal, rice, and pasta group.
   d. 2 to 3 servings of the meat, poultry, fish, beans, egg, and nut group.

2. In general, nutrient or food interactions with drugs can result in all of the following except
   a. enhancing drug absorption.
   b. decreasing drug bioavailability.
   c. increasing a nutrient requirement.
   d. all of the above options can happen.

3. During the first 24 hours of starvation, the order in which the body obtains substrate for energy is
   a. glycogen, skeletal protein.
   b. visceral protein, fat stores, glycogen.
   c. fat stores, skeletal protein, visceral protein.
   d. liver protein, muscle protein, visceral protein.

4. An elderly patient with a recent stroke is exhibiting signs of severe dysphagia. The optimal form of nutrition support at this time would be
   a. TPN.
   b. regular diet.
   c. nasoenteric tube feedings.
   d. nothing by mouth (NPO) until dysphagia resolves.

5. A nutritionally stressed patient weighing 60 kg is NPO and receiving TPN. In evaluating the patient's nutritional intake, the nurse calculates that the daily TPN solution should provide
   a. 40 g fat.
   b. 80 g protein.
   c. 20 calories per kilogram.
   d. 1000 calories from carbohydrate.

6. One advantage of a percutaneous endoscopic gastrostomy tube placement relative to NG feedings for the patient receiving long-term enteral nutrition is that
   a. it increases patient comfort.
   b. it eliminates the risk of aspiration.
   c. feedings can be initiated before bowel sounds are present.
   d. more calories can be delivered compared with NG feeding.

7. The obesity aspect that is most often associated with cardiovascular health problems is
   a. primary obesity.
   b. secondary obesity.
   c. gynoid fat distribution.
   d. android fat distribution.

8. A morbidly obese patient has undergone Roux-en-Y gastric bypass surgery. In planning postoperative care, the nurse anticipates that the patient
   a. may have severe diarrhea early in the postoperative period.
   b. will require nasogastric suction until healing of the site occurs.
   c. will not be allowed to ambulate for 5 to 7 days postoperatively.
   d. may have only liquids orally, and in very limited amounts, during the early postoperative period.

9. The nurse recognizes that the major goal of treatment for a patient with anorexia nervosa is being met when the patient
   a. demonstrates a rapid weight gain.
   b. consumes the required daily intake of nutrients.
   c. commits to long-term individual and family counseling.
   d. verbalizes feelings regarding self-image and fears of becoming obese.

REFERENCES

1. Fiscella K et al: Does patient educational level affect office visits to family physicians? *J Natl Med Assoc* 94:157, 2002.
2. Lutz CA, Przytulski KR: *Nutrition and diet therapy,* ed 3, Philadelphia, 2001, FA Davis.
3. Frazao E: America's eating habits: changes and consequences, *Agriculture Information Bulletin* No. 750, May 1999.
4. ASPEN Board of Directors: Guidelines for the use of parenteral and enteral nutrition in adult and pediatric patients: 2001 revision, *J Parenter Enteral Nutr* 26 (suppl 1):1SA, 2002.
5. Shopbell JM, Hopkins B, Shronts EP: Nutrition screening and assessment. In Gottschlich MM, editor: *The science and practice of nutrition support,* Dubuque, Iowa, 2001, Kendall/Hunt.
6. Thomas DR et al: Nutritional management in long-term care: development of a clinical guideline, *J Gerontol Med Sci* 55A:M725, 2000.
7. Wilmore DW: *The metabolic management of the critically ill,* New York, 1977, Plenum Publishing.
8. Institute of Medicine, Food, and Nutrition Board: *Dietary reference intakes: vitamin A, vitamin K, arsenic, boron, chromium, copper, iodine, iron, manganese, molybdenum, nickel, silicon, vanadium, and zinc,* Washington DC, 2001, National Academy Press.
9. American Dietetic Association: ADA's definition for nutrition screening and assessment, *J Am Diet Assoc* 94:838, 1994.
10. Project of the American Academy of Family Physicians, The American Dietetic Association, and National Council on Aging: *Nutrition interventions manual for professional caring for older Americans,* Washington DC, 1994, Nutrition Screening Initiative.
*11. Kovacevich DS et al: Nutrition risk classification: a reproducible and valid tool for nurses, *Nutr Clin Pract* 12:20, 1997.
*12. Keller JJ, Hirdes JP: Using the minimum data set to determine the prevalence of nutrition problems in an Ontario population of chronic care patients, *Can J Diet Pract Res* 61:165, 2000.
13. US Dept of Agriculture and US Dept of Health and Human Services: *Dietary guidelines for Americans,* ed 4, Home and garden bulletin. No. 232. Washington DC, 1995, US Government Publishing Office.
*14. Keele AM et al: Two phase randomized controlled clinical trial of postoperative oral dietary supplements in surgical patients, *Gut* 40:393, 1997.
15. Guenter P: Tube feeding administration. In Guenter P, Silkroski M, editors: *Tube feeding: practical guidelines and nursing protocols,* Gaithersburg, Md, 2001, Aspen.

*Nursing research–based reference.

16. Edwards SJ, Metheny NA: Measurement of gastric residual volume: state of the science, *MedSurg Nurs* 9:125, 2000.
17. Guenter P: Nursing care of patients with enteral feeding devices. In Guenter P, Silkroski M, editors: *Tube feeding: practical guidelines and nursing protocols*, Gaithersburg, Md, 2001, Aspen.
18. National Advisory Group on Standards and Practice Guidelines for Parenteral Nutrition: Safe practices for parenteral nutrition formulations, *JPEN* 22:49, 1998.
19. Shuster MH: Parenteral nutrition. In Hennessey KA, Orr ME, editors: *Nutrition support nursing core curriculum*, ed 3, Silver Spring, Md, 1996, Aspen.
20. Krzywda EA, Andris DA, Edmiston CE: Catheter infections: diagnosis, etiology, treatment, and prevention. *Nutr Clin Pract* 14:178, 1999.
21. Flegal KM et al: Overweight and obesity in the United States: prevalence and trends 1960-1994, *Int J Obes Relat Metab Disord* 22:39, 1998.
22. Bray G: Obesity: part 1—pathogenesis, *West J Med* 149:431, 1988.
23. Dwyer J: Medical evaluation and class of obesity. In Blackburn GL, Kanders BS, editors: *Obesity pathophysiology, psychology and treatment*, New York, 1994, Chapman & Hall.
24. Apovian CM: Medical management of obesity and the role of pharmacotherapy: an update, *Nutr Clin Pract* 15:5, 2000.
25. Yanovski SZ, Yanovski JA: Drug therapy: obesity, *N Engl J Med* 346:591, 2002.
26. Pi-Sunyer FX: Obesity. In Shils ME, Olsen JA, Ross CA, editors: *Modern nutrition in health and disease*, ed 9, Baltimore, 1999, Williams & Wilkins.
27. Shikora SA: Surgical treatment for severe obesity: the state-of-the-art for the new millennium, *Nutr Clin Pract* 15:13, 2000.
28. American Dietetic Association: Position of the ADA: Nutrition intervention in the treatment of anorexia nervosa, bulimia nervosa, and eating disorders not otherwise specified, *J Am Diet Assoc* 101:810, 2001.
29. Muse DM, Lucas AR: Behavioral disorders affecting food intake: anorexia nervosa, bulimia nervosa and other psychiatric conditions. In Shils ME, Olsen JA, Ross CA, editors: *Modern nutrition in health and disease*, ed 9, Baltimore, 1999, Williams & Wilkins.

RESOURCES

Academy for Eating Disorders
6728 Old McLean Village Drive
McLean, VA 22101
703-556-9222
Fax: 703-556-8729
www.aedweb.org/

American Dietetic Association
216 West Jackson Blvd.
Chicago, IL 60606-6995
800-877-1600
312-899-0040
www.eatright.org

American Society for Bariatric Surgery
7328 West University Avenue, Suite F
Gainesville, FL 32607
352-331-4900
Fax: 352-331-4975
www.asbs.org

American Society for Parenteral and Enteral Nutrition
8630 Fenton Street, Suite 412
Silver Spring, MD 20910
800-727-4567
301-587-6315
Fax: 301-587-2365
www.nutritioncare.org

Council for Nutrition Clinical Strategies in Long-Term Care
Programs in Medicine
3415 West Chester Pike
Newtown Square, PA 19073

FDA Center for Food Safety and Applied Nutrition (CFSAN)
5100 Paint Branch Parkway
College Park, MD 20740-3835
www.cfsan.fda.gov

Healthy People 2010
Office of Disease Prevention and Health Promotion
Hubert H. Humphrey Building, Room 738G
200 Independence Avenue SW
Washington, DC 20201
Fax: 202-205-9478
www.health.gov/healthypeople/

National Association of Anorexia Nervosa and Associated Disorders (ANAD)
PO Box 7
Highland Park, IL 60035
847-831-3438
Fax: 847-433-4632
www.anad.org/

National Center for Complementary and Alternative Medicine (NCCAM)
National Institutes of Health
Bethesda, MD 20892
http://nccam.nih.gov

National Eating Disorder Information Centre
CW 1-211, 200 Elizabeth Street
M5G 2C4
Toronto, Canada
866-NEDIC-20
416-340-4156
Fax: 416-340-4736
E-mail: nedic@uhn.on.ca
www.nedic.ca/

National Eating Disorders Association
603 Stewart Street, Suite 803
Seattle, WA 98101
800-931-3327
206-382-3587
Fax: 206-829-8501
www.nationaleatingdisorders.org

OLEY Foundation
214 Hun Memorial, A-28
Albany Medical Center
Albany, NY 12208-3478
800-776-OLEY
518-262-5079
Fax: 518-262-5528
http://c4isr.com/oley/

Overeaters Anonymous Headquarters
PO Box 44020
Rio Rancho, NM 87174-4020
505-891-2664
Fax: 505-891-4320
www.overeatersanonymous.org/

For additional Internet resources, see the website for this book at *http://evolve.elsevier.com/Lewis/medsurg/*.

CHAPTER *40*

NURSING MANAGEMENT
Upper Gastrointestinal Problems

Margaret McLean Heitkemper

LEARNING OBJECTIVES

1. Describe the etiology, complications, collaborative care, and nursing management of nausea and vomiting.
2. Describe the etiology, clinical manifestations, and treatment of common oral inflammations and infections.
3. Describe the etiology, clinical manifestations, complications, collaborative care, and nursing management of oral cancer.
4. Explain the types, pathophysiology, clinical manifestations, complications, and collaborative care including surgical therapy and nursing management of gastroesophageal reflux disease and hiatal hernia.
5. Describe the pathophysiology, clinical manifestations, complications, and collaborative care of esophageal cancer, diverticula, achalasia, and esophageal strictures.
6. Differentiate between acute and chronic gastritis, including the etiology, pathophysiology, collaborative care, and nursing management.
7. Explain the common etiology, clinical manifestations, collaborative care, and nursing management of upper gastrointestinal bleeding.
8. Compare and contrast gastric and duodenal ulcers, including etiology and pathophysiology, clinical manifestations, complications, collaborative care, and nursing management.
9. Describe the clinical manifestations, collaborative care, and nursing management of gastric cancer.
10. Identify the common types of food poisoning and the nursing responsibilities related to food poisoning.

KEY TERMS

achalasia, p. 1019
Barrett's esophagus, p. 1012
dysphagia, p. 1009
esophageal cancer, p. 1017
esophageal diverticula, p. 1019
esophagitis, p. 1012
gastric cancer, p. 1044
gastritis, p. 1020
gastroesophageal reflux disease, p. 1011

hiatal hernia, p. 1015
leukoplakia, p. 1009
Mallory-Weiss tear, p. 1023
nausea, p. 1003
peptic ulcer disease, p. 1028
physiologic stress ulcers, p. 1031
vomiting, p. 1003

NAUSEA AND VOMITING

Nausea and vomiting are the most common manifestations of gastrointestinal (GI) diseases. **Nausea** is a feeling of discomfort in the epigastrium with a conscious desire to vomit. **Vomiting** is the forceful ejection of partially digested food and secretions (*emesis*) from the upper GI tract. Vomiting is a complex act that requires the coordinated activities of several structures: closure of the glottis, deep inspiration with contraction of the diaphragm in the inspiratory position, closure of the pylorus, relaxation of the stomach and lower esophageal sphincter, and contraction of the abdominal muscles with increasing intraabdominal pressure. These simultaneous activities force the stomach contents up through the esophagus, into the pharynx, and out the mouth. Although nausea and vomiting can occur independently, they are usually closely related and usually treated as one problem.

Etiology and Pathophysiology

Nausea and vomiting are found in a wide variety of GI disorders, as well as in conditions that are unrelated to GI disease. These include pregnancy, infectious diseases, central nervous system (CNS) disorders (e.g., meningitis, CNS tumor), cardiovascular problems (e.g., myocardial infarction, congestive heart failure), metabolic disorders (e.g., Addison's disease, uremia), side effects of drugs (e.g., narcotics, digitalis), and psychologic factors (e.g., stress, fear).

Generally, nausea occurs before vomiting and is characterized by contraction of the duodenum and by slowing of gastric motility and emptying. A single episode of nausea accompanied by vomiting may not be significant. However, if vomiting occurs several times, it is important that the cause be identified.

A vomiting center in the brainstem coordinates the multiple components involved in vomiting. This center receives input from various stimuli. Neural impulses reach the vomiting center via afferent pathways through branches of the autonomic nervous system. Visceral receptors for these afferent fibers are located in the GI tract, kidneys, heart, and uterus. When stimulated, these receptors relay information to the vomiting center, which then initiates the vomiting reflex (Fig. 40-1).

In addition, the chemoreceptor trigger zone (CTZ) located on the floor of the fourth ventricle in the brain responds to chemical stimuli of drugs and toxins. The CTZ also plays a role in vomiting when it is due to labyrinthine stimulation (e.g., motion sickness). Once stimulated, the CTZ transmits impulses directly to the vomiting center.

Vomiting also can occur when the GI tract becomes overly irritated, excited, or distended. It can be a protective mechanism to rid the body of spoiled or irritating foods and liquids. Immediately

---

Reviewed by Marilee Schmelzer, RN, PhD, Associate Professor, University of Texas at Arlington, Arlington, Tex.

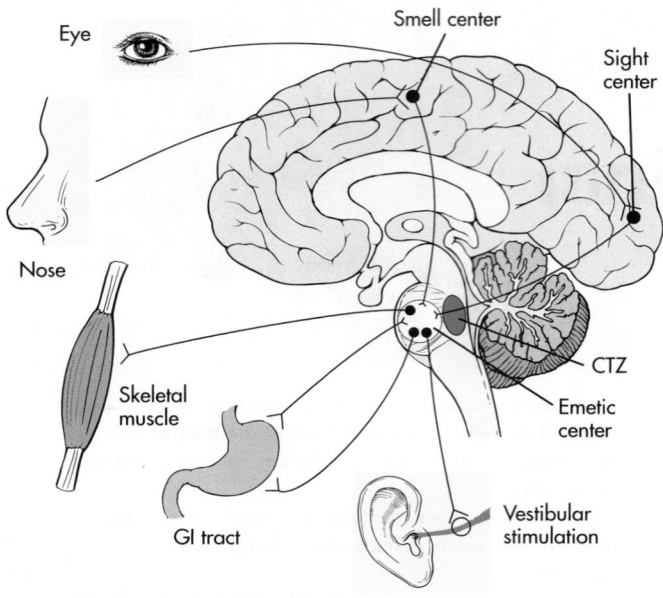

FIG. 40-1 Stimuli involved in the act of vomiting. *CTZ*, Chemoreceptor trigger zone; *GI*, gastrointestinal.

before the act of vomiting, the person becomes aware of the need to vomit. The autonomic nervous system is activated, resulting in both parasympathetic and sympathetic nervous system stimulation. Sympathetic activation produces tachycardia, tachypnea, and diaphoresis. Parasympathetic stimulation causes relaxation of the lower esophageal (cardiac) sphincter, an increase in gastric motility, and a pronounced increase in salivation. These manifestations are experienced immediately before vomiting.

Clinical Manifestations

Nausea is a subjective complaint. *Anorexia* (lack of appetite) usually accompanies nausea and is brought on by unpleasant stimulation involving any of the five senses. When nausea and vomiting are prolonged, dehydration can rapidly occur. In addition to water, essential electrolytes (e.g., potassium, sodium, chloride, hydrogen) are also lost. As vomiting persists, there may be severe electrolyte imbalances, loss of extracellular fluid volume, decreased plasma volume, and eventually circulatory failure. Metabolic alkalosis can result from loss of gastric hydrochloric acid (HCl). Metabolic acidosis can occur because of the loss of bicarbonate when contents from the small intestine are vomited. However, metabolic acidosis as a result of severe vomiting is less common than metabolic alkalosis. Weight loss resulting from fluid loss is evident in a short time when vomiting is severe.

The threat of pulmonary aspiration is a concern when vomiting occurs in the patient who is elderly, is unconscious, or has other conditions that impair the gag reflex. The patient who cannot adequately manage self-care should be put in a semi-Fowler's or side-lying position to prevent aspiration.

Collaborative Care

The goals of collaborative care are to determine and treat the underlying cause of the nausea and vomiting and to provide symptomatic relief of nausea and vomiting. Determining the cause is often difficult because nausea and vomiting are manifes-

tations of many conditions of the GI tract and of disorders of other body systems.

A careful history must elicit important information regarding times when the vomiting occurs, precipitating factors, and a description of the contents of the vomitus or emesis. There are ethnic and gender differences in risk for nausea and vomiting associated with both surgical procedures and motion sickness.[1] Asian Americans, Middle Easterners, and African Americans are more likely to experience nausea and vomiting than whites. Women are more likely than men to experience nausea and vomiting.

In all patients, differentiation must be made between vomiting, regurgitation, and projectile vomiting. *Regurgitation* is a process in which partially digested food is slowly brought up from the stomach. Retching or vomiting seldom precedes it. *Projectile vomiting* is a very forceful expulsion of stomach contents without nausea and is characteristic of CNS tumors.

The presence of fecal odor and bile after prolonged vomiting indicates intestinal obstruction below the level of the pylorus. The presence of bile in the emesis may suggest obstruction below the ampulla of Vater or bile reflux gastritis. The presence of partially digested food several hours after a meal is indicative of gastric outlet obstruction or delay in gastric emptying.

The color of the emesis aids in determining the presence and source of bleeding. Vomitus with a "coffee ground" appearance is associated with bleeding in the stomach, where blood changes to dark brown as a result of its interaction with gastric acid. Bright red blood indicates active bleeding, which is suggestive of a tear in the mucosal lining of the lower esophagus or fundus of stomach, bleeding gastric or duodenal ulcer or neoplasm, or bleeding esophageal varices.

The time of day at which the vomiting occurs is often helpful in determining the cause. Early morning vomiting is a frequent occurrence in pregnancy. Emotional stressors with no evident pathologic disorder may elicit vomiting during or immediately after the ingestion of a meal.

Drug Therapy. The use of drugs in the treatment of nausea and vomiting depends on the cause of the problem. Many different drugs can be used (Table 40-1). Because the cause cannot always be readily determined, drugs must be used with caution. The use of antiemetics before the cause of the vomiting is established can mask the underlying disease process and delay diagnosis and treatment. Many of the antiemetic drugs act on the CNS at the level of the CTZ. In general, they block the neurochemicals that appear to trigger nausea and vomiting.

Drugs that control nausea and vomiting include antimuscarinics (e.g., scopolamine), antihistamines (e.g., diphenhydramine [Benadryl]), and phenothiazines (e.g., chlorpromazine [Thorazine], prochlorperazine [Compazine]). Because many of these drugs have anticholinergic actions, they are contraindicated for the patient with glaucoma, prostatic hyperplasia, pyloric or bladder neck obstruction, or biliary obstruction. They share many common side effects, which include dry mouth, hypotension, sedative effects, rashes, and GI disturbances such as constipation. Consultation with a pharmacist may be indicated before administering these drugs to the patient with multiple medical problems.

Other drugs with antiemetic properties include metoclopramide (Reglan) and domperidone (Motilium). These drugs act both centrally and peripherally on dopamine receptors. Peripherally they enhance the release of acetylcholine, resulting in increased gastric emptying. Because of this effect, these drugs are

TABLE 40-1 Drug Therapy
Nausea and Vomiting

CLASSIFICATION	DRUG
Antiemetic and antipsychotic	chlorpromazine (Thorazine)
	haloperidol (Haldol)
	perphenazine (Trilafon)
	prochlorperazine (Compazine)
	promazine (Sparine)
	trifluoperazine (Stelazine)
	triflupromazine (Vesprin)
Antihistamine	buclizine (Bucladin-S)
	cyclizine (Marezine)
	dimenhydrinate (Dramamine)
	diphenhydramine (Benadryl)
	hydroxyzine (Vistaril)
	meclizine (Antivert, Bonine)
	promethazine (Phenergan)
Prokinetic	domperidone (Motilium)
	metoclopramide (Reglan)
Serotonin antagonist	dolasetron (Anzemet)
	granisetron (Kytril)
	ondansetron (Zofran)
Antimuscarinic	scopolamine transdermal (Transderm-Scop)
Others	benzquinamide (Emete-Con)
	dexamethasone (Decadron)
	diphenidol (Vontrol)
	dronabinol (Marinol)
	thiethylperazine (Torecan)
	trimethobenzamide (Tigan)

considered *prokinetics*. However, about 10% to 20% of patients taking metoclopramide experience CNS side effects ranging from anxiety to hallucinations. Extrapyramidal side effects including tremor and dyskinesias similar to Parkinson's disease may also occur. Domperidone does not cross the blood-brain barrier, resulting in fewer side effects compared with metoclopramide.

Antagonists to specific serotonin (5-HT) receptors have been found to act both centrally and peripherally to reduce nausea and vomiting. In particular, antagonists to the 5-HT$_3$ receptors are effective in reducing cancer chemotherapy–induced vomiting, vomiting caused by total body radiation, GI motility disturbances, carcinoid syndrome, and nausea and vomiting related to migraine headache and anxiety. Serotonin antagonists including ondansetron (Zofran), granisetron (Kytril), and dolasetron (Anzemet) act centrally in the vomiting center, as well as peripherally to enhance gastric emptying.

Dexamethasone (Decadron) is used in the management of cancer chemotherapy–induced emesis, usually in combination with other antiemetics. Dexamethasone alone or in combination with ondansetron reduces both acute and delayed chemotherapy-induced nausea and vomiting. Dronabinol (Marinol) is an orally active cannabinoid. It can be used alone or in combination with other antiemetics for the prevention of chemotherapy-induced emesis. Because of the potential for abuse, as well as CNS side

effects including drowsiness and sedation, this drug is used when other therapies are ineffective.

Nutritional Therapy. The patient with severe vomiting requires intravenous (IV) fluid therapy with electrolyte and glucose replacement until able to tolerate oral intake. In some cases a nasogastric (NG) tube and suction are used to decompress the stomach. Once the symptoms have subsided, oral nourishment beginning with clear liquids is started. Extremely hot or cold liquids are not usually well tolerated. Carbonated beverages at room temperature and with the carbonation gone and warm tea are more easily tolerated. The addition of dry toast or crackers may alleviate the feeling of nausea and help prevent vomiting. Although broth and Gatorade have been used widely for the patient with severe vomiting, these substances are high in sodium and should be administered with caution. Water is the initial fluid of choice for rehydration by mouth.

As the patient's condition improves, a diet high in carbohydrates and low in fatty foods should be provided. Items such as a baked potato, plain gelatin, cereal with milk and sugar, and hard candy may be added. Foods that are known to be poorly tolerated include coffee, spicy foods, and highly acidic foods. Food should be eaten slowly and in small amounts to prevent overdistention of the stomach. When solid foods have been reintroduced, fluids should be taken between meals rather than with meals. It is advised that the patient remain quietly relaxed for approximately 1 hour after meals. A dietitian may be consulted regarding appropriate foods that have nutritional value and are well tolerated by the patient during the recovery process.

NURSING MANAGEMENT
NAUSEA AND VOMITING

■ Nursing Assessment

Each patient with a history of prolonged and persistent nausea or vomiting requires a thorough nursing assessment before a specific plan of care is developed. Although the conditions associated with nausea and vomiting are numerous, the nurse should have a basic understanding of the more common conditions and should be able to identify the patient who is at high risk. Knowledge of the physiologic mechanisms involved in nausea and vomiting and the demonstration of a genuine regard for the patient are essential. Table 40-2 presents subjective and objective data that should be obtained from a patient with nausea and vomiting, regardless of the underlying cause.

COMPLEMENTARY & ALTERNATIVE THERAPIES
Ginger

Clinical Uses
Dyspepsia, nausea and vomiting, and motion sickness.

Effects
Analgesic and sedative effects. Reduction of GI motility. May also decrease the effects of acid-inhibiting drugs. Overdoses can cause CNS depression and cardiac arrhythmias.

Nursing Implications
Should not be taken if using anticoagulant therapy, digoxin, or hypoglycemic agents. Should not be used if patient has gallstones or heart failure.

CNS, Central nervous system; *GI,* gastrointestinal.

TABLE 40-2	Nursing Assessment Nausea and Vomiting

Subjective Data

Important Health Information

Past health history: GI disorders, chronic indigestion, food allergies, pregnancy, infection, CNS disorders, recent travel, bulimia, metabolic disorders, cancer, cardiovascular disease, renal disease

Medications: Use of antiemetics, digitalis, opiates, ferrous sulfate, aspirin, aminophylline, alcohol, antibiotics; general anesthesia; chemotherapy

Surgery or other treatments: Recent surgery

Functional Health Patterns

Nutritional-metabolic: Amount, frequency, character, and color of vomitus; dry heaves; anorexia; weight loss

Activity-exercise: Weakness, fatigue

Cognitive-perceptual: Abdominal tenderness or pain

Coping–stress tolerance: Stress, fear

Objective Data

General

Lethargy, sunken eyeballs

Integumentary

Pallor, dry mucous membranes, poor skin turgor

Gastrointestinal

Amount, frequency, character (e.g., projectile), content (undigested food, blood, bile, feces), and color of vomitus (red, "coffee ground," green-yellow)

Urinary

Decreased output, concentrated urine

Possible Findings

Altered serum electrolytes (especially hypokalemia), metabolic alkalosis, abnormal upper GI findings on endoscopy or abdominal x-rays

CNS, Central nervous system; *GI,* gastrointestinal.

■ Nursing Diagnoses

Nursing diagnoses for the patient with nausea and vomiting may include, but are not limited to, those presented in NCP 40-1.

■ Planning

The overall goals are that the patient with nausea and vomiting will (1) experience minimal or no nausea and vomiting, (2) have normal electrolyte levels and hydration status, and (3) return to a normal pattern of fluid balance and nutrient intake.

■ Nursing Implementation

Acute Intervention. The majority of individuals with nausea and vomiting can be managed at home. However, when nausea and vomiting persist regardless of home treatment strategies, hospitalization may be necessary for diagnosis of the underlying problem. Until a diagnosis is confirmed, the patient is kept on nothing-by-mouth (NPO) status and given IV fluids. An NG tube connected to suction may be necessary for the patient with persistent vomiting, as well as for the patient in whom the possible diagnosis may be bowel obstruction or paralytic ileus. Keeping the stomach empty reduces the stimulus to vomit. The NG tube should be stabilized to eliminate its movement in the nose and back of the throat because this can stimulate nausea and vomiting.

With prolonged vomiting, there is a probability of dehydration and acid-base and electrolyte imbalances. The nurse plans care that includes accurate recording of intake and output, monitoring vital signs, assessing for signs of dehydration, proper positioning to prevent possible aspiration in the susceptible patient, and observing for changes in the patient's general physical comfort and mentation. The nurse takes responsibility for providing physical and emotional support; maintaining a quiet, odor-free environment; and giving explanations regarding any diagnostic tests or procedures performed.

Patients who are hospitalized for other health problems may be prone to episodes of nausea and vomiting. These individuals include the postoperative patient who is recovering from the effects of a surgical procedure, anesthesia, and pain. Nausea and vomiting are common side effects in the cancer patient receiving chemotherapeutic drugs. (Nursing care of the cancer patient is found in Chapter 15.)

Ambulatory and Home Care. The patient and family may need instructions on (1) how to deal successfully with the unpleasant sensations of nausea, (2) methods of preventing nausea and vomiting, and (3) strategies to maintain fluid and nutritional intake. The occurrence of nausea or vomiting may be minimized if measures are taken to keep the immediate environment quiet, free of noxious odors, and well ventilated. The avoidance of sudden changes of position and unnecessary activity is also helpful. Use of relaxation techniques, frequent rest periods, and diversional tactics help prevent nausea and vomiting or facilitate a more rapid recovery from their effects. Cleansing the face and hands with a cool washcloth and mouth care between episodes increase the person's comfort level. When the symptoms occur, all foods and drugs should be stopped until the acute phase is past.

If a medication is suspected as the cause, the health care provider should be notified immediately so that either the dosage can be altered or a new drug can be prescribed. The patient should be reminded that stopping the drug without consulting the health care provider may eliminate the immediate cause of the nausea and vomiting but that omission of the prescribed drug may have detrimental effects on health or the disease state.

When food is identified as the precipitating cause of nausea and vomiting, the nurse should help the patient solve the problem. What food was it? When was it eaten? Has this food caused problems in the past? Is anyone else in the family sick?

When the patient believes some foods and fluids can be tolerated, the nurse might suggest that it would be helpful to begin with clear liquids or warm cola beverages, Gatorade, tea or broth, dry crackers or toast, and then plain gelatin. Bland foods, such as pasta, rice, and cooked chicken, are generally well tolerated in small amounts. An antiemetic drug should be taken only if prescribed by the health care provider. Taking over-the-counter (OTC) drugs for relief of symptoms may make the condition worse.

■ Evaluation

The expected outcomes are that the patient with nausea and vomiting will

- be comfortable with minimal or no nausea and vomiting
- maintain body weight
- have electrolyte levels within normal range
- be able to maintain adequate intake of fluids and nutrients

NURSING CARE PLAN 40-1

Patient with Nausea and Vomiting

EXPECTED PATIENT OUTCOMES	NURSING INTERVENTIONS and *RATIONALES*
NURSING DIAGNOSIS	**Nausea** *related to* multiple etiologies *as manifested by* episodes of nausea and vomiting
• Minimal or no nausea • Verbalization of satisfaction with care	• Assess duration, frequency, and nature of nausea and vomiting and aggravating and alleviating factors *to plan appropriate interventions.* • Remove visual stimuli and source of odors *to avoid precipitating triggers of nausea and/or vomiting.* • Provide mouth care; change soiled gown and linens *to ensure patient comfort.* • Maintain quiet environment, restrict visitors, and avoid unnecessary procedures or activities *to minimize triggers of vomiting.* • Administer antiemetic as ordered. • Instruct patient to take several deep breaths; prevent sudden changes in position; keep head of bed elevated *to decrease stimulation of the vomiting center.* • Instruct patient to avoid foods and beverages *that stimulate nausea and vomiting.*
NURSING DIAGNOSIS	**Deficient fluid volume** *related to* prolonged vomiting and inability to ingest, digest, or absorb food and fluids *as manifested by* decreased urine output and increased urine concentration, increased pulse rate, hypotension (postural), decreased intake, decreased skin turgor, dry skin and mucous membranes
• No signs of dehydration	• Assess for signs of dehydration *to plan appropriate care.* • Administer and monitor amount and type of IV fluid *to maintain fluid and electrolyte balance.* • Administer antiemetic as prescribed. • Provide small amounts of clear liquids when vomiting stops *to maintain hydration.* • Record amount and frequency of vomitus; maintain accurate intake and output records; weigh daily in acute phase *to monitor fluid balance accurately.* • Monitor laboratory results of serum sodium, potassium, chloride, and bicarbonate *as indicators of electrolyte balance.*
NURSING DIAGNOSIS	**Imbalanced nutrition: less than body requirements** *related to* nausea and vomiting *as manifested by* lack of interest in or aversion to food, perceived or actual inability to ingest food, weight loss
• Gradual return to usual weight and eating habits	• Assess patient's interest in food, ability to ingest food, and weight *to determine if a problem is present.* • Assure patient that appetite will return when nausea and vomiting are controlled. • Maintain IV feedings or total parenteral nutrition until oral intake is possible *to provide necessary fluids, electrolytes, calories, and protein intake.* • Instruct patient to resume eating cautiously with bland, nonirritating foods in small amounts *to avoid irritating the stomach and initiating recurrence of nausea and vomiting.*

■ Gerontologic Considerations: Nausea and Vomiting

The older patient experiencing nausea and vomiting requires careful assessment and monitoring, particularly during periods of fluid loss and subsequent rehydration therapy. Older patients are more likely to have cardiac or renal insufficiency that places them at greater risk for life-threatening fluid and electrolyte imbalances. In addition, excessive replacement of fluid and electrolytes may result in adverse consequences for the elderly person who has congestive heart failure or renal disease. Finally, the older adult with a decreased level of consciousness may be at high risk for aspiration of vomitus. Close monitoring of the patient's physical status and level of consciousness during episodes of vomiting must be a primary concern for the nurse.

In addition, the elderly are particularly susceptible to the CNS side effects of antiemetic drugs; these drugs may produce confusion. Dosages should be reduced and efficacy closely evaluated. Safety precautions also should be instituted for these patients. ■

ORAL INFLAMMATIONS AND INFECTIONS

Oral infections and inflammations may be specific mouth diseases, or they may occur in the presence of some systemic diseases such as leukemia or vitamin deficiency. When oral inflammations and infections are present, they can severely impair the ingestion of food and fluids. Common inflammations and infections of the oral cavity are presented in Table 40-3. The patient who is immunosuppressed (e.g., patient with acquired immunodeficiency syndrome or receiving chemotherapy) is most susceptible to oral infections. Patients receiving corticosteroid inhalant treatment for asthma are at risk for oral infections, especially candidiasis.

Oral infections may predispose to infections in other body organs. For example, the oral cavity can be considered a potential reservoir for respiratory pathogens. In addition, oral pathogens have also been associated with heart disease.

An important element in reducing oral infections and inflammation is good oral hygiene. Management of oral infections and

CULTURAL & ETHNIC CONSIDERATIONS
Oral, Pharyngeal, and Esophageal Problems

- Periodontal disease is more prevalent among African Americans than among whites.
- Cancers of the oral cavity and pharynx are the fourth leading cause of death in African American men 35 to 54 years of age.
- Death rates as a result of oral cancer are decreasing in whites but increasing in non-whites.
- Esophageal cancer has a higher incidence among African Americans and Asian Americans than among whites.
- Esophageal cancer has a higher incidence in Alaska Natives compared with whites.
- Asian Americans, Middle Easterners, and African Americans are more likely to experience nausea and vomiting than whites.

inflammation is focused on identification of the cause, elimination of infection, provision of comfort measures, and maintenance of nutritional intake.

ORAL CANCER

Oral (or oropharyngeal) cancer may occur on the lips or anywhere within the mouth (e.g., tongue, floor of the mouth, buccal mucosa, hard palate, soft palate, pharyngeal walls, and tonsils). Oral cancer is diagnosed in 30,100 Americans annually, and it is estimated that 7800 persons a year die from the disease.[1] It is more common after 40 years of age, with 60 years being the average age at onset. Oral cancer occurs in all ethnic groups. It is more common in men (male-to-female ratio of 2:1). Squamous cell carcinoma is the most common oral malignant tumor (more than 90%). Mortality rates have been decreasing since the early 1980s. The 5-year survival for all stages of cancer of the oral cavity and pharynx combined is 53%, and the 10-year rate is 43%.[2]

TABLE 40-3   Infections and Inflammation of the Mouth

CONDITION	ETIOLOGY	CLINICAL MANIFESTATIONS	TREATMENT
• Gingivitis	Neglected oral hygiene, malocclusion, missing or irregular teeth, faulty dentistry, eating of soft rather than fibrous foods	Inflamed gingivae and interdental papillae; bleeding during toothbrushing; development of pus; formation of abscess with loosening of teeth (periodontitis)	Prevention through health teaching, dental care, gingival massage, professional cleaning of teeth, fibrous foods, conscientious brushing habits with flossing
• Vincent's infection (acute necrotizing ulcerative gingivitis, trench mouth)	Fusiform bacteria; Vincent spirochetes; predisposing factors of stress, excessive fatigue, poor oral hygiene, nutritional deficiencies (B and C vitamins)	Painful, bleeding gingivae; eroding necrotic lesions of interdental papillae; ulcerations that bleed; increased saliva with metallic taste; fetid mouth odor; anorexia, fever, and general malaise	Rest (physical and mental); avoidance of smoking and alcoholic beverages; soft, nutritious diet; correct oral hygiene habits; topical applications of antibiotics; mouth irrigations with hydrogen peroxide and saline solutions
• Oral candidiasis (moniliasis or thrush)	*Candida albicans* (a yeastlike fungus), debilitation, prolonged high-dose antibiotic or corticosteroid therapy	Pearly, bluish white "milk-curd" membranous lesions on mucosa of mouth and larynx; sore mouth; yeasty halitosis	Nystatin or amphotericin B as oral suspension or buccal tablets, good oral hygiene
• Herpes simplex (cold sore, fever blister)	Herpes simplex virus, type I or II; predisposing factors of upper respiratory infections, excessive exposure to sunlight, food allergies, emotional tension, onset of menstruation	Lip lesions, mouth lesions, vesicle formation (single or clustered), shallow, painful ulcers	Spirits of camphor, corticosteroid cream, mild antiseptic mouthwash, viscous lidocaine; removal or control of predisposing factors, antiviral agents (e.g., acyclovir [Zovirax]; penciclovir [Denavir])
• Aphthous stomatitis (canker sore)	Recurrent and chronic form of infection secondary to systemic disease, trauma, stress, or unknown causes	Ulcers of mouth and lips, causing extreme pain; ulcers surrounded by erythematous base	Corticosteroids (topical or systemic), tetracycline oral suspension
• Parotitis (inflammation of parotid gland, surgical mumps)	Usually *Staphylococcus* species, *Streptococcus* species occasionally, debilitation and dehydration with poor oral hygiene, NPO status for an extended time	Pain in area of gland and ear, absence of salivation, purulent exudate from gland, erythema, ulcers	Antibiotics, mouthwashes, warm compresses; preventive measures such as chewing gum, sucking on hard candy (lemon drops), adequate fluid intake
• Stomatitis (inflammation of mouth)	Trauma; pathogens; irritants (tobacco, alcohol); renal, liver, and hematologic diseases; side effect of many cancer chemotherapy drugs and radiation	Excessive salivation, halitosis, sore mouth	Removal or treatment of cause, oral hygiene with soothing solutions, topical medications; soft bland diet

Most of the oral malignant lesions occur on the lower lip in men. Other common sites are the lateral border and undersurface of the tongue, the labial commissure, and the buccal mucosa. Carcinoma of the lip has the most favorable prognosis of any of the oral tumors. This is probably because lip lesions are more apparent to the patient than other oral lesions and are usually diagnosed earlier.

Etiology and Pathophysiology

Although the definitive cause of oral cancer is unknown, there are a number of predisposing factors (Table 40-4). Factors that influence the development of oral cancer include tobacco use (e.g., cigar, cigarette, pipe, snuff), excessive alcohol intake, and chronic irritation such as from a jagged tooth or poor dental care. A positive history of tobacco and alcohol use, in the past or currently, is the most significant etiologic factor in oral cancer.[2] Constant overexposure to ultraviolet radiation from the sun is also a factor in the development of cancer of the lip. Irritation from the pipe stem resting on the lip is a factor in pipe smokers.

Clinical Manifestations

The common manifestations of oral cancer are leukoplakia, erythroplakia, ulcerations, a sore that bleeds easily and does not heal, and a rough area (felt with the tongue). **Leukoplakia,** called "white patch" or "smoker's patch," is often considered a precancerous lesion, although less than 5% of these lesions actually transform into malignant cells. It is a whitish patch on the mucosa of the mouth or tongue. The patch becomes *keratinized* (hard and leathery) and is sometimes described as hyperkeratosis. Leukoplakia is the result of chronic irritation, especially from smoking. *Erythroplasia* (erythroplakia), which is seen as a red velvety patch on the mouth or tongue, is also considered a precancerous lesion. Areas of erythroplakia have a 90% chance of becoming malignant. Later symptoms of oral cancer are pain, **dysphagia** (difficulty swallowing), and difficulty in moving the jaw (e.g., chewing and speaking).

Cancer of the lip usually appears as an indurated, painless ulcer on the lip. The first sign of carcinoma of the tongue is an ulcer or area of thickening. Soreness or pain of the tongue may occur, especially when eating hot or highly seasoned foods. Cancerous lesions are most likely to develop in the proximal half of the tongue. Some patients experience limitation of movement of the tongue. Later symptoms of cancer of the tongue include increased salivation, slurred speech, dysphagia, toothache, and earache. Approximately 30% of patients with oral cancer have an asymptomatic neck mass.

Diagnostic Studies

Biopsy of the suspected lesion with cytologic examination is the best definitive diagnostic study for oral cancer. Oral exfoliative cytology involves scraping the suspicious lesion and spreading this scraping on a slide. Unlike biopsy, a negative cytologic smear does not reliably rule out the possibility of a malignant condition, but it may be used as an initial screening test. The toluidine blue test may also be used as a screening test for oral cancer. Toluidine blue is applied topically to stain an area, and cancer cells preferentially take up the dye. However, the definitive diagnosis of cancer is based on biopsy and histology.[3]

Collaborative Care

Collaborative care of oral carcinoma usually consists of surgery, radiation, chemotherapy, or a combination of these (Table 40-5).

TABLE 40-5	*C*ollaborative Care **Oral Cancer**
Diagnostic	
History and physical examination	
Biopsy	
Oral exfoliative cytology	
Toluidine blue test	
CT and MRI scans	
Collaborative Therapy*	
Surgery	
Surgical excision of the tumor	
Radical neck dissection	
Radiation (internal or external)	
Combined surgical resection with radiation	
Chemotherapy	

*Any of the following approaches may be used, depending on the primary lesion and the extent of metastasis.
CT, Computed tomography; *MRI,* magnetic resonance imaging.

TABLE 40-4	**Types and Characteristics of Oral Cancer**		
LOCATION	**PREDISPOSING FACTORS**	**CLINICAL MANIFESTATIONS**	**TREATMENT**
• Lip	Constant overexposure to sun, ruddy and fair complexion, recurrent herpetic lesions, irritation from pipe stem, syphilis, immunosuppression	Indurated, painless ulcer	Surgical excision, radiation
• Tongue	Tobacco, alcohol, chronic irritation, syphilis	Ulcer or area of thickening; soreness or pain; increased salivation, slurred speech, dysphagia, toothache, earache (later signs)	Surgery (hemiglossectomy or glossectomy), radiation
• Oral cavity	Poor oral hygiene, tobacco usage (pipe and cigar smoking, snuff, chewing tobacco), chronic alcohol intake, chronic irritation (jagged tooth, ill-fitting prosthesis, chemical or mechanical irritants)	Leukoplakia; erythroplakia; ulcerations; sore spot; rough area; pain, dysphagia, difficulty in chewing and speaking (later signs)	Surgery (mandibulectomy, radical neck dissection, resections of buccal mucosa), internal and external radiation

Surgical Therapy. Surgery remains the most effective treatment, especially for removing the central core of the tumor. Many of the operations are radical procedures involving extensive resections. Various surgical procedures may be performed, depending on the location and extent of the tumor. Some examples are partial *mandibulectomy* (removal of the mandible), *hemiglossectomy* (removal of half of the tongue), *glossectomy* (removal of the tongue), resections of the buccal mucosa and floor of the mouth, and radical neck dissection. Composite resections, which are combinations of the various surgical procedures, may be performed.

Because cancers of the oral cavity metastasize early to the cervical lymph nodes, a radical neck dissection is commonly performed. It includes wide excision of the involved primary lesion with removal of the regional lymph nodes, the deep cervical lymph nodes, and their lymphatic channels. In addition, the following structures may also be removed or transected (depending on the extent of the primary lesion): sternocleidomastoid muscle and other closely associated muscles, internal jugular vein, mandible, submaxillary gland, part of the thyroid and parathyroid glands, and spinal accessory nerve. A tracheostomy is commonly performed along with the radical neck dissection. Drainage tubes are inserted into the surgical area and connected to suction to remove fluid and blood.

Nonsurgical Therapy. Chemotherapy and radiation therapy are used together when the lesions are more advanced or involve several structures of the oral cavity. Chemotherapy may also be used when surgery and radiation therapy fail or as the initial therapy for smaller tumors. Chemotherapeutic agents used include 5-fluorouracil (5-FU), cyclophosphamide (Cytoxan), bleomycin (Blenoxane), vinblastine (Velban), hydroxyurea (Hydrea), and cisplatin (Platinol) (see Chapter 15).

Palliative treatment may be the best management when the prognosis is poor, the cancer is inoperable, or the patient decides against surgery. Palliation aims to treat the symptoms and make the patient more comfortable. If it becomes difficult for the patient to swallow, a gastrostomy may be performed to allow for adequate nutritional intake (see Gastrostomy in Chapter 39). Analgesic medication should be given freely to this patient. Frequent suctioning of the oral cavity becomes necessary when swallowing becomes difficult. (Other nursing measures for the terminally ill patient are discussed in Chapter 15.)

Nutritional Therapy. Because of depression, alcoholism, or presurgery radiation treatment, patients may be malnourished even before surgery. After radical neck surgery, the patient may be unable to take in nutrients through the normal route of ingestion because of swelling, location of sutures, or difficulty with swallowing. Parenteral fluids will be given for the first 24 to 48 hours. After this time, tube feedings are usually given via an NG or nasointestinal tube that was placed during surgery. Sometimes a temporary feeding gastrostomy may be used. (NG and gastrostomy feedings are described in Chapter 39.) Cervical esophagostomy and pharyngostomy have also been used. The nurse must observe for tolerance of the feedings and adjust the amount, time, and formula if nausea, vomiting, diarrhea, or distention occurs. The patient is instructed about the tube feedings. When the patient can swallow, small amounts of water are given. Close observation for choking is essential. Suctioning may be necessary to prevent aspiration.

NURSING MANAGEMENT
ORAL CANCER

■ Nursing Assessment

Subjective and objective data that should be obtained from a patient with oral cancer are presented in Table 40-6.

■ Nursing Diagnoses

Nursing diagnoses for the patient with oral cancer may include, but are not limited to, the following:
- Imbalanced nutrition: less than body requirements *related to* oral pain, difficulty chewing and swallowing, surgical resection, and radiation treatment
- Chronic pain *related to* the tumor and surgical radiation
- Anxiety *related to* diagnosis of cancer, uncertain future, potential for disfiguring surgery, potential for recurrence, and prognosis
- Ineffective coping *related to* body image change
- Ineffective health maintenance *related to* lack of knowledge of disease process and therapeutic regimen and unavailability of a support system

■ Planning

The overall goals are that the patient with carcinoma of the oral cavity will (1) have a patent airway, (2) be able to communicate, (3) have adequate nutritional intake to promote wound healing, and (4) have relief of pain and discomfort.

TABLE 40-6	Nursing Assessment Oral Cancer

Subjective Data
Important Health Information
Past health history: Recurrent oral herpetic lesions, syphilis, exposure to sunlight
Medications: Immunosuppressants
Surgery or other treatments: Removal of prior tumors or lesions
Functional Health Patterns
Health perception–health management: Use of alcohol and tobacco, pipe smoking; poor oral hygiene
Nutritional-metabolic: Reductions in oral intake, weight loss; difficulty in chewing food; increased salivation; intolerance to certain foods or temperatures of food
Cognitive-perceptual: Mouth or tongue soreness or pain, toothache, earache, neck stiffness, dysphagia, difficulty speaking
Objective Data
Integumentary
Indurated, painless ulcer on lip; painless neck mass
Gastrointestinal
Areas of thickening or roughness, ulcers, leukoplakia, or erythroplakia on the tongue or oral mucosa; limited movement of the tongue; increased salivation, drooling; slurred speech; foul breath odor
Possible Findings
Positive exfoliative smear cytology (microscopic examination of cells removed by scraping); positive biopsy

■ Nursing Implementation

Health Promotion. The nurse has a significant role in early detection and treatment of oral cancer. The nurse needs to provide the patient with information regarding predisposing factors, such as constant overexposure to the sun, tobacco, and other irritants. Smoking and the long-term use of smokeless tobacco are the major risk factors for oral cancer. A patient identified as a smoker should be informed about smoking cessation programs available in the community. (Smoking cessation is discussed in Chapter 11 and Tables 11-13 and 11-14).

It is important that adolescents and teenagers be informed about the danger of using snuff, or chewing tobacco. In addition, oral cancers have an increased chance of recurrence if risk factors are not reduced. The nurse should also teach correct oral hygiene and dental care and encourage the patient to seek preventive dental care. Risk factors should be identified. Because early detection of oral cancer is important, the patient should be taught to examine the mouth and to recognize danger signals of oral cancer. If any of these signals are present, the patient should be instructed to visit a health care provider. Danger signals include unexplained pain or soreness in the mouth, unusual bleeding from the oral cavity, dysphagia, and swelling or lump in the neck.

Any individual with an ulcerative lesion that does not heal within 2 to 3 weeks should be referred to a health care provider, and a biopsy of the lesion should probably be performed. The nurse should inspect the patient's oral cavity to detect suspicious lesions.

Acute Intervention. Preoperative care for the patient who is to have a radical neck dissection involves consideration of the patient's physical and psychosocial needs. Physical preparation is the same as for any major surgery, with special emphasis on oral hygiene. Thorough assessment of alcohol intake should be done, and measures to assess and treat withdrawal if it is a problem should be implemented early. Explanations and emotional support are of special significance and should include postoperative measures relating to communication and feeding. The surgical procedure should be explained to the patient, and the nurse should make sure that the patient understands the information. Radical neck dissection and related nursing management are discussed in Chapter 26 and NCP 26-2.

■ Evaluation

The expected outcomes are that the patient with oral cancer will

- have no respiratory complications
- be able to communicate
- participate in regular follow-up examinations
- maintain an adequate nutritional intake to promote wound healing
- experience minimal pain and discomfort with eating, drinking, and talking

Esophageal Disorders

GASTROESOPHAGEAL REFLUX DISEASE

Etiology and Pathophysiology

Gastroesophageal reflux disease (GERD) is not a disease but a syndrome. The term *GERD* is defined as any clinically significant symptomatic condition or histopathologic alter-

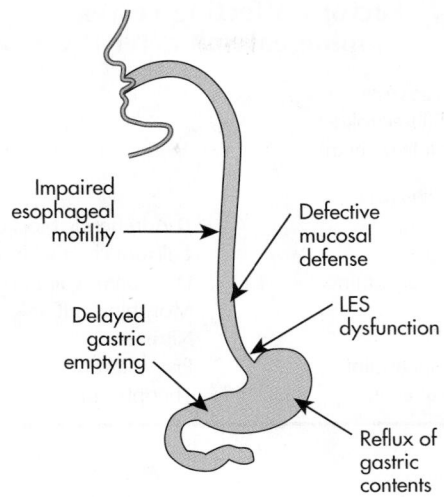

FIG. 40-2 Factors involved in the pathogenesis of gastroesophageal reflux disease (GERD). *LES,* Lower esophageal sphincter.

ation presumed to be secondary to reflux of gastric contents into the lower esophagus. Approximately 5% to 7% of the world's population experience GERD. More than 60 million Americans periodically experience symptoms of gastroesophageal reflux, and approximately 17.5 million (or 7%) experience daily symptoms.[4]

There is no one single cause of GERD. Several factors or combination of factors can be involved (Fig. 40-2). It results when the defenses of the lower esophagus are overwhelmed by the reflux of stomach acidic contents into the esophagus. Predisposing conditions include hiatal hernia, incompetent lower esophageal sphincter (LES), decreased esophageal clearance (ability to clear liquids or food from the esophagus into the stomach) resulting from impaired esophageal motility, and decreased gastric emptying. The acidic gastric secretions that reflux up into the lower esophagus result in esophageal irritation and inflammation (esophagitis). In addition, the presence of the gastric enzyme pepsin and intestinal enzymes (e.g., trypsin) and bile salts are also corrosive to the esophageal mucosa. The degree of inflammation depends on the amount and composition of gastric reflux and on the ability of the esophagus to clear the acidic contents.

One of the primary factors in GERD is an incompetent LES. An incompetent LES results in a decrease in pressure in the distal portion of the esophagus. As a result, gastric contents are able to move from an area of higher pressure (stomach) to an area of lower pressure (esophagus) when the patient is in a supine position or has an increase in intraabdominal pressure. Decreased LES pressure can be due to certain foods (e.g., caffeine, chocolate) and drugs (e.g., anticholinergics). A common cause of GERD is a hiatal hernia, which is discussed in the next section.

Clinical Manifestations

The symptoms of GERD vary from individual to individual. Heartburn *(pyrosis)* from gastroesophageal reflux is the most common clinical manifestation. It is caused by irritation of the esophagus by the gastric secretions. Heartburn is described as a

TABLE 40-7	Factors Affecting Lower Esophageal Sphincter Pressure

Increase Pressure
bethanechol (Urecholine)
metoclopramide (Reglan)

Decrease Pressure

Alcohol	β-Adrenergic blockers
Anticholinergics	Calcium channel blockers
Chocolate (theobromine)	Diazepam (Valium)
Fatty foods	Morphine sulfate
Nicotine	Nitrates
Peppermint, spearmint	Progesterone
Tea, coffee (caffeine)	Theophylline

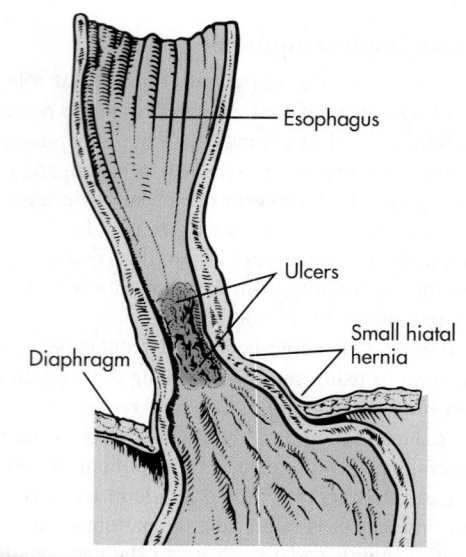

FIG. 40-3 Esophagitis with esophageal ulcerations.

burning, tight sensation that is felt intermittently beneath the lower sternum and spreads upward to the throat or jaw. The majority of individuals have mild symptoms including heartburn after a meal that occurs about once a week with no evidence of mucosal damage. However, the persistence of mild symptoms for a period of 5 years or more or symptoms associated with difficulty swallowing should be evaluated. In addition, heartburn that occurs more frequently than once a week, becomes more severe, or occurs at night and wakes a person from sleep may be a sign of a more serious condition, and consultation with a health care provider is advised.[5]

Heartburn may occur following ingestion of food or drugs that decrease the LES pressure or are directly irritating to the esophageal mucosa (Table 40-7). Heartburn is relieved with milk, alkaline substances, or water. An individual with GERD may also report respiratory symptoms including wheezing, coughing, and dyspnea. Otolaryngologic symptoms include hoarseness, sore throat, a globus sensation (sense of a lump in the throat), and choking. *Regurgitation* (effortless return of food or gastric contents from the stomach into esophagus or mouth) is a fairly common manifestation of GERD. It is often described as hot, bitter, or sour liquid coming into the throat or mouth. Gastric symptoms including early satiety, postmeal bloating, nausea, and vomiting are related to delayed gastric emptying.

Complications

Complications of GERD are related to the direct local effects of gastric acid on the esophageal mucosa. **Esophagitis** (inflammation of the esophagus) is a frequent complication of GERD. Other risk factors for esophagitis include hiatal hernia, chemical irritation from lye or physical irritants such as smoking, cold or hot liquids, and excessive alcoholic intake. Trauma to the esophagus may also produce inflammation. Esophagitis with esophageal ulcerations is shown in Fig. 40-3.

Repeated exposure may cause scar tissue formation and decreased distensibility (*esophageal stricture*) of the esophagus. This may result in dysphagia.

Another complication of GERD is **Barrett's esophagus** (esophageal metaplasia). Barrett's esophagus is considered a precancerous lesion, which places the patient at risk for esophageal cancer. In Barrett's esophagus there is replacement of the normal squamous epithelium of the esophagus with columnar epithelium. These cell changes are thought to be related to chronic reflux esophagitis. Signs and symptoms of Barrett's esophagus can range from none to mild to bleeding and perforation. Because patients with Barrett's esophagus are at higher risk for adenocarcinoma, they may need to be monitored on a regular basis (every 1 to 3 years) by endoscopy and biopsy.

Respiratory complications of GERD include bronchospasm, laryngospasm, and cricopharyngeal spasm. These complications are due to irritation of the upper airway by gastric secretions. With GERD there is also the potential for pneumonia as a result of aspiration of gastric contents into the respiratory system. Dental erosion, especially in the posterior teeth, may result from acid reflux into the mouth.

Diagnostic Studies

Diagnostic studies are performed to determine the cause of the GERD (e.g., hiatal hernia) (Table 40-8). Barium swallow is done to determine if there is protrusion of the upper part of the stomach (called the *gastric fundus*). Endoscopy is useful in assessing the competence of the LES and the extent of inflammation (if present), potential scarring, and strictures. Biopsy and cytologic specimens can be taken to differentiate carcinoma of the stomach or esophagus from Barrett's esophagus. Esophageal manometric studies are performed to measure pressure in the esophagus, as well as in the LES. The determination of pH using specially designed probes in the laboratory or using ambulatory monitoring systems may demonstrate the presence of acid in the normally alkaline esophagus. Radionuclide tests may also be performed to detect reflux of gastric contents and the rate of esophageal clearance.

Because of the cost and discomfort of diagnostic procedures, it has been suggested that high-dose proton pump inhibitor (PPI) treatment (explained under Drug Therapy) for a short period (2 weeks) can be used as a first step in the diagnosis of GERD.[6] In patients with GERD, PPI treatment should result in a marked reduction or elimination of symptoms.[7]

TABLE 40-8	Collaborative Care

Gastroesophageal Reflux Disease (GERD) and Hiatal Hernia

Diagnostic
History and physical examination
Upper GI endoscopy with biopsy and cytologic analysis
Barium swallow
Motility (manometry) studies
pH monitoring (laboratory or 24 hr ambulatory)

Collaborative Therapy
Conservative
Elevation of head of bed on 4- to 6-inch blocks
High-protein, low-fat diet with avoidance of foods that decrease LES pressure or irritate acid-sensitive esophagus
Antacids
Antisecretory agents
  H₂-receptor blockers*
  Proton pump inhibitors*
Prokinetic drug therapy*
Cholinergic drugs
Surgical
Nissen fundoplication
Toupet fundoplication
Hill gastropexy
Belsey fundoplication
Endoscopic
Stretta device

*See Table 40-9.
LES, Lower esophageal sphincter.

Collaborative Care

Most patients with GERD can be successfully managed by lifestyle modifications and drug therapy. These are long-term approaches requiring patient teaching and compliance with therapies. When these therapies are ineffective, surgery is an option (see Table 40-8).

Lifestyle Modifications. The patient with GERD is taught to avoid factors that aggravate symptoms. Particular attention is given to diet and drugs that may affect the LES, acid secretion, or gastric emptying. Patients who smoke are encouraged to stop. Cigarette smoking has been associated with decreased acid clearance from the lower esophagus.[8]

Nutritional Therapy. Diet does not cause GERD, but food can aggravate symptoms. No specific diet is necessary, but foods that cause reflux should be avoided. Fatty foods stimulate the release of cholecystokinin, a hormone from the duodenum that decreases LES pressure. High-fat foods also decrease the rate of gastric emptying. Foods that decrease LES pressure, such as chocolate, peppermint, coffee, and tea (see Table 40-7), should be avoided because they predispose to reflux. Milk products should be avoided, especially at bedtime, because milk increases gastric acid secretion. Small, frequent meals are advised to prevent overdistention of the stomach. The patient should avoid late evening meals and nocturnal snacking. Fluids should be taken between rather than with meals to reduce gastric distention. Cer-

tain foods (e.g., tomato-based products, orange juice) may irritate the acid-sensitive esophagus and may need to be avoided. To reduce intraabdominal pressure, weight reduction is recommended if the patient is overweight.

Drug Therapy. Drug therapy for GERD is focused on improving LES function, increasing esophageal clearance, decreasing volume and acidity of reflux, and protecting the esophageal mucosa (Table 40-9). There are two approaches to drug therapy. The first is the "step-up" approach, which means starting with antacids and OTC histamine-2 receptor (H₂R) blockers and increasing to prescription H₂R blockers and, finally, proton pump inhibitors (PPIs). The "step-down" approach involves starting with a PPI and over time titrating down to prescription H₂R blockers and, finally, OTC H₂R blockers and antacids.

Antacids produce quick but short-lived relief of heartburn. They act by neutralizing HCl. They should be taken 1 to 3 hours after meals and at bedtime. OTC antacids with or without alginic acid (e.g., Gaviscon) may be useful in patients with mild, intermittent heartburn. The alginic acid reacts with sodium bicarbonate and forms a viscous solution that floats to the surface of the gastric contents and coats the esophagus, acting as a mechanical barrier to reflux. However, in patients with moderate to severe or frequent symptoms or patients with documented esophagitis, these regimens are not effective in relieving symptoms or healing erosive lesions.

Antisecretory agents decrease the secretion of HCl acid by the stomach. H₂R blockers (e.g., cimetidine [Tagamet], ranitidine [Zantac], famotidine [Pepcid], nizatidine [Axid]) are available in OTC and prescription formulations. OTC preparations (e.g., Pepcid AC, Tagamet HB, Zantac 75, Axid AR) have lower drug dosages compared with prescription drugs (e.g., Zantac 75 has 75 mg compared with 150 mg in prescription Zantac). Some formulations include an H₂R plus antacid combinations. For example, Pepcid Complete includes famotidine, calcium carbonate, and magnesium hydroxide. In prescription doses, H₂R blockers reduce symptoms and promote esophageal healing in approximately 50% of patients. Patients frequently relapse (i.e., GERD symptoms return) with discontinuance of the drug.

PPIs such as omeprazole (Prilosec), esomeprazole (Nexium), pantoprazole (Protonix), lansoprazole (Prevacid), and rabeprazole (Aciphex) also decrease stomach HCl acid secretion. These agents act by inhibiting the proton pump mechanism responsible for the secretion of H⁺ ions. PPIs promote esophageal healing in approximately 80% to 90% of patients but are more expensive than H₂R blockers. PPIs may also be beneficial in decreasing the incidence of esophageal strictures, a complication of chronic GERD.

Another drug that may be used to treat GERD is sucralfate (Carafate), an antiulcer drug used for its cytoprotective properties. Cholinergic drugs, such as bethanechol (Urecholine), may be used to increase LES pressure, improve esophageal emptying in the supine position, and increase gastric emptying. However, the value of current cholinergic agents is limited because they also stimulate HCl acid secretion. Prokinetic (motility-enhancing) drugs such as metoclopramide (Reglan) promote gastric emptying and reduce the risk of gastric acid reflux (see Table 40-9).

Surgical Therapy. Surgical therapy (antireflux surgery) may be necessary if long-term conservative therapy fails; if a hiatal hernia is present; or if complications, such as esophageal stricture and stenosis (narrowing), chronic esophagitis, and

TABLE 40-9 Drug Therapy — Gastroesophageal Reflux Disease (GERD)

MECHANISM OF ACTION	EXAMPLES
Increase LES Pressure Cholinergic	bethanecol (Urecholine)
Promotility Prokinetic	metoclopramide (Reglan)
Acid Neutralizing Antacids	Gelusil, Maalox, Mylanta
Antisecretory H₂-receptor blockers	cimetidine (Tagamet) famotidine (Pepcid) nizatidine (Axid) ranitidine (Zantac)
Proton pump inhibitors (PPIs)	esomeprazole (Nexium) lansoprazole (Prevacid) omeprazole (Prilosec) pantoprazole (Protonix) rabeprazole (Aciphex)
Cytoprotective Alginic acid-antacid Acid-protective	Gaviscon sucralfate (Carafate)

LES, Lower esophageal sphincter.

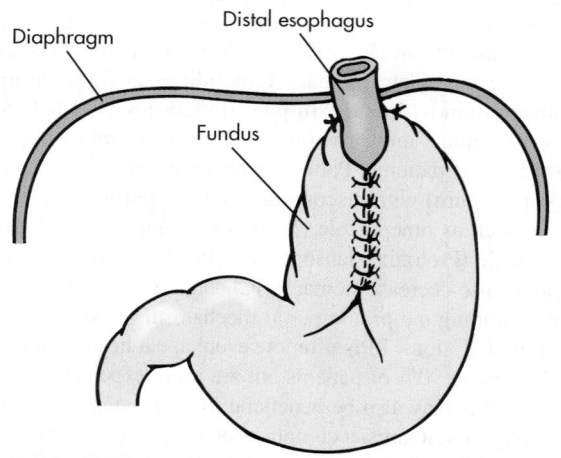

FIG. 40-4 Nissen fundoplication for repair of hiatal hernia. Fundus of stomach is wrapped around distal esophagus and sutured to itself.

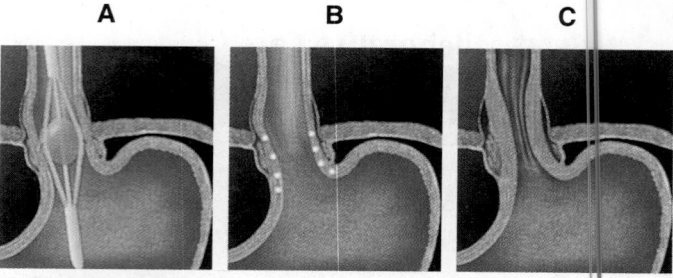

FIG. 40-5 Stretta procedure used to treat GERD. **A,** Catheter positioned. **B,** Multiple sites treated with radiofrequency energy. **C,** Remodeling occurs with collagen formation.

bleeding, exist. Most surgical procedures are performed laparoscopically. The objective of surgical interventions for GERD is to reduce reflux of gastric contents by enhancing the integrity of the LES. Surgical interventions for GERD are called *antireflux* procedures. In these procedures the fundus of the stomach is wrapped around the lower portion of the esophagus in varying positions.

The Nissen fundoplication is shown in Fig. 40-4. Laparoscopically performed Nissen and Toupet fundoplications have become the standard antireflux surgeries.[9] The use of laparoscopic antireflux surgery for GERD has reduced complications, overall morbidity, and the cost of hospitalization compared with a thoracic or open abdominal approach.

Endoscopic Therapy. Recently the Food and Drug Administration approved the use of the Stretta device, which is a balloon-tipped four-needle catheter that delivers radiofrequency energy to the smooth muscle of the gastroesophageal junction for the management of GERD[10] (Fig. 40-5). The radiofrequency energy induces collagen contraction, which helps to form a barrier against acid reflux. This procedure can be performed endoscopically under conscious sedation. The Stretta procedure can be used in patients who have breakthrough symptoms while receiving drug therapy, are intolerant to drug therapy, are candidates for antireflux surgery but desire a less invasive option, or are not surgical candidates because of comorbidities. At this time, the long-term benefit of this approach remains to be determined.

Enteryx, a permanently implanted device, can be inserted endoscopically into the wall of the lower esophagus. This device is a solution that solidifies into spongy material that prevents reflux.

NURSING MANAGEMENT
GASTROESOPHAGEAL REFLUX DISEASE

Patients with GERD must avoid factors that cause reflux. A patient teaching guide is provided in Table 40-10. The patient who is a smoker should stop smoking. Smoking causes an almost immediate drop in LES pressure and decreases the ability to clear acid from the esophagus. The patient may need to be referred to other members of the health care team or to community resources for assistance in stopping smoking. (See Chapter 11 for additional information related to smoking cessation.) Substances that decrease LES pressure and tone should be avoided (see Table 40-7). If stress seems to cause symptoms, measures to cope with stress should be discussed. (See Chapter 8 for stress management techniques.) The patient should also be taught possible side effects of drugs.

Nursing care for the patient who is having acute symptoms consists mainly of encouraging the patient to follow the necessary regimen. The nurse should ensure that the head of the bed is elevated to approximately 30 degrees (usually on 4- to 6-inch blocks) and that the patient does not lie down during the first 2 to 3 hours after eating. Teaching the patient to avoid food and activities that cause reflux is important (e.g., late-night eating should be avoided). The patient may be taking drugs to relieve heartburn, so the nurse must observe for side effects, as well as

TABLE
40-10

*P*atient & Family Teaching Guide
Prevention of Gastroesophageal Reflux Disease (GERD)

The following are teaching guidelines for the patient and family:
1. Explain the rationale for a high-protein, low-fat diet.
2. Encourage the patient to eat small, frequent meals to prevent gastric distention.
3. Explain the rationale for avoiding alcohol, smoking (causes an almost immediate, marked decrease in LES pressure), and beverages that contain caffeine.
4. Teach the patient not to lie down for 2 to 3 hours after eating, wear tight clothing around the waist, or bend over (especially after eating).
5. Encourage the patient to sleep with head of bed elevated on 4- to 6-inch blocks (gravity fosters esophageal emptying).
6. Teach information regarding drugs, including rationale for their use and common side effects.
7. Discuss strategies for weight reduction if appropriate.
8. Encourage patient and family to share concerns about lifestyle changes and living with a chronic problem.

evaluate their effectiveness. Even when symptoms are brought under control, the patient may need to continue drugs because the underlying problem is still present. Because of the link between GERD and metaplastic changes in the lower esophagus (Barrett's esophagus), patients are instructed to see their health care provider if symptoms persist.

The nurse needs to observe for and instruct the patient about side effects of the drugs being taken. Side effects with H_2R blockers and PPIs are rare. Antacids have minimal side effects. Antacids that contain aluminum tend to cause constipation, whereas those that contain magnesium tend to cause diarrhea. Several of the antacids are combinations of aluminum and magnesium designed to minimize these side effects. If the patient is taking bethanechol, side effects to observe for include urinary urgency, increased salivation, abdominal cramping with diarrhea, nausea, vomiting, and hypotension. Such side effects often limit the effectiveness of cholinergic agents in the treatment of GERD. Side effects of metoclopramide include restlessness, anxiety, insomnia, and hallucinations. Side effects of sucralfate include drowsiness, dizziness, nausea, vomiting, constipation, urticaria, and rash.

Postoperative care focuses on concerns related to prevention of respiratory complications, maintenance of fluid and electrolyte balance, and prevention of infection. If a thoracic approach is used, a chest tube is inserted. Assessment and management related to closed chest drainage are important (see Chapter 27).

If an open abdominal incision is used, respiratory complications can occur in a patient because of the high abdominal incision. Respiratory assessment should include respiratory rate and rhythm, pulse rate and rhythm, and signs of pneumothorax (e.g., dyspnea, chest pain, cyanosis). Deep breathing is essential to fully expand the lungs.

The patient receives IV fluids and electrolytes until the return of peristalsis. Care should be taken to maintain patency of the NG tube (if present) to prevent the need to reinsert the tube. It is dangerous to attempt to replace the tube because of the possibility of perforation of the surgical repair. Immediately after the surgical procedure, the patient cannot voluntarily vomit or belch, and this may cause the bloating and abdominal discomfort. When peristalsis returns, only fluids are given initially. Solids are added gradually so that the stomach is not overdistended. The nurse must maintain an accurate recording of intake and output and observe for fluid and electrolyte imbalances (see Chapter 16). (Care of the patient undergoing a laparotomy procedure is described in NCP 41-2 on p. 1063.)

After surgical therapy, there should be no symptoms of gastric reflux. However, the recurrence rate may range from 10% to 30% over a 20-year period following surgery. The patient should be instructed to report symptoms such as heartburn and regurgitation. Such problems may be temporary and resolve with time. In the first month after surgery the patient may report mild dysphagia caused by edema, but it should resolve.[5] The patient should report persistent dysphagia, epigastric fullness, and bloating. A normal diet is gradually resumed. The patient should avoid foods that are gas forming and should try to prevent gastric distention. Food should be chewed thoroughly.

HIATAL HERNIA

Hiatal hernia is herniation of a portion of the stomach into the esophagus through an opening, or hiatus, in the diaphragm. It is also referred to as diaphragmatic hernia and esophageal hernia. The incidence of hiatal hernia is difficult to determine. However, it is the most common abnormality found on x-ray examination of the upper GI tract. Hiatal hernias are common in older adults and occur more often in women than in men.

Types

Hiatal hernias are classified into the following two types (Fig. 40-6):
1. *Sliding:* The junction of the stomach and esophagus is above the hiatus of the diaphragm, and a part of the stomach slides through the hiatal opening in the diaphragm. The stomach "slides" into the thoracic cavity when the patient is supine and usually goes back into the abdominal cavity when the patient is standing upright. This is the most common type of hiatal hernia.
2. *Paraesophageal or rolling:* The esophagogastric junction remains in the normal position, but the fundus and the greater curvature of the stomach roll up through the diaphragm, forming a pocket alongside the esophagus.

Etiology and Pathophysiology

The actual cause of hiatal hernia is unknown. Many factors contribute to the development of hiatal hernia. Structural changes, such as weakening of the muscles in the diaphragm around the esophagogastric opening, are usually contributing factors. Factors that increase intraabdominal pressure, including obesity, pregnancy, ascites, tumors, tight corsets, intense physical exertion, and heavy lifting on a continual basis, may also predispose to development of a hiatal hernia. Other predisposing factors are increased age, trauma, poor nutrition, and a forced recumbent position, as when a prolonged illness confines the person to bed. In some cases, congenital weakness is a contributing factor.

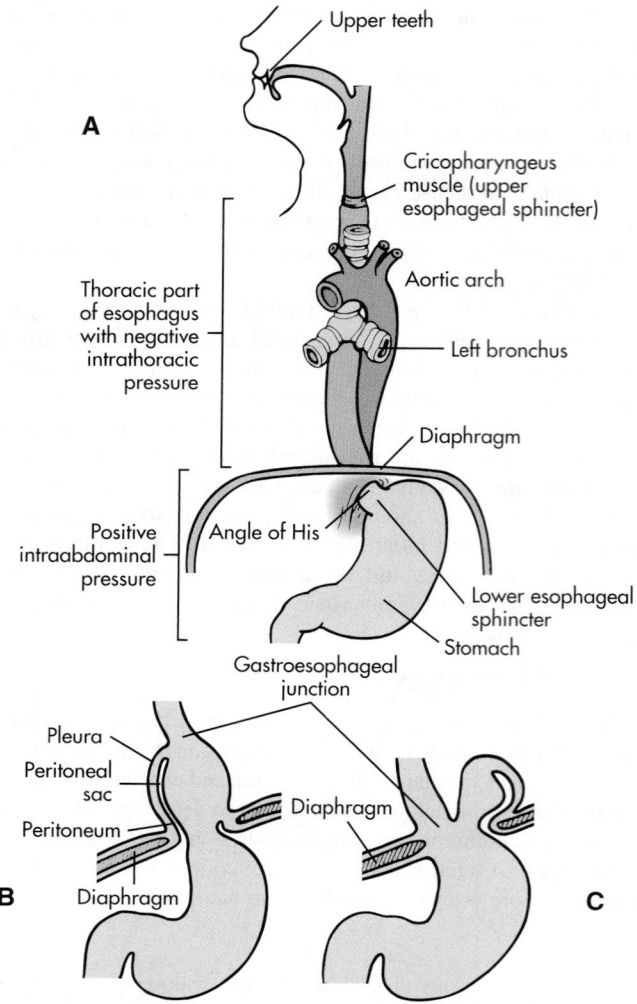

FIG. 40-6 A, Normal esophagus. B, Sliding hiatal hernia. C, Rolling or paraesophageal hernia.

Clinical Manifestations

Persons with hiatal hernia may be asymptomatic. When present, the signs and symptoms of hiatal hernia are similar to those described for GERD. Heartburn, especially after a meal or after lying supine, is a common symptom. Patients may complain of dysphagia. Frequently the symptoms of hiatal hernia mimic gallbladder disease, peptic ulcer disease, and angina. However, some patients with hiatal hernia have no symptoms. Reflux and discomfort are also associated with position, occurring soon or several hours after lying down. Bending over may cause a severe burning pain, which is usually relieved by sitting or standing. Other common precipitating factors of pain include large meals, alcohol, and smoking. Nocturnal symptoms of heartburn are common, especially if the person has eaten before going to sleep.

Complications

Complications that may occur with hiatal hernia include GERD, hemorrhage from erosion, stenosis (narrowing of the esophagus), ulcerations of the herniated portion of the stomach, strangulation of the hernia, and regurgitation with tracheal aspiration. Patients with a history of hiatal hernia are more at risk for hospitalization for respiratory disease.[11]

Diagnostic Studies

A barium swallow is an important diagnostic measure that may show the protrusion of gastric mucosa through the esophageal hiatus in the patient with hiatal hernia. Endoscopic visualization of the lower esophagus provides information on the degree of mucosal inflammation or other abnormalities. Other tests are similar to those described in Table 40-8.

NURSING *and* COLLABORATIVE MANAGEMENT HIATAL HERNIA

■ Conservative Therapy

Conservative therapy of hiatal hernia is similar to that described under GERD, including lifestyle modifications (e.g., reduction of intraabdominal pressure by eliminating constricting garments, avoiding lifting and straining, eliminating alcohol and smoking, elevating the head of the bed), and the use of antacids and antisecretory agents (PPIs, H₂R blockers). Elevation of the bed on 4- to 6-inch blocks assists gravity in maintaining the stomach in the abdominal cavity and also helps prevent reflux and tracheal aspiration. If overweight, the patient should be encouraged to lose weight.

■ Surgical Therapy

The objective of surgical interventions for hiatal hernia is to reduce reflux by enhancing the integrity of the LES. There are four slightly varied procedures: the Nissen fundoplication, the Toupet fundoplication or technique, the Hill gastropexy, and the Belsey fundoplication. These surgical procedures are all variations of fundoplication, which involves "wrapping" the fundus of the stomach around the lower portion of the esophagus in varying positions. These procedures reduce the hernia, provide an acceptable LES pressure, and prevent movement of the gastroesophageal junction. The Nissen fundoplication is shown in Fig. 40-4. Similar to GERD, laparoscopically performed Nissen and Toupet techniques have become the standard antireflux surgeries for hiatal hernia.[9] A thoracic or open abdominal approach may also be used in selected cases.

■ Gerontologic Considerations: GERD and Hiatal Hernia

The incidence of both GERD and hiatal hernia increases with age. It is associated with weakening of the diaphragm, obesity, kyphosis, and use of corsets or other factors that increase intraabdominal pressure. Some older adults with hiatal hernia are asymptomatic. The first indications may include esophageal bleeding secondary to esophagitis or respiratory complications (e.g., aspiration pneumonia) related to aspiration of gastric contents. The LES may become less competent with aging in some individuals.

The clinical course and management of GERD and hiatal hernia in the older adult are similar to that for the younger adult. With the increased use of laparoscopic procedures, surgical risks have been reduced. However, an older adult with cardiovascular and pulmonary problems may not be a good candidate for surgical intervention. In addition, changes in lifestyle, including elimination of dietary factors, such as caffeine-containing beverages and chocolate, and elevating the head of the bed on blocks, may be more difficult for the older adult.

ESOPHAGEAL CANCER

Esophageal cancer (a rare malignant neoplasm of the esophagus) is unique in its geographic distribution. There are parts of Asia in which the rate of esophageal cancer is extremely high, whereas in Western societies the incidence is relatively low. For example, esophageal cancer is the second most common type of cancer in China. In the United States in 2002 there were 13,100 cases of esophageal cancer (9800 were men) and 12,600 Americans died from esophageal cancer. Because esophageal cancer is rarely diagnosed in early stages, the 5-year survival rate is 12%.[2]

Estimates of the percentage of esophageal cancer that are adenocarcinomas range from 30% to 70% with the remainder being squamous cell. The incidence of squamous cell esophageal cancer is currently decreasing in the United States, whereas the incidence of adenocarcinoma of the distal esophagus is increasing.[2] In the last 30 years, the incidence of adenocarcinoma has increased sevenfold.[12] Adenocarcinomas arise from the glands lining the esophagus and resemble cancers of the stomach and small intestine. The incidence of esophageal cancer increases with age. There is a higher incidence of esophageal cancer in African Americans relative to whites. The incidence of esophageal cancer is also higher in Alaska Native men and women compared with whites.

One risk factor for esophageal adenocarcinoma is Barrett's esophagus. At this time, it is estimated that 1 of 200 cases of Barrett's esophagus will progress to esophageal cancer. Barrett's esophagus is described earlier under GERD.

Etiology and Pathophysiology

The cause of esophageal cancer is unknown. Two important risk factors are smoking and excessive alcohol intake. Diets that are low in fruits and vegetables and certain minerals and vitamins may increase the risk of this cancer. Lye that is found in strong cleaners like drain cleaners can burn and destroy esophageal cells. As a result, a person who has swallowed lye has a higher risk of squamous cell cancer. A patient with a history of *achalasia,* a condition in which there is delayed emptying of the lower esophagus, is also at greater risk for squamous cell cancer. Other risk factors include exposure to asbestos and metal.[2]

The majority of esophageal tumors are located in the middle and lower portions of the esophagus. The malignant tumor usually appears as an ulcerated lesion and has often advanced by the time the patient experiences symptoms. The tumor may penetrate the muscular layer and even extend outside the wall of the esophagus. Obstruction of the esophagus occurs in the later stages.

Clinical Manifestations

The onset of symptoms is usually late in relation to the extent of the tumor. Progressive dysphagia is the most common symptom and may be expressed as a substernal feeling (globus sensation) as if food is not passing. Initially the dysphagia occurs only with meat, then with soft foods, and eventually with liquids.

Pain develops late and is described as occurring in the substernal, epigastric, or back areas and usually increases with swallowing. The pain may radiate to the neck, jaw, ears, and shoulders. If the tumor is in the upper third of the esophagus, symptoms such as sore throat, choking, and hoarseness may occur. Weight loss is fairly common. When esophageal stenosis is severe, regurgitation of blood-flecked esophageal contents is common.

Complications

Hemorrhage may occur if the cancer erodes through the esophagus and into the aorta. Esophageal perforation with fistula formation into the lung or trachea sometimes develops. The tumor may enlarge enough to cause esophageal obstruction. There is spread via the lymph system, with the liver and lung being common sites of metastasis.

Diagnostic Studies

Barium swallow with fluoroscopy may demonstrate a narrowing of the esophagus at the site of the tumor (Table 40-11). Sometimes a crater is visible. Endoscopy with biopsy is necessary to make a definitive diagnosis of carcinoma by identification of malignant cells. Endoscopic ultrasonography is an important tool used to stage esophageal cancer. A bronchoscopic examination may be performed to detect malignant involvement of the lung. Computed tomography (CT) scanning and magnetic resonance imaging (MRI) are also used to assess the extent of the disease.

Collaborative Care

The treatment of esophageal cancer depends on the location of the tumor and whether invasion or metastasis has occurred (see Table 40-11). Esophageal cancer has a poor prognosis, mainly because it is not usually diagnosed until the disease is advanced. The best results may be obtained with a combination of surgery, chemotherapy, and radiation.

The types of surgical procedures that can be performed are (1) removal of part or all of the esophagus (*esophagectomy*) with use of a Dacron graft to replace the resected part, (2) resection of a portion of the esophagus and anastomosis of the remaining portion to the stomach (*esophagogastrostomy*), and (3) resection of a portion of the esophagus and anastomosis of a segment of colon to the remaining portion (*esophagoenterostomy*). The surgical approaches may be thoracic or both abdominal and thoracic.

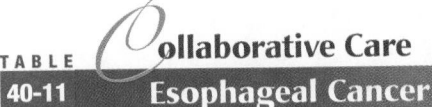

TABLE 40-11   *Collaborative Care* **Esophageal Cancer**
Diagnostic
History and physical examination
Endoscopy of esophagus with biopsy
Barium swallow
Endoscopic ultrasonography
Bronchoscopy
CT and MRI
Collaborative Therapy
Surgical resection
Esophagectomy
Esophagogastrostomy
Esophagoenterostomy
Radiation
Chemotherapy
Palliative
Dilation
Stent or prosthesis
Laser therapy
Gastrostomy

Surgery may not be performed if the patient is an older adult or in poor physical health.

Chemotherapeutic agents cisplatin (Platinol), paclitaxel (Taxol), and 5-FU in combination with radiation before and/or after surgery are currently used.[13] If the tumor is in the cervical section (upper third) of the esophagus, radiation is usually indicated. A tumor in the lower third of the esophagus is usually resected surgically.

Palliative therapy consists of restoration of the swallowing function and maintenance of nutrition and hydration. Dilation, stent placement, or both can relieve obstruction. Dilation is done with various types of dilators (e.g., Celestin tube). Dilation often relieves dysphagia and allows for improved nutrition. Placement of a stent or prosthesis may help when dilation is no longer effective. The prostheses are composed of silicone rubber or nylon-reinforced latex tubes with distal and proximal collars. The prosthesis is placed in the esophagus so that food and fluids can pass through the stenotic segment of the esophagus. The prosthesis can be placed endoscopically.

Endoscopic laser therapy or vaporization of the tumor may be used in combination with dilation. Obstruction recurs as the tumor grows, but laser therapy can be repeated. Sometimes these procedures are combined with radiation therapy. Other measures for palliation include gastrostomy or esophagostomy tube placements for nutrition support and pain management.

Nutritional Therapy. After esophageal surgery, parenteral fluids are given. When fluids are allowed after bowel sounds have returned, 30 to 60 ml of water are given hourly, with gradual progression to small, frequent bland meals. The patient should be in an upright position to prevent regurgitation of the fluid. The patient is observed for signs of intolerance to the feeding or leakage of the feeding into the mediastinum. Symptoms that indicate leakage are pain, increased temperature, and dyspnea. Symptoms of food intolerance include vomiting and abdominal distention. A gastrostomy may be performed for the purpose of feeding the patient. (Gastrostomy and tube feedings are discussed in Chapter 39.)

NURSING MANAGEMENT
ESOPHAGEAL CANCER

■ Nursing Assessment

The patient should be asked about any history of GERD, hiatal hernia, achalasia, or Barrett's esophagus. The patient is also questioned regarding tobacco and alcohol use. The patient should be assessed for progressive dysphagia and *odynophagia* (burning, squeezing pain while swallowing). The nurse should question the patient regarding the type of substances ingested that cause dysphagia, such as meat, soft foods, and liquids. The patient is also assessed for pain (substernal, epigastric, or back areas), choking, heartburn, hoarseness, cough, anorexia, weight loss, and regurgitation (sometimes bloody).

■ Nursing Diagnoses

Nursing diagnoses for the patient with esophageal cancer include, but are not limited to, the following:

- Imbalanced nutrition: less than body requirements *related to* dysphagia, odynophagia, weakness, chemotherapy, and radiation therapy
- Chronic pain *related to* the tumor
- Deficient fluid volume *related to* inadequate intake

- Risk for aspiration *related to* impaired esophageal function
- Anxiety *related to* diagnosis of cancer, uncertain future, and poor prognosis
- Anticipatory grieving *related to* diagnosis of life-threatening malignancy
- Ineffective health maintenance *related to* lack of knowledge of disease process and therapeutic regimen, unavailability of a support system, and chronic debilitating disease

■ Planning

The overall goals are that the patient with esophageal cancer will (1) have relief of symptoms including pain and dysphagia, (2) achieve optimal nutritional intake, (3) understand the prognosis of the disease, and (4) experience a quality of life appropriate to disease progression.

■ Nursing Implementation

Health Promotion. Patients with diagnosed GERD and hiatal hernia need to be counseled regarding regular follow-up evaluation. Health counseling should focus on elimination of smoking and excessive alcohol intake, as well as other risk factors for GERD. Maintenance of good oral hygiene and dietary habits (intake of fresh fruits and vegetables) may also be helpful.

Patients diagnosed with Barrett's esophagus need to be monitored because this is considered a premalignant condition. Early diagnosis of esophageal tumors is important but difficult because the onset of symptoms is usually late. Patients are encouraged to seek medical attention for any esophageal problems, especially dysphagia. Patients who are at risk for esophageal adenocarcinoma, such as those with evidence of Barrett's esophagus and a diagnosis of achalasia (discussed later under Other Esophageal Disorders), may need regular endoscopic screening with biopsy and cytologic study.

Acute Intervention

Preoperative care. In addition to general preoperative teaching and preparation, particular attention to the patient's nutritional needs and oral care is important. Many patients are poorly nourished because of the inability to ingest adequate amounts of food and fluids before surgery. A high-calorie, high-protein diet is recommended. It may have to be in liquid form. Some patients may need IV fluid replacement or total parenteral nutrition. The patient and/or family member is instructed on how to keep an intake and output record and assess for signs of fluid and electrolyte imbalance. Some treatment protocols necessitate preoperative radiation and chemotherapy.

Meticulous oral care is essential. The mouth, including tongue, gingivae, and teeth or dentures, must be cleaned thoroughly. It may be necessary to use swabs or a gauze pad and to really scrub the mouth, including the tongue. Milk of magnesia with mineral oil may be used to remove crust formation. A mixture of mouthwash, ice, and water makes a refreshing rinse for the patient.

Teaching should include information about chest tubes (if a thoracic approach is used), IV lines, NG tube, gastrostomy feeding, turning, coughing, and deep breathing. (General preoperative care is presented in Chapter 17.)

Postoperative care. The patient usually has an NG tube in place, and there may be bloody drainage for 8 to 12 hours. The drainage gradually changes to greenish yellow. Assessment of the drainage, maintenance of the tube, and oral and nasal care are nursing responsibilities. The NG tube should not be repositioned or reinserted without consulting with the surgeon.

Because of the location of the incision and the general condition of the patient, special emphasis must be placed on prevention of respiratory complications. Turning and deep breathing should be done every 2 hours. Use of an incentive spirometer helps to prevent respiratory complications.

The patient should be positioned in a semi-Fowler's or Fowler's position to prevent reflux and aspiration of gastric secretions. When the patient can drink fluids or eat, the upright position should be maintained for at least 2 hours after eating to assist the movement of food through the GI tract.

Ambulatory and Home Care. Many patients require long-term follow-up care after surgery for esophageal cancer. The patient may undergo chemotherapy and radiation treatment following surgery. The patient needs encouragement and assistance in maintaining adequate nutrition. The patient may need a permanent feeding gastrostomy. The patient usually has fears and anxieties about a diagnosis of cancer. The nurse should know what the health care provider has told the patient regarding the prognosis and then provide appropriate counseling.

Referral to a home health nurse may be necessary for continued care of the patient (e.g., gastrostomy teaching, follow-up wound care). (See Chapter 10 for management of the terminally ill patient and Chapter 15 for the cancer patient.)

■ Evaluation

The expected outcomes are that the patient with esophageal cancer will
- maintain a patent airway
- have relief of pain
- be able to swallow comfortably
- consume adequate nutritional intake
- understand the prognosis of the disease
- experience quality of life appropriate to disease progression

OTHER ESOPHAGEAL DISORDERS

Esophageal Diverticula

Esophageal diverticula are saclike outpouchings of one or more layers of the esophagus. They occur in three main areas: (1) above the upper esophageal sphincter (*Zenker's diverticulum*), which is the most common location; (2) near the esophageal midpoint (traction diverticulum); and (3) above the LES (epiphrenic diverticulum) (Fig. 40-7). Pharyngeal pouches (Zenker's diverticula) occur most commonly in elderly patients (over 70 years), and typical symptoms include dysphagia, regurgitation, chronic cough, aspiration, and weight loss.[14] Traction diverticulum may not cause signs and symptoms. The patient frequently complains of tasting sour food and smelling a foul odor caused by the stagnant food. Complications include malnutrition, aspiration, and perforation. A diagnosis is easily established by barium studies.

There is no specific treatment for diverticula. Some patients find they can empty the pocket of food that collects by applying pressure at a point on the neck. The diet may have to be limited to foods that pass more readily (e.g., blenderized foods). Treatment of the diverticulum may be necessary if nutrition becomes disrupted. Treatment is surgical via an endoscopic or external cervical approach and should include a cricopharyngeal myotomy. Open approaches have been associated with significant

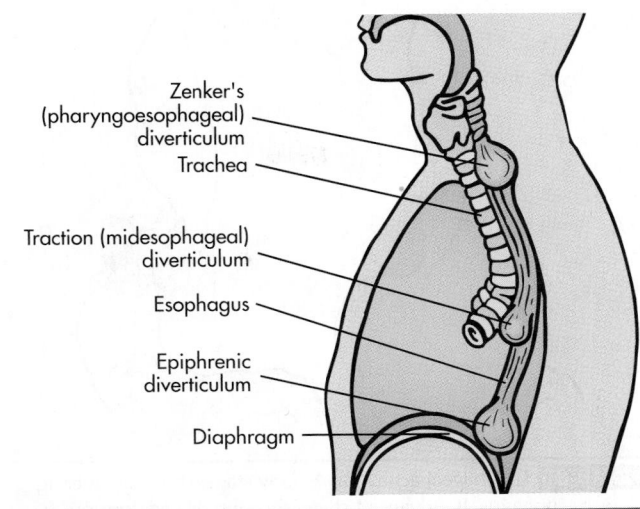

FIG. 40-7 Possible sites for the occurrence of esophageal diverticula. These hollow outpouchings may occur just above the upper esophageal sphincter (Zenker's, the most common type of pulsion diverticulum), near the midpoint of the esophagus (traction), and just above the lower esophageal sphincter (epiphrenic).

morbidity because the majority of patients are elderly and often have general medical problems. Treatment by endoscopic stapling diverticulotomy has become increasingly popular with its distinct advantages related to decreased complications, although long-term results are not yet available.[14]

Esophageal Strictures

The most common causes of esophageal strictures are strong acids or alkalis that have been ingested and reflux of gastric juices. Trauma such as throat lacerations and gunshot wounds may also lead to strictures as a result of scar formation (collagen deposition) from healing. The strictures usually develop over a long time. Strictures can be dilated endoscopically using *bougies* (dilating instruments). Another technique is balloon dilation, which is done under endoscopy and does not require fluoroscopy. Surgical excision with anastomosis is sometimes necessary. The patient may have a temporary or permanent gastrostomy.

Achalasia

In **achalasia** (cardiospasm), peristalsis of the lower two thirds (smooth muscle) of the esophagus is absent. Pressure in the LES is increased, along with incomplete relaxation of the LES. Obstruction of the esophagus at or near the diaphragm occurs. Food and fluid accumulate in the lower esophagus. The result of this condition is dilation of the lower esophagus (Fig. 40-8). The altered peristalsis is a result of impairment of the neurons that innervate the lower esophagus. There is a selective loss of inhibitory neurons, resulting in unopposed excitation of the LES. Achalasia affects all ages and both genders. The course of the disease is chronic.

Dysphagia (difficulty swallowing) is the most common symptom and occurs with both liquids and solids. Patients may report a globus sensation (a lump in the throat). Substernal chest pain (similar to the pain of angina) occurs during or immediately after a meal. *Halitosis* (foul-smelling breath) and the inability to eructate (belch) are other symptoms. Another common symptom is re-

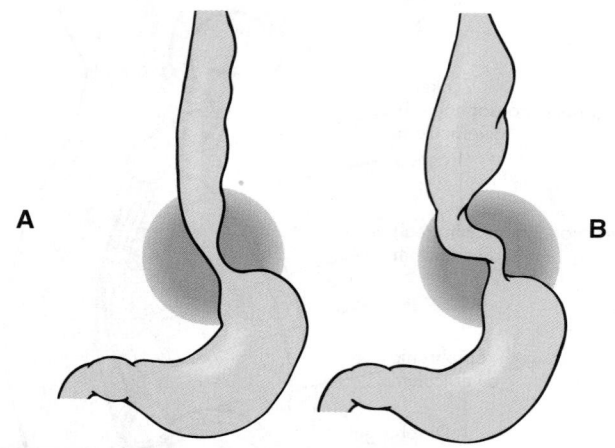

FIG. 40-8 Esophageal achalasia. **A,** Early stage, showing tapering of lower esophagus. **B,** Advanced stage, showing dilated, tortuous esophagus.

gurgitation of sour-tasting food and liquids, especially when the patient is in a horizontal position. Patients with achalasia also report symptoms (e.g., heartburn) of GERD. Weight loss is typical.

Diagnosis usually involves radiologic studies, manometric studies of the lower esophagus, and endoscopy. The exact cause of achalasia is not known, so treatment is focused on symptom management. Treatment consists of dilation, surgery, and use of drugs. All these therapies are directed at relieving the stasis caused by the increased LES pressure, nonrelaxing LES, and aperistaltic esophagus. Symptomatic treatment consists of a semisoft bland diet, eating slowly and drinking fluid with meals, and sleeping with the head elevated.

Esophageal dilation *(bougienage)* is an effective treatment measure for many patients. Pneumatic dilation of the LES with a balloon-tipped dilator passed orally is usually used. A variety of different dilators are available for this procedure. All depend on forcible expansion of a balloon in the LES (Fig. 40-9). The force-

ful dilation does not restore normal esophageal motility, but it does provide for emptying of the esophagus into the stomach.

Surgical intervention may become necessary. An esophagomyotomy may be performed. In this procedure the muscle fibers that enclose the narrowed area of the esophagus are divided. This allows the mucosa to pouch out through the division in the muscle layer so that food can be swallowed without obstruction.

A similar procedure is Heller myotomy (cardiomyotomy), which disrupts the LES and reduces LES pressure. An antireflux procedure is often done with the myotomy. This procedure can be performed laparoscopically, reducing the potential for postoperative complications.[15]

Drug therapy is used to manage early achalasia when there is no significant esophageal dilation. Drug therapy is used as a short-term measure and is considered as an alternative only in patients unfit to undergo pneumatic dilation or surgery. Endoscopic injection of botulinum toxin (Botox) into the LES is gaining acceptance.[16] It works by inhibiting the release of acetylcholine from nerve endings, thereby promoting relaxation of the smooth muscle. This treatment does not carry the risk of perforation that can occur with pneumatic dilation. However, symptomatic improvement with botulinum toxin only lasts a few months. Therefore either repeated injections are required or the patient must be switched to other therapy. There may be, however, subsets of patients, such as elderly patients or those with multiple medical problems who are poor candidates for more invasive procedures, for whom Botox injection is the preferred approach. Other classes of drugs used in the management of achalasia include anticholinergics, calcium channel blockers (e.g., nifedipine [Procardia]), and long-acting nitrates, which act by relaxing the smooth muscle.

Esophageal Varices

Esophageal varices are dilated, tortuous veins occurring in the lower portion of the esophagus as a result of portal hypertension. Esophageal varices are a common complication of liver cirrhosis and are discussed in Chapter 42.

Disorders of the Stomach and Upper Small Intestine

GASTRITIS

Types

Gastritis, an inflammation of the gastric mucosa, is one of the most common problems affecting the stomach. Gastritis may be acute or chronic and may be diffuse or localized. Chronic gastritis has been further divided into three subtypes including (1) autoimmune, which involves the body and fundus of the stomach; (2) diffuse antral, which primarily affects the antrum; and (3) multifocal, which is diffuse throughout the stomach. Presently, the causes of gastritis and its relationship to other gastric disorders, such as *Helicobacter pylori* infection and gastric cancer, are the focus of ongoing research.

Etiology and Pathophysiology

Gastritis occurs as the result of a breakdown in the normal gastric mucosal barrier. This mucosal barrier normally protects the stomach tissue from autodigestion by HCl acid and the proteolytic enzyme pepsin. When the barrier is broken, HCl acid can diffuse back into the mucosa. The acid back diffusion results in

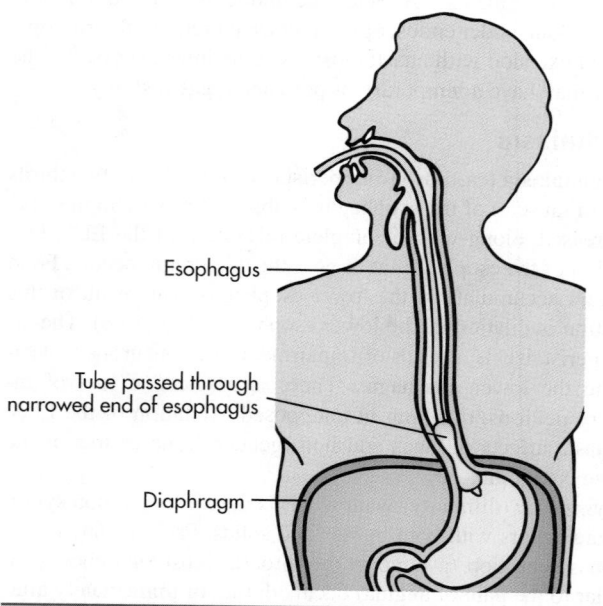

FIG. 40-9 Pneumatic dilation attempts to treat achalasia by maintaining an adequate lumen and decreasing lower esophageal sphincter (LES) tone.

Esophagus

Tube passed through narrowed end of esophagus

Diaphragm

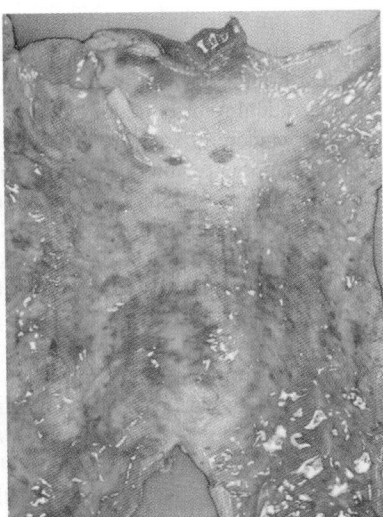

FIG. 40-10 Acute erosive gastritis is shown in the opened stomach. The mucosa appears hyperemic, and the foci of superficial ulceration are manifest as scattered, small, red areas termed erosions.

TABLE 40-12 **Causes of Gastritis**

Drugs
Aspirin
Corticosteroid drugs
Nonsteroidal antiinflammatory drugs

Diet
Alcohol
Spicy, irritating food

Microrganisms
Helicobacter pylori
Salmonella
Staphylococcus organisms

Environmental Factors
Radiation
Smoking

Pathophysiologic Conditions
Burns
Large hiatal hernia
Physiologic stress
Reflux of bile and pancreatic secretions
Renal failure (uremia)
Sepsis
Shock

Other Factors
Endoscopic procedures
Nasogastric suction
Psychologic stress

tissue edema, disruption of capillary walls with loss of plasma into the gastric lumen, and possible hemorrhage (Fig. 40-10).

Causes of gastritis are listed in Table 40-12. Drugs such as aspirin, nonsteroidal antiinflammatory drugs (NSAIDs), and digitalis have direct irritating effects on the gastric mucosa. For example, the ingestion of even small amounts of aspirin by the susceptible person is known to result in asymptomatic GI bleeding manifested by positive stool tests for occult blood. In addition, corticosteroids and NSAIDs are known to inhibit the synthesis of prostaglandins that are protective to the gastric mucosa. This leaves the gastric mucosa more susceptible to mucosal damage. NSAID-related gastritis is associated with many of the older drugs, including piroxicam (Feldene), naproxen (Naprosyn), sulindac (Clinoril), indomethacin (Indocin), diclofenac (Voltaren), and ibuprofen (Motrin, Advil). The use of cyclooxygenase-2 (COX-2) inhibitors (e.g., celecoxib [Celebrex], rofecoxib [Vioxx], valdecoxib [Bextra]) has been associated with fewer GI side effects as compared to nonselective NSAIDs. However, even these agents are associated with an increased risk of upper GI inflammation and bleeding. Risk factors for NSAID-induced gastritis include being female, being over the age of 60, and taking other ulcerogenic drugs including corticosteroids and anticoagulants (warfarin [Coumadin]).[17]

Dietary indiscretions can also result in acute gastritis. After an alcoholic drinking binge, acute damage to the gastric mucosa can range from local destruction of superficial epithelial cells to desquamation and destruction of the mucosa, with mucosal congestion, edema, and hemorrhage. Prolonged damage induced by repeated alcohol abuse can result in chronic gastritis. Eating large quantities of spicy, irritating foods and metabolic conditions such as uremia can also cause acute gastritis.

An important causative factor in chronic gastritis, in particular, diffuse antral and multifocal, is *H. pylori* infection. *H. pylori*–associated gastritis is a common problem in adults, many of whom do not have symptoms of gastritis. It is currently thought that *H. pylori* infection is acquired in childhood and is able to survive in the hostile environment of the gastric lumen. For reasons not clearly understood, *H. pylori* is capable of promoting the breakdown of the gastric mucosal barrier, given certain "trig-

gers" or conditions. Thus, given time, *H. pylori* will eventually have a destructive effect on its host environment. This is consistent with the finding that the incidence of chronic gastritis increases with age. However, studies also have shown that not all persons infected with *H. pylori* go on to develop chronic gastritis or peptic ulcer disease. Thus a combination of factors may be at work to "turn on" the virulent process by which *H. pylori* damage the gastric mucosal barrier. The role of *H. pylori* in ulcer development is discussed in greater detail on pp. 1030-1031.

Autoimmune atrophic gastritis is a form of chronic gastritis that affects both the fundus and body of the stomach and is associated with an increased risk of gastric cancer. Approximately 30% of patients with *H. pylori* infection are also found to have antigastric antibodies. Thus there may be a link between the host's response to the presence of *H. pylori* and the development of autoimmune chronic gastritis.

Although not as common, other causes of chronic gastritis have been identified. Bacterial, viral, and fungal infections including *Mycobacterium,* cytomegalovirus, and syphilis are associated with chronic gastritis. Gastritis can occur from reflux of bile salts from the duodenum into the stomach as a result of anatomic changes following surgical procedures such as gastroduodenostomy and gastrojejunostomy. Prolonged vomiting may also cause reflux of bile salts. Intense emotional responses and CNS lesions may also produce inflammation of the mucosal lining as a result of hypersecretion of HCl acid or corticosteroids (Cushing syndrome).

Progressive gastric mucosal atrophy from chronic alterations in the protective mucosal barrier causes the chief and parietal cells to die eventually. With the decrease in the number of acid-secreting parietal cells and atrophy of the gastric mucosa, *hypochlorhydria* (decreased acid secretion) or *achlorhydria* (lack of acid secretion) occurs.

Clinical Manifestations

The symptoms of acute gastritis include anorexia, nausea and vomiting, epigastric tenderness, and a feeling of fullness. Hemorrhage is commonly associated with alcohol abuse and at times may be the only symptom. Acute gastritis is self-limiting, lasting from a few hours to a few days, with complete healing of the mucosa expected.

The manifestations of chronic gastritis are similar to those described for acute gastritis. Some patients have no symptoms directly associated with the gastric lesion. However, when the acid-secreting cells are lost or do not function as a result of atrophy, the source of intrinsic factor is also lost. The loss of *intrinsic factor,* a substance secreted by the gastric mucosa that is essential for the absorption of cobalamin (vitamin B_{12}) in the terminal ileum, ultimately results in cobalamin deficiency. With time, the body's storage of cobalamin in the liver is depleted, and a deficiency state exists. Lack of this important vitamin, which is essential for the growth and maturation of red blood cells (RBCs), results in the development of anemia and neurologic complications. (Cobalamin deficiency anemia is discussed in Chapter 30.)

Diagnostic Studies

Diagnosis of acute gastritis is most often based on a history of drug and alcohol use. The diagnosis of chronic gastritis may be delayed or completely missed because the symptoms are nonspecific. Endoscopic examination with biopsy is necessary to obtain a definitive diagnosis. Breath, urine, serum, or gastric tissue biopsy tests are available for the determination of *H. pylori.* These tests are described under Peptic Ulcer Disease. Radiologic studies are not helpful because the superficial mucosa is generally involved, and changes will not show clearly on x-ray. A complete blood count (CBC) may demonstrate the presence of anemia from blood loss or lack of intrinsic factor. Stools are tested for the presence of occult blood. A gastric analysis, although currently not used as much, demonstrates the amount of HCl acid present, with achlorhydria being a common sign of severe atrophic gastritis. Serum tests for antibodies to parietal cells and intrinsic factor may be performed. Tissue biopsy with cytologic examination is necessary to rule out gastric carcinoma.

NURSING *and* COLLABORATIVE MANAGEMENT GASTRITIS

■ Acute Gastritis

Eliminating the cause and preventing or avoiding it in the future are generally all that is needed to treat acute gastritis. The plan of care is supportive and similar to that described for nausea and vomiting. If vomiting accompanies acute gastritis, bed rest, NPO status, and IV fluids may be prescribed. Dehydration can occur rapidly in acute gastritis with vomiting. Fluids and electrolytes lost through vomiting and, occasionally, diarrhea are replaced. Antiemetics are given for nausea and vomiting (see Table 40-1). In severe cases of acute gastritis an NG tube may be used,

either for lavage of the precipitating agent from the stomach or in conjunction with suction to keep the stomach empty and free of noxious stimuli. Clear liquids are resumed when acute symptoms have subsided, with gradual reintroduction of solid, bland foods.

If hemorrhage is considered likely, frequent checking of vital signs and testing the vomitus for blood are indicated. All of the management strategies discussed in the section on upper GI bleeding also apply to the patient with severe gastritis.

Drug therapy is focused on reducing irritation of the gastric mucosa and providing symptomatic relief. Antacids are beneficial in the relief of abdominal discomfort by raising intragastric pH to above 6. H_2R blockers (e.g., ranitidine [Zantac], cimetidine [Tagamet]) or PPIs (e.g., omeprazole [Prilosec], lansoprazole [Prevacid]) may be used to reduce gastric HCl acid secretion. An agent that contains an H_2R blocker plus bismuth (ranitidine bismuth citrate [Tritec]) has been shown to reduce bleeding and promote healing of erosive gastritis. It is essential that the nurse have knowledge of the action and therapeutic effects of PPIs and H_2R blockers to teach the patient and to monitor the effects of the drugs.

■ Chronic Gastritis

The treatment of chronic gastritis focuses on evaluating and eliminating the specific cause (e.g., cessation of alcohol intake, abstinence from drugs, *H. pylori* eradication). Currently, antibiotic and antisecretory agent combinations are used to eradicate infection with *H. pylori* (Table 40-13). For the patient with pernicious anemia, regular injections of cobalamin are needed (see Chapter 30). Discussion of the continued need for this essential vitamin must be included in the plan of care.

The patient undergoing treatment for chronic gastritis may have to adapt to many lifestyle changes and adopt a strict adherence to a drug regimen. A nonirritating diet consisting of six small feedings a day and the use of an antacid after meals may help provide symptomatic relief. Smoking is contraindicated in

TABLE 40-13 **Drug Therapy** *Helicobacter pylori* **Infection**		
TREATMENT	**DURATION**	**ERADICATION RATE**
Triple Drug Therapy Proton pump inhibitor* or ranitidine bismuth citrate (Tritec) amoxicillin clarithromycin (Biaxin)	7 days	>90%
Dual Therapy ranitidine bismuth citrate (Tritec) clarithromycin (Biaxin)	7 days	>90%
Quadruple Therapy Proton pump inhibitor* bismuth tetracycline metronidazole (Flagyl)	14 days	60%–80%

*See Table 40-9.

all forms of gastritis. An interdisciplinary team approach in which the physician, nurse, dietitian, and pharmacist provide consistent information and support may increase the patient's success in making these alterations. Because the incidence of gastric cancer is higher in the patient who has a history of chronic gastritis, especially atrophic gastritis, close medical follow-up should be stressed.

UPPER GASTROINTESTINAL BLEEDING

In the United States there are approximately 150,000 to 200,000 hospital admissions each year for upper GI bleeding.[18,19] Despite advances in intensive care, hemodynamic monitoring, and endoscopy, there has been little change in the mortality rate for upper GI bleeding, which has remained approximately 6% to 10% for the past 40 years. This is due in part to the greater incidence of upper GI bleeding in older adults, especially women, related to the use of NSAIDs.

Etiology and Pathophysiology

Although the most serious loss of blood from the upper GI tract is characterized by a sudden onset, insidious occult bleeding can also be a major problem. The severity of bleeding depends on whether the origin is venous, capillary, or arterial. (Types of upper GI bleeding are presented in Table 40-14.) Bleeding from an arterial source is profuse, and the blood is bright red. The bright red color indicates that the blood has not been in contact with the stomach's acid secretions. In contrast, "coffee ground" vomitus reveals that the blood and other contents have been in the stomach for some time and have been changed by contact with gastric secretions. A massive upper GI hemorrhage is generally defined as a loss of more than 1500 ml of blood or a loss of 25% of intravascular blood volume. *Melena* (black, tarry stools) indicates slow bleeding from an upper GI source. The longer the passage of blood through the intestines, the darker the color of the stool as a result of the degradation of hemoglobin and the release of iron.

Discovering the cause of the bleeding is not always an easy task. A variety of areas in the GI tract may be involved, and there may be many different reasons for the blood loss. Table 40-15 lists the common causes of bleeding. Although systemic diseases (e.g., leukemia, blood dyscrasias) that interfere with normal

TABLE 40-14 Types of Upper Gastrointestinal Bleeding

TYPE	CLINICAL MANIFESTATIONS
Obvious bleeding	
▪ Hematemesis	Bloody vomitus appearing as fresh, bright red blood or "coffee ground" appearance (dark, grainy digested blood)
▪ Melena	Black, tarry stools (often foul smelling) caused by digestion of blood in the GI tract. The black appearance is from the presence of iron
Occult bleeding	Small amounts of blood in gastric secretions, vomitus, or stools not apparent by appearance; detectable by guaiac test

TABLE 40-15 Common Causes of Upper Gastrointestinal Bleeding

Drug Induced
Corticosteroids
Nonsteroidal antiinflammatory drugs
Salicylates

Esophagus
Esophageal varices
Esophagitis
Mallory-Weiss tear

Stomach and Duodenum
Gastric cancer
Hemorrhagic gastritis
Peptic ulcer disease
Polyps
Stress ulcer

Systemic Diseases
Blood dyscrasias (e.g., leukemia, aplastic anemia)
Renal failure (uremia)

blood clotting must be considered whenever upper GI bleeding occurs, the most common sites are the esophagus, stomach, and duodenum.

Esophageal Origin. Bleeding from an esophageal source is most likely the result of chronic esophagitis, bleeding from a tear in the mucosa near the esophagogastric junction (Mallory-Weiss tear), or esophageal varices. Chronic esophagitis can be caused by the ingestion of chemicals, including drugs irritating to the mucosa. Alcohol and smoking are known irritants of the esophageal mucosa. GERD with or without a hiatal hernia can lead to chronic irritation and erosion. A **Mallory-Weiss tear** is usually caused by severe retching and vomiting. This tear occurs in the esophageal mucosa at the junction of the esophagus and stomach and results in severe bleeding.

Esophageal varices usually occur secondary to cirrhosis of the liver. Branches of the vena cava and the azygos vein from the systemic circulation converge with the smaller vessels of the lower esophagus. These vessels are inelastic and become engorged and tortuous because of increased pressure exerted on them secondary to portal hypertension. Anything that may increase the pressure (e.g., coughing, sneezing, trauma) or cause mechanical irritation (e.g., vomiting, irritation, erosion) may result in sudden, massive bleeding. (Esophageal varices are discussed in Chapter 42.)

Stomach and Duodenal Origin. Bleeding ulcers account for the majority of cases of upper GI bleeding.[20] Erosion of a blood vessel by an ulcer located in the stomach or duodenum must always be considered as a possible cause of upper GI bleeding. A gastric ulcer may penetrate the left gastric artery, and a duodenal ulcer may penetrate the superior pancreaticoduodenal artery. Most bleeding ulcers are related to the presence of *H. pylori* or drug use.[21]

Acute gastritis produced by ingestion of drugs or alcohol or the reflux of bile from the small intestine can result in bleeding. Drugs, either prescribed by the health care provider or OTC, are a major cause of upper GI bleeding. For example, the patient who regularly takes aspirin or aspirin-containing compounds may be at risk for bleeding episodes. Aspirin, NSAIDs (e.g., ibuprofen), and corticosteroids can cause irritation and disruption of the gastric mucosal barrier. Aspirin-containing products are sold without prescriptions as OTC drugs. It is not unusual for a patient to deny the use of aspirin yet be self-medicating with aspirin-containing drugs, such as Alka-Seltzer, Bufferin, and Excedrin. A careful history of all commonly used drugs is therefore necessary whenever upper GI bleeding is suspected.

Physiologic stress ulcers, which may occur after severe burn, trauma, or major surgery, erode more superficial blood vessels than does a peptic ulcer. In one study, mucosal injury was found to be present in 70% of patients in an intensive care unit.[18] The combination of hypoperfusion and gastric irritants (HCl and pepsin) likely contributes to this mucosal damage. Gastric cancer can also result in upper GI bleeding. Gastric cancer can be the cause of a steady blood loss as it grows and ulcerates through the mucosa and blood vessels located in its path.

Emergency Assessment and Management

Although approximately 80% to 85% of patients who have massive hemorrhage spontaneously stop bleeding, the cause must be identified and treatment initiated immediately. Although a complete history of events leading to the bleeding episode is important in discovering the cause of the blood loss, it should be deferred until emergency care has been initiated. The immediate physical examination must include a systemic evaluation of the patient's condition with emphasis on blood pressure, rate and character of pulse, peripheral perfusion with capillary refill, and observation for the presence or absence of neck vein distention. Vital signs should be monitored every 15 to 30 minutes. Signs and symptoms of shock must be evaluated, and treatment should be started as soon as possible (see Chapter 65). The patient's respiratory status is carefully assessed, along with a thorough abdominal examination. The presence or absence of bowel sounds should be assessed and noted. A tense, rigid, boardlike abdomen may indicate a perforation and peritonitis.

Once the immediate interventions have begun, the patient or family should answer the following questions. Is there a history of previous bleeding episodes? Has weight loss been a recent problem? Has the patient received blood transfusions in the past, and were there any transfusion reactions? Is there a religious preference that prohibits the use of blood or blood products? Are there any other illnesses that may contribute to bleeding or interfere with treatment (e.g., congestive heart failure, diabetes mellitus)?

Laboratory studies are ordered, including a CBC, blood urea nitrogen (BUN), serum electrolytes, blood glucose, prothrombin time, liver enzymes, arterial blood gases (ABGs), and a type and crossmatch for possible blood transfusions. All vomitus and stools should be tested for the presence of gross and occult blood. A urinalysis provides information on the presence of blood in the urine, and the specific gravity gives an immediate indication of the patient's hydration status.

IV lines, preferably two, with a 16- or 18-gauge needle should be established for fluid and blood replacement. The type and amount of fluids infused are dictated by physical and laboratory findings. It is generally best to begin with an isotonic crystalloid solution (e.g., lactated Ringer's solution). Whole blood, packed RBCs, and fresh frozen plasma may be used for replacement of lost volume in massive hemorrhage. Because of the potential for fluid overload and immunologic reactions, packed RBCs are often preferred over whole blood. (The use of blood transfusions and volume expanders is discussed in Chapter 30.) The hemoglobin and hematocrit values are not of immediate assistance in estimating the degree of blood loss, but they provide a baseline for guiding further treatment. The initial hematocrit may be normal and may not reflect the loss until 4 to 6 hours after fluid replacement has taken place, since initially the loss of plasma and RBCs is equal. When upper GI bleeding is less profuse, infusion of isotonic saline solution followed by packed RBCs permits restoration of the hematocrit more quickly and does not create complications related to fluid volume overload. The use of supplemental oxygen delivered by face mask or nasal cannula may help increase blood oxygen saturation.

For most patients who are bleeding profusely, an indwelling urinary catheter is inserted so that urine volume can be accurately assessed hourly. A central venous pressure line may be inserted so that the patient's fluid volume status can be monitored easily. When a history of valvular heart disease, coronary artery disease, or congestive heart failure is elicited or when pulmonary edema is a factor, the use of a pulmonary artery catheter may be necessary to monitor the patient.

Most endoscopists advocate endoscopy without prior lavage to avoid delays in treatment. However, others prefer an NG tube to be placed and lavage with room temperature water or saline to be initiated before endoscopy. In this case a large tube passed through the mouth may be more beneficial than a small one passed through the nose. Passage through the mouth is easier, but no tube should ever be advanced against resistance because of the likelihood of damaging the gastric mucosa or causing perforation. Aspiration of stomach contents through a large-bore tube such as an Ewald tube facilitates the removal of clots from the stomach and alleviates the patient's need to vomit. Gastric lavage with water or saline may be initiated to ensure that blood will not interfere with emergency endoscopic visualization of the gastric mucosa. If used, the usual procedure for gastric lavage is to instill approximately 50 to 100 ml of tap water or saline solution each time, leave it in place for several minutes, and then allow drainage by gravity or low suction. This procedure may be repeated every 30 to 45 minutes.

Diagnostic Studies

In addition to using endoscopic procedures to stop bleeding, these procedures also allow direct visualization of the bleeding site. Endoscopy is quite accurate in identifying the specific source of the bleeding. When a skilled practitioner performs the procedure, bleeding from severe gastritis can be easily distinguished from that of a gastric or duodenal ulcer.

Angiography is used in diagnosing upper GI bleeding only when endoscopy cannot be done. It is an invasive procedure requiring preparation and setup time and may not be appropriate for a high-risk, unstable patient. In this procedure a catheter is placed into the left gastric or superior mesenteric artery and advanced until the site of bleeding is discovered.

Barium contrast studies are of little value in the identification of major bleeding sites during the acute phase of treatment. After the acute bleeding phase, barium studies can document an actual lesion but cannot verify that it is the bleeding source.

Collaborative Care

Endoscopic Therapy. The goal of endoscopic hemostasis is to coagulate or thrombose the bleeding artery and then reduce the necessity of a surgical procedure. This procedure has proven useful in stopping the bleeding of gastritis, Mallory-Weiss tear, esophageal and gastric varices, bleeding peptic ulcers, and polyps. Several techniques are used, including (1) thermal (heat) probe, (2) multipolar and bipolar electrocoagulation probe, and (3) neodymium:yttrium-aluminum-garnet (Nd:YAG) laser. Multipolar electrocoagulation and thermal probe are the two most commonly used procedures. The heat probe coagulates tissue by directly applying a heating element to the bleeding site. Overall, endoscopic therapy is more effective than medical management alone in reducing bleeding episodes.[18]

Surgical Therapy. Surgical intervention is indicated when bleeding continues regardless of the therapy provided and when the site of the bleeding has been identified. A high percentage of patients are known to have another massive hemorrhage within 5 years after the first bleeding episode. Some physicians regard surgical therapy as necessary when the patient continues to bleed after rapid transfusion of up to 2000 ml of whole blood or remains in shock after 24 hours. The site of the hemorrhage determines the choice of operation. In addition, the surgeon must consider the age of the patient because mortality rates increase considerably over the age of 60 years. It is essential that the operation be performed as soon as the need has been established.

Drug Therapy. During the acute phase, drugs are used to decrease bleeding, decrease HCl acid secretion, and neutralize the HCl acid that is present. Drug therapy to decrease bleeding is administered during endoscopy. Injection therapy with absolute alcohol (ethanol) or epinephrine (1:10,000 dilution) is effective for acute hemostasis. These agents produce tissue edema and, ultimately, pressure on the source of bleeding. To prevent rebleeding, injection therapy is often combined with other therapies (e.g., thermocoagulation or laser treatment). A *sclerosant* (an agent that produces inflammation and results in fibrosis of the tissues) such as ethanolamine (Ethamolin) or morrhuate (Scleromate) may be used, especially if the cause of bleeding is esophageal varices.

For variceal bleeding, vasopressin (Pitressin), which is posterior pituitary extract, can be used to produce vasoconstriction. It is used to treat upper GI bleeding in those patients who do not respond to other therapies and are poor surgical risks. It is administered systemically through a vein or intraarterially at the local site of actual bleeding. Side effects of intravenously administered vasopressin include decreased myocardial contractility and decreased coronary blood flow. The patient undergoing vasopressin therapy must be closely monitored for its myocardial, visceral, and peripheral ischemic side effects. Vasopressin should be used with caution in the patient with a known history of vascular disease.

Efforts are made to reduce acid secretion because the acidic environment can alter platelet function, as well as interfere with clot stabilization. H_2R blockers (e.g., cimetidine [Tagamet]) or PPIs (e.g., pantoprazole [Protonix]) are administered intravenously to decrease acid secretion. Table 40-16 reviews the mechanism of action of H_2R blockers and PPIs. Although these drugs have no proven ability to control active bleeding, they have become part of standard treatment protocols.

In patients with upper GI bleeding, early administration of the somatostatin analog octreotide (Sandostatin) may be used. The drug reduces splanchnic blood flow, as well as acid secretion. This drug is given in IV boluses up to 5 to 6 days after the initiation of bleeding.

Antacids have long been known to neutralize HCl acid and continue to be used as an adjunct therapy for peptic ulcer disease. Because antacids neutralize HCl acid and increase the pH of gas-

TABLE 40-16 Drug Therapy — Gastrointestinal Bleeding		
DRUG	**SOURCE OF GI BLEEDING**	**MECHANISM OF ACTION**
Antacids*	Duodenal ulcer, gastric ulcer, acute gastritis (corrosive, erosive, and hemorrhagic)	Neutralizes acid and maintains gastric pH above 5.5; elevated pH inhibits activation of pepsinogen
H_2-receptor blockers cimetidine (Tagamet) famotidine (Pepcid) nizatidine (Axid) ranitidine (Zantac)	Duodenal ulcer, gastric ulcer, esophagitis, acute gastritis (especially hemorrhagic)	Inhibits action of histamine at H_2-receptors on parietal cells and decreases HCl acid secretion
Proton pump inhibitors omeprazole (Prilosec) esomeprazole (Nexium) lansoprazole (Prevacid) pantoprazole (Protonix)	—	Inhibits the cellular pump, which is necessary for secretion of HCl acid
vasopressin (Pitressin)	Acute gastritis (corrosive, erosive, and hemorrhagic), esophageal varices	Causes vasoconstriction and increases smooth muscle activity of the GI tract; reduces pressure in the portal circulation and arrests bleeding
octreotide (Sandostatin)	Upper gastrointestinal bleeding, esophageal varices	Somatostatin analog that decreases splanchnic blood flow; decreases HCl acid secretion via decrease in release of gastrin

*See Table 40-21.

tric contents to above 5, there is inhibition of the conversion of pepsinogen to its active form pepsin. The most frequently used antacid preparations are magnesium hydroxide, magnesium trisilicate, aluminum hydroxide, calcium carbonate, and sodium bicarbonate (see Table 40-21 later in this chapter). Aluminum hydroxide and magnesium trisilicate are the most useful because they are nonabsorbable. Calcium carbonate and sodium bicarbonate are absorbable, and prolonged use can lead to systemic alkalosis.

Sedatives to control agitation and restlessness should be administered cautiously. They make accurate assessment of the patient's condition more difficult. Anticholinergic drugs are contraindicated in acute upper GI bleeding episodes.

NURSING MANAGEMENT
UPPER GASTROINTESTINAL BLEEDING

■ Nursing Assessment

As the nurse begins care of the patient admitted with upper GI bleeding, a thorough and accurate nursing assessment is an essential first step. Subjective and objective data that should be obtained from the patient or significant others are presented in Table 40-17.

The patient experiencing upper GI bleeding may not be able to provide specific information about the cause of the bleeding until the immediate physical needs are met. An immediate nursing assessment is performed while getting the patient ready for initial treatment. The assessment includes the patient's level of consciousness, vital signs, appearance of neck veins, skin color, and capillary refill. The abdomen is checked for distention, guarding, and peristalsis. Immediate determination of vital signs indicates whether the patient is in shock from blood loss and also provides a baseline blood pressure and pulse by which to monitor the progress of treatment. Signs and symptoms of shock include low blood pressure; rapid, weak pulse; increased thirst; cold, clammy skin; and restlessness. Vital signs are monitored every 15 to 30 minutes, and the health care provider should be informed of any significant changes.

When obtaining vital signs, the nurse considers the patient's age and physical condition. Taking the blood pressure and pulse with the patient lying down and then sitting will indicate postural changes that occur after acute blood loss. The older the patient, the more changes in vital signs should be expected.

■ Nursing Diagnoses

Nursing diagnoses for the patient with upper GI bleeding include, but are not limited to, the following:

- Deficient fluid volume *related to* acute loss of blood, as well as gastric secretions
- Ineffective tissue perfusion *related to* loss of circulatory volume
- Anxiety *related to* upper GI bleeding, hospitalization, uncertain outcome, source of bleeding
- Ineffective coping *related to* situational crisis and personal vulnerability
- Risk of aspiration *related to* active bleeding and altered level of consciousness
- Decreased cardiac output *related to* loss of blood

■ Planning

The overall goals are that the patient with upper GI bleeding will (1) have no further GI bleeding, (2) have the cause of the bleeding identified and treated, (3) experience a return to a nor-

TABLE 40-17	Nursing Assessment — Upper Gastrointestinal Bleeding

Subjective Data

Important Health Information

Past health history: Precipitating events before bleeding episode, previous bleeding episodes and treatment, peptic ulcer disease, esophageal varices, esophagitis, acute and chronic gastritis, stress ulcers

Medications: Use of aspirin, nonsteroidal antiinflammatory drugs, corticosteroids, anticoagulants

Functional Health Patterns

Health perception–health management: Family history of bleeding, smoking, alcohol use

Nutritional-metabolic: Nausea, vomiting, weight loss; thirst

Elimination: Diarrhea; black, tarry stools; decreased urinary output; sweating

Activity-exercise: Weakness, dizziness, fainting

Cognitive-perceptual: Epigastric pain, abdominal cramps

Coping–stress tolerance: Acute or chronic stressors

Objective Data

General

Fever

Integumentary

Clammy, cool, pale skin; pale mucous membranes, nailbeds, and conjunctivae; spider angiomas; jaundice; peripheral edema

Respiratory

Rapid, shallow respirations

Cardiovascular

Tachycardia, weak pulse, orthostatic hypotension, slow capillary refill

Gastrointestinal

Red or "coffee ground" vomitus; tense, rigid abdomen, ascites; hypoactive or hyperactive bowel sounds; black, tarry stools

Urinary

Decreased urinary output, concentrated urine

Neurologic

Agitation, restlessness; decreasing level of consciousness

Possible Findings

↓ Hematocrit and hemoglobin; hematuria; guaiac-positive stools, emesis, or gastric aspirate; ↓ levels of clotting factors; ↑ liver enzymes; abnormal upper GI studies or endoscopy results

mal hemodynamic state, and (4) experience minimal or no symptoms of pain or anxiety.

■ Nursing Implementation

Health Promotion. Although not all cases of upper GI bleeding can be anticipated and prevented, the nurse shares responsibility with the health care provider in trying to identify the patient who is at high risk. The patient with a history of chronic gastritis or peptic ulcer disease should always be considered in the high-risk category because of the increased incidence of bleeding associated with chronic irritation or chronic ulcers. The patient who has had one major bleeding episode is more likely to have another bleed. The patient is instructed to avoid gastric irritants such as alcohol and smoking, to prevent or decrease stress-inducing situations at home or at work, and to take only prescribed medications. OTC drugs can be harmful because they may contain ingredients (e.g., aspirin) that have potentially irritating effects on the mucosa. The patient is instructed in the methods of testing vomitus or stools for the presence of occult blood. Positive results should be promptly reported to the health care provider or the nurse.

The patient who requires regular administration of ulcerogenic drugs, such as aspirin, corticosteroids, or NSAIDs, needs instruction regarding the potential adverse effects that these agents may have on the GI mucosa. These drugs are avoided if at all possible. However, if aspirin must be prescribed, enteric-coated tablets can be substituted for regular tablets. Taking the drugs with meals or snacks lessens the potential irritating effects. For patients who must take NSAIDs, a change to a preparation with less GI toxicity may be considered. Cyclooxygenase-2 (COX-2) inhibitors (e.g., rofecoxib [Vioxx], celecoxib [Celebrex], valdecoxib [Bextra]) have less of an effect on the production of tissue prostaglandins and are associated with fewer GI side effects.[22] The co-administration of an NSAID with a PPI can reduce bleeding risk. For the patient at risk for gastric ulcers because of NSAID use, misoprostol (Cytotec) may also be prescribed. This prostaglandin analog inhibits acid secretion and reduces upper GI bleeding episodes associated with NSAID use. However, the drug has several important side effects, including uterine cramping in women and diarrhea. Because of its effects on the uterus, it is contraindicated in women of childbearing age.

When the nurse is working with the patient who has a history of liver cirrhosis with esophageal varices, the instructions must be specific regarding the importance of avoiding known irritants, such as alcohol and smoking. The prompt treatment of an upper respiratory tract infection should be stressed. Severe coughing or sneezing can create increased pressure on the already fragile varices and may result in massive hemorrhage.

The patient who is known to have blood dyscrasias (e.g., aplastic anemia) or liver dysfunction or who is taking cancer chemotherapeutic drugs has a potential bleeding problem because of altered hemostasis caused by a decrease in clotting factors and platelets. When these patients also have a history of ulcer disease, gastritis, varices, or drug and alcohol abuse, they should be carefully instructed regarding their disease process and drugs, and they should be closely observed for bleeding.

Acute Intervention. The patient should be approached in a calm and assured manner to help decrease the level of anxiety. Caution should be used before administering sedatives for restlessness because it is one of the warning signs of shock and may be masked by the drugs.

Once an infusion has been started, the IV line must be maintained for fluid or blood replacement. An accurate intake and output record is essential so that the patient's hydration status can be assessed. Urine output should be measured hourly. A rate of at least 0.5 ml/kg per hour indicates adequate renal perfusion. Lesser amounts may indicate renal ischemia secondary to loss of blood volume. Urine specific gravity should be measured because it gives additional information regarding the patient's hydration status. Consistent readings greater than 1.025 (normal is 1.005 to 1.025) indicate that the urine is extremely concentrated and that there is probably a low blood volume. The health care provider must be kept informed of these important parameters so that the IV solutions can be increased or decreased accordingly. If the patient has a central venous pressure line or pulmonary artery catheter in place, readings should be recorded every 1 to 2 hours. Hemodynamic monitoring provides an accurate and quick assessment of blood flow and pressure within the cardiovascular system (see Chapter 64).

The older adult or the patient with a history of cardiovascular problems should be observed closely for signs of fluid overload. However, the threat of volume overload and pulmonary edema must be a constant concern in all patients who are receiving large amounts of IV fluids within a short time. Therefore auscultation of breath sounds and close observation of respiratory effort are important. Electrocardiographic (ECG) monitoring can also be used to evaluate cardiac function.

Foods such as beets or even swallowed mouthwash can give vomitus a bloody appearance. Unless the contents of the vomitus are checked for occult blood, false information may be recorded. Swallowed blood from a nosebleed must also be accurately noted to avoid misdiagnosis of an upper GI bleeding episode. When an NG tube is inserted, the nurse must pay special attention to keeping it in proper position and observing the aspirate for blood.

The majority of upper GI bleeding episodes cease spontaneously, even without intervention. Although the use of room temperature, cool, or iced gastric lavage is used in some institutions, its effectiveness is of questionable value. Water has the advantage of being able to break up large clots more easily than saline solution, is less expensive, and is always available. A disadvantage of tap water is that it may create more electrolyte imbalances than would an isotonic saline solution.

When lavage is used, approximately 50 to 100 ml of fluid is instilled at a time into the stomach. The lavage fluid may be aspirated from the stomach or drained by gravity. When aspiration is the method used, it is important not to aspirate if resistance is felt. The tip of the NG tube may be up against the gastric mucosal lining. The constant pressure from attempts to aspirate the lavage fluid may cause erosion of the mucosa. When resistance is a factor, the nurse should use gravity as the alternative method of gastric drainage. Close monitoring of vital signs, especially in the patient with cardiovascular disease, is important because arrhythmias may occur. Keeping the patient warm and the head of the bed elevated provides comfort and prevents possible aspiration problems.

The nurse caring for a patient with upper GI bleeding should be well informed as to what constitutes blood in the stools. Black, tarry stools are not usually associated with a brisk hemorrhage but are indicative of the presence of bleeding of prolonged duration. Bright red blood in the stool is usually from a source in the lower bowel. Menses and bleeding hemorrhoids should be ruled out as possible sources of blood in the stools. When vomitus contains blood but the stool contains no gross or occult blood, the hemorrhage is considered to have been of short duration.

Monitoring the patient's laboratory studies enables the nurse to estimate the effectiveness of therapy. The hemoglobin and hematocrit are usually evaluated about every 4 to 6 hours if the patient is actively bleeding. At first the hematocrit level may not accurately reflect the amount of blood lost or the amount of blood replaced and will appear falsely high or low. The patient's BUN level is assessed. It is generally elevated with a significant hemorrhage because blood proteins are broken down by GI tract bacteria. However, renal disease may also result in an elevated BUN level. Many patients receive oxygen by mask or nasally to ensure that the circulating blood has an adequate oxygen content.

When oral nourishment is begun, the patient is observed for symptoms of nausea and vomiting and a recurrence of bleeding.

Feedings initially consist of clear fluids or milk and are given hourly until tolerance is determined. These feedings help neutralize the gastric secretions and assist in the mucosal repair. Gradual introduction of foods follows if the patient exhibits no signs of discomfort.

The patient in whom hemorrhage was the result of chronic alcohol abuse requires close observation for the beginning of delirium tremens as withdrawal from alcohol takes place. Symptoms indicating the beginning of delirium tremens are agitation, uncontrolled shaking, sweating, and vivid hallucinations. (Alcohol withdrawal is discussed in Chapter 11.)

Ambulatory and Home Care. The patient and family must be taught how to avoid future bleeding episodes. Ulcer disease, drug or alcohol abuse, and liver and respiratory diseases can all result in upper GI bleeding. The patient and family must be made aware of the consequences of noncompliance with diet and drug therapy. It must be emphasized that no drugs (especially aspirin, NSAIDs) other than those prescribed by the health care provider should be taken. Smoking and alcohol should be eliminated because they are sources of irritation and interfere with tissue repair. The need for long-term follow-up care may be necessary because of the possibility of another bleeding episode. The patient and family should be instructed on what to do if an acute hemorrhage occurs in the future.

■ Evaluation

The expected outcomes are that the patient with upper GI bleeding will

- have no upper GI bleeding
- maintain normal fluid volume
- experience a return to a normal hemodynamic state
- experience absence or tolerable levels of pain and is comfortable
- understand potential etiologic factors and make appropriate lifestyle modifications

PEPTIC ULCER DISEASE

Peptic ulcer disease is a condition characterized by erosion of the GI mucosa resulting from the digestive action of HCl acid and pepsin. Any portion of the GI tract that comes into contact with gastric secretions is susceptible to ulcer development, including the lower esophagus, stomach, duodenum, and margin of gastrojejunal anastomosis after surgical procedures. It is estimated that approximately 10% of men and 4% of women in the United States will have ulcers during their lifetimes.

Types

Peptic ulcers can be classified as acute or chronic, depending on the degree and duration of mucosal involvement (Fig. 40-11), and gastric or duodenal, according to the location. The *acute ulcer* (see Fig. 40-11) is associated with superficial erosion and minimal inflammation. It is of short duration and resolves quickly when the cause is identified and removed. A chronic ulcer (Fig. 40-12) is one of long duration, eroding through the muscular wall with the formation of fibrous tissue. It is present continuously for many months or intermittently throughout the person's lifetime. A chronic ulcer is at least four times as common as acute erosion.

Gastric and duodenal ulcers, although defined as peptic ulcers, are different in their etiology and incidence (Table 40-18). Generally, the treatment of all types of ulcers is quite similar.

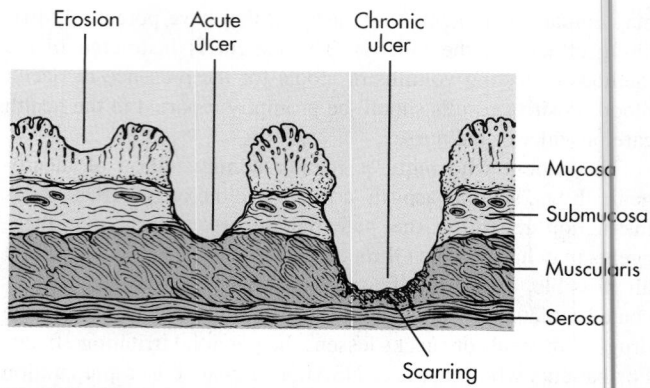

FIG. 40-11 Peptic ulcers, including an erosion, acute ulcer, and chronic ulcer. Both the acute and chronic ulcer may penetrate the entire wall of the stomach.

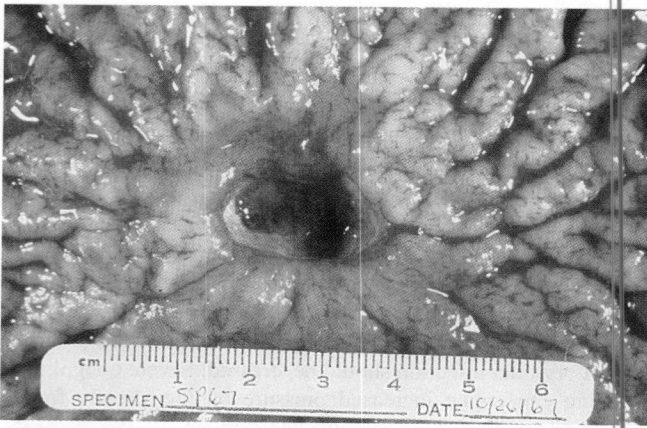

FIG. 40-12 Photograph of a chronic peptic ulcer located in the lesser curvature of stomach.

Etiology and Pathophysiology

Peptic ulcers develop only in the presence of an acid environment. It has been well established that the patient with pernicious anemia and achlorhydria rarely has gastric ulcers. An excess of gastric acid may not be necessary for ulcer development. The typical person with a gastric ulcer has normal to less than normal gastric acidity compared with the person with a duodenal ulcer. However, some intraluminal acid does seem to be essential for a gastric ulcer to occur.

Pepsinogen, the precursor of pepsin, is activated to pepsin in the presence of HCl acid and a pH of 2 to 3. The secretion of HCl acid by the parietal cells has a pH of 0.8. After mixing with the stomach contents, the pH reaches 2 to 3, a highly favorable range of acidity for pepsin activity. When the stomach acid level is neutralized by the presence of food or antacids or acid secretion is blocked by drugs, the pH is increased to 3.5 or more. At a pH of 3.5 or more, pepsin has little or no proteolytic activity.

The stomach is normally protected from autodigestion by the gastric mucosal barrier. The GI tract has a high cell turnover rate, and the surface mucosa of the stomach is renewed about every 3 days. As a result of this high turnover rate, the mucosa can continually repair itself except in extreme instances when the cell breakdown surpasses the cell renewal rate. Normally, water, electrolytes, and water-soluble substances (e.g., glucose) can easily

TABLE 40-18	Comparison of Gastric and Duodenal Ulcers	
	GASTRIC ULCERS	**DUODENAL ULCERS**
Lesion	Superficial; smooth margins; round, oval, or cone shaped	Penetrating (associated with deformity of duodenal bulb from healing of recurrent ulcers)
Location of lesion	Predominantly antrum, also in body and fundus of stomach	First 1-2 cm of duodenum
Gastric secretion	Normal to decreased	Increased
Incidence	• Greater in women • Peak age 50-60 yr • More common in persons of lower socioeconomic status and in unskilled laborers • Increased with smoking, drug, and alcohol use • Increased with incompetent pyloric sphincter and bile reflux • Increased with stress ulcers after severe burns, head trauma, and major surgery	• Greater in men, but increasing in women, especially postmenopausal • Peak age 35-45 yr • Associated with psychologic stress • Increased with smoking, drug, and alcohol use • Associated with other diseases (e.g., chronic obstructive pulmonary disease, pancreatic disease, hyperparathyroidism, Zollinger-Ellison syndrome, chronic renal failure)
Clinical manifestations	• Burning or gaseous pressure in high left epigastrium and back and upper abdomen • Pain 1-2 hr after meals; if penetrating ulcer, aggravation of discomfort with food • Occasional nausea and vomiting, weight loss	• Burning, cramping, pressurelike pain across midepigastrium and upper abdomen; back pain with posterior ulcers • Pain 2-4 hr after meals and midmorning, midafternoon, middle of night, periodic and episodic • Pain relief with antacids and food; occasional nausea and vomiting
Recurrence rate	High	High
Complications	Hemorrhage, perforation, outlet obstruction, intractability	Hemorrhage, perforation, obstruction

pass through the barrier. However, the mucosal barrier prevents the back diffusion of acid from the gastric lumen through the mucosal layers to the underlying tissue.

Under specific circumstances the mucosal barrier can be impaired and back diffusion of acid can occur (Fig. 40-13). When the barrier is broken, HCl acid freely enters the mucosa and injury to the tissues occurs. This results in cellular destruction and inflammation. Histamine is released from the damaged mucosa, resulting in vasodilation and increased capillary permeability. The released histamine is then capable of stimulating further secretion of acid and pepsin.

As described in the section on gastritis, a variety of agents are known to destroy the mucosal barrier. By generating ammonia in the mucous layer, *H. pylori* may create a condition of chronic inflammation, rendering the mucosa especially vulnerable to other noxious substances. Ulcerogenic drugs, such as aspirin and NSAIDs, inhibit synthesis of prostaglandins and cause abnormal permeability. Corticosteroids have the ability to decrease the rate of mucosal cell renewal and thereby decrease its protective effects. Lipid-soluble cytotoxic drugs can pass through the barrier and destroy it.

When the mucosal barrier is disrupted, there is a compensatory increase in blood flow (Fig. 40-14). This phenomenon can occur in several ways. Prostaglandin-like substances and histamine act as vasodilators, thus increasing capillary blood flow. As blood flow increases within the affected mucosa, hydrogen ions are rapidly removed from the area, buffers are delivered to help neutralize the hydrogen ions present, nutrients necessary for cell function arrive, and the rate of mucosal cell replication increases. When the increase is sufficient to dilute, buffer, and remove the excess hydrogen ions, tissue damage may be minimal or may result in no injury at all. When blood flow is not sufficient to carry out these events, tissue injury results. Fig. 40-14 shows a repre-

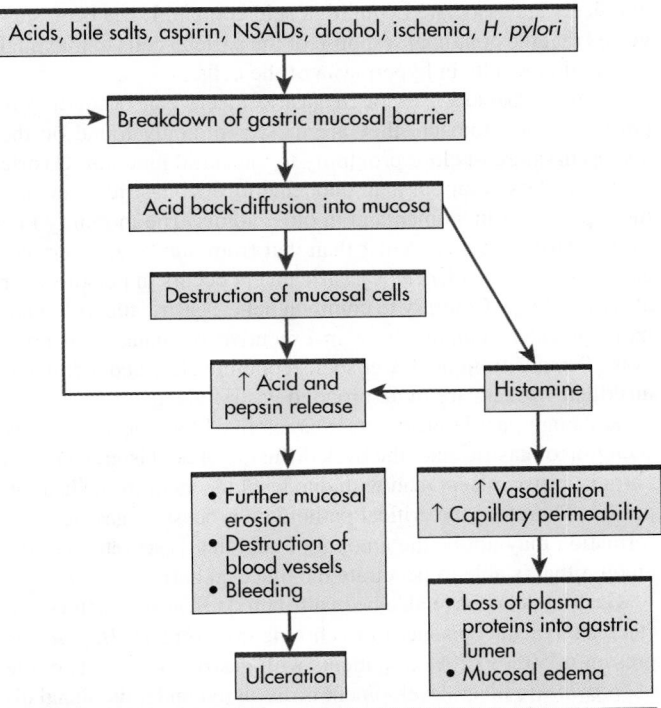

FIG. 40-13 Disruption of gastric mucosa and pathophysiologic consequences of back-diffusion of acids.

sentation of the interrelationship between the mucosal blood flow and disruption of the gastric mucosal barrier.

There are two mechanisms that protect against damage. First, mucus is secreted by superficial mucous cells and forms a layer that can entrap or slow the diffusion of hydrogen ions across the

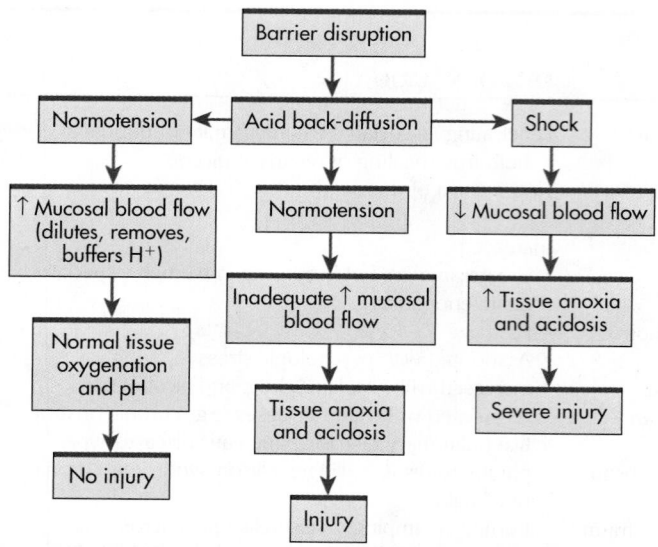

FIG. 40-14 Relationship between mucosal blood flow and disruption of the gastric mucosal barrier.

mucosal barrier in the stomach. Second, bicarbonate is secreted by the gastric and duodenal mucosa, and this helps neutralize HCl acid in the lumen of the GI tract.

Increased vagal nerve stimulation from a variety of causes (e.g., emotions) results in hypersecretion of HCl acid. Increased concentrations of HCl acid can alter the mucosal barrier. Duodenal ulcers are associated with high acid content. It has been suggested that the continual response of the parietal cells to maximal stimulation results in hyperplasia of the cells.

Gastric Ulcers. Although gastric ulcers can occur in any portion of the stomach, they are most commonly found on the lesser curvature in close proximity to the antral junction. Gastric ulcers are less common than duodenal ulcers. Gastric ulcers are more prevalent in women and in older adults. The mortality rate from gastric ulcers is greater than that from duodenal ulcers because the peak incidence of gastric ulcers occurs in persons over 50 years of age. Contrary to common belief, gastric ulcers are not more prevalent among those in executive or managerial positions. Persons from the lower socioeconomic class and manual or unskilled workers are more prone to gastric ulcers.

Although gastric ulcers are characterized by a normal to low secretion of gastric acid, the back diffusion of acid is greater with chronic gastric ulcers than with duodenal ulcers or in the healthy person. Therefore the critical pathologic process in gastric ulcer formation may not be the amount of acid that is secreted but the amount that is able to penetrate the mucosal barrier.

Gastric ulcers have also been attributed to various factors that can lead to acute episodes or to chronic involvement. *H. pylori* is present in 50% to 70% of patients with gastric ulcers.[22] The role of *H. pylori* in ulcer development is discussed under duodenal ulcers. It is thought that destruction of the gastric mucosa by noxious agents such as drugs or smoking may be enhanced by the presence of *H. pylori,* which further promotes gastric mucosal destruction.

Drugs can cause acute gastric ulcers and in some cases can lead to the development of chronic ulcers. The drugs most often implicated include aspirin, corticosteroids, NSAIDs (e.g., ibuprofen), and reserpine (Serpasil). It is estimated that 1% to 3% of pa-

tients taking NSAIDs for 1 year experience serious GI complications, including gastritis, gastric ulcer, upper GI hemorrhage, or perforation. It is estimated that approximately 10 million Americans use NSAIDs, and 100,000 to 300,000 GI adverse events associated with NSAID use are reported each year.[21] Other known causative factors of gastric ulcer formation are chronic alcohol abuse, chronic gastritis, and bile reflux gastritis from an incompetent pyloric sphincter. Cigarette smoking is positively linked with gastric ulcers. Nicotine seems to enhance reflux of duodenal contents into the antrum of the stomach. The ingestion of hot, rough, or spicy foods has been suggested as a causative factor, but there is no evidence to substantiate this claim.

Duodenal Ulcers. Duodenal ulcers account for about 80% of all peptic ulcers. Although duodenal ulcers still affect more men than women, the incidence of duodenal ulcers has followed a downward trend in men and a steady increase in women. The explanation for this change has not been clearly identified. Duodenal ulcers may occur at any age, but the incidence is especially high between the ages of 35 and 45 years. Duodenal ulcers can develop in anyone, regardless of occupation or socioeconomic group.

The development of duodenal ulcers is associated with a high HCl acid secretion. Several diseases have been identified with a high risk of duodenal ulcer development, including chronic obstructive pulmonary disease, cirrhosis of the liver, chronic pancreatitis, hyperparathyroidism, chronic renal failure, and the Zollinger-Ellison syndrome. (*Zollinger-Ellison syndrome* is a rare condition characterized by severe peptic ulceration, gastric acid hypersecretion, elevated serum gastrin levels, and gastrinoma of the pancreas or duodenum.) It is possible that the treatments used for these conditions may also promote ulcer development. Alcohol ingestion and heavy smoking habits are also associated with duodenal ulcer formation because both are known stimulants of acid secretion.

Although many factors are thought to contribute to the formation of duodenal ulcers, *H. pylori* has been identified as playing a key role. *H. pylori* is found in approximately 90% to 95% of patients with duodenal ulcers.[22] However, a clear-cut direct causal relationship between *H. pylori* and duodenal ulcer formation has not yet been proven. Not all individuals with evidence of *H. pylori* go on to develop ulcers, suggesting that additional factors are needed to produce these conditions. *H. pylori* survives in the human upper GI tract for a long time as a result of its ability to move in mucus and attach to mucosal cells. In addition, it secretes a substance called *urease,* which buffers the area around the bacterium and protects it from destruction in an acidic environment.

Infection with *H. pylori* is highest in underdeveloped countries and in persons of low socioeconomic status. Although the routes of transmission are largely unknown, it is thought that infection occurs during childhood via transmission from family members to the child, possibly through a fecal-oral and/or oral-oral route. In the United States and Canada, persons born before 1940 have a significantly higher risk of carrying *H. pylori* than persons in younger age groups. This enhanced prevalence in older persons has been attributed to the presence of crowded living conditions and poor sanitation practices, which were more common in the first half of the last century.

Research into a genetic cause for ulcers has shown that some members of the same family are more prone to develop gastric or duodenal ulcers. Supporting a genetic etiology is the fact that persons with blood group O have an increased incidence of duodenal ulcers. This may be related to increased susceptibility to *H. pylori*. Evidence is not complete, however, and the ulcer development could just as well be due to the sharing of the same environment.

Physiologic Stress Ulcers. **Physiologic stress ulcers** are acute ulcers that develop following a major physiologic insult such as trauma or surgery. A physiologic stress ulcer is a form of erosive gastritis. It is believed that the gastric mucosa of the body of the stomach undergoes a period of transient ischemia in association with hypotension, severe injury, extensive burns, and complicated surgery. The ischemia is due to decreased capillary blood flow or shunting of blood away from the GI tract so that blood flow bypasses the gastric mucosa. This occurs as a compensatory mechanism in hypotension or shock. The decrease in blood flow produces an imbalance between the destructive properties of HCl acid and pepsin and protective factors of the stomach's mucosal barrier, especially in the fundic portion, resulting in ulceration. Multiple superficial erosions result, and these may bleed. Risk factors for development of stress ulcer bleeding are respiratory failure and coagulopathy. These patients should receive prophylaxis with antisecretory agents. The diagnosis of stress gastritis is made on endoscopy, and treatment is with aggressive reduction of gastric acid secretions using H$_2$R blockers or PPIs.

Clinical Manifestations

It is common for the person with gastric or duodenal ulcers to have no pain or other symptoms. The gastric and duodenal mucosas are not rich in sensory pain fibers, which may account for this phenomenon. When pain does occur with duodenal ulcer, it is described as "burning" or "cramplike." It is most often located in the midepigastric region beneath the xiphoid process. The pain associated with gastric ulcers is located high in the epigastrium and occurs spontaneously about 1 to 2 hours after meals. The pain is described as "burning" or "gaseous." The pain can occur when the stomach is empty or when food has been ingested. If the ulcer has eroded through the gastric mucosa, food tends to aggravate rather than alleviate the pain. Some persons do not experience any pain until the presence of the ulcer is demonstrated through a serious complication such as hemorrhage or perforation.

Ulcers located on the posterior aspect of the duodenum can be manifested by back pain. The pain usually occurs 2 to 4 hours after meals. It is relieved by antacids alone or in combination with an H$_2$R blocker and sometimes by foods that neutralize and dilute the HCl acid. A characteristic of duodenal ulcer is its tendency to occur continuously for a few weeks or months and then disappear for a time, only to recur some months later. Some patients claim their symptoms worsen in the spring and fall of the year, thus strengthening the concept of a seasonal trend in occurrence.

Complications

The three major complications of chronic peptic ulcer disease are hemorrhage, perforation, and gastric outlet obstruction. All are considered emergency situations and are initially treated conservatively. However, surgery may become necessary at any time during the course of the therapy.

Hemorrhage. Hemorrhage is the most common complication of peptic ulcer disease. It develops from erosion of the granulation tissue found at the base of the ulcer during healing or from erosion of the ulcer through a major blood vessel. Duodenal ulcers account for a greater percentage of upper GI bleeding episodes than gastric ulcers.

Perforation. Perforation is considered the most lethal complication of peptic ulcer. Perforation is commonly seen in large penetrating duodenal ulcers that have not healed and are located on the posterior mucosal wall (Fig. 40-15). Perforated gastric ulcers are most often located on the lesser curvature of the stomach. Even though duodenal ulcers are more prevalent and perforate more frequently, mortality rates associated with perforation of gastric ulcers are higher. The older age of the patient with gastric ulcers, who often has other concurrent medical problems, is thought to be the crucial factor in the higher mortality rates.

Perforation of a peptic ulcer occurs when the ulcer penetrates the serosal surface, with spillage of either gastric or duodenal contents into the peritoneal cavity. The size of the perforation is directly proportional to the length of time the patient has had the ulcer. The larger the perforation, the longer the history of the ulcer. Small perforations seal themselves and result in a cessation of symptoms; larger perforations require immediate surgical closure. Spontaneous sealing occurs as a result of large amounts of fibrin being produced in response to the perforation. This leads to fibrinous fusion of the duodenum or gastric curvature to adjacent tissue, mainly the liver.

The clinical manifestations of perforation are characterized by their sudden and dramatic onset. The patient experiences sudden, severe upper abdominal pain that quickly spreads throughout the abdomen. The visceral and parietal layers of the peritoneum have an abundance of pain receptors, and this contributes to the abrupt, intense pain experienced. There may be shoulder pain if the spillage causes irritation to the phrenic nerve. The abdominal muscles contract, appearing rigid and boardlike as they attempt to protect the abdomen from further injury. The patient's respirations become shallow and rapid. Bowel sounds are usually absent. Nausea and vomiting may occur but are generally absent. Many patients report a history of ulcer disease or recent symptoms of indigestion.

The contents entering the peritoneal cavity from the stomach or duodenum contain a variety of ingredients that include air, saliva, food particles, HCl acid, pepsin, bacteria, bile, and pancreatic fluid and enzymes. Bacterial peritonitis may occur within

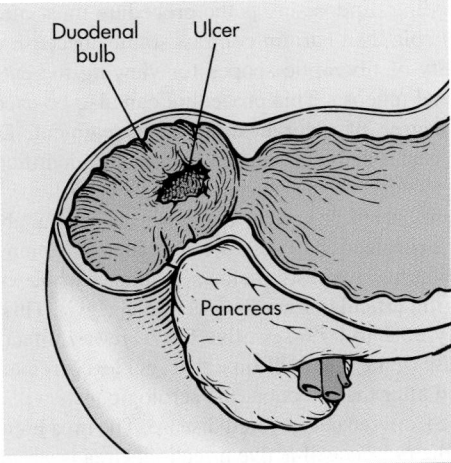

FIG. 40-15 Duodenal ulcer of the posterior wall penetrating into the head of the pancreas, resulting in walled-off perforation.

6 to 12 hours. The intensity of the peritonitis is proportional to the amount and duration of the spillage through the perforation. It is difficult to determine from the sudden onset of symptoms whether gastric or duodenal ulcer is the cause because the clinical characteristics of intestinal perforation are the same (see Chapter 41).

Gastric Outlet Obstruction. Ulcers located in the antrum and the prepyloric and pyloric areas of the stomach and the duodenum can predispose to gastric outlet obstruction. In the early phase of obstruction (often referred to as the compensated phase), gastric emptying is normal to near normal. Over time, increased contractile force needed to empty the stomach results in hypertrophy of the stomach wall. After long-standing obstruction the stomach enters the decompensated phase, which results in dilation and atony. The obstruction is not totally due to fibrous scar tissue because active ulcer formation is associated with edema, inflammation, and pylorospasm, all of which contribute to the narrowing of the pylorus.

The patient with gastric outlet obstruction generally has a long history of ulcer pain. Ulcerlike pain of short duration or complete absence of pain is more indicative of a malignant obstruction. The pain progresses to a more generalized upper abdominal discomfort that becomes worse toward the end of the day as the stomach fills and dilates. Relief may be obtained by belching or by self-induced vomiting. Vomiting is common and often projectile. The vomitus contains food particles that were ingested many hours or even a day or two before the vomiting episode. There is often an offensive odor if the contents have been dormant in the stomach for a time. The patient who vomits frequently will be anorectic, with evident weight loss, and will complain of thirst and an unpleasant taste in the mouth. Constipation is a common complaint that usually results from dehydration and lack of roughage in the diet.

The patient with gastric outlet obstruction may show a swelling in the upper abdomen indicating dilation of the stomach. Loud peristalsis can be heard, and visible peristaltic waves are often observed passing across the abdomen from left to right. If the stomach is grossly dilated, it is possible to palpate it as well.

Diagnostic Studies

The diagnostic measures used to determine the presence and location of a peptic ulcer are similar to those used for acute upper GI bleeding. Endoscopy is the procedure most often used. It is more reliable than barium contrast studies because of the maneuverability of fiberoptic scopes for viewing the entire gastric and duodenal mucosa. This procedure can also be used to determine the degree of ulcer healing after treatment. During endoscopy, tissue specimens can be obtained for identification of *H. pylori* and to rule out gastric cancer.

There are currently several diagnostic tests available to confirm *H. pylori* infection. These are classified as noninvasive and invasive. Noninvasive tests include serum or whole blood antibody tests, in particular, immunoglobulin G (IgG). This test is approximately 90% to 95% sensitive for *H. pylori* infection. However, because of the length of time that IgG levels remain elevated in the blood after the infection, the serologic tests will not distinguish active from recently treated disease. The urea breath test can determine the presence of active infection. Urea is a by-product of the metabolism of *H. pylori* bacteria. Invasive tests involve biopsy of the stomach and include the rapid urease test, as well as other

histologic markers of infection. These tests have greater sensitivity and specificity but involve an endoscopic procedure.[22]

Barium contrast studies, although widely used, are not accurate in identifying shallow, superficial ulcers because of failure of the barium to properly fill the ulcer crater. X-ray studies are also ineffective in differentiating a peptic ulcer from a malignant tumor. In addition, x-rays do not as readily demonstrate the degree of healing that can be visually determined with the endoscope. Barium studies are of benefit in the diagnosis of gastric outlet obstruction. Barium normally should pass from the stomach within 2 hours, but with gastric outlet obstruction, 50% of the barium remains on follow-up films up to 6 hours later.

Gastric analysis has questionable value in the diagnosis of peptic ulcer disease because in many patients gastric secretions are normal in amount and composition. However, it can provide important data in (1) identifying a possible gastrinoma (Zollinger-Ellison syndrome), (2) determining the degree of gastric hyperacidity, and (3) evaluating the results of therapy such as vagotomy and antisecretory drug therapy. Gastric analysis procedure is described in Table 38-12.

Laboratory analyses, including a CBC, urinalysis, liver enzyme studies, serum amylase determination, and stool examination, should be performed. A CBC may indicate the presence of anemia secondary to bleeding from the ulcer. Liver enzyme studies help determine any liver problems, such as cirrhosis, that may complicate the treatment of the ulcer. Urine and stool are routinely tested for the presence of blood. A serum amylase determination is frequently ordered to provide information on pancreatic function in patients in whom posterior penetration of the pancreas is suspected.

Collaborative Care: Conservative Therapy

When the patient's clinical manifestations and health history suggest the diagnosis of peptic ulcer disease and diagnostic studies confirm it, a medical regimen is instituted (Table 40-19). The regimen consists of adequate rest, dietary modifications, drug therapy, elimination of smoking, and long-term follow-up care. The aim of the treatment program is to decrease the degree of gastric acidity, enhance mucosal defense mechanisms, and minimize the harmful effects on the mucosa.

Patients are generally treated in ambulatory care clinics. The healing of a peptic ulcer requires many weeks of therapy. Pain disappears after 3 to 6 days, but ulcer healing is much slower. Complete healing may take 3 to 9 weeks, depending on ulcer size and the treatment regimen employed. Healing of the ulcer should be assessed by means of x-rays or endoscopic examination. Barium contrast films provide a rough estimate of the degree of ulcer healing. However, it should be noted that endoscopic examination is the only accurate method to monitor for ulcer healing.

Adequate rest, both physical and emotional, is important in the treatment process. A quiet, calm environment at home or on the job is not easy to achieve and may require some modifications in the patient's daily routine. The benefits derived from the elimination or reduction of stressors help decrease the stimulus for overproduction of HCl acid. Moderation in daily activity is essential.

Aspirin and nonselective NSAIDs with GI side effects may be discontinued or NSAIDs that are COX-2 inhibitors are used.[23] When aspirin or nonselective NSAIDs must be continued, enteric-coated preparations or co-administration with a PPI or misoprostol (Cytotec) should be considered.

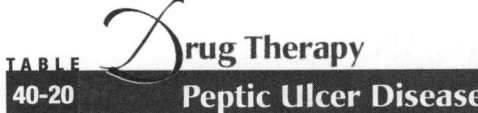

TABLE 40-19 Collaborative Care
Peptic Ulcer Disease

Diagnostic
History and physical examination
Upper GI endoscopy with biopsy
H. pylori testing of breath, urine, blood, tissue
Upper GI barium contrast study
Complete blood count
Urinalysis
Liver enzymes
Serum electrolytes

Collaborative Therapy
Conservative Therapy
Adequate rest
Bland diet (six small meals a day)
Cessation of smoking
Drug therapy
  H₂-receptor blockers (see Table 40-20)
  Proton pump inhibitors (see Table 40-20)
  Antibiotics for *H. pylori* (see Table 40-13)
  Antacids (see Table 40-21)
  Anticholinergics
  Cytoprotective drugs
Stress reduction
Acute Exacerbation without Complications
NPO
NG suction
Adequate rest
Cessation of smoking
IV fluid replacement
Drug therapy
  H₂-receptor blockers
  Proton pump inhibitors
  Antacids
  Anticholinergics
  Sedatives
Acute Exacerbation with Complications (Hemorrhage, Perforation, Obstruction)
NPO
NG suction
Bed rest
IV fluid replacement (lactated Ringer's solution)
Blood transfusions
Stomach lavage (possible)
Surgical Therapy
Perforation—simple closure with omentum graft
Gastric outlet obstruction—pyloroplasty and vagotomy
Ulcer removal/reduction
  Billroth I and II
  Vagotomy and pyloroplasty

GI, Gastrointestinal; *IV,* intravenous; *NG,* nasogastric; *NPO,* nothing by mouth.

TABLE 40-20 Drug Therapy
Peptic Ulcer Disease

Antisecretory
H₂-receptor blockers
  cimetidine (Tagamet)
  ranitidine (Zantac)
  famotidine (Pepcid)
  nizatidine (Axid)
Proton pump inhibitors
  omeprazole (Prilosec)
  lansoprazole (Prevacid)
  esomeprazole (Nexium)
  pantoprazole (Protonix)
Anticholinergics

Antisecretory and Cytoprotective
misoprostol (Cytotec)

Cytoprotective
sucralfate (Carafate)
bismuth subsalicylate (Pepto-Bismol)

Neutralizing
Antacids*

Antibiotics for *H. pylori*
amoxicillin
metronidazole (Flagyl)
tetracycline
clarithromycin (Biaxin)

Others
Tricyclic antidepressants
  imipramine (Tofranil)
  doxepin (Sinequan)

*See Table 40-21.

dered, and the expected benefits. Strict adherence to the prescribed regimen of drugs is important. Drug therapy includes the use of antacids, H₂R blockers, PPIs, antibiotics, antacids, anticholinergics, and cytoprotective therapy (Tables 40-19 through 40-22).

Because recurrence of peptic ulcer is frequent, interruption or discontinuation of therapy can have detrimental results. The patient must be encouraged to comply with therapy and continue with follow-up care for at least 1 year. If changes in lifestyle are part of the prescribed therapy, they should be maintained. Antacids, H₂R blockers, and PPIs may be stopped after the ulcer has healed or may be prescribed in the form of low-dose maintenance therapy. No other drugs, unless prescribed by the health care provider, should be taken because they may have an ulcerogenic effect. Finally, the patient and family should be told what to do in the event that pain and discomfort recur or blood is noted in the vomitus or stools.

Histamine-2 receptor blockers. H₂R blockers, cimetidine (Tagamet), ranitidine (Zantac), famotidine (Pepcid), and nizatidine (Axid), are frequently used in the management of peptic ulcer disease. These drugs block the action of histamine on the H₂ receptors and thus reduce HCl acid secretion. This decreases the conversion of pepsinogen to pepsin, and accelerates ulcer heal-

Smoking has an irritating effect on the mucosa, increases gastric motility, and delays mucosal healing. It should be eliminated completely or severely reduced. The combination of adequate rest and abstinence from smoking accelerates ulcer healing.

Drug Therapy. Drugs are a vital part of therapy. The patient must be well informed about each drug prescribed, why it is or-

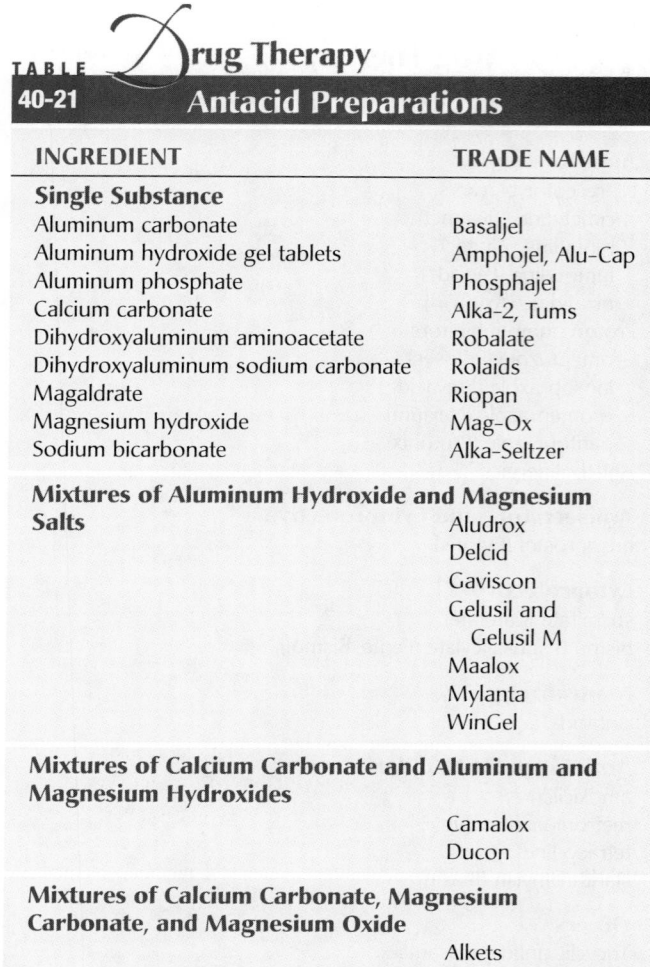

TABLE 40-21

Drug Therapy

Antacid Preparations

INGREDIENT	TRADE NAME
Single Substance	
Aluminum carbonate	Basaljel
Aluminum hydroxide gel tablets	Amphojel, Alu-Cap
Aluminum phosphate	Phosphajel
Calcium carbonate	Alka-2, Tums
Dihydroxyaluminum aminoacetate	Robalate
Dihydroxyaluminum sodium carbonate	Rolaids
Magaldrate	Riopan
Magnesium hydroxide	Mag-Ox
Sodium bicarbonate	Alka-Seltzer
Mixtures of Aluminum Hydroxide and Magnesium Salts	
	Aludrox
	Delcid
	Gaviscon
	Gelusil and
	Gelusil M
	Maalox
	Mylanta
	WinGel
Mixtures of Calcium Carbonate and Aluminum and Magnesium Hydroxides	
	Camalox
	Ducon
Mixtures of Calcium Carbonate, Magnesium Carbonate, and Magnesium Oxide	
	Alkets

TABLE 40-22

Drug Therapy

Side Effects of Antacid Therapy

ANTACID	REACTIONS
Aluminum hydroxide gels	Constipation, phosphorus depletion with chronic use
Calcium carbonate	Constipation or diarrhea, hypercalcemia, milk-alkali syndrome, renal calculi
Magnesium preparations	Diarrhea, hypermagnesemia
Sodium preparations	Milk-alkali syndrome if used with large amounts of calcium; used with caution in patients on sodium restrictions

ing. (Antihistamine drugs used to treat allergies are H_1R blockers and have no effect on gastric acid secretion.)

H_2R blocker drugs may be administered orally or intravenously. Depending on the specific drug, therapeutic effects last up to 12 hours. However, the onset of action (i.e., symptom relief) is longer than antacids. H_2R blockers have demonstrated capabilities in the healing of gastric and duodenal ulcers. Famotidine, ranitidine, and nizatidine have longer half-lives than cimetidine, thus requiring fewer doses and providing nocturnal HCl acid suppression. More side effects are associated with cimetidine. These include granulocytopenia, gynecomastia, diarrhea, fatigue, dizziness, rash, and mental confusion in the older adult. However, the rate of these side effects is low. Famotidine and nizatidine are considered more potent at reduced dosage levels as compared with cimetidine, and side effects are minimal. There are OTC forms of H_2R blockers currently available. Such preparations are at a lower dose than drugs that are prescribed. H_2Rs are used in combination with antibiotics to treat ulcers related to *H. pylori*.

Proton pump inhibitors. PPIs, such as omeprazole (Prilosec), lansoprazole (Prevacid), pantoprazole (Protonix), and esomeprazole (Nexium), block the ATPase enzyme that is important for the secretion of HCl acid. These agents are more effective than H_2R blockers in reducing gastric acid secretion and promoting ulcer healing. PPIs are also used in combination with antibiotics to treat ulcers caused by *H. pylori*.

Antibiotic therapy. Antibiotics to eradicate *H. pylori* infection are prescribed. The treatment of *H. pylori* is the most important element of treating ulcer disease in patients positive for *H. pylori*. When *H. pylori* is present, ulcer recurrence rates with H_2R blockers alone can be as high as 75% to 90%, whereas with antibiotic treatment the recurrence rate may be less than 10%. Antibiotic therapy for *H. pylori* is shown in Table 40-13.

Once the presence of *H. pylori* has been determined, antibiotic treatment is instituted. The regimen of choice is based on the antibiotic susceptibility of the *H. pylori* organism, patient compliance, side effects, and costs. Most drug regimens involve treatment for 7 to 14 days. No single agents have been effective in eliminating *H. pylori* (see Table 40-13). Bismuth subsalicylate (Pepto-Bismol) or bismuth combined with an H_2R (Tritec) is used as part of one therapy to facilitate healing. Bismuth is nonabsorbable and causes black stools.

Antacids. Antacids are used as adjunct therapy for peptic ulcer disease. They increase gastric pH by neutralizing the acid. As a result, the acid content of chyme reaching the duodenum is reduced. In addition, some antacids, such as aluminum hydroxide, can bind to bile salts, thus decreasing the detrimental effects of bile on the gastric mucosa. Patients who are vulnerable for physiologic stress ulcer formation may be treated prophylactically with antacids along with an antisecretory agent.

Antacids consist of systemic and nonsystemic types. Systemic antacids, such as sodium bicarbonate, are extremely soluble and are absorbed into the circulation. Their long-term use can lead to systemic alkalosis; therefore they are rarely used in ulcer treatment. The nonsystemic antacids are insoluble and poorly absorbed. The common commercial nonsystemic antacids consist of magnesium hydroxide or aluminum hydroxide as single preparations or in various combinations (see Table 40-21).

The antacid preparation may be in liquid or tablet form. A large number of tablets may be required to equal the same dose of a liquid preparation. Because the tablets are chewable, some of the drug is left coating the teeth and gingivae instead of the stomach.

The neutralizing effects of antacids taken on an empty stomach last only 20 to 30 minutes because they are quickly evacuated. When antacids are taken after meals, the effects may last as long as 3 to 4 hours. Therapy recommending frequent dosing (e.g., hourly) often results in poor compliance.

After the acute phase of bleeding has diminished, antacids are generally administered hourly, either orally or through the NG tube. If the tube is in place, the stomach contents should be aspirated and tested periodically for pH level. If pH is less than 5, intermittent suction may be used, or the frequency or dosage of the antacid may be increased.

The type and dosage of antacid prescribed depends on side effects (see Table 40-22), as well as potential drug interactions. Preparations high in sodium (e.g., Titralac) should be used with caution in older adults and in the patient with liver cirrhosis, hypertension, congestive heart failure, and renal disease. Magnesium preparations should not be prescribed for the patient with renal failure because of the risk of magnesium toxicity. The most frequent side effect experienced with magnesium antacids is diarrhea. Aluminum hydroxide causes constipation. An antacid combination of aluminum and magnesium salts seems to lessen the side effects of both.

Antacids have the capacity to interact unfavorably with some drugs. They can enhance the absorption of drugs such as dicumarol and amphetamines. The action of digitalis preparations can be potentiated when taken in combination with calcium or magnesium antacids. In some instances, antacids may decrease the absorption rates of prescribed drugs, such as tetracycline. Therefore it is important to inform the health care provider of any drugs that are being taken before antacid therapy is begun.

Anticholinergic drugs. Anticholinergic drugs are only occasionally ordered in the treatment of peptic ulcer disease. These drugs decrease cholinergic (vagal) stimulation of HCl acid. There is divided opinion concerning their efficacy in preventing recurrences and their therapeutic effectiveness in alleviating symptoms and preventing complications. Because of their tendency to decrease gastric motility, they should not be used for gastric ulcers in which stasis of secretions increases the patient's pain and discomfort. Anticholinergics are associated with a high number of side effects, such as dry mouth and skin, flushing, thirst, tachycardia, dilated pupils, blurred vision, and urine retention. Anticholinergics must be prescribed with caution in the patient with narrow-angle glaucoma, benign prostatic hyperplasia, and gastric outlet obstruction.

Cytoprotective drug therapy. Sucralfate (Carafate) is used for the short-term treatment of ulcers. It has proven to be cytoprotective of the esophagus, stomach, and duodenum. Its ability to accelerate ulcer healing is thought to be a result of the formation of an ulcer-adherent complex covering the ulcer and thereby protecting it from erosion caused by pepsin, acid, and bile salts. Sucralfate does not have acid-neutralizing capabilities. Its action is most effective at a low pH, and it should be given at least 30 minutes before or after an antacid. Adverse side effects are minimal. However, it does bind with cimetidine, digoxin, warfarin (Coumadin), phenytoin (Dilantin), and tetracycline, causing reduced bioavailability of these drugs.

Misoprostol (Cytotec) is a synthetic prostaglandin analog. It has protective and some antisecretory effects on gastric mucosa. Misoprostol is the only drug approved in the United States for the prevention of gastric ulcers induced by NSAIDs and aspirin. A major advantage of misoprostol is that it does not interfere with the therapeutic effects of aspirin and NSAIDs. Persons who require chronic NSAID therapy, such as those with osteoarthritis, may benefit from the use of misoprostol. All NSAIDs, even COX-2 inhibitors, impair ulcer healing.

Other drugs. Tricyclic antidepressants (e.g., imipramine [Tofranil], doxepin [Sinequan]) and serotonin reuptake inhibitors may be prescribed for patients with ulcer disease. Antidepressants may contribute to overall pain relief through their effects on afferent pain fiber transmission. In addition, tricyclic antidepressants have, to varying degrees, some anticholinergic properties, which results in reduced acid secretion.

Nutritional Therapy. Dietary modifications may be necessary so that foods and beverages irritating to the patient can be avoided or eliminated. A nonirritating or bland diet consisting of six small meals a day may be recommended for the patient during the symptomatic phase. However, there is considerable controversy over the actual therapeutic benefits derived from a bland diet because the rationale is not supported by scientific evidence. Each patient should be instructed to eat and drink foods and fluids that do not cause any distressing symptoms. Alcohol and caffeine-containing products should be eliminated because of their irritating effects.

Dietary instructions should include a sample diet with a list of foods that usually cause distress and should therefore be eliminated from the diet. Foods known to irritate the gastric mucosa include hot, spicy foods and pepper, alcohol, carbonated beverages, tea, coffee, and broth (meat extract). These foods also have limited buffering ability in addition to stimulating gastric acid secretion. Foods high in roughage, such as raw fruit, salads, and vegetables, may irritate an inflamed mucosa. If these foods are well chewed, this seems to be less of a problem.

Protein is considered the best neutralizing food, but it also stimulates gastric secretions. Carbohydrates and fats are the least stimulating to HCl acid secretion, but they do not neutralize well. The patient must determine a suitable combination of these essential nutrients without causing undue distress.

Historically, milk was an essential part of ulcer therapy until it was learned that milk proteins and calcium stimulate gastric acid production. For this reason, milk as part of diet therapy for ulcers was out of favor for a time. However, milk is again used as part of the diet plan because it can neutralize gastric acidity and contains prostaglandins and growth factors, both of which may protect the GI mucosa from injury.

Therapy Related to Complications of Peptic Ulcer Disease

Acute exacerbation. The patient with an acute exacerbation of peptic ulcer can usually be treated with the same regimen used for conservative therapy. However, the situation is considered more serious because of the possible complications of perforation, hemorrhage, and gastric outlet obstruction.

An acute exacerbation is frequently accompanied by bleeding, increased pain and discomfort, and nausea and vomiting. If the patient experiences recurrent vomiting or gastric outlet obstruction, an NG tube is placed into the stomach with intermittent suction for about 24 to 48 hours.

If there is a history of an incompetent pyloric sphincter allowing reflux of duodenal contents into the stomach, an NG tube will remove intestinal contents from the stomach. This period of stomach rest eliminates any causative factors that may have precipitated the acute exacerbation and permits the resolution of edema and inflammation of the mucosa. Fluids and electrolytes are replaced by IV infusion until the patient is able to tolerate oral feedings without distress.

Management is similar to that described for upper GI bleeding. Blood or blood products may be administered. Careful monitoring of the vital signs, intake and output, laboratory studies, and signs of impending shock are important during this acute episode.

Endoscopic evaluation is performed to reveal the degree of inflammation or bleeding, as well as the ulcer location. It is important to ascertain the presence of a prepyloric or pyloric ulcer that can cause gastric outlet obstruction. When endoscopic examination reveals no major problems and the patient's physical condition stabilizes, the plan of care for the patient should follow the same regimen of diet, activity, and drugs used in conservative therapy. A 5-year follow-up program is recommended after acute exacerbation. An increase in the healing rate is achieved after conservative treatment, but the treatment plan cannot prevent the scar formation that can result in gastric outlet obstruction.

Perforation. The immediate focus of management of a patient with a perforation is to stop the spillage of gastric or duodenal contents into the peritoneal cavity and restore blood volume. An NG tube is inserted into the stomach to provide continuous aspiration and gastric decompression to halt spillage through the perforation. Although duodenal aspiration is not achieved as promptly, placement of the tube as near to the perforation site as possible facilitates decompression.

Circulating blood volume must be replaced with lactated Ringer's and albumin solutions. These solutions substitute for the fluids lost from the vascular and interstitial space as the peritonitis develops. Blood replacement in the form of packed RBCs may be necessary. Unless contraindicated, a central venous pressure line and an indwelling urinary catheter should be inserted and monitored hourly. The patient with a history of cardiac disease requires ECG monitoring or placement of a pulmonary artery catheter for more accurate assessment of left ventricular function. Broad-spectrum antibiotic therapy should be started immediately to treat bacterial peritonitis. Administration of pain medications provides comfort.

The operative procedure involving the least risk to the patient is simple oversewing of the perforation and reinforcement of the area with a graft of omentum. The excess gastric contents are suctioned from the peritoneal cavity during the surgical procedure. There is controversy regarding the need for more definitive surgical treatment of a perforated ulcer than can be achieved with simple closure. Other types of surgical procedures depend on the location of the peptic ulcer and the surgeon's preference. If cure of the ulcer is the ultimate goal, the surgical procedures may include gastric resection or vagotomy and pyloroplasty.

Gastric outlet obstruction. The aim of therapy for obstruction is to decompress the stomach, correct any existing fluid and electrolyte imbalances, and improve the patient's general state of health. An NG tube is inserted into the stomach and attached to continuous suction to remove excess fluids and undigested food particles. With continuous decompression for several days, the stomach has the opportunity to regain its normal muscle tone, the ulcer can begin healing, and the inflammation and edema will subside.

The tube is clamped after several days of suction, and gastric residue is measured periodically. The frequency and amount of time the tube remains clamped are proportional to the amount of aspirate obtained and the comfort level of the patient. A method commonly followed is to clamp the tube overnight for approximately 8 to 12 hours and to measure the gastric residue in the morning. When the aspirate falls below 200 ml, it is considered

to be within a normal range and the patient can begin oral intake of clear liquids. Initially, oral fluids are begun at 30 ml per hour and then gradually increased in amount. The patient must be watched carefully for signs of distress or vomiting. As the amount of gastric residue decreases, solid foods are added and the tube is removed.

IV fluids and electrolytes are administered according to the degree of dehydration, vomiting, and electrolyte imbalance indicated by laboratory studies. Pain relief results from the decompression measures, and analgesics are usually not necessary. Antacids and antisecretory drug therapy (i.e., H_2R blockers, PPIs) are an integral part of treatment if the obstruction has been determined on endoscopic examination to be the result of an active ulcer. Pyloric obstruction may be treated nonsurgically by balloon dilations performed through the endoscope. Surgical intervention may be necessary to remove scar tissue.

NURSING MANAGEMENT
PEPTIC ULCER DISEASE

■ Nursing Assessment

Subjective and objective data that should be obtained from a patient with peptic ulcer disease are presented in Table 40-23.

TABLE 40-23	Nursing Assessment Peptic Ulcer Disease

Subjective Data
Important Health Information
Past health history: Chronic renal failure, pancreatic disease, chronic obstructive pulmonary disease, serious illness or trauma, hyperparathyroidism, cirrhosis of the liver, Zollinger-Ellison syndrome
Medications: Use of aspirin, corticosteroids, nonsteroidal anti–inflammatory drugs
Surgery or other treatments: Complicated or prolonged surgery
Functional Health Patterns
Health perception–health management: Chronic alcohol abuse, smoking, caffeine use; family history of peptic ulcer disease
Nutritional-metabolic: Weight loss, anorexia; nausea and vomiting, hematemesis; dyspepsia, heartburn, belching
Elimination: Black, tarry stools
Cognitive–perceptual: Duodenal ulcers—burning, midepigastric or back pain occurring 2 to 4 hours after meals and relieved by food; nocturnal pain common; Gastric ulcers—high epigastric pain occurring 1 to 2 hours after meals; pain may be precipitated or aggravated by food
Coping-stress tolerance: Acute or chronic stress

Objective Data
General
Anxiety, irritability
Gastrointestinal
Epigastric tenderness
Possible Findings
Anemia; guaiac-positive stools; gastric analysis indicating high gastric acid secretion; positive blood, urine, breath, or stool tests for *H. pylori;* abnormal upper gastrointestinal endoscopic and barium studies

■ Nursing Diagnoses

Nursing diagnoses related to peptic ulcer disease may include, but are not limited to, those presented in NCP 40-2.

■ Planning

Overall goals are that the patient with peptic ulcer disease will (1) comply with the prescribed therapeutic regimen, (2) experience a reduction or absence of discomfort related to peptic ulcer disease, (3) exhibit no signs of GI complications related to the ulcerative process, (4) have complete healing of the peptic ulcer, and (5) make appropriate lifestyle changes to prevent recurrence.

■ Nursing Implementation

Health Promotion. Nurses need to be involved in identifying patients at risk for ulcer development. Early detection and treatment of ulcers are important aspects of reducing morbidity associated with ulcers. Patients who are taking ulcerogenic drugs such as aspirin and NSAIDs are at risk for ulcer development. Patients need to be encouraged to take these drugs with food or milk. Patients should be taught to report symptoms related to gastric irritation, including epigastric pain, to their health care provider.

Acute Intervention. During the acute exacerbation of an ulcer, the patient generally complains of increased pain and nausea and vomiting, and some may have evidence of bleeding. Initially many patients attempt to cope with the symptoms at home before seeking medical assistance.

During this acute phase the patient may be maintained on NPO status for a few days, have an NG tube inserted and connected to intermittent suction, and have fluids replaced intravenously. The rationale for this therapy must be conveyed to the anxious patient and family. They must understand that the advantages far outweigh any temporary discomfort imposed by the presence of the tube. Regular mouth care alleviates the dry mouth. Cleansing and lubrication of the nares facilitate breathing and decrease soreness. Gastric contents may be analyzed for pH, blood, bile, or other irritating substances. When the stomach is kept empty of gastric secretions, the ulcer pain diminishes and ulcer healing begins. Usually this form of intervention is effective.

Because the patient is on NPO status, IV fluids are ordered. The type and amount administered are directly related to the fluid lost; the manifestations exhibited by the patient; and the results of the hemoglobin, hematocrit, and electrolyte determinations. The nurse should be aware of any other current health problem that could be adversely affected by the type of fluid used or the rate of the infusion. Repeated monitoring of these parameters provides information on the hydration status and the effectiveness of treatment. Vital signs are initially taken at least hourly so that shock can be detected and treated.

Physical and emotional rest are conducive to ulcer healing. The patient's immediate environment should be quiet and restful. The use of a mild sedative or tranquilizer has beneficial effects when the patient is anxious and apprehensive. The nurse must use good judgment before sedating a person who is becoming increasingly restless. There is danger that the drug will mask the signs of shock secondary to upper GI bleeding.

If the patient's condition improves without progression of symptoms (e.g., increased pain, vomiting, and hemorrhage), the regimen outlined for conservative therapy is followed. However, complications such as hemorrhage, perforation, and obstruction can occur.

Hemorrhage. Changes in the vital signs and an increase in the amount and redness of the aspirate often signal massive upper GI bleeding. When there is an increased amount of blood in the gastric contents, the patient's pain is often decreased because the blood helps to neutralize the acidic gastric contents. It is important to maintain the patency of the NG tube so that blood clots do not obstruct the tube. If the tube becomes blocked, the patient can develop abdominal distention. Similar interventions to those described for upper GI bleeding on pp. 1025-1026 are used. The nurse needs to monitor the results of the hemoglobin and hematocrit determinations.

Perforation. When there is sudden, severe abdominal pain unrelated in intensity and location to the pain that brought the patient to the hospital, the nurse must recognize the possibility of ulcer perforation. When any person with an ulcer, particularly a chronic duodenal ulcer, demonstrates these manifestations, perforation should be suspected and the health care provider notified immediately.

Perforation is indicated by a rigid, boardlike abdomen; severe generalized abdominal and shoulder pain; drawing up of the knees; and shallow, grunting respirations. The bowel sounds that may have been previously normal or hyperactive may diminish and become absent.

Vital signs are important parameters and should be promptly taken and recorded every 15 to 30 minutes. The nurse should temporarily stop all oral or NG drugs and feedings until the health care provider can be notified and a definitive diagnosis made. If perforation does exist, anything taken internally can add to the spillage into the peritoneal cavity and increase discomfort. If IV fluids are being administered at the time of the perforation, the rate should be maintained or increased to replace the depleted plasma volume.

When perforation is confirmed, the nurse should ensure that any known patient allergies have been recorded on the chart. This is important because antibiotic therapy is usually started, and careful observation for allergic reactions must be made. When the perforation fails to seal spontaneously, surgical closure is necessary and is performed as soon as possible. There is often little time to prepare the patient and family thoroughly for the surgical intervention, yet some instructions can be carried out while the immediate therapy is begun. If major reconstructive surgery is anticipated, the patient and family may question the need when the problem is only a small hole.

Gastric outlet obstruction. Gastric outlet obstruction can occur at any time and is most likely to occur in the patient whose ulcer is located close to the pylorus. Because the onset of symptoms is usually gradual, the condition is not generally as serious an emergency as hemorrhage or perforation. Relief of symptoms may be achieved by constant NG aspiration of stomach contents. This allows edema and inflammation to subside and then permits normal flow of gastric contents through the pylorus.

Obstruction can also occur during the treatment of an acute episode of peptic ulcer exacerbation. If these symptoms are experienced while the patient is still on NPO status, the patency of the NG tube should be suspected. Regular irrigation of the tube with a saline solution facilitates proper functioning. It may be helpful to reposition the patient from side to side so that the tube tip is not constantly lying against the mucosal surface.

NURSING CARE PLAN 40-2

Patient with Peptic Ulcer Disease

EXPECTED PATIENT OUTCOMES	NURSING INTERVENTIONS and *RATIONALES*

CONSERVATIVE MANAGEMENT

NURSING DIAGNOSIS | **Acute pain** *related to* increased gastric secretions, decreased mucosal protection, and ingestion of gastric irritants *as manifested by* burning cramplike pain in epigastrium and abdomen; pain onset ½ to 2 hr after meals with gastric ulcer; pain onset 2 to 4 hr after meals (midmorning, midafternoon) and middle of night with duodenal ulcer.

- Verbalization of satisfaction with pain control

- Determine pain characteristics from verbal description and physical assessment data *so that appropriate interventions can be planned.*
- Administer antacids, H₂-receptor blockers, proton pump inhibitors, anticholinergics, and cytoprotective agents as ordered *to reduce pain.*
- Teach patient to avoid smoking and ingesting spicy, hot or cold foods, coffee, tea and cola drinks, and alcoholic beverages *to prevent irritation and increasing acid production.*
- Teach patient stress reduction *as relaxation results in decreased acid production and reduction in pain.*

NURSING DIAGNOSIS | **Ineffective therapeutic regimen management** *related to* lack of knowledge of long-term management of peptic ulcer disease and consequences of not following treatment plan and unwillingness to modify lifestyle *as manifested by* frequent questions about home care, incorrect responses to questions about peptic ulcer disease, noncompliance with medical regimen.

- Verbalization of plan to modify lifestyle and incorporate therapeutic regimen into lifestyle

- Explain peptic ulcer disease process at patient's level *to foster understanding.*
- Help patient identify stressors and initiate modifications in daily routine *as stress causes hypersecretion of HCl acid and pepsin, which can alter the mucosal barrier.*
- Discuss diet plan and assist with implementation at home and in work setting.
- Explain rationale for the elimination of alcohol, spicy foods, coffee, tea, and colas from diet; explain the harmful effects of smoking *as these agents increase acid production and directly irritate gastric mucosa.*
- Provide information on actions and side effects of drug therapy *to ensure safe self-administration.*
- Inform patient what to do if symptoms related to ulcers recur *to ensure early initiation of treatment.*

EXACERBATION MANAGEMENT

NURSING DIAGNOSIS | **Acute pain** *related to* exacerbation of disease process and inadequate comfort measures *as manifested by* verbalization of increase in pain, nonverbal indicators of pain (e.g., moaning, crying, doubling up).

- Expression of satisfaction with pain management

- Encourage bed rest or light activity *to conserve energy and promote comfort.*
- Provide quiet, relaxed environment and limit visitors *to decrease stress and other factors that increase acid secretion.*
- Administer medications as ordered *to relieve pain.*

NURSING DIAGNOSIS | **Nausea** *related to* acute exacerbation of disease process *as manifested by* episodes of nausea and/or vomiting (See NCP 40-1).

When oral feedings have been resumed and symptoms of obstruction are observed, the health care provider should be promptly informed. Generally, all that is necessary to treat the problem is to resume gastric aspiration so that the edema and inflammation resulting from the acute episode have time to resolve. IV fluids with electrolyte replacement keep the patient hydrated during this period. The NG tube can be clamped and gastric fluids can be aspirated to check for retention. It is important to maintain accurate intake and output records, especially of the gastric aspirate. The patient should be kept aware of why these symptoms are being experienced. In some instances in which treatment is not successful, surgery may be performed after the acute phase has passed.

Ambulatory and Home Care. The patient in whom peptic ulcer disease has been diagnosed has specific needs that must be met to prevent and avoid recurrence or complications. General instructions should cover aspects of the disease process itself, drugs, possible changes in lifestyle (including diet), and regular follow-up care. Table 40-24 provides a patient and family teaching guide for the patient with peptic ulcer disease.

Knowing the cause of the ulcer and understanding the disease process may motivate the patient to become more involved in care and increase compliance with therapy. The patient must understand the dietary modifications and why they are important for recovery and health maintenance. The nurse and the dietitian should elicit a dietary history from the patient and plan for ways that dietary modifications can be easily incorporated into the patient's home and work setting. The patient who is following a diet prescribed for another illness needs to know how to balance the two so that neither condition is harmed by dietary interventions.

NURSING CARE PLAN 40-2

Patient with Peptic Ulcer Disease—cont'd

COLLABORATIVE PROBLEMS

NURSING GOALS	NURSING INTERVENTIONS AND RATIONALES
POTENTIAL COMPLICATION • Monitor for signs of hemorrhage • Carry out medical and nursing interventions if hemorrhage occurs	**Hemorrhage** secondary to eroded mucosal tissue. • Assess for evidence of hematemesis, bright red or melena stool, abdominal pain or discomfort, symptoms of shock (e.g., decreased blood pressure; cool, clammy skin; dyspnea; tachycardia; decreased urine output) *to plan appropriate interventions.* • If ulcer is actively bleeding, observe NG tube aspirate or emesis for amount and color *to assess degree of bleeding.* • Take vital signs every 15 to 30 minutes *to determine patient's hemodynamic status and as indicators of shock.* • Maintain IV infusion line *to provide ready access for blood and fluid replacement.* • If RBC transfusion is given, observe for transfusion reaction *so that appropriate actions can be taken immediately.* • Monitor hematocrit and hemoglobin *as indicators of severity of hemorrhage and need for fluid and blood replacement.* • Record intake and output *to monitor fluid balance.* • Reassure patient and family to decrease their anxiety. • Remain calm and confident in plan of care *to foster calm and confidence in patient and family.* • Prepare patient for possible endoscopy or surgery.
POTENTIAL COMPLICATION • Monitor for signs of perforation • Carry out appropriate medical and nursing interventions	**Perforation of GI mucosa** secondary to impaired mucosal tissue integrity. • Observe for manifestations of perforation (e.g., sudden, severe abdominal pain; rigid, boardlike abdomen; radiating pain to shoulders; increasing distention; decreasing bowel sounds) *to ensure early recognition and intervention.* • Take vital signs every 15 to 30 minutes *to determine patient's hemodynamic status and as indicators of shock.* • Maintain NG tube to suction *to provide continuous aspiration and gastric decompression to prevent further leakage of gastric fluid through the perforation.* • Administer pain medication *to promote comfort and reduce anxiety.* • Prepare patient for emergency diagnostic tests and possible surgery *to foster timely intervention.*

The patient does not always give the health care provider accurate information regarding habitual use of alcohol or cigarettes. The nurse should provide useful information about the detrimental effects of alcohol and cigarettes on ulcer disease and ulcer healing.

The nurse should teach the patient about prescribed drugs, including their actions, side effects, and inherent dangers if omitted for any reason. The patient should know why OTC drugs (e.g., aspirin) should not be taken unless approved by the health care provider. Because antacids and some H_2R blockers may be bought without a prescription, the patient must be informed that interchanging brands without checking with the health care provider or nurse can lead to harmful side effects.

Efforts should be made to obtain more information about the patient's psychosocial status. Knowledge of lifestyle, occupation, and coping behaviors can be helpful to the plan of care. The patient may be reluctant to talk about personal subjects, the stress experienced at home or on the job, the usual methods of coping, or dependence on drugs or alcohol. Unfortunately, the patient does not often see the relationship between lifestyle or occupation and ulcer disease. It is important to listen for subtle clues from the patient's statements and to observe for behaviors that broaden this database.

The need for long-term follow-up care must be stressed. Because successful treatment is frequently followed by a recurrence of the ulcer disease, the patient should be encouraged to seek immediate intervention if symptoms of the disease come back. The patient who has recurrence of ulcer disease following initial healing must learn to live with a disease that is chronic. The patient may be angry and frustrated, especially if the prescribed mode of therapy has been faithfully followed yet has failed to prevent the recurrence or extension of the disease process.

Unfortunately, many patients do not comply with the plan of care originally designed, and they experience repeated exacerbations. Patients quickly learn that they often experience no discomfort when they omit prescribed drugs or indulge in occasional dietary indiscretions. Consequently, they make no or little alteration in lifestyle. After an acute exacerbation the patient is often more amenable to following the plan of care and open to suggestions for changes in lifestyle. Changes, such as smoking cessation and alcohol abstinence, are difficult for many people and may be met with resistance. The patient may fare better from

TABLE 40-24 Patient & Family Teaching Guide

Peptic Ulcer Disease

The following are teaching guidelines for the patient and family:

1. Explain dietary modifications, including avoidance of foods that cause epigastric distress. This may include black pepper, spicy foods, and acidic foods. Small frequent meals are better tolerated than large meals.
2. Explain the rationale for avoiding cigarettes. In addition to promoting ulcer development, smoking will delay ulcer healing.
3. Encourage the need to reduce or eliminate alcohol ingestion.
4. Explain the rationale for avoiding OTC drugs unless approved by the patient's care provider. Many preparations contain ingredients, such as aspirin, that should not be taken unless approved by the health care provider. Check with the care provider regarding the use of nonsteroidal antiinflammatory drugs.
5. Explain the rationale for not interchanging brands of antacids and H$_2$-receptor blockers that can be purchased OTC without checking with the health care provider. This can lead to harmful side effects.
6. Teach the need to take all medications as prescribed. This includes both antisecretory and antibiotic drugs. Failure to take medications as prescribed can result in relapse.
7. Explain the importance of reporting any of the following:
   - Increased nausea and/or vomiting
   - Increase in epigastric pain
   - Bloody emesis or tarry stools
8. Explain the relationship between symptoms and stress. Stress-reducing activities or relaxation strategies are encouraged.
9. Encourage patient and family to share concerns about lifestyle changes and living with a chronic illness.

OTC, Over-the-counter.

a reduction in his or her use of these substances rather than from total elimination. Although alcohol and smoking are known to interfere with ulcer healing, they frequently serve as coping mechanisms. From the patient's point of view, the distress caused by their total elimination may outweigh the benefits to be gained from abstention. The goal, however, should always be total cessation. A patient with chronic ulcers must be aware of the complications that may result from the disease, the clinical manifestations indicating their presence, and what to do until the health care provider can be seen.

■ Evaluation

Expected outcomes for the patient with a peptic ulcer disease are addressed in NCP 40-2.

Collaborative Therapy: Surgical Therapy for Peptic Ulcer Disease

Less than 20% of patients with ulcers need surgical intervention. Because there is a high recurrence rate for both duodenal and gastric ulcers and complications increase with the duration of the ulcer, many health care providers believe that surgery is

necessary after therapy has been tried and has proven unsuccessful. The following criteria are used as general indications for surgical intervention:

- Intractability: failure of the ulcer to heal or recurrence of the ulcer after therapy
- History of hemorrhage or increased risk of bleeding during treatment
- Prepyloric or pyloric ulcers (both have high recurrence rates)
- Concurrent condition, such as severe burns, trauma, or sepsis
- Multiple ulcer sites
- Drug-induced ulcers, especially when withdrawal from the drug may put the person at risk
- Possible existence of a malignant ulcer
- Obstruction

A variety of surgical procedures are used to treat ulcer disease. They usually involve a partial gastrectomy, vagotomy, or pyloroplasty. Partial gastrectomy with removal of the distal two thirds of the stomach and anastomosis of the gastric stump to the duodenum is called a *gastroduodenostomy* or *Billroth I* operation (Fig. 40-16). Partial gastrectomy with removal of the distal two thirds of the stomach and anastomosis of the gastric stump to the jejunum is called a *gastrojejunostomy* or *Billroth II* operation. In both procedures the antrum and the pylorus are removed. Because the duodenum is bypassed, the Billroth II operation is the preferred surgical procedure to prevent recurrence of duodenal ulcers.

Vagotomy is the severing of the vagus nerve, either totally (truncal) or selectively at some point in its innervation to the stomach. In a truncal vagotomy both the anterior and posterior trunks are severed. *Selective vagotomy* consists of cutting the nerve at a particular branch of the vagus nerve, resulting in denervation of only a portion of the stomach, such as the antrum or the parietal cell mass.

Pyloroplasty consists of surgical enlargement of the pyloric sphincter to facilitate the easy passage of contents from the stomach. It is most commonly done after vagotomy or to enlarge an opening that has been constricted from scar tissue. A vagotomy decreases gastric motility and, subsequently, gastric emptying. A pyloroplasty accompanying vagotomy increases gastric emptying.

The combination of a Billroth I or II procedure with vagotomy has the advantage of eliminating the ulcer and the stimulus for acid secretion. Surgical removal of the antrum results in removal of the source of gastrin secretion. (Gastrin normally stimulates parietal and chief cells.) Vagotomy eliminates the stimulus of HCl acid and gastrin hormone secretion caused by vagal stimulation.

Postoperative Complications. The most common postoperative complications from peptic ulcer surgery are (1) dumping syndrome, (2) postprandial hypoglycemia, and (3) bile reflux gastritis.

Dumping syndrome. *Dumping syndrome* is the direct result of surgical removal of a large portion of the stomach and the pyloric sphincter. These changes drastically reduce the reservoir capacity of the stomach. Although dumping syndrome is more commonly experienced after a Billroth II procedure, it can occur after any gastric reconstruction and vagotomy.

Dumping syndrome is associated with meals having a hyperosmolar composition. Normally, gastric chyme enters the small intestine in small amounts, and shifts in fluid from the extracellular space are minimal. After surgery, however, the stomach no longer has control over the amount of gastric chyme entering the

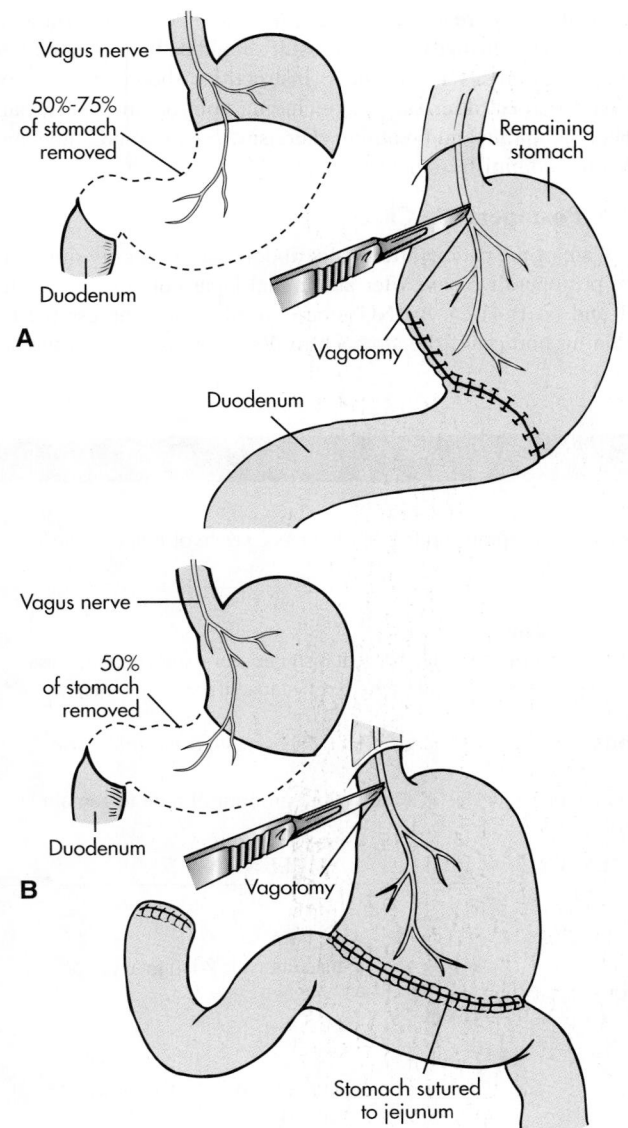

Postprandial hypoglycemia. *Postprandial hypoglycemia* is considered a variant of the dumping syndrome because it is the result of uncontrolled gastric emptying of a bolus of fluid high in carbohydrate into the small intestine. The bolus of concentrated carbohydrate results in hyperglycemia and the release of excessive amounts of insulin into the circulation. A secondary hypoglycemia then occurs, with symptoms appearing about 2 hours after meals. The symptoms experienced are the ones observed in any hypoglycemic reaction and include sweating, weakness, mental confusion, palpitations, tachycardia, and anxiety.

Bile reflux gastritis. Gastric surgery that involves the pylorus, either reconstruction or removal, can result in reflux alkaline gastritis. Prolonged contact of bile, especially bile salts, causes damage to the gastric mucosa. Chronic gastritis of this form may result in the back diffusion of hydrogen ions through the gastric mucosa. Paradoxically, peptic ulcer may recur after surgical treatment that was intended as a cure.

The symptoms associated with reflux alkaline gastritis are continuous epigastric distress that increases after meals. Vomiting relieves the distress but only temporarily. The administration of cholestyramine (Questran), either before or with meals, has met with success. Cholestyramine binds with the bile salts that are the source of irritation in this condition. Aluminum hydroxide antacids have also been used in the treatment of this condition.

Nutritional Therapy. Discharge planning and instruction should be started as soon as the immediate postoperative period is successfully passed. Dietary instructions may be given by the dietitian and reinforced by the nursing staff. Because the stomach's reservoir has been greatly diminished after gastric resection, the meal size must be reduced accordingly. The patient should be advised to eliminate drinking fluids with meals. Dry foods with a low-carbohydrate content and moderate protein and fat content are better tolerated initially. These dietary changes, with the incorporation of a short rest period after each meal, reduce the likelihood of dumping syndrome. Reassurance that following these dietary measures will result in cessation of these symptoms within a few months is essential to long-term compliance.

Postprandial hypoglycemic reaction can be avoided if these dietary instructions are followed. The immediate ingestion of sugared fluids or candy relieves the hypoglycemic symptoms. The treatment of this type of hypoglycemia is similar to that of dumping syndrome. To avoid similar occurrences the patient should be instructed to limit the amount of sugar consumed with each meal and to eat small, frequent meals with moderate amounts of protein and fat. Although only a small percentage of patients experience bile reflux gastritis, the patient must be cautioned to notify the health care provider of any continuous epigastric distress after meals that is similar to that felt before surgery.

With regard to dumping syndrome, the symptoms are self-limiting and often disappear within several months to a year after surgery. Interventions prescribed for the patient are diet instruction, rest, and reassurance. The diet should consist of small dry feedings daily that are low in carbohydrate, are restricted in refined sugars, and contain moderate amounts of protein and fat. Sample menu plans are presented in Table 40-25. Fluids should be taken between meals but not with the meal, and the patient should plan rest periods of at least 30 minutes after each meal. The recumbent position is the most beneficial if the patient can arrange it. Reassuring the patient that the unpleasant symptoms are usually of short duration is helpful in gaining cooperation. A

FIG. 40-16 A, Billroth I procedure (subtotal gastric resection with gastroduodenostomy anastomosis). **B,** Billroth II procedure (subtotal gastric resection with gastrojejunostomy anastomosis).

small intestine. Consequently, a large bolus of hypertonic fluid enters the intestine and results in fluid being drawn into the bowel lumen. This creates a decrease in plasma volume. A secondary consequence of this fluid shift is distention of the bowel lumen, which stimulates intestinal motility and the urge to defecate.

Approximately one third to one half of patients experience dumping syndrome after peptic ulcer surgery. The onset of symptoms occurs at the end of a meal or within 15 to 30 minutes after eating. The patient usually describes feelings of generalized weakness, sweating, palpitations, and dizziness. These symptoms are attributed to the sudden decrease in plasma volume. The patient complains of abdominal cramps, borborygmi (audible abdominal sounds produced by hyperactive intestinal peristalsis), and the urge to defecate. These manifestations usually last for no longer than an hour after meals.

small percentage of patients experience long-term problems and may require further reconstructive surgery.

NURSING MANAGEMENT
SURGICAL THERAPY FOR PEPTIC ULCER DISEASE

■ Preoperative Care

When surgery is planned with the goal of curing the ulcer disease, the surgeon should provide necessary information about the procedure and the expected outcome so that the patient can make an informed decision. The nurse can help the patient and family by clarifying and interpreting their questions. A discussion of the surgical procedure accompanied by a diagram or picture showing the anatomic changes that will result should be incorporated into the preoperative teaching plan. Instructions should be clear on what to expect after surgery, including comfort measures, pain relief, coughing and breathing exercises, use of an NG tube, and IV fluid administration (see Chapter 17).

■ Postoperative Care

Care of the patient after major abdominal surgery is similar to the postoperative care after abdominal laparotomy (see Chapter 41 and NCP 41-2). An NG tube is used to decompress the remaining portion of the stomach to decrease pressure on the su-

---

TABLE 40-25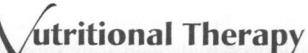

Nutritional Therapy
Postgastrectomy Dumping Syndrome

Purpose
To slow the rapid passage of food into the intestine; to control symptoms of the dumping syndrome (dizziness, sense of fullness, diarrhea, tachycardia), which sometimes occur following a partial or total gastrectomy

Diet Principles
1. Meals are divided into six small feedings to avoid overloading intestines at mealtimes.
2. Fluids should not be taken with meals but at least 30–45 minutes before or after meals; this helps prevent distention or a feeling of fullness.
3. Concentrated sweets (e.g., honey, sugar, jelly, jam, candies, sweet pastries, sweetened fruit) are avoided because they sometimes cause dizziness, diarrhea, and a sense of fullness.
4. Protein and fats are increased to promote rebuilding of body tissues and to meet energy needs. Meat, cheese, eggs, and milk products are specific foods to increase in the diet.
5. Amount of time these restrictions should be followed varies. The health care provider decides the proper amount of time to remain on this prescribed diet according to the patient's clinical condition and progress.

EXCHANGES	SAMPLE MENU 1	SAMPLE MENU 2	SAMPLE MENU 3
Breakfast			
1 meat	1 poached egg	1 fried egg	1 oz ham
1 starch	1 slice toast	1 corn tortilla	2 biscuits with 2 tsp gravy
Fat	2 sausage	2 slices bacon	
	Margarine	Margarine	
10 AM snack			
1 starch	¾ cup dry cereal	½ cup atole	½ cup grits with 2 tbs margarine
½ cup milk	½ cup milk	½ cup milk	added
1 fruit	½ fresh banana	2 unsweetened canned peach halves	⅓ cantaloupe
	Sugar substitute	Sugar substitute	½ cup buttermilk
Lunch			
2 meat	Grilled cheese sandwich with 2 oz	1 burrito with 1 oz meat, 1 oz	2 oz fried fish
2 starch	cheese, lettuce	cheese, ½ cup pinto beans,	½ cup buttered rice
1 vegetable	2 unsweetened pear halves	1 flour tortilla	½ cup mustard greens
1 fruit		½ diet gelatin dessert with fruit	1 fresh apple
Fat		cocktail added	1 slice bread
2 PM snack			
1 meat or substitute	½ cup plain yogurt	½ cup cottage cheese	2 tsp peanut butter
1 starch	2 graham crackers	5 soda crackers	1 slice bread
Dinner			
2 meat	2 oz tomato meatloaf	2 tamales	2 oz fried pork chop
1 starch	½ cup mashed potatoes with	½ cup buttered corn	½ cup black-eyed peas
Vegetable	gravy	1 fresh orange	½ cup buttered carrots
1 fruit	½ cup buttered green beans		1 fresh plum
Fat	½ cup unsweetened apple sauce		
8 PM snack			
1 meat	½ sandwich with 1 slice bread,	1 corn tortilla with 1 oz melted	½ sandwich with 1 slice bread,
1 starch	1 oz roast beef, lettuce,	cheese and green chili	1 slice salami, lettuce,
Vegetable	mayonnaise		mayonnaise
Fat			

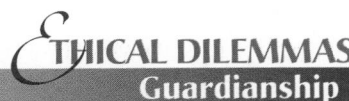

ETHICAL DILEMMAS
Guardianship

Situation

A 32-year-old man, institutionalized almost all of his life for profound developmental disabilities, is hospitalized for his fourth aspiration-related pneumonia in the last year. His health care provider believes that a feeding tube would solve the problem of aspiration and wants the family to agree to the procedure. The family believes his life span should not be extended by artificial means and refuses to give consent. The hospital is considering seeking a court-appointed guardian because the family is not acting in the best interest of the patient.

Important Points for Consideration

- Before making an ethical or legal decision, it is important that all contextual factors relating to the case be explored, such as possible reasons for the increase in aspiration pneumonia. These may include the technique used to feed the patient, how the patient is positioned during and after feedings, and how the patient might respond to the placement of a feeding tube.
- In most cases, families are considered in the best position to make treatment decisions for incompetent patients, unless there is some evidence they are not acting in the best interests of the patient. Courts are usually reserved as a last resort for treatment decisions in these situations.
- Two standards are used in decision-making for incompetent patients including substituted judgment and best interest. *Substituted judgment* is basing the decision on what previously competent patients would have decided for themselves. The *best interest standard* involves making the best decision possible under the circumstances using experiences from the patient's life that are meaningful or bring satisfaction to the patient, if known.
- A consultation with an ethics committee may be helpful to clarify the issues or assist the health care team to understand quality of life from the perspective of the patient and family.

Critical Thinking Questions

1. What are your thoughts and beliefs about the two opposing positions of preserving life in all circumstances versus maintaining an adequate quality of life?
2. In your opinion, who is in the best position to define quality of life for this patient?

---

ture line and to allow for resolution of edema and inflammation resulting from surgical trauma.

The gastric aspirate must be carefully observed for color, amount, and odor during the immediate postoperative period. The color of the aspirate is expected to be bright red at first, with a gradual darkening within the first 24 hours after surgery. Normally the color changes to yellow-green within 36 to 48 hours. If the tube becomes clogged during this period, the health care provider may order periodic gentle irrigations with normal saline solution. It is essential that the NG suction is working and that the tube remains patent so that accumulated gastric secretions do not put a strain on the anastomosis. This can lead to distention of the remaining portion of the stomach and result in (1) rupture of the sutures, (2) leakage of gastric contents into the peritoneal cavity, (3) hemorrhage, and (4) possible abscess formation. If the

tube must be replaced or repositioned, the health care provider must be called to perform this task because of the danger of perforating the gastric mucosa or disrupting the suture line.

The nurse observes the patient for signs of decreased peristalsis and lower abdominal discomfort that may indicate impending intestinal obstruction. Accurate intake and output records must be kept. Vital signs are monitored and recorded every 4 hours.

The patient is kept comfortable and free of pain by the administration of the prescribed drugs and by frequent changes in position. The incision is relatively high in the epigastrium and may interfere with deep-breathing and coughing measures. Splinting the area with a pillow while gently and persistently encouraging the patient to put forth the best efforts possible helps prevent pulmonary complications. Splinting also protects the abdominal suture line from rupturing during coughing. The dressing must be observed for signs of bleeding or odor and drainage indicative of an infection. Ambulation is encouraged and is increased daily.

While the NG tube is connected to suction, IV therapy is maintained. Potassium and vitamin supplements are added to the infusion until oral feedings are resumed. Before the NG tube is removed, the patient is started on oral feedings of clear liquids to determine the tolerance level. The stomach is aspirated within 1 or 2 hours to assess the amount remaining and its color and consistency. When fluids are well tolerated, the tube is removed and fluids are increased in frequency with a slow progression to regular foods. The regimen of six small meals a day is begun.

Pernicious anemia is a long-term complication of total gastrectomy and may occur after partial gastrectomy. Pernicious anemia is caused by the loss of intrinsic factor, which is produced by the parietal cells. Depending on the amount of parietal cell mass removed in surgery, the patient may eventually require regular injections of cobalamin (vitamin B_{12}). (Cobalamin deficiency and pernicious anemia are discussed in Chapter 30.)

Peptic ulcer disease is a chronic problem, and ulcers can recur especially at the site of the anastomosis. Adequate rest, nutrition, and avoidance of known irritants and stressors are keys to complete recovery. Avoiding the use of drugs not prescribed by the health care provider is reemphasized, along with restrictions on smoking and alcohol use. If the patient is willing to make these kinds of adjustment in lifestyle, a successful rehabilitation is more likely.

■ Gerontologic Considerations: Peptic Ulcer Disease

The incidence of peptic ulcers and, in particular, gastric ulcers in patients over 60 years of age is increasing. This is related to the increased use of NSAIDs. In the elderly patient, pain may not be the first symptom associated with an ulcer. For some patients the first manifestation may be frank gastric bleeding (e.g., hematemesis, melena) or a decrease in hematocrit. The morbidity and mortality rates associated with gastric ulcers in the elderly patient are higher than those for younger adults because of concomitant health problems (e.g., cardiovascular, pulmonary) and a decreased ability to withstand hypovolemia.

The treatment and management of ulcers in older adults are similar to that in younger adults. An emphasis is placed on prevention of both gastritis and peptic ulcers. This includes teaching the patient to take NSAIDs and other gastric-irritating drugs with food, milk, or antacids. The patient may be treated with antisecretory agents (i.e., PPIs or H$_2$R blockers). The patient should be instructed to avoid irritating substances, such as alcohol and smoking, and to report abdominal pain or discomfort to his or her health care provider.

GASTRIC CANCER

Gastric cancer is an adenocarcinoma of the stomach wall. The rate of gastric cancer has been steadily declining in the United States since the 1930s. However, it still accounts for more than 12,400 deaths and 21,600 new cancer cases annually.[1] Worldwide gastric adenocarcinoma is the second most common malignant growth. Gastric cancer is more prevalent in men of the lower socioeconomic class, primarily those living in urban areas. Gastric or stomach cancer is typically at an advanced stage when diagnosed and is not usually amenable to surgical resection. Only 10% to 20% of patients develop disease confined to the stomach. The five-year survival rate is 75% in patients with early stages of gastric cancer and less than 30% in those with advanced disease.

Etiology and Pathophysiology

Many factors have been implicated in the development of gastric cancer, yet no single causative agent has been identified. It is believed that a diet of smoked, highly salted, or spiced foods may have a carcinogenic effect. At the same time there appears to be a negative association between fresh fruits and the development of gastric cancer. A genetic etiology has been postulated because of the greater than normal occurrence of stomach cancer in immediate family members. However, at the present time there is no universally accepted genetic basis for gastric cancer.

Gastric carcinogenesis probably begins with a nonspecific mucosal injury as a result of aging, autoimmunity, or repeated exposure to irritants such as bile, antiinflammatory agents, or alcohol. Nutritional or other undetermined genetic deficiencies may impede mucosal repair, resulting in chronic gastritis and subsequent proliferation of *H. pylori*. Infection with *H. pylori,* especially at an early age, is considered a definite risk factor for gastric cancer. It is possible that *H. pylori* and resulting metabolic changes can induce a sequence of transitions from dysplasia to carcinoma in situ.

Other predisposing factors associated with a high incidence of gastric cancer are atrophic gastritis, pernicious anemia, adenomatous polyps, hyperplastic polyps, and achlorhydria. The relationship between chronic gastric ulcers and the development of gastric cancer is still controversial. Malignant transformation of a benign chronic ulcer does occur but accounts for less than 5% of all gastric cancers. It is known that the person with achlorhydria or pernicious anemia is more likely to develop gastric cancer than is the person with normal gastric acid production.

Gastric cancers often spread to adjacent organs before any distressing symptoms occur. The tumor may grow to large dimensions without obstructing the lumen of the stomach simply because the lumen itself is so large. The mean interval from onset of symptoms to consultation with a health care provider may be as long as 6 months. This long delay is largely attributed to the vague, intermittent abdominal distress experienced by the patient. Unfortunately, most healthy persons at one time or another experience these symptoms as a result of dietary indiscretions, nervous tension, and anxiety.

Gastric cancer can occur in any portion of the stomach. Tumors located at the cardia and fundus are associated with a poor prognosis. These tumors typically infiltrate rapidly to the surrounding tissue, regional lymph nodes, and liver. The patient with tumor growth along the lesser curvature has a better survival rate. Adenocarcinomas account for more than 95% of the cancers, and sarcomas (comprising lymphomas and leiomyomas) make up the rest.

The tumor growth is insidious and follows a pattern of continuous infiltration. Gastric cancer may spread by direct extension along the mucosal surface and infiltrate through the stomach wall. The rich lymphatic plexuses in the stomach facilitate distant metastasis. Seeding of tumor cells into the peritoneal cavity may occur late in the course of the disease. Evidence of spread to the peritoneal cavity is manifested by ascites and by spread to the ovaries.

Clinical Manifestations

The clinical manifestations exhibited by persons with gastric cancer can be categorized by signs and symptoms of anemia, peptic ulcer disease, or indigestion. Anemia is a common occurrence with stomach cancer. It is caused by chronic blood loss as the lesion erodes through the mucosa or as a direct result of pernicious anemia, which develops when intrinsic factor is lost. The person appears pale and weak and complains of fatigue, weakness, dizziness, and, in extreme cases, shortness of breath. The stool may be positive for occult blood.

The symptoms of gastric cancer are sometimes identical to those of peptic ulcer disease. The pain and discomfort may be alleviated by belching and by the use of antacids, antisecretory agents, and diet modifications. Manifestations related to indigestion include vague epigastric fullness with feelings of early satiety after meals. Weight loss, dysphagia, and constipation frequently accompany epigastric distress. When nausea, vomiting, and hematemesis occur, they may indicate gastric outlet obstruction or may be a warning of impending hemorrhage.

With more advanced disease, the physical examination may reveal that the patient is pale and lethargic if anemia is present. When the appetite has been poor and weight loss has been considerable, the patient may appear cachectic. A mass can often be detected beneath the abdominal wall and is seen to move with each inspiration. On palpation the mass may be felt in the epigastrium. Masses that are predominantly in the antrum of the stomach are generally found to the left of the midline. Masses located to the right of midline usually tend to be metastases to the liver or indicate involvement of the perigastric lymph nodes. Supraclavicular lymph nodes that are hard and enlarged and located on the left side are suggestive of metastasis via the thoracic duct from the stomach lesion. The presence of ascites is a poor prognostic sign.

Diagnostic Studies

The diagnostic studies for gastric cancer are presented in Table 40-26. Upper GI barium studies may demonstrate alterations in gastric contractility and emptying. On x-ray examination the malignant ulcer crater is more irregular around the edges and more elevated than the craters found with benign peptic ulcers. Barium studies do not always detect small lesions of the cardia and fundus.

Endoscopic examination of the stomach remains the best diagnostic tool. Lesions that go undetected on x-ray can be more easily viewed and a biopsy performed when endoscopy is used.

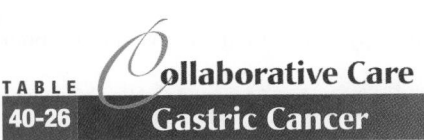

TABLE 40-26 **Collaborative Care**
Gastric Cancer

Diagnostic
History and physical examination
Upper GI barium study
Endoscopy and biopsy
Exfoliative cytology
Endoscopic ultrasonography
Upper GI barium study
Complete blood count
Urinalysis
Stool examination
Liver enzymes
Serum amylase
Tumor markers
   Carcinoembryonic antigen (CEA)
   Carbohydrate antigen (CA) 19-9

Collaborative Therapy
Surgery
Subtotal gastrectomy—Billroth I or II procedure
Total gastrectomy with esophagojejunostomy
Adjuvant therapy
Radiation therapy
Chemotherapy
Combination radiation therapy and chemotherapy

GI, Gastrointestinal.

The stomach can be distended with air during the procedure so that the mucosal folds can be stretched. Fixation of the mucosa is indicative of malignancy.

Blood chemistry studies assist in the determination of anemia and its severity. Elevations in liver enzymes and serum amylase levels may indicate liver and pancreatic involvement. Stool examination provides evidence of occult or gross bleeding.

Several tumor markers are often present in patients with gastric cancer. These include carcinoembryonic antigen (CEA) and carbohydrate antigen (CA) 19-9.[24] Serum tests for these markers are commonly performed before surgery for gastric cancer. Studies have shown that serum levels of these markers are correlated with the degree of invasion, liver metastasis, and cure rate.[24] Serum markers are not used as the only diagnostic tools for gastric cancer because elevations may be related to other factors such as smoking and the presence of benign lesions. (CEA and other tumor markers are discussed in Chapter 15.)

Collaborative Care

When the diagnosis of gastric cancer has been confirmed, the treatment of choice is surgical removal of the tumor. The preoperative management of the patient with gastric cancer focuses on the correction of nutritional deficits, treatment of anemia, and replacement of blood volume.

Transfusions of packed RBCs correct the anemia. If a gastric lesion has been located at or near the pylorus and is causing gastric outlet obstruction, gastric decompression may be necessary before surgery. When the tumor has extended into the transverse colon and partial colon resection is also required, special preparation of the bowel is necessary. This preparation may include a

low-residue diet, enemas to cleanse the bowel, and the use of antibiotics to reduce the intestinal bacteria. Correction of malnutrition is important if surgery is planned. Malnutrition is associated with increased postoperative complications and mortality rates.

Surgical Therapy. The surgical intervention used in the treatment of gastric cancer may be the same surgical procedures used for peptic ulcer disease. Surgical resection is curative in less than 40% of cases of gastric cancer.[25] The location and extent of the lesion, the patient's physical condition, and preference of the surgeon determine the specific surgery employed. When metastasis is widespread at the time of diagnosis, surgical intervention may be only palliative.

The surgical aim is to remove as much of the stomach as necessary to remove the tumor and a margin of normal tissue. When the lesion is located in the cardia or high in the fundus, a total gastrectomy with esophagojejunostomy is performed. This procedure involves anastomosis of the lower end of the esophagus to the jejunum (Fig. 40-17). Lesions located in the antrum or the pyloric region are generally treated by either a Billroth I or Billroth II procedure. When metastasis has occurred to adjacent organs, such as the spleen, ovaries, or bowel, the surgical procedures must be modified and extended as necessary.

The chance of a complete cure by surgical means is decreased considerably when the lymph nodes are involved. Survival rates are considerably shortened when organs adjacent to the stomach show evidence of invasion at the time of surgery.

Adjuvant Therapy. Surgery is the only definitive means of achieving a cure. However, when the patient cannot physically withstand a surgical procedure or when surgical cure is not feasible, radiation or chemotherapy alone or in combination may be used. Neither radiation therapy nor chemotherapeutic agents have been very successful when used as the primary mode of treatment. Because the radiosensitivity of gastric cancers is low, radiation therapy has proven to be of little value. When radiation

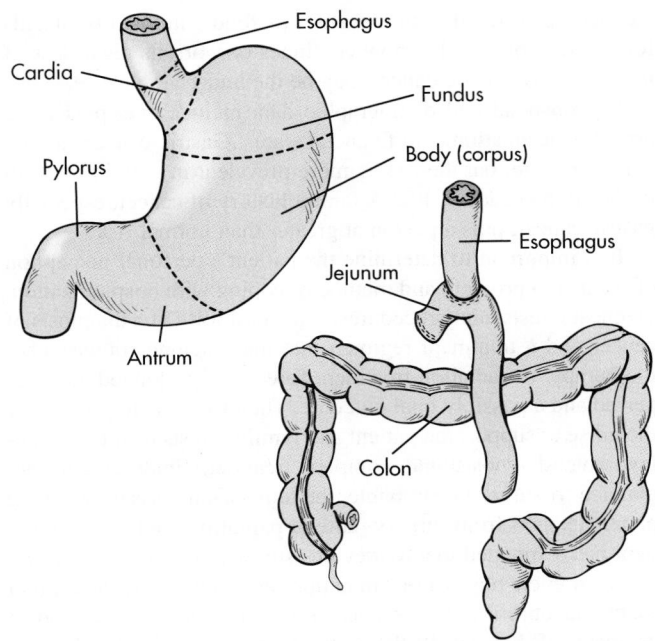

FIG. 40-17 Total gastrectomy for gastric cancer (total gastrectomy with esophagojejunostomy).

is used as a palliative measure, the tumor mass can be decreased, with temporary relief of the cardia or pyloric obstruction.

The combination of chemotherapy and radiation is now being used for patients who are at high risk for disease recurrence following surgery. Until recently, single-agent chemotherapy for gastric cancer has proven to be of little value. Agents that have been identified as having some effect on gastric cancer are 5-FU, BCNU, methyl-CCNU, and doxorubicin (Adriamycin). Combination of radiation and chemotherapy involving 5-FU and leucovorin following surgical resection increases survival. Additional therapies including intraperitoneal administration of chemotherapeutic agents are undergoing evaluation. The role of biologic therapy is still under investigation for use in gastric cancer. (These therapies are discussed in Chapter 15.)

NURSING MANAGEMENT
GASTRIC CANCER

■ Nursing Assessment

The assessment of a person with possible gastric cancer is similar to that done for peptic ulcer disease (see Table 40-23). Important data to be obtained from the patient and the family should include a nutritional assessment, a psychosocial history, the patient's perceptions of the health problem and need for hospitalization, and the physical examination of the patient.

The nutritional assessment must elicit information regarding appetite and changes in eating patterns over the previous 6 months. It is necessary to determine the patient's normal weight and any changes that may have occurred in the past few months. Unexplained weight loss is common in many types of cancer before diagnosis. A history of vague symptoms of dyspepsia, early satiety, feeling full after consuming even a small amount of food, or reporting symptoms of gas pain should help the nurse differentiate these typical gastric cancer symptoms from those of peptic ulcer. The nurse should determine whether pain is present, where and when it occurs, and how it is relieved. When the pain has been controlled with ingestion of foods, fluids, or antacids for a period of time but now continues or worsens regardless of interventions, gastric cancer may be the underlying cause.

Psychosocial and demographic data include age, present or previous occupation, and financial status. Gastric cancer can occur at any age, but the risk is more prevalent in men in the fifth to the sixth decade of life. A family history of cancer, especially gastric cancer, puts a person at greater than normal risk.

It is important to determine the patient's personal perception of the health problem and method of coping with hospitalization, diagnostic tests, and procedures. The possibility of a diagnosis of cancer and a treatment regimen that may include surgery, chemotherapy, or radiation treatment forecast a prolonged stressful period and a possibly fatal outcome. Therefore it is important for the nurse to support the patient and family if tests result in an unfavorable diagnosis and complex treatment interventions are planned. If surgery is probable, the nurse should assess what the patient expects from surgery (cure or palliation) and how that patient has responded to any previous surgical procedures.

A complete physical examination reveals the patient's current functional abilities, the presence of other health problems, and an estimate of how well the patient may respond to therapy. Cachexia may be evident if the nutritional state has been compromised for an extended time. A malnourished patient does not respond well to chemotherapy or radiation therapy and is a poor surgical risk.

■ Nursing Diagnoses

Nursing diagnoses for the patient with gastric cancer include, but are not limited to, the following:

- Imbalanced nutrition: less than body requirements *related to* inability to ingest, digest, or absorb nutrients
- Activity intolerance *related to* generalized weakness, abdominal discomfort, and nutritional deficits
- Anxiety *related to* lack of knowledge of diagnostic tests, unknown diagnostic outcome, disease process, and therapeutic regimen
- Acute pain *related to* underlying disease process and side effects of surgery, chemotherapy, or radiation therapy
- Anticipatory grieving *related to* perceived unfavorable diagnosis and impending death

■ Planning

The overall goals are that the patient with gastric cancer will (1) experience minimal discomfort, (2) achieve optimal nutritional status, and (3) maintain a degree of spiritual and psychologic well-being appropriate to the disease stage.

■ Nursing Implementation

Health Promotion. The nursing role in the early detection of cancer of the stomach is focused primarily on identification of the patient at risk because of specific disorders such as pernicious anemia and achlorhydria. The nurse should be aware of symptoms associated with gastric cancer, method of spread, and the significant findings on physical examination. The nurse should understand that the cure rate is often quite dismal because symptoms arise late in the course of the disease process, are vague, and often mimic other conditions, such as peptic ulcer disease.

The nurse must be alert to problems suggesting gastric cancer, such as poor appetite, weight loss, fatigue, and persistent gastric distress. If any of these manifestations are present, medical attention should be obtained and the necessary diagnostic tests performed.

In addition, any patient with a positive family history of gastric cancer should be encouraged to undergo diagnostic evaluation if manifestations of anemia, peptic ulcer, or vague epigastric distress are present. It is important that the nurse recognize the possible existence of stomach cancer in a patient who is treated for peptic ulcer and who fails to have relief after 3 weeks of prescribed therapy. The ulcer, if it is benign, should show signs of healing on x-ray examination.

Acute Intervention

Preoperative care. When the diagnostic tests confirm the presence of a malignancy, the patient and the family generally react with shock, disbelief, and depression, regardless of how thoroughly they may have been prepared for this possible outcome. Throughout this period the nurse must give emotional and physical support, provide information, clarify test results, and maintain a positive attitude with respect to the patient's immediate recovery and long-term survival.

On admission to the hospital, the patient may be in poor physical condition. Surgery may have to be delayed while the patient becomes more physically able to withstand the strain of major surgery. A positive nutritional state enhances wound healing, as well as the ability to withstand infection and other possible postoperative complications. Often the patient is better able to tolerate several small meals a day rather than three regular meals. The diet may be supplemented by a variety of commercial liquid supplements (see Chapter 39) and vitamins. The nurse is challenged to find innovative ways of persuading the patient to eat when lack of appetite and state of mind make eating difficult and unrewarding. Getting the patient's family to assist with meals and encourage intake may be beneficial. If the patient is unable to ingest oral feedings, it may be necessary to provide for nutritional needs with tube feedings or parenteral nutrition.

If needed, blood replacement and fluid volume restoration may be carried out in the preoperative period. Because anemia is usually present, packed RBCs may be administered. Close observation for reactions to the transfusions is important. Monitoring the hemoglobin and hematocrit levels provides information on the progress of therapy.

The preoperative teaching plan before gastric surgery for cancer is much the same as that for peptic ulcer surgery (see the previous section, Surgical Therapy for Peptic Ulcer Disease).

Postoperative care. Postoperative care of the patient with gastric carcinoma is similar to that following a Billroth I or II procedure (see the previous section, Surgical Therapy for Peptic Ulcer Disease). When the surgical intervention has involved a total gastrectomy, the plan of care is somewhat different. The operation performed usually requires some resecting of the lower esophagus along with the removal of the entire stomach and anastomosis of the esophagus to the jejunum. The chest cavity must be entered, and drainage is accomplished by the insertion of chest tubes. (Chest surgery and drainage tubes are discussed in Chapter 27.) After total gastrectomy, the NG tube does not drain a large quantity of secretions because removal of the stomach has eliminated the reservoir capacity. The NG tube is removed after several days, when intestinal peristalsis has resumed. Small amounts of clear fluid may then be started. The patient requires close observation for signs of leakage of the fluids at the anastomosis as evidenced by an elevation in the temperature and increasing dyspnea. When fluids are well tolerated without distress, the amount may be increased along with the addition of some solid foods.

As a consequence of a total gastrectomy, a patient experiences the symptoms of the dumping syndrome. Unfortunately, weight loss is very common, and poor nutritional intake often contributes. Postoperative wound healing may be impaired because of inadequate dietary intake. This necessitates the IV or oral replacement of vitamins C, D, K, and the B complex vitamins and intramuscular administration of cobalamin. Because these vitamins (with the exception of cobalamin) are absorbed primarily in the upper part of the small intestine, they must be replaced because the duodenum has been bypassed in the surgical procedure.

A patient who has had a Billroth I or II operative procedure should receive the same postoperative care as someone who has had peptic ulcer surgery. This patient is also subject to the same type of postoperative complications such as the dumping syndrome and postprandial hypoglycemia.

The patient with advanced malignant disease can be offered only palliative treatment. The chemotherapy agent found most useful for controlling symptoms of gastric cancer is 5-FU. When this drug or any of the combination drugs is prescribed, the nurse must have current information regarding the action and side effects of the drugs. The patient should be made aware of the potential benefits and hazards that can result from the chemotherapy. (The care of the patient receiving chemotherapy is discussed in detail in Chapter 15.)

Radiation therapy can be used as an adjuvant to surgery or for palliation. A patient is generally quite fearful of radiation and may develop many misconceptions regarding its value and dangers. To reassure the patient and ensure completion of the designated number of treatments, the nurse must provide detailed instruction. Because most therapy is completed on an outpatient basis, the nurse should assess the patient's knowledge of radiation, care of the skin, the need for good nutrition and fluid intake during therapy, and the appropriate use of antiemetic drugs. (Specific care of the patient receiving radiation therapy is discussed in Chapter 15.)

Ambulatory and Home Care. Before the patient is discharged, the need for teaching should be reviewed. Most dietary measures useful after peptic ulcer surgery are applicable after surgery for gastric carcinoma. Plans should be made for the relief of pain, including comfort measures and the judicious use of analgesics. Wound care, if needed, must be taught to the primary caregiver in the home situation. Dressings, special equipment, or special services may be required for the patient's continued care at home. A list of community agencies that are available for assistance can be provided before the patient goes home. The services of the American Cancer Society are especially helpful.

When treatment in the form of chemotherapy or radiation therapy is to be continued after discharge, a referral to the home health nurse may be beneficial. The home health nurse can assist with recovery, determine the degree of patient compliance, and be a sympathetic health care provider with whom the patient can consult.

Long-term follow-up must be stressed. The patient must be encouraged to comply with the prescribed dietary and drug regimens, to keep appointments for chemotherapy administration or radiation treatments, and to keep the physician informed of changes in physical condition. (Long-term management of the cancer patient is discussed in Chapter 15.)

■ Evaluation

Expected outcomes are that the patient with gastric cancer will

- experience no or minimal discomfort, pain, or nausea
- achieve optimal nutritional status
- maintain a degree of psychologic well-being appropriate to the disease stage

FOOD POISONING

Food poisoning is a nonspecific term that describes acute GI symptoms such as nausea, vomiting, diarrhea, and colicky abdominal pain caused by the intake of contaminated food. Food most commonly causes illness if it is contaminated with microorganisms or their products. The GI tract is frequently the portal of entry for the microorganisms. The epidemiology of foodborne illness is changing. There are new organisms, and many have spread worldwide. The two main types of food poisoning are (1) acute gastroenteritis from bacteria and (2) neurologic symptoms from botulism. The most common bacterial food poisonings are presented in Table 40-27.

TABLE 40-27 Bacterial Food Poisoning

TYPE	CAUSATIVE AGENT	SOURCES	ONSET OF SYMPTOMS	MANIFESTATIONS	TREATMENT	PREVENTION
Staphylococcal	Toxin from *Staphylococcus aureus*	Meat, bakery products, cream fillings, salad dressings, milk; skin and respiratory tract of food handlers	30 min–7 hr	Vomiting, nausea, abdominal cramping diarrhea	Symptomatic, fluid and electrolyte replacement, antiemetics	Immediate refrigeration of foods, monitoring of food handlers
Clostridial	*Clostridium perfringens*	Meat or poultry dishes cooked at lower temperature (stew or pot pie), rewarmed meat dishes, gravies, improperly canned vegetables	8–24 hr	Diarrhea, nausea, abdominal cramps, vomiting (rare); midepigastrium pain	Symptomatic, fluid replacement	Correct preparation of meat dishes, serving of food immediately after cooking or rapid cooling of food
Salmonella	*Salmonella typhimurium* (grows in gut)	Improperly cooked poultry, pork, beef, lamb, and eggs	8 hr–several days	Nausea and vomiting, diarrhea, abdominal cramps, fever and chills	Symptomatic, fluid and electrolyte replacement	Correct preparation of food
Botulism	Toxin from *Clostridium botulinum*, ingested toxin absorbed from gut and blocks acetylcholine at neuromuscular junction	Improperly canned or preserved food, home-preserved vegetables (most common), preserved fruits and fish, canned commercial products	12–36 hr	GI symptoms of nausea, vomiting, abdominal pain, constipation, distention. Central nervous system symptoms of headache, dizziness, muscular incoordination, weakness, inability to talk or swallow, diplopia, breathing difficulties, paralysis, delirium, coma	Maintenance of ventilation, polyvalent antitoxin, guanidine hydrochloric acid (enhances acetylcholine release)	Correct processing of canned foods, boiling of suspected canned foods for 15 min before serving
Escherichia coli	*E. coli* serotype 0157:H7	Contaminated beef, pork, milk, cheese, fish	Varies by strain: 8 hr–1 wk	Bloody stools, hemolytic uremic syndrome, abdominal cramping profuse diarrhea	Symptomatic, fluid and electrolyte replacement	Correct preparation of food

Poisonous chemicals, such as mercury, arsenic, zinc, and potassium chlorate, may contaminate foods. Poisoning can also occur from ingestion of poisonous plants (e.g., certain mushroom species).

Prevention of occurrence is the focus of interventions. Teaching should include correct food preparation and cleanliness, adequate cooking, and refrigeration. If the patient is hospitalized, care focuses on correction of fluid and electrolyte imbalance from diarrhea and vomiting. With botulism, additional assessment and care relative to neurologic symptoms are indicated (see Chapter 59).

Escherichia coli 0157:H7 Poisoning

Of recent importance is the increase in number of cases of hemorrhagic colitis caused by the presence of the bacterial strain *Escherichia coli 0157:H7*. Widespread outbreaks in the United States, Canada, and Japan have increased the public's awareness of this organism. Poisoning with *E. coli* 0157:H7 can be life threatening, particularly in the very young and the elderly. *E. coli* 0157:H7 is found primarily in undercooked meats, such as hamburger, roast beef, ham, and turkey. However, other sources include cheese sandwiches, apple cider, and unpasteurized milk. *E. coli* 0157:H7 can also be transmitted from person to person, particularly in settings such as nursing homes and day care centers. *E. coli* 0157:H7 may be responsible for 0.6% to 2.4% of all nonbloody diarrhea and 15% to 36% of all cases of bloody diarrhea.

The clinical manifestations of *E. coli* 0157:H7 vary from mild diarrhea to bloody diarrhea and systemic complications, including hemolytic uremia and thrombocytopenic purpura and even death. The diarrhea may start out as watery but may progress to bloody. Treatment involves supportive care to maintain intravascular volume. Other therapies may include dialysis and plasmapheresis. The use of antibiotics remains controversial.

CRITICAL THINKING EXERCISES

Case Study
Hiatal Hernia
Patient Profile. Mary, a 63-year-old white elementary school teacher, has had a sliding hiatal hernia for 10 years. Mary is admitted to the hospital for a hiatal hernia repair.

Subjective Data
- Reports increasing heartburn, especially at night
- Is currently on a bland diet and taking antacids
- Complains of substernal pain and heartburn
- Reports some problems with regurgitation

Objective Data
Physical Examination
- 5 feet 2 inches tall and weighs 195 pounds

Diagnostic Study
- Barium swallow and an endoscopy revealed a large sliding hiatal hernia.

Collaborative Care
- Mary had a Nissen fundoplication through a laparoscopic approach.

CRITICAL THINKING QUESTIONS

1. Explain the pathophysiology of a hiatal hernia. What is the difference between a sliding and a paraesophageal hiatal hernia?
2. What are the characteristic symptoms of a hiatal hernia? Which of these did Mary have?
3. Describe a Nissen fundoplication procedure. What is the objective of this surgical procedure? Why was a laparoscopic approach used?
4. What are potential postoperative complications, and what nursing measures prevent them?
5. What should be included in a teaching plan for Mary?
6. Based on the assessment data presented, write one or more nursing diagnoses. Are there any collaborative problems?

Nursing Research Issues

1. What are the most effective topical methods to relieve pain related to stomatitis secondary to infection?
2. Are dietary interventions successful in improving symptoms in the patient with gastroesophageal reflux disease?
3. What are optimal strategies to promote multiple lifestyle changes in a patient with peptic ulcer disease?
4. What are environmental manipulations that could be used to promote decreased nausea in patients receiving chemotherapy?
5. What sensory stimuli in the environment, including sight, smell, and sound, could promote optimal nutrient intake in the chemotherapy patient who is experiencing nausea?
6. What is the most effective way to obtain a nutritional assessment from a patient with gastric carcinoma?

REVIEW QUESTIONS

The number of the question corresponds to the same-numbered objective at the beginning of the chapter.

1. Mrs. Jones calls to tell you that her elderly mother, who is 85 years of age, has been nauseated all day and has vomited twice. Before you hang up and telephone the health care provider to communicate your assessment data, you instruct Mrs. Jones to
   a. administer antispasmodic drugs and observe skin turgor.
   b. give her mother sips of water and elevate the head of her bed to prevent aspiration.
   c. offer her mother a high-protein liquid supplement to drink to maintain her nutritional needs.
   d. offer her mother large quantities of Gatorade to drink because elderly people are at risk for sodium depletion.

2. The nurse explains to the patient with Vincent's infection that treatment will include
   a. smallpox vaccinations.
   b. viscous lidocaine rinses.
   c. amphotericin B suspension.
   d. topical application of antibiotics.

3. The nurse is involved in health promotion related to oral cancer. Teaching of adolescents regarding behaviors that put them at risk for oral cancer includes
   a. avoiding use of perfumed lip gloss.
   b. discouraging use of chewing gum.
   c. avoiding use of smokeless tobacco.
   d. discouraging drinking of carbonated beverages.

4. The nurse explains to the patient with gastroesophageal reflux disease that this disorder
   a. results in acid erosion and ulceration of the esophagus caused by the frequent vomiting.
   b. will require surgical wrapping or repair of the pyloric sphincter to control the symptoms.
   c. is the protrusion of a portion of the stomach into the esophagus through an opening in the diaphragm.
   d. often involves relaxation of the lower esophageal sphincter, allowing stomach contents to back up into the esophagus.

5. A patient who has undergone an esophagectomy for esophageal cancer develops increasing pain, fever, and dyspnea when a full liquid diet is started postoperatively. The nurse recognizes that these symptoms are most indicative of
   a. an intolerance to the feedings.
   b. extension of the tumor into the aorta.
   c. leakage of fluid or foods into the mediastinum.
   d. esophageal perforation with fistula formation into the lung.

6. The pernicious anemia that may accompany gastritis is due to which of the following?
   a. Chronic autoimmune destruction of cobalamin stores in the body
   b. Progressive gastric atrophy from chronic breakage in the mucosal barrier and blood loss
   c. A lack of intrinsic factor normally produced by acid-secreting cells of the gastric mucosa
   d. Hyperchlorhydria resulting from an increase in acid-secreting parietal cells and degradation of RBCs

7. Your teaching plan for the patient being discharged following an acute episode of GI bleeding will include information concerning the importance of
   a. taking only drugs prescribed by the health care provider.
   b. avoiding taking aspirin with acidic beverages such as orange juice.
   c. taking all drugs 1 hour before mealtime to prevent further bleeding.
   d. reading all OTC drug labels to avoid those containing stearic acid and calcium.

8. You are teaching your patient and her family about possible causative factors for peptic ulcers. You explain that ulcer formation is
   a. caused by a stressful lifestyle and other acid-producing factors such as *C. pylori*.
   b. inherited within families and reinforced by bacterial spread of *Staphylococcus aureus* in childhood.
   c. promoted by factors that tend to cause oversecretion of acid, such as excess dietary fats, smoking, and *B. pylori*.
   d. promoted by a combination of possible factors that may result in erosion of the gastric mucosa, including certain drugs and alcohol.

9. An optimal teaching plan for an outpatient with gastric carcinoma receiving radiation therapy should include information about
   a. cancer support groups, alopecia, and stomatitis.
   b. avitaminosis, ostomy care, and community resources.
   c. prosthetic devices, skin conductance, and grief counseling.
   d. wound and skin care, nutrition, drugs, and community resources.

10. Several patients are seen at an urgent care center with symptoms of nausea, vomiting, and diarrhea that began 2 hours ago while attending a large family reunion potluck dinner. The nurse questions the patients specifically about foods they ingested containing
   a. beef.
   b. meat and milk.
   c. poultry and eggs.
   d. home-preserved vegetables.

REFERENCES

1. McLauchlan R et al: Ethnic variation in fluorescein angiography induced nausea and vomiting, *Eye* 15(Pt 2):159, 2001.
2. American Cancer Society: *Cancer facts and figures 2001*, Atlanta, Ga, 2001, American Cancer Society.
3. Handlers JP: Diagnosis and management of oral soft-tissue lesions: the use of biopsy, toluidine blue staining, and brush biopsy, *J Calif Dent Assoc* 29:602, 2001.
4. Bjorkman DJ: Community issues in gastroesophageal reflux disease: what we know and what we do not know, *Am J Gastroenterol* 96(8 suppl):S34, 2001.
5. Richter JE: Noncardiac (unexplained) chest pain, *Curr Treat Options Gastroenterol* 3:329, 2000.
6. Fass R et al: Clinical and economic assessment of the omeprazole test in patients with symptoms suggestive of gastroesophageal reflux disease, *Arch Intern Med* 159:2161, 1999.
7. Kaynard A, Flora K: Gastroesophageal reflux disease: control of symptoms, prevention of complications, *Postgrad Med* 110:42, 2001.
8. Smit CF et al: Effect of cigarette smoking on gastropharyngeal and gastroesophageal reflux, *Ann Otol Rhinol Laryngol* 110:190, 2001.
9. Livingston CD et al: Laparoscopic hiatal hernia repair in patients with poor esophageal motility or paraesophageal herniation, *Am Surg* 67:987, 2001.
10. Richards WO et al: Initial experience with the Stretta procedure for the treatment of gastroesophageal reflux disease, *J Laparoendosc Adv Surg Tech* 11:267, 2001.
11. Ruhl CE, Sonnenberg A, Everhart JE: Hospitalization with respiratory disease following hiatal hernia and reflux esophagitis in a prospective, population-based study, *Ann Epidemiol* 11:477, 2001.
12. Bollschweiler E et al: Demographic variations in the rising incidence of esophageal adenocarcinoma in white males, *Cancer* 92:549, 2001.
13. Ajani JA et al: A three-step strategy of induction chemotherapy then chemoradiation followed by surgery in patients with potentially resectable carcinoma of the esophagus or gastroesophageal junction, *Cancer* 92:279, 2001.
14. Siddiq MA, Sood S, Strachan D: Pharyngeal pouch (Zenker's diverticulum), *Postgrad Med J* 77:506, 2001.
15. Diener U et al: Laparoscopic Heller myotomy relieves dysphagia in patients with achalasia and low LES pressure following pneumatic dilatation, *Surg Endosc* 15:687, 2001.
16. Bruley des Varannes S, Scarpignato C: Current trends in the management of achalasia, *Dig Liver Dis* 33:266, 2001.
17. Huang JP, Hunt RH: Treatment of acute gastric and duodenal ulcers. In MM Wolfe, editor: *Therapy of digestive diseases*, Philadelphia, 2000, WB Saunders.
18. Yacyshyn BR, Thomson A: Critical review of acid suppression in nonvariceal, acute, upper gastrointestinal bleeding, *Dig Dis* 18:117, 2000.
19. Lichtenstein DR: Nonvariceal upper GI hemorrhage. In MM Wolfe, editor: *Therapy of digestive diseases*, Philadelphia, 2000, WB Saunders.
20. Chan HL et al: Is non-*Helicobacter pylori*, non-NSAID peptic ulcer a common cause of upper GI bleeding? A prospective study of 977 patients, *Gastrointest Endosc* 53:438, 2001.
21. Fennerty MB: NSAID-related gastrointestinal injury: evidence-based approach to a preventable complication, *Postgrad Med* 110:87, 2001.
22. Knigge KL: The role of *H pylori* in gastrointestinal disease: a guide to identification and eradication, *Postgrad Med* 110:71, 2001.
23. Giercksky KE, Haglund U, Rask-Madsen J: Selective inhibitors of COX-2—are they safe for the stomach? *Scand J Gastroenterol* 35:1121, 2000.
24. Ishigami S et al: Clinical importance of preoperative carcinoembryonic antigen and carbohydrate antigen 19-9 levels in gastric cancer, *J Clin Gastroenterol* 32:41, 2001.
25. Macdonald JS et al: Chemoradiotherapy after surgery compared with surgery alone for adenocarcinoma of the stomach or gastroesophageal junction, *N Engl J Med* 345:725, 2001.

RESOURCES

American College of Gastroenterology
4900 B South 31st Street
Arlington, VA 22206
703-820-7400
Fax: 703-931-4520
www.acg.gi.org/

American Gastroenterological Association
7910 Woodmont Avenue, 7th Floor
Bethesda, MD 20814
301-654-2055
Fax: 301-652-3890
www.gastro.org/

American Society for Gastrointestinal Endoscopy
1520 Kensington Road, Suite 202
Oak Brook, IL 60523
630-573-0600
Fax: 630-573-0691
www.asge.org/

Digestive Disease National Coalition
711 2nd Street, NE, Suite 200
Washington, DC 20002
202-544-7497
Fax: 202-546-7105
www.ddnc.org/

Digestive Health Resource Center
www.gastro.org/public/digestinfo.html

National Digestive Diseases Information Clearinghouse
2 Information Way
Bethesda, MD 20892-3570
800-891-5389 or 301-654-3810
Fax: 301-907-8906
www.niddk.nih.gov/health/digest/nddic.htm

National Heartburn Alliance
877-471-2081
www.heartburnalliance.org/

National Institute of Diabetes & Digestive & Kidney Diseases (NIDDK)
Building 31, Room 9A-52
Bethesda, MD 20892
301-496-5877
www.niddk.nih.gov/index.htm

Society of Gastroenterology Nurses and Associates (SGNA)
401 North Michigan Avenue
Chicago, IL 60611-4267
800-245-7462 or 312-321-5165
Fax: 312-527-6658
www.sgna.org

For additional Internet resources, see the website for this book at *http://evolve.elsevier.com/Lewis/medsurg/*.

CHAPTER 41

NURSING MANAGEMENT
Lower Gastrointestinal Problems

Donna Zimmaro Bliss
Lynda Sawchuk

LEARNING OBJECTIVES

1. Explain the common etiologies, collaborative care, and nursing management of diarrhea, fecal incontinence, and constipation.
2. Describe common causes of acute abdominal pain and nursing management of the patient following an exploratory laparotomy.
3. Describe the collaborative care and nursing management of acute appendicitis, peritonitis, and gastroenteritis.
4. Compare and contrast ulcerative colitis and Crohn's disease, including pathophysiology, clinical manifestations, complications, collaborative care, and nursing management.
5. Differentiate among mechanical, neurogenic, and vascular bowel obstructions, including causes, collaborative care, and nursing management.
6. Describe the clinical manifestations and collaborative management of colorectal cancer.
7. Explain the anatomic and physiologic changes and nursing management of the patient with an ileostomy and colostomy.
8. Differentiate between diverticulosis and diverticulitis, including clinical manifestations, collaborative care, and nursing management.
9. Compare and contrast the types of hernias, including etiology and surgical and nursing management.
10. Describe the types of malabsorption syndrome and collaborative care of sprue syndrome, lactase deficiency, and short bowel syndrome.
11. Describe the types, clinical manifestations, collaborative care, and nursing management of anorectal conditions.

KEY TERMS

anal fissure, p. 1100
anal fistula, p. 1101
appendicitis, p. 1064
constipation, p. 1057
Crohn's disease, p. 1076
diarrhea, p. 1052
diverticulum, p. 1093
fecal impaction, p. 1056
fecal incontinence, p. 1055
gastroenteritis, p. 1067
hemorrhoids, p. 1099
hernia, p. 1095
inflammatory bowel disease, p. 1067

intestinal obstruction, p. 1078
irritable bowel syndrome, p. 1064
lactase deficiency, p. 1098
nontropical sprue, p. 1097
ostomy, p. 1087
paralytic (adynamic) ileus, p. 1078
peritonitis, p. 1066
pilonidal sinus, p. 1101
pseudoobstruction, p. 1078
short bowel syndrome, p. 1098
steatorrhea, p. 1096
ulcerative colitis, p. 1068
Valsalva maneuver, p. 1057

DIARRHEA

Diarrhea—the frequent passage of loose, watery stools—is not a disease but a symptom. The term *diarrhea* may mean different things to different patients. It is commonly used to denote an increase in stool frequency or volume and an increase in the looseness of stool.

Etiology and Pathophysiology

Causes of diarrhea can be divided into the general classifications of decreased fluid absorption, increased fluid secretion, motility disturbances, or a combination of these (Table 41-1). Causes of acute infectious diarrhea are listed in Table 41-2.

Clinical Manifestations

Diarrhea may be acute or chronic. Acute diarrhea most commonly results from infection. Bacterial or viral infection of the intestine may result in explosive watery diarrhea, *tenesmus* (spasmodic contraction of anal sphincter with pain and persistent desire to defecate), and abdominal cramping pain. Perianal skin irritation may also develop. Systemic manifestations include fever, nausea, vomiting, and malaise. Leukocytes, blood, and mucus may be present in the stool, depending on the causative agent (see Table 41-2). Acute diarrhea is often self-limiting in the adult. Symptoms continue until the irritant or causative agent is excreted. The mucous membrane lining of the gastrointestinal (GI) tract is composed of epithelial cells, which regenerate following the inflammatory response.

Diarrhea is considered chronic when it persists for at least 2 weeks or when it subsides and returns more than 2 to 4 weeks after the initial episode. Severe diarrhea may be debilitating and life threatening. A patient may have severe dehydration (water and sodium loss) and electrolyte disturbances (e.g., hypokalemia). Malabsorption and malnutrition are also sequelae of chronic diarrhea. Throughout the world, diarrhea is one of the major causes of death.

Diagnostic Studies

Accurate diagnosis and management require a thorough history, physical examination, and, when indicated, laboratory tests. A history of travel, medication use, diet, previous surgery, interpersonal contacts, and family history should be obtained. Blood tests may identify anemia, elevated white blood cell (WBC) count, iron and folate deficiencies, elevated liver enzyme levels, and electrolyte disturbances. Stools may be examined for the

Reviewed by Marilee Schmelzer, RN, PhD, Associate Professor, University of Texas at Arlington, Arlington, Tex.

presence of blood, mucus, WBCs, and parasites. Stool cultures help to identify infectious organisms.

In a patient with chronic diarrhea, measurement of stool electrolytes, pH, and osmolality may help determine whether the diarrhea is related to decreased fluid absorption or increased fluid secretion (secretory diarrhea). Measurement of stool fat and undigested muscle fibers may indicate fat and protein malabsorption conditions, including pancreatic insufficiency. Elevated serum levels of GI hormones such as vasoactive intestinal polypeptide and gastrin may be present in some patients with secretory diarrhea. Endoscopy may be used to examine the mucosa and to obtain specimens via biopsy for examination. Upper and lower radiologic studies with barium contrast may be helpful in detecting mucosal disease, as well as structural abnormalities.

Collaborative Care

The treatment of diarrhea is based on the cause and is aimed at replacing fluid and electrolytes and decreasing the number, volume, and frequency of stools. Oral solutions containing glucose and electrolytes (e.g., Gatorade, Pedialyte) may be sufficient to replace losses from mild diarrhea. In situations of severe diarrhea, parenteral administration of fluids, electrolytes, vitamins, and nutrition is warranted.

Once the cause of the diarrhea has been determined, antidiarrheal agents may be given to coat and protect mucous membranes, absorb irritating substances, inhibit GI motility, decrease intestinal secretions, and decrease central nervous system stimulation of the GI tract (Table 41-3). Antiperistaltic agents are not given to a patient who has infectious diarrheal syndromes because of the potential of prolonging exposure to the infectious agent. Regardless of the cause of diarrhea, antidiarrheal drugs should not be given for a prolonged time.

Antibiotics are reserved for treating specific bacterial organisms. Antibiotics can cause diarrhea by altering the normal bowel flora. Patients receiving antibiotics (e.g., clindamycin [Cleocin]) are susceptible to *Clostridium difficile* (*C. difficile*) infection. Health care workers who do not adhere to infection control precautions can transmit *C. difficile* from patient to patient. Some

TABLE 41-1   Causes of Diarrhea

Decreased Fluid Absorption
Oral intake of poorly absorbable solutes (e.g., laxatives)
Maldigestion and malabsorption
Mucosal damage: tropical sprue, celiac disease, Crohn's disease, radiation injury, ulcerative colitis, ischemic bowel disease
Pancreatic insufficiency
Intestinal enzyme deficiencies (e.g., lactase)
Bile salt deficiency
Decreased surface area (e.g., intestinal resection)

Increased Fluid Secretion
Infectious: bacterial endotoxins (e.g., *Cholera, Escherichia coli, Shigella, Salmonella, Staphylococcus, Clostridium difficile*, viral agents [rotavirus], and parasitic agents [*Giardia lamblia*])
Drugs: laxatives, antibiotics, suspensions or elixirs containing sorbitol (e.g., valproic acid syrup [Depakene])
Foods: candy, gum, and mints containing sorbitol
Hormonal: vasoactive intestinal polypeptide secretion from adenoma of the pancreas; gastrin secretion caused by Zollinger-Ellison syndrome; calcitonin secretion from carcinoma of the thyroid
Tumor: Villous adenoma

Motility Disturbances
Irritable bowel syndrome: ↑ visceral sensitivity and transit
Diabetic enteropathy: ↑ transit secondary to peripheral neuropathy
Gastrectomy: ↑ transit as a result of dumping syndrome

TABLE 41-2   Causes of Acute Infectious Diarrhea

	ONSET	DURATION	SYMPTOMS AND SIGNS
Viral			
Rotavirus, Norwalk	18-24 hr	24-48 hr	Explosive, watery diarrhea; nausea; vomiting; abdominal cramps
Bacterial			
Escherichia coli	4-24 hr	3-4 days	Four or five loose stools per day, nausea, malaise, low-grade fever
Enterohemorrhagic *E. coli* (0157:H7)	4-24 hr	4-9 days	Bloody diarrhea, severe cramping, fever
Shigella	24 hr	7 days	Watery stools containing blood and mucus, tenesmus, urgency, severe cramping, fever
Salmonella	6-48 hr	2-5 days	Watery diarrhea, nausea, vomiting, abdominal cramps, fever
Campylobacter species	24 hr	<7 days	Profuse, watery diarrhea; malaise, nausea, abdominal cramps, low-grade fever
Clostridium perfringens	8-12 hr	24 hr	Watery diarrhea, abdominal cramps, vomiting
Clostridium difficile	4-9 days after start of antibiotics	24 hr	Associated with antibiotic treatment; symptoms range from mild, watery diarrhea to severe abdominal pain, fever, leukocytosis, leukocytes in stool
Parasitic			
Giardia lamblia	1-3 wk	Few days to 3 months	Sudden onset; malodorous, explosive, watery diarrhea; flatulence, epigastric pain and cramping, nausea
Entamoeba histolytica	4 days	Weeks to months	Frequent soft stools with blood and mucus (in severe cases, watery stools), flatulence, distention, abdominal cramps, fever, leukocytes in stool
Cryptosporidium	2-10 days	1-6 months	Watery diarrhea, nausea, vomiting, abdominal cramps, weight loss in AIDS

AIDS, Acquired immunodeficiency syndrome.

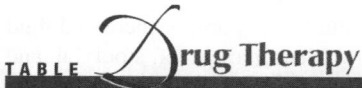

TYPE	MECHANISM OF ACTION	EXAMPLES
Demulcent	Soothes, coats, and protects mucous membranes	bismuth subsalicylate* (Pepto-Bismol); calcium polycarbophil (Mitrolan-OTC); activated charcoal; kaolin,† pectin, hyoscyamine sulfate, and hyoscine hydrobromide (Donnagel)*†; Donnagel and opium (Donnagel-PG)*†
Anticholinergic	Inhibits GI motility	Donnagel,*† Donnagel-PG,*† diphenoxylate with atropine sulfate (Lomotil, Colonaid), loperamide (Imodium)†‡
Antisecretory	Decreases intestinal secretion	octreotide (Sandostatin), a synthetic analog of somatostatin
Narcotic	Decreases CNS stimulation of GI tract motility and secretion; directly inhibits GI motility	camphorated tincture of opium (paregoric); Donnagel-PG†; paregoric, pectin, and kaolin (Parepectolin)†; tincture of opium, homatropine methylbromide, and pectin (Dia-Quel liquid OTC)§

*Also inhibits bacterial activity.
†Also absorbent, which contributes to the adhesiveness of the stool.
‡Has cholinergic and noncholinergic actions.
§Also an anticholinergic
CNS, Central nervous system; GI, gastrointestinal.

strains of *C. difficile* release a toxin that causes mucosal damage, resulting in cramping, pain, and diarrhea that may be bloody. *C. difficile* infection can also result in pseudomembranous enterocolitis and intestinal perforation.[1] Vancomycin (Vancocin) or metronidazole (Flagyl) is used to treat *C. difficile*.

NURSING MANAGEMENT
ACUTE INFECTIOUS DIARRHEA

■ Nursing Assessment

Nursing assessment should begin with a thorough history and physical examination (Table 41-4). The patient should be asked to describe the stool pattern and associated symptoms. Questions should focus on the duration, frequency, character, and consistency of stool. A medication history should include use of antibi-

otics, laxatives, and other drugs known to cause diarrhea. Recent travel, stress, and health and family illnesses should be discussed. Dietary history should include questions about eating habits, appetite, and food intolerances, especially milk and dairy products, and food preparation practices.

Physical examination begins with obtaining vital signs, height, and weight. The patient's skin should be inspected for decreased turgor, dryness, and areas of breakdown. The abdomen should be inspected for distention, auscultated for bowel sounds, and palpated for tenderness.

■ Nursing Diagnoses

Nursing diagnoses for the patient with acute infectious diarrhea may include, but are not limited to, those presented in NCP 41-1 on the facing page.

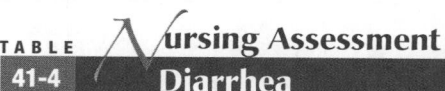

Subjective Data
Important Health Information
Past health history: Recent travel, infections, stress; diverticulitis or malabsorption; metabolic disorders; inflammatory bowel disease; irritable bowel syndrome
Medications: Use of laxatives, magnesium-containing antacids, sorbitol-containing suspensions or elixirs, antibiotics, methyldopa, digitalis, colchicine; OTC antidiarrheal medications
Surgery or other treatments: Stomach or bowel surgery, radiation
Functional Health Patterns
Health perception–health management: Chronic laxative abuse, malaise
Nutritional-metabolic: Ingestion of coarse and spicy foods, food intolerances; anorexia, nausea, vomiting; weight loss; thirst
Elimination: Increased stool frequency, volume, and looseness; change in color and character of stools; abdominal bloating; decreased urinary output
Cognitive-perceptual: Abdominal tenderness, abdominal pain and cramping; tenesmus

Objective Data
General
Lethargy, sunken eyeballs, fever, malnutrition
Integumentary
Pallor, dry mucous membranes, poor skin turgor, perianal irritation
Gastrointestinal
Frequent soft to liquid stools that may alternate with constipation; altered stool color; abdominal distention, hyperactive bowel sounds; presence of pus, blood, mucus, or fat in stools; fecal impaction
Urinary Tract
Decreased output, concentrated urine
Possible Findings
Abnormal serum electrolyte levels; anemia; leukocytosis; eosinophilia, hypoalbuminemia; positive stool cultures; presence of ova, parasites, leukocytes, blood, or fat in stool; abnormal sigmoidoscopic or colonoscopic findings; abnormal lower GI series

GI, Gastrointestinal; OTC, over-the-counter.

NURSING CARE PLAN 41-1

Patient with Acute Infectious Diarrhea

EXPECTED PATIENT OUTCOMES	NURSING INTERVENTIONS and *RATIONALES*
NURSING DIAGNOSIS	**Diarrhea** *related to* acute infectious process *as manifested by* frequent loose, watery stools
• Normal bowel elimination • Afebrile	• Monitor frequency, amount, color, and consistency of stools *to determine severity of diarrhea and need for intervention.* • Follow hospital procedure for infection control precautions; use strict medical asepsis when handling bedpan, linens, or patient *to prevent spread of infection.* • Administer antiinfective and antidiarrheal medications as ordered *to treat bacterial infection and relieve diarrhea.*
NURSING DIAGNOSIS	**Deficient fluid volume** *related to* excessive fluid loss and decreased fluid intake secondary to diarrhea *as manifested by* dry skin and mucous membranes, poor skin turgor, hypotension, tachycardia, decreased urine output, electrolyte imbalances
• Normal vital signs • Normal skin turgor • Moist mucous membranes • Urine output >0.5 ml/kg/hr • Normal serum electrolytes	• Assess for skin turgor changes, sunken eyes, rapid pulse, and anorexia *as indicators of fluid volume deficit.* • Monitor intake and output *to determine fluid balance.* • Monitor serum sodium and potassium levels *so that abnormalities can be reported to the health care provider.* • Monitor vital signs q4hr *because changes can indicate hypovolemia.* • Weigh patient daily *to monitor fluid loss.* • Administer IV fluids as ordered and increase intake of fluids as tolerated to at least 3000 ml/day *to replace fluids and electrolytes lost in stools.* • Assess mouth for dryness and note patient's complaints of thirst *because dry mucous membranes and thirst are indicators of dehydration.* • If patient is not vomiting, administer oral fluids, such as Gatorade or Pedialyte, *to replace electrolytes lost in stools.*
NURSING DIAGNOSIS	**Impaired skin integrity** *related to* contact with diarrheal stools and inadequate perianal hygiene *as manifested by* redness, irritation, swelling, possible ulceration of skin, pain during defecation and urination
• No evidence of skin breakdown in perianal area	• Assess skin of perianal area *to plan appropriate interventions.* • Cleanse area with warm water after each bowel movement, rinse well, and dry with a soft towel *to prevent skin breakdown and promote patient comfort.* • Apply ointment (e.g., A and D, zinc oxide) *to protect skin and promote healing.* • Use an anesthetic ointment or spray foam *to decrease local discomfort.*

▪ Planning

The overall goals are that the patient with diarrhea will (1) not transmit the microorganism causing the infectious diarrhea, (2) cease having diarrhea and resume normal bowel patterns, (3) have normal fluid and electrolyte and acid-base balance, (4) have normal nutritional intake, and (5) have no perianal skin breakdown.

▪ Nursing Implementation

Adherence to infection control precautions for infectious diseases (see Table 12-19) is important because some cases of acute diarrhea are infectious. All cases of acute diarrhea should be considered infectious until the cause is determined. The use of precautions is effective in reducing the spread of infectious diarrhea.

Hand washing is the most important measure in preventing the transfer of microorganisms. Hands should be washed before and after contact with each patient and when body fluids of any kind are handled. The patient should be taught the principles of hygiene, infection control precautions, and the potential dangers of an illness that is infectious to themselves and others. Proper handling, cooking, and storage of food should be discussed with the patient suspected of having infectious diarrhea.

FECAL INCONTINENCE

Etiology and Pathophysiology

Fecal incontinence, or the involuntary passage of stool, may be due to multiple causes (Table 41-5). It is important to have an understanding of normal fecal continence to understand fecal incontinence. Normally, fecal contents pass from the sigmoid colon into the rectum, causing rectal distention. Sensory (stretch) receptors in the muscles surrounding the rectum provide the sensation of rectal filling. This causes a reflex relaxation of the internal anal sphincter and contraction of the external anal sphincter. Sensory receptors in the epithelium of the anal canal can usually distinguish among solid, liquid, and gas. The combination of contraction of the abdominal muscles, relaxation of the pelvic muscles, squatting (which straightens the anorectal angle), and voluntary relaxation of the external anal sphincter allows for

TABLE 41-5 Causes of Fecal Incontinence

Traumatic
Anorectal surgery
Fistulectomy
Hemorrhoidectomy
Postabdominal surgery

Neurologic
Degenerative diseases
Dementia
Diabetes mellitus (secondary to neuropathic changes)
Multiple sclerosis
Spinal cord injuries
Spinal cord tumor
Stroke

Inflammatory
Infection
Radiation
Trauma

Other
Diarrhea
Fecal impaction
Loss of rectal elasticity

Pelvic Floor Dysfunction
Medications
Rectal prolapse

Functional
Physical or mobility impairments affecting toileting ability

---

elimination of feces. Therefore motor (contraction of muscles) or sensory (ability to perceive presence of stool or to experience the urge to defecate) problems or their combination can result in fecal incontinence. In addition, fecal incontinence can be secondary to **fecal impaction,** which is an accumulation of hardened feces in the rectum or sigmoid colon that the individual is unable to move. Fecal incontinence caused by fecal impaction is a common problem in older adults.

Diagnostic Studies and Collaborative Care

The diagnosis and effective management of fecal incontinence require a thorough health history and physical examination with appropriate diagnostic studies. In all cases a rectal examination should be performed, followed by examination with a flexible sigmoidoscope. Fecal impaction, internal prolapse, increased perineal descent, and rectocele may be identified by rectal examination. If the impaction is higher in the colon, an abdominal x-ray may be helpful. Flexible sigmoidoscopy may identify inflammation, tumors, fissures, and other sigmoid-rectum pathologic conditions. Other studies may include barium enema, colonoscopy, and anorectal manometry.

Treatment of incontinence depends on the underlying cause. If fecal incontinence is related to noninfectious diarrhea, antidiarrheal agents may be prescribed. For example, loperamide (Imodium) may be useful in reducing diarrhea and increasing sphincter tone.

Fecal impaction usually resolves after manual disimpaction and cleansing enemas. To prevent recurrence, a high-fiber diet (see Table 41-9 later in this chapter), along with increased fluid intake, should be given unless contraindicated. Dietary fiber supplements or bulk-forming laxatives (e.g., psyllium in Metamucil) can improve continence by increasing stool bulk, firming consistency, and promoting sensation of rectal filling.[2] Perianal pouching or disposable pads or briefs provide containment of stool, protect skin, and promote comfort and dignity.

Biofeedback therapy is aimed at improving awareness of rectal sensation and coordination of the internal and external anal sphincters and increasing the strength of contraction of the external sphincter.[3] Biofeedback training requires adequate mental status and motivation to learn. Components of biofeedback include education, reinforcement, and concentration. It is a safe, painless, and inexpensive treatment for fecal incontinence. (Biofeedback is discussed further in Chapter 7.)

Surgery (e.g., sphincter repair procedures) should be considered only when conservative treatment fails, in cases of full-thickness prolapse, and when the sphincter needs repair.

NURSING MANAGEMENT
FECAL INCONTINENCE

■ Nursing Assessment

Fecal incontinence is not only an embarrassment to the patient but also a potential hazard to normal skin integrity. An assessment of the patient's general condition is necessary to identify the best alternative for managing the patient with fecal incontinence. The health care provider should identify normal bowel habits and current symptoms, including stool frequency and consistency. Information about the passage of blood or mucus, pain during defecation, and a feeling of incomplete evacuation is sought. The health care provider determines whether the patient has defecation urgency and is aware of leaking stool. The coexistence of urinary incontinence should be determined.[4]

A neurologic assessment that includes evaluation of mental status can be helpful in identifying the most effective treatment for the patient. Assessment should also include history of multiple or traumatic childbirths, previous anorectal surgery, and injury.

■ Nursing Diagnoses

Nursing diagnoses for the patient with fecal incontinence include, but are not limited to, the following:
- Bowel incontinence *related to* inability to control bowel function
- Toileting self-care deficit *related to* inability to manage bowel evacuation voluntarily
- Risk for situational low self-esteem *related to* inability to control bowel movements
- Risk for impaired skin integrity *related to* incontinence of stool
- Social isolation *related to* inability to control bowel functions

■ Planning

The overall goals are that the patient with fecal incontinence will (1) have normal bowel control, (2) maintain perianal skin integrity, and (3) not suffer any self-esteem problems related to problems with bowel control.

■ Nursing Implementation

Prevention and treatment of fecal incontinence may be managed by implementing a bowel training program. Bowel training is effective in many patients because once the bowel is empty the rectum does not fill until the next day. The lack of stool in the rectum reduces the likelihood of incontinence. The patient should be put on a bedpan, assisted to a bedside commode, or walked to the bathroom at a regular time daily to assist with reestablishment of bowel regularity. A good time to establish this pattern is within 30 minutes after breakfast. Most individuals experience an urge to defecate following the first meal of the day because of the gastrocolic reflex. If the usual bowel habits differ from this pattern, efforts should be made to adhere to the patient's individual timing.

If these techniques are ineffective in reestablishing bowel regularity, a bisacodyl (Dulcolax), glycerin suppository, or a small phosphate enema may be administered 15 to 30 minutes before the usual evacuation time. These preparations stimulate the anorectal reflex and often can be discontinued when a regular pattern is reestablished.

Maintenance of skin integrity is of utmost importance, especially in the bedridden and older adult patient. Nursing management may necessitate the use of drainage tubes or catheters, incontinence briefs, and meticulous skin care. Rectal tubes and catheters are usually not recommended because their use for an extended period may decrease responsiveness of the rectal sphincter and cause ulceration of the rectal mucosa. Use of incontinence briefs may be helpful in maintaining skin integrity if changed frequently, but this can be demeaning and humiliating to the patient. Meticulous cleaning after each stool is required. Washing, rinsing, thorough drying, and application of a protective barrier are essential to the maintenance of skin integrity. Because the patient may have several stools each day, maintaining skin integrity is a time-consuming task for the nurse and the family.

Perianal pouching is an alternative in the management of fecal incontinence. Pouching provides skin protection and fecal containment, as well as comfort and dignity. Because odor is often a problem, deodorant sprays and room deodorizers may be used. For the patient who is ambulatory, a regular chair or special commode wheelchair may be used. Regardless of the patient's mobility, the nurse must make sure the skin is clean, odorless, and intact.

CONSTIPATION

Constipation is a decrease in frequency of bowel movements from what is "normal" for the individual; hard, difficult-to-pass stools; a decrease in stool volume; and retention of feces in the rectum. Normal bowel elimination may vary from three times a day to once every 3 days.[4] Because of this variability, it is important to determine the severity of constipation on the basis of the patient's normal pattern of elimination. It is important to remember that changes in bowel habits may also indicate bowel obstruction produced by a tumor.

Etiology and Pathophysiology

Often constipation may be due to insufficient dietary fiber, inadequate fluid intake, medications, and lack of exercise. If proper preventive measures are subsequently taken, constipation should

TABLE 41-6	Causes of Constipation
Colonic Disorders	**Systemic Disorders**
Luminal or extraluminal obstructing lesions	*Metabolic/Endocrine*
Inflammatory strictures	Diabetes mellitus
Volvulus	Hypothyroidism
Intussusception	Pregnancy
Irritable bowel syndrome	Hypercalcemia/ hyperparathyroidism
Diverticular disease	Pheochromocytoma
Rectocele	*Collagen Vascular Disease*
	Systemic sclerosis (scleroderma)
Drug Induced	Amyloidosis
Antacids (calcium and aluminum)	*Neurologic Disorders*
Antidepressants	Hirschsprung's megacolon
Anticholinergics	Neurofibromatosis
Antipsychotics	Autonomic neuropathy (secondary to diabetes mellitus)
Antihypertensives	
Barium sulfate	Multiple sclerosis
Iron supplements	Parkinson's disease
Bismuth	Spinal cord lesions or injury
Calcium supplements	Stroke
Laxative abuse	

not recur. Constipation may also be due to sociocultural beliefs, environmental constraints, ignoring the urge to defecate, chronic laxative abuse, and multiple organic causes (Table 41-6). Changes in diet, mealtime, or daily routines are a few environmental factors that may cause constipation. Depression and stress can also result in constipation. For many patients with constipation, however, it is not possible to identify the underlying cause.[5]

Some patients believe that they are constipated if they do not have a daily bowel movement. This can result in chronic laxative use and subsequent cathartic colon syndrome. In this condition, the colon becomes dilated and *atonic* (lacking muscle tone).

Ignoring the urge to defecate for a period of time causes the muscles and mucosa in the rectal area to become insensitive to the presence of feces. In addition, the prolonged retention of feces in the rectum results in drying of stool because of the absorption of water. The harder and drier the feces, the more difficult it is to expel.

Clinical Manifestations

The clinical presentation of constipation may vary from a chronic discomfort to an acute event mimicking an "acute abdomen." Other clinical manifestations are presented in Table 41-7. Hemorrhoids are the most common complication of chronic constipation. They result from venous engorgement caused by repeated Valsalva maneuvers (straining) and venous compression from hard impacted stool.

Valsalva maneuver, which occurs during straining to pass a hardened stool, may cause serious problems in patients with congestive heart failure, cerebral edema, hypertension, and coronary artery disease. During straining, the patient takes a deep inspiration, the breath is held, and the glottis closes and traps the air. The abdominal muscles contract and try to push against the colon. Increases in intraabdominal pressure and in-

TABLE 41-7	Clinical Manifestations of Constipation

Abdominal distention/bloating
Abdominal pain
Anorexia
Decreased frequency of bowel movements
Hard, dry stool
Headache
Increased flatulence
Increased rectal pressure
Nausea
Palpable mass
Stone or rock–shaped stool
Stool with blood
Straining
Tenesmus

cannot compensate for sudden overload of blood flow returning to the heart.

Diverticulosis is another potential complication of chronic constipation. This is a relatively common complication in an older adult. Diverticula or outpouchings of the colon wall are thought to be due to the increased intraluminal pressure needed to expel hard stool. Diverticulosis and diverticulitis are described later in this chapter.

In the presence of *obstipation,* or fecal impaction secondary to constipation, colonic perforation may occur. Perforation, which is life threatening, causes abdominal pain, nausea, vomiting, fever, and an elevated WBC count. An abdominal x-ray shows the presence of free air, which is diagnostic of perforation. Rectal mucosal ulcers may also occur as a result of stool stasis or straining. These complications are most common in older patients.

Diagnostic Studies and Collaborative Care

A thorough history and physical examination should be performed so that the underlying cause of constipation can be identified and treatment started. Abdominal x-rays, barium enema, colonoscopy, sigmoidoscopy, and anorectal manometry may be helpful in the diagnosis. Most cases of constipation can be managed with diet therapy including fiber and fluids and an exercise program. Laxatives (Table 41-8) should always be used cautiously because with chronic overuse they may become a cause of constipation. A stepwise approach for laxative use that pro-

trathoracic pressure occur, reducing venous return to the heart. The heart slows temporarily (bradycardia), the cardiac output is decreased, and there is a transient drop in arterial pressure. When the patient relaxes, there is decreased thoracic pressure and a sudden flow of blood into the heart, causing distention and an increase in heart rate. Immediately the arterial pressure rises momentarily. These changes may be fatal for the patient who

TABLE 41-8	*D*rug Therapy Cathartic Agents			
CATEGORY	**MECHANISMS OF ACTION**	**EXAMPLE**	**ONSET OF ACTION**	**COMMENTS**
▪ Bulk forming	Absorbs water; increases bulk, thereby stimulating peristalsis	Metamucil, Perdiem, Konsyl, Hydrocil, Citrucel, FiberCon	Usually within 24 hr	Contraindicated in patients with abdominal pain, nausea, and vomiting and in patients suspected of having appendicitis, biliary tract obstruction, or acute hepatitis; must be taken with fluids
▪ Stool softeners and lubricants	Lubricate intestinal tract and soften feces, making hard stools easier to pass; do not affect peristalsis	Mineral oil, dioctyl sodium, sulfosuccinate, Colace, Peri-Colace, Doxidan	Softeners up to 72 hr, lubricants up to 8 hr	Can block absorption of fat-soluble vitamins such as vitamin K, which may increase risk of bleeding in patients on anticoagulants
▪ Saline and osmotic solutions	Cause retention of fluid in intestinal lumen caused by osmotic effect	Magnesium salts: magnesium citrate, Milk of Magnesia Sodium phosphates: Fleet enema, Phospho-Soda Lactulose Polyethylene glycol saline solutions Go-Lytely, Colyte	15 min to 3 hr	Magnesium-containing products may cause hypermagnesemia in patients with renal insufficiency
▪ Stimulants	Increase peristalsis by irritating colon wall and stimulating enteric nerves	Antraquinone drugs: cascara sagrada, senna Phenolphthalein drugs: Ex-Lax, Correctol, Feen-a-Mint, bisacodyl, Dulcolax	Usually within 12 hr	Cause melanosis coli (brown or black pigmentation of colon); are most widely abused laxatives; should not be used in patients with impaction or obstipation

gresses from bulk-forming fiber preparations to stimulants is recommended, depending on the acuteness of the constipation episode.[6] Enemas are fast acting and are beneficial in the immediate treatment of constipation, but they should be limited in their use for long-term treatment of constipation. Soapsuds enemas should be avoided because they may lead to inflammation of colon mucosa. Excessive hypotonic enemas with tap water can cause water excess, and sodium phosphate enemas have been associated with electrolyte imbalances. Oil-retention enemas may be used to soften fecal impactions. Biofeedback therapy may benefit patients who are constipated as a result of *anismus* (uncoordinated contraction of the anal sphincter during straining).[7]

For the patient in whom perceived constipation is related to rigid beliefs regarding bowel function, the nurse should initiate a discussion about these beliefs with the patient. Appropriate information on normal bowel function needs to be given and discussed along with the adverse consequences of excessive use of laxatives and enemas.

A patient with severe constipation related to bowel motility or mechanical disorders may require more intensive treatment. Diagnostic studies such as anorectal manometry, GI tract transit studies, and sigmoidoscopic rectal biopsies should be performed before treatment. In a patient with unrelenting constipation, a subtotal colectomy with ileorectal anastomosis is the procedure of choice.

Nutritional Therapy. Diet is an important factor in the prevention of constipation. Many patients experience an improvement in their symptoms when they simply increase their intake of dietary fiber and fluids.[8] Dietary fiber is found in two forms: insoluble and soluble in water. Both are contained in most foods, but some foods are higher in soluble fiber (Table 41-9).

Insoluble fiber, which is found in higher concentrations in whole wheat and bran, remains essentially unchanged by the time it reaches the colon. Soluble fibers form gel-like substances that add viscosity to the digested contents, causing decreased gastric emptying and increased transit in the small intestine. When these fibers are fermented, they increase stool bulk, promoting defecation and sequestering fluid, which softens stools. Soluble fiber is found in oat bran, fruits, vegetables, and psyllium. Patients should be told that initially fiber will increase gas production but that this effect decreases with time.

The diet should also include a fluid intake of at least 3000 ml per day, unless contraindicated by cardiac or renal disease. Increasing fiber intake without increasing fluids may predispose the patient to impaction or obstruction. The nurse should encourage the selection of foods that the patient likes, is able to prepare, and can afford. The patient's understanding of the diet and the importance of dietary fiber is important to ensure compliance.

NURSING MANAGEMENT
CONSTIPATION

■ Nursing Assessment

Subjective and objective data that should be obtained from a patient with constipation are presented in Table 41-10.

■ Nursing Diagnoses

Nursing diagnosis for the patient with constipation includes, but is not limited to, the following:

- Constipation *related to* inadequate intake of dietary fiber and fluid and decreased physical activity

TABLE 41-9   Nutritional Therapy — High-Fiber Foods*

	FIBER PER SERVING (G)	SIZE OF SERVING	CALORIES PER SERVING
Vegetables			
Asparagus	3.5	½ cup	18
Beans			
Navy	8.4	½ cup	80
Kidney	9.7	½ cup	94
Lima	8.3	½ cup	63
Pinto	8.9	½ cup	78
String	2.1	½ cup	18
Broccoli	3.5	½ cup	18
Carrots, raw	1.8	½ cup	15
Corn	2.6	½ medium ear	72
Peas, canned	6.7	½ cup	63
Potatoes			
Baked	1.9	½ medium	72
Sweet	2.1	½ medium	79
Squash			
Acorn	7.0	1 cup	82
Tomato, raw	1.5	1 small	18
Fruits			
Apple	2.0	½ large	42
Banana	1.5	½ medium	48
Blackberries	6.7	¾ cup	40
Orange	1.6	1 small	35
Peach	2.3	1 medium	38
Pear	2.0	½ medium	44
Raspberries	9.2	1 cup	42
Strawberries	3.1	1 cup	45
Grain Products			
Bread			
Rye	0.8	1 slice	62
White	0.7	1 slice	64
Whole wheat	1.3	1 slice	59
Cereal			
All Bran (100%)	8.4	⅓ cup	70
Corn Flakes	2.6	¾ cup	70
Shredded Wheat	2.8	1 biscuit	70
Crackers			
Graham	1.4	2 squares	53
Popcorn	3.0	3 cups	62
Rice			
Brown	1.6	⅓ cup	72
White	0.5	⅓ cup	76

*Recommended for patients with diverticulosis, irritable bowel syndrome, constipation, hemorrhoids, colon cancer, atherosclerosis, hyperlipidemia, and diabetes mellitus.

■ Planning

The overall goals are that the patient with constipation will (1) increase dietary intake of fiber and fluids; (2) have the passage of soft, formed stools; and (3) not have any complications, such as bleeding hemorrhoids.

TABLE 41-10 Nursing Assessment — Constipation

Subjective Data

Important Health Information*

Past health history: Colorectal disease, neurologic dysfunction, bowel obstruction, environmental changes, cancer, irritable bowel syndrome

Medications: Use of aluminum and calcium antacids, anticholinergics, antidepressants, antihistamines, antipsychotics, diuretics, narcotics, iron, laxatives, enemas

Functional Health Patterns

Health perception–health management: Chronic laxative or enema abuse; rigid beliefs regarding bowel function; malaise

Nutritional-metabolic: Changes in diet or mealtime; inadequate fiber and fluid intake; anorexia, nausea

Elimination: Change in usual elimination patterns; hard, difficult-to-pass stool, decrease in frequency and amount of stools; flatus, abdominal distention; tenesmus, rectal pressure; fecal incontinence (if impacted)

Activity-exercise: Change in daily activity routines; immobility; sedentary lifestyle

Cognitive-perceptual: Dizziness, headache, anorectal pain; abdominal pain on defecation

Coping–stress tolerance: Acute or chronic stress

Objective Data

General

Lethargy

Integumentary

Anorectal fissures, hemorrhoids, abscesses

Gastrointestinal

Abdominal distention; hypoactive or absent bowel sounds; palpable abdominal mass; fecal impaction; small, hard, dry stool; stool with blood

Possible Findings

Guaiac-positive stools; abdominal x-ray demonstrating stool in lower colon

*See Table 41–6.

■ Nursing Implementation

Nursing management should be based on the patient's symptoms (see Table 41-7) and the assessment of the patient (see Table 41-10). An important role of the nurse is teaching the patient the importance of dietary measures to prevent constipation. A patient and family teaching guide for constipation is presented in Table 41-11. Emphasis should be placed on maintenance of a high-fiber diet, increasing fluid intake, and a regular exercise program. The patient should be taught to establish a regular time to defecate and not to suppress the urge to defecate. In many persons the urge to defecate occurs after breakfast because of the stimulation of the gastrocolic reflex. The patient should be discouraged from using laxatives and enemas to achieve fecal elimination.

Proper position is important when defecating. For a patient in bed, the bedpan should be placed and the head of the bed should be elevated as high as the patient can tolerate. For the person who can sit on a toilet, a footstool may be placed in front of the toilet. Placing the feet on the footstool promotes flexion of the thighs, which assists in defecation.

The patient with poor muscle tone should be encouraged to exercise the abdominal muscles and can be taught to contract the abdominal muscles several times a day. Sit-ups and straight leg raises can also be used to improve abdominal muscle tone.

TABLE 41-11 Patient & Family Teaching Guide — Constipation

The following are teaching guidelines for the patient and family:

1. **Eat dietary fiber**

   Eat 20 to 30 g of fiber per day. Gradually increase the amount of fiber eaten over 1 to 2 weeks. Fiber softens hard stools and adds bulk to stool, promoting evacuation.
   - Foods high in fiber: raw vegetables and fruits, beans, breakfast cereals (All Bran, oatmeal)
   - Fiber supplements: Metamucil, Citrucel, FiberCon

2. **Drink fluids**

   Drink 3 quarts per day. Drink water or fruit juices; avoid caffeinated coffee, tea, and cola. Fluid softens hard stools; caffeine stimulates fluid loss through urination.

3. **Exercise regularly**

   Walk, swim, or bike at least 3 times per week. Contract and relax abdominal muscles when standing or by doing sit-ups to strengthen muscles and prevent straining. Exercise stimulates bowel motility and moves stool through the intestine.

4. **Establish a regular time to defecate**

   First thing in the morning or after the first meal of the day is a good time because people often have the urge to defecate at this time.

5. **Do not delay defecation**

   Respond to the urge to have a bowel movement as soon as possible. Delaying defecation results in hard stools and a decreased "urge" to defecate. Water is absorbed from stool by the intestine over time. The intestine becomes less sensitive to the presence of stool in the rectum.

6. **Record your bowel elimination pattern**

   Develop a habit of recording when you have a bowel movement on your calendar. Regular monitoring of bowel movement will assist in early identification of a problem.

7. **Avoid laxatives and enemas**

   Do not overuse laxatives and enemas because they can actually cause constipation. The normal motility of the bowel is interrupted, and bowel movements slow or stop.

ACUTE ABDOMINAL PAIN

Etiology and Pathophysiology

The causes of an acute onset of abdominal pain are varied (Table 41-12).

Clinical Manifestations

Pain is the most common presenting symptom. The patient may also complain of abdominal tenderness, vomiting, diarrhea, constipation, flatulence, fatigue, fever, and an increase in abdominal girth.

TABLE 41-12	Causes of Acute Abdominal Pain
Abdominal penetrating trauma	Pancreatitis
Acute ischemic bowel injury	Pelvic inflammatory disease
Appendicitis	Peptic ulcer
Bowel obstruction with perforation or necrosis	Perforated gastrointestinal malignancy
Cholecystitis	Peritonitis
Crohn's disease	Ruptured abdominal aneurysm
Diverticulitis with peritonitis	Ruptured ectopic pregnancy
Foreign body perforation	Ruptured ovarian cyst
Gastritis	Ulcerative colitis
Gastroenteritis	Uterine rupture
Mesenteric adenitis	Volvulus

Diagnostic Studies and Collaborative Management

Many disorders must be ruled out before a diagnosis is confirmed. Diagnosis begins with a complete history and physical examination. Physical examination should include a rectal and pelvic examination. A complete blood count (CBC), urinalysis, abdominal x-ray, and an electrocardiogram are done initially. Pregnancy tests should be performed in women of childbearing age who have acute abdominal pain to rule out ectopic pregnancy. The findings of these studies may provide some information about the cause of the acute abdomen.

Emergency management of the patient with acute abdominal pain is presented in Table 41-13. The goal of management is to identify and treat the cause. The health care provider attempts to make a differential diagnosis when the patient is seen with an acute abdomen because many causes of abdominal pain do not require surgery (see Table 41-12). It was previously thought that pain medication should be withheld because analgesics might obscure progression of clinical manifestations and impede diagnosis. Appropriate pain management that does not result in altered consciousness (e.g., ketorolac [Toradol]) can decrease diffuse pain and abdominal rigidity and help localize the pain. This can lead to earlier diagnosis and treatment.[9]

In addition to being a therapeutic measure, surgery can also be diagnostic. Operative exploration is usually done after a careful examination of the patient and is justified when "look and see" is better than "wait and see." The surgical procedure is an *ex-*

TABLE 41-13	Emergency Management	Acute Abdominal Pain

ETIOLOGY	ASSESSMENT FINDINGS	INTERVENTIONS
Inflammation Appendicitis Cholecystitis Crohn's disease Gastritis Pancreatitis Pyelonephritis Ulcerative colitis **Vascular Problems** Ruptured aortic aneurysm Mesenteric vascular occlusion **Gynecologic Problems** Pelvic inflammatory disease Ruptured ectopic pregnancy Ruptured ovarian cyst **Infectious Disease** *Giardia* *Salmonella* **Other** Obstruction or perforation of abdominal organ Gastrointestinal bleeding Trauma	**Abdominal/Gastrointestinal Findings** ▪ Diffuse, localized, dull, burning, or sharp abdominal pain or tenderness ▪ Rebound tenderness ▪ Abdominal distention ▪ Abdominal rigidity ▪ Nausea and vomiting ▪ Diarrhea ▪ Hematemesis ▪ Melena **Hypovolemic Shock** ▪ ↓ Blood pressure ▪ ↓ Pulse pressure ▪ Tachycardia ▪ Cool, clammy skin ▪ ↓ Level of consciousness	**Initial** ▪ Ensure patent airway. ▪ Administer oxygen via nasal cannula or nonrebreather mask. ▪ Establish IV access with large-bore catheter and infuse warm normal saline or lactated Ringer's solution. Insert additional large-bore catheter if shock present. ▪ Obtain blood for CBC and electrolytes. ▪ Anticipate order for amylase level, pregnancy tests, clotting studies, and type and crossmatch as appropriate. ▪ Insert indwellng urinary catheter. ▪ Obtain urinalysis. ▪ Insert NG tube as needed. **Ongoing Monitoring** ▪ Monitor vital signs, level of consciousness, O₂ saturation, and intake/output. ▪ Assess quality and amount of pain. ▪ Assess amount and character of emesis. ▪ Anticipate surgical intervention. ▪ Keep NPO.

CBC, Complete blood count; *IV,* intravenous; *NG,* nasogastric; *NPO,* nothing by mouth.

ploratory laparotomy, in which an opening is made through the abdominal wall into the peritoneal cavity to determine the cause of acute abdominal pain. If the cause of the acute abdomen can be surgically removed (e.g., inflamed appendix) or surgically repaired (e.g., ruptured abdominal aneurysm), surgery is considered definitive therapy.

NURSING MANAGEMENT
ACUTE ABDOMINAL PAIN

■ Nursing Assessment

Vital signs should be taken immediately. Blood pressure and pulse rate should be obtained to determine hypovolemic changes. An elevated temperature may indicate an inflammatory or infectious process. The abdomen should be inspected for distention, masses, abnormal pulsation, rashes, scars, and pigmentation changes. Bowel sounds should be auscultated. Bowel sounds that are diminished or absent in a quadrant may indicate a complete bowel obstruction, acute peritonitis, or paralytic ileus. Palpation should be gentle.

A thorough assessment of the patient's symptoms should be made to determine the onset, location, intensity, duration, frequency, and character of pain. The nurse should determine whether the pain has spread or moved to new locations (quadrants), as well as what makes the pain worse or better. It should also be determined whether the pain is associated with other symptoms, such as nausea, vomiting, changes in bowel and bladder habits, or vaginal discharge in women. Assessment of vomiting should include the amount, color, consistency, and odor of the vomitus. Bowel patterns and habits should also be assessed carefully.

■ Nursing Diagnoses

Nursing diagnoses for the patient with acute abdominal pain include, but are not limited to, the following:

- Acute pain *related to* inflammation of the peritoneum and abdominal distention
- Risk for deficient fluid volume *related to* collection of fluid in peritoneal cavity secondary to inflammation or infection
- Imbalanced nutrition: less than body requirements *related to* anorexia, nausea, and vomiting
- Anxiety *related to* uncertainty of cause or outcome of condition and pain

■ Planning

The overall goals are that the patient with acute abdominal pain will have (1) resolution of inflammation, (2) relief of abdominal pain, (3) freedom from complications (especially hypovolemic shock), and (4) normal nutritional status.

■ Nursing Implementation

Nursing interventions are based on the diagnosis and medical or surgical management of the patient. General care for the patient involves management of fluid and electrolyte imbalances, pain, and anxiety.

Acute Intervention

Preoperative care. Emergency preparation of the patient with acute abdominal pain is usually limited to a CBC, typing and crossmatching of blood, and clotting studies. Catheterization, preparation of the abdominal skin, and the passage of a nasogas-

tric (NG) tube may be done in the emergency department or operating room. (General care of the preoperative patient is discussed in Chapter 17.)

Postoperative care. Postoperative care depends on the type of surgical procedure performed. The increased use of laparoscopic procedures has reduced the risk of postoperative complications related to wound care and altered GI motility. These procedures generally result in shorter hospital stays.

A general nursing care plan for the postoperative patient is presented in Chapter 19. Nursing care for the patient following a laparotomy is presented in NCP 41-2.

An NG tube may or may not be present in the patient returning from surgery. If present, the NG tube is connected to suction as ordered. The purpose of the NG tube is to empty the stomach of secretions and gas to prevent gastric dilation. GI peristaltic activity is often impaired because of the manipulative procedures of the surgery and anesthesia. Low intermittent suctioning is ordered to prevent trauma to the gastric mucosa.

If the upper GI tract has been entered, drainage from the NG tube may be dark brown to dark red for the first 12 hours. Later it should be light yellowish brown, or it may have a greenish tinge because of the presence of bile. If a dark red color continues or if bright red blood is observed, the health care provider should be notified at once of the possibility of hemorrhage. "Coffee ground" granules in the drainage are due to the presence of small amounts of blood that have been chemically acted on by gastric secretions.

The NG tube is checked frequently for patency. The tube may become obstructed with mucus, sediment, or blood clots. An order is usually written to irrigate the tube with 20 to 30 ml of normal saline solution if needed. Repositioning the tube may facilitate drainage.

An accurate record of intake and output, including emesis and gastric drainage, is essential. The nurse assesses serum electrolyte values and acid-base balance because prolonged gastric suctioning can result in loss of sodium, chloride, potassium, water, and hydrochloric acid.

The NG tube is removed when intestinal peristalsis returns, usually 24 to 72 hours after surgery. Motility of the stomach normally returns within 24 to 48 hours. Motility of the small intestine usually resumes within 24 hours, whereas return of large intestine motility may take as long as 3 to 5 days. Peristaltic activity is assessed by auscultation for bowel sounds.

Mouth care and nasal care are essential. The patient tends to breathe through the mouth while the NG tube is in place. In addition, increased nasal secretions and crusting result from mechanical stimulation of the NG tube.

Parenteral fluids are administered to provide the patient with fluids and electrolytes until bowel sounds return. Occasionally, ice chips may be ordered because they aid in the flow of saliva and prevent a dry mouth. When bowel sounds return, fluids and food are increased gradually. The diet may be supplemented with multivitamins and iron.

Nausea and vomiting are not uncommon after abdominal surgery. These problems are often self-limiting. Observation is important in determining the cause. Antiemetics such as promethazine (Phenergan), ondansetron (Zofran), prochlorperazine (Compazine), or trimethobenzamide (Tigan) may be ordered.

Abdominal distention and gas pains are also common after surgery; these are due to swallowed air and impaired peristalsis

NURSING CARE PLAN 41-2

Patient Following Laparotomy

EXPECTED PATIENT OUTCOMES	NURSING INTERVENTIONS and *RATIONALES*
NURSING DIAGNOSIS	**Acute pain** *related to* surgical incision and inadequate pain control measures *as manifested by* complaints of pain, body posturing, unwillingness to move in bed or to ambulate
▪ Satisfactory level of pain control	▪ Assess for pain and give pain medication every 3 to 4 hr as ordered for first 72 hr *to treat pain appropriately.* ▪ Splint incision with pillows during coughing, deep breathing, and moving *to relieve pain while performing these activities.* ▪ Position patient comfortably *to relieve pain.*
NURSING DIAGNOSIS	**Nausea** *related to* decreased GI motility, GI distention, and narcotics *as manifested by* nausea, vomiting, lack of or diminished bowel sounds, abdominal distention
▪ Relief of nausea and vomiting.	▪ Administer antiemetic medications (as ordered) *to relieve nausea and vomiting.* ▪ Assess response to pain medications *to determine if this is a possible cause of nausea and vomiting.* ▪ Maintain patency of NG tube (if present) *to prevent accumulation of gastric secretions and subsequent vomiting.* ▪ Assess for bowel sounds and abdominal distention *to determine return of peristalsis.* ▪ Keep patient on NPO status until bowel sounds return *to prevent vomiting.* ▪ Limit unpleasant sights, smells, and stimuli *to prevent initiating episodes of nausea and vomiting.*
NURSING DIAGNOSIS	**Constipation** *related to* immobility, pain, medication, and decreased GI motility *as manifested by* decreased or absent bowel sounds, abdominal pain, abdominal distention, inability to pass flatus or stool
▪ Normal bowel sounds within 72 hr after surgery ▪ Soft, formed bowel movement within 4 days	▪ Assess abdomen for distention and bowel sounds every 8 hours *to determine need for intervention.* ▪ Administer stool softener (if ordered) *to soften fecal mass or promote elimination.* ▪ Encourage frequent position changes and ambulation as tolerated *to increase peristalsis.* ▪ Encourage increased fluid intake as tolerated *to soften fecal material.*

*General nursing care for the postoperative patient is presented in the NCP 19-1 in Chapter 19 on pp. 402-403.

resulting from immobility, manipulation of abdominal contents during surgery, and side effects of anesthesia. The pain can be so uncomfortable that drugs to stimulate peristalsis, such as bethanechol (Urecholine) or neostigmine methylsulfate (Prostigmin), may be given. A rectal tube or moist heat on the abdomen may be effective in relieving distention. The health care provider should be informed of abdominal distention and rigidity. Gradually, as intestinal activity increases, distention and gas pains decrease.

Ambulatory and Home Care. Preparation for discharge begins when the patient returns from the operating room. Instructions to the patient and the family should include any modifications in activity, care of the incision, diet, and drug therapy. Small, frequent meals high in calories should be taken initially, with a gradual increase in intake of food as tolerated.

Normal activities should be resumed gradually, with planned rest periods. The patient should be aware of possible complications after surgery and should notify the health care provider immediately if vomiting, pain, weight loss, incisional drainage, or changes in bowel function occur.

▪ Evaluation

The expected outcomes are that the patient with acute abdominal pain will have (1) resolution of the cause of the acute abdominal pain; (2) relief of abdominal pain and discomfort; (3) freedom from complications (especially hypovolemic shock and septicemia); and (4) normal fluid, electrolyte, and nutritional status.

Chronic Abdominal Pain

Chronic abdominal pain may originate from abdominal structures or may be referred from a site with the same or a similar nerve supply. Some common causes are irritable bowel syndrome (IBS), peptic ulcer disease, diverticulitis, chronic pancreatitis, hepatitis, cholecystitis, pelvic inflammatory disease, and vascular insufficiency.

Diagnosis of chronic abdominal pain presents a challenge. Assessment should begin with a thorough history and identification of the specific pain pattern. Character and severity of pain, location, duration, and onset should be determined. The assessment should also include the relationship of pain to meals, defecation, and activity and factors that increase or decrease the pain. Chronic abdominal pain is often described as dull, aching, or diffuse.

Endoscopy, computed tomography (CT) scans, magnetic resonance imaging, laparoscopy, and radiologic barium studies have decreased the need for exploratory laparotomy. Treatment for chronic abdominal pain is comprehensive and directed toward palliation of symptoms using analgesics and antiemetics, as well as psychologic or behavioral therapies (e.g., relaxation therapies).

IRRITABLE BOWEL SYNDROME

Irritable bowel syndrome (IBS) is a symptom complex characterized by intermittent and recurrent abdominal pain associated with an alteration in bowel function (diarrhea or constipation). Other symptoms commonly found include abdominal distention, excessive flatulence, bloating, urge to defecate, urgency, and sensation of incomplete evacuation. IBS is a common problem affecting approximately 15% to 20% of the population in the United States.[10] In western societies, approximately 2 to 3 times as many women as men seek health care services for IBS. Stress, psychologic factors, and specific food intolerances have been identified as major factors that precipitate IBS symptoms.

The key to accurate diagnosis is a thorough history and physical examination. Emphasis should be on symptoms, past health history (including psychosocial aspects such as physical or sexual abuse), family history, and drug and dietary history. Diagnostic tests should be selectively used to rule out more serious life-threatening disorders with symptoms similar to those of IBS, such as colorectal cancer, peptic ulcer disease, inflammatory bowel disease, and malabsorption disorders. Symptom-based criteria for IBS have been standardized and are referred to as the Rome criteria.[10]

The health care provider should establish a trusting relationship with the patient at the onset of treatment. The patient should be encouraged to verbalize concerns and anxiety. A diet containing at least 20 g per day of dietary fiber should be initiated (see Table 41-9). This may also include the addition of psyllium-containing products (e.g., Metamucil).

The patient whose primary symptoms are abdominal distention and increased flatulence should be advised to eliminate common gas-producing foods such as broccoli and cabbage from the diet and to substitute yogurt for milk products if there is lactose intolerance. Anticholinergic agents, such as dicyclomine (Bentyl), may be helpful if taken before meals to alleviate the pain associated with ingestion of food. Alosetron (Lotronex) is used to treat IBS that causes diarrhea and severe pain in women who have failed other therapies. Its use must be monitored closely because of side effects. Tegaserod (Zelnorm) recently has been approved to treat women with IBS whose primary bowel symptom is constipation. It increases the movement of stools through the colon. Other therapies include relaxation and stress management techniques, acupuncture, and Chinese herbs although no single therapy has been found to be effective for all patients with IBS.

ABDOMINAL TRAUMA

Etiology and Pathophysiology

Injuries to the abdominal area most often occur as a result of blunt trauma (e.g., motor vehicle accident) or penetration injuries, primarily gunshot wounds or stab wounds to the abdomen. Blunt trauma is most common. Regardless of whether it is a blunt or penetration injury, the result is often the same damage to or alteration of the internal organs.

Common injuries of the abdomen include lacerated liver, ruptured spleen, pancreatic trauma, mesenteric artery tears, diaphragmatic rupture, urinary bladder rupture, great vessel tears, renal injury, and stomach or intestinal rupture. These injuries may result in massive blood loss and hypovolemic shock. Surgery must be performed as early as possible to repair the damaged organs and to stop the bleeding. Common sequelae of intraabdominal trauma are peritonitis and sepsis, particularly when the bowel is perforated.

Clinical Manifestations

Clinical manifestations of abdominal trauma are (1) guarding and splinting of the abdominal wall; (2) a hard, distended abdomen (indicating intraabdominal bleeding); (3) decreased or absent bowel sounds; (4) contusions, abrasions, or bruising over the abdomen; (5) abdominal pain; (6) pain over the scapula caused by irritation of the phrenic nerve by free blood in the abdomen; (7) hematemesis or hematuria; and (8) signs of hypovolemic shock (Table 41-14). An ecchymotic discoloration around the umbilicus (Cullen sign) can indicate intraabdominal or retroperitoneal hemorrhage.

Intraabdominal injuries are often associated with low rib fractures, fractured femur, fractured pelvis, and thoracic injury. If any of these injuries are present, the patient should be observed for abdominal trauma.

Diagnostic Studies

Specific diagnostic procedures include CBC, urinalysis, x-ray of the abdomen, CT scan, and peritoneal lavage. In peritoneal lavage the abdomen below the umbilicus is locally anesthetized, and a large angiocatheter or peritoneal dialysis catheter is inserted into the abdomen. A syringe is attached to the catheter, and an attempt is made to gently aspirate any blood. If less than 10 ml of blood is aspirated, a liter of saline solution is then infused into the abdomen and drained. The fluid is observed for gross abnormalities, especially blood, and is sent to the laboratory for microscopic evaluation. Positive findings may include (1) red blood cell count greater than $100,000/\mu l$; (2) WBC count greater than $500/\mu l$; (3) high amylase level; and (4) presence of bacteria, bile, or fecal material. If the results are positive, immediate surgery is indicated. If the results are negative, continued observation of the patient is warranted. An impaled object should never be removed until skilled care is available. Removal may cause further injury and bleeding.

NURSING *and* COLLABORATIVE MANAGEMENT
ABDOMINAL TRAUMA

Emergency management of abdominal trauma focuses on establishing a patent airway and adequate breathing, fluid replacement, and prevention of hypovolemic shock (see Table 41-14). IV lines are inserted, and volume expanders or blood is given if the patient is hypotensive. An NG tube is inserted to decompress the stomach and prevent the aspiration of vomitus.

Regardless of the mechanism of injury, physical evidence of abdominal trauma in a patient who is hemodynamically unstable mandates immediate laparotomy. In other cases the indications for laparotomy must be correlated with the mechanism of injury. For example, if an individual has a gunshot wound or impaled object, surgery is usually indicated. If surgery is performed, the postoperative nursing care is similar to the care of the patient after laparotomy (see NCP 41-2).

Inflammatory Disorders

APPENDICITIS

Appendicitis is an inflammation of the appendix, a narrow blind tube that extends from the inferior part of the cecum. Appendicitis occurs in 7% to 12% of the world's population. Peak incidence is between the ages of 11 and 19 years, and males in this age group are afflicted more often than females.[11]

TABLE 41-14 Emergency Management
Abdominal Trauma

ETIOLOGY	ASSESSMENT FINDINGS	INTERVENTIONS
Blunt Falls Motor vehicle collisions Pedestrian event Assault with blunt object Crush injuries Explosions **Penetrating** Knife Gunshot wounds Other missiles	**Hypovolemic Shock** • ↓ Level of consciousness • Tachypnea • Tachycardia • ↓ Blood pressure • ↓ Pulse pressure **Surface Findings** • Abrasions or ecchymoses on abdominal wall, flank, or peritoneum • Open wounds: lacerations, eviscerations, puncture wounds, gunshot wounds • Impaled object • Healed incisions or old scars **Abdominal/Gastrointestinal Findings** • Nausea and vomiting • Bloody urine • Abdominal distention • Abdominal rigidity • Abdominal pain with palpation • Rebound tenderness • Pain radiation to shoulder and back	**Initial** • Ensure patent airway. • Administer O_2 via non-rebreather mask. • Control external bleeding with direct pressure or sterile pressure dressing. • Establish IV access with two large-bore catheters and infuse warm normal saline or lactated Ringer's solution. • Obtain blood for type and crossmatch and CBC. • Remove clothing. • Stabilize impaled objects with bulky dressing—*do not remove*. • Cover protruding organs or tissue with sterile, saline dressing. • Insert indwelling urinary catheter if there is no blood at the meatus, pelvic fracture, or boggy prostate. • Obtain urine for urinalysis. • Insert NG tube if no evidence of facial trauma. • Anticipate diagnostic peritoneal lavage. **Ongoing Monitoring** • Monitor vital signs, level of consciousness, O_2 saturation, and urine output. • Maintain patient warmth using blankets, warm IV fluids, or warm humidified oxygen.

CBC, Complete blood count; *IV,* intravenous; *NG,* nasogastric.

Etiology and Pathophysiology

The most common causes of appendicitis are obstruction of the lumen by a *fecalith* (accumulated feces) (Fig. 41-1), foreign bodies, tumor of the cecum or appendix, or intramural thickening caused by hypergrowth of lymphoid tissue. Obstruction results in distention, venous engorgement, and the accumulation of mucus and bacteria, which can lead to gangrene and perforation.[10]

Clinical Manifestations

Appendicitis typically begins with periumbilical pain, followed by anorexia, nausea, and vomiting. The pain is persistent and continuous, eventually shifting to the right lower quadrant and localizing at McBurney's point (located halfway between the umbilicus and the right iliac crest). Further assessment of the patient reveals localized tenderness, rebound tenderness, and muscle guarding. The patient usually prefers to lie still, often with the right leg flexed. Low-grade fever may or may not be present, and coughing aggravates pain. Rovsing's sign may be elicited by palpation of the left lower quadrant, causing pain to be felt in the right lower quadrant. Complications of acute appendicitis are perforation, peritonitis, and abscesses.

Diagnostic Studies and Collaborative Care

Examination of the patient includes a complete history and physical examination (particularly palpation of the abdomen) and a differential WBC count. A urinalysis may be done to rule

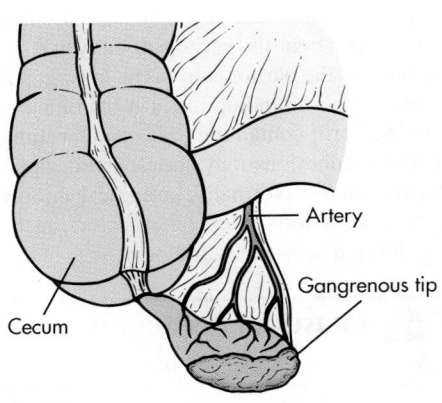

Artery

Gangrenous tip

Cecum

FIG. 41-1 In appendicitis the blood supply of the appendix is impaired by inflammation and bacterial infection in the wall of the appendix, which may result in gangrene.

out genitourinary conditions that mimic the manifestations of appendicitis.

The treatment of appendicitis is immediate surgical removal (appendectomy) if the inflammation is localized. If the appendix has ruptured and there is evidence of peritonitis or an abscess, conservative treatment, consisting of antibiotic therapy and parenteral fluids, may be used to prevent sepsis and dehydration for 6 to 8 hours before an appendectomy is performed.

NURSING MANAGEMENT
APPENDICITIS

The patient with abdominal pain is encouraged to see a health care provider and to avoid self-treatment, particularly the use of laxatives and enemas. The increased peristalsis from them may cause perforation of the appendix. Until the patient is seen by a health care provider, nothing should be taken by mouth (NPO) to ensure that the stomach is empty in the event that surgery is needed. An ice bag may be applied to the right lower quadrant to decrease the flow of blood to the area and impede the inflammatory process. Heat is never used because it may cause the appendix to rupture. Surgery is usually performed as soon as a diagnosis is made.

Postoperative nursing management is similar to postoperative care of the patient after laparotomy (see NCP 41-2). In addition, the patient should be observed for evidence of peritonitis. Ambulation begins the day of surgery or the first postoperative day. The diet is advanced as tolerated. The patient is usually discharged on the first or second postoperative day, and normal activities are resumed 2 to 3 weeks after surgery.

PERITONITIS
Etiology and Pathophysiology

Peritonitis results from a localized or generalized inflammatory process of the peritoneum. Causes of peritonitis are listed in Table 41-15. Peritonitis may appear in acute and chronic forms, and trauma or rupture of an organ containing chemical irritants or bacteria (which are released into the peritoneal cavity) may cause it. Examples of a chemical peritonitis include peptic ulcer perforation and ruptured ectopic pregnancy. A chemical peritonitis is commonly followed by bacterial invasion. Bacterial peritonitis can be caused by a traumatic injury (e.g., gunshot wound, ruptured appendix), or it can be secondary to other diseases or conditions (e.g., pancreatitis, peritoneal dialysis).

The response of the peritoneum to the leakage of GI contents is localization of the offending agent by attempting to "wall it off" by exuding fibrin-containing fluids and swelling. Adhesions may form. These adhesions may shrink and disappear when the infection is eliminated. Normally, peritoneal injuries heal without formation of adhesions unless other factors, such as infection, ischemia, or foreign substances, are present.

Clinical Manifestations

Abdominal pain is the most common symptom of peritonitis.[9] A universal sign of peritonitis is tenderness over the involved area. Rebound tenderness, muscular rigidity, and spasm are other major signs of irritation of the peritoneum. Abdominal distention or ascites, fever, tachycardia, tachypnea, nausea, vomiting, and altered bowel habits may also be present. These manifestations vary, depending on severity and acuteness of the underlying cause. Complications of peritonitis include hypovolemic shock, septicemia, intraabdominal abscess formation, paralytic ileus, and organ failure.

Diagnostic Studies

A CBC is done to determine elevations in WBC and hemoconcentration (Table 41-16). Peritoneal aspiration may be performed and the fluid analyzed for blood, bile, pus, bacteria, fungus, and amylase content. An x-ray of the abdomen may show dilated loops of bowel consistent with paralytic ileus, free air if perforation has occurred, or air and fluid levels if an obstruction is present. Ultrasound and CT scans may be useful in identifying the presence of ascites and abscesses. *Peritoneoscopy* (an endoscope is placed through a stab wound in the abdomen to inspect the peritoneum) may be helpful in the patient without ascites. Direct examination of the peritoneum can be obtained, along with biopsy specimens for diagnosis.

TABLE 41-15	Causes of Peritonitis
PRIMARY	**SECONDARY**
Blood-borne organisms	Appendicitis with rupture
Genital tract organisms	Blunt or penetrating trauma to abdominal organs
Cirrhosis with ascites	Diverticulitis with rupture
	Ischemic bowel disorders
	Obstruction in the gastrointestinal tract
	Pancreatitis
	Perforated peptic ulcer
	Peritoneal dialysis
	Postoperative (breakage of anastomosis)

TABLE 41-16 *Collaborative Care*
Peritonitis

Diagnostic
History and physical examination
CBC
Serum electrolytes
Abdominal x-ray
Abdominal paracentesis and culture of fluid
CT scan or ultrasound
Peritoneoscopy

Collaborative Therapy
Preoperative or Nonoperative
NPO status
Fluid replacement
Antibiotic therapy
NG suction
Analgesics
Preparation for surgery to include the above and total parenteral nutrition

Postoperative
NPO status
NG tube to low-intermittent suction
Semi-Fowler's position
IV fluids with electrolyte replacement
Total parenteral nutrition as needed
Antibiotic therapy
Blood transfusions as needed
Sedatives and narcotics

CBC, Complete blood count; *CT,* computed tomography; *IV,* intravenous; *NG,* nasogastric; *NPO,* nothing by mouth.

Collaborative Care

The goals of management of peritonitis are to identify and eliminate the cause, combat infection, and prevent complications. Patients with milder cases of peritonitis or those who are poor surgical risks may be managed nonsurgically. Treatment consists of antibiotics, NG suction, analgesics, and IV fluid administration. Patients who require surgery need preoperative preparation as previously described. Those patients may be placed on total parenteral nutrition (TPN) because of increased nutritional requirements.

NURSING MANAGEMENT
PERITONITIS

■ Nursing Assessment

Assessment of the patient's pain, including the location, is important and may help in determining the cause of peritonitis. The patient should be assessed for the presence and quality of bowel sounds, increasing abdominal distention, abdominal guarding, nausea, fever, and manifestations of hypovolemic shock.

■ Nursing Diagnoses

Nursing diagnoses for the patient with peritonitis include, but are not limited to, the following:

- Acute pain *related to* inflammation of the peritoneum and abdominal distention
- Risk for deficient fluid volume *related to* collection of fluid in peritoneal cavity secondary to trauma, infection, or ischemia
- Imbalanced nutrition: less than body requirements *related to* anorexia, nausea, and vomiting
- Anxiety *related to* uncertainty of cause or outcome of condition and pain

■ Planning

The overall goals are that the patient with peritonitis will have (1) resolution of inflammation, (2) relief of abdominal pain, (3) freedom from complications (especially hypovolemic shock), and (4) normal nutritional status.

■ Nursing Implementation

The patient with peritonitis is extremely ill and needs skilled supportive care. The patient is monitored for pain and response to analgesic therapy. The patient may be positioned with knees flexed to increase comfort. The nurse should provide rest and a quiet environment. Sedatives may be given to allay anxiety.

Accurate monitoring of fluid intake and output and electrolyte status is necessary to determine replacement therapy. Vital signs are monitored frequently. Antiemetics may be administered to decrease nausea and vomiting and further fluid losses. The patient is on NPO status and may have an NG tube in place to decrease gastric distention.

If the patient has an open surgical procedure, drains are inserted to remove purulent drainage and excessive fluid. Postoperative care of the patient is similar to the care of the patient with an exploratory laparotomy (see NCP 41-2).

GASTROENTERITIS

Gastroenteritis is an inflammation of the mucosa of the stomach and small intestine. Clinical manifestations include nausea, vomiting, diarrhea, abdominal cramping, and distention. Fever, increased WBC, and blood or mucus in the stool may be present. Causative agents are varied (see Table 41-2). Most cases are self-limiting and do not require hospitalization. However, older adults and chronically ill patients may be unable to consume sufficient fluids orally to compensate for fluid loss. Until vomiting has ceased, the patient should be on NPO status. If dehydration has occurred, IV replacement of fluids may be necessary. As soon as tolerated, fluids containing glucose and electrolytes (e.g., Pedialyte) should be given. If the causative agent is identified, appropriate antibiotic, antimicrobial, or antiinfective drugs are given.

NURSING MANAGEMENT
GASTROENTERITIS

Accurate monitoring of intake and output is important for successful replacement of lost fluid. Strict medical asepsis and infection control precautions should be instituted when indicated. The patient should be instructed in the importance of proper food handling and preparation of food to prevent infections such as salmonellosis and trichinosis (see Chapter 40, Table 40-27).

Symptomatic nursing care is given for nausea, vomiting, and diarrhea. The importance of rest and increased fluid intake should be stressed. The nurse should assess complaints of pain, vomiting, and diarrhea because gastroenteritis is often confused with appendicitis. To allay the patient's apprehension, the nurse should explain that gastroenteritis usually runs an acute course with no sequelae.

Inflammatory Bowel Disease

Crohn's disease and ulcerative colitis are immunologically related disorders that are referred to as **inflammatory bowel disease** (IBD). These disorders are characterized by chronic, recurrent inflammation of the intestinal tract. For both conditions, the clinical manifestations are varied, with long periods of remission interspersed with episodes of acute inflammation. Both diseases can be debilitating.

Although there has been extensive research on the etiology of IBD, the cause of both ulcerative colitis and Crohn's disease remains unknown. Possible causes include (1) an infectious agent (e.g., virus, bacteria) because IBD produces mucosal changes in the colon similar to those of infectious diarrhea, although no consistent pathogen has been identified; (2) an autoimmune reaction from the presence of other immune-related disorders, such as systemic lupus erythematosus, ankylosing spondylitis, and erythema nodosum in patients with IBD; (3) food allergies (al-

---

CULTURAL & ETHNIC CONSIDERATIONS
Colon Disorders

- Inflammatory bowel disease (IBD) is more common among whites than African Americans and Asian Americans.
- IBD is more common among Jewish people and those of middle European origin.
- Colorectal cancer is higher in the United States and Canada than in Japan, Finland, or Africa.
- Incidence of colorectal cancer is declining in the United States except for African American men.

though this has not been substantiated); and (4) heredity. Both Crohn's disease and ulcerative colitis occur more commonly in families. It is likely that more than one of the above factors may be involved in the pathogenesis of IBS. For example, a patient who is genetically susceptible to IBD may develop active IBD after a viral GI infection. Studies of identical twins and siblings with IBS support that there is a genetic predisposition to IBD.[12]

ULCERATIVE COLITIS

Ulcerative colitis is characterized by inflammation and ulceration of the colon and rectum. It may occur at any age but peaks between the ages of 15 and 25 years. There is a second, smaller peak onset between 60 and 80 years of age. Ulcerative colitis equally affects both sexes.[13] It is more common in Jewish and upper-middle-class urban populations.

Etiology and Pathophysiology

The inflammation of ulcerative colitis is diffuse and involves the mucosa and submucosa, with alternate periods of exacerbations and remissions (Table 41-17). The disease usually begins in the rectum and sigmoid colon and spreads up the colon in a continuous pattern.

The mucosa of the colon is hyperemic and edematous in the affected area (Fig. 41-2). Multiple abscesses develop in the crypts of Lieberkühn (intestinal glands). As the disease advances, the abscesses break through the crypts into the submucosa, leaving ulcerations. These ulcerations also destroy the mucosal epithelium, causing bleeding and diarrhea. Losses of fluid and electrolytes occur because of the decreased mucosal surface area for absorption. Breakdown of cells results in protein loss through the stool. Areas of inflamed mucosa form pseudopolyps, tonguelike

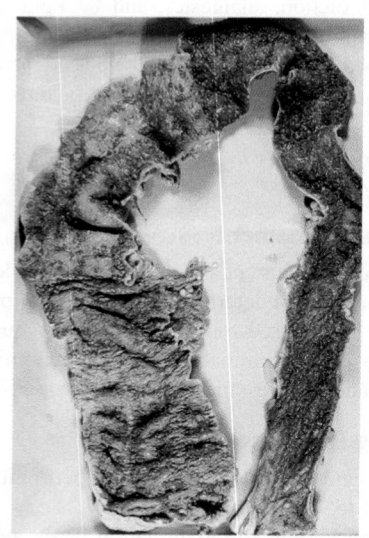

FIG. 41-2 Acute ulcerative colitis. Colitis with extensive mucosal ulceration involving the entire colon.

TABLE 41-17 Comparison of Ulcerative Colitis and Crohn's Disease

CHARACTERISTIC	ULCERATIVE COLITIS	CROHN'S DISEASE
Clinical		
Usual age at onset	Young to middle age	Young
Diarrhea	Common	Common
Abdominal cramping pain	Possible	Common
Fever (intermittent)	During acute attacks	Common
Weight loss	Common	Severe
Rectal bleeding	Common	Infrequent
Tenesmus	Severe	Rare
Malabsorption and nutritional deficiencies	Minimal incidence	Common
Pathologic		
Location	Starts distally and spreads in a continuous pattern up the colon	Occurs anywhere along GI tract in characteristic skip lesions; most frequent site is terminal ileum
Distribution	Continuous	Segmental
Depth of involvement	Mucosa and submucosa	Entire thickness of bowel wall (transmural)
Granulomas	Absent	Common
Cobblestoning of mucosa	Rare	Common
Pseudopolyps	Common	Rare
Small bowel involvement	Minimal	Common
Complications		
Fistulas	Rare	Common
Strictures	Rare	Common
Anal abscesses	Rare	Common
Perforation	Common	Common
Toxic megacolon	Common	Rare
Carcinoma	Increased incidence after 10 yr of disease	Slightly greater than general population
Recurrence after surgery	Cure with colectomy	40% to 60% or more recurrence after segmental resections of small or large intestine

projections into the bowel lumen. Granulation tissue develops, and the mucosa musculature becomes thickened, shortening the colon.

Although the precipitating factors involved in ulcerative colitis are poorly understood, it is clear that once initiated the inflammatory response is involved. Specific proinflammatory cytokines such as tumor necrosis factor-alpha (TNF-α) have been implicated in promoting this inflammatory response.

Clinical Manifestations

Ulcerative colitis may appear as an acute fulminating crisis or, more commonly, as a chronic disorder with mild to severe acute exacerbations that occur at unpredictable intervals over many years. The major symptoms of ulcerative colitis are bloody diarrhea and abdominal pain. Pain may vary from the mild lower abdominal cramping associated with diarrhea to the severe, constant abdominal pain that may be associated with acute perforations. With mild disease, diarrhea may consist of one or two semiformed stools containing small amounts of blood per day. The patient may have no other systemic manifestations. In moderate ulcerative colitis there is increased stool output (four to five stools per day), increased bleeding, and systemic symptoms (fever, malaise, anorexia). In severe cases, diarrhea is bloody, contains mucus, and occurs 10 to 20 times a day. In addition, fever, weight loss greater than 10% of total body weight, anemia, tachycardia, and dehydration are present. Acute fulminant colitis is present in only 6% to 10% of patients with severe ulcerative colitis.[14]

Complications

Complications of ulcerative colitis may be classified into those that are intestinal and those that are extraintestinal. Intestinal complications of ulcerative colitis include hemorrhage, strictures, perforation, toxic megacolon, and colonic dilation. Hemorrhage is a result of inflamed, ulcerated mucosa and is usually controlled with conservative therapy. Massive hemorrhage is unusual and requires emergency surgery. Strictures are less common in ulcerative colitis than in Crohn's disease and are seen most often in patients with severe, long-standing disease. *Toxic megacolon* (dilation and paralysis of the colon) occurs in approximately 5% of patients with ulcerative colitis.[14] Colonic dilation, most often in the transverse colon, occurs as a result of severe acute inflammation of the entire colon wall. Perforation is most often associated with toxic megacolon but may occur alone. Most cases of perforation occur in the left side of the colon.

A patient who has had ulcerative colitis for more than 10 years is at greater risk of colorectal cancer. The risk of cancer depends on age at onset, duration, and extent of disease. The patient should be periodically screened with colonoscopy. During this procedure, biopsy specimens should be taken every 10 cm throughout the entire colon.

Extraintestinal complications may be directly related to the colitis and small intestinal pathologic conditions (malabsorption), or they may be nonspecific complications mediated by a disturbance in the immune system (Table 41-18). Colitis-related complications are associated with active inflammation and often respond to treatment of the underlying bowel disease. These manifestations can involve the joints, skin, mouth, and eyes, as well as disturbances of the hematologic system including anemia, leukocytosis, and thrombocytosis.[14] Skin lesions such as

TABLE 41-18	Extraintestinal Complications of Ulcerative Colitis

Colitis Related
Joints
  Peripheral arthritis (colitic)
  Ankylosing spondylitis
  Sacroiliitis
  Finger clubbing
Skin
  Erythema nodosum
  Pyoderma gangrenosum
Mouth
  Aphthous ulcers
Eye
  Conjunctivitis
  Uveitis
  Episcleritis

Related to Small Bowel Pathology
Malabsorption
Gallstones
Kidney stones

Nonspecific
Liver disease—primary sclerosing cholangitis
Osteoporosis
Amyloidosis
Peptic ulcer disease

erythema nodosum and pyoderma gangrenosum are among the most frequently seen extraintestinal manifestations. Uveitis is the most common eye problem. Hepatobiliary disease may accompany ulcerative colitis.[15]

Diagnostic Studies

Several studies are appropriate for diagnosis of ulcerative colitis (Table 41-19). Blood studies should include a CBC, serum electrolyte levels, and serum protein levels. A CBC typically shows iron deficiency anemia from blood loss. An elevated WBC count may indicate toxic megacolon or perforation. Decreases in serum electrolytes, such as sodium, potassium, chloride, bicarbonate, and magnesium, are due to fluid and electrolyte losses from diarrhea and vomiting. Hypoalbuminemia is present with severe disease and is due to protein loss from the bowel. The stool should be examined for blood, pus, and mucus. Stool cultures should be obtained to rule out infectious causes of inflammation.

Examinations with a sigmoidoscope and a colonoscope allow direct examination of the mucosa of the large intestine. Using a sigmoidoscope the health care provider can view the rectum, the sigmoid colon, and the descending colon. The colonoscope allows for examination of the entire large intestine. The extent of inflammation, ulcerations, pseudopolyps, strictures, and lesions may be identified. Biopsy specimens should be taken for definitive diagnosis.

A double-contrast barium enema may show areas of granular inflammation with ulcerations. The colon may appear narrow and shortened, and pseudopolyps may be present. A double-contrast study (in which air is introduced into the bowel after the expul-

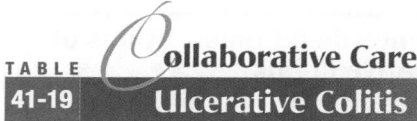

TABLE 41-19   Collaborative Care
Ulcerative Colitis

Diagnostic
History and physical examination
Colonoscopy
Sigmoidoscopy
Barium enema
CBC
Testing of stool for occult blood
Culture and sensitivity testing of stool

Collaborative Therapy
Mild and Moderate Disease
Low-roughage diet and no milk or milk products
Antimicrobial therapy*
5-Aminosalicylates*
Corticosteroids*
Anticholinergic therapy*
Antidiarrheal agents*
Severe (Fulminant) Disease
IV fluids with electrolytes
Blood transfusions
NPO status
NG tube to low suction
Antimicrobial therapy*
Immunosuppressants*
Immunomodulators*
Corticosteroids*
Parenteral nutritional therapy
Surgery if no improvement (colon resection with ileostomy)

*See Table 41-20.
CBC, Complete blood count; *IV,* intravenous; *NG,* nasogastric; *NPO,* nothing by mouth.

sion of barium) is effective in detecting mucosal abnormalities in ulcerative colitis.

Collaborative Care

The goals of treatment are to (1) rest the bowel, (2) control the inflammation, (3) combat infection, (4) correct malnutrition, (5) alleviate stress, and (6) provide symptomatic relief using drug therapy. The mainstays of drug therapy are sulfasalazine (Azulfidine) and corticosteroids. Hospitalization is indicated if the patient fails to respond to corticosteroid therapy or if complications are suspected.

Drug Therapy. Drug therapy is an extremely important aspect of treatment[15] (Table 41-20). Sulfasalazine, a combination of sulfapyridine and 5-aminosalicylic acid (5-ASA), is the principal drug used. It is effective in the maintenance of clinical remission and in the treatment of mild to moderately severe attacks. After remission is obtained, therapy is continued with a gradual reduction over several months. The maintenance dose is usually continued for at least 1 year.

During active disease, 5-ASA (the active form of sulfasalazine) and 4-ASA, given as retention enemas, are effective in the treatment of left-sided ulcerative colitis and proctitis. Topical salicylate therapy is the treatment of choice in patients with localized disease. 5-ASA (mesalamine [Rowasa]) can also be administered orally. The acrylic-coated tablets provide delivery of the drug more distally in the intestine.

Corticosteroids are of proven benefit in the management of active ulcerative colitis. Oral prednisone or prednisolone is effective in treatment of mild to moderate disease without systemic manifestations. If remission is not achieved, the patient requires hospitalization and IV corticosteroid therapy. The patient is placed on a regimen of bowel rest. Fluids and electrolytes are administered intravenously. For *proctitis* (inflammation of the rectum and anus), hydrocortisone enemas, rectal foams, or suppositories are effective in the treatment of inflammation. Rectal foams are usually administered in 5-ml volumes and are generally preferred over enemas because of the ease of administration. However, enemas are the preferred choice if the disease spreads beyond the sigmoid colon. Retention enemas have been shown to deliver drugs into the descending colon and beyond in patients with active disease. Although corticosteroids are reported to bring remission in 60% to 89% of cases, they do not necessarily prolong remission.[16] The patient taking corticosteroids needs to be monitored for signs of Cushing syndrome, hypertension, hirsutism, and mood swings.

Immunosuppressive drugs (e.g., 6-mercaptopurine [6-MP]) have been used in severe cases of ulcerative colitis when a patient has failed to respond to any of the usual drugs and before surgery is considered. Side effects of 6-MP, including bone marrow suppression and increased risk of infection, necessitate that it be used cautiously in these patients. Patients receiving this drug need to maintain an adequate fluid intake of 1800 to 2400 ml to reduce the risk of nephrotoxicity. The drug should be taken with food and milk to reduce gastric irritation. Cyclosporine (discussed in Chapter 13) and methotrexate have been evaluated for their effectiveness in the treatment of severe ulcerative colitis that is unresponsive to corticosteroid treatment. Although the monoclonal antibody against TNF-α (infliximab [Remicade]) is used more often in Crohn's disease, it has been used in patients with refractory ulcerative colitis.

Epidemiologic studies showing a low incidence of ulcerative colitis among smokers has led to investigation of nicotine transdermal patches or delayed-release nicotine capsules to induce remission.[16] For distal ulcerative colitis, rectal enemas containing short-chain fatty acids have been evaluated for their antiinflammatory effects. Short-chain fatty acids are important fuels supporting colonic cell function and are naturally produced from fiber fermentation.[17]

Surgical Therapy. Approximately 80% to 85% of patients with ulcerative colitis go into remission with conservative therapy and nursing management, but 15% to 20% require surgery. Surgery is indicated if (1) the patient fails to respond to treatment; (2) exacerbations are frequent and debilitating; (3) massive bleeding, perforation, strictures, or obstruction occur; (4) tissue changes that suggest that dysplasia is occurring; or (5) carcinoma develops.

Surgical procedures used to treat chronic ulcerative colitis include (1) total proctocolectomy with permanent ileostomy, (2) total proctocolectomy with continent ileostomy (Kock pouch), and (3) total colectomy with rectal mucosal stripping and ileoanal reservoir.

Total proctocolectomy with permanent ileostomy. *Total proctocolectomy with a permanent ileostomy* is a one-stage operation involving the removal of the colon, rectum, and anus with closure of the anus. The end of the terminal ileum is brought out through the abdominal wall and forms a stoma, or ostomy. The stoma is usually placed in the right lower quadrant below the belt line.

TABLE 41-20   Drug Therapy
Inflammatory Bowel Disease

CATEGORY	ACTION	EXAMPLES
Antimicrobial	Prevent or treat secondary infection	metronidazole (Flagyl)

5-Aminosalicylates (5-ASA)	Decrease GI inflammation*	*Systemic:*
		    sulfasalazine (Azulfidine)
		    mesalamine (Rowasa)
		    olsalazine (Dipentum)
		    balsalazide (Colazal)
		Rectal suppository:
		    mesalamine (Canasa)

Corticosteroids	Decrease inflammation	*Systemic:* corticosteroids (cortisone, prednisone, budesonide [Entocort]) *Enemas:* hydrocortisone (Cortenema) *Rectal suppository:* Cortifoam
Anticholinergics	Decrease GI motility and secretions and relieve smooth muscle spasms†	methantheline bromide (Banthine) propantheline (Pro-Banthine) oxyphencyclimine (Daricon)
Sedatives	Reduce anxiety and restlessness	diazepam (Valium) flurazepam (Dalmane)
Antidiarrheal	Decrease GI motility†	diphenoxylate (Lomotil)
Immunosuppressants	Suppress immune response	azathioprine (Imuran), cyclosporine
Immunomodulators	Inhibit the cytokine tumor necrosis factor-alpha (TNF-α)	infliximab (Remicade)
	Block lymphocyte adhesion to blood vessel walls and subsequent migration into tissues	natalizumab (Antegren)
Hematinics and vitamins	Correct iron deficiency anemia and promote healing	oral ferrous sulfate, ferrous gluconate; iron dextran injection (Imferon) cobalamin, zinc

*Mechanism of action unknown, possibly antimicrobial, as well as antiinflammatory.
†Used with caution during severe disease because of potential to produce toxic megacolon.
CNS, Central nervous system; *GI,* gastrointestinal.

Total proctocolectomy with continent ileostomy. *Total proctocolectomy with continent ileostomy* (Kock pouch) is a variation from the traditional ileostomy (Fig. 41-3). This method eliminates the need for the patient to wear an external pouch over the stoma. The stoma is usually covered with a cap or dressing in case of mucous leakage. This procedure is considered curative for ulcerative colitis but has a higher complication rate than the traditional ileostomy.

In this procedure an internal pouch in the distal segment of the ileum is made surgically, the intestine is split, a fold is made, and a one-way nipple valve is created and sutured into place on the abdomen. The pouch acts as a reservoir and is drained at regular intervals by insertion of a catheter. During surgery, a catheter is inserted into the pouch to allow suture lines to heal and to allow fixation of scar tissue around the valve to prevent slippage. Postoperative irrigations are performed every 2 to 4 hours to rinse mucus from the pouch. The catheter may stay in place for up to 3 to 4 weeks. Once the catheter is removed, insertion of a catheter to remove contents begins every 2 hours and is gradually decreased until it is needed only 3 to 6 times a day. The patient eventually determines the frequency by the changes in sensation of pressure in the pouch. A continuous leakage of fluid is prevented by the one-way valve created at the internal end of the ileum from the stoma to the ileal pouch. Pressure created when the pouch fills with feces forces the valve to close. The majority of complications that arise are a result of valve failure, which has been reported to be as high as 40%.

The primary late complications of the procedure include pouchitis, fistula development, and nipple valve extrusion. These complications affect function by increasing intubation frequency and compromising pouch continence. Manifestations of pouchitis are increased stool frequency, *hematochezia* (passage of blood), urgency, abdominal cramping, and, occasionally, fever, malaise, and pelvic pain.[18] The lining appears red and inflamed, and the biopsy result shows nonspecific inflammation. Patients usually respond to treatment with metronidazole (Flagyl). Patients who require repeated treatment or whose inflammation is unresponsive to therapy are considered to have chronic pouchitis.

Total colectomy and ileal anal reservoir. A more widely performed procedure involves total colectomy and ileoanal anastomosis with the formation of an ileal anal reservoir (Fig. 41-4). The ileoanal surgical procedure is usually a combination of two procedures performed approximately 8 to 12 weeks apart. The initial procedure includes colectomy, rectal mucosectomy, ileal reservoir construction, ileoanal anastomosis, and temporary ileostomy. The second surgery involves closure of the ileostomy, which functionalizes the reservoir. Adaptation of the reservoir occurs over the next 3 to 6 months, which usually results in the ability to control and have decreased numbers of bowel movements over a 24-hour period.

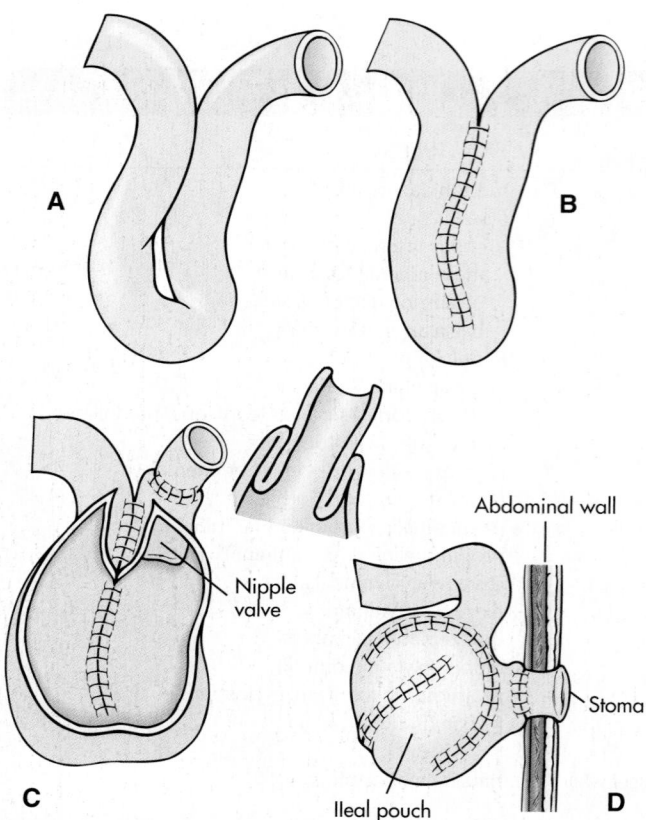

FIG. 41-3 Surgical formation of continent ileostomy (Kock pouch). **A,** Loop of terminal ileum. **B,** Both limbs sutured together and incised in a U *shape.* **C,** Pouch created with nipple valve. **D,** Pouch sutured to abdominal wall.

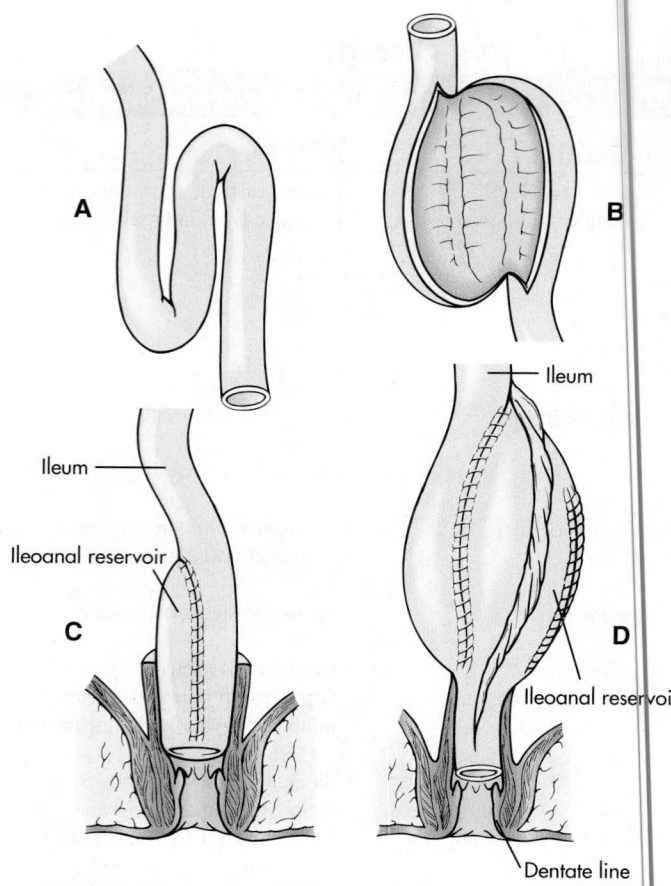

FIG. 41-4 Ileoanal reservoir. **A,** Formation of a reservoir. **B,** Posterior suture lines completed. **C,** J-shaped configuration for ileoanal reservoir. **D,** S-shaped configuration for ileoanal reservoir.

Patient selection criteria include absence of colorectal cancer, small intestine free of disease (e.g., Crohn's disease), competent anorectal sphincter, and physical status adequate to permit lengthy surgery. In addition, the patient needs to be motivated and capable of understanding self-care instructions.

Postoperative care. Postoperative care following surgical procedures to treat ulcerative colitis includes routine observations for patients who have had abdominal surgery. Stoma viability, mucocutaneous juncture (the area where the mucous membrane of the bowel interfaces with the skin), and peristomal skin integrity must be monitored. Because a more proximal portion of the bowel is used to create the ileostomy, output initially may be as high as 1500 to 2000 ml per 24 hours. The patient must be observed for signs of hemorrhage, abdominal abscess, small bowel obstruction, dehydration, and other related complications. If an NG tube is used, it will be removed when bowel function returns and oral intake is instituted. Drainage of serosanguineous fluid from the abdominal drain site may vary from 100 to 150 ml per 24 hours. The drain is usually removed within 4 days of surgery. The urinary catheter is removed 2 to 5 days after surgery. Systemic antibiotics are discontinued within 24 hours of the operation, and corticosteroids, if used, are tapered.

Transient incontinence of mucus is a result of intraoperative manipulation of the anal canal. The patient should be reassured before the operation regarding this potential transient problem. Kegel exercises are recommended later on (several weeks postopera-

tively) to strengthen the pelvic floor and sphincter muscles. They are not recommended in the immediate postoperative period. Perianal skin care must be implemented to protect the epidermis from mucous drainage and maceration. The patient should be instructed to gently rinse the skin with water and dry thoroughly. A moisture barrier ointment may be used, and a perineal pad may be required.

The most frequent type of ileostomy that is constructed is a loop. This often presents a pouching challenge because it retracts or drains inferiorly, resulting in effluent contact with the skin and predisposing to a denuded epidermis. An enterostomal therapy (ET) nurse should help with these challenging problems. Self-care instructions should be reviewed and written information provided before discharge. Stoma care is presented later in this chapter (see p. 1089).

Nutritional Therapy. An important component in the treatment of ulcerative colitis is diet. The dietitian is an important member of the team and should be consulted regarding dietary recommendations. The goals of diet management are to provide adequate nutrition without exacerbating symptoms, to correct and prevent malnutrition, to replace fluid and electrolyte losses, and to prevent weight loss. The diet for each patient must be individualized.

Traditionally during the acute phase the patient may be on NPO status. When food is permitted, a high-calorie, high-protein, low-residue diet with vitamin and iron supplements is frequently prescribed. (A low-residue diet is presented in Table 41-21.) Special dietary restrictions are not usually necessary. Some health care providers allow the patient to eat anything that does not

TABLE 41-21 Nutritional Therapy

Low-Residue Diet

Purpose
Low-residue diet provides foods low in fiber, which will result in a reduced amount of fecal material in the lower intestinal tract.

General Principles
1. This diet eliminates foods that are indigestible or stimulating to the intestinal tract to reduce the amount of residue in the colon. Foods should be included or excluded according to the following list.
2. Hot and cold foods should be eaten slowly.
3. Milk products are limited to 2 cups daily. For a more restricted-residue diet, milk should be eliminated.

FOOD	FOODS INCLUDED	FOODS EXCLUDED
Beverages	Carbonated drinks, coffee, tea, cocoa, strained fruit juices	Alcohol, fruit juices with pulp
Bread	White bread, rolls, rusk, melba toast, crackers	Bread and crackers containing whole grain flour or bran; any hot breads such as biscuits, muffins, waffles, or pancakes
Cereals	Cooked, refined, or strained cereals: Cream of Wheat, Cream of Rice, farina, grits, dry cereals without bran, noodles, spaghetti, and macaroni	Whole grain cereals; cereals containing bran, nuts, and raisins; Shredded Wheat
Meat	Lean, tender ground beef, lamb, pork, veal or fish, broiled, stewed, or baked; canned tuna or salmon; shellfish; crisp bacon, chicken or turkey without skin, liver; creamy peanut butter	Fried, smoked, pickled, or cured meats, highly seasoned ham, fried fish, luncheon meats
Egg	All but fried	Fried or uncooked eggs
Cheese	Milk, cheese (American, cheddar), cottage cheese	All other cheeses
Milk	Limit to 1-2 cups (if tolerated), including that used in cooking; plain yogurt	Fruit yogurt
Fats	Butter, margarine, cream, oil, crisp bacon, mayonnaise, plain gravy	Any other; rich or spiced gravies
Soup	Cream and vegetable soups made from foods allowed and with milk allowed, bouillon, broth; strained vegetable juices	Cream and vegetable soups from foods not allowed (peas and dried beans)
Vegetables	Tender carrots, beets, or asparagus; strained vegetables; potatoes without skins; vegetable juices	Raw vegetables, all vegetables not strained, dried beans, peas, and legumes
Fruits	Strained fruit juices, ripe bananas, applesauce, pears, peaches, peeled apricots, Napoleon cherries, baked apple (no skin)	Raw fruits, fruits with skins, seeds
Desserts	Plain desserts (custards and puddings, plain ice cream for milk allowance), sherbet, plain gelatin desserts, angel food cake, sponge cake, plain butter cake, plain cookies	Nuts, coconut, raisins, rich desserts (pies, rich cakes, cobblers)
Condiments	Allspice, cinnamon, mace, paprika, salt, ground thyme, sugar, vinegar, lemon juice	All others

BREAKFAST	LUNCH	DINNER
Sample Menu Plan		
½ cup applesauce	Roast beef sandwich on 2 slices white bread (no lettuce or tomato)	Baked chicken
½ cup Cream of Wheat		Mashed potato
Scrambled egg	1 tbs mayonnaise	Cooked carrots
White toast	2 sugar cookies	White bread
Butter or jelly	Canned peach halves	Butter
1 cup milk	Coffee	Angel food cake
Coffee		1 cup milk
		Coffee

cause symptoms. Cold foods, high-residue foods (whole-wheat bread, cereal with bran, nuts, raw fruit), and smoking increase GI motility and should be avoided. Fish oil preparations have been evaluated for their ability to reduce inflammation in active ulcerative colitis. However, their palatability has been low.[17]

Often enteral supplements and parenteral nutrition are necessary. Patients with systemic manifestations, significant fluid and electrolyte losses, or malabsorption may need parenteral nutrition or enteral feedings, such as elemental diets. Elemental diets are high in calories and nutrients, lactose free, and absorbed in the proximal small intestine, which allows the more distal bowel to rest.

Parenteral nutrition allows for a positive nitrogen balance while resting the bowel. Vitamins, minerals, electrolytes, and other important nutrients (e.g., glucose, amino acids) can be administered to promote healing and correct nutritional deficiencies. (TPN is discussed in Chapter 39.)

Supplemental iron (ferrous sulfate or ferrous gluconate) may be necessary to prevent or treat iron deficiency anemia resulting from chronic blood loss. Parenteral iron may be needed for patients who cannot tolerate oral iron. Iron dextran (Imferon) intramuscularly by Z-track or intravenously may be necessary if anemia is severe. In patients receiving long-term sulfasalazine therapy, folic acid deficiency may develop, and supplementation may be necessary. Potassium supplements may be necessary if corticosteroid therapy is used because retention of sodium and loss of potassium can result in hypokalemia and subsequent toxic megacolon. Zinc deficiency can result from severe or chronic diarrhea, and supplementation may be necessary.

NURSING MANAGEMENT
ULCERATIVE COLITIS

■ Nursing Assessment

Subjective and objective data that should be obtained from a patient with ulcerative colitis are presented in Table 41-22.

■ Nursing Diagnoses

Nursing diagnoses for the patient with ulcerative colitis include, but are not limited to, those presented in NCP 41-3.

■ Planning

The overall goals are that the patient with ulcerative colitis will (1) experience a decrease in number and severity of acute exacerbations, (2) maintain normal fluid and electrolyte balance, (3) be free from pain or discomfort, (4) comply with medical regimens, and (5) maintain nutritional balance.

■ Nursing Implementation

During the acute phase, attention is focused on hemodynamic stability, pain control, fluid and electrolyte balance, and nutritional support. Accurate intake and output records must be maintained. The number and appearance of stools are monitored. Nursing care of the patient with ulcerative colitis is directed toward an intensive therapeutic and supportive program (see NCP 41-3). It is important that the nurse establishes a good working relationship and encourages the patient to talk about self and daily activities. Honesty, patience, and understanding are crucial in the relationship with the patient. An explanation of all procedures and treatment is necessary and may allay some apprehension.

Psychotherapy may be indicated if the patient is experiencing emotional problems, but the nurse must recognize that the patient's behavior may result from factors other than emotional ones. Any person who has 10 to 20 bowel movements a day and has rectal discomfort may be anxious, frustrated, discouraged, and depressed. Along with other team members, the nurse can assist the patient to accept the chronic condition and to have an optimistic view with the possibility of cure after surgery. The nurse may find that inadequate coping mechanisms in the patient with ulcerative colitis are due to early onset of the disease (often at 10 to 15 years of age), which may have interfered with usual growth, development, and maturation.

Restricted physical activity and possibly bed rest may be ordered if the patient has a severe exacerbation. Nursing interventions to prevent complications of immobility should be instituted. A sedative or tranquilizer may be prescribed to ensure rest. Teaching related to treatment, drugs, diet, diagnostic tests, and the disease and its management is important.

Rest is important in the management of ulcerative colitis. Patients may lose much sleep because of frequent episodes of diarrhea and abdominal pain. Nutritional deficiencies and anemia leave the patient feeling weak and listless. Activities should be scheduled around rest periods. The nurse should also set limits and follow through because the patient can be demanding. The patient needs to know and understand that the nurse wants to help and does not consider the care repugnant.

Until diarrhea is controlled, the patient must be kept clean, dry, and free of odor. A bedpan and wipes should be kept within reach of the patient. The bedpan should be emptied as soon as possible. A deodorizer should be placed in the room. Antidiarrheal agents should be administered as ordered. If the patient has continuous diarrhea, the ET nurse may give helpful suggestions. Meticulous perianal skin care using plain water (no harsh soap) is necessary to treat and prevent skin breakdown. Dibucaine (Nupercainal), witch

TABLE 41-22	Nursing Assessment Ulcerative Colitis
Subjective Data	**Objective Data**
Important Health Information	**General**
Past health history: Infection, autoimmune disorders	Intermittent fever; emaciated appearance
Medications: Use of antidiarrheal medications	**Integumentary**
Functional Health Patterns	Pale skin with poor turgor, dry mucous membranes; rash, nodules, or blisters; anorectal irritation
Health perception–health management: Family history of ulcerative colitis; fatigue, malaise	**Gastrointestinal**
Nutritional-metabolic: Nausea, vomiting; anorexia; weight loss	Abdominal distention, hyperactive bowel sounds
Elimination: Frequent bloody stools containing mucus and pus	**Cardiovascular**
Cognitive-perceptual: Lower abdominal pain (worse before defecation), cramping, tenesmus	Tachycardia, hypotension
	Possible Findings
	Anemia; leukocytosis; electrolyte imbalance; hypoalbuminemia; vitamin and trace metal deficiencies; guaiac-positive stool; abnormal sigmoidoscopic, colonoscopic, and barium enema findings

NURSING CARE PLAN 41-3

Patient with Ulcerative Colitis

EXPECTED PATIENT OUTCOMES	NURSING INTERVENTIONS and *RATIONALES*

NURSING DIAGNOSIS   **Diarrhea** *related to* irritated bowel and intestinal hyperactivity *as manifested by* frequent diarrheal stools (>10 per day).

- Fewer, firmer stools
  - Monitor frequency and character of stools *to evaluate effectiveness of therapy and dietary restrictions.*
  - Maintain food and fluid restrictions *to rest bowel during exacerbations.*
  - Teach patient to avoid smoking, caffeine, and foods or fluids that *are irritating to bowel or cause increased motility.*

NURSING DIAGNOSIS   **Anxiety** *related to* possible social embarrassment, unfamiliar environment, diagnostic tests, and treatment *as manifested by* expression of concerns about effect of disease on social relationships, questions about disease and treatment.

- Decreased anxiety
  - Monitor for signs of anxiety *to plan appropriate interventions.*
  - Encourage open discussion of feelings about diagnosis *to demonstrate acceptance and concern for patient and allow verbalization of concerns.*
  - Explain disease treatments, diagnostic tests, and drugs *because understanding may reduce anxiety.*
  - Provide privacy *to reduce embarrassment and anxiety associated with frequent bowel movements.*

NURSING DIAGNOSIS   **Imbalanced nutrition: less than body requirements** *related to* decreased intake, decreased absorption, and increased nutrient loss through diarrhea *as manifested by* anorexia, weight loss, weakness, lethargy, anemia.

- Maintenance of body weight within normal range
- Adequate nutritional intake
- Increased strength and activity tolerance
  - Assess for signs of malnutrition (e.g., hair loss, fatigue) *to direct plan for treating the problem.*
  - Record daily weights *to evaluate nutritional status and response to treatment.*
  - Perform ongoing calorie counts *to determine adequacy of caloric intake.*
  - Administer IV fluids and TPN as ordered *to allow for a positive nitrogen balance while resting the bowel.*
  - Give and instruct patient on high-caloric, nonspicy, caffeine-free, low-residue diet with small, frequent feedings *to reduce discomfort associated with eating.*
  - Administer nutritional supplements (as ordered) *to provide additional calories, protein, and fluid.*

NURSING DIAGNOSIS   **Impaired skin integrity** *related to* diarrhea and altered nutritional status *as manifested by* erythema of perianal area, discomfort around perianal area during and after evacuation.

- No evidence of skin breakdown in the perianal area
  - Assess skin for signs of breakdown *to ensure early intervention.*
  - Cleanse perianal area after each bowel movement with mild soap and warm water and dry thoroughly *to remove bacteria, provide comfort, and stimulate circulation to treat and prevent skin breakdown.*
  - Provide sitz baths for comfort and hygiene and apply protective ointment.
  - Instruct patient and family on proper skin care techniques *to enable them to participate fully in treatment plan.*

NURSING DIAGNOSIS   **Ineffective coping** *related to* chronic disease, lifestyle changes, stress, and pain *as manifested by* inability to express feelings and concerns; display of dependent, attention-getting behavior.

- Development of healthy coping behaviors
  - Identify ineffective behaviors and institute plan *to assist patient in learning more effective behaviors.*
  - Encourage patient's expression of feelings *to provide support as patient explores areas of concern and add to patient's feelings of self-worth.*
  - Offer reassurance and psychologic support *to demonstrate caring and concern.*
  - Know limitations and refer to counseling when appropriate *because more intensive treatment may be required to deal with specific stress/problem areas.*

NURSING DIAGNOSIS   **Ineffective therapeutic regimen management** *related to* lack of knowledge of course of disease, appropriate lifestyle adjustments, and nutritional and drug therapy *as manifested by* questioning about disease and treatment, poor decisions about activities of daily living.

- Able to repeat correct information about disease and treatment
  - Provide information about the disease *to ensure that patient has adequate knowledge about the disease and treatment.*
  - Refer to dietitian if complex dietary changes are necessary *to provide patient with expert counseling.*
  - Teach about the relationships of stress to the disease *because stress may stimulate hyperreactivity of the colon in susceptible persons.*
  - Teach stress-reduction techniques *to assist patient in developing positive ways to reduce stress.*
  - Recommend regular colorectal cancer screening *because of increased risk of cancer.*

hazel, or other soothing compresses or prescribed ointment and sitz baths may reduce irritation and relieve discomfort of the anus.

■ Evaluation

The expected outcomes for the patient with ulcerative colitis are presented in NCP 41-3.

CROHN'S DISEASE

Crohn's disease is a chronic, nonspecific inflammatory bowel disorder of unknown origin that can affect any part of the GI tract from the mouth to the anus. It was once thought to be a disease specific to the small intestine and was called regional enteritis.

Crohn's disease may occur at any age but occurs most often between the ages of 15 and 30 years. When it occurs in older adults, the morbidity and mortality rates are higher because of other chronic problems that may be present. Both genders are affected, with a slightly higher incidence in women. Similar to ulcerative colitis, it occurs more often in Jewish and upper-middle-class urban populations. The incidence of Crohn's disease is slightly lower than that of ulcerative colitis.

Etiology and Pathophysiology

Crohn's disease is characterized by inflammation of segments of the GI tract. It can affect any part of the GI tract but is most often seen in the terminal ileum, jejunum, and colon. Involvement of the esophagus, stomach, and duodenum is rare. The inflammation involves all layers of the bowel wall (i.e., transmural). Areas of involvement are usually discontinuous *skip lesions,* with segments of normal bowel occurring between diseased portions (see Table 41-17). Typically, ulcerations are deep and longitudinal and penetrate between islands of inflamed edematous mucosa, causing the classic cobblestone appearance (Fig. 41-5). Thickening of the bowel wall occurs, as well as narrowing of the lumen with stricture development. The areas of inflammation can extend through all layers of the bowel wall. Abscesses or fistula tracts that communicate with other loops of bowel, skin, bladder, rectum, or vagina may develop. Histologically, granulomas are present in 50% of patients and may be located in any layer of the bowel wall.

TNF-α may be directly related to the pathogenesis of Crohn's disease. Levels of TNF-α are elevated in the stools of patients with Crohn's disease and correlate with disease activity. Treatment with the TNF-α blocker (discussed later under

Drug Therapy) decreases endoscopic and histologic disease activity in Crohn's colitis.[19] Other proinflammatory cytokines may also be involved in the pathophysiology of Crohn's disease (e.g., interleukin-1 [IL-1], interleukin-6 [IL-6]).

Clinical Manifestations

The manifestations depend largely on the anatomic site of involvement, extent of the disease process, and presence or absence of complications. The onset of Crohn's disease is usually insidious, with nonspecific complaints such as diarrhea, fatigue, abdominal pain, weight loss, and fever. Early diagnosis may be more difficult than for ulcerative colitis. The principal manifestations of Crohn's disease are diarrhea and abdominal pain. Diarrhea is usually nonbloody and is a result of the inflammatory process or malabsorption. Pain may be severe and intermittent or constant, depending on the cause. Other manifestations include abdominal cramping and tenderness, abdominal distention, fever, and fatigue. Similar to ulcerative colitis, extraintestinal complications may be directly related to the GI inflammation and small intestinal pathologic conditions (malabsorption), or they may be nonspecific complications mediated by a disturbance in the immune system. Extraintestinal manifestations, such as arthritis and finger clubbing, may precede the onset of bowel disease. As the disease progresses, there is weight loss, malnutrition, dehydration, electrolyte imbalances, anemia, increased peristalsis, and pain around the umbilicus and right lower quadrant.

Crohn's disease is a chronic disorder with unpredictable periods of recurrence and remission. Attacks are intermittent, usually recurring over a period of several weeks to months, with diarrhea and abdominal pain subsiding spontaneously.

Complications

Complications, both GI and extragastrointestinal, are common in Crohn's disease. Scar tissue from the inflammation narrows the lumen of the intestine and may cause strictures and obstruction, a frequent complication. Fistulas are a cardinal feature and may develop between segments of bowel. Cutaneous fistulas, common in the perianal area, and rectovaginal fistulas also occur. Fistulas communicating with the urinary tract may cause urinary tract infections. Inflammation of the intestines may involve all layers, predisposing the patient to perforation and the formation of intraabdominal abscesses and peritonitis.

Impaired absorption causing various nutritional abnormalities may occur as a result of damage to areas of the intestinal mucosa. Fat malabsorption causes a deficiency in the fat-soluble vitamins (A, D, E, and K). The patient may have an intolerance to gluten (a protein found in barley, rye, and wheat).

Systemic complications are similar to those of ulcerative colitis and include arthritis, liver disease, cholelithiasis (especially with ileal involvement), ankylosing spondylitis, pyoderma gangrenosum, erythema nodosum, and uveitis. Renal disorders are common, especially nephrolithiasis (kidney stones) secondary to increased oxalate absorption.

Diagnostic Studies

Diagnosis of Crohn's disease can be made by means of a thorough history and physical examination to establish clinical signs and symptoms, barium studies, and endoscopy with biopsy (Table 41-23). Laboratory studies may determine electrolyte disturbances and the presence of anemia. Barium studies are useful in determining location and extent of the disease and may reveal

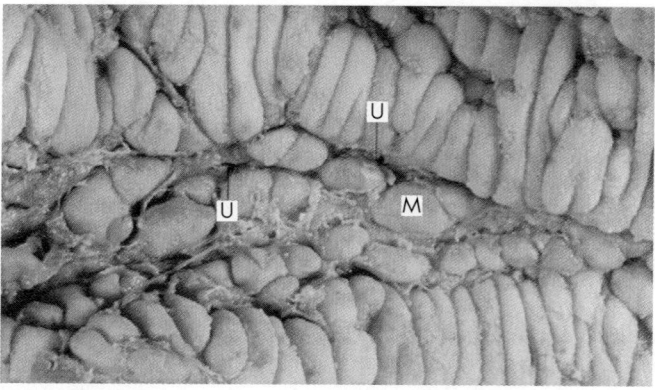

FIG. 41-5 Crohn's disease. The mucosa in Crohn's disease demonstrates a cobblestone pattern as a result of fissured ulcers *(U)* with intervening areas of edematous mucosa *(M).*

classic findings, such as stricturing of the ileum (string sign), cobblestoning of the mucosa, fistulas, and areas of abnormal and normal mucosa. Endoscopic studies, such as colonoscopy and sigmoidoscopy, are useful in detecting such early mucosal changes as patchy inflammation, small ulcerations, and skip areas that may not be seen radiologically. Biopsies may be performed to determine the presence of *granulomas* (chronic inflammatory lesions). Barium studies are performed to determine the degree of ileal involvement. Upper GI barium studies are done to diagnose upper gastroduodenal disease.

Collaborative Care

The goal of collaborative care is to control the inflammatory process, relieve symptoms, correct metabolic and nutritional problems, and promote healing. Drug therapy and nutritional support are the mainstays of treatment. Balloon dilation of strictures may be effective in relieving symptoms in some patients. This is usually performed through a colonoscope or under fluoroscopic guidance. Strictures most often dilated are those in the colon or small bowel.

Drug Therapy. Drug therapy for Crohn's disease is presented in Table 41-20. Sulfasalazine is effective when the disease involves the large intestine but is much less effective when only the small intestine is involved. Corticosteroid therapy is effective in reducing inflammation and suppressing disease. The dosage and the route of administration depend on the severity of the illness and the area involved. Once clinical symptoms subside, the dosage should be tapered. Immunosuppressive agents (6-MP, azathioprine) may be tried if repeated trials with corticosteroids fail. Patients require close monitoring because of the serious side effects of these drugs. Metronidazole (Flagyl) is useful in treating Crohn's disease of the perianal area. Marked exacerbations have been reported when the drug is stopped. In patients with Crohn's disease in remission, fish oil preparations have been evaluated for their ability to prevent recurrence of inflammation; however, their palatability has been low.

Biologic drug therapies of Crohn's disease include monoclonal antibodies to TNF-α (infliximab [Remicade]) and to a leukocyte adhesion molecule (natalizumab [Antegren]). Infliximab (by blocking the action of TNF-α) has been shown to reduce the degree of inflammation in patients who are refractory to other drug therapies. However, not all patients with Crohn's disease respond to infliximab. Natalizumab, on the other hand, works by interrupting the movement of lymphocytes into the endothelial layer of the gut wall. By reducing the migration of lymphocytes, the inflammatory process can be decreased.

Nutritional Therapy. Elemental diets and parenteral nutrition may be used in the patient with Crohn's disease (see Chapter 39). Parenteral nutrition may be given to patients with severe disease, small bowel fistulas, or short bowel syndrome (described later in this chapter). It is given before and after surgery to promote wound healing, reduce complications, and hasten recovery. The elemental diet provides a high-calorie, high-nitrogen, fat-free, no-residue substrate that is absorbed in the proximal small bowel. This diet can be given to most patients with Crohn's disease, even during acute exacerbations.

The diet should otherwise be low in residue, roughage, and fat but high in calories and protein. It may be difficult to maintain adequate absorption during periods of disease exacerbation and even during periods of remission. Milk and milk products may have to be excluded from the diet. Lactose, the primary disaccharide found in milk, may not be adequately digested because of the inability of the damaged intestinal mucosa to produce sufficient amounts of lactase. High-fat diets are poorly tolerated because of the loss of absorbing mucosa and altered bile salt metabolism and absorption.

Vitamin deficiencies may develop as a result of malabsorption. Cobalamin (vitamin B_{12}) injections every month may be needed because of the inability of the terminal ileum (if affected) to absorb this vitamin.

Surgical Therapy. Surgery is used in patients with severe symptoms that are unresponsive to therapy and in those with life-threatening complications. The majority of patients with Crohn's disease eventually require surgery at least once in the course of their disease. Indications for surgery are outlined in Table 41-24. Unlike ulcerative colitis, which can be cured by total proctocolectomy, Crohn's disease is not cured by surgery. The recurrence rate after surgery is high. The surgical procedure depends on the affected area and the condition of the patient. Conservative intestinal resection with anastomosis of healthy bowel is the procedure of choice.

TABLE 41-23	Collaborative Care Crohn's Disease

Diagnostic
History and physical examination
CBC
Serum chemistries
Testing of stool for occult blood
Radiologic studies with barium contrast
Sigmoidoscopy and colonoscopy with biopsy

Collaborative Therapy
High-calorie, high-vitamin, high-protein, low-residue, milk-free diet
Antimicrobial agents*
Corticosteroid drugs*
Immunosuppressants*
Immunomodulators*
Supplementary parenteral nutrition
Elemental diet
Physical and emotional rest
Surgery†

*See Table 41-20.
†See Table 41-24.
CBC, Complete blood count.

TABLE 41-24	Indications for Surgical Therapy of Crohn's Disease

- Drainage of abdominal abscess
- Failure to respond to conservative therapy
- Fistulas
- Inability to decrease corticosteroids
- Intestinal obstruction
- Massive hemorrhage
- Perforation
- Secondary hydronephrosis
- Severe anorectal disease
- Suspicion of carcinoma

NURSING MANAGEMENT
CROHN'S DISEASE

Care of the patient is similar to that of the patient with ulcerative colitis (see NCP 41-3 and p. 1075). As the patient's condition improves, the nurse should allow for more self-care, provide frequent rest periods, and advise the patient of the importance of rest and avoidance or control of emotional stress. Initially this may be difficult for the patient when told the nature of the disease and the limitations of the treatment. Patients who have perianal fistulas or abscesses may need special skin care. Postoperative care should be the same as for exploratory laparotomy (see pp. 1062-1063).

In the majority of patients with Crohn's disease the course is chronic and intermittent, regardless of the site of involvement. The patient and significant others may need help in setting realistic short-term and long-term goals. Teaching is important and should include (1) the importance of rest and diet management, (2) perianal care, (3) action and side effects of drugs, (4) symptoms of recurrence of disease, (5) when to seek medical care, and (6) use of diversional activities to reduce stress.

■ Gerontologic Considerations: Inflammatory Bowel Disease

Although inflammatory bowel diseases (i.e., ulcerative colitis and Crohn's disease) are considered diseases of young adults, a second peak in the distribution of these inflammatory conditions occurs around the age of 70 years. The pathogenesis, natural history, and clinical course of ulcerative colitis and Crohn's disease in older adults are similar to those observed in younger patients. However, the distribution of the inflammation appears to be somewhat different. In the older patient with ulcerative colitis, the distal colon (proctitis) is usually involved. In the older patient with Crohn's disease, the colon rather than the small intestine tends to be involved. There is less recurrence of Crohn's disease in older patients treated with surgical resection. The degree of inflammation associated with both conditions tends to be less in the older adult than in the younger patient.

Collaborative care of the older patient with one of these conditions is similar to care of the younger patient. However, because of increased risk of cardiovascular and pulmonary complications, older adults tend to have increased morbidity associated with surgical procedures.

In addition to Crohn's disease and ulcerative colitis, older adults are also vulnerable to inflammation of the colon (colitis) from medication use and systemic vascular disease. Drugs such as nonsteroidal antiinflammatory drugs (NSAIDs), digitalis, vasopressin, estrogen, and allopurinol (Zyloprim) have been associated with colitis development in the elderly patient. Colitis may also be secondary to ischemic bowel disease related to atherosclerosis and congestive heart failure.

Inflammation of the colon as a result of Crohn's disease or ulcerative colitis results in diarrhea, which may be bloody. The loss of fluid and electrolytes and possibly blood may leave the older adult more vulnerable to problems related to volume depletion and dehydration. This may be particularly problematic in the patient with diminished renal and cardiovascular function. Thus nursing management is focused on careful assessment of fluid and electrolyte status and evaluation of the replacement therapies.

INTESTINAL OBSTRUCTION

Intestinal obstruction occurs when intestinal contents cannot pass through the GI tract, and it requires prompt treatment. The obstruction may be partial or complete. The causes of intestinal obstruction can be classified as mechanical or nonmechanical.

Types of Intestinal Obstruction

Mechanical. *Mechanical obstruction* may be caused by an occlusion of the lumen of the intestinal tract. Most intestinal obstructions occur in the small intestine, most often in the ileum. Mechanical obstruction accounts for 90% of all intestinal obstructions[20] (Fig. 41-6). Adhesions account for 50%, hernias for 15%, and neoplasms for 15% of obstructions of the small intestine. Adhesions can develop after abdominal surgery. Obstruction can occur within days of surgery or years later. Carcinoma is the most common cause of large bowel obstruction, followed by volvulus and diverticular disease.

Nonmechanical. A *nonmechanical obstruction* may result from a neuromuscular or vascular disorder. **Paralytic (adynamic) ileus** (lack of intestinal peristalsis) is the most common form of nonmechanical obstruction. It occurs to some degree after any abdominal surgery. Other causes of paralytic ileus include inflammatory responses (e.g., acute pancreatitis, acute appendicitis), electrolyte abnormalities, and thoracic or lumbar spinal fractures.

Pseudoobstruction is an apparent mechanical obstruction of the intestine without demonstration of obstruction by radiologic methods. Collagen vascular diseases and neurologic and endocrine disorders may cause pseudoobstruction, but mostly it is found to be idiopathic.

Vascular obstructions are rare and are due to an interference with the blood supply to a portion of the intestines. The most common causes are emboli and atherosclerosis of the mesenteric arteries. The celiac, inferior, and superior mesenteric arteries supply blood to the bowel. Emboli may originate from thrombi in patients with chronic atrial fibrillation, diseased heart valves, and prosthetic valves. Venous thrombosis may be seen in low-blood-flow states, such as heart failure and shock.

Etiology and Pathophysiology

Normally 6 to 8 L of fluid enters the small bowel daily. Most of the fluid is absorbed before it reaches the colon. Approximately 75% of intestinal gas is swallowed air. Bacterial metabolism produces methane and hydrogen gases. Fluid, gas, and intestinal contents accumulate proximal to the intestinal obstruction. This causes distention, and the distal bowel may collapse. The distention reduces the absorption of fluids and stimulates intestinal secretions. As the fluid increases, so does the pressure in the lumen of the bowel. The increased pressure leads to an increase in capillary permeability and extravasation of fluids and electrolytes into the peritoneal cavity. Edema, congestion, and necrosis from impaired blood supply and possible rupture of the bowel may occur. The retention of fluid in the intestine and peritoneal cavity can lead to a severe reduction in circulating blood volume and result in hypotension and hypovolemic shock.

The electrolyte-rich fluids, which are normally absorbed in the bowel, are retained in the bowel and subsequently lost into the peritoneal cavity. The location of the obstruction determines the extent of fluid, electrolyte, and acid-base imbalances. If the ob-

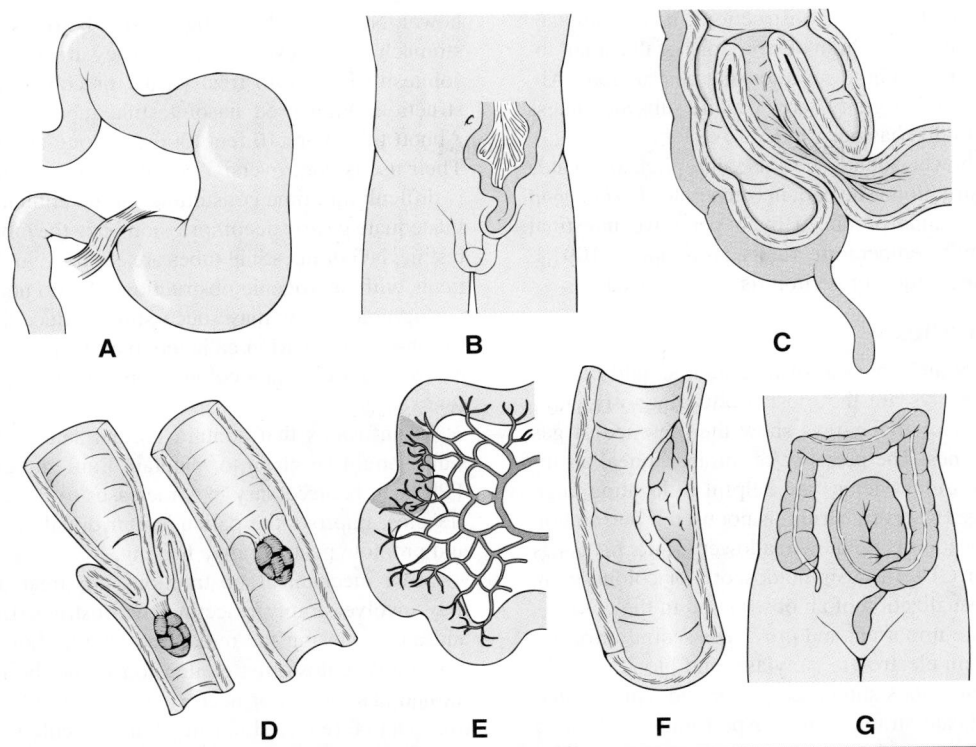

FIG. 41-6 Bowel obstructions. **A,** Adhesions. **B,** Strangulated inguinal hernia. **C,** Ileocecal intussus-ception. **D,** Intussusception from polyps. **E,** Mesenteric occlusion. **F,** Neoplasm. **G,** Volvulus of the sigmoid colon.

struction is high, as in the pylorus, metabolic alkalosis may result from the loss of hydrochloric acid from the stomach through vomiting or NG intubation.

When the obstruction is located in the small bowel, dehydration occurs rapidly. Dehydration and electrolyte imbalances do not occur early in large bowel obstruction. If the obstruction is below the proximal colon, most GI fluids have been absorbed before reaching the point of the obstruction. Solid fecal material accumulates until symptoms of discomfort appear. Reverse peristalsis may cause vomiting of fecal material very late in the bowel obstruction.

Simple obstructions of the intestine involve blockage of the lumen in one spot. A closed-loop obstruction occurs when the lumen is blocked in two different spots (e.g., *volvulus*). This results in an isolated segment of bowel and obstruction proximal to that segment. Strangulation and gangrene are likely to develop if treatment is not immediate. A strangulated obstruction occurs when the circulation to the obstructed intestine is impaired. This is the most dangerous form of obstruction because it may lead to necrosis of the intestine (*incarcerated*). Volvulus, hernias, or adhesions are the most common causes.

Clinical Manifestations

The clinical manifestations of intestinal obstruction vary, depending on the location of the obstruction, and include nausea, vomiting, abdominal pain, distention, inability to pass flatus, and obstipation (Table 41-25). Obstruction located high in the small intestine produces rapid-onset, sometimes projectile vomiting with bile-containing vomitus. Vomiting from more distal obstructions of the small intestine is more gradual in onset. The

TABLE 41-25	Clinical Manifestations of Small and Large Intestinal Obstructions	
CLINICAL MANIFESTATION	**SMALL INTESTINE**	**LARGE INTESTINE**
Onset	Rapid	Gradual
Vomiting	Frequent and copious	Rare
Pain	Colicky, cramplike, intermittent	Low-grade, cramping abdominal pain
Bowel movement	Feces for a short time	Absolute constipation
Abdominal distention	Minimally increased	Greatly increased

vomitus may be orange-brown and foul smelling because of bacterial overgrowth. Vomiting may be entirely absent in large bowel obstruction if the ileocecal valve is competent; otherwise, the patient may eventually vomit fecal material.

Vomiting usually relieves abdominal pain in high intestinal obstructions. Persistent, colicky abdominal pain is seen with lower intestinal obstruction. A characteristic sign of mechanical obstruction is pain that comes and goes in waves. This is due to intestinal peristalsis trying to move bowel contents past the obstructed area. In contrast, paralytic ileus produces a more constant generalized discomfort. Strangulation causes severe, constant pain that is rapid in onset. Abdominal distention is a common manifestation of intestinal obstructions. It is usually absent or minimally noticeable in high obstructions of the small intestine and greatly increased in lower intestinal obstructions. Abdominal tenderness and rigidity are usually absent unless strangulation or peritonitis has occurred.

Auscultation of bowel sounds reveals high-pitched sounds above the area of obstruction. The patient often notes *borborygmi* (audible abdominal sounds produced by hyperactive intestinal motility). The patient's temperature rarely rises above 100° F (37.8° C) unless strangulation or peritonitis has occurred.

Diagnostic Studies

A thorough history and physical examination should be performed. Abdominal x-rays are the most useful diagnostic aids. Upright and lateral abdominal x-rays show the presence of gas and fluid in the intestines. The presence of intraperitoneal air indicates perforation. Barium enemas are helpful in locating large intestinal obstructions. However, barium is not used if perforation is suspected. If the location is unknown, a lower GI tract study is done before an upper GI series. Sigmoidoscopy or colonoscopy may provide direct visualization of an obstruction in the colon.

Laboratory tests are important and provide essential information. A CBC and serum electrolyte, amylase, and blood urea nitrogen (BUN) determinations should be performed. An elevated WBC count may indicate strangulation or perforation; elevated hematocrit values may reflect hemoconcentration. Decreased hemoglobin and hematocrit values may indicate bleeding from a neoplasm or strangulation with necrosis. Serum electrolytes should be monitored frequently. They provide essential information on the patient's fluid and electrolyte balance. Serum sodium, potassium, and chloride concentrations are decreased in small bowel obstruction. The BUN value may be increased because of dehydration. The stool should be checked for occult blood.

Collaborative Care

Treatment is directed toward decompression of the intestine by removal of gas and fluid, correction and maintenance of fluid and electrolyte balance, and relief or removal of the obstruction. NG or intestinal tubes (Fig. 41-7) may be used to decompress the bowel. NG tubes should be inserted before surgery to empty the stomach and relieve distention. They are also used instead of nasointestinal tubes to treat partial or complete small bowel obstruction. When used, nasointestinal tubes (e.g., Cantor or Miller-Abbott tubes) are 10 feet (300 cm) long and mercury weighted. Their use is controversial because passing a long intestinal tube is difficult and time consuming. Some clinicians believe there is inadequate gastric decompression once the tube is in the small intestine. NG or intestinal tubes are effective in the treatment of patients with neurogenic obstruction who do not require surgery.

Sigmoidoscopy may successfully reduce a sigmoid volvulus. Colon-decompression catheters may be passed through partially obstructed areas via a colonoscope to decompress the bowel before surgery.

IV infusions that contain normal saline solution and potassium should be given to maintain fluid and electrolyte balance. TPN may be necessary in some cases to correct nutritional deficiencies, improve the patient's nutritional status before surgery, and promote postoperative healing.

Most mechanical obstructions are treated surgically. They may involve simply resecting the obstructed segment of bowel and anastomosing the remaining healthy bowel. Partial or total colectomy, colostomy, or ileostomy may be required when extensive obstruction or necrosis is present. Occasionally obstructions can be removed nonsurgically. A colonoscope can be used to remove polyps, dilate strictures, and remove and destroy tumors with a laser.

NURSING MANAGEMENT
INTESTINAL OBSTRUCTION

■ Nursing Assessment

Intestinal obstruction is a potentially life-threatening condition. Nursing assessment must begin with a detailed patient history and physical examination. The type and location of obstruction usually cause characteristic symptoms. The nurse should determine the location, duration, intensity, and frequency of abdominal pain and whether abdominal tenderness or rigidity is present. Onset, frequency, color, odor, and amount of vomitus

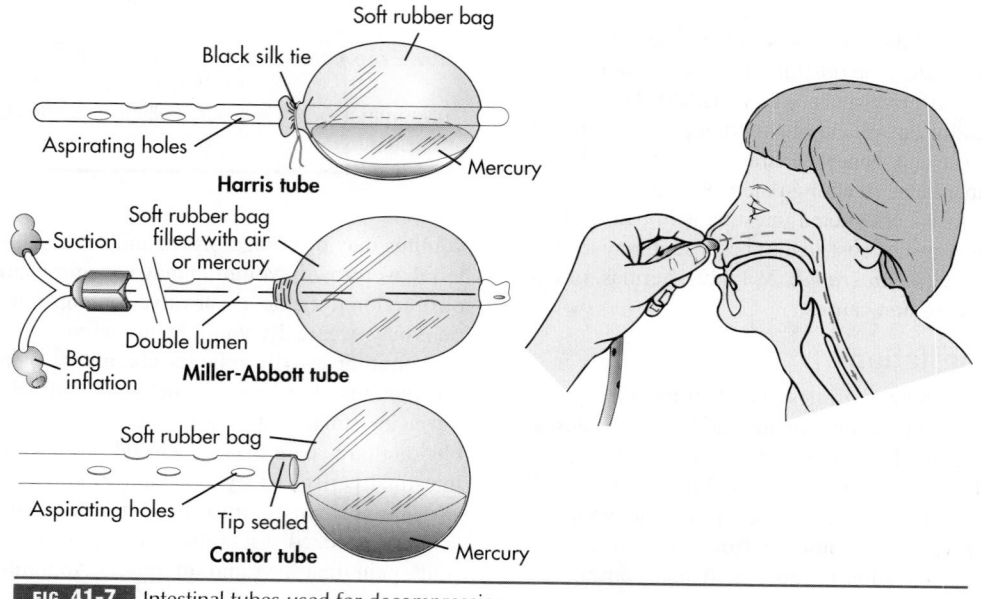

FIG. 41-7 Intestinal tubes used for decompression.

should be recorded. Bowel function, including passage of flatus, should be determined. The nurse auscultates for bowel sounds and documents the character and location; inspects the abdomen for scars, palpable masses, and distention; and observes for muscle guarding and tenderness.

■ Nursing Diagnoses

Nursing diagnoses for the patient with intestinal obstructions include, but are not limited to, the following:

- Acute pain *related to* abdominal distention and increased peristalsis
- Deficient fluid volume *related to* decrease in intestinal fluid absorption and loss of fluids secondary to vomiting
- Imbalanced nutrition: less than body requirements *related to* intestinal obstruction and vomiting

■ Planning

The overall goals are that the patient with an intestinal obstruction will have (1) relief of the obstruction and return to normal bowel function, (2) minimal to no discomfort, and (3) normal fluid and electrolyte status.

■ Nursing Implementation

The patient should be monitored closely for signs of dehydration and electrolyte imbalance. A strict intake and output record should be maintained. All vomitus and tube drainage should be included. IV fluids should be administered as ordered. Serum electrolyte levels should be monitored closely. A patient with a high obstruction is more likely to have metabolic alkalosis; a patient with a low obstruction is at greater risk of metabolic acidosis. The patient is often restless and constantly changes position to relieve the pain. Analgesics may be withheld until the obstruction is diagnosed because they may mask other signs and symptoms and decrease intestinal motility. The nurse should provide comfort measures, promote a restful environment, and keep distractions and visitors to a minimum. Nursing care of the patient after surgery for an intestinal obstruction is similar to care of the patient after a laparotomy (see NCP 41-2 and p. 1063).

Care of Nasogastric and Nasointestinal Tubes. Although the health care provider usually inserts intestinal tubes, the nurse assists with the procedure. Insertion is easier if the patient relaxes, takes deep breaths, and swallows when instructed. If insertion of the tube to the small intestine is desired, the patient may be instructed or positioned to lie on the right side to facilitate tube passage through the pylorus. In some situations a prokinetic drug such as metoclopramide (Reglan) may be used to facilitate tube movement.

Once the tube is in place, mouth care is extremely important. Vomiting leaves a terrible taste in the patient's mouth, and fecal odor may be present. When an NG or nasointestinal tube is in place, the patient breathes through the mouth, drying the mouth and lips. The nurse should encourage and assist the patient to brush the teeth frequently. Mouthwash and water for the patient to use in rinsing the mouth and petroleum jelly or water-soluble lubricant for the lips should be provided at the bedside.

The patient's nose should be checked for signs of irritation from the NG or nasointestinal tube. This area should be cleaned and dried daily with application of a water-soluble lubricant and retaping of the tube. NG and intestinal tubes should be checked every 4 hours for patency. The patient may be placed on a schedule to clamp the tube for 1 hour out of every 3 hours or for 3 out of every 4 hours before removal of the tube.

POLYPS OF THE LARGE INTESTINE

Colonic polyps arise from the mucosal surface of the colon and project into the lumen. They may be *sessile* (flat, broad based, and attached directly to the intestinal wall) or *pedunculated* (attached to the intestinal wall by a thin stalk). Polyps tend to be sessile when small and become pedunculated as they enlarge, especially if they are in the left or descending colon (Fig. 41-8). They may be found anywhere in the large intestine but are most commonly found in the rectosigmoid area. Although most polyps are asymptomatic, rectal bleeding or occult blood in the stool are the most common manifestations.

Types of Polyps

The most common types of polyp are hyperplastic and adenomatous. *Hyperplastic polyps* originate from the epithelium and are nonneoplastic growths. They rarely grow larger than 5 mm in size and never cause clinical symptoms. Other benign (nonneoplastic) polyps include inflammatory polyps, lipomas, and juvenile polyps (Table 41-26).

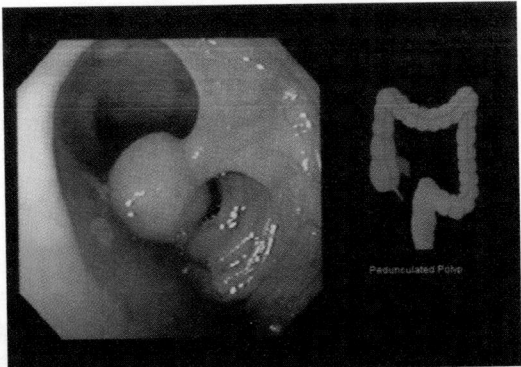

FIG. 41-8 Endoscopic image of pedunculated polyp in descending colon.

TABLE 41-26 Types of Polyps of the Large Intestine

Neoplastic
Epithelial polyps (adenomatous)
   Tubular adenoma
   Tubular villous adenoma
   Villous adenoma
Hereditary polyposis syndromes (adenomatous polyposis syndrome)
   Familial adenomatous polyposis

Nonneoplastic
Epithelial polyps (hyperplastic)
Hereditary polyposis syndromes
   Familial juvenile polyposis
Inflammatory polyps
   Pseudopolyps
   Benign lymphoid polyp
Submucosal
   Lipomas
   Leiomyomas
   Fibromas

Adenomatous polyps are characterized by neoplastic changes in the epithelium. They are closely linked to colorectal adenocarcinoma. Structurally, there are three types, with tubular adenomas being the most prevalent. The risk of cancer in the polyp increases with polyp size and villous structure. Villous adenomas have a higher risk of turning cancerous than tubular adenomas. Removing adenomatous polyps has been reported to decrease the occurrence of subsequent colorectal cancer by 90%.[21]

Although there are several polyposis syndromes, they are relatively rare. Of these, *familial adenomatous polyposis (FAP)* is the most common (see the Genetics in Clinical Practice box below. This disorder is characterized by multiple polyps that at times number in the thousands and that are located in the large intestine and sometimes in other areas of the GI tract. Patients with a history of FAP have a lifetime risk of developing colorectal cancer that approaches 100%. They also develop cancer at an earlier age (i.e., 40 years of age) than patients with non-FAP colorectal cancer. For children of patients with FAP, screening must be initiated at puberty and then conducted annually. There is a 50% risk for these children to develop FAP. When there is indication of disease, total colectomy with ileostomy is the treatment of choice.[22]

Diagnostic Studies and Collaborative Care

Barium enema, sigmoidoscopy, and colonoscopy are used to diagnose polyps. All polyps are considered abnormal and should be removed. In patients whose polyps are identified through barium enema, removal (polypectomy) should be done through a colonoscope or a sigmoidoscope. If the polyp is not removable, a biopsy specimen should be taken for tissue examination. Surgery

is not indicated unless carcinoma is present or certain cases of polyposis syndromes warrant it. The patient should be observed for rectal bleeding, fever, severe abdominal pain, and abdominal distention, which may indicate hemorrhage or perforation.

COLORECTAL CANCER

Colorectal cancer is the third most common cause of cancer death in the United States. Colorectal cancer in the United States accounts for an estimated 56,600 deaths each year. In 2002, there were approximately 148,300 new cases of colorectal cancer in the United States. Colorectal cancer may occur at any age but is most prevalent over the age of 50 years. The 5-year survival rate is 90% for early, localized colorectal cancers and 64% for cancer that has spread to adjacent organs and lymph nodes.[23]

The incidence of colorectal cancer at specific sites varies (Fig. 41-9). In both sexes, the incidence of right colon cancers has increased and cancers in the rectum have decreased. The highest percentages of colorectal cancers in the United States are currently located in the rectum, ascending colon, and sigmoid colon. Approximately 20% of colorectal cancers are within reach of the examining finger, and 50% are within reach of the sigmoidoscope.

Etiology and Pathophysiology

The causes of colorectal cancer remain unclear. Groups at high risk of colorectal cancer have been identified (Table 41-27). For at least 6% of patients who develop colorectal cancer there is a clear genetic predisposition (see the Genetics in Clinical Practice boxes at left and on p. 1083). Age is a risk factor in both men and women. The risk for development in the general population increases slightly after the age of 40 years and then rises rapidly in the following decades. Diet, especially the high-calorie, high-fat Western diet, has been associated with development of colorectal cancer.

Adenocarcinoma is the most common type of colorectal cancer. Most colorectal cancers appear to arise from adenomatous polyps. All tumors tend to spread through the walls of the intestine and into the lymphatic system. Tumors commonly spread to

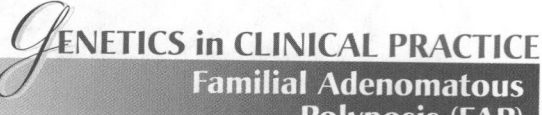

GENETICS in CLINICAL PRACTICE
Familial Adenomatous Polyposis (FAP)

Genetic Basis
- Autosomal dominant disorder
- Mutation in adenomatous polyposis coli (APC) gene located on chromosome 5

Incidence
- 1 in 5000-7500 people
- Men and women affected equally

Genetic Testing
- DNA testing available to detect APC gene mutation

Clinical Implications
- FAP is characterized by the presence of colorectal polyps (usually >1000).
- Polyps are not present at birth but appear during adolescence and early adulthood.
- FAP accounts for at least 1% of all colorectal cancers.
- If untreated, FAP almost always results in the development of colon cancer before the age of 40.
- With FAP, there is also increased incidence of gastric and small intestinal polyps.
- Many deaths related to FAP could be prevented with early and aggressive monitoring and treatment including frequent colonoscopies and total colectomy.
- Individuals with a family history of FAP could benefit from genetic counseling and teaching.

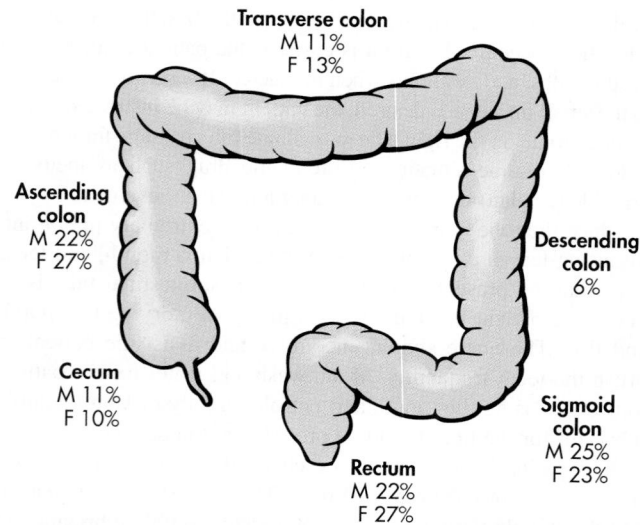

FIG. 41-9 Incidence of cancer. Approximately one half of all colon cancers occur in the rectosigmoid area. Percentages are listed for males (*M*) and females (*F*).

Transverse colon
M 11%
F 13%

Ascending colon
M 22%
F 27%

Descending colon
6%

Cecum
M 11%
F 10%

Sigmoid colon
M 25%
F 23%

Rectum
M 22%
F 27%

TABLE 41-27	Risk Factors for Colorectal Cancer

- Age >50 years
- Familial polyposis
- Colorectal polyps
- Chronic inflammatory bowel disease
- Family history of colorectal cancer or adenomas
- Previous history of colorectal cancer
- History of ovarian or breast cancer (women)
- High-fat and/or low-fiber diet (controversial)

GENETICS in CLINICAL PRACTICE
Hereditary Nonpolyposis Colorectal Cancer (HNPCC)

Genetic Basis
- Autosomal dominant disorder
- Mutations in genes that error-check DNA (repair genes)

Incidence
- 1 in 500 to 2000 people

Genetic Testing
- DNA testing available

Clinical Implications
- HNPCC accounts for 5% of all colorectal cancers.
- Individuals with gene mutation have 80% to 90% lifetime risk of developing colorectal cancer.
- Average age of diagnosis is in the mid-40s.
- Cancer arises from single colorectal lesion in absence of polyposis.
- Cancers tend to occur on right side of colon.
- HNPCC is less aggressive, and survival rates are longer than colon cancers that develop without known risk factors.
- Persons with gene mutation are also at high risk of developing other cancers, including uterine, ovarian, ureter, pancreas, stomach, and small intestinal cancer.
- Individuals with known gene mutations should be monitored with colonoscopy every year. Examination by pelvic ultrasound and endometrial biopsy should also be considered for women.

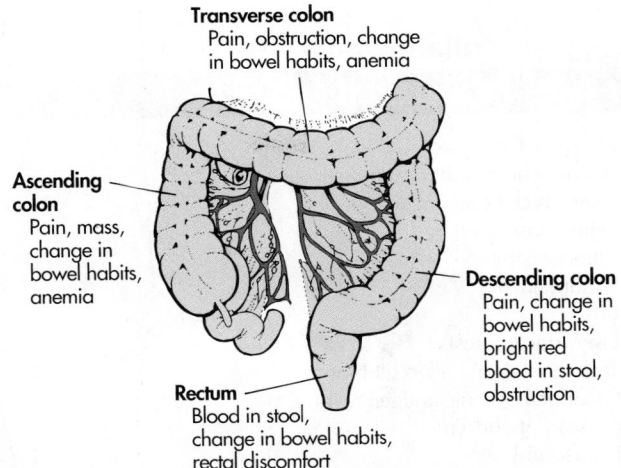

FIG. 41-10 Signs and symptoms of colorectal cancer by location of primary lesion.

the liver because the venous blood flow from the colorectal tumor is through the portal vein.

Clinical Manifestations

Clinical manifestations of colorectal cancer are usually non-specific or do not appear until the disease is advanced. Cancer on the right side of the colon gives rise to clinical manifestations that are different from those on the left side of the colon.[24] Rectal bleeding, the most common symptom of colorectal cancer, is most often seen with left-sided lesions. Other commonly seen manifestations of left-sided lesions include alternating constipation and diarrhea, change in stool caliber (narrow, ribbonlike), and sensation of incomplete evacuation. Obstruction symptoms appear earlier with left-sided lesions because of the smaller lumen size (Fig. 41-10).

Cancers of the right side of the colon are usually asymptomatic. Vague abdominal discomfort or crampy, colicky abdomi-

nal pain may be present. Iron deficiency anemia and occult bleeding dictate further investigation. Weakness and fatigue result from anemia.

Diagnostic Studies

A thorough history with close attention to family history should be obtained, and a physical examination should be performed initially (Table 41-28). The digital rectal examination is the most important aspect of the physical examination because many rectal cancers are within reach of the finger. In the asymptomatic person who is 50 years or older with no risk factors (other than age), fecal occult blood testing once a year and flexible sigmoidoscopy every 5 years beginning at age 50 are important aspects of the examination.[24] (Screening options for colorectal cancer are presented in Table 15-7.) If colorectal cancer is suspected, examinations with the flexible sigmoidoscope and a double-contrast barium enema (in combination) are often performed. Colonoscopy is the gold standard for colorectal cancer screening. If not used as the primary screening method, it is the procedure of choice if a questionable lesion is seen on barium enema or sigmoidoscopy. Other procedures include endorectal ultrasonography and a CT scan of the abdomen and pelvis to localize the lesion or determine its size. Synchronous lesions may be present at other sites in the colon, and tissue diagnosis may be made by brushing or biopsy during the procedure.

Fecal occult blood tests have been used for over 30 years to screen for colorectal cancer and continue to be widely used in North America. Patients need to be taught to abstain from red meat and NSAIDs before testing to avoid false positives. Newer, more sensitive stool tests are undergoing clinical evaluation. These include the presence of cancer cell markers (e.g., neoplasm specific DNA alterations).[25]

Laboratory studies should include a CBC to check for anemia, clotting studies, and liver function tests. A CT scan of the abdomen may be helpful in detecting liver metastases, retroperitoneal and pelvic disease, and depth of penetration of tumor into the bowel wall. A CT scan should be done before surgery. Liver function tests are performed to determine liver metastases.

A carcinoembryonic antigen (CEA) test is often performed, although it is not specific for colorectal cancer. A normal level of

TABLE 41-28 Collaborative Care — Colorectal Cancer

Diagnostic
History and physical examination
Digital rectal examination
Sigmoidoscopy
Colonoscopy
Barium enema
CBC
Liver function tests
Testing of stool for occult blood
Carcinoembryonic antigen test (CEA)
CT scan of abdomen
Ultrasound

Collaborative Therapy
Surgery
  Right hemicolectomy
  Left hemicolectomy
  Abdominal-perineal resection
  Laparoscopic colectomy
Radiation
Chemotherapy
  5-fluorouracil (5-FU)
  leucovorin (Wellcovorin)
  leucovorin-modulated 5-FU (Orzel)
  irinotecan (Camptosar)
  capecitabine (Xeloda)
  levamisole (Ergamisol)
  oxaliplatin (Eloxatin)
  raltitrexed (Tomudex)

CBC, Complete blood count.

TABLE 41-29 Dukes' Staging System for Colorectal Cancer

CLASSIFICATION	DESCRIPTION
A	Negative nodes, limitation of lesion to mucosa
B_1	Negative nodes, extension of lesion through mucosa but still within bowel wall
B_2	Negative nodes, extension through entire bowel wall
C_1	Positive nodes, limitation of lesion to bowel wall
C_2	Positive nodes, extension of lesion through entire bowel wall
D	Presence of distant, unresectable metastases

TABLE 41-30 Tumor–Node–Metastasis (TNM) Classification of Colorectal Cancer

T	PRIMARY TUMOR
T_X	Primary tumor cannot be assessed
T_0	No evidence of primary tumor
T_{is}	Carcinoma in situ
T_1	Tumor invades submucosa
T_2	Tumor invades muscularis propria
T_3	Tumor invades through the muscularis propria into the subserosa or into nonperitonealized pericolic or perirectal tissues
T_4	Tumor perforates the visceral peritoneum or directly invades other organs or structures

N	REGIONAL LYMPH NODE INVOLVEMENT
N_X	Regional lymph node cannot be assessed
N_0	No regional lymph node metastasis
N_1	Metastasis in one to three pericolic or perirectal lymph nodes
N_2	Metastasis in four or more pericolic or perirectal lymph nodes
N_3	Metastasis in any lymph node along the course of a named vascular trunk

M	DISTANT METASTASIS
M_X	Presence of distant metastasis cannot be assessed
M_0	No distant metastasis
M_1	Distant metastasis

STAGE	TNM		
0	T_{is}	N_0	M_0
IA	T_1	N_0	M_0
IB	T_2	N_0	M_0
II	T_1	N_2	M_0
	T_2	N_1	M_0
	T_3	N_0	M_0
IIIA	T_2	N_2	M_0
	T_3	N_{1-2}	M_0
IIIB	T_4	N_{0-1}	M_0
IV	T_4	N_2	M_0
	T_{1-4}	N_{0-2}	M_1

CEA does not exclude the possibility of a malignant condition. This test is used most effectively in following the progress of a patient after surgery. Return to normal of a previously elevated CEA indicates successful removal of the tumor. In contrast, persistent postoperative elevated or increasing CEA levels suggest residual tumor or tumor spread.

Collaborative Care

Prognosis and treatment correlate with pathologic staging of the disease. Several methods of staging are currently being used. The most widely known is Dukes' classification (Table 41-29). Surgical removal of the primary lesion is the treatment for Dukes' stages A, B, and C. The 5-year survival rate for Dukes' stage A is 90% to 100%, compared with less than 15% for Dukes' stage D.

Another classification system for colorectal cancer is the TNM system (Table 41-30), which is based on pathologic assessment and includes data from the history and physical examination and presurgical endoscopic and laboratory evaluations. Colorectal cancer can also be divided into stages, with stage 0 representing cancer in situ, stage I corresponding to Dukes' A and B_1, stage II corresponding to B_2, stage III corresponding to C_1 and C_2, and stage IV corresponding to Dukes' D.

Several noninvasive procedures may be performed through a colonoscope to effectively treat certain types of colorectal cancer.

Endoscopic polypectomy is a highly effective and safe procedure. Adequate treatment can be obtained if the resected margin of the polyp is free of cancer, the cancer is well differentiated, and there is no apparent lymphatic or blood vessel involvement. Laser therapy may be used to ablate nonresectable tumors. This is usually used only as palliative therapy in patients with obstructive symptoms.

Surgical Therapy. Surgery is the only curative treatment of colorectal cancer. The location and extent of the cancer determine the type of surgery performed. Success of surgery depends on resection of the tumor with an adequate margin of healthy bowel and resection of the regional lymph nodes.

Right hemicolectomy is performed when the cancer is located in the cecum, ascending colon, hepatic flexure, or transverse colon to the right of the middle colic artery. A portion of the terminal ileum, the ileocecal valve, and the appendix are removed, and an ileotransverse anastomosis is performed. A left hemicolectomy involves resection of the left transverse colon, the splenic flexure, the descending colon, the sigmoid colon, and the upper portion of the rectum.

Clear margins are most difficult to obtain with rectal carcinoma. Location of the rectal lesion determines the surgical procedure to be performed. There must be enough rectum left to ensure a secure anastomosis, or an abdominal-perineal resection is indicated. Abdominal-perineal resection is most often performed when the cancer is located within 5 cm of the anus.

In the abdominal-perineal resection, an abdominal incision is made, and the proximal sigmoid is brought through the abdominal wall in a permanent colostomy. The distal sigmoid, rectum, and anus are removed through a perineal incision. The perineal wound may be closed around a drain or left open with packing to allow healing by granulation. Complications that can occur are delayed wound healing, hemorrhage, persistent perineal sinus tracts, infections, and urinary tract and sexual dysfunctions.

Low anterior resection may be indicated for tumors of the rectosigmoid and the mid-to-upper rectum. The use of EEA (end-to-end anastomosis) staplers has allowed lower and more secure anastomoses. The stapler is passed through the anus, where the colon is stapled to the rectum. This technique has made it possible to resect lesions as low as 5 cm from the anus.

Sphincter-sparing procedures are being performed on the patient who is a poor operative risk and for the patient with early disease. The number of these procedures may increase with continued early detection and surveillance. In these procedures a local resection is performed, and the anal sphincters are left intact.

Laparoscopic colectomy is being evaluated for its effectiveness in eliminating cancer and improving survival. Potential benefits are faster return of bowel function, fewer incisional infections, shortened hospital stay, and improved cosmetic appearance.[26]

Chemotherapy and Radiation Therapy. Chemotherapy is recommended when a patient has positive lymph nodes at the time of surgery or has metastatic disease. Chemotherapy is used both as an adjuvant therapy following colon resection and as primary treatment for nonresectable colorectal cancer.[27] At present, the combination of 5-fluorouracil (5-FU) plus leucovorin and irinotecan (Camptosar) is approved as first-line chemotherapy for patients with metastatic colorectal cancer. Additional treatment protocols include the use of 5-FU and levamisole (Ergamisol) with or without leucovorin (Wellcovorin). For patients who are not considered appropriate candidates for this triple therapy, ei-

ther leucovorin-modulated 5-FU (Orzel) or capecitabine (Xeloda) is used as an acceptable alternative first-line treatment. New agents being examined for adjuvant therapy of colorectal cancer include oxaliplatin (Eloxatin), raltitrexed (Tomudex), and monoclonal antibodies.[27]

Radiation may be used postoperatively as an adjuvant to colon resection and chemotherapy or as a palliative measure for patients with advanced lesions. As a palliative measure, its primary objective is to reduce tumor size and provide symptomatic relief. (For discussion on radiation therapy, see Chapter 15.)

NURSING MANAGEMENT
COLORECTAL CANCER

■ Nursing Assessment

Subjective and objective data that should be obtained from a patient with colorectal cancer are presented in Table 41-31.

■ Nursing Diagnoses

Nursing diagnoses for the patient with cancer of the colon or rectum include, but are not limited to, the following:

- Diarrhea or constipation *related to* altered bowel elimination patterns
- Acute pain *related to* difficulty in passing stools because of partial or complete obstruction from tumor
- Fear *related to* diagnosis of colorectal cancer, surgical or therapeutic interventions, and possible terminal illness
- Ineffective coping *related to* diagnosis of cancer and side effects of treatment

TABLE 41-31	*Nursing Assessment* **Colorectal Cancer**

Subjective Data
Important Health Information
Past health history: Previous breast or ovarian cancer, familial polyposis, villous adenoma, adenomatous polyps, inflammatory bowel disease
Medications: Use of any medications affecting bowel function (e.g., cathartics, antidiarrheal drugs)
Functional Health Patterns
Health perception–health management: Family history of colorectal, breast, or ovarian cancer; weakness, fatigue
Nutritional-metabolic: High-calorie, high-fat, low-fiber diet; anorexia, weight loss; nausea and vomiting
Elimination: Change in bowel habits; alternating diarrhea and constipation, defecation urgency; rectal bleeding; mucoid stools; black, tarry stools; increased flatus, decrease in stool caliber; feelings of incomplete evacuation
Cognitive-perceptual: Abdominal and low back pain, tenesmus

Objective Data
General
Pallor, cachexia, lymphadenopathy (later signs)
Gastrointestinal
Palpable abdominal mass, distention, ascites, and hepatomegaly (liver metastasis)
Possible Findings
Anemia; guaiac-positive stools, palpable mass on digital rectal examination; positive sigmoidoscopy, colonoscopy, barium enema, or CT scan; positive biopsy

NURSING RESEARCH
Demands of Colorectal Cancer

Citation Klemm P, Miller MA, Fernsler J: Demands of illness in people treated for colorectal cancer, *Oncol Nurs Forum* 27:633, 2000.

Purpose To describe the most common and intense demands of illness in patients with colorectal cancer.

Methods Patients who were treated for colorectal cancer were recruited through online computer postings. Patients (n = 121) were mailed Demands of Illness Inventory and demographic questionnaires that were returned to the investigators. Respondents were from 35 states and 5 countries.

Results and Conclusions Overall the greatest demands reported were related to psychosocial and existential concerns. The demands of illness were greatest in the personal meaning domain with 93% of patients reporting that they thought about the value of life and how long they might live and 83% reported uncertainty. Younger patients (<45 years of age) reported more demands than older patients. Time since treatment, perception of illness, and activity level all influenced the demands of illness scores.

Implications for Nursing Practice Patients with colorectal cancer experience a number of physical and psychologic challenges, especially the younger patients. Nurses need to address these concerns with patients, as well as provide interventions to reduce the psychologic distress associated with the diagnosis and treatment of colorectal cancer.

■ Planning

The overall goals are that the patient with colorectal cancer will have (1) normal bowel elimination patterns, (2) quality of life appropriate to disease progression, (3) relief of pain, and (4) feelings of comfort and well-being.

■ Nursing Implementation

Health Promotion. The current recommendations from the American Cancer Society for colorectal cancer screening in patients who are not at high risk include annual digital rectal examination beginning at the age of 50 years. Starting at the age of 50 years, fecal testing for occult blood should be done every year, and flexible sigmoidoscopy should be performed every 5 years. Positive findings should be followed with colonoscopy or double-contrast barium enema.[24]

Screening for high-risk patients should begin before age 50, usually beginning with colonoscopy and continuing at more frequent intervals that vary according to risk factors.[24] Participation in early cancer screening is effective in decreasing mortality, but barriers exist, including lack of information and fear of diagnosis.[28]

Recent epidemiology studies reported that use of NSAIDs (e.g., sulindac [Clinoril], ibuprofen [Motrin])[29] or long-term use of aspirin (four to six tablets per day)[30] may reduce the risk of colorectal cancer.

Acute Intervention

Preoperative care. Acute nursing care for the patient with a colon resection is similar to care of the patient having a laparotomy (see NCP 41-2). In addition to general preoperative teaching and ostomy care instructions, the patient undergoing abdominal-perineal resection should be informed of the extent of the surgical procedure and the amount of care necessary to facilitate complete wound healing. The patient should be taught side-to-side positioning and made to understand that short walks are better than sitting. The nurse should teach and assist the patient in proper positioning for taking a sitz bath. The patient may not know that the sitz bath and positioning are sources of comfort. The patient may experience phantom rectal sensation because the sympathetic nerves responsible for rectal control are not severed during the surgery. The nurse must be astute in distinguishing phantom sensations from perineal abscess pain.

Postoperative care. After an abdominal-perineal resection, there are two wounds, and a stoma is surgically constructed in the left lower quadrant. There is an abdominal incision through which the colon is resected, and an incision is made in the perineum. The management of a perineal incision differs depending on the type of wound. Three techniques are used: (1) packing of the entire open wound, (2) partial closure with Penrose drains for open drainage, and (3) primary closure of the perineal wound with closed-suction drainage of the pelvic cavity. The type of management of the perineal wound is individualized. The open and packed method is used in patients with extensive surgery or uncontrollable bleeding in the pelvic wound. When infection or contamination is minimal, a partial closure with drains is used. Wound sites connected to low intermittent suction or a Jackson-Pratt or Hemovac suction placed in the perineal wound is commonly used to provide drainage of the operative site during the

EVIDENCE-BASED PRACTICE
Follow-up for Patients with Colorectal Cancer

Clinical Problem

Does intensive follow-up of patients with nonmetastatic colorectal cancer improve survival?

Best Clinical Practice

- Considerable controversy exists about how often patients should be seen and what tests should be performed after surgery for colorectal cancer in patients with no evidence of metastatic disease at the time of surgery.
- Results of a review of five randomized controlled clinical trials suggest there is an overall survival benefit for intensifying the follow-up of patients, including visits to health care provider and diagnostic studies (e.g., liver imaging).
- Ongoing clinical trials will investigate the best combination and frequency of clinical visits, blood tests, endoscopic procedures, and other diagnostic tests to maximize the outcomes for these patients.

Implication for Nursing Practice

Patients may assume their surgery was "curative" and not feel the necessity to return for periodic follow-up evaluations. It is very important that nurses emphasize the value of follow-up visits to a health care provider after surgery for colorectal cancer.

Reference for Evidence

Jeffery GM, Hickey BE, Hider P: Follow-up strategies for patients treated for non-metastatic colorectal cancer, *Cochrane Database of Systematic Reviews*, Issue 2, 2002.

early postoperative period. This usually remains until drainage is less than 50 ml per 24 hours, which occurs after approximately 3 to 5 days.

A patient who has open and packed wounds requires meticulous postoperative care. During the immediate postoperative period the perineal dressing is reinforced and changed frequently because drainage can be profuse for several hours after surgery. All drainage is carefully assessed for amount, color, and consistency. The drainage is usually serosanguineous.

The packing is usually left in place for 2 to 3 days. Packing the pelvic cavity for prolonged periods may result in sepsis and rigidity of the cavity wall and thus impede the healing process. The nurse should examine the wound regularly and record bleeding, excessive drainage, and unusual odor. The perineal wound is usually irrigated with a normal saline solution when the dressings are changed. Dressings are changed several times a day, and aseptic technique is always used.

If the wound is partially closed and drains are in place, the nurse assesses the incision for suture integrity and signs and symptoms of wound inflammation and infection. The drainage is examined for amount, color, and characteristics. When the primary closure technique is used, the catheters are left in place for approximately 3 to 5 days, and during this time the drainage is examined and observations recorded. The area around the catheter is observed for signs of inflammation and kept clean and dry. The nurse should observe for signs of edema, erythema, drainage around the suture line, fever, and elevated WBC count. If the perineal wound was not closed, warm sitz baths at 100.4° to 106° F (38° to 41° C) for 10 to 20 minutes three to four times a day assist in tissue debridement, provide comfort, and increase circulation to the area. Moist heat causes vasodilation, which allows more oxygen to flow to the affected area. Sitz baths of more than 20 minutes may result in too much vasodilation, causing congestion and discomfort.

The patient may complain of pain and itching in and around the wound. There is no physiologic explanation of sensations that are felt, but a careful examination should be made to rule out delayed wound healing. Antipruritic agents and sitz baths are usually ordered. Use of a pressure-reducing chair cushion provides comfort when sitting. Sitting on a toilet for prolonged periods is discouraged until the perineal wound is well healed.

Sexual dysfunction is a possible complication of an abdominal-perineal resection and should be included in the plan of care. Although the effect of the procedure depends on the technique used, the surgeon should discuss the subject intelligently and tactfully, with follow-up as necessary by other members of the health care team. The nurse should understand that erection, ejaculation, and orgasm involve different nerve pathways and that a dysfunction of one does not mean total sexual dysfunction. The ET nurse is an important member of the team and can often provide correct and factual information concerning sexual dysfunction resulting from an abdominal-perineal resection.

Ambulatory and Home Care. Psychologic support for the patient and family is important. The recovery period is long, and the possibility of recurrence of cancer is always present. The overall 5-year survival rate for all patients undergoing resection for colorectal cancer is less than 50%. This presents a problem for the patient and health care providers because of the often painful, debilitating, and demoralizing manifestations produced by the recurrent disease and the lack of any effective palliative

therapy. Chemotherapy may be used as an adjuvant measure for the patient with evidence of local or distant metastasis. (The special needs of the cancer patient are discussed in Chapter 15.)

The perineal wound may not be completely healed before discharge. After discharge the health care provider, the home health nurse, and the ET nurse in an outpatient clinic usually see the patient. The wound is usually irrigated and debrided. The skin around the wound should be assessed for loose hair. Shaving may be necessary to prevent the development of a chronic draining sinus. The nurse should report the drainage because it may also indicate the presence of a foreign body, fistula, or rectal tissue not removed during surgery. The patient and significant others are taught management of the wound and the procedure to take a sitz bath at home. The patient and the family should be aware of all community services available for assistance.

■ Evaluation

The expected outcomes for the patient with colorectal cancer are that the patient will have
- minimal alterations in bowel elimination patterns
- relief of pain
- balanced nutritional intake
- quality of life appropriate to disease progression
- feelings of comfort and well-being

OSTOMY SURGERY

Types

An **ostomy** is a surgical procedure in which an opening is made to allow the passage of intestinal contents from the bowel to an incision or stoma. The stoma, which is the opening on the surface of the abdomen, is created when the intestine is brought through the abdominal wall and sutured to the skin. It may be permanent or temporary. Fecal matter is diverted through the stoma to the outside of the abdominal wall.

An *ileostomy* is an opening from the ileum through the abdominal wall and is also referred to as a conventional or Brooke ileostomy (Fig. 41-11). It is most commonly used in surgical treatment of ulcerative colitis, Crohn's disease, and familial polyposis.

A *cecostomy* is an opening between the cecum and the abdominal wall. Both cecostomies and ascending colostomies are uncommon. They are usually temporary and most often are used for fecal diversion before surgery or for palliation.

A *colostomy* is an opening between the colon and the abdominal wall. The proximal end of the colon is sutured to the skin. Locations for colostomies are shown in Fig. 41-11. A temporary colostomy is usually performed to protect an end-to-end anastomosis after a bowel resection or is an emergency measure following bowel obstruction (e.g., malignant tumor), abdominal trauma (e.g., gunshot wound), or a perforated diverticulum. Temporary colostomies are usually located in the transverse colon. Loop colostomy (Fig. 41-12) and double-barrel colostomy (see Fig. 41-11) are most commonly performed as temporary colostomies, but they may be permanent. A comparison of colostomies and ileostomy is shown in Table 41-32.

Surgical Therapy

End stoma. An end stoma is surgically constructed by dividing the bowel and bringing out the proximal end as a single stoma. The distal portion of the GI tract is surgically removed, or the distal segment is oversewn and left in the abdominal cavity with its

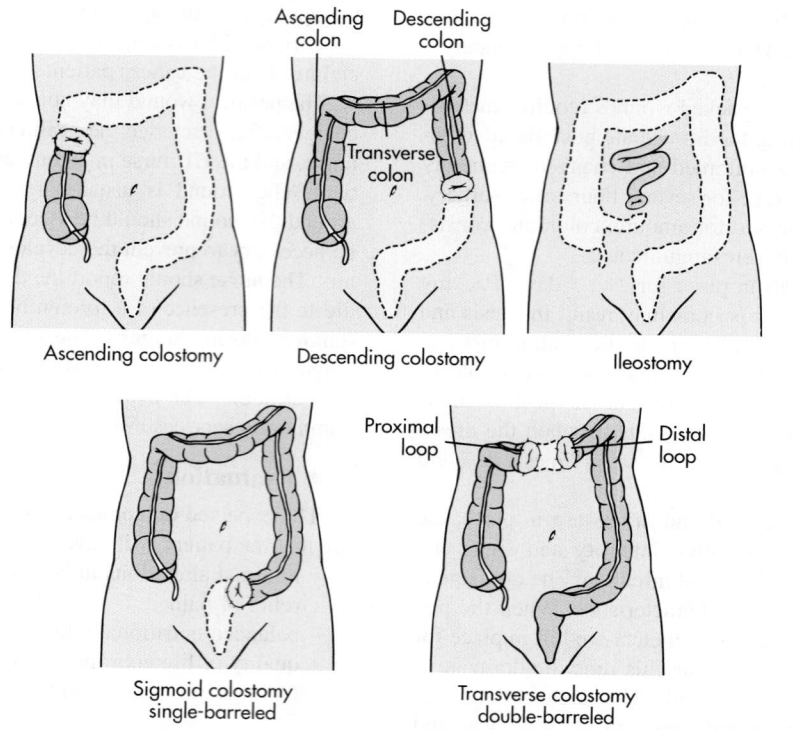

Ascending colon   Descending colon

Transverse colon

Ascending colostomy   Descending colostomy   Ileostomy

Proximal loop   Distal loop

Sigmoid colostomy
single-barreled

Transverse colostomy
double-barreled

FIG. 41-11 Types of ostomies.

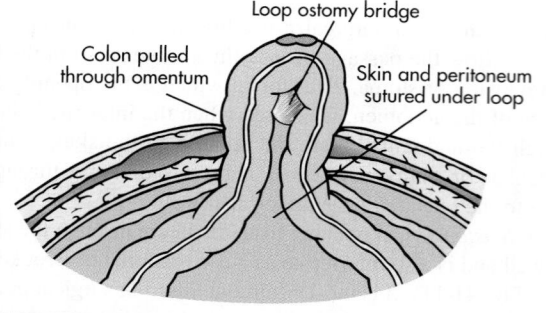

Loop ostomy bridge

Colon pulled
through omentum

Skin and peritoneum
sutured under loop

FIG. 41-12 Loop colostomy.

mesentery intact. An end colostomy or ileostomy is then constructed. When the distal bowel is oversewn rather than removed, the procedure is known as a Hartmann's pouch (Fig. 41-13). If the distal bowel is removed, the stoma is permanent; if the distal bowel remains intact and oversewn, the potential exists for the bowel to be reanastomosed and the stoma to be closed (referred to as a *takedown*).

Loop stoma. A loop stoma is constructed by bringing a loop of bowel to the abdominal surface and then opening the anterior wall of the bowel to provide fecal diversion. This results in one stoma with a proximal and distal opening and an intact posterior

TABLE 41-32   Comparison of Colostomies and Ileostomy

| | COLOSTOMY | | | |
	ASCENDING	TRANSVERSE	SIGMOID	ILEOSTOMY
Stool consistency	Semiliquid	Semiliquid to semiformed	Formed	Liquid to semiliquid
Fluid requirement	Increased	Possibly increased	No change	Increased
Bowel regulation	No	Uncommon	Yes (if there is a history of a regular bowel pattern)	No
Pouch and skin barriers	Yes	Yes	Dependent on regulation	Yes
Irrigation	No	No	Possible every 24–48 hr (if patient meets criteria)	No
Indications for surgery	Perforating diverticulitis in lower colon; trauma; inoperable tumors of colon, rectum, or pelvis; rectovaginal fistula	Same as for ascending; birth defect	Cancer of the rectum or rectosigmoidal area; perforating diverticulum; trauma	Ulcerative colitis, Crohn's disease, diseased or injured colon, birth defect, familial polyposis, trauma, cancer

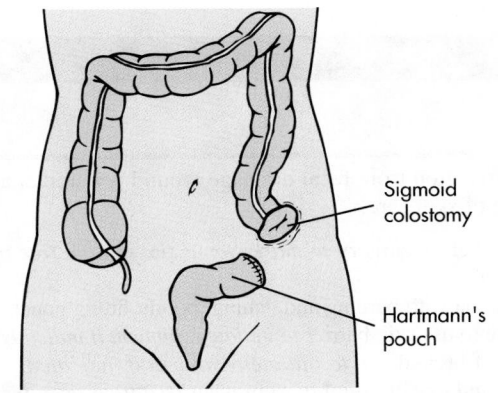

FIG. 41-13 Sigmoid colostomy. Distal bowel is oversewn and left in place to create Hartmann's pouch.

Sigmoid colostomy

Hartmann's pouch

wall that separates the two openings. The loop of bowel is frequently held in place with a plastic rod for 7 to 10 days after surgery to prevent it from slipping back into the abdominal cavity (see Fig. 41-12). A loop stoma is usually temporary.

Double-barrel stoma. When the bowel is divided, both the proximal and distal ends are brought through the abdominal wall as two separate stomas (see Fig. 41-11). The proximal one is the functioning stoma; the distal, nonfunctioning stoma is referred to as the mucus fistula. The double-barrel stoma is usually temporary.

Kock pouch. As described previously in this chapter (see pp. 1071-1072), the *Kock pouch* is a continent ileostomy, which is a variation from the traditional ileostomy (see Fig. 41-3).

Ileoanal reservoir. As previously described in this chapter (pp. 1071-1072), this procedure involves total colectomy and ileoanal anastomosis with the formation of an ileal reservoir (see Fig. 41-4).

NURSING MANAGEMENT
OSTOMY SURGERY

■ Preoperative Care

It is important to review the information the patient has received from the health care provider. Psychologic preparation is very important. The family and the patient usually have many questions concerning the procedures. If available, an ET nurse should visit with the patient and the family. The nurse or ET nurse must determine the patient's ability to perform self-care, identify support systems, and determine potential adverse factors that could be modified to facilitate learning during rehabilitation. Preoperative assessment must be comprehensive and include physical, psychologic, social, cultural, and educational components. Assessment is ongoing, including both the patient and family. The ET nurse marks the stoma site before surgery. An improperly placed stoma complicates rehabilitation by increasing time and expense of pouch change routine. It can also contribute to skin irritation and poor adaptation. The patient and the family should understand the extent of surgery, the type of stoma, and its care.

If the patient desires a referral and the health care provider agrees, a trained ostomy visitor from the United Ostomy Association can provide meaningful psychologic support. The patient has the opportunity to see a person who has adjusted well and who has experienced some of the same feelings and concerns. The family will also benefit from the visit.

Bowel preparation before surgery decreases the chance of a postoperative infection by cleansing the bowel of feces and bacteria. Orally administered osmotic lavages (e.g., Go-Lytely) have shortened the classic 72-hour preparation with clear liquids, cathartics, and enemas. IV and oral antibiotics are given. Nonabsorbable neomycin and erythromycin are given orally to decrease the number of intracolonic bacteria.

■ Colostomy Care

Postoperative nursing care should focus on assessing the stoma, protecting the skin, selecting the pouch, and assisting the patient to adapt psychologically to a changed body. Nursing care for the patient with a colostomy is presented in NCP 41-4.

The stoma should be pink. A dusky blue stoma indicates ischemia, and a brown-black stoma indicates necrosis. The nurse should assess and document stoma color every 8 hours. There is mild to moderate swelling of the stoma the first 2 to 3 weeks after surgery (Table 41-33). A skin barrier should be applied to protect the peristomal skin surrounding the stoma. Solid skin barriers include Stomahesive (Convatec), Coloplast, and Hollister skin barriers. The skin should be washed with mild soap, rinsed with warm water, and dried thoroughly before the barrier is applied.

TABLE 41-33	**Characteristics of Stoma**
CHARACTERISTIC	**DESCRIPTION OR CAUSE**
Color*	
Rose to brick red	Viable stoma mucosa
Pale	May indicate anemia
Blanching, dark red to purple	Indicates inadequate blood supply to the stoma or bowel from adhesions, low flow state, or excessive tension on the bowel at the time of construction
Edema†	
Mild to moderate edema	Normal in the initial postoperative period
	Trauma to the stoma
	Any medical condition that results in edema
Moderate to severe edema	Obstruction of the stoma
	Allergic reaction to food
	Gastroenteritis
Bleeding	
Small amount	Oozing from the stoma mucosa when touched is normal because of its high vascularity
Moderate to large amount‡	Moderate to large amount‡ of bleeding from the stoma mucosa could indicate coagulation factor deficiency; stomal varices secondary to portal hypertension
	Moderate to large amount from intestinal stoma opening could indicate lower gastrointestinal bleeding

*Sustained color changes must be reported to surgeon.
†Closely observe and report to the surgeon and adjust the stoma opening size in the pouch.
‡Report moderate to large amounts of bleeding to surgeon.

NURSING CARE PLAN 41-4

Patient with a Colostomy/Ileostomy

EXPECTED PATIENT OUTCOMES	NURSING INTERVENTIONS and *RATIONALES*
NURSING DIAGNOSIS	**Risk for impaired skin integrity** *related to* irritation from fecal drainage around peristomal area, irritation of appliance, and lack of knowledge of skin care.
• Normal skin integrity • Intact pouch seal	• Have enterostomal therapy nurse see patient before surgery *to mark stoma site in area free of creases and folds for better seal of the pouch.* • After surgery, assess peristomal skin for erythema with burning and itching, poorly fitting pouch with leakage, lack of adequate skin care, and failure to use skin barrier *to initiate treatment if indicated.* • During pouch change, assess skin for signs of breakdown *to initiate treatment if indicated.* • Clean area with mild soap and water, rinse, and dry thoroughly *to prevent irritation from intestinal contents or pouch adhesive.* • Apply skin barrier *to protect skin and prevent direct contact with intestinal contents.* • Teach patient proper skin and appliance care *to ensure proper technique for long-term care.* • Plan for outpatient or home visit *for continued teaching and monitoring.* • Empty pouch when it is one third to one half full or inflated with gas *to prevent the pouch from leaking.*
NURSING DIAGNOSIS	**Disturbed body image** *related to* presence of ostomy and malodor *as manifested by* verbalization of embarrassment or shame caused by malodor or presence of stoma.
• Adjustment to altered body image • Satisfactory plan for control of odor	• Assess patient's attitude toward ostomy *to determine if problem is present* and, if indicated, *plan appropriate intervention.* • Instruct patient on measures for odor control, use of odor-proof pouch, pouch deodorants, use of room deodorants when pouch is emptied, and avoidance of foods that are known to increase odor *to minimize embarrassing odors from drainage.* • Discuss normal emotional response to stoma and encourage patient to express feelings *to assist patient in adjusting to change in body.* • Provide patient with information on local United Ostomy Association *to offer patient and family an opportunity for education and support.* • Prepare patient to do own stoma and appliance care *to increase independence and enhance self-esteem/image.*
NURSING DIAGNOSIS	**Imbalanced nutrition: less than body requirements** *related to* lack of knowledge of appropriate foods and decreased appetite *as manifested by* weight loss, vitamin and mineral deficiencies, inability to tolerate certain foods.
• Adequate dietary intake to maintain weight at optimum level	• Assess nutritional intake *to determine need for intervention.* • Gradually introduce foods one at a time *to identify individual foods that may be problematic* and begin with low-residue diet, *which is usually well-tolerated.* • Teach patient to chew food slowly and thoroughly *to facilitate digestion and prevent gas.* • Give list of foods (high roughage) that have potential for obstruction to ileostomy patients *so that patient has a ready source for reference.* • Arrange visit with dietitian if indicated.
NURSING DIAGNOSIS	**Ineffective sexuality patterns** *related to* perceived loss of sexual appeal and possibility of accidental seepage of fecal material during sexual activity *as manifested by* verbalization of concern about intimate relations with spouse or significant other.
• Confidence in ability to resume previous sexual activity	• Assess patient's attitude about impact of ostomy on sexual functioning *to determine if a problem exists and if there is a need to plan interventions.* • Encourage discussion of meaning of sexuality to patient and significant other *to allow patient opportunity to discuss sensitive topic in a nonthreatening situation.* • Discuss ways to avoid seepage and conceal stoma and/or appliance during intimate relations *to decrease fear of embarrassment or withdrawal from intimate situations because of anxiety over "accidents."* • If appropriate, arrange visit with person of same sex and condition *to discuss sexual concerns and share potential solutions; to provide an opportunity to ask questions; and to get practical, realistic answers from a supportive, understanding other.* • Encourage use of perfumes or fragrant body oils during sexual activity *to decrease fear of having an offensive body odor.*

NURSING CARE PLAN 41-4

Patient with a Colostomy/Ileostomy—cont'd

EXPECTED PATIENT OUTCOMES	NURSING INTERVENTIONS and *RATIONALES*
NURSING DIAGNOSIS	**Risk for deficient fluid volume** *related to* excess fluid loss from ileostomy or diarrhea with a colostomy and inadequate oral intake.
▪ Normal serum electrolytes ▪ Normal vital signs ▪ Good skin turgor ▪ Urine output >0.5 ml/kg/hr	▪ Assess for signs of weakness, poor skin turgor, sunken eyes, hypotension, tachycardia, hypokalemia, hyponatremia, oliguria *to determine presence of fluid volume deficit and, if present, plan appropriate interventions.* ▪ Record intake and output and include ileostomy drainage *to have an accurate record of fluid balance.* ▪ Ensure fluid intake of at least 3000 ml/day in the initial postoperative period *to prevent dehydration.* ▪ Instruct patient to maintain high fluid intake and to increase it during very hot weather, when patient is perspiring excessively, and during episodes of diarrhea *to ensure adequate fluid intake in various situations.* ▪ Monitor serum electrolytes *to detect any imbalances.* ▪ Instruct patient on signs and symptoms of sodium, potassium, and fluid deficits *to ensure early reporting and correction of underlying problem.*

With an open-ended, transparent, plastic, odor-proof pouch, it is easy to protect the skin and to observe and collect the drainage. The pouch must fit snugly to prevent leakage around the stoma. The size of the stoma is determined with a stoma-measuring card. Although the pouch is applied after surgery, the colostomy functions when peristalsis has been adequately restored. When a temporary colostomy is performed and the stoma is opened in the operating room with no bowel preparation being done previously, the stoma functions immediately.

The volume, color, and consistency of the drainage are recorded. Each time the pouch is changed, the condition of the skin is observed for irritation. A pouch should never be placed directly on irritated skin without the use of a skin barrier.

A colostomy in the ascending and transverse colon has semiliquid stools. The patient needs to be instructed to use a drainable pouch. A colostomy in the sigmoid or descending colon has semiformed or formed stools and can sometimes be regulated by the irrigation method. The patient may or may not wear a drainage pouch. A nondrainable pouch should have a gas filter.

For most patients with colostomies, there are few, if any, dietary restrictions. A well-balanced diet and adequate fluid intake are important. The patient's medical and surgical history must be considered when individualizing dietary instructions. Table 41-34 lists foods and their effects on stoma output.

Colostomy Irrigations. Colostomy irrigations are intended to regulate bowel function, treat constipation, or prepare the bowel for surgery. When done to achieve a regular bowel pattern, the irrigations stimulate the bowel to function at a specific time every day or every other day. If control is achieved, there should be little or no spillage between irrigations. The patient who establishes regularity may need to wear only a pad or small pouch over the stoma. The patient who cannot or chooses not to establish regularity by irrigations must wear a pouch at all times. The procedure for colostomy irrigation is presented in Table 41-35.

All equipment should be assembled before the irrigation. A commercially obtained irrigation set usually has all the equipment needed. The nurse should encourage the patient to watch

TABLE 41-34	Nutritional Therapy **Effects of Food on Stoma Output**

Odor Producing*	**Diarrhea Causing***
Eggs	Alcohol
Garlic	Beer
Onions	Cabbage family
Fish	Spinach
Asparagus	Green beans
Cabbage	Coffee
Broccoli	Spicy foods
Alcohol	Fruits (raw)
Gas Forming*	**Potential Obstruction in Ileostomy†**
Beans	Nuts
Cabbage family	Raisins
Onions	Popcorn
Beer	Seeds
Carbonated beverages	Vegetables (raw)
Cheeses (strong)	Celery
Sprouts	Corn

*The effect of food on stoma output is individual. Patients are not discouraged from eating the above-listed foods and beverages.
†Patients are encouraged to chew high-roughage food well and initially limit the amount, and to drink increased amounts of fluids.

the procedure and should explain each step to the patient. The cone tip on the tubing controls the depth of insertion and prevents the water from coming out from the stoma and not going into the colon. If resistance is met, force should not be used because perforation of the intestine can result. However, this is unlikely when using a stoma cone. A hard plastic catheter is not recommended because of the risk of intestinal perforation. The procedure should not be rushed; the patient should feel relaxed. The patient or family member must be instructed in the procedure and

Patient & Family Teaching Guide

TABLE 41-35   **Colostomy Irrigation**

Equipment
Lubricant
Irrigation set (1000- to 2000-ml container, tubing with irrigating stoma cone, clamp)
Irrigating sleeve with adhesive or belt
Toilet tissue to clean around the stoma
Disposal sack for soiled dressing

Procedure
1. Place 500 to 1000 ml of lukewarm water (not to exceed 105° F [40.5° C]) in container. The volume is titrated for the individual; use enough irrigant to distend the bowel but not enough to cause cramping pain. Most adults use 500 to 1000 ml of water.
2. Ensure comfortable position. Patient may sit in chair in front of toilet or on the toilet if the perineal wound is healed.
3. Clear tubing of all air by flushing it with fluid.
4. Hang container on hook or IV pole (18 to 24 inches) above stoma (about shoulder height).
5. Apply irrigating sleeve and place bottom end in toilet bowl.
6. Lubricate stoma cone, insert cone tip gently into the stoma, and hold tip securely in place.
7. Allow irrigation solution to flow in steadily for 5 to 10 minutes.
8. If cramping occurs, stop the flow of solution for a few seconds, leaving the cone in place.
9. Clamp the tubing and remove irrigating cone when the desired amount of irrigant has been delivered or when the patient senses colonic distention.
10. Allow 30 to 45 minutes for the solution and feces to be expelled. Initial evacuation is usually complete in 10 to 15 minutes. Close off the irrigating sleeve at the bottom to allow ambulation.
11. Clean, rinse, and dry peristomal skin well.
12. Replace the colostomy drainage pouch or desired stoma covering.
13. Wash and rinse all equipment and hang to dry.

Patient & Family Teaching Guide

TABLE 41-36   **Ostomy Self-Care**

The following are guidelines to include for patient and family teaching:
1. Explain the following principles of ostomy and pouch care
   - Apply and change pouch to collect intestinal drainage.
   - Empty pouch before it is one-third full to prevent leakage.
   - Cleanse skin and use skin barriers and deodorizers to prevent skin breakdown and malodor.
   - Irrigate colostomy to regulate bowel elimination (optional).
   - Explain how to contact the enterostomal therapy nurse with questions.
   - Explain how to obtain additional supplies.
2. Teach the following dietary and fluid intake guidelines
   - Identify a well-balanced diet and dietary supplements to prevent nutritional deficiencies.
   - Identify foods to avoid to reduce diarrhea, gas, or obstruction (with ileostomy).
   - Drink at least 3000 ml/day of fluid to prevent dehydration (unless contraindicated).
   - Increase fluid intake during hot weather, excessive perspiration, and diarrhea to replace losses and prevent dehydration.
   - Explain how to contact registered dietitian with questions.
3. Describe potential resources to assist with emotional and psychologic adjustment
   - Identify persons available to provide emotional support.
   - Identify community resources for psychologic counseling.
   - Contact United Ostomy Association for information or peer support.
   - Inform that treatment for potential depression is available if needed.
4. Explain the importance of follow-up care
   Report signs and symptoms of:
   - Fluid and electrolyte deficits
   - Fever
   - Diarrhea
   - Skin irritation
   - Other stoma problems, including a change in appearance of the stoma or its function, a change in the peristomal area, tenderness, erythema, or pain

must be able to demonstrate the ability to irrigate before being independent. This can be done in the outpatient setting.

The patient should be able to perform a pouch change, care for skin, control odor, care for the stoma, and identify signs and symptoms of complications. The patient should know the importance of fluids and food in the diet, have names and addresses of the United Ostomy Association, and know when to seek medical care. Home care and outpatient follow-up by an ET nurse is highly recommended. Patients should be discharged with written instructions for pouch change, teaching literature relevant to the type of stoma they have, a list of equipment they use, a list of equipment retailers (including names and phone numbers), outpatient follow-up appointments with the surgeon and ET nurse, and the phone numbers of the surgeon and nurse. The patient and family teaching guidelines are included in Table 41-36.

■ Ileostomy Care

Care of the ileostomy is presented in NCP 41-4. An ileostomy stoma protrusion of at least 1 to 1.5 cm makes care easier. When the stoma is flat, seepage occurs, resulting in altered skin integrity. Drainage is frequent and extremely irritating to the skin. Regularity cannot be established. A pouch must be worn at all times. An open-ended, drainable pouch is worn by the patient so that drainage can be emptied when one-third full. The drainable pouch is usually worn for 4 to 7 days before being changed as long as leakage does not occur around the stoma. If pouch leakage occurs, the pouch should be promptly removed, the skin should be cleansed, and a new pouch placed. A solid skin barrier should always be used. A transparent pouch should be used in the initial postoperative period to facilitate assessment of stoma viability and ease of pouch application by the patient.

Immediately after surgery, intake and output must be accurately monitored. The patient should be observed for signs and symptoms of fluid and electrolyte imbalance, particularly potassium, sodium, and fluid deficits. In the first 24 to 48 hours after surgery the amount of drainage from the stoma may be negligible. A person with an ileostomy has lost the absorptive functions provided by the colon, as well as the delay feature provided by the ileocecal valve. Once peristalsis returns, the patient may experience a period of high-volume output of 1000 to 1800 ml per day. Later on, the average amount can be 800 ml daily because the proximal small bowel adapts. If the small bowel has been shortened as a result of surgical resections, the drainage from the ileostomy may be greater. The patient must understand the importance of fluid and electrolyte balance.

The patient should be instructed to drink at least 2 to 3 L of fluid daily; more may be necessary when diarrhea occurs and when perspiration is increased. Diarrhea from an ileostomy produces acidosis from the loss of bicarbonate. The health care provider may instruct the patient to take an electrolyte solution at home (e.g., 1 teaspoon of salt and 1 teaspoon of baking soda in 1 quart of water). Fluids rich in electrolytes should be encouraged.

Usually a low-roughage diet is ordered initially. Fiber-containing foods are reintroduced gradually. Later there are no dietary restrictions. It is important to limit the amount of high-roughage foods (e.g., popcorn), chew them well, and accompany them with fluids. The goal for the patient is a return to a normal, presurgical diet.

The stoma may bleed easily when it is touched because it has a high vascular supply. The patient should be told that minimal oozing of blood is normal. If the terminal ileum has been removed, the patient may need cobalamin (vitamin B_{12}) injections.

■ Adaptation to an Ostomy

Adaptation to the ostomy is a gradual process. The patient experiences a grief reaction to the loss of a body part and an alteration in body image. Each person uses different coping mechanisms. The adjustment period for the person depends on the individual. Psychologic support during the grieving process is needed. There are concerns about body image, sexual activity, family responsibilities, and changes in lifestyle. The patient may become resentful and have fears of odor or soiling. Supportive measures by nurses include helping the patient acquire knowledge, providing or recommending support services, and identifying coping mechanisms that are effective. The nurse provides support by responding to the physiologic needs of stoma care and the psychosocial needs of self-esteem.

The patient should not be forced to learn to care for the stoma. The nurse should watch for clues that the patient is ready. Teaching at the appropriate time is an important part of the care and can contribute to a smooth adjustment process.

Activities of daily living are resumed within 6 to 8 weeks. Heavy lifting should be avoided. The patient's physical condition determines when sports may be resumed. Bathing and swimming are not prohibited. Water does not harm the stoma.

■ Sexual Dysfunction after Ostomy Surgery

Discussion of sexuality and sexual function must be incorporated in the plan of care. The nurse can help the patient understand that sexual function or sexual activity may be affected, but sexuality does not have to be altered.

Pelvic surgery can disrupt nerve and vascular supply to the genitals. Radiation, chemotherapy, and medications can also alter sexual function. Hormones and overall physical health of the patient influence desire. Certain pain medications and antiemetics can lower the sex drive. Generalized fatigue caused by illness can also influence desire. By communicating this information to patients, they can plan sexual activity around a drug schedule and energy levels. Any pelvic surgery that removes the rectum has the potential of damaging the parasympathetic nerve plexus. Erection in men depends on the parasympathetic nerves that control blood flow and vascular supply to the pelvis and the pudendal nerves that transmit sensory responses from the genital area. Nerve-sparing surgical techniques are used when possible to preserve sexual function. Radiation therapy to the pelvis can reduce blood vascularity to the pelvis by causing scarring in the small blood vessels. A woman's sexual functioning after healing includes expansion and lubrication of the vagina. Pelvic surgery usually does not affect a woman's arousal unless part of or the entire vagina is removed. Radiation therapy can affect vaginal expansion and lubrication.

Muscular contraction and genital pleasure that occur during orgasm are not disrupted by pelvic surgery. If the sympathetic nerves in the presacral area are damaged, the male mechanism of emission can be disrupted. This can occur in an abdominal-perineal resection. Orgasms can occur in both men and women who have had stoma surgery, although other aspects of the sexual response may be affected.

The psychologic impact of the stoma and how it affects the patient's body image and self-esteem must be discussed. Emotional factors can contribute to sexual problems. A life-threatening illness can override concerns about sexual function. The nurse can assist a patient to identify ways of coping with depression and anxiety resulting from illness, surgery, or postoperative problems.

The social impact of the stoma is interrelated with the psychologic, physical, and sexual aspects. Concerns of people with stomas include the ability to resume sexual activity, altering clothing styles, the effect on daily activities, sleeping while wearing a pouch, passing gas, the presence of odor, cleanliness, and deciding when or if to tell others about the stoma. The fear of rejection from a partner or the fear that others will not find them desirable as a sexual partner can be a concern. The nurse should encourage open communication about feelings and should realize that the patient needs time to adjust to the pouch and to body changes before feeling secure in his or her sexual functioning.

Although pregnancy is possible, the health care provider may recommend a limited number of pregnancies on the basis of the patient's physical condition. The person with an ostomy who becomes pregnant should have regular medical care.

DIVERTICULOSIS AND DIVERTICULITIS

A **diverticulum** is a saccular dilation or outpouching of the mucosa through the circular smooth muscle of the intestinal wall. Clinically, diverticular disease occurs in two forms: diverticulosis and diverticulitis. Multiple noninflamed diverticula are present with *diverticulosis*. The patient is most often free of symptoms but may have some abdominal discomfort. In *diverticulitis*, inflammation of the diverticula occurs (Fig. 41-14). Diverticula may occur at any point within the GI tract but are most commonly found in the sigmoid colon.

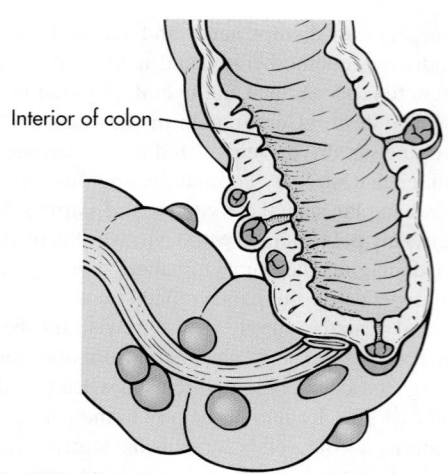

FIG. 41-14 Diverticula are outpouchings of the colon. When they become inflamed, the condition is diverticulitis. The inflammatory process can spread to the surrounding area in the intestine.

Etiology and Pathophysiology

Diverticular disease is a common GI disorder that affects 5% of the population by the age of 40 years and 50% by the age of 80 years.[31] It affects men and women equally, but men seem to have a higher complication rate. Although it affects almost 30 million Americans, most are asymptomatic.

There is no known cause of diverticular disease, but deficiency in dietary fiber has been associated with it. The disease is more prevalent in Western populations that consume diets low in fiber and high in refined carbohydrates, and it is virtually unknown in areas of the world, such as rural Africa, where high-fiber diets are consumed.

When diverticula form, the smooth muscle of the colon wall becomes thickened (Fig. 41-15). Lack of dietary fiber slows transit time, and more water is absorbed from the stool, making it more difficult to pass through the lumen. Decreased bulk of the stool, combined with a more narrowed lumen in the sigmoid colon, causes high intraluminal pressures. These factors are believed to contribute to the formation of diverticula.

The cause of diverticulitis is related to the retention of stool and bacteria in the diverticulum, forming a hardened mass called a *fecalith*. This causes inflammation and usually small perfora-

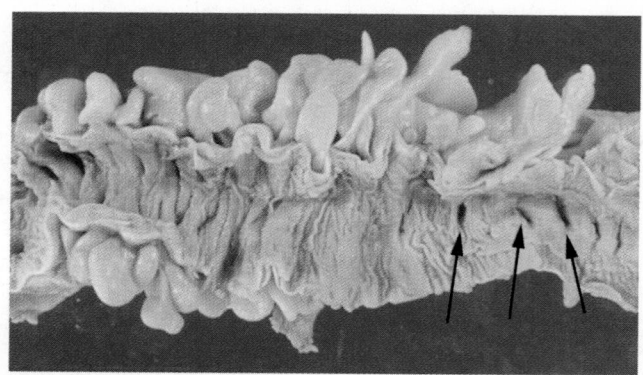

FIG. 41-15 In diverticular disease, the outpouches *(arrows)* of mucosa appear as slitlike openings from the mucosal surface of the open bowel.

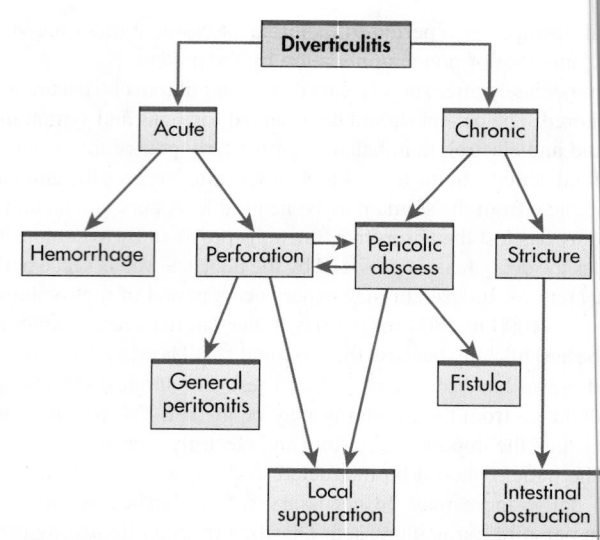

FIG. 41-16 Complications of diverticulitis.

tions. Inflammation of the diverticulum spreads to the surrounding area in the intestines (Fig. 41-16), causing the tissue to become edematous. Abscesses may form, or complete perforation with peritonitis may occur.

Clinical Manifestations

The majority of patients with diverticulosis have no symptoms. Those with symptoms typically have crampy abdominal pain located in the left lower quadrant that is usually relieved by passage of flatus or bowel movement. Alternating constipation and diarrhea may be present.

Approximately 15% of patients with diverticulosis progress to acute diverticulitis. In patients with diverticulitis, abdominal pain is localized over the involved area of the colon. A tender, left lower quadrant mass may be felt on palpation of the abdomen. Fever, chills, nausea, anorexia, and elevated WBC may be present. Elderly patients with diverticulitis are frequently afebrile, with a normal WBC, and little, if any, abdominal tenderness.

Complications of diverticulitis include perforation with peritonitis, abscess and fistula formation, bowel obstruction, ureteral obstruction, and bleeding. Bleeding is a common complication of diverticulitis and is manifested by *hematochezia* (maroon stools). Bleeding usually stops spontaneously.

Diagnostic Studies

A CT scan with oral contrast is the test of choice for diverticulitis.[31] A CBC, urinalysis, and fecal occult blood test should be performed (Table 41-37). A barium enema is used to determine narrowing or obstruction of the colonic lumen. A colonoscopy may be performed to rule out possible hidden polyps or lesions. A patient with acute diverticulitis should not have a barium enema or colonoscopy because of the possibility of perforation and peritonitis.

NURSING *and* COLLABORATIVE MANAGEMENT
DIVERTICULOSIS AND DIVERTICULITIS

Uncomplicated diverticular disease is treated with a high-fiber diet (see Table 41-9) and bulk laxatives, such as psyllium hydrophilic mucilloid (Metamucil). Anticholinergic drugs such as

TABLE 41-37	Collaborative Care Diverticulosis and Diverticulitis

Diagnostic
History and physical examination
Testing of stool for occult blood
Barium enema
Sigmoidoscopy
Colonoscopy
CBC
Urinalysis
Blood culture

Collaborative Therapy
Ambulatory and Home Care
High-residue diet
Dietary fiber supplements
Stool softeners
Anticholinergics
Mineral oil
Bed rest
Clear liquid diet
Oral antibiotics
Bulk laxatives
Acute Care: Diverticulitis
Antibiotics
NPO status
IV fluids
Possible colon resection for obstruction or hemorrhage
Bed rest
NG suction

CBC, Complete blood count; *IV,* intravenous; *NG,* nasogastric; *NPO,* nothing by mouth.

dicyclomine (Bentyl) and Donnatal may be used to relieve discomfort from spasm of the bowel (see Table 41-37).

Fluids should be increased because fibers retain water, thus decreasing the amount absorbed by the body. If the patient is obese, a reduction in weight is needed. Increased intraabdominal pressure should be avoided because it may precipitate an attack. Factors that increase intraabdominal pressure are straining at stool, vomiting, bending, lifting, and tight, restrictive clothing.

In acute diverticulitis, the goal of treatment is to allow the colon to rest and the inflammation to subside. The patient is kept on NPO status and bed rest and is given parenteral fluids. An NG tube may be necessary. The patient should be observed for signs of possible peritonitis. In acute diverticulitis, broad-spectrum antibiotic therapy is required. The WBC count is monitored.

When the acute attack subsides, oral fluids progressing to a semisolid diet are allowed. Ambulation is also permitted. At this stage the patient should be observed for a recurrent attack. If the patient has a bowel resection or colostomy, the nursing care is the same as for these procedures.

Approximately 30% of patients with acute diverticulitis require surgical intervention. Patients with complicated diverticular disease often require surgery. Surgical intervention is necessary to drain abscesses or to resect an obstructing inflammatory mass. The usual surgical procedures involve resection of the involved colon with a temporary diverting colostomy. The colostomy is reanastomosed after the colon is healed.

The patient should be provided with a full explanation of the condition. The better the patient understands the disease process and adheres to the prescribed regimen, the less likely the exacerbation of the disease and the onset of complications.

HERNIAS

A **hernia** is a protrusion of a viscus through an abnormal opening or a weakened area in the wall of the cavity in which it is normally contained. A hernia may occur in any part of the body, but it usually occurs within the abdominal cavity. If the hernia can be placed back into the abdominal cavity, it is known as *reducible.* The hernia can be reduced by manipulation, or it can occur without manipulation when the person lies down. If the hernia cannot be placed back into the abdominal cavity, it is known as *irreducible,* or incarcerated. In this situation the intestinal flow may be obstructed. When the hernia is irreducible and the intestinal flow and blood supply are obstructed, the hernia is strangulated. The result is an acute intestinal obstruction.

Types

The *inguinal hernia* is the most common type of hernia and occurs at the point of weakness in the abdominal wall where the spermatic cord in men and the round ligament in women emerge (Fig. 41-17). When the protrusion escapes through the inguinal ring and follows the spermatic cord or the round ligament, it is termed an *indirect* hernia. When it escapes through the posterior inguinal wall, it is a *direct* hernia. An inguinal hernia is more common in men.

A femoral hernia occurs when there is a protrusion through the femoral ring into the femoral canal. It occurs below the inguinal (Poupart's) ligament as a bulge. It becomes strangulated easily and occurs more often in women. The umbilical hernia occurs when the rectus muscle is weak or the umbilical opening fails to close after birth.

Ventral, or incisional, hernia is due to weakness of the abdominal wall at the site of a previous incision. It is found most commonly in patients who are obese, who have had multiple surgical procedures in the same area, and who have had inadequate wound healing because of poor nutrition or infection.

Clinical Manifestations

A hernia commonly occurs over the involved area when the patient stands or strains. There may be some discomfort as a result of tension. Severe pain is caused if the hernia becomes strangulated. In this situation, the clinical manifestations of a bowel obstruction, such as vomiting, crampy abdominal pain, and distention, are found.

NURSING *and* COLLABORATIVE MANAGEMENT HERNIAS

Diagnosis is based on history and physical examination findings. Surgery is the treatment of choice for hernias to prevent the possible complication of strangulation. The surgical repair of a hernia is known as a *herniorrhaphy.* The reinforcement of the weakened area with wire, fascia, or mesh is known as a *hernioplasty.* When there is strangulation, necrosis and gangrene may develop if immediate care is not given. A bowel resection of the involved area or a temporary colostomy may be needed to treat a strangulated hernia.

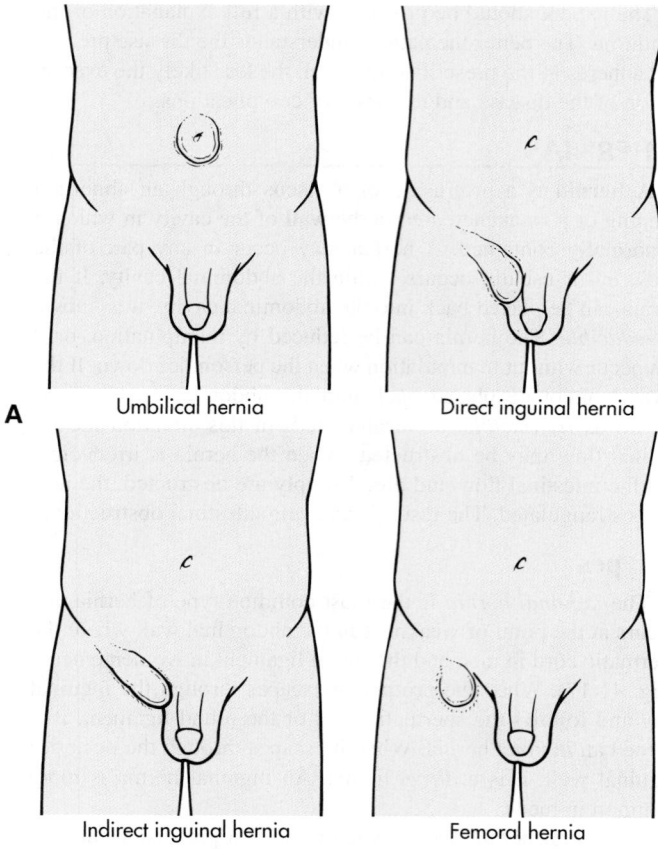

A   Umbilical hernia   Direct inguinal hernia

Indirect inguinal hernia   Femoral hernia

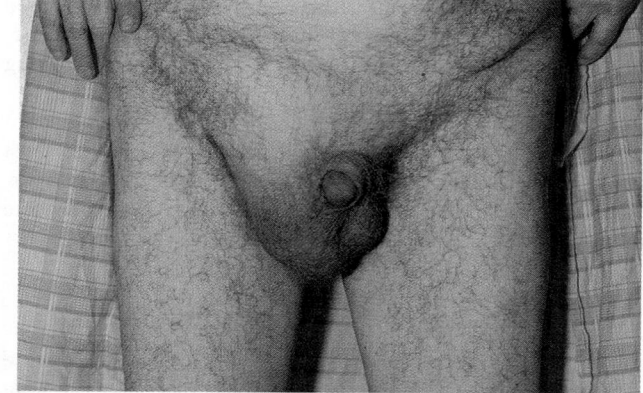

B

FIG. 41-17   **A,** Types of hernias. **B,** Indirect inguinal hernia.

Some patients with hernias wear a *truss,* a pad placed over the hernia and held in place with a belt. The truss is worn to keep the hernia from protruding. If a patient wears a truss, the nurse should check for skin irritation caused by the continual rubbing of the truss.

After a hernia repair, the patient may have difficulty voiding. Therefore the nurse should observe for a distended bladder. An accurate intake and output record is important. Scrotal edema is a painful complication after an inguinal hernia repair. A scrotal support with application of an ice bag may help relieve pain and edema. Coughing is not encouraged, but deep breathing and turning should be done. If the patient needs to cough or sneeze, the incision should be splinted during coughing, and sneezing should be done with the mouth open.

After discharge the patient may be restricted from heavy lifting for 6 to 8 weeks. Some surgeons do not put any limitations on physical activities.

Malabsorption Syndrome

Malabsorption results from impaired absorption of fats, carbohydrates, proteins, minerals, and vitamins. The stomach, small intestine, liver, and pancreas regulate normal digestion and absorption. Digestive enzymes ordinarily break down nutrients so that absorption can take place through the intestinal mucosa and nutrients can get into the bloodstream. If there is an interruption in this process at any point, malabsorption may occur. Several problems can cause malabsorption (Table 41-38). They can be classified into malabsorptions caused by (1) biochemical or enzyme deficiencies, (2) bacterial proliferation, (3) disruption of small intestine mucosa, (4) disturbed lymphatic and vascular circulation, or (5) surface area loss. Lactose intolerance is the most common malabsorption disorder, followed by inflammatory bowel disease, nontropical (celiac) and tropical sprue, and cystic fibrosis.

The most common clinical manifestation of malabsorption is **steatorrhea** (bulky, foul-smelling, yellow-gray, greasy stools with puttylike consistency). Bulky, foul-smelling stools that float in water and are difficult to flush are characteristic of steatorrhea (Table 41-39). However, steatorrhea does not occur with lactose intolerance.

Screening tests available for malabsorption include qualitative examination of stool for fat (Sudan stain), a 72-hour stool

TABLE 41-38   Common Causes of Malabsorption
Biochemical or Enzyme Deficiencies
Lactase deficiency
Biliary tract obstruction
Pancreatic insufficiency
Cystic fibrosis
Chronic pancreatitis
Zollinger-Ellison syndrome
Bacterial Proliferation
Tropical sprue
Parasitic infection
Small Intestinal Mucosal Disruption
Celiac disease
Whipple's disease
Crohn's disease
Disturbed Lymphatic and Vascular Circulation
Lymphoma
Ischemia
Lymphangiectasia
Heart failure
Surface Area Loss
Billroth II gastrectomy
Short bowel syndrome
Distal ileal resection, disease, or bypass

TABLE 41-39 Clinical Manifestations of Malabsorption

MANIFESTATIONS	PATHOPHYSIOLOGY
Gastrointestinal	
Weight loss	Malabsorption of fat, carbohydrates, and protein leading to loss of calories; marked reduction in caloric intake or increased use of calories
Diarrhea	Impaired absorption of water, sodium, fatty acids, bile, or carbohydrates
Flatulence	Bacterial fermentation of unabsorbed carbohydrates
Steatorrhea	Undigested and unabsorbed fat
Glossitis, cheilosis, stomatitis	Deficiency of iron, riboflavin, cobalamin, folic acid, and other vitamins
Hematologic	
Anemia	Impaired absorption of iron, cobalamin, and folic acid
Hemorrhagic tendency	Vitamin C deficiency
	Vitamin K deficiency inhibiting production of clotting factors II, VII, IX, and X
Musculoskeletal	
Bone pain	Osteoporosis from impaired calcium absorption
	Osteomalacia secondary to hypocalcemia, hypophosphatemia, inadequate vitamin D
Tetany	Hypocalcemia, hypomagnesemia
Weakness, muscle cramps	Anemia, electrolyte depletion (especially potassium)
Muscle wasting	Protein malabsorption
Neurologic	
Altered mental status	Dehydration
Paresthesias	Cobalamin deficiency
Peripheral neuropathy	Cobalamin deficiency
Night blindness	Thiamine deficiency
	Vitamin A deficiency
Integumentary	
Bruising	Vitamin K deficiency
Dermatitis	Fatty acid deficiency, zinc deficiency, niacin and other vitamin deficiencies
Brittle nails	Iron deficiency
Hair thinning and loss	Protein deficiency
Cardiovascular	
Hypotension	Dehydration
Tachycardia	Hypovolemia, anemia
Peripheral edema	Protein malabsorption, protein loss in diarrhea

collection for quantitative measurement of fecal fat, and the D-xylose absorption-excretion test, which is a good screening test for carbohydrate absorption (see Table 38-12). Other diagnostic studies include three different kinds of breath tests: (1) the bile acid breath test, which is used to evaluate bile salt malabsorption or malabsorption from bacterial overgrowth; (2) the triolein breath test, which measures carbon dioxide excretion after ingestion of a radioactive triglyceride; and (3) the excretion of breath hydrogen after ingestion of lactose, which is a sensitive, specific, and noninvasive test for detection of lactase deficiency. The rationale for the hydrogen breath test is that undigested lactose, which when metabolized by bacteria in the colon produces an increase in hydrogen production, is excreted via the lungs.

A pancreatic secretion test may be performed to rule out pancreatic insufficiency. Endoscopy may be used to obtain a small bowel biopsy specimen for diagnosis. Radiologic studies of the esophagus, stomach, and small intestine may be indicated. A small bowel barium enema is often performed to identify abnormal mucosal patterns.

Laboratory studies that are frequently ordered include a CBC, determination of prothrombin time, serum vitamin A and carotene levels, serum electrolytes, cholesterol, and calcium.

SPRUE

Two closely related malabsorption conditions are nontropical sprue and tropical sprue. Tropical and nontropical sprue are found in adults. **Nontropical sprue** is most commonly referred to as celiac sprue (especially in children) but is also called adult celiac disease and gluten-induced enteropathy.

Etiology and Pathophysiology

In celiac disease there is marked atrophy and flattening of the villi. As a result, absorption within the small intestine is reduced. The proposed reason for the injury to the villi is a hypersensitivity response initiated by gluten and *gliadin* (a breakdown product of gluten). *Gluten* is a protein found in wheat, rye, barley, and oats. The hypersensitivity leads to an inflammatory response of the mucosa.

Tropical sprue is a chronic disorder acquired in endemic tropical areas. The exact cause is unknown, but the disorder has been linked to an infectious agent. Folate deficiency is also believed to play a role in the development of this disease. Clinically, it resembles nontropical sprue.

Clinical Manifestations

A patient may become symptomatic at any age with celiac sprue, but the incidence peaks in childhood when gluten is first introduced and then during the fourth and fifth decades.[32] Symptoms include steatorrhea, diarrhea, weight loss, abdominal distention, and excessive flatulence. There may also be signs of multiple vitamin deficiencies (e.g., glossitis, cheilosis).

Diagnostic Studies and Collaborative Care

Diagnosis of sprue may be made by stool content analyses or intestinal biopsy. Barium enema may demonstrate abnormalities, including obliteration of intestinal folds. Treatment of sprue syndrome is based on the underlying cause. In nontropical sprue, a gluten-free diet usually leads to clinical recovery. Wheat, barley, oats, and rye products should be avoided. Soybean flours may be used. Foods must be scrutinized for the gluten content. Additives such as hydrolyzed vegetable proteins are often derived from cereal grains, including wheat. For those patients who are unresponsive to dietary exclusion therapy (gluten-free diet), corticosteroids may be used to treat nontropical sprue. The basis for this treatment is that the inflammatory response is mediated by an immunologic response.

Tropical sprue is treated with broad-spectrum antibiotics (e.g., tetracycline) in conjunction with folic acid therapy. The patient who responds to this therapy and achieves a remission is usually maintained on folic acid.

LACTASE DEFICIENCY

Lactase deficiency is a condition in which the lactase enzyme is deficient or absent. *Lactase* is the enzyme that breaks down lactose into two simple sugars—glucose and galactose. Although primary lactase deficiency seems to be hereditary, milk intolerance may not become clinically evident until late adolescence or early adulthood. About 5% of the adult population has primary lactase deficiency. The highest incidence is found in African Americans, Native Americans, Mexican Americans, Asian Americans, and persons of Jewish descent. Acquired lactase deficiency is often seen in other GI diseases in which the mucosa has been damaged, including ulcerative colitis, Crohn's disease, gastroenteritis, and tropical and nontropical sprue.

Clinical Manifestations

The symptoms of lactose intolerance include bloating, flatulence, crampy abdominal pain, and diarrhea. They may occur within a half hour to several hours after drinking a glass of milk or ingesting a milk product. The diarrhea of lactose intolerance results from fluid secretion into the small intestines, responding to the osmotic action of undigested lactose.

NURSING *and* COLLABORATIVE MANAGEMENT
LACTASE DEFICIENCY

Many lactose-intolerant persons are aware of their milk intolerance and avoid milk. A lactose intolerance test can be performed to rule out milk allergies. The patient is given 50 g of lactose orally. Blood samples are drawn before the consumption of lactose and at 15-, 30-, 60-, and 90-minute intervals. Failure of the blood glucose level to increase more than 20 mg/dl is suggestive of lactase deficiency. Results of the hydrogen breath test after ingestion of lactose are abnormal.

Treatment consists of eliminating lactose from the diet by avoiding milk and milk products. A lactose-free diet is given initially and is gradually advanced to a low-lactose diet as tolerated by the patient. The objective of care is to teach the importance of adherence to the diet. Many lactose-intolerant persons may not exhibit symptoms if lactose is taken in small amounts. In some persons, lactose may be tolerated better if taken with meals.

The patient needs to be aware that milk, ice cream, cottage cheese, and cheese have a high lactose content. If the milk has been fermented (e.g., cultured buttermilk, yogurt, sour cream), the patient with low lactase levels may tolerate it better.

Lactase enzyme (Lactaid) is available commercially as an over-the-counter (OTC) product. It is mixed with milk and breaks down the lactose before the milk is ingested.

SHORT BOWEL SYNDROME

Short bowel syndrome (SBS) results from extensive resection of the small intestine. Rapid intestinal transit, impaired digestive and absorption processes, and fluid and electrolyte losses characterize the syndrome. In adults, resection of the small intestine may be necessary for bowel infarction because of vascular thrombosis or insufficiency, abdominal trauma, cancer, radiation enteritis, or Crohn's disease.

The length and portions of small bowel resected are associated with the number and severity of symptoms. Resections of up to 50% of the small intestine cause little disturbance of bowel function, especially if the terminal ileum and ileocecal valve remain intact. After large resections, the remaining intestine undergoes adaptive changes that are more pronounced in the ileum. The villi and crypts increase in size, and absorptive capacity of the remaining intestine increases. Intestinal adaptation is enhanced by the presence of food, fiber, bile, and pancreatic secretions in the lumen and continues for up to 2 years. Resection of the ileum, ileocecal valve, or colon results in a rapid intestinal transit, decreasing absorption time. Ileal resection causes malabsorption of cobalamin, bile salts, and fat, resulting in steatorrhea.

Clinical Manifestations

The predominant manifestations of SBS are diarrhea or steatorrhea.[33] There may be signs of malnutrition and multiple vitamin and mineral deficiencies (e.g., weight loss, cobalamin and zinc deficiency, hypocalcemia). The patient may develop lactase deficiency and bacterial overgrowth. Oxalate kidney stones may form from increased colonic absorption of oxalate.

Collaborative Care

The overall goals are that the patient with SBS will have fluid and electrolyte balance, normal nutritional status, and control of diarrhea. In the period immediately following massive bowel resection, patients receive TPN to replace fluid, electrolyte, and nutrient losses and to rest the bowel. Hypersecretion of gastric acid, for which the cause is unknown, is reduced by proton pump inhibitors (e.g., omeprazole [Prilosec]).

A diet high in carbohydrate and low in fat is recommended. A high-carbohydrate, low-fat diet supplemented with soluble fiber, pectin, the amino acid glutamine, and parenteral growth hormone improves nutrient absorption, decreases stool output, and enables patients to wean off parenteral nutrition.[33] The patient with SBS is encouraged to eat at least six meals per day to increase the time of contact between food and the intestine. Oral intake can be supplemented with elemental nutrient formulas and tube feeding during the night. For patients with severe malabsorption, TPN may be reinstituted. Oral supplements of calcium, zinc, and multivitamins are typically recommended.

Narcotic antidiarrheal drugs are the most effective in decreasing intestinal motility (see Table 41-3). For patients with limited ileal resections (<100 cm), cholestyramine (Questran) reduces diarrhea resulting from unabsorbed bile acids and increases their excretion in feces. Bile acids stimulate intestinal fluid secretion and reduce colonic fluid absorption.

Anorectal Problems

HEMORRHOIDS

Hemorrhoids are dilated hemorrhoidal veins. They may be *internal* (occurring above the internal sphincter) or *external* (occurring outside the external sphincter) (Fig. 41-18). Symptoms of hemorrhoids, including bleeding, pruritus, prolapse, and pain, are common in all age groups. In affected persons, hemorrhoids appear periodically, depending on amount of anorectal pressure.

Etiology and Pathophysiology

Hemorrhoids are thought to develop as a result of shearing forces during defecation. This force damages supporting muscles. When supporting tissues in the anal canal weaken, usually as a result of straining at defecation, venules become dilated. In addition, blood flow through the veins of the hemorrhoidal

plexus is impaired. An intravascular clot in the venule results in a thrombosed external hemorrhoid. They are the most common cause of bleeding with defecation. The amount of blood lost at one time may be small but may lead to iron deficiency anemia over time.

Hemorrhoids may be precipitated by many factors, including pregnancy, prolonged constipation, straining in an effort to defecate, heavy lifting, prolonged standing and sitting, and portal hypertension (as found in cirrhosis).

Clinical Manifestations

The patient with internal hemorrhoids may be asymptomatic. However, when internal hemorrhoids become constricted, the patient will report pain. Internal hemorrhoids can bleed, resulting in blood on toilet paper after defecation or blood on the outside of stool. The patient may report a chronic, dull aching discomfort, particularly when the hemorrhoids have prolapsed.

External hemorrhoids are reddish blue and seldom bleed or cause pain unless a vein ruptures. If the blood clots in external hemorrhoids, they become inflamed and painful and are said to be thrombosed. External hemorrhoids cause intermittent pain, pain on palpation, itching, and burning. Patients also report bleeding associated with defecation. Constipation or diarrhea can aggravate these symptoms.

Diagnostic Studies and Collaborative Care

Internal hemorrhoids are diagnosed by digital examination, anoscopy, or sigmoidoscopy. External hemorrhoids can be diagnosed by visual inspection and digital examination. Therapy should be directed toward the causes and the patient's symptoms. A high-fiber diet and increased fluid intake prevent constipation and reduce straining, which allows engorgement of the veins to subside. Ointments such as Nupercainal; creams, suppositories, and impregnated pads that contain antiinflammatory agents (e.g., hydrocortisone); or astringents and anesthetics (e.g., witch hazel, pramoxine, benzocaine) may be used to shrink the mucous membranes and relieve discomfort. Stool softeners may be ordered to keep the stools soft, and sitz baths may be ordered to relieve pain.

Application of ice packs for a few hours, followed by warm packs, may be used for thrombosed external hemorrhoids. Another conservative treatment involves use of a sclerosing solution such as 5% phenol in oil, or a combined solution of quinine and urea may be injected into the submucosal tissue surrounding the hemorrhoids, causing a fibrosing and shrinking of the supporting tissues. Topical nitroglycerin has been shown to be effective in reducing acute hemorrhoidal thrombosis.

For internal hemorrhoids, one of four nonsurgical approaches (band ligation, infrared coagulation, cryotherapy, laser treatment) can be used. The first is *band ligation*. Through an anoscope the hemorrhoid is identified and then ligated with a rubber band. The constrictive effect impairs circulation, and the tissue becomes necrotic, separates, and sloughs off. There is some local discomfort with this procedure, but no anesthetic is required. Aspirin or propoxyphene (Darvon) is usually given for discomfort. *Infrared coagulation* can be used to treat bleeding internal hemorrhoids. In this procedure, either infrared or electrical current produces local inflammation. *Cryotherapy* involves rapid freezing of the hemorrhoid. Because this method can result in acute pain, it is used less often. Finally, *laser treatment* can be used to treat internal hemorrhoids. This procedure involves expensive equip-

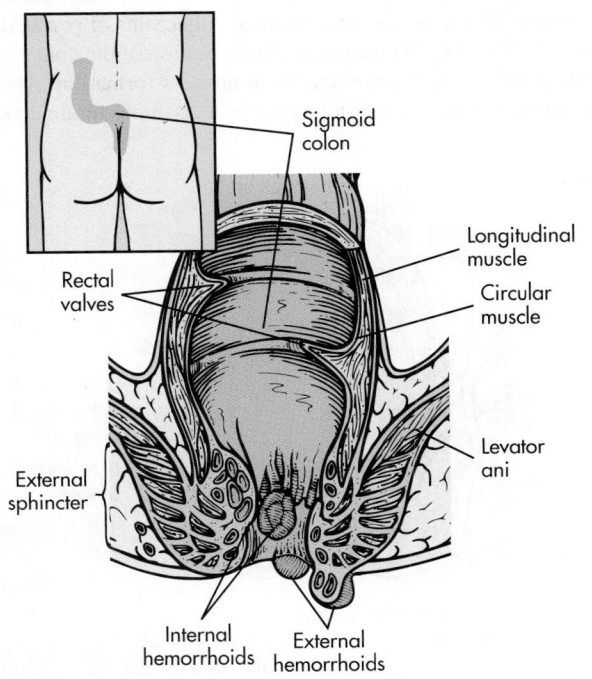

FIG. 41-18 Anatomic structures of the rectum and anus with external and internal hemorrhoids.

Labels in figure:
Sigmoid colon
Longitudinal muscle
Circular muscle
Rectal valves
Levator ani
External sphincter
Internal hemorrhoids
External hemorrhoids

ment and tends to be more costly compared with band ligation and coagulation therapies.

A *hemorrhoidectomy* is the surgical excision of hemorrhoids. Surgery is indicated when there is prolapse, excessive pain or bleeding, or large hemorrhoids. In general, hemorrhoidectomy is reserved for patients with severe symptoms related to multiple thrombosed hemorrhoids or marked protrusion. Surgical removal may be done by cautery, clamp, or excision. One surgical approach is to leave the area open so that healing takes place by secondary intention. In another approach the hemorrhoids are removed, the tissue is sutured, and healing takes place by primary-intention wound healing.

NURSING MANAGEMENT
HEMORRHOIDS

Conservative nursing management for the patient with hemorrhoids includes teaching measures to prevent constipation, avoidance of prolonged standing or sitting, proper use of OTC drugs available for hemorrhoidal symptoms, and the need to seek medical care for severe symptoms of hemorrhoids (e.g., excessive pain and bleeding, prolapsed hemorrhoids) when necessary. Sitz baths (15 to 20 minutes) two to three times each day for 7 to 10 days may be helpful to reduce discomfort and swelling associated with hemorrhoids.

Pain caused by sphincter spasm is a common problem after a hemorrhoidectomy. The nurse must be aware that although the procedure is minor, the pain is severe. Narcotics are usually given initially. Postoperatively, topical nitroglycerin preparations may be used to decrease pain and subsequent narcotic use.[34]

Sitz baths are started 1 to 2 days after surgery. A warm sitz bath provides comfort and keeps the anal area clean. A sponge ring in the sitz bath helps relieve pressure on the area. Initially the patient should not be left alone because of the possibility of weakness or fainting.

Packing may be inserted into the rectum to absorb drainage. A T-binder may hold the dressing in place. If packing is inserted, it usually is removed on the first or second postoperative day. The nurse should assess for rectal bleeding. The patient may be embarrassed when the dressing is changed, and privacy should be provided. The patient usually dreads the first bowel movement and often resists the urge to defecate. Pain medication may be given before the bowel movement to reduce discomfort.

A stool softener such as docusate (Colace) is usually ordered for the first few postoperative days. If the patient does not have a bowel movement within 2 to 3 days, an oil-retention enema is given.

Patients are taught the importance of diet, care of the anal area, symptoms of complications (especially bleeding), and avoidance of constipation and straining. Sitz baths are recommended for 1 to 2 weeks. The health care provider may order a stool softener to be taken for a time. Hemorrhoids may recur. Occasionally, anal strictures develop and dilation is necessary. Regular checkups are important in the prevention of any further problems.

ANAL FISSURE

An **anal fissure** is a skin ulcer or a crack in the lining of the anal wall that is caused by trauma, local infection, or inflammation. Fissures are considered either primary or secondary based

on their etiology. Primary fissures usually occur as a result of local trauma associated with defecation. When there is high pressure in the internal anal sphincter, it can result in ischemia, which can lead to fissuring. Thus conditions that promote constipation are likely to be associated with fissure development. Secondary fissures are due to a variety of conditions, including inflammatory bowel disease (Crohn's disease, ulcerative colitis), prior anal surgery, infection (syphilis, tuberculosis, chlamydia, gonorrhea, herpes simplex virus), and human immunodeficiency virus infection.

The most common clinical manifestations are painful spasms of the anal sphincter and severe, burning pain during defecation. Some bleeding may occur, and constipation results because of fear of pain associated with bowel movements.

Anal fissures are diagnosed through physical examination. Treatment of anal fissures is directed at correcting the underlying conditions, such as hard stools. Most acute fissures require 2 to 4 weeks to heal. Conservative treatment consists of bowel regulation with mineral oil and stool softeners. Warm sitz baths (15 to 20 minutes, 3 times a day) and anal anesthetic suppositories (Anusol) are also ordered. The application of nitroglycerin topical ointment before and immediately after a bowel movement can reduce pain. More recently, injection of botulinum toxin (Botox), which results in reversible paralysis of the internal anal sphincter, has been performed to promote fissure healing.[34] This treatment is transient (i.e., effects last approximately 6 weeks) and invasive. Side effects of Botox include transient incontinence and perianal thrombosis.

For chronic fissures, other invasive procedures may be needed. These include coagulation therapy or surgical treatment (sphincterotomy). Surgical treatment involves excision of the fissure. Postoperative nursing care is the same as the care for the patient who has had a hemorrhoidectomy.

ANORECTAL ABSCESS

Anorectal abscesses are undrained collections of perianal pus (Fig. 41-19). They are the result of obstruction of the anal glands, leading to infection and subsequent abscess formation. Abscess formation can occur secondary to anal fissures, trauma, or in-

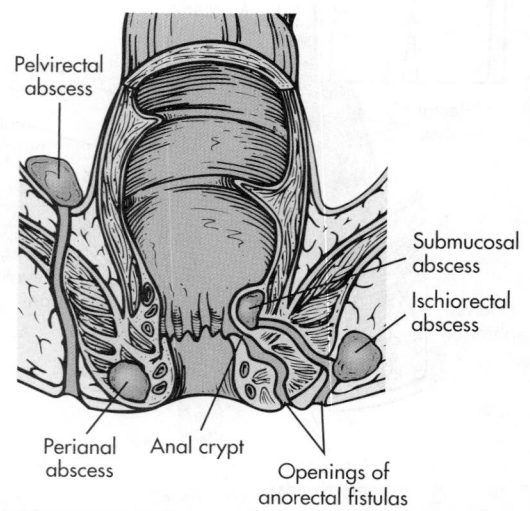

Pelvirectal abscess

Submucosal abscess

Ischiorectal abscess

Perianal abscess

Anal crypt

Openings of anorectal fistulas

FIG. 41-19   Common sites of anorectal abscesses and fistula formation.

flammatory bowel disease. The most common causative organisms are *Escherichia coli*, staphylococci, and streptococci. Clinical manifestations include local pain and swelling, foul-smelling drainage, tenderness, and elevated temperature. Sepsis can occur as a complication. Anorectal abscesses are diagnosed by rectal examination.

Surgical therapy consists of drainage of abscesses. If packing is used, it should be impregnated with petroleum jelly, and the area should be allowed to heal by granulation. The packing is changed every day, and moist, hot compresses are applied to the area. Care must be taken to avoid soiling the dressing during urination or defecation. A low-residue diet is given. The patient may leave the hospital with the area open. Discharge teaching should include wound care, the importance of sitz baths, thorough cleaning after bowel movements, and follow-up visits to a health care provider.

ANAL FISTULA

An **anal fistula** is an abnormal tunnel leading out from the anus or rectum. It may extend to the outside of the skin, vagina, or buttocks. Anal fistulas are a complication of Crohn's disease. This condition often precedes an anorectal abscess.

Feces may enter the fistula and cause an infection. There may be persistent, blood-stained, purulent discharge or stool leakage from the fistula. The patient may have to wear a pad to prevent staining of clothes.

Surgical therapy involves a fistulotomy or a fistulectomy. In a *fistulotomy* the fistula is opened, and healthy tissue is allowed to granulate. A *fistulectomy* is an excision of the entire fistulous tract. Gauze packing is inserted, and the wound is allowed to heal by granulation. Care is the same as that given after a hemorrhoidectomy.

PILONIDAL SINUS

A **pilonidal sinus** is a small tract under the skin between the buttocks in the sacrococcygeal area. It is thought to be of congenital origin. It may have several openings and is lined with epithelium and hair, thus given the name *pilonidal* ("a nest of hair").

The skin is moist, and movement of the buttocks causes the short, wiry hair to penetrate the skin. The irritated skin becomes infected and forms a pilonidal cyst or abscess. There are no symptoms unless there is an infection. If it becomes infected, the patient complains of pain and swelling at the base of the spine.

The formed abscess requires incision and drainage. The wound may be closed or left open to heal by secondary intention. The wound is packed, and sitz baths are ordered.

Nursing care includes hot, moist heat applications when an abscess is present. The patient is usually more comfortable lying on the abdomen or side. The patient should be instructed to avoid contaminating the dressing when urinating or defecating and to avoid straining whenever possible.

CRITICAL THINKING EXERCISES

Case Study
Colorectal Cancer

Patient Profile. Joseph Sandoval, a 58-year-old Native American, is from a Pueblo tribe in northern New Mexico. Mr. Sandoval's wife and family drove 50 miles to take him to the Indian Health Service Hospital because of his deteriorating health.

Subjective Data
- Complains of bright red bleeding during a bowel movement
- Family states that he has become thinner over the past several months and has little appetite
- Describes feeling weak and being easily fatigued; he appears ill
- Complains of abdominal pain and a feeling of fullness
- Bowel pattern has episodes of constipation followed by diarrhea
- No prior screening for colorectal cancer; family history of colorectal cancer is unknown

Objective Data

Physical Examination
- Temperature: 100.4° F (38° C)
- Heart rate is 100 beats/min; BP is 120/74 mm Hg
- Weight: 140 lb (63.6 kg); height: 5 feet 9 inches (172.5 cm)
- Mild palpation over transverse and descending colon elicits pain
- Digital rectal exam revealed a mass

Laboratory Tests
- Double-contrast barium enema showed two medium-sized tumors
- Hct: 26%
- Hb: 9 g/dl (90 g/L)

CRITICAL THINKING QUESTIONS

1. What are the signs and symptoms of colorectal cancer that Mr. Sandoval manifests?
2. What is the significance of Mr. Sandoval's tachycardia?
3. What types of diagnostic information are available from a colonoscopy versus a double-contrast barium enema?
4. What nursing interventions are indicated for Mr. Sandoval at this stage of his illness?
5. What is a culturally sensitive way for the nurse to support Mr. Sandoval and his family in making decisions about his continued health care?
6. Based on the assessment data, write one or more nursing diagnoses. Are there any collaborative problems?

Nursing Research Issues

1. What are the primary problems related to sexuality and sexual function in patients with an ostomy?
2. Are the psychologic responses and coping strategies of younger patients receiving an ostomy different from those of older patients?
3. What can a nurse do to help improve the self-image of patients with ostomies?
4. Do psychosocial factors have a significant role in the exacerbation of IBD?
5. Which sources of dietary fiber are most effective in treating fecal incontinence and IBS?

REVIEW QUESTIONS

The number of the question corresponds to the same-numbered objective at the beginning of the chapter.

1. The appropriate collaborative therapy for the patient with acute diarrhea caused by rotavirus is to
   a. increase fluid intake.
   b. administer an antibiotic.
   c. administer antimotility drugs.
   d. quarantine the patient to prevent spread of the virus.

2. During the assessment of a patient with acute abdominal pain, the nurse should
   a. perform deep palpation before auscultation.
   b. obtain blood pressure and pulse rate to determine hypervolemic changes.
   c. auscultate bowel sounds because hyperactive bowel sounds suggest paralytic ileus.
   d. measure body temperature because an elevated temperature may indicate an inflammatory or infectious process.

3. The nurse would increase the comfort of the patient with appendicitis by
   a. having the patient lie prone.
   b. flexing the patient's right knee.
   c. sitting the patient upright in a chair.
   d. turning the patient onto his or her left side.

4. In planning care for the patient with Crohn's disease, the nurse recognizes that a major difference between ulcerative colitis and Crohn's disease is that Crohn's disease
   a. frequently results in toxic megacolon.
   b. causes fewer nutritional deficiencies than does ulcerative colitis.
   c. often recurs after surgery, whereas ulcerative colitis is curable with a colectomy.
   d. is manifested by rectal bleeding and anemia more frequently than is ulcerative colitis.

5. The nurse performs a detailed assessment of the abdomen of a patient with a possible bowel obstruction, knowing that a manifestation of an obstruction in the large intestine is
   a. a largely distended abdomen.
   b. diarrhea that is loose or liquid.
   c. persistent, colicky abdominal pain.
   d. profuse vomiting that relieves abdominal pain.

6. A patient with metastatic colorectal cancer is scheduled for both chemotherapy and radiation therapy. Patient teaching regarding these therapies for this patient would include an explanation that
   a. chemotherapy can be used to cure colorectal cancer.
   b. radiation is routinely used as adjuvant therapy following surgery.
   c. both chemotherapy and radiation can be used as palliative treatments.
   d. the patient should expect few if any side effects from chemotherapeutic agents.

7. The nurse explains to the patient undergoing ostomy surgery that the procedure that maintains the most normal functioning of the bowel is
   a. a sigmoid colostomy.
   b. a transverse colostomy.
   c. a descending colostomy.
   d. an ascending colostomy.

8. In contrast to diverticulitis, the patient with diverticulosis
   a. has rectal bleeding.
   b. often has no symptoms.
   c. has localized crampy pain.
   d. frequently develops peritonitis.

9. A nursing intervention that is most appropriate to decrease postoperative edema and pain following an inguinal herniorrhaphy is
   a. applying a truss to the hernia site.
   b. allowing the patient to stand to void.
   c. supporting the incision during routine coughing.
   d. elevating the scrotum with a support or small pillow.

10. The nurse determines that the goals of dietary teaching have been met when the patient with nontropical sprue selects from the menu
    a. scrambled eggs and sausage.
    b. buckwheat pancakes with syrup.
    c. oatmeal, skim milk, and orange juice.
    d. yogurt, strawberries, and rye toast with butter.

11. Which of the following should a patient be taught after a hemorrhoidectomy?
    a. Do not use the Valsalva maneuver.
    b. Eat a low-fiber diet to rest the colon.
    c. Administer oil-retention enema to empty the colon.
    d. Use prescribed pain medication before a bowel movement.

REFERENCES

1. Miller MA et al: Morbidity, mortality, and healthcare burden of nosocomial *Clostridium difficile*-associated diarrhea in Canadian hospitals, *Infect Control Hosp Epidemiol* 23:137, 2002.
*2. Bliss DZ et al: Supplementation with dietary fiber improves fecal incontinence, *Nurs Res* 50:203, 2001.
3. Cooper ZR, Rose S: Fecal incontinence: a clinical approach, *M Sinai J Med* 67:96, 2000.
4. Norton C, Chelvanayagam S: A nursing assessment tool for adults with fecal incontinence, *J WOCN* 27: 279, 2000.
5. Camilleri M et al: Insights into the pathology and mechanisms of constipation, irritable bowel syndrome, and diverticulosis in older people, *JAGS* 48:1142, 2000.

*6. Hinrichs M, Huseboe J: Research-based protocol: management of constipation, *J Gerontol Nurs* 27:17, 2001.
7. Thompson WG: Constipation: a physiological approach, *Can J Gastroenterol* 14:155D, 2000.
8. Muller-Lissner S: General geriatrics and gastroenterology: constipation and faecal incontinence, *Best Pract Res Clin Gastroenterol* 16:115, 2002.
9. Wolfe JM et al: Analgesic administration to patients with an acute abdomen: a survey, *Am J Emerg Med* 18:250, 2000.
10. Heitkemper M, Jarrett M: It's not all in your head: irritable bowel syndrome, *AJN* 101:26, 2001.
11. Gauf CL: Diagnosing appendicitis across the life span, *J Am Acad Nurse Pract* 12:129, 2000.
12. van Heel DA et al: Inflammatory bowel disease: progress toward a gene, *Can J Gastroenterol* 14:207, 2000.
13. Andres PG, Friedman LS: Epidemiology and the natural course of inflammatory bowel disease, *Gastroenterol Clin North Am* 28:255, 1999.

*Nursing research–based reference.

14. Worley J: Diagnosis and management of inflammatory bowel disease, *J Am Acad Nurs Pract* 11:23, 1999.

15. Hugot JP et al: Etiology of the inflammatory bowel diseases, *Int J Colorect Dis* 14:2, 1999.

16. Guslandi M: Nicotine treatment for ulcerative colitis, *J Clin Pharmacol* 48:481, 1999.

17. Wachtershauser A, Stein J: Rationale for the luminal provision of butyrate in intestinal diseases, *Eur J Nutr* 39:164, 2000.

18. Collins J, Corless CL, Deveney K: Pouchitis, *Clin Perspect Gastroent* 5:156, 2002.

19. Sandborn WJ: Transcending conventional therapies: the role of biologic and other novel therapies, *Inflamm Bowel* (Suppl 1):S9, 2001.

20. McCloy C et al: The etiology of intestinal obstruction in patients without prior laparotomy or hernia, *Am Surg* 64:19, 1998.

21. Bond JH: Clinical evidence for the adenoma-carcinoma sequence, and the management of patients with colorectal adenomas, *Semin Gastrointest Dis* 11:176, 2000.

22. Read TE, Kodner IJ: Colorectal cancer: risk factors and recommendations for early detection, *Am Fam Physician* 59:3083, 1999.

23. American Cancer Society: *Cancer facts and figures 2002*, Atlanta, 2002, American Cancer Society.

24. Pontieri-Lewis V: Colorectal cancer: prevention and screening, *Medsurg Nurs* 9:9, 2000.

25. Ahlquist DA, Shuber AP: Stool screening for colorectal cancer: evolution from occult blood to molecular markers, *Clin Chim Acta* 315:157, 2002.

26. Gibson M et al: Laparoscopic colon resections: a five-year retrospective review, *Am Surg* 66:245, 2000.

27. Royce ME, Hoff PM, Pazdur R: Progress in colorectal cancer chemotherapy: how far have we come, how far to go? *Drugs Aging* 17:201, 2000.

28. Beeker C et al: Colorectal cancer screening in older men and women: qualitative research findings and implications for intervention, *J Community Health* 25:263, 2000.

29. Moran EM: Epidemiological and clinical aspects of nonsteroidal antiinflammatory drugs and cancer risks, *J Environ Pathol Toxicol Oncol* 2:193, 2002.

30. Reddy BS, Rao CV: Novel approaches for colon cancer prevention by cyclooxygenase-2 inhibitors, *J Environ Pathol Toxicol Oncol* 2:155, 2002.

31. Carter JJ, Whelan RL: Evaluation and medical management of diverticular disease, *Sem Colon Rectal Surg* 11:196, 2000.

32. Green PHR et al: Characteristics of adult celiac disease in the USA: results of a national survey, *Am J Gastroenterol* 96:126, 2001.

33. Lord LM et al: Management of the patient with short bowel syndrome, *AACN Clin Iss* 11:604, 2000.

34. Lysy J et al: Topical nitrates potentiate the effect of botulinum toxin in the treatment of patients with refractory anal fissure, *Gut* 48:221, 2001.

RESOURCES

American Cancer Society
1599 Clifton Road NE
Atlanta, GA 30329
800-ACS-2345
www.cancer.org

American Gastroenterological Association
7910 Woodmont Avenue, Seventh Floor
Bethesda, MD 20814
301-654-2055
Fax: 301-654-5920
www.gastro.org

American Society for Gastrointestinal Endoscopy (ASGE)
1520 Kensington Road, Suite 202
Oak Brook, IL 60523
630-573-0600
Fax: 630-573-0691
www.asge.org

Crohn's & Colitis Foundation of America (CCFA)
386 Park Avenue South, 17th Floor
New York, NY 10016
800-932-2423
Fax: 212-779-4098
E-mail: info@ccfa.org
www.ccfa.org

Crohn's & Colitis Foundation of Canada (CCFC)
60 St. Clair Avenue East, Suite 600
Toronto, ON
M4T 1N5 Canada
800-387-1479 or 416-920-5035
Fax: 416-929-0364
www.ccfc.ca

International Ostomy Association
c/o British Colostomy Association
15 Station Road
Reading Berks
RG1 1LG England
44 1189 391537
Fax: 44 1189 569095
www.ostomyinternational.org

Society of Gastroenterology Nurses and Associates
401 North Michigan Avenue
Chicago, IL 60611-4267
800-245-7462 or 312-321-5165
Fax: 312-527-6658
www.sgna.org

United Ostomy Association (UOA)
19772 MacArthur Boulevard, Suite 200
Irvine, CA 92612-2405
800-826-0826
www.uoa.org

Wound, Ostomy and Continence Nurses Society
WOCN National Office
4700 West Lake Avenue
Glenview, IL 60025
888-224-WOCN or 866-615-8560
Fax: 866-615-8560
www.wocn.org

For additional Internet resources, see the website for this book at *http://evolve.elsevier.com/Lewis/medsurg/.*

CHAPTER 42

NURSING MANAGEMENT
Liver, Biliary Tract, and Pancreas Problems

Margaret McLean Heitkemper

LEARNING OBJECTIVES

1. Define jaundice and describe signs and symptoms that may occur with the different types of jaundice.
2. Differentiate among the types of viral hepatitis, including etiology, pathophysiology, clinical manifestations, complications, and collaborative care.
3. Describe the nursing management of the patient with viral hepatitis.
4. Explain the etiology, pathophysiology, clinical manifestations, complications, and collaborative care of the patient with cirrhosis of the liver.
5. Describe the nursing management of the patient with cirrhosis.
6. Describe the clinical manifestations and management of liver cancer.
7. Describe the pathophysiology, clinical manifestations, complications, and collaborative care of acute and chronic pancreatitis.
8. Describe the nursing management of the patient with pancreatitis.
9. Explain the clinical manifestations and collaborative care of the patient with pancreatic cancer.
10. Explain the pathophysiology, clinical manifestations, complications, and collaborative care, including surgical therapy, of gallbladder disorders.
11. Describe the nursing management of the patient undergoing conservative or surgical treatment of cholecystitis and cholelithiasis.

KEY TERMS

acute pancreatitis, p. 1133	fulminant viral hepatitis, p. 1109
ascites, p. 1118	hepatic encephalopathy, p. 1120
asterixis, p. 1120	hepatitis, p. 1105
cholecystitis, p. 1141	hepatorenal syndrome, p. 1120
cholelithiasis, p. 1141	jaundice, p. 1104
chronic pancreatitis, p. 1138	paracentesis, p. 1121
cirrhosis, p. 1116	portal hypertension, p. 1118
esophageal varices, p. 1118	pseudocyst, p. 1134
fetor hepaticus, p. 1120	spider angiomas, p. 1117
fulminant hepatic failure, p. 1131	

JAUNDICE

Jaundice, a yellowish discoloration of body tissues, results from an alteration in normal bilirubin metabolism or flow of bile into the hepatic or biliary duct systems. It is a symptom rather than a disease. Jaundice results when the concentration of bilirubin in the blood becomes abnormally increased. The bilirubin level has to be approximately 3 times the normal levels (2 to 3 mg/dl [34 to 51 mol/L]) for jaundice to occur. Jaundice can usually first be detected in the sclera and skin (Fig. 42-1).

Most of the body's bilirubin is formed from the breakdown of hemoglobin (from erythrocytes) by macrophages (see Fig. 38-6). This unconjugated (indirect) bilirubin is released into the circulation bound to albumin and is not water soluble. Because it is not water soluble and cannot be filtered in the kidneys, unconju-

gated bilirubin is not excreted in the urine. In the liver the unconjugated bilirubin is conjugated with glucuronic acid to form conjugated (direct) bilirubin, which is water soluble. Conjugated bilirubin is secreted into bile, which flows through the hepatic and biliary duct system into the small intestine. In the large intestine, bilirubin is converted to stercobilinogen and urobilinogen by bacterial action. Stercobilinogen gives the characteristic brown color to feces. Some urobilinogen is reabsorbed into the portal circulation and returned to the liver. Normally a very small amount of urobilinogen is excreted in urine.

The three types of jaundice are classified as hemolytic, hepatocellular, and obstructive. Diagnostic findings associated with these types of jaundice are shown in Table 42-1.

Hemolytic Jaundice

Hemolytic (prehepatic) jaundice is due to an increased breakdown of red blood cells (RBCs), which produces an increased amount of unconjugated bilirubin in the blood (Table 42-1). The liver is unable to handle this increased load. Causes of hemolytic jaundice include blood transfusion reactions, sickle cell crisis, and hemolytic anemia.

Hepatocellular Jaundice

Hepatocellular (hepatic) jaundice results from the liver's altered ability to take up bilirubin from the blood or to conjugate or excrete it. Initially both unconjugated and conjugated bilirubin serum levels are increased (see Table 42-1). In hepatocellular disease the hepatocytes are damaged and leak bilirubin, thus increasing levels of conjugated bilirubin. In severe disease, both unconjugated and conjugated bilirubin are elevated as a result of both the inability of hepatocytes to conjugate bilirubin

Reviewed by Anne Croghan, RN, MN, ARNP, Nurse Practitioner, Hepatology, VA Puget Sound Health Care System, Seattle, Wash.

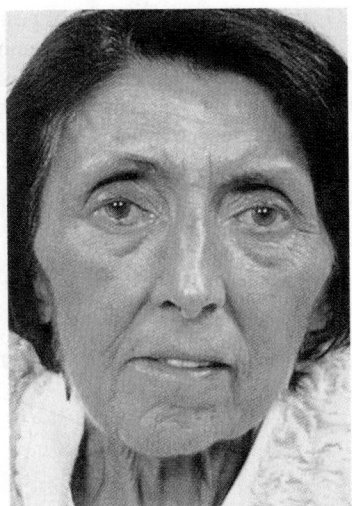

FIG. 42-1 Severe jaundice.

TABLE 42-1	Diagnostic Findings in Jaundice		
	Hemolytic	**Hepatocellular**	**Obstructive**
Serum bilirubin			
Unconjugated (indirect)	↑	↑	Somewhat ↑
Conjugated (direct)	Normal	↑↓	Moderately ↑
Urine bilirubin	Negative	↑	↑
Urobilinogen			
Stool	↑	Normal to ↓	↓
Urine	↑	Normal to ↑	↓

and continued cell leaking of conjugated bilirubin. As the number of unhealthy hepatocytes increases, the ability to conjugate bilirubin will eventually decrease. Because conjugated bilirubin is water soluble, it is excreted in the urine. The most common causes of hepatocellular jaundice are hepatitis, cirrhosis, and hepatic carcinoma.

Obstructive Jaundice

Obstructive (posthepatic) jaundice is due to impeded or obstructed flow of bile through the liver or biliary duct system. The obstruction may be intrahepatic or extrahepatic. Intrahepatic obstructions are due to swelling or fibrosis of the liver's canaliculi and bile ducts. This can be caused by damage from liver tumors, hepatitis, or cirrhosis. Causes of extrahepatic obstruction include common bile duct obstruction from a stone, sclerosing cholangitis, and carcinoma of the head of the pancreas. Laboratory findings show an elevation of both unconjugated and conjugated bilirubin and urine bilirubin (see Table 42-1). Because bilirubin does not enter the intestines, there is decreased to no fecal or urinary urobilinogen. With complete obstruction, the stools are clay colored.

Disorders of the Liver

HEPATITIS

Hepatitis is an inflammation of the liver. Acute viral hepatitis is the most common cause of hepatitis. The types of infectious viral hepatitis are A, B, C, D, E, and G. Hepatitis may also be caused by drugs (including alcohol), chemicals (see Table 38-6), and autoimmune liver disease. Rarely, hepatitis is caused by bacteria, such as streptococci, salmonellae, and *Escherichia coli*.

Viral hepatitis is a major public health concern in the United States. Approximately 152,000 cases of hepatitis A occur annually in the United States, and 10 million, worldwide.[1] It is nearly universal during childhood in developing countries. Worldwide, nearly 300 million people are infected with the hepatitis B virus (HBV). Of these approximately 50% to 75% have active viral replication or chronic active infection. There are an estimated 80,000 new cases of hepatitis B annually in the United States.[1] In the 1990s the incidence of hepatitis B decreased overall because of the widespread use of the HBV vaccine. Today, the highest rate of the disease occurs in those 20 to 49 years of age. Currently, 1.25 million Americans are chronically infected with HBV, 20% to 30% of whom acquired the infection in childhood.[1-3]

Worldwide, approximately 170 million people are infected with hepatitis C virus (HCV). In the United States it is estimated that 4 million individuals (1.8% of the population) have been exposed, with 3 million of them chronically infected.[4] Of these nearly 50% are not aware of their infection.[1] Currently, an estimated 25,000 new cases are diagnosed annually.[1] HCV accounts for 45% of all cases of chronic viral hepatitis, and it is the most common liver disease in the United States.[1] Approximately 20% of patients with chronic HCV will progress to cirrhosis within 20 years. It is estimated that 8000 to 10,000 individuals in the United States die each year from complications of end-stage liver disease secondary to chronic HCV.[2,5] The characterization of the virus and the introduction of transfusion blood and blood product testing along with safer needle-using practices by injecting drug users has resulted in a drop in new cases since the late 1980s. However, because of the 15- to 20-year delay between infection and the clinical appearance of liver damage, it is likely that the long-term effects of HCV infection will pose important health care challenges for the next 20 years.[5-7]

Coinfection of HCV and human immunodeficiency virus (HIV) is increasing. Approximately 40% of HIV-infected patients also have HCV. This high rate of coinfection is primarily related

CULTURAL & ETHNIC CONSIDERATIONS
Disorders of the Liver, Pancreas, and Gallbladder

- Mortality from cirrhosis occurs more frequently among African Americans than in other ethnic groups.
- Primary hepatic cancer has a higher incidence among African Americans, Asian Americans, and Eskimos than whites.
- Pancreatic cancer occurs more frequently among African Americans and Asian Americans than whites.
- Whites and Native Americans have a higher incidence of gallbladder disease than African Americans or Asian Americans.

to intravenous (IV) drug use. The presence of both HIV and HCV places the patient at greater risk for end-stage liver disease.

Etiology

Viral hepatitis can be caused by one of five major viruses: A, B, C, D, and E. Hepatitis G has recently been described. Other viruses known to produce liver inflammation and damage include cytomegalovirus, Epstein-Barr virus, herpesvirus, coxsackie-virus, and rubella virus.

The only definitive way to distinguish among the various forms of viral hepatitis is by the presence of the antigens and antigenic subtypes and the subsequent development of antibodies to them. Outbreaks of hepatitis are consistently caused by hepatitis A virus (HAV). Approximately 50% of acute viral hepatitis cases in adults in the United States are hepatitis B, 20% are hepatitis C, and 30% are hepatitis A.[1] Infection with each virus provides immunity to that virus (homologous immunity). However, the patient can still develop another type of viral hepatitis. Characteristics of hepatitis viruses are summarized in Table 42-2.

Hepatitis A Virus. HAV is an RNA virus that is transmitted through the fecal-oral route. It frequently occurs in small outbreaks caused by fecal contamination of food or drinking water. It is found in feces 2 or more weeks before the onset of symptoms and up to 1 week after the onset of jaundice (Fig. 42-2). It is present in the blood only briefly. Anti-HAV (antibody to HAV) immunoglobulin M (IgM) appears in the serum as the stool becomes negative for the virus. Detection of IgM anti-HAV indicates acute

hepatitis, and IgG anti-HAV is an indicator of past infection. The presence of IgG antibody provides lifelong immunity.

The mode of transmission of HAV is predominantly fecal-oral (mainly by ingestion of food or liquid infected with the virus) and rarely parenteral. Poor hygiene, crowded situations, and poor san-

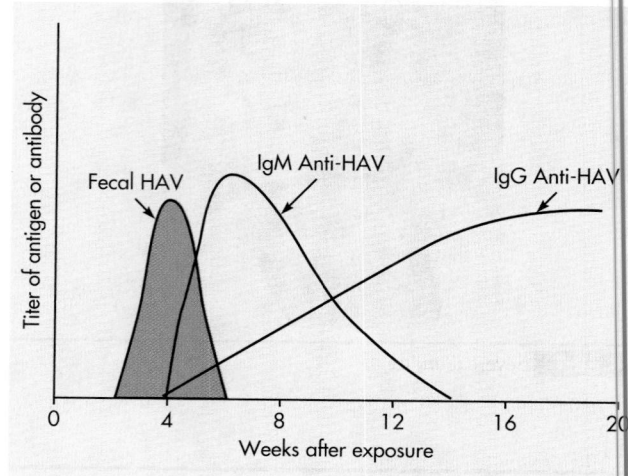

FIG. 42-2 Serologic events of a typical patient infected with hepatitis A virus (HAV). Elevated alanine aminotransferase (ALT) levels are present by 4 weeks, and jaundice appears by about 5 weeks after exposure to the virus.

TABLE 42-2 Characteristics of Hepatitis Viruses

	INCUBATION PERIOD	MODE OF TRANSMISSION	SOURCES OF INFECTION AND SPREAD OF DISEASE	INFECTIVITY
Hepatitis A virus (HAV)	15-50 days (average 28)	Fecal-oral (fecal contamination and oral ingestion)	Crowded conditions; poor personal hygiene; poor sanitation; contaminated food, milk, water, and shellfish; persons with subclinical infections; infected food handlers; sexual contact	Most infectious during 2 weeks before onset of symptoms; infectious until 1-2 weeks after symptoms start
Hepatitis B virus (HBV)	45-180 days (average 56-96)	Percutaneous (parenteral)/permucosal exposure to blood or blood products; Sexual contact; Perinatal transmission	Contaminated needles, syringes, and blood products; sexual activity with infected partners; asymptomatic carriers; Tattoo/body piercing, bites	Before and after symptoms appear; infectious for 4-6 months; in carriers continues for patient's lifetime
Hepatitis C virus (HCV)	14-180 days (average 56)	Percutaneous (parenteral)/permucosal exposure to blood or blood products; High-risk sexual contact; Perinatal contact	Blood and blood products, needles and syringes, sexual activity with infected partners	1-2 weeks before symptoms; continues during clinical course; 75%-85% go on to develop chronic hepatitis
Hepatitis D virus (HDV)	2-26 weeks; HBV must precede HDV; chronic carriers of HBV are always at risk	Can cause infection only together with HBV; routes of transmission same as for HBV	Same as HBV	Blood is infectious at all stages of HDV infection
Hepatitis E virus (HEV)	15-64 days (average 26-42 days in different epidemics)	Fecal-oral; Outbreaks associated with contaminated water supply in developing countries	Contaminated water; poor sanitation; found in Asia, Africa, and Mexico; not common in the United States and Canada	Not known; may be similar to HAV

itary conditions are all factors related to hepatitis A. Transmission occurs between family members, institutionalized individuals, children in day care centers, and from common-source outbreaks. The disease occurs more frequently in underdeveloped countries. Food-borne hepatitis A outbreaks are usually due to contamination of food during preparation by an infected food handler.

There is no chronic carrier state for HAV. The virus is present in feces during the incubation period, so it can be carried and transmitted by persons who have undetectable, subclinical infections. The greatest risk of transmission occurs before clinical symptoms are apparent. It can also be transmitted by patients with *anicteric* (nonjaundice) hepatitis A.

Hepatitis B Virus. HBV is a DNA virus that is transmitted by percutaneous (e.g., IV drug use, accidental needle-stick punctures) or permucosal exposure to infectious blood, blood products, or other body fluids (e.g., semen, vaginal secretions, saliva). Transmission occurs when infected blood or other body fluids enter the body of a person who is not immune to the virus. Perinatal transmission from mother to infant can occur. Approximately 90% of infants infected at birth go on to develop chronic hepatitis B.[1] In persons who have HBV, hepatitis B surface antigen (HBsAg) has been detected in almost every body fluid, including vaginal secretions, menstrual fluids, semen, saliva, respiratory secretions, tears, gastric juice, synovial fluid, and cerebrospinal fluid. Infected semen and saliva contain much lower concentrations of HBV than blood, but the virus can be transmitted via these secretions. If gastrointestinal (GI) bleeding occurs, feces can be contaminated with the virus from the blood. There is no evidence that urine, feces (without GI bleeding), breast milk, tears, and sweat are infective. In 20% to 30% of patients with acute hepatitis B, there are no readily identifiable risk factors.

Hepatitis B is a sexually transmitted disease. Approximately 30% of HBV cases are related to heterosexual activity (e.g., unprotected sex with an infected person). Male homosexuals (especially those practicing unprotected anal intercourse) are at risk for HBV infection. Although there is a much lower risk of transmission, kissing and sharing of food items may spread the virus via saliva. Other at-risk individuals include those who have household contacts with chronically infected persons, hemodialysis patients, and health care and public safety workers. The HBV can live on a dry surface for at least 7 days. HBV is much more infectious than HIV.

HBV is a complex structure with three distinct antigens: the surface antigen (HBsAg), the core antigen (HBcAg), and the e antigen (HBeAg). The persistence of HBsAg in the serum for 6 to 12 months or longer after infection with the virus indicates a carrier state of hepatitis B. Each antigen has a corresponding antibody that may be elicited during acute viral hepatitis B. These antibodies can be detected in the serum of persons with prior exposure to the antigenic virus (Fig. 42-3). The presence of hepatitis B surface antibody (anti-HBs or HBsAB) indicates immunity from the HBV vaccine or from past HBV infection.

From 2% to 10% of adults who become infected with HBV become chronic HBV carriers and may transmit the virus.[1] The HBsAg level remains detectable in chronic carriers (HBsAg positive on at least two occasions at least 6 months apart). With chronic carrier states, liver enzyme values may be normal or elevated. Patients with chronic HBV may have a normal liver, low-grade disease, or severe liver disease. They are also at higher risk of developing hepatocellular carcinoma.

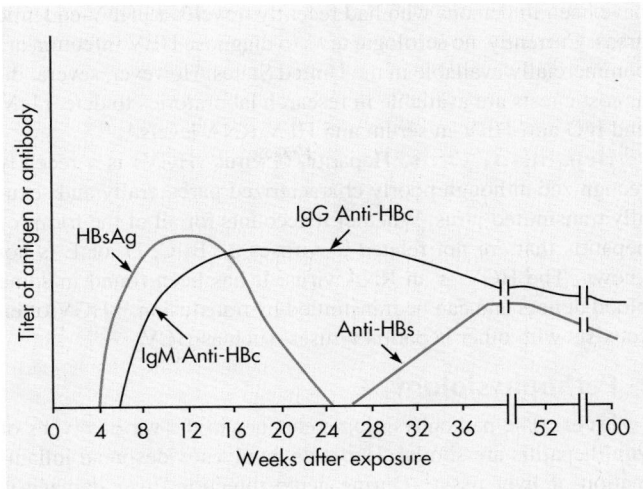

FIG. 42-3 Clinical and serologic events of a typical patient infected with acute hepatitis B virus (HBV). Elevated alanine aminotransferase (ALT) levels are present by about 8 weeks, and jaundice appears by about 10 weeks after exposure to the virus. *HBc,* Hepatitis B core antigen; *HBsAg,* hepatitis B surface antigen.

Hepatitis C Virus. HCV is an RNA virus that is primarily transmitted percutaneously. The major risk factor for infection is direct percutaneous exposure, such as injecting drugs, transfusion of infected blood products, hemodialysis, high-risk sexual behavior (e.g., unprotected sex, multiple partners), organ transplants, and exposure to blood and blood products by health care workers. In the United States IV drug use is the most common method of transmission, accounting for approximately 60% of all cases, and in Canada this number approaches 90%.[8-10] In the United States, approximately 20% of all cases are thought to be due to sexual transmission and another 10% to occupational exposure, hemodialysis, and perinatal transmission. However, 10% of patients with HCV cannot identify a source. A reliable antibody test for HCV was not widely available before 1992, so any patients given blood or blood products before then are at risk for chronic HCV infection and should be tested. Additional data are needed regarding the risks of body piercings, tattooing, and intranasal (e.g., cocaine) drug use in the transmission of HCV.

Hepatitis D Virus. Hepatitis D virus (HDV), also called *delta virus,* is a defective single-stranded RNA virus that cannot survive on its own. HDV requires the helper function of HBV to replicate. The importance of HDV relates to its clinical virulence. HDV infection can be acquired as a coinfection with HBV, often resulting in a superinfection; that is, patients with HBV-HDV coinfection may have more severe acute disease and a greater risk of fulminant hepatitis (2% to 20%) compared with those infected with HBV alone. However, in HBV patients coinfected with HDV, chronic HBV is less likely to develop. HDV is transmitted percutaneously, similar to HBV. However, the risk of transmission via sexual activity is much less.[1]

Hepatitis E Virus. Hepatitis E virus (HEV) is an RNA virus that is transmitted by the fecal-oral route. The most common mode of transmission is drinking contaminated water. Hepatitis E occurs primarily in developing countries. There have been reported epidemics in India, Asia, Mexico, and Africa. Only a few cases have been reported in the United States, and these cases have been in persons who had recently traveled to HEV-endemic areas. Currently, no serologic tests to diagnose HEV infection are commercially available in the United States. However, several diagnostic tests are available in research laboratories to detect IgM and IgG anti-HEV in serum and HEV RNA levels.[1]

Hepatitis G Virus. Hepatitis G virus (HGV) is a recently recognized although poorly characterized parenterally and sexually transmitted virus. Whether it accounts for all of the forms of hepatitis that are not related to viruses A, B, C, D, or E is not known. The HGV is an RNA virus. It has been found in some blood donors and can be transmitted by transfusion.[11] HGV often coexists with other hepatitis viruses, such as HCV.

Pathophysiology

Liver. The pathophysiologic changes in the various types of viral hepatitis are similar. Hepatitis involves widespread inflammation of liver tissue. During acute infection, liver damage is mediated by cytotoxic cytokines and natural killer cells that cause lysis of infected hepatocytes. Liver cell damage results in hepatic cell necrosis. There is proliferation and enlargement of the Kupffer cells. Inflammation of the periportal areas may interrupt bile flow. Cholestasis may occur. The liver cells can regenerate in an orderly manner, and if no complications occur, they should resume their normal appearance and function.

Systemic Effects. The antigen-antibody complexes between the virus and its corresponding antibody form a circulating immune complex in the early phases of hepatitis. The circulating immune complexes activate the complement system (see Chapter 13). The clinical manifestations of this activation are rash, angioedema, arthritis, fever, and malaise. *Cryoglobulinemia* (abnormal proteins found in the blood), glomerulonephritis, and vasculitis have also been found secondary to immune complex activation.

Clinical Manifestations

A large number of patients have no symptoms. For example, 30% of patients with acute HBV and 80% of patients with acute HCV will be asymptomatic. The clinical manifestations of viral hepatitis may be classified into three phases: (1) preicteric or prodromal phase, (2) icteric phase, and (3) posticteric or convalescent phase (Table 42-3).

Preicteric Phase. The preicteric phase precedes jaundice and lasts from 1 to 21 days. This is the period of maximal infectivity for hepatitis A. Hepatitis B patients who are HBsAg positive and patients with HCV can be infective for years. GI symptoms include anorexia, nausea, abdominal (right upper quadrant) discomfort, and sometimes vomiting, constipation, or diarrhea. The anorexia is frequently severe and may be due to cytokines or other chemicals produced by the infected liver. The patient may find food repugnant and, if a smoker, may have a distaste for cigarettes. There is also a decreased sense of smell. Weight loss occurs during the preicteric phase. Other symptoms during this phase are malaise, headache, low-grade fever, arthralgias, and skin rashes. Physical examination reveals hepatomegaly, lymphadenopathy, and sometimes splenomegaly.

Icteric Phase. The icteric phase lasts 2 to 4 weeks and is characterized by jaundice. Jaundice results when bilirubin diffuses into the tissues. The urine may darken because of excess bilirubin being excreted by the kidneys. If conjugated bilirubin cannot flow out of the liver because of obstruction or inflamma-

TABLE 42-3	Clinical Manifestations of the Phases of Hepatitis	
PREICTERIC	**ICTERIC**	**POSTICTERIC**
Anorexia	Jaundice	Malaise
Nausea, vomiting	Pruritus	Easy fatigability
Right upper quadrant discomfort	Dark urine	Hepatomegaly
	Bilirubinuria	
	Light stools	
Constipation or diarrhea	Fatigue	
Decreased sense of taste and smell	Continued hepatomegaly with tenderness	
	Weight loss	
Malaise		
Headache		
Fever		
Arthralgias		
Urticaria		
Hepatomegaly		
Splenomegaly		
Weight loss		

tion of the bile ducts, the stools will be light or clay colored. Pruritus sometimes accompanies the jaundice, especially if cholestasis is present. The pruritus occurs as a result of the accumulation of bile salts beneath the skin.

When jaundice occurs, the fever usually subsides. The GI symptoms usually remain, and some fatigue may continue. The liver is usually enlarged and tender.

Posticteric Phase. The convalescent stage of the posticteric phase begins as jaundice is disappearing and lasts weeks to months, with an average of 2 to 4 months. During this period the patient's major complaint is malaise and easy fatigability. Hepatomegaly remains for several weeks, but splenomegaly subsides during this period. Relapses may occur, and the disappearance of jaundice does not mean the patient has totally recovered.

General Considerations. Not all patients with viral hepatitis have jaundice. This is termed *anicteric hepatitis*. A high percentage of persons with HAV are anicteric and do not have symptoms.

There is some slight variation in manifestations between the types of hepatitis. In hepatitis A the onset is more acute, and the symptoms are usually mild, flulike manifestations. In hepatitis B the onset is more insidious, and the symptoms are usually more severe, but there may be fewer GI symptoms. In hepatitis C the majority of cases are asymptomatic or mild. However, HCV has a high rate of persistence and can induce chronic liver disease.

Complications

Most patients with acute viral hepatitis recover completely with no complications. The overall mortality rate for acute hepatitis is less than 1%. The mortality rate is higher in older adults and those with underlying debilitating illnesses (including chronic liver disease). Complications that can occur include fulminant hepatic failure, chronic hepatitis, cirrhosis of the liver, and hepatocellular carcinoma.

HAV infection can cause fulminant hepatic failure but does not cause chronic hepatitis. HBV can also cause fulminant hepatic failure and results in chronic infection in approximately 10% of those infected. Chronic HBV is identified by the persistence of HBsAg for longer than 6 months. Patients with chronic HBV are evaluated by assessment of liver function tests, HBV DNA (which measures the level of circulating HBV), and the presence of HBeAg and anti-HBe. A liver biopsy may be required to assess for the degree of inflammation and the presence and degree of fibrosis. Fibrosis may progress to cirrhosis in some patients. Chronic hepatitis B is a risk factor for the development of hepatocellular carcinoma.

It is not known what factors contribute to the persistence of the virus in some patients. Chronic HBV is more likely to develop in infants born to infected mothers and those who acquire the infection as children (e.g., before the age of 5) compared with those who acquire the virus over the age of 5. Alterations in the patient's cellular immune response may be important in the development of the chronic HBsAg carrier state and consequent progression from acute hepatitis B to chronic active hepatitis. These immune system alterations may explain why the patient with chronic renal failure who is undergoing dialysis when hepatitis B develops is more at risk for chronic hepatitis. (Persons with chronic renal failure are known to have a depressed cellular immune response.)

There is a greater risk for HCV infection to become chronic compared with HBV. Approximately 75% to 85% of patients who acquire HCV will go on to develop chronic infection.[2] Approximately 20% of patients with HCV will develop cirrhosis over 20 to 30 years; of these, 20% will develop liver failure. The prognosis of chronic HCV has greatly increased the demand for liver transplants. Risk factors for progression to cirrhosis include male gender, heavy alcohol consumption, and excess iron deposition in the liver. Steatorrhea, obesity, and diabetes mellitus are also risk factors for the progression of HCV to chronic liver disease. Patients who have cirrhosis caused by HCV are at risk for hepatocellular carcinoma.

Fulminant Hepatitis. **Fulminant viral hepatitis** is a clinical syndrome that results in severe impairment or necrosis of liver cells and potential liver failure. Fulminant viral hepatitis develops in a small percentage of patients. The disorder may occur as a complication of hepatitis B, particularly hepatitis B accompanied by infection with delta virus (HDV). Fulminant hepatitis occurs much less frequently with HCV. Toxic reactions to drugs and congenital metabolic disorders may also cause fulminant hepatitis and liver failure. Hepatocellular failure with death usually occurs.

Diagnostic Studies

Tests for the different types of viral hepatitis are presented in Table 42-4. In viral hepatitis many of the liver function tests show significant abnormalities. The common abnormalities are identified in Table 42-5.

Several tests are available to determine the presence of HCV. Unlike HAV and HBV, antibodies to hepatitis C are not protective and may be an indicator of chronic disease. For the patient who has a positive anti-HCV test by enzyme immunoassay, or if the HCV is suspected and there is a false positive antibody test (approximately 90% of patients with HCV are positive for anti-HCV), more sensitive testing is required. The HCV recombinant immunoblot assay is a more sensitive antibody test. To detect active disease (the presence of circulating HCV), HCV RNA polymerase chain reaction (PCR) is performed. This may be particularly helpful in the immunocompromised patient (e.g., patient with HIV) whose antibody production is very low (below the detection level of the antibody tests). In addition, this test may be helpful in identifying the presence of the virus in exposed individuals (e.g., health care workers) before the development of antibodies. However, HCV RNA PCR testing is not done as the initial testing for HCV infection.

For those patients who test positive for HCV, genotyping of the virus may also be done. Genotyping does not influence the type of treatment but may be used to guide length of treatment.

TABLE 42-4	Tests for Viral Hepatitis	
VIRUS	**TESTS**	**SIGNIFICANCE**
A	Anti-HAV IgM	Acute infection
	Anti-HAV IgG	Previous infection and long-term immunity
B	HBsAg (hepatitis B surface antigen)	Current infection (but not necessarily acute)*
		Positive in chronic carriers
	Anti-HBs (antibody to surface antigen)	Indicates previous infection with hepatitis B or immunization
		Marker of response to vaccine
	HBeAg (hepatitis B e antigen)	Indicates high infectivity; present in acute, active infection
	Anti-HBe (antibody to e antigen)	Indicates previous infection
	HBcAg (hepatitis B core antigen)	Ongoing infection with hepatitis B
	Anti-HBc IgM	Acute infection*
	Anti-HBc IgG (antibody to HB core antigen)	Indicates previous infection or ongoing infection with hepatitis B
		Does not appear after vaccination
	HBV DNA	Indicates active ongoing viral replication
		Best indicator of viral replication
C	Anti-HCV (antibody to hepatitis C)	Marker for acute or chronic infection with HCV
	Enzyme immunoassay (EIA)	Used in initial screening for HCV
	Recombinant immunoblot assay (RIBA)	More sensitive antibody test
	HCV RNA (RNA polymerase chain reaction [PCR] assay)	Indicates active ongoing viral replication
D	Anti-HDV	Present in past or current infection with hepatitis D

*If positive HBsAg and anti-HBc IgM, it indicates the presence of acute infection.
A, Hepatitis A virus (HAV); *B,* hepatitis B virus (HBV); *C,* hepatitis C virus (HCV); *D,* hepatitis D virus (HDV); *DNA,* deoxyribonucleic acid; *RNA,* ribonucleic acid.

TABLE 42-5	Diagnostic Findings in Acute Hepatitis	
TEST	**ABNORMAL FINDING**	**ETIOLOGY**
Transaminases (aminotransferases)		
Aspartate aminotransferase (AST)	Elevation in preicteric phase; decrease as jaundice disappears	Liver cell injury
Alanine aminotransferase (ALT)	Elevation in preicteric phase; decrease as jaundice disappears	Liver cell injury
γ-Glutamyl transpeptidase (GGT)	Elevation	Liver cell injury
Alkaline phosphatase	Some elevation	Impaired excretory function of the liver
Serum proteins		
γ-Globulin	Normal or increased	Impaired clearance of the liver
Albumin	Normal or decreased	Liver damage
Serum bilirubin (total)	Elevation to about 8-15 mg/dl (137-257 μmol/L)	Liver cell damage
Urinary bilirubin	Elevation	Conjugated hyperbilirubinemia
Urinary urobilinogen	Elevation 2-5 days before jaundice	Diminished reabsorption of urobilinogen
Prothrombin time	Prolonged	Decreased absorption of vitamin K in intestine with decreased production of prothrombin by liver

Genotype 1, the most common form in the United States, Canada, and other Western countries, is more resistant to treatment than genotypes 2 through 6.[6]

Physical assessment reveals hepatic tenderness, hepatomegaly, and splenomegaly. The liver is palpable. A liver biopsy is not indicated in acute hepatitis unless the diagnosis is in doubt. In chronic persistent hepatitis a liver biopsy may be performed to assess the degree of liver damage.

Patients with chronic HBV and HCV may undergo liver biopsy. Biopsy of liver tissue allows for histologic examination of liver cells and characterization of the degree of inflammation, fibrosis, or cirrhosis that may be present.[12] A patient who has a bleeding disorder may not be an appropriate candidate for biopsy because of the risk of bleeding.

Collaborative Care

There is no specific treatment or therapy for acute viral hepatitis. Most patients can be managed at home. Emphasis is on measures to rest the body and assist the liver in regenerating (Table 42-6). Adequate nutrients and rest seem to be most beneficial for healing and liver cell (hepatocyte) regeneration. Dietary emphasis is on a well-balanced diet that the patient can tolerate. Rest reduces the metabolic demands on the liver and promotes cell regeneration. Bed rest may be indicated while the patient is symptomatic. The degree of rest ordered depends on the severity of symptoms, but usually alternating periods of activity and rest are adequate. Counseling should include the importance of avoiding alcohol and notification of possible contacts for testing and prophylaxis, if indicated.

Drug Therapy. There are no specific drug therapies for the treatment of acute viral hepatitis. Supportive drug therapy may include antiemetics, such as dimenhydrinate (Dramamine) or trimethobenzamide (Tigan). Phenothiazines should not be used because of their possible cholestatic and hepatotoxic effects. If the patient requires a sedative or hypnotic drug, diphenhydramine (Benadryl) or chloral hydrate may be used.

Chronic hepatitis B. Drug therapy for chronic HBV is focused on decreasing the viral load, decreasing the rate of disease progression, and decreasing the rate of drug-resistant HBV. At the moment, several drugs are useful in suppressing viral activity

TABLE 42-6	Collaborative Care — Viral Hepatitis

Diagnostic
History and physical examination
Liver function studies
   Alanine aminotransferase (ALT)
   Aspartate aminotransferase (AST)
Hepatitis testing
  Anti-HAV—IgM and IgG
  HBsAg (HBeAg in some cases)
  Anti-HBs
  Anti-HBc—IgM and IgG
  HBV DNA
  Anti-HCV
  HCV RNA
  Anti-HDV

Collaborative Therapy
Acute and Chronic
High-calorie, high-protein, high-carbohydrate, low-fat diet
Vitamin supplements
Rest—degree of strictness varies
Avoid alcohol intake and drugs detoxified by the liver
Chronic HBV and HCV
α-Interferon (Peg-Intron, Pegasys)
Antiviral agents (lamivudine [Epivir], ribavirin [Rebetol])

DNA, Deoxyribonucleic acid; *HAV*, hepatitis A virus; *HB*, hepatitis B; *HBV*, hepatitis B virus; *HCV*, hepatitis C virus; *HDV*, hepatitis D virus; *RNA*, ribonucleic acid.

and decreasing viral load in patients with chronic HBV. However, the percentage of patients seroconverting (developing antibodies against the virus) remains relatively low.

Lamivudine (Epivir, 3TC), a reverse transcriptase inhibitor, is used to treat chronic HBV. This drug taken orally for 1 year has beneficial effects in terms of reducing viral load, decreasing liver damage, and decreasing liver enzymes in approximately two thirds of patients.[13,14] However, seroconversion occurs in less than 20% of patients. When lamivudine is stopped, the majority of patients (except those who have seroconverted)

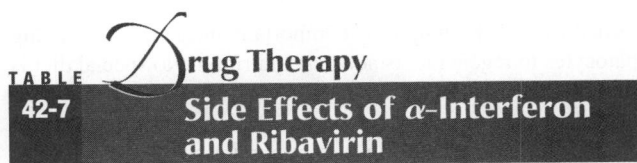

TABLE 42-7	Drug Therapy Side Effects of α-Interferon and Ribavirin

α-Interferon

Flulike Symptoms
Arthralgia
Asthenia (loss of strength)
Fatigue
Headache
Myalgia
Nausea/anorexia

Other Effects
Anemia
Decline in platelet and neutrophil counts
Depression
Hair loss (alopecia)
Insomnia
Rash
Thyroid dysfunction
Weight loss

Less Common Effects
Diarrhea
Peripheral neuropathy
Retinopathy
Seizures
Vasculitis

Ribavirin
Anemia (hemolytic)
Anorexia
Cough
Dyspnea
Insomnia
Pruritus
Rash
Teratogenicity (interferes with normal fetal development)

have HBV DNA and inflammation levels that return to pretreatment levels. Approximately 20% to 30% of patients develop resistance to the drug. Lamivudine has been used along with HBV immunoglobulin to reduce viral activity in patients who have a liver transplant for HBV. Other drugs in this class undergoing investigation include famciclovir (Famvir) and ganciclovir (Cytovene).[13]

α-Interferon is an important drug in the treatment of chronic HBV. A 4-month course of treatment with α-interferon results in a significant reduction of serum HBV DNA levels, normalization of alanine aminotransferase (ALT) level, and loss of HBV antigen (HBeAg) in 30% to 40% of those treated.[11] In addition, the development of cirrhosis and hepatocellular cancer appears to be decreased in those who receive α-interferon treatment. α-Interferon treatment is associated with a number of side effects (Table 42-7). These side effects are dose related and tend to decrease in severity with continued treatment.

Adefovir dipivoxil (Hepsera) can be used for the treatment of chronic HBV in patients with active viral replication and either elevations of serum ALT or AST, or histologically active disease. Hepsera slows the progression of chronic HBV by interfering with viral replication.

Chronic hepatitis C. Drug therapy is directed at reducing the viral load, decreasing progression of the disease, and promoting seroconversion. Treatment for HCV includes monotherapy with α-interferon alone or the combination of ribavirin (Rebetol) and α-interferon. Approximately 40% to 50% of patients will initially respond to α-interferon alone (monotherapy) with a decrease in HCV RNA levels. However, approximately 50% of these patients will relapse in 6 months, indicating that α-interferon monotherapy is effective in less than 25% of patients with chronic HCV. Currently there are pegylated formulas of α-interferon (e.g., Peg-Intron, Pegasys) that allow for once weekly administration as opposed to three injections weekly. In these formulations polyethylene glycol is attached to the interferon, providing a protective barrier against its breakdown. With pegylated forms of α-interferon, the blood levels of the drug remain sustained over a longer period and provide more constant suppression of HCV.[15]

Ribavirin, given in combination with α-interferon, has a synergistic effect and has been used to reduce the rate of relapse following α-interferon therapy for HCV. Combination therapy (α-interferon plus ribavirin) has been shown to be more effective than monotherapy in the treatment of HCV.[16] Patients who have advanced fibrosis or cirrhosis can be treated with drug therapy as long as liver decompensation (e.g., ascites, esophageal hemorrhage, jaundice, wasting, encephalopathy) is not present. Ribavirin has a number of side effects, as shown in Table 42-7.

An increasing number of patients with HIV also have HCV. Patients who have stable HIV and relatively intact immune systems (CD4+ counts >200) are treated for HCV with the goal of eradicating HCV and enhancing quality of life. However, for those with advanced liver disease, the goal of HCV treatment is to delay disease progress.

The drug treatment of HIV in patients with coexisting HCV requires close attention to liver function. Treatment of HCV in patients with HIV requires close attention to lymphocyte and white and red blood cell counts. HCV treatment with ribavirin and α-interferon may reduce CD4+ counts, increase leukopenia, and increase the patient's risk for anemia (ribavirin effects). Drug interactions may also occur in patients being treated for both HIV and HCV. Depending on the degree of liver damage associated with HCV, drug therapy for HIV may need to be altered because of the decreased ability of the liver to metabolize the drugs.

Prevention
Hepatitis A. Both hepatitis A vaccine and immune globulin (IG) are used for prevention of hepatitis A. The vaccine is used for preexposure prophylaxis, and IG can be used either before or after exposure. IG provides temporary (6 to 8 weeks) passive immunity and is effective for preventing hepatitis A if given within 1 to 2 weeks after exposure. IG is recommended for persons who do not have anti-HAV antibodies and are exposed to hepatitis A from close (household, day care center) contact with persons who have HAV or food-borne exposure.[17] Because patients with hepatitis A are most infectious just before the onset of symptoms, those exposed through household contact or food-borne outbreaks should be given IG within 1 to 2 weeks of exposure. Although IG may not prevent infection in all persons, it may modify the illness to a subclinical infection. It may also be used as a prophylactic measure for travelers to countries that have a high incidence of hepatitis A.

There are currently several forms of the hepatitis A vaccine, including Havrix, Vaqta, and Avaxim. Active immunization is an important and effective means of controlling hepatitis A from a public health perspective. Primary immunization consists of a single dose administered intramuscularly in the deltoid muscle. A booster is recommended any time between 6 and 12 months after the initiation of the primary dose to ensure adequate antibody titers and long-term protection. However, a primary immunization provides immunity within 30 days after a single dose. The vaccine may be administered concomitantly with IG, although the ultimate antibody titer obtained is likely to be lower than if the vaccine is given alone.

Twinrix, a combined HAV and HBV vaccine, is available for persons over the age of 18 years.[18] The primary immunization consists of three doses, given on a 0-, 1-, and 6-month schedule, the same schedule as that used for the single HBV vaccine. Twinrix may be given to high-risk individuals, including patients with chronic liver disease, users of illicit injectable drugs, men who have sex with men, and persons with clotting factor disorders who receive therapeutic blood products. The side effects of the vaccine are mild and are usually limited to soreness and redness at the injection site.

Hepatitis B. Immunization with hepatitis B vaccine is the most effective method of preventing HBV infection. Recommendations from the Centers for Disease Control and Prevention (CDC) Immunization Practices Advisory Committee include making hepatitis B vaccine a part of routine vaccination schedules for all newborns and adolescents.

In addition to immunizing newborns and adolescents, it is important to vaccinate adults in the major risk groups, such as IV drug users and household members living with a hepatitis B carrier. It is hoped that universal vaccination will lead to eventual prevention and control of hepatitis B.

Hepatitis B vaccine is produced through recombinant DNA technology (see Fig. 13-15). The vaccines are Recombivax HB and Engerix-B. The vaccine is given in a series of three intramuscular injections in the deltoid muscle. The second dose is administered within 1 month of the first one, and the third one within 6 months of the first. The vaccine is greater than 95% effective. Successful vaccination should result in Anti-HBs titers of 10 mIU/ml or greater. However, it has not been definitely determined what level of antibody is required to provide protection. Therefore it remains to be determined how frequently boosters (additional doses) are necessary. Only minor adverse reactions have been reported with vaccination, including transient fever and soreness at the injection site. The vaccine is not contraindicated in pregnancy.

For postexposure prophylaxis, the vaccine and hepatitis B immune globulin (HBIG) are used. HBIG contains antibodies to HBV and confers temporary passive immunity. HBIG is prepared from plasma of donors with a high titer of anti-HBs and is expensive. HBIG is recommended for postexposure prophylaxis in cases of needle stick, mucous membrane contact, or sexual exposure and for infants born to mothers who are positive for HBsAg. It should be given after exposure, preferably within 24 hours. The vaccine series should also be started.

Hepatitis C. Currently there are no products to prevent HCV. However, several vaccines are in development. The CDC does not recommend IG or antiviral agents such as α-interferon for postexposure prophylaxis (e.g., needle-stick exposure from an infected patient) for HCV infection. Following an acute exposure (e.g., needle stick), the person (i.e., the source) should have anti-HCV testing done.[19] For the person exposed to HCV, baseline anti-HCV and ALT levels should be measured. Follow-up testing should be done at 4 to 6 months for anti-HCV and ALT activity. Testing for HCV RNA may be performed at 4 to 6 weeks. It is not known if antiviral therapy initiated after exposure has any positive effect.

Nutritional Therapy. An important measure in assisting hepatocytes to regenerate is adequate nutrition. No special diet is required in the treatment of viral hepatitis. However, a diet high in carbohydrates and proteins with low fat content is usually recommended. Adequate calories are important because the patient usually loses weight. If fat content is poorly tolerated because of decreased bile production, it should be reduced. Basically, the specific foods in the diet are dictated by the patient. Vitamin supplements, particularly B-complex vitamins and vitamin K, are frequently used. If anorexia, nausea, and vomiting are severe, IV solutions of glucose or supplemental tube feedings may be used. Fluid and electrolyte balance must be maintained.

NURSING MANAGEMENT
HEPATITIS

■ Nursing Assessment

Subjective and objective data that should be obtained from a person with hepatitis are presented in Table 42-8.

TABLE 42-8	Nursing Assessment Hepatitis

Subjective Data
Important Health Information
Past health history: Hemophilia; exposure to infected persons; ingestion of contaminated food or water; exposure to benzene, carbon tetrachloride, or other hepatotoxic agents; crowded, unsanitary living conditions; exposure to contaminated needles; recent travel; organ transplant recipient; exposure to new drug regimens
Medications: Use and misuse of acetaminophen, phenytoin, halothane, methyldopa

Functional Health Patterns
Health perception–health management: IV drug and alcohol abuse; malaise, distaste for cigarettes (in smokers), high-risk sexual behaviors
Nutritional-metabolic: Weight loss, anorexia, nausea, vomiting; feeling of fullness in right upper quadrant
Elimination: Dark urine; light-colored stools, constipation or diarrhea; skin rashes, hives
Activity-exercise: Fatigue, arthralgias, myalgias
Cognitive-perceptual: Right upper quadrant pain and liver tenderness, headache; pruritus
Role-relationship: Exposure as health care worker, chronic care institution resident, incarceration

Objective Data
General
Low-grade fever, lethargy, lymphadenopathy
Integumentary
Rash, angioedema, jaundice, icteric sclera, injection sites
Gastrointestinal
Hepatomegaly, splenomegaly
Possible Findings
Abnormal liver enzyme studies; ↑ serum total bilirubin, hypoalbuminemia, anemia, bilirubin in urine and increased urobilinogen, prolonged prothrombin time, positive tests for hepatitis including anti-HAV IgM, anti-HAV IgG, HBsAg, HBeAg, HBcAg, anti-HBc IgM, HBV DNA, anti-HCV, HCV RNA, anti-HDV; abnormal liver scan; positive liver biopsy

DNA, Deoxyribonucleic acid; *HAV,* hepatitis A virus; *HB,* hepatitis B; *HBV,* hepatitis B virus; *HCV,* hepatitis C virus; *HDV,* hepatitis D virus; *RNA,* ribonucleic acid.

▪ Nursing Diagnoses

Nursing diagnoses for the patient with hepatitis may include, but are not limited to, those presented in NCP 42-1.

▪ Planning

The overall goals are that the patient with viral hepatitis will (1) have relief of discomfort, (2) be able to resume normal activities, and (3) return to normal liver function without complications.

▪ Nursing Implementation

Health Promotion. Viral hepatitis is a community health problem. The nurse must assume a significant role in the control and prevention of this disease. It is helpful to first understand the epidemiology of the different types of viral hepatitis before considering appropriate control measures.

Hepatitis A. Vaccination is the best protection against HAV. Vaccination is recommended for persons 2 years of age and older who travel to areas with increased rates of hepatitis A, men who have sex with men, injecting and noninjecting drug users, per-

sons with clotting factor disorders (e.g., hemophilia), persons with chronic liver disease, and children living in regions of the United States with consistently increased rates of hepatitis A.

Outbreaks of viral hepatitis are usually due to HAV. In the United States there is usually one major outbreak per decade, the last being in 1995.[1] Preventive measures include personal and environmental hygiene and health education to promote good sanitation (Table 42-9). Hand washing is essential and is probably the most important precaution. Health teaching should include careful hand washing after bowel movements and before eating. When hepatitis A occurs in a food handler, IG should be administered to all other food handlers at the establishment. Patrons may also need to be given IG.

Isolation is not required for hepatitis A. For a patient with hepatitis A, infection control precautions should be used (see Table 12-19). A private room is indicated if the patient is incontinent of stool or has poor personal hygiene.

Hepatitis B. The use of the hepatitis B vaccine is the best means of protection. Control and prevention of hepatitis B also focus on identification of possible exposure via percutaneous and sexual transmission (see Table 42-9). The nurse must be aware of

---

NURSING CARE PLAN 42-1

Patient with Acute Viral Hepatitis

EXPECTED PATIENT OUTCOMES	NURSING INTERVENTIONS and *RATIONALES*
NURSING DIAGNOSIS	**Imbalanced nutrition: less than body requirements** *related to* anorexia, nausea, and reduced metabolism of nutrients by liver *as manifested by* inadequate food intake; perceived inability to ingest food.
▪ Adequate nutritional intake ▪ Progression toward or maintenance of normal body weight	▪ Collaborate with health care provider, dietitian, and family to provide appropriate diet *so the proper nutritional requirements can be provided.* ▪ Assess patient's appetite and adequacy of intake *so appropriate interventions can be planned.* ▪ Offer frequent small meals, provide oral care before *meals to enhance patient's dietary intake.* ▪ Allow patient to choose food items; serve high-carbohydrate and high-protein foods at time of day the patient feels most like eating *to increase likelihood of adequate intake.* ▪ Provide attractively served meals in pleasant surroundings *to stimulate patient's appetite.* ▪ Take weight daily on same scale, at same time, with same clothing *to monitor weight loss secondary to poor appetite.*
NURSING DIAGNOSIS	**Activity intolerance** *related to* fatigue and weakness *as manifested by* verbal report of fatigue or weakness, altered response to activity (as measured by BP, pulse, respiratory rate).
▪ Increased tolerance for activity	▪ Provide rest periods. ▪ Increase patient's activity gradually as allowed and tolerated *so previous activity pattern can be resumed.* ▪ Conserve patient's strength by careful monitoring of activity *to prevent increasing weakness and fatigue.* ▪ Teach patient to monitor and control activities that provoke fatigue *so patient can be an active participant in plan.*
NURSING DIAGNOSIS	**Ineffective therapeutic regimen management** *related to* lack of knowledge of follow-up care *as manifested by* frequent questions about transmission of disease, activities allowed, and general follow-up care.
▪ Verbalization of understanding of follow-up care ▪ Able to explain methods of transmission and methods of preventing transmission to others	▪ Teach patient basic facts about illness, modes of transmission, diet, activities allowed, avoidance of alcohol, and need for follow-up care *so appropriate follow-up care will be planned and carried out.* ▪ Teach patient to watch for and report signs of complications such as muscle cramps, bleeding gums or stools, worsening of symptoms *to enable prompt intervention.* Emphasize the importance of adequate rest *to enable liver to repair itself and to prevent relapse.* ▪ Teach use of infection control precautions *to reduce risk of cross-contamination.*

TABLE 42-9	Preventive Measures for Viral Hepatitis	
HEPATITIS A	**HEPATITIS B AND C**

General Measures
Hand washing
Proper personal hygiene
Environmental sanitation
Control and screening (signs, symptoms) of food handlers
Serologic screening while carrying virus
Active immunization: HAV vaccine to anyone over age 2
	Percutaneous Transmission
	Screening of donated blood
	  B—HBsAg
	  C—anti-HCV
	Use of disposable needles and syringes
	
	Sexual Transmission
	Acute exposure: HBIG administration to sexual partner of HBsAg-positive person
	Administer hepatitis B vaccine series to uninfected sexual partners
	Use condoms for sexual intercourse

Use of Immune Globulin Early administration (1-2 wk after exposure) to those exposed Prophylaxis for travelers to areas where hepatitis A is common if not vaccinated with HAV vaccine	**General Measures** Hand washing Avoid sharing toothbrushes and razors HBIG administration for one-time exposure (needle stick, contact of mucous membranes with infectious material) Active immunization: HBV vaccine

the individuals at high risk of contracting hepatitis B and teach methods to reduce risks. These include patients receiving frequent transfusions or hemodialysis, workers in hemodialysis units and laboratories where blood is handled, IV drug users, persons with multiple sexual partners, prisoners, and household members and sexual partners of HBV carriers.[1,19]

Good hygienic practices, including hand washing and the use of gloves when expecting contact with blood, are important. A condom is advised for sexual intercourse, and the partner should be vaccinated. Razors, toothbrushes, and other personal items should not be shared. Close contacts of the patient with hepatitis B who are HBsAg negative and antibody negative should be vaccinated.

According to CDC guidelines, infection control precautions should be followed for the patient with hepatitis B. This includes the use of disposable needles and syringes, which should be disposed of in puncture-resistant disposal units without recapping, bending, or breaking. (See Table 12-19 for various types of infection control precautions.)

Hepatitis C. There is no vaccine currently available. The primary measures to prevent HCV transmission are screening of blood, organ, and tissue donors; use of infection control precautions; and modification of high-risk behavior. Similar to HBV prevention, the nurse should identify individuals at high risk for contracting HCV and teach methods to reduce risks. Individuals at risk include those who use IV drugs (or have ever used, even once many years ago), patients who received blood or blood products before 1992, patients who are or have been on hemodialysis, workers in hemodialysis units and laboratories in which blood is handled, persons with multiple sexual partners, prisoners, and sexual partners of individuals with HCV. Infection with HCV often coexists with HIV infection.

The use of gloves when expecting contact with blood is important. A condom is advised for sexual intercourse with an individual with HCV. Razors, toothbrushes, and other personal items should not be shared. Preventive and control measures for hepatitis A, B and C are summarized in Table 42-9.

Acute Intervention

Jaundice. The nurse should assess for the degree of jaundice. In light-skinned persons the jaundice is usually observed first in the sclera of the eyes and later in the skin. In dark-skinned persons, jaundice is observed in the hard palate of the mouth and inner canthus of the eyes. Ictotest reagent tablets may be used to detect urinary bilirubin. The urine may have a dark brown or brownish red color because of the presence of bilirubin. Comfort measures to relieve pruritus (if present), headache, and arthralgias are helpful (see NCP 42-1).

Ensuring that the patient receives adequate nutrients is not always easy. The anorexia and extreme distaste for food cause nutritional problems. Dietary assessment must be considered. The nurse should try to determine whether there is something that appeals to the patient in spite of the anorexia. Small, frequent meals may be preferable to three large ones and may also help prevent nausea. Often, a patient with hepatitis finds that anorexia is not as severe in the morning, so it is easier to eat a good breakfast than a large dinner. Measures to stimulate the appetite, such as mouth care, antiemetics, and attractively served meals in pleasant surroundings, should be included in the nursing care plan. Other measures that may be tried to counteract the anorexia are carbonated beverages and avoidance of very hot or very cold foods. Adequate fluid intake (2500 to 3000 ml per day) is important.

Rest. Rest is essential and is an important factor in promoting liver cell regeneration. The nurse must assess the patient's response to the rest and activity plan and modify it accordingly. If the patient is on strict bed rest, measures to prevent respiratory and circulatory complications should be initiated. Assessment of the liver function tests and symptoms should continue as a guide to activity.

Psychologic and emotional rest is as essential as physical rest. Strict bed rest may produce anxiety and extreme restlessness in some patients and may be more damaging than reasonable ambulation. Diversional activities, such as reading and hobbies (e.g., knitting, stamp collecting), may help the patient.

Ambulatory and Home Care. Most patients with viral hepatitis will be cared for at home, so the nurse must assess the patient's knowledge of nutrition and provide the necessary dietary teaching. Rest and adequate nutrition are especially important until studies show that liver function has returned to normal. The patient must be cautioned about overexertion and the need to follow the physician's advice about when it is safe to return to work. The nurse must also teach the patient and family about preventive measures and how to prevent transmission to other family members. The patient should know what symptoms should be reported to the health care provider.

The patient should be assessed for any manifestations indicative of complications. Bleeding tendencies with increasing prothrombin time values, symptoms of encephalopathy, or abnormal liver function tests indicate problems, and the patient should be assessed and treated promptly.

The patient should be instructed to have regular follow-up for at least 1 year after the diagnosis of hepatitis. Because relapses are fairly common with hepatitis B and C, the patient should be instructed about the symptoms of recurrence and the need for follow-up evaluations. All patients with chronic HBV or HCV should avoid alcohol.

A patient who remains positive for HBsAg is a chronic carrier and should never be a blood donor. A patient who tests positive for the HCV antibody should also not donate blood. The patient with HBV and HCV should also be instructed to use a condom when engaging in sexual intercourse.

The patient who is receiving α-interferon for the treatment of hepatitis B or C requires education regarding this drug. α-Interferon is administered intramuscularly or subcutaneously, and thus the patient or family member needs to be taught how to administer the drug. There are numerous side effects with the therapy, including flulike symptoms (e.g., fever, malaise, fatigue, chills). The physician may recommend that acetaminophen be administered 30 to 60 minutes before injection to reduce these symptoms. Other significant side effects include thrombocytopenia, neutropenia, psychologic disturbances (e.g., mood swings, depression), and limited alopecia (see Table 42-7).

(Additional information on α-interferon is presented in Chapters 13 and 15.)

■ **Evaluation**

Expected outcomes for the patient with hepatitis are addressed in NCP 42-1.

Control of Hepatitis in Health Care Personnel

Hepatitis A. Hepatitis A is rarely transmitted from patients to health care personnel. When this does occur, it is associated with patients with undiagnosed hepatitis A who are treated for other problems. Usually these patients are incontinent of feces. The use of infection control precautions should prevent transmission of HAV to health care personnel.

Hepatitis B. Health care workers may be exposed to HBV from needle sticks or blood contamination to mucous membranes or nonintact skin. If a health care worker is exposed to HBV through a needle stick and does not receive the vaccine, there is a 6% to 30% chance of infection with hepatitis B.[1] Vaccination is the most effective method to prevent HBV in health care workers. Employers are required by the Occupational Safety and Health Administration to provide free HBV immunization to employees at risk for infection.

The principal mode of transmission of HBV for health care personnel is parenteral. Examples of parenteral transmission include accidental needle sticks and, rarely, transfusion of contaminated blood or blood products. Because all blood and blood products are tested for HBV and anti-HCV, there is diminishing risk of this latter mode of transmission. Other forms of transmission include contamination of fresh cutaneous scratches or abrasions, burns, and contamination of mucosal surfaces with infective blood, blood products, saliva, or semen.

Hepatitis C. Transmission is usually due to percutaneous needle exposure or other blood exposure and undetected parenteral transmission. Measures to prevent transmission of the viruses from patients to health care personnel are presented in Table 42-10. Very rarely do health care workers infect patient contacts.

TABLE 42-10   **Measures to Prevent Transmission of Hepatitis Viruses from Patients to Health Care Personnel***

HEPATITIS A	HEPATITIS B	HEPATITIS C
Always maintain good personal hygiene.	Use infection control precautions.[†]	Use infection control precautions.[†]
Wash hands after contact with a patient or removal of gloves.	Wash hands.	Wash hands.
Use infection control precautions.[†]	Reduce contact with blood or blood-containing secretions.	Reduce contact with blood or blood-contaminated secretions.
	Handle the blood of patients as potentially infective.	Handle the blood of patients as potentially infective.
	Dispose of needles properly.	Dispose of needles properly.
	Administer HBV vaccine to all health care personnel.	Use needleless IV access devices when available.
	Use needleless IV access devices when available.	

*A suggested guideline for general practice to prevent the nurse from contracting viral hepatitis from diagnosed and undiagnosed patients and carriers is for the nurse to wear disposable gloves, goggles, gowns (sometimes) when fecal or blood contamination is likely in handling (1) soiled bedpans, urinals, and catheters and (2) patient's bed linens soiled by body excreta or secretions.
†See Table 12-19.
IV, Intravenous.

TOXIC AND DRUG-INDUCED HEPATITIS

Liver injury and death may occur after the inhalation, parenteral injection, or ingestion of certain chemical substances (see
Table 38-6). The two major types of chemical hepatotoxicity are
toxic and drug-induced hepatitis. Agents producing toxic hepatitis are generally systemic poisons (e.g., carbon tetrachloride,
gold compounds) or are converted in the liver to toxic metabolites (e.g., acetaminophen). Liver necrosis generally occurs
within 2 to 3 days of acute exposure to a toxic substance.

Idiosyncratic drug reactions produce drug-induced hepatitis.
Such agents as halothane (Fluothane), isoniazid (INH), chloro-
thiazides (e.g., Diuril), methotrexate, and methyldopa (Aldomet)
may produce idiosyncratic reactions because of patient susceptibility (metabolic reactivity) to these agents or immunologically
mediated hypersensitivity responses. Liver injury may occur at
any time during or shortly after exposure. Some responses occur
2 to 5 weeks after exposure.

Older patients are particularly vulnerable to drug-induced
hepatitis. This is due to several factors, including increased use
of prescription and over-the-counter drugs, which can lead to
drug interactions and potential drug toxicity. Age-related decreases in liver function caused by decreased liver blood flow and
enzyme activity result in decreased drug metabolism. In addition,
with aging there is a decreased ability of the liver to recover from
drug-induced injury.

Toxic and drug-induced hepatitis are similar to viral hepatitis
in the pathophysiologic changes in the liver and the clinical manifestations. The usual presenting clinical findings are anorexia,
nausea, vomiting, hepatomegaly, splenomegaly, and abnormal
liver function studies. Treatment is largely supportive as in acute
viral hepatitis. Recovery may be rapid if the hepatotoxin is identified and removed. Liver transplantation may be necessary.

AUTOIMMUNE HEPATITIS

Chronic hepatitis may also occur in a number of patients who
have no known risk factors for the development of viral hepatitis.
This form of hepatitis is idiopathic; that is, the cause is unknown.
However, because many of these patients often have a number of
systemic problems, including glomerulonephritis and arthritis,
the disease is thought to be autoimmune. The presenting signs
and symptoms are variable and similar to viral hepatitis. Laboratory tests (elevation of liver enzymes) reveal liver inflammation
without evidence of viral antigens. The majority (70% to 80%) of
patients who are diagnosed with autoimmune hepatitis are
women. The course of the disease is also variable, with the majority of the patients exhibiting chronic active hepatitis.

Unlike viral hepatitis, autoimmune hepatitis (in which there is
evidence of necrosis and cirrhosis) is treated with corticosteroids
or other immunosuppressive agents. Daily treatment with methylprednisolone alone or in combination with azathioprine (Imuran)
will induce remission in approximately 80% of patients. If these
drugs do not work, other immunosuppressive therapies (e.g., cyclosporine, tacrolimus [Prograf], or mycophenolate mofetil [Cell-
Cept]) are initiated. Liver transplant is indicated for liver failure.

CIRRHOSIS OF THE LIVER

Cirrhosis is a chronic progressive disease of the liver characterized by extensive degeneration and destruction of the liver
parenchymal cells (Fig. 42-4). The liver cells attempt to regenerate, but the regenerative process is disorganized, resulting in ab-

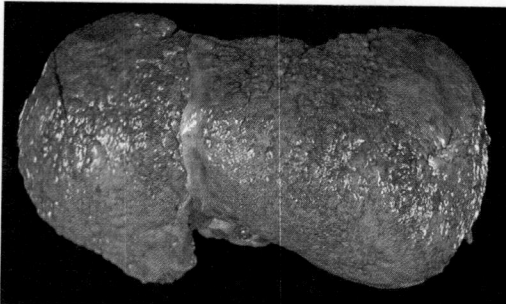

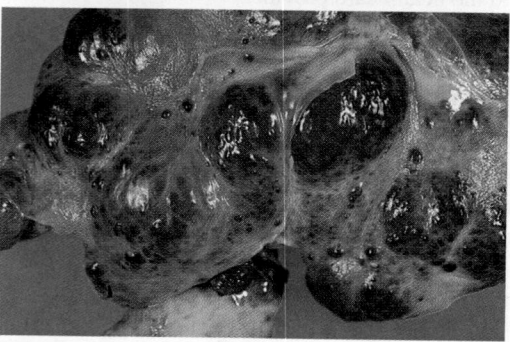

FIG. 42-4   Cirrhosis. **A,** Micronodular cirrhosis. **B,** Macronodular
cirrhosis.

normal blood vessel and bile duct relationships from the fibrosis.
The overgrowth of new and fibrous connective tissue distorts the
liver's normal lobular structure, resulting in lobules of irregular
size and shape with impeded vascular flow. Cirrhosis may have
an insidious, prolonged course.

Cirrhosis is ranked as the ninth leading cause of death in the
United States and the fourth leading cause of death in persons between 35 and 54 years of age. The highest incidence occurs between the ages of 40 and 60, and it is twice as common in men
as in women. Excessive alcohol ingestion is the single most common cause of cirrhosis.

Etiology and Pathophysiology

The four types of cirrhosis, in order of incidence, are as follows:
1. *Alcoholic* (previously called *Laënnec's*) *cirrhosis,* also
   called *portal* or *nutritional cirrhosis,* is usually associated
   with alcohol abuse. The first change in the liver from excessive alcohol intake is an accumulation of fat in the liver
   cells. Uncomplicated fatty changes in the liver are potentially reversible if the person stops drinking alcohol. If the
   alcohol abuse continues, widespread scar formation occurs
   throughout the liver.
2. *Postnecrotic cirrhosis* is a complication of viral, toxic, or
   idiopathic (autoimmune) hepatitis. Broad bands of scar tissue form within the liver.
3. *Biliary cirrhosis* is associated with chronic biliary obstruction and infection. There is diffuse fibrosis of the liver with
   jaundice as the main feature.
4. *Cardiac cirrhosis* results from long-standing, severe right-
   sided heart failure in patients with cor pulmonale, constrictive pericarditis, and tricuspid insufficiency.

In cirrhosis, cell necrosis occurs, and the destroyed liver cells
are replaced by scar tissue. The normal lobular architecture becomes nodular. Eventually, irregular, disorganized regeneration

poor cellular nutrition; and hypoxia caused by inadequate blood flow and scar tissue result in decreased functioning of the liver.

The specific cause of cirrhosis may not be determined in all patients. It is known that cirrhosis occurs with greatest frequency among alcoholics.[20] There continues to be some controversy as to whether the cause is the alcohol or the malnutrition that frequently coexists with chronic ingestion of alcohol. A common problem in alcoholics is protein malnutrition. There have been cases of nutritional cirrhosis resulting from extreme dieting or malnutrition. It is believed that the combined impact of malnutrition and alcohol is especially damaging to hepatocytes. Alcohol alone has a direct hepatotoxic effect. It is known to produce necrosis of cells and fatty infiltration. Some persons seem to have a predisposition to cirrhosis, regardless of their dietary or alcohol intake.

Approximately 20% of patients with chronic hepatitis C and 10% to 20% of those with chronic hepatitis B will develop cirrhosis. Chronic inflammation and cell necrosis result in fibrosis and, ultimately, cirrhosis. The combination of chronic hepatitis and alcohol ingestion is synergistic in terms of accelerating liver damage.

Clinical Manifestations

Early Manifestations. The onset of cirrhosis is usually insidious. Occasionally there is an abrupt onset of symptoms. GI disturbances are common early symptoms and include anorexia, dyspepsia, flatulence, nausea and vomiting, and change in bowel habits (diarrhea or constipation). These symptoms occur as a result of the liver's altered metabolism of carbohydrates, fats, and proteins. The patient may complain of abdominal pain described as a dull, heavy feeling in the right upper quadrant or epigastrium. The pain may be due to swelling and stretching of the liver capsule, spasm of the biliary ducts, and intermittent vascular spasm. Other early manifestations are fever, lassitude, slight weight loss, and enlargement of the liver and spleen. The liver is palpable in many patients with cirrhosis.

Later Manifestations. Later symptoms may be severe and result from liver failure and portal hypertension. Jaundice, peripheral edema, and ascites develop gradually. Other late symptoms include skin lesions, hematologic disorders, endocrine disturbances, and peripheral neuropathies (Fig. 42-5). In the advanced stages the liver becomes small and nodular.

Jaundice. Jaundice results from the functional derangement of liver cells and compression of bile ducts by connective tissue overgrowth. Jaundice occurs as a result of the decreased ability to conjugate and excrete bilirubin (hepatocellular jaundice). The jaundice may be minimal or severe, depending on the degree of liver damage. If obstruction of the biliary tract occurs, obstructive jaundice may also occur and is usually accompanied by pruritus. The pruritus is due to an accumulation of bile salts underneath the skin.

Skin lesions. Various skin manifestations are commonly seen in cirrhosis. **Spider angiomas** (*telangiectasia* or *spider nevi*) are small, dilated blood vessels with a bright red center point and spi-

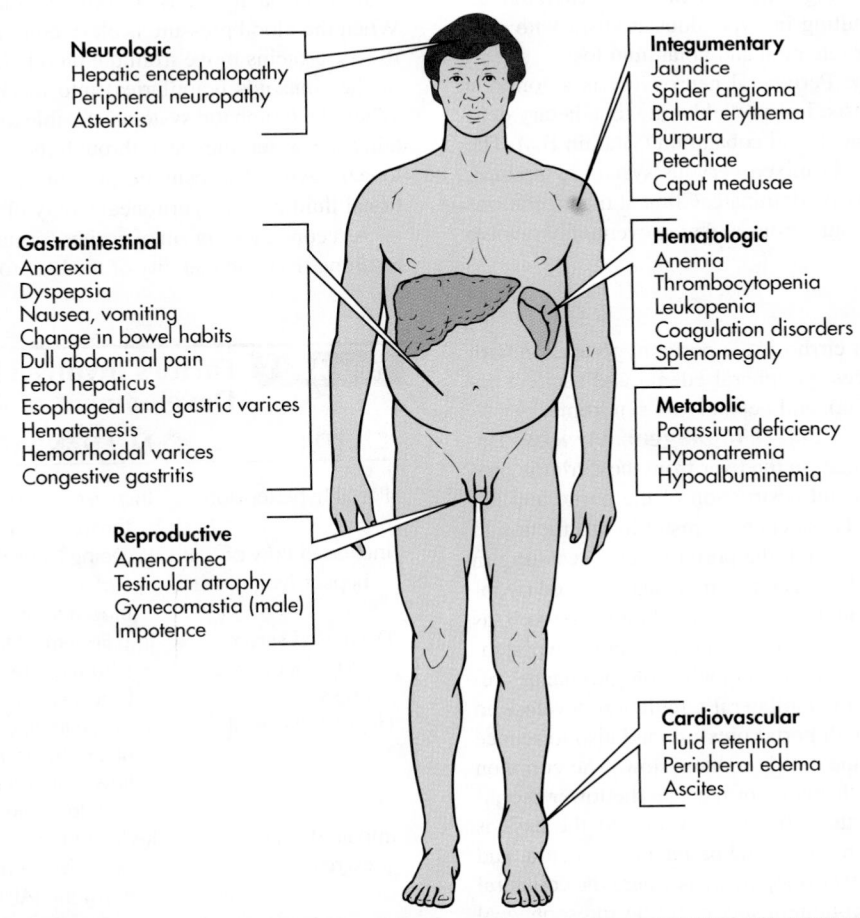

Neurologic
Hepatic encephalopathy
Peripheral neuropathy
Asterixis

Gastrointestinal
Anorexia
Dyspepsia
Nausea, vomiting
Change in bowel habits
Dull abdominal pain
Fetor hepaticus
Esophageal and gastric varices
Hematemesis
Hemorrhoidal varices
Congestive gastritis

Reproductive
Amenorrhea
Testicular atrophy
Gynecomastia (male)
Impotence

Integumentary
Jaundice
Spider angioma
Palmar erythema
Purpura
Petechiae
Caput medusae

Hematologic
Anemia
Thrombocytopenia
Leukopenia
Coagulation disorders
Splenomegaly

Metabolic
Potassium deficiency
Hyponatremia
Hypoalbuminemia

Cardiovascular
Fluid retention
Peripheral edema
Ascites

FIG. 42-5   Systemic clinical manifestations of liver cirrhosis.

derlike branches. They occur on the nose, cheeks, upper trunk, neck, and shoulders. *Palmar erythema* (a red area that blanches with pressure) is located on the palms of the hands. Both of these lesions are attributed to an increase in circulating estrogen as a result of the damaged liver's inability to metabolize steroid hormones.

Hematologic problems. Hematologic problems include thrombocytopenia, leukopenia, anemia, and coagulation disorders. Thrombocytopenia, leukopenia, and anemia are probably caused by the splenomegaly. Splenomegaly results from backup of blood from the portal vein into the spleen. Overactivity of the enlarged spleen results in increased removal of blood cells from circulation. The anemia is also due to inadequate RBC production and survival. Other factors involved in the anemia relate to poor diet, poor absorption of folic acid, and bleeding from varices.

The coagulation problems result from the liver's inability to produce prothrombin and other factors essential for blood clotting. Coagulation problems are manifested by hemorrhagic phenomena or bleeding tendencies, such as epistaxis, purpura, petechiae, easy bruising, gingival bleeding, and heavy menstrual bleeding.

Endocrine disturbances. Several signs and symptoms relating to the metabolism and inactivation of adrenocortical hormones, estrogen, and testosterone occur in cirrhosis. Normally the liver metabolizes these hormones. When the damaged liver is unable to do this, various manifestations occur. In men, gynecomastia, loss of axillary and pubic hair, testicular atrophy, and impotence with loss of libido may occur as a result of estrogen accumulation. In younger women amenorrhea may occur, and in older females there may be vaginal bleeding. The liver fails to metabolize aldosterone adequately, resulting in hyperaldosteronism with subsequent sodium and water retention and potassium loss.

Peripheral neuropathy. Peripheral neuropathy is a common finding in alcoholic cirrhosis. It is probably due to a dietary deficiency of thiamine, folic acid, and cobalamin (vitamin B_{12}). The neuropathy usually results in mixed nervous system symptoms, but sensory symptoms may predominate. Clinical manifestations of cirrhosis of the liver are numerous and may eventually involve the total body (see Fig. 42-5).

Complications

Major complications of cirrhosis are portal hypertension with resultant esophageal varices, peripheral edema and ascites, hepatic encephalopathy (coma), and hepatorenal syndrome.

Portal Hypertension and Esophageal Varices. Because of the structural changes in the liver from the cirrhotic process, there is compression and destruction of the portal and hepatic veins and sinusoids. These changes result in obstruction to the normal flow of blood through the portal system, resulting in portal hypertension. **Portal hypertension** is characterized by increased venous pressure in the portal circulation, as well as splenomegaly, large collateral veins, ascites, systemic hypertension, and esophageal varices. Many pathophysiologic changes result from portal hypertension. Collateral circulation develops in an attempt to reduce this high portal pressure and also to reduce the increased plasma volume and lymphatic flow. The common areas where the collateral channels form are in the lower esophagus (the anastomosis of the left gastric vein and the azygos veins), the anterior abdominal wall, the parietal peritoneum, and the rectum. Varicosities may develop in areas where the collateral and systemic circulations communicate, resulting in esophageal

and gastric varices, *caput medusae* (ring of varices around the umbilicus), and hemorrhoids.

Esophageal varices are a complex of tortuous veins at the lower end of the esophagus, enlarged and swollen as a result of portal hypertension. Esophageal varices are a common complication of cirrhosis, occurring in two thirds to three fourths of patients with cirrhosis. These collateral vessels contain little elastic tissue and are quite fragile. They tolerate the high pressure poorly, and the result is distended veins that bleed easily. Large varices are more likely to bleed.

Bleeding esophageal varices are the most life-threatening complication of cirrhosis. Approximately 30% to 50% of patients with cirrhosis die within 6 weeks of their first esophageal bleed.[21] The varices rupture and bleed in response to ulceration and irritation. Factors producing ulceration and irritation include alcohol ingestion; swallowing of poorly masticated food; ingestion of coarse food; acid regurgitation from the stomach; and increased intraabdominal pressure caused by nausea, vomiting, straining at stool, coughing, sneezing, or lifting heavy objects. The patient may have melena or hematemesis. There may be slow oozing or massive hemorrhage. Massive hemorrhage is a medical emergency.

Peripheral Edema and Ascites. Peripheral edema sometimes precedes ascites, but in some patients its development coincides with or occurs after ascites. Edema results from decreased colloidal oncotic pressure from impaired liver synthesis of albumin and increased portocaval pressure from portal hypertension. Peripheral edema occurs as ankle and presacral edema.

Ascites is the accumulation of serous fluid in the peritoneal or abdominal cavity. It is a common manifestation of cirrhosis. When the blood pressure is elevated in the liver, as occurs in cirrhosis, proteins move from the blood vessels via the larger pores of the sinusoids (capillaries) into the lymph space (Fig. 42-6). When the lymphatic system is unable to carry off the excess proteins and water, they leak through the liver capsule into the peritoneal cavity. The osmotic pressure of the proteins pulls additional fluid into the peritoneal cavity (Table 42-11).

A second mechanism of ascites formation is hypoalbuminemia resulting from the inability of the liver to synthesize albumin. The

TABLE 42-11   Factors Involved in the Development of Ascites

FACTOR	MECHANISM
Portal hypertension	Increase in resistance of blood flow through liver
Increased flow of hepatic lymph	Weeping of protein-rich lymph from surface of cirrhotic liver, intrahepatic blockage of lymph channels
Decreased serum colloidal oncotic pressure	Impairment of liver synthesis of albumin, loss of albumin into peritoneal cavity
Hyperaldosteronism	Increase in aldosterone secretion stimulated by decreased renal blood flow; impairment of liver metabolism of aldosterone
Impaired water excretion	Reduction in renal vascular flow and excessive serum levels of antidiuretic hormone (ADH)

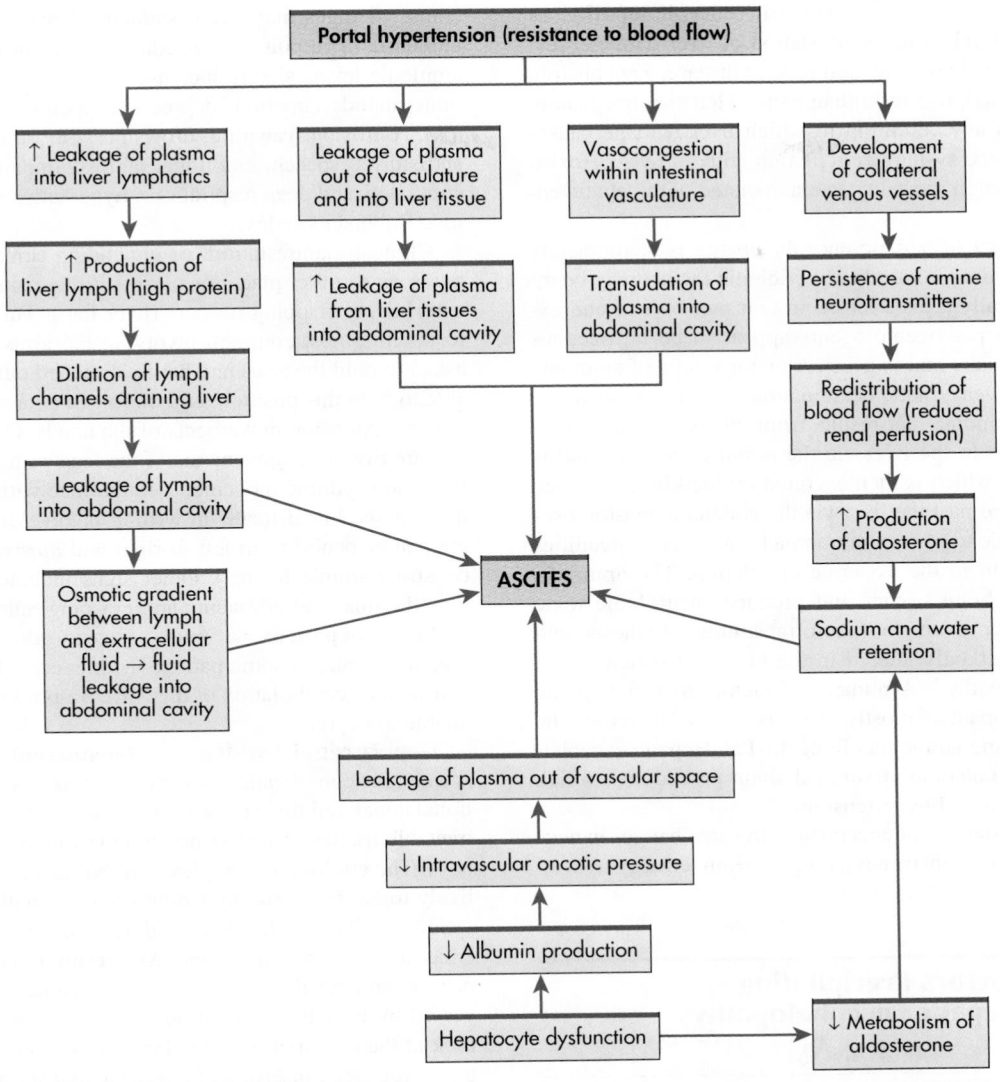

FIG. 42-6 Mechanisms for development of ascites.

hypoalbuminemia results in decreased colloidal oncotic pressure. A third mechanism of ascites, hyperaldosteronism, results when aldosterone is not metabolized by damaged hepatocytes. The increased level of aldosterone causes increased sodium reabsorption by the renal tubules. This retention of sodium, as well as an increase in antidiuretic hormone, causes additional water retention in these patients. Because of edema formation there is decreased intravascular volume and, subsequently, decreased renal blood flow and glomerular filtration.

Ascites is manifested by abdominal distention with weight gain (Fig. 42-7). If the ascites is severe, the umbilicus may be everted. Abdominal striae with distended abdominal wall veins may be present. The patient has signs of dehydration (e.g., dry tongue and skin, sunken eyeballs, muscle weakness). There is also a decrease in urinary output. Hypokalemia is common and is due to an excessive loss of potassium because of the effects of aldosterone. Low potassium levels can also result from diuretic therapy used to treat the ascites.

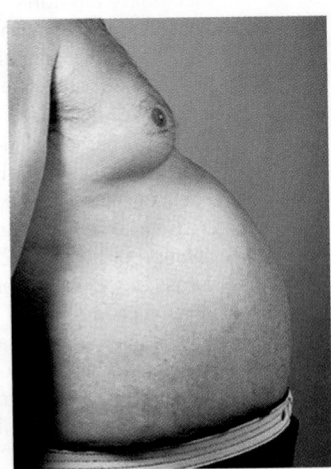

FIG. 42-7 Ascites and gynecomastia associated with cirrhosis of the liver. Photograph was taken after a paracentesis was performed.

Hepatic Encephalopathy. **Hepatic encephalopathy,** or coma, is a neuropsychiatric manifestation of liver damage. It is considered a terminal complication in liver disease. Encephalopathy is a more descriptive term than coma. Hepatic encephalopathy can occur in any condition in which liver damage causes ammonia to enter the systemic circulation without liver detoxification. There is a high mortality rate associated with hepatic encephalopathy.

The pathogenesis of hepatic encephalopathy is incompletely understood at this time. A number of etiologic factors may be involved. It is basically a disorder of protein metabolism and excretion. The main pathogenic agents appear to be nitrogenous ammonia and aromatic amino acids. A major source of ammonia is the bacterial and enzymatic deamination of amino acids in the intestines. The ammonia that results from this deamination process normally goes to the liver via the portal circulation and is converted to urea, which is then excreted by the kidneys. When the blood is shunted past the liver via the collateral anastomoses or the liver is unable to convert ammonia to urea, large quantities of ammonia remain in the systemic circulation. The ammonia crosses the blood-brain barrier and produces neurologic toxic manifestations. For example, neurotransmitter synthesis and degradation are markedly altered in the brains of patients with hepatic encephalopathy.[22] A number of factors may precipitate hepatic encephalopathy, mostly because they increase the amount of circulating ammonia (Table 42-12). Hepatic encephalopathy is also an outcome of surgical shunt procedures, which are used to reduce portal hypertension.[23]

Clinical manifestations of encephalopathy are changes in neurologic and mental responsiveness, ranging from lethargy to deep coma. Changes may occur suddenly because of an increase in ammonia in response to bleeding varices or gradually as blood ammonia levels slowly increase. In the early stages, manifestations include euphoria, depression, apathy, irritability, memory loss, confusion, yawning, drowsiness, insomnia, agitation, slow and slurred speech, emotional lability, impaired judgment, hiccups, slow and deep respirations, hyperactive reflexes, and a positive Babinski's reflex.

Clinical manifestations of impending coma include disorientation as to time, place, or person. A characteristic symptom is **asterixis,** or flapping tremors (liver flap). This may take several forms, the most common involving the arms and hands. When asked to hold the arms and hands stretched out, the patient is unable to hold this position, and there will be a series of rapid flexion and extension movements of the hands. Other signs of asterixis are rhythmic movements of the legs with dorsiflexion of the foot and rhythmic movements in the face with strong closure of the eyelids. Impairments in writing involve difficulty in moving the pen or pencil from left to right and *apraxia* (the inability to construct simple figures). Other signs include hyperventilation, hypothermia, and grimacing and grasping reflexes.

Fetor hepaticus—a musty, sweet odor of the patient's breath—occurs in some patients with encephalopathy. This odor is from the accumulation of digestive by-products that the liver is unable to degrade.

Hepatorenal Syndrome. **Hepatorenal syndrome** (HRS) is a serious complication of cirrhosis. It is characterized by functional renal failure with advancing azotemia, oliguria, and intractable ascites. There is no structural abnormality of the kidneys. The etiology is complex, but the final common pathway is likely to be that portal hypertension along with liver decompensation results in splanchnic and systemic vasodilation and decreased arterial blood volume. As a result, renal vasoconstriction occurs, and renal failure occurs. This renal failure can be reversed by liver transplantation. Current efforts are underway to look at the potential use of splanchnic vasoconstrictors and volume expanders, insertion of a transjugular intrahepatic portosystemic shunt radiologically, and improved forms of dialysis to manage this severe complication. In the patient with cirrhosis, HRS frequently follows diuretic therapy, GI hemorrhage, or paracentesis.[24]

Diagnostic Studies

In cirrhosis there are abnormalities in most of the liver function studies. Enzyme levels, including alkaline phosphatase, aspartate aminotransferase (AST) (serum glutamic-oxaloacetic transaminase [SGOT]), alanine aminotransferase (ALT) (serum glutamate pyruvate transaminase [SGPT]), and γ-glutamyl transferase (GGT), are elevated because of the release of these enzymes from damaged liver cells. Protein metabolism tests show decreased total protein, decreased albumin, and increased globulin levels. The liver does not synthesize γ-globulins but does synthesize albumin. γ-Globulins (antibodies) are produced by B lymphocytes. The globulin level often increases in cirrhosis and indicates increased synthesis or decreased removal. Fat metabolism abnormalities are reflected by decreased cholesterol levels. The prothrombin time is prolonged, and bilirubin metabolism is altered (Table 42-13). Liver biopsy may be performed to identify liver cell changes and alterations in the lobular structure. Differential analysis of ascitic fluid may be helpful in establishing a diagnosis.

TABLE 42-12	**Factors Precipitating Hepatic Encephalopathy**
FACTOR	**MECHANISM**
GI hemorrhage	Increase in ammonia in GI tract
Constipation	Increase in ammonia from bacterial action on feces
Hypokalemia	Potassium ions are needed by brain to metabolize ammonia
Hypovolemia	Increase in blood ammonia by causing hepatic hypoxia; impairment of cerebral, hepatic, and renal function because of decreased blood flow
Infection	Increase in catabolism, increase in cerebral sensitivity to toxins
Cerebral depressants (e.g., narcotics)	No detoxification by liver, causing increase in cerebral depression
Metabolic alkalosis	Facilitation of transport of ammonia across blood-brain barrier, increase in renal production of ammonia
Paracentesis	Loss of sodium and potassium ions, decrease in blood volume
Dehydration	Potentiation of ammonia toxicity
Increased metabolism	Increase in workload of liver
Uremia (renal failure)	Retention of nitrogenous metabolites

GI, Gastrointestinal.

TABLE 42-13	Bilirubin Metabolism Abnormalities in Cirrhosis*	
TYPE	**FINDING**	
Serum bilirubin		
Unconjugated	↑	
Conjugated	↑↓	
Urine bilirubin	↑	
Urobilinogen		
Stool	Normal, ↓	
Urine	Normal, ↑	

*Bilirubin metabolism abnormalities occurring with hepatocellular jaundice, the most frequent type of jaundice with cirrhosis.

Collaborative Care

Rest. Although there is no specific therapy for cirrhosis, certain measures can be taken to promote liver cell regeneration and prevent or treat complications (Table 42-14). Rest is significant in reducing metabolic demands of the liver and allowing for recovery of liver cells. At various times during the progress of cirrhosis, the rest may have to take the form of complete bed rest.

Ascites. Management of ascites is focused on sodium restriction, diuretics, and fluid removal. The amount of sodium restriction is based on the degree of ascites. Initially the patient may be encouraged to limit sodium intake to 2 g per day. Patients with severe ascites may need to restrict their sodium intake to 250 to 500 mg per day. Very low sodium intake can result in reduced nutritional intake and subsequent problems associated with malnutrition. The patient is usually not on restricted fluids unless severe ascites develops. There should be accurate assessment and control of fluid and electrolyte balance. Bed rest initially produces diuresis, which increases fluid excretion. Salt-poor albumin may be used to help maintain intravascular volume and adequate urinary output by increasing plasma colloid osmotic pressure.

Diuretic therapy is an important part of management. Often a combination of drugs that work at multiple sites in the nephron is more effective. Spironolactone (Aldactone) is an effective diuretic, even in patients with severe sodium retention. Spironolactone is an antagonist of aldosterone and is potassium sparing. Other potassium-sparing diuretics include amiloride (Midamor) and triamterene (Dyrenium). A high-potency loop diuretic, such as furosemide (Lasix), is frequently used in combination with a potassium-sparing drug. Chlorothiazide (Diuril) or hydrochlorothiazide (HydroDiuril) may also be used, but the thiazide diuretics are not as potent as the loop diuretics.

A **paracentesis** (needle puncture of the abdominal cavity) may be performed to remove ascitic fluid. However, it is reserved for the patient with impaired respiration or abdominal pain caused by severe ascites. It is only a temporary measure because the fluid tends to reaccumulate.

Peritoneovenous shunt. *Peritoneovenous shunt* is a surgical procedure that provides continuous reinfusion of ascitic fluid into the venous system. One type, the LaVeen peritoneovenous shunt, consists of a tube and a one-way valve. The tube runs from the abdominal cavity through the peritoneum, under the subcutaneous tissue, and into the jugular vein or superior vena cava (Fig. 42-8). The valve opens when the pressure in the peritoneal cavity is 3 to 5 cm H_2O higher than that in the superior vena cava. This allows the ascitic fluid to flow into the venous system. The patient's inspiration increases the intraperitoneal pressure, causing the valve to open. This shunting of the ascitic fluid causes an improvement

TABLE 42-14	Collaborative Care Cirrhosis of the Liver	

Diagnostic	**Ascites**
History and physical examination	Administration of 3000-calorie, high-carbohydrate, protein
Liver function studies	(depends on stage), low-fat diet, low sodium for ascites
Liver biopsy (percutaneous needle)	Diuretics
Esophagogastroduodenoscopy	spironolactone (Aldactone)
Angiography (percutaneous transhepatic portography)	amiloride (Midamor)
Liver scan	triamterene (Dyrenium)
Liver ultrasound	furosemide (Lasix)
Serum electrolytes	Paracentesis (if indicated)
Prothrombin time	Peritoneovenous shunt (if indicated)
Serum albumin	***Esophageal Varices***
CBC	β-Adrenergic blockers
Testing of stool for occult blood	vasopressin (Pitressin)
Upper GI barium swallow	Endoscopic sclerotherapy or ligation
Collaborative Therapy	Balloon tamponade
Conservative Therapy	octreotide (Sandostatin)
Administration of B-complex vitamins	Surgical shunting procedure
Rest	Transjugular intrahepatic portosystemic shunt (TIPS)
Avoidance of alcohol and aspirin	***Hepatic Encephalopathy***
	Antibiotics to decrease bacterial flora in GI tract
	lactulose (Cephulac)

CBC, Complete blood count; *GI,* gastrointestinal.

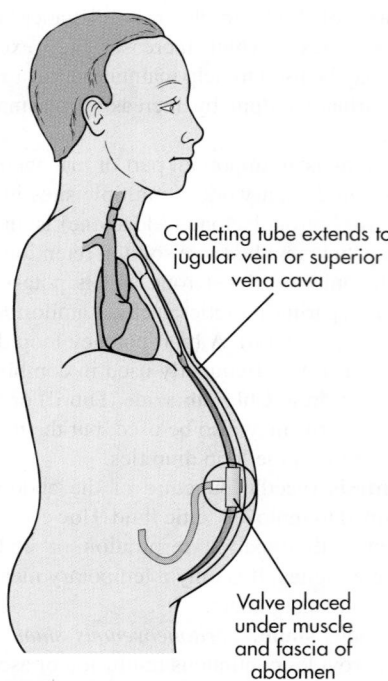

Collecting tube extends to
jugular vein or superior
vena cava

Valve placed
under muscle
and fascia of
abdomen

FIG. 42-8 Peritoneovenous shunt.

in hemodynamic factors and increases sodium and fluid excretion. Urine output is also increased.

Peritoneovenous shunt is not a first-line therapy for ascites because of the number of complications associated with it, including thrombosis formation at the venous tip of the shunt, infection, fluid overload, disseminated intravascular coagulopathy, variceal hemorrhage, and shunt occlusion. In addition, peritoneovenous shunts do not improve patient survival rates. Transjugular intrahepatic portosystemic shunt (TIPS) (discussed later in this section) is used increasingly to alleviate ascites.

Esophageal Varices. The main therapeutic goal related to esophageal varices is avoidance of bleeding and hemorrhage. Risk factors for esophageal bleeding include variceal size, decreased wall thickness, and degree of liver dysfunction. The patient who has esophageal varices should avoid ingesting alcohol, aspirin, and irritating foods. Upper respiratory infections should be treated promptly, and coughing should be controlled. For patients who have not bled from esophageal varices, prophylactic treatment with nonselective β-blockers (e.g., propranolol [Inderal]) has been shown to reduce the risk of bleeding, as well as bleeding-related deaths.[25]

Management of bleeding esophageal varices includes emergency, therapeutic, and prophylactic interventions. Management, which involves a combination of drug and endoscopic therapy, is more successful than either approach alone.[25] Drug therapy may include octreotide (Sandostatin), vasopressin (VP), nitroglycerin (NTG), and β-adrenergic blockers. Endoscopic therapies include sclerotherapy, ligation of varices, and shunt therapy.

When esophageal variceal bleeding occurs, the first step is to stabilize the patient and manage the airway. IV therapy is initiated and may include administration of blood products. The diagnosis of esophageal variceal bleeding is made by endoscopic examination as soon as possible. At the time of endoscopy, sclerotherapy

or banding of the varices may be performed. The main goal of drug therapy is to stop bleeding so that treatment measures can be done. The initial measures to stop the bleeding include IV administration of VP, which produces vasoconstriction of the splanchnic arterial bed, decreases portal blood flow, and decreases portal hypertension. It has many side effects, including decreased coronary blood flow and heart rate and increased blood pressure. Current drug therapy in some institutions is a combination of VP and NTG. The NTG reduces the detrimental effects of the VP while enhancing its beneficial effect. VP should be avoided or used cautiously in the older adult because of the risk of cardiac ischemia.[26]

Endoscopic sclerotherapy is a treatment method for both acute and chronic bleeding varices in many institutions. The sclerosing agent, introduced via endoscopy, thromboses and obliterates the distended veins.

Another procedure for managing acute variceal bleeding is endoscopic ligation or banding of the varices. A small rubber band (elastic O-ring) is slipped around the base of the varix. Endoscopic variceal ligation can be done using clips instead of the O-rings (endoscopic clipping). Endoscopic ligation is as effective as endoscopic sclerotherapy with fewer complications. A combination of endoscopic sclerotherapy and ligation may be used and seems to be more effective than either treatment alone.

Balloon tamponade may be used in patients with brisk esophageal or gastric variceal hemorrhage that cannot be controlled on initial endoscopy. Balloon tamponade controls the hemorrhage by mechanical compression of the varices. The Minnesota or Sengstaken-Blakemore tube is used for this purpose (Fig. 42-9). These tubes have two balloons: gastric and esophageal. The Sengstaken-Blakemore tube has three lumens: one for the gastric balloon, one for the esophageal balloon, and one for gastric aspiration. The Minnesota tube has an esophageal aspiration port. When inflated, the gastric and esophageal balloons put mechanical compression on the varices. The gastric balloon anchors the tube in position and also applies pressure to any bleeding gastric varices.

Supportive measures during an acute variceal bleed include administration of fresh frozen plasma and packed RBCs, vitamin K (AquaMEPHYTON), and histamine (H_2)–receptor blockers such as cimetidine (Tagamet). Lactulose (Cephulac) and neomycin administration may be started to prevent hepatic encephalopathy from breakdown of blood and the release of ammonia in the intestine.

Long-term management. Long-term management of patients who have had an episode of bleeding includes β-adrenergic blockers, repeated sclerotherapy, endoscopic ligation, and portosystemic shunts. There is a high incidence of recurrent bleeding with a high mortality risk with each bleeding episode, so continued therapy is necessary. Repeated endoscopic sclerotherapy and ligation are commonly used.

Propranolol (Inderal), a β-adrenergic blocker, can be given orally to prevent recurrent GI bleeding. It reduces portal venous pressure. This effect is due to reduced cardiac output and, possibly, constriction of splanchnic vessels. However, because it reduces hepatic blood flow, it can enhance the possibility of hepatic encephalopathy.

Shunting procedures. Surgical and nonsurgical methods of shunting blood away from the esophageal varices are available. Shunting procedures tend to be used more after a second major bleeding episode than an initial bleeding episode. *Transjugular intrahepatic portosystemic shunt (TIPS)* is a nonsurgical procedure

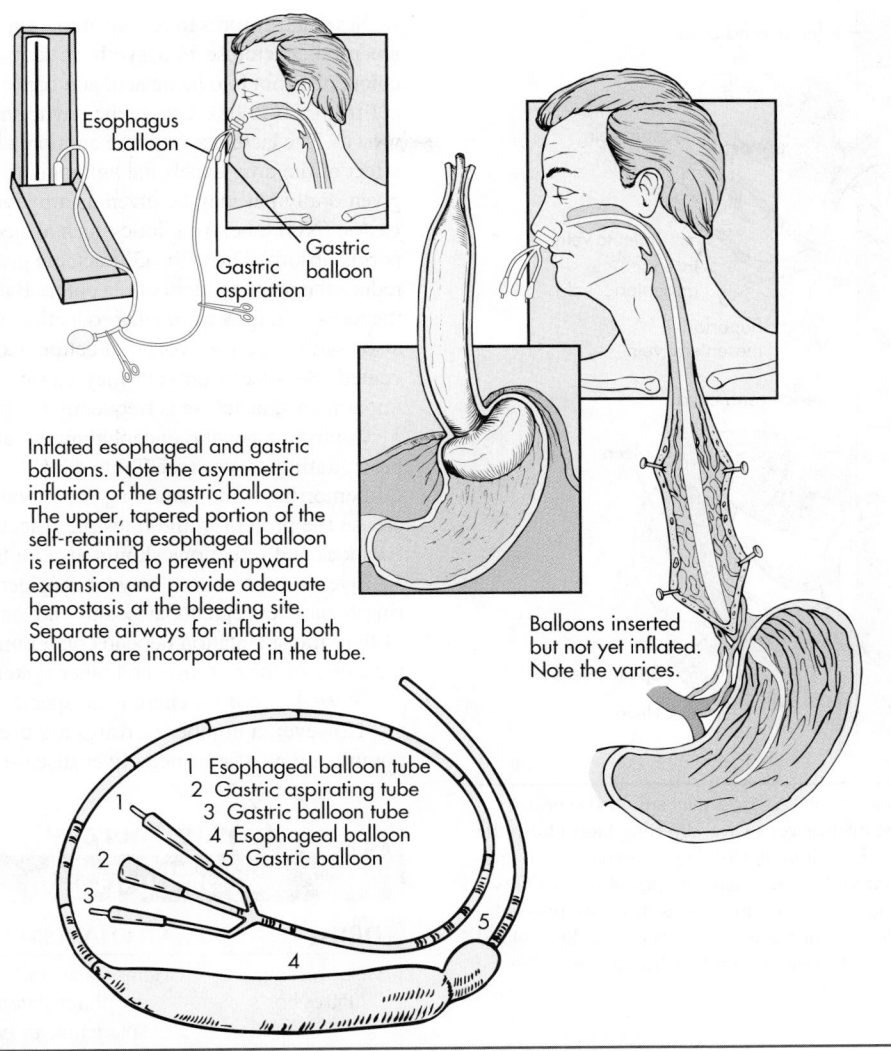

Inflated esophageal and gastric balloons. Note the asymmetric inflation of the gastric balloon. The upper, tapered portion of the self-retaining esophageal balloon is reinforced to prevent upward expansion and provide adequate hemostasis at the bleeding site. Separate airways for inflating both balloons are incorporated in the tube.

Balloons inserted but not yet inflated. Note the varices.

1 Esophageal balloon tube
2 Gastric aspirating tube
3 Gastric balloon tube
4 Esophageal balloon
5 Gastric balloon

FIG. 42-9 Esophageal tamponade accomplished with Sengstaken-Blakemore tube.

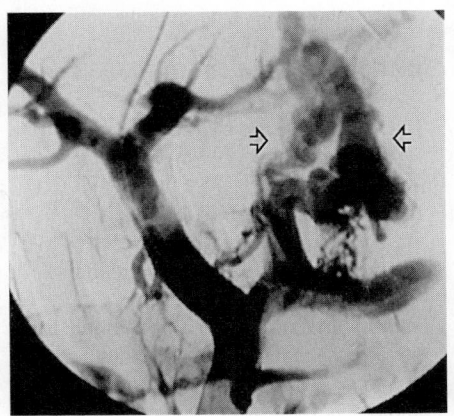

A

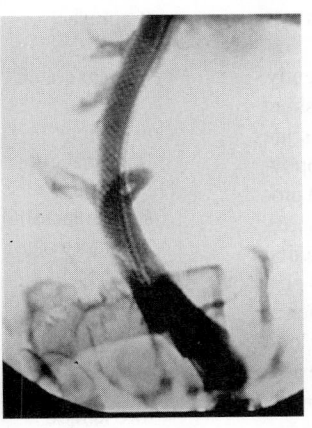

B

FIG. 42-10 Total portal diversion after transjugular intrahepatic portosystemic shunt (TIPS). **A,** Portal venogram before TIPS shows filling of large esophageal varices *(arrows).* **B,** After insertion of a TIPS, flow to varices is eliminated. Intrahepatic portal vein flow is now reversed, with the direction of intrahepatic flow toward the TIPS.

in which a tract (shunt) between the systemic and portal venous systems is created to redirect portal blood flow (Fig. 42-10). A catheter is placed in the jugular vein and then threaded through the superior and inferior vena cava to the hepatic vein. The wall of the hepatic vein is punctured and the catheter is directed to the portal vein. Stents are positioned along the passageway, overlapping in the liver tissue and extending into both veins.

This procedure reduces portal venous pressure and decompresses the varices, thus controlling bleeding. This procedure does not interfere with future liver transplantation. Limitations of the

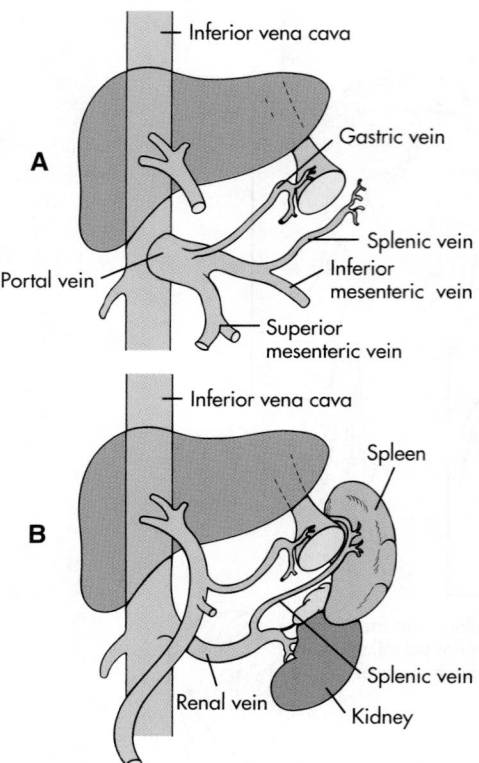

FIG. 42-11 Portosystemic shunts. **A,** Portacaval shunt. The portal vein is anastomosed to the inferior vena cava, diverting blood from the portal vein to the systemic circulation. **B,** Distal splenorenal shunt. The splenic vein is anastomosed to the renal vein. The portal venous flow remains intact while esophageal varices are selectively decompressed. (The short gastric veins are decompressed.) The spleen conducts blood from the high pressure of the esophageal and gastric varices to the low-pressure renal vein.

TIPS procedure include the increased risk of hepatic encephalopathy and stenosis of the stent.

Various surgical shunting procedures may be used to decrease portal hypertension by diverting some of the portal blood flow while at the same time allowing adequate liver perfusion. Currently, the surgical shunts most commonly used are the portacaval shunt and the distal splenorenal shunt (Fig. 42-11). Surgical shunts are more likely to be used in emergency situations. Although a prophylactic portacaval shunt decreases bleeding episodes, it does not prolong life. Patients die of hepatic encephalopathy caused by the diversion of the ammonia past the liver and into the systemic circulation. The distal splenorenal shunt (Warren shunt) leaves portal venous flow intact (see Fig. 42-11), so it has a lower incidence of hepatic encephalopathy. However, with time the flow of blood through the liver decreases. Similar to TIPS, surgical stents are also prone to occlusion, necessitating angiography and stent dilation.

Hepatic Encephalopathy. The goal of management of hepatic encephalopathy is the reduction of ammonia formation. This consists mainly of protein restriction and reduction of ammonia formation in the intestines. The degree of protein restriction is determined by the severity of mental change. The protein restriction may range from 0 to 40 g per day. With improvement of mental function, dietary protein content is increased gradually over days.

Several measures to reduce ammonia formation in the intestines are used. Lactulose is a synthetic keto-analog of lactose. In the colon, it is split into lactic acid and acetic acid, which decreases the pH from 7.0 to 5.0. The acidic environment discourages bacterial growth. The lactulose traps the ammonia in the gut, and the laxative effect of the drug expels the ammonia from the colon. It is usually given orally but may be given as a retention enema or via a nasogastric (NG) tube. Antibiotics such as neomycin sulfate, which are poorly absorbed from the GI tract, are given orally or rectally. They reduce the bacterial flora of the colon. Bacterial action on protein in the feces results in ammonia production. Cathartics and enemas are also used to decrease bacterial action. Constipation should be prevented. Because neomycin may cause renal toxicity and hearing impairments, lactulose is frequently the preferred drug.

Control of hepatic encephalopathy also involves treatment of precipitating causes (see Table 42-12). This involves controlling GI hemorrhage and removing the blood from the GI tract to decrease the protein in the intestine. Electrolyte and acid-base imbalances and infections should also be treated.

Liver transplantation may be considered in patients with recurring hepatic encephalopathy and end-stage liver disease. The use of liver transplantation depends on a number of factors, including the cause of the cirrhosis and other systemic medical problems.[27]

Drug Therapy. There is no specific drug therapy for cirrhosis. However, a number of drugs are used to treat symptoms and complications of advanced liver disease (Table 42-15).

TABLE 42-15   *Drug* Therapy
Cirrhosis

DRUG	MECHANISM OF ACTION
vasopressin (Pitressin)	Hemostasis and control of bleeding in esophageal varices, constriction of splanchnic arterial bed
propranolol (Inderal)	Reduction of portal venous pressure, reduction of esophageal varices bleeding
lactulose (Cephulac)	Acidification of feces in bowel and trapping of ammonia, causing its elimination in feces
neomycin sulfate	Decrease in bacterial flora, decreasing formation of ammonia
cimetidine (Tagamet)	Decrease in gastric acidity
Diuretics	
spironolactone (Aldactone)	Blocking of action of aldosterone, potassium sparing
amiloride (Midamor)	Inhibits reabsorption of sodium and secretion of potassium
chlorothiazide (Diuril)	Thiazide that acts on proximal tubule to decrease reabsorption of sodium and water
furosemide (Lasix)	Rapid action on distal tubule and loop of Henle to prevent reabsorption of sodium and water
triamterene (Dyrenium)	Inhibits reabsorption of sodium and secretion of potassium
magnesium sulfate	Magnesium replacement; hypomagnesemia occurs with liver dysfunction
Vitamin K	Correction of clotting abnormalities

Nutritional Therapy. The diet for the patient with cirrhosis without complications is high in calories (3000 kcal per day) with high carbohydrate content and moderate to low fat levels. The amount of protein varies depending on the degree of liver damage and the potential for encephalopathy. When the patient is symptomatic (e.g., ascites, edema, mental changes), a low-protein diet is indicated. When there is reduced risk of encephalopathy, 1.5 g of protein per kilogram of body weight may be ordered to maintain plasma osmotic balance and promote liver cell regeneration. Foods high in protein include meat, fish, poultry, eggs, and dairy

products. High-protein nourishment in the form of eggnogs, milkshakes, or protein supplements may be used, particularly for the patient who is malnourished. Vitamin supplements are usually given.

The patient with hepatic encephalopathy is on a very-low-protein to no-protein diet (Table 42-16). Foods allowed include toast, cereal, rice, tea, fruit juices, and hard candies. Sufficient carbohydrate intake must be provided to maintain an intake of 1500 to 2000 calories to prevent hypoglycemia and catabolism. Glucose polymer (Polycose) is protein free and can be used as a source of

TABLE 42-16	**Nutritional Therapy** Low-Protein Diet for Hepatic Failure*		

General Principles
Limit protein to 20 g per day at onset of severe hepatic failure.
Protein must be from protein sources with high biologic value.
Diet must be high in calories.
Fat is limited only to prevent early satiety.
Protein is increased in diet by 10-g increments as tolerated without causing signs and symptoms of hepatic encephalopathy.
Sodium is also usually restricted, as well as fluid when edema and ascites are present.

MEAL	MENU PLAN 1	MENU PLAN 2	MENU PLAN 3
Breakfast 1 fruit, calorie supplement 1 low-protein bread 1 egg (protein) Fat, calorie supplement ¼ cup milk (2 g protein)	½ cup grape juice with 2 tbs Polycose powder† French toast made with low-protein bread, 1 egg, 3 tsp salt-free butter and syrup ¼ cup milk	¼ cup cranberry juice with 2 tbs Polycose powder Low-protein toast with 3 tsp salt-free butter and 2 tsp jelly 1-egg omelet with 3 tsp salt-free butter ¼ cup milk	¼ cup prune juice with 2 tbs Polycose powder Low-protein toast with 3 tsp salt-free butter 1 egg fried in 3 tsp salt-free butter ¼ cup milk
Snack Calorie supplement	Jelly beans	Hard candy	Sugar mints
Lunch 2 starch (4 g protein) 1 vegetable (2 g protein) 1 fruit, calorie supplement Fat, calorie supplement	¼ cup half and half ½ cup Cream of Wheat with 3 tsp salt-free butter Applesauce with whipped topping or Lipomul‡ Small tossed salad with 3 tbs oil and vinegar§ Peas with 3 tsp salt-free butter	¼ cup half and half ½ cup cornmeal (atole) with 3 tsp salt-free butter Small guacamole salad Gelatin with whipped topping or Lipomul Corn with 3 tsp salt-free butter	¼ cup half and half ½ cup grits with 3 tsp salt-free butter Cucumbers in sour cream Peaches with whipped topping or Lipomul Sweet potatoes with brown sugar and 3 tsp salt-free butter
Snack Calorie supplement	Low-protein cookies	Low-protein bread cubes with whipped cream and strawberries	Popsicles made with Polycose
Dinner 1 starch (2 g protein) 1 vegetable (2 g protein) 1 low-protein bread ¼ cup milk (2 g protein) Fat, calorie supplement	½ baked potato 3 tsp salt-free butter Low-protein bread ¼ cup sour cream ½ cup green beans with 3 tsp salt-free butter and 2 tsp jelly ¼ cup milk	½ cup fried potatoes with 1 tsp melted salt-free butter ½ cup zucchini with 3 tsp salt-free butter Low-protein toast with 3 tsp salt-free butter and 2 tsp marmalade ¼ cup milk	½ cup mashed potatoes ½ cup fried okra Low-protein toast with 3 tsp salt-free butter and 2 tsp jam ¼ cup milk

*The diet plan contains approximately 20 g protein.
†Polycose is a brand-name product made by Ross Laboratories.
‡Lipomul is a fat emulsion made by Upjohn.
§Crisp food should be avoided because of the possibility of esophageal varices.

calories. It can be given orally or via NG tube. A patient with alcoholic cirrhosis frequently has protein-calorie malnutrition. For the patient with protein malnutrition, enteral formulas such as Travasorb Hepatic or Hepatic-Aid may be used. These supplements contain protein from branched-chain amino acids that are metabolized by the muscles. They provide protein but put less burden on the liver. TPN or tube feedings may be required.

The patient with ascites and edema is on a low-sodium diet. The degree of sodium restriction varies depending on the patient's condition. The patient needs instruction regarding the degree of restriction. Table salt is the most common source of sodium. Sodium is also present in baking soda and baking powder. Foods that are high in sodium content include canned soups and vegetables, salted snacks such as potato chips, nuts, smoked meats and fish, crackers, breads, olives, pickles, ketchup, and beer.

Sodium is also present in many over-the-counter drugs (e.g., antacids). However, most antacids are now lower in sodium than previously. Carbonated beverages tend to be high in sodium, and low-sodium and sodium-free carbonated drinks are available. The patient should be advised to read labels. Foods high in protein usually have large amounts of sodium. Alternative protein supplements that are low in sodium may have to be used. The patient and the family need assistance to make the diet more palatable by the use of seasonings such as garlic, parsley, onion, lemon juice, and spices.

NURSING MANAGEMENT
CIRRHOSIS

■ Nursing Assessment

Subjective and objective data that should be obtained from an individual with cirrhosis are presented in Table 42-17.

■ Nursing Diagnoses

Nursing diagnoses for the patient with cirrhosis include, but are not limited to, those presented in NCP 42-2.

■ Planning

The overall goals are that the patient with cirrhosis will (1) have relief of discomfort, (2) have minimal to no complications (ascites, esophageal varices, hepatic encephalopathy), and (3) return to as normal a lifestyle as possible.

■ Nursing Implementation

Health Promotion. The common etiologies of cirrhosis are alcohol, malnutrition, hepatitis, biliary obstruction, and right-sided heart failure. Prevention and early treatment of cirrhosis must focus on the primary cause. Alcoholism must be treated. Patients should be urged to avoid alcohol ingestion, and their efforts should be supported. Adequate nutrition, especially for the alcoholic and other individuals at risk for cirrhosis, is essential to promote liver regeneration. Acute hepatitis must be identified and treated early so that it does not progress to chronic hepatitis. Biliary disease must be treated so that the stones do not cause obstruction and infection. The underlying cause (e.g., chronic lung disease) of right-sided heart failure must be treated so that the heart failure does not lead to cirrhosis.

Acute Intervention. The focus of nursing care for the patient with cirrhosis is on conserving the patient's strength (see NCP 42-2). Rest enables the liver to restore itself. Complete bed rest may not always be necessary. When the patient requires complete bed rest, measures to prevent pneumonia, thromboembolic problems, and pressure ulcers should be taken. The activity and rest schedule may be modified according to

TABLE 42-17	Nursing Assessment
	Cirrhosis

Subjective Data	Objective Data
Important Health Information	**General**
Past health history: Previous viral, toxic, or idiopathic hepatitis; chronic biliary obstruction and infection; severe right-sided heart failure	Fever, cachexia, wasting of extremities
	Integumentary
Medications: Adverse reaction to any medication; use of anticoagulants, aspirin, acetaminophen	Icteric sclera, jaundice, petechiae, ecchymoses, spider angiomas, palmar erythema, alopecia, loss of axillary and pubic hair, peripheral edema
Functional Health Patterns	**Respiratory**
Health perception–health management: Chronic alcoholism; weakness, fatigue	Shallow, rapid respirations, epistaxis
	Gastrointestinal
Nutritional-metabolic: Anorexia, weight loss, dyspepsia, nausea and vomiting; gingival bleeding	Abdominal distention, ascites, distended abdominal wall veins, palpable liver and spleen, foul breath; hematemesis; black, tarry stools; hemorrhoids
Elimination: Dark urine, decreased urinary output; light-colored or black stools, flatulence, change in bowel habits; dry, yellow skin, bruising	**Neurologic**
	Altered mentation, asterixis
Cognitive-perceptual: Dull, right upper quadrant or epigastric pain; numbness, tingling of extremities; pruritus	**Reproductive**
Sexuality-reproductive: Impotence, amenorrhea	Gynecomastia and testicular atrophy (men), impotence (men), loss of libido (men and women), amenorrhea or heavy menstrual bleeding (women)
	Possible Findings
	Anemia, thrombocytopenia; leukopenia; ↓ serum albumin, ↓ potassium; abnormal liver function studies; ↑ coagulation studies, ammonia, and bilirubin levels; abnormal abdominal ultrasound and liver scan; positive liver biopsy

NURSING CARE PLAN 42-2

Patient with Cirrhosis

EXPECTED PATIENT OUTCOMES	NURSING INTERVENTIONS and *RATIONALES*
NURSING DIAGNOSIS	**Imbalanced nutrition: less than body requirements** *related to* anorexia, impaired use and storage of nutrients, nausea, and loss of nutrients from vomiting *as manifested by* lack of interest in food, aversion to eating, reported inadequate food intake.
▪ Adequate intake of nutrients ▪ Maintenance of normal body weight	▪ Monitor weight *to evaluate nitrogen balance.* ▪ Provide oral care before meals *to remove foul tastes and improve taste of food.* ▪ Administer antiemetics as ordered *to relieve vomiting.* ▪ Provide small, frequent meals with nourishments *to prevent feeling of fullness and maintain nutritional status.* ▪ Determine food preferences and allow these whenever possible *to increase nutritional appeal for patient since a low- or no-protein diet is unpalatable.*
NURSING DIAGNOSIS	**Impaired skin integrity** *related to* edema, ascites, and pruritus *as manifested by* complaints of itching; areas of excoriation caused by scratching; taut, shiny skin over edematous areas; areas of skin breakdown.
▪ Maintenance of skin integrity ▪ Relief of pruritus	▪ Restrict sodium intake as ordered *to prevent additional fluid retention.* ▪ Restrict fluids if ordered *to reduce fluid retention.* ▪ Administer prescribed diuretics *to prevent fluid retention and promote diuresis.* ▪ Monitor intake and output *to maintain necessary fluid restrictions and assess renal function.* ▪ Assess location and extent of edema by weighing patient at the same time each day, taking daily measurements of extremities and of abdominal girth (same location each time) *to determine patient's response to treatment.* ▪ Provide meticulous skin care *as edematous tissues are easily traumatized and subject to breakdown.* ▪ Reposition patient at least q2hr *to relieve pressure over bony prominences.* ▪ Elevate edematous areas *to promote venous drainage.* ▪ Have patient use pressure-relieving devices, such as alternating–air pressure or egg crate mattress *to reduce the risk of skin breakdown from prolonged pressure.* ▪ Clip patient's nails short and keep clean *to prevent excoriation caused by pruritus secondary to deposit of bile salts on skin.* ▪ Administer antipruritic medication as ordered *to relieve itching.* ▪ Provide diversions and distractions *to assist patient in coping with the discomfort of itching and edema.*
NURSING DIAGNOSIS	**Ineffective breathing pattern** *related to* pressure on diaphragm and reduced lung volume secondary to ascites *as manifested by* dyspnea, cyanosis, cough, changes in pulse or respiratory rate, depth, or pattern.
▪ Able to breathe with minimal difficulty ▪ Effective breathing pattern ▪ Absence of cyanosis and other signs and symptoms of hypoxia	▪ Place patient in semi-Fowler's or Fowler's position; support the arms and chest with pillows *to facilitate breathing by relieving pressure on diaphragm.* ▪ Auscultate chest for crackles *to identify collection of fluid in lungs.* ▪ Assess respiratory rate and rhythm *to identify increasing dyspnea.*
NURSING DIAGNOSIS	**Risk for injury** *related to* diminished sensory perception secondary to peripheral neuropathy.
▪ No injury caused by decreased sensory perception	▪ Assess for numbness and tingling of lower extremities, decreased sensation in lower extremities *to determine risk of injury.* ▪ Prevent excess stimulation or trauma to extremities *because patient may not be able to detect harmful stimuli.* ▪ Do not use restrictive bed linens *because they reduce circulation and place pressure on edematous tissue.* ▪ Instruct patient to avoid tight clothing *because it impedes circulation.* ▪ Use care with heat and cold applications *because patient's ability to perceive temperature is impaired.* ▪ Assist with ambulation *to assess patient's ability to safely ambulate and to prevent injury.*

Continued

NURSING CARE PLAN 42-2

Patient with Cirrhosis—cont'd

EXPECTED PATIENT OUTCOMES	NURSING INTERVENTIONS and *RATIONALES*
NURSING DIAGNOSIS	**Risk for infection** *related to* leukopenia and increased susceptibility to environmental pathogens.
• No signs or symptoms of infections	• Use appropriate infection control measures. • Assess patient for evidence of risk factors, including leukopenia, altered immune response, and altered circulation *to ensure early identification of infection.* • Monitor patient's temperature every 2 to 4 hours *because fever is an indicator of infection.* • Observe for any local and systemic manifestations of infection *to enable early diagnosis and treatment.* • Protect patient from others with infections *to reduce the risk of infection secondary to decreased resistance.* • Monitor white blood cell count *to assess patient's response to treatment.*

COLLABORATIVE PROBLEMS

NURSING GOALS	NURSING INTERVENTIONS and *RATIONALES*
POTENTIAL COMPLICATION	**Hepatic encephalopathy** *related to* increased formation of ammonia and aromatic amino acids.
• Monitor for signs of hepatic encephalopathy • Report deviation from acceptable parameters • Carry out appropriate medical and nursing interventions	• Monitor for encephalopathy by assessing patient's general behavior, orientation to time and place, speech, blood pH, and ammonia levels *because liver is unable to convert accumulating ammonia to urea for renal excretion.* • Encourage fluids (if not restricted) and give laxatives and enemas as ordered *to decrease production of ammonia.* • Provide low-protein or no-protein diet as ordered *because ammonia (a breakdown product of protein) is responsible for mental changes.*
POTENTIAL COMPLICATION	**Hemorrhage** *related to* bleeding tendency secondary to altered clotting factors and rupture of esophageal or gastric varices.
• Monitor for signs of hemorrhage • Initiate appropriate medical and nursing interventions	• Limit physical activity *because exercise produces ammonia as a by-product of metabolism.* • Monitor for hemorrhage by assessing for epistaxis, purpura, petechiae, easy bruising, gingival bleeding, heavy menstrual bleeding, hematuria, melena *because liver disease results in impaired synthesis of clotting factors.* • Provide gentle nursing care *to minimize the risk of tissue trauma.* • Observe for bleeding from body orifices, urine, and stool *to detect bleeding early and allow prompt intervention.* • Use smallest-gauge needle possible when giving injection and apply gentle but prolonged pressure after injection *to minimize risk of bleeding into tissue.* • Advise use of soft-bristle toothbrush and avoidance of irritating food *to reduce trauma because mucous membranes have increased risk of injury as a result of high vascularity.* • Teach patient to avoid straining at stool, vigorous blowing of nose, and coughing *to reduce risk of hemorrhage from these areas.* • Observe for bruising on the forearms, axillae, and skin. • Monitor laboratory results (hematocrit, hemoglobin, and prothrombin time) *as indicators of anemia, active bleeding, or impending complications.*

signs of clinical improvement (e.g., decreasing jaundice, improvement in liver function studies). Major concerns of the nurse in determining appropriate nursing care measures to meet the need for rest involve regulation of the physical, emotional, and social climate.

Anorexia, nausea and vomiting, pressure from ascites, and poor eating habits all create problems in maintaining an adequate intake of nutrients. The nursing measures relating to nutrition for patients with hepatitis also apply here. Oral hygiene before meals may improve the patient's taste sensation. Between-meal nourishments should be available so that they can be provided at times when the patient can best tolerate them. Food preferences should be provided whenever possible. The reason for any dietary restrictions should be explained to the patient and family.

Nursing assessment and care should include the patient's physiologic response to cirrhosis. Is jaundice present? Where is it observed—sclera, skin, hard palate? What is the progression of jaundice? If the jaundice is accompanied by pruritus, measures to relieve itching should be carried out. Cholestyramine (Questran) may be ordered to help relieve the pruritus. The color of the urine and stools should be noted. With jaundice the urine is often dark brown and foamy when shaken. The stool is gray or tan.

Edema and ascites are frequent manifestations of cirrhosis and require nursing assessments and interventions. Accurate calculation and recordings of intake and output, daily weights, and measurements of extremities and abdominal girth help in the ongoing assessment of the location and extent of the edema. If the patient can assume a kneeling position when abdominal girth measurement is taken, the abdominal fluid will go to the most dependent part of the abdomen. This gives the best measurement of abdominal girth. For many patients, girth must be measured in the standing or lying position. Where the measurements are taken should be recorded and should be a part of the nursing care plan.

When a paracentesis is done, the nurse must have the patient void immediately before the procedure to prevent puncture of the bladder. The patient should sit on the side of the bed or be placed in high-Fowler's position. Following the procedure the nurse should monitor for hypovolemia and electrolyte imbalances and check the dressing for bleeding and leakage.

Dyspnea is a frequent problem for the patient with ascites. A semi-Fowler's or Fowler's position allows for maximal respiratory efficiency. Pillows can be used to support the arms and chest and may increase the patient's comfort and ability to breathe.

Meticulous skin care is essential because the edematous tissues are subject to breakdown. An alternating–air pressure mattress or other special mattress should be used. A turning schedule (minimum of every 2 hours) must be adhered to rigidly. The abdomen may be supported with pillows. If the abdomen is taut, cleansing must be done very gently. This patient tends to move very little because of the abdominal discomfort and dyspnea. Therefore range-of-motion exercises are helpful, and measures such as coughing and deep breathing to prevent respiratory problems should be implemented. The lower extremities may be elevated. If scrotal edema is present, a scrotal support provides some comfort.

When the patient is taking diuretics, the serum levels of sodium, potassium, chloride, and bicarbonate should be monitored. The patient should be observed for signs of fluid and electrolyte imbalance, especially hypokalemia. Hypokalemia may be manifested by cardiac arrhythmias, hypotension, tachycardia, and generalized muscle weakness. Water excess is manifested by muscle cramping, weakness, lethargy, and confusion.

Observations and nursing care in relation to hematologic disorders (bleeding tendencies, anemia, increased susceptibility to infection) are the same as for the patient with advanced liver disease (see NCP 42-2).

The nurse must assess the patient's response to altered body image resulting from jaundice, spider angiomas, palmar erythema, ascites, and gynecomastia. The patient may experience a great deal of anxiety regarding these changes. The nurse should explain these phenomena and should be a supportive listener. Nursing care with concern and warmth regardless of physical changes helps the patient maintain self-esteem.

Bleeding esophageal varices. If the patient has esophageal varices in addition to cirrhosis, the nurse must observe for any signs of bleeding from the varices, such as hematemesis and melena. If hematemesis occurs, the nurse should assess the patient for hemorrhage, call the physician, and be ready to assist with whatever treatment is used to control the bleeding. The patient will be admitted to the intensive care unit (ICU). The patient's airway must be maintained. To stop the bleeding the physician may perform sclerotherapy or ligation procedures.

Balloon tamponade is not used as first-line therapy for bleeding esophageal varices. However, it is used in those patients who have refractory bleeding that is unresponsive to sclerotherapy or ligation. When balloon tamponade is used, the initial nursing task related to insertion of the tube is to explain the use of the tube and how it will be inserted. The balloons should be checked for patency. It is usually the physician's responsibility to insert the tube. It may be inserted via the nose or the mouth (see Fig. 42-9). Then the gastric balloon is inflated with approximately 250 ml of air, and the tube is retracted until resistance (gastroesophageal junction) is felt. The tube is secured by placement of a piece of sponge or foam rubber at the nostrils (nasal cuff). For continued bleeding the esophageal balloon is then inflated. A sphygmomanometer is used to measure and maintain the desired pressure at 20 to 40 mm Hg. The position of the balloons is verified by x-ray.

Sometimes saline lavage is used to remove blood from the stomach. (Nursing care of upper GI bleeding is discussed in Chapter 40.) This helps prevent the blood from degrading to ammonia, leading to encephalopathy. The esophageal balloon should be deflated every 8 to 12 hours to avoid necrosis. Each lumen must be labeled to avoid confusion. The NG lumen may be connected to suction to remove blood and keep the stomach empty to reduce the risk of aspiration. The most common complication of balloon tamponade therapy is aspiration pneumonia.

Nursing care includes monitoring for complications of rupture or erosion of the esophagus, regurgitation and aspiration of gastric contents, and occlusion of the airway by the balloon. If the gastric balloon breaks or is deflated, the esophageal balloon will slip upward, obstructing the airway and causing asphyxiation. If this happens, the nurse must cut the tube or deflate the esophageal balloon. Scissors should be kept at the bedside. Regurgitation can be minimized by oral and pharyngeal suctioning and by keeping the patient in a semi-Fowler's position.

The patient is unable to swallow saliva because of the inflated esophageal balloon occluding the esophagus. With the Minnesota tube, which has an esophageal aspiration lumen, this problem can be alleviated. The nurse should encourage the patient to expectorate and should provide an emesis basin and tissues. Frequent oral and nasal care provides relief from the taste of blood and irritation from mouth breathing.

Hepatic encephalopathy. The focus of nursing care of the patient with hepatic encephalopathy is on sustaining life and assisting with measures to reduce the formation of ammonia. The nurse should assess (1) the patient's level of responsiveness (e.g., reflexes, pupillary reactions, orientation), (2) sensory and motor abnormalities (e.g., hyperreflexia, asterixis, motor coordination), (3) fluid and electrolyte imbalances, (4) acid-base imbalances, and (5) the effect of treatment measures.

The neurologic status, including an exact description of the patient's behavior, should be assessed and recorded at least every 2 hours. Care of the patient with neurologic problems should be based on the severity of the encephalopathy.

Nursing measures to prevent constipation should be instituted to decrease ammonia production. Drugs, laxatives, and enemas should be given as ordered. Encouragement of fluids may also help if not contraindicated. The patient should not strain at stool because this may cause bleeding of hemorrhoidal varices. Any GI bleeding may worsen the coma. The patient who is taking lactulose should be assessed for diarrhea and excessive fluid and electrolyte losses. Some physicians have diarrhea as a goal because diarrhea increases ammonia expulsion from the colon. Because lactulose can cause severe purging, the nurse should observe the patient for excessive fluid and electrolyte losses.

Factors that are known to precipitate coma should be controlled as much as possible. Because exercise produces ammonia as a by-product of metabolism, the physical activity of the patient must be limited. Hypokalemia should be controlled.

The patient is on either a very low-protein or a no-protein diet, neither of which is very palatable. Vegetable protein is better tolerated than meat protein. Foods and fluids high in carbohydrate should be given because the liver is not synthesizing and storing glucose. The patient may require tube feedings if an adequate diet cannot be ingested.

Ambulatory and Home Care. The patient with cirrhosis may be faced with a prolonged course and the possibility of serious, life-threatening problems and complications. The nurse should be a resource person in helping the patient achieve the highest level of wellness. The patient and the family need to understand the importance of continuous health care and medical supervision. They should be taught symptoms of complications and when to seek

medical attention. Patients with cirrhosis should avoid activities that place them at risk for contracting viral hepatitis.

Measures to achieve and maintain a remission should be encouraged. These include proper diet, rest, avoidance of potentially hepatotoxic over-the-counter drugs such as acetaminophen, and abstinence from alcohol. Abstinence from alcohol is important and results in improvement in most patients. The nurse must realize the difficulty this poses for some patients. The nurse's own attitude regarding the patient whose cirrhosis is attributed to alcohol abuse should be explored. Care should be given without rejection and moralizing. The alcoholic patient should be treated with a caring attitude (see Chapter 11).

Cirrhosis is a chronic disease. The patient is affected not only physically but also psychologically, socially, and economically. Major adjustments may be required to make lifestyle changes, especially if alcohol abuse is the primary etiologic factor. The nurse should provide information regarding community support programs, such as Alcoholics Anonymous, for help with alcohol abuse.

Adequate explanations, along with written instructions, related to fluid or dietary restrictions should be given to the patient and the family (Table 42-18). Other health teaching should include instruction about adequate rest periods, how to detect early signs of complications, skin care, drug therapy precautions, observation for bleeding, and protection from infection. Counseling information regarding sexual problems may be needed. Referral to a community or home health nurse may be helpful to ensure adequate patient compliance with prescribed therapy. The emphasis of home care for the patient with cirrhosis should be on helping the patient maintain the highest level of wellness possible and initiate and maintain necessary lifestyle changes.

■ Evaluation

Expected outcomes for the patient with cirrhosis are addressed in NCP 42-2.

ETHICAL DILEMMAS
Rationing

Situation
A 43-year-old patient with cirrhosis of the liver is frequently admitted to the hospital. She has been told that her continued drinking will inevitably lead to her death. Now she has been admitted for GI bleeding and needs blood transfusions. She has a rare blood type, and it is frequently difficult to get compatible blood. Should the nurse call an ethics consultation?

Important Points for Consideration
- Rationing or the distribution of scarce resources is a difficult ethical problem. The needs of an individual patient or group of patients are weighed against the needs of many patients who may have a greater chance of recovery and the availability of the needed resources.
- Because alcoholism has a behavioral component, health care providers sometimes view these patients as noncompliant and not deserving of aggressive treatment.
- Whether blood transfusions at this point will alter the course of the patient's disease, extend her life, or improve the quality of her life are important questions to determine if this treatment is medically futile.
- Triage is the basis for rationing decisions. The amount of blood supply available, the number of people needing the blood, and the degree to which their condition can be effectively treated by blood transfusions should provide the justification for treatment decisions.
- An ethics consultation could assist in determining who would receive the greatest benefit from the scarce resource, rather than a health care provider deciding for a particular patient.

Critical Thinking Questions
1. What are your feelings about patients with disorders such as substance abuse, which have a behavioral component? Are these patients deserving of aggressive treatment?
2. How would you proceed to make a decision in this case? Would you request an ethics committee consult?

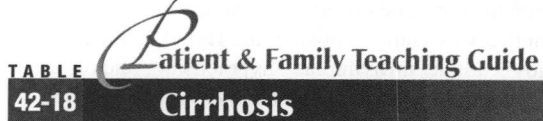

| TABLE 42-18 | **Patient & Family Teaching Guide** **Cirrhosis** |

1. Explain to the patient and family the importance of continuous health care so that they understand that cirrhosis is a chronic illness.
2. Teach the patient and family symptoms of complications and when to seek medical attention to enable prompt treatment of complications.
3. Teach proper diet because a low-protein, high-carbohydrate diet is usually indicated and can be difficult to follow.
4. Teach the patient to avoid potentially hepatotoxic over-the-counter drugs because the diseased liver is unable to metabolize these drugs.
5. Encourage abstinence from alcohol because continued use of alcohol will increase the risk of liver complications.
6. Instruct the patient to avoid aspirin and control coughing to prevent hemorrhage when esophageal or gastric varices are present.
7. Teach the patient to avoid spicy and rough foods and activities that increase portal pressure, such as straining at stool, coughing, sneezing, and retching and vomiting because hemorrhage is a danger as a result of the inability of the liver to produce clotting factors.

FULMINANT HEPATIC FAILURE

Fulminant hepatic failure is a clinical syndrome characterized by severe impairment of liver function associated with hepatic encephalopathy. In fulminant hepatic failure the encephalopathy occurs within 8 weeks of the first symptoms. The most common cause is viral hepatitis, in particular HBV, but it may also occur with HAV and less frequently with HCV.

Drugs are the second most common cause of fulminant hepatic failure. Acetaminophen in combination with alcohol is a common offending agent. Persons who abuse alcohol are particularly susceptible to detrimental effects of acetaminophen on the liver. Other drugs include isoniazid (INH), halothane (Fluothane), sulfa-containing drugs, and nonsteroidal antiinflammatory drugs.

The patient has jaundice and signs of encephalopathy. Laboratory tests reveal elevated liver function tests, prolonged prothrombin time, and increased bilirubin. Depending on the degree of liver failure, treatment may involve liver transplantation.

LIVER CANCER

Primary liver cancer (originating in the liver) is rare. In 2002 in the United States there were 16,600 new cases of liver cancer and 14,100 deaths related to liver cancer.[28] Of these, the majority occur in males. Hepatocellular carcinoma is the most common primary liver cancer. The remaining primary tumors are cholangiomas or bile duct carcinomas. A high percentage of patients with primary cell carcinoma have cirrhosis of the liver. Hepatocellular carcinoma is often associated with chronic liver diseases including chronic hepatitis B or C. Metastatic carcinoma of the liver is more common than primary carcinoma. The liver is a common site of metastatic growth because of its high rate of blood flow and extensive capillary network. Cancer cells in other parts of the body are commonly carried to the liver via the portal circulation.

The malignant cells cause the liver to be enlarged and misshapen. Hemorrhage and necrosis in the liver are common (Fig. 42-12). Lesions may be singular or numerous and nodular or diffusely spread over the entire liver. Some tumors infiltrate into other organs such as the gallbladder or into the peritoneum or diaphragm. Primary liver tumors commonly metastasize to the lung.

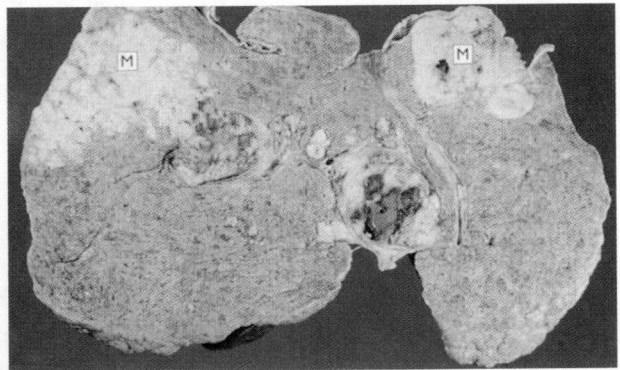

FIG. 42-12 Hepatocellular carcinoma. Macroscopically, hepatocellular carcinoma may be single or multifocal. They usually develop in a liver already affected by cirrhosis. Tumor appears as an abnormal mass (*M*) within the liver.

Clinical Manifestations and Diagnostic Studies

It is difficult to diagnose liver cancer. It is particularly difficult to differentiate it from cirrhosis in its early stages because many of the clinical manifestations (e.g., hepatomegaly, weight loss, peripheral edema, ascites, portal hypertension) are similar. Other common manifestations include dull abdominal pain in the epigastric or right upper quadrant region, jaundice, anorexia, nausea and vomiting, and extreme weakness. Patients frequently have pulmonary emboli. Tests used to assist in the diagnosis are a liver scan, computed tomography (CT), magnetic resonance imaging, hepatic arteriography, endoscopic retrograde cholangiopancreatography (ERCP), and a liver biopsy. The test for α-fetoprotein (AFP) may be positive in hepatocellular carcinoma. AFP is elevated in approximately 70% of patients with hepatocellular carcinoma and helps to distinguish primary cancer from metastatic cancer. (AFP is discussed in Chapter 15.)

NURSING *and* COLLABORATIVE MANAGEMENT LIVER CANCER

Treatment of liver cancer is largely palliative. Overall the management is similar to liver cirrhosis. Surgical excision (lobectomy) is sometimes performed if the tumor is localized to one portion of the liver. Only 30% to 40% of patients have surgically resectable disease. Usually surgery is not feasible because the cancer is too far advanced when it is detected. Surgical excision of the entire tumor offers the best chance for cure of liver cancer. Other treatment options are ablation with radiofrequency, cryosurgery, or alcohol injection, and chemotherapy and/or chemoembolization.

In *radiofrequency* treatment electrical energy is used to create heat in a specific location for a limited amount of time. The end result is destruction of liver tumors. This procedure can be done percutaneously, laparoscopically, or through an open incision. This therapy, while not ideal for all patients, can be used both for tumors that are considered resectable as well as for palliative purposes. Complications are not common but can include infection, bleeding, arrhythmias, and skin burn.

Cryosurgery is another procedure used for patients whose tumors are considered unresectable but who do not have signs of metastasis. Cryosurgery involves an open surgical approach. Cryoprobes are placed directly into the liver, and liquid nitrogen/argon gas flows through the probe and freezes the liver tissue. The tissue in the area surrounding the probe is destroyed. Cryosurgery is not used for metastatic liver disease.

Percutaneous ethanol injection (PEI) is used to treat unresectable liver cancer that has not metastasized outside the liver. This is an outpatient procedure in which a catheter is guided to the liver using ultrasound. Ethanol is injected for six to eight treatments over a 3- to 4-week period, with two to three injections each week. The most common side effect is transient pain following the procedure. Other, less frequent adverse events include intraperitoneal hemorrhage, hepatic insufficiency, bile duct necrosis, hepatic infarction, and transient hypotension.

Chemotherapy is used for patients with hepatocellular cancer who are not likely to benefit from other procedures (e.g., surgery, transplantation, ablation). A variety of chemotherapeutic agents (e.g., 5-fluorouracil [5-FU] and leucovorin) administered either systemically or regionally has been used to treat liver cancer.

Other chemotherapeutic drugs include raltitrexed (Tomudex) and experimental drugs. However, the overall response has been poor. Regional chemotherapy includes portal vein or hepatic artery perfusion with 5-FU or other chemotherapeutic agents. Chemotherapy delivered directly to the liver is referred to as hepatic arterial infusion therapy. With the patient under general anesthesia, a catheter is placed in the hepatic artery and a pump is implanted percutaneously for administration of chemotherapy. Systemic chemotherapy may also be given along with hepatic administration.

Chemoembolization is a minimally invasive procedure frequently performed in the interventional radiology department. In this procedure a catheter is placed in the arteries to the tumor and an embolic agent is administered, often mixed with a chemotherapeutic agent(s). The embolic agent reduces the blood supply, thus allowing greater exposure of liver cells to the chemotherapy drugs.

Liver transplantation is an option for patients with liver cancer that has not spread beyond the liver. However, there is a limited availability of organs.

Nursing intervention for the patient with liver cancer focuses on keeping the patient as comfortable as possible. Because this patient manifests the same problems as any patient with advanced liver disease, the nursing interventions discussed for cirrhosis of the liver apply. (See Chapter 15 for care of the patient with cancer.)

The prognosis for patients with liver cancer is poor. The cancer grows rapidly, and death may occur within 4 to 7 months as a result of hepatic encephalopathy or massive blood loss from GI bleeding.

LIVER TRANSPLANTATION

The first human liver transplant was performed in 1963 at the University of Colorado by Thomas Starzl. Liver transplantation has become a practical therapeutic option for many people with irreversible liver disease. It improves the quality of life for end-stage liver patients and is an accepted treatment modality for these patients. Indications for liver transplantation include congenital biliary abnormalities, inborn errors of metabolism, hepatic malignancy (confined to the liver), sclerosing cholangitis, and chronic end-stage liver disease. Liver disease related to chronic viral hepatitis is the leading indication for liver transplantation.[27] Liver transplants are not recommended for the patient with widespread malignant disease.

The major postoperative complications are rejection and infection. Rejection is not as major a problem as it is in kidney transplants. The liver seems to be less susceptible to rejection than the kidney. Cyclosporine is an effective immunosuppressant drug. The use of cyclosporine has been a major factor in the success rates of liver transplantation. The mechanism of action and side effects of cyclosporine are discussed in Chapter 13 and Table 13-17. It does not cause bone marrow suppression and does not impede wound healing. Other immunosuppressants used include azathioprine (Imuran), corticosteroids, tacrolimus (Prograf), and the monoclonal antibody OKT3 (see Table 13-17). Newer agents including the interleukin-2 receptor antagonists basiliximab (Simulect) and daclizumab (Zenapax) are being used in combination with other immunosuppressive agents to reduce rejection. Other factors in the improved success rate are advances in surgical techniques, better selection of potential recipients, and improved management of the underlying liver disease before surgery.

Patients who have liver disease secondary to viral hepatitis often experience reinfection of the transplanted liver with hepatitis B or C. HCV recurrence as evidence by histologic damage is almost universal after transplant. Approximately 20% to 30% of patients will develop cirrhosis of the transplanted liver by the fifth year posttransplant.[27] Antiviral therapy for HCV initiated posttransplant even before the development of histologic evidence of recurrence has failed to alter this recurrence pattern.[27]

The patient who has had a liver transplant requires competent and highly skilled nursing care, either in an ICU or in some other specialized unit. Postoperative nursing care includes assessing neurologic status; monitoring for signs of hemorrhage; preventing pulmonary complications; monitoring drainage, electrolyte levels, and urinary output; and monitoring for signs and symptoms of infection and rejection. Common respiratory problems are pneumonia, atelectasis, and pleural effusions. The nurse should have the patient use measures such as coughing, deep breathing, incentive spirometry, and repositioning to prevent these complications. Drainage from the Jackson-Pratt drain, NG tube, and T tube should be measured, and the color and consistency of drainage noted. A critical aspect of nursing care following liver transplantation is monitoring for infection. The first 2 months after the surgery are critical. Infection can be viral, fungal, or bacterial. Fever may be the only sign of infection. Emotional support and teaching the patient and family are essential.

NURSING RESEARCH
Physical Activity and Liver Transplant

Citation   Painter P et al: Physical activity and health-related quality of life in liver transplant recipients, *Liver Transpl* 7:213, 2001.

Purpose   This study was conducted to determine the relationship between physical activity and health-related quality of life in patients following a liver transplant.

Methods   The Medical Outcomes Study Short Form-36 (SF-36) Health Status Questionnaire was sent to patients who were 5 years or more posttransplantation. Data obtained related to coexisting medical problems and participation in regular physical activity. Regression analyses were performed.

Results and Conclusions   Patients who participated in regular physical activity had significantly higher scores on all physical scales and the physical component scale. The regression model, which included age, sex, time posttransplantation, retransplantation, recurrence of hepatitis C, number of comorbid conditions, and physical activity participation, showed that the number of comorbid conditions and participation in physical activity were significant independent contributors to the physical functioning scale. This study indicates that physical activity is related to quality of life following liver transplant.

Implications for Nursing Practice   There are many positive benefits of physical activity for patients following a liver transplant. These patients should be encouraged to engage in physical activity for the potential benefits related to their cardiovascular health and to enhance their overall physical functioning.

Disorders of the Pancreas

ACUTE PANCREATITIS

Acute pancreatitis is an acute inflammatory process of the pancreas. The degree of inflammation varies from mild edema to severe hemorrhagic necrosis. Acute pancreatitis is most common in middle-aged men and women, but it affects more men than women. The severity of the disease varies according to the extent of pancreatic destruction. Some patients recover completely, others have recurring attacks, and chronic pancreatitis develops in others. Acute pancreatitis can be life threatening.

Etiology and Pathophysiology

Many factors can cause injury to the pancreas. The primary etiologic factors are biliary tract disease and alcoholism. In the United States the most common cause is alcoholism, followed by gallbladder disease. Other, less common causes of acute pancreatitis include trauma (postsurgical, abdominal), viral infections (mumps, coxsackievirus B), penetrating duodenal ulcer, cysts, abscesses, cystic fibrosis, Kaposi's sarcoma, certain drugs (corticosteroids, thiazide diuretics, oral contraceptives, sulfonamides, nonsteroidal antiinflammatory drugs), and metabolic disorders (hyperparathyroidism, hyperlipidemia, renal failure). Pancreatitis may occur after surgical procedures on the pancreas, stomach, duodenum, or biliary tract. Pancreatitis can also occur after ERCP. In some cases the cause is not known (idiopathic).

The most common pathogenic mechanism is believed to be autodigestion of the pancreas (Fig. 42-13). The etiologic factors cause injury to pancreatic cells or activation of the pancreatic enzymes in the pancreas rather than in the intestine. It is not clear how the activation of pancreatic enzymes occurs. One possible cause is believed to be the reflux of bile acids into the pancreatic ducts through an open or distended sphincter of Oddi. This reflux may occur because of gallstones impacted at the ampulla of Vater, atony and edema of the sphincter, or obstruction of pancreatic ducts and pancreatic ischemia.

Trypsinogen is an inactive proteolytic enzyme produced by the pancreas. Normally it is released into the small intestine via the pancreatic duct. In the intestine it is activated to trypsin by enterokinase. Normally, trypsin inhibitors in the pancreas and plasma bind and inactivate any trypsin that is inadvertently produced. In pancreatitis, activated trypsin is present in the pancreas. This enzyme can digest the pancreas and can activate other proteolytic enzymes such as elastase and phospholipase A.

Elastase and phospholipase A play a major role in autodigestion of the pancreas. Elastase causes hemorrhage by producing dissolution of the elastic fibers of blood vessels. Phospholipase A is probably activated by trypsin and bile acids and causes fat necrosis.

It is not entirely clear how alcohol causes acute pancreatitis. One theory is that it stimulates secretion and excess production of hydrochloric acid. A decrease in the gastric pH results in the release of the hormone secretin from the intestinal mucosa. This hormone then stimulates pancreatic secretions. Alcohol may also cause regurgitation of duodenal contents into the pancreatic duct, resulting in inflammation.

The pathophysiologic involvement of acute pancreatitis ranges from *edematous pancreatitis* (which is mild and self-limiting) to *necrotizing pancreatitis* (in which the degree of necrosis correlates with the severity of manifestations) (Fig. 42-14).

Clinical Manifestations

Abdominal pain is the predominant symptom of acute pancreatitis. The pain is usually located in the left upper quadrant, but it may be in the midepigastrium. It commonly radiates to the back because of the retroperitoneal location of the pancreas. The pain has a sudden onset and is described as severe, deep, piercing, and continuous or steady. It is aggravated by eating and frequently has its onset when the patient is recumbent; it is not relieved by vomiting. The pain may be accompanied by flushing,

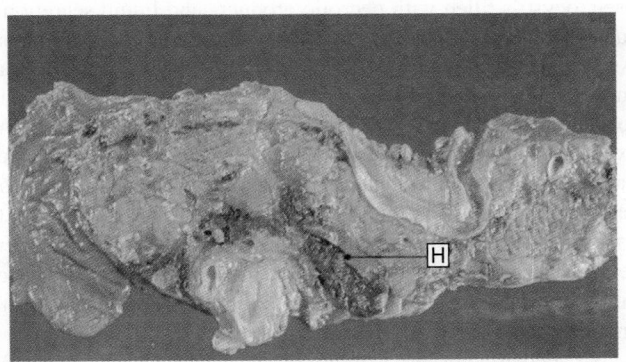

FIG. 42-14 In acute pancreatitis, the pancreas appears edematous and is commonly hemorrhagic *(H)*.

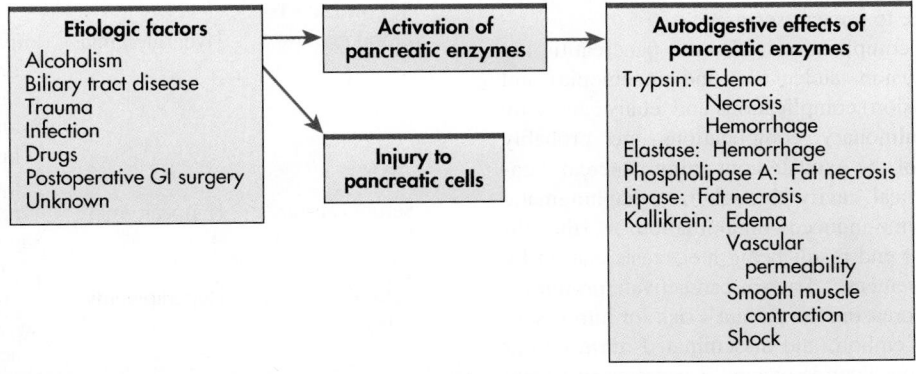

FIG. 42-13 Pathogenic process of acute pancreatitis. *GI,* Gastrointestinal.

cyanosis, and dyspnea. The patient may assume various positions involving flexion of the spine in an attempt to relieve the severe pain. The pain is due to distention of the pancreas, peritoneal irritation, and obstruction of the biliary tract.

Other manifestations of acute pancreatitis include nausea and vomiting, low-grade fever, leukocytosis, hypotension, tachycardia, and jaundice. Abdominal tenderness with muscle guarding is common. Bowel sounds may be decreased or absent. Ileus may occur and causes marked abdominal distention. The lungs are frequently involved, with crackles present. Intravascular damage from circulating trypsin may cause areas of cyanosis or greenish to yellow-brown discoloration of the abdominal wall. Other areas of ecchymoses are the flanks (*Grey Turner spots or sign,* a bluish flank discoloration) and the periumbilical area (*Cullen's sign,* a bluish periumbilical discoloration). These result from seepage of blood-stained exudate from the pancreas and may occur in severe cases.

Shock may occur because of hemorrhage into the pancreas or toxemia from the activated pancreatic enzymes. The increased formation of kinin peptides (activated by trypsin), such as kallikrein and bradykinin, causes vasodilation, increased capillary permeability, and altered vasomotor tone. Hypovolemia also occurs as a result of exudation of blood and plasma proteins into the retroperitoneal space (massive fluid shifts).

Complications

Two significant local complications of acute pancreatitis are pseudocyst and abscess. A pancreatic **pseudocyst** is a cavity continuous with or surrounding the outside of the pancreas. The pseudocyst is filled with necrotic products and liquid secretions, such as plasma, pancreatic enzymes, and inflammatory exudates. As pancreatic enzymes escape from the pseudocyst, the serosal surfaces next to the pancreas become inflamed, with subsequent formation of granulation tissue leading to encapsulation of the exudate. Manifestations of pseudocyst are abdominal pain, palpable epigastric mass, nausea, vomiting, and anorexia. The serum amylase level frequently remains elevated. These cysts usually resolve spontaneously within a few weeks but may perforate, causing peritonitis, or rupture into the stomach or duodenum. Treatment consists of an internal drainage procedure with an anastomosis between the pancreatic duct and the jejunum.

A pancreatic abscess is a large fluid-containing cavity within the pancreas. It results from extensive necrosis in the pancreas. It may become infected or perforate into adjacent organs. Manifestations of an abscess include upper abdominal pain, abdominal mass, high fever, and leukocytosis. Pancreatic abscesses require prompt surgical drainage to prevent sepsis.

The main systemic complications of acute pancreatitis are pulmonary (pleural effusion, atelectasis, and pneumonia) and cardiovascular (hypotension) complications and tetany caused by hypocalcemia. The pulmonary complications are probably caused by the passage of the exudate containing pancreatic enzymes from the peritoneal cavity through transdiaphragmatic lymph channels. Enzyme-induced inflammation of the diaphragm occurs with an end result being atelectasis caused by reduced diaphragm movement.[29] Trypsin can activate prothrombin and plasminogen, increasing the patient's risk for intravascular thrombi, pulmonary emboli, and disseminated intravascular coagulation.[29] When hypocalcemia occurs, it is a sign of severe disease. It is due in part to the combining of calcium and fatty acids during fat necrosis. The exact mechanisms of how or why hypocalcemia occurs are not well understood.

Diagnostic Studies

The primary diagnostic tests for acute pancreatitis are serum amylase and lipase and urinary amylase levels (Table 42-19). The serum amylase level is the criterion most commonly used. It may be elevated to levels greater than 200 U/L (3.34 μkat/L). The serum amylase is usually elevated early and remains elevated for 24 to 72 hours.

The serum lipase is also elevated in acute pancreatitis and is a helpful complementary test because other disorders (e.g., mumps, cerebral trauma, renal transplantation) may also cause an increase in serum amylase. The serum lipase level may be especially useful in patients with alcohol-induced acute pancreatitis.[30]

There is an increase in urinary amylase, which may persist several days beyond the elevation of serum amylase. Urinary amylase may be increased to more than 3600 U per day. Normally a timed collection (e.g., a 2-hour collection) is a more dependable measure than a randomly collected urinary specimen. The renal amylase-creatinine clearance test estimates the amount of blood cleared of amylase by the kidney per minute. The finding that the renal clearance of amylase is higher than the creatinine clearance in acute pancreatitis has led to the suggestion that the amylase-creatinine clearance ratio is a more specific test than urinary amylase levels alone. A new urinary test strip that uses trypsinogen-2 is being investigated for its use in diagnosing acute pancreatitis.[30]

Other laboratory abnormalities include hyperglycemia, hyperlipidemia, and hypocalcemia (see Table 42-19). There is a high incidence of hyperlipidemia with recurrent pancreatitis.

TABLE 42-19	**Diagnostic Studies** **Acute Pancreatitis**		
LABORATORY TEST	**ABNORMAL FINDING**	**ETIOLOGY**
Primary Tests		
Serum amylase	Increased (>200 U/L [3.34 μkat/L])	Pancreatic cell injury
Serum lipase	Elevated	Pancreatic cell injury
Urinary amylase	Elevated	Pancreatic cell injury
Secondary Tests		
Blood glucose	Hyperglycemia	Impairment of carbohydrate metabolism due to β-cell damage and decrease in insulin secretion and increase in glucagon release
Serum calcium	Hypocalcemia	Saponification of calcium by fatty acids in areas of fat necrosis
Serum triglycerides	Hyperlipidemia	Release of free fatty acids by lipase

Diagnostic evaluation of acute pancreatitis is also directed at determining the cause. An abdominal ultrasound, x-ray, or CT can be used to identify pancreatic problems. The CT scan can also determine the presence of pseudocysts and abscesses. ERCP is the definitive diagnostic test for gallstones, pancreatic cysts, and abscesses. Endoscopic ultrasound and magnetic resonance cholangiopancreatography are being used with greater frequency. A combination of laboratory studies and ERCP is usually used to help make the diagnosis.

Collaborative Care

Objectives of collaborative care for acute pancreatitis include (1) relief of pain; (2) prevention or alleviation of shock; (3) reduction of pancreatic secretions; (4) control of fluid and electrolyte imbalance; (5) prevention or treatment of infections; and (6) removal of the precipitating cause, if possible (Table 42-20).

Conservative Therapy. Treatment is principally focused on supportive care including aggressive hydration, pain management, management of metabolic complications, and minimizing pancreatic stimulation. A primary consideration in the treatment of acute pancreatitis is the relief and control of pain. Meperidine (Demerol) was once the preferred pain medication because it causes less spasm of the smooth muscles of the ducts than morphine. However, IV morphine may be used because of its longer half-life. Pain medications may be combined with an antispasmodic. However, atropine-like drugs should be avoided when paralytic ileus is present because they may contribute to the problem. Other medications that relax smooth muscles (spasmolytics), such as nitroglycerin or papaverine, may be used.

If shock is present, blood volume replacements are used. Plasma or plasma volume expanders such as dextran or albumin may be given. Fluid and electrolyte imbalances are corrected with lactated Ringer's solution or other electrolyte solutions. Central venous pressure readings may be used to assist in determination of fluid replacement requirements. Vasoactive drugs such as dopamine (Intropin) may be used to increase systemic vascular resistance in patients with ongoing hypotension.

It is important to reduce or suppress pancreatic enzymes to decrease stimulation of the pancreas and allow it to rest. This is accomplished in several ways. First, the patient is allowed to take nothing by mouth (NPO). Second, NG suction may be used to reduce vomiting and gastric distention and to prevent gastric acidic contents from entering the duodenum. These measures suppress pancreatic secretion. Certain drugs may also be used for this purpose (Tables 42-20 and 42-21).

The inflamed and necrotic pancreatic tissue is a good medium for bacterial growth. Therefore it is important to prevent infections. There is some controversy about the prophylactic use of antibiotics. It is important to monitor the patient closely so that antibiotic therapy can be instituted early if infection occurs.

Peritoneal lavage or dialysis has been used to remove the kinin and phospholipase A–containing exudate from the peritoneal cavity. This has proved beneficial in some cases of severe acute pancreatitis. It prevents early death but has little effect on overall mortality rate.

Surgical Therapy. When the acute pancreatitis is related to the presence of gallstones, an urgent ERCP plus endoscopic sphincterotomy may be performed. This may be followed by laparoscopic cholecystectomy to reduce the potential for recurrence. Surgical intervention may also be indicated when the diagnosis is uncertain and in patients who do not respond to conservative therapy. Surgery is necessary for an abscess, acute pseudocyst, and severe peritonitis. Percutaneous drainage of a pseudocyst can be performed, and a drainage tube is left in place.

Drug Therapy. Several different drugs may be used in the treatment of both acute and chronic pancreatitis (see Table 42-21). A number of drugs are used in an effort to suppress pancreatic secretion, but these drugs have not proved effective in the management of pancreatitis.

Nutritional Therapy. Initially the patient with acute pancreatitis is on NPO status to reduce pancreatic secretion. When food is allowed, small, frequent feedings are given. The diet is usually high in carbohydrate content because that is the least stimulating to the exocrine portion of the pancreas. The diet is bland, with no stimulants (e.g., caffeine) or alcohol. Supplemental fat-soluble vitamins may be given. The patient may require enteral feeding via jejunal feeding tube. If severe nutritional deficiencies exist, total parenteral nutrition (TPN) may be used (see Chapter 39).

TABLE 42-20 *C*ollaborative Care
Acute Pancreatitis

Diagnostic
History and physical examination
Serum amylase
Serum lipase
Two-hour urinary amylase and renal amylase clearance
Blood glucose
Serum calcium
Triglycerides
Flat plate of the abdomen
Abdominal ultrasound
Endoscopic ultrasound
CT scan of the pancreas
Magnetic resonance cholangiopancreatography
ERCP
Chest x-rays

Collaborative Therapy
Pain medication (meperidine, morphine)
NPO with NG tube to suction
Albumin (if shock present)
IV calcium gluconate (10%) (if tetany present)
Lactated Ringer's solution
cimetidine (Tagamet) or omeprazole (Prilosec)
Antibiotics (if necrotizing pancreatitis)

CT, Computed tomography; *ERCP,* endoscopic retrograde cholangiopancreatography; *IV,* intravenous; *NG,* nasogastric; *NPO,* nothing by mouth.

NURSING MANAGEMENT
ACUTE PANCREATITIS

■ Nursing Assessment

Subjective and objective data that should be obtained from a person with acute pancreatitis are presented in Table 42-22.

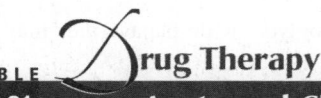

TABLE 42-21   Drug Therapy
Acute and Chronic Pancreatitis

DRUG	MECHANISM OF ACTION
Acute Pancreatitis	
meperidine (Demerol), morphine	Relief of pain
nitroglycerin or papaverine	Relaxation of smooth muscles and relief of pain
Antispasmodics (e.g., dicyclomine [Bentyl], propantheline bromide [Pro-Banthine])	Decrease of vagal stimulation, motility, pancreatic outflow (inhibition of volume and concentration of bicarbonate and enzymatic secretion); contraindicated in paralytic ileus
Carbonic anhydrase inhibitor (acetazolamide [Diamox])	Reduction in volume and bicarbonate concentration of pancreatic secretion
Antacids	Neutralization of gastric HCl secretion and subsequent decrease in secretin, which stimulates production and secretion of pancreatic secretions
Histamine H_2-receptor antagonists (cimetidine [Tagamet], ranitidine [Zantac]); proton pump inhibitors (omeprazole [Prevacid])	Decrease in HCl secretion (HCl stimulates pancreatic activity)
Chronic Pancreatitis	
pancreatin (Viokase), pancrelipase (Cotazym)	Replacement therapy for pancreatic enzymes
Insulin	Treatment for diabetes mellitus if it occurs or for hyperglycemia

HCl, Hydrochloric acid.

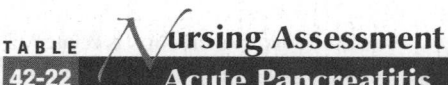

TABLE 42-22   Nursing Assessment
Acute Pancreatitis

Subjective Data

Important Health Information

Past health history: Biliary tract disease, alcohol use, abdominal trauma, duodenal ulcers, infection, metabolic disorders

Medications: Use of thiazides, nonsteroidal antiinflammatory drugs

Surgery or other treatments: Surgical procedures on the pancreas, stomach, duodenum, or biliary tract; endoscopic retrograde cholangiopancreatography

Functional Health Patterns

Health perception–health management: Alcohol abuse; weakness

Nutritional-metabolic: Nausea and vomiting; anorexia

Activity-exercise: Dyspnea

Cognitive-perceptual: Severe midepigastric or left upper quadrant pain that may radiate to the back, aggravated by food and alcohol intake and unrelieved by vomiting

Objective Data

General

Restlessness, anxiety, low-grade fever

Integumentary

Flushing, diaphoresis, discoloration of abdomen and flanks, cyanosis, jaundice; decreased skin turgor, dry mucous membranes

Respiratory

Tachypnea, basilar crackles

Cardiovascular

Tachycardia, hypotension

Gastrointestinal

Abdominal distention, tenderness, and muscle guarding; diminished bowel sounds

Possible Findings

↑ Serum amylase and lipase, leukocytosis, hyperglycemia, ↑ urine amylase, hyperlipidemia, hypocalcemia, abnormal ultrasound and CT scans of pancreas, abnormal ERCP

CT, Computed tomography; *ERCP,* endoscopic retrograde cholangiopancreatogram.

■ **Nursing Diagnoses**

Nursing diagnoses for the patient with acute pancreatitis may include, but are not limited to, those presented in NCP 42-3.

■ **Planning**

The overall goals are that the patient with acute pancreatitis will have (1) relief of pain, (2) normal fluid and electrolyte balance, (3) minimal to no complications, and (4) no recurrent attacks.

■ **Nursing Implementation**

Health Promotion. The major factors involved in health promotion are assessment of the patient for predisposing and etiologic factors of pancreatitis and encouragement of early treatment of these factors to prevent occurrence of acute pancreatitis. The nurse should encourage the early diagnosis and treatment of biliary tract disease, such as cholelithiasis. The patient should be encouraged to eliminate alcohol intake, especially if there have been

NURSING CARE PLAN 42-3

Patient with Acute Pancreatitis

EXPECTED PATIENT OUTCOMES	NURSING INTERVENTIONS and *RATIONALES*
NURSING DIAGNOSIS	**Acute pain** *related to* distention of pancreas, peritoneal irritation, obstruction of biliary tract, and ineffective pain and comfort measures *as manifested by* communication of pain descriptors, guarding behavior, behaviors indicative of pain (e.g., moaning), diaphoresis, changes in blood pressure, pulse, and respiratory rate.
• Minimal to no pain	• Assess degree and nature of pain *to plan appropriate interventions.* • Give ordered analgesic and antispasmodic medications before pain gets too severe *to ensure more effective relief of pain.* • Ascertain how long the medication provides relief *to adjust pain medication administration to provide ongoing relief of pain.* • Provide comfort measures, such as positioning patient comfortably with frequent changes in position and diversional activities *to assist in reducing the restlessness that usually accompanies the pain and to demonstrate caring behaviors by the nurse.*
NURSING DIAGNOSIS	**Deficient fluid volume** *related to* nausea, vomiting, NG suction, and restricted oral intake *as manifested by* thirst, increased fluid output, altered intake, dry skin and mucous membranes, decreased skin turgor, decreased oral intake.
• Normal skin turgor • Moist mucous membranes • Stable weight • Normal serum electrolyte levels	• Give antiemetics as ordered *to reduce fluid loss by preventing vomiting.* • Measure and describe emesis *as indicators of replacement needs and effectiveness of treatment.* • Observe for manifestations of electrolyte imbalances such as confusion, irritability, tachycardia, nausea, vomiting, muscle cramps, and tetany caused by loss of chloride, sodium, potassium, and calcium *so that appropriate replacements can be started promptly.*
NURSING DIAGNOSIS	**Imbalanced nutrition: less than body requirements** *related to* anorexia, dietary restrictions, nausea, loss of nutrients from vomiting, and impaired digestion resulting in decreased use of nutrients *as manifested by* weight loss, weakness, fatigue, weight below normal for height and age.
• Weight appropriate for height • No further weight loss • Normal stool	• Monitor weight and laboratory values *as indicators of patient's response to treatment.* • Observe stools for steatorrhea, *which may develop from incomplete digestion of fats.* • Administer nasointestinal tube feedings or total parenteral nutrition (if severe pancreatitis) if ordered *to provide carbohydrates, lipids, and amino acids to prevent negative nitrogen balance.* • Implement measures to reduce pain and nausea *to increase patient's desire to eat.* • Provide oral care before and after meals *to decrease foul taste and odor that inhibit appetite.* • If oral intake is allowed, provide small portions of high-carbohydrate, low-fat foods *to decrease stimulation of pancreas.*
NURSING DIAGNOSIS	**Ineffective therapeutic regimen management** *related to* lack of knowledge of preventive measures, diet restrictions, restriction of alcohol intake, and follow-up care *as manifested by* verbalization of the problem, request for information, inaccurate follow-through on instructions.
• Verbalization of understanding of condition or disease process and treatment • Initiation of lifestyle changes • Participation in treatment regimen	• Teach patient to (1) abstain from alcohol *to prevent the patient from experiencing future attacks of acute pancreatitis and development of chronic pancreatitis,* (2) restrict fats and avoid rich and stimulating foods *to decrease stimulation of the pancreas and allow it to rest,* (3) use more carbohydrates in diet *because these are less stimulating to pancreas,* and (4) correctly measure blood glucose levels and observe for steatorrhea *because high blood glucose and fatty stools indicate destruction of pancreatic tissue or loss of viable pancreatic tissue.* • Assess patient's understanding of prescribed regimen; provide details on follow-up care *to increase likelihood of successful convalescence and to minimize the possibility of recurrence.* • Suggest follow-up if alcohol use problematic *because continued use of alcohol will result in additional attacks of acute pancreatitis and eventual chronic pancreatitis.*

any previous episodes of pancreatitis. Attacks of pancreatitis become milder or disappear with the discontinuance of alcohol use.

Acute Intervention. During the acute phase, it is important to monitor vital signs. Hemodynamic stability may be compromised by hypotension, fever, and tachypnea, which may result in fluid volume deficit. IV fluids are ordered, and the response to

therapy is monitored. A vital part of the nursing care plan for this patient is observation for electrolyte imbalances. Frequent vomiting, along with gastric suction, may result in decreased chloride, sodium, and potassium levels.

Respiratory failure may develop in the patient with severe acute pancreatitis. It is important that respiratory function be assessed (e.g., lung sounds). If acute respiratory distress syndrome develops, the patient may require intubation and mechanical ventilatory support.

Because hypocalcemia can also occur, the nurse must observe for symptoms of tetany, such as jerking, irritability, and muscular twitching. Numbness or tingling around the lips and in the fingers is an early indicator of hypocalcemia. The patient should be assessed for a positive Chvostek or Trousseau sign (see Chapter 16). Calcium gluconate (as ordered) should be given to treat symptomatic hypocalcemia. In addition, hypomagnesemia may develop, necessitating the observation of serum magnesium levels.

Because abdominal pain is a prominent symptom of pancreatitis, a major focus of nursing care is the relief of pain (see NCP 42-3). Giving the prescribed medications before the pain becomes too severe makes the medication more effective. Morphine or meperidine may be used for pain relief. The nurse should ascertain how long the pain medication provides relief. Measures such as comfortable positioning, frequent changes in position, and relief of nausea and vomiting assist in reducing the restlessness that usually accompanies the pain. Some patients experience lessened pain by assuming positions that flex the trunk and draw the knees up to the abdomen. A side-lying position with the head elevated 45 degrees decreases tension on the abdomen and may help ease the pain. It is important to control the pain and restlessness because they increase body metabolism and subsequent stimulation of pancreatic secretions.

Nursing measures for the patient who is on NPO status or has an NG tube should be employed. Frequent oral and nasal care to relieve the dryness of the mouth and nose is comforting to the patient. Oral care is essential to prevent parotitis. If the patient is taking anticholinergics to decrease GI secretions, there will be additional dryness of the mouth caused by the side effects of the drug. If the patient is taking antacids to suppress secretions, they should be sipped slowly or inserted in the NG tube. The nurse must regularly assess the functioning of the suction.

The patient with acute pancreatitis is susceptible to infections. The nurse should observe for fever and other manifestations of infection. Respiratory infections are common because the retroperitoneal fluid raises the diaphragm, which causes the patient to take shallow, guarded abdominal breaths. Measures to prevent respiratory infections include turning, coughing, deep breathing, and assuming a semi-Fowler's position.

Other important assessments are observation for signs of paralytic ileus, renal failure, and mental changes. Determination of the blood glucose level should be done to assess damage to the β-cells of the islets of Langerhans in the pancreas.

After pancreatic surgery the patient may require special wound care for an anastomotic leak or a fistula. Measures to prevent skin irritation should be used. These include skin barriers such as Stomahesive, Karaya paste, or Colly-Seel; pouching; and drains. In addition to protecting the skin, pouching also provides a more accurate determination of fluid and electrolyte losses and increases patient comfort. Sterile pouching systems are available. The nurse may want to consult with a clinical specialist or an enterostomal therapy nurse, if available.

Ambulatory and Home Care. After acute pancreatitis, most patients will need home care follow-up. The patient may have lost physical reserve and muscle strength. Physical therapy may be needed. Continued care to prevent infection and detect any complications is important. Because frequent doses of narcotics may be required for this patient during the acute stage, follow-up for assessment of possible narcotic addiction may be indicated. This is a more likely problem with chronic pancreatitis than in the patient with acute pancreatitis. Counseling regarding abstinence from alcohol is important to prevent the patient from experiencing future attacks of acute pancreatitis and development of chronic pancreatitis. Beverages with caffeine should not be consumed. Because smoking and stressful situations can overstimulate the pancreas, they should be avoided.

Dietary teaching should include restriction of fats because they stimulate the secretion of cholecystokinin, which then stimulates the pancreas. Carbohydrates are less stimulating to the pancreas, so they should be encouraged. The patient should be instructed to avoid crash dieting and bingeing because they can precipitate attacks.

The patient and the family should be given instructions regarding the recognition and reporting of symptoms of infection, diabetes mellitus, or steatorrhea (foul-smelling, frothy stools). These changes indicate possible destruction of pancreatic tissue. The nurse should make sure the patient fully understands the prescribed regimen. Each aspect must be explained. The importance of taking the required medications and following the recommended diet should be stressed.

■ Evaluation

Expected outcomes for the patient with acute pancreatitis are presented in NCP 42-3.

CHRONIC PANCREATITIS

Chronic pancreatitis is progressive destruction of the pancreas with fibrotic replacement of pancreatic tissue. Strictures and calcifications may also occur in the pancreas.

Etiology and Pathophysiology

There are several types of chronic pancreatitis, but they all have a common underlying pathophysiologic disorder. The two major types are *chronic obstructive pancreatitis* and *chronic calcifying pancreatitis*. Chronic pancreatitis may follow acute pancreatitis, but it may also occur in the absence of any history of an acute condition.

Chronic obstructive pancreatitis is associated with biliary disease. The most common cause is inflammation of the sphincter of Oddi associated with cholelithiasis. Cancer of the ampulla of Vater, duodenum, or pancreas can also cause this type of chronic pancreatitis.

In chronic calcifying pancreatitis there is inflammation and sclerosis, mainly in the head of the pancreas and around the pancreatic duct. This type of chronic pancreatitis is the most common form. It is also called alcohol-induced pancreatitis. Increases in heavy social drinking have produced a higher incidence in countries in which the disease was previously considered rare. In the United States, chronic pancreatitis is found almost exclusively in alcoholics. As with cirrhosis there seems to be a metabolic abnormality that predisposes a person who drinks to the direct toxic effect of the alcohol on the pancreas.

In chronic calcifying pancreatitis the ducts are obstructed with protein precipitates. These precipitates block the pancreatic duct and eventually calcify. This is followed by fibrosis and glandular atrophy. Pseudocysts and abscesses commonly develop.

Clinical Manifestations

As with acute pancreatitis, a major manifestation of chronic pancreatitis is abdominal pain. The patient may have episodes of acute pain, but it usually is chronic (recurrent attacks at intervals of months or years). The attacks may become more and more frequent until they are almost constant, or they may diminish as the pancreatic fibrosis develops. The pain is located in the same areas as in acute pancreatitis but is usually described as a heavy, gnawing feeling or sometimes as burning and cramplike. The pain is not relieved with food or antacids.

Other clinical manifestations include symptoms of pancreatic insufficiency, including malabsorption with weight loss, constipation, mild jaundice with dark urine, steatorrhea, and diabetes mellitus. The steatorrhea may become severe, with voluminous, foul, fatty stools. Urine and stool may be frothy. Some abdominal tenderness may be present.

Diagnostic Studies

In chronic pancreatitis the levels of serum amylase and lipase may be elevated slightly or not at all, depending on the degree of pancreatic fibrosis. Increased serum bilirubin and increased alkaline phosphatase levels may be present. There is usually mild leukocytosis and an elevated sedimentation rate.

The secretin stimulation test is used to assess pancreatic function. In the normal pancreas secretin stimulates HCO_3^- secretion. In the stimulation test secretin is given intravenously, and gastric-duodenal secretions are collected with a double-lumen tube for separate gastric and duodenal aspiration. In chronic pancreatitis there is reduced volume of secretions and reduced bicarbonate concentration (less than 90 mEq/L). Normally, secretin stimulates the production of pancreatic fluid high in bicarbonate content.

Other abnormal diagnostic findings are hyperglycemia and fatty stools (steatorrhea). Stools are examined for fecal fat content. Arteriography and x-rays may demonstrate fibrosis and calcification.

ERCP involves cannulation and visualization of the pancreatic and common bile ducts through an endoscope that is inserted into the esophagus and then into the duodenum. The common bile duct and the pancreatic duct are then cannulated. Contrast dye can be injected into the ducts for visualization. Changes in the pancreatic ductal system, such as gross dilation and microcysts, can be visualized through the use of ERCP.

Imaging studies such as CT, MRI, transabdominal ultrasound, and endoscopic ultrasound are useful in patients with chronic pancreatitis. Transabdominal ultrasonography, CT, and MRI show a variety of changes including calcifications, ductal dilation, pseudocysts, and pancreatic enlargement.

Collaborative Care

When the patient with chronic pancreatitis is experiencing an acute attack, the therapy is identical to that for acute pancreatitis. At other times the focus is on prevention of further attacks, relief of pain, and control of pancreatic exocrine and endocrine insufficiency. It sometimes takes large, frequent doses of analgesics to relieve the pain.

Diet, pancreatic enzyme replacement, and control of the diabetes are measures used to control the pancreatic insufficiency. The diet is bland, low in fat, and high in carbohydrate. The patient does not tolerate fatty, rich, and stimulating foods, and these should be avoided to decrease pancreatic secretions and demands on the pancreas. Alcohol must be totally eliminated.

Pancreatic enzymes such as pancreatin (Viokase) and pancrelipase (Cotazym) contain amylase, lipase, and trypsin and are used to replace the deficient pancreatic enzymes. They are usually enteric coated to prevent their breakdown or inactivation by gastric acid. Bile salts are sometimes given to facilitate the absorption of the fat-soluble vitamins (A, D, E, and K) and prevent further fat loss. If diabetes develops, it is controlled with insulin or oral hypoglycemic agents. Acid-neutralizing (e.g., antacids) and acid-inhibiting drugs (e.g., H_2-receptor blockers, proton pump inhibitors, anticholinergics) may be given to decrease hydrochloric acid but have little overall effect on the outcome of the disease.

Treatment of chronic pancreatitis sometimes requires surgery. When biliary disease is present or if obstruction or pseudocyst develops, surgery may be indicated. Surgical procedures can divert bile flow or relieve ductal obstruction. A choledochojejunostomy diverts bile around the ampulla of Vater, where there may be spasm or hypertrophy of the sphincter. In this procedure the common bile duct is anastomosed into the jejunum. If the pancreatic sphincter is fibrotic, a sphincterotomy enlarges it. Pancreatic drainage procedures relieve ductal obstruction. One type is the Roux-en-Y pancreatojejunostomy, in which the pancreatic duct is opened and an anastomosis is made with the jejunum.

NURSING MANAGEMENT
CHRONIC PANCREATITIS

Except during an acute episode, the focus of nursing management is on chronic care and health promotion. The patient should be instructed to take measures to prevent further attacks. Dietary control, along with consistency of other treatment measures, such as taking pancreatic enzymes, is essential. The pancreatic extracts are usually given with meals or can be given with a snack. The nurse should observe the patient's stools for steatorrhea to help determine the effectiveness of the enzymes. The patient and the family need instructions regarding observation of stools.

If diabetes has developed, the patient will need instruction regarding testing of blood glucose levels and drugs (see Chapter 47). The nurse should make sure that the patient who is taking antacids takes them as ordered to control gastric acidity. Antacids should be taken after meals.

Alcohol must be avoided, and the patient may need assistance with this problem. If the patient has developed a dependence on alcohol, referral to other agencies or resources may be necessary (see Chapter 11).

PANCREATIC CANCER

In the United States in 2002 30,300 people were diagnosed with pancreatic cancer and 29,700 died of pancreatic cancer. It is the fourth leading cause of death from cancer in the United States and Canada. The risk increases with age, with the peak incidence occurring between 65 and 80 years of age.[28]

Most of the pancreatic tumors are adenocarcinomas originating from the epithelium of the ductal system. More than half the tumors occur in the head of the pancreas. As the tumor grows, the common bile duct becomes obstructed, and obstructive jaundice develops. Tumors starting in the body or tail often remain silent until their growth is advanced. The majority of cancers have metastasized at the time of diagnosis. The signs and symptoms of pancreatic cancer are often similar to chronic pancreatitis. The prognosis of a patient with cancer of the pancreas is poor. The majority of patients die within 5 to 12 months of the initial diagnosis, and the 5-year survival rate is only about 10%.[31] The prognosis is related to the location of the tumor.

Etiology and Pathophysiology

The cause of pancreatic cancer remains unknown. There may be some relationship among cancer, diabetes mellitus, and chronic pancreatitis. However, it is not clear whether the cancer follows these diseases or whether these diseases occur as a result of pancreatic cancer. It is known that pancreatic cancer can be induced with chemicals such as nitrosoureas. Major risk factors seem to be cigarette smoking, high-fat diet, diabetes, and exposure to chemicals such as benzidine and coke. The most firmly established risk factor is cigarette smoking. Pancreatic cancer develops twice as often in persons with a history of heavy cigarette use (more than two packs a day) than in nonsmokers. The carcinogens from the tobacco probably reach the pancreatic ducts by bile reflux or via the bloodstream. Another risk factor is the Western diet, particularly the high-fat content. High consumption of meat has also been implicated.

Clinical Manifestations

Common manifestations of pancreatic cancer include abdominal pain (dull, aching), anorexia, rapid and progressive weight loss, nausea, and jaundice. Pain is common and is related to the location of malignancy. Extreme, unrelenting pain is related to extension of the cancer into the retroperitoneal tissues and nerve plexuses. The pain is frequently located in the upper abdomen or left hypochondrium and often radiates to the back. It is commonly related to eating, and it also occurs at night. Weight loss is due to poor digestion and absorption caused by lack of digestive enzymes from the pancreas.

Diagnostic Studies

Better diagnostic measures are needed for detection of pancreatic cancer because most of the current methods detect only advanced stages. Transabdominal ultrasound and CT are the most commonly used diagnostic imaging techniques for pancreatic diseases including cancer. CT scan is often the initial study and provides information on metastasis and vascular involvement. ERCP is the "gold standard" for visualization of the pancreatic duct and biliary system.[31] When ERCP is used, pancreatic secretions, as well as tissue, can be collected for analysis of different tumor markers. Endoluminal ultrasound involves imaging the pancreas with the use of an endoscope positioned in the stomach and duodenum. This procedure also allows for fine needle aspiration of the tumor.

Tumor markers are used both for establishing the diagnosis of pancreatic adenocarcinoma and for monitoring the response to treatment. CA19-9 is most frequently increased in pancreatic cancer but may also be elevated in gallbladder cancer, as well as in benign conditions such as acute and chronic pancreatitis, hepatitis, and biliary obstruction.[31] Carcinoembryonic antigen (CEA) is a protein expressed in the colon during embryonic development and is used as a tumor marker in pancreatic cancer. However, CEA is best known as a tumor marker for colon cancer and is less specific for pancreatic cancer.

Collaborative Care

Surgery provides the most effective treatment of cancer of the pancreas. The classic surgery is a *radical pancreaticoduodenectomy,* or *Whipple's procedure* (Fig. 42-15). This entails resection of the proximal pancreas (proximal pancreatectomy), the adjoining duodenum (duodenectomy), the distal portion of the stomach (partial gastrectomy), and the distal segment of the common bile duct. An anastomosis of the pancreatic duct, common bile duct, and stomach to the jejunum is done. A total pancreatectomy is performed in some institutions for cancers of the head of the pancreas. Sometimes a simple bypass procedure, such as a cholecystojejunostomy to relieve biliary obstruction, may be used as a palliative measure. Some surgeons suggest a more radical resection, such as a total pancreaticoduodenectomy with splenectomy. Biliary stents (e.g., Cotton-Leung stent) can be used as a palliative measure when tumors compress the bile duct.

Radiation therapy alters survival rates little but is effective for pain relief. External radiation is usually used, but implantation of internal radiation seeds into the tumor has also been used. The current role of chemotherapy in pancreatic cancer is limited. Chemotherapy usually consists of 5-FU and gemcitabine (Gemzar) either alone or in combination.[32,33] However, response rates are below 15% with minor effects on overall survival. Because of the aggressive nature of pancreatic cancer, current emphasis of new experimental chemotherapy is also focused on clinical benefits including reductions in pain. Several oral formulations of 5-FU, such as capecitabine (Xeloda) and eniluracil with 5-FU, have been developed to simulate long-term continuous infusion. Response rates of these formulations are comparable to those of 5-FU continuous infusion and 5-FU bolus injections. Combinations of drugs such as 5-FU and carmustine (BCNU) produce a better response than single chemotherapeutic agents. Gemcitabine is currently a main treatment for pancreatic

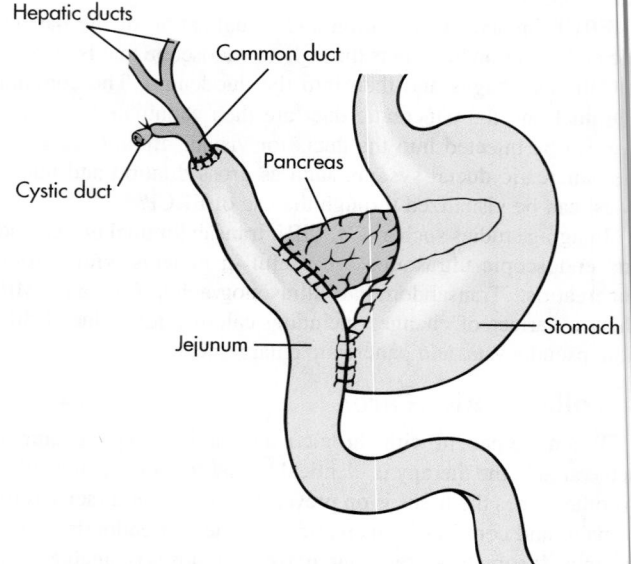

FIG. 42-15 Whipple procedure or radical pancreaticoduodenectomy. This surgical procedure involves resection of the proximal pancreas, adjoining duodenum, distal portion of the stomach, and distal portion of the common bile duct. An anastomosis of the pancreatic duct, common bile duct, and stomach to the jejunum is done.

cancer that has metastasized. Adjuvant therapy, which uses surgical resection, radiation, and chemotherapy, is believed by some to be the most effective way to manage cancer of the pancreas.

NURSING MANAGEMENT
PANCREATIC CANCER

Because the patient with pancreatic cancer has many of the same problems as the patient with pancreatitis, nursing care includes the same measures (see NCP 42-3). The nurse should provide symptomatic and supportive nursing care. Medications and comfort measures to relieve pain should be provided before the patient reaches the peak of pain. Psychologic support is essential, especially during times of anxiety or depression, which seem to occur frequently in these patients.

Adequate nutrition is an important part of the nursing care plan. Frequent and supplemental feedings may be necessary. Measures to stimulate the appetite as much as possible and to overcome anorexia, nausea, and vomiting should be included in the nursing care. Because bleeding can result from impaired vitamin K production, the nurse should assess for bleeding from body orifices and mucous membranes. If the patient is undergoing radiation therapy, the nurse must observe for adverse reactions, such as anorexia, nausea, vomiting, and skin irritation.

The prognosis for a patient with pancreatic cancer is not good. A significant component of the nursing care is helping the patient and the family or significant others through the grieving process.

Disorders of the Biliary Tract
CHOLELITHIASIS AND CHOLECYSTITIS

The most common disorder of the biliary system is **cholelithiasis** (stones in the gallbladder) (Figs. 42-16 and 42-17). **Cholecystitis** (inflammation of the gallbladder) is usually associated with cholelithiasis. The stones may be lodged in the neck of the gallbladder or in the cystic duct. Cholecystitis may be acute or chronic. These conditions usually occur together.

Gallbladder disease is a common health problem in the United States. It is estimated that 8% to 10% of the adults in the United States have cholelithiasis. The actual number is not known because many persons are asymptomatic with stones. *Cholecystec-*

tomy (removal of the gallbladder) ranks among the most common surgical procedures performed in the United States. The incidence of cholelithiasis is higher in women, multiparous women, and persons over 40 years of age. Postmenopausal women on estrogen therapy are at somewhat greater risk of having gallbladder disease than are women who are taking birth control pills. Oral contraceptives alter the character of bile, resulting in increased cholesterol saturation. Other factors that seem to increase the occurrence of gallbladder disease are a sedentary lifestyle, a familial tendency, and obesity. Obesity causes increased secretion of cholesterol in bile. Gallbladder disease is more common in whites than in Asian Americans and African Americans. There is an especially high incidence in the Native American population, particularly in the Navajo and Pima tribes.

Etiology and Pathophysiology

Cholecystitis. Cholecystitis is most commonly associated with obstruction caused by gallstones or biliary sludge. When cholecystitis occurs in the absence of obstruction (acalculous cholecystitis), it is most often in older adults and in patients who have trauma, extensive burns, or recent surgery. Acalculous cholecystitis can also occur as a result of prolonged immobility and fasting, prolonged total parenteral nutrition, and diabetes mellitus. Bacteria reaching the gallbladder via the vascular or lymphatic route, or chemical irritants in the bile can also produce cholecystitis. *Escherichia coli* is the most common bacteria involved. Streptococci and salmonellae are also common causative bacteria. Other etiologic factors include adhesions, neoplasms, anesthesia, and narcotics.[34]

Inflammation is the major pathophysiologic condition and may be confined to the mucous lining or involve the entire wall of the gallbladder. During an acute attack of cholecystitis the gallbladder is edematous and hyperemic. It may be distended with bile or pus. The cystic duct is also involved and may become occluded. The wall of the gallbladder becomes scarred after an acute attack. Decreased functioning occurs if large amounts of tissue are fibrosed.

Cholelithiasis. The actual cause of gallstones is unknown. Basically, cholelithiasis develops when the balance that keeps cholesterol, bile salts, and calcium in solution is altered so that precipitation of these substances occurs. Conditions that upset this balance include infection and disturbances in the metabolism

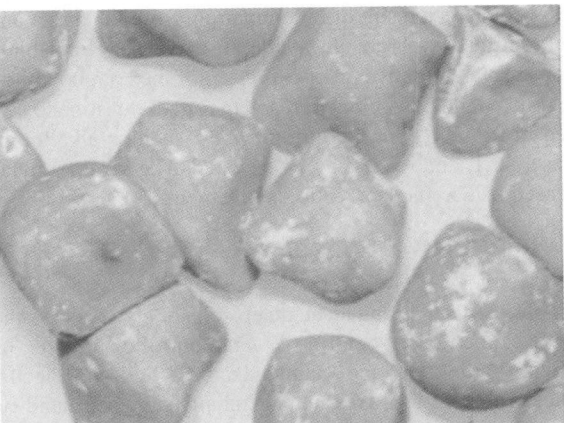

FIG. 42-16 Gallstones.

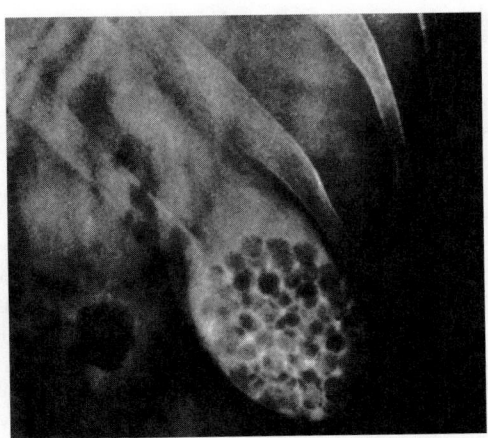

FIG. 42-17 X-ray of a gallbladder with gallstones.

of cholesterol. It is known that in patients with cholelithiasis the bile secreted by the liver is supersaturated with cholesterol (lithogenic bile). The bile in the gallbladder also becomes supersaturated with cholesterol. Whenever bile is supersaturated with cholesterol, precipitation of cholesterol will occur.

A high percentage of gallstones are precipitates of cholesterol. Other components of bile that precipitate into stones are bile salts, bilirubin, calcium, and protein. The stones sometimes have a mixed consistency. Mixed cholesterol stones, which are predominantly cholesterol, are the most common gallstones.

The changes in the composition of bile are probably significant in the formation of gallstones. Stasis of bile leads to progression of the supersaturation and changes in the chemical composition of the bile. Immobility, pregnancy, and inflammatory or obstructive lesions of the biliary system decrease bile flow. Hormonal factors during pregnancy may cause delayed emptying of the gallbladder.

The stones may remain in the gallbladder or migrate to the cystic duct or to the common bile duct. They cause pain as they pass through the ducts, and they may lodge in the ducts and produce an obstruction. Small stones are more likely to move into a duct and cause obstruction. Table 42-23 depicts the changes and manifestations that occur when the stones obstruct the common bile duct. If the blockage occurs in the cystic duct, the bile can continue to flow into the duodenum directly from the liver. However, when the bile in the gallbladder cannot escape, this stasis of bile may lead to cholecystitis.

Clinical Manifestations

Manifestations of cholecystitis vary from indigestion to moderate to severe pain, fever, and jaundice. Initial symptoms of acute cholecystitis include indigestion and pain and tenderness in the right upper quadrant, which may be referred to the right shoulder and scapula. The pain may be acute and be accompanied by nausea and vomiting, restlessness, and diaphoresis. Manifestations of inflammation include leukocytosis and fever. Physical findings include right upper quadrant tenderness and abdominal rigidity. Symptoms of chronic cholecystitis include a history of fat intolerance, dyspepsia, heartburn, and flatulence.

Cholelithiasis may produce severe symptoms or none at all. Many patients have "silent cholelithiasis." The severity of symptoms depends on whether the stones are stationary or mobile and whether obstruction is present. When a stone is lodged in the ducts or when stones are moving through the ducts, spasms may result. The gallbladder spasms occur in response to the stone. This sometimes produces severe pain, which is termed *biliary colic* even though the pain is rarely colicky; it is more often steady. The pain can be excruciating and accompanied by tachycardia, diaphoresis, and prostration. The severe pain may last up to an hour, and when it subsides there is residual tenderness in the right upper quadrant. The attacks of pain frequently occur 3 to 6 hours after a heavy meal or when the patient assumes a recumbent position. When total obstruction occurs, symptoms related to bile blockage are manifested (see Table 42-23).

Complications

Complications of cholecystitis include subphrenic abscess, pancreatitis, *cholangitis* (inflammation of biliary ducts), biliary cirrhosis, fistulas, and rupture of the gallbladder, which can produce bile peritonitis.

Many of the same complications can occur from cholelithiasis, including cholangitis, biliary cirrhosis, carcinoma, and peritonitis. *Choledocholithiasis* (stone in the common bile duct) may occur, producing symptoms of obstruction.

Diagnostic Studies

Ultrasonography is probably the best means of diagnosing gallstones (see Table 38-12). It is 90% to 95% accurate in detecting stones. It is especially useful for patients with jaundice (because it does not depend on liver function) and for patients who are allergic to contrast medium. ERCP allows for visualization of the gallbladder, cystic duct, common hepatic duct, and common bile duct. Bile taken during ERCP is sent for culture to identify any possible infecting organism.

Percutaneous transhepatic cholangiography may be used to diagnose obstructive jaundice and to locate stones within the bile ducts. Laboratory tests may demonstrate abnormalities in some of the liver function tests and an increased white blood cell (WBC) count as a result of inflammation. Both the direct and indirect bilirubin levels are elevated, as is the urinary bilirubin level if there is an obstructive process present. If the common bile duct is obstructed, no bilirubin will reach the small intestine to be converted to urobilinogen. Serum enzymes, such as alkaline phosphatase, ALT, and AST, may be elevated. The serum amylase is increased if there is pancreatic involvement.

Collaborative Care

Conservative Therapy

Cholecystitis. During an acute episode of cholecystitis the focus of treatment is on control of pain, control of possible infection with antibiotics, and maintenance of fluid and electrolyte balance (Table 42-24). Treatment is mainly supportive and symptomatic. If nausea and vomiting are severe, gastric decompression may be used to prevent further gallbladder stimulation. An

TABLE 42-23	Clinical Manifestations Caused by Obstructed Bile Flow	
CLINICAL MANIFESTATION	**ETIOLOGY**
Obstructive jaundice	No bile flow into duodenum
Dark amber urine, which foams when shaken	Soluble bilirubin in urine
No urobilinogen in urine	No bilirubin reaching small intestine to be converted to urobilinogen
Clay-colored stools	Same as above
Pruritus	Deposition of bile salts in skin tissues
Intolerance for fatty foods (nausea, sensation of fullness, anorexia)	No bile in small intestine for fat digestion
Bleeding tendencies	Lack of or decreased absorption of vitamin K, resulting in decreased production of prothrombin
Steatorrhea	No bile salts in duodenum, preventing fat emulsion and digestion

TABLE 42-24   Collaborative Care

Cholelithiasis and Acute Cholecystitis

Diagnostic
History and physical examination
Ultrasound
Liver function studies
WBC count
Serum bilirubin
ERCP

Collaborative Therapy
Conservative Therapy
IV fluid
NPO with NG tube, later progressing to low-fat diet
Antiemetics
Analgesics (e.g., meperidine)
Fat-soluble vitamins (A, D, E, and K)
Anticholinergics (antispasmodics)
Antibiotics (for secondary infection)
ERCP with sphincterotomy (papillotomy)
Extracorporeal shock-wave lithotripsy
Dissolution Therapy
ursodeoxycholic acid (UDCA)
ursodiol (Actigall)
chenodeoxycholic acid (CDCA)
Surgical Therapy*
Laparoscopic cholecystectomy
Incisional cholecystectomy

*See Table 42-25.
ERCP, Endoscopic retrograde cholangiopancreatography; *IV,* intravenous; *NG,* nasogastric; *NPO,* nothing by mouth; *WBC,* white blood cell.

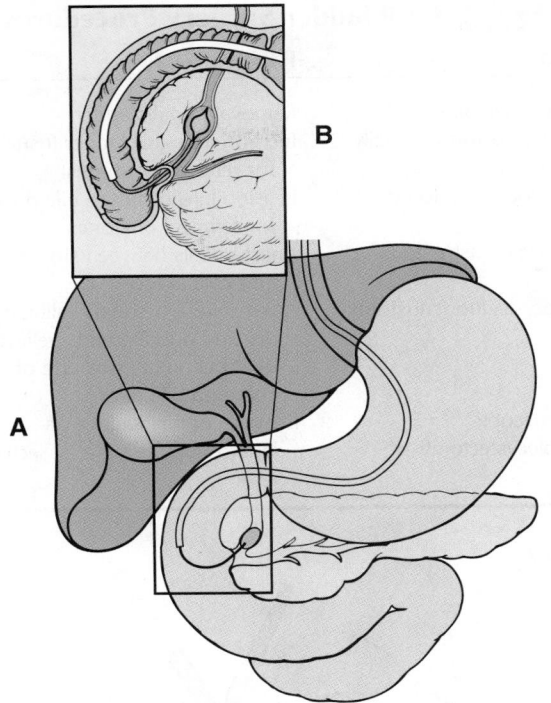

FIG. 42-18 **A,** During endoscopic sphincterotomy, an endoscope is advanced through the mouth and stomach until its tip sits in the duodenum opposite the common bile duct. **B,** After widening the duct mouth by incising the sphincter muscle, the physician advances a basket attachment into the duct and snags the stone.

ticholinergics to decrease secretions (which prevents biliary contraction) and counteract smooth muscle spasms may be administered. Analgesics are given to decrease the pain.

Cholelithiasis. There are two nonsurgical approaches for biliary stone removal. Most patients are treated by means of ERCP. Standard ERCP techniques will clear stones from the biliary tree in approximately 90% of patients. This procedure allows for visualization of the biliary system, as well as the placement of stents and sphincterotomy (papillotomy) if warranted. Endoscopic sphincterotomy is especially effective in removing common bile duct stones (Fig. 42-18). The endoscope is passed to the duodenum. With an electrodiathermy knife attached to the endoscope, the sphincter of Oddi is widened by incision of the sphincter muscle (sphincterotomy). A basket is used to retrieve the stone. The stone may be removed in the basket, but more commonly it is left in the duodenum and will be passed naturally in the stool.

If the stone is too large to pass through the duct, the endoscopist can crush the stone (mechanical lithotripsy). The limitation of this procedure is ERCP-induced acute pancreatitis. In approximately 10% of patients, nonstandard management, including peroral or percutaneous mechanical, electrohydraulic, or laser lithotripsy, will be needed. Other options for cholelithiasis include cholesterol solvents such as methyl tertiary terbutyl ether (MTBE), oral drugs that dissolve stones, endoscopic sphincterotomy, extracorporeal shock-wave lithotripsy (ESWL), and surgery. A direct-contact dis-

solving agent such as MTBE can be instilled into the gallbladder via a percutaneous catheter. MTBE dissolves cholesterol stones within hours. The gallstones may recur. Oral bile acids are also used to dissolve stones.

In ESWL a biliary lithotriptor uses high-energy shock waves to disintegrate gallstones. The patient must have a functioning gallbladder. An ultrasound scan is first done to locate the stones and to determine where to direct the shock waves. The shock waves are directed through the abdomen as a water-filled cushion is pressed against the area. It usually takes 1 to 2 hours to disintegrate the stones. After they are broken up, the fragments pass through the common bile duct and into the small intestine. There has been mixed success with ESWL.

Supportive treatment, similar to that given for cholecystitis, may also be necessary. If the stones cause an obstruction, additional treatment consists of replacement of fat-soluble vitamins, administration of bile salts to facilitate digestion and vitamin absorption, and a low-fat diet.

Surgical Therapy. Surgical intervention for cholelithiasis is often indicated and may consist of any one of several procedures (Table 42-25). The procedure of choice for most patients is still a cholecystectomy. This is a safe procedure with minimal morbidity, and it requires only a brief hospitalization. One procedure is removal of the gallbladder through a right subcostal incision. A T tube is inserted into the common bile duct during surgery when a common bile duct exploration is part of the surgical procedure (Fig. 42-19). This ensures patency of the duct until the edema produced by the trauma of exploring and probing the duct has sub-

TABLE 42-25	Gallbladder Surgery Procedures
NAME	**DESCRIPTION**
Cholecystectomy	Removal of gallbladder
Cholecystostomy (usually an emergency)	Incision into gallbladder (usually for removal of stones)
Choledocholithotomy	Incision into common bile duct for removal of stones
Cholecystogastrostomy	Anastomosis between stomach and gallbladder
Cholecystoduodenostomy	Anastomosis between gallbladder and duodenum to relieve obstruction at distal end of common bile duct
Laparoscopic cholecystectomy	Removal of gallbladder via laparoscopy using a dissecting laser

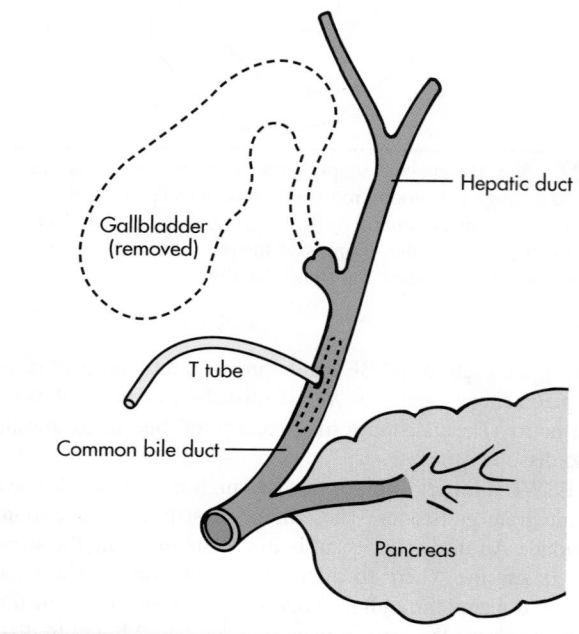

FIG. 42-19   Placement of T tube. Dotted lines indicate parts removed.

may vary.) Using closed-circuit monitors to view the abdominal cavity, the surgeon retracts and dissects the gallbladder and removes it with grasping forceps.

This procedure is relatively minor with few complications. Most patients experience minimal postoperative pain and are discharged the day of surgery or the day after. In most cases they are able to resume normal activities and return to work within 1 week.

Advantages of the laparoscopic cholecystectomy include decreased postoperative pain, shorter hospital stay, and earlier return to work and full activity. The main complication is injury to the common bile duct. There are few contraindications to laparoscopic cholecystectomy. The primary ones are peritonitis, cholangitis, gangrene or perforation of the gallbladder, portal hypertension, and serious bleeding disorders.

Transhepatic Biliary Catheter. The transhepatic biliary catheter can be used preoperatively in biliary obstruction and in hepatic dysfunction secondary to obstructive jaundice. It can also be inserted when inoperable liver, pancreatic, or bile duct carcinoma obstructs bile flow. The catheter is inserted under fluoroscopy and involves percutaneous insertion across the liver parenchyma into the common bile duct and duodenum. It decompresses obstructed extrahepatic bile ducts so that bile can flow freely. After insertion, the catheter is connected to a drainage bag. The skin around the catheter insertion site has to be cleansed daily with an antiseptic. It is important to observe for bile leakage at the insertion site. Depending on the reason the catheter was inserted, the patient may be discharged with it in place.

Drug Therapy. The most common drugs used in the treatment of gallbladder disease are analgesics, anticholinergics (antispasmodics), fat-soluble vitamins, and bile salts. Meperidine (Demerol) is used if a narcotic analgesic is required. This causes less spasm in the ducts than opiates such as morphine. Anticholinergics such as atropine and other antispasmodics may be used to relax the smooth muscle and decrease ductal tone.

If the patient has chronic gallbladder disease or any biliary tract obstruction, fat-soluble vitamins (A, D, E, and K) will probably be given. Bile salts may be administered to facilitate digestion and vitamin absorption.

For treatment of pruritus, cholestyramine (Questran) may provide relief. This is a resin that binds bile salts in the intestine, increasing their excretion in the feces. Cholestyramine is administered in powder form and should be mixed with milk or juice. Side effects include nausea, vomiting, diarrhea or constipation, and skin reactions.

Medical dissolution therapy is recommended for patients with small radiolucent stones who are mildly symptomatic and are poor surgical risks. Ursodeoxycholic acid (UDCA), ursodiol (Actigall), and chenodeoxycholic acid (CDCA, chenodiol, Chenix) may be used to dissolve the stones. The main side effects of CDCA are cramps and diarrhea, but these are usually not severe. A more serious side effect is hepatotoxicity. UDCA has fewer side effects than CDCA. Dissolution therapy may take anywhere from 6 months to 2 years for dissolution of the stones, and low-dose therapy is recommended to prevent recurrence. The drugs to dissolve the gallstones are not used as much currently because of high use of laparoscopic cholecystectomy and ERCP.

Nutritional Therapy. The major dietary modification for a patient with cholelithiasis and cholecystitis is a low-fat diet (see Table 33-4). If obesity is a problem, a reduced-calorie diet is indicated. The low-fat diet decreases stimulation of the gallbladder.

sided. It also allows the excess bile to drain while the small intestine is adjusting to receiving a continuous flow of bile.

The *laparoscopic cholecystectomy* has become the treatment of choice for cholecystectomy. Currently, approximately 92% of all cholecystectomies are performed laparoscopically. In this procedure the gallbladder is removed through one of four small punctures in the abdomen. A 1 cm puncture is made slightly above the umbilicus, and the surgeon inflates the abdominal cavity with 3 to 4 L of CO_2 to improve visibility. A laparoscope, which has a camera attached, is then inserted into the abdomen. Two additional punctures are made just below the ribs, one on the right anterior axillary line and the other on the right midclavicular line. These punctures are used for insertion of grasping forceps. A dissection laser is inserted into the fourth puncture, which is made just right of the midsection. (The incision sites

Foods that are avoided include dairy products such as whole milk, cream, butter, whole milk cheese, and ice cream; fried foods; rich pastries; gravies; and nuts. Many patients have fewer problems if they eat smaller, more frequent meals.

After a laparoscopic cholecystectomy the patient is instructed to have liquids for the rest of the day and eat light meals for a few days. If an incisional cholecystectomy is done, the patient will progress from liquids to a bland diet once bowel sounds have returned. The amount of fat in the postoperative diet depends on the patient's tolerance of fat. A low-fat diet may be helpful if the flow of bile is reduced (usually only in the early postoperative period) or if the patient is overweight. Sometimes the patient is instructed to restrict fats for 4 to 6 weeks. Otherwise, no special dietary instructions are needed other than to eat nutritious meals and avoid excessive fat intake.

NURSING MANAGEMENT
GALLBLADDER DISEASE

▪ Nursing Assessment

Subjective and objective data that should be obtained from a person with gallbladder disease are presented in Table 42-26.

▪ Nursing Diagnoses

Nursing diagnoses for the patient with gallbladder disease treated surgically include, but are not limited to, the following:
- acute pain *related to* surgical procedure
- ineffective therapeutic regimen management *related to* lack of knowledge of diet and postoperative management

▪ Planning

The overall goals are that the patient with gallbladder disease will have (1) relief of pain and discomfort, (2) no complications postoperatively, and (3) no recurrent attacks of cholecystitis or cholelithiasis.

▪ Nursing Implementation

Health Promotion. The nurse should assume responsibility for recognition of predisposing factors of gallbladder disease in general health screening. Ethnic groups in which the disease is

COMPLEMENTARY & ALTERNATIVE THERAPIES
Milk Thistle

Clinical Uses
Liver conditions including hepatitis and cirrhosis and following liver transplant or mushroom poisoning. Also used in gallbladder disease.

Effects
Protects liver cells from toxic damage, promotes regeneration of liver cells, and has antiinflammatory and antioxidant effects. Can increase the secretion and flow of bile from the gallbladder. May have a laxative effect in some people.

Nursing Implications
In general, it is a safe herb when administered appropriately. People with allergies to ragweed, marigolds, daisies, and other plants of the Asteraceae family may have mild allergic reactions with use of milk thistle. Should not be used in combination with phenothiazines or haloperidol (Haldol).

more common, such as Native Americans, should be taught initial manifestations and instructed to seek medical care if these manifestations occur. The patient with chronic cholecystitis does not have acute symptoms and may not seek help until jaundice and biliary obstruction occur. Earlier detection in these patients is beneficial so that they can be managed with a low-fat diet and monitored more closely.

Acute Intervention. Nursing objectives for the patient undergoing conservative therapy include relieving pain, relieving nausea and vomiting, providing comfort and emotional support, maintaining fluid and electrolyte balance and nutrition, making accurate assessments for effectiveness of treatment, and observing for complications.

The patient with acute cholecystitis or cholelithiasis is frequently experiencing severe pain. The medications ordered to relieve the pain should be given as required by the patient and before the pain becomes more severe. The nurse should assess what medications relieve the pain and how much medication is required. Observations for side effects of the medications must be part of the continued assessment. Nursing comfort measures,

TABLE 42-26	**Nursing Assessment** **Cholecystitis or Cholelithiasis**

Subjective Data	**Objective Data**
Important Health Information	**General**
Past health history: Obesity, multiparity, infection, cancer, extensive fasting, pregnancy	Fever, restlessness
Medications: Use of estrogen or oral contraceptives	**Integumentary**
Surgery or other treatments: Previous abdominal surgery	Jaundice, icteric sclera; diaphoresis
Functional Health Patterns	**Respiratory**
Health perception–health management: Positive family history; sedentary lifestyle	Tachypnea, splinting during respirations
Nutritional-metabolic: Weight loss, anorexia; indigestion, fat intolerance, nausea and vomiting, dyspepsia; chills	**Cardiovascular** Tachycardia
Elimination: Clay-colored stools, steatorrhea, flatulence; dark urine	**Gastrointestinal** Palpable gallbladder, abdominal guarding and distention
Cognitive-perceptual: Moderate to severe pain in right upper quadrant that may radiate to the back or scapula; pruritus	**Possible Findings** ↑ Serum liver enzymes and bilirubin, absence of urobilinogen in urine, ↑ urinary bilirubin; leukocytosis, abnormal gallbladder ultrasound

such as a clean bed, comfortable positioning, and oral care, are appropriate.

Some patients have more severe nausea and vomiting than others. For these patients it may be necessary to use gastric decompression. The elimination of intake of food and fluids also prevents further stimulation of the gallbladder. Oral hygiene, care of nares, accurate intake and output measurements, and maintenance of suction should be a part of the nursing care plan for this patient. For patients with less severe nausea and vomiting, antiemetics are usually adequate. When the patient is vomiting, comfort measures such as frequent mouth rinses should be provided. Any vomitus should be immediately removed from the patient's view.

If pruritus occurs with jaundice, measures to relieve itching are necessary. Such measures include baking soda or Alpha Keri baths; lotions, such as those containing calamine; antihistamines; soft, old linen; and control of the temperature (not too hot and not too cold). The patient's nails should be kept short and clean. Patients should be taught to rub with their knuckles rather than scratch with their nails when they cannot resist scratching.

A significant portion of the nursing care plan for this patient centers on accurate assessment of progression of the symptoms and development of complications. The nurse must be knowledgeable of and observe for signs of obstruction of the ducts by stones. These include jaundice; clay-colored stools; dark, foamy urine; steatorrhea; fever; and increased WBC count.

When symptoms of obstruction are present (see Table 42-23), the nurse must be aware of the possibility of bleeding as a result of decreased prothrombin production. Common sites to observe for bleeding are the mucous membranes of the mouth, nose, gingivae, and injection sites. If injections are given, a small-gauge needle should be used and gentle pressure applied after the injection. The nurse should know the patient's prothrombin time and use this as a guide in the assessment process.

Assessment for infections includes monitoring of vital signs. A temperature elevation with chills and jaundice may indicate choledocholithiasis.

Nursing care of the patient after endoscopic papillotomy includes assessment to detect complications such as pancreatitis, perforation, infection, and bleeding. The patient's vital signs should be monitored. Abdominal pain and fever may indicate pancreatitis. The patient should be on bed rest for several hours and should have nothing by mouth until the gag reflex returns.

Postoperative care. Postoperative nursing care following a laparoscopic cholecystectomy includes monitoring for complications such as bleeding, making the patient comfortable, and preparing the patient for discharge. A common postoperative problem is referred pain to the shoulder because of the CO_2 that was not released or absorbed by the body. The CO_2 can irritate the phrenic nerve and the diaphragm, causing some difficulty breathing. Placing the patient in Sims' position (left side with right knee flexed) helps move the gas pocket away from the diaphragm. Deep breathing should be encouraged, along with movement and ambulation. There is usually minimal pain that can be relieved by narcotic analgesics such as oxycodone (Oxycontin) or codeine. The patient is allowed clear liquids and can walk to the bathroom to void. Many patients go home the same day, but some will stay overnight.

Postoperative nursing care for incisional cholecystectomy focuses on adequate ventilation and prevention of respiratory com-

---

TABLE 42-27

Patient & Family Teaching Guide
Postoperative Laparoscopic Cholecystectomy

1. Instruct patient to remove the bandages on the puncture site the day after surgery and bathe or shower.
2. Explain the need to report the following signs and symptoms:
   - Redness, swelling, bile-colored drainage or pus from any incision
   - Severe abdominal pain, nausea, vomiting, fever, chills
3. Explain that normal activities can be resumed gradually.
4. Instruct that returning to work can occur within 1 week of surgery.
5. Instruct to resume usual diet; may need to be a low-fat diet for several weeks following surgery.

---

plications. Other nursing care is the same as general postoperative nursing care (see Chapter 19).

If the patient has a T tube (see Fig. 42-19), part of the nursing care plan is related to maintaining bile drainage and observation of the T-tube functioning and drainage. The T tube is connected to a closed gravity drainage system. If the Penrose or Jackson-Pratt drain or the T tube is draining large amounts, it is helpful to use a sterile pouching system to protect the skin.

Ambulatory and Home Care. When the patient has conservative therapy, long-term nursing management depends on symptoms and on whether surgical intervention is being planned. Dietary teaching is usually necessary. The diet is usually low in fat, and sometimes a weight-reduction diet is also recommended. The patient may need to take fat-soluble vitamin supplements. The nurse should provide instructions regarding observations that the patient should make indicating obstruction (stool and urine changes, jaundice, and pruritus). Continued health care is important, and its significance should be explained and stressed.

The patient who undergoes a laparoscopic cholecystectomy is discharged soon after the surgery, so home care is important. Teaching is essential (Table 42-27).

After an open-incision cholecystectomy, the patient may be discharged as soon as 2 to 3 days. The patient should be instructed to avoid heavy lifting for 4 to 6 weeks. Usual sexual activities, including intercourse, can be resumed as soon as the patient feels ready unless given other instructions by the physician.

Sometimes the patient is required to remain on a low-fat diet for 4 to 6 weeks. If so, a dietary teaching plan is necessary. A weight-reduction program may be helpful if the patient is overweight. Most patients tolerate a regular diet with no difficulties but should avoid excessive fats.

■ Evaluation

The overall expected outcomes are that the patient with gallbladder disease will
- appear comfortable and verbalize pain relief
- verbalize knowledge of activity level and dietary restrictions

GALLBLADDER CANCER

Primary cancer of the gallbladder is uncommon. The majority of gallbladder carcinomas are adenocarcinomas. There seems to be a definite relationship between cancer of the gallbladder and chronic cholecystitis and cholelithiasis. The early symptoms of carcinoma of the gallbladder are insidious and are similar to those of chronic cholecystitis and cholelithiasis, which makes diagnosis difficult. Later symptoms are usually those of biliary obstruction.

Diagnosis and staging of gallbladder cancer is done using endoscopic ultrasound, transabdominal ultrasound, CT, MRI, and/or MR cholangiopancreatography. Unfortunately, gallbladder cancer often presents with advanced disease.[35] When found early, surgery can be curative. Several factors influence suc-cessful surgical outcomes, including the depth of cancer invasion, extent of liver involvement, presence of venous or lymphatic invasion, and lymph node metastasis. Extended cholecystectomy with lymph node dissection has improved the outcomes for patients with gallbladder cancer. When surgery is not an option, endoscopic stenting of the biliary tree to reduce obstructive jaundice may be warranted. Adjuvant therapies including radiation therapy and chemotherapy may be used depending on the disease state. Overall cancer of the gallbladder has a poor prognosis.

Nursing management involves supportive care with special attention to nutrition, hydration, skin care, and pain relief. Many of the nursing care measures used for patients with cholecystitis and cholelithiasis are frequently applied, as well as nursing care measures for the patient with cancer (see Chapter 15).

CRITICAL THINKING EXERCISES

Case Study
Cirrhosis of the Liver

Patient Profile. Mr. Begay is a 55-year-old Native American man admitted with a diagnosis of cirrhosis of the liver.

Subjective Data
- Has had cirrhosis for 12 years
- Acknowledges that he had been drinking heavily for 20 years but has been sober for the past 2 years
- Complains of anorexia, nausea, and abdominal discomfort

Objective Data
Physical Examination
- Thin and malnourished
- Has moderate ascites
- Has jaundice of sclera and skin
- Has 4+ pitting edema of the lower extremities
- Liver and spleen are palpable

Laboratory Values
- Total bilirubin: 15 mg/dl (257 mmol/L)
- Serum ammonia: 220 mg/dl (122 mmol/L)
- AST: 190 U/L (3.2 μkat/L)
- ALT: 210 U/L (3.5 μkat/L

CRITICAL THINKING QUESTIONS

1. What are possible causes of cirrhosis? What type of cirrhosis does Mr. Begay probably have?
2. Describe the pathophysiologic changes that occur in the liver as cirrhosis develops.
3. List Mr. Begay's clinical manifestations of liver failure. For each manifestation, explain the pathophysiologic basis.
4. Explain the significance of the results of his laboratory values.
5. If Mr. Begay begins to manifest signs and symptoms of hepatic encephalopathy, what would you monitor? What measures should be instituted to control or decrease the ammonia level?
6. Mr. Begay was being closely observed for the possibility of gastrointestinal bleeding. Why is this considered a possible complication?
7. In the early stages of cirrhosis, what can be done to control the disease?
8. Based on the assessment data presented, write one or more nursing diagnoses. Are there any collaborative problems?

Nursing Research Issues

1. What is the most effective way to assess jaundice in a dark-skinned person?
2. What are the most significant psychosocial problems experienced by a patient with viral hepatitis?
3. What are the best ways to treat pruritus associated with jaundice in patients with hepatitis?
4. What is the quality of life for a patient after a liver transplant?
5. Can nutritional support improve outcomes in patients with alcohol-related cirrhosis?
6. What support resources are needed by the family of a patient with pancreatic cancer?

REVIEW QUESTIONS

The number of the question corresponds to the same-numbered objective at the beginning of the chapter.

1. During assessment of a patient with obstructive jaundice the nurse would expect to find
   a. clay-colored stools.
   b. dark urine and stools.
   c. pyrexia and severe pruritus.
   d. elevated urinary urobilinogen.

2. A patient with hepatitis A is in the prodromal (pre-icteric) phase. The nurse plans care for the patient based on the knowledge that
   a. pruritus is a common problem with jaundice in this phase.
   b. the patient is most likely to transmit the disease during this phase.
   c. gastrointestinal symptoms are not as severe in hepatitis A as they are in hepatitis B.
   d. extrahepatic manifestations of glomerulonephritis and polyarteritis are common in this phase.

3. A patient with hepatitis B is being discharged in 2 days. The nurse includes in the discharge teaching plan instructions to
   a. avoid alcohol for 3 weeks.
   b. use a condom during sexual intercourse.
   c. have family members get an injection of immunoglobulin.
   d. follow a low-protein, moderate-carbohydrate, moderate-fat diet.

4. The patient with advanced cirrhosis asks the nurse why his abdomen is so swollen. The nurse's response to the patient is based on the knowledge that
   a. a lack of clotting factors promotes the collection of blood in the abdominal cavity.
   b. portal hypertension and hypoalbuminemia cause a fluid shift into the peritoneal space.
   c. decreased peristalsis in the GI tract contributes to gas formation and distention of the bowel.
   d. bile salts in the blood irritate the peritoneal membranes, causing edema and pocketing of fluid.

5. When caring for a patient with hepatic encephalopathy, the nurse may give enemas, provide a low-protein diet, and limit physical activity. These measures are done to
   a. promote fluid loss.
   b. decrease portal pressure.
   c. eliminate potassium ions.
   d. decrease the production of ammonia.

6. In planning care for a patient with metastatic cancer of the liver, the nurse includes interventions that
   a. focus primarily on symptomatic and comfort measures.
   b. reassure the patient that chemotherapy offers a good prognosis for recovery.
   c. promote the patient's confidence that surgical excision of the tumor will be successful.
   d. provide information necessary for the patient to make decisions regarding liver transplantation.

7. The nurse explains to the patient with acute pancreatitis that the most common pathogenic mechanism of the disorder is
   a. cellular disorganization.
   b. overproduction of enzymes.
   c. lack of secretion of enzymes.
   d. autodigestion of the pancreas.

8. Nursing management of the patient with acute pancreatitis includes
   a. checking for signs of hypercalcemia.
   b. observing stools for signs of steatorrhea.
   c. providing a diet low in carbohydrates with moderate fat.
   d. monitoring for infection, particularly respiratory infection.

9. A patient with pancreatic cancer is admitted to the hospital for evaluation for treatment. The patient asks the nurse to explain the Whipple procedure the surgeon has described. The nurse's explanation includes the information that a Whipple procedure involves
   a. creating a bypass around the obstruction caused by the tumor by joining the gallbladder to the jejunum.
   b. resection of the entire pancreas and the distal portion of the stomach, with anastomosis of the common bile duct and stomach into the duodenum.
   c. removal of part of the pancreas, part of the stomach, the duodenum, and the gallbladder, with joining of the pancreatic duct, common bile duct, and stomach into the jejunum.
   d. radical removal of the pancreas, duodenum, and spleen, attaching the stomach to the jejunum, which requires oral supplementation of pancreatic digestive enzymes and insulin replacement therapy.

10. The nursing management of the patient with cholecystitis associated with cholelithiasis is based on the knowledge that
    a. a low-fat diet is recommended.
    b. gallstones once removed tend not to recur.
    c. meperidine is to be avoided in the management of pain.
    d. the disorder can be successfully treated with oral bile salts that dissolve gallstones.

11. Teaching in relation to home management following a laparoscopic cholecystectomy should include
    a. keeping the bandages on the puncture sites for 48 hours.
    b. reporting any bile-colored drainage or pus from any incision.
    c. using over-the-counter antiemetics if nausea and vomiting occur.
    d. emptying and measuring the contents of the bile bag from the T tube every day.

REFERENCES

1. National Center for Infection Control: Hepatitis. Available at *www.cdc.gov/ ncidod/diseases/hepatitis.* Site last accessed December 28, 2002.
2. Alter MJ et al: The epidemiology of hepatitis C. In Liang TJ, Hoofnagle JH, editors: *Hepatitis C,* Boston, 2000, Academic Press.
3. Wasley A, Alter MJ: Epidemiology of hepatitis C: geographic differences and temporal trends, *Semin Liver Dis* 20:1, 2000.
4. Rehermann B: Immunopathogenesis of hepatitis C. In Liang TJ, Hoofnagle JH, editors: *Hepatitis C,* Boston 2000, Academic Press.
5. Wong JB et al: Estimating future hepatitis C morbidity, mortality, and costs in the United States, *Am J Public Health* 90:1562, 2000.
6. Williams I: Epidemiology of hepatitis C in the United States, *Am J Med* 27:2S, 1999.
7. Goldman M, Spurll G: Hepatitis C lookback, *Curr Opin Hematol* 7:392, 2000.
8. Patrick DM et al: Public health and hepatitis C, *Can J Public Health* 91(suppl 1):S18, 2000.
9. Thorpe LE et al: Hepatitis C virus infection: prevalence, risk factors, and prevention opportunities among young injection drug users in Chicago, 1997-1999, *J Infect Dis* 182:1588, 2000.
10. Diaz T et al: Several factors associated with prevalent hepatitis C virus infection differ among young adult injection drug users in lower and upper Manhattan, New York City, *Am J Public Health* 91:23, 2001.
11. Giulivi A et al: Prevalence of GBV-C/hepatitis G virus viremia and anti-E2 in Canadian blood donors, *Vox Sang* 79:201, 2000.
12. Dougherty AS, Dreher HM: Hepatitis C: current treatment strategies for an emerging epidemic, *Medsurg Nurs* 10:9, 2001.
13. Torresi J, Locarnini S: Antiviral chemotherapy for the treatment of hepatitis B virus infections, *Gastroenterology* 118:S83, 2000.
14. Dienstag JL et al: Lamivudine as initial treatment for chronic hepatitis B in the United States, *N Engl J Med* 341:1256, 1999.
15. Perry CM, Jarvis B: Peginterferon-alpha-2a (40kD): a review of its use in the management of chronic hepatitis C, *Drugs* 61:2263, 2001.
16. Wilkinson T: Hepatitis C virus: prospects for future therapies, *Curr Opin Investig Drugs* 2:1516, 2001.
17. Prevention of hepatitis A through active or passive immunization: recommendations of the Advisory Committee on Immunization Practices, *MMWR Morb Mortal Wkly Rep* 48(RR12):1, 1999.
18. FDA approval for a combined hepatitis A and B vaccine, *MMWR Morb Mortal Wkly Rep* 50:806, 2001.
19. Beltrami EM et al: Risk and management of bloodborne infections in health-care workers, *Clin Microbiol Rev* 13:385, 2000.
20. Riley TR, Bhatti AM: Preventive strategies in chronic liver disease: alcohol, vaccines, toxic medications and supplements, diet and exercise, *Am Fam Physician* 64:1555, 2001.
21. McCormick PA, O'Keefe C: Improving prognosis following a first variceal haemorrhage over four decades, *Gut* 49:682, 2001.
22. Butterworth RF: Neurotransmitter dysfunction in hepatic encephalopathy: new approaches and new findings, *Metab Brain Dis* 16:55, 2001.
23. Klempnaue J, Schrem H: Review: surgical shunts and encephalopathy, *Metab Brain Dis* 16:21, 2001.
24. Wong F, Blendis L: New challenge of hepatorenal syndrome: prevention and treatment, *Hepatology* 34:1242, 2001.
25. Brandenburger LA et al: Variceal hemorrhage, *Curr Treat Options Gastroenterol* 5:73, 2002.
26. Anand BS: Drug treatment of the complications of cirrhosis in the older adult, *Drugs Aging* 18:575, 2001.
27. Rosen HR: Hepatitis B and C in the liver transplant recipient: current understanding and treatment, *Liver Transpl* 7(11 suppl 1):S87, 2001.
28. American Cancer Society: *Facts and figures 2002,* Atlanta, Ga, 2002. Available at *www.cancer.org.* (accessed Dec 28, 2002).
29. Cole L: Unraveling the mystery of acute pancreatitis, *Nursing* 31:58, 2001.
30. Smotkin J, Tenner S: Laboratory diagnostic tests in acute pancreatitis, *J Clin Gastroenterol* 34:459, 2002.
31. Brand R: The diagnosis of pancreatic cancer, *Cancer J* 7:287, 2001.
32. Kozuch P, Grossbard ML, Barzdins A: Irinotecan combined with gemcitabine, 5-fluorouracil, leucovorin, and cisplatin (G-FLIP) is an effective and noncrossresistant treatment for chemotherapy refractory metastatic pancreatic cancer, *Oncologist* 6:488, 2001.
33. Heinemann V: Gemcitabine-based combination treatment of pancreatic cancer, *Semin Oncol* 29:25, 2002.
34. Farrar JA: Acute cholecystitis, *Am J Nurs* 101:35, 2001.
35. Dawes LG: Gallbladder cancer, *Cancer Treat Res* 109:145, 2001.

RESOURCES

American Association for the Study of Liver Diseases (AASLD)
1729 King Street, Suite 200
Alexandria, VA 22314
703-299-9766
Fax: 703-299-9622
www.aasld.org

American Gastroenterological Association
7910 Woodmont Avenue, Seventh Floor
Bethesda, MD 20814
301-654-2055
Fax: 301-652-3890
www.gastro.org

American Liver Foundation
75 Maiden Lane, Suite 603
New York, NY 10038
800-GO-LIVER (465-4837)
www.liverfoundation.org

United Ostomy Association
19772 MacArthur Boulevard, Suite 200
Irvine, CA 92612-2405
800-826-0826
www.uoa.org

For additional Internet resources, see the website for this book at *http://evolve.elsevier.com/Lewis/medsurg/.*

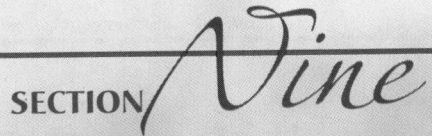
Problems of Urinary Function

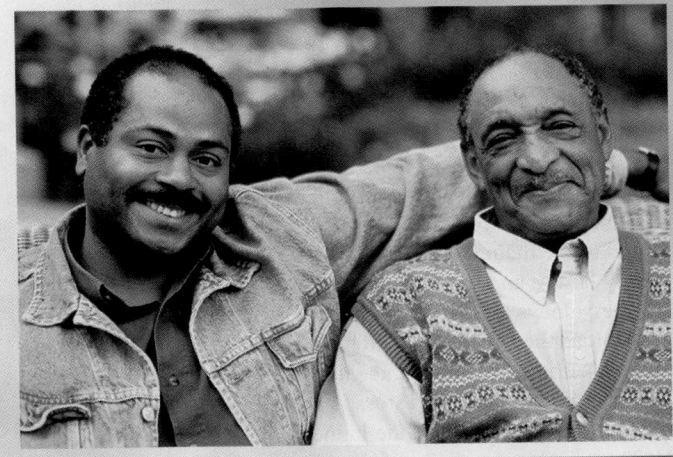

CHAPTER 43
NURSING ASSESSMENT
Urinary System

Mikel Gray

LEARNING OBJECTIVES

1. Describe the anatomic location and functions of the kidneys, ureters, bladder, and urethra.
2. Explain the physiologic events involved in the formation and passage of urine from glomerular filtration to voiding.
3. Identify the significant subjective and objective data related to the urinary system that should be obtained from a patient.
4. Describe age-related changes in the urinary system and differences in assessment findings.
5. Describe the appropriate techniques used in the physical assessment of the urinary system.
6. Differentiate normal from common abnormal findings of a physical assessment of the urinary system.
7. Describe the purpose, significance of results, and nursing responsibilities related to diagnostic studies of the urinary system.
8. Describe the normal physical and chemical characteristics of urine.

KEY TERMS

costovertebral angle, p. 1161
creatinine, p. 1166
cystometrogram, p. 1170
cystoscopy, p. 1169
glomerular filtration rate, p. 1154
glomerulus, p. 1153

intravenous pyelogram, p. 1167
nephron, p. 1152
renal arteriogram, p. 1168
renal biopsy, p. 1169
retrograde pyelogram, p. 1167
urinalysis, p. 1162

"Bones can break, muscles can atrophy, glands can loaf, even the brain can go to sleep without immediate danger to survival. But should the kidneys fail . . . neither bone, muscle, gland, nor brain could carry on."[1] This statement underlines the importance of kidneys to our lives. Adequate functioning of the kidneys is essential to the maintenance of a healthy body. If there is complete kidney failure and treatment is not given, death is inevitable.

The kidneys are the principal organs of the urinary system. In addition to the two kidneys, the urinary system consists of two ureters, a urinary bladder, and a urethra (Fig. 43-1). The other organs can be thought of as storage and drainage channels for the urine after it is formed by the kidneys.

The primary functions of the kidneys are (1) to regulate the volume and composition of extracellular fluid (ECF) and (2) excrete waste products from the body. Additional functions of the kidneys include blood pressure control, erythropoietin production, vitamin D activation, and acid-base balance regulation.

STRUCTURES AND FUNCTIONS OF THE URINARY SYSTEM

Kidneys

Macrostructure. The paired kidneys are bean-shaped organs that are retroperitoneal (behind the peritoneum) on either side of the vertebral column at about the level of the twelfth thoracic (T12) vertebra to the third lumbar (L3) vertebra. Each kidney weighs 4 to 6 ounces (115 to 175 g) and is about 5 inches (12 cm) long. The right kidney, with the liver above it, is lower than the left. The right kidney is at the level of the twelfth rib. An adrenal gland lies on top of each kidney.

Each kidney is surrounded by a considerable amount of fat and connective tissue that serves to support and maintain its position. The surface of the kidney is covered by a thin, smooth layer of fibrous membrane called the *capsule*. These structures protect the kidney and serve as a shock absorber should the kidney be subjected to a sudden force from a blunt object striking the abdomen or back. The *hilus* on the medial side of the kidney serves as the entry site for the renal artery and nerves, as well as the exit site for the renal vein and ureter.

On a longitudinal section of the kidney (Fig. 43-2), the parenchyma (actual tissue) of the kidney can be visualized. The outer layer is termed the *cortex*, and the inner layer is called the *medulla*. The medulla consists of a number of pyramids. The apices of these pyramids are called *papillae*, through which urine passes to enter the calyces. The minor calyces widen and merge to form major calyces, which form a funnel-shaped sac called the *renal pelvis*. The minor and major calyces transport urine to the renal pelvis in preparation for transportation to the bladder via the ureter. The pelvis of the kidney can store a small volume of urine (3 to 5 ml).

Microstructure. The functional unit of the kidney is termed the **nephron.** Each kidney has more than 1 million nephrons. A nephron is composed of a glomerulus, Bowman's capsule, and tubular system. The tubular system consists of the proximal convoluted tubule, the loop of Henle, and the distal convoluted tubule (Fig. 43-3). Several nephrons converge into a collecting duct, which eventually merges into a pyramid and empties via the papilla into a minor calyx.

The glomeruli, Bowman's capsule, proximal tubule, and distal tubule are located in the cortex of the kidney. The loop of Henle and the collecting ducts are located in the medulla.

Blood Supply. A blood supply of about 1200 ml per minute, which is 20% to 25% of the cardiac output, flows to the two kidneys. Blood reaches the kidneys via the renal artery, which arises from the aorta and enters the kidney through the hilus. The renal artery divides into secondary branches and then into still smaller branches,

Reviewed by Vicki Y. Johnson, RN, PhD, FN, CUCNS, Assistant Professor, University of Alabama, School of Nursing, Birmingham, Ala.

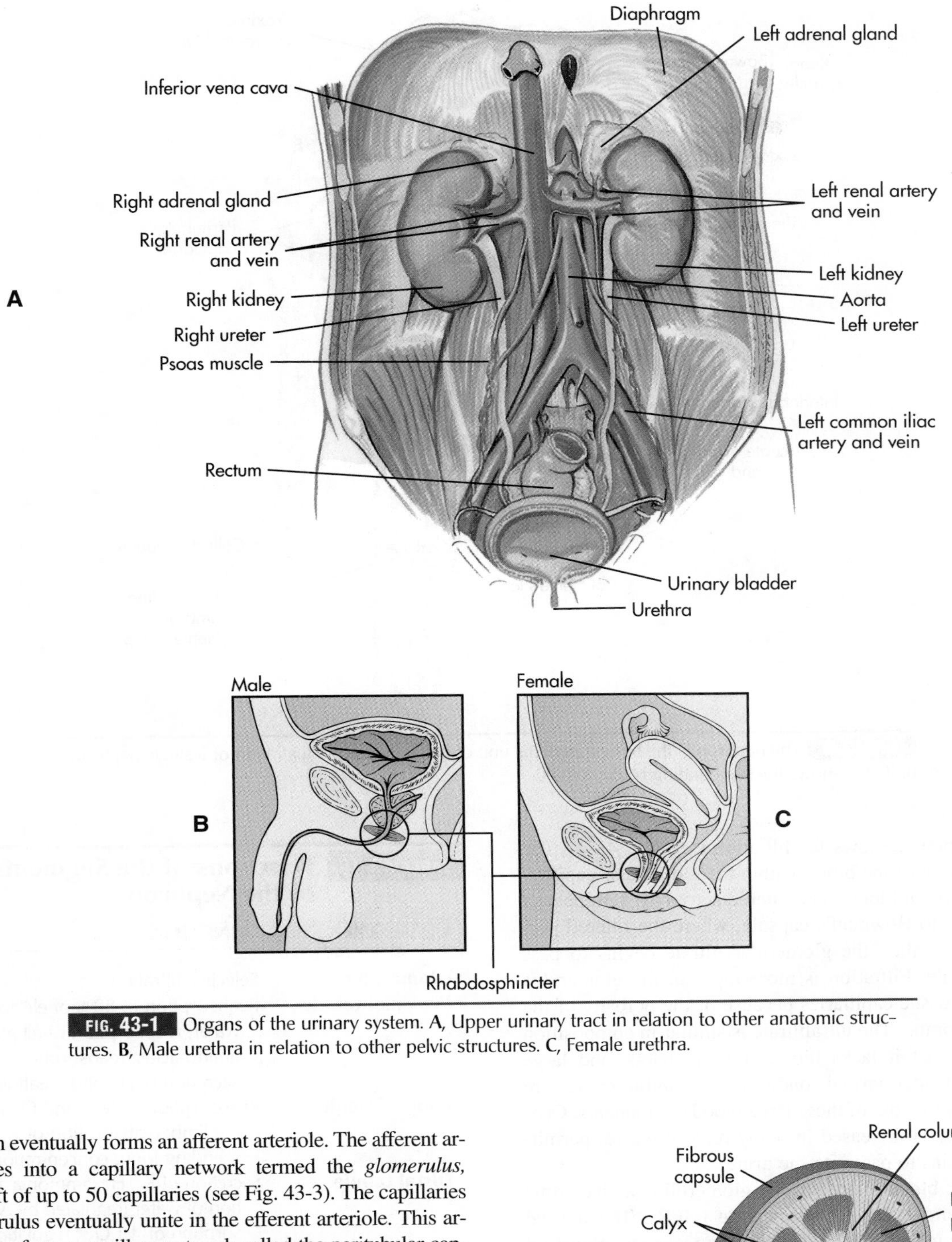

A

Diaphragm
Left adrenal gland
Inferior vena cava
Right adrenal gland
Right renal artery and vein
Left renal artery and vein
Right kidney
Left kidney
Right ureter
Aorta
Psoas muscle
Left ureter
Rectum
Left common iliac artery and vein
Urinary bladder
Urethra

Male

Female

B

C

Rhabdosphincter

FIG. 43-1   Organs of the urinary system. A, Upper urinary tract in relation to other anatomic structures. B, Male urethra in relation to other pelvic structures. C, Female urethra.

each of which eventually forms an afferent arteriole. The afferent arteriole divides into a capillary network termed the *glomerulus,* which is a tuft of up to 50 capillaries (see Fig. 43-3). The capillaries of the glomerulus eventually unite in the efferent arteriole. This arteriole splits to form a capillary network called the peritubular capillaries, which, as the name suggests, surround the tubular system. All peritubular capillaries eventually drain into the venous system. The renal vein empties into the inferior vena cava.

Physiology of Urine Formation. The process of urine formation is extremely complex. It represents the outcome of a multistep process of filtration, reabsorption, secretion, and excretion of water, electrolytes, and metabolic waste products. Although urine formation is the result of this process, the primary function of the kidneys is to filter the blood and maintain the body's internal homeostasis.[2]

Glomerular function. Urine formation starts at the glomerulus, where blood is filtered. The **glomerulus,** which is a semi-

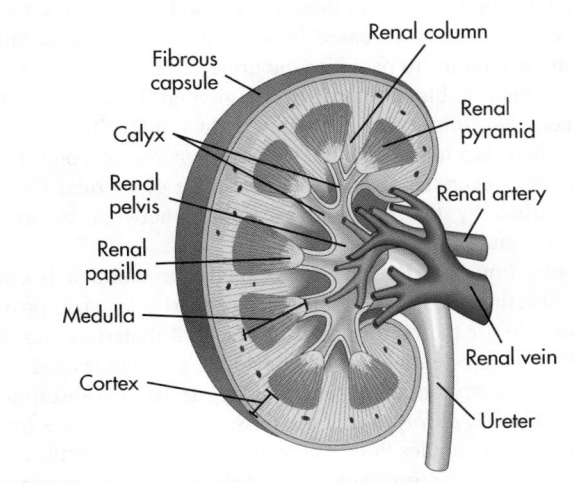

Fibrous capsule
Renal column
Renal pyramid
Calyx
Renal pelvis
Renal artery
Renal papilla
Medulla
Renal vein
Cortex
Ureter

FIG. 43-2   Longitudinal section of the kidney.

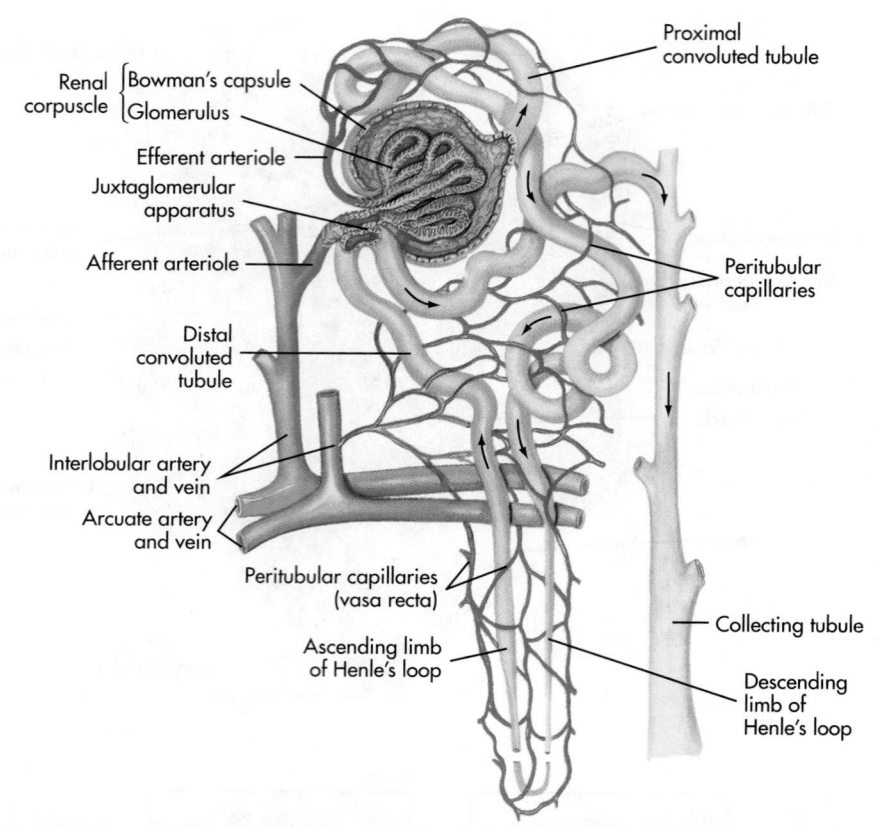

Renal corpuscle { Bowman's capsule, Glomerulus

Proximal convoluted tubule

Efferent arteriole

Juxtaglomerular apparatus

Afferent arteriole

Peritubular capillaries

Distal convoluted tubule

Interlobular artery and vein

Arcuate artery and vein

Peritubular capillaries (vasa recta)

Collecting tubule

Ascending limb of Henle's loop

Descending limb of Henle's loop

FIG. 43-3 The nephron is the basic functional unit of the kidney. This illustration of a single nephron unit also shows the surrounding blood vessels.

permeable membrane, allows for filtration (see Fig. 43-3). The hydrostatic pressure of the blood within the glomerular capillaries causes a portion of blood to be filtered across the semipermeable membrane into Bowman's capsule, where the filtered portion of the blood called the glomerular filtrate begins to pass down to the tubule. Filtration is more rapid in the glomerulus than in ordinary tissue capillaries because of the porosity of the glomerular membrane. The ultrafiltrate is similar in composition to blood except that it lacks blood cells, platelets, and large plasma proteins. Under normal conditions the capillary pores are too small to allow the loss of these large blood components. Capillary permeability is increased in many renal diseases, permitting plasma proteins to pass into the urine.

The amount of blood filtered by the glomeruli in a given time is termed the **glomerular filtration rate** (GFR). The normal GFR is about 125 ml per minute. However, on average, only 1 ml per minute is excreted as urine because most glomerular filtrate is reabsorbed by the peritubular capillary network before it reaches the end of the collecting duct.

Tubular function. Because the glomerular membrane is a selective filtration membrane that filters primarily by size, provision is made for the reabsorption of essential materials and the excretion of nonessential ones (Table 43-1). The tubules and collecting ducts carry out these functions by means of reabsorption and secretion. *Reabsorption* is the passage of a substance from the lumen of the tubules through the tubule cells and into the capillaries. This process involves both active and passive transport. Tubular *secretion* is the passage of a substance from the capillaries through the tubular cells into the lumen of the tubule. Reab-

TABLE 43-1	Functions of the Segments of the Nephron
COMPONENT	**FUNCTION**
Glomerulus	Selective filtration
Proximal tubule	Reabsorption of 80% of electrolytes and water; reabsorption of all glucose and amino acids; reabsorption of HCO_3^-; secretion of H^+ and creatinine
Loop of Henle	Reabsorption of Na^+ and Cl^- in ascending limb; reabsorption of water in descending loop; concentration of filtrate
Distal tubule	Secretion of K^+, H^+, ammonia; reabsorption of water (regulated by ADH); reabsorption of HCO_3^-; regulation of Ca^{2+} and PO_4^{2-} by parathyroid hormone, regulation of Na^+ and K^+ by aldosterone
Collecting duct	Reabsorption of water (ADH required)

ADH, Antidiuretic hormone; Ca^{2+}, calcium; Cl^-, chloride; H^+, hydrogen; HCO_3^-, bicarbonate; K^+, potassium; Na^+, sodium; PO_4^{2-}, phosphate.

sorption and secretion occur along the entire length of the tubule, causing numerous changes in the composition of the glomerular filtrate as it moves through the tubules.

In the proximal convoluted tubule, about 80% of the electrolytes are reabsorbed. Normally, all the glucose, amino acids, and small proteins are reabsorbed. For the most part, reabsorption occurs by active transport. Hydrogen ions (H^+) and creatinine are secreted into the filtrate.[3]

The loop of Henle is important in conserving water and thus concentrating the filtrate. In the loop of Henle, reabsorption continues. The descending loop is permeable to water and moderately permeable to sodium, urea, and other solutes. In the ascending limb, chloride ions (Cl^-) are actively reabsorbed, followed passively by sodium ions (Na^+). About 25% of the filtered sodium is reabsorbed here.

Two important functions of the distal convoluted tubules are final regulation of water balance and acid-base balance. Antidiuretic hormone (ADH), released by the posterior pituitary gland, is required for water reabsorption. The stimuli for ADH release are increased serum osmolality and decreased blood volume. ADH makes the distal convoluted tubules and the collecting ducts permeable to water, allowing it to be reabsorbed into the peritubular capillaries and to be eventually returned to circulation. In the absence of ADH the tubules are practically impermeable to water, and any water in the tubules leaves the body as urine.

In the presence of aldosterone (released from the adrenal cortex) acting on the distal tubule, reabsorption of Na^+ and water occurs. In exchange for Na^+, potassium ions (K^+) are excreted. The secretion of aldosterone is influenced by both circulating blood volume and plasma concentrations of Na^+ and K^+.

Acid-base regulation involves reabsorbing and conserving most of the bicarbonate (HCO_3^-) and secreting excess H^+. The distal tubule functions in different ways to maintain the pH of ECF within a range of 7.35 to 7.45 (see Chapter 16).

Atrial natriuretic factor (ANF) is a hormone secreted from cells in the right atrium when right atrial blood pressure increases. ANF inhibits the secretion and effect of ADH and results in a large volume of dilute urine (see Chapter 46).

Parathyroid hormone is released from the parathyroid gland in response to low serum calcium levels. It causes increased tubular reabsorption of calcium ions (Ca^{2+}) and decreased tubular reabsorption of phosphate ions (PO_4^{2-}). Therefore serum Ca^{2+} levels are increased.

The basic function of nephrons is to clean or clear blood plasma of unnecessary substances. After the glomerulus has filtered the blood, the tubules separate the unwanted from the wanted portions of tubular fluid. The necessary portions are returned to the blood, and the unnecessary portions pass into urine.

Other Functions of the Kidney. In addition to their function in regulating the volume and composition of ECF, the kidneys also have other vital functions, including the production of erythropoietin, production and secretion of renin, and activation of vitamin D.

Erythropoietin is produced and released in response to hypoxia and decreased renal blood flow. Erythropoietin stimulates the production of red blood cells (RBCs) in the bone marrow. A deficiency of erythropoietin leads to anemia in renal failure.

Vitamin D is a hormone that can be obtained in the diet or synthesized by the action of ultraviolet radiation on cholesterol in the skin. These forms of vitamin D are inactive and require two more steps to become metabolically active. The first step in activation occurs in the liver. The second step occurs in the kidneys. Active vitamin D is essential for the absorption of calcium from the gastrointestinal (GI) tract. The patient with renal failure has a deficiency of the active metabolite of vitamin D and manifests problems of altered calcium and phosphate balance (see Chapter 45).

Renin is important in the regulation of blood pressure. Renin is released from the *juxtaglomerular apparatus* of the nephron (Fig. 43-4). Renin is released in response to decreased arterial blood pressure, renal ischemia, ECF depletion, increased norepinephrine, and increased urinary Na^+ concentration. Renin catalyzes the splitting of the plasma protein angiotensinogen (from the liver) into angiotensin I, which is subsequently converted to angiotensin II by a converting enzyme made in the lungs. Angiotensin II stimulates the release of aldosterone from the adrenal cortex, which causes Na^+ and water retention, leading to an increased ECF volume. Angiotensin II also causes increased peripheral vasoconstriction. The increase in ECF and vasoconstriction causes an elevation in blood pressure, which should inhibit renin release. Excessive renin production caused by impaired re-

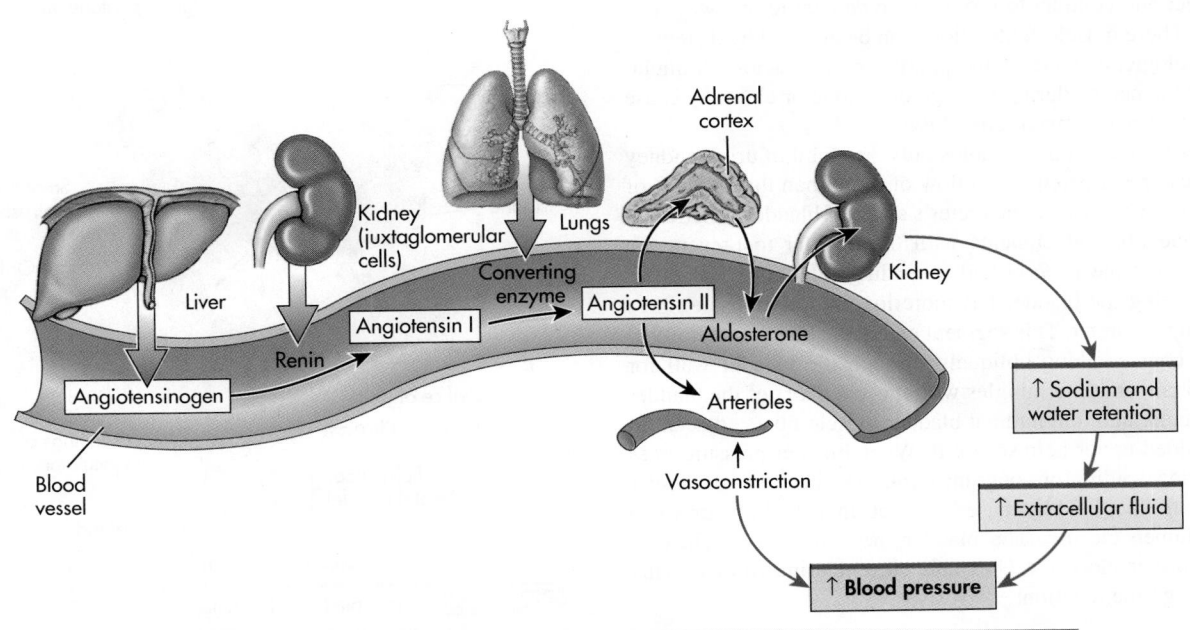

FIG. 43-4 Renin-angiotensin-aldosterone system.

nal perfusion may be a contributing factor in the etiology of hypertension (see Chapters 32 and 45).

Prostaglandins (PGs) are synthesized by most body tissues from the precursor, arachidonic acid, in response to appropriate stimuli. PGs, which are involved in the regulation of cell function and host defenses, exert their influence primarily on cells or tissues that are close to the site where they are synthesized. (See Chapter 12 and Fig. 12-7 for a more detailed discussion of PGs.)

In the kidney, PG synthesis (primarily PGE_2 and PGI_2) occurs primarily in the medulla. These PGs have a vasodilating action in addition to increasing renal blood flow and promoting Na^+ excretion. They counteract the vasoconstrictor effect of substances such as angiotensin and norepinephrine. Renal PGs may have a systemic effect in lowering blood pressure by decreasing systemic vascular resistance.[4]

The significance of these PGs is related to the role of the kidneys in causing hypertension. In renal failure with a loss of functioning tissue, these renal vasodilator factors are also lost. This may be one factor that contributes to the common finding of hypertension in renal failure (see Chapter 45).

Ureters

The ureters are tubes approximately 10 to 12 inches (25 to 35 cm) long and 0.08 to 0.3 inch (0.2 to 0.8 cm) in diameter that carry urine from the renal pelvis to the bladder (see Fig. 43-1). The narrow area where the ureter joins the renal pelvis is termed the *ureteropelvic junction*. After coursing down along the psoas muscle, the ureter crosses over the pelvic brim and iliac artery and inserts into the base of the bladder at the *ureterovesical junction* (UVJ). The ureteral lumen is narrowest at these junctions; consequently, they are often the sites of urinary stone (calculi) obstruction. Because the lumen of the ureter is narrow, it can be easily occluded internally (e.g., calculi) or externally (e.g., tumors, adhesions, inflammation).

Sympathetic and parasympathetic nerves, along with the vascular supply, surround the mucosal lining of the ureter. Circular and longitudinal smooth muscle fibers are arranged in a meshlike outer layer and contract to promote the peristaltic one-way flow of urine. These muscle contractions can be affected by distention and neurologic, endocrine, and pharmacologic factors. Stimulation of these nerves during passage of a stone or clot may cause acute, severe pain termed *renal colic*.

Because the renal pelvis holds only 3 to 5 ml of urine, kidney damage can result from a backflow of more than that amount of urine. The UVJ relies on the ureter's angle of bladder penetration and muscle fiber attachments with the bladder to prevent the backflow of urine *(reflux)* and ascending infection. The distal ureter entering the bladder has more longitudinal muscle fibers than the upper ureter. This segment enters the bladder laterally at its base, courses along obliquely through the bladder wall for about 1.5 cm, and intermingles with muscle fibers of the bladder base. Circular and longitudinal bladder muscle fibers adjacent to the imbedded ureter help secure it. When bladder pressure rises (e.g., during voiding or coughing), muscle fibers that the ureter shares with the bladder base contract first to help promote ureteral lumen closure. The bladder then contracts against its base to further close the UVJ and prevent urine from moving back through the junction.

Bladder

The urinary bladder is a distensible organ positioned behind the symphysis pubis and anterior to the vagina and rectum (Fig. 43-5). Its primary functions are to serve as a reservoir for urine and to help the body eliminate waste products. Normal adult urine output is approximately 1500 ml per day, which varies with food and fluid intake. The volume of urine produced at night is less than half of that formed during the day because of hormonal influences (e.g., ADH). This diurnal pattern of urination is normal. Most people urinate five to six times during the day and occasionally at night.

The triangular area formed by the two ureteral openings and the bladder neck at the base of the bladder is termed the *trigone*. It is affixed to the pelvis by many ligaments, and it does not change its shape during bladder filling or emptying. The bladder muscle, termed the *detrusor*, is composed of layers of intertwined smooth muscle fibers and is capable of considerable distention during bladder filling and contraction during emptying. It is affixed to the abdominal wall by an umbilical ligament. Consequently, as the bladder fills, it rises toward the umbilicus. The dome, anterior, and lateral aspects of the bladder expand and contract. When the bladder is empty, it appears as multiple folds within the pelvis.

On the average, 200 to 250 ml of urine in the bladder causes moderate distention and the urge to urinate. When the quantity of urine reaches about 400 to 600 ml, the person feels uncomfortable. Bladder capacity varies with the individual, usually ranging from 600 to 1000 ml. Evacuation of urine is termed *urination*, *micturition*, or *voiding*.

The bladder has the same mucosal lining as that of the renal pelvis, ureter, and bladder neck. It is called transitional cell epithelium or urothelium and is unique to the urinary tract. Transitional cell epithelium is resistant to absorption of urine. Therefore urinary wastes produced by the kidneys do not leak out of the urinary system after they leave the kidneys. Microscopically, transitional cell epithelium is several cells deep. These cells

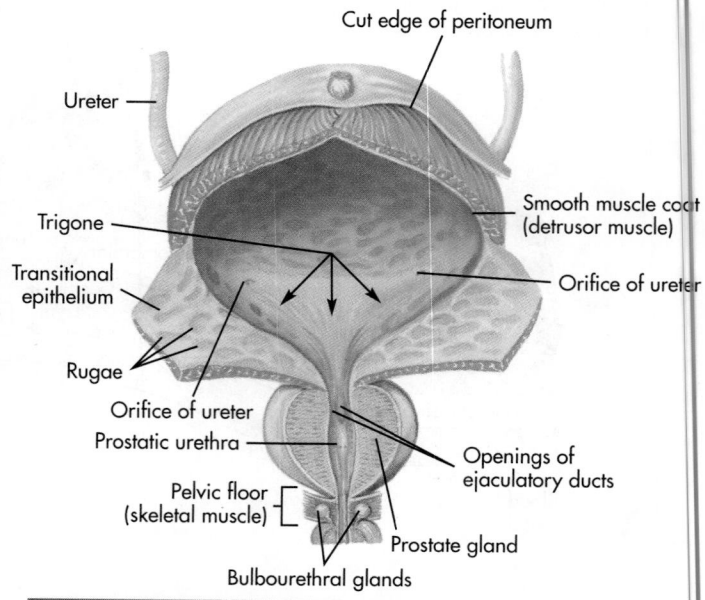

FIG. 43-5 Urinary bladder of a male.

stretch out in the bladder to only a few cells deep as it accommodates filling. As the bladder empties, the epithelium resumes its multicellular layer formation.

Because the lining is the same, transitional cell tumors that occur in one section of the urinary tract can easily metastasize to other urinary tract areas. Malignant cells may move down from upper urinary tract tumors and imbed in the bladder, or large bladder tumors can invade the ureter. Tumor recurrence within the bladder is common. Intact urothelium also has phagocytic properties, although the exact mechanism is unknown.

Urethra

The urethra is a small muscular tube that leads from the bladder neck to the external meatus. Its primary function is to serve as a conduit for urine to the bladder and then to the outside of the body.

The urothelium and submucosal layers are the same as that of the bladder. Smooth muscle fibers extend from the bladder neck down into the urethra and are further supported by circular smooth muscle fibers around the urethra. Special C-shaped striated muscle fibers (the rhabdosphincter, or external sphincter) surround a portion of the urethra and voluntarily contract and prevent leaking when bladder pressure increases.

The female urethra is 1 to 2 inches (3 to 5 cm) long and lies behind the symphysis pubis but anterior to the vagina (see Fig. 43-1, *C*). The rhabdosphincter encircles the middle third of the urethra. The short urethra is a contributing factor to the increased incidence of urinary tract infections in women.

The male urethra, which is about 8 to 10 inches (20 to 25 cm) long, originates at the bladder neck and extends the length of the penis (see Fig. 43-1, *B*). It is often separated into three parts. The prostatic urethra extends from the bladder neck through the prostate to the urogenital diaphragm. The membranous urethra passes through the urogenital diaphragm. The rhabdosphincter encircles this portion. Because of the concentrated muscular support, this short portion is not as expandable; consequently, stricture formation in this area after instrumentation is common. The penile urethra continues through the corpus spongiosum, a cavernous penile body, from the urogenital diaphragm to a distal dilated area, the fossa navicularis, before terminating at the meatus.

Urethrovesical Unit Function

Together, the bladder, urethra, and pelvic floor muscles form what is called the urethrovesical unit. Normal voluntary control of this unit is defined as *continence*. Various areas of the brain send stimulating and inhibiting impulses to the thoracolumbar (T11 to L2) and sacral (S2 to S4) areas of the spinal cord to control voiding. Distention of the bladder stimulates stretch receptors within the bladder wall. Impulses are transmitted to the sacral spinal cord and then to the brain, causing a desire to urinate. If the time to void is not appropriate, inhibitor impulses in the brain are stimulated and transmitted back to the thoracolumbar and sacral nerves innervating the bladder. In a coordinated fashion, the detrusor accommodates to the pressure (does not contract) while the sphincter and pelvic floor muscles tighten to resist bladder pressure. If voiding is appropriate, cerebral inhibition is voluntarily suppressed, and impulses are transmitted via the spinal cord for the bladder neck, sphincter, and pelvic floor muscles to relax and for the bladder to contract. The sphincter

closes and the detrusor muscle relaxes when the bladder is empty.

Any disease or trauma that affects function of the brain, spinal cord, or nerves that directly innervate the bladder, bladder neck, external sphincter, or pelvic floor can affect bladder function. These conditions include diabetes mellitus, paraplegia, and tetraplegia (quadriplegia). Drugs affecting nerve transmission also can affect bladder function.

■ Gerontologic Considerations: Effects of Aging on the Urinary System

Anatomic changes in the aging kidney include a 20% to 30% decrease in size and weight between the ages of 30 and 90 years. This loss in renal mass is predominantly in the cortex. The aging nephron fails as a unit because glomerular and tubular function appears to decrease at the same rate. By the seventh decade of life, 30% to 50% of glomeruli have lost their function. Despite losing this original kidney volume, older individuals maintain body fluid homeostasis unless they encounter diseases or other physiologic stressors.[5]

Blood flow to and within the kidneys also decreases. There is no evidence that atherosclerotic vascular disease is primarily responsible for the age-related changes in the kidneys.

Physiologic changes in the aging kidney include decreased renal blood flow, decreased GFR, and decreased ability to conserve Na^+, dilute or concentrate urine, and excrete an acid load. Under normal conditions, the aging kidney is able to maintain homeostasis, but after abrupt changes in blood volume, acid load, or other insults, the kidney may not be able to function effectively because much of its renal reserve has been lost.[6]

Physiologic changes also occur in the aging bladder and urethra. Estrogen receptors exist in the female urethra, bladder, vagina, and pelvic floor. As estrogen levels decrease with age, tissues become less elastic, thin, and less vascular. Periurethral striated muscle fibers and muscles supporting the bladder relax. Consequently, older women are more prone to urethral irritation, urethral and bladder infections, and urinary incontinence.

Men's prostates enlarge as they age, and because the prostate surrounds the proximal urethra, increasing prostate size may affect urinary patterns in men, causing hesitancy, retention, slow stream, and bladder infections.

Constipation, a complaint often expressed by the elderly, can also affect urination. Partial urethral obstruction may occur because of the rectum's close proximity to the urethra.

Age-related changes in the urinary system and differences in assessment findings are presented in Table 43-2. ■

ASSESSMENT OF THE URINARY SYSTEM

Subjective Data

Important Health Information

Past health history. The patient should be questioned about the presence or history of diseases that are known to be related to renal or other urologic problems. Some of these diseases are hypertension, diabetes mellitus, gout and other metabolic problems, connective tissue disorders (e.g., systemic lupus erythematosus, systemic sclerosis [scleroderma]), skin or upper respiratory infections of streptococcal origin, tuberculosis, viral hepatitis, con-

TABLE 43-2 Gerontologic Differences in Assessment — Urinary System

CHANGES	DIFFERENCES IN ASSESSMENT FINDINGS
Kidney	
↓ Amount of renal tissue	Less palpable
↓ Number of nephrons and renal blood vessels; thickened basement membrane of Bowman's capsule and glomeruli	↓ Creatinine clearance, ↑ BUN level
↓ Function of loop of Henle and tubules	Alterations in drug excretion; nocturia; loss of normal diurnal excretory pattern because of ↓ ability to concentrate urine; less concentrated urine
Ureter, Bladder, and Urethra	
↓ Elasticity and muscle tone	Palpable bladder after urination because of retention
Weakening of urinary sphincter	Stress incontinence (especially during Valsalva maneuver), dribbling of urine after urination
↓ Bladder capacity and sensory receptors	Frequency, urgency, nocturia, overflow incontinence
Estrogen deficiency leading to thin, dry vaginal tissue	Stress or overactive bladder, dysuria
↑ Prevalence of unstable bladder contractions	Overactive bladder
Prostatic enlargement	Hesitancy, frequency, urgency, nocturia, straining to urinate, retention, dribbling

BUN, Blood urea nitrogen.

TABLE 43-3 Potentially Nephrotoxic Agents

ANTIBIOTICS	OTHER AGENTS
amikacin (Amikin)	captopril (Capoten)
amphotericin B	cimetidine (Tagamet)
bacitracin	cisplatin (Platinol)
Cephalosporins	cocaine
gentamicin	Contrast medium
kanamycin	cyclosporine
neomycin	Ethylene glycol
polymyxin B	Gold
streptomycin	Heavy metals
Sulfonamides	Heroin
tobramycin (Nebcin)	lithium
vancomycin	methotrexate
	Nitrosoureas (e.g., carmustine)
	Nonsteroidal antiinflammatory drugs (e.g., ibuprofen, indomethacin)
	phenacetin
	quinine
	rifampin
	Salicylate (large quantities)

genital disorders, neurologic conditions (e.g., stroke, back injury), or trauma. Specific urinary problems such as cancer, infections, benign prostatic hyperplasia, and calculi should be noted.

Medications. An assessment of the patient's current and past use of medications is important. This should include over-the-counter drugs, as well as prescription medications and herbs. Drugs affect the urinary tract in several ways. Many drugs are known to be nephrotoxic (Table 43-3). Certain drugs may alter the quantity and character of urine output (e.g., diuretics). Numerous drugs such as phenazopyridine (Pyridium) and nitrofurantoin (Macrodantin) change its color. Anticoagulants may cause hematuria. Many antidepressants, calcium channel blockers, antihistamines, and drugs used for neurologic and musculoskeletal disorders affect the ability of the bladder or sphincter to contract or relax normally.

Surgery or other treatments. The patient should also be questioned about any previous hospitalizations related to renal or urologic diseases and all urinary problems during past pregnancies. The duration, severity, and patient's perception of any problem and its treatment should be elicited. Past surgeries, particularly pelvic surgeries, or urinary tract instrumentation should be documented. Information should be obtained from the patient about any radiation or chemotherapy treatment for cancer.

Functional Health Patterns. Key questions to ask a patient with problems related to the urinary system are listed in Table 43-4.

Health perception–health management pattern. The nurse should ask about the patient's general health, particularly when disease affecting the kidneys is suspected. Sometimes responses such as "feeling tired all of the time," changes in weight or appetite, excess thirst, fluid retention, and complaints of headache, pruritus, or blurred vision may be related to abnormal kidney function. Similarly, the elderly patient may report malaise and nonlocalized abdominal discomfort as the only symptoms of a urinary tract infection.[7]

An occupational history should be taken. Exposure to certain chemicals can affect the kidneys and urinary tract system. Phenol and ethylene glycol are examples of nephrotoxic chemicals. Aromatic amines and certain organic chemicals may increase the risk of bladder cancers. Textile workers, painters, hairdressers, and industrial workers have a high incidence of bladder tumors.

TABLE 43-4	Health History — Urinary System

Health Perception–Health Management Pattern
- How is your energy level compared with a year ago?
- Do you notice any visual changes?*
- Have you ever smoked? If yes, how many packs per day?

Nutritional-Metabolic Pattern
- How is your appetite?
- Has your weight changed over the past year?*
- Do you take vitamin or mineral supplements?*
- How much and what kinds of fluids do you drink daily?
- How many dairy products or meat do you eat?
- Do you drink coffee? Colas?
- Do you eat chocolate?
- Do you spice your food heavily?*

Elimination Pattern
- Are you able to sit through a 2-hour meeting or ride in a car for 2 hours without urinating? Do you awaken at night with the desire to urinate? If so, how many times does this occur during an average night?
- Do you ever notice blood in your urine?* If so, at what point in the urination does it occur?
- Do you find it difficult to postpone urination when you feel the urge to urinate?*
- Do you ever leak urine? If so, what causes urine leakage? Do you leak when you cough, walk, run, or lift a heavy object? Do you leak if you are unable to reach a toilet right away? Do you ever find that you have leaked without awareness of doing so?
- Do you use special devices or supplies for urine elimination or control?*
- Do you ever have pain when you urinate?* If so, where is the pain?
- How often do you move your bowels? Do you ever experience constipation (hardened stools that are difficult to pass or a sensation that you are unable to completely evacuate your bowels)?
- Do you frequently experience diarrhea (high-volume, loose watery stools)? Do you ever have problems controlling your bowels? If so, do you have problems controlling the passage of gas? Watery or liquid stool? Solid stool?

Activity-Exercise Pattern
- Have you noticed any changes in your ability to do your usual daily activities?*
- Do certain activities aggravate your urinary problem?*
- Has your urinary problem caused you to alter or stop any activity or exercise?*
- Do you require assistance in moving or getting to the bathroom?*

Cognitive-Perceptual Pattern
- Describe any pain you have in relation to urination.

Self-Perception–Self-Concept Pattern
- How does your urinary problem make you feel about yourself?
- Do you perceive your body differently since you have developed a urinary problem?

Role-Relationship Pattern
- Does your urinary problem interfere with your relationships with family or friends?*
- Has your urinary problem caused a change in your job status or affected your ability to carry out job-related responsibilities?*

Sexuality-Reproductive Pattern
- Has your urinary problem caused any change in your sexual pleasure or performance?*
- Do you have hygiene problems related to sexual activities that cause you concern?*

Coping–Stress Tolerance Pattern
- Do you feel able to manage the problems associated with your urinary problem? If not, explain.
- What strategies are you using to cope with your urinary problem?

Values-Beliefs Pattern
- Has your present illness affected your belief system?*
- Are your treatment decisions related to your urinary problem in conflict with your value system?*

*If yes, describe.

A smoking history should be obtained. Cigarette smoking is a major factor in the risk for bladder cancer. Tumors occur four times more frequently in cigarette smokers than in nonsmokers.

Places where a patient has lived may be important information to obtain. It has been shown that persons living in certain parts of the United States (Great Lakes, Southwest, Southeast) have a higher than normal incidence of urinary calculi. This may be caused by the higher mineral content of the soil and water. A person living in Middle Eastern countries or Africa can acquire certain parasites that can cause cystitis or bladder cancer.

The presence of certain renal or urologic problems in a family history increases the likelihood of similar problems occurring in the patient. The nurse should ask about family members who have had any of the diseases referred to in the past health history, as well as polycystic renal disease and congenital urinary tract abnormalities, such as Alport syndrome (congenital nephritis).

Nutritional-metabolic pattern. The usual quantity and types of fluid a patient drinks are important information related to urinary tract disease. Dehydration may contribute to urinary infections, calculi formation, and renal failure. Large intake of particular foods, such as dairy products or foods high in proteins, may also lead to calculi formation. Coffee, alcohol, carbonated beverages, or spicy foods often aggravate urinary inflammatory diseases. An unexplained weight gain may be the result of fluid retention secondary to a renal problem. Anorexia, nausea, and vomiting can dramatically affect fluid status and require careful assessment. Information on vitamin and mineral supplements and herbal therapies should be obtained. The patient may not think of these supplements and therapies when listing over-the-counter drugs; supplements are often considered part of nutritional intake.

Elimination pattern. Questions about urine elimination patterns are the cornerstone of the health history in the patient with a lower urinary tract disorder. This line of inquiry begins with a question of how the patient manages urine elimination. The majority of patients eliminate urine by spontaneous voiding, and they should be asked about daytime (diurnal) voiding frequency and the frequency of nocturia. Patients should also be queried about additional bothersome lower urinary tract symptoms, including urgency, incontinence, or urinary retention. Table 43-5 lists some of the common clinical manifestations of urinary tract disorders. Changes in the color and appearance of urine are often significant and should be evaluated. If blood is visible in the urine, it should be determined if it occurs at the beginning, throughout, or at the end of urination.

Bowel function should also be investigated. Problems with fecal incontinence may signal neurologic causes for bladder problems because of shared nerve pathways. Constipation and fecal impaction can partially obstruct the urethra, causing inadequate bladder emptying, overflow incontinence, and infection.

The nurse should find out the patient's method of handling a urinary problem. A patient may already be using a catheter or collection device. Sometimes a patient has to assume a particular position to urinate or perform such maneuvers as pressing on the lower abdomen (Credé method), straining (Valsalva maneuver), or stretching the rectum to empty the bladder.

Activity-exercise pattern. The patient's level of activity should be assessed. A sedentary person is more likely than an active individual to have stasis of urine, which can predispose to infection and calculi. Demineralization of bones in a person with limited physical activity causes increased urine calcium precipitation.

An active person may find that increasing activity aggravates the urinary problem. The patient who has had prostate surgery or who has weakened pelvic floor muscles may leak urine when attempting particular activities such as running. Some men may develop chronic inflammatory prostatitis or epididymitis after heavy lifting or long-distance driving.

Sleep-rest pattern. Nocturia is a common and a particularly bothersome lower urinary tract symptom that often leads to sleep deprivation, daytime sleepiness, and fatigue. It occurs in multiple disorders affecting the lower urinary tract, including urinary incontinence, urinary retention, and interstitial cystitis. Nocturia also may be attributable to polyuria owing to renal disease, poorly controlled diabetes mellitus, alcoholism, excessive fluid intake, or obstructive sleep apnea. When asking about nocturia, it is helpful to determine whether it is the desire to urinate that causes the person to arise from sleep or whether pain or some other symptom interrupts sleep and the person urinates as a matter of habit before returning to bed. Up to one episode of nocturia is considered normal in younger adults, and up to two episodes are acceptable among adults age 65 years or older. Sleep problems associated with a urinary disorder should be documented. The older adult may awaken many times during the night to urinate and may need to be assured that this may be normal. However, a complete assessment should be made to rule out any problem.

Cognitive-perceptual pattern. Level of mobility, visual acuity, and dexterity are important factors to determine for a patient with urologic problems when managing his or her own care at home, particularly when urine retention or incontinence is a problem. It should be determined if the patient is alert, able to understand instructions, and can recall the instructions when necessary.

If urinary incontinence is present, a thorough history of the problem should be elicited to assist in determining the type of incontinence. It is important to document what the patient has previously tried to manage the problem. Incontinence is a distressing problem and calls for great sensitivity on the part of the nurse if accurate information is to be obtained.

Pain is a frequent symptom of urinary tract disease. Types of pain associated with renal and urologic problems include dysuria, groin pain, costovertebral pain, and suprapubic pain. If present, the location, character, and duration should be assessed. The absence of pain when other urinary symptoms exist is also significant. Many urinary tract tumors are painless in the early stages.

Self-perception–self-concept pattern. Problems associated with the urinary system, such as incontinence, urinary diversion

TABLE 43-5	Clinical Manifestations of Disorders of the Urinary System

General Manifestations

Fatigue	Itching
Headaches	Excess thirst
Blurred vision	Chills
Elevated blood pressure	Change in body weight
Anorexia	Change in mentation
Nausea and vomiting	

Related to Urinary System

Pain	*Changes in Urine Output*
Dysuria	Polyuria
Flank or costovertebral angle	Oliguria
Groin	Anuria
Suprapubic	*Changes in Urine Composition*
Changes in Patterns of Urination	Hematuria
Frequency	Pyuria
Nocturia	Concentrated
Dysuria	Dilute
Hesitancy of stream	Color (red, brown, yellowish green)
Change in stream	*Edema*
Overactive bladder	Facial (periorbital)
Urgency	Ankle
Retention	Ascites
Incontinence	Anasarca
Stress incontinence	Sacral
Dribbling	

procedures, and chronic fatigue, can result in loss of self-esteem and a negative body image. Sensitive questioning may elicit cues to problems in this area.

Role-relationship pattern. Urinary problems can affect many aspects of a person's life, including the ability to work and relationships with others. These factors will have important implications on future treatment and management. The nurse must be aware of cues from the patient.

Urinary system problems may be serious enough to cause problems in job-related and social situations. Chronic dialysis therapy often makes regular employment or full-time homemaking difficult. Also, concurrent poor health and negative body image can seriously alter existing roles. The nurse should assess this area to plan appropriate interventions.

Sexuality-reproductive pattern. The patient should be questioned about the effect of a renal or urologic problem on her or his sexual patterns and satisfaction. Problems related to personal hygiene and fatigue can seriously affect a sexual relationship. Although urinary incontinence is not directly associated with sexual dysfunction, it often has a devastating effect on self-esteem and social and intimate relationships. Counseling of both the patient and partner may be indicated.

Objective Data

Physical Examination

Inspection. The nurse should assess for changes in the following:

Skin: pallor, yellow-gray cast, excoriations, changes in turgor, bruises, texture (e.g., rough, dry skin)

Mouth: stomatitis, ammonia breath odor

Face and extremities: generalized edema, peripheral edema, bladder distention, masses, enlarged kidneys

Abdomen: skin changes described earlier, as well as striae, abdominal contour for midline mass in lower abdomen (may indicate urinary retention) or unilateral mass (occasionally seen in adult, indicating enlargement of one or both kidneys from large tumor or polycystic kidney)

Weight: weight gain secondary to edema; weight loss and muscle wasting in renal failure

General state of health: fatigue, lethargy, and diminished alertness

Palpation. The kidneys are posterior organs protected by the abdominal organs, the ribs, and the heavy back muscles. A landmark useful in locating the kidneys is the **costovertebral angle** (CVA) formed by the rib cage and the vertebral column. The normal-sized left kidney is rarely palpable because the spleen lies directly on top of it. Occasionally the lower pole of the right kidney is palpable.

To palpate the right kidney, the examiner's left hand is placed behind and supports the patient's right side between the rib cage and the iliac crest (Fig. 43-6). The right flank is elevated with the left hand, and the right hand is used to palpate deeply for the right kidney. The lower pole of the right kidney may be felt as a smooth, rounded mass that descends on inspiration. If the kidney is palpable, its size, contour, and tenderness should be noted. Kidney enlargement is suggestive of neoplasm or other serious renal pathologic conditions.

The urinary bladder is normally not palpable unless it is distended with urine. If the bladder is full, it may be felt as a smooth, round, firm organ and is sensitive to palpation.

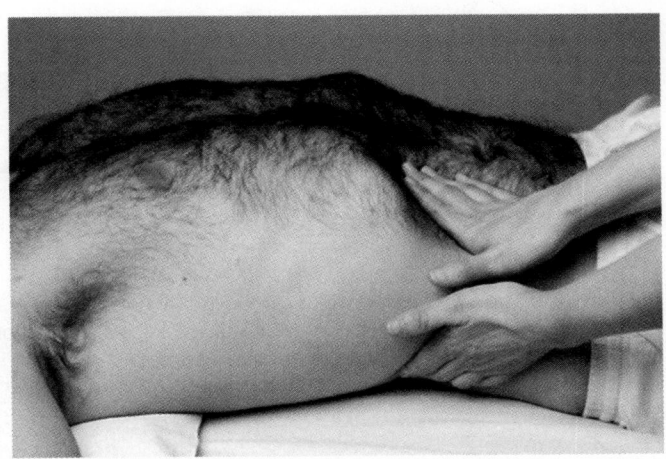

FIG. 43-6 Palpating the right kidney.

TABLE 43-6   **Normal Physical Assessment of the Urinary System**

No costovertebral angle tenderness
Nonpalpable kidney and bladder
No palpable masses

Percussion. Tenderness in the flank area may be detected by fist percussion. This technique is performed by striking the fist (kidney punch) of one hand against the dorsal surface of the other hand, which is placed flat along the posterior CVA margin. Normally a firm blow in the flank area should not elicit pain. If CVA tenderness and pain are present, it may indicate a kidney infection or polycystic kidney disease.

Normally a bladder is not percussible until it contains 150 ml of urine. If the bladder is full, dullness is heard above the symphysis pubis. A distended bladder may be percussed as high as the umbilicus.

Auscultation. The diaphragm of the stethoscope may be used to auscultate over both CVAs and in the upper abdominal quadrants. With this technique, the abdominal aorta and renal arteries are auscultated for a bruit (an abnormal murmur), which indicates impaired blood flow to the kidneys.

Table 43-6 shows how to record the normal physical assessment findings of the urinary system. Table 43-7 presents common assessment abnormalities of the urinary system. Normally, assessment findings may vary in the older adult. Table 43-2 shows the age-related changes in the urinary system and differences in assessment findings.

DIAGNOSTIC STUDIES OF THE URINARY SYSTEM

Table 43-8 discusses diagnostic studies common to the urinary system. Diagnostic studies are important in locating and understanding problems of the urinary system. The accuracy of the results is influenced by (1) adherence to the proper procedures related to the study and (2) cooperation of the patient in restrict-

TABLE 43-7

Common Assessment Abnormalities
Urinary System

FINDING	DESCRIPTION	POSSIBLE ETIOLOGY AND SIGNIFICANCE
Dysuria	Painful or difficult urination	Sign of urinary tract infection and interstitial cystitis and wide variety of pathologic conditions
Frequency	Increased incidence of urinating	Acutely inflamed bladder, retention with overflow, excess fluid intake
Enuresis	Involuntary nocturnal urinating	Symptomatic of lower urinary tract disorder
Hesitancy	Delay or difficulty in initiating urination	Partial urethral obstruction
Urgency	Strong desire to urinate	Inflammatory lesions in bladder or urethra, acute bacterial infections
Hematuria	Blood in the urine	Cancer of genitourinary tract, blood dyscrasias, renal disease, urinary tract infection, stones in kidney or ureter, medications (anticoagulants)
Burning on urination	Stinging pain in urethral area	Urethral irritation, urinary tract infection
Pneumaturia	Passage of urine containing gas	Fistula connections between bowel and bladder, gas-forming urinary tract infections
Retention	Inability to urinate, even though bladder contains excessive amount of urine	Finding after pelvic surgery, childbirth, catheter removal; urethral stricture or obstruction; neurogenic bladder; postanesthesia
Pain	Presence over suprapubic area (related to bladder), urethral pain (irritation of bladder neck), flank (CVA) pain	Infection, urinary retention, foreign body in urinary tract, urethritis, pyelonephritis, renal colic or stones
Incontinence	Inability to voluntarily control discharge of urine	Neurogenic bladder, bladder infection, injury to external sphincter
Stress incontinence	Involuntary urination with increased pressure (sneezing or coughing)	Weakness of sphincter control
Nocturia	Frequency of urination at night	Renal disease with impaired concentrating ability, bladder obstruction, congestive heart failure, diabetes mellitus, finding after renal transplant
Polyuria	Large volume of urine in a given time	Diabetes mellitus, diabetes insipidus, chronic renal failure, diuretics, excess fluid intake
Anuria	Technically no urination (24-hr urine output <100 ml)	Acute renal failure, end-stage renal disease, bilateral ureteral obstruction
Oliguria	Diminished amount of urine in a given time (24-hr urine output of 100–400 ml)	Severe dehydration, shock, transfusion reaction, kidney disease, end-stage renal disease

CVA, Costovertebral angle.

ing fluids, collecting urine specimens, lying quietly on the examination table, or following other instructions.

Many radiologic studies require the use of a bowel preparation the evening before the study to clear the lower GI tract of feces and flatus. Because the kidneys lie in a retroperitoneal location, the contents of the colon may obstruct visualization of the urinary tract. If a bowel preparation is not properly done, the study may be unsuccessful and have to be rescheduled. Commonly used bowel preparations include enemas, castor oil, magnesium citrate, and bisacodyl (Dulcolax) tablets or suppositories. Some bowel preparations, such as magnesium citrate and Fleet enema, are contraindicated in the patient with renal failure. Magnesium cannot be excreted by patients with renal failure (see Chapter 45).

When a patient has repeated diagnostic studies on consecutive days, it is important to prevent dehydration. It is not uncommon to have a patient take nothing by mouth (NPO) after midnight, spend all morning in the x-ray department, be too tired to eat, sleep all afternoon, and be on NPO status after midnight again because of studies scheduled for the next day. Severe dehydration, especially in a diabetic, debilitated, or older patient, may lead to acute renal failure. The nurse is responsible for ensuring that a patient undergoing diagnostic studies is properly hydrated and given adequate nourishment between studies. The nurse should also check with the health care provider regarding the insulin dose for the diabetic patient who is NPO.

Urine Studies

Urinalysis. In evaluating disorders of the urinary tract, one of the first studies done is a **urinalysis** (Tables 43-8 and 43-9). This test may provide information about possible abnormalities, indicate what further studies need to be done, and supply information on the progression of a diagnosed disorder.

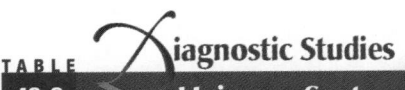

TABLE 43-8

Diagnostic Studies

Urinary System

STUDY	DESCRIPTION AND PURPOSE	NURSING RESPONSIBILITY
Urine Studies		
▪ Urinalysis	Study is a general examination of urine to establish baseline information or provide data to establish a tentative diagnosis and determine whether further studies are to be ordered (see Table 43-9).	Try to obtain first urinated morning specimen. Ensure that specimen is examined within 1 hr of urinating. Wash perineal area if soiled with menses or fecal material.
▪ Creatinine clearance	Creatinine is a waste product of protein breakdown (primarily body muscle mass). Clearance of creatinine by the kidney approximates the GFR. *Normal finding* is 85-135 ml/min.	Collect 24-hr urine specimen. Discard first urination when test is started. Save urine from all subsequent urinations for 24 hr. Instruct patient to urinate at end of 24 hr and add specimen to collection. Ensure that serum creatinine is determined during 24-hr period.
▪ Urine culture ("clean catch," "midstream")	Study is done to confirm suspected urinary tract infection and identify causative organisms. *Normally,* bladder is sterile, but urethra contains bacteria and a few WBCs. If properly collected, stored, and handled: <10,000 organisms/ml usually indicates no infection; 10,000-100,000/ml is usually not diagnostic, and test may have to be repeated; >100,000/ml indicates infection.	Use sterile container for collection of urine. Touch only outside of container. For women, separate labia with one hand and clean meatus with other hand, using at least three sponges (saturated with cleansing solution) in a front-to-back motion. For men, retract foreskin (if present) and cleanse glans with at least three cleansing sponges. After cleaning, instruct patient to start urinating and then continue voiding in sterile container. (The initial voided urine flushes out most contaminants in the urethra and perineal area.) Catheterization may be needed if patient is unable to cooperate with this procedure.
▪ Concentration test	Study evaluates renal concentration ability. Concentration is measured by specific gravity readings. *Normal finding* is 1.020-1.035.	Instruct patient to fast after given time in evening (in usual procedure). Collect three urine specimens at hourly intervals in morning.
▪ Residual urine	Study determines amount of urine left in bladder after urinating. Finding may be abnormal in problems with bladder innervation, sphincter impairment, BPH, or urethral strictures. *Normal finding* is ≤50 ml urine (increases with age).	If residual urine test is ordered, catheterize patient immediately after urinating or use bladder ultrasound equipment. If a large amount of residual urine is obtained, health care provider may want catheter left in bladder.
▪ Protein determination Dipstick (Albustix, Combistix)	Test detects protein (primarily albumin) in urine. *Normal finding* is 0-trace.	Dip end of stick in urine and read result by comparison with color chart on label as directed. Grading is from 0 to 4+. Interpret with caution. A positive result may not indicate significant proteinuria; some medications may give false-positive readings.
Quantitative test for protein	A 12- or 24-hr collection gives a more accurate indication of the amount of protein in urine. Persistent proteinuria usually indicates glomerular renal disease. *Normal finding* is <150 mg/24 hr (<0.15 g/24 hr), consisting mainly of albumin.	Perform 12- or 24-hr urine collection.
▪ Urine cytology	Study is used to identify changes in cellular structure indicative of malignancy, especially bladder cancer.	Obtain urine and send immediately to lab. The first morning specimen should *not* be used.
Blood Chemistries		
▪ BUN	Study is most commonly used to identify presence of renal problems. Concentration of urea in blood is regulated by rate at which kidney excretes urea. *Normal finding* is 10-30 mg/dl (1.8-7.1 mmol/L).	Be aware that when interpreting BUN, nonrenal factors may cause increase (e.g., rapid cell destruction from infections, fever, GI bleeding, trauma, athletic activity and excessive muscle breakdown, corticosteroid therapy).
▪ Creatinine	Study is more reliable than BUN as a determinant of renal function. Creatinine is end product of muscle and protein metabolism and is liberated at a constant rate. *Normal finding* is 0.5-1.5 mg/dl (44-133 μmol/L). Results are higher in men.	Explain test and watch for postpuncture bleeding.
▪ BUN/creatinine ratio	*Normal finding* is 10:1.	

BPH, Benign prostatic hyperplasia; *BUN,* blood urea nitrogen; *GI,* gastrointestinal; *GFR,* glomerular filtration rate; *WBC,* white blood cell.

Continued

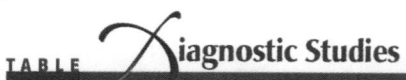

TABLE 43-8   Diagnostic Studies
Urinary System—cont'd

STUDY	DESCRIPTION AND PURPOSE	NURSING RESPONSIBILITY
Blood Chemistries—cont'd		
• Uric acid	Study is used as a screening test primarily for disorders of purine metabolism but can indicate kidney disease as well. Values depend on renal function and rate of purine metabolism and dietary intake of food rich in purines. *Normal finding* is 2.5-5.5 mg/dl (149-327 μmol/L) for women and 4.5-6.5 mg/dl (268-387 μmol/L) for men.	Explain test and watch for postpuncture bleeding.
• Sodium (Na$^+$)	Sodium is main extracellular electrolyte determining blood volume. Usually, values stay within normal range until late stages of renal failure. *Normal finding* is 135-145 mEq/L (135-145 mmol/L).	Explain test and watch for postpuncture bleeding.
• Potassium (K$^+$)	Kidneys are responsible for excreting majority of body's potassium. In renal disease, K$^+$ determinations are critical because K$^+$ is one of the first electrolytes to become abnormal. Elevated K$^+$ levels of >6 mEq/L can lead to muscle weakness and cardiac arrhythmias. *Normal finding* is 3.5-5.5 mEq/L (3.5-5.5 mmol/L).	Explain test and watch for postpuncture bleeding.
• Calcium (Ca^{2+})	Calcium is main mineral in bone and aids in muscle contraction, neurotransmission, and clotting. In renal disease, decreased reabsorption of Ca^{2+} leads to renal osteodystrophy. *Normal finding* is 9-11 mg/dl (4.5-5.5 mEq/L, 2.25-2.74 mmol/L).	Explain test and watch for postpuncture bleeding.
• Phosphorus	Phosphorus balance is inversely related to Ca^{2+} balance. In renal disease, phosphorus levels are elevated because the kidney is the primary excretory organ. *Normal finding* is 2.8-4.5 mg/dl (0.95-1.45 mmol/L)	Explain test and watch for postpuncture bleeding.
• Bicarbonate (HCO$_3^-$)	Most patients in renal failure have metabolic acidosis and low serum HCO$_3^-$ levels. *Normal finding* is 20-30 mEq/L (20-30 mmol/L).	Explain test and watch for postpuncture bleeding.
Radiologic Procedures		
• Kidneys, ureters, bladder (KUB)	Study involves x-ray examination of abdomen and pelvis and delineates size, shape, and position of kidneys.	Perform bowel preparation (if ordered).
• Intravenous pyelogram (IVP)	X-ray examination visualizes urinary tract after IV injection of contrast material.	Evening before procedure, give cathartic or enema to empty colon of feces and gas. Keep patient on NPO status 8 hr before procedure. Before procedure, assess patient for iodine sensitivity to avoid anaphylactic reaction. Inform patient that procedure involves lying on table and having serial x-rays taken. After procedure, force fluids (if permitted) to flush out contrast material.
• Nephrotomogram	X-ray is taken with rotating tubes. Test delineates segments of the kidney at different levels. Multiple exposures are taken to visualize specific sections of the kidney after IV injection of contrast material.	Explain procedure and prepare patient as for IVP.
• Retrograde pyelogram	X-ray of urinary tract is taken after injection of contrast material into kidneys. Cystoscope is inserted, and ureteral catheters are inserted through it into renal pelvis. Contrast material is injected through catheters.	Prepare patient as for IVP. Inform patient that pain may be experienced from distention of pelvis and discomfort from cystoscope. Inform patient that anesthesia may be given for procedure.
• Renal arteriogram (angiogram)	Study is performed by injecting contrast material into renal artery via catheter inserted into femoral artery. Purpose is to visualize renal blood vessels.	Prepare patient evening before procedure by giving cathartic or enema. Before injection of contrast material, test for iodine sensitivity. After procedure, check insertion site for bleeding and take peripheral pulses in involved leg every 30-60 min to detect occluded blood flow.

NPO, Nothing by mouth.

TABLE
43-8

Diagnostic Studies
Urinary System—cont'd

STUDY	DESCRIPTION AND PURPOSE	NURSING RESPONSIBILITY
Radiologic Procedures—cont'd		
▪ Renal ultrasound	Small external ultrasound probe is placed on patient's skin. Conductive gel is applied to the skin. Noninvasive procedure involves passing sound waves into body structures and recording images as they are reflected back. Computer interprets tissue density based on sound waves and displays it in picture form. Study is most valuable in detection of renal or perirenal masses, differential diagnosis of renal cysts, solid masses, and identification of obstructions. It can be used safely in patients with renal failure.	Explain procedure to patient.
▪ CT scan	Study provides excellent visualization of kidneys. Kidney size can be evaluated; tumors, abscesses, suprarenal masses (e.g., adrenal tumors, pheochromocytomas), and obstructions can be detected. Advantage of CT over ultrasound is its ability to distinguish subtle differences in density. Use of IV-administered contrast media during CT accentuates density of renal tissue and helps differentiate masses.	Explain procedure to patient. Ask patient about iodine sensitivity.
▪ MRI	Computer-generated films rely on radiofrequency waves and alteration in magnetic field. Useful for visualization of kidneys. Not proven useful for detecting urinary calculi or calcified tumors.	Explain procedure to patient. Have patient remove all metal objects. Patients with a history of claustrophobia may need to be sedated.
▪ Cystogram	Contrast material is instilled into bladder via cystoscope or catheter. Purpose is to visualize bladder and evaluate vesicoureteral reflux.	Explain procedure to patient. If done via cystoscope, follow nursing care related to cystoscopy.
Renal Radionuclide Imaging		
▪ Renal scan	Radioactive isotopes are injected IV. Radiation detector probes are placed over kidney, and scintillation counter monitors radioactive material in kidney. Purpose is to show blood flow, glomerular filtration, tubular function, and excretion. Radioisotope distribution in kidney is scanned and mapped. Test is useful in showing location, size, and shape of kidney and, in general, assessing blood perfusion and its ability to secrete urine. Abscesses, cysts, and tumors may appear as cold spots because of presence of nonfunctioning tissue.	Requires no dietary or activity restriction. Inform patient that no pain or discomfort should be felt during test.
Renal Biopsy	Technique is usually done as a skin (percutaneous) biopsy through needle insertion into lower lobe of kidney. Can be performed with CT or ultrasound guidance. Purpose is to obtain renal tissue for examination to determine type of renal disease or to follow progress of renal disease.	Before procedure, ascertain coagulation status through patient history, medication history, CBC, hematocrit, prothrombin time, and bleeding and clotting time. Type and crossmatch patient for blood. Ensure consent form is signed. After procedure, apply pressure dressing to biopsy site and check frequently for bleeding. Take vital signs frequently. Observe urine for gross bleeding. Determine microscopic bleeding by use of dipstick. Assess patient for flank pain. Monitor hematocrit levels.

CBC, Complete blood count; *CT,* computed tomography; *MRI,* magnetic resonance imaging.

Continued

TABLE 43-8   Diagnostic Studies Urinary System—cont'd

STUDY	DESCRIPTION AND PURPOSE	NURSING RESPONSIBILITY
Endoscopy • Cystoscopy	Study involves use of tubular lighted scope to inspect bladder. Lithotomy position is used. It may be done using local or general anesthesia, depending on needs and condition of patient.	Before procedure, force fluids or give IV fluids if general anethesia is to be used. Ensure consent form is signed. Explain procedure to patient. Give preoperative medication. After procedure, explain that burning on urination, pink-tinged urine, and urinary frequency are expected effects after cystoscopy. Do not let patient walk alone immediately after procedure because orthostatic hypotension may occur. Offer warm sitz baths, heat, mild analgesics to relieve discomfort.
Urodynamics • Cystometrogram	Study involves insertion of catheter and instillation of water or saline solution into bladder. Measurements of pressure exerted against bladder wall are recorded. Purpose is to evaluate bladder tone, sensations of filling, and bladder (detrusor) stability.	Explain procedure to patient. Observe patient for manifestations of urinary infection after procedure.

For a routine urinalysis, a specimen may be collected at any time of the day. However, it is best to obtain the first specimen urinated in the morning. This concentrated specimen is more likely to contain abnormal constituents if they are present in the urine. The specimen should be examined within 1 hour of urinating. If it is not, bacteria multiply rapidly, RBCs hemolyze, casts (molds of renal tubules) disintegrate, and the urine becomes alkaline as a result of urea-splitting bacteria. If it is not possible to send the specimen to the laboratory immediately, it should be refrigerated. However, to obtain the best results, the nurse should coordinate specimen collection with routine laboratory hours.

Multiple reagent strips (also called urine dipsticks) are commonly used by laboratories and in outpatient settings to provide chemical analysis of urine along with a microscopic interpretation. The results of a urinalysis usually include a description of the appearance, specific gravity (mass and density), pH, glucose, ketones, and protein in the urine and a microscopic examination of urine sediment for white blood cells (WBCs), RBCs, crystals, and casts (see Table 43-9).

Composite Urine Collections. Composite urine specimens are collected over a period that may range from 2 to 24 hours. The purpose of a composite specimen is to examine or measure specific components, such as electrolytes, glucose, protein, 17-ketosteroids, catecholamines, creatinine, and minerals. These specimens may have to be refrigerated, or preservatives may have to be added to the container used for collecting urine.

For collection of a composite urine specimen, the patient is instructed to urinate and discard this first urine specimen. This time is noted as the start of the test. All urine from subsequent urinations is saved in a container for the designated period. Finally, at the end of the period, the patient is asked to urinate, and this urine is added to the container. Incomplete collections do not provide valid results. Reminding the patient to save all urine during the study period is critical.

Creatinine Clearance. One of the most common composite indicators used to analyze urinary system disorders is creatinine clearance. **Creatinine** is a waste product produced by muscle breakdown. Urinary excretion of creatinine is a measure of the amount of active muscle tissue in the body, not of body weight. Therefore people with larger muscle mass have higher values. Because almost all creatinine in the blood is normally excreted by the kidneys, creatinine clearance is the most accurate indicator of renal function. The result of a creatinine clearance test closely approximates that of the GFR.[8] A blood specimen for serum creatinine determination should be obtained during the period of urine collection. Creatinine clearance is calculated as follows:

$$\text{Creatinine clearance (ml/min)} = \frac{\text{Urine creatinine (mg/ml)} \times \text{Urine volume (ml/min)}}{\text{Serum creatinine (mg/ml)}}$$

Creatinine levels remain remarkably constant for each person because they are not significantly affected by protein ingestion, muscular exercise, water intake, or rate of urine production. Normal creatinine clearance values range from 85 to 135 ml per minute. After age 40, the creatinine clearance rate decreases at a rate of about 1 ml per minute per year.

Urine Cytology. Urine can be checked for abnormal cellular structures that occur with bladder cancer. Specimens may be obtained by voiding, catheterization, or bladder irrigation (bladder washing). The first morning's voided specimen should not be used because epithelial cells may change in appearance in urine held in the bladder overnight. As with urinalysis, the specimen should be fresh or brought to the lab within the hour. An alcohol-based fixative is then added to preserve the cellular structure. Urine cytology is used for detection of and following the prognosis of bladder cancer.

Radiologic Studies (See Table 43-8)

Kidney, Ureter, and Bladder Film. The kidney, ureter, and bladder (KUB) film is an abdominal view taken without using a contrast medium to show the renal outline, psoas shadow, and the bladder, if full. Radiopaque stones and foreign bodies can

TABLE 43-9   Urinalysis Findings

TEST	NORMAL	ABNORMAL FINDING AND SIGNIFICANCE
Color	Amber yellow	• Dark, smoky color suggests hematuria. Yellow-brown to olive green indicates excessive bilirubin. Orange-red or orange-brown caused by phenazopyridine (Pyridium). Cloudiness of freshly voided urine indicates infection. Colorless urine indicates excessive fluid intake, renal disease, or diabetes insipidus.
Smell	Aromatic	• On standing, urine becomes more ammonia-like in smell. In urinary tract infections, urine smells unpleasant.
Protein	0-150 mg/24 hr 0-18 mg/dl	• Persistent proteinuria is characteristic of acute and chronic renal disease, especially involving glomeruli. In absence of disease, positive reading may be caused by high-protein diet, strenuous exercise, dehydration, fever, or emotional stress. Vaginal secretions may contaminate urine specimen and give positive reading.
Glucose	None	• Glycosuria indicates diabetes mellitus or low renal threshold for glucose reabsorption (if blood glucose level is normal). Small amounts may be found after glucose loading (e.g., glucose tolerance test).
Ketones	None	• Altered carbohydrate and fat metabolism indicates diabetes mellitus and starvation. Findings can also be seen in dehydration, vomiting, and severe diarrhea.
Bilirubin	None	• Presence of bilirubinuria is as significant as jaundice in detection of liver disorders. Bilirubin may appear in urine before jaundice becomes visible or may be present in persons with hepatic disorders who do not have recognizable jaundice.*
Specific gravity	1.003-1.030	• Specific gravity of morning urine specimen reflects maximum concentrating ability of kidney and is 1.025-1.030. Low specific gravity indicates dilute urine and possibly excessive diuresis. High specific gravity indicates dehydration. If it becomes fixed at about 1.010, this indicates renal inability to concentrate urine, suggesting that kidney is progressing to end-stage renal disease.
Osmolality	300-1300 mOsm/kg (300-1300 mmol/kg)	• Measurement is a more accurate method than specific gravity for determining diluting and concentrating ability of kidneys. Deviations from normal indicate tubular dysfunction. Findings indicate if kidney has lost ability to concentrate or dilute urine. (Not part of routine urinalysis.)
pH	4.0-8.0 (average, 6.0)	• If >8.0, finding may be the result of standing of urine or urinary tract infections because bacteria decompose urea to form ammonia. If <4.0, may indicate respiratory or metabolic acidosis.
RBC	0-4/hpf	• Bleeding in urinary tract is caused by calculi, cystitis, neoplasm, glomerulonephritis, tuberculosis, kidney biopsy, or trauma.
WBC	0-5/hpf	• Increased number of WBCs in urine (pyuria) indicates urinary tract infection or inflammation.
Casts	None-occasional hyaline	• Casts are molds of the renal tubules and may contain protein, WBCs, RBCs, or bacteria. Noncellular casts are hyaline in appearance, and a few may be found in normal urine. Casts indicate renal dysfunction or upper urinary tract infections.
Culture for organisms	No organisms in bladder, <10⁴ organisms/ml result of normal urethral flora	• Bacteria counts >10⁵/ml indicate urinary tract infection. Organisms most commonly found in urinary tract infections are *Escherichia coli*, enterococci, *Klebsiella*, *Proteus*, and streptococci.

*See Chapter 42 for further discussion.
hpf, High-powered field.

be seen on this x-ray. The form, size, and position of the kidneys can also be seen. Abscesses, tumors, and cysts may distort anatomic relationships on the KUB. Sometimes nephrotomograms (sectional views that focus on a single plane of the kidney) are ordered at the same time as the KUB x-ray to maximize visualization of the kidneys.

Intravenous Pyelogram. The **intravenous pyelogram** (IVP), or excretory urogram, allows visualization of the urinary tract. The presence, position, size, and shape of the kidneys, ureters, and bladder can be evaluated. Cysts, tumors, lesions, and obstructions cause a distortion in the normal appearance of these structures.

The procedure consists of injecting an intravenous dose of contrast material, which circulates in the blood and is excreted by the kidneys into the urine. During injection, the patient may experience warmth, a flushed face, and a salty taste. After injection, films are taken sequentially. The sequencing of films is planned so that contrast excretion can be followed from the cortex of the kidney to the bladder. The presence of bladder atony or outlet obstruction also can be detected by a film taken after urination, which shows the residual volume of urine in the bladder.

The patient with significantly decreased renal function should not have an IVP because the contrast material will not be properly excreted by the kidneys. Contrast medium can also be nephrotoxic and can worsen renal function.

Retrograde Pyelogram. A **retrograde pyelogram** is an x-ray visualization of the kidneys, ureter, and bladder after direct injection of a contrast material into the kidney via a ureteral catheter introduced through a cystoscope. It may be done if an IVP does not visualize the urinary tract or if the patient is allergic to the contrast material or has decreased renal function. The dangers associated with a retrograde pyelogram are similar to those related to cystoscopy, including the risk of infection and the use of anesthesia.

Antegrade Pyelogram. Sometimes an antegrade pyelogram is done to evaluate the upper urinary tract when there is allergy to contrast media or decreased renal function and when abnormalities prevent passage of a ureteral catheter. Contrast media may be injected percutaneously into the renal pelvis or via a nephrostomy tube that is already in place (also called a nephrostogram) when determining tube function or ureteral integrity after trauma or surgery. Complications of an antegrade pyelogram include hematuria, infection, and hematoma.

Renal Ultrasound. A renal ultrasound uses high-frequency waves to image the kidneys, ureter, and bladder. Because radiation exposure is avoided, a number of images can be obtained, and repeat studies over a brief period of time can be done. Images can be obtained from both the prone and supine positions. A bowel preparation is not required for a renal ultrasound.

Computed Tomography Scan. Computed tomography (CT) scan of the abdomen and pelvis may be done to detect tumors and possible metastases. The CT scan can differentiate these from cysts or abscesses. Contrast material may be used to help visualize urinary structures more clearly in the computer-generated images. The patient is instructed to lie very still during the procedure while the machine takes precise transaxial images. Sedation may be required if the patient is unable to cooperate.

Renal Arteriogram. The purpose of a **renal arteriogram** (angiogram) is to visualize the renal blood vessels. The findings of an arteriogram can assist in diagnosing renal artery stenosis (Fig. 43-7), additional or missing renal blood vessels, and renovascular hypertension and can assist in differentiating between a

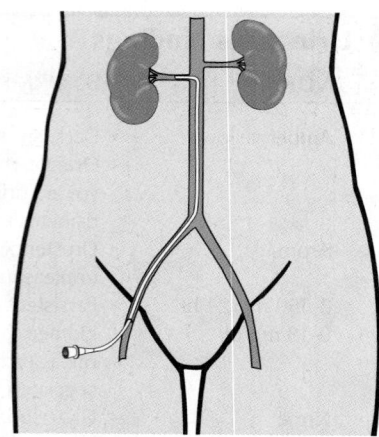

FIG. 43-8   Catheter insertion for a renal arteriogram.

renal cyst and a renal tumor. Renal arteriograms are also included in the workup of a potential renal transplant donor.

The patient is given a local anesthetic at the site of catheter insertion. A catheter is usually inserted into the femoral artery and passed up the aorta to the level of the renal arteries (Fig. 43-8). Contrast media is then injected to outline the renal blood supply, and x-rays are taken. The patient may experience a transient warm feeling along the course of the blood vessel when the contrast material is injected. As with all contrast studies, possible iodine and shellfish allergies should be determined before the study.

After the catheter is removed, a pressure dressing is placed over the femoral injection site. It is important to observe the site for bleeding. Bed rest is usually prescribed with the affected leg straight. Peripheral pulses in the involved leg should be taken at least every 30 to 60 minutes to detect occlusion of blood flow caused by a thrombus. Complications that may result from a renal arteriogram include thrombus, embolus, local inflammation, and hematoma. The patient with baseline renal insufficiency may experience a decrease in renal function secondary to the nephrotoxic contrast material.

Cystogram. The purpose of a cystogram is to outline and visualize the bladder and evaluate the UVJ for reflux. In addition to suspected vesicoureteral reflux, indications for a cystogram include a neurogenic bladder and recurrent urinary tract infections. A cystogram can also delineate abnormalities of the bladder, such as diverticula, calculi, and tumors. The procedure involves instillation of a contrast material into the bladder, which may be done via a cystoscope or catheter.

A *voiding cystourethrogram* (VCUG) is a voiding study of the bladder opening (bladder neck) and urethra. The bladder is filled with contrast material. During urination, films are taken to visualize the bladder and urethra. After urination, another film is taken to assess for residual urine. A VCUG can detect abnormalities of the lower urinary tract, urethral stenosis, bladder neck obstruction, and prostatic enlargement.[9]

Urethrogram. A urethrogram is similar to a cystogram. Contrast material is injected retrograde into the urethra to identify strictures, diverticula, or other urethral pathologic conditions. When urethral trauma is suspected, a urethrogram is done before catheterization.

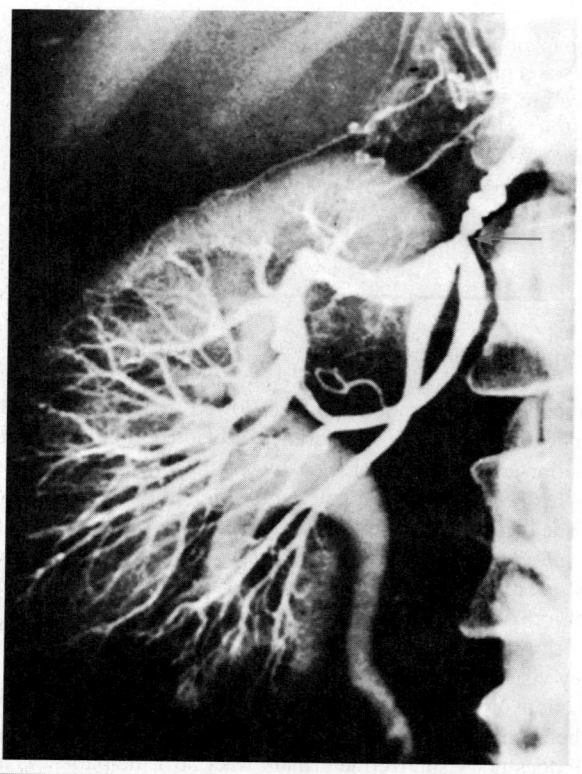

FIG. 43-7   Renal arteriogram showing stenosis of the right renal artery.

Loopogram. A loopogram is used to detect obstructions, anastomotic leaks, stones, reflux, and other uropathologic features when a patient has a urinary pouch or ileal conduit. Because urinary diversions are created with bowel, there is risk of contrast absorption. The patient should be closely monitored for reactions to the contrast media.

Renal Radionuclide Imaging. Renal scans involving the use of radionuclides are useful in evaluating the anatomic structures, perfusion, and function of the kidneys. The results reveal the difference between the two kidneys with respect to blood flow, tubular function, and excretion. A normal scan shows symmetric functioning of both kidneys. Normally the distribution of activity is recorded throughout the kidneys. A lesion (e.g., a tumor) is indicated by the absence of radioactivity in the involved area and the appearance of the resultant defect on the scan. This study is particularly useful in detecting renal vascular disease, acute renal failure, and upper urinary tract obstruction. It is also useful in monitoring the function of a transplanted kidney.

Renal Biopsy. The purpose of a **renal biopsy** is to determine the nature and extent of renal disease. This information can be used in establishing a diagnosis or following the progression of renal disease. Biopsy material can be obtained through an open biopsy or a closed percutaneous needle biopsy. An open biopsy is rarely performed because it requires a surgical procedure with anesthesia. A percutaneous needle biopsy is more commonly done.

Absolute contraindications to a percutaneous renal biopsy are bleeding disorders, the presence of a single kidney, and uncontrolled hypertension. Relative contraindications include suspected renal infection, hydronephrosis, and possible vascular lesions. The patient who is going to have a biopsy done should not be taking aspirin or warfarin (Coumadin) before the procedure.

The procedure consists of having the patient lie prone with a pillow or sandbag to elevate the abdomen and kidneys. The position of the kidney is marked on the body using CT, IVP, or ultrasound guidance. Local anesthesia is used, and a biopsy needle is inserted into the kidney just below the twelfth rib. The patient is instructed to hold his or her breath while the biopsy specimen is being taken.

After the procedure, a pressure dressing is applied, and the patient is kept prone for 30 to 60 minutes. Usually bed rest is prescribed for 24 hours. Vital signs should be taken every 5 to 10 minutes during the first hour and then with decreasing frequency, if no problems are noted. The biopsy site should be inspected frequently for bleeding. Serial urine specimens should be assessed for gross and microscopic hematuria. A dipstick can be used to test for bleeding, even when hematuria is not obvious. The physician may order all urine sent for laboratory analysis to detect possible hematuria. The patient should also be assessed for flank pain, hypotension, decreasing hematocrit, and temperature elevation. The patient should be observed for chills, urinary frequency, and dysuria.

Complications of a renal biopsy include renal hemorrhage, hematoma, and infection. Even if no complications occur, the patient should be instructed to avoid lifting heavy objects for 5 to 7 days. The patient should be instructed not to take any anticoagulant drugs until permission is given by the physician who performed the biopsy.

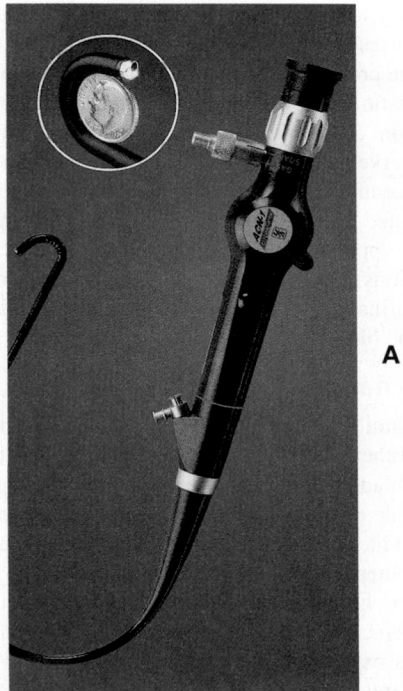

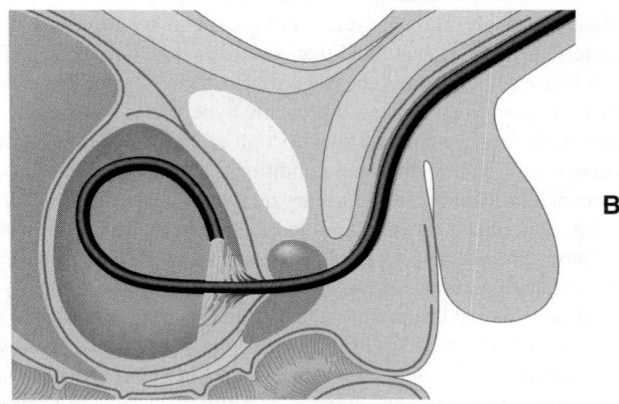

FIG. 43-9 Cystoscopic examination of the bladder in a man. A, Flexible Cysto Nephroscope. B, Scope inserted into bladder.

Endoscopy

Cystoscopy. The main purpose of **cystoscopy** is to inspect the interior of the bladder with a tubular lighted scope called a cystoscope (Fig. 43-9). Cystoscopes can be used to insert ureteral catheters, remove calculi, obtain biopsy specimens of bladder lesions, and treat bleeding lesions. In most cases, bladder disorders can be determined by cystoscopic examination.

Cystoscopy is usually done in a cystoscopy room in the x-ray department, in urology clinics, or in the operating room. Most of the pain associated with cystoscopy results from spasms and contractions of bladder and sphincter. Relaxation and deep breathing by the patient may alleviate some of the bladder and sphincter spasms. A local anesthetic is instilled into the urethra before scope insertion. During the examination, saline solution is instilled slowly to distend the bladder. This allows better visualization but causes an urge to urinate.

After the procedure the patient can expect to have some burning on urination, blood-tinged urine, and urinary frequency from the irritation of scope insertion and manipulation. The nurse should observe for bright red bleeding, which is not normal. After the procedure the nurse is responsible for keeping the patient well hydrated, administering mild analgesics, providing sitz baths, and applying heat to decrease the patient's discomfort. Complications that may result from cystoscopy include urinary retention, urinary tract hemorrhage, bladder infection, and perforation of the bladder.

Urodynamics

Urodynamics is a set of tests that are designed to measure urinary tract function. Urodynamic tests study the storage of urine within the bladder and the flow of urine through the urinary tract to the outside of the body. A combination of techniques may be used to provide a detailed urinary incontinence assessment of urinary incontinence.[10]

Urinary Flow Study. The urinary flow study (uroflow) measures urine volume in a single voiding expelled in a period of time and is expressed as milliliters per second. As the patient voids, the stream pattern is depicted graphically on a printout.

The patient is asked to start the test with a comfortably full bladder, urinate into a special container, and try to empty completely. A graph is generated that compares flow rate to time. This test is used to (1) assess the degree of outflow obstruction caused by such conditions as benign prostatic hyperplasia or stricture, (2) assess bladder or sphincter dysfunction effects on voiding such as occurs with neuropathologic conditions, and (2) evaluate the effects of treatment for lower urinary tract problems. A residual urine volume should be measured immediately after a urinary flow study because this will help to identify the degree of chronic urinary retention that is often associated with abnormal flow patterns.

A normal maximum flow rate for men is about 20 to 25 ml per second and about 25 to 30 ml per second for women. However, the volume voided and the patient's age can affect the flow rate, so normal variations are common. Graphic displays can illustrate straining and intermittent flow patterns or other abnormal voiding disorders.

Cystometrogram. A **cystometrogram** evaluates the compliance (elastic property) and stability of the detrusor muscle of the bladder. It is a measurement of intravesical pressure during the course of bladder filling. It is usually ordered if a patient has incontinence or neurogenic bladder. The procedure consists of insertion of a specially designed catheter while the patient is in a supine position. If abdominal pressure is measured, a second tube is inserted into the rectum or vagina. This tube is typically attached to a small fluid-filled balloon to allow pressure recording. Saline or sterile water for irrigation or contrast used for a cystogram is infused into the bladder, and pressures are measured. During the infusion, the patient is asked about sensations of bladder filling, usually including the first desire (urge) to urinate, a strong desire to urinate, and perception of bladder fullness.

Sphincter Electromyography (EMG). An EMG is a recording of the electrical activity created when the nervous system stimulates motor units within a muscle. By placing needles, percutaneous wires, or patches near the urethra, the pelvic floor muscle activity can be assessed. During the filling cystometrogram, the sphincter EMG is used to identify voluntary pelvic floor muscle contractions and the response of these muscles to bladder filling, coughing, and other provocative maneuvers.

Voiding Pressure Flow Study. The voiding pressure flow study combines a urinary flow rate, cystometric pressures (intravesical, abdominal, and detrusor pressures), and a sphincter EMG for detailed evaluation of micturition. It is completed by assisting the patient to a specialized toilet and allowing the person to urinate while the various pressure tubes and EMG apparatus remain in place.

Videourodynamics. *Videourodynamics* is a combination of the filling cystometrogram, sphincter EMG, and/or urinary flow study with anatomic imaging of the lower urinary tract, typically via fluoroscopy. This combination is used in selected cases to identify an obstructive lesion and characterize anatomic changes in the bladder and lower urinary tract.

Whitaker Study. The Whitaker study is used to measure the pressure differential between the renal pelvis and the bladder. The presence of a ureteral obstruction can be assessed. Percutaneous access is gained to the renal pelvis by placing a catheter in the renal pelvis. A catheter is also placed in the bladder. Fluid is perfused through the percutaneous tube or needle at a rate of 10 ml per minute. Pressure data are then collected. These pressure measurements are combined with fluoroscopic imaging to identify the level of obstruction.

REVIEW QUESTIONS

The number of the question corresponds to the same-numbered objective at the beginning of the chapter.

1. A renal stone in the pelvis of the kidney will alter the function of the kidney by interfering with
   a. the structural support of the kidney.
   b. regulation of the concentration of urine.
   c. the entry and exit of blood vessels at the kidney.
   d. collection and drainage of urine from the kidney.

2. A patient with renal disease has oliguria and a creatinine clearance of 40 ml per minute. The nurse recognizes that these findings most directly reflect abnormal function of
   a. tubular secretion.
   b. glomerular filtration.
   c. capillary permeability.
   d. concentration of filtrate.

3. The nurse identifies a risk for urinary calculi in a patient who relates a past health history that includes
   a. measles.
   b. gastric ulcer.
   c. diabetes mellitus.
   d. hyperparathyroidism.

4. Normal changes associated with aging of the urinary system that the nurse expects to find include
   a. decreased levels of BUN.
   b. urine postvoiding residual.
   c. increased bladder capacity.
   d. more easily palpable kidneys.

5. During physical assessment of the urinary system, the nurse
   a. percusses the flank area with a firm blow.
   b. palpates an empty bladder as a small nodule.
   c. positions the patient prone to palpate the kidneys.
   d. uses auscultation to determine the level of urine in the bladder.

6. Normal findings expected by the nurse on physical assessment of the urinary system include
   a. nonpalpable left kidney.
   b. auscultation of renal artery bruit.
   c. CVA tenderness elicited by a kidney punch.
   d. palpable bladder to the level of the pubic symphysis.

7. An important nursing responsibility after an IVP is to
   a. assess the patient for flank pain.
   b. encourage extra oral fluid intake.
   c. observe urine for remaining contrast material.
   d. encourage ambulation 2 to 3 hours after the study.

8. On reading the urinalysis results of a dehydrated patient, the nurse would expect to find
   a. a pH of 8.4.
   b. RBC of 4/hpf.
   c. color: yellow, cloudy.
   d. specific gravity of 1.035.

REFERENCES

1. Smith HW: *Fish to philosopher,* Boston, 1953, Little, Brown.
2. Gray ML: Physiology of voiding. In Doughty DB, editor: *Urinary and fecal incontinence: nursing management,* St Louis, 2000, Mosby.
3. McCance KL, Huether SE: *Pathophysiology: the biologic basis for disease in adults and children,* ed 4, St Louis, 2002, Mosby.
4. Guyton AC: *Textbook of medical physiology,* Philadelphia, 2000, Saunders.
5. Hazzard WR: Aging kidneys in an aging population: how does this impact nephrology and nephrologists? *Geriatr Nephrol Urol* 9:177, 1999.
6. Muhlberg W, Platt D: Age-dependent changes of the kidneys: pharmacological implications, *Gerontology* 45:243, 1999.
7. Greenberg A: *Primer on kidney disease,* San Diego, 2001, Academic Press.
8. Manjunath G, Sarnak MJ, Levey AS: Estimating the glomerular filtration rate: dos and don'ts for assessing kidney function, *Postgrad Med* 110:55, 2001.
9. Gordon D, Groutz A: Evaluation of female lower urinary tract symptoms: overview and update, *Curr Opin Obstet Gynecol* 13:521, 2001.
10. Gray M: Urodynamics in the clinical management of urinary incontinence in men and women, *Topics in Geriatric Rehabilitation* 15:42, 2000.

RESOURCES

Resources for this chapter are listed in Chapter 44 on page 1209 and Chapter 45 on page 1246.

CHAPTER 44

NURSING MANAGEMENT
Renal and Urologic Problems

Mikel Gray

LEARNING OBJECTIVES

1. Describe the pathophysiology, clinical manifestations, collaborative care, and drug therapy of cystitis, urethritis, and pyelonephritis.
2. Explain the nursing management of urinary tract infections.
3. Describe the immunologic mechanisms involved in glomerulonephritis.
4. Explain the clinical manifestations and nursing and collaborative management of acute poststreptococcal glomerulonephritis, Goodpasture syndrome, and chronic glomerulonephritis.
5. Describe the common causes, clinical manifestations, collaborative care, and nursing management of nephrotic syndrome.
6. Compare and contrast the etiology, clinical manifestations, collaborative care, and nursing management of various types of urinary calculi.

7. Explain the common causes and management of renal trauma, renal vascular problems, and hereditary renal problems.
8. Describe the mechanisms of renal involvement in metabolic and connective tissue disorders.
9. Describe the clinical manifestations and collaborative care of kidney and bladder cancer.
10. Describe the common causes and management of bladder dysfunctions.
11. Differentiate among ureteral, suprapubic, nephrostomy, and urethral catheters with regard to indications for use and nursing responsibilities.
12. Explain the nursing management of the patient undergoing nephrectomy or urinary diversion surgery.

KEY TERMS

calculus, p. 1186
cystitis, p. 1173
glomerulonephritis, p. 1180
Goodpasture syndrome, p. 1182
hydronephrosis, p. 1184
hydroureter, p. 1184
ileal conduit, p. 1203
interstitial cystitis, p. 1179
lithotripsy, p. 1188
nephrolithiasis, p. 1185

nephrosclerosis, p. 1191
nephrotic syndrome, p. 1183
polycystic kidney disease, p. 1192
pyelonephritis, p. 1173
renal artery stenosis, p. 1191
renal vein thrombosis, p. 1191
stricture, p. 1189
urethritis, p. 1173
urinary incontinence, p. 1195
urinary retention, p. 1195

Renal and urologic disorders encompass a wide spectrum of clinical problems. The diverse causes of these disorders may involve infectious, immunologic, obstructive, metabolic, collagen-vascular, traumatic, congenital, neoplastic, and neurologic mechanisms. This chapter discusses specific disorders of the kidneys, ureters, bladder, and urethra. Acute renal failure and chronic kidney disease are discussed in Chapter 45. Female reproductive problems are discussed in Chapter 52. Male genitourinary problems are discussed in Chapter 53.

Infectious and Inflammatory Disorders of the Urinary System

URINARY TRACT INFECTION

Urinary tract infections (UTIs) are the second most common bacterial disease. UTIs account for more than 8 million office visits per year. More than 100,000 people are hospitalized annu-

ally because of UTIs. More than 15% of patients who develop gram-negative bacteremia die, and one third of these are caused by bacterial infections originating in the urinary tract.[1]

Inflammation of the urinary tract may be attributable to a variety of disorders, but bacterial infection is by far the most common.[2] In the majority of healthy persons, the bladder and its contents are free from bacteria. Nevertheless, a minority of otherwise healthy individuals, including many young adult women and older women and men, have some bacteria colonizing the bladder. This condition is called *asymptomatic bacteriuria* and does not justify treatment. In contrast, an infection of the urinary system is diagnosed when bacterial invasion of the urinary tract occurs.

Escherichia coli (E. coli) (Table 44-1) is the most common pathogen leading to a UTI. Bacterial counts of 10^5 colony-forming units per milliliter (CFU/ml) or higher typically indicate a clinically significant UTI. However, counts as low as 10^2 to 10^3 CFU/ml in a person with signs and symptoms are indicative of UTI. Although fungal and parasitic infections may also cause UTIs, they are uncommon. UTIs from these causes are sometimes observed in patients who are immunosuppressed, have diabetes mellitus, or have undergone multiple courses of antibiotic

CULTURAL & ETHNIC CONSIDERATIONS
Urologic Disorders

- Urinary tract calculi are more common among whites than African Americans.
- Jewish men have a high incidence of uric acid stones.
- Bladder cancer has a higher incidence among white men than African American men.
- In all ethnic groups, bladder cancer affects men about three times more often than women.

Reviewed by Vicki Y. Johnson, RN, PhD, FN, CUCNS, Assistant Professor, University of Alabama, School of Nursing, Birmingham, Ala.

TABLE 44-1	Common Microorganisms Causing Urinary Tract Infections

*Escherichia coli**	*Proteus*
Enterococcus	*Pseudomonas*
Klebsiella	*Staphylococcus*
Enterobacter	*Candida*
Serratia	

*Causes about 80% of cases in persons who do not have urinary tract structural abnormalities or calculi.

therapy. They also may be seen in persons living in or having traveled to certain third world countries.

Classification

Several classification systems can be used for UTIs.[2,3] For example, a UTI can be broadly classified as an upper or lower UTI according to its location within the urinary system (Fig. 44-1). Infection of the upper urinary tract (involving the renal parenchyma, pelvis, and ureters) typically causes fever, chills, and flank pain, whereas a UTI confined to the lower urinary tract does not usually have systemic manifestations. Specific terms are used to further delineate the location of a UTI or inflammation. For example, **pyelonephritis** implies inflammation (usually due to infection) of the renal parenchyma and collecting system, **cystitis** indicates inflammation of the bladder wall, and **urethritis** means inflammation of the urethra.

Classifying a UTI as complicated or uncomplicated is also useful. *Uncomplicated* infections are those that occur in an otherwise normal urinary tract.[4] *Complicated* infections include those with coexisting presence of obstruction, stones, or catheters; existing di-

abetes or neurologic diseases; or an infection that is recurrent. The individual with a complicated infection is at risk for renal damage.

UTIs can also be classified according to their natural history. An *initial infection* (sometimes called a first or isolated infection) refers to an uncomplicated UTI in a person who has never had an infection or experiences one that is remote from any previous UTI (usually separated by a period of years). In contrast, a *recurrent UTI* is a reinfection in a person who experienced a previous infection that was successfully eradicated. If a recurrent UTI occurs because the original infection is not adequately eradicated, it is classified as unresolved bacteriuria or bacterial persistence. *Unresolved bacteriuria* occurs when bacteria are initially resistant to the antibiotic used to treat an infection, when the antibiotic agent fails to achieve adequate concentrations in the urine or bloodstream to kill bacteria, or when the drug is discontinued before the underlying bacteriuria is completely eradicated. *Bacterial persistence* also may occur when bacteria develop resistance to the antibiotic agent selected for treatment or when a foreign body in the urinary system serves as a harbor or anchor allowing bacteria to survive despite appropriate therapy.

Etiology and Pathophysiology

The urinary tract above the urethra is normally sterile. Several physiologic and mechanical defense mechanisms assist in maintaining sterility and preventing UTIs. These defenses include normal voiding with complete emptying of the bladder, normal antibacterial ability of the bladder mucosa and urine, ureterovesical junction competence, and peristaltic activity that propels urine toward the bladder. An alteration in any of these defense mechanisms increases the risk of contracting a UTI. Table 44-2 lists predisposing factors to UTIs.

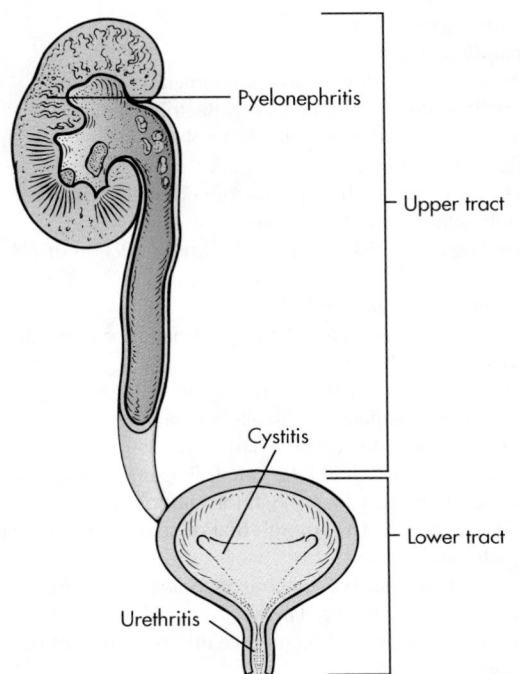

FIG. 44-1   Sites of infectious processes in the urinary tract.

TABLE 44-2	Predisposing Factors to Urinary Tract Infections

Factors Increasing Urinary Stasis
- Intrinsic obstruction (stone, tumor of urinary tract)
- Extrinsic obstruction (tumor, fibrosis compressing urinary tract)
- Urinary retention (including neurogenic bladder and low bladder wall compliance)

Foreign Bodies
- Urinary calculi
- Indwelling catheter
- Ureteral stent

Anatomic Factors
- Congenital defects leading to obstruction or urinary stasis
- Fistula (abnormal opening) exposing urinary stream to skin, vagina, or fecal stream
- Shorter female urethra

Factors Compromising Immune Response
- Human immunodeficiency virus infection
- Diabetes mellitus

Functional Disorders
- Constipation
- Voiding dysfunction with detrusor sphincter dyssynergia

The organisms that usually cause UTIs are introduced via the ascending route from the urethra. Other less common routes are via the bloodstream or lymphatic system. Most infections are due to gram-negative bacilli normally found in the gastrointestinal (GI) tract, although gram-positive organisms such as streptococci, enterococci, and *Staphylococcus saprophyticus* can also cause urinary infections. A common factor contributing to ascending infection is urologic instrumentation (e.g., catheterization, cystoscopic examinations). Instrumentation allows bacteria that are normally present at the opening of the urethra to enter the urethra or bladder. Sexual intercourse promotes "milking" of bacteria from the vagina and perineum and may cause minor urethral trauma that predisposes women to UTIs.

Rarely do UTIs result from a hematogenous route, where blood-borne bacteria secondarily invade the kidneys, ureters, or bladder from elsewhere in the body. For a kidney infection to occur from hematogenous transmission, there must be prior injury to the urinary tract, such as obstruction of the ureter, damage caused by stones, or renal scars.

An important source of UTIs is hospital-acquired, or *nosocomial,* infection. The cause of nosocomial infection is often *E. coli* and, less frequently, *Pseudomonas* organisms. Urologic instrumentation, particularly with an indwelling urinary catheter, is the most common predisposing factor.

Clinical Manifestations

Bothersome lower urinary tract symptoms are seen in UTIs of the upper urinary tracts, as well as those confined to the lower tract. These symptoms include dysuria, frequent urination (more often than every 2 hours), urgency, and suprapubic discomfort or pressure. The urine may contain grossly visible blood (hematuria) or sediment, giving it a cloudy appearance. Flank pain, chills, and the presence of a fever indicate an infection involving the upper urinary tract (pyelonephritis). It is important to remember that these symptoms, considered characteristic of a UTI, are often absent in older adults. Older adults tend to experience nonlocalized abdominal discomfort rather than dysuria and suprapubic pain.[2] In addition, they may have cognitive impairment.[4] Older adults are also less likely to experience a fever with infection of the upper urinary tract. Patients over age 80 years may experience a slight decline in temperature. People with significant bacteriuria may have no symptoms or may have nonspecific symptoms such as fatigue or anorexia.

Multiple factors may produce bothersome lower urinary tract symptoms similar to a UTI. For example, patients with bladder tumors or those receiving intravesical chemotherapy or pelvic radiation usually experience urinary frequency, urgency, and dysuria. Interstitial cystitis, a chronic inflammatory condition of unknown etiology, also produces bothersome urinary symptoms that are sometimes confused with a UTI. (Interstitial cystitis is discussed later in this chapter.)

Diagnostic Studies

Dipstick urinalysis should be obtained initially to identify the presence of nitrites (indicating bacteriuria), white blood cells (WBCs), and leukocyte esterase (an enzyme present in WBCs). These findings can be confirmed by microscopic urinalysis. Following confirmation of bacteriuria and pyuria, a urine culture may be obtained. A urine culture is indicated in complicated or nosocomial UTIs, persistent bacteria, or frequently recurring UTIs (more than two to three episodes per year). Urine also may

be cultured when the infection is unresponsive to empiric therapy or the diagnosis is questionable.[5] A voided midstream technique yielding a clean-catch urine sample is preferred for obtaining a urine culture in most circumstances. (See Table 43-8 for an explanation of this technique.) However, a specimen obtained by catheterization or suprapubic needle aspiration provides more accurate results and may be necessary when an adequate clean-catch specimen cannot be readily obtained.

A urine culture is accompanied by *sensitivity testing* to determine the bacteria's susceptibility to a variety of antibiotic drugs. The results of this test allow the health care provider to select an antibiotic known to be capable of destroying the bacterial strain producing a UTI in a specific patient.

Imaging studies of the urinary tract are indicated in selected cases. For example, an intravenous pyelogram (IVP) or abdominal computed tomography (CT) scan may be obtained when obstruction of the urinary system is suspected of causing a UTI.

Collaborative Care and Drug Therapy

Once a UTI has been diagnosed, appropriate antimicrobial therapy is initiated. An antibiotic may be selected based on the health care provider's best judgment (empiric therapy) or the

TABLE 44-3
Collaborative Care
Urinary Tract Infection

Diagnostic
History and physical examination
Urinalysis
Urine for culture and sensitivity (if indicated)
Imaging studies of urinary tract (e.g., IVP, cystoscopy) (if indicated)

Collaborative Therapy
Uncomplicated UTI
Antibiotic: 1- to 3-day treatment regimen
  trimethoprim-sulfamethoxazole (Bactrim, Septra)
  nitrofurantoin (Macrodantin, Macrobid)
Adequate fluid intake
Urinary analgesic such as phenazopyridine (Pyridium) or combination agent (e.g., Urised)
Counseling about risk of recurrence and reduction of risk factors

Recurrent, Uncomplicated UTI
Repeat urinalysis and consideration of need for urine culture and sensitivity testing
Antibiotic: 3- to 5-day treatment regimen
  trimethoprim-sulfamethoxazole (Bactrim, Septra)
  nitrofurantoin (Macrodantin, Furadantin)
  Sensitivity-guided antibiotic (ampicillin, amoxicillin, first-generation cephalosporin, fluoroquinolone)
Consideration of 3- to 6-month trial of suppressive antibiotics
Adequate fluid intake
Urinary analgesic such as phenazopyridine (Pyridium) or combination agent (e.g., Urised)
Counseling about risk of recurrence and reduction of risk factors
Imaging study of urinary tract in selected cases

IVP, Intravenous pyelogram; *UTI,* urinary tract infection.

results of sensitivity testing. The collaborative care and drug therapy of cystitis are summarized in Table 44-3. Uncomplicated cystitis can be treated by a short-term course of antibiotics, typically for 1 to 3 days. In contrast, complicated UTIs require longer-term treatment, lasting 7 to 14 days or even longer.[6,7]

Trimethoprim-sulfamethoxazole (TMP-SMX) or nitrofurantoin (Macrodantin) is often used to empirically treat uncomplicated or initial UTIs. TMP-SMX has the advantages of being relatively inexpensive and is taken twice daily. Nitrofurantoin is normally given 3 to 4 times daily, but a long-acting preparation (Macrobid) is available that is taken twice daily. Ampicillin or amoxicillin are not frequently selected when empirically treating a noncomplicated UTI because they must be administered 3 to 4 times daily. In addition to these agents, the fluoroquinolones (including ciprofloxacin [Cipro], levofloxacin [Levaquin], norfloxacin [Noroxin], ofloxacin [Floxin], or gatifloxacin [Tequin]) may be used to treat complicated UTIs.

A number of over-the-counter (OTC) or prescription drugs may be used in combination with antibiotic agents to relieve the discomfort associated with a UTI. Phenazopyridine (Pyridium) is an OTC drug that provides a soothing effect on the urinary tract mucosa. It also stains the urine a reddish orange that may be mistaken for blood in the urine, and it may permanently stain underclothing. Although this drug is typically effective in relieving the transient acute discomfort associated with a UTI, patients should be advised to avoid long-term use of phenazopyridine because it can produce hemolytic anemia. Combination agents such as Urised (methenamine, phenylsalicylate, atropine, hyoscyamine) may also be used to relieve the pain associated with a UTI. The patient taking a combination agent such as Urised should be advised that preparations containing methylene blue are expected to tint the urine blue or green.

Prophylactic or *suppressive antibiotics* are sometimes administered to patients who experience repeated UTIs. A low dose of TMP-SMX, nitrofurantoin, or another antibiotic may be administered on a daily basis in an attempt to prevent recurring UTIs, or a single dose may be taken before an event likely to provoke a UTI, such as intercourse. However, although suppressive therapy is often effective on a short-term basis, this strategy is limited because of the risk of antibiotic resistance ultimately leading to breakthrough infections with increasingly virulent pathogens.[8]

NURSING MANAGEMENT
URINARY TRACT INFECTION

■ Nursing Assessment

Subjective and objective data that should be obtained from a patient with a UTI are presented in Table 44-4.

■ Nursing Diagnoses

Nursing diagnoses for the patient with a UTI may include, but are not limited to, those presented in NCP 44-1.

■ Planning

The overall goals are that the patient with a UTI will have (1) relief from bothersome lower urinary tract symptoms, (2) prevention of upper urinary tract involvement, and (3) prevention of recurrence.

■ Nursing Implementation

Health Promotion. Health promotion measures include recognizing individuals who are at risk for a UTI. Debilitated persons, older adults, patients with underlying diseases (e.g., cancer, human immunodeficiency virus [HIV], or diabetes mellitus) that compromise host immune responses, and patients treated with immunosuppressive drugs or corticosteroids are at high risk for UTIs. Especially for these individuals, health promotion activities can help decrease the frequency of infections and promote early detection of infection. Health promotion activities include teaching preventive measures, such as (1) emptying the bladder regularly and completely, (2) evacuating the bowel regularly, (3) wiping the perineal area from front to back after urination and defecation, and (4) drinking an adequate amount of liquid each day. The recommended daily liquid intake for the ambulatory adult is approximately 15 ml per pound of body weight per day. Thus a 150-pound person would require 2250 ml each day. Because the person will obtain approximately 20% of this fluid from food, this leaves 1800 ml obtained by drinking, or just over seven 8-ounce glasses of fluid. Although suppressive antibiotics are not generally recommended, daily intake of cranberry juice (consumed as pure juice, 8 ounces twice daily) or cranberry essence tablets may reduce the risk of certain UTIs.[9] In addition, it is important to teach the patient to seek early treatment once symptoms are identified.

TABLE 44-4	Nursing Assessment Urinary Tract Infection

Subjective Data

Important Health Information

Past health history: Previous urinary tract infections; urinary calculi, stasis, reflux, strictures, or retention; neurogenic bladder; pregnancy; prostatic hyperplasia; sexually transmitted disease; bladder cancer

Medications: Use of antibiotics, anticholinergics, antispasmodics

Surgery or other treatments: Recent urologic instrumentation (catheterization, cystoscopy, surgery)

Functional Health Patterns

Health perception–health management: Urinary hygiene practices; lassitude, malaise

Nutritional-metabolic: Nausea, vomiting, and anorexia; chills

Elimination: Urinary frequency, urgency, hesitancy; nocturia

Cognitive-perceptual: Suprapubic or low back pain, costovertebral tenderness; bladder spasms, dysuria, burning on urination

Objective Data

General

Fever

Urinary

Hematuria; cloudy, foul-smelling urine; tender, enlarged kidney

Possible Findings

Leukocytosis; urinalysis positive for bacteria, pyuria, RBCs, and WBCs; positive urine culture; IVP, CT scan, ultrasound, voiding cystourethrogram and cystoscopy demonstrating abnormalities of urinary tract

CT, Computed tomography; *IVP,* intravenous pyelogram; *RBCs,* red blood cells; *WBCs,* white blood cells.

NURSING CARE PLAN 44-1

Patient with a Urinary Tract Infection

NURSING DIAGNOSIS **Acute pain** *related to* inflammation of mucosal tissue of urinary tract *as manifested by* pain on urination, flank pain, suprapubic pain, lower back pain, bladder spasms.

OUTCOMES—NOC	INTERVENTIONS—NIC and *RATIONALES*
Pain Control (1605)	*Pain Management (1400)*
▪ Uses nonanalgesic relief measures ____	▪ Perform a comprehensive assessment of pain to include location, characteristics, onset and duration, frequency, quality, intensity or severity, and precipitating factors *to establish history and baseline pain level.*
▪ Uses analgesics appropriately ____	▪ Provide the patient optimal pain relief by administering analgesics such as phenazopyridine (Pyridium) or combination agents (e.g., Urised) as ordered *to promote comfort.*
	▪ Alert patient that phenazopyridine will color urine orange and combination agents containing methylene blue will color urine blue or green *to prevent concern over unusual appearance of urine.*
Outcome Scale	▪ Teach the use of nonpharmacologic techniques (e.g., heating pad to suprapubic area or lower back, warm showers) during painful episodes along with other relief measures *to supplement pain medication and increase pain relief.*
1 = Never demonstrated	
2 = Rarely demonstrated	
3 = Sometimes demonstrated	
4 = Often demonstrated	
5 = Consistently demonstrated	

NURSING DIAGNOSIS **Impaired urinary elimination** *related to* urinary tract infection (UTI) *as manifested by* bothersome urgency, daytime voiding frequency, nocturia, or hematuria and verbalization of concern over altered elimination pattern.

OUTCOMES—NOC	INTERVENTIONS—NIC and *RATIONALES*
Urinary Elimination (0503)	*Urinary Elimination Management (0590)*
▪ Elimination pattern IER ____	▪ Monitor urinary elimination including frequency, consistency, odor, volume, and color (as appropriate) *to assess elimination status.*
▪ Urine passes without urgency ____	▪ Obtain midstream voided specimen for culture and sensitivity (as appropriate) *to determine pathogen causing UTI or to monitor effectiveness of treatment.*
▪ Urine free of blood ____	▪ Administer antimicrobial drugs as ordered *to eliminate symptoms by inhibiting bacterial growth.*
▪ Digestion of adequate fluids ____	▪ Teach patient signs and symptoms of UTI *to monitor effectiveness of treatment and recognize symptoms of recurrence.*
Outcome Scale	▪ Encourage adequate fluid *to help prevent infection and dehydration.*
1 = Extremely compromised	
2 = Substantially compromised	
3 = Moderately compromised	
4 = Mildly compromised	
5 = Not compromised	

IER, In expected range.

The nurse can play a major role in the prevention of nosocomial infections. Avoidance of unnecessary catheterization and early removal of indwelling catheters are the most effective means for reducing nosocomial UTIs. All patients undergoing instrumentation of the urinary tract are at risk for developing a nosocomial UTI. Aseptic technique must always be followed during these procedures. Washing hands before and after contact with each patient and wearing gloves for care involving the urinary system are especially important. When a catheter has been inserted, special measures must be employed as explained in the section on urethral catheterization later in this chapter.

Routine and thorough perineal hygiene is important for all hospitalized patients, especially when a bedpan is used. Incontinent episodes should be avoided by answering the call light quickly or offering the bedpan or urinal at frequent intervals to the bedridden patient.

Acute Intervention. Acute intervention for a patient with a UTI includes ensuring adequate fluid intake if it is not con-traindicated. It is sometimes difficult to get the patient to maintain an adequate fluid intake because the person may think it will worsen the discomfort and frequency associated with a UTI. The patient needs to be told that fluids will increase frequency of urination at first but will also dilute the urine, making the bladder less irritable. Fluids will help flush out bacteria before they have a chance to colonize in the bladder. Caffeine, alcohol, citrus juices, chocolate, and highly spiced foods or beverages should be avoided because they are potential bladder irritants.

Application of local heat to the suprapubic area or lower back may relieve the discomfort associated with a UTI. The patient can be advised to apply a heating pad (turned to its lowest setting) against the back or suprapubic area. A warm shower or sitting in a tub of warm water filled above the waist can also be effective in providing temporary relief.

The patient should be instructed about the prescribed drug therapy, including side effects. The nurse should emphasize the importance of taking the full course of antibiotics. Often patients stop antibiotic therapy once symptoms disappear. This practice can lead to inadequate treatment and recurrence of infection or to bacterial resistance to antibiotics. Sometimes a second drug or a reduced dose of drug is ordered after the initial course to suppress bacterial growth in certain patients susceptible to recurrent UTI. The patient should be instructed to watch for any changes in the color or consistency of the urine and a decrease in or cessation of symptoms as a sign of the effectiveness of therapy. The patient should be counseled that persistence of bothersome lower urinary tract symptoms beyond the antibiotic treatment course or the onset of flank pain or fever should be reported promptly to a health care provider.

Ambulatory and Home Care. Home care for the patient with a UTI should emphasize the patient's compliance with the drug regimen. The nurse's responsibility is to teach the patient about the need for ongoing care (Table 44-5). This includes taking antimicrobial drugs as ordered, maintaining adequate daily fluid intake, regular voiding (approximately every 2 to 4 hours), urinating after intercourse, and temporarily discontinuing the use of a diaphragm (if used).

The patient must understand the need for follow-up care with urine culture to determine if the infection has been adequately treated. Recurrent symptoms because of bacterial persistence or inadequate treatment typically occur within 1 to 2 weeks after completion of therapy. If the patient has been compliant, a relapse indicates the need for further evaluation.

■ Evaluation

The expected outcomes for the patient with a UTI are presented in NCP 44-1.

TABLE 44-5

Patient & Family Teaching Guide
Urinary Tract Infection

The following are important to teach to the patient with a UTI to prevent recurrence:

1. Explain importance of taking all antibiotics as prescribed. Symptoms may improve after 1 to 2 days of therapy, but organisms may still be present.
2. Instruct the patient on appropriate hygiene, including the following:
   a. Careful cleansing of perineal region
   b. Wiping from front to back after urinating
   c. Cleansing with soap and water after each bowel movement
3. Explain the importance of emptying the bladder before and after intercourse.
4. Instruct the patient to urinate regularly, approximately every 2 to 4 hours during the day.
5. Instruct the patient about the need to maintain adequate fluid intake (one-half ounce per pound of body weight per day).
6. Instruct the patient to avoid harsh soaps, bubble baths, powders, and sprays in the perineal area.
7. Advise the patient to report symptoms or signs of recurrent UTI (e.g., cloudy urine, pain on urination, urgency, frequency).

UTI, Urinary tract infection.

ACUTE PYELONEPHRITIS
Etiology and Pathophysiology

Pyelonephritis is an inflammation of the renal parenchyma and collecting system (including the renal pelvis). The most common cause is bacterial infection, but fungi, protozoa, or viruses sometimes infect the kidney.[10]

Urosepsis is a systemic infection arising from a urologic source. Its prompt diagnosis and effective treatment are critical because it can lead to septic shock and death in 15% of cases unless promptly eradicated. Septic shock is the outcome of unresolved bacteremia involving a gram-negative organism. (Septic shock is discussed in Chapter 65.)

Pyelonephritis usually begins with colonization and infection of the lower urinary tract via the ascending urethral route. Bacteria normally found in the intestinal tract, such as *E. coli, Proteus, Klebsiella,* or *Enterobacter* species, frequently cause pyelonephritis. A preexisting factor is often present, such as *vesicoureteral reflux* (retrograde or backward movement of urine from lower to upper urinary tract) or dysfunction of lower urinary tract function such as obstruction from benign prostatic hyperplasia, a stricture, or urinary stone.

Acute pyelonephritis commonly starts in the renal medulla and spreads to the adjacent cortex. Recurring episodes of pyelonephritis, especially in the presence of obstructive abnormalities, can lead to a scarred, poorly functioning kidney and a condition called *chronic pyelonephritis.*

Clinical Manifestations and Diagnostic Studies

The clinical manifestations of acute pyelonephritis vary from mild fatigue to the sudden onset of chills, fever, vomiting, malaise, flank pain, and the bothersome lower urinary tract symptoms characteristic of cystitis. *Costovertebral tenderness* is typically present on the affected side. The clinical manifestations usually subside within a few days, even without specific therapy, but bacteriuria and pyuria usually persist.

Urinalysis shows pyuria, bacteriuria, and varying degrees of hematuria. White blood cell (WBC) casts may be found in the urine, indicating involvement of the renal parenchyma. A complete blood count will show leukocytosis and a shift to the left with an increase in immature neutrophils (bands). Urine cultures must be obtained when pyelonephritis is suspected. In patients with more severe illness who are hospitalized, blood cultures are also obtained.

Imaging studies, such as an IVP or CT scan, requiring intravenous injection of contrast materials are usually not obtained in the early stages of pyelonephritis to prevent the possible spread of infection. Alternatively, ultrasonography of the urinary system may be obtained to identify anatomic abnormalities or the presence of an obstructing stone. Imaging studies are also used to assess for complications of pyelonephritis such as impaired renal function, scarring, chronic pyelonephritis, or abscesses.

Urosepsis is characterized by bacteriuria and bacteremia (presence of bacteria in blood). If bacteremia is a possibility, close observation and vital sign monitoring are essential. Prompt recognition and treatment of septic shock may prevent irreversible damage or death.

Collaborative Care and Drug Therapy

The diagnostic tests and collaborative therapy of acute pyelonephritis are summarized in Table 44-6. Patients with severe infections or complicating factors such as nausea and vomiting with dehydration require hospital admission.

The patient with mild symptoms may be treated as an outpatient with antibiotics for 14 to 21 days (see Table 44-6). Parenteral antibiotics are often given initially in the hospital to rapidly establish high serum and urinary drug levels. When initial treatment resolves acute symptoms and the patient is able to tolerate oral fluids and drugs, the person may be discharged on a regimen of oral antibiotics for an additional 14 to 21 days. Symptoms and signs typically improve or resolve within 48 to 72 hours after starting therapy.[11,12]

Relapses may be treated with a 6-week course of antibiotics. Reinfections may be treated as individual episodes of disease or managed with long-term antibiotic therapy. Antibiotic prophylaxis may also be used for recurrent infections. The effectiveness of therapy is evaluated in accordance with the presence or absence of bacterial growth on urine culture.

TABLE 44-6 Collaborative Care — Acute Pyelonephritis

Diagnostic

History and physical examination
Urinalysis
Urine for culture and sensitivity
Ultrasound (initially), IVP, VCUG, radionuclide imaging, CT scan
CBC count with WBC differential
Blood culture (if bacteremia is suspected)
Palpation for flank pain

Collaborative Therapy

Mild Symptoms

Outpatient management or short hospitalization for IV antibiotics
- Empirically selected broad-spectrum antibiotics (ampicillin, vancomycin) combined with an aminoglycoside (e.g., tobramycin [Nebcin], gentamicin [Garamycin])
- Switch to sensitivity-guided therapy (when results available) for 14 to 21 days
  trimethoprim–sulfamethoxazole (Bactrim, Septra)
  Fluoroquinolones (ciprofloxacin [Cipro], ofloxacin [Floxin], norfloxacin [Noroxin], gatifloxacin [Tequin])
Adequate fluid intake
Nonsteroidal antiinflammatory drugs or antipyretic drugs
Urinary analgesics (e.g., phenazopyridine [Pyridium])
Follow-up urine culture and imaging studies

Severe Symptoms

Hospitalization
Parenteral antibiotics
- Empirically selected broad-spectrum antibiotics (e.g., ampicillin, vancomycin) combined with an aminoglycoside (e.g., tobramycin, gentamicin)
- Switch to sensitivity-guided antibiotic therapy when results of urine and blood culture are available
Oral antibiotics when patient tolerates oral intake; administer for 7 to 21 days
Adequate fluid intake (parenteral initially, switched to oral fluids as nausea, vomiting, and dehydration subside)
Nonsteroidal antiinflammatory or antipyretic drugs to reverse fever and relieve discomfort
Urinary analgesics (e.g., to relieve bothersome lower urinary tract symptoms)
Follow-up urine culture and imaging studies

CBC, Complete blood count; *CT,* computed tomography; *IVP,* intravenous pyelogram; *VCUG,* voiding cystourethrogram; *WBC,* white blood cell.

NURSING MANAGEMENT ACUTE PYELONEPHRITIS

■ Nursing Assessment

Subjective and objective data that should be obtained from a patient with pyelonephritis are presented in Table 44-4.

■ Nursing Diagnoses

Nursing diagnoses for the patient with pyelonephritis include, but are not limited to, those for the patient with UTI (see NCP 44-1).

■ Planning

The overall goals are that the patient with pyelonephritis will have (1) relief of pain, (2) normal body temperature, (3) no complications, (4) normal renal function, and (5) no recurrence of symptoms.

■ Nursing Implementation

Health Promotion. Health promotion and maintenance measures are similar to those for cystitis (see p. 1175). In addition, it is important that the patient receive early treatment for cystitis to prevent ascending infections. Because the patient with structural abnormalities of the urinary tract is at high risk for infection, the need for regular medical care should be stressed to these patients.

Acute Intervention and Home Care. Nursing interventions vary depending on the severity of symptoms. These interventions include teaching the patient about the disease process with emphasis on (1) the need to continue drugs as prescribed, (2) the need for a follow-up urine culture to ensure proper management, and (3) identification of risk for recurrence or relapse (see Table 44-5 and NCP 44-1). In addition to antibiotic therapy, the patient should be encouraged to drink at least eight glasses of fluid every day, even after the infection has been treated. Rest is often indicated to increase patient comfort. The patient with frequent relapses or reinfections may be treated with long-term, low-dose antibiotics. Understanding the rationale for therapy is important to enhance patient compliance.

■ Evaluation

The expected outcomes for the patient with pyelonephritis are presented in NCP 44-1.

CHRONIC PYELONEPHRITIS

Chronic pyelonephritis is a term used to describe a kidney that has become shrunken and has lost function owing to scarring or fibrosis.[13] It usually occurs as the outcome of recurring infections involving the upper urinary tract. However, it also may occur in the absence of an existing infection and a recent or remote history of UTIs. Alternative terms used to describe this condition include *interstitial nephritis,* chronic atrophic pyelonephritis, or reflux nephropathy (when scarring occurs in the presence of vesicoureteral reflux).

Chronic pyelonephritis is diagnosed by radiologic imaging and histologic testing rather than clinical features. Imaging studies reveal a small, contracted kidney with a thinned parenchyma. The collecting system may be small or hydronephrotic. Pathologic analysis reveals loss of functioning nephrons, infiltration of the parenchyma with inflammatory cells, and fibrosis.

The level of renal function in chronic pyelonephritis varies, depending on whether one or both kidneys are affected, the magnitude of scarring, and the presence of coexisting infection. Chronic pyelonephritis often progresses to end-stage renal disease when both kidneys are involved, even if the underlying infection is successfully eradicated. (Nursing and collaborative management of the patient with chronic kidney disease is discussed in Chapter 45.)

URETHRITIS

Urethritis is an inflammation of the urethra. Causes of urethritis include a bacterial or viral infection, *Trichomonas* and monilial infection (especially in women), chlamydia, and gonorrhea (especially in men). Among men, the causes of urethritis are usually sexually transmitted. In men, purulent discharge usually indicates a gonococcal urethritis, whereas a clear discharge typically signifies a nongonococcal urethritis.[14] (Sexually transmitted diseases are discussed in Chapter 51). Urethritis also produces bothersome lower urinary tract symptoms, including dysuria and frequent urination, similar to those seen with cystitis.

In women, urethritis is difficult to diagnose. It frequently produces bothersome lower urinary tract symptoms as described previously, but urethral discharge may not be present. Cultures on split urine collections (taken at beginning of urine flow and then midstream) or any urethral discharge may confirm a diagnosis of urethral infection.

Treatment is based on identifying and treating the cause and providing symptomatic relief. Sulfamethoxazole with trimethoprim or nitrofurantoin are examples of drugs used for bacterial infections. Metronidazole (Flagyl) and clotrimazole (Mycelex) may be used for treating *Trichomonas*. Drugs such as nystatin (Mycostatin) or fluconazole (Diflucan) may be prescribed for monilial infections. In chlamydial infections, doxycycline (Vibramycin) may be used. Women with negative urine cultures and no pyuria do not usually respond to antibiotics. Hot sitz baths may temporarily relieve bothersome symptoms. The patient should be instructed to avoid the use of vaginal deodorant sprays, properly cleanse the perineal area after bowel movements and urination, and avoid intercourse until symptoms subside.

INTERSTITIAL CYSTITIS

Interstitial cystitis (IC) is a chronic, painful inflammatory disease of the bladder. It is thought to affect as many 700,000 Americans. The average age at onset is 40 years. The ratio of women to men with IC is 10-12:1. Although the etiology of IC remains unknown, probable contributing factors include chronic inflammation with mast cell invasion of the bladder wall (possibly provoked by an infection or an autoimmune disorder), defects of the glycosaminoglycan layer that protects the bladder mucosa from the irritating effects of urine exposure, abnormal constituents in the urine, dysfunction of the sympathetic innervation of the lower urinary tract, or a reflex sympathetic dystrophy.[15]

The two primary clinical manifestations that characterize IC include pain and bothersome lower urinary tract symptoms (e.g., frequency, urgency). The pain associated with IC is usually located in the suprapubic area but may involve the vagina, labia, or entire perineal region. It varies from moderate to severe in intensity and is exacerbated by bladder filling, postponing urination, physical exertion, pressure against the suprapubic area, dietary intake of certain foods, or emotional distress. The pain is transiently relieved by urination. Bothersome lower urinary tract symptoms are very similar to a UTI, and the condition is often misdiagnosed as a recurring or chronic UTI. The pain and bothersome voiding symptoms produced by IC remit and exacerbate over time. Some patients experience an onset of symptoms that disappears altogether after a period of weeks to months, whereas others have persistent symptoms over a period of months to years.

IC is a diagnosis of exclusion. The condition is suspected whenever a patient experiences symptoms of a UTI despite the absence of bacteriuria, pyuria, or a positive urine culture. A careful history and physical examination are necessary to exclude a variety of disorders that may produce somewhat similar symptoms, such as UTI or endometriosis. This evaluation must include at least one negative urine culture during a period of active symptoms. Cystoscopic examination may reveal a small bladder capacity and superficial ulcerations with bladder filling called *glomerulations,* but these findings are frequently absent and are not unique to IC. Criteria for diagnosing IC are presented in Table 44-7.

Collaborative Care and Drug Therapy

Because the etiology of IC is unknown, no single treatment has been identified that consistently reverses or relieves symptoms. Various therapies have been effective in alleviating or relieving bothersome symptoms in most patients.[15]

Dietary and lifestyle alterations are used to relieve pain and diminish voiding frequency and nocturia. Dietary alterations in-

---

TABLE 44-7   Clinical Criteria for the Diagnosis of Interstitial Cystitis

Inclusion Criteria
- Pain with bladder filling or postponing urination
- Bothersome urinary urgency
- Small bladder capacity on urodynamic testing
- Cystoscopic evidence of ulcerations or glomerulations (*not* specific to interstitial cystitis)

Exclusion Criteria
- Bladder capacity >350 ml on urodynamic testing
- Overactive bladder contractions on urodynamic testing
- Daytime voiding frequency <8 times per day
- Active genital herpes
- History of chemotherapy, particularly if treated with cyclophosphamide (Cytoxan)
- Tubercular cystitis
- History of pelvic radiation
- Bladder tumor

clude elimination of foods and beverages likely to exacerbate the symptoms. A diet low in acidic foods and avoiding beverages such as coffee, tea, and carbonated and alcoholic drinks can be helpful in reducing IC symptoms. Patients may be advised that an OTC dietary supplement called calcium glycerophosphate (Prelief) alkalinizes the urine and can provide relief from the irritating effects of certain foods. This agent may be particularly helpful when dining away from home where the patient has less control over the preparation of foods.

Two tricyclic antidepressants, amitriptyline (Elavil) and nortriptyline (Doxepin), are used to reduce the burning pain and urinary frequency. Pentosan (Elmiron) is a drug used to enhance the protective effects of the glycosaminoglycan layer of the bladder. It is thought to relieve pain associated with IC by reducing the irritative effects of urine on the bladder wall. Drugs that provide modest relief from IC symptoms in certain cases include nifedipine (Procardia), which is a calcium channel blocker. These drugs are effective over time (weeks to months), but they do not provide immediate relief that may be needed when a patient experiences an acute exacerbation of symptoms. In this case, a short course of opioid analgesics may be given.

Several agents may be instilled directly into the bladder through a small catheter. Dimethyl sulfoxide probably acts by desensitizing pain receptors in the bladder wall. Heparin and hyaluronic acid also may be instilled into the bladder to relieve IC symptoms. Like pentosan, they are thought to enhance the protective properties of the glycosaminoglycan layer of the bladder. These drugs are often administered with lidocaine, which rapidly desensitizes the bladder wall, rendering the patient better able to tolerate instillation of additional heparin or hyaluronic acid and providing transient relief from pain. Bacille Calmette-Guérin (BCG), an attenuated form of the *Mycobacterium bovis,* administered intravesically is now in clinical trials. The mechanism of action of BCG is unclear, but it may alleviate a possible autoimmune disorder provoking the chronic inflammation characteristic of the disorder.

Distention of the bladder during endoscopic examination relieves IC-related pain and voiding frequency, probably by temporarily disrupting sensory nerve endings in the bladder wall. Several surgical procedures have been used in an attempt to relieve severe, debilitating pain.[15] Urinary diversion is an approach that can be used when other measures fail. Unfortunately, some patients have reported pain within the urinary diversion, possibly indicating that components of the urine may contribute to IC in certain cases.

NURSING MANAGEMENT
INTERSTITIAL CYSTITIS

Assessment focuses on characterization of the pain associated with IC. The patient is asked about specific dietary or lifestyle factors known to exacerbate or alleviate pain and about the intensity of the pain. Objective data collection includes a bladder log or voiding diary kept over a period of at least 3 days to determine diurnal voiding frequency and patterns of nocturia. A simultaneous pain record may be useful.

Reassurance that IC is a real condition experienced by others and that it can be effectively treated may relieve the anxiety, anger, guilt, and frustration related to experiences of chronic pain and voiding dysfunction in the absence of a clear-cut diagnosis and treatment strategy. A UTI may occur during the course of IC management. A UTI is likely to produce an acute exacerbation of bothersome lower urinary tract symptoms and urinary frequency, as well as dysuria (not typically associated with IC) and odorous urine, possibly with hematuria.

The patient also must be given instruction about the need to maintain good nutrition, particularly in light of the broad dietary restrictions often necessary to control IC-related pain. Specifically, the patient may be advised to take a multivitamin containing no more than the recommended dietary allowance for essential vitamins and to avoid high-potency vitamins because these formulations may irritate the bladder. The patient is also assisted to obtain information from the Interstitial Cystitis Association, which includes recipes and menus for a well-balanced diet that is specifically designed to avoid bladder-irritating foods and beverages.

Elimination of a variety of foods and beverages from the diet that are likely to irritate the bladder typically provides modest to profound relief from symptoms. Typical bladder irritants include caffeine, alcohol, citrus products, aged cheeses, nuts, foods containing vinegar, curries or hot peppers, and foods or beverages likely to lower urinary pH. In addition, the patient should be taught to self-use Prelief. The patient is advised to avoid clothing that creates suprapubic pressure, including pants with tight belts or restrictive waistlines.

Written educational materials concerning diet, coping with the need for frequent urination, and strategies for coping with the emotional burden of IC are available from the Interstitial Cystitis Association (www.ichelp.com). Providing such materials provides an excellent opportunity for the nurse to introduce the patient to the existence of this patient advocacy group and to participate in local support groups when desired.

RENAL TUBERCULOSIS

Renal tuberculosis (TB) is rarely a primary lesion. It is usually secondary to TB of the lung. In a small percentage of patients with pulmonary TB, the tubercle bacilli reach the kidneys via the bloodstream. Onset occurs 5 to 8 years after the primary infection. The patient is often asymptomatic when the kidney is initially infiltrated with bacilli. Sometimes the patient complains of fatigue and develops a low-grade fever. As the lesions ulcerate, infection descends to the bladder, and the patient experiences frequent urination, burning on voiding, and epididymitis (in men). Symptoms of a UTI are the first sign in the majority of patients with renal TB. Renal lesions may calcify as they heal. Infrequently, renal colic, lumbar and iliac pain, and hematuria may be present. A diagnosis is based on localization of tubercle bacilli in the urine and on IVP findings.[16]

Long-term complications of renal TB depend on the duration of the disease before treatment. Scarring of the renal parenchyma and the development of ureteral strictures occur. The earlier treatment is initiated, the less likely renal failure will develop. Reduced bladder volume may be irreversible in advanced disease. The patient may require long-term urologic follow-up. (Nursing and collaborative management for the patient with TB is discussed in Chapter 27.)

Immunologic Disorders of the Kidney
GLOMERULONEPHRITIS

Immunologic processes involving the urinary tract predominantly affect the renal glomerulus. The disease process results in **glomerulonephritis** (inflammation of the glomeruli), which affects both kidneys equally. Although the glomerulus is the primary site of inflammation, tubular, interstitial, and vascular changes also occur. Glomerulonephritis is divided into a number of classifications, which may describe (1) the extent of damage (diffuse or focal), (2) the initial cause of the disorder (systemic lupus erythematosus, systemic sclerosis [scleroderma], streptococcal infection), or (3) the extent of changes (minimal or widespread).

Etiology and Pathophysiology

Two types of antibody-induced injury can initiate glomerular damage. In the first type, the antibodies have specificity for antigens within the glomerular basement membrane (GBM). These are termed anti-GBM antibodies. Immunoglobulins and complement are deposited along the basement membrane. The mechanism that causes a person to develop antibodies against its GBM is not known. Production of autoantibodies (antibodies to one's own tissue) may be stimulated by a structural alteration in the GBM or by a reaction of the basement membrane with an exogenous agent (e.g., hydrocarbon, viruses).

In the second type of immune process, the antibodies react with circulating nonglomerular antigens and are randomly deposited as immune complexes along the GBM. On electron microscopy of renal tissue sections, the deposits appear "lumpy-bumpy." In this immune complex process, the antigens do not come from the glomeruli but from either endogenous circulating native deoxyribonucleic acid (DNA) or exogenous sources (e.g., bacteria, viruses, chemicals, drugs). Bacterial products appear to be important in poststreptococcal glomerulonephritis. Viral agents have been recognized in certain cases of glomerulonephritis that develop after hepatitis B or C and rubella (measles).

All forms of immune complex disease are characterized by an accumulation of antigen, antibody, and complement in the glomeruli, which can result in tissue injury. The immune complexes activate complement (see Chapters 12 and 13). Complement activation results in the release of chemotactic factors that attract polymorphonuclear leukocytes and causes the release of histamine and other inflammatory mediators. The end result of these processes is glomerular injury as a result of inflammation.

Clinical Manifestations

Clinical manifestations of glomerulonephritis include varying degrees of hematuria (ranging from microscopic to gross) and urinary excretion of various formed elements, including red blood cells (RBCs), WBCs, and casts. Proteinuria and elevated blood urea nitrogen (BUN) and serum creatinine levels are other manifestations. In most cases, recovery from the acute illness is complete. However, if progressive involvement occurs, the result is destruction of renal tissue and marked renal insufficiency.

The patient's history provides important information related to glomerulonephritis. It is necessary to assess exposure to drugs, immunizations, microbial infections, and viral infections such as hepatitis. It is also important to evaluate the patient for more generalized conditions involving immune disorders, such as systemic lupus erythematosus and systemic sclerosis.

ACUTE POSTSTREPTOCOCCAL GLOMERULONEPHRITIS

Acute poststreptococcal glomerulonephritis (APSGN) is most common in children and young adults, but all age groups can be affected. APSGN develops 5 to 21 days after an infection of the pharynx or skin (e.g., streptococcal sore throat, impetigo) by certain nephrotoxic strains of group A β-hemolytic streptococci. The person produces antibodies to the streptococcal antigen. Although the specific mechanism is not known, the antigen-antibody complexes are deposited in the glomeruli and activate complement.[17] Complement activation causes an inflammatory reaction to the injury. The response to the injury is also a decrease in the filtration of metabolic waste products from the blood and an increase in the permeability of the glomerulus to larger protein molecules.

Clinical Manifestations and Complications

The clinical manifestations of APSGN appear as a variety of signs and symptoms, which may include generalized body edema, hypertension, oliguria, hematuria with a smoky or rusty appearance, and proteinuria. Fluid retention occurs as a result of decreased glomerular filtration. The edema appears initially in low-pressure tissues, such as around the eyes (periorbital edema), but later progresses to involve the total body as ascites or peripheral edema in the legs. Smoky urine indicates bleeding in the upper urinary tract. The degree of proteinuria varies with the severity of the glomerulonephropathy. Hypertension primarily results from increased extracellular fluid volume. The patient with APSGN may have abdominal or flank pain. At times the patient has no symptoms, with the problem found on routine urinalysis.

More than 95% of patients with APSGN recover completely or improve rapidly with conservative management. Chronic glomerulonephritis develops in 5% to 15% of the affected persons, and irreversible renal failure occurs in less than 1% of patients.[17]

Diagnostic Studies

The diagnosis of APSGN is based on a complete history and physical examination and laboratory studies (Table 44-8) to determine the presence or history of a group A β-hemolytic streptococcus in a throat or skin lesion. An immune response to the streptococcus is often demonstrated by assessment of antistreptolysin O (ASO) titers. The finding of decreased complement components (especially C3 and CH50) indicates an immune-mediated response. A renal biopsy may be performed to confirm the presence of the disease.

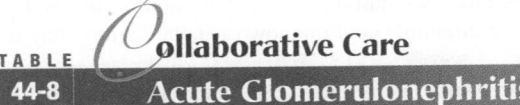

TABLE 44-8	**Collaborative Care** **Acute Glomerulonephritis**

Diagnostic
History and physical examination
Urinalysis
CBC
BUN, serum creatinine, and albumin
Complement levels and ASO titer
Renal biopsy (if indicated)

Collaborative Therapy
Rest
Sodium and fluid restriction
Diuretics
Antihypertensive therapy
Adjustment of dietary protein intake to level of proteinuria
  and uremia

ASO, Antistreptolysin O; *BUN*, blood urea nitrogen; *CBC*, complete blood count.

Dipstick and urine sediment microscopy will reveal the presence of erythrocytes in significant numbers. Erythrocyte casts are highly suggestive of acute glomerulonephritis. Proteinuria may range from mild to severe. Screening blood tests include BUN and serum creatinine to assess the extent of renal impairment.

NURSING and COLLABORATIVE MANAGEMENT ACUTE POSTSTREPTOCOCCAL GLOMERULONEPHRITIS

The management of APSGN focuses on symptomatic relief (see Table 44-8). Rest is recommended until the signs of glomerular inflammation (proteinuria, hematuria) and hypertension subside. Edema is treated by restricting sodium and fluid intake and by administrating diuretics. Severe hypertension is treated with antihypertensive drugs. Dietary protein intake may be restricted if there is evidence of an increase in nitrogenous wastes (e.g., elevated BUN value). The restriction varies with the degree of proteinuria. (Low-protein, low-sodium, fluid-restricted diets are discussed in Chapter 45.)

Antibiotics should be given only if the streptococcal infection is still present. Corticosteroids and cytotoxic drugs have not been shown to be of value.

One of the most important ways to prevent the development of APSGN is to encourage early diagnosis and treatment of sore throats and skin lesions. If streptococci are found in the culture, treatment with appropriate antibiotic therapy (usually penicillin) is essential. The patient must be encouraged to take the full course of antibiotics to ensure that the bacteria have been eradicated. Good personal hygiene is an important factor in preventing the spread of cutaneous streptococcal infections.

GOODPASTURE SYNDROME

Goodpasture syndrome, an example of cytotoxic (type II) autoimmune disease, is characterized by the presence of circulating antibodies against GBM and alveolar basement membrane.[18] Although the primary target organ is the kidney, the lungs are also involved. The pathologic nature of the syndrome results when binding of the antibody causes an inflammatory reaction mediated by complement fixation and activation (see Chapters 12 and 13). The causative factors for development of autoantibody production are unknown, although type A influenza viruses, hydrocarbons, penicillamine, and unknown genetic factors may be involved.

Goodpasture syndrome is a rare disease that is seen mostly in young male smokers. The clinical manifestations include hemoptysis, pulmonary insufficiency, crackles, rhonchi, renal involvement with hematuria and renal failure, weakness, pallor, and anemia. Pulmonary hemorrhage usually occurs and may precede glomerular abnormalities by weeks or months. Abnormal diagnostic findings include low hematocrit and hemoglobin levels, elevated BUN and serum creatinine levels, hematuria, and proteinuria. Circulating serum anti-GBM antibodies parallel the activity of the renal disease and are diagnostic of this syndrome.

NURSING and COLLABORATIVE MANAGEMENT GOODPASTURE SYNDROME

Until recently, the prognosis for the patient with Goodpasture syndrome was poor.[19] Management consists of corticosteroids, immunosuppressive drugs (e.g., cyclophosphamide [Cytoxan],

azathioprine [Imuran]), plasmapheresis (see Chapter 13), and dialysis. Plasmapheresis removes the circulating anti-GBM antibodies, and immunosuppressive therapy inhibits further antibody production. Renal transplantation can be attempted after the circulating anti-GBM antibody titer decreases. Although recurrences may develop, the disease is not a contraindication to transplantation. In selected patients with severe pulmonary hemorrhage, bilateral nephrectomy has been helpful. The exact mechanism for improvement has not been determined.

Nursing management appropriate for a critically ill patient who is experiencing symptoms of acute renal failure and respiratory distress is instituted. Death is often secondary to hemorrhage in the lungs and respiratory failure. (Nursing interventions for a patient in acute renal failure are discussed in Chapter 45, and nursing interventions for a patient with respiratory failure are discussed in Chapter 66.) Because this syndrome is rare and primarily affects previously healthy young adults, support and understanding of the patient and family are of major importance. The patient and family need instructions concerning current therapy, drugs, and complications of the disease process.

RAPIDLY PROGRESSIVE GLOMERULONEPHRITIS

Rapidly progressive glomerulonephritis (RPGN) is glomerular disease associated with rapid, progressive loss of renal function over days to weeks. Renal failure may occur within weeks to months in contrast to chronic glomerulonephritis, which develops insidiously and progresses over many years. The manifestations of RPGN are hypertension, edema, proteinuria, hematuria, and RBC casts.

RPGN can occur in a variety of situations: (1) as a complication of inflammatory or infectious disease (e.g., APSGN), (2) as a complication of a multisystemic disease (e.g., systemic lupus erythematosus, Goodpasture syndrome), (3) as an idiopathic disease, or (4) in association with the use of certain drugs (e.g., penicillamine).

Treatment is directed toward correction of fluid overload, hypertension, uremia, and inflammatory injury to the kidney. Treatment includes corticosteroids, cytotoxic agents, and plasmapheresis. Dialysis therapy and transplantation are used as maintenance therapy for the patient with RPGN. Following renal transplantation, RPGN may recur.

CHRONIC GLOMERULONEPHRITIS

Chronic glomerulonephritis is a syndrome that reflects the end stage of glomerular inflammatory disease. Most types of glomerulonephritis and nephrotic syndrome can eventually lead to chronic glomerulonephritis.

The syndrome is characterized by proteinuria, hematuria, and the slow development of uremic syndrome (see Chapter 45) as a result of decreasing renal function. Chronic glomerulonephritis does not usually follow an acute course. It progresses insidiously toward renal failure over a few to as many as 30 years.

Chronic glomerulonephritis is often found coincidentally when an abnormality on a urinalysis or elevated blood pressure is detected. It is common to find that the patient has no recollection or history of acute nephritis or any renal problems. A renal biopsy may be performed to determine the exact cause and nature of the glomerulonephritis. However, ultrasound and CT scanning are generally preferred as diagnostic measures.

Treatment is supportive and symptomatic. Hypertension and UTIs should be treated vigorously. Protein and phosphate restrictions may slow the rate of progression of kidney disease. (Management of chronic kidney disease is discussed in Chapter 45.)

NEPHROTIC SYNDROME

Etiology and Clinical Manifestations

Nephrotic syndrome describes a clinical course that can be associated with a number of disease conditions. Some of the more common causes of nephrotic syndrome are listed in Table 44-9. In adults about one third of patients with nephrotic syndrome will have a systemic disease such as diabetes or systemic lupus erythematosus. The remainder will be categorized as having idiopathic nephrotic syndrome.[20]

The characteristic manifestations include peripheral edema, massive proteinuria, hyperlipidemia, and hypoalbuminemia. Characteristic blood chemistries include decreased serum albumin, decreased total serum protein, and elevated serum cholesterol. The increased glomerular membrane permeability found in nephrotic syndrome is responsible for the massive excretion of protein in the urine. This results in decreased serum protein and subsequent edema formation. Ascites and anasarca develop if there is severe hypoalbuminemia.

The diminished plasma oncotic pressure from the decreased serum proteins stimulates hepatic lipoprotein synthesis, which results in hyperlipidemia. Initially, cholesterol and low-density lipoproteins are elevated. Later the triglyceride level is also increased. Fat bodies (fatty casts) commonly appear in the urine.

Immune responses, both humoral and cellular, are altered in nephrotic syndrome. As a result, infection is an important cause of morbidity and mortality. Calcium and skeletal abnormalities may occur, including hypocalcemia, blunted calcemic response to parathyroid hormone, hyperparathyroidism, and osteomalacia.

TABLE 44-9   ### Causes of Nephrotic Syndrome

Primary Glomerular Disease
Membraneous proliferative glomerulonephritis
Primary nephrotic syndrome
Focal glomerulonephritis
Inherited nephrotic disease

Extrarenal Causes
Multisystem Disease
Systemic lupus erythematosus
Diabetes mellitus
Amyloidosis
Infections
Bacterial (streptococcal, syphilis)
Viral (hepatitis, human immunodeficiency virus infection)
Protozoal (malaria)
Neoplasms
Hodgkin's disease
Solid tumors of lungs, colon, stomach, breast
Leukemias
Allergens (e.g., bee sting, pollen)
Drugs
Penicillamine
Nonsteroidal antiinflammatory drugs
captopril (Capoten)
Heroin

With nephrotic proteinuria, loss of clotting factors can result in a relative hypercoagulable state. Hypercoagulability with thromboembolism is potentially the most serious complication of nephrotic syndrome. The renal vein is the site most commonly involved for thrombus formation. Pulmonary emboli occur in about 40% of nephrotic patients with thrombosis.

Collaborative Care

Treatment of nephrotic syndrome is symptomatic.[20] The goals are to relieve edema and cure or control the primary disease. Management of the edema includes the cautious use of angiotensin-converting enzyme inhibitors, nonsteroidal antiinflammatory drugs, and a low-sodium (2 to 3 g per day), low- to moderate-protein diet (0.5 to 0.6 kg per day). Dietary salt restrictions are a key to managing edema. In some individuals, thiazide or loop diuretics may be needed. If urine protein loss exceeds 10 g per 24 hours, additional dietary protein may be needed.

The treatment of hyperlipidemia is often unsuccessful. However, treatment with lipid-lowering agents, such as colestipol (Colestid) and lovastatin (Mevacor), may result in moderate decreases in serum cholesterol levels. If thrombosis is detected, anticoagulant therapy may be necessary for up to 6 months.

Corticosteroids and cyclophosphamide (Cytoxan) may be used for the treatment of severe cases of nephrotic syndrome. Prednisone has been effective to varying degrees in persons with lipoid nephrosis, membranous glomerulonephritis, proliferative glomerulonephritis, and lupus nephritis. Management of diabetes and treatment of edema are the only measures used for nephrotic syndrome related to diabetes.

NURSING MANAGEMENT
NEPHROTIC SYNDROME

A major nursing intervention for a patient with nephrotic syndrome is related to edema. It is important to assess the edema by weighing the patient daily, accurately recording intake and output, and measuring abdominal girth or extremity size. Comparing this information daily provides the nurse with a tool for assessing the effectiveness of treatment. The edematous skin must be cleaned carefully. Trauma should be avoided, and the effectiveness of diuretic therapy must be monitored.

The patient with nephrotic syndrome has the potential to become malnourished from the excessive loss of protein in the urine. Maintaining a low- to moderate-protein diet that is also low in sodium is not always easy. The patient is usually anorexic. Serving small, frequent meals in a pleasant setting may encourage better dietary intake.

Because the patient is susceptible to infection, measures should be taken to avoid exposure to persons with known infections. The person with nephrotic syndrome is often ashamed of an edematous appearance and needs support in dealing with an altered body image.

RENAL DISEASE AND ACQUIRED
IMMUNODEFICIENCY SYNDROME

The patient with HIV infection can have a variety of renal manifestations, ranging from mild fluid and electrolyte abnormalities to progressive renal impairment resulting in end-stage renal disease. The incidence of renal disease associated with HIV infection is about 10% and is highest among IV drug users.

HIV-associated renal syndromes include the following:

1. *Proteinuria and nephrotic syndrome,* which occurs in about 10% of patients with HIV infection. It may be the initial sign of HIV infection in some persons.

2. *HIV-associated nephropathy,* which is characterized by proteinuria, progressive azotemia, absence of hypertension, large kidney size on renal imaging studies, and unusually rapid progression to end-stage renal disease.

3. *Acute renal failure,* which is most commonly seen in the patient with acquired immunodeficiency syndrome (AIDS) who is critically ill with HIV-related infection or malignancy. The natural cause of acute renal failure secondary to AIDS is similar to acute renal failure associated with other acute illnesses (see Chapter 45). Survival and recovery usually depend on the treatment of the primary cause of renal failure and support of renal function by dialysis. (HIV infection is discussed in Chapter 14.)

Obstructive Uropathies

Urinary obstruction refers to any anatomic or functional condition that blocks or impedes the flow of urine (Fig. 44-2). It may be congenital or acquired. Obstruction may be due to intrinsic causes such as anomalies, diverticula, tumors, or benign growth within the urinary tract; extrinsic causes such as tumors, adhesions, retroperitoneal fibrosis, or prolapsed adjacent organs; or functional causes as a result of neurologic or psychogenic factors. Some common intrinsic obstructions are narrowing of the ureteropelvic junction (UPJ), bladder neck contracture, benign prostatic hyperplasia, urethral stricture, and urethral meatal stenosis. Common extrinsic causes include pelvic and abdominal tumors or a prolapsed uterus. Examples

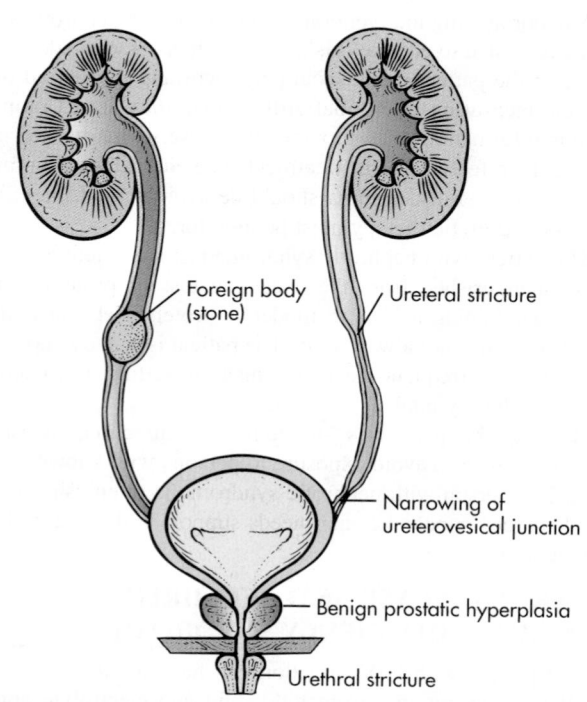

FIG. 44-2 Common causes of urinary tract obstruction.

Foreign body (stone)
Ureteral stricture
Narrowing of ureterovesical junction
Benign prostatic hyperplasia
Urethral stricture

of functional causes are neurogenic bladder and vesicosphincter dyssynergia (disturbance in muscle coordination) after spinal cord injury.

Damaging effects from urinary tract obstruction affect the system above the level of the obstruction. The severity of these effects depends on the location, duration of obstruction, amount of pressure or dilation, presence of urinary stasis, and whether infection is present. Infection increases the risk of irreversible damage.

Although obstruction distal to the prostate in men or the bladder neck in women causes mucosal scarring and a slower stream, it rarely results in major obstructive uropathy because the urethral wall pressure is less than that of the bladder neck and bladder. Urethral obstruction may contribute to outlet resistance and cause lower or upper urinary tract damage when other obstructive or dysfunctional factors are also present. For example, there is an increased risk of compromised renal function in the patient with a spinal cord injury with vesicosphincter dyssynergia.

When obstruction occurs at the level of the bladder neck or prostate, significant bladder changes can occur. Detrusor muscle fibers *hypertrophy* (increase in size) to contract harder to push urine out a narrower pathway. Over a long period, the detrusor loses its ability to compensate for this resistance. Muscle bundles separate and become less compliant. This separation is called *trabeculation.* Trabeculation is caused by the deposition of collagen in the bladder wall that separates the smooth muscle fascicles. Trabeculation may hasten the decompensation of the detrusor. The areas between these muscle bundles are called *cellules.* Because these areas have no muscle support, the bladder mucosa can herniate between detrusor muscle bundles, forming sacs that drain poorly, called *diverticula.* Residual urine can be very high in a noncompensating bladder.

Pressure increases during bladder filling or storage and can be transmitted to the ureter when *bladder outlet obstruction* is present. This pressure overcomes the normal peristaltic pressure and leads to *reflux* (a backflow of urine); ureteral dilation, kinking, and tortuosity; **hydroureter** (dilation of the renal pelvis); vesicoureteral reflux (backflow or backward movement of urine from the lower to upper urinary tracts); and **hydronephrosis** (dilation or enlargement of the renal pelves and calyces) (Fig. 44-3), and consequent chronic pyelonephritis and renal atrophy. If only one kidney is obstructed, the other kidney may try to compensate by hypertrophy, but the ureter will not be dilated on this contralateral side.

Partial obstruction may occur in the ureter or at the UPJ. If the pressure remains low or moderate, the kidney may continue to dilate with no noticeable loss of function. There is an increased risk of pyelonephritis because of urinary stasis and reflux. If only one kidney is involved and the other kidney is functioning, the patient may be free of symptoms. If both kidneys or only one functioning kidney is involved (e.g., if the patient has only one kidney), alterations in renal function (e.g., increased BUN or serum creatinine levels) are found. If the obstruction progresses, oliguria or anuria develops. Often episodes of oliguria are followed by polyuria if the obstruction is a stone that becomes dislodged. Treatment requires location and relief of the blockage. This can include insertion of a tube (e.g., urethral or ureteral), surgical correction of the disease process, or diversion of the urinary stream above the level of blockage.

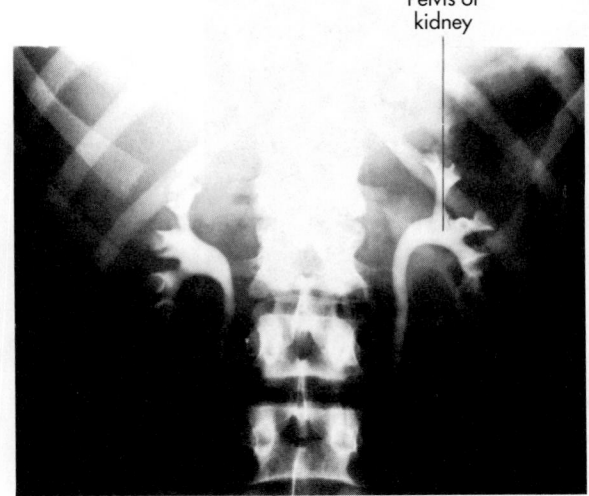

Pelvis of kidney

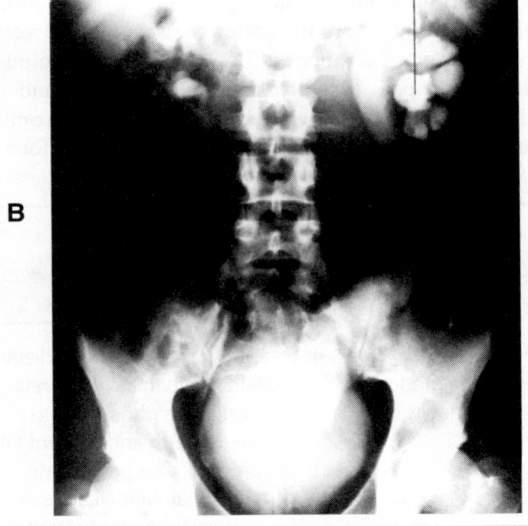

Distended pelvis and kidney secondary to hydronephrosis

FIG. 44-3 A, Normal intravenous pyelogram (IVP). B, IVP showing hydronephrosis and hydroureter.

URINARY TRACT CALCULI

Each year an estimated 500,000 people in the United States have **nephrolithiasis** (kidney stone disease). Many of these people require hospitalization. In the United States the incidence of urinary stone disease is highest in the Southeast and Southwest, followed by the Midwest. Except for struvite (magnesium-ammonium phosphate) stones associated with UTI, stone disorders are more common in men than in women.[21] The majority of patients are between 20 and 55 years of age. Stone formation is more frequent in whites than in African Americans. The incidence is also higher in persons with a family history of stone formation. Recurrence of stones can occur in up to 50% of patients.[22] There is seasonal variation, with stone formation occurring more often in the summer months, thus supporting the role of dehydration in this process. Stone formation

in the kidney also seems to increase in incidence as countries become more industrialized, whereas the incidence of bladder stones decreases.

Etiology and Pathophysiology

Many factors are involved in the incidence and type of stone formation, including metabolic, dietary, genetic, climatic, lifestyle, and occupational influences (Table 44-10). Many theories have been proposed to explain the formation of stones in the urinary tract. No single theory can account for stone formation in all cases. Crystals, when in a supersaturated concentration, can precipitate and unite to form a stone. Keeping urine dilute and free flowing reduces the risk of recurrent stone formation in many individuals. It is known that a mucoprotein is formed (the matrix for the stone) in the kidneys that form stones. Urinary pH, solute load, and inhibitors in the urine affect the formation of stones. The higher the pH, the less soluble are calcium and phosphate. The lower the pH, the less soluble are uric acid and cystine.

Other important factors in the development of stones include obstruction with urinary stasis and urinary infection with urea-splitting bacteria (e.g., *Proteus, Klebsiella, Pseudomonas,* and some species of staphylococci). These bacteria cause the urine to become alkaline and contribute to the formation of struvite (calcium-magnesium-ammonium phosphate) stones.[23] Infected stones, when they are entrapped in the kidney, may assume a staghorn configuration as they enlarge (Fig. 44-4). Infected stones are frequent in the patient with an external urinary diversion, long-term indwelling catheter, neurogenic bladder, or urinary retention. Genetic factors may also contribute to urine stone formation. Cystinuria is an autosomal recessive disorder. In this disorder there is a marked increased excretion of cystine.

TABLE 44-10   Risk Factors for the Development of Urinary Tract Calculi

Metabolic
Abnormalities that result in increased urine levels of calcium, oxaluric acid, uric acid, or citric acid

Climate
Warm climates that cause increased fluid loss, low urine volume, and increased solute concentration in urine

Diet
Large intake of dietary proteins that increases uric acid excretion
Excessive amounts of tea or fruit juices that elevate urinary oxalate level
Large intake of calcium and oxalate
Low fluid intake that increases urinary concentration

Genetic Factors
Family history of stone formation, cystinuria, gout, or renal acidosis

Lifestyle
Sedentary occupation, immobility

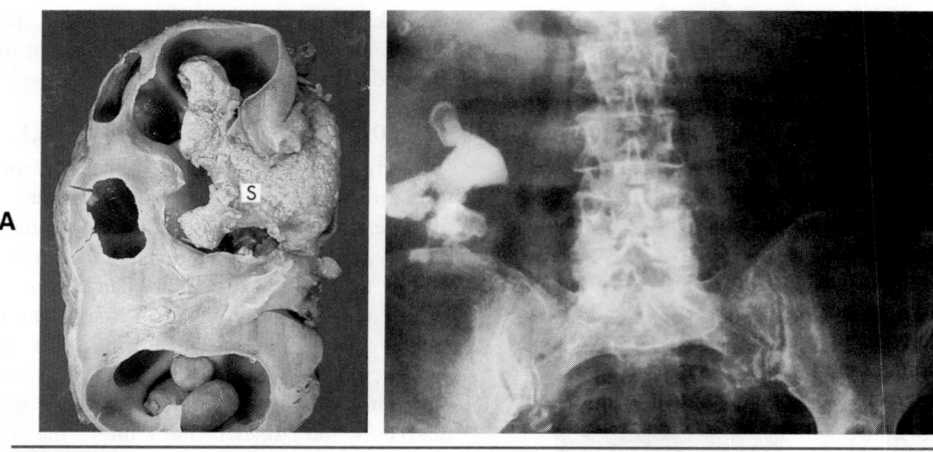

FIG. 44-4 **A,** Renal staghorn calculus. The renal pelvis is filled with a large calculus that is shaped to its contours, resembling the horn of a stag *(S)*. **B,** Staghorn calculus as seen on an intravenous pyelogram (IVP).

Types

The term **calculus** refers to the stone, and *lithiasis* refers to stone formation. The five major categories of stones are (1) calcium phosphate, (2) calcium oxalate, (3) uric acid, (4) cystine, and (5) struvite (magnesium-ammonium phosphate) (Table 44-11). Stone composition may be mixed, although calcium stones are the most common. Calculi can be found in various locations in the urinary tract (Fig. 44-5).

Clinical Manifestations

Urinary stones cause clinical manifestations when they obstruct urinary flow. Common sites of complete obstruction are at the UPJ (the point where the ureter crosses the iliac vessels) and at the ureterovesical junction (UVJ). Symptoms include abdominal or flank pain (usually severe), hematuria, and renal colic. The pain may be associated with nausea and vomiting. The type of pain is determined by the location of the stone (see

TABLE 44-11	Types of Urinary Tract Calculi			
URINARY STONE	**INCIDENCE (%)**	**CHARACTERISTICS**	**PREDISPOSING FACTORS**	**THERAPEUTIC MEASURES**
Calcium oxalate*	35–40	Small, often possible to get trapped in ureter; more frequent in men than in women	Idiopathic hypercalciuria, hyperoxaluria, independent of urinary pH, family history	Increase hydration. Reduce dietary oxalate.‡ Give thiazide diuretics. Give cellulose phosphate to chelate calcium and prevent GI absorption. Give potassium citrate to maintain alkaline urine. Give cholestyramine to bind oxalate. Give calcium lactate to precipitate oxalate in GI tract.
Calcium phosphate	8–10	Mixed stones (typically), with struvite or oxalate stones	Alkaline urine, primary hyperparathyroidism	Treat underlying causes and other stones.
Struvite ($MgNH_4PO_4$)	10–15	Three to four times as common in women than men, always in association with urinary tract infections, large staghorn type (usually)†	Urinary tract infections (usually *Proteus* organisms)	Administer antimicrobial agents, acetohydroxamic acid. Use surgical intervention to remove stone. Take measures to acidify urine.
Uric acid	5–8	Predominant in men, high incidence in Jewish men	Gout, acid urine, inherited condition	Reduce urinary concentration of uric acid. Alkalinize urine with potassium citrate. Administer allopurinol. Reduce dietary purines.‡
Cystine	1–2	Genetic autosomal recessive defect, defective absorption of cystine in GI tract and kidney, excess concentrations causing stone formation	Acid urine	Increase hydration. Give α-penicillamine and tiopronin to prevent cystine crystallization. Give potassium citrate to maintain alkaline urine.

*Calcium stones can exist as calcium oxalate, calcium phosphate, or a mixture of both. Calcium stones account for the majority of all stones.
†See Figure 44-4.
‡See Table 44-12.
GI, Gastrointestinal.

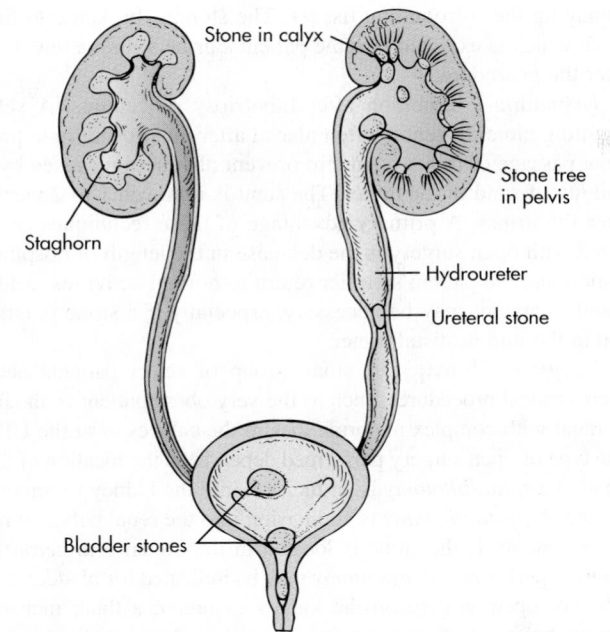

Stone in calyx

Stone free in pelvis

Staghorn

Hydroureter

Ureteral stone

Bladder stones

FIG. 44-5 Location of calculi in the urinary tract.

Fig. 44-5). If the stone is nonobstructing, pain may be absent. If the obstruction is in a calyx or at the UPJ, the patient may experience dull costovertebral flank pain or even colic. Pain resulting from the passage of a calculus down the ureter is intense and colicky. The patient may be in mild shock with cool, moist skin. As a stone nears the UVJ, pain will be felt in the lateral flank and sometimes down into the testicles, labia, or groin. Other clinical manifestations include the presence of urinary infection accompanied by fever, vomiting, nausea, and chills.

Diagnostic Studies

Diagnostic studies useful in the evaluation and management of renal lithiasis include urinalysis, urine culture, IVP, retrograde pyelogram, ultrasound, and cystoscopy. A plain film of the abdomen and renal ultrasound will identify larger, radiopaque stones. An IVP or retrograde pyelogram is used to localize the degree and site of obstruction or to confirm the presence of a radiolucent stone, such as a uric acid or cystine calculus (see Fig. 44-4, *B*). Ultrasonography can be used to identify a radiopaque or radiolucent calculus in the renal pelvis, calyx, or proximal ureter. It is less useful when attempting to locate stones trapped in the midureter. A CT scan may be used to differentiate a nonopaque stone from a tumor.

Retrieval and analysis of the stones are important in the diagnosis of the underlying problem contributing to stone formation. The patient's BUN and serum creatinine levels are also measured to assess renal function. A careful history, including previous stone formation, prescribed and OTC medications and dietary supplements, and family history of urinary calculi is useful. Measurement of urine pH is useful in the diagnosis of struvite stones and renal tubular acidosis (tendency to alkaline pH) and uric acid stones (tendency to acidic pH).[24]

Collaborative Care

Evaluation and management of a patient with renal lithiasis consist of two concurrent approaches. The first approach is directed toward management of the acute attack. This involves treating the symptoms of pain, infection, or obstruction as indicated for the individual patient. At frequent intervals, narcotics are typically required for relief of renal colic pain. Many stones pass spontaneously. However, stones larger than 4 mm are unlikely to pass through the ureter.

The second approach is directed toward evaluation of the cause of the stone formation and the prevention of further development of stones. Information to be obtained from the patient includes family history of stone formation, geographic residence, nutritional assessment including the intake of vitamins A and D, activity pattern (active or sedentary), history of periods of prolonged illness with immobilization or dehydration, and any history of disease or surgery involving the GI or genitourinary tract.

Therapy for people who are active stone formers requires a concerted management approach, with primary emphasis on teaching and on developing a therapeutic regimen with which the patient can comply. Adequate hydration, dietary sodium restrictions, dietary changes (Table 44-12), and the use of drugs minimize urinary stone formation. Various drugs are prescribed, depending on the specific problem underlying stone formation. These drugs prevent stone formation in various ways, including altering urine pH, preventing excessive urinary excretion of a substance, or correcting a primary disease (e.g., hyperparathyroidism).

Treatment of struvite stones requires control of infection. This may be difficult if the stone remains in place. In addition to antibiotics, acetohydroxamic acid may be used in the treatment of kidney infections that result in the continual formation of struvite stones. Acetohydroxamic acid, an inhibitor of the chemical action caused by the persistent bacteria, can be used effectively to retard struvite stone formation.[25] If the infection cannot be controlled, the stone may have to be removed surgically.

Indications for endourologic, lithotripsy, or open surgical stone removal include the following:
1. Stones too large for spontaneous passage
2. Stones associated with bacteriuria or symptomatic infection
3. Stones causing impaired renal function
4. Stones causing persistent pain, nausea, or ileus
5. Inability of patient to be treated medically
6. Patient with one kidney

TABLE 44-12	*N*utritional Therapy **Urinary Tract Calculi**

The following is a list of foods high in purine, calcium, or oxalate content.

Purine
High: Sardines, herring, mussels, liver, kidney, goose, venison, meat soups, sweetbreads
Moderate: Chicken, salmon, crab, veal, mutton, bacon, pork, beef, ham

Calcium
Milk, cheese, ice cream, yogurt, sauces containing milk; all beans (except green beans), lentils; fish with fine bones (e.g., sardines, kippers, herring, salmon); dried fruits, nuts; chocolate, cocoa, Ovaltine

Oxalate
Spinach, rhubarb, asparagus, cabbage, tomatoes, beets, nuts, celery, parsley, runner beans; chocolate, cocoa, instant coffee, Ovaltine, tea; Worcestershire sauce

Endourologic Procedures. If the stone is located in the bladder, a cystoscopy is done to remove small stones. For large stones a *cystolitholapaxy* is done. In this procedure, large stones can be broken up with an instrument called a lithotrite (stone crusher). The bladder is then irrigated and the crushed stones washed out. A *cystoscopic lithotripsy* uses an ultrasonic lithotrite to pulverize stones. Complications associated with these cystoscopic procedures include hemorrhage, retained stone fragments, and infection.

Flexible *ureteroscopes,* inserted via a cystoscope, can be used to remove stones from the renal pelvis and upper urinary tract. Ultrasonic, laser, or electrohydraulic lithotripsy can be used in conjunction with the ureteroscope to pulverize and break the stone into fragments.

In *percutaneous nephrolithotomy* a nephroscope is inserted through a sinus tract from the skin into the kidney pelvis. Stones can be fragmented using ultrasound, electrohydraulic, or laser lithotripsy. The stone fragments are removed and the pelvis irrigated. A percutaneous nephrostomy tube is usually left in place to ensure that the ureter is not obstructed. Complications include bleeding, injury to adjacent structures, and infection.

Lithotripsy. **Lithotripsy** is a procedure used to eliminate calculi from the urinary tract. Lithotripsy techniques include percutaneous ultrasonic lithotripsy, electrohydraulic lithotripsy, laser lithotripsy, and extracorporeal shock-wave lithotripsy.[26] Extracorporeal shock-wave lithotripsy and laser lithotripsy are the most common. In *percutaneous ultrasonic lithotripsy* an ultrasonic probe is placed in the renal pelvis via a percutaneous nephroscope (inserted through a small incision in the flank) and is positioned against the stone. (The patient is given general or spinal anesthesia for this procedure.) The probe produces ultrasonic waves, which break the stone into sandlike particles. Percutaneous lithotripsy is not used as much as a primary approach to renal or upper ureteral stones unless the stone is large and other lithotripsy procedures have failed.

The *electrohydraulic lithotripsy* probe is also placed directly on a stone, but it breaks the stone into small fragments that are removed by forceps or by suction. A continuous saline irrigation flushes out the stone particles, and all outflow drainage is strained so that the particles can be analyzed. The calculi can also be removed by forceps or basket extraction. Complications are rare but include hemorrhage, sepsis, and abscess formation. Postoperatively, the patient usually complains of moderate to severe colicky pain. The first few voids are bright red; as the bleeding subsides, the urine becomes dark red or turns a smoky color. Antibiotics are usually given for 2 weeks to reduce the risk of infection.

Laser lithotripsy probes are used to fragment lower ureteral and large bladder stones. A holmium laser medium is preferred; it fragments stones but does not injure the surrounding tissue.

In *extracorporeal shock-wave lithotripsy,* a noninvasive procedure, the patient is anesthetized (spinal or general) and placed in a water bath. Anesthesia is necessary to keep the patient very still during the procedure. Some of the newer-generation lithotripters do not require submersion and use other means of initiating shock waves. The lithotripters are categorized as electrohydraulic, electromagnetic, and piezoelectric. The second-generation lithotripters use less power to fragment stones. Lower power reduces a patient's pain, but usually some sedation or analgesia is necessary.

Fluoroscopy or ultrasound is used to focus the lithotripter on the affected kidney, and a high-voltage spark generator produces high-energy acoustic shock waves that shatter the stone without damaging the surrounding tissues. The stone is broken into fine sand, which is excreted into the patient's urine within a few days after the procedure.

Hematuria is common after lithotripsy procedures. A self-retaining ureteral stent is often placed after the procedure to promote passage of this sand and to prevent obstruction caused by a buildup of sand in the ureter. The stent is removed 1 to 2 weeks after lithotripsy. A primary advantage of these techniques compared with open surgery is the decrease in the length of hospitalization and the patient's earlier return to normal activities. Additional treatment may be necessary, especially if a stone is large and in the mid or distal ureter.

Surgical Therapy. A small group of select patients need open surgical procedures, such as the very obese patient or the individual with complex abnormalities in the calyces or at the UPJ. The type of open surgery performed depends on the location of the stone. A *nephrolithotomy* is an incision into the kidney to remove a stone. A *pyelolithotomy* is an incision into the renal pelvis to remove a stone. If the stone is located in the ureter, a *ureterolithotomy* is performed. A *cystotomy* may be indicated for bladder calculi. For open surgery on the kidney or ureter, a flank incision directly below the diaphragm and across the side is usually the preferred surgical approach. Complications related to hemorrhage are the most common following these surgical procedures.

Nutritional Therapy. When managing an obstructing stone, the patient is advised to drink adequate fluids to avoid dehydration. Forcing fluids is avoided because this strategy has not proved effective in assisting the patient to spontaneously "pass" (excrete) the stone via the urine. In addition, forcing fluids may exacerbate the colic associated with this episode.

A high fluid intake (approximately 3000 ml per day) is recommended after an episode of urolithiasis to produce a urine output of at least 2 L per day. High urine output prevents supersaturation of minerals (i.e., dilutes the concentration) and flushes them out before the minerals have a chance to precipitate and form a stone. Increasing the fluid intake is especially important for the patient who is active in sports, lives in a dry climate, performs physical exercise, has a family history of stone formation, or works in an occupation that requires outdoor work or a great deal of physical activity that can lead to dehydration. Water is the preferred fluid, and consumption of colas, coffee, and tea should be limited because high intake of these beverages tends to increase rather than diminish the risk of recurring urinary calculi.[27]

Dietary intervention may be important in the management of urolithiasis. In the past, calcium restriction was routinely implemented for the patient with kidney stones. However, more recent research suggests that a high dietary calcium intake, which was previously thought to contribute to kidney stones, may actually lower the risk by reducing the urinary excretion of oxalate, a common factor in many stones.[28] Initial nutritional management should include limiting oxalate-rich foods and thereby reducing oxalate excretion. Foods high in calcium, oxalate, and purines are presented in Table 44-12.

NURSING MANAGEMENT
RENAL CALCULI

■ Nursing Assessment

Subjective and objective data that should be obtained from a patient with urinary tract lithiasis are presented in Table 44-13.

TABLE 44-13	Nursing Assessment
	Urinary Tract Calculi

Subjective Data

Important Health Information

Past health history: Recent or chronic UTI; bed rest; immobilization; previous urinary tract stones, obstruction, or kidney disease with urinary stasis; gout; prostatic hyperplasia; hyperparathyroidism

Medications: Prior use of medication for prevention of stones or treatment of UTI; allopurinol, analgesics

Surgery or other treatments: External urinary diversion, long-term indwelling urinary catheter

Functional Health Patterns

Health perception–health management: Family history of renal calculi; sedentary lifestyle

Nutritional-metabolic: Nausea, vomiting; dietary intake of purines, calcium, oxalates, phosphates; low fluid intake; chills

Elimination: Decreased urinary output, urinary urgency, frequency, feeling of bladder fullness

Cognitive-perceptual: Acute, severe, colicky pain in flank, back, abdomen, groin, or genitalia; burning on urination, dysuria, anxiety

Objective Data

General

Guarding, fever

Integumentary

Warm, flushed skin or pallor with cool, moist skin (mild shock)

Gastrointestinal

Abdominal distention, absence of bowel sounds

Urinary

Oliguria, hematuria, tenderness on palpation of renal areas, passage of stone or stones

Possible Findings

↑ BUN and serum creatinine levels; RBCs, WBCs, pyuria, crystals, casts, minerals, bacteria on urinalysis; ↑ uric acid, calcium, phosphorus, oxalate, or cystine values on 24-hr urine sample; calculi or anatomic changes on IVP or KUB x-ray; direct visualization of obstruction on cystoureteroscopy

BUN, Blood urea nitrogen; *IVP,* intravenous pyelogram; *KUB,* kidneys, ureters, bladder; *RBCs,* red blood cells; *UTI,* urinary tract infection; *WBCs,* white blood cells.

■ **Nursing Diagnoses**

Nursing diagnoses for the patient with urinary tract lithiasis include, but are not limited to, those presented in NCP 44-2.

■ **Planning**

The overall goals are that the patient with urinary tract calculi will have (1) relief of pain, (2) no urinary tract obstruction, and (3) an understanding of measures to prevent further recurrence of stones.

■ **Nursing Implementation**

A program to prevent stone recurrence always includes adequate fluid intake to produce a urine output of approximately 2 L per day, and it may include measures to alleviate metabolic or secondary risk factors. The nurse should consult with the health care provider concerning recommendations for fluid intake in a given patient. In the modestly active, ambulatory person, this re-

quires the patient to drink about 2000 to 2200 ml per day with the residual 20% to 30% of fluids gained through consumption of foods. The volume of fluids will be higher in the highly active patient who works outdoors or who regularly engages in demanding athletic activities. In contrast, fluid intake will be less for the very sedentary or immobile person. Preventive measures related to the person who is on bed rest or is relatively immobile for a prolonged time include maintaining an adequate fluid intake, turning the patient every 2 hours, and helping the patient to sit or stand, if possible, to maximize urinary flow.[29]

Additional preventive measures focus on reducing metabolic or secondary risk factors. For example, dietary restriction of purines may be helpful to the patient at risk for developing uric acid stones. Reduced intake of oxalates may be indicated in the person with recurring calcium oxalate calculi. The patient is taught the dosage, scheduling, and potential side effects of drugs used to reduce the risk of stone formation. Selected patients may be taught to self-monitor urinary pH, or they may be asked to measure urinary output.

Pain management and patient comfort are primary nursing responsibilities when managing an obstructing stone and renal colic (see NCP 44-2). It is important to ensure that the patient retrieves any spontaneously passed stones. All urine voided by the patient should be strained through gauze or a special urine strainer in an effort to detect the stone. The high fluid intake necessary for stone prevention is avoided, but consumption should be adequate to meet daily needs and avoid dehydration. Ambulation is generally encouraged to promote the movement of the stone from the upper to lower urinary tract, but the patient should not walk unattended when experiencing acute colic, particularly if opioid analgesics are being used.

■ **Evaluation**

The expected outcomes for the patient with urinary calculi are presented in NCP 44-2.

STRICTURES

A **stricture** is a narrowing of the lumen of the ureter or urethra.

Ureteral Strictures

Ureteral strictures can affect the entire length of the ureter, from the UPJ to UVJ.[30] These strictures are usually an unintended result of surgical intervention, usually secondary to adhesions or scar formation. Depending on its severity, ureteral obstruction can threaten the function of the kidney. Clinical manifestations of a ureteral stricture include mild to moderate colic; this pain may be of moderate to severe intensity if the patient consumes a large volume of fluids (such as alcohol) over a brief period. Infection is unusual unless a calculus or foreign object such as a stent or nephrostomy tube is present.

The discomfort and obstruction of a ureteral stricture may be temporarily bypassed by placing a stent under endoscopic control or by diverting urinary flow via a nephrostomy tube inserted into the renal pelvis of the affected kidney. Definitive correction requires dilation with a balloon or catheter. If the stricture is severe or recurs after initial balloon or catheter dilation, it may be incised under endoscopic control (*endoureterotomy*). In selected cases, an open surgical approach may be required to excise the stenotic area and reanastomose the ureter to the contralateral ureter (*ureteroureterostomy*) or to the renal pelvis. Alternatively,

NURSING CARE PLAN 44-2

Patient with Acute Renal Lithiasis

EXPECTED PATIENT OUTCOMES	NURSING INTERVENTIONS and *RATIONALES*
NURSING DIAGNOSIS	**Acute pain** *related to* irritation of stone and inadequate pain control or comfort measures *as manifested by* complaints of pain, facial grimacing, restlessness.
▪ Minimal or no pain ▪ Decrease in pain and satisfaction with pain control	▪ Assess for pain location and severity *to plan appropriate interventions.* ▪ Encourage fluid intake unless contraindicated *to promote passage of stone, dilute the urine, and reduce risk of additional stone formation.* ▪ Administer pain medication as ordered *to promote comfort.* ▪ Apply heat to flank area as needed *because heat reduces reflex muscle spasm and promotes comfort.*
NURSING DIAGNOSIS	**Anxiety** *related to* uncertain outcome and lack of knowledge regarding possible surgery *as manifested by* expressions of concern about future treatments.
▪ Relief of anxiety ▪ Expression of confidence in treatment plan	▪ Assess cause and level of anxiety *to plan appropriate interventions.* ▪ Explain surgical or nonsurgical procedure (include insertion of urethral catheters) *because accurate information often decreases anxiety and fosters control.* ▪ Encourage patient to express feelings of anxiety, fear of surgery *to validate feelings and provide support.*
NURSING DIAGNOSIS	**Ineffective therapeutic regimen management** *related to* lack of knowledge about prevention of recurrence, diet, fluid requirements, and symptoms of recurrence *as manifested by* questions that indicate inadequate knowledge of disorder.
▪ Verbalization of correct self-care measures ▪ Able to list symptoms of recurrence	▪ Instruct patient during initial hospital stay regarding increasing fluids unless contraindicated and diet restrictions and rationale *to prepare for home self-care.* ▪ Inform patient about rationale, dose, frequency, and side effects of medication *to foster adherence to medication regimen.* ▪ Tell patient to strain all urine through a urine strainer or piece of gauze (if necessary) *to determine if stones are passed* and to bring stone to physician for analysis. ▪ Teach patient about symptoms of recurrence (e.g., hematuria, flank pain) *to ensure early reporting and initiation of treatment.*
NURSING DIAGNOSIS	**Impaired urinary elimination** *related to* trauma or blockage of ureters or urethra *as manifested by* decrease in urinary output, bloody urine.
▪ Free flow of urine ▪ Minimal to no hematuria ▪ Maintains balanced intake and output	▪ Monitor urine amount and character *to ensure patency in urinary system and that hematuria is not excessive.* ▪ Encourage increased fluid intake *as increased hydration flushes bacteria and blood and may facilitate passage of stone fragments.*
NURSING DIAGNOSIS	**Risk for infection** *related to* introduction of bacteria following manipulations of the urinary tract and obstructed urinary flow.
▪ No urinary tract infections	▪ Assess for elevation in temperature; chills; cloudy, foul-smelling urine *as indicators of potential infection.* ▪ Monitor vital signs and observe for fever *because abnormalities may indicate infection.* ▪ Encourage high fluid intake unless contraindicated *because stones form more readily in concentrated urine and increased fluids help the stone fragments pass down urinary tract.*

distal ureteral strictures may be managed by a *ureteroneocystostomy* (reimplantation of the ureter into the bladder wall).

Urethral Stricture

A *urethral stricture* is the result of fibrosis or inflammation of the urethral lumen.[31] Causes of urethral strictures include trauma, urethritis (particularly following gonococcal infection), iatrogenic (following surgical intervention), or a congenital defect in the canalization of the urethra. Once the process of inflammation and fibrosis begins, the lumen of the urethra narrows, and its

compliance (ability to close or open in response to bladder filling or micturition) is compromised. Meatal stenosis, a narrowing of the urethral opening, is also common. A urethral stricture creates symptoms when it creates voiding dysfunction or bladder outlet obstruction.[32]

Clinical manifestations associated with a urethral stricture include a diminished force of the urinary stream, spraying, or a split urine stream. The patient may report feelings of incomplete bladder emptying with urinary frequency and nocturia. Moderate to severe obstruction of the bladder outlet may lead to acute urinary retention. The patient may report a history of urethritis, difficulty with placement of a urinary catheter, or trauma involving the penis or perineum. However, many patients are unable to recall any such events, thus leading to a diagnosis of an idiopathic stricture. A history of a UTI is not uncommon, particularly if the stricture involves the distal urethra.

Initial management of a stricture may be based on dilation. A metal instrument (urethral sound) may be placed, or a series of progressively enlarging stents can be placed into the urethra (filiforms and followers) to expand its lumen in a stepwise fashion. While initially successful, recurring stenosis is frequent. Recurrences may be managed by teaching the patient to repeatedly dilate the urethra by self-catheterization every few days. Alternatively, an endoscopic or open surgical procedure may be completed to provide a more durable solution to an obstructive urethral stricture. Shorter strictures may be managed by resection of the fibrotic area with primary reanastomosis. Longer strictures may require autotransplantation of a substitute segment such as a skin flap.

Renal Trauma

A continual increase in the incidence of traumatic renal injuries is related to an increase in the mechanization and speed of transportation and to the increase in violent crimes and injuries. The majority of incidents occur in men younger than 30 years of age. Blunt trauma is the most common cause. Injury to the kidney should be considered in multiple or sports injuries, traffic accidents, and falls. It is especially likely when the patient injures the abdomen, flank, or back. Penetrating injuries may result from violent encounters (e.g., gunshot or stabbing incidents) or from iatrogenic injuries.

Clinical findings include a history of trauma to the area of the kidneys. Gross or microscopic hematuria may be present. Diagnostic studies include urinalysis, IVP with cystography, ultrasound, CT, or magnetic resonance imaging (MRI) evaluation. Renal arteriography may also be used. Both the injured kidney and the noninvolved kidney should be evaluated to provide information for further management.

The severity of renal trauma depends on the extent of the injury. Treatments range from bed rest, fluids, and analgesia to surgical exploration and repair or nephrectomy.

Nursing interventions vary with the type and extent of associated injuries. Specific interventions related to renal trauma include ensuring increased fluid intake, providing comfort measures, monitoring intake and output, observing for hematuria, determining the presence of myoglobinuria, assessing the cardiovascular status, and monitoring potentially nephrotoxic antibiotics.

Renal Vascular Problems

Vascular problems involving the kidney include (1) nephrosclerosis, (2) renal artery stenosis, and (3) renal vein thrombosis.

NEPHROSCLEROSIS

Nephrosclerosis consists of sclerosis of the small arteries and arterioles of the kidney. There is decreased blood flow, which results in patchy necrosis of the renal parenchyma. Ischemic necrosis and destruction of glomeruli with subsequent fibrosis also occur.

Benign nephrosclerosis usually occurs in adults 30 to 50 years of age. It is caused by vascular changes resulting from hypertension and from the atherosclerosis process. Atherosclerotic vascular changes account for most of the loss of renal function associated with aging. There is a direct relation between the degree of nephrosclerosis and the severity of hypertension. The patient with benign nephrosclerosis may have normal renal function in the early stages. The only detectable abnormality may be hypertension.

Accelerated nephrosclerosis, or *malignant nephrosclerosis,* is associated with malignant hypertension, a complication of hypertension characterized by a sharp increase in BP with a diastolic pressure greater than 130 mm Hg. The patient is usually a young adult, with a male-to-female predominance of 2:1. Renal insufficiency progresses rapidly.

Treatment for benign nephrosclerosis is the same as that for essential hypertension (see Chapter 32). Malignant nephrosclerosis is treated with aggressive antihypertensive therapy (see Chapter 32). The availability and use of antihypertensives have improved the prognosis for the patient with benign and malignant nephrosclerosis. Renal dysfunction and renal failure (in some persons) constitute two of the major complications of hypertension. The prognosis for the patient with malignant hypertension is poor, with the major cause of death related to renal failure.

RENAL ARTERY STENOSIS

Renal artery stenosis is a partial occlusion of one or both renal arteries and their major branches. It can be due to atherosclerotic narrowing or fibromuscular hyperplasia. Renal artery stenosis accounts for 1% to 2% of all cases of hypertension.

When hypertension develops rather abruptly, renal artery stenosis should be considered as a possible cause, especially in the patient under 30 or over 50 years of age and in the patient with no familial history of hypertension. This contrasts with the age distribution for essential hypertension, which is 30 to 50 years of age. A renal arteriogram is the best diagnostic tool for identifying renal artery stenosis.

The goals of therapy are control of BP and restoration of perfusion to the kidney. Percutaneous transluminal renal angioplasty is the procedure of first choice, especially in older patients who are poor surgical risks. Surgical revascularization of the kidney is indicated when blood flow is decreased enough to cause renal ischemia or when evidence indicates that renovascular hypertension is present and surgical intervention may result in the patient becoming normotensive. The surgical procedure usually involves anastomoses between the kidney and another major artery, usually the splenic artery or aorta. In selected cases of unilateral renal involvement with high renin production, unilateral nephrectomy may be indicated.

RENAL VEIN THROMBOSIS

Renal vein thrombosis may occur unilaterally or bilaterally. Trauma, extrinsic compression (e.g., tumor, aortic aneurysm), renal cell carcinoma, pregnancy, contraceptive use, and nephrotic syndrome are associated with renal vein thrombosis.

The patient has symptoms of flank pain, hematuria, or fever or has nephrotic syndrome. Anticoagulation is important in treatment because there is a high incidence of pulmonary emboli. Corticosteroids may be used for the patient with nephrosis. Sur-

	ADULT	CHILD
Genetic basis	• Autosomal dominant	• Autosomal recessive
Incidence	• 1 in 500 to 1000	• 1 in 6000 to 40,000
Gene location	• Chromosomes 4 and 16	• Chromosome 6
Genetic testing	• DNA testing available	• DNA testing available
Age of onset	• Third to fourth decade of life	• Infancy or childhood
Clinical implications	• Multisystem involvement	• Up to 30% to 50% of affected newborns die shortly after birth
	• Systemic hypertension occurs in 60% to 80% of patients	
	• Families at risk should be screened	

gical thrombectomy may be performed instead of or along with anticoagulation.

Hereditary Renal Diseases

Hereditary renal diseases involve developmental abnormalities of the renal parenchyma. These abnormalities are either isolated or part of more complex malformation syndromes. The majority of inherited structural abnormalities are cystic. However, cysts may also develop as a result of obstructive uropathies, metabolic derangements, or neurologic diseases. Cysts may be evaluated to rule out any tumor content.

POLYCYSTIC KIDNEY DISEASE

Polycystic kidney disease (PKD) is one of the most common genetic diseases, affecting 600,000 people in the United States.[33] There are two forms of hereditary polycystic renal disease. It may be manifested in childhood or adulthood. The childhood form of PKD is a rare autosomal recessive disorder that is often rapidly progressive (see the Genetics in Clinical Practice box).

The adult form of PKD is an autosomal dominant disorder. It is latent for many years and is usually manifested between 30 and 40 years of age. However, PKD has also been found in newborns. It involves both kidneys and occurs in both men and women. The cortex and the medulla are filled with thin-walled cysts that are several millimeters to several centimeters in diameter (Fig. 44-6). The cysts enlarge and destroy surrounding tissue by compression. They are filled with fluid and may contain blood or pus.

Clinical Manifestations

In the patient with PKD, symptoms appear when the cysts begin to enlarge. A common early symptom of adult PKD is abdominal or flank pain, which is steady and dull or abrupt in onset, as well as episodic and colicky. This pain is often caused by bleeding into the cysts. On physical examination, palpable bilateral enlarged kidneys are often found (Fig. 44-7). Other clinical manifestations include hematuria (from rupture of cysts), UTI, and hypertension.

Diagnosis is based on clinical manifestations, family history, IVP, ultrasound, or CT scan. Usually the disease progresses to end-stage renal failure, although some individuals have relatively mild disease and die from unrelated problems. Loss of kidney function to the point of end-stage renal disease occurs by age 60 in 50% of patients.[33]

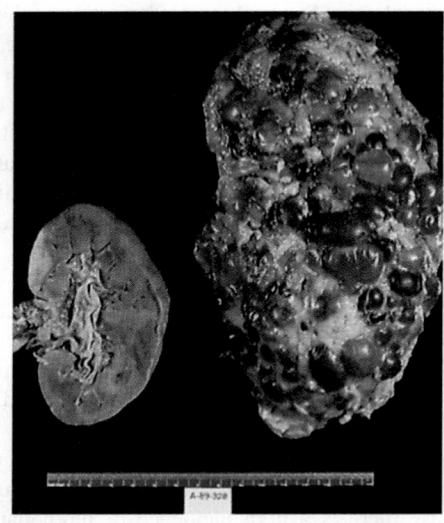

FIG. 44-6 Comparison of polycystic kidney with normal kidney.

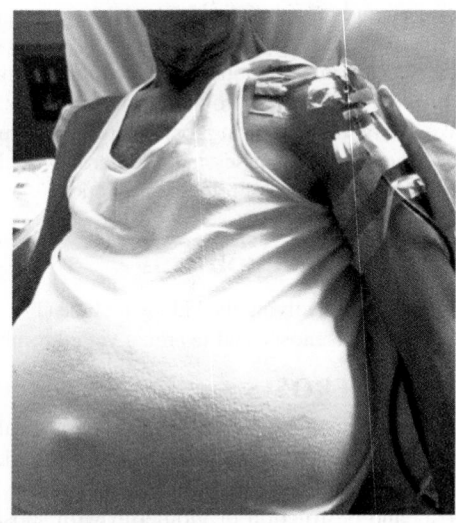

FIG. 44-7 Man with a 24-pound polycystic kidney.

Collaborative Care

There is no specific treatment for PKD. A major aim of treatment is to prevent infections of the urinary tract and/or to treat them with appropriate antibiotics if they occur. Nephrectomy may be necessary if pain, bleeding, or infection becomes a chronic, serious problem.

When the patient begins to experience progressive renal failure, the interventions are determined by the remaining renal function. Nursing measures are those used for management of end-stage renal disease (see Chapter 45). They include diet modification, fluid restriction, drugs (e.g., antihypertensives), assisting the patient to accept the chronic disease process, and assisting the patient and family to deal with financial concerns and other issues related to the hereditary nature of the disease.

The patient who has adult polycystic disease often has children by the time the disease is diagnosed. Each child of a parent with PKD has a 50% chance of having the disease. The patient will need appropriate counseling regarding plans for having more children. In addition, genetic counseling resources should be provided for the children.

MEDULLARY CYSTIC DISEASE

Medullary cystic disease is a hereditary disorder that occurs in two forms. The *autosomal recessive form* is associated with renal failure before age 20; the *autosomal dominant form* is associated with renal failure after age 20. Most cysts are located in the medulla. The kidneys are asymmetric in shape and are significantly scarred. There are defects in the concentration ability of the kidneys. Polyuria, progressive renal failure, severe anemia, metabolic acidosis, and poor sodium conservation are common. Hypertension can be a terminal event. Genetic counseling may be helpful in family planning. Treatment measures are those related to end-stage renal disease (see Chapter 45).

ALPORT SYNDROME

Alport syndrome is also known as *chronic hereditary nephritis*. Two forms of the disease exist: (1) classic Alport syndrome, which is inherited as a sex-linked disorder with hematuria, sensorineural deafness, and deformities of the anterior surface of the lens, and (2) nonclassical Alport syndrome, which is inherited as an autosomal trait that causes hematuria but not deafness or lens deformities.[34] Men are affected earlier and more severely than women. The disease is often diagnosed in the first decade of life. The basic defect is altered synthesis of the GBM. The patient most commonly has hematuria and progressive uremia. Treatment is supportive. Corticosteroids and cytotoxic drugs are not effective. The disease does not recur after kidney transplantation.

Renal Involvement in Metabolic and Connective Tissue Diseases

Various metabolic and connective tissue disease processes may have an effect on renal function. The pathophysiologic effects on the renal parenchyma are not always specific to each process. The clinical course of renal involvement is that of chronic progressive nephropathy, which can result in uremia and death. Management includes treatment of the primary disorder along with symptomatic relief of renal involvement. If renal involvement progresses to end-stage renal disease, management includes dialysis or transplantation (see Chapter 45). Nursing interventions include teaching the patient about the primary disease process, the renal involvement, and the resulting need to comply with dietary and fluid restrictions and drug regimens.

Diabetic nephropathy is the primary cause of end-stage renal failure in the United States. Diabetes mellitus may affect the kidneys in several ways. Microangiopathic changes in diabetes consist of diffuse glomerulosclerosis, involving thickening of the glomerular basement membrane (GBM), and nodular glomerulosclerosis (Kimmelstiel-Wilson syndrome), which is characterized by nodular lesions. Nodular glomerulosclerosis is reasonably specific for type 1 diabetes mellitus. The diabetic patient prone to glomerulonephropathy (e.g., the presence of trace proteinuria or retinopathy) requires careful monitoring of glucose levels and insulin requirements. (Diabetes mellitus is discussed in Chapter 47.)

Gout is a syndrome of acute attacks of arthritis caused by hyperuricemia (see Chapter 63). Monosodium urate crystals deposited in joints are responsible for the syndrome. Renal disease may develop as a result of damage caused by deposition of uric acid crystals in the renal interstitium and tubules.

Amyloidosis is a group of disorders manifested by impaired organ function from the infiltration of tissues with a hyaline substance (amyloid). The hyaline consists largely of protein. Kidney involvement is common in amyloidosis. Proteinuria is often the first clinical manifestation.

Systemic lupus erythematosus is a connective tissue disorder characterized by the involvement of several tissues and organs, particularly the joints, skin, and kidneys. (Systemic lupus erythematosus is discussed in Chapter 63). Clinical manifestations of lupus nephritis are similar to those of other forms of glomerulonephritis. Renal failure frequently occurs in systemic lupus erythematosus and has a poor prognosis.

Systemic sclerosis (scleroderma) is a disease of unknown etiology characterized by widespread alterations of connective tissue and by vascular lesions in many organs (see Chapter 63). In the kidney, vascular lesions are associated with fibrosis. An immune complex mechanism has been postulated as a possible etiologic factor. The severity of renal involvement varies. The patient who develops severe renal lesions has a poor prognosis.

Urinary Tract Tumors

KIDNEY CANCER

In 2002 in the United States 31,800 new cases of kidney cancer were diagnosed and 11,600 people died from kidney cancer.[35] Kidney cancers arise from the cortex or pelvis (and calyces). Tumors arising from both areas may be benign or malignant. However, malignant tumors are more frequent. Renal cell carcinoma (adenocarcinoma) is the most common type. Adenocarcinoma occurs twice as often in men as in women and is typically discovered when the person is 50 to 70 years old. Cigarette smoking is the most significant risk factor for the development of renal cell carcinoma. Other risk factors are obesity and the use of phenacetin-containing analgesics and exposure to asbestos, cadmium, and gasoline.[36]

TABLE 44-14   Robson's System of Staging Renal Carcinoma

STAGE	DESCRIPTION
I	Limitation to renal capsule
II	Spreading to perirenal fat but confined within fascia; includes metastasis to adrenal gland
III	Regional lymph node involvement, tumor thrombus in renal vein or vena cava, involvement of renal vein or vena cava
IV	Presence of distant metastases

There are no characteristic early symptoms. Generalized symptoms of weight loss, weakness, and anemia are the earliest manifestations. The classic manifestations of gross hematuria, flank pain, and a palpable mass are those of advanced disease. The most common sites of metastases include the lungs, liver, and long bones. Local extension of kidney cancer into the renal vein and vena cava is common. Renal cystic disease and renal-associated carcinomas may develop in the patient with end-stage renal disease who is receiving maintenance renal dialysis (see Chapter 45).

Several studies are used to diagnose kidney cancer. IVP with nephrotomography is the primary examination by which most masses are detected and evaluated. Ultrasounds have improved the ability to differentiate between a tumor and a cyst. Angiography, percutaneous needle aspiration, CT, and MRI are also used in the diagnosis of renal tumors. Small renal tumors are found earlier because of the increased use of CT scans and MRI. Radionuclide isotope scanning is used to detect metastases.

Robson's system of staging renal carcinoma is presented in Table 44-14. The treatment of choice is a radical nephrectomy. Radical nephrectomy is the removal of the kidney, adrenal gland, surrounding fascia, part of the ureter, and draining lymph nodes. Radiation therapy is used palliatively in inoperable cases and when there are metastases to bone or lungs. No effective chemotherapy is available for metastatic renal cell carcinoma. Biologic therapy, including α-interferon and interleukin-2 (IL-2), is most promising in the treatment of metastatic disease.[37,38] Side effects of IL-2 include capillary leakage syndrome, fever, chills, fatigue, and hypotension.

BLADDER CANCER

In 2002 there were about 56,500 new cases of bladder cancer and 12,600 deaths related to bladder cancer. Bladder cancer accounts for nearly 1 in every 20 cancers diagnosed in the United States.[35] The most frequent malignant tumor of the urinary tract is transitional cell carcinoma of the bladder. Most bladder tumors are papillomatous growths within the bladder. Cancer of the bladder is most common between the ages of 60 and 70 years and is at least three times as common in men as in women. Risk factors for bladder cancer include cigarette smoking, exposure to dyes used in the rubber and cable industries, and chronic abuse of phenacetin-containing analgesics. Women treated with radiation for cervical cancer and patients receiving cyclophosphamide (Cytoxan) also have increased risk, but the reason is unknown.

Individuals with chronic, recurrent stones (often bladder) and chronic lower urinary infections have an increased risk of squamous cell cancer of the bladder. Patients who have indwelling catheters for long periods can develop these chronic conditions.

Clinical Manifestations and Diagnostic Studies

Gross, painless hematuria (chronic or intermittent) is the most common clinical finding. Bladder irritability with dysuria, frequency, and urgency may also occur. When cancer is suspected, urine specimens for cytology can be obtained to determine the presence of neoplastic or atypical cells. Exfoliated cells from the epithelial surface of the bladder can readily be detected in voided specimens. Other recent urine tests assess for specific factors associated with bladder cancer, such as bladder tumor antigens. Bladder cancers can be detected using IVP, ultrasound, CT, or MRI. However, the presence of cancer is confirmed by cystoscopy and biopsy.

The clinical staging of carcinoma of the bladder is determined by the depth of invasion of the bladder wall and surrounding tissue. The Jewett-Strong-Marshall classification system broadly classifies bladder cancer as superficial (carcinoma in situ [CIS], O, A), invasive (B1, B2, C), or metastatic (D1 to D4) disease. Pathologic grading systems are also used to classify the malignant potential of tumor cells, indicating a scale from well-differentiated to anaplastic categories. Low-stage, low-grade bladder cancers are the most responsive to treatment and are more easily cured.

NURSING *and* COLLABORATIVE MANAGEMENT BLADDER CANCER

Collaborative care of bladder cancer is outlined in Table 44-15.

■ Surgical Therapy

Surgical therapies include a variety of procedures. *Transurethral resection with fulguration* (electrocautery) is used for the diagnosis and treatment of superficial lesions with a low recurrence rate. This procedure is also used to control bleeding in the patient who is a poor operative risk or who has advanced tumors. With this technique the tumor mass is excised by means of a blade inserted through the cystoscope. The remaining portions of the tumor are cauterized.

A second technique, *laser photocoagulation,* is also used to treat superficial bladder cancers. This procedure can be repeated a number of times for recurrence. The advantages of laser include bloodless destruction of the lesion, minimal risk of perforation, and lack of need for a urinary catheter. The primary disadvantage is destruction of the tumor, so pathologic evaluation for grading and staging cannot be completed.

A third technique used is *open loop resection* (snaring of polyp types of lesion) *with fulguration.* It is used for the control of bleeding, for large superficial tumors, and for multiple lesions. Treatment of large lesions entails a segmental resection of the bladder *(segmental cystectomy).*

Postoperative management of the patient who has had any of these surgical procedures includes instructions to drink a large volume of fluid each day for the first week following the procedure and to avoid intake of alcoholic beverages. The patient is taught to self-monitor the urine. It is anticipated to be pink during the first several days after the procedure, but it should not be bright red or contain blood clots. Approximately 7 to 10 days following tumor resection or ablation, the patient may observe dark red or rust-colored flecks in the urine. These are anticipated and represent

TABLE 44-15   Collaborative Care
Bladder Cancer

Diagnostic
History and physical examination
Urinalysis
Intravenous pyelogram
Cystoscopy with biopsy
Cytology studies
Ultrasound
CT scan

Collaborative Therapy
Surgical treatment
   Transurethral resection with fulguration
   Laser photocoagulation
   Open loop resection or fulguration
   Segmental cystectomy
   Radical cystectomy
Radiation
Intravesical immunotherapy
   Bacille Calmette-Guérin (BCG)
   α-Interferon
Intravesical chemotherapy
   thiotepa
   mitomycin (Mutamycin)
   doxorubicin (Adriamycin)
   valrubicin (Valstar)
Systemic chemotherapy

CT, Computed tomography.

scabs from the healing tumor resection sites. Opioid analgesics may be required for a brief period after the procedure, along with stool softeners. The patient can be encouraged to take a 15- to 20-minute sitz bath two to three times a day to promote muscle relaxation and to reduce the risk of urinary retention. The nurse should also help the patient and family cope with fears about cancer, surgery, and sexuality and should emphasize the importance of regular follow-up care. Frequent routine cystoscopies are required.

When the tumor is invasive or when it involves the trigone (the area where the ureters insert into the bladder) and the patient is free from metastasis beyond the pelvic area, a partial or radical cystectomy with urinary diversion is the treatment of choice (see the following section on urinary diversion). A *partial cystectomy* includes resection of that portion of the bladder wall containing the tumor, along with a margin of normal tissue. A *radical cystectomy* involves removal of the bladder, prostate, and seminal vesicles in men and the bladder, uterus, cervix, urethra, and ovaries in women.[39]

■ Radiation Therapy and Chemotherapy

Radiation therapy is used with cystectomy or as the primary therapy when the cancer is inoperable or when surgery is refused. Increasingly, radiation therapy is being combined with systemic chemotherapy. Sometimes combination systemic chemotherapy is used for bladder cancer, usually preoperatively or before radiation therapy, or is used to treat distant metastases. Chemotherapy drugs used in treating invasive bladder cancer include cisplatin (Platinol), vinblastine (Velban), doxorubicin (Adriamycin), and methotrexate.

■ Intravesical Therapy

Chemotherapy with local instillation of chemotherapeutic or immune-stimulating agents can be delivered directly into the bladder by a urethral catheter. Protocols vary, but *intravesical* therapy is usually initiated at weekly intervals for 6 to 12 weeks. The chemotherapeutic agents are instilled directly into the patient's bladder and retained for about 2 hours. The patient's position may be changed every 15 minutes for maximum contact in all areas of the bladder, especially if the tumor occurred on the bladder dome. The use of maintenance therapy after the initial induction regimen may be beneficial.

BCG, a weakened strain of *Mycobacterium bovis,* is the treatment of choice for carcinoma in situ. BCG stimulates the immune system rather than acting directly on cancer cells in the bladder. When BCG fails, α-interferon in addition to BCG may be used. Other treatments that can be used when BCG fails include thiotepa, an alkylating agent, and valrubicin (Valstar), an antineoplastic antibiotic.

Most patients have irritative voiding symptoms and hemorrhagic cystitis following intravesical therapy. Thiotepa (when absorbed into circulation from the bladder wall) can significantly reduce WBC and platelet counts in some individuals. BCG may cause flulike symptoms, hematuria, or systemic infection. Other side effects usually associated with chemotherapy, such as nausea, vomiting, and hair loss, are not experienced with intravesical chemotherapy.

Nursing responsibilities include encouraging the patient to increase the daily fluid intake and to quit smoking, assessing the patient for secondary UTI, and stressing the need for routine urologic follow-up. The patient may have fears or concerns about sexual activity or bladder function that will need to be addressed.[40]

URINARY INCONTINENCE AND RETENTION

Urinary incontinence (UI) is defined as an uncontrolled loss of urine that is of sufficient magnitude to be a problem. Approximately 13 million people living in the United States suffer from UI. Among younger adults, UI affects far more women than men. Estimates of UI prevalence in working older women exceed 50%. In contrast, UI affects 2% to 9% of working older men.[41,42] Although the prevalence of incontinence is higher among older women and older men, it is not a natural consequence of aging. Although UI has traditionally been viewed as a social or hygienic problem, it is now known to affect quality of life, as well as contribute to serious health problems in older adults.[41]

Anything that interferes with bladder or urethral sphincter control can result in UI. Causes may be transient (e.g., caused by confusion or depression, infection, drugs, restricted mobility, or stool impaction). Congenital disorders that produce incontinence include exstrophy of the bladder, epispadias, spina bifida with myelomeningocele, and ectopic ureteral orifice. Acquired disorders are described in Table 44-16. Patients may have more than one type of incontinence.

Urinary retention is the inability to empty the bladder despite micturition or the accumulation of urine in the bladder because of an inability to urinate.[43] In certain cases, it is associated with dribbling urinary leakage called overflow UI. *Acute urinary retention* is the total inability to pass urine via micturition; it is a medical emergency. *Chronic urinary retention* is defined as incomplete bladder emptying despite urination. The postvoid residual volumes in patients with chronic urinary retention vary widely; values of 150 to 200 ml or higher generally require fur-

TABLE 44-16   Acquired Disorders Causing Urinary Incontinence

TYPE AND DESCRIPTION	CAUSES	TREATMENT
Stress Incontinence* Sudden increase in intraabdominal pressure causes involuntary passage of urine. It can occur during coughing, heavy lifting, straining, or laughing.	Condition is found most commonly in women with relaxed pelvic musculature (frequently from obstetric complications or multiple pregnancies). Structures of the female urethra atrophy when estrogen decreases. Prostate surgery for benign prostatic hyperplasia or prostatic carcinoma.	Perineal muscle exercises (e.g., Kegel exercises), weight loss if patient is obese, insertion of vaginal pessary, estrogen vaginal creams, condom catheters or penile clamp, surgery Urethral inserts, patches, or bladder neck support devices to correct underlying problem
Urge Incontinence* Condition occurs randomly when involuntary urination is preceded by warning of few seconds to few minutes. Leakage is periodic but frequent. Nocturnal frequency and incontinence are common. Condition may appear with varying severity during psychologic stress.	Condition is caused by uncontrolled contraction or overactivity of detrusor muscle. Bladder escapes central inhibition and contracts reflexively. Conditions include central nervous system disorders (e.g., cerebrovascular disease, Alzheimer's disease, brain tumor, Parkinson's disease), bladder disorders (e.g., carcinoma in situ, radiation effects, interstitial cystitis), interference with spinal inhibitory pathways (e.g., malignant growth in spinal cord, spondylosis), and bladder outlet obstruction, as well as conditions of unknown etiology.	Treatment of underlying cause, instruction to have patient urinate more frequently or on time schedule, anticholinergic drugs (e.g., propantheline [Pro-Banthine]), imipramine (Tofranil) at bedtime, calcium channel blockers, condom catheters, vaginal estrogen creams
Overflow Incontinence Condition occurs when the pressure of urine in overfull bladder overcomes sphincter control. Leakage of small amounts of urine is frequent throughout the day and night. Urination may also occur frequently in small amounts. Bladder remains distended and is usually palpable.	Disorder is caused by outlet obstruction (prostatic hyperplasia, bladder neck obstruction, urethral stricture) or by underactive detrusor muscle caused by myogenic or neurogenic factors (e.g., herniated disk, diabetic neuropathy). It may also occur after anesthesia and surgery (especially procedures such as hemorrhoidectomy, herniorrhaphy, cystoscopy). Neurogenic bladder (flaccid type) is another cause.	Urinary catheterization to decompress bladder, implementation of Credé or Valsalva maneuver, α-adrenergic blocker (e.g., prazosin [Minipress]) to decrease outlet resistance, bethanechol (Urecholine) to enhance bladder contractions, intermittent catheterization, surgery to correct underlying problem
Reflex Incontinence Condition occurs when no warning or stress precedes periodic involuntary urination. Urination is frequent, is moderate in volume, and occurs equally during the day and night.	Spinal cord lesion above S2 interferes with central nervous system inhibition. Disorder results in detrusor hyperreflexia and interferes with pathways coordinating detrusor contraction and sphincter relaxation.	Treatment of underlying cause, bladder decompression to prevent ureteral reflux and hydronephrosis, intermittent self-catheterization, α-adrenergic blocker (e.g., prazosin [Minipress]) to relax internal sphincter, diazepam or baclofen to relax external sphincter, prophylactic antibiotics, surgical sphincterotomy
Incontinence After Trauma or Surgery Vesicovaginal or urethrovaginal fistula may occur in women. Alteration in continence control in men involves proximal urethral sphincter (bladder neck and prostatic urethra) and distal urethral sphincter (external striated muscle).	Fistulas may occur during pregnancy, after delivery of baby, as a result of hysterectomy or invasive cancer of cervix, or after radiation therapy. Incontinence is found as postoperative complication after transurethral, perineal, or retropubic prostatectomy.	Surgery to correct fistula, urinary diversion surgery to bypass urethra and bladder, external condom catheter, penile clamp, placement of artificial implantable sphincter
Functional Incontinence Loss of urine resulting from problems of patient mobility or environmental factors.	Elderly often have problems that affect balance and mobility.	Modifications of environment or care plan that facilitate regular, easy access to toilet and promote patient safety (e.g., better lighting, ambulatory assistance equipment, clothing alterations, timed voiding, different toileting equipment)

*Patients can have combination of stress and urge incontinence that is referred to as mixed incontinence.

ther evaluation. Even smaller volumes may justify evaluation when they produce bothersome lower urinary tract symptoms or occur in a context of recurring UTIs.

Urinary retention is caused by two different dysfunctions of the urinary system: bladder outlet obstruction and deficient detrusor contraction strength. Obstruction leads to urinary retention when the blockage is sufficiently severe so that the bladder can no longer evacuate its contents despite a detrusor contraction. A common cause of obstruction in men is an enlarged prostate. Deficient detrusor contraction strength leads to urinary retention when the muscle is no longer able to contract with enough force or for a sufficient period of time to completely empty the bladder.

Common causes of deficient detrusor contraction strength are neurologic diseases affecting sacral segments 2, 3, and 4; long-standing diabetes mellitus; overdistention; chronic alcoholism; and drugs (e.g., anticholinergic drugs).

Diagnostic Studies

The basic evaluation for UI and urinary retention includes a focused history, physical assessment, and a bladder log or voiding record whenever possible. Information should be obtained on the onset of UI, factors that provoke urinary leakage, and associated conditions. The nurse should pay special attention to factors known to produce transient UI, particularly when a relatively sudden onset of urine loss is reported.[44] The physical examination begins with an assessment of general health and functional issues associated with urinary function, including mobility, dexterity, and cognitive function. A pelvic examination includes careful inspection of the perineal skin for signs of erosion or rashes related to UI. Local innervation and pelvic muscle strength should also be evaluated. Whenever possible, the patient is asked to keep a bladder log or voiding diary documenting the timing of urinations, episodes of urinary leakage, and frequency of nocturia for a period of 1 to 7 days. This record can be kept by nursing staff if the person is in an inpatient facility.

The urinalysis is used to identify possible factors contributing to transient UI or urinary retention (e.g., urinary infection, diabetes mellitus). A postvoid residual urine must be measured in the patient undergoing evaluation for urinary retention and UI. The postvoid residual volume is obtained by asking the patient to urinate, followed by catheterization within a relatively brief period (preferably 5 to 10 minutes). Alternatively, a bladder scan device can be used to estimate the residual volume. Although less accurate than the catheterized residual measurement, this technique avoids catheterization with its associated discomfort and risk of UTI. Urodynamic testing is indicated in selected cases of UI and urinary retention.[45] Imaging studies of the upper urinary tract (e.g., ultrasound, IVP) are obtained when retention or UI is associated with UTIs or when there is evidence of upper urinary tract involvement.

Collaborative Care: Urinary Incontinence

An estimated 80% of incontinence can be cured or significantly improved. Transient, reversible factors are corrected initially, followed by management of established UI (see Table 44-16). In general, less invasive treatments are attempted before more invasive methods (e.g., surgery) are used. Nevertheless, the choice of initial treatment is highly individualized and based on patient preference, the type and severity of UI, and associated anatomic defects.

Several behavioral therapies may be employed to improve urinary continence. Pelvic muscle training (Kegel exercises) is used to manage stress, urge, or mixed UI. Biofeedback is used to assist the

patient to identify, isolate, contract, and relax the pelvic muscles (see the Complementary and Alternative Therapies box). Strength training is used to improve the efficiency of the sphincter. Neuromuscular education is used to teach patients how and when to contract the pelvic floor muscles to maximize continence. Bladder training or habit training involves rigidly scheduled toileting intervals designed to enhance bladder capacity and reduce the frequency and volume of urine loss. *Prompted toileting* is a behavioral technique used in patients with functional UI. In this case, the patient with impaired cognitive function is regularly reminded to urinate, assisted to the toilet, and offered praise for successful toileting.

COMPLEMENTARY & ALTERNATIVE THERAPIES
Biofeedback for Urinary Incontinence

Clinical Uses
Kegel exercises help to strengthen the pelvic floor muscles. Biofeedback helps to isolate muscle groups in the pelvis.

Effects
Sensors for biofeedback are placed in the vagina or on the skin outside of the vagina. These sensors measure electrical signals produced when muscles contract. Biofeedback training develops an awareness of and control of the pelvic floor muscles.

Nursing Implications
If done correctly, pelvic floor exercise is effective treatment for mild to moderate urinary incontinence and other conditions related to pelvic floor weakness. Unfortunately, many women do not do these exercises correctly. Biofeedback is a tool to make sure that these exercises are done correctly. Most insurance companies cover the cost of biofeedback.

EVIDENCE-BASED PRACTICE
Pelvic Floor Muscle Training for Incontinence

Clinical Problem
Pelvic floor muscle training is a commonly recommended treatment for women with stress incontinence. Is pelvic floor muscle training effective for women with symptoms or urodynamic diagnoses of stress, urge, or mixed incontinence?

Best Clinical Practice
- Pelvic floor muscle training is an effective treatment for adult women with stress or mixed incontinence.
- Pelvic floor muscle training is better than no treatment or placebo treatments.
- Evidence for the effectiveness of pelvic floor muscle training for urge incontinence is inconclusive.

Nursing Implications
- Women who have problems with incontinence should be taught how to do Kegel exercises.
- It is important that patients learn the correct technique for pelvic floor muscle training to avoid squeezing the wrong muscles.
- It is recommended that Kegel exercises be done 5 minutes twice a day, once the correct technique has been established.

Reference for Evidence
Hay-Smith EJC et al: Pelvic floor muscle training for urinary incontinence in women. (Systematic review) Cochrane Incontinence Group, *Cochrane Database of Systematic Reviews*, issue 4, 2002.

Electrical stimulation of the pelvic floor muscles relies on very low-voltage and low-frequency pulses to stimulate muscle contraction and diminish overactive bladder contractions. It can be used as monotherapy for the treatment of urge or mixed UI or in conjunction with pelvic muscle training in the management of stress UI. Minimally invasive electrical stimulation uses a transvaginal or transrectal probe, or a device can be surgically implanted near the pelvic nerve roots.

Drug Therapy. Drug therapy varies according to the UI type (Table 44-17). Drugs have a very limited role in the management of stress UI. α-Adrenergic agonists can be used to increase urethral resistance at the level of the sphincter mechanism. Unfortunately, they exert a limited beneficial effect, and they are associated with adverse effects including exacerbation of hypertension and tachycardia. Drugs play a more central role in the management of urge or reflex UI. Antimuscarinic (also called anticholinergic or antispasmodic) drugs relax the bladder muscle and inhibit overactive detrusor contractions. Two preparations, long-acting tolterodine (Detrol LA) and oxybutynin in a releasing capsule (Ditropan XL) are preferred because of their efficacy and modest incidence of side effects compared with older antimuscarinic agents. Oxybutynin transdermal system (Oxytrol) is a transdermal patch designed to deliver the drug continuously over a 3- to 4-day period.

Surgical Therapy. Surgical techniques also vary according to the type of UI.[46,47] The Marshall-Marchetti procedure involves suspending the urethra and bladder neck by suturing the anterior vaginal wall on each side to the periosteum of the pubic bones and lower rectum through an abdominal incision. The Pereyra procedure and subsequent modifications involve suspending the tissues adjacent to the bladder neck to the abdominal fascia, mainly through a transvaginal approach. Placement of a suburethral sling, using autologous fascia, cadaveric fascia, or a synthetic material, is also used to correct stress UI in women. An artificial urethral sphincter can be used in women or men with intrinsic sphincter deficiency and severe stress UI. Bolsters can also be implanted in men with stress UI to increase urethral resistance. This procedure is technically similar to the suburethral sling surgery often performed in women.

Alternatively, one of several bulking agents can be injected underneath the mucosa of the urethra to correct stress UI in women or men.[48] Bulking agents include glutaraldehyde cross-linked bovine collagen (GAX collagen), small silicone beads (Durasphere), or polytetrafluoroethylene (Teflon). Because of the risk of migration of Teflon particles, GAX collagen or Durasphere injections are most commonly used today. Although treatment with suburethral compounds avoids the risk associated with open surgery, reinjection after a period of several years is typically required.

NURSING MANAGEMENT
URINARY INCONTINENCE

The nurse must recognize both the physical and the emotional problems associated with UI. The patient's dignity, privacy, and feelings of self-worth must be maintained or enhanced. This often

TABLE 44-17	**Drug Therapy** Urinary Incontinence*	
DRUG CLASS AND MECHANISM OF ACTION	**DRUG**
Muscarinic Receptor Antagonists and Anticholinergics Reduce overactive bladder contractions	oxybutynin (Ditropan IR, Ditropan XL) oxybutynin transdermal system (Oxytrol) tolterodine (Detrol IR, Detrol LA) hyoscyamine (Levsin, Levbid) dicyclomine (Bentyl) flavoxate (Urispas) propantheline (Pro-Banthine)
α-Adrenergic Antagonists Reduce urethral sphincter resistance to urinary outflow	doxazosin (Cardura) terazosin (Hytrin) tamsulosin (Flomax)
α-Adrenergic Agonists Increase urethral resistance	Phenylpropanolamine
Tricyclic Antidepressants Reduce sensory urgency and burning pain of interstitial cystitis Reduce overactive bladder contractions	imipramine (Tofranil) desipramine (Norpramin) nortriptyline (Aventyl)
Calcium Channel Blockers Reduces smooth muscle contraction strength May reduce burning pain of interstitial cystitis	nifedipine (Adalat) diltiazem (Cardizem) verapamil (Calan, Isoptin)
Hormone Replacement Therapy Local application reduces urethral irritation and increases host defenses against UTI	Premarin cream Estrace cream EST ring Vagifem

*The type of drug therapy depends on the type of incontinence.
UTI, Urinary tract infection.

includes a two-step approach comprising containment devices to manage existing urinary leakage and a definitive plan of management designed to reduce or resolve the factors leading to UI.

Management includes instructing the patient on consumption of an adequate volume of fluids and reduction or elimination of bladder irritants (particularly caffeine and alcohol) from the diet. The patient is advised to maintain a regular, flexible schedule of urination (usually every 2 to 3 hours while awake). In addition, patients are strongly advised to quit smoking because this habit increases the risk of stress incontinence. Patients should also be counseled about the relationship among constipation, UI, and urinary retention. Aggressive management of constipation, beginning with ensuring adequate fluid intake, increasing dietary fiber, light exercise, and judicious use of stool softeners, is recommended. (The management of constipation is discussed in Chapter 41.)

The nurse should assess strategies the patient uses to contain UI and offer advice concerning alternative devices when indicated. When attempting to manage UI, many women use feminine hygiene pads, and many men and women use household products such as rags, paper towels, or folded toilet tissue. Unfortunately, none of these products are adequately designed to wick urine away from the skin, prevent soiling of clothing, and reduce or eliminate odor. Instead, the nurse should share information on products specifically designed to contain urine. For example, patients with mild to moderate UI often benefit from incontinent pads containing Superabsorbent, a material specifically designed to absorb many times its weight in water. Patients with higher volume urine loss or those with double urinary and fecal incontinence may benefit from disposable or reusable incontinence briefs or pad/pant systems designed for more severe cases.

Several behavioral interventions are used in the management of UI. Habit training or prompted toileting are useful for patients with urge, mixed, and functional UI, respectively. Habit training uses the results of a voiding diary or bladder log to determine patterns of daytime voiding frequency. The patient and nurse then negotiate a goal for voiding frequency, usually ranging from 2 to 3 hours. The patient is taught to schedule rigidly during waking hours according to the baseline urinary frequency identified on the bladder log. At night the person is advised to urinate as normal if awakened from sleep with the desire to void. This interval is increased in a stepwise fashion to the goal negotiated with the nurse, usually over a period of 2 to 6 weeks. Habit training may be combined with pelvic muscle training, focusing on techniques such as urge suppression. Prompted toileting is indicated for patients with altered cognitive function and functional UI (usually coexisting with urge UI). In this case, caregivers are taught to remind the patient to toilet on a regular basis (usually every 2 to 3 hours), and the patient is assisted to the toilet and given praise for successful toileting. A trial of prompted toileting, in conjunction with a urologic evaluation, is used to predict the ultimate success of such a program.

In the hospital, nursing management includes maximizing toilet access. This assistance may take the form of offering the urinal or bedpan or assisting the patient to the bathroom every 2 to 3 hours or at scheduled times. The nurse ensures that patient toilets are accessible to patients and that adequate privacy occurs to allow effective urine elimination.

Collaborative Care: Urinary Retention

Behavioral therapies also may be used in the management of urinary retention.[49] Scheduled toileting and double voiding may be effective in chronic urinary retention with moderate postvoid residual volumes. However, for acute or chronic urinary retention, catheterization may be required. Ideally, intermittent catheterization is used to manage urinary retention. It allows the patient to remain free of an indwelling catheter with its associated risk of UTI and urethral irritation. Despite these potential advantages, an indwelling catheter is preferred in certain cases (e.g., the patient who is unwilling or unable to perform intermittent catheterization). An indwelling catheter is also used when urethral obstruction renders intermittent catheterization uncomfortable or unfeasible.

Drug Therapy. Several drugs may be administered to promote bladder evacuation. For the patient with obstruction at the level of the bladder neck, an α-adrenergic blocker may be prescribed. These drugs relax the smooth muscle of the bladder neck, prostatic urethra, and possibly dual innervated rhabdosphincter, diminishing urethral resistance. Examples of α-adrenergic blocking agents are listed in Table 44-17. They are indicated in patients with benign prostatic hyperplasia, bladder neck dyssynergia, or detrusor sphincter dyssynergia. Finasteride (Proscar) is a 5-α-reductase enzyme inhibitor that reduces prostate size by inhibiting the conversion of testosterone to dihydrotestosterone. Finasteride is also useful for the hematuria that occasionally complicates symptomatic benign prostatic hyperplasia in older men. Bethanechol chloride (Urecholine) is sometimes prescribed to promote contractility in the weakened detrusor muscle.[50]

Surgical Therapy. Surgical interventions are often useful when managing urinary retention caused by obstruction. Transurethral or open surgical techniques are used to treat benign or malignant prostatic enlargement, bladder neck contracture, urethral strictures, or dyssynergia of the bladder neck in selected patients. Pelvic reconstruction using an abdominal or transvaginal approach can be used to correct bladder outlet obstruction in women with severe pelvic organ prolapse.

Unfortunately, surgery plays little role in the management of urinary retention caused by deficient detrusor contraction strength. Attempts to create a bladder stimulator (implanted device capable of stimulating micturition) have proved largely unsuccessful because of the difficulty achieving a coordinated detrusor contraction associated with pelvic muscle and striated sphincter relaxation.

NURSING MANAGEMENT
URINARY RETENTION

Acute urinary retention is a medical emergency that requires prompt recognition and bladder drainage. The nurse should insert a catheter (as prescribed) unless otherwise directed. A catheter with a retention balloon is used in anticipation of the need for an indwelling catheter.

The patient with acute urinary retention (as well as the patient predisposed to these episodes) should be taught strategies to minimize risk, including avoiding intake of large volumes of fluid over a brief period. Instead, the patient is advised to drink small volumes throughout the day. The patient is advised to warm up before attempting urination when chilled and to avoid large volumes of alcohol intake because it leads to polyuria and a diminished awareness of the need to urinate until the bladder is distended. A patient who is unable to urinate is advised to drink a cup of coffee or brewed tea containing caffeine to create or maximize urinary urgency and to sit in a tub of warm water or take a warm shower and attempt to urinate while in the bath tub or shower. The patient can be reassured that he or she can easily bathe immediately following bladder evacuation. If this does not lead to successful urination, the patient is advised to seek immediate care.

Patients with chronic urinary retention may be managed by behavioral methods, indwelling or intermittent catheterization, surgery, or drugs.[49] Scheduled toileting and double voiding are the primary behavioral interventions used for chronic retention. Scheduled toileting is used to reduce rather than expand bladder capacity. In this case, patients are asked to void every 3 to 4 hours regardless of the desire to urinate. This intervention is particularly useful in the patient with chronic overdistention, diabetes mellitus, or chronic alcoholism characterized by a large bladder capacity and diminished or delayed sensations of bladder filling and urgency. Double voiding is an attempt to maximize bladder evacuation. The patient is asked to urinate, sit on the toilet for 3 to 4 minutes, and urinate again before exiting the bathroom.

INSTRUMENTATION

Reasons for urinary catheterization are listed in Table 44-18. Two reasons that are not indications for catheterization are (1) routine acquisition of a urine specimen for laboratory analysis and (2) convenience of the nursing staff or the patient's family. The risks of nosocomial infection are too high to allow catheterization of a patient for the convenience of hospital personnel or family members. Catheterization for sterile urine specimens may occasionally be indicated when patients have a history of complicated urinary infection. These specimens have to be as free of contaminants as possible. A catheter should be the final means of providing the patient with a dry environment for prevention of skin breakdown and protection of dressings or skin lesions.

Urinary catheterization is commonly used in the management of the hospitalized patient. However, it is not without serious risks. The urinary tract is the most common site of nosocomial infections. Urinary catheterization is a major cause of UTIs. Scrupulous aseptic technique is mandatory when a urinary catheter is inserted. After insertion, maintenance and protection of the closed drainage system are major nursing responsibilities. Irrigation of the catheter should not be routinely performed.

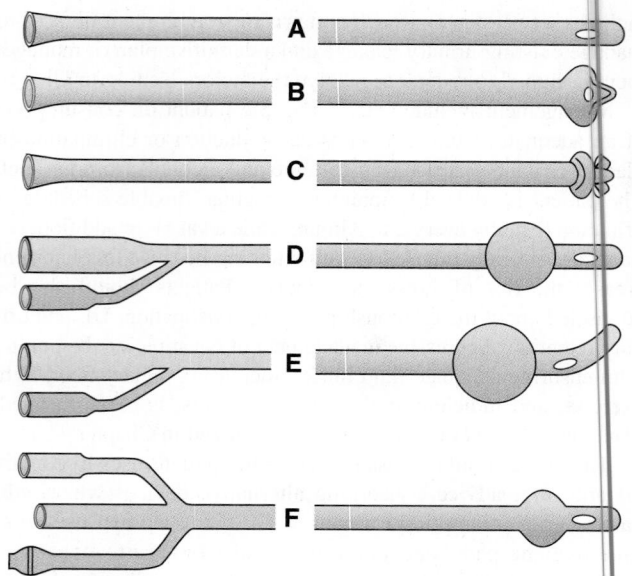

FIG. 44-8 Different types of commonly used catheters. **A**, Simple urethral catheter. **B**, Mushroom or Pezzar (can be used for suprapubic catheterization). **C**, Winged-tip or Malecot. **D**, Indwelling with inflated balloon. **E**, Indwelling with Coudé tip or Tiemann. **F**, Three-way indwelling (the third lumen is used for irrigation of the bladder).

While the patient has a catheter in place, nursing actions should include maintaining patency of the catheter, managing fluid intake, providing for the comfort and safety of the patient, and preventing infection. Attention should be given to the psychologic implications of urinary drainage. Concerns of the patient can include embarrassment related to exposure of the body, an altered body image, and fear concerning the care of the catheter that results in increased dependency.

Catheters vary in construction materials, tip shape (Fig. 44-8), and size of the lumen. Catheters are sized according to the French scale. Each French unit equals 0.33 mm of diameter. The diameter measured is the internal diameter of the catheter. The size used varies with the size of the individual and the purpose for catheterization. In women, urethral catheter sizes 12F to 14F are the most common; in men, sizes 14F to 16F are used. The primary problem resulting from too large a catheter is tissue erosion secondary to excessive pressure on the meatus or urethra. Four routes are used for urinary tract catheterization: urethral, ureteral, suprapubic, and via a nephrostomy tube.

Urethral Catheterization

The most common route of catheterization is insertion of the catheter through the external meatus into the urethra, past the internal sphincter, and into the bladder. Principles that should be considered in the management of the patient with a urethral catheter include the following:

1. The catheterized patient, particularly the person who is ambulatory, should receive appropriate instruction regarding catheter care.
2. A sterile, closed drainage system should always be used in short-term catheterization. The distal urinary catheter and the proximal drainage tube should not be disconnected except for necessary catheter irrigation. Unobstructed down-

TABLE 44-18	Indications for Urinary Catheterization

1. Relief of urinary retention caused by lower urinary tract obstruction, paralysis, or inability to void
2. Bladder decompression preoperatively and operatively for lower abdominal or pelvic surgery
3. Facilitation of surgical repair of urethra and surrounding structures
4. Splinting of ureters or urethra to facilitate healing after surgery or other trauma in area
5. Instillation of medications into bladder
6. Accurate measurement of urinary output in critically ill patient
7. Measurement of residual urine after urination
8. Study of anatomic structures of urinary system
9. Urodynamic testing
10. Collection of sterile urine sample in selected situations

hill flow must be maintained. The collecting bag should be emptied regularly and kept below the level of the bladder. A poorly functioning catheter should be replaced. The leg bag should not be used for the short-term patient in the hospital setting because the risk of bacterial infection is great when the catheter is disconnected and the drainage bags are exchanged.

3. Perineal care (one to two times per day and when necessary) should include cleaning of the meatus-catheter junction with soap and water. Following this, an antimicrobial ointment may be applied. Lotion or powder should not be used near the catheter. The catheter should be properly secured to the leg to prevent movement and urethral traction.

4. Sterile technique must be used whenever the collecting system is opened. Catheter irrigation is performed only when obstruction or blood clots are suspected or, in the case of long-term catheterization, to reduce sediment buildup. If frequent irrigations are necessary in short-term catheterization for catheter patency, a triple-lumen catheter may be preferable, permitting continuous irrigations within a closed system. Small volumes of urine for culture can be aspirated from the distal catheter by means of a sterile syringe and a 21-gauge needle after the drainage tubing is clamped. The puncture site must first be prepared with a tincture of iodine or alcohol solution. Many drainage systems are now equipped with a sampling port. Silicone or plastic catheters do not self-seal. Urine for chemical analysis (e.g., electrolytes) can be obtained from the drainage bag.

5. When the patient is catheterized for less than 2 weeks, routine catheter change is not necessary. For long-term use of an indwelling catheter, regular replacement is necessary. With long-term use of a catheter, a leg bag may be used. If the collection bag is reused, it should be washed in soap and water and rinsed thoroughly. When not reused immediately, it should be filled with ½ cup of vinegar and drained. The vinegar is effective against *Pseudomonas* and other organisms and eliminates odors.

Ureteral Catheters

The ureteral catheter is placed through the ureters into the renal pelvis. The catheter is inserted either (1) by being threaded up the urethra and bladder to the ureters under cystoscopic observation or (2) by surgical insertion through the abdominal wall into the ureters. The ureteral catheter is used after surgery to splint the ureters and to prevent them from being obstructed by edema. The urine volume from the ureteral catheter should be recorded separately from other urinary catheters. The patient is usually kept on bed rest while a ureteral catheter is in place until specific orders indicate that ambulation is permissible. The self-retaining ureteral catheter is often inserted after a lithotripsy procedure or when ureteral obstruction from adjacent tumors or fibrosis threatens renal function. The double-J ureteral catheter is often used and allows the patient to ambulate. One end coils up in the kidney pelvis, while the other coils in the bladder.

The placement of the ureteral catheter should be checked frequently, and tension on the catheter should be avoided. The catheter drains urine from the renal pelvis, which has a capacity of 3 to 5 ml. If the volume of urine in the renal pelvis increases, tissue damage to the pelvis will result from pressure. Therefore the ureteral catheter should not be clamped. If the physician orders irrigation of the ureteral catheter, strict aseptic technique is required. If output is decreased, the physician should be notified immediately. Drainage should be checked often (at least every 1 to 2 hours). It is normal for some urine to drain around the ureteral catheter into the bladder. Accurate recording of urine output from both the ureters and the urethral catheter is essential. Sometimes a ureteral catheter may be used as a stent and is not expected to drain. It is important to check with the physician as to the type of catheter and what to expect.

Suprapubic Catheters

Suprapubic catheterization is the simplest and oldest method of urinary diversion. The two methods of insertion of a suprapubic catheter into the bladder are (1) through a small incision in the abdominal wall and (2) by the use of a trocar. A suprapubic catheter is placed while the patient is under general anesthesia for another surgical procedure or at the bedside with a local anesthetic. The catheter may be sutured into place. The nursing responsibility includes taping the catheter to prevent dislodgment. The care of the tube and catheter is similar to that of the urethral catheter. A pectin-base skin barrier (e.g., Stomahesive) is effective around the insertion site in protecting the skin from breakdown.

The suprapubic catheter is used in temporary situations such as bladder, prostate, and urethral surgery. The suprapubic catheter is also used long term in selected patients (e.g., male tetraplegic (quadriplegic) patient who tends to form penoscrotal fistulas).

A suprapubic catheter is prone to poor drainage because of mechanical obstruction of the catheter tip by the bladder wall, sediment, and clots. Nursing interventions to ensure patency of the tube include (1) preventing tube kinking by coiling the excess tubing and maintaining gravity drainage, (2) having the patient turn from side to side, and (3) milking the tube. If these measures are not effective, the catheter is irrigated with sterile technique after a physician's order has been obtained.

If the patient experiences bladder spasms that are difficult to control, urinary leakage may result. Oxybutynin (Ditropan) or other oral antispasmodics or belladonna and opium (B&O) suppositories may be prescribed to decrease bladder spasms.

Nephrostomy Tubes

The nephrostomy tube (catheter) is inserted on a temporary basis to preserve renal function when a complete obstruction of the ureter is present. It is inserted directly into the pelvis of the kidney and attached to connecting tubing for closed drainage. The principle is the same as with the ureteral catheter; that is, the catheter should never be kinked, laid or leaned on, or clamped. If the patient complains of excessive pain in the area or if there is excessive drainage around the tube, the catheter should be checked for patency. If irrigation is ordered, strict aseptic technique is required. No more than 5 ml of sterile saline solution is gently instilled at one time to prevent overdistention of the kidney pelvis and renal damage. Infection and secondary stone formation are complications associated with the insertion of a nephrostomy tube.

Intermittent Catheterization

An alternative approach to a long-term indwelling catheter is intermittent catheterization.[51] It is being used with increasing frequency in conditions characterized by neurogenic bladder (e.g., spinal cord injuries, chronic neurologic diseases) or bladder outlet obstruction in men. This type of catheterization may also be used in the oliguric and anuric phases of acute renal failure to reduce the possibility of infection from an indwelling catheter. Intermittent catheterization is also used postoperatively, often after a surgical procedure for female incontinence or radioactive seed implantation into the prostate for cancer. The main goal of intermittent catheterization is to prevent urinary retention, stasis, and compromised blood supply to the bladder caused by prolonged pressure.

The technique consists of inserting a urethral catheter into the bladder every 3 to 5 hours. Some patients do intermittent catheterization only once or twice a day to measure residual urine and to ensure an empty bladder. Patients should be instructed to wash and rinse the catheter and their hands with soap and water before and after catheterization. Lubricant is necessary for men and may make catheterization more comfortable for women. The catheter may be inserted by the patient or the care provider. The bladder is emptied and the catheter is removed. The catheter can be dried and placed in a carrying pouch or purse or folded in a paper towel until it is next needed. The same catheter can be used for weeks at a time. In general, patients should change the catheter every 2 to 4 weeks.

In the hospital, sterile technique is used. For home care, a clean technique that includes good hand washing with soap and water is used. There has been no significant increase in infection with the use of an appropriate clean technique as compared with sterile technique. The patient is taught to observe for signs of UTI so that treatment can be instituted early. If indicated, some patients are placed on a regimen of prophylactic antibiotics.

Surgery of the Urinary Tract

RENAL AND URETERAL SURGERY

The most common indications for nephrectomy are a renal tumor, polycystic kidneys that are bleeding or severely infected, massive traumatic injury to the kidney, and the elective removal of a kidney from a donor. Surgery involving the ureters and kidneys is most commonly performed to remove calculi that become obstructive, correct congenital anomalies, and divert urine when necessary.

Preoperative Management

The basic needs of the patient undergoing renal and ureteral surgery are similar to those of any patient who experiences surgery (see Chapters 17 through 19). In addition, it is especially important preoperatively to ensure adequate fluid intake and a normal electrolyte balance. The patient should be told that there will probably be a flank incision on the affected side and that surgery will require a hyperextended, side-lying position. This position frequently causes the patient to experience muscle aches after surgery. If a nephrectomy is planned, the patient must be assured that one working kidney is sufficient to maintain normal renal function.

Postoperative Management

Specific postoperative needs of a patient are related to urine output, respiratory status, and abdominal distention.

Urine Output. In the immediate postoperative period, urine output should be determined at least every 1 to 2 hours. Drainage from various catheters should be recorded separately. The catheter or tube should not be clamped or irrigated without a specific order. The total urine output should be at least 0.5 ml/kg per hour. It is also important to assess for urine drainage on the dressing and to estimate the amount. Daily weighing of the patient is important. The same scale should be used and properly balanced, and the patient should wear similar clothing and dressings each time.

It is important to observe and monitor the color and consistency of urine. Urine with increased amounts of mucus, blood, or sediment may occlude the drainage tubing or catheter.

Respiratory Status. Renal surgery is often performed through a flank incision just below the diaphragm and often involves removal of the twelfth rib. Postoperatively, it is important to ensure adequate ventilation. The patient is often reluctant to turn, cough, and deep breathe because of the incisional pain. Adequate pain medication should be given to ensure the patient's comfort and ability to perform coughing and deep-breathing exercises. Frequently, additional respiratory devices such as an incentive spirometer are used every 2 hours while the patient is awake. In addition, early and frequent ambulation assists in maintaining adequate respiratory function.

Abdominal Distention. Abdominal distention is present to some degree in most patients who have had surgery on their kidneys or ureters. It is most commonly due to paralytic ileus caused by manipulation and compression of the bowel during surgery. Oral intake is restricted until bowel sounds are present (usually 24 to 48 hours after surgery). IV fluids are given until the patient can take oral fluids. Progression to a regular diet follows.

Laparoscopic Nephrectomy

Laparoscopic nephrectomy can be performed in selected situations to remove a diseased kidney. Laparoscopic nephrectomy can also be used to obtain a kidney from a living donor to be transplanted into a person with end-stage renal disease. In contrast to the open incision of about 7 inches (18 cm) required in a conventional nephrectomy, a laparoscopic nephrectomy is performed using five puncture sites. One incision is to view the kidney and another is to dissect it. The laparoscope contains a miniature camera so that the surgeons can watch what they are doing on a video monitor. Once dissected, the kidney is maneuvered into a nylon impermeable sack, and its contents can then be safely removed from the patient. Compared with conventional nephrectomy, the laparoscopic approach is less painful and requires no sutures or staples, involves a shorter hospital stay, and has a much faster recovery.

URINARY DIVERSION

Urinary diversion may be performed with and without cystectomy. Urinary diversion procedures are performed to treat cancer of the bladder, neurogenic bladder, congenital anomalies, strictures, trauma to the bladder, and chronic infections with deterioration of renal function. Numerous urinary diversion techniques and bladder substitutes are possible, including an incontinent urinary diversion, continent urinary diversion catheterized by patient, or an orthotopic bladder so that the patient voids urethrally.[52] Types of these surgical procedures are presented in Table 44-19 and Fig. 44-9.

TABLE 44-19	Types of Urinary Diversion Surgery Requiring Collection Devices			
TYPE	DESCRIPTION	ADVANTAGES	DISADVANTAGES	SPECIAL CONSIDERATIONS
Ileal Conduit	Ureters are implanted into part of ileum or colon that has been resected from intestinal tract. Abdominal stoma is created.	Relatively good urine flow with few physiologic alterations	External appliance necessary to continually collect urine	Surgical procedure is more complex. Postoperative complications may be increased. Reabsorption of urea by ileum occurs. Meticulous attention is necessary to care for stoma and collecting device.
Cutaneous Ureterostomy	Ureters are excised from bladder and brought through abdominal wall, and stoma is created. Ureteral stomas may be created from both ureters, or ureters may be brought together and one stoma created.	No need for major surgery as required with ileal conduit	External appliance necessary because of continuous urine drainage; possibility of stricture or stenosis of small stoma	Periodic catheterizations may be required to dilate stomas to maintain patency.
Nephrostomy	Catheter is inserted into pelvis of kidney. Procedure may be done to one or both kidneys and may be temporary or permanent. It is most frequently done in advanced disease as palliative procedure.	No need for major surgery	High risk of renal infection; predisposition to calculus formation from catheter	Nephrostomy tube may have to be changed every month. Catheter must never be clamped.

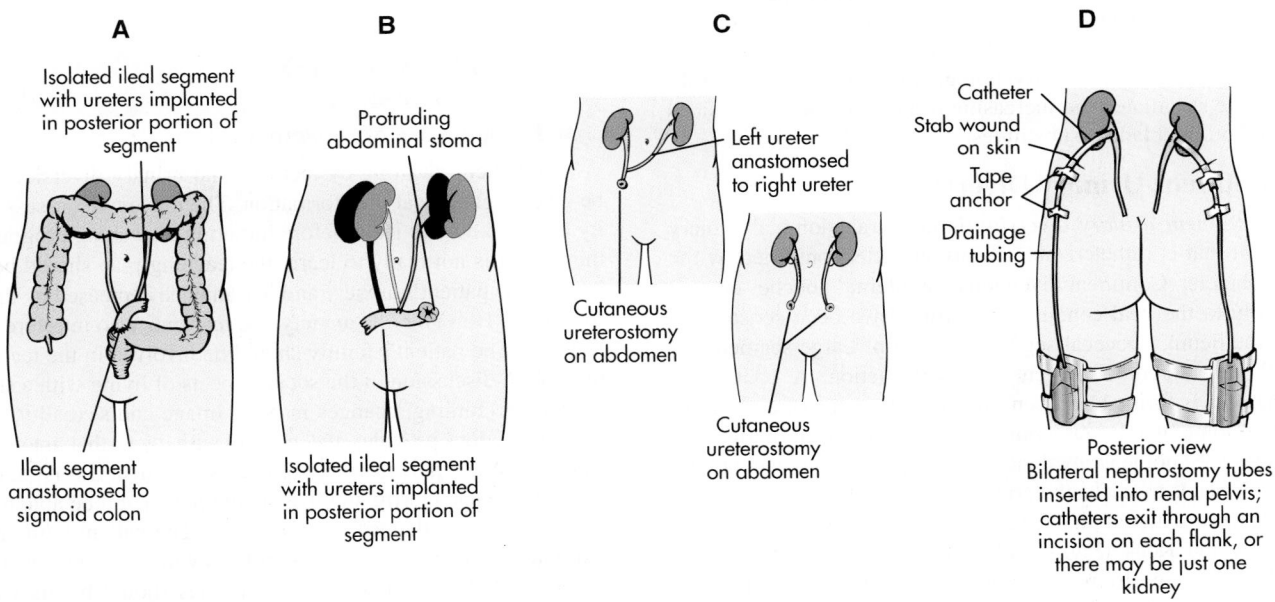

FIG. 44-9 Methods of urinary diversion. **A,** Ureteroileosigmoidostomy. **B,** Ileal loop (or ileal conduit). **C,** Ureterostomy (transcutaneous ureterostomy and bilateral cutaneous ureterostomies). **D,** Nephrostomy.

Incontinent Urinary Diversion

Incontinent urinary diversion is diversion to the skin, requiring an appliance. The simplest form is the cutaneous ureterostomy, but scarring and strictures of the ureter have led to the use of ileal or colonic conduits. The most commonly performed in-

continent urinary diversion procedure is the **ileal conduit** (ileal loop). In this procedure a 6- to 8-inch (15- to 20-cm) segment of the ileum is converted into a conduit for urinary drainage. The colon (colon conduit) can be used instead of the ileum. The ureters are anastomosed into one end of the conduit, and

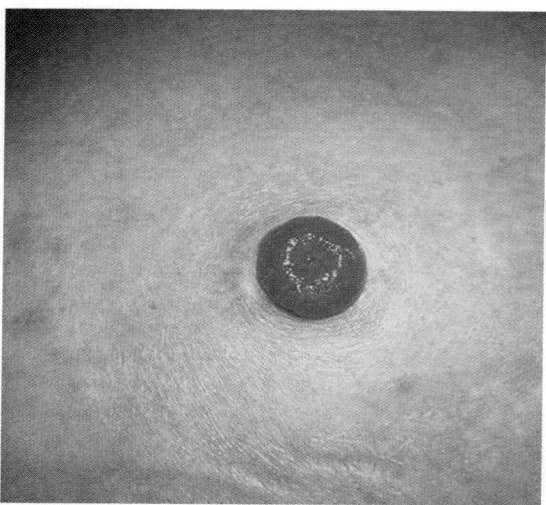

FIG. 44-10 Ideal urinary stoma. It is symmetric, has no skin breakdown, and protrudes about 1.5 cm; the mucosa is a healthy red, and the configuration is flat when the patient is upright and supine.

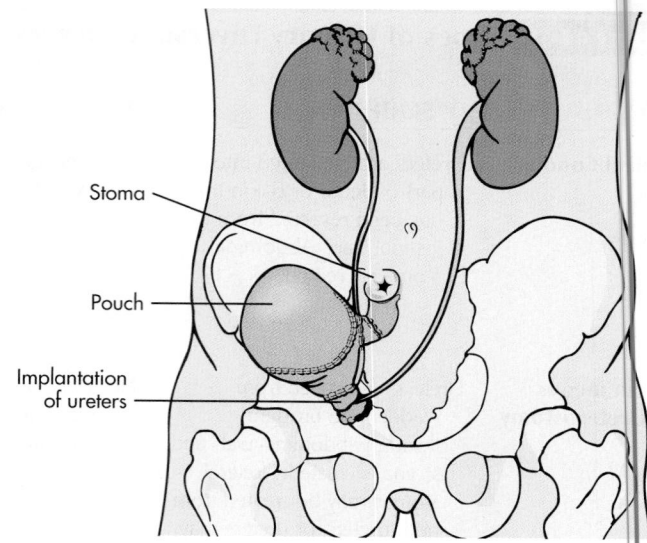

FIG. 44-11 Creation of a Kock pouch with implantation of ureters into one intussuscepted portion of the pouch and creation of a stoma with the other intussuscepted portion.

the other end of the bowel is brought out through the abdominal wall to form a stoma (Fig. 44-10). Although the segment of bowel remains supported by the mesentery, it is completely isolated from the intestinal tract. The bowel is anastomosed and continues to function normally. Because there is no valve and no voluntary control over the stoma, drops of urine flow from the stoma every few seconds, requiring the use of a permanent external collecting device. The visible stoma and the need for external collection devices are obvious disadvantages of this procedure. The lifelong care and dealing with the stoma and collection devices may be psychologically difficult. These problems have stimulated the increasing use of continent diversions and orthotopic bladder substitutes.

Continent Urinary Diversions

A *continent urinary diversion* is an intraabdominal urinary reservoir that is catheterizable or has an outlet controlled by the anal sphincter. Continent diversions are internal pouches created similarly to the ileal conduit. Reservoirs have been constructed from the ileum, ileocecal segment, or colon. Large segments of bowel are altered to prevent peristaltic action. A continence mechanism is formed between this large, low-pressure reservoir and the stoma by intussuscepting a portion of bowel. In this way, a patient does not leak involuntarily. The patient with a continent reservoir needs to self-catheterize every 4 to 6 hours but does not need to wear external attachments. Examples of continent diversions are the Kock (Fig. 44-11), Mainz, Indiana, and Florida pouches. A main difference among the various diversions is the segment of bowel used. For example, the Indiana pouch uses the right colon as a reservoir and has become a popular form of continent urinary diversion.

Orthotopic Bladder Substitution

Orthotopic bladder substitutes can be derived from various segments of the intestines. An isolated segment of the distal ileum is often preferred. Various procedures include the hemi-Kock pouch, Studer pouch, and the ileal W-neobladder. In these procedures the bowel is surgically reshaped to become a neobladder. The ureters and urethra are sutured into the neobladder. Orthotopic bladder substitution has been more commonly done in men because in women the urethra is usually removed when the bladder is resected.[53] The advantage of orthotopic bladder substitution is that it allows for natural micturition. Incontinence is a possible problem with this technique, and intermittent catheterization may be required.

NURSING MANAGEMENT
URINARY DIVERSION

■ Preoperative Management

The patient awaiting cystectomy and urinary diversion must be given a great deal of information. The nurse must assess ability and readiness to learn before initiating a teaching program. If the patient is not ready to learn, the teaching plan should be adjusted. The patient's anxiety and fear may be decreased by the information. However, the anxiety and fear may also interfere with learning. The patient's family should be involved in the teaching process. A discussion of the social aspects of living with a stoma (including clothing, changes in body image and sexuality, exercise, and odor) provides the patient with facts that may allay some fears. The patient who will have a continent diversion must be taught to catheterize and irrigate the pouch and be able to adhere to a strict catheterization schedule. The patient with an orthotopic neobladder may have problems with incontinence. Concerns about the effect on sexual activities should be discussed. The enterostomal therapy nurse should be involved in the preoperative phase of the patient's care. A visit from an ostomate or enterostomal therapy nurse can be helpful. Additional interventions are presented in NCP 44-3.

■ Postoperative Management

Nursing interventions during the postoperative period (see NCP 44-3 for care after an ileal conduit) should be planned to prevent surgical complications such as postoperative atelectasis and shock (see Chapter 19). After pelvic surgery, there is an in-

NURSING CARE PLAN 44-3

Patient with an Ileal Conduit

EXPECTED PATIENT OUTCOMES	NURSING INTERVENTIONS and *RATIONALES*
NURSING DIAGNOSIS	**Anxiety** *related to* effects of ileal conduit on lifestyle and relationships; lack of knowledge regarding surgical procedure, appliance, and its use *as manifested by* frequent questions about surgical procedure, restlessness, inability to sleep.
• Knowledgeable about preoperative, operative, and postoperative procedures, including both stoma and appliance	• Instruct patient in preoperative, operative, and postoperative procedures including diet, drugs, nasogastric tube, IVs, NPO status, pain management, turning, deep breathing, and leg exercises *to reduce anxiety and facilitate patient's progress through postoperative recovery.* • Demonstrate how to apply appliance and use equipment *because knowledge before surgery reduces patient's postoperative concerns.* • Answer questions honestly and provide emotional support *to reduce fear of the unknown and convey a caring attitude.* • Arrange for visit with person with an ileal conduit or with enterostomal therapy nurse *to provide patient with significant information related to ostomy care.*
NURSING DIAGNOSIS	**Risk for infection** *related to* surgical procedure, ureteral obstruction, chronic use of external appliance, and incorrect or inadequate stoma care.
• No urinary tract infection	• Assess patient for elevation in body temperature, pain in back or abdomen, bloody or cloudy urine, decrease in urinary output *to ensure early detection of UTI.* • Empty appliance q2-3hr or when one-third to one-half full of urine *to reduce risk of urinary reflux.* • Use bedside drainage bag at night *to prevent reflux of urine into conduit.* • Instruct patient about symptoms to be reported *as indicators of possible infection.*
NURSING DIAGNOSIS	**Disturbed body image** *related to* effects of change in body function on lifestyle or relationships *as manifested by* negative feelings about self, refusal to look at or touch stoma or participate in self-care, expression of concern about effect on family and lifestyle.
• Acceptance of changes in body image and function	• Encourage patient to share feelings *to provide opportunity to assist with issues and misconceptions and plan appropriate interventions.* • Demonstrate willingness to listen and answer questions *to convey interest in the patient's concerns and to provide needed information.* • Determine the need for additional support (e.g., psychiatric support, visit by an ostomate) *because these persons may provide new information and suggestion of ways to modify lifestyle.* • Encourage gradual involvement in self-care *because independence in self-care helps to improve self-esteem.*
NURSING DIAGNOSIS	**Ineffective therapeutic regimen management** *related to* lack of knowledge regarding stoma and appliance care *as manifested by* expression of concern about how to manage ileal conduit, frequent questions or inaccurate responses regarding stoma care.
• Able to change stoma bag and clean stoma • Able to maintain permanent appliance	• Demonstrate proper method of changing stoma bag and have patient give return demonstration *to teach correct care and evaluate learning.* • Teach measures such as high fluid intake, regular activity, and urine acidification *to prevent urinary calculi and infection.* • Teach practices such as proper stoma and pouch care; empty or change pouch when one-third to one-half full; avoid odor-producing foods such as onions, fish, eggs, cheese; drink cranberry juice or use a liquid appliance deodorant *to enable satisfactory self-care.*
NURSING DIAGNOSIS	**Risk for impaired skin integrity** *related to* ill-fitting appliance, inadequate hygiene, and lack of knowledge regarding stoma care.
• Intact, viable stoma • Clean and intact skin surrounding stoma	• Assess skin for improperly fitted appliance, reddened and irritated skin around stoma *to ensure prompt identification of the problem.* • Check appliance position *to prevent leakage of caustic drainage onto skin.* • Observe stoma for any bleeding or eroded areas *for early identification and treatment of complications.* • Cleanse stoma as ordered *to reduce encrustations and bacterial contact with the stoma and surrounding skin.* • Allow no tight clothing or binders over stoma *to enable unobstructed circulation of blood and flow of urine.*

IVs, Intravenous lines; *NPO,* nothing by mouth; *UTI,* urinary tract infection.

Continued

NURSING CARE PLAN 44-3

Patient with an Ileal Conduit—cont'd

EXPECTED PATIENT OUTCOMES	NURSING INTERVENTIONS and *RATIONALES*
NURSING DIAGNOSIS	**Ineffective sexuality patterns** *related to* perceived or actual effects of surgery on sexual activity *as manifested* by verbalizing concerns about sexuality and unwillingness to discuss sexual issues with partner.
• Satisfaction with sexual practices	• Assess patient's concerns related to sexuality such as future sexual functioning and lack of understanding by significant other *to determine presence and extent of problem.* • Provide accurate information related to sexual activity *so that patient will know the effect of this surgery on sexual activities and practices.*

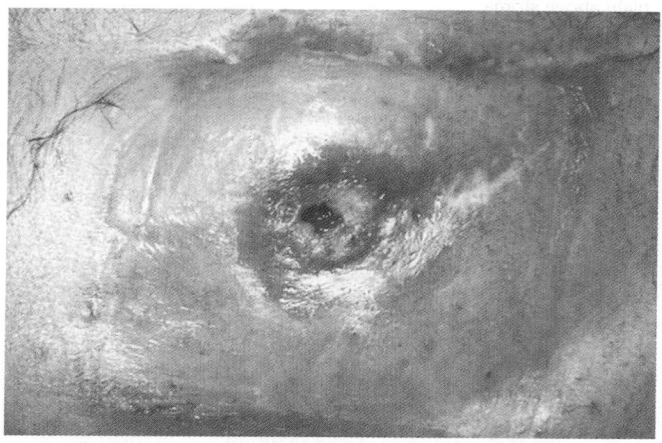

FIG. 44-12 Ammonia salt encrustation secondary to alkaline urine.

creased incidence of thrombophlebitis. With removal of part of the bowel, the incidence of paralytic ileus and small bowel obstruction is increased, the patient is NPO, and a nasogastric tube is necessary for 3 to 5 days.

Specific attention should be given to preventing injury to the stoma and maintaining urine output. Mucus is present in the urine because it is secreted by the intestines as a result of the irritating effect of the urine. The patient should be told that this is a normal occurrence. A high fluid intake is encouraged to "flush" the ileal conduit or continent diversion.

When an ileal conduit is created, the skin around the stoma requires meticulous care. Alkaline encrustations with dermatitis may occur when alkaline urine comes in contact with exposed skin (Fig. 44-12). Other common peristomal skin problems include yeast infections, product allergies, and shearing-effect excoriations. Changing appliances (pouches) is described in Table 44-20. A properly fitting appliance is essential to prevent

TABLE 44-20 *Patient & Family Teaching Guide*
Changing Ileal Conduit Appliances

Temporary Appliance
1. Cut hole in pouch to fit over stoma (pouch 3.2 mm [⅛ in] larger than stoma).
2. Remove old pouch.
3. Clean area gently and remove old adhesive.
4. Wash area with warm water.
5. Place wick (rolled-up 4 × 4–in pad) over stoma to keep area dry during rest of procedure.
6. Dry skin around stoma.
7. Apply tincture of benzoin or other skin protectant around stoma to area where pouch will be placed.
8. Apply pouch by first smoothing its edges toward side and lower portion of body.
9. Remove wick and complete application of bag.
10. If patient is usually in bed, apply bag so that it lies toward side of body.
11. If patient is ambulatory, apply bag so that it lies vertically.
12. Connect drainage tubing to pouch.
13. Keep drainage pouch on same side of bed as stoma.

Permanent Appliance*
1. Keep appliance in place for 2 to 14 days.
2. Change appliance when fluid intake has been restricted for several hours.
3. Have patient sit or stand in front of mirror.
4. Moisten edge of faceplate with adhesive solvent and gently remove.
5. Clean skin with adhesive solvent.
6. Wash skin with warm water. (Patient may shower.)
7. Dry skin and inspect.
8. Place wick (rolled-up 4 × 4–in pad) over stoma to keep skin free of urine.
9. Apply skin cement to faceplate and skin.
10. Place appliance over stoma.
11. Wash removed appliance with soap and lukewarm water; soak in distilled vinegar; rinse with lukewarm water and air dry.

*Many disposable appliances with self-adhesive backing are used as permanent appliances.

skin problems. The appliance should be about 0.1 inch (0.2 cm) larger than the stoma. It is normal for the stoma to shrink within the first few weeks after surgery. The urine is kept acidic to prevent alkaline encrustations.

Acceptance of the surgery and of alterations in body image is needed to ensure the patient's best adjustment. Concerns of the patient include fear that the stoma will be offensive to others and will interfere with sexual, personal, professional, and recreational activities. The patient should know that few activities, if any, will be restricted as a result of the urinary diversion.

Discharge planning after an ileal conduit includes teaching the patient symptoms of obstruction or infection and care of the ostomy. The patient with an ileal conduit is fitted for a permanent appliance 7 to 10 days after surgery and may need to be refitted at a later time, depending on the degree of stoma shrinkage. Appliances are made of a variety of products, including natural and synthetic rubbers, plastics, and metals. Most appliances have a faceplate that adheres to the skin, a collecting pouch, and an opening to drain the pouch. The faceplate may be secured to the skin with glues, adhesives, or adhering synthetic wafers. Some appliances do not require adhesives, but their design relies on pressure to keep the pouch in place. If improperly fitted or applied, the faceplate may cause skin problems (Fig. 44-13). The patient needs information on

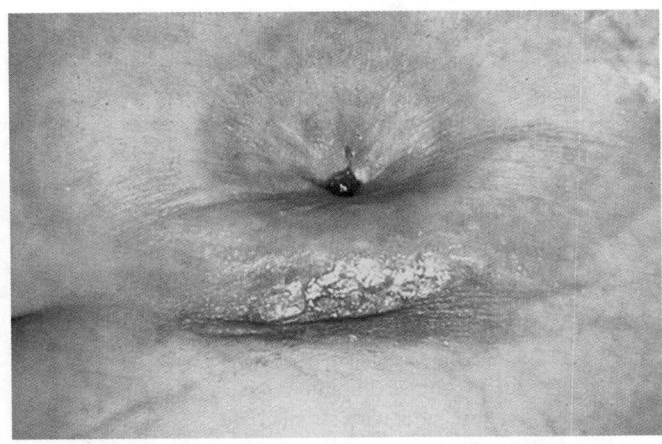

FIG. 44-13 Retracted urinary stoma with pressure sore from faceplate above stoma.

where to purchase supplies, emergency telephone numbers, location of ostomy clubs, and follow-up visits with an enterostomal therapist. Physician follow-up is imperative to monitor and correct homeostatic abnormalities and to prevent complications and renal function deterioration.

CRITICAL THINKING EXERCISES

Case Study
Urinary Tract Infection

Patient Profile. Suzanna, a 28-year-old Hispanic woman, was seen in the nurse practitioner's office for a history of painful, frequent urination.

Subjective Data
- Has had a history of painful, frequent urination with passage of small volumes of urine for 3 days
- Has had intermittent fever, chills, and back pain during these 3 days
- Was frightened when she saw blood in her urine
- Is anxious because her father died of kidney cancer

Objective Data

Physical Examination
- Complains of bilateral flank pain and abdominal tenderness to palpation
- Temperature is 100.4° F (38° C)

Diagnostic Study
- Urinalysis: pyuria and hematuria

CRITICAL THINKING QUESTIONS

1. What are the most common organisms that cause UTIs?
2. What factors predispose a patient to a UTI?
3. What is the difference between upper and lower UTIs?
4. What nursing interventions will help Suzanna cope with her symptoms?
5. What can the nurse do to help Suzanna prevent another UTI?
6. Based on the data presented, write one or more appropriate nursing diagnoses. Are there any collaborative problems?

Nursing Research Issues

1. In the patient with UTI, what are the most effective methods to ensure compliance with therapy and follow-up care?
2. What therapeutic measures are most effective in treating stress incontinence?
3. What are the differences in quality of life of the patient with an ileal conduit compared with the patient with a continent urinary diversion?
4. What are the most effective ways to manage pain following lithotripsy?
5. Does biofeedback improve the effectiveness of pelvic muscle exercises?

REVIEW QUESTIONS

The number of the question corresponds to the same-numbered objective at the beginning of the chapter.

1. In teaching a patient with pyelonephritis about the disorder, the nurse informs the patient that the organisms that cause pyelonephritis most commonly reach the kidneys through
   a. the bloodstream.
   b. the lymphatic system.
   c. a descending infection.
   d. an ascending infection.

2. The nurse teaches the female patient who has frequent UTIs that she should
   a. urinate after sexual intercourse.
   b. take tub baths with bubble bath.
   c. take prophylactic sulfonamides for the rest of her life.
   d. restrict fluid intake to prevent the need for frequent voiding.

3. The immunologic mechanisms involved in glomerulonephritis include
   a. tubular blocking by precipitates of bacteria and antibody reactions.
   b. deposition of immune complexes and complement along the GBM.
   c. thickening of the GBM from autoimmune microangiopathic changes.
   d. destruction of glomeruli by proteolytic enzymes contained in the GBM.

4. One of the most important roles of the nurse in relation to acute poststreptococcal glomerulonephritis is to
   a. promote early diagnosis and treatment of sore throats and skin lesions.
   b. encourage patients to request antibiotic therapy for all upper respiratory infections.
   c. teach patients with APSGN that long-term prophylactic antibiotic therapy is necessary to prevent recurrence.
   d. monitor patients for respiratory symptoms that indicate that the disease is affecting the alveolar basement membrane.

5. The edema that occurs in nephrotic syndrome is due to
   a. decreased aldosterone secretion from adrenal insufficiency.
   b. increased hydrostatic pressure caused by sodium retention.
   c. increased fluid retention caused by decreased glomerular filtration.
   d. decreased colloidal osmotic pressure caused by loss of serum albumin.

6. A patient is admitted to the hospital with severe renal colic caused by renal lithiasis. The nurse's first priority in management of the patient is to
   a. administer narcotics as prescribed.
   b. obtain supplies for straining all urine.
   c. encourage fluid intake of 3 to 4 L per day.
   d. keep the patient NPO in preparation for surgery.

7. The nurse recommends genetic counseling for the children of a patient with
   a. nephrotic syndrome.
   b. chronic pyelonephritis.
   c. malignant nephrosclerosis.
   d. adult-onset polycystic renal disease.

8. The nurse encourages strict diabetic control in the patient prone to diabetic nephropathy knowing that the renal tissue changes that may occur in this condition include
   a. uric acid calculi and nephrolithiasis.
   b. renal sugar-crystal calculi and cysts.
   c. lipid deposits in the glomeruli and nephrons.
   d. thickening of the GBM and glomerulosclerosis.

9. The nurse identifies a risk factor for kidney and bladder cancer in a patient who relates a history of
   a. aspirin use.
   b. tobacco use.
   c. chronic alcohol abuse.
   d. use of artificial sweeteners.

10. In planning nursing interventions to increase bladder control in the patient with urinary incontinence, the nurse includes
    a. restricting fluids to diminish the risk of urinary leakage.
    b. counseling the patient concerning choice of incontinence containment device.
    c. clamping and releasing a catheter to increase bladder tone.
    d. teaching the patient biofeedback mechanisms to suppress the urge to void.

11. A patient with a ureterolithotomy returns from surgery with a nephrostomy tube in place. Postoperative nursing care of the patient includes
    a. encouraging the patient to drink fruit juices and milk.
    b. forcing fluids of at least 2 to 3 L per day after nausea has subsided.
    c. notifying the physician if nephrostomy tube drainage is more than 30 ml per hour.
    d. irrigating the nephrostomy tube with 10 ml of normal saline solution as needed.

12. A patient has had a cystectomy and ileal conduit diversion performed. Four days postoperatively, mucous shreds are seen in the drainage bag. The nurse should
    a. notify the physician.
    b. notify the charge nurse.
    c. irrigate the drainage tube.
    d. chart it as a normal observation.

REFERENCES

1. Moore KN, Day RA, Albers M: Pathogenesis of urinary tract infections, *J Clin Nurs* 11:568, 2002.
2. Warren JW: Practice guidelines for the treatment of uncomplicated cystitis, *Curr Urol Rep* 2:326, 2001.
3. Bjerklund Johansen TE: Diagnosis and imaging in urinary tract infections, *Curr Opin Urol* 12:39, 2002.
4. Bostwick JM: The many faces of confusion: timing and collateral history often hold the key to diagnosis, *Postgrad Med* 108:60, 2000.
5. Graham JC, Galloway A: ACP best practice no 167: the laboratory diagnosis of urinary tract infection, *J Clin Pathol* 54:911, 2001.

6. Gupta K, Hooton TM, Stamm WE: Increasing antimicrobial resistance and the management of uncomplicated community-acquired urinary tract infections, *Ann Intern Med* 135:41, 2001.
7. Nicolle LE: A practical guide to antimicrobial management of complicated urinary tract infection, *Drugs Aging* 18:243, 2001.
8. Schaeffer AJ: Urinary tract infections: antimicrobial resistance, *Curr Opin Urol* 10:23, 2000.
9. Kontiokari T et al: Randomized trial of cranberry-lingonberry juice and Lactobacillus GG drink for the prevention of urinary tract infections in women, *BMJ* 322:1571, 2001.
10. Kincaid-Smith P: Acute pyelonephritis. In Brumfitt W, Hamilton-Miller JMT, Bailey RR, editors: *Urinary tract infection,* London, 1998, Chapman & Hall Medical.
11. Roberts JA: Management of pyelonephritis and upper urinary tract infections, *Urol Clin North Am* 26:753, 1999.
12. Nickel JC: The management of acute pyelonephritis in adults, *Can J Urol* 8(suppl 1):29, 2001.
13. Roberts JA: Management of pyelonephritis and upper urinary tract infections, *Urol Clin North Am* 26:753, 1999.
14. Nickel P, Naher H: Nongonococcal urethritis, *Curr Probl Dermatol* 24:97, 1996.
15. Gray M, Albo M, Hufstuttler S: Interstitial cystitis: a guide to recognition, evaluation and management for nurse practitioners, *J Wound Ostomy Continence Nurs* 29:93, 2002.
16. Eastwood JB, Corbishley CM, Grange JM: Tuberculosis and the kidney, *J Am Soc Nephro* 12:1307, 2001.
17. Watanabe T, Yoshizawa N: Recurrence of acute poststreptococcal glomerulonephritis, *Pediatr Nephrol* 16:598, 2001.
18. Turner AN: Goodpasture's disease, *Nephrol Dial Transplant* 16(suppl 6):52, 2001.
19. Salama AD et al: Goodpasture's disease, *Lancet* 358:917, 2001.
20. Schwarz A: New aspects of the treatment of nephrotic syndrome, *J Am Soc Nephrol* 12(suppl 17):S44, 2001.
21. Bushinsky DA: Kidney stones, *Adv Intern Med* 47:219, 2001.
22. Morton AR, Iliescu EA, Wilson JW: Nephrology: investigation and treatment of recurrent kidney stones, *CMAJ* 166:213, 2002.
23. Wilkinson H: Clinical investigation and management of patients with renal stones, *Ann Clin Biochem* 38:180, 2001.
24. Lindbloom EJ: What is the best test to diagnose urinary tract stones? *J Fam Pract* 50:657, 2001.
25. Blair B, Fabrizio M: Pharmacology for renal calculi, *Expert Opin Pharmacother* 1:435, 2000.
26. Painter D, Keeley FX: New concepts in the treatment of ureteral calculi, *Curr Opin Urol* 11:373, 2001.
27. Colussi G, et al: Medical prevention and treatment of urinary stones, *J Nephrol* 13(suppl 3):S65, 2000.
28. Jenkins AD: Calculus formation. In Gillenwater JY et al, editors: *Adult and pediatric urology,* ed 4, Philadelphia, 2002, Lippincott Williams & Wilkins.
29. Pearle MS: Prevention of nephrolithiasis, *Curr Opin Nephrol Hypertens* 10:203, 2001.
30. Clayman RV et al: Endourology of the upper urinary tract: noncalculous applications. In Gillenwater JY et al, editor: *Adult and pediatric urology,* ed 4, Philadelphia, 2002, Lippincott Williams & Wilkins.
31. Andrich DE, Mundy AR: Urethral strictures and their surgical management, *BJU Int* 86:571, 2000.
32. Valchanov K et al: An unusual cause of acute renal failure: urethral stricture in a female, *Nephron* 87:89, 2001.
33. Igarashi P, Somlo S: Genetics and pathogenesis of polycystic kidney disease, *J Am Soc Nephrol* 13:9, 2002.
34. Tachibana M: Alport syndrome, *Adv Otorhinolaryngol* 56:19, 2000.
35. American Cancer Society: *2002 Cancer facts and figures,* Atlanta, Ga, 2002, ACS.
36. Godley P, Kim SW: Renal cell carcinoma, *Curr Opin Oncol* 14:280, 2002.
37. Tian GG, Dawson NA: New agents for the treatment of renal cell carcinoma, *Expert Rev Anticancer Ther* 1:546, 2001.
38. Fishman M, Seigne J: Immunotherapy of metastatic renal cell cancer, *Cancer Control* 9:293, 2002.
39. Sarosdy MF, Machtens S: Advanced bladder cancer: where are we now and where are we going? *World J Urol* 20:143, 2002.
40. Roodhouse A: Management of bladder cancer: a nursing view, *Prof Nurse* 16:987, 2000.
41. Wells M: Meeting the needs of people with urinary incontinence, *Community Nurse* 6:35, 2000.
42. Miller JA: Urinary incontinence: a classification system and treatment protocols for the primary care provider, *J Am Acad Nurse Pract* 12:374, 2000.
43. Gray M: Urinary retention: management in the acute care setting (part 1), *Am J Nurs* 100:40, 2000.
44. Vickerman J: Thorough assessment of functional incontinence, *Nurs Times* 98:58, 2002.
45. Glazener CM, Lapitan MC: Urodynamic investigations for management of urinary incontinence in adults, *Cochrane Database Syst Rev* 3:CD003195, 2002.
46. Jarvis GJ: Surgery for urinary incontinence, *Best Pract Res Clin Obstet Gynecol* 14:315, 2000.
47. Leng WW, McGuire EJ: Reconstructive surgery for urinary incontinence, *Urol Clin North Am* 26:61, 1999.
48. Kershen RT, Atala A: New advances in injectable therapies for the treatment of incontinence and vesicoureteral reflux, *Urol Clin North Am* 26:81, 1999.
49. Gray M: Urinary retention: management in the acute care setting, part 2. *Am J Nurs* 100:36, 2000.
50. De Wachter S, Wyndaele JJ: Does bladder tone influence sensation of filling and electro-sensation in the bladder? A blind controlled study in young healthy volunteers using bethanechol, *J Urol* 165:802, 2001.
51. Hollander JB, Biokno AC: Clean intermittent catheterization: an update, *Infect Urol* 9:118, 1996.
52. Turner WH, Studer UE: Cystectomy and urinary diversion, *Semin Surg Oncol* 13:350, 1997.
53. Montie JE, Park JM: Orthotopic diversion in women, *Semin Urol Oncol* 15:184, 1997.

RESOURCES

American Urological Association
1120 North Charles Street
Baltimore, MD 21201
410-727-1100
Fax: 410-223-4370
www.auanet.org

Bladder Health Council
American Foundation for Urologic Disease
1128 North Charles Street
Baltimore, MD 21201
800-242-2383 or 410-727-2908
www.afud.org/education/bladder.html

National Association for Continence (NAFC)
PO Box 8310
Spartanburg, SC 29305-8310
800-BLADDER (252-3337) or 864-579-7900
Fax: 864-579-7902
www.nafc.org

Society of Urological Nurses and Associates
East Holly Avenue, Box 56
Pitman, NJ 08071-0056
888-TAP-SUNY or 856-256-2335
Fax: 856-589-7463
www.suna.org

United Ostomy Association
19772 MacArthur Boulevard, Suite 200
Irvine, CA 92612-2405
800-826-0826
www.uoa.org

Wound, Ostomy and Continence Nurses Society
4700 West Lake Avenue
Glenview, IL 60025
888-224-WOCN or 866-615-8560
Fax: 866-615-8560
www.wocn.org

Also see Resources for Chapter 45 on page 1246.

For additional Internet resources, see the website for this book at *http://evolve.elsevier.com/Lewis/medsurg.*

CHAPTER *45*

NURSING MANAGEMENT
Acute Renal Failure
and Chronic Kidney Disease

Mary Jo Holechek

LEARNING OBJECTIVES

1. Differentiate between acute renal failure and chronic kidney disease.
2. Differentiate among the causes of prerenal, intrarenal, and postrenal acute renal failure.
3. Describe the clinical course of reversible acute renal failure.
4. Explain the collaborative care and nursing management of a patient with acute renal failure.
5. Describe the systemic manifestations of chronic kidney disease.
6. Explain the conservative collaborative care and the related nursing management of the patient with chronic kidney disease.
7. Differentiate between peritoneal dialysis and hemodialysis in terms of purpose, indications, advantages and disadvantages, and nursing responsibilities.
8. Describe common vascular access sites used for hemodialysis.
9. Compare dialysis and renal transplantation as methods of treatment for end-stage renal disease.
10. Describe the nursing management of patients in the preoperative, intraoperative, and postoperative stages of kidney transplantation.
11. Discuss the potential long-term problems of the patient with a kidney transplant.

KEY TERMS

acute renal failure, p. 1210	continuous renal replacement therapy, p. 1236
acute tubular necrosis, p. 1211	dialysis, p. 1228
arteriovenous grafts, p. 1232	end-stage renal disease, p. 1217
automated peritoneal dialysis, p. 1230	hemodialysis, p. 1228
azotemia, p. 1210	oliguria, p. 1212
chronic kidney disease, p. 1217	peritoneal dialysis, p. 1228
continuous ambulatory peritoneal dialysis, p. 1230	renal osteodystrophy, p. 1220
	uremia, p. 1210, 1218

Renal failure is the partial or complete impairment of kidney function. There is an inability to excrete metabolic waste products and water, as well as functional disturbances of all body systems. Renal failure is classified as acute or chronic. Acute renal failure (ARF) has a rapid onset. Although ARF is potentially reversible, the mortality rate for intrarenal ARF remains at about 50% despite advances in treatment over the last 30 years.[1]

Chronic kidney disease usually develops slowly over months to years and necessitates the initiation of dialysis or transplantation for long-term survival. The focus in chronic kidney disease has changed from treating a terminally ill patient to caring for a person with a manageable chronic disease that requires long-term care. The change in focus is a result of technical advances, improved surgical techniques, and more effective immunosuppressive therapy.

ACUTE RENAL FAILURE

Acute renal failure (ARF) is a clinical syndrome characterized by a rapid loss of renal function with progressive **azotemia** (an accumulation of nitrogenous waste products such as blood urea nitrogen [BUN]) and increasing levels of serum creatinine.

Uremia is the condition in which renal function declines to the point that symptoms develop in multiple body systems. ARF is often associated with oliguria, which is a decrease in urinary output to less than 400 ml per day. In about 50% of the cases there is normal or increased urinary output. Patients with oliguric ARF have a higher mortality rate.[2]

ARF usually develops over hours or days with progressive elevations of BUN, creatinine, and potassium with or without oliguria. Most commonly, ARF follows severe, prolonged hypotension or hypovolemia or exposure to a nephrotoxic agent.

Etiology and Pathophysiology

The causes of ARF are multiple and complex. They are categorized according to similar pathogenesis into prerenal, intrarenal (or intrinsic), and postrenal causes (Table 45-1).

Prerenal ARF is due to factors external to the kidneys that reduce renal blood flow and lead to decreased glomerular perfusion

CULTURAL & ETHNIC CONSIDERATIONS
Chronic Kidney Disease

- Chronic kidney disease has a disproportionate impact on minority populations, especially African Americans and Native Americans. A history of hypertension and diabetes mellitus is also more common in these high-risk groups.
- The rate of chronic kidney disease is six times higher among Native Americans with diabetes than among other ethnic groups with diabetes.
- The risk of chronic kidney disease as a complication of hypertension is significantly increased in African Americans.
- African Americans live longer and have better outcomes on chronic dialysis than whites.

TABLE 45-1	Common Causes of Acute Renal Failure	
PRERENAL	**INTRARENAL**	**POSTRENAL**

• Hypovolemia
  Dehydration
  Hemorrhage
  GI losses (diarrhea, vomiting)
  Excessive diuresis
  Hypoalbuminemia
  Burns
• Decreased cardiac output
  Cardiac arrhythmias
  Cardiogenic shock
  Congestive heart failure
  Myocardial infarction
  Pericardial tamponade
  Pulmonary edema
  Valvular heart disease
• Decreased peripheral vascular resistance
  Anaphylaxis
  Antihypertensive drugs
  Neurologic injury
  Septic shock
• Decreased renovascular blood flow
  Bilateral renal vein thrombosis
  Embolism
  Hepatorenal syndrome
  Renal artery thrombosis
	• Prolonged prerenal ischemia
	• Nephrotoxic injury
	  Drugs (aminoglycosides [gentamicin, amikacin],
	    amphotericin B)
	  Radiocontrast agents
	  Hemolytic blood transfusion reaction
	  Severe crush injury
	  Chemical exposure (ethylene glycol, lead, arsenic,
	    carbon tetrachloride)
	• Acute glomerulonephritis
	• Thrombotic disorders
	• Toxemia of pregnancy
	• Malignant hypertension
	• Systemic lupus erythematosus
	• Interstitial nephritis
	  Allergies (antibiotics [sulfonamides, rifampin],
	    nonsteroidal antiinflammatory drugs, ACE in-
	    hibitors)
	  Infections (bacterial [acute pyelonephritis], viral
	    [CMV], fungal [candidiasis])
		• Benign prostatic hyperplasia
		• Bladder cancer
		• Calculi formation
		• Neuromuscular disorders
		• Prostate cancer
		• Spinal cord disease
		• Strictures
		• Trauma (back, pelvis, perineum)

ACE, Angiotensin–converting enzyme; *CMV,* cytomegalovirus; *GI,* gastrointestinal.

and filtration. Hypovolemia, decreased cardiac output, decreased peripheral vascular resistance, and vascular obstruction all can decrease the effective circulating volume of the blood. Prerenal ARF can lead to intrarenal disease if renal ischemia is prolonged. Prerenal causes account for approximately 55% to 60% of all cases of ARF.[1]

Intrarenal causes include conditions that cause direct damage to the renal tissue (parenchyma), resulting in impaired nephron function. Intrarenal causes account for approximately 35% to 40% of all cases of ARF.[1] Intrarenal ARF is usually due to prolonged ischemia, nephrotoxins (e.g., aminoglycoside antibiotics, contrast media), hemoglobin released from hemolyzed red blood cells (RBCs), or myoglobin released from necrotic muscle cells. Nephrotoxins can cause obstruction of intrarenal structures by crystallization or actual damage to the epithelial cells of the tubules. Hemoglobin and myoglobin block the tubules and cause renal vasoconstriction. Primary renal diseases such as acute glomerulonephritis and systemic lupus erythematosus may also cause ARF.

Acute tubular necrosis (ATN) is a type of intrarenal ARF caused by ischemia, nephrotoxins, or pigments.[3] Ischemic and nephrotoxic ATN are responsible for 90% of intrarenal ARF cases.[1]

Postrenal causes involve mechanical obstruction of urinary outflow. As the flow of urine is obstructed, urine refluxes into the renal pelvis, impairing kidney function. The most common causes are benign prostatic hyperplasia, prostate cancer, calculi, trauma, and extrarenal tumors. Postrenal causes of ARF account for less than 5% of the cases.[3] Postrenal ARF is almost always treatable if identified before permanent kidney damage occurs.

The two most common causes of ARF are prolonged renal ischemia and nephrotoxic injury, which lead to ATN (Fig. 45-1). Severe renal ischemia causes a disruption in the basement membrane and patchy destruction of the tubular epithelium. Nephrotoxic agents cause necrosis of tubular epithelial cells, which slough off and plug the tubules. Nephrotoxic injury usually leaves the basement membrane intact. ATN is potentially reversible if the basement membrane is not destroyed and the tubular epithelium regenerates.

Possible pathologic processes involved in ATN include the following:

1. Hypovolemia and decreased renal blood flow stimulate renin release, which activates the renin-angiotensin-aldosterone system (see Fig. 43-4) and results in constriction of the peripheral arteries and the renal afferent arterioles. With decreased renal blood flow, there is decreased glomerular capillary pressure and glomerular filtration rate (GFR), as well as tubular dysfunction and, ultimately, oliguria.

2. Ischemia alters glomerular epithelial cells and decreases glomerular capillary permeability. This reduces the GFR, which significantly reduces blood flow and leads to tubular dysfunction.

3. When tubules are damaged, interstitial edema occurs, and necrotic epithelial cells accumulate in the tubules. The debris lowers the GFR by obstructing the tubules and increasing intratubular pressure.

4. Glomerular filtrate leaks back into plasma through holes in the damaged tubular membranes, which decreases intratubular fluid flow.

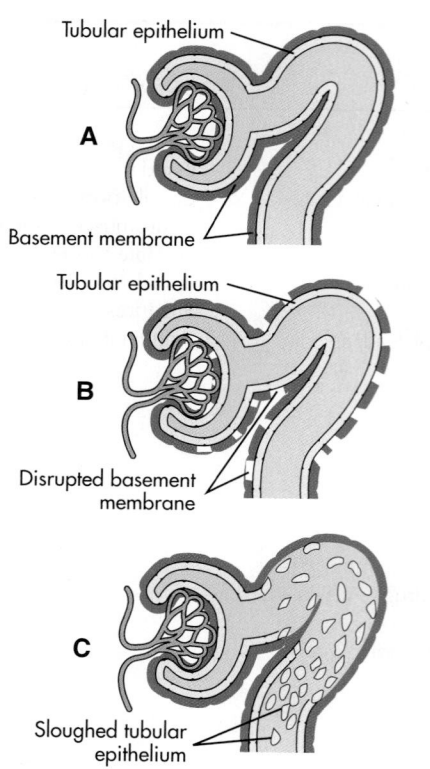

FIG. 45-1 Nephron destruction in acute renal failure. **A,** Normal nephron. **B,** Damage from renal ischemia results in patchy necrosis of the tubule. The lumen may also be blocked by casts. **C,** Damage from nephrotoxic agents.

Clinical Course

Prerenal and postrenal ARF resolve quickly with correction of the cause, but intrarenal disease with ATN has a prolonged course of recovery because actual parenchymal damage has occurred. Clinically, ARF may progress through four phases: initiating, oliguric, diuretic, and recovery. In some situations, the patient does not recover from ARF, and chronic kidney disease results.

Initiating Phase. This begins at the time of the insult and continues until the signs and symptoms become apparent. It can last hours to days.

Oliguric Phase. The most common initial manifestation of ARF is oliguria caused by a reduction in the GFR. **Oliguria** (<400 ml of urine in 24 hours) usually occurs within 1 to 7 days of the causative event. If the cause is ischemia, oliguria may occur within 24 hours. When nephrotoxic drugs are involved, the onset may be delayed for as long as a week. About 50% of the patients will not demonstrate oliguria, making the initial diagnosis more difficult.[3] The duration of the oliguric phase lasts on average about 10 to 14 days but can last months in some cases. The longer the oliguric phase lasts, the poorer the prognosis for recovery of complete renal function.

It is important to distinguish prerenal oliguria from the oliguria of intrarenal ARF. In prerenal oliguria there is no damage to the renal tissue. The oliguria is caused by a decrease in circulating blood volume (e.g., as a result of severe dehydration, decreased cardiac output, burns) and is usually reversible. With a decrease in circulating blood volume, autoregulatory mechanisms that increase angiotensin II, aldosterone, norepinephrine,

and antidiuretic hormone attempt to preserve blood flow to essential organs. Vasoconstriction occurs along with sodium and water retention. Prerenal oliguria is characterized by urine with a high specific gravity (>1.015) and a low sodium concentration (<10 to 20 mEq/L [10 to 20 mmol/L]).

In contrast, oliguria of intrarenal failure is characterized by urine with a normal specific gravity (1.010) and a high sodium concentration (>40 mEq/L [>40 mmol/L]), indicating that the injured tubules cannot respond to autoregulatory mechanisms. In addition, the oliguria of intrarenal failure caused by ATN from ischemia or toxins is characterized by the presence of tubular, RBC, and white blood cell (WBC) casts in the urine. The casts are formed from mucoprotein impressions of the necrotic renal tubular epithelial cells, which detach or slough into the tubules.

The manifestations of the oliguric phase are changes in urinary output, fluid and electrolyte abnormalities, and uremia. The nurse must be alert for the signs and symptoms of these changes.

Urinary changes. Urinary output decreases to less than 400 ml per 24 hours for about 50% of the patients. A urinalysis may show casts, RBCs, WBCs, a specific gravity fixed at around 1.010, and urine osmolality at about 300 mOsm/kg (300 mmol/kg). This is the same specific gravity and osmolality as for plasma, reflecting tubular damage with a loss of concentrating ability by the kidney. Proteinuria may be present if the renal failure is related to glomerular membrane dysfunction.

Fluid volume excess. When urinary output decreases, fluid retention occurs. The severity of the symptoms depends on the extent of the fluid overload. The neck veins may become distended with a bounding pulse. Edema and hypertension may develop. Fluid overload can eventually lead to congestive heart failure (CHF), pulmonary edema, and pericardial and pleural effusions.

Metabolic acidosis. In renal failure, the kidneys cannot synthesize ammonia, which is needed for hydrogen ion excretion, or excrete acid products of metabolism. The serum bicarbonate level decreases because bicarbonate is used up in buffering hydrogen ions. In addition, defective reabsorption and regeneration of bicarbonate occurs. The patient may develop Kussmaul respirations (rapid, deep respirations) to increase the excretion of carbon dioxide. Lethargy and stupor will occur if treatment is not started.

Sodium balance. Damaged tubules cannot conserve sodium. Consequently, the urinary excretion of sodium may increase, resulting in normal or below normal levels of serum sodium. Excessive intake of sodium should be avoided because it can lead to volume expansion, hypertension, and CHF. Uncontrolled hyponatremia or water excess can lead to cerebral edema.

Potassium excess. The serum potassium levels increase because the normal ability of the kidneys to excrete 80% to 90% of the body's potassium is impaired. If the ARF is caused by massive tissue trauma, the damaged cells release additional potassium into the extracellular fluid. Bleeding and blood transfusions cause cellular destruction, releasing more potassium into the extracellular fluid. Acidosis worsens hyperkalemia as hydrogen ions enter the cells and potassium is driven out of the cells into the extracellular fluid.

When potassium levels exceed 6 mEq/L (6 mmol/L) or arrhythmias are identified, treatment must be initiated immediately. Before clinical signs of hyperkalemia are apparent, the electrocardiogram (ECG) will show tall, peaked T waves; widening of the QRS complex; and ST depression. Progressive changes in the ECG, which are related to increasing potassium levels, are depicted in Fig. 16-14. The cardiac muscle is very intolerant of acute increases in potassium.

Hematologic disorders. Several hematologic disorders are seen in ARF. Anemia occurs because renal failure results in impaired erythropoietin production. The anemia may be compounded by platelet abnormalities that can lead to bleeding from multiple sources (intestines, brain). WBCs are also altered, causing immunodeficiency. This leaves the patient susceptible to numerous systemic and local infections. Infection is the major cause of death in ARF.[1]

Calcium deficit and phosphate excess. A low serum calcium level results from decreased gastrointestinal (GI) absorption of calcium. To absorb calcium from the GI tract, activated vitamin D must be present. Only functioning kidneys can activate vitamin D, allowing absorption to occur. When hypocalcemia occurs, the parathyroid gland secretes parathyroid hormone (PTH), which stimulates bone demineralization, thereby releasing calcium from the bones. Phosphate is released as well, worsening the hyperphosphatemia. Elevated serum phosphate levels are also a result of its decreased excretion by the kidneys. Normally plasma calcium is found ionized or free (physiologically active form) or bound to protein. In renal failure it is unusual for hypocalcemia to be symptomatic. The reason for this is that in the acidotic state associated with renal failure, more calcium is in the ionized form rather than bound to protein. However, a low ionized calcium level can lead to tetany.

Waste product accumulation. The kidneys are the primary excretory organs for urea, an end product of protein metabolism, and creatinine, an end product of endogenous muscle metabolism. The BUN and serum creatinine levels are elevated in kidney failure. An elevated BUN level must be interpreted with caution because dehydration, corticosteroids, and catabolism resulting from infections, fever, severe injury, or GI bleeding can also elevate BUN. The best serum indicator of renal failure is creatinine because it is not significantly altered by other factors. Measuring creatinine clearance with a 24-hour urine study or using radioactive tracer is the best method for assessing renal function. But clinically, serum creatinine is most commonly used.

Neurologic disorders. Neurologic changes can occur as the nitrogenous waste products accumulate in the brain and other nervous tissue. The symptoms can be as mild as fatigue and difficulty concentrating and escalate to seizures, stupor, and coma.

Eventually all body systems become involved in the acute uremic syndrome (Table 45-2). The extrarenal manifestations are generally similar to those found in the patient with chronic uremia (see Fig. 45-3 later in this chapter).

Diuretic Phase. The diuretic phase begins with a gradual increase in daily urine output to 1 to 3 L per day, but it may reach 3 to 5 L or more per day. Although urine output is increasing, the nephrons are still not fully functional. The high urine volume is caused by osmotic diuresis from the high urea concentration in the glomerular filtrate and the inability of the tubules to concentrate the urine. In this phase the kidneys have recovered their ability to excrete wastes, but not to concentrate the urine. Hypovolemia and hypotension can occur from massive fluid losses.

At this stage the uremia may still be severe, as reflected by low creatinine clearances, elevated serum creatinine and BUN levels, and persistent signs and symptoms. Because of the large losses of fluid and electrolytes, the patient must be monitored for hyponatremia, hypokalemia, and dehydration. The diuretic phase may last 1 to 3 weeks. Near the end of this phase the patient's

TABLE 45-2	**Manifestations of Acute Renal Failure**
BODY SYSTEM	**CLINICAL MANIFESTATIONS**
Urinary	↓ Urinary output
	Proteinuria
	Casts
	↓ Specific gravity
	↓ Osmolality
	↑ Urinary sodium
Cardiovascular	Volume overload
	Congestive heart failure
	Hypotension (early)
	Hypertension (after development of fluid overload)
	Pericarditis
	Pericardial effusion
	Arrhythmias
Respiratory	Pulmonary edema
	Kussmaul respirations
	Pleural effusions
Gastrointestinal	Nausea and vomiting
	Anorexia
	Stomatitis
	Bleeding
	Diarrhea
	Constipation
Hematologic	Anemia (development within 48 hr)
	↑ Susceptibility to infection
	Leukocytosis
	Defect in platelet functioning
Neurologic	Lethargy
	Seizures
	Asterixis
	Memory impairment
Metabolic	↑ BUN
	↑ Creatinine
	↓ Sodium
	↑ Potassium
	↓ pH
	↓ Bicarbonate
	↓ Calcium
	↑ Phosphate

BUN, Blood urea nitrogen.

acid-base, electrolyte, and waste product (BUN, creatinine) values begin to normalize.

Recovery Phase. The recovery phase begins when the GFR increases, allowing the BUN and serum creatinine levels to plateau and then decrease. Although the major improvements occur in the first 1 to 2 weeks of this phase, renal function may take up to 12 months to stabilize.

The outcome of ARF is influenced by the patient's overall health, the severity of renal failure, and the number and type of complications. Some individuals do not recover and progress to chronic kidney disease. The older adult patient is less likely to recover full kidney function than the younger patient. Among the individuals who recover, the majority achieves clinically normal kidney function with no complications (e.g., hypertension).

Diagnostic Studies. A thorough history is essential for diagnosing the etiology of ARF. Prerenal causes should be considered when there is a history of dehydration, blood loss, or severe heart disease. Intrarenal causes may be suspected if the patient has been taking potentially nephrotoxic drugs or has a recent history of prolonged hypotension or hypovolemia. Postrenal ARF is suggested by a history of changes in urinary stream, stones, benign prostatic hyperplasia, or cancer of the bladder or prostate.

Urinalysis is an important diagnostic test. Urine sediment containing abundant cells, casts, or proteins suggests intrarenal disorders. The urine osmolality, sodium content, and specific gravity help to differentiate the three different types of ARF. Urine sediment may be normal in both prerenal and postrenal ARF. Hematuria, pyuria, and crystals may be seen with postrenal ARF.

To establish a diagnosis of ARF, other testing may be required. A renal ultrasound is often the first test done and provides information about anatomy and function. A renal scan can assess renal blood flow and the integrity of the collecting system. A computed tomography (CT) scan and magnetic resonance imaging can identify masses, collections, and vascular anomalies.

Collaborative Care

Because ARF is potentially reversible, the primary goals of treatment are to eliminate the cause, manage the signs and symptoms, and prevent complications while the kidneys recover (Table 45-3). The first step is to determine if there is adequate intravascular volume and cardiac output to ensure adequate perfusion of the kidneys. Diuretic therapy is often administered along with volume expanders to prevent fluid overload. Diuretic therapy usually includes loop diuretics (e.g., furosemide [Lasix]), bumetanide [Bumex]), or an osmotic diuretic (e.g., mannitol). If ARF is already established, forcing fluids and diuretics will not be effective and may, in fact, be harmful. Conservative therapy may be all that is necessary until renal function improves. The general trend is to initiate early and frequent dialysis to minimize symptoms and prevent complications.

Fluid intake must be closely monitored during the oliguric phase. The general rule for calculating the fluid restriction is to add all losses for the previous 24 hours (e.g., urine, diarrhea, emesis, blood) plus 600 ml for insensible losses (e.g., respiration, diaphoresis). For example, if a patient excreted 300 ml of urine on Tuesday with no other losses, the fluid restriction on Wednesday would be 900 ml.

Hyperkalemia is one of the most serious complications in ARF because it can cause life-threatening cardiac arrhythmias. The various therapies used to treat elevated potassium levels are listed in Table 45-4. Both insulin and sodium bicarbonate temporarily shift potassium into the cells, but it will eventually shift back out. Calcium gluconate raises the threshold at which arrhythmias will occur. Only sodium polystyrene sulfonate (Kayexalate) and dialysis actually remove potassium from the body. Sodium polystyrene sulfonate should never be given to a patient with a paralytic ileus because bowel necrosis can occur.

TABLE 45-3   Collaborative Care
Acute Renal Failure

Diagnostic
History and physical examination
Identification of precipitating cause
Serum creatinine and BUN levels
Serum electrolytes
Urinalysis
Renal ultrasound
Renal scan (as indicated)
CT scan or MRI (as indicated)
Retrograde pyelogram (as indicated)

Collaborative Therapy
Treatment of precipitating cause
Fluid restriction (600 ml plus previous 24-hour fluid loss)
Nutritional therapy
  ▪ Adequate protein intake (0.6 to 2 g/kg per day) depending
    on degree of catabolism
  ▪ Potassium restriction
  ▪ Phosphate restriction
  ▪ Sodium restriction
Measures to lower potassium (if elevated)*
Calcium supplements or phosphate-binding agents
Total parenteral nutrition (if indicated)†
Enteral nutrition (if indicated)†
Initiation of dialysis (if necessary)
Continuous renal replacement therapy (if necessary)

BUN, Blood urea nitrogen; *CT*, computed tomography; *MRI*, magnetic resonance imaging.
*See Table 45-4.
†Renal formulations of these two forms of nutrition are available.

TABLE 45-4   Therapies to Treat Elevated Potassium Levels

1. **Regular Insulin Administration IV**
   Potassium moves into cells when insulin is given. Glucose is given concurrently to prevent hypoglycemia. When effects of insulin diminish, potassium shifts back out of cells.

2. **Sodium Bicarbonate**
   Therapy can correct acidosis and causes shift of potassium into cells.

3. **Calcium Gluconate IV**
   Therapy is given IV and generally used in advanced cardiac toxicity. Calcium raises the threshold for excitation, resulting in arrhythmias.

4. **Dialysis**
   Hemodialysis can bring potassium levels to normal within 30 min to 2 hr.

5. **Sodium Polystyrene Sulfonate (Kayexalate)**
   Cation-exchange resin is administered by mouth or retention enema. When resin is in the bowel, potassium is exchanged for sodium. Therapy removes 1 mEq of potassium per gram of drug. It is mixed in water with sorbitol to produce osmotic diarrhea, allowing for evacuation of potassium-rich stool from body.

6. **Dietary Restriction**
   Daily potassium intake is limited to 40 mEq.

IV, Intravenous.

The most common indications for dialysis in ARF include (1) volume overload, resulting in compromised cardiac and/or pulmonary status; (2) elevated potassium level with ECG changes; (3) metabolic acidosis (serum bicarbonate level less than 15 mEq/L [15 mmol/L]); (4) BUN level greater than 120 mg/dl (43 mmol/L); (5) significant change in mental status; and (6) pericarditis, pericardial effusion, or cardiac tamponade. Laboratory values are only rough parameters, and clinical assessment is the most important guide in determining the need for dialysis.

If dialysis is required, two options are available: hemodialysis (HD) and peritoneal dialysis (PD). HD is the method of choice when rapid changes are required in a short time. It is technically more complicated because specialized staff and equipment and vascular access are required. Anticoagulation therapy may be necessary to prevent blood clotting when blood contacts the foreign membrane material in the dialysis blood circuit. Rapid fluid shifts during HD may cause hypotension. HD is preferred for the hypercatabolic patient and for the individual who has had abdominal or thoracic trauma or surgery. PD is much simpler than HD, but it carries the risk of peritonitis, is less efficient in the catabolic patient, and requires longer treatment times. PD may be preferred for the individual with intracranial bleeding or cardiovascular instability. (HD and PD are discussed later in this chapter.)

Continuous renal replacement therapy (CRRT) may also be used in the treatment of ARF. (CRRT is discussed later in this chapter.) In the hemodynamically unstable patient, CRRT provides gradual removal of excess fluid and solutes. It is technically similar to HD and requires extracorporeal blood circulation via cannulation of two veins or an artery and vein. Blood removed from the artery or vein passes through a hemofilter where solutes and water are removed, and then the blood is returned to the patient. CRRT runs continuously and requires at least 12 to 24 hours to accomplish what can be done with 3 to 4 hours of HD. Larger amounts of fluid may be removed than with intermittent HD. It is the preferred treatment in the hemodynamically unstable patient with mild to moderate ARF with fluid overload.

Nutritional Therapy. The challenge of nutritional management in renal failure is to provide adequate calories to prevent catabolism despite the restrictions required to prevent electrolyte and fluid disorders and azotemia. If the patient does not receive adequate nutrition, catabolism of body protein will occur.[4] This process causes increased urea, phosphate, and potassium levels. Adequate energy should be provided from carbohydrate and fat sources to prevent ketosis from endogenous fat breakdown and gluconeogenesis from muscle protein breakdown.[5] The daily caloric intake should be about 30 to 35 kcal/kg of body weight. Protein intake is generally 1.2 to 1.3 g/kg but can be as high as 2 g/kg if the patient is catabolic.[6] Essential amino acid supplements (e.g., Amin-Aid) can be given for amino acid and caloric supplementation.

Potassium and sodium are regulated in accordance with plasma levels. Sodium is restricted as needed to prevent edema, hypertension, and CHF. Dietary fat intake is increased so that the patient receives at least 30% to 40% of total calories from fat. Fat emulsion IV infusions can also be given as a nutritional supplement and provide a good source of nonprotein calories (see Chapter 39). If a patient cannot maintain adequate oral intake, enteral nutrition is the preferred route for nutritional support (see Chapter 39). When the GI tract is not functional, total parenteral nutrition (TPN) is necessary for the provision of adequate nutrition. The patient treated with TPN may need daily HD or CRRT to remove the excess fluid. Concentrated TPN formulas are available to minimize fluid volume.[7]

NURSING MANAGEMENT
ACUTE RENAL FAILURE

■ Nursing Assessment

An assessment of the patient in ARF includes the specific areas presented in Table 45-2. It is important to monitor the vital signs and intake and output. The urine should be examined for color, specific gravity, glucose, protein, blood, or sediment. The patient's general appearance should be assessed, including skin color, peripheral edema, neck vein distention, and bruises.

If the patient is receiving dialysis, the access site should be observed for signs of inflammation. The patient's mental status and level of consciousness should also be evaluated. The oral mucosa should be examined for dryness and inflammation. The lungs should be auscultated for crackles and rhonchi or diminished breath sounds. The heart should be monitored for the presence of an S_3, other murmurs, or a pericardial friction rub. ECG readings should be assessed for the presence of arrhythmias. Laboratory values and diagnostic test results should be reviewed. All of the previous data are essential for developing a collaborative plan of care.

■ Nursing Diagnoses

Nursing diagnoses and potential complications for the patient with ARF include, but are not limited to, the following:

- Excess fluid volume *related to* renal failure and fluid retention
- Risk for infection *related to* invasive lines, uremic toxins, and altered immune responses secondary to kidney failure
- Imbalanced nutrition: less than body requirements *related to* altered metabolic state and dietary restrictions
- Disturbed thought processes *related to* effects of uremic toxins on central nervous system (CNS)
- Fatigue *related to* anemia, metabolic acidosis, and uremic toxins
- Anxiety *related to* disease process, therapeutic interventions, and uncertainty of prognosis
- Potential complication: arrhythmias *related to* electrolyte imbalances
- Potential complication: metabolic acidosis *related to* inability to excrete H^+, impaired HCO_3^- reabsorption, and decreased synthesis of ammonia

■ Planning

The overall goals are that the patient with ARF will (1) completely recover without any loss of kidney function, (2) be maintained in normal fluid and electrolyte balance, (3) have decreased anxiety, and (4) comply with and understand the need for careful follow-up care.

■ Nursing Implementation

Health Promotion. Prevention of ARF is essential because of the high mortality rate and is primarily directed toward identifying and monitoring high-risk populations, controlling nephrotoxic drugs and industrial chemicals, and preventing prolonged episodes of hypotension and hypovolemia. In the hospital, the factors that increase the risk for developing ARF are advanced age, massive trauma, major surgical procedures, extensive burns, cardiac failure, sepsis, obstetric complications, or baseline renal insufficiency caused by hypertension or diabetes mellitus. Careful monitoring of intake and output and fluid and electrolyte balance is essential. Extrarenal losses of fluid from vomiting, diarrhea, and hemorrhage and increased insensible losses must be assessed and recorded. Prompt replacement of significant fluid losses will help prevent ischemic tubular damage associated with trauma, burns, and extensive surgery. Intake and output records and the patient's weight provide valuable indicators of fluid volume status. Aggressive diuretic therapy for the patient with fluid overload resulting from any cause can lead to inadequate renal vascular perfusion.

Streptococcal infections must be identified and treated with antibiotics. Compliance with the antibiotic regimen is critical to eliminate the source of infection and prevent complications such as acute poststreptococcal glomerulonephritis and rheumatic heart disease.

For the older adult or diabetic patient who is undergoing diagnostic studies requiring intravenous (IV) contrast media, special attention must be given to prevent a nephrotoxic injury secondary to the dye. Adequate hydration before and after the test is critical. Patients with urinary tract infections need prompt treatment and careful follow-up care. Chemotherapeutic drugs that cause hyperuricemia also can put a patient at risk for renal injury.

The individual who is taking drugs that are potentially nephrotoxic (see Table 43-3) must have renal function monitored. Nephrotoxic drugs should be used sparingly in the high-risk patient. When these drugs must be used, they should be given in the smallest effective doses for the shortest possible periods. The patient should be cautioned about the abuse of over-the-counter analgesics (especially nonsteroidal antiinflammatory drugs [NSAIDs]) because some of these may worsen renal function in the patient with borderline renal insufficiency by decreasing glomerular pressure. Angiotensin-converting enzyme (ACE) inhibitors can also decrease perfusion pressure and cause hyperkalemia and are contraindicated in renal insufficiency. Industrial and agricultural chemicals and products (organic solvents, insecticides, cleaning agents) must be monitored regularly to assess their safety for employees and the general population.

Acute Intervention. The patient with ARF is critically ill and suffers not only from the effects of renal disease but also from the effects of comorbid diseases or conditions (e.g., diabetes, cardiovascular disease) that also affect renal function. The nurse must focus on the patient as a total person with many physical and emotional needs. Usually the changes caused by ARF come on suddenly. Both the patient and the family need assistance in understanding that the functioning of the whole body can be disrupted by renal failure but that these changes are generally reversible with time.

The nurse has an important role in managing fluid and electrolyte balance during the oliguric and diuretic phases. Observing and recording accurate intake and output are essential. Daily weights measured with the same scale at the same time each day allow for the evaluation and detection of excessive gains or losses of body fluid (1 kg is equivalent to 1000 ml of fluid). The nurse must be knowledgeable about the common signs and symptoms of hypervolemia (in the oliguric phase) or hypovolemia (in the diuretic phase), potassium and sodium disturbances, and other electrolyte imbalances that may occur in ARF (see Chapter 16). Hyperkalemia is a leading cause of death in the oliguric phase of

ARF. Most typically, hyperkalemia is manifested by arrhythmias and impairment of neuromuscular function including muscle weakness, abdominal cramps, flaccid paralysis, and absence of deep tendon reflexes. Cardiac conduction abnormalities to watch for include a prolonged PR interval, prolonged QRS interval, peaked T wave, and depressed ST segment.

Because infection is the leading cause of death overall in ARF, meticulous aseptic technique is critical. The patient should be protected from other individuals with infectious diseases. The nurse should be alert for local manifestations of infection (e.g., swelling, redness, pain) and systemic manifestations (e.g., malaise, leukocytosis) because an elevated temperature may not be present. Patients with renal failure have a blunted febrile response to an infection (e.g., pneumonia). If antibiotics are used to treat an infection, the type, frequency, and dosage must be carefully considered because the kidneys are the primary route of excretion for many antibiotics. Nephrotoxic drugs (see Table 43-3) should not be used unless there is no other alternative.

Respiratory complications, especially pneumonitis, can be prevented. Humidified oxygen, incentive spirometry; coughing, turning, and deep breathing; and ambulation are measures the nurse can use to help maintain adequate respiratory ventilation.

Skin care and measures to prevent pressure ulcers should be performed because the patient usually develops edema, as well as decreased muscle tone. Mouth care is important to prevent stomatitis, which develops when ammonia (produced by bacterial breakdown of urea) in saliva irritates the mucous membranes.

Ambulatory and Home Care. Recovery from ARF is highly variable and depends on the underlying illness, the general condition and age of the patient, the length of the oliguric phase, and the severity of nephron damage. Good nutrition, rest, and activity are necessary. The diet should be high in calories. Protein and potassium intake should be regulated in accordance with renal function. Follow-up care and regular evaluation of renal function are necessary. The patient should be taught the signs and symptoms of recurrent kidney disease. Measures to prevent the recurrence of ARF must be emphasized.

The long-term convalescence of 3 to 12 months may cause psychosocial and financial hardships for the family, and appropriate counseling and social work and psychiatry referrals should be made as indicated. If the kidneys do not recover, the patient will eventually need dialysis and transplantation.

■ Evaluation

The expected outcomes are that the patient with ARF will
- regain and maintain normal fluid and electrolyte balance
- comply with treatment regimen
- experience no infectious complications
- have complete recovery

■ Gerontologic Considerations: Acute Renal Failure

The older adult is more susceptible than the younger adult to ARF as the number of functioning nephrons decrease with age. Impaired function of other organ systems (e.g., cardiovascular disease, impaired pancreas function) can increase the risk of developing ARF. The aging kidney is less able to compensate for changes in fluid volume, solute load, and cardiac output. Common causes of ARF in the older adult include dehydration, hypotension, diuretic therapy, aminoglycoside therapy, obstructive disorders (e.g., prostatic hyperplasia), surgery, infection, and radiocontrast agents. The prognosis after an episode of ARF is generally worse in the older adult than in the younger person. The mortality rate of ARF is 5% to 25% higher in the older adult than in the younger adult, and death is usually caused by infection, GI hemorrhage, or myocardial infarction.[2] ■

CHRONIC KIDNEY DISEASE

Chronic kidney disease (CKD) involves progressive, irreversible destruction of the nephrons in both kidneys. Among individuals with CKD, the stages are defined based on the level of kidney function (Table 45-5). The last stage of kidney failure (**end-stage renal disease [ESRD]**) occurs when the GFR is less than 15 ml per minute. At this point, renal replacement (dialysis or transplantation) is required. Although there are many different causes of chronic kidney disease (Fig. 45-2), the end result is a systemic disease involving every body organ. (The specific disease processes are discussed in Chapter 44.)

The kidneys have remarkable functional reserve. Up to 80% of the GFR (reflected in creatinine clearance measurements) may be lost with few overt changes in the functioning of the body. A person is born with about 2 million nephrons and can survive without dialysis until almost 90% of the nephrons are lost. In the majority of cases the individual passes through the early stages of CKD without recognizing the disease state because the remaining nephrons hypertrophy to compensate. The prognosis and course of CKD are highly variable depending on the etiology, patient's condition and age, and adequacy of medical follow-up. Some individuals live normal, active lives with compensated renal failure, whereas others may rapidly progress to end-stage renal failure. When the creatinine clearance falls below 15 ml per minute (from the normal range of 85 to 135 ml per minute for the average adult), some form of dialysis or transplantation is required for survival.

In the United States at the end of 2002, over 345,000 individuals with ESRD were being treated for CKD. Of these, more than 245,000 were dialysis patients, and more than 100,000 had a functioning kidney transplant. Over the past 5 years, the number of new patients with kidney failure has averaged about 80,000 annually.

This number of patients with ESRD is expected to reach 660,000 by 2010. Each year about 70,000 people die from causes related to renal failure. At least 40 million Americans are at risk for CKD. In the United States the leading causes of ESRD are diabetes mellitus and hypertension[8] (see Fig. 45-2). In Canada, the primary causes are diabetes mellitus and glomerulonephritis.

In 1973, dramatic legislative changes related to chronic kidney disease occurred when the federal government enacted a law providing financial assistance through Medicare to all eligible persons who had ESRD and required treatment. Under this law, Medicare pays 80% of the cost of health care for ESRD patients who have worked long enough to qualify for benefits.

Since 1973 many deaths have been prevented through the use of maintenance dialysis and renal transplantation. Most patients are treated with dialysis because (1) there is a lack of donated organs, (2) some patients are physically or mentally unsuitable for transplantation, or (3) some patients do not want transplants. With the advancement of medical science, an increasing number of individuals are receiving maintenance dialysis, including the elderly and those with complex medical problems. Every patient with ESRD, regardless of age, should be offered dialysis unless

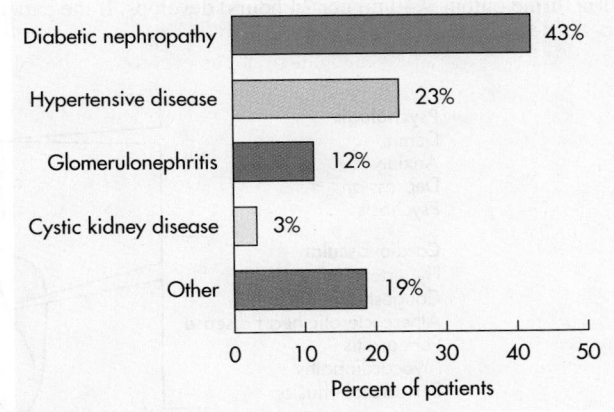

FIG. 45-2 Incidence of primary renal disease leading to end-stage renal disease (United States Renal Data Systems).

TABLE 45-5	Stages and Descriptions of Chronic Kidney Disease*		
	DESCRIPTION	**GFR (ml/min/1.73 m²)**	**ACTION†**
	At increased risk for CKD	≥90 (with CKD risk factors)	Screening CKD risk reduction
Stage 1	Kidney damage with normal or ↑ GFR	≥90	Diagnosis and treatment Treatment of comorbid conditions CVD risk reduction
Stage 2	Kidney damage with mild ↓ GFR	60-89	Estimation of progression
Stage 3	Moderate ↓ GFR	30-59	Evaluation and treatment of complications
Stage 4	Severe ↓ GFR	15-29	Preparation for renal replacement therapy
Stage 5	Kidney failure	<15 (or dialysis)	Renal replacement (if uremia present)

Source: Kidney/Disease Outcomes Quality Initiative clinical practice guidelines for chronic kidney disease: evaluation, classification, and stratification, National Kidney Foundation.
Stages 1 to 5 identify patients who have chronic kidney disease.
*Chronic kidney disease is defined as either kidney damage or GFR <60 ml/min/1.73 m² for ≥3 months. Kidney damage is defined as pathologic abnormalities or markers of damage, including abnormalities in blood or urine tests or imaging studies.
†Includes actions from preceding stages.
GFR, Glomerular filtration rate; *CKD,* chronic kidney disease; *CVD,* cardiovascular disease.

it is medically contraindicated or the patient refuses treatment. If a patient is not covered by Medicare, a variety of state and private programs are available to provide financial assistance.

Clinical Manifestations

As renal function progressively deteriorates, every body system becomes affected. The clinical manifestations are a result of retained substances, including urea, creatinine, phenols, hormones, electrolytes, water, and many other substances. **Uremia** is a syndrome that incorporates all the signs and symptoms seen in the various systems throughout the body in chronic kidney disease (Fig. 45-3). It is important to recognize that the manifestations of uremia vary among patients, according to the cause of the kidney disease, comorbid conditions, age, and degree of compliance with the prescribed medical regimen. Many patients are very tolerant of the changes that occur because they develop gradually.

Urinary System. In the early stage of renal insufficiency, polyuria results from the inability of the kidneys to concentrate urine. This happens most often at night, and the patient must arise several times to urinate (nocturia). Because of the decrease in renal concentrating ability, the specific gravity of urine gradually becomes fixed at around 1.010 (the osmolar concentration of plasma). As CKD worsens, oliguria develops and eventually anuria (urine output <40 ml per 24 hours) develops. If the patient is still producing urine, proteinuria, casts, pyuria, and hematuria could be present depending on the cause of the kidney disease.

Metabolic Disturbances

Waste product accumulation. As the GFR decreases, the BUN and serum creatinine levels increase. The BUN is increased not only by the kidney failure but also by protein intake, fever, corticosteroids, and catabolism. For this reason, serum creatinine and creatinine clearance determinations are considered more accurate indicators of kidney function than BUN. As the BUN increases, nausea, vomiting, lethargy, fatigue, impaired thought processes, and headaches become common as a result of the presence of waste products in the CNS and GI tissues.

The serum creatinine level in an older adult patient with ESRD will be lower than in a younger person with the same degree of renal dysfunction. Decreased muscle mass and decreased muscle activity from aging account for this finding because creatinine is an end product of muscle metabolism.

Altered carbohydrate metabolism. Defective carbohydrate metabolism is caused by impaired glucose use resulting from cellular insensitivity to the normal action of insulin. The exact nature of this insulin resistance is unclear, but it may be related to circulating insulin antagonists, alterations in hormone receptors, or abnormalities of transport mechanisms. Moderate hyperglycemia, hyperinsulinemia, and abnormal glucose tolerance

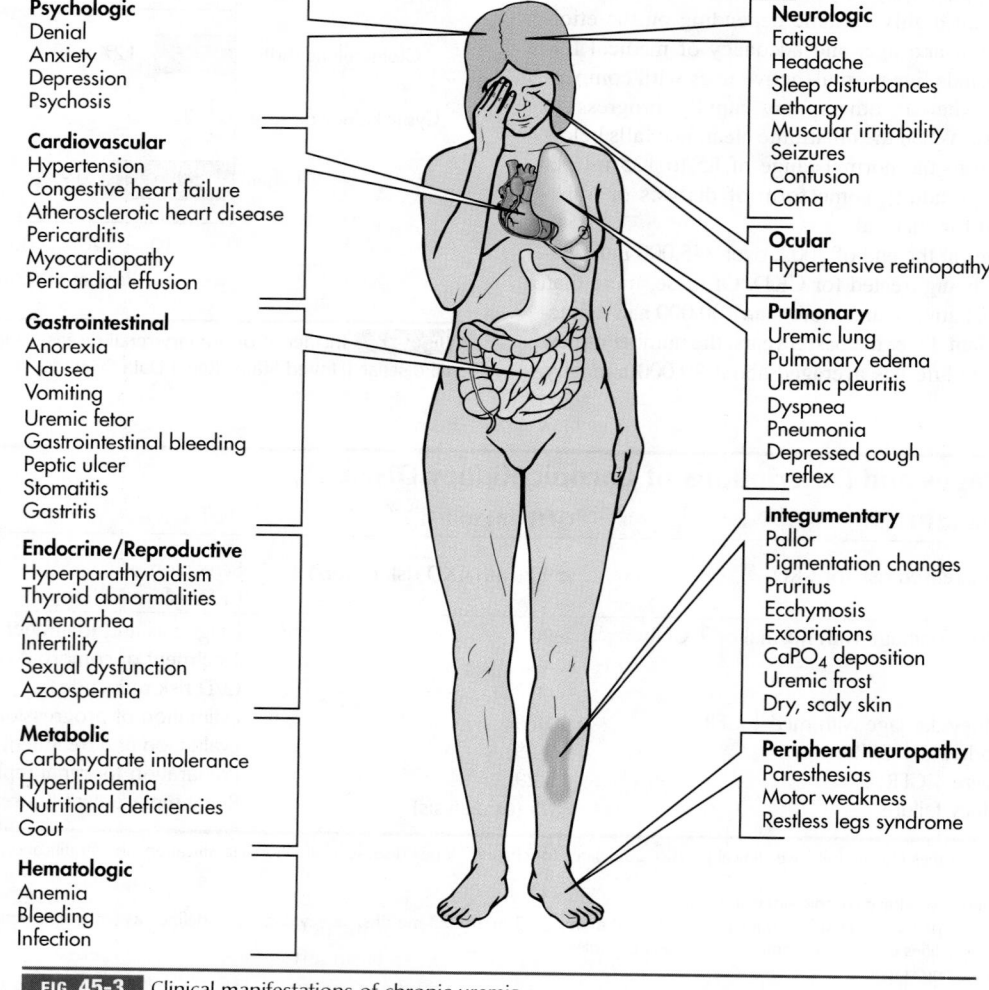

Psychologic
Denial
Anxiety
Depression
Psychosis

Cardiovascular
Hypertension
Congestive heart failure
Atherosclerotic heart disease
Pericarditis
Myocardiopathy
Pericardial effusion

Gastrointestinal
Anorexia
Nausea
Vomiting
Uremic fetor
Gastrointestinal bleeding
Peptic ulcer
Stomatitis
Gastritis

Endocrine/Reproductive
Hyperparathyroidism
Thyroid abnormalities
Amenorrhea
Infertility
Sexual dysfunction
Azoospermia

Metabolic
Carbohydrate intolerance
Hyperlipidemia
Nutritional deficiencies
Gout

Hematologic
Anemia
Bleeding
Infection

Neurologic
Fatigue
Headache
Sleep disturbances
Lethargy
Muscular irritability
Seizures
Confusion
Coma

Ocular
Hypertensive retinopathy

Pulmonary
Uremic lung
Pulmonary edema
Uremic pleuritis
Dyspnea
Pneumonia
Depressed cough
  reflex

Integumentary
Pallor
Pigmentation changes
Pruritus
Ecchymosis
Excoriations
$CaPO_4$ deposition
Uremic frost
Dry, scaly skin

Peripheral neuropathy
Paresthesias
Motor weakness
Restless legs syndrome

FIG. 45-3 Clinical manifestations of chronic uremia.

tests may be seen. Insulin and glucose metabolism may improve (but not to normal values) after the initiation of dialysis.

Diabetics who become uremic may require less insulin than before the onset of chronic kidney disease. This is because insulin, which is dependent on the kidneys for excretion, remains in circulation longer. The insulin dosing must be individualized and glucose levels monitored carefully.

Elevated triglycerides. Hyperinsulinemia stimulates hepatic production of triglycerides. Almost all patients with uremia develop hyperlipidemia, with elevated very-low-density lipoproteins (VLDLs), normal or decreased low-density lipoproteins (LDLs), and lowered high-density lipoproteins (HDLs). The reason for the altered lipid metabolism is related to decreased levels of the enzyme lipoprotein lipase that is important in the breakdown of lipoproteins. Hyperlipidemia is a definite risk factor for accelerated atherosclerosis (see Chapter 33). This can worsen atherosclerotic changes in diabetics with ESRD.

The serum level of triglycerides does not usually decrease after dialysis is started. For patients receiving chronic PD, the level frequently becomes higher as a result of the increased amounts of glucose absorbed from the peritoneal dialysate fluid. Elevated glucose levels lead to increased insulin levels. Insulin stimulates the liver to produce triglycerides.

Electrolyte and Acid-Base Imbalances

Potassium. Hyperkalemia is the most serious electrolyte disorder associated with kidney disease. Fatal arrhythmias can occur when the serum potassium level reaches 7 to 8 mEq/L (7 to 8 mmol/L). Hyperkalemia results from the decreased excretion by the kidneys, the breakdown of cellular protein, bleeding, and metabolic acidosis. Potassium may also come from the food consumed, dietary supplements, drugs, and IV infusions.

Sodium. Sodium may be normal or low in renal failure. Because of impaired sodium excretion, sodium along with water is retained. If large quantities of body water are retained, dilutional hyponatremia occurs. Sodium retention can contribute to edema, hypertension, and congestive heart failure. Sodium intake must be individually determined but is generally restricted to 2 g per 24 hours.

Calcium and phosphate. Calcium and phosphate alterations are discussed in the section on ARF (p. 1213) and in the section on the musculoskeletal system (p. 1220).

Magnesium. Magnesium is primarily excreted by the kidneys. Hypermagnesemia is generally not a problem unless the patient is ingesting magnesium (e.g., milk of magnesia, magnesium citrate, antacids containing magnesium). Clinical manifestations of hypermagnesemia can include absence of reflexes, decreased mental status, cardiac arrhythmias, hypotension, and respiratory failure.

Metabolic acidosis. Metabolic acidosis results from the impaired ability of the kidneys to excrete the acid load (primarily ammonia) and from defective reabsorption and regeneration of bicarbonate. The average adult produces 80 to 90 mEq of acid per day. In renal failure, plasma bicarbonate, which is an indirect measure of acidosis, usually falls to a new steady state at around 16 to 20 mEq/L (16 to 20 mmol/L). It generally does not progress below this level because hydrogen ion production is usually balanced by buffering from demineralization of the bone (the phosphate buffering system). Although Kussmaul respiration is uncommon in CRF, this breathing pattern reduces the severity of acidosis by increasing carbon dioxide excretion.

Hematologic System

Anemia. The anemia associated with CKD is classified as normocytic, normochromic. It is due to decreased production of the hormone erythropoietin by the kidneys, resulting in decreased erythropoiesis by the bone marrow.[9] Erythropoietin stimulates precursor cells in the bone marrow to produce RBCs. Other factors contributing to anemia are nutritional deficiencies, decreased RBC life span, increased hemolysis of RBCs, frequent blood samplings, and bleeding from the GI tract. For patients receiving maintenance HD, blood loss in the dialyzer may also contribute to the anemic state. Elevated levels of PTH (produced to compensate for low serum calcium levels) can inhibit erythropoiesis, shorten survival of RBCs, and cause bone marrow fibrosis, which can result in decreased numbers of hematopoietic cells.

Sufficient iron stores are needed for erythropoiesis. Many patients with renal failure are iron deficient and require iron replacement. Folic acid, which is essential for RBC maturation, is dialyzable. If it is not adequately replaced in the diet or by drugs, megaloblastic anemia may develop in a patient receiving chronic HD.

Bleeding tendencies. The most common cause of bleeding in uremia is a qualitative defect in platelet function. This dysfunction is caused by impaired platelet aggregation and impaired release of platelet factor 3. In addition, alterations in the coagulation system with increased concentrations of both factor VIII and fibrinogen are found in the serum of these patients. The altered platelet function, hemorrhagic tendencies, and GI bleeding can usually be corrected with regular HD or PD.

Infection. Infectious complications are caused by changes in leukocyte function and altered immune response and function. There is a diminished inflammatory response because of an altered chemotactic response by both neutrophils and monocytes. This impairment significantly decreases the accumulation of WBCs at the site of injury or infection. Both cellular and humoral immune responses are suppressed. Characteristic clinical findings include lymphopenia, lymphoid tissue atrophy (especially of the thymus), decreased antibody production, and suppression of the delayed hypersensitivity response. Other factors contributing to the increased risk of infection include malnutrition, hyperglycemia, and external trauma (e.g., catheters, needle insertions into vascular access sites).

Increased incidence of cancer. There is a significant increase in the incidence of neoplasms in the patient with renal failure who has not had a transplant compared with the general population. Lung, breast, uterus, colon, prostate, and skin malignancies are most commonly found.

Cardiovascular System.
The most common cardiovascular abnormality is hypertension, which usually exists pre-ESRD and is worsened by sodium retention and increased extracellular fluid volume. In some individuals, increased renin production contributes to the problem (see Fig. 43-4). Hypertension accelerates atherosclerotic vascular disease, produces intrarenal arterial spasm, and eventually leads to left ventricular hypertrophy and congestive heart failure.[10] Hypertension also causes retinopathy, encephalopathy, and nephropathy.

The vascular changes from long-standing hypertension and the accelerated atherosclerosis from elevated triglyceride levels are responsible for many cardiovascular complications (e.g., myocardial infarction, stroke). These are leading causes of death for patients receiving chronic dialysis. Diabetes mellitus is a major risk factor for the development of vascular problems.

CHF from left ventricular hypertrophy can lead to pulmonary edema. Peripheral edema is often present. Cardiac arrhythmias may result from hyperkalemia, hypocalcemia, and decreased coronary artery perfusion.

Uremic pericarditis can develop and occasionally progresses to pericardial effusion and cardiac tamponade. Pericarditis is manifested by a friction rub, chest pain, and low-grade fever.

Respiratory System. Respiratory changes include Kussmaul respiration, dyspnea from fluid overload, pulmonary edema, uremic pleuritis (pleurisy), pleural effusion, and a predisposition to respiratory infections, which may be related to decreased pulmonary macrophage activity. The sputum is thick and tenacious. The cough reflex is depressed. "Uremic lung," or uremic pneumonitis, is typically found in CKD and shows up as interstitial edema on chest x-ray. This condition usually responds to vigorous fluid removal during dialysis treatments.

Gastrointestinal System. Every part of the GI system is affected as a result of inflammation of the mucosa caused by excessive urea. Mucosal ulcerations, found throughout the GI tract, are caused by the increased ammonia produced by bacterial breakdown of urea. Stomatitis with exudates and ulcerations, a metallic taste in the mouth, and *uremic fetor* (a urinous odor of the breath) are commonly found. Anorexia, nausea, and vomiting caused by irritation of the GI tract by waste products contribute to weight loss and malnutrition. Diabetic gastroparesis can compound these problems for patients with diabetes. GI bleeding is also a risk because of irritation of the mucosa by waste products coupled with the platelet defect. Diarrhea may occur because of hyperkalemia and altered calcium metabolism. Constipation may be due to the ingestion of iron salts and/or calcium-containing phosphate binders. Constipation can be made worse by the limited fluid intake and inactivity.

Neurologic System. Neurologic changes are expected as renal failure progresses. They are attributed to increased nitrogenous waste products, electrolyte imbalances, metabolic acidosis, and axonal atrophy and demyelination of nerve fibers.[11] High levels of uremic toxins have been implicated in axonal damage.

In renal failure a general depression of the CNS results in lethargy, apathy, decreased ability to concentrate, fatigue, irritability, and altered mental ability. Seizures and coma may result from a rapidly increasing BUN and hypertensive encephalopathy. Dialysis encephalopathy (dialysis dementia), a progressive neurologic impairment associated with aluminum toxicity, is characterized by speech disturbances, dementia, lack of muscle coordination, and myoclonic seizures. Aluminum toxicity is now uncommon as aluminum-based drugs have been replaced.

Peripheral neuropathy is initially manifested by a slowing of nerve conduction to the extremities. The patient complains of restless legs syndrome and may describe it as "bugs crawling inside the leg." Paresthesias are most often in the feet and legs and may be described by the patient as a burning sensation. Eventually, motor involvement may lead to bilateral foot drop, muscular weakness and atrophy, and loss of deep tendon reflexes. Muscle twitching, jerking, *asterixis* (hand-flapping tremor), and nocturnal leg cramps also occur. In patients with diabetes, uremic neuropathy is compounded by the neuropathy associated with diabetes mellitus.

The treatment for neurologic problems is dialysis or transplantation. Altered mental status is often the signal that dialysis must be initiated. Dialysis should improve the general CNS symptoms and may slow or halt the progression of neuropathies. However, motor neuropathy may not be reversible.

Musculoskeletal System. **Renal osteodystrophy** is a syndrome of skeletal changes found in chronic kidney disease.[12] This syndrome is a result of alterations in calcium and phosphate metabolism (Fig. 45-4). Normally the calcium/phosphate ratio maintains the electrolytes in a soluble state. As the GFR decreases, urinary phosphate excretion is impaired, and the serum phosphate increases.

The kidneys metabolize vitamin D (formed in the skin or ingested) to its active form. The active form of vitamin D is needed for calcium absorption from the GI tract. In renal failure the kidneys fail to activate vitamin D, calcium absorption is impaired, and serum calcium decreases. Low serum calcium stimulates the release of PTH, which causes resorption of calcium and phosphate from the bone. This release increases serum calcium, as well as serum phosphate. The excess phosphate will bind with calcium, leading to the formation of insoluble metastatic calcifications that are deposited throughout the body. Common sites are the blood vessels, joints, lungs, muscles, myocardium, and eyes.[13] "Uremic red eye" is caused by the irritation from deposits in the eye. Metastatic calcifications in the arteries of the fingers and toes may cause gangrene. Intracardiac calcifications can disrupt the conduction system and cause cardiac arrest.

Two types of renal osteodystrophy are associated with ESRD:

1. *Osteomalacia.* This condition results from lack of mineralization of newly formed bone. It can be a result of hypocalcemia. It can also be caused by aluminum accumulation because the primary route for aluminum excretion is through the kidneys. The primary source of aluminum is aluminum-based phosphate binders. Over the past decade, there has been a decreased use of aluminum-based phosphate binders and a concomitant decrease in the incidence of osteomalacia.

2. *Osteitis fibrosa.* This condition results from calcium resorption from the bone and replacement with fibrous tissue. Osteitis fibrosa is primarily a result of markedly elevated levels of PTH that cause bone resorption.

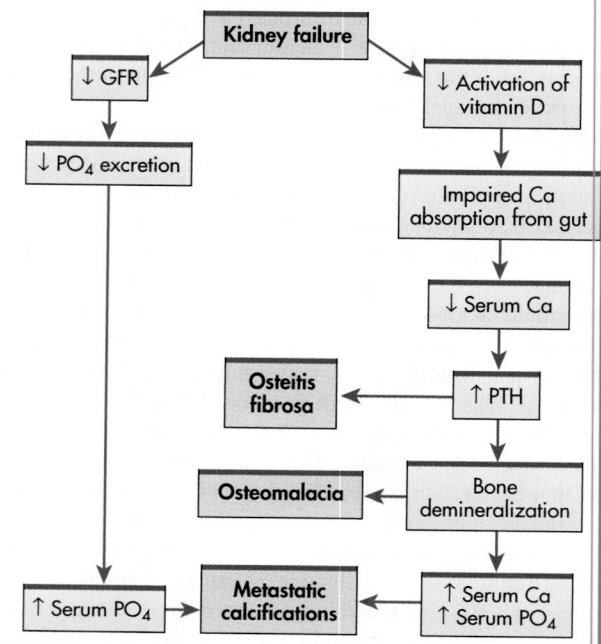

FIG. 45-4 Mechanisms of renal osteodystrophy. *GFR,* Glomerular filtration rate.

Integumentary System. The most noticeable change in the integumentary system is a yellow-gray discoloration of the skin. This change is a result of the absorption and retention of urinary pigments that normally give the characteristic color to urine. The skin also appears pale as a result of anemia and is dry and scaly because of a decrease in oil and sweat gland activity. Decreased perspiration results from a decrease in the size of the sweat glands.

Pruritus most commonly results from a combination of the dry skin, calcium-phosphate deposition in the skin, and sensory neuropathy. The itching may be so intense that it can lead to bleeding or infection secondary to scratching. Uremic frost is a rare condition in which urea crystallizes on the skin and is usually seen only when BUN levels are extremely high. It occurs when a patient refuses dialysis or is withdrawn from dialysis.

The hair is dry and brittle and may fall out. The nails are thin, brittle, and ridged. Petechiae and ecchymoses may be present and are due to platelet abnormalities.

Reproductive System. Both sexes characteristically experience infertility and a decreased libido. Women usually have decreased levels of estrogen, progesterone, and luteinizing hormone, causing anovulation and menstrual changes (usually amenorrhea). Menses and ovulation may return after dialysis is started. Men experience loss of testicular consistency, decreased testosterone levels, and low sperm counts. Sexual dysfunction in both sexes may also be caused by anemia, which causes fatigue and decreased libido. In addition, peripheral neuropathy can cause impotence in men and anorgasmy in women. Additional factors that may cause changes in sexual function are psychologic problems (e.g., anxiety, depression), physical stress, and side effects of drugs.

Sexual function may improve with maintenance dialysis and may become normal with successful transplantation. Pregnant dialysis patients have been able to carry a fetus to term, but there is significant risk to the mother and infant. Pregnancy in transplant patients is more common, but there is also a risk to both the mother and fetus.

Endocrine System. Many patients with chronic kidney disease exhibit some clinical manifestations of hypothyroidism. Tests of thyroid function may yield low to low-normal levels for serum triiodothyronine (T_3) and thyroxine (T_4) levels. Neither the clinical significance nor the exact cause of these findings is known.

Psychologic Changes. Personality and behavioral changes, emotional lability, withdrawal, and depression are commonly observed. Fatigue and lethargy contribute to the feeling of illness. The changes in body image caused by edema, integumentary disturbances, and access devices (e.g., fistulas, catheters) lead to further anxiety and depression. Decreased ability to concentrate and slowed mental activity can give the appearance of dullness and disinterest in the environment. There are also significant changes in lifestyle, occupation, family responsibilities, and financial status that must be dealt with by the patient. Long-term survival depends on drugs, dietary restrictions, dialysis, and possibly transplantation. The patient will also grieve the loss of renal function. This can be a prolonged process for some individuals.

Diagnostic Studies

Adverse outcomes of CKD can often be prevented or delayed through early detection and treatment. Early stages of CKD can be detected through routine laboratory measurements (Table 45-6).

TABLE 45-6	Collaborative Care — Conservative Therapy of Chronic Kidney Disease

Diagnostic
History and physical examination
Identification of reversible renal disease
   Renal ultrasound
   Renal scan
   CT scan
   Renal biopsy
BUN, serum creatinine, and creatinine clearance levels
Serum electrolytes
Protein-to-creatinine ratio in first morning voided specimen
Urinalysis and urine culture
Hematocrit and hemoglobin levels

Collaborative Therapy
Correction of extracellular fluid volume overload or deficit
Nutritional therapy*
Erythropoietin therapy
Calcium supplementation, phosphate binders, or both
Antihypertensive therapy
Measures to lower potassium†
Adjustment of drug dosages to degree of renal function

BUN, Blood urea nitrogen; *CT*, computed tomography.
*See Tables 45-7 and 45-8.
†See Table 45-4.

Serum creatinine is used to estimate GFR. A protein-to-creatinine ratio or albumin-to-creatinine ratio in a first morning or random urine specimen can be done. A urinalysis can be done to detect RBCs, WBCs, protein, and glucose. Imaging of the kidneys is usually done by ultrasound.

Collaborative Care: Conservative Therapy of Chronic Kidney Disease

When a patient is diagnosed as having CKD, conservative therapy is attempted before maintenance dialysis begins (see Table 45-6). Every effort is made to detect and treat potentially reversible causes of renal failure (e.g., cardiac failure, dehydration, infections, nephrotoxins, urinary tract obstruction, renal artery stenosis). A renal biopsy may be necessary to provide a definitive diagnosis. The goals of conservative therapy are to preserve existing renal function, treat the clinical manifestations, prevent complications, and provide for the patient's comfort. Drug and nutritional therapy and supportive care are essential components of the conservative treatment plan.

Drug Therapy

Hyperkalemia. There are multiple strategies for managing hyperkalemia (see Table 45-4). Every effort is made to control hyperkalemia with the restriction of high-potassium foods and drugs. Acute hyperkalemia may require treatment with IV glucose and insulin or IV 10% calcium gluconate. Sodium polystyrene sulfonate (Kayexalate), a cation-exchange resin, is commonly used to lower potassium levels and can be administered on an outpatient basis. The patient should be told to expect some diarrhea because this preparation contains sorbitol, a bulk laxative that ensures evacuation of the potassium from the bowel. It should never be given to a patient with a hypoactive bowel (paralytic ileus) because fluid shifts could lead to bowel necrosis. As sodium polystyrene sulfonate exchanges sodium ions for potassium ions, the patient should be observed for sodium and water retention. If life-threatening arrhythmias are present, dialysis may be required.

Hypertension. The progression of chronic kidney disease can be delayed by controlling hypertension.[14] Treatment of hypertension initially consists of sodium and fluid restriction and the administration of antihypertensive drugs. The antihypertensive drugs most commonly used are diuretics (e.g., furosemide [Lasix]), β-adrenergic blockers (e.g., metoprolol [Lopressor]), calcium channel blockers (e.g., nifedipine [Procardia], and ACE inhibitors (e.g., captopril [Capoten], enalapril [Vasotec]) (see Chapter 32). Diuretics and β-adrenergic blockers are the recommended initial therapy. β-Adrenergic blockers also decrease the incidence of cardiovascular events and mortality from myocardial infarction.[15] ACE inhibitors decrease proteinuria and delay the progression of renal failure. They must be used cautiously when ESRD occurs because they can further decrease the GFR and increase serum potassium levels.

The BP should periodically be measured in supine, sitting, and standing positions to effectively monitor the effect of antihypertensive drugs. The patient should be taught how to monitor the blood pressure (BP) at home and what BP readings require immediate intervention. BP control is essential to slow atherosclerotic changes that could further impair renal function.

Renal osteodystrophy. Phosphate intake is generally restricted to less than 1000 mg per day, but usually dietary control is not adequate. Calcium-based phosphate binders such as calcium carbonate (e.g., Tums) and calcium acetate (e.g., PhosLo) are used to bind the phosphate, which is then excreted in the stool. Giving a calcium-based binder when the phosphate levels are still high (6 mg/dl [1.98 mmol/L]) may cause the formation of calcium-phosphate deposits. Sevelamer (Renagel) is a new phosphate binder that does not contain either calcium or aluminum. It has the added benefits of lowering cholesterol and LDLs.[16]

Because dementia and bone disease (osteomalacia) are associated with excessive absorption of aluminum, aluminum hydroxide gels or antacids (e.g., Alu-Caps, Amphojel, Basaljel, Alternagel) should not be used to bind phosphate. Magnesium-containing antacids (Maalox, Mylanta) should not be given because magnesium is dependent on the kidneys for excretion. Phosphate binders should be administered with each meal to be effective because most phosphate is absorbed within 1 hour after eating. Hypercalcemia may occur with calcium supplementation and is associated with increased cardiac calcifications and mortality in ESRD patients. Constipation is a frequent side effect of phosphate binders and may necessitate the use of stool softeners.

Hypocalcemia is often a problem because of the inability of the GI tract to absorb calcium in the absence of vitamin D. If hypocalcemia persists in the setting of controlled serum phosphate levels and supplemental calcium, the active form of vitamin D should be given. It is commercially available in oral preparations such as calcitriol (Rocaltrol) and in IV form as calcitriol (Calcijex). Paricalcitol (Zemplar) and doxercalciferol (Hectorol) are new synthetic vitamin D_2 analogs that are designed to reduce PTH levels. They cause less hypercalcemia and hyperphosphatemia than the older analogs.[16] It is important to lower the phosphate level before administering calcium or vitamin D be-

cause these drugs may contribute to soft tissue calcification if both calcium and phosphate levels are elevated.

If renal osteodystrophy remains severe despite conservative therapy, a subtotal parathyroidectomy may be performed to decrease the synthesis and secretion of PTH. In some situations a total parathyroidectomy is performed, and some parathyroid tissue is transplanted into the forearm. The transplanted cells produce PTH as needed. If production of PTH becomes excessive, some of the cells can be removed from the forearm using local anesthesia.

The most common methods for evaluating the status of the bone disease are skeletal x-rays, bone scans, bone biopsy, and bone densitometry. PTH and alkaline phosphatase levels should also be measured. Alkaline phosphatase is elevated when there is demineralization of the bone but can also be increased by liver disease.

Anemia. The most important cause of anemia is a decreased production of erythropoietin. With the use of recombinant deoxyribonucleic acid (DNA) technology (see Fig. 13-15), erythropoietin (Epogen, Procrit) is made in large amounts and is available for the treatment of anemia.[9] It can be administered intravenously or subcutaneously. It has been very effective in treating anemia. A significant increase in hematocrit is usually not seen for 2 to 3 weeks. The patient who is receiving erythropoietin has improved cardiac performance and exercise tolerance and an enhanced quality of life. Darbepoetin (Aranesp) is a long-acting form of erythropoietin that is now available.

A common adverse effect of exogenous erythropoietin is the development or acceleration of hypertension. The underlying mechanism is related to the hemodynamic changes (e.g., increased whole blood viscosity) that occur as the anemia is corrected. Another side effect of erythropoietin therapy is the development of functional iron deficiency resulting from the increased demand for iron to support erythropoiesis. Most patients receive oral iron supplements. The GI side effects of iron, including gastric irritation and constipation, may lead to noncompliance. Orally administered iron should not be taken at the same time as phosphate binders because calcium binds the iron. The patient should be advised that iron may make the stool dark in color. Parenteral iron (Venofer, Ferrlecit) is used if iron deficiencies persist in spite of oral iron intake. Supplemental folic acid (1 mg daily) is usually given because it is needed for RBC formation and is removed by dialysis.

Blood transfusions should be avoided in treating anemia unless the patient experiences an acute blood loss or has symptomatic anemia (i.e., dyspnea, excess fatigue, tachycardia, palpitations, chest pain). Undesirable effects of transfusions are the suppression of erythropoiesis as a result of a decrease in the hypoxic stimulus, the possible transmission of hepatitis B or C or human immunodeficiency virus (HIV), and the possibility of iron overload because each unit of blood contains about 250 mg of iron.

Complications of drug therapy. Many drugs are partially or totally excreted by the kidneys. Drug toxicity is a serious problem in the patient with uremia. Delayed and decreased elimination lead to an accumulation of drugs in the body. Drug doses and frequency of administration must be adjusted based on the severity of the kidney disease. Increased sensitivity may result as drug levels increase in the blood and tissues. Drugs of particular concern include digitalis preparations, antibiotics, and pain medication.

Digitalis preparations are excreted largely by the kidneys. Loading doses may not have to be changed, but maintenance doses and frequency may have to be adjusted. Many patients require only 0.125 mg every other day. Dialysis does not affect body levels of digoxin, but it does affect potassium levels. Hypokalemia can potentiate the action of digitalis.

Aminoglycosides (gentamicin, amikacin), penicillin in high doses, and tetracyclines are potentially nephrotoxic and require dose and frequency adjustments. The frequency and dose of vancomycin and gentamicin must be decreased because they are dependent on the kidney for excretion. These drugs can accumulate to toxic levels if appropriate adjustments are not made.

Meperidine (Demerol) should never be administered to a patient with CKD because the liver metabolizes it to normeperidine, which is dependent on the kidneys for excretion. If normeperidine accumulates, seizures can result. Other pain medications may be given, but less frequently and in smaller doses (e.g., oxycodone with acetaminophen, morphine sulfate).

Patients should be advised to avoid NSAIDs. These drugs block the synthesis of the renal prostaglandins that promote vasodilation. This can worsen renal hypoperfusion. Many NSAIDs are available over the counter, so it is essential that the patient be cautioned. Acetaminophen can be substituted.

Nutritional Therapy

Protein restriction. The current diet is designed to be as normal as possible to maintain good nutrition (Table 45-7). Protein is restricted because BUN is an end product of protein metabolism. For the patient who is not undergoing dialysis, one guide is to restrict protein intake to 0.6 to 0.75 g/kg of ideal body weight (IBW) per day when the creatinine clearance is less than 25 ml per minute.[17] Some treatment centers use a routine 40-g protein diet. Because this diet is deficient in vitamins and water-soluble vitamins are lost through dialysis, multivitamins are prescribed.

Protein restriction may reduce the decline of renal function in the patient with chronic renal insufficiency. A low-protein (0.6 to 0.8 g/kg body weight per day), low-phosphorus diet supplemented with amino acids and their ketoanalogues can slow the progression of renal failure.[18] Keto acids of essential amino acids

are a dietary supplement. The rationale for using this treatment is that in the body, nonessential amino acids transfer amine groups to the essential keto acids synthesizing essential amino acids. The nitrogen present in nonessential amino acids is used, and the total nitrogen intake is kept to an absolute minimum. Keto acid supplements are available in liquid preparations. Modest protein restriction (0.6 to 0.8 g/kg per day) appears to be a relatively safe therapeutic option for patients with moderate renal insufficiency. For patients with more severe renal insufficiency, low-protein diets should be used with caution because these patients are at risk for developing malnutrition.

Once the patient starts dialysis, protein intake can be increased to 1.2 to 1.3 g/kg of IBW per day. Dietary protein guidelines for PD differ from those for HD because excessive amounts of protein are lost in the dialysate. The protein intake must be high enough to compensate for the losses so that the nitrogen balance is maintained. The recommended protein intake is at least 1.2 g/kg of IBW per day and can be increased depending on the individual needs of the patient. At least 50% of protein intake should have high biologic value containing all of the essential amino acids (e.g., eggs, milk, meat, poultry).

Sufficient calories from carbohydrates and fat are needed to minimize catabolism of body protein and to maintain body weight. Therefore 100 g of carbohydrates and an appropriate amount of fat are prescribed to maintain an intake of 30 to 35 kcal/kg body weight per day. See Table 45-7 for specific guidelines.

For patients with malnutrition or inadequate caloric intake, commercially prepared products that are high in calories and low in protein, sodium, and potassium are available. Liquid and powder preparations include Nepro, Microlipid, SumaCal, Suplena, and Polycose. Products containing only the essential amino acids (Amin-Aid) can also be used as dietary supplements.

Water restriction. Water intake depends on the daily urine output. Generally, 600 ml (from insensible loss) plus an amount equal to the previous day's urine output is allowed for a patient with chronic kidney disease who is not receiving dialysis. Foods that are liquid at room temperature (e.g., gelatin, ice cream) should be counted as fluid intake. The fluid allotment should be

TABLE 45-7   Nutritional Therapy: Daily Requirements for the Patient with Chronic Kidney Disease

	CONSERVATIVE MANAGEMENT	HEMODIALYSIS	PERITONEAL DIALYSIS
Fluid allowance	Urine output plus 600 ml	Urine output plus 600 ml	Often no restriction
Protein*	0.6-0.75 g/kg body weight	1.2-1.3 g/kg IBW	≥1.2-1.3 g/kg IBW
Calories	30-35 kcal/kg EDW	30-35 kcal/kg EDW[†]	30-35 kcal/kg IBW[†]
Fat	Determined by caloric requirement	Determined by caloric requirement	Determined by caloric requirement
Carbohydrate	Unlimited intake of sugars, starches; bread and cereal products limited due to protein restriction	Same as for conservative management	Dependent on individual patient needs
Iron	Variable	Variable	Variable
Potassium	2-3 g	2-3 g	3-4 g, no restrictions
Sodium	2-3 g	2-3 g	2-4 g
Phosphorus	800-1000 mg	1000 mg	1000 mg
Calcium	Variable	1000-1500 mg	1000-1500 mg
Folic acid	1 mg supplement	1 mg supplement	1 mg supplement

EDW, Estimated dry weight; *IBW,* ideal body weight.
*At least 50% of protein intake should be of high biologic value (e.g., coming from eggs, milk, meat).
[†]Includes dialysate calories.

TABLE 45-8	Nutritional Therapy — High-Potassium Foods	
Fruits/Fruit Juices	**Vegetables**	**Cereal**
Apple juice	Beans, white and pinto*	All-bran*
Grapefruit juice	Broccoli	Raisin bran*
Orange juice*	Carrots	**Meat and Poultry**
Prune juice*	Lima beans, cooked*	Beef*, pork, cooked
Tomato juice*	Mushrooms, fresh*	Chicken
Oranges	Potato, baked*	Turkey
Tomatoes	Squash, baked*	**Miscellaneous**
Honeydew melons*	Spinach, cooked*	Chocolate
Raisins*	**Dairy**	Molasses
Avocados*	Milk*	Sunflower seeds*
Bananas*	Yogurt*	
Prunes*		

*Greater than 10 mEq of potassium per serving.

spaced throughout the day so that the patient does not become thirsty. For the chronic HD patient, fluid intake is adjusted so that weight gains are no more than 1 to 3 kg between dialyses.

Sodium and potassium restriction. The sodium and potassium restriction depends on the ability of the kidneys to excrete these electrolytes. Sodium-restricted diets may vary from 2 to 4 g depending on the degree of edema and hypertension. Sodium and salt should not be equated because the sodium content in 1 g of sodium chloride is equivalent to 400 mg of sodium. The patient should be instructed to avoid high-sodium foods such as cured meats, pickled foods, canned soups and stews, frankfurters, cold cuts, soy sauce, and salad dressings (see Tables 34-9 through 34-11). Most salt substitutes should not be used because they contain potassium chloride.

Dietary restrictions for potassium range from about 2 to 4 g (39 mg = 1 mEq). Some PD patients do not need potassium restrictions. Some foods with high potassium content that should be avoided are oranges, bananas, melons, tomatoes, prunes, raisins, deep green and yellow vegetables, beans, and legumes (Table 45-8).

Phosphate restriction. Phosphate should be limited to approximately 1000 mg a day. Foods that are high in phosphate include dairy products (e.g., milk, ice cream, cheese, yogurt) or foods containing dairy products (pudding). Most foods that are high in phosphate are also high in calcium. Restricting phosphate will restrict calcium intake.

NURSING MANAGEMENT
CONSERVATIVE THERAPY OF CHRONIC KIDNEY DISEASE

■ Nursing Assessment

The nurse should obtain a complete history of any existing renal disease or family history of renal disease because some renal disorders have a hereditary basis. Information on long-term health problems such as hypertension, diabetes, recurrent urinary tract infections, and systemic lupus erythematosus should be ob-

tained. Because many drugs are potentially nephrotoxic, both current and past use of prescription and over-the-counter drugs must be reviewed.

The nurse should assess the patient's dietary habits and discuss any problems. The height and weight should be measured, and any recent weight changes must be evaluated.

Clinical manifestations of CKD are apparent in multiple body systems (see Fig. 45-3). Fatigue, lethargy, and pruritus are often the early symptoms of CKD. Hypertension and changes in urine characteristics are often the first signs.

Support systems should be assessed. The chronicity of renal disease and the long-term nature of treatment modalities affect every area of a person's life, including family relationships, social and work activities, and self-image. The choice of treatment modality may be related to support systems available to the patient. Recognition that CKD is a lifelong illness will facilitate the care.

■ Nursing Diagnoses

Nursing diagnoses for CKD may include, but are not limited to, those presented in NCP 45-1.

■ Planning

The overall goals are that a patient with CKD will (1) demonstrate knowledge and ability to comply with the therapeutic regimen, (2) participate in decision making for the plan of care and future treatment modality, (3) demonstrate effective coping strategies, and (4) continue with activities of daily living within physiologic limitations.

■ Nursing Implementation

Health Promotion. Individuals at risk for CKD must be identified. These include people with a history (or a family history) of renal disease, hypertension, diabetes mellitus, and repeated urinary tract infection. These individuals should have regular checkups including serum creatinine, BUN, and urinalysis. They should be advised that any changes in urine appearance (color, odor), frequency, or volume must be reported to the health care provider. If a patient must be prescribed a potentially nephrotoxic drug, it is important to monitor renal function with serum creatinine and BUN.

Individuals identified as at risk need to take measures to prevent or delay the progression of CKD. These include glycemic control for patients with diabetes (see Chapter 47), BP control, and early and definitive treatment of urinary tract infections.

Acute Intervention. The specific nursing management of the patient with CKD is detailed in NCP 45-1. It is important to teach the patient and family because diet, drugs, and follow-up medical care are the responsibilities of the patient (Table 45-9). The patient should check a daily weight; learn to take daily BPs; and be able to identify signs and symptoms of fluid overload, hyperkalemia, and other electrolyte imbalances. The patient and family must understand the importance of strict dietary adherence. The dietitian should meet with the patient and family on a regular basis for diet planning. A diet history and consideration of cultural variations will facilitate diet planning and adherence.

The patient needs a complete understanding of the drugs, the dosages, and the common side effects. It may be helpful to make

NURSING CARE PLAN 45-1

Patient with Chronic Kidney Disease

EXPECTED PATIENT OUTCOMES	NURSING INTERVENTIONS and *RATIONALES*
NURSING DIAGNOSIS	**Excess fluid volume** *related to* inability of kidneys to excrete fluid, inadequate dialysis, and excessive fluid intake *as manifested by* edema, hypertension, bounding pulse, weight gain, shortness of breath, pulmonary edema.
• No edema • No evidence of dyspnea • Dry weight remaining within 4 lb (2 kg) of patient's dry weight • BP and pulse within limits for patient	• Monitor for increase in BP, periorbital sacral and peripheral edema, dyspnea, and pericardial friction rub, *which are indicators of fluid excess.* • Teach patient how to maintain a low-sodium diet *to help control edema and hypertension.* • Teach patient fluid control measures and importance of daily weights *to help monitor and control fluid overload and related hypertension.*
NURSING DIAGNOSIS	**Impaired skin integrity** *related to* decrease in oil and sweat gland activity, hyperphosphatemia, deposition of calcium-phosphate precipitates, capillary fragility, excess fluid, and neuropathy *as manifested by* itching, bruising, dry skin, edema, excoriation.
• No itching or skin dryness • Intact, clean skin • No calcium-phosphate deposits	• Assess skin for changes in color, texture, turgor, and vascularity *to provide information for appropriate interventions.* • Inspect patient for bruises, purpura, and signs of infection *to detect early signs of problems.* • Provide skin care with tepid water, bath oils, super-fatted soaps, or oatmeal *to relieve itching and moisturize dry skin.* • Apply ointments or creams (lanolin, Aquaphor) following bath or shower *to relieve itching and promote comfort.* • Administer antihistamines and antipruritics as prescribed *to relieve itching.* • Monitor serum calcium and phosphate levels *because elevated blood levels may lead to severe pruritus and calcium-phosphate precipitation in the skin.*
NURSING DIAGNOSIS	**Risk for injury** (fracture) *related to* alterations in the absorption of calcium and excretion of phosphate, altered vitamin D metabolism.
• Slowing of bone disease • Serum calcium levels >8 mg/dl (2 mmol/L) and phosphate levels <5.5 mg/dl (1.8 mmol/L) • No bone fractures	• Assess for hypocalcemia and hyperphosphatemia *to determine degree of bone demineralization and potential risk for injury.* • Provide safe environment *to reduce the risk of injury.* • Administer calcium supplements, vitamin D, and phosphate binders as ordered *to prevent and/or treat the bone demineralization.* • Give calcium supplement or phosphate binder with meals *to increase effectiveness.* • Ensure that patient understands and follows phosphate restrictions and can state the purpose of phosphate binders, calcium supplements, and vitamin D supplements. • Observe for hypercalcemia when using calcium supplements. • Explain to patient the potential for fracture *to reduce the risk of unsafe practices that might result in a traumatic or pathologic fracture.*
NURSING DIAGNOSIS	**Activity intolerance** *related to* anemia and neuropathy *as manifested by* fatigability, shortness of breath, pallor, dyspnea, tachycardia.
• Hematocrit and hemoglobin levels in acceptable range • Transferrin percent saturation and ferritin in acceptable range • Able to perform activities of daily living without undue fatigue	• Monitor hematocrit and hemoglobin levels *as an indicator of the patient's oxygen-carrying capacity.* • Monitor response of hematocrit and hemoglobin to erythropoietin (if ordered). • Monitor transferrin percent saturation and ferritin as indicators of iron available for erythropoiesis. • Administer oral iron between meals and IV iron (as ordered) and erythropoietin (as ordered) *to maintain normal erythropoiesis and stimulate production of RBCs.* • Administer folic acid after hemodialysis *because folic acid is dialyzable and would be lost in the dialysate.* • Provide adequate periods of rest *to enable patient to recuperate from past activities and participate in future activity.* • Teach patient to plan activities *to avoid fatigue.*

Continued

NURSING CARE PLAN 45-1

Patient with Chronic Kidney Disease—cont'd

EXPECTED PATIENT OUTCOMES	NURSING INTERVENTIONS and *RATIONALES*
NURSING DIAGNOSIS	**Imbalanced nutrition: less than body requirements** *related to* restricted intake of nutrients (especially protein), nausea, vomiting, anorexia, and stomatitis *as manifested by* loss of appetite and weight.
▪ Maintenance of ideal body weight ▪ Prealbumin, transferrin, and albumin within acceptable limits	▪ Monitor weight, BUN, serum creatinine, prealbumin, total protein, and serum electrolytes *as indicators of effectiveness of dialysis, nutritional status, and response to treatment.* ▪ Provide frequent mouth care *to prevent stomatitis, remove bad taste, and increase patient's comfort.* ▪ Provide small, frequent meals *to reduce nausea and vomiting.* ▪ Administer H$_2$ histamine blockers (e.g., famotidine [Pepcid]), proton pump inhibitors (e.g., omeprazole [Prilosec]), and GI promotility agents (e.g., metoclopramide [Reglan]) (as ordered) *to minimize GI irritation and facilitate motility.* ▪ Allow patient freedom in choosing food and fluid intake within limitations *to increase the patient's sense of control.* ▪ Provide at least 30-35 kcal/kg body weight/day with a high carbohydrate intake *to minimize catabolism of body protein and maintain body weight.* ▪ Restrict protein and phosphate to prescribed amount *to decrease the metabolic end products of urea, potassium, phosphate, and hydrogen.* ▪ Provide hard candy, gum, and lollipops *to improve taste and increase carbohydrate/calorie intake. If diabetic, sugar-free gum or hard candy may be substituted.*
NURSING DIAGNOSIS	**Anticipatory grieving** *related to* loss of kidney function *as manifested by* expression of feelings of sadness, anger, inadequacy, hopelessness.
▪ Acceptance of chronic disease	▪ Listen to the concerns of patient *to convey a caring attitude and foster a relationship to determine how patient is handling the situation.* ▪ Allow patient time to mourn loss of body function *so that patient can deal with feelings and identify ways of coping with losses more effectively.* ▪ Include family members in discussions of patient's concerns *to enable them to assist the patient and foster their support and understanding.*
NURSING DIAGNOSIS	**Risk for infection** *related to* suppressed immune system, access sites, and malnutrition secondary to dialysis and uremia.
▪ No infections ▪ WBC within normal range	▪ Assess for local (pain on urination, hematuria, cloudy urine; redness, swelling, or drainage in areas of skin breaks) and systemic (chills, fever, tachycardia) manifestations of infection *to ensure early identification and treatment.* ▪ Instruct patient to avoid exposure to people with infections *to decrease risk of infection.* ▪ Maintain aseptic technique when performing dialysis or other invasive procedures (IV insertion, urinary catheter insertion) *to prevent the introduction of organisms.*

COLLABORATIVE PROBLEMS

NURSING GOALS	NURSING INTERVENTIONS and *RATIONALES*
POTENTIAL COMPLICATION	**Hypertension** *related to* sodium and water retention and alterations of renin-angiotensin system.
▪ Monitor for hypertension ▪ Report deviations from acceptable parameters ▪ Carry out appropriate medical and nursing interventions	▪ Assess patient for elevated BP, headache, dizziness, shortness of breath, chest pain, and edema *to identify the presence and effects of hypertension.* ▪ Take vital signs *to provide a database for ongoing analysis of patient's response to treatment.* ▪ Administer antihypertensive drugs (as ordered) after checking BP. ▪ Observe for orthostatic hypotension and other side effects of antihypertensive drugs *because overtreatment may cause problems.* ▪ Instruct patient to change positions slowly *to minimize dizziness caused by orthostatic hypotension.* ▪ Explain the actions and side effects of antihypertensive drugs and risks of uncontrolled hypertension (e.g., stroke) *to foster adherence to drug regimen.*

NURSING CARE PLAN 45-1

Patient with Chronic Kidney Disease—cont'd

COLLABORATIVE PROBLEMS—cont'd

NURSING GOALS	NURSING INTERVENTIONS and *RATIONALES*
POTENTIAL COMPLICATION ▪ Monitor for signs of hyperkalemia ▪ Report deviations from acceptable parameters ▪ Carry out appropriate medical and nursing interventions	**Hyperkalemia** *related to* decreased renal function, increased tissue catabolism, and shift of potassium into extracellular fluid secondary to metabolic acidosis. ▪ Assess for manifestations of hyperkalemia such as serum potassium >5.5 mEq/L (5.5 mmol/L), muscle weakness, arrhythmias (peaked T waves, widened QRS, depressed ST segment on ECG), paresthesias, abdominal cramping, and diarrhea *to ensure early identification and treatment.* ▪ Do not administer IV solutions, drugs (e.g., potassium penicillin IV), or nutritional supplements that contain potassium. ▪ Discuss importance of following prescribed diet and avoiding foods high in potassium and receiving regular dialysis *to prevent complications of hyperkalemia.* ▪ Monitor serum potassium and notify physician of elevated levels and abnormal ECG results *because elevated potassium can cause life-threatening cardiac arrhythmias.* ▪ Be prepared to administer treatment for hyperkalemia *because this is a medical emergency requiring prompt treatment.* (See Table 45-4 for treatments.)
POTENTIAL COMPLICATION ▪ Monitor for peripheral neuropathies ▪ Report deviations from acceptable parameters ▪ Carry out appropriate medical and nursing interventions	**Peripheral neuropathy** *related to* effects of uremia on peripheral nerves. ▪ Assess patient for decreased sensation in feet, numbness and burning of feet, muscle cramps, restlessness of legs, loss of muscle strength, footdrop *to identify the presence of peripheral neuropathy.* ▪ Explain to patient the reason for neuropathy *to increase understanding and decrease anxiety.* ▪ Prevent trauma and excess stimulation to extremities *because areas with diminished sensation are extremely prone to injury.* ▪ Teach patient to examine areas of decreased sensation *to observe for injury.* ▪ In collaboration with physical therapy department, develop exercise regimen *to maintain prescribed level of activity.*

a list of the drugs and the times of administration that can be posted in the home. The patient must be instructed to avoid certain over-the-counter drugs such as NSAIDs and magnesium-based laxatives and antacids. The patient should also be aware that meperidine and ACE inhibitors may be harmful because of renal insufficiency.

Motivation to assume the primary role in the management of their disease is essential. The period of conservative management provides an opportunity to evaluate each patient's ability to manage the disease. This knowledge will be helpful when determining the treatment modality.

Ambulatory and Home Care. The length of time that a patient can receive conservative therapy is highly variable and depends on the progression of renal failure and the presence of other comorbid conditions. When conservative therapy is no longer effective, HD, PD, and transplantation are the available treatment options.

While the patient is receiving conservative therapy, the decision regarding future therapies should be made. This should be done before complications such as mental status changes, bleeding, progressive neuropathies, and fluid overload occur.[19]

The patient and family need a clear explanation of what is involved in dialysis and transplantation. If alternative treatments are presented early in the course of therapy, there will be an opportunity to carefully consider choices. Providing information about the treatment options will allow the patient to be active in

TABLE 45-9

Patient & Family Teaching Guide

Chronic Kidney Disease

1. Explain dietary (protein, sodium, potassium, phosphate) and fluid restrictions.
2. Encourage discussion of difficulties in modifying diet and fluid intake.
3. Explain signs and symptoms of electrolyte imbalance, especially high potassium.
4. Teach alternative ways of reducing thirst, such as sucking on ice cubes, lemon, or hard candy.
5. Explain the rationale for prescribed drugs and common side effects. Examples:
   Phosphate binders should be taken with meals.
   Iron supplements should be taken between meals.
6. Explain the importance of reporting any of the following:
   Weight gain greater than 4 lb (2 kg)
   Increasing BP
   Shortness of breath
   Edema
   Increasing fatigue or weakness
   Confusion or lethargy
7. Encourage patient and family to share concerns about lifestyle changes, living with a chronic illness, and decisions about type of dialysis or transplantation.

NURSING RESEARCH
Uncertainty and Coping in Family Members of Patients with End-Stage Renal Disease

Citation Pelletier-Hibbert M, Sohi P: Sources of uncertainty and coping strategies used by family members of individuals living with end-stage renal disease, *Nephrology Nursing J* 28:411, 2000.

Purpose To describe sources of uncertainty and common coping strategies used by family members of patients with end-stage renal disease (ESRD).

Methods Using a qualitative-descriptive-exploratory design, 41 family members of patients receiving dialysis in eastern Canada were interviewed in focus groups. They were asked to describe the experience of living with a loved one who required dialysis. Open-ended questions were used during the audiotaped sessions. The interviews were analyzed by thematic analysis.

Results and Conclusions Family members reported that uncertainty was a major source of stress. There were four themes identified as sources of uncertainty: (1) patient's health, (2) dialysis treatment, (3) potential loss, and (4) availability of renal transplant. Coping strategies included "living each day as it comes," finding positive meaning in the illness and treatment, hoping for a transplant, and believing in God. Uncertainty was attributed to the unpredictability of ESRD and its effects on all aspects of life. Uncertainty was felt most intensely by those who live day-to-day with the patient. Family members used coping strategies that included day-to-day rather than long-term planning.

Implications for Nursing Practice It is essential that the nurses caring for ESRD patients recognize potential sources of uncertainty for both patients and the family members. Teaching and care can be directed at alleviating sources of uncertainty and assisting in the development of effective coping strategies for the patient and the family members.

the decision-making process and give a sense of control over life-altering decisions. The patient should be informed that if dialysis is chosen, the option of transplantation still remains. It should be emphasized that if a transplanted organ fails, the patient can return to dialysis. The patient should also be counseled that retransplantation is also an option.

■ Evaluation

The expected outcomes for the patient with chronic kidney disease are presented in NCP 45-1.

Dialysis

Dialysis is the movement of fluid and molecules across a semipermeable membrane from one compartment to another. Clinically, dialysis is a technique in which substances move from the blood through a semipermeable membrane and into a dialysis solution (dialysate). It is used to correct fluid and electrolyte imbalances and to remove waste products in renal failure. It can also be used to treat drug overdoses. The two methods of dialysis available are **peritoneal dialysis** (PD) and **hemodialysis** (HD) (Table 45-10). In PD the peritoneal membrane acts as the semipermeable membrane. In HD an artificial membrane (usually made of cellulose-based or synthetic materials) is used as the semipermeable membrane and is in contact with the patient's blood.

Dialysis is begun when the patient's uremia can no longer be adequately managed conservatively. Generally dialysis is initiated when the GFR (or creatinine clearance) is less than 15 ml per minute. This criterion can vary widely in different clinical situations and the physician will determine when to start dialysis based on the patient's clinical status. Certain uremic complications, including encephalopathy, neuropathies, uncontrolled hyperkalemia, pericarditis, and accelerated hypertension, indicate a need for immediate dialysis.

TABLE 45-10	Comparison of Peritoneal Dialysis and Hemodialysis		
PERITONEAL DIALYSIS		**HEMODIALYSIS**	
ADVANTAGES	**DISADVANTAGES**	**ADVANTAGES**	**DISADVANTAGES**
Immediate initiation in almost any hospital	Bacterial or chemical peritonitis	Rapid fluid removal	Vascular access problems
Less complicated than hemodialysis	Protein loss into dialysate	Rapid removal of urea and creatinine	Dietary and fluid restrictions
Portable system with CAPD	Exit site and tunnel infections	Effective potassium removal	Heparinization may be necessary
Fewer dietary restrictions	Self-image problems with catheter placement	Less protein loss	Extensive equipment necessary
Relatively short training time	Hyperglycemia	Lowering of serum triglycerides	Hypotension during dialysis
Usable in the patient with vascular access problems	Aggravated hyperlipidemia	Home dialysis possible	Added blood loss that contributes to anemia
Less cardiovascular stress	Surgery for catheter placement	Temporary access can be placed at bedside	Specially trained personnel necessary
Home dialysis possible	Contraindication in the patient with multiple abdominal surgeries, trauma, unrepaired hernia		Surgery for permanent access placement
Preferable for the diabetic patient	Specially trained personnel needed		Self-image problems with permanent access
	Catheter can migrate		

CAPD, Continuous ambulatory peritoneal dialysis.

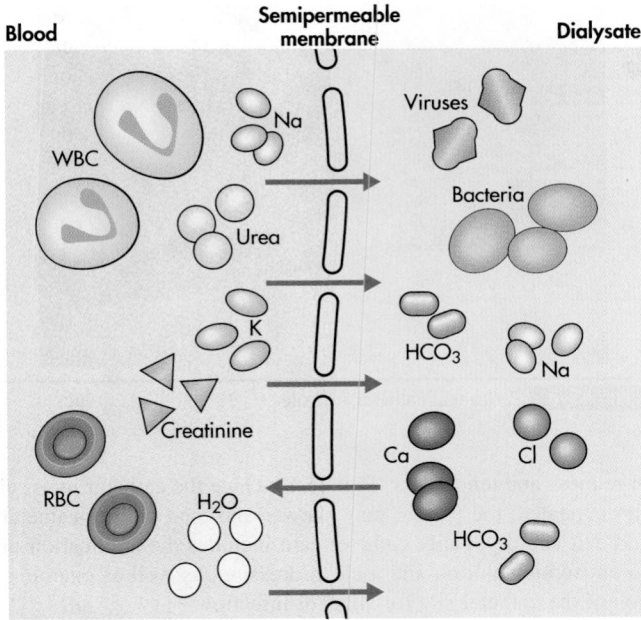

FIG. 45-5 Osmosis and diffusion across a semipermeable membrane.

General Principles of Dialysis

Solutes and water move across the semipermeable membrane from the blood to the dialysate or from the dialysate to the blood in accordance with concentration gradients. The principles of diffusion, osmosis, and ultrafiltration are involved in dialysis (Fig. 45-5). *Diffusion* is the movement of solutes from an area of greater concentration to an area of lesser concentration. In renal failure, urea, creatinine, uric acid, and electrolytes (potassium, phosphate) move from the blood to the dialysate with the net effect of lowering their concentration in the blood. RBCs, WBCs, and plasma proteins are too large to diffuse through the pores of the membrane. Bacteria and viruses that may be present in the dialysate are too large to migrate through the pores into the blood.

Osmosis is the movement of fluid from an area of lesser to an area of greater concentration of solutes. Glucose is added to the dialysate and creates an osmotic gradient across the membrane, pulling excess fluid from the blood.

Ultrafiltration (water and fluid removal) results when there is an osmotic gradient or pressure gradient across the membrane. In PD, excess fluid is removed by increasing the osmolality of the dialysate (osmotic gradient) with the addition of glucose. In HD, the gradient is created by increasing pressure in the blood compartment (positive pressure) or decreasing pressure in the dialysate compartment (negative pressure). Extracellular fluid moves into the dialysate because of the pressure gradient. The excess fluid is removed by creating a pressure differential between the blood and the dialysate solution with a combination of positive pressure in the blood compartment or a negative pressure in the dialysate compartment.

PERITONEAL DIALYSIS

Although PD was first used in 1923, it did not come into widespread use for chronic treatment until the 1970s with the development of soft, pliable peritoneal solution bags and the intro-

duction of the concept of continuous PD. In the United States, approximately 10% of patients receiving dialysis treatments are on PD.[8] In Canada, approximately 36% of patients are receiving PD because of the decreased availability of HD. In recent years the use of PD to treat chronic kidney disease has decreased in the United States.

Catheter Placement

Peritoneal access is obtained by inserting a catheter through the anterior abdominal wall (Fig. 45-6). The prototype of the catheter that is used was developed by Tenckhoff in 1968 and is made of silicone rubber tubing. The catheters are about 60 cm long and have two Dacron cuffs on the subcutaneous and peritoneal portions of the catheter that act as anchors and prevent the migration of microorganisms down the shaft from the skin. Within a few weeks, fibrous tissue grows into the Dacron cuff, holding the catheter in place and preventing bacterial penetration into the peritoneal cavity. The tip of the catheter rests in the peritoneal cavity and has many perforations spaced along the distal end of the tubing to allow fluid to flow in and out of the catheter. Bent or "swan neck" catheters with curled, "pigtail" ends are preferred because they prevent catheter migration and kinking and allow for easier fills and drains. There are numerous variations of the Tenckhoff catheter, including the Toronto-Western, Purdue Column-Disc, and Gore-Tex catheters (Fig. 45-7).

The technique for catheter placement varies. Although it is possible to place a permanent catheter in the peritoneal cavity at the bedside with a trocar, it is usually done via surgery so that its placement can be directly visualized, minimizing potential complications. Preparation of the patient for catheter insertion includes emptying the bladder and bowel, weighing the patient, and obtaining a signed consent form.

In the nonsurgical (bedside) approach, an area approximately 2 cm below the umbilicus is numbed with a local anesthetic, and a small stab wound is made. A stylet is inserted, and the abdomen is distended with dialysis solution. The catheter is then placed

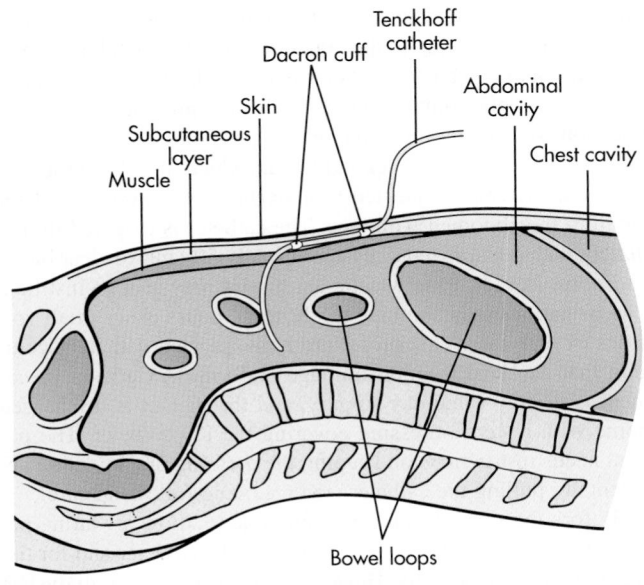

FIG. 45-6 Tenckhoff catheter used in peritoneal dialysis.

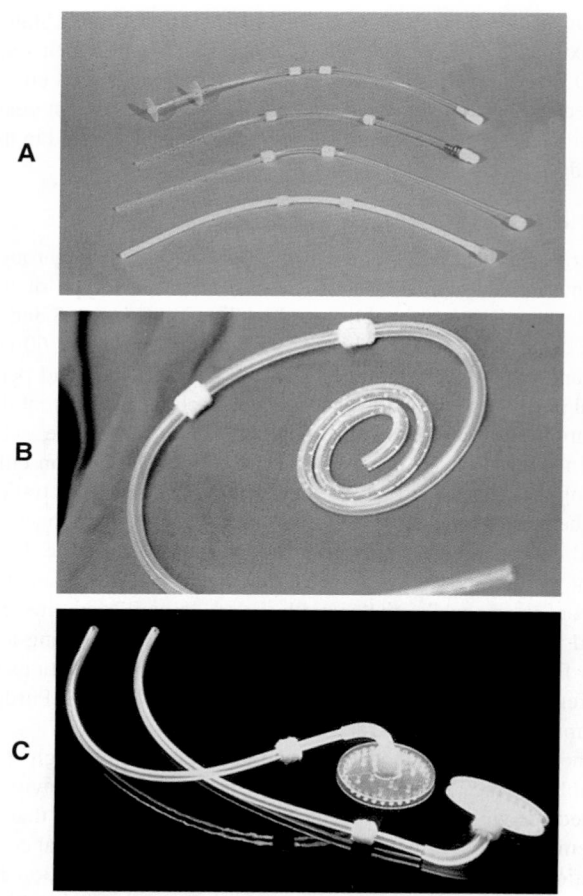

FIG. 45-7 **A,** Peritoneal catheters used for peritoneal dialysis. **B,** Bent neck, curl catheters. **C,** Disc catheters.

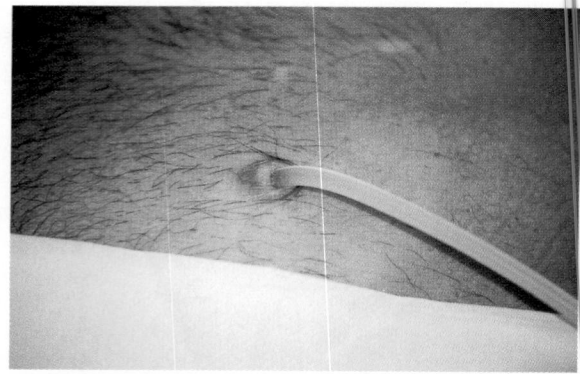

FIG. 45-8 Peritoneal catheter exit site.

into the peritoneal cavity. When the patient feels pressure in the rectal area and has the urge to defecate, the catheter is in place.

In the surgical approach, a midline umbilical incision is made, and a small puncture is made to one side and below this incision. The distal end of the catheter is placed in the peritoneum, and it is tunneled under the skin to the puncture site. The tunnel helps prevent peritonitis. After the catheter is inserted, the skin is cleaned with an antiseptic solution, and a sterile dressing is applied. Complications of catheter insertion include perforation of the bladder, the bowel, or a blood vessel and the introduction of bacteria.

The catheter is connected to a sterile tubing system and secured to the abdomen with tape. The catheter is irrigated immediately with heparinized dialysate (usually 500 ml) to clear blood and fibrin from it. Prophylactic antibiotics may also be instilled. The irrigations may continue for 12 to 24 hours using small volumes of dialysate. This procedure helps prevent catheter occlusion that can lead to poor drainage and inflow. Catheter placement is usually same-day surgery, and the patient is discharged home with a sterile dressing covering the PD catheter. The patient needs instructions on keeping the dressing dry, avoiding accidentally pulling the catheter, and receiving follow-up care.

Before the start of PD, it is preferable to allow a waiting period of 7 to 14 days for proper sealing of the catheter and for tissue to grow into the cuffs. However, some centers start dialysis 5 to 7 days after catheter insertion. About 2 to 4 weeks after catheter implantation, the exit site should be clean, dry, and free

of redness and tenderness (Fig. 45-8). Once the catheter incision site is healed, the patient may shower and then pat the catheter and exit site dry. Daily catheter care includes the application of an antiseptic solution and a clean dressing, as well as examination of the catheter site for signs of infection.

Dialysis Solutions and Cycles

Dialysis solutions are available commercially in 1- or 2-L (and sometimes smaller or larger volume) plastic bags (Dianeal, Inpersol) with glucose concentrations of 1.5%, 2.5%, and 4.25%. The electrolyte composition is similar to that of plasma. The dialysis solution is warmed to body temperature using dry heat to increase peritoneal clearance, prevent hypothermia, and enhance comfort.

Ultrafiltration (fluid removal) during PD depends on osmotic forces, with glucose being the most effective osmotic agent currently available. However, the problems arising from high rates of peritoneal glucose absorption, such as obesity, hypertriglyceridemia, and difficult control of blood glucose in the diabetic patient, have led to a search for alternative osmotic agents, including amino acid solutions. Many of these agents are currently under investigation.

The three phases of the PD cycle are *inflow* (fill), *dwell* (equilibration), and *drain*. The three phases are called an *exchange*. The patient dialyzing at home will receive about four exchanges per day. An acutely ill hospitalized patient may receive 12 to 24 exchanges per day. During inflow, a prescribed amount of solution, usually 2 L, is infused through an established catheter over about 10 minutes. The flow rate may be decreased if the patient has pain. After the solution has been infused, the inflow clamp is closed before air enters the tubing.

The next part of the cycle is the dwell phase, or equilibration, during which diffusion and osmosis occur between the patient's blood and the peritoneal cavity. The duration of the dwell time can last 20 to 30 minutes to 8 or more hours, depending on the method of PD. Drain time takes 15 to 30 minutes and may be facilitated by gently massaging the abdomen or changing position. The cycle starts again with the infusion of another 2 L of solution. For manual PD, a period of about 30 to 50 minutes is required to complete an exchange.

Peritoneal Dialysis Systems

Two types of PD currently being used are **automated peritoneal dialysis** (APD) and **continuous ambulatory peritoneal dialysis** (CAPD).

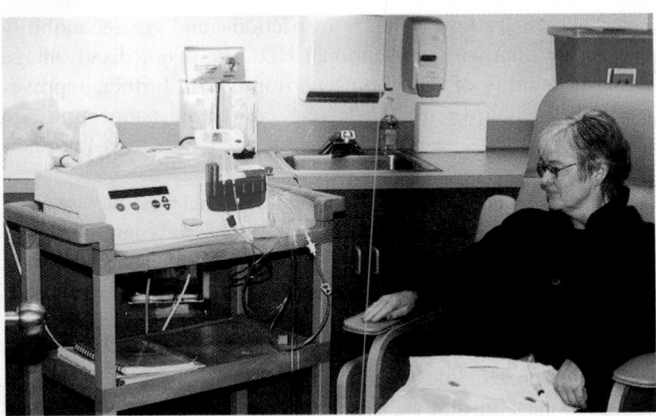

FIG. 45-9 Automated peritoneal dialysis cycler, which can be used while the patient is sleeping at night or for hospitalized patients who require frequent exchanges.

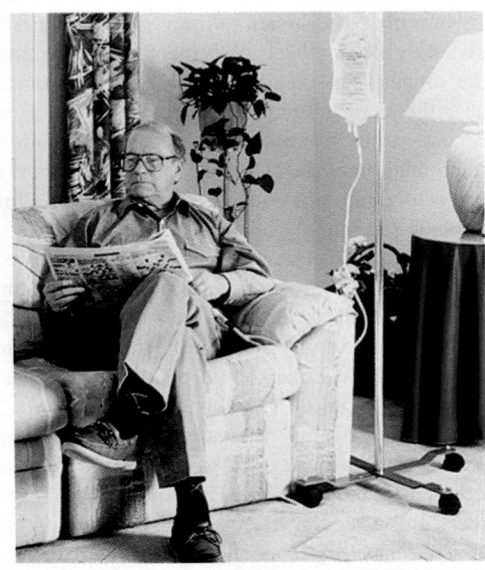

FIG. 45-10 Infusion period for a continuous ambulatory peritoneal dialysis patient.

Automated Peritoneal Dialysis. An automated device called a cycler is used to deliver the dialysate for APD (Fig. 45-9). The automated cycler times and controls the fill, dwell, and drain phases. The machine cycles four or more exchanges per night with 1 to 2 hours per exchange. Alarms and monitors are built into the system to make it safe for the patient to dialyze while sleeping. It may be easier to teach the patient and family to use the PD machine at home compared with the HD machine. The patient disconnects from the machine in the morning and usually leaves fluid in the abdomen during the day. One to two daytime manual exchanges may also be prescribed to ensure adequate dialysis. It is difficult to achieve the required solute and fluid clearance with solely nighttime APD. Older cyclers were quite large. With new technology cyclers are now about the size of a VCR or DVD player and have longer tubing to allow greater mobility.

Continuous Ambulatory Peritoneal Dialysis. CAPD is carried out manually by exchanging 1.5 to 3 L (usually 2 L) of peritoneal dialysate at least four times daily with dwell times of 4 to 10 hours. For example, one schedule starts the exchanges at 7 AM, 12 noon, 5 PM, and 10 PM. In this procedure the person instills 2 L of dialysate from a collapsible plastic bag into the peritoneal cavity through a disposable plastic tube.

Technical advances in CAPD systems allow the bag and line to be disconnected after the instillation of the fluid, decreasing the risk of peritonitis. After the equilibration period, the line is reconnected to the catheter, the dialysate (effluent) is drained from the peritoneal cavity, and a new 2-L bag of dialysate solution is infused (Fig. 45-10). It is critical in PD to maintain aseptic technique to avoid peritonitis. Several tubing connections and devices are commercially available to help maintain an aseptic system.

Contraindications for PD include the following:
1. History of multiple abdominal surgical procedures or severe abdominal pathologic condition (e.g., severe pancreatitis, diverticulitis)
2. Recurrent abdominal wall or inguinal hernias
3. Excessive obesity with large abdominal wall and fat deposits
4. Preexisting vertebral disease (e.g., chronic back problems)
5. Severe obstructive pulmonary disease

Complications of Peritoneal Dialysis

Exit Site Infection. Infection of the peritoneal catheter exit site is most commonly caused by *Staphylococcus aureus* or *S. epidermidis* (from skin flora). Superficial exit site infections caused by these organisms are generally resolved with antibiotic therapy. Clinical manifestations of an exit site infection include redness at site, tenderness, and drainage. If not treated immediately, subcutaneous tunnel infections usually result in abscess formation and may cause peritonitis, necessitating catheter removal.

Peritonitis. Peritonitis results from contamination of the dialysate or tubing or from progression of an exit site or tunnel infection. Less commonly, peritonitis results from bacteria in the intestine crossing over into the peritoneal cavity. Peritonitis is usually caused by *S. aureus* or *S. epidermidis*.[20] The primary clinical manifestation of peritonitis is a cloudy peritoneal effluent that has a WBC count of over 100 cells/μl (particularly neutrophils). GI manifestations may also be present, including diffuse abdominal pain, diarrhea, vomiting, abdominal distention, and hyperactive bowel sounds. Fever may or may not be present. Cultures, Gram stain, and a cell count with WBC differential of the peritoneal effluent are used to confirm the diagnosis of peritonitis. Antibiotics can be given by mouth, IV, or intraperitoneal. The patient is usually treated on an outpatient basis. Repeated infections may require the removal of the peritoneal catheter and termination of PD. The formation of adhesions in the peritoneum can result from repeated infections and interferes with the peritoneal membrane's ability to act as a dialyzing surface.

Abdominal Pain. Although not severe, pain is a common complication caused by the low pH of the dialysate solution, peritonitis, intraperitoneal irritation (which usually subsides in 1 to 2 weeks), and placement of the catheter. Pain can also occur when the tip of the catheter touches the bladder, bowel, or peritoneum. A change in the position of the catheter should correct this problem. Accidental infusion of air or infusing the dialysate too rapidly may cause referred pain in the shoulder. If the infusion rate is decreased, the pain usually subsides.

Outflow Problems. When outflow is less than 80% of inflow immediately after catheter placement, it may be caused by a kink in the tunnel segment of the catheter, omentum wrapped around the catheter, or migration of the catheter out of the pelvic region. Persistent outflow problems may require radiologic or surgical manipulation of the catheter. Outflow problems after the catheter has settled into place are often the result of a full colon. Bowel evacuation frequently relieves the problem.

Hernias. Because of increased intraabdominal pressure secondary to the dialysate infusion, hernias can develop in predisposed individuals such as multiparous women and older men. However, in most situations after hernia repair, PD can be resumed after several days using small dialysate volumes and by keeping the patient supine.

Lower Back Problems. Increased intraabdominal pressure can cause or aggravate lower back pain. The lumbosacral curvature is increased by intraperitoneal infusion of dialysate. Orthopedic binders and a regular exercise program for strengthening the back muscles have been beneficial for some patients.

Bleeding. Effluent drained after the first few exchanges may be pink or slightly bloody because of the trauma of catheter insertion. Bloody effluent over several days or the new appearance of blood in the effluent can indicate active intraperitoneal bleeding. If this occurs, the BP and hematocrit should be checked. Blood may also be present in the effluent of women who are menstruating or ovulating, and this requires no intervention.

Pulmonary Complications. Atelectasis, pneumonia, and bronchitis may occur from repeated upward displacement of the diaphragm, resulting in decreased lung expansion. The longer the dwell time, the greater the likelihood of pulmonary problems. Frequent repositioning and deep-breathing exercises can help. When lying in bed, elevation of the head of the bed may prevent these problems.

Protein Loss. The peritoneal membrane is permeable to plasma proteins, amino acids, and polypeptides. These substances are lost in the dialysate fluid. The amount of loss may be as much as 5 to 15 g per day. This loss may increase up to 40 g per day during episodes of peritonitis as the membrane becomes more permeable. Positive nitrogen balance can be maintained with adequate protein intake.

Carbohydrate and Lipid Abnormalities. Dialysate glucose is absorbed via the peritoneum and may be as much as 100 to 150 g per day. Continuous absorption of glucose results in increased insulin secretion and increased plasma insulin levels. The hyperinsulinemia stimulates hepatic production of triglycerides.

Encapsulating Sclerosing Peritonitis and Loss of Ultrafiltration. *Encapsulating sclerosing peritonitis* is a term applied to the development of a thick fibrous membrane that surrounds and compresses the bowel. Intestinal obstruction and strangulation are common complications. This condition generally necessitates changing the patient to HD because of the loss of ultrafiltration. It can occur for unknown reasons or from accidental infusion of disinfecting agents. Loss of ultrafiltration is associated with rapid glucose absorption.

Effectiveness of and Adaptation to Chronic Peritoneal Dialysis

The technique is associated with a short training program, independence, and ease of traveling. Clinically, the patient receiving PD does as well as the patient receiving HD and sometimes better. There are fewer dietary restrictions, and greater mobility is possible than with conventional HD. The major disadvantage is the possibility of developing peritonitis. As further improvements in techniques are made (e.g., improved connecting and sterilizing devices, in-line filters, improved catheters), the incidence of peritonitis should decrease.

PD is especially indicated for the individual who has vascular access problems or responds poorly to the hemodynamic stresses of HD (e.g., the older adult patient with diabetes and cardiovascular disease). The diabetic patient with ESRD does better with PD than with HD. The advantages of PD for the diabetic patient include better BP control, less hemodynamic instability because fluid shifts are gradual, better control of blood glucose by using intraperitoneal insulin (which can often eliminate the need for subcutaneous insulin), and prevention of retinal hemorrhage because heparin is not required as it is in HD.

HEMODIALYSIS

In 1943 Willem Kolff in the Netherlands performed the first successful dialysis on a human being with the use of a rotating-drum dialyzer. He initiated dialysis treatment in the United States in 1948.[21] Tremendous technologic advances have been made in HD since the 1940s, allowing for safer, shorter treatments using sophisticated equipment.

Vascular Access Sites

Obtaining vascular access is one of the most difficult problems associated with HD. To carry out HD, a very rapid blood flow is required, and access to a large blood vessel is essential. The types of vascular access in current use include arteriovenous fistulas (AVFs) and grafts (AVGs), temporary and semipermanent catheters, subcutaneous ports, and shunts.

Shunts. In the past external shunts were used, but today they are rarely used except with CRRT because of the numerous complications associated with them. The shunt consists of a U-shaped Silastic tube divided at the midpoint, and each of the two ends is placed in an artery and a vein (Fig. 45-11, *A*).

Internal Arteriovenous Fistulas and Grafts. In 1966 the use of the subcutaneous internal arteriovenous native (using the person's own blood vessels) fistula (see Fig. 45-11, *B*) was introduced. An arteriovenous native fistula (AVF) is created most commonly in the forearm with an anastomosis between an artery (usually radial or ulnar) and a vein (usually cephalic). The fistula provides for arterial blood flow through the vein. The arterial blood flow is essential to provide the rapid blood flow required for HD. The increased pressure of the arterial blood flow through the vein makes the vein dilate and become tough, making it amenable to repeated venipuncture. The vein is accessed using two large-gauge needles.

Native fistulas have the best overall patency rates and least number of complications of all vascular accesses. However, they are suitable only for the patient with relatively healthy blood vessels.[22] AVFs may not be possible in patients with a history of severe hypertension, peripheral vascular disease, diabetes, prolonged IV drug use, or previous multiple IV procedures in the forearm.

For these individuals a synthetic graft is usually required. **Arteriovenous grafts** (AVGs), first introduced in 1976, are made of synthetic materials (polytetrafluoroethylene [PTFE], Teflon) and form a "bridge" between the arterial and venous blood supplies.

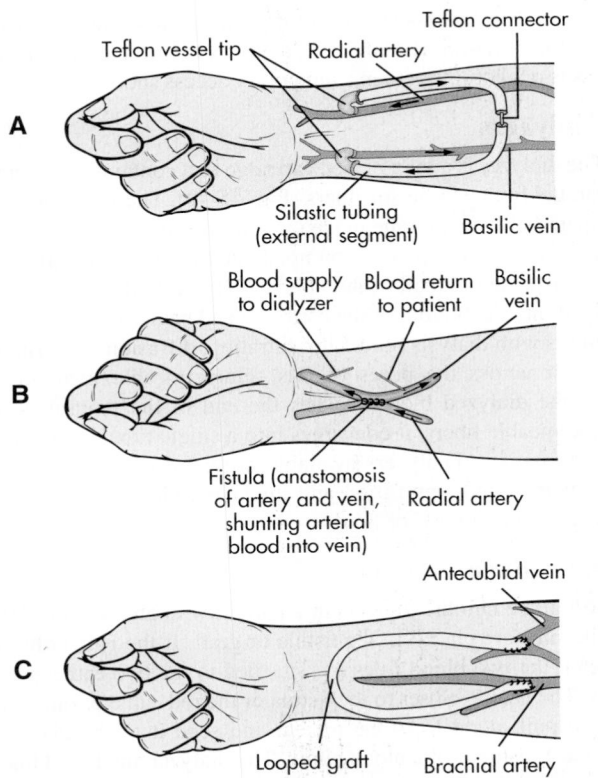

FIG. 45-11 Vascular access for hemodialysis. **A**, External shunt. **B**, Internal arteriovenous fistula. **C**, Internal arteriovenous graft.

Grafts are surgically anastomosed between an artery (usually brachial) and a vein (usually antecubital) (see Fig. 45-11, *C*). The graft, like the fistula, is under the skin and accessed using two large-gauge needles. The graft material is self-healing, meaning it should close over any puncture site after the needle is removed. Because grafts are made of artificial materials, they can become infected easily and are thrombogenic.

The AVF requires 4 to 6 weeks to mature (dilate and toughen) sufficiently for use. When an AVG is placed, an interval of 2 to 4 weeks is usually necessary to allow the graft to heal, but some centers may use it earlier.

Two 14- to 16-gauge needles are inserted into the fistula or graft to obtain vascular access. One needle is placed to pull blood from the circulation to the HD machine, and the other needle is used to return the dialyzed blood to the patient. The needles are attached via tubing to dialysis lines. Normally, a *thrill* can be felt by palpating the area of anastomosis, and a *bruit* can be heard with a stethoscope. The bruit and thrill are created by arterial blood rushing into the vein. BPs, IV insertion, and venipuncture should not be performed on the affected extremity. This prevents infection and clotting of the vascular access. Vascular access can be difficult to obtain for patients with ESRD. Protection of the vascular access site is of paramount importance.

The AVF is much less likely to clot and become infected than a graft. Thrombosis in AVGs is common but can often be corrected with interventional radiology techniques or a surgical procedure. AVGs can cause the development of distal ischemia (*steal syndrome*) because too much of the arterial blood is being shunted or "stolen" from the distal extremity. This is usually seen soon after surgery and may require surgical correction.

Aneurysms can also develop at the fistula site and can rupture if left untreated. AVG infections are not uncommon, and immediate treatment is essential to salvage the graft and prevent bacteremia. Severe AVG infections may necessitate graft removal.

Temporary Vascular Access. In some situations when immediate vascular access is required, percutaneous cannulation of the internal jugular or femoral vein is performed. In the past, the subclavian vein was often cannulated, but the central stenosis that can occur with this approach has made it the option of last resort. A flexible Teflon, silicone rubber, or polyurethane catheter is inserted at the bedside into one of these large veins and provides access to circulation without surgery (Fig. 45-12, *A*). The catheters usually have a double external lumen with an internal septum separating the two internal segments (Fig. 45-12, *B*). One lumen is used for blood removal and the other for blood return. Temporary catheters in the jugular or subclavian veins can be left in place for 1 to 3 weeks. Femoral vein cannulas can remain in place for up to 1 week.

Jugular vein cannulation is associated with a low incidence of thrombosis. That is the primary reason this method is preferred over subclavian cannulation. Short-term jugular vein access with stiff catheters may be uncomfortable and restrict neck movement. Bent catheters can ease this problem (see Fig. 45-12, *A*). In addition to vessel thrombosis and stenosis, subclavian vein cannulation has been associated with pneumothorax, brachial plexus neuropathies, and hemothorax. Both types of catheter placements pose the risk of infection.

Disadvantages of femoral vessel cannulation include the following: (1) the catheter can remain in place only a short time, (2) the location encourages catheter kinking, and (3) the groin is not a clean site. Potential complications of femoral catheterization are femoral vein thrombosis with pulmonary emboli (especially if the treatment is prolonged), infections, immobility, and inad-

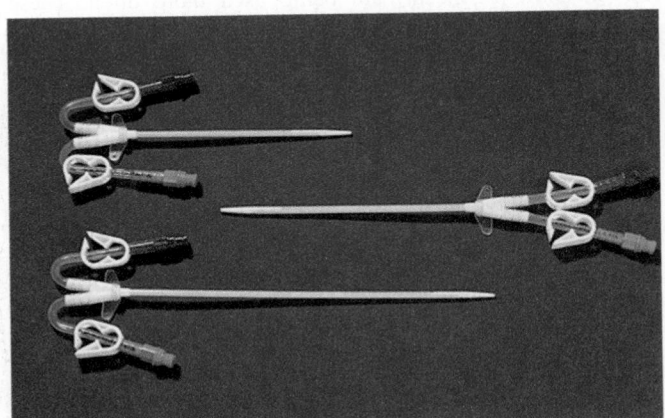

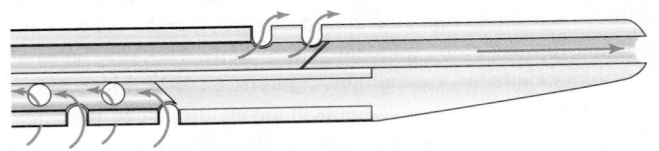

FIG. 45-12 Temporary double-lumen vascular access catheter for acute hemodialysis. **A**, Soft, flexible dual-lumen tube is attached to a Y hub. **B**, Blood is withdrawn continuously through the red lumen (upstream) and returned through the blue lumen (downstream), thus reducing recirculation.

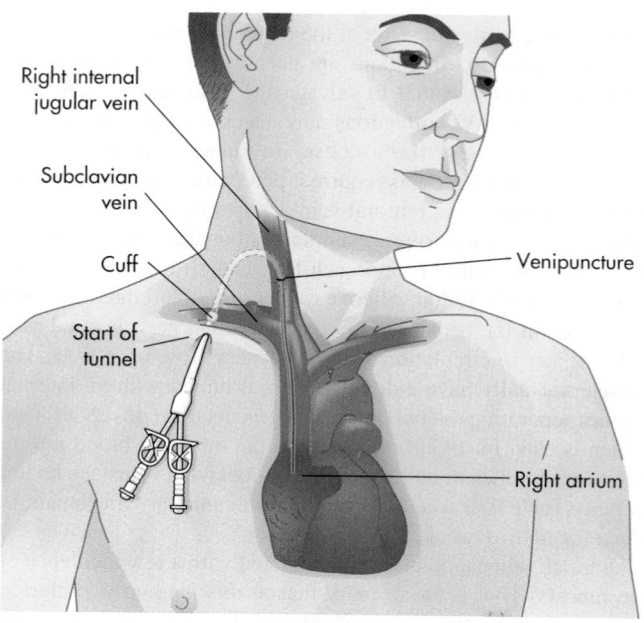

Right internal jugular vein

Subclavian vein

Cuff

Start of tunnel

Venipuncture

Right atrium

FIG. 45-13 Right internal jugular placement for a tunneled, cuffed semipermanent catheter.

vertent blood vessel punctures with hematoma formation. The patient must be on bed rest while the femoral catheter is in place to prevent trauma to the vessel.

For all temporary catheters, no drugs should be administered or blood withdrawn via the catheter by nondialysis staff. This is to minimize the risk of infection, catheter loss, and accidental injection of heparin. Trained dialysis staff will instill heparin into the lumens of the catheter at the end of each treatment to ensure patency and withdraw it before the next treatment.

Semipermanent, soft, flexible Silastic double-lumen catheters (Davol, Bard, Permcath) are being used more often. These catheters can be used as temporary access while awaiting fistula placement and development or as long-term access when other forms of access have failed. This type of catheter exits on the upper chest wall and is tunneled subcutaneously to the internal or external jugular vein (Fig. 45-13). The catheter tip rests in the right atrium. It has one or two subcutaneous Dacron cuffs that prevent infection from tracking along the catheter and anchor the catheter, eliminating the need for sutures.

Several new semipermanent silicone and polyurethane catheters are now available. The aim of all of the new catheters is to increase blood flow rates while decreasing rates of infections and catheter loss from clotting or the development of fibrin sheaths on the catheter exterior. The Tesio catheters involve two tunneled cuffed catheters that are placed through separate tunnels. Both catheter tips are in the right atrium. The Ash Split catheter is a single tunneled cuffed catheter, but the internal and external lumens are split into two lumens.[23] The separate catheters or lumens are thought to improve blood flows. A system called LifeSite uses two subcutaneous implanted ports that are accessed using 14-gauge needles. The implanted ports are attached to internal silicone catheters that are usually tunneled into the internal or external jugular vein.[24]

Advance planning is essential for management of the patient with renal failure who is approaching end-stage disease and dialysis. Several months before the estimated start of dialysis, a per-

manent dialysis access should be created to allow time for healing and maturation. If dialysis is required before the permanent access is ready for use, then a temporary access should be placed.

Dialyzers

The dialyzer is a long plastic cartridge that contains thousands of parallel hollow tubes or fibers (Fig. 45-14). The fibers are the semipermeable membrane made of cellulose-based or other synthetic materials. The blood is pumped into the top of the cartridge and is dispersed into all of the fibers. Dialysis fluid (dialysate) is pumped into the bottom of the cartridge and bathes the outside of the fibers with dialysis fluid. Ultrafiltration, diffusion, and osmosis occur across the pores of this semipermeable membrane. When the dialyzed blood reaches the end of the thousands of semipermeable fibers, it converges into a single tube that returns it to the patient. Dialyzers available differ in regard to surface area, membrane composition and thickness, clearance of waste products, and removal of fluid.

Procedure

To initiate chronic dialysis in a patient with an AVG or AVF, two needles are placed in the fistula or graft. If the patient has a catheter, the two blood lines are attached to the two catheter lumens. The needle closer to the fistula or the red catheter lumen is used to pull blood from the patient and send it to the dialyzer with the assistance of a blood pump. The dialyzer and blood lines are usually primed with up to 1000 ml of saline solution to eliminate air from the system. Heparin is added to the blood as it flows into the dialyzer because any time blood contacts a foreign substance it has a tendency to clot. When the blood enters the extracorporeal circuit, it is propelled through the top of the dialyzer by a blood pump at a flow rate of 200 to 500 ml per minute, while the dialysate (warmed to body temperature) circulates in the opposite direction at a rate of 300 to 900 ml per minute. Blood is returned from the dialyzer to the patient through the second needle or blue catheter lumen.

In addition to the dialyzer, there is a dialysate delivery and monitoring system (Fig. 45-15). This system pumps the dialysate through the dialyzer, countercurrent to the blood flow. Adjustments can be made for ultrafiltration by creating a positive pressure on the blood side or a negative pressure on the dialysate side or by a combination of both. The newest dialysis delivery systems have ultrafiltration controllers that equalize negative and positive pressures for the removal of the precise amount of fluid per hour. The dialysis system has alarm systems to warn of blood leaking into the dialysate or air leaking into the blood; alterations in dialysate temperature, concentration, or pressure; and extremes in BP readings.

Dialysis is terminated by flushing the dialyzer with saline solution to return all blood through the access. The needles are then removed from the patient, and firm pressure is applied to the venipuncture sites until the bleeding stops. On occasion the access site can begin to bleed again. If this occurs, pressure should be reapplied, but not so firmly that flow is occluded because this could cause thrombosis. For patients with a catheter, the blood lines are clamped and removed from the catheter lumens.

Before beginning treatment, the nurse must complete an assessment that includes fluid status (weight, BP, peripheral edema, lung and heart sounds), condition of vascular access, temperature, and general skin condition. The difference between the last

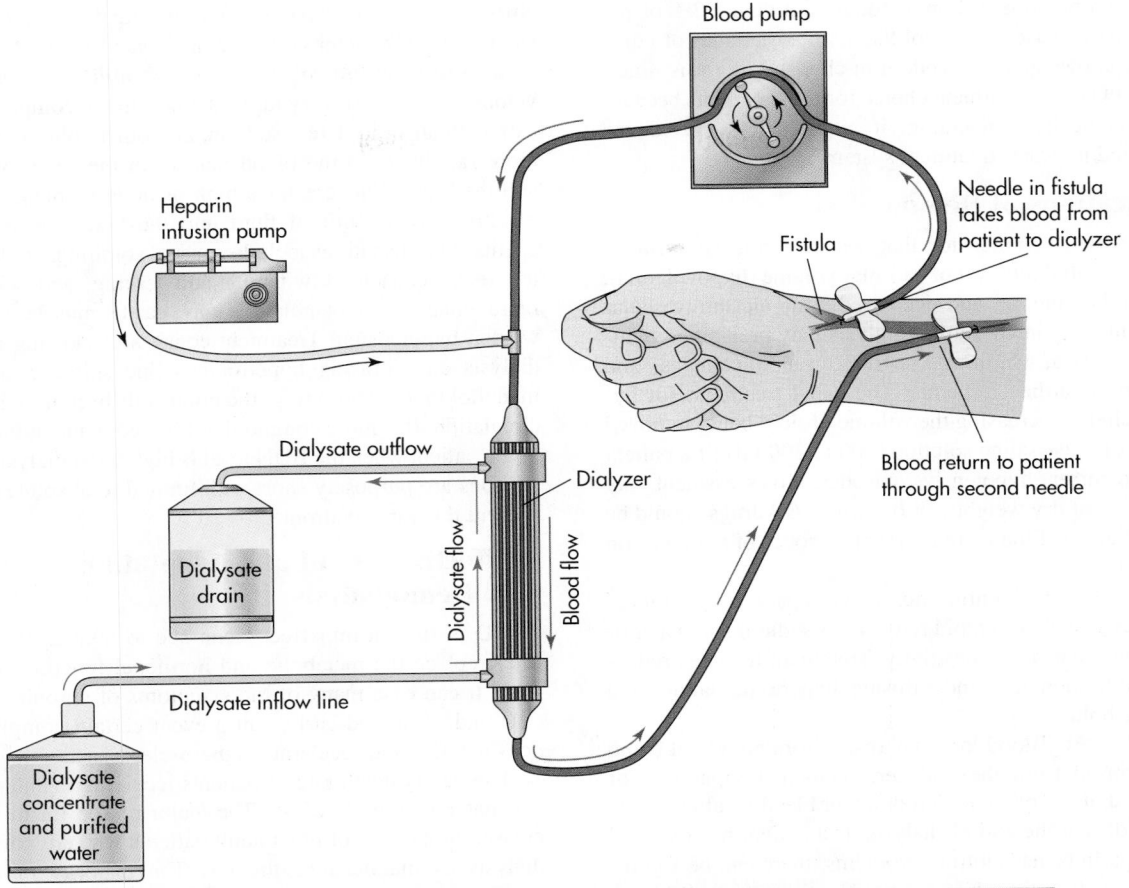

FIG. 45-14 Components of a hemodialysis system. Blood is removed via a needle inserted in a fistula or via catheter lumen. It is propelled to the dialyzer by a blood pump. Heparin is infused to prevent clotting. Dialysate is pumped in and flows in the opposite direction of the blood. The dialyzed blood is returned to the patient through a second needle or catheter lumen. Old dialysate and ultrafiltrate are drained and discarded.

postdialysis weight and the present predialysis weight determines the ultrafiltration or the amount of weight to be removed. Ideally, no more than 1 to 1.5 kg should be gained between treatments to avoid causing hypotension associated with the removal of larger volumes of fluid. Many patients gain 2 to 3 kg between treatments, and this volume usually can be removed if their BP is not labile. While the patient is on dialysis, vital signs should be taken at least every 30 to 60 minutes because rapid changes may occur in the BP.

Most maintenance dialysis units use reclining chairs that allow for elevation of the feet if hypotension develops. Most people sleep, read, talk, or watch television during dialysis. Treatments usually last 3 to 5 hours and are done three times per week to achieve adequate clearance and maintain fluid balance.

Settings for Hemodialysis. HD can be done in an inpatient (hospital) or outpatient (clinic or hospital) setting. Inpatient dialysis is used for treating hospitalized patients. In outpatient dialysis the patient comes to the unit for treatment. The patient may choose to do self-care with backup support from trained personnel if needed. Self-care patients put in the dialysis needles, set up the machine, and monitor the course of the treatment.

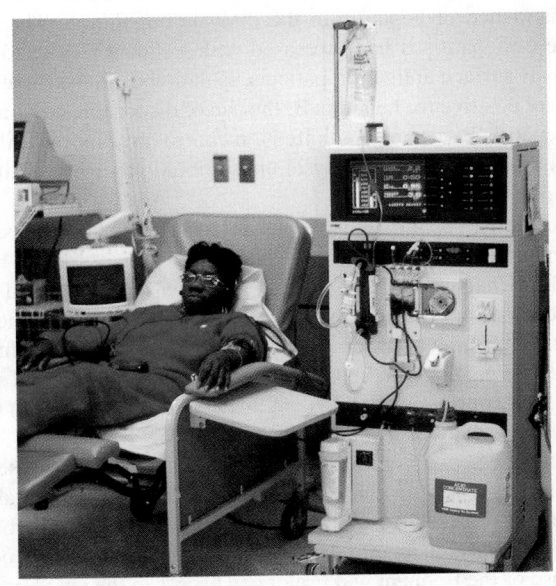

FIG. 45-15 Patient receiving in-center hemodialysis.

HD can also be done at home. Today less than 1.3% of patients receiving HD use it.[8] One of the main advantages of home HD is that it allows greater freedom in choosing dialysis times. Today home PD is the treatment choice for more patients because it is less technically demanding, it requires less specialized equipment, and no water treatment system is needed.

Complications of Hemodialysis

Hypotension. Hypotension that occurs during HD primarily results from rapid removal of vascular volume (hypovolemia), decreased cardiac output, and decreased systemic intravascular resistance. The drop in BP during dialysis may precipitate lightheadedness, nausea, vomiting, seizures, vision changes, and chest pain from cardiac ischemia. The usual treatment for hypotension includes decreasing the volume of fluid being removed and infusion of 0.9% saline solution (100 to 300 ml). If a patient experiences recurrent hypotensive episodes, a reassessment may have to be done of dry weight and BP drugs. BP drugs should be held before dialysis if there are frequent episodes of hypotension during dialysis.

Muscle Cramps. Painful muscle cramps are a common problem. They result from rapid removal of sodium and water or from neuromuscular hypersensitivity. Treatment includes reducing the ultrafiltration rate and infusing hypertonic saline or a normal saline bolus.

Loss of Blood. Blood loss may result from blood not being completely rinsed from the dialyzer, accidental separation of blood tubing, dialysis membrane rupture, or bleeding after the removal of needles at the end of dialysis. If a patient has received too much heparin or has clotting problems, there can be significant postdialysis bleeding. It is essential to rinse back all blood, to closely monitor heparinization to avoid excess anticoagulation, and to hold firm but nonocclusive pressure on access sites until the risk of bleeding has passed.

Hepatitis. The causes of hepatitis B and C in dialysis patients include blood transfusions or the lack of adherence to precautions used to prevent the spread of infection. As blood is now screened for hepatitis B and C, blood is an unlikely source of infection. IV drug abuse and unprotected sex can also contribute to the incidence of hepatitis in the dialysis population. The incidence of hepatitis B has decreased with frequent testing for hepatitis B surface antigen in patients, isolation of dialysis patients who are positive for hepatitis B, the use of disposable equipment, the hepatitis B vaccine, and infection control precautions. All patients and personnel in dialysis units should receive hepatitis B vaccine.

Currently, hepatitis C is responsible for the majority of cases of hepatitis in dialysis patients. (Hepatitis is discussed in more detail in Chapter 42.) The Centers for Disease Control and Prevention does not recommend isolation of the HD patient who has hepatitis C. Infection control precautions are mandated in the care of the patient with hepatitis C to protect the patient and staff. (Infection control precautions are discussed in Chapter 12.) Currently, no vaccine is available for hepatitis C.

Sepsis. Sepsis is most often related to infections of vascular access sites. Bacteria can also be introduced during the dialysis treatment as a result of poor technique or interruption of blood tubing or dialyzer membranes. Bacterial endocarditis can occur because of the frequent and prolonged access to the vascular system. Aseptic technique is essential to prevent this problem.

Nurses must monitor patients for signs and symptoms of sepsis such as fever, hypotension, and an elevated WBC.

Disequilibrium Syndrome. *Disequilibrium syndrome* develops as a result of very rapid changes in the composition of the extracellular fluid. Urea, sodium, and other solutes are removed more rapidly from the blood than from the cerebrospinal fluid and the brain. This creates a high osmotic gradient in the brain resulting in the shift of fluid into the brain, causing cerebral edema. Manifestations include nausea, vomiting, confusion, restlessness, headaches, twitching and jerking, and seizures. The rapid changes in osmolality may cause muscle cramps and worsen hypotension. Treatment consists of slowing or stopping dialysis and infusing hypertonic saline solution, albumin, or mannitol to draw fluid from the brain cells back into the systemic circulation. It is more commonly observed in the initial treatment of the patient when the BUN level is high. First dialysis treatment sessions are purposely short with limited total solute removal to prevent this rare syndrome.

Effectiveness of and Adaptation to Hemodialysis

HD is still an imperfect technique to treat ESRD. It cannot fully replace the metabolic and hormonal functions of the kidneys. It can ease many of the symptoms of chronic kidney disease and, if started early, can prevent certain complications. It does not alter the accelerated atherosclerosis.

The yearly death rate of patients receiving maintenance dialysis has increased to 22%.[8] The major reason for this is the increased proportion of older adult patients who are now receiving dialysis as maintenance therapy. The majority of deaths are caused by cardiovascular disease (stroke or myocardial infarction). Infectious complications are the second leading cause of death.

Individual adaptation to maintenance HD varies considerably. Initially many patients feel positive about the dialysis because it makes them feel better and keeps them alive, but there is often great ambivalence about whether it is worthwhile. Dependence on a machine is a reality, and some have dreams about being tied to the machine. In response to their illness, dialysis patients may demonstrate noncompliance, depression, and suicidal tendencies. The primary nursing goals are to help the patient regain or maintain positive self-esteem and control of his or her life and to continue to be productive in society.[25]

CONTINUOUS RENAL REPLACEMENT THERAPY

Continuous renal replacement therapy (CRRT) is an alternative or adjunctive method for treating ARF. CRRT provides a means by which solutes and a large volume of fluid can be removed slowly and continuously from a hemodynamically unstable patient. Continuous renal replacement therapies are contraindicated if a patient has life-threatening manifestations of uremia (hyperkalemia, pericarditis) that require rapid resolution.[26] CRRT can be used in conjunction with HD for continuous fluid removal.

There are several technical variations of CRRT. Both fluid and solute removal can be achieved with continuous therapies. There are two types of CRRT differentiated by whether arterial or venous access is required and if a blood pump is needed (Table 45-11). The continuous arteriovenous therapies (CAVTs) require arterial

TABLE 45-11	Types of Continuous Renal Replacement Therapies	
ACRONYM	**THERAPY**	**PURPOSE**
SCUF (AV)	Slow continuous ultrafiltration	Fluid removal via ultrafiltration
CVVU (VV)	Continuous venovenous ultrafiltration	Solute loss via convection
CAVH (AV)	Continuous arteriovenous hemofiltration	Fluid removal via ultrafiltration
CVVH (VV)	Continuous venovenous hemofiltration	Solute loss via convection; hemodilution using replacement fluid
CAVHD (AV)	Continuous arteriovenous hemodialysis	Fluid removal via ultrafiltration and osmosis
CVVHD (VV)	Continuous venovenous hemodialysis	Solute loss via convection and diffusion

AA, Arteriovenous; *VV,* venovenous.

access because the arterial pressure is needed to pump blood through the circuit that is placed between the arterial and venous catheters (Fig. 45-16). Vascular access is usually achieved by cannulation of the femoral artery and femoral, jugular, or subclavian vein. Rarely, an external shunt may be placed. The CAVTs include slow continuous ultrafiltration (SCUF), continuous arteriovenous hemofiltration (CAVH), and continuous arteriovenous hemodialysis (CAVHD). There are other more complex mixed modalities.

Continuous venovenous therapies (CVVTs) achieve the same goals as CAVT but use venous dual-lumen catheters for access, necessitating the use of a blood pump to propel the blood through the circuit (Fig. 45-17). The CVVTs include continuous venovenous ultrafiltration (CVVU), continuous venovenous hemofiltration (CVVH), and continuous venovenous hemodialysis (CVVHD). In many clinical situations, CVVT is preferred because it is difficult to obtain and maintain arterial access for long periods.

In CRRT a highly permeable, hollow fiber hemofilter placed between the two catheter lumens removes plasma water and nonprotein solutes, which are collectively termed *ultrafiltrate.* Under the influence of hydrostatic pressure and osmotic pressure, water and nonprotein solutes pass out of the filter into the extracapillary space and drain through the ultrafiltrate port into a collection device (see Fig. 45-16). The remaining fluid continues through the filter and returns to the patient through the second catheter or catheter lumen. While the ultrafiltrate drains out of the hemofilter, fluid and electrolyte replacements can be infused into the venous line infusion port. This fluid is designed to replace volume and solutes such as sodium, chloride, bicarbonate, and glucose. It will also further dilute intravascular fluid, decreasing the concentration of unwanted solutes such as BUN, creatinine, and potassium. The infusion rate of replacement fluid is determined by the degree of fluid and electrolyte imbalance. Replacement fluid may also be infused into the arterial line infusion port. This method allows for greater clearance of urea and can decrease filter clotting.

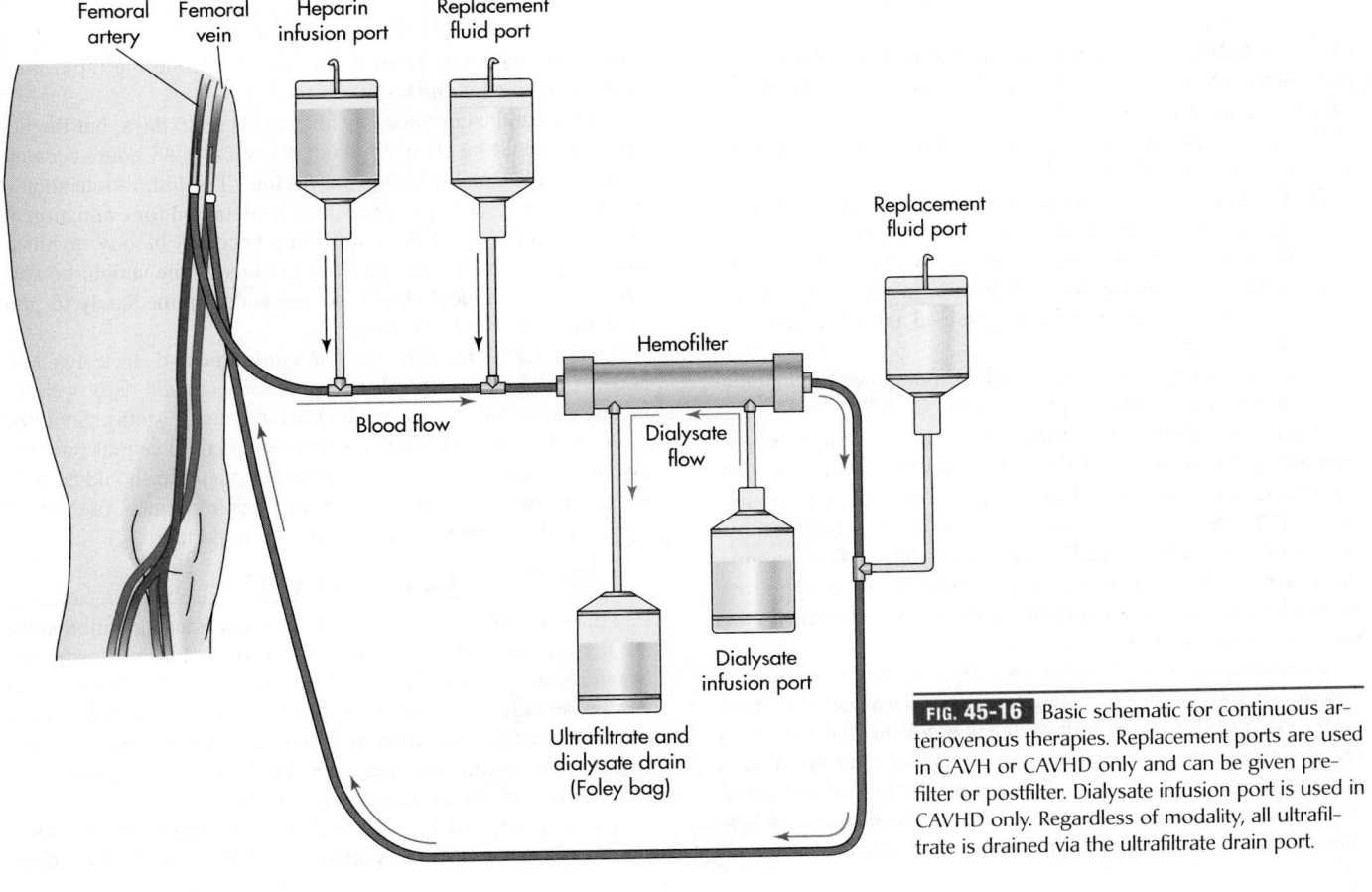

FIG. 45-16 Basic schematic for continuous arteriovenous therapies. Replacement ports are used in CAVH or CAVHD only and can be given prefilter or postfilter. Dialysate infusion port is used in CAVHD only. Regardless of modality, all ultrafiltrate is drained via the ultrafiltrate drain port.

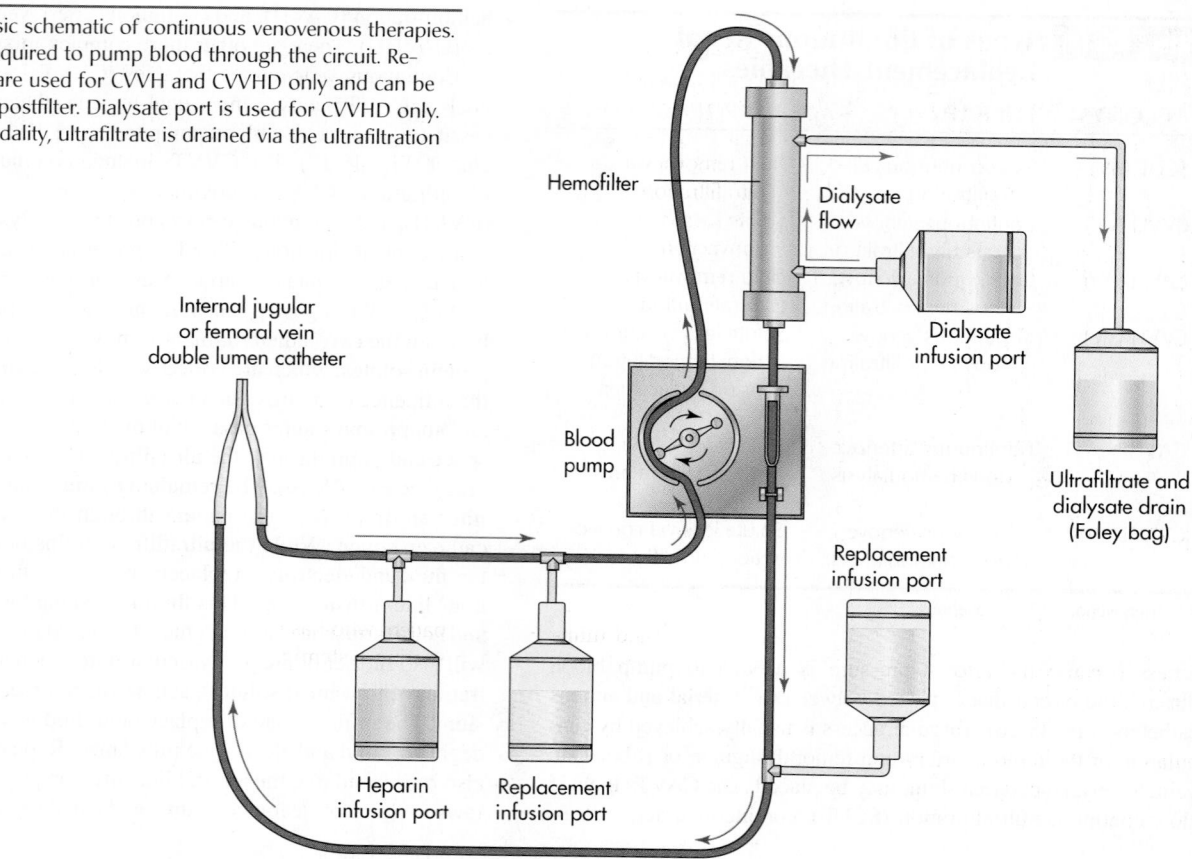

FIG. 45-17 Basic schematic of continuous venovenous therapies. Blood pump is required to pump blood through the circuit. Replacement ports are used for CVVH and CVVHD only and can be given prefilter or postfilter. Dialysate port is used for CVVHD only. Regardless of modality, ultrafiltrate is drained via the ultrafiltration drain port.

Labels in figure: Hemofilter; Dialysate flow; Dialysate infusion port; Ultrafiltrate and dialysate drain (Foley bag); Internal jugular or femoral vein double lumen catheter; Blood pump; Replacement infusion port; Heparin infusion port; Replacement infusion port

Like HD, CRRT provides for the removal of fluid, electrolytes, and solutes. However, several of its features differ from HD, including the following:

1. It is continuous rather than intermittent. Large volumes can be removed over days versus hours.
2. Solute removal can occur by *convection* (no dialysate required) in addition to osmosis and diffusion.
3. It causes less hemodynamic instability (e.g., hypotension).
4. It does not require constant monitoring by a specialized HD nurse but does require a trained intensive care unit (ICU) nurse.
5. It does not require complicated HD equipment, but a modified blood pump is required for the CVVTs.

Regardless of whether the modality is arteriovenous or venovenous, each modality has three therapies that have equivalent outcomes. SCUF and CVVU are strictly for ultrafiltration or fluid removal. There is some convective loss of solutes, but no diffusion or osmosis is involved. CAVH and CVVH involve the introduction of replacement fluids. Large volumes of fluid are removed hourly (600 to 900 ml), and then a portion of this fluid is replaced (500 to 800 ml).

Ultrafiltration and convective losses occur, and solute concentrations in the blood are diluted with the replacement fluid. CAVHD and CVVHD use dialysate. Peritoneal dialysate bags are attached to the distal end of the hemofilter, and the fluid is pumped countercurrent to the blood flow. As in dialysis, diffusion of solutes and ultrafiltration via hydrostatic pressure and osmosis occur. This is an ideal treatment for a patient who needs both fluid and solute control but cannot tolerate the rapid fluid shifts associated with HD.[27]

CRRT can be continued as long as 30 to 40 days, but the hemofilter should be changed about every 24 to 48 hours because of loss of filtration efficiency or clotting. The ultrafiltrate should be clear yellow, and specimens may be obtained for evaluation of serum chemistries. If the ultrafiltrate becomes bloody or blood tinged, a possible rupture in the filter membrane should be suspected, and treatment should be suspended immediately to prevent blood loss and infection.

During CRRT the nurse must monitor fluid and electrolyte balance. Hourly intake and output measurements and daily weights must be recorded. Vital signs and hemodynamic status should be monitored hourly. Although reductions in central venous pressure and pulmonary artery pressure are expected, there should be little change in mean arterial pressure or cardiac output. Assessment and care of the vascular access sites are important.

KIDNEY TRANSPLANTATION

Major progress has been made in organ transplantation since the first kidney transplant was performed in 1954 in Boston between identical twins. The advances made in organ procurement and preservation, surgical techniques, tissue typing and matching, understanding the immune system, immunosuppressant therapy, and preventing and treating rejection have dramatically increased the success of organ transplantation.

The disparity between the supply and demand for organs is significant. Over 245,000 patients are receiving dialysis. Over

54,000 patients are currently awaiting cadaveric kidney transplants, but only about 8000 cadaveric transplants were performed in 2002. Over 5200 living donor kidney transplants were done in 2002. Transplantation from a cadaver donor usually requires a prolonged waiting period, with median waiting times of 18 months to 4 years depending on blood type and other factors. Blood types B and O have the longest waiting times.[28]

Kidney transplantation is extremely successful, with 1-year graft survival rates of about 90% for cadaver transplants and 95% for live donor transplants.[28] An advantage of kidney transplantation when compared with dialysis is that it reverses many of the pathophysiologic changes associated with renal failure when normal kidney function is restored. It also eliminates the dependence on dialysis and the accompanying dietary and lifestyle restrictions. Transplantation is also less expensive than dialysis after the first year.

Recipient Selection

Appropriate recipient selection is important for a successful outcome. Candidacy is determined by a variety of medical and psychosocial factors that vary among transplant centers. A careful evaluation is completed in an attempt to identify and minimize potential complications after transplantation. Certain patients, particularly those with cardiovascular disease and diabetes mellitus, are considered high risk. With careful evaluation and monitoring, high-risk patients can achieve the same success rates as other patients.[29] Some patients who are approaching ESRD can receive a transplant before dialysis is required if they have a living donor. This approach is most advantageous for patients with diabetes, who have a much higher mortality rate on dialysis than nondiabetics.

Contraindications to transplantation include disseminated malignancies, refractory or untreated cardiac disease, chronic respiratory failure, extensive vascular disease, chronic infection, and unresolved psychosocial disorders (e.g., noncompliance with medical regimens, alcoholism, drug addiction). The presence of hepatitis B or C is not a contraindication to transplantation.

Surgical procedures may be required before transplantation based on the results of the recipient evaluation. Coronary artery bypass may be indicated for advanced coronary artery disease. Cholecystectomy may be necessary for patients with a history of gallstones, biliary obstruction, or cholecystitis. On rare occasions, bilateral nephrectomies may be done for patients with refractory hypertension, recurrent urinary tract infections, or grossly enlarged kidneys resulting from polycystic kidney disease.

Histocompatibility Studies

Histocompatibility testing is discussed in Chapter 13 on p. 256.

Donor Sources

Kidneys for transplantation may be obtained from compatible blood type cadaver donors, blood relatives, emotionally related living donors (e.g., spouses, friends), and altruistic living donors who are unknown to the recipient. Expanding the living donor pool is one of the best possibilities for decreasing the size of the cadaveric waiting list and reducing waiting times.

Live Donors. Live donors must undergo an extensive multidisciplinary evaluation to be certain that they are in good health and have no history of disease that would place them at risk for

*E*THICAL DILEMMAS
Allocation of Resources

Situation

A transplant nurse coordinator is considering her feelings about two patients who are being evaluated for placement on the cadaveric kidney transplant waiting list. One patient is a 40-year-old African American school teacher. She is married and has two children. The other patient is a 22-year-old unemployed white male who is actively using cocaine. He misses 3 to 4 dialysis treatments per month and does not take his phosphate binders or antihypertensive drugs consistently.

Important Points for Consideration

- It is tempting to believe that nurses can be neutral, basing allocation of scarce resources on need rather than worth. However, it is difficult to practice patient-neutral care.
- Psychologic, physiologic, and adherence factors are included in the assessment process for eligibility for organ transplantation.
- In kidney transplantation, the organ is transplanted into the patient who has received the most points based on a scoring system, regardless of the health care provider's opinion of the patient's worth. If a patient is denied transplant candidacy on this basis, he or she must be given a chance to change or improve the problem or condition in a specified period.
- The national organ procurement system is designed to be unbiased about the patient in all respects. Once a patient is placed on the list for transplantation, that patient is deemed of no greater or lesser worth than any other patient.
- Because organ donation is voluntary and altruistic in the United States, any concerns that the system of procurement and transplantation is not fair may negatively affect the pool of available organs.

Critical Thinking Questions

1. What does the 2001 American Nurses Association (ANA) Code of Ethics say about how nurses should view patients?
2. What are your feelings about which of the patients should receive the next available organ?

developing kidney failure or operative complications. Psychosocial and financial evaluations are done as well. Crossmatches are done at the time of the evaluation and about a week before the transplant to ensure that no antibodies to the donor are present or that the antibody titer is below the allowed level. Advantages of a live donor kidney include better patient and graft survival rates regardless of histocompatibility match, immediate organ availability, immediate function because of minimal cold time (kidney out of body and not getting blood supply), and the opportunity to have the recipient in the best possible medical condition because the surgery is elective.

As a result of advances in technology and immunology, living donors do not necessarily need to be ABO compatible with the recipient. Plasmapheresis can be used to remove the antibodies to the incompatible blood group, and potent immunosuppression and immunomodulation with IV immune globulin dampen the response to the antibody. It is also possible to have some antibodies to the donor human leukocyte antigens (HLA) present and still proceed with the transplant. These antibodies can also be removed with plasmapheresis and the antibody level reduced with significant immunosuppression and immunomodulation. ABO incompatibility or the presence of antibody to the donor's HLA complicates the transplant process. However, because the donor shortage is severe, complex measures are necessary to ensure that as many patients as possible are transplanted.

The donor will see a nephrologist for a complete history and physical and laboratory and diagnostic studies. Laboratory studies include a 24-hour urine study for creatinine clearance and total protein, complete blood count, and chemistry and electrolyte profiles. Hepatitis B and C, HIV, and cytomegalovirus (CMV) testing are done to assess for the presence of any transmissible diseases. An ECG and chest x-ray are also done. A renal ultrasound and a renal arteriogram or three-dimensional CT are performed to ensure that the blood vessels supplying each kidney are adequate and that there are no anomalies and to determine which kidney will be removed.

A transplant psychologist or social worker will determine if the individual is emotionally stable and able to deal with the issues related to organ donation. All donors must be informed about the risks and benefits of donation, the potential short-term and long-term complications, and what can be expected during the hospitalization and recovery phases. Although the cost of the evaluation and surgery are covered by the recipient's insurance, there is no compensation available for lost wages during the posthospitalization recovery period. This period can last 6 weeks or longer. The laparoscopic donor nephrectomy procedure shortens the amount of time before a person can return to work or other usual activities.[30]

Cadaver Donors. Cadaver kidney donors are relatively healthy individuals who have suffered an irreversible brain injury. The most common causes of injury are cerebral trauma from motor vehicle accidents or gunshot wounds, intracerebral or subarachnoid hemorrhage, and anoxic brain damage caused by cardiac arrest. The brain-dead donor must have effective cardiovascular function and be supported on a ventilator to preserve the organs. The age range of most suitable kidney donors is from 2 to 70 years. The age of the donor is less important than the quality of kidney function. The donor must be free of active IV drug abuse; severe hypertension; long-standing diabetes mellitus; malignancies; sepsis; and communicable diseases, including HIV, hepatitis B and C, syphilis, and tuberculosis. Permission from the donor's legal next-of-kin is required after brain death is determined even if the donor carried a signed donor card.

The kidneys are removed and preserved. They can be preserved for up to 72 hours, but most transplant surgeons prefer to transplant kidneys before the cold time reaches 24 hours. Experience has shown that prolonged cold time increases the likelihood that the kidney will not function immediately, and the transplant recipient will require dialysis until the ATN from the extended cold time resolves.

Cadaveric kidneys are distributed by the United Network for Organ Sharing using an objective computerized point system. The ABO group, HLA typing, age, antibody level, and length of time waiting are entered into the national computer for each candidate when they are listed. When a donor becomes available, the donor's HLA data, ABO type, and other key information are compared with the data of all patients awaiting transplantation locally and nationwide. Donors and recipients must have the same blood type. Points are given for how close the HLA match is, how long the patient has been waiting, if the antibody level is

unusually high, and if the recipient is less than 19 years old. Extra points are given for high antibody levels because this can severely limit the number of donors with which the patient will not have a positive crossmatch. The kidney is offered to the recipient with the most points in the local area. If there are no patients in the local area who are suitable, the organ is then offered in the region and then to the nation. When a kidney arrives at the recipient's transplant center, a final crossmatch is done. The final crossmatch must be negative for the cadaveric transplant to proceed. (Crossmatching is discussed in Chapter 13.)

The only exception to the previous plan is if a patient needs an emergency transplant or if a donor and recipient do not mismatch on any of the six HLA antigens (zero antigen mismatch). In these situations, the patient meeting either one of these criteria goes to the top of the list. Emergency transplants are given priority because the patient is facing imminent death if not transplanted (for example, a patient who had no vascular access sites left and can no longer dialyze). Zero antigen mismatches are given priority because statistically these grafts have much better survival rates. If a zero antigen mismatch patient is identified nationally, one of the donor kidneys must be sent to that recipient's transplant center regardless of location.

Surgical Procedure

Live Donor. The donor nephrectomy is performed by a urologist or transplant surgeon. The donor's surgery begins an hour or two before the recipient's surgery is started. The recipient is surgically prepared for the kidney transplant in a nearby operating room. For a conventional nephrectomy, the donor is placed in the lateral decubitus position on the operating table so that the flank is presented laterally. An incision is made at the level of the eleventh rib. The rib may have to be removed to provide adequate visualization of the kidney. After removal of the kidney, it is flushed with a chilled, sterile electrolyte solution and prepared for immediate transplant into the recipient. The nephrectomy takes about 3 hours. The short cold time is the primary reason for the success of living donor transplants.

Laparoscopic donor nephrectomy is an alternative to a conventional nephrectomy. (Laparoscopic nephrectomy is discussed in Chapter 44.) This procedure is now being used as the primary method of live kidney procurement. The laparoscopic approach significantly decreases the hospital stay, pain, operative blood loss, debilitation, and length of time off work. For these reasons, the number of people willing to donate a kidney has increased significantly.[31]

Kidney Transplant Recipient

The transplanted kidney is usually placed extraperitoneally in the iliac fossa. The right iliac fossa is preferred to facilitate anastomoses and minimize the occurrence of ileus.

Before any incisions are made, a urinary catheter is placed into the bladder. An antibiotic solution is instilled to distend the bladder and decrease the risk of infection. A crescent-shaped incision is made extending from the iliac crest to the symphysis pubis (Fig. 45-18). The peritoneum is left intact. The iliac and hypogastric vessels are dissected free.

Rapid revascularization is critical to prevent ischemic injury to the kidney. The donor artery is anastomosed to the recipient's internal iliac (hypogastric) or external iliac artery. The donor vein is anastomosed to the recipient's external iliac vein. Kidney transplants with living donors can be technically more difficult because the blood vessel lengths can be shorter than in cadaveric transplants.

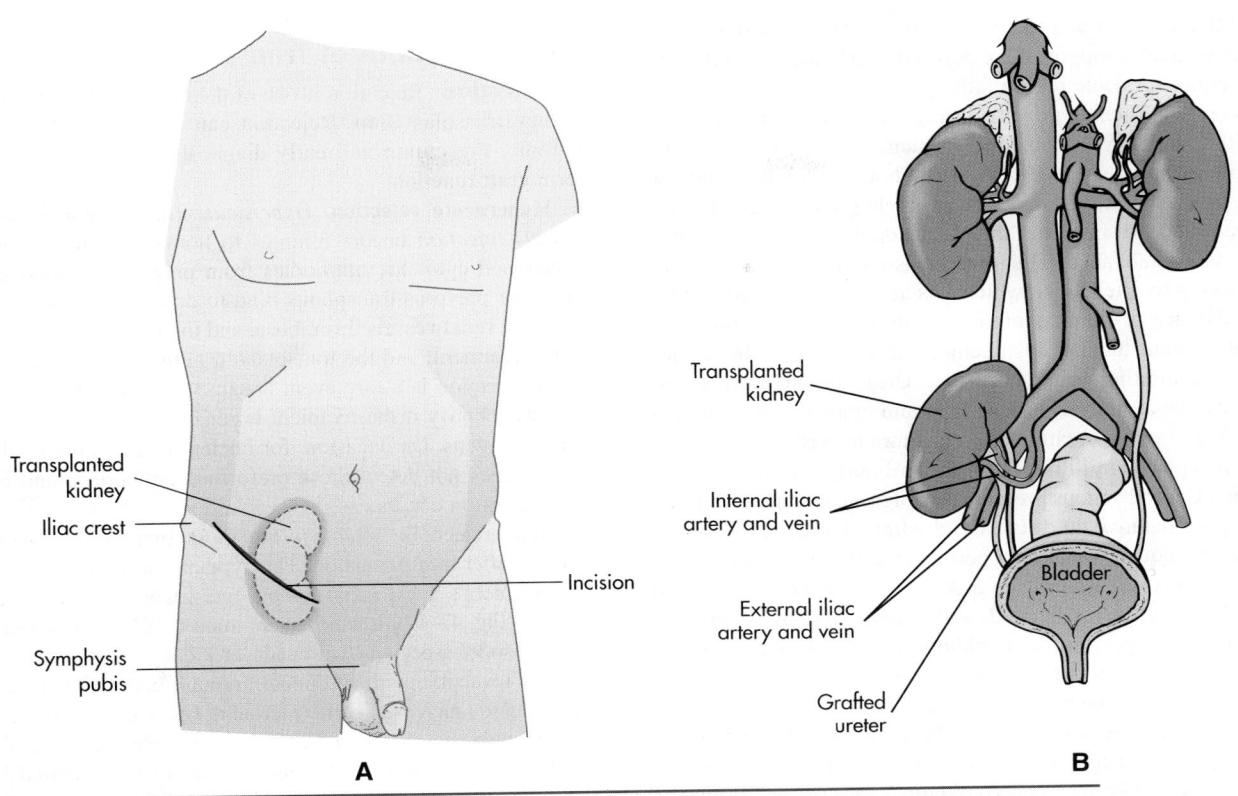

FIG. 45-18 **A,** Surgical incision for a renal transplant. **B,** Surgical placement of transplanted kidney.

When the anastomoses are complete, the clamps are released, and blood flow to the kidney is reestablished. The kidney should become firm and pink. Urine may begin to flow from the ureter immediately. Mannitol or furosemide (Lasix) may be administered to promote diuresis.

The donor ureter in most cases is then tunneled through the bladder submucosa before entering the bladder cavity and being sutured in place. This approach is called *ureteroneocystostomy.* This allows the bladder wall to compress the ureter as it contracts for micturition, thereby preventing reflux of urine up the ureter into the transplanted kidney. The transplant surgery takes approximately 3 to 4 hours.

NURSING MANAGEMENT
KIDNEY TRANSPLANT RECIPIENT

The successful recovery and rehabilitation of the recipient are made possible with careful nursing assessment, diagnosis, intervention, and evaluation of all body systems. With a hospital length of stay averaging 4 to 5 days, discharge planning and teaching needs must be identified and addressed early in the hospital course.

■ Preoperative Care

Nursing care of the patient in the preoperative phase includes emotional and physical preparation for surgery. Because the patient and family may have been waiting years for the kidney transplant, a review of the operative procedure and what can be expected in the immediate postoperative recovery period is necessary. It is important to stress that there is a chance the kidney may not function immediately, and dialysis may be required for

days to weeks. The need for immunosuppressive drugs and measures to prevent infection must be reviewed.

To ensure the patient is in optimal physical condition for surgery, an ECG, chest x-ray, and laboratory studies are ordered. Dialysis may be required before surgery for any significant abnormality such as fluid overload or hyperkalemia. A patient on PD must empty the peritoneal cavity of all dialysate solution before going to surgery. Because dialysis may be required after transplant, the patency of the vascular access must be maintained. The vascular access extremity should be labeled "dialysis access, no procedures" to prevent use of the affected extremity for BP measurement, blood drawing, or IV infusions.

■ Postoperative Care

Live Donor. The usual postoperative care for the donor is similar to that following conventional or laparoscopic nephrectomy (see Chapter 44). Close monitoring of renal function to assess for impairment and of the hematocrit to assess for bleeding is essential. The creatinine should be less than 1.4 mg/dl, and the hematocrit should not fall more than 3 to 6 points. The pain that a donor who has had a conventional nephrectomy experiences is greater than that of the donor who had a laparoscopic procedure. Generally, all donors have more pain than their recipients. Conventional donors are ready to be discharged from the hospital in 4 to 7 days and can usually return to work in 6 to 8 weeks. Laparoscopic donors are able to be discharged from the hospital in 2 to 4 days and can return to work in 4 to 6 weeks. The donor is seen by the surgeon 1 to 2 weeks after discharge.

Nurses caring for the living donor need to acknowledge the precious gift that this person has given. The donor has taken physical, emotional, and financial risks to assist the recipient. It is vital that they not be forgotten postoperatively. The donor will need even greater support if the donated organ does not work immediately or for some reason fails.

Recipient. The first priority during this period is maintenance of fluid and electrolyte balance. In many centers, kidney transplant recipients spend the first 12 to 24 hours in the ICU because of the close monitoring required. Very large volumes of urine may be produced soon after the blood supply to the transplanted kidney is reestablished. This diuresis is due to (1) the new kidney's ability to filter BUN, which acts as an osmotic diuretic; (2) the abundance of fluids administered during the operation; and (3) initial renal tubular dysfunction, which inhibits the kidney from concentrating urine normally. Urine output during this phase may be as high as 1 L per hour and gradually decreases as the BUN and serum creatinine levels return toward normal. Urine output is replaced milliliter for milliliter hourly for the first 12 to 24 hours. Central venous pressure readings are essential for monitoring postoperative fluid status. Dehydration must be avoided to prevent subsequent renal hypoperfusion and renal tubular damage. Electrolyte monitoring to assess for the hyponatremia and hypokalemia often associated with rapid diuresis is critical. Treatment with potassium supplements or 0.9% normal saline solution infusion may be indicated. IV sodium bicarbonate may also be required if the patient becomes acidotic.

Acute tubular necrosis (ATN) is becoming more common because of prolonged cold times and the use of marginal donors. The ischemic damage from extended cold times causes ATN. While the patient is in ATN, dialysis is required to maintain fluid and electrolyte balance. Some patients have high-output ATN with the ability to excrete fluid, but not metabolic wastes or electrolytes. Other patients have oliguric or anuric ATN. These patients are at risk for fluid overload in the immediate postoperative period and must be assessed closely for the need for dialysis. The period of ATN can last anywhere from days to weeks, with gradually improving kidney function. Most patients with ATN will be discharged from the hospital on dialysis. This is extremely discouraging for the patient, who will need reassurance that renal function usually improves. Dialysis will be discontinued when urine output increases and serum creatinine and BUN begin to normalize.

A sudden decrease in urine output in the early postoperative period is a cause for concern. It may be due to dehydration, rejection, a urine leak, or obstruction. A common cause of early obstruction is a blood clot in the urinary catheter. Catheter patency must be maintained as the catheter remains in the bladder for 3 to 5 days to allow the bladder anastomosis to heal. If blood clots are suspected, gentle catheter irrigation with an order from the health care provider can reestablish patency.

Postoperative teaching should include the prevention and treatment of rejection, infection, and complications of surgery and the purpose and side effects of immunosuppression. Patients should be aware that rejection is a common occurrence during the first 3 months after transplant. Frequent blood tests and clinic visits help detect rejection early. Patient education to ensure a smooth transition from hospital to home is an integral part of the nursing care.[32]

Immunosuppressive Therapy

The goal of immunosuppression is to adequately suppress the immune response to prevent rejection of the transplanted kidney while maintaining sufficient immunity to prevent overwhelming infection. Immunosuppressive therapy is discussed in Chapter 13 and in Table 13-17.

Complications of Transplantation

Rejection. Rejection is one of the major problems following kidney transplantation. Rejection can be hyperacute, acute, or chronic. Prevention and early diagnosis are essential for long-term graft function.

Hyperacute rejection. *Hyperacute (antibody-mediated, humoral) rejection* occurs minutes to hours after transplantation. Preformed cytotoxic antibodies from pregnancy, blood transfusions, or previous transplants bind to donor antigens in the kidney. The renal vessels thrombose, and the kidney necroses. There is no treatment, and the transplanted kidney is removed. Hyperacute rejection is a rare event because the final crossmatch will usually identify if the recipient is sensitized to any of the donor HLA antigens. On occasion, for unclear reasons, the final crossmatch does not detect these preformed antibodies, and hyperacute rejection occurs.

Acute rejection. *Acute rejection* most commonly occurs days to months after transplantation. This type of rejection is mediated by the recipient's T cytotoxic lymphocytes, which attack the foreign kidney (Fig. 45-19). It is not uncommon to have at least one rejection episode, especially with cadaver kidneys. These episodes are usually reversible with additional immunosuppressive therapy that may include increased corticosteroid doses or polyclonal or monoclonal antibodies. Signs of rejection include elevated creatinine and BUN, fever, weight gain, decreased urine output, increased BP, and tenderness over the transplanted kidney. It is sometimes difficult to distinguish between acute rejection and nephrotoxicity caused by high cyclosporine or tacrolimus (Prograf) levels.

Chronic rejection. *Chronic rejection* is a process that occurs over months or years and is irreversible. The kidney is infiltrated with large numbers of T and B cells characteristic of an ongoing,

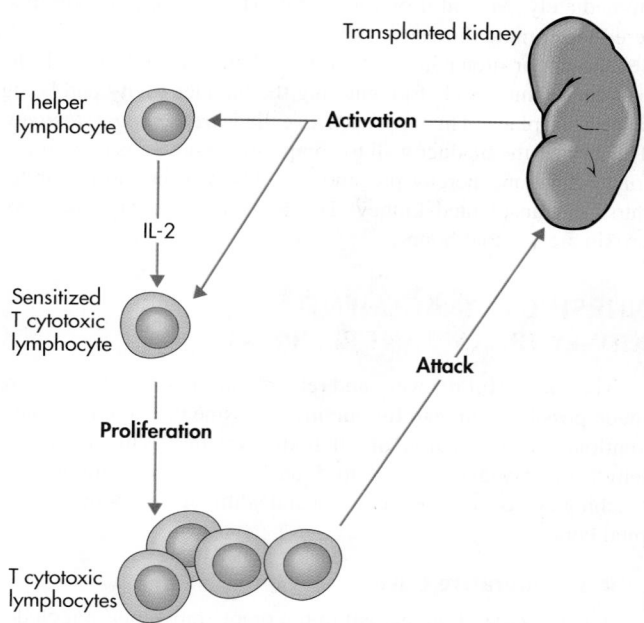

FIG. 45-19 Mechanism of action of T cytotoxic lymphocyte activation and attack of renal transplanted tissue. The transplanted kidney is recognized as foreign and activates the immune system. T helper cells are activated to produce IL-2, and T cytotoxic lymphocytes are sensitized. After these T cytotoxic cells proliferate, they attack the transplanted kidney.

low-grade immune-mediated injury. Chronic rejection is associated with a gradual occlusion of the renal blood vessels. Signs include proteinuria, hypertension, and increasing serum creatinine levels. There is no definitive therapy for this type of rejection. Changing immunosuppressive therapy to include tacrolimus or mycophenolate mofetil (CellCept) has brought some improvement for some patients who were not previously taking these drugs. Treatment is mainly supportive. This type of rejection is difficult to manage and is not associated with the optimistic prognosis of acute rejection. Patients with chronic rejection should be put on the transplant list in the hope that they can be retransplanted before dialysis is required.

Infection. Infection remains a significant cause of morbidity and mortality after transplantation.[33] The transplant recipient is at risk for infection because of suppression of the body's normal defense mechanisms by surgery, immunosuppressive drugs, and the effects of ESRD. Underlying systemic illness such as diabetes mellitus or systemic lupus erythematosus, malnutrition, and older age can further compound the negative effects on the immune response. At times the signs and symptoms of infection can be subtle. Nurses caring for transplant recipients must be astute in their observation and assessment because prompt diagnosis and treatment of infections will improve patient outcomes.

The most common infections observed in the first month after transplantation are similar to those acquired by any postoperative patient, such as pneumonia, wound infections, IV line and drain infections, and urinary tract infections. Fungal and viral infections are not uncommon because of the patient's immunosuppressed state. Fungal infections can include *Candida, Cryptococcus, Aspergillus,* and *Pneumocystis carinii.* Fungal infections are difficult to treat, require prolonged treatment periods, and often involve the administration of nephrotoxic drugs. Transplant recipients usually receive prophylactic antifungal drugs to prevent these infections, such as clotrimazole (Mycelex), fluconazole (Diflucan), and sulfamethoxazole-trimethoprim (Bactrim).

Viral infections including CMV, Epstein-Barr virus, herpes simplex virus (HSV), varicella-zoster virus, and polyomavirus (e.g., BK virus) can be primary or reactivation of existing disease.[34,35] Primary infections occur as new infections after transplantation from an exogenous source such as the donated organ or blood transfusion. Reactivation occurs when a virus exists in a patient and becomes reactivated after transplantation because of immunosuppression.

CMV is one of the most common viral infections. If a recipient has never had CMV and receives an organ from a donor with a history of CMV, antiviral prophylaxis will be administered (ganciclovir IV, valganciclovir [Valcyte]). If a primary active CMV infection is diagnosed or there is symptomatic reactivation of CMV, IV ganciclovir will be given along with an immune globulin that contains CMV antibodies. To prevent HSV infections, oral acyclovir is given for several months after the transplant.

Cardiovascular Disease. Transplant recipients have an increased incidence of atherosclerotic vascular disease. Cardiovascular disease is the leading cause of death after renal transplantation.[8] Hypertension, hyperlipidemia, diabetes mellitus, smoking, rejection, infections, and increased homocysteine levels can all contribute to cardiovascular disease. Immunosuppressants can worsen hypertension and hyperlipidemia. It is important that the patient be taught to control risk factors such as elevated cholesterol, triglycerides, and blood glucose and weight gain. Adherence to the prescribed antihypertensive regimen is essential not only to prevent cardiovascular events but also to prevent damage to the new kidney. (Hypertension is discussed in Chapter 32.)

Malignancies. The overall incidence of malignancies in kidney transplant recipients is about 6%, which is 100 times greater than in the general population. The primary cause of this increased incidence is the immunosuppressive therapy. Not only do immunosuppressants suppress the immune system, but they also suppress the ability to fight infection and the production of abnormal cells such as cancer cells. The malignancies include cancer of the skin, lips, kidney, hepatobiliary system, vulva, and perineum; lymphomas; and Kaposi's sarcoma and other sarcomas. Regular screening for cancer is an important part of the transplant recipient's preventive care. The patient must also be advised to avoid sun exposure by using protective clothing and sunscreens to minimize the incidence of skin cancers.

Recurrence of Original Renal Disease. Recurrence of the original disease that destroyed the native kidneys occurs in some kidney transplant recipients. It is most common with certain types of glomerulonephritis, IgA nephropathy, diabetes mellitus, and focal segmental sclerosis. Disease recurrence can result in the loss of a functioning kidney transplant. Patients must be advised before transplant if they have a disease known to recur.

Corticosteroid-Related Complications. Aseptic necrosis of the hips, knees, and other joints can result from chronic corticosteroid therapy and renal osteodystrophy. Other significant problems related to corticosteroids include peptic ulcer disease, glucose intolerance and diabetes, cataracts, hyperlipidemia, and an increased incidence of infections and malignancies. In the first year after transplant, corticosteroid doses are usually decreased to 5 to 10 mg a day. The use of tacrolimus and cyclosporine has allowed for the corticosteroid doses to be much lower than they were in the past. Some patients have been successfully withdrawn from corticosteroids 1½ to 2 years after transplantation, thus eliminating these problems. Vigilant monitoring for side effects of corticosteroids and early treatment is essential.

■ Gerontologic Considerations: Chronic Kidney Disease

The incidence of ESRD in the United States and Canada is increasing most rapidly in older patients. The mean age of the United States ESRD population has increased. Recent data indicate that of all the patients who have ESRD about 48% are 65 or older.[8] The most common diseases leading to renal failure in the older adult are hypertension and diabetes. Medicare and non-Medicare expenditures can be expected to increase as the ESRD population ages and as a result has a greater number of comorbid conditions.

The care of the geriatric ESRD patient is particularly challenging, not only because of the normal physiologic changes of aging that occur but also because of the number of comorbid conditions that develop.[36] Physiologic changes of clinical importance in the older ESRD patient include diminished cardiopulmonary function, bone loss, immunodeficiency, altered protein synthesis, impaired cognition, and altered drug metabolism. Malnutrition is common in the older ESRD patient for a variety of reasons, including lack of mobility, lack of understanding of basic nutritional requirements, social isolation, physical disability, impaired cognitive function, and malabsorption problems.[37,38]

The older patient needs to consider what is the best treatment modality based on his or her health, personal preferences, and support available. Home PD allows the patient to be more mobile and to enjoy an increased sense of control over the illness. PD causes less hemodynamic instability than HD but does require self-care or assistance from another person. The older adult may not have adequate help in the home to provide assistance. Establishing vascular access for HD may be difficult in an older patient because of atherosclerotic changes. Travel to and from the HD unit may also be problematic if the patient does not drive or have access to reliable public transportation. Although transplantation is an option, elderly patients must be carefully screened to ensure that the benefits outweigh the risks. A living donor is preferable so that there is not a prolonged waiting time.

The most common cause of death in the elderly ESRD patient is cardiovascular disease (MI, stroke) followed by withdrawal from dialysis. If a competent patient decides to withdraw from dialysis, it is essential to support the patient and family. Ethical issues (see the Ethical Dilemmas box) to be considered in this situation include patient competency, benefit versus burden of treatment, and futility of treatment.[36] Withdrawal from treatment is not a failure if the patient is well informed and comfortable with the decision.

The increasing number of elderly, debilitated ESRD patients receiving dialysis has raised a number of ethical concerns about the use of scarce resources in a population with a limited life expectancy. Substantial evidence exists showing success of dialysis (especially PD) in the elderly. Quality of life has also been reported to be good to excellent in many older ESRD patients. There appears to be no justification for excluding the older adult from dialysis programs. Rationing dialysis on the basis of age alone is not supported based on current outcome and quality-of-life data. ■

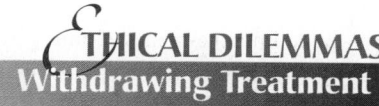

ETHICAL DILEMMAS
Withdrawing Treatment

Situation

A 70-year-old patient with diabetes mellitus and chronic renal failure who has been receiving dialysis for 10 years tells the nurse that he wants to discontinue his dialysis. His quality of life has diminished during the past 2 years since his wife died. He is not a prospective transplant patient.

Important Points for Consideration

- Quality of life is an important consideration for patients when weighing whether to begin or discontinue treatment.
- Quality-of-life decisions often weigh the benefit against the burden of treatment. When a treatment becomes too burdensome, the patient (if competent) may request to withdraw the treatment.
- A determination must be made if there is some other treatable problem such as depression that may be clouding the patient's judgment.
- Patient autonomy, or the patient's right to self-determination regarding treatment decisions, applies both to initiating and discontinuing treatment.
- If a decision is made to withdraw treatment, the health care team, patient, and family should develop an appropriate follow-up plan that includes palliative care and hospice support.

Critical Thinking Questions

1. How should the nurse respond to the patient's request?
2. What is the ANA's position on withdrawing or withholding treatment that no longer benefits the patient or causes suffering?

CRITICAL THINKING EXERCISES

Case Study
Chronic Kidney Disease

Patient Profile. Juanita, a 46-year-old Native American school teacher, has been treated for type 2 diabetes mellitus since the age of 25. She has been observed by her nephrologist for the past several years for manifestations of progressive chronic kidney disease. Eight weeks ago she had an arteriovenous fistula created in preparation for starting hemodialysis. Over the past week she has experienced anorexia, nausea, vomiting, problems with concentration, and pruritus.

Subjective Data
- Complains of swelling in her feet and hands
- Has gained 10 lb (4.5 kg) in the past 2 weeks
- Complains of dyspnea and weakness when walking

Objective Data

Laboratory Data
- Creatinine clearance: 8.2 ml/min
- Serum creatinine: 12.8 mg/dl (1132 mmol/L)
- BUN: 125 mg/dl (45 mmol/L)
- Potassium: 6 mEq/L (6 mmol/L)
- Hematocrit: 20%

Chest X-ray
- Pulmonary edema

CRITICAL THINKING QUESTIONS

1. Explain the basic pathophysiologic changes that resulted in the development of her diabetic nephropathy.
2. What are the indications for dialysis in this patient?
3. Identify the abnormal diagnostic study results and why each would occur.
4. Explain why Juanita developed each of her clinical manifestations.
5. What are important nursing interventions for Juanita and her family?
6. Based on the assessment data provided, write one or more nursing diagnoses. Are there any collaborative problems?

Nursing Research Issues

1. What is the psychosocial impact of dialysis on the spouse and family?
2. What nursing strategies promote compliance in the dialysis patient?
3. Are the stressors for older (>65 years) dialysis patients different from those of younger patients?
4. What is the quality of life for a living-related donor following surgery?
5. What are the needs of the family when a patient chooses to withdraw from dialysis treatment?

REVIEW QUESTIONS

The number of the question corresponds to the same-numbered objective at the beginning of the chapter.

1. A patient is admitted to the hospital with chronic kidney disease. The nurse understands that this condition is characterized by
   a. progressive irreversible destruction of the kidneys.
   b. a rapid decrease in urinary output with an elevated BUN.
   c. an increasing creatinine clearance with a decrease in urinary output.
   d. prostration, somnolence, and confusion with coma and imminent death.

2. Prerenal causes of ARF include
   a. prostate cancer and calculi formation.
   b. hypovolemia and myocardial infarction.
   c. acute glomerulonephritis and neoplasms.
   d. septic shock and nephrotoxic injury from drugs.

3. During the oliguric phase of ARF, the nurse monitors the patient for
   a. hypernatremia and CNS depression.
   b. pulmonary edema and ECG changes.
   c. Kussmaul respirations and hypotension.
   d. urine with high specific gravity and low sodium concentration.

4. If a patient is in the diuretic phase of ARF, the nurse must monitor for which serum electrolyte imbalances?
   a. Hyperkalemia and hyponatremia
   b. Hyperkalemia and hypernatremia
   c. Hypokalemia and hyponatremia
   d. Hypokalemia and hypernatremia

5. A systemic effect of chronic kidney disease that is usually reversed by the initiation of dialysis is
   a. anemia.
   b. hyperlipidemia.
   c. psychologic changes.
   d. nausea and vomiting.

6. Measures indicated in the conservative therapy of chronic kidney disease include
   a. decreased fluid intake, carbohydrate intake, and protein intake.
   b. increased fluid intake, decreased carbohydrate intake and protein intake.
   c. decreased fluid intake and protein intake, increased carbohydrate intake.
   d. decreased fluid intake and carbohydrate intake, increased protein intake.

7. One of the major disadvantages of peritoneal dialysis is that
   a. hypotension is a constant problem because of continuous fluid removal.
   b. blood loss can be extensive because of the use of heparin to keep the catheter patent.
   c. solutes are removed more rapidly from the blood than from the CNS, causing disequilibrium syndrome.
   d. high glucose concentrations of the dialysate necessary for ultrafiltration cause carbohydrate and lipid abnormalities.

8. To assess the patency of a newly placed arteriovenous graft for dialysis, the nurse should
   a. irrigate the graft daily with low-dose heparin.
   b. monitor for any increase in BP in the affected arm.
   c. listen with a stethoscope over the graft for the presence of a bruit.
   d. frequently monitor the pulses and neurovascular status distal to the graft.

9. A patient in ESRD receiving hemodialysis is considering asking a relative to donate a kidney for transplant. In assisting the patient to make a decision about treatment, the nurse informs the patient that
   a. successful transplantation usually provides better quality of life than that offered by dialysis.
   b. if rejection of the transplanted kidney occurs, no further treatment for the renal failure is available.
   c. the immunosuppressive therapy that is required following transplantation causes fatal malignancies in many patients.
   d. hemodialysis replaces the normal functions of the kidneys and patients do not have to live with the continual fear of rejection.

10. Following a kidney transplant, the nurse teaches the patient that signs of rejection include
    a. fever, weight loss, increased urinary output, increased BP.
    b. fever, weight gain, increased urinary output, increased BP.
    c. fever, weight loss, increased urinary output, decreased BP.
    d. fever, weight gain, decreased urinary output, increased BP.

11. Most of the long-term problems that occur in the patient with a kidney transplant are a result of
    a. chronic rejection.
    b. immunosuppressive therapy.
    c. recurrence of the original renal disease.
    d. failure of the patient to follow the prescribed regimen.

REFERENCES

1. Brady H et al: Acute renal failure. In Brenner BM, editor: *The kidney,* Philadelphia, 2000, WB Saunders.
2. Agrawal M, Swartz R: Acute renal failure, *Am Fam Physician* 61:2077, 2000.
3. Johnson DC, Anderson RJ: Acute renal failure, part 2: zeroing in on the diagnosis: early remedial efforts can stop disease progression, *J Crit Illn* 17:301, 2002.
4. Bozfakioglu S: Nutrition in patients with acute renal failure, *Nephrol Dial Transplant* 16:S6, 2001.
5. Richard C: Renal disorders. In Lancaster L, editor: *Core curriculum for nephrology nursing,* ed 4, New Jersey, 2001, Anthony Janetti.
6. Druml W: Nutritional management of acute renal failure, *Am J Kidney Dis* 37:S89, 2001.
7. Greene JH, Hoffart N: Nutrition in renal failure, dialysis, and transplant. In Lancaster L, editor: *Core curriculum for nephrology nursing,* ed 4, New Jersey, 2001, Anthony Janetti.
8. US Renal Data System: USRDS 2001 annual data report: Atlas of end-stage renal disease, Bethesda, MD, 2001, National Institutes of Health, National Institute of Diabetes & Digestive and Kidney Diseases.

9. Foret JP: Diagnosing and treating anemia and iron deficiency in hemodialysis patients, *Nephrol Nurs J* 29:292, 2002.

10. Levin A, Stevens L, McCullough P: Cardiovascular disease and the kidney: tracking a killer in chronic kidney disease, *Postgrad Med* 111:53, 2002.

11. Laaksonen S et al: Does dialysis therapy improve autonomic and peripheral nervous system abnormalities in chronic uraemia? *J Intern Med* 248:21, 2000.

12. Lancaster L: Systemic manifestations of renal failure. In Lancaster L, editor: *Core curriculum for nephrology nursing,* ed 4, New Jersey, 2001, Anthony Janetti.

13. Roth C, Culp K: Renal osteodystrophy in older adults with end-stage renal disease, *J Gerontol Nurs* 27:46, 2001.

14. Andrews L, Gibbs M: Antihypertensive medications and renal disease, *Nephrol Nurs J* 29:379, 2002.

15. Chorzempa A, Tabloski P: Post myocardial infarction: treatment in the older adult, *Nurse Pract* 26:36, 2001.

16. Markauskas I: The complexities of renal bone disease, *Nephrol News Issues* 15:41, 2001.

17. Kopple J: National Kidney Foundation K/DOQI clinical practice guidelines for nutrition in chronic renal failure, *Am J Kidney Dis* 37(suppl 2):S66, 2001.

18. Hartley GH: Nutritional status, delaying progression and risks associated with protein restriction, *Edtna-Erca Journal* 27:101, 2001.

19. Compton A, Provenzano R, Johnson C: The nephrology nurse's role in improved care of patients with chronic kidney disease, *Nephrol Nurs J* 29:331, 2002.

20. Finkelstein ES et al: Patterns of infection in patients maintained on long-term peritoneal dialysis therapy with multiple episodes of peritonitis, *Am J Kidney Dis* 39:1278, 2002.

21. Work J: Introduction: advances in hemodialysis access, *Adv Ren Replac Ther* 9:71, 2002.

22. Trerotola S: Hemodialysis catheter placement and management, *Radiology* 215:651, 2000.

23. Richard HM et al: A randomized, prospective evaluation of the Tesio, Ash Split, and Opti-flow hemodialysis catheters, *J Vasc Interv Radiol* 12:431, 2001.

24. Beathard GA, Posen GA: Initial clinical results with Life-site® hemodialysis access system, *Kidney Int* 58:2221, 2000.

25. Morgan L: A decade review: methods to improve adherence to the treatment regimen among hemodialysis patients, *Nephrol Nurs J* 27:299, 2000.

26. Kaplow R, Richard B: Continuous renal replacement therapies: a more gentle blood filtering technique allows for fewer complications, *Am J Nsg* 102:26, 2002.

27. Bellmann R et al: Elimination of levofloxacin in critically ill patients with renal failure: influence of continuous veno-venous hemofiltration, *Int J Clin Pharmacol Ther* 40:142, 2002.

28. United Network for Organ Sharing: 2001 Annual report: the US scientific registry of transplant recipients and the organ procurement and transplantation network, 2001, Department of Health and Human Services.

29. Dabbs A et al: Rejection after organ transplantation: a historical review, *Am J Crit Care* 9:419, 2000.

30. Connerney I et al: Laparoscopic nephrectomy program boosts successful outcomes at university, *Inside Case Management* 6:6, 1999.

31. Ratner LE, Montgomery RA, Kavoussi LR: Laparoscopic live-donor nephrectomy: the four year Johns Hopkins University experience, *Nephrol Dial Transplant* 14:2090, 1999.

32. Manuel P et al: Strategies to improve long-term outcomes after renal transplantation, *N Engl J Med* 346:580, 2002.

33. Andany M, Kasiske B: Care of the kidney transplant recipient: vigilant monitoring creates the best outcome, *Postgrad Med* 112:93, 2002.

34. Pellegrin I et al: New molecular assays to predict occurrence of cytomegalovirus disease in renal transplant recipients, *J Infect Dis* 182:36, 2000.

35. Hopwood P, Crawford DH: The role of EBV in post-transplant malignancies: a review, *J Clin Pathol* 53:248, 2000.

36. Brown WW: The geriatric dialysis patient. In Henrick WL, editor: *Principles and practice of dialysis,* ed 2, Baltimore, 1999, Lippincott Williams & Wilkins.

37. Wolfson M: Nutrition in elderly dialysis patients, *Seminars in Dialysis* 15:113, 2002.

38. Thomas LK et al: Identification of the factors associated with compliance to therapeutic diets in older adults with end stage renal disease, *Journal of Renal Nutrition* 11:80, 2001.

RESOURCES

American Association of Kidney Patients (AAKP)
3505 East Frontage Road, Suite 315
Tampa, FL 33607
800-749-2257
Fax: 813-636-8122
www.aakp.org

American Kidney Fund (AKF)
6110 Executive Boulevard, Suite 1010
Rockville, MD 20852
800-638-8299
www.akfinc.org

American Nephrology Nurses' Association
ANNA National Office
East Holly Avenue, Box 56
Pitman, NJ 08071-0056
888-600-ANNA (2662) or 856-256-2320
Fax: 856-589-7463
http://anna.inurse.com

American Organ Transplant Association
P.O. Box 441766
Houston, TX 77244
281-493-2047
Fax: 281-493-2099
www.a-o-t-a.org

International Society of Nephrology (ISN)
www.isn-online.org

International Transplant Nurses Society
1739 East Carson Street, Box 351
Pittsburgh, PA 15203
412-343-ITNS
Fax: 412-343-3959
www.itns.org

Kidney Transplant/Dialysis Association, Inc.
P.O. Box 51362 GMF
Boston, MA 02205-1362
781-641-4000
http://users.rcn.com/ktda1

National Association of Transplant Coordinators (NATCO)
P.O. Box 15384
Lenexa, KS 66285-5384
913-492-3600
Fax: 913-599-5340
www.natco1.org

National Institute of Diabetic and Digestive and Kidney Diseases Information (NIDDK)
Office of Communications and Public Liaison
NIH, Building 31, Room 9A04
31 Center Drive MSC 2560
Bethesda, MD 20892-2560
www.niddk.nih.gov/

National Kidney Foundation
30 East 33rd Street, Suite 1100
New York, NY 10016
800-622-9010 or 212-889-2210
Fax: 212-689-9261
www.kidney.org

RENALNET
www.renalnet.org

RenalWEB Patient Education
www.renalweb.com/topics/patiented/patiented.htm

United Network for Organ Sharing
1100 Boulders Parkway, Suite 500
Richmond, VA 23225-8770
888-TX-INFO-1 or 804-330-8541
www.unos.org

For additional Internet resources, see the website for this book at *http://evolve.elsevier.com/Lewis/medsurg/*.

Problems Related to Regulatory Mechanisms

CHAPTER 46
NURSING ASSESSMENT
Endocrine System

Jean Foret Giddens

LEARNING OBJECTIVES

1. Identify the common characteristics and functions of hormones.
2. Identify the locations of the endocrine glands.
3. Describe the functions of hormones secreted by the pituitary, thyroid, parathyroid, and adrenal glands and the pancreas.
4. Describe the locations and roles of hormone receptors.
5. Identify the significant subjective and objective assessment data related to the endocrine system that should be obtained from a patient.
6. Describe the appropriate technique used in the physical assessment of the thyroid gland.
7. Describe age-related changes in the endocrine system and differences in assessment findings.
8. Differentiate normal from common abnormal findings in the assessment of the endocrine system.
9. Describe the purpose, significance of results, and nursing responsibilities related to diagnostic studies of the endocrine system.

KEY TERMS

aldosterone, p. 1255
antidiuretic hormone, p. 1253
calcitonin, p. 1254
catecholamines, p. 1254
corticosteroid, p. 1255
cortisol, p. 1255
glucagon, p. 1255
growth hormone, p. 1253
hormone, p. 1248

insulin, p. 1255
islets of Langerhans, p. 1255
negative feedback, p. 1249
oxytocin, p. 1254
parathyroid hormone, p. 1254
target tissue, p. 1248
thyroxine, p. 1254
triiodothyronine, p. 1254
tropic hormones, p. 1252

The endocrine system and the nervous system are two of the primary communicating and coordinating systems in the body. The nervous system communicates through nerve impulses; the endocrine system communicates through chemical substances known as hormones, and it plays a role in reproduction, growth and development, and regulation of energy. The endocrine system is composed of glands or glandular tissues that produce, store, and secrete hormones that travel through the blood to specific target cells throughout the body.

The endocrine glands include the hypothalamus, pituitary, thyroid, parathyroids, adrenals, pancreas, ovaries, testes, pineal, and thymus (Fig. 46-1). The thymus gland is important in the function of the immune system and is discussed in Chapter 13. The pineal gland, which secretes melatonin, is not discussed in this chapter, because the significance of this gland in humans is not well understood.[1] In addition to the endocrine glands, other body organs secrete hormones. For example, the kidneys secrete erythropoietin, the heart secretes atrial natriuretic hormone, and the gastrointestinal tract secretes numerous peptide hormones (e.g., gastrin). These hormones are discussed in their respective assessment chapters.

Reviewed by Rebecca B. Griffin, RN, MS, Instructor, McLennan Community College, Waco, Tex.

STRUCTURES AND FUNCTIONS OF THE ENDOCRINE SYSTEM

Glands

The organs of the endocrine system are referred to as *glands*. Endocrine glands produce chemical substances called *hormones* and secrete them into blood, where they eventually affect specific target tissues. A **target tissue** is the body tissue or organ that the hormone has its effect on. For example, the thyroid (gland) synthesizes thyroxine (the hormone), which influences all body tissues (target tissue). It is important to note that not all glands in the body belong to the endocrine system. There are two types of glands—*exocrine glands* and *endocrine glands*. Exocrine glands secrete their substances into ducts that then empty into a body cavity or onto a surface (e.g., skin). For example, salivary glands produce saliva, which is secreted through salivary ducts into the mouth. By contrast, endocrine glands do not have ducts. They secrete their substances directly into the blood.

Hormones

Classifications and Functions. A **hormone** is a chemical substance synthesized and secreted by a specific organ or tissue. Most hormones have common characteristics, including (1) secretion in small amounts at variable but predictable rates, (2) circulation through the blood, and (3) binding to specific cellular receptors either in the cell membrane or within the cell.

Hormones are classified by their chemical structure: lipid-soluble hormones and water-soluble (protein-based) hormones. Lipid-soluble hormones include steroid hormones (all hormones produced by the adrenal cortex and sex glands) and thyroid hormones. All other hormones are water soluble.[2] The differences in solubility become important in understanding how the hormone interacts with the target cell.

As mentioned previously, the hormones control a number of physiologic activities. Important hormonal functions are related to reproduction, response to stress and injury, electrolyte balance, energy metabolism, growth, maturation, and aging. Hormones also play a role in nervous system function. Some hormones have a regulatory effect on nervous tissue. For example, catechol-

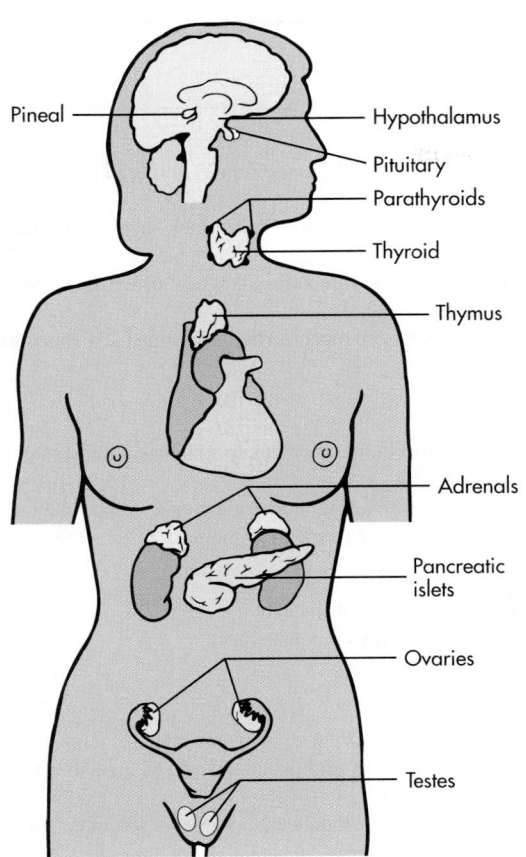

FIG. 46-1 Location of the major endocrine glands. The parathyroid glands actually lie on the posterior surface of the thyroid.

Labels in Fig. 46-1: Pineal, Hypothalamus, Pituitary, Parathyroids, Thyroid, Thymus, Adrenals, Pancreatic islets, Ovaries, Testes

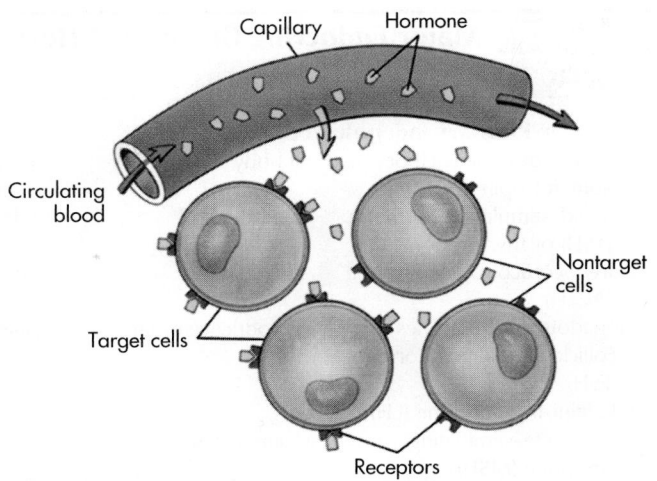

FIG. 46-2 The target cell concept. Hormones act only on cells that have receptors specific to that hormone, because the shape of the receptor determines which hormone can react with it. This is an example of the lock–and–key model of biochemical reactions.

Labels in Fig. 46-2: Capillary, Hormone, Circulating blood, Nontarget cells, Target cells, Receptors

amines are hormones when they are secreted by the adrenal medulla, but act as neurotransmitters when secreted by nerve cells in the brain and peripheral nervous system. When epinephrine travels through the blood, it is a hormone and affects target tissues. When it travels across synaptic junctions, it acts as a neurotransmitter. Hormones can also influence behavior.[3] For example, excess growth hormone, cortisol, and parathyroid hormone can cause mood swings. Depression has been associated with adrenal insufficiency. Table 46-1 summarizes the major hormones, glands or tissues from which they are synthesized, target organs or tissues, and functions.

Hormone Transport. Hormones are carried by the blood to other sites in the body where their actions are exerted. Some hormones (e.g., steroid and thyroid hormones) are not water soluble. Therefore these types of hormones are bound to plasma proteins for transport in the blood. Although hormones are inactive when bound to plasma proteins, they can be released when appropriate and immediately exert their action at the target tissue. Water-soluble hormones (e.g., protein hormones, catecholamines) circulate freely in the blood and are not dependent upon proteins for transport.

Targets and Receptors. As mentioned above, hormones exert their effects on target tissue. The hormone recognizes the target tissue through receptors (the site that interacts with the hormone) on or within cells of the target tissue. The specificity of hormone–target cell interaction is determined by receptors in a "lock-and-key" type of mechanism. Thus a hormone will act only on cells that have a receptor specific for that hormone (Fig. 46-2). It is important to note there are two types of receptors: those that are within the cell (e.g., steroid and thyroid hormone receptors) and those that are on the cell membrane (e.g., protein-type hormone receptors). The location of the receptor sites affects the mechanism of action for the hormone.

Steroid hormone receptors. Steroid and thyroid hormone receptors are located inside the cell. Because these hormones are lipid soluble, they pass through the target cell membrane by passive diffusion and bind to receptor sites located in the cytoplasm or nucleus of the target cell.[4] Intracellular hormone-receptor complexes, such as those seen in steroid hormone action, bind to specific sites on deoxyribonucleic acid (DNA) to stimulate or inhibit the synthesis of messenger ribonucleic acid (mRNA). When new mRNA is synthesized, it migrates to the cytoplasm, where it stimulates the synthesis of new protein. These new proteins produce specific effects in the target cell (Fig. 46-3).

Protein hormone receptors. Protein hormone action is a two-step process. The receptor is located in the target cell membrane; thus the hormone itself acts as a "first messenger." The hormone-receptor interaction stimulates the production of a "second messenger" such as cyclic adenosine monophosphate (cAMP). cAMP works by activating enzymes to regulate intracellular activity (see Fig. 46-3).

Regulation of Hormonal Secretion. The regulation of endocrine activity is controlled by specific mechanisms of varying levels of complexity. These mechanisms stimulate or inhibit hormone synthesis and secretion and include simple feedback, complex feedback, nervous system control, and physiologic rhythms.

Simple feedback. The regulation of hormone levels in the blood depends on a highly specialized mechanism called *feedback*. Feedback is based on the blood level of a particular substance. This substance may be a hormone or other chemical compound regulated by, or responsive to, a hormone. With **negative feedback,** the most common type of feedback system, the gland responds by increasing or decreasing the secretion of a hormone based on feedback from various factors.[5] Negative

TABLE 46-1   Major Endocrine Glands and Hormones

HORMONES	TARGET TISSUE	FUNCTIONS
Anterior Pituitary (adenohypophysis)		
Growth hormone (GH) or somatotropin	All body cells	Promotes protein anabolism (growth, tissue repair) and lipid mobilization and catabolism
Thyroid-stimulating hormone (TSH) or thyrotropin	Thyroid gland	Stimulates synthesis and release of thyroid hormones, growth and function of thyroid gland
Adrenocorticotropic hormone (ACTH)	Adrenal cortex	Fosters growth of adrenal cortex; stimulates secretion of corticosteroids
Gonadotropic hormones • Follicle-stimulating hormone (FSH) • Luteinizing hormone (LH)	Reproductive organs	Stimulates sex hormone secretion, reproductive organ growth, reproductive processes
Melanocyte-stimulating hormone (MSH)	Melanocytes in skin	Increases melanin production in melanocytes to make skin darker in color
Prolactin	Ovary and mammary glands in females	Stimulates milk production in lactating women; increases response of follicles to LH and FSH; has unclear function in men
Posterior Pituitary (neurohypophysis)		
Oxytocin	Uterus; mammary glands	Stimulates milk secretion, uterine contractility
Antidiuretic hormone (ADH) or vasopressin	Renal tubules, vascular smooth muscle	Promotes reabsorption of water, vasoconstriction
Thyroid		
Thyroxine (T_4)	All body tissues	Precursor to T_3
Triiodothyronine (T_3)	All body tissues	Regulates metabolic rate of all cells and processes of cell growth and tissue differentiation
Calcitonin	Bone tissue	Regulates calcium and phosphorus blood levels; decreases serum Ca^{2+} levels
Parathyroids		
Parathyroid hormone (PTH) or parathormone	Bone, intestine, kidneys	Regulates calcium and phosphorus blood levels; promotes bone demineralization and increases intestinal absorption of Ca^{2+}; increases serum Ca^{2+} levels
Adrenal Medulla		
Epinephrine (Adrenaline)	Sympathetic effectors	Response to stress; enhances and prolongs effects of sympathetic nervous system
Norepinephrine	Sympathetic effectors	Response to stress; enhances and prolongs effects of sympathetic nervous system
Adrenal Cortex		
Corticosteroids (e.g., cortisol, hydrocortisone)	All body tissues	Promotes metabolism, response to stress
Androgens (e.g., testosterone, androsterone) and estrogen	Reproductive organs	Promotes masculinization in men, growth and sexual activity in women
Mineralocorticoids (e.g., aldosterone)	Kidney	Regulates sodium and potassium balance and thus water balance
Pancreas		
Islets of Langerhans		
Insulin (from beta cells)	General	Promotes movement of glucose out of blood and into cells
Glucagon (from alpha cells)	General	Promotes movement of glucose from glycogen (glycogenolysis) and into blood
Somatostatin	Pancreas	Inhibits insulin and glucagon secretion
Pancreatic polypeptide	General	Influences regulation of pancreatic exocrine function and metabolism of absorbed nutrients
Gonads		
Women: Ovaries		
Estrogen	Reproductive system, breasts	Stimulates development of secondary sex characteristics, preparation of uterus for fertilization and fetal development; stimulates bone growth
Progesterone	Reproductive system	Maintains lining of uterus necessary for successful pregnancy
Men: Testes		
Testosterone	Reproductive system	Stimulates development of secondary sex characteristics, spermatogenesis

A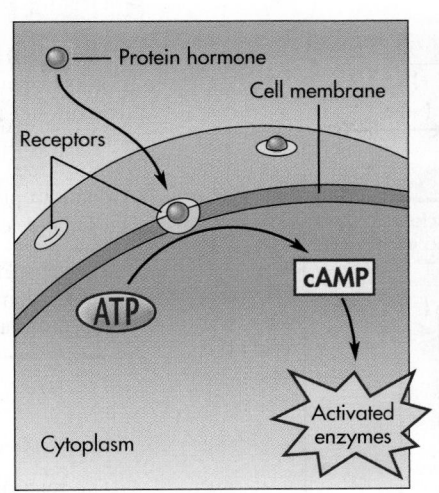

B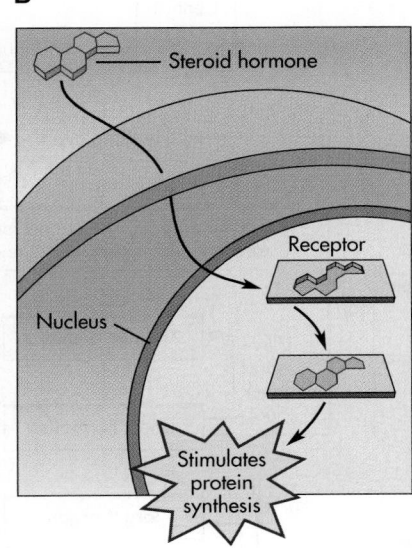

FIG. 46-3 **A,** Protein hormones bind to receptors located on the surface of the cell membrane. The hormone-receptor interaction stimulates the formation of cAMP, thereby activating various cell processes. **B,** Steroid hormones penetrate the cell membrane and interact with intracellular receptors. The hormone-receptor complex activates the cell by stimulating protein synthesis.

feedback is similar to the functioning of a thermostat in which cold air in a room activates the thermostat to release heat, and hot air turns off the thermostat to prevent more warm air from entering the room.

The pattern of insulin secretion is a physiologic example of negative feedback between glucose and insulin. Elevated blood glucose levels stimulate the secretion of insulin from the pancreas. As blood glucose levels decrease, the stimulus for insulin secretion also decreases (Fig. 46-4). The homeostatic mechanism is considered negative feedback because it reverses the change in blood glucose level. Another example of negative feedback is the relationship between calcium and parathyroid hormone (PTH). Low blood levels of calcium stimulate the parathyroid gland to release PTH, which acts on bone, the intestine, and kidneys to increase blood calcium levels. The increased blood calcium levels then inhibit further PTH release (Fig. 46-5).

Complex feedback. Another level of complexity exists in feedback systems. An example of this is regulation of thyroid hormones (Fig. 46-6). The synthesis and release of thyroid stimulating hormone (TSH) or thyrotropin from the anterior pituitary is stimulated by thyrotropin-releasing hormone (TRH), which is secreted by the hypothalamus. The thyroid hormones, T_3 and T_4, have an inhibitory effect on the secretion of both TRH from the hypothalamus and TSH from the anterior pituitary.

Nervous system control. In addition to chemical regulation, some endocrine glands are directly affected by the activity of the nervous system. Pain, emotion, sexual excitement, and stress can stimulate the nervous system to modulate hormone secretion. Neural involvement is initiated by the central nervous system (CNS) and implemented by the sympathetic nervous system (SNS). For example, stress is sensed by the CNS, and the SNS secretes catecholamines that increase heart rate and blood pressure to deal with stress more effectively. (Effects of stress are discussed in Chapter 8.)

Rhythms. Another regulatory mechanism affecting many hormonal secretions involves the rhythms of secretions. These rhythms originate in brain structures. A common physiologic rhythm is the *circadian rhythm,* in which a hormone level fluctuates predictably during a 24-hour period.[6] These rhythms may be

A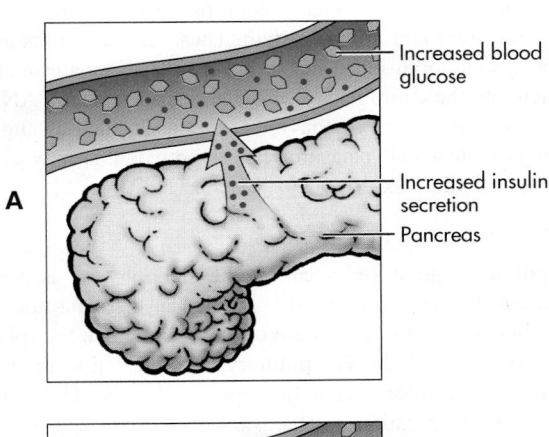

B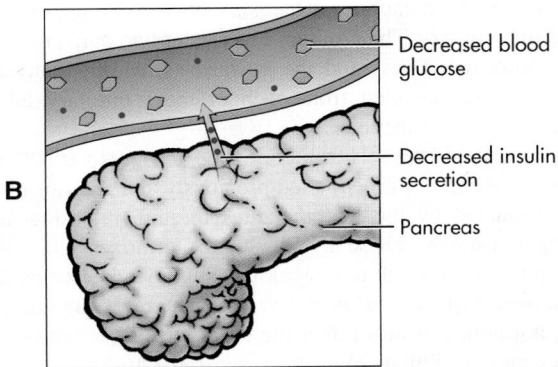

FIG. 46-4 Feedback mechanism between blood glucose and insulin. Increased blood glucose stimulates increased insulin secretion from the pancreas. As blood glucose levels decline, insulin secretion decreases.

↓ Calcium → ↑ PTH → ↑ Calcium absorption (intestine)
↑ Calcium resorption (bone) → ↑ Calcium → ↓ PTH
↓ Calcium excretion (kidneys)
↑ Calcium reabsorption (kidneys)

FIG. 46-5 Feedback mechanism between parathyroid hormone (PTH) and calcium.

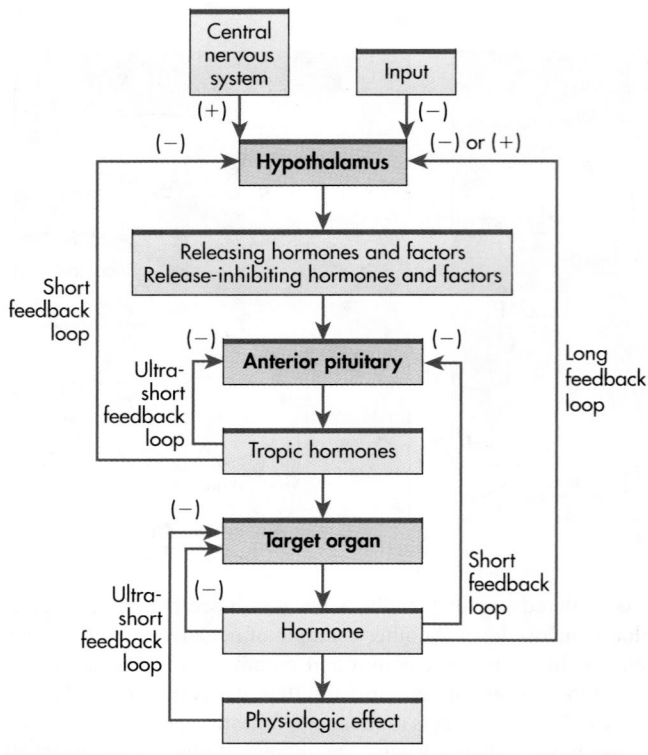

FIG. 46-6 General model for control and negative feedback to hypothalamus-pituitary target organ systems. Negative feedback regulation is possible at three levels: target organ (ultrashort feedback), anterior pituitary (short feedback), and hypothalamus (long feedback).

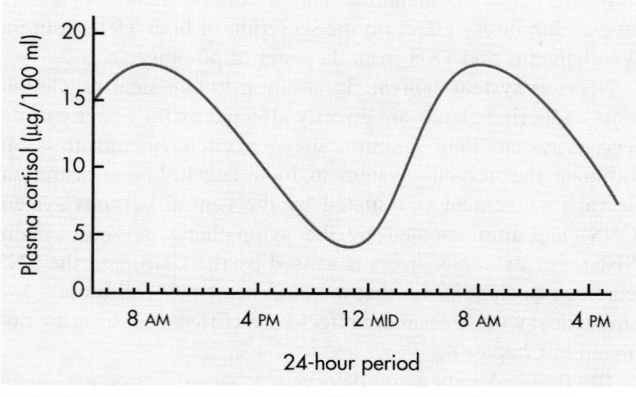

FIG. 46-7 Circadian rhythm of cortisol secretion.

related to sleep-wake or dark-light cycles. For example, cortisol rises early in the day, declines toward evening, and rises again toward the end of sleep to peak by morning (Fig. 46-7). Growth hormone (GH) and prolactin secretion peak during sleep. TSH secretion is also maximal during sleep and ebbs 3 hours after a person awakens in the morning. The menstrual cycle is an example of a body rhythm that is longer than 24 hours (*ultradian*). These rhythms must be considered when interpreting hormone levels on laboratory results. (See diagnostic studies section in this chapter and Chapter 49.)

TABLE 46-2	Hormones of the Hypothalamus

Releasing Hormones
Corticotropin-releasing hormone (CRH)
Thyrotropin-releasing hormone (TRH)
Growth hormone–releasing factor or somatotropin-releasing hormone
Gonadotropin-releasing hormone (GnRH)
Prolactin-releasing hormone

Inhibiting Hormones
Somatostatin (inhibits growth hormone release)
Prolactin-inhibiting hormone

Hypothalamus

The relationship between the hypothalamus and the pituitary gland is one of the most important aspects of the endocrine system. Although the pituitary gland has been referred to as the "master gland," most of its functions rely on an interrelationship with the hypothalamus. The hypothalamus and pituitary gland integrate communication between nervous and endocrine systems.

The hypothalamus is located in the most central part of the diencephalon area of the brain (see Fig. 46-1). Although it is really part of the brain, the hypothalamus secretes many hormones. Two important groups of hormones from the hypothalamus are *releasing* hormones and *inhibiting* hormones. The function of these hormones is to either stimulate (release) or inhibit the secretion of hormones from the anterior pituitary (Table 46-2).

The hypothalamus also contains neurons, which receive input from the brainstem and limbic system. These neurons influence the limbic system, brainstem, and spinal cord. This creates a circuit to facilitate the coordination of the endocrine system, ANS, and expression of complex behavioral responses, such as anger and feelings of fear and pleasure. The hypothalamus may also have a role in libido (sex drive).[7]

Pituitary

The pituitary gland (also called the hypophysis) is very small—about the size of a pea. It is located in the sella turcica under the hypothalamus at the base of the brain above the sphenoid bone (see Fig. 46-1). The pituitary is connected to the hypothalamus by the infundibular (hypophyseal) stalk. This stalk serves as a communication mechanism between the hypothalamus and the pituitary. The pituitary consists of two parts, the *anterior* (adenohypophysis) and the *posterior* (neurohypophysis) lobes. Hormones secreted from each of these pituitary lobes serve very different functions.

Anterior Pituitary. The anterior lobe accounts for 80% of the gland by weight. As mentioned previously, the anterior pituitary is regulated by the hypothalamus through releasing and inhibiting hormones. These hypothalamic hormones reach the anterior pituitary through a network of capillaries known as the *hypothalamus-hypophyseal portal system.* The releasing and inhibiting hormones in turn affect the secretion of six hormones from the anterior pituitary (Fig. 46-8; see Table 46-2).

Tropic hormones. Several hormones secreted by the anterior pituitary are referred to as **tropic hormones.** These are hormones that control the secretion of hormones by other glands.

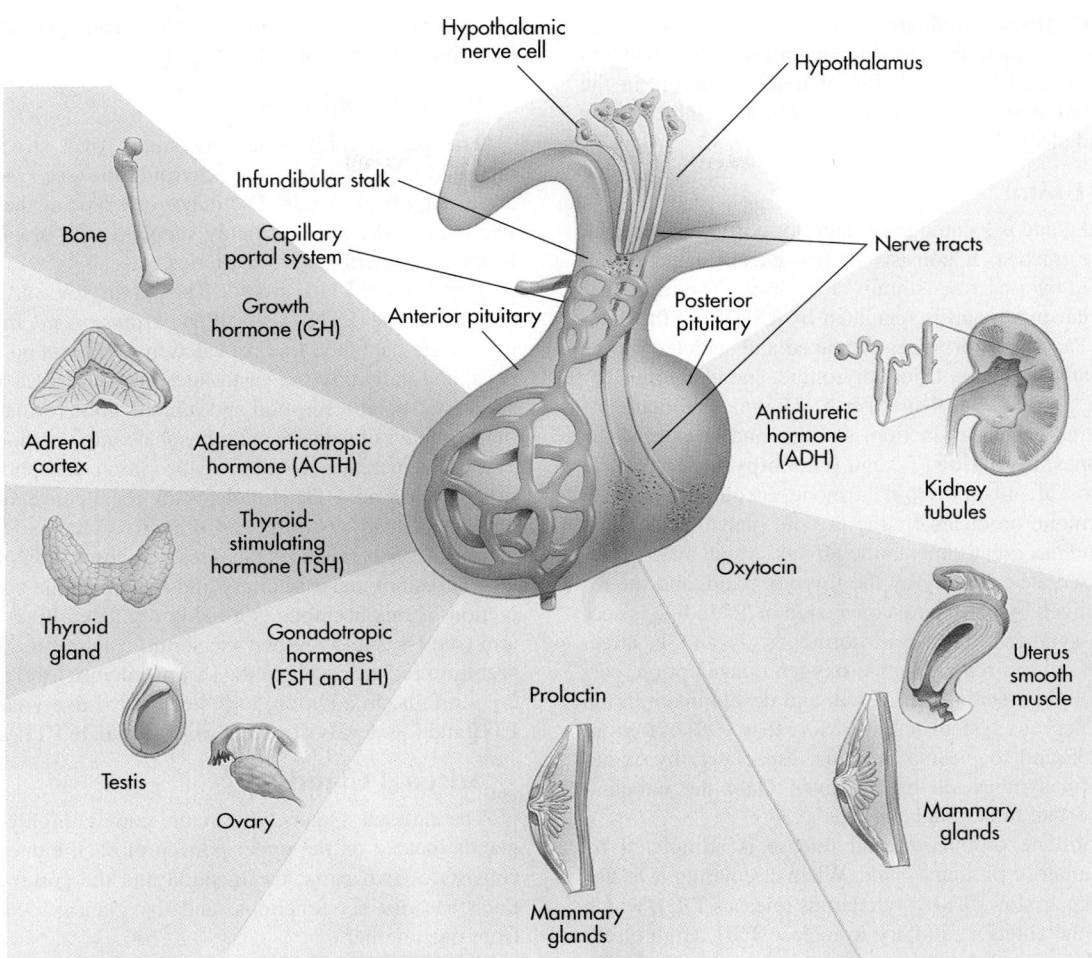

Hypothalamic nerve cell

Hypothalamus

Infundibular stalk

Bone

Capillary portal system

Nerve tracts

Growth hormone (GH)

Anterior pituitary

Posterior pituitary

Adrenal cortex

Adrenocorticotropic hormone (ACTH)

Antidiuretic hormone (ADH)

Kidney tubules

Thyroid-stimulating hormone (TSH)

Oxytocin

Thyroid gland

Gonadotropic hormones (FSH and LH)

Prolactin

Uterus smooth muscle

Testis

Ovary

Mammary glands

Mammary glands

FIG. 46-8 Relationship between the hypothalamus, pituitary, and target organs. The hypothalamus communicates with the anterior pituitary via a capillary system and with the posterior pituitary via nerve tracts. The anterior and posterior pituitary hormones are shown with their target tissues.

Thyroid-stimulating hormone (TSH) stimulates the thyroid gland to secrete thyroid hormones. Adrenocorticotropic hormone (ACTH) stimulates the adrenal cortex to secrete corticosteroids. Follicle-stimulating hormone (FSH) stimulates secretion of estrogen and the development of ova in the female and sperm development in the male. Luteinizing hormone (LH) stimulates ovulation in the female and secretion of sex hormones in both the male and female.

Growth hormone. Growth hormone (GH) has effects on all body tissue. GH, as its name suggests, affects the growth and development of skeletal muscles and long bones, affecting a person's size and height. It also has numerous biologic actions, including a role in protein, fat, and carbohydrate metabolism.[8]

Prolactin. Prolactin is a hormone that stimulates breast development necessary for lactation after childbirth. Prolactin is also referred to as lactogenic hormone.

Posterior Pituitary. The posterior pituitary is composed of nerve tissue and is essentially an extension of the hypothalamus. The communication between the hypothalamus and posterior pituitary occurs through nerve tracts known as the *median eminence*. The hormones secreted by the posterior pituitary, **antidiuretic hormone** (ADH) and oxytocin, are actually produced in the hypo-

thalamus. These hormones travel down the nerve tracts from the hypothalamus to the posterior pituitary and are stored until their release is triggered by the appropriate stimuli (see Fig. 46-8).

Antidiuretic hormone. The major physiologic role of ADH is regulation of fluid volume by stimulating reabsorption of water in the renal tubules. ADH, also called vasopressin, is also a potent vasoconstrictor.

The most important stimulus to ADH secretion is plasma osmolality (a measure of solute concentration of circulating blood). Plasma osmolality will increase when there is a decrease in extracellular fluid or an increase in solute concentration. The increased plasma osmolality activates osmoreceptors, which are extremely sensitive, specialized neurons in the hypothalamus. These activated osmoreceptors stimulate ADH release. ADH secretion is also stimulated by decreased blood volume, orthostatic changes in blood pressure, hypotension, pain, nausea, vomiting, and many drugs (e.g., anesthetic drugs, narcotics).[2] When ADH is released, the renal tubules reabsorb water, creating a more concentrated urine. The release of ADH is inhibited by an increase in fluid volume, β-adrenergic agonists, and alcohol. When ADH release is inhibited, renal tubules do not reabsorb water, thus creating a more dilute urine.

Oxytocin. Oxytocin stimulates ejection of milk into mammary ducts and contraction of uterine smooth muscle. Oxytocin secretion is increased by stimulation of touch receptors in the nipples of lactating women. Oxytocin secretion is inhibited by endorphins and alcohol.

Thyroid Gland

The thyroid gland is located in the anterior portion of the neck in front of the trachea. It consists of two encapsulated lateral lobes connected by a narrow isthmus (Fig. 46-9). The thyroid is a highly vascular organ and is regulated by TSH from the anterior pituitary. The three hormones produced and secreted by the thyroid gland are thyroxine, triiodothyronine, and calcitonin.

Thyroxine and Triiodothyronine. The major function of the thyroid gland is the production, storage, and release of the thyroid hormones, **thyroxine** (T_4) and **triiodothyronine** (T_3). T_4 is by far the most abundant thyroid hormone, accounting for 90% of thyroid hormone produced by the thyroid gland. T_3 is much more potent and has greater metabolic effects. About 10% of circulating T_3 is secreted directly by the thyroid gland, and the remainder is obtained by peripheral conversion of T_4. Iodine is necessary for the synthesis of thyroid hormones. T_4 and T_3 affect metabolic rate, caloric requirements, oxygen consumption, carbohydrate and lipid metabolism, growth and development, brain functions, and nervous system activity. More than 99% of thyroid hormones are bound to plasma proteins, especially thyroxine-binding globulin synthesized by the liver. Only the unbound "free" hormones are biologically active.

Thyroid hormone production and release is stimulated by TSH from the anterior pituitary gland. When circulating levels of thyroid hormone are low, the hypothalamus releases TRH, which in turn causes the anterior pituitary to release TSH. High circulating thyroid hormone levels have an inhibitory effect on the secretion of both TRH from the hypothalamus and TSH from the anterior pituitary.[9]

Calcitonin. Calcitonin is a hormone produced by C cells (parafollicular cells) of the thyroid gland in response to high circulating calcium levels. Calcitonin inhibits calcium *resorption* (loss of substance) from bone, increases calcium storage in bone, and increases renal excretion of calcium and phosphorus, thereby lowering serum calcium levels.[2]

Parathyroid Glands

The parathyroid glands are small, oval structures usually arranged in pairs behind each thyroid lobe (see Fig. 46-9). There are usually four glands. The major cell type of the glands is epithelial, and the gland is richly supplied with blood from the inferior and superior thyroid arteries.

Parathyroid Hormone. The parathyroids secrete **parathyroid hormone** (PTH), also called *parathormone*. Its major role is to regulate the blood level of calcium. PTH acts on bone, the kidneys, and indirectly the gastrointestinal (GI) tract. In bone, PTH stimulates bone resorption and inhibits bone formation, resulting in the release of calcium and phosphate into the blood. In the kidney, PTH increases calcium reabsorption and phosphate excretion. In addition, PTH stimulates the renal conversion of vitamin D to its most active form (1,25-dihydroxyvitamin D_3). This active vitamin D then enhances the intestinal absorption of calcium.

PTH is not under pituitary and hypothalamic control. The secretion of this hormone is directly regulated by a feedback system (see Fig. 46-5). When the serum calcium level is low, PTH secretion increases; when the serum calcium level rises, PTH secretion falls. In addition, high levels of active vitamin D inhibit PTH and low levels of magnesium stimulate PTH secretion.

Adrenal Glands

The adrenal glands are small, paired, highly vascularized glands located on the upper portion of each kidney. Each gland consists of two parts, the medulla and the cortex (Fig. 46-10). Each has distinct functions, and the glands act independently from one another.

Adrenal Medulla. The adrenal medulla constitutes 10% to 20% of the gland and consists of sympathetic postganglionic neurons. The medulla secretes the catecholamines epinephrine (the major hormone [75%]), norepinephrine (25%), and dopamine. **Catecholamines,** usually considered neurotransmitters, are hormones when secreted by the adrenal medulla, because they are released into the circulation and transported to their target organs.

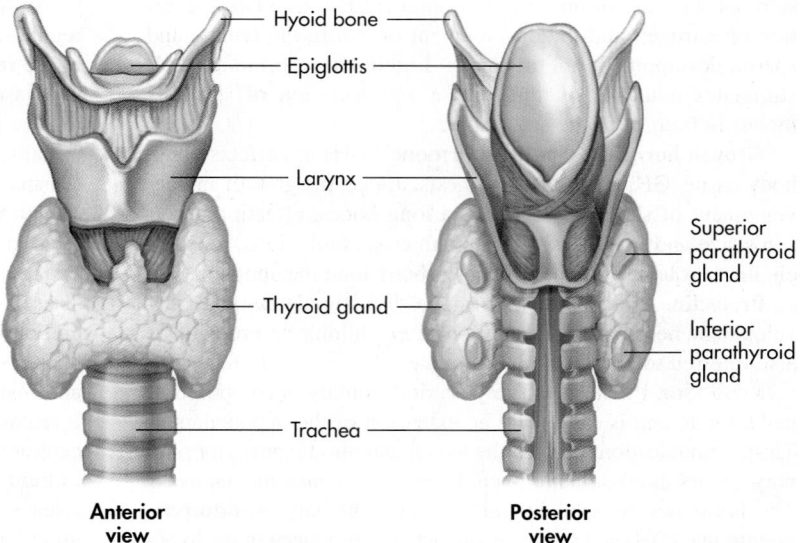

FIG. 46-9 Thyroid and parathyroid glands. Note the surrounding structures.

Anterior view

Posterior view

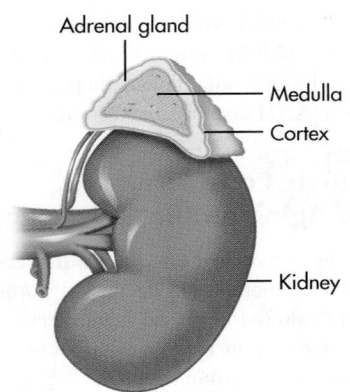

FIG. 46-10 The adrenal gland is composed of the adrenal cortex and the adrenal medulla.

Catecholamines exert their effects after binding to adrenergic receptors on cells, and they have widespread effects on all body systems. Catecholamines are an essential part of the body's response to stress (see Chapter 8).

Adrenal Cortex. The adrenal cortex, the outer part of the adrenal gland, constitutes 80% to 90% of the gland. It secretes more than 50 steroid hormones, which are classified as glucocorticoids, mineralocorticoids, and androgens. Cholesterol is the precursor for steroid hormone synthesis. Glucocorticoids (e.g., cortisol) are named for their effects on glucose metabolism. Mineralocorticoids (e.g., aldosterone) are essential for the maintenance of fluid and electrolyte balance. Adrenal androgens are produced and secreted in small but significant amounts. The term **corticosteroid** refers to any of the hormones synthesized by the adrenal cortex (excluding androgens).

Cortisol. Cortisol, the most abundant and potent glucocorticoid, is necessary to maintain life. One major function of cortisol is the regulation of blood glucose concentration. Cortisol increases blood glucose through facilitation of hepatic gluconeogenesis by promoting conversion of amino acids to glucose and inhibiting protein synthesis.[5] Cortisol also decreases peripheral glucose use in the fasting state. Additionally, glucocorticoids stimulate lipolysis in adipose tissue, thereby mobilizing glycerol and free fatty acids.

Another major effect of glucocorticoids is their antiinflammatory action and supportive actions in response to stress. A marked increase in the rate of cortisol secretion by the adrenal cortex aids the body in coping more effectively with stressful situations (see Chapter 8). Cortisol decreases the inflammatory response by stabilizing the membranes of cellular lysosomes and preventing increased capillary permeability. The lysosomal stabilization reduces the release of proteolytic enzymes and thereby their destructive effects on surrounding tissue. Cortisol can also inhibit production of prostaglandins, thromboxanes, and leukotrienes (see Chapter 12, Fig. 12-7) and alter the cell-mediated immune response.

Cortisol helps maintain vascular integrity and fluid volume. It has a mineralocorticoid effect because it can bind to mineralocorticoid receptor.

Cortisol is secreted in a diurnal pattern (see Fig. 46-7). The major control of cortisol is by means of a negative feedback mechanism that involves the secretion of corticotropin-releasing hormone (CRH) from the hypothalamus. CRH stimulates the secretion of ACTH by the anterior pituitary. Cortisol levels are also increased by surgical stress, burns, infection, fever, psychoses, acute anxiety, and hypoglycemia.

Aldosterone. Aldosterone is a potent mineralocorticoid that maintains extracellular fluid volume. It acts at the renal tubule to promote renal reabsorption of sodium and excretion of potassium and hydrogen ions. Aldosterone synthesis and secretion are stimulated by angiotensin II, hyponatremia, and hyperkalemia and inhibited by atrial natriuretic hormone and hypokalemia.

Adrenal androgens. The third class of steroids synthesized and secreted by the adrenal cortex are the androgens. Normally, the adrenal cortex secretes small amounts of androgens. Adrenal androgens stimulate pubic and axillary hair growth and sex drive in females. In the female, androgens are converted to estrogen in the peripheral tissues. In postmenopausal women the major source of estrogen is from the peripheral conversion of adrenal androgen to estrogen. The effects of adrenal androgen in men are negligible in comparison with testosterone secreted by the testes.

Pancreas

The pancreas is a long, tapered, lobular, soft gland located behind the stomach and anterior to the first and second lumbar vertebrae. The pancreas has both exocrine and endocrine functions (see Chapter 38). The hormone-secreting portion of the pancreas is referred to as the **islets of Langerhans.** The islets account for less than 2% of the gland and consist of four types of hormone-secreting cells: alpha, beta, delta, and F cells. Alpha cells produce and secrete the hormone glucagon. Insulin is produced and secreted by beta cells. Somatostatin is produced and secreted by the delta cells. Pancreatic polypeptide is secreted by the F (or PP) cells.

Glucagon. Glucagon is synthesized and released from pancreatic alpha cells in response to low levels of blood glucose, protein ingestion, and exercise. It increases blood glucose by stimulating glycogenolysis, gluconeogenesis, and ketogenesis. Usually, glucagon and insulin function in a reciprocal manner to maintain normal blood glucose levels. The exception is after ingestion of a high-protein carbohydrate-free diet, in which case both hormones are secreted. In this instance, glucagon counteracts the inhibitory effect of insulin on gluconeogenesis, and normal blood glucose levels are maintained.

Insulin. Insulin is the principal regulator of the metabolism and storage of ingested carbohydrates, fats, and proteins. Insulin facilitates glucose transport across cell membranes in most tissues. However, the brain, nerves, the lens of the eye, hepatocytes, erythrocytes, and cells in the intestinal mucosa and kidney tubules are not dependent on insulin for glucose uptake. An increased blood glucose level is the major stimulus for insulin synthesis and secretion. Other stimuli to insulin secretion are increased amino acid levels and vagal stimulation. Insulin secretion is usually inhibited by low blood glucose levels, glucagon, somatostatin, hypokalemia, and catecholamines (Table 46-3).

A major effect of insulin on glucose metabolism occurs in the liver, where the hormone enhances glucose incorporation into glycogen and triglycerides by altering enzymatic activity and inhibiting gluconeogenesis. Another major effect occurs in peripheral tissues where insulin facilitates glucose transport into cells, transport of amino acids across muscle membranes and their synthesis into protein, and transport of triglycerides into adipose tissue. Thus insulin is a storage, or *anabolic,* hormone.

The endocrine system is concerned with the regulation of body processes and the maintenance of internal homeostasis despite

TABLE 46-3   Factors Influencing Insulin Secretion

Stimulate Secretion	Inhibit Secretion
↑ Glucose levels	↓ Glucose levels
↑ Amino acid levels	↓ Amino acid levels
↑ Gastrointestinal hormone levels	↓ Potassium levels
	↑ Corticosteroid hormone levels
↑ Vagal stimulation	↑ Catecholamine levels
↑ Fats	↑ Somatostatin levels
	↑ Glucagon levels (usually)
	↑ Insulin levels

vastly changing substrates, as is seen in glucose homeostasis after food ingestion. After a meal, insulin is responsible for the storage of nutrients (anabolism). In the fasting state (during which ingested glucose is not readily available), hormones such as catecholamines, cortisol, and glucagon break down stored complex fuels (catabolism) to provide simple glucose as fuel for energy.

Heart

Atrial Natriuretic Hormone. *Natriuretic hormones* are a family of peptides; the most abundant is atrial natriuretic hormone (ANH). ANH is produced from cells in the right atrium in response to an increase in the stretch of the atrial wall caused by an abnormally high blood volume or blood pressure. These receptors in the atrium are also stimulated by high serum sodium levels. ANH acts on the kidneys to increase sodium loss. Increased loss of urinary sodium pulls water into the urine, result-

ing in a decrease in blood volume and a decrease in blood pressure.[10] ANH also inhibits renin, ADH, and the action of angiotensin II on the adrenal glands, thereby suppressing aldosterone secretion. ANH also causes vasodilation.

■ Gerontologic Considerations: Effects of Aging on the Endocrine System

Normal aging has many effects on the endocrine system (Table 46-4). These include (1) decreased hormone production and secretion, (2) altered hormone metabolism and biologic activity, (3) decreased responsiveness of target tissues to hormones, and (4) alterations in circadian rhythms.

Assessment of the effects of aging on the endocrine system is difficult because the subtle changes of aging often mimic manifestations of endocrine disorders. Some endocrine changes associated with aging are obvious; others are subtle. The nurse must be aware that endocrine problems may manifest differently in an older adult than in a younger person. Additionally, symptoms of endocrine dysfunction such as fatigue, constipation, or mental impairment in the older adult are often missed because they are attributed solely to aging.[11] It is important that the nurse consider age-related endocrine changes when assessing the older adult.[12-14] ■

ASSESSMENT OF THE ENDOCRINE SYSTEM

Hormones affect every body tissue and system, causing great diversity in the signs and symptoms of endocrine dysfunction.[3] Therefore assessment of the endocrine system is often difficult and requires keen clinical skills to detect manifestations of disorders. Endocrine dysfunction may result from deficient or ex-

TABLE 46-4   Gerontologic Differences in Assessment — Effects of Aging on the Endocrine System

GLAND	CHANGES	CLINICAL SIGNIFICANCE
Thyroid	Atrophy of thyroid gland. TSH and T₃ secretion is decreased	Increased incidence of hypothyroidism with aging. However, most older adults maintain adequate thyroid function
Parathyroid	Increased basal level of PTH and increased secretion	Increased calcium resorption from bone; hypercalcemia, hypercalciuria
Adrenal cortex	Adrenal cortex becomes more fibrotic and slightly smaller	Unknown. Possibly contributes to a decreased response to sodium restriction and upright posture
	Higher plasma levels of cortisol	
	Decreased plasma levels of adrenal androgens and aldosterone	
Adrenal medulla	Increased secretion and basal level of norepinephrine	Decreased responsiveness to β-adrenergic agonists and receptor blockers
	No change in plasma epinephrine levels with aging	May partly explain increased incidence of hypertension with aging
	Decreased β-adrenergic receptor response to norepinephrine	
Pancreas	Increase in fibrosis and fatty deposits in pancreas	May partly contribute to increased incidence of diabetes mellitus with advanced aging
	Increased glucose intolerance and decreased sensitivity to insulin	
Gonads	*Females:* decline in estrogen secretion	Women experience symptoms associated with menopause and have increased risk for atherosclerosis and osteoporosis
	Males: decline in testosterone secretion	Men may or may not experience symptoms

PTH, Parathyroid hormone; *TSH,* thyroid–stimulating hormone; T_3, triiodothyronine; T_4, thyroxine.

cessive hormone secretion, transport abnormalities, an inability of the target tissue to respond to a hormone, or inappropriate stimulation of the target-tissue receptor.

Endocrine disorders may have specific or nonspecific (vague) clinical manifestations. Specific signs and symptoms such as the classic "polys" (polyuria, polydipsia, and polyphagia) in diabetes mellitus make the assessment easier; nonspecific signs and symptoms such as tachycardia, palpitations, fatigue, or altered mood are more problematic. Nonspecific changes should alert the health care provider to the possibility of an endocrine disorder. The most common nonspecific symptoms, fatigue and depression, often are accompanied by other manifestations such as changes in energy level, alertness, sleep patterns, mood, affect, weight, skin, hair, personal appearance, and sexual function (Table 46-5).

TABLE 46-5 Health History — Endocrine System

Health Perception–Health Management
- What is your usual day like?
- Have you noticed any changes in your ability to perform your usual activities compared with last year? 5 years ago?*

Nutritional-Metabolic
- What is your weight and height?
- How much do you want to weigh?
- Have there been any changes in your appetite or weight?*
- Have you noticed any changes in the distribution of the hair anywhere on your body?*
- Have you noticed any changes in the color of your skin, particularly on your face, neck, hands, or body creases?*
- Has the texture of your skin changed? For example, does it seem thicker and drier than it used to?*
- Have you noticed any difficulty swallowing, or are your shirts more difficult to button?*
- Do you feel more nervous than you used to? Do you notice your heart pounding, or that you sweat when you do not think you should be sweating?
- Do you have difficulty holding things because of shakiness of your hands?*
- Do you feel that most rooms are too hot or too cold? Do you frequently have to put on a sweater, or feel as though you need to open windows when others in the room seem comfortable?*

Elimination
- Do you have to get up at night to urinate? If so, how many times? Do you keep water by your bed at night?
- Have you ever had a kidney stone?*
- Describe your usual bowel pattern. Have you noted any bowel changes?*
- Do you use anything, such as laxatives, to help you move your bowels?*

Activity-Exercise
- What is your usual activity pattern during a typical day?
- Do you have a planned exercise program? If yes, what is it and have you had to make any changes in this routine lately? If so, why and what kinds of changes?
- Do you experience fatigue with or without activity?*

Sleep-Rest
- How many hours do you sleep at night? Do you feel rested on awakening?
- Are you ever awakened by sweating during the night?*
- Do you have nightmares?*
- Does anyone in your family complain about your snoring?*

Cognitive-Perceptual
- How is your memory? Have you noticed any changes?
- How long can you concentrate on any one thing? Has this changed lately?
- Have you experienced any blurring or double vision?*
- When was your last eye examination?

Self-Perception–Self Concept
- Have you noticed any changes in your physical appearance or size?*
- Are you concerned about your weight?*
- Do you feel you are able to do what you think you should be capable of doing? If not, why not?
- Does your health problem affect how you feel about yourself?*

Role-Relationship
- Are you married? Do you have any children? Do you think you are able to take care of your family, home? If no, why not?
- Where do you work? What kind of work do you do? Are you able to do what is expected of you and what you expect of yourself?
- If retired, what do you do with your time? What did you do before you retired?
- If unemployed, are you looking for work?
- Is your income adequate for your needs?

Sexuality-Reproductive
Women
- When did you start to menstruate? Was this earlier or later than other women in your family? Do you have scant, heavy, or irregular menstrual flows?
- How many children have you had? How much did they weigh at birth? Were you told you had diabetes during any pregnancy?*
- Were you able to nurse your children if you wanted to?
- Are you attempting to get pregnant but cannot?*

Men
- Have you noticed any changes in your ability to have an erection?*
- Are you trying to have children but cannot?*

Coping–Stress Tolerance
- What kind of stressors do you have?
- How do you deal with stress or problems?
- What is your support system? To whom do you turn when you have a problem?

Value-Belief
- Do you think medicine should still be taken even though you feel OK?
- Do any of your prescribed therapies cause any conflict in your value-belief system?*

*If yes, describe.

TABLE 46-6	Common Assessment Abnormalities	
	Endocrine System	

FINDING	DESCRIPTION	POSSIBLE ETIOLOGY AND SIGNIFICANCE
Head, Neck		
Visual changes	Decreased visual acuity and/or decreased peripheral vision	Enlargement of pituitary gland or pituitary tumor can result in pressure on the optic nerve.
Exophthalmos	Protrusion of the eyeballs from the orbits	Classic finding associated with hyperthyroidism; results from fluid accumulation in the eye and retroorbital tissues.
Moon face	Periorbital edema and facial fullness	Classic finding associated with Cushing syndrome.
Myxedema	Puffiness, periorbital edema, masklike affect	Accumulation of hydrophilic mucopolysaccharides in the dermis; associated with long-standing hypothyroidism.
Goiter	Enlargement of the thyroid gland	Thyroid dysfunction or iodine deficiency; seen in hyperthyroidism and hypothyroidism.
Integument		
Hyperpigmentation	Darkening of the skin, particularly in creases and skinfolds	Addison's disease caused by increased secretion of melanocyte-stimulating hormone.
Striae	Purplish red marks below the skin surface—usually seen on abdomen, breasts, and buttocks	Cushing syndrome.
Changes in skin texture	Thick, cold, dry skin	Hypothyroidism.
	Thick, leathery, oily skin	Growth hormone excess (acromegaly).
	Warm, smooth, moist skin	Hyperthyroidism.
Changes in hair distribution	Hair loss	Hypothyroidism, hyperthyroidism, decreased pituitary secretion.
	Diminished axillary and pubic hair	Cortisol deficiency.
	Hirsutism (excessive facial hair on women)	Cushing syndrome, prolactinoma (a pituitary tumor).
Skin ulceration	Areas of ulcerated skin, most commonly found on the legs and feet	Peripheral neuropathy and peripheral vascular disease are contributory factors in the development of diabetic foot ulcers.
Musculoskeletal		
Changes in muscular strength or muscle mass	Generalized weakness and/or fatigue	Common symptoms associated with many endocrine problems, including pituitary, thyroid, parathyroid, and adrenal dysfunctions; diabetes mellitus; diabetes insipidus.
	Decreased muscle mass	Specifically seen in those with growth hormone deficiency and in Cushing syndrome secondary to protein wasting.
Enlargement of bones and cartilage	Coarsening of facial features; increases in size of hand and feet over a period of several years	Gradual enlargement and thickening of bony tissue occurs with growth hormone excess in adults as seen in acromegaly.
Nutrition		
Changes in weight	Weight loss	Hyperthyroidism due to increases in metabolism.
	Weight gain	Hypothyroidism, Cushing syndrome.
Altered glucose levels	Increased serum glucose	Diabetes mellitus, Cushing syndrome, growth hormone excess.
Neurologic		
Lethargy	State of mental sluggishness or somnolence	Hypothyroidism.
Tetany	Intermittent involuntary muscle spasms usually involving the extremities	Severe calcium deficiency that can occur with hypoparathyroidism.
Seizure	Sudden involuntary contraction of muscles	Consequence of a pituitary tumor; fluid and electrolyte imbalance associated with excessive ADH secretion; complications of diabetes mellitus; severe hypothyroidism.
Gastrointestinal		
Constipation	Passage of infrequent hard stools	Hypothyroidism; hyperparathyroidism due to calcium imbalances.

ADH, Antidiuretic hormone.

TABLE 46-6   Common Assessment Abnormalities
Endocrine System—cont'd

FINDING	DESCRIPTION	POSSIBLE ETIOLOGY AND SIGNIFICANCE
Reproductive		
Changes in reproductive function	Menstrual irregularities, decreased libido, decreased fertility, impotence	Reproductive function is significantly affected by various endocrine abnormalities, including pituitary hypofunction, growth hormone excess, thyroid dysfunction, and adrenocortical dysfunction.
Other		
Polyuria	Excessive urinary output	Diabetes mellitus (secondary to hyperglycemia) or diabetes insipidus (associated with decreased ADH).
Polydipsia	Excessive thirst	Extreme water losses in diabetes mellitus (with severe hyperglycemia) and diabetes insipidus.
Thermoregulation	Cold insensitivity Heat intolerance	Hypothyroidism caused by a slowing of metabolic processes. Hyperthyroidism caused by excessive metabolism.

Subjective Data

The lack of clear-cut manifestations of endocrine problems requires a conscientious and detailed health history. A careful health history will yield data to help sort out possible causes and the effect of the problem on the person's life (Table 46-6).

Important Health Information

Past health history. During an assessment, the patient should be questioned about the general state of health and if there have been any changes. In addition, the patient or significant other should be specifically questioned about previous or current endocrine abnormalities and abnormal patterns of growth and development.

Medications. The patient should be questioned about the use of all medications (both prescription and over-the-counter drugs) and the use of herbs and dietary supplements. The patient should be asked the reason for taking the drug, dose, and the length of time taken. The patient should specifically be asked about the use of hormone replacements. Information that the patient is currently taking hormone replacements such as insulin, thyroid, or corticosteroids (e.g., prednisone) helps direct the nurse regarding possible problems associated with the use of these agents. For example, corticosteroids may cause glucose intolerance in the susceptible patient by increasing glycogenolysis and insulin resistance. The side and adverse effects of many nonhormone medications can contribute to problems affecting endocrine function. For example, many drugs can affect blood glucose levels (see Chapter 47, Table 47-8).

Surgery or other treatments. The nurse should inquire about previous hospitalizations, surgery, chemotherapy, and radiation therapy (especially of the neck). Surgery of the brain or a severe blow to the head could have resulted in pituitary or hypothalamic alterations.

Functional Health Patterns

Health perception–health management pattern. Inquiry should be made about the patient's general health care and health care behaviors. Such an inquiry might result in the identification of vague, nonspecific symptoms that could suggest an endocrine problem.

Heredity can play a major role in the occurrence of endocrine problems. The patient should be questioned about the following conditions in family members: diabetes mellitus or insipidus; hyperthyroidism or hypothyroidism, goiter; hypertension or hypotension; obesity; infertility; growth problems; pheochromocytoma (neoplastic tumor of the adrenal medulla or sympathetic ganglia); autoimmune diseases (e.g., Addison's disease); and adrenal hyperplasia. Further information may be elicited by asking additional questions such as the following: Are there any other members of your family who have, or have had, a similar problem? This frequently uncovers evidence of a familial tendency.

Nutritional-metabolic pattern. Because a major function of the endocrine system is regulating metabolism and maintaining homeostasis, the patient with endocrine dysfunction will often experience alterations in nutritional-metabolic patterns. Reported changes in appetite and weight can indicate endocrine dysfunction. Weight loss with increased appetite may indicate hyperthyroidism or diabetes mellitus, particularly type 1. Weight loss with decreased appetite may indicate hypopituitarism, hypocortisolism, or gastroparesis (decreased gastric motility and emptying) from diabetes mellitus. Weight gain may indicate hypothyroidism and, if the weight gain is concentrated in the truncal area, hypercortisolism. In addition, weight gain in a genetically susceptible patient may increase the risk for type 2 diabetes mellitus.

Difficulty swallowing or a change in neck size may indicate a thyroid disorder or inflammation. Questions related to increased sympathetic nervous system activity (e.g., nervousness, palpitations, sweating, tremors) may assist the nurse in identifying a thyroid disorder or pheochromocytoma. Heat or cold intolerance may indicate hyperthyroidism or hypothyroidism, respectively.

The patient should be questioned about dietary intake. This record should be examined for the presence of foods that contain thyroid-inhibiting substances (goitrogens) (see Chapter 48, Table 48-8).

The patient should also be asked about changes to his or her skin or hair. Hair distribution and skin and hair color and texture can all indicate endocrine dysfunction. Hair loss can indicate hypopituitarism, hypothyroidism, hypoparathyroidism, or increased testosterone and other androgens. Increased body hair may indicate hypercortisolism. Decreased skin pigmentation can occur in hypopituitarism, hypothyroidism, and hypoparathyroidism, whereas increased skin pigmentation, particularly in sun-exposed areas, can indicate hypocortisolism. A patient with hypothyroidism or excess growth hormone may complain of coarse, leathery skin. A patient with hyperthyroidism may comment about fine, silky hair.

Elimination pattern. Because maintenance of fluid balance is a major role of the endocrine system, questions related to elimination patterns may uncover endocrine dysfunction. For example, increased thirst and urination can indicate diabetes mellitus or insipidus. The patient should be asked about the frequency and consistency of bowel movements. Frequent defecation may indicate hyperthyroidism. Large-volume, watery stools or fecal incontinence may indicate autonomic neuropathy of diabetes mellitus. Constipation is also seen in the patients with diabetes mellitus, as well as in hypothyroidism, hypoparathyroidism, and hypopituitarism.

Activity-exercise pattern. The nurse should ask about energy levels, particularly as compared with the patient's past energy level. Fatigue and hyperactivity are two common problems associated with endocrine problems. The major effect of endocrine dysfunction on activity-exercise pattern is an inability to maintain previous activity levels.

Sleep-rest pattern. It is important that the nurse obtain a detailed sleep history. Sleep disturbances are frequently seen in endocrine dysfunction. The patient with diabetes mellitus or insipidus will complain of nocturia, which can severely disrupt normal sleep patterns. The patient with type 1 diabetes mellitus on a tight glucose control regimen who complains of sweating or nightmares may be experiencing hypoglycemia. The hyperthyroid patient may complain of inability to sleep, as may one with hypercortisolism. The patient with hypothyroidism, hypocortisolism, or hypopituitarism may tell the nurse of sleeping all the time, yet still being fatigued.

Cognitive-perceptual pattern. A patient with an endocrine dysfunction will frequently manifest apathy and depression. The nurse can question both the patient and significant other to determine if any cognitive changes are present. Memory deficits and an inability to concentrate are common in endocrine disorders. A patient report of visual changes such as blurring or double vision could be an indication of endocrine problems.

Self-perception–self-concept pattern. Endocrine disorders may affect the patient's self-perception because of associated physical changes affecting appearance. Changes in weight, size, and level of fatigue should be determined. The chronicity of many endocrine disorders and need for continued therapy can affect the patient's self-perception. The patient can be asked to describe the effects of the present illness on self-perception.

Role-relationship pattern. The nurse should ask whether there have been any changes in the patient's ability to maintain roles at home, at work, or in the community. Often the patient with an endocrine disorder will be unable to sustain life's roles. However, in most cases the patient can be advised that, with adequate management, previous roles can be resumed. This can be very reassuring for the patient and family.

Sexuality-reproductive pattern. The development of abnormal secondary sex characteristics (e.g., facial hair in a woman or decreased need for shaving in a man) should be documented. Problems with menstruation and pregnancy in a woman may indicate an endocrine disorder. Consequently, a detailed history of menstruation and pregnancy should be obtained. Menstrual irregularities are seen in disorders of the ovaries, pituitary, thyroid, and adrenal glands. A female patient with a history of large ba-

bies may have had undiagnosed gestational diabetes, which may put her at a higher risk to develop diabetes mellitus. A history of inability to lactate may indicate a pituitary disorder.

Male sexual dysfunction is also frequently seen in endocrine disorders. It usually takes the form of impotence, although retrograde ejaculation can occur. Infertility in either sex warrants a full reproductive and endocrine workup.

Coping–stress tolerance pattern. Stressors of all kinds affect the endocrine system. Areas that can cause a great deal of stress should be investigated. The patient should be asked about place of employment, kind of work, ability to meet job requirements, and the amount of stress involved. The nurse should ask whether the job provides an adequate income in order to identify financial stressors. Usual coping patterns are also discussed. The nurse then determines whether previous coping patterns are still successful. It is often useful to ask family members or a significant other about the patient's coping strategies and reaction to stress.

Value-belief pattern. When dealing with a patient with a chronic condition, identification of the patient's value-belief patterns can assist the health care team to identify appropriate regimens. This is particularly important in a condition such as diabetes mellitus, which may require major lifestyle changes for successful management. Other endocrine disorders, such as hypothyroidism or hypocortisolism, can be easily managed with oral medication taken faithfully. Identification of a patient's ability to make lifestyle changes or take daily medication (and increase this medication as indicated) is an important nursing function.

Objective Data

Most endocrine glands are inaccessible to direct examination. With the exception of the thyroid and male gonads, the glands are deeply encased in the body, protected against injury and trauma. However, assessment can be accomplished using a variety of objective data. It is imperative that the nurse understand the actions of hormones so that the function of a gland can be assessed by monitoring the target tissue.

Physical Examination. It is important to keep in mind that the endocrine system affects every body system. Clinical manifestations of endocrine function vary significantly depending on the gland involved. Specific clinical findings for the various endocrine problems are discussed in Chapters 47 and 48. Regardless of the type of endocrine dysfunction, the following general examination procedure should be followed.

Vital signs. A full set of vital signs is taken at the beginning of the examination. Variations in temperature may be associated with thyroid dysfunction. Cardiovascular changes such as tachycardia, bradycardia, hypotension, or hypertension may be seen with a variety of endocrine-related problems.

Height and weight. Assessment of the endocrine system includes a history of growth and development patterns, weight distribution and changes, and comparisons of these factors with normal findings. Growth pattern abnormalities suggest problems associated with growth hormone. Changes in weight also may be associated with endocrine dysfunction. Thyroid disorders and diabetes mellitus are examples of endocrine disorders that can affect body weight. Body mass index (BMI) is a height-to-weight ratio used to assess nutritional status (see Chapter 39, Fig. 39-6).

It may also be helpful to compare the patient's current body weight to her or his usual body weight in order to assess changes. Weight change (%) is calculated by dividing the current body weight by usual body weight and multiplying by 100. Weight change greater than 5% in 1 month, 7.5% in 3 months, or 10% in 6 months is considered significant.[15]

Mental-emotional status. Throughout the examination the patient's orientation, alertness, memory, affect, personality, anxiety, and appropriateness of dress and speech pattern should be objectively assessed. Endocrine disorders can commonly cause changes in mental and emotional status.

Integument. The nurse should note the color and texture of the skin, hair, and nails. The overall skin color should be noted, as well as pigmentation and possible ecchymosis. Hyperpigmentation of the skin (particularly on the knuckles, elbows, knees, genitalia, and palmar creases) is a classic finding in Addison's disease, but also is seen with ACTH-producing tumors and acromegaly.[3] The skin should be palpated for skin texture and presence of moisture. The hair distribution should be examined not only on the head, but also on the face, trunk, and extremities. The appearance and texture of the hair should be examined. Dull, brittle hair; excessive hair growth; or hair loss may indicate endocrine dysfunction.

Head. The size and contour of the head should be inspected. Facial features should be symmetric. Eyes should be inspected for position, symmetry, shape and eye movement, opacity over the lens, lid lag, and edema. Visual acuity should also be checked because changes may be associated with a pituitary tumor. In the mouth, the nurse should inspect the buccal mucosa and the condition of teeth, malocclusion and mottling, tongue size, and fasciculations (localized, uncoordinated, uncontrollable twitching of a single muscle group).

Neck. When inspecting the thyroid gland, observation should be made first in the normal position (preferably with side lighting), then in slight extension, and then as the patient swallows some water. The trachea should be midline and the neck should appear symmetric. Any unusual bulging over the thyroid area should be noted. If there is no noticeable enlargement of the thyroid gland, palpation can be done. (Because palpation can trigger the release of thyroid hormones, palpation should be deferred in the patient with a visibly enlarged thyroid gland.) When an enlarged thyroid is noted, the lateral lobes should be auscultated with the stethoscope bell to determine the presence of a bruit.

The thyroid gland is difficult to palpate. Thyroid palpation requires considerable practice, as well as validation by a more experienced examiner. Water should always be available for the patient to swallow as part of this examination. There are two acceptable approaches to thyroid palpation: anterior or posterior. For anterior palpation the nurse stands in front of the patient, with the patient's neck flexed. The nurse places the thumb horizontally with the upper edge along the lower border of the cricoid cartilage. The thumb is then moved over the isthmus as the patient swallows water. The fingers are then placed laterally to the anterior border of the sternocleidomastoid muscle, and each lateral lobe is palpated before and while the patient swallows water.

For posterior palpation the examiner stands behind the patient. With the thumbs of both hands resting on the nape of the patient's neck, the nurse uses the index and middle fingers of both hands to feel for the thyroid isthmus and for the anterior surfaces of the lateral lobes. To facilitate the examination of each lobe and to relax the neck muscles, the nurse asks the patient to flex the neck slightly forward and to the right. The thyroid cartilage is displaced to the right by the left hand and fingers. The nurse palpates with the right hand after placing the thumb deep

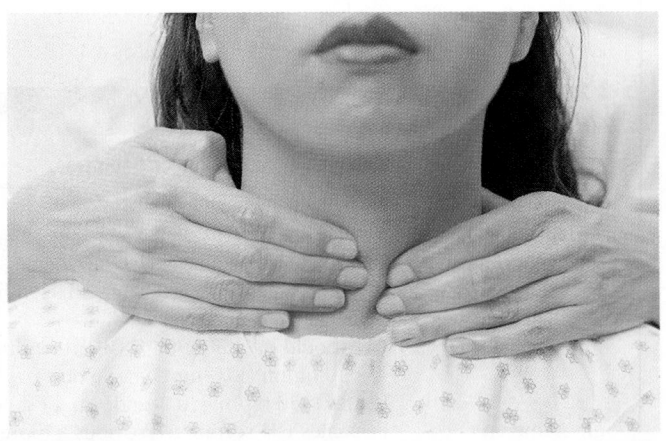

Posterior palpation of the thyroid gland.

and behind the sternocleidomastoid muscle with the index and middle fingers in front of it; the area is palpated with the right hand (Fig. 46-11). While this is done, the patient is asked to swallow water. This procedure is then repeated on the left side. The thyroid is palpated for its size, shape, symmetry, and tenderness and for any nodules.

In a normal person the thyroid is often not palpable. If palpable, it usually feels smooth, with a firm consistency, and is not tender with gentle pressure. Nodules, enlargement, asymmetry, or hardness is abnormal, and the patient should be referred for further evaluation.

Thorax. The thorax should be inspected for shape and characteristics of the skin. The presence of gynecomastia in men should be noted. Lung sounds and heart sounds are auscultated, noting the presence of adventitious lung sounds or extra heart sounds.

Abdomen. There are no specific abdominal examination findings for endocrine dysfunction other than skin characteristics and hyperactive or hypoactive bowel sounds.

Extremities. The size, shape, symmetry, and general proportion of hand and feet size should be assessed. The skin should be inspected for changes in pigmentation and presence of lesions and edema. Muscle strength should be evaluated, as well as deep tendon reflexes. In the upper extremities, the presence of tremors is assessed by placing a piece of paper in the outstretched fingers, palm down.

Genitalia. The hair distribution pattern should be inspected. A diamond pattern in women is an abnormal finding and may indicate endocrine dysfunction. For males, the testes should be palpated; for females, any clitoral enlargement should be noted.

Common assessment abnormalities related to the endocrine system are presented in Table 46-6.

DIAGNOSTIC STUDIES OF THE ENDOCRINE SYSTEM

Accurately performed laboratory tests and radiologic examinations contribute to the diagnosis of an endocrine problem. Laboratory tests usually involve blood and urine testing. Radiologic tests include regular x-ray, computed tomography (CT), and magnetic resonance imaging (MRI). With all diagnostic testing, the nurse is responsible for explaining the procedure to the patient and family. Diagnostic studies common to the endocrine system are presented in Table 46-7.

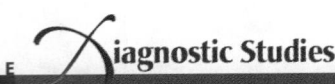

TABLE
46-7

iagnostic Studies
Endocrine System

STUDY	PURPOSE AND DESCRIPTION	NURSING RESPONSIBILITY
Pituitary Studies		
Serum Studies		
▪ Growth hormone (GH) (Somatotropin)	Evaluates GH secretion. Used to identify GH deficiency or GH excess. GH levels are affected by time of day, food intake, and stress. GH should be <5 ng/ml (5.0 μg/L) in men and <10 ng/ml (10.0 μg/L) in women. Values >50 ng/ml (50.0/μg/L) suggest acromegaly.	Make sure that patient has been fasting and has not recently been emotionally or physically stressed. Indicate patient fasting status and recent activity level on the laboratory slip. Send blood sample to laboratory immediately.
▪ Somatomedin C (insulin-like growth factor 1 [IGF-1])	Evaluates GH secretion. Provides a more accurate reflection of mean plasma concentration of GH because it is not subject to circadian rhythm and fluctuations. *Normal values* are 135-250 ng/ml; low levels indicate GH deficiency, all high levels indicate GH excess.	Overnight fasting is preferred but not necessary.
▪ Growth hormone stimulation test	Needed to adequately diagnose GH deficiency. Measures GH secretion in response to stimulation (insulin, arginine). For insulin, baseline blood levels for GH, glucose, and cortisol are obtained. Insulin is then administered intravenously; blood samples for GH are obtained 30, 60, and 90 minutes after insulin is administered; blood glucose levels are monitored at 15- to 30-minute intervals. Blood glucose should drop to less than 40 mg/dl for effective testing. GH level should rise twofold to threefold over baseline levels. Response is subnormal or absent in GH deficiency.	Ensure patient/family understands this procedure. Patient must be NPO after midnight. Water is permitted on morning of the test. IV access is established for administration of medications and frequent blood sampling. Nurse must continually assess for hypoglycemia and hypotension. 50% dextrose and 5% dextrose IV solution should be kept at the bedside in case severe hypoglycemia occurs.
▪ Gonadotropin levels Follicle-stimulating hormone (FSH) Luteinizing hormone (LH)	Useful in distinguishing primary gonadal problems from pituitary insufficiency. Normal levels vary according to age and sex. In women, there are marked differences during menstrual cycle and in postmenopausal period. Levels are low in pituitary insufficiency and high in primary gonadal failure. In women, values for FSH are basal rate—2-15 mIU/ml (2-15 IU/L); ovulatory surge—8-40 mIU/ml (8-40 IU/L); and postmenopausal level—greater than 50 mIU/ml (50 IU/L). In women, values for LH are basal rate—2-20 mIUml (2-20 IU/L); ovulatory surge—30-140 mIU/ml (30-140 IU/L); and postmenopausal level—greater than 50 mIU/ml (50 IU/L). In men, values for FSH are 2-15 mIU/ml (2-15 IU/L) and values for LH are 3-25 mIU/ml (3-25 IU/L).	There is no special preparation of the patient. Only one blood tube is needed for both FSH and LH. Note on the laboratory slip time of menstrual cycle or whether she is postmenopausal.
▪ Water deprivation test	Used to differentiate causes of polyuria, including central diabetes insipidus (DI), nephrogenic DI, syndrome of inappropriate antidiuretic hormone (SIADH), and psychogenic polydipsia. ADH or vasopressin is administered intravenously or subcutaneously. In normal patients and those with psychogenic DI, urine osmolality and plasma osmolality are normal after ADH administration. In patients with central DI, urine osmolality increases after ADH administration. In patients with nephrogenic DI, there is little or no response to ADH.	Have patient discontinue fluids and smoking after midnight. Obtain baseline weight and urine and plasma osmolality. Weigh patient and take three postural BP measurements (lying and standing BP measurements separated by 2 minutes) hourly. Assess urine hourly for volume and specific gravity. Send hourly samples for urine osmolality. Draw sample for plasma osmolality when (1) urine samples are collected and (2) orthostatic hypotension and postural tachycardia appear. Assess weight at 4, 6, 7, and 8 hours. Patients must be very closely supervised during this test.

BP, Blood pressure; *IV,* intravenous; *NPO,* nothing by mouth.

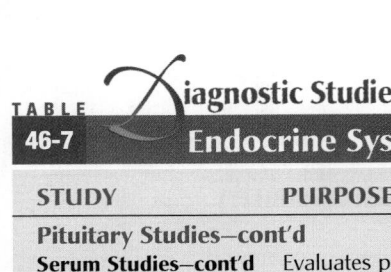

TABLE 46-7   Diagnostic Studies

Endocrine System—cont'd

STUDY	PURPOSE AND DESCRIPTION	NURSING RESPONSIBILITY
Pituitary Studies—cont'd		
Serum Studies—cont'd • Prolactin level	Evaluates prolactin levels. Decreased levels in postpartum women attempting to nurse may be associated with Sheehan syndrome. *Normal values* <20 ng/ml (<20 μg/L) (nonlactating); levels >200 ng/ml (200 μg/L) indicate pituitary tumors.	Draw blood within 3-4 hours after patient awakens. Specimen must be sent to the laboratory immediately. If there is a delay, the specimen is placed on ice.
Radiologic Studies • Magnetic resonance imaging (MRI)	Examination of choice for radiologic evaluation of the pituitary gland and hypothalamus. Useful in identification of tumors involving the hypothalamus or pituitary.	Inform patient of the need to lie as still as possible during the test; explain that tests are painless and noninvasive.
Thyroid Studies		
Serum Studies • Thyroid-stimulating hormone (TSH)	Measures levels for TSH. *Normal values* are 0.3-5.4 μU/ml (0.3-5.4 mU/L). Considered the most sensitive method for evaluating thyroid disease. Generally recommended as first diagnostic test for thyroid dysfunction.	Explain blood draw procedure to the patient. No specific preparations are necessary.
• Thyroxine (T_4)	Measures total serum level of T_4. Useful in evaluating thyroid function and monitoring thyroid therapy. *Normal values* are 5-12 μg/dl (51-142 nmol/L).	See above.
• Triiodothyronine (T_3)	Measures serum levels of T_3. It is helpful in diagnosing hyperthyroidism if T_4 levels are normal. *Normal values* are 65-195 ng/dl (1.0-3.0 nmol/L).	See above.
• Free T_4	Measures active component of total T_4. *Normal values* are 1.0-3.5 ng/dl (12.9-45.0 pmol/L). Because level remains constant, this is considered better indication of thyroid function than T_4.	See above.
• T_3 resin uptake (T_3RU)	Indirectly measures binding capacity of thyroid-binding globulin. *Normal values* are 25%-35%.	See above.
Radiologic Studies • Radioactive iodine uptake (RAIU)	Provides direct measure of thyroid activity. Useful for evaluation of functional activity of solitary thyroid nodules. Patient is given radioactive iodine either orally or intravenously. The uptake by the thyroid gland is measured with a scanner at several time intervals such as 2 to 4 hours and at 24 hours. The values of RAIU are expressed in percentage of uptake. For 2-4 hours *normal values* are 3%-19%; for 24 hours, they are 11%-30%.	Patient should be NPO for 6-8 hours before test, but can resume eating 1 hour after oral iodine dose is taken. Patient should not have supplemental iodine for several weeks before the test. Thyroid medications interfere with test results.
• Thyroid scan	Used to evaluate nodules of the thyroid. Radioactive isotopes are given orally or intravenously. Scanner passes over thyroid and makes graphic record of radiation emitted. Normal thyroid scan reveals homogeneous pattern with symmetric lobes. Benign nodules appear as warm spots because they take up the radionuclide; malignant tumors appear as cold spots because they tend not to take up the radionuclide.	Explain procedure to the patient; be sure patient understands that radioactive iodine taken orally is harmless. No special preparation is required.

Continued

TABLE
46-7

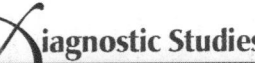

Diagnostic Studies

Endocrine System—cont'd

STUDY	PURPOSE AND DESCRIPTION	NURSING RESPONSIBILITY
Parathyroid Studies **Serum Studies**		
• Parathyroid hormone (PTH)	Measures PTH level in serum. Normal range depends on assay used (check with laboratory). This study must be interpreted in terms of concomitantly drawn serum calcium level.	Fasting specimen preferred. Inform patient that blood sample will be drawn. Sample must be kept on ice. Observe venipuncture site for bleeding or hematoma formation.
• Total serum calcium	Measures total serum calcium to help detect bone and parathyroid disorders. Hypercalcemia can indicate primary hyperparathyroidism, and hypocalcemia can indicate hypoparathyroidism. *Normal values* are 9.0-11.0 mg/dl or 4.5-5.5 mEq/L (2.25-2.74 mmol/L).	Fasting specimen preferred. Inform patient that blood sample will be drawn. Observe venipuncture site for bleeding or hematoma formation. Ensure that prolonged tourniquet application does not cause falsely elevated values.
• Serum phosphate	Measures inorganic phosphorus. Hyperphosphatemia indicates primary hypoparathyroidism or secondary causes (e.g., renal failure); hypophosphatemia indicates hyperparathyroidism. Phosphorus and calcium levels are inversely related. *Normal values* are 2.8-4.5 mg/dl (0.90-1.45 mmol/L).	Need for fasting varies with laboratory. Determine fasting requirement. Inform patient that blood sample will be drawn. Observe venipuncture site for bleeding or hematoma formation.
Adrenal Studies **Serum Studies**		
• Cortisol	Measures amount of total cortisol in serum and evaluates status of adrenal cortex function. *Normal values* are 5-25 μg/dl (0.14-0.69 μmol/L) at 8 AM, 10 mg/dl (0.28 mmol/L) at 8 PM.	Cortisol has diurnal variation—levels are higher in the morning than in evening. Sample should be drawn in morning—evening samples may also be ordered. Mark time of blood draw on laboratory slip. Patient anxiety should be minimized.
• Aldosterone	Aldosterone levels are drawn to evaluate for hyperaldosteronism. *Normal values* are 5-20 ng/dl (140-556 pmol/L) (upright posture) and 8.5 ng/dl (237 pmol/L) (supine position).	Usually morning blood sample is preferred. Indicate patient position (supine, sitting, standing) during venipuncture.
• Adrenocorticotropic hormone (ACTH, corticotropin)	Measures the plasma level of ACTH. Although ACTH is a pituitary hormone, it controls adrenal cortex secretion, thus helps to determine if underproduction or overproduction of cortisol is caused by dysfunction of the adrenal gland or pituitary gland. *Normal values* are morning: <80 pg/ml (18 pmol/L); evening: <50 pg/ml (<11 pmol/L).	Patient should be NPO after midnight before morning blood draw. Minimize stress. Diurnal levels correspond with variation of cortisol levels; that is, levels are higher in morning, lower in evening. ACTH is very unstable; blood tube must be placed on ice and sent to laboratory immediately.
• ACTH stimulation with cosyntropin	Used to evaluate adrenal function. After baseline samples are drawn, 250 mg cosyntropin (synthetic ACTH) is given as IV or IM bolus; samples are drawn 30 and 50 minutes after bolus. Baseline ACTH sample is often drawn in case results are abnormal. Plasma cortisol at 60 minutes should be (1) greater than baseline and (2) greater than 20 μg/dl.	Obtain baseline cortisol level at beginning of cosyntropin infusion. Inject cosyntropin with a plastic syringe and collect blood samples in plastic heparinized tubes. Administer test with continuous-infusion method. Monitor site and rate of IV infusion. Ensure sample collection at appropriate times.
• ACTH suppression (dexamethasone suppression)	Assesses adrenal function and is especially helpful if hyperactivity is suspected. Useful in evaluation of Cushing syndrome. Dexamethasone (Decadron) 2 mg is given at 11 PM to suppress secretion of corticotropin-releasing hormone. Plasma cortisol sample is drawn at 8 AM. Cortisol level <5 μg/dl (138 nmol/L) indicates normal adrenal response (50% decrease in cortisol production).	Ensure that patient has fasted. Inform patient that blood sample will be taken. Observe venipuncture site for bleeding and hematoma formation. Do not test acutely ill patients; those under stress are not tested. ACTH may override suppression. Screen patient for drugs such as estrogen and glucocorticoids, which may give false-positive results. Ensure accurate timing of medication and sample collection.

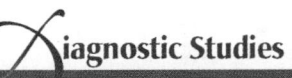

TABLE 46-7   **Diagnostic Studies**

Endocrine System—cont'd

STUDY	PURPOSE AND DESCRIPTION	NURSING RESPONSIBILITY
Urine Studies		
• 17-Ketosteroids	Measures androgen metabolites in urine and evaluates adrenocortical and gonadal function. *Normal values* are 10-22 mg/day (35-76 μmol/day) for men and 6-16 mg/day (21-55 μmol/day) for women.	Instruct patient regarding 24-hour urine collection. Tell patient that specimen must be kept refrigerated or iced during collection. Determine whether preservative is required for method used.
• Aldosterone	Measures urinary aldosterone level to evaluate adrenal function. Useful in determining therapy for hypertension. *Normal values* are 2-26 μg/24 hours (5.5-72 nmol/day).	Ensure that patient is on unrestricted diet with normal salt intake and no medication for 3 weeks before collection. Instruct patient regarding 24-hour urine collection.
• Free cortisol	Measures free (unbound) cortisol. Preferred test to evaluate hypercortisolism. *Normal values* are <100 μg/24 hours.	Instruct patient about 24-hour urine collection and avoidance of stressful situations and excessive physical exercise. Some drugs (e.g., reserpine, diuretics, phenothiazines, amphetamines) may elevate levels. Ensure that patient is on low-sodium diet.
• Vanillylmandelic acid	Measures urinary excretion of catecholamine metabolite and is helpful in diagnosing pheochromocytoma. *Normal values* are <8 mg/24 hours (40 μmol/day); pheochromocytoma is indicated with values of 10-250 mg/24 hours (51-126 μmol/day).	Keep 24-hour urine collection at pH of less than 3.0 with hydrochloric acid as preservative. Know that newer methods are not affected by dietary intake. Consult with laboratory or physician about patient discontinuing any drugs 3 days before urine collection.
Radiologic Tests		
• Computed tomography (CT)	Abdominal CT is the radiologic examination of choice for the adrenal gland. Used to detect tumor and size of tumor mass or metastatic spread. Oral and/or IV contrast medium may be used.	Inform patient of procedure. Patient must lie still during the procedure. If IV contrast is used, check for iodine allergy.
Pancreatic Studies		
Serum Studies		
• Fasting blood sugar (FBS) level	Measures circulating glucose level. *Normal values* for adults are 70-110 mg/dl (3.9-6.7 mmol/L); for pregnant women they are 60-90 mg/dl (3.3-5 mmol/L).	Patient should fast for at least 4-8 hours—water intake is permitted. If patient has an IV infusion containing dextrose, test is not considered valid.
• Oral glucose tolerance	A. 2-hour test used to diagnose diabetes mellitus if FBS is equivocal. Patient drinks 75 g of glucose; samples for glucose are drawn immediately and at 30, 60, and 120 minutes. *Normal values* are <200 mg/dl (11.1 mmol/L) at 30, 60, and 90 minutes and <140 mg/dl (7.8 mmol/L) at 120 minutes. B. 5-hour test used to evaluate hypoglycemia. Patient drinks 100 g of glucose; samples of glucose are drawn immediately and at 30, 60, 90, 120, 180, 240, and 300 minutes. Baseline cortisol level test is done if patient becomes symptomatic. Patients with reactive hypoglycemia have adrenergic symptoms and glucose <60 mg/dl (3.3 mmol/L) between 30 minutes and 5 hours after glucose ingestion.	Ensure that tests are not done on patients who are malnourished, confined to bed for over 3 days, or severely stressed. Instruct patient to refrain from smoking and caffeine and to fast for 12 hours before test. Ensure that patient's diet 3 days before test included 150-300 g of carbohydrate with intake of at least 1500 calories per day. Screen for estrogens, phenytoin (Dilantin), and corticosteroids, and check for hypokalemia, which may impair glucose tolerance. Simultaneously monitor glucose levels with capillary glucose monitoring.
• Capillary glucose monitoring	Used to give immediate glucose values with glucose oxidase or electrochemical methods. Capillary values (whole blood) are usually 10%-15% less than serum values.	Obtain large drop of blood from clean finger, touch strip to drop of blood (not finger), time accurately, and compare colors in good lighting, if using visual method. Use digital readout if available. Use automatic finger-puncture device if available. Be sure to change section of device that touches patient's fingers between patients.
• Glycosylated hemoglobin (Hb A$_{1c}$ [A1C])	Measures degree of glucose control during previous 3 months (life span of hemoglobin molecule). *Normal values* are 4%-6% (values vary widely; check with laboratory).	Inform patient that fasting is not necessary and that blood sample will be drawn. Observe venipuncture site for bleeding or hematoma formation.

Continued

TABLE 46-7	Diagnostic Studies Endocrine System—cont'd	
STUDY	**PURPOSE AND DESCRIPTION**	**NURSING RESPONSIBILITY**
Urine Studies		
• Glucose	Estimate amount of glucose in urine by using an enzymatic method. Dipstick is dipped into the urine and read for color changes after 1 minute. Normal results will show negative glucose in the urine.	Use freshly voided urine specimen collected at appropriate time. Know that many different drugs alter glucose readings and that errors are great if directions for timing are not followed exactly. Follow package directions.
• Ketones	Measures amount of acetone excreted in urine as result of incomplete fat metabolism. Tested with a dipstick as described above. Normal value is negative or trace ketone. Positive result can indicate lack of insulin and diabetic acidosis.	Use freshly voided urine specimen. Test is often done with glucose test. Directions must be followed exactly. Certain drugs can produce false-positive and false-negative results.
Radiologic Tests		
• Computed tomography (CT)	Abdominal CT is the radiologic examination of choice for pancreas. Used to identify tumors or cysts. Oral and/or intravenous contrast medium may be ordered.	Inform patient of procedure. Patient must lie still during the procedure. If IV contrast is used, check for iodine allergy.

Laboratory Studies

Laboratory studies used to diagnose endocrine problems may include direct measurement of the hormone level, or they may involve an indirect indication of gland function by evaluating blood or urine components affected by the hormone (e.g., electrolytes).

Hormones with fairly constant basal levels (e.g., T_4) require only a single measurement. Notation of sample time on the laboratory slip and sample is important for hormones with circadian or sleep-related secretion (e.g., cortisol). Evaluation of other hormones may require multiple blood sampling such as in suppression (e.g., dexamethasone) and stimulation (e.g., glucose tolerance) tests. In these situations, it is often necessary to obtain intravenous access to administer medications and fluids and to draw multiple blood samples.

Nursing interventions common to all patients requiring venipuncture for blood sampling include explaining the procedure to the patient, use of sterile technique, and applying pressure to the venipuncture site to minimize development of a hematoma. Many tests of endocrine function require the patient to fast and require the elimination of as many environmental stimuli as possible.[16] Normal values and collection procedures vary among laboratories. It is therefore important to refer to institutional policy and procedure for collection and handling of the various laboratory specimens, as well as established normal values for test results.

Pituitary Studies. Disorders associated with the pituitary gland can manifest in a wide variety of ways because of the number of hormones produced. There are many diagnostic studies that evaluate these hormones either directly or indirectly. The studies used to assess function of the anterior pituitary hormones relate to growth hormone, prolactin, follicle-stimulating hormone, luteinizing hormone, thyroid-stimulating hormone (TSH), and adrenocorticotropic hormone.

Thyroid Studies. There are a number of tests available to evaluate thyroid function. The most sensitive and accurate laboratory test is measurement of TSH; thus it is often recommended as a first diagnostic test for evaluation of thyroid function.[9] Common additional tests ordered in the presence of abnormal

TSH include total serum thyroxine (T_4), free T_4, and total serum triiodothyronine (T_3). Free T_4 is the unbound thyroxine and is a more accurate reflection of thyroid function than total T_4. Less common tests that help in the differentiation of various types of thyroid disease include T_3, free T_3 resin uptake, thyroid autoantibodies, thyroid scanning, ultrasound, and biopsy. These tests are done to help differentiate various types of thyroid disorders.

Parathyroid Studies. The only hormone secreted by the parathyroid glands is parathyroid hormone (PTH). Because the function of PTH is to regulate serum calcium and phosphate levels, abnormalities in PTH secretion are reflected in the calcium and phosphate levels.[16] For this reason, diagnostic tests for the parathyroid gland typically include PTH, serum calcium, and serum phosphate.

Adrenal Studies. Diagnostic tests associated with the adrenal glands focus on the three types of hormones secreted: glucocorticoids, mineralocorticoids, and androgens. These hormone levels can be measured both in blood plasma and in urine. If urine studies are done, these will usually be done as 24-hour urine collection. The major advantage of a 24-hour urine sample is that the short-term fluctuations in hormone levels seen in plasma samples are eliminated.[17]

Pancreatic Studies. The tests found in Table 46-7 are geared toward evaluating the metabolism of glucose. The best way to diagnose diabetes mellitus is the oral glucose tolerance test. However, other tests listed are useful in management of diabetes. (Diagnostic studies for diabetes are discussed in Chapter 47.)

Radiologic Studies

A variety of radiologic studies are done to evaluate the endocrine system. Basic x-ray, CT, MRI, and radiologic isotope tests are examples of procedures commonly done. These studies are helpful in identifying the size of the gland or the presence of lesions or tumor on the gland, and in some cases the function of the gland. Nursing interventions common for patients undergoing radiologic testing include explaining the procedure to the patient. Some procedures may involve injection of a contrast medium; therefore the nurse must check for allergies.

REVIEW QUESTIONS

The number of the question corresponds to the same-numbered objective at the beginning of the chapter.

1. A characteristic common to all hormones is that they
   a. circulate in the blood bound to plasma proteins.
   b. influence cellular activity of specific target tissues.
   c. accelerate the metabolic processes of all body cells.
   d. enter cells to alter the cell's metabolism or gene expression.

2. A patient is receiving radiation therapy for cancer of the kidney. The nurse monitors the patient for signs and symptoms of damage to the
   a. pancreas.
   b. thyroid gland.
   c. adrenal glands.
   d. posterior pituitary gland.

3. A patient has a serum sodium level of 152 mEq/L (152 mmol/L). The normal hormonal response to this situation is
   a. release of ADH.
   b. release of renin.
   c. secretion of aldosterone.
   d. secretion of corticotropin-releasing hormone.

4. All cells in the body are believed to have intracellular receptors for
   a. insulin.
   b. glucagon.
   c. growth hormone.
   d. thyroid hormone.

5. When obtaining subjective data from a patient during assessment of the endocrine system, the nurse asks specifically about
   a. energy level.
   b. intake of vitamin C.
   c. employment history.
   d. frequency of sexual intercourse.

6. An appropriate technique to use during physical assessment of the thyroid gland is
   a. asking the patient to hyperextend the neck during palpation.
   b. percussing the neck for dullness to define the size of the thyroid.
   c. having the patient swallow water during inspection and palpation of the gland.
   d. using deep palpation to determine the extent of a visibly enlarged thyroid gland.

7. Endocrine disorders often go unrecognized in the older adult because
   a. symptoms are often attributed to aging.
   b. older adults rarely have identifiable symptoms.
   c. endocrine disorders are relatively rare in the older adult.
   d. older adults usually have subclinical endocrine disorders that minimize symptoms.

8. An abnormal finding by the nurse during an endocrine assessment would be
   a. blood pressure of 100/70.
   b. soft, formed stool every other day.
   c. excessive facial hair on a woman.
   d. 5 lb weight gain over last 6 months.

9. A patient has a total serum calcium level of 3 mg/dl (1.5 mEq/L). If this finding reflects hypoparathyroidism, the nurse would expect further diagnostic testing to reveal
   a. decreased serum PTH.
   b. increased serum ACTH.
   c. increased serum glucose.
   d. decreased serum cortisol levels.

REFERENCES

1. Molitch M: Neuroendocrinology. In Felig P, Frohman LA, editors: *Endocrinology and metabolism,* ed 4, New York, 2001, McGraw-Hill.
2. McCance KL, Huether SE: *Pathophysiology: the biologic basis for disease in children and adults,* ed 4, St Louis, 2002, Mosby.
3. Frohman LA, Felig P: The clinical manifestations of endocrine disease. In Felig P, Frohman LA, editors: *Endocrinology and metabolism,* ed 4, New York, 2001, McGraw-Hill.
4. Rasenick MM, Jaffe RC: Molecular mechanism of hormone action: biology of signal transduction. In Felig P, Frohman LA, editors: *Endocrinology and metabolism,* ed 4, New York, 2001, McGraw-Hill.
5. Herlihy B, Maebius NK: *The human body in health and illness,* Philadelphia, 2000, WB Saunders.
6. Becker KL, editor: *Principles and practice of endocrinology and metabolism,* ed 3, Philadelphia, 2001, Lippincott Williams & Wilkins.
7. Cooper PE: Physiology and pathophysiology of the endocrine brain and hypothalamus. In Becker KL, editor: *Principles and practice of endocrinology and metabolism,* ed 3, Philadelphia, 2001, Lippincott Williams & Wilkins.
8. Baumann G: Growth hormone and its disorders. In Becker KL, editor: *Principles and practice of endocrinology and metabolism,* ed 3, Philadelphia, 2001, Lippincott Williams & Wilkins.
9. Larson J, Anderson EH, Koslawy M: Thyroid disease: a review for primary care, *J Am Acad Nurse Pract* 12:226, 2000.
10. McCance KL, Huether SE: *Pathophysiology: the biologic basis for disease in children and adults,* ed 4, St Louis, 2002, Mosby.
11. Gruenewald DA: Endocrinology and aging. In Becker KL, editor: *Principles and practice of endocrinology and metabolism,* ed 3, Philadelphia, 2001, Lippincott Williams & Wilkins.
12. Fletcher KR: Physical and laboratory assessment. In Stone JT, Wyman JF, Salisbury SA, editors: *Clinical gerontological nursing,* ed 2, Philadelphia, 1999, WB Saunders.
13. Dellasega C, Yonushonis ME, Johnson AD: The aging endocrine system. In Stanley M, Beare PG: *Gerontological nursing,* ed 2, Philadelphia, 1999, FA Davis.
14. Kessenich CR, Cichon MJ: Hormonal decline in elderly men and male menopause, *Geriatr Nurs* 22:24, 2001.
15. Wilson SF, Giddens JF: *Health assessment for nursing practice,* ed 2, St Louis, 2001, Mosby.
16. Pagana KD, Pagana TJ: *Diagnostic and laboratory test reference,* ed 5, St Louis, 2001, Mosby.
17. Corbett JG: *Laboratory tests and diagnostic procedures with nursing diagnoses,* ed 5, Upper Saddle River, NJ, 2000, Prentice-Hall.

RESOURCES

Resources for this chapter are listed in Chapter 47 on page 1302 and Chapter 48 on page 1338.

CHAPTER 47

NURSING MANAGEMENT
Diabetes Mellitus

Susan Semb

LEARNING OBJECTIVES

1. Describe the pathophysiology and clinical manifestations of diabetes mellitus.
2. Describe the differences between type 1 and type 2 diabetes mellitus.
3. Describe the collaborative care of the patient with diabetes mellitus.
4. Describe the role of nutrition and exercise in the management of diabetes mellitus.
5. Describe the nursing management of a patient with newly diagnosed diabetes mellitus.
6. Describe the nursing management of the patient with diabetes mellitus in the ambulatory and home care settings.
7. Identify the pathophysiology and clinical manifestations of acute and chronic complications of diabetes mellitus.
8. Explain the collaborative care and nursing management of the patient with acute and chronic complications of diabetes mellitus.

KEY TERMS

angiopathy, p. 1296
diabetes mellitus, p. 1268
diabetic ketoacidosis, p. 1271
diabetic nephropathy, p. 1297
diabetic neuropathy, p. 1298
diabetic retinopathy, p. 1297
hyperosmolar hyperglycemic nonketotic syndrome, p. 1293
hypoglycemic unawareness, p. 1295
impaired fasting glucose, p. 1272
impaired glucose tolerance, p. 1271

insulin pump, p. 1276
insulin resistance, p. 1271
insulin resistance syndrome, p. 1271
intensive insulin therapy, p. 1277
lipodystrophy, p. 1278
prediabetes, p. 1271
self-monitoring of blood glucose, p. 1283
Somogyi effect, p. 1278

Diabetes Mellitus

Diabetes mellitus is a multisystem disease related to abnormal insulin production, impaired insulin utilization, or both. Diabetes mellitus is a serious health problem throughout the world. In the United States an estimated 17 million people, or 6.2% of the population, have diabetes mellitus. More than 2 million Canadians have diabetes. About one third of the people with diabetes mellitus are not diagnosed, and these individuals are unaware that they have the disease. Diabetes mellitus is the fifth leading cause of death in the United States, with 210,000 deaths annually. Nearly 20% of people over age 65 years have diabetes. The incidence of diabetes is expected to increase 165% in the next 50 years.[1]

Diabetes is the leading cause of heart disease, stroke, adult blindness, and nontraumatic lower limb amputations. People with diabetes mellitus have at least a twofold risk for the devel-

opment of coronary artery disease, and more than 65% have hypertension. The staggering annual cost due to medical expenditures attributable to diabetes is estimated at $98 billion. Hospitalization costs account for the greatest proportion of medical costs.[1] These dollar amounts do not reflect the impact that this disease has on the quality of the lives of the affected people and their families.

Etiology and Pathophysiology

Current theories link the causes of diabetes, singly or in combination, to genetic, autoimmune, viral, and environmental factors (e.g., obesity, stress). Regardless of its cause, diabetes is primarily a disorder of glucose metabolism related to absent or insufficient insulin supplies and/or poor utilization of the insulin that is available.

Although the American Diabetes Association (ADA) recognizes 11 different classifications of the disease, most of these types

CULTURAL & ETHNIC CONSIDERATIONS
Diabetes Mellitus

- The highest incidence of diabetes is among Native Americans, 15% of whom are treated for diabetes.
- Pima Indians in Arizona have the highest rate of diabetes in the world, with 50% of adults having diabetes.
- Complications of diabetes are more common in Native Americans and African Americans than in whites.
- Complications from diabetes are the major causes of death in most Native American populations.
- The rate of end-stage renal failure is six times higher among Native Americans than among other people with diabetes.
- Amputation rates among Native Americans are three to four times higher than in other populations with diabetes.
- The incidence of diabetes is higher among African Americans and Hispanics than whites, with 10% of Hispanics and 13% of African Americans having diabetes.
- Type 2 diabetes tends to affect a younger-age population in nonwhites than in whites.

Reviewed by Elizabeth Alden, RNC, BSN, CDE, Clinical Diabetic Educator, Diabetes Disease Management Team, University of New Mexico Hospital, Albuquerque, N.M.; and M. Susan Grinslade, RN, PhD(c), Assistant Professor, School of Nursing, University of Texas Health Science Center, San Antonio, Tex.

TABLE 47-1	Characteristics of Type 1 and Type 2 Diabetes Mellitus	
FACTOR	**TYPE 1 DIABETES MELLITUS**	**TYPE 2 DIABETES MELLITUS**
Age at onset	More common in young person but can occur at any age	Usually age 35 yr or older but can occur at any age Incidence is increasing in children
Type of onset	Signs and symptoms abrupt, but disease process may be present for several years	Insidious
Prevalence	Accounts for 5%-10% of all types of diabetes	Accounts for 90% of all types of diabetes
Environmental factors	Virus, toxins	Obesity, lack of exercise
Islet cell antibodies	Often present at onset	Absent
Endogenous insulin	Minimal or absent	Possibly excessive; adequate but delayed secretion or reduced utilization
Nutritional status	Thin, catabolic state	Obese or possibly normal
Symptoms	Thirst, polyuria, polyphagia, fatigue	Frequently none or mild
Ketosis	Prone at onset or during insulin deficiency	Resistant except during infection or stress
Nutritional therapy	Essential	Essential, possibly sufficient for glycemic control
Insulin	Required for all	Required for some
Oral hypoglycemic agents	Not beneficial	Usually beneficial
Vascular and neurologic complications	Frequent	Frequent

are rarely encountered in routine nursing practice (Table 47-1).[2] The two most common types of diabetes are classified as type 1 or type 2 diabetes mellitus. Gestational diabetes and secondary diabetes are other classifications of diabetes commonly seen in clinical practice (discussed later in this chapter).

Normal Insulin Metabolism. Insulin is a hormone produced by the β cells in the islets of Langerhans of the pancreas. Under normal conditions, insulin is continuously released into the bloodstream in small pulsatile increments (a basal rate), with increased release (bolus) when food is ingested (Fig. 47-1). The activity of released insulin lowers blood glucose and facilitates a stable, normal glucose range of approximately 70 to 120 mg/dl (3.9 to 6.66 mmol/L). The average amount of insulin secreted daily by an adult is approximately 40 to 50 U, or 0.6 U/kg of body weight.

Other hormones (glucagon, epinephrine, growth hormone, and cortisol) work to oppose the effects of insulin and are often referred to as *counterregulatory hormones*. These hormones work to increase blood glucose levels by stimulating glucose production and output by the liver and by decreasing the movement of glucose into the cells. Insulin and these counterregulatory hormones provide a sustained but regulated release of glucose for energy during food intake and periods of fasting and usually maintain blood glucose levels within the normal range. An abnormal production of any or all of these hormones may be present in diabetes.

Insulin is released from the pancreatic β cells as its precursor, proinsulin, and is then routed through the liver. Proinsulin is composed of two polypeptide chains, chain A and chain B, which are linked by the C-peptide chain. Insulin is formed when enzymes cleave C off, leaving the A and B chains. The presence of C peptide in serum and urine is a useful indicator of β cell function.

Insulin promotes glucose transport from the bloodstream across the cell membrane to the cytoplasm of the cell. The rise in plasma insulin after a meal stimulates storage of glucose as glycogen in liver and muscle, inhibits gluconeogenesis, enhances

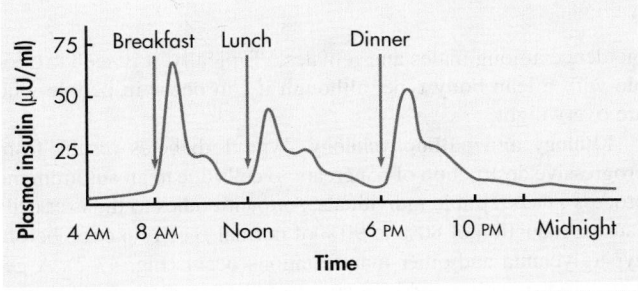

FIG. 47-1 Normal endogenous insulin secretion. In the first hour or two after meals, insulin concentrations rise rapidly in blood and peak at about 1 hour. After meals, insulin concentrations promptly decline toward preprandial values as carbohydrate absorption from the gastrointestinal tract declines. After carbohydrate absorption from the gastrointestinal tract is complete and during the night, insulin concentrations are low and fairly constant, with a slight increase at dawn.

fat deposition in adipose tissue, and increases protein synthesis. The fall in insulin level during normal overnight fasting facilitates the release of stored glucose from the liver, protein from muscle, and fat from adipose tissue. For this reason insulin is known as the *anabolic* or storage hormone.

Skeletal muscle and adipose tissue have specific receptors for insulin and are considered insulin-dependent tissues. Other tissues (e.g., brain, liver, blood cells) do not directly depend on insulin for glucose transport but require an adequate glucose supply for normal function. Although liver cells are not considered insulin-dependent tissue, insulin receptor sites on the liver facilitate the hepatic uptake of glucose and its conversion to glycogen.

Type 1 Diabetes Mellitus. Formerly known as "juvenile onset" or "insulin dependent" diabetes, *type 1 diabetes mellitus* most often occurs in people who are under 30 years of age, with a peak onset between ages 11 and 13. The rate of type 1 diabetes is 1.5 to 2 times higher in whites than nonwhites, with a similar

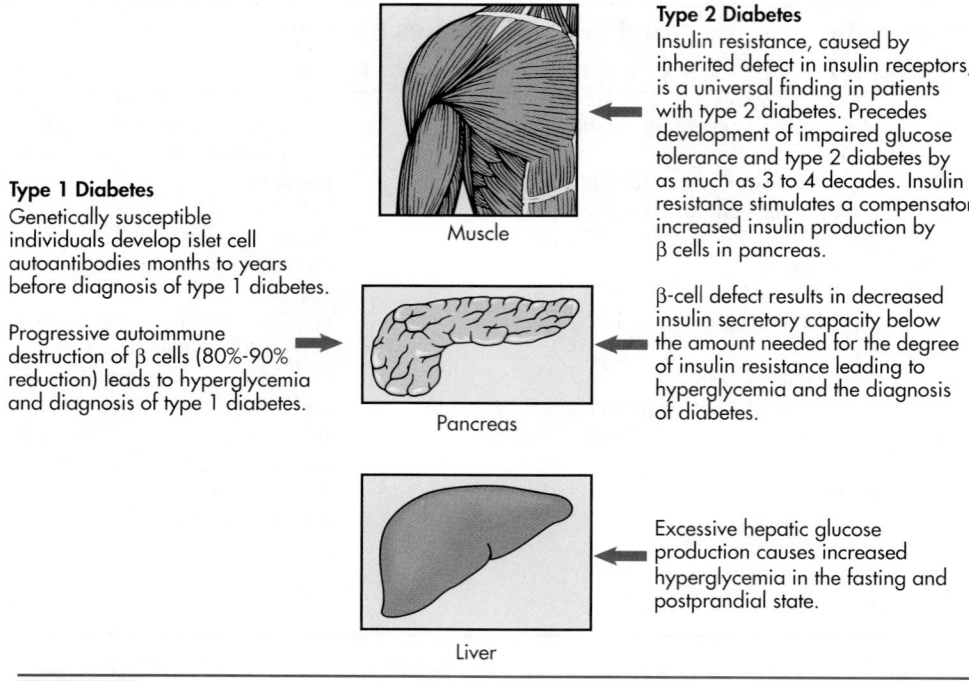

Type 1 Diabetes
Genetically susceptible individuals develop islet cell autoantibodies months to years before diagnosis of type 1 diabetes.

Progressive autoimmune destruction of β cells (80%-90% reduction) leads to hyperglycemia and diagnosis of type 1 diabetes.

Type 2 Diabetes
Insulin resistance, caused by inherited defect in insulin receptors, is a universal finding in patients with type 2 diabetes. Precedes development of impaired glucose tolerance and type 2 diabetes by as much as 3 to 4 decades. Insulin resistance stimulates a compensatory increased insulin production by β cells in pancreas.

β-cell defect results in decreased insulin secretory capacity below the amount needed for the degree of insulin resistance leading to hyperglycemia and the diagnosis of diabetes.

Excessive hepatic glucose production causes increased hyperglycemia in the fasting and postprandial state.

Muscle

Pancreas

Liver

FIG. 47-2   Altered mechanisms in type 1 and type 2 diabetes mellitus.

incidence among males and females.[3] Typically, it is seen in people with a lean body type, although it can occur in people who are overweight.

Etiology and pathophysiology. Type 1 diabetes results from progressive destruction of pancreatic β cells due to an autoimmune process in susceptible individuals. Autoantibodies to the islet cells cause a reduction of 80% to 90% of normal β cell function before hyperglycemia and other manifestations occur (Fig. 47-2). A genetic predisposition and exposure to a virus are factors that may contribute to the pathogenesis of type 1 diabetes.

Predisposition to type 1 diabetes is believed to be related to human leukocyte antigens (HLAs). (See Chapter 13 for a discussion of HLAs and disease associations). Theoretically, when an individual with certain HLA types is exposed to viral infections, the β cells of the pancreas are destroyed, either directly or through an autoimmune process. The HLA types associated with an increased risk for type 1 diabetes include HLA-DR3 and HLA-DR4 (see Genetics in Clinical Practice box).

Onset of disease. Type 1 diabetes is associated with a long preclinical period. The islet cell autoantibodies responsible for β cell destruction are present for months to years before the onset of symptoms. Manifestations of type 1 diabetes develop when the person's pancreas can no longer produce insulin. Once this occurs, the onset of symptoms is usually rapid, and the patient comes to the emergency department with impending or actual ketoacidosis. The patient usually has a history of recent and sudden

𝒢ENETICS in CLINICAL PRACTICE
Types 1 and 2 Diabetes Mellitus

	TYPE 1 DIABETES MELLITUS	TYPE 2 DIABETES MELLITUS
Genetic basis	Associations between specific human leukocyte antigens (HLA-DR3, HLA-DR4)	Polygenic
	Possible mutation in insulin gene on chromosome 11	Major genes have not yet been identified
		Maturity-onset diabetes of the young (MODY)
		MODY1—linked to chromosome 20
		MODY2—linked to chromosome 7
		MODY3—linked to chromosome 12
Incidence	Accounts for about 5%-10% of cases in the United States	Accounts for about 90% of cases in the United States
Risk to offspring	Risk to offspring of diabetic mothers is only 1%-3%	Risk to first-degree relatives is 10%-15%
	Risk to offspring of diabetic fathers is 4%-6%	Identical twin concordance often exceeds 90%
	Identical twin concordance is 30%-50%	
Genetic testing	Currently under investigation	Currently under investigation
Clinical implications	Most individuals with type 1 diabetes do not have a first-degree relative with disorder	Most important risk factors include family history and obesity

weight loss, as well as the classic symptoms of *polydipsia* (excessive thirst), *polyuria* (frequent urination), and *polyphagia* (excessive hunger).

The individual with type 1 diabetes requires a supply of insulin from an outside source *(exogenous insulin),* such as an injection, in order to sustain life. Without insulin, the patient will develop **diabetic ketoacidosis** (DKA), a life-threatening condition resulting in metabolic acidosis. Newly diagnosed patients with type 1 diabetes often experience a remission, or "honeymoon period," soon after treatment is initiated. During this time, the patient requires very little injected insulin because β cell mass remains sufficient for glucose control as the progressive destruction continues to occur. Eventually, as more β cells are destroyed, blood glucose levels increase, more insulin is needed, and the honeymoon period ends. The honeymoon period usually lasts 3 to 12 months, after which the person will require insulin on a permanent basis.

Type 2 Diabetes Mellitus. *Type 2 diabetes mellitus* is, by far, the most prevalent type of diabetes, accounting for over 90% of patients with diabetes. Type 2 diabetes usually occurs in people over 40 years of age, and 80% to 90% of patients are overweight at the time of diagnosis. It has a tendency to run in families and probably has a genetic basis (see Genetics in Clinical Practice box). Prevalence of this type of diabetes is greater in some ethnic populations. The highest rates occur among Native Americans, who are about three times as likely to have type 2 diabetes as non-Hispanic whites of similar age. Hispanics also have higher rates, being about twice as likely to have diabetes as age-matched white counterparts. African Americans are about 1.7 times as likely to have diabetes as non-Hispanic whites of similar age.[1]

Prevalence of type 2 diabetes increases with age, with about half of the people diagnosed being older than 55. In the past, type 2 diabetes was known as "adult onset" diabetes. This term is no longer considered appropriate because the disease is now being seen in a rapidly growing number of children and adolescents.

Etiology and pathophysiology. In type 2 diabetes, the pancreas usually continues to produce some *endogenous* (self-made) insulin. However, the insulin that is produced is either insufficient for the needs of the body and/or is poorly utilized by the tissues. In contrast, there is a virtual absence of endogenous insulin in type 1 diabetes. The presence of endogenous insulin is the major pathophysiologic distinction between type 1 and type 2 diabetes.

Genetic mutations that lead to insulin resistance and a higher risk for obesity have been found in many people with type 2 diabetes. It is likely that multiple genes are involved in this complex, multifactorial disorder (see Genetics in Clinical Practice box).

Three major metabolic abnormalities have a role in the development of type 2 diabetes. The first factor is **insulin resistance,** which is a condition in which body tissues do not respond to the action of insulin. This is due to insulin receptors that are either unresponsive to the action of insulin and/or insufficient in number. Most insulin receptors are located on skeletal muscle, fat, and liver cells. When insulin is not properly used, the entry of glucose into the cell is impeded, resulting in hyperglycemia. In the early stages of insulin resistance, the pancreas responds to high blood glucose by producing greater amounts of insulin (if β cell function is normal). This creates a temporary state of hyperinsulinemia that coexists with the hyperglycemia.

A second factor in the development of type 2 diabetes is a marked decrease in the ability of the pancreas to produce insulin, as the β cells become fatigued from the compensatory overproduction of insulin. **Impaired glucose tolerance** (IGT), often called **prediabetes,** usually occurs when the alteration in β cell function is mild. IGT is a condition in which blood glucose levels are higher than normal but not high enough for a diagnosis of diabetes. Most people with IGT are at increased risk for developing type 2 diabetes and will develop it within 10 years. It is estimated that about 16 million Americans have IGT.

A third factor is inappropriate glucose production by the liver. Instead of properly regulating the release of glucose in response to blood levels, the liver does so in a haphazard way that does not correspond to the body's needs at the time. However, this is not considered a primary factor in the development of type 2 diabetes. Figure 47-2 depicts the altered mechanisms in type 1 and type 2 diabetes.

Insulin resistance syndrome (also known as *syndrome X,* metabolic syndrome, and cardiovascular dysmetabolic syndrome) is a cluster of abnormalities that act synergistically to greatly increase the risk for cardiovascular disease. Insulin resistance syndrome is characterized by elevated insulin levels, high levels of triglycerides, decreased levels of high-density lipoproteins (HDLs), increased levels of low-density lipoproteins (LDLs), and hypertension. Risk factors for insulin resistance syndrome include central obesity, sedentary lifestyle, polycystic ovary syndrome, urbanization/Westernization, ethnicity (Native Americans, Hispanics, and African Americans), family history, gestational diabetes, and increased age. Overweight people with IGT can prevent or delay the onset of diabetes through a program of weight loss and regular physical activity.[4]

Onset of disease. Disease onset in type 2 diabetes is usually gradual. The person may go for many years with undetected hyperglycemia that might produce few, if any, symptoms. If the patient with type 2 diabetes has marked hyperglycemia (e.g., 500 to 1000 mg/dl [27.6 to 55.1 mmol/L]), a sufficient endogenous insulin supply may prevent DKA from occurring. However, osmotic fluid and electrolyte loss related to hyperglycemia may become severe and lead to hyperosmolar coma. (Complications of diabetes are discussed later in this chapter.)

Gestational Diabetes. *Gestational diabetes* develops during pregnancy and occurs in about 4% of pregnancies in the United States. It is detected at 24 to 28 weeks of gestation, usually following an oral glucose tolerance test (OGTT). Women with gestational diabetes have a higher risk for cesarean delivery, perinatal death, and neonatal complications. Although most women with gestational diabetes will have normal glucose levels within 6 weeks postpartum, their risk for developing type 2 diabetes in 5 to 10 years is increased. Nutritional therapy is considered to be the first-line therapy. If nutritional therapy alone does not achieve desirable fasting blood glucose levels, insulin therapy is usually indicated. Gestational diabetes and management of the pregnant patient with diabetes is a specialized area not covered in detail in this chapter. The reader is advised to consult an obstetric text for information about this area.

Secondary Diabetes. Diabetes occurs in some people because of another medical condition or due to the treatment of a medical condition that causes abnormal blood glucose levels. Conditions that may cause secondary diabetes include Cushing syndrome, hyperthyroidism, and the use of parenteral nutrition.

Commonly used medications that can induce diabetes in some people include corticosteroids (prednisone), phenytoin (Dilantin), and atypical antipsychotics (e.g., clozapine [clozapril]). Secondary diabetes usually resolves when the underlying condition is treated. (Drugs that can alter blood glucose levels are listed in Table 47-8 later in this chapter.)

Clinical Manifestations

Type 1 Diabetes Mellitus. Because the onset of type 1 diabetes is rapid, the initial manifestations are usually acute. The classic symptoms are *polyuria* (frequent urination), *polydipsia* (excessive thirst), and *polyphagia* (excessive hunger). The osmotic effect of glucose produces the manifestations of polydipsia and polyuria. Polyphagia is a consequence of cellular malnourishment when insulin deficiency prevents utilization of glucose for energy. Weight loss may occur as the body cannot get glucose and turns to other energy sources, such as fat and protein. Weakness and fatigue may also be experienced, as body cells lack needed energy from glucose. Ketoacidosis, a complication associated with untreated type 1 diabetes, is associated with additional clinical manifestations that are discussed later in this chapter.

Type 2 Diabetes Mellitus. The clinical manifestations of type 2 diabetes are often nonspecific, although it is possible that an individual with type 2 diabetes will experience some of the classic symptoms associated with type 1. Some of the more common manifestations associated with type 2 diabetes include fatigue, recurrent infections, prolonged wound healing, and visual changes. Unfortunately the clinical manifestations appear so gradually that before the person knows it, he or she may have complications.

Complications

Complications of diabetes are discussed in detail later in this chapter.

Diagnostic Studies

Regardless of the type, the diagnosis of diabetes mellitus can be made through one of three methods. Whichever method is used, diagnosis of diabetes must be confirmed on a subsequent day by any of the three methods.[2] These methods and their criteria for diagnosis are as follows:

- Fasting plasma glucose level exceeding 126 mg/dl (7.0 mmol/L).
- Random, or casual, plasma glucose measurement exceeding 200 mg/dl (11.1 mmol/L), plus manifestations of diabetes, such as polyuria, polydipsia, and unexplained weight loss. *Casual* is defined as any time of day without regard to the time of the last meal.
- Two-hour OGTT level exceeding 200 mg/dl (11.1 mmol/L), using a glucose load of 75 g.

The fasting plasma glucose (FPG) test, confirmed by repeat testing on another day, is the preferred method of diagnosis. When overt symptoms of hyperglycemia (polyuria, polydipsia, and polyphagia) coexist with fasting plasma glucose levels of 126 mg/dl (7.0 mmol/L) or greater, further testing using the oral glucose tolerance test (OGTT) may not be necessary to make a diagnosis.[2]

When OGTT is used, the accuracy of test results depends on adequate patient preparation and attention to the many factors that may influence the outcome of such tests. For example, factors that can cause falsely elevated values include recent severe restrictions of dietary carbohydrate, acute illness, medications (e.g., contraceptives, glucocorticosteroids), and restricted activity such as bed rest. A patient with impaired gastrointestinal absorption may also have false-negative test results.

Impaired glucose tolerance (IGT) and impaired fasting glucose (IFG) each represent an intermediate stage between normal glucose homeostasis and diabetes. When the fasting blood glucose level is greater than 110 mg/dl (6.1 mmol/L) but less than 126 mg/dl (7.0 mmol/L), the individual is considered to have **impaired fasting glucose.** *Impaired glucose tolerance* is classified as a 2-hour plasma glucose level higher than normal but lower than that considered diagnostic for diabetes mellitus (between 140 mg/dl [7.8 mmol/L] and 200 mg/dl [11.1 mmol/L]).[2] IGT and IFG are risk factors for diabetes, as well as cardiovascular disease.

Measurement of glycosylated hemoglobin, also known as the *hemoglobin A_{1c}* (A1C) test, is useful in determining glycemic levels over time. The test works by showing the amount of glucose that has been attached to hemoglobin molecules over their life span. When blood glucose is elevated over time, the amount of glucose attached to the hemoglobin molecule increases and remains attached to the red blood cell (RBC) for the life of the cell (approximately 120 days). Therefore a glycosylated hemoglobin test indicates the overall glucose control for the previous 90 to 120 days. All patients with diabetes should have regular assessments of A1C done. Major studies have demonstrated that people with diabetes who can maintain near-normal A1C levels over time have a greatly reduced risk for the development of retinopathy, nephropathy, and neuropathy. For people with diabetes, the ideal A1C goal is 7.0% or less. Diseases affecting RBCs (e.g., sickle cell anemia) can affect the A1C results and should be taken into consideration in the interpretation of this test result.

Collaborative Care

The goals of diabetes management are to reduce symptoms, promote well-being, prevent acute complications of hyperglycemia, and delay the onset and progression of long-term complications. These goals are most likely to be met when the patient is able to maintain blood glucose levels as near to normal as possible. Patient teaching, which enables the patient to become the most active participant in his or her own care, is essential for a successful treatment plan. Nutritional therapy, drug therapy, exercise, and self-monitoring of blood glucose are the tools used in the management of diabetes (Table 47-2). The two types of glucose-lowering agents (GLAs) used in the treatment of diabetes are insulin and oral agents (OAs). All individuals with type 1 diabetes require insulin. For some people with type 2 diabetes, a regimen of proper nutrition, regular physical activity, and maintenance of desirable body weight will be sufficient to attain an optimal level of blood glucose control. For the majority, however, drug therapy will be necessary.

Drug Therapy: Insulin

Exogenous (injected) insulin is needed when a patient has inadequate insulin to meet specific metabolic needs and the combination of nutritional therapy, exercise, and OAs cannot maintain a satisfactory blood glucose level. Exogenous insulin is required for the management of type 1 diabetes. Exogenous insulin may be prescribed for the patient with type 2 diabetes who

TABLE 47-2	Collaborative Care
	Diabetes Mellitus

Diagnostic

History and physical examination

Blood tests, including fasting blood glucose, postprandial blood glucose, glycosylated hemoglobin (A1C), lipid profile, blood urea nitrogen and serum creatinine, electrolytes

Urine for complete urinalysis, microalbuminuria, glucose and acetone (if indicated)

Funduscopic examination—dilated eye examination

Neurologic examination, including monofilament test for sensation to lower extremities

ECG

Blood pressure

Monitoring of weight

Doppler scan (if indicated)

Dental examination

Foot (podiatric) examination

Collaborative Therapy

Nutritional therapy (see Table 47-9)

Exercise therapy (see Tables 47-10 and 47-11)

Drug therapy

- Insulin (see Fig. 47-3 and Tables 47-3 and 47-4)
- Oral agents (see Table 47-7)
- Enteric-coated aspirin (325 mg)
- Angiotension-converting enzyme (ACE) inhibitors (see Table 32-8)
- Antilipidemic drugs (if indicated) (see Chapter 33, Table 33-6)

Self-monitoring of blood glucose (SMBG)

Patient and family teaching and follow-up programs

ECG, Electrocardiogram.

cannot control blood glucose by other means, especially during periods of severe stress, such as illness or surgery.[5]

Types of Insulin. In the past, purified preparations of insulin made from beef and pork pancreas were used. However, human insulin is now the most widely used type of insulin. Human insulin is not directly harvested from human organs, but is derived from common bacteria (e.g., *Escherichia coli*) or yeast cells using recombinant DNA technology (see Chapter 13, Fig. 13-15). Although some patients who have had diabetes for many years may still be using animal insulin, newly diagnosed patients using insulin use the synthetically derived human insulin. The major advantage of human insulin is cost-effectiveness and decreased likelihood of causing an allergic reaction to animal insulin or additives to regular insulin.

Insulins differ in regard to onset, peak action, and duration (Fig. 47-3). The specific properties of each type of insulin are matched with the patient's diet and activity. Different combinations of these insulins can be used to tailor treatment to the patient's specific pattern of blood glucose levels, lifestyle, eating, and activity patterns. Different types of insulin are listed in Table 47-3. All insulin preparations start with regular insulin as a base. By adding zinc, acetate buffers, and protamine to insulin in various ways, the onset of activity, peak, and duration times can be manipulated. Zinc is added to make lente insulin, and zinc and protamine are added to make NPH. These additives can cause an allergic reaction at the injection site.

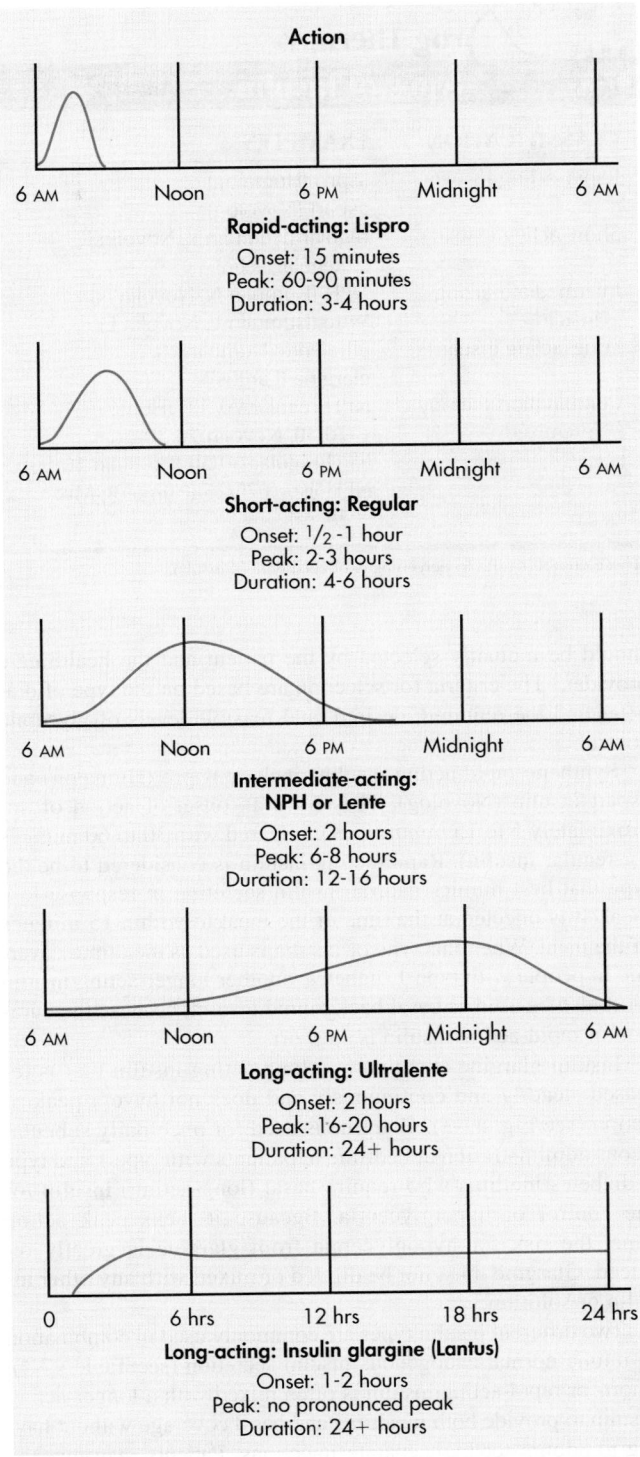

Action

Rapid-acting: Lispro
Onset: 15 minutes
Peak: 60-90 minutes
Duration: 3-4 hours

Short-acting: Regular
Onset: ½-1 hour
Peak: 2-3 hours
Duration: 4-6 hours

Intermediate-acting: NPH or Lente
Onset: 2 hours
Peak: 6-8 hours
Duration: 12-16 hours

Long-acting: Ultralente
Onset: 2 hours
Peak: 16-20 hours
Duration: 24+ hours

Long-acting: Insulin glargine (Lantus)
Onset: 1-2 hours
Peak: no pronounced peak
Duration: 24+ hours

FIG. 47-3 Commercially available insulin preparations showing onset, peak, and duration of action.

The timing of insulin administration in relation to meals is important. Regular insulin should be taken 30 to 45 minutes before meals to ensure the onset of action in conjunction with meal absorption. Examples of insulin combination regimens, onset, peak, and descriptions of the advantages and disadvantages of each regimen are presented in Table 47-4. Ideally, regimens

TABLE 47-3 Drug Therapy — Types of Insulin

CLASSIFICATION	EXAMPLES
Rapid-acting insulin	lispro (Humalog)
	aspart (Novolog)
Short-acting insulin	regular (Humulin R, Novolin R, Regular Iletin)
Intermediate-acting insulin	NPH (Humulin N, Novolin N)
	lente (Humulin L, Novolin L)
Long-acting insulin	ultralente (Humulin U)
	glargine (Lantus)
Combination therapy (premixed)	NPH/regular 70/30* (Humulin 70/30, Novolin 70/30)
	NPH/regular 50/50 (Humulin 50/50)
	NPH/lispro 75/25 (Humalog Mix 75/25)

*These numbers refer to percentages of each type of insulin.

should be mutually selected by the patient and the health care provider.[6] The criteria for selection are based on the type of diabetes and the required, desired, and feasible levels of glycemic control.

Synthetic rapid-acting insulins include lispro (Humalog) and aspart insulin (Novolog). They have an onset of action of approximately 5 to 15 minutes (as compared with 30 to 60 minutes for regular insulin). Rapid-acting insulin is considered to be the type that best mimics natural insulin secretion in response to a meal. It is injected at the time of the meal to within 15 minutes of the meal. When this type of insulin is used as mealtime coverage in people with type 1 diabetes, another longer-acting insulin must also be used as basal background insulin, because the duration of rapid-acting insulin is so short.

Insulin glargine (Lantus) is a long-acting insulin that is released steadily and continuously and does not have a peak of action (see Fig. 47-3). Glargine is used for once-daily subcutaneous administration at bedtime in patients with type 1 and type 2 diabetes mellitus who require basal (long-acting) insulin for the control of hyperglycemia. Because it lacks peak action time, the risk for hypoglycemia from glargine is greatly reduced. Glargine must not be diluted or mixed with any other insulin or solution.[7]

Two different insulin types are commonly used in combination to mimic normal endogenous insulin secretion (see Table 47-4). Short- or rapid-acting insulin is often mixed with a longer-acting insulin to provide both mealtime and basal coverage without having to administer two separate injections. Patients may mix the two types of insulin themselves or may use a commercially premixed formula (see Table 47-3). These offer convenience to patients and are especially helpful to those who lack the visual, manual, or cognitive skills to mix insulin themselves. However, the convenience of these formulas sacrifices the potential for optimal blood glucose control, because there is less opportunity for flexible dosing based on need.

As a protein, insulin requires special storage considerations. Heat and freezing alter the insulin molecule. Insulin vials that the patient is currently using may be left at room temperature for up to 4 weeks unless the room temperature is higher than 86° F (30° C) or below freezing (less than 37° F [2° C]). Prolonged exposure to direct sunlight should be avoided. Extra insulin may be stored in the refrigerator. The same principles apply for a patient who is traveling. Insulin can be stored in a thermos or cooler to keep it cool (not frozen) if the patient is traveling in hot climates.

Prefilled syringes are stable for up to 30 days when stored in the refrigerator. This may be beneficial to patients who are sight impaired or who lack the manual dexterity to fill their own syringes at home. In these cases family members, friends, and caregivers may prefill syringes on a periodic basis. Syringes prefilled with a cloudy solution should be stored in a vertical position with the needle pointed up to avoid clumping of suspended insulin binders in the needle.[8] When stored properly, prefilled syringes with mixed insulins should maintain potency for 30 days. Likewise, commercially prepared mixtures may be prefilled and stored for later use. Some insulin combinations are not appropriate for prefilling and storage because the mixture can alter the onset, action, and/or peak times of either of the types. Pharmacy references should be consulted as needed when mixing and prefilling different types of insulin. Prefilled syringes should be gently rolled between the palms before injection to warm the refrigerated insulin and to resuspend the particles.

Administration of Insulin. Because insulin is inactivated by gastric juices, it cannot be taken orally. Injection is the only route of administration currently approved for self-administration. Routine administration of insulin is most commonly done by means of subcutaneous (SQ) injection, although intravenous (IV) administration of regular insulin can be done when immediate onset of action is desired.

Injection. The steps in administering an SQ insulin injection are outlined in Table 47-5. The technique should be taught to new insulin users and reviewed periodically with long-term users. It should never be assumed that because insulin is being used, the patient knows and practices the correct insulin injection technique. Inaccurate preparation is often caused by poor eyesight. Air bubbles in the syringe may not be seen, or the scale on the syringe may be read improperly.

The patient receiving mixed insulins (e.g., regular and an intermediate-acting insulin) needs to learn the proper technique for combining both in the same syringe if commercially prepared premixed insulins are not used (Fig. 47-4). Insulins should not be mixed if they differ in purity or species origin.

The speed with which peak serum concentrations are reached varies with the anatomic site for injection. The fastest absorption is from the abdomen, followed by the arm, thigh, and buttock. Appropriate sites for insulin injection are noted in Fig. 47-5, although the abdomen is the preferred site. The patient should be cautioned about injecting into a site that is to be exercised. For example, the patient should not inject insulin into the thigh and then go jogging. Exercise of the area containing the injection site together with the increased body heat generated by the exercise may increase the rate of absorption and speed the onset of insulin action.

Before purified human insulins were widely used, patients were advised to rotate anatomic injection sites to prevent *lipodystrophy,* a condition that produces lumps and dents in the skin from repeated injection in the same spot. The use of

Drug Therapy

TABLE 47-4 Insulin Regimens

REGIMEN	TYPE OF INSULIN USED	TIME ADMINISTERED AND EXPECTED TIME-ACTION CURVE*	ADVANTAGES	DISADVANTAGES
Single dose	Intermediate insulin (I)	7 AM (I), Noon, 6 PM, Midnight, 7 AM	One injection should cover noon and PM meal. Hypoglycemia during sleep is not a problem.	No fasting, breakfast, or nighttime coverage of hyperglycemia is available.
Split-mixed dose (70/30 premix)	Intermediate and regular or Humalog insulin (I + R or I + H)	7 AM (I + R)(I + H), Noon, 6 PM (I + R)(I + H), Midnight, 7 AM	Two injections provide coverage for 24 hr.	Two injections are required. Patient must adhere to a set meal pattern.
Split-mixed dose	Intermediate and regular or Humalog insulin (I + R or I + H)	7 AM (I + R)(I + H), Noon, 7 PM (R)(H), 9 PM (I), Midnight, 7 AM	Three injections provide coverage for 24 hr, particularly during early AM hours. Potential is reduced for 2-3 AM hypoglycemia.	Three injections are required.
Multiple dose	Intermediate and regular or Humalog insulin (I + R or I + H)	7 AM (R)(H), Noon (R)(H), 7 PM (R)(H), 9 PM (I), 7 AM	More flexibility is allowed at mealtimes and for amount of food intake.	Four injections are required. Premeal blood glucose checks, establishing and following individualized algorithm are necessary. Patients with type 1 will require basal insulin (I or LA) during the day.
Multiple dose† (split dose long-acting insulin [ultralente])	Regular or Humalog and long-acting insulin (R + LA or H + LA)	7 AM (H + LA)(R + LA), Noon (H)(R), 7 PM (H + LA)(R + LA), Midnight, 7 AM	Insulin delivery pattern more closely simulates normal endogenous insulin pattern. Some flexibility is allowed in food intake pattern. Regimen gives a basal insulin coverage and regular or Humalog insulin covers meal blood glucose excursions.	Required three or four injections and blood glucose check premeal and on retiring. Establishing and following individualized algorithm are necessary.

H, lispro (Humalog) or rapid-acting insulin (R) = _____; I, intermediate insulin = ----------; LA, long-acting insulin = – – – –; R, regular insulin = _____.
†Insulin delivery through a pump is similar to this regimen.

TABLE 47-5 *Patient & Family Teaching Guide*
Insulin Therapy

1. Wash hands thoroughly.
2. Roll intermediate or long-acting insulin bottle between palms of hands to mix insulin. *Note:* Always inspect insulin bottle before using it. Make sure that it is of proper type and concentration, expiration date has not passed, and top of bottle is in perfect condition.
3. Prepare insulin injection in same manner as for any injection.
4. Select proper injection site and inject following procedure for any SQ injection (see Fig. 47-5). In sites where SQ tissue is adequate, inject commercial insulin needles at 90-degree angle. For sites with minimal SQ tissue, pinch up skin and insert needle at 45-degree angle.
5. If blood appears in syringe after needle is inserted, select new site for injection. Aspiration of syringe is not necessary.
6. After injecting insulin, apply some pressure with dry cotton ball (or 2 × 2 gauze pad) at site when withdrawing needle.
7. Hold ball in place for a few seconds but do not massage.
8. Destroy and dispose of single-use syringe safely. *Note:* When instructing patient to self-inject insulin, use the following guidelines (if appropriate):
   - Aspiration does not need to be done before injection.
   - The injection site does not need to be cleansed with alcohol.

SQ, Subcutaneous.

1 Wash hands.
2 Gently rotate NPH insulin bottle.
3 Wipe off tops of insulin vials with alcohol sponge.
4 Draw back amount of air into the syringe that equals total dose.

5 Inject air equal to NPH dose into NPH vial. Remove syringe from vial.

6 Inject air equal to regular dose into regular vial.

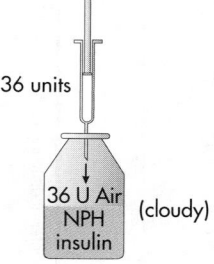

36 units

36 U Air NPH insulin (cloudy)

12 units

12 U Air Regular insulin (clear)

7 Invert regular insulin bottle and withdraw regular insulin dose.

8 Without adding more air to NPH vial, carefully withdraw NPH dose.

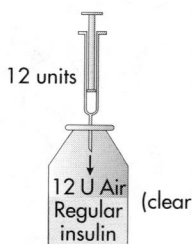

Regular insulin (clear)

Regular insulin   12 units

NPH insulin (cloudy)

NPH insulin
Regular insulin   36 units
48 units (total dose)

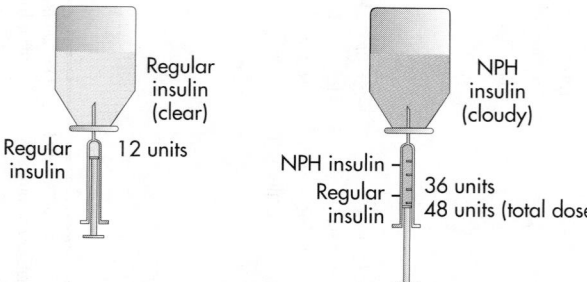

FIG. 47-4 Mixing insulins. This step-order process avoids the problem of contaminating regular insulin with intermediate-acting insulin.

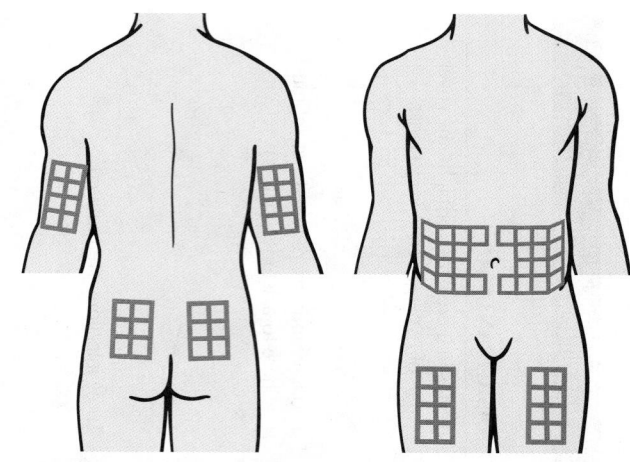

FIG. 47-5 Injection sites for insulin.

human insulin reduces the risk for lipodystrophy. Because of this, and because rotating sites causes variability in insulin absorption, rotation of injection sites to different anatomic sites is no longer the recommended practice. Instead, patients are advised to rotate the injection within one particular site, such as the abdomen. Sometimes it is helpful to think of the entire abdomen as a checkerboard, with each square representing an injection site as the patient rotates sites systematically across the board.

Most commercial insulin is available as U100, indicating that 1 ml contains 100 U of insulin. U100 insulin must be used with a U100-marked syringe. Disposable plastic insulin syringes are available in a variety of sizes, including 1, 0.5, and 0.3 ml. The 0.5 ml size may be used for doses of 50 U or less, and the 0.3 ml syringe can be used for doses of 30 U or less. Smaller syringes offer a number of advantages. The major benefit is increased accuracy and reliability when delivering smaller doses because wider line markings are easier to see. Patients should be cautioned to check dosage lines carefully when changing syringe types because some use a scale of 1 U increments and others use a 2 U increment.

Recapping should *only* be done by the person using the syringe. The nurse must never recap a needle that has been used by a patient. The use of an alcohol swab on the site before self-injection is no longer recommended. Routine hygiene such as washing with soap and rinsing with water is adequate. This applies primarily to patient self-injection technique. When injection occurs in a health care facility, policy may dictate site preparation with alcohol to prevent nosocomial infection.

An insulin pen is a compact portable device that serves the same function as a needle and syringe but is handier to use (Fig. 47-6, *A*). The pen usually comes preloaded with insulin. One of the advantages of insulin pens is that they are less "medical" looking. A new type of pen is the InDuo, which combines an insulin pen and a blood glucose monitor (Fig. 47-6, *B*).

Alternate delivery methods. Continuous subcutaneous insulin infusion can be administered using an **insulin pump,** a small battery-operated device that resembles a standard paging device in size and appearance (Fig. 47-7). Usually worn on the belt, the pump is connected via a small plastic tube to a catheter inserted into the subcutaneous tissue in the abdominal wall.

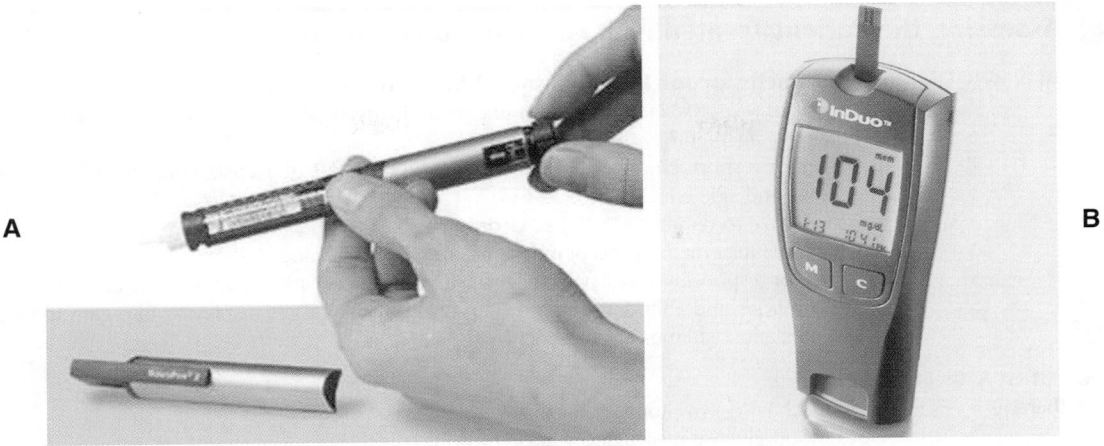

FIG. 47-6   **A,** NovoPen insulin pen. **B,** Blood glucose monitor by InDuo is used to measure blood glucose levels.

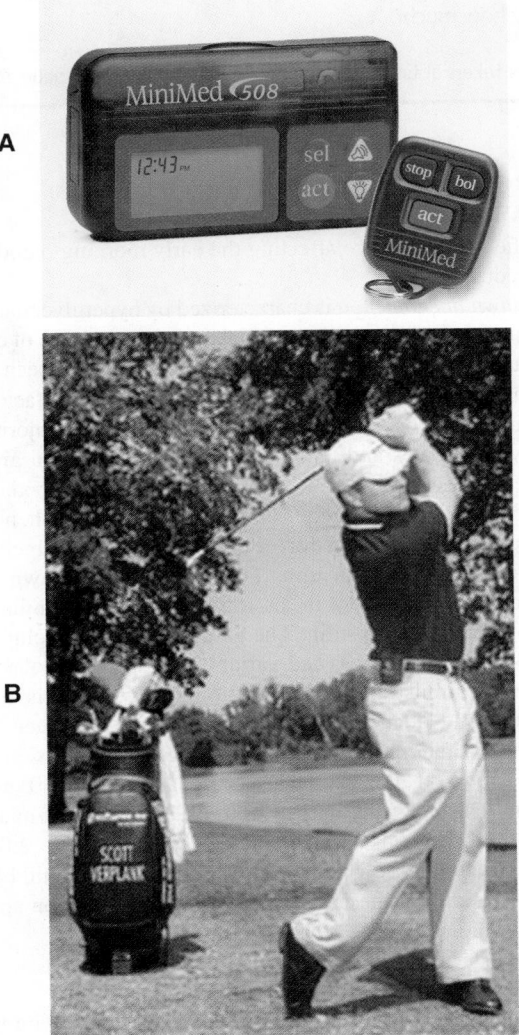

FIG. 47-7   **A,** MiniMed insulin pump. **B,** Professional golfer Scott Verplank wearing his MiniMed pump at the Ryder Cup 2002.

Every 2 to 3 days the insertion site is changed and the pump is refilled with insulin and reprogrammed. The device is programmed to deliver a continuous infusion of short-acting insulin 24 hours a day, known as the "basal rate." At mealtime, the user programs the pump to deliver a bolus infusion of insulin appropriate to the amount of carbohydrate ingested and to bring down high premeal blood glucose, if necessary. A major advantage of the insulin pump is the potential for tight glucose control.[9] This is possible because insulin delivery becomes very similar to the normal physiologic pattern. Pumps also offer the benefit of a more normal lifestyle, allowing users more flexibility with meal and activity patterns. The insertion site should be checked daily for redness and swelling.[10]

An alternative to the insulin pump is **intensive insulin therapy,** which consists of multiple daily insulin (MDI) injections together with frequent self-monitoring of blood glucose. The goal is to achieve a near-normal glucose level of 80 to 120 mg/dl (4.45 to 6.7 mmol/L) before meals. The Diabetes Control and Complications Trial (DCCT) demonstrated that people with type 1 diabetes who have tight glucose control through intensive management develop fewer and less severe complications.[11] Studies have shown comparable control outcomes in patients receiving intensive therapy and patients with an insulin pump. The disadvantages of MDI are that three or more injections are needed daily. In addition, intermediate- and long-acting insulins (NPH, lente, ultralente, glargine) must be used as the basal component.

Problems with Insulin Therapy. Hypoglycemia, allergic reactions, lipodystrophy, and Somogyi effect are the problems associated with insulin therapy. Hypoglycemia is discussed in detail later in this chapter. (Guidelines for assessing patients treated with insulin are presented in Table 47-6.)

Allergic reactions. Local inflammatory reactions to insulin may occur, such as itching, erythema, and burning around the injection site. Local reactions may be self-limiting within 1 to 3 months or may improve with a low dose of antihistamine. A true insulin allergy is a systemic response with urticaria and possibly anaphylactic shock generally resulting from the use of animal

TABLE 47-6	Assessing the Patient Treated with Glucose-Lowering Agents

For Patient with Newly Diagnosed Diabetes or for Reevaluation of Medication Regimen

Cognitive	Is patient or responsible other able to understand why insulin or OAs are being used as part of diabetes management?
	Is patient or responsible other able to understand concepts of asepsis, combining insulins, insulin-OA actions, and side effects?
	Is patient able to remember to take >1 dose/day?
	Does patient take medications at right times in relation to meals?
Psychomotor	Is patient or responsible other physically able to prepare and administer accurate doses of the medication?
Affective	What emotions and attitudes are patient and responsible others displaying in regard to diagnosis of diabetes and insulin or OA treatment?

For Follow-up of GLA-treated Patient

Effectiveness of therapy	Is patient having symptoms of hyperglycemia?
	Does blood glucose record show good or poor control?
	Is glycosylated hemoglobin consistent with glucose records?
Side effects of therapy	Is atrophy or hypertrophy present at injection sites?
	Has patient had hypoglycemic episodes? If so, how often? What time of day?
	Are there complaints of nightmares, night sweats, or early morning headaches?
	Has patient had skin rash or GI upset since taking OA?
Self-management behaviors	If patient is having hypoglycemic episodes, how are those episodes managed?
	How much insulin or OA is the patient taking and at what time of day? Is patient adjusting insulin or OA dose? Under what circumstances and by how much?
	Has exercise pattern changed?
	Is patient adhering to the meal plan? Are meals taken at times corresponding to peak insulin action?

GI, Gastrointestinal; *GLA*, glucose-lowering agent; *OAs*, oral agents.

insulins. Fortunately, this type of allergy is rare, particularly since human insulin has become available.

Lipodystrophy. **Lipodystrophy** (hypertrophy or atrophy of SQ tissue) may occur if the same injection sites are used frequently. Hypertrophy, a thickening of the SQ tissue, eventually regresses if the patient does not use the site for at least 6 months. The use of hypertrophied sites may result in erratic insulin absorption. Lipodystrophies have been most commonly associated with beef or beef and pork insulin and rarely with human insulin. Site rotation on a daily or weekly basis is not necessary with human insulin.

Somogyi effect and dawn phenomenon. Wide differences in early morning (low) and fasting (high) glucose levels characterize the **Somogyi effect** (Fig. 47-8). Usually occurring during the hours of sleep, the Somogyi effect produces a decline in blood glucose level in response to too much insulin. Counterregulatory hormones are released, stimulating lipolysis, gluconeogenesis, and glycogenolysis, which in turn produce rebound hyperglycemia and ketosis. The danger of this effect is that when blood glucose levels are measured in the morning, hyperglycemia is apparent and the patient (or the health care professional) may increase the insulin dose. The Somogyi effect is associated with the occurrence of undetected hypoglycemia during sleep, although it can happen at any time.

The patient may report headaches on awakening and may recall night sweats or nightmares. If the Somogyi effect is suspected as a cause for early morning high blood glucose, the patient may be advised to check blood glucose levels between 2:00 and 4:00 AM to determine if hypoglycemia is present at that time.

If it is, the insulin dosage affecting the early morning blood glucose is reduced.

The *dawn phenomenon* is characterized by hyperglycemia that is present on awakening in the morning due to the release of counterregulatory hormones in the predawn hours. It has been suggested that growth hormone and/or cortisol are possible factors in this occurrence. The dawn phenomenon affects the majority of people with diabetes and tends to be most severe when growth hormone is at its peak in adolescence and young adulthood.

Careful assessment is required to document each phenomenon because the treatment for each differs. The treatment for Somogyi effect is less insulin. The treatment for dawn phenomenon is an adjustment in the timing of insulin administration or an increase in insulin. The assessment must include insulin dose, injection sites, and variability in the time of meals or insulin administration. In addition, the patient is asked to measure and document bedtime, nighttime (between 2:00 and 4:00 AM), and morning fasting blood glucose levels on several occasions. If the predawn levels are below 60 mg/dl (3.3 mmol/L) and signs and symptoms of hypoglycemia are present, the insulin dosage should be reduced. If the 2:00 to 4:00 AM blood glucose is high, the insulin dosage should be increased. In addition, the patient should be counseled on appropriate bedtime snacks.

Drug Therapy: Oral Agents

Oral agents (OAs) are not insulin, but they work to improve the mechanisms by which insulin and glucose are produced and used by the body. For any of the OAs to be effective, the patient

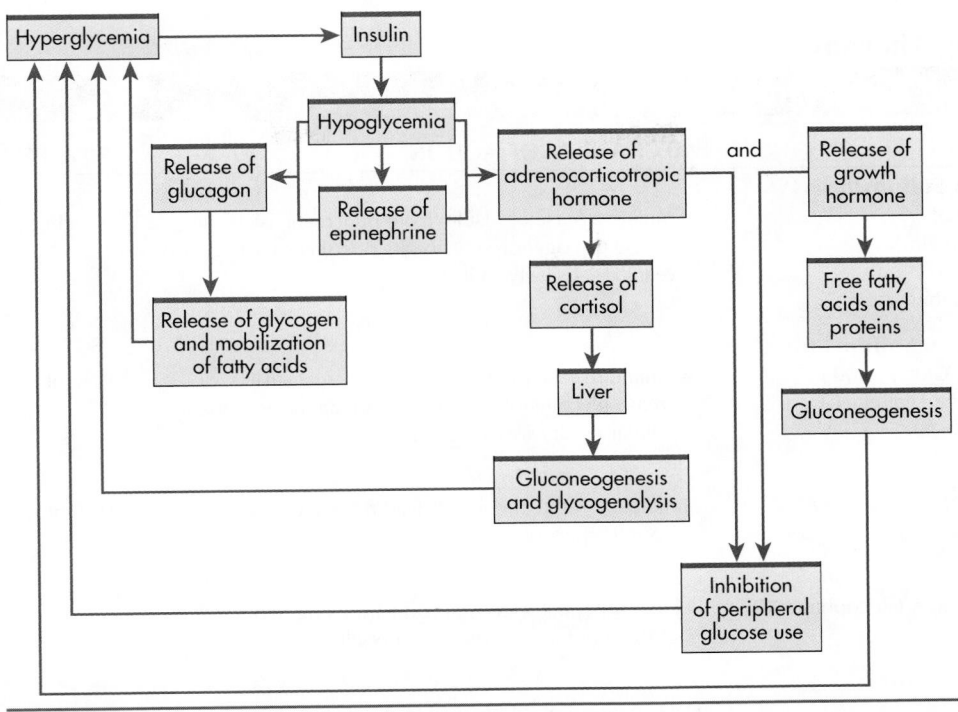

FIG. 47-8   The Somogyi effect.

must have some circulating endogenous insulin. There are currently no OAs for the treatment of type 1 diabetes. OAs may be used in combination with agents from other classes or with insulin to achieve blood glucose targets. Guidelines for assessing patients receiving OAs are shown in Table 47-6.

Currently, five classes of oral medications are available to improve diabetes control for patients with type 2 diabetes.[12] These agents are listed in Table 47-7.

Sulfonylureas. Sulfonylureas have been widely used to treat type 2 diabetes since the 1950s. They are called *first generation* or *second generation* depending on when they were introduced into clinical use in the United States. The first generation of these drugs used in the treatment of diabetes mellitus includes tolbutamide (Orinase), acetohexamide (Dymelor), tolazamide (Tolinase), and chlorpropamide (Diabinese). The second generation of sulfonylureas includes glipizide (Glucotrol, Glucotrol XL), glyburide (Micronase, DiaBeta, Glynase), and glimepiride (Amaryl). Second-generation drugs have fewer adverse effects and are more potent by weight, but they are more expensive.

The primary action of the sulfonylureas is to increase insulin production from the pancreas. Therapy with sulfonylureas is generally more effective early in the course of type 2 diabetes. About 10% of patients will experience decreased effectiveness of these medications after prolonged use.[13]

Meglitinides. Like the sulfonylureas, repaglinide (Prandin) and nateglinide (Starlix) increase insulin production from the pancreas. But because they are more rapidly absorbed and eliminated, they offer a reduced potential for hypoglycemia. When taken just before meals, pancreatic insulin production increases during and after the meal, mimicking the normal blood glucose response to eating. Patients should be instructed to take meglitinides anytime from 30 minutes before each meal right up to the time of the meal.

Biguanides. Metformin (Glucophage) is a biguanide glucose-lowering agent. It can be used alone or with sulfonylureas, other OAs, or insulin to treat type 2 diabetes. The primary action of metformin is to reduce glucose production by the liver. It also enhances insulin sensitivity at the tissue level and improves glucose transport into the cells. Besides being an effective blood glucose–lowering agent, metformin has other advantages. Unlike sulfonylureas and insulin, metformin does not promote weight gain. It also has beneficial effects on plasma lipids. Metformin is also used to treat prediabetes, especially in individuals who are obese and have diabetes.

Combination therapy that combines metformin with another drug is available as one tablet. These combinations include metformin with glyburide (Glucovance), with rosiglitazone (Avandia), and with glipizide (Metaglip).[6]

α-Glucosidase inhibitors. Also known as "starch blockers," these drugs work by slowing down the absorption of carbohydrate in the small intestine. Acarbose (Precose) and miglitol (Glyset) are the available drugs in this class. Taken with the first bite of each main meal, they are most effective in lowering postprandial blood glucose. Effectiveness of these medications is measured by checking 2-hour postprandial glucose levels. Medications from this class are not effective against fasting hyperglycemia.[13]

Thiazolidinediones. Sometimes referred to as "insulin sensitizers," these agents include pioglitazone (Actos) and rosiglitazone (Avandia). They are most effective for people who have insulin resistance. They improve insulin sensitivity, transport, and

Drug Therapy

TABLE
47-7

Oral Agents for Diabetes Mellitus

TYPE	MECHANISM OF ACTION	SIDE EFFECTS
First-Generation Sulfonylureas* tolbutamide (Orinase) acetohexamide (Dymelor) tolazamide (Tolinase) chlorpropamide (Diabinese)	Stimulate release of insulin from pancreatic islets; decrease glycogenolysis and gluconeogenesis; enhance cellular sensitivity to insulin	Weight gain, hypoglycemia
Second-Generation Sulfonylureas glipizide (Glucotrol, Glucotrol XL) glyburide (Micronase, DiaBeta, Glynase) glimepiride (Amaryl)	Stimulate release of insulin from pancreatic islets; decrease glycogenolysis and gluconeogenesis; enhance cellular sensitivity to insulin	Weight gain, hypoglycemia
Meglitinides repaglinide (Prandin) nateglinide (Starlix)	Stimulate a rapid and short-lived release of insulin from the pancreas	Weight gain, hypoglycemia
Biguanide metformin (Glucophage, Glucophage XR)	↓ Rate of hepatic glucose production; augments glucose uptake by tissues, especially muscles	Diarrhea, lactic acidosis
α-Glucosidase Inhibitors acarbose (Precose) miglitol (Glyset)	Delay absorption of glucose from GI tract	Gas, abdominal pain, diarrhea
Thiazolidinediones pioglitazone (Actos) rosiglitazone (Avandia)	↑ Glucose uptake in muscle; ↓ endogenous glucose production	Weight gain, edema
Combination Therapy Glucovance Avandamet Metaglip	Combination of metformin and glyburide Combination of rosiglitazone and metformin Combination of metformin and glipizide	Nausea, diarrhea, abdominal pain, lactic acidosis, weight gain, hypoglycemia

*These drugs are not commonly used because they have been replaced by the second-generation sulfonylureas.

utilization at target tissues. Because they do not increase insulin production, thiazolidinediones will not cause hypoglycemia when used alone, but the risk is still present when a thiazolidinedione is used in combination with a sulfonylurea or insulin. Patients taking these medications may experience a secondary benefit of improved lipid profiles and blood pressure levels.[13,14]

Other Drugs Affecting Blood Glucose Levels. Both the patient and the health care provider must be aware of drug interactions that can potentiate hypoglycemic and hyperglycemic effects. For example, β-adrenergic blockers can mask symptoms of hypoglycemia and prolong the hypoglycemic effects of insulin. Thiazide and loop diuretics can potentiate hyperglycemia by inducing potassium loss, although low-dose therapy with a thiazide is usually considered safe. A list of medications that may influence glycemic control is presented in Table 47-8.

Nutritional Therapy

Although nutritional therapy is the cornerstone of care for the person with diabetes, it is also the most challenging for many people. Achieving nutritional goals requires a coordinated team effort that takes into account the behavioral, cognitive, socioeco-

nomic, cultural, and religious aspects of the person. Because of these complexities it is recommended that a diabetes nurse educator and a registered dietitian, with expertise in diabetes management, be members of the team.

Many people, both lay and professional, are misinformed about the nutritional management of diabetes. Although it is still used in many settings, the term "ADA diet" is no longer recommended because the American Diabetes Association (ADA) no longer endorses a single meal plan. Instead, nutritional therapy for the management of diabetes is based on a plan of healthy eating that is appropriate and beneficial to most people, whether they have diabetes or not. In an institutional setting, the prescribed diet is often labeled "ADA," indicating that the meal plan follows the ADA's current nutritional recommendations.

Recently issued guidelines from the ADA indicate that within the context of an overall healthy eating plan, a person with diabetes can eat the same foods as a person who does not have diabetes. This means that the same principles of good nutrition that apply to the general population also apply to the person with diabetes. The Food Guide Pyramid (see Chapter 39, Fig. 39-1) summarizes and illustrates nutritional guidelines and nutrient needs. These are also appropriate in guiding the food choices of

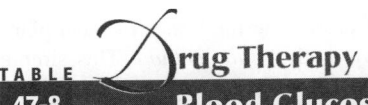

TABLE 47-8 Drug Therapy: Blood Glucose Level Effects

Glucose-Lowering Effect

acetaminophen (Tylenol)	Monoamine oxidase inhibitors
allopurinol (Zyloprim)	phenylbutazone
α-Glucosidase inhibitors	Potassium salts
Anabolic steroids	probenecid
β-Adrenergic blockers	Salicylates in large doses
Biguanides	Sulfonylureas
chloramphenicol	Thiazolidinediones
clofibrate (Atromid)	Tricyclic antidepressants
Insulin	Urinary acidifiers

Glucose-Raising Effect

acetazolamide (Diamox)	Glucagon
Alcohol	Glucose
asparaginase (Elspar)	Glycerin
Caffeine in large doses	Glycerol
Arginine	levodopa
Barbiturates	lithium
Birth control pills	Niacin
calcitonin	Marijuana
Calcium channel blockers	Nicotine
cholestyramine (Questran)	nifedipine (Procardia)
clonidine (Catapres)	phenobarbital
Corticosteroids	Phenothiazines
cyclosporine	phenytoin (Dilantin)
ethacrynic acid (Edecrin)	rifampin
morphine	tacrolimus (Prograf)
epinephrine	Thiazide diuretics
furosemide (Lasix)	Urinary alkalizing agents

people with diabetes. Tools used to measure the effectiveness of nutritional therapy include blood glucose, A1C and lipid values, tests of renal status, and clinical measurements such as body weight and blood pressure.[15] Table 47-9 describes nutritional therapy for type 1 and type 2 diabetes.

According to the ADA, the overall goal of nutritional therapy is to assist people with diabetes in making changes in nutrition and exercise habits that will lead to improved metabolic control. Additional specific goals include the following:[16]

1. Maintain blood glucose levels to as near normal as safely possible to prevent or reduce the risk for complications of diabetes.
2. Achieve lipid profiles and blood pressure levels that reduce the risk for cardiovascular disease.
3. Modify lifestyle as appropriate for the prevention and treatment of obesity, dyslipidemia, cardiovascular disease, and nephropathy.
4. Improve health through healthy food choices and physical activity.
5. Address individual nutritional needs while taking into account personal and cultural preferences and respecting the individual's willingness to change.

Type 1 Diabetes Mellitus. Meal planning should be based on the individual's usual food intake and balanced with insulin and exercise patterns. The insulin regimen should be developed with the patient's eating habits and activity pattern in mind. Patients using rapid-acting insulin can make adjustments in dosage before the meal based on the current blood glucose level and the carbohydrate content of the meal. Intensified insulin therapy, such as multiple daily injections or the use of an insulin pump, allows considerable flexibility in food selection and can be adjusted for deviations from usual eating and exercise habits.

Type 2 Diabetes Mellitus. The emphasis for nutritional therapy in type 2 diabetes should be placed on achieving glucose, lipid, and blood pressure goals. Because 80% to 90% of people with type 2 diabetes are overweight, calorie reduction is a goal.[17]

There is no one proven strategy or method that can be uniformly recommended. A nutritionally adequate meal plan with a reduction of total fat, especially saturated fats, and simple sugars can bring about decreased calorie and carbohydrate consumption. Spacing meals is another strategy that can be adopted to spread nutrient intake throughout the day. A weight loss of 5% to 7% of body weight often improves glycemic control, even if desirable body weight is not achieved. Weight loss is best attempted by a moderate decrease in calories and an increase in caloric expenditure. Regular exercise and learning new behaviors and attitudes can help facilitate long-term lifestyle changes. Monitoring of blood glucose levels, A1C, lipids, and blood pressure provide

TABLE 47-9 Nutritional Therapy: Diabetes Mellitus

FACTOR	TYPE 1 DIABETES MELLITUS	TYPE 2 DIABETES MELLITUS
Total calories	Increase in caloric intake possibly necessary to achieve desirable body weight and restore body tissues	Reduction in caloric intake desirable for overweight or obese patient
Effect of diet	Diet and insulin necessary for glucose control	Diet alone possibly sufficient for glucose control
Distribution of calories	Equal distribution of carbohydrates through meals or adjustment of carbohydrates for insulin activity	Equal distribution recommended; low-fat diet desirable; consistency of carbohydrate at meals desirable
Consistency in daily intake	Necessary for glucose control	Desirable for weight reduction and moderation of blood glucose levels
Uniform timing of meals	Crucial for NPH/lente insulin programs; flexibility with multidose rapid-acting insulin	Desirable but not essential
Intermeal and bedtime snacks	Frequently necessary	Not usually recommended
Nutritional supplement for exercise programs	Carbohydrates 20 g/hr for moderate physical activities	May be necessary if patient controlled on sulfonylurea or insulin

feedback on how well the goals of nutritional therapy are being met.

Food Composition. The meal plan for people with diabetes does not prohibit the consumption of any one type of food. All food groups should be represented in a daily meal plan that is nutritionally balanced. Although an individualized meal plan should be developed with a dietitian, general guidelines and recommendations for people with diabetes include the following:[15]

- *Protein*—15% to 20% of total daily calories. Those with nephropathy should limit protein intake to 10%.
- *Fat*—less than 10% of daily calories from saturated fat. Cholesterol intake should be less than 300 mg/day.
- *Carbohydrate*—should constitute the remaining percentage of calories after determining protein and fat needs. Carbohydrates should include whole grains, fresh vegetables, and fresh fruits. Although overall intake of simple sugar should be limited as much as possible, its consumption is acceptable in moderate amounts when counted as part of total carbohydrate intake.
- *Sodium*—intake should be less than 2400 mg/day.
- *Fiber*—approximately 25 to 30 g/day from a variety of food sources.

Alcohol. Alcohol is high in calories, has no nutritive value, and promotes hypertriglyceridemia. In addition, it has detrimental effects on the liver (see Chapter 42). The inhibitory effect of alcohol on glucose production by the liver can cause severe hypoglycemia in patients on insulin or oral hypoglycemic medications that increase insulin secretion. Patients should be cautioned to honestly discuss the use of alcohol with their health care providers because its use can make blood glucose more difficult to control.

Alcohol can also cause other serious adverse effects when used in conjunction with certain oral medications used to treat diabetes. For example, it may produce a disulfiram (Antabuse) effect (nausea and vomiting, flushing, respiratory distress, chest pain) when ingested with some sulfonylurea medications, such as chlorpropamide (Diabinese). It can also increase the risk of lactic acidosis in patients who use metformin (Glucophage).

Moderate alcohol consumption can sometimes be safely incorporated into the meal plan if blood glucose levels are well controlled and if the patient is not on medications that will cause adverse effects. A patient can reduce the risk for alcohol-induced hypoglycemia by eating carbohydrates when drinking alcohol. One drink has approximately 135 calories. The patient with diabetes should drink alcohol with food, use sugar-free mixes, and drink dry, light wines.

Diet Teaching. Most often, the dietitian initially teaches the principles of the nutrition therapy prescription. Whenever possible, nurses should be prepared to work with dietitians as part of an interdisciplinary diabetes care team. In some instances, access to a dietitian is not possible for patients with limited insurance coverage or who live in remote areas. In these cases, nurses often assume responsibility for teaching basic dietary management to patients with diabetes.

The Food Guide Pyramid is an appropriate teaching tool for people with diabetes (see Chapter 39, Fig. 39-1). The pyramid helps the patient visualize the recommended amounts of foods that should be eaten from each group on a daily basis. For many people, the graphic representation of the pyramid makes this method of meal planning more approachable and easier to understand than exchange lists.

An alternative method of presenting the basics of meal planning is to use what is known as the *plate method*. This simple method helps the patient visualize the amount of vegetables, starch, and meat that should fill a 9-inch plate. For lunch and dinner one half of the plate is filled with nonstarchy vegetables, one fourth is filled with a starch, and one fourth is filled with 2 to 3 oz of lean meat. A glass of low-fat milk and a small piece of fresh fruit complete the meal. The breakfast plate is filled halfway with starch, and one fourth of the plate contains an optional protein. Low-fat milk and fresh fruit complete the breakfast. Assuming low-fat and nonfat foods are selected, following the plate method will provide 1200 to 1400 calories per day and a properly balanced meal plan.[18]

Diet teaching should include the patient's family and significant others whenever possible. It is most effective to direct teaching efforts to the person who will be cooking. It is important, however, that the responsibility for maintaining a diabetic diet not fall to someone other than the patient with diabetes. Reliance on another person to make health decisions fosters dependence and should be avoided except in special situations.

Exercise

Regular, consistent exercise is considered an essential part of diabetes management. Exercise increases insulin sensitivity and can have a direct effect on lowering the blood glucose levels. It also contributes to weight loss, which also decreases insulin resistance. The therapeutic benefits of regular physical activity may result in a decreased need for diabetes medicines in order to reach target blood glucose goals. Regular exercise may also help reduce triglyceride and LDL cholesterol levels, reduce blood pressure, and improve circulation.[19]

Patients who use insulin, sulfonylureas, or meglitinides are at increased risk for hypoglycemia when there is an increase in physical activity, especially if the patient exercises at the time of peak drug action or if food intake has not been sufficient to maintain adequate blood glucose levels. This can also occur if a normally sedentary patient with diabetes has an unusually active day. The glucose-lowering effects of exercise can last up to 48 hours after the activity, so it is possible for hypoglycemia to occur for that long after the activity. It is recommended that patients who use medications that can cause hypoglycemia schedule exercise about 1 hour after a meal, or that they have a 10 to 15 g carbohydrate snack before exercising. Several small carbohydrate snacks can be taken every 30 minutes during exercise to prevent hypoglycemia.[15] Patients using medications that place them at risk for hypoglycemia should always carry a fast-acting source of carbohydrate, such as glucose tablets or hard candies, when exercising. Table 47-10 gives guidelines on the number of calories burned per hour for different activities.

Although exercise is generally beneficial to blood glucose levels, strenuous activity can be perceived by the body as a stress, causing a release of counterregulatory hormones that results in a temporary elevation of blood glucose. As a result, hyperglycemia may occur in cases of poorly controlled type 2 diabetes or in patients with type 1 diabetes who exercise at a time of day when insulin action is waning. Some patients may have to inject a small bolus of rapid-acting or regular insulin if the blood glucose level is elevated before exercising to prevent progressive hyperglycemia. Furthermore, patients should exercise with caution if the blood glucose is greater than 300 mg/dl and there are no ketones, or if the blood glucose is greater than 250 mg/dl and ke- tones are present in the urine.[20] Additional information about ex- ercise and diabetes that is important for both the patient and the health care provider is provided in the patient and family teach- ing guide (Table 47-11).

Monitoring Blood Glucose

Self-monitoring of blood glucose (SMBG) is a cornerstone of diabetes management. By providing a current blood glucose read- ing, SMBG enables the patient to make self-management deci- sions regarding diet, exercise, and medication. SMBG is also im- portant for detecting episodic hyperglycemia and hypoglycemia. In the past, monitoring was accomplished by checking for the presence and degree of glucose in the urine. This is rarely used anymore because urine testing does not provide current blood glu- cose levels, making it much less useful for self-management de- cisions and the early detection and treatment of hypoglycemia.

Portable blood glucose meters are used at the hospital bedside and by patients who perform SMBG. A wide variety of blood glu- cose meters are available. Disposable lancets are usually used to ob- tain a small drop of capillary blood (usually from a finger stick) that is placed onto a reagent strip. After a specified time, the meter dis- plays a digital reading of the blood glucose. The technology of SMBG is a rapidly changing field with newer and more convenient systems being introduced every year. Newer systems allow the user to collect blood from alternative sites such as the forearm. Nonin- vasive approaches to blood glucose monitoring have also been de- veloped. The G2 Biographer from GlucoWatch is a device worn on the wrist. It pulls glucose through the skin using low electric cur- rent. It then measures glucose levels for 13 hours and sends an alarm if the reading is abnormal. Another device already in use in Europe measures glucose using infrared rays directed at the skin.

The blood glucose level reported by a laboratory is sometimes higher than the patient's home glucose monitor or the hospital's portable meter. This is because some meters give capillary blood glucose values from whole blood (via finger stick), whereas ve- nous samples taken in the laboratory provide plasma readings. Plasma samples, or venous samples, are approximately 10% to 12% higher. Some meters are automatically calibrated to give a "plasma" test result (although whole blood was used for the sam- ple) so that the home readings can be more readily compared with laboratory values. The literature accompanying a meter will identify if that particular meter is calibrated to give plasma or whole blood readings.

Instructions for using a blood glucose meter also accompany each product. Because errors in monitoring technique can cause errors in management strategies, thorough patient training is cru- cial. Initial training should be followed up at regular intervals with reassessment. In addition, patients must be taught to use and interpret calibration and control solutions that are a part of each blood glucose monitoring kit.[20] Table 47-12 lists the steps that should be taught to the patient learning to perform SMBG.

TABLE 47-10 Activities That Affect Caloric Expenditure

LIGHT ACTIVITY (100-200 kcal/hr)	MODERATE ACTIVITY (200-350 kcal/hr)	VIGOROUS ACTIVITY (400-900 kcal/hr)
Driving a car	Active housework	Aerobic exercise
Fishing	Bicycling (light)	Bicycling (vigorous)
Light housework	Bowling	Hard labor
Secretarial work	Dancing	Ice skating
Teaching	Gardening	Outdoor sports
Walking casually	Golf	Running
	Roller skating	Soccer
	Walking briskly	Tennis
		Wood chopping

TABLE 47-11 Patient & Family Teaching Guide — Exercise for Patients with Diabetes Mellitus

1. Exercise does not have to be vigorous to be effective. The blood glucose–reducing effects of exercise can be attained with exercise such as brisk walking. The exercises selected should be enjoyable to foster regularity.
2. Exercise is best done after meals, when the blood glucose level is rising.
3. Exercise plans should be individualized for each patient and monitored by the health care provider.
4. It is important to self-monitor blood glucose levels before, during, and after exercise to determine the effect exercise has on blood glucose level at particular times of the day.
5. Be alert to the possibility of delayed exercise-induced hy- poglycemia, which may occur several hours after the com- pletion of exercise.
6. Taking a glucose-lowering medication does not mean that planned or spontaneous exercise cannot occur.
7. It is important to compensate for extensive planned and spontaneous activity by monitoring blood glucose level to make adjustments in the insulin dose (if taken) and food intake.

TABLE 47-12 Patient & Family Teaching Guide — Self-Monitoring of Blood Glucose (SMBG)

1. Wash hands in warm water. It is not necessary to clean the site with alcohol, and it may interfere with test results.
2. If it is difficult to obtain an adequate drop of blood for testing, warm the hands in warm water or let the arms hang dependently for a few minutes before the finger puncture is made.
3. If the puncture is made on the finger, use the side of the finger pad rather than near the center. Fewer nerve endings are along the side of the finger pad. If an alternative site is used (e.g., forearm), special equipment may be needed. Refer to manufacturer's instructions for alternative site use.
4. The puncture should be only deep enough to obtain a suf- ficiently large drop of blood. Unnecessarily deep punctures may cause pain and bruising.

The chief advantage of SMBG is that it supplies immediate information about blood glucose levels that can be used to make adjustments in food intake, activity patterns, and medication dosages. It also produces accurate records of daily glucose fluctuations and trends, as well as alerting the patient to acute episodes of hyperglycemia and hypoglycemia. Furthermore, it provides patients with a tool for achieving and maintaining specific glycemic goals. SMBG is recommended for all insulin-treated patients with diabetes. Other patients with diabetes frequently use SMBG to help achieve and maintain glycemic goals, as well as monitor for acute fluctuations in blood glucose.

The frequency of monitoring depends on several factors, including the patient's glycemic goals, the type of diabetes that the patient has, the patient's ability to perform the test independently, and the patient's willingness to test. Patients with type 1 diabetes typically test four times per day (before meals and at bedtime). Those using an insulin pump may test more frequently. Patients with type 2 diabetes will have more variable and individualized testing regimens.

Testing is most often done before meals, but certain situations warrant more frequent monitoring. For example, the patient should be instructed to test blood glucose before and after exercise to determine its effects on metabolic control. This is especially important in the patient with type 1 diabetes. Blood glucose testing should also be performed whenever hypoglycemia is suspected so that immediate action can be taken if necessary. When the person with diabetes is ill, the blood glucose should be tested at 4-hour intervals to determine the effects of this stressor on the blood glucose level.[20]

SMBG is an empowering tool that allows the patient to be an active partner in the treatment of diabetes. Achieving the desired level of patient participation does require time and effort from the health care professional. The nurse involved in this aspect of management should anticipate a close working relationship with patients as they refine their techniques and learn appropriate decision making about managing their diabetes. A patient who is visually impaired, cognitively impaired, or limited in manual dexterity needs careful evaluation of the degree to which SMBG can be performed independently. Nurses working in home health and outpatient settings may need to identify caregivers who can assume this responsibility. Adaptive devices are available to help patients with certain limitations. These include talking meters and other equipment for the visually impaired, as well as devices to stabilize insulin vials and syringes for those with limitations affecting dexterity.

Pancreas Transplantation. Pancreas transplantation is used as a treatment option for patients with type 1 diabetes mellitus who have end-stage renal disease and who have had or plan to have a kidney transplant. Kidney and pancreas transplants are often done together. If renal failure is not present, the ADA recommends that pancreas transplantation should only be considered for patients who exhibit the following three criteria: (1) a history of frequent, acute, and severe metabolic complications (e.g., hypoglycemia, hyperglycemia, ketoacidosis) requiring medical attention; (2) clinical and emotional problems with exogenous insulin therapy that are so severe as to be incapacitating; and (3) consistent failure of insulin-based management to prevent acute complications.

Successful pancreas transplantation can improve the quality of life of people with diabetes, primarily by eliminating the need for exogenous insulin, frequent daily blood glucose measurements, and many of the dietary restrictions imposed by the disorder. Transplantation can also eliminate the acute complications commonly experienced by patients with type 1 diabetes (e.g., hypoglycemia, hyperglycemia). However, pancreas transplantation is only partially successful in reversing the long-term renal and neurologic complications of diabetes.

Patients who undergo pancreas transplantation require immunosuppression to prevent rejection of the graft and potential recurrence of the autoimmune process that might again destroy pancreatic islet cells. (Immunosuppressive therapy is discussed in Chapter 13.)

Pancreatic islet cell transplantation is another potential treatment measure. However, at this time, islet cell transplantation is an experimental procedure.

New Developments in Diabetic Therapy

Many new insulin delivery systems are being researched. However, these products are still not approved by the Food and Drug Administration. These include the following: (1) *inhaled insulin,* which delivers a dose of liquid or dry powder insulin through the mouth and directly into the lungs, where it enters the blood as rapid-acting insulin; (2) a *skin patch* containing a reservoir of insulin, which can be changed after 12 to 24 hours of wear; (3) an *oral spray,* which is a liquid aerosol version of insulin that is absorbed by mucous membranes in cheeks, tongue, and throat; and (4) *insulin pills* with a special delivery system that prevents enzymatic breakdown as they go through the digestive system. The insulin in the pills is then absorbed in the small intestine, enters the circulation, and is available for use.

■ Culturally Competent Care: Diabetes Mellitus

Because culture can have a strong influence on dietary preferences and meal preparation practices, culturally competent care has special relevance for the care of the patient with diabetes. This is especially pertinent when considering the prevalence of diabetes in such diverse cultural groups as Hispanics, Native Americans, and African Americans. The influences of culture on food choices and meal planning should be explored with the patient as part of the health history. When giving diet instructions, efforts should be made to consider the food preferences of the cultural group. Nutritional resources specifically designed for members of different cultural groups are available from the American Diabetes Association and the American Dietetic Association. ■

NURSING MANAGEMENT
DIABETES MELLITUS

■ Nursing Assessment

Table 47-13 provides initial subjective and objective data that might be obtained from a person with diabetes mellitus. After the initial assessment, periodic patient assessments should be done on a regular basis.

■ Nursing Diagnoses

Nursing diagnoses related to diabetes mellitus may include, but are not limited to, those found in NCP 47-1.

| TABLE 47-13 | Nursing Assessment | Diabetes Mellitus |

Subjective Data

Important Health Information

Past health history: Mumps, rubella, coxsackievirus or other viral infections; recent trauma, infection, or stress; pregnancy, gave birth to infant >9 lb; chronic pancreatitis; Cushing syndrome, acromegaly; family history of type 1 or type 2 diabetes mellitus

Medications: Use of and compliance with insulin or OAs; use of corticosteroids, diuretics, phenytoin (Dilantin)

Surgery or other treatments: Any recent surgery

Functional Health Patterns

Health perception–health management: Positive family history; malaise; date of last eye and dental examination

Nutritional-metabolic: Obesity; weight loss (type 1), weight gain (type 2): thirst, hunger; nausea and vomiting; poor healing especially involving the feet, compliance with diet in patients with previously diagnosed diabetes

Elimination: Constipation or diarrhea; frequent urination, nocturia, urinary incontinence; skin infections

Activity-exercise: Muscle weakness, fatigue

Cognitive-perceptual: Abdominal pain, headache; blurred vision; numbness or tingling of extremities; pruritus

Sexuality-reproductive: Impotence; frequent vaginal infections; decreased libido

Coping–stress tolerance: Depression, irritability, apathy

Value-belief: Commitment to lifestyle changes involving diet, medication, and activity patterns

Objective Data

Eyes
Soft, sunken eyeballs; vitreal hemorrhages, cataracts

Integumentary
Dry, warm, inelastic skin; pigmented lesions (on legs); ulcers (especially on feet), loss of hair on toes

Respiratory
Rapid, deep respirations (Kussmaul respirations)

Cardiovascular
Hypotension; weak, rapid pulse

Gastrointestinal
Dry mouth, vomiting, fruity breath

Neurologic
Altered reflexes, restlessness, confusion, stupor, coma

Musculoskeletal
Muscle wasting

Possible Findings
Serum electrolyte abnormalities; fasting blood glucose level ≥126 mg/dl (7.0 mmol/L); glucose tolerance test ≥200 mg/dl (11.1 mmol/L); leukocytosis; ↑ blood urea nitrogen, creatinine, triglycerides, cholesterol, LDL, VLDL; ↓ HDL; glycosylated hemoglobin ≥6%; glycosuria; ketonuria; albuminuria; acidosis

HDL, High-density lipoprotein; *LDL,* low-density lipoprotein; *OA,* oral agents; *VLDL,* very-low-density lipoprotein.

■ Planning

The overall goals for the patient with diabetes mellitus include the following: (1) to be an active participant in the management of the diabetes regimen; (2) to experience few or no episodes of acute hyperglycemic emergencies or hypoglycemia; (3) to maintain blood glucose levels at normal or near-normal levels; (4) to prevent, minimize, or delay the occurrence of chronic complications of diabetes; and (5) to adjust lifestyle to accommodate diabetes regimen with a minimum of stress.

■ Nursing Implementation

Health Promotion. The role of the nurse in health promotion and maintenance relates to the identification, monitoring, and education of the patient at risk for the development of diabetes mellitus. Obesity is the number one predictor of type 2 diabetes mellitus. The Diabetes Prevention Program found that a modest weight loss of 5% to 7% of body weight and regular exercise of 30 minutes five times a week lowered the risk of developing type 2 diabetes up to 58%.[1]

The ADA recommends routine screening for diabetes for all overweight adults over age 45. If normal, it should be repeated at 3-year intervals. The FPG is the preferred method for screening in clinical settings, although the OGTT is also suitable. Testing should be considered at a younger age or be carried out more frequently in individuals who meet the criteria listed in Table 47-14.[2] It is important to know where an individual is on the glucose continuum (Fig. 47-9).

Acute Intervention. Acute situations involving the patient with diabetes include hypoglycemia, diabetic ketoacidosis (DKA), and hyperosmolar hyperglycemic nonketotic syndrome (HHNS). Nursing management for these situations is discussed in more detail later in this chapter. Other areas of acute intervention relate to management during stress, such as during acute illness and surgery.

Stress of acute illness and surgery. Both emotional and physical stress can increase the blood glucose level and result in hyperglycemia. Because it is impossible to avoid stress totally in life, certain situations may require more intense management, such as extra insulin, to maintain glycemic goals and avoid hyperglycemia.

Acute illness, injury, and surgery are situations that may evoke a counterregulatory hormone response resulting in hyperglycemia. Even minor illnesses such as a viral upper respiratory infection or the flu can cause this. When patients with diabetes are ill, they should continue with the regular meal plan while increasing the intake of noncaloric fluids, such as broth, water, and other decaffeinated beverages. They should also continue taking oral agents and insulin as prescribed and check blood glucose at least every 4 hours. If the glucose is greater than 240 mg/dl (13.3 mmol/l), urine should be tested for ketones every 3 to 4 hours. Patients should report moderate to large ketone levels to the health care provider.

When the illness causes the patient to eat less than normal, she or he should continue to take oral hypoglycemic medications and/or insulin as prescribed while supplementing food

NURSING CARE PLAN 47-1

Patient with Diabetes Mellitus

NURSING DIAGNOSIS **Ineffective therapeutic regimen management** *related to* inadequate knowledge *as manifested by* continued hyperglycemia, inaccurate statements regarding diabetes and its management, and self-professed confusion regarding the pathophysiology of diabetes and its treatment.

OUTCOMES—NOC	INTERVENTIONS—NIC and *RATIONALES*
Knowledge: Diabetes Management (1820)	*Teaching: Disease Process (5602)*
▪ Description of insulin function _____	▪ Assess the patient's current level of knowledge related to specific disease process *to determine the scope and extent of required teaching.*
▪ Description of role of nutrition in controlling blood glucose level _____	▪ Describe the disease process and treatment recommendations *to enable patient to better understand rationale behind treatment regimen and lifestyle changes.*
▪ Description of hyperglycemia and related symptoms _____	▪ Discuss lifestyle changes that may be required to control the disease process *to encourage patient to actively participate in determining changes that will be acceptable.*
▪ Description of target blood glucose range _____	▪ Describe possible chronic complications *to increase awareness of the long-term effects of inadequate control of disease process.*
▪ Identification of actions to be taken in relation to blood glucose levels _____	▪ Plan individualized exercise program with patient *because exercise is an integral part of diabetes management.*
▪ Demonstration of proper technique to draw up and administer insulin _____	▪ Review steps to prevent hyperglycemia and hypoglycemia *because activity changes can cause changes in insulin needs.*
	▪ Review insulin administration (if used); have patient give return demonstration of insulin injection *to ensure proper technique.*

Outcome Scale
1 = None
2 = Limited
3 = Moderate
4 = Substantial
5 = Extensive

NURSING DIAGNOSIS **Fatigue** *related to* nutritional deficits secondary to mismanaged diabetes *as manifested by* inability to perform ADLs secondary to malaise, desire for frequent naps during the daytime, and lethargy that is unrelieved by sleep.

OUTCOMES—NOC	INTERVENTIONS—NIC and *RATIONALES*
Endurance (0001)	*Energy Management (0180)*
▪ Performance of usual routine _____	▪ Assist the patient in assigning priority to activities to accommodate energy levels *so that the most energy costly activities are performed during periods of peak energy.*
▪ Lethargy not present _____	▪ Assist the patient to identify tasks that family and friends can perform in the home *to prevent fatigue and to relieve patient stress regarding activities of daily living.*
▪ Concentration _____	
▪ Rested appearance _____	*Hyperglycemia Management (2120)*
▪ Energy restored after rest _____	▪ Monitor for signs and symptoms of hyperglycemia: polyuria, polydipsia, polyphagia, weakness, lethargy, malaise, blurring of vision, or headache *to alert patient to glucose/insulin imbalance and need for treatment.*
	▪ Anticipate situations in which insulin requirements will increase (e.g., times of stress and illness) *to allow patient to adjust insulin dosage appropriately and avoid undue fatigue.*
	▪ Facilitate diet and exercise regimen *to promote and preserve energy balance.*
	▪ Restrict exercise when blood glucose levels are >250 mg/dl *to decrease the body's requirement for already unavailable glucose.*

Outcome Scale
1 = Extremely compromised
2 = Substantially compromised
3 = Moderately compromised
4 = Mildly compromised
5 = Not compromised

ADLs, Activities of daily living.

intake with carbohydrate-containing fluids. Examples include soups, juices, and regular decaffeinated soft drinks.[20] The health care provider should be notified promptly if the patient is unable to keep anything down. The patient should understand that medication for diabetes, including insulin, should not be withheld during times of illness because counterregulatory mechanisms often increase the blood glucose level dramatically. Food intake is also important during this time because the body requires extra energy to deal with the stress of the illness. Extra insulin may be necessary to meet this demand and to prevent the onset of DKA in the patient with type 1 diabetes.[21]

During the intraoperative period adjustments in the diabetes regimen can be planned to ensure glycemic control. The patient

NURSING CARE PLAN 47-1

Patient with Diabetes Mellitus—cont'd

NURSING DIAGNOSIS   **Risk for infection** *related to* compromised immune system secondary to diabetes and decreased sensory percpetion secondary to diminished peripheral vascular circulation.

OUTCOMES—NOC	INTERVENTIONS—NIC and *RATIONALES*
Immune Status (0702)	**Skin Surveillance (3590)**
• Skin integrity _____	• Observe extremities for color, warmth, swelling, pulses, texture, edema, and ulcerations *to detect early signs and symptoms of infection and decreased circulation.*
• Recurrent infections not present _____	• Monitor skin for excessive dryness and moistness *to prevent conditions that favor skin breakdown.*
• Chronic fatigue not present _____	
	Infection Protection (6550)
	• Promote sufficient nutritional intake *to prevent illness and encourage wound healing.*
	• Encourage fluid intake *to maintain adequate hydration and blood viscosity.*
	• Encourage rest periods *to allow the body to rejuvenate itself and decrease stress.*
Outcome Scale	• Encourage increased mobility and exercise *to promote and increase circulation to prevent the formation of pressure ulcers and to improve the efficiency of the body's use of insulin.*
1 = Extremely compromised	• Teach patient and family about signs and symptoms of infection (and ask for return demonstration) and when to report them to health care provider *to promote early detection.*
2 = Substantially compromised	
3 = Moderately compromised	
4 = Mildly compromised	
5 = Not compromised	

NURSING DIAGNOSIS   **Powerlessness** *related to* sudden change in lifestyle and restrictions placed on normal eating habits secondary to diagnosis of diabetes *as manifested by* anger and statements alluding to lack of control over the situation.

OUTCOMES—NOC	INTERVENTIONS—NIC and *RATIONALES*
Health Beliefs (1700)	**Self-Responsibility Facilitation (4480)**
• Perceived importance of taking action _____	• Hold patient responsible for own behavior *to encourage patient to view self as responsible for health outcomes.*
• Perceived threat from inaction _____	• Encourage verbalization of feelings, perceptions, and fears about assuming responsibility *to identify barriers to patient assuming responsibility for health care.*
• Perceived ability to perform action _____	• Monitor level of responsibility that patient assumes *to determine whether changes need to be made.*
• Perceived absence of barriers to action _____	• Discuss consequences of not dealing with own responsibilities *so that patient will have realistic knowledge of the health implications of inaction.*
Outcome Scale	• Provide positive feedback for accepting additional responsibility *to reinforce positive behavior.*
1 = Very weak	
2 = Weak	
3 = Moderate	
4 = Strong	
5 = Very strong	

is given IV fluids and insulin immediately before, during, and after surgery when there is no oral intake. The type 2 diabetic patient who uses OAs is usually instructed to discontinue them 48 hours before surgery and is treated with insulin during the surgical period. The patient should understand that this is a temporary measure and is not to be interpreted as a worsening of diabetes.

The nurse caring for an unconscious surgical patient receiving insulin must be alert for hypoglycemic signs such as sweating, tachycardia, and tremors. Frequent monitoring of blood glucose will prevent episodes of severe hypoglycemia in this patient.

Ambulatory and Home Care. Successful management of diabetes requires ongoing interaction among the patient, the family,

and the health care team. It is important that a diabetes nurse educator be involved in the care of the patient and the family. This person provides expertise in many areas of specialized care needs.

Because diabetes is a complex, chronic condition, a great deal of patient contact takes place in outpatient and home settings. The major goal of patient care in these settings is to enable the patient or caregiver to reach an optimal level of independence in self-care activities. Unfortunately, many patients with diabetes face challenges in reaching these goals. Diabetes increases the risk for other chronic conditions that can affect self-care activities. These include visual impairment, lower extremity problems that affect mobility, and other functional limitations related to cerebrovascular disease. Therefore important nursing

TABLE 47-14 Criteria for Testing in Asymptomatic, Undiagnosed Individuals

Type 1 Diabetes Mellitus

Testing presumably healthy individuals for the presence of any immune markers (e.g., HLA), outside of a clinical trials setting, is not recommended.

Type 2 Diabetes Mellitus

In asymptomatic, undiagnosed individuals, testing for diabetes should be considered in all individuals at age 45 years and above and, if normal, it should be repeated at 3-year intervals.

Testing* should be considered at a younger age, or be carried out more frequently, in individuals who

- are overweight (body mass index [BMI] ≥25 kg/m²).
- have a first-degree relative with diabetes.
- are members of a high-risk ethnic population (African American, Hispanic, Native American, Asian American, Pacific Islander).
- have delivered a baby weighing >9 lb or were diagnosed with gestational diabetes mellitus.
- are hypertensive (≥140/90 mm Hg).
- have an HDL cholesterol level ≤35 mg/dl (0.90 mmol/L) and/or a triglyceride level ≥250 mg/dl (2.82 mmol/L).
- on previous testing, had impaired glucose tolerance or increased fasting glucose.

Adapted from American Diabetes Association Clinical Practice Recommendations.
*Testing may include fasting plasma glucose (FPG) or oral glucose tolerance test (OGTT). The FPG is the recommended diagnostic test because of its ease of administration, convenience, acceptability to patients, and lower cost.
HDL, High-density lipoprotein.

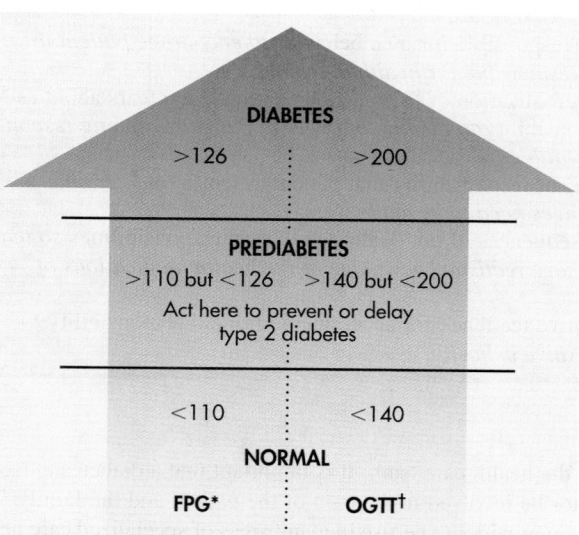

* The fasting plasma glucose (FPG) test: After an overnight fast, blood glucose is measured in the morning.

† The 2-hour oral glucose tolerance test (OGTT): Includes a fasting blood glucose test and glucose measurements 2 hours after drinking a glucose-containing solution.

Note: The American Diabetes Association and the National Institute of Diabetes and Digestive and Kidney Diseases believe either test is appropriate to measure prediabetes and diabetes.

FIG. 47-9 The glucose continuum. Numbers represent blood glucose levels in mg/dl.

functions are to assess the ability of patients and caregivers in such activities as SMBG and insulin injection techniques. Assistive devices for self-administration of insulin include syringe magnifiers, vial stabilizers, and dosing aids for the visually impaired. In some cases, the nurse will make referrals to others who can help the patient achieve the self-care goal. These may include an occupational therapist, a social worker, a home health aid, or a dietitian.

A diagnosis of diabetes affects the patient in many profound ways. Patients with diabetes must continually contend with lifestyle choices that affect the food they eat, the activity they engage in, and demands on their time and energy. In addition, they face the potential of becoming victim to the devastating complications of this disease. Careful assessment of what it means to the patient to have diabetes should be the starting point of patient teaching. The nurse can help patients make adjustments by displaying an attitude that is supportive and nonjudgmental. The goals of teaching should be mutually determined by the patient and the nurse based on individual needs, as well as therapeutic requirements.

The patient's support system must be identified. If this is the family, they need to be involved in teaching so they can care for the patient when self-care is no longer possible. The family and significant others need to be encouraged to provide emotional support and encouragement as the patient deals with the reality of living with a chronic disease.

Insulin therapy. Nursing responsibilities for the patient receiving insulin include proper administration, assessment of the

EVIDENCE-BASED PRACTICE

Self-Management Education of Type 2 Diabetes Mellitus

Clinical Problem

What is the effectiveness of diabetes self-management education in patients with type 2 diabetes mellitus?

Best Clinical Practice

- Self-management education in patients with type 2 diabetes mellitus is effective.
- Interventions involving active participation have been effective in improving diabetes knowledge, self-monitoring of blood glucose levels, self-reported dietary habits, and glycemic control.
- Interventions involving active patient participation are more effective than didactic interventions.

Implications for Nursing Practice

- The nurse needs to realize that patients need to be in control of their own health and encourage patients to assume this role.
- Knowledge can empower a person to take a central role in his or her own health care.
- Teaching should involve getting the patient actively involved in the learning process (see Chapter 4).

References for Evidence

Norris SL, Engelgau MM, Venkat Narayan KM: Effectiveness of self-management training in type 2 diabetes. A systematic review of randomized controlled trials, *Diabetes Care* 24:561, 2001.
Review: self-management training in type 2 diabetes mellitus is effective in the short term, *ACP Journal* 135:45, 2001.

patient's response to insulin therapy, and education of the patient regarding administration, adjustment to, and side effects of insulin (see Table 47-5). Table 47-6 lists guidelines for the nurse assessing a patient using glucose-lowering agents, including insulin and OAs.

Assessment of the patient who is new to insulin must include an evaluation of his or her ability to manage this therapy safely. This includes the ability to understand the interaction of insulin, diet, and activity and to be able to recognize and treat the symptoms of hypoglycemia appropriately. If the patient does not have the cognitive skills to do these things, another responsible person must be identified and trained. The patient or caregiver must also have the cognitive and manual skills needed to prepare and inject the insulin. If the patient or family lacks these, additional resources will be needed to assist the patient.

Many patients are fearful when they first begin using insulin. Some patients find it difficult to self-inject because they are afraid of needles or the pain associated with an injection. Some are afraid they will hurt themselves by giving too much or too little insulin. And in some cases, the patient believes that using insulin is a "last ditch" effort and that he or she is now in the final stages of the disease process. Therefore it is important to explore the patient's underlying fears before beginning the teaching.

Follow-up assessment of the patient who has been using insulin therapy includes an inspection of injection sites for signs of lipodystrophy and other reactions, review of insulin preparation and injection technique, a history pertaining to the occurrence of hypoglycemic episodes, and the patient's method for handling hypoglycemic episodes. A review of the patient's recorded blood glucose tests is also important in assessing overall glycemic control.

Oral agents. Nursing responsibilities for the patient taking OAs are similar to those for the patient taking insulin. Proper administration, assessment of the patient's use of and response to the OA, and education of the patient and the family about OAs are all part of the nurse's function.

The nurse's assessment can be extremely valuable in determining the most appropriate OA for a patient. Factors such as the patient's mental status, eating habits, home environment, attitude toward diabetes, and medication history all play a significant role in determining the most appropriate OA for the individual patient. For example, frail older adults who live alone are at high risk for severe hypoglycemia because low blood glucose is frequently undetected and/or untreated in this population. This is especially true if the patient has a short-term memory deficit. In these cases, an OA that does not cause hypoglycemia, or a shorter-acting OA, would be most appropriate.

Patient teaching is an essential nursing function when caring for the patient who uses OAs for blood glucose control. Some patients may assume that their diabetes is not a serious condition if they are taking only a pill for glycemic control. Therefore the patient should be instructed that these agents will help keep blood glucose controlled and will help prevent serious long- and short-term complications of diabetes. Patients should be instructed that OAs are used in addition to diet and activity as therapy for diabetes and that they should continue with their meal and activity plans. Patients should not take extra pills if overeating has occurred, unless specifically instructed to do so by their health care

provider. If the patient uses sulfonylureas, instructions should be given with regard to prevention, symptom recognition, and management of hypoglycemia.

The patient should also be instructed to contact a health care provider if periods of illness or extreme stress occur. During such a period, insulin therapy may be required to prevent or treat hyperglycemic symptoms and avoid an acute hyperglycemia emergency.

Personal hygiene. The potential for microvascular complications and infections requires diligent skin and dental hygiene practices on the part of the patient. Because of the susceptibility to periodontal disease, daily brushing and flossing should be encouraged in addition to regular visits to the dentist. When dental work must be done, the dentist should be informed that the patient has diabetes.

Routine care should include regular bathing, with particular emphasis given to foot care. Problems associated with the feet and lower extremities are presented later in this chapter. If cuts, scrapes, or burns occur, they should be treated promptly and monitored carefully. The area should be washed, and a nonabrasive or nonirritating antiseptic ointment may be applied. The area should be covered with a dry, sterile pad. If the injury does not begin to heal within 24 hours or if signs of infection develop, the health care provider should be notified immediately.

Medical identification and travel. The patient should be instructed to carry medical identification at all times indicating that he or she has diabetes. Police, paramedics, and many private citizens are aware of the need to look for this identification when working with sick or unconscious persons. Every person with diabetes should wear a medical alert bracelet or necklace. An identification card (Fig. 47-10) can supply valuable information, such as the name of the health care provider and the type and dose of insulin or OA.

Travel for a patient with diabetes requires advance planning. The patient should have a full set of diabetes care supplies in the carry-on luggage when traveling by plane, train, or bus. This includes blood glucose monitoring equipment, insulin, and syringes. When syringes and lancing devices are carried onto a

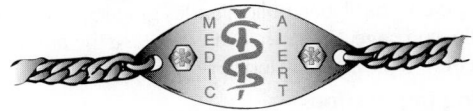

FIG. 47-10 Medical alerts. A patient with diabetes should carry a card and wear a bracelet or necklace that indicates diabetes. If the patient with diabetes is unconscious, these measures will ensure prompt and appropriate attention.

commercial airliner, a letter from the prescribing health care provider indicating medical necessity may prevent delays at security checkpoints. For patients who use insulin or an OA that can cause hypoglycemia, snack items and a quick-acting carbohydrate source for treating hypoglycemia should be included in the carry-on luggage. Extra insulin should be available in case a bottle breaks or gets lost. In addition, the patient should carry a full day's supply of food in the event of cancelled flights, delayed meals, or closed restaurants. If the patient is planning a trip out of the country, it is wise to have a letter from the health care provider explaining that the patient has diabetes and requires all the materials, particularly syringes, for ongoing health care.

Some travel involves time changes such as traveling coast to coast or across the International Date Line. The patient should contact the health care provider to plan an appropriate insulin schedule. Many patients find it easier and more predictable to take only regular insulin every 4 to 6 hours to cover insulin needs while on long airplane trips instead of trying to anticipate the peak of intermediate insulin and the availability of meals. During travel, most patients find it helpful to keep watches set to the time of the city of origin until they reach their destination. The key to travel when taking insulin is to know the type of insulin being taken, its onset of action, the anticipated peak time, and meal times.

Patient and family teaching. The goals of diabetes self-management education are to enable the patient to become the most active participant in his or her care, while matching level of self-management to the ability of the individual patient. Patients who actively manage their diabetes care have better outcomes than those who do not. For this reason, an educational approach that facilitates informed decision making on the part of the patient is widely advocated. Sometimes this is referred to as the *empowerment approach* to education.

Unfortunately, patients can encounter a variety of physical, psychologic, and emotional barriers when it comes to effectively managing their diabetes. These barriers may include feelings of inadequacy about one's own abilities, unwillingness to make the necessary behavioral changes, ineffective coping strategies, and cognitive deficits. If the patient is not able to manage the disease, a family member may be able to assume part of this role. If the patient or the family cannot

make decisions related to diabetes management, the nurse may refer the patient to a social worker or other resources within the community. These resources can assist the patient and the family in outlining a feasible treatment program that meets their capabilities. Patient and health care provider resources are listed at the end of this chapter.

An assessment of the patient's knowledge of diabetes and lifestyle preferences is useful in planning a teaching program. Table 47-15 presents guidelines to use for patient teaching. The nurse should assess the patient's knowledge base frequently so that gaps in knowledge or incorrect or inaccurate ideas can be quickly corrected.

The ADA and the American Association of Diabetes Educators offer pamphlets, booklets, and a bimonthly magazine called *Diabetes Forecast.* Affiliates of the ADA are located in all states and most can be reached by dialing 1-800-DIABETES. The ADA also publishes materials and sponsors conferences for health care professionals concerned with diabetes education, research, and management of patients. This organization also gives recognition to education programs that meet the national standards of diabetes education and can provide a list of these programs. Drug companies manufacturing diabetes-related products also have free educational materials for patients and health care providers.

■ Evaluation

The expected outcomes for the patient with diabetes mellitus are addressed in NCP 47-1.

Acute Complications of Diabetes Mellitus

The acute complications of diabetes mellitus arise from events associated with hyperglycemia and insufficient insulin. A problem that may arise from too much insulin or an excessive dose of an OA is *hypoglycemia* (also referred to as *insulin reaction* or *low blood glucose*). It is important for the health care provider to be able to distinguish between hyperglycemia and hypoglycemia because hypoglycemia worsens rapidly and constitutes a serious threat if action is not immediately taken. Table 47-16 compares the manifestations, causes, management, and prevention of hyperglycemia and hypoglycemia.

DIABETIC KETOACIDOIS

Etiology and Pathophysiology

Diabetic ketoacidosis (DKA), also referred to as *diabetic acidosis* and *diabetic coma*, is caused by a profound deficiency of insulin and is characterized by hyperglycemia, ketosis, acidosis, and dehydration. It is most likely to occur in people with type 1 diabetes but may be seen in type 2 in conditions of severe illness or stress when the pancreas cannot meet the extra demand for insulin. Precipitating factors include illness and infection, inadequate insulin dosage, undiagnosed type 1 diabetes, poor self-management, and neglect.

When the circulating supply of insulin is insufficient, glucose cannot be properly used for energy so that the body breaks down fat stores as a secondary source of fuel (Fig. 47-11). Ketones are acidic by-products of fat metabolism that can cause serious prob-

---

COMPLEMENTARY & ALTERNATIVE THERAPIES
Herbs That Affect Glucose Levels

Effects
Herbs can affect glycemic control. Herbs that can increase the antidiabetic effect of medications (i.e., lower blood glucose) include bay, basil, bee pollen, garlic, ginger, ginseng, milk thistle, and sage. Herbs that can decrease the antidiabetic effect of medications include St. John's wort.

Nursing Implications
It is very important that patients with diabetes consult with their health care provider before using herbs or nutritional supplements. Patients who use herbs should monitor their blood glucose levels carefully and regularly.

TABLE 47-15	Patient & Family Teaching Guide

General Guidelines for Management of Diabetes Mellitus

	DO	DON'T
Blood glucose	• Monitor your blood glucose at home and record results in a log. • Take your insulin or OA as prescribed. • Obtain a hemoglobin A1C blood test every 3-6 mo as an indicator of your long-term blood glucose control. • Carry some form of glucose at all times so you can treat hypoglycemia quickly. • Instruct family members in the use of glucagon administration in the case of emergencies due to hypoglycemia.	• Skip doses of your insulin, especially when you are sick. • Run out of insulin. • Enroll in a fad diet. • Rub the area where insulin was administered.
Exercise	• Learn how exercise and food affect your blood glucose levels. • Begin a medically supervised exercise program.	• Forget that exercise will lower your blood glucose level. • Exercise if your blood glucose levels are very elevated. This may lead to a temporary worsening of your blood glucose levels.
Diet	• Follow your diet, eating regular meals at regular times. • Eat slowly and chew food thoroughly. • Choose foods low in saturated fats. • Limit the amount of alcohol you drink. • Learn your cholesterol level.	• Drink excessive amounts of alcohol because this may lead to unpredictable low blood glucose reactions. • Eat fried foods.
Other guidelines	• Obtain an annual eye examination by an ophthalmologist. • Obtain annual urine testing for protein. • Examine your feet at home. • Wear comfortable, well-fitting shoes to help prevent foot injury. Break in new shoes gradually. • Always carry identification that says you have diabetes. • Have other medical problems treated, especially high blood pressure. • Know the symptoms of hypoglycemia and hyperglycemia. • Quit smoking.	• Smoke. • Apply hot or cold directly to your feet. • Go barefoot. • Ignore the symptoms of hypoglycemia and hyperglycemia. • Put baby oil or lotion between your toes.

OA, Oral agent.

lems when they become excessive in the blood. Ketosis alters the pH balance, causing metabolic acidosis to develop. Ketonuria is a process that begins when ketone bodies are excreted in the urine. During this process, electrolytes become depleted as cations are eliminated along with the anionic ketones in an attempt to maintain electrical neutrality.

Insulin deficiency impairs protein synthesis and causes excessive protein degradation. This results in nitrogen losses from the tissues. Insulin deficiency also stimulates the production of glucose from amino acids (from proteins) in the liver and leads to further hyperglycemia. But because there is a deficiency of insulin, the additional glucose cannot be used and the blood glucose level rises further, adding to the osmotic diuresis. Untreated, this leads to severe depletion of sodium, potassium, chloride, magnesium, and phosphate. Vomiting caused by the acidosis results in more fluid and electrolyte losses. Eventually, hypovolemia followed by shock will ensue.

Renal failure may eventually occur from hypovolemic shock. This causes the retention of ketones and glucose, and the acidosis progresses. Untreated, the patient becomes comatose as a result of dehydration, electrolyte imbalance, and acidosis. If the condition is not treated, death is inevitable.

Clinical Manifestations

Signs and symptoms of DKA include manifestations of dehydration such as poor skin turgor, dry mucous membranes, tachycardia, and orthostatic hypotension. Early symptoms may include lethargy and weakness. As the patient becomes severely dehydrated, the skin becomes dry and loose, and the eyeballs become soft and sunken. Abdominal pain is another symptom of DKA that may be accompanied by anorexia and vomiting. Finally, Kussmaul respirations (rapid, deep breathing associated with dyspnea) are the body's attempt to reverse metabolic acidosis through the exhalation of excess carbon dioxide. Acetone is noted on the breath as a sweet, fruity odor. (See Chapter 16 for a discussion of respiratory compensation of metabolic acidosis.) Laboratory findings include a blood glucose level above 250 mg/dl, arterial blood pH below 7.35, serum bicarbonate level less than 15 mEq/L, and ketones in the blood and urine.[21]

Collaborative Care

Before the advent of self-monitoring of blood glucose, patients with DKA required hospitalization for treatment. Today, hospitalization may not be required. In instances where fluid and

TABLE 47-16 Comparison of Hyperglycemia and Hypoglycemia

HYPERGLYCEMIA	HYPOGLYCEMIA	HYPERGLYCEMIA	HYPOGLYCEMIA
Manifestations*		**Treatment**	
Elevated blood glucose†	Blood glucose <50 mg/dl (2.8 mmol/L)	Physician's attention	Immediate ingestion of 5-20 g of simple carbohydrates
Increase in urination	Cold, clammy skin	Continuance of diabetes medication as ordered	Ingestion of another 5-20 g of simple carbohydrates in 15 min if no relief obtained
Increase in appetite followed by lack of appetite	Numbness of fingers, toes, mouth	Frequent checking of blood and urine specimens and recording of results	Contacting of physician if no relief obtained
Weakness, fatigue	Rapid heartbeat		
Blurred vision	Emotional changes	Hourly drinking of fluids	Discussion with physician about medication dosage
Headache	Headache		
Glycosuria	Nervousness, tremors		
Nausea and vomiting	Faintness, dizziness		
Abdominal cramps	Unsteady gait, slurred speech	**Preventive Measures**	
Progression to DKA or HHNS	Hunger	Taking prescribed dose of medication at proper time	Taking prescribed dose of medication at proper time
	Changes in vision		Accurate administration of insulin/OA
	Seizures, coma	Accurate administration of insulin/OA	
Causes		Maintenance of diet	Ingestion of all ordered diet foods at proper time
Too much food	Alcohol intake without food	Maintenance of good personal hygiene	Provision of compensation for exercise
Too little or no diabetes medication	Too little food—delayed, omitted, inadequate intake	Adherence to sick-day rules when ill	Ability to recognize and know symptoms and treat them immediately
Inactivity	Too much diabetic medication	Checking of blood for glucose as ordered	Carrying of simple carbohydrates
Emotional, physical stress	Too much exercise without compensation	Contacting of physician regarding ketonuria	Education of friends, family, fellow employees about symptoms and treatment
Poor absorption of insulin	Diabetes medication or food taken at wrong time	Wearing of diabetic identification	Checking blood glucose as ordered
	Loss of weight without change in medication		Wearing medical alert (diabetic) identification
	Use of β-adrenergic blockers interfering with recognition of symptoms		

*There is usually a gradual onset of symptoms in hyperglycemia and a rapid onset in hypoglycemia.
†Specific clinical manifestations related to elevated levels of blood glucose vary according to the patient.
DKA, Diabetic ketoacidosis; *HHNS,* hyperosmolar hyperglycemic nonketotic syndrome; *OA,* oral agent.

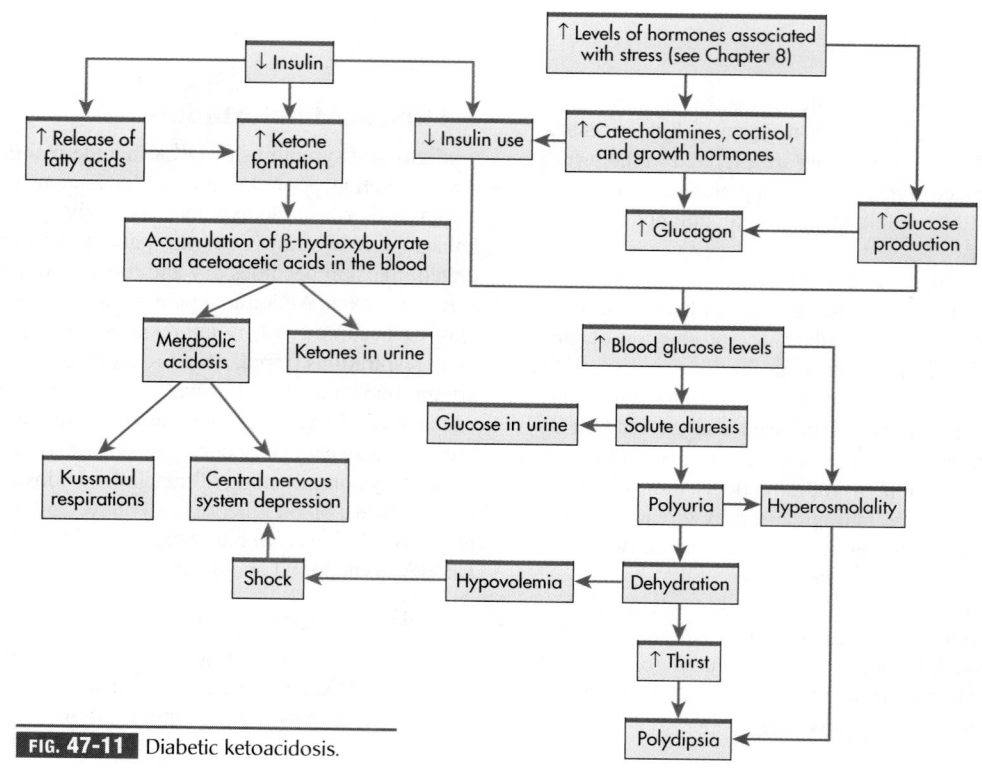

FIG. 47-11 Diabetic ketoacidosis.

electrolyte imbalances are not severe and blood glucose levels can be safely monitored at home, less severe forms of DKA may be managed on an outpatient basis (Table 47-17). However, other factors must be considered as to the location of where the patient is managed. These include the presence of fever, nausea, vomiting, and diarrhea; altered mental status; nature of the cause of the ketoacidosis; and availability of frequent communication with the health care provider (every few hours).

TABLE **47-17**

*C*ollaborative Care

Diabetic Ketoacidosis (DKA) and Hyperosmolar Hyperglycemic Nonketotic Syndrome (HHNS)

Diagnostic
History and physical examination
Blood studies, including immediate blood glucose, complete blood count, ketones, pH, electrolytes, blood urea nitrogen, arterial blood gases
Urinalysis, including specific gravity, pH, glucose, acetone

Collaborative Therapy
Intravenous administration of rapid-acting insulin
Administration of intravenous fluids
Electrolyte replacement
Assessment of mental status
Recording of intake and output
Central venous pressure monitoring (if indicated)
Assessment of blood glucose levels
Assessment of blood and urine for ketones
ECG monitoring
Assessment of cardiovascular and respiratory status

ECG, Electrocardiogram.

Regardless of the setting in which it occurs, DKA is a serious condition that proceeds rapidly and must be treated promptly. (See Table 47-18 for the emergency management of a patient with DKA.) Because fluid imbalance is potentially life threatening, the initial goal of therapy is to establish intravenous access and begin fluid and electrolyte replacement. Typically, an infusion of 0.45% or 0.9% NaCl at a rate to restore urine output to 30 to 60 ml/hr and to raise blood pressure constitutes the initial fluid therapy regimen. When blood glucose levels approach 250 mg/dl (13.9 mmol/L), 5% dextrose is added to the fluid regimen to prevent hypoglycemia.[22]

The aim of fluid and electrolyte therapy is to replace extracellular and intracellular water and to correct deficits of sodium, chloride, bicarbonate, potassium, phosphate, magnesium, and nitrogen. Early potassium replacement is essential because hypokalemia is a significant cause of unnecessary and avoidable death during treatment of DKA. Although initial serum potassium may be normal or high, levels can rapidly decrease once therapy starts as insulin drives potassium into the cells, leading to life-threatening hypokalemia.

IV insulin administration is therapy directed toward correcting hyperglycemia and hyperketonemia. Insulin therapy is withheld until fluid resuscitation is underway, because insulin allows water to enter the cell along with glucose and can lead to a depletion of vascular volume. Initially a bolus of insulin is delivered, followed by a continuous infusion.

HYPEROSMOLAR HYPERGLYCEMIC NONKETOTIC SYNDROME

Hyperosmolar hyperglycemic nonketotic syndrome (HHNS) is a life-threatening syndrome than can occur in the patient with diabetes who is able to produce enough insulin to prevent DKA but not enough to prevent severe hyperglycemia, osmotic diuresis, and extracellular fluid depletion (Fig. 47-12). The main difference be-

TABLE **47-18**

*E*mergency Management

Diabetic Ketoacidosis

ETIOLOGY	ASSESSMENT FINDINGS	INTERVENTIONS
• Undiagnosed diabetes mellitus • Inadequate treatment of existing diabetes mellitus • Insulin not taken as presribed • Infection • Change in diet, insulin, or exercise regimen	• Dry mouth • Thirst • Abdominal pain • Nausea and vomiting • Gradually increasing restlessness, confusion, lethargy • Flushed, dry skin • Eyes appear sunken • Breath odor of ketones • Rapid, weak pulse • Labored breathing (Kussmaul respirations) • Fever • Urinary frequency • Serum glucose >300 mg/dl (16.7 mmol/L) • Glucosuria and ketonuria	**Initial** • Ensure patent airway. • Administer oxygen via nasal cannula or non-rebreather mask. • Establish IV access with large-bore catheter. • Begin fluid resuscitation with 0.9% NaCl solution 1 L/hr until BP stabilized and urine output 30-60 ml/hr. • Begin continuous regular insulin drip 0.1 U/kg/hr. • Identify history of diabetes, time of last food, and time/amount of last insulin injection. **Ongoing Monitoring** • Monitor vital signs, level of consciousness, cardiac rhythm, oxygen saturation, and urine output. • Assess breath sounds for fluid overload. • Monitor serum glucose and serum potassium. • Administer potassium to correct hypokalemia. • Administer sodium bicarbonate if severe acidosis (pH <7.0).

BP, Blood pressure; IV, intravenous.

tween HHNS and DKA is that the patient with HHNS usually has enough circulating insulin so that ketoacidosis does not occur. Because HHNS produces fewer symptoms in the earlier stages, blood glucose levels can climb quite high before the problem is recognized. The higher blood glucose levels increase serum osmolality and produce more severe neurologic manifestations, such as somnolence, coma, seizures, hemiparesis, and aphasia. HHNS often occurs in the older adult patient with type 2 diabetes and is often related to impaired thirst sensation and/or a functional inability to replace fluids. There is usually a history of inadequate fluid intake, increasing mental depression, and polyuria. Laboratory values in HHNS include blood glucose greater than 400 mg/dl and a marked increase in serum osmolality. Ketone bodies are absent or minimal in both blood and urine.

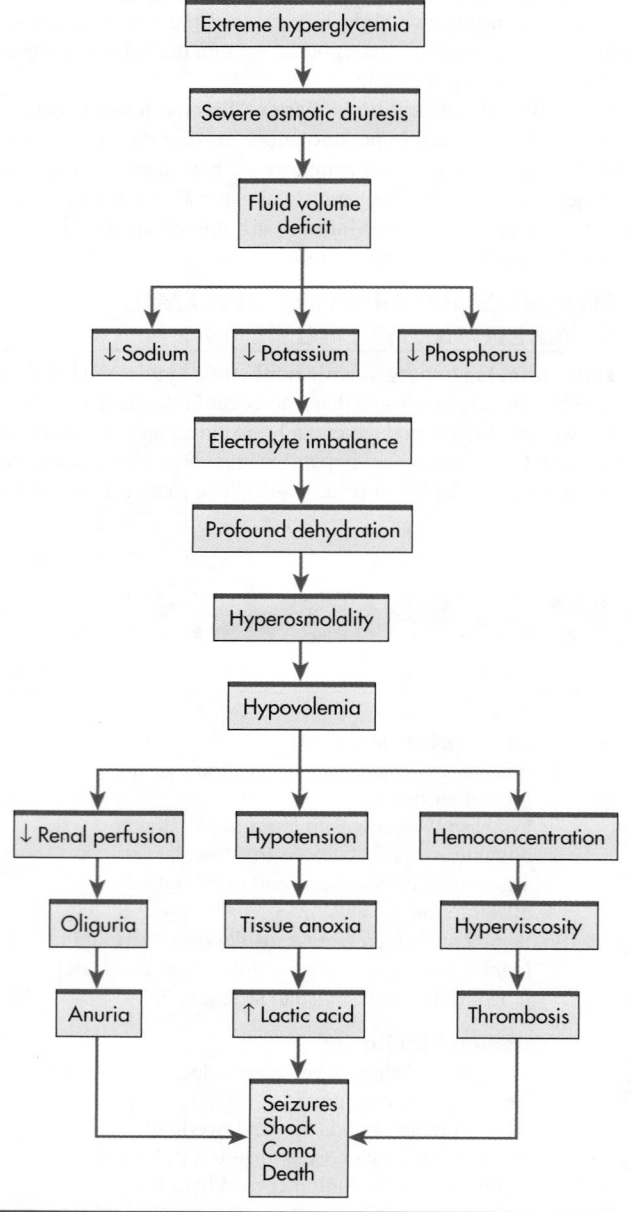

FIG. 47-12 Pathophysiology of hyperosmolar hyperglycemic nonketotic syndrome (HHNS).

Collaborative Care

HHNS constitutes a medical emergency and has a high mortality rate. Therapy is similar to that for the treatment of DKA and includes immediate IV administration of either 0.9% or 0.45% NaCl at a rate that is dependent on cardiac status and the degree of fluid volume deficit. Regular insulin is given by IV bolus, followed by an infusion after fluid replacement therapy is instituted to aid in reducing the hyperglycemia. When blood glucose levels fall to approximately 250 mg/dl (13.9 mmol/L), IV fluids containing glucose are administered to prevent hypoglycemia. Electrolytes are monitored and replaced as needed. Hypokalemia is not as significant in HHNS as it is in DKA, although fluid losses may result in milder potassium deficits that require replacement. Vital signs, intake and output, tissue turgor, laboratory values, and cardiac monitoring are assessed to monitor the efficacy of fluid and electrolyte replacement. Patients with renal or cardiac compromise require special monitoring to avoid fluid overload during fluid replacement. This includes monitoring of serum osmolality and frequent assessment of cardiac, renal, and mental status.

The management for both DKA and HHNS is similar, except that HHNS requires greater fluid replacement (see Table 47-17). Once the patient is stabilized, attempts to detect and correct the underlying precipitating cause should be initiated.

NURSING MANAGEMENT
DIABETIC KETOACIDOSIS AND HYPEROSMOLAR HYPERGLYCEMIC NONKETOTIC SYNDROME

When hospitalized, the patient is closely monitored with appropriate blood and urine tests. The nurse is responsible for monitoring blood glucose and urine for output and ketones, as well as using laboratory data to direct care.

Areas that must be monitored are administration of IV fluids to correct dehydration, administration of insulin therapy to reduce blood glucose and serum acetone, administration of electrolytes to correct electrolyte imbalance, assessment of renal status, assessment of the cardiopulmonary status related to hydration and electrolyte levels, and monitoring of the level of consciousness.

The nurse must also monitor the signs of potassium imbalance resulting from hypoinsulinemia and osmotic diuresis (see Chapter 16). When treatment for hyperglycemia is begun with insulin, serum potassium levels may decrease rapidly as potassium moves into the cells once insulin becomes available. This movement of potassium into and out of extracellular fluid influences cardiac functioning. Cardiac monitoring is a useful aid in detecting hyperkalemia and hypokalemia because characteristic changes indicating potassium excess or deficit are observable on ECG tracings (see Chapter 16, Fig. 16-14). Vital signs should be assessed often to determine the presence of fever, hypovolemic shock, tachycardia, and Kussmaul breathing.

HYPOGLYCEMIA

Hypoglycemia, or low blood glucose, occurs when there is too much insulin in proportion to available glucose in the blood. This causes the blood glucose level to drop to less than 70 mg/dl (3.9 mmol/L). Because the brain requires a constant supply of glucose in sufficient quantities to function properly, hypoglycemia can affect mental functioning. Common manifestations of hypoglycemia include confusion, irritability, diaphoresis, tremors, hunger, weakness, and visual disturbances. Manifestations of hypoglycemia can mimic alcohol intoxication. Untreated hypoglycemia can progress to loss of consciousness, seizures, coma, and death.

Hypoglycemic unawareness is a condition in which a person does not experience the warning signs and symptoms of hypoglycemia, increasing his or her risk for dangerously low blood glucose levels. This is often related to autonomic neuropathy of diabetes that interferes with the secretion of counterregulatory hormones that produce these symptoms. Elderly patients and patients who use β-adrenergic blockers are also at risk for hypoglycemic unawareness. It is usually not safe for patients with risk factors for hypoglycemic unawareness to aim for tight blood glucose control, because a major drawback of intensive treatment is hypoglycemia. These patients are usually managed with blood glucose goals that are somewhat higher than patients who are able to detect and manage the onset of hypoglycemia.

Hypoglycemic symptoms may occur when a very high blood glucose level falls too rapidly (e.g., a blood glucose level of 300 mg/dl [16.7 mmol/L] falling quickly to 180 mg/dl [10 mmol/L]). Although the blood glucose level is above normal by definition and measurement, the sudden metabolic shift can evoke hypoglycemic symptoms. Too vigorous management of hyperglycemia with insulin can induce this type of situation.

Causes of hypoglycemia are often related to a mismatch in the timing of food intake and the peak action of insulin or oral hypoglycemic agents that increase endogenous insulin secretion. The balance between blood glucose and insulin can be disrupted by the administration of too much insulin or medication, the ingestion of too little food, delaying the time of eating, and performing unusual amounts of exercise. Insulin reactions can occur at any time, but most reactions occur when the OA or insulin is at its peak of action or when the patient's daily routine is disrupted without adequate adjustments in diet, medications, and activity. Although hypoglycemia is more common with insulin therapy, it can occur with OAs and may be severe and persist for an extended time because of the longer duration of action.

NURSING and COLLABORATIVE MANAGEMENT
HYPOGLYCEMIA

With effective treatment, hypoglycemia can usually be quickly reversed. At the first sign of hypoglycemia, the blood glucose should be checked if possible (Table 47-19). If it is below 70 mg/dl (3.9 mmol/L), the patient should immediately begin treatment for hypoglycemia. If the blood glucose is above 70 mg/dl (3.9 mmol/L), other causes of the signs and symptoms should be investigated. If the patient has manifestations of hypoglycemia and monitoring equipment is not available, hypoglycemia should be assumed and treatment should be initiated.

Hypoglycemia is treated by ingesting 10 to 15 g of a simple (fast-acting) carbohydrate, such as 4 to 8 oz of fruit juice or regular (non-diet) soft drink or 8 oz of low-fat milk. Commercial products such as gels or tablets containing specific amounts of glucose are convenient for carrying in a purse or pocket to be used in such situations.

TABLE 47-19	Collaborative Care: Hypoglycemia

Diagnostic
Stat blood glucose
History (if possible) and physical examination

Collaborative Therapy
Determination of cause of hypoglycemia (after correction of condition)

Conscious Patient
Administration of 15-20 g of quick-acting carbohydrate (e.g., 6-8 oz of regular soda, 8-10 LifeSavers, 1 tb syrup or honey, 4 tsp jelly, 4-6 oz orange juice, 8 oz low-fat milk, commercial dextrose products [per label instructions])
Repetition of treatment in 15 min (if no improvement)
Administration of additional food of longer-acting carbohydrate (e.g., slice of bread, crackers) after symptoms subside
Immediate notification of health care provider or emergency service (if patient outside hospital) if symptoms do not subside after two to three administrations of quick-acting carbohydrate

Worsening Symptoms or Unconscious Patient
Subcutaneous or intramuscular injection of 1 mg glucagon
Intravenous administration of 50 ml 50% glucose

Treatment with sweet foods that also contain fat, such as candy bars, cookies, and ice cream, should be avoided because the fat in them will slow down the absorption of the sugar and delay the response to treatment. Overtreatment with large quantities of quick-acting carbohydrates should also be avoided so that a rapid fluctuation to hyperglycemia does not occur. A prompt but moderate approach is best. Blood glucose should be checked about 15 minutes following the initial treatment for hypoglycemia, and treatment should be repeated if the blood glucose remains below 70 mg/dl (3.9 mmol/L). Once the blood glucose is greater than 70 mg/dl (3.9 mmol/L), the patient should eat the regularly scheduled meal or a snack to prevent hypoglycemia from recurring. Good snacks include peanut butter and cheese and crackers. Blood glucose should also be checked again about 45 minutes after treatment to ensure that hypoglycemia is not recurring.

If there is no significant improvement in the patient's condition after two to three doses of 10 to 15 g of simple carbohydrate, or if the patient is not alert enough to swallow, 1 mg of glucagon may be administered by intramuscular (IM) or SQ injection. An IM injection in a site such as the deltoid muscle will result in a quicker response. Glucagon stimulates a strong hepatic response to convert glycogen to glucose and therefore makes glucose rapidly available. Rebound hypoglycemia is a potential adverse effect of glucagon. Having the patient ingest a complex carbohydrate after recovery may prevent this from happening.

Once the acute hypoglycemia has been reversed, the nurse should explore with the patient the reasons why the situation developed. This assessment may indicate the need for additional education of the patient and the family to avoid future episodes of hypoglycemia. The danger of hypoglycemic reactions must be stressed because memory and learning impairment can result from repeated episodes of severe hypoglycemia.

Chronic Complications of Diabetes Mellitus

Chronic complications of diabetes are primarily those of end-organ disease that result from damage to the large and small blood vessels from chronic hyperglycemia. Several theories exist as to how and why chronic hyperglycemia damages cells and tissues. Possible causes include (1) the accumulation of damaging by-products of glucose metabolism, such as sorbitol, which is associated with damage to nerve cells; (2) the formation of abnormal glucose molecules in the basement membrane of small blood vessels such as those that circulate to the eye and kidney; and (3) a derangement in red blood cell function that leads to a decrease in oxygenation to the tissues.

The Diabetes Control and Complication Trial (DCCT) was a landmark study that has greatly influenced diabetes management since its results were announced in 1993.[23] This study demonstrated that in patients with type 1 diabetes the risk for microvascular complications could be significantly reduced by keeping blood glucose levels as near to normal as possible for as much of the time as possible (tight glucose control). In this study, patients were randomly assigned to one of two groups: intensive or standard treatment. The intensive treatment group took three or more insulin injections a day or used an insulin pump. The patients in the standard treatment group took one to two injections a day and tested their blood glucose once or twice a day. The average A1C in the intensive treatment group was 7.2% and in the standard treatment group was 9%. (The normal range for A1C in a person without diabetes is 4.0% to 6.05%.)

In addition, the results found that the subjects in the intensive therapy group reduced their risk for the development of retinopathy and nephropathy. The main adverse effect associated with intensive therapy was an increase in cases of severe hypoglycemia.

Based on the findings of the DCCT, the ADA issued recommendations for the management of diabetes that included treatment goals to maintain blood glucose levels as near to normal as possible. Specific targets for individual patients must take into account the risk for severe or undetected hypoglycemia as a side effect of tight glucose control.

More recently, the United Kingdom Prospective Diabetes Study (UKPDS) demonstrated that intensive treatment of type 2 diabetes can also significantly lower the risk for developing diabetes-related eye, kidney, and neurologic problems. The findings from this study included a 25% reduction of microvascular disease in subjects who maintained long-term glycemic control.[24]

Because of the devastating effects of long-term complications, patients with diabetes require scheduled and ongoing monitoring for the detection and prevention of chronic complications.[25] The ADA recommendations for ongoing evaluation are listed in Table 47-20. It is imperative that patients understand the importance of participating in regular follow-up examinations.

ANGIOPATHY

Angiopathy, or blood vessel disease, is estimated to account for the majority of deaths among patients with diabetes. These chronic blood vessel dysfunctions are divided into two categories: macrovascular complications and microvascular complications.

Macrovascular Complications

Macrovascular complications are diseases of the large and medium-sized blood vessels that occur with greater frequency and with an earlier onset in people with diabetes. Although atherosclerotic plaque formation is believed to have a genetic origin, its development seems to be promoted by the altered lipid metabolism common to diabetes. Tight glucose control may help delay the atherosclerotic process.[23] Macrovascular diseases include cerebrovascular, cardiovascular, and peripheral vascular disease. Although genetic makeup cannot be altered, a patient with diabetes can diminish other risk factors associated with macroangiopathy, such as obesity, smoking, hypertension, high fat intake, and sedentary lifestyle. Smoking, which is detrimental to health in general, is especially injurious to people with diabetes. Smoking significantly increases the risk for blood vessel disease in people with diabetes and increases the risk for cardiovascular disease, stroke, and lower extremity amputation.

Insulin resistance seems to play an important role in the development of cardiovascular disease and is implicated in the pathogenesis of essential hypertension and dyslipidemia. The term *insulin resistance syndrome* is applied to the clinical associ-

---

TABLE 47-20   Prevention, Detection, and Monitoring of Long-Term Complications of Diabetes Mellitus*

COMPLICATION	TYPE OF EXAMINATION	FREQUENCY
Retinopathy	• Funduscopic–dilated eye examination	• Annually
Nephropathy	• Urinalysis for microalbuminuria	• Annually
Neuropathy (foot and lower extremities)	• Visual examination of foot	• Daily by patient; every visit by health care provider
	• Comprehensive foot examination: —Visual examination —Sensory examination with monofilament and tuning fork —Palpation (pulses, temperature, callus formation)	• Annually
Cardiovascular disease	• Blood pressure	• Every visit
	• Lipid panel	• Annually
	• Exercise stress testing (may include stress ECG, stress echocardiogram, perfusion imaging)	• As needed based on risk factors

ECG, Electrocardiogram.
*Based on the recommendations of the American Diabetes Association.

ation of insulin resistance, hypertension, and increased very-low-density lipoprotein (VLDL) and decreased high-density lipoprotein (HDL) cholesterol concentrations. The role of insulin resistance in the pathogenesis of cardiovascular disease is not well understood, but it seems to combine with dyslipidemia in contributing to greater risk of cardiovascular disease in patients with diabetes mellitus.[22] All patients with diabetes should be screened for dyslipidemia at the time diabetes is diagnosed. These abnormalities typically include an elevated triglyceride level and reduced HDL cholesterol.

Microvascular Complications

Microvascular complications result from thickening of the vessel membranes in the capillaries and arterioles in response to conditions of chronic hyperglycemia. They differ from the macrovascular complications in that they are specific to diabetes. Although microangiopathy can be found throughout the body, the areas most noticeably affected are the eyes (retinopathy), the kidneys (nephropathy), and the skin (dermopathy). Thickening of the basement membrane has been found in some persons with diabetes before or at the time of diagnosis or before the onset of symptoms of diabetes mellitus. However, clinical manifestations usually do not appear until 10 to 20 years after the onset of diabetes.

DIABETIC RETINOPATHY

Etiology and Pathophysiology

Diabetic retinopathy refers to the process of microvascular damage to the retina as a result of chronic hyperglycemia in patients with diabetes. After 15 years with diabetes mellitus, nearly all patients with type 1 diabetes and 80% with type 2 diabetes will have some degree of retinal disease. Diabetic retinopathy is estimated to be the most common cause of new cases of blindness in people ages 20 to 74 years.[26]

Retinopathy can be classified as nonproliferative or proliferative. In *nonproliferative retinopathy,* the most common form, partial occlusion of the small blood vessels in the retina causes the development of microaneurysms in the capillary walls. The walls of these microaneurysms are so weak that capillary fluid leaks out, causing retinal edema and eventually hard exudates or intraretinal hemorrhages. Vision may be affected if the macula is involved.

Proliferative retinopathy, the most severe form, involves the retina and the vitreous. When retinal capillaries become occluded, the body compensates by forming new blood vessels to supply the retina with blood, a pathologic process known as *neovascularization.* These new vessels are extremely fragile and hemorrhage easily, producing vitreous contraction. Eventually light is prevented from reaching the retina as the vessels become torn and bleed into the vitreous cavity. The patient sees black or red spots or lines. If these new blood vessels pull the retina while the vitreous contracts, causing a tear, partial or complete retinal detachment will occur. If the macula is involved, vision is lost. Without treatment, more than half of patients with proliferative diabetic retinopathy will be blind.

Collaborative Care

The earliest and most treatable stages of diabetic retinopathy often produce no changes in the vision. Because of this, the patient with diabetes must have regular dilated eye examinations by an ophthalmologist or a specially trained optometrist for early detection and treatment.

The most common forms of treatment for diabetic retinopathy are early photocoagulation of the retina, cryotherapy (cryoprexy), and vitrectomy. Photocoagulation by laser destroys the ischemic areas of the retina that produce growth factors that encourage neovascularization.[27] (Photocoagulation is discussed in Chapter 21.)

Cryotherapy (cryoprexy) is sometimes used to treat peripheral areas of the retina that cannot be reached with lasers or when retinal hemorrhage prevents complete photocoagulation. In this procedure, topical anesthesia is used so that a cryoprobe can be placed directly on the surface of the eye. When the probe is properly located, its tip creates a frozen area that extends through the external tissue through the eyeball until it reaches a specific point on the retina. Multiple points on the retina can be treated in this way. (Cryotherapy is discussed in Chapter 21.)

Vitrectomy is the aspiration of blood, membrane, and fibers from the inside of the eye through a small incision just behind the cornea. Vitrectomy is indicated when there is vitreal hemorrhage that does not clear in 6 months or when there is threatened or actual retinal detachment. (Vitrectomy is discussed in Chapter 21.)

Persons with diabetes are also prone to other visual problems. Glaucoma occurs as a result of the occlusion of the outflow channels secondary to neovascularization. This type of glaucoma is difficult to treat and often results in blindness. Cataracts develop at an earlier age and progress more rapidly in people with diabetes.

NEPHROPATHY

Diabetic nephropathy is a microvascular complication associated with damage to the small blood vessels that supply the glomeruli of the kidney. It is the leading cause of end-stage renal disease (ESRD) in the United States. The risk of nephropathy is about the same in patients with either type 1 or type 2 diabetes. Risk factors for the development of diabetic nephropathy include hypertension, genetic predisposition, smoking, and chronic hyperglycemia. Results of the DCCT and UKPDS studies have demonstrated that kidney disease can be significantly reduced when near-normal blood glucose control is achieved and maintained.[11,24]

Hypertension significantly accelerates the progression of diabetic nephropathy. Therefore aggressive blood pressure management is indicated for all patients with diabetes. Angiotensin-converting enzyme (ACE) inhibitor drugs (e.g., lisinopril [Prinivil, Zestril]) are commonly prescribed to patients with diabetes because they are effective blood pressure–lowering agents with few side effects. In addition, ACE inhibitors are often prescribed to patients with diabetes even when they are not hypertensive. This is because drugs in this class have a protective effect on the kidney that prevents the progression of diabetic nephropathy independent of hypertension control.[28] Angiotensin II receptor antagonists (e.g., losartan [Cozaar]) may also be used for their kidney-protective benefits. (See Chapter 32 for a discussion of hypertension and Chapter 45 for a discussion of renal failure.)

Standards for the prevention and detection of nephropathy in patients with diabetes include yearly screening for the presence of microalbuminuria (MAU) in the urine. This test detects kidney damage at an earlier stage than the standard dipstick test for urine protein. The presence of protein in the urine as detected by MAU urinalysis should be followed with an albumin/creatinine ratio or 24-hour urine collection for determination of creatinine clearance and serum creatinine.

NEUROPATHY

Diabetic neuropathy is nerve damage that occurs because of the metabolic derangements associated with diabetes mellitus. About 60% to 70% of patients with diabetes have some degree of neuropathy, with neurologic complications occurring equally in type 1 and type 2 diabetes.[1,29] The most common type of neuropathy affecting persons with diabetes is sensory neuropathy. This can lead to the loss of protective sensation in the lower extremities, and, coupled with other factors, this significantly increases the risk for complications that result in a lower limb amputation.

Etiology and Pathophysiology

The pathophysiologic processes of diabetic neuropathy are not well understood. Several theories exist, including metabolic, vascular, and autoimmune elements. The prevailing theory suggests that persistent hyperglycemia leads to an accumulation of sorbitol and fructose in the nerves that causes damage by an unknown mechanism. The result is reduced nerve conduction and demyelinization. Ischemia in blood vessels damaged by chronic hyperglycemia that supply the peripheral nerves is also implicated in the development of diabetic neuropathy. Neuropathy can precede, accompany, or follow the diagnosis of diabetes.

Classification

The two major categories of diabetic neuropathy are *sensory neuropathy,* which affects the peripheral nervous system, and *autonomic neuropathy.* Each of these types can take on several forms.

Sensory Neuropathy. The most common form of sensory neuropathy is distal symmetric neuropathy, which affects the hands and/or feet bilaterally. This is sometimes referred to as "stocking-glove neuropathy." Characteristics of distal symmetric neuropathy include loss of sensation, abnormal sensations, pain, and paresthesias. The pain, which is often described as burning, cramping, crushing, or tearing, is usually worse at night and may occur only at that time. The paresthesias may be associated with tingling, burning, and itching sensations. The patient may report a feeling of walking on pillows or numb feet. At times the skin becomes so sensitive (hyperesthesia) that even light pressure from bedsheets cannot be tolerated. Complete or partial loss of sensitivity to touch and temperature is common. Foot injury and ulcerations can occur without the patient ever having pain (Fig. 47-13). Neuropathy can also cause atrophy of the small muscles of the hands and feet, causing deformity and limiting fine movement.

Control of blood glucose is the only treatment for diabetic neuropathy. It is effective in many, but not all, cases. Drug therapy may be used to treat neuropathic symptoms, particularly pain. Medications commonly used include topical creams (e.g., capsaicin [Zostrix]), tricyclic antidepressants (e.g., amitriptyline [Elavil]), and antiseizure medications (e.g., gabapentin [Neurontin]). Capsaicin is a moderately effective topical cream made from chili peppers. It depletes the accumulation of pain-mediating chemicals in the peripheral sensory neurons. The cream is applied three to four times a day. There is usually an increase in symptoms at the start of therapy, which is followed by relief of pain in 2 to 3 weeks.[29] Tricyclic antidepressants are also moderately effective in treating the symptoms of diabetic neuropathy. They work by inhibiting the reuptake of norepinephrine and serotonin, which are

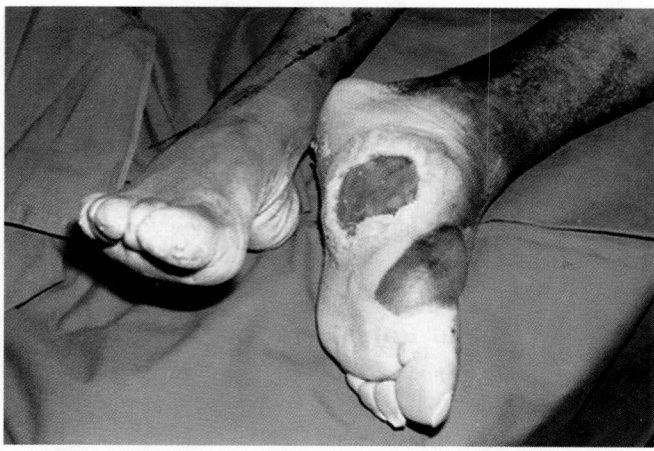

FIG. 47-13 Neuropathy: neurotrophic ulceration.

neurotransmitters that are believed to play a role in the transmission of pain through the spinal cord.[29] Although gabapentin has been found to be effective in treating the pain of diabetic neuropathy, its mechanism of action is not well understood.

Autonomic Neuropathy. Autonomic neuropathy can affect nearly all body systems and lead to hypoglycemic unawareness, bowel incontinence and diarrhea, and urinary retention. Delayed gastric emptying (gastroparesis) is a complication of autonomic neuropathy that can produce anorexia, nausea, vomiting, gastroesophageal reflux, and persistent feelings of fullness. Gastroparesis can trigger hypoglycemia by delaying food absorption. Cardiovascular abnormalities associated with autonomic neuropathy are postural hypotension, resting tachycardia, and painless myocardial infarction. A patient with postural hypotension should be instructed to change from a lying or sitting position slowly.

Diabetes can affect sexual function in men and women. Erectile dysfunction associated with diabetes mellitus is believed to result from damage to the sacral parasympathetic nerves. Determining whether this problem is of organic or psychologic origin is an important part of the assessment. Decreased libido is a problem with some women with diabetes. Monilial and nonspecific vaginitis are also common. Organic impotence or sexual dysfunctioning in either the male or the female patient requires sensitive therapeutic counseling for both the patient and the patient's partner. (See Chapter 53 for a further discussion of impotence.)

A neurogenic bladder may develop as sensation in the inner bladder wall decreases, causing urinary retention. A patient with retention has infrequent voiding, difficulty in voiding, and a weak stream of urine. Emptying the bladder every 3 hours in a sitting position helps prevent stasis and subsequent infection. Tightening the abdominal muscles during voiding and using the Credé maneuver (mild massage downward over the lower abdomen and bladder) may also help with complete bladder emptying. Cholinergic agonist drugs such as bethanechol (Urecholine) may be used. The patient may also have to learn self-catheterization (see Chapter 44).

COMPLICATIONS OF THE FOOT AND LOWER EXTREMITY

Foot complications are the most common cause of hospitalization in the person with diabetes.[30] The development of diabetic foot complications is a multifactoral process. They result from a combination of microvascular and macrovascular diseases that place the patient at risk for injury and serious infection that may lead to amputation. Sensory neuropathy and peripheral vascular disease (PVD) are risk factors, and clotting abnormalities, impaired immune function, and autonomic neuropathy also play important roles. Smoking is deleterious to the health of lower extremity blood vessels and increases the risk for amputation.

PVD increases the risk for amputation by causing a reduction in blood flow to the lower extremities. When blood flow is decreased, oxygen, white blood cells, and vital nutrients are not available to the tissues. Therefore wounds take longer to heal and the risk for infection increases. Signs of PVD include intermittent claudication, pain at rest, cold feet, loss of hair, delayed capillary filling, and dependent rubor (redness of the skin that occurs when the extremity is in a dependent position). The disease is diagnosed by history, Doppler findings, and angiography. Management includes control or reduction of risk factors, particularly smoking, high cholesterol intake, and hypertension. Bypass or graft surgery is indicated in some patients. Proper care of the feet is essential for the patient with PVD. Guidelines for patient teaching are listed in Table 47-21.

Sensory neuropathy is a major risk factor for lower extremity amputation in the person with diabetes. Loss of protective sensation (LOPS) often prevents the patient from becoming aware that a foot injury has occurred. Improper footwear and injury from stepping on foreign objects while barefoot are common causes of undetected foot injury in the person with LOPS. Because the primary risk factor for lower extremity amputation is LOPS, annual screening using a *monofilament* is an extremely important preventive measure. This is done by applying a thin, flexible filament to several spots on the plantar surface of the foot and asking the patient to report if it is felt. Insensitivity to a 10 g Semmes-Weinstein monofilament has been shown to greatly increase the risk for diabetic foot ulcers that can lead to amputation. If the patient has LOPS, aggressive measures must be taken to teach the patient how to prevent foot ulceration. These measures include the selection of proper footwear, including prescription shoes. Other measures are to carefully avoid injury to the foot, to practice diligent skin and nail care, to inspect the foot thoroughly each day, and to treat small problems promptly.

The Doppler instrument is used to diagnose the presence or degree of PVD. Similar to an electronic stethoscope, this device amplifies sound. The procedure is noninvasive and can measure blood pressure in the lower extremities and blood flow velocity. It can indicate areas of stenosis or occlusion and is useful as an indicator of the need for additional vascular tests.

Neuropathic arthropathy, or *Charcot foot,* results in ankle and foot changes that ultimately lead to joint dysfunction and footdrop. These changes occur gradually and promote an abnormal distribution of weight over the foot, further increasing the chances of developing a foot ulcer as new pressure points emerge. Neuropathic ulcers resemble a "BB shot" or "punched out" wound and are usually painless. Infection is a danger and necessitates the long-term use of antibiotics and weeks of avoidance of weight bearing on the affected limb.

INTEGUMENTARY COMPLICATIONS

Skin disorders such as diabetic dermopathy and necrobiosis lipoidica diabeticorum are attributed to microangiopathy. Shin spots are brown spots located on the anterior surfaces of the lower extremities. They are harmless and painless and initially measure less than 1 cm in diameter. *Necrobiosis lipoidica dia-*

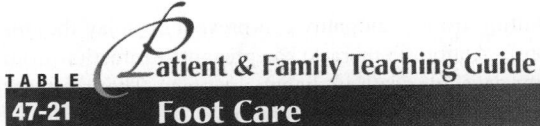

TABLE 47-21 ***Patient & Family Teaching Guide***

Foot Care

1. Wash feet daily with a mild soap and *warm* water. Test water temperature with hands first.
2. Pat feet dry gently, especially between toes.
3. Examine feet daily for cuts, blisters, swelling, and red, tender areas. Do not depend on feeling sores. If eyesight is poor, have others inspect feet.
4. Use lanolin on feet to prevent skin from drying and cracking. Do not apply between toes.
5. Use mild foot powder on sweaty feet.
6. Do not use commercial remedies to remove calluses or corns.
7. Cleanse cuts with *warm* water and mild soap, covering with clean dressing. Do not use iodine, rubbing alcohol, or strong adhesives.
8. Report skin infections or nonhealing sores to health care provider immediately.
9. Cut toenails even with rounded contour of toes. Do not cut down corners. The best time to trim nails is after a shower or bath.
10. Separate overlapping toes with cotton or lamb's wool.
11. Avoid open-toe, open-heel, and high-heel shoes. Leather shoes are preferred to plastic ones. Wear slippers with soles. Do not go barefoot. Shake out shoes before putting on.
12. Wear clean, absorbent (cotton or wool) socks or stockings that have not been mended. Colored socks must be colorfast.
13. Do not wear clothing that leaves impressions, hindering circulation.
14. Do not use hot water bottles or heating pads to warm feet. Wear socks for warmth.
15. Guard against frostbite.
16. Exercise feet daily either by walking or by flexing and extending feet in suspended position. Avoid prolonged sitting, standing, and crossing of legs.

beticorum is believed to be the result of the breakdown of collagen in the skin. It usually appears as red-yellow lesions, with atrophic skin that becomes shiny and transparent revealing tiny blood vessels under the surface. Because the thin skin is prone to injury, special care must be taken to protect affected areas from injury and ulceration. This condition is not common, but it may appear before other clinical signs or symptoms of diabetes. It is more frequently seen in young women.

INFECTION

A patient with diabetes is more susceptible to infections than other patients. The mechanisms for this phenomenon include a defect in the mobilization of inflammatory cells and an impairment of phagocytosis by neutrophils and monocytes. Recurring or persistent infections such as *Candida albicans,* as well as boils and furuncles, in the undiagnosed patient often lead the health care provider to suspect diabetes. Loss of sensation (neuropathy) may delay the detection of an infection.

Persistent glycosuria may predispose to bladder infections, especially in patients with a neurogenic bladder. Decreased circulation resulting from angiopathy can prevent or delay the immune response. Antibiotic therapy has prevented infection from being a major cause of death in diabetic patients. The treatment of infections must be prompt and vigorous.

■ Gerontologic Considerations: Diabetes Mellitus

Diabetes is more prevalent in older populations. A major reason for this is that the process of aging involves insulin resistance and glucose intolerance, which are believed to be precursors to type 2 diabetes.[31] Aging is also associated with a number of conditions that are more likely to be treated with medications that impair insulin action (e.g., corticosteroids, antihypertensives, phenothiazines). Undiagnosed and untreated diabetes is more common in the elderly, partly because many of the normal physiologic changes of aging resemble those of diabetes, such as visual changes and decreased glomerular filtration.

Although good glycemic control is important to people of all ages with diabetes, several factors are taken into account when determining glycemic goals for an older adult. One is that hypoglycemic unawareness is more common in this age-group, making these patients more likely to suffer adverse consequences from blood glucose–lowering therapy. They may also have delayed psychomotor function that could interfere with the ability to treat hypoglycemia. Other factors to consider in establishing glycemic goals for the older patient include the patient's own desire for treatment and other coexisting medical problems such as cognitive impairment. Although it is generally agreed that treatment is indicated for older adults with diabetes to prevent acute complications and avoid unpleasant symptoms, strict glycemic control may be difficult to achieve.[32,33]

As with any group, diet and exercise are recommended as therapy for older adult patients with diabetes. This should take into account functional limitations that may interfere with physical activity and the ability to prepare meals. Because of the physiologic changes that occur with aging, the therapeutic outcome for the older adult with diabetes who receives OAs may be altered. First-generation sulfonylureas, such as tolazamide (Tolinase), are generally avoided in this age-group because the long half-life of these drugs increases the risk for hypoglycemia. The second-generation sulfonylurea drugs (e.g., glyburide [Micronase]) are usually well tolerated and have increased potency but appear to have fewer side effects and fewer drug interaction problems when compared with the first-generation agents. Other OAs described earlier in this chapter may also be used in older patients with diabetes. Insulin therapy may be instituted if OAs fail. However, it is important to recognize that elderly patients are more likely to have limitations in manual dexterity and visual acuity, both of which are necessary for accurate insulin administration.

Patient teaching should be based on the individual's needs, using a slower pace with simple printed or audio materials. It is important to include family or a support person in the teaching. The patient education issues for the older patient include those related to vision, mobility, mental status, functional ability, financial and social situation, the effect of multiple medications, eating habits, the potential for undetected hypoglycemia, and quality-of-life issues.[34] ■

CRITICAL THINKING EXERCISES

Case Study
Diabetic Ketoacidosis

Patient Profile. John, a 34-year-old Native American man, was admitted to the emergency department after he was found comatose in his apartment by his wife.

Subjective Data (provided by wife)
- Was diagnosed with diabetes mellitus 12 months ago
- Was taking 48 U of insulin daily: 12 U of regular insulin plus 20 U of NPH before breakfast, 8 U of regular insulin before dinner, and 8 U of NPH at bedtime
- Has history of flu for 1 week with vomiting and anorexia
- Stopped taking insulin 2 days ago when he was unable to eat

Objective Data

Physical Examination
- Breathing is deep and rapid
- Acetone smell on breath
- Skin flushed and dry

Diagnostic Studies
- Blood glucose level of 730 mg/dl (40.5 mmol/L)
- Blood pH of 7.26

CRITICAL THINKING QUESTIONS

1. Briefly explain the pathophysiology of the development of diabetic ketoacidosis (DKA) in this patient.
2. What clinical manifestations of DKA does this patient exhibit?
3. What factors precipitated this patient's DKA?
4. What distinguishes this case history from one of hyperosmolar hyperglycemic nonketotic syndrome (HHNS) or hypoglycemia?
5. What teaching should be done with this patient and his family?
6. What role should John's wife have in the management of his diabetes?
7. Based on the assessment data presented, write one or more appropriate nursing diagnoses. Are there any collaborative problems?

Nursing Research Issues

1. What degree of pain does the patient associate with capillary blood glucose monitoring?
2. How often does the patient make phone contact with a diabetes nurse educator when this service is available free as compared with when there is a charge?
3. What factors contribute to a patient's willingness to maintain tight glycemic control in the present to prevent chronic complications from diabetes in the future?
4. Does the frequency of review of major diabetes education issues affect the frequency of occurrence of acute complications of diabetes?

REVIEW QUESTIONS

The number of the question corresponds to the same-numbered objective at the beginning of the chapter.

1. The polydipsia and polyuria related to diabetes mellitus are primarily caused by
   a. the release of ketones from cells during fat metabolism.
   b. fluid shifts resulting from the osmotic effect of hyperglycemia.
   c. damage to the kidneys from exposure to high levels of glucose.
   d. changes in RBCs resulting from attachment of excessive glucose to hemoglobin.

2. When a patient with type 2 diabetes mellitus is admitted to the hospital with pneumonia, the nurse recognizes that the patient
   a. must receive insulin therapy to prevent the development of ketoacidosis.
   b. has islet cell antibodies that have destroyed the ability of the pancreas to produce insulin.
   c. has minimal or absent endogenous insulin secretion and requires daily insulin injections.
   d. may have sufficient endogenous insulin to prevent ketosis but is at risk for development of hyperosmolar hyperglycemic nonketotic syndrome.

3. Effective collaborative management of diabetes includes
   a. using insulin with all patients to achieve glycemic goals.
   b. relying on the health care provider as the central figure in the program for good control.
   c. relying solely on nutritional therapy as the initial treatment modality for all patients with diabetes.
   d. aiming for a balance of diet, activity, and medications together with appropriate monitoring and patient and family teaching.

4. The nurse assists the patient with nutritional therapy of diabetes with the knowledge that a "diabetic diet" is designed
   a. to be used only for type 1 diabetes.
   b. for use during periods of high stress.
   c. to normalize blood glucose by elimination of sugar.
   d. to help normalize blood glucose through a balanced diet.

5. In teaching a newly diagnosed type 1 diabetic "survival skills," the nurse includes information about
   a. weight loss measures.
   b. elimination of sugar from diet.
   c. need to reduce physical activity.
   d. self-monitoring of blood glucose.

6. An appropriate teaching measure for the patient with diabetes mellitus related to care of the feet is to
   a. use heat to increase blood supply.
   b. avoid softening lotions and creams.
   c. inspect all surfaces of the feet daily.
   d. use iodine to disinfect cuts and abrasions.

7. A diabetic patient has a serum glucose level of 824 mg/dl (45.7 mmol/L) and is unresponsive. Following assessment of the patient, the nurse suspects diabetic ketoacidosis rather than hyperosmolar hyperglycemic nonketotic syndrome based on the finding of
   a. polyuria.
   b. severe dehydration.
   c. rapid, deep respirations.
   d. decreased serum potassium.

8. Which of the following is not an appropriate therapy for patients with diabetes mellitus?
   a. Use of diuretics to treat renal problems
   b. Use of ACE inhibitors to treat renal problems
   c. Use of laser photocoagulation to treat retinopathy
   d. Use of regular insulin for a patient with type 2 diabetes during the intraoperative period

REFERENCES

1. American Diabetes Association: Available at *www.ada.org* (accessed Nov 1, 2002).
2. Report of the expert committee on the diagnosis and classification of diabetes mellitus, *Diabetes Care* 25(suppl 1):5, 2002.
3. Edelman SV, Henry RR: *Diagnosis and management of type 2 diabetes,* ed 3, Caddo, Okla, 1999, Professional Communications.
4. National Institute of Diabetes and Digestive and Kidney Disease: Diet and exercise dramatically delay type 2 diabetes: diabetes medication metformin also effective. Available at *www.niddk.nih.gov* (accessed Nov 1, 2002).
5. Stoller WA: Individualizing insulin management: three practical cases, rules for regimen adjustment, *Postgrad Med* 111:51, 2002.
6. Mayerson AB, Inzucchi SE: Type 2 diabetes therapy: a pathophysiologically based approach, *Postgrad Med* 111:83, 2002.
7. Aventis Pharmaceuticals: Lantus prescribing information. Available at *www.aventispharma-us.com* (accessed Nov 1, 2002).
8. American Diabetes Association: Position statement: insulin administration, *Diabetes Care* 25(suppl 1):112, 2002.
9. Bode BW, Tamborlane WV, Davidson PC: Insulin pump therapy in the 21st century: strategies for successful use in adults, adolescents, and children with diabetes, *Postgrad Med* 111:69, 2002.
10. Fain JA: Delivering insulin 'round the clock, *Nursing* 32:54, 2002.
11. American Diabetes Association: Position statement: implications of the Diabetes Control and Complication Trial, *Diabetes Care* 25(suppl 1):25, 2002.
12. Ahmann AJ, Riddle MC: Current oral agents for type 2 diabetes: many options, but which to choose when? *Postgrad Med* 111:32, 2002.
13. Funnell MM, Barlage DL: Saying a mouthful about oral diabetes drugs, *Nursing* 30:34, 2000.
14. Takeda Pharmaceuticals America, Eli Lilly and Company: Actos product insert, no date.
15. American Diabetes Association: Position statement: nutritional recommendations and principles for people with diabetes mellitus, *Diabetes Care* 25(suppl 1):61, 2002.
16. American Diabetes Association: Position statement: evidence-based nutrition principles and recommendations for the treatment and prevention of diabetes and related complications, *Diabetes Care* 25:50, 2002.
17. American Diabetes Association: *Medical management of type 2 diabetes,* ed 4, Alexandria, Va., 1998, American Diabetes Association.
18. Funnell MM et al: *Life with diabetes,* ed 2, Alexandria, Va., 2000, American Diabetes Association.
19. Flood L, Constance A: Diabetes and exercise safety, *Am J Nurs* 102:47, 2002.

20. American Diabetes Association: *The diabetes ready-reference guide for health care professionals,* Alexandria, Va., 2000, American Diabetes Association.

21. Konick-McMahan J: Riding out a diabetic emergency, *Nursing* 29:9, 1999.

22. American Diabetes Association: Position statement: insulin administration, *Diabetes Care* 25(suppl 1):112, 2002.

23. Diabetes Control and Complications Trial Research Group: The effect of intensive treatment of diabetes on the development and progression of long-term complications in insulin-dependent diabetes mellitus, *N Engl J Med* 329:977, 1993.

24. American Diabetes Association: Position statement: implications of the United Kingdom Prospective Diabetes Study, *Diabetes Care* 25(suppl 1):28, 2002.

25. American Diabetes Association: Position statement: standards of medical care for patients with diabetes mellitus, *Diabetes Care* 25(suppl 1):33, 2002.

26. American Diabetes Association: Position statement: diabetic retinopathy, *Diabetes Care* 25(suppl 1):90, 2002.

27. Grand MG et al: Eye disease. In Levin ME, Pfeifer MA, editors: *The uncomplicated guide to diabetes complications,* Alexandria, Va., 1998, American Diabetes Association.

28. American Diabetes Association: Position statement: diabetic nephropathy, *Diabetes Care* 25(suppl 1):85, 2002.

29. Vinik AI: Diagnosis and management of diabetic neuropathy, *Advances in the Care of Older People with Diabetes* 15:293, 1999.

30. Mulder GD: Evaluating and managing the diabetic foot, *Adv Skin Wound Care* 13:33, 2000.

31. Barzilai N et al: Advances in diabetes management: application to the geriatric patient, *Ann Long Term Care* 8:58, 2000.

32. Chau D, Edelman SV: Clinical management of diabetes in the elderly, *Clinical Diabetes* 19:172, 2001.

33. Gabriely I, Barzilai N: Management of insulin resistance in the elderly patient with diabetes, *Clin Geriatr* 10:38, 2002.

34. Strachan M: Cognitive decline and the older patient with diabetes, *Clin Geriatr* 10:29, 2002.

RESOURCES

American Association of Diabetes Educators
100 West Monroe Street, Suite 400
Chicago, IL 60603
800-338-3633
Fax: 312-424-2427
www.aadenet.org/

American Diabetes Association
1701 North Beauregard Street
Alexandria, VA 22311
800-DIABETES (342-2383)
Fax: 703-549-6995
www.diabetes.org/

American Dietetic Association
216 West Jackson Boulevard
Chicago, IL 60606-6995
800-877-1600 or 312-899-0040
www.eatright.org/

Juvenile Diabetes Research Foundation International
120 Wall Street
New York, NY 10005-4001
800-533-CURE (2873) or 212-785-9500
Fax: 212-785-9595
www.jdrf.org/index.php

National Diabetes Information Clearinghouse
1 Information Way
Bethesda, MD 20892-3560
301-654-3327
Fax: 301-907-8906
www.niddk.nih.gov/

For additional Internet resources, see the website for this book at *http://evolve.elsevier.com/Lewis/medsurg/.*

CHAPTER 48

NURSING MANAGEMENT
Endocrine Problems

Jean Foret Giddens

LEARNING OBJECTIVES

1. Describe the pathophysiology, clinical manifestations, collaborative care, and nursing management of the patient with an imbalance of hormones produced by the anterior pituitary gland.
2. Describe the pathophysiology, clinical manifestations, collaborative care, and nursing management of the patient with an imbalance of antidiuretic hormone secretion.
3. Describe the pathophysiology, clinical manifestations, collaborative care, and nursing management of the patient with thyroid dysfunction.
4. Describe the pathophysiology, clinical manifestations, collaborative care, and nursing management of the patient with an imbalance of the hormone produced by the parathyroid glands.

5. Describe the pathophysiology, clinical manifestations, collaborative care, and nursing management of the patient with an imbalance of hormones produced by the adrenal cortex.
6. Describe the pathophysiology, clinical manifestations, collaborative care, and nursing management of the patient with an excess of hormones produced by the adrenal medulla.
7. Describe the side effects of corticosteroid therapy.
8. List common nursing assessments, interventions, rationales, and expected outcomes related to patient teaching for management of chronic endocrine problems.

KEY TERMS

acromegaly, p. 1303
Addison's disease, p. 1331
cretinism, p. 1319
Cushing syndrome, p. 1326
diabetes insipidus, p. 1309
exophthalmos, p. 1312
goiter, p. 1311
goitrogens, p. 1317
Graves' disease, p. 1311
hyperaldosteronism, p. 1334
hyperparathyroidism, p. 1323
hyperthyroidism, p. 1311

hypoparathyroidism, p. 1325
hypopituitarism, p. 1306
hypothyroidism, p. 1319
myxedema, p. 1320
pheochromocytoma, p. 1335
syndrome of inappropriate antidiuretic hormone, p. 1307
tetany, p. 1324
thyroiditis, p. 1318
thyrotoxic crisis, p. 1312
thyrotoxicosis, p. 1311

Disorders of the Anterior Pituitary Gland

GROWTH HORMONE EXCESS

Etiology and Pathophysiology

Growth hormone (GH), an anabolic hormone, promotes protein synthesis and mobilizes glucose and free fatty acids. GH is produced by the anterior pituitary and stimulates the liver to produce insulin-like growth factor–1 (IGF-1), also known as somatomedin C. IGF-1 stimulates growth of bones and soft tissues. Normally IGF-1 also signals the anterior pituitary to reduce GH

production. Overproduction of GH is almost always caused by a benign pituitary adenoma (tumor). The pituitary tumor secretes GH despite elevated IGF-1 levels, leading to unwanted growth of bones and other soft tissue. Overproduction of GH also causes elevation of blood glucose through insulin antagonism. Prolonged elevated glucose levels associated with elevation in GH leads to glucose intolerance.

In children, excessive secretion of GH results in *gigantism*. When the onset of GH excess occurs before closure of the epiphyses, the long bones are still capable of longitudinal growth. The excessive growth is usually proportional. These children may grow as tall as 8 feet (240 cm) and weigh more than 300 lb (136 kg).

In adults, excessive secretion of GH results in acromegaly. **Acromegaly** is characterized by an overgrowth of the bones and soft tissues. Because the problem develops after epiphyseal closure in adults, the bones are unable to grow longer. Instead, the bones increase in thickness and width. Acromegaly is relatively rare. Only three out of every 1 million adults in the United States is diagnosed with this disease each year, with a prevalence of 40 to 60 out of every 1 million individuals.[1] Both genders are affected equally.

Untreated, acromegaly leads to a number of changes in the body. Effects on the cardiovascular system include cardiomegaly, left ventricular hypertrophy, and hypertension. For this reason, disease of the cardiovascular system is associated with increased mortality rates in these individuals. Other systems that undergo changes include the gastrointestinal, genitourinary, musculoskeletal, and nervous systems.

Clinical Manifestations

Manifestations of acromegaly begin gradually, usually in the third and fourth decades of life. Typically there is an average of 7 to 9 years between the initial onset of symptoms and final diagnosis. Individuals experience enlargement of the hands and

Reviewed by Karla Jones, RN, MS, Nursing Faculty, Treasure Valley Community College, Ontario, Ore.; JoAnne Konick-McMahan, RN, MSN, CCRN, Advance Practice Nurse, School of Nursing, University of Pennsylvania, Philadelphia, Pa.; Debra A. Morgan, RN, EdD, Assistant Professor, College of Health Sciences and Human Services, Midwestern State University, Wichita Falls, Tex.

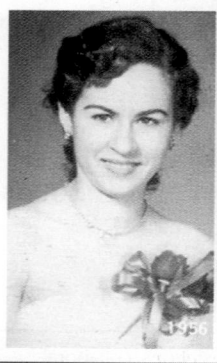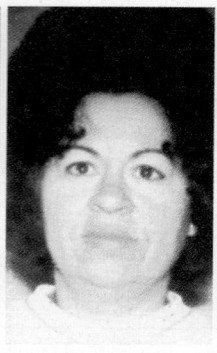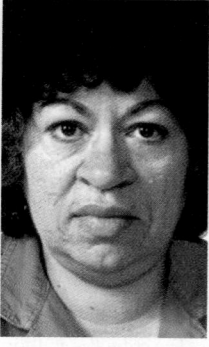

FIG. 48-1 Progressive development of facial features of acromegaly.

feet. The fingertips develop a tufted or clubbed-like appearance. The enlargement of the bones and cartilage may cause symptoms that range from mild joint pain to deforming, crippling arthritis. Changes in physical appearance occur with thickening and enlargement of bony and soft tissue on the face and head (Fig. 48-1). Enlargement of the mandible causes the jaw to jut forward. The paranasal and frontal sinuses enlarge, as does the bony tissue of the forehead. Enlargement of soft tissue around the eyes, nose, and mouth results in a coarsening of facial features. Enlargement of the tongue results in speech difficulties, and the voice deepens as a result of hypertrophy of the vocal cords.

Sleep apnea may also occur and is thought to be related to upper airway narrowing resulting from changes in pharyngeal soft tissues.[2] The skin becomes thick, leathery, and oily. Persons with acromegaly may also experience peripheral neuropathy and proximal muscle weakness. Women may develop menstrual disturbances. The patient may also exhibit manifestations of diabetes mellitus such as polydipsia and polyuria. Cardiovascular disease may manifest as hypertension, angina pectoris, and congestive heart failure.

The enlarged pituitary tumor gland can exert pressure on surrounding structures within the brain, leading to visual disturbances and headaches. Because GH mobilizes stored fat for energy, it increases free fatty acid levels in the blood and predisposes the patient to atherosclerosis. The hormone also antagonizes the action of insulin and causes hyperglycemia. Prolonged secretion of GH leads to glucose intolerance.

Diagnostic Studies

In addition to the history and physical examination, diagnosis of GH excess requires evaluation of plasma GH, plasma IGF-1 levels, IGF binding protein–3 (IGFBP-3) levels, and GH response to an oral glucose challenge. A single measurement of serum GH is of limited value in the diagnosis of acromegaly because GH levels normally fluctuate. IGF-1 levels are more constant and thus provide a more reliable measure than GH levels. The definitive test for acromegaly is the oral glucose challenge test. Normally GH concentration falls during an oral glucose tolerance test. In acromegaly, these levels do not fall.[3]

Magnetic resonance imaging (MRI) is indicated for the identification, localization, and determination of the extension of the pituitary tumor into surrounding tissue. High-resolution computed tomography (CT) scanning with contrast media may also be used to localize the tumor. A complete ophthalmologic examination, including visual fields, is typically done because the tu-

mor (especially a macroadenoma larger than 10 mm) potentially causes pressure on the optic chiasm or optic nerves.

Collaborative Care

The therapeutic goal in acromegaly is to return GH levels to normal. This is accomplished by surgery, radiation, drug therapy, or a combination of these therapies. The prognosis depends on age at onset, age when treatment is initiated, and tumor size. Usually bone growth can be arrested and soft tissue hypertrophy can be reversed. However, sleep apnea and diabetic and cardiac complications may persist in spite of treatment.

Surgical Therapy. Surgery (hypophysectomy) is the treatment of choice and offers the best hope for a cure, especially for smaller tumors (microadenomas smaller than 10 mm). More than 97% of surgeries done to remove pituitary tumors associated with acromegaly are accomplished with the *transsphenoidal* approach.[4] With this procedure, an incision is made in the inner aspect of the upper lip and gingiva. The sella turcica is entered through the floor of the nose and sphenoid sinuses (Fig. 48-2).

The goal of transsphenoidal surgery is to remove only the tumor that is causing GH secretion. This procedure produces an immediate reduction in GH levels followed by a drop in IGF-1 levels within a few weeks. Although 94% of these procedures are effective, some patients (especially those with larger tumors or those with GH levels greater than 50 ng/ml) do not obtain a cure with the surgery and require adjunctive radiation or drug therapy to control GH hypersecretion.[4] In some cases, the entire pituitary gland is removed during surgery *(hypophysectomy),* resulting in a permanent absence of pituitary hormones. Rather than replacing the pituitary (tropic) hormones, which requires parenteral administration, the essential hormones produced by target organs (glucocorticoids, thyroid hormone, and sex hormones) can be given orally. Hormone replacement must be continued throughout life.

Radiation Therapy. Irradiation of the tumor is considered a secondary treatment option. It is indicated when surgery has failed to produce complete remission. External radiation can successfully reduce GH levels in 30% to 70% of patients, but the primary disadvantage is the long delay (months to years) for GH levels to normalize.[4] Because of the length of time it takes to achieve GH reduction, radiation therapy is usually offered in combination

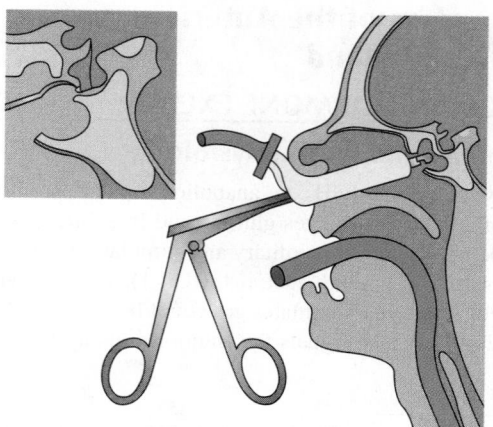

FIG. 48-2 Surgery on the pituitary gland is most commonly performed with the transsphenoidal approach. An incision is made in the inner aspect of the upper lip and gingiva. The sella turcica is entered through the floor of the nose and sphenoid sinuses.

with drugs that reduce GH levels. If a tumor is large or has extensive spread, surgery may be followed by radiation. Radiation has also been used to reduce the size of a tumor before surgery. Depending on the amount of radiation and the patient's susceptibility, the patient may experience local skin changes, alopecia, or oral complications. Hypopituitarism commonly results from radiation therapy and requires hormone replacement therapy.

Stereotactic radiosurgery (gamma surgery) may be used for small, surgically inaccessible pituitary tumors (see Chapter 55). This procedure consists of radiation delivered to a single site from multiple angles and can be used to occlude blood vessels feeding the tumor, thereby starving it.[5,6]

Drug Therapy. Three groups of agents are used in the treatment of acromegaly: somatostatin analogs, dopamine agonists, and GH receptor antagonists. These drugs reduce GH levels and are often used as initial treatment or as adjunct therapy to surgery or radiation. The use of drug therapy as primary treatment has been considered, but the safety and cost of long-term drug treatment have yet to be established.[5]

The most common drug used for acromegaly is octreotide (Sandostatin), a somatostatin analog that reduces GH levels to within the normal range in many patients. Octreotide is given by subcutaneus injection three times a week. Two newer long-acting analogs, octreotide (Depot, Sandostatin LAR) and lanreotide SR (Ipstyl), are now available that are administered as intramuscular (IM) injections every 2 to 4 weeks. Another group of agents, dopamine agonists, are useful in the treatment of acromegaly because these agents suppress GH secretion. Cabergoline (Dostinex) has essentially replaced bromocriptine (Parlodel) because it is more effective and is associated with fewer side effects.

A GH receptor antagonist, pegvisomant (Somavert), has recently been developed for use in the treatment of acromegaly and is considered an alternative to dopamine agonists or somatostatin analogs. This agent is best used to control disease for patients who have received radiation therapy, but still have hypersecretion of GH.[7] It is not considered appropriate for primary treatment because this agent only blocks hormone action rather than acting on the tumor.

NURSING MANAGEMENT
GROWTH HORMONE EXCESS

■ Nursing Assessment

The nurse needs to assess for signs and symptoms of abnormal tissue growth and evaluate changes in the physical size of each patient. The adult should be questioned about increases in hat, ring, glove, and shoe sizes. The patient can be questioned about changes in appearance. Photographs are helpful to evaluate any changes. Because physical changes occur slowly and over a long period of time, it is possible that the individual is not even aware of such changes. The patient needs unconditional acceptance by health care workers and considerable emotional support during the periods of diagnosis and treatment.

■ Nursing Diagnoses

Nursing diagnoses for the patient with GH excess include, but are not limited to, the following:

- Disturbed body image *related to* enlargement of the hands, feet, jaw, and soft body tissue
- Deficient fluid volume *related to* polyuria
- Disturbed sleep pattern *related to* soft tissue swelling
- Disturbed sensory perception (visual) *related to* enlarged pituitary gland

■ Planning

The overall goals are that the patient with GH excess will (1) accept and cope effectively with altered body image, (2) maintain adequate fluid volume, (3) experience restful sleep patterns, (4) develop no complications, and (5) obtain long-term follow-up care.

■ Nursing Implementation

Acute Intervention. Patients typically have many questions and concerns regarding surgery. It is important for the nurse to offer reassurance and to provide accurate information regarding this process. An explanation regarding hormonal replacement, should it be necessary, is also important.

The individual treated surgically needs skilled neurosurgical nursing care and must be prepared before surgery for postoperative care. Nursing interventions include preoperative installation of antibiotic nose drops, discussion of mouth breathing, mouth care, ambulation, pain control, activity, and hormone replacement. The patient should be instructed to avoid vigorous coughing, sneezing, and straining at stool (Valsalva maneuver) to prevent cerebrospinal fluid leakage from the point at which the sella turcica was entered.

After surgery in which a transsphenoidal approach has been used, the head of the patient's bed should be elevated at a 30-degree angle at all times. This elevation avoids pressure on the sella turcica and decreases headaches, a frequent postoperative problem. Monitoring neurologic status, including pupillary response, should be done in order to detect neurologic complications.

Any clear nasal drainage should be sent to the laboratory to be tested for glucose. A glucose level greater than 30 mg/dl (1.67 mmol/L) indicates cerebrospinal fluid leakage from an open connection to the brain. If this happens, the patient is at an increased risk for meningitis. Complaints of persistent and severe generalized or supraorbital headache may indicate cerebrospinal fluid leakage into the sinuses. A cerebrospinal fluid leak usually resolves within 72 hours when treated with head elevation and bed rest. If the leak persists, daily spinal taps may be done to reduce pressure to below-normal levels and allow the fossa to heal. Intravenous (IV) antibiotics are usually administered when there is a cerebrospinal fluid leak to prevent meningitis. If the leak does not respond to treatment in 72 hours, surgical intervention may be required.

Mild analgesia is given for headaches. The nurse should perform mouth care every 4 hours to keep the surgical area clean and free of debris and to promote patient comfort. Toothbrushing should be avoided for at least 10 days to prevent disrupting the suture line and to avoid discomfort.

If stereotactic radiosurgery is used, the patient is usually moved from the specialized radiation center to the neurosurgical nursing unit for overnight observation. The patient will be in a stereotactic head frame. Vital signs, neurologic status, and fluid volume status must be carefully monitored. Possible complications include increased headaches, seizures, nausea, and vomiting. The patient with a history of seizures is at increased risk for seizures for at least 24 hours after the procedure. All staff should know how to remove a stereotactic frame in case of an emergency. The patient may experience discomfort at the pin sites. Pin-site care should be done according to institutional policy. Family members can be instructed in pin-site care if the patient is discharged the day after the procedure.

A possible postoperative complication is transient diabetes insipidus (DI). This may occur because of the loss of antidiuretic hormone (ADH), which is stored in the posterior lobe of the pituitary gland, or cerebral edema related to manipulation of the pituitary during surgery. To assess for DI, urine output and serum and urine osmolarity must be closely monitored. Clinical manifestations and treatment of DI are discussed in more detail later in this chapter.

Ambulatory and Home Care. If a hypophysectomy is performed or the pituitary is damaged, hormone replacement will be necessary. ADH, cortisol, and thyroid hormone replacement will be needed. Because these medications need to be taken for life, careful patient teaching is essential when replacement of these hormones is necessary.

Because surgery may result in permanent hormone deficiencies and possible decreased fertility, the patient needs assistance in working through the grieving process associated with these losses. The need for continued drug therapy reduces the patient's perception of independence and requires considerable emotional adjustment. The nurse must consider the emotional impact of a hypophysectomy when counseling the patient and planning the educational program related to hormone replacement.

■ Evaluation

The expected outcomes are that the patient with GH excess will
- experience no complications postoperatively
- know how and when to take hormone replacements (if indicated)
- state symptoms requiring immediate attention and appropriate actions
- state the importance of long-term follow-up
- have a follow-up medical appointment

EXCESSES OF OTHER TROPIC HORMONES

Excesses of tropic hormones and overproduction of a single anterior pituitary hormone usually produce syndromes related to hormone excess from the target organ. If adrenocorticotropic hormone (ACTH) is increased, Cushing's disease results; if thyroid-stimulating hormone (TSH) levels are excessive, hyperthyroidism develops.

Prolactinomas (prolactin-secreting adenomas) are the most frequently occurring pituitary tumor, accounting for 40% to 60% of all hyperfunctioning pituitary tumors.[8] Common manifestations experienced by women with prolactinomas include galactorrhea, ovulatory dysfunction (anovulation, infertility), menstrual dysfunction (oligomenorrhea or amenorrhea), decreased libido, and hirsutism. In men, impotence and decreased libido and sperm density may result. The affected patient may also experience headaches and visual problems. The visual problems are secondary to pressure on the optic chiasm. Because prolactinomas do not typically progress in size, drug therapy is usually the first-line treatment.[8] Dopamine agonists such as bromocriptine (Parlodel), cabergoline (Dostinex), and pergolide (Permax) have successfully been used to treat this disorder. Surgery using the transsphenoidal approach (discussed previously) may be considered depending on the size and extent of the tumor. Use of radiation for treatment of prolactinomas has been somewhat limited, but is mainly used in those patients who have failed to respond to medical or surgical therapy.

HYPOFUNCTION OF THE PITUITARY GLAND

Hypopituitarism is a rare disorder that involves a decrease in one or more of the pituitary hormones. The anterior pituitary gland secretes ACTH, TSH, follicle-stimulating hormone (FSH), luteinizing hormone (LH), GH, and prolactin; the posterior pituitary gland secretes ADH and oxytocin. A deficiency of only one pituitary hormone is referred to as *selective hypopituitarism*. Total failure of the pituitary gland results in deficiency of all pituitary hormones—a condition referred to as *panhypopituitarism*. The most common hormone deficiencies associated with hypopituitarism involve GH and gonadotropins. TSH, ACTH, and ADH are less frequently involved.[9]

Etiology and Pathophysiology

The most common cause of pituitary hypofunction is a pituitary tumor. Autoimmune disorders, infections, pituitary infarction (Sheehan syndrome), or destruction of the pituitary gland (as a result of trauma, radiation, and surgical procedures) also can cause hypopituitarism. *Sheehan syndrome* is a postpartum condition of pituitary necrosis and hypopituitarism after circulatory collapse resulting from uterine hemorrhaging.

Hormone deficiencies involving anterior pituitary hormones lead to end-organ failure; thus the effects of hypopituitarism depend on the specific pituitary hormone or hormones that are lacking. For example, infertility may be the first indication of pituitary hypofunction associated with a pituitary tumor. Deficiencies of TSH and ACTH are life threatening. ACTH deficiency causes a tendency toward shock and may result in an episode of acute adrenal insufficiency (refractory and life-threatening shock from sodium and water depletion). (Adrenal shock is discussed later in this chapter.)

Clinical Manifestations

The signs and symptoms associated with pituitary hypofunction vary with the degree and speed of onset of pituitary dysfunction and are related to hyposecretion of the target glands and/or a growing pituitary tumor. Common symptoms associated with a space-occupying lesion include headaches, visual changes (decreased peripheral vision or decreased visual acuity), *anosmia* (loss of the sense of smell), and seizures.

Adults with GH deficiency often have subtle nonspecific clinical findings. They have truncal obesity and decreased muscle mass causing reduced strength, decreased energy, and reduced exercise capability. Decreased bone density and pathologic fractures may occur.[10] They may have a flat affect or appear depressed. Impaired psychologic well-being is a common finding associated with GH deficiency in adults.

FSH and LH deficiencies in the adult woman are first manifested as menstrual irregularities, diminished libido, and changes in secondary sex characteristics (e.g., decreased breast size). Men with FSH and LH deficiencies experience testicular atrophy, diminished spermatogenesis, loss of libido, impotence, and decreased facial hair and muscle mass.

Deficiency of ACTH and cortisol often produce a nonspecific clinical picture. Signs and symptoms may include weakness, fatigue, headache, dry and pale skin, and diminished axillary and pubic hair. Individuals may have postural hypotension, fasting hypoglycemia, diminished tolerance for stress, and poor resistance to infection.

The clinical presentations of individuals with thyroid hormone deficiency associated with hypopituitarism are similar (although usually milder) to those seen with primary hypothyroidism. Common symptoms include cold intolerance, constipation, fatigue, lethargy, and weight gain. (Hypothyroidism is discussed in greater detail later in this chapter.)

Diagnostic Studies

In addition to conducting a history and physical examination, diagnostic studies are useful in the diagnosis and treatment of hypopituitarism. Radiologic tests such as MRI and CT are indicated to determine the presence of a pituitary tumor. The laboratory tests indicated for hypopituitarism vary widely, but generally involve the direct measurement of pituitary hormones or an indirect determination of the hormone level. Diagnostic tests are also used to evaluate the effectiveness of therapy. See Chapter 46 for more information regarding diagnostic studies.

Collaborative Care

Treatment of hypopituitarism consists of surgery or radiation for tumor removal, followed by permanent hormone replacement. Surgery and radiation of pituitary tumors are discussed earlier in this chapter. Hormone replacement therapy is carried out with the appropriate hormone needed (e.g., GH, corticosteroids, thyroid hormone, and sex hormones). Hormone replacement therapies for thyroid hormone and corticosteroids are discussed later in this chapter.

Somatropin (Genotropin, Humatrope) is used for GH replacement therapy. Adults with GH deficiency respond well to GH replacement and experience increased energy, increased lean body mass, a feeling of well-being, and improved body image. The side effects most commonly reported by adults include swelling in the feet and hands, pain in the joints, and headache. Somatropin is given as a subcutaneous injection. The dosing is variable because it is adjusted based on relief of symptoms, IGF-1 levels, and the development of adverse effects.

Although gonadal deficiency is not life threatening, replacement therapy is offered to improve sexual function and general well-being. This therapy, however, is contraindicated in individuals with certain medical conditions, such as breast cancer, phlebitis, and pulmonary embolism in women and prostate cancer in men. Testosterone is used to treat men with gonadotropin deficiency. The benefits achieved with testosterone therapy include a return of male secondary sex characteristics, improvement in libido, and increase in muscle mass, bone mass, and bone density. Testosterone can be administered via a transdermal patch, topical gel, self-administered IM injection, or orally. Because oral preparations are often ineffective and have more side effects, their use is limited.[9] Dosing is adjusted to keep serum testosterone levels within a normal range.

Estrogen and progesterone replacement therapy may be indicated for hypogonadal women to treat hot flashes, vaginal dryness, and decreased libido. Hormone replacement for women is discussed in greater detail in Chapter 52.

NURSING MANAGEMENT
HYPOFUNCTION OF THE PITUITARY GLAND

A primary nursing role in anterior pituitary insufficiency is assessment and recognition of signs and symptoms associated with hypopituitarism. Nursing management is directed at providing interventions associated with problems that result from hormone deficiency. The nurse also plays a pivotal role in teaching the patient about diagnostic procedures, the disease process, and collaborative care options. Because of the need for lifelong hormonal therapy, patient teaching is important regarding hormonal administration, side effects, and follow-up therapy. Because individuals with hypopituitarism incur a number of health-related costs and are more likely to take sick days compared with the general population, the nurse should also explore concerns associated with finances and role performance at both home and work.[11]

Disorders Associated with Antidiuretic Hormone Secretion

The two primary conditions associated with antidiuretic hormone (ADH) secretion are a result of either overproduction or underproduction of ADH. Overproduction or oversecretion of ADH results in a condition known as *syndrome of inappropriate antidiuretic hormone* (SIADH). Underproduction or undersecretion of ADH results in a condition referred to as *diabetes insipidus* (DI).

ADH, also referred to as *arginine vasopressin* (AVP), is synthesized in the hypothalamus and then transported and stored in the posterior pituitary gland. It plays a major role in the regulation of water balance and osmolarity (see Chapter 46).

SYNDROME OF INAPPROPRIATE ANTIDIURETIC HORMONE

Etiology and Pathophysiology

Syndrome of inappropriate antidiuretic hormone (SIADH) occurs when ADH is released despite normal or low plasma osmolarity (Fig. 48-3). SIADH results from an abnormal production or sustained secretion of ADH and is characterized by fluid retention, serum hypoosmolality, dilutional hyponatremia, hypochloremia, concentrated urine in the presence of normal or increased intravascular volume, and normal renal function. This syndrome occurs more commonly in older adults. SIADH is thought to be the most common cause of hyponatremia in older adults.[12]

SIADH has various causes (Table 48-1). The most common cause is malignancy, especially small cell lung cancer. These cancerous cells are capable of producing, storing, and releasing ADH.[13]

SIADH tends to be self-limiting when caused by head trauma or drugs but is chronic in nature when associated with tumors or metabolic diseases. Treatment of the underlying cause or discontinuing the causal medication is indicated to improve the clinical course.

Clinical Manifestations

The excess ADH increases distal tubule and collecting duct permeability and reabsorption of water into the circulation. Consequently, extracellular fluid volume expands, plasma osmolality declines, the glomerular filtration rate increases, and sodium levels decline (dilutional hyponatremia). Hyponatremia causes muscle cramps and weakness. The patient with SIADH will experience low urinary output and increased body weight.[14] As the serum sodium level falls (usually less than 120 mEq/L [120 mmol/L]),

Syndrome of Inappropriate Antidiuretic Hormone (SIADH)

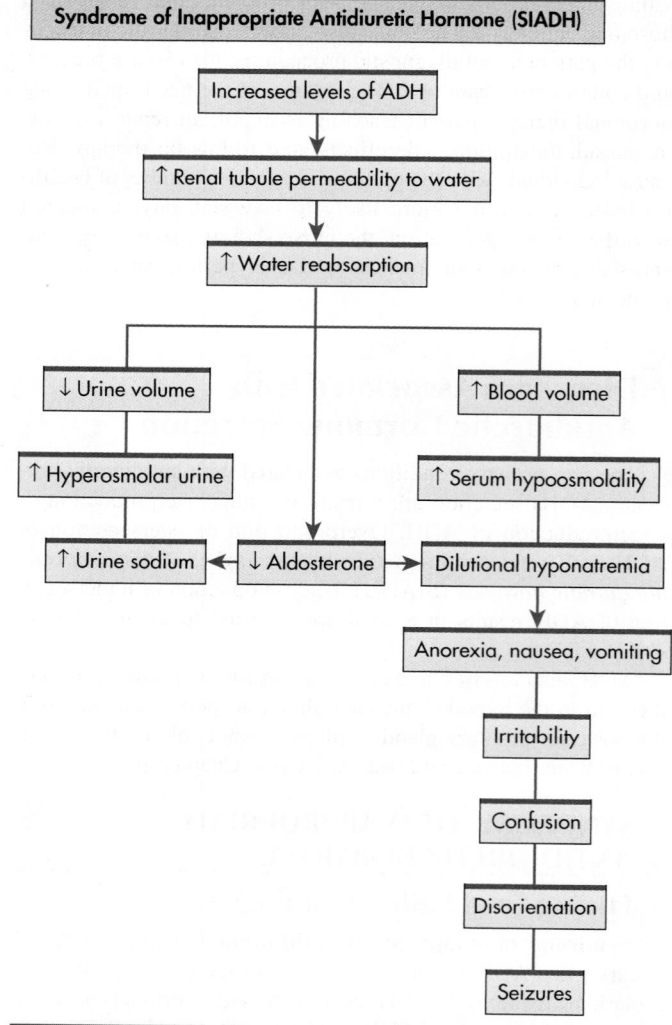

FIG. 48-3 Pathophysiology of syndrome of inappropriate antidiuretic hormone (SIADH).

TABLE 48-1	Causes of Syndrome of Inappropriate Antidiuretic Hormone

Malignant Tumors
Small cell carcinoma of the lung
Pancreatic cancer
Lymphoid cancers (Hodgkin's disease, non-Hodgkin's lymphoma, lymphocytic leukemia)
Thymus cancer
Prostate cancer
Colorectal cancer

Central Nervous System Disorders
Head injury (skull fracture, subdural hematoma, subarachnoid hemorrhage)
Cerebrovascular injury
Brain tumors
Infection (encephalitis, meningitis)
Cerebral atrophy
Guillain-Barré syndrome
Systemic lupus erythematosus

Drug Therapy
carbamazepine (Tegretol)
chlorpropamide (Diabinese)
General anesthesia agents
Opioids
Oxytocin
Thiazide diuretics
Tricyclic antidepressants
Antineoplastic agents (vincristine [Oncovin], vinblastine [Velban], cyclophosphamide [Cytoxan])

Miscellaneous Conditions
Hypothyroidism
Lung infection (pneumonia, tuberculosis, lung abscess)
Chronic obstructive pulmonary disease
Positive pressure mechanical ventilation

manifestations become more severe and include vomiting, abdominal cramps, muscle twitching, and seizures. As plasma osmolality and serum sodium levels continue to decline, cerebral edema may occur, leading to lethargy, anorexia, confusion, headache, seizures, and coma.

Diagnostic Studies

The diagnosis of SIADH is made by simultaneous measurements of urine and serum osmolality. The dilutional hyponatremia is indicated by a serum sodium less than 134 mEq/L, serum osmolality less than 280 mOsm/kg (280 mmol/kg), and a urine specific gravity greater than 1.005. A serum osmolality much lower than the urine osmolality indicates the inappropriate excretion of concentrated urine in the presence of dilute serum. Initially, thirst, dyspnea on exertion, fatigue, and dulled sensorium may be evident. Other laboratory findings are decreased blood urea nitrogen, creatinine clearance, hemoglobin, and hematocrit.

Collaborative Care

Once SIADH is identified, treatment is directed at the underlying cause of the disorder. Medications that stimulate the release of ADH should be avoided or discontinued. The immediate treatment goal is to restore normal fluid volume and osmolality. If symptoms are mild and serum sodium is greater than 125 mEq/L (125 mmol/L), the only treatment may be restriction of fluids to 800 to 1000 ml per day. This restriction should result in gradual, daily reductions in weight, a progressive rise in serum sodium concentration and osmolality, and symptomatic improvement. In cases of severe hyponatremia (less than 120 mEq/L), especially in the presence of neurologic symptoms such as seizures, intravenous hypertonic saline solution (3% to 5%) may be administered. Hypertonic saline requires a very slow infusion rate on an infusion pump to avoid too rapid a rise in sodium. A diuretic such as furosemide (Lasix) may be used to promote diuresis, but only if the serum sodium is at least 125 mEq/L (125 mmol/L), because it may promote further loss of sodium. Because furosemide increases potassium excretion, potassium supplements may be needed. A fluid restriction of 500 ml per day is also indicated for those with severe hyponatremia.

In chronic SIADH, water restriction of 800 to 1000 ml per day is recommended. Because this degree of restriction may not be tolerated, demeclocycline (Declomycin) and lithium may be administered. These agents block the effect of ADH on the renal tubules, thereby allowing a more dilute urine.

NURSING MANAGEMENT
SYNDROME OF INAPPROPRIATE ANTIDIURETIC HORMONE

The nurse can be instrumental in the early detection and treatment of SIADH. An appropriate nursing assessment (Table 48-2) should be conducted for those at risk and those who have confirmed SIADH. Specifically, the nurse should be alert for low urinary output with a high specific gravity, a sudden weight gain, or a serum sodium decline. Nursing management of acute onset of SIADH is presented in Table 48-2.

When SIADH is chronic, the patient must learn to self-manage treatment regimens. Fluids are restricted to 800 to 1000 ml per day. Sucking on hard candy or ice chips can help decrease thirst.[14] If drinking liquids is an aspect of socialization, the patient should be assisted in planning fluid intake so liquid allowances are saved for social occasions. The patient may be treated with a diuretic to remove excess fluid volume. The diet should be supplemented

---

TABLE 48-2	**Nursing Assessment and Management: Syndrome of Inappropriate Antidiuretic Hormone**

Assessment
- Hourly vital signs
- Hourly intake (oral and parenteral) and output
- Hourly measurement of urine specific gravity
- Daily weights
- Level of consciousness
- Observe for signs of hyponatremia (e.g., decreased neurologic function, seizures, nausea and vomiting, muscle cramping)
- Monitor heart and lung sounds

Management
- Restrict total fluid intake to no more than 1000 ml/day (including that taken with medications)
- Position head of bed flat or with no more than 10 degrees of elevation to enhance venous return to heart and increase left atrial filling pressure, reducing ADH release
- Protect from injury (i.e., assist with ambulation, side rails up on bed) because of potential alterations in mental status
- Seizure precautions
- Frequent turning, positioning, and range-of-motion exercise (if patient is bedridden)
- Frequent oral hygiene
- Provide distractions to decrease the discomfort of thirst related to fluid restrictions

ADH, Antidiuretic hormone.

---

with sodium and potassium, especially if diuretics are prescribed. Solutions of these electrolytes must be well diluted to prevent gastrointestinal (GI) irritation or damage. They are best taken at mealtime to allow mixing with and dilution by food. The patient should be taught the symptoms of fluid and electrolyte imbalances, especially those involving sodium and potassium, so that responses to treatment can be monitored (see Chapter 16). If a patient is to be treated with demeclocycline (Declomycin), the need for close follow-up care should be stressed because of the nephrotoxic side effects and the potential for fungal infections associated with this drug.

DIABETES INSIPIDUS

Etiology and Pathophysiology

Diabetes insipidus (DI) is a group of conditions associated with a deficiency of production or secretion of ADH or a decreased renal response to ADH. The decrease in ADH results in fluid and electrolyte imbalances caused by increased urinary output and increased plasma osmolality (Fig. 48-4). Depending on the cause, DI may be transient or a chronic lifelong condition.

There are several classifications of DI (Table 48-3). *Central DI* (also known as *neurogenic DI*) occurs when any organic lesion of the hypothalamus, infundibular stem, or posterior pituitary interferes with ADH synthesis, transport, or release.

Nephrogenic DI (NDI) describes conditions in which there is adequate ADH, but there is a decreased response to ADH in the kidney. Lithium is one of the most common causes of drug-induced NDI.[15,16]

Dispogenic DI, a less common condition, is associated with excessive water intake. This can be caused by a structural lesion in the thirst center or may be caused by a psychologic disorder most commonly associated with schizophrenia.[17]

Clinical Manifestations

DI is characterized by increased thirst (polydipsia) and increased urination (polyuria) (see Fig. 48-4). The primary characteristic of DI is the excretion of large quantities of urine (5 to 20 L per day) with a very low specific gravity (less than 1.005) and urine osmolality of <100 mOsm/kg (<100 mmol/kg). Serum osmolality is elevated (usually greater than 295 mOsm/kg [295 mmol/kg]) as a result of hypernatremia due to pure water loss in the kidney. In partial central DI, urinary output may be lower (2 to 4 L per day). Most patients compensate for fluid loss by drinking great amounts of water so that serum osmolality is normal or only moderately elevated. The patient with central DI particularly favors cold or iced drinks. The patient may be fatigued from nocturia and may experience generalized weakness.

Central DI usually occurs suddenly with excessive fluid loss. After intracranial surgery, DI usually has a triphasic pattern: the acute phase with abrupt onset of polyuria; an interphase, where urine volume apparently normalizes; and a third phase, where central DI is permanent. The third phase is usually apparent within 10 to 14 days postoperatively. Central DI that results from head trauma is usually self-limiting and improves with treatment of the underlying problem. DI following cranial surgery is more likely to be permanent. Although the clinical manifestations of NDI are similar, the onset and amount of fluid losses are less dramatic.

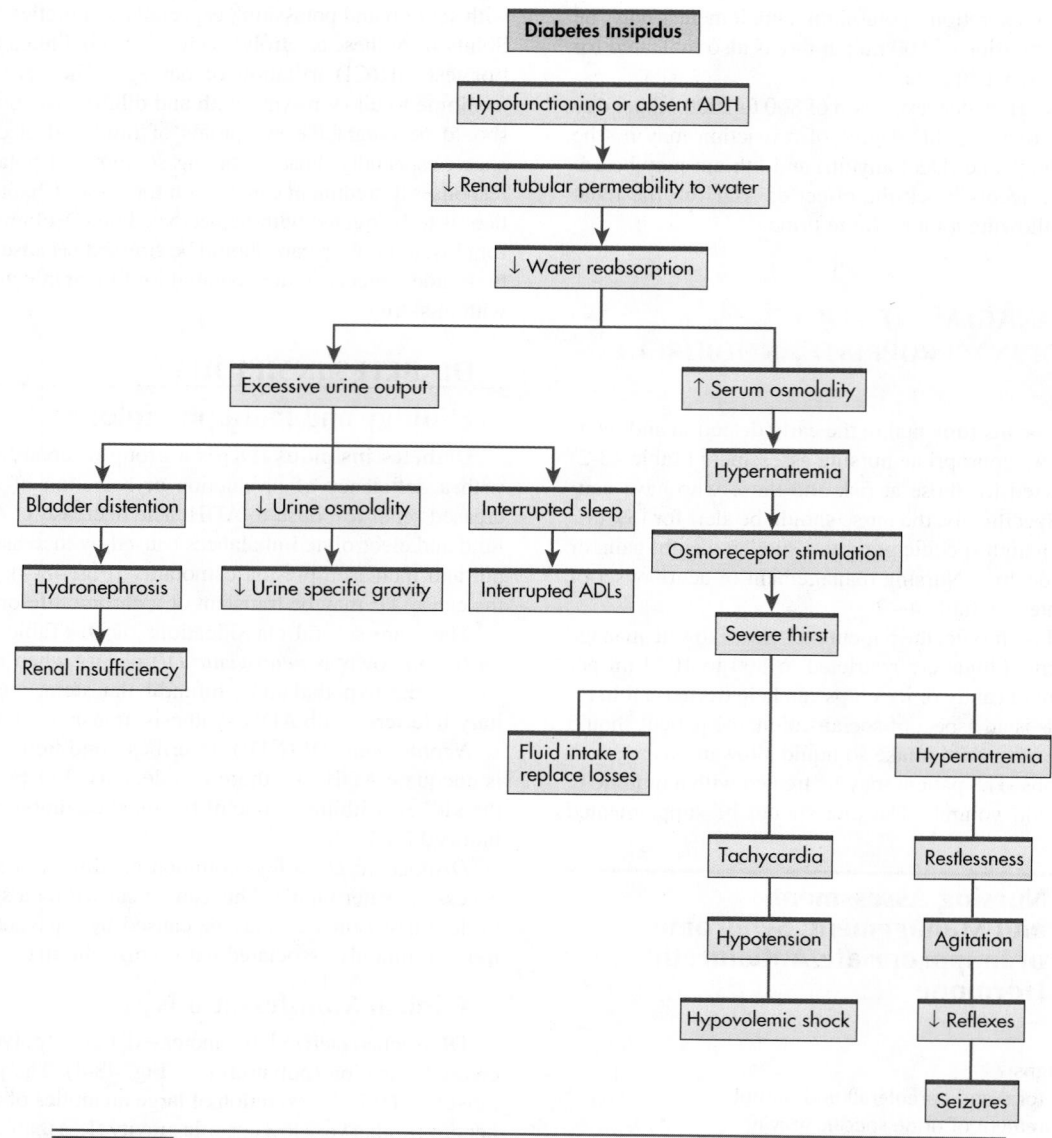

FIG. 48-4 Pathophysiology of diabetes insipidus (DI). *ADH,* Antidiuretic hormone; *ADLs,* activities of daily living.

TABLE 48-3	Types and Causes of Diabetes Insipidus (DI)
TYPES	**CAUSES**
Central DI	Problem stems from an interference with ADH synthesis or release. Multiple causes include brain tumor, head injury, brain surgery, CNS infections.
Nephrogenic DI	Problem stems from inadequate renal response to ADH despite presence of adequate ADH. Caused by drug therapy (especially lithium), renal damage, or hereditary renal disease.
Dispogenic DI	Problem stems from excessive water intake. Caused by structural lesion in thirst center or psychologic disorder.

ADH, Antidiuretic hormone; *CNS,* central nervous system.

If oral fluid intake cannot keep up with urinary losses, severe fluid volume deficit results. This deficit is manifested by weight loss, constipation, poor tissue turgor, hypotension, tachycardia, and shock. In addition, the patient shows central nervous system (CNS) manifestations, ranging from irritability and mental dullness to coma. These manifestations are related to increasing serum osmolality and hypernatremia. Because of the polyuria, severe dehydration and hypovolemic shock may occur.

Diagnostic Studies

Because DI may be central, nephrogenic, or dispogenic in origin, identification of the cause is the initial step. A complete history and physical is done. Dispogenic DI is associated with overhydration and hypervolemia rather than with dehydration and hypovolemia seen in other forms of DI. A water deprivation test is usually done to confirm the diagnosis of central DI. Before a water deprivation test is done, the patient's baseline weight, pulse, urine and plasma osmolalities, specific gravity of urine, and blood pressure are obtained. All fluids are withheld for 8 to 16 hours. The patient may be anxious and should be reassured that the test will be stopped if fluid volume deficit becomes severe. The patient should be observed throughout the test because of the craving to drink. During the test, the patient's blood pressure, weight, and urine osmolality are assessed hourly. The test continues until urine osmolalities stabilize (hourly increase less than 30 mOsm/kg [30 mmol/kg] in 2 consecutive hours) or body weight declines by 5%, or orthostatic hypotension develops. ADH is then given, and urine osmolality is measured 1 hour later. In central DI, the rise in urinary osmolality after vasopressin exceeds 9%.

Collaborative Care

Determining and treating the primary cause is central to the collaborative management of DI. The therapeutic goal is maintenance of fluid and electrolyte balance.

For central DI, fluid and hormonal replacement is the cornerstone of treatment. In acute DI, hypotonic saline is administered intravenously, titrated to replace urinary output.[17] Hormone replacement is necessary because of the lack of ADH production or secretion. Desmopressin acetate (DDAVP), an analog of ADH, is the hormone replacement of choice for central DI. DDAVP can be administered orally, intravenously, or as a nasal spray. Several other drugs are available for ADH replacement, including aqueous vasopressin (Pitressin), vasopressin tannate, and lysine vasopressin (Diapid). Several drugs can be used for the treatment of partial central DI, including chlorpropamide (Diabinese), clofibrate (Atromid), and carbamazepine (Tegretol). Chlorpropamide, thought to potentiate the action of ADH and stimulate endogenous release, is considered the most consistently effective and safest of these agents.

Hormone replacement and chlorpropamide have little effect in the treatment of NDI because the kidney is unable to respond to ADH. Instead, the treatment for NDI revolves around dietary measures (low-sodium diet) and thiazide diuretics. Limiting sodium intake to no more than 3 g per day is thought to help decrease urine output.[17] Interestingly, thiazide diuretics are used in the treatment of NDI. Although it seems paradoxic to treat a condition associated with polyuria with a diuretic, thiazides produce a net decrease in urine output. The thiazides are able to slow the glomerular filtration rate, allowing the kidney to reabsorb more water in the loop of Henle and distal tubles.[18] Thiazide diuretics most commonly used are hydrochlorothiazide (HydroDiuril) and chlorothiazide (Diuril). When low-sodium diet and thiazides are not effective, indomethacin (Indocin) may be prescribed. Indomethacin, a nonsteroidal antiinflammatory agent, helps increase renal responsiveness to ADH.

NURSING MANAGEMENT
DIABETES INSIPIDUS

Nursing management of the patient with DI revolves around early detection, maintenance of adequate hydration, and patient teaching for long-term management.

During acute DI, the nurse administers fluids and hormone replacement. Fluids are replaced orally or intravenously, depending on the patient's condition and ability to drink copious amounts of fluids. Adequate fluids should be kept at the bedside. If IV glucose solutions are used, urine should be assessed for glucose. If urine is positive for glucose, the health care provider should be notified, because glucosuria causes an osmotic diuresis, which increases the fluid volume deficit. Accurate records of intake and output, urine specific gravity, and daily weights are mandatory in the assessment of fluid volume status.

Nursing interventions also include the administration of DDAVP. The patient should be assessed for weight gain, headache, restlessness, and chest pain. The adequacy of treatment is assessed by monitoring fluid intake and output and by urine specific gravity. Increased urine volume with low specific gravity is related to an inadequate pharmacologic effect, and the health care provider should be notified immediately.

The patient with chronic DI requiring long-term ADH replacement needs instruction in self-management. DDAVP can be taken orally or intranasally. Nasal irritation, headache, and nausea may indicate overdosage, whereas failure to improve may indicate underdosage. The patient should be instructed to report any of these symptoms. Patients taking DDAVP should be instructed to monitor their weight daily. Increases in weight may indicate fluid retention. The need for close follow-up should be stressed.

Disorders of the Thyroid Gland

Thyroid hormones, thyroxine (T_4) and triiodothyronine (T_3), regulate energy metabolism and growth and development. Thyroid disorders include hyperfunction, hypofunction, inflammation, and enlargement of the thyroid. Thyroid enlargement is referred to as **goiter.** A goiter may interfere with surrounding structures and can be associated with increased, normal, or decreased hormone production.

HYPERTHYROIDISM

Hyperthyroidism is a clinical syndrome in which there is a sustained increase in synthesis and release of thyroid hormones by the thyroid gland. The term **thyrotoxicosis** refers to the physiologic effects of hypermetabolism that result from excess circulating levels of T_4, T_3, or both. Hyperthyroidism and thyrotoxicosis usually occur together as in Graves' disease. However, in some forms of thyroiditis, thyrotoxicosis may occur without hyperthyroidism.[19]

Hyperthyroidism occurs in approximately 2% of women and only 0.2% men; the highest frequency is in the 30- to 50-year-old age group. The most common form of hyperthyroidism is Graves' disease. Other causes include toxic nodular goiter, thyroiditis, exogenous iodine excess, pituitary tumors, and thyroid cancer.[19]

Etiology and Pathophysiology

Graves' Disease. Graves' disease is an autoimmune disease of unknown etiology marked by diffuse thyroid enlargement and excessive thyroid hormone secretion. Precipitating factors such as insufficient iodine supply, infections, and stressful life events may interact with genetic factors that control the immune response and metabolic abnormalities to cause Graves' disease. A concordance rate of 50% in identical twins indicates genetic and environmental components in the expression of the disease.

Graves' disease accounts for 75% of the cases of hyperthyroidism. The patient develops antibodies to the TSH receptor. These antibodies attach to the receptors and stimulate the thyroid gland to release T_3, T_4, or both. The excessive release of thyroid hormones leads to the clinical manifestations associated with thyrotoxicosis.

The disease is characterized by remissions and exacerbations, with or without treatment. It may progress to destruction of thyroid tissue, causing hypothyroidism.

Toxic Nodular Goiters. Nodular goiters are characterized by thyroid hormone–secreting nodules that are independent of TSH stimulation. If associated with signs of hyperthyroidism, a nodule is termed *toxic*. There may be multiple nodules (multinodular goiter) or a single nodule (solitary autonomous nodule). The nodules are usually benign follicular adenomas. Toxic nodular goiters occur equally in men and women. Although they can appear at any age, the frequency of toxic multinodular goiter is greatest in people over 40 years of age. Small solitary autonomous nodules do not usually secrete enough thyroid hormone to cause clinical thyrotoxicosis. However, larger nodules (greater than 3 cm) may result in clinical disease.

Clinical Manifestations

The clinical manifestations of hyperthyroidism are related to the effects of excess thyroid hormones in two ways. The first is the direct effect of hormones on increasing metabolism. The second is increased tissue sensitivity to stimulation by the sympathetic nervous system. Thyroid hormones increase the number of β-adrenergic receptors, thereby increasing sensitivity to the action of catecholamines (epinephrine and norepinephrine). However, the absolute levels of these hormones are not elevated.

Palpation of the thyroid gland may reveal a goiter. When the thyroid gland is excessively large, a goiter may be noted on inspection. Auscultation of the thyroid gland may reveal bruits. Another common finding associated with hyperthyroidism is *ophthalmopathy,* a term used to describe abnormal eye appearance or function. A classic finding in Graves' disease is **exophthalmos,** a protrusion of the eyeballs from the orbits (Fig. 48-5). Exophthalmos is a type of infiltrative ophthalmopathy that is due to impaired venous drainage from the orbit, which causes increased fat deposits and fluid (edema) in the retroorbital tissues. Because of increased pressure, the eyeballs are forced outward and protrude. This sign is seen in 20% to 40% of patients with Graves' disease. It is usually bilateral but can be unilateral or asymmetric. In non-infiltrative ophthalmopathy, the upper lids are usually retracted and elevated, with the sclera visible above the iris. When the eyelids do not close completely, the exposed corneal surfaces become dry and irritated. Serious consequences, such as corneal ulcers and eventual loss of vision, can occur.

Other common manifestations of thyroid hyperfunction are summarized in Table 48-4. A patient with advanced disease may exhibit many of the manifestations, whereas a patient in the early stages of hyperthyroidism may exhibit only weight loss and increased nervousness. Symptoms in the elderly patient with this disorder may be very different (referred to as *apathetic hyperthyroidism*) and may include anorexia, apathy, lassitude, depression, and confusion.[20] Table 48-5 compares features of hyperthyroidism in younger and older adult patients.

Complications

Thyrotoxic crisis (also called *thyroid storm*) is an acute, rare condition in which all hyperthyroid manifestations are heightened. Although it is considered a life-threatening emergency, death is rare when treatment is vigorous and initiated early. The cause is presumed to be stressors (e.g., infection, trauma, surgery) in a patient with preexisting hyperthyroidism, either diagnosed or undiagnosed. The physiologic factor or factors that initiate thyrotoxic crisis are unknown.[19]

Manifestations include severe tachycardia, heart failure, shock, hyperthermia (up to 105.3° F [40.7° C]), restlessness, agitation, seizures, abdominal pain, nausea, vomiting, diarrhea, delirium, and coma. Aggressive measures must be taken to prevent death. Treatment is aimed at reducing circulating thyroid hormone levels and the clinical manifestations of this disorder by appropriate drug therapy. Therapy is directed at fever reduction, fluid replacement, and elimination or management of the initiating stressor(s).

Diagnostic Studies

The two primary laboratory findings used to confirm the diagnosis of hyperthyroidism are decreased TSH levels and elevated free thyroxine (FT_4) levels.[21] Total T_3 and T_4 may also be assessed, but these are not as useful. Measurements of total T_3 and T_4 measure both free and bound (to protein) hormone levels. In the body, the free hormone is the only form of the hormone that is biologically active.

The radioactive iodine uptake (RAIU) test is indicated to differentiate Graves' disease from other forms of thyroiditis. The patient with Graves' disease will show a diffuse, homogeneous uptake of 35% to 95%, whereas the patient with thyroiditis will show an uptake of less than 2%. The person with nodular goiter will show an uptake in the high-normal range (Table 48-6).

Collaborative Care

The overall goal in the treatment of hyperthyroidism is to block the adverse effects of thyroid hormones and stop their oversecretion. The three primary treatment options for the patient with hyperthyroidism are antithyroid medications, radioactive iodine therapy, and subtotal thyroidectomy (see Table 48-6). In general, the treatment of choice in nonpregnant adults is radioac-

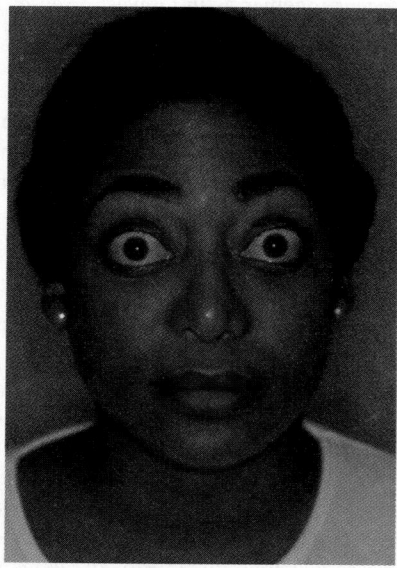

FIG. 48-5 Graves' disease. This woman has a diffuse goiter and exophthalmos.

TABLE 48-4   Clinical Manifestations: Thyroid Hormone Dysfunction

HYPOFUNCTION	HYPERFUNCTION	HYPOFUNCTION	HYPERFUNCTION
Cardiovascular System Increased capillary fragility Decreased rate and force of contraction Varied changes in blood pressure Cardiac hypertrophy Distant heart sounds Anemia Tendency to develop congestive heart failure, angina, myocardial infarction	Systolic hypertension Increased rate and force of cardiac contractions Bounding, rapid pulse Increased cardiac output Cardiac hypertrophy Systolic murmurs Arrhythmias Palpitations Atrial fibrillation (more common in the older adult) Angina	**Musculoskeletal System** Fatigue Weakness Muscular aches and pains Slow movements Arthralgia	Fatigue Muscle weakness Proximal muscle wasting Pretibial myxedema Dependent edema Osteoporosis
Respiratory System Dyspnea Decreased breathing capacity	Increased respiratory rate Dyspnea on mild exertion	**Nervous System** Apathy Lethargy Fatigue Forgetfulness Slowed mental processes Hoarseness Slow, slurred speech Prolonged relaxation of deep tendon muscles Stupor, coma Paresthesias Anxiety, depression Polyneuropathy	Difficulty in focusing eyes Nervousness Fine tremor (of fingers and tongue) Insomnia Lability of mood, delirium Restlessness Personality changes of irritability, agitation Exhaustion Hyperreflexia of tendon reflexes Depression, fatigue, apathy (in the older adult) Lack of ability to concentrate Stupor, coma
Gastrointestinal System Decreased appetite Nausea and vomiting Weight gain Constipation Distended abdomen Enlarged, scaly tongue	Increased appetite, thirst Weight loss Increased peristalsis Diarrhea, frequent defecation Increased bowel sounds Splenomegaly Hepatomegaly		
		Reproductive System Prolonged menstrual periods or amenorrhea Decreased libido Infertility	Menstrual irregularities Amenorrhea Decreased libido Impotence in men Gynecomastia in men Decreased fertility
Integumentary System Dry, thick, inelastic, cold skin Thick, brittle nails Dry, sparse, coarse hair Poor turgor of mucosa Generalized interstitial edema Puffy face Decreased sweating Pallor	Warm, smooth, moist skin Thin, brittle nails detached from nailbed (onycholysis) Hair loss (may be patchy) Clubbing of fingers Palmar erythema Fine silky hair Premature graying (in men) Diaphoresis Vitiligo	**Other** Increased susceptibility to infection Increased sensitivity to narcotics, barbiturates, anesthesia Intolerance to cold Decreased hearing Sleepiness Goiter	Intolerance to heat Increased sensitivity to stimulant drugs Elevated basal temperature Lid lag, stare Eyelid retraction Exophthalmos Goiter Rapid speech

TABLE 48-5   Comparison of Hyperthyroidism in Younger and Older Adults

	YOUNGER ADULT	OLDER ADULT
Common causes	Graves' disease in >90% of cases	Graves' disease or toxic nodular goiter
Common symptoms	Nervousness, irritability, weight loss, heat intolerance, warm, moist skin	Anorexia, weight loss, apathy, lassitude, depression, confusion
Goiter	Present in >90% of cases	Present in about 50% of cases
Ophthalmopathy	Exophthalmos present in 20%–40% of cases	Exophthalmos less common
Cardiac features	Tachycardia and palpitations common, but without heart failure	Angina, arrhythmia, congestive heart failure may occur

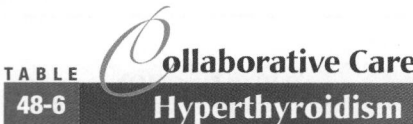

TABLE 48-6	Collaborative Care — Hyperthyroidism

Diagnostic
History and physical examination
Ophthalmologic examination
ECG
Laboratory tests
• Serum free T_4, TSH levels
• TRH stimulation test
Radioactive iodine uptake (RAIU)

Collaborative Therapy
Drug Therapy
Antithyroid drugs
• propylthiouracil (PTU)
• methimazole (Tapazole)
Iodine
β-Adrenergic blockers (e.g., propranolol [Inderal]
Radiation Therapy
Radioactive iodine
Surgical Therapy
Subtotal thyroidectomy
Nutritional Therapy
High-calorie diet
High-protein diet
Frequent meals

ECG, Electrocardiogram; *TRH*, thyrotropin-releasing hormone; *TSH*, thyroid-stimulating hormone.

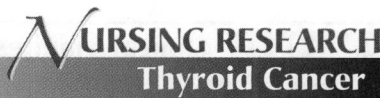

NURSING RESEARCH
Thyroid Cancer

Citation
Stajduhar KI et al: Thyroid cancer: patients' experiences of receiving I[131] therapy, *Oncol Nurs Forum* 27:1213, 2000.

Purpose
To enhance the understanding of experiences and needs of patients with thyroid cancer receiving iodine-131 therapy.

Methods
Data for this qualitative study were collected through focus groups, telephone interviews, and field notes. Tape recordings were made of the interviews. Data were subjected to thematic analysis.

Results and Conclusions
Four major themes emerged from data analysis: recognizing the totality of the cancer experience, isolation, recognizing the totality of the treatment experience, and understanding barriers to treatment. Based on the data, it was concluded that health care workers involved with patients with thyroid cancer lack an understanding of thyroid disease and the effects of therapy. Educational programs are needed to adequately prepare both nurses and patients.

Implications for Nursing Practice
An improvement in the care and education provided to patients receiving I[131] therapy is needed. Nurse education, as well as patient education, is needed. In order for nurses to provide comprehensive cancer care, psychosocial and physical needs must be addressed, requiring a collaborative approach among patient, nurses, and other health care professionals.

tive iodine therapy. However, the choice of treatment is influenced by the patient's age, severity of the disorder, complicating features (including pregnancy), and patient's preferences. If surgery is to be performed, the patient is usually given antithyroid drugs and iodine to produce a euthyroid state and possibly β-adrenergic blockers to relieve symptoms preoperatively.

Drug Therapy. Drugs used in the treatment of hyperthyroidism include antithyroid drugs, iodine, and β-adrenergic blockers. It is important to note that although these drugs are useful in the treatment of thyrotoxic states, they are not considered curative. Radiation therapy or surgery may ultimately be required.

Antithyroid drugs. The first-line antithyroid drugs used in the treatment of hyperthyroidism are propylthiouracil (PTU) and methimazole (Tapazole). These drugs inhibit the synthesis of thyroid hormones. PTU also blocks peripheral conversion of T_4 to T_3. Although there is considerable individual variation, improvement usually begins 1 to 2 weeks after the initiation of therapy, and good results are seen within 4 to 8 weeks. Therapy is usually continued for 6 months to 2 years to allow for spontaneous remission. These drugs are not curative. The major disadvantages of these drugs are patient noncompliance and a high rate of recurrence of hyperthyroidism when the drugs are discontinued. In addition, agranulocytosis may occur in rare situations. Indications for use of antithyroid drugs include Graves' disease in the young patient, hyperthyroidism during pregnancy, and the need to attain a euthyroid state before surgery or radiation therapy.

Iodine. Iodine is useful in conjunction with other antithyroid drugs in the preparation of a patient for thyroidectomy or for treatment of thyrotoxic crisis. The administration of iodine in

large doses rapidly inhibits synthesis of T_3 and T_4 and blocks the release of these hormones into circulation. It also decreases the vascularity of the thyroid gland, making surgery safer and easier. The maximal effect of iodine is usually seen within 1 to 2 weeks. After that time, a reduction in the therapeutic effect may be seen. For this reason, long-term iodine therapy is not effective in controlling hyperthyroidism. Iodine is available in the form of saturated solution of potassium (SSKI) and Lugol's solution.

β-Adrenergic blockers. β-Adrenergic blockers are used for symptomatic relief of thyrotoxicosis that results from increased β-adrenergic receptor stimulation caused by excess thyroid hormones. Propranolol (Inderal), the most frequently used β-adrenergic blocker, is usually administered with other antithyroid agents and rapidly provides symptomatic relief. Atenolol (Tenormin) is the preferred β-adrenergic blocker for use in the hyperthyroid patient with asthma or heart disease.

Radioactive Iodine Therapy. As mentioned previously, radioactive iodine therapy (RAI) is the treatment of choice for most nonpregnant adults. (A pregnancy test is done on all women who experience menstrual cycles before initiation of therapy.) RAI damages or destroys thyroid tissue, thus limiting thyroid hormone secretion. Radioactive iodine has a delayed response, and maximum effects may not be seen for 2 to 3 months. For this reason, the patient is usually treated with antithyroid drugs and propranolol before and during the first 3 months after the initiation of RAI until the effects of irradiation become apparent. Although this method of treatment is usually effective, the biggest disadvantage is the high incidence of posttreatment hypothyroidism, resulting in the need for lifelong thyroid hormone replacement.[21]

Surgical Therapy. Another effective treatment option for the individual with hyperthyroidism is a thyroidectomy. A *subtotal thyroidectomy* is the preferred surgical procedures and involves the removal of a significant portion of the thyroid gland. For subtotal thyroidectomy to be effective, approximately 90% of thyroid tissue must be removed. If too much tissue is taken, the gland will not regenerate after surgery and hypothyroidism will result. Thyroidectomy is indicated for individuals who have been unresponsive to antithyroid therapy, for individuals with very large goiters causing tracheal compression, and for individuals with a possible malignancy. Additionally, this surgery may be done when an individual is not a good candidate for RAI or does not want to take RAI.[22,23] One advantage thyroidectomy has over RAI is a more rapid reduction in T_3 and T_4 levels.

Endoscopic thyroidectomy is a minimally invasive procedure. It is an appropriate procedure for patients with small nodules (less than 3 cm) where there is no evidence of malignancy. An advantage of endoscopic thyroidectomy over the traditional approach is less scarring, less pain, and a faster return to normal activity.

Before surgery, antithyroid drugs, iodine, and β-adrenergic blockers may be administered to achieve a euthyroid state and to control symptoms. Iodine reduces vascularization of the gland, reducing the risk of hemorrhage. Other associated disorders such as cardiac disease or diabetes mellitus must also be controlled. Postoperative complications include hypothyroidism, damage to or inadvertent removal of parathyroid glands causing hypoparathyroidism and hypocalcemia, hemorrhage, injury to the recurrent or superior laryngeal nerve, thyrotoxic crisis, and infection.

Nutritional Therapy. The potential for nutritional deficits is high when an increased metabolic rate is present. A high-calorie diet (4000 to 5000 kcal/day) may be ordered to satisfy hunger and prevent tissue breakdown. This is accomplished with six full meals a day and snacks high in protein, carbohydrates, minerals, and vitamins, particularly vitamin A, thiamine, vitamin B_6, and vitamin C. The protein allowance should be 1 to 2 g/kg of ideal body weight. Increased carbohydrates should compensate for disturbed metabolism, provide energy, and spare body protein stores. Highly seasoned and high-fiber foods should be avoided because they stimulate the already hyperactive gastrointestinal tract. Substitutes should be provided for caffeine-containing liquids such as coffee, tea, and cola because the stimulating effects of these fluids increase restlessness and sleep disturbances. Milk is an excellent food source that provides calcium and protein. A dietitian should be consulted for guidance in meeting the nutritional needs of a patient with hyperthyroidism.

NURSING MANAGEMENT
HYPERTHYROIDISM

■ Nursing Assessment

Subjective and objective data that should be obtained from an individual with hyperthyroidism are presented in Table 48-7.

■ Nursing Diagnoses

Nursing diagnoses for the patient with hyperthyroidism include, but are not limited to, those presented in NCP 48-1.

■ Planning

The overall goals are that the patient with hyperthyroidism will (1) experience relief of symptoms, (2) have no serious complications related to the disease or treatment, and (3) cooperate with the therapeutic plan.

TABLE 48-7	Nursing Assessment Hyperthyroidism

Subjective Data

Important Health Information

Past health history: Preexisting goiter; recent infection or trauma, immigration from iodine-deficient area, autoimmune disease

Medications: Use of thyroid hormones

Functional Health Patterns

Health perception–health management: Positive family history of thyroid or autoimmune disorders

Nutritional-metabolic: Insufficient iodine intake; weight loss; increased appetite, thirst; nausea

Elimination: Diarrhea; polyuria; sweating

Activity-exercise: Dyspnea on exertion; palpitations; muscle weakness, fatigue

Sleep-rest: Insomnia

Cognitive-perceptual: Chest pain; nervousness; heat intolerance; pruritus

Sexuality-reproductive: Decreased libido; impotence; gynecomastia (in men); amenorrhea (in women)

Coping–stress tolerance: Emotional lability, irritability, restlessness, personality changes, delirium

Objective Data

General Observation

Agitation, rapid speech and body movements; hyperthermia, enlarged or nodular thyroid gland

Eyes

Exophthalmos, eyelid retraction; infrequent blinking

Integumentary

Warm, diaphoretic, velvety skin; thin, loose nails; fine, silky hair and hair loss; palmar erythema; clubbing; white pigmentation of skin (vitiligo), diffuse edema of legs and feet

Respiratory

Tachypnea

Cardiovascular

Tachycardia, bounding pulse, systolic murmurs, arrhythmias, hypertension

Gastrointestinal

Increased bowel sounds; hepatosplenomegaly

Neurologic

Hyperreflexia; diplopia; fine tremors of hands, tongue, eyelids; stupor; coma

Musculoskeletal

Muscle wasting

Reproductive

Menstrual irregularities, infertility; impotence, gynecomastia in men

Possible Findings

↑ T_3, ↑ T_4; ↑ T_3 resin uptake; ↓ serum thyroid-stimulating hormone (TSH); chest x-ray showing enlarged heart

NURSING CARE PLAN 48-1

Patient with Hyperthyroidism

EXPECTED PATIENT OUTCOMES	NURSING INTERVENTIONS and *RATIONALES*
NURSING DIAGNOSIS	**Activity intolerance** *related to* fatigue, exhaustion, and heat intolerance secondary to hypermetabolism *as manifested by* complaints of weakness, hyperactivity, short attention span, memory lapses, dyspnea, tachycardia, irritability.
▪ Decreased perception of weakness and fatigue	▪ Assess for signs of activity intolerance *because hyperthyroidism results in protein catabolism, overactivity, and increased metabolism leading to exhaustion.* ▪ Monitor vital signs q4hr and before and after activities *because tachycardia and BP elevations can indicate excessive thyroid hormone activity.* ▪ Assist patient with self-care as needed *to make certain patient's daily needs are met.* ▪ Schedule activities of daily living and treatments *to promote adequate rest periods.*
NURSING DIAGNOSIS	**Risk for injury** (corneal ulceration) *related to* decreased blinking or inability to close eyelids secondary to exophthalmos.
▪ No evidence of corneal damage	▪ Assess patient for complaints of eye pain, feeling of grittiness or "sand" in eyes, inability to close eyelids completely, lid lag, lid retraction, visible sclera above iris, and "stare" *to determine if risk factors are present for corneal ulcers and initiate appropriate interventions.* ▪ Teach patient to exercise extraocular muscles daily *to maintain flexibility.* ▪ Cover patient's eyes with mask or tape shut if eyes will not close *to prevent corneal drying and, at night, to promote sleep.* ▪ Apply methylcellulose eyedrops (artificial tears) *to soothe and moisten conjunctival membranes.*
NURSING DIAGNOSIS	**Imbalanced nutrition: less than body requirements** *related to* hypermetabolism and inadequate diet *as manifested by* complaints of weight loss; less than optimal body weight.
▪ Maintenance of weight (or gain weight) ▪ Alleviation (or prevention) of nutritional deficiency	▪ Assess patient's eating habits and weight pattern *to determine extent of the problem and plan appropriate interventions.* ▪ Teach and provide high-calorie, high-vitamin, high-mineral diet that includes between-meal and bedtime snacks *because hyperthyroidism increases metabolic rate.* ▪ Weigh patient daily *to evaluate effectiveness of nutritional plan.* ▪ Arrange dietary consultation if indicated.
NURSING DIAGNOSIS	**Anxiety** *related to* lack of knowledge about management and course of disease and hypermetabolism *as manifested by* verbalization of inability to cope with stress.
▪ Verbalization of knowledge of management and course of disease ▪ Verbalization of decrease in anxiety	▪ Teach patient about disease management, including medication regimen, potential for hypertension, chronic nature of disease, and dietary implications, *because knowledge decreases anxiety and increases a sense of control.* ▪ Promote rest and relaxation *because anxiety often causes difficulty with rest and sleep.* ▪ Teach patient strategies for coping with stress *to prevent increasing anxiety.* ▪ Administer medications as ordered *because decrease in clinical manifestations will decrease anxiety.*

▪ Nursing Implementation

Acute Intervention. Individuals who have hyperthyroidism are usually treated in an outpatient setting. However, patients who develop acute thyrotoxicosis or those who undergo thyroidectomy require hospitalization and acute care.

Acute thyrotoxicosis. Acute thyrotoxicosis is a systemic syndrome that requires aggressive treatment, often in an intensive care unit. The nurse needs to administer medications (previously discussed) that block thyroid hormone production. Nursing management also includes provisions for supportive therapy. Having an understanding of the major organ response to the hypermetabolic state is a critical aspect of nursing management. Supportive therapy includes monitoring for cardiac arrhythmias and decompensation, ensuring adequate oxygenation, and administration of

intravenous fluids to replace fluid and electrolyte losses. This is especially important in the patient who develops vomiting and diarrhea.[24,25]

A calm, quiet room should be provided because increased metabolism causes sleep disturbances. Provision of adequate rest may be a challenge because of the patient's irritability and restlessness. Specific interventions may include (1) placing the patient in a cool room, away from very ill patients and noisy, high-traffic areas; (2) using light bed coverings and changing the linen frequently if the patient is diaphoretic; (3) encouraging and assisting with exercise involving large muscle groups (tremors can interfere with small-muscle coordination) to allow the release of nervous tension and restlessness; (4) restricting visitors who upset the patient; and (5) establishing a supportive, trusting relationship to help the patient cope with aggravating events and lessen anxiety.

If exophthalmos is present, there is a potential for corneal injury related to irritation and dryness. The patient may also have orbital pain. Nursing interventions to relieve eye discomfort and prevent corneal ulceration include applying artificial tears to soothe and moisten conjunctival membranes. Salt restriction may help reduce periorbital edema. Elevation of the patient's head promotes fluid drainage from the periorbital area; the patient should sit upright as much as possible. Dark glasses reduce glare and prevent irritation from smoke, air currents, dust, and dirt. If the eyelids cannot be closed, they should be lightly taped shut for sleep. To maintain flexibility, the patient should be taught to exercise the intraocular muscles several times a day by turning the eyes in the complete range of motion. Good grooming can be helpful in reducing the loss of self-esteem that can result from an altered body image. If the exophthalmos is severe, treatment may involve suturing the eyelids together, administering corticosteroids, radiation of retroorbital tissues, orbital decompression, or corrective lid or muscle surgery.

Thyroid surgery. When subtotal thyroidectomy is the treatment of choice, the patient must be adequately prepared to avoid postoperative complications. The signs and symptoms of thyrotoxicosis must be alleviated as much as possible, and cardiac problems must be controlled before surgery. If iodine is used to relieve hyperthyroid symptoms, it should be mixed with water or juice, sipped through a straw, and administered after meals. The patient must be assessed for signs of iodine toxicity such as swelling of buccal mucosa and other mucous membranes, excessive salivation, nausea and vomiting, and skin reactions. If toxicity occurs, iodine administration should be discontinued and the physician notified.

Preoperative teaching should include comfort and safety measures in which the patient can participate. Coughing, deep breathing, and leg exercises should be practiced and their importance explained. The patient should be taught how to support the head manually while turning in bed, because this maneuver minimizes stress on the suture line after surgery. Range-of-motion exercises of the neck should be practiced. The nurse should explain routine postoperative care such as IV infusions. The patient should be told that talking is likely to be difficult for a short time after surgery.

The hospital room must be prepared before the patient's return from surgery. Oxygen, suction equipment, and a tracheostomy tray should be readily available. A tracheostomy tray is required in case airway obstruction occurs. Although this rarely occurs, it is an emergency situation the nurse must be prepared for. Recurrent laryngeal nerve damage leads to vocal cord paralysis. If there is paralysis of both cords, spastic airway obstruction will occur, requiring an immediate tracheostomy.

Respiration may also become difficult because of excess swelling of the neck tissues, hemorrhage, hematoma formation, and laryngeal stridor. *Laryngeal stridor* (harsh, vibratory sound) may occur during inspiration and expiration as a result of tetany, which occurs if the parathyroid glands are removed or damaged during surgery. To treat tetany, calcium salts such as calcium gluconate and calcium chloride should be readily available for IV administration.

After a thyroidectomy the nurse should do the following:

1. Assess the patient every 2 hours for 24 hours for signs of hemorrhage or tracheal compression such as irregular breathing, neck swelling, frequent swallowing, sensations of fullness at the incision site, choking, and blood on the anterior or posterior dressings.

2. Place the patient in a semi-Fowler position and support the patient's head with pillows, avoiding flexion of the neck and any tension on the suture lines.

3. Monitor vital signs. Complete the initial assessment by checking for signs of tetany secondary to hypoparathyroidism (e.g., tingling in toes, fingers, or around the mouth; muscular twitching; apprehension) and by evaluating difficulty in speaking and hoarseness. Trousseau's sign and Chvostek's sign should be monitored for 72 hours (see Chapter 16, Fig. 16-15). Some hoarseness is to be expected for 3 to 4 days after surgery because of edema.

4. Control postoperative pain by giving medication.

If postoperative recovery is uneventful, the patient is ambulated within hours after surgery, is permitted to take fluid as soon as tolerated, and eats a soft diet the day after surgery.

The appearance of the incision may be highly distressing to the patient. The patient can be reassured that the scar will fade in color and eventually look like a normal neck wrinkle. A scarf, jewelry, high collar, or other covering can effectively camouflage a fresh scar.

Ambulatory and Home Care

Postoperative care. Discharge teaching for the patient following surgery is an important aspect of nursing care. The patient and family need to be aware that thyroid hormone balance should be monitored periodically to ensure that normal function has returned. Most patients experience a period of relative hypothyroidism soon after surgery because of the substantial reduction in the size of the thyroid. However, the remaining tissue usually hypertrophies, recovering the capacity to produce the hormone needed by the body, but this takes time. The administration of thyroid hormone is avoided because exogenous hormone inhibits pituitary production of TSH and delays or prevents the restoration of normal gland function and thyroid tissue regeneration.

The patient can do a great deal to prevent complications and promote a return to normal function during the hypothyroid period after surgery. Caloric intake must be reduced substantially below the amount that was required before surgery to prevent weight gain. The patient may be advised to avoid **goitrogens** (foods that contain thyroid-inhibiting substances) (Table 48-8). Adequate iodine is necessary to promote thyroid function, but excesses inhibit the thyroid. Seafood once or twice a week or normal use of iodized salt should provide sufficient intake.

Regular exercise helps stimulate the thyroid gland and should be encouraged. High environmental temperature should be avoided because it inhibits thyroid regeneration.

Regular follow-up care is necessary. The patient should be seen biweekly for a month and then at least semiannually to assess for the development of hypothyroidism. If a complete thyroidectomy has been performed, the patient needs instruction in lifelong thyroid replacement. Failure of thyroid function is considered the normal end stage of Graves' disease. The patient should be taught the signs and symptoms of progressive thyroid failure and instructed to seek medical care if these develop.

TABLE 48-8	Common Exogenous Goitrogens	
Foods	**Drugs**
Potent Goitrogens	***Thyroid Inhibitors***
Turnips	propylthiouracil (PTU)
Rutabagas	methimazole (Tapazole)
Soybeans	Iodine in large doses
Skins of peanuts	***Others***
Milk from kale-fed cattle	Sulfonamides
Less Potent Goitrogens	Salicylates
Seafood	p-Aminosalicylic acid
Green leafy vegetables	phenylbutazone (Butazolidin)
Peanuts	lithium
Peaches	amiodarone (Cardarone)
Peas	
Strawberries	
Carrots	
Cabbage	
Mustard seed	
Radishes	

Hypothyroidism is relatively easy to manage with oral administration of thyroid replacement.

Radioactive iodine therapy. Radioactive iodine therapy is administered on an outpatient basis and is the therapy of choice for the nonpregnant adult. Because the therapeutic dose of radioactive iodine is low, no radiation safety precautions are necessary. The patient should be instructed that radiation thyroiditis and parotiditis are possible and may cause dryness and irritation of the mouth and throat. Relief may be obtained with frequent sips of water, ice chips, or the use of a salt and soda gargle three or four times per day. This gargle is made by dissolving 1 teaspoon of salt and 1 teaspoon of baking soda in 2 cups of warm water. The discomfort should subside in 3 to 4 days. If dryness and irritation persist, the patient should contact his or her health care provider. Because of the high frequency of hypothyroidism after radioactive iodine therapy, the patient and significant others should be taught the symptoms of hypothyroidism and instructed to seek medical help if these symptoms occur.

■ **Evaluation**

The expected outcomes are that the patient with hyperthyroidism will
■ experience relief of symptoms
■ have no serious complications related to the disease or treatment
■ cooperate with the therapeutic plan

THYROID ENLARGEMENT

Goiter is hypertrophy of the thyroid gland caused by excess TSH stimulation, which in turn can be caused by inadequate circulating thyroid hormones. Goiter may also be caused by growth-stimulating immunoglobulins and other growth factors. Goitrogens (see Table 48-8), which inhibit synthesis of thyroid hormone, can cause goiter but usually only in the individual who lives in an iodine-deficient area (endemic goiter). A goiter is also commonly found in patients with Graves' disease.

TSH and T$_4$ levels are measured to determine whether a goiter is associated with hyperthyroidism, hypothyroidism, or nor-

mal thyroid function. Thyroid antibodies are measured to assess for thyroiditis. Treatment with thyroid hormone may prevent further thyroid enlargement. Surgery to remove large goiters may be necessary.

THYROID NODULES

A thyroid nodule, a palpable deformity of the thyroid gland, may be benign or malignant. Benign nodules are usually not dangerous, but they can cause tracheal compression if they become too large. Malignant tumors of the thyroid gland are not common. The American Cancer Society estimated 20,700 new cases of thyroid cancer were diagnosed in 2002.[26] The four major types of thyroid cancer are papillary, follicular, medullary, and anaplastic. The major sign of thyroid cancer is the presence of a hard, painless nodule or nodules on an enlarged thyroid gland.

Nodular enlargement of the thyroid gland or palpation of a mass usually requires radiologic evaluation. Ultrasound is often the first radiologic test used in the diagnostic workup of a thyroid nodule. Computed tomography (CT), magnetic resonance imaging (MRI), and ultrasound-guided fine-needle aspiration (FNA) are other diagnostic options. FNA is indicated when a tissue sample for pathologic examination is necessary. FNA is considered one of the most effective methods to identify malignancy.[27] A thyroid scan may also be done to evaluate for possible malignancy. The scan shows whether nodules on the thyroid are "hot" or "cold." Thyroid tumors may or may not take up radioactive iodine. Tumors that take up the radioactive iodine are called "hot" nodules and are nearly always benign. If the nodule does not take up the radioactive iodine, it appears as "cold" and has a higher risk of being malignant. Measurement of serum calcitonin is also helpful in diagnosis, because increased levels are associated with medullary thyroid carcinoma.

Surgical removal of the tumor is usually indicated in the treatment of thyroid cancer. Surgical procedures may range from unilateral total lobectomy with removal of the isthmus to total thyroidectomy with bilateral lobectomy. Many thyroid cancers are TSH dependent, and thyroid hormone in hyperphysiologic doses is often prescribed to inhibit pituitary secretion of TSH. Radiation therapy may also be indicated to prolong survival.

Nursing care for the patient with thyroid tumors is similar to care for the patient who has undergone thyroidectomy and also includes general nursing measures for the patient with cancer (see Chapter 15).

THYROIDITIS

Thyroiditis is an inflammatory process in the thyroid and can have several causes. *Subacute granulomatous thyroiditis* (de Quervain's thyroiditis), which causes thyrotoxicosis, is thought to be caused by a viral infection. *Acute thyroiditis* is due to bacterial or fungal infection. Subacute and acute forms of thyroiditis have abrupt onsets and the thyroid gland is painful. *Chronic autoimmune thyroiditis* (Hashimoto's thyroiditis), leading to hypothyroidism, is insidious in onset. Hashimoto's thyroiditis is a chronic autoimmune disease in which thyroid tissue is replaced by lymphocytes and fibrous tissue. It is the most common cause of goiterous hypothyroidism in the United States. *Silent thyroiditis,* a form of lymphocytic thyroiditis, has a variable onset. In women, this condition may occur in the postpartal period. It is believed to be an autoimmune disease and may be early Hashimoto's thyroiditis.

T_4 and T_3 are initially elevated in subacute, acute, and silent thyroiditis but may become depressed with time. TSH levels are low and then elevated. Thyroid hormone levels are usually low in chronic Hashimoto's thyroiditis, and TSH is high. Suppression of RAIU is seen in subacute and silent thyroiditis. Antithyroid antibodies are present in Hashimoto's thyroiditis.

Recovery from thyroiditis may be complete in weeks or months without treatment. If the condition is bacterial in origin, treatment may include specific antibiotics or surgical drainage. In subacute and acute forms, salicylates and nonsteroidal antiinflammatory drugs are used. If there is no response to these drugs in 48 hours, corticosteroids are given. Propranolol (Inderal) or atenolol (Tenormin) may be used for the cardiovascular symptoms of a hyperthyroid condition. Thyroid hormone replacement is indicated if the patient is hypothyroid.

Nursing care of the patient with thyroiditis depends, in part, on the therapeutic management. Education regarding treatment and encouraging compliance are important for all types of thyroiditis. The patient should be instructed to remain under close health care supervision so that progress can be monitored and to report any change in symptoms to the health care provider.

The patient with thyroiditis of autoimmune origin may be susceptible to other autoimmune diseases such as Addison's disease, pernicious anemia, premature gonadal failure, or Graves' disease. The patient should be taught the signs and symptoms of these disorders, particularly Addison's disease. The patient should also be given a list of common goitrogens (see Table 48-8) and encouraged to avoid them as much as possible. A patient receiving thyroid hormone replacement must be taught the expected side effects of these drugs and measures to manage them. This information is covered in greater detail in the following section. The patient treated surgically needs care similar to that given to the person undergoing thyroidectomy.

HYPOTHYROIDISM

Etiology and Pathophysiology

Hypothyroidism is one of the most common medical disorders in the United States, affecting 8% of women and 2% of men over 50 years of age.[28] Hypothyroidism results from insufficient circulating thyroid hormone as a result of a variety of abnormalities. Hypothyroidism can be primary (related to destruction of thyroid tissue or defective hormone synthesis) or secondary (related to pituitary disease with decreased TSH secretion or hypothalamic dysfunction with decreased thyrotropin-releasing hormone [TRH] secretion). It may also be transient, related to thyroiditis or discontinuance of thyroid hormone therapy.[19]

Iodine deficiency is the most common cause of hypothyroidism worldwide and is most prevalent in iodine-deficient areas of the world. In areas where iodine intake is adequate, such as the United States, the most common cause of primary hypothyroidism in the adult is atrophy of the thyroid gland. This atrophy is the end result of Hashimoto's thyroiditis and Graves' disease. These autoimmune diseases destroy the thyroid gland. Hypothyroidism also may develop as a consequence of treatment for hyperthyroidism, specifically the surgical removal of the thyroid glands, or radioactive iodine therapy. Occasionally, hypothyroidism develops as a result of the ingestion of excessive amounts of goitrogens (see Table 48-7).

Although the typical patient with hypothyroidism is a woman over 50 years of age, the disease can occur at any age and in either sex. Hypothyroidism that develops in infancy (termed **cretinism**) is caused by thyroid hormone deficiencies during fetal or early neonatal life.

Clinical Manifestations

All hypothyroid states have certain features in common, regardless of the cause. Manifestations vary depending on the severity and the duration of thyroid deficiency, as well as the patient's age at onset of the deficiency.[29]

Hypothyroidism has systemic effects characterized by an insidious and nonspecific slowing of body processes. The clinical presentation can range from a patient with no symptoms to a patient with classic symptoms and physical changes easily detected on examination (Fig. 48-6). Unless hypothyroidism occurs after thyroidectomy or thyroid ablation, or during treatment with antithyroid drugs, the onset of symptoms may occur over months to years. The development of symptoms is so slow and subtle that medical attention is seldom sought. The patient's family and friends are often unaware of the changes. The severity of symptoms experienced depends on the degree of thyroid hormone deficiency and the long-term physiologic effects of thyroid hormone deficiency. Long-term effects may involve any body system but are more pronounced in the neurologic, cardiovascular, GI, reproductive, and hematologic systems.

The adult with hypothyroidism often is fatigued, lethargic, and experiences personality and mental changes.[29] The mental changes seen in hypothyroidism include impaired memory, slowed speech, decreased initiative, and somnolence. Many individuals with hypothyroidism appear depressed. Although the patient with hypothyroidism sleeps long periods of time, the stages of sleep are altered.

Although hypothyroidism affects cardiac function, it is usually significant only in the presence of coexisting cardiac disease. Hypothyroidism is associated with decreased cardiac output and decreased cardiac contractility. Thus the patient may experience

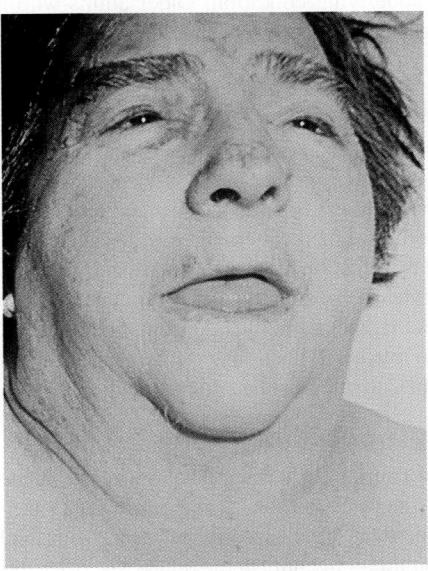

FIG. 48-6 Myxedema facies with dull, puffy skin; coarse, sparse hair; periorbital edema; and prominent tongue.

low exercise tolerance and shortness of breath on exertion. In the patient with a preexisting cardiovascular condition, hypothyroidism may cause significant hemodynamic compromise. Anemia is a common feature of hypothyroidism. Erythropoietin levels may be low or normal. Oxygen demand is decreased, and there is a hypocellular bone marrow. The result is a low hematocrit. Other hematologic problems are related to cobalamin, iron, and folate deficiencies. The patient may bruise easily. Increased serum cholesterol and triglyceride levels and the accumulation of mucopolysaccharides in the intima of small blood vessels can result in coronary atherosclerosis. This accumulation is seldom symptomatic (i.e., characterized by angina) because of the decreased myocardial oxygen consumption that has been observed in hypothyroidism.

GI motility is decreased in hypothyroidism, and achlorhydria (absence or decrease of hydrochloric acid) is common. Constipation, which is a common complaint, may progress to obstipation and, rarely, to intestinal obstruction. The underlying metabolic disease makes the individual a high risk candidate for intestinal surgery.

Other physical changes include cold intolerance, hair loss, dry and coarse skin, brittle nails, hoarseness, muscle weakness and swelling, and weight gain.[29] Weight gain is most likely a result of decreased metabolic rate. Those with severe long-standing hypothyroidism may display **myxedema,** the accumulation of hydrophilic mucopolysaccharides in the dermis and other tissues (see Fig. 48-6). This mucinous edema causes the characteristic facies of hypothyroidism (i.e., puffiness, periorbital edema, and masklike affect). Individuals with hypothyroidism may describe an impaired self-image in regard to their disabilities and altered appearance. Women with hypothyroidism frequently complain of menorrhagia. Some affected individuals have been treated for menorrhagia for years and may have undergone hysterectomy before the hypothyroidism was diagnosed. In addition, anovulatory cycles with subsequent infertility may occur.

In the older adult, the typical manifestations of hypothyroidism (including fatigue, cold and dry skin, hoarseness, hair loss, constipation, and cold intolerance) may be attributed to normal aging. For this reason, these symptoms may not raise suspicion of an underlying condition. Older adults who have confusion, lethargy, and depression should be evaluated for thyroid disease.

Complications

The mental sluggishness, drowsiness, and lethargy of hypothyroidism may progress gradually or suddenly to a notable impairment of consciousness or coma. This situation, termed *myxedema coma,* constitutes a medical emergency. Myxedema coma can be precipitated by infection, drugs (especially narcotics, tranquilizers, and barbiturates), exposure to cold, and trauma. It is characterized by subnormal temperature, hypotension, and hypoventilation. For the patient to live, vital functions must be supported and IV thyroid hormone replacement must be administered.

Diagnostic Studies

The most common and reliable laboratory tests used to evaluate thyroid function are those that measure TSH and FT_4. These values, correlated with symptoms gathered from the history and physical examination, confirm the diagnosis.[29] Serum TSH levels help determine the cause of hypothyroidism. Serum TSH is high when the defect is in the thyroid and low when it is in the pitu-

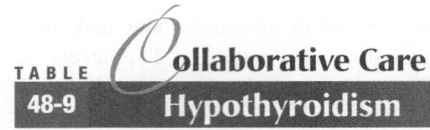

TABLE 48-9   Collaborative Care   Hypothyroidism

Diagnostic
History and physical examination
Serum TSH and free T_4
Serum T_3 and T_4
TRH stimulation test

Collaborative Therapy
Thyroid hormone replacement (e.g., levothyroxine)
Monitor thyroid hormone levels and adjust dosage (if needed)
Nutritional therapy to promote weight loss
Patient and family teaching (see Table 48-10)

TRH, Thyrotropin-releasing hormone; *TSH,* thyroid-stimulating hormone.

itary or hypothalamus. An increase in TSH after TRH injection suggests hypothalamic dysfunction, whereas no change suggests anterior pituitary dysfunction (Table 48-9). Other abnormal laboratory findings are elevated cholesterol and triglycerides, anemia, and increased creatine kinase.

Collaborative Care

The overall goal for treatment in a patient with hypothyroidism is restoration of a euthyroid state as safely and rapidly as possible with hormone replacement therapy. A low-calorie diet is indicated to promote weight loss.

Levothyroxine (Synthroid, Levothroid) is the drug of choice to treat hypothyroidism.[19] In the young and otherwise healthy patient, the maintenance replacement dose can be started at once. The typical initial adult dose usually starts at 0.05 mg taken orally daily. The maintenance dose is adjusted according to the patient's response and laboratory findings. In the older adult patient and the person with compromised cardiac status, a smaller initial dose (0.0125 to 0.025 mg/day) is recommended because the usual dose may increase myocardial oxygen demand. The increased oxygen demand may cause angina and cardiac arrhythmias. Any chest pain experienced by a patient starting thyroid replacement should be reported immediately, and electrocardiogram (ECG) and serum cardiac enzyme tests must be performed. In the patient without side effects the dose is increased at 1- to 4-week intervals. It is important that the patient take replacement medication regularly. Lifelong thyroid replacement therapy is usually required.

NURSING MANAGEMENT
HYPOTHYROIDISM

■ Nursing Assessment

The nurse plays an important role in the detection of hypothyroidism. Careful assessment may reveal the early and subtle changes that indicate dysfunction, particularly when caring for the patient with a condition that may predispose him or her to endocrine dysfunction. Assessment of the patient who is suspected of having hypothyroidism should include questions about weight gain, mental changes, fatigue, slowed and slurred speech, cold intolerance, skin changes such as increased dryness or thickening, constipation, and dyspnea. In addition, the nurse should assess for recent introduction of iodine-containing medications or ingestion of large amounts of goitrogens (see Table 48-8). The patient should be assessed for bradycardia; distended abdomen; dry, thick, cold skin; thick, brittle nails; paresthesias; and muscular aches and pains.

■ Nursing Diagnoses

Nursing diagnoses for the patient with hypothyroidism may include, but are not limited to, those presented in NCP 48-2.

■ Planning

The overall goals are that the patient with hypothyroidism will (1) experience relief of symptoms, (2) maintain a euthyroid state, (3) maintain a positive self-image, and (4) comply with lifelong thyroid replacement therapy.

■ Nursing Implementation

Health Promotion. There is currently no consensus regarding thyroid function screening. Although hypothyroidism is relatively common, particularly among women over age 50, there does not appear to be strong justification to screen the general population. However, some research indicates that it might be reasonable to screen certain adult populations such as individuals with family history of thyroid disease, those with history of neck radiation, women over 50, and all persons over 60.[30,31]

Acute Intervention. Most individuals with hypothyroidism do not require acute nursing care, because most are managed on an outpatient basis. However, the patient who develops

---

NURSING CARE PLAN 48-2

Patient with Hypothyroidism

EXPECTED PATIENT OUTCOMES	NURSING INTERVENTIONS and *RATIONALES*
NURSING DIAGNOSIS	**Hypothermia** *related to* cold intolerance *as manifested by* complaints of feeling cold, shivering.
▪ Satisfaction with temperature of environment ▪ Personal comfort	▪ Provide extra clothing, blankets, warm environment *to increase patient's comfort.* ▪ Explain to patient and significant others that decreased heat production causes discomfort *to increase patient's understanding of disease.*
NURSING DIAGNOSIS	**Imbalanced nutrition: more than body requirements** *related to* hypometabolism *as manifested by* weight gain.
▪ Maintenance of weight in usual range	▪ Provide low-calorie, high-protein diet; include foods high in cobalamin (vitamin B_{12}), folic acid, iron, and vitamin C *to reduce tendency for weight gain while preventing muscle wasting and anemia.* ▪ Explain the need for fewer calories *so patient will be more agreeable to dietary restrictions.* ▪ Assist patient to develop method of monitoring weight and caloric intake *so excess weight gain can be avoided.* ▪ Encourage small, frequent meals *because eating frequently will prevent feelings of hunger and overeating.*
NURSING DIAGNOSIS	**Constipation** *related to* gastrointestinal hypomotility *as manifested by* irregular, hard stools.
▪ Regular soft, formed stool	▪ Assess bowel pattern and characteristics *to plan appropriate interventions.* ▪ Provide 2-3 L of fluids per day *to maintain soft stool.* ▪ Offer foods high in bulk and roughage *to increase fecal mass.* ▪ Encourage activity *to stimulate peristalsis.* ▪ Administer laxatives or stool softeners if necessary *to stimulate GI motility.*
NURSING DIAGNOSIS	**Activity intolerance** *related to* decreased metabolic rate and mucin deposits in joints and interstitial spaces *as manifested by* generalized weakness and muscle and joint stiffness.
▪ Able to participate in self-care activities with minimal discomfort and fatigue	▪ Assess ability to participate in self-care activities *to determine extent of problem and plan appropriate interventions.* ▪ Monitor vital signs and comfort level *to determine effect of activities and plan activity increases.* ▪ Administer thyroid hormone replacement as ordered *to correct hypometabolic state.* ▪ Plan frequent rest periods *to improve patient's tolerance and comfort level.* ▪ Pace activities to match patient's abilities *to allow maximum participation.*
NURSING DIAGNOSIS	**Disturbed thought processes** *related to* diminished cerebral blood flow secondary to decreased cardic output *as manifested by* forgetfulness, memory loss, and personality changes.
▪ Maintenance of orientation to reality to highest level possible	▪ Assess thinking processes such as memory, attention span, orientation *to enable appropriate planning.* ▪ Repeat information to patient *because he or she requires more time to comprehend.* ▪ Explain cause of problems to patient and family *to reduce anxiety and frustration.* ▪ Provide clock and calendar *to maintain orientation to time and day.* ▪ Provide written handouts with all instructions *to help patient adhere to regimen.*

myxedema coma requires acute nursing care, often in an intensive care setting. Mechanical respiratory support is frequently necessary, and the patient will require cardiac monitoring. The nurse will administer thyroid hormone replacement therapy and all other medications intravenously because the paralytic ileus associated with myxedema coma causes unreliable absorption of oral medications. If the patient is hyponatremic, hypertonic saline may be administered until the serum sodium reaches at least 130 mEq/L (130 mmol/L). The nurse should monitor core temperature because the patient with myxedema coma is often hypothermic.[25]

For assessment of the patient's progress, vital signs, body weight, fluid intake and output, and visible edema should be monitored. Cardiac assessment is especially important because the cardiovascular response to the hormone determines the medication regimen. Energy level and mental alertness should be noted. These should increase within 2 to 14 days and continue to rise steadily to normal levels.

Ambulatory and Home Care. Patient teaching is imperative for the patient with hypothyroidism. A patient and family teaching guide is provided in Table 48-10. Initially the hypothyroid patient needs more time than usual to comprehend all of the necessary information. It is important to provide written instructions, repeat the information often, and assess the patient's comprehension level regularly.

The need for lifelong drug therapy must be stressed. The patient should be instructed in expected and unexpected side effects. Specifically, the signs and symptoms of hypothyroidism or hyperthyroidism that indicate hormone imbalance should be included in the teaching plan. Toxic symptoms should be clearly defined. Table 48-4 lists signs of hyperthyroidism that are the same as toxic symptoms of thyroid hormone replacement.

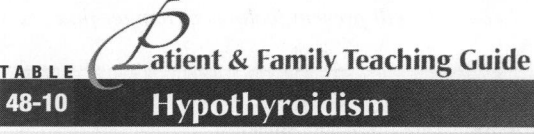

TABLE 48-10   Patient & Family Teaching Guide
Hypothyroidism

1. Explain the nature of thyroid hormone deficiency and self-care practices necessary to prevent complications. Patient and family must understand thyroid replacement therapy. It is especially important to emphasize the need for lifelong replacement, the need to continually take the medication, and the need for regular follow-up care.
2. Emphasize the need for a comfortable, warm environment because of intolerance to cold.
3. Teach measures to prevent skin breakdown. Soap should be used sparingly and lotion applied to skin.
4. Caution the patient to avoid sedatives. If they must be used, suggest that the lowest dose be used. Family members should closely monitor mental status, level of consciousness, and respirations.
5. Discuss with the patient measures to minimize constipation. Suggestions should include a gradual increase in activity and exercise, increased fiber in diet, use of stool softeners, and maintenance of a regular bowel elimination time. Use of enemas should be avoided because they produce vagal stimulation, which can be hazardous if cardiac disease is present.

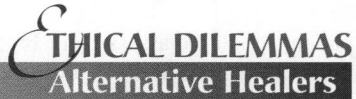

The patient must be taught to contact a health care provider immediately if signs of overdose such as orthopnea, dyspnea, rapid pulse, palpitations, nervousness, or insomnia appear. The patient with diabetes mellitus should test his or her capillary blood glucose at least daily because return to the euthyroid state frequently increases insulin requirements. In addition, thyroid preparations potentiate the effects of other common drug groups, such as anticoagulants, antidepressants, and digitalis compounds. Thus the patient should be taught the toxic signs and symptoms of these medications and should remain under close medical observation until stable.

It is sometimes difficult for the patient to recognize signs of overdosage or underdosage of drug therapy; therefore a family member or friend should be included in the instruction process. Handouts for the patient should be written in understandable language and should accompany verbal instruction. The handouts should be reviewed with the patient and family to assess understanding, and information should be clarified when necessary.

With treatment, striking transformations occur in both appearance and mental function. Most adults return to a normal state. Cardiovascular conditions and (occasionally) psychosis may persist despite corrections of the hormonal imbalance. Relapses occur if treatment is interrupted.

■ **Evaluation**

The expected outcomes are that the patient with hypothyroidism will
- have relief from symptoms
- maintain a euthyroid state as evidenced by normal thyroid hormone and TSH levels
- state the need for and a plan to adhere to lifelong therapy

Disorders of the Parathyroid Glands

HYPERPARATHYROIDISM

Etiology and Pathophysiology

Hyperparathyroidism is a condition involving increased secretion of parathyroid hormone (PTH). PTH helps regulate calcium and phosphate levels by stimulating bone resorption of calcium, renal tubular reabsorption of calcium, and activation of vitamin D. Thus oversecretion of PTH is associated with increased serum calcium levels. Hyperparathyroidism affects approximately 0.1% of the general population.[32]

Hyperparathyroidism is classified as primary, secondary, or tertiary. *Primary hyperparathyroidism* is due to an increased secretion of PTH leading to disorders of calcium, phosphate, and bone metabolism. The most common cause is a benign neoplasm or a single adenoma (80% of cases) in the parathyroid gland. Primary hyperparathyroidism is more common in women and usually occurs between 30 and 70 years of age.[32] The peak incidence is in the fifth and sixth decades of life. Patients who have previously undergone head and neck radiation may have an increased predisposition to the development of parathyroid adenoma.

Secondary hyperparathyroidism appears to be a compensatory response to states that induce or cause hypocalcemia, the main stimulus of PTH secretion. Disease conditions associated with secondary hyperparathyroidism include vitamin D deficiencies, malabsorption, chronic renal failure, and hyperphosphatemia. *Tertiary hyperparathyroidism* occurs when there is hyperplasia of the parathyroid glands and a loss of negative feedback from circulating calcium levels. Thus there is autonomous secretion of PTH, even with normal calcium levels. It is observed in the patient who has had a kidney transplant after a long period of dialysis treatment for chronic renal failure (see Chapter 45).

The excessive levels of circulating PTH usually lead to hypercalcemia and hypophosphatemia, creating a multisystem effect (Table 48-11). In the bones, subperiosteal bone resorption, decreased bone density, cyst formation, and general weakness can occur as a result of the effect of PTH on osteoclastic (bone resorption) and osteoblastic (bone formation) activity. In the kidneys, the excess calcium cannot be reabsorbed, leading to increased levels of calcium in the urine (hypercalciuria). This urinary calcium, along with a large amount of urinary phosphate, can lead to calculi formation. In addition, PTH stimulates the synthesis of a biologically active form of vitamin D, a potent stimulator of calcium transport in the intestine. In this way, PTH indirectly increases GI absorption of calcium, contributing further to the high serum calcium levels.

Clinical Manifestations and Complications

Clinical manifestations of hyperparathyroidism range from the asymptomatic individual (who is diagnosed through testing for unrelated problems) to the patient with overt symptoms. Most clinical manifestations are associated with hypercalcemia and are summarized in Table 48-11. The major manifestations include weakness, loss of appetite, constipation, increased need for sleep, emotional disorders, and shortened attention span. Major signs include loss of calcium from bones (osteoporosis), fractures, and kidney stones (nephrolithiasis). Neuromuscular abnormalities are characterized by muscle weakness, particularly in the proximal muscles of the lower extremities. Asymptomatic cases are being identified with increasing frequency with routine calcium screening. Serious complications of hyperparathyroidism are renal failure; pancreatitis; cardiac changes; and long bone, rib, and vertebral fractures.

Diagnostic Studies

PTH, as measured by radioimmunoassay, is elevated with hyperparathyroidism. Serum calcium levels usually exceed 10 mg/dl (2.50 mmol/L). Because of its inverse relation with calcium, the serum phosphorus level is usually below 3 mg/dl (0.1 mmol/L). Elevations in other laboratory tests include urine calcium, serum chloride, uric acid, creatinine, amylase (if pancreatitis is present), and alkaline phosphatase (in the presence of bone disease). Bone density measurements may also be used to detect bone loss. Imaging, such as MRI, CT scanning, and ultrasound, may be used for localization of the adenoma.

Collaborative Care

The treatment objectives are to relieve the manifestations and prevent complications caused by excess PTH. The choice of therapy depends on the urgency of the clinical situation, the degree of hypercalcemia, the underlying disorder, renal and hepatic function, the clinical presentation of the patient, and the particular advantages and disadvantages of the different therapeutic modalities.

Surgical Therapy. The most effective treatment of primary and secondary hyperparathyroidism is surgical intervention.[19] Parathyroidectomy leads to rapid reduction of chronically high calcium levels. Criteria for surgery include serum calcium levels greater than 12 mg/dl (3.0 mmol/L), hypercalciuria (greater than 400 mg/day), markedly reduced bone mineral density, overt symptoms (i.e., neuromuscular effects, nephrolithiasis), or those under age 50.[33] The surgical procedure involves partial or complete removal of the parathyroid glands. In the past, this surgery always involved an open surgical approach. However, this procedure is now being done using an endoscope on an outpatient basis in many health care facilities. Autotransplantation of normal parathyroid tissue in the forearm or near the sternocleidomastoid muscle may be done, allowing PTH secretion to continue with normalization of calcium levels. If autotransplantation is not possible, or if it fails, the patient will need to take calcium supplements for life.

Nonsurgical Therapy. If the patient does not meet the criteria for surgical intervention, or if the patient is elderly or at increased surgical risk from other health problems, a conservative management approach is used. This includes an annual examination with tests for serum PTH, calcium, phosphorus, and alkaline phosphatase levels; renal function; x-rays to assess for metabolic bone disease; and measurement of urinary calcium excretion. Continued ambulation and the avoidance of immobility are critical aspects of management. Dietary measures also include maintenance of a high fluid intake and a moderate calcium intake. The diet should contain 8 to 10 g of sodium per day to replace losses from increased urine output.

Phosphorus is usually supplemented unless contraindicated by an increased risk for urinary calculi formation. Several drugs currently used in the treatment of hyperparathyroidism are helpful in

TABLE 48-11	Clinical Manifestations: Parathyroid Dysfunction	
SYSTEM	**HYPOFUNCTION**	**HYPERFUNCTION**
Cardiovascular	Decreased contractility of heart muscle Decreased cardiac output Prolongation of QT and ST intervals on ECG Arrhythmias	Arrhythmias Shortened QT interval on ECG Hypertension
Gastrointestinal	Abdominal cramps Fecal incontinence (in older adult)	Vague abdominal pain Anorexia Nausea and vomiting Constipation Pancreatitis Peptic ulcer disease Cholelithiasis Weight loss
Integumentary	Dry, scaly skin Hair loss on scalp and body Brittle nails, transverse ridging Changes in developing teeth, lack of tooth enamel	Skin necrosis Moist skin
Musculoskeletal	Fatigue Weakness Painful muscle cramps Skeletal x-ray changes, osteosclerosis Soft tissue calcification Difficulty in walking	Skeletal pain Backache Weakness, fatigue Pain on weight bearing Osteoporosis Pathologic fractures of long bones Compression fractures of spine Decreased muscle tone
Neurologic	Personality changes Psychiatric manifestations of depression, anxiety Irritability Memory impairment Headache Seizures Positive Chvostek's sign or Trousseau's phenomenon Tremor Paresthesias of perioral area, hands, feet Hyperactive deep-tendon reflexes Disorientation, confusion (in older adult)	Personality disturbances Emotional irritability Memory impairment Psychosis Delirium, confusion, coma Incoordination Hyperactive deep-tendon reflexes Abnormalities of gait Psychomotor retardation Headache
Renal	Urinary frequency Urinary incontinence	Hypercalciuria Kidney stones (nephrolithiasis) Urinary tract infections Polyuria
Other	Eye changes, including lenticular opacities, cataracts, papilledema	Corneal calcification on slit-lamp examination

ECG, Electrocardiogram.

lowering calcium levels, but do not, in themselves, treat the underlying problem. Bisphosphonates (e.g., alendronate [Fosamax]) inhibit osteoclastic bone resorption and rapidly normalize serum calcium levels. Estrogen or progestin therapy can reduce serum and urinary calcium levels in the postmenopausal woman and may retard demineralization of the skeleton. Oral phosphate may be used to inhibit the calcium-absorbing effects of vitamin D in the intestine. Phosphates should only be used if the patient has normal renal function and low serum phosphate levels. Diuretics may be given to increase the urinary excretion of calcium.

Calcimimetic agents (such as R-586) are a new class of drugs that increase the sensitivity of the calcium receptor on the parathyroid gland, resulting in decreased PTH secretion and calcium

blood levels, thus sparing calcium stores in the bone. Although these agents are still under clinical investigation, initial studies have been encouraging.[34,35]

NURSING MANAGEMENT
HYPERPARATHYROIDISM

Nursing management of the patient with hyperparathyroidism is somewhat dependent on the collaborative treatment strategy. Nursing care for the patient following a parathyroidectomy is similar to that for a patient after thyroidectomy. The major postoperative complications are associated with hemorrhage and fluid and electrolyte disturbances. **Tetany,** a condition of neuromuscular hyperexcitability associated with sudden decrease in calcium levels, is another concern. It is usually apparent early in the postoperative period but may develop over several days. Mild tetany, characterized by unpleasant tingling of the hands and around the mouth, may be present but should abate without problems. If tetany becomes more severe (e.g., muscular spasms or laryngospasms develop), IV calcium may be given. IV calcium gluconate should be readily available for patients following parathyroidectomy in the event that acute tetany occurs.

Strict monitoring of intake and output is necessary to evaluate fluid status. Calcium, potassium, phosphate, and magnesium levels are assessed frequently, as well as Chvostek's and Trousseau's signs (see Chapter 16, Fig. 16-15). Mobility is encouraged to promote bone calcification.

If surgery is not performed, treatment to relieve symptoms and prevent complications is initiated. The nurse can assist the patient with hyperparathyroidism to adapt the meal plan to his or her lifestyle. A referral to a dietitian may be useful. Because immobility can aggravate the bone loss, the nurse can assist the patient to implement an exercise program and identify resources, such as shopping malls and YMCAs as places to exercise safely. The patient should be encouraged to keep the regular appointments, and the tests being performed should be explained. The patient should also be instructed in the symptoms of hypocalcemia or hypercalcemia and to report these should they occur. Hypocalcemia and hypercalcemia are discussed in Chapter 16.

HYPOPARATHYROIDISM

Etiology and Pathophysiology

Hypoparathyroidism, a condition associated with inadequate circulating PTH, is uncommon. It is characterized by hypocalcemia resulting from a lack of PTH to maintain serum calcium levels. PTH resistance at the cellular level may also occur (pseudohypoparathyroidism). This is caused by a genetic defect resulting in hypocalcemia in spite of normal or high PTH levels and is often associated with hypothyroidism and hypogonadism.

The most common cause of hypoparathyroidism is iatrogenic. This may include accidental removal of the parathyroids or damage to the vascular supply of the glands during neck surgery (e.g., thyroidectomy, radical neck surgery). Idiopathic hypoparathyroidism resulting from the absence, fatty replacement, or atrophy of the glands is a rare disease that usually occurs early in life and may be associated with other endocrine disorders. Affected patients may have antiparathyroid antibodies. Severe hypomagnesemia also leads to a suppression of PTH secretion.[36]

Clinical Manifestations

The clinical features of acute hypoparathyroidism are due to a low serum calcium level (see Table 48-11). Sudden decreases in calcium concentration cause tetany. This state is characterized by tingling of the lips, fingertips, and occasionally feet and increased muscle tension leading to paresthesias and stiffness. Painful tonic spasms of smooth and skeletal muscles (particularly of the extremities and face), dysphagia, a constricted feeling in the throat, and laryngospasms are also present. Chvostek's sign and Trousseau's sign are usually positive. Respiratory function may be severely compromised by accessory muscle spasm and laryngospasm-induced airway obstruction. Patients are usually anxious and apprehensive. Abnormal laboratory findings include de-

creased serum calcium and PTH levels and increased serum phosphate levels. Other causes of chronic hypocalcemia include chronic renal failure, vitamin D deficiency, and hypomagnesemia.

NURSING *and* COLLABORATIVE MANAGEMENT HYPOPARATHYROIDISM

The primary management objectives for a patient with hypoparathyroidism are to treat acute complications such as tetany, maintain normal serum calcium levels, and prevent long-term complications. Emergency treatment of tetany requires the administration of IV calcium. Generally, in adults, 10 to 20 ml of a 10% solution of calcium gluconate is infused over 10 minutes.[37] Calcium must be infused slowly because high blood levels can cause hypotension, serious cardiac arrhythmias, or cardiac arrest. Thus ECG monitoring is indicated when calcium is administered. The patient who takes digoxin is particularly vulnerable. In addition, IV calcium can cause venous irritation and inflammation. Extravasation may cause cellulitis, necrosis, and tissue sloughing. IV patency should be assessed before administration.

Rebreathing may partially alleviate acute neuromuscular symptoms associated with hypocalcemia such as generalized muscle cramps or mild tetany. The patient who can cooperate should be instructed to breathe in and out of a paper bag or breathing mask. This reduces carbon dioxide excretion from the lungs, increases carbonic acid levels in the blood, and lowers the pH.

Calcium is present in serum as free calcium (ionized), bound to protein, or complexed with phosphate, citrate, or carbonate. The free (ionized form) of calcium is the biologically active form. Because an acidic environment enhances the degree of ionization of calcium, the proportion of total body calcium available in the active form is increased, temporarily relieving the manifestations of hypocalcemia.

The patient with hypoparathyroidism needs instruction in the management of long-term drug therapy and nutrition. Oral calcium supplements of at least 1 g per day in divided doses for the patient under 40 years of age and 2 g per day in divided doses for the patient more than 40 years of age are usually prescribed. Specific hormone replacement of PTH is not used to treat hypoparathyroidism because of expense and the need for parenteral administration. Vitamin D is used in chronic and resistant hypocalcemia to enhance intestinal calcium absorption and bone resorption. The preferred preparations are dihydrotachysterol (Hytakerol) and 1,25-dihydroxycholecalciferol (calcitriol [Rocaltrol]). These drugs raise calcium levels rapidly and are quickly metabolized. Rapid metabolism is desired because vitamin D is a fat-soluble vitamin and toxicity can cause irreversible renal impairment. Ergocalciferol (Calciferol) may also be prescribed.

A high-calcium meal plan includes foods such as dark green vegetables, soybeans, and tofu. The patient should be told that foods containing oxalic acid (e.g., spinach, rhubarb), phytic acid (e.g., bran, whole grains), and phosphorus reduce calcium absorption.

The patient should be instructed about the need for lifelong treatment and follow-up care. The patient's calcium levels should be monitored three to four times a year. Treatment modification is often necessary because hypercalcemia can develop without apparent cause. The patient must also be taught to recognize signs and symptoms of hypocalcemia and hypercalcemia, and to contact the health care provider if they occur.

Disorders of the Adrenal Cortex

There are three main classifications of adrenal steroid hormones. Glucocorticoids regulate metabolism, increase blood glucose levels, and are critical in the physiologic stress response. In humans the primary glucocorticoid is cortisol. Mineralocorticoids regulate sodium and potassium balance. The primary mineralocorticoid is aldosterone. Androgens contribute to growth and development in both genders and to sexual activity in adult women. The term *corticosteroid* refers to any one of these three types of hormones produced by the adrenal cortex.

CUSHING SYNDROME

Etiology and Pathophysiology

Cushing syndrome is a spectrum of clinical abnormalities caused by excess corticosteroids, particularly glucocorticoids. Several conditions can cause Cushing syndrome (Table 48-12). The most common cause is iatrogenic administration of exogenous corticosteroids (e.g., prednisone). Approximately 85% of endogenous Cushing syndrome is due to an ACTH-secreting pituitary tumor (Cushing's disease). Other causes of Cushing syn-

---

TABLE 48-12   Causes of Cushing Syndrome

- Prolonged administration of high doses of corticosteroids
- ACTH-secreting pituitary tumor (Cushing's disease)
- Cortisol-secreting neoplasm within the adrenal cortex that can be either carcinoma or adenoma
- Excess secretion of ACTH from carcinoma of the lung or other malignant growth outside the pituitary or adrenal glands

ACTH, Adrenocorticotropic hormone.

---

drome include adrenal tumors and ectopic ACTH production by tumors outside the hypothalamic-pituitary-adrenal axis (usually of the lung or pancreas). Cushing's disease and primary adrenal tumors are more common in women in the 20- to 40-year age-group; ectopic ACTH production is more common in men.

Clinical Manifestations

The clinical manifestations of Cushing syndrome can be seen in most body systems and are related to excess levels of corticosteroids (Table 48-13). Although manifestations of glucocorticoid excess usually predominate, symptoms of mineralocorticoid and androgen excess may also be seen.

Corticosteroid excess causes pronounced changes in physical appearance (Fig. 48-7). Weight gain, the most common feature, results from the accumulation of adipose tissue in the trunk, face, and cervical area (Fig. 48-8). Transient weight gain from sodium and water retention may be present because of the mineralocorticoid effects of cortisol. Hyperglycemia occurs because of glucose intolerance (associated with cortisol-induced insulin resistance) and increased gluconeogenesis by the liver.

Protein wasting is caused by the catabolic effects of cortisol on peripheral tissue. Muscle wasting leads to muscle weakness, especially in the extremities. Loss of protein matrix in bone leads to osteoporosis with subsequent pathologic fractures (e.g., vertebral compression fractures) and bone and back pain. Loss of collagen makes the skin weaker and thinner. Therefore the skin bruises easier. Catabolic processes predominate, and wound healing is delayed. Mood disturbances (irritability, anxiety, euphoria), insomnia, irrationality, and occasionally psychosis may occur.

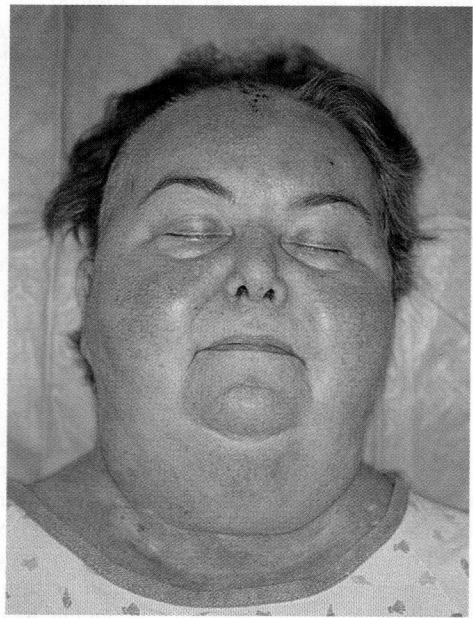

FIG. 48-7 Cushing syndrome. Facies include a rounded face ("moon face") with thin, reddened skin. Hirsutism may also be present.

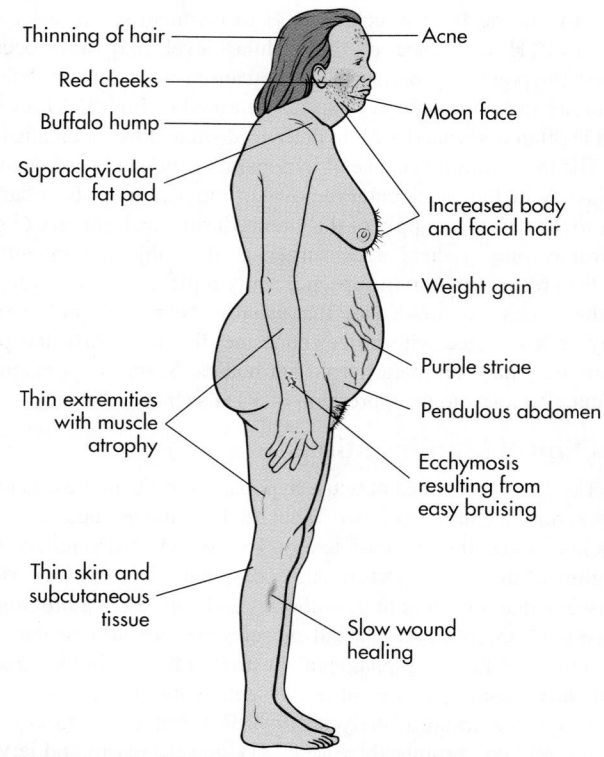

FIG. 48-8 Common characteristics of Cushing syndrome.

TABLE 48-13	Clinical Manifestations: Adrenocortical Hormone Dysfunction	
SYSTEM	**HYPOFUNCTION (ADDISON'S DISEASE)**	**HYPERFUNCTION (CUSHING SYNDROME)**
Glucocorticoids		
General appearance	Weight loss	Truncal (centripedal) obesity, thin extremities, rounding of face (moon face), fat deposits on back of neck and on shoulders ("buffalo hump")
Integumentary	Bronzed or smoky hyperpigmentation of face, neck, hands (especially creases), buccal membranes, nipples, genitalia, and scars (if pituitary function normal); vitiligo, alopecia	Thin, fragile skin; purplish red striae; petechial hemorrhages; bruises; florid cheeks (plethora); acne; poor wound healing
Cardiovascular	Hypotension, tendency to develop refractory shock, vasodilation	Hypervolemia, hypertension, edema of lower extremities
Gastrointestinal	Anorexia, nausea and vomiting, cramping abdominal pain, diarrhea	Increase in secretion of pepsin and hydrochloric acid, anorexia
Urinary		Glycosuria, hypercalciuria, kidney stones
Musculoskeletal	Fatigability	Muscle wasting in extremities, proximal muscle weakness, fatigue, osteoporosis, awkward gait, back and joint pain, weakness
Immune	Propensity toward co-existing autoimmune diseases	Inhibition of immune response, suppression of allergic response, inhibition of inflammation
Hematologic	Anemia, lymphocytosis	Leukocytosis, lymphopenia, polycythemia, increased coagulability
Fluids and electrolytes	Hyponatremia, hypovolemia, dehydration, hyperkalemia	Sodium and water retention, edema, hypokalemia
Metabolic	Hypoglycemia, insulin sensitivity, fever	Hyperglycemia, negative nitrogen balance, dyslipidemia
Emotional	Neurasthenia, depression, exhaustion or irritability, confusion, delusions	Psychic stimulation, euphoria, irritability, hypomania to depression, emotional lability
Mineralocorticoids		
Fluid and electrolytes	Sodium loss, decreased volume of extracellular fluid, hyperkalemia, salt craving	Marked sodium and water retention, tendency toward edema, marked hypokalemia
Cardiovascular	Hypovolemia, tendency toward shock, decreased cardiac output, decreased heart size	Hypertension, hypervolemia
Androgens		
Integumentary	Decreased axillary and pubic hair (in women)	Hirsutism, acne
Reproductive	No effect in men, decreased libido in women	Menstrual irregularities and enlargement of clitoris (in females); gynecomastia and testicular atrophy (in males)
Musculoskeletal	Decrease in muscle size and tone	Muscle wasting and weakness

Mineralocorticoid excess may cause hypertension (secondary to fluid retention), whereas adrenal androgen excess may cause pronounced acne, virilization in women, and feminization in men. Menstrual disorders and hirsutism in women and gynecomastia and impotence in men are seen more commonly in adrenal carcinomas.

The clinical presentation, as revealed by the history and physical examination, is the first indication of Cushing syndrome. Of particular importance are (1) centripedal (truncal) obesity or generalized obesity; (2) "moon facies" (fullness of the face) with facial plethora; (3) purplish red striae, which are usually depressed below the skin surface, on the abdomen, breast, or buttocks; (4) hirsutism in women; (5) menstrual disorders in women; (6) hypertension; and (7) unexplained hypokalemia.

Diagnostic Studies

When Cushing syndrome is suspected, a 24-hour urine collection for free cortisol and a low-dose dexamethasone suppression test are done (see Chapter 46). If these results are borderline, a high-dose dexamethasone suppression test is done. False-positive results can occur in patients with depression, those under acute stress, and those who are active alcoholics. Plasma cortisol (the primary glucocorticoid) levels may be elevated, with loss of diurnal variation. CT scanning and MRI may be used for tumor localization.

Other findings on diagnostic tests associated with, but not diagnostic of, Cushing syndrome include granulocytosis, lymphopenia, eosinopenia, hyperglycemia, glycosuria, hypercalciuria, and osteoporosis. Hypokalemia and alkalosis are seen in ectopic

ACTH syndrome and adrenal carcinoma. Plasma ACTH levels may be low, normal, or elevated depending on the underlying problem. High or normal levels indicate ACTH-dependent Cushing's disease, whereas low or undetectable levels indicate an adrenal or exogenous etiology.

Collaborative Care

The primary goal of treatment for Cushing's disease is to normalize hormone secretion. The specific treatment is dependent on the underlying cause (Table 48-14). If the underlying cause is a pituitary adenoma, the standard treatment is surgical removal of the pituitary tumor using the transsphenoidal approach.[38] (Transsphenoidal approach is discussed earlier in this chapter.) Radiation to the pituitary adenoma may be necessary if surgical outcomes are not optimal or if the patient is not a good surgical candidate. Adrenalectomy is indicated for Cushing syndrome caused by adrenal tumors or hyperplasia. Occasionally, bilateral adrenalectomy is necessary. Laparoscopic adrenalectomy is considered an appropriate surgical approach except for patients with known or suspected malignant adrenal tumors. An open surgical adrenalectomy is the treatment of choice for adrenal cancer.[39] Patients with ectopic ACTH-secreting tumors are managed by treating the primary neoplasm.

TABLE 48-14	Collaborative Care — Cushing Syndrome
Diagnostic	
History and physical examination	
Mental status examination	
Plasma cortisol levels for diurnal variations	
Plasma ACTH level	
Complete blood count	
Blood chemistries for sodium, potassium, glucose	
Dexamethasone suppression test	
24-hour urine for free cortisol	
Examination of visual field	
CT scan, MRI	

Collaborative Therapy*
Adrenocortical Adenoma, Carcinoma, or Hyperplasia
Adrenalectomy (open or laparoscopic)
Drug therapy
- mitotane (Lysodren)
- metyrapone
- ketoconazole (Nizoral)
- aminoglutethimide (Cytaden)

Pituitary Adenoma
Transsphenoidal resection
Radiation therapy

Ectopic ACTH-secreting Tumor
Treatment of the tumor responsible (surgical removal or radiation)

Exogenous Corticosteroid Therapy
Discontinuance of or alteration in administration of exogenous corticosteroids

*Treatment is based on underlying cause.
ACTH, Adrenocorticotropic hormone; *CT*, computed tomography; *MRI*, magnetic resonance imaging.

Drug therapy as a treatment measure for Cushing syndrome is usually indicated when surgery is contraindicated. The goal of drug therapy is the inhibition of adrenal function. Mitotane (Lysodren) suppresses cortisol production, alters peripheral metabolism of cortisol, and decreases plasma and urine corticosteroid levels. This drug essentially results in a "medical adrenalectomy." Metyrapone, ketoconazole (Nizoral), and aminoglutethimide (Cytaden) are used to inhibit cortisol synthesis. The relatively common side effects of these agents include anorexia, nausea and vomiting, GI bleeding, depression, vertigo, skin rashes, and diplopia. The GI side effects may be minimized by administering mitotane (Lysodren) with meals and with a bedtime snack.

If Cushing syndrome has developed during the course of prolonged administration of corticosteroids (e.g., prednisone), one or more of the following alternatives may be tried: (1) gradual discontinuance of corticosteroid therapy, (2) reduction of the corticosteroid dose, and (3) conversion to an alternate-day regimen. Gradual tapering of the corticosteroids is necessary to avoid potentially life-threatening adrenal insufficiency. An alternate-day regimen is one in which twice the daily dosage of a shorter-acting corticosteroid is given every other morning to minimize hypothalamic-pituitary-adrenal suppression, growth suppression, and altered appearance. This regimen is not used when the corticosteroids are given as endocrine replacement therapy.

NURSING MANAGEMENT
CUSHING SYNDROME

■ Nursing Assessment

Subjective and objective data that should be obtained from a patient with Cushing syndrome are presented in Table 48-15.

■ Nursing Diagnoses

Nursing diagnoses for the patient with Cushing syndrome may include, but are not limited to, those presented in the NCP 48-3.

■ Planning

The overall goals are that the patient with Cushing syndrome will
- experience relief of symptoms
- have no serious complications
- maintain a positive self-image
- actively participate in the therapeutic plan

■ Nursing Implementation

Health Promotion. Health promotion is focused on identifying patients at risk for Cushing syndrome. Patients receiving long-term, exogenous cortisol for a variety of diseases are at risk. Patient teaching related to the medication use and monitoring of side effects are important preventive measures.

Acute Intervention. The patient with Cushing syndrome is seriously ill. Because the therapeutic interventions have many side effects, the focus of daily assessment is on signs and symptoms of hormone and drug toxicity and complicating conditions such as cardiovascular disease, diabetes mellitus, infection, nephrolithiasis, and pathologic fractures. Nursing assessment should include monitoring of vital signs, daily weight, glucose, possible infection (especially pain, loss of function, and purulent drainage, because other signs and symptoms of inflammation such as fever and redness may be minimal or absent), and signs

TABLE 48-15	Nursing Assessment
	Cushing Syndrome

Subjective Data	Objective Data
Important Health Information	**General**
Past health history: Pituitary tumor (Cushing's disease); adrenal, pancreatic or pulmonary neoplasms; GI bleeding; frequent infections	Truncal obesity, supraclavicular fat pads, buffalo hump, moon facies
Medications: Use of corticosteroids	**Integumentary**
Functional Health Patterns	Plethora; hirsutism of body and face, thinning of head hair; thin, friable skin; acne; petechiae; purpura; hyperpigmentation; purplish red striae on breasts, buttocks, and abdomen; edema of lower extremities
Health perception–health management: Malaise	
Nutritional-metabolic: Weight gain, anorexia	**Cardiovascular**
Elimination: Polyuria; prolonged wound healing, easy bruising	Hypertension
Activity-exercise: Weakness, fatigue	**Musculoskeletal**
Sleep: Insomnia, poor sleep quality	Muscle wasting, thin extremities, awkward gait
Cognitive-perceptual: Headache; back, joint, bone, and rib pain; poor concentration and memory	**Reproductive**
Self-perception–self concept: Negative feelings regarding changes in personal appearance	Gynecomastia, testicular atrophy (in men), enlarged clitoris (in women)
Sexuality-reproductive: Amenorrhea, impotence, decreased libido	**Possible Findings**
Coping–stress tolerance: Anxiety, mood disturbances, emotional lability, psychosis	Hypokalemia, hyperglycemia, dyslipidemia; polycythemia, granulocytosis, lymphocytopenia, eosinopenia; ↑ plasma cortisol; high, low, or normal ACTH levels; abnormal dexamethasone suppression test; ↑ urine free cortisol, 17-ketosteroids; glycosuria, hypercalciuria; osteoporosis on x-ray

ACTH, Adrenocorticotropic hormone; *GI,* gastrointestinal.

and symptoms of abnormal thromboembolic phenomena, such as sudden chest pain, dyspnea, or tachypnea.

Another important focus of nursing care is emotional support. Changes in appearance such as centripedal obesity, multiple bruises, hirsutism in women, and gynecomastia in men can be distressing. The patient may feel unattractive, repulsive, or unwanted.[40] The nurse can help by remaining sensitive to the patient's feelings and offering respect and unconditional acceptance. The patient can be reassured that the physical changes and much of the emotional lability will resolve when hormone levels return to normal.

If treatment involves surgical removal of a pituitary adenoma, an adrenal tumor, or one or both adrenal glands, nursing care will have an additional focus on preoperative and postoperative care.

Preoperative care. Before surgery the patient should be brought to optimal physical condition. Hypertension and hyperglycemia must be controlled, and hypokalemia is corrected with diet and potassium supplements. A high-protein meal plan helps correct the protein depletion. Preoperative teaching will depend on the type of surgical approach planned (hypophysectomy or adrenalectomy), but should include information regarding the postoperative care the patient should anticipate. In the postoperative period (for both open and laparoscopic adrenalectomy), patients will probably have a nasogastric tube, urinary catheter, intravenous therapy, central venous pressure monitoring, and leg sequential compression devices to prevent emboli.[38]

Postoperative care. Surgery on glands poses risks beyond those of other types of operations. Because glands are highly vascular, the risk of hemorrhage is increased. Manipulation of glandular tissue during surgery may release large amounts of hormone into the circulation, producing marked fluctuations in the metabolic processes affected by these hormones. Postopera-

tively, blood pressure, fluid balance, and electrolyte levels tend to be unstable because of these hormone fluctuations. High doses of corticosteroids (e.g., hydrocortisone [Solu-Cortef]) are administered intravenously during surgery and for several days afterward to ensure adequate responses to the stress of the procedure. If large amounts of endogenous hormone have been released into the systemic circulation during surgery, the patient is likely to develop hypertension, increasing the risk of hemorrhage. High levels of corticosteroids also increase susceptibility to infection and delay wound healing.

Any rapid or significant changes in blood pressure, respirations, or heart rate should be reported. Fluid intake and output should be monitored carefully and assessed for potential imbalances. The critical period for circulatory instability ranges from 24 to 48 hours after surgery. IV corticosteroids are given, and the dose and rate of flow are adjusted to the patient's clinical manifestations and fluid and electrolyte balance. Oral doses are given as tolerated. The IV line may be kept in place after IV corticosteroids are withdrawn to keep a line open for quick administration of corticosteroids or vasopressors. Morning urine levels of cortisol (obtained at the same time each morning) are measured to evaluate the effectiveness of the surgery.

If corticosteroid dosage is tapered too rapidly after surgery, acute adrenal insufficiency may develop. Vomiting, increased weakness, dehydration, and hypotension may indicate hypocortisolism. In addition, the patient may complain of painful joints, pruritus, or peeling skin and may experience severe emotional disturbances. These signs and symptoms should be reported so that drug doses can be adjusted. The nurse must constantly be alert for signs of corticosteroid imbalance. After surgery the patient is usually maintained on bed rest until the blood pressure stabilizes. The nurse must be alert for subtle signs of postopera-

NURSING CARE PLAN 48–3

Patient with Cushing Syndrome

EXPECTED PATIENT OUTCOMES	NURSING INTERVENTIONS and *RATIONALES*
NURSING DIAGNOSIS	**Risk for infection** *related to* lowered resistance to stress and suppression of immune system.
• No infection • Early detection and treatment of any infectious process	• Assess for inadequate protein stores, proteinuria, muscle wasting, poor wound healing *as indicators of risk for infection.* • Assess potential infection sites such as urinary and respiratory tracts, skin, and IV lines *so infection can be detected early and treatment initiated promptly.* • Note pain, loss of function, and purulent drainage and teach patient and family to be aware of these signs *because other signs and symptoms of infecton may be minimal or absent.* • Provide private room, if possible; maintain meticulous asepsis and prevent contact with contagious individuals *to reduce the risk of cross-contamination.* • Instruct patient in self-care practices *to avoid infection (e.g., hand washing).* • Refer patient to dietitian for high-protein diet instruction *to help correct the protein depletion caused by excess corticosteroids.*
NURSING DIAGNOSIS	**Imbalanced nutrition: more than body requirements** *related to* increased appetite, high caloric content of foods, and inactivity *as manifested by* statement of increased appetite; weight 10% or more than optimum for height.
• Maintenance of body weight if appropriate or no more than 1 to 2 lb loss per week	• Obtain dietary consult for instruction in low-calorie, high-nutrition diet (including protein and calcium) *because excess corticosteroids produce weight gain and calcium and protein loss.* • Assist with appropriate menu choices *to reinforce dietary instructions.* • Provide low-calorie, high-vitamin snacks.
NURSING DIAGNOSIS	**Disturbed self-esteem** *related to* altered body image, emotional lability, and diminished physical capabilities *as manifested by* verbalization of negative feelings regarding personal appearance and inability to perform usual activities.
• Verbalization of acceptance of appearance by patient and family • Self-care methods to improve appearance	• Explain to patient and family that physical and emotional changes are related to hormone imbalance and that most will disappear when hormone imbalance is corrected *to increase their understanding and assist with coping.* • Accept and respect patient as a person *to maintain patient's self-worth.* • Encourage good grooming and use of attractive attire *to improve patient's appearance and self-esteem.* • Compliment patient when appropriate *to boost morale by providing positive feedback.*
NURSING DIAGNOSIS	**Impaired skin integrity** *related to* excess corticosteroids, immobility, and altered skin fragility *as manifested by* edema; thin, fragile skin; impaired healing.
• Intact skin	• Assess skin *for early detection of trauma.* • Protect patient from bumping and bruising *to prevent injury to easily traumatized tissue.* • Change patient's position frequently *to minimize pressure over bony prominences and improve circulation in edematous tissue.* • Provide good skin care, particularly to edematous areas and areas over bony prominences *because these areas have decreased circulation.*

tive infections because the usual inflammatory responses are suppressed. Meticulous care must be used when changing the dressing and during any other procedures that necessitate access to body cavities, circulation, or areas under the skin so that infection is prevented.

Ambulatory and Home Care. Discharge instructions are based on the patient's lack of endogenous corticosteroids and resulting inability to react to stressors physiologically. Patients should wear Medic Alert bracelets at all times and carry medical identification and instructions in a wallet or purse. Exposure to extremes of temperature, infections, and emotional disturbances should be avoided as much as possible. Stress may produce or precipitate acute adrenal insufficiency because the remaining adrenal tissue cannot meet an increased hormonal demand. Many patients can be taught to adjust their corticosteroid replacement therapy in accordance with their stress levels. The nurse should consult with each patient's health care provider to determine the parameters for dosage changes if this plan is feasible. If the patient cannot adjust his or her own medication or if weakness, fainting, fever, or nausea and vomiting occur, the patient should contact the health care provider for a possible adjustment in corticosteroid dosage. Lifetime replacement therapy is required by many patients. However, it may take several months to adjust the hormone dose satisfactorily, and patients should be prepared for this.

■ Evaluation

Expected outcomes for the patient with Cushing's syndrome are addressed in NCP 48-3.

ADRENOCORTICAL INSUFFICIENCY

Etiology and Pathophysiology

Adrenocortical insufficiency (hypofunction of the adrenal cortex) may be from a primary cause (known as **Addison's disease**) or a secondary cause (lack of pituitary ACTH secretion). In Addison's disease, all three classes of adrenal corticosteroids (glucocorticoids, mineralocorticoids, and androgens) are reduced. In secondary adrenocortical insufficiency, corticosteroids and androgens are deficient but mineralocorticoids rarely are. ACTH deficiency may be caused by pituitary disease or suppression of the hypothalamic-pituitary axis as a result of the administration of exogenous corticosteroids.

The most common cause of Addison's disease is an autoimmune response. Adrenal tissue is destroyed by antibodies against the patient's own adrenal cortex. Often, other endocrine conditions are present and Addison's disease is considered a component of *polyendocrine deficiency syndrome*. Tuberculosis can cause Addison's disease, but this is now rare. Other causes include infarction, fungal infections (e.g., histoplasmosis), acquired immunodeficiency syndrome (AIDS), and metastatic cancer. Iatrogenic Addison's disease may be due to adrenal hemorrhage, often related to anticoagulant therapy, antineoplastic chemotherapy, ketoconazole (Nizoral) therapy for AIDS, or bilateral adrenalectomy. Although adrenal insufficiency most often occurs in adults between 30 and 60 years of age and affects both genders equally, Addison's disease caused by an autoimmune response is most common in white females.[41]

Clinical Manifestations

Because manifestations do not tend to become evident until 90% of the adrenal cortex is destroyed, the disease is often advanced before it is diagnosed. The manifestations have a very slow (insidious) onset and include progressive weakness, fatigue, weight loss, and anorexia as primary features. Skin hyperpigmentation, a striking feature, is seen primarily in sun-exposed areas of the body, at pressure points, over joints, and in creases, especially palmar creases. It is most likely due to increased secretion of β-lipotropin (which contains melanocyte-stimulating hormone [MSH]) or ACTH. These tropic hormones are increased because of decreased negative feedback and subsequent low corticosteroid levels. Other frequent manifestations are hypotension, hyponatremia, hyperkalemia, nausea and vomiting, and diarrhea.

Patients with secondary adrenocortical hypofunction may have many signs and symptoms in common with patients with Addison's disease but are characteristically not hyperpigmented because ACTH and related peptide levels are low. When severe dehydration, hyponatremia, and hyperkalemia are present, a diagnosis of primary adrenocortical insufficiency is favored because of the mineralocorticoid insufficiency associated with this disorder.

Complications

Patients with adrenocortical insufficiency are at risk for an acute adrenal insufficiency (addisonian crisis), a life-threatening emergency caused by insufficient adrenocortical hormones or a sudden sharp decrease in these hormones. Addisonian crisis is triggered by stress (e.g., from infection, surgery, trauma, hemorrhage, or psychologic distress); following sudden withdrawal of corticosteroid hormone replacement therapy (which is often done by a patient who lacks knowledge of the importance of replacement therapy); after adrenal surgery; or following sudden pituitary gland destruction.

During acute adrenal insufficiency, severe manifestations of glucocorticoid and mineralocorticoid deficiencies are exhibited, including hypotension (particularly postural), tachycardia, dehydration, hyponatremia, hyperkalemia, hypoglycemia, fever, weakness, and confusion. Hypotension may lead to shock. Circulatory collapse associated with adrenal insufficiency is often unresponsive to the usual treatment (vasopressors and fluid replacement). GI manifestations include nausea, vomiting, diarrhea, and vague abdominal pain.

Diagnostic Studies

In addition to clinical features, a diagnosis of Addison's disease can be made when cortisol levels are subnormal or fail to rise over basal levels with an ACTH stimulation test. A failure of cortisol levels to rise in response to ACTH stimulation indicates primary adrenal disease. A positive response to ACTH stimulation indicates a functioning adrenal gland and points to a probable pituitary disease (see Chapter 46). Other abnormal laboratory findings include hyperkalemia, hypochloremia, hyponatremia, hypoglycemia, anemia, and increased blood urea nitrogen levels. Urine levels of free cortisol are low. An ECG may show low voltage and a vertical QRS axis. In addition, peaked T waves caused by hyperkalemia may be evident. CT scans and MRI are used to localize tumors or identify adrenal calcifications or enlargement (Table 48-16).

Collaborative Care

Treatment of adrenocortical insufficiency is focused on management of the underlying cause when possible. The mainstay of treatment for adrenocortical insufficiency is replacement therapy (see Table 48-16). Hydrocortisone, the most commonly used form of replacement therapy, has both glucocorticoid and mineralocorticoid properties. During situations associated with physi-

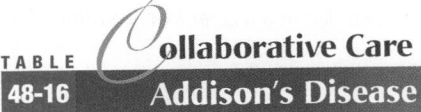

TABLE 48-16   Collaborative Care
Addison's Disease

Diagnostic
History and physical examination
Plasma cortisol levels
Serum electrolytes
ACTH-stimulation test
CT scan, MRI

Collaborative Therapy
Daily glucocorticoid replacement (two thirds on awakening in morning, one third in late afternoon)*
Daily mineralocorticoid in morning*
Salt additives for excess heat or humidity

*For conditions of normal daily stress in individuals with usual daytime activity.
ACTH, Adrenocorticotropic hormone; *CT,* computed tomography; *MRI,* magnetic resonance imaging.

ologic stress, glucocorticoid dosage must be increased to prevent addisonian crisis.[42]

Addisonian crisis is a life-threatening emergency requiring aggressive management. Treatment must be directed toward shock management and high-dose hydrocortisone replacement. Large volumes of 0.9% saline solution and 5% dextrose are administered to reverse hypotension and electrolyte imbalances until blood pressure returns to normal.[41]

NURSING MANAGEMENT
ADDISON'S DISEASE

■ Nursing Implementation

Acute Intervention. When the patient with Addison's disease is hospitalized, whether for diagnosis, an acute crisis, or some other health problem, frequent nursing assessment is necessary. Vital signs and signs of fluid volume deficit and electrolyte imbalance should be assessed every 30 minutes to 4 hours for the first 24 hours depending on the patient's instability. In addition, daily weights, diligent corticosteroid administration, protection against exposure to infection, and complete assistance with daily hygiene should be practiced. The patient should be protected from noise, light, and environmental temperature extremes. The patient cannot cope with these stresses because he or she cannot produce corticosteroids.

If the hospitalization was due to adrenal crisis, the patient usually responds by the second day and can start oral corticosteroid replacement. Because discharge frequently occurs before the usual maintenance dose of corticosteroids is reached, the patient should be instructed on the importance of keeping scheduled follow-up appointments.

Ambulatory and Home Care. The nurse has an important role in the long-term management of Addison's disease. The serious nature of the disease and the need for lifelong replacement therapy necessitate a well-organized and carefully presented teaching plan. Table 48-17 outlines the major areas that must be included in the teaching plan.

Glucocorticoids are usually given in divided doses, two thirds in the morning and one third in the afternoon. Mineralocorticoids are given once daily, preferably in the morning. This dosage schedule reflects normal circadian rhythm in endogenous hormone secretion and decreases the side effects associated with corticosteroid replacement therapy. A hormone-deficit patient receiving glucocorticoid replacement is less apt to exhibit harmful symptoms from the medication than a patient receiving pharmacologic doses of these drugs. Because the aim of replacement therapy is to return to normal hormone levels, nursing care is designed to help the patient maintain hormone balance and manage the medication regimen.

Because the patient with Addison's disease is unable to tolerate physical or emotional stress without additional exogenous corticosteroids, long-term care revolves around recognizing the need for extra medication and techniques for stress management. The need for corticosteroid hormone is proportional to stress levels. A patient who cannot produce endogenous hormone must adjust the dose of exogenous hormone to the stress level. Examples of situations requiring corticosteroid adjustment are fever, influenza, extraction of teeth, and rigorous physical activity, such as playing tennis on a hot day or running a marathon. Doses are usually doubled when minor stress occurs (e.g., a respiratory infection, dental work) and tripled when major stress occurs. When in doubt, it is better to err on the side of overreplacement. If vomiting or diarrhea occurs, as may happen with influenza, the health care provider must be notified immediately because electrolyte replacement may be necessary. In addition, these manifestations may be early indicators of crisis. Overall, patients who take their medications consistently can anticipate a normal life expectancy.

Patients must be taught the signs and symptoms of corticosteroid deficiency and excess and to report to their clinicians so that the dose can be adjusted to each patient's need. It is critical that the patient wear an identification bracelet (Medic Alert) and carry a wallet card stating that the patient has Addison's disease so that appropriate therapy can be initiated in case of an unexpected trauma, accident, or crisis. The patient should be instructed and given handouts related to other medications that cause a need to increase glucocorticoid dosage (e.g., phenytoin [Dilantin], barbiturates, rifampin [Rifadin], and antacids). Estrogen inhibits steroid metabolism. Patients using mineralocorticoid therapy should be instructed how to take their blood pressure and given parameters to report to their health care providers, because untoward changes may indicate a need for dosage adjustment.

The patient should carry an emergency kit at all times. The kit should consist of 100 mg of IM hydrocortisone, syringes, and instructions for use. The patient and significant others should be instructed in how to give an IM injection in case the replacement therapy cannot be taken orally. The patient should verbalize instructions, practice IM injections with saline, and have written instructions as to when to alter the dose.

CORTICOSTEROID THERAPY

Cortisol and related glucocorticoids are used to relieve the signs and symptoms associated with many diseases (Table 48-18). The long-term administration of corticosteroids in therapeutic doses of-

---

TABLE 48-17 Patient & Family Teaching Guide
Addison's Disease

The following should be included in a teaching plan for the patient and family.
1. Names and dosages of drugs
2. Actions of drugs
3. Symptoms of overdosage and underdosage
4. Conditions requiring increased medication (e.g., trauma, infection, surgery, emotional crisis)
5. Course of action to take relative to changes in medication
   a. Increase in dose of corticosteroid
   b. Administration of large dose of corticosteroid intramuscularly, including demonstration and return demonstration
   c. Consultation with health care provider
6. Prevention of infection and need for prompt and vigorous treatment of existing infections
7. Need for lifelong replacement therapy
8. Need for lifelong medical supervision
9. Need for medical identification device

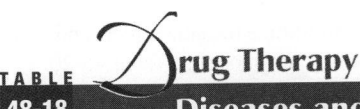

TABLE 48-18 — Drug Therapy: Diseases and Disorders Treated with Corticosteroids

Hormone Replacement
Adrenal insufficiency
Congenital adrenal hyperplasia

Therapeutic Effect
Allergic reactions
- Anaphylaxis
- Bee stings
- Contact dermatitis
- Drug reactions
- Serum sickness
- Urticaria

Collagen diseases
- Giant cell arteritis
- Mixed connective tissue disorders
- Polymyositis
- Polyarteritis nodosa
- Rheumatoid arthritis
- Systemic lupus erythematosus

Inflammation
Gastrointestinal diseases
- Inflammatory bowel disease
- Nontropical sprue

Endocrine diseases
- Hypercalcemia
- Hashimoto's thyroiditis
- Thyroid storm

Immunosuppression (after organ transplantation)
Liver diseases
- Alcoholic hepatitis
- Autoimmune hepatitis

Nephrotic syndrome
Neurologic disease
- Prevention of cerebral edema and increased intracranial pressure
- Head trauma

Pulmonary diseases
- Aspiration pneumonia
- Asthma
- Chronic obstructive pulmonary disease

Skin diseases
Malignancies, leukemia, lymphoma

TABLE 48-19 — Drug Therapy: Side Effects of Corticosteroids

- Hypokalemia may develop.
- Predisposition to peptic ulcer disease.
- Skeletal muscle atrophy and weakness occurs.
- Mood and behavior changes may be observed.
- Glucose intolerance predisposes to diabetes mellitus.
- Fat from extremities is redistributed to trunk and face.
- Hypocalcemia related to anti–vitamin D effect may occur.
- Healing is delayed. At increased risk for wound dehiscence.
- Susceptibility to infection is increased. Infection develops more rapidly and spreads more widely.
- Suppression of pituitary ACTH synthesis occurs. Corticosteroid deficiency is likely if hormones are withdrawn abruptly.
- Increased blood pressure occurs because of excess blood volume and potentiation of vasoconstrictor effects. Hypertension predisposes to heart failure.
- Protein depletion decreases bone formation, density, and strength. Predisposes to pathologic fractures, especially compression fractures of the vertebrae (osteoporosis).

ACTH, Adrenocorticotropic hormone.

well. The expected effects of corticosteroid therapy include the following:

1. *Antiinflammatory action.* Corticosteroids decrease the number of circulating lymphocytes, monocytes, and eosinophils. They enhance the release of polymorphonuclear leukocytes from bone marrow, inhibit the accumulation of leukocytes at the site of inflammation, and inhibit the release of substances involved in the inflammatory response (e.g., kinins, prostaglandins, histamine) from the leukocytes. Therefore manifestations of inflammation, including redness, tenderness, heat, swelling, and local edema, are suppressed.

2. *Immunosuppression.* Corticosteroids cause atrophy of lymphoid tissue, suppress the cell-mediated immune responses, and decrease the production of antibodies.

3. *Maintenance of normal blood pressure.* Corticosteroids potentiate the vasoconstrictor effect of norepinephrine and act on the renal tubules to increase sodium reabsorption and enhance potassium and hydrogen excretion. Retention of sodium (and subsequently water) increases blood volume and helps maintain blood pressure. Mineralocorticoids have a direct effect on sodium reabsorption in the distal tubule of the kidney and as a result increase sodium and water retention.

4. *Carbohydrate and protein metabolism.* Corticosteroids antagonize the effects of insulin and can induce glucose intolerance by increasing hepatic glycogenolysis and insulin resistance. They also stimulate the breakdown of protein for gluconeogenesis, which can lead to skeletal muscle wasting. Although corticosteroids mobilize free fatty acids and redistribute fat in cushingoid patterns, the mechanism for this process is unknown.

Complications Associated with Corticosteroid Therapy

As mentioned previously, the effects of corticosteroids can prove to be beneficial or harmful based on the physiologic actions. A beneficial effect in one situation may be a harmful one

ten leads to serious complications and side effects (Table 48-19). For this reason, corticosteroid therapy is not recommended for minor chronic conditions. Therapy should be reserved for diseases in which there is a risk of death or permanent loss of function and conditions in which short-term therapy is likely to produce remission or recovery. The potential benefits of treatment must always be weighed against the risks.

Effects of Corticosteroid Therapy

There are multiple effects of corticosteroid therapy. Although these actions can prove to be beneficial and therapeutic in some situations, they can also contribute to adverse effects as in another. For example, the vasopressive effect of the hormone is critical in enabling the organism to function in stressful situations but can produce hypertension when used for drug therapy. Suppression of inflammation and the immune response may help save the lives of the victim of anaphylaxis and the transplant recipient, but it causes reactivation of latent tuberculosis and greatly reduces resistance to other infections. In addition, corticosteroids inhibit the antibody response to vaccines. Specific side effects related to corticosteroid therapy are listed in Table 48-19.

NURSING and COLLABORATIVE MANAGEMENT
CORTICOSTEROID THERAPY

Many patients receive corticosteroid therapy, in particular glucocorticoid therapy, for nonendocrine reasons (see Table 48-18). Thorough instruction is necessary to ensure patient compliance. When corticosteroids are used as nonreplacement therapies, they are taken once daily or once every other day. They should be taken early in the morning with food to decrease gastric irritation. Because exogenous corticosteroid administration may suppress endogenous ACTH and therefore endogenous cortisol (suppression is time and dose dependent), the danger of abrupt cessation of corticosteroid therapy must be emphasized to patients and significant others.

Because patients often receive corticosteroid treatment for prolonged periods of time (greater than 3 months), corticosteroid-induced osteoporosis is an important concern. Therapies to reduce the resorption of bone may include increased calcium intake, vitamin D supplementation, bisphosphonates (e.g., alendronate [Fosamax]), and institution of a low-impact exercise program. Further

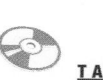

TABLE 48-20

Patient & Family Teaching Guide
Corticosteroid Therapy

The nurse needs to teach the patient and family the following:
1. Plan a diet high in protein, calcium (at least 1500 mg per day), and potassium but low in fat and concentrated simple carbohydrates such as sugar, honey, syrups, and candy.
2. Identify measures to ensure adequate rest and sleep, such as daily naps and avoidance of caffeine late in the day.
3. Develop and maintain an exercise program to help maintain bone integrity.
4. Recognize edema and ways to restrict sodium intake to less than 2000 mg per day if edema occurs.
5. Monitor glucose levels and recognize symptoms and signs of hyperglycemia (e.g., polydipsia, polyuria, blurred vision) and glycosuria (glucose in the urine). The patient should be instructed to report hyperglycemic symptoms or capillary glucose levels greater than 180 mg/dl (10 mmol/L) or urine positive for glucose.
6. Notify health care provider if experiencing postprandial heartburn or epigastric pain that is not relieved by antacids.
7. See an eye specialist yearly to assess development of possible cataracts.
8. Use safety measures such as getting up slowly from bed or a chair and use good lighting to avoid accidental injury.
9. Maintain good hygiene practices and avoid contact with persons with colds or other contagious illnesses to avoid infection.

instruction and interventions to minimize the side effects and complications of corticosteroid therapy are shown in Table 48-20.

HYPERALDOSTERONISM
Etiology and Pathophysiology

Hyperaldosteronism is characterized by excessive aldosterone secretion. The main effects of aldosterone are sodium retention and potassium and hydrogen ion excretion. Thus the hallmark of this disease is hypertension with hypokalemic alkalosis. *Primary hyperaldosteronism* (PA) is most commonly caused by a small solitary aldosterone-producing adenoma of the adrenal zona glomerulosa. Occasionally multiple lesions are involved and are associated with adrenal hyperplasia. PA affects both genders equally and occurs most frequently between 30 and 50 years of age.[43] It is estimated that approximately 1 of every 200 cases of hypertension is caused by PA.[44] *Secondary hyperaldosteronism* occurs in response to a nonadrenal cause of elevated aldosterone levels such as renal artery stenosis, renin-secreting tumors, and chronic renal disease.

Clinical Manifestations

Elevated levels of aldosterone are associated with sodium retention and elimination of potassium. Sodium retention leads to hypernatremia, hypertension, and headache. Edema does not usually occur because the rate of sodium excretion increases, which prevents more severe sodium retention. The potassium wasting leads to hypokalemia, which causes generalized muscle weakness, fatigue, cardiac arrhythmias, glucose intolerance, and metabolic alkalosis that may lead to tetany.[43]

Diagnostic Studies

The diagnosis of hyperaldosteronism should be suspected in all hypertensive patients with hypokalemia who are not being treated with diuretics. PA is associated with elevated plasma aldosterone levels, elevated sodium levels, decreased serum potassium levels, and decreased plasma renin activity.[44] An IV saline infusion test is often performed. In this test, 2 L of normal saline is infused over 4 hours, with plasma aldosterone levels measured at the beginning and end of the infusion. If aldosterone levels fail to decrease (i.e., levels are >10 ng/dl [277 pmol/L]), the patient probably has hyperaldosteronism. Adenomas are localized by means of a CT scan. If a tumor is not found, plasma 18-hydroxycorticosterone is measured after overnight bed rest. A level >50 ng/dl (1387 pmol/L) indicates an adenoma.

NURSING and COLLABORATIVE MANAGEMENT
PRIMARY HYPERALDOSTERONISM

The preferred treatment for PA is surgical removal of the adrenal gland that has the adenoma (adrenalectomy). Although this surgery can be done as an open procedure, laparoscopic adrenalectomy is increasingly performed because of the benefits this minimally invasive surgery offers.[44] Before surgery, patients should be treated with a low-sodium diet, potassium-sparing diuretics (spironolactone [Aldactone], eplerenone [Inspra]), and antihypertensive agents to normalize serum potassium levels and blood pressure. Spironolactone and eplerenone block the binding of aldosterone to the mineralocorticoid receptor in the terminal distal tubules and collecting ducts of the kidney, thus increasing the excretion of sodium and water and retention of potassium.

Oral potassium supplements and sodium restrictions are also necessary. Potassium supplementation and a potassium-sparing diuretic should not be started simultaneously because of the danger of hyperkalemia.

Patients with bilateral adrenal hyperplasia are treated with spironolactone; amiloride (Midamor), which is another potassium-sparing diuretic; or aminoglutethimide (Cytadren), which blocks aldosterone synthesis. Calcium channel blockers may also be used to control blood pressure. A new drug that is available for the treatment of hyperaldosteronism is eplerenone (Inspra). Eplerenone is the first agent of a new class of drugs known as selective aldosterone receptor antagonists.[45]

Nursing care includes careful assessment for signs of fluid and electrolyte balance (especially potassium) and cardiovascular status. Blood pressure should be monitored frequently before and after surgery because unilateral adrenalectomy is successful in controlling hypertension in only 50% of patients with adenoma. Patients receiving maintenance therapy with spironolactone or amiloride need instruction about the possible side effects of gynecomastia, impotence, and menstrual disorders, as well as knowledge about the signs and symptoms of hypokalemia and hyperkalemia. Patients should be taught how to monitor their own blood pressure and the need for frequent monitoring. The need for continued health supervision should be stressed.

Disorders of the Adrenal Medulla

PHEOCHROMOCYTOMA

Etiology and Pathophysiology

Pheochromocytoma is a rare condition characterized by a tumor of the adrenal medulla that produces excessive catecholamines (epinephrine, norepinephrine). Pheochromocytoma can occur at any age and in either gender, but it is found most commonly in young to middle-aged adults. In most cases affecting adults, the tumor is benign, encapsulated, unilateral, and solitary.[46] Occasionally bilateral tumors are found. The secretion of excessive catecholamines results in severe hypertension. If undiagnosed and untreated, pheochromocytoma may be fatal.

Clinical Manifestations

The most striking clinical features of pheochromocytoma include severe, episodic hypertension accompanied by the classic triad of severe, pounding headache, tachycardia, and profuse sweating. Attacks of episodic hypertension are due to sympathetic nervous system stimulation and are often accompanied by anxiety and palpitations. Attacks may be provoked by many medications, including antihypertensives, opioids, radiologic contrast media, and tricyclic antidepressants. The duration of the attacks may vary from a few minutes to several hours. Untreated, pheochromocytoma may lead to diabetes mellitus, cardiomyopathy, manifestations of uncontrolled hypertension, and death.

Diagnostic Studies

Although pheochromocytoma is associated with a number of symptoms, correct diagnosis is often missed. Pheochromocytoma is an uncommon cause of hypertension, accounting for only 0.1% of all cases of hypertension.[47] This condition should be considered in patients who do not respond to traditional hypertensive treatments.

The measurement of urinary metanephrines (catecholamine metabolites), usually done as a 24-hour urine collection, is the simplest and most reliable test. Values are elevated in at least 90% of persons with pheochromocytoma. Vanillylmandelic acid (VMA) may also be measured in a 24-hour urine sample. However, this test has more false negatives than urine metanephrines. Plasma catecholamines are also elevated. It is preferable to measure serum catecholamines during an "attack." CT scans and MRI are used for tumor localization.

NURSING *and* COLLABORATIVE MANAGEMENT
PHEOCHROMOCYTOMA

The primary treatment consists of surgical removal of the tumor. Before surgery the patient is hospitalized for treatment to correct cardiovascular complications to decrease the risk of surgery. Preoperatively, sympathetic blocking agents (e.g., phenoxybenzamine [Dibenzyline], prazosin [Minipress], terazosin [Hytrin], or doxazosin [Cardura]) are administered to reduce the blood pressure and alleviate other symptoms of catecholamine excess. Because this management may result in orthostatic hypotension, the patient must be advised to make postural changes cautiously. Calcium channel blockers may be used to treat the hypertension and to avoid problems with orthostatic hypotension in patients with preexisting cardiovascular disease.

Surgery is done via laparoscopic adrenalectomy or by open abdominal incision. Complete removal of the adrenal tumor cures the hypertension in the majority of individuals, but hypertension persists in approximately 10% to 30% of patients.[47] For these individuals, blood pressure management involves standard antihypertensive drug therapy. If surgery is not an option, metyrosine is used to diminish catecholamine production by the tumor and simplify chronic management.

Case finding is an important nursing function. Any patient with hypertension accompanied by symptoms of sympathoadrenal discharge should be referred to a health care provider for definitive diagnosis. An important part of the nursing assessment is observation of the patient for the classic triad of symptoms of pheochromocytoma (severe pounding headache, tachycardia, and profuse sweating). Blood pressure should be monitored immediately if the patient is experiencing an "attack." The nurse should be prepared to check blood pressure when any of the drugs that might precipitate an attack are given.

The nurse should attempt to make the patient with pheochromocytoma as comfortable as possible. All diagnostic samples should be collected appropriately. Capillary blood glucose levels should be monitored to assess for diabetes mellitus. Patients should be monitored closely if any medications are used that may precipitate an "attack." Patients need rest, nourishing food, and emotional support during this period. Preoperative and postoperative care is similar to that for any patient undergoing adrenalectomy except that blood pressure fluctuations from catecholamine excesses tend to be severe and must be carefully monitored. Because hypertension may persist even when the tumor is removed, the nurse should stress the importance of follow-up care and routine blood pressure monitoring. If metyrosine is being used, the patient should be instructed to rise slowly and hold onto a secure object, because this medication can cause orthostatic hypotension.

CRITICAL THINKING EXERCISES

Case Study
Graves' Disease
Patient Profile. Sally C., a 43-year-old white woman, was admitted to the hospital with a high fever. Following an endocrine workup, she was diagnosed as having Graves' disease.

Subjective Data
- Reports recent job loss because of inability to cope with job stress
- Reports symptoms including fatigue, unintentional weight loss, insomnia, palpitations, and heat intolerance

Objective Data

Physical Examination
- Has a fever of 104° F (40° C)
- Has blood pressure of 150/78, pulse of 118, and respiratory rate of 24
- Has hot, moist skin
- Has fine tremors of the hands
- Has 4+ deep tendon reflexes and muscle strength of 1 to 2

Collaborative Care
- Subtotal thyroidectomy planned for 2 months later
- Started on propylthiouracil (PTU) and propranolol (Inderal)

CRITICAL THINKING QUESTIONS
1. What is the etiology of the patient's symptoms?
2. What diagnostic studies were probably ordered? What would the results have been to establish the diagnosis of Graves' disease?
3. Why was surgery delayed?
4. What was the purpose of the drug therapy?
5. What are the patient's immediate learning needs and her learning needs preoperatively and postoperatively?
6. What are the nursing interventions for successful long-term management of this patient after the subtotal thyroidectomy?
7. Based on the assessment data presented, write one or more appropriate nursing diagnoses pertinent to this patient while hospitalized. Are there any collaborative problems?

Nursing Research Issues
1. Is sucking on hard candy or ice chips more effective in decreasing the subjective sensation of thirst in patients with SIADH?
2. What is the difference in the mental status of hypothyroid patients before and after thyroid replacement therapy?
3. What are the symptoms of infection in patients with Cushing syndrome?
4. Is a nurse-directed dosage adjustment more effective than a patient-directed dosage adjustment in preventing symptoms in the patient lacking endogenous cortisol who is exposed to stress?
5. Does regular exercise prevent bone loss in patients receiving glucocorticoid therapy?

REVIEW QUESTIONS

The number of the question corresponds to the same-numbered objective at the beginning of the chapter.

1. Following a hypophysectomy for treatment of acromegaly, a patient develops hypopituitarism. The nurse teaches the patient that
   a. hormone replacement with ACTH, TSH, FSH, and LH will be necessary.
   b. permanent ADH replacement will be needed if the postoperative diabetes insipidus does not reverse.
   c. frequent monitoring of blood and urine glucose is needed to identify the development of diabetes mellitus.
   d. the elimination of the source of excess growth hormone will reverse the physiologic effects of acromegaly.

2. A patient with a head injury develops SIADH. Symptoms the nurse would expect to find include
   a. edema.
   b. weight gain.
   c. urine specific gravity of 1.004.
   d. serum sodium of 140 mEq/L (140 mmol/L).

3. The health care provider prescribes levothyroxine for a patient with myxedema. Following teaching regarding this therapy, the nurse determines that further instruction is needed when the patient says,
   a. "I can expect to return to normal function with the use of this drug."
   b. "I can expect the medication dose to be increased every several weeks."
   c. "I will only need to take this medication until my symptoms are improved."
   d. "I will report any chest pain or difficulty breathing to the doctor right away."

4. Following thyroid surgery, the nurse suspects damage or removal of the parathyroid glands when the patient develops
   a. laryngeal stridor.
   b. muscle weakness.
   c. hoarseness and difficulty swallowing.
   d. hyperthermia and severe tachycardia.

Continued

REVIEW QUESTIONS—cont'd

5. An important nursing intervention when caring for a patient with Cushing syndrome is to
   a. restrict protein intake.
   b. observe for signs of hypotension.
   c. administer medication in equal doses.
   d. protect the patient from exposure to infection.

6. After an adrenalectomy for pheochromocytoma, the patient is most likely to experience
   a. hypokalemia.
   b. hyperglycemia.
   c. marked sodium and water retention.
   d. marked fluctuations in blood pressure.

7. To control the side effects of pharmacologic corticosteroid therapy, the nurse teaches the patient to
   a. increase calcium intake to 1500 mg per day.
   b. perform glucose monitoring for hypoglycemia.
   c. carry an emergency kit of hydrocortisone in case of severe stress.
   d. avoid abrupt position changes because of orthostatic hypotension.

8. The nurse teaches the patient that the best time to take corticosteroids for replacement purposes is
   a. once a day at bedtime.
   b. every other day on awakening.
   c. on arising and in the late afternoon.
   d. at consistent intervals every 6 to 8 hours.

REFERENCES

1. Sachse D: Acromegaly: early recognition of this rare multisystem disorder results in considerable benefit to patients, *Am J Nurs* 101:69, 2001.
2. Dostalova S et al: Craniofacial abnormalities and their relevance for sleep apnea syndrome aetiopathogenesis in acromegaly, *Eur J Endocrinol* 144:491, 2001.
3. Quabbe HJ, Plockinger U: Somatotroph adenomas. In Thapar K et al, editors: *Diagnosis and management of pituitary tumors,* Totowa, NJ, 2001, Humana Press.
4. Laws ER, Vance ML, Thapar K: Pituitary surgery for the management of acromegaly, *Horm Res* 53(suppl 3):71, 2000.
5. Darzy DH, Shalet SM: Evolving therapeutic strategies for acromegaly, *J Endocinol Invest* 24:468, 2001.
6. Zhang N et al: Radiosurgery for growth hormone-producing pituitary adenomas, *J Neurosurg* 93(suppl 3):6, 2000.
7. van der Lely AJ et al: Long-term treatment of acromegaly with pegvisomant, a growth hormone receptor antagonist, *Lancet* 358:1754, 2001.
8. Abbound CF, Ebersold MJ: Prolactinomas. In Thaper K et al: *Diagnosis and management of pituitary tumors,* Totowa, NJ, 2001, Humana Press.
9. Pinzone JJ: Hypopituitarism. In Becker KL, editor: *Principles and practice of endocrinology and metabolism,* ed 3, Philadelphia, 2001, Lippincott Williams & Wilkins.
10. Wuster C: Fracture rates in patients with growth hormone deficiency, *Horm Res* 54(suppl 1):31, 2000.
11. Ehrnborg C et al: Cost of illness in adult patients with hypopituitarism, *Pharmacoeconomics* 17:621, 2000.
12. Anpalahan M: Chronic idopathic hyponatremia in older people due to syndrome of inappropriate antidiuretic hormone secretion (SIADH) possibly related to aging, *J Am Geriatr Soc* 49:788, 2001.
13. Abrams C: ADH-associated pathologies, *Medical Laboratory Observer* 32:24, 2000.
14. Terpstra TL, Terpstra TL: Syndrome of inappropriate antidiuretic hormone secretion: recognition and management, *Medsurg Nurs* 9:61, 2000.
15. Bendz H, Aurell M: Drug-induced diabetes insipidus: incidence, prevention and management, *Drug Safety* 21:449, 1999.
16. Bichet DG: Nephrogenic diabetes insipidus, *Am J Med* 105:431, 1998.
17. Nickolaus MJ: Diabetes insipidus: a current perspective, *Crit Care Nurse* 19:18, 1999.
18. Magaldi AJ: New insights into the paradoxical effects of thiazides in diabetes insipidus therapy, *Nephrol Dial Transplant* 15:1903, 2000.
19. Trotto NE: Hypothyroidsm, hyperthyroidism, hyperparathyroidism, *Patient Care* 33:186, 1999.
20. Bailes BK: Hyperthyroidism in elderly patients, *AORN J* 69:254, 1999.
21. Larson J, Anderson EH, Koslawy M: Thyroid disease: a review for primary care, *J Am Acad Nurse Pract* 12:226, 2000.
22. Clement B: Thyrotoxicosis, *Semin Periop Nurs* 7:152, 1998.
23. Burman KD: Hyperthyroidism. In Becker KL, editor: *Principles and practice of endocrinology and metabolism,* ed 3, Philadelphia, 2001, Lippincott Williams & Wilkins.
24. Dahlen R: Managing patients with acute thyrotoxicosis, *Crit Care Nurse* 22:62, 2002.
25. Rignel MD: Management of hypothyroidism and hyperthyroidism in the intensive care unit, *Crit Care Clin* 17:59, 2001.
26. American Cancer Society: CA facts and figures 2002. Available at *www.cancer.org* (accessed Feb 26 2003)
27. Weber AL, Randolph G, Askoy FG: The thyroid and parathyroid glands: CT and MR imaging and correlation with pathology and clinical findings, *Radiol Clin North Am* 38:1005, 2000.
28. Canaris GJ et al: The Colorado thyroid disease prevalence study, *Arch Intern Med* 160:526, 2000.
29. Elliott B: Diagnosing and treating hypothyroidism, *Nurse Pract* 25:92, 2000.
30. American College of Physicians: Screening for thyroid disease: clinical guide part 1, *Ann Intern Med* 129:141, 1998.
31. Helfand M, Redfern CC: Screening for thyroid disease: clinical guide part 2, *Ann Intern Med* 129:144, 1998.
32. Silverberg SJ: Natural history of primary hyperparathyroidism, *Endocrinol Metab Clin North Am* 29:451, 2000.
33. National Institutes of Health consensus development conference statement on primary hyperparathyroidism, *J Bone Miner Res* 6(suppl 2):S9, 1991.
34. Strewler GJ: Medical approaches to primary hyperparathyroidism, *Endocrinol Metab Clin North Am* 29:523, 2000.
35. Weigel RJ: Nonoperative management of hyperparathyroidism: present and future, *Curr Opin Oncol* 13:33, 2001.
36. Dacey MJ: Hypomagnesemic disorders, *Crit Care Clin* 17:155, 2001.
37. DeBeur SM, Streeten EA, Levine MA: Hypoparathyroidism and other causes of hypocalcemia. In Becker KL, editor: *Principles and practice of endocrinology and metabolism,* ed 3, Philadelphia, 2001, Lippincott Williams & Wilkins.

38. Williams M: Disorders of the adrenal gland, *Semin Periop Nurs* 7:179, 1998.
39. Gill IS: The case for laparoscopic adrenalectomy, *J Urol* 166:429, 2001.
40. Gotch P: Cushing's syndrome from the patient's perspective, *Endocrinol Metab Clin North Am* 23:607, 1994.
41. Leuken K: Clinical manifestations and management of Addison's disease, *J Am Acad Nurse Pract* 11:151, 1999.
42. Oelkers W, Diederich S, Bahr V: Therapeutic strategies in adrenal insufficiency, *Ann Endocrinol* 62:212, 2001.
43. Gill JR: Hyperaldosteronism. In Becker KL, editor: *Principles and practice of endocrinology and metabolism,* ed 3, Philadelphia, 2001, Lippincott Williams & Wilkins.
44. Rossi H, Kim A, Prinz R: Primary hyperaldosteronism in the era of laparoscopic adrenalectomy, *Am Surg* 68:253, 2002.
45. Pitt OL, Young WF, MacDonald TM: A review of the medical treatment of primary aldosteronism, *J Hypertens* 19:353, 2001.
46. Landsberg L, Young JB: Pheochromocytoma. In *Harrison's online,* 2002, McGraw-Hill. Available at *www.harrisonsonline.com* (accessed Feb 26, 2003)
47. Lo CY et al: Adrenal pheochromocytoma remains a frequently overlooked diagnosis, *Am J Surg* 179:212, 2000.

RESOURCES

American Association of Clinical Endocrinologists (AACE)
1000 Riverside Avenue, Suite 205
Jacksonville, FL 32204
904-353-7878
Fax: 904-353-8185
www.aace.com

American Society for Bone and Mineral Research
2025 M Street, NW, Suite 800
Washington, DC 20036-3309
202-367-1161
Fax: 202-367-2161
www.asbmr.org

American Thyroid Association
6066 Leesburg Pike, Suite 650
Falls Church, VA 22041
703-998-8890
Fax: 703-998-8893
www.thyroid.org

Endocrine Nurses Society (ENS)
4350 East West Highway, Suite 500
Bethesda, MD 20814-4410
301-941-0249
Fax: 301-941-0259
www.endo-nurses.org

Endocrine Society
4350 East West Highway, Suite 500
Bethesda, MD 20814-4426
301-941-0200
Fax: 301-941-0259
www.endo-society.org

National Institute of Diabetes and Digestive and Kidney Diseases (Addison's Disease)
2 Information Way
Bethesda, MD 20892-3570
www.niddk.nih.gov

Pituitary Tumor Network Association
P.O. Box 1958
Thousand Oaks, CA 91358
805-499-9973
Fax: 805-480-0633
www.pituitary.com

Thyroid Federation International
96 Mack Street
Kingston, ON
K7L 1N9 Canada
613-544-8364
Fax: 613-544-9731
www.thyroid-fed.org

For additional Internet resources, see the website for this book at *http://evolve.elsevier.com/Lewis/medsurg/.*

CHAPTER 49
NURSING ASSESSMENT
Reproductive System

Jean Foret Giddens

LEARNING OBJECTIVES

1. Describe the structures and functions of the male and female reproductive systems.
2. Explain the functions of the major hormones essential for the structure and function of the reproductive systems.
3. Describe the physiologic and psychologic changes of a man and of a woman during the stages of sexual response.
4. Describe age-related changes in the reproductive systems and differences in assessment findings.
5. Identify significant subjective and objective data related to the reproductive systems and information about sexual function that should be obtained from a patient.
6. Describe noninvasive techniques used in the physical assessment of the reproductive systems.
7. Differentiate normal from abnormal findings obtained from a physical assessment of the reproductive systems.
8. Describe the purpose, significance of results, and nursing responsibilities related to diagnostic studies of the reproductive systems.

KEY TERMS

amenorrhea, p. 1345	menarche, p. 1344
clitoris, p. 1343	menopause, p. 1345
ductus deferens, p. 1339	menstrual cycle, p. 1345
dyspareunia, p. 1350	mons pubis, p. 1342
epididymis, p. 1339	nulliparous, p. 1341
gonads, p. 1339	spermatogenesis, p. 1339

STRUCTURES AND FUNCTIONS OF THE MALE AND FEMALE REPRODUCTIVE SYSTEMS

The reproductive system of both males and females consists of primary (or essential) organs and secondary (or accessory) organs. The primary reproductive organs are referred to as **gonads.** The female gonads are the ovaries; the male gonads are the testes. The primary responsibility of the gonads is secretion of hormones and production of gametes (ova and sperm). Secondary or accessory organs are responsible for transporting and nourishing the ova and sperm, as well as preserving and protecting the fertilized eggs.

Male Reproductive System

The three primary roles of the male reproductive system are (1) production and transportation of sperm, (2) deposit of sperm in the female reproductive tract, and (3) secretion of hormones. The primary reproductive organs in the male are the testes. Secondary reproductive organs include ducts (epididymis, ductus deferens, ejaculatory duct, and urethra), sex glands (prostate gland, Cowper's glands, and seminal vesicles), and the external genitalia (scrotum and penis)[1] (Fig. 49-1).

Testes. The paired testes are ovoid, smooth, firm organs measuring 3.5 to 5.5 cm long and 2 to 3 cm wide. They are within the scrotum—a pouchlike structure composed of a thin, loose outer layer of skin over a tough connective tissue layer. Within the testes coiled structures known as seminiferous tubules form *spermatozoa* (immature sperm). The process of sperm production is called **spermatogenesis.** Interstitial cells of the testes lie between the seminiferous tubules and produce the male sex hormone testosterone.

Ducts. Sperm formed in the seminiferous tubules move through a series of ducts. These ducts transport the sperm from the testes to the outside of the body. As sperm exit the testes they enter and pass through the epididymis, ductus deferens, ejaculatory duct, and urethra.

The **epididymis** is a comma-shaped structure located on the top and behind each testis inside the scrotum (Figs. 49-1 and 49-2). It is a very long, tightly coiled structure that measures about 20 feet in length.[1] The epididymis transports the sperm as they mature. Sperm exit the epididymis through a long, thick tube known as the ductus deferens.

The **ductus deferens** (also known as the *vas deferens*) is continuous with the epididymis within the scrotal sac. It travels upward through the scrotum and continues through the inguinal ring into the abdominal cavity. The spermatic cord is a connective tissue sheath that encloses the ductus deferens, arteries, veins, nerves, and lymph vessels as it ascends up through the inguinal canal (see Fig. 49-2). In the abdominal cavity, the ductus deferens travels up, over, and behind the bladder. Behind the bladder the ductus deferens joins the seminal vesicle to form the ejaculatory duct (see Fig. 49-1).

The ejaculatory duct passes downward through the prostate gland, connecting with the urethra. The urethra extends from the bladder, through the prostate, and ends in a slitlike opening (the meatus) on the ventral side of the *glans,* the tip of the penis. During the process of ejaculation, sperm travels through the urethra and out of the body.

Glands. The seminal vesicles, prostate gland, and Cowper's (bulbourethral) glands are the accessory glands of the male repro-

Reviewed by Susan K. Goebel, RNC, MS, WHNP, SANE, Assistant Professor of Nursing, Mesa State College, Grand Junction, Colo.; Nurse Practitioner, Mesa County Health Department.

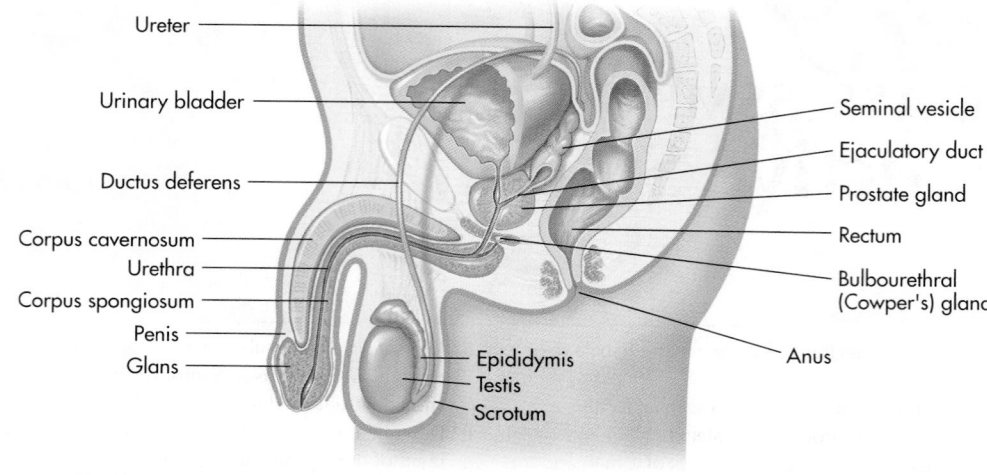

FIG. 49-1   External and internal male sex organs.

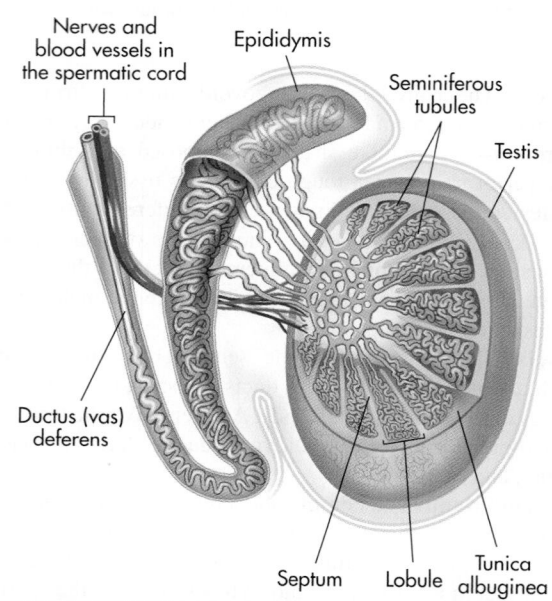

FIG. 49-2   Seminiferous tubules, testis, epididymis, and ductus (vas) deferens.

ductive system. These glands produce and secrete seminal fluid (semen), which surrounds the sperm and forms the *ejaculate.*

The seminal vesicles lie just behind the bladder and between the rectum and the bladder. The ducts of the seminal vesicles fuse with the ductus deferens to form the ejaculatory ducts that enter the prostate gland. The prostate gland lies underneath the bladder. Its posterior surface approximates the rectal wall. The prostate normally measures 2 cm wide and 3 cm long and is divided into the right and left lateral lobes and an anteroposterior median lobe. Cowper's glands lie on each side of the urethra and slightly posterior to it, just below the prostate. The ducts of these glands enter directly into the urethra.

The secretion from the seminal vesicles and prostate makes up most of the fluid in the ejaculate. By comparison, the seminal vesicles and Cowper's glands contribute a minimum amount of fluid to the ejaculate. These various secretions serve as a medium

for the transport of sperm and create an alkaline, nutritious environment that promotes sperm motility and survival.

External Genitalia. The external genitalia consist of the penis and the scrotum. The penis consists of a shaft, and the tip is known as the glans. The glans is covered by a fold of skin, the prepuce (or foreskin), that forms at the junction of the glans and the shaft of the penis. In circumcised men the prepuce has been removed. The broadened segment of the glans at the junction is the corona. The shaft of the penis consists of erectile tissue composed of the corpus cavernosum, the corpus spongiosum, the fibrous sheath that encases the erectile tissue, and the urethra. The skin covering the penis is thin, loose, and essentially hairless.

Female Reproductive System

The three primary roles of the female reproductive system are (1) production of ova (eggs), (2) secretion of hormones, and (3) protection and facilitation of the development of the fetus in a pregnant female. Like the male, the female has primary and secondary reproductive organs. The primary reproductive organs in the female are the paired ovaries. Secondary reproductive organs include ducts (fallopian tubes), the uterus, the vagina, sex glands (Bartholin's glands and breasts), and the external genitalia (vulva).

Pelvic Organs

Ovaries. The ovaries are usually located on either side of the uterus, just behind and below the fallopian (uterine) tubes (Figs. 49-3 and 49-4). The ovaries are firm and solid, approximately 1.5 cm wide, and 3 cm long. Their functions include *ovulation,* as well as secretion of the two major reproductive hormones, estrogen and progesterone. The outer zone of the ovary contains follicles with germ cells, or *oocytes.* Each follicle contains a primordial (immature) oocyte surrounded by granulosa and theca cells. These two layers protect and nourish the oocyte until the follicle reaches maturity and ovulation occurs. However, not all follicles reach maturity. In a process termed *atresia,* most of the primordial follicles become smaller and are reabsorbed by the body; thus the number of follicles declines from 2 million to 4 million at birth to approximately 300,000 to 400,000 at menarche. This number continues to de-

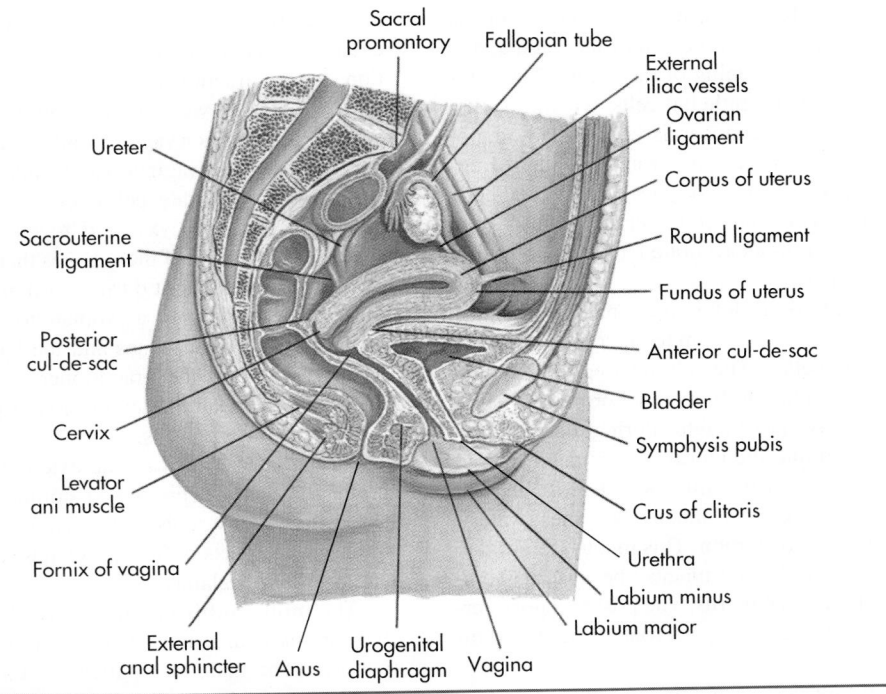

FIG. 49-3 Female reproductive tract and related organs.

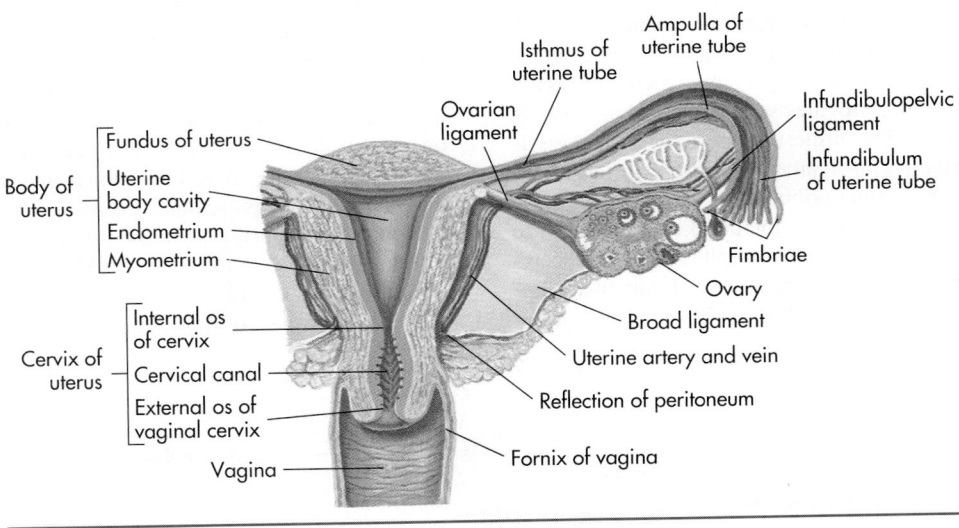

FIG. 49-4 Female reproductive tract: anterior view.

crease throughout a woman's reproductive years. Fewer than 500 oocytes are actually released by ovulation during the reproductive years of the normal healthy woman.

Fallopian tubes. Normally, each month during a woman's reproductive years, one ovarian follicle reaches maturity, and the ovum is ovulated, or expelled, from the ovary through the stimulus of the gonadotropic hormones, follicle-stimulating hormone (FSH) and luteinizing hormone (LH). The ovum then travels up a fallopian tube where fertilization by sperm may occur, if they are present. An ovum can be fertilized up to 72 hours after its release.

The distal ends of the fallopian tubes consist of fingerlike projections called *fimbriae* that "massage" the ovaries at ovulation to help extract the mature ovum. The tubes, which average 4.8 inches (12 cm) in length, extend from the fimbriae to the superior lateral

borders of the uterus. Fertilization usually takes place within the outer one third of the fallopian tubes.

Uterus. The uterus is a pear-shaped, hollow, muscular organ (see Figs. 49-3 and 49-4). It is located between the bladder and the rectum. In the mature **nulliparous** (never pregnant) female, the uterus is approximately 6 cm long and 4 cm wide. The uterine walls consist of an outer serosal layer, the perimetrium; a middle muscular layer, the myometrium; and an inner mucosal layer, the endometrium.

The uterus consists of the fundus, body (or corpus), and cervix (see Fig. 49-4). The body makes up about 80% of the uterus and connects with the cervix at the isthmus, or neck. The cervix is the lower portion of the uterus that projects into the anterior wall of the vaginal canal. It makes up about 15% to 20% of the uterus in the nulliparous female. The cervix consists of the *ectocervix,* the outer portion that protrudes into the vagina, and the *endocervix,* the canal in the opening of the cervix. The ectocervix is covered with squamous epithelial cells, which give it a smooth, pinkish appearance. The endocervix contains a lining of columnar epithelial cells, which give it a rough, reddened appearance. The junction at which the two types of epithelial cells meet is termed the *squamocolumnar junction* and contains the optimal types of cells needed for an accurate Papanicolaou (Pap) smear to screen for malignancies.

The cervical canal is 2 to 4 cm long and is relatively tightly closed. The cervix, however, allows sperm to enter the uterus and also allows menses to be expelled. The columnar epithelium, under hormonal influence, provides elasticity at labor for the cervix to stretch to allow for the passage of a fetus during the birth process. The entrance of sperm into the uterus is facilitated by mucus produced by the cervix under the influence of estrogen. Under normal conditions, the cervical mucus becomes watery, stretchy, and more abundant at ovulation. This mucus, referred to as *spinnbarkeit,* is considered "fertile mucus" because it facilitates the passage of sperm into the uterus. The postovulatory cervical mucus, under the influence of progesterone, is thick and inhibits sperm passage.

The anterior and posterior peritoneal covering of the uterus is called the *broad ligament.* It separates the uterus from the bladder and the rectum but does not provide support for the uterus or the *adnexa* (ovaries and tubes). The cardinal ligaments, which extend from the isthmus of the uterus to the pelvic wall, also offer only minimal support. The round ligament, which extends anteriorly to the labia majora, provides some support but is easily weakened by pregnancy. The firmest support for the uterus is provided by the uterine sacral ligaments, which pull the uterus back and away from the vaginal orifice.

Vagina. The vagina is a tubular structure 3 to 4 inches (8 to 10 cm) long that is lined with squamous epithelium. The secretions of the vagina consist of cervical mucus, desquamated epithelium, and, during sexual stimulation, a direct transudate se-

cretion. These fluids protect against vaginal infection. The muscular and erectile tissue of the vaginal walls allows enough dilation and contraction to accommodate the passage of the fetus during labor, as well as penetration of the penis during intercourse. The anterior vaginal wall lies along the urethra and bladder. The posterior vaginal wall is adjacent to the rectum.

Pelvis. The female pelvis consists of four bones (two hipbones, sacrum, coccyx) held together by several strong ligaments. The sections of these bones that lie below the iliopectineal line are very important during birth and are often a factor determining the ability of a woman to deliver a child vaginally. Knowledge of these bones and the landmarks that they form in the pelvis allows the practitioner to estimate pelvic measurements and the potential for a woman's pelvis to accommodate the birth of a full-term fetus.

External Genitalia. The external portion of the female reproductive system (Fig. 49-5), commonly called the *vulva,* consists of the mons pubis, labia majora, labia minora, clitoris, urethral meatus, ducts of Skene's glands, vaginal introitus (opening), and Bartholin's glands.

The **mons pubis** is a fatty layer lying over the pubic bone. It contains coarse hair that lies in an upside-down triangular pattern. (The male hair pattern is diamond shaped.) The labia majora are folds of adipose tissue that form the outer borders of the vulva. These hair-covered folds contain sweat glands and sebaceous glands. The hairless labia minora form the borders of the vaginal orifice and extend anteriorly to enclose the clitoris.[2]

The *vestibule* is a boat-shaped fossa between the labia minora, extending from the clitoris at the anterior end to the vaginal opening at the posterior end. The perineum is the area between the vagina and the anus. The vaginal introitus is surrounded by thin membranous tissue called the *hymen.* In the adult female, the hymen usually appears as folds or hymenal tags and separates the external genitalia from the vagina. Although all females have this structure, there is wide anatomic variation in its morphology. At the posterior aspect of the vagina, a tense band of mucous mem-

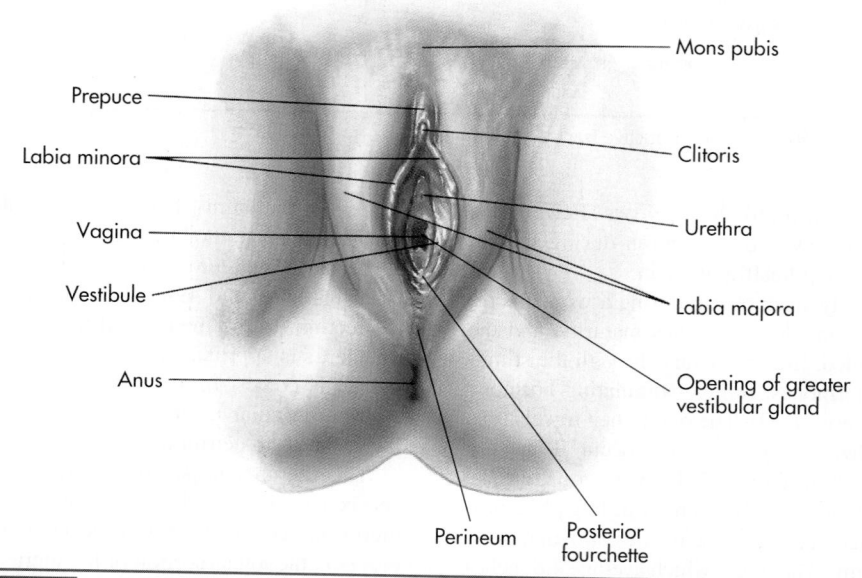

Prepuce

Labia minora

Vagina

Vestibule

Anus

Mons pubis

Clitoris

Urethra

Labia majora

Opening of greater vestibular gland

Perineum   Posterior fourchette

FIG. 49-5 External female genitalia.

brane connecting the posterior ends of the labia minora is referred to as the *posterior fourchette*.

The **clitoris** is erectile tissue that becomes engorged during sexual excitation. It lies anterior to the urethral meatus and the vaginal orifice and is usually covered by the prepuce, or hood.[2] Clitoral stimulation is an important part of sexual activity for many women.

Ducts of the Skene's glands lie alongside the urinary meatus and are thought to help lubricate the urinary meatus.[3] The Bartholin's glands, located at the posterior and lateral aspects of the vaginal orifice, secrete a thin, mucoid material believed to contribute slightly to lubrication during sexual intercourse. These glands are not usually palpable unless sebaceous-like cysts form or in the presence of an infection, such as a sexually transmitted disease.

Breasts. The breasts are a secondary sex characteristic that develops during puberty in response to estrogen and progesterone. Cyclic hormonal changes lead to regular changes in breast tissue to prepare it for lactation when fertilization and pregnancy occur. The breasts are also considered a major organ of sexual stimulation and response in some cultures.

The breasts extend from the second to the sixth ribs, with the tail reaching the axilla (Fig. 49-6). The fully mature breast is dome shaped and contains a pigmented center termed the *areola*. The areolar region contains Montgomery's tubercles, which are similar to sebaceous glands and assist in lubricating the nipple. During lactation, the alveoli, or acini, secrete milk. The milk then flows into a ductal system and is transported to the lactiferous sinuses. The nipple contains 15 to 20 tiny openings through which the milk flows during breastfeeding. The fibrous and fatty tissue that supports and separates the channels of the mammary duct system is primarily responsible for the varying sizes and shapes of the breasts in different individuals.

The breast's rich lymphatic network drains primarily into the axillary, infraclavicular, and supraclavicular channels (Fig. 49-7). Superficial lymph nodes are located in the axilla and are accessible to

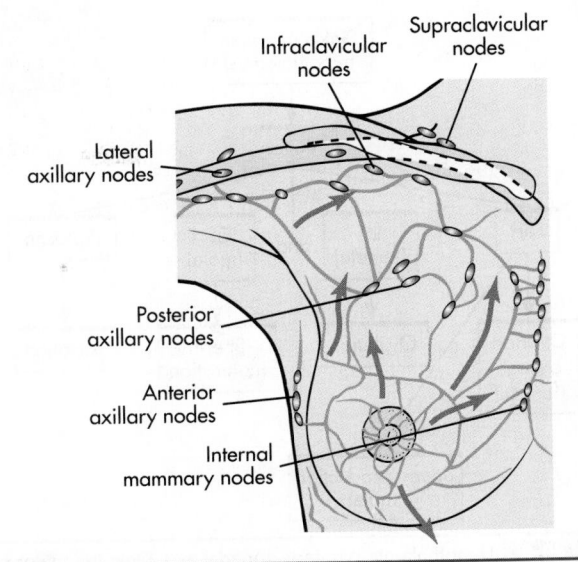

FIG. 49-7 Lymphatic drainage of the breast. *Arrows* indicate direction of drainage.

examination. This system is often responsible for the metastasis of a malignant tumor from the breast to other parts of the body.

Neuroendocrine Regulation of the Reproductive System

The hypothalamus, the pituitary gland, and the gonads secrete numerous hormones (Fig. 49-8). (Endocrine hormones are discussed in Chapter 46.) These hormones regulate the processes of ovulation, spermatogenesis (formation of sperm), and fertilization and the formation and function of the secondary sex characteristics. The amounts of hormones secreted by the anterior pituitary gland cause cyclic changes in the ovaries. The hypothalamus

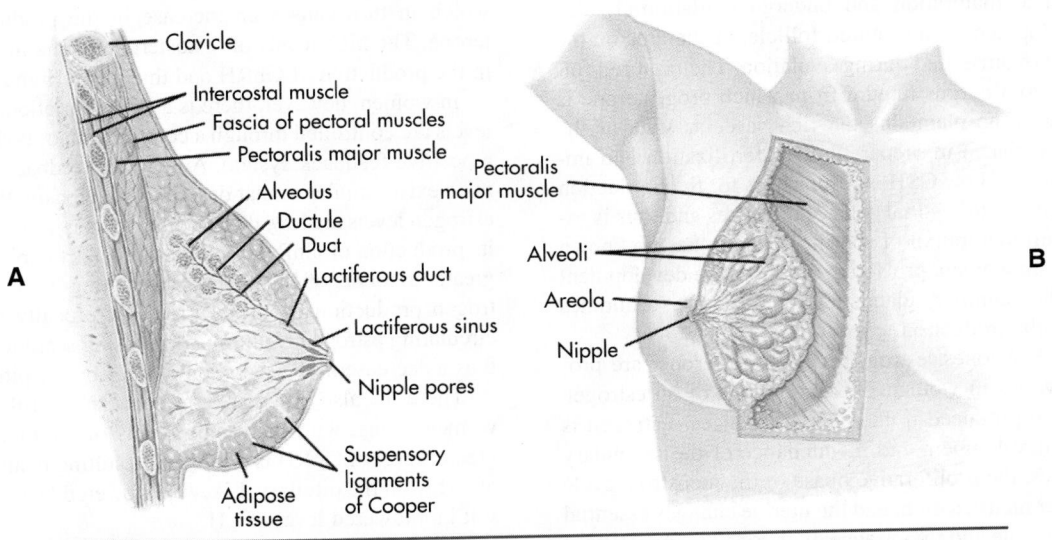

FIG. 49-6 The female breast. **A,** Sagittal section of a lactating breast. Notice how the glandular structures are anchored to the overlying skin and to the pectoral muscle by suspensory ligaments of Cooper. Each lobule of glandular tissues is drained by a lactiferous duct that eventually opens through the nipple. **B,** Anterior view of a lactating breast. In nonlactating breasts, the glandular tissue is much less prominent with adipose tissue making up most of each breast.

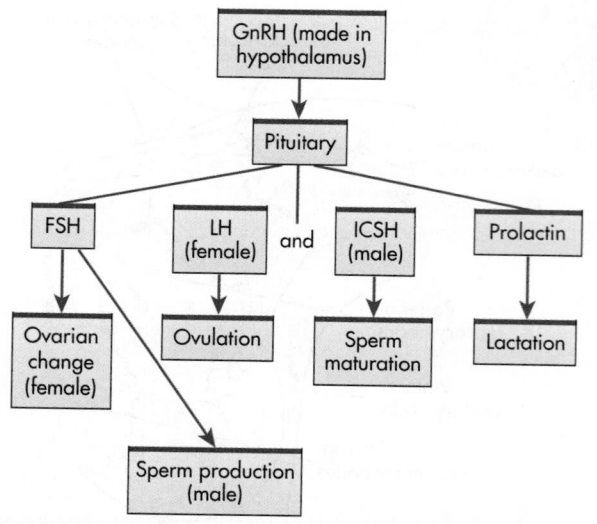

TABLE 49-1	**Gonadal Feedback Mechanisms**			
Negative Feedback				
↓ Estrogen →	↑ GnRH (hypothalamus)	→	↑ FSH (pituitary)	→ ↑ Estrogen (ovaries)
Positive Feedback				
↑ Estrogen →	↑ GnRH (hypothalamus)	→	↑ LH (pituitary)	
Testes (Negative Feedback)				
↓ Testosterone →	↑ GnRH (hypothalamus)	→	↑ FSH and ICSH (pituitary)	→ ↑ Testosterone (testes)

FSH, Follicle-stimulating hormone; *GnRH*, gonadotropin-releasing hormone; *ICSH*, interstitial cell–stimulating hormone; *LH*, luteinizing hormone.

secretes gonadotropin-releasing hormone (GnRH), which stimulates the pituitary gland to secrete its hormones, including FSH and LH. LH in males is sometimes called interstitial cell–stimulating hormone (ICSH). The gonadal hormones are estrogen, progesterone, and testosterone.

In women, FSH production by the anterior pituitary stimulates the growth and maturity of the ovarian follicles necessary for ovulation. The mature follicle produces estrogen, which in turn suppresses the release of FSH. Another hormone, inhibin, is also secreted by the ovarian follicle and inhibits both GnRH and FSH secretion. In men, FSH stimulates the seminiferous tubules to produce sperm.

LH contributes to the ovulatory process because it causes follicles to complete maturation and undergo ovulation. It also causes the development of a ruptured follicle, or the area on the ovum where the ovum exited during ovulation. The ruptured follicle develops into a corpus luteum from which progesterone is secreted. Progesterone maintains the rich vascular state of the uterus (secretory phase) in preparation for fertilization and implantation. In men, LH or ICSH is responsible for the production of testosterone by the interstitial cells of the testes and thus is essential for the full maturation of sperm. Prolactin has no known function in men. In women, prolactin stimulates the development and growth of the mammary glands. During lactation, it initiates and maintains milk production.

The gonadal hormones, estrogen and progesterone, are produced by the ovaries in women. Small amounts of an estrogen precursor are also produced in the adrenal cortices. Estrogen is essential to the development and maintenance of the secondary sex characteristics, the proliferative phase of the menstrual cycle immediately after menstruation, and the uterine changes essential to pregnancy. The role and importance of estrogen in men are not well understood. In men, estrogen is produced predominantly in the adrenal cortex.

Progesterone plays a major role in the menstrual cycle but most specifically in the secretory phase. Like estrogen, progesterone is involved in the bodily changes associated with pregnancy. Adequate progesterone is necessary to maintain an implanted egg.

The major gonadal hormone of men, testosterone, is produced by the testes. Testosterone is responsible for the development and maintenance of secondary sex characteristics, as well as for adequate spermatogenesis. Androgens are produced in females by the adrenal glands and ovaries in small amounts.

The circulating levels of gonadal hormones are controlled primarily by a negative feedback process. Receptors within the hypothalamus and pituitary are sensitive to the circulating blood levels of the hormones (Table 49-1). Increased levels of hormones stimulate a hypothalamic response to decrease the high circulating levels. Likewise, low circulating levels provoke a hypothalamic response that increases the low circulating levels. For example, if the circulating level of testosterone in men is low, the hypothalamus is stimulated to secrete GnRH. This stimulates the anterior pituitary to secrete greater amounts of FSH and ICSH, which in turn causes an increase in the production of testosterone. The high levels of testosterone then stimulate a decrease in the production of GnRH and thus of FSH and ICSH.

In women, however, there is a slight variation. The circulating levels are controlled through a combination of both a negative and a positive feedback system. A negative feedback control mechanism exists similar to that described previously. When circulating estrogen levels are low, the hypothalamus is stimulated to increase its production of GnRH. GnRH stimulates the pituitary to secrete greater amounts of FSH and LH, resulting in higher levels of estrogen production by the ovaries. Reciprocally higher levels of circulating estrogen result in a decreasing secretion of GnRH and thus a decrease in the secretion of FSH by the pituitary.

There is also a positive feedback control mechanism in women. Thus, with increasing levels of circulating estrogen, a greater level of GnRH is produced, resulting in an increased level of LH from the pituitary. Likewise, lowered levels of estrogen result in a lowered level of LH.

Menarche

Menarche is the first episode of menstrual bleeding, indicating that a female has reached puberty. This usually occurs at approximately 12 to 13 years of age, although normal onset can be as early as 10 years of age in some individuals.[4] As puberty approaches, there are changes associated with the elevated rate of estrogen and progesterone secretion by the ovaries. These changes include the development of breast buds and pubic hair, and later the development of axillary hair. During this time, there is a decrease in the sensitivity of the hypothalamic-pituitary axis that allows for increased secretion of FSH and LH and a resultant increase in estrogen. It is during this time that the adult pattern of gonadotropin secretion occurs, resulting in the menstrual cycle. Menstrual cycles are often irregular for the first 1 to 2 years following menarche because of *anovulatory cycles* (cycles without ovulation).[4]

Menstrual Cycle

The major functions of the ovaries are ovulation and the secretion of hormones. These functions are accomplished during the normal **menstrual cycle,** a monthly process mediated by the hormonal activity of the hypothalamus, pituitary gland, and ovaries. Menstruation occurs during each month in which an egg is not fertilized (Fig. 49-9). The endometrial cycle is divided into three phases labeled in relation to uterine and ovarian changes: (1) the *proliferative* or *follicular phase,* (2) the *secretory* or *luteal phase,* and (3) the *menstrual* or *ischemic phase.* The length of the menstrual cycle ranges from 20 to 40 days, the average being 28 days.

The menstrual cycle begins on the first day of menstruation, which usually lasts 3 to 7 days. Table 49-2 includes characteristics of the menstrual cycle and related patient teaching. During this time, estrogen and progesterone levels are low, but FSH levels begin to increase. During the follicular phase, a single follicle matures fully under the stimulation of FSH. (The mechanism that ensures that usually only one follicle reaches maturity is not known.) The mature follicle stimulates estrogen production, causing a negative feedback with resulting decreased FSH secretion.

Although the initial stage of follicular maturation is stimulated by FSH, complete maturation and ovulation occur only with the presence of LH. When estrogen levels peak on about the twelfth day of the cycle, there is a surge of LH, which triggers ovulation a day or two later. After ovulation (maturation and release of an ovum), LH promotes the development of the corpus luteum.

The fully developed corpus luteum continues to secrete estrogen and initiates progesterone secretion. If fertilization occurs, high levels of estrogen and progesterone continue to be secreted as a result of the continued activity of the corpus luteum from stimulation by human chorionic gonadotropin (hCG). If fertilization does not take place, menstruation occurs because of a decrease in estrogen production and progesterone withdrawal.

During the follicular phase, the endometrial lining of the uterus also undergoes change. As larger amounts of estrogen are produced, the endometrial lining undergoes proliferative changes, and there is an increase in cellular growth, including an increase in the length of blood vessels and glandular tissue.

With ovulation and the resulting increased levels of progesterone, the luteal (or secretory) phase begins. In this phase, the blood vessels begin to coil, increasing the surface area of the vascular supply. The glandular tissues mature and secrete a glycogen-rich substance, and the glandular ducts dilate. If the corpus luteum regresses (when fertilization does not occur) and estrogen and progesterone levels fall, the endometrial lining can no longer be supported. As a result, the blood vessels contract, and tissue begins to slough (fall away). This sloughing results in the menses and the start of the menstrual phase.

Menopause

Menopause is the physiologic cessation of menses associated with declining ovarian function. It is usually considered complete after 1 year of **amenorrhea** (absence of menstruation).[5] (Menopause is discussed in Chapter 52.)

Phases of the Sexual Response

The sexual response is a complex interplay of psychologic and physiologic phenomena and is influenced by a number of variables, including daily stress, illness, and crisis. The changes that occur during sexual excitement are similar for men and women. Masters and Johnson described the sexual response in terms of the excitement, plateau, orgasmic, and resolution phases.[6]

Male Sexual Response. The penis and the urethra are essential to the transport of sperm into the vagina and the cervix during intercourse. This transport is facilitated by penile erection in response to sexual stimulation during the excitement phase. Erection results from the filling of the large venous sinuses within the erectile tissue of the penis. In the flaccid state the sinuses hold only a small amount of blood, but during the erection stage they are congested with blood. Because the penis is richly endowed with sympathetic, parasympathetic, and pudendal nerve endings, it is readily stimulated to erection. The loose skin of the

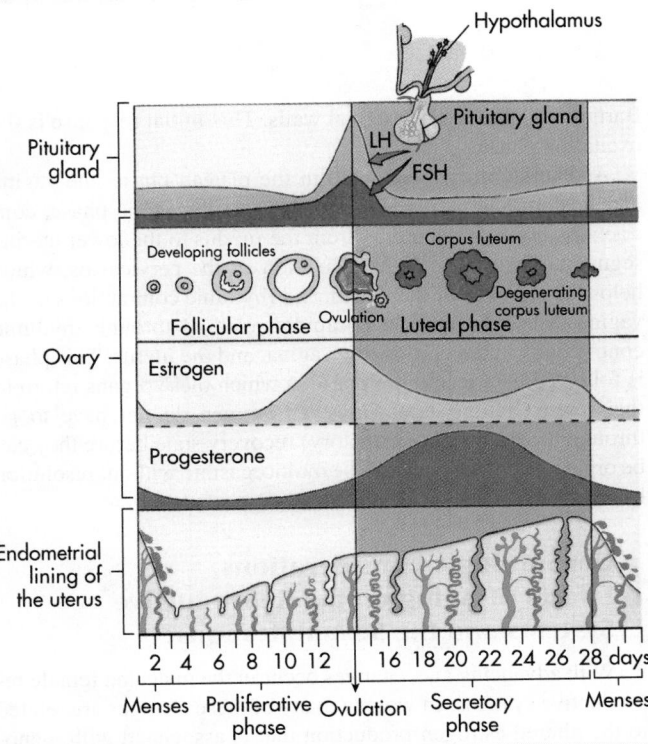

FIG. 49-9 Events of the menstrual cycle. The various lines depict the changes in blood hormone levels, the development of the follicles, and the changes in the endometrium during the cycle. *FSH,* Follicle-stimulating hormone; *LH,* luteinizing hormone.

TABLE 49-2	**Patient & Family Teaching Guide**
	Characteristics of Menstruation

CHARACTERISTIC	PATIENT TEACHING
Menarche Occurs between ages 9 and 16 yr; average age at onset is 12 or 13 yr.	See health care provider regarding possible endocrine or developmental abnormality when delayed.
Interval Usually is 21-35 days, but regular cycles as short as 17 or as long as 45 days are considered normal if pattern is consistent for individual.	Keep written record to identify own pattern of menstrual cycle. Expect some irregularity in premenopausal period. Be aware that drugs (phenothiazines, narcotics, contraceptives) and stressful life events can result in missed periods.
Duration Menstrual flow generally lasts 2-8 days.	Realize that pattern is fairly constant but that wide variations do exist.
Amount Menstrual flow varies from 20-80 ml per menses; average is 30 ml; amount varies among women and in the same woman at different times; it is usually heaviest first 2 days.	Count pads or tampons used per day. The average tampon or pad, when completely saturated, absorbs 20-30 ml. Very heavy flow is indicated by complete soaking of two pads in 1-2 hr. Flow increases and then gradually decreases in premenopausal period. IUD or drugs such as anticoagulants and thiazides can produce heavy menses.
Composition Menstrual discharge is mixture of endometrium, blood, mucus, and vaginal cells; it is dark red and less viscous than blood and usually does not clot.	Clots indicate heavy flow or vaginal pooling.

IUD, Intrauterine device.

penis becomes taut as a result of the intense venous congestion. This erectile tautness allows for easy insertion into the vagina.

As the man reaches the plateau phase, the erection is maintained, and a small increase in diameter occurs as a result of a slight increase in vasocongestion. There is also an increase in testicle size. Sometimes a change in color occurs in the glans penis, which becomes more reddish-purple.

The subsequent contraction of the penile and urethral musculature during the orgasmic phase propels the sperm outward through the meatus. In this process, termed *ejaculation,* sperm are released into the ductus deferens during contractions. Sperm advance through the urethra, where fluids from the prostate and seminal vesicles are added to the ejaculate. The sperm continue their path through the urethra, receiving a small amount of fluid from the Cowper's glands, and are finally ejaculated through the urinary meatus. Orgasm is characterized by the rapid release of the vasocongestion and muscular tension (myotonia) that have developed. The rapid release of muscular tension (through rhythmic contractions) occurs primarily in the penis, prostate gland, and seminal vesicles. After ejaculation, a man enters the resolution phase. During this phase the penis undergoes involution, gradually returning to its unstimulated, flaccid state.

Female Sexual Response. The changes that occur in a woman during sexual excitement are similar to those in a man. In response to stimulation the clitoris becomes congested and vaginal lubrication increases from secretions from the cervix,

Bartholin's glands, and vaginal walls. This initial response is the excitation phase.

As excitation is maintained in the plateau phase, the vagina expands and the uterus is elevated. In the orgasmic phase, contractions occur in the uterus from the fundus to the lower uterine segment. There is a slight relaxation of the cervical os, which helps the entrance of the sperm, and rhythmic contractions of the vagina. Muscular tension is rapidly released through rhythmic contractions in the clitoris, the vagina, and the uterus. This phase is followed by a resolution phase in which these organs return to their preexcitation state. However, women do not have to go through the resolution (refractory) recovery state before they can be orgasmic again. They can be multiorgasmic without resolution between orgasms.

■ Gerontologic Considerations: Effects of Aging on the Reproductive Systems and the Sexual Response

With advancing age, changes occur in the male and female reproductive systems. In women many of these changes are related to the altered estrogen production that is associated with menopause. A reduction in circulating estrogen along with an increase in androgens in postmenopausal women is associated with breast and genital atrophy, reduction in bone mass, and increased rate of atherosclerosis.[7] The decrease in estrogen also contributes to dry,

TABLE 49-3 Gerontologic Differences in Assessment: Reproductive Systems

CHANGES	DIFFERENCES IN ASSESSMENT FINDINGS
Male	
Penis	
Decreased subcutaneous fat, decreased skin turgor	Easily retractable foreskin (if uncircumcised); decrease in size; fewer sustained erections
Testes	
Decreased testosterone production	Decrease in size; change in position (lower); increase in firmness
Prostate	
Benign hyperplasia	Enlargement
Breasts	
Enlargement	Gynecomastia (abnormal enlargement)
Female	
Breasts	
Decreased subcutaneous fat, increased fibrous tissue, decreased skin turgor	Less resilient, looser, more pendulous tissue; decreased size; duct around nipple may feel like stringy strand
Vulva	
Decreased skin turgor	Atrophy; decreased amount of pubic hair; decreased size of clitoris and labia
Vagina	
Atrophy of tissue, decreased muscle tone	Pale and dry mucosa; relaxation of outlets; mucosa thins; vagina narrower and shorter
Urethra	
Decreased muscle tone	Cystocele (protrusion of bladder through vaginal wall)
Uterus	
Decreased thickness of myometrium	Decrease in size; uterine prolapse
Ovaries	
Decreased ovarian function	Nonpalpable ovaries; decreased size

TABLE 49-4 Gerontologic Differences in Assessment: Sexual Function

Male
Increased stimulation necessary for erection
Decreased ability to attain erection
Possible decreased response to sexual stimuli

Female
Decreased vaginal lubrication
Possible decreased response to sexual stimuli

effects of these changes, as well as the negative social attitude toward sexuality in older adults, can affect the sexual practices of people in this age-group. Nurses have an important role in providing accurate and unbiased information about sexuality and age. Nurses should emphasize the normalcy of sexual activity in older adults. Counseling may be necessary to help older patients accommodate to these normal physiologic changes. ■

ASSESSMENT OF THE MALE AND FEMALE REPRODUCTIVE SYSTEMS

Subjective Data

Important Health Information. In addition to general health information, the nurse needs to elicit information specifically relating to the reproductive system. Reproduction and sexual issues are often considered extremely personal and private. The nurse must develop trust to elicit such information. A professional demeanor is important when taking a reproductive or sexual history. The nurse needs to be sensitive, ask gender-neutral questions, and maintain an awareness of a patient's culture and beliefs.[10] It is helpful if the nurse begins with the least sensitive information (e.g., menstrual history) before asking questions about more sensitive issues such as sexual practices or sexually transmitted diseases.

Past health history. The past health history should include information about major illnesses, hospitalizations, and surgeries for both men and women.[2] The nurse should also inquire about any infections involving the reproductive system, including sexually transmitted diseases. Women should also have a complete obstetric and gynecologic history taken.

Common pediatric illnesses that affect reproductive function are mumps and rubella. The occurrence of mumps in young men has been associated with an increase in sterility. Bilateral testicular atrophy can occur secondary to mumps-related orchitis. In the health history the nurse should ask if male patients have had mumps, have been immunized with mumps vaccine, or have any indications of sterility.

Rubella is of primary concern to women of childbearing age. If rubella occurs during the first 3 months of pregnancy, the possibility of congenital anomalies is increased. For this reason, nurses should encourage immunization for all women of childbearing age who have not been immunized for rubella or have not already had the disease. However, women should not be immunized if they are already pregnant. Women are also advised not to conceive for at least 3 months after immunization.

The nurse should also question the patient regarding the patient's current health status and the presence of any acute or

friable vaginal mucosa, causing many women to experience dyspareunia.[8] A gradual hormonal decline in elderly men also occurs and is sometimes referred to as male menopause. Manifestations of hormonal decline in men can be physical, psychologic, or sexual. Some of the changes include an increase in prostate size, decreased testosterone level, decreased sperm production, decreased muscle tone of the scrotum, and a decrease in the size and firmness of the testicles. Impotence and sexual dysfunction occur in some men as a result of these changes.[9] Age-related changes in the reproductive systems and differences in assessment findings are presented in Table 49-3.

Gradual changes resulting from advancing age occur in the sexual responses of men and women (Table 49-4). These changes occur at different rates and to varying degrees. The cumulative

chronic health problems. Problems in other body systems are often related to problems with the reproductive system. Questions relating to possible endocrine disorders, particularly diabetes mellitus (DM), hypothyroidism, and hyperthyroidism, must be asked, because these disorders directly interfere with women's menstrual cycles and with sexual performance. Men who have DM may experience impotence and retrograde ejaculation. In women with uncontrolled DM, pregnancy and the use of oral contraceptives may constitute significant risks to health. Many other chronic illnesses such as cardiovascular disease, respiratory disorders, anemia, cancer, and kidney and urinary tract disorders may affect the reproductive system and sexual functioning.

A history of a stroke should be determined. In men, strokes may cause physiologic or psychologic impotence. Men who have suffered a myocardial infarction (MI) may experience impotence because of the fear of precipitating another heart attack resulting from sexual activity. This same concern is shared by the woman both as a partner of someone who has had an MI and as the person recovering from an MI. Although most patients have concerns about sexual activity following an MI, many are not comfortable expressing these concerns to the nurse.[11] The nurse must be sensitive to this concern. In women, a history of cardiovascular disease (e.g., hypertension, thrombophlebitis, angina) causes a higher incidence of morbidity and mortality with pregnancy or oral contraceptive use.

Medications. A list of all prescription and over-the-counter medications that the patient is taking should be documented, including reason for the medication, the dosage, and the length of time that the medication has been taken. All drugs taken by female patients should be evaluated for possible teratogenic effects in women of childbearing age. The patient should be asked about the use of herbal products and dietary supplements.

Particularly relevant in the assessment of the reproductive system is the use of diuretics (sometimes prescribed for premenstrual edema), psychotropic agents (which may interfere with sexual performance), and antihypertensives (some of which may cause impotence). Thus patients who use drugs such as methyldopa (Aldomet), clonidine (Catapres), guanethidine (Ismelin), and hydralazine (Apresoline) must be closely assessed for these problems. The nurse must also note the use of drugs such as alcohol, marijuana, barbiturates, amphetamines, or phencyclidine hydrochloride (PCP; also called "angel dust"), which can have serious behavioral or physiologic effects on the functioning of the reproductive system.

In women, the use of oral contraceptives or other hormones should be noted. The use of hormone replacement therapy (HRT) is relevant for women because of its potential benefit in preventing osteoporosis. Estrogen may also have beneficial effects on memory and cognitive function in older women. In women with a uterus, the concurrent use of progesterone should be documented. The use of estrogen alone in women who have a uterus has been shown to increase the incidence of endometrial cancer.[5]

Oral contraceptive use can aggravate the symptoms of certain neurologic disorders, such as seizures or migraine headaches. However, the use of lower doses of estrogen in current contraceptives makes these side effects less problematic and may actually be therapeutic. A history of cholecystitis and hepatitis is important information because these conditions may be contraindications for oral contraceptives; cholecystitis is often aggravated by oral contraceptives, and chronic active inflammation of the liver generally precludes the use of estrogen products because they are metabolized by the liver. Chronic obstructive pulmonary disease may be a contraindication to oral contraceptive use because progesterone thickens respiratory secretions.

Surgery or other treatments. Any surgical procedures should be noted in the health history. Surgical procedures involving the reproductive system are listed in Table 49-5. Therapeutic or spontaneous abortions should also be documented.

TABLE 49-5	Surgeries of the Reproductive Systems
SURGERY	**DESCRIPTION**
Male	
Herniorrhaphy	Repair of hernia
Orchiectomy	Removal of one or both testes
Prostatectomy	Removal of prostate gland
Repair of testicular torsion	Correction of axial rotation of spermatic cord, which cuts off blood supply to the testicle, epididymis, and other structures
Varicocelectomy	Repair of varicose vein of scrotum
Vasectomy	Removal of part of ductus (vas) deferens; can be an elective procedure for sterilization or contraception
Female	
Cryosurgery	Use of subfreezing temperature to destroy tissue, especially in treatment of abnormal cells
Dilation and curettage	Dilation of uterus and scraping of endometrium, performed to diagnose disease of uterus, correct heavy or prolonged vaginal bleeding, or empty uterus of products of conception; also used in the treatment of infertility to correlate state of endometrium and time of cycle
Hysterectomy	Removal of uterus
Mastectomy	Removal of one or both breasts
Oophorectomy	Removal of one or both ovaries
Repair of cystocele	Correction of protrusion of urinary bladder through vaginal wall
Repair of rectocele	Correction of protrusion of rectum into vagina
Salpingectomy	Removal of one or both fallopian tubes
Tubal sterilization	Ligation of fallopian tubes

Functional Health Patterns. The key questions to ask a patient with a reproductive problem are presented in Table 49-6.

Health perception–health management pattern. Two of the primary focuses of this health pattern are the patient's perception of his or her own health and measures that the patient takes to maintain health. Specifically, it is important to ask about self-examination practices and screenings. Monthly breast self-examination (BSE), mammography according to age-specific guidelines (see Chapter 50), and routine Pap smears are integral to a woman's health. Testicular self-examination (TSE) should be practiced by all men, starting in adolescence. Regular prostate examination should be encouraged as well. The American Cancer Society recommends that men over age 50 have digital rectal examination (DRE) yearly.[12]

Family history is also a component of this health pattern. The nurse should inquire about a history of cancer, particularly cancer of the reproductive organs. First-degree relatives who have cancer of the breast, ovaries, uterus, or prostate significantly increases the risk of cancer for the patient. Determination of a familial tendency for diabetes mellitus, hypothyroidism, hyperthyroidism, hypertension, stroke, angina, myocardial infarction, endocrine disorders, or anemia is also important.

Assessment of the reproductive system is incomplete without a knowledge of the patient's lifestyle choices. The nurse should know whether a woman uses cigarettes, alcohol, caffeine, or other drugs because these substances can be detrimental to both mother and fetus. Cigarette smoking may delay conception. Cigarette smoking also can increase the risk of morbidity in women using oral contraceptives and is associated with early menopause. These substances may also adversely affect the sperm count in men and cause impotence or decreased libido.

TABLE 49-6	**Health History** **Reproductive System**

Health Perception–Health Management
- How would you describe your overall health?
- *Women:* Explain how you examine your breasts. When was your last Pap smear? Mammogram? What were the results?
- *Men:* Explain how you examine your testes. When was your last prostate examination?
- Describe the health of your family members. Any history of breast, uterine, ovarian, or prostate cancer?
- Do you use tobacco products, alcohol, or drugs?*

Nutritional-Metabolic
- Describe what you usually eat and drink.
- Have you experienced any changes in weight?*
- How do you feel about your current weight?
- Do you take any nutritional supplements such as calcium or vitamins?*
- Do you have any dietary restrictions?*

Elimination
- Do you experience problems with urination (e.g., pain, burning, dribbling, incontinence, frequency)?*
- Have you had bladder infections? If so, when? How often?
- Do you experience problems with bowel movements?* Do you use laxatives?*

Activity-Exercise
- What activities do you typically do each day?
- Do you have enough energy for your desired activities?
- Can you dress yourself? Feed yourself? Walk without help?

Sleep-Rest
- How many hours do you typically sleep each night?
- Do you feel rested after sleep?
- Do you experience any problems associated with sleeping?*

Cognitive-Perceptual
- Are you able to read and write?
- Do you experience problems with dizziness?*
- Do you experience pain? If yes, where?
- Do you experience pain during sexual activity or intercourse?*

Self-Perception–Self-Concept
- How would you describe yourself?
- Have there been any changes recently that have made you feel differently about yourself?*
- Are you experiencing any problems that are affecting your sexuality?*

Role-Relationship
- Describe your living arrangements. Who do you live with?
- Do you have a significant other? If yes, is this relationship satisfying?
- Are you experiencing any role-related problems in your family?* At work?*
- What are the relationships among your family members?

Sexuality-Reproductive
- Are you sexually active? If so, how many partners do you have?
- What kind of sex do you engage in (e.g., oral, vaginal, rectal)?
- How do you protect yourself against sexually transmitted disease and unwanted pregnancy?
- Are you satisfied with your present means of sexual expression? If no, explain.
- Have you experienced any recent changes in your sexual practices?*
- *Women:* date of last menstruation, description of menstrual flow, problems with menstruation, age of menarche, age of menopause.
- *Women:* pregnancy history—number of times pregnant, number of living children, number of miscarriages/abortions.

Coping–Stress Tolerance
- Have there been any major changes in your life within the last couple of years?*
- What is stressful in your life right now?
- How do you handle health problems when they occur?

Value-Belief
- What beliefs do you have about your health and illnesses?
- Do you use home remedies?*
- Is religion an important part of your life?*
- Do you feel that any of your personal beliefs or values may be compromised because of your treatment?*

*If yes, describe.

The nurse must determine if the patient is allergic to sulfon-amides, penicillin, rubber, or latex. Sulfonamides and penicillin are used frequently in the treatment of reproductive and geni-tourinary problems such as vaginitis and gonorrhea. Rubber and latex are commonly used in diaphragms and condoms. An allergy to these substances precludes their use as contraceptive methods.

Nutritional-metabolic pattern. Anemia is a common prob-lem in women in their reproductive years, particularly during pregnancy and the postpartum period. The adequacy of the diet should be evaluated with this condition in mind.

A thorough nutritional and psychologic history should be taken to assess for the presence of an eating disorder. Anorexia can cause amenorrhea and the subsequent problems, such as os-teoporosis, that are related to estrogen cessation. The nurse has the opportunity to help prevent the debilitating condition of os-teoporosis. From early adolescence, women can be counseled re-garding adequate calcium intake and the role of calcium in the prevention of osteoporosis. The patient's daily calcium intake should be estimated to determine whether there is a need for sup-plementation. Folic acid intake for women in their reproductive years should be evaluated because a deficiency can result in spina bifida and other neural tube defects in the fetus.[13]

Elimination pattern. Many gynecologic problems can result in genitourinary problems. Stress and urge incontinence are com-mon in older women because of relaxation of the pelvic muscu-lature caused by multiple births or advancing age. Vaginal infec-tions predispose patients to chronic or recurrent urinary tract infections. The proximity of the reproductive organs and the gen-itourinary tract makes metastasis of malignant tumors to this site a possibility to be considered. Benign prostatic hyperplasia is a common problem of older men. It can alter normal urination, causing retention and difficulty in initiating the urinary stream.

Activity-exercise pattern. The amount, type, and intensity of activity and exercise should be documented. Lack of stress on bones secondary to lack of exercise is an important factor in the development of osteoporosis. Weight-bearing exercise decreases the risk of osteoporosis in women. Women who engage in exces-sive exercise may experience amenorrhea. This may result from decreased estrogen related to a low percentage of body fat be-cause estrogen is stored in fat cells. Anemia can result in fatigue and activity intolerance and can interfere with satisfactory per-formance of the activities of daily living.

Sleep-rest pattern. Sleep patterns may be affected during the postpartum period and also while raising young children. The hot flashes and sweating often present during the perimenopause can cause serious sleep interruption when the woman is awakened in a drenching sweat. The need to change her nightgown and bed-ding further disrupts her sleep. Insomnia is also a common com-plaint of perimenopausal women. Daytime fatigue often results from such nighttime awakenings. In men, sleep disturbances may be caused by frequent urination at night associated with prostate enlargement.

Cognitive-perceptual pattern. Pelvic pain is associated with various gynecologic disorders such as pelvic inflammatory dis-ease, ovarian cysts, and endometriosis. **Dyspareunia** (painful in-tercourse) can be particularly problematic for a woman. The pain associated with intercourse can make her reluctant to participate in sexual activity and strain her relationship with her sexual part-ner. The woman should be referred to her health care provider if dyspareunia is present.

Self-perception–self-concept pattern. The reproductive changes of aging such as pendulous breasts and vaginal dryness in women and decreased size of the penis in men may lead to emotional dis-tress. The subtle changes associated with sexuality and advancing age may alter the self-concept of many persons.

Role-relationship pattern. The nurse needs to obtain infor-mation regarding the family structure and occupation. Questions regarding recent changes in work-related relationships or family conflicts should be asked. It is important to ascertain the pa-tient's role in the family as a starting point in determining fam-ily dynamics.

Roles and relationships are affected by changes within the family. The addition of a new baby into the family may change family dynamics. Role-relationship patterns change as children begin their careers and move away from home. Another change occurs when people retire.

Sexuality-reproductive pattern. The extent and depth of the in-terview about a patient's sexuality depend primarily on the exper-tise of the interviewer and on the needs and the willingness of the patient. Before taking a sexual history, interviewers should assess their own comfort with their sexuality, because any discomfort in questioning becomes obvious to the patient. Interviews must be carried out in an environment that provides reassurance, confiden-tiality, and a nonjudgmental attitude. It is best to begin with the least sensitive areas and then move to more sensitive areas.

For women, it is important to obtain a menstrual and an ob-stetric history. The menstrual history includes the date of the last menstrual period, description of menstrual flow, age of menarche, and, if applicable, age at menopause. Menstrual history data are used in the detection of pregnancy, infertility, and numerous other gynecologic concerns. Changes in the usual menstrual pattern must be explicitly described to determine whether the change is transient and unimportant or connected with a more serious gyne-cologic problem. *Metrorrhagia* (spotting or bleeding between menstruations), *menorrhagia* (excessive menstrual bleeding), *amenorrhea* (lack of menstruation), and *postcoital bleeding* are examples of such problems. Changes in menstrual patterns asso-ciated with the use of contraceptive pills, intrauterine devices (IUDs), subdermal estrogen-only implant (Norplant), or medroxy-progesterone (Depo-Provera) injections must be identified. Con-traceptive pills usually decrease the amount and duration of flow, whereas some IUDs may cause an increase in the amount and du-ration. Some IUDs also increase the severity of dysmenorrhea. However, newer IUDs contain progestin and may be therapeutic. The obstetric history includes the number of pregnancies, full-term births, preterm births, and live births. Other obstetric infor-mation should include information about any ectopic pregnancies or abortions, either spontaneous or therapeutic. Any problems that occurred with pregnancy should be documented.

A sexual history should include information regarding sexual activity, beliefs, and practices. Sexual preference (heterosexual, homosexual, bisexual), the frequency and type of sexual activity (penile-vaginal, penile-rectal, recipient rectal, oral), and the num-ber of partners and protective measures against sexually trans-mitted disease and pregnancy should be explored. The patient's knowledge of safe sexual practices should be determined. A his-tory of multiple sex partners and unprotected sex increases the risk of contracting a sexually transmitted disease. For a woman, this can increase the risk of pelvic inflammatory disease, which can compromise her ability to become pregnant.

TABLE 49-7	Sexual History Format

- How long have you been sexually active?
- Are you currently in a relationship that involves sexual intercourse? If yes, do you have one or multiple partners?
- How frequently do you engage in sexual activities? Are you and your partner(s) satisfied with the sexual relationship?
- How many sexual partners have you had in the past 6 months?
- Do you prefer relationships with men, women, or both? (If the patient is gay or lesbian, inquire if he or she is in a significant relationship and has a partner.)
- Has your sex life changed during the past year? If yes, how?
- Have you ever had a sexually transmitted disease? If yes, what?
- What are you doing to protect yourself from sexually transmitted diseases? If protection is used, what type? Do you use protection every time you have intercourse?
- Are you currently using any birth control measures? If yes, what type? How long have you been using this product? How effective do you feel this has been?
- Have you ever been in a relationship with anyone who hurt you? Have you ever been forced into sexual acts as a child or an adult?
- How often have you experienced impotence (male) or difficulty with vaginal lubrication (female) or pain with intercourse?

Adapted from Wilson SF, Giddens JF: *Health assessment for nursing practice,* ed 2, St Louis, 2001, Mosby.

Table 49-7 outlines specific questions for a sexual history. It should be noted that only a skilled interviewer should approach some of the questions presented in Table 49-7, and then only with discretion.

Both men and women should be asked about their general satisfaction with sexuality. The patient's satisfaction with the opportunities for sexual gratification is important information that should be elicited. The patient should be questioned about sexual beliefs and practices and whether orgasm is achieved. Any unexplained change in sexual practices or performance should be explored. Problems of the reproductive system can cause physiologic or psychologic problems that can lead to painful intercourse, impotence, sexual dysfunction, or infertility. Both the cause and the effect of such problems should be determined.

Coping–stress tolerance pattern. The stress related to situations such as pregnancy or menopause may cause an increased dependence on support systems. It is essential for the nurse to ascertain who the support people are in the patient's life. The diagnosis of a sexually transmitted disease can cause stress to the patient and the partner. Means to manage such stress should be explored.

Value-belief pattern. Sexual and reproductive functioning is closely related to cultural, religious, moral, and ethical values. The nurse should be aware of his or her own beliefs in these areas and should recognize and sensitively react to the patient's personal beliefs associated with reproductive and sexuality issues.

Objective Data

Physical Examination: Male. The examination of the male external genitalia includes inspection and palpation. An examination may be performed with the patient lying or standing. The standing position is generally preferred. The examiner should be seated in front of the standing patient. Gloves should be used during examination of the male genitalia.

Pubis. The nurse observes the distribution and general characteristics of the pubic hair and the skin. Normally, the hair is in a diamond-shaped pattern. The hair is usually coarser than scalp hair. The absence of hair is not a normal finding. The skin is also evaluated.

Penis. The nurse notes the size and skin texture of the penis and any lesions, scars, or swelling. The location of the urethral meatus, as well as the presence or absence of a foreskin, should be noted. If present, the foreskin should be retracted to note cleanliness and replaced over the glans after observation. The glans is compressed to note any discharge and its amount, color, and odor if present. The nurse also palpates the penile shaft for tenderness or masses and observes the ventral and dorsal aspects.

Scrotum and testes. The nurse performs a complete skin examination by lifting each testis to inspect all sides of the scrotal sac. Palpation of the scrotum is done to note changes in consistency or the presence of masses. It is important to note if the testes are descended. The left testis usually hangs lower than the right. Undescended testis is a major risk factor for testicular cancer, as well as a potential cause of male infertility.

Inguinal region and spermatic cord. The examiner inspects the skin overlying the inguinal regions for rashes or lesions. The patient should be asked to bear down or cough. While he is straining, the inguinal area should be inspected for the presence of a bulge. No bulging should be seen.

Examination of the inguinal area continues with palpation. The right and left inguinal rings should be palpated using the index finger or middle finger. The finger should be inserted into the lower aspect of the scrotum and should follow the spermatic cord upward through the triangular, slitlike opening of the inguinal ring. At this point, the patient should be asked to bear down and cough. The nurse determines whether the strain produces a bulging of the intestines through the ring, indicating the presence of a hernia, a condition that requires follow-up. The inguinal lymph nodes should also be palpated. Enlargement of the lymph nodes (termed *lymphadenopathy*) could suggest a pelvic organ infection or malignancy.

Anus and prostate. The anal sphincter and perineal regions are inspected for lesions, masses, and hemorrhoids. A DRE is required for all men who have symptoms of prostate trouble, such as difficulty in initiating the flow and the urge to void frequently. This examination should be performed annually for all men over 50 years of age.

Physical Examination: Female. Physical examination of women often begins with inspection and palpation of the breasts and then proceeds to the abdomen and genitalia. Examination of the abdomen provides an opportunity to detect pain or any masses that may involve the genitourinary system. Abdominal examination is discussed in Chapter 38.

Breasts. Breasts are examined first by visual inspection. The nurse, with the patient seated, observes the breasts for symmetry, size, shape, skin color and texture, vascular patterns, dimpling, and the presence of unusual lesions. The patient is asked to put her arms at her sides, arms overhead, lean forward, and press hands on hips. The nurse observes for any abnormalities during these maneuvers. The axillae and the clavicular areas are then palpated for enlarged lymph nodes.

TABLE 49-8   Normal Physical Assessment of the Reproductive System

MALE	FEMALE
External Genitalia Diamond-shaped hair distribution. Penis circumcised, no lesions or discharge noted. Scrotum symmetric, no masses, descended testes. No inguinal hernia.	**Breasts** Symmetric without dimpling. Nipples soft; no drainage, retraction, or lesions noted. No masses or tenderness; no lymphadenopathy.
Anus No hemorrhoids, fissures, or lesions noted.	**External Genitalia** Triangular hair distribution. Genitalia dark pink, no lesions, redness, swelling, or inflammation in perineal region. No vaginal discharge noted. No tenderness with palpation of Skene's ducts and Bartholin's glands.
	Anus No hemorrhoids, fissures, or lesions noted.

TABLE 49-9   *C*ommon Assessment Abnormalities   Breast

FINDING	DESCRIPTION	POSSIBLE ETIOLOGY AND SIGNIFICANCE
Nipple inversion or retraction	Recent onset, erythematous, pain, unilateral	Abscess, inflammation, cancer
	Recent onset (usually within past year), unilateral presentation, lack of tenderness	Neoplasm
Nipple secretions		
▪ Galactorrhea (female)	Milky, no relationship to lactation, unilateral or bilateral or intermittent or consistent presentation	Drug therapy, particularly phenothiazines, tricyclic anti-depressants, methyldopa; hypofunction or hyperfunction of thyroid or adrenal glands; tumors of hypothalamus or pituitary gland; excessive estrogen; prolonged suckling or breast foreplay
▪ Galactorrhea (male)	Milky, bilateral presentation	Chorioepithelioma of testes, manifestation of pituitary tumor
▪ Purulent	Gray-green or yellow color; frequent unilateral presentation; association with pain, erythema, induration, nipple inversion	Puerperal (after birth) mastitis (inflammatory condition of breast) or abscess
	Same as above but usually without nipple inversion	Infected sebaceous cyst
▪ Serous discharge	Clear appearance, unilateral or bilateral or intermittent or consistent presentation	Intraductal papilloma
▪ Dark green or multicolored discharge	Thick, sticky, and frequently bilateral	Ductal ectasia (dilation of mammary ducts)
▪ Serosanguineous or bloody drainage	Unilateral presentation	Papillomatosis (widespread development of nipplelike growths), intraductal papilloma, carcinoma (male and female)
Scaling or irritation of nipple	Unilateral or bilateral presentation, crusting, possible ulceration	Paget's disease, eczema, infection
Nodules, lumps, or masses	Multiple, bilateral, well-delineated, soft or firm, mobile cysts; pain; premenstrual occurrence	Fibrocystic changes
	Rubbery consistency, fluid-filled interior, pain	Ductal ectasia
	Soft, mobile, well-delineated cyst, absence of pain	Lipoma, fibroadenoma
	Erythema, tenderness, induration	Infected sebaceous cysts, abscesses
	Usually singular, hard irregularly shaped, poorly delineated, nonmobile	Neoplasm
Dimpling of breast	Unilateral, recent onset, no pain	Neoplasm

After the patient assumes a supine position, a pillow is placed under the back on the side to be examined. The patient is asked to put her arm above and behind her head. These maneuvers flatten breast tissue and make palpation easier. The breast is then palpated in a systematic fashion using a vertical line, a clockwise, or a spoke approach. The nurse should use the distal finger pads for palpation. The tail of Spence should be included in the examination because this area and the upper outer quadrant are the areas where most breast malignancies develop. Finally, the nurse should palpate the area around the areolae for masses. The nipple should be compressed to determine the presence of discharge or any masses. The color, consistency, and odor of any discharge should be documented.

External genitalia. The nurse uses gloves for examination of the external genitalia. The mons pubis, labia majora, labia minora, posterior fourchette, perineum, and anal region are inspected for characteristics of skin, hair distribution, and contour. Lesions, inflammation, swelling, and discharge are noted. The nurse must separate the labia to fully inspect the clitoris, urethral meatus, and vaginal orifice.

Internal pelvic examination. During the speculum examination, the nurse observes the walls of the vagina and the cervix for inflammation, discharge, polyps, and suspicious growths. During this examination, it is possible to take a Pap smear and collect secretions for culture and microscopic examination. After the speculum examination, a bimanual examination is performed to allow assessment of the size, shape, and consistency of the uterus, ovaries, and tubes. The tubes are not normally palpable.

Pelvic and bimanual examinations are considered advanced skills and are not usually within the scope of the nurse general-ist.[14] For this reason, these parts of the examination are not included in this text. Pelvic and bimanual examinations are described in physical assessment textbooks.

Table 49-8 provides an example of a recording format for the physical assessment findings for the male and female reproductive systems. Tables 49-9 through 49-11 summarize common assessment abnormalities of the breasts, female reproductive system, and male reproductive system, respectively.

DIAGNOSTIC STUDIES OF THE REPRODUCTIVE SYSTEMS

Table 49-12 summarizes the most commonly used diagnostic studies in the assessment of the reproductive systems and the nurse's responsibility regarding these diagnostic tests.

Urine Studies

Pregnancy Testing. Occurrence of pregnancy is generally validated by measuring human chorionic gonadotropin (hCG) in the urine. A solution containing monoclonal antibodies specific for hCG is mixed with a small amount of urine. The presence of hCG causes a change in color of the tested urine.

Home pregnancy test kits use the same assay principle described in the preceding paragraph. Positive results are based on the presence of hCG in urine. Some tests can detect pregnancy as early as the first day following a missed menstrual period. These tests are 98% accurate if the test is performed exactly per instructions. A second test is recommended within a week if the first test is negative (assuming menses has not yet occurred).[15]

Hormone Studies. Although estrogen studies are performed on urine, the results are frequently inaccurate because of

TABLE 49-10	Common Assessment Abnormalities — Female Reproductive System	
FINDING	**DESCRIPTION**	**POSSIBLE ETIOLOGY AND SIGNIFICANCE**
• Vulvar discharge	Plaque-like consistency, frequent itching and inflammation, lack of odor or yeast-like smell	Candidiasis (*Candida* or yeast infection), vaginitis
	Grayish color, copious flow, frothy appearance, vulvar irritation	Bacterial vaginosis infection
	Grayish green or yellow color; malodorous or "fishy" odor	*Trichomonas vaginalis*
	Bloody color	*Chlamydia trachomatis* or *Neisseria gonorrhoeae* infection, menstruation, trauma, cancer
• Vulvar erythema	Bright or beefy red color, itching	*Candida albicans*, allergy, chemical vaginitis
	Reddened base, painful vesicles or ulcerations	Genital herpes
	Macules or papules, itching	Chancroid (STD), contact dermatitis, scabies, pediculosis
• Vulvar growths	Soft, fleshy growth; nontender	Condyloma acuminatum
	Flat and warty appearance, nontender	Condyloma latum
	Same as either of above, possible pain	Neoplasm
	Reddened base, vesicles, and small erosions; pain	Lymphogranuloma venereum, genital herpes, chancroid
	Indurated, firm ulcers; lack of pain	Chancre (syphilis), granuloma inguinale
• Abdominal pain or tenderness	Intermittent or consistent tenderness in right or left lower quadrant	Salpingitis (infection of fallopian tube), ectopic pregnancy, ruptured ovarian cyst, PID, tubal or ovarian abscess
	Periumbilical location, consistent occurrence	Cystitis, endometritis (inflammation of endometrium), ectopic pregnancy

PID, Pelvic inflammatory disease; *STD,* sexually transmitted disease.

TABLE 49-11

Common Assessment Abnormalities
Male Reproductive System

FINDING	DESCRIPTION	POSSIBLE ETIOLOGY AND SIGNIFICANCE
• Penile growths or masses	Indurated, smooth, disklike appearance; absence of pain; singular presentation	Chancre
	Papular to irregularly shaped ulceration with pus, lack of induration	Chancroid
	Ulceration with induration and nodularity	Cancer
	Flat, wartlike nodule	Condyloma latum
	Elevated, fleshy, moist, elongated projections with single or multiple projections	Condyloma acuminatum
	Localized swelling with retracted, tight foreskin	Paraphimosis (inability to replace foreskin to its normal position after retraction), trauma
• Vesicles, erosions, or ulcers	Painful, erythematous base; vesicular or small erosions	Genital herpes, balanitis (inflammation of glans penis), chancroid
	Painless, singular, small erosion with eventual lymphadenopathy	Lymphogranuloma venereum, cancer
• Scrotal masses	Localized swelling with tenderness, unilateral or bilateral presentation	Epididymitis (inflammation of epididymis), testicular torsion, orchitis (mumps)
	Swelling, tenderness	Incarcerated hernia
	Unilateral or bilateral presentation; swelling without pain; translucent, cordlike or wormlike appearance	Hydrocele (accumulation of fluid in outer covering of testes), spermatocele (firm, sperm-containing cyst of epididymis), varicocele (dilation of veins that drain testes), hematocele (accumulation of blood within scrotum)
	Firm, nodular testes or epididymis; frequent unilateral presentation	Tuberculosis, cancer
• Penile discharge	Clear to purulent color, minimal to copious flow	Urethritis or gonorrhea, *Chlamydia trachomatis* infection, trauma
• Penile or scrotal erythema	Macules and papules	Scabies, pediculosis
• Inguinal masses	Bulging, unilateral presentation during straining	Inguinal hernia
	Shotty, 1-3 cm nodules	Lymphadenopathy

variable estrogen levels during the normal cycle and the difficulty in estimating the day of the cycle in women with irregular menses. Adrenal androgens are precursors of estrogens and can be measured in the urine of both men and women. FSH can be measured in a 24-hour urine specimen. Increased and decreased FSH levels can indicate gonadal failure resulting from pituitary dysfunction. For more information regarding hormone studies, see Chapter 46.

Blood Studies

Hormone Studies. A common serum hormone test, hCG, is used to identify pregnancy. Serum assays for hCG can detect pregnancy before a woman misses her menstrual period.[16] The prolactin assay is used primarily in the workup of a patient with amenorrhea. High levels of prolactin are normally associated with low levels of estrogen, such as those that occur during lactation. However, the same finding can occur with pituitary adenomas, especially with otherwise unexplained *galactorrhea* (excessive secretion of breast milk). Serum progesterone and estradiol are sometimes measured in ovarian function assessment, particularly for amenorrhea. In addition, hormonal blood studies are essential components of a thorough fertility workup.

Tumor Markers. Biologic tumor markers are substances associated with malignant disease. Measurement of these markers is useful in monitoring therapy (marker levels rise as disease progresses and fall with disease regression) because marker levels may rise months before new disease or metastasis is evident. α-Fetoprotein (AFP) and hCG are sometimes used as tumor markers for testicular malignancy. A specific tumor antigen such as prostate-specific antigen (PSA) is another type of tumor marker frequently used.[15]

Serology Tests for Syphilis. The Venereal Disease Research Laboratory (VDRL) test and the rapid plasma reagin (RPR) detect the presence of antibodies in the serum of patients infected with syphilis. These tests are inexpensive and reliable but have high levels of false-positive results. The fluorescent treponemal antibody absorption (FTA-ABS) test is highly reliable and should be used after a positive VDRL or RPR, even if it is weakly positive or questionable.[15]

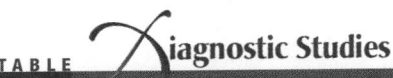

TABLE
49-12 Diagnostic Studies
Male and Female Reproductive Systems

STUDY	DESCRIPTION AND PURPOSE	NURSING RESPONSIBILITY
Urine Studies		
▪ hCG	hCG is detected in urine to ascertain whether a woman is pregnant. Hydatidiform mole and chorioepithelioma (in men and women) may also be detected using hCG.	Obtain thorough menstrual history from patient, including birth control methods. Determine presence or absence of presumptive signs of pregnancy (e.g., breast changes, increased whitish vaginal discharge).
▪ Testosterone levels	Tumors and developmental anomalies of the testes can be detected.	Instruct patient to collect 24 hr urine specimen. Keep it refrigerated.

▪ Follicle-stimulating hormone (FSH) assay	Indicates gonadal failure because of pituitary dysfunction.
	Female:
	  Follicular phase: 2-5 IU/24 hr
	  Midcycle: 8-40 IU/24 hr
	  Luteal phase: 2-10 IU/24 hr
	  Postmenopause: 35-100 IU/24 hr
	Male: 2-15 IU/24 hr
		Instruct patient to collect 24 hr urine specimen. Indicate phase of menstrual cycle, if menopausal, and if on oral contraceptives or hormones.

Blood Studies		
▪ Prolactin assay	Detects pituitary dysfunction that can cause amenorrhea.	Observe venipuncture site for bleeding or hematoma formation.
▪ Prostate specific antigen (PSA)	Used to detect prostate cancer. Also a sensitive test for monitoring response to therapy. Normal finding is <4 ng/ml (<4 μg/L).	No food or fluid restrictions. Collect 5 ml blood. Observe venipuncture site for bleeding.
▪ Serum hCG assay	hCG is detected in serum to ascertain whether a woman is pregnant; can also be used as a tumor marker for testicular malignancy.	Instruct patient to have blood drawn in laboratory. Elicit where she is in her menstrual cycle, whether she has missed menses, and if so, how late she is.
▪ Serum androstenedione and testosterone levels	Ascertain whether elevated androgens are due to adrenal or ovarian dysfunction. Serum testosterone is also drawn to assess cause of amenorrhea.	Collect health history to eliminate potential sources of interference with accuracy of results (e.g., use of corticosteroids or barbiturates, presence of hypothyroidism or hyperthyroidism).
▪ Serum progesterone	Frequently used to detect functioning corpus luteum cyst.	Observe venipuncture site for bleeding or hematoma formation. Include last menstrual period and trimester of pregnancy because progesterone levels vary with gestation.
▪ Serum estradiol	Measures ovarian function. Particularly useful in assessing estrogen-secreting tumors and states of precocious female puberty. Normal values depend on laboratory that performs test and should be obtained from that laboratory. May be used to confirm perimenopausal status. Increased serum estradiol levels in men may be indicative of testicular tumors.	Observe venipuncture site for bleeding or hematoma formation.

▪ Serum FSH	Indicates gonadal failure due to pituitary dysfunction; used to validate menopausal status.
	Female:
	  Follicular phase: 2-15 mIU/ml
	  Midcycle: 8-40 mIU/ml
	  Luteal phase: 2-15 mIU/ml
	  Postmenopause: 50-250 mIU/ml
	Male: 2-15 mIU/ml
		No food or fluid restrictions required. State phase of menstrual cycle, if menopausal, or if on oral contraceptive or hormones.

▪ Venereal Disease Research Laboratory (VDRL) (flocculation)	Nonspecific antibody tests used to screen for syphilis. Positive readings can be made within 1-2 wk after appearance of primary lesion (chancre) or 4-15 wk after initial infection.	Observe venipuncture site for bleeding or hematoma formation.
▪ Rapid plasma reagin (RPR) (agglutination)		Obtain data to determine presence or absence of problems such as hepatitis, pregnancy, and autoimmune diseases that may interfere with the accuracy of results.

hCG, Human chorionic gonadotropin.

Continued

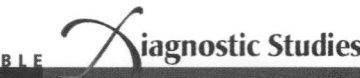

TABLE 49-12 **Diagnostic Studies**

Male and Female Reproductive Systems—cont'd

STUDY	DESCRIPTION AND PURPOSE	NURSING RESPONSIBILITY
Blood Studies—cont'd		
• Fluorescent treponemal antibody absorption (FTA-ABS)	Detects syphilis antibodies. Also detects early syphilis with great accuracy. Usually performed if results of above nonspecific tests are questionable.	Inform patient that blood sample will be drawn. Observe venipuncture site for bleeding or hematoma formation.
Cultures and Smears		
• Dark-field microscopy	Direct examination of specimen obtained from potential syphilitic lesion (chancre) is performed to detect *Treponema pallidum*.	Avoid direct skin contact with open lesion.
• Wet mounts	Direct microscopic examination of specimen of vaginal discharge is performed immediately after collection. Determines presence or absence and number of *Trichomonas* organisms, bacteria, white and red blood cells, and candidal buds or hyphae. Other clues or causes of inflammation or infection may be determined.	Explain procedure and purpose to patient. Instruct patient not to douche before examination. Prepare for collection of specimens (glass slide, 10%-20% potassium hydroxide [KOH] solution, sodium chloride [NaCl] solution, and cotton-tipped applicators).
• Cultures	Specimens of vaginal, urethral, or cervical discharge are cultured and used to assess presence of gonorrhea or chlamydia. Rectal and throat cultures may also be taken, depending on data obtained from sexual history.	Obtain specific contact and sexual history inclusive of oral and rectal intercourse. Instruct against douching before examination. Obtain urethral specimen from men before they void. Instruct women who are sexually active with multiple partners to have at least a yearly culture for gonorrhea and chlamydia. Instruct sexually active men to have any discharge evaluated immediately to rule out gonorrhea strains that do not cause classic symptoms of dysuria.
• Gram stain	Used for rapid detection of gonorrhea. Presence of gram-negative intracellular diplococci generally warrants initiation of treatment. Not highly accurate for women. Has also been shown as accurate alternative for *Chlamydia* testing.	Same as above.
Cytologic Studies		
• Pap smear	Microscopic study of exfoliated cells via special staining and fixation technique detects abnormal cells. Cells most commonly studied are those obtained directly from endocervix, cervix, vaginal pool, and endometrial lining of uterine cavity.	Instruct women who are sexually active and who are over age 18 to have Pap smears according to American Cancer Society guidelines. Arrange for smear at midcycle time. Instruct patients not to douche for at least 24 hr before examination. Collect careful menstrual and gynecologic history.
• Nipple discharge test	Cytologic study of nipple discharge is performed.	Indicate whether hormonal preparations or other drugs are being taken, breastfeeding, or history of amenorrhea. Instruct patient during demonstration of breast self-examination or examination of breasts that nipple discharge should always be evaluated.
Radiologic Studies		
• Mammography	Low-dose x-ray image of breast tissue on radiographic film is used to assess breast tissue.	Instruct patient about advantages of the examination. Instruct regarding American Cancer Society recommendations for screening (see Chapter 50).
• Ultrasound	Measures and records high-frequency sound waves as they pass through tissues of variable density. It is very useful in detecting masses greater than 3 cm, such as ectopic pregnancies, IUDs, ovarian cysts, and hydatidiform moles. In men, is used to detect testicular torsion or masses.	Instruct patient that a full bladder may be required depending on the reason for the study.

IUDs, Intrauterine devices.

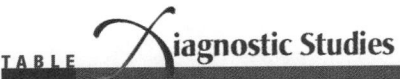

TABLE
49-12   **Male and Female Reproductive Systems—cont'd**

STUDY	DESCRIPTION AND PURPOSE	NURSING RESPONSIBILITY
Radiologic Studies—cont'd		
• Computed tomography (CT) of pelvis	Pelvic CT is used to detect tumor within the pelvis.	Inform patient of procedure. Patient must lie still during the procedure. If intravenous contrast is used, check for iodine allergy.
Invasive Procedures		
• Breast biopsy	Histologic examination of excised breast tissue is performed, either by needle-aspiration or excisional biopsy.	Before surgery, instruct patient about operative procedures and sedation. After surgery, perform wound care and instruct patient about breast self-examination.
• Hysterosalpingogram	Involves instillation of contrast media through cervix into uterine cavity and subsequently through and out fallopian tubes. Spot x-ray images are taken to detect abnormalities of uterus and its adnexa (ovaries and tubes) as contrast progresses through them. Test may be most useful in diagnostic assessment of fertility (e.g., to detect adhesions near ovary, an abnormal uterine shape, blockage of tubal pathways).	Inform patient about procedure and that it may be fairly uncomfortable. Determine possibility of iodine allergy.
• Colposcopy	Direct visualization of cervix with binocular microscope that allows magnification and study of cellular dysplasia and vascular and tissue abnormalities of cervix. This test is used as a follow-up study for abnormal Pap smears and for examination of women exposed to DES in utero. Biopsy of cervix may be taken during colposcopic examination. This test is valuable in decreasing number of false-negative cervical biopsies.	Instruct patient about this outpatient procedure. Inform patient that this examination is similar to speculum examination. Explain purpose of procedure and prepare patient for it.
• Conization	Cone-shaped sample of squamocolumnar tissue of cervix is removed for direct study.	Explain purpose and method of procedure and that it requires use of surgical facilities and anesthesia. Instruct patient to rest for at least 3 days after procedure. Also discuss necessity for 3 wk follow-up check.
• Loop electrosurgical excision of transformation zone (LEETZ)	Excision of cervical tissue via an electrosurgical instrument.	Explain purpose and method of procedure and that it may be done in the physician's office for further diagnostic testing.
• Loop electrosurgical excision procedure (LEEP)	Same as above.	Same as above.
• Culdotomy, culdoscopy, and culdocentesis	Culdotomy is an incision made through posterior fornix of cul-de-sac and allows visualization of peritoneal cavity (i.e., uterus, tubes, and ovaries). Culdoscope can then be used to study these structures closely. This technique is valuable in fertility evaluations. Withdrawal of fluid (culdocentesis) allows examination of fluid characteristics.	Explain purpose and method of procedure. Prepare patient for vaginal operation with preoperative instruction and sedation. Perform assessment of bleeding and discomfort after surgery.
• Laparoscopy (peritoneoscopy)	Allows visualization of pelvic structures via fiberoptic scopes inserted through small abdominal incisions. Instillation of carbon dioxide into cavity improves visualization. This technique is used in diagnostic assessment of uterus, tubes, and ovaries. Can be used in conjunction with tubal sterilization.	Explain purpose and method of procedure. Before surgery, instruct patient about procedure, prepare abdomen, and reassure patient about sedation. Tell patient to rest for 1-3 days after surgery. Inform patient of probability of shoulder pain because of air in the abdomen.
• Dilation and curettage	The operative procedure dilates cervix and allows curetting of endometrial lining. This test is used in assessment of abnormal bleeding patterns and cytologic evaluation of lining.	Before surgery, instruct patient about procedure and sedation. Perform postoperative assessment of degree of bleeding (frequent pad check during first 24 hr).

DES, Diethylstilbestrol.

Continued

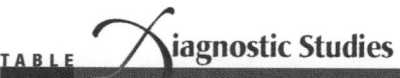

TABLE 49-12	Diagnostic Studies — Male and Female Reproductive Systems—cont'd	
STUDY	**DESCRIPTION AND PURPOSE**	**NURSING RESPONSIBILITY**
Fertility Studies		
▪ Semen analysis	Semen is assessed for volume (2-5 ml), viscosity, sperm count (>20 million/ml), sperm motility (60% motile), and percent of abnormal sperm (60% with normal structure).	Instruct patient to bring in fresh specimen within 2 hr after ejaculation.
▪ Basal body temperature assessment	This measurement indicates indirectly whether ovulation has occurred. (Temperature rises at ovulation and remains elevated during secretory phase of normal menstrual cycle.)	Instruct woman to take her temperature using special basal temperature thermometer (calibrated in tenths of degrees) every morning before getting out of bed. Tell woman to record temperature on graph.
▪ Huhner test or Sims-Huhner	Mucus sample of cervix is examined within 2-8 hr after intercourse. Total number of sperm is assessed in relation to number of live sperm. This test is performed to determine whether cervical mucus is "hostile" to passage of sperm from vagina into uterus.	Instruct couples to have intercourse at estimated time of ovulation and be present for test within 2-8 hr after intercourse.
▪ Endometrial biopsy	Small curette is used to obtain piece of endometrial lining to assess endometrial changes common to progesterone secretion after ovulation.	Tell patient that test must be performed postovulation. Explain that procedure should cause only short period of uterine cramping.
▪ Hysterosalpingogram	Same as operative procedures.	Same as operative procedures.
▪ Serum progesterone	Same as blood studies.	Same as blood studies.

Cultures and Smears

Cultures and smears are most frequently employed in the diagnosis of sexually transmitted disease. Specimens for cultures and smears are most commonly taken from the vagina, endocervix, and rectum for females and the urethra and rectum for males. For a culture, the specimen is placed on a special culture medium; a smear involves rubbing the specimen on a slide for direct examination. Gram stain smears have been shown to be effective in the diagnosis of chlamydia infection.[17] Dark-field microscopy involves the direct examination of a specimen obtained from a syphilitic chancre for the diagnosis of syphilis.

Cytologic Studies

Cytology involves the study of cells under microscopic examination. The Pap smear is a screening test to detect abnormal cells obtained from the cervix or vagina. It is performed by obtaining cells from the cervical canal, preferably the endocervix, as well as from the vagina, and placing these cells in a fixative for examination by a cytologist for cellular abnormalities. Pap smears are more accurate if performed at midcycle or during the secretory phase of the menstrual cycle because there is a greater likelihood that abnormal cells will be detected during these times. A Pap smear should be performed annually or more frequently in women with a history of dysplasia. Pap smears are necessary in women who have had a hysterectomy because abnormal vaginal

cells (if present) can sometimes be detected. Although a Pap smear is highly accurate in detecting cervical cancer, a negative Pap test does not rule out endometrial cancer.

Cytologic study is also indicated for nipple discharge. Cytologic examination discharge can detect the presence of malignant cells as opposed to a discharge associated with infection.

Radiologic Studies

Mammography. Mammography has become one of the most frequently used diagnostic tools in reproductive system assessment. It is used to detect breast masses. Mammography can detect breast masses before they are palpable. Mammography and screening guidelines for mammography are discussed in Chapter 50.

Ultrasound. Ultrasound has many applications for diagnostic study. Pelvic ultrasound is used to obtain images of the pelvic organs. It is used to detect pregnancy in the uterus, ectopic pregnancy, ovarian cysts, and other pelvic masses. Breast ultrasound is useful in the detection of fluid-filled masses. In men, ultrasound is used to detect testicular masses and testicular torsion. Transrectal ultrasound is useful in locating prostate tumors.

Pelvic Computed Tomography (CT) and Magnetic Resonance Imaging (MRI). Pelvic CT or MRI is used to detect primary or metastatic tumors of the reproductive organs. Contrast medium may be used in conjunction with the CT procedure.

REVIEW QUESTIONS

The number of the question corresponds to the same-numbered objective at the beginning of the chapter.

1. A normal reproductive function that may be altered in a patient who undergoes a prostatectomy is
   a. sperm production.
   b. production of testosterone.
   c. production of seminal fluid.
   d. release of sperm from the epididymis.

2. Estrogen production by the mature ovarian follicle causes
   a. decreased secretion of FSH and LH.
   b. increased production of GnRH and FSH.
   c. release of GnRH and increased secretion of LH.
   d. decreased release of FSH and decreased progesterone production.

3. Male orgasm is the result of
   a. clitoral swelling and increased vaginal lubrication.
   b. vaginal enlargement and secretion with penile insertion.
   c. clitoral swelling, vaginal lubrication, and uterine elevation.
   d. rapid release of vasocongestion and muscular tension in the reproductive structures.

4. An age-related finding noted by the nurse during assessment of the older woman's reproductive system is
   a. gynecomastia.
   b. increased vaginal discharge.
   c. decreased amount of pubic hair.
   d. soft, nontender, fleshy vulvar lesions.

5. Significant information about a patient's past medical history related to the reproductive system should include
   a. extent of sexual activity.
   b. general satisfaction with sexuality.
   c. previous sexually transmitted diseases.
   d. self-image and relationships with others.

6. The examination technique used to evaluate the prostate involves
   a. palpation.
   b. percussion.
   c. inspection.
   d. auscultation.

7. An abnormal finding noted during physical assessment of the male reproductive system is
   a. slight clear urethral discharge.
   b. the glans covered with prepuce.
   c. rubbery feeling of the testes on palpation.
   d. urethral meatus on the ventral side of the glans.

8. The screening criteria for assessing prostate cancer include a
   a. baseline ultrasound of the prostate at age 40.
   b. baseline ultrasound of the prostate at age 50.
   c. yearly digital rectal examination for men over age 30.
   d. yearly digital rectal examination for men over age 50.

REFERENCES

1. Thibodeau GA, Patton KT: *The human body in health and disease,* ed 3, St Louis, 2002, Mosby.
2. Di Saia PJ: Clinical anatomy of the female. In Scott JR et al, editors: *Danforth's obstetrics and gynecology,* ed 8, Philadelphia, 1999, Lippincott Williams & Wilkins.
3. McCance KL, Huether SE: *Pathophysiology: the biologic basis for disease in adults and children,* ed 4, St Louis, 2002, Mosby.
4. Arvidson CR: The adolescent gynecologic exam, *Pediatr Nurs* 25:71, 1999.
5. Hammond CB: Climacteric. In Scott JR et al, editors: *Danforth's obstetrics and gynecology,* ed 8, Philadelphia, 1999, Lippincott Williams & Wilkins.
6. Masters WH, Johnson E: *Human sexual response,* Boston, 1966, Little, Brown.
7. Dougherty JD, Knutesen P: The aging female reproductive system. In Stanley M, Beare PG, editors: *Gerontological nursing,* ed 2, Philadelphia, 1999, FA Davis.
8. Stone JT, Wyman JF, Salisburg SA: *Clinical gerontologic nursing: guide to advanced practice,* ed 2, Philadelphia, 1999, WB Saunders.
9. Kessenich CR, Cichon MJ: Hormonal decline in elderly men and male menopause, *Geriatr Nurs* 22:24, 2001.
10. Warner PH, Rowe T, Whipple B: Shedding light on the sexual history, *Am J Nurs* 99:34, 1999.
11. Steinke EE: Sexual counseling after myocardial infarction, *Am J Nurs* 100:38, 2000.
12. American Cancer Society: Prostate cancer reference information. Available at *www.cancer.org* (accessed Feb 20, 2003).
13. Grodner M, Anderson SL, DeYoung S: *Foundations and clinical applications of nutrition: a nursing approach,* ed 2, St Louis, 2000, Mosby.
14. Wilson S, Giddens JF: *Health assessment for nursing practice,* ed 2, St Louis, 2001, Mosby.
15. Corbett JV: *Laboratory tests and diagnostic procedures with nursing diagnosis,* ed 5, Upper Saddle River, NJ, 2000, Prentice Hall.
16. Pagana KD, Pagana TJ: *Mosby's diagnostic and laboratory test reference,* ed 5, St Louis, 2001, Mosby.
17. Mysiuk L, Romanowski B, Brown M: Endocervical Gram stain smears and their usefulness in the diagnosis of *Chlamydia trachomatis, Sexually Transmitted Infections* 77:103, 2001.

RESOURCES

Resources for this chapter are listed in Chapter 52 on p. 1434 and Chapter 53 on p. 1462.

CHAPTER *50*
NURSING MANAGEMENT
Breast Disorders

Shannon Ruff Dirksen

LEARNING OBJECTIVES

1. Assess breast tissue by inspection and palpation using appropriate examination techniques.
2. Teach breast health awareness and breast self-examination, including rationale, technique, and reasons for referral.
3. Describe the types, causes, clinical manifestations, collaborative care, and nursing management of common benign breast disorders.
4. Identify the known risk factors for breast cancer.
5. Describe the pathophysiology, clinical manifestations, and collaborative care of breast cancer.

6. Identify the types of, indications for, and complications of surgical interventions for breast cancer.
7. Explain the physical and psychologic preoperative and postoperative aspects of nursing management for the patient undergoing a mastectomy.
8. Describe the indications for reconstructive breast surgery; types, potential risks, and complications of reconstructive breast surgery; and nursing management after reconstructive breast surgery.

KEY TERMS

ductal ectasia, p. 1365	lymphedema, p. 1370
fibroadenoma, p. 1364	mammoplasty, p. 1378
fibrocystic changes, p. 1364	mastalgia, p. 1363
galactorrhea, p. 1365	mastectomy, p. 1369
gynecomastia, p. 1365	mastitis, p. 1363
intraductal papilloma, p. 1365	Paget's disease, p. 1367
lumpectomy, p. 1370	

Breast disorders are a significant health concern for women. Although most breast pain is of a benign nature, in a woman's lifetime there is a one in eight chance that she will be diagnosed with breast cancer.[1] Whether benign or malignant, intense feelings of shock, fear, and denial often accompany the initial discovery of a lump or change in the breast. These feelings can be associated both with the fear of death and with the possible loss of a breast. Throughout history, the female breast has been regarded as a symbol of beauty, femininity, sexuality, and motherhood. The potential loss of a breast, or part of a breast, may be devastating for many women because of the significant psychologic, social, sexual, and body image implications associated with it. The most frequently encountered breast disorders in women are fibrocystic changes, breast cancer, fibroadenoma, intraductal papilloma, and ductal ectasia. In men, gynecomastia is the most common breast disorder.

ASSESSMENT OF BREAST DISORDERS

It is critical that breast disorders be detected early, diagnosed accurately, and treated promptly.[2] The essential factors in the early detection of breast cancer and other breast-related problems are the regular performance of routine mammography, regular clinical breast examination (CBE), and breast self-examination

(BSE). The frequency of these examinations is determined by the woman's age, the presence of significant risk factors, and her past medical history (Table 50-1). The American Cancer Society's new guidelines for the early detection of breast cancer are:[3,4]

1. Yearly mammograms starting at age 40 and continuing for as long as a woman is in good health.
2. Clinical breast exams (CBE) should be part of a periodic health exam, about every three years for women in their 20s and 30s and every year for women 40 and over.
3. Women should report any breast change promptly to their health care providers.
4. Breast self-exam (BSE) is an option for women starting in their 20s.
5. Women at increased risk (e.g., family history, genetic tendency, past breast cancer) should talk with their doctors about the benefits and limitations of starting mammography screening earlier, having additional tests (e.g., breast ultrasound, MRI), or having more frequent exams.

The NCI is currently reviewing guidelines on mammography screening for healthy women to determine the best schedule for screening.[4] The benefits of early detection of breast cancer are well established. The use of screening mammography has significantly improved early and accurate detection of breast malignancies. Mammography can identify breast abnormalities that may be cancer before physical symptoms appear.

Breast Self-Examination

Providing education and encouraging women to perform BSE are recommended to decrease mortality rates from breast cancer. In recent years there has been some controversy regarding the value of BSE and its role in reducing mortality rates from breast cancer in women.[5] Until the issue is resolved, women should continue doing BSE with regular screening by mammography and CBE.

Although the reasons that women report for failing to practice regular BSE have changed somewhat over the years, many women still do not regularly examine their breasts. Some reasons cited by women for not practicing BSE are embarrassment, fear of finding a lump, lack of confidence in ability to do BSE, inade-

Reviewed by Rebecca Crane-Okada, RN, PhD, AOCN, Clinical Researcher and Oncology Clinical Nurse Specialist, Joyce Eisenberg Keefer Breast Center, John Wayne Cancer Institute, Saint John's Health Center, Santa Monica, Calif.

TABLE 50-1	Risk Factors for Breast Cancer	
INCREASED RISK	**COMMENTS**
Female	Women account for 99% of breast cancer cases.
Age 50 or over	Majority of breast cancers are found in postmenopausal women.
Family history	Breast cancer in a first-degree relative, particularly when premenopausal or bilateral, increases risk. Gene mutations (BRCA-1 or BRCA-2) play a role in 5%-10% of breast cancer cases.
Personal history of breast cancer, colon cancer, endometrial cancer, ovarian cancer	Personal history significantly increases risk of breast cancer, risk of cancer in other breast, and recurrence.
Early menarche (< age 12); late menopause (> age 55)	A long menstrual history increases the risk of breast cancer.
First full-term pregnancy after age 30; nulliparity	Prolonged exposure to unopposed estrogen increases risk for breast cancer.
Benign breast disease with atypical epithelial hyperplasia	Atypical changes in breast biopsy increase the risk of breast cancer.
Obesity after menopause	Fat cells store estrogen.
Exposure to ionizing radiation	Radiation damages DNA (e.g., prior treatment for Hodgkin's disease).

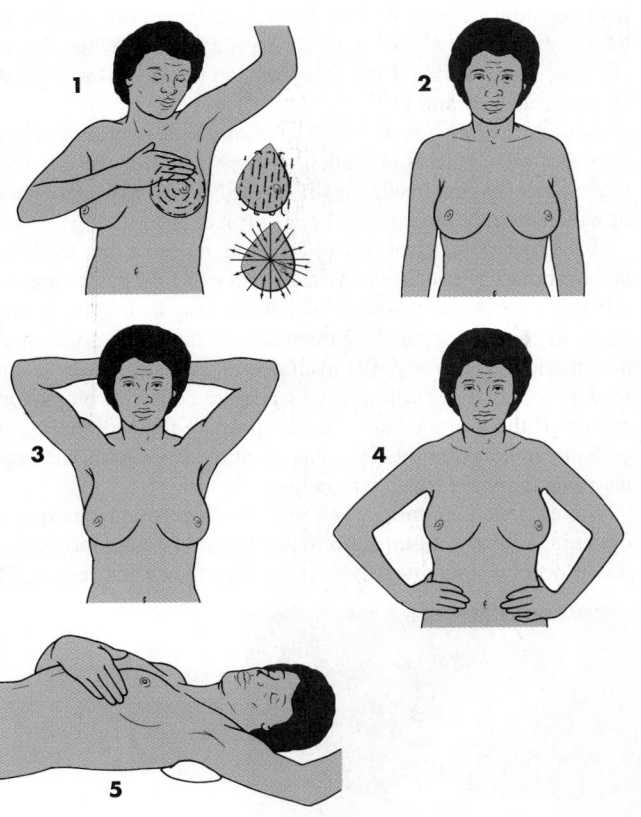

FIG. 50-1 Breast self-examination and patient instruction. *1,* While in the shower or bath, when the skin is slippery with soap and water, examine your breasts. Use the pads of your second, third, and fourth fingers to firmly press every part of the breast. While examining your left breast, use your right hand, and use your left hand to examine your right breast. Using the pads of the fingers on your left hand, examine the entire breast using small circular motions in a spiral or in an up-and-down motion so that the entire breast area is examined. Repeat the procedure using your right hand to examine your left breast. Repeat pattern of palpation under the arm. Check for any lump, hard knot, or thickening of the tissue. *2,* Look at your breasts in a mirror. Stand with your arms at your side. *3,* Raise your arms overhead and check for any changes in the shape of your breasts, dimpling of the skin, or any changes in the nipple. *4,* Next, place your hands on your hips and press down firmly, tightening the pectoral muscles. Observe for asymmetry or changes, keeping in mind that your breasts probably do not exactly match. *5,* While lying down, feel your breasts as described in step 1. When examining your right breast, place a folded towel under your right shoulder and put your right hand behind your head. Repeat the procedure while examining your left breast. Mark your calendar that you have completed your BSE; note any changes or unique characteristics you want to check with your health care provider.

quate knowledge of the procedure, and not remembering to do BSE. Factors that increase BSE compliance include positive beliefs about screening, lower perceived risk, history of breast biopsies, family history of breast cancer, and BSE demonstration.[6]

The nurse who is teaching BSE should emphasize that early detection and treatment enhance survival rates. Efforts must be directed toward teaching women the importance of BSE, how to perform it, and what to do if a problem is detected. BSE teaching techniques should include allowing time for the woman to ask questions about the procedure and to perform a return demonstration. The technique for BSE has been established by the ACS (available on the Internet at *www.cancer.org*) and the NCI

(Fig. 50-1). BSE should be done monthly at a regular time when the breasts are not tender. In premenopausal women, the best time is 7 days after the start of menstruation. At this time, hormonal stimulation of the breasts is at its lowest point. In most women, nodularity and tenderness will be minimal. For women taking oral contraceptives (about 20% to 25% of women ages 15 to 45) the first day of a new package may be a helpful reminder. Postmenopausal women and women who have had hysterectomies should set a regular date for monthly BSE. Many women use the monthly date of a birthday or the first day of the month.

BSE should be done in good light and should include inspection before a mirror and careful, systematic palpation. The entire breast, axilla, and clavicle should be examined. The woman should be taught the BSE procedure by a health care provider using the woman's own hand on her breast. A gentle circular motion over wet, soapy skin is particularly useful if she is in the shower. The woman should be told what to look for, such as a lump, nipple discharge, nipple retraction, redness, pain or tenderness, dimpling of the skin, or edema. Some teaching techniques involve using silicone breast models that simulate normal and abnormal breast tissue to help women learn to identify problems. The woman should be shown the normal variations in her own breasts so that she will be able to detect changes. Finally, she should be reminded that most breast problems are not related to malignancy. At every annual physical examination the health care provider should ask the woman to demonstrate how she performs BSE.

If a problem is suspected such as nipple discharge or finding a lump, the woman should see her primary care provider or contact a comprehensive breast center as soon as possible so that additional diagnostic studies can be promptly initiated. If the problem is not serious, the woman's anxiety can be quickly relieved. If a serious problem is suspected or diagnosed, definitive treatment should not be delayed.

Even when a woman faithfully practices BSE, she should have an annual breast examination by a qualified health care provider and a mammogram if age appropriate. The care and attention to detail shown by the clinician in performing CBE reinforce the practice of BSE by the patient.

Diagnostic Studies

Several techniques can be used to screen for breast disease or provide a diagnosis of a suspicious physical finding. *Mammography* is a method used to visualize the internal structure of the breast using low-dose x-rays (Fig. 50-2). This simple, safe procedure can detect tumors and cysts that cannot be felt by palpation. Improved imaging techniques have reduced the radiation that accompanies mammography to insignificant levels.

Digital mammography has been recently approved by the Food and Drug Administration. In this procedure x-ray images are digitally coded into a computer. This allows for a clearer and more accurate image than conventional mammography x-ray film.

The minimum size of a tumor detectable by physical examination is 1 cm. It may take 10 years or longer for a tumor to grow to this size. Mammography can detect masses of 0.5 cm.

Calcifications are the most easily recognized mammogram abnormality. These deposits of calcium crystals form in the breast for many reasons, such as inflammation, trauma, and aging. Although most calcifications are benign, they also may be associated with preinvasive cancer.[7]

A comparison of current and prior mammograms may show early cancer tissue changes. Because some tumors metastasize late in the preclinical course, early detection by mammography allows for early treatment and the prevention of metastasis of these smaller lesions. In younger women mammography is less sensitive because of the greater density of breast tissue, resulting in more false-negative results.[8] From 10% to 15% of breast cancers cannot be seen on mammography and are detected only by palpation. Suspicious masses should be biopsied even if mammogram findings are unremarkable.

Ultrasound is another diagnostic procedure that can be used to differentiate a benign tumor from a malignant tumor. It is particularly useful in women with fibrocystic changes whose breasts are very dense. Unlike a mammogram, an ultrasound will not detect microcalcifications.

A definitive diagnosis of a suspicious area is often made by means of histologic examination of biopsied tissue. Biopsy techniques include fine-needle aspiration (FNA) biopsy, stereotactic or handheld core biopsy, and open surgical biopsy.

FNA biopsy is performed by inserting a needle into the lesion and aspirating tissue into a syringe. Three or four passes are usually made. FNA and cytologic evaluation may be helpful in making a diagnosis and planning treatment. It should be done only if an experienced cytologist is available and all suspicious lesions read as negative are followed with a more definitive biopsy procedure. If the aspirated specimen is positive for malignancy, the patient can be given this information at the same visit and begin learning about the treatment options.

Stereotactic core biopsy is a reliable diagnostic technique for obtaining a biopsy of an abnormality seen on a mammogram. In this procedure mammography is used to locate the lesion. The

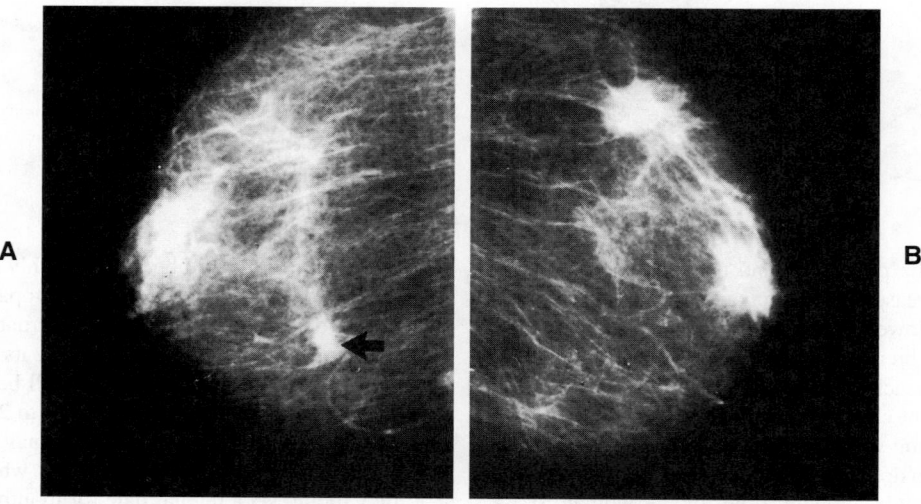

FIG. 50-2 Mammogram showing bilateral invasive ductal carcinoma. **A,** Left breast. The larger left mass was palpable. The smaller right mass was not palpable *(arrow).* **B,** Right breast. Multiple masses are shown.

skin is anesthetized, and a small skin incision is made to allow the entrance of a biopsy gun device. The gun is fired and removes a core sample of the lesion. This is repeated several times, and the core samples are sent for pathologic analysis. This technique has several advantages over an open surgical biopsy, including minimal scarring, the use of local anesthesia, outpatient procedure, reduced cost, and shorter recovery time.[9]

Benign Breast Disorders

MASTALGIA

Mastalgia (breast pain) is the most common breast-related complaint in women. It affects up to 70% of all women.[10] The most common form is *cyclic mastalgia,* which coincides with the menstrual cycle. It is described as diffuse breast tenderness or heaviness. Breast pain may last 2 to 3 days or most of the month. The pain is related to hormonal sensitivity. The symptoms often decrease with menopause. *Noncyclic mastalgia* has no relationship to the menstrual cycle and can continue into menopause.[11] It may be constant or intermittent throughout the month and last for several years. Symptoms include a burning, aching, or soreness in the breast. The etiology of the pain may be due to trauma, fat necrosis, or duct ectasia.

Mammography is frequently done to exclude cancer and provide information on the etiology of mastalgia. Some relief may occur with caffeine and dietary fat reduction; taking vitamins E, A, and B complex and gamma-linolenic acid (evening primrose oil); and the continual wearing of a support bra. Hormonal therapy may be recommended, including oral contraceptives and danazol (Danocrine).

BREAST INFECTIONS

Mastitis

Mastitis is an inflammatory condition of the breast that occurs most frequently in lactating women (Table 50-2). *Lactational mastitis* manifests as a localized area that is erythematous, painful, and tender to palpation. Fever is usually present. The infection develops when organisms, usually staphylococci, gain access to the breast through a cracked nipple. In its early stages, mastitis can be cured with antibiotics. Breastfeeding should continue unless an abscess is forming or a purulent drainage is noted. The mother may wish to use a nipple shield or to hand-express milk from the involved breast until the pain subsides. The woman should see her health care provider promptly to begin a course of antibiotic therapy. Any breast that remains red, tender, and not responsive to antibiotics requires follow-up care and evaluation for inflammatory breast cancer.

Lactational Breast Abscess

If lactational mastitis persists after several days of antibiotic therapy, a lactational breast abscess may have developed. In this condition the skin may become red and edematous over the involved breast, often with a corresponding palpable mass, and the patient may have an elevated temperature. Antibiotics alone constitute insufficient treatment for a breast abscess. Surgical incision and drainage are necessary. The drainage is cultured, sensi-

TABLE 50-2   Differential Diagnosis of Selected Benign Breast Disorders

DISORDER	RISK FACTORS	CLINICAL MANIFESTATIONS
Lactation mastitis	Lactating woman Occurs spontaneously in approximately 2% of all postpartum lactating mothers (both primipara and multipara), usually 2-4 wk after birth	Warm to touch Indurated Usually unilateral Most common etiology is *Staphylococcus aureus*
Nonlactation mastitis	Rare condition Usually women in late adolescence or middle age	Palpable mass Usually an obscure organism Should rule out syphilis or tuberculosis
Fibrocystic breast changes	Most common between ages 35 and 50	Not usually discrete masses, nodularity instead; usually accompanied by cyclic pain and tenderness; mass(es) usually cyclic in occurrence (movable, soft)
Cysts	Most common between ages 30 and 50	Palpable mass (movable, soft); may have multiple microcysts
Fibroadenoma	Peak age range between ages 15 and 25 Most occur before age 30 Most common among African American women	Often bilateral Palpable mass (movable, firm) Most common size at diagnosis is 2-3 cm Rapid growth Accounts for 2%-3% of all breast masses
Fat necrosis	50% report previous history of trauma to breast	Usually a hard, tender, mobile, indurated mass with irregular borders
Intraductal papilloma	Affects women ages 40-60	Usually associated with serous, serosanguineous, or bloody nipple discharge on affected side
Ductal ectasia	Perimenopausal woman—most common in women in their fifties Previous lactation Inverted nipples	Fixation of nipple Usually accompanied by nipple discharge of thick gray material Often associated with breast pain

tivities are obtained, and therapy with an appropriate antibiotic is begun. Often the woman will find it necessary to express and discard milk from the affected breast until the abscess is resolved.

FIBROCYSTIC CHANGES

Fibrocystic changes in the breast constitute a benign condition characterized by changes in breast tissue (see Table 50-2). The changes include the development of excess fibrous tissue, hyperplasia of the epithelial lining of the mammary ducts, proliferation of mammary ducts, and cyst formation. These changes produce pain by nerve irritation from edema in connective tissue and by fibrosis from nerve pinching. The use of the term *fibrocystic disease* is incorrect because the cluster of problems is actually an exaggerated response to hormonal influence. It has been suggested that the term *fibrocystic condition* or *fibrocystic complex* be used. Fibrocystic changes do not increase the risk of breast cancer for the majority of patients. Masses or nodularities can appear in both breasts and are often found in the upper, outer quadrants and usually occur bilaterally. It is the most frequently occurring breast disorder.

Fibrocystic changes occur most frequently in women between 35 and 50 years of age but often begin in women as young as 20 years of age. Pain and nodularity often increase over time but tend to subside after menopause unless high doses of estrogen replacement are used. The cause of these fibrocystic changes is thought to be heightened responsiveness of breast parenchyma and stroma to circulating estrogen and progesterone. Fibrocystic changes most commonly occur in women with premenstrual abnormalities, nulliparous women, women with a history of spontaneous abortion, nonusers of oral contraceptives, and women with early menarche and late menopause. Symptoms related to fibrocystic changes often worsen in the premenstrual phase and subside after menstruation.

Manifestations of fibrocystic breast changes include one or more palpable lumps that are usually round, well delineated, and freely movable within the breast. Some lumps are fibrous and do not contain cysts. There may be accompanying discomfort ranging from tenderness to pain. The lump is usually observed to increase in size and perhaps in tenderness before menstruation. Cysts may enlarge or shrink rapidly. Nipple discharge associated with fibrocystic breasts is often milky, watery-milky, yellow, or green.

Mammography may be helpful in distinguishing fibrocystic changes from breast cancer. However, in some women the breast tissue is so dense that it is difficult to obtain a worthwhile mammogram study. In these situations, ultrasound may be more useful in differentiating a cystic mass from a solid mass.

NURSING *and* COLLABORATIVE MANAGEMENT
FIBROCYSTIC CHANGES

With the initial discovery of a discrete mass in the breast by a woman or her health care provider, aspiration or surgical biopsy may be indicated. A wait of 7 to 10 days may be planned if the nodularity is recurrent to note changes as the menstrual cycle changes. With large or frequent cysts, surgical removal may be favored over repeated aspiration. An excisional biopsy should be done if no fluid is found on aspiration, if the fluid that is found is hemorrhagic, or if a residual mass remains. This surgery is performed in an office or day surgery unit with the patient under local anesthesia.

Biopsies in women with fibrocystic disease may be indicated for women with an increased risk for breast cancer (see Table 50-1).

Hyperplastic changes approximating the histologic appearance of carcinoma in situ (atypical hyperplasia) and a family history of breast cancer increase the probability of developing breast cancer.

The woman with cystic changes should be encouraged to return regularly for follow-up examinations throughout her life. She should also be taught BSE to self-monitor the problem. Severe fibrocystic changes may make palpation of the breast more difficult. Any new lumps or changes in the breasts should be evaluated, and changes in symptoms should be reported and investigated.

Many types of treatment have been suggested for a fibrocystic condition. These include the use of a good support bra, dietary therapy (low-salt diet, restriction of methylxanthines such as coffee and chocolate), vitamin E therapy, analgesics, danazol (Danocrine), diuretics, hormone therapy, and antiestrogen therapy.[12] Because stress can be a contributing factor in breast discomfort, efforts should also be directed toward the reduction of stress. Although many of these treatments have not been scientifically proven to be beneficial, many women report less discomfort with these nonsurgical measures. Danazol has been used for patients with severe pain. It decreases follicle-stimulating hormone (FSH) and luteinizing hormone (LH), resulting in reduced estrogen production and subsequent decreased pain and nodularity. The androgenic side effects of danazol (acne, edema, hirsutism) often make this therapy intolerable for many women.

The role of the nurse in the care of the patient with fibrocystic breast changes is primarily one of teaching. A woman with fibrocystic breasts should be told that she may expect recurrence of the cysts in one or both breasts until menopause and that cysts may enlarge or become painful just before menstruation. Additionally, she should be reassured that cysts do not "turn into" cancer. Any new lump that does not respond in a cyclic manner over 1 to 2 weeks should be examined by a health care provider promptly. The woman should be carefully instructed in BSE, using her own breasts. The use of silicone breast models can also aid instruction.

FIBROADENOMA

Fibroadenoma is a common cause of discrete benign breast lumps in young women. It generally occurs in women between 15 and 25 years of age and is the most frequent cause of breast masses in women under 25 years of age. Fibroadenomas tend to develop more frequently and at a younger age in African American women.[13] The possible cause of fibroadenoma may be increased estrogen sensitivity in a localized area of the breast. Fibroadenomas are usually small (but can be large, 2 to 3 cm), painless, round, well delineated, and very mobile. They may be soft but are usually solid, firm, and rubbery in consistency. There is no accompanying retraction or nipple discharge. The lump is often painless. The fibroadenoma may appear as a single unilateral mass, although multiple bilateral fibroadenomas have been reported. Growth is slow and often ceases when size reaches 2 to 3 cm. Size is not affected by menstruation. However, pregnancy can stimulate dramatic growth. Fibroadenomas are rarely associated with cancer.

NURSING *and* COLLABORATIVE MANAGEMENT
FIBROADENOMA

Fibroadenomas are easily detected by physical examination and are often visible on mammography. Definitive diagnosis, however, requires biopsy and tissue examination by a pathologist. Treatment of fibroadenomas can include surgical excision, which is not urgent in women under 25 years of age. In women over 35 years of age all new lesions should be examined using an excisional biopsy. Fibroadenomas are not reduced by radiation and are not affected by hormone therapy.

As an alternative to surgery, tumor removal can be accomplished using *cryoablation.* In this procedure a cryoprobe is inserted into the tumor using ultrasound guidance. Extremely cold gas is piped into the tumor. The frozen tumor dies and gradually shrinks.

The nurse frequently has the opportunity to counsel a young woman with fibroadenomas. During this contact the benign nature of the lesion should be stressed and follow-up examinations and BSE should be encouraged.

NIPPLE DISCHARGE

Nipple discharge may occur spontaneously or as a result of nipple manipulation. A milky secretion is due to inappropriate lactation (termed **galactorrhea**) as a result of such problems as drug therapy, endocrine problems, and neurologic disorders. Nipple discharge may also be idiopathic.

Secretions can also be serous, grossly bloody, or brown to green. These may be caused by either benign or malignant disease. A slide can be made of the secretion to detect specific disease. Diseases associated with nipple discharge include malignancies, cystic disease, intraductal papilloma, and ductal ectasia. Treatment depends on identification of the cause. In most cases, nipple discharge is not related to malignancy. If galactorrhea is accompanied by amenorrhea, various gynecologic endocrinopathies should be explored.

Intraductal Papilloma

An **intraductal papilloma** is a benign, wartlike growth found in the mammary ducts, usually near the nipple. Typically, there is an associated bloody nipple discharge, a mass, or both. Intraductal papillomas usually affect women 40 to 60 years of age. A single duct or several ducts may be involved. Treatment includes excision of the papilloma and the involved duct or duct system.

Ductal Ectasia

Ductal ectasia is a benign breast disease of perimenopausal and postmenopausal women involving the ducts in the subareolar area. It usually involves several bilateral ducts. Nipple discharge is the primary symptom. This discharge is multicolored and sticky. Ductal ectasia is initially painless but may progress to burning, itching, and pain around the nipple, as well as swelling in the areolar area. Inflammatory signs are often present, the nipple may retract, and the discharge may become bloody in more advanced disease. Ductal ectasia is not associated with malignancy. If an abscess develops, warm compresses and antibiotics are usually effective treatments. Therapy consists of close follow-up examinations or surgical excision of the involved ducts.

GYNECOMASTIA IN MEN

Gynecomastia, a transient, noninflammatory enlargement of one or both breasts, is the most common breast problem in men (Fig. 50-3). The condition is usually temporary and benign. Gynecomastia in itself is not an established risk factor for breast cancer. The most common cause of gynecomastia is a disturbance of the normal ratio of active androgen to estrogen in plasma or within the breast itself.

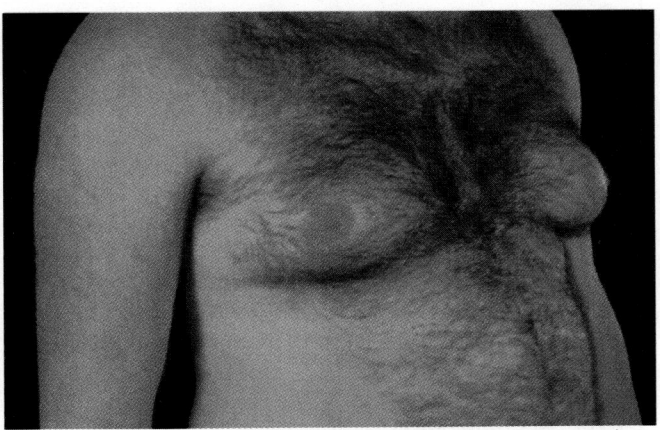

FIG. 50-3 Gynecomastia.

Gynecomastia may also be a symptom of other problems. It is seen accompanying developmental abnormalities of the male reproductive organs. It may also accompany organic diseases, including testicular tumors, cancer of the adrenal cortex, pituitary adenomas, hyperthyroidism, and liver disease.[14] Gynecomastia may occur as a side effect of drug therapy, particularly with administration of estrogens and androgens, digitalis, isoniazid (INH), ranitidine (Zantac), and spironolactone (Aldactone). Use of heroin and marijuana can also cause gynecomastia.

Pubertal Gynecomastia

Pubertal gynecomastia caused by increased estrogen production is seen most often in boys between ages 13 and 17. It is usually limited, although occasionally the localized hyperplasia may measure 2 to 3 cm in size. Pubertal gynecomastia is almost always self-limiting, and disappears within 4 to 6 months of onset. Parents and the affected boy should be reassured that in almost all cases this is a normal physiologic phenomenon that will disappear spontaneously and will require no treatment. Rarely, unilateral gynecomastia in the young male may be marked and fail to regress. This is the only indication for surgical intervention.

Senescent Gynecomastia

Senescent gynecomastia occurs in 40% of older men. A probable cause is the elevation in plasma estrogen in older adult men as the result of increased conversion of androgens to estrogens in peripheral circulation. Although initially unilateral, the tender, firm, centrally located enlargement may become bilateral. When gynecomastia is characterized by a discrete, circumscribed mass, it must be diagnosed to differentiate it from the rarer breast cancer in males. Senescent hyperplasia requires no treatment and generally regresses within 6 to 12 months.

■ Gerontologic Considerations: Age-Related Breast Changes

Loss of subcutaneous fat and structural support and atrophy of mammary glands often result in pendulous breasts in the postmenopausal woman. The nurse should encourage older women to wear a well-fitting bra. Adequate support can improve physical appearance and reduce pain in the back, shoulders, and neck. It can also prevent *intertrigo* (dermatitis caused by friction between opposing surfaces of skin). Surgical lifting of sagging breasts is possible and may be desirable when reconstruction after a mastectomy is performed.

The decrease in glandular tissue in older women makes a breast mass easier to palpate. This decreased density is probably age related and occurs even with women on hormone replacement therapy. Rib margins may be palpable in the older adult woman and can be confused with a mass. As a woman becomes more familiar with her own breasts and is reassured about her findings, the anxiety about this finding should decrease. The nurse should encourage the older woman to continue BSE and to have annual mammograms and clinical examinations because the incidence of breast cancer increases with age. ■

BREAST CANCER

Breast cancer is the most common malignancy in American women except for skin cancer. It is second only to lung cancer as the leading cause of death from cancer in women. An estimated 203,500 new cases of breast cancer were diagnosed in women in the United States in 2002. About 1500 new cases were diagnosed in men.[1] Each year in the United States, approximately 40,000 deaths (39,600 women and 400 men) occur related to breast cancer. The number of deaths of women from breast cancer appears to be leveling off. The largest decreases have been noted in younger women, both African American and white.

Research indicates that 96% of patients diagnosed with localized breast cancer with little or no axillary node involvement will be alive in 5 years. Conversely, only 21% of patients diagnosed with advanced-stage breast cancer with metastases to distant sites will survive 5 years.[2]

Etiology and Risk Factors

Although the etiology is not completely understood, a number of factors are thought to relate to the cause of breast cancer. Heredity or genetically related susceptibility is considered to play a role. Hormonal regulation of the breast is related to the development of breast cancer, but the mechanisms are poorly understood. Sex hormones may act as tumor promoters

CULTURAL & ETHNIC CONSIDERATIONS
Breast Cancer

- African American women have lower survival rates from breast cancer than white women, even when diagnosed at an early stage.
- African American women are diagnosed at a later stage of breast cancer than white women, but this fact alone does not account for the higher mortality rate.
- White women have a higher incidence of breast cancer than nonwhites.
- Breast cancer is the most commonly diagnosed cancer among Hispanic women.
- Hispanic women, especially Mexican Americans, have the lowest rate of cancer screening of any ethnic group.
- Hispanic women tend to have larger, more advanced tumors, which may relate to their higher mortality rate compared with white women.
- Hispanic women are more likely to be diagnosed at a later stage of breast cancer than white women.

if initiating agents have induced malignant changes. Additional factors under study include physical inactivity, dietary fat intake, obesity, and alcohol intake.[2] Environmental factors such as chemical, pesticide, and radiation exposure may also play a role.

Some factors that place a woman at higher risk for breast cancer have been identified (see Table 50-1). Women are at far greater risk than men because 99% of breast cancers occur in women. Increasing age also increases the risk of developing breast cancer. The incidence of breast cancer in women under 25 years of age is very low and increases gradually until age 60. After age 60 the incidence increases dramatically. Positive family history is an important risk factor, especially if the involved member with breast cancer was premenopausal, had bilateral disease, and is a first-degree relative (i.e., mother, sister, daughter). Having any first-degree relative with breast cancer increases a woman's risk of breast cancer 1.5 to 3 times, depending on age. Controversy exists as to whether hormone replacement therapy (HRT), primarily estrogen, in postmenopausal women increases breast cancer risk. Some studies suggest that risk increases only with prolonged HRT use.[15] Limited long-term data suggest that adding progesterone to the estrogen may cause an even higher risk than estrogen therapy alone.[16] The Nurses' Health Study has linked long-term oral contraceptive use to an increased risk of breast cancer.[17]

Risk factors appear to be cumulative and interacting. Therefore the presence of other risk factors may greatly increase the overall risk, especially for those with a positive family history. Identification of risk factors indicates an increased need for careful clinical surveillance of the patient and participation in cancer screening measures. Most women who develop breast cancer have none of the identifiable risk factors.

As many as 5% to 10% of all breast cancer patients may have inherited a specific genetic abnormality contributing to the development of their breast cancer. The first genetic alteration to be identified was in the tumor suppressor gene, p53. The BRCA-1 gene, located on chromosome 17, is a tumor suppressor gene that inhibits tumor development when functioning normally. Women who have BRCA-1 mutations have a 50% to 85% lifetime chance of developing breast cancer.[18] The BRCA-2 gene, located on chromosome 11, is another tumor suppressor gene, and women with a mutation of this gene have a similar risk of breast cancer. Mutations in BRCA genes may cause as many as 10% to 40% of all inherited breast cancers. As many as 1 in 200 to 400 women in the United States may be carriers. These women are also at high risk for developing ovarian cancer.[19] Routine screening for genetic abnormalities in women without evidence of a strong family history of breast cancer is not warranted. Genetic screening is expensive, time consuming, and often not covered by health care insurance.

In women with BRCA-1 or BRCA-2 mutations, prophylactic bilateral oophorectomy can decrease the risk of breast cancer and ovarian cancer.[20,21] In deciding whether to undergo this surgical procedure, women should take into account how long they wish to maintain fertility. In addition, they should receive counseling about the risks and benefits of prophylactic oophorectomy.

A woman who has a high risk of developing breast cancer, related to factors such as family history and prior tissue biopsies, may choose (in consultation with her physician) to undergo pro-

GENETICS in CLINICAL PRACTICE
Breast Cancer

Genetic Basis
- Mutations in genes BRCA-1 and BRCA-2
- Autosomal dominant transmission

Incidence
- Approximately 5% to 10% of breast cancers are related to BRCA-1 and BRCA-2 gene mutations.
- Women with BRCA-1 and BRCA-2 gene mutations have a 50% to 85% lifetime risk of developing breast cancer.
- BRCA-1 and BRCA-2 gene mutations are associated with early-onset breast cancer.
- Family history of both breast and ovarian cancer increases the risk of having a BRCA mutation.

Genetic Testing
- DNA testing is available for BRCA-1 and BRCA-2.

Clinical Implications
- Bilateral oophorectomy reduces the risk of breast cancer in women with BRCA-1 and BRCA-2 mutations.
- Genetic counseling and testing for BRCA mutations should be considered for women whose personal or family history puts them at high risk for a genetic predisposition to breast cancer.

phylactic bilateral mastectomy. This surgery may reduce a women's breast cancer risk by 90%.[22]

Predisposing risk factors in men include states of hyperestrogenism, a family history of breast cancer, and radiation exposure. A thorough examination of the male breast should be a routine part of a physical examination.

Pathophysiology

Various types of breast cancer have been identified based on their histologic characteristics and growth patterns (Table 50-3). The main components of the breast are lobules (milk-producing glands) and ducts (milk passages that connect the lobules and the nipple). In general breast cancer arises from the epithelial lining of the ducts (ductal carcinoma) or from the epithelium of the lobules (lobular carcinoma). Breast cancers may be invasive or in situ. Most breast cancers arise from the ducts and are invasive.

TABLE 50-3	Types of Breast Cancer	
TYPE	**FREQUENCY OF OCCURRENCE**
Infiltrating ductal carcinoma	70%–80%
• Colloid (mucinous)	
• Inflammatory	
• Paget's disease	
• Medullary	
• Papillary	
• Tubular	
Infiltrating lobular carcinoma	10%–15%
Noninvasive	4%–6%
• Ductal carcinoma in situ	

The natural history of breast cancer varies considerably from patient to patient. Cancer growth rate can range from slow to rapid. Factors that affect cancer prognosis are size, axillary node involvement (the more nodes involved, the worse the prognosis), tumor differentiation, DNA content (characteristics of malignant cells), and estrogen and progesterone receptor status. The histologic type of breast cancer seems to have little prognostic significance once the cancer has metastasized.

Noninvasive Breast Cancer. The increased use of screening mammography has led to more women being diagnosed with noninvasive breast cancer. These intraductal cancers include *ductal carcinoma in situ* (DCIS) and *lobular carcinoma in situ* (LCIS). DCIS tends to be unilateral and most likely would progress to invasive breast cancer (usually infiltrating ductal cell carcinoma) if left untreated. LCIS appears to be more of a premalignant breast cancer, and women with this condition have a higher risk of later developing an invasive breast cancer in the same or opposite breast.

Although the management of these two disorders can be controversial, patients with DCIS and LCIS should discuss all treatment options with their physician, including local excision, mastectomy with breast reconstruction, breast-conserving treatment (lumpectomy), radiation therapy, and/or tamoxifen (Nolvadex).

Paget's Disease. **Paget's disease** is a breast malignancy characterized by a persistent lesion of the nipple and areola with or without a palpable mass. Itching, burning, bloody nipple discharge with superficial erosion, and ulceration may be present. Diagnosis of Paget's disease is confirmed by pathologic examination of the erosion. Nipple changes are often diagnosed as an infection or dermatitis, which can lead to treatment delays. (This is different from Paget's disease of the bone, which is discussed in Chapter 62.) The treatment of Paget's disease is a simple or modified radical mastectomy. Prognosis is good when the cancer remains in the nipple only. The nursing care for the patient with Paget's disease is the same as the care for a patient with breast cancer.

Inflammatory Breast Cancer. Inflammatory breast cancer, the most malignant form of all breast cancers, is rare. It is an aggressive and fast-growing cancer. The skin of the breast looks red, feels warm, and has a thickened appearance that is often described as resembling an orange peel (peau d'orange). Sometimes the breast develops ridges and small bumps that look like hives. The inflammatory changes, often mistaken for an infection, are caused by cancer cells blocking lymph channels. Metastases occur early and widely. Radiation, chemotherapy, and hormone therapy are more likely to be used for treatment than surgery.

Clinical Manifestations

Breast cancer is detected as a single lump or mammographic abnormality in the breast. It occurs most often in the upper, outer quadrant of the breast because it is the location of most of the glandular tissue (Fig. 50-4). The rate at which the lesion grows varies considerably. Slow-growing lesions are often associated with a lower mortality rate. If palpable, breast cancer is characteristically hard, irregularly shaped, poorly delineated, nonmobile, and nontender.

A small percentage of breast cancers cause nipple discharge. The discharge is usually unilateral and may be clear or bloody.

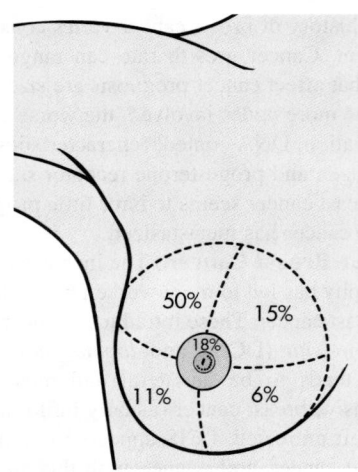

FIG. 50-4 Distribution of where breast cancer occurs.

liver). However, metastatic disease can be found in any distant site.

Widely disseminated or metastatic disease involves the growth of colonies of cancerous breast cells in parts of the body distant from the breast. Metastases primarily occur through the lymphatic chains, principally those of the axilla (see Chapter 49, Fig. 49-7). However, the cancer can spread to other parts of the body without invading the axillary nodes even when the primary breast tumor is small. Even in node-negative breast cancer, there is a possibility of distant metastasis.

Diagnostic Studies

In addition to studies used to diagnose breast cancer (see earlier in chapter), other tests are useful in predicting the risk of recurrence or metastatic breast disease. These tests include axillary lymph node status, tumor size, estrogen and progesterone receptor status, DNA content analysis (ploidy status), and cell proliferative indices. Many of these diagnostic studies are useful prognostic indicators of the disease.

Axillary lymph node involvement is one of the most important prognostic factors in early-stage breast cancer.[23] The presence of metastasis in axillary nodes can be determined by pathologic examination of as few as 6 to 10 nodes. The more nodes involved, the greater the risk of recurrence. Patients with four or more positive nodes have the greatest risk of recurrence.

Studies are examining improved methods to assess tumor growth in the regional lymph nodes. This information is important when considering possible adjuvant systemic therapy. A newer surgical technique called *lymphatic mapping* and *sentinel lymph node dissection* (SLND) helps the surgeon identify the lymph

Nipple retraction may occur. Peau d'orange may occur due to the plugging of the dermal lymphatics. In large cancers, infiltration, induration, and dimpling (pulling in) of the overlying skin may also be noted.

Complications

The main complication of breast cancer is recurrence (Table 50-4). Recurrence may be local or regional (skin or soft tissue near the mastectomy site, axillary or internal mammary lymph nodes) or distant (most commonly involving the bone, lung, brain, and

TABLE 50-4	Common Sites of Breast Cancer Recurrence and Metastasis
SITE	**CLINICAL PRESENTATION**
Local Recurrence	
Skin	Firm, discrete nodules; occasionally pruritic, usually painless
Regional Recurrence	
Lymph nodes	Enlarged nodes in axilla or supraclavicular area, usually nontender, superior vena caval obstruction from enlarged supraclavicular nodes (oncologic emergency), pain in shoulder and arm of affected side
Distant Metastases	
Skeletal metastasis	Localized pain of gradually increasing intensity, percussion tenderness at involved sites, pathologic fracture caused by involvement of bone cortex, hypercalcemia from skeletal metastasis or endocrine therapy
Spinal cord metastasis	Progressive back pain, localized and radicular; muscular weakness, usually in lower extremities; paresthesias in one or more extremities; bowel or bladder sphincter dysfunction; paralysis from epidural spinal cord compression
Brain metastasis	Headache, unilateral sensory loss, focal muscular weakness, hemiparesis, incoordination (ataxia), visual defects, speech disorder (dysphasia), impaired cognition, behavioral or mental changes, loss of sphincter control, papilledema, persistent nausea and vomiting, seizure activity, progressive decrease in level of consciousness
Pulmonary metastasis (including lung nodules and pleural effusions)	Dependent on sites and extent of pulmonary metastases; chest pain, dyspnea on exertion, shortness of breath, tachypnea, nonproductive cough (not present in all patients); adventitious breath sounds, dullness to percussion, restricted chest-wall expansion on affected side with pleural effusion
Liver metastasis	Abdominal distention; right lower quadrant abdominal pain sometimes with radiation to scapular area; nausea and vomiting, anorexia, weight loss; weakness and fatigue; hepatomegaly, ascites, jaundice; peripheral edema; elevated liver enzymes
Bone marrow metastasis	Anemia; infection; increased bleeding, bruising, petechiae; weakness and fatigue; mild confusion, light-headedness; dyspnea

node dissection (SLND) helps the surgeon identify the lymph node(s) that drain first from the tumor site (sentinel node).[24] A radioisotope and/or blue dye is injected into the tumor site, and intraoperatively, it is determined in which node(s) the radioisotope and/or blue dye is located. A local incision is made, and the surgeon dissects the blue-stained sentinel node and/or the radioactive lymph node. The node is then subsequently analyzed by pathologic studies. Assessment of this node can be used to determine if tumor spread has occurred related to the entire axillary area. SLND has been associated with lower morbidity rates and greater accuracy as compared with complete axillary node dissection.[24] National clinical research trials are evaluating whether standard lymph node dissection can be avoided if SLND is performed.

Tumor size is a valuable prognostic variable: the larger the tumor, the poorer the prognosis. The wide variety of histologic types of breast cancer explains the heterogeneity of the disease. In general, the more well differentiated the tumor, the less aggressive it is. Poorly differentiated tumors appear morphologically disorganized and are more aggressive.

Another diagnostic test useful both for treatment decisions and prediction of prognosis is estrogen and progesterone receptor status. Receptor-positive tumors commonly (1) show histologic evidence of being well differentiated, (2) frequently have a *diploid* (more normal) DNA content and low proliferative indices, (3) have a lower chance for recurrence, and (4) are frequently hormone dependent and responsive to hormonal therapy. Receptor-negative tumors (1) are often poorly differentiated histologically, (2) have a high incidence of *aneuploidy* (abnormally high or low DNA content) and higher proliferative indices, (3) frequently recur, and (4) are usually unresponsive to hormonal therapy.

Ploidy status correlates with tumor aggressiveness. Diploid tumors have been shown to have a significantly lower risk of recurrence than aneuploid tumors.

Cell-proliferative indices indirectly measure the rate of tumor cell proliferation. The percent of tumor cells in the S phase of the cell cycle (see Chapter 15, Fig. 15-1) is another important prognostic indicator. Patients with cells that have high S-phase fractions have a higher risk for recurrence and earlier cancer death.

Another prognostic indicator is the genetic marker HER-2/neu (also called c-erb-B2 or neu). Amplification and overexpression of this gene have been associated with a greater risk for recurrence and a poorer prognosis in breast cancer.[25] The presence of this gene assists in the selection and sequence of chemotherapy and predicting patient response to treatment.

Collaborative Care

Historically, a radical **mastectomy** (removal of breast, pectoral muscles, axillary lymph nodes, and all fat and adjacent tissue) was the standard of care. Presently a wide range of treatment options is available to both the patient and the care providers attempting to make critical decisions about what treatment to select (Table 50-5). Prognostic factors are considered when treatment decisions are made about a specific breast cancer. Some of these factors also enter into the staging of breast cancer. The most widely accepted staging method for breast cancer is the American Joint Committee on Cancer's TNM system (Table 50-7).[26] This system uses tumor size (T), nodal involvement (N), and presence of metastasis (M) to determine the stage of disease. The stages range from I to IV, with stage I being very small tumors

(less than 2 cm) with no lymph node involvement and no metastasis. Further classification within these stages depends on the size of the tumor and the number of lymph nodes involved. Stage IV indicates the presence of metastatic spread, regardless of tumor size or lymph node involvement. The therapeutic regimen is

TABLE 50-5	*C*ollaborative Care Breast Cancer

Diagnostic
History including risk factors
Physical examination including breast and lymphatics
Mammography
Ultrasound
Biopsy
MRI (if indicated)

Staging Workup
Complete blood count, platelet count
Calcium and phosphate levels
Liver function tests
Sentinel lymph node dissection
Chest x-ray
Bone scan
CT scan of chest, abdomen, pelvis
MRI (if indicated)

Collaborative Therapy
Surgery
  Breast-conserving (lumpectomy) with sentinel lymph node biopsy/dissection and/or axillary lymph node dissection
  Modified radical mastectomy (may include reconstruction)
Radiation therapy
  Primary radiotherapy
  Adjuvant radiotherapy
  High-dose brachytherapy
  Palliative radiotherapy
Chemotherapy
  Adjuvant chemotherapy
  Chemotherapy for recurrent disease
Hormonal therapy (Table 50-6)
Biologic therapy

CT, Computed tomography; *MRI,* magnetic resonance imaging.

TABLE 50-6	*D*rug Therapy Hormonal Therapy for Breast Cancer

MECHANISM OF ACTION	EXAMPLES
Blocks estrogen receptors	tamoxifen (Nolvadex)
	toremifene (Fareston)
Destroys estrogen receptors	fulvestrant (Faslodex)
Prevents production of estrogen by inhibiting aromatase	anastrozole (Arimidex)
	letrozole (Femara)
	exemestane (Aromasin)
	vorozole (Rizivor)
	aminoglutethimide (Cytadren)

TABLE 50-7 **TNM Classification of Breast Cancer**

Primary Tumor (T)

T_0	No evidence of primary tumor
T_{is}	Carcinoma in situ
T_1	Tumor <2 cm
T_2	Tumor 2-5 cm
T_3	Tumor >5 cm
T_4	Extension to chest wall, inflammation

Regional Lymph Nodes (N)

N_0	No tumor in regional lymph nodes
N_1	Metastasis to movable ipsilateral nodes
N_2	Metastasis to matted or fixed ipsilateral nodes
N_3	Metastasis to ipsilateral internal mammary nodes

Distant Metastasis (M)

M_0	No distant metastasis
M_1	Distant metastasis (includes spread to ipsilateral supraclavicular nodes)

Stage Grouping

Stage 0	T_{is}	N_0	M_0
Stage I	T_1	N_0	M_0
Stage IIA	T_0	N_1	M_0
	T_1	N_1	M_0
	T_2	N_0	M_0
Stage IIB	T_2	N_1	M_0
	T_3	N_0	M_0
Stage IIIA	T_0	N_2	M_0
	T_1	N_2	M_0
	T_2	N_2	M_0
	T_3	N_1, N_2	M_0
Stage IIIB	T_4	Any N	M_0
	Any T	N_3	M_0
Stage IV	Any T	Any N	M_1

(Side effects and appropriate nursing management of general treatment modalities for cancer are discussed in Chapter 15.)

In spite of the advent of new prognostic indicators such as determination of DNA content and analysis of cell-cycle phases, the single most powerful prognostic factor related to local recurrence or metastasis after primary therapy is still the presence or absence of malignant cells in axillary lymph nodes.

Surgical Therapy. Breast conservation surgery with radiation therapy and modified radical mastectomy with or without reconstruction are currently the most common options for resectable breast cancer. Most women diagnosed with early-stage breast cancer (tumors smaller than 4 to 5 cm) are candidates for either treatment choice. The overall survival rate with lumpectomy and radiation is about the same as that with modified radical mastectomy.[18]

Axillary node dissection. Axillary lymph node dissection is often performed regardless of the treatment option selected. Examination of nodes provides the most powerful prognostic data currently available and helps determine further treatment (chemotherapy, hormone therapy, or both). For all cases of invasive breast cancer, a typical lymph node dissection has always in-

volved the removal of 10 to 15 lymph nodes. However, this technique may not be necessary or appropriate for some women with very small invasive breast cancers or with noninvasive (in situ) cancers. Sentinel lymph node dissection shows promise for reducing unnecessary lymph node dissection. If the sentinel node does not show any signs of cancer, further lymph nodes may not be removed, depending on the health care setting.

Lymphedema (accumulation of lymph in soft tissue) can occur as a result of the excision or radiation of lymph nodes.[27] When the axillary nodes cannot return lymph fluid to the central circulation, the fluid accumulates in the arm, causing obstructive pressure on the veins and venous return. The patient may experience heaviness, pain, impaired motor function in the arm, and numbness and paresthesia of the fingers as a result of lymphedema. Cellulitis and progressive fibrosis can result from lymphedema.

Although lymphedema is not always preventable, it can be controlled somewhat after surgery or radiation. Frequent and sustained elevation of the arm, performing hand and arm exercises daily, and avoidance of clothing that constricts the arm are all helpful in preventing and reducing lymphedema.[28]

Breast conservation surgery. Breast conservation surgery (termed **lumpectomy**) involves the removal of the entire tumor along with a margin of normal tissue. Following surgery, radiation therapy is delivered to the entire breast, ending with a boost to the tumor bed. If there is evidence of systemic disease, chemotherapy may be given before radiation therapy. Contraindications to breast conservation surgery include breast size too small to yield an acceptable cosmetic result, masses and calcifications that are multifocal (within the same breast quadrant), masses that are multicentric (in more than one quadrant), or diffuse calcifications in more than one quadrant.

One of the main advantages of breast conservation surgery and radiation is that it preserves the breast, including the nipple. The goal of the combined surgery and radiation is to maximize the benefits of both cancer treatment and cosmetic outcome while minimizing risks. Disadvantages of this surgery include the increased cost of the surgery plus radiation over surgery alone and the possible side effects of radiation. Table 50-8 describes treatment options, side effects, complications, and patient issues related to the most common surgical procedures currently used to treat breast cancer.

Modified radical mastectomy. A modified radical mastectomy includes removal of the breast and axillary lymph nodes, but it preserves the pectoralis major muscle. This surgery would be selected over breast conservation therapy if the tumor is too large to excise with good margins and attain a reasonable cosmetic result. Some patients may select this surgical procedure over lumpectomy when presented with the choice of either procedure.

When a modified radical mastectomy is performed, the patient has the option of breast reconstruction. If the patient chooses to have reconstructive surgery, it can be performed immediately following the mastectomy or it can be delayed until postoperative recovery is complete (about 6 months).

Follow-up care. After surgery, the woman must be followed up for the rest of her life at regular intervals. Most women have professional examinations every 6 months for 2 years and then annually thereafter. In addition, the woman must continue to practice monthly BSE on both breasts or the remaining breast and the mastectomy site. The most common site of recurrence of

TABLE 50-8   Breast Cancer: Surgical Procedures, Side Effects, Complications, and Patient Issues

PROCEDURES	DESCRIPTION	SIDE EFFECTS	POTENTIAL COMPLICATIONS	PATIENT ISSUES
Modified radical mastectomy	Removal of breast, preservation of pectoralis muscle, axillary node dissection	Chest wall tightens Phantom breast sensations Arm swelling Sensory changes	Short term: skin flap necrosis, seroma, hematoma, infection Long term: sensory loss, muscle weakness, lymphedema	Loss of breast Incision Body image Need for prosthesis Impaired arm mobility
Breast conservation surgery (lumpectomy) with radiation therapy	Wide excision of tumor, sentinel lymph node dissection (SLND) and/or axillary lymph node dissection (ALND), radiation therapy	Breast soreness Breast edema Skin reactions Arm swelling Sensory changes in breast and arm Fatigue	Short term: moist desquamation,* hematoma, seroma, infection Long term: fibrosis, lymphedema,† myositis, pneumonitis,* rib fractures*	Prolonged treatment* Impaired arm mobility† Change in texture and sensitivity of breast
Tissue expansion and breast implants	Expander used to slowly stretch tissue; saline gradually injected into reservoir over weeks to months Insertion of implant under musculofascial layer of chest wall	Discomfort Chest wall tightness	Short term: skin flap necrosis, wound separation, seroma, hematoma, infection Long term: capsular contractions, displacement of implant	Body image Prolonged physician visits to expand implants Additional surgeries for nipple construction, symmetry
Musculocutaneous flap procedures	A musculocutaneous flap (muscle, skin, blood supply) is transposed from latissimus dorsi to transverse rectus abdominis to chest wall‡	Pain related to two surgical sites and extensive surgery	Short term: delayed wound healing, infection, skin flap necrosis, abdominal hernia, hematoma	Prolonged postoperative recovery

*Specific to radiation therapy.
†If ALND (less likely with SLND).
‡Concurrent with mastectomy.

breast cancer is at the surgical site. The woman should also have yearly mammography of the remaining breast or breast tissue.

Postmastectomy pain syndrome. *Postmastectomy pain syndrome* can occur in patients following a mastectomy or axillary node dissection. Common symptoms include chest and upper arm pain, tingling down the arm, numbness, shooting or pricking pain, and unbearable itching that persist beyond the normal 3-month healing time. The pain syndrome is caused by a number of factors including injury to nerves and tissue as a result of surgery, radiation therapy, chemotherapy, or secondary neuroma development. The most common theory for its onset is the injury to intercostobrachial nerves, which are sensory nerves that exit chest wall muscles and provide sensation to the shoulder and upper arm.

Treatments include nonsteroidal antiinflammatory drugs, antidepressants, topical lidocaine patches, EMLA (eutectic mixture of local anesthetics: lidocaine and prilocaine), and antiseizure drugs (e.g., gabapentin [Neurontin]). Other possible treatment modalities include guided imagery training, biofeedback, physical therapy to prevent "frozen shoulder" syndrome as a result of inadequate movement, and psychologic counseling with a person trained in the management of chronic pain syndromes.

Adjuvant Therapy. The decision to recommend adjuvant (additional) therapy after surgery depends on the stage of the disease (number of involved nodes and tumor size), menstrual status and age, cell characteristics, presence or absence of estrogen receptors, and other preexisting health problems that can complicate treatment. Adjuvant therapies include radiation therapy after breast conservation surgery and systemic therapies such as chemotherapy and hormonal therapy.[29]

Radiation therapy. The three situations in which radiation therapy may be used for breast cancer are (1) as the primary treatment to destroy the tumor or as a companion to surgery to prevent local recurrence, (2) to shrink a large tumor to operable size, and (3) as the palliative treatment for pain caused by local recurrence and metastases. Lumpectomy is almost always followed by radiation.

Primary radiation therapy. When radiation therapy is the primary treatment, it is usually performed after local excision of the breast mass. The breast (and the regional lymph nodes in some cases) is radiated daily over the course of approximately 5 to 6 weeks. An external beam of radiation is used to deliver an approximate total dose of 4500 to 5000 cGy (4500 to 5000 rads; 1 rad = 1 cGy). A "boost" treatment to the full breast may also be given, either before or after therapy has been completed. The boost is a dose of radiation delivered to the area in which the original tumor was located. It can be given by external beam and usually adds 10 treatments to the total number given. Fatigue, skin changes, and breast edema may be temporary side effects of external beam radiation therapy. Radiation of the axilla is also effective in decreasing the incidence of axillary recurrence. Chemotherapy may be used systemically to enhance the local effects of radiation. (Nursing management of the patient receiving radiation therapy is discussed in Chapter 15.)

Radiation therapy as adjunct to surgery. Although an uncommon treatment mode, preoperative radiation therapy can be used to reduce the size of a large tumor mass to operable proportions by destroying the cancer cells. Additionally, because the malignant cells are partially or completely destroyed, the rate of local recurrence decreases.

The decision to use radiation therapy after mastectomy is based on the probability of the presence of local residual cancer cells (related to size of cancer and number of involved lymph nodes). Radiating the area will not prevent the appearance of distant metastasis at a later date. The site of radiation therapy (lymph nodes, chest wall, or both) depends on the degree of possible spread of the cancer.

High-dose brachytherapy. High-dose brachytherapy is a new procedure that is an alternative to traditional radiation treatment for early-stage breast cancer. The technique uses a balloon catheter to insert radioactive seeds into the breast after the tumor is removed (Fig. 50-5). The seeds deliver a concentrated dose of radiation directly to the site where the cancer is most likely to occur. Traditional radiation treatments can take 5 to 6 weeks. In contrast, high-dose brachytherapy may require only 5 days.

Palliative radiation therapy. In addition to reducing the primary tumor mass with a resultant decrease in pain, radiation therapy is also used to stabilize symptomatic metastatic lesions in such sites as bone, soft tissue organs, brain, and chest. Radiation therapy relieves pain and is often successful in controlling recurrent or metastatic disease for long periods.

Systemic therapy. The goal of systemic therapy is to destroy tumor cells that may have spread undetected to distant sites. Systemic therapy as an adjuvant to primary local treatment, in the absence of demonstrable metastases, can decrease the rate of recurrence and increase the length of survival.[18] Because of the high risk for recurrent disease, nearly all women with evidence of node involvement, particularly those who are hormone-receptor negative, will have some type of systemic therapy. Certain women, particularly those who are premenopausal, are known to be at higher risk for recurrent or metastatic disease. These women are often recommended for systemic therapy even when no evidence of node involvement is found. Weighing the different risk factors to determine the need for adjuvant therapy in a node-negative patient is a complex process.

Chemotherapy. Chemotherapy refers to the use of cytotoxic drugs to destroy cancer cells. The greatest benefits from chemotherapy have been achieved among premenopausal women with node findings that are positive for malignancy.

In some instances chemotherapy is used preoperatively. Preoperative chemotherapy may be more convenient than postoperative administration and can decrease the size of the primary tumor, possibly permitting less extensive surgery. Also, it has been shown that preoperative chemotherapy suppresses tumor growth and prolongs survival.

Breast cancer is one of the solid tumors that is the most responsive to chemotherapy. The use of combinations of drugs is clearly superior to the use of a single drug. The benefit of combination treatment results from the use of drugs that have different actions on cell growth and division. The more common combination-therapy protocols are cyclophosphamide (Cytoxan), methotrexate, and 5-fluorouracil (5-FU), referred to as

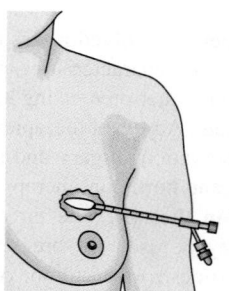

Step 1: During the lumpectomy or shortly thereafter, a deflated balloon is placed inside the cavity created by removal of the tumor.

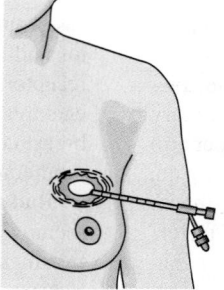

Step 2: Patient returns to clinic for 1 to 5 days of outpatient treatment, where a radioactive seed is inserted through a catheter into the balloon twice a day for 10 minutes each time. The seed targets radiation to the area where tumors are more likely to recur, while minimizing exposure to healthy tissue.

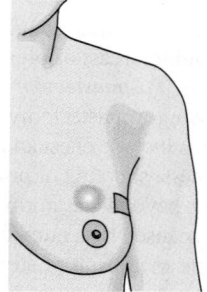

Step 3: The balloon is deflated and the catheter is removed. No source of radiation remains in the patient's body between treatments or after the final procedure.

FIG. 50-5 High-dose brachytherapy for breast cancer.

CMF; and cyclophosphamide and doxorubicin (Adriamycin), referred to as AC, with or without the addition of a taxane such as paclitaxel (Taxol) or docetaxel (Taxotere); or cyclophosphamide, 5-FU, and epirubicin (Ellence) or doxorubicin, referred to as CEF or CAF, respectively. Paclitaxel, docetaxel, and capecitabine (Xeloda) are used in women whose metastatic breast cancer has not responded to standard chemotherapy.[29] Vinorelbine (Navelbine), a relatively new chemotherapeutic drug for treating metastatic breast cancer, is well tolerated with fewer and milder side effects than other chemotherapy drugs.

Because healthy cells are also affected by chemotherapy, a variety of side effects accompany this treatment modality. The incidence and severity of predictable and commonly observed side effects will be influenced by the specific drug combination, drug schedule, and dose intensity of the drug or drugs. Usually body organs with rapidly growing cells are the most strongly affected. The most common side effects involve the gastrointestinal tract, bone marrow, and hair follicles, resulting in nausea, anorexia, weight loss, bone marrow suppression and subsequent fatigue, and alopecia (hair loss).

Hormonal therapy. Estrogen can promote the growth of breast cancer cells if the cells are estrogen-receptor positive. Hormonal therapy removes or blocks the source of estrogen, thus promoting tumor regression.

Two advances have increased the use of hormone therapy in breast cancer. First, hormone receptor assays, which are reliable diagnostic tests, have been developed to identify women who are likely to respond to hormone therapy. Both estrogen and progesterone receptor status of the tumor can be determined. The importance of these assays is their ability to predict whether hormonal therapy is a treatment option for women with breast cancer, either at the time of initial therapy or if the cancer recurs. Second, drugs have been developed that can inactivate the hormone-secreting glands as effectively as surgery or radiation. Premenopausal and perimenopausal women are more likely to have tumors that are not hormone dependent, whereas women who are postmenopausal are more likely to have hormone-dependent tumors. Chances of tumor regression are significantly greater in women whose tumors contain estrogen and progesterone receptors.

Estrogen deprivation can occur by destroying the ovaries by surgery or radiation therapy or drug therapy (see Table 50-6). Hormonal therapy can (1) block or destroy the estrogen receptors or (2) suppress estrogen synthesis through inhibiting aromatase, an enzyme needed for endogenous estrogen synthesis.[30] Hormonal therapy is widely used to treat recurrent or metastatic cancer but may also be used as an adjuvant to primary treatment.

Tamoxifen (Nolvadex) is the hormonal agent of choice in postmenopausal, estrogen receptor–positive women with or without lymph node involvement. Tamoxifen, an antiestrogen drug, blocks the estrogen receptor sites of malignant cells and thus inhibits the growth-stimulating effects of estrogen. It is commonly used in advanced and early-stage breast cancer to prevent or treat recurrent disease. Tamoxifen may also be used to prevent breast cancer in high risk individuals.[31] Side effects of tamoxifen are minimal but include hot flashes, nausea, vomiting, vaginal discharge, and other effects commonly associated with decreased estrogen. It also increases the risk of blood clots, cataracts, and endometrial cancer in postmenopausal women.[32]

Toremifene (Fareston), an antiestrogen agent similar to tamoxifen, is indicated as first-line treatment for metastatic breast cancer in postmenopausal women with estrogen receptor–positive or estrogen receptor–unknown tumors.

Fulvestrant (Faslodex) may be given to women with advanced breast cancer who no longer respond to tamoxifen. This drug slows cancer progression by destroying estrogen receptors in the breast cancer cells. Fulvestrant is given intramuscularly on a monthly basis.

Aromatase inhibitor drugs, which interfere with the enzyme that synthesizes endogenous estrogen, are used in the treatment of advanced breast cancer in postmenopausal women with disease progression. These drugs include anastrozole (Arimidex), letrozole (Femara), vorozole (Rizivor), exemestane (Aromasin), and aminoglutethimide (Cytadren).

Raloxifene (Evista), a drug used to prevent bone loss, may also reduce the risk of breast cancer without stimulating endometrial growth. Raloxifene acts as an estrogen antagonist at the hormone-sensitive tissues of breast cancer and bone. (Raloxifene is discussed in the section on osteoporosis in Chapter 62.)

Additional drugs that may be used to suppress hormone-dependent breast tumors include megestrol acetate (Megace), diethylstilbestrol (DES), and fluoxymesterone (Halotestin). Less common hormone-deprivation strategies include bilateral oophorectomy, adrenalectomy, and hypophysectomy.

Biologic Therapy. The use of biologic therapy represents an attempt to stimulate the body's natural defenses to recognize and attack cancer cells. Trastuzumab (Herceptin) is an antibody to HER-2/neu, an antigen that often appears on the surface of breast cancer cells. After the antibody attaches to the antigen, it is taken into the cells and eventually kills them. It can be used alone or in combination with other chemotherapy to treat patients with metastatic breast cancer whose tumors overexpress the HER-2 gene. Current research is examining the effectiveness of trastuzumab on early-stage breast cancer.[25] (The use of biologic therapies is discussed in Chapter 15.)

Bone Marrow and Stem Cell Transplantation. Autologous bone marrow or peripheral stem cell transplantation combined with high-dose chemotherapy has been used to treat patients with advanced metastatic breast cancer. In this technique patients donate their own bone marrow or peripheral blood from which stem cells are harvested. Then they receive high doses of chemotherapy, which causes bone marrow suppression. The patient subsequently undergoes autologous bone marrow or stem cell transplantation. These treatments remain under investigation. (Bone marrow and stem cell transplantation are discussed in Chapter 15.)

NURSING MANAGEMENT
BREAST CANCER

■ Nursing Assessment

Many factors need to be considered when a nurse is assessing a patient with a breast problem. The history of the breast disorder assists in establishing the diagnosis. The presence of nipple discharge, pain, rate of growth of the lump, breast asymmetry, and correlation with the menstrual cycle should all be investigated.

The size and location of the lump or lumps should be carefully documented, and the physical characteristics of the lesion, such as consistency, mobility, and shape, should be assessed. If nipple discharge is present, the color and consistency should be noted, as well as whether it occurs from one or both breasts.

Subjective and objective data that should be obtained from an individual suspected of having or diagnosed as having breast cancer are presented in Table 50-9.

TABLE 50-9 Nursing Assessment — Breast Cancer

Subjective Data

Important Health Information

Past health history: Benign breast disease with atypical changes; previous unilateral breast cancer; menstrual history (early menarche with late menopause); pregnancy history (nulliparity or first full-term pregnancy after age 30); previous endometrial, ovarian, or colon cancer; hyperestrogenism and testicular atrophy (in men)

Medications: Use of hormones, especially as postmenopausal hormone replacement therapy and in oral contraceptives, infertility treatments

Surgery or other treatments: Exposure to excessive radiation (e.g., thyroid radiation)

Functional Health Patterns

Health perception–health management: Family history (especially mother or sister); mammography history; palpable change found on BSE; alcohol use

Nutritional-metabolic: Obesity; anorexia (possible indicator of metastasis); dietary habits

Cognitive-perceptual: Headache, back, arm, or bone pain (possible indicators of metastasis)

Sexuality-reproductive: Unilateral nipple discharge (clear, milky, or bloody); change in breast contour, size, or symmetry

Coping–stress tolerance: Chronic psychologic stress

Self-perception–self-concept: Anxiety regarding threat to self-esteem

Objective Data

General

Axillary and supraclavicular lymphadenopathy

Integumentary

Firm, discrete nodules at mastectomy site (possible indicator of local recurrence); peripheral edema (possible indicator of metastasis)

Respiratory

Pleural effusions (possible indicator of metastasis)

Gastrointestinal

Hepatomegaly, jaundice; ascites (possible indicators of liver metastasis)

Reproductive

Hard, irregular, nonmobile breast lump most often in upper, outer sector, possibly fixated to fascia or chest wall; nipple inversion or retraction, erosion; edema ("orange peel"), erythema, induration, infiltration, or dimpling (in later stages)

Possible Findings

Finding of mass or change in tissue on breast examination; positive results of mammography or ultrasonography; positive results of FNA or surgical biopsy or similar results with a needle biopsy

BSE, Breast self-examination; *FNA,* fine-needle aspiration.

■ Nursing Diagnoses

Nursing diagnoses related to the care of a patient diagnosed with breast cancer vary. Following diagnosis and before a treatment plan has been selected, the following diagnoses would apply:

- Decisional conflict *related to* lack of knowledge about treatment options and their effects
- Fear *related to* diagnosis of breast cancer
- Disturbed body image *related to* anticipated physical and emotional effects of treatment modalities

If a mastectomy is planned, the nursing diagnoses may include, but are not limited to, those presented in NCP 50-1.

■ Planning

The overall goals are that the patient with breast cancer will (1) actively participate in the decision-making process related to treatment options, (2) fully comply with the therapeutic plan, (3) manage the side effects of adjuvant therapy, and (4) be satisfied with the support provided by significant others and health care providers.

■ Nursing Implementation

Acute Intervention. The time between the diagnosis of breast cancer and the selection of a treatment plan is a difficult period for the woman and her family. Although the primary care provider has discussed treatment options, the woman often relies on the nurse to clarify and expand on these options. During this time, the woman may be very self-focused, verbalizing her conflict and indecision frequently. Appropriate nursing interventions during this period include exploring the woman's usual decision-making patterns, helping the woman accurately evaluate the advantages and disadvantages of the options, providing information relevant to the decision, and supporting the patient once the decision is made.

During this period the woman may exhibit signs of distress or tension, such as tachycardia, increased muscle tension, sleep disturbances, and restlessness, whenever she focuses on the decision to be made. The nurse should assess the woman's body language, motor activity, and affect during periods of high stress and indecision so that appropriate interventions can be carried out.

Regardless of the surgery planned, the patient must be provided with sufficient information to ensure informed consent. Some patients seek extensive, detailed information, whereas others avoid information.[33] Sensitivity to an individual's need for information is essential. Teaching in the preoperative phase includes instruction in turning, coughing, and deep breathing; a review of postoperative exercises; a pain management plan; and an explanation of the recovery period from the time of surgery until discharge.

The woman who has breast conservation surgery usually has an uneventful postoperative course with only a moderate amount of pain. If an axillary lymph node dissection (ALND) has been done or if a woman has had a modified radical mastectomy, specific interventions will be needed.

Restoring arm function on the affected side after mastectomy and axillary lymph node dissection is one of the most important goals of nursing activities. The woman should be placed in a semi-Fowler position with the arm on the affected side elevated on a pillow. Flexing and extending the fingers should begin in the recovery room with progressive increases in activity encouraged. (Information pertaining to arm exercises and care applies to women who have had an axillary node dissection after lumpectomy or total mastectomy.) Postoperative arm and shoulder exercises are instituted gradually at the surgeon's direction (Fig. 50-6). These exercises are designed to prevent contractures and muscle shortening, maintain muscle tone, and improve lymph and blood circulation. The difficulty and pain encountered by the woman in performing the previously simple tasks included in the exercise program may cause frustration and depression. The goal of all exercise is a gradual return to full range of motion within 4 to 6 weeks.

NURSING CARE PLAN 50-1

Patient after a Modified Radical Mastectomy*

EXPECTED PATIENT OUTCOMES	NURSING INTERVENTIONS and *RATIONALES*
NURSING DIAGNOSIS	**Acute pain** *related to* surgical procedure *as manifested by* verbalization regarding presence and degree of pain at operative area.
• Absence of or tolerable level of pain • Satisfaction with pain control	• Administer analgesics as prescribed *to relieve pain*. Position arm *to prevent tension on suture line and provide support.* • Encourage use of noninvasive pain management strategies such as distraction, imagery, and relaxation *to complement analgesics and decrease need for analgesia.*
NURSING DIAGNOSIS	**Fear** *related to* diagnosis of cancer *as manifested by* insomnia, crying, and questioning of prognosis.
• Verbalization of fear • Support of significant others • Confidence in ability to cope • Early recognition of recurrent or metastatic disease	• Encourage woman to talk about feelings and diagnosis of cancer *to promote successful resolution of fear and establish effective coping mechanisms.* • Provide opportunity for significant others to discuss situation and learn about support groups *because their fear about the diagnosis and outcome can decrease their effectiveness as a support system.* • Reinforce importance of annual mammogram *because it is a recommended screening technique for identification of local recurrence after mastectomy and for assessing other breast.* • Provide information about signs and symptoms to report to health care provider (i.e., new and persistent problems such as skin changes at surgical site, new changes in breast or chest wall).
NURSING DIAGNOSIS	**Disturbed body image** *related to* loss of body part *as manifested by* verbalization of concern about appearance and feelings of loss of femininity, and refusal to view incision.
• Verbalization of feelings about surgery and change in body image • Indication of beginning of resolution of negative feelings toward self • Acceptance of altered body image	• Assess degree of self-esteem disturbance *so appropriate interventions can be initiated.* • Arrange for Reach to Recovery visitor or similar community resource *to serve as a role model and provide hope for recovery and a normal future.* • Provide information regarding prosthesis fitting and breast reconstruction (if patient is interested) *so patient can make informed decisions regarding options.* • Assist patient to verbalize feelings and encourage open communication with significant others *to promote grief work and maintain support from family and friends.*
NURSING DIAGNOSIS	**Ineffective therapeutic regimen management** *related to* lack of knowledge regarding postoperative care and breast self-examination (BSE).
• Able to change dressings with minimal assistance • Practice of monthly BSE	• Demonstrate to patient and significant other how to take care of incision and apply new dressing as appropriate. Have patient return demonstration. • Teach or evaluate BSE performance *to ensure that patient is performing correctly.*
NURSING DIAGNOSIS	**Impaired physical mobility** *related to* pain *as manifested by* limitation in movement or upper extremity on surgical side.
• Return to usual arm and shoulder function	• Assess degree of mobility impairment *to provide baseline data and to plan appropriate interventions.* • Treat pain *to promote participation in exercise plan.* • Carry out exercises *to prevent contractures and muscle shortening, maintain muscle tone, and improve lymph and blood circulation.* • Assist woman to resume activities of daily living as tolerated or as directed by physician *to reduce dependent behaviors, raise self-esteem, and maintain mobility of affected arm.* • Emphasize bilateral activity of upper extremities *to prevent guarding of operative side and loss of function.*

*These nursing diagnoses may also be applicable to the patient who has had a lumpectomy with an axillary lymph node dissection.   *Continued*

NURSING CARE PLAN 50-1

Patient after a Modified Radical Mastectomy—cont'd

COLLABORATIVE PROBLEM

NURSING GOALS	NURSING INTERVENTIONS and *RATIONALES*
POTENTIAL COMPLICATION - Monitor for signs of lymphedema - Report deviations from acceptable parameters - Carry out appropriate medical and nursing interventions	**Lymphedema** *related to* impaired lymphatic drainage and lack of knowledge of preventive measures. - Assess woman for signs of lymphedema such as edema in hand and/or arm on operative side, heaviness, and/or localized pain *to enable early diagnosis and intervention to prevent and treat the complication.* - Instruct patient about self-care strategies and precautions to reduce risk of lymphedema *so patient will be an active, informed participant in self-care.* - Do not perform venipunctures or take blood pressure measurements on affected arm *to reduce risk of constriction, infection, and lymphedema in affected arm.* - Avoid dependent arm position *to allow proper wound healing and decrease stress to incision site.* - Use elastic sleeve if ordered *to apply mechanical pressure to reduce fluid collection in affected arm and promote venous return.*

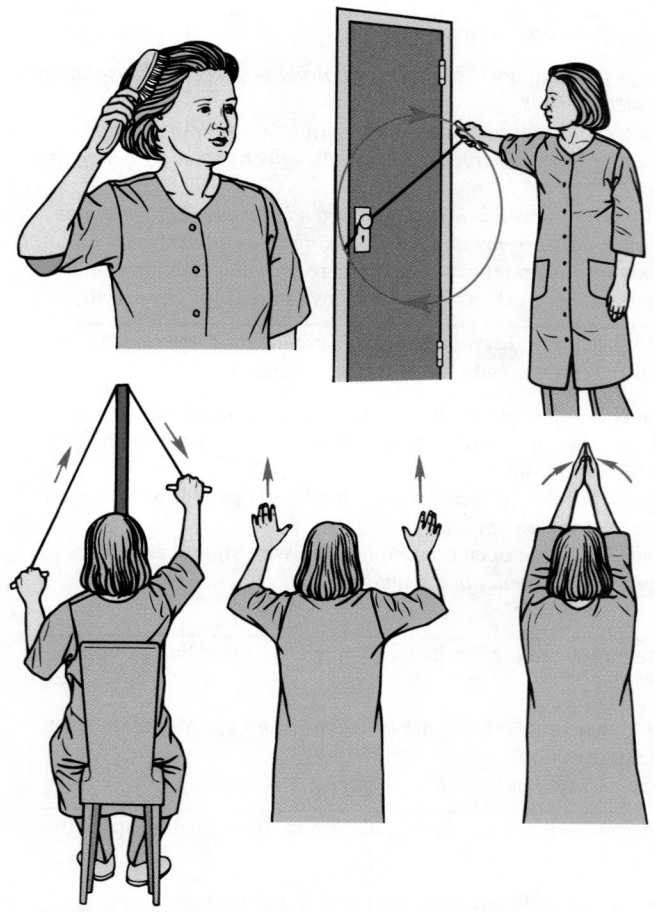

FIG. 50-6 Postoperative exercises for patient with a mastectomy or lumpectomy with axillary lymph node dissection.

Postoperative discomfort can be minimized by administering analgesics about 30 minutes before initiating exercises. When showering is appropriate, the flow of warm water over the involved shoulder often has a soothing effect and reduces joint stiffness. Whenever possible, the same nurse should work with the woman so that progress can be monitored and problems can be identified.

Measures to prevent or reduce lymphedema after ALND must be used by the nurse and taught to the woman. The affected arm should never be dependent, even while the person is sleeping. Blood pressure readings, venipunctures, and injections should not be done on the affected arm. Elastic bandages should not be used in the early postoperative period because they inhibit collateral lymph drainage. The woman must be instructed to protect the arm on the operative side from even minor trauma such as a pinprick or sunburn. If trauma to the arm occurs, the area should be washed thoroughly with soap and water. A topical antibiotic ointment and a bandage or other sterile dressing should be applied. The surgeon must be advised of the trauma, and the site of injury must be observed closely for evidence of inflammation. The patient must know and understand that she is at risk of developing lymphedema for the rest of her life.[27]

When lymphedema is acute, an intermittent pneumatic compression sleeve may be prescribed. This device applies mechanical massage to the arm. Manual massage is also effective in mobilizing subcutaneous accumulations of fluid. Elevation of the arm so that it is level with the heart, diuretics, and isometric exercises may be recommended to reduce the fluid volume in the arm. The patient may need to wear a fitted elastic pressure-gradient sleeve during waking hours, to maintain maximum volume reduction, and preventively, during air travel.

Psychologic care. Throughout interactions with a woman with breast cancer, the nurse must keep in mind the extensive psychologic impact of the disease. All aspects of care must include sensitivity to the woman's efforts to cope with a life-threatening disease. An open relationship in which the woman can express her fears and feelings is essential. The nurse can help meet the woman's psychologic needs by doing the following:

1. Assisting her to develop a positive but realistic attitude
2. Helping her identify sources of support and strength to her, such as her partner, family, and spiritual practices
3. Encouraging her to verbalize her anger and fears about her diagnosis and the impact it will have on her life

COMPLEMENTARY & ALTERNATIVE THERAPIES
Imagery

Imagery, or visualization, is the process of using mental images to create a desired state.

Clinical Uses

Imagery has many uses, including managing pain, stress, anxiety, asthma, menstrual disorders, gastrointestinal disorders, arthritis, hypertension, and headaches.

Effects

Imagery can promote relaxation, decrease stress, lower blood pressure, relieve pain, reduce side effects of chemotherapy, improve immune function, enhance performance, and enhance wound healing. This behavioral intervention has few side effects.

Nursing Implications

Imagery should be individualized. Images should be avoided that are distressing. People can invent their own imagery or use those that have been created by others. Imagery is well suited as a self-care technique because almost anyone can use it.

4. Promoting open communication of thoughts and feelings between the patient and her family
5. Providing accurate and complete answers to questions about her disease, treatment options, and reproductive or lactation issues (if appropriate)
6. Offering information about community resources, such as Reach to Recovery, Y-Me, CanSurmount, Encore, and local support organizations and groups

The nurse can promote the woman's recovery by arranging a visit from a woman who had similar treatment, such as a Reach to Recovery volunteer, if the service is available. The Reach to Recovery program of the American Cancer Society is a rehabilitation program for women who have had breast surgery. It is designed to help them meet their psychologic, physical, and cosmetic needs. The volunteers, who are all women who have had breast cancer, can answer questions about what to expect at home, how to tell people about the surgery, and what prosthetic devices are available. If a Reach to Recovery volunteer is not available, it is the nurse's responsibility to be knowledgeable about the needs of the woman after breast surgery. The American Cancer Society and the National Cancer Institute can provide excellent materials to assist the nurse in meeting the special needs of women with breast cancer.

The professional staff must never underestimate the tremendous psychologic impact that a diagnosis of cancer and subsequent breast surgery can have on a woman. Emotional complications are common. The nurse's accepting, concerned attitude can do a great deal to relieve the feelings of anger and depression experienced by many patients.

Ambulatory and Home Care. The nurse should explain the follow-up routine to the patient and emphasize the importance of beginning and continuing BSE and annual mammography. Referral to a mental health provider to address individual and family support in addition to coping needs may be indicated. Immediately after surgery, symptoms that should be reported to the clinician include fever, inflammation at the surgical site, erythema, postoperative constipation, and unusual swelling. Other changes to report in the future are new back pain, weakness, shortness of breath, and confusion. If adjuvant therapy is to be used, the woman should have specific instructions about appointment times and treatment locations and management of side effects.

For women who have had a mastectomy, the nurse should stress the importance of wearing a well-fitting prosthesis. A variety of products are available to meet the specific needs of the individual woman. After surgery a temporary camisole prosthesis may be used. A well-trained salesperson can help the woman select a suitable, more permanent weighted prosthesis and bra, generally at 6 weeks postoperatively. There are both physical and psychologic advantages to the use of a prosthesis. The return of a normal external appearance is especially important to most women.

The implications of the loss of a breast on the sexual identity and relationships of the woman vary. A preoperative sexual assessment provides helpful baseline data that the nurse can use to plan postoperative interventions. Often the husband, sexual partner, or family members may need assistance in dealing with their emotional reactions to the diagnosis and surgery for them to act as effective means of support for the patient.[34] There are no physical reasons for a mastectomy to prevent sexual satisfaction. The woman taking tamoxifen may have a decreased sexual drive or vaginal dryness. She may need to use lubrication to prevent discomfort during intercourse. If difficulty in adjustment or other problems develop, counseling may be necessary to deal with the emotional component of a mastectomy and the diagnosis of cancer.

Depression and anxiety may occur with the continued stress and uncertainty of a cancer diagnosis. A woman's self-esteem and identity may also be threatened. Special nursing interventions are necessary, in terms of both psychologic support and self-care teaching, if a recurrence of cancer is found. The support of family and friends and participation in a cancer support group are important aspects of care that are helpful in improving quality of life and have been found to have a clinically significant impact on survival.[35]

■ Evaluation

The expected outcomes for the patient after a modified radical mastectomy are presented in NCP 50-1.

■ Culturally Competent Care: Breast Cancer

Breast cancer does not respect the boundaries of ethnicity or culture. However, there are differences in various ethnic groups related to breast cancer (see Cultural and Ethnic Considerations box on p. 1366 and Nursing Research box on p. 1378). The differences may be due to dietary factors and insufficient use of early detection procedures such as BSE and mammograms.

Cultural values will strongly influence how women will respond to and cope with breast cancer and treatment. It is important for the nurse to be aware of the cultural value of breasts. In addition, the nurse needs to explore cultural factors that relate to the disease of breast cancer. A possible reason that some women may delay treatment after they have discovered a large breast lump is their belief in fatalism—an acceptance of disease as inevitable fate or "God's will." ■

⋀URSING RESEARCH
Issues of African American Breast Cancer Survivors

Citation
Wilmoth M, Sanders LD: Accept me for myself: African American women's issues after breast cancer, *Oncol Nurs Forum* 28:875, 2001.

Purpose
To identify personal issues and concerns of African American women who are breast cancer survivors.

Methods
Women (*n* = 24) were recruited to participate in two focus group sessions, which were held in a community library. The specific aim of the sessions was to learn the women's perception of the impact that breast cancer had on their personal lives. All sessions were audiotaped and transcribed.

Results and Conclusions
Five themes were identified through content analysis: (1) body appearance (keloid formation and unable to find appropriate color of prosthesis); (2) social support (viewed as both positive and negative); (3) health activism (a need to inform other women of color about the risk); (4) menopause (health care providers had not provided enough information); and (5) learning to live with chronic illness (a sense of survival with a change in priorities).

Implications for Nursing Practice
Nurses play an important role in helping African American women develop awareness of the availability of prostheses and wigs to match their skin tones and hair. Breast cancer survivors should be supported in their own outreach efforts to inform other women in the African American community about breast cancer risk and screening. Providing information to women about the potential for menopausal symptoms should be clearly addressed by health care providers at the same time that other chemotherapy side effects are discussed.

MAMMOPLASTY

Mammoplasty is the surgical change in the size or shape of the breast. It may be done electively for cosmetic purposes to either enlarge or reduce the size of the breasts. It may also be done to reconstruct the breast after a mastectomy.

Health care providers should remain nonjudgmental toward women who desire mammoplasty. The desire to alter the appearance of the breasts has special significance for each woman as she attempts to alter or re-create her body image. It is important for the nurse to be aware of the cultural value placed on the breast by the woman. It is important that the woman have a realistic idea about what mammoplasty can accomplish and about possible complications, such as hematoma formation, hemorrhage, and infection. If an implant is involved, capsular contracture and loss of the implant are possible.

Breast Augmentation

In augmentation mammoplasty (the procedure to enlarge the breasts), an implant is placed in a surgically created pocket between the capsule of the breast and the pectoral fascia, or ideally under the pectoral muscle. Most implants are silicone envelopes filled with a fluid such as dextran, saline, or silicone. Because of their resemblance to the human breast, implants filled with silicone were the most widely used. In 1992 the Food and Drug Administration suspended the routine use of silicone implants in response to potential hazards related to silicone leakage. Allegations of associated immune-related diseases caused or exacerbated by the presence of silicone gel implants have caused considerable controversy and litigation. Currently the use of silicone implants is approved only when medically prescribed in clinical trials.

In the United States saline-filled implants are usually used. Saline-filled implants are silicone shells filled with normal saline. Soybean oil implants are an alternative form of implant. This implant has an outer shell of silicone that is filled with highly refined soybean oil. A major advantage of soybean implants is that it is easier for x-rays to penetrate the implant, so better visualization of the underlying breast tissue is possible with mammography.

Breast Reduction

For some women, large breasts can be a source of pain and embarrassment. They can interfere with normal daily activities such as walking, typing, and driving a car. Overly large breasts can interfere with self-esteem and self-image and can lead to back, shoulder, and neck problems, including degenerative nerve changes. They may make stylish dressing more difficult. Reduction in the size of the breasts can have positive effects on both the psychologic and the physical health of the patient. Reduction mammoplasty is performed by resecting wedges of tissue from the upper and lower quadrants of the breast. The excess skin is removed, and the areola and nipple are relocated on the breast. Lactation can usually be accomplished if massive amounts of tissue are not removed and the nipples are left connected during surgery.

NURSING MANAGEMENT
BREAST AUGMENTATION AND REDUCTION

Breast augmentation and breast reduction may be done in the outpatient surgical area, or it may involve overnight hospitalization. General anesthesia is used. Drains are generally placed in the surgical site to prevent hematoma formation and then removed 2 to 3 days after surgery or when drainage is under 20 ml per day. The drainage must be examined for color and odor to detect postoperative infection or hemorrhage. The woman's temperature should also be monitored. Dressings should be changed as necessary and prescribed using sterile technique. After surgery the woman should be assured that the appearance of the breast will improve when healing is completed. Depending on physician instructions, the patient may be instructed to wear a bra that provides good support continuously for 2 to 3 days after breast reduction or augmentation. Depending on the extent of the operation, most women can resume normal activities within 2 to 3 weeks. Strenuous exercise may not be appropriate until several weeks later.

Breast Reconstruction

Breast reconstructive surgery may be done simultaneously with a mastectomy or some time afterward to achieve symmetry and to restore or preserve body image.[36] The timing of reconstruction surgery should be individualized, based on the psychologic needs of the patient. Immediate breast reconstruction after mastectomy is commonly being performed. The advantages to immediate reconstruction are only one surgical procedure, one anesthesia induction, and one recovery period. Also, surgery takes place before the development of scar tissue or adhesions. Early reconstruction does not delay or influence further treatment or adversely affect predicted survival.

Indications. The main indication for breast reconstruction is to improve the woman's self-image and regain a sense of normality.[37] Present techniques cannot restore lactation, nipple sensation, or erectility. Therefore the erotic functions of the breast are not present. Although the breast will not fully resemble its premastectomy appearance, the reconstructed appearance usually represents an improvement over the mastectomy scar (Fig. 50-7). The contour of the breast is restored without the use of an external prosthesis.

Types of Reconstruction

Breast implants and tissue expansion. Breast implants are placed in a pocket under the pectoralis muscle, which protects the implant and provides soft tissue coverage over the implant. Implants can be placed either at the time of mastectomy or later. Because many mastectomy patients have insufficient tissue, simple placement of an implant may lead to small breast reconstruction that is tight or firm. Autologous tissue reconstruction may then be recommended.

A tissue expander can be used to stretch the skin and muscle at the mastectomy site before inserting implants (Fig. 50-8). The use of tissue expanders and breast implants is the most common breast reconstruction technique currently used.[28] Placement of the expander can be performed at the time of mastectomy or at a later date. The tissue expander, which is minimally inflated at the time of surgery, is gradually filled by weekly injections of sterile water or saline solution, which stretch the skin and muscle. Once the tissue is adequately stretched and the anticipated breast size is reached, the expander is surgically removed and a permanent implant is inserted. Some expanders are designed to remain in place and become the implant, eliminating the need for a second surgical procedure. Tissue expansion does not work well in individuals with extensive scar tissue from surgery or radiation therapy.

The body's natural response to the presence of a foreign substance is the formation of a fibrous capsule around the implant. If excessive capsular formation occurs as a result of infection, hematoma, trauma, or reaction to a foreign body, a contracture can develop, resulting in a deformed breast. Surgeons differ in their approaches to the prevention of contracture formation, although gentle manual massage around the implant is routine. Prevention of the problems that cause excessive capsule formation is critical. Other postoperative complications include skin ulceration, hypertrophic scar formation, intercostal neuralgia, and wound infection.

Musculocutaneous flap procedure. If insufficient muscle is left after mastectomy or if the chest wall has been radiated, the person's own tissue may be used to repair the soft tissue defects. Musculocutaneous flaps are most often taken from the back (latissimus dorsi muscle) or the abdomen (transverse rectus abdominis muscle). In the latissimus dorsi musculocutaneous flap, a block of skin and muscle from the patient's back is used to replace tissue removed during mastectomy.[38] A small implant may

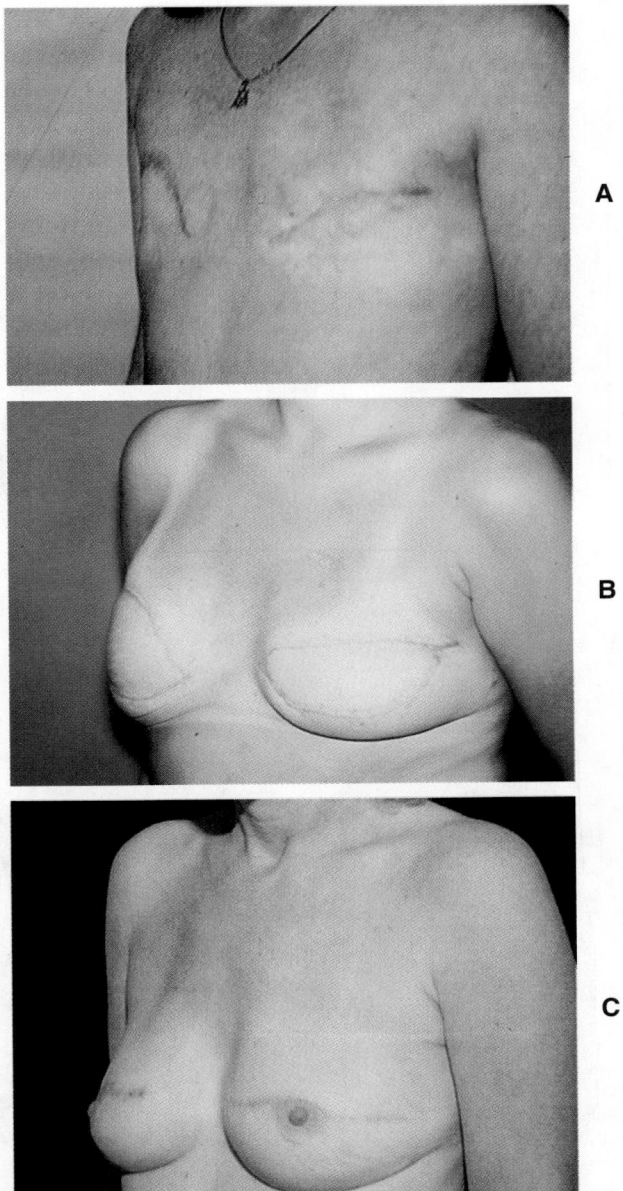

FIG. 50-7   A, Appearance of chest following bilateral mastectomy. B, Postoperative breast reconstruction before nipple–areolar reconstruction. C, Postoperative breast reconstruction after nipple–areolar reconstruction.

be needed beneath the flap to gain reasonable breast shape and size. A disadvantage of this technique is an additional scar on the back.

The *transverse rectus abdominis musculocutaneous* (TRAM) flap is the most frequently used flap operation. The rectus abdominis muscles are paired flat muscles running from the rib cage down to the pubic bone. Arteries running inside the muscle provide branches at many levels, and these branches supply the fat and skin across a large expanse of the abdomen. With this technique the surgeon elevates a large block of tissue from the lower abdominal area, but leaves it attached to the rectus muscle (Fig. 50-9). This tissue is then tunneled or placed as "free flaps"

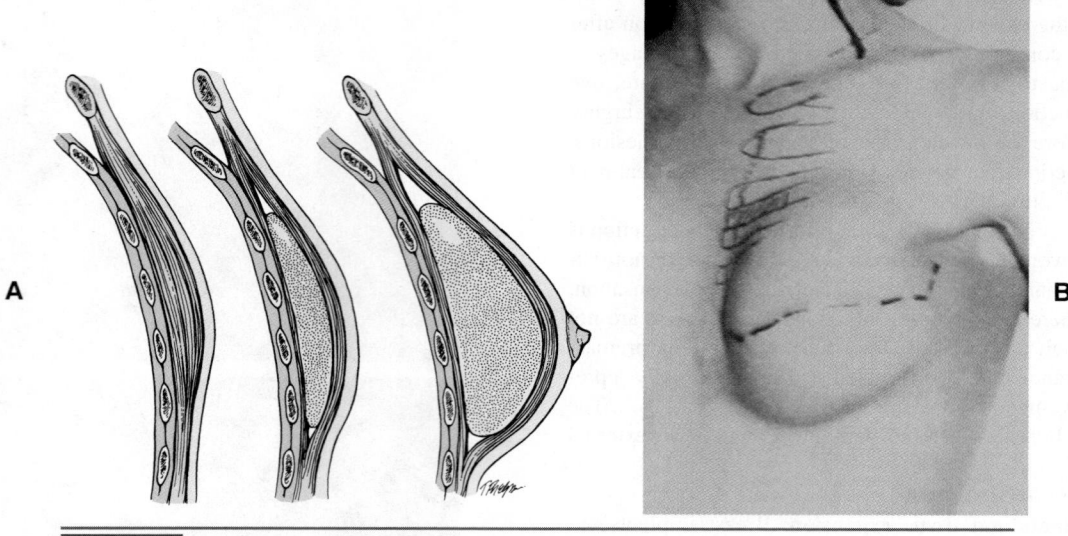

FIG. 50-8   **A,** Tissue expander with gradual expansion. **B,** Tissue expander in place after mastectomy.

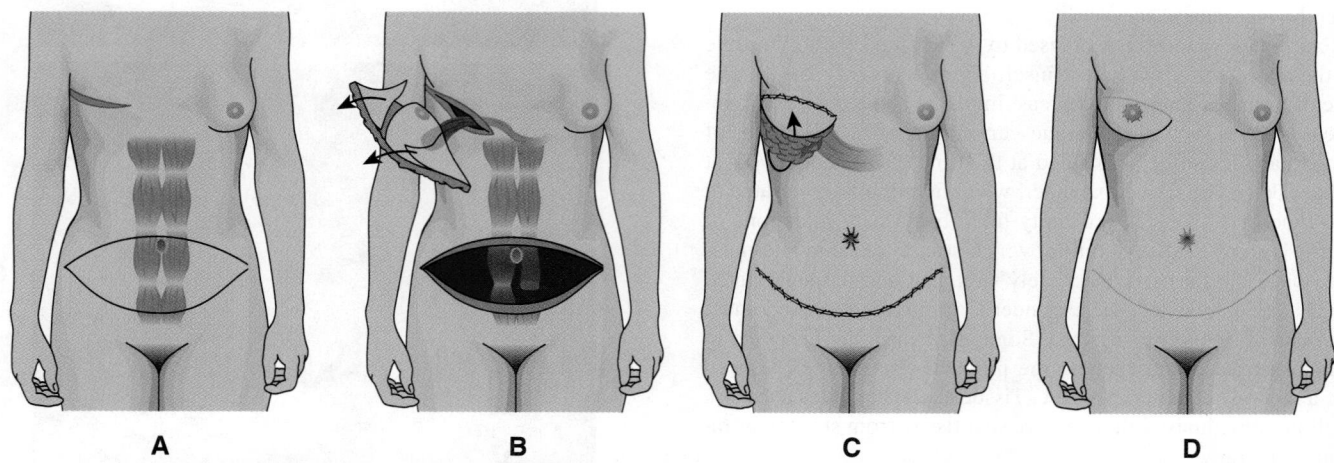

FIG. 50-9   TRAM flap. **A,** TRAM flap is planned. **B,** The abdominal tissue, while attached to the rectus muscle, nerve, and blood supply, is tunneled through the abdomen to the chest. **C,** The flap is trimmed to shape the breast. The lower abdominal incision is closed. **D,** Nipple and areola are reconstructed after the breast is healed.

under the skin up to the area where the breast will be reconstructed. Then it is molded and fashioned to form a breast. The abdominal incision is closed, giving the patient a result that is similar to having an abdominoplasty. This surgical procedure can last 2 to 8 hours, with recovery taking 4 to 6 weeks. Complications include bleeding, hernia, and infection. An implant may be used in addition to the flap if the flap does not provide the desired cosmetic result alone.

Nipple-areolar reconstruction. The majority of patients who have breast reconstruction also have nipple-areolar reconstruc-

tion. Nipple reconstruction gives the reconstructed breast a much more natural appearance. Nipple-areolar reconstruction is usually done a few months after breast reconstruction. Tissue to construct a nipple may be taken from the opposite breast or from a small flap of tissue on the reconstructed breast mound. The areola may be grafted from the labia, skin in area of the groin, or lower abdominal skin, or it may be tattooed with a permanent pigmented dye. In some patients a small implant may be placed under the completed nipple areolar reconstruction to add additional projection.

CRITICAL THINKING EXERCISES

Case Study

Breast Cancer

Patient Profile. Susan Paulson, a 52-year-old white woman, found a large lump in the upper outer quadrant of her left breast while showering.

Subjective Data

- Has family history of breast cancer—mother diagnosed at age 48 and sister diagnosed at age 45
- Had onset of menarche at age 11
- Has two daughters
- Has no prior history of breast cancer
- States she is afraid she has cancer

Objective Data

- Palpable 1.5 cm mass in upper outer quadrant of left breast
- Left breast mass confirmed by mammogram
- Otherwise normal physical examination
- Fine-needle aspiration biopsy of mass indicates diagnosis of breast cancer

Collaborative Care

- Scheduled for lumpectomy and sentinel lymph node dissection

CRITICAL THINKING QUESTIONS

1. What characteristics of malignancy could be determined by palpation of Susan's breast mass?
2. What in Susan's breast cancer experience with her family members might influence her coping response?
3. What information would the nurse provide to Susan about her planned therapy?
4. What are the possible complications the patient may face after a lumpectomy?
5. What are common postoperative exercises that Susan will need to practice if she has an axillary lymph node dissection?
6. What community resources are available to help Susan and her family adjust to the change in her body and to cope with the diagnosis of cancer? How can the nurse access these resources?
7. What information about breast cancer risks is important to provide to Susan and her daughters? What early detection measures are important for them to know?
8. Based on the assessment data presented, write one or more appropriate nursing diagnoses. Are there any collaborative problems?

Nursing Research Issues

1. What are the major concerns of women who are long-term survivors of breast cancer?
2. Do elderly women experience more or fewer sensory changes after breast surgery than young women?
3. Does perceived susceptibility to breast cancer increase a woman's motivation to participate in breast cancer screening?
4. What effect does dietary intake of caffeine have on a woman's perception of the severity of fibrocystic changes in the breast?
5. What influence does immediate versus delayed reconstruction have on the psychosocial adjustment of a woman after a mastectomy?
6. What is the influence of individualized teaching by a health professional on the frequency of breast self-examination practice in women?

REVIEW QUESTIONS

The number of the question corresponds to the same-numbered objective at the beginning of the chapter.

1. The nurse teaches a patient that BSE involves both the palpation of the breast tissue and
   a. palpation of cervical lymph nodes.
   b. hard squeezing of the breast tissue.
   c. a mammogram to evaluate breast tissue.
   d. inspection of the breasts for any changes.

2. An occupational health nurse is planning a program on BSE for women in the company. To best promote learning and compliance of the participants, the nurse includes
   a. a movie that demonstrates the procedure of BSE.
   b. distribution of detailed written instructions for use at home.
   c. explanations emphasizing the value of early detection of breast cancer.
   d. an opportunity to practice BSE on themselves with individual guidance from the nurse.

3. In teaching a patient with painful fibrocystic breast changes about the condition, the nurse explains that
   a. all discrete breast lumps must be biopsied to rule out malignant changes.
   b. the symptoms will probably subside following menopause unless hormone replacement is used.
   c. the lumps will become progressively larger and more painful, eventually necessitating surgical removal.
   d. restrictions of coffee and chocolate and supplements of vitamin E may relieve the discomfort for many patients.

4. While discussing risk factors for breast cancer with a group of women, the nurse stresses that the greatest known risk factor for breast cancer is
   a. being a woman over age 60.
   b. experiencing menstruation for 40 years or more.
   c. using estrogen replacement therapy during menopause.
   d. having a paternal grandmother with postmenopausal breast cancer.

Continued

REVIEW QUESTIONS—cont'd

5. A patient has an excisional biopsy of a breast nodule that is positive for cancer. The nurse explains that of the other tests done to determine the risk for cancer recurrence or spread, the result that supports the most favorable prognosis is
   a. cells with low S-phase fractions.
   b. absence of an HER-2/neu genetic marker.
   c. absence of axillary lymph node involvement.
   d. estrogen and progesterone receptor–positive tumors.

6. A patient diagnosed with breast cancer has been offered the treatment choice of breast conservation surgery with radiation or a modified radical mastectomy. When questioned by the patient about these options, the nurse informs the patient that the lumpectomy with radiation
   a. preserves the normal appearance and sensitivity of the breast.
   b. provides a shorter treatment period with fewer long-term complications.
   c. has about the same 10-year survival rate as the modified radical mastectomy.
   d. reduces the fear and anxiety that accompany the diagnosis and treatment of cancer.

7. Postoperatively the nurse teaches the patient with a modified radical mastectomy to prevent lymphedema by
   a. using a sling to keep the arm flexed at the side.
   b. exposing the arm to sunlight to increase circulation.
   c. wrapping the arm with elastic bandages during the night.
   d. avoiding unnecessary trauma (e.g., venipuncture, blood pressure measurement) to the arm on the operative side.

8. To prevent capsular formation following breast reconstruction with implants, the nurse teaches the patient to
   a. gently massage the area around the implant.
   b. bind the breasts tightly with elastic bandages.
   c. exercise the arm on the affected side to promote drainage.
   d. avoid strenuous exercise until implant healing has occurred.

REFERENCES

1. Jemal A et al: Cancer statistics 2002, *CA Cancer J Clin* 52:23, 2002.
2. American Cancer Society: *Cancer facts and figures 2002,* Atlanta, 2002, American Cancer Society.
3. Smith RA et al: American Cancer Society Guidelines for Breast Cancer Screening: Update 2003, *CA: A Cancer Journal for Clinicians* 53: 141-169, 2003.
4. American Cancer Society (http://www.cancer.org).
*5. Kuyl M: The value of breast self-examination: meta analysis of the literature, *Oncol Nurs Forum* 28:815, 2001.
*6. Lauver D et al: Engagement in breast cancer screening behaviors, *Oncol Nurs Forum* 26:545, 1999.
7. Harvard Women's Health Watch: *Benign breast conditions 5:4,* Boston, 1998, Harvard Women's Health.
8. National Cancer Institute: Cancer facts: questions and answers about screening. Available at *http://cis.nci.nin.gov/fact* (accessed Feb. 15, 2002).
9. Cleveland Clinic: Minimally invasive breast biopsy–stereotactic breast biopsy. Available at *www.clevelandclinic.org/breastcenter/services* (accessed Aug 12, 2002).
10. Padden D: Mastalgia: evaluation and treatment, *Nurse Pract Forum* 11:213, 2000.
11. Arona A: Mastalgia. In Hindle W: *Breast care: a clinical guidebook for women's primary health care providers,* New York, 1999, Springer.
12. Cady B et al: Evaluation of common breast problems: guidance for primary care providers, *CA Cancer J Clin* 48:49, 1998.
13. McCance KL, Huether SE, editors: *Pathophysiology: biologic basis for disease in adults and children,* ed 4, St Louis, 2002, Mosby.
14. Jarvis C: *Physical examination and health assessment,* ed 4, St Louis, 2004, WB Saunders.
15. American Cancer Society: *Breast cancer facts and figures 2001-2002,* Atlanta, 2001, American Cancer Society.
16. Schairer C et al: Menopausal estrogen and estrogen-progestin replacement therapy and breast cancer risk, *JAMA* 283:485, 2000.
17. Nurses' Health Study: Risks and benefits of oral contraceptives and postmenopausal hormones, *Nurses' Health Study Newsletter* 5:6, 1998.
18. Giuliano A: Breast. In Tierney L, McPhee S, Papadakis M, editors: *Current medical diagnosis and treatment 2001,* ed 40, New York, 2001, Lange.
19. Vogel V: Breast cancer prevention: a review of current evidence, *CA Cancer J Clin* 50:156, 2000.
20. Kauff ND et al: Risk-reducing salpingo-oophorectomy in women with a BRCA-1 or BRCA-2 mutation, *N Engl J Med* 346:1609, 2002.
21. Rebbeck TR et al: Prophylactic oophorectomy in carriers of BRCA-1 or BRCA-2 mutation, *N Engl J Med* 346:1609, 2002.
22. Hartmann LC, Schaid DJ, Woods JE: Efficiency of bilateral prophylactic mastectomy in women with a family history of breast cancer, *N Engl J Med* 340:77, 1999.
23. Westendorp J: Sentinel lymph node dissection in breast cancer, *Innovations in Breast Cancer Care* 5:94, 2001.
24. Hsueh E, Hansen N, Giuliano A: Intraoperative lymphatic mapping and sentinel lymph node dissection in breast cancer, *CA Cancer J Clin* 50:279, 2000.
25. Hubbard S, Goodman M, Knobf MT: HER-2, herceptin, and breast cancer, *Oncology Nursing Updates* 7:1, 2000.
26. American Joint Committee on Cancer: *Manual for staging of cancer,* ed 4, Philadelphia, 1992, Lippincott.
27. Petrek J, Pressman P, Smith R: Lymphedema: current issues in research and management, *CA Cancer J Clin* 50:292, 2000.
28. Hamolsky D, Facione N: Infiltrating breast cancer. In Miaskowski C, Buchsel P: *Oncology nursing: assessment and clinical care,* St Louis, 1999, Mosby.
29. Aikin J: Adjuvant therapy for breast cancer: choices and challenges, *Innovations in Breast Cancer Care* 5:3, 2000.
30. National Institutes of Health: Adjuvant therapy for breast cancer, *NIH Consensus Statement 2000* 17:1, Nov 2000. Available at *http://consensus.nih.gov* (accessed Dec 28, 2002).
31. Dunn B, Ford L: Breast cancer prevention: results of the National Surgical Adjuvant Breast and Bowel Project (NSABP) breast cancer prevention trial, *Eur J Cancer* 36(suppl 4):S49, 2000.
32. Machia J: Breast cancer: risk, prevention and tamoxifen, *Am J Nurs* 101:26, 2001.
33. Rees C, Bath P: Information-seeking behaviors of women with breast cancer, *Oncol Nurs Forum* 28:899, 2001.
34. Hosleins C, Haber J: Adjusting to breast cancer, *Am J Nurs* 100:26, 2000.
35. Ferrell B et al: Quality of life in breast cancer survivors: implications for developing support services, *Oncol Nurs Forum* 25:887, 1998.

*Nursing research–based reference.

36. Fortunato N, McCullough SM: *Plastic and reconstructive surgery,* St Louis, 1998, Mosby.

*37. Neil K, Armstrong N, Burnett C: Choosing reconstruction after mastectomy: a qualitative analysis, *Oncol Nurs Forum* 25:743, 1998.

38. Thomas S, Greifzu S: Breast reconstruction, *RN* 63:45, 2000.

RESOURCES

American Cancer Society—Reach to Recovery
1599 Clifton Road NE
Atlanta, GA 30329
800-ACS-2345
www.cancer.org

American Society of Plastic Surgeons
Plastic Surgery Education Foundation
444 East Algonquin Road
Arlington Heights, IL
888-475-2784
www.plasticsurgery.org

Breast Cancer Information Center
www.feminist.org/other/bc/bchome.html

Living Beyond Breast Cancer
Survivors' helpline: 888-753-5222
610-645-4567
www.lbbc.org

National Alliance of Breast Cancer Organizations
9 East 37th Street, 10th Floor
New York, NY 10016
888-80-NABCO
212-889-0606
Fax: 212-689-1213
www.nabco.org

National Breast Cancer Coalition
1707 L Street, NW, Suite 1060
Washington, DC 20036
202-296-7477
Fax: 202-265-6854
www.natlbcc.org/

National Cancer Institute
Suite 3036A
6116 Executive Boulevard, MSC8322
Bethesda, MD 20892-8322
800-4-CANCER
www.nci.nih.gov

National Coalition for Cancer Survivorship (NCCS)
1010 Wayne Avenue, Suite 770
Silver Spring, MD 20910
877-622-7936
301-650-9127
Fax: 301-565-9670
www.cansearch.org/

National Lymphedema Network (NLN)
Latham Square
1611 Telegraph Avenue, Suite 1111
Oakland, CA 94612-2138
Hotline: 800-541-3259 or 510-208-3200
Fax: 510-208-3110
www.lymphnet.org/

OncoLink (cancer information site)
University of Pennsylvania Cancer Center
www.oncolink.upenn.edu

Oncology Nursing Society
501 Holiday Drive
Pittsburgh, PA 15220
412-921-7373
Fax: 412-921-6565
www.ons.org

Sisters Network (a national support group for African American breast cancer patients)
8787 Woodway Drive, Suite 4206
Houston, TX 77063
713-781-0255
Fax: 713-780-8998
www.sistersnetworkinc.org

Susan G. Komen Breast Cancer Foundation
800-462-9273
www.komen.org

Y-me National Breast Cancer Organization
212 West Van Buren, Suite 500
Chicago, IL 60607
800-221-2141
312-986-8338
Fax: 312-294-8597
www.Y-me.org

For additional Internet resources, see the website for this book at *http://evolve.elsevier.com/Lewis/medsurg/.*

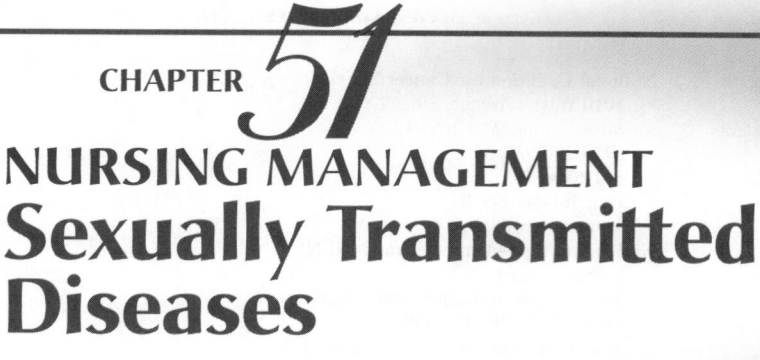

CHAPTER 51

NURSING MANAGEMENT
Sexually Transmitted Diseases

Shannon Ruff Dirksen

LEARNING OBJECTIVES

1. Identify the factors contributing to the high incidence of sexually transmitted diseases.
2. Explain the etiology, clinical manifestations, complications, and diagnostic abnormalities of gonorrhea, syphilis, chlamydial infections, genital herpes, and genital warts.
3. Compare primary genital herpes with recurrent genital herpes.
4. Explain the collaborative care and drug therapy of gonorrhea, syphilis, chlamydial infections, genital herpes, and genital warts.

5. Identify the nursing assessment and nursing diagnoses for patients who have a sexually transmitted disease.
6. Describe the nursing role in the prevention and control of sexually transmitted diseases.
7. Describe the nursing management of patients with sexually transmitted diseases.

KEY TERMS

chancres, p. 1387
chlamydial infections, p. 1390
genital herpes, p. 1392
gonorrhea, p. 1385
gummas, p. 1388
lymphogranuloma venereum, p. 1391
sexually transmitted diseases, p. 1384
syphilis, p. 1387
tabes dorsalis, p. 1389
venereal diseases, p. 1384

Sexually Transmitted Diseases

Sexually transmitted diseases (STDs) are infectious diseases transmitted most commonly through sexual contact (Table 51-1). Historically they have been referred to as **venereal diseases.** Many of the agents causing STDs are easily inactivated by drying, heating, and washing. These infections can be bacterial (gonorrhea, chlamydia, syphilis) and/or viral (genital herpes, genital warts). Most infections start as lesions on the genitalia and other sexually exposed mucous membranes. Wide dissemination to other areas of the body can then occur. A latent or subclinical phase is present with all STDs. This can lead to a long-term persistent infection and the transmission of disease from an asymptomatic (but infected) person to another contact. Different STDs can coexist within one person. For example, if a person has gonorrhea, chlamydial infection may also be present.

In the United States all cases of gonorrhea and syphilis, and in most states chlamydial infection, must be reported to the state or local public health authorities. In spite of this requirement, there are many unreported cases of these infections. An estimated 65 million Americans are currently infected with one or more STDs.[1] Every year an additional 15 million Americans are newly infected with an STD.[2] Diseases that are associated with sexual

transmission can also be contracted by other routes such as through blood, blood products, and autoinoculation.

The more commonly diagnosed STDs are discussed in this chapter. Human immunodeficiency virus (HIV) infection and related problems are discussed in Chapter 14. Hepatitis B infection and related problems are discussed in Chapter 42.

Factors Affecting Incidence of Sexually Transmitted Diseases

Many contributing factors are related to the current STD rates. Earlier reproductive maturity and increased longevity have resulted in a longer sexual life span. The increase in the total population has resulted in an increase in the number of susceptible hosts. Other factors include greater sexual freedom, changing roles of women, decreased social control by religious institu-

TABLE 51-1	Microorganisms Responsible for Diseases Transmitted by Sexual Activity
ORGANISM	**DISEASE**
Chlamydia trachomatis	Nongonococcal urethritis (NGU); cervicitis; lymphogranuloma venereum
Cytomegalovirus (CMV)	Multiple diseases
Hepatitis B virus	Hepatitis B
Herpes simplex virus (HSV)	Genital herpes
Human immunodeficiency virus (HIV)	HIV infection, acquired immunodeficiency syndrome (AIDS)
Human papillomavirus	Genital warts
Poxvirus	Molluscum contagiosum
Neisseria gonorrhoeae	Gonorrhea
Treponema pallidum	Syphilis

Reviewed by Dana Rosdahl, RN-C, PhD(c), FNP, Instructor, Arizona State University, Tempe, Ariz.

tions, and an increased emphasis in the media on sexuality. In addition, increased leisure time, inexpensive travel, and urbanization have brought together people with varying social behaviors and value systems.

Changes in the methods of contraception are also reflected in the incidence of STDs. The condom is considered to be the only contraceptive device that is prophylactic in regard to STDs. Although condom use is increasing in selected populations, it is not used frequently in the general population. Commonly used oral contraceptives cause the secretions of the cervix and the vagina to become more alkaline. This change produces a more favorable environment for the growth of organisms that cause STDs at these sites. Women who take oral contraceptives have a lower risk of pelvic inflammatory disease (PID) as a result of the ability of the cervical mucus to act as a barrier against bacteria. However, the proliferation of chlamydia, the leading cause of non-gonococcal PID, may be enhanced by oral contraceptive use. Whether or not intrauterine device (IUD) users are at increased risk of PID is controversial, but it is clear that IUDs confer no protection against STDs.[3] Long-acting contraceptives such as levonorgestrel (Norplant) and medroxyprogesterone (Depo-Provera) have been shown to lower the concurrent use of condoms, even among women with risk factors for STDs.[4] Both Norplant and Depo-Provera confer no protection against STDs. Lack of awareness of this fact may be a factor leading to STDs in people using these products.

Bacterial Infections

GONORRHEA

Gonorrhea is the second most frequently occurring STD. Following a 73.9% decline in the reported rate of gonorrhea from 1975 to 1997, the gonorrhea rate increased in 1998.[5] The overall rate of gonorrhea in the United States since 1998 has remained essentially unchanged even though true increases may have occurred in some populations and geographic areas. In 2000, 358,995 cases of gonorrhea were reported in the United States. The incidence of gonorrhea is highest among people under 24 years old living in high-density urban areas who have multiple sex partners and unprotected sexual intercourse. Increases have also been noted among men who have sex with men. Most states have enacted laws that permit examination and treatment of minors without parental consent.

Etiology and Pathophysiology

Gonorrhea is caused by *Neisseria gonorrhoeae,* a gram-negative diplococcus. The disease is spread by direct physical contact with an infected host, usually during sexual activity (vaginal, oral, or anal). Mucosa with columnar epithelium is susceptible to gonococcal infection. This tissue is present in the genitalia (urethra in men, cervix in women), the rectum, and the oropharynx. Neonates can develop a gonococcal infection during delivery from an infected mother. The delicate gonococcus is easily killed by drying, heating, or washing with an antiseptic solution. Consequently, indirect transmission by instruments or linens is rare. The incubation period is 3 to 4 days. The disease confers no immunity to subsequent reinfection. Gonococcal infection elicits an inflammatory response, which, if left untreated, leads to the formation of fibrous tissue and adhesions. This fi-

brous scarring is subsequently responsible for many complications in women such as strictures and tubal abnormalities, which can lead to tubal pregnancy, chronic pelvic pain, and infertility.

Clinical Manifestations

Men. The initial site of infection in heterosexual men is usually the urethra. Symptoms of urethritis consist of dysuria and profuse, purulent urethral discharge developing 2 to 5 days after infection (Fig. 51-1). Painful or swollen testicles may also occur. Men generally seek medical evaluation early in the disease because their symptoms are usually obvious and distressing. It is unusual for men with gonorrhea to be asymptomatic.

Women. Most women who contract gonorrhea are asymptomatic or have minor symptoms that are often overlooked, making it possible for them to remain a source of infection. A few women may complain of vaginal discharge, dysuria, or frequency of urination. Changes in menstruation may be a symptom, but these changes are often disregarded by the woman. After the incubation period, redness and swelling occur at the site of contact, which is usually the cervix or urethra (Fig. 51-2). A purulent exudate often develops with a potential for abscess formation. The disease may remain local or can spread by direct tissue extension to the uterus, fallopian tubes, and ovaries. Although the vulva and vagina are uncommon sites for a gonorrheal infection, they may become involved when little or no estrogen is present, as is the case in prepubertal girls and postmenopausal women. Because the vagina acts as a natural reservoir for infectious secretions,

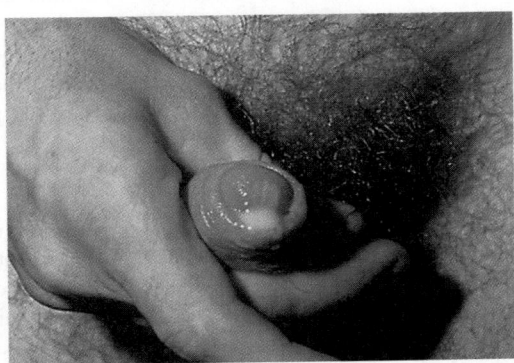

FIG. 51-1 Gonococcal urethritis. Profuse, purulent drainage.

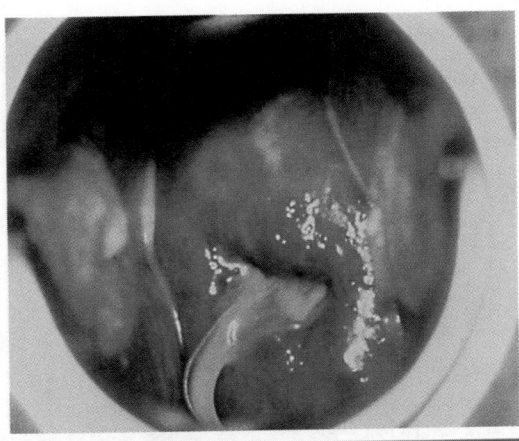

FIG. 51-2 Endocervical gonorrhea. Cervical redness and edema with discharge.

transmission is often more efficient from men to women than it is from women to men.

General. Anorectal gonorrhea may be present and is usually caused by anal intercourse. Symptoms may include soreness, itching, and discharge. Most patients with rectal infections and infections in the throat have few symptoms. A small percentage of individuals develop gonococcal pharyngitis resulting from orogenital sexual contact. When the gonococcus can be demonstrated by a laboratory culture, individuals of either gender are infectious to their sexual partners.

Complications

Because men often seek treatment early in the course of the disease, they are less likely to develop complications. The complications that do occur in men are prostatitis, urethral strictures, and sterility from orchitis or epididymitis. Because women who are asymptomatic seldom seek treatment, complications are more common and usually constitute the reason for seeking medical attention. Pelvic inflammatory disease (PID), Bartholin's abscess, ectopic pregnancy, and infertility are the main complications of gonorrhea in women. A small percentage of infected persons, mainly women, may develop a disseminated gonococcal infection (DGI). In DGI the appearance of skin lesions, fever, arthralgia, or arthritis usually causes the patient to seek medical help (Fig. 51-3).

Eye Infections in Newborns. Almost all states have a health department regulation or law requiring the instillation of a prophylactic drug such as erythromycin (0.5%) ophthalmic ointment or silver nitrate (0.1%) aqueous solution into the eyes of all newborns in a single application. The incidence of gonorrheal eye infections in newborns *(ophthalmia neonatorum)* is therefore relatively rare today. Untreated infected infants develop permanent blindness.

Diagnostic Studies

The immediate identification of *N. gonorrhoeae* is usually made with a Gram stain of smears made from the exudate. The slides should be interpreted by an experienced technician so that a correct diagnosis is made initially, because some patients fail to return for follow-up care. A reliable way to confirm gonococcal infection is to isolate the organism in culture. Cultures of the discharge or secretion can provide a definitive diagnosis after

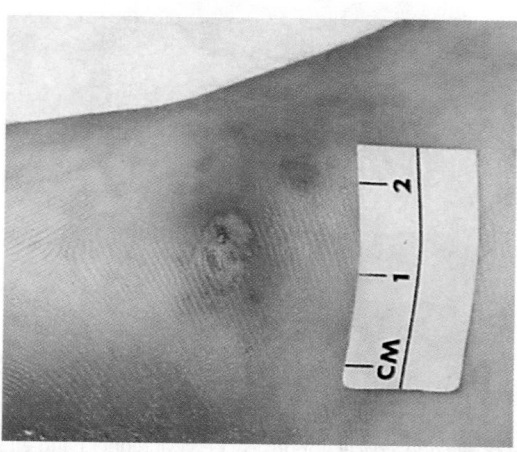

FIG. 51-3 Disseminated gonococcal infection. Skin lesion with gray, necrotic center on erythematous base.

incubation for 24 to 48 hours. Whenever practical, the swab from any mucosal site should be inoculated immediately onto a special growth medium (Thayer-Martin medium) at room temperature, and then placed promptly in an enriched CO_2 environment and incubated. However, various nonnutrient transport media are adequate if the specimen can be transported to the laboratory without refrigeration and inoculated onto the growth medium within 6 hours.

For men, a presumptive diagnosis of gonorrhea is made if there is a history of sexual contact with a new or infected partner followed within a few days by a urethral discharge. Typical clinical manifestations, combined with a positive finding in a Gram-stained smear of the purulent discharge from the penis, gives an almost certain diagnosis. A culture of the discharge is indicated for men whose smears are negative in the presence of strong clinical evidence.

Making a diagnosis of gonorrhea in women on the basis of symptoms is difficult because most women are symptom free or have complaints that may be confused with other conditions. Smears and purulent discharge do not establish a diagnosis of gonorrhea because the female genitourinary tract normally harbors a large number of organisms that resemble *N. gonorrhoeae.* A culture must be performed to confirm the diagnosis. Although the cervix is the most common site of sampling, specimens for culture may also be taken from the urethra, anus, or oropharynx to confirm the diagnosis. The Centers for Disease Control and Prevention (CDC) recommends that all women treated for gonorrhea have a rectal culture done.

A new technique, DNA amplification using polymerase chain reaction (PCR) or ligase chain reaction (LCR), is being used to diagnose gonorrhea. (PCR is discussed in Chapter 13.) This testing technique does not involve culture and is a quicker approach to detecting infection. DNA amplification has a high rate of sensitivity and specificity. The test can be performed on urine, vaginal fluid or discharge, or urethral secretions. This eliminates the need for a urethral swab in male patients and potentially the necessity for pelvic examination in female patients.

Collaborative Care

Drug Therapy. Because of a short incubation period and high infectivity, treatment is generally instituted without awaiting culture results, even in the absence of any signs or symptoms. The treatment of gonorrhea in the early stage is curative. Traditionally, the drug of choice for gonorrheal therapy had been penicillin, but changes have been made because of resistant strains of *N. gonorrhoeae.* As a result of penicillin-resistant strains, ceftriaxone (Rocephin), a penicillinase-resistant cephalosporin, or cefixime (Suprax), ciprofloxacin (Cipro), ofloxacin (Floxin), or levofloxacin (Levaquin) has become part of the treatment plan (Table 51-2). The recommended drug regimen has resulted in a success rate of at least 95% in eliminating uncomplicated urogenital and anorectal gonococcal infections.[6] Resistance to the fluoroquinolones, such as ciprofloxacin (Cipro), has been reported, and although still somewhat rare, is a cause for concern. The high frequency (up to 20% in men and 40% in women) of coexisting chlamydial and gonococcal infections has led to the addition of azithromycin (Zithromax) or doxycycline (Vibramycin) to the treatment regimen. Patients with coexisting syphilis are likely to be cured by the same drugs used for gonorrhea.

All sexual contacts of patients with gonorrhea must be evaluated and treated to prevent reinfection after resumption of sexual

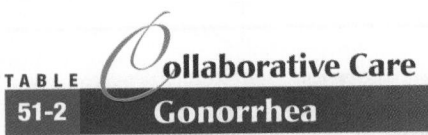

TABLE 51-2   Collaborative Care — Gonorrhea

Diagnostic
History and physical examination
Gram-stained smears of urethral or endocervical exudate
Cultures for *N. gonorrhoeae*
DNA amplification to detect *N. gonorrhoeae*
Testing for other STDs (syphilis, HIV, chlamydia)

Collaborative Therapy
Uncomplicated gonorrhea: cefixime (Suprax) 400 mg orally in
   a single dose or ceftriaxone (Rocephin) 125 mg IM in a
   single dose or ciprofloxacin (Cipro) 500 mg orally in a
   single dose or ofloxacin (Floxin) 400 mg orally in a single
   dose or levofloxacin (Levaquin) 250 mg orally in a single
   dose
If chlamydial infection is not ruled out: azithromycin (Zithromax) 1 g orally in a single dose or doxycycline (Vibramycin)
   100 mg orally twice a day for 7 days
Patients who are allergic to cephalosporins or quinolones
   should be treated with spectinomycin
Patients who have uncomplicated gonorrhea and who are
   treated with any of the above therapies may not need to
   return to confirm that they are cured
Case finding
Treatment of sexual contacts
Instruction on abstinence from sexual intercourse and alcohol
Reexamination if symptoms persist or recur after completion
   of treatment

Modified from Centers for Disease Control and Prevention: STD treatment guide-lines, *MMWR* 51(RR-6):1, 2002.
HIV, Human immunodeficiency virus; *IM,* intramuscular; *STD,* sexually transmitted disease.

relations. The "ping-pong" effect of reexposure, treatment, and reinfection can cease only when infected partners are treated simultaneously. Additionally, the patient should be counseled to abstain from sexual intercourse and alcohol during treatment. Sexual intercourse allows the infection to spread and can delay complete healing. Alcohol has an irritant effect on the healing urethral walls. Men should be cautioned against squeezing the penis to look for further discharge. Follow-up examination and reculture may be done at least once after treatment, usually in 4 to 7 days. Reinfection, rather than treatment failure, is the main cause for infections identified after treatment has ended.

SYPHILIS

The incidence of **syphilis** reported in the United States in 2000 is at its lowest rate since reporting started in 1941.[7] In 2000 only 5979 cases of syphilis were reported in the United States. The credit for this decline is a national effort that began in 1999 that focuses on community-based prevention programs, faster response to outbreaks, and better access to clinics.[8] However, syphilis remains an important health problem.

Etiology and Pathophysiology

The causative organism of syphilis is *Treponema pallidum,* a spirochete. This bacterium is thought to enter the body through very small breaks in the skin or mucous membranes. Its entry is facilitated by the minor abrasions that often occur during sexual

intercourse. Syphilis is a complex disease in which many organs and tissues of the body can become infected by *T. pallidum.* The infection causes the production of antibodies that also react with normal tissues. After a short period of protection, the antibody levels decrease, and a person is susceptible to reinfection.[9] Not all people who are exposed to syphilis acquire the disease; about one third become infected after intercourse with an infected person. In addition to sexual contact, syphilis may be spread through contact with infectious lesions and sharing of needles among intravenous (IV) drug users. *T. pallidum* is extremely fragile and easily destroyed by drying, heating, or washing. The incubation period for syphilis ranges from 10 to 90 days (average 21 days). Congenital syphilis is transmitted from an infected mother to the fetus in utero after the tenth week of pregnancy. The rate of infant death is up to 40% of women untreated for syphilis.[10]

More so than for gonorrhea, those with untreated syphilis tend to be young persons of a low educational and socioeconomic level who have limited access to health care. Racial disparities also exist, with African Americans having syphilis at a rate 30 times greater than the rate for whites.[1]

There is an association between syphilis and HIV infection. Persons at high risk for acquiring syphilis are also at an increased risk for acquiring HIV. Often, both infections may be present in the same person. The presence of syphilitic lesions on the genitals enhances HIV transmission. HIV-infected patients with syphilis appear to be at greatest risk for clinically significant central nervous system (CNS) involvement and may require more intensive treatment with penicillin than do other patients with syphilis. Therefore the evaluation of all patients with syphilis should also include testing for HIV with the patient's consent.

Clinical Manifestations

Syphilis has a variety of signs and symptoms that can mimic a number of other diseases. Consequently, compared with other STDs, it is more difficult to recognize syphilis. If it is not treated, specific clinical stages are characteristic of the progression of the disease (Table 51-3). In the *primary stage* of the bacterial invasion (Fig. 51-4), **chancres** appear. These are painless indurated lesions on the penis, vulva, lips, mouth, vagina, and rectum. They frequently occur 10 to 90 days after inoculation. The chancre lasts 3 to 6 weeks, eventually healing on its own. During this time the draining of the microorganisms into the lymph nodes causes regional lymphadenopathy. Genital ulcers may also be present. Without treatment the infection progresses to the secondary stage.

The *secondary stage* of syphilis is systemic. The stage begins a few weeks after the chancres are first seen. During this stage blood-borne bacteria spread to all major organ systems. Manifestations characteristic of the secondary stage can include cutaneous eruptions, fever, alopecia (hair loss), sore throat, headaches, weight loss, tiredness, and generalized adenopathy. The cutaneous eruptions (Fig. 51-5) include a bilateral, symmetric rash usually involving the palms and soles; mucous patches in the mouth, tongue, or cervix; and condylomata lata (moist, weeping papules) in the anal and genital area.

The *latent* or *hidden stage* of syphilis follows the secondary stage and is a period during which the immune system is able to suppress the infection. The latent stage can be further divided into an early stage, in which the infection has been acquired in the preceding year, and a late stage, in which the infection has been present for greater than 1 year. There are no signs or symptoms of syphilis during this time. During the latent stage, the di-

TABLE 51-3	Stages of Syphilis		
CLINICAL STAGE	**CHARACTERISTIC FINDINGS**	**COMMUNICABILITY**	**DURATION OF STAGE**
Primary	Chancre	Exudate from chancre highly infectious; blood is infectious	3-8 wk
Secondary	Cutaneous eruptions, alopecia, systemic symptoms (malaise, arthralgia, headache, occasionally liver and kidney dysfunction), regional adenopathy 6-12 wk after chancre	Exudate from skin and mucous membrane lesions highly infectious	1-2 yr
Latent	Absence of signs or symptoms	Noninfectious after 4 yr, possible placental transmission	Throughout life or progression to late stage
Late*	Appearance 3-20 yr after initial infection	Noninfectious	Chronic (without treatment), possibly fatal
Benign	Gummas (chronic, destructive lesions affecting any organ of body, especially skin, bone, liver, mucous membranes)	Spinal fluid possibly containing organism	
Cardiovascular	Aortic valve insufficiency or saccular aneurysm of thoracic aorta, aortitis		
Neurosyphilis	General paresis (personality changes from minor to psychotic, tremors, physical and mental deterioration)		
	Tabes dorsalis (ataxia, areflexia, paresthesias, lightning pains, damaged joints [Charcot's joints])		

*Several forms such as cardiovascular and neurosyphilis occur together in approximately 25% of untreated cases.

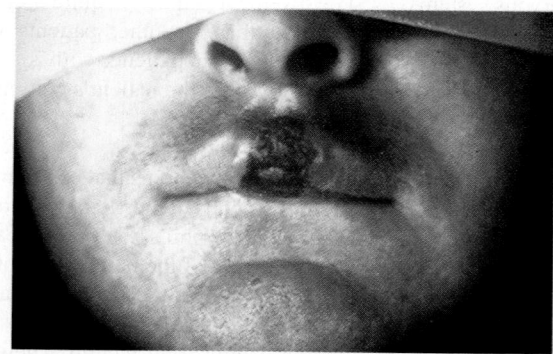

FIG. 51-4 Primary syphilis chancre on upper lip.

agnosis is established by a positive specific treponemal antibody test for syphilis together with a normal cerebrospinal fluid (CSF) examination and the absence of clinical manifestations on physical examination and chest x-rays. About 70% of untreated patients with latent syphilis never develop clinically evident, third-stage syphilis, but the occurrence of a spontaneous cure of syphilis is doubtful.[11]

The *third stage* of syphilis (also called *late* or *tertiary* syphilis) is the most severe stage of the disease. Because antibiotics can cure syphilis, manifestations of late syphilis are rare. However, when it does occur, it is responsible for significant morbidity and mortality rates. The pathogenesis of the manifestations of this stage is unclear. **Gummas** (destructive skin, bone, and soft tissue nodular lesions associated with late syphilis) are probably caused by a severe hypersensitivity reaction to the microorganism. Within the cardiovascular system late syphilis may cause aneurysms, heart valve insufficiency, and heart failure. Within the CNS the presence of *T. pallidum* in CSF may cause manifestations of *neurosyphilis* (general paresis) (see Table 51-3).

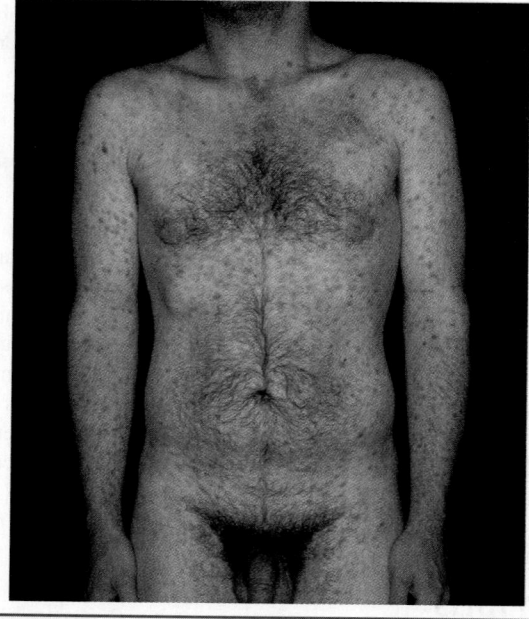

FIG. 51-5 Secondary syphilis. Bilateral, symmetric cutaneous lesions.

Complications

Complications of the disease occur mostly in late syphilis. The gummas of benign late syphilis may produce irreparable damage to bone, liver, or skin but seldom result in death. In cardiovascular syphilis, the resulting aneurysm may press on structures such as the intercostal nerves, causing pain. The possibility of a rupture exists as the aneurysm increases in size. Scarring of the aortic valve results in aortic valve insufficiency and eventually heart failure.

Neurosyphilis is responsible for degeneration of the brain with mental deterioration. Evidence of other neurologic deficits may be present. Problems related to sensory nerve involvement are a result of **tabes dorsalis** (progressive locomotor ataxia). There may be sudden attacks of pain anywhere in the body, which can confuse the diagnosis with other conditions. Loss of vision and sense of position in the feet and legs can also occur. Walking may become even more difficult as joint stability is lost. (Late syphilis is also discussed in Chapter 57.)

Diagnostic Studies

The first step in diagnosis is to obtain a detailed and accurate sexual history. A physical examination should be done to identify any suspicious lesions, as well as to note other significant signs and symptoms.

The presence of spirochetes on dark-field microscopy and direct fluorescent antibody tests of lesion exudate or tissue can confirm a clinical diagnosis of syphilis. However, syphilis is more commonly diagnosed by a serologic test. Tests for syphilis may be classified as those performed for screening and those per-

formed for confirmation of a positive screening test. Nonspecific antitreponemal antibodies can be detected by tests such as the Venereal Disease Research Laboratory (VDRL) test and the rapid plasma reagin (RPR) test. These nontreponemal tests are suitable for screening purposes and usually become positive 10 to 14 days after the appearance of a chancre. The fluorescent treponemal antibody absorption (FTA-ABS) test and the microhemagglutination (MHA) test detect specific antitreponemal antibodies and are suitable for confirming the diagnosis.

False-negative and false-positive test results do occur with the nontreponemal tests (VDRL, RPR). A false-negative result may be obtained during primary syphilis if the test is done before the individual has had time to produce antibodies. A false-positive finding may occur with other diseases or conditions such as hepatitis, infectious mononucleosis, after smallpox vaccination, collagen diseases (e.g., systemic lupus erythematosus), pregnancy, or aging. Positive nontreponemal test results should be confirmed by more specific treponemal tests to rule out other causes. In the CSF, changes such as increased white blood cell count, increased total protein, and a positive treponemal antibody test are diagnostic of asymptomatic neurosyphilis.

If a patient is treated with antibiotics early in the course of the disease on the basis of the history and the symptoms, the serologic testing may not indicate the presence of syphilis. Once a person has positive serologic findings for syphilis, indicating the presence of antibodies, these findings may remain positive for an indefinite period in spite of successful treatment.

Collaborative Care

Drug Therapy. Management of syphilis is aimed at eradication of all syphilitic organisms (Table 51-4). However, treatment cannot reverse damage that is already present in the late stage of the disease. Benzathine penicillin G (Bicillin) or aqueous procaine penicillin G remains the treatment of choice for all stages of syphilis. To date, after four decades of use, there is no evidence to suggest a decrease in the effectiveness of penicillin against *T. pallidum*. Table 51-5 describes therapy for the various stages of syphilis and is in accordance with U.S. Public Health Service recommendations. All stages of syphilis should be

TABLE 51-4 Collaborative Care — Syphilis

Diagnostic
History and physical examination
Dark-field microscopy
Nontreponemal or treponemal serologic testing
Testing for other STDs (HIV, gonorrhea, chlamydia)

Collaborative Therapy
Appropriate drug therapy (see Table 51-5)
Confidential counseling and testing for HIV infection
Case finding
Surveillance
 Repeat of quantitative nontreponemal tests at 3, 6, and 12 mo
 Examination of cerebrospinal fluid at 1 year if treatment involves alternative antibiotics or treatment failure has occurred

HIV, Human immunodeficiency virus; *STD,* sexually transmitted disease.

TABLE 51-5 Drug Therapy — Syphilis

STAGE	TYPE OF PENICILLIN	OTHER ANTIBIOTICS*
Early syphilis (primary, secondary, and early latent)	2.4 million U IM of penicillin G benzathine (Bicillin) in a single dose	doxycycline (Vibramycin) 100 mg orally twice a day for 2 wk, or tetracycline 500 mg orally four times a day for 2 wk
Re-treatment, if needed	7.2 million U of Bicillin total, given as 3 doses of 2.4 million U IM of Bicillin each, at 1 wk intervals	
Late latent syphilis	7.2 million U total of Bicillin given as 3 doses of 2.4 million U IM of Bicillin each at 1 wk intervals	doxycycline or tetracycline given for 4 wk at same dosage/routes as early syphilis
Tertiary syphilis		
Gumma, cardiovascular	Same as for re-treatment and late latent stage	Same as for late latent stage
Neurosyphilis	Aqueous crystalline penicillin G 18-24 U IV daily, given as 3-4 million U every 4 hr for 10-14 days	procaine penicillin 2.4 million U IM once daily plus probenecid (Benemid) 500 mg orally 4 times a day; both drugs given for 10-14 days

Modified from Centers for Disease Control and Prevention: STD treatment guidelines, *MMWR* 51(RR-6):1, 2002.
*Given when penicillin is contraindicated.
IM, Intramuscular; *IV,* intravenous.

treated. Patients having persistent or recurring symptoms after drug therapy has ended should be re-treated. All patients with neurosyphilis must be carefully monitored, with periodic serologic testing, clinical evaluation at 6-month intervals, and repeat CSF examinations for at least 3 years. Specific management is based on the symptoms.

Appropriate penicillin treatment according to the stage of syphilis before the eighteenth week of pregnancy prevents maternal transmission to the fetus. Appropriate treatment after 18 weeks of pregnancy usually cures both mother and fetus because the antibiotics can cross the placental barrier. Treatment administered in the second half of pregnancy may pose a risk of premature labor and fetal distress. Some authorities recommend hospitalization and fetal monitoring of women at 20 weeks of gestation or greater.[12]

CHLAMYDIAL INFECTIONS

Chlamydial infections are the most prevalent bacterial STDs in the United States today. More than 650,000 cases are reported annually, and three of every four cases reported occurred in persons under age 25.[13] As many as 3 million Americans per year may be infected with chlamydia. Underreporting is substantial because most people are asymptomatic and do not seek testing. Chlamydial infections are a major contributor to PID, ectopic pregnancy, infertility among women, and nongonococcal urethritis in men.

Etiology and Pathophysiology

Chlamydial infections are caused by *Chlamydia trachomatis,* a gram-negative bacterium. Chlamydia can be transmitted during vaginal, anal, or oral sex. Numerous different serotypes, or strains, of *C. trachomatis* cause urogenital infections (e.g., nongonococcal urethritis [NGU] in men and cervicitis in women), ocular trachoma, and lymphogranuloma venereum. Women with chlamydial infections during the second week of pregnancy are two to three times more likely to have a preterm birth.[14]

Chlamydia is largely underreported because most people infected are asymptomatic and do not seek health care.[5] By age 30, it is estimated that at sometime during their lives 50% of all sexually active women have had a chlamydial infection. Women with chlamydia may also be at high risk for acquiring HIV from an infected partner.

Because chlamydial infections are closely associated with gonococcal infections, clinical differentiation may be difficult (Table 51-6). Therefore both infections are usually treated concurrently even without diagnostic evidence. The incubation period of 1 to 3 weeks for chlamydial infection is longer than that for gonorrhea, and the symptoms are often milder. The high incidence of recurrence may be because of failure to treat the sexual partners of infected persons. Table 51-7 lists the risk factors for chlamydial infection. Because of the high prevalence of asymptomatic infections, screening of high risk populations is needed to identify those infected.

Clinical Manifestations and Complications

Chlamydia is known as a silent disease because symptoms may be absent or minor in most infected women and in many men. As with gonorrhea, chlamydial infections result in a superficial mucosal infection that can become more invasive. Signs and symptoms in men include urethritis (dysuria, urethral dis-

charge), epididymitis (unilateral scrotal pain, swelling, tenderness, fever), and proctitis (rectal discharge and pain during defecation) (Fig. 51-6). Signs and symptoms in women include cervicitis (mucopurulent discharge and hypertrophic ectopy [area that is edematous and bleeds easily]), urethritis (dysuria, frequent urination, and pyuria), bartholinitis (purulent exudate), PID (abdominal pain, nausea, vomiting, fever, malaise, abnormal vaginal bleeding, and menstrual abnormalities), and perihepatitis (fever, nausea, vomiting, and right upper quadrant pain). A large number of women with chlamydial cervicitis have been found to have a male partner with NGU.

Complications often develop from poorly managed, inaccurately diagnosed, or undiagnosed chlamydial infections. The infection is often not diagnosed until complications appear. Complications in men may result in epididymitis, with possible

TABLE 51-6	**Comparison of Gonorrhea and Chlamydia**	
SITE OF INFECTION	**N. GONORRHOEAE**	**C. TRACHOMATIS**
Men		
Urethra	Urethritis	Nongonococcal urethritis; post-gonococcal urethritis
Epididymis	Epididymitis	Epididymitis
Rectum	Proctitis	Proctitis
Conjunctiva	Conjunctivitis	Conjunctivitis
Systemic	Disseminated gonococcal infection	Reiter syndrome
Women		
Urethra	Acute urethral syndrome	Acute urethral syndrome
Bartholin's gland	Bartholinitis	Bartholinitis
Cervix	Cervicitis	Cervicitis; atypical cervical cells
Fallopian tube	Salpingitis	Salpingitis
Conjunctiva	Conjunctivitis	Conjunctivitis
Liver capsule	Perihepatitis	Perihepatitis
Systemic	Disseminated gonococcal infection	Arthritis-dermatitis syndrome

Data from Holmes KK, et al, editors: *Sexually transmitted diseases,* ed 2, New York, 1990 McGraw-Hill. In McCance KL, Huether SE: *Pathophysiology: the biologic basis for disease in adults and children,* ed 4, St Louis, 2002, Mosby.

TABLE 51-7	**Risk Factors for Chlamydial Infection**

- Women and adolescents
- New or multiple sex partners
- Sex partners who have had multiple partners
- History of STDs and cervical ectopy
- Patients with other STDs
- Lack of barrier contraception

Data from United States Preventive Services Task Force: Screening for chlamydial infection: recommendations and rationale, *Am J Prev Med* 20(3 suppl):90, 2001. *STDs,* Sexually transmitted diseases.

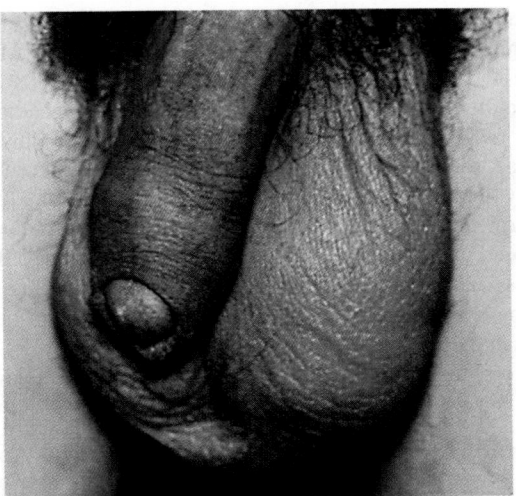

FIG. 51-6 Chlamydial epididymitis. Red, swollen scrotum.

infertility and Reiter's disease (a systemic condition characterized by urethritis, conjunctivitis, arthritis, and mucocutaneous lesions). Complications from chlamydial infections in women may result in PID, which can lead to chronic pelvic pain and infertility. For this reason the CDC recommends that all females younger than 20 years of age be routinely screened for chlamydia at their annual gynecologic examination. They further advise annual screening of all sexually active women older than 20 years of age with one or more risk factors for the disease.[15]

Diagnostic Studies and Collaborative Care

Chlamydial infections in men can be diagnosed by excluding gonorrhea. The cervical or urethral discharge appears to be less purulent, watery, and painful in chlamydial infections than in gonorrhea. If no gram-negative diplococci are found on the Gram-stained smear of male urethral discharge or the sediment of a first-catch urine specimen, a culture for both *C. trachomatis* and *N. gonorrhoeae* may be appropriate. If both cultures are negative and signs of inflammation are present (e.g., polymorphonuclear leukocytes [PMNs] on the Gram-stained smear), a diagnosis of NGU chlamydia infection can be made.

The availability of nonculture tests has allowed for the screening and confirmation of diagnoses in both men and women. Direct fluorescent antibody (DFA) tests, enzyme immunoassay (EIA), and DNA amplification do not require special handling of specimens and are easier to perform than cell cultures. DNA amplification tests are the most sensitive diagnostic methods available. In addition, they can be used with urine samples rather than urethral and cervical swabs.

Drug Therapy. When diagnosed, chlamydia can be easily treated and cured. Chlamydial infections respond to treatment with doxycycline (Vibramycin) or azithromycin (Zithromax).[16] For doxycycline, the dosage is 100 mg two times a day for 7 days. Azithromycin (1 g in a single dose) offers the advantage of ease of administration. Alternative regimens include erythromycin, ofloxacin (Floxin), or levofloxacin (Levaquin). Follow-up care should include advising the patient to return if the symptoms persist or recur, treatment of sex partners, and encouraging the use of condoms during all sexual contacts.

Lymphogranuloma Venereum

Lymphogranuloma venereum (LGV) is an STD caused by specific strains of *C. trachomatis*. LGV is rare in the United States, but it is endemic in other areas of the world, including Africa, India, Southeast Asia, South America, and the Caribbean.

The strain of *C. trachomatis* that causes LGV is transmitted through intercourse or through contact with exudate from active lesions. LGV begins as a genital lesion and spreads via the lymph nodes of the genital-rectal areas. It may also spread systemically through the bloodstream and enter the CNS. Penile, vulvar, and anal infection can lead to inguinal and femoral lymphadenopathy. Marked inflammation occurs, resulting in necrosis, *buboes* (greatly enlarged, inflamed lymph nodes), abscesses of inguinal lymph nodes, and infection of surrounding tissue. Healing occurs by fibrosis after several weeks or months and can result in chronic scarring, which damages the lymph nodes and disrupts nodal function.

Constitutional symptoms that occur during the stage of regional lymphadenopathy include fever, chills, headache, *meningismus* (meningitis-like symptoms), anorexia, myalgia, and arthralgia. Complications of untreated anorectal infection include strictures, fissures, constipation, perirectal abscesses, and rectovaginal and perianal fistulas. LGV is generally treated with doxycycline (Vibramycin), 100 mg orally twice a day, for 21 days. Also effective is erythromycin 500 mg orally four times a day for

21 days. Buboes may require aspiration to prevent inguinal and femoral ulcerations from occurring. Sex partners should also be treated.

Viral Infections

GENITAL HERPES

Because **genital herpes** is not a reportable disease in most states, its true incidence is difficult to determine. It is estimated that more than 45 million people in the United States are infected with genital herpes.[3] Since the late 1970s the prevalence of herpes simplex virus type 2 (HSV-2) has risen by 30%.

Etiology and Pathophysiology

The herpes simplex virus (HSV) enters through the mucous membranes or breaks in the skin during contact with an infected person (Fig. 51-7). HSV then reproduces inside the cell and spreads to the surrounding cells. The virus next enters the peripheral or autonomic nerve endings and ascends to the sensory or autonomic nerve ganglion, where it often becomes dormant. Viral reactivation (recurrence) may occur when the virus descends down to the initial site of infection, either the mucous membranes or skin. When a person is infected with HSV, the virus usually persists within the individual for life. Shedding of the virus even in the absence of an identifiable lesion is a well-established phenomenon.

Two different strains of HSV cause infection. In general, HSV type 1 (HSV-1) causes infection above the waist, involving the gingivae, the dermis, the upper respiratory tract, and the CNS. HSV type 2 (HSV-2) most frequently infects the genital tract and the perineum (i.e., locations below the waist). However, either strain can cause disease on the mouth or the genitals. Because HSV is readily inactivated at room temperature and by drying, airborne and fomitic (nonliving objects) spread have not been documented as significant means of transmission. Most people infected with HSV-1 or HSV-2 are asymptomatic or unaware of their infection.[17]

Clinical Manifestations

In the *primary (initial) episode* of genital herpes the patient may complain of burning or tingling at the site of inoculation. Vesicular lesions, which may occur on the penis, scrotum, vulva, perineum, perianal region, vagina, or cervix, contain large quantities of infectious viral particles (Fig. 51-8). The lesions rupture and form shallow, moist ulcerations. Finally, crusting and epithelialization of the erosions occur. Primary infections tend to be associated with local inflammation and pain, accompanied by sys-

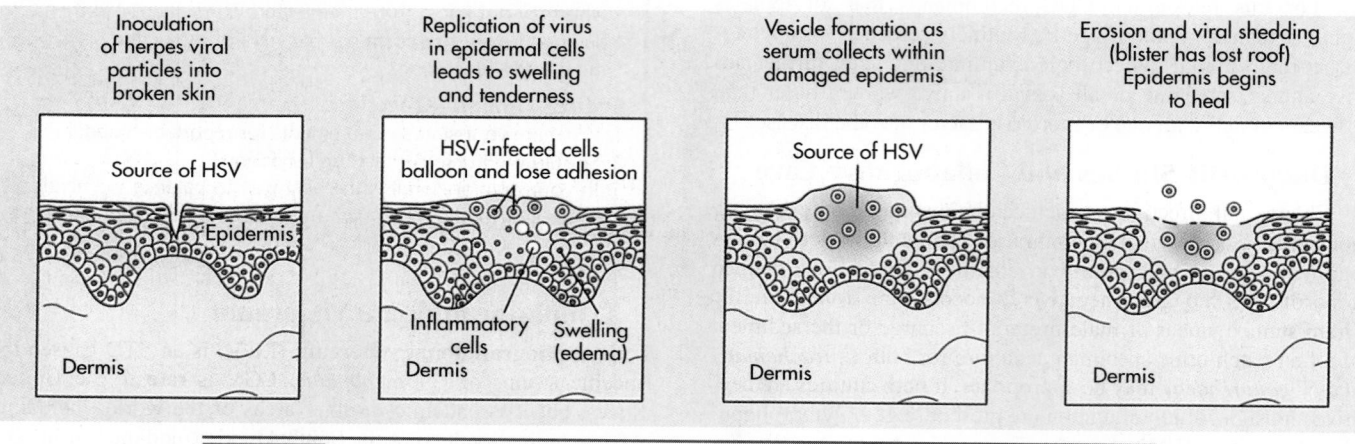

| Inoculation of herpes viral particles into broken skin | Replication of virus in epidermal cells leads to swelling and tenderness | Vesicle formation as serum collects within damaged epidermis | Erosion and viral shedding (blister has lost roof) Epidermis begins to heal |

FIG. 51-7 Infection with herpes simplex virus (HSV).

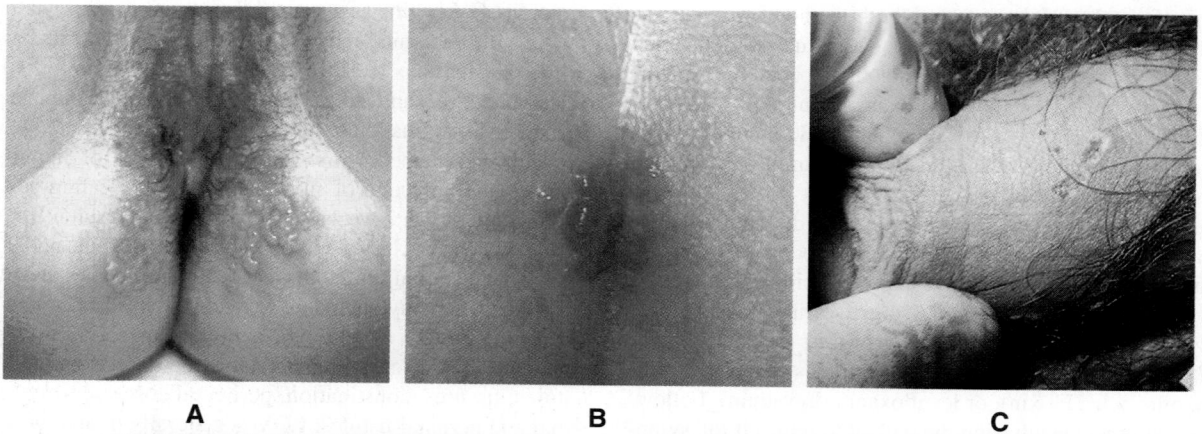

FIG. 51-8 Unruptured vesicles of herpes simplex virus (HSV) type 2. **A,** Vulvar area. **B,** Perianal area. **C,** Penile herpes simplex, ulcerative stage.

temic manifestations of fever, headache, malaise, myalgia, and regional lymphadenopathy.

Urination may be painful from the urine touching active lesions. Urinary retention may occur as a result of HSV urethritis or cystitis. A purulent vaginal discharge may develop with HSV cervicitis. The duration of symptoms is longer and the frequency of complications is greater in women. Primary lesions are generally present for 17 to 20 days, but new lesions sometimes continue to develop for 6 weeks. The lesions heal spontaneously unless secondary infection occurs.

Recurrent genital herpes occurs in about 50% to 80% of individuals during the year following the primary episode. Stress, fatigue, sunburn, and menses are commonly noted trigger factors. Many patients can predict a recurrence by noticing the early prodromal symptoms of tingling, burning, and itching at the site where the lesions will eventually appear. The symptoms of recurrent episodes are less severe, and the lesions usually heal within 8 to 12 days. With time the recurrent lesions will generally occur less frequently.

Women with recurrent symptomatic genital herpes can shed the virus up to 1% of the time even when no visible lesions are present. Suppressive therapy with antiviral agents can reduce but not eradicate asymptomatic shedding.[18] Barrier forms of contraception, especially condoms, used during asymptomatic periods may decrease transmission of the virus. When lesions are present, the patient should avoid sexual activity altogether because even barrier protection is not satisfactory in eliminating disease transmission.

Complications

Although most infections are of a relatively benign nature, complications of genital herpes may involve the CNS, causing aseptic meningitis and lower motor neuron damage. Neuron damage may result in atonic bladder, impotence, and constipation. Another complication is *autoinoculation* of the virus to extragenital sites such as the lips, breasts, and, most commonly, the fingers (herpetic whitlow) (Fig. 51-9).

Herpes Simplex Virus Infection in Pregnancy. Studies indicate no difference in the length or severity of symptoms between pregnant and nonpregnant women. Women with a primary

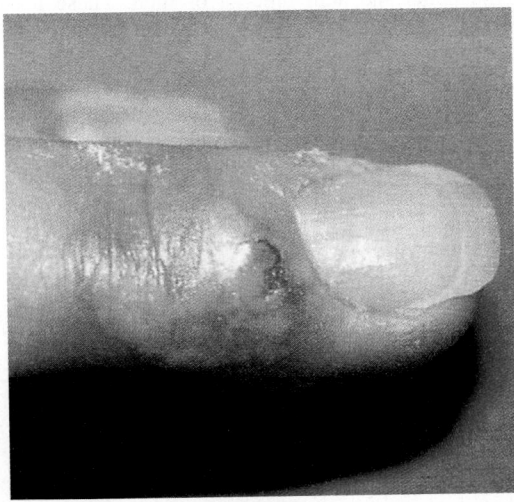

FIG. 51-9 Autoinoculation of herpes simplex virus (HSV), herpetic whitlow.

episode of HSV near the time of delivery have the highest risk of transmitting genital herpes to the neonate. The risk of transmission is lowest for women who acquire HSV early in the pregnancy or have a history of recurrent HSV. Although women with recurrent HSV infections are not at higher risk for transmitting the virus to their infants, an active genital lesion at the time of delivery is usually an indication for cesarean section delivery, because most infections to neonates occur during birth.[19]

Diagnostic Studies

A diagnosis of genital herpes is usually based on the patient's symptoms and history. The diagnosis can be confirmed through isolation of the virus from active lesions by means of tissue culture. Tzanck- or Pap-stained smears from lesions may show the cellular characteristics of viral infection, including multinucleated giant cells and intranuclear inclusions. HSV infection can be confirmed by isolation of the virus in culture. Other techniques to detect HSV include direct immunofluorescence and EIA. In addition, DNA amplification can be performed to detect HSV. These tests permit more rapid identification of HSV than a culture. Highly accurate serologic methods for detecting the HSV type are available.

Collaborative Care

Drug Therapy. Three antiviral agents are available for the treatment of HSV: acyclovir (Zovirax), valacyclovir (Valtrex), and famciclovir (Famvir). These drugs inhibit herpetic viral replication and are prescribed for primary and recurrent infections (Table 51-8). Acyclovir, valacyclovir, and famciclovir are also used to suppress frequent recurrences (more than six episodes per year). Although not a cure, these drugs shorten the duration of viral shedding and the healing time of genital lesions and reduce outbreaks by 75%.[15] Continued use of oral acyclovir as suppressive therapy for up to 5 years is safe and effective. Adverse reactions are mild and include headache, occasional nausea and vomiting, and diarrhea. The safety of these drugs for treatment of pregnant women has not been established. Acyclovir ointment appears to have no clinical benefit in the treatment of recurrent lesions, either in speed of healing or in resolution of pain, and is not commonly recommended. IV acyclovir is reserved for severe or life-threatening infections in which hospitalization is required for the treatment of disseminated infections, CNS infections (meningitis), or pneumonitis. Nephrotoxicity has been observed with high-dose IV use.

Symptomatic Care. Symptomatic treatment such as good genital hygiene and the wearing of loose-fitting cotton undergarments should be encouraged. The lesions should be kept clean and dry. To ensure complete drying of the perineal area, women may use a hair dryer set on a cool setting. Frequent sitz baths may soothe the area and reduce inflammation. Drying agents such as colloidal oatmeal (Aveeno) and aluminum salts (Burow's solution) may provide some relief from the burning and itching. Techniques to reduce pain on urination include pouring a pitcher of water onto the perineal area while voiding to dilute the urine, and voiding in a warm tub of water or shower. Pain may require a local anesthetic such as lidocaine (Xylocaine) or systemic analgesics such as codeine and aspirin. Sexual transmission of HSV has been documented during asymptomatic periods, and the use of barrier methods, especially condoms, should be encouraged.

TABLE
51-8

Collaborative Care
Genital Herpes

Diagnostic
History and physical examination
Viral isolation by tissue culture
Antibody assay for specific HSV viral type

Collaborative Therapy
Primary Infection
acyclovir (Zovirax) 400 mg three times a day or acyclovir
  200 mg five times a day or famciclovir (Famvir) 250 mg
  three times a day or valacyclovir (Valtrex) 1 g twice a day.
  All drugs are given orally for 7 to 10 days.

Recurrent Episodic Infection
acyclovir 400 mg three times a day or acyclovir 200 mg five
  times a day or acyclovir 800 mg two times a day or famciclovir 125 mg twice a day or valacyclovir 500 mg twice a
  day or valacyclovir 1 g once a day. Drugs are given orally
  for 5 days.
Attempt to identify trigger mechanisms.
Yearly Pap smear.
Abstinence from sexual contact while lesions are present;
  however, virus may be shed without lesions.
Symptomatic care.
Confidential counseling and testing for HIV.

Suppressive Therapy for Frequent Recurrence
acyclovir 400 mg two times a day or famciclovir 250 mg two
  times a day or valacyclovir 500 mg twice a day or valacyclovir 1 g once a day.

Severe Infection
acyclovir 5 to 10 mg/kg IV every 8 hours for 2 to 7 days or
  until clinical improvement, followed by oral antiviral therapy
  to complete at least 10 days of treatment.

Modified from Centers for Disease Control and Prevention: STD treatment guidelines, *MMWR* 51(RR–6):1, 2002.
HIV, Human immunodeficiency virus; *HSV,* herpes simplex virus.

GENITAL WARTS

Genital warts *(condylomata acuminata)* are caused by the human papillomavirus (HPV). Visible genital warts are usually
caused by HPV types 6 and 11. These types can also cause warts
on the anus, urethra, and vagina. Other HPV types in the genital

region (e.g., types 16, 18, 31, 33, and 35) are associated with
vaginal, anal, and cervical dysplasia. HPV is a highly contagious
STD seen frequently in young, sexually active adults. An estimated 20 million people are currently infected with HPV.[1] It is
found 25% of the time in conjunction with other STDs.[20]

Minor trauma during intercourse can cause abrasions that
allow HPV to enter the body. The epithelial cells infected with
HPV undergo transformation and proliferation to form a warty
growth. The incubation period of the virus is generally 1 to
6 months, but may be longer. Prevention is hampered by a
high proportion of asymptomatic infections and lack of curative treatment. In most states, genital warts is not a reportable
disease.

Clinical Manifestations and Complications

Genital warts are discrete single or multiple papillary
growths that are white to gray and pink-flesh colored. They
may grow and coalesce to form large, cauliflower-like masses.
Most patients have from 1 to 10 genital warts. In men, the warts
may occur on the penis and scrotum, around the anus, or in the
urethra. In women, the warts may be located on the vulva,
vagina, or cervix and in the perianal area (Fig. 51-10). There
are usually no other signs or symptoms. Itching may occur with
anogenital warts. Bleeding on defecation may occur with anal
warts.

During pregnancy, genital warts tend to grow rapidly. An infected mother may transmit the condition to her newborn. Cesarean delivery is not routinely indicated unless the birth canal
becomes blocked by massive warts.

Subclinical Human Papillomavirus Infections. HPV
infection has been linked with cervical and vulvar cancer in
women and with anorectal and squamous cell carcinoma of the
penis in men. To date more than 100 types of HPV have been
identified, at least 33 of which invade the genital tract.[21] Some of
these types appear to be harmless and self-limiting (e.g., types 6
and 11 commonly found in genital warts), whereas others are
thought to have oncogenic (cancer-causing) potential (e.g., types
16 and 18). Up to two thirds of the early lesions caused by HPV
are undetectable by visual examination. Flat subclinical lesions
are commonly found on the cervix and anal mucosa of women
and on the penis and anal mucosa of men. These lesions are
strongly associated with the development of dysplasia and neoplasia at these sites.

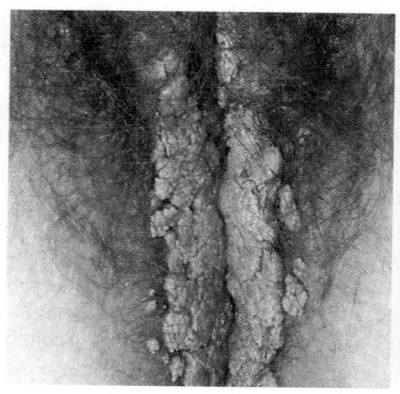
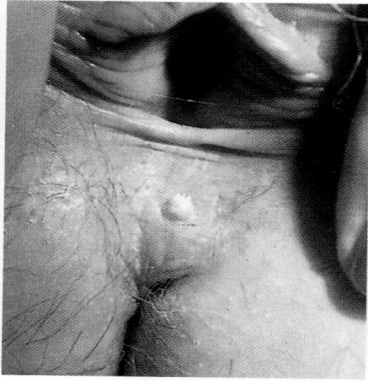
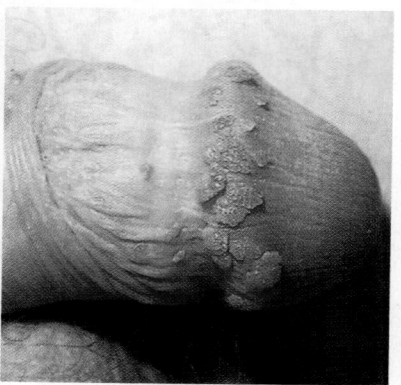

A   **B**   **C**

FIG. 51-10 Genital warts. **A,** Severe vulvular warts. **B,** Perineal wart. **C,** Multiple genital warts of the
glans penis.

Diagnostic Studies and Collaborative Care

A diagnosis of genital warts can be made on the basis of the gross appearance of the lesions. However, the warts may be confused with condylomata lata of secondary syphilis, carcinoma, or benign neoplasms. Serologic and cytologic testing should be done to rule out these conditions. If dysplasia is confirmed by the Papanicolaou (Pap) smear, a colposcopic examination and biopsies should be performed. Virapap, a test that uses DNA amplification techniques, can be used to determine some molecular types of HPV present in a lesion. Currently, HPV cannot be confirmed by culture.

The primary goal when treating visible genital warts is the removal of symptomatic warts. The removal may or may not decrease infectivity. Genital warts are difficult to treat and often require multiple office visits with a variety of treatment modalities. None of the treatments are superior to other treatments. Many patients will have a course of therapy rather than one treatment. The therapy should be modified if a patient has not improved after three treatments or if after six treatments the warts have not completely disappeared. One common treatment is the use of 80% to 90% trichloroacetic acid (TCA) or bichloroacetic acid (BCA) applied directly to the wart surface. Petroleum jelly is applied to the surrounding normal skin to minimize irritation before a small amount of TCA is applied to the wart with a cotton swab. A sharp stinging pain is often felt with initial acid contact, but this quickly subsides. TCA is not washed off after treatment. It can be used in pregnant women.

Podophyllin resin (10% to 25%), a cytotoxic agent, is recommended therapy for small external genital warts. When podophyllin is used, it is applied carefully to each wart, with normal tissue being avoided, and is then thoroughly washed off in 1 to 4 hours. This substance encourages the sloughing off of skin containing viral particles. Podophyllin has local (e.g., pain, burning) and systemic (e.g., nausea, dizziness, leukopenia, respiratory distress) toxic symptoms. It is contraindicated in pregnant women. In general, warts located on moist surfaces respond better to topical treatment (e.g., TCA, podophyllin) than do warts on drier surfaces.

Patient-managed treatment is also an option. Podofilox liquid and gel are available by prescription (Condylox and Condylox Gel). The patient applies the solution or gel for 3 successive days followed by 4 days of no treatment. Treatment can be repeated for up to 4 weeks or until resolution of the lesions. Imiquimod cream (Aldara) is an immune response modifier that is applied once daily at bedtime, three times a week for up to 16 weeks. None of these treatments is recommended for use during pregnancy or lactation.

If the warts do not regress with any of these therapies, treatments such as cryotherapy with liquid nitrogen, electrocautery, laser therapy, intralesional use of interferon, and surgical excision may be indicated.[22] Because treatment does not destroy the virus, merely the infected tissue, recurrences and reinfection are possible, and careful long-term follow-up is advised.

NURSING MANAGEMENT SEXUALLY TRANSMITTED DISEASES

■ Nursing Assessment

Subjective and objective data that should be obtained from a person with an STD are presented in Table 51-9.

■ Nursing Diagnoses

Nursing diagnoses for the patient with an STD include, but are not limited to, the following:

- Risk for infection *related to* lack of knowledge about mode of transmission, inadequate personal and genital hygiene, and failure to practice precautionary measures
- Anxiety *related to* impact of condition on relationships, disease outcome, and lack of knowledge of disease
- Ineffective health maintenance *related to* lack of knowledge about disease process, appropriate follow-up measures, and possibility of reinfection

TABLE 51-9	Nursing Assessment Sexually Transmitted Disease

Subjective Data

Important Health Information

Past health history: Contact with individuals with STDs, multiple sexual partners, pregnancy

Medications: Use of oral contraceptives; allergy to any antibiotics, especially penicillin

Functional Health Patterns

Health perception–health management: Shared needles during IV drug use; malaise

Nutritional-metabolic: Nausea, vomiting, anorexia; pharyngitis, oral lesions, itching at infected site; chills; alopecia

Elimination: Dysuria, urinary frequency, retention; urethral discharge; tenesmus, proctitis

Cognitive-perceptual: Arthralgia; headache; painful, burning lesions

Sexuality-reproductive: Dyspareunia; vaginal discharge, menstrual abnormalities; presence of genital or perianal lesions

Objective Data

General

Fever, lymphadenopathy (generalized or inguinal)

Integumentary

Syphilis: Primary: painless, indurated genital, oral, or perianal lesions; secondary: bilateral, symmetric rash on palms, soles, or entire body, mucous patches on mouth or tongue, alopecia

Genital herpes: Painful genital or anal vesicular lesions

Genital warts: Single or multiple gray or white genital or anal warts (possibly becoming massive)

Gastrointestinal

Purulent rectal discharge (indicator of gonorrhea), rectal lesions, proctitis

Urinary

Urethral discharge, erythema

Reproductive

Cervical discharge, lesions, inflamed Bartholin's glands

Possible Findings

Gonorrhea: Positive Gram stain, smears, cultures, and DNA amplification for *N. gonorrhoeae*

Syphilis: Positive findings on VDRL and RPR, spirochetes on dark-field microscopy

Chlamydia: Positive culture or DNA amplification for *Chlamydia* organism

Genital herpes: Positive tissue culture for HSV-2 or anti–HSV-2 antibody assay

HSV-2, Herpes simplex virus type 2; *IV,* intravenous; *RPR,* rapid plasma reagin; *STD,* sexually transmitted disease; *VDRL,* Venereal Disease Research Laboratory.

■ Planning

The overall goals are that the patient with an STD will (1) demonstrate understanding of the mode of transmission of STDs and the risk posed by STDs, (2) complete treatment and return for appropriate follow-up, (3) notify or assist in notification of sexual contacts about their need for testing and treatment, (4) abstain from intercourse until infection is resolved, and (5) demonstrate knowledge of safer sex practices.

■ Nursing Implementation

Health Promotion. Many approaches to curtailing the spread of STDs have been advocated and have met with varying degrees of success. Nurses should be prepared to discuss practices with all patients, not only those who are perceived to be at risk. These "safe" sex practices include abstinence, monogamy with an uninfected partner, avoidance of certain high risk sexual practices, and use of condoms and other barriers to limit contact with potentially infectious body fluids or lesions. Sexual abstinence is a certain method of avoiding all STDs, but few adults consider this a feasible alternative to sexual expression. Limiting sexual intimacies outside of a well-established monogamous relationship can reduce the risk of contracting an STD. A patient and family teaching guide related to the patient with an STD is presented in Table 51-10.

All sexually active women should be screened for cervical cancer. Women with a history of STDs are at greater risk for cervical cancer than women without this history. Pap smears are discussed in Chapter 52.

Measures to prevent infection. An inspection of the sexual partner's genitals before coitus is recommended. The presence of discharge, sores, blisters, or rash should be viewed with concern. A patient who is aware of specific signs and symptoms of infection can intelligently make the decision to continue the sexual interaction with modifications or elect not to have sexual relations. The patient should remember that, when engaging in sex, there is exposure to the infections of everyone with whom the partner has ever had sex. Men should be told that some protection is provided if they void immediately following intercourse and wash their genitalia and the adjacent areas with soap and water. Women may also benefit from postcoital voiding and washing. However, it should not be assumed that this provides adequate protection against STDs after exposure to infection. Although spermicidal jellies and creams have a mild detergent effect that may reduce the risk of contracting STDs, this has not been proven. These same barriers can serve as supplementary lubrication, thereby decreasing irritation and friction and chances for development of a minor laceration that could serve as an entry point for the organism.

Proper use of a latex condom provides a highly effective mechanical barrier to infection. The condom should be undamaged and correctly in place throughout all phases of sexual activity. It is unknown if a condom lubricated with a spermicide such as nonoxynol-9 further reduces the risk of STDs. Vaginal spermicides, when used alone without a condom, reduce the risk for chlamydia and gonorrhea.[15] A deterrent to condom usage is alcohol and drug use. Studies continue to document that IV drug users do not consistently use condoms.[23] Use of barrier contraceptives requires planning and motivation, both of which are impaired with alcohol or drug ingestion. The patient should be

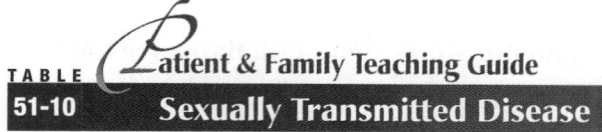

TABLE 51-10 Patient & Family Teaching Guide
Sexually Transmitted Disease

1. Instruct patient in hygienic measures, such as washing and urinating after intercourse to destroy many causative organisms.
2. Explain the importance of taking all antibiotics as prescribed. Symptoms will improve after 1-2 days of therapy, but organisms may still be present.
3. Teach patient about the need for treatment of sexual partners with antibiotics to prevent transmission of disease.
4. Instruct patient to abstain from sexual intercourse during treatment and to use condoms when sexual activity is resumed to prevent spread of infection and prevent reinfection.
5. Explain the importance of follow-up examination and reculture at least once after treatment if appropriate to confirm complete cure and prevent relapse.
6. Allow patient and partner to verbalize concerns to clarify areas that need explanation.
7. Instruct patient about symptoms of complications and need to report problems to ensure proper follow-up and early treatment of reinfection.
8. Explain precautions to take, such as being monogamous; asking potential partners about sexual history; avoiding sex with partners who use IV drugs or who have visible oral, inguinal, genital, perineal, or anal lesions; using condoms; voiding and washing genitalia after coitus to reduce the occurrence of reinfection.
9. Inform patient regarding state of infectivity to prevent a false sense of security, which might result in careless sexual practices and poor personal hygiene.

given specific verbal and written instructions on the proper use of condoms (see Chapter 14, Figs. 14-6 and 14-7). The objections to condom usage, such as interference with spontaneity and the presence of a barrier, should be discussed by the partners. Information about the mechanics of sexual arousal and incorporating a condom into lovemaking can help in overcoming patient or partner resistance to its use. Female condoms are lubricated polyurethane sheaths with a ring at each end designed for vaginal wear (see Chapter 14, Fig. 14-7). Laboratory studies indicate that it is an effective barrier to microorganisms, including viruses, but clinical trials are currently lacking for STDs.

Sexual contact with persons known or suspected to have HIV infection should be avoided (see Chapter 14). Among couples with one infected partner, consistent and scrupulous condom use can reduce transmission to the uninfected partner. A sexually active homosexual man can reduce risk by minimizing the number of sexual contacts. Unprotected anal intercourse and other high risk behaviors should be eliminated, and condoms should be used if sexual contact continues.

The nurse can initiate an interview to establish the patient's risk for contracting an STD. Questions to ask include number of partners, type of birth control used, use of condoms, use of IV drugs, and sexual preference. Patient education can be planned based on the response to these questions. Interpersonal skills necessary for this interview include respect, compassion, and a nonjudgmental attitude. Counseling should be tailored to the individual patient.

Screening programs. Screening programs that are used to detect infected patients can also help prevent certain STDs. For many years, there have been various screening programs to find cases of syphilis. With the decline of infection rates across the United States, many states have eliminated laws requiring premarital testing for syphilis. Many institutions offer voluntary prenatal HIV and syphilis testing and counseling for pregnant women.

Screening programs have been developed and implemented for detection of gonorrhea and chlamydia. These programs are targeted to women because women are more likely to have asymptomatic gonorrhea and thereby serve as sources of infection. Routine gonorrheal and chlamydial testing during pelvic examinations and prenatal visits are being performed as a major part of these programs. Their effectiveness is well documented.[24] Mass application of screening programs for genital chlamydial infections, genital herpes, and HPV infections (warts) may also be possible with the advent of rapid, cost-effective tests.

Case finding. Interviewing and case finding are other processes used to control STDs. These activities are directed toward locating and examining all contacts of each known patient with an STD as soon after sexual exposure as possible, so that effective treatment can be initiated. Trained interviewers may often find cases even if they are supplied with only limited information. The caseworkers, who are often nurses, are aware of the social implications of these diseases and the need for discretion. Sexual contacts are often not informed about the origin of the information naming them as a contact so that greater cooperation and privacy is ensured.

Educational and research programs. Nurses can actively encourage their communities to provide better education about STDs for their citizens. Teenagers, who are known to have a high incidence of infection, should be a prime target for such educational programs. Hot-line services, school nurses, nurse practitioners, nurse midwives, and outreach programs sponsored by the CDC in the United States and Canada's Health Protection Branch are effective. The National Gay Task Force and the Herpes Resource Center were established to provide education and support. Knowledge and understanding can decrease the STD epidemic. Currently, efforts are being made to develop vaccines for syphilis, gonorrhea, genital herpes, HPV, and HIV. The development of effective vaccines is viewed by many clinicians as a prerequisite for eradication of STDs.

Acute Intervention

Psychologic support. The diagnosis of an STD may be met with a variety of emotions, such as shame, guilt, anger, and a desire for vengeance. The nurse should provide counseling and try to help the patient verbalize feelings. Couples in marital or committed relationships are confronted with an added problem when an STD is diagnosed. The implication of sexual activity by one of the partners with a person outside the relationship must be faced. Other concerns relative to their relationship are present, and the acute problem may serve as an incentive for further problem solving. Support and counseling for the couple are needed. A referral for professional counseling to explore the ramifications of an STD in their relationship may be indicated.

EVIDENCE-BASED PRACTICE
Sexually Transmitted Diseases and Cervical Cancer

Clinical Problem
What is the effectiveness of health education interventions to promote sexual risk reduction behaviors among women in order to reduce the transmission of human papillomavirus (HPV)?

Best Clinical Practice
- Evidence summarized from 30 studies showed a positive effect of educational interventions on sexual risk reduction behavior, typically with increased use of condoms for vaginal intercourse.
- The positive effects of the interventions lasted up to 3 months after the intervention.

Implications for Nursing Practice
- Educational interventions can promote sexual risk reduction behavior.
- These interventions have the potential to reduce the transmission of HPV and possibly reduce the incidence of cervical carcinoma.

Reference for Evidence
Sheperd J et al: Interventions for encouraging sexual lifestyles and behaviors intended to prevent cervical cancer, *Cochrane Database of Systematic Reviews* (2), CD001035, 2000.

A patient who has genital herpes is faced with the fact that repeated infections can occur and that no cure is available. This can be frustrating and disruptive to the patient's physical, emotional, social, and sexual lives. Helping the patient identify and avoid any factors that may precipitate the condition is indicated. Informing the patient that the incidence and severity of recurrences will decrease over time may provide some support.

HPV infections involve a prolonged course of treatment. The patient can become frustrated and distressed because of frequent office visits, associated costs, potential for unpleasant side effects as a result of treatment, and effects of the infection on future health and sexual relationships. Tremendous support and a willingness to listen to the patient's concerns are needed.

Compliance and follow-up. A nurse working in public health facilities, clinics, or other outpatient settings may care for a patient with an STD more often than a nurse in a hospital. This nurse is in a position to explain and interpret treatment measures such as the purpose and possible side effects of prescribed drugs and the need for follow-up care.

Frequently, single-dose treatment for gonorrhea, chlamydial infection, and syphilis helps prevent the problems associated with noncompliance with drug therapy. The patient requiring multiple-dose therapy should be given special instructions in completing the prescribed regimen and should be informed about problems resulting from noncompliance. All patients should return to the treatment center for a repeat culture from the infected sites or for serologic testing at designated times to determine the effectiveness of the treatment. Informing the patient that cures are not always obtained on the first treatment can reinforce the need for a follow-up visit. The patient should also be advised to inform sexual partners of the need for testing and treatment, regardless of whether they are free of symptoms or experiencing symptoms.

Hygiene measures. The patient with an STD should have certain hygiene measures emphasized. An important measure is frequent hand washing and bathing. Bathing and cleaning of the involved areas can provide local comfort and prevent secondary infection. Douching may spread the infection or undermine local immune responses and is therefore contraindicated. The synthetic materials used in most undergarments frequently increase or exacerbate local irritations by trapping moisture. Cotton undergarments provide better absorption and are cooler and more comfortable for the patient with an STD.

Sexual activity. Sexual abstinence is indicated during the communicable phase of the disease. If sexual activity occurs before treatment of the patient has been completed, the use of condoms may prevent the spread of infection and reinfection. Condom usage after treatment should be encouraged to prevent future exposure to infection. The patient can also choose to relate to a partner in an intimate way that avoids both coitus and oral-genital contact. It is important to note that even single-dose treatments can take up to 1 week to be effective and thus the patient is infective during this period.

Ambulatory and Home Care. Because many STDs are cured with a single dose or short course of antibiotic therapy, many persons are casual about the outcome of these diseases. The consequences of this attitude can include delays in treatment, noncompliance with instructions, and subsequent development of complications. The complications are serious and costly; they can result in disfigurement and destruction of important tissues and organs.

Surgery and prolonged therapy are indicated for many patients with disease-related complications. Major surgical procedures such as resection of an aneurysm or aortic valve replacement may be necessary to treat cardiovascular problems caused by syphilis. Pelvic surgery and procedures to correct fertility problems secondary to an STD may include lysis of adhesions, dilation of strictures, reconstructive tuboplasty, and in vitro fertilization.

■ Evaluation

Expected outcomes for the patient with an STD are that the patient will
- describe modes of transmission
- use appropriate hygienic measures
- experience no reinfection
- demonstrate compliance with follow-up protocol

CRITICAL THINKING EXERCISES

Case Study
Chlamydia

Patient Profile. Jade K. is a 17-year-old female who visits the outpatient Teen Clinic seeking birth control pills.

Subjective Data
- Had first-time intercourse with boyfriend 2 weeks ago
- Did not use condom or spermicide
- Has not asked boyfriend about his sexual practices
- Denies any symptoms

Objective Data
- Has cervical ectopy noted during Pap test
- Tests positive for *Chlamydia*
- Crying and very upset when informed of positive test result

Collaborative Care
- Doxycycline 100 mg bid for 7 days

CRITICAL THINKING QUESTIONS

1. What were Jade's risk factors for acquiring chlamydial infection?
2. What complications could have occurred if Jade's infection had not been detected?
3. What impact is her diagnosis likely to have on Jade's self-image? On her relationship with her boyfriend?
4. What instructions should Jade receive to ensure successful treatment? To prevent reinfection? To prevent further transmission of the infection?
5. What does she need to know about other STDs? What other testing would you recommend?
6. Based on the assessment data presented, write one or more nursing diagnoses. Are there any collaborative problems?

Nursing Research Issues
1. What are the best strategies for encouraging safer sex practices and condom use among high risk populations?
2. What is the level of teens' knowledge of risk, transmission, and impact of STDs? How can teaching about STDs best be adapted to their developmental level?
3. Does education about safer sex practices increase preventive behaviors?

REVIEW QUESTIONS

The number of the question corresponds to the same-numbered objective at the beginning of the chapter.

1. The individual with the lowest risk for sexually transmitted pelvic inflammatory disease is a woman who
   a. uses oral contraceptives.
   b. uses barrier methods of contraception.
   c. uses an intrauterine device for contraception.
   d. uses a Norplant implant or injectible Depo-Provera for contraception.

2. While obtaining subjective assessment data from a woman reported as a sexual contact of a man with chlamydia, the nurse understands that symptoms of chlamydial infections in women
   a. are frequently absent.
   b. mimic those of genital herpes.
   c. include a macular palmar rash in later stages.
   d. may involve chancres hidden inside the vagina.

REVIEW QUESTIONS—cont'd

3. A primary HSV infection differs from recurrent episodes in that
   a. it is of shorter duration than recurrent episodes.
   b. only primary infections are sexually transmissible.
   c. systemic manifestations such as fever and myalgia are more common.
   d. transmission of the virus to a fetus is less likely during primary infection.

4. The nurse explains to a patient with gonorrhea that treatment will include both ceftriaxone and doxycycline because
   a. most patients do not respond to ceftriaxone alone.
   b. coverage with more than one antibiotic prevents reinfection.
   c. no single agent successfully eradicates all strains of gonorrhea.
   d. the high rate of coexisting chlamydia and gonorrhea indicates dual coverage.

5. A patient with an STD who is most likely to have a nursing diagnosis of disturbed body image that hinders future sexual relationships is the patient with
   a. syphilis.
   b. gonorrhea.
   c. genital warts.
   d. chlamydial infection.

6. Teaching by the nurse to prevent infection and transmission of STDs includes explanations of
   a. the appropriate use of birth control pills.
   b. sexual positions used to avoid infection.
   c. sexual practices that are considered high risk.
   d. the necessity of annual Pap smears for patients with HPV.

7. An appropriate nursing intervention to provide emotional support to a patient with an STD is to
   a. use concerned listening when the patient expresses negative feelings.
   b. reassure the patient that the disease is curable with appropriate treatment.
   c. offer many alternatives that the patient can use to change sexual relationships.
   d. help the patient who is an innocent sexual partner forgive the infecting partner.

REFERENCES

1. Centers for Disease Control and Prevention, Division of STD Prevention: *Tracking the hidden epidemics, 2000,* Atlanta, 2000, Centers for Disease Control and Prevention.
2. Centers for Disease Control and Prevention, Divisions of HIV/AIDS Prevention: *Prevention and treatment of sexually transmitted diseases as an HIV prevention strategy. Fact sheet,* Atlanta, 1998, Centers for Disease Control and Prevention.
3. Sarma SP, Garafalo K, Graves WL: Use of intrauterine device by inner city women, *Arch Fam Med* 7:130, 1998.
4. Cushman L et al: Condom use among women choosing long-term hormonal contraception, *Fam Plann Perspect* 30:240, 1998.
5. Centers for Disease Control and Prevention, Division of STD Prevention: *Sexually transmitted disease surveillance, 1999,* Atlanta, 2000, Centers for Disease Control and Prevention.
6. Bignell C et al: National guidelines for the management of gonorrhea in adults, *Sex Transm Dis* (suppl 1):S13, 1999.
7. Centers for Disease Control and Prevention: Primary and secondary syphilis—United States, 1999, *MMWR* 50:7, 2001.
8. Centers for Disease Control and Prevention, Division of STD Prevention: *National plan to eliminate syphilis from the United States,* Atlanta, 1999, National Center for HIV, STD and TB Prevention.
9. Jacobs R: Infectious diseases—spirochetal. In Tierney L et al, editors: *Current medical diagnosis and treatment,* ed 40, New York, 2001, Lange/McGraw-Hill.
10. Centers for Disease Control and Prevention, Division of Sexually Transmitted Diseases: *Syphilis elimination—history in the making,* media release, Atlanta, Nov 28, 2001.
11. Lukehart SA, Holmes KK: Syphilis. In Fauci AS et al, editors: *Harrison's principles of internal medicine,* ed 15, New York, 2000, McGraw-Hill.
12. Centers for Disease Control and Prevention, Division of Sexually Transmitted Diseases: *Syphilis elimination—history in the making. Fact sheets,* Atlanta, May 2001, Centers for Disease Control and Prevention.
13. Centers for Disease Control and Prevention: *Chlamydia trachomatis* genital infections—United States, 1999, *MMWR* 48:1, 2001.
14. Andrews W et al: The preterm prediction study: association of second trimester genitourinary chlamydia infection with subsequent spontaneous birth, *Am J Obstet Gynecol* 183:662, 2000.
15. Centers for Disease Control and Prevention: *1998 guidelines for treatment of sexually transmitted diseases,* Atlanta, 1998, Centers for Disease Control and Prevention.
16. Centers for Disease Control and Prevention: STD treatment guidelines, *MMWR* 51(RR-6):1, 2002.
17. Sacks S: Improving the management of genital herpes, *Hosp Pract* 34:41, 1999.
18. Herpes Simplex Advisory Panel: National guidelines for the management of genital herpes, *Sex Transm Infect* (suppl 1):S24, 1999.
19. Thomas D: Sexually transmitted viral infections: epidemiology and treatment, *JOGNN* 30:316, 2001.
20. Wright T: Genital warts: their etiology and treatment, *Nurs Times* 94:52, 1998.
21. Centers for Disease Control and Prevention, Division of STD Prevention: *Prevention of genital HPV infection and sequelae,* Atlanta, 1999, Centers for Disease Control and Prevention.
22. McKay S: Why we need to worry about warts, *RN* 63:68, 2000.
23. Metsch L et al: Alternative strategies for sexual risk reduction used by active drug users, *AIDS and Behavior* 5:75, 2001.
24. Centers for Disease Control and Prevention: *Recommendations for the prevention and management of* Chlamydia trachomatis *infections, 1998,* Atlanta, 1998, Centers for Disease Control and Prevention.

RESOURCES

Herpes Resource Center
American Social Health Association
P.O. Box 13827
Research Triangle Park, NC 27709
919-361-8400
Fax: 919-361-8425
www.ashastd.org
www.iwannaknow.org (for teens)
National STD/AIDS Hotline
800-342-2437 (800-342-AIDS)
Sexuality Information and Education Council of the United States
130 West 42nd Street, Suite 350
New York, NY 10036-7802
212-819-9770
Fax: 212-819-9776
www.siecus.org

For additional Internet resources, see the website for this book at *http://evolve.elsevier.com/Lewis/medsurg/.*

CHAPTER **52**

NURSING MANAGEMENT
Female Reproductive Problems

Nancy J. MacMullen
Laura Dulski

LEARNING OBJECTIVES

1. Identify causes of infertility and the strategies for diagnosis and treatment of infertility.
2. Discuss the nursing management of women who miscarry or terminate a pregnancy.
3. Describe the etiology, clinical manifestations, and collaborative and nursing management of menstrual problems and irregular vaginal bleeding.
4. Identify the risk factors, clinical manifestations, and collaborative care of ectopic pregnancy.
5. Discuss the changes related to menopause and the collaborative and nursing management of the patient with menopausal symptoms.
6. Identify the clinical manifestations of sexual assault and the appropriate collaborative and nursing management of the patient who has been sexually assaulted.
7. Differentiate among the common problems that affect the vulva, vagina, and cervix and the related collaborative care and nursing management.

8. Describe the assessment, collaborative care, and nursing management of women with pelvic inflammatory disease.
9. Describe the clinical manifestations, complications, collaborative care, and nursing management of endometriosis.
10. Describe the clinical manifestations and collaborative care of benign tumors of the female reproductive system.
11. Identify the clinical manifestations, diagnostic studies, collaborative care, and surgical therapy for cervical, endometrial, ovarian, and vulvar cancers.
12. Describe the preoperative and postoperative nursing management for the patient requiring surgery of the female reproductive system.
13. Describe common problems that occur with cystoceles, rectoceles, and fistulas and the related collaborative and nursing management.

KEY TERMS

abortion, p. 1402	metrorrhagia, p. 1406
amenorrhea, p. 1406	pelvic inflammatory disease,
cystocele, p. 1431	p. 1416
dysmenorrhea, p. 1405	perimenopause, p. 1409
ectopic pregnancy, p. 1408	postmenopause, p. 1409
endometriosis, p. 1418	premenstrual syndrome (PMS),
hysterectomy, p. 1419	p. 1404
infertility, p. 1400	rectocele, p. 1431
leiomyomas, p. 1419	sexual assault, p. 1412
menopause, p. 1409	uterine prolapse, p. 1430
menorrhagia, p. 1406	

INFERTILITY

Infertility is the inability to achieve a pregnancy after at least 1 year of regular intercourse without contraception.[1] Approximately 15% of couples in North America are infertile. Assessment and therapy measures can be invasive, expensive, and lengthy. Understandably, infertility can constitute a physical and emotional crisis.

Etiology and Pathophysiology

Infertility may be caused by either female, male, or combined factors. Conditions that cause male infertility are discussed in Chapter 53. In up to 20% of the couples evaluated, the cause of infertility may not be identified.[1] The most frequent female causes of infertility include factors associated with ovulation (anovulation or inadequate corpus luteum), tubal obstruction or dysfunction (endometriosis or damage from pelvic infection), and uterine or cervical factors (fibroid tumors or structural anomalies). Risk factors for infertility include tobacco and illicit drug use, infection of the reproductive tract, and specific occupational and environmental exposures. In women the risk for infertility increases with age.[1]

Diagnostic Studies

A detailed history and general physical examination of the woman and her partner provide the basis for selecting diagnostic studies (Table 52-1). The possibility of medical or gynecologic diseases is explored before tests are performed to determine problems affecting general health, as well as fertility. These tests include ovulatory studies, tubal patency studies, and postcoital studies.

Ovulatory Studies. A basal body temperature record is kept to determine whether there is regular ovulation (Fig. 52-1). The woman is instructed to take and graph her temperature, referred to as *basal body temperature*, on awakening before any ac-

Reviewed by Susan K. Goebel, RNC, MS, WHNP, SANE, Assistant Professor of Nursing, Mesa State College, Grand Junction, Colo.; Nurse Practitioner, Mesa County Health Department.

TABLE 52-1 Collaborative Care

Infertility

Diagnostic
History and physical examination of both partners, including psychosocial functioning
Review of menstrual history
Assessment of possible sexually transmitted diseases
Basal body temperature record
Serum hormone levels (e.g., FSH, LH, prolactin)
Urinary LH
Sperm penetration assay
Papanicolaou test
Semen analysis
Postcoital test
Endometrial biopsy
Hysterosalpingogram
Pelvic ultrasound

Collaborative Therapy
Hormone supplement therapy
Drug therapy (see Table 52-2)
Intrauterine insemination
Assisted reproductive technologies (ARTs)

FSH, Follicle-stimulating hormone; *LH,* luteinizing hormone.

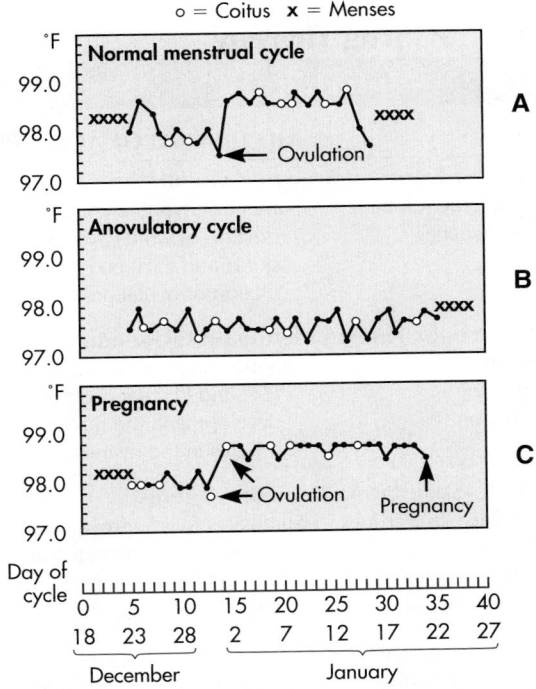

FIG. 52-1 Basal body temperature chart. **A,** Typical biphasic temperature curve indicative of ovulation and normal progesterone effect. **B,** Irregular monophasic curve characteristic of anovulatory cycles. **C,** Ovulatory curve with sustained temperature elevation following conception and the first missed period.

tivity. The same site (e.g., oral, rectal) for taking the temperature should be used each time. Any cause for variation, such as sleeplessness or illness, should be noted. As ovulation approaches, the production of estrogen increases. This may cause a drop in temperature. When ovulation occurs, progesterone is produced, causing a rise in temperature. The temperature graph thus helps detect ovulation and suggests the timing of intercourse if pregnancy is desired. Rigid adherence to a schedule for intercourse can produce psychologic stress sufficient to inhibit sexual relations.

Ovulation prediction kits are now available for use by women at home. These kits are generally used daily to measure luteinizing hormone (LH) levels in urine samples. Ovulation occurs about 28 to 36 hours after the first rise of LH, so intercourse can be timed accordingly. Other tests for ovulation include cervical and vaginal smears, endometrial biopsy, and plasma progesterone levels.

Tubal Patency Studies. Tubal factors (occlusion or deformity) are assessed most commonly by means of hysterosalpingogram. This procedure consists of the radiographic visualization of the uterus and tubes by injecting a radiopaque dye through the cervix. Tubal patency, shape, position, and any distortions of the endometrial cavity can be determined. Laparoscopy may be used when hysterosalpingogram is contraindicated or other pelvic pathology appears likely.

Postcoital Studies. Examination of the cervical mucus can reveal whether it undergoes favorable changes at ovulation, enabling penetration, survival, and normal motility of the sperm. A postcoital test can determine whether the cervical environment is favorable for the sperm. The couple is asked to have intercourse about the time ovulation is expected and 2 to 12 hours before the office visit. Douching or bathing should be avoided before the

test. The cervical and vaginal secretions are aspirated and examined for the number and motility of sperm present. Other screening tests for infertility include semen analysis, endometrial biopsy, and laser laparoscopy.

NURSING *and* COLLABORATIVE MANAGEMENT INFERTILITY

The management of infertility problems depends on the cause. If infertility is secondary to an alteration in ovarian function, supplemental hormone therapy to restore and maintain ovulation may be attempted.[2] Drug therapy used to treat infertility is presented in Table 52-2. Chronic cervicitis and inadequate estrogenic stimulation are cervical factors causing infertility. Antibiotic therapy is indicated for cervicitis. Inadequate estrogenic stimulation is treated by the administration of estrogens.

When a couple has not succeeded in conceiving while under infertility management, an option is intrauterine insemination with sperm from the partner or a donor. If this technique does not succeed, assisted reproductive technologies (ARTs) may be used. ARTs include in vitro fertilization (IVF), gamete intrafallopian transfer (GIFT), zygote intrafallopian transfer (ZIFT), donor gametes, and embryo cryopreservation. IVF is the removal of mature oocytes from the woman's ovarian follicle via laparoscopy, followed by in vitro fertilization of the ova with the partner's sperm. When fertilization and cleavage have occurred, the resulting embryos are transferred into the woman's uterus. The procedure requires 2 to 3 days to complete and is used in cases of fallopian tube obstruction, diminished sperm count, and unexplained

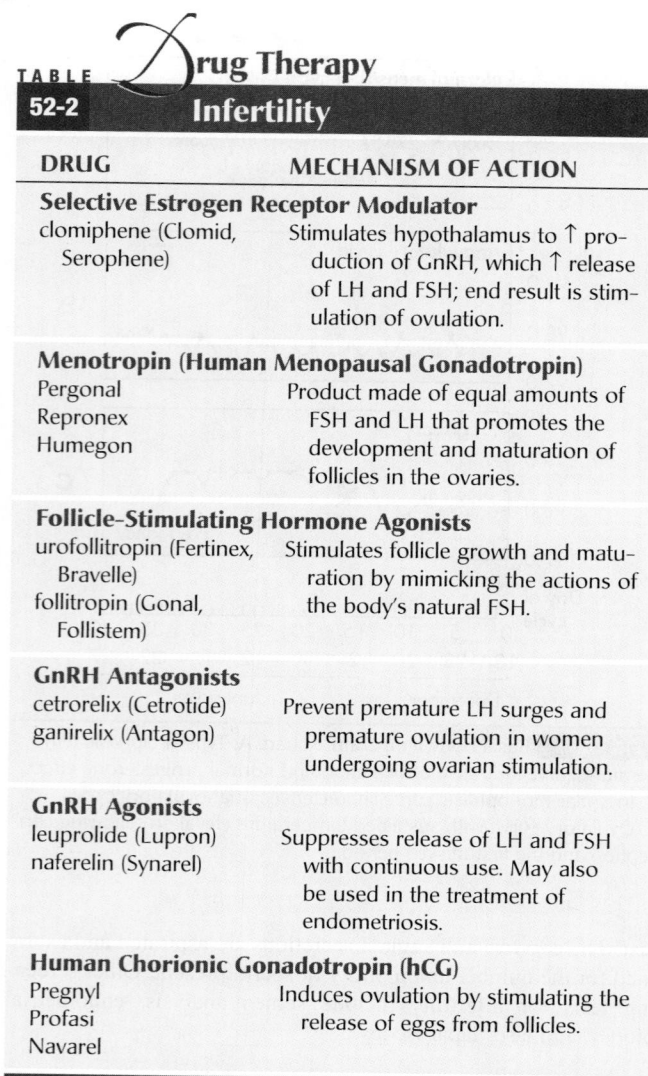

TABLE 52-2 Drug Therapy Infertility

DRUG	MECHANISM OF ACTION
Selective Estrogen Receptor Modulator	
clomiphene (Clomid, Serophene)	Stimulates hypothalamus to ↑ production of GnRH, which ↑ release of LH and FSH; end result is stimulation of ovulation.
Menotropin (Human Menopausal Gonadotropin)	
Pergonal Repronex Humegon	Product made of equal amounts of FSH and LH that promotes the development and maturation of follicles in the ovaries.
Follicle-Stimulating Hormone Agonists	
urofollitropin (Fertinex, Bravelle) follitropin (Gonal, Follistem)	Stimulates follicle growth and maturation by mimicking the actions of the body's natural FSH.
GnRH Antagonists	
cetrorelix (Cetrotide) ganirelix (Antagon)	Prevent premature LH surges and premature ovulation in women undergoing ovarian stimulation.
GnRH Agonists	
leuprolide (Lupron) naferelin (Synarel)	Suppresses release of LH and FSH with continuous use. May also be used in the treatment of endometriosis.
Human Chorionic Gonadotropin (hCG)	
Pregnyl Profasi Navarel	Induces ovulation by stimulating the release of eggs from follicles.

FSH, Follicle-stimulating hormone; *GnRH,* gonadotropin-releasing hormone; *LH,* luteinizing hormone.

infertility. IVF is costly and emotionally stressful, but it has become a recognized and accepted method of therapy for infertile couples.

With the increasing sophistication of ART, couples will have an increased potential for pregnancy. However, the use of ART poses many ethical, legal, and social concerns.

Nurses can assist women experiencing infertility by providing information about the physiology of reproduction, infertility evaluation, and addressing the psychologic and social distress that can accompany infertility. Reducing psychologic stress can improve the emotional climate, making it more conducive to achieving a pregnancy.

The nurse has a major responsibility for teaching and providing emotional support throughout infertility testing and treatment. Feelings of anger, frustration, grief, and helplessness may heighten as additional diagnostic tests are performed. Infertility can generate great tension in a marriage as the couple exhausts financial and emotional resources. Few insurance carriers cover the high cost of infertility testing or expensive in-

fertility treatment. Recognizing and taking steps to deal with the psychologic factors that surface can assist the couple to better cope with the situation. Couples should be encouraged to participate in a support group for infertile couples, as well as individual therapy.

ABORTION

An **abortion** is the loss or termination of a pregnancy before the fetus has developed to a state of viability. Abortions are classified as *spontaneous* (those occurring naturally) or *induced* (those occurring as a result of mechanical or medical intervention). *Miscarriage* is the common term for the unintended loss of a pregnancy. *Habitual abortion* is defined as a history of three or more abortions.

Spontaneous Abortion

Spontaneous abortion is the natural loss of pregnancy before 20 weeks of gestation. Fetal chromosomal anomalies account for 50% of miscarriages before 8 weeks of gestation. Other causes of spontaneous abortions include endocrine abnormalities, maternal infection, acquired anatomic abnormalities (e.g., uterine fibroids, endometriosis), immunologic factors, and environmental factors. About 10% to 15% of all pregnancies end as a result of spontaneous abortion.[3]

Uterine cramping coupled with vaginal bleeding often indicates a spontaneous abortion. Cramping is usually absent if the vaginal bleeding is caused by other conditions, such as polyps. Serial serum β–human chorionic gonadotropin hormone (hCG) and vaginal ultrasound examination of the pelvis are the most reliable indicators of pregnancy with an early abortion. The gestational sac can be visualized using ultrasound as early as 6 weeks of gestation.

Treatment for a possible spontaneous abortion is limited. Although bed rest and avoiding vaginal intercourse are often recommended, there is no evidence that these measures improve the outcome. The woman is advised to report any bleeding to her health care provider. An estimated 80% of patients proceed to abortion regardless of treatment. If the products of conception do not pass completely or bleeding becomes excessive, a *dilation and curettage* (D&C) procedure is generally performed. The D&C involves dilating the uterine cervix and scraping the endometrium of the uterus to empty the uterus of the products of conception.

Women who are experiencing bleeding and cramping during pregnancy may be admitted to the hospital. Nurses need to attend to both the physical and the emotional needs of patients. Vital signs and estimated blood loss are monitored. Any tissue or blood clots that might contain tissue are examined for products of conception. Women are very distressed and experience both physical and emotional pain. Nurses should use comfort measures to provide the needed physical and mental rest. Arranging for someone to stay with the patient provides important emotional support. The nurse should be aware of the grieving process that results from pregnancy loss. Support of the patient and her family is essential.

Induced Abortion

Induced abortion is an intentional termination of a pregnancy. Induced abortion is done for personal reasons (at the request of the woman) and for medical reasons. Several techniques are used to induce abortion, including menstrual extraction, suction curettage, dilation and evacuation (D&E), and drug therapy. Deciding which technique to use to terminate a pregnancy depends on the gestational length of the pregnancy and the woman's condition. Suction curettage may be performed up to 14 weeks of gestation and accounts for more than 90% of abortion procedures.[3] Table 52-3 lists current techniques for abortion.

Drug therapy to induce abortion (medical abortion) early in pregnancy is also available. These agents must be given within the first 49 days of pregnancy (day 1 being the first day of the last menstrual period). Mifepristone (Mifeprex) (also known as

TABLE 52-3	**Methods for Inducing Abortion**			
METHOD	**LENGTH OF PREGNANCY**	**PROCEDURE**	**ADVANTAGES**	**DISADVANTAGES**
Early Abortion				
Menstrual extraction	Usually up to 2 wk after first missed period	Catheter is inserted through cervix into uterus, and suction is applied. Endometrium and contents of uterus are aspirated.	Low cost, simple, done at outpatient facility without anesthesia or cervical dilation, minimally traumatic	Continuation of pregnancy possible, potential for uterine injury and bleeding
Suction curettage	Up to 14 wk	Cervix is usually dilated, uterine aspirator is introduced, and suction is applied, removing endometrial tissue and implanted pregnancy.	Outpatient procedure, most often involving local anesthesia, 1- to 2-day recovery period	Infection, uterine perforation possible
Dilation and evacuation (D&E)	10-16 wk (approximate)	Cervix is dilated, and products of conception are removed by vacuum cannula and the use of other instruments as needed.	Safe and effective procedure for more advanced pregnancy, outpatient procedure with general anesthesia, 2-day recovery period	More psychologic trauma, more expensive, greater risk with general anesthesia and more invasive procedure
mifepristone (Mifeprex) (RU 486) with misoprostol (Cytotec)	Up to 7 wk	Mifepristone is administered orally. Misoprostol is administered orally or intravaginally 2 days later.	Safe, effective, does not require surgical procedure	Very expensive; prolonged bleeding possible
methotrexate with misoprostol	Up to 7 wk	Methotrexate is administered intramuscularly. Misoprostol is given intravaginally 5-7 days later.	Safe, effective, does not require surgical procedure	Not considered as effective as mifepristone; prolonged bleeding possible
Late Abortion				
Instillation of drugs • Hypertonic saline solution	After 16 wk	About 200 ml of amniotic fluid is withdrawn, and a similar amount of 20% normal saline solution is injected. Uterus is irritated and begins to contract within 12-36 hr. Contractions may be assisted with IV oxytocin.	Inexpensive, readily available, feticidal	Hypernatremia, infection, hemorrhage, disseminated intravascular coagulation, more emotional trauma because of time required
• Prostaglandins	After 16 wk	Amniocentesis is done, and 8 ml of prostaglandin is inserted into amniotic sac, resulting in stimulation of smooth muscle of uterus. Expulsion of uterine contents occurs within 24 hr.	Fast induction, no need for surgery	Nausea and vomiting, abdominal cramps, cervical laceration, possible delivery of live fetus, high cost
Hysterotomy	16-20 wk	Miniature cesarean section is performed. Incision is made into uterus and contents are removed.	Concurrent sterilization procedure possible	More difficult and expensive in time and money, surgical incision with possible complications

IV, Intravenous.

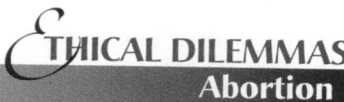

ETHICAL DILEMMAS
Abortion

Situation

A recently married, 39-year-old woman is informed that the results of her amniocentesis indicate that her fetus has major chromosomal abnormalities and is expected to have severe physical and mental disabilities. The patient has no children, but her husband has three children from a previous marriage. She asks the nurse what she should do. How would the nurse respond?

Important Points for Consideration

- Decisions about whether to continue a pregnancy with a child who has severe disabilities are extremely personal and emotional. The woman and her husband will need support and information to explore their options and their values.
- Pregnancy counseling is warranted about the woman's choices, her feelings about the pregnancy, her desire to have a child with her husband, her concerns about raising a child with severe disabilities, her feelings about abortion, and concerns about possible future pregnancies.
- Patient autonomy ensures that a woman decide for herself whether or not to continue a pregnancy.
- The Supreme Court decision in 1973, *Roe v. Wade,* legalized abortion in the United States. In the first trimester, abortion is a private matter between a woman and her physician. In the second trimester, the state may regulate abortion services for safety reasons. In the third trimester, abortions may only be performed when the life or health of the woman is endangered by the pregnancy.
- The role of the health care professional in these difficult situations is to provide education and support, to facilitate a decision consistent with the patient's values.

Critical Thinking Questions

1. How would your feelings about abortion affect your ability to care for this patient?
2. How would you proceed in this case?

RU 486) works by blocking progesterone, a hormone needed for pregnancy to continue. It is given in combination with misoprostol (Cytotec), an agent that produces uterine contractions resulting in expulsion of the products of conception.[4]

Methotrexate, also given in combination with misoprostol, is another option for medically induced abortions. Methotrexate induces abortion because of its toxicity to trophoblastic tissue; misoprostol induces uterine contractions.

Once the decision is made to have an abortion, the woman and her significant others need support and acceptance. The patient should be prepared for what to expect both emotionally and physically. Grief and sadness are normal emotions after an abortion. The patient needs to understand the procedure, including instructions for preprocedure and postprocedure care. The nurse's caring attitude can be a positive factor in the patient's experience.

Follow-up care includes instructions on signs and symptoms of possible complications, including abnormal vaginal bleeding, severe abdominal cramping, fever, and foul drainage. Avoiding intercourse, tampons, and douching until reexamination should be stressed. The patient needs to return for reexamination in 2 weeks. Contraception can be started the day of the procedure

or during the patient's return visit in accordance with her needs and desires.

Problems Related to Menstruation

The normal menstrual cycle is discussed in Chapter 49. The hormonal influences related to the menstrual cycle are shown in Fig. 49-9. Menstruation may be irregular during the first few years after menarche and the years preceding menopause. Once established, a woman's menstrual cycles usually have a predictable pattern. However, considerable normal variation exists among women in cycle length, as well as in the duration, amount, and character of the menstrual flow (see Table 49-2).

PREMENSTRUAL SYNDROME

Premenstrual syndrome (PMS) is a common disorder in women in which a group of physical and psychologic symptoms occur during the last few days of the menstrual cycle and before the onset of menstruation. The symptoms can be severe enough to impair interpersonal relationships or interfere with usual activities. Because many symptoms are associated with PMS, it is difficult to concisely define it. However, PMS symptoms always occur cyclically during the luteal phase before the onset of menstruation and are not present at other times of the month.

Etiology and Pathophysiology

The etiology and pathophysiology are not well understood. PMS is thought to have a biologic trigger with compounding psychosocial factors. Some women may have a genetic predisposition to PMS. Other proposed causes of PMS include estrogen and progesterone imbalances and nutritional deficiencies of pyridoxine (vitamin B_6) or magnesium.[5] *Premenstrual dysphoric disorder* (PMD-D) is the term applied to a type of PMS. Women with PMD-D have a severe mood disorder in addition to PMS.

Clinical Manifestations

PMS is extremely variable in its clinical manifestation. Variation is common between women and, for an individual woman, from one cycle to another. Commonly occurring physical symptoms include breast discomfort, peripheral edema, abdominal bloating, sensation of weight gain, episodes of binge eating, and headache. Abdominal bloating and breast swelling are caused by fluid shifts because total body weight does not generally change. Symptoms of autonomic nervous system arousal (e.g., heart palpitations, dizziness) have been reported by women with PMS. Anxiety, depression, irritability, and mood swings are some of the emotional symptoms that women may experience.

Diagnostic Studies and Collaborative Care

PMS can be diagnosed only when other possible causes for the symptoms have been eliminated. A focused health history and physical examination are done to identify any underlying conditions, such as thyroid dysfunction, uterine fibroids, or depression, that may account for the symptoms. No definitive diagnostic test is available for PMS. When PMS or PMD-D is a possible diagnosis, a woman is given a symptom diary to record her symptoms prospectively for two or three menstrual cycles. Diagnosis is based on an evaluation of the woman's symptoms.

Nonpharmacologic and pharmacologic strategies can relieve some PMS symptoms (Table 52-4). However, no single treatment

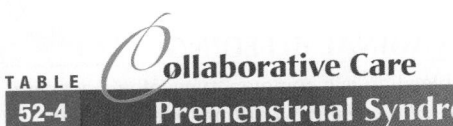

TABLE 52-4	Collaborative Care Premenstrual Syndrome

Diagnostic
History and physical examination
Symptom diary

Collaborative Therapy
Stress management and relaxation therapy
Nutritional therapy
- Avoid caffeine and alcohol
- Reduce refined carbohydrates
- Vitamin B₆
- Limit salt intake before menstruation
Aerobic exercise
Drug therapy
- Diuretics
- Prostaglandin inhibitors (e.g., ibuprofen [Advil, Motrin])
- buspirone (Buspar)
- Tricyclic antidepressants (e.g., amitriptyline [Elavil])
- fluoxetine (Sarafem)
- Selective serotonin reuptake inhibitors (e.g., sertraline [Zoloft])
- Combined oral contraceptives

is available. The goal of treatment is to reduce the severity of symptoms and enhance the woman's sense of control and quality of life.

Several conservative approaches to managing PMS symptoms are considered helpful, including stress management, diet changes, exercise, education, and counseling.[5] Techniques for stress reduction include yoga, meditation, imagery, and biofeedback training. To decrease autonomic nervous system arousal, women should avoid caffeine, reduce refined carbohydrates, exercise on a regular basis, and practice relaxation techniques. Eating complex carbohydrates with high fiber, foods rich in vitamin B₆, and sources of tryptophan (dairy and poultry) are thought to promote serotonin production, which improves the symptoms. Vitamin B₆ may be found in such foods as pork, milk, egg yolk, and legumes. Although no strongly supportive data exist, limiting salt intake before menstruation and increasing calcium intake have been proposed to alleviate fluid retention, weight gain, bloating, breast swelling, and tenderness.

Exercise results in a release of endorphins, leading to mood elevation. Aerobic exercise can also have a relaxing effect. Because fatigue tends to exaggerate the symptoms of PMS, adequate rest in the premenstrual period is a priority.

Explanations about PMS help the woman understand the complexity of the disorder and ways that she can regain a better sense of control. The patient needs to be assured that her symptoms are real, PMS exists, and she is not "crazy." Acknowledgment of having PMS can itself be therapeutic. Teaching the woman's partner about the nature of PMS assists the partner to better understand PMS and to provide support to the woman in making lifestyle changes to reduce the symptoms of PMS.

Drug Therapy. Drug therapy is considered when symptoms persist. Presently, no single drug can treat PMS symptoms. One therapy may be tried for a time, and if no improvement is observed, another approach is tried. Some treatments are symptom specific. For fluid retention, diuretics such as spironolactone (Aldactone) are used. For reducing cramps, backache, and headache, prostaglandin inhibitors such as ibuprofen (Motrin, Advil) are used. To improve negative mood, vitamin B₆ supplementation (50 mg daily) may be used. For anxiety, buspirone (Buspar) taken during the luteal phase has helped some women. Women with PMD-D may benefit from antidepressants, including fluoxetine (Sarafem) and tricyclic antidepressants (e.g., amitriptyline [Elavil]).

Other pharmacologic treatments are directed at PMS in general. Selective serotonin reuptake inhibitors (SSRIs) (e.g., sertraline [Zoloft]) have provided significant relief to women with severe PMS. Other general treatments include oral contraceptives containing estrogen and progesterone. Evening primrose oil, an herb, may help some women.

DYSMENORRHEA

Dysmenorrhea is abdominal cramping pain or discomfort associated with menstrual flow. The degree of pain and discomfort varies with the individual. The two types of dysmenorrhea are primary, when no pathology exists, and secondary, when pelvic disease is the underlying cause. Dysmenorrhea is one of the most common gynecologic problems, affecting approximately 50% of all women.[6]

Etiology and Pathophysiology

Primary dysmenorrhea is not a disease; rather it is caused by an excess of prostaglandin F₂α (PGF₂α) and/or an increased sensitivity to it. The sequential stimulation of the endometrium by estrogen, followed by progesterone, results in a dramatic increase in prostaglandin production by the endometrium. With the onset of menses, degeneration of the endometrium releases prostaglandin. Locally, prostaglandins increase myometrial contractions and constriction of small endometrial blood vessels with consequent tissue ischemia and increased sensitization of the pain receptors, resulting in menstrual pain. Prostaglandins absorbed into the circulatory system may be responsible for symptoms of headache, diarrhea, and vomiting. Primary dysmenorrhea begins in the few years after menarche, typically with the onset of regular ovulatory cycles.

Secondary dysmenorrhea is usually acquired after adolescence, occurring most commonly at 30 to 40 years of age. Common pelvic conditions that cause secondary dysmenorrhea include endometriosis, chronic pelvic inflammatory disease, and uterine fibroids. Because secondary dysmenorrhea is caused by multiple conditions, symptoms vary. However, painful menses is present in all situations.[6]

Clinical Manifestations

Primary dysmenorrhea starts 12 to 24 hours before the onset of menses. The pain is most severe the first day of menses and rarely lasts more than 2 days. Characteristic manifestations include lower abdominal pain that is colicky in nature, frequently radiating to the lower back and upper thighs. The abdominal pain is often accompanied by nausea, diarrhea, loose stools, fatigue, headache, and light-headedness.

Secondary dysmenorrhea usually occurs after the woman has experienced problem-free periods for some time. The pain, which may be unilateral, is generally more constant in nature and usually continues longer than in primary dysmenorrhea. Depending on the cause, symptoms such as *dyspareunia* (painful intercourse), painful defecation, or irregular bleeding may occur at times other than menstruation.

Collaborative Care

Evaluation begins with distinguishing primary from secondary dysmenorrhea. A complete health history with special attention to menstrual and gynecologic history should be obtained. A pelvic examination is also performed. If the history reveals an onset shortly after menarche and symptoms only associated with menses in addition to normal pelvic examination findings, the probable diagnosis is primary dysmenorrhea. If any specific cause of dysmenorrhea is evident, the diagnosis is secondary dysmenorrhea.

Treatment for primary dysmenorrhea includes heat, exercise, and drug therapy. Heat is applied to the lower abdomen or back. Regular exercise is thought to be beneficial because it may reduce endometrial hyperplasia and subsequently reduce prostaglandin production. The primary drug therapy is nonsteroidal antiinflammatory drugs (NSAIDs) such as ibuprofen, which has antiprostaglandin activity. NSAIDs should be started at the first sign of menses and continued every 4 to 8 hours to maintain a sufficient level of the drug to inhibit prostaglandin synthesis for the usual duration of discomfort. Birth control pills may also be used. They decrease dysmenorrhea by reducing endometrial hyperplasia.

Acupuncture and transcutaneous nerve stimulation also provide varying degrees of relief. (See Chapter 7 for a discussion of acupuncture.) These methods may be used for women who obtain inadequate relief from medications or who prefer not to take medications. Patients who are unresponsive to these treatments should be evaluated for chronic pelvic pain.

Treatment of secondary dysmenorrhea depends on the cause. Some individuals with secondary dysmenorrhea will be helped by the approaches used for primary dysmenorrhea. Depending on the underlying causes of dysmenorrhea, additional drug or surgical interventions are used.

NURSING MANAGEMENT
DYSMENORRHEA

One of the primary roles of the nurse is teaching. Women should be taught why dysmenorrhea occurs, as well as how to treat it. Teaching and supportive therapy can provide women with a foundation for coping with this common occurrence and increase feelings of control and self-reliance.

Women often ask the nurse what can be done for minor discomforts associated with menstrual cycles. Women should be advised that during acute pain, relief may be obtained by lying down for short periods, drinking hot beverages, applying heat to the abdomen or back, and taking an antiinflammatory drug for analgesia. The nurse can also suggest noninvasive pain-relieving practices such as distraction and guided imagery.

Other health care measures can reduce the discomfort of dysmenorrhea. These include regular exercise and proper nutritional habits. Avoiding constipation, maintaining good body mechanics, and eliminating stress and fatigue, particularly during the time preceding menstrual periods, can also decrease discomfort. Staying active and interested in activities may also help.

IRREGULAR VAGINAL BLEEDING

Irregular vaginal bleeding is a common gynecologic concern. Irregularities include *oligomenorrhea* (long intervals between menses), **amenorrhea** (absence of menstruation), **menorrhagia** (excessive menstrual bleeding), and **metrorrhagia** (irregular bleeding or bleeding between menses). The cause of irregular bleeding may vary from anovulatory menstrual cycles to more serious causes such as ectopic pregnancy or endometrial cancer. The age of the woman provides direction for identifying the cause of bleeding. For example, a postmenopausal woman with irregular bleeding must always be evaluated for endometrial cancer but does not need to be evaluated for possible pregnancy. For a 20-year-old woman with irregular bleeding, the possibility of pregnancy must always be considered and the possibility of endometrial cancer would be unlikely.

Irregular bleeding may be caused by dysfunction of the hypothalamic-pituitary-ovarian axis such as a pituitary adenoma. Another cause may be infection. Changes in lifestyle such as marriage, recent moves, a death in the family, financial stress, and other emotional crises can also cause irregular bleeding. Because psychologic factors can influence endocrine function, they should be considered when the patient is evaluated.

Types of Irregular Bleeding

Oligomenorrhea and Secondary Amenorrhea. Anovulation is the most common cause for missing menses once pregnancy has been ruled out. Additional causes of amenorrhea are listed in Table 52-5. *Primary amenorrhea* refers to the failure of menstrual cycles to begin by age 16 years or by age 14 years if secondary sex characteristics are present. *Secondary amenorrhea,* on the other hand, refers to cessation of menstrual cycles once established.

Ovulation is often erratic for several years following menarche and before menopause. Thus oligomenorrhea due to anovulation is common for women at the beginning and end of menstruation. In anovulatory cycles, the corpus luteum that produces progesterone does not form. This may result in a situation referred to as *unopposed estrogen.* When unopposed by progesterone, estrogen can cause excessive buildup of the endometrium. Persistent overgrowth of the endometrium increases a woman's risk for endometrial cancer. To reduce this risk, progesterone or birth control pills are prescribed to ensure that the patient's endometrial lining will be shed at least four to six times per year.

Menorrhagia. Excessive bleeding associated with menorrhagia may be an increased duration (more than 7 days), increased amount (more than 80 ml), or both. Anovulatory uterine bleeding is the most common cause of menorrhagia. An unopposed estrogen state continues to build up the endometrium until it becomes unstable, resulting in menorrhagia. For young women with excessive bleeding, clotting disorders must be considered. Uterine fibroids (also called *leiomyomas*) are a common cause of menorrhagia for women in their thirties and forties.

Metrorrhagia. Metrorrhagia, also referred to as *spotting* or *breakthrough bleeding,* is bleeding between menstrual periods. For all reproductive-age women, pregnancy complications such as spontaneous abortion or ectopic pregnancy must be considered as a possible cause. Other causes include cervical or endometrial polyps, infection, and carcinoma. Spotting is common during the first three cycles of birth control pills. If spotting continues past

TABLE 52-5	Causes of Amenorrhea

Hypothalamic-Pituitary Axis
Reversible CNS-mediated causes (e.g., emotional stress,
   anorexia nervosa or severe dieting, strenuous exercise, post-
   pill syndrome, chronic or acute illness)
Prolactinoma and other causes of hyperprolactinemia (e.g., drugs)
Craniopharyngioma and other brainstem or parasellar tumors
Congenital conditions (e.g., isolated gonadotropin
   deficiency)*
Trauma (e.g., head injury with hypothalamic contusion)
Infiltrative processes (e.g., sarcoidosis)
Vascular disease (e.g., hypothalamic vasculitis)
Pituitary tumors
Sheehan syndrome

Ovaries
Autoimmune disease (often involving thyroid, adrenal, and
   islet cells)
Premature menopause (idiopathic) or resistant-ovary syndrome
Polycystic ovary disease
Tumors
Congenital or genetic conditions (e.g., Turner syndrome)*
Infection (e.g., mumps oophoritis)
Toxins (especially alkylating chemotherapeutic agents)
Radiation
Trauma, torsion (rare)

Uterovaginal Outflow Tract
Asherman syndrome (postcurettage loss of endometrium)
Müllerian dysgenesis*

Hormonal Synthesis and Action
Male pseudohermaphroditism (e.g., testicular feminization)*
17-Hydroxylase deficiency*

*Usually manifests as primary amenorrhea.
CNS, Central nervous system.

the woman's third cycle using birth control pills, a different pill formulation can be prescribed when other causes of metrorrhagia have been ruled out. Spotting with long-acting progestin therapy, such as Depo-Provera or Norplant, is also common. For post-menopausal women, endometrial cancer must be considered whenever spotting is experienced. In postmenopausal women, exogenous estrogen administration during hormone replacement therapy is a common cause of metrorrhagia. *Menometrorraghia* is excessive bleeding that occurs at irregular intervals. It may be caused by endometrial cancer or uterine fibroids.

Diagnostic Studies and Collaborative Care

Because irregular vaginal bleeding has multiple causes, diagnostic and collaborative care vary as well. A health history and physical examination directed at the most likely causes of vaginal bleeding for the woman's age-group is the first step. These findings will provide the basis for selecting the necessary laboratory tests and diagnostic procedures. Treatment depends on the nature of the problem (e.g., menorrhagia, amenorrhea), degree of threat to the patient's health, and whether children are desired in the future.

Combined oral contraceptives may be prescribed for a woman with amenorrhea to ensure regular shedding of endome-trium if she also wants contraception. If she does not need birth control, progesterone may be prescribed to ensure a shedding of the endometrial lining four to six times per year. On the other hand, if she wants to become pregnant, a fertility drug may be prescribed.

The treatment goal for women with menorrhagia is to minimize further blood loss. If menorrhagia is the result of anovulatory cycles, the endometrium must be stabilized by a combination of oral estrogen and progesterone.

A new therapy for treating menorrhagia has recently become available. Balloon therapy is a technique that involves the introduction of a soft, flexible balloon into the uterus; the balloon is then inflated with sterile fluid (Fig. 52-2). The fluid in the balloon is heated and maintained for 8 minutes, thus causing ablation (removal) of the uterine lining. When the treatment is completed, the fluid is withdrawn from the balloon and the catheter is removed from the uterus. The uterine lining sloughs off in the following 7 to 10 days. Uterine balloon therapy is contraindicated for women desiring future fertility and for women with any suspected uterine abnormalities such as fibroids, suspected endometrial carcinoma, previous classical cesarean section, or myomectomy.[7] With severe bleeding, hospitalization is indicated. All patients with menorrhagia should be evaluated for anemia and treated as indicated.

Surgical Therapy. Surgery may be indicated depending on the underlying cause of the irregular vaginal bleeding. Dilation and curettage (D&C) was once a common therapy for excessive bleeding or for spotting in perimenopausal women. Now D&C is used only in extreme cases of bleeding or for older women when endometrial biopsy and ultrasonography have not provided the necessary diagnostic information. Endometrial ablation done by laser or electrosurgical technique has been successful with many patients with uncontrolled menorrhagia. If menorrhagia is caused by uterine fibroids, a hysterectomy may be performed. A *myomectomy* (removal of fibroids without removal of the uterus) may be performed if the patient wants to preserve her uterus. Hormonal regimens, ablative techniques, and embolization of blood vessels supplying the fibroid are newer options.[8]

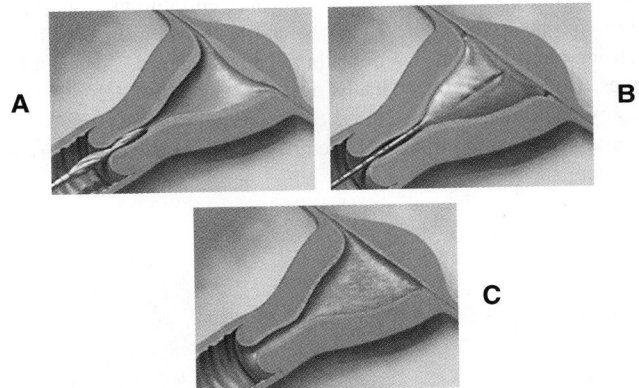

FIG. 52-2 Balloon thermotherapy for treatment of menorrhagia. **A,** Balloon-tipped catheter is inserted into the uterus through the vagina and cervix. **B,** The balloon is inflated with a sterile fluid that expands to fit the size and shape of the uterus. The fluid is heated to 188° F (87° C) and maintained for 8 minutes while the uterine lining is treated. **C,** Fluid is withdrawn from the balloon and the catheter is removed.

NURSING MANAGEMENT
IRREGULAR VAGINAL BLEEDING

For some women, infrequent or no menses might seem a desirable state. Teaching women about the characteristics of the menstrual cycle will assist them to identify normal variations.

Table 49-2 includes characteristics of the menstrual cycle and related patient teaching. This knowledge can diminish apprehension and dispel misconceptions about the menstrual cycle. If the patient's menstrual cycle pattern does not fall within the normal range, the nurse should urge her to visit her health care provider. Myths concerning activities allowed during menstruation are common. The nurse should be prepared to clarify the facts. The patient should be assured that bathing and hair washing are safe. A daily warm tub bath may actually relieve some of the associated pelvic discomfort. Women can swim, exercise, have intercourse, and basically continue their usual daily activities.

Frequent changing of tampons or pads meets comfort and hygiene needs during menstruation. The selection of internal or external sanitary protection is a matter of personal preference. Tampons are convenient and make menstrual hygiene easier, whereas pads may provide better protection. Using a combination of tampons and pads and avoiding prolonged use of superabsorbent tampons may decrease the risk of *toxic shock syndrome* (TSS).[8] TSS is an acute condition caused by a toxin from *Staphylococcus aureus*. TSS causes high fever, vomiting, diarrhea, weakness, myalgia, and a sunburn-like rash.

Whenever excessive, the amount of the patient's vaginal bleeding should be assessed as accurately as possible. The number and size of pads or tampons used and the degree of saturation should be reported and recorded. The patient's fatigue level, along with variations in blood pressure and pulse, should be monitored because anemia and hypovolemia may be present. If a surgical procedure is indicated, the nurse should provide appropriate preoperative and postoperative care.

ECTOPIC PREGNANCY

An **ectopic pregnancy** is the implantation of the fertilized ovum anywhere outside the uterine cavity (Fig. 52-3). Between 97% and 98% of ectopic pregnancies occur in the fallopian tube. The remaining 2% to 3% may be ovarian, abdominal, or cervical (Fig. 52-4). Ectopic pregnancy is a life-threatening condition. Earlier identification has contributed to a decrease in mortality rates. However, 40 to 50 deaths occur as a result of ectopic pregnancy each year in the United States. Ectopic pregnancy is the leading cause of maternal death among African American women.[9]

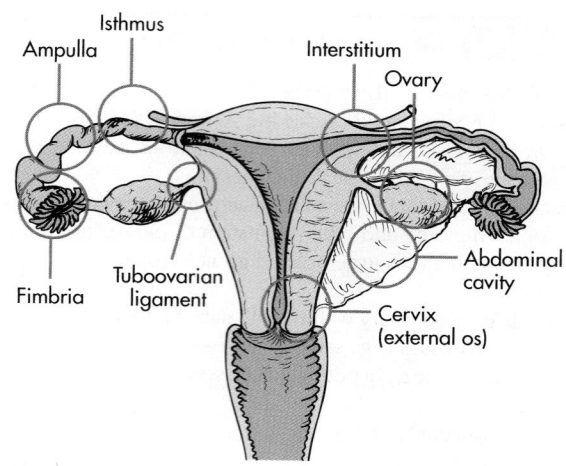

FIG. 52-4 Sites of implantation of ectopic pregnancies. Order of frequency of occurrence is ampulla, isthmus, interstitium, fimbria, tuboovarian ligament, ovary, abdominal cavity, and cervix (external os).

Etiology and Pathophysiology

Any blockage of the tube or reduction of tubal peristalsis that impedes or delays the zygote passing to the uterine cavity can result in tubal implantation. After implantation, the growth of the gestational sac expands the tubal wall. Eventually the tube ruptures, causing acute peritoneal symptoms. Less acute symptoms usually begin within 6 to 8 weeks after the last normal menstrual period and weeks before rupture would occur.

Risk factors for ectopic pregnancy include a history of pelvic inflammatory disease, prior ectopic pregnancy, current progestin-releasing intrauterine device (IUD), progestin-only birth control failure, and prior pelvic or tubal surgery. Additional risk factors for ectopic pregnancy include procedures used in infertility treatment, including in vitro fertilization procedures, embryo transfer, and ovulation induction.

Clinical Manifestations

The classic symptoms of ectopic pregnancy are abdominal or pelvic pain, missed menses, and irregular vaginal bleeding. Other symptoms include amenorrhea, morning sickness, breast tenderness, gastrointestinal disturbance, malaise, and syncope. Pain is almost always present and is caused by distention of the fallopian tube. It may start unilaterally and then spread to become bilateral. The character of the pain varies among women and can be colicky or vague. If tubal rupture occurs, the pain is intense and may be referred to the shoulder as a result of irritation of the

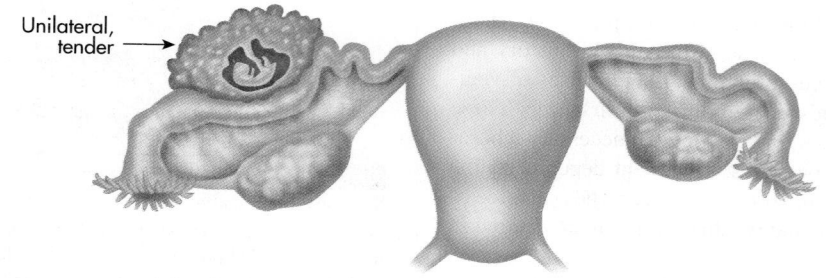

FIG. 52-3 Ruptured tubal pregnancy.

diaphragm by blood released into the abdominal cavity. Symptom severity does not necessarily correlate with the extent of external bleeding present. With rupture, the risk of hemorrhage and hypovolemic shock is present. Suspected rupture is treated as an emergency.

The vaginal bleeding that may accompany ectopic pregnancy is usually described as spotting. However, it is also possible that bleeding may be heavier and can be confused with menses. The woman may also experience irregular bleeding.

Diagnostic Studies

Because of the life-threatening nature of ectopic pregnancy, it should be considered whenever pregnancy is even remotely possible. Ectopic pregnancy can be a diagnostic challenge because of its similarity to other pelvic and abdominal disorders, such as salpingitis, spontaneous abortion, ruptured ovarian cyst, appendicitis, and peritonitis. A sensitive serum pregnancy test should be performed. If the test is negative, an ectopic pregnancy is not likely. If ectopic pregnancy cannot be excluded by the pregnancy test, further evaluation is warranted. If the patient is in a stable condition, a combination of serial β–human chorionic gonadotropin (β-hCG) and vaginal ultrasonography is used. β-hCG is expected to double about every 48 hours in a normal pregnancy. If the hCG level fails to double, the patient may have an ectopic pregnancy. Ultrasound can be used to confirm the presence of an intrauterine pregnancy once the β-hCG level has reached 2000 mIU/ml.

Absence of a normal intrauterine pregnancy means that the diagnosis is probably spontaneous abortion or ectopic pregnancy. With a spontaneous abortion, serial β-hCG levels will decrease over time. A complete blood count is obtained when there is any concern regarding the amount of blood loss or if surgery is contemplated. A gradually decreasing hematocrit may indicate internal bleeding.

NURSING *and* COLLABORATIVE MANAGEMENT ECTOPIC PREGNANCY

Surgery remains the primary approach for treating ectopic pregnancies and should be performed immediately. However, medical management with methotrexate (Folex) is being used with increasing success with patients who are hemodynamically stable and have a mass less than 3 cm in size. A conservative surgical approach limits damage to the reproductive system as much as possible. Removal of the pregnancy from the tube is preferred to removing the tube. Laparoscopy is preferable to laparotomy, because it decreases blood loss and the length of the hospital stay. If the tube ruptures, conservative surgical approaches may not be possible. The patient may need a blood transfusion and supplemental intravenous (IV) fluid therapy to relieve shock and restore a satisfactory blood volume for safe anesthesia and surgery. The use of microsurgery techniques has resulted in fewer repeated ectopic pregnancies and a higher rate of future successful pregnancies.

Nursing care depends on the condition of the patient. Before the diagnosis has been confirmed, the nurse should be alert to signs of increasing pain and vaginal bleeding, which may indicate that rupture of the tube has occurred. Vital signs are monitored closely, along with observation for signs of shock. Explanations and preparation for diagnostic procedures are given when

appropriate. Preparation of the patient for abdominal surgery may follow rapidly. The patient's emotional status should be assessed. Reassurance and support for the surgery should be given to the patient and her family. Postoperatively, the patient may express a fear of future ectopic pregnancies and have many questions about the impact of this experience on her future fertility.

PERIMENOPAUSE AND POSTMENOPAUSE

The **perimenopause** is a normal life transition that begins with the first signs of change in menstrual cycles and ends after cessation of menses. **Menopause** is the physiologic cessation of menses associated with declining ovarian function. It is usually considered complete after 1 year of *amenorrhea* (absence of menstruation). Menopause starts gradually and is usually associated with changes in menstruation, including menstrual flows that are increased, decreased, and/or irregular. Cessation of menses finally occurs. **Postmenopause** is a term that refers to the time in a woman's life after menopause.

The age at which menopause occurs ranges from 45 to 55 years but may occur earlier due to illness, surgical removal of the uterus or both ovaries, side effects of radiation therapy or chemotherapy, or drugs. The age at which menopause occurs is not affected by age at menarche, race, physical characteristics, number of pregnancies, date of last pregnancy, socioeconomic status, or oral contraceptive use. However, cigarette smoking, chemotherapy, and radiation have been linked to acceleration of menopause.[10]

Changes in the ovary start the cascade of events that finally result in menopause. The regression of the follicles within each ovary begins with puberty and accelerates after age 35. With age, fewer and fewer follicles remain that are responsive to follicle-stimulating hormone (FSH). FSH normally stimulates the dominant follicle to secrete estrogen. When the follicles can no longer respond to FHS, ovarian production of estrogen and progesterone declines. However, perimenopausal women can get pregnant until menopause has occurred.

With decreased ovarian function there are decreased levels of estrogen that cause a gradual increase in FSH and LH as a result of the negative feedback process. By the time menopause occurs, there is a tenfold to twentyfold increase in FSH. The elevated FSH level may take several years to return to the premenopausal level. The reduced estrogen level also causes a decrease in the frequency of ovulation and results in changes in the secondary sex characteristics (e.g., decreased skin elasticity).

Clinical Manifestations

Clinical manifestations of perimenopause and postmenopause are presented in Table 52-6. The perimenopause is a time of erratic hormonal fluctuation. Irregular vaginal bleeding is common. With decreasing estrogen, hot flashes and other symptoms begin. The signs and symptoms of diminished estrogen are listed in Table 52-7. The loss of estrogen plays a significant role in the cause of age-related alterations. Changes most critical to a woman's well-being are the increased risks for coronary artery disease and osteoporosis secondary to bone density loss. Other changes include a redistribution of fat, a tendency to gain weight more easily, muscle and joint pain, loss of skin elasticity, changes in hair amount and distribution, and atrophy of external genitalia and breast tissue.

Hallmarks of the perimenopause include *vasomotor instability* (hot flashes) and irregular menses. A hot flash is described as a

TABLE 52-6   Clinical Manifestatons of Perimenopause and Postmenopause

PERIMENOPAUSE	POSTMENOPAUSE
Irregular menses	Cessation of menses
Vasomotor instability (hot flashes and night sweats)	Occasional vasomotor symptoms
Atrophy of genitourinary tissue (e.g., vaginal epithelium)	Atrophy of genitourinary tissue with decreased support
Stress and urge incontinence	Stress and urge incontinence
Breast tenderness	Osteoporosis
Mood changes	

TABLE 52-7   Signs and Symptoms of Estrogen Deficiency

Vasomotor
Hot flashes
Night sweats
Genitourinary
Atrophic vaginitis
Dyspareunia secondary to poor lubrication
Incontinence
Psychologic
Emotional lability
Change in sleep pattern
Decreased REM sleep
Skeletal
Increased fracture rate, particularly of vertebral bodies but also of humerus, distal radius, and upper femur
Cardiovascular
Decreased high–density lipoproteins (HDL)
Increased low–density lipoproteins (LDL)
Dermatologic
Diminished collagen content of skin
Breast tissue changes

REM, Rapid eye movement.

sensation of warmth in the upper part of the chest, neck, and face followed by profuse perspiration and sometimes chilling. These sensations last from several seconds to 5 minutes and occur most often at night, thereby disturbing sleep. The cause of hot flashes, or vasomotor instability, is not clearly understood. It has been theorized that temperature regulators in the brain are in proximity to the area where gonadotropin-releasing hormone (GnRH) is released. However, lowered estrogen levels are correlated with dilation of cutaneous blood vessels resulting in hot flashes and increased sweating. The more sudden the withdrawal of estrogen (e.g., surgical removal of the ovaries), the more likely the symptoms will be severe if no hormone replacement is provided. These symptoms subside over time with or without hormone replacement therapy. Hot flashes can be triggered by situations that affect body temperature, such as eating a hot meal, hot weather, drinking an alcoholic beverage, stress, or warm clothing.

Atrophic vaginal changes secondary to decreased estrogen include thinning of the vaginal mucosa and disappearance of rugae. Vaginal secretions also decrease and become more alkaline. As a result of these changes, the vagina is easily traumatized and susceptible to infection. *Dyspareunia* (painful intercourse) may also occur. This can lead to unnecessary and premature cessation of sexual activity. Dryness is a problem that can be easily corrected with water-soluble lubricants or, if needed, with hormonal creams or systemic hormone replacement therapy. In general, the extent and severity of the symptoms of menopause vary and are not easily predicted, even with a detailed history of family patterns.

Atrophic changes in the lower urinary tract also occur with a decrease in estrogen. Bladder capacity decreases and the bladder and urethral tissue lose tone. These changes can cause symptoms that mimic a bladder infection (e.g., dysuria, urgency, frequency) when no infection is present.

Whether decreasing estrogen is responsible for the psychologic changes associated with perimenopause is unclear. The attributed depression, irritability, and cognitive problems could result from life stressors or sleep deprivation from hot flashes. Research has not found a statistically significant relationship between perimenopause and depression.[11] Women who are most likely to be depressed believe that depression is related to menopause, are concerned about menopause and aging, or have a previous history of depression or unemployment.[11]

Collaborative Care

The diagnosis of perimenopause should be made only after careful consideration of other possible causes for the woman's symptoms. Depression, thyroid dysfunction, anemia, or anxiety reactions could be responsible for the same symptoms. Because of the hormonal fluctuations that occur before menopause, routine testing of the serum FSH level is not indicated. After age 50, postmenopause can be diagnosed by an FSH of 30 mIU/ml or greater if the woman is not on any hormonal medication.

Nonhormonal Therapy. The frequency and severity of hot flashes can be reduced by avoiding things that increase heat production and by promoting heat loss. Keeping a cool environment and reducing caffeine and alcohol intake reduce heat production. Behavioral changes, such as relaxation techniques, also help. To promote heat loss at night when hot flashes can disrupt sleep, increasing air circulation in the room and avoiding bedding that traps the heat (e.g., heavy quilts) may help. Loose-fitting clothes do not retain body heat, as do clothes with tight necks and wrists. Cool cloths applied to flushed areas also aid heat loss. Daily intake of vitamin E in doses up to 600 IU may help reduce hot flashes.[12]

Dry skin can be improved by the use of moisturizing soaps and body lotions. Kegel exercises can decrease stress incontinence. Dyspareunia related to vaginal dryness can be managed with a water-soluble lubricant.

Improving nutrition, exercise, and sleep can improve anxiety and depression. Sleep may be improved by avoiding alcohol and controlling hot flashes. Stress reduction techniques can improve sleep by decreasing anxiety.

Hormonal Therapy. Hormone replacement therapy (HRT) includes estrogen for women without a uterus or estrogen and progesterone for women with a uterus. Some HRT regimens include low-dose testosterone to increase libido. HRT helps retard bone loss and may help prevent osteoporosis. HRT also minimizes atrophic changes to the genitourinary tissues. Although observational studies have suggested that estrogen replacement in women may reduce the risk of Alzheimer's disease, there are no definitive research findings to support the use of estrogen to prevent Alzheimer's disease.[13]

Known or suspected breast cancer is generally a contraindication to estrogen use.[14] In addition to known or suspected breast cancer, other absolute contraindications to HRT include abnormal vaginal bleeding, pregnancy, active thrombophlebitis, thromboembolic disorder, and liver dysfunction. Long-term use of HRT increases the risk for endometrial cancer, but this increased risk is decreased with 12 or more days of progesterone per month. The risk for endometrial cancer is present only in those women who still have a uterus. Some women will have an increase in hyperlipidemia with progesterone. However, this is not a contraindication to HRT. The lowest dose of progesterone is used, and serum lipid levels are monitored.

Many different regimens of HRT are available, from continuous combined estrogen-progesterone therapy to various sequential and cyclic patterns. The choice of using HRT or not, and if using, which regimen to use, is tailored to the individual woman. Factors for consideration include concern about cancer, previously used regimens, tolerance of hormonal side effects, and presence of perimenopausal symptoms (see Evidence-Based Practice box).

EVIDENCE-BASED PRACTICE

Hormone Replacement Therapy (HRT) and Coronary Artery Disease

Clinical Problem
Does long-term use of estrogen therapy prevent coronary artery disease?

Best Clinical Practice
- Combination estrogen-medroxyprogesterone (Prempro) does not have a protective effect for coronary artery disease.
- Prempro should not be prescribed to postmenopausal women for prevention of cardiovascular problems.
- Women taking Prempro have an increased risk of breast cancer and cardiovascular disease (myocardial infarction and stroke) but lower risk of fractures and colorectal cancer.
- Because of the differences in estrogen potency and product composition, the extent to which these findings can be generalized to other combination estrogen-progesterone products is not known.

Implications for Nursing Practice
- Based on their individual risk factors and health care needs, women should discuss the benefits and risks of using HRT with their health care provider.
- If a woman and her health care provider believe that the use of HRT is important to manage symptoms of menopause, the best recommendation is to use HRT on a short-term basis.
- Herb and dietary supplements may be used to reduce the symptoms of menopause (see Complementary and Alternative Therapies box on p. 1412).

Reference for Evidence
Writing Group for the Women's Health Initiative Investigators: Risks and benefits of estrogen plus progestin in healthy postmenopausal women: principal results from the Women's Health Initiative randomized controlled trial, *JAMA* 288:321, 2002.

The side effects of estrogen include nausea, fluid retention, headache, and breast enlargement. Side effects of progesterone include increased appetite, weight gain, irritability, depression, spotting, and breast tenderness. To minimize these unwanted side effects, the lowest possible dose of each should be used.

A commonly used estrogen preparation is 0.625 mg of conjugated estrogen (Premarin) daily. For symptom relief, a higher dose may be needed. To receive the protective benefit of progesterone, 5 to 10 mg of medroxyprogesterone (Provera) is indicated for 12 days of each month on a cyclic regimen or 2.5 mg if on a continuous regimen. If the estrogen is to be increased for symptom relief, the progesterone should also be increased. Other forms of progesterone include norethindrone (Aygestin) and micronized progesterone (Prometrium). Estrogen comes in a variety of forms including oral tablets, vaginal creams, dermal patches, rings placed around the cervix, and subcutaneous pellets. Vaginal creams are especially useful for urogenital symptoms (e.g., dryness). Transdermal (skin patch) estrogen has the advantage of bypassing the liver, but has the disadvantage of causing skin irritation.

Selective estrogen receptor modulators (SERMs) are also used in treating menopausal problems. These drugs have some of the positive benefits of estrogen, such as preventing bone loss, without the negative effects such as endometrial hyperplasia. Raloxifene (Evista) competes with estrogen for estrogen receptor sites. It decreases bone loss and serum cholesterol but has minimal effects on breast and uterine tissue. SERMs are also discussed, with respect to their role in the management of osteoporosis, in Chapter 62.

Nutritional Therapy. Good nutrition can decrease the risk of cardiovascular disease and osteoporosis in addition to assisting with vasomotor symptoms. A daily intake of about 30 kcal/kg of body weight with maintenance of sound nutrition is recommended. A decrease in metabolic rate and careless eating habits can cause the weight gain and fatigue often attributed to menopause. An adequate intake of calcium and vitamin D helps maintain healthy bones and counteracts loss of bone density. Postmenopausal women who are not receiving supplemental estrogen should have a daily calcium intake of at least 1500 mg; those who are taking estrogen replacement need at least 1000 mg per day. Calcium supplements are best absorbed when taken with meals. Either dietary calcium or calcium supplements may be used (see Chapter 62, Tables 62-12 and 62-13).

The diet should be high in complex carbohydrates and vitamin B complex, especially B_6. Phytoestrogens from plant sources have been shown to be beneficial in some women.[15] Examples of foods containing phytoestrogens include soy, tofu, chick peas, and sunflower seeds. Herbal remedies have become popular in treating menopausal symptoms (see Complementary and Alternative Therapies box). Consultation with an experienced herbal practitioner is recommended before initiating therapy. Many herbs can cause serious adverse effects.[11]

■ Culturally Competent Care: Menopause

Nurses must be aware of the differences in attitudes and beliefs regarding menopause among women from various ethnic backgrounds. Menopause is a significant milestone in a woman's life. The way in which she approaches this life change is embedded in her own personality and her culture. American culture is

COMPLEMENTARY &ALTERNATIVE THERAPIES
Herbs and Supplements for Menopause

Phytoestrogens
Phytoestrogens are found in plants and may act similar to estrogen produced naturally in the body. The food that is richest in phytoestrogens is soybeans.

Clinical Uses
Menopausal symptoms such as hot flashes, night sweats, insomnia, mood swings, dry skin, and vaginal mucosa

Effects
Soy: May lower cholesterol, decrease hot flashes, and promote bone strength.
Black cohosh: Reduces hot flashes; possible positive effect on bone and cardiovascular health and mood. Can cause minor upset stomach. May interact with antihypertensive medication. Large amounts may cause toxicity.
Dong quai: Chinese herb promoted as being able to reduce hot flashes and improve cardiovascular health. May be toxic. Increases the effects of oral anticoagulants. Can cause photosensitivity.

Nursing Implications
- Women who have had a history of breast cancer should consult with their health care provider before using any of these herbs and supplements.
- Increasing consumption of soy products in the diet appears to be an effective treatment modality for postmenopausal women.

COMPLEMENTARY &ALTERNATIVE THERAPIES
Valerian

Clinical Uses
Insomnia, anxiety, restlessness, urinary tract disorders

Effects
Mild tranquilizer, muscle relaxant, sedative, or sleep aid. May cause hepatotoxicity when combined with other herbs such as skullcap or mistletoe.

Nursing Implications
Valerian should not be taken with alcohol, drugs that depress the central nervous system, or Antabuse. Valerian should not be used on a regular basis. Liver function should be assessed if used on a long-term basis.

generally negative toward aging and places a high value on youth. Many ethnic groups have their traditions and beliefs regarding childbirth and menopause. Research has found that African American women are more positive in attitude toward menopause than other ethnic groups.[16] African American women are more likely than white American women to experience hot flashes.[17]

NURSING MANAGEMENT
PERIMENOPAUSE AND POSTMENOPAUSE

Nurses can play a key role in helping women to understand perimenopausal changes and options to minimize unwanted symptoms. Women can decrease their risk for cardiovascular disease and osteoporosis. Nurses can foster a positive image of perimenopause as a time of vitality and attractiveness. Perimenopause can provide women with an incentive to enhance self-care.

Nurses should provide teaching and reassurance to perimenopausal women distraught by their symptoms. They should be taught that the symptoms are normal and only temporary. Nonpharmacologic approaches to managing symptoms should be discussed. The nurse should dispel misconceptions about menopause. This can reduce unnecessary anxiety.

A regular program of exercise and physical activity can improve circulation, maintain good muscle tone, and delay some aspects of aging for postmenopausal women. Regular aerobic exercise stimulates osteoblastic activity, thereby stimulating calcium deposition into bone and delaying osteoporosis.

Sexual function can continue with little change in the vast majority of postmenopausal women. Cessation of menstruation and ability to bear children should not be equated with cessation of sexual capability; in fact it may be liberating. Femininity and libido do not disappear with menopause. Atrophic changes in vaginal epithelium associated with decreased estrogen may lead to dyspareunia. A water-soluble lubricant (e.g., Replens, Astroglide, K-Y jelly) is often effective in managing this problem. An active sex life helps increase lubrication and maintains the pliability of vaginal tissues. The patient should be given an opportunity to candidly discuss concerns related to sexual functioning.

SEXUAL ASSAULT

Sexual assault is defined as the forcible perpetration of a sexual act on a person without his or her consent. It can include any of the following actions: sodomy, forced anal intercourse, oral copulation, forced copulation of mouth or anus of another, assault with a foreign object, and serial battery. Sexual assault can dramatically disrupt the roles normally performed by the adult woman.

Clinical Manifestations

Physical. Of the women who seek help immediately after the assault, between one half and two thirds will not have any evidence of physical trauma. Evidence of trauma may be limited because women do not resist for fear of physical danger and injury. When present, physical injuries may include bruising and lacerations to the perineum, hymen, vulva, vagina, cervix, and anus. Fractures, subdural hematomas, cerebral concussions, and intraabdominal injuries have resulted in the need for hospitalization. Sexual assault also places women at risk for sexually transmitted diseases (STDs) and pregnancy.

Psychologic. Immediately after the assault, women may show shock, numbness, denial, or withdrawal. Some women may seem unnaturally calm; others may cry or express anger. Feelings of humiliation, degradation, embarrassment, anger, self-blame, and fear of another assault are commonly expressed. These symptoms usually decrease after 2 weeks, and victims may appear to have adjusted. Yet any time from 2 to 3 weeks to months to years after the assault, symptoms may return and become more severe. The rape-trauma syndrome is a classification of posttraumatic stress disorder. Flashbacks, intrusive recall, sleep disturbances, and numbing of feelings are common initial symptoms. Women will feel embarrassment, self-blame, and powerlessness.

Later symptoms include mood swings, irritability, and anger. Feelings of despair, shame, and hopelessness are often the cause of the anger. These feelings may be internalized and expressed as depression. Suicidal ideations may also occur.

Collaborative Care

In the acute care of an assault survivor, ensuring the woman's emotional and physical safety has the highest priority. Table 52-8 outlines the emergency management of the patient who has been sexually assaulted. Most emergency departments (EDs) have identified personnel who have received special training in order to work with women who have been assaulted. Many crime-fighting agencies within communities have created the position of the Sexual Assault Nurse Examiner (SANE).[18] The SANE is a registered nurse who is certified to provide care to victims of sexual assault, while ensuring evidence is safeguarded. Special procedures are followed in taking the history and conducting the examination in order to preserve all evidence in case of future prosecution.

When the survivor of an assault is admitted to the ED or clinic, a specific chain of events occurs (Table 52-9). A signed informed consent is obtained from the woman before any data are collected. All materials gathered are well documented, labeled, and given to the appropriate person, such as the pathologist or a police officer. The materials are handled by as few people as possible, and signatures of all responsible for keeping and handling the data are obtained. Many items can be used as evidence if the victim chooses to file a complaint. Consequently, the integrity of the material must be maintained. The nurse's involvement in the medicolegal process depends on the policies of the individual institution and state law.

A gynecologic and sexual history and an account of the assault (who, what, when, and where), as well as a general physical and pelvic examination, add further information about the rape incident. Laboratory tests are done primarily to determine the presence of sperm in the vagina and to identify any existing STDs or pregnancy.

Follow-up physical and psychologic care is essential. Women should return weekly for the first month following the assault. This includes the time period when women's psychologic reactions may be the most severe. Providers should have the telephone numbers and names of contact persons for local resources for sexual assault survivors, including rape crisis centers, legal and law enforcement authorities, and human services.

NURSING MANAGEMENT
SEXUAL ASSAULT

Nurses can assist all women in becoming aware of prevention tactics (Table 52-10). They should also be encouraged to learn some basic techniques of self-defense. Local high schools and the

---

TABLE 52-8	**Emergency Management**	
Sexual Assault		
ETIOLOGY	**ASSESSMENT FINDINGS**	**INTERVENTIONS**
Sexual molestation Sodomy Assault involving genitalia (male or female) without consent	• Emotional or physical manifestations of shock • Hysteria • Crying • Anger • Silence • Decreased level of consciousness • Hyperventilation • Oral, vaginal, and rectal injuries • Extragenital injuries • Pain in genital area or extragenital area	**Initial** • Treat shock and other urgent medical problems, (e.g., head injury, hemorrhage, wounds, fractures). • Assess emotional state. • Contact support person (i.e., social worker, rape advocate, sexual assault nurse examiner). • Do *not* clean the patient until all evidence is collected. Make sure the patient does not wash, douche, urinate, brush teeth, or gargle. • Place sheet on floor. Then have patient stand on sheet to remove clothing. Place sheet with clothing in paper bag. • Obtain forensic evidence per local protocol (i.e., body hair, nail scrapings, tissue, dried semen, vaginal washing, blood samples). • Maintain chain of evidence for all legal specimens. Clearly label evidence and keep in locked cabinet until given to law enforcement agency. • Obtain baseline HIV, syphilis, and other STD screening. • Determine method of contraception, date of last menstrual period, and date of last tetanus immunization. • Consider tetanus prophylaxis if lacerations contain soil/dirt. • Vaccinate with hepatitis B if not immunized. **Ongoing Monitoring** • Monitor vital signs and emotional status. • Provide clothing as needed. • Counsel patient regarding confidential HIV and STD testing.

HIV, Human immunodeficiency virus; *STD,* sexually transmitted disease.

TABLE 52-9   Evaluation of Alleged Sexual Assault

1. Medicolegal
Valid written consent for examination, photographs, laboratory tests, release of information, and laboratory samples
Appropriate "chain of evidence" documentation

2. History
History of assault (who, what, when, where)
Penetration, ejaculation, extragenital acts
Activities since assault (e.g., changed clothes, bathed, douched)
Inquire about safety
Menstrual and contraceptive history
Medical history
Emotional status
Current symptoms

3. General Physical Examination
Vital signs and general appearance
Extragenital trauma—mouth, breasts, neck
Cuts, bruises, scratches (photograph taken)

4. Pelvic Examination
Vulvar trauma, erythema; hymen, anal, and rectal status
Matted hairs or free hairs
Vaginal examination with unlubricated speculum for discharge, blood, lacerations
Uterine size
Adnexa, especially hematomas

5. Laboratory Samples
Vaginal vault content sampling
Vaginal smears—microscope evaluation for trichomonads and semen
Oral or rectal swabs and smears, if indicated
Blood samples—VDRL serology, pregnancy test; serologic testing for HIV and hepatitis B infection
Freeze serum sample for later testing
Cultures—cervix and other areas (if indicated) for gonorrhea and chlamydia
Fingernail scrapings
Pubic hair scrapings
Clipping of matted pubic hairs

6. Treatment
Care of injuries and emotional trauma
Prophylaxis for STDs, tetanus, and hepatitis B (see appropriate chapters)
Follow-up for pregnancy test in 2-3 wk (if appropriate)
Testing for HIV, syphilis, and hepatitis B may be done at 6-8 wk
Protection of legal rights
Recommendation of continued follow-up and services of rape crisis center

HIV, Human immunodeficiency virus; *STDs,* sexually transmitted diseases; *VDRL,* Venereal Disease Research Laboratory.

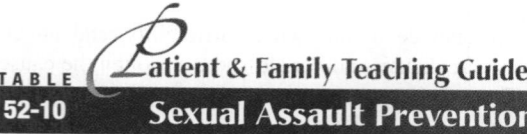

TABLE 52-10   Patient & Family Teaching Guide — Sexual Assault Prevention

1. See that there are lights at all entrances to your home.
2. Keep your doors locked and do not open them to a stranger; ask for identification if a service person comes to the door.
3. Do not advertise that you live alone; list only your initials with your last name in the telephone directory or on the mailbox; never reveal to a caller that you are home alone.
4. Avoid walking alone in deserted areas; walk to the parking lot with a friend; be sure you see each other leave.
5. Have your keys ready as you approach your car or home.
6. Keep all doors locked and windows up when driving.
7. Never get on an elevator with a suspicious person; pretend you have forgotten something and get off.
8. Say what you mean in social situations; be sure your voice and body language reflect your response.
9. Carry a loud whistle and use it when you think you are in danger.
10. Yell "fire" if you are attacked and run toward a lighted area.

the examinations that follow. The patient should not be left alone. Whenever possible, the same nurse should remain with her throughout her stay and provide needed emotional support. The patient's actions and words as she describes the incident may be inconsistent, confused, and inappropriate. The nurse should maintain a nonjudgmental attitude.

The patient usually has many feelings and thoughts about the assault and generally wants to talk about them to an interested listener. Talking may help the patient feel better and gain understanding of her reactions to the incident. When the nurse listens carefully, the patient feels that she is not alone and is better able to gain control over the situation.

The nurse should assess the patient's stress level before preparing her for the various procedures that will follow. The patient's coping mechanisms are supported when she knows what to expect and what is expected of her, as well as why the particular procedure must be done. Because the pelvic examination may trigger a flashback of the attack, the nurse should answer all related questions before the examination and be a supportive presence during the examination.

Following the examinations, the patient's physical comfort needs should be considered. She will need a change of clothing, because her original garments may be torn or soiled, or kept as evidence. Most women who have been sexually assaulted feel dirty and would appreciate a place to wash, as well as use a mouthwash, especially if oral sex was involved. Food and drink may also provide comfort to the victim.

Many sexual assault survivors are unaware of the availability of financial compensation (a law in most states) and appreciate information about the application process. This compensation is to assist them in paying for emergency services and for emotional injuries that may temporarily interfere with their ability to work.

When the patient is discharged, the nurse should make certain the patient has transportation home. If friends or family members

YWCA usually have self-defense classes in which formal instruction is given. Practicing the various techniques with a friend builds up a woman's confidence in her ability to fight back. Learning self-defense can make the woman less vulnerable and more self-reliant.

When a sexual assault survivor is brought to the clinic or ED, a quiet, private area should be used for the initial assessment and

are not available, the hospital or clinic should make arrangements with an appropriate community resource. The patient should not be sent home alone. The victim's partner and family have a tremendous potential for both negative and positive influence. They can "revictimize" her and increase her burden in resolving the sexual assault, or they can provide her with support and find support themselves in resolving a shared crisis.

Many communities today have crisis centers. These public service organizations have trained professional and nonprofessional volunteers who provide an emotional support system for survivors on request. Their programs provide advocacy to ensure dignified treatment throughout the medical and police procedures, short-term counseling for the woman and her family, and court assistance and public education on rape-related issues. The nurse should be able to give the patient the names and local telephone numbers of such organizations.

CONDITIONS OF THE VULVA, VAGINA, AND CERVIX

Etiology and Pathophysiology

Infection and inflammation of the vagina, cervix, and vulva tend to occur when the natural defenses of the acid vaginal secretions (maintained by sufficient estrogen levels) and the presence of *Lactobacillus* are disrupted. The woman's resistance may

also be decreased as a result of aging, poor nutrition, and the use of drugs (e.g., antibiotics) that alter the bacterial flora or mucosa. Organisms gain entrance to the areas through contaminated hands, clothing, and douche tips and during intercourse, surgery, and childbirth. Table 52-11 relates the specific etiologic factors, clinical manifestations and diagnostic methods, and collaborative care of common inflammations and infections.

Most lower genital tract infections are related to sexual intercourse. Intercourse can transmit organisms, injure tissues, and alter the acid-base balance of the vagina. Vulvar infections caused by viruses such as herpes and genital warts can be sexually transmitted when no lesions are apparent. Oral contraceptives, antibiotics, and corticosteroids may produce changes in the vaginal pH and trigger an overgrowth of the organisms present. For example, *Candida albicans* may be present in small numbers in the vagina. An overgrowth of this organism causes vulvovaginitis.

Clinical Manifestations

Abnormal vaginal discharge and vulvar lesions are the two main clinical manifestations. In addition to a thick white curdy discharge, women with vulvovaginal candidiasis (VVC) often experience intense itching and dysuria, which is the result of urine coming into contact with fissures and irritated areas on the vulva. The hallmark of bacterial vaginosis is the fishy odor of

TABLE 52-11   Infections of the Lower Genital Tract

INFECTION/ETIOLOGY	CLINICAL MANIFESTATIONS AND DIAGNOSTIC METHODS	DRUG THERAPY
Vulvovaginal Candidiasis (VVC) (Monilial Vaginitis)		
Candida albicans (fungus)	Commonly found in mouth, gastrointestinal tract, and vagina; pruritus, thick white curdy discharge; KOH microscopic examination—pseudohyphae; pH 4.0-4.7	Antifungal agents (e.g., Monistat, Gyne-Lotrimin, Myclex [available over the counter]) available in cream or suppository
Trichomoniasis		
Trichomonas vaginalis (protozoa)	Sexually transmitted; pruritus; frothy greenish or gray discharge; hemorrhagic spots on cervix or vaginal walls; saline microscopic examination—swimming trichomonads; pH 5.0-7.0	Metronidazole (Flagyl) orally in single dose for patient and partner
Bacterial Vaginosis		
Gardnerella vaginalis *Corynebacterium vaginale*	Watery discharge with fishy odor; may or may not have other symptoms; saline microscopic examination—epithelial cells; pH 5.0-5.5	Sexually transmitted; metronidazole (Flagyl) 500 mg orally or clindamycin (Cleocin) 300 mg orally bid for 7 days; examine and treat partner
Cervicitis		
Chlamydia trachomatis *Neisseria gonorrhoeae* *Staphylococcus aureus*	Sexually transmitted; mucopurulent discharge with postcoital spotting from cervical inflammation; culture for chlamydia and gonorrhea	Azithromycin (Zithromax) PO single dose or doxycycline PO bid for 7 days and ciprofloxacin (Cipro) PO single dose or ceftriaxone (Rocephin) IM in single dose; treat partners with same drugs
Severe Recurrent Vaginitis		
Candida albicans (most often)	May be indication of HIV infection; all women who are unresponsive to first-line treatment should be counseled and offered HIV testing	Drug appropriate to opportunistic organism

HIV, Human immunodeficiency virus; *IM,* intramuscular.

the discharge. Women with cervicitis may notice spotting after intercourse.

Common vulvar lesions include herpes infection and genital warts. Initial or primary herpes infections may be extremely painful. Herpes begins as a small vesicle followed by a superficial red ulcer. Most herpes lesions are painful. Dysuria is common when urine touches the lesion. Genital warts, caused by the human papillomavirus, vary in appearance. Irregularly shaped "cauliflower" lesions are common. Genital warts are painless unless traumatized. (Herpes infection and genital warts are discussed in Chapter 51.)

Older women may develop gynecologic problems such as lichen sclerosis.[19] This condition is associated with intense itching. The lesions are white initially, although scratching produces changes in the appearance.

Collaborative Care

Genital problems are evaluated by taking a history, performing a physical examination, and obtaining the appropriate laboratory and diagnostic studies. Because many problems relate to sexual activity, a sexual history is essential. The nature of the problem directs specific aspects of the evaluation. Ulcerative lesions should be cultured for herpes. A blood test for syphilis may be done when ulcerative lesions are present. Genital warts are usually identified by their clinical appearance. Vulva dystrophies may be examined via colposcopy. A biopsy is taken for diagnosis.

Problems involving vaginal discharge are evaluated by microscopy and cultures. The most common vaginal conditions (bacterial vaginosis, VVC, and trichomoniasis) are diagnosed by a procedure called a *wet mount*. The findings characteristic of each condition are shown in Table 52-11. To assess for cervicitis, endocervical cultures are obtained for chlamydia and gonorrhea. If purulent discharge is observed coming from the cervix, a sample of endocervical cells may be taken to conduct a Gram stain. The Gram-stained slide is examined on high power to identify white blood cells and gram-negative diplococci (indicative of gonorrhea). (STDs are discussed in Chapter 51.)

Drug therapy is based on the diagnosis and is shown in Table 52-11.[20] Antibiotics taken as directed will cure bacterial infections. Antifungal preparations, usually creams, are indicated for VVC. Women with vaginal conditions or cervical infection should abstain from intercourse for at least 1 week. Douching should be avoided. Douching disrupts the normal protective mechanisms within the vagina and may force the pathogens higher into the genital tract. Sexual partners must be evaluated and treated if the patient is diagnosed with trichomoniasis, chlamydia, gonorrhea, or syphilis.

Treatment of vulvar dystrophies is symptomatic because no cures are available. Treatment involves controlling the itching and hence the scratching. Interrupting the "itch-scratch cycle" prevents further secondary damage to the skin.

NURSING MANAGEMENT
CONDITIONS OF THE VULVA, VAGINA, AND CERVIX

Nurses have the opportunity to teach women about common genital conditions and how to reduce their risks. Recognizing symptoms that indicate a problem helps women seek care in a

timely manner. Discussing problems concerning one's genitals or sexual intercourse is frequently difficult. The nurse's nonjudgmental attitude makes women feel more comfortable and empowers them to ask questions seeking accurate information.

When a woman is diagnosed with a genital condition, the nurse should ensure that she fully understands the directions for treatment. Taking the full course of medication is especially important to decrease the chance of relapse. Because genitalia are such a private area, use of graphs and models is especially helpful for patient teaching. When a woman will be using a vaginal medication for the first time, showing her the applicator and how to fill it is important. The woman should be taught where and how the applicator should be inserted using visual aids or models. Vaginal creams should be inserted before going to bed so that the medication will remain in the vagina for a long period of time. Women using vaginal creams or suppositories may wish to use panty liners during the day, when the residual medication may drain out.

PELVIC INFLAMMATORY DISEASE

Pelvic inflammatory disease (PID) is an infectious condition of the pelvic cavity that may involve infection of the fallopian tubes (salpingitis), ovaries (oophoritis), and pelvic peritoneum (peritonitis). A tubo-ovarian abscess may also form. PID is referred to as "silent" when women do not perceive any symptoms. Other women with PID will be in acute distress.

Etiology and Pathophysiology

PID is often the result of untreated cervicitis. The organism infecting the cervix ascends higher into the uterus, fallopian tubes, ovaries, and peritoneal cavity (Fig. 52-5). *Chlamydia tra-*

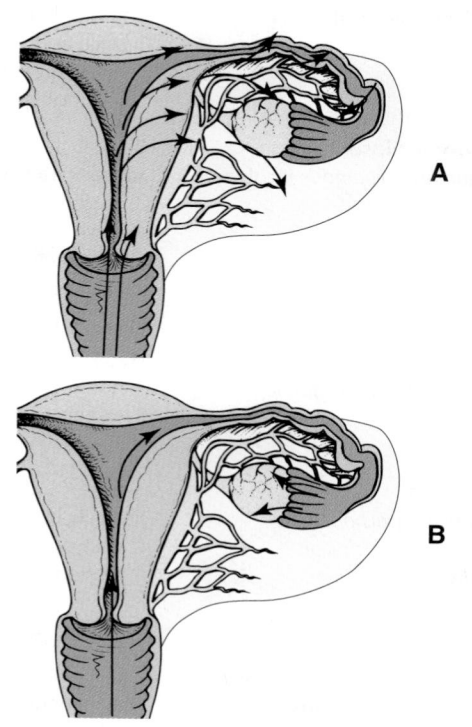

FIG. 52-5 Common routes of the spread of pelvic inflammatory disease. **A,** Direct spread of bacterial infection other than *Neisseria gonorrhoeae.* **B,** Direct spread of *Neisseria gonorrhoeae.*

chomatis and *Neisseria gonorrhoeae* are the most common causative organisms of PID. These organisms, as well as mycoplasma, streptococci, and anaerobes, gain entrance during sexual intercourse or after pregnancy termination, pelvic surgery, or childbirth. It is important to remember that not all cases of PID are the result of an STD.

Women at increased risk for chlamydia infections (younger than 24 years of age, have multiple sex partners, or a new sex partner) should be routinely tested for chlamydia. Chlamydial infections can be asymptomatic and unknowingly transmitted during intercourse. Silent PID can cause damage that cannot be reversed. PID remains a major cause of female infertility.

Clinical Manifestations

Women with PID usually go to a health care provider because they are experiencing lower abdominal pain. The pain typically starts gradually and is constant. The intensity may vary from mild to severe. Movement such as walking can increase the pain; pain is also frequently associated with intercourse. Spotting after intercourse and abnormal vaginal discharge are common. Fever and chills may also be present. Women with less acute symptoms notice increased cramping pain with menses, irregular bleeding, and some pain with intercourse. Women who have mild symptoms may go untreated either because they did not seek care or the health care provider misdiagnosed their complaints.

PID is a clinical diagnosis based on the patient's signs and symptoms. The diagnosis of PID is based on data obtained during the bimanual portion of the pelvic examination.[20] Women with PID have lower abdominal tenderness, bilateral adnexal tenderness, and positive cervical motion tenderness. Additional criteria useful for diagnosis include fever and abnormal discharge (vaginal or cervical). Cultures for gonorrhea and chlamydia are obtained from the endocervix. A pregnancy test should be done. Drug therapy begins when minimal diagnostic criteria are met, thus treatment is not delayed for culture results. When the patient's pain or obesity compromises the pelvic examination and a tubo-ovarian abscess may be present, a vaginal ultrasound is indicated. This patient meets the minimal criteria for diagnosing and treating PID. If a tubo-ovarian abscess is present, hospitalization is necessary.

Complications

Immediate complications of PID include septic shock and *Fitz-Hugh–Curtis syndrome,* which occurs when PID spreads to the liver and causes acute perihepatitis. The patient will have symptoms of right upper quadrant pain, but liver function tests will be normal. Pelvic and tubo-ovarian abscesses may "leak" or rupture, resulting in pelvic or generalized peritonitis. As the general circulation is flooded with bacterial endotoxins from the infected areas, septic shock may result. Embolisms may occur as the result of thrombophlebitis of the pelvic veins.

Long-term complications include ectopic pregnancy, infertility, and chronic pelvic pain. PID can cause adhesions and strictures to develop in the fallopian tubes. Ectopic pregnancy may result when a tube is partially obstructed because the sperm can pass through the stricture but the fertilized ovum cannot reach the uterus. After one episode of PID, the risk of having an ectopic pregnancy increases tenfold. Further damage can obstruct the fallopian tubes and cause infertility.

Collaborative Care

PID is usually treated on an outpatient basis. The patient is given a combination of antibiotics such as cefoxitin (Mefoxin) and doxycycline (Vibramycin) to provide broad coverage against the causative organisms. With effective antibiotic therapy, the pain should subside. The patient must have no intercourse for 3 weeks. Her partner(s) must be examined and treated. An important part of care is physical rest and oral fluids. Reevaluation in 48 to 72 hours, even if symptoms are improving, is an essential part of outpatient care.

If outpatient treatment is unsuccessful or if the patient is acutely ill or in severe pain, admission to the hospital is indicated. Maximum doses of parenteral antibiotics are given in the hospital. Some providers believe that the addition of corticosteroids to the antibiotic regimen reduces the inflammation, allowing for faster recovery and improvement in subsequent fertility. Application of heat to the lower abdomen or sitz baths may be used to improve circulation and decrease pain. Bed rest in the semi-Fowler position promotes drainage of the pelvic cavity by gravity and may prevent the development of abscesses high in the abdomen. Analgesics to relieve pain and IV fluids to prevent dehydration are also prescribed.

An indication for surgery is the presence of abscesses that fail to resolve with IV antibiotics. The abscess may be drained by laparoscopy or laparotomy. In extreme cases, a hysterectomy may be performed. When surgery is necessary, the capacity for childbearing is preserved whenever possible.

NURSING MANAGEMENT
PELVIC INFLAMMATORY DISEASE

Subjective and objective data that should be obtained from the woman with PID are presented in Table 52-12. Prevention, early recognition, and prompt treatment of vaginal and cervical infections can help prevent PID and its serious complications. Nurses can provide accurate information about factors that place a woman at increased risk for PID. Nurses should urge women to seek medical attention for any unusual vaginal discharge or possible infection of their reproductive organs. Women should be helped to understand that not all discharge is indicative of infection, but that early diagnosis and treatment of an infection, if present, can prevent serious complications. Women should be informed of the methods to decrease the risk of getting STDs and to recognize the signs of infection in their partner(s).

The patient may have guilt feelings about having PID, especially if it was associated with an STD. She may also be concerned about the complications associated with PID, such as adhesions and strictures of the fallopian tubes, infertility, and the increased incidence of ectopic pregnancy. Discussion with the patient regarding her feelings and concerns can assist her to cope more effectively with them.

For patients requiring hospitalization, nurses have an important role in implementing drug therapy, monitoring the patient's health status, and providing symptom relief and patient teaching. Vital signs and the character, amount, color, and odor of the vaginal discharge should be recorded. Explanations about the need for limited activity, being in a semi-Fowler position, and increased fluid intake should increase patient cooperation. Assessing the degree of abdominal pain will provide information about the effectiveness of drug therapy.

TABLE 52-12 · Nursing Assessment — Pelvic Inflammatory Disease

Subjective Data

Important Health Information

Past health history: Use of IUD; previous PID, gonorrhea, or chlamydia; multiple sexual partners; exposure to partner with urethritis; infertility

Medications: Use of and allergy to any antibiotics

Surgery or other treatments: Recent abortion or pelvic surgery

Functional Health Patterns

Health perception-health management: Malaise

Nutritional-metabolic: Nausea, vomiting; chills

Elimination: Urinary frequency, urgency

Cognitive-perceptual: Lower abdominal and pelvic pain; low back pain; pain on fundal palpation and cervical motion; onset of pain just after a menstrual cycle; dysmenorrhea, dyspareunia, dysuria, vulvar pruritus

Sexuality-reproductive: Abnormal vaginal bleeding and menstrual irregularity; vaginal discharge

Objective Data

General

Fever

Reproductive

Mucopurulent cervicitis, vulvar maceration, vaginal discharge (heavy and purulent to thin and mucoid), tenderness on motion of cervix and uterus; presence of inflammatory masses on palpation

Possible Findings

Leukocytosis; ↑ erythrocyte sedimentation rate; positive culture of secretions or endocervical fluid; pelvic inflammation and positive endometrial biopsy on laparoscopic examination; abscess or inflammation on ultrasonography

IUD, Intrauterine device; *PID,* pelvic inflammatory disease.

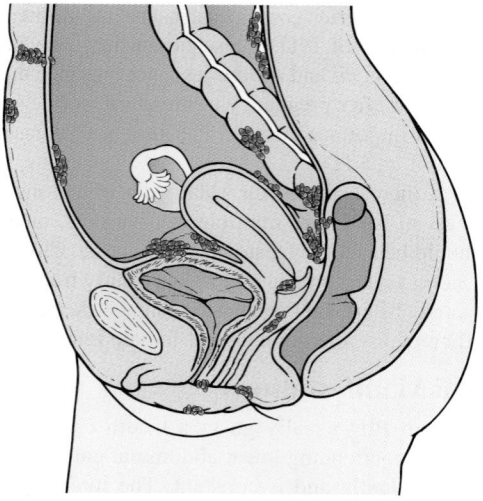

FIG. 52-6 Common sites of endometriosis.

ENDOMETRIOSIS

Endometriosis is the presence of normal endometrial tissue in sites outside the endometrial cavity. The most frequent sites are in or near the ovaries, the uterosacral ligaments, and the uterovesical peritoneum (Fig. 52-6). However, endometrial tissues can be in many other locations such as the stomach, lungs, intestines, and spleen. The tissue responds to the hormones of the ovarian cycle and undergoes a "mini–menstrual cycle" similar to the uterine endometrium.

Endometriosis is found equally among whites and African Americans, but is slightly more prevalent in Asian women. It occurs across all socioeconomic groups. However, most typically, the patient with endometriosis will be in her late twenties or early thirties, white, and never had a full-term pregnancy. Although it is not a life-threatening condition, endometriosis is responsible for considerable pain and loss of work time. Endometriosis is found in 5% to 10% of women of reproductive age.[21]

Etiology and Pathophysiology

The etiology is not well understood, and many theories about the cause of endometriosis have been proposed. A widely held view is that retrograde menstrual flow passes through the fallopian tubes carrying viable endometrial tissues into the pelvis. The tissue attaches to various sites shown in Fig. 52-6. Another theory suggests that undifferentiated embryonic peritoneal cavity cells remain dormant in the pelvic tissue until the ovaries produce sufficient hormones to stimulate their growth. Other proposed causes are a genetic predisposition and altered immune function.

Clinical Manifestations

In patients with endometriosis a wide range of clinical manifestations and severity exists. The magnitude of a woman's symptoms does not necessarily correlate with the clinical extent of her endometriosis. Dysmenorrhea after years of relatively pain-free menses and infertility may serve as clues to the presence of endometriosis. The most common manifestations are secondary dysmenorrhea, infertility, pelvic pain, dyspareunia, and irregular bleeding. Less common manifestations include backache, painful bowel movements, and dysuria. These symptoms may or may not correspond to the woman's menstrual cycles. With menopause, estrogen is no longer produced in the ovaries. This may lead to the disappearance of the symptoms.

When the ectopic endometrial tissues "menstruate," the blood collects in cystlike nodules that have a characteristic bluish black color. Nodules in the ovaries are sometimes called *chocolate cysts* because of the thick, chocolate-colored material they contain. When a cyst ruptures, the pain may be acute and the resulting irritation promotes the formation of adhesions, which fix the affected area to another pelvic structure. The adhesions may become severe enough to cause a bowel obstruction or painful micturition. Adhesions involving the uterus, tubes, or ovaries may result in infertility.

Collaborative Care

Endometriosis may be suspected from a woman's history of the characteristic symptoms and the health care provider's palpation of firm nodular lumps in the adnexa on bimanual examination. However, laparoscopy is necessary for a definitive diagnosis. The treatment of endometriosis is influenced by the patient's age, desire for pregnancy, symptom severity, and extent and location of the disease. When symptoms are not disruptive, a watch and wait approach is used. When endometriosis is identified as a probable cause of infertility, therapy proceeds more rapidly.

Surgical Therapy. The only cure for endometriosis is surgical removal of all the endometrial implants. Surgical therapy may be conservative or definitive. Conservative surgery is done to confirm the diagnosis or to remove implants. It involves removal or destruction of endometrial implants and lysing or excision of adhesions by means of laparoscopic laser surgery or laparotomy. Gonadotropin-releasing hormone (GnRH) agonist therapy (e.g., leuprolide [Lupron]) can be administered for 4 to 6 months to reduce the size of the lesions before surgery. By reducing the extent of the surgery, this preoperative drug treatment helps reduce the development of adhesions that may further threaten fertility.

For women wishing to get pregnant, conservative surgical therapy is used to remove implants blocking the fallopian tube. Adhesions are removed from the tubes, ovaries, and pelvic structures. Efforts are made to conserve all tissues necessary to maintain fertility.

Definitive surgery involves removal of the uterus, tubes, ovaries, and as many endometrial implants as possible. The individual woman should be actively involved in making the decision about preserving part or all of her ovaries, if surgically possible. Her feelings about maintaining her cyclic ovarian function need to be explored. The health care provider should assess the woman's risk for ovarian cancer and provide this information for her consideration.

Drug Therapy. Drug therapy is used to reduce symptoms. Drugs are selected to inhibit estrogen production by the ovary so that the endometrial tissue will shrink. The various drugs used imitate a state of pregnancy or menopause. Continuous use (for 9 months) of combined oral contraceptives causes regression of endometrial tissue. Ovulation is suppressed and *pseudopregnancy* (hyperhormonal amenorrhea) is produced by progestin agents such as Depo-Provera. Another approach to hormonal treatment is danazol (Danocrine), a synthetic androgen that inhibits the anterior pituitary. This drug produces a *pseudomenopause* (ovarian suppression) with atrophy of ectopic endometrial tissue. Subjective relief of symptoms is noted within 6 weeks of danazol use. Side effects include weight gain, acne, hot flashes, and hirsutism. These side effects and the expense of this drug restrict its use.

Another class of drugs used is GnRH agonists (e.g., leuprolide [Lupron], nafarelin [Synarel]). These drugs cause a hypoestrogenic state resulting in amenorrhea. The side effects reported by patients are usually the same as menopause (hot flashes, vaginal dryness, and emotional lability). Loss of bone density has also been reported in women who remain on the therapy longer than 6 months. Endometriosis is controlled but not cured by hormonal therapy. Persistent lesions give rise to subsequent recurrences once the menstrual cycle is reestablished.

NURSING MANAGEMENT
ENDOMETRIOSIS

Education of the patient and reassurance that a life-threatening situation does not exist may permit her to accept a conservative and progressive treatment. When the symptoms are less severe, teaching about nondrug comfort measures may be helpful. Nurses need to assist patients to understand the drugs that have been ordered to treat their condition. The action of the prescribed drug should be explained, as well as the possible side effects. Psychologic support may be needed for women experiencing se-

vere disabling pain, sexual difficulties secondary to dyspareunia, and infertility.

If conservative surgery is the treatment selected, the nursing care is similar to the general preoperative and postoperative care of a patient undergoing laparotomy (see Chapter 41, p. 1063). If definitive surgery is planned, the nursing care is similar to the patient undergoing an abdominal **hysterectomy** (surgical removal of the uterus) (NCP 52-1). The nurse must know the extent of the procedure so that appropriate preoperative teaching can be done.

Benign Tumors of the Female Reproductive System

LEIOMYOMAS

Etiology and Pathophysiology

Leiomyomas (uterine fibroids) are benign smooth-muscle tumors that occur within the uterus. Leiomyomas are the most common benign tumors of the female genital tract (Fig. 52-7). By 30 years of age, 10% of white women and 30% of African American women have uterine leiomyomas. The cause of leiomyomas is unknown. They appear to depend on ovarian hormones because they grow slowly during the reproductive years and undergo atrophy after menopause.

Clinical Manifestations

The majority of women with leiomyomas do not have any symptoms. Of the women who develop symptoms, the most common include abnormal uterine bleeding, pain, and symptoms associated with pelvic pressure. Increased bleeding is thought to be associated with increased endometrial surface area that is associated with leiomyomas. Pain is thought to be associated with infection or twisting of the pedicle from which the tumor is growing. Devascularization and blood vessel compression are also thought to contribute to pain. Pressure on surrounding organs may result in rectal, bladder, and lower abdominal discomfort. Large tumors may

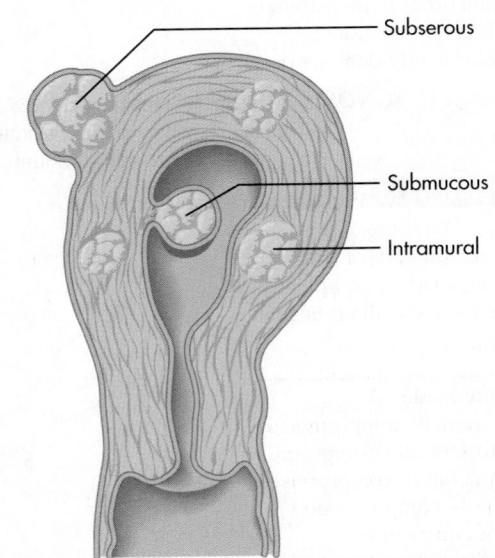

FIG. 52-7 Leiomyomas. Uterine section showing whorl-like appearance and locations of leiomyomas, which are also called *uterine fibroids.*

NURSING CARE PLAN 52-1

Patient with Abdominal Hysterectomy

NURSING DIAGNOSIS   **Acute pain** *related to* incision and manipulation of internal organs *as manifested by* statements about pain, guarding of incision, reluctance to ambulate, and facial grimacing.

OUTCOMES–NOC	INTERVENTIONS–NIC and *RATIONALES*
Pain Control (1605) • Reports pain control _____ • Uses preventive measures _____ • Uses analgesics appropriately _____	*Pain Management (1400)* • Perform a compressive assessment of pain to include location, characteristics, onset/duration, frequency, quality, intensity or severity, and precipitating factors *to plan appropriate interventions and establish a baseline pain level.* • Use therapeutic communication strategies *to acknowledge the pain experience and convey acceptance of the patient's response to pain.* • Use pain control measures before pain becomes severe by providing medication at a given intensity level that has been decided with the patient before having pain *so that appropriate medications and dosages can be used.* • Teach the use of nonpharmacologic techniques, such as splinting the incision with a pillow when coughing or moving and/or relaxation techniques, *to help minimize pain.*
Outcome Scale 1 = Never demonstrated 2 = Rarely demonstrated 3 = Sometimes demonstrated 4 = Often demonstrated 5 = Consistently demonstrated	*Medication Administration (2300)* • Give medication using appropriate technique and route *to provide the appropriate relief of pain.* • Document medication administration and patient responsiveness.

NURSING DIAGNOSIS   **Disturbed body image** *related to* perceived loss of femininity and future inability to conceive *as manifested by* crying, weeping, depression; verbalization of perceived loss of femininity and/or ability to conceive.

OUTCOMES–NOC	INTERVENTIONS–NIC and *RATIONALES*
Sexual Identify: Acceptance (1207) • Affirmation of self as a sexual being _____ • Challenges negative images of sexual self _____	*Body Image Enhancement (5220)* • Determine patient's body image expectations based on developmental stage *to establish need and plan for interventions.* • Assist patient to discuss changes caused by surgery, as appropriate, *to clarify any misunderstandings.* • Determine patient's and family's perceptions of the alteration in body image versus reality *to provide accurate facts and decrease fear of consequences of hysterectomy.* • Identify support groups available to patient *to minimize emotional impact of hysterectomy through open discussion.* • Assist the patient to discuss stressors affecting body image due to surgery (e.g., surgical menopause) *so patient is informed about possible treatment* (e.g., hormone replacement therapy).
Outcome Scale 1 = Never demonstrated 2 = Rarely demonstrated 3 = Sometimes demonstrated 4 = Often demonstrated 5 = Consistently demonstrated	

NURSING DIAGNOSIS   **Urinary retention** *related to* loss of bladder tone, uncomfortable urinating position, and pain *as manifested by* patient's statement, "I can't pass my water when I feel I need to," distention of bladder, and voiding small amounts.

OUTCOMES–NOC	INTERVENTIONS–NIC and *RATIONALES*
Urinary Elimination (0503) • Elimination pattern IER _____ • Empties bladder completely _____ • Urine passes without hesitancy _____	*Urinary Retention Care (0620)* • Monitor intake and output *to determine if satisfactory fluid balance is maintained.* • Monitor degree of bladder distention by palpation and percussion *to detect distention.* • Provide time for bladder emptying while providing patient's privacy *to assist urinary flow.* • Catheterize *to determine amount of residual,* as appropriate. • Provide Credé maneuver, as necessary, *to help flow of urine.* • Stimulate the bladder by applying cold to the abdomen, stroking the inner thigh, running water, and providing the patient with an upright position to void, as appropriate, *to allow for bladder emptying.*
Outcome Scale 1 = Extremely compromised 2 = Substantially compromised 3 = Moderately compromised 4 = Mildly compromised 5 = Not compromised	

IER, In expected range.

cause a general enlargement of the lower abdomen. These tumors are sometimes associated with miscarriage and infertility.

Collaborative Care

Clinical diagnosis is based on the characteristic pelvic findings of an enlarged uterus distorted by nodular masses. Treatment depends on the symptoms, the age of the patient, her desire to bear children, and the location and size of the tumor or tumors. If the symptoms are minor, the provider may elect to follow the patient closely for a time. If the woman is experiencing menorrhagia, the use of aspirin is discouraged because of its effect on platelets.

Persistent heavy menstrual bleeding causing anemia and large or rapidly growing tumors are indications for surgery. The leiomyomas are removed by hysterectomy or myomectomy. A myomectomy is performed for women who wish to have children. In this case, only the fibroids are removed to preserve the uterus. Small tumors may be removed using a hysteroscope and laser resection instruments.[22] Embolization of the fibroid blood supply and cryosurgery are other options. In cases of large leiomyomas, a GnRH agonist (e.g., leuprolide [Leupron]) may be used preoperatively to shrink the size of the tumor. However, the risks and benefits of this drug should be fully discussed, including the potential for irreversible loss of bone mass.

CERVICAL POLYPS

Cervical polyps are benign pedunculated lesions that generally arise from the endocervical mucosa and are seen protruding through the cervical os during a speculum examination. Polyps are a characteristic bright cherry red and are soft and fragile in consistency. They are generally small, measuring less than 3 cm in length, and may be single or multiple. Their cause is unknown. Symptoms are usually not present, but metrorrhagia and bleeding after straining and coitus can occur. Polyps are prone to infection. When the polyp is small, it can be excised in an outpatient procedure. If the point of attachment of the polyp cannot be identified and is not accessible to cautery, a polypectomy is performed in an operating room. All tissue removed is sent for pathologic review because polyps occasionally undergo malignant changes.

BENIGN OVARIAN TUMORS

There are many different types of benign tumors. The cause of most of them is unknown. They can be divided into cysts and neoplasms. *Cysts* are usually soft, surrounded by a thin capsule, and may be detected during the reproductive years (Fig. 52-8). Follicle and corpus luteum cysts are common ovarian cysts. Multiple small ovarian follicles may occur in a condition called *polycystic ovary syndrome* (PCOS) (discussed in the next section). Epithelial ovarian neoplasms may be cystic or solid, small or extremely large. Cystic teratomas, or dermoid cysts, originate from germ cells and can contain bits of any type of body tissue, such as hair or teeth.

Ovarian masses are often asymptomatic until they are large enough to cause pressure in the pelvis. Constipation, menstrual irregularities, urinary frequency, a full feeling in the abdomen, anorexia, and peripheral edema may occur, depending on the size and location of the tumor. There may be an increase in abdominal girth. Pelvic pain may be present if the tumor is growing rapidly. Severe pain results when the cyst twists on its pedicle (ovarian torsion).

Pelvic examination reveals a mass or an enlarged ovary that demands further investigation. If the mass is cystic and smaller

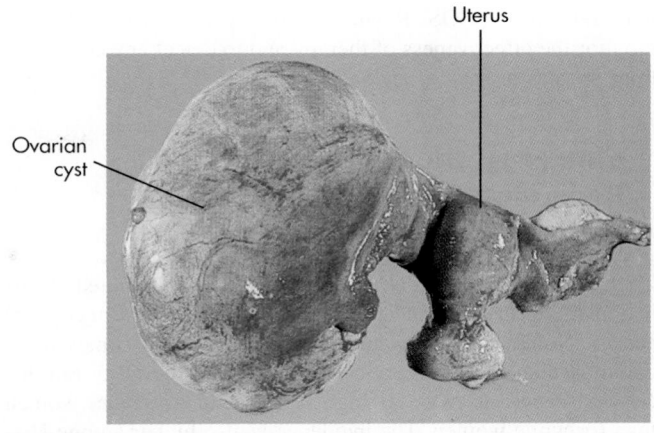

FIG. 52-8 Large ovarian cyst.

than 8 cm, the patient is asked to return for reexamination in 4 to 6 weeks. If the mass is cystic and greater than 8 cm or is solid, laparoscopic surgery or laparotomy is performed. Immediate surgery is necessary if ovarian torsion occurs, causing the ovary to rotate and cutting off circulation. Surgical techniques are used to save as much of the ovary as possible.

Polycystic Ovary Syndrome

Polycystic ovary syndrome (PCOS), also known as Stein-Leventhal syndrome, is a chronic disorder in which many benign cysts form on the ovaries. It most commonly occurs in women under 30 years old. It affects about 5% of women of reproductive age. PCOS is caused by increased production of LH and decreased FSH. This imbalance prevents the ovaries from releasing an egg each month. The ovaries produce estrogen and excess testosterone but not progesterone. Small cysts develop in the ovaries related to chronic failure of the ovaries to release eggs. Recent research suggests a familial or genetic basis and a close association with obesity.[23]

Clinical manifestations include irregular menstrual periods (particularly long cycles), amenorrhea or oligomenorrhea, dysfunctional uterine bleeding, infertility, hirsutism, obesity, and acne. Many start with normal menstrual periods and then, after 1 to 2 years, the periods become irregular and then infrequent. If left untreated, cardiovascular disease, abnormal insulin metabolism with type 2 diabetes mellitus, and ovarian and endometrial cancers may develop.

Successful management includes early diagnosis and treatment to improve quality of life and decrease the risk of complications. Pelvic ultrasound will reveal enlarged ovaries with multiple small cysts. Oral contraceptives are useful in regulating menstrual cycles.

Hyperandrogenism can be treated with flutamide (Eulexin) and a GnRH agonist such as leuprolide (Lupron). Metformin (Glucophage) has been shown to improve hyperandrogenism and restore ovulation. For women desiring to become pregnant, fertility drugs (e.g., clomiphene [Clomid]) may be used to induce ovulation. If all other treatments are unsuccessful, a hysterectomy with bilateral salpingectomy and oophorectomy may be performed.

Patient teaching for the patient with PCOS includes the importance of weight management. Obesity exacerbates the problems related to PCOS. Regular follow-up care is important to monitor the effectiveness of therapy and to detect any complications such as ovarian or endometrial cancer.

Cancer of the Female Reproductive System

CERVICAL CANCER

In 2002 approximately 13,000 women in the United States had invasive cervical cancer and 4100 women died from cervical cancer. Noninvasive cervical cancer is about four times more common than invasive cervical cancer.[24] The mortality rate for cervical cancer is twice as high for African American women than for white women. The incidence is also higher among Hispanic women than white women. An increased risk of cervical cancer is associated with low socioeconomic status, early sexual activity (before 17 years of age), multiple sexual partners, infection with human papillomavirus, and smoking.[25]

The number of deaths from cervical cancer has fallen steadily over the past 40 years. This is attributable to better and earlier diagnosis with the widespread use of the Papanicolaou (Pap) test. In addition to cancer, the Pap test detects precancerous changes. By treating precancerous lesions, progression to cervical cancer can be prevented. The American Cancer Society recommends annual Pap tests beginning with the onset of sexual activity. After three negative Pap tests, less frequent tests may be recommended by the health care provider.

Etiology and Pathophysiology

The progression from normal cervical cells to dysplasia and then to cervical cancer appears to be related to repeated injuries to the cervix. The progression occurs slowly over years rather than months. There is a relationship between certain subtypes of human papillomavirus (HPV) and cervical cancer.[25] However, a cofactor such as smoking is thought to be needed in addition to the specific subtype of HPV. Women who smoke have a 50% higher risk for developing cervical cancer than nonsmokers. This risk is greatest in those with longer duration of smoking, increased number of cigarettes smoked, and use of unfiltered cigarettes.[24]

CULTURAL & ETHNIC CONSIDERATIONS
Cancer of the Female Reproductive System

- Japanese women have a low incidence of ovarian cancer. However, second- and third-generation Japanese women in the United States have much higher rates, similar to those of white women born in the United States. Dietary practices may explain this difference.
- Although the incidence of endometrial cancer is higher for white women and African American women, the mortality rate for African American women is nearly twice as high as that for white women.
- Cervical cancer has a higher incidence among Hispanic, African American, and Native American women than white women.
- Mortality rates from cervical cancer are more than twice as high among African American women as among white women.

Clinical Manifestations

Precancerous changes are asymptomatic. This highlights the importance of routine screening. The peak incidence of noninvasive cervical cancer is in women in their early thirties. The average age for women with invasive cervical cancer is 50. Early cervical cancer is generally asymptomatic, but leukorrhea and intermenstrual bleeding eventually occur. The discharge is usually thin and watery but becomes dark and foul smelling as the disease advances, suggesting the presence of an infection. The vaginal bleeding is initially only spotting, but as the tumor enlarges, it becomes heavier and more frequent. Pain is a late symptom and is followed by weight loss, anemia, and cachexia.

Diagnostic Studies

The Pap test, the Schiller iodine test, colposcopy, and biopsy are used to diagnose cervical cancer. These diagnostic tests are described in Chapter 49. Various classification systems are used to interpret the cytologic findings. The current trend is to use the Bethesda system because it improves accuracy and quality of diagnosis by standardizing diagnostic reports (Table 52-13). Pap tests are less than 100% accurate. There are problems with both

---

TABLE 52-13   Bethesda Classification System for Reporting Pap Test Results

Negative for Intraepithelial Lesion or Malignancy
Organisms
- *Trichomonas vaginalis*
- Fungal organisms morphologically consistent with *Candida* species
- Shift in flora suggestive of bacterial vaginosis
- Bacteria morphologically consistent with *Actinomyces* species
- Cellular changes consistent with herpes simplex virus
Other nonneoplastic findings
- Reactive cellular changes associated with inflammation, radiation, or intrauterine contraceptive device
- Glandular cells status posthysterectomy
- Atrophy

Epithelial Cell Abnormalities
Squamous cell
- Atypical squamous cells (ASC) of undetermined significance (ASC-US) cannot exclude HSIL (ASC-H)
- Low-grade squamous intraepithelial lesion (LSIL) encompassing: human papillomavirus/mild dysplasia/cervical intraepithelial neoplasia (CIN) 1
- High-grade squamous intraepithelial lesion (HSIL) encompassing: moderate and severe dysplasia, carcinoma in situ; CIN 2 and CIN 3
- Squamous cell carcinoma
Glandular cell
- Atypical glandular cells (AGC)
- Atypical glandular cells, favor neoplastic
- Endocervical adenocarcinoma in situ (AIS)
- Adenocarcinoma

Other
Endometrial cells in a woman ≥40 years of age

Source: Solomon D et al: The 2001 Bethesda System: terminology for reporting results of cervical cytology, *JAMA* 287:2114, 2002.

false-positive and false-negative reports. New techniques for cervical cancer screening are being explored. A new technique for Pap smears, Thin Prep, has reduced the amount of equivocal or limited Pap smear results. Recent research indicates that HPV testing may be more effective than the Pap test in identifying patients at risk for cervical cancer.[26]

Collaborative Care

The finding of an abnormal Pap smear indicates the need for follow-up. The type of follow-up depends on the findings. Women with minor changes may be followed with a repeated Pap test in 3 to 4 months. Up to 80% may revert to normal spontaneously. Women with more prominent changes will receive additional procedures, such as colposcopy and biopsy, before a definitive diagnosis can be made. Colposcopy involves examination of the cervix with a binocular microscope with low levels of magnification ($10\times$ to $40\times$). The procedure helps in the identification of possible epithelial abnormalities and suggests areas for biopsy. Biopsies are sent to pathology for evaluation. Colposcopy and biopsy have improved diagnosis and allow more focused treatments to be selected.

The type and extent of the biopsy vary with the abnormality seen. A punch biopsy may be done on an outpatient basis with special punch biopsy forceps. The excision of a cone-shaped section of the cervix may be used for both diagnosis and treatment. Conization is accomplished using one of several techniques. The choice of procedure is determined by the health care provider's experience and the availability of equipment. Cryotherapy (freezing) and laser cone vaporization destroy the tissue. Laser cone excision and loop electrosurgery excision procedure (LEEP) remove the identified tissue and allow for histologic examination to ensure that all microinvasive tissue has been removed. These procedures can be performed in the office with mild analgesics or sedation. Complications of these procedures include excessive bleeding and possible cervical stenosis after healing.

Treatment of cancer of the cervix is guided by the stage of the tumor and the patient's age and general state of health (Table 52-14). There are four procedures in which fertility can be preserved. Conization may be the only type of therapy needed for noninvasive cervical cancer if analysis of removed tissue demonstrates that a wide area of normal tissue surrounds the excised tissue. Laser treatments can be used in which a directed infrared beam is employed to destroy abnormal tissue. Alternatively, cautery and cryosurgery may also be used.

Invasive cancer of the cervix is treated with surgery, radiation, or a combination of the two. Surgical procedures include hysterectomy, radical hysterectomy (involving adjacent structures), and, rarely, pelvic exenterations. (Surgical therapy is discussed on pp. 1426-1428.) Radiation may be external (e.g., cobalt) or internal (e.g., cesium, radium). Standard radiation treatment is 4 to 6 weeks of external radiation followed with one or two treatments with internal implants. (Radiation therapy is discussed in Chapter 15.)

ENDOMETRIAL CANCER

Cancer of the endometrium is the most common gynecologic malignancy, accounting for nearly 50% of female genital tract neoplasms. Approximately 39,300 newly diagnosed cases of endometrial cancer and 6600 deaths occur each year. Endometrial cancer has a relatively low mortality rate, with a survival rate of 94% if the cancer has not spread at the time of diagnosis.[27] About 25% of the cases of endometrial cancer are diagnosed before women reach menopause. The average age at the time of diagnosis is 61 years old.[27]

TABLE 52-14	**International Classification of Clinical Stages of Cervical Cancer**	
STAGE	**EXTENT**	**TREATMENT**
Stage 0	In situ, intraepithelial	Cervical conization, total hysterectomy, cryosurgery, laser surgery
Stage I	Strict confinement to cervix (no consideration of extension to corpus)	
Stage IA	Microinvasive (early stromal invasion)	Radiation or surgery
Stage IB	All other cases of stage I	Radiation, Wertheim's hysterectomy
Stage II	Extension beyond cervix but not to pelvic wall, involvement of vagina, but not as far as lower third	
Stage IIA	No obvious parametrial involvement	Radiation, Wertheim's hysterectomy
Stage IIB	Obvious parametrial involvement	Radiation; if this fails, pelvic exenteration may be required
Stage III	Extension to pelvic wall, no cancer-free space between tumor and pelvic wall on rectal examination, involvement of lower third of vagina, hydronephrosis or nonfunctioning kidney	Radiation
Stage IIIA	No extension to pelvic wall	
Stage IIIB	Extension to pelvic wall or hydronephrosis or nonfunctioning kidney	
Stage IV	Extension beyond true pelvis or clinical involvement of the mucosa of bladder or rectum, no stage IV classification with bullous edema alone	Radiation, surgery (e.g., exenteration)
Stage IVA	Spread to adjacent organs	
Stage IVB	Spread to distant organs	

Etiology and Pathophysiology

The major risk factor for endometrial cancer is estrogen, especially unopposed estrogen. Additional risk factors include increasing age, nulliparity, obesity, hypertension, diabetes mellitus, and having a personal or family history of hereditary nonpolyposis colorectal cancer. Obesity is a risk factor because adipose cells store estrogen. This increases endogenous estrogen and increases its availability. Pregnancy and birth control pills are protective factors.

Endometrial cancer arises from the lining of the endometrium. Most tumors are adenocarcinomas. The precursor may be a hyperplasic state that progresses to invasive carcinoma. Hyperplasia occurs when estrogen is not counteracted by progesterone. The cancer directly extends into the cervix and through the uterine serosa. As invasion of the myometrium occurs, regional lymph nodes, including the paravaginal and paraaortic, become involved. Hematogenous metastases develop concurrently. The usual sites of metastases are lung, bone, liver, and eventually the brain. Malignant cells can be found in the peritoneal cavity, presumably by tubal transport, and their presence is included in staging. Prognostic factors include histologic differentiation, uterine size at time of diagnosis, myometrial invasion, peritoneal cytology, lymph node and adnexal metastases, and tumor size. Endometrial cancer grows slowly, metastasizes late, and is amenable to therapy if diagnosed early.

Clinical Manifestations

The first sign of endometrial cancer is abnormal uterine bleeding, usually in postmenopausal women. Because perimenopausal women have sporadic periods for a time, it is important that this sign not be ignored or attributed to menopause. Pain occurs late in the disease process, and other symptoms that may arise are related to metastasis to other organs.

Collaborative Care

Endometrial biopsy is the primary diagnostic procedure for endometrial cancer. Endometrial biopsy, which is done on an outpatient basis, involves obtaining endometrial tissue from the uterus. Any occurrence of spotting or unexpected bleeding in a postmenopausal woman mandates obtaining a tissue sample to exclude endometrial cancer. The American Cancer Society recommends that an endometrial biopsy be performed at menopause and then periodically in women who are at risk. The Pap test is not a reliable diagnostic tool for endometrial cancer, but it can rule out cervical cancer.

Treatment of endometrial cancer is a total hysterectomy and bilateral salpingo-oophorectomy with lymph node biopsies. Although they are not in widespread use, molecular markers help identify high risk groups that could benefit from postoperative adjuvant therapy. These markers include p53 and p16 overexpression, markers of high proliferative activity, and the expression of estrogen and/or progesterone receptors by the tumor cells. The absence of estrogen and progesterone receptors is a poor prognostic indicator.

Most cases of endometrial cancer are diagnosed at an early stage when surgery alone may result in cure. Surgery may be followed by radiation, either to the pelvis or abdomen externally or intravaginally, to decrease local recurrence. Treatment of advanced or recurrent disease is difficult. Progesterone hormonal therapy (e.g., megestrol [Megace]) is the treatment of choice when the progesterone receptor status is positive and the tumor is well differentiated. Tamoxifen (Novaldex), either alone or in combination with progesterone therapy, is also effective in women with advanced or recurrent endometrial cancer. Chemotherapy is considered when progesterone therapy is unsuccessful. The most common agents used are doxorubicin (Adriamycin), cisplatin (Platinol), carboplatin (Paraplatin), and paclitaxel (Taxol).[25]

OVARIAN CANCER

Ovarian cancer is a malignant neoplasm of the ovaries. In 2002 there were 23,300 new cases of ovarian cancer in the United States, and 13,900 women died from the disease.[28] It is the fifth leading cause of cancer deaths in the United States. Because most women with ovarian cancer have advanced disease at diagnosis, it causes more deaths than any other cancer of the female reproductive system. It occurs most frequently in women between 55 and 65 years of age. White women of North American or European descent are at greater risk for ovarian cancer as compared with African American women.

Etiology and Pathophysiology

The cause of ovarian cancer is not known. Women who have mutations of the BRCA genes have increased susceptibility for ovarian cancer.[28] The BRCA genes are tumor suppressor genes that inhibit tumor growth when functioning normally. When they mutate, they lose their tumor suppressor ability, and hence there is increased risk for women to develop ovarian or breast cancer (see the Genetics in Clinical Practice box).

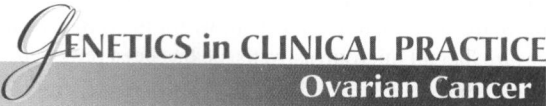

ℊENETICS in CLINICAL PRACTICE
Ovarian Cancer

Genetic Basis
- Mutations in genes BRCA-1 and BRCA-2
- Autosomal dominant transmission
- Mutations can be passed down from either mother or father

Incidence
- About 10% of cases of ovarian cancer are genetically related.
- Women with BRCA-1 mutations have a 25% to 40% lifetime risk of developing ovarian cancer.
- Women with BRCA-2 mutations have a 10% to 20% lifetime risk of developing ovarian cancer.
- Family history of both breast and ovarian cancer increases the risk of having a BRCA mutation.
- BRCA mutations occur in 10% to 20% of patients with ovarian cancer who have no family history of breast or ovarian cancer.
- Family of genes associated with hereditary nonpolyposis colorectal cancer accounts for 10% of ovarian cancers.

Genetic Testing
- DNA testing is available for BRCA-1 and BRCA-2.

Clinical Implications
- Bilateral oophorectomy reduces the risk of ovarian cancer in women with BRCA-1 and BRCA-2 mutations.
- Genetic counseling and testing for BRCA mutations should be considered for women whose personal or family history puts them at high risk for a genetic predisposition to ovarian cancer.

The greatest risk factor for ovarian cancer is family history (one or more first-degree relatives). Having a family history of breast or colon cancer is also a risk factor. Other risk factors include a personal history of breast or colon cancer and hereditary nonpolyposis colorectal cancer. Women who have never been pregnant (nulliparity) are also at higher risk. Other risk factors include increasing age, high-fat diet, increased number of ovulatory cycles (usually associated with early menarche and late menopause), hormone replacement therapy, and use of infertility drugs. The use of oral contraceptives is associated with lower ovarian cancer risk.

Breast-feeding, multiple pregnancies, oral contraceptive use (greater than 5 years), and early age at first birth seem to reduce the risk of ovarian cancer. It is thought that these factors have a protective effect because they reduce the number of ovulatory cycles, and thus reduce the exposure to estrogen.[29]

About 90% of ovarian cancers are epithelial carcinomas that arise from malignant transformation of the surface epithelial cells. Germ cell tumors account for another 10%. Histologic grading is an important prognostic determinant. Tumors are graded according to how well differentiated they are. These include well differentiated (grade I), moderately well differentiated (grade II), and poorly differentiated (grade III). Grade III lesions carry a poorer prognosis than the other grades.

Ovarian cancer can metastasize directly by shedding malignant cells, which frequently implant on the uterus, bladder, bowel, and omentum. In addition, ovarian cancer can metastasize by lymphatic spread. Primary lymphatic drainage of the ovary is through the retroperitoneal lymph nodes, but drainage also can occur through the iliac and inguinal lymph nodes.

Clinical Manifestations

In its early stages, ovarian cancer is usually asymptomatic. Clinical manifestations may include general abdominal discomfort (gas, indigestion, pressure, bloating, cramps), sense of pelvic heaviness, loss of appetite, feeling of fullness, and change in bowel habits. Pain is not an early symptom. As the malignancy grows, a variety of manifestations, such as an increase in abdominal girth, bowel and bladder dysfunction, persistent pelvic or abdominal pain, menstrual irregularities, and ascites, can occur. An ovarian malignancy should be considered when abnormal vaginal bleeding occurs.

Diagnostic Studies

Unlike the Pap test used to screen for cervical cancer, no screening test exists for ovarian cancer. Because early ovarian cancer is usually asymptomatic, yearly bimanual pelvic examinations should be performed to identify the presence of an ovarian mass. Postmenopausal women should not have palpable ovaries, so a mass of any size should be suspected as possible ovarian cancer. An abdominal or vaginal ultrasound can be used to detect ovarian masses. Color Doppler imaging, in conjunction with ultrasonography, can be used to visualize vascular changes associated with malignancy.

For women with a high risk for ovarian cancer, screening using a combination of the tumor marker, CA-125, and ultrasound is recommended in addition to a yearly pelvic examination. CA-125 is positive in 80% of women with epithelial ovarian cancer and is used to monitor the course of the disease.[25] However, levels of CA-125 may be elevated with other non-

ovarian malignancies or with benign conditions such as fibroids or endometriosis.

Collaborative Care

Women identified as being at high risk based on family and health history may require counseling regarding options such as prophylactic oophorectomy and birth control pills. It is important to note that although oophorectomy will significantly reduce the risk of ovarian cancer, it will not completely eliminate the possibility of disease.

If a diagnosis of ovarian cancer is made, staging is critical for guiding treatment decisions. Because of the numerous metastatic pathways for ovarian cancer, accurate staging usually involves multiple biopsies. Stage I describes disease limited to the ovaries; stage II, disease limited to the true pelvis; stage III, disease limited to the abdominal cavity; and stage IV, distant metastatic disease. The usual treatment for stage I malignancies is a total abdominal hysterectomy and bilateral salpingo-oophorectomy with removal of as much of the tumor as possible (i.e., tumor debulking). The remaining tissues in the abdomen and pelvis are carefully scruti-

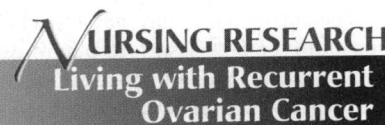

NURSING RESEARCH
Living with Recurrent Ovarian Cancer

Citation
Fitch MI, Gray RE, Frannsen EM: Women's perspectives regarding the impact of ovarian cancer: implications for nursing practice, *Cancer Nurs* 23:359, 2000.

Purpose
The purpose of this study was to gain knowledge about the experiences of women living with recurrent ovarian cancer.

Methods
The study was conducted using a survey instrument developed by the authors. Surveys were distributed to 1068 women with ovarian cancer. Respondents were divided into two groups: those with recurrent disease ($n = 93$) and those without recurrent disease ($n = 170$).

Results and Conclusions
A greater proportion of women with recurrent ovarian cancer reported bowel problems, fear of dying, pain, mobility problems, and self-blame than women without recurrent disease. These women did not feel that they were receiving adequate help for bowel problems and problems with sexual function. They rated their quality of life lower than women without recurrent disease and indicated a greater need to talk about their problems. Women with recurrent disease reported dissatisfaction with the information they received regarding emotional reactions to their disease and treatment. Nurses were identified as helpful by women with recurrent ovarian cancer.

Implications for Nursing Practice
This study identified a patient population whose needs are not being met. Nurses working with ovarian cancer patients need to assess them carefully and plan educational interventions based on their needs. Referrals to community resources are important. Further research is needed to find ways to identify methods to meet the unmet needs of patients with ovarian cancer.

nized. Ascitic fluid is submitted for cytologic study, and appropriate biopsies are performed to determine the stage of the disease.

The addition of chemotherapy or the instillation of intraperitoneal radioisotopes is usually suggested for stage I disease. The patient with stage II disease may receive external abdominal and pelvic radiation, intraperitoneal radiation, or systemic combined chemotherapy after tumor-reducing surgery. After completion of systemic chemotherapy in the patient who is clinically free of symptoms, a "second-look" surgical procedure is often performed to determine whether there is any evidence of disease. This option does not necessarily improve the outcome. If no disease is found, the patient is monitored for recurrent disease.

Chemotherapy (e.g., cisplatin [Platinol], carboplatin [Paraplatin]) is used for the treatment of stage III and stage IV diseases. Altretamine (Hexalen) is used for palliative treatment of persistent, recurrent ovarian cancer. Paclitaxel (Taxol) and topotecan (Hycamtin) are used to treat metastatic ovarian cancer. Surgical debulking is often done in conjunction with chemotherapy for advanced disease. Intraperitoneal chemotherapy, although associated with substantial side effects, is coming into wider use for the patient who has minimum residual disease after surgery.

The malignancy may have metastasized to the peritoneum, omentum, or bowel surface before discovery of the tumors. In these situations the prognosis is poor. Recurrent pleural effusion causing shortness of breath and discomfort may require frequent paracentesis, but the fluid accumulates again. Radiation and chemotherapy may be used to shrink the size of the tumor, relieving pressure and pain.

VAGINAL CANCER

Primary vaginal cancers are rare, with 2000 new cases reported in 2002.[27] The peak incidence is between 50 and 70 years of age. Vaginal tumors are usually secondary sites or metastases of other cancers such as cervical or endometrial cancer. The most common type of vaginal cancer is squamous cell carcinoma. Intrauterine exposure to diethylstilbestrol (DES) places a woman at risk for clear cell adenocarcinoma of the vagina. Treatment of vaginal cancer depends on the type of cells involved and the stage of the disease, the size of the tumor, and the location of the tumor. Squamous cell carcinomas can be treated with both surgery and radiation.

VULVAR CANCER

Cancer of the vulva is relatively rare, with 3800 new cases reported in 2002.[27] Similar to cervical cancer, preinvasive lesions referred to as vulvar intraepithelial neoplasia (VIN) precede invasive vulvar cancer (Fig. 52-9). The invasive form occurs mainly in women over 60 years of age with the highest incidence being in women in their seventies.[25] Patients with vulvar neoplasia may have symptoms of vulvar itching or burning, pain, bleeding, or discharge. Women who are immunosuppressed and/or have diabetes mellitus, hypertension, or chronic vulvar dystrophies are at a higher risk for developing vulvar cancers. Several subtypes of human papillomavirus have been identified in some but not all vulvar cancers.[22]

Diagnosis of vulvar cancer is determined by the pathology report on the biopsy of the suspicious lesion. VIN is managed by eradicating the lesion medically with 5-fluorouracil (5-FU) or surgical excision. Larger lesions may require more extensive surgery and skin graft. The traditional treatment for vulvar can-

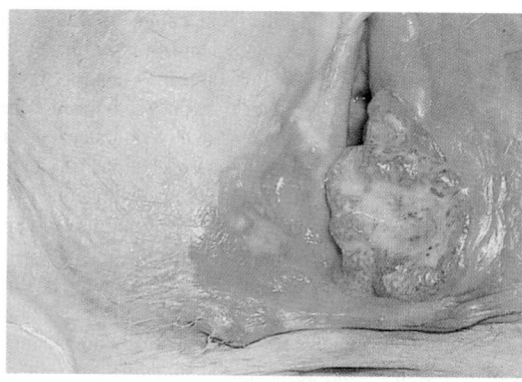

FIG. 52-9 Ulcerative squamous cell carcinoma of the vulva.

cer has been radical vulvectomy. However, the procedure results in extensive morbidity related to scarring and wound breakdown. For this reason, more conservative surgical techniques such as radical hemivulvectomy are being used. Cure rates are comparable between the radical vulvectomy and hemivulvectomy. Morbidity and loss of function have been significantly decreased with the hemivulvectomy.

SURGICAL PROCEDURES: FEMALE REPRODUCTIVE SYSTEM

A variety of surgical procedures are performed when benign or malignant tumors of the genital tract are found (Table 52-15). A hysterectomy may be done either vaginally or abdominally. A

TABLE 52-15 Surgical Procedures Involving the Female Reproductive System

TYPE OF SURGERY	DESCRIPTION
Subtotal hysterectomy	Removal of uterus without cervix (rarely done today)
Total hysterectomy	Removal of uterus and cervix
Panhysterectomy (TAH-BSO)	Removal of uterus, cervix, fallopian tubes, and ovaries
Simple vulvectomy	Excision of vulva and wide margin of skin
Radical vulvectomy	Excision of tissue from anus to few cm above symphysis pubis (skin, labia majora and minora, and clitoris) with superficial and deep lymph node dissection
Vaginectomy	Removal of vagina
Radical hysterectomy (Wertheim)	Panhysterectomy, partial vaginectomy, and dissection of lymph nodes in pelvis
Pelvic exenteration	Radical hysterectomy, total vaginectomy, removal of bladder with diversion of urinary system and resection of bowel with colostomy
Anterior pelvic exenteration	Above operation without bowel resection
Posterior pelvic exenteration	Above operation without bladder removal

TAH-BSO, Total abdominal hysterectomy and bilateral salpingo-oophorectomy.

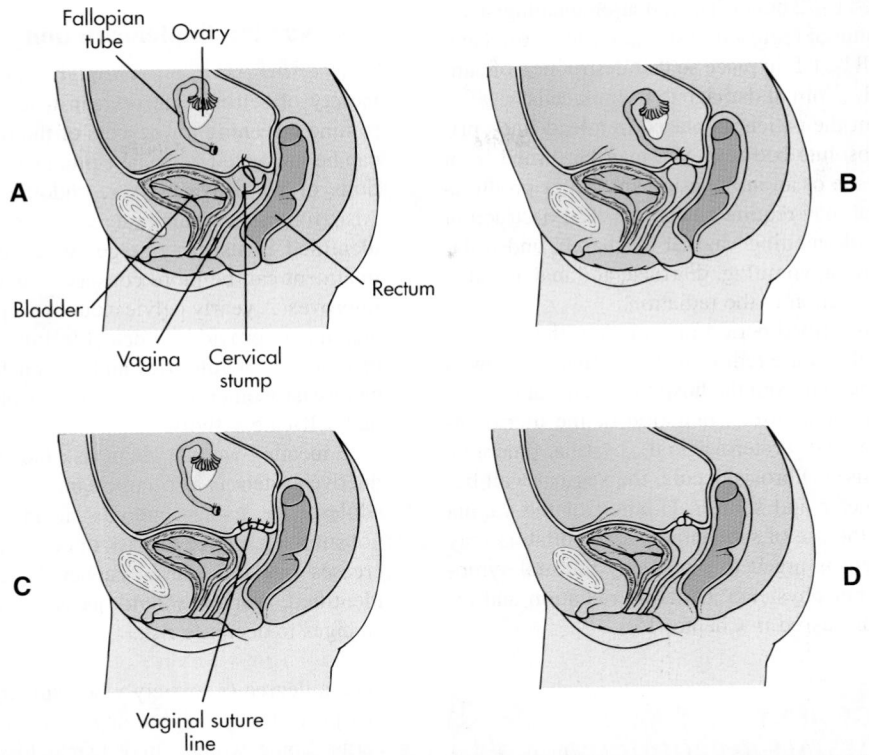

FIG. 52-10 **A,** Cross section of subtotal hysterectomy. Note that cervical stump, fallopian tubes, and ovaries remain. **B,** Cross section of total hysterectomy. Note that fallopian tubes and ovaries remain. **C,** Cross section of vaginal hysterectomy. Note that fallopian tubes and ovaries remain. **D,** Total hysterectomy, salpingectomy, and oophorectomy. Note that uterus, fallopian tubes, and ovaries are completely removed.

vaginal route is often used when vaginal repair is to be done in addition to removal of the uterus. The abdominal route is used when large tumors are present and the pelvic cavity is to be explored or when the tubes and ovaries are to be removed at the same time (Fig. 52-10). The abdominal route can present more postoperative problems because it involves an incision and the opening of the abdominal cavity. In both vaginal and abdominal hysterectomies, the ligaments that support the uterus are attached to the vaginal cuff so that normal depth of the vagina is maintained. A combined approach using laparoscopy with vaginal hysterectomy is becoming more common. This surgical technique decreases morbidity associated with abdominal hysterectomy.

RADIATION THERAPY: CANCERS OF THE FEMALE REPRODUCTIVE SYSTEM

Radiation is used to cure, control, or act as a palliative measure for cancers of the female reproductive system either alone or in combination with other treatments. The goal of radiation therapy is to deliver a specific amount of high-energy (or ionizing) radiation to the cancer and with minimal damage to the normal surrounding tissue.[25] Radiation therapy may be external or internal.

External Radiation Therapy

With external radiation therapy, a source outside of the body delivers electromagnetic radiation in the form of waves. (External radiation therapy is discussed in Chapter 15.)

Internal Radiation Therapy

Use of internal radiation therapy allows the radiation to be placed near or into the tumor. This method can deliver a high dose of radiation directly to the tumor. The dose decreases sharply the farther away from the source, causing less damage to the surrounding normal tissue. A variety of forms are used to deliver internal radiation, including wires, capsules, needles, tubes, and seeds. Internal radiation is used in the management of cervical and endometrial cancer because of the accessibility of these body parts and the favorable results obtained. Radium and cesium are two commonly used isotopes. In preparation of the patient for the treatment, a cleansing enema is given to prevent straining at stool, which could cause displacement of the isotope. An indwelling catheter is inserted to prevent a distended bladder from coming into contact with the radioactive source.

A variety of applicators have been developed for intrauterine treatment. Applicators are inserted into the endometrial cavity and vagina of an anesthetized patient in the operating room. When the applicator contains the radioactive material, this is known as preloading. In afterloading, the applicator is implanted in the operating room but is not loaded with the radioactive material until its correct placement is verified and the patient has been returned to her room. Radiation exposure to the patient is precisely controlled. The radiation exposure to the physician and other personnel involved in the implantation is reduced when the afterload technique is used. The applicator is secured with vaginal packing and is left in place for 24 to 72 hours. The radiation oncologist determines the exact amount of radioactive substance to be used and the length of time it will be left in place so that destruction of cancer cells can occur with minimal damage to normal cells.

During the treatment the patient is placed in a lead-lined private room and is on absolute bed rest. She may be turned from side to side. The presence of an intrauterine applicator produces uterine contractions that may require analgesics. The destruction of cells results in a foul-smelling vaginal discharge, and a deodorizer is helpful. Nausea, vomiting, diarrhea, and malaise may develop as a systemic reaction to the radiation.

At the end of the prescribed period of radiation, the radioactive material and the catheter are removed. The patient is allowed off bed rest and is discharged from the hospital when stable. Late complications that may arise after irradiation of the uterus include fistulas (vesicovaginal, ureterovaginal), cystitis, phlebitis, hemorrhage, and fibrosis. If fibrosis occurs, the vaginal wall becomes smaller in diameter and shorter. Dilation of the vagina through intercourse or the use of sequentially sized dilators may be indicated. The patient is urged to report any unusual symptoms or complaints to her physician. (Internal radiation and related nursing care are discussed in Chapter 15.)

NURSING MANAGEMENT
CANCERS OF THE FEMALE REPRODUCTIVE SYSTEM

■ Nursing Assessment

Malignant tumors of the female reproductive system can be found in the cervix, endometrium, ovaries, vagina, and vulva. The patient with any of these malignant tumors may experience a variety of clinical manifestations, including leukorrhea, irregular vaginal bleeding, vaginal discharge, increase in abdominal pain and pressure, bowel and bladder dysfunction, and vulvar itching and burning. Assessment for these signs and symptoms is an important nursing responsibility.

■ Nursing Diagnoses

Nursing diagnoses for the female patient with cancer of the reproductive system include, but are not limited to, the following:
- Anxiety *related to* threat of a malignancy and lack of knowledge about the disease process and prognosis
- Acute pain *related to* pressure secondary to enlarging tumor
- Disturbed body image *related to* loss of body part and loss of good health
- Ineffective sexuality patterns *related to* physiologic limitations and fatigue
- Ineffective breathing pattern *related to* presence of ascites and effusions
- Anticipatory grieving *related to* poor prognosis of advanced disease

■ Planning

The overall goals are that the patient with a malignant tumor of the female reproductive system will (1) actively participate in treatment decisions, (2) achieve satisfactory pain and symptom management, (3) recognize and report problems promptly, (4) maintain preferred lifestyle as long as possible, and (5) continue to practice cancer detection strategies.

■ Nursing Implementation

Health Promotion. Through their contact with women in a variety of settings, nurses can teach women the importance of routine screening for cancers of the reproductive system. Cancer can be prevented when screening can reveal precancerous conditions of the vulva, cervix, endometrium, and, rarely, ovaries. Also, routine screening increases the chance that a cancer will be identified in its early stage. When cancer is identified earlier, treatment can be more conservative and the woman's prognosis improves. A yearly pelvic examination and Pap test will allow the health care provider to detect lesions on the vulva or any uterine or ovarian irregularities and screen for cervical cancer. Nurses can assist women to view routine cancer screening as an important self-care activity.

Educating women about risk factors for cancers of the reproductive system is also important. Limiting sexual activity during adolescence, using condoms, having fewer sexual partners, and not smoking reduce the risk of cervical cancer. A high-fat diet increases risk for ovarian cancer. When high risk behaviors are identified, nurses should assist women to identify lifestyle changes to decrease risk.

Acute Intervention Related to Surgery. All patients experience a degree of anxiety when surgery is contemplated, but the prospect of major gynecologic surgery may heighten these concerns. Some women may fear a loss of femininity and worry about possible changes in their secondary sex characteristics. Others may experience feelings of guilt, anger, or embarrassment. Still others may focus on the effect the surgery will have on their reproductive and sexual functions. Some women view the whole process as annoying, whereas others are relieved by the thought of no longer having menstrual periods or becoming pregnant. Each patient must be understood in light of her fears and concerns and must be approached and evaluated individually. The nurse who exhibits interest and a willingness to listen can provide considerable psychologic support.

Hysterectomy. Preoperatively, the patient is prepared physically for surgery with the standard perineal or abdominal preparation. A vaginal douche and enemas may be given, according to the preference of the surgeon. The bladder should be emptied before the patient is sent to the operating room. An indwelling catheter is commonly inserted preoperatively.

After surgery the patient who has had a hysterectomy will have an abdominal dressing (abdominal hysterectomy) or a sterile perineal pad (vaginal hysterectomy). (See NCP 52-1 for care of the patient after a total abdominal hysterectomy.) The dressing should be observed frequently for any sign of bleeding during the first 8 hours after surgery. A moderate amount of serosanguineous drainage on the perineal pad is expected following a vaginal hysterectomy.

The patient may experience urinary retention postoperatively because of temporary bladder atony resulting from edema or nerve trauma. This problem is more acute when a radical hysterectomy has been performed. At times an indwelling catheter is used for 1 to 2 days postoperatively to maintain constant drainage of the bladder and prevent strain on the suture line. If an indwelling catheter is not used, catheterization may be necessary if the patient has not urinated for 8 hours postoperatively. If residual urine is suspected after the removal of an indwelling catheter, catheterization is done to prevent bladder infection caused by pooling of urine. Accidental ligation of a ureter is a serious surgical complication. Any complaint of backache or decreased urine output should be reported to the surgeon.

Abdominal distention may develop from the sudden release of pressure on the intestines when a large tumor is removed or from paralytic ileus secondary to anesthesia and pressure on the bowel. Food and fluids may be restricted if the patient is nauseated. A rectal tube may be prescribed to relieve abdominal flatus, and ambulation is encouraged. A Fleet enema or suppository is frequently given on the third postoperative day.

Special care must be taken to prevent the development of deep vein thrombosis (DVT). Frequent changes of position, avoidance of the high Fowler position, and avoidance of pressure under the knees minimize stasis and pooling of blood. Special attention must be given to patients with varicosities. Leg exercises to promote circulation and the use of elastic gradient compression stockings or elastic bandages can be helpful.

The loss of the uterus may bring about grief responses similar to any great personal loss. The ability to bear children is central to society's image of being a woman. Although not experienced by all women, grief over this loss is normal. Eliciting the woman's feelings and concerns about her surgery will provide the needed information to give understanding care. When surgery removes the ovaries as well, women experience surgical menopause. Estrogen is no longer available from the ovaries, so symptoms of estrogen deficiency will arise. To counter this, hormone replacement therapy may be initiated in the early postoperative period.

Discharge teaching should prepare the patient for what to expect following surgery (e.g., she will not menstruate). Teaching should include specific activity restrictions. Intercourse should be avoided until the wound is healed (about 4 to 6 weeks). However, intercourse is not contraindicated once healing is complete. If a vaginal hysterectomy is performed, the woman needs to know that there may be a temporary loss of vaginal sensation. She should be reassured that sensation will return in several months.

Physical restrictions are limited for a short time. Heavy lifting should be avoided for 2 months. Activities that may increase pelvic congestion, such as dancing and walking swiftly, should be avoided for several months, whereas activities such as swimming may be both physically and mentally helpful. Wearing a girdle is allowed and may provide comfort. Once the patient has been assured that healing is complete, all previous activity can be resumed.

Salpingectomy and oophorectomy. Postoperative care of the woman who has undergone removal of a fallopian tube (salpingectomy) or an ovary (oophorectomy) is similar to that for any patient having abdominal surgery. One exception is that if a large ovarian cyst is removed, there may be abdominal distention caused by the sudden release of pressure in the intestines. An abdominal binder may provide relief until the distention subsides.

When both ovaries are removed (bilateral oophorectomy), surgical menopause results. The symptoms are similar to those of regular menopause but may be more severe because of the sudden withdrawal of hormones. Attempts may be made to leave at least a portion of an ovary.

Vulvectomy. Although cancer of the vulva is relatively uncommon, it is important that the nurse recognize the extent of the vulvectomy and the significant effect it is likely to have on the patient's life. An honest, open attitude with the patient and her partner preoperatively can be most helpful in the postoperative period.

After a vulvectomy the patient returns to the unit with a wound in the perineal area extending to the groin. The wound may be covered or left exposed and frequently has drains attached to portable suction (e.g., Hemovac). A heavy pressure dressing is often in place for the first 24 to 48 hours. The wound is cleaned with normal saline solution or an antiseptic twice daily. Solutions can be applied with an aseptic bulb syringe or a Water Pik machine. A heat lamp or a hair dryer is then used to dry the area. Wound care must be meticulous to prevent infection, which results in delayed healing.

Special attention to bowel and bladder care is needed. A low-residue diet and stool softeners prevent straining and wound contamination. An indwelling catheter is used to provide urinary drainage. Great care is taken not to dislodge the catheter because extensive edema makes its reinsertion difficult. Heavy, taut sutures are often used to close the wounds, resulting in severe discomfort for the patient. In other instances the wound may be allowed to heal by granulation. Analgesics may be required frequently to control pain. Careful positioning of the patient through the use of strategically placed pillows provides comfort. Ambulation is usually begun on the second postoperative day, but this varies with the preference of the surgeon. Anticoagulant therapy to prevent DVTs is common.

Because the surgery causes mutilation of the perineal area and the healing process is slow, the patient is likely to become discouraged. Opportunities for the patient to express her feelings and concerns about the operation should be provided. The patient needs specific instructions in self-care before she is discharged. She should be told to report any unusual odor, fresh bleeding, breakdown of incision, or perineal pain. Home care nursing can benefit the patient during her adjustment period. Sexual function is often retained. Whether clitoral sensation is retained may be critical to some women, particularly if it was a primary source of orgasmic satisfaction. A discussion of alternative methods of achieving sexual satisfaction may also be indicated.

Pelvic exenteration. When other forms of therapy are ineffective in controlling the spread of cancer and no metastases have been found outside of the pelvis, pelvic exenteration may be performed. Although different types are done, this radical surgery usually involves removal of the uterus, ovaries, fallopian tubes, vagina, bladder, urethra, and pelvic lymph nodes (Fig. 52-11). In

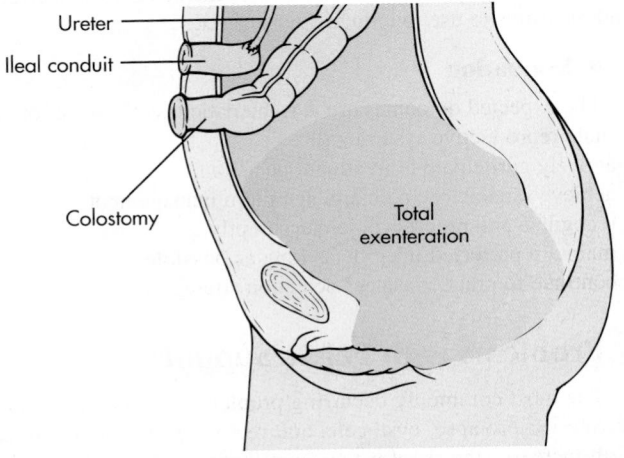

FIG. 52-11 Total exenteration is removal of all pelvic organs with creation of an ileal conduit and colostomy.

some situations, the descending colon, rectum, and anal canal may also be removed. Candidates for this procedure are selected on the basis of their likelihood of surviving the surgery and their ability to adjust to and accept the resulting limitations.

The postoperative care involves that of a patient who has had a radical hysterectomy, an abdominal perineal resection, and an ileostomy or colostomy. The physical, emotional, and social adjustments to life on the part of the woman and her family are great. There are urinary or fecal diversions in the abdominal wall, a reconstructed vagina, and the onset of menopausal symptoms.

The patient's rehabilitative process should keep pace with her acceptance of the situation. Much understanding and support is needed from the nursing staff during a long recovery period. The patient should be gently encouraged to regain her independence. She needs to verbalize her feelings about her altered body structure. Inclusion of the family in the plan of care is important.

The patient will need to return to her health care provider at specified intervals. Early recurrence of the cancer may be identified and treated. At this time the patient's physical and emotional adjustment to the changes in body image produced by the surgery and her ability to carry out any treatment measures can also be assessed. Additional teaching and counseling can then be provided.

Acute Intervention with Radiation Therapy. Nursing management of the patient receiving internal radiation therapy requires special considerations. The nurse should not stay in the immediate area any longer than is necessary to give proper care and attention. No individual nurse should attend the patient for more than 30 minutes per day. The nurse should stay at the foot of the bed or at the entrance to the room to minimize radiation exposure. Visitors need to be told to stay 6 feet away from the bed and limit visits to less than 3 hours a day. Efficient organization of nursing care is essential, so that the nurse does not stay in the immediate area of the patient any longer than is necessary. The reasons for these precautions must be explained fully to the patient and her visitors. (A more detailed discussion of nursing care of the patient with an internal implant is given in Chapter 15.)

When the patient is to receive external radiation, she should be told to urinate immediately before the treatment to minimize radiation exposure to the bladder. She should be advised about radiation side effects, including enteritis and cystitis. These are natural reactions to radiotherapy and do not indicate an overdose. The patient should be fully informed of the possible side effects and measures to use to reduce their impact.

■ **Evaluation**

The expected outcomes are that the patient with cancer of the female reproductive system will
- actively participate in treatment decisions
- achieve satisfactory pain and symptom management
- recognize and report problems promptly
- maintain preferred lifestyle as long as possible
- continue to practice cancer detection strategies

Problems with Pelvic Support

The most commonly occurring problems with pelvic support are uterine prolapse, cystocele, and rectocele. Although vaginal birth increases the risk for these problems, these conditions can occur in women who have never experienced childbirth. Obesity, chronic coughing, and straining during bowel movements can in-

crease the likelihood of these problems. The decreased estrogen that normally accompanies the perimenopause also reduces some connective tissue support.

UTERINE PROLAPSE

Uterine prolapse is the downward displacement of the uterus into the vaginal canal (Fig. 52-12). Prolapse is rated by degrees. In first-degree prolapse, the cervix rests in the lower part of the vagina. Second-degree prolapse means the cervix is at the vaginal opening. A third-degree prolapse means the uterus protrudes through the introitus. Symptoms vary with the degree of prolapse. The patient may describe a feeling of "something coming down." She may have dyspareunia, a dragging or heavy feeling in the pelvis, backache, and bowel or bladder problems if cystocele or rectocele is also present. Stress incontinence is a common and troubling problem. When third-degree uterine prolapse occurs, the protruding cervix and vaginal walls are subjected to constant irritation, and tissue changes may occur.

Therapy depends on the degree of prolapse and how much the woman's daily activities have been affected. Pelvic muscle strengthening exercises (Kegel exercises) may be effective for some women. If not, a pessary may be used. A *pessary* is a device that is placed in the vagina to help support the uterus. A wide variety of shapes exist, including rings, arches, and balls. Most are made of plastic or wire coated with plastic. When a woman first receives a pessary, she needs instructions for its cleaning and follow-up. Pessaries that are left in place for long periods are associated

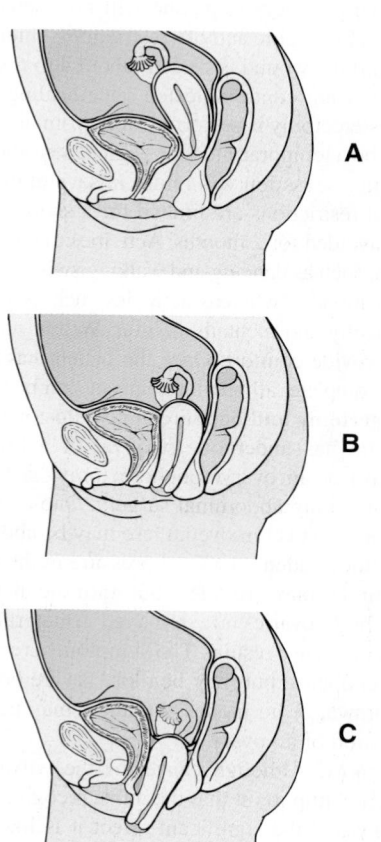

FIG. 52-12 Uterine prolapse. **A,** First-degree prolapse. **B,** Second-degree prolapse. **C,** Third-degree prolapse.

with erosion, fistulas, and an increased incidence of vaginal carcinoma. If more conservative measures are not successful, surgery is indicated. Surgery generally involves a vaginal hysterectomy with anterior and posterior repair of the vagina and underlying fascia.

CYSTOCELE AND RECTOCELE

Cystocele occurs when support between the vagina and bladder is weakened (Fig. 52-13). Similarly, a **rectocele** results from weakening between the vagina and rectum. These problems are common and asymptomatic in many women. With large cystoceles, complete emptying of the bladder can be difficult, predisposing women to bladder infections. A woman with a large rectocele may not be able to completely empty her rectum when defecating unless she helps push the stool out by putting her fingers in her vagina.

As with uterine prolapse, Kegel exercises may be used to strengthen the weakened perineal muscles if the cystocele or rectocele is not too problematic. A pessary may be helpful for cystoceles. Surgery designed to tighten the vaginal wall is generally the method of treatment. A cystocele is corrected with a procedure called an anterior colporrhaphy, whereas a posterior colporrhaphy is done for a rectocele. If further surgery is needed to relieve stress incontinence, procedures to support the urethra and restore the proper angle between the urethra and the posterior bladder wall are used.

NURSING MANAGEMENT
PROBLEMS WITH PELVIC SUPPORT

Nurses can assist women to avoid or decrease problems with pelvic support by teaching them how to do Kegel exercises. Women of all ages can benefit from these exercises. However, Kegel exercises are especially important following childbirth or whenever women begin to have incontinence. To instruct a patient in this exercise, she should be told to pull in or contract her muscles as if she were trying to stop the flow of urine. She should hold the contraction for several seconds and then relax. Sets of 5 to 10 contractions each should be done several times daily.

If vaginal surgery is necessary, the preoperative preparation usually includes a cleansing douche the morning of surgery. A cathartic and a cleansing enema are usually given when a rectocele repair is scheduled. A perineal shave is done.

In the postoperative period, the goals of care are to prevent wound infection and pressure on the vaginal suture line. This necessitates perineal care at least twice a day and after each urination or defecation. An ice pack applied locally may relieve the initial perineal discomfort and swelling. A disposable glove filled with ice and covered with a cloth works well in these instances. Later, sitz baths may be used.

After an anterior colporrhaphy, an indwelling catheter is usually left in the bladder for 4 days to allow the local edema to subside. The catheter keeps the bladder empty, preventing strain on the sutures. Catheter care with an antiseptic is generally done twice daily. After posterior colporrhaphy, straining at stool is avoided by means of a low-residue diet and the prevention of constipation. A stool softener is usually given each night.

Discharge instructions should be reviewed before the patient leaves the hospital. They include the use of douches or a mild laxative as needed; restriction of heavy lifting and prolonged standing, walking, or sitting; and avoidance of intercourse until the physician gives permission. There may be a loss of vaginal sensation, which can last for several months. The patient needs to be reassured that this situation is temporary.

FISTULA

A *fistula* is an abnormal opening between internal organs or between an organ and the exterior of the body (Fig. 52-14). Gynecologic procedures cause 75% of urinary tract fistulas.[22] Other causes include injury during childbirth and disease processes, such as carcinoma. They may develop between the vagina and the bladder, urethra, ureter, or rectum. When vesicovaginal fistulas (between the bladder and the vagina) develop, some urine leaks into the vagina, whereas with rectovaginal fistulas (between

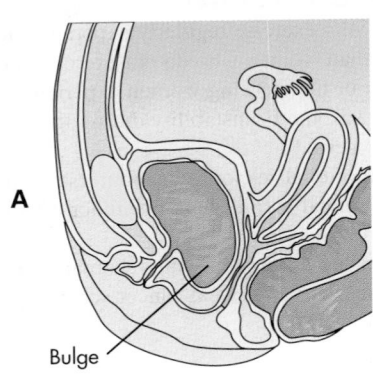

A

Bulge

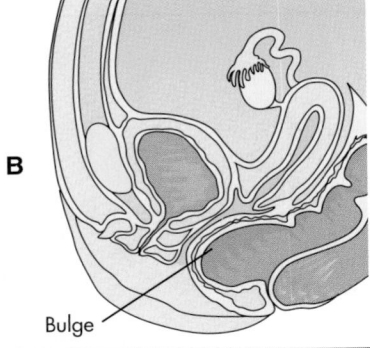

B

Bulge

FIG. 52-13 A, Cystocele. B, Rectocele.

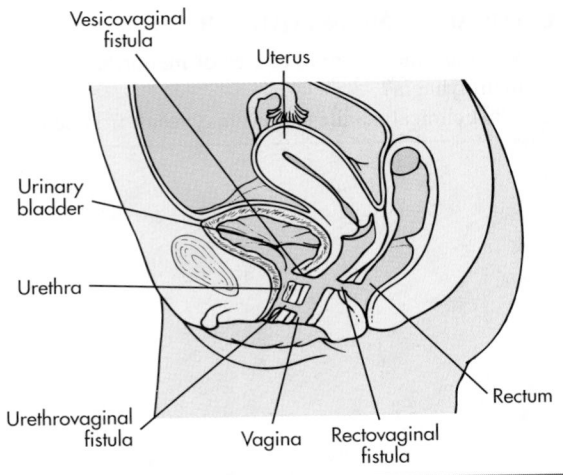

Vesicovaginal fistula

Uterus

Urinary bladder

Urethra

Rectum

Urethrovaginal fistula

Vagina

Rectovaginal fistula

FIG. 52-14 Common fistulas involving the vagina.

the rectum and the vagina), flatus and feces escape into the vagina. In both instances, excoriation and irritation of the vaginal and vulvar tissues occur and may lead to severe infections. In addition to wetness, offensive odors may develop, causing embarrassment and severely limiting socialization.

Because small fistulas may heal spontaneously within a matter of months, treatment may not be needed. If the fistula does not heal, surgical excision is required. Inflammation and tissue edema must be eliminated before surgery is attempted. This may involve a wait of up to 6 months for the surgery. The fistulectomy may result in the patient's having an ileal conduit or temporary colostomy.

NURSING MANAGEMENT
FISTULA

Perineal hygiene is of great importance, both preoperatively and postoperatively. The perineum should be cleansed every 4 hours. Warm sitz baths should be taken three times daily if pos-

sible. Perineal pads should be changed frequently. The patient should be encouraged to maintain an adequate fluid intake. Encouragement and reassurance are needed in helping the patient cope with her problems.

Postoperatively, nursing care emphasis is on avoidance of stress on the repaired areas and prevention of infection. Care should be taken so that the indwelling catheter, usually in place for 7 to 10 days, is draining at all times. Oral fluids should be urged to provide for internal catheter irrigation. Minimal pressure and strict asepsis are used if catheter irrigation becomes necessary. The first stool after bowel surgery may be purposely delayed to prevent contamination of the wound. Later, stool softeners or mild laxatives may be given. See Chapter 44 for care of a patient with an ileal conduit and Chapter 41 for care of a patient with a colostomy. Surgical repair of fistulas is not always effective, even in the best conditions. Therefore supportive nursing care for the patient and her significant others is especially important.

CRITICAL THINKING EXERCISES

Case Study
Total Abdominal Hysterectomy

Patient Profile. Marion P., a 40-year-old Hispanic woman with two children, consulted her health care provider about experiencing menorrhagia and occasionally metrorrhagia for the past 5 months. She was diagnosed with leiomyomas, and a total abdominal hysterectomy was recommended.

Subjective Data
- Was initially reluctant about surgery
- States she wants no more children
- Concerned that she may have uterine cancer

Objective Data

Physical Examination
- Has several large, firm masses in body of uterus thought to be leiomyomas
- Had otherwise normal physical examination

Postoperative Status
- Returned to room with indwelling urinary catheter in place
- Legs wrapped in full-length elastic compression gradient stockings

CRITICAL THINKING QUESTIONS

1. What are the common causes of menorrhagia and metrorrhagia?
2. What clinical manifestations may result from leiomyomas?

3. What physical and psychologic preoperative preparation should be given to this patient?
4. What observation should be made in the patient's immediate postoperative period?
5. What possible complications, including their basis for development, can arise after abdominal hysterectomy?
6. Based on the assessment data, write one or more appropriate nursing diagnoses. Are there any collaborative problems?

Nursing Research Issues

1. Do women who exercise regularly experience less dysmenorrhea than women who do not exercise regularly?
2. Do working or nonworking women experience more episodes of vasomotor instability during the perimenopausal period?
3. Does the emotional response of the nurse caring for a victim of sexual assault help or hinder effective intervention?
4. What factors are associated with a woman's decision to participate in regular cervical cancer screening?

REVIEW QUESTIONS

The number of the question corresponds to the same-numbered objective at the beginning of the chapter.

1. In telling a patient with infertility what she and her partner can expect, the nurse explains that
   a. the cause should be diagnosed by the second visit.
   b. a hysterosalpingogram is a common diagnostic study.
   c. the cause will remain unexplained for 50% of couples.
   d. if postcoital studies are normal, infection tests will be done.

2. A patient with a spontaneous abortion is more likely than a patient with an induced abortion to have
   a. a D&C.
   b. feelings of loss and grief.
   c. physical complications such as infection.
   d. emotional support from family and friends.

3. An appropriate question to ask the patient with painful menstruation to differentiate primary from secondary dysmenorrhea is,
   a. "Does your pain become worse with activity or overexertion?"
   b. "Have you had a recent personal crisis or change in your lifestyle?"
   c. "Is your pain relieved by nonsteroidal antiinflammatory medications?"
   d. "When in your menstrual history did the pain with your period begin?"

4. In caring for a patient after an ectopic pregnancy was surgically removed, the nurse advises the patient that
   a. most ectopic pregnancies attach to the ovary.
   b. she will not be able to get pregnant in the future.
   c. bed rest must be maintained for 24 hours to assist healing.
   d. having one ectopic pregnancy increases her risk for another.

5. To prevent or decrease age-related changes that occur after menopause in a patient who chooses not to take hormone therapy, the nurse teaches the patient that the most important self-care measure is
   a. maintaining usual sexual activity.
   b. increasing the intake of dairy products.
   c. performing regular aerobic, weight-bearing exercise.
   d. taking vitamin E and B-complex vitamin supplements.

6. The first nursing intervention for the patient who has been sexually assaulted is to
   a. treat urgent medical problems.
   b. contact support person for the patient.
   c. provide supplies for the patient to cleanse self.
   d. document bruises and lacerations of the perineum and cervix.

7. The patient's history indicating thick, white, and curd-like vaginal discharge and vulvar pruritus is most consistent with
   a. trichomoniasis.
   b. monilial vaginitis.
   c. bacterial vaginosis.
   d. chlamydial cervicitis.

8. The nurse caring for a patient with pelvic inflammatory disease places her in semi-Fowler position. The rationale for this measure is to
   a. relieve pain.
   b. prevent the complication of sterility.
   c. promote drainage to prevent abscesses.
   d. improve circulation and promote healing.

9. In planning care for the patient receiving medical management of endometriosis, the nurse includes teaching regarding the side effect of
   a. estrogen supplementation.
   b. long-term use of an NSAID.
   c. large doses of vitamins A and E.
   d. hormonal suppression of ovulation.

10. A 31-year-old woman who wishes to have children is diagnosed with leiomyoma. The nurse plans care for the patient based on the knowledge that
    a. a hysterectomy will be necessary to treat the tumor.
    b. a myomectomy may be performed to maintain fertility.
    c. aspirin and other NSAIDs used to control pain may cause fetal defects.
    d. hormonal therapy to shrink the tumor and increase fertility can be used.

11. A 52-year-old woman who has not had a menstrual period for 18 months tells the nurse that she has recently had some spotting. The nurse advises the patient that
    a. she should keep a menstrual calendar for the next 6 months.
    b. this problem should be further investigated by an endometrial biopsy.
    c. this is a common, but not serious, problem that can occur after menopause.
    d. warm douching is recommended to promote healing of fragile vaginal tissue.

12. The nurse plans early and frequent ambulation for the patient who has undergone an abdominal hysterectomy in order to
    a. prevent urinary retention.
    b. promote pelvic circulation.
    c. relieve abdominal distention.
    d. maintain a sense of normalcy.

13. Nursing responsibilities related to the patient receiving internal radiation for endometrial cancer include
    a. maintaining absolute bed rest.
    b. allowing the patient bathroom privileges only.
    c. limiting an individual nurse's contact with the patient to 1 hour per day.
    d. allowing visitors to stay as long as desired if they stay 6 feet (2 meters) from the bed.

REFERENCES

1. McKinney ES et al: *Maternal-child nursing,* ed 2, Philadelphia, 2000, WB Saunders.
2. Leibowitz D, Hoffman J: Fertility drug therapies: past, present and future, *JOGNN* 29:201, 2000.
3. Henshaw SK, Singh D, Haas T: The incidence of abortion worldwide, *Fam Plann Perspect Digest* 25(suppl):S30, 1999.
4. Papp D et al: Biological mechanisms underlying the clinical effects of mifepristone (RU 486) on the endometrium, *Early Pregnancy* 4:230, 2000.
5. Moline M, Zendell SM: Evaluating and managing premenstrual syndrome, *Medscape Women's Health* 5:1, 2000.
6. Proctor M, Farquhar D: Dysmenorrhoea, *Clinical Evidence* 7:1639, 2002.
7. Excessive menstrual bleeding: what you can expect. Available at *www.ethiconinc.com* (accessed Feb 18, 2003).
8. Shoupe D: Hysterectomy or an alternative? *Hosp Pract* 35:52, 2000.
9. Soriano D et al: Diagnosis and treatment of heterotopic pregnancy compared with ectopic pregnancy, *Journal of the American Association of Gynecologic Laparoscopists* 9:352, 2002.
10. McCoy NL: Longitudinal study of menopause and sexuality, *Acta Obstet Gynecol Scand* 81:617, 2002.
11. Kass-Annese B: *Management of the perimenopausal and postmenopausal woman: a total wellness program,* Philadelphia, 1999, Lippincott Williams & Wilkins.
12. Warren MP, Shortle B, Dominguez JE: Use of alternative therapies in menopause, *Best Practice and Research in Clinical Obstetrics and Gynaecology* 16:411, 2002.
13. Mayhew MS, Hersey LC, McMullen PC: Hormone replacement therapy. In Edmunds MW, Mayhew MS, editors: *Pharmacology for the primary care provider,* St Louis, 2000, Mosby.
14. Arcangelo VP, Nichols A: Menopause and hormone replacement therapy. In Arcangelo VP, Peterson AM, editors: *Pharmacotherapeutics for advanced practice: a practical approach,* Philadelphia, 2001, Lippincott.
15. Ewiss AA: Phytoestrogens in the management of the menopause: up-to-date, *Obstet Gynecol Surv* 57:306, 2002.
16. Sommer B et al: Attitudes toward menopause and aging across ethnic/racial groups, *Psychosom Med* 61:868, 1999.
17. Grisso JA et al: Racial differences in menopause information and the experiences of hot flashes, *J Gen Intern Med* 14:98, 1999.
18. The Mamouth County S.A.N.E. program. Available at *www.wcmcnj.org* (accessed Nov 10, 2002).
19. Staats DO: Geriatric gynecology in long-term care settings, *Ann Long Term Care* 8:52, 2000.
20. Centers for Disease Control and Prevention: 2002 guidelines for treatment of sexually transmitted diseases, *MMWR* 47, 2002.
21. Attaran M, Falcone T, Goldberg J: Endometriosis: still tough to diagnose and treat, *Cleve Clin J Med* 69:647, 2002.
22. MacKay H, Trent MD: Gynecology. In Tierney LM, McPhee SJ, Papadakis M, editors: *Current medical diagnosis and treatment,* ed 41, Stamford, CT, 2002, Appleton & Lange.
23. Markle ME: Polycystic ovary syndrome: implications for the advanced practice nurse in primary care, *J Am Acad Nurse Pract* 13:160, 2001.
24. Reproductive Health Outlook: Cervical cancer. Available at *www.rho.org* (accessed Feb 18, 2003).
25. Moore-Higgs GJ et al: *Women and cancer: a gynecologic oncology nursing perspective,* ed 2, Boston, 2000, Jones & Bartlett.
26. Mandelblatt JS et al: Benefits and costs of using HPV testing to screen for cervical cancer, *JAMA* 287:2372, 2002.
27. American Cancer Society: *Cancer facts and figures: 2002,* Atlanta, 2002, American Cancer Society.
28. Harris LL: Ovarian cancer: screening for early detection, *Am J Nurs* 102:46 2002.
29. Tiedeman D: Oncology today: ovarian cancer, *RN* 63:36, 2000.

RESOURCES

American Cancer Society
1599 Clifton Road, NE
Atlanta, GA 30329
800-ACS-2345 or 404-320-3333
www.cancer.org

American College of Obstetricians and Gynecologists
409 12th Street SW
P.O. Box 96920
Washington, DC 20090-6920
202-863-2518
Fax: 202-484-1595
www.acog.org

American Urological Association
1120 North Charles Street
Baltimore, MD 21201
410-727-1100
Fax: 410-223-4370
www.auanet.org

Hysterectomy Educational Resources and Services (HERS) Foundation
422 Bryn Mawr Avenue
Bala Cynwyd, PA 19004
888-750-HERS (4377)
610-667-7757
Fax: 610-667-8096
www.hersfoundation.com

Sexuality Information and Education Council of the United States (SIECUS)
130 West 42nd Street, Suite 350
New York, NY 10036-7802
212-819-9770
Fax: 212-819-9776
www.siecus.org

For additional Internet resources, see the website for this book at *http://evolve.elsevier.com/Lewis/medsurg/.*

CHAPTER 53
NURSING MANAGEMENT
Male Reproductive Problems

Jean Foret Giddens

LEARNING OBJECTIVES

1. Describe the pathophysiology, clinical manifestations, and collaborative care of benign prostatic hyperplasia.
2. Discuss the nursing management of benign prostatic hyperplasia.
3. Describe the pathophysiology, clinical manifestations, and collaborative care of prostate cancer.
4. Discuss the nursing management of prostate cancer.

5. Describe the pathophysiology, clinical manifestations, and collaborative and nursing management of problems of the penis, problems of the scrotum, and prostatitis.
6. Discuss the nursing management of problems related to male sexual functioning.
7. Identify the psychologic and emotional implications related to male reproductive problems.

KEY TERMS

benign prostatic hyperplasia, p. 1435	prostate cancer, p. 1444
epididymitis, p. 1452	prostate-specific antigen, p. 1444
epispadias, p. 1451	prostatitis, p. 1450
erectile dysfunction, p. 1456	radical prostatectomy, p. 1446
hydrocele, p. 1453	spermatocele, p. 1453
hypospadias, p. 1451	testicular torsion, p. 1453
orchitis, p. 1453	transurethral resection of the prostate, p. 1438
paraphimosis, p. 1451	varicocele, p. 1453
phimosis, p. 1451	vasectomy, p. 1455

Problems of the male reproductive system can involve a variety of structures, including the prostate, penis, urethra, ejaculatory duct, scrotum, testes, epididymis, vas deferens, and rectum (Fig. 53-1).

Problems of the Prostate Gland

BENIGN PROSTATIC HYPERPLASIA

Benign prostatic hyperplasia (BPH) is an enlargement of the prostate gland resulting from an increase in the number of epithelial cells and stromal tissue. It is the most common problem of the adult male reproductive system. BPH occurs in about 50% of men over 50 years of age and in over 80% of men over 80 years of age. Approximately 25% of men require some form of treatment by the time they reach age 80.[1] Prostate hyperplasia does not predispose to the development of prostate cancer.

Etiology and Pathophysiology

Although the cause of BPH is not completely understood, it is thought that BPH results from endocrine changes associated with the aging process. Possible causes include excessive accumula-

tion of dihydroxytestosterone (the principal intraprostatic androgen), stimulation by estrogen, and local growth hormone action.[1]

Typically BPH develops in the inner part of the prostate. (Prostate cancer is most likely to develop in the outer part.) This enlargement gradually compresses the urethra, eventually leading to partial or complete obstruction (Fig. 53-2). It is the compression of the urethra that ultimately leads to the development of clinical symptoms. There is no direct relationship between the size of the prostate and degree of obstruction. It is the location of the enlargement that is most significant in the development of obstructive symptoms. For example, it is possible for mild hyperplasia to cause severe obstruction; likewise, it is possible for extreme hyperplasia to cause few obstructive symptoms.

Risk factors for BPH include a family history (particularly involving first-degree relatives), environment, and diet. Although men from both Western and Eastern cultures develop BPH disease at about the same rates, men from Western cultures are

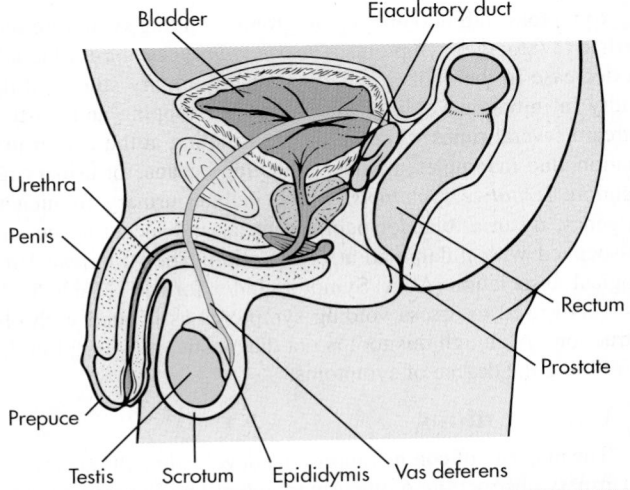

FIG. 53-1 Areas of the male reproductive system in which problems are likely to develop.

Reviewed by Judy L. Goodhart, RN, MSN, Professor of Nursing, Mesa State College, Grand Junction, Colo.

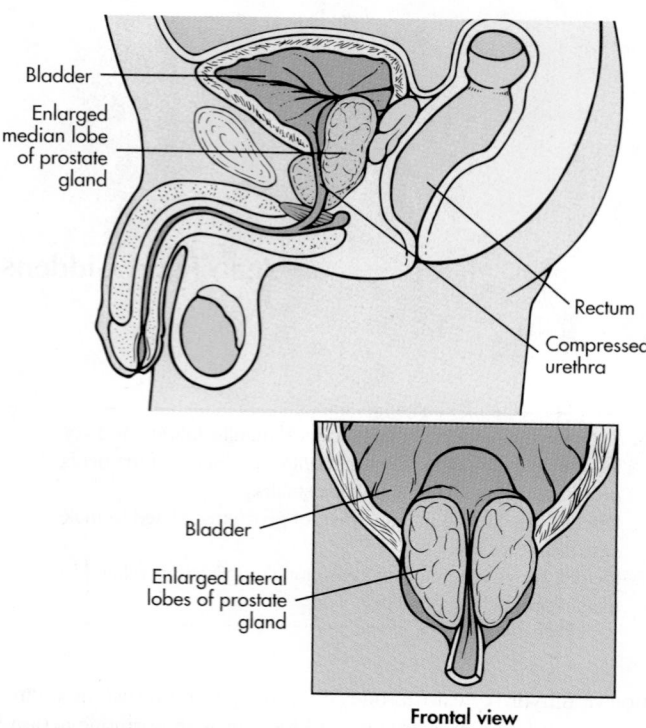

Bladder

Enlarged median lobe of prostate gland

Rectum

Compressed urethra

Bladder

Enlarged lateral lobes of prostate gland

Frontal view

FIG. 53-2 Benign prostatic hyperplasia.

much more likely to develop obstructive problems. Higher risk for BPH has been found in association with a diet high in zinc, butter, and margarine, whereas individuals who eat lots of fruits are thought to have a lower risk for BPH.

Clinical Manifestations

The symptoms of BPH experienced by the patient result from urinary obstruction. Symptoms are usually gradual in onset and may not be noticed until prostatic enlargement has been present for some time. Early symptoms are usually minimal because the bladder can compensate for a small amount of resistance to urine flow. The symptoms gradually worsen as the degree of urethral obstruction increases.

Symptoms fall into one of two groups: voiding symptoms and irritative (storage) symptoms. *Classic voiding symptoms* include a decrease in the caliber and force of the urinary stream, difficulty in initiating voiding, intermittency (stopping and starting stream several times while voiding), dribbling at the end of urination, and incomplete bladder emptying because of urinary retention. *Irritative symptoms,* which include urinary frequency, urgency, dysuria, bladder pain, nocturia, and incontinence, are associated with inflammation or infection. The American Urological Association (AUA) Symptom Index for BPH (Table 53-1) is a tool used to assess voiding symptoms associated with obstruction.[2] Although this tool is not diagnostic, it is useful in determining the degree of symptoms.

Complications

The majority of complications that develop in BPH are related to urinary obstruction. Acute urinary retention is a common complication and is an indication for surgical intervention in about

25% to 30% of patients.[3] Another common complication is urinary tract infection (UTI) and potentially sepsis secondary to UTI. Incomplete bladder emptying (associated with partial obstruction) results in residual urine, providing a favorable environment for bacterial growth. Calculi may develop in the bladder because of the alkalinization of the residual urine. Although bladder stones are eight times more common in men with BPH, risk of renal calculi is not significantly increased.[3] Other less common but potential complications include renal failure caused by *hydronephrosis* (distention of pelvis and calyces of kidney by urine that cannot flow through the ureter to the bladder), pyelonephritis, and bladder damage if treatment for acute urinary retention is delayed.

Diagnostic Studies

The primary methods used to diagnose BPH include a history and physical examination. The prostate can be palpated by digital rectal examination (DRE). Using DRE, the health care provider can estimate the size, symmetry, and consistency of the prostate gland. In BPH the prostate is symmetrically enlarged, firm, and smooth.

Additional diagnostic tests may be indicated, depending on the type and severity of symptoms and clinical findings. Diagnostic tests are typically done to determine the presence of complications or for differential diagnosis. A urinalysis with culture is routinely done to determine the presence of infection. The presence of bacteria, white blood cells, or microscopic hematuria is an indication of infection or inflammation. The prostate-specific antigen (PSA) blood level is usually measured to rule out prostate cancer. However, PSA levels may be slightly elevated in patients with BPH. Serum creatinine may be ordered to rule out renal insufficiency.

In patients with an abnormal DRE and elevated PSA, a *transrectal ultrasound* (TRUS) scan is typically indicated. This examination allows for accurate assessment of prostate size and is helpful in differentiating BPH from prostate cancer.[4] Biopsies can be taken during the ultrasound procedure. *Uroflometry,* a study that measures the volume of urine expelled from the bladder per second, is helpful in determining the extent of uretheral blockage and thus the type of treatment needed. Postvoid residual urine volume is often measured to determine the degree of urine flow obstruction. Cystourethroscopy, a procedure allowing internal visualization of the urethra and bladder, is performed if the diagnosis is uncertain and in patients who are scheduled for prostatectomy.[5] Diagnostic studies are outlined in Table 53-2.

Collaborative Care

The goals of collaborative care are to restore bladder drainage, relieve the patient's symptoms, and prevent or treat the complications of BPH. Treatment is generally based on the degree to which the symptoms bother the patient or the presence of complications rather than the size of the prostate. The numerous treatment options for BPH can be categorized as conservative (including drug therapy) and invasive therapy.

The most conservative initial treatment for BPH is referred to as "watchful waiting." When there are no symptoms or only mild ones (AUA symptom scores less than 7), a wait-and-see approach is taken. Because symptoms may come and go, a con-

TABLE 53-1	American Urological Association Symptom Index to Determine Severity of Prostatic Problems

QUESTIONS TO BE ANSWERED	AMERICAN UROLOGICAL ASSOCIATION (AUA) SYMPTOM SCORE* (CIRCLE 1 NUMBER ON EACH LINE)					
	NOT AT ALL	LESS THAN 1 TIME IN 5	LESS THAN HALF THE TIME	ABOUT HALF THE TIME	MORE THAN HALF THE TIME	ALMOST ALWAYS
Over the past month, 1. How often have you had a sensation of not emptying your bladder completely after you finished urinating?	0	1	2	3	4	5
2. How often have you had to urinate again, less than 2 hr after you finished urinating?	0	1	2	3	4	5
3. How often have you found you stopped and started again several times when you urinated?	0	1	2	3	4	5
4. How often have you found it difficult to postpone urination?	0	1	2	3	4	5
5. How often have you had a weak urinary stream?	0	1	2	3	4	5
6. How often have you had to push or strain to begin urination?	0	1	2	3	4	5
7. How many times did you most typically get up to urinate from the time you went to bed at night until the time you got up in the morning?	0 (None)	1 (1 time)	2 (2 times)	3 (3 times)	4 (4 times)	5 (5 times or more)
Sum of circled numbers (AUA Symptom Score):* _____						

From Barry B et al: The American Urological Association symptom index for benign prostatic hyperplasia, *J Urol* 148:1547, 1992. Used with permission.
*Score is interpreted as: 0-7, mild; 8-19, moderate; 20-35, severe.

servative approach has value. Dietary changes (decreasing intake of caffeine and artificial sweeteners, limiting spicy or acidic foods), avoiding medication such as decongestants and anticholinergics, and restricting evening fluid intake may result in improvement of symptoms. A timed voiding schedule may reduce or eliminate symptoms, thus negating the need for further intervention. If the patient begins to have signs or symptoms that indicate an increase in obstruction, further treatment is indicated.

Drug Therapy. Drugs that have been used to treat BPH with variable degrees of success include 5α-reductase inhibitors and α-adrenergic receptor blockers.

5α-Reductase inhibitors. These drugs work by reducing the size of the prostate gland. Finasteride (Proscar) blocks the enzyme 5α-reductase, which is necessary for the conversion of testosterone to dihydroxytestosterone, the principal intraprostatic androgen. This drug results in regression of hyperplastic tissue through suppression of androgens. Finasteride is an appropriate treatment option for individuals who score between 12 and 26 on the AUA Symptom Index for BPH (see Table 53-1).

Although 40% to 50% of those treated show improvement, it takes between 3 and 6 months to be effective, and the medication must be taken on a continuous basis to maintain therapeutic results. Duasteride (Duagen) is a dual inhibitor of 5α-reductase type 1 and 2 isoenzymes. (Finasteride inhibits only the type 2 isoenzyme.) Side effects of 5 α-reductase inhibitors include decreased libido, decreased volume of ejaculate, and erectile dysfunction.

α-Adrenergic receptor blockers. Another drug treatment option for BPH is agents that block α_1-adrenergic receptors. Although this group of drugs is more commonly used for treatment of hypertension, these drugs promote smooth muscle relaxation in the prostate. α_1-Adrenergic receptors are abundant in the prostate and are increased in hyperplastic prostate tissue. Relaxation of the smooth muscle ultimately facilitates urinary flow through the urethra. Currently, the α-adrenergic blockers are the most widely prescribed drug for the patient with BPH who is experiencing moderate symptoms without the presence of other complications. These agents demonstrate a 50% to 60% efficacy in improvement of symptoms. Improvement of symptoms occurs

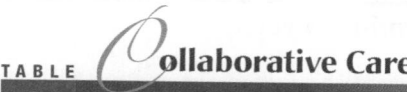

TABLE	Collaborative Care
53-2	**Benign Prostatic Hyperplasia**

Diagnostic
History and physical examination
Digital rectal examination (DRE)
Urinalysis with culture
Serum creatinine
Prostate-specific antigen (PSA)
Postvoid residual
Uroflowmetry
Transrectal ultrasound (TRUS)
Cystourethroscopy

Collaborative Therapy
Conservative therapy ("watchful waiting")
Drug therapy
- 5α–Reductase inhibitors
- α–Adrenergic receptor blockers
- Herb therapy
Invasive therapy
- Transurethral resection of the prostate (TURP)
- Simple open prostatectomy
- Transurethral incision of the prostate (TUIP)
- Transurethral microwave thermotherapy (TUMT)
- Transurethral needle ablation (TUNA)
- Laser prostatectomy
- Transurethral electrovaporization of the prostate (TUVP)
- Urethral stents.

COMPLEMENTARY & ALTERNATIVE THERAPIES
Saw Palmetto

Clinical Uses
Benign prostatic hyperplasia (BPH), urinary tract infections.

Effects
Extract of saw palmetto (Serenoa repens) is considered an antiandrogen herb. Improves urinary symptoms and urinary flow measures. Side effects are mild and infrequent. May cause gastrointestinal disturbances (e.g., diarrhea) and headache or dizziness. May cause increase in blood pressure in some people.

Nursing Implications
Men should see a physician for the correct diagnosis of BPH. Self-treatment is not recommended. Prostate-specific antigen levels should be done before starting this herb. The long-term effectiveness and ability to prevent complications are not currently known. Should not take if on hormonal replacement therapy.

within 2 to 3 weeks. The most important side effects are orthostatic hypotension and dizziness.

Several α-adrenergic blockers, including doxazosin (Cardura), terazosin (Hytrin), tamsulosin (Flomax), and alfuzosin (UroXatral) are currently being used. Side effects, including postural hypotension, dizziness, and fatigue, can be problematic, especially if the patient is also taking cardiac or other antihypertensive medication. It must be pointed out that although these drugs offer symptomatic relief of BPH, they do not treat hyperplasia.

Herbal therapy. Herbs extracted from plants have been used in the management of BPH. In particular, plant extracts, such as saw palmetto (Serenoa repens), have been used. Saw palmetto has been shown to improve urinary symptoms and urinary flow measures. However, the long-term effectiveness and ability to prevent complications are currently unknown (see the Complementary and Alternative Therapies box on this page).

Invasive Therapy. Invasive therapy is indicated when there is a decrease in urine flow sufficient to cause discomfort, persistent residual urine, acute urinary retention because of obstruction with no reversible precipitating cause, or hydronephrosis. Intermittent catheterization or insertion of an indwelling catheter can temporarily reduce symptoms and bypass the obstruction. However, long-term catheter use should be avoided because of the increased risk of infection.

Invasive treatment of symptomatic BPH primarily involves resection or ablation of the prostate. The choice of the treatment approach depends on the size and location of the prostatic en-

largement, as well as patient factors such as age and surgical risk. Various invasive treatments are summarized in Table 53-3.

Transurethral resection of the prostate. Transurethral resection of the prostate (TURP) is a surgical procedure involving the removal of prostate tissue using a resectoscope inserted through the urethra. TURP has long been considered the "gold standard" surgical treatment for obstructing BPH. Although this procedure remains by far the most common operation performed, there has been a decrease in the number of TURP procedures done in recent years due to the development of less invasive technologies.[6]

The TURP is performed under a spinal or general anesthetic. No external surgical incision is made. A resectoscope is inserted through the urethra to excise and cauterize obstructing prostatic tissue (Fig. 53-3). A large three-way indwelling catheter with a 30 ml balloon is inserted into the bladder after the procedure to provide hemostasis and to facilitate urinary drainage. The bladder is irrigated, either continuously or intermittently, usually for the first 24 hours to prevent obstruction from mucus and blood clots.

The outcome for 80% to 90% of patients is excellent, with marked improvements in symptoms and urinary flow rates. TURP is a surgical procedure with relatively low risk. Some of the postoperative complications include bleeding, clot retention, and dilutional hyponatremia associated with irrigation. Because bleeding is a common complication, patients taking aspirin or warfarin (Coumadin) must discontinue these medications several days before surgery.

Transuretheral microwave thermotherapy. Transuretheral microwave thermotherapy (TUMT) is an outpatient procedure that involves the delivery of microwaves directly to the prostate through a transurethral probe in order to raise the temperature of the prostate tissue to about 113° F (45° C).[7] The heat causes necrosis and death of tissue, thus relieving the obstruction. A rectal temperature probe is used during the procedure to ensure that the rectal temperature is kept below 110° F (43.5° C) to prevent rectal tissue damage. Although infrequent, serious thermal injuries can occur as a consequence of TUMT as a result of incor-

TABLE 53-3	Invasive Treatment Options for Benign Prostatic Hyperplasia		
TREATMENT	**DESCRIPTION**	**ADVANTAGES**	**DISADVANTAGES**
Transurethral resection of the prostate (TURP)	Use of excision and cauterization to remove prostate tissue cystoscopically. Considered the most effective treatment of BPH.	Best long-term relief of prostatic obstruction Erectile dysfunction unlikely	Bleeding Retrograde ejaculation
Open prostatectomy	Surgery of choice for men with large prostates. Involves external incision with three possible approaches (see Fig. 53-4).	Complete visualization of prostate and surrounding tissue Usually only indicated if prostate gland is very large	Erectile dysfunction Bleeding Postoperative pain Risk of infection
Transurethral incision of the prostate (TUIP)	Involves making transurethral slits or incisions into prostatic tissue to relieve obstruction. Effective for men with relatively little prostatic enlargement.	Outpatient procedure Minimal complications Good for high risk patients No erectile dysfunction or retrograde ejaculation	Considered temporary solution to obstructive problem Urinary catheter needed after procedure
Transurethral microwave thermotherapy (TUMT)	Use of microwave radiating heat to produce coagulative necrosis of the prostate.	Outpatient procedure Short procedure Erectile dysfunction and retrograde ejaculation are rare	Potential for damage to surrounding tissue Urinary catheter needed after procedure
Transurethral needle ablation of the prostate (TUNA)	Low-wave radiofrequency used to heat the prostate causing necrosis.	Short outpatient procedure Erectile dysfunction and retrograde ejaculation are rare Precise delivery of heat to desired area Very little pain experienced by patient	Urinary retention common Irritative voiding symptoms Hematuria
Laser prostatectomy	Procedure uses a laser beam to cut or destroy part of the prostate. Different techniques are available: Visual laser ablation of prostate (VLAP) Contact laser technique Interstitial laser coagulation (ILC)	Short procedure Minimal bleeding Fast recovery time Very effective	Postprocedure catheterization (up to 7 days) needed because of edema and urinary retention Delayed sloughing of tissue Takes several weeks to reach optimal effect Retrograde ejaculation
Transurethral electrovaporization of prostate (TUVP)	Electrosurgical vaporization and desiccation are used together to destroy prostatic tissue.	Minimal risks Minimal bleeding and sloughing	Retrograde ejaculation Intermittent hematuria
Urethral stents	Insertion of self-expandable metallic stent into the urethra where enlarged area of prostate occurs.	Safe and effective Low risk	Stent may move Long-term experience is limited

rect placement of the transurethral probe or rectal temperature probe.[8]

Postoperative urinary retention is a common complication. Thus the patient is generally sent home with an indwelling catheter for 2 to 7 days to maintain urinary flow and to facilitate the passing of small clots or necrotic tissue. Antibiotics, pain medication, and bladder antispasmodic medications are used to treat and prevent postprocedure problems. The procedure is not appropriate for men with rectal problems. Anticoagulant therapy should be stopped 10 days before treatment. Mild side effects include occasional problems of bladder spasm, hematuria, dysuria, and retention.

Transuretheral needle ablation. Transuretheral needle ablation (TUNA) is another procedure that increases the tempera-

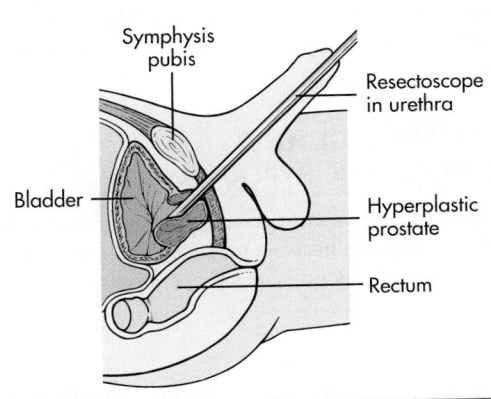

FIG. 53-3 Transurethral resection of the prostate.

ture of prostate tissue, thus causing localized necrosis. TUNA differs from TUMT in that low-wave radiofrequency is used to heat the prostate, and only prostate tissue in direct contact with the needle is affected, allowing greater precision in removal of the target tissue. The extent of tissue removed by this process is determined by the amount of tissue contact (needle length), amount of energy delivered, and duration of treatment. Seventy percent of patients undergoing TUNA report an improvement in symptoms, making this an attractive treatment option for men with BPH.[9]

This procedure is performed in an outpatient unit or physician's office using local anesthesia and intravenous or oral sedation. The TUNA procedure typically lasts only 30 minutes. The patient typically experiences little pain and an early return to regular activities. Complications include urinary retention, urinary tract infection, and irritative voiding symptoms (e.g., frequency, urgency, dysuria). Some patients require a urinary catheter for a short duration. Patients typically have hematuria for up to a week.

Laser prostatectomy. The use of laser therapy has recently been developed to treat BPH. The laser beam is delivered transurethrally through a fiber instrument and is used for cutting, coagulation, and vaporization of prostatic tissue. There are a variety of laser procedures using different sources, wavelengths, and delivery systems. A common laser procedure is laser coagulation of the prostate, often referred to as visual laser ablation of the prostate (VLAP). VLAP uses the laser beam to produce deep coagulation necrosis of the prostate. The affected prostate tissue gradually sloughs in the urinary stream. It takes several weeks before the patient reaches optimal results following this type of laser therapy. At the completion of VLAP, a urinary catheter is inserted to allow for drainage.

Contact laser technique involves the direct contact of the laser to the prostate tissue. This produces an immediate vaporization of the prostate tissue. Blood vessels near the laser tip immediately are cauterized, thus bleeding during the procedure is rare. A three-way catheter with slow-drip irrigation is placed immediately after the procedure for a short time. Typically the catheter is removed within 6 to 8 hours after the procedure. Advantages of this procedure over TURP include minimal bleeding both during and after the procedure, faster recovery time, and ability to perform the surgery on patients taking anticoagulants.

Another approach to laser prostatectomy is interstitial laser coagulation (ILC). The prostate is viewed through a cytoscope. A laser is used to quickly treat precise areas of the enlarged prostate by placement of interstitial light guides directly into the prostate tissue.

NURSING MANAGEMENT
BENIGN PROSTATIC HYPERPLASIA

Because the nurse is most directly involved with care of patients with BPH having invasive procedures, the focus of nursing management in this section is on preoperative and postoperative care.

■ Nursing Assessment

Subjective and objective data that should be obtained from a patient with BPH are presented in Table 53-4.

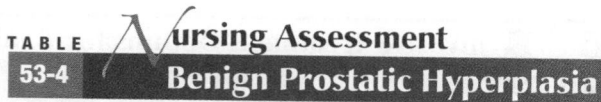

| TABLE 53-4 | Nursing Assessment Benign Prostatic Hyperplasia |

Subjective Data

Important Health Information
Medications: Estrogen or testosterone supplementation
Surgery or other treatments: Previous treatment for BPH

Functional Health Patterns
Health perception–health management: Knowledge of the condition
Nutritional-metabolic: Voluntary fluid restriction
Elimination: Urinary urgency, diminution in caliber and force of urinary stream; hesitancy in initiating voiding; postvoiding dribbling; urinary retention; incontinence
Sleep: Nocturia
Cognitive-perceptual: Dysuria, sensation of incomplete voiding; bladder discomfort
Sexuality-reproductive: Anxiety about sexual dysfunction

Objective Data

General
Older adult male

Urinary
Distended bladder on palpation; smooth, firm, elastic enlargement of prostate on rectal examination

Possible Findings
Enlarged prostate on ultrasonography; vesicle neck obstruction on cystourethroscopy; residual urine with postvoiding catheterization; presence of white blood cells, bacteria, or microscopic hematuria with infection; ↑ serum creatinine levels with renal involvement

BPH, Benign prostatic hyperplasia.

■ Nursing Diagnoses

Nursing diagnoses for the patient with BPH may include, but are not limited to, those presented in NCP 53-1.

■ Planning

The overall preoperative goals for the patient having invasive procedures are to have (1) restoration of urinary drainage, (2) treatment of any urinary tract infection, and (3) understanding of the upcoming procedure, implications for sexual functioning, and urinary control. The overall postoperative goals are to have (1) no complications, (2) restoration of urinary control, (3) complete bladder emptying, and (4) satisfying sexual expression.

■ Nursing Implementation

Health Promotion. The cause of BPH is largely attributed to the aging process. The focus of health promotion is on early detection and treatment. The American Cancer Society, along with the AUA, recommends a yearly medical history and DRE for men over 50 years of age in an effort to provide early detection of prostate problems. When symptoms of prostatic hyperplasia become evident, further diagnostic screening may be necessary (see Table 53-2).

Some men find that the ingestion of alcohol and caffeine tends to increase prostatic symptoms because the diuretic effect of these substances increases bladder distention. Compounds found in common cough and cold remedies such as pseudoephedrine (in Sudafed) and phenylephrine (in Allerest and Coricidin prepa-

NURSING CARE PLAN 53–1

Patient Undergoing Prostate Surgery*

EXPECTED PATIENT OUTCOMES	NURSING INTERVENTIONS and *RATIONALES*

PREOPERATIVE

NURSING DIAGNOSIS

Acute pain *related to* bladder distention secondary to enlarged prostate *as manifested by* complaints of discomfort caused by inability to void, palpable bladder, no urine output, diaphoresis, restlessness.

- No complaints of pain

- Assist with insertion of indwelling catheter (usually done by urologist) *to reduce pain by providing urinary drainage of urine from bladder.*
- Monitor intake and output *to evaluate fluid balance.*
- Percuss bladder for distention *to validate adequate emptying of the bladder.*
- Maintain patency of catheter *to ensure continuous flow of urine from the bladder.*
- Assess comfort status *to continue or revise plan as necessary.*

NURSING DIAGNOSIS

Risk for infection (urinary tract) *related to* indwelling catheter, environmental pathogens, and urinary stasis.

- No evidence of urinary tract infection

- Assess for elevated temperature and cloudy, foul-smelling urine *to identify manifestations of infection and initiate appropriate interventions.*
- Obtain urinalysis for culture (if ordered) *to determine presence and cause of infection.*
- Give patient 8 oz of water every waking hour *to prevent urinary stasis and dilute the urine.*
- Observe strict aseptic technique for catheter care *to minimize the risk of introducing an infectious organism.*

NURSING DIAGNOSIS

Fear *related to* actual or potential sexual dysfunction, possible diagnosis of cancer, and lack of knowledge regarding surgical procedure and postoperative care *as manifested by* verbalization of fear about impact of surgery on sexuality; questioning or inaccurate comments about surgical course.

- Decreased fear about effect of surgery on sexuality and surgical course
- Correct responses to questions
- Calm demeanor

- Perform preoperative teaching *to provide information regarding the preoperative and postoperative routines.*
- Assess patient's concerns related to sexual functioning and correct misconceptions and inaccuracies *to plan appropriate interventions that address unique concerns.*
- Provide opportunity for private conversation for patient to ask personal questions *because a private setting facilitates open discussion.*

POSTOPERATIVE

NURSING DIAGNOSIS

Acute pain *related to* irrigations and clots, presence of catheter, and surgical procedure *as manifested by* expression of pain; nonverbal signs of pain such as moaning, crying, legs drawn to abdomen.

- Decreased or no pain

- Maintain patency of catheter *because clots cause obstruction of urine flow resulting in bladder spasms.*
- Irrigate catheter if occluded with clots (according to aseptic technique and institution protocols) *so urine can flow freely.*
- Instruct patient to try not to urinate around catheter *because this increases the occurrence of spasm.*
- Give belladonna and opium suppository as needed; instruct patient in relaxation techniques such as deep breathing exercises, distraction therapy, and visual imagery *to relieve pain and decrease spasm.*

NURSING DIAGNOSIS

Ineffective therapeutic regimen management *related to* lack of knowledge regarding need for follow-up care and activity restriction postoperatively *as manifested by* questioning or inaccurate comments about postoperative activity.

- No postoperative bleeding because of performing activities that increase intraabdominal pressure

- Teach patient to avoid heavy lifting (>10 lb [45 kg]), straining during defecation, prolonged periods of travel, stair climbing, driving, and sexual activity until surgeon approves such activity *to prevent increases in intraabdominal pressure and the possibility of bleeding.*
- Teach patient about the need for follow-up care *to evaluate prostate (if present) and overall health.*

*The specific nursing management will vary depending on the type of surgical intervention for BPH or prostate cancer.

Continued

NURSING CARE PLAN 53-1

Patient Undergoing Prostate Surgery—cont'd

POSTOPERATIVE—cont'd

EXPECTED PATIENT OUTCOMES	NURSING INTERVENTIONS and *RATIONALES*
NURSING DIAGNOSIS	**Urge urinary incontinence** *related to* poor sphincter control *as manifested by* inappropriate leakage of urine.
• Absence of or satisfactory control of dribbling	• Teach patient Kegel exercises *to strengthen sphincter tone.* • Advise patient about devices to control dribbling *so patient is aware of various devices and can make an informed decision among alternatives.*
NURSING DIAGNOSIS	**Risk for infection** *related to* indwelling catheter, bladder irrigations, environmental pathogens, inadequate oral intake, and poor catheter care.
• No evidence of infection	• Assess for fever, diaphoresis, self-restriction of fluid intake, cloudy urine *to determine if risk factors and/or signs and symptoms of infection are present.* • Monitor temperature q4hr first 48 hr postoperatively *because fever is an indicator of infection.* • Give patient 8 oz of water hourly while awake *to maintain good urine flow and dilute the urine.* • Observe strict aseptic technique for catheter care and bladder irrigations *to prevent introducing infectious organisms.*

COLLABORATIVE PROBLEM

NURSING GOALS	NURSING INTERVENTIONS and *RATIONALES*
POTENTIAL COMPLICATION	**Hemorrhage** *related to* surgical procedure.
• Monitor for and report signs of hemorrhage • Carry out appropriate medical and nursing interventions	• Observe urinary drainage and report bright red bleeding in larger than expected quantities *because this could indicate hemorrhage and the need for immediate intervention.* • Monitor blood pressure, pulse, and respirations and report abnormalities *because increasing pulse and respirations and decreasing blood pressure can indicate hemorrhage and possible shock.* • Maintain catheter drainage *to prevent obstruction and allow monitoring of bleeding and urine flow.* • Do not perform rectal treatments such as enemas or rectal temperatures (except belladonna and opium suppositories for bladder spasms) *because bleeding could be initiated.*

rations) often worsen the symptoms of BPH. These drugs are α-adrenergic agonists that cause smooth muscle contraction. If this happens, the patient should avoid these drugs.

The patient with obstructive symptoms should be advised to urinate every 2 to 3 hours and when first feeling the urge. This will minimize urinary stasis and acute urinary retention. Fluid intake should be maintained at a normal level to avoid dehydration or fluid overload. The patient may believe that if he restricts his fluid intake, symptoms will be less severe, but this only increases the chances of an infection. However, if the patient increases his intake too rapidly, bladder distention can develop because of the prostatic obstruction.

Acute Intervention

Preoperative care. Urinary drainage must be restored before surgery. Prostatic obstruction may result in acute retention or inability to void. A urethral catheter such as a Coudé (curved-tip) catheter may be needed to restore drainage. In many health care settings, 10 ml of sterile 2% lidocaine gel is injected into the urethra before insertion of the catheter. The lidocaine gel not only acts as a lubricant, but also provides local anesthesia and helps open the urethral lumen.[10] If a sizable obstruction of the urethra exists, a urologist may insert a filiform catheter with sufficient rigidity to pass the obstruction. Aseptic technique is important at all times to avoid introducing bacteria into the bladder. (Urinary catheters are discussed in Chapter 44.)

Antibiotics are usually administered before any invasive procedure. Any infection of the urinary tract must be treated before surgery. Restoring urine drainage and encouraging a high fluid intake (2 to 3 L/day unless contraindicated) are also helpful in managing the infection.

The patient is often concerned about the impact of the impending surgery on his sexual functioning. Data gathered from the health history relating to sexual activities will identify possible problem areas. The nurse should provide an opportunity for the patient and partner to express their concerns. The patient needs to know how the surgery may affect sexual functioning. All types of prostatic surgery generally result in some degree of retrograde ejaculation. The patient should be informed that the ejaculate may be decreased in amount or totally absent. This may decrease orgasmic sensations felt during ejaculation. Retrograde ejaculation is not harmful because the semen is eliminated during the next urination.

Postoperative care. The main complications following surgery are hemorrhage, bladder spasms, urinary incontinence, and infection. The plan of care should be adjusted to the type of surgery, the reasons for surgery, and the patient's response to surgery.

After surgery the patient will have a standard catheter or a triple-lumen catheter. Bladder irrigation is typically done to remove clotted blood from the bladder and ensure drainage of urine. The bladder is irrigated either manually on an intermittent basis or more commonly as a continuous bladder irrigation (CBI) with sterile normal saline solution or another prescribed solution. If the bladder is manually irrigated (if ordered), 50 ml of irrigating solution should be instilled and then withdrawn with a syringe to remove clots that may be in the bladder and catheter. Painful bladder spasms often occur as a result of manual irrigation. With CBI, irrigating solution is continuously infused and drained from the bladder. The rate of infusion is based on the color of drainage. Ideally the urine drainage should be light pink without clots. The inflow and outflow of irrigant must be continuously monitored. If outflow is less than inflow, the catheter patency should be assessed for kinks or clots. If the outflow is blocked and patency cannot be reestablished by manual irrigation, the CBI is stopped and the physician notified.

Careful aseptic technique should be used when irrigating the bladder because bacteria can easily be introduced into the urinary tract. Proper care of the catheter is important. To prevent urethral irritation and minimize the risk of bladder infection, the catheter must be secured to the leg or abdomen with tape or catheter strap. The catheter should be connected to a closed-drainage system and should not be disconnected unless it is being removed, changed, or irrigated. The secretions that accumulate around the meatus can be cleansed daily with soap and water.

Blood clots are expected after prostate surgery for the first 24 to 36 hours. However, large amounts of bright red blood in the urine can indicate hemorrhage. Postoperative hemorrhage may occur from displacement of the catheter, dislodging a large clot, or increases in abdominal pressure. Release or displacement of the catheter dislodges the balloon that provides counterpressure on the operative site. Traction on the catheter may be applied to provide counterpressure (tamponade) on the bleeding site in the prostate, thereby decreasing bleeding. Such traction can result in local necrosis if pressure is applied for too long. Pressure should therefore be relieved on a scheduled basis by qualified personnel. Activities that increase abdominal pressure, such as sitting or walking for prolonged periods and straining to have a bowel movement (Valsalva maneuver), should be avoided in the postoperative recovery period.

Bladder spasms are a distressing complication for the patient after transurethral procedures. They occur as a result of irritation of the bladder mucosa from the insertion of the resectoscope, presence of a catheter, or clots leading to obstruction of the catheter. The patient should be instructed not to urinate around the catheter because this increases the likelihood of spasm. If bladder spasms develop, the catheter should be checked for clots. If present, the clots should be removed by irrigation so that urine can flow freely. Belladonna and opium suppositories, or other antispasmodics (e.g., oxybutynin [Ditropan]) along with relaxation techniques, are used to relieve the pain and decrease spasm. The catheter is often removed 2 to 4 days after surgery. The patient should urinate within 6 hours after catheter removal. If he cannot, a catheter is reinserted for a day or two. If the problem continues, the nurse may need to instruct the patient in clean intermittent self-catheterization (see Chapter 44).

Sphincter tone may be poor immediately after catheter removal, resulting in urinary incontinence or dribbling. This is a common but distressing situation for the patient. Sphincter tone can be strengthened by having the patient practice Kegel exercises (pelvic floor muscle technique) 10 to 20 times per hour while awake. The patient should be encouraged to practice start-

ing and stopping the stream several times during urination. This facilitates learning the pelvic floor exercises. It usually takes several weeks to achieve urinary continence. In some instances, control of urine may never be fully regained. Continence can improve for up to 12 months. If continence has not been achieved by that time, the patient may be referred to a continence clinic. A variety of methods, including biofeedback, have been used to achieve positive results. The patient can also be instructed to use a penile clamp, condom catheter, or incontinence pads or briefs to avoid embarrassment from dribbling. In severe cases, an occlusive cuff that serves as an artificial sphincter can be surgically implanted to restore continence. The nurse should assist the patient in finding ways to manage the problem that will allow him to continue socializing and interacting with others.

The patient should be observed for signs of postoperative infection. If an external wound is present (from an open prostatectomy), the area should be observed for redness, heat, swelling, and purulent drainage. Special care must be taken if a perineal incision is present because of the proximity of the anus. Rectal procedures, such as taking rectal temperatures and administering enemas, should be avoided. The insertion of well-lubricated belladonna and opium suppositories is acceptable.

Dietary intervention and stool softeners are important in the postoperative period to prevent the patient from straining while having bowel movements. Straining increases the intraabdominal pressure, which can lead to bleeding at the operative site. A diet high in fiber facilitates the passage of stool.

Ambulatory and Home Care. Discharge planning and home care issues are important aspects of care after prostate surgery. Instructions include (1) caring for an indwelling catheter (if one is left in place); (2) managing urinary incontinence; (3) maintaining oral fluids between 2000 and 3000 ml per day; (4) observing for signs and symptoms of urinary tract and wound infection; (5) preventing constipation; (6) avoiding heavy lifting (more than 10 lb [4.5 kg]); and (7) refraining from driving or intercourse after surgery as directed by the physician.

The patient may experience a change in sexual functioning following surgery. Many men experience retrograde ejaculation because of trauma to the internal sphincter. Semen is discharged into the bladder at orgasm and may produce cloudy urine when the patient urinates after orgasm. Physiologic erectile dysfunction (ED) may occur if the nerves are cut or damaged during surgery. The patient may experience anxiety over the change due to a perceived loss of his sex role, self-esteem, or quality of sexual interaction with his partner. The nurse should discuss these changes with the patient and his partner and allow them to ask questions and express their concerns. Sexual counseling and treatment options may be necessary if ED becomes a chronic or permanent problem. ED is discussed later in the chapter. It should be pointed out that although some patients experience concerns regarding change in sexual function, this is not a universal concern. Many men are comfortable with such changes and view them as appropriate for their age. If this is the case, nurses should be careful not to impose concern in their enthusiastic attempts to pursue such problems.[11]

The bladder may take up to 2 months to return to its normal capacity. The patient should be instructed to drink at least 2 L of fluid per day and urinate every 2 to 3 hours to flush the urinary tract. Bladder irritants such as caffeine products, citrus juices, and alcohol should be avoided or limited to small amounts.

Because the patient may be experiencing incontinence or dribbling, he may incorrectly believe that decreasing fluid intake will relieve this problem. Urethral strictures may result from instrumentation or catheterization. Treatment may include teaching the patient intermittent clean catheterization or having a urethral dilation.

The patient must be advised that he should continue to have a yearly DRE if he has had any procedure other than complete removal of the prostate. Hyperplasia or cancer can occur in the remaining prostatic tissue.

■ Evaluation

Expected outcomes for the patient with BPH are presented in NCP 53-1.

PROSTATE CANCER

Prostate cancer is a malignant tumor of the prostate gland. It is estimated that 189,000 new cases of prostate cancer were diagnosed in 2002, and 30,200 men died from the disease.[12] One of every five men will develop prostate cancer at some point during their lives. Prostate cancer is the most common cancer among men, excluding skin cancer. It is the second leading cause of cancer death in men (exceeded only by lung cancer). The majority (more than 75%) of cases occur in men over age 65. However, many cases occur in younger men who sometimes have a more aggressive type of cancer. There was a large increase in the incidence of newly diagnosed cases of prostate cancer between 1988 and 1992. This increase in number was attributed to the widespread use of prostate-specific antigen (PSA) as a screening procedure, allowing early detection of prostate cancer. The incidence of prostate cancer appears to have peaked and has now leveled off.[12]

Etiology and Pathophysiology

Prostate cancer is an androgen-dependent adenocarcinoma. The majority of tumors occur in the outer aspect of the prostate gland. Prostate cancer is usually slow growing. It can spread by three routes: direct extension, through the lymph system, or through the bloodstream. Spread by direct extension involves the seminal vesicles, urethral mucosa, bladder wall, and external sphincter. The cancer later spreads through the lymphatic system

CULTURAL & ETHNIC CONSIDERATIONS
Cancer of the Male Reproductive System

- Prostate cancer occurs twice as frequently among African American men as among white men.
- African American men tend to be diagnosed with prostate cancer at an earlier age, have more advanced disease at the time of diagnosis, and have a higher mortality rate than do white men. Although the mortality rate among African American men is higher than that among whites, the mortality rate is declining.
- Hispanic and Asian American men have a lower incidence of prostate cancer and lower mortality rates as compared with white men.
- Testicular cancer occurs most frequently among whites compared with other ethnic groups and is rare in African Americans.

to the regional lymph nodes. The veins from the prostate seem to be the mode of spread to the pelvic bones, head of the femur, lower lumbar spine, liver, and lungs.

Age, ethnicity, and family history are three nonmodifiable risk factors for prostate cancer. The incidence of prostate cancer rises markedly after age 50; more than 80% of men diagnosed are older than 65.[13] African Americans have the highest incidence of prostate cancer of any ethnic group, with a rate twice that of white men. In addition, they are more likely to have prostate cancer at a younger age, have more aggressive tumors at diagnosis, and have higher mortality rates.[14] A family history of prostate cancer, especially first-degree relatives (fathers, brothers), is also associated with an increased risk. Genetic mutations in certain genes may contribute to the risk of prostate cancer in susceptible men.

A high-fat diet is thought to be associated with an increased risk of prostate cancer.[15,16] Although occupational exposure to chemicals (e.g., cadmium) may be associated with higher prostate cancer risk, this possible risk continues to be studied.[13,14] A history of BPH is not a risk factor for prostate cancer.

Clinical Manifestations and Complications

Prostate cancer is usually asymptomatic in the early stages. Eventually the patient may have symptoms similar to those of BPH, including dysuria, hesitancy, dribbling, frequency, urgency, hematuria, nocturia, retention, interruption of urinary stream, and inability to urinate. Pain in the lumbosacral area that radiates down to the hips or legs, when coupled with urinary symptoms, may indicate metastasis.

Early recognition and treatment is required to control growth, prevent metastasis, and preserve quality of life. The tumor can spread to pelvic lymph nodes, bones, bladder, lungs, and liver. Once the tumor has spread to distant sites, the major problem becomes the management of pain. As the cancer spreads to the bones (a common site of metastasis), pain can become severe, especially in the back and the legs because of compression of the spinal cord and destruction of bone.

Diagnostic Studies

Improved diagnostic techniques have greatly enhanced the detection of prostate cancer. The two primary screening tools are DRE and a blood test for **prostate-specific antigen** (PSA), a glycoprotein produced by the prostate. On DRE the prostate may feel hard and have asymmetric enlargement with areas of induration or nodules.

Elevated levels of PSA (normal level, 0 to 4 ng/ml [0 to 4 μg/L]) indicate prostatic pathology, although not necessarily prostate cancer. Mild elevations in PSA may occur in BPH, acute or chronic prostatitis, or urinary retention, or after long bike rides. In addition, cystoscopy, indwelling urethral catheters, and prostate biopsies may produce an elevation. When prostate cancer exists, serum PSA levels are a useful marker of tumor volume (i.e., the higher the PSA level, the greater the tumor mass). Some men with prostate cancer have normal PSA levels.

PSA is not only used to detect prostate cancer, but it is also used to monitor the success of treatment. When the treatment has been successful in removing prostate cancer, PSA levels should fall to undetectable levels. Regular measurement of PSA levels following treatment is important to evaluate the effectiveness of treatment and possible recurrence of prostate cancer.

Elevated levels of prostatic isoenzyme of serum acid phosphatase (prostatic acid phosphatase [PAP]) is another indication of prostate cancer, especially if there is extracapsular spread. With advanced prostate cancer, serum alkaline phosphatase is increased as a result of bone metastasis. Investigation is now under way to locate a serum marker for prostate cancer similar to CA-125, which is a useful marker in ovarian cancer. (Ovarian cancer is discussed in Chapter 52.)

Neither PSA nor DRE is a definitive diagnostic test for prostate cancer. If PSA levels are elevated or if the DRE is abnormal, biopsy of the prostate tissue is indicated. Biopsy of prostate tissue is necessary to confirm the diagnosis of prostate cancer. The biopsy is typically done using TRUS because it allows the physician to visualize the prostate and pinpoint abnormalities. When a suspicious area is located, a special biopsy needle is inserted into the prostate to obtain a tissue sample. A pathologic examination of the tissue specimen is done to assess for malignant changes. Other tests used to determine the location and extent of the spread of the cancer may include bone scan, computed tomography (CT), magnetic resonance imaging (MRI) using an endorectal probe, and TRUS.

The Prostascint scan is a single-photon emission computed tomography (SPECT) imaging technique that uses a monoclonal antibody to target prostate-specific membrane antigens. This procedure is able to detect spread of prostate cancer to the pelvic lymph nodes.

Collaborative Care

Early-stage prostate cancer is a curable disease in the majority of men. Based on findings from diagnostic studies, the prostate cancer is staged and graded. Two common classification systems used for staging prostate cancer, the Whitmore-Jewett and tumor, node, metastasis (TNM) systems, are both based on the size (volume) of the tumor and spread (Table 53-5). It is estimated that 80% of patients with prostate cancer are initially diagnosed when the cancer is in either a local or regional stage. The 5-year survival rate with an initial diagnosis at this stage is 100%.[12]

Grading of the tumor is done based on tumor histology using the Gleason scale. With this scale, tumors are graded from 1 to 5 based on the degree of glandular differentiation. Grade 1 represents the most well differentiated (most like the original cells) and grade 5 represents the most poorly differentiated (undifferentiated). Gleason grades are given to the two most commonly occurring patterns of cells and added together. The Gleason score is a number from 2 to 10. This scale is used to predict how quickly the cancer will progress.

The collaborative care of the patient with prostate cancer depends on the stage of the cancer and the overall health of the patient. At all stages, there is more than one possible treatment option. The decision of which treatment course to pursue is made jointly by the patient and the physician based on a careful analysis of the facts and the patient's preference.[17] Table 53-6 summarizes the various treatment options available.

Conservative Therapy. Prostate cancer is relatively slow growing. Therefore a conservative approach to management of prostate cancer is "watchful waiting" (also known as "deferred treatment"). The decision to adopt a strategy of watchful waiting is appropriate when there is (1) a life expectancy of less than 10 years, (2) presence of significant comorbid disease, and (3) presence of a low-grade, low-stage tumor. These patients are

---

TABLE 53-5   Whitmore-Jewett Staging Classification of Prostate Cancer

Stage A: Clinically Unrecognized

A1	<5% of prostatic tissue neoplastic
A2	>5% of prostatic tissue neoplastic, all high-grade tumors

Stage B: Clinically Intracapsular

B1	Nodule <2 cm and surrounded by palpably normal tissue
B2	Nodule >2 cm or multiple nodules

Stage C: Clinically Extracapsular, Localized to Periprostatic Area

C1	Minimal extracapsular extension
C2	Large tumors involving seminal vesicles, adjacent structures, or both

Stage D: Metastatic Disease

D1	Pelvic lymph node metastases or ureteral obstruction causing hydronephrosis
D2	Distant metastases to bone, viscera, or other soft tissue structures

---

TABLE 53-6   Collaborative Care   Prostate Cancer

Diagnostic
History and physical examination
Digital rectal examination (DRE)
Prostate-specific antigen (PSA)
Prostatic acid phosphatase (PAP)
Transrectal ultrasound
Biopsy of prostate and lymph nodes
Computed tomography (CT), magnetic resonance imaging (MRI), bone scan (to evaluate for metastatic disease)

Collaborative Therapy
Stage A
Watchful waiting with annual PSA and DRE
Radical prostatectomy
Radiation therapy
• External beam
• Brachytherapy
Stage B
Radical prostatectomy
Radiation therapy
Stage C
Radical prostatectomy
Radiation therapy
Hormone therapy
Orchiectomy
Stage D
Hormone therapy
Orchiectomy
Chemotherapy
Radiation therapy to metastatic bone areas

typically followed with frequent PSA measurements, along with DRE, to monitor the progress of the disease. Significant changes in either PSA, DRE, or the development of symptoms warrant a reevaluation of treatment options, whether they be definitive or palliative.

Surgical Therapy

Radical prostatectomy. With **radical prostatectomy,** the entire prostate gland, seminal vesicles, and part of the bladder neck (ampulla) are removed. The entire prostate is removed because the cancer tends to be in many different locations within the gland. In addition, a retroperitoneal lymph node dissection is usually done. A radical prostatectomy is the surgical procedure considered the most effective treatment for long-term survival. Thus it is the preferred treatment for men younger than 70 years of age who are in good health and with the cancer confined to the prostate (stages A and B).[17] Surgery is usually not considered an option for stage D cancer (except to relieve symptoms associated with obstruction) because metastasis has already occurred. The two most common approaches for radical prostatectomy are retropubic and perineal resection (Fig. 53-4). With the *retropubic*

approach, a low midline abdominal incision is made to access the prostate gland, and the pelvic lymph nodes can be dissected. With the *perineal* resection, an incision is made between the scrotum and anus. This procedure cannot remove lymph nodes. A laparoscopic approach to prostatectomy is being used in some settings. It has the potential to offer technologic improvement, less bleeding, less pain, and faster recovery compared with traditional approaches, but the long-term benefits are still being investigated.[18]

After surgery, the patient has a large indwelling catheter with a 30 ml balloon placed in the bladder via the urethra. This catheter is typically left in place for 1 to 2 weeks. A drain is left in the surgical site to aid in the removal of drainage from the area. This drain is typically removed after a couple of days. Because the perineal approach has a higher risk of postoperative infection (due to of the location of the incision related to the anus), careful dressing changes and perineal care after each bowel movement are important for comfort and to prevent infection. The typical length of hospital stay postoperatively is 3 days.

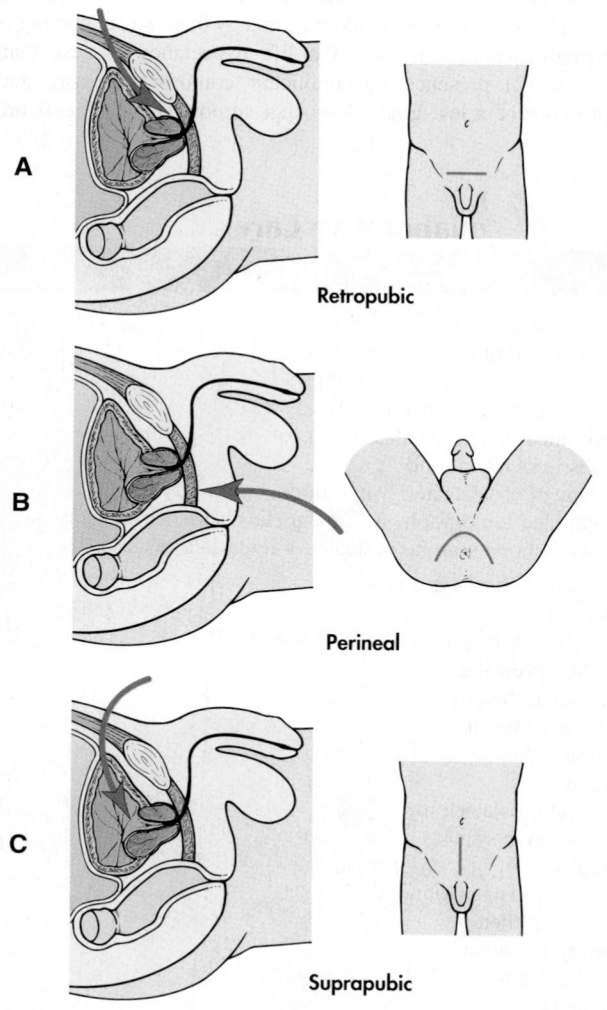

FIG. 53-4 Three approaches used to perform a prostatectomy. **A,** Retropubic approach involves a midline abdominal incision. **B,** Perineal approach involves an incision between the scrotum and anus. **C,** Suprapubic approach involves an abdominal incision.

NURSING RESEARCH
Incontinence and Impotence after Prostatectomy for Prostate Cancer

Citation
Maliski SL, Heilemann MV, McCorkle R: Mastery of post-prostatectomy incontinence and impotence: his work, her work, our work, *Oncol Nurs Forum* 28:985, 2001.

Purpose
To describe couples' experiences of incontinence and impotence following prostatectomy for prostate cancer.

Method
This qualitative design involved a sample of 20 couples from a clinical trial of a Standardized Nursing Intervention Protocol Postprostatectomy. The couples were interviewed using a semistructured guide to discuss their experiences with incontinence and impotence as a result of prostatectomy. Data were analyzed using grounded theory techniques.

Results and Conclusions
The men focused on gaining an understanding of incontinence, mastering incontinence, networking, confronting impotency, and putting these issues in perspective. Wives were supportive by managing anxiety, encouraging mastery, putting impotence into perspective, and reassuring their spouses. The couples found nurses to be a source of information, support, and affirmation. Both men and women worked through incontinence and impotence in the context of surviving cancer and maintaining a loving relationship. Mastery emerged as a key concept from the findings.

Implications for Nursing Practice
Incontinence and impotence that result from prostectectomy affect both the man and his wife. The wife can play a key role in dealing with these issues. Nursing interventions that promote mastery, as well as helping couples place these issues in the context of cancer survival, are an important aspect of helping couples cope with incontinence and impotence. Nurses can help couples regain a sense of mastery by providing information, encouraging the attainment of self-care skills, confirming progress, and providing emotional support.

The two major complications following a radical prostatectomy are erectile dysfunction and incontinence.[19] Because this procedure destroys the nerves needed for erection, erectile dysfunction occurs. The incidence of erectile dysfunction is dependent on the patient's age, preoperative sexual functioning, whether nerve-sparing surgery was performed, and the expertise of the surgeon. Problems with urinary control occur in nearly all men for the first few months following surgery because the bladder must be reattached to the urethra after the prostate is removed. Over time, the bladder adjusts and most men regain control. One study reported that only 6.4% were incontinent 18 months after surgery.[20] Other common complications associated with surgery include hemorrhage, urinary retention, infection, wound dehiscence, deep vein thrombosis, and pulmonary emboli.

Nerve-sparing procedure. Many men desire to retain sexual function following radical prostatectomy. In such cases a nerve-sparing procedure that spares the nerves responsible for erection may be possible. This procedure is the preferred choice for most men undergoing prostatectomy in the early stage of the disease. Nerve-sparing prostatectomy is indicated only for patients with cancer confined within the prostate gland. Although the risk of erectile dysfunction is significantly reduced with this procedure, there is no guarantee that potency will be maintained. Because the nerves lie directly beneath the prostate gland, the risk of damage is very high. The percent of success reported varies.[20]

Cryosurgery. Prostatic cryosurgery is a surgical technique that destroys cancer cells by freezing the tissue. It has been used both as an initial treatment and as a second-line treatment after radiation treatment failures. A transrectal ultrasound probe is inserted to visualize the prostate gland. Probes containing liquid nitrogen are then inserted into the prostate. Liquid nitrogen delivers freezing temperatures, destroying the tissue. The treatment takes about 2 hours under general or spinal anesthesia and does not involve an abdominal incision. Possible complications of prostatic cryosurgery include damage to the urethra, and, in rare cases, a urethrorectal fistula (an opening between the urethra and the rectum) or a urethrocutaneous fistula (an opening between the urethra and the skin). Tissue sloughing, erectile dysfunction, urinary incontinence, prostatitis, and hemorrhage have also been reported.

Radiation Therapy. Radiation therapy is a common treatment option for prostate cancer, especially for men over 70, patients who are poor surgical risks, or those who wish to avoid surgery. The long-term outcome of radiation therapy is dependent on the stage of the cancer. Because many of the men choosing radiation therapy are older and perhaps not in as good health as those undergoing prostatectomy, comparisons are difficult.[21] Radiation therapy may be offered as the only treatment, or it may be offered in combination with surgery or with hormonal therapy.

External beam radiation. External beam is the most widely used method of delivering radiation treatments for those with prostate cancer. This therapy can be used to treat patients with prostate cancer confined to the prostate and/or surrounding tissue (stages A, B, and C). Patients are treated on an outpatient basis 5 days a week for 6 to 8 weeks. Each treatment lasts only a few minutes. Side effects from radiation can be acute (occurring during treatment or within 90 days that follow) or delayed (occur-

ring months or years after treatment). Common side effects involve the skin (dryness, redness, irritation, pain), gastrointestinal tract (diarrhea, abdominal cramping, bleeding), urinary tract (dysuria, frequency, hesitancy, urgency, nocturia), sexual functioning (erectile dysfunction), fatigue, and bone marrow suppression.[21] These problems usually resolve 2 to 3 weeks after the completion of radiation therapy. In patients with clinically localized disease, cure rates with external beam radiation are comparable to those with radical prostatectomy.

Brachytherapy. Brachytherapy involves the implantation of radioactive seed implants into the prostate gland, allowing higher radiation doses directly in the tissue while sparing the surrounding tissue (rectum and bladder). The radioactive seeds are placed in the prostate gland with a needle through a grid template guided by transrectal ultrasound (Fig. 53-5). The grid template and ultrasound ensure accurate placement of the seeds.[21] Because brachytherapy is a one-time outpatient procedure, many patients find this more convenient than external beam radiation treatment. Brachytherapy is best suited for patients with stage A or B prostate cancer.[17] The most common side effect is the development of urinary irritative or obstructive problems. The AUA Symptom Index (see Table 53-1) can be used to measure urinary function for patients undergoing brachytherapy and can be incorporated into postoperative nursing management.[22] For those with more advanced tumors, brachytherapy may be offered in combination with external beam radiation treatment. Brachytherapy is discussed further in Chapter 15.

Drug Therapy. The forms of drug therapy available for the treatment of prostate cancer are hormonal therapy, chemotherapy, or a combination of both.

Hormonal therapy. Prostate cancer growth is largely dependent on the presence of androgens. Therefore androgen deprivation is the primary therapeutic approach for men with prostatic cancer. Hormone therapy is focused on reducing the levels of circulating androgens in order to reduce the tumor growth. Hormone or antiandrogen therapy can also be used as adjunct therapy before surgery or radiation therapy to reduce tumor size, and in men with locally advanced disease (stage C). One of the biggest challenges with hormonal therapy is the development of hormone-refractory disease. The duration of response to initial hormonal therapy averages from 18 to 24 months.[23] Androgen ablation can be produced by interference with androgen production (e.g.,

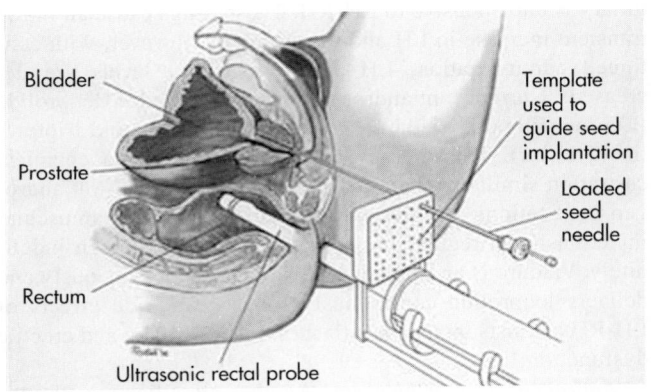

Bladder

Prostate

Rectum

Ultrasonic rectal probe

Template used to guide seed implantation

Loaded seed needle

FIG. 53-5 Prostate brachytherapy. Radioactive seeds are implanted with a needle guided by ultrasound and a template grid.

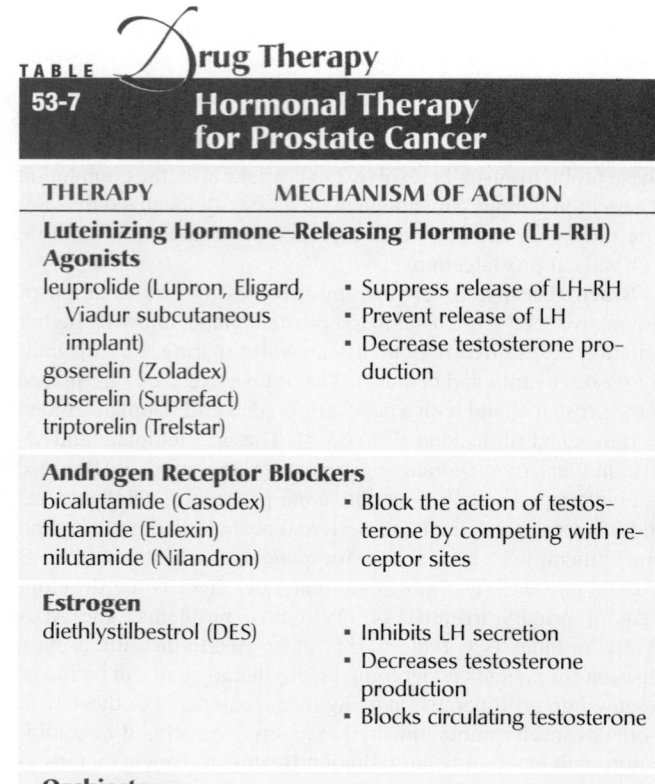

TABLE 53-7 Drug Therapy Hormonal Therapy for Prostate Cancer	
THERAPY	**MECHANISM OF ACTION**
Luteinizing Hormone–Releasing Hormone (LH-RH) Agonists	
leuprolide (Lupron, Eligard, Viadur subcutaneous implant) goserelin (Zoladex) buserelin (Suprefact) triptorelin (Trelstar)	• Suppress release of LH-RH • Prevent release of LH • Decrease testosterone production
Androgen Receptor Blockers	
bicalutamide (Casodex) flutamide (Eulexin) nilutamide (Nilandron)	• Block the action of testosterone by competing with receptor sites
Estrogen	
diethlystilbestrol (DES)	• Inhibits LH secretion • Decreases testosterone production • Blocks circulating testosterone
Orchiectomy	
Surgical removal of testicles	• Removes 95% of testosterone source

LH, Luteinizing hormone.

luteinizing hormone–releasing hormone [LH-RH] agonists, orchiectomy) or androgen receptor blockers (Table 53-7).

Luteinizing hormone–releasing hormone agonists. Luteinizing hormone–releasing hormone (LH-RH) is released from the hypothalamus to stimulate the anterior pituitary to produce luteinizing hormone (LH) and follicle-stimulating hormone (FSH). LH stimulates the testicular Leydig cells to produce testosterone. The LH-RH agonists superstimulate the pituitary. This ultimately results in downregulation of the LH-RH receptors, leading to a refractory condition in which the anterior pituitary is unresponsive to LH-RH. These drugs cause an initial transient increase in LH and testosterone. However, with continued administration, LH and testosterone levels are decreased. Current antiandrogen therapy includes leuprolide (Lupron, Eligard, Viadure), goserelin (Zoladex), and triptorelin (Trelstar). This therapy essentially produces a chemical castration similar to the effects of an orchiectomy. Antiandrogen medications are given by subcutaneous or intramuscular injections on a regular basis, and they must be taken indefinitely. Viadure is an implant that is placed subcutaneously and delivers leuprolide continuously for 1 year. Side effects of LH-RH agonists include hot flashes, loss of libido, and erectile dysfunction.

Androgen receptor blockers. Another classification of antiandrogens are drugs that compete with circulating androgens at the receptor sites. Flutamide (Eulexin), nilutamide (Nilandron),

and bicalutamide (Casodex) are nonsteroidal androgen receptor blockers. They can be used in combination with goserelin or leuprolide. The combination has been found to be safe and well tolerated as a potency-sparing, androgen-ablative therapy. Adverse effects of androgen receptor blockers include loss of libido, erectile dysfunction, and hot flashes. Breast pain and gynecomastia may also occur in men treated with androgen receptor blockers.

Estrogen. Estrogen (e.g., diethylstilbestrol) has been used as a form of androgen deprivation therapy. However, estrogen treatment is declining in popularity because of cardiovascular complications (e.g., myocardial infarction, deep vein thrombosis, cerebrovascular disease), and the development of more effective hormone therapies.

Orchiectomy. A bilateral orchiectomy is the surgical removal of the testes that may be done alone or in combination with prostatectomy. For advanced stages of prostate cancer (stage D) an orchiectomy is one treatment option for cancer control. Testosterone, produced by the testes, stimulates growth of the prostate cancer. An orchiectomy reduces the circulating testosterone levels by 90%.[18] Another possible benefit of this procedure is the rapid relief of bone pain associated with advanced tumors. Orchiectomy may also induce sufficient shrinkage of the prostate to relieve urinary obstruction in later stages of disease when surgery is not an option.

Side effects of orchiectomy include hot flashes, erectile dysfunction, loss of sex drive, and irritability. Weight gain and loss of muscle mass, which are also common, can alter a man's physical appearance. Osteoporosis has also been reported as a consequence of orchiectomy. These physical changes can affect self-esteem, leading to grief and depression. Although this procedure is permanent and cost effective (compared with chemical hormone manipulation using LH-RH agonists), many men prefer drug therapy to orchiectomy.

Chemotherapy. The use of chemotherapeutic agents has primarily been limited to treatment for those with hormone-resistant prostate cancer (HRPC) in late-stage disease. In HRPC the cancer is progressing despite treatment. This occurs in patients who have taken an antiandrogen for a certain period of time. Historically, prostate cancer has been poorly responsive to chemotherapy and has not been shown to improve survival. Thus the goal of chemotherapy is palliation.[24] Some of the more commonly used chemotherapy drugs include mitoxantrone (Novantrone), cyclosphophamide (Cytoxan), idarubicin (Idamycin), epirubicin (Ellence), and estramustine (Emcyt).

Bisphosphonates. Patients with advanced prostate cancer have a high risk of developing bone complication such as pain, fractures, and spinal cord compression. Bisphosphonates can be used to prevent and treat bone complications in advanced prostate cancer. Bisphosphonates include zolendronate (Zomex), risendronate (Actonel), etidronate (Didronel), and alendronate (Fosamax).

■ Culturally Competent Care: Prostate Cancer

Nurses must be aware of not only the epidemiologic differences that occur with prostate cancer, but also the differences that exist in health promotion practice. Demographic characteristics should be considered when providing information about the risk for prostate cancer and screening recommendations.

African American men suffer higher mortality rates than white men, in part because their prostate cancer often is more advanced at the time of diagnosis. Despite the availability of early screening measures (PSA and DRE), African American men and those in lower socioeconomic groups frequently do not use such services. This is partially related to actual and perceived knowledge levels of prostate cancer.[25] One study found that men are most likely to take part in regular screenings when a health care provider informed them of their risk of prostate cancer and screening options.[26] Although exposure to electronic and print media is successful in informing some men about prostate cancer, significant differences of effectiveness exist based on demographic variables such as ethnicity, age, education level, and socioeconomic level. Ideally, no man should be unaware of the risks associated with prostate cancer and screening methods available. The nurse must consider the best method to communicate this information to men of all cultures that will result in the greatest degree of understanding and participation in prostate cancer screening. ■

NURSING MANAGEMENT
PROSTATE CANCER

■ Nursing Assessment

Subjective and objective data that should be obtained from a patient with prostate cancer are presented in Table 53-8.

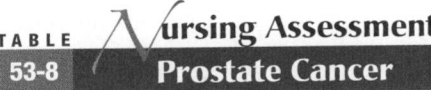

TABLE 53-8	Nursing Assessment Prostate Cancer

Subjective Data
Important Health Information
Medications: Testosterone supplements; use of any medications affecting urinary tract such as morphine, anticholinergics, monoamine oxidase inhibitors, and tricyclic antidepressants
Functional Health Patterns
Health perception–health management: Positive family history; increasing fatigue and malaise
Nutritional-metabolic: High-fat diet; anorexia, weight loss (possible indicators of metastasis)
Elimination: Hesitancy or straining to start stream, urinary urgency, frequency, retention with dribbling, weak stream, hematuria
Sleep: Nocturia
Cognitive-perceptual: Dysuria; low back pain radiating to legs or pelvis, bone pain (possible indicators of metastasis)
Self-perception–self-concept: Anxiety regarding self-concept

Objective Data
General
Older adult male; pelvic lymphadenopathy (late sign)
Urinary
Distended bladder on palpation; unilaterally hard, enlarged, fixed prostate on rectal examination
Musculoskeletal
Pathologic fractures (metastasis)
Possible Findings
↑ Serum PSA; ↑ serum PAP (metastasis); nodular and irregular prostate on ultrasonography, positive biopsy results; anemia

PAP, Prostatic acid phosphatase; *PSA,* prostate-specific antigen.

EVIDENCE-BASED PRACTICE
Urinary Incontinence after Prostatectomy

Clinical Problem
Does pelvic floor muscle training for patients with urinary incontinence as a result of radical prostatectomy have any beneficial effects?

Best Clinical Practice
▪ Pelvic floor training (biofeedback and Kegel exercises*) decreases the duration and degree of incontinence.
▪ Pelvic floor training should be considered as a primary treatment option in male patients with incontinence following a prostatectomy.

Implications for Nursing Practice
▪ Urinary incontinence is a common complication after radical prostatectomy. Following surgery, spontaneous recovery of normal urinary control can take 1 to 2 years.
▪ Pelvic floor muscle training using Kegel exercises and biofeedback can decrease the duration and degree of incontinence.
▪ Lifestyle adjustments, including decreasing or eliminating caffeine, physical exercise, and cessation of smoking, are also important in treating incontinence.

Reference for Evidence
Van Kampen M et al: Effect of pelvic-floor re-education on duration and degree of incontinence after radical prostatectomy: a randomized controlled trial, *Lancet* 355:98, 2000.

*Kegel exercises are discussed in Chapter 44.

■ Nursing Diagnoses

Nursing diagnoses for the patient with prostate cancer depend on the stage of the cancer. General nursing diagnoses, which may or may not apply to every patient with cancer of the prostate, may include, but are not limited to, the following:
▪ Decisional conflict *related to* numerous alternative treatment options
▪ Acute pain *related to* surgery, prostatic enlargement, bone metastasis, and bladder spasms
▪ Urinary retention *related to* obstruction of urethra or bladder neck by the prostate, blood clots, and loss of bladder tone
▪ Impaired urinary elimination *related to* bladder neck sphincter damage
▪ Constipation or diarrhea *related to* treatment interventions
▪ Sexual dysfunction *related to* effects of treatment
▪ Anxiety *related to* uncertain outcome of disease process on life and lifestyle and effect of treatment on sexual functioning

■ Planning

The overall goals are that the patient with prostate cancer will (1) be an active participant in the treatment plan, (2) have satisfactory pain control, (3) follow the therapeutic plan, (4) accept the effect of the therapeutic plan on sexual function, and (5) find a satisfactory way to manage the impact on bladder or bowel function.

■ Nursing Implementation

Health Promotion. One of the most important roles for nurses in relation to prostate cancer is to encourage patients to have an annual prostate screening (PSA and DRE) starting at age 50 or younger if risk factors are present. Because of their increased risk of prostate cancer, African American men and other men with a family history of prostate cancer should have an annual PSA and DRE beginning at age 45.[27]

Acute Intervention. Preoperative and postoperative phases of radical prostatectomy are similar to surgical procedures for BPH (see pp. 1441-1443). Nursing interventions for the patient who undergoes radiation therapy and chemotherapy are discussed in Chapter 15. An additional consideration is the psychologic response of the patient to a diagnosis of cancer. The nurse should provide sensitive, caring support for the patient and his family to help them cope with the diagnosis of cancer. Prostate support groups are available for men and their families to encourage them to be active, informed participants in their own care.

Ambulatory and Home Care. If the patient is discharged with an indwelling catheter in place, the nurse must teach appropriate catheter care. The patient should be instructed to clean the urethral meatus with soap and water once a day; maintain a high fluid intake; keep the collecting bag lower than the bladder at all times; keep the catheter securely anchored to the inner thigh or abdomen; and report any signs of bladder infection, such as bladder spasms, fever, or hematuria. If urinary incontinence is a problem, patients should be encouraged to practice pelvic floor muscle exercises (Kegel exercises) at every urination and throughout the day. Continuous practice during the 4- to 6-week healing process improves the success rate. Products used for incontinence specifically designed for men are available through home care product catalogs and many retail stores.

Although prostate cancer has a high cure rate if detected and treated early, prognosis for stage D prostate cancer is very unfavorable. Hospice care is often appropriate and beneficial to the patient and family. (Hospice care is discussed in Chapter 6.) Common problems experienced by the patient with advanced prostate cancer include fatigue, bladder outlet obstruction and ureteral obstruction (caused by compression of the urethra and/or ureters from tumor mass or lymph node metastasis), severe bone pain and fractures (caused by bone metastasis), spinal cord compression (from spinal metastasis), and leg edema (caused by lymphedema, deep vein thrombosis, and other medical conditions). Nursing interventions must focus on all of these problems. However, management of pain is one of the most important aspects of nursing care for these patients. Pain control is managed through ongoing pain assessment, administration of prescribed medications (both narcotic and nonnarcotic agents), and the use of nonpharmacologic methods of pain relief. (Pain management is discussed further in Chapter 9.)

■ **Evaluation**

Evaluation is based on expected outcomes. The outcomes are that the patient with prostate cancer will
- be an active participant in the treatment plan
- have satisfactory pain control
- follow the therapeutic plan
- accept the effect of the treatment on sexual function
- find a satisfactory way to manage the impact on bladder or bowel function

PROSTATITIS

Etiology and Pathophysiology

Prostatitis is a broad term that describes a group of inflammatory conditions affecting the prostate gland. It is the most common urologic problem in men younger than 50 years of age.

Nearly 2 million men are treated for prostatitis each year.[28] Historically, this condition has lacked a strong agreement regarding the cause, diagnosis, and optimal treatment. To bring greater consistency in approaching this common condition, the National Institutes of Health established consensus classifications of prostatitis syndromes. The consensus classifications include four categories: (1) acute bacterial prostatitis, (2) chronic bacterial prostatitis, (3) chronic prostatitis/chronic pelvic pain syndrome, and (4) asymptomatic inflammatory prostatitis.[29]

Both acute and chronic bacterial prostatitis generally result from organisms reaching the prostate gland by one of the following routes: ascending from the urethra, descending from the bladder, and invasion via the bloodstream or the lymphatic channels. Common causative organisms are *Escherichia coli, Klebsiella, Pseudomonas, Enterobacter, Proteus, Chlamydia trachomatis, Neisseria gonorrhoeae,* and group D streptococci. Chronic bacterial prostatitis differs from acute prostatitis in that it involves recurrent episodes of infection.[29]

Chronic prostatitis/chronic pelvic pain syndrome is a new term that describes the syndrome with prostate and urinary pain in the absence of an obvious infectious process. The etiology of chronic prostatitis/chronic pelvic pain syndrome is unclear. It may occur after a viral illness, or it may be associated with sexually transmitted diseases (STDs), particularly in a younger adult. The etiology is not known, and a culture reveals no causative organisms. However, leukocytes may be found in prostatic secretions.

Asymptomatic inflammatory prostatitis is usually diagnosed in individuals who have no symptoms, but are found to have an inflammatory process in the prostate. These patients are usually diagnosed during the evaluation of other genitourinary tract problems. Leukocytes are present in the seminal fluid from the prostate, but the cause of this process is unclear.

Clinical Manifestations and Complications

Common clinical manifestations of acute bacterial prostatitis include fever, chills, back pain, and perineal pain, along with acute urinary symptoms such as dysuria, urinary frequency, urgency, and cloudy urine. The patient may also have acute urinary retention caused by prostatic swelling. With DRE, the prostate is extremely swollen, very tender, and firm. The complications of prostatitis are epididymitis and cystitis. Sexual functioning may be affected as manifested by postejaculation pain, libido problems, and erectile dysfunction. Prostatic abscess is also a potential, but uncommon, complication.

Chronic bacterial prostatitis and chronic prostatitis/pelvic pain syndrome manifest with similar symptoms that are generally milder than those associated with acute bacterial prostatitis. These include irritative voiding symptoms (frequency, urgency, dysuria), backache, perineal/pelvic pain, and ejaculatory pain. Obstructive symptoms are uncommon unless the patient has coexisting BPH. With DRE, the prostate feels enlarged and firm (often described as boggy) and is slightly tender with palpation. Chronic prostatitis can predispose the patient to recurrent urinary tract infections.

The clinical features of prostatitis can be mimicked by urinary tract infection. However, acute cystitis is not common in men.

Diagnostic Studies

Because patients with prostatitis have urinary symptoms, a urinalysis (UA) and urine culture are indicated; often white blood cells (WBCs) and bacteria are present. If the patient has a fever,

WBC count and blood cultures are also indicated. The PSA test may be done to rule out prostate cancer. However, PSA levels are often elevated with prostatic inflammation. Thus it is not considered diagnostic in itself.

Microscopic evaluation and culture of expressed prostate secretion (EPS) is considered useful in the diagnosis of prostatitis. EPS is obtained using a premassage and postmassage test. The patient is asked to void into a specimen cup just before and just after a vigorous prostate massage. Prostatic massage (for EPS) should be avoided if acute bacterial prostatitis is suspected, because compression is extremely painful and can increase the risk of bacteria spread.[30] TRUS has not been particularly useful in the diagnosis of prostatitis. However, transabdominal ultrasound or MRI may be done to rule out an abscess on the prostate.

NURSING and COLLABORATIVE MANAGEMENT
PROSTATITIS

Antibiotics commonly used for acute and chronic bacterial prostatitis include trimethoprim-sulfamethoxazole (Bactrim), ciprofloxacin (Cipro), and floxacin (Floxin). Doxycycline (Vibramycin) or tetracycline may be prescribed for those patients with multiple sex partners. Antibiotics are usually given orally for up to 4 weeks for acute bacterial prostatitis. However, if the patient has high fever or other signs of impending sepsis, hospitalization and intravenous antibiotics are prescribed. Patients with chronic bacterial prostatitis are given oral antibiotic therapy for 4 to 16 weeks. A short course of oral antibiotics is usually prescribed for those with chronic prostatitis/chronic pelvic pain syndrome. However, antibiotic therapy often is ineffective for these patients.

Although patients with acute and chronic bacterial prostatitis tend to experience a great amount of discomfort, the pain resolves as the infection is treated. Pain management for patients with chronic prostatitis/chronic pelvic pain syndrome is more difficult because the pain persists for weeks to months. Antiinflammatory agents are the most common agents used for pain control in prostatitis, but these provide only moderate pain relief. Narcotic pain medications can be used, but because this pain is chronic in nature, the use of narcotics should be approached cautiously.

Acute urinary retention can develop in acute prostatitis requiring bladder drainage with suprapubic catheterization. Passage of a catheter through an inflamed urethra is contraindicated in acute prostatitis. Repetitive prostatic massage is thought to be therapeutic for most types of prostatitis, but it is not an appropriate measure for acute bacterial prostatitis. This measure relieves congestion within the prostate by squeezing out excess prostatic secretions, thus providing pain relief. Prostatic massage is performed by using the index finger of a gloved hand and pressing down on the prostate, covering the entire gland's surface in longitudinal strokes. This is done two to three times a week for 6 weeks.[30] Measures to stimulate ejaculation (masturbation and intercourse) help drain the prostate as well and are encouraged.

Because the prostate can serve as a source of bacteria, fluid intake should be kept at a high level for all patients experiencing prostatitis. Nursing interventions are aimed at encouraging the patient to drink plenty of fluids. This is especially important for those with acute bacterial prostatitis because of the increased fluid needs associated with fever and infection. Management of fever is also an important nursing intervention.

Problems of the Penis

Health problems of the penis are rare if sexually transmitted infectious diseases are excluded (see Chapter 51). Problems of the penis may be classified as congenital, problems of the prepuce, problems with the erectile mechanism, and cancer.

CONGENITAL PROBLEMS

Hypospadias is a urologic abnormality in which the urethral meatus is located on the ventral surface of the penis anywhere from the corona to the perineum. Hormonal influences in utero, environmental factors, and genetic factors are possible causes. Surgical repair of hypospadias may be necessary if it is associated with *chordee* (a painful downward curvature of the penis during erection) or if it prevents intercourse or normal urination. Surgery may also be done for cosmetic reasons or emotional well-being.

Epispadias, an opening of the urethra on the dorsal surface of the penis, is a complex birth defect that is usually associated with other genitourinary tract defects. Corrective surgery to place the urethra in a normal position in the penis is usually done in early childhood.

PROBLEMS OF THE PREPUCE

Problems of the prepuce in the United States are rare because circumcision has been a routine procedure for most male infants for many years. Circumcision, the surgical removal of the foreskin of the penis, is a procedure done to male infants for religious or cultural reasons. It is believed to prevent problems such as *phimosis* (tightness of the foreskin resulting in the inability to retract it), *paraphimosis* (tightness of the foreskin resulting in the inability to pull it forward from a retracted position), and cancer of the penis. A recent trend is that fewer parents are having their infants circumcised, which may result in an increased incidence of problems in the future.

Phimosis is a constriction of the uncircumcised foreskin around the head of the penis, making retraction difficult. It is caused by edema or inflammation of the foreskin, usually associated with poor hygiene techniques that allow bacterial and yeast organisms to become trapped under the foreskin.

Paraphimosis is edema of the retracted uncircumcised foreskin, preventing normal return over the glans. This can occur when the foreskin is pulled back during bathing, use of urinary catheters, or intercourse and is not placed back in the forward position. Antibiotics, warm soaks, and sometimes circumcision or dorsal slit of the prepuce may be required. Careful cleaning followed by replacement of the foreskin generally prevents these problems.

PROBLEMS OF THE ERECTILE MECHANISM

Priapism is a painful erection lasting longer than 6 hours. Causes of priapism include thrombosis of the corpus cavernosal veins, leukemia, sickle cell anemia, diabetes mellitus, degenerative lesions of the spine, neoplasms of the brain or spinal cord, prolonged foreplay, injection of vasoactive medications into the corpus cavernosa, and cocaine use. Treatment may include sedatives, injection of smooth muscle relaxants directly into the penis, aspiration and irrigation of the corpora cavernosa with a large-bore needle, or the surgical creation of a shunt to drain the corpora. Prolonged priapism constitutes a medical emergency. Complications may include penile tissue necrosis caused by lack of blood flow or hydronephrosis from bladder distention. After an episode of priapism, the patient may be unable to achieve a normal erection.

Peyronie's disease, sometimes referred to as curved or crooked penis, is caused by plaque formation in one of the corpora cavernosa of the penis. The palpable, nontender, hard plaque formation is usually found on the posterior surface. It may result from trauma to the penile shaft or may occur spontaneously. The plaque prevents adequate blood flow into the spongy tissue, which results in a curvature during erection. The condition is not dangerous but can result in painful erections, erectile dysfunction, or embarrassment. If conservative measures do not correct the problem, surgery may be necessary.

CANCER OF THE PENIS

Cancer of the penis is rare apart from cancers associated with the STD human papillomavirus (HPV) and in men who were not circumcised as infants.[31] The tumor may appear as a superficial ulceration or a pimple-like nodule. The nontender warty lesion may be mistaken for a venereal wart. The majority of malignancies (95%) are well-differentiated squamous cell carcinomas. Treatment in the early stages is laser removal of the growth. A radical resection of the penis may be done if the cancer has spread. Surgery, radiation, or chemotherapy may be tried depending on the extent of the disease, lymph node involvement, or metastasis.

Problems of the Scrotum and Testes

INFLAMMATORY AND INFECTIOUS PROBLEMS

Skin Problems

The skin of the scrotum is susceptible to a number of common skin diseases. The most common conditions of the scrotal skin are fungal infections, dermatitis (neurodermatitis, contact dermatitis, seborrheic dermatitis), and parasitic infections (scabies, lice). These conditions involve discomfort for the patient but are associated with few, if any, severe complications (see Chapter 23).

Epididymitis

Epididymitis is an inflammatory process of the epididymis (Fig. 53-6), usually secondary to an infectious process (sexually or nonsexually transmitted), trauma, or urinary reflux down the vas deferens. When the problem is associated with prostatitis, it is usually painful. Swelling may progress to the point that the epididymis and testis are indistinguishable. In men younger than 35 years of age, the most common cause is through sexual transmission of either gonorrhea or chlamydia. The use of antibiotics is important for both partners if the transmission is through sexual contact. Patients should be encouraged to refrain from sexual intercourse during the acute phase. If they do engage in intercourse, a condom should be used. Conservative treatment consists of bed rest with elevation of the scrotum, use of ice packs, and analgesics. Ambulation places the scrotum in a dependent position and increases pain. Most tenderness subsides within 1 week, although swelling may last for weeks or months.

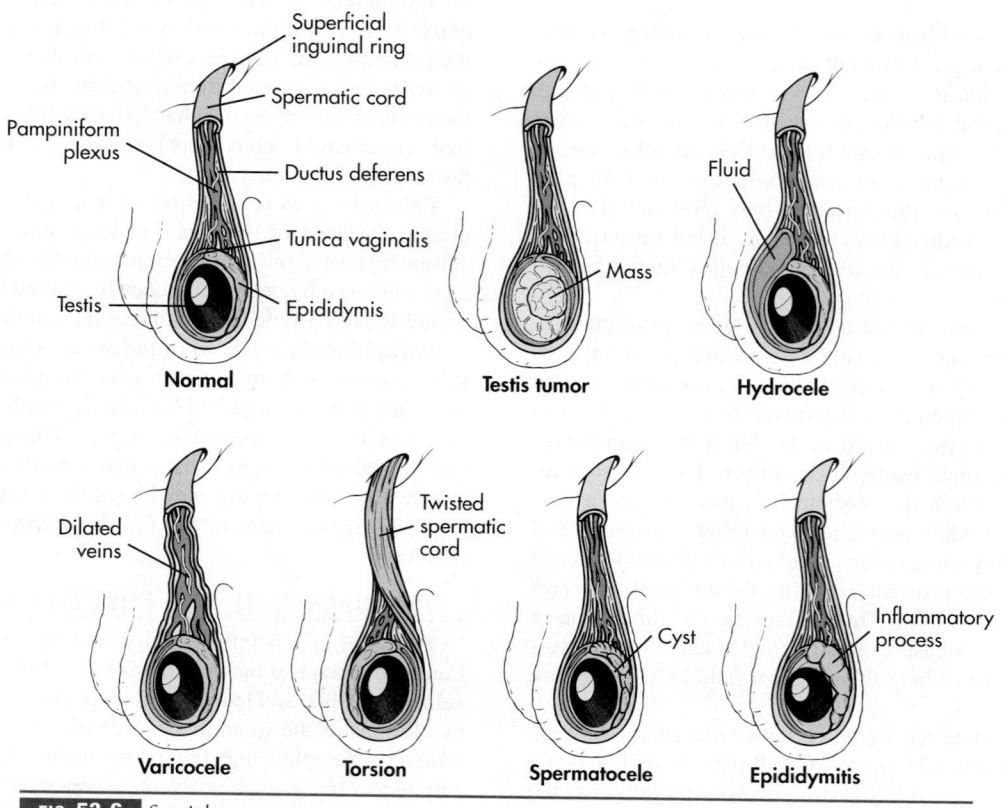

FIG. 53-6 Scrotal masses.

Orchitis

Orchitis refers to an acute inflammation of the testis. In orchitis, the testis is painful, tender, and swollen. It generally occurs after an episode of bacterial or viral infections such as mumps, pneumonia, tuberculosis, or syphilis. It can also be a side effect of epididymitis, prostatectomy, trauma, infectious mononucleosis, influenza, catheterization, or complicated urinary tract infection. Mumps orchitis is a condition contributing to infertility and could easily be decreased by childhood vaccination against mumps. Treatment involves the use of antibiotics (if the organism is known), pain medications, or bed rest with the scrotum elevated on an ice pack.

CONGENITAL PROBLEMS

Cryptorchidism (undescended testes) is failure of the testes to descend into the scrotal sac before birth. It is the most common congenital testicular condition. It may occur bilaterally or unilaterally and may be the cause of infertility if corrective surgery is not done by 2 years of age. The incidence of testicular cancer is also higher if the condition is not corrected before puberty. Surgery is performed to locate and suture the testis or testes to the scrotum.

Absence of the vas deferens is a rare condition associated most often with cystic fibrosis. With the advent of advanced techniques to treat infertility, this defect can be circumvented by aspirating the sperm directly from the testis.

"DES sons" are the male children of women who took diethylstilbestrol (DES) during pregnancy. The effects of DES on males can include undescended or underdeveloped testes, small penis, varicocele, or epididymal cysts. These males also have an increased risk of infertility and testicular cancer.[32]

ACQUIRED PROBLEMS

Hydrocele

A **hydrocele** is a nontender, fluid-filled mass that results from interference with lymphatic drainage of the scrotum and swelling of the tunica vaginalis that surrounds the testis (Figs. 53-6 and 53-7). Diagnosis is fairly simple because the mass can be seen by shining a flashlight through the scrotum (transillumination). No treatment is indicated unless the swelling becomes very large and uncomfortable, in which case aspiration or surgical drainage of the mass is performed.

Spermatocele

A **spermatocele** is a firm, sperm-containing, painless cyst of the epididymis that may be visible with transillumination (see Fig. 53-6). The cause is unknown, and surgical removal is the treatment. It is important for the patient to see his doctor if he feels any scrotal lumps. He would be unable to distinguish this cyst from cancer when performing self-examination.

Varicocele

A **varicocele** is a dilation of the veins that drain the testes (Figs. 53-6 and 53-8). The scrotum feels wormlike when palpated. The cause of the problem is unknown. The varicocele is usually located on the left side of the scrotum as a consequence of retrograde blood flow from the left renal vein. Surgery is indicated if the patient is infertile, because persistent varicoceles are

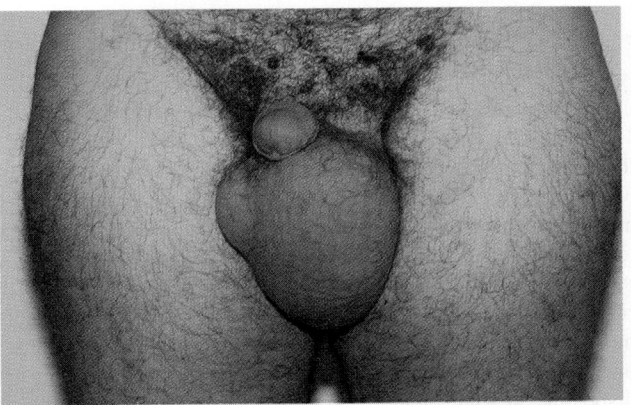

FIG. 53-7 Hydrocele.

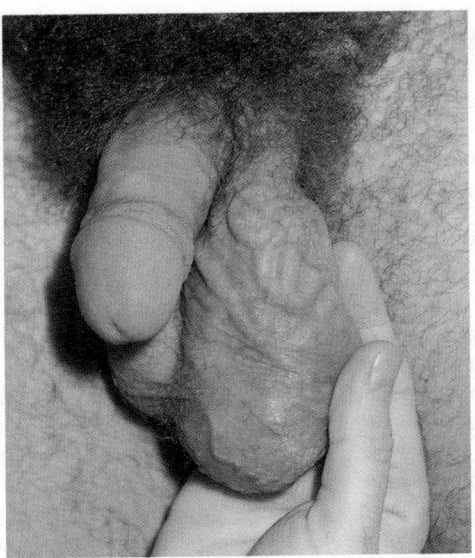

FIG. 53-8 A large varicocele.

associated with 40% to 50% of cases of infertility. Repair of the varicocele may be through injection of a sclerosing agent or by surgical ligation of the spermatic vein.

Testicular Torsion

Testicular torsion involves a twisting of the spermatic cord that supplies blood to the testes and epididymis (see Fig. 53-6). It is most commonly seen in males younger than age 20. The patient experiences severe scrotal pain, tenderness, swelling, nausea, and vomiting. Urinary symptoms, fever, and WBCs or bacteria in the urine are absent. The pain does not usually subside with rest or elevation of the scrotum. Nuclear technetium scan of the testes or Doppler ultrasound is typically performed to assess blood flow within the testicle. A decrease or absence in blood flow confirms the diagnosis.[33] Unless it resolves spontaneously, surgery to untwist the cord and restore the blood supply must be performed immediately. Torsion constitutes a surgical emergency because if the blood supply to the affected testicle is not restored within 4 to 6 hours, ischemia to the testis will occur, leading to necrosis and the possible need for removal.

TESTICULAR CANCER

Etiology and Pathophysiology

Testicular cancer is relatively rare, accounting for less than 1% of all cancers found in males. However, testicular cancer is the most common type of cancer in young men between 15 and 35 years of age. In the United States in 2002, 7500 new cases of and 400 deaths from testicular cancer occurred. The incidence of testicular cancer is four times higher in white males than in African American males, and it occurs more commonly in the right testicle than the left.[31] Testicular tumors are also more common in males who have had undescended testes (cryptorchidism) or a family history of testicular cancer or anomalies. Other predisposing factors include orchitis, human immunodeficiency virus infection, maternal exposure to DES, and testicular cancer in the contralateral testis.

Most testicular cancers develop from embryonic germ cells. The two types of germ cell cancers are seminomas and nonseminomas. Although seminoma germ cell cancers are the most common, they are the least aggressive. Nonseminoma testicular germ cell tumors are rare, but are very aggressive. Non–germ cell tumors arise from other testicular tissue and include Leydig cell and Sertoli cell tumors. These account for less than 10% of testicular cancers.

Clinical Manifestations and Complications

Testicular cancer may have a slow or rapid onset depending on the type of tumor. The patient may notice a lump in his scrotum, as well as scrotal swelling and a feeling of heaviness. The scrotal mass usually is nontender and is very firm. Some patients complain of a dull ache or heavy sensation in the lower abdomen, perianal area, or scrotum. Acute pain is the presenting symptom in about 10% of patients. Manifestations associated with metastasis to other systems are varied and include back pain, cough, dyspnea, hemoptysis, dysphagia (difficulty swallowing), alterations in vision or mental status, papilledema, and seizures.

Diagnostic Studies

Palpation of the scrotal contents is the first step in diagnosing testicular cancer. A cancerous mass is firm and does not transilluminate. Ultrasound of the testes is indicated whenever testicular cancer is suspected (e.g., palpable mass) or when persistent or painful testicular swelling is present. If a testicular neoplasm is suspected, blood is obtained to determine the serum levels of α-fetoprotein (AFP) and human chorionic gonadotropin (hCG). (These tumor markers are discussed in Chapter 15.) A chest x-ray and CT scan of the abdomen and pelvis are done to detect metastasis.

NURSING *and* COLLABORATIVE MANAGEMENT TESTICULAR CANCER

■ Testicular Self-Examination

As with many forms of cancer, the survival of the patient is closely associated with early recognition of the tumor. The scrotum is easily examined, and beginning tumors are usually palpable. Every male at puberty should be taught and encouraged to perform a monthly testicular self-examination for the purpose of detecting testicular tumors or other scrotal abnormalities such as varicoceles. The nurse should teach the patient how to perform

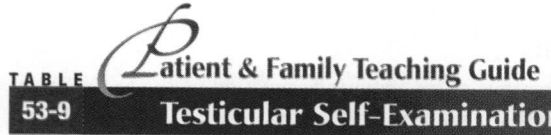

TABLE 53-9 Patient & Family Teaching Guide — Testicular Self-Examination

1. During a shower or bath is the easiest time to examine the testes. Warm temperatures make the testes hang lower in the scrotum (see Fig. 53-9).
2. Use both hands to feel each testis. Roll the testis between the thumb and first three fingers until the entire surface has been covered. Palpate each one separately.
3. Identify the structures. The testis should feel round and smooth, like a hard-boiled egg. Differentiate the testis from the epididymis. The epididymis is not as smooth as the egg-shaped testis. One testis may be larger than the other. Size is not as important as texture. Check for lumps, irregularities, pain in the testes, or a dragging sensation. Locate the spermatic cord, which is usually firm and smooth and goes up toward the groin.
4. Choose a consistent day of the month, such as a birth date, that is easy to remember to examine the testes. The examination can be performed more frequently if desired.
5. Notify the health care provider at once if any abnormalities are found.

self-examination with a particular emphasis on males with a history of an undescended testis or a previous testicular tumor.

The procedure for self-examination is not difficult. The man may indicate some reluctance to examine his own genitals, but with encouragement he can learn this simple procedure. He should be encouraged to perform self-examinations frequently until he is comfortable with the procedure. The scrotum should then be examined once a month. Videotapes and illustrations on shower hangers are available as teaching aids and ideally should be introduced during high school or college physical education classes. Free information is available through the American Cancer Society and on various medical websites.

Guidelines for self-examination of the scrotum are presented in Table 53-9 and Fig. 53-9. The nurse should make this procedure as simple and uncomplicated for the man as possible. The man should choose a technique that is comfortable and consistent for him.

■ Collaborative Care

Collaborative care of testicular cancer generally involves an orchiectomy or a radical orchiectomy (surgical removal of the affected testis, spermatic cord, and regional lymph nodes). Postorchiectomy treatment involves surveillance, radiation therapy, or chemotherapy, depending on the stage of the cancer. Chemotherapy protocols use combination therapy including cisplatin (Platinol), etoposide (VePesid), and/or bleomycin (Blenoxane). (Testicular germ cell tumors are more sensitive to systemic chemotherapy than any other adult solid tumor.)

The prognosis for patients with testicular cancer has improved, and 95% of the patients obtain complete remission if the disease is detected in the early stages. As a result of treatment successes, the majority of men with testicular cancer are long-term survivors and treatment-related toxicity is a significant issue. All patients with testicular cancer, regardless of pathology or stage, require meticulous follow-up and regular physical exami-

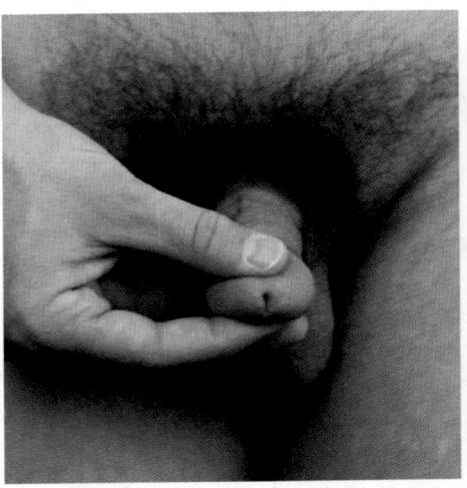
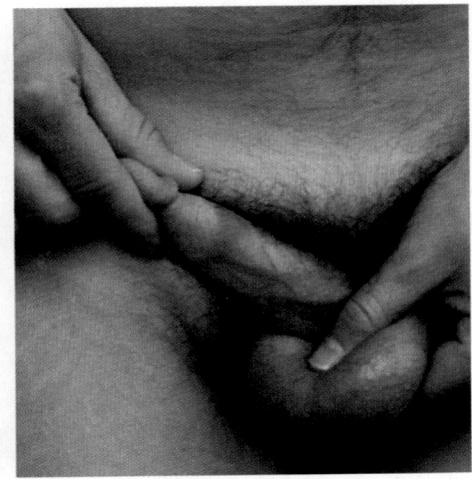

FIG. 53-9 Testicular self-examination.

nations, chest x-rays, CT scans, and assessment of hCG and AFP. The goal is to detect relapse when the tumor burden is minimal. Secondary malignancies that occur as a result of chemotherapy and radiation are described in Chapter 15.

The man with testicular cancer should have the opportunity to discuss fertility and sperm banking before any treatment. The nurse should be sensitive to any psychosocial problems this type of cancer can have on a man's feelings of maleness or self-worth.[34] Treatment has the potential to interfere with both erections and fertility.

Sexual Functioning

VASECTOMY

Vasectomy is the bilateral surgical ligation or resection of the vas deferens performed for the purpose of sterilization (Fig. 53-10). The procedure requires only 15 to 30 minutes and is usually performed with the patient under local anesthesia on an outpatient

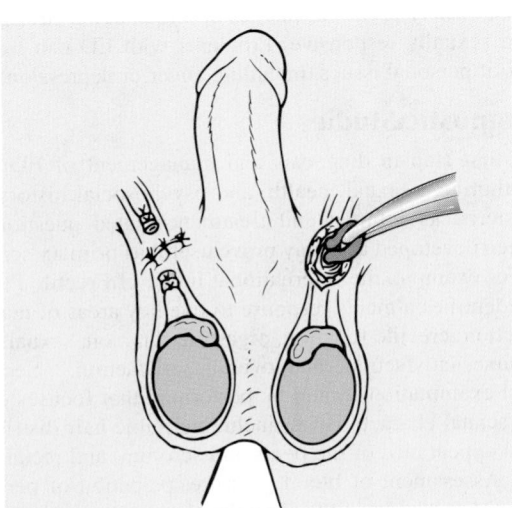

FIG. 53-10 Vasectomy procedure. The vas deferens is ligated or resected for the purpose of sterilization.

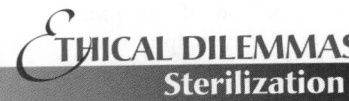

ETHICAL DILEMMAS
Sterilization

Situation

A 43-year-old male patient is requesting a vasectomy and informs the nurse that he does not wish to discuss this with his wife. The physician's policy is to have the spouse or partner sign a form acknowledging the patient's desire to be sterilized. This patient explains that although his wife wants to have more children, the one they already have is all he wants.

Important Points for Consideration

- Patient autonomy suggests that matters of reproduction are left to the privacy and discretion of the individual. Competent adults may legally choose to be sterilized for medical reasons or convenience.
- To prevent possible future harm, this man should include his wife in the decision to permanently eliminate his ability to procreate.
- In most states, women can terminate a pregnancy without proof that their husbands are aware of their intentions. Sterilization, on the other hand, is a more permanent decision that has consequences for both parties in the relationship.
- This physician's standard is to have evidence of the spouse's or significant other's knowledge of the intent for sterilization. This is not a state requirement. The nurse should inform the man of the standard in this particular physician's practice and the benefits to the integrity of his marriage.
- If the patient is still unwilling to discuss the matter with his wife, either the nurse or the physician should inform the man that they will not participate in deception and he is free to select another physician to perform the procedure.

Critical Thinking Questions

1. How would you approach this situation?
2. Should the nurse tell the wife of her husband's plans?
3. Are there ever circumstances in which deception of a patient or family would be justified?

basis. Vasectomy is considered a permanent form of sterilization, although some successful reversals (vasovasotomy) have been reported.

After vasectomy, the patient should not notice any difference in the look or feel of the ejaculate, because its major component is seminal and prostatic fluid. The patient will need to use an alternative form of contraception until semen examination reveals no sperm. This usually requires at least 10 ejaculations or 6 weeks to evacuate sperm distal to the surgical site. Sperm cells continue to be produced by the testes but are absorbed by the body rather than being passed through the vas deferens. Occasionally postoperative hematoma and swelling of the scrotum occur.

Vasectomy does not affect the production of hormones, ability to ejaculate, or physiologic mechanisms related to erection or orgasm. Psychologic adjustment may be a problem after surgery. It may be difficult for the patient to separate vasectomy from castration at a subconscious level. Some men may develop erectile dysfunction or may feel the need to become much more sexually active than they were in the past to prove their masculinity. Careful discussion of the procedure and its outcome before the surgery can be helpful in detecting patients who may have problems with psychologic adjustment. Surgery should be delayed for these patients.

ERECTILE DYSFUNCTION

Erectile dysfunction (ED) is the inability to attain or maintain an erect penis that allows satisfactory sexual performance. Although sexual function is a topic that many individuals are uncomfortable discussing, health care providers must be able and willing to address ED. This topic has been more visible in recent years, partially due to the improvements in treatment with the introduction of sildenafil (Viagra).

The effects of ED potentially interfere with a man's self-esteem, confidence, relationships, and overall sense of well-being. ED is a condition that is significant because of its prevalence; it is estimated that 20 million to 30 million men in the United States experience ED.[35] ED can occur at any age, although the incidence increases with age. In fact, it is estimated that about 50% of all men between ages 40 and 70 have at least some degree of ED.[35] The problem is increasing in all segments of the sexually active male population and affects both the man and his partner. In younger men the increase is attributed to substance abuse, such as recreational drugs and alcohol. Middle-aged men are affected by medical conditions such as diabetes, hypertension, renal disease, organ transplants, coronary artery bypass surgeries, and cancer, or the therapy for these problems. The older population (men over 70 years of age) are living longer, fuller lives and expect to remain sexually active, regardless of any existing medical conditions. Stress factors associated with modern lifestyles are affecting men of all ages and contribute greatly to the overall causes of erectile failure.

Etiology and Pathophysiology

Normal erectile function is a parasympathetic reflex initiated mainly by certain tactile, visual, and mental stimuli. It consists of dilation of the arteries and arterioles of the penis, which in turn fills and distends spaces in its erectile tissue and compresses veins. When this occurs, more blood enters the penis through the dilated arteries than leaves it through the constricted veins. The penis then becomes larger and rigid, or, in other words, erection occurs. Problems occur when these spaces (corporeal bodies) fail to fill when desired or when they empty before orgasm. A functional erection requires not only the desire but also adequate blood supply, nerve innervation, and hormone balance.

ED can result from a number of factors in two general categories: physiologic (organic) and psychogenic. From 80% to 90% of cases of ED are attributed to physiologic causes.[36] *Physiologic ED* can result from a number of etiologic factors (Table 53-10). Common causes include diabetes mellitus, vascular disease, side effects from medications, result of surgery (such as prostatectomy), trauma, chronic illness, and Peyronie's disease. *Psychologic ED* can be caused by a number of issues but is most often associated with stress, difficulty in a relationship, depression, or low self-esteem.

Normal physiologic age-related changes are associated with changes in erectile function and may be an underlying cause of ED for some men. Table 53-11 lists normal age-related changes in sexual performance. Explanation of these age-related changes may be necessary to reassure an anxious older man regarding normal changes in his sexual abilities.

Clinical Manifestations and Complications

A patient's self-report of problems associated with sexual performance is the typical symptom of ED. The patient usually describes an inability to attain or maintain an erection. The symptoms may occur only occasionally, or may be constant with an onset occurring gradually over time, or very rapidly. A gradual onset of symptoms usually is associated with physiologic ED, whereas sudden or rapid onset of symptoms is typically associated with ED caused by psychologic issues.

Although the patient may specifically seek help to alleviate the problem, many men have misconceptions about ED that make them less likely to present this as their chief complaint. More often ED is identified from the history-taking process. This underscores the need for nurses to conduct interviews that address sexuality with men of all ages.

The major complication of ED is that the man's inability to perform sexually can cause great distress in his interpersonal relationships and may interfere with his concept of himself as a man. Our society promotes images of a man being strong, capable, and sexually responsive. Problems with ED can lead to a number of personal issues, including anger or depression.

Diagnostic Studies

The first step in diagnosis and management of ED begins with a thorough sexual, health, and psychosocial history. Self-administered assessment and treatment-related questionnaires have been developed and may prove useful as primary screening tools. For example, the International Index of Erectile Function (IIEF) identifies a man's response to five key areas of male sexual function: erectile function, orgasmic function, sexual desire, intercourse satisfaction, and overall satisfaction.[37] Second, a physical examination should be performed that focuses on secondary sexual characteristics, including pubic hair distribution, size and appearance of the penis and scrotum, and rectal examination. Assessment of blood pressure, palpation of peripheral pulses, and sensation of the genitalia should also be included.

Further examination or diagnostic testing is typically based on findings from the history and physical examination. A serum glu-

TABLE 53-10   Risk Factors for Erectile Dysfunction

Anatomic
Congenital deformities of the penis (e.g., hypospadias)
Peyronie's disease

Cardiorespiratory
Angina pectoris
Atherosclerosis
Emphysema
Hypertension
Myocardial infarction
Post-cardiac surgery

Drug Induced
5α-Reductase inhibitors (finasteride [Proscar])
Alcohol
Antiandrogens
Antilipidemic agents
Antihypertensives
Caffeine
Diuretics (chlorothiazide [Diuril]; spironolactone [Aldactone])
Drugs for Parkinson's disease (carbidopa-levodopa [Sinemet])
Estrogens
Major tranquilizers (diazepam [Valium]; alprazolam [Xanax])
Marijuana, cocaine, LSD
Narcotics
Nicotine
Tricyclic antidepressants (amitriptyline [Elavil])

Endocrine
Addison's disease
Diabetes mellitus
High levels of prolactin
Obesity
Pituitary tumor
Testosterone deficiency
Thyrotoxicosis

Genitourinary
Cystectomy
Hydrocele
Perineal or suprapubic prostatectomy
Phimosis
Post–kidney transplant
Postpriapism
Prostatitis
Renal failure
Varicocele

Neurologic and Nerve Conduction
Central nervous system disorders
Electroshock therapy
Multiple sclerosis
Parkinson's disease
Peripheral neuropathic conditions
Spina bifida
Stroke
Sympathectomy
Trauma to the spinal cord
Tumors or transection of spinal cord

Psychogenic
Depression
Excessive stress in family, work, or interpersonal relationships
Fatigue
Fear of failure to perform

Vascular
Aortic aneurysm
Aortofemoral bypass surgery
Atherosclerosis of pelvic blood vessels

cose and lipid profile is recommended to rule out diabetes mellitus. Hormonal levels for testosterone, prolactin, and thyroid may help identify endocrine-related problems, and other blood chemistries and complete blood count may be helpful in identifying unrecognized systemic diseases.

Other diagnostic tests may be conducted to diagnose ED. Nocturnal penile tumescence and rigidity testing is a noninvasive method that involves the continuous measurement of penile circumference and axial rigidity during sleep. Such measurements are used to differentiate between physiologic or psychogenic causes of ED, as well as to evaluate the effectiveness of drug therapy. Vascular studies including penile arteriography, penile blood flow study, and duplex Doppler ultrasound studies are used to assess penile blood inflow and outflow. Such studies help assess vascular problems interfering with erection.

Collaborative Care

The goal of ED therapy is for the patient and his partner to achieve a satisfactory sexual relationship. The treatment for ED is based on the underlying cause. A step-wise treatment approach with a ranking of treatment options is advocated (Table 53-12).[37]

TABLE 53-11   Effects of Aging on Sexual Performance

- Time lag between perceiving sexual opportunity and full erection
- Diminished size and rigidity of the penis at full erection
- Increased time interval to ejaculation
- Changed nature of ejaculation with less spurting and lessened intensity of feeling
- Shortened period between ejaculation and flaccidity
- Increase in time to next reaction to sexual stimulation

The results of these interventions are usually most satisfactory when both partners are involved in the decision-making process and have realistic expectations of the treatment.

It is important to determine if ED is reversible before treatment is started. For example, if ED appears to be a side effect of prescribed drugs, alternative agents and/or treatments should be explored. When there is an established diagnosis of testicular

TABLE 53-12	**Collaborative Care** **Erectile Dysfunction**

Diagnostic
History and physical examination
Sexual history
Serum glucose and lipid profile
Testosterone, prolactin, and thyroid hormone levels
Nocturnal penile tumescence and rigidity testing
Vascular studies

Collaborative Therapy
Modify reversible causes
First-line interventions
- sildenafil (Viagra), vardenafil (Levitra), tadalafil (Cialis)
- Vacuum constriction device (VCD)
- Sexual therapy
Second-line interventions
- Intraurethral medication pellet
- Intracavernosal self-injection
- Topical gels
Third-line interventions
- Penile implants

failure (hypogonadism), androgen replacement therapy may sometimes be effective in improving erectile function. For individuals who have ED that is psychogenic in nature, counseling for the patient (and possibly his partner) is recommended.[38] This counseling should be carried out by a qualified therapist.

First-Line Interventions

Oral drug therapy. Sildenafil (Viagra), tadalafil (Cialis), and vardenafil (Nuviva) are erectogenic drugs. Because these drugs have been found to be safe and effective for the treatment of most types of ED, they are considered first-line treatment. These drugs cause smooth muscle relaxation and increased arterial inflow with corporal venoocclusion resulting in an erection. They are taken orally about 1 hour before sexual activity, but not more than once a day. Because they potentiate the hypotensive effect of nitrates, they are contraindicated for individuals taking nitrates (such as nitroglycerin). The success of these drugs has had a revolutionary

impact on drug therapy for ED, resulting in an explosive area for further research.[39]

Vacuum constriction device. A second option that is considered a first-line intervention is the vacuum constriction device (VCD). Suction devices applied to the flaccid penis produce an erection by pulling blood up into the corporeal bodies. A penile ring or constrictive band is placed around the base of the penis to retain venous blood, thereby preventing the erection from subsiding (Fig. 53-11). Special care must be taken in using these devices to prevent tissue bruising.

Sexual therapy. Treatment of ED may include sexual therapy. This therapy addresses psychologic or interpersonal factors that may enhance sexual expression, as well as other factors that are of concern. The therapy can be effective for the individual patient, but it is typically preferred to include his partner, particularly if he is involved in a long-term relationship.

Second-Line Interventions. The second-line therapies are indicated for patients for whom first-line interventions fail, or based on patient preference. These interventions include the use of vasoactive drugs administered as topical gel, an injection into the penis (intracavernosal self-injection) (Fig. 53-12, *B*), or insertion of a medication pellet (alprostadil) into the urethra (intraurethral) using a medicated urethral system for erection (MUSE) device (Fig. 53-12, *A*). These vasoactive drugs enhance blood flow into the penile arteries. Current vasoactive medications include papaverine (topical gel or injection), alprostadil

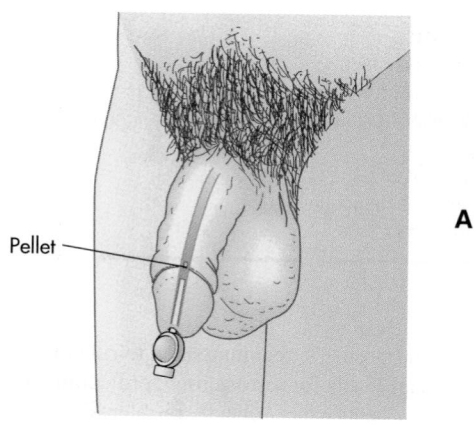

Pellet

A

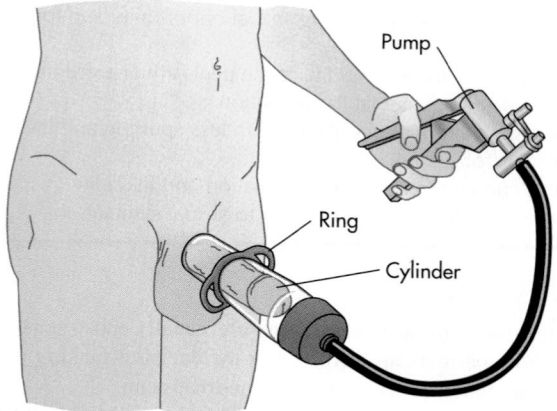

Pump

Ring

Cylinder

FIG. 53-11 Vacuum constriction device. With the vacuum device in place, blood can be drawn into the penis by means of a hand pump. This creates an erection. For intercourse, the ring is slipped to the base of the penis and the cylinder removed.

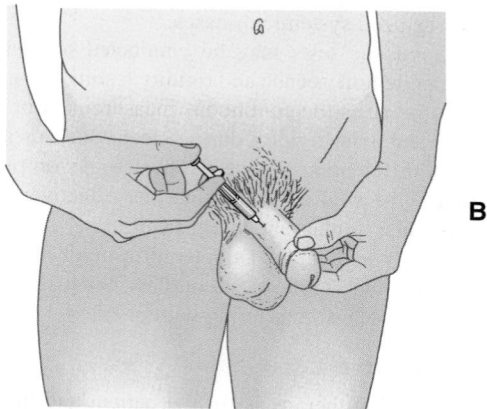

B

FIG. 53-12 A, Intraurethral insertion of medicated pellet (alprostadil) using a medicated urethral system for erection (MUSE) device. B, Intracavernosal self-injection. Self-injection therapy involves injecting a medication directly into the penis. This increases blood flow and causes an erection.

(Caverject) (topical gel, transurethral pellet, or injection), and phentolamine (Vasomax).

The vasoactive medication dose is regulated on an individual basis to prevent side effects. Side effects may include penile pain, priapism, corporal fibrosis, fibrotic nodules, and hypotension. It is important to instruct patients carefully on the specific administration techniques and precautions for any of the vasoactive medications.

Home injection therapy instruction is given to those men who are suitable candidates for the therapy. The injection is nearly painless and generally begins to work in 20 to 30 minutes. Success rates have been high when there is adequate patient teaching and follow-up. This treatment is not suitable for men with severe vascular problems, intolerance for transient hypotension, severe psychiatric disease, poor manual dexterity, or poor vision or those receiving anticoagulant therapy. The man may discontinue treatment if he perceives a lack of spontaneity, has a needle phobia, or wants a more permanent treatment option.

Third-Line Interventions. Surgical implantation of semirigid or inflatable penile prostheses are third-line interventions (Fig. 53-13). These surgical procedures are highly invasive and associated with many potential complications. Thus they are usually indicated for men with severe ED in which first- and second-line interventions are ineffective.

Penile implants have provided surgical management of ED for more than 25 years. The devices are implanted into the corporeal bodies to provide an erection firm enough for penetration. All implants provide a usable erection and should be chosen carefully based on the man's mental and physical capabilities, surgical risk factors, personal lifestyle, insurance, and financial resources.

The semirigid malleable implant is displayed in Fig. 53-13, *A*. The inflatable implant consists of cylinders in the penis, a small pump in the scrotum, and a reservoir in the lower abdomen (Fig. 53-13, *B*). The main problems associated with penile prostheses are mechanical failure, infection, and erosions.

For essentially healthy men the surgical procedure may be performed on an outpatient basis, with patients also being monitored on an outpatient basis. Complete recovery time varies from 4 to 6 weeks. Patients considered to be at high risk for complications include those with uncontrolled diabetes mellitus and those with severe circulatory problems.

Patients should be advised that none of the options will restore ejaculation or tactile sensations if they were absent before treatment. Sexual counseling is often recommended before and after treatment. The ability to please both partners enhances satisfaction levels.

NURSING MANAGEMENT
ERECTILE DYSFUNCTION

The man experiencing ED requires a great deal of emotional support for both himself and his partner. Men often do not feel comfortable discussing their problems with others because of society's expectations of a man's sexual abilities. The man may experience and demonstrate isolation from support systems, and he may also lose self-esteem.

The patient needs reassurance that confidentiality will be maintained. In conjunction with medical treatment, it often becomes necessary to provide counseling and therapy for the couple to establish realistic expectations and develop meaningful communication patterns. The majority of men delay seeking medical assistance. They are often highly motivated and expect immediate solutions to their problems. The health care team should provide a support system and accurate information as soon as possible.

Nurses are in a unique position of conducting routine health assessments on men seeking any form of medical treatment. It provides an opportunity to ask questions pertaining to general health, as well as sexual health and function. Given the opportunity, men will be less hesitant to answer these questions when they know that someone cares and can provide them with answers.

INFERTILITY

Infertility in a couple is defined as the inability to achieve conception despite 1 year of frequent unprotected intercourse. Infertility is a disorder of a couple, not of one individual. For this reason, both partners must be involved in determining the cause of infertility. The primary cause of infertility is due to factors involving the man in about 33% of the cases. Male infertility can

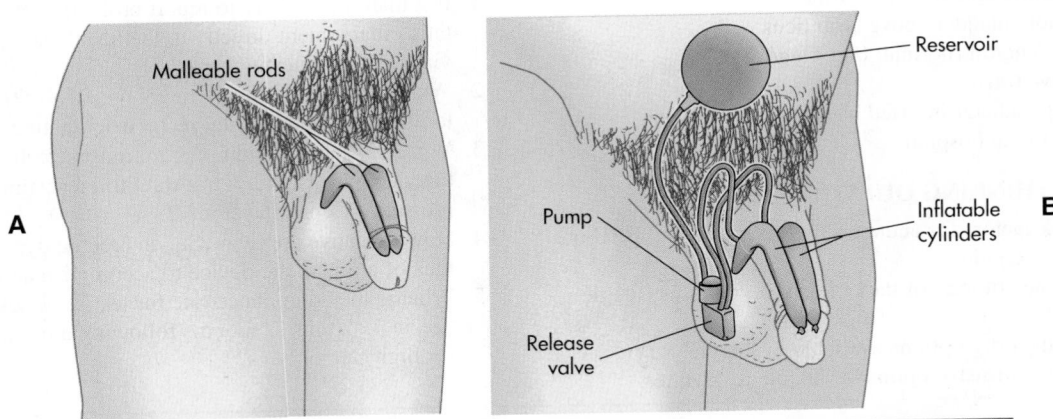

FIG. 53-13 Penile implants. **A,** Malleable implant is always erect but can be bent close to body for concealment. **B,** Inflatable implant consists of cylinders in the penis, a small pump in the scrotum, and a reservoir in the lower abdomen. When activated, the pump fills the cylinders with fluid from the reservoir. A small release valve permits the fluid to drain back into the reservoir after intercourse.

be caused by disorders of the hypothalamic-pituitary system, disorders of the testes, and abnormalities of the ejaculatory system.

The physical causes are generally divided into three categories: pretesticular, testicular, and posttesticular. The pretesticular or endocrine causes occur only in about 3% of the cases and can generally be treated with medication or surgery. Testicular problems make up 50% of the cases. The most common cause of male infertility is a varicocele. Other factors that influence the testes include infection (e.g., mumps virus, STDs, bacterial infections), congenital anomalies, medications, radiation, substance abuse (alcohol, nicotine, drugs), and environmental hazards. Posttesticular causes account for approximately 5% to 7% of the cases, with obstruction, infection, or the result of a surgical procedure being the primary causes. The remaining 40% are classified as *idiopathic,* or of unknown causes.

A careful health history and examination may reveal the cause of a patient's infertility. Thus the history is a starting point for determining cause and treatment. The history should include age; occupation; past injury, surgery, or infections to the genital tract; lifestyle issues such as hot tubs, weight training, or wearing tight undergarments; sexual practices; frequency of intercourse; and emotional factors such as stress levels and the desire for children. The use of drugs, such as chemotherapeutic agents, anabolic steroids (testosterone), sulfasalazine (Azulfidine), cimetidine (Tagamet), and recreational drugs, should be documented because these can reduce sperm count. A physical examination can disclose a varicocele, Peyronie's disease, or other physical abnormalities.

The first test in an infertility study is a semen analysis. The test determines the sperm concentration (count greater than 20 million/ml), forward progressive motility (at least 60% with a grade greater than 2), and morphology (at least 60% have normal oval head and long tail).[40] Additional tests that may be helpful in determining the etiology include plasma testosterone and serum LH and FSH measurements. A test for sperm penetration abilities may also be done. The specific cause of infertility is often not determined.

The nurse should be concerned and tactful in dealing with the male patient undergoing infertility studies. For many men, fertility and masculinity are equated. The nurse must be sensitive to the problem of gender identity in the infertile man.

Treatment options for the man include medications, conservative lifestyle changes (e.g., avoidance of scrotal heat, substance abuse, high stress), in vitro fertilization techniques, and corrective surgery. Achievement of pregnancy varies from 8% to 60% and ranges in cost from several hundred to several thousand dollars. Infertility can seriously strain a marriage, and the couple may require counseling and discussion of alternatives if conception is not achieved. (Female infertility is discussed in Chapter 52.)

CRITICAL THINKING EXERCISES

Case Study
Benign Prostatic Hyperplasia
Patient Profile. Reggie Keller, a 71-year-old African American married man, comes to the emergency department because of an inability to void for the past 12 hours.

Subjective Data
- Complains of severe bladder pain and pressure
- Is very restless and agitated
- Relates history of three cans of beer the previous evening; has not voided since then

Objective Data
- Has prostate enlargement on digital rectal examination
- Has hematuria and WBCs in urine
- Has palpable bladder above umbilicus
- PSA test: 6 ng/ml (normal: 0 to 4 ng/ml)

Collaborative Care
- Indwelling catheter inserted by a urology resident
- Admitted to the hospital

CRITICAL THINKING QUESTIONS
1. What risk factors for acute urinary retention and BPH are present in Reggie?
2. Explain the etiology of the objective symptoms Reggie exhibited.
3. Discuss the drug options available to Reggie.
4. Discuss the invasive options available to Reggie.

5. Reggie asks you about the effect of the various treatment options on his ability to have sex. How would you respond?
6. Write one or more appropriate nursing diagnoses based on the assessment data presented. Are there any collaborative problems?
7. On further assessment, you note that Reggie has a nursing diagnosis of decisional conflict. How would you help him resolve this conflict related to treatment options?

Nursing Research Issues
1. Is a man more likely to report problems related to prostatic enlargement directly to the health care provider or via a printed questionnaire?
2. What is the best strategy to get men over 50 years of age to have an annual digital rectal examination?
3. What relaxation techniques are most effective in relieving bladder spasms after a transurethral resection of the prostate or a prostatectomy?
4. How receptive are men with an erectile dysfunction to the idea of a prosthetic device to accomplish an erection?
5. What is the compliance rate for testicular self-examination at 3, 6, and 12 months following a training program for high school boys?

REVIEW QUESTIONS

The number of the question corresponds to the same-numbered objective at the beginning of the chapter.

1. A patient with BPH experiences hesitancy in initiating voiding and a feeling of incomplete bladder emptying. In assessing for complications related to these symptoms, the nurse asks specifically about the presence of
   a. constipation.
   b. dysuria and urgency.
   c. gross blood in the urine.
   d. decreased force of the urinary stream.

2. Postoperatively, a patient who has had a transurethral prostatectomy has continuous bladder irrigation with a three-way Foley with a 30 ml balloon and traction applied. The patient complains that he feels the urge to void even with the catheter in place. The nurse should
   a. hand-irrigate the catheter to ensure that it is patent.
   b. deflate the catheter balloon to 10 ml to decrease bulk in the bladder.
   c. encourage the patient to try to have a bowel movement to relieve colon pressure.
   d. explain that this feeling is normal and that he should not try to urinate around the catheter.

3. In teaching health promotion related to early detection of prostate cancer, the nurse advises that beginning at middle age men should have an annual
   a. urinalysis.
   b. prostatic ultrasound.
   c. digital rectal examination.
   d. prostatic acid phosphatase (PAP).

4. A patient scheduled for a prostatectomy for prostate cancer expresses the fear that he will be impotent. In responding to the patient, the nurse must keep in mind that
   a. impotence is a possibility even with a nerve-sparing procedure.
   b. the most common complication of this surgery is postoperative urinary retention.
   c. pain control will be a more important factor than sexual function or the long-term consideration of his condition.
   d. a penile implant is the best method to treat erectile dysfunction and should be considered after he has recovered from his surgery.

5. The nurse advises the patient with chronic prostatitis that management includes
   a. a permanent indwelling catheter.
   b. regular injection of sclerosing agents.
   c. sexual activities that result in ejaculation.
   d. aspiration or surgical drainage of abscesses.

6. Discharge teaching for the patient who has had a vasectomy includes explaining that
   a. the procedure blocks the production of sperm.
   b. the ejaculate will be about half the volume it was before the procedure.
   c. an alternative form of contraception will be necessary for 6 to 8 weeks.
   d. erectile dysfunction is temporary and will return with continued sexual activity.

7. A nursing measure that can decrease the patient's discomfort over care involving his reproductive organs includes
   a. relating his sexual concerns to his sexual partner.
   b. arranging to have only male nurses care for the patient.
   c. maintaining a nonjudgmental attitude toward his sexual practices.
   d. using only technical terminology when discussing reproductive function.

REFERENCES

1. Partin AW: Benign prostatic hyperplasia. In Lepor H, editor: *Prostatic diseases,* Philadelphia, 2000, WB Saunders.
2. Barry B et al: The American Urologic Association symptom index for benign prostatic hyperplasia, *J Urol* 148:1549, 1992.
3. Barry MJ, Meigo JB: The natural history of benign prostatic hyperplasia. In Lepor H, editor: *Prostatic diseases,* Philadelphia, 2000, WB Saunders.
4. Hamper UM: Elevated PSA and/or abnormal prostate physical exam. In Bluth EI et al, editors: *Ultrasonography in urology,* New York, 2001, Thieme.
5. Nelson DA, Schumann L. Continuing education forum. Differentiating prostate disorders, *J Am Acad Nurse Pract* 10:415, 1998.
6. Nobel MJ, Mebust WK: Transurethral resection of the prostate. In Resnick MI, Thomson IM, editors: *Advanced therapy of prostate disease,* Hamilton, Ontario, 2000, Decker.
7. DeWildt M, DeLa Rosette J: Transurethral microwave thermotherapy. In Koshiba K et al, editors: *Treatment of benign prostatic hyperplasia,* Toyko, 2000, Springer.
8. Henney JE: Microwave therapy warning, *JAMA* 284:2711, 2000.
9. Schulman CC, Zlotta AR: Transurethral needle ablation of the prostate for treatment of benign prostate hyperplasia. In Resnick MI, Thomson IM, editors: *Advanced therapy of prostate disease,* Hamilton, Ontario, 2000, Decker.
10. Gray M: Urinary retention: management in the acute care setting, *Am J Nurs* 100:36, 2000.
11. Pateman B, Johnson M: Men's lived experiences following transuretheral prostatectomy for benign prostatic hypertrophy, *J Adv Nurs* 31:51, 2000.
12. *Cancer facts and figures,* Atlanta, 2002, American Cancer Society.
13. *Prostate cancer,* Rochester, 2000, Mayo Foundation for Medical Education and Research.
14. Brawley OW, Barnes S: The epidemiology of prostate cancer in the United States, *Semin Oncol Nurs* 17:72, 2001.
15. Kolonel LN, Nomura MNY, Cooney RV: Dietary fat and prostate cancer: current status, *J Natl Cancer Inst* 91:414, 1999.
16. Hayes RB et al: Dietary factors and risk for prostate cancer among blacks and whites in the United States, *Cancer Epidemiol Biomarkers Prev* 8:25, 1999.
17. Hines S: Treating early prostate cancer: difficult decisions abound, *Patient Care for the Nurse Practitioner* 2:18,1999.
18. Marschke PS: The role of surgery in the treatment of prostate cancer, *Semin Oncol Nurs* 17:85, 2001.
19. Moore KN, Estey A: The early postoperative concerns of men after radical prostatectomy, *J Adv Nurs* 29:1121, 1999.
20. Stanford JL et al: Urinary and sexual function after radical prostatectomy for clinically localized prostate cancer, *JAMA* 283:354, 2000.
21. Iwamoto RR, Maher KE: Radiation therapy for prostate cancer, *Semin Oncol Nurs* 17:90, 2001.
22. Abel LJ et al: The role of urinary assessment scores in the nursing management of patients receiving prostate brachytherapy, *Clin J Oncol Nurs* 4:126, 2000.
23. Stempkowski L: Hormonal therapy. In Held-Warmkessel J, editor: *Contemporary issues in prostate cancer: a nursing perspective,* Boston, 2000, Jones & Bartlett.
24. Held-Warmkessel J: Treatment of advanced prostate cancer, *Semin Oncol Nurs* 17:118, 2001.
25. Agho AO, Lewis MA: Correlates of actual and perceived knowledge of prostate cancer among African Americans, *Cancer Nurs* 24:165, 2001.
26. Nivens AS et al: Cues to participation in prostate cancer screening: a theory for practice, *Oncol Nurs Forum* 28:1449, 2001.
27. McDougall GJ: The controversy of prostate screening, *Geriatr Nurs* 21:245, 2000.
28. Ridner SL: Prostatitis: an advanced nursing practice guideline, *Geriatr Nurs* 21:49, 2000.
29. Krieger JN, Nyberg L, Nickel JC: NIH consensus definition and classification of prostatitis, *JAMA* 282:236, 1999.
30. Gleich P: Prostatitis: a state-of-the-art review of diagnosis and therapy, *Consultant* 38:345, 1998.
31. Epperson WJ, Frank WL: Male genital cancers, *Prim Care* 25:459, 1998.
32. McLachlan JA et al: Are estrogens carcinogenic during development of the testes? *AOMIS* 106:240, 1998.
33. Blaivas M, Batts M, Lambert M: Ultrasonographic diagnosis of testicular torsion by emergency physicians, *J Emerg Med* 18:198, 2000.
34. Arai Y et al: Psychosocial aspects in long-term survivors of testicular cancer, *J Urol* 155:574, 1996.
35. Laumann EO, Paik A, Rosen C: Sexual dysfunction in the United States. Prevalence and predictors, *JAMA* 281:537, 1999.
36. Althof S: The patient with erectile dysfunction: psychological issues, *Nurse Pract* 25(suppl):11, 2000.
37. Rosen RC et al: The international index of erectile function (IIEF): a multidimensional scale for assessment of erectile dysfunction, *Urology* 49:822, 1997.
38. Padma-Nathan H, Forrest C: Diagnosis and treatment of erectile dysfunction: the process of care model, *Nurse Pract* 25(suppl):4, 2000.
39. Padma-Nathan H, Giuliano F: Oral pharmacotherapy. In Mulcahy JJ, editor: *Current clinical urology: male sexual function: a guide to clinical management,* Totowa, NJ, 2001, Humana Press.
40. Jequier AM: *Male infertility: a guide for the clinician,* London, 2000, Blackwell Science.

RESOURCES

American Cancer Society
1599 Clifton Road NE
Atlanta, GA 30329-4251
800-ACS-2345
www.cancer.org

American Urological Association
1120 North Charles Street
Baltimore, MD 21201
410-727-1100
Fax: 410-223-4370
www.auanet.org

National Prostate Cancer Coalition
1158 15th Street NW
Washington, DC 20005
888-245-9455 or 202-463-9455
Fax: 202-463-9456
www.4npcc.org

Sexuality Information and Education Council of the United States
130 West 42nd Street, Suite 350
New York, NY 10036-7802
212-819-9770
Fax: 212-819-9776
www.siecus.org

Urologic Oncology Program
University of Michigan Comprehensive Cancer Center
1500 East Medical Center Drive
Ann Arbor, MI 48109-0944
Cancer Information Line: 800-865-1125
www.cancer.med.umich.edu/prostcan/prostcan.html

For additional Internet resources, see the website for this book at *http://evolve.elsevier.com/Lewis/medsurg.*

SECTION *Eleven*

Problems Related to Movement and Coordination

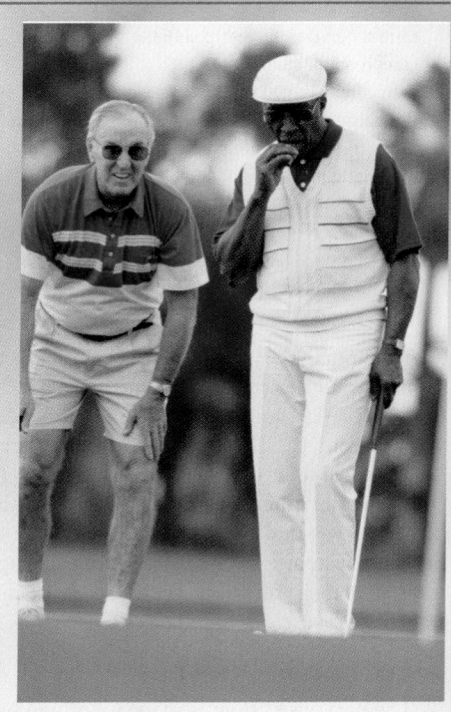

CHAPTER 54

NURSING ASSESSMENT
Nervous System

Judith M. Ozuna

LEARNING OBJECTIVES

1. Describe the functions of neurons and neuroglia.
2. Explain the electrochemical aspects of nerve impulse transmission.
3. Explain the anatomic location and functions of the cerebrum, brainstem, cerebellum, spinal cord, peripheral nerves, and cerebrospinal fluid.
4. Identify the major arteries supplying the brain.
5. Describe the functions of the 12 cranial nerves.
6. Compare the functions of the two divisions of the autonomic nervous system.
7. Describe age-related changes in the neurologic system and differences in assessment findings.
8. Identify the significant subjective and objective data related to the nervous system that should be obtained from a patient.
9. Describe the techniques used in the physical assessment of the nervous system.
10. Differentiate normal from common abnormal findings of a physical assessment of the nervous system.
11. Describe the purpose, significance of results, and nursing responsibilities related to diagnostic studies of the nervous system.

KEY TERMS

autonomic nervous system, p. 1473	neuroglia, p. 1464
	neuron, p. 1464
blood-brain barrier, p. 1475	neurotransmitter, p. 1466
central nervous system, p. 1464	peripheral nervous system, p. 1464
cerebrospinal fluid, p. 1470	
cranial nerves, p. 1473	reflex, p. 1468
dermatome, p. 1472	synapse, p. 1466
lower motor neurons, p. 1468	upper motor neurons, p. 1468
meninges, p. 1476	

STRUCTURES AND FUNCTIONS OF THE NERVOUS SYSTEM

The human nervous system is a highly specialized system responsible for the control and integration of the body's many activities. The nervous system can be divided into the central nervous system (CNS) and the peripheral nervous system (PNS). The **central nervous system** consists of the brain and spinal cord. The **peripheral nervous system** consists of the cranial and spinal nerves and the peripheral components of the autonomic nervous system (ANS). Before considering higher-order structures and their functions, cellular elements and nerve impulse transmission are discussed.

Cells of the Nervous System

The nervous system is made up of two types of cells: neurons and neuroglia. Although neuroglial cells are more numerous, they are mainly supportive to the **neuron** (the primary functional unit of the nervous system). Neurons are generally nonmitotic; that is, they do not replicate and cannot replace themselves if they are irreversibly damaged. However, the brain is capable of generating new neurons from stem cells located in certain regions of the brain.[1] Neuroglia are mitotic and can replicate themselves.

Neurons. The neurons of the nervous system come in many different shapes and sizes, but they all share common characteristics: (1) excitability, or the ability to generate a nerve impulse; (2) conductivity, or the ability to transmit the impulse to other portions of the cell; and (3) the ability to influence other neurons, muscle cells, and glandular cells by transmitting nerve impulses to them.

A typical neuron consists of a cell body, an axon, and several dendrites (Fig. 54-1). The cell body containing the nucleus and cytoplasm is the metabolic center of the neuron. Dendrites are short processes extending from the cell body. They receive nerve impulses from the axons of other neurons and conduct impulses toward the cell body. The nerve axon projects varying distances from the cell body, ranging from several micrometers to more than a meter. Its function is to carry nerve impulses to other neurons or to end organs. The end organs are smooth and striated muscles and glands. Axons may be myelinated or unmyelinated. Many axons present in the CNS and the PNS are covered by a segmentally interrupted myelin sheath composed of a white, lipid substance that acts as an insulator for the conduction of impulses. Generally, the smaller fibers are unmyelinated.

Neuroglia. Neuroglia, or glial cells, provide support, nourishment, and protection to neurons. They constitute almost half the brain and spinal cord mass and are 5 to 10 times more numerous than neurons. Different types of glial cells, including oligodendrocytes, astrocytes, ependymal cells, and microglia, have specific functions. *Oligodendrocytes* are specialized cells that produce the myelin sheath of nerve fibers in the CNS (Schwann cells myelinate the nerve fibers in the periphery) and are primarily found in the white matter of the CNS.

Astrocytes provide structural support to neurons and their delicate processes, form the blood-brain barrier with the endothelium of the blood vessels, and play a role in synaptic transmission (conduction of impulses between neurons). They are found primarily in gray matter. When the brain is injured, astrocytes act

---

Reviewed by Mary S. Baird, RN, MN, CNRN, ARNP, Nurse Practitioner, Northwest Neuromuscular Association, Olympia, Wash.

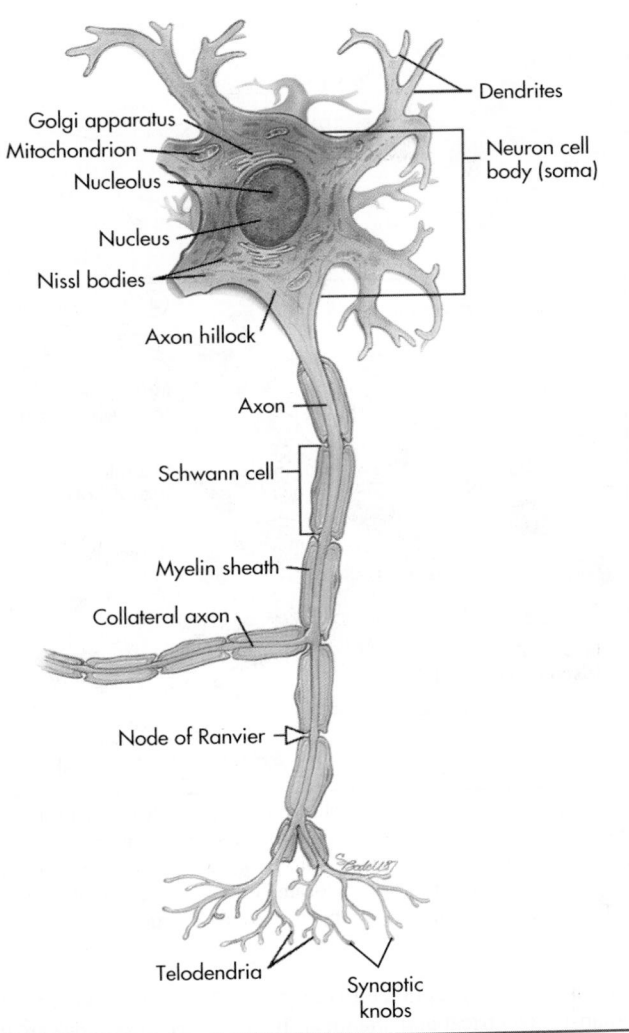

FIG. 54-1   Structural features of neurons: dendrites, cell body, and axons.

Labels on figure:
Golgi apparatus
Mitochondrion
Nucleolus
Nucleus
Nissl bodies
Axon hillock
Axon
Schwann cell
Myelin sheath
Collateral axon
Node of Ranvier
Telodendria
Synaptic knobs
Dendrites
Neuron cell body (soma)

protective myelin sheath of the supporting Schwann cells if the cell body is intact. The final result of nerve regeneration depends on the number of axon sprouts that join with the appropriate Schwann cell columns and reinnervate appropriate end organs.

Nerve Impulse

The purpose of a neuron is to initiate, receive, and process messages about events both within and outside the body. The initiation of a neuronal message (nerve impulse) involves the generation of an action potential. Once an action potential is initiated, a series of action potentials travel along the axon. When the impulse reaches the end of the nerve fiber, it is transmitted across the junction between nerve cells (synapse) by a chemical interaction involving neurotransmitters. This chemical interaction generates another set of action potentials in the next neuron. These events are repeated until the nerve impulse reaches its destination.

Action Potential. When nerve cells are in a resting (nonactive) state, the inside of the cell carries a negative electric charge relative to the outside of the cell. Sodium ions (Na^+) are in high concentration outside the cell, and potassium ions (K^+) are in high concentration inside the cell. The difference in electric charge across the cell membrane is termed the *resting membrane potential* (Fig. 54-2). An action potential occurs when a stimulus is of sufficient magnitude to alter the membrane potential.

During the action potential, the cell membrane becomes more permeable to Na^+, allowing the Na^+ to move readily into the cell. The resulting change in the voltage across the cell membrane is called *depolarization.* The inside of the cell temporarily becomes positive relative to the outside. After rapid depolarization, *repo-*

as phagocytes for neuronal debris. They help restore the neurochemical milieu and provide support for repair. Proliferation of astrocytes contributes to the formation of scar tissue (gliosis) in the CNS. *Ependymal cells* line the brain ventricles and aid in the secretion of cerebrospinal fluid (CSF). *Microglia*, a type of macrophage, are relatively rare in normal CNS tissue. They are phagocytes and are important in host defense.

Most primary CNS tumors involve neuroglia. Primary malignancies involving neurons are rare because these cells are not usually mitotic.

Nerve Regeneration

If the axon of the nerve cell is damaged, the cell attempts to repair itself. When damaged, all nerve cells attempt to grow back to their original destinations by sprouting many branches from the damaged ends of their axons. Unfortunately, axons in the CNS are less successful than peripheral axons in regenerating. This difference may be because of scar formation and lack of trophic factors within the CNS.[2] Regenerating nerve fibers grow 4 mm per day.

In the PNS (outside the brain and the spinal cord), injured nerve fibers can successfully regenerate by growing within the

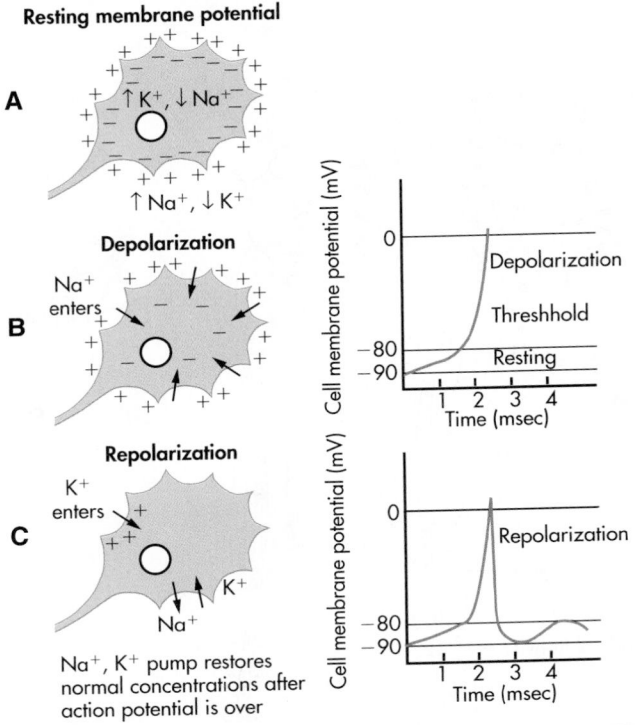

Figure labels:
Resting membrane potential
$\uparrow K^+, \downarrow Na^+$
$\uparrow Na^+, \downarrow K^+$

Depolarization
Na^+ enters

Repolarization
K^+ enters
K^+
Na^+
Na^+, K^+ pump restores normal concentrations after action potential is over

Cell membrane potential (mV)
Depolarization
Threshhold
Resting
Time (msec)
0
−80
−90

Repolarization
Time (msec)
0
−80
−90

FIG. 54-2   **A,** Resting membrane potential. **B,** Depolarization. **C,** Repolarization.

larization (the inside of the cell becoming negative relative to the outside) is facilitated by a slower increase in K⁺ permeability, which in turn is caused by the depolarization associated with entry of Na⁺ into the cell. The whole process of depolarization and repolarization of the nerve cell membrane takes only 1 to 2 milliseconds. With repeated action potentials the cells accumulate Na⁺. An active metabolic process within the cell is required to move Na⁺ out of and K⁺ back into the cell. This metabolic process is accomplished by the Na⁺-K⁺ pump, which requires energy from the breakdown of adenosine triphosphate (ATP).

The action potential has an all-or-none quality; that is, once the cell depolarizes enough to cause an action potential, the size of the action potential is independent of the strength of the stimulus. When an action potential is initiated at one point of a neuron, it is transmitted along the axon without losing its intensity.

Because of its insulating capacity, myelination of nerve axons facilitates the conduction of an action potential. Many peripheral nerve axons have gaps, termed *nodes of Ranvier*, at regular intervals in the myelin sheath surrounding them. An action potential traveling down one of these axons hops from node to node without traversing the insulated membrane segment between nodes, making the action potential travel much faster than it would otherwise. This is called *saltatory* (hopping) conduction. In an unmyelinated fiber the wave of depolarization traverses the entire length of the axon, with each portion of the membrane becoming depolarized in turn. Fig. 54-3 compares nerve impulse transmission of myelinated and unmyelinated fibers.

Synapse. A **synapse** is the structural and functional junction between two neurons. It is the point at which the nerve impulse is transmitted from one neuron to another or from neuron to glands or muscles. The essential structures of synaptic transmission are a presynaptic terminal, a synaptic cleft, and a receptor

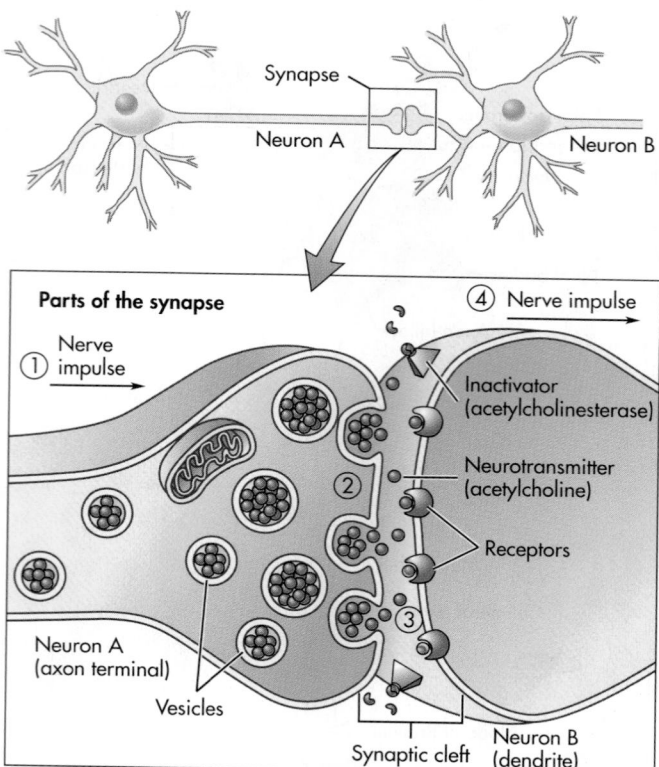

FIG. 54-4   The synapse is located in the space between neuron A and neuron B. Parts of the synapse include the neurotransmitters, inactivators, and receptors. The neurotransmitters are located in the vesicles of neuron A. The inactivators are located on the membrane of neuron B. The receptors are located on the membrane of neuron B.

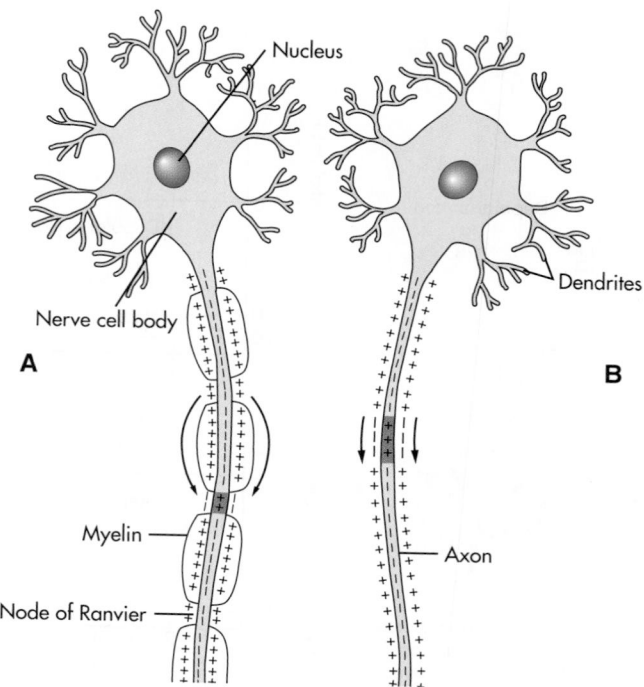

FIG. 54-3   A, Saltatory conduction in a myelinated nerve. B, Depolarization in an unmyelinated fiber.

site on the postsynaptic cell (Fig. 54-4). There are two types of synapses: electrical and chemical. In an electrical synapse an action potential moves from neuron to neuron directly by allowing electrical current to flow between neurons. In a chemical synapse an action potential reaches the end of the axon (presynaptic terminal); then it causes release of a chemical substance (neurotransmitter) from tiny vesicles within the axon terminal. This release depends on influx of calcium, initiated by depolarization of the nerve terminal. The neurotransmitter then crosses the microscopic space (synaptic cleft) between the two neurons and attaches to receptor sites of the receiving (postsynaptic) neuron. This causes a change in the permeability of the postsynaptic cell membrane to specific ions such as Na⁺ and K⁺ and a change in the electric potential of the membrane.

Neurotransmitters. A **neurotransmitter** is a chemical agent involved in the transmission of an impulse across the synaptic cleft. Some neurotransmitters are excitatory: they cause an increase in Na⁺ permeability at the postsynaptic cell membrane, increasing the likelihood that an action potential will be generated. This type of synaptic input results in an excitatory postsynaptic potential. Other neurotransmitters are inhibitory: they cause an increase in permeability of K⁺ and chloride (Cl⁻) ions, decreasing the likelihood that an action potential will be generated. This type of synaptic input results in an inhibitory postsynaptic potential.

Each of the hundreds to thousands of synaptic connections of a single neuron has an influence on that neuron. The net effect of the input is sometimes excitatory and sometimes inhibitory. In general, the net effect depends on the number of presynaptic neurons that are releasing neurotransmitters on the postsynaptic cell. A presynaptic cell that releases an excitatory neurotransmitter does not always cause the postsynaptic cell to depolarize enough to generate an action potential. However, when many presynaptic cells release excitatory neurotransmitters on a single neuron, the sum of their input is enough to generate an action potential. The presynaptic input can be summed by the number of presynaptic cells firing *(spatial summation)* or by the frequency of firing of a single presynaptic cell *(temporal summation).* Summation usually occurs by both events.

The effect of an excitatory or inhibitory neurotransmitter depends on which ion channels in the postsynaptic membrane are influenced by that neurotransmitter. The neurotransmitters that are known to generally have an excitatory influence are acetylcholine, norepinephrine, serotonin, dopamine, glutamate, and histamine. The neurotransmitters that generally have an inhibitory influence are gamma-aminobutyric acid (GABA) and glycine.

Neurotransmitters continue to combine with the receptor sites at the postsynaptic membrane until they are inactivated by enzymes, are taken up by the presynaptic endings, or diffuse away from the synaptic region. In addition, neurotransmitters can be affected by drugs and toxins, which can modify their function or block their attachment to receptor sites on the postsynaptic membrane. Enkephalins and endorphins are also considered neurotransmitters. These substances have opiate-like properties. They are found in multiple areas of the CNS and PNS and act to inhibit pain perception (see Chapter 9).

Central Nervous System

Major structural components of the CNS are the spinal cord and brain. The brain consists of the cerebral hemispheres, cerebellum, and brainstem.

Spinal Cord. The spinal cord is continuous with the brainstem and exits from the cranial cavity through the foramen magnum. A cross section of the spinal cord reveals gray matter that is centrally located in an H shape and is surrounded by white matter (Fig. 54-5). The gray matter contains the cell bodies of

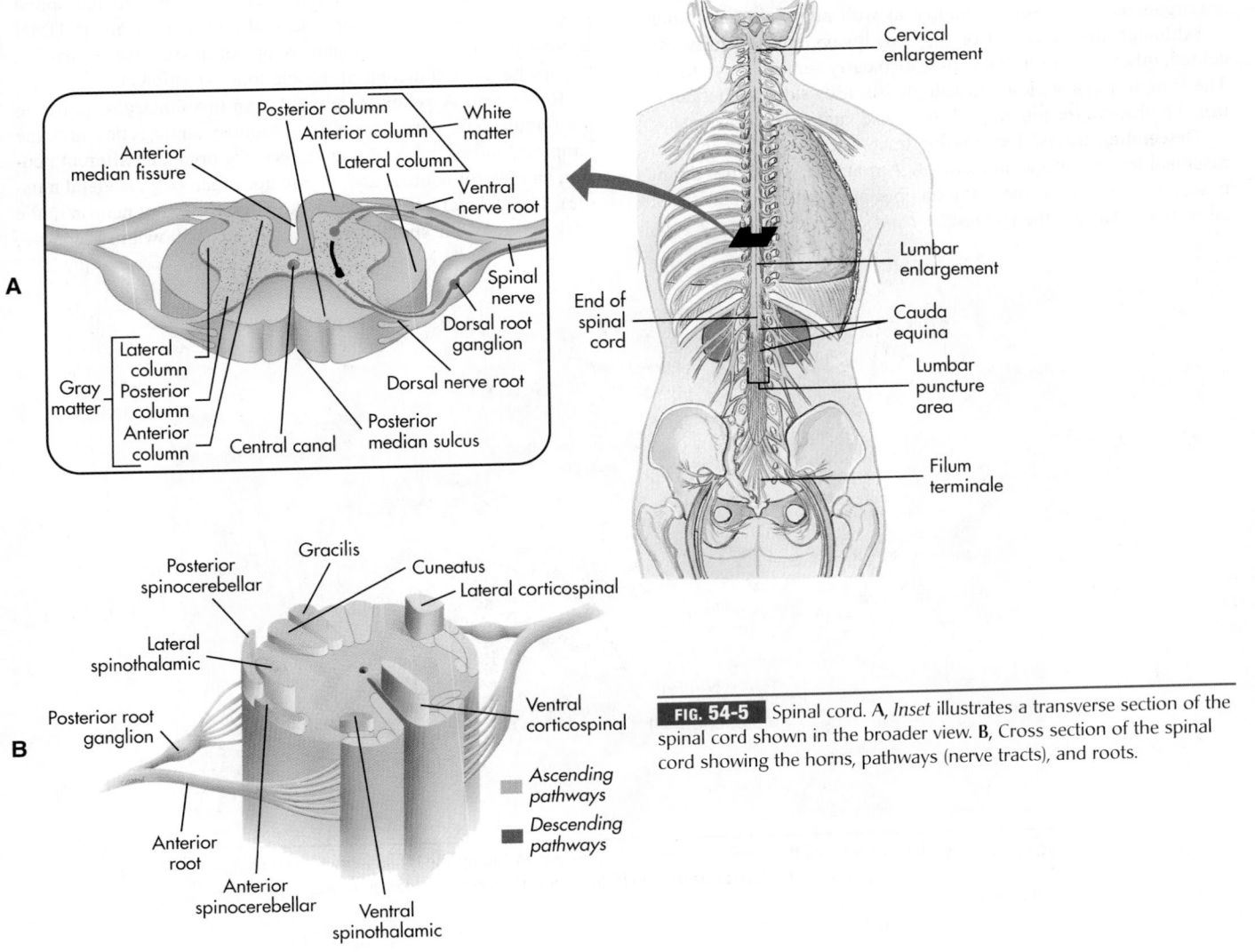

FIG. 54-5 Spinal cord. **A,** *Inset* illustrates a transverse section of the spinal cord shown in the broader view. **B,** Cross section of the spinal cord showing the horns, pathways (nerve tracts), and roots.

voluntary motor neurons and preganglionic autonomic motor neurons, as well as cell bodies of association neurons (interneurons). The white matter contains the axons of the ascending sensory and the descending (suprasegmental) motor fibers. The myelin surrounding these fibers gives them their white appearance. Specific ascending and descending pathways in the white matter can be identified. The spinal pathways or tracts are named for the point of origin and the point of destination (e.g., spinocerebellar tract [ascending], corticospinal tract [descending]). The major spinal pathways are presented in Fig. 54-5.

Ascending tracts. In general, the ascending tracts carry specific sensory information to higher levels of the CNS. This information comes from special sensory endings (receptors) in the skin, muscles and joints, viscera, and blood vessels and enters the spinal cord by way of the dorsal roots of the spinal nerves. The fasciculus gracilis and the fasciculus cuneatus (commonly called the dorsal or posterior columns) carry information and transmit impulses concerned with touch, deep pressure, vibration, position sense, and kinesthesia (appreciation of movement, weight, and body parts). The *spinocerebellar tracts* carry subconscious information about muscle tension and body position to the cerebellum for coordination of movement. This information is not consciously perceived. The *spinothalamic tracts* carry pain and temperature sensations. Therefore the ascending tracts are organized by sensory modality, as well as by anatomy.

Although the functions of these pathways are generally accepted, other ascending tracts may also carry sensory modalities. The symptoms of various neurologic diseases suggest that additional pathways for touch, position sense, and vibration exist.

Descending tracts. Descending tracts carry impulses that are responsible for muscle movement. Among the most important descending tracts are the corticobulbar and corticospinal tracts, collectively termed the *pyramidal tract*. These tracts carry voli-

tional (voluntary) impulses from the cortex to the cranial and peripheral nerves, respectively. Another group of descending motor tracts carries impulses from the extrapyramidal system, which includes all motor systems (except the pyramidal system) concerned with voluntary movement. It includes descending pathways originating in the brainstem, basal ganglia, and cerebellum. The motor output exits the spinal cord by way of the ventral roots of the spinal nerves.

Lower and upper motor neurons. Lower motor neurons (LMNs) are the final common pathway through which descending motor tracts influence skeletal muscle, the effector organ for movement. The cell bodies of LMNs, which send axons to innervate the skeletal muscles of the arms, trunk, and legs, are located in the anterior horn of the corresponding segments of the spinal cord (e.g., cervical segments contain LMNs for the arms). LMNs for skeletal muscles of the eyes, face, mouth, and throat are located in the corresponding segments of the brainstem. These cell bodies and their axons make up the somatic motor components of the cranial nerves. LMN lesions generally cause weakness or paralysis, denervation atrophy, hyporeflexia or areflexia, and decreased muscle tone (flaccidity).

Upper motor neurons (UMNs) originate in the cerebral cortex and project downward. The corticobulbar tract ends in the brainstem, and the corticospinal tract descends into the spinal cord. These neurons influence skeletal muscle movement. UMN lesions generally cause weakness or paralysis, disuse atrophy, hyperreflexia, and increased muscle tone (spasticity).

Reflex arc. A **reflex** is defined as an involuntary response to a stimulus. The components of a monosynaptic reflex arc (the simplest kind of reflex arc) are a receptor organ, an afferent neuron, an effector neuron, and an effector organ (e.g., skeletal muscle). The afferent neuron synapses with the efferent neuron in the gray matter of the spinal cord. A reflex arc is shown in Fig. 54-6.

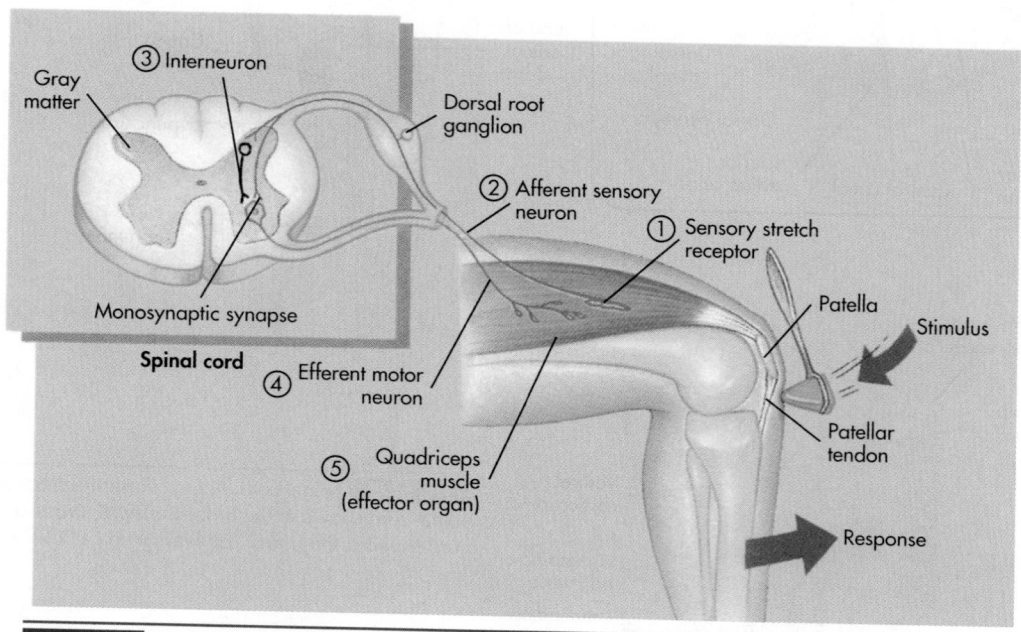

FIG. 54-6   Basic diagram of the patellar "knee-jerk" reflex arc, including the *(1)* sensory stretch receptor, *(2)* afferent sensory neuron, *(3)* interneuron, *(4)* efferent motor neuron, and *(5)* quadriceps muscle (effector organ).

More complex reflex arcs have other neurons (interneurons) in addition to the afferent neuron influencing the effector neuron. In the spinal cord, reflex arcs play an important role in maintaining muscle tone, which is essential for body posture.

Brain. The brain can be divided into three major components: cerebrum, brainstem, and cerebellum.

Cerebrum. The *cerebrum* is composed of the right and left hemispheres. Both hemispheres can be further divided into four major lobes: frontal, temporal, parietal, and occipital (Fig. 54-7). These divisions are useful to delineate portions of the neocortex (gray matter), which makes up the outer layer of the cerebral hemispheres. Neurons in specific parts of the neocortex are essential for various highly complex and sophisticated aspects of mental functioning, such as language, memory, and appreciation of visual-spatial relationships.

The functions of the cerebrum are multiple and complex. Specific areas of the cerebral cortex are associated with specific functions. Table 54-1 summarizes the location and function of the parts of the cerebrum.

The basal ganglia, thalamus, hypothalamus, and limbic system are also located in the cerebrum. The basal ganglia are a group of paired structures located centrally in the cerebrum and midbrain; most of them are on both sides of the thalamus. The function of the basal ganglia is to modulate the initiation, execution, and completion of voluntary movements and automatic movements associated with skeletal muscle activity, such as swinging of the arms while walking, swallowing saliva, and blinking.

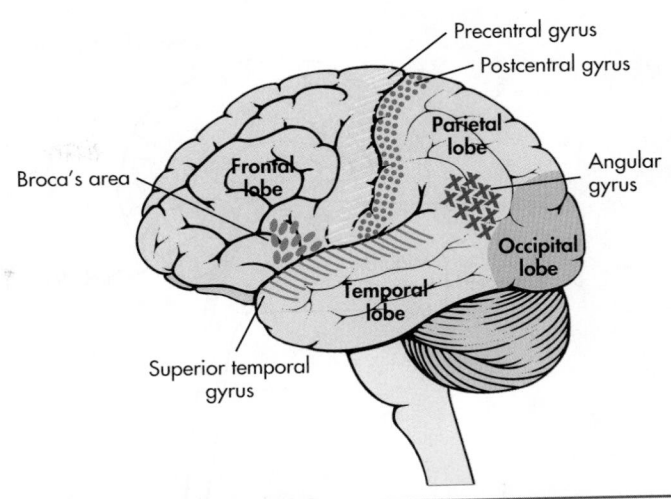

FIG. 54-7 Left hemisphere of cerebrum, lateral surface, showing major lobes and areas of the brain.

The thalamus (part of the diencephalon) lies directly above the brainstem (Fig. 54-8) and is the major relay center for sensory and other afferent (i.e., cerebellar) inputs to the cerebral cortex. The hypothalamus is located just inferior to the thalamus and slightly in front of the midbrain. It regulates the ANS and the endocrine system. The limbic system is, phylogenetically, an old part of the human cerebrum. It is located near the inner surfaces

TABLE 54-1   Location and Function of the Parts of the Cerebrum

PART	LOCATION	FUNCTION
Cortical areas		
Motor		
Primary	Precentral gyrus	Controls initiation of movement on opposite side of body
Supplemental	Anterior to precentral gyrus	Facilitates proximal muscle activity, including activity for stance and gait, and spontaneous movement and coordination
Sensory		
Somatic	Postcentral gyrus	Registers body sensations (e.g., temperature, touch, pressure, pain) from opposite side of body
Visual	Occipital lobe	Registers visual images
Auditory	Superior temporal gyrus	Registers auditory inputs
Association areas	Parietal lobe	Integrates somatic and special sensory inputs
	Posterior temporal lobe	Integrates visual and auditory inputs for language comprehension
	Anterior temporal lobe	Integrates past experiences
	Anterior frontal lobe	Controls higher-order processes (e.g., judgment, insight, reasoning, problem solving, planning)
Language		
Comprehension	Wernicke's area	Integrates auditory language (understanding of spoken words)
Expression	Broca's area	Regulates verbal expression
Basal ganglia	Near lateral ventricles of both cerebral hemispheres	Controls and facilitates learned and automatic movements
Thalamus	Below basal ganglia	Relays sensory and motor inputs to cortex and other parts of cerebrum
Hypothalamus	Below thalamus	Regulates endocrine and autonomic functions (e.g., feeding, sleeping, emotional and sexual responses)
Limbic system	Lateral to hypothalamus	Influences affective (emotional) behavior and basic drives such as feeding and sexual behavior

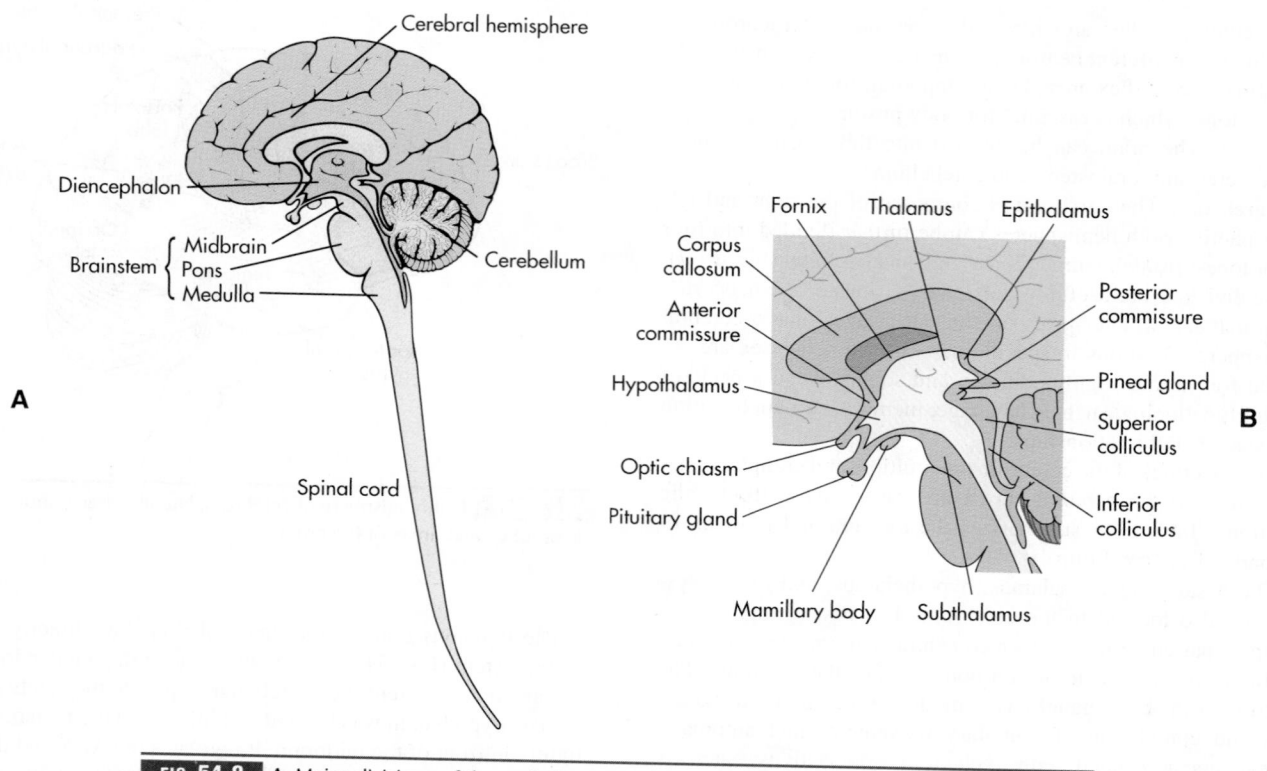

FIG. 54-8   A, Major divisions of the central nervous system (CNS). B, Diencephalon (thalamus and hypothalamus).

of the cerebral hemispheres (Fig. 54-9) and is concerned with emotion, aggression, feeding behavior, and sexual response.

Brainstem. The *brainstem* includes the midbrain, pons, and medulla (see Fig. 54-8). Ascending and descending fibers pass through the brainstem going to and from the cerebrum and cerebellum. The cell bodies, or nuclei, of cranial nerves III through XII are in the brainstem. Also located in the brainstem is the *reticular formation,* a diffusely arranged group of neurons and their axons that extends from the medulla to the thalamus and hypothalamus. The functions of the reticular formation include relaying sensory information, influencing excitatory and inhibitory control of spinal motor neurons, and controlling vasomotor and respiratory activity. The reticular activating system is part of the reticular formation and is the regulatory system for arousal, a component of consciousness.

The vital centers concerned with respiratory, vasomotor, and cardiac function are located in the medulla. The brainstem also contains the centers for sneezing, coughing, hiccupping, vomiting, sucking, and swallowing.

Cerebellum. The cerebellum is located in the posterior part of the cranial fossa, along with the brainstem, under the occipital lobe of the cerebrum. The function of the cerebellum is to coordinate voluntary movement and to maintain trunk stability and equilibrium. It influences motor activity through its axonal connections to the motor cortex, brainstem nuclei, and their descending pathways. To perform these functions, the cerebellum receives information from the cerebral cortex, muscles, joints, and inner ear.

Ventricles and cerebrospinal fluid. Several supporting structures located within the CNS are important in regulating neuronal

function and physical support of the brain. The ventricles are four fluid-filled cavities within the brain that connect with one another and with the spinal canal. The lower portion of the fourth ventricle becomes the central canal in the lower part of the brainstem. The spinal canal is located in the center and extends the full length of the spinal cord. Fig. 54-10 shows the ventricles and the flow of CSF in the CNS.

Cerebrospinal fluid (CSF) circulates within the subarachnoid space that surrounds the brain, brainstem, and spinal cord. This fluid provides cushioning for the brain and spinal cord, allows fluid shifts from the cranial cavity to the spinal cavity, and carries nutrients. The formation of CSF in the choroid plexus in the ventricles involves both passive diffusion and active transport of substances. CSF resembles an ultrafiltrate of blood. Although CSF is continually being formed, many physiologic factors influence its rate of absorption and formation. The ventricles and central canal are normally filled with an average of 135 ml of CSF.

The CSF circulates throughout the ventricles and seeps into the subarachnoid space surrounding the brain and spinal cord. It is absorbed primarily through the *arachnoid villi* (tiny projections into the subarachnoid space), into the intradural venous sinuses, and eventually into the venous system. The analysis of CSF composition provides useful diagnostic information relating to certain nervous system diseases. CSF pressure is sometimes measured in patients with actual or suspected intracranial diseases. Increases in intracranial pressure, indicated by increased CSF pressure, can lead to herniation of the brain and compression of vital brainstem structures. The

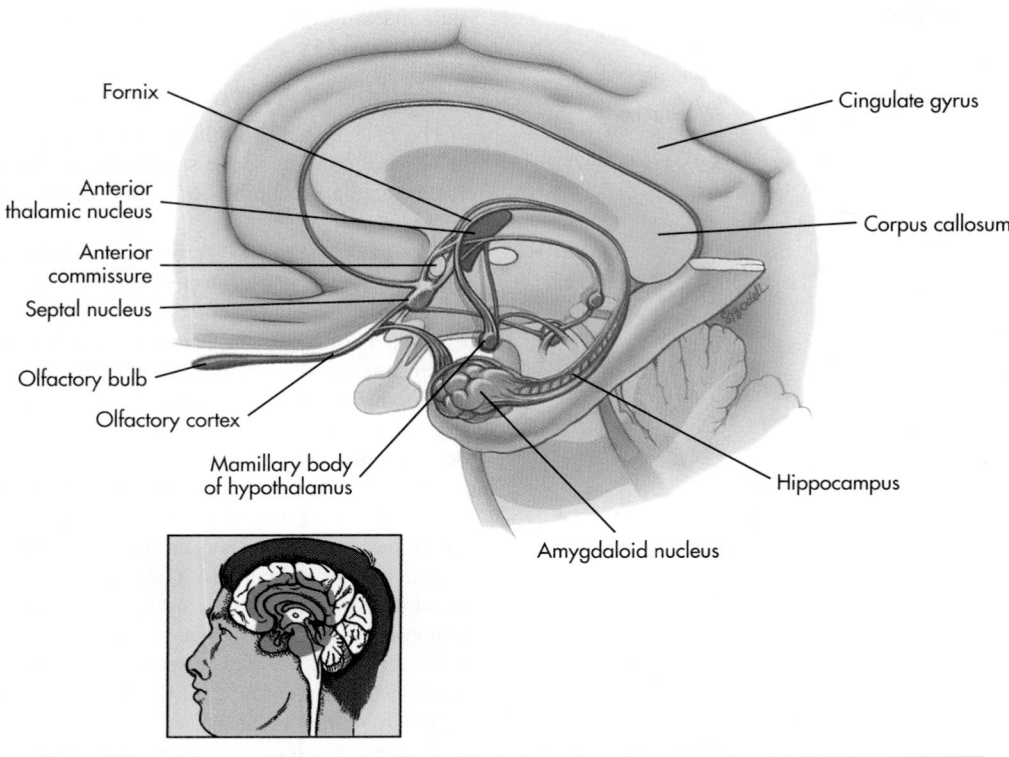

FIG. 54-9 Structures of the limbic system.

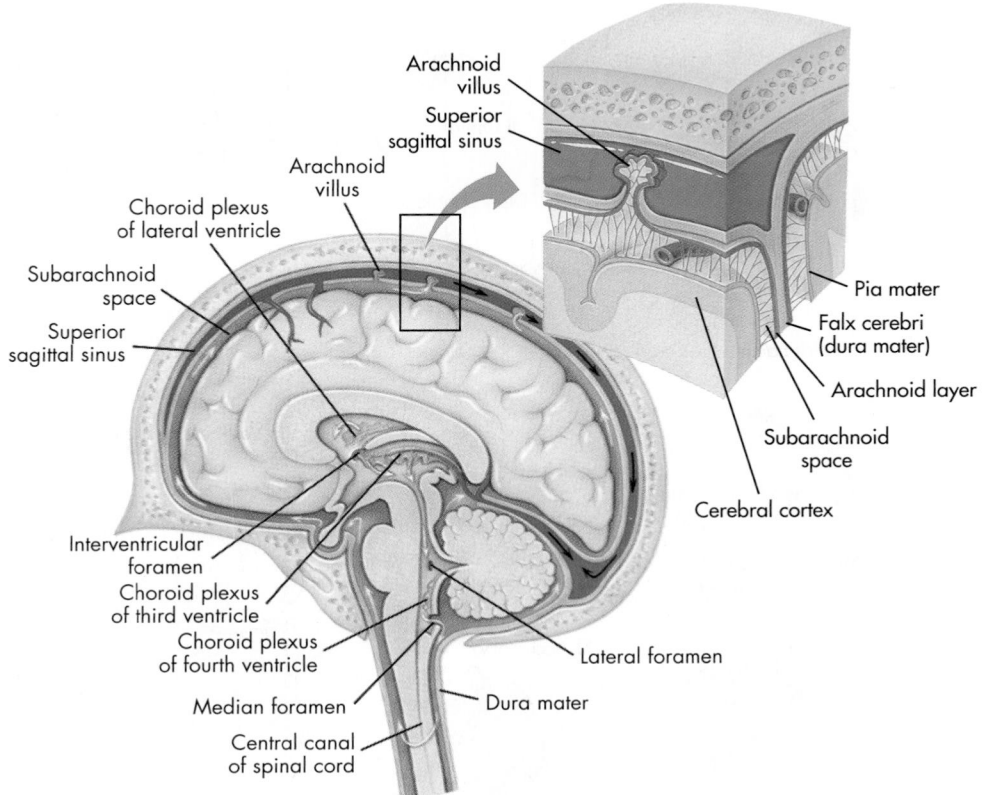

FIG. 54-10 Flow of cerebrospinal fluid (CSF). The fluid produced by filtration of blood by the choroid plexus of each ventricle flows inferiorly through the lateral ventricles, interventricular foramen, third ventricle, cerebral aqueduct, fourth ventricle, and subarachnoid space and to the blood.

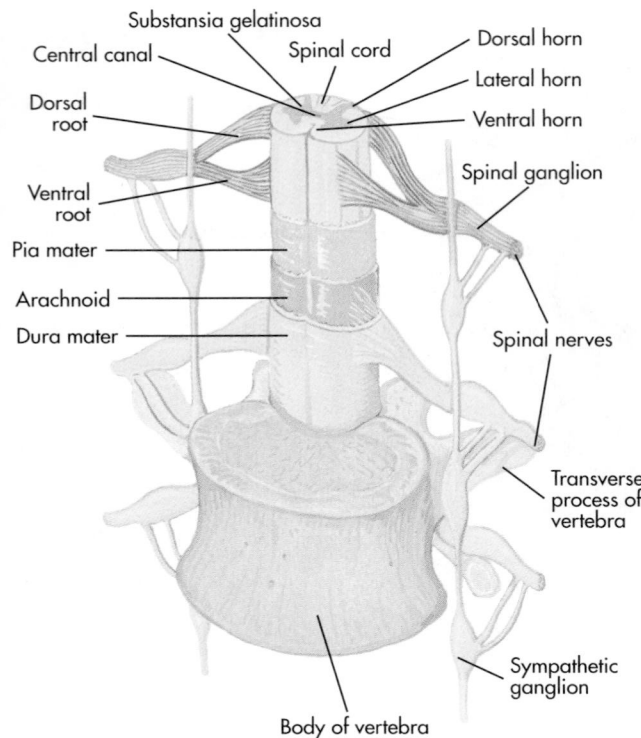

FIG. 54-11 Cross section of spinal cord showing attachments of spinal nerves and coverings of the spinal cord.

signs marking this event are part of the herniation syndrome (see Chapter 55).

Peripheral Nervous System

The PNS includes all the neuronal structures that lie outside the CNS. It consists of the spinal and cranial nerves, their associated ganglia (groupings of cell bodies), and portions of the ANS.

Spinal Nerves. The spinal cord can be seen as a series of spinal segments, one on top of another. In addition to the cell bodies, each segment contains a pair of dorsal (afferent) sensory nerve fibers or roots and ventral (efferent) motor fibers or roots, which innervate a specific region of the neck, trunk, or limbs. This combined motor-sensory nerve is called a *spinal nerve* (Fig. 54-11). The cell bodies of the voluntary motor system are located in the anterior horn of the spinal cord gray matter. The cell bodies of the autonomic (involuntary) motor system are located in the anterolateral portion of spinal cord gray matter. The cell bodies of sensory fibers are located in the dorsal root ganglia just outside the spinal cord. On exiting the spinal column, each spinal nerve divides into ventral and dorsal rami, a collection of motor and sensory fibers that eventually goes to peripheral structures (e.g., skin, muscles, viscera). The sympathetic ganglia are attached to the ventral rami of the spinal nerves by gray and white rami communicantes.

A **dermatome** is the area of skin innervated by the sensory fibers of a single dorsal root of a spinal nerve. The dermatomes

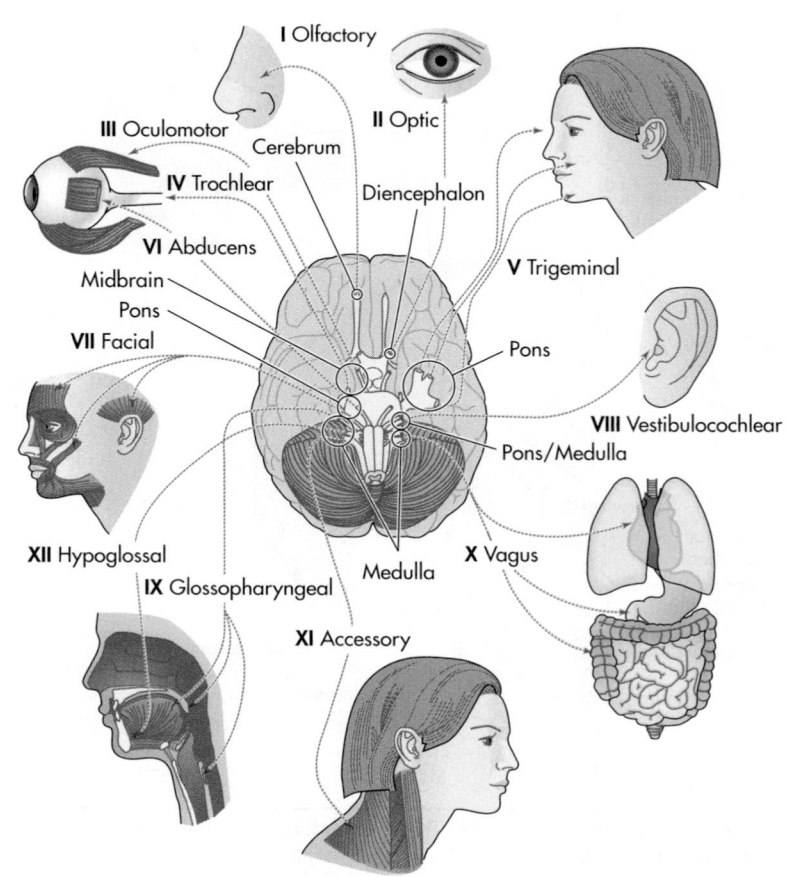

FIG. 54-12 The cranial nerves are numbered according to the order in which they leave the brain.

give a general picture of somatic sensory innervation by spinal segments. A *myotome* is a muscle group innervated by the primary motor neurons of a single ventral root. These are simple components in the embryonic stage of human development. However, the dermatomes and myotomes of a given spinal segment overlap with those of adjacent segments because of the development of ascending and descending collateral branches of nerve fibers.

Cranial Nerves. The **cranial nerves** (CNs) are the 12 paired nerves composed of cell bodies with fibers that exit from the cranial cavity. Unlike the spinal nerves, which always have both afferent sensory and efferent motor fibers, some CNs have only afferent and some only efferent fibers; others have both. Table 54-2 summarizes the motor and sensory components of the CNs. Fig. 54-12 shows the position of the CNs in relation to the brain and spinal cord. Just as the cell bodies of the spinal nerves are located in specific segments of the spinal cord, so are the cell bodies (nuclei) of the CNs located in specific segments of the brain. Exceptions are the nuclei of the olfactory and optic nerves. The primary cell bodies of the olfactory nerve are located in the nasal epithelium, and those of the optic nerve are in the retina. CN XI is a spinal nerve, and its efferent fibers migrate upward before exiting the neuroaxis at the level of the medulla.

Autonomic Nervous System. The **autonomic nervous system** (ANS) governs involuntary functions of cardiac muscle, smooth (involuntary) muscle, and glands.

The ANS is divided into two components, sympathetic and parasympathetic, which are anatomically and functionally different. These two systems function together to maintain a relatively balanced internal environment. The ANS is both an efferent and afferent system. It consists of preganglionic nerves and postganglionic nerves.

The preganglionic cell bodies of the *sympathetic nervous system* (SNS) are located in spinal segments T1 through L2. The sympathetic ganglia, which contain the cell bodies of the postganglionic neurons, lie close to the spinal column, along the vertebral bodies in the rami communicantes. These ganglia and the connecting nerves are called the paravertebral chain. The major neurotransmitter released by the postganglionic fibers of the SNS is norepinephrine, and the neurotransmitter released by the preganglionic fibers is acetylcholine.

In contrast, the preganglionic cell bodies of the *parasympathetic nervous system* (PSNS) are located in the brainstem and in the sacral spinal segments (S2 through S4). The parasympathetic ganglia are located in or near the structures that they innervate. Acetylcholine is the neurotransmitter released at both preganglionic and postganglionic nerve endings.

The ANS provides dual and often reciprocal innervation to many structures. For example, the SNS increases the rate and force of the heart contraction, and the PSNS decreases the rate and force. The SNS dilates bronchi and bronchioles of the lungs, and the PSNS constricts them. Some structures are innervated by only one system (e.g., the hair follicles and the sweat glands,

---

TABLE 54-2   Cranial Nerves

NERVE	CONNECTION WITH BRAIN	FUNCTION
I Olfactory nerves and tract	Anterior ventral cerebrum	*Sensory:* from olfactory epithelium of superior nasal cavity
II Optic nerve	Lateral geniculate body of the thalamus	*Sensory:* from retina of eyes
III Oculomotor nerve	Midbrain	*Motor:* to four eye movement muscles and levator palpebrae Parasympathetic: smooth muscle in eyeball
IV Trochlear nerve	Midbrain	*Motor:* to one eye movement muscle, the superior oblique
V Trigeminal nerve		
Ophthalmic branch	Pons	*Sensory:* from forehead, eye, superior nasal cavity
Maxillary branch	Pons	*Sensory:* from inferior nasal cavity, face, upper teeth, mucosa of superior mouth
Mandibular branch	Pons	*Sensory:* from surfaces of jaw, lower teeth, mucosa of lower mouth, and anterior tongue *Motor:* to muscles of mastication
VI Abducens nerve	Pons	*Motor:* to one eye movement muscle, the lateral rectus
VII Facial nerve	Junction of pons and medulla	*Motor:* to facial muscles of expression and cheek muscle, the buccinator *Sensory:* taste from anterior two thirds of tongue
VIII Vestibulocochlear nerve		
Vestibular branch	Junction of pons and medulla	*Sensory:* from equilibrium sensory organ, the vestibular apparatus
Cochlear branch	Junction of pons and medulla	*Sensory:* from auditory sensory organ, the cochlea
IX Glossopharyngeal nerve	Medulla	*Sensory:* from pharynx and posterior tongue, including taste *Motor:* superior pharyngeal muscles
X Vagus nerve	Medulla	*Sensory:* much of viscera of thorax and abdomen *Motor:* larynx and middle and inferior pharyngeal muscles Parasympathetic: heart, lungs, most of digestive system
XI Accessory nerve	Medulla and superior spinal segments	*Motor:* to several neck muscles, sternocleidomastoid and trapezius
XII Hypoglossal nerve	Medulla	*Motor:* to intrinsic and extrinsic muscles of tongue

| | **TABLE 54-3** | **Effect of Sympathetic and Parasympathetic Nervous Systems** | |

VISCERAL EFFECTOR	EFFECT OF SYMPATHETIC NERVOUS SYSTEM*	EFFECT OF PARASYMPATHETIC NERVOUS SYSTEM†
Heart	Increase in rate and strength of heartbeat (β-receptors)	Decrease in rate and strength of heartbeat
Smooth muscle of blood vessels		
Skin blood vessels	Constriction (α-receptors)	No effect
Skeletal muscle blood vessels	Dilation (β-receptors)	No effect
Coronary blood vessels	Dilation (β-receptors), constriction (α-receptors)	Dilation
Abdominal blood vessels	Constriction (α-receptors)	No effect
Blood vessels of external genitals	Ejaculation (contraction of smooth muscle in male ducts [e.g., epididymis, ductus deferens])	Dilation of blood vessels causing erection in male
Smooth muscle of hollow organs and sphincters		
Bronchi	Dilation (β-receptors)	Constriction
Digestive tract, except sphincters	Decrease in peristalsis (β-receptors)	Increase in peristalsis
Sphincters of digestive tract	Contraction (α-receptors)	Relaxation
Urinary bladder	Relaxation (β-receptors)	Contraction
Urinary sphincters	Contraction (α-receptors)	Relaxation
Eye		
Iris	Contraction of radial muscle, dilation of pupil	Contraction of circular muscle, constriction of pupil
Ciliary	Relaxation, accommodation for far vision	Contraction, accommodation for near vision
Hairs (pilomotor muscles)	Contraction producing goose pimples or piloerection (α-receptors)	No effect
Glands		
Sweat	Increase in sweat (neurotransmitter, acetylcholine)	No effect
Digestive (e.g., salivary, gastric)	Decrease in secretion of saliva; not known for others	Increase in secretion of saliva and gastric HCl acid
Pancreas, including islets	Decrease in secretion	Increase in secretion of pancreatic juice and insulin
Liver	Increase in glycogenolysis (β-receptors), increase in blood glucose level	No effect
Adrenal medulla‡	Increase in epinephrine secretion	No effect

Modified from Thibodeau GA, Patton KT: *Anatomy and physiology,* ed 5, St Louis, 2003, Mosby.
*Neurotransmitter is norepinephrine unless otherwise stated.
†Neurotransmitter is acetylcholine unless otherwise stated.
‡Sympathetic preganglionic axons terminate in contact with secreting cells of the adrenal medulla. Thus the adrenal medulla functions as a "giant sympathetic postganglionic neuron."

which are innervated only by the SNS). Table 54-3 compares the SNS and PSNS.

The result of SNS stimulation is activation of mechanisms required for the "fight or flight" response that occurs throughout the body. In contrast, the PSNS is geared to act in localized and discrete regions. It serves to conserve and restore the energy stores of the body.

Cerebral Circulation

The blood supply of the brain arises from the internal carotid arteries (anterior circulation) and the vertebral arteries (posterior circulation), which are shown in Fig. 54-13. Knowledge of the distribution of the major arteries of the brain and the area supplied is essential for understanding and evaluating the signs and symptoms of cerebrovascular disease and trauma.

Each internal carotid artery supplies the ipsilateral hemisphere, whereas the basilar artery, formed by the junction of the two vertebral arteries, supplies structures within the posterior fossa (cerebellum and brainstem). The *circle of Willis* arises from the basilar artery and the two internal carotid arteries (Fig. 54-14). This vascular circle may act as a safety valve when differential pressures are present in these arteries. It also may function as an anastomotic pathway when occlusion of a major artery on one side of the brain occurs. In general, the two anterior cerebral arteries supply the medial portion of the frontal lobes. The two middle cerebral arteries supply the outer portions of the frontal, parietal, and superior temporal lobes. The two posterior cerebral arteries supply the medial portions of the occipital and inferior temporal lobes. Fig. 54-13 shows the major cerebral arteries. Venous blood drains from the brain through the

FIG. 54-13 Arteries of the head and neck. **A,** Brachiocephalic artery, right common carotid artery, right subclavian artery, and their branches. The major arteries to the head are the common carotid and vertebral arteries. **B,** Inferior view of the brain showing the vertebral, basilar, and internal carotid arteries and their branches.

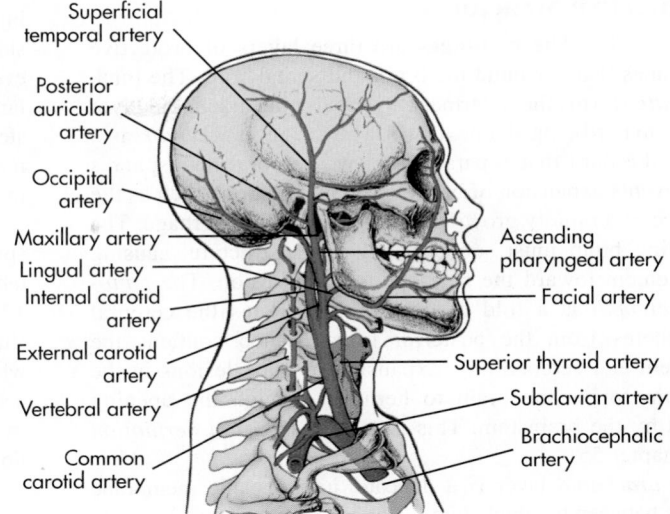

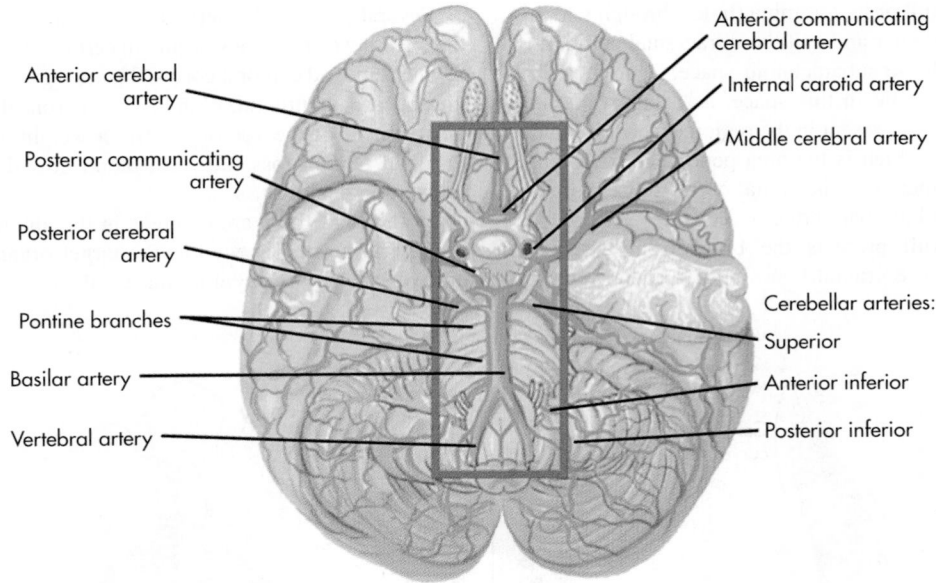

dural sinuses, which form channels that drain into the two jugular veins.

Blood-Brain Barrier. The **blood-brain barrier** is a physiologic barrier between blood capillaries and brain tissue. The structure of brain capillaries differs from that of other capillaries. Some substances that normally pass readily into most tissues are prevented from entering brain tissue. This barrier protects the brain from certain potentially harmful agents, while allowing nutrients and gases to enter. Because the blood-brain barrier affects the penetration of drugs, only certain ones can enter the CNS from the bloodstream. Lipid-soluble compounds enter the brain easily, whereas water-soluble and ionized drugs enter the brain and spinal cord slowly. Damage to the blood-brain barrier results in the penetration of drugs and other substances into brain tissue.

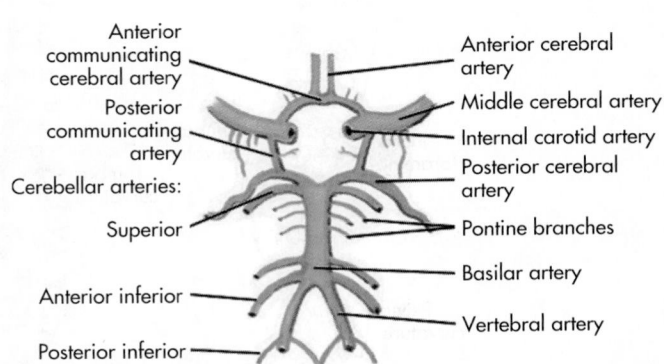

FIG. 54-14 Arteries at the base of the brain. The arteries that compose the circle of Willis are the two anterior cerebral arteries joined to each other by the anterior communicating cerebral artery and to the posterior cerebral arteries by the posterior communicating arteries.

Protective Structures

Meninges. The **meninges** are three layers of protective membranes that surround the brain and spinal cord. The thick *dura mater* forms the outermost layer, with the arachnoid layer and pia mater being the next two layers. The *falx cerebri* is a fold of the dura that separates the two cerebral hemispheres and prevents expansion of brain tissue in situations such as the presence of a rapidly growing tumor or acute hemorrhage. The expanding brain must squeeze under this structure, causing displacement toward the side opposite the lesion. The *tentorium cerebelli* is a fold of dura that separates the cerebral hemispheres from the posterior fossa (which contains the brainstem and cerebellum). Expansion of mass lesions in the cerebrum forces the brain to herniate through the opening created by the brainstem. This is termed *tentorial herniation* (see Chapter 55).

The *arachnoid* layer is a delicate, impermeable membrane that lies between the thick dura mater and the pia mater. The *subarachnoid space* lies between the arachnoid layer and the pia mater. This space is filled with CSF. Structures passing to and from the brain and the skull or its foramina (holes through which blood vessels and nerves enter and exit the intracranial compartment) must pass through the subarachnoid space. Therefore all cerebral arteries and veins lie in this space, as do the CNs. A larger subarachnoid space is present in the region of the third and fourth lumbar vertebrae, which is the area penetrated to obtain CSF during a lumbar puncture. (The spinal cord itself ends between the first and second lumbar vertebrae.)

Skull. The bony skull protects the brain from external trauma. It is composed of 8 cranial bones and 14 facial bones.

The structure of the skull cavity explains the physiology of head injuries (see Chapter 55). Although the top and sides of the inside of the skull are relatively smooth, the bottom surface is uneven. It has many ridges, prominences, and foramina. The largest hole is the foramen magnum, through which the brainstem extends to the spinal cord. This foramen offers the only major space for the expansion of brain contents when increased intracranial pressure occurs.

Vertebral Column. The vertebral column protects the spinal cord, supports the head, and provides flexibility. The vertebral column is made up of 33 individual vertebrae: 7 cervical, 12 thoracic, 5 lumbar, 5 sacral (fused into one), and 4 coccygeal (fused into one). Each vertebra has a central opening through which the spinal cord passes. The vertebrae are held together by a series of ligaments. Intervertebral disks occupy the spaces between vertebrae. Fig. 54-15 shows the vertebral column in relation to the trunk.

■ Gerontologic Considerations: Effects of Aging on the Nervous System

Several parts of the nervous system are affected by aging. In the CNS, loss of neurons occurs in certain areas of the brainstem, cerebellum, and cerebral cortex. This is a gradual process that begins in early adulthood. With loss of neurons there is widening or enlargement of the ventricles. Brain weight also decreases as a result of neuron loss. Cerebral blood flow decreases, and CSF production declines.

In the PNS there are changes in the anterior horn cells and peripheral nerves, as well as the target organ, muscle. Degenerative changes in myelin cause a decrease in nerve conduc-

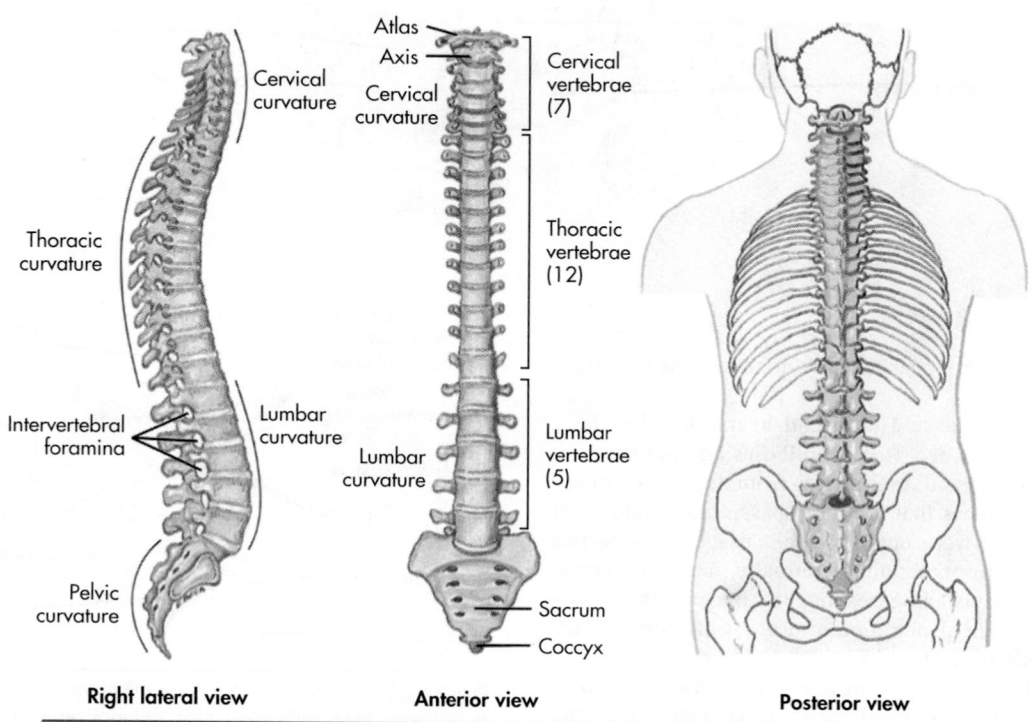

Right lateral view   Anterior view   Posterior view

FIG. 54-15 Vertebral column (three views).

tion. Coordinated neuromuscular activity, such as the maintenance of blood pressure in response to changing from a lying to a standing position, is altered with aging. As a result, older adults are more vulnerable to problems with orthostatic hypotension. Similarly, coordination of neuromuscular activity to maintain body temperature is also less efficient with aging. Older adults are less able to adapt to extremes in environmental temperature and are more vulnerable to both hypothermia and hyperthermia.

Additional relevant changes associated with aging include decreases in memory, vision, hearing, taste, smell, vibration and position sense, muscle strength, and reaction time.[3] Sensory changes including decreases in taste and smell perception may result in decreased dietary intake in the older adult. Reduced hearing and vision can result in perceptual confusion. Problems with balance and coordination can put the older adult at risk for falls and subsequent fractures.

Changes in assessment findings result from age-related alterations in the various components of the nervous system. Age-related changes in the nervous system and differences in assessment findings are presented in Table 54-4. ■

ASSESSMENT OF THE NERVOUS SYSTEM

Subjective Data

Important Health Information

Past health history. Three points should be considered in taking the history of a patient with neurologic problems. First, avoid suggesting certain symptoms to the patient or asking leading questions such as, "Is your headache throbbing?" or

---

TABLE 54-4　Gerontologic Differences in Assessment　Nervous System

COMPONENT	CHANGES	DIFFERENCES IN ASSESSMENT FINDINGS
Central Nervous System		
Brain	Reduction in cerebral blood flow and metabolism	Alterations in selected mental functioning
	Decrease in efficiency of temperature-regulating mechanism	Decrease in body temperature, impairment of ability to adapt to environmental temperature
	Decrease in neurotransmitter content, disruption in integration as result of loss of neurons	Repetitive movements, tremors
	Decrease in oxygen supply, changes in basal ganglia caused by vascular changes	Changes in gait and ambulation (e.g., extrapyramidal, Parkinson-like gait); diminished kinesthetic sense
Peripheral Nervous System		
Cranial and spinal nerves	Loss of myelin and decrease in conduction time in some nerves	Decrease in reaction time in specific nerves
	Cellular degeneration, death of neurons	Decrease in speed and intensity of neuronal reflexes
Functional Divisions		
Motor	Decrease in muscle bulk	Diminished strength and agility
	Decrease in electrical activity	Decrease in reactions and movement time
Sensory*	Decrease in sensory receptors caused by degenerative changes and involution of fine corpuscles of nerve endings	Diminished sense of touch; inability to localize stimuli; decrease in appreciation of touch, temperature, and peripheral vibrations
	Decrease in electrical activity	Slowing of or alteration in sensory reception
	Atrophy of taste buds	Signs of malnutrition, weight loss
	Degeneration and loss of fibers in olfactory bulb	Diminished sense of smell
	Degenerative changes in nerve cells in vestibular system of inner ear, cerebellum, and proprioceptive pathways in nervous system	Poor ability to maintain balance, widened gait
Reflexes	Possible decrease in deep tendon reflexes	Below-average reflex score
	Decrease in sensory conduction velocity as result of myelin sheath degeneration	Sluggish reflexes, slowing of reaction time
Reticular Formation		
Reticular activating system	Modification of hypothalamic function, reduction in stage IV sleep	Increase in frequency of spontaneous awakening together with tiredness, interrupted sleep, insomnia
Autonomic Nervous System		
SNS and PSNS	Morphologic features of ganglia, slowing of ANS responses	Orthostatic hypotension, systolic hypertension

*Specific changes related to the eye are in Table 20-1 and specific changes related to the ear are in Table 20-7.
ANS, Autonomic nervous system; *PSNS,* parasympathetic nervous system; *SNS,* sympathetic nervous system.

"Are you weak on the right side?" It is better to ask open-ended questions such as, "What is your headache like?" or "Is there anything about your right side that bothers you?" Second, the mode of onset and the course of the illness are especially important aspects of the history. Often the nature of a neurologic disease process can be described by these facts alone, and the nurse should obtain all pertinent data in the history of the present illness, especially data related to the characteristics and progression of the symptoms. Third, because many neurologic diseases affect a patient's mental functioning, mental status must be assessed accurately before assuming that the history is factual. If the patient is not considered a reliable historian, obtain the history from a person who has firsthand knowledge of the patient's problems and complaints. Many times a health history cannot be obtained, and the nurse must proceed with only objective data.

The health history helps guide the approach for the neurologic examination; that is, it can direct the health care provider toward the parts of the nervous system that need to be closely assessed. If the patient's primary complaint is dizziness, the examination may be focused on visual, vestibular, and cerebellar functions rather than on somatic motor and sensory functions.

Medications. Special attention should be given to obtaining a careful medication history, especially the use of sedatives, narcotics, tranquilizers, and mood-elevating drugs. Many other drugs can also cause neurologic adverse effects.

Surgery or other treatments. The nurse should inquire about any surgery involving any part of the nervous system, such as the head, spine, or sensory organs. If a patient had surgery, the date, cause, procedure, recovery, and current status should be investigated.

The perinatal history may reveal exposure to toxic agents such as viruses, alcohol, tobacco, drugs, and radiation, which are known to adversely influence the development of the nervous system. The history may reveal a difficult labor and delivery, which can cause brain damage as a result of hypoxia, forceps delivery, or Rh incompatibility.

Growth and developmental history can be important in ascertaining whether nervous system dysfunction was present at an early age. The nurse should specifically inquire about major developmental tasks such as walking and talking. Successes at school or identified problems in an educational setting are other important developmental data to gather. Often this information is not available when the older patient is interviewed.

Functional Health Patterns. Key questions to ask a patient with a neurologic problem are presented in Table 54-5.

Health perception–health management pattern. The nurse should ask about the patient's health practices related to the nervous system, such as avoidance of substance abuse and smoking, maintenance of adequate nutrition, safe participation in physical and recreational activities, use of seat belts and helmets, and control of hypertension. The nurse should ask about previous hospitalizations for neurologic problems. A careful family history may determine whether the neurologic problem has a hereditary or congenital background.

If the patient has an existing neurologic problem, the nurse should ask about how it affects daily living and the ability to carry out self-care. After a careful review of information, the nurse should ask someone who knows the patient well whether any mental or physical changes have been noticed in the patient. The patient with a neurologic problem may not be aware of it or may be unable to provide enough specific data to aid in the diagnosis.[4]

Nutritional-metabolic pattern. Neurologic problems can result in problems of inadequate nutrition. Problems related to chewing, swallowing, facial nerve paralysis, and muscle coordination could make it difficult for the patient to ingest adequate nutrients. Also, certain vitamins such as thiamine (B_1), niacin, and pyridoxine (B_6) are essential for the maintenance and health of the CNS. Deficiencies in one or more of these vitamins could result in such nonspecific complaints as depression, apathy, neuritis, weakness, mental confusion, and irritability.

Elimination pattern. Bowel and bladder problems are often associated with neurologic problems, such as stroke, head injury, spinal cord injury, multiple sclerosis, and dementia. It is important to determine if the bowel or bladder problem was present before or after the neurologic event to plan appropriate interventions. Incontinence of urine and feces and urinary retention are the most common elimination problems associated with a neurologic problem. Careful documentation of the details of the problem, such as number of episodes, accompanying sensations or lack of sensations, and measures to control the problem, is important.

Activity-exercise pattern. Many neurologic disorders can cause problems in the patient's mobility, strength, and coordination. These problems can result in changes in the patient's usual activity and exercise patterns. Falls can also result from such problems. Many aspects of daily living such as getting out of a bed or chair, ambulating, preparing meals, and performing personal hygiene can be affected and should be assessed. The ability to perform fine motor tasks may be affected, which increases the possibility of personal injury.

Sleep-rest pattern. Sleep can be disrupted by many neurologically related factors. Discomfort from pain and inability to move and change to a position of comfort because of muscle weakness and paralysis could interfere with sound sleep. Hallucinations resulting from dementia or drugs can also interrupt sleep. The nurse should carefully document the sleep problem and the patient's methods of dealing with the problem.

Cognitive-perceptual pattern. Because the nervous system controls cognition and sensory integration, many neurologic disorders affect these functions. The nurse should assess memory, language, calculation ability, problem-solving ability, insight, and judgment. Often a structured mental status questionnaire is used to evaluate these functions and provide baseline data.

Information about sensory changes related to hearing, sight, and touch should be sought. In addition, the patient should be questioned about problems with vertigo and sensitivity to heat and cold.

Ability to both use and understand language is a cognitive function that the nurse should also assess. Appropriateness of responses is a useful indicator of cognitive and perceptual ability.

Pain is a common event associated with many health problems. It is often the reason a patient seeks health care. A careful assessment of the patient's pain should be carried out (see Chapter 9).

Neurologic problems and their treatment can be complex and confusing. The patient's understanding and ability to carry out necessary treatments should be determined. Cognitive changes

TABLE 54-5

Health History
Nervous System

Health Perception–Health Management Pattern
- What are your usual daily activities?
- Do you use any recreational drugs?*
- What safety practices do you perform in a car? On a motorcycle? On a bicycle?
- Do you have hypertension? If so, is it controlled?
- Have you ever been hospitalized for a neurologic problem?*
- How does it affect your daily living?

Nutritional–Metabolic Pattern
- Give a 24-hour dietary recall.
- Do you have any problems getting adequate nutrition because of chewing or swallowing difficulties, facial nerve paralysis, or poor muscle coordination?*
- Are you able to feed yourself?

Elimination Pattern
- Do you have incontinence of bowel or bladder? If yes, explain in detail the onset and pattern of the problem.
- What measures have you used to control the incontinence?
- Do you ever experience problems with hesitancy, urgency, retention?*
- Do you postpone defecation?*
- Does a neurologic problem make it difficult to reach a toilet when needed?
- Do you take any medication to manage neurologic problems? If so, what?

Activity-Exercise Pattern
- Describe any problems you experience with usual activities and exercise as a result of a neurologic problem.
- Do you have weakness or lack of coordination caused by a neurologic problem?*
- Does a neurologic problem keep you from performing your personal hygiene needs independently?*

Sleep-Rest Pattern
- Describe any problems you have with sleep.
- If you have trouble falling asleep, what do you do about it? (Ask specifically about use of sleep-inducing drugs.)

Cognitive-Perceptual Pattern
- Have you noticed any changes in your memory?*
- Do you experience vertigo, heat or cold sensitivity, numbness, or tingling?*
- Describe any pain you have experienced during the past 6 months.
- Do you have any difficulty with verbal or written communication?*

Self-Perception–Self-Concept Pattern
- What effect has your neurologic problem had on how you feel about yourself? Your abilities? Your body?
- Describe your general emotional pattern.

Role-Relationship Pattern
- Have you experienced changes in roles such as spouse, parent, or breadwinner because of neurologic disease?*
- How do you feel about these changes?

Sexuality-Reproductive Pattern
- Are you satisfied with sexual functioning? Describe any problems you experience related to your sexuality and sexual functioning.
- Are problems related to sexual functioning causing tension in an important relationship?*
- Do you feel the need for professional counseling related to your sexual functioning?*
- Do you use alternative methods of achieving sexual satisfaction?

Coping–Stress Tolerance Pattern
- Describe your usual coping pattern.
- Do you think your present coping pattern is adequate to meet the stressors of your neurologic problem?*
- Is your support system adequate to meet your needs? If not, what needs are unmet?

Value-Belief Pattern
- Describe any culturally specific beliefs and attitudes that may influence the treatment of this neurologic problem.

*If yes, describe.

associated with the problem can also interfere with understanding and compliance.[5]

Self-perception–self-concept pattern. Neurologic disease can drastically alter control over one's life and create dependency on others for daily needs. Also, the patient's physical appearance and emotional control can be affected. The nurse should ask about the patient's evaluation of self-worth, perception of abilities, body image, and general emotional pattern.

Role-relationship pattern. The patient should be asked if changes in roles, such as spouse, parent, or breadwinner, resulting from a neurologic problem have occurred. Physical impairments such as weakness and paralysis can alter or limit participation in usual roles and activities. Cognitive changes, however, can permanently change a person's ability to maintain previous roles. These changes can dramatically affect both the patient and significant others. Dependent relationships can develop.

Sexuality-reproductive pattern. The ability to participate in sexual activity should be assessed because many nervous system disorders can affect sexual response. Cerebral lesions may inhibit the desire phase or the reflex responses of the excitement phase. Brainstem and spinal cord lesions may partially or completely interrupt the connections between the brain and effector systems necessary for intercourse.

Neuropathies and spinal cord lesions that affect sensation, especially in the erotic zones, may decrease desire. Autonomic neuropathies and lesions of the sacral cord and cauda equina may prevent reflex activities of the sexual response. The nurse should determine if the patient and the spouse or significant other are satisfied with their sexual activity. The use or need for alternative methods of achieving sexual satisfaction should be explored. Despite neurologic-related changes in sexual functioning, many persons can achieve satisfying expression of intimacy and affection.

Coping–stress tolerance pattern. The physical sequelae of a neurologic problem can seriously strain a patient's coping patterns. Often the problem is chronic and may require that the patient learn new coping skills. The nurse should assess the patient's usual coping pattern to determine if coping skills are adequate to meet the stress of a problem.

When the problem is a decrease in cognitive functioning, both the patient and the caregiver can be seriously stressed. The nurse should assess for the potential for suicide, abuse, and burnout. The presence of an adequate support system in this type of situation should be assessed.

Value-belief pattern. Many neurologic problems have serious, long-term, life-changing effects. These effects can strain the patient's belief system and should be assessed. The nurse should also determine if any religious or cultural beliefs could interfere with the planned treatment regimen.

Objective Data

Physical Examination. The standard neurologic examination helps determine the presence, location, and nature of disease of the nervous system. The examination assesses six categories of functions: mental status, function of CNs, motor function, cerebellar function, sensory function, and reflex function. The choice of particular parts of the examination depends on the purpose for which it is done. If a comprehensive baseline assessment of neurologic functioning is desired, all components of the examination are done. However, if a specific problem is to be evaluated, only certain components may be assessed. For example, if a patient's primary complaint is lack of feeling in the feet, the examination may be focused only on movement and sensation of the lower limbs. Similarly, if a patient comes into the emergency department after a head injury and is unconscious, a limited examination is conducted because the patient is not able to respond to verbal instructions.[6]

A different approach to the neurologic examination has been proposed for nursing purposes.[7] The primary purposes of the nursing neurologic examination are to determine the effects of neurologic dysfunction on daily living in relation to the patient's and the family's ability to cope with the neurologic deficits. Although the method of gathering data may be the same, the interpretation of the data differs from the medical model. The standard medical model of the neurologic examination can also be used for nursing purposes. Health care providers share the responsibility for assessing life-threatening neurologic dysfunction.

Mental status. Assessment of mental status (cerebral functioning) gives an indication of how the patient is functioning as a whole and how the patient is adapting to the environment. It involves determination of complex and high-level cerebral functions that are governed by many areas of the cerebral cortex. Much of the area covered in this part of the examination is assessed during the history and therefore does not need to be evaluated further. For example, language and memory can be assessed when the patient is asked for details of the illness and significant past events. The patient's cultural and educational background should be taken into account when evaluating mental status.

The components of the mental status examination are as follows:

- *General appearance and behavior.* This component includes motor activity, body posture, dress and hygiene, facial expression, and speech.
- *State of consciousness.* The patient must be conscious before other functions can be determined. The nurse should note orientation to time, place, person, and situation, as well

as memory, general knowledge, insight, judgment, problem solving, and calculation. Common questions are "Who were the last three presidents?" "What does 'a stitch in time saves nine' mean?" "Subtract 7 from 100, and keep subtracting 7." The nurse should consider whether the patient's plans and goals match the physical and mental capabilities. Problems with memory may have implications for the ability to retain patient education.

- *Mood and affect.* The nurse should note agitation, anger, depression, or euphoria and the appropriateness of these states. Questions should be directed to bring out the feelings of the patient.
- *Thought content.* The nurse should note illusions, hallucinations, delusions, or paranoia.
- *Intellectual capacity.* The nurse should note retardation, dementia, and intelligence.

Cranial nerves. Testing of each CN is an essential component of the neurologic examination (see Table 54-2).

Olfactory nerve. After determining that both nostrils are patent, the olfactory nerve (CN I) is tested by asking the patient to close one nostril, close both eyes, and sniff from a bottle containing coffee, spice, soap, or some other readily recognized odor. The same is done for the other nostril. Generally, olfaction is not tested unless the patient has some disturbance with smell. Chronic rhinitis, sinusitis, and heavy smoking can often decrease the sense of smell. Disturbance in ability to smell may be associated with a tumor involving the olfactory bulb, or it may be the result of a basilar skull fracture that has damaged the olfactory fibers as they pass through the delicate cribriform plate of the skull.

Optic nerve. Visual fields and visual acuity are assessed to test the function of the optic nerve (CN II). Visual fields are assessed by confrontation. The examiner, positioned directly opposite the patient, asks the patient to close one eye, look directly at the bridge of the examiner's nose, and indicate when an object (finger, pencil tip, head of pin) presented from the periphery of each of the four visual field quadrants is seen (Fig. 54-16). The same test is repeated for the other eye. The examiner is used as a control because both examiner and patient are sharing the same visual field. It is important to remember that the nasal side of the visual field is narrower because of the nasal bridge. Visual field defects may arise from lesions of the optic nerve, optic chiasm, or tracts that extend through the temporal, parietal, or occipital lobes. Visual field changes resulting from brain lesions are usually either a *hemianopsia* (one half of the visual field is affected), a *quadrantanopsia* (one fourth of the visual field is affected), or monocular.

Visual acuity is tested by asking the patient to read a Snellen chart from 20 feet away. The number on the lowest line that the patient can read with 50% accuracy is recorded. The patient who wears glasses should wear them during testing, unless they are used only for reading. The eyes should be tested individually and together. If a Snellen chart is not available, the patient should be asked to read newsprint for a gross assessment of acuity. The distance from the patient to the newsprint required for accurate reading should be recorded. Acuity may not be testable by these means if the patient does not read English or is aphasic.

Funduscopy reveals the physical condition of the optic disc (head of the optic nerve), as well as the retina and blood vessels. This procedure is routinely performed when the optic nerve is tested. Optic nerve atrophy and papilledema can be detected by this method.

on the examiner's finger as it moves toward the patient's nose. Another function of the oculomotor nerve is to keep the eyelid open. Damage to the nerve can cause *ptosis* (drooping eyelid), pupillary abnormalities, and eye muscle weakness.

Trigeminal nerve. The sensory component of the trigeminal nerve (CN V) is tested by having the patient identify light touch (cotton) and pinprick in each of the three divisions (ophthalmic, maxillary, and mandibular) of the nerve on both sides of the face. The patient's eyes should be closed during this part of the examination. The motor component is tested by asking the patient to clench the teeth and palpating the masseter muscles just above the mandibular angle. The corneal reflex test evaluates CN V and CN VII simultaneously. It involves applying a cotton wisp strand to the cornea. The sensory component of this reflex (corneal sensation) is innervated by the ophthalmic division of CN V. The motor component (eye blink) is innervated by the facial nerve (CN VII). This reflex is not normally tested in patients who are awake and alert because other tests evaluate these two nerves. However, for patients with a decreased level of consciousness, the corneal reflex test provides an opportunity to evaluate the integrity of the brainstem at the level of the pons because the fibers of CN V and CN VII have connections in this area.

Facial nerve. The facial nerve (CN VII) innervates the muscles of facial expression. Its function is tested by asking the patient to raise the eyebrows, close the eyes tightly, purse the lips, draw back the corners of the mouth in an exaggerated smile, and frown. The examiner should note any asymmetry in the facial movements because they can indicate damage to the facial nerve. Although taste discrimination of salt and sugar in the anterior two thirds of the tongue is a function of this nerve, it is not routinely tested unless a peripheral nerve lesion is suspected.

Acoustic nerve. The cochlear portion of the acoustic (vestibulocochlear) nerve (CN VIII) is tested by having the patient close the eyes and indicate when a ticking watch or the rustling of the examiner's fingertips is heard as the stimulus is brought closer to the ear. Each ear is tested individually, and the distance from the patient's ear to the sound source when first heard is recorded. This test identifies only gross deficits in hearing. For more precise assessment of hearing, an audiometer is used (see Chapter 20). The vestibular portion of this nerve is not routinely tested unless the patient complains of dizziness, vertigo, or unsteadiness or has auditory dysfunction. If this is the case, caloric testing, which is beyond the scope of routine testing, may be done.

Glossopharyngeal and vagus nerves. The glossopharyngeal and vagus nerves are tested together because both innervate the pharynx. The glossopharyngeal nerve (CN IX) is primarily sensory. In the gag reflex (bilateral contraction of the palatal muscles initiated by stroking or touching either side of the posterior pharynx or soft palate with a tongue blade), the sensory component is mediated by CN IX and the major motor component by the vagus nerve (CN X). It is important to assess the gag reflex in patients who have a decreased level of consciousness, a brainstem lesion, or a disease involving the throat musculature. If the reflex is weak or absent, the patient is in danger of aspirating food or secretions. The strength and efficiency of swallowing are important to test in these patients for the same reason. Another test for the awake, cooperative patient is to have the patient phonate by saying "ah" and to note the bilateral symmetry of elevation of the soft palate. Any asymmetry can indicate weakness or paralysis. Swallowing is also assessed by lightly holding the examiner's

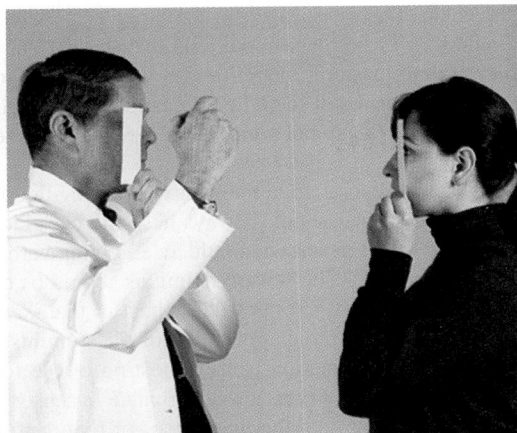

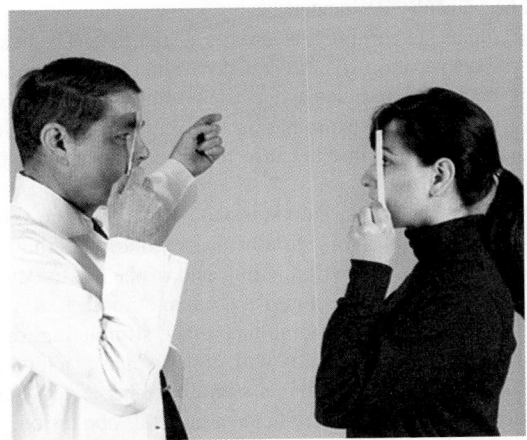

FIG. 54-16 Assessment of visual fields by gross confrontation.

Oculomotor, trochlear, and abducens nerves. Because the oculomotor (CN III), trochlear (CN IV), and abducens (CN VI) nerves all help move the eye, they are tested together. The patient is asked to follow the examiner's finger as it moves horizontally and vertically (making a cross) and diagonally (making an X). If there is weakness or paralysis of one of the eye muscles, the eyes do not move together, and the patient has a *disconjugate gaze*. The presence and direction of *nystagmus* (fine, rapid jerking movements of the eyes) are observed at this time, even though this condition most often indicates vestibulocerebellar problems.

Other functions of the oculomotor nerve are tested by checking for pupillary constriction and for *convergence* (eyes turning inward) and *accommodation* (pupils constricting with near vision). To test pupillary constriction, the examiner shines a light into the pupil of one eye and looks for ipsilateral constriction of the same pupil and contralateral (consensual) constriction of the opposite eye. The size and shape of the pupils are also noted. The optic nerve must be intact for this reflex to occur. Testing for pupillary constriction is an important component of the neurologic assessment of patients at risk for herniation syndrome (see Chapter 55). Because the oculomotor nerve exits at the top of the brainstem at the tentorial notch, it can be easily compressed by expanding mass lesions in the cerebral hemispheres. The result is a pupil that does not constrict to light; it may become dilated because the sympathetic input to the pupil acts unopposed. Convergence and accommodation are tested by having the patient focus

hands on either side of the patient's throat and asking the patient to swallow. Any asymmetry is noted.

Spinal accessory nerve. The spinal accessory nerve (CN XI) is tested by asking the patient to shrug the shoulders against resistance and to turn the head to either side against resistance. There should be smooth contraction of the sternomastoid and trapezius muscles. Symmetry, atrophy, or fasciculation of the muscle should also be noted.

Hypoglossal nerve. The hypoglossal nerve (CN XII) is tested by asking the patient to protrude the tongue. It should protrude in the midline. The patient should also be able to push the tongue to either side against the resistance of a tongue blade. Again, any asymmetry, atrophy, or fasciculation should be noted.

Motor system. The motor system examination includes assessment of bulk, tone, and power of the major muscle groups of the body, as well as assessment of balance and coordination. The examiner tests strength by asking the patient to push and pull against the resistance of the examiner's arm as it opposes flexion and extension of the patient's muscle. The patient should be asked to offer resistance at the shoulder, elbow, wrist, hips, knees, and ankles. The patient's grip strength can also be tested. Mild weakness of the upper extremities may be tested by having the patient extend both arms forward at shoulder height with palms up while the eyes are closed. Mild weakness of the arm is demonstrated by downward drifting of the arm or pronation of the palm (pronator drift). Any weakness or asymmetry of strength between the same muscle groups of the right and left side should be noted.[8]

Tone is tested by passively moving the limbs through their range of motion; there should be a slight resistance to these movements. Abnormal tone is described as hypotonia (flaccidity) or hypertonia (spasticity). Involuntary movements (e.g., tics, tremor, myoclonus [spasm of muscles], athetosis [slow, writhing, involuntary movements of extremities], chorea [involuntary, purposeless, rapid motions], dystonia [impairment of muscle tone]) should be noted.

Cerebellar function is tested by assessing balance and coordination. A good screening test for both balance and muscle strength is to observe the patient's stature (posture while standing) and gait. The examiner should note the pace and rhythm of the gait and observe the arm swing. (The arms should move symmetrically and in the opposite direction of the leg on the same side.) The patient's ability to ambulate is a key factor in determining the amount of nursing care that is needed and the risk of injury from falling. A patient with cerebellar disease may have an ataxic or staggering gait, in which the feet are placed wide apart and the steps are unsteady.

Coordination can be easily tested in several ways. The finger-to-nose test involves having the patient alternately touch the nose with the index finger, then touch the examiner's finger. The examiner repositions the finger while the patient is touching the nose so that the patient must adjust to a new distance each time the examiner's finger is touched. These movements should be performed smoothly and accurately. Other tests include asking the patient to pronate and supinate both hands rapidly and to do a shallow knee bend, first on one leg and then on the other. Dysarthria or slurred speech should be noted because it is a sign of incoordination of the speech muscles.

The heel-to-shin test involves having the patient place one heel on the opposite shin below the knee and moving the heel down the shin to the ankle. This is repeated for the other leg. These movements should flow smoothly without jerking or hesitation.

Sensory system. Several modalities are tested in the somatic sensory examination. Each modality is carried by a specific ascending pathway in the spinal cord before it reaches the sensory cortex.

There are some general guidelines for performing the sensory examination. The patient should always have the eyes closed to avoid visual clues. The examiner should avoid giving verbal cues such as, "Is this sharp?" The sensory stimulus should be applied in such a way that the patient does not expect it; that is, the examiner should avoid rhythmic application of the stimulus. In the routine neurologic examination, sensory testing of the four extremities is sufficient. However, if a disturbance in sensory function of the skin is identified, the boundaries of that dysfunction should be carefully delineated.

Light touch. Light touch is usually tested first. The examiner gently strokes a cotton wisp over each of the four extremities and asks the patient to indicate when the stimulus is felt by saying "touch." (The sensory examination of the trigeminal nerve may be delayed until this time because the same material for testing sensation is used.)

Pain and temperature. Pain is tested by touching the skin with the sharp end of a pin. This stimulus is irregularly alternated with a simple touch stimulus with the dull end of the pin to determine whether the patient can distinguish the two stimuli. Extinction or inhibition is assessed by simultaneously stimulating opposite sides of the body symmetrically with either a pain or a touch stimulus. Normally, the simultaneous stimuli are perceived (sensed); perception of only one may indicate a parietal lobe lesion.

The sensation of temperature is tested by applying tubes of warm and cold water to the skin and asking the patient to identify the stimuli with the eyes closed. If pain sensation is intact, assessment of temperature sensation may be omitted because both sensations are carried by the same ascending pathways.

Vibration sense. Vibration sense is assessed by applying a vibrating C128 tuning fork to the fingernails and the bony prominences of the hands, legs, and feet with the patient's eyes closed. The examiner asks the patient if the vibration or "buzz" is felt. The examiner then asks the patient to indicate when the vibration ceases. The examiner stops the vibration with the hand as desired.

Position sense. Position sense is assessed by placing the thumb and forefinger on either side of the patient's forefinger or great toe and gently moving the finger up or down. The patient is asked to indicate the direction in which the digit is moved.

Another test of position sense of the lower extremities is the Romberg test. The patient is asked to stand with the feet together and then close his or her eyes. If the patient is able to maintain balance with the eyes open but sways or falls with the eyes closed (i.e., a positive Romberg test), this may indicate disease in the posterior columns of the spinal cord. It is important that the nurse be aware of patient safety during this test.

Cortical sensory functions. Several tests evaluate cortical integration of sensory perceptions (which occurs in the parietal lobes). Two-point discrimination is assessed by placing the two points of a calibrated compass on the tips of the fingers and toes. The minimum recognizable separation is 4 to 5 mm in the fingertips and a greater degree of separation elsewhere. This test is important in diagnosing diseases of the sensory cortex and peripheral nervous system.

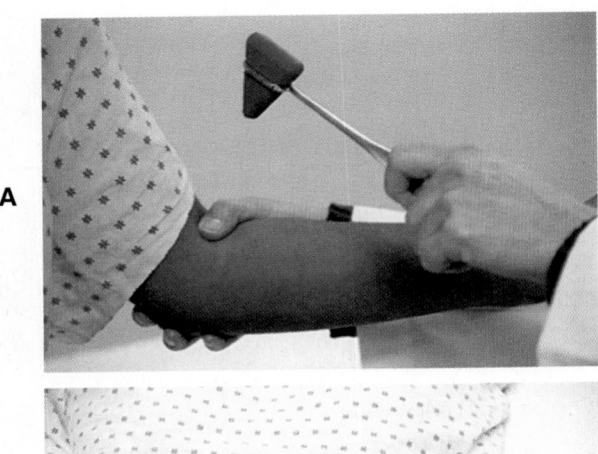

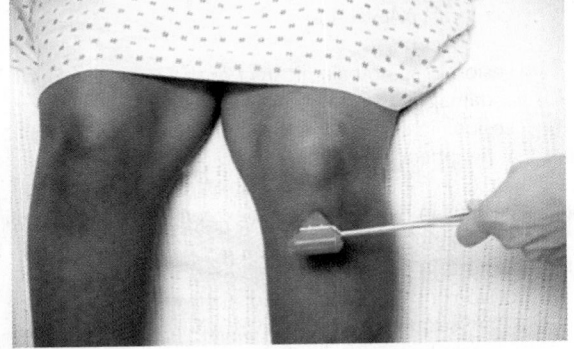

FIG. 54-17 The examiner strikes a swift blow over a stretched tendon to elicit a stretch reflex. **A**, Biceps reflex. **B**, Patellar reflex.

Graphesthesia (ability to feel writing on skin) is tested by having the patient identify numbers traced on the palm of the hands. *Stereognosis* (ability to perceive the form and nature of objects) is tested by having the patient identify the size and shape of easily recognized objects (e.g., coins, keys, a safety pin) placed in the hands. Sensory extinction or inattention is evaluated by touching both sides of the body simultaneously. An abnormal response occurs when the patient perceives the stimulus only on one side. The other stimulus is "extinguished."

Reflexes. Tendons attached to skeletal muscles have receptors that are sensitive to stretch. A reflex contraction of the skeletal muscle occurs when the tendon is stretched. A simple muscle stretch reflex is initiated by briskly tapping the tendon of a stretched muscle, usually with a reflex hammer (Fig. 54-17). The response (muscle contraction of the corresponding muscle) is measured as follows: 0/5 absent, 1/5 weak response, 2/5 normal response, 3/5 exaggerated response, 4/5 hyperreflexia with clonus. *Clonus,* an abnormal response, is a continued rhythmic contraction of the muscle with continuous application of the stimulus.

In general, the biceps, triceps, brachioradialis, and patellar and Achilles tendon reflexes are tested. The examiner elicits the biceps reflex by placing the thumb over the biceps tendon in the antecubital space and striking the thumb with a hammer. The patient should have the arms partially flexed at the elbow with the palms up. The normal response is flexion of the arm at the elbow or contraction of the biceps muscle that can be felt by the examiner's thumb.

The triceps reflex is elicited by striking the triceps tendon above the elbow while the patient's arm is flexed. The normal response is extension of the arm or visible contraction of the triceps.

TABLE 54-6 Normal Physical Assessment of the Nervous System*

Mental Status
Alert and oriented, orderly thought processes, appropriate mood and affect

Cranial Nerves†
Smell intact to soap and coffee; visual fields full to confrontation; visual acuity 20/20 in both eyes; intact extraocular movements; no nystagmus; pupils equal, round, reactive to light and accommodation; intact facial sensation to touch and pinprick; facial movements full; intact gag and swallow reflexes; symmetric elevation of soft palate; full strength with head turning and shrugging of shoulders against resistance; midline protrusion of tongue

Motor System
Normal gait and station; normal tandem walk; negative Romberg test; normal and symmetric muscle bulk, tone, strength; smooth performance of finger-nose, heel-shin movements

Sensory System
Intact sensation to light touch, position sense, vibration, pinprick, heat and cold, two-point discrimination; intact stereognosis and graphesthesia

Reflexes‡
Biceps, triceps, brachioradialis, patellar, and Achilles tendon reflexes 2+ bilaterally; downgoing toes with plantar stimulation

*If some portion of the neurologic examination was not done, this should be indicated (e.g., "Smell not tested").
†May also be recorded as "CN I to XII intact."
‡May also be recorded as drawing of stick figure indicating reflex strength at appropriate sites.

The brachioradialis reflex is elicited by striking the radius 3 to 5 cm above the wrist while the patient's arm is relaxed. The normal response is flexion and supination at the elbow or visible contraction of the brachioradialis muscle.

The patellar reflex is elicited by striking the patellar tendon just below the patella. The patient can be sitting or lying as long as the leg being tested hangs freely. The normal response is extension of the leg with contraction of the quadriceps.

The Achilles tendon reflex is elicited by striking the Achilles tendon while the patient's leg is flexed at the knee and the foot is dorsiflexed at the ankle. The normal response is plantar flexion at the ankle.

Table 54-6 is an example of a normal neurologic assessment. Common abnormal assessment findings of the neurologic system are presented in Table 54-7.

DIAGNOSTIC STUDIES OF THE NERVOUS SYSTEM

Diagnostic studies provide important information to the nurse in monitoring the patient's condition and planning appropriate interventions. These studies are considered to be objective data. Diagnostic studies used to assess the nervous system are presented in Table 54-8.

TABLE 54-7   *Common Assessment Abnormalities*

Nervous System

FINDING	DESCRIPTION	POSSIBLE ETIOLOGY AND SIGNIFICANCE
Altered consciousness	Inability to speak, obey commands, open eyes appropriately with verbal or painful stimulus	Intracranial lesions, metabolic disorder, psychiatric disorders
Anisocoria	Inequality of pupil size	Lesion, injury, or intracranial pressure in area of midbrain
Agnosia	Inability to determine meaning or significance of sensory stimulus	Cerebral cortex lesion
Apraxia	Inability to perform learned movements, defect in motor planning	Cerebral cortex lesion
Aphasia	Loss of language faculty (language comprehension, language expression, or both)	Cerebral cortex lesion
Analgesia	Loss of pain sensation	Lesion in spinothalamic tract or thalamus, lack of or damage to sensory nerve endings
Anesthesia	Absence of sensation	Lesions in spinal cord, thalamus, sensory cortex, or peripheral sensory nerve
Hyperesthesia	Increase in sensation	
Hypoesthesia	Decrease in sensation	
Anosognosia	Inability to recognize bodily defect or disease	Lesions in right parietal cortex, common in right-brain stroke
Astereognosis	Inability to recognize form of object by touch	Lesions in parietal cortex
Ataxia	Lack of coordination of movement	Lesions of sensory or motor pathways, cerebellum; antiseizure drugs, sedative, hypnotic drug toxicity (including alcohol)
Muscle atrophy (disuse or denervation atrophy)	Wasting away or diminution in size of muscle	Suprasegmental (upper motor neuron) lesions, segmental (lower motor neuron) lesions
Bladder dysfunction		
Atonic (autonomous)	Absence of muscle tone and contractility, enlargement of capacity, no sensation of discomfort, overflow with large residual, inability to voluntarily empty or empty by reflex	Early stage of spinal cord injury
Hypotonic	More ability than atonic bladder but less than normal	Interruption of afferent pathways from bladder
Hypertonic	Increase in muscle tone, diminished capacity, reflex emptying, dribbling, incontinence	Lesions in pyramidal tracts (efferent pathways)
Diplopia	Double vision	Lesions affecting nerves of extraocular muscles, cerebellar damage
Dysarthria	Lack of coordination in articulating speech	Lesions in cerebellum or pathway of cranial nerves (including brainstem); antiseizure drug, sedative, or hypnotic drug toxicity (including alcohol)
Dyskinesia	Impairment of power of voluntary movement, resulting in fragmentary or incomplete movements	Disorders of basal ganglia, idiosyncratic reaction to psychotropic drugs
Dysphagia	Difficulty in swallowing	Lesions involving motor pathways of CN IX, X (including lower brainstem)
Extensor plantar response (Babinski's sign)	Upgoing toes with plantar stimulation	Suprasegmental or upper motor neuron lesion
Homonymous hemianopsia	Loss of vision in one side of visual field	Injury or lesions in area of optic tract or its radiations to occipital cortex
Hemiplegia	Paralysis on one side	Stroke and other lesions involving motor cortex
Nystagmus	Jerking or bobbing of eyes as they track moving object	Lesions in cerebellum, brainstem, vestibular system; antiseizure, sedative, hypnotic toxicity (including alcohol)
Ophthalmoplegia	Paralysis of eye muscles	Lesions in brainstem or CN III, IV, VI
Opisthotonus	Extreme arching of back with retraction of head	Meningitis, tonic phase of grand mal seizure
Papilledema	"Choked disc," swelling of optic nerve head	Increase in intracranial pressure
Paraplegia	Paralysis of lower extremities	Spinal cord transection or mass lesion (thoracolumbar region)
Tetraplegia (quadriplegia)	Paralysis of all extremities	Spinal cord transection or mass lesion (cervical region) or brainstem

TABLE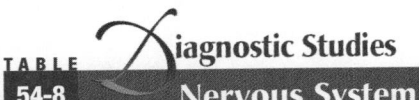

54-8 **Nervous System**

STUDY	DESCRIPTION AND PURPOSE	NURSING RESPONSIBILITY
Cerebrospinal Fluid Analysis		
▪ Lumbar puncture	CSF is aspirated by needle insertion in L3–4 or L4–5 interspace to assess many CNS diseases. (See Table 54-9.)	Assist patient to assume and maintain lateral recumbent position with knees flexed. Ensure maintenance of strict aseptic technique. Ensure labeling of CSF specimens in proper sequence. Keep patient flat for at least a few hours depending on physician preference. Encourage fluids. Monitor neurologic and VS. Administer analgesia as needed.
Radiologic		
▪ Skull and spine x-rays	Simple x-ray of skull and spinal column is done to detect fractures, bone erosion, calcifications, abnormal vascularity.	Explain that procedure is noninvasive. Explain positions to be assumed.
▪ Cerebral angiography	Serial x-ray visualization of intracranial and extracranial blood vessels is performed to detect vascular lesions and tumors of brain. Contrast medium is used.	Withhold preceding meal. Explain that patient will have hot flush of head and neck when contrast medium is injected. Administer premedication. Explain need to be absolutely still during procedure. Monitor neurologic and VS every 15–30 min first 2 hr, every hour next 6 hr, then every 2 hr for 24 hr. Maintain pressure dressing and ice to injection site. Maintain bed rest until patient is alert and VS are stable. Report any signs of change in neurologic status.
▪ Computed tomography (CT) scan	Computer-assisted x-ray of several levels or thin cross sections of body parts are done to detect problems such as hemorrhage, tumor, cyst, edema, infarction, brain atrophy, and other abnormalities.	Explain that procedure is noninvasive (if no contrast medium used). Observe for allergic reaction and note puncture site (if contrast medium used). Explain appearance of scanner. Instruct patient on need to remain absolutely still during procedure.
▪ Magnetic resonance imaging (MRI)	Imaging of brain, spinal cord, and spinal canal by means of magnetic energy. Used in detection of strokes, multiple sclerosis, tumors, trauma, herniation, and seizures. No invasive procedures are required. Gadolinium contrast media may be used to enhance visualization.	Screen patient for metal parts and pacemaker in body. Instruct patient on need to lie very still for up to 1 hr. Sedation may be necessary if patient is claustrophobic.
▪ Magnetic resonance angiography (MRA)	Uses differential signal characteristics of flowing blood to evaluate extracranial and intracranial blood vessels. Provides both anatomic and hemodynamic information. Can be used in conjunction with contrast media (contrast-enhanced MRA [cMRA]). Rapidly replacing cerebral angiography for use in diagnosing cerebrovascular diseases.	Similar to MRI (see above).
▪ Magnetic resonance spectroscopy (MRS)	Provides information about chemical composition of tissue. Used to study brain diseases, including brain tumors, Alzheimer's disease, strokes, acquired immunodeficiency syndrome, seizure disorders, and multiple sclerosis. Markers of neuronal integrity (e.g., N-acetyl aspartate) used to determine loss of neurons.	Similar to MRI (see above).
▪ Functional MRI (fMRI)	Use of MRI to detect changes in cerebral metabolism or blood flow, volume, or oxygenation response to specific tasks, consisting of periods of activity and periods of rest. Can functionally map brain.	Similar to MRI (see above).
▪ Myelography	X-ray of spinal cord and vertebral column after injection of contrast medium into subarachnoid space is used to detect spinal lesions (e.g., ruptured disk, tumor).	Administer preprocedure sedation as ordered. Instruct patient to empty bladder. Inform patient that test is performed with patient on tilting table that is moved during test. Encourage fluids. Monitor neurologic and VS.

CSF, Cerebrospinal fluid; *CNS,* central nervous system; *IV,* intravenous; *VS,* vital signs.

Continued

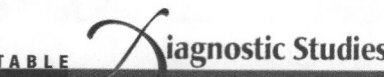

TABLE 54-8 **Diagnostic Studies**

Nervous System—cont'd

STUDY	DESCRIPTION AND PURPOSE	NURSING RESPONSIBILITY
Radiologic—cont'd		
Positron emission tomography (PET)	Measures metabolic activity of brain regions to assess cell death or damage. Uses radioactive material that shows up as a bright spot on the image.	Explain procedure to patient. Explain that two IV lines will be inserted. Instruct patient not to take sedatives or tranquilizers. Empty bladder before procedure. May be asked to perform different activities during test.
Single-photon emission computed tomography (SPECT)	A method of scanning similar to PET, but it uses more stable substances and different detectors. Radiolabeled compounds are injected and their photon emissions can be detected. Images made are accumulation of labeled compound. Used to visualize blood flow or oxygen or glucose metabolism in the brain. Useful in diagnosing strokes, brain tumors, and seizure disorders.	Similar to PET (see above)
Electrographic		
Electroencephalography (EEG)	Electrical activity of brain is recorded by scalp electrodes to evaluate cerebral disease, CNS effects of systemic diseases, brain death.	Inform patient that procedure is painless and without danger of electric shock. Withhold stimulants. Inform that patient may be asked to perform various activities such as hyperventilation during test. Determine whether any medications (e.g., tranquilizers, antiseizure drugs) should be withheld. Resume medications after test. Assist patient to wash electrode paste out of hair.
Magnetoencephalography (MEG)	Uses a sensitivity machine called a biomagnetometer, which detects very small magnetic fields generated by neural activity. It can accurately pinpoint the part of the brain involved in a stroke, seizure, or other disorder or injury. Measures extracranial magnetic fields, as well as scalp electric field (EEG).	MEG, a passive sensor, does not make physical contact with patient. Explain procedure to patient.
Electromyography (EMG) and nerve conduction	Electrical activity associated with nerve and skeletal muscle is recorded by insertion of needle electrodes to detect muscle and peripheral nerve disease.	Inform patient of slight discomfort associated with insertion of needles.
Evoked potentials	Electrical activity associated with nerve conduction along sensory pathways is recorded by electrodes placed on skin and scalp. Stimulus generates the impulse. Procedure is used to diagnose disease, locate nerve damage, and monitor function intraoperatively.	Explain procedure to patient.
Visual evoked potentials	Electrical activity in visual pathway is recorded with rapidly reversing checkerboard pattern on television screen. One eye is tested at a time.	Explain procedure to patient.
Brainstem auditory evoked potentials	Electrical activity in auditory pathway is recorded with earphones that produce clicking sounds. One ear is tested at a time.	Explain procedure to patient.
Somatosensory evoked potentials	Electrical activity in certain nerve pathways is recorded with mild electrical pulse (several per second).	Inform patient that stimulus may cause mild discomfort or muscle twitch.
Ultrasound		
Carotid duplex studies	Sound waves determine blood flow velocity, which indicates presence of occlusive vascular disease.	Explain procedure to patient.
Transcranial Doppler	Same technology as carotid duplex, but evaluates intracranial vessels.	Explain procedure to patient.

TABLE 54-9	Normal Cerebrospinal Fluid Values	
PARAMETER	**NORMAL VALUE**	
Specific gravity	1.007	
pH	7.35	
Appearance	Clear, colorless	
RBCs	None	
WBCs	0–8/μl (0–0.008/L)	
Protein		
Lumbar	15–45 mg/dl (0.15–0.45 g/L)	
Cisternal	15–25 mg/dl (0.15–0.25 g/L)	
Ventricular	5–15 mg/dl (0.05–0.15 g/L)	
Glucose	45–75 mg/dl (2.5–4.2 mmol/L)	
Microorganisms	None	
Opening pressure with lumbar puncture	60–150 mm H_2O	

RBCs, Red blood cells; *WBCs,* white blood cells.

Cerebrospinal Fluid Analysis. CSF analysis provides information about a variety of CNS diseases. Normal CSF fluid is clear, colorless, and free of red blood cells and contains little protein. Normal CSF values are listed in Table 54-9.

Lumbar Puncture. Lumbar puncture is the most common method of obtaining CSF for analysis. It is contraindicated in the presence of increased intracranial pressure or infection at the site of puncture.

Nurses often assist in this procedure because it is usually performed in the patient's room. Before the procedure, the nurse should have the patient empty the bladder. The patient should lie in the lateral recumbent position, with the back as near as possible to the edge of the bed. The nurse should assist the patient to draw up the knees to the abdomen and flex the head to the chest. This helps separate the vertebrae so that the needle can be inserted more easily.

Using strict sterile technique, the physician inserts a long needle below the third lumbar vertebra. This may cause some local discomfort. There is no danger of injuring the spinal cord because the cord terminates between the first and second lumbar vertebrae. However, the patient may have some pain radiating down the leg or muscle twitching if the needle irritates the spinal root. The nurse can assure the patient that this is temporary and that the patient is not in danger of being paralyzed.

A manometer is attached to the needle, and CSF pressure is determined after the patient is asked to relax and extend the legs. If this is not done, the pressure appears abnormally high. CSF is withdrawn in a series of tubes and sent for analysis. Some examiners believe that the patient should be kept lying flat for at least a few hours after the procedure to avoid a spinal headache, which is presumably caused by loss of the cushioning effect of CSF as a result of leakage of CSF at the puncture site. The prone position may be effective in preventing CSF leakage. Others do not believe that the lying position is necessary because headache seems to develop in some patients despite precautions. Meningeal irritation (nuchal rigidity) or signs and symptoms of local trauma (e.g., hematoma, pain) may develop in some patients.

Radiologic Studies

Cerebral Angiography. Cerebral angiography is indicated when vascular lesions or tumors are suspected. A catheter is inserted into the femoral (sometimes brachial) artery. It is then passed up the artery to the aortic arch and into the base of a carotid or a vertebral artery for injection of radiopaque contrast medium. A series of x-rays is taken in a timed sequence so that pictures of the arteries, smaller vessels, and veins can be obtained (Fig. 54-18). This study can help to localize and determine the presence of abscesses, aneurysms, hematomas, arteriovenous malformations, arterial spasm, and certain tumors.

Because this is an invasive procedure, adverse reactions may occur. The patient may have an allergic (anaphylactic) reaction to the contrast medium. This reaction usually occurs immediately after injection of the contrast medium and may require emergency resuscitation measures in the procedure room. The most common precaution for nurses to take in caring for the patient after the return to the room is observation for bleeding at the catheter puncture site (usually the groin). A pressure dressing and ice are usually placed on the site to promote hemostasis and prevent swelling.

Computed Tomography. Computed tomography (CT) is a noninvasive procedure, although intravenous injection of contrast medium may be used to enhance visualization of the blood vessels and identify disruptions in the blood-brain barrier. CT scans can be done on an outpatient basis. A number of x-rays scanning different levels of the brain are compiled with computer assistance and presented in a series of black-and-white pictures. These pictures, which illustrate "slices" of the brain, can show hemorrhages, tumors, cysts, edema, infarction, brain atrophy, and hydrocephalus. CT scans do not illustrate structures in the posterior fossa and the base of the brain as clearly as does magnetic resonance imaging (MRI).

Magnetic Resonance Imaging. Rather than using x-rays, MRI involves two kinds of magnetism. The patient is placed within a giant magnetic field that aligns the protons of the hydrogen ions in the cells of the body (Fig. 54-19). Bursts of radiofrequency magnetism are introduced to flip the protons out of

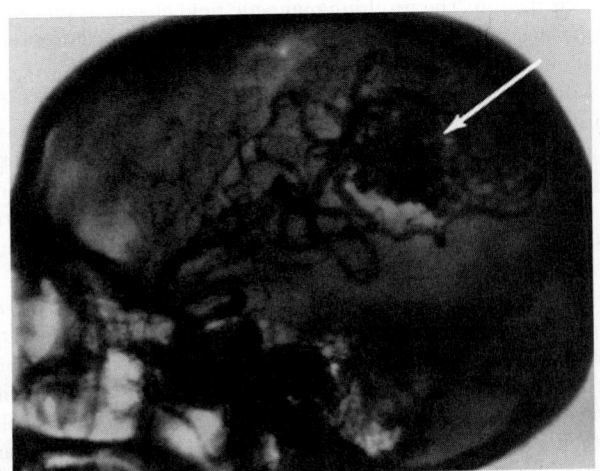

FIG. 54-18 Cerebral angiogram illustrating an arteriovenous malformation (*arrow*).

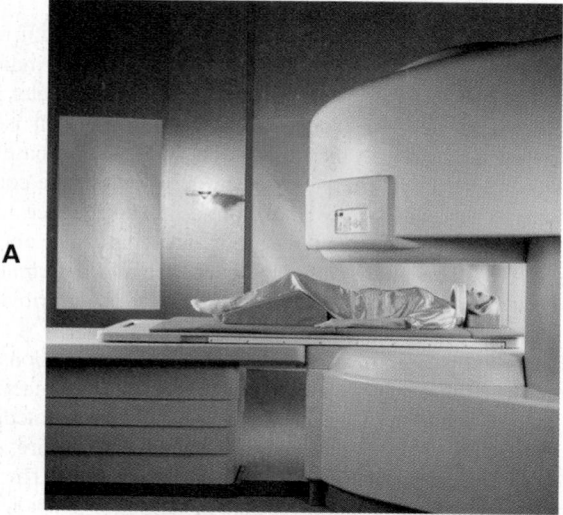

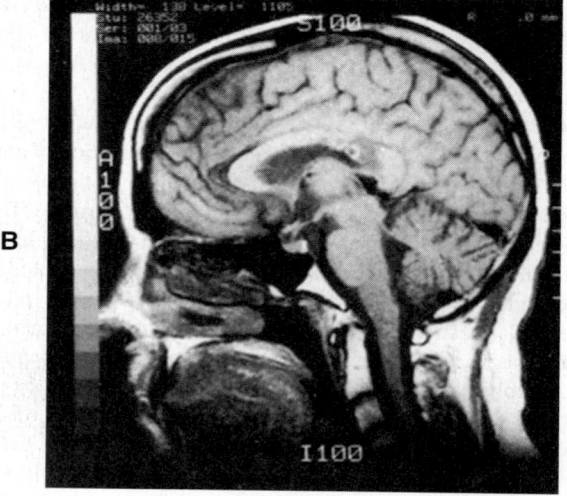

FIG. 54-19 A, Clinical setting for magnetic resonance imaging (MRI). B, Midline sagittal view of the brain using MRI.

alignment. When the radiofrequency magnetism is turned off, the protons realign. The resulting magnetic field change is picked up by the machine and processed by a computer. Vivid black-and-white pictures are then produced.

MRI is useful in evaluating brain and spinal cord edema, hemorrhage, infarction, blood vessels, tumors, herniation, and bone lesions. It is used in the detection of early strokes and multiple sclerosis. Intravenous injection of gadolinium can enhance the images obtained with MRI. Because MRI yields greater contrast in the images of soft tissue structures than does the CT scan, it is the diagnostic test of choice for many neurologic diseases.

Positron Emission Tomography. *Positron emission tomography* (PET) is used to determine regional metabolism in the brain. PET provides a noninvasive means of determining biochemical processes that occur in the brain. There is increasing clinical use of PET scanning to monitor patients with stroke, Alzheimer's disease, seizure disorders, epilepsy, tumors, and Parkinson's disease.

Myelography. *Myelography* is used to visualize the spinal column and the subarachnoid space when a spinal lesion is sus-

pected. The most common lesion for which this test is used is a herniated or protruding intervertebral disk. Other lesions include spinal tumors, adhesions, syringomyelia, bony deformations, and arteriovenous malformations. The test involves x-rays of the spinal column after injection of the contrast medium into the subarachnoid space via a catheter. Water-soluble iodine contrast materials such as iopamidol (Isovue) are used most often because they are absorbed into the bloodstream and excreted by the kidneys.

Preparation for this procedure is the same as for lumbar puncture. Before the contrast material is injected, patients must be asked whether they have any allergies, specifically whether they have had any anaphylactic or hypotensive episodes from other contrast media. After myelography the patient should lie flat for a few hours.

Headache is the most common complaint after myelography. It may be accompanied by nausea and occasionally by vomiting. The nurse should observe the patient for any changes in neurologic status and provide a quiet, comfortable environment after the procedure.

Electrographic Studies

Electroencephalography. The technique of *electroencephalography (EEG)* involves the recording of the electrical activity of the surface cortical neurons of the brain by 8 to 16 electrodes placed on specific areas of the scalp. This test is done to evaluate not only cerebral disease but also the CNS effects of many metabolic and systemic diseases and to determine brain death. Among the cerebral diseases assessed by EEG are epilepsy, mass lesions (e.g., tumor, abscess, hematoma), cerebrovascular lesions, and brain injury (Fig. 54-20). The procedure is noninvasive. Patients sometimes have the misconception that the recording electrodes will give them an electric shock. They should be assured that this is not true and that the procedure is similar to electrocardiography.

Electromyography and Nerve Conduction Studies. *Electromyography (EMG)* is the recording of electrical activity associated with innervation of skeletal muscle. The recording is displayed on a computer screen and may be played on a loudspeaker for simultaneous analysis. Needle electrodes are inserted into the muscle to record specific motor units because recording from the skin is not sufficient. Normal muscle at rest shows no electrical activity. Typical electrical activity occurs when the muscle contracts. This activity may be altered in diseases of muscle itself (e.g., myopathic conditions) or in disorders of muscle innervation (e.g., segmental or LMN lesions, peripheral neuropathic conditions). Fibrillations are spontaneous, independent contractions of individual muscle fibers that can be detected only by EMG. They appear on EMG 1 to 3 weeks after a muscle has lost its nerve supply.

Nerve conduction studies involve application of a brief electrical stimulus to a distal portion of a sensory or mixed nerve and recording the resulting wave of depolarization at some point proximal to the stimulation. For example, a stimulus can be applied to the forefinger and a recording electrode placed over the median nerve at the wrist. The time between the onset of the stimulus and the initial wave of depolarization at the recording electrode is measured. This is termed *nerve conduction velocity.* Damaged nerves have slower conduction velocities.

Evoked Potentials. *Evoked potentials* are recordings of electrical activity associated with nerve conduction along sen-

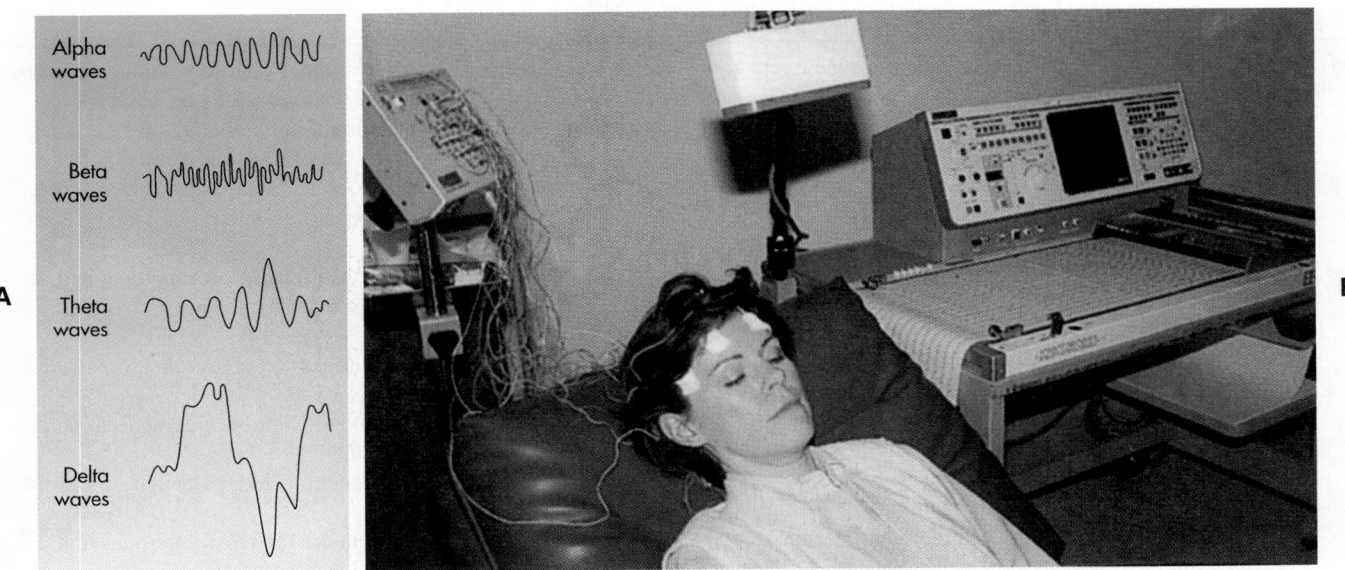

FIG. 54-20 Electroencephalogram (EEG). **A,** Examples of alpha, beta, theta, and delta waves seen on an EEG. **B,** Photograph showing a person undergoing an EEG test. Notice the scalp electrodes that detect voltage fluctuations within the cranium.

sory pathways. The activity is generated by a specific sensory stimulus related to the type of study (e.g., checkerboard patterns for visual evoked potentials, clicking sounds for auditory evoked potentials, mild electrical pulses for somatosensory evoked potentials). Electrodes placed on specific areas of the skin and scalp record the electrical activity, which is stored and averaged by a computerized instrument. A wave pattern appears on a screen and is printed on paper. Peaks in the wave pattern correspond to conduction of the stimulus through certain points along the sensory pathway (e.g., peripheral nerve, brainstem, cortical areas). Increases in the normal time from stimulus onset to a given peak (latency) indicate slowed nerve conduction or nerve damage. This technique is useful in diagnosing abnormalities of the visual or auditory systems because it reveals whether a sensory impulse is reaching the appropriate part of the brain. Indications for these tests include evaluation of the optic nerve in conditions such as multiple sclerosis (optic neuritis) and the vestibulocochlear nerve in acoustic neuroma.

Combined Doppler and Ultrasound (Duplex) Studies

Carotid Duplex. A duplex study uses combined ultrasound and pulsed Doppler technology. A technician places a probe on the skin over the carotid artery and slowly moves the probe along the course of the common carotid to the bifurcation of the external and internal carotid arteries. The ultrasound signal emitted from the probe reflects off the moving blood cells within the vessel. The frequency of the reflected signal corresponds to the blood velocity. This response is amplified and is registered on a graphic record and also as sound. The graphic record registers blood velocity. Increased blood flow velocity can indicate stenosis of a vessel. Duplex scanning is a noninvasive study that evaluates the degree of stenosis of the carotid and vertebral arteries.

Transcranial Doppler Sonography. Transcranial Doppler (TCD) sonography uses the same technology as duplex studies, except that it records blood flow velocities of the intracranial blood vessels. The probe is placed on the skin at various "windows" in the skull (areas in the skull that have only a thin bony covering) to register velocities of the middle cerebral artery, anterior cerebral artery, posterior cerebral artery, terminal carotid artery, and occasionally the anterior and posterior communicating arteries. The temporal, orbital, and suboccipital sites are used. The ultrasound signal received is recorded graphically as a waveform. Peak blood flow velocities and systolic-diastolic ratios can be calculated from this information. TCD sonography is a noninvasive technique that is useful in assessing vasospasm associated with subarachnoid hemorrhage, altered intracranial blood flow dynamics associated with occlusive vascular disease, presence of emboli, and cerebral autoregulation.

REVIEW QUESTIONS

The number of the question corresponds to the same-numbered objective at the beginning of the chapter.

1. In a patient with a disease that affects the myelin sheath of nerves, such as multiple sclerosis, the glial cells that are affected are the
   a. microglia.
   b. astrocytes.
   c. oligodendrocytes.
   d. ependymal cells.

2. A state of hypoxia alters the repeated action potentials necessary for transmission of nerve impulses because energy is required for
   a. repolarization of the cell membrane.
   b. creation of cell membrane permeability.
   c. movement of sodium into the nerve cell.
   d. maintenance of the resting membrane potential.

3. Drugs or diseases that impair the function of the extrapyramidal system may cause loss of
   a. sensations of pain and temperature.
   b. regulation of the autonomic nervous system.
   c. integration of somatic and special sensory inputs.
   d. automatic movements associated with skeletal muscle activity.

4. An obstruction of the anterior cerebral arteries will affect functions of
   a. visual imaging.
   b. balance and coordination.
   c. judgment, insight, and reasoning.
   d. visual and auditory integration for language comprehension.

5. Paralysis of lateral gaze indicates a lesion of cranial nerve
   a. II.
   b. III.
   c. IV.
   d. VI.

6. A result of stimulation of the parasympathetic nervous system is
   a. dilation of skin blood vessels.
   b. increased secretion of insulin.
   c. increased blood glucose levels.
   d. relaxation of the urinary sphincters.

7. Assessment of muscle strength of older adults cannot be compared with that of younger adults because
   a. stroke is more common in older adults.
   b. nutritional status is better in young adults.
   c. most young people exercise more than older people.
   d. aging leads to a decrease in muscle bulk and strength.

8. Data regarding mobility, strength, coordination, and activity tolerance are important for the nurse to obtain because
   a. many neurologic diseases affect one or more of these areas.
   b. patients are less able to identify other neurologic impairments.
   c. these are the first functions to be affected by neurologic disease.
   d. aspects of movement are the most important functions of the nervous system.

9. During neurologic testing the patient is able to perceive pain elicited by pinprick. Based on this finding, the nurse may omit testing for
   a. position sense.
   b. patellar reflexes.
   c. temperature perception.
   d. heel-to-shin movements.

10. A patient's eyes jerk as they follow the nurse's moving finger. The nurse records this finding as
    a. nystagmus.
    b. normal tracking.
    c. ophthalmoplegia.
    d. ophthalmic dyskinesia.

11. Nursing responsibilities for lumbar puncture include
    a. ensuring the patient has a full bladder.
    b. placing the patient in the lateral recumbent position.
    c. straightening the patient's legs just before the puncture.
    d. having the patient cough when the needle has been inserted.

REFERENCES

1. Kempermann G, Gage FH: Neurogenesis in the adult hippocampus, *Novartis Found Symp* 231:231, 2000.
2. Kandel ER, Schwartz JH, Jessell TM, editors: *Principles of neural science*, New York, 2000, McGraw-Hill.
3. Odenheimer GL: Geriatric neurology, *Neurol Clin* 16:561, 1998.
4. Motyka KM, Yanuck SF: Expanding the neurological examination using functional neurologic assessment: part 1: methodological considerations, *International Journal of Applied Kinesiology & Kinesiologic Medicine* 7:28, 2000.
5. Lower J: Facing neuro assessment fearlessly, *Nursing* 32:58, 2002.
6. Beckerman B: Nervous energy: conducting a neurologic assessment in the field, *Emerg Med Serv* 29:45, 2000.
7. Mitchell PH et al: *Neurologic assessment for nursing practice*, Reston, Va, 1984, Reston.
8. Baker RA, Andrew MJ, Knight JL: Evaluation of neurologic assessment and outcomes in cardiac surgical patients, *Semin Thorac Cardiovasc Surg* 13:149, 2001.

RESOURCES

CHAPTER **55**

NURSING MANAGEMENT
Acute Intracranial Problems

Mary Kerr
Elizabeth A. Crago

LEARNING OBJECTIVES

1. Identify the physiologic mechanisms that maintain normal intracranial pressure.
2. Identify the common etiologies, clinical manifestations, and collaborative care of the patient with increased intracranial pressure.
3. Describe the collaborative and nursing management of the patient with increased intracranial pressure.
4. Differentiate types of head injury by mechanism of injury and clinical manifestations.
5. Describe the collaborative care and nursing management of the patient with a head injury.

6. Compare the types, clinical manifestations, and collaborative care of brain tumors.
7. Discuss the nursing management of the patient with a brain tumor.
8. Describe the nursing management of the patient undergoing cranial surgery.
9. Compare the primary causes, collaborative care, and nursing management of meningitis, encephalitis, and brain abscess.

KEY TERMS

brain abscess, p. 1522	Glasgow Coma Scale, p. 1500
cerebral edema, p. 1493	head injury, p. 1505
coma, p. 1494	intracerebral hematoma, p. 1508
concussion, p. 1507	intracranial pressure, p. 1491
contusion, p. 1507	meningitis, p. 1518
diffuse axonal injury, p. 1507	nuchal rigidity, p. 1518
encephalitis, p. 1521	subdural hematoma, p. 1507
epidural hematoma, p. 1507	unconsciousness, p. 1495

Acute intracranial problems include diseases and disorders that can increase intracranial pressure (ICP). This chapter discusses the mechanisms that maintain normal ICP, increased ICP, head injury, brain tumors, and cerebral inflammatory disorders.

INTRACRANIAL PRESSURE

Understanding the mechanisms associated with ICP is important in caring for patients with many different neurologic problems. The skull is like a closed box with three essential volume components: brain tissue, blood, and cerebrospinal fluid (CSF) (Fig. 55-1). The total volume in the skull is 1900 ml. The intracellular and extracellular fluids of brain tissue make up approximately 78% of this volume. Blood in the arterial, venous, and capillary network makes up 12% of the volume, and the remaining 10% is the volume of the CSF. Under normal conditions, in which intracranial volume remains relatively constant, the balance among these components maintains the ICP. Factors that influence ICP under normal circumstances are changes in (1) arterial pressure, (2) venous pressure, (3) intraabdominal and intrathoracic pressure, (4) posture, (5) temperature, and (6) blood gases, particularly CO_2 levels. The degree to which these factors increase

or decrease the ICP depends on the ability of the brain to accommodate to the changes.

Regulation and Maintenance of Intracranial Pressure

Normal Intracranial Pressure. **Intracranial pressure** (ICP) is the hydrostatic force measured in the brain CSF compartment. Normal ICP is the pressure exerted by the total volume from the three components within the skull: brain tissue, blood, and CSF. The modified Monro-Kellie doctrine describes the relatively constant volume of these three components within the rigid skull structure. If the volume in any one of the three components increases within the cranial vault and the volume from another component is displaced, the total intracranial volume will not change.[1] This hypothesis is not applicable in situations in which the skull is not rigid (e.g., in neonates, in adults with unfused skull fractures).

Normal Compensatory Adaptations. In applying the modified Monro-Kellie doctrine, the body can adapt to changes

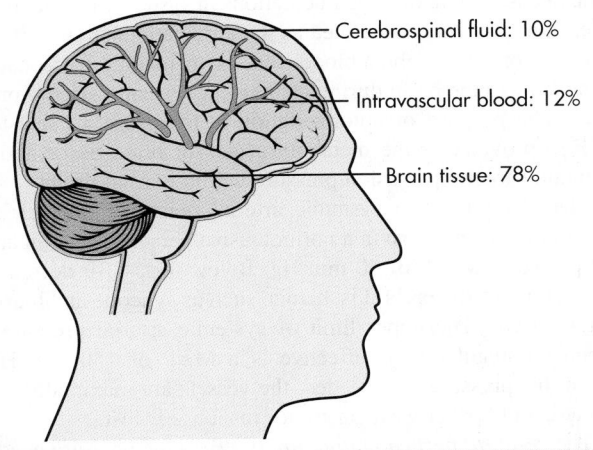

Cerebrospinal fluid: 10%

Intravascular blood: 12%

Brain tissue: 78%

FIG. 55-1 Components of the brain.

Reviewed by Sherry Garrett Hendrickson RN, PhD, CNS, Assistant Professor of Clinical Nursing, University of Texas at Austin School of Nursing, Austin, Tex.

in the volume of components of the skull to maintain a normal ICP. Initial compensatory mechanisms include changes in the CSF volume by altering CSF absorption or production and displacement of CSF into the spinal subarachnoid space. Alterations in intracranial blood volume occur through the collapse of cerebral veins and dural sinuses, regional cerebral vasoconstriction or dilation, and changes in venous outflow. Tissue brain volume compensates through dispensability of the dura or compression of brain tissue. Initially, an increase in volume produces no increase in ICP as a result of these compensatory mechanisms. However, these compensatory adaptations to changes in volume are limited; as the volume increase continues, the ICP rises and decompensation occurs, resulting in compression and ischemia.[1]

Measuring ICP. ICP can be measured in the ventricles, subarachnoid space, subdural space, epidural space, or brain parenchymal tissue using a water manometer or a pressure transducer. Normal intracranial ICP ranges from 0 to 15 mm Hg with the use of the pressure transducer. A sustained pressure above the upper limit is considered abnormal. ICP may become elevated because of head trauma, stroke, subarachnoid hemorrhage, brain tumor, inflammation, hydrocephalus, or brain tissue damage from other causes. Any patient who becomes acutely unconscious, regardless of the cause, is managed as if there were actual or potential elevations in the ICP. Patients with or at risk for elevated ICP usually receive invasive ICP monitoring in an intensive care unit (ICU), except those with irreversible problems or advanced neurologic disease. Goals for nursing management of an elevated ICP include preservation of cerebral perfusion, early identification of neurologic changes, and prevention of complications.

Cerebral Blood Flow

Cerebral blood flow (CBF) is the amount of blood in milliliters passing through 100 g of brain tissue in 1 minute. The global CBF is approximately 50 ml per minute per 100 g of brain tissue. There is a difference in flow between the white and gray matter of the brain. The white matter has a slower blood flow, approximately 25 ml per minute per 100 g, and the gray matter has a faster blood flow, approximately 75 ml per minute per 100 g.[2] The maintenance of blood flow to the brain is critical because the brain requires a constant supply of oxygen and glucose. The brain uses 20% of the body's oxygen and 25% of its glucose.

Autoregulation of Cerebral Blood Flow. The brain has the ability to regulate its own blood flow in response to its metabolic needs in spite of wide fluctuations in systemic arterial pressure. *Autoregulation* is defined as the automatic alteration in the diameter of the cerebral blood vessels to maintain a constant blood flow to the brain during changes in systemic arterial pressure.[3] The purpose of autoregulation is to ensure a consistent CBF to provide for the metabolic needs of brain tissue and to maintain cerebral perfusion pressure within normal limits.

The lower limit of systemic arterial pressure at which autoregulation is effective in a normotensive person is a mean arterial pressure (MAP) of 50 mm Hg. Below this, CBF decreases, and symptoms of cerebral ischemia, such as syncope and blurred vision, occur. The upper limit of systemic arterial pressure at which autoregulation is effective is a MAP of 150 mm Hg.[2] When this pressure is exceeded, the vessels are maximally constricted, and further vasoconstrictor response is lost.

The *cerebral perfusion pressure* (CPP) is the pressure needed to ensure blood flow to the brain. CPP is equal to the MAP mi-

---

TABLE 55-1 Calculation of Cerebral Perfusion Pressure

CPP = MAP − ICP

$$MAP = DBP + \tfrac{1}{3}(SBP - DBP) \text{ or } \frac{SBP + 2(DBP)}{3}$$

Example: Systemic blood pressure = 122/84
    MAP = 97
    ICP = 12 mm Hg
    CPP = 85 mm Hg

CPP, Cerebral perfusion pressure; *DBP,* diastolic blood pressure; *ICP,* intracranial pressure; *MAP,* mean arterial pressure; *SBP,* systolic blood pressure.

---

nus the ICP (CPP = MAP − ICP) (see example in Table 55-1). This formula is clinically useful, although it does not consider the effect of systemic vascular resistance. Cerebral vascular resistance, generated by the arterioles within the cranium, links CPP and blood flow as follows:

$$CPP = Flow \times Resistance$$

Noninvasive techniques used in intensive care to monitor changes in cerebrovascular resistance include transcranial Doppler.

As the CPP decreases, autoregulation fails and CBF decreases. Normal CPP is 70 to 100 mm Hg. At least 50 to 60 mm Hg is necessary for adequate cerebral perfusion. CPP less than 50 mm Hg is associated with ischemia and neuronal death. A CPP below 30 mm Hg results in cellular ischemia and is incompatible with life. Under normal circumstances, autoregulation maintains an adequate CBF and perfusion pressure primarily by cerebral vasoreactivity and metabolic adjustments that impact ICP. It is of paramount importance to maintain MAP when ICP is elevated. It should be remembered that CPP does not reflect perfusion pressure in all parts of the brain. There may be local areas of swelling and compression limiting regional perfusion pressure. Thus a higher CPP may be needed for these patients to prevent localized tissue damage.

Pressure Changes. The relationship of pressure to volume is depicted in the pressure-volume curve. The curve is affected by the brain's elastance and compliance. *Elastance* is the brain's ability to accommodate changes in volume. It represents the stiffness of the brain. With high elastance, large increases in pressure occur with small increases in volume.

$$Elastance = Pressure/Volume$$

Compliance is the inverse of elastance and is the expandability of the brain. It is represented as the volume increase for each unit increase in pressure. Low compliance is the same as high elastance. With low compliance, high changes in pressure result from small changes in volume.

$$Compliance = Volume/Pressure$$

The concept of the pressure-volume curve can be used to represent the stages of increased ICP (intracranial hypertension) (Fig. 55-2). At stage 1 on the curve, there is high compliance and low elastance. The brain is in total compensation, with accommodation and autoregulation intact. An increase in volume (in any of the three volume components) does not increase the ICP. At stage 2, the compliance is lower and elastance is increasing. An increase in volume places the patient at risk of increased ICP.

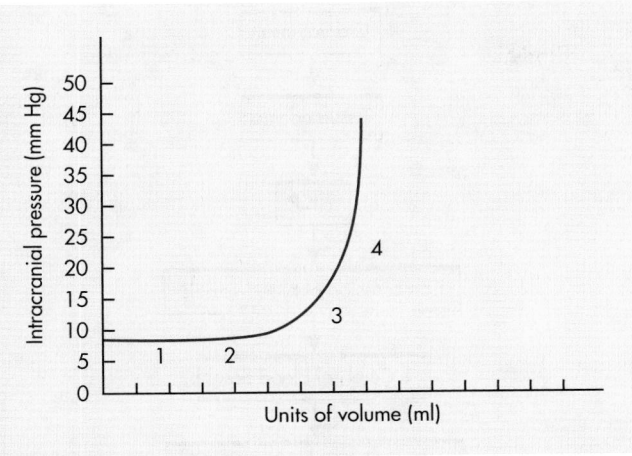

FIG. 55-2 Intracranial volume-pressure curve. (See text for descriptions of *1, 2, 3,* and *4.*)

At stage 3, there is high elastance and low compliance. Any small addition of volume causes a great increase in pressure. Compensatory mechanisms fail, there is a loss of autoregulation, and the patient may exhibit symptoms indicating increased ICP, such as changes in mentation or level of consciousness, headache, or pupillary responsiveness.

With a loss of autoregulation and a rise in systolic blood pressure as a result of the Cushing response, decompensation occurs. The Cushing triad includes systolic hypertension with an increased pulse pressure, bradycardia, and irregular respiratory rate.

As the patient enters stage 4, the ICP rises to terminal levels with little increase in volume. Herniation occurs as the brain tissue shifts from the compartment of greater pressure to a compartment of lesser pressure.

Factors Affecting Cerebral Blood Flow. Carbon dioxide, oxygen, and hydrogen ion concentration affect cerebral vessel tone. The partial pressure of arterial carbon dioxide ($PaCO_2$) is a potent vasoactive agent. An increase in $PaCO_2$ relaxes smooth muscle, dilates cerebral vessels, decreases cerebrovascular resistance, and increases CBF. Alternately, a decrease in $PaCO_2$ reverses this process and decreases CBF. Cerebral oxygen tension below 50 mm Hg results in cerebral vascular dilation. This dilation decreases cerebral vascular resistance, increases CBF, and raises oxygen tension. However, if oxygen tension is not raised, anaerobic metabolism begins, resulting in an accumulation of lactic acid. As lactic acid increases and hydrogen ions accumulate, the environment becomes more acidic. Within this acidic environment, further vasodilation occurs in a continued attempt to increase blood flow. The combination of a severely low arterial oxygen pressure ($PaCO_2$) and an elevated hydrogen ion concentration (acidosis), which are both potent cerebral vasodilators, may produce a state wherein autoregulation is lost and compensatory mechanisms fail to meet tissue metabolic demands.[1]

CBF can be globally affected by cardiac or respiratory arrest, systemic hemorrhage, and other pathophysiologic states (e.g., diabetic coma, encephalopathies, infections, toxicities). Regional CBF can also be affected by trauma, tumors, cerebral hemorrhage, or stroke. When regional or global autoregulation is lost, CBF is no longer maintained at a constant level but is directly in-

fluenced by changes in systemic blood pressure, hypoxia, or catecholamines.

INCREASED INTRACRANIAL PRESSURE

Increased ICP is a life-threatening situation that results from an increase in any or all of the three components (brain tissue, blood, CSF) of the skull. Cerebral edema is an important factor contributing to increased ICP.

Cerebral Edema

As shown in Table 55-2 there are a variety of causes of **cerebral edema** (increased accumulation of fluid in the extravascular spaces of brain tissue). Regardless of the cause, cerebral edema results in an increase in tissue volume that carries the potential for increased ICP. The extent and severity of the original insult are factors that determine the degree of cerebral edema.

Three types of cerebral edema have been distinguished: vasogenic, cytotoxic, and interstitial edema.[3] More than one type may result from a single insult in the same patient.

Vasogenic Cerebral Edema. *Vasogenic cerebral edema,* the most common type of edema, occurs mainly in the white matter and is attributed to changes in the endothelial lining of cerebral capillaries. These changes allow leakage of macromolecules from the capillaries into the surrounding extracellular space, resulting in an osmotic gradient that favors the flow of water from the intravascular to the extravascular space. A variety of insults, such as brain tumors, abscesses, and ingested toxins, may cause an increase in the permeability of the blood-brain barrier and produce an increase in the extracellular fluid volume. The speed and extent of the spread of the edema fluid are influenced by the systemic blood pressure, the site of the brain injury, and the extent of the blood-brain barrier defect. This edema may produce a con-

TABLE 55-2   Causes of Cerebral Edema

Mass Lesions
Brain abscess
Brain tumor (primary or metastatic)
Hematoma (intracerebral, subdural, epidural)
Hemorrhage (intracerebral, cerebellar, brainstem)

Head Injuries
Contusion
Hemorrhage
Posttraumatic brain swelling

Brain Surgery

Cerebral Infections
Meningitis
Encephalitis

Vascular Insult
Anoxic and ischemic episodes
Cerebral infarction (thrombotic or embolic)
Venous sinus thrombosis

Toxic or Metabolic Encephalopathic Conditions
Lead or arsenic intoxication
Hepatic encephalopathy
Uremia

tinuum of symptoms ranging from focal neurologic deficits to disturbances in consciousness, including **coma** (profound state of unconsciousness).

Cytotoxic Cerebral Edema. *Cytotoxic cerebral edema* results from local disruption of the functional or morphologic integrity of cell membranes and occurs most often in the gray matter. Cytotoxic cerebral edema develops from destructive lesions or trauma to brain tissue resulting in cerebral hypoxia or anoxia, sodium depletion, and syndrome of inappropriate antidiuretic hormone (SIADH). Cerebral edema results as fluid and protein shift from the extracellular space directly into the cells, with subsequent swelling and loss of cellular function.

Interstitial Cerebral Edema. *Interstitial cerebral edema* is the result of periventricular diffusion of ventricular CSF in a patient with uncontrolled hydrocephalus. It can also be caused by enlargement of the extracellular space as a result of systemic water excess (hyponatremia). Fluid moves into the cells to equilibrate with the hypoosmotic interstitial fluid. Regardless of the cause of cerebral edema, manifestations of increased ICP result, unless compensation is adequate.

Mechanisms of Increased Intracranial Pressure

Elevated ICP (above the threshold of 20 mm Hg) is clinically significant because it diminishes CPP, increases risks of brain ischemia and infarction, and is associated with a poor prognosis.[4] Increased ICP can be caused by several clinical problems, including a mass lesion (e.g., hematoma, contusion, abscess, tumor), cerebral edema (associated with brain tumors, hydrocephalus, head injury, or brain inflammation), or metabolic insult. These cerebral insults may result in hypercapnia, cerebral acidosis, impaired autoregulation, and systemic hypertension, which promote the formation and spread of cerebral edema. This edema distorts brain tissue, further increasing the ICP, which leads to even more tissue hypoxia and acidosis. Fig. 55-3 illustrates the progression of increased ICP.

Crucial to preservation of tissue is maintenance of CBF. Elevations in pressure that are more evenly distributed throughout the brain or slow increases in ICP (e.g., an enlarging brain lesion) preserve blood flow better than a rapid increase, as in primary brain injury. Sustained increases in ICP result in brainstem compression and herniation of the brain from one compartment to another.

Displacement and herniation of brain tissue cause a potentially reversible pathophysiologic process to become irreversible. Ischemia and edema are further increased, compounding the preexisting problem. Compression of the brainstem and cranial nerves may be fatal. Fig. 55-4 illustrates herniation. Herniations force the cerebellum and brainstem downward through the foramen magnum. If compression of the brainstem is unrelieved, respiratory arrest may occur.

Clinical Manifestations

The clinical manifestations of increased ICP can take many forms, depending on the cause, location, and rate at which the pressure increase occurs (Fig. 55-5). The earlier the condition is recognized and treated, the better the prognosis. The clinical manifestations of increased ICP are discussed below.

Change in Level of Consciousness. The *level of consciousness* (LOC) is a sensitive and important indicator of the pa-

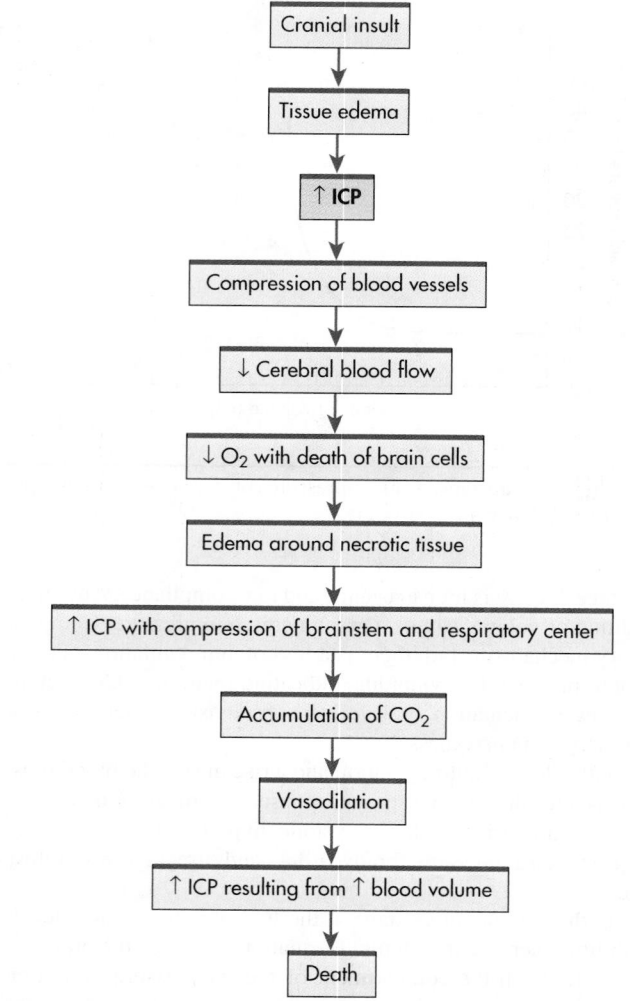

FIG. 55-3 Progression of increased intracranial pressure.

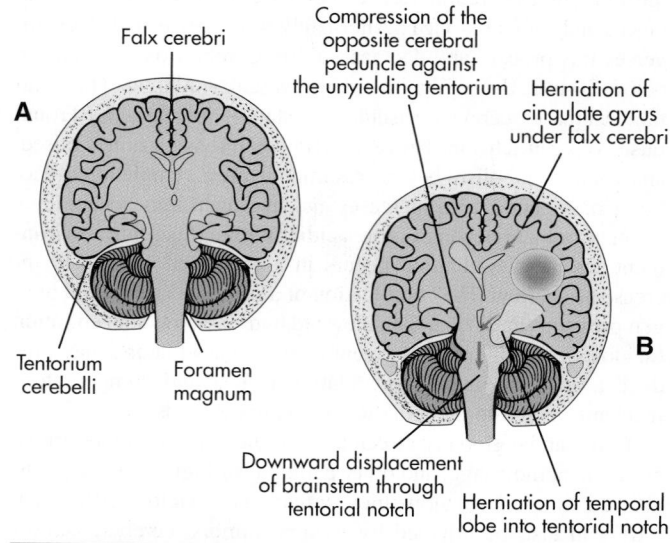

FIG. 55-4 Herniation. **A,** Normal relationship of intracranial structures. **B,** Shift of intracranial structures.

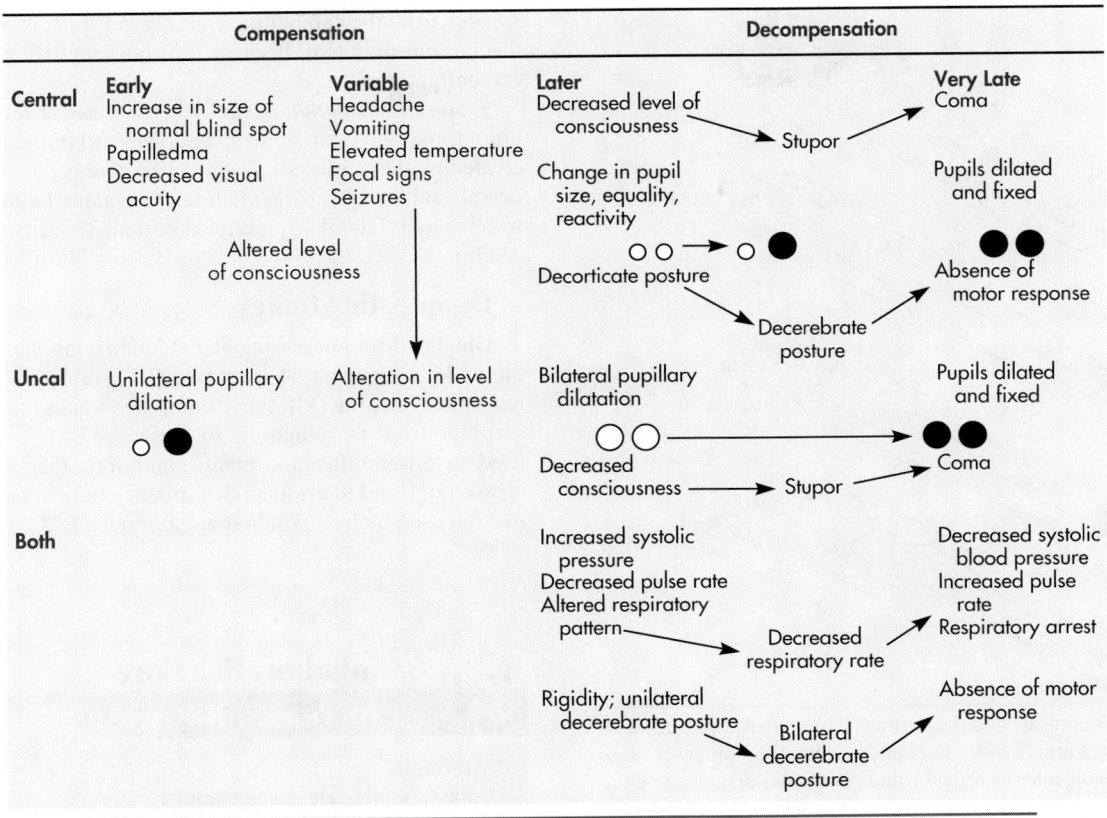

	Compensation		Decompensation	
Central	**Early** Increase in size of normal blind spot Papilledma Decreased visual acuity	**Variable** Headache Vomiting Elevated temperature Focal signs Seizures	**Later** Decreased level of consciousness → Stupor Change in pupil size, equality, reactivity Decorticate posture → Decerebrate posture	**Very Late** Coma Pupils dilated and fixed Absence of motor response
		Altered level of consciousness		
Uncal	Unilateral pupillary dilation	Alteration in level of consciousness	Bilateral pupillary dilatation Decreased consciousness → Stupor → Coma	Pupils dilated and fixed Coma
Both			Increased systolic pressure Decreased pulse rate Altered respiratory pattern → Decreased respiratory rate Rigidity; unilateral decerebrate posture → Bilateral decerebrate posture	Decreased systolic blood pressure Increased pulse rate Respiratory arrest Absence of motor response

FIG. 55-5   Clinical manifestations of increased intracranial pressure.

tient's neurologic status. Changes in LOC are a result of impaired CBF, which affects the cells of the cerebral cortex and the reticular activating system (RAS). The RAS is located in the brainstem with neural connections to many parts of the nervous system. An intact RAS can maintain a state of wakefulness even in the absence of a functioning cerebral cortex.

Interruptions of impulses from the RAS or alteration of the functioning of the cerebral hemispheres can cause **unconsciousness** (abnormal state of complete or partial unawareness of self or environment).

The patient's state of consciousness is defined by both the behavior and the pattern of brain activity recorded by an electroencephalogram (EEG). The change in consciousness may be dramatic, as in coma, or subtle, such as a flattening of affect, change in orientation, or decrease in level of attention. In the deepest state of unconsciousness (i.e., coma), the patient does not respond to painful stimuli. Corneal and pupillary reflexes are absent. The patient cannot swallow or cough and is incontinent of urine and feces. The EEG pattern demonstrates decreased or absent neuronal activity.

Changes in Vital Signs. Changes in vital signs are caused by increasing pressure on the thalamus, hypothalamus, pons, and medulla. Manifestations such as Cushing triad consisting of increasing systolic pressure (widening pulse pressure), bradycardia with a full and bounding pulse, and irregular respiratory pattern may be present but often do not appear until ICP has been increased for some time or markedly increased suddenly (e.g., head trauma). A change in body temperature may also be noted.

Ocular Signs. Compression of the oculomotor nerve (cranial nerve [CN] III) results in dilation of the pupil ipsilateral to the mass or lesion, sluggish or no response to light, inability to move the eye upward, and ptosis of the eyelid. These signs can be the result of a shifting of the brain from the midline, a process that compresses the trunk of CN III, paralyzing the pupil sphincter. A fixed, unilaterally dilated pupil is a neurologic emergency that indicates herniation of the brain. Other cranial nerves may also be affected, such as the optic (CN II), trochlear (CN IV), and abducens (CN VI) nerves. Signs of dysfunction of these cranial nerves include blurred vision, diplopia, and changes in extraocular eye movements. Central herniation may initially manifest as sluggish but equal pupil response. Uncal herniation may cause a dilated unilateral pupil. *Papilledema*, a choked optic disc seen on retinal examination, is also noted and is a nonspecific sign associated with long-standing increased ICP.

Decrease in Motor Function. As the ICP continues to rise, the patient manifests changes in motor ability. A contralateral hemiparesis or hemiplegia may be seen, depending on the location of the source of the increased ICP. If painful stimuli are used to elicit a motor response, the patient may exhibit localization to the stimuli or a withdrawal from the stimuli. *Decorticate* (flexor) and *decerebrate* (extensor) posturing may also be elicited by noxious stimuli (Fig. 55-6). Decorticate posture consists of internal rotation and adduction of the arms with flexion of the elbows, wrists, and fingers as a result of interruption of voluntary motor tracts. Extension of the legs may also be seen. A decerebrate posture may indicate more serious damage and results from

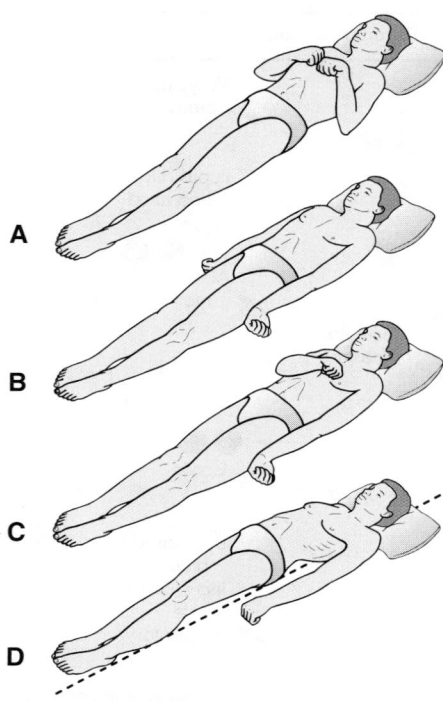

FIG. 55-6 Decorticate and decerebrate posturing. **A**, Decorticate response. Flexion of arms, wrists, and fingers with adduction in upper extremities. Extension, internal rotation, and plantar flexion in lower extremities. **B**, Decerebrate response. All four extremities in rigid extension, with hyperpronation of forearms and plantar flexion of feet. **C**, Decorticate response on right side of body and decerebrate response on left side of body. **D**, Opisthotonic posturing.

disruption of motor fibers in the midbrain and brainstem. In this position, the arms are stiffly extended, adducted, and hyperpronated. There is also hyperextension of the legs with plantar flexion of the feet.

Headache. Although the brain itself is insensitive to pain, compression of other intracranial structures, such as the walls of arteries and veins and the cranial nerves, can produce headache. The headache is often continuous but worse in the morning. Straining or movement may accentuate the pain.

Vomiting. Vomiting, usually not preceded by nausea, is often a nonspecific sign of increased ICP. This is called unexpected vomiting and is related to pressure changes in the cranium. Projectile vomiting may also be seen and is related to increased ICP.

It is often difficult to identify increased ICP as the cause of coma. Loss of consciousness also confuses the interpretation of clinical signs, making it difficult to follow the progression of the increasing ICP.

Complications

The major complications of uncontrolled increased ICP are inadequate cerebral perfusion and cerebral herniation (see Fig. 55-4). To better understand cerebral herniation, two important structures in the brain must be described. The *falx cerebri* is a thin wall of dura that folds down between the cortex, separating the two cerebral hemispheres. The *tentorium cerebelli* is a rigid fold of dura that separates the cerebral hemi-

spheres from the cerebellum (see Fig. 55-4). It is called the tentorium (meaning tent) because it forms a tentlike cover over the cerebellum.

Tentorial herniation occurs when a mass lesion in the cerebrum forces the brain to herniate downward through the opening created by the brainstem. *Uncal herniation* occurs when there is lateral and downward herniation. *Cingulate herniation* occurs when there is lateral displacement of brain tissue beneath the falx cerebri.

Diagnostic Studies

Diagnostic studies are aimed at identifying the presence and the underlying cause of increased ICP (Table 55-3). Magnetic resonance imaging (MRI) and computed tomography (CT) have revolutionized the diagnosis of increased ICP. These tests are used to differentiate the many conditions that can cause increased ICP and to evaluate therapeutic options. Other tests that may be used include cerebral angiography, EEG, ICP measure-

TABLE 55-3	*C*ollaborative Care — Increased Intracranial Pressure

Diagnostic
History and physical examination
Vital signs, neurologic assessments, ICP measurements
Skull, chest, and spinal x-ray studies
MRI, CT scan, PET, EEG, angiography
Transcranial Doppler studies
Laboratory studies, including CBC, coagulation profile, electrolytes, creatinine, ABGs, ammonia level, general drug and toxicology screen, CSF analysis for protein, cells, glucose
ECG

Collaborative Therapy
Elevation of head of bed to 30 degrees with head in a neutral position
ICP monitoring
Intubation and mechanical ventilation
Maintenance of PaO₂ at 100 mm Hg or greater
Maintenance of fluid balance and assessment of osmolality
Maintenance of systolic arterial pressure between 100 and 160 mm Hg
Maintenance of CPP >70 mm Hg
Reduction of cerebral metabolism (e.g., high-dose barbiturates)
Drug therapy
  Osmotic diuretics (mannitol)
  Loop diuretics (e.g., furosemide [Lasix], ethacrynic acid [Edecrin])
  Antiseizure drugs (e.g., phenytoin [Dilantin])
  Corticosteroids (dexamethasone [Decadron])
  Histamine H₂-receptor antagonist (e.g., cimetidine [Tagamet]) or proton pump inhibitor (e.g., omeprazole [Prilosec]) to prevent GI ulcers and bleeding

ABGs, Arterial blood gases; *CBC*, complete blood count; *CPP*, cerebral perfusion pressure; *CSF*, cerebrospinal fluid; *CT*, computed tomography; *ECG*, electrocardiogram; *EEG*, electroencephalogram; *GI*, gastrointestinal; *ICP*, intracranial pressure; *MRI*, magnetic resonance imaging; *PaO₂*, partial pressure of arterial oxygen; *PET*, positron emission tomography.

ment, transcranial Doppler studies, near-infrared spectroscopy for regional cerebral oxygenation, and evoked potential studies. Positron emission tomography (PET) is also used to diagnose the cause of increased ICP. In general, a lumbar puncture is not performed when increased ICP is suspected because of the possibility of cerebral herniation from the sudden release of the pressure in the skull from the area above the lumbar puncture.

Measurement of ICP

Indications for ICP Placement. ICP monitoring is used to guide clinical care when the patient is at risk for or has elevations in ICP. It may be used in patients with a variety of neurologic insults, including hemorrhage, stroke, tumor, infection, or traumatic brain injury. ICP should be monitored if patients are admitted with a Glasgow Coma Scale (GCS) score of 8 or less and an abnormal CT scan (hematomas, contusion, edema, or compressed basal cisterns).[5]

Methods of Measuring ICP. Multiple methods and devices are available to monitor ICP (Fig. 55-7).

The "gold standard" for monitoring ICP is the ventriculostomy, whereby a catheter is inserted into the lateral ventricle and coupled to an external transducer. This technique directly measures the pressure within the ventricles, facilitates removal and/or sampling of CSF, and allows for intraventricular drug administration. As with fluid-coupled blood pressure monitoring systems, signals can be distorted by excessive tube length or bubbles in the line. In these systems, the transducer is external, and its position must remain constant with respect to the patient's head to produce comparable pressures. An alternative technology, the fiberoptic catheter, uses a sensor transducer located within the catheter tip. The sensor tip is placed within the ventricle or the brain tissue and provides a direct measurement of brain pressure. Other less commonly used transducers include pneumatic systems and intracranial strain gauges. Similar to the fiberoptic system, these systems produce excellent quality waveforms, do not require repositioning with patient movement, and usually cannot be rezeroed.

Infection is a serious consideration with ICP monitoring. Infection rates are highest in fluid-coupled systems, with incidence rates ranging from 1% to 30%.[6] Prophylactic systemic antibiotics may be administered to reduce the chances of infection. Factors that contribute to the development of infection include ICP monitoring greater than 5 days, use of a ventriculostomy, the presence of a CSF leak, and a concurrent systemic infection. Routine care may include regular diagnostic testing for CSF organism growth.

ICP should be measured as a mean pressure at the end of expiration. If a CSF drainage device is in place, the drain must be closed for at least 6 minutes to ensure an accurate reading. The waveform strip should be recorded along with other pressure monitoring waveforms. The normal ICP waveform is shaped somewhat like an arterial pressure trace (Fig. 55-8, A), although the pressures are in a much lower range. This is because arterial pressure is transmitted to the choroid plexus and then to the CSF in the ventricular and subarachnoid spaces. When the waveform is monitored so that components in synchrony with the cardiac cycle can be visualized, the normal ICP waveform has three phases (Table 55-4).

It is important that the nurse monitor the ICP waveform, as well as mean CPP. It has been noted that when the height of P2 is higher than P1, the intracranial space may be noncompliant and the patient is at risk for development of elevated ICP (see Fig. 55-8, B). It is important to consider the rate at which changes occur and the patient's clinical condition. Neurologic deterioration might not occur until ICP elevation is pronounced and sustained. Any indication of ICP elevation, either as a mean increase in pressure or as an abnormal waveform configuration, should be reported to the health care provider immediately.

Inaccurate ICP readings can be caused by CSF leaks around the monitoring device, obstruction of the intraventricular catheter or bolt (from tissue or blood clot), difference between the height of the bolt and the transducer, and kinks in the tubing. In fluid-coupled systems, bubbles or air in the tubing also dampens the waveform.

CSF Drainage. With the ventricular catheter and certain fiberoptic systems, it is possible to control ICP by removing CSF.

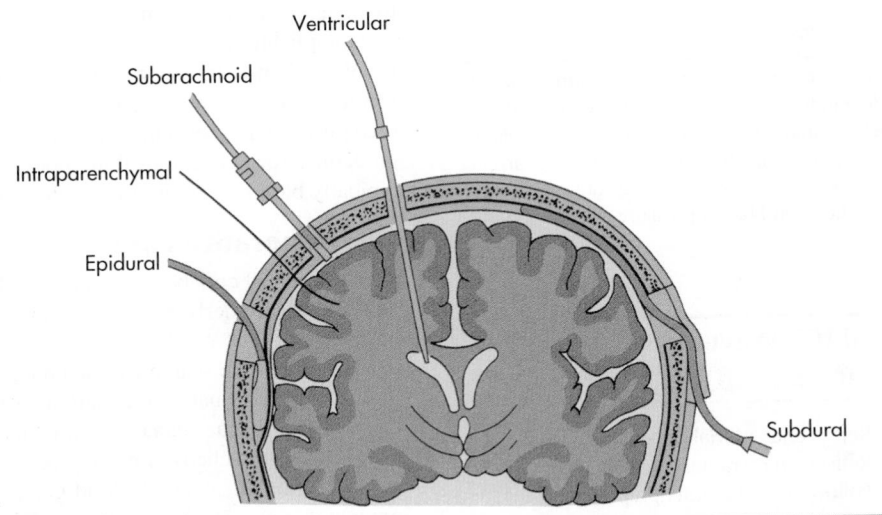

FIG. 55-7   Coronal section of brain showing potential sites for placement of ICP monitoring devices.

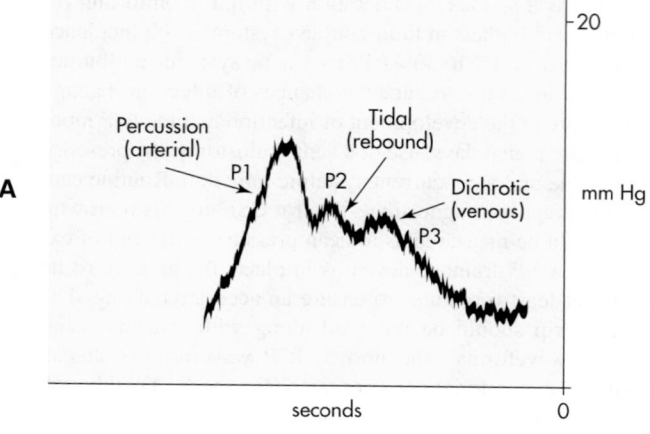

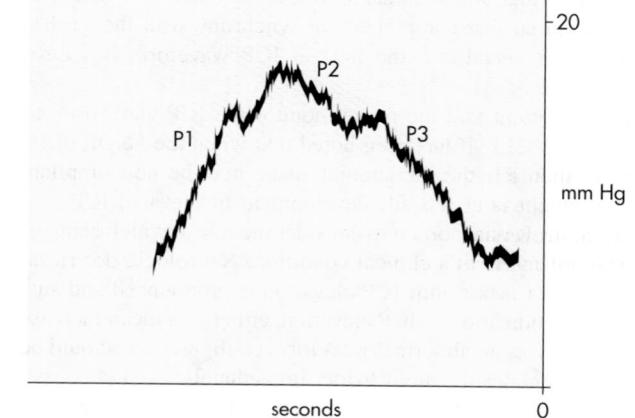

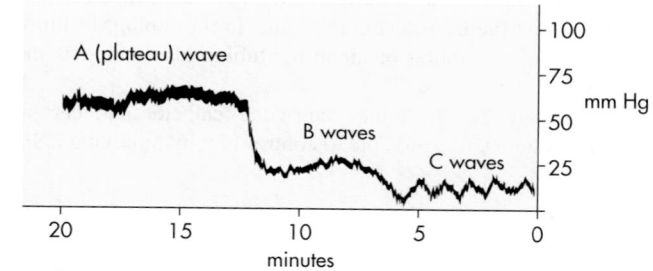

FIG. 55-8   A, Normal intracranial pressure (ICP) waveform as noted on a fast time scale recording indicating P1, P2, P3 (see Table 55-4). B, Abnormal ICP waveform indicating high pressure and noncompliant brain. C, Pathologic ICP waveforms. A (plateau) waves indicate sharp increases in ICP. B waves often precede A waves. C waves are related to normal fluctuations in respirations and blood pressure.

TABLE 55-4	Normal ICP Waveforms*
WAVEFORM	**MEANING**
P1 percussion wave	Represents arterial pulsations
P2 rebound wave	Reflects intracranial compliance
P3 dicrotic wave	Follows dicrotic notch; represents venous pulsations

*See Fig. 55-8.

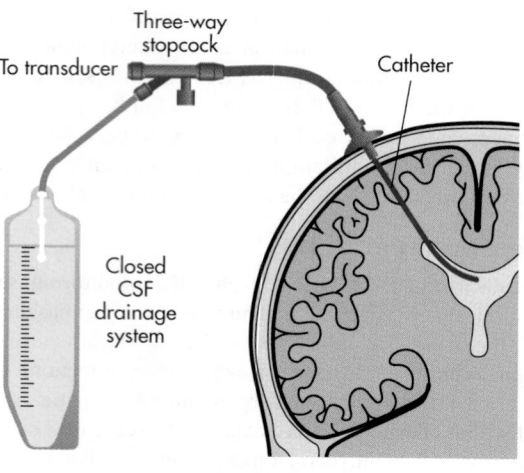

Intraventricular catheter

FIG. 55-9   Intermittent drainage system. CSF is drained via a ventriculostomy when ICP exceeds the upper pressure parameter set by the physician. The three-way stopcock is opened to allow CSF to flow into the draining bag for brief periods (30 to 120 seconds) until the pressure is below the upper pressure parameters.

To do this, a Y connector is inserted in the line (Fig. 55-9). Using a closed system, elevations in ICP are controlled by removal of CSF by gravity drainage and by adjusting the height of the drip chamber and drainage bag relative to the patient's ventricular reference point. Typically a point 15 cm above the ear canal (foramen of Monroe) is selected. Raising the system diminishes drainage, whereas lowering the system increases drainage volume. Careful monitoring of the volume of CSF drained is essential, keeping in mind that normal adult CSF production is about 20 to 30 ml per hour, with a total CSF volume of 90 to 150 ml within the ventricles and subarachnoid space. The level of the ICP to initiate drainage, amount of fluid to be drained, height of the system, and frequency of drainage are ordered by the physician. Prevention of infection by use of strict aseptic technique during dressing changes or sampling of CSF is imperative. The system must remain intact to ensure that the ICP readings are accurate because treatment is initiated on the basis of the level of the pressures.

Complications of this type of drainage system include ventricular collapse, infection, and herniation or subdural hematoma formation from rapid decompression. Although it is generally recognized that CSF removal decreases ICP and improves CPP, guidelines for CSF removal are not universally accepted but are typically based on institution or physician preference.[7]

Collaborative Care

The goals of collaborative care (see Table 55-3) are to identify and treat the underlying cause of increased ICP and to support brain function. A careful history is an important diagnostic aid that can direct the search for the underlying cause.

Ensuring adequate oxygenation to support brain function is the first step in the management of increased ICP. An endotracheal tube or tracheostomy may be necessary to maintain adequate ventilation. Arterial blood gas (ABG) analysis guides the oxygen therapy. The goal is to maintain the PaO_2 at 100 mm Hg or greater. It may be necessary to maintain the patient on a mechanical ventilator to ensure adequate oxygenation.

If the condition is caused by a mass lesion, such as a tumor or hematoma, surgical removal of the mass is the best management (see Brain Tumors and Cranial Surgery later in this chapter). Nonsurgical intervention for the reduction of tissue volume related to cerebral tissue swelling and cerebral edema includes the use of diuretics and corticosteroids.

Drug Therapy. Drug therapy plays an important part in the management of increased ICP. Mannitol (Osmitrol), glycerol, and urea are used as osmotic diuretics. Mannitol (25%) is the most widely used agent and is given intravenously. Mannitol acts to decrease the ICP in two ways: plasma expansion and osmotic effect. There is an immediate plasma-expanding effect that reduces the hematocrit and blood viscosity, thereby increasing CBF and cerebral oxygen delivery. A vascular osmotic gradient is created by mannitol. Thus fluid moves from the tissues into the blood vessels. Therefore the ICP is reduced by a decrease in the total brain fluid content. Fluid and electrolyte status must be monitored when osmotic diuretics are used. Mannitol may be contraindicated if renal disease is present and if serum osmolality is elevated.[8]

Loop diuretics such as furosemide (Lasix), bumetanide (Bumex), and ethacrynic acid (Edecrin) may also be used in the management of increased ICP. These diuretics inhibit sodium and chloride reabsorption in the ascending limb of the loop of Henle and thus reduce blood volume and, ultimately, tissue volume. In addition, these agents cause a reduction in the rate of CSF production, which also contributes to the reduction in ICP.[3]

Corticosteroids (e.g., dexamethasone [Decadron]) are thought to control the vasogenic edema surrounding tumors and abscesses but appear to have limited value in the management of head-injured patients. The mode of action of corticosteroids is not completely known. It is theorized that they act by their stabilizing effect on the cell membrane and by inhibiting the synthesis of prostaglandins (see Chapter 12, Fig. 12-7), thus preventing the formation of proinflammatory mediators. Corticosteroids are also thought to improve neuronal function by improving CBF and restoring autoregulation.

Complications associated with the use of corticosteroids include hyperglycemia, increased incidence of infections, gastrointestinal (GI) bleeding, and hyponatremia. Fluid intake and sodium and glucose levels should be monitored regularly. Patients receiving corticosteroids should concurrently be given antacids or histamine H_2 receptor blockers (e.g., cimetidine [Tagamet]) or proton pump inhibitors (e.g., omeprazole [Prilosec]) to prevent GI ulcers and bleeding.

Drug therapy for reducing cerebral metabolism may be an effective strategy to control ICP. The reduction in the metabolic rate decreases the CBF and therefore the ICP. High-dose barbiturates (e.g., pentobarbital [Nembutal], thiopental [Pentothal]) are used in patients with increased ICP refractory to treatment. Barbiturates produce a decrease in cerebral metabolism and a subsequent decrease in ICP. A secondary effect is a reduction in cerebral edema and production of a more uniform blood supply to the brain.[3] Capabilities to monitor the patient's ICP, blood flow, EEG, and metabolism should be available when this treatment is used. Antiseizure drugs such as phenytoin (Dilantin) may be used because seizures can further increase ICP.

Hyperventilation Therapy. In the past, aggressive hyperventilation ($PaCO_2$ <25 mm Hg) had been a mainstay treatment of elevated ICP. The lowering of the $PaCO_2$ leads to constriction of the cerebral blood vessels, reducing CBF and thereby decreasing the ICP. More recent evidence suggests that aggressive hyperventilation increases the risk of focal cerebral ischemia and may adversely affect outcomes.[3] Prolonged aggressive hyperventilation therapy should be avoided in the absence of increased ICP, particularly during the first 24 hours following a head injury or when CBF is low. Brief periods of hyperventilation therapy may be useful for refractory intracranial hypertension.[3,5]

Nutritional Therapy. All patients must have their nutritional needs met, regardless of their state of consciousness or health. Early feeding following brain injury improves outcomes[9] (see the Evidence-Based Practice box). The patient with increased ICP is in a hypermetabolic and hypercatabolic state that increases the need for glucose to provide the necessary fuel for metabolism of the injured brain. If the patient cannot maintain an adequate oral intake, other means of meeting the nutritional requirements, such as enteral feedings or total parenteral nutrition, should be initiated. Nutritional replacements should begin within 3 days after injury to reach full nutritional replacement within 7 days after injury.[9] Because malnutrition promotes continued cerebral edema, maintenance of optimal nutrition is imperative. (Nutritional therapy is discussed in Chapter 39.) Feedings or supplements should be guided by the patient's fluid and electrolyte status, as well as the patient's metabolic needs.

It is controversial as to whether patients should be maintained in a state of moderate dehydration. On one hand, moderate dehydration is thought to be effective in reducing cerebral edema; in this case, fluids are restricted to 65% to 75% of normal requirements. However, the concern is that hypovolemia may result in a decrease in cardiac output and blood pressure, which may affect cerebral perfusion and the amount of oxygen delivered to the brain. There is additional concern that dehydrated patients do not respond well to vasoactive drugs. Because of this, the current therapy is directed at keeping patients normovolemic. The use of

---

$\mathcal{E}$VIDENCE-BASED PRACTICE
Nutritional Support Following Head Injury

Clinical Problem
Does nutritional support following head injury affect mortality and morbidity?

Best Clinical Practice
- Early feeding is associated with better outcomes in terms of survival and disability.
- Nutritional support can include parenteral nutrition or enteral nutrition (nasogastric or nasojejunal), depending on the condition of the patient and presence of bowel sounds.

Implications for Nursing Practice
- Head injury increases the body's metabolic responses and therefore nutritional demands.
- Provision of an adequate supply of nutrients is associated with improved outcome.
- The nurse must assess the nutritional status of the patient with a head injury and ensure that the patient receives adequate nutrition.

Reference for Evidence
Yanagawa T et al: Nutritional support for head-injured patients, *Cochrane Database Syst Rev,* Issue 3, 2002.

fluid restriction to reduce tissue volume should be evaluated on the basis of clinical factors such as urine output, insensible fluid loss, serum and urine osmolality, and the condition of the patient. Intravenous (IV) 0.45% or 0.9% sodium chloride is the preferred solution for administration of piggyback medications because a lowering of serum osmolarity and an increase in cerebral edema occur if 5% dextrose in water is used.

NURSING MANAGEMENT
INCREASED INTRACRANIAL PRESSURE

■ Nursing Assessment

Subjective data about the patient with increased ICP can be obtained from the patient or family members or other persons who are familiar with the patient. The nurse must learn appropriate assessment techniques and describe the LOC by noting the specific behaviors observed. When a deviation from the normal state of consciousness occurs, a more structured method of observation should be initiated. This type of systematic approach to nursing assessment is illustrated in Fig. 55-10 and consists of assessing the LOC by the GCS (Table 55-5) and by body functions. Adequate circulation and respiration are the most vital and should always be the first body functions assessed.

Glasgow Coma Scale. Because of the confusion and ambiguity that surround terms describing altered states of consciousness, the GCS was developed in 1974. The **Glasgow Coma Scale** is a quick, practical, and standardized system for assessing the degree of consciousness impairment. The three areas assessed in the GCS correspond to the definition of coma as the inability of a patient to speak, obey commands, or open the eyes when a verbal or painful stimulus is applied.[10] Specific assessments evaluate the patient's response to varying degrees of stimuli. Three indicators of response are evaluated: (1) opening of the eyes, (2) the best verbal response, and (3) the best motor response (see Table 55-5). Specific behaviors that are seen as responses to the testing stimulus in each of these three areas are given a numeric value and can be plotted on a graph. The nurse's responsibility is to elicit the best response on each of the scales: the higher the scores, the higher the level of brain functioning. A graph can be used to determine whether the patient is stable, improving, or deteriorating. The subscale scores are particularly important if a patient is untestable in one area. For example, severe periorbital edema may make eye opening impossible. The total GCS score is a sum of the numeric values assigned to each of the three areas evaluated. The highest GCS score is 15 for a fully alert person, and the lowest possible score is 3. A GCS score of 8 or less is generally indicative of coma.[11]

The GCS offers several advantages in the assessment of the unconscious patient. It is specific and structured, allowing different health care professionals to arrive at the same conclusion regarding the patient's status. It saves time for the assessor because the ratings are done with numbers rather than with lengthy descriptions.

The GCS is also specific enough to discriminate between different or changing states. The GCS is used to assess the arousal aspect of consciousness. Other components of the neurologic assessment include pupillary checks, extremity strength testing, and, if appropriate, corneal reflex testing.

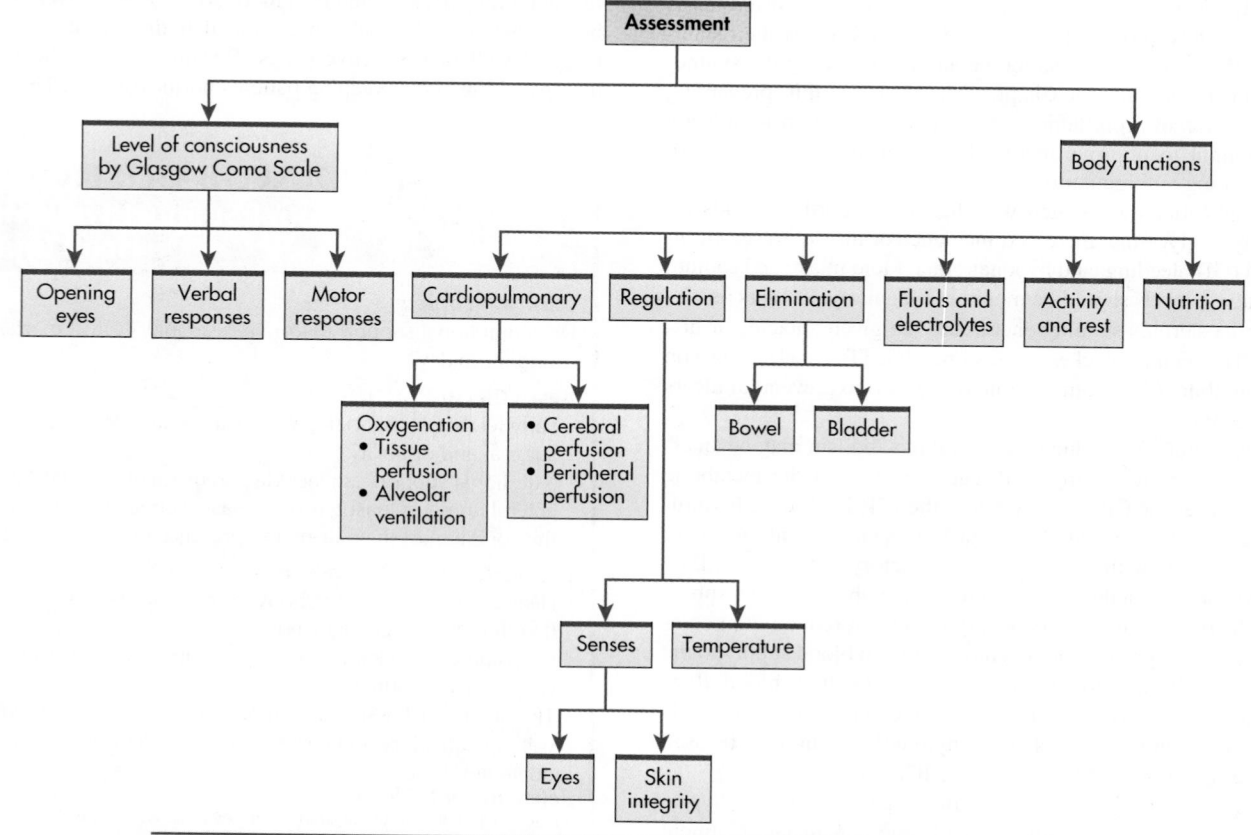

FIG. 55-10 Systematic approach to nursing assessment of the unconscious patient.

TABLE 55-5   Glasgow Coma Scale

CATEGORY OF RESPONSE	APPROPRIATE STIMULUS	RESPONSE	SCORE
Eyes Open	• Approach to bedside • Verbal command • Pain	Spontaneous response	4
		Opening of eyes to name or command	3
		Lack of opening of eyes to previous stimuli but opening to pain	2
		Lack of opening of eyes to any stimulus	1
		Untestable	U
Best Verbal Response	• Verbal questioning with maximum arousal	Appropriate orientation, conversant, correct identification of self, place, year, and month	5
		Confusion, conversant, but disorientation in one or more spheres	4
		Inappropriate or disorganized use of words (e.g., cursing), lack of sustained conversation	3
		Incomprehensible words, sounds (e.g., moaning)	2
		Lack of sound, even with painful stimuli	1
		Untestable	U
Best Motor Response	• Verbal command (e.g., "raise your arm, hold up two fingers") • Pain (pressure on proximal nailbed)	Obedience of command	6
		Localization of pain, lack of obedience but presence of attempts to remove offending stimulus	5
		Flexion withdrawal,* flexion of arm in response to pain without abnormal flexion posture	4
		Abnormal flexion, flexing of arm at elbow and pronation, making a fist	3
		Abnormal extension, extension of arm at elbow usually with adduction and internal rotation of arm at shoulder	2
		Lack of response	1
		Untestable	U

*Added to the original scale by many centers.

Neurologic Assessment. The pupils are compared to one another for size, movement, and response (Fig. 55-11). If the oculomotor nerve is compressed, the pupil on the affected side (ipsilateral) becomes larger until it fully dilates. If ICP continues to increase, both pupils dilate.

Pupillary reaction is tested with a flashlight. The normal reaction is brisk constriction when the light is shone directly into the eye. A consensual response (a slight constriction in the opposite pupil) should also be noted at the same time. A sluggish reaction can indicate early pressure on cranial nerve III. A fixed pupil shows no response to light stimulus, which usually indicates increased ICP.

Evaluation of other cranial nerves can be included in the neurologic check. Eye movements controlled by cranial nerves III, IV, and VI can be examined in the patient who is awake and can be used to assess the function of the brainstem. In the unconscious patient, extraocular eye movements are not specifically tested. Testing the corneal reflex gives information on the functioning of cranial nerves V and VII. If this reflex is absent, routine eye care should be initiated to prevent corneal abrasion (see Chapters 20 and 21).

Eye movements of the uncooperative or unconscious patient can be elicited by reflex with the use of head movements (oculocephalic) and caloric stimulation (oculovestibular) (see Chapters 20 and 21). To test the oculocephalic reflex (doll's head or doll's

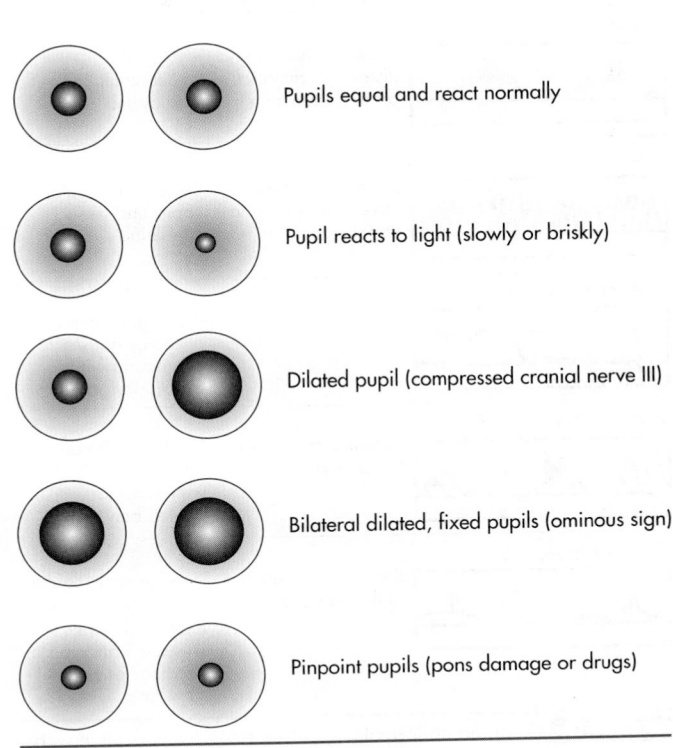

Pupils equal and react normally

Pupil reacts to light (slowly or briskly)

Dilated pupil (compressed cranial nerve III)

Bilateral dilated, fixed pupils (ominous sign)

Pinpoint pupils (pons damage or drugs)

FIG. 55-11 Pupillary check for size and response.

eyes phenomenon), the nurse rotates the patient's head briskly while holding the eyelids open. A positive response is movement of the eyes across the midline in the direction opposite that of the rotation. Next, the nurse quickly flexes and then extends the neck. Eye movement should be opposite to the direction of head movement—up when the neck is flexed and down when it is extended. Abnormal responses can aid in locating the intracranial lesion. This test should not be attempted if a cervical spine problem is suspected. (The oculovestibular reflex is discussed in Chapter 20.)

Motor strength is tested by asking the awake patient to squeeze the nurse's hands to compare strength in the hands. The palmar drift test is an excellent measure of strength in the upper extremities. The patient raises the arms in front of the body with the palmar surface facing upward. If there is any weakness in the upper extremity, the palmar surface turns downward and the arm drifts downward. Asking the patient to raise the foot from the bed or to bend the knees up in bed is a good assessment of lower extremity strength. All four extremities should be tested for strength and evaluated for any asymmetry in strength or movement.

The motor strength of the unconscious or uncooperative patient can be assessed by observation of spontaneous movement. If no spontaneous movement is possible, a pain stimulus should be applied to the patient, and the response should be noted. Resistance to movement during passive range-of-motion exercises is another measure of strength.

The vital signs, including blood pressure, pulse, respiratory rate, and temperature, should also be systematically recorded. The nurse must be aware of Cushing triad because this indicates severe increased ICP. Besides recording respiratory rate, the nurse should also note the respiratory pattern (Fig. 55-12).

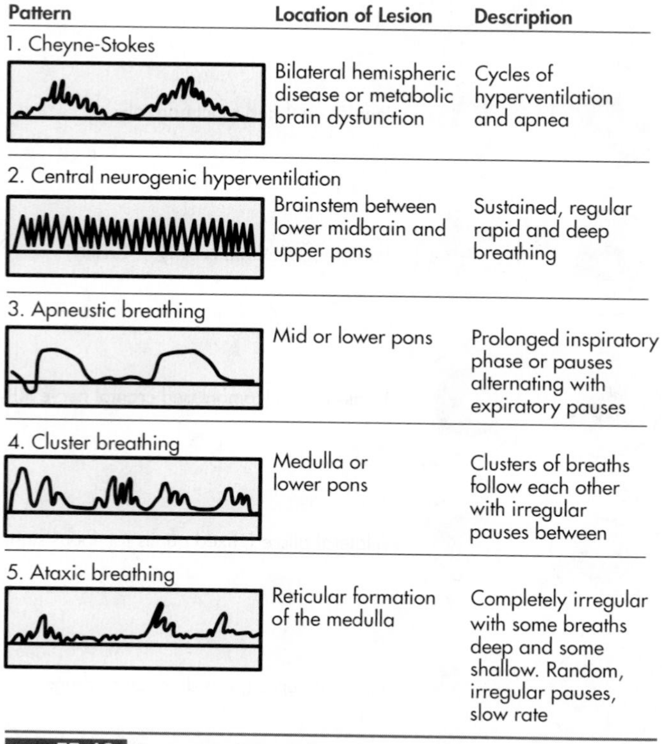

Pattern	Location of Lesion	Description
1. Cheyne-Stokes	Bilateral hemispheric disease or metabolic brain dysfunction	Cycles of hyperventilation and apnea
2. Central neurogenic hyperventilation	Brainstem between lower midbrain and upper pons	Sustained, regular rapid and deep breathing
3. Apneustic breathing	Mid or lower pons	Prolonged inspiratory phase or pauses alternating with expiratory pauses
4. Cluster breathing	Medulla or lower pons	Clusters of breaths follow each other with irregular pauses between
5. Ataxic breathing	Reticular formation of the medulla	Completely irregular with some breaths deep and some shallow. Random, irregular pauses, slow rate

FIG. 55-12 Common abnormal respiratory patterns associated with coma.

■ Nursing Diagnoses

Nursing diagnoses for the patient with increased ICP include, but are not limited to, those presented in NCP 55-1.

■ Planning

The overall goals are that the patient with increased ICP will (1) have ICP within normal limits, (2) maintain a patent airway, (3) demonstrate normal fluid and electrolyte balance, and (4) have no complications secondary to immobility and decreased LOC.

■ Nursing Implementation

Acute Intervention

Respiratory function. Maintenance of a patent airway is critical in the patient with increased ICP and is a primary nursing responsibility. As the LOC decreases, the patient is at increased risk of airway obstruction from the tongue dropping back and occluding the airway or from accumulation of secretions. Altered breathing patterns may become evident. Airway patency can be aided by keeping the patient lying on one side, with frequent position changes. Snoring sounds, which may indicate obstruction, should be noted. Accumulated secretions should be removed by suctioning, as needed. An oral airway facilitates breathing and provides an easier suctioning route in the comatose patient.

The nurse must use measures to prevent hypoxia and hypercapnia. Proper positioning of the head is important. Elevation of the head of the bed by 30 degrees enhances respiratory exchange and aids in decreasing cerebral edema. Suctioning and coughing can cause transient decreases in the PaO_2 and increases in the ICP. Suctioning should be kept to a minimum and should be less than 10 seconds in duration, with administration of 100% oxygen before and after to prevent decreases in the PaO_2.[12] To avoid cumulative increases in the ICP with suctioning, suctioning should be limited to two passes per suction procedure. Patients with elevated ICP are at risk for lower CPP during suctioning.[13]

Abdominal distention can interfere with respiratory function and should be prevented. Insertion of a nasogastric tube to aspirate the stomach contents can prevent distention, vomiting, and possible aspiration. However, in patients with facial and skull fractures, a nasogastric tube is contraindicated, and oral insertion of a gastric tube is preferred.

Pain, anxiety, and fear from the initial injury, therapeutic procedures, or noxious stimuli can increase ICP and blood pressure, complicating the management and recovery of the brain-injured patient. The appropriate choice or combination of sedatives, paralytics, and analgesics for symptom management presents a challenge to the ICU team. Administration of these agents may alter the neurologic state, masking true neurologic changes. It may be necessary to temporarily suspend pharmacologic therapy to appropriately assess neurologic status. The choice, dose, and combination of agents may vary depending on the patient's history, neurologic state, and overall clinical presentation.

Narcotics, such as morphine sulfate, fentanyl (Actig, Duragesic), and sufentanil (Sufenta), are rapid-onset analgesics with minimal effect on CBF or oxygen metabolism. The IV anesthetic sedative propofol (Diprivan) has gained popularity in the management of pain and anxiety in the ICU because of its rapid onset, short half-life, and oxygen-saving properties. Unlike narcotics, it decreases the ICP, CBF, and oxygen metabolism. Nondepolarizing

NURSING CARE PLAN 55-1

Patient with Increased Intracranial Pressure

EXPECTED PATIENT OUTCOMES	NURSING INTERVENTIONS and *RATIONALES*
NURSING DIAGNOSIS	**Ineffective airway clearance** *related to* decreased level of consciousness (LOC), immobility, and inability to mobilize secretions *as manifested by* ineffective cough, inability to clear secretions, crackles on auscultation, thick secretions.
• Demonstration of increased air exchange as measured by ABGs within normal limits • Normal breath sounds in all lobes of the lungs	• Maintain patient's side-lying position, keeping head of bed elevated *to prevent aspiration and tongue from blocking airway.* • Suction frequently *to remove accumulated secretions, reduce risk of aspiration, and ensure patent airway.* • Perform chest physical therapy at least q4hr *to improve ventilation and prevent pulmonary complications.* • Monitor patient for signs of decreased oxygenation, including changes in LOC, decreased PaO_2 or SaO_2, and increased respiratory rate *as low as PaO_2 and a high hydrogen ion concentration (acidosis) are potent cerebral blood vasodilators that increase cerebral blood flow and may increase ICP.*
NURSING DIAGNOSIS	**Ineffective tissue perfusion (cerebral)** *related to* cerebral edema *as manifested by* Glasgow Coma Scale <8; agitation; elevated systolic blood pressure, bradycardia, and widened pulse pressure; intracranial pressure >20 mm Hg, CPP <60 mm Hg.
• No further deterioration in LOC • ICP <20 mm Hg, CPP >60 mm Hg • Stable vital signs	• Monitor patient's neurologic status at least every hour initially; assess LOC and document *to evaluate patient's response to treatment and modify if necessary.* • Monitor ICP and calculate CPP *to evaluate adequacy of cerebral blood perfusion and detect patient's response to treatment.* • Limit care activities that increase ICP (e.g., suctioning) *to prevent increases in ICP.* • Provide comfort measures *as pain or agitation increase ICP.* • Elevate head of bed 30 to 45 degrees *to facilitate reduction of cerebral edema.* • Monitor reactions to all medications (especially diuretics and sedatives) *to evaluate for signs (e.g., change in LOC) of reduced cerebral edema.* • Calibrate and maintain intracranial monitoring device *to provide an accurate indicator of ICP.*
NURSING DIAGNOSIS	**Impaired skin integrity** *related to* nutritional deficit, self-care deficit, and immobility *as manifested by* inability to move or change position, dry skin, weight loss >10 lb (4.5 kg), abrasions or lacerations.
• Absence of skin breakdown • Intact skin	• Assess skin frequently, especially over bony prominences and around genitalia and buttocks *to identify potential or actual skin problems and initiate a plan of care.* • Turn patient at least q2hr as indicated *as prolonged pressure decreases circulation and leads to tissue ischemia and necrosis.* • Use low-air-loss beds as indicated *to reduce pressure to bony prominences by distributing body weight evenly.* • Cleanse all abrasions and lacerations *to reduce risk of infection*; massage skin as indicated *to stimulate circulation.*
NURSING DIAGNOSIS	**Self-care deficit (total)** *related to* altered LOC *as manifested by* inability to follow commands or move purposefully, inability to perform ADLs.
• All ADLs met by caregivers until self-care is possible	• Assess level of motor and sensory abilities at least q4hr *to determine level of care needed.* • Bathe patient daily *to maintain hygienic needs.* • Perform ROM exercises at least q4hr as tolerated *to maintain joint ROM and muscle strength.* • Begin bowel program as soon as possible *to resume usual bowel elimination pattern and prevent constipation and impaction.* • Provide urinary catheter care *to reduce risk of infection.*

Continued

NURSING CARE PLAN 55-1

Patient with Increased Intracranial Pressure—cont'd

EXPECTED PATIENT OUTCOMES	NURSING INTERVENTIONS and *RATIONALES*
NURSING DIAGNOSIS	**Interrupted family processes** *related to* comatose family member *as manifested by* inability to adapt to health crisis of family member, lack of communication or miscommunication among family members.
• Verbalization of feelings by family members • Participation in care of ill member by family members • Use of appropriate referrals	• Assess effect of ill family member on family as a whole *to determine extent of problems and to plan appropriate interventions.* • Teach and assist family members to provide care to ill family members *to enable the family to be an integral part of patient's care.* • Facilitate family communication and realistic planning for needs of ill family member *so patient's care needs are met with minimal disruption to lives of other family members.* • Provide accurate information to family regarding patient's situation *to promote understanding and facilitate effective coping.* • Initiate referrals as indicated *so specialized care and instruction are provided as needed.*

COLLABORATIVE PROBLEM

NURSING GOALS	NURSING INTERVENTIONS and *RATIONALES*
POTENTIAL COMPLICATION	**Increased ICP** *related to* cerebral edema.
• Monitor for signs of increased ICP • Report deviations from acceptable parameters • Carry out appropriate medical and nursing interventions	• Assess for signs of increased ICP (e.g., altered LOC, headache, pupil inequality, decreased respirations and pulse rate, elevated systolic blood pressure with widened pulse pressure *to enable immediate reporting and initiation of treatment.* • Report significant changes *to enable prompt intervention and to prevent serious complications.* • Calibrate and maintain ICP monitoring equipment in functioning condition *to ensure accurate readings.* • Administer diuretics and corticosteroids as ordered *to reduce cerebral edema.* • Position patient with head of bed elevated to 30 degrees *to promote venous drainage from head, reducing cerebral edema.* • Manage elevated temperature *as elevated temperature increases cerebral metabolism and causes increased ICP.* • Use measures to decrease agitation and hyperactivity *to reduce risk of self-injury and to prevent increased ICP.*

neuromuscular blocking agents (e.g., vecuronium [Norcuron], pancuronium [Pavulon]) are useful for ventilatory management and treatment of refractory intracranial hypertension. Because these agents paralyze muscles without blocking pain or noxious stimuli, they are used in combination with sedatives, analgesics, or benzodiazepines. Benzodiazepines, although useful for symptom management and ventilatory support, are usually avoided in the management of the patient with increased ICP because of the hypotension effect and long half-life, unless used as an adjunct to neuromuscular blocking agents.

ABGs should be measured and evaluated regularly (see Chapter 25). The nurse should frequently monitor the ABG values and maintain the levels within prescribed or acceptable parameters. The appropriate ventilatory support can be ordered on the basis of the PaO_2 and $PaCO_2$ values.

Fluid and electrolyte balance. Fluid and electrolyte disturbances can have an adverse effect on ICP. IV fluids should be closely monitored with the use of a limited-volume device or a volume-control apparatus for accuracy. Intake and output, with insensible losses and daily weights taken into account, are important parameters in the assessment of fluid balance.

Electrolyte determinations should be made daily, and any abnormal values should be discussed with the physician. It is especially important to monitor serum glucose, sodium, potassium, and osmolality. Urinary output is monitored to detect problems related to *diabetes insipidus* (e.g., increased urinary output related to a decrease in antidiuretic hormone secretion) and SIADH (syndrome of inappropriate antidiuretic hormone), which results in decreased urinary output. Besides urinary output, the serum sodium and osmolality are also used to diagnose diabetes insipidus and SIADH. Diabetes insipidus may result in severe dehydration unless treated. The usual treatment is fluid replacement, vasopressin (Pitressin), or desmopressin acetate (DDAVP) (see Chapter 48). SIADH results in a dilutional hyponatremia that may produce cerebral edema, changes in LOC, seizures, and coma. (Treatment of SIADH is described in Chapter 48.)

Monitoring intracranial pressure. The measurement of ICP enhances clinical decision-making by detecting early signs of intracranial hypertension and response to therapy. ICP monitoring is used in combination with other physiologic parameters to guide the care of the patient and assess the patient's response to routine care. Valsalva maneuver, coughing, sneezing, hypoxemia, and arousal from sleep are factors that can increase ICP. Nurses should be alert to these factors and should attempt to minimize them. Nursing management of the patient with increased ICP is one of the most important aspects of the care provided these patients.

Body position. The patient with increased ICP should be maintained in the head-up position. The nurse must take care to prevent extreme neck flexion, which can cause venous obstruction and contribute to elevated ICP. The body position should be adjusted to decrease the ICP maximally and to improve the CPP. Traditional practice has been to elevate the head of the bed to 30 degrees, unless a concurrent cervical neck injury has been identified. Research now suggests there is an inconsistent response of the ICP and the CPP to head elevation.[3,14] Elevation of the head of the bed reduces sagittal sinus pressure, promotes venous drainage from the head via the valveless jugular system, and decreases the vascular congestion that can produce cerebral edema. However, raising the head of the bed above 30 degrees may decrease the CPP. There is no evidence, however, that head-of-bed elevation decreases cerebral tissue oxygenation.[3] Careful evaluation of the effects of elevation of the head of the bed on both the ICP and the CPP is required. The bed should be positioned so that it lowers the ICP while maintaining the CPP and other indices of cerebral oxygenation.

Care should be taken to turn the patient with slow, gentle movements because rapid changes in position may increase the ICP. Caution should be used to prevent discomfort in turning and positioning the patient because pain or agitation also increases pressure. Increased intrathoracic pressure contributes to increased ICP by impeding the venous return. Thus coughing, straining, and the Valsalva maneuver should be avoided. Extreme hip flexion should be avoided to decrease the risk of raising the intraabdominal pressure, which can restrict movement of the diaphragm and cause respiratory distress. The patient should be turned at least every 2 hours.

Decorticate or decerebrate posturing is a reflex response in some patients with increased ICP. Turning, skin care, and even passive range of motion can elicit the posturing reflexes. Attempts should be made to provide needed physical care activities to minimize complications of immobility, such as atelectasis and contractures. In cases of severe posturing reflexes, these activities may have to be done less frequently because posturing can cause increases in ICP.

Protection from injury. The patient with increased ICP and a decreased LOC needs protection from self-injury. Confusion, agitation, and the possibility of seizures can put the patient at risk for injury. Restraints should be used judiciously in the agitated patient. If restraints are absolutely necessary to keep the patient from removing tubes or falling out of bed, they should be secure enough to be effective, and the skin area under the restraints should be observed regularly for irritation. Agitation may increase with the use of restraints, which indicates the need for other measures to protect the patient from injury. Light sedation with agents such as haloperidol (Haldol) or lorazepam (Ativan) may be needed. Having a family member stay with the patient may have a calming effect. For the patient with seizures or the patient at risk for seizure activity, seizure precautions should be instituted. These include padded side rails, an airway at the bedside, accurate and timely administration of antiseizure drugs, and close observation.

The patient can benefit from a quiet, nonstimulating environment. The nurse should always use a calm, reassuring approach.

Touching and talking to the patient, even one who is in a coma, is always appropriate care. The nurse must create a balance between sensory deprivation and overload for the patient with increased ICP.

Psychologic considerations. Besides the carefully planned physical care provided patients with increased ICP, the nurse must also be aware of the psychologic well-being of the patients and their families. Anxiety over the diagnosis and the prognosis for the patient with neurologic problems can be distressing to the patient, the family, and the nursing staff. The nurse's competent and assured manner in performing the care needed by the patient is reassuring to everyone involved. Short, simple explanations are appropriate and allow the patient and the family to acquire the amount of information they desire. There is a need for support, information, and education of both patients and families. The nurse should assess the family members' desire and need to assist in providing care for the patient and allow for their participation as appropriate.

■ **Evaluation**

The expected outcomes for the patient with ICP are addressed in NCP 55-1.

HEAD INJURY

Head injury includes any trauma to the scalp, skull, or brain. The term *head trauma* is used primarily to signify craniocerebral trauma, which includes an alteration in consciousness, no matter how brief.

Statistics regarding the occurrence of head injuries are incomplete because many victims die at the scene of the accident or because the condition is considered minor and health care services are not sought. In the United States an estimated 1 million persons are treated and released with traumatic brain injury (TBI) in hospital emergency departments. Fifty thousand people die and 230,000 persons are hospitalized with TBI. Of individuals hospitalized, 22% of the patients die.[15] It is estimated that there has been a 21% decline in fatalities related to head injury since 1976.[16] In the past, motor vehicle accidents and falls were the most common causes of head injury in both Canada and the United States. More recently, in the United States, deaths from motor vehicle accidents and falls have decreased, whereas firearm-related head injury death rates have increased.[16] Other causes of head injury include assaults, sports-related injuries, and recreational accidents.

Head trauma has a high potential for poor outcome.[16] Deaths from head trauma occur at three time points after injury: immediately after the injury, within 2 hours after injury, and approximately 3 weeks after injury. Factors that predict a poor outcome include the presence of an intracranial hematoma, increasing age of the patient, abnormal motor responses, impaired or absent eye movements or pupil light reflexes, early sustained hypotension, hypoxemia or hypercapnia, and ICP levels higher than 20 mm Hg.[17] The majority of deaths after a head injury occur immediately after the injury, either from the direct head trauma or from massive hemorrhage and shock. Deaths occurring within a few hours of the trauma are caused by progressive worsening of the head injury or from internal bleeding. An immediate note of changes in neurologic status and surgical intervention are critical in the prevention of deaths at this point. Deaths occurring 3 weeks or more after injury result from multisystem failure. Expert nursing care in the weeks following the injury is crucial in decreasing mortality.

Types of Head Injuries

Scalp Lacerations. *Scalp lacerations* are the most minor type of head trauma. Because the scalp contains many blood vessels with poor constrictive abilities, most scalp lacerations are associated with profuse bleeding. The major complication associated with scalp laceration is infection.

TABLE 55-6 Types of Skull Fractures	
DESCRIPTION	**CAUSE**
Linear Break in continuity of bone without alteration of relationship of parts	Low-velocity injuries
Depressed Inward indentation of skull	Powerful blow
Simple Linear or depressed skull fracture without fragmentation or communicating lacerations	Low-to-moderate impact
Comminuted Multiple linear fractures with fragmentation of bone into many pieces	Direct, high-momentum impact
Compound Depressed skull fracture and scalp laceration with communicating pathway to intracranial cavity	Severe head injury

TABLE 55-7 Clinical Manifestations of Different Types of Skull Fractures	
LOCATION	**SYNDROME OR SEQUELAE**
Frontal fracture	Exposure of brain to contaminants through frontal air sinus, possible association with air in forehead tissue, CSF rhinorrhea, or pneumocranium
Orbital fracture	Periorbital ecchymosis (raccoon eyes)
Temporal fracture	Boggy temporal muscle because of extravasation of blood, oval-shaped bruise behind ear in mastoid region (Battle's sign), CSF otorrhea
Parietal fracture	Deafness, CSF or brain otorrhea, bulging of tympanic membrane caused by blood or CSF, facial paralysis, loss of taste, Battle's sign
Posterior fossa fracture	Occipital bruising resulting in cortical blindness, visual field defects; rare appearance of ataxia or other cerebellar signs
Basilar skull fracture	CSF or brain otorrhea, bulging of tympanic membrane caused by blood or CSF, Battle's sign, tinnitus or hearing difficulty, facial paralysis, conjugate deviation of gaze, vertigo

CSF, Cerebrospinal fluid.

Skull Fractures. *Skull fractures* frequently occur with head trauma. There are several ways to describe skull fractures: (1) linear or depressed; (2) simple, comminuted, or compound; and (3) closed or open (Table 55-6). Fractures may be closed or open, depending on the presence of a scalp laceration or extension of the fracture into the air sinuses or dura. The type and severity of a skull fracture depend on the velocity, the momentum, the direction of injuring agent, and the site of impact.

The location of the fracture alters the presentation of the manifestations (Table 55-7). For example, a specialized type of linear fracture is seen when the fracture occurs at the base of the skull, a basilar skull fracture. Manifestations include facial paralysis, Battle's sign (Fig. 55-13), and conjugate deviation of gaze. This fracture generally crosses a sinus and tears the dura (e.g., the frontal or the temporal) and is associated with leakage of CSF. Rhinorrhea (CSF leakage from the nose) or otorrhea (CSF leakage from the ear) generally confirms that the fracture has traversed the dura (Fig. 55-14).

Two methods of testing can be used to determine whether the fluid leaking from the nose or ear is CSF. The first method is to

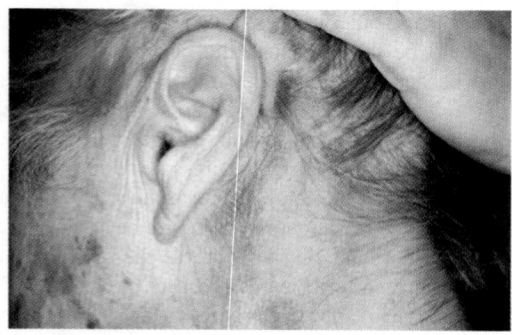

FIG. 55-13   Battle's sign.

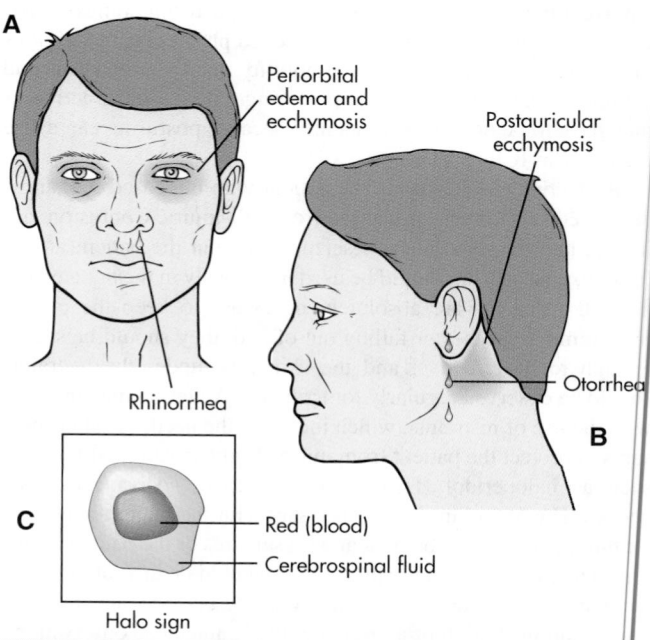

FIG. 55-14   **A,** Raccoon eyes and rhinorrhea. **B,** Battle's sign (postauricular ecchymosis) with otorrhea. **C,** Halo or ring sign (see text).

test the leaking fluid with a Dextrostix or Tes-Tape strip to determine whether glucose is present. CSF gives a positive reading for glucose. If blood is present in the fluid, testing for the presence of glucose is unreliable because blood contains glucose. In this event, the nurse should look for the "halo" or "ring" sign (see Fig. 55-14, *C*). To perform this test, the nurse allows the leaking fluid to drip onto a white pad (4 x 4) or towel and observes the drainage. Within a few minutes the blood coalesces into the center, and a yellowish ring encircles the blood if CSF is present. The color, appearance, and amount of leaking fluid must be noted because both tests can give false-positive results.

The major potential complications of skull fractures are intracranial infections and hematoma, as well as meningeal and brain tissue damage.

Minor Head Trauma. Brain injuries are categorized as being minor or major. **Concussion** (a sudden transient mechanical head injury with disruption of neural activity and a change in the LOC) is considered a minor head injury. The patient may not lose total consciousness with this injury.

Signs of concussion include a brief disruption in LOC, amnesia regarding the event (retrograde amnesia), and headache. The manifestations are generally of short duration. If the patient has not lost consciousness, or if the loss of consciousness lasts less than 5 minutes, the patient is usually discharged from the care facility with instructions to notify the health care provider if symptoms persist or if behavioral changes are noted.

The *postconcussion* syndrome is seen anywhere from 2 weeks to 2 months after the concussion. Symptoms include persistent headache, lethargy, personality and behavioral changes, shortened attention span, decreased short-term memory, and changes in intellectual ability. This syndrome can significantly affect the patient's abilities to perform the activities of daily living.

Although concussion is generally considered benign and usually resolves spontaneously, the symptoms may be the beginning of a more serious, progressive problem. At the time of discharge, it is important to give the patient and the family instructions for observation and accurate reporting of symptoms or changes in neurologic status.

Major Head Trauma. Major head trauma includes cerebral contusions and lacerations. Both injuries represent severe trauma to the brain. Contusions and intracerebral lacerations are generally associated with closed injuries.

A **contusion** is the bruising of the brain tissue within a focal area that maintains the integrity of the pia mater and arachnoid layers. A contusion develops areas of hemorrhage, infarction, necrosis, and edema. A contusion frequently occurs at the site of a fracture. With contusion, the phenomenon of *coup-contrecoup injury* is often noted. Damage from coup-contrecoup injury occurs because of mass movement of the brain inside the skull. Contusions or lacerations occur both at the site of the direct impact of the brain on the skull (*coup*) and at a secondary area of damage on the opposite side away from injury (*contrecoup*), leading to multiple contused areas. Bleeding around the contusion site is generally minimal, and the blood is reabsorbed slowly. Neurologic assessment demonstrates focal findings and a generalized disturbance in the LOC. Seizures are a common complication of brain contusion.

Lacerations involve actual tearing of the brain tissue and often occur in association with depressed and compound fractures and penetrating injuries. Tissue damage is severe, and surgical repair of the laceration is impossible because of the texture of the brain tissue. If bleeding is deep into the brain parenchyma, focal and generalized signs are noted.

When major head trauma occurs, many delayed responses are seen, including hemorrhage, hematoma formation, seizures, and cerebral edema. Intracerebral hemorrhage is generally associated with cerebral laceration. This hemorrhage manifests as a space-occupying lesion accompanied by unconsciousness, hemiplegia on the contralateral side, and a dilated pupil on the ipsilateral side. As the hematoma expands, symptoms of increased ICP become more severe. Prognosis is generally poor for the patient with a large intracerebral hemorrhage. Subarachnoid hemorrhage and intraventricular hemorrhage can also occur secondary to head trauma.

Pathophysiology

Diffuse axonal injury (DAI) is widespread axonal damage occurring after a mild, moderate, or severe TBI. The damage occurs primarily around axons in subcortical white matter of the cerebral hemispheres, basal ganglia, thalamus, and brainstem.[18] Initially, DAI was believed to occur from the tensile forces of trauma that sheared axons, resulting in axonal disconnection. There is increasing evidence that axonal damage is not preceded by an immediate tearing of the axon from the traumatic impact, but rather the trauma changes the function of the axon, resulting in axon swelling (axonal ballooning) and disconnection. This process takes approximately 12 to 24 hours to develop and may persist longer. The clinical signs and symptoms include a decreased LOC, increased ICP, decerebration or decortication, and global cerebral edema.

Complications

Epidural Hematoma. An **epidural hematoma** results from bleeding between the dura and the inner surface of the skull. An epidural hematoma is a neurologic emergency and is usually associated with a linear fracture crossing a major artery in the dura, causing a tear. It can have a venous or an arterial origin. Venous epidural hematomas are associated with a tear of the dural venous sinus and develop slowly. With arterial hematomas, the middle meningeal artery lying under the temporal bone is often torn. Hemorrhage occurs into the epidural space, which lies between the dura and the inner surface of the skull (Fig. 55-15, *A*). Because this is an arterial hemorrhage, the hematoma develops rapidly and under high pressure. Symptoms typically include unconsciousness at the scene, with a brief lucid interval followed by a decrease in LOC. Other symptoms may be a headache, nausea and vomiting, or focal findings. Rapid surgical intervention to prevent cerebral herniation dramatically improves outcomes.[19] Patients over 65 years of age with increased ICP have a higher mortality rate than younger patients.[15]

Subdural Hematoma. A **subdural hematoma** occurs from bleeding between the dura mater and the arachnoid layer of the meningeal covering of the brain. A subdural hematoma usually results from injury to the brain substance and its parenchymal vessels (see Fig. 55-15, *B*). The veins that drain from the surface of the brain into the sagittal sinus are the source of most subdural hematomas. Because a subdural hematoma is usually venous in origin, the hematoma is much slower to develop into a mass large enough to produce symptoms. However, a subdural hematoma may be caused by an arterial hemorrhage, in which

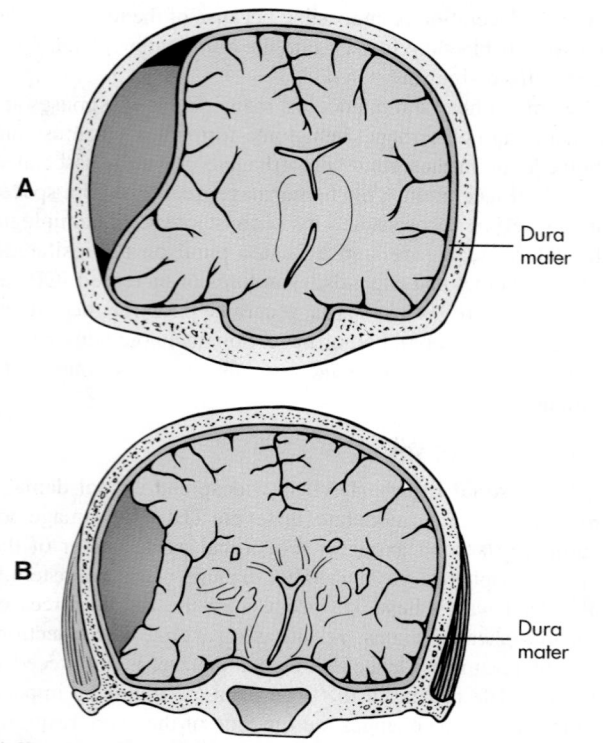

FIG. 55-15 A, Epidural hematoma in the temporal fossa, usually a result of laceration of the middle meningeal artery. B, Subdural hematoma, usually a result of laceration of the subdural veins.

life when a potentially larger subdural space is available as a result of brain atrophy. With atrophy, the brain remains attached to the supportive structures, but tension is increased, and it is subject to tearing. The larger size of the subdural space also accounts for the presenting complaint to be the focal symptoms, rather than the signs of increased ICP. Chronic alcoholics are also prone to cerebral atrophy and subsequent development of subdural hematoma.

Delay in diagnosis of a subdural hematoma in the older adult can be attributed to symptoms that mimic other health problems in persons of this age-group, such as vascular disease and senile dementia. Somnolence, confusion, lethargy, and memory loss are associated with health problems other than subdural hematoma.

Intracerebral Hematoma. Intracerebral hematoma occurs from bleeding within the parenchyma and occurs in approximately 16% of head injuries. It usually occurs within the frontal and temporal lobes, possibly from the rupture of intracerebral vessels at the time of injury. A "burst" lobe is an intracerebral or intracerebellar hematoma that is an extension of a subarachnoid hemorrhage. This type of intracerebral hematoma is thought to result from hemorrhage of supracortical vessels.

Diagnostic Studies and Collaborative Care

CT scan is considered the best diagnostic test to determine craniocerebral trauma because it allows for rapid diagnosis and intervention. MRI, PET, and evoked potential studies may also be used in the diagnosis and differentiation of head injuries. An MRI scan is more sensitive in detecting small DAI lesions than the CT scan because of the lack of gross pathologic changes in brain tissue. Transcranial Doppler studies allow for the measurement of CBF velocity. A cervical spine x-ray may also be indicated. In general, the diagnostic studies are similar to those used for a patient with increased ICP (see Table 55-3). The GCS can be used to classify head injury as mild (score of 13 to 15), moderate (score of 9 to 12), or severe (score of 3 to 8).

Emergency management of the patient with a head injury is presented in Table 55-9. In addition to measures to prevent secondary injury by treating cerebral edema and managing increased ICP, the principal treatment of head injuries is timely diagnosis and surgery if necessary. For the patient with concussion and contusion, observation and management of increased ICP are the primary management strategies.

The treatment of skull fractures is usually conservative. For depressed fractures and fractures with loose fragments, a craniotomy is necessary to elevate the depressed bone and remove the free fragments. If large amounts of bone are destroyed, the bone

case it develops more rapidly. Subdural hematomas may be acute, subacute, or chronic (Table 55-8).

An *acute subdural hematoma* manifests signs within 48 hours of the injury. The signs and symptoms are similar to those associated with brain tissue compression in increased ICP and include decreasing LOC and headache. The patient appears drowsy and confused. The ipsilateral pupil dilates and becomes fixed.

A *subacute subdural hematoma* usually occurs within 2 to 14 days of the injury. Failure to regain consciousness may point to this possibility. After the initial bleeding, a subdural hematoma may appear to enlarge over time as the breakdown products of the blood draw fluid into the subdural space to reach isotonicity.

A *chronic subdural hematoma* develops over weeks or months after a seemingly minor head injury. The peak incidence of chronic subdural hematoma is in the sixth and seventh decades of

TABLE 55-8	**Types of Subdural Hematomas**		
TYPE	**OCCURRENCE AFTER INJURY**	**PROGRESSION OF SYMPTOMS**	**TREATMENT**
Acute	24–48 hr after severe trauma	Immediate deterioration	Craniotomy, evacuation and decompression
Subacute	48 hr–2 wk after severe trauma	Initial unconsciousness, gradual improvement, deterioration over hours, dilation of pupils, ptosis	Evacuation and decompression
Chronic	Weeks, months, usually >20 days after injury; often injury seemed trivial or forgotten by patient	Nonspecific, nonlocalizing progression; progressive alteration in LOC	Evacuation and decompression, membranectomy

LOC, Level of consciousness.

may be removed (craniectomy) and a cranioplasty will be needed at a later time (see Cranial Surgery later in this chapter).

In cases of acute subdural and epidural hematomas, the blood must be removed. A craniotomy is generally performed to visualize the bleeding vessels so that the bleeding can be controlled. Burr-hole openings may be used in an extreme emergency for a more rapid decompression, followed by a craniotomy to stop all bleeding. A drain is generally placed postoperatively for several days to prevent any reaccumulation of blood.

NURSING MANAGEMENT
HEAD INJURY

■ Nursing Assessment

The patient with a head injury is always considered to have the potential for developing increased ICP. Increased ICP is associated with higher mortality rates and poorer functional out-

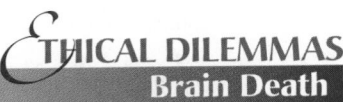

ETHICAL DILEMMAS
Brain Death

Situation

The emergency nurse receives a radio call from emergency medical service (EMS) personnel about a young man who has been involved in a motorcycle crash. The patient was not wearing a helmet and has a large open skull fracture with obvious gray matter oozing from the area. Transport from the accident scene was delayed by 45 minutes as a result of a severe thunderstorm and traffic congestion. On the way to the hospital the patient has fixed, dilated pupils and a cardiac arrest. Estimated arrival at the hospital is still an additional 45 minutes as a result of the severe weather. EMS personnel request permission to stop cardiopulmonary resuscitation (CPR) efforts.

Important Points for Consideration

- Brain death occurs when the cerebral cortex stops functioning or is irreversibly destroyed.
- Since technology has been developed that assists in supporting life, controversies have arisen related to an exact definition of death.
- Criteria for brain death include coma or unresponsiveness, absence of brainstem reflexes, and apnea (see Chapter 10). Specific assessments by a physician are required to validate each of the criteria.
- The patient's clinical manifestations indicate that brain death has occurred.
- Although there is a slight chance that the patient's heart function could be resuscitated and supported with mechanical ventilation, there is no obligation to provide medically futile care for a patient with brain death.
- Brain death criteria do not address patients in permanent vegetative state because the brainstem activity in these patients is adequate to maintain heart and lung function.

Critical Thinking Questions

1. What are your feelings about cessation of brain function versus cessation of heart and lung function as the criteria for death of a patient?
2. What are your state's laws or practices about stopping CPR efforts by EMS personnel in the field?

comes.[6] The most important aspects of the objective data are noting the GCS score (see Table 55-5), assessing and monitoring the neurologic status (see Fig. 55-10), and determining whether a CSF leak has occurred. (Nursing assessment related to increased ICP is on pp. 1500-1502.)

■ Nursing Diagnoses

Nursing diagnoses and potential complication for the patient who has sustained a head injury may include, but are not limited to, the following:

- Ineffective tissue perfusion (cerebral) *related to* interruption of CBF associated with cerebral hemorrhage, hematoma, and edema
- Hyperthermia *related to* increased metabolism, infection, and loss of cerebral integrative function secondary to possible hypothalamic injury
- Acute pain (headache) *related to* trauma and cerebral edema
- Impaired physical mobility *related to* decreased LOC and treatment-imposed bed rest
- Anxiety *related to* abrupt change in health status, hospital environment, and uncertain future
- Potential complication: increased ICP *related to* cerebral edema and hemorrhage

■ Planning

The overall goals are that the patient with an acute head injury will (1) maintain adequate cerebral perfusion; (2) remain normothermic; (3) be free from pain, discomfort, and infection; and (4) attain maximal cognitive, motor, and sensory function.

■ Nursing Implementation

Health Promotion. One of the best ways to prevent head injuries is to prevent car and motorcycle accidents. The nurse can be active in campaigns that promote driving safety and can speak to driver education classes regarding the dangers of unsafe driving and of driving after drinking alcohol. The use of seat belts in cars and the use of helmets for riding on motorcycles are the most effective measures for increasing survival after accidents. Increasingly, individual states are passing legislation requiring the use of automobile safety devices for both children and adults. The wearing of protective helmets by lumberjacks, construction workers, miners, horseback riders, bicycle riders, snowboarders, and skydivers is also recommended. The nurse should be familiar with data on outcomes with and without safety devices in working with groups who oppose safety legislation as an infringement of personal freedom.

Acute Intervention. Management at the scene of the accident can have a significant impact on the outcome of the head injury. Emergency management of head injury is discussed in Table 55-9. The general goal of nursing management of the head-injured patient is to maintain cerebral perfusion and prevent secondary cerebral ischemia. Surveillance or monitoring for changes in neurologic status is critically important because the patient's condition may deteriorate rapidly, necessitating emergency surgery. Appropriate preoperative and postoperative nursing interventions are initiated if surgery is anticipated. Because of the close association between hemodynamic status and cerebral perfusion, the nurse must be aware of any coexisting injuries or conditions. In the acute injury period, treating other life-threatening conditions (i.e., hemorrhage, hypoxia) may take initial priority in nursing care.

TABLE 55-9   Emergency Management — Head Injury

ETIOLOGY	ASSESSMENT FINDINGS	INTERVENTIONS
Blunt Motor vehicle collision Pedestrian event Fall Assault Sports injury	**Surface Findings** • Scalp lacerations • Fracture or depressions in skull • Bruises or contusions on face, Battle's sign (bruising behind ears) • Raccoon eyes (dependent bruising around eyes)	**Initial** • Ensure patent airway. • Stabilize cervical spine. • Administer O_2 via nasal cannula or non-rebreather mask. • Establish IV access with two large-bore catheters to infuse normal saline or lactated Ringer's solution. • Control external bleeding with sterile pressure dressing. • Assess for rhinorrhea, otorrhea, scalp wounds. • Remove patient's clothing.
Penetrating Gunshot wound Arrow	**Respiratory** • Central neurogenic hyperventilation • Cheyne-Stokes respirations • Decreased O_2 saturation • Pulmonary edema	
	Central Nervous System • Unequal or dilated pupils • Asymmetric facial movements • Garbled speech, abusive speech • Confusion • Decreased level of consciousness • Combativeness • Involuntary movements • Seizures • Bowel and bladder incontinence • Flaccidity • Depressed or hyperactive reflexes • Decerebrate or decorticate posturing • Glasgow Coma Scale score <12 • CSF leaking from ears or nose	**Ongoing Monitoring** • Maintain patient warmth using blankets, warm IV fluids, overhead warming lights, warm humidified O_2. • Monitor vital signs, level of consciousness, O_2 saturation, cardiac rhythm, Glasgow Coma Scale score, pupil size and reactivity. • Anticipate need for intubation if gag reflex is absent. • Assume neck injury with head injury. • Administer fluids cautiously to prevent fluid overload and increasing ICP.

CSF, Cerebrospinal fluid; *ICP,* intracranial pressure; *IV,* intravenous.

TABLE 55-10   Patient & Family Teaching Guide — Head Injury

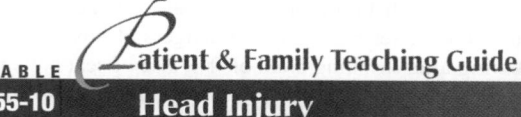

Teaching guidelines for the patient and family during the initial 2 to 3 days after a head injury include the following:

1. Notify your health care provider immediately if experiencing signs and symptoms that may indicate complications. These include:
   - Increased drowsiness (e.g., difficulty arousing, confusion)
   - Nausea and/or vomiting
   - Worsening headache or stiff neck
   - Seizures
   - Vision difficulties (e.g., blurring)
   - Behavioral changes (e.g., irritability, anger)
   - Motor problems (e.g., clumsiness, difficulty walking, slurred speech, weakness in arms or legs)
   - Sensory disturbances (e.g., numbness)
   - Decreased heart rate
2. Have someone stay with the patient.
3. Abstain from alcohol.
4. Check with your health care provider before taking drugs that may increase drowsiness, including muscle relaxants, tranquilizers, and narcotic pain medications.
5. Avoid driving, using heavy machinery, playing contact sports, and taking warm baths.

The nurse should explain the need for frequent neurologic assessments to both the patient and the family. Behavioral manifestations associated with head injury can result in a frightened, disoriented patient who is combative and resists help. The nurse's approach should be calm and gentle. A family member may be available to stay with the patient and thus prevent increasing anxiety and fear. Other teaching points are presented in Table 55-10.

The nurse should perform neurologic assessments at intervals based on the patient's condition. The GCS is useful in assessing the level of arousal (see Table 55-5). Indications of a deteriorating neurologic state, such as a decreasing LOC or a lessening of motor strength, should be reported to the health care provider, and the patient's condition should be closely monitored.

The major focus of nursing care for the brain-injured patient relates to increased ICP (see NCP 55-1). However, there may be specific problems that require nursing intervention.

Eye problems may include loss of the corneal reflex, periorbital ecchymosis and edema, and diplopia. Loss of the corneal reflex may necessitate administering lubricating eye drops, taping the eyes shut, or suturing the eyelids to prevent abrasion. Periorbital ecchymosis and edema disappear spontaneously, but cold and, later, warm compresses provide comfort and hasten the process. Diplopia can be relieved by use of an eye patch.

Hyperthermia may occur from injury to or inflammation of the hypothalamus. Elevations in body temperature can result in increased CBF, cerebral blood volume, and ICP.[3] Increased metabolism secondary to hyperthermia increases metabolic waste, which in turn produces further cerebral vasodilation. The nurse should attempt to control hyperthermia and maintain normothermia in the head-injured patient. There is some evidence to suggest that therapeutic hypothermia (32° to 35° C) may be beneficial during the first 24 hours following injury.[3]

If CSF rhinorrhea or otorrhea occurs, the nurse should inform the physician immediately. The patient should lie flat in bed unless this is contraindicated because of increased ICP. The head of the bed may be raised to decrease the CSF pressure so that a tear can seal. A loose collection pad may be placed under the nose or over the ear. No dressing should be placed into the nasal or ear cavities. The patient should be cautioned not to sneeze or blow the nose. Nasogastric tubes should not be used, and nasotracheal suctioning should not be performed on these patients.

Nursing measures specific to the care of the immobilized patient, such as those related to bladder and bowel function, skin care, and infection, are also indicated. Nausea and vomiting may be a problem and can be alleviated by antiemetic drugs. Headache can usually be controlled with acetaminophen or small doses of codeine.

If the patient's condition deteriorates, intracranial surgery may be necessary (see Cranial Surgery later in this chapter). A burr-hole opening or craniotomy may be indicated, depending on the underlying injury that is causing the symptoms. The emergency nature of the surgery may hasten the usual careful preoperative preparation. The nurse should consult with the neurosurgeon to determine specific preoperative nursing measures.

The patient is often unconscious before surgery, making it necessary for a family member to sign the consent form for surgery. This is a difficult and frightening time for the patient's family and requires sensitive nursing management. The suddenness of the situation makes it especially difficult for the family to cope.

Ambulatory and Home Care. Once the condition has stabilized, the patient is usually transferred for acute rehabilitation management to prepare the patient for reentry into the community. As with any craniocerebral problem, there may be chronic problems related to motor and sensory deficits, communication, memory, and intellectual functioning. Many of the principles of nursing management of the patient with a stroke are appropriate (see Chapter 56). Conditions that may require nursing and collaborative management include poor nutritional status, bowel and bladder management, spasticity, dysphagia, neurogenic heterotopic ossification (overgrowth of bone), deep vein thrombosis, and hydrocephalus. With time and patience, many of the chronic problems subside or disappear. The patient's outward appearance is not a good indicator of how well the patient will function in the home or work environment.

Seizure disorders are seen in approximately 5% of patients with a nonpenetrating head injury. The most vulnerable time for seizures to develop is during the first week after the head injury. Some patients may not develop a seizure disorder until years after the initial injury. Some health care providers recommend that antiseizure drugs be used prophylactically. Others may not institute treatment until a seizure is witnessed or an EEG demonstrates seizure activity. Phenytoin (Dilantin) is the antiseizure drug of choice in posttraumatic seizure activity.

The mental and emotional sequelae of brain trauma are often the most incapacitating problems. Many of the patients with head injuries who have been comatose for more than 6 hours undergo some personality change. They may suffer loss of concentration and

memory and defective memory processing. Personal drive may decrease; apathy and apparent laziness may increase. Euphoria and mood swings, along with a seeming lack of awareness of the seriousness of the injury, may occur. The patient's behavior may indicate a loss of social restraint, judgment, tact, and emotional control.

Progressive recovery may continue for 6 months or more before a plateau is reached and a prognosis for recovery can be made. Specific nursing management in the posttraumatic phase depends on specific residual deficits.

In all cases the family must be given special consideration. They need to understand what is happening and taught appropriate interaction patterns. The nurse must give guidance and referrals for financial aid, child care, and other personal needs and must assist the family in involving the patient in family activities whenever possible. Assisting the patient and family in developing and maintaining hope and keeping communication open are strategies perceived as supportive by families.[20,21]

The family often has unrealistic expectations of the patient as the coma begins to recede. The family expects full return to pretrauma status. In reality, the patient experiences a reduced awareness and ability to interpret environmental stimuli. The nurse must prepare the family for the emergence of the patient from coma and must explain that the process of awakening often takes several weeks.

When the time for discharge planning arrives, the family and the patient may benefit from very specific posthospital instructions to avoid family-patient friction.[22] Special "no" policies that may be appropriately suggested by the neurosurgeon, neuropsychologist, and nurse include no drinking of alcoholic beverages, no driving, no use of firearms, no work with hazardous implements and machinery, and no unsupervised smoking.[16] Family members, particularly spouses, go through role transition as the role changes from one of spouse to that of caregiver.

■ Evaluation

The expected outcomes are that the patient with a head injury will

- maintain normal cerebral perfusion pressure
- achieve maximal cognitive, motor, and sensory function
- experience no infection, hyperthermia, or pain

BRAIN TUMORS

The annual rate of newly diagnosed brain tumors in the United States is 17,000, with an estimated 13,100 deaths related to brain tumors.[22] The brain is also a frequent site for metastasis from other sites. Brain tumors rank fourth as cause of death from cancer in individuals 35 to 54 years of age. The incidence of

CULTURAL & ETHNIC CONSIDERATIONS
Brain Tumors

- Whites have a higher incidence of malignant brain tumors compared with African Americans.
- White males have the highest incidence of malignant brain tumors.
- African Americans have a higher incidence of benign brain tumors (e.g., meningiomas) compared with whites.
- Meningiomas are the most common brain tumor in many areas of Africa.

brain tumors has increased in the past 20 years, especially in older adults.[23]

Types

Brain tumors can occur in any part of the brain or spinal cord. Tumors of the brain may be *primary,* arising from tissues within the brain, or *secondary,* resulting from a metastasis from a malignant neoplasm elsewhere in the body. Secondary brain tumors are the most common type. Brain tumors are generally classified according to the tissue from which they arise. The most common primary brain tumors originate in astrocytes. These tumors are called gliomas (astrocytoma, glioblastoma multiforme) and account for 65% of primary brain tumors (Table 55-11). Glioblastoma multiforme is the most common primary brain tumor, followed by meningioma and astrocytoma. More than half of the brain tumors are malignant; they infiltrate the brain parenchyma and are not amenable to complete surgical removal. Other tumors may be histologically benign but are located such that complete removal is not possible. Brain tumors are more commonly seen in middle-aged persons, but they may occur at any age.

Unless treated, all brain tumors eventually cause death from increasing tumor volume leading to increased ICP. Brain tumors rarely metastasize outside the central nervous system (CNS) because they are contained by structural (meninges) and physiologic (blood-brain) barriers. Table 55-11 compares the major brain tumors. A glioblastoma and meningioma are depicted in Fig. 55-16.

Clinical Manifestations

The clinical manifestations of brain tumors depend mainly on the location and size of the tumor. The rate of growth and the appearance of manifestations depend on the location, size, and mitotic rate of the cells of tissue of origin. Fig. 55-17 illustrates the functional areas of the cerebral cortex and can be used as a guide to correlate manifestations with the location of the tumor.

Wide ranges of possible clinical manifestations are associated with brain tumors. Headache is a common problem. Tumor-related headaches tend to be worse at night and may awaken the patient. The headaches are usually dull and constant but occasionally throbbing. Seizures are common in gliomas and brain metastases. Brain tumors can cause nausea and vomiting from increased ICP. Cognitive dysfunction, including memory problems and mood or

TABLE 55-11	**Types of Brain Tumors**	
TYPE	**TISSUE OF ORIGIN**	**CHARACTERISTICS**
Gliomas		
• Astrocytoma	Supportive tissue, glial cells and astrocytes	Can range from low-grade to moderate-grade malignancy
• Glioblastoma multiforme	Primitive stem cell (glioblast)	Highly malignant and invasive; among the most devastating of primary brain tumors
• Oligodendroglioma	Oligodendrocytes	Benign (encapsulation and calcification)
• Ependymoma	Ependymal epithelium	Range from benign to highly malignant; most are benign and encapsulated
• Medulloblastoma	Primitive neuroectodermal cell	Highly malignant and invasive; metastatic to spinal cord and remote areas of brain
Meningioma	Meninges	Can be benign or malignant; most are benign
Acoustic neuroma (Schwannoma)	Cells that form myelin sheath around nerves; commonly affects cranial nerve VIII	Many grow on both sides of the brain; usually benign or low-grade malignancy
Pituitary adenoma	Pituitary gland	Usually benign
Hemangioblastoma	Blood vessels of brain	Rare and benign; surgery is curative
Primary central nervous system lymphoma	Lymphocytes	Increased incidence in transplant recipients and acquired immunodeficiency syndrome (AIDS) patients
Metastatic tumors	Lungs, breast, kidney, thyroid, prostate	Malignant

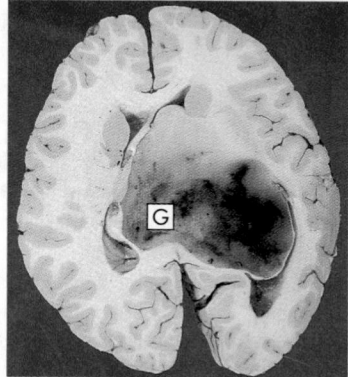
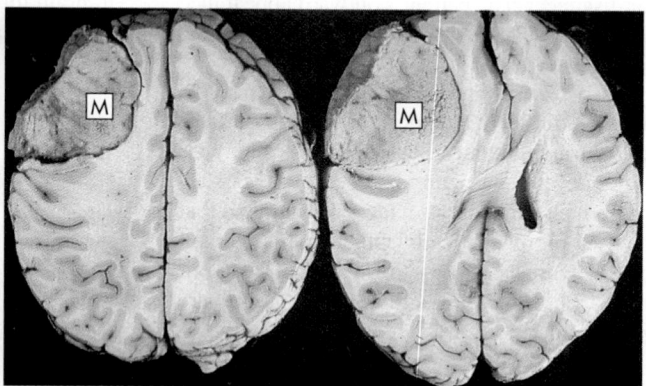

FIG. 55-16 **A,** Glioblastoma. A large glioblastoma (*G*) arises from one cerebral hemisphere and has grown to fill the ventricular system. **B,** Meningioma. These two different sections from different levels in the same brain show a meningioma (*M*) compressing the frontal lobe and distorting underlying brain.

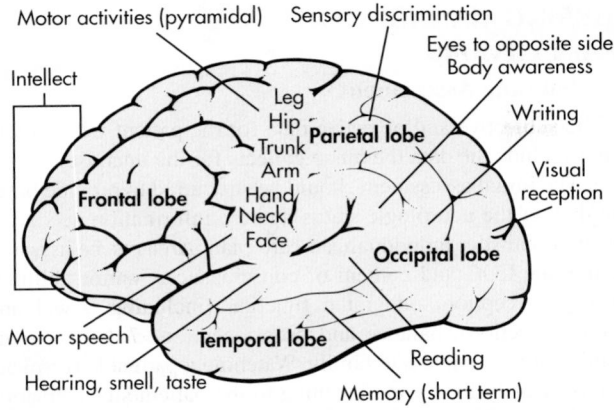

Motor activities (pyramidal)   Sensory discrimination
Eyes to opposite side
Body awareness
Intellect
Leg
Hip   **Parietal lobe**
Trunk   Writing
Arm
Frontal lobe   Hand   Visual
Neck   reception
Face
Occipital lobe
Motor speech   **Temporal lobe**
Hearing, smell, taste   Reading
Memory (short term)

FIG. 55-17 Each area of the brain controls a particular activity.

personality changes, is another common manifestation, especially in patients with brain metastases. Muscle weakness, sensory losses, aphasia, and visuospatial dysfunction are also manifestations of brain tumors. As the brain tumor expands, it may also produce manifestations of increased ICP, cerebral edema, or obstruction of the CSF pathways. Manifestations may clearly indicate the location of the tumor by an alteration in the function controlled by the affected area (Table 55-12).

Complications

If the tumor mass obstructs the ventricles or occludes the outlet, ventricular enlargement (hydrocephalus) can occur. Surgical treatment is necessary to relieve the pressure and involves placement of a ventriculoatrial or a ventriculoperitoneal shunt. A catheter with one-way valves is placed in the lateral ventricle and then tunneled through the skin to drain CSF into the right atrium or the peritoneum. Rapid decompression of ICP can cause prostration and headache that may be prevented by gradually introducing the patient to the upright position. The patient should be instructed to avoid contact sports that may result in a blow to the valve or shearing of the catheter. The health care provider should be notified if signs of increased ICP occur, such as decreasing LOC, restlessness, headache, blurred vision, or vomiting without nausea. Signs of an infected shunt, such as high fever, persistent headache, and stiff neck, warrant investigation.

Diagnostic Studies

An extensive history and a comprehensive neurologic examination must be done in the workup of a patient with a suspected brain tumor. A careful history and physical examination may provide data with respect to location. Diagnostic studies are similar to those used for a patient with increased ICP (see Table 55-3). The sensitivity of techniques such as MRI and PET allows for detection of very small tumors and may provide more reliable diagnostic information. CT and brain scanning are used to diagnose the location of the lesion. Other tests include magnetic resonance spectroscopy, functional MRI, PET scans, and single photon emission computed tomography (SPECT). The EEG is useful but of less importance. A lumbar puncture is seldom diagnostic and carries with it the risk of cerebral herniation. Angiography can be used to determine blood flow to the tumor and further localize the tumor. Other studies are done to rule out a primary lesion elsewhere in the body. Endocrine studies are helpful when a pituitary adenoma is suspected (see Chapter 48).

The correct diagnosis of a brain tumor can be made by obtaining tissue for histologic study. In most patients, tissue is obtained at the time of surgery. A smear or frozen section can be performed in the operating room for a preliminary interpretation of the histologic type. With this information, the neurosurgeon can make a better decision about the extent of surgery. In some cases, immunohistochemical stains or electron microscopy may be necessary to ascertain the correct diagnosis. Determination of the MIB-1 index, a measure of mitotic rate, is often helpful in assessing the mitotic activity of a given tumor.

Collaborative Care

Treatment goals are aimed at (1) identifying the tumor type and location, (2) removing or decreasing tumor mass, and (3) preventing or managing increased ICP.

TABLE 55-12   Brain Tumor Locations and Presenting Manifestations

TUMOR LOCATION	PRESENTING MANIFESTATIONS
Cerebral hemisphere	
• Frontal lobe (unilateral)	Unilateral hemiplegia, seizures, memory deficit, personality and judgment changes, visual disturbances
• Frontal lobe (bilateral)	Symptoms associated with unilateral frontal lobe tumors; ataxic gait
• Parietal lobe	Speech disturbance (if tumor is in the dominant hemisphere: inability to write, spatial disorders, unilateral neglect)
• Occipital lobe	Blindness and seizures
• Temporal lobe	Few symptoms; seizures, dysphagia
Subcortical	Hemiplegia; other symptoms may depend on area of infiltration
Meningeal tumors	Symptoms are associated with compression of the brain and depend on tumor location
Metastatic tumors	Headache, nausea, or vomiting because of ↑ ICP; other symptoms depend on tumor location
Thalamus and sellar tumors	Headache, nausea, vision disturbances, papilledema, and nystagmus occur from ↑ ICP; diabetes insipidus may occur
Fourth ventricle and cerebellar tumors	Headache, nausea, and papilledema from ↑ ICP; ataxic gait and changes in coordination
Cerebellopontine tumors	Tinnitus and vertigo, deafness
Brainstem tumors	Headache on awakening, drowsiness, vomiting, ataxic gait, facial muscle weakness, hearing loss, dysphagia, dysarthria, "crossed eyes" or other visual changes, hemiparesis

ICP, Intracranial pressure.

Surgical Therapy. Surgical removal is the preferred treatment for brain tumors (see Cranial Surgery later in this chapter). Stereotactic surgical techniques are used with greater frequency to perform a biopsy and remove small brain tumors. The outcome of surgical therapy depends on the type, size, and location of the tumor. Meningiomas and oligodendrogliomas can usually be completely removed, whereas the more invasive gliomas and medulloblastomas can be only partially removed. Computer-guided stereotactic biopsy, ultrasound, functional MRI, and cortical mapping can be used to localize brain tumors intraoperatively. Complete surgical removal is not always possible because the tumor is not always accessible or it has involved vital parts of the brain. Surgery can reduce tumor mass, which decreases ICP and provides relief of symptoms with an extension of survival time. Tumors located in the deep central areas of the dominant hemisphere, the posterior corpus callosum, or the upper brainstem cause extensive neurologic damage and are considered probably inoperable.

Radiation Therapy and Radiosurgery. Radiation therapy is commonly used as a follow-up measure after surgery. Radiation seeds can also be implanted into the brain. Cerebral edema and rapidly increasing ICP may be a complication of radiation therapy, but they can be managed with high doses of corticosteroids (dexamethasone [Decadron], prednisone, or methylprednisolone [Solu-Medrol]). (Radiation therapy is discussed in Chapter 15.)

Stereotactic radiosurgery is a method of delivering a high concentrated dose of radiation precisely directed at a location within the brain. Stereotactic radiosurgery may be used when conventional surgery has failed or is not an option because of the tumor location. (Radiosurgery is discussed on p. 1516.)

Chemotherapy. The effectiveness of chemotherapy has been limited by difficulty getting drugs across the blood-brain barrier, tumor cell heterogeneity, and tumor cell drug resistance. A group of chemotherapeutic drugs called the nitrosoureas (e.g., carmustine [BCNU], lomustine [CCNU]) are particularly effective in treating brain tumors. Normally the blood-brain barrier prohibits the entry of most drugs into the brain. The most malignant tumors cause a breakdown of the blood-brain barrier in the area of the tumor, allowing chemotherapeutic agents to be used to treat the malignancy. Chemotherapy-laden biodegradable wafers (e.g., Gliadel wafer [polifeprosan with carmustine implant]) implanted at the time of surgery can deliver chemotherapy directly to the tumor site. Other drugs being used include methotrexate and procarbazine (Matulane). Two methods used to deliver chemotherapeutic drugs directly to the CNS are via an Ommaya reservoir (see Chapter 15) and intrathecal administration.

Temozolomide (Temodar) is the first oral chemotherapeutic agent found to cross the blood-brain barrier. In contrast with many traditional chemotherapies, which require metabolic activation to exert their effects, temozolomide has the ability to convert spontaneously to a reactive agent that directly interferes with tumor growth. It does not interact with other drugs commonly taken by patients with brain tumors such as antiseizure medications, corticosteroids, and antiemetics.

Many techniques to control and treat brain tumors are currently under investigation. These include local hyperthermia and biologic therapy. Although progress in treatment has increased length and quality of survival of patients with gliomas, outcomes still remain poor.[24]

NURSING MANAGEMENT
BRAIN TUMORS

■ Nursing Assessment

The subjective and objective data for the patient with a brain tumor include the data the nurse collects for the unconscious patient. The initial assessment should be structured to provide baseline data of the neurologic status and the information needed to design a realistic, individualized care plan. Areas to be assessed include the LOC and content of consciousness, motor abilities, sensory perception, integrated function (including bowel and bladder function), balance and proprioception, and the coping abilities of the patient and family. Watching a patient perform activities of daily living and listening to the patient's conversation are convenient ways to perform part of the neurologic assessment. Having the patient or the family explain the problem can be helpful in determining the patient's limitations and can also provide the nurse with information about the patient's insight into the problems. All initial data should be accurately recorded to provide a baseline for comparison to determine whether the patient's condition is improving or deteriorating.

Interview data are as important as the actual physical assessment. Questions concerning medical history, intellectual abilities and educational level, and history of nervous system infections and trauma should be asked. Determination of the presence of seizures, syncope, nausea and vomiting, pain, and headaches or other pain is important in planning care for the patient.

■ Nursing Diagnoses

Nursing diagnoses for the patient with a brain tumor may include, but are not limited to, the following:

- Impaired tissue perfusion (cerebral) *related to* cerebral edema
- Acute pain (headache) *related to* cerebral edema and increased ICP
- Self-care deficits *related to* altered neuromuscular function secondary to tumor growth and cerebral edema
- Anxiety *related to* diagnosis and treatment
- Potential complication: seizures *related to* abnormal electrical activity of the brain
- Potential complication: increased ICP *related to* presence of tumor and failure of normal compensatory mechanisms

■ Planning

The overall goals are that the patient with a brain tumor will (1) maintain normal ICP, (2) maximize neurologic functioning, (3) be free from pain and discomfort, and (4) be aware of the long-term implications with respect to prognosis and cognitive and physical functioning.

■ Nursing Implementation

A primary or metastatic tumor of the frontal lobe can cause behavioral and personality changes. Loss of emotional control, confusion, disorientation, memory loss, and depression may be signs of a frontal lobe lesion. These behavioral changes are often not perceived by the patient but can be disturbing and even frightening to the family. These changes can also cause a distancing to occur between the family and the patient. Assisting the family in understanding what is happening to the patient and supporting the family through this diagnostic phase are important roles for the nurse.

The confused patient with behavioral instability can be a challenge. Protecting the patient from self-harm is an important part of nursing care. At times when the patient manifests rage and aggression, the nurse must also be concerned about self-protection. Close supervision of activity, use of side rails, judicious use of restraints, padding of the rails and the area around the bed, and a calm, reassuring approach to care are all essential techniques in the care of these patients.

Perceptual problems associated with frontal lobe and parietal lobe tumors contribute to a patient's disorientation and confusion. Minimization of environmental stimuli, creation of a routine, and use of reality orientation can be incorporated into the care plan for the confused patient.

Seizures often occur with brain tumors. These are managed with antiseizure drugs. Seizure precautions should be instituted for the protection of the patient. Some behavioral changes seen in the patient with a brain tumor are a result of seizure disorders and can improve with control of the seizures by means of drugs (see Chapter 57).

Motor and sensory dysfunctions are problems that interfere with the activities of daily living. Alterations in mobility must be managed, and the patient should be encouraged to provide as much self-care as physically possible. Self-image often depends on the patient's ability to participate in care within the limitations of the physical deficits.

Language deficits can also occur in patients with brain tumors. Motor (expressive) or sensory (receptive) dysphasia may occur. The disturbance in communication can be frustrating for the patient and may interfere with the nurse's ability to meet the patient's needs. Attempts should be made to establish a communication system that can be used by both the patient and the staff.

Nutritional intake may be decreased because of the patient's inability to eat, loss of appetite, or loss of desire to eat. Assessing the nutritional status of the patient and ensuring adequate nutritional intake are important aspects of care. The patient may need encouragement to eat or, in some cases, may have to be fed orally, by gastrostomy or nasogastric tube, or by total parenteral nutrition. The patient with a brain tumor who undergoes cranial surgery requires complex nursing care. This is discussed in the next section.

■ Evaluation

The expected outcomes are that the patient with a brain tumor will

- be free of pain, vomiting, and other discomforts
- maintain ICP within normal limits
- demonstrate maximal neurologic function (cognitive, motor, sensory) with regard to the location and extent of the tumor
- maintain optimal nutritional status
- accept the long-term consequences of the tumor and its treatment

CRANIAL SURGERY

The cause or indication for cranial surgery may be related to a brain tumor, CNS infection (e.g., abscess), vascular abnormalities, craniocerebral trauma, epilepsy, or intractable pain (Table 55-13).

TABLE 55-13   Indications for Cranial Surgery

INDICATION	CAUSE	MANIFESTATIONS	PROCEDURE
Intracranial infection	Bacteria	*Early findings:* stiff neck, headache, fever, weakness, seizures *Later findings:* seizures, hemiplegia, speech disturbances, ocular disturbances, change in LOC	Excision or drainage of abscess
Hydrocephalus	Overproduction of CSF, obstruction to flow, defective reabsorption	*Early findings:* mental changes, disturbances in gait *Later findings:* memory impairment, urinary incontinence, increased tendon reflexes	Placement of ventriculoatrial or ventriculoperitoneal shunt
Brain tumors	Benign or malignant cell growth	Change in LOC, pupillary changes, sensory or motor deficit, papilledema, seizures, personality changes	Excision or partial resection of tumor
Intracranial bleeding	Rupture of cerebral vessels because of trauma or stroke	*Epidural:* momentary unconsciousness; lucid period, then rapid deterioration *Subdural:* headache, seizures, pupillary changes	Surgical evacuation through burr holes or craniotomy
Skull fractures	Trauma to skull	Headache, CSF leakage, cranial nerve deficit	Debridement of fragments and necrotic tissue, elevation and realignment of bone fragments
Arteriovenous (AV) malformation	Congenital tangle of arteries and veins (frequently in middle cerebral artery)	Headache, intracranial hemorrhage, seizures, mental deterioration	Excision of malformation
Aneurysm repair	Dilation of weak area in arterial wall (usually near anterior portion of circle of Willis)	*Before rupture:* headache, lethargy, visual disturbance *After rupture:* violent headache, decreased LOC, visual disturbances, motor deficit	Dissection and clipping or coiling of aneurysm

CSF, Cerebrospinal fluid; *LOC,* level of consciousness.

Types

Various types of cranial surgical procedures are presented in Table 55-14.

Stereotactic Surgery. Stereotactic surgery is neurosurgery using a precision apparatus (often computer-guided) to assist the surgeon to precisely target an area of the brain (Fig. 55-18). Stereotactic biopsy can be performed to obtain tissue samples for histologic examination. CT scanning and MRI are used to image the targeted tissue. With the patient under general or local anesthesia, the surgeon drills a burr hole or creates a bone flap for an entry site and then introduces a probe and biopsy needle. Stereotactic procedures are used for removal of small brain tumors and abscesses, drainage of hematomas, ablative procedures for extrapyramidal diseases (e.g., Parkinson's disease), and repair of arteriovenous malformations. A major advantage of the stereotactic approach is a reduction in damage to surrounding tissue.

Stereotactic radiosurgery is a procedure that involves closed-skull destruction of an intracranial target using ionizing radiation focused with the assistance of an intracranial guiding device. A sophisticated computer program is used while the patient's head is held still in a stereotactic frame. Radiosurgical techniques can use linear accelerator or a gamma knife. In the gamma knife procedure, a high dose of cobalt radiation is delivered to precisely targeted tumor tissue. The dose of radiation can be delivered over a single 4- to 6-hour treatment time. In some situations, some tumors are treated over several weeks.

In combination with stereotactic procedures to identify and localize tumor sites, surgical lasers can be used to destroy tumors. Stereotactic procedures are used to identify the tumor site. Three surgical lasers currently used include the carbon dioxide, argon, and neodymium: yttrium-aluminum-garnet (Nd:YAG) lasers. All three work by creating thermal energy, which destroys the tissue on which it is focused. Laser therapy also provides the benefit of reducing damage to surrounding tissue.

Craniotomy. Depending on the location of the pathologic condition, a craniotomy may be frontal, parietal, occipital, temporal, or a combination of any of these. A set of burr holes is drilled, and a saw is used to connect the holes to remove the bone flap. Sometimes operating microscopes are used to magnify the site. After surgery the bone flap is wired or sutured. Sometimes drains are placed to remove fluid and blood. Patients are usually cared for in an ICU until stable.

TABLE 55-14	Types of Cranial Surgery
TYPE	**DESCRIPTION**
Burr hole	Opening into the cranium with a drill; used to remove localized fluid and blood beneath the dura
Craniotomy	Opening into the cranium with removal of a bone flap and opening the dura to remove a lesion, repair a damaged area, drain blood, or relieve increased ICP
Craniectomy	Excision into the cranium to cut away a bone flap
Cranioplasty	Repair of a cranial defect resulting from trauma, malformation, or previous surgical procedure; artificial material used to replace damaged or lost bone
Stereotaxis	Precision localization of a specific area of the brain using a frame or a frameless system based on three-dimensional coordinates; procedure is used for biopsy, radiosurgery, or dissection
Shunt procedures	Alternate pathway to redirect cerebrospinal fluid from one area to another using a tube or implanted device; examples include ventriculoperitoneal shunt and Ommaya reservoir

ICP, Intracranial pressure.

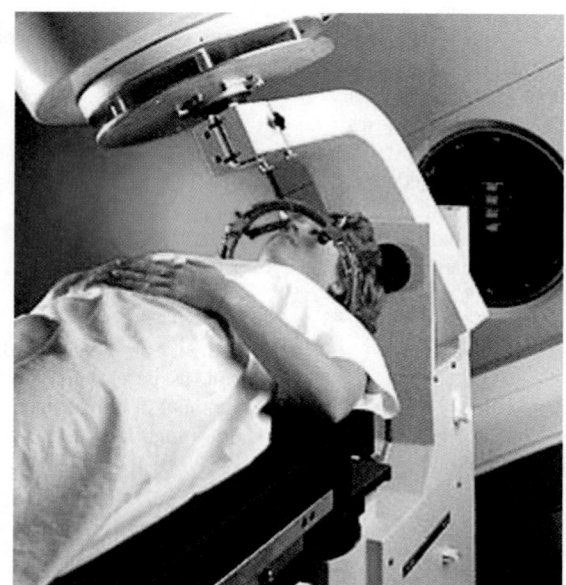

FIG. 55-18 Stereotactic frame.

NURSING MANAGEMENT
CRANIAL SURGERY

■ Nursing Assessment

The nursing assessment of the patient undergoing cranial surgery would be similar to that for the patient with increased ICP (see pp. 1500-1502).

■ Nursing Diagnoses

Nursing diagnoses for the patient with cranial surgery are similar to that for the patient with increased ICP and may include, but are not limited to, those presented in NCP 55-1.

■ Planning

The overall goals are that the patient with cranial surgery will (1) return to normal consciousness, (2) be free from pain and discomfort, (3) maximize neuromuscular functioning, and (4) be rehabilitated to maximum ability.

■ Nursing Implementation

Acute Intervention. The general preoperative and postoperative nursing care for the patient undergoing cranial surgery is similar regardless of the cause. Nursing management is presented in NCP 55-1. The patient (if conscious and coherent) and the family will be gravely concerned about the potential physical and emotional problems that can result from surgery. The uncertainty regarding prognosis and outcome requires compassionate nursing care in the preoperative period.

Preoperative teaching is important in allaying the fears of the patient and the family and also in preparing them for the postoperative period. The patient and the family should be given general information concerning the type of operation that will be performed and what can be expected immediately after the operation. Explaining that some hair is shaved to allow for better exposure and prevention of contamination may prevent unnecessary concern over this task. The hair is usually removed in the operating room after induction of anesthesia. The family should also be informed that the patient will be taken to an ICU or to a special care unit after the operation.

The primary goal of care after cranial surgery is prevention of increased ICP. (Nursing management of the patient with increased ICP is presented on pp. 1502-1505.) Frequent assessment of the neurologic status of the patient is essential during the first 48 hours. In addition to the neurologic functions, fluids, electrolyte levels, and osmolality are monitored closely to detect changes in sodium regulation, the onset of diabetes insipidus, or severe hypovolemia. The turning and positioning of the patient sometimes depend on the site of the operation. If the surgical approach is in the posterior fossa, the patient is generally kept flat or at a slight elevation (10 to 15 degrees). Lying on the back will be prevented as much as possible, and flexion of the neck will be avoided to protect the suture line. The maximum swelling in the operative area occurs within 24 to 48 hours after the surgery.

The dressing is usually in place for 3 to 5 days. With an incision over the skull in the anterior or middle fossa, the patient will return from the operating room with the head elevated at an angle of 30 to 45 degrees. If a bone flap has been removed (craniectomy), care should be taken not to have the patient positioned on the operative side. The dressing should be observed for color, odor, and amount of drainage. The health care provider should be notified immediately of any excessive bleeding or clear drainage. Checking drains for placement and assessing the area around the dressing are also important Scalp care should include meticulous care of the incision to prevent wound infection. The area should be cleansed with povidone iodine (Betadine) or a similar antiseptic disinfectant. Cleansing should be followed by application of an antibiotic ointment according to procedure. Once the dressing is removed, use of an antiseptic soap for washing the scalp may also be beneficial. The psychologic impact of hair removal can be alleviated by the use of a wig, turban, scarves, or cap after the incision has completely healed. For the patient who is receiving radiation, use of a sunblock and head covering should be advocated if any exposure to the sun is anticipated.

Ambulatory and Home Care. The rehabilitative potential for a patient after cranial surgery depends on the reason for the surgery, the postoperative course, and the patient's general state of health. Nursing interventions must be based on a realistic appraisal of these factors. An overall goal for the nurse is to foster independence for as long as possible and to the highest degree possible.

Specific rehabilitation potential cannot be determined until cerebral edema and increased ICP subside postoperatively. Care must be taken to maintain as much function as possible through measures such as careful positioning, meticulous skin and mouth care, regular range-of-motion exercises, bowel and bladder care, and adequate nutrition.

Referrals may be made to other specialists on the health care team. For example, the speech therapist may be helpful to the patient who has a speech problem, or the physical therapist may provide an exercise plan to regain functional deficits. The needs and problems of each patient should be addressed individually because many variables affect the plan.

The mental and physical deterioration of the patient, including seizures, personality disorganization, apathy, and wasting, is difficult for both family and health professionals to endure. Mental and emotional residual deficits are often more difficult for the patient and the family to accept than are motor and sensory losses. Although progress is continually being made to help the patient with a brain tumor by means of chemotherapy, conventional and interstitial radiation, and biologic therapies, the prognosis remains grim. The nurse can provide much help and support during the adjustment phase and in long-range planning.

ETHICAL DILEMMAS
Withholding Treatment

Situation

A 26-year-old patient in a permanent vegetative state is diagnosed with her fifteenth bladder infection. Her home care nurse must determine whether or not to seek antibiotics for this infection. The family members have expressed a concern that no heroic measures be used to extend the biologic life of the patient, but they have been unwilling to withdraw the existing treatment, which is enteral nutrition through a gastrostomy tube. Should antibiotics be withheld?

Important Points for Consideration

- Patients in persistent vegetative state do not recover.
- Providing nutrition and hydration, even if by artificial means, can have significant cultural, religious, and psychologic meaning to patients and families.
- Clarification with the family about the goals of treatment and the patient's wishes, when she was competent and if they are known, is imperative. It is important to know whether treatment for an infection would be considered heroic based on the family's perspective of what the patient would want.
- The family's concerns about pain, suffering, and quality of life for the patient must be explored within the context of the overall plan of care.
- Withholding treatment is morally acceptable when a competent patient consents to it, if there is no medical benefit to the patient, if the treatment merely prolongs life, or if the burden of treatment outweighs the benefit to the patient.

Critical Thinking Questions

1. How would you approach the patient's family?
2. What are your feelings about providing nutrition, hydration, and treatments that will prolong life in a patient for whom there is no hope of recovery?

■ **Evaluation**

The expected outcomes are that the patient who has had cranial surgery will

- regain maximal cognitive, motor, and sensory function possible
- be free of infection
- have pain and discomfort alleviated
- be free of seizures
- have optimal nutritional intake

Inflammatory Conditions of the Brain

Meningitis, encephalitis, and brain abscesses are the most common inflammatory conditions of the brain and spinal cord. Inflammation can be caused by bacteria, viruses, fungi, and chemicals (e.g., contrast media used in diagnostic tests or blood in the subarachnoid space) (Table 55-15). CNS infections may occur via the bloodstream, by extension from a primary site, or along cranial and spinal nerves. The mortality rate is approximately 15% in the general population, with higher rates in elderly patients. Up to 15% of those who recover have long-term neurologic deficits.[25]

BACTERIAL MENINGITIS

Etiology and Pathophysiology

Meningitis is an acute inflammation of the pia mater and the arachnoid membrane surrounding the brain and the spinal cord. Therefore meningitis is always a cerebrospinal infection. Bacterial meningitis is considered a medical emergency. Untreated bacterial meningitis has a mortality rate approaching 100%. The organisms usually gain entry to the CNS through the upper respiratory tract or the bloodstream, but they may enter by direct extension from penetrating wounds of the skull or through fractured sinuses in basal skull fractures.

Meningitis usually occurs in the fall, winter, or early spring and is often secondary to viral respiratory disease. Older adults and persons who are debilitated are more often affected than is the general population. *Streptococcus pneumoniae* and *Neisseria meningitidis* are the leading causes of bacterial meningitis. *Haemophilus influenzae* was once the most common cause. However, the use of *H. influenzae* vaccine has resulted in a significant decrease in meningitis related to this organism.

The inflammatory response to the infection tends to increase CSF production, with a moderate increase in ICP. In bacterial meningitis the purulent secretions produced quickly spread to other areas of the brain through the CSF. If this process extends into the brain parenchyma or if concurrent encephalitis is present, cerebral edema and increased ICP become more of a problem. All patients with meningitis must be observed closely for manifestations of increased ICP, which is thought to be a result of swelling around the dura, and increased CSF volume.

Clinical Manifestations

Fever, severe headache, nausea, vomiting, and **nuchal rigidity** (resistance to flexion of the neck) are key signs of meningitis. A positive Kernig sign, a positive Brudzinski sign (see Chapter 54), photophobia, a decreased LOC, and signs of increased ICP may also be present. Coma is associated with a poor prognosis and occurs in 5% to 10% of patients with bacterial meningitis. Seizures occur in 20% of all cases.[26] With meningitis the headache be-

TABLE 55-15	**Comparison of Cerebral Inflammatory Conditions**		
	MENINGITIS	**ENCEPHALITIS**	**BRAIN ABSCESS**
Causative Organisms	Bacteria (*Streptococcus pneumoniae*, *Neisseria meningitidis*, group B streptococcus, viruses, fungi)	Bacteria, fungi, parasites, herpes simplex virus (HSV), other viruses (e.g., West Nile virus)	Streptococci, staphylococci through bloodstream
CSF			
Pressure (normal, 60-150 mm H$_2$O)	Increased	Normal to slight increase	Increased
WBC count (normal, 0-8/μl)	*Bacterial:* >1000/μl (mainly PMN) *Viral:* 25-500/μl (mainly lymphocytes)	500/μl, PMN (early), lymphocytes (later)	25-300/μl (PMN)
Protein (normal, 15-45 mg/dl [0.15-0.45 g/L])	*Bacterial:* >500 mg/dl *Viral:* 50-500 mg/dl	Slight increase	Normal
Glucose (normal, 45-75 mg/dl [2.5-4.2 mmol/L])	*Bacterial:* decreased *Viral:* normal or low	Normal	Low or absent
Appearance	*Bacterial:* turbid, cloudy *Viral:* clear or cloudy	Clear	Clear
Diagnostic Studies	Gram stain, smear, culture, PCR*	EEG, MRI, PET, PCR, IgM antibodies to virus in serum or CSF	CT scan, EEG, skull x-ray
Treatment	Antibiotics, supportive care, prevention of ↑ ICP	Supportive care, prevention of ↑ ICP, acyclovir (Zovirax) for HSV	Antibiotics, incision and drainage Supportive care

*PCR is used to detect viral RNA or DNA.
CSF, Cerebrospinal fluid; *CT,* computed tomography; *EEG,* electroencephalogram; *ICP,* intracranial pressure; *MRI,* magnetic resonance imaging; *PCR,* polymerase chain reaction; *PET,* positron emission tomography; *PMN,* polymorphonuclear cells; *WBC,* white blood cell.

comes progressively worse and may be accompanied by vomiting and irritability. If the infecting organism is a meningococcus, a skin rash is common and petechiae may be seen.

Complications

The most common acute complication of bacterial meningitis is increased ICP. More than 90% of patients will have increased ICP, and it is the major cause of unconsciousness. Another complication of bacterial meningitis is residual neurologic dysfunction. Cranial nerve dysfunction often occurs with cranial nerves III, IV, VI, VII, or VIII in bacterial meningitis. The dysfunction usually disappears within a few weeks. However, hearing loss may be permanent after bacterial meningitis.

Cranial nerve irritation can have serious sequelae. The optic nerve (CN II) is compressed by increased ICP. Papilledema is often present, and blindness may occur. When the oculomotor (CN III), trochlear (CN IV), and abducens (CN VI) nerves are irritated, ocular movements are affected. Ptosis, unequal pupils, and diplopia are common. Irritation of the trigeminal nerve (CN V) is evidenced by sensory losses and loss of the corneal reflex, and irritation of the facial nerve (CN VII) results in facial paresis. Irritation of the vestibulocochlear nerve (CN VIII) causes tinnitus, vertigo, and deafness.

Hemiparesis, dysphasia, and hemianopsia may also occur. These signs usually resolve over time. If resolution does not occur, a cerebral abscess, subdural empyema, subdural effusion, or persistent meningitis is suggested. Acute cerebral edema may occur with bacterial meningitis, causing seizures, CN III palsy, bradycardia, hypertensive coma, and death.

A noncommunicating hydrocephalus may occur if the exudate causes adhesions that prevent the normal flow of the CSF from the ventricles. CSF reabsorption by the arachnoid villi may also be obstructed by the exudate. Surgical implantation of a shunt is the only treatment.

A complication of meningococcal meningitis is the Waterhouse-Friderichsen syndrome. The syndrome is manifested by petechiae, disseminated intravascular coagulation (DIC), and adrenal hemorrhage. DIC is a serious complication of meningitis. (DIC is discussed in Chapter 30.) DIC is the cause of death in about 1% of patients with meningitis.

Diagnostic Studies

When a patient presents with manifestations suggestive of bacterial meningitis, a blood culture should be done. Diagnosis is usually verified by doing a lumbar puncture and analysis of the CSF. Variations in the CSF depend on the causative organism. Protein levels in the CSF are usually elevated and are higher in bacterial than in viral meningitis. Decreased CSF glucose concentration is common in bacterial meningitis and may be normal in viral meningitis. The CSF is purulent and turbid in bacterial meningitis; it may be the same or clear in viral meningitis. The predominant white blood cell type in the CSF during bacterial meningitis is polymorphonuclear cells (see Table 55-15). Specimens of the CSF, sputum, and nasopharyngeal secretions are taken for culture before the start of antibiotic therapy to identify the causative organism. A Gram stain is done to detect bacteria.

X-rays of the skull may demonstrate infected sinuses. CT scans and MRI may be normal in uncomplicated meningitis. In other cases, CT scans may reveal evidence of increased ICP or hydrocephalus.

Collaborative Care

Bacterial meningitis is a medical emergency. Rapid diagnosis based on history and physical examination is crucial because the patient is usually in a critical state when health care is sought. When meningitis is suspected, antibiotic therapy is instituted after the collection of specimens for cultures, even before the diagnosis is confirmed (Table 55-16). The fundus of the eye should be examined via ophthalmoscope for papilledema before lumbar puncture for identification of possible increased ICP.

Ampicillin, penicillin, cefuroxime (Ceftin), cefotaxime (Claforan), ceftriaxone (Rocephin), ceftizoxime (Cefizox), and ceftazidime (Ceptaz) are the drugs of choice for treating meningitis. These drugs are effective because of their ability to penetrate the blood-brain barrier.

NURSING MANAGEMENT
BACTERIAL MENINGITIS

■ Nursing Assessment

Initial assessment should include vital signs, neurologic evaluation, fluid intake and output, and evaluation of the lungs and skin (see Fig. 55-10).

■ Nursing Diagnoses

Nursing diagnoses for the patient with bacterial meningitis may include, but are not limited to, those presented in NCP 55-2.

■ Planning

The overall goals are that the patient with bacterial meningitis will have (1) return to maximal neurologic functioning, (2) resolution of infection, and (3) decreased pain and discomfort.

TABLE 55-16	Collaborative Care Bacterial Meningitis

Diagnostic
History and physical examination
Analysis of CSF for protein, glucose, WBC, Gram stain, and culture
CBC, coagulation profile, electrolyte levels, glucose, platelet count
Blood culture
CT scan, MRI, PET scan
Skull x-ray studies

Collaborative Therapy
Bed rest
IV fluids
Antibiotics IV
  ampicillin, penicillin
  cephalosporin (e.g., cefotaxime [Claforan], ceftriaxone [Rocephin])
Codeine for headache
Acetaminophen or aspirin for temperature above 100.4° F (38° C)
Hypothermia
Clear liquids as desired or tolerated
phenytoin (Dilantin) IV
furosemide (Lasix) or mannitol IV for diuresis

CBC, Complete blood count; *CSF,* cerebrospinal fluid; *CT,* computed tomography; *IV,* intravenous; *MRI,* magnetic resonance imaging; *PET,* positron emission tomography; *WBC,* white blood cell.

NURSING CARE PLAN 55-2

Patient with Bacterial Meningitis

EXPECTED PATIENT OUTCOMES	NURSING INTERVENTIONS and *RATIONALES*
NURSING DIAGNOSIS	**Disturbed sensory perception** *related to* decreased LOC *as manifested by* inaccurate interpretation of environment, signs of fear or anxiety, disorientation, and restlessness.
▪ Minimal disorientation ▪ Lack of evidence of agitation	▪ Assess LOC *to determine extent of the problem.* ▪ Administer sedative medication as ordered *to reduce fear and anxiety.* ▪ Keep room quiet and lights dim; use calm, reassuring approach *to avoid stimulating or frightening the patient.* ▪ Assist and support patient during uncomfortable or frightening diagnostic procedures; have family member at bedside when possible *to assist with orientation and reduce anxiety.*
NURSING DIAGNOSIS	**Acute pain** *related to* headache and muscle and joint aches *as manifested by* general discomfort of head, joints, and muscles; apathy; grimacing on movement.
▪ Satisfaction with pain relief ▪ Increased participation in treatment plan	▪ Administer mild analgesia as needed; assist patient to position of comfort in bed *to relieve pain.* ▪ Encourage gentle range-of-motion and leg exercises *to reduce joint stiffness and promote circulation.* ▪ Massage muscles as needed or requested *to promote comfort and show a caring attitude.* ▪ Control environment to encourage rest *because pain can be exhausting to the patient.*
NURSING DIAGNOSIS	**Hyperthermia** *related to* infection and abnormal temperature regulation by hypothalamus from increased ICP *as manifested by* increased temperature and chills.
▪ Normal body temperature	▪ Carry out general measures of care for patient with a fever.* ▪ If prescribed, use hypothermia blanket to reduce temperature *because an elevated temperature increases brain metabolism and increases the risk of seizures or increased ICP.* ▪ Reduce temperature gradually *to prevent shivering, which can cause a rebound effect and raise rather than lower the temperature.*
NURSING DIAGNOSIS	**Ineffective therapeutic regimen management** *related to* possible sequelae of condition *as manifested by* motor or sensory problems and activity limitations.
▪ Satisfactory management of condition by self or others	▪ Monitor for residual effects of condition such as vision, hearing, activity, and cognitive problems *to determine appropriate referrals.* ▪ Inform patient and others that residual problems often improve over time *to reduce anxiety.* ▪ Arrange for post-discharge care if required *so that patient's needs are met.*

COLLABORATIVE PROBLEMS

NURSING GOALS	NURSING INTERVENTIONS and *RATIONALES*
POTENTIAL COMPLICATION	**Seizure activity** *related to* cerebral irritation.
▪ Monitor for seizure activity ▪ Carry out appropriate medical and nursing interventions ▪ Report and record any seizure activity	▪ Monitor for seizure activity *so that interventions can be initiated immediately.* ▪ Keep side rails up and padded *to protect patient if a seizure occurs.* ▪ Administer sedative and antiseizure drugs as ordered *to control or prevent seizure activity.* ▪ Reduce fever *to decrease brain's oxygen demand.* ▪ Carry out interventions to treat underlying causes of inflammatory brain condition *to prevent seizure activity.*
POTENTIAL COMPLICATION	**Increased ICP** *related to* presence of infectious exudate, increased production of CSF.†

*See the Nursing Care Plan for the Patient with a Fever (NCP 12-1) on p. 219.
†See NCP 55-1 on p. 1503.
CSF, Cerebrospinal fluid; *ICP,* intracranial pressure; *LOC,* level of consciousness.

■ Nursing Implementation

Health Promotion. Prevention of respiratory infections through vaccination programs for pneumococcal pneumonia and influenza should be supported by nurses.[27] In addition, early and vigorous treatment of respiratory and ear infections is important. Persons who have close contact with anyone who has bacterial meningitis should be given prophylactic antibiotics.

Acute Intervention. The patient with bacterial meningitis is usually acutely ill. The fever is high, and head pain is severe. Irritation of the cerebral cortex may result in seizures. The changes in mental status and LOC depend on the degree of increased ICP. Assessment of vital signs, neurologic evaluation, fluid intake and output, and evaluation of lung fields and skin should be performed at regular intervals based on the patient's condition and recorded carefully.

Head pain and neck pain secondary to movement require attention. Codeine provides some pain relief without undue sedation for most patients. The patient should be assisted to a position of comfort, often curled up with the head slightly extended. The head of the bed should be slightly elevated, when permitted after lumbar puncture. A darkened room and a cool cloth over the eyes relieve the discomfort of photophobia.

For the delirious patient, additional low lighting may be necessary to decrease hallucinations. All patients suffer some degree of mental distortion and hypersensitivity and may be frightened and misinterpret the environment. Every attempt should be made to minimize environmental stimuli and prevent injury. Restraints should be avoided. Armboards, secured with multiple layers of stretch gauze (e.g., Kerlix), protect the IV infusion site. The presence of a familiar person at the bedside has a calming effect. The nurse must be efficient with care but also should project an attitude of caring and of unhurried gentleness. The use of touch and a soothing voice to give simple explanations of activities is helpful. If seizures occur, appropriate observations should be made and protective measures should be taken. Antiseizure drugs such as phenytoin (Dilantin) are administered as ordered. Problems associated with increased ICP are also managed (see Increased ICP earlier in this chapter).

Fever must be vigorously managed because it increases cerebral edema and the frequency of seizures. In addition, neurologic damage may result from an extremely high temperature over a prolonged time. Acetaminophen or aspirin may be used to reduce fever. However, if the fever is resistant to aspirin or acetaminophen, more vigorous means are necessary, such as an automatic cooling blanket. Care should be taken not to reduce the temperature too rapidly because shivering may result, causing a rebound effect and increasing the temperature. The extremities should be wrapped in sheepskin, soft towels, or a blanket covered with a sheet to protect them from "frostbite." Care of the skin should be frequent to prevent breaks in the skin. If a cooling blanket is not available or desirable, tepid sponge baths with water may be effective in lowering the temperature. The skin must be protected from excessive drying and injury.

Because high fever greatly increases the metabolic rate and thus insensible fluid loss, the patient should be assessed for dehydration and adequacy of fluid intake. Diaphoresis further increases fluid losses, which should be estimated and included in an intake and output record. Replacement fluids should be calculated as 800 ml per day for respiratory losses and 100 ml for each degree of temperature above 100.4° F (38° C). Supplemental feeding to maintain adequate nutritional intake via tube or oral feedings may be necessary. The designated antibiotic schedule must be followed to maintain therapeutic blood levels. Observations should be made for side effects of the drugs used.

In most cases, meningitis does not require isolation, with the exception of meningococcal meningitis. However, good aseptic technique is essential to protect the patient and the nurse.

Ambulatory and Home Care. After the acute period has passed, the patient requires several weeks of convalescence before normal activities can be resumed. In this period, good nutrition should be stressed, with an emphasis on a high-protein, high-calorie diet in small, frequent feedings.

Muscle rigidity may persist in the neck and the backs of the legs. Progressive range-of-motion exercises and warm baths are useful. Activity should be gradually increased as tolerated, but adequate bed rest and sleep should be encouraged.

Residual effects are uncommon in meningococcal meningitis, but pneumococcal meningitis can result in sequelae such as dementia, seizures, deafness, hemiplegia, and hydrocephalus. Vision, hearing, cognitive skills, and motor and sensory abilities should be assessed after recovery, with appropriate referrals as indicated. Meningitis in infancy may have "silent" neurologic sequelae, which are manifested as learning and behavioral problems when the child reaches school age.

Throughout the acute and convalescent periods the nurse should be aware of the anxiety and stress experienced by individuals close to the patient.

■ Evaluation

The expected outcomes for the patient with bacterial meningitis are addressed in NCP 55-2.

VIRAL MENINGITIS

The most common causes of viral meningitis are enteroviruses, arboviruses, human immunodeficiency virus, and herpes simplex virus (HSV). Viral meningitis usually presents as a headache, fever, photophobia, and stiff neck. The fever may be moderate or high. There are usually no symptoms of brain involvement.

The most important diagnostic test is examination of the CSF. The typical finding is lymphocytosis (see Table 55-15). Organisms are not seen on Gram stain or acid-fast smears. Polymerase chain reaction (PCR) used to detect viral-specific DNA or RNA is the most important method for diagnosing CNS viral infections.

Viral meningitis is managed symptomatically because the disease is self-limiting. Antiviral therapy is not used. Full recovery from viral meningitis is expected. Rare sequelae include persistent headaches, mild mental impairment, and incoordination.

ENCEPHALITIS

Encephalitis, an acute inflammation of the brain, is a serious, and sometimes fatal, disease. In the United States, encephalitis is responsible for about 20,000 cases and 1400 deaths annually.[28]

Etiology and Pathophysiology

Encephalitis is usually caused by a virus. Many different viruses have been implicated in encephalitis, some of them associated with certain seasons of the year and endemic to certain geographic areas. Ticks and mosquitoes transmit epidemic encephalitis. Examples include Eastern equine encephalitis, Japanese encephalitis (rarely seen in the United States at this time), LaCrosse encephalitis, St. Louis encephalitis, West Nile virus, and Western equine encephalitis. Nonepidemic encephalitis may occur as a complication of measles, chickenpox, or mumps. HSV encephalitis is the most common cause of acute nonepidemic viral encephalitis. Cytomegalovirus encephalitis is one of the common complications in patients with acquired immunodeficiency syndrome (AIDS).

The West Nile virus was first identified in North America in New York City in the summer of 1999. Advanced age is the primary risk factor for encephalitis and mortality associated with this virus. The incubation period of West Nile Virus is from 3 to 14 days. Most cases are mild flulike symptoms. However, about 1 in 150 infections will result in severe neurologic disease, with encephalitis more commonly seen than meningitis.[29]

Clinical Manifestations and Diagnostic Studies

The onset of infection is typically nonspecific with fever, headache, nausea, and vomiting. It can be acute or subacute. Signs of encephalitis appear on day two or three and may vary from minimal alterations in mental status to coma. Virtually any CNS abnormality can occur, including hemiparesis, tremors, seizures, cranial nerve palsies, personality changes, memory impairment, amnesia, and dysphasia.

Early diagnosis and treatment of viral encephalitis are essential for favorable outcomes. Diagnostic findings related to viral encephalitis are shown in Table 55-15. Brain imaging techniques include MRI and PET. PCR tests for HSV DNA and RNA levels in CSF allow for early detection of HSV viral encephalitis.[30] West Nile virus should be strongly considered in adults over 50 years old who develop encephalitis or meningitis in summer or early fall. The best diagnostic test for West Nile virus is IgM antibody to the virus in serum or CSF collected within 8 days of illness onset. Because IgM dose not cross the blood-brain barrier, IgM antibody in the CSF strongly suggests CNS infection.

The clinical distinction between meningitis and encephalitis is based on brain function. Patients with meningitis may be uncomfortable, lethargic, or distracted by headache, but their cerebral function remains normal. In encephalitis, however, abnormalities in brain function are common, including altered mental status, motor or sensory deficits, and speech or movement disorders.

NURSING and COLLABORATIVE MANAGEMENT
VIRAL ENCEPHALITIS

To prevent encephalitis, mosquito control should be practiced, including cleaning rain gutters, removing old tires, draining bird baths, and removing water where mosquitoes can breed. In addition, insect repellant should be used during mosquito season.

Collaborative and nursing management of encephalitis is symptomatic and supportive. Cerebral edema is a major problem, and diuretics (mannitol) and corticosteroids (dexamethasone [Decadron]) are used to control it. In the initial stages of encephalitis, many patients require intensive care.

Acyclovir (Zovirax) and vidarabine (Vira-A) are used to treat encephalitis caused by HSV infection. Acyclovir has fewer side effects than vidarabine and is often the preferred treatment. Use of these antiviral agents has been shown to reduce mortality rates although neurologic complications may not be reduced. For maximal benefit, antiviral agents should be started before the onset of coma. Seizure disorders should be treated with antiseizure drugs (see Table 57-9). Prophylactic treatment with antiseizure drugs may be used in severe cases of encephalitis. Treatment of cytomegalovirus encephalitis in AIDS patients is discussed in Chapter 14.

BRAIN ABSCESS

Brain abscess is an accumulation of pus within the brain tissue that can result from a local or a systemic infection. Direct extension from ear, tooth, mastoid, or sinus infection is the primary cause. Other causes for brain abscess formation include spread from a distant site (e.g., pulmonary infection, bacterial endocarditis) skull fracture, and a prior brain trauma or surgery. Streptococci and *Staphylococcus aureus* are the primary infective organisms.

Manifestations are similar to those of meningitis and encephalitis and include headache, fever, and nausea and vomiting. Signs of increased ICP may include drowsiness, confusion, and seizures. Focal symptoms may be present and reflect the local area of the abscess. For example, visual field defects or psychomotor seizures are common with a temporal lobe abscess, whereas an occipital abscess may be accompanied by visual impairment and hallucinations. Computed tomography (CT) and MRI are used to diagnose a brain abscess.

Antimicrobial therapy is the primary treatment for brain abscess. Other manifestations are treated symptomatically. If drug therapy is not effective, the abscess may need to be drained, or removed if it is encapsulated. In untreated cases, the mortality rate approaches 100%. Nursing measures are similar to those for management of meningitis or increased ICP. If surgical drainage or removal is the treatment of choice, nursing care is similar to that described under cranial surgery.

Other infections of the brain include subdural empyema, osteomyelitis of the cranial bones, epidural abscess, and venous sinus thrombosis after periorbital cellulitis.

CRITICAL THINKING EXERCISES

Case Study
Head Injury

Patient Profile. T.J. is a 43-year-old white man who was the driver of a motorcycle that ran into an automobile. He was sedated, paralyzed, and intubated by paramedics at the scene before transport by helicopter. He was brought to the emergency department with a diagnosis of closed head injury with skull fracture.

Subjective Data

He was reportedly unresponsive at the scene with a Glasgow Coma Scale score = 3, hypotension, tachycardia, and shallow irregular respirations.

Objective Data

At the Scene

- Unresponsive with obvious deformity to the left side of the skull
- Respirations were shallow and irregular

- O_2 saturations ranged from 90% to 95%
- Systolic blood pressure ranged from 50 to 80 mm Hg
- Heart rate ranged from 100 to 130 beats/min

In the ED

- Right pupil, 4 mm nonreactive; left pupil, 3 mm nonreactive
- Glasgow Coma Scale score = 3
- Hypotension and tachycardia continued in spite of fluid resuscitation

Diagnostic Studies

- CT of the head was positive for left skull fracture, left subdural hematoma, bilateral intraventricular and subarachnoid hemorrhage, and cerebral edema.
- CT of the abdomen/pelvis showed a lacerated liver, multiple infarcts to the right kidney, fluid around the duodenum and pancreas, and multiple left pelvic fractures.
- C-spine series was negative.

CRITICAL THINKING EXERCISES—cont'd

- Chest x-ray showed a right lung contusion and pneumo-mediastinum and subcutaneous emphysema.

CRITICAL THINKING QUESTIONS

1. What could be the cause of T.J.'s hypoxia, hypotension, and tachycardia?
2. How could the injuries impact his neurologic condition?
3. What area of the brain do T.J.'s clinical manifestations suggest may be injured?
4. What nursing interventions should be implemented? What are the priorities?
5. Based on the assessment data presented, write one or more nursing diagnoses. Are there any collaborative problems?

Nursing Research Issues

1. What type of information and education do families need at each stage of recovery for the head-injured patient?
2. What is the effect of nursing activities or interventions on intracranial pressure, cerebral perfusion pressure, cerebral blood flow, and cerebral tissue oxygenation?
3. What is the most valid noninvasive or continuous method for real-time monitoring of cerebral tissue perfusion and oxygenation?
4. Do cognitive stimulation programs decrease the frequency of cognitive and behavioral changes that occur after minor head injury?

REVIEW QUESTIONS

The number of the question corresponds to the same-numbered objective at the beginning of the chapter.

1. Vasogenic cerebral edema increases intracranial pressure by
   a. shifting fluid in the gray matter.
   b. altering the endothelial lining of cerebral capillaries.
   c. leaking molecules from the intracellular fluid to the capillaries.
   d. altering the osmotic gradient flow into the intravascular component.

2. A patient with intracranial pressure monitoring has pressure of 12 mm Hg. The nurse understands that this pressure reflects
   a. a severe decrease in cerebral perfusion pressure.
   b. an alteration in the production of cerebrospinal fluid.
   c. the loss of autoregulatory control of intracranial pressure.
   d. a normal balance between brain tissue, blood, and cerebrospinal fluid.

3. The nurse plans care for the patient with increased intracranial pressure with the knowledge that the best way to position the patient is to
   a. keep the head of the bed flat.
   b. elevate the head of the bed to 30 degrees.
   c. maintain patient on left side with head supported on pillow.
   d. use a continuous-rotation bed to continuously change patient position.

4. The nurse is alerted to a possible acute subdural hematoma in the patient who
   a. has a linear skull fracture crossing a major artery.
   b. has focal symptoms of brain damage with no recollection of a head injury.
   c. develops decreased level of consciousness and a headache within 48 hours of a head injury.
   d. has an immediate loss of consciousness with a brief lucid interval followed by decreasing level of consciousness.

5. During admission of a patient with a severe head injury to the emergency department, the nurse places the highest priority on assessment for
   a. patency of airway.
   b. presence of a neck injury.
   c. neurologic status with the Glasgow Coma Scale.
   d. cerebrospinal fluid leakage from the ears or nose.

6. A patient is suspected of having a cranial tumor. The signs and symptoms include memory deficits, visual disturbances, weakness of right upper and lower extremities, and personality changes. The nurse recognizes that the tumor is most likely located in the
   a. frontal lobe.
   b. parietal lobe.
   c. occipital lobe.
   d. temporal lobe.

7. Nursing management of a patient with a brain tumor includes
   a. discussing with the patient methods to control inappropriate behavior.
   b. using diversion techniques to keep the patient stimulated and motivated.
   c. assisting and supporting the family in understanding any changes in behavior.
   d. limiting self-care activities until the patient has regained maximum physical functioning.

8. The primary goal of nursing care after a craniotomy is
   a. preventing infection.
   b. ensuring patient comfort.
   c. avoiding the need for secondary surgery.
   d. preventing increased intracranial pressure.

9. A nursing measure that is indicated to reduce the potential for seizures and increased intracranial pressure in the patient with bacterial meningitis is
   a. administering codeine for relief of head and neck pain.
   b. controlling fever with prescribed drugs and cooling techniques.
   c. keeping the room darkened and quiet to minimize environmental stimulation.
   d. maintaining the patient on strict bed rest with the head of the bed slightly elevated.

REFERENCES

1. Cushing H: *Studies in intracranial physiology and surgery,* London, 1925, Oxford University Press.
2. Cold GE: Measurement of cerebral blood flow and oxygen consumption, and the regulation of cerebral circulation, *ACTA Neurochir Suppl* 49:1, 1990.
3. Wong FWH: Prevention of secondary brain injury, *Crit Care Nurs* 20:18, 2000.
4. Juul N et al: Intracranial hypertension and cerebral perfusion pressure: influence on neurological deterioration and outcome in severe head injury, *J Neurosurg* 92:1, 2000.
5. Bullock R et al: The Brain Trauma Foundation. The American Association of Neurological Surgeons. The Joint Section on Neurotrauma and Critical Care. Recommendations for intracranial pressure monitoring technology, *J Neurotrauma* 17:497, 2000.
6. Rebuck JA et al: Infection related to intracranial pressure monitors in adults: analysis of risk factors and antibiotic prophylaxis, *J Neurol Neurosurg Psychiatry* 69:381, 2000.
7. Kerr ME et al: Dose response to cerebrospinal fluid drainage on cerebral perfusion in traumatic brain-injured adults, *Neurosurg Focus* 11:Article 2, 2001.
8. Nau R: Osmotherapy for elevated intracranial pressure: a critical reappraisal, *Clin Pharmacokin* 38:23, 2000.
9. Yanagawa T et al: Nutritional support for head-injured patients (Cochrane Review), *Cochrane Database Syst Rev* 3:CD001530, 2002.
10. Jennett B, Teasdale G: Aspects of coma after severe head injury, *Lancet* 23:878, 1977.
11. Plum F, Posner J: *The diagnosis of stupor and coma,* ed 3, Philadelphia, 1980, FA Davis.
*12. Kerr ME et al: Effect of short-duration hyperventilation during endotracheal suctioning on intracranial pressure in severe head injured adults, *Nurs Res* 48:195, 1997.
13. Gemma M et al: Intracranial effects of endotracheal suctioning in the acute phase of head injury, *J Neurosurg Anesthesiol* 14:50, 2002.
14. Moraine JJ, Berre J, Melot C: Is cerebral perfusion pressure a major determinant of cerebral blood flow during head elevation in comatose patients with severe intracranial lesions? *J Neurosurg* 92:606, 2000.
15. Traumatic brain injury in the United States: a report to congress, 1999, Centers for Disease Control.
16. Traumatic brain injury in the United States, Centers for Disease Control. Available at www.cdc.gov/ncipc/didop/tbi (accessed August 22, 2002).
17. Marmarou A et al: Impact of ICP instability and hypotension on outcome in patients with severe head trauma, *J Neurosurg* 75:S59, 1991.
18. Meythaler JM et al: Current concepts: diffuse axonal injury-associated traumatic brain injury, *Arch Phys Med Rehabil* 82:1461, 2001.
19. Walleck C: Patients with head injury and brain dysfunction. In Clochesy JM et al, editors: *Critical Care Nursing,* ed 2, Philadelphia, 1996, WB Saunders.
20. Machamer J, Temkin N, Dikmen S: Significant other burden and factors related to it in traumatic brain injury, *J Clin Exp Neuropsychol* 24:420, 2002.
21. Boyle GJ, Haines S: Severe traumatic brain injury: some effects on family caregivers, *Psychol Rep* 90:415, 2002.

22. Paterson B, Kieloch B, Gmiterek J: "They never told us anything": post-discharge instruction for families of persons with brain injuries, *Rehabil Nurs* 26:48, 2001.
23. *Cancer Facts and Figures 2002,* Atlanta, 2002, American Cancer Society.
24. Stafford SI et al: Meningioma radiosurgery: tumor control, outcomes, and complications among 190 consecutive patients, *Neurosurgery* 49:1029, 2001.
25. Miner JR et al: Presentation, time to antibiotics, and mortality of patients with bacterial meningitis at an urban county medical center, *J Emerg Med* 21:387, 2001.
26. Choi C: Bacterial meningitis in aging adults, *Clin Infect Dis* 33:1380, 2001.
27. Patel M, Lee CK: Polysaccharide vaccines for preventing serogroup A meningococcal meningitis, *Cochrane Database Syst Rev* 3:CD001093, 2001.
28. Khetsuriani N, Holman RC, Anderson LJ: Burden of encephalitis-associated hospitalizations in the United States, 1988-1997, *Clin Infect Dis* 15; 35:175, 2002.
29. West Nile virus encephalitis, *N Engl J Med* 347:1225, 2002.
30. Simko JP et al: Differences in laboratory findings for cerebrospinal fluid specimens obtained from patients with meningitis or encephalitis due to herpes simplex virus (HSV) documented by detection of HSV DNA, *Clin Infect Dis* 35:414, 2002.

---

*Nursing research–based reference.

RESOURCES

American Brain Tumor Association
2720 River Road
Des Plaines, IL 60018
800-886-2282 or 847-827-9910
Fax: 847-827-9918
www.abta.org

Brain Injury Association of America
105 North Alfred Street
Alexandria, VA 22314
800-444-6443 (family helpline) or 703-236-6000
Fax: 703-236-6001
www.biausa.org

Brain Tumor Center
Massachusetts General Hospital/Harvard Medical School
Cox-315, 100 Blossom Street
Boston, MA 02114
617-724-8770
Fax: 617-724-8769
http://btc.mgh.harvard.edu

National Brain Tumor Foundation
414 Thirteenth Street, Suite 700
Oakland, CA 94612-2603
800-934-CURE (2873) (Brian Tumor Information Line) or
510-839-9777
Fax: 510-839-9779
www.braintumor.org

For additional Internet resources, see the website for this book at *http://evolve.elsevier.com/Lewis/medsurg/.*

CHAPTER **56**

NURSING MANAGEMENT
Stroke

Catherine Kirkness

LEARNING OBJECTIVES

1. Describe the incidence of and risk factors for stroke.
2. Explain mechanisms that affect cerebral blood flow.
3. Compare and contrast the etiology and pathophysiology of ischemic and hemorrhagic strokes.
4. Correlate the clinical manifestations of stroke with the underlying pathophysiology.
5. Identify diagnostic studies performed for patients with strokes.
6. Describe the collaborative care, drug therapy, and nutritional therapy for a patient with a stroke.
7. Describe the acute nursing management of the patient with a stroke.
8. Describe the rehabilitative nursing management of the patient with a stroke.
9. Explain the psychosocial impact of a stroke on the patient and family.

KEY TERMS

aneurysm, p. 1529
aphasia, p. 1531
dysarthria, p. 1531
dysphasia, p. 1531
embolic stroke, p. 1529
hemorrhagic strokes, p. 1529
intracerebral hemorrhage, p. 1529

ischemic strokes, p. 1528
lacunar stroke, p. 1529
stroke, p. 1525
subarachnoid hemorrhage, p. 1529
thrombotic stroke, p. 1528
transient ischemic attack, p. 1527

Stroke occurs when there is *ischemia* (inadequate blood flow) to a part of the brain or hemorrhage into the brain that results in death of brain cells. Functions, such as movement, sensation, or emotions, that were controlled by the affected area of the brain are lost or impaired. The severity of the loss of function varies according to the location and extent of the brain involved.

Stroke is a major public health concern. An estimated 700,000 to 750,000 persons in the United States and 50,000 in Canada suffer a stroke annually.[1,2] Stroke is the third most common cause of death in the United States and Canada, behind cancer and heart disease.[2,3] Stroke is also a leading cause of serious, long-term disability. There are an estimated 4.5 million stroke survivors in the United States and up to 300,000 in Canada.[2,3] With an aging population, a further increase in stroke incidence can be expected.

Approximately 25% of individuals who have an initial stroke die within 1 year.[3] The percentage is higher for people age 65 and older. Of those who survive, 50% to 70% will be functionally independent, and 15% to 30% will live with permanent disability.[3] Common long-term disabilities include hemiparesis, inability to walk, complete or partial dependence in activities of daily living (ADLs), and aphasia. Over a lifetime, four out of five families will be affected by stroke.[4]

In addition to the physical, cognitive, and emotional impact of stroke on stroke survivors and their families, stroke also has an enormous financial impact. The direct and indirect costs of strokes are estimated to be greater than $51 billion per year in the United States and $2.7 billion per year in Canada.[1,2]

ETIOLOGY AND PATHOPHYSIOLOGY

Risk Factors for Stroke

The most effective way to decrease the burden of stroke is prevention. Awareness and control of modifiable risk factors can contribute to reducing the incidence and burden of stroke. Risk factors can be divided into nonmodifiable and modifiable. Stroke risk increases several-fold with multiple risk factors.

Nonmodifiable risk factors include age, gender, race, and heredity. Stroke risk increases with age, doubling each decade after 55 years of age. Two thirds of all strokes occur in individuals over 65 years, but stroke can occur at any age. The overall incidence and prevalence of stroke are almost equal for men and women, but women die more often from stroke than men.[3] Because women tend to live longer than men, they have more opportunity to suffer a stroke. African Americans have a higher incidence of stroke, as well as a higher death rate from stroke, than whites.[1] This may be related in part to a higher incidence of hypertension, obesity, and diabetes mellitus in African Americans. Hispanics, American Indians/Alaska Natives, and Asian Americans also have a higher stroke incidence than whites. A family history of stroke, a prior transient ischemic attack, or a prior stroke also increases the risk of stroke.[1]

CULTURAL & ETHNIC CONSIDERATIONS
Cerebrovascular Disease

- African Americans have a higher incidence of stroke and higher death rates from strokes than whites. This may be related to a higher incidence of hypertension, obesity, and diabetes mellitus in African Americans.
- Hispanics, Native Americans, and Asian Americans have a higher stroke incidence than whites.

Reviewed by Patricia A. Blissitt, RN, PhD, CCRN, CNRN, CCM, CS, Staff Nurse, Neurosurgical Intensive Care Unit, Harborview Medical Center, Seattle, Wash.

TABLE 56-1	Modifiable Risk Factors for Stroke

- Asymptomatic carotid stenosis
- Diabetes mellitus
- Heart disease, atrial fibrillation
- Heavy alcohol consumption
- Hypercoagulability
- Hyperlipidemia
- Hypertension
- Obesity
- Oral contraceptive use
- Physical inactivity
- Sickle cell disease
- Smoking

Modifiable risk factors are those that can potentially be altered through lifestyle changes and medical treatment, thus reducing the risk of stroke (Table 56-1). Hypertension is the single most important modifiable risk factor, but it is still often undetected and inadequately treated.[4] Increases in systolic and diastolic blood pressure independently increase the risk of stroke. Stroke risk can be reduced by up to 42% with appropriate treatment of hypertension.[5]

Heart disease, including atrial fibrillation, myocardial infarction, cardiomyopathy, cardiac valve abnormalities, and cardiac congenital defects, is also a risk factor for stroke. Of these, atrial fibrillation is the most important treatable cardiac-related risk factor.[6] The incidence of atrial fibrillation increases with age. Approximately 25% of strokes in patients over 80 years of age are due to atrial fibrillation.[7] Following myocardial infarction, nearly 8% of men and 11% of women will have a stroke within 6 years. Diabetes mellitus is a significant risk for stroke.[8,9] Although tight control of hypertension in diabetics significantly decreases stroke risk, tight control of blood glucose has not been shown to reduce stroke risk.[9]

Increased serum cholesterol is another risk factor for stroke.[10,11] Smoking nearly doubles the risk of stroke.[1,12] Fortunately, the risk associated with smoking decreases over time after quitting smoking and is reduced to that of nonsmokers by 5 years.[12] Asymptomatic carotid stenosis, which can be detected by the presence of a cervical bruit or by ultrasound testing, is another risk factor.[13]

Other modifiable risk factors include lifestyle habits such as excessive alcohol consumption, obesity, physical inactivity, poor diet, and drug abuse. The effect of alcohol on stroke risk appears to depend on the amount consumed. Moderate alcohol consumption (≤ 2 drinks/day) may be protective, but heavy alcohol consumption (>2 drinks/day) is associated with increased risk.[14,15] Abdominal obesity in men increases stroke risk, and obesity and weight gain in women increase the risk of ischemic stroke but not hemorrhagic stroke.[16] In addition, obesity is also associated with conditions such as hypertension, high blood glucose, and elevated blood lipid levels, which also increase stroke risk.

An association of physical inactivity and increased stroke risk is present in both men and women, regardless of ethnicity. Benefits of physical activity can occur with even light-to-moderate regular activity and may be in part related to the beneficial effect of exercise on other risk factors. The effect of diet on stroke risk is not clear, although a diet high in saturated fat and low in fruits and vegetables may increase stroke risk. Illicit drug use, commonly cocaine, has been associated with stroke risk.[17,18]

Older, high-dose estrogen oral contraceptives are strongly associated with increased stroke risk. A meta-analysis of studies looking at the relationship between low-dose (<50 μg) estrogen oral contraception and ischemic stroke concluded that low-dose estrogen use is associated with an increased risk of ischemic stroke, but the absolute risk is low, given a low incidence of stroke in this group of individuals.[19] The presence of other risk factors, particularly smoking and hypertension, in women taking oral contraceptives can increase stroke risk.[20] In 2002, data from the Women's Health Initiative (longitudinal intervention trial in middle-aged women) showed an increased risk of strokes in women taking estrogen plus progestin compared with those not receiving hormone replacement therapy. These data suggest that postmenopausal hormone replacement therapy does not protect against stroke.[21] Other conditions that may increase stroke risk include migraine headaches, inflammatory states, and hyperhomocysteinemia.

Hypercoagulation disorders predispose to vascular occlusive diseases including ischemic strokes, especially in younger adults.[22] Sickle cell disease is another known stroke risk factor for stroke.[1]

Pathophysiology

Anatomy of Cerebral Circulation. Blood is supplied to the brain by two major pairs of arteries: the internal carotid arteries (anterior circulation) and the vertebral arteries (posterior circulation). The carotid arteries branch to supply most of the frontal, parietal, and temporal lobes; the basal ganglia; and part of the diencephalon (thalamus and hypothalamus). The major branches of the carotid arteries are the middle cerebral and the anterior cerebral arteries. The vertebral arteries join to form the basilar artery, which branches to supply the middle and lower part of the temporal lobes, the occipital lobes, cerebellum, brainstem, and part of the diencephalon. The main branch of the basilar artery is the posterior cerebral artery. The anterior and posterior cerebral circulation is connected at the circle of Willis by the anterior and posterior communicating arteries (Fig. 56-1). Anomalies in this area are common, and all connecting vessels may not be present.

Regulation of Cerebral Blood Flow. The brain requires a continuous supply of blood to provide the oxygen and glucose that neurons need to function. Blood flow must be maintained at 750 to 1000 ml per minute (55 ml per 100 g of brain tissue), or 20% of the cardiac output, for optimal brain functioning. If blood flow to the brain is totally interrupted (e.g., cardiac arrest), neurologic metabolism is altered in 30 seconds, metabolism stops in 2 minutes, and cellular death occurs in 5 minutes.

The brain is normally well protected from changes in mean systemic arterial blood pressure over a range from 50 and 150 mm Hg by a mechanism known as *cerebral autoregulation.* This involves changes in the diameter of cerebral blood vessels in response to changes in pressure so that the blood flow to the brain stays constant. Cerebral autoregulation may be impaired following cerebral ischemia, and cerebral blood flow then changes directly in response to changes in blood pressure. Carbon dioxide is a potent cerebral vasodilator, and changes in arterial carbon dioxide levels have a dramatic effect on cerebral blood flow (increased carbon dioxide levels increase cerebral blood flow and vice versa). Very low arterial oxygen levels (partial pressure of arterial oxygen <50 mm Hg) or an increase in hydrogen ion concentration also increase cerebral blood flow.

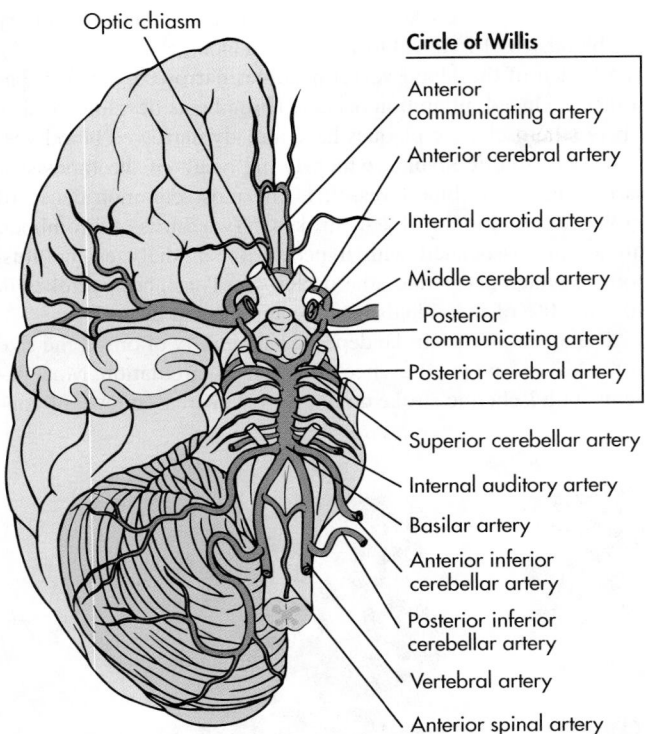

FIG. 56-1 Cerebral arteries and the circle of Willis. The tip of the temporal lobe has been removed to show the course of the middle cerebral artery.

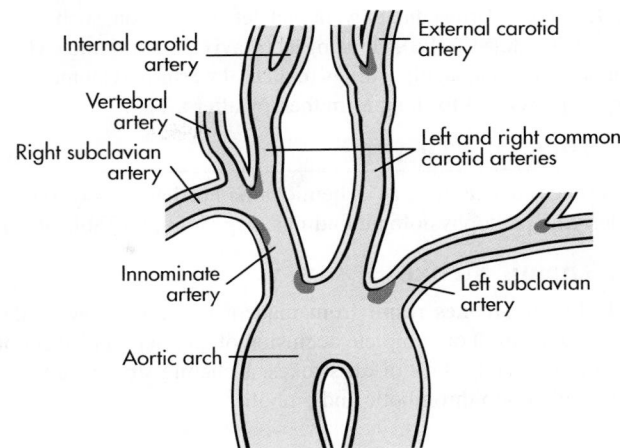

FIG. 56-2 Common sites for the development of atherosclerosis in extracranial and intracranial arteries. The main locations are just above the common carotid bifurcation (most common site) and the start of the branches from the aorta, innominate, and subclavian arteries.

Factors that affect blood flow to the brain include systemic blood pressure, cardiac output, and blood viscosity. During normal activity, oxygen requirements vary considerably, but changes in cardiac output, vasomotor tone, and distribution of blood flow normally maintain adequate blood flow to the head. Cardiac output has to be reduced by one third before cerebral blood flow is reduced. Changes in blood viscosity affect cerebral blood flow, with decreased viscosity increasing flow.

Collateral circulation may develop to compensate for a decrease in cerebral blood flow. Because of the connections between arteries at the circle of Willis, an area of the brain can potentially receive blood supply from another blood vessel if its original blood supply is cut off (e.g., because of thrombosis). Individual differences in collateral circulation partly determine the degree of brain damage and functional loss when a stroke occurs.

Intracranial pressure (ICP) also influences cerebral blood flow (see Chapter 55). Increased ICP causes brain compression and reduced cerebral blood flow.

Atherosclerosis. Atherosclerosis (hardening and thickening of arteries) is a major cause of stroke. It can lead to thrombus formation and contribute to emboli. (The role of atherosclerosis in thrombosis and emboli development is discussed in Chapter 33 and shown in Fig. 33-4.) Initially there is abnormal infiltration of lipids in the intimal layer of the artery. This fatty streak further develops into a plaque. Plaques often develop in areas of increased turbulence of the blood, such as at the bifurcation of an artery or a tortuous area (Fig. 56-2). Calcified, brittle plaques may rupture or fissure. Platelet and fibrin stick to the roughened plaque surface. Plaques lead to narrowing or occlusion of the artery. Also, parts of the plaque or thrombus can break off and travel to a nar-

rower distal artery. Cerebral infarction occurs when an artery becomes blocked and blood supply to the brain beyond the blockage is cut off.

In response to ischemia a series of metabolic events, termed the *ischemic cascade*, occur, including inadequate adenosine triphosphate (ATP) production, loss of ion homeostasis, release of excitatory amino acids (e.g., glutamate), free radical formation, and cell death.[23] Around the core area of ischemia is a border zone of reduced blood flow where ischemia is potentially reversible. If adequate blood flow can be restored early (e.g., within 3 hours) and the ischemic cascade can be interrupted, there may be less brain damage and less neurologic function lost. Research is ongoing to identify thrombolytic and neuroprotective therapies to reestablish blood flow and protect neurons from further ischemic damage.

Transient Ischemic Attack

A **transient ischemic attack** (TIA) is a temporary focal loss of neurologic function caused by ischemia of one of the vascular territories of the brain, lasting less than 24 hours and often lasting less than 15 minutes. Most TIAs resolve within 3 hours. TIAs may be due to microemboli that temporarily block the blood flow. TIAs are a warning sign of progressive cerebrovascular disease. The signs and symptoms of a TIA depend on the blood vessel that is involved and the area of the brain that is ischemic. If the carotid system is involved, patients may have a temporary loss of vision in one eye *(amaurosis fugax),* a transient hemiparesis, numbness or loss of sensation, or a sudden inability to speak. Signs of a TIA involving the vertebrobasilar system may include tinnitus, vertigo, darkened or blurred vision, diplopia, ptosis, dysarthria, dysphagia, ataxia, and unilateral or bilateral numbness or weakness.

Evaluation must be done to confirm that the signs and symptoms of a TIA are not related to other brain lesions, such as a developing subdural hematoma or an increasing tumor mass. Computed tomography (CT) of the brain without contrast is the most important initial diagnostic study. Cardiac monitoring and tests may reveal an underlying cardiac condition that is responsible for clot formation. Drugs that prevent platelet aggregation, such as aspirin, ticlopidine (Ticlid), clopidogrel (Plavix), dipyridamole (Persantine), and anticoagulant drugs (e.g., oral warfarin [Coumadin]), may be prescribed for long-term therapy after a TIA.

TYPES OF STROKE

Strokes are classified as ischemic or hemorrhagic based on the underlying pathophysiologic findings (Fig. 56-3 and Table 56-2).

Ischemic Stroke

Ischemic strokes result from inadequate blood flow to the brain from partial or complete occlusion of an artery and account for approximately 85% of all strokes. Ischemic strokes are further divided into thrombotic and embolic.

Thrombotic Stroke. Thrombosis occurs in relation to injury to a blood vessel wall and formation of a blood clot (Fig. 56-3, *A*). The lumen of the blood vessel becomes narrowed, and if it becomes occluded, infarction occurs. Thrombosis develops readily where atherosclerotic plaques have already narrowed blood vessels. **Thrombotic stroke,** which is the result of thrombosis or narrowing of the blood vessel, is the most common cause of stroke, accounting for 61% of strokes.[24] Two thirds of thrombotic strokes are associated with hypertension or diabetes mellitus, both of which accelerate atherosclerosis. Thrombotic strokes in 30% to 50% of individuals have been preceded by a TIA.

The extent of the stroke depends on rapidity of onset, the size of the lesion, and the presence of collateral circulation. Most patients with ischemic stroke do not have a decreased level of con-

A

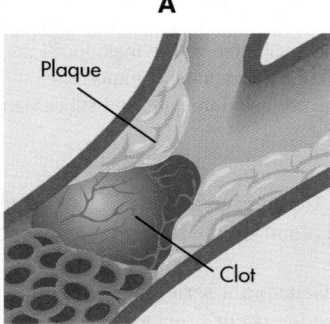

Thrombotic stroke. Cerebral thrombosis is a narrowing of the artery by fatty deposits called *plaque*. Plaque can cause a clot to form, which blocks the passage of blood through the artery.

B

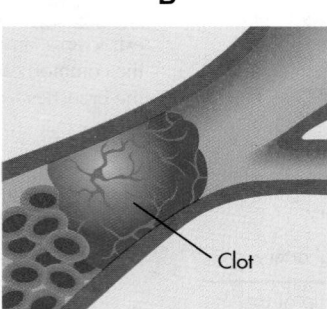

Embolic stroke. An embolus is a blood clot or other debris circulating in the blood. When it reaches an artery in the brain that is too narrow to pass through, it lodges there and blocks the flow of blood.

C

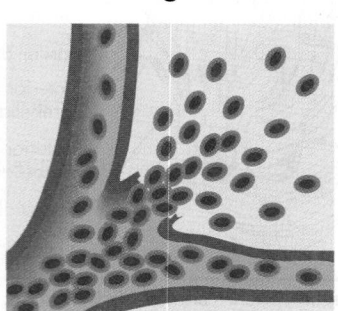

Hemorrhagic stroke. A burst blood vessel may allow blood to seep into and damage brain tissues until clotting shuts off the leak.

FIG. 56-3   Major types of stroke.

TABLE 56-2	Types of Stroke			
TYPE	**GENDER/AGE**	**WARNING**	**TIME OF ONSET**	**COURSE/PROGNOSIS**
Ischemic				
Thrombotic	Men more than women, oldest median age	TIA (30%–50% of cases)	During or after sleep	Stepwise progression, signs and symptoms develop slowly, usually some improvement, recurrence in 20%–25% of survivors
Embolic	Men more than women	TIA (uncommon)	Lack of relationship to activity, sudden onset	Single event, signs and symptoms develop quickly, usually some improvement, recurrence common without aggressive treatment of underlying disease
Hemorrhagic				
Intracerebral	Slightly higher in women	Headache (25% of cases)	Activity (often)	Progression over 24 hr; poor prognosis, fatality more likely with presence of coma
Subarachnoid	Slightly higher in women, youngest median age	Headache (common)	Activity (often), sudden onset Most commonly related to head trauma	Single sudden event usually, fatality more likely with presence of coma

TIA, Transient ischemic attack.

sciousness in the first 24 hours, unless it is due to a brainstem stroke or other conditions such as seizures, increased ICP, or hemorrhage. Ischemic stroke symptoms may progress in the first 72 hours as infarction and cerebral edema increase.

A **lacunar stroke** refers to a stroke from occlusion of a small penetrating artery with development of a cavity in the place of the infarcted brain tissue. This most commonly occurs in the basal ganglia, thalamus, internal capsule, or pons. Although a large percentage of lacunar strokes are asymptomatic, when present, symptoms can cause considerable deficits. These include pure motor hemiplegia, pure sensory stroke (contralateral loss of all sensory modalities), contralateral leg and face weakness with arm and leg ataxia, and isolated motor or sensory stroke. Multiple small vessel infarcts may also result in a decrease in cognitive function (i.e., multiinfarct dementia) (see Chapter 58).[25]

Embolic Stroke. **Embolic stroke** occurs when an embolus lodges in and occludes a cerebral artery, resulting in infarction and edema of the area supplied by the involved vessel (Fig. 56-3, B). Embolism is the second most common cause of stroke, accounting for about 24% of strokes.[24] The majority of emboli originate in the endocardial (inside) layer of the heart, with plaque breaking off from the endocardium and entering the circulation. The embolus travels upward to the cerebral circulation and lodges where a vessel narrows or bifurcates. Heart conditions associated with emboli include atrial fibrillation, myocardial infarction, infective endocarditis, rheumatic heart disease, valvular prostheses, and atrial septal defects. Less common causes of emboli include air and fat from long bone (femur) fractures.

The patient with an embolic stroke commonly has a rapid occurrence of severe clinical symptoms. Embolic strokes can affect any age group. Rheumatic heart disease is one cause of embolic stroke in young to middle-aged adults. An embolus arising from an atherosclerotic plaque is more common in older adults. Warning signs are less common with embolic than with thrombotic stroke. The onset of an embolic stroke is usually sudden and may or may not be related to activity. The patient usually remains conscious although may have a headache. Prognosis is related to the amount of brain tissue deprived of its blood supply. The effects of the emboli are initially characterized by severe neurologic deficits, which can be temporary if the clot breaks up and allows blood to flow. Smaller emboli then continue to obstruct smaller vessels, which in turn involve smaller portions of the brain with fewer deficits noted. The embolic stroke often occurs rapidly, and the body does not have time to accommodate by developing collateral circulation. Recurrence of embolic stroke is common unless the underlying cause is aggressively treated.

Hemorrhagic Stroke

Hemorrhagic strokes account for approximately 15% of all strokes and result from bleeding into the brain tissue itself (intracerebral or intraparenchymal hemorrhage) or into the subarachnoid space or ventricles (subarachnoid hemorrhage or intraventricular hemorrhage).

Intracerebral Hemorrhage. **Intracerebral hemorrhage** is bleeding within the brain caused by a rupture of a vessel (Fig. 56-3, C). Hypertension is the most important cause of intracerebral hemorrhage. Other causes include cerebral amyloid angiopathy, vascular malformations, coagulation disorders, anticoagulant and thrombolytic drugs, trauma, brain tumors, and ruptured aneurysms. Hemorrhage commonly occurs during periods of activity. There is most often a sudden onset of symptoms, with progression over minutes to hours because of ongoing bleeding. Symptoms include neurologic deficits, headache, nausea, vomiting, decreased level of consciousness (in about 50% of patients), and hypertension. The extent of the symptoms varies depending on the amount and duration of the bleeding. A blood clot within the closed skull can result in a mass that causes pressure on brain tissue, displaces brain tissue, and decreases cerebral blood flow, leading to ischemia and infarction.

Approximately half of intracerebral hemorrhages occur in the putamen and internal capsule, central white matter, thalamus, cerebellar hemispheres, and pons. Initially, patients experience a severe headache with nausea and vomiting. Clinical manifestations of putaminal and internal capsule bleeding include weakness of one side (including the face, arm, and leg) slurred speech, and deviation of the eyes. Progression of symptoms related to a severe hemorrhage includes hemiplegia, fixed and dilated pupils, abnormal body posturing, and coma. Thalamic hemorrhage results in hemiplegia with more sensory than motor loss. Bleeding into the subthalamic areas of the brain leads to problems with vision and eye movement. Cerebellar hemorrhages are characterized by severe headache, vomiting, loss of ability to walk, dysphagia, dysarthria, and eye movement disturbances. Hemorrhage in the pons is the most serious because basic life functions (e.g., respiration) are rapidly affected. Hemorrhage in the pons can be characterized by hemiplegia leading to complete paralysis, coma, abnormal body posturing, fixed pupils, hyperthermia, and death. The prognosis of patients with intracerebral hemorrhage is poor, with over 50% of patients dying soon after the hemorrhage occurs and only about 20% being functionally independent at 6 months.[26]

Subarachnoid Hemorrhage. **Subarachnoid hemorrhage** occurs when there is intracranial bleeding into the cerebrospinal fluid–filled space between the arachnoid and pia mater membranes on the surface of the brain. Subarachnoid hemorrhage is commonly caused by rupture of a cerebral **aneurysm** (congenital or acquired weakness and ballooning of vessels). Aneurysms may be saccular or berry aneurysms ranging from a few millimeters to 20 to 30 mm in size or fusiform atherosclerotic aneurysms. The majority of aneurysms are in the circle of Willis. Other causes of subarachnoid hemorrhage include arteriovenous malformations (AVMs), trauma, and illicit drug (cocaine) abuse. The annual incidence of subarachnoid hemorrhage caused by ruptured aneurysm is 6 to 16 per 100,000.[27] The incidence increases with age and is higher in women than men.

The patient may have warning symptoms if the ballooning artery applies pressure to brain tissue or minor warning symptoms from leaking of an aneurysm before major rupture. The characteristic presentation of a ruptured aneurysm is the sudden onset of a severe headache that is different from a previous headache and typically the "worst headache of one's life." Loss of consciousness may or may not occur, and the patient's level of consciousness may range from alert to comatose, depending on the severity of the bleed. Other symptoms include focal neurologic deficits (including cranial nerve deficits), nausea, vomiting, seizures, and stiff neck. Despite improvements in surgical techniques and management, many patients with subarachnoid hemorrhage die, and many are left with significant morbidity, including cognitive difficulties.[27]

Complications of aneurysmal subarachnoid hemorrhage include rebleeding before surgery or other therapy is initiated and cerebral vasospasm (narrowing of the large blood vessels at the base of the brain), which can result in cerebral infarction. Cerebral vasospasm is most likely due to an interaction between the metabolites of blood and the vascular smooth muscle. During the lysis of subarachnoid blood clots, metabolites are released. These metabolites can cause endothelial damage and vasoconstriction. In addition, release of *endothelin* (a potent vasoconstrictor) may play a major role in the induction of cerebral vasospasm after subarachnoid hemorrhage.

The most frequent surgical procedure to prevent rebleeding is clipping of the aneurysm (Fig. 56-4). Endovascular techniques may also be used. In the procedure known as *coiling,* a metal coil can be inserted into the lumen of the aneurysm via interventional neuroradiology (Fig. 56-5). This results in thrombus formation around the coil, resulting in blockage of the aneurysmal sac. Interventions to treat cerebral vasospasm either before or following aneurysm clipping or coiling include administration of the calcium channel blocker nimodipine (Nimotop). Following aneurysmal occlusion, hyperdynamic therapy, including hemodilution, induced hypertension using vasoconstricting agents (e.g., phenylephrine or dopamine [Intropin]), and hypervolemia, may be instituted in an effort to increase the mean arterial pressure and increase cerebral perfusion. Volume expansion is achieved via crystalloid or colloid solution.

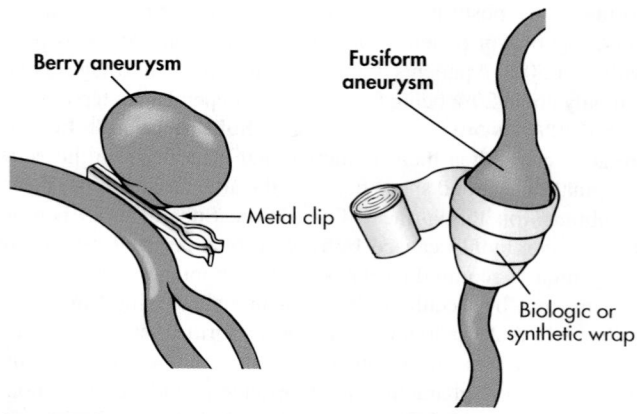

FIG. 56-4 Clipping and wrapping of aneurysms.

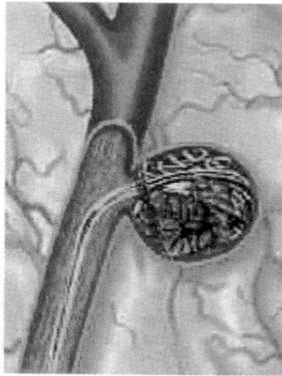

FIG. 56-5 Coil is used to occlude an aneurysmal sac. Soft platinum coil is attached to a stainless steel delivery wire. The softness allows the coil to conform to the often irregular shape of intracranial aneurysms.

Clinical Manifestations

A stroke can have an effect on many body functions, including motor activity, elimination, intellectual function, spatial-perceptual alterations, personality, affect, sensation, and communication. The functions affected are directly related to the artery involved and area of the brain it supplies (Table 56-3). Manifestations related to right- and left-brain damage differ somewhat and are shown in Fig. 56-6.

The term *brain attack* is increasingly being used to describe stroke and communicate the urgency of recognizing stroke symptoms and treating their onset as a medical emergency, similar to what would be done with a *heart attack.* Following the onset of stroke symptoms, immediate medical attention is crucial to reduce disability and death.

TABLE 56-3	**Clinical Manifestations: Specific Cerebral Artery Involvement**

Middle Cerebral Artery Involvement
Contralateral weakness (hemiparesis) or paralysis (hemiplegia)
Contralateral hemianesthesia; loss of proprioception, fine touch, localization
Dominant hemisphere: aphasia
Nondominant hemisphere: neglect of opposite side, anosognosia
Homonymous hemianopsia

Anterior Cerebral Artery Involvement
Occlusion of stem*
Occlusion distal to anterior communicating artery
- Contralateral sensory and motor deficits of foot and leg, greatest distally
- Contralateral weakness of proximal upper extremity
- Urinary incontinence (possibly unrecognized by patient)
- Sensory loss (discrimination, proprioception)
- Contralateral grasp and sucking reflexes may be present
- Apraxia
- Personality change: flat affect, loss of spontaneity, loss of interest in surroundings, distractibility, slowness in responding
- Possible cognitive impairment

Posterior Cerebral Artery and Vertebrobasilar Involvement†
Alert to comatose
Unilateral or bilateral sensory loss
Contralateral or bilateral weakness
Dysarthria
Dysphagia
Hoarseness
Ataxia
Horner syndrome: miosis, ptosis, decreased sweating
Vertigo
Unilateral hearing loss
Nausea, vomiting
Visual disturbances (blindness, homonymous hemianopsia, nystagmus, diplopia)

*There is usually no problem if the stem is occluded near the anterior communicating artery because perfusion from the opposite side is maintained.
†The site of occlusion, the origin of the basilar arteries, and the arrangement of the circle of Willis are involved in the type of deficit seen. This can occur from a thrombus or embolus.

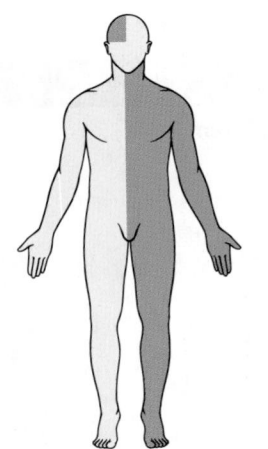
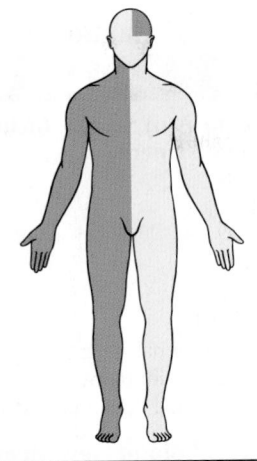

Right-brain damage
(stroke on right side of the brain)
- Paralyzed left side: hemiplegia
- Left-sided neglect
- Spatial-perceptual deficits
- Tends to deny or minimize problems
- Rapid performance, short attention span
- Impulsive, safety problems
- Impaired judgment
- Impaired time concepts

Left-brain damage
(stroke on left side of the brain)
- Paralyzed right side: hemiplegia
- Impaired speech/language aphasias
- Impaired right/left discrimination
- Slow performance, cautious
- Aware of deficits: depression, anxiety
- Impaired comprehension related to language, math

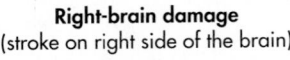 **FIG. 56-6** Manifestations of right-brain and left-brain stroke.

Motor Function. Motor deficits are the most obvious effect of stroke. Motor deficits include impairment of (1) mobility, (2) respiratory function, (3) swallowing and speech, (4) gag reflex, and (5) self-care abilities. Symptoms are caused by the destruction of motor neurons in the pyramidal pathway (nerve fibers from the brain and passing through the spinal cord to the motor cells). The characteristic motor deficits include loss of skilled voluntary movement *(akinesia)*, impairment of integration of movements, alterations in muscle tone, and alterations in reflexes. The initial *hyporeflexia* (depressed reflexes) progresses to *hyperreflexia* (hyperactive reflexes) for most patients.

Motor deficits after a stroke follow certain specific patterns. Because the pyramidal pathway crosses at the level of the medulla, a lesion on one side of the brain affects motor function on the opposite side of the brain (contralateral). The arms and legs of the affected side may be weakened or paralyzed to different degrees depending on which part of and to what extent the cerebral circulation was compromised. A stroke affecting the middle cerebral artery leads to a greater weakness in the upper extremity than the lower extremity. The affected shoulder tends to rotate internally, and the hip rotates externally. The affected foot is plantar flexed and inverted. An initial period of flaccidity may last from days to several weeks and is related to nerve damage. Spasticity of the muscles follows the flaccid stage and is related to interruption of upper motor neuron influence.

Communication. The left hemisphere is dominant for language skills in right-handed persons and in most left-handed per-

sons. Language disorders involve expression and comprehension of written and spoken words. The patient may experience **aphasia** (total loss of comprehension and use of language) when a stroke damages the dominant hemisphere of the brain. **Dysphasia** refers to difficulty related to the comprehension or use of language and is due to partial disruption or loss. Patterns of dysphasia may differ as the stroke affects different portions of the brain. Dysphasias can be classified as *nonfluent* (minimal speech activity with slow speech that requires obvious effort) or *fluent* (speech is present but contains little meaningful communication). Most dysphasias are mixed with impairment in both expression and understanding. A massive stroke may result in *global aphasia,* in which all communication and receptive function is lost.

Strokes affecting Wernicke's area of the brain exhibit symptoms of *receptive aphasia,* when neither the sounds of speech nor its meaning can be understood. This results in impairment of the patient's comprehension of both spoken and written language. Strokes affecting Broca's area of the brain cause *expressive aphasia* (difficulty in speaking and writing).

Many stroke patients also experience **dysarthria,** a disturbance in the muscular control of speech. Impairments may involve pronunciation, articulation, and phonation. Dysarthria does not affect the meaning of communication or the comprehension of language, but it does affect the mechanics of speech. Some patients experience a combination of aphasia and dysarthria.

Affect. Patients who have had a stroke may have difficulty controlling their emotions. Emotional responses may be exaggerated or unpredictable. Depression and feelings associated with changes in body image and loss of function can make this worse. Patients may also be frustrated by mobility and communication problems. An example of unpredictable affect is as follows. A reserved professional engineer has returned home from the hospital following a stroke. During meals with his family, he becomes frustrated and begins to cry because of the difficulty getting food into his mouth and chewing, something that he was able to do easily before his stroke.

Intellectual Function. Both memory and judgment may be impaired as a result of stroke. These impairments can occur with strokes affecting either side of the brain. A left-brain stroke is more likely to result in memory problems related to language. Patients with a left-brain stroke often are very cautious in making judgments. The patient with a right-brain stroke tends to be impulsive and to move quickly. An example of behavior with right-brain stroke is the patient who tries to rise quickly from the wheelchair without locking the wheels or raising the foot rests. The patient with a left-brain stroke would move slowly and cautiously from the wheelchair. Patients with either type of stroke may have difficulty making generalizations, which interferes with their ability to learn.

Spatial-Perceptual Alterations. A stroke on the right side of the brain is more likely to cause problems in spatial-perceptual orientation, although this can also occur with left-brain stroke. Spatial-perceptual problems may be divided into four categories. The first is related to the patient's incorrect perception of self and illness. This deficit follows damage to the parietal lobe. Patients may deny their illnesses or their own body parts. The second category concerns the patient's erroneous perception of self in space. The patient may neglect all input from the affected side. This may be worsened by *homonymous hemianopsia,* in which blindness occurs in the same half of the visual fields of both eyes. The patient also has difficulty with spatial orientation, such as judging distances. The third spatial-perceptual deficit is *agnosia*, the inability to recognize an object by sight, touch, or hearing. The fourth deficit is *apraxia*, the inability to carry out learned sequential movements on command. Patients may or may not be aware of their spatial-perceptual alterations.

Elimination. Fortunately, most problems with urinary and bowel elimination occur initially and are temporary. When a stroke affects one hemisphere of the brain, the prognosis for normal bladder function is excellent. At least partial sensation for bladder filling remains, and voluntary urination is present. Initially, the patient may experience frequency, urgency, and incontinence. Although motor control of the bowel is usually not a problem, patients are frequently constipated. Constipation is associated with immobility, weak abdominal muscles, dehydration, and diminished response to the defecation reflex. Urinary and bowel elimination problems may also be related to inability to express needs and to manage clothing.

Diagnostic Studies

When symptoms of a stroke occur, diagnostic studies are done to (1) confirm that it is a stroke and not another brain lesion, such as a subdural hematoma, and (2) identify the likely cause of the stroke (Table 56-4). Tests also guide decisions about therapy to prevent a secondary stroke. CT is the primary diagnostic test used after a stroke. CT can indicate the size and location of the lesion and differentiate between ischemic and hemorrhagic stroke. CT angiography (CTA) provides visualization of vasculature and can be performed at the same time as the CT scan. CTA allows detection of intracranial or extracranial occlusive disease. Serial CT scans may be used to assess the effectiveness of treatment and to evaluate recovery.

Magnetic resonance imaging (MRI) is used to determine the extent of brain injury. MRI has greater specificity compared with CT. Diffusion-weighted MRI is a more sensitive MRI that better delineates ischemic brain injury early after a stroke when CT and standard MRI may appear normal. Use of MRI may be restricted in patients with claustrophobia or with devices such as pacemakers that would be affected by the magnetic field. Magnetic resonance angiography (MRA) is a noninvasive method of assessing vascular occlusive disease in the head or neck, similar to CTA.

Other tests used to diagnose stroke and assess the extent of tissue damage include positron emission tomography (PET), magnetic resonance spectroscopy (MRS), xenon CT, single photon emission computed tomography (SPECT), and cerebral angiography. PET shows the metabolic activity of the brain and provides a depiction of the extent of tissue damage after a stroke. Less active or diseased tissue appears darker than healthy, active cells. MRS detects biochemical changes that may be present before physical changes are apparent. Its value in the clinical evaluation of stroke remains to be determined.

Angiography is the gold standard for imaging the carotid arteries. Angiography can identify cervical and cerebrovascular occlusion, atherosclerotic plaques, and malformation of vessels. Intraarterial digital subtraction angiography (DSA) reduces the dose of contrast material, uses smaller catheters, and shortens the length of the procedure compared with conventional angiography. DSA involves the injection of a contrast agent to visualize blood vessels in the neck and the large vessels of the circle of Willis. It is considered safer than cerebral angiography because

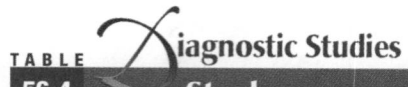

TABLE 56-4	Diagnostic Studies — Stroke
Diagnosis of Stroke, Including Extent of Involvement	
CT, CTA	
MRI, MRA	
SPECT	
PET	
MRS	
Xenon CT	
Electroencephalogram	
Cerebral angiography	
Cerebrospinal fluid analysis*	
Cerebral Blood Flow Measures	
Cerebral angiography	
Digital subtraction angiography	
Doppler ultrasonography	
Transcranial Doppler	
Carotid duplex	
Carotid angiography	
Cardiac Assessment	
Electrocardiogram	
Chest x-ray	
Cardiac enzymes	
Echocardiography (transthoracic, transesophageal)	
Holter monitor (evaluation of arrhythmias)	
Additional Studies	
Complete blood count	
Platelets, prothrombin time, activated partial thromboplastin time	
Electrolytes, blood glucose	
Renal and hepatic studies	
Lipid profile	
Arterial blood gases (if hypoxia suspected)	

*A lumbar puncture to obtain cerebrospinal fluid is avoided if increased intracranial pressure is suspected.
CT, Computed tomography; *CTA,* computed tomography angiography; *MRA,* magnetic resonance angiography; *MRI,* magnetic resonance imaging; *MRS,* magnetic resonance spectroscopy; *PET,* positron emission tomography; *SPECT,* single photon emission computed tomography.

less vascular manipulation is required. Risks of angiography include dislodging an embolus, vasospasm, inducing further hemorrhage, and allergic reaction to contrast media.

Transcranial Doppler (TCD) ultrasonography is a noninvasive study that measures the velocity of blood flow in the major cerebral arteries. TCD has been shown to be effective in detecting microemboli and vasospasm. Other neurodiagnostic tests such as skull x-rays, brain scan, lumbar puncture, and electroencephalogram (EEG) are currently used much less in the diagnosis of stroke. A skull x-ray result is usually normal after a stroke, but there may be a pineal gland shift with a massive infarction.

A lumbar puncture may be done to look for evidence of red blood cells in the cerebrospinal fluid if a subarachnoid hemorrhage is suspected but the CT does not show hemorrhage. A lumbar puncture is avoided if there are signs of increased ICP because of the danger of herniation of the brain downward leading to pressure on cardiac and respiratory centers in the brainstem and potentially death. An EEG may show low-voltage, slow-wave activity suggestive of ischemic infarction. If the stroke is due to a hemorrhage, the EEG may show high-voltage slow waves. If the suspected cause of the stroke includes emboli from the heart, diagnostic cardiac tests should be done (see Table 56-4).

Blood tests are also done to help identify conditions contributing to stroke and to guide treatment (see Table 56-4).

Collaborative Care

Prevention. Primary prevention is a priority for decreasing morbidity and mortality from stroke (Table 56-5). The goals of stroke prevention include health management for the well individual and education and management of modifiable risk factors to prevent a primary or secondary stroke. Health management focuses on (1) healthy diet, (2) weight control, (3) regular exercise, (4) no smoking, (5) limiting alcohol consumption, and (6) routine health assessments. Patients with known risk factors such as diabetes mellitus, hypertension, obesity, high serum lipids, or cardiac dysfunction require close management.

TABLE 56-5	Collaborative Care Stroke

Diagnostic*
History and physical examination

Collaborative Therapy
Prevention
Control of hypertension
Control of diabetes mellitus
Treatment of underlying cardiac problem
Anticoagulation therapy for patients with atrial fibrillation
No smoking
Platelet inhibitors (e.g., aspirin)
Limiting alcohol intake
Surgical interventions for patients with aneurysms at risk of bleeding
Carotid endarterectomy
Stenting
Transluminal angioplasty
Extracranial-intracranial bypass
Acute Care
Maintenance of airway
Fluid therapy
Ischemic Stroke
Tissue plasminogen activator (tPA)
Anticoagulation
Ischemic and Hemorrhagic Stroke
Treatment of cerebral edema
Hemorrhagic Stroke
Surgical decompression if indicated
Subarachnoid Hemorrhage
Surgical obliteration (dependent on size and location of hemorrhage)
Embolic Stroke
Treatment of underlying cause

*Diagnostic studies are presented in Table 56-4.

Drug therapy. Measures to prevent the development of a thrombus or embolus are used in patients at risk for stroke. Antiplatelet drugs are usually the chosen treatment to prevent further stroke in patients who have had a TIA related to atherosclerosis.[28] Aspirin is the most frequently used antiplatelet agent, commonly at a dose of 50 to 325 mg per day. Other drugs include ticlopidine (Ticlid), clopidogrel (Plavix), dipyridamole (Persantine), and combined dipyridamole and aspirin (Aggrenox). Oral anticoagulation using warfarin is the treatment of choice for individuals with atrial fibrillation who have had a TIA.[28]

Surgical therapy. Surgical interventions for the patient with TIAs from carotid disease include carotid endarterectomy, transluminal angioplasty, stenting, and extracranial-intracranial (EC-IC) bypass. In a carotid endarterectomy (CEA), the atheromatous lesion is removed from the carotid artery to improve blood flow[29] (Fig. 56-7).

Transluminal angioplasty is the insertion of a balloon to open a stenosed artery and improve blood flow. Stenting involves intravascular placement of a stent in an attempt to maintain patency of the artery. These procedures are still being evaluated as options to CEA.

EC-IC bypass involves anastomosing (surgically connecting) a branch of an extracranial artery to an intracranial artery (most commonly, superficial temporal to middle cerebral artery) beyond an area of obstruction with the goal of increasing cerebral perfusion. This procedure is generally reserved for those patients who do not benefit from other forms of therapy.[30] Further study is needed to determine the benefit of this therapy over medical therapy.

Acute Care. The goals for collaborative care during the acute phase are preserving life, preventing further brain damage, and reducing disability. Treatment differs according to the type of stroke and changes as the patient progresses from the acute to the rehabilitation phase.

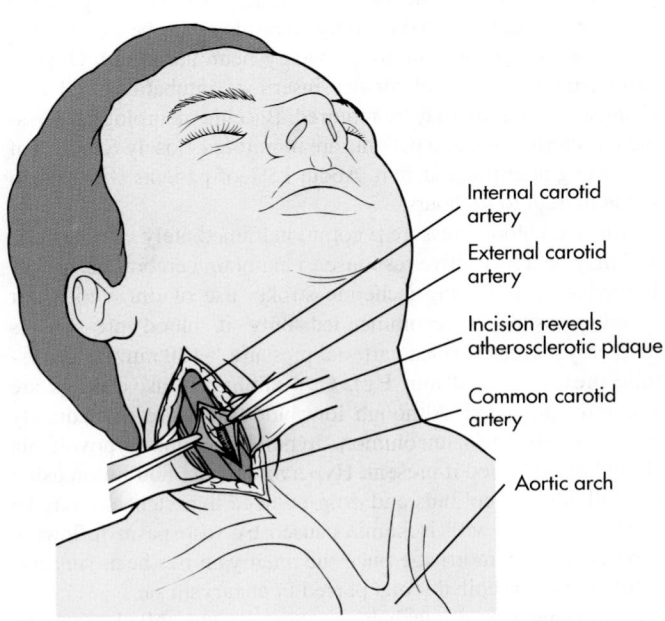

Internal carotid artery

External carotid artery

Incision reveals atherosclerotic plaque

Common carotid artery

Aortic arch

FIG. 56-7 Carotid endarterectomy. Atherosclerotic plaque in the internal carotid artery is removed to prevent impending cerebral infarction.

TABLE 56-6   Emergency Management

Stroke

ETIOLOGY	ASSESSMENT FINDINGS	INTERVENTIONS
• Sudden vascular compromise causing disruption of blood flow to the brain • Thrombosis • Trauma • Aneurysm • Embolism • Hemorrhage	• Altered level of consciousness • Weakness, numbness, or paralysis of portion of body • Speech or visual disturbances • Severe headache • Increased or decreased heart rate • Respiratory distress • Unequal pupils • Hypertension • Facial drooping on affected side • Difficulty swallowing • Seizures • Bladder or bowel incontinence • Nausea and vomiting • Vertigo	**Initial** • Ensure patent airway. • Remove dentures. • Perform pulse oximetry. • Maintain adequate oxygenation (SaO_2 >92%) with supplemental O_2, if necessary. • Establish IV access with normal saline. • Maintain BP according to guidelines (e.g., Advanced Cardiac Life Support).* • Remove clothing. • Obtain CT scan immediately. • Perform baseline laboratory tests, including blood glucose immediately, and treat if hypoglycemic. • Position head midline. • Elevate head of bed 30 degrees if no symptoms of shock or injury. • Institute seizure precautions. • Anticipate thrombolytic therapy for ischemic stroke. **Ongoing Monitoring** • Monitor vital signs and neurologic status, including level of consciousness (Glasgow Coma Scale), motor and sensory function, pupil size and reactivity, O_2 saturation, and cardiac rhythm. • Reassure patient and family.

BP, Blood pressure; *CT*, computed tomography; *IV*, intravenous.
*See Chapter 35.

Table 56-6 outlines the emergency management of the patient with a stroke. Acute care begins with managing the ABCs. Patients may have difficulty keeping an open and clear airway because of a decreased level of consciousness or decreased or absent gag and swallowing reflexes. Maintaining adequate oxygenation is important. Both hypoxia and hypercarbia are to be avoided because they can contribute to secondary neuronal injury. Oxygen administration, artificial airway insertion, intubation, and mechanical ventilation may be required. Baseline neurologic assessment is carried out, and patients are monitored closely for signs of increasing neurologic deficit. About 25% of patients will worsen in the first 24 to 48 hours.

Elevated blood pressure is common immediately after a stroke and may be a protective response to maintain cerebral perfusion. Immediately following ischemic stroke, use of drugs to lower blood pressure is recommended only if blood pressure is markedly increased (mean arterial pressure >130 mm Hg or systolic pressure >220 mm Hg). Oral antihypertensive drugs are generally preferred. Although low blood pressure immediately following stroke is uncommon, hypotension and hypovolemia should be corrected if present. Hypervolemic hemodilution using crystalloids and colloids and drug-induced hypertension may be used in patients with ischemia caused by vasospasm following subarachnoid hemorrhage once the aneurysm has been successfully clipped or coiled (coils placed in aneurysm sac).

Fluid and electrolyte balance must be controlled carefully. The goal generally is to keep the patient adequately hydrated to promote perfusion and decrease further brain injury. Overhydra-tion may compromise perfusion by increasing cerebral edema. Adequate fluid intake during acute care via oral, intravenous (IV), or tube feedings should be 1500 to 2000 ml per day. Urine output is monitored. If secretion of antidiuretic hormone (ADH) increases in response to the stroke, urine output decreases and fluid is retained. Low serum sodium (hyponatremia) may occur. IV solutions with glucose and water are avoided because they are hypotonic and may further increase cerebral edema and ICP. In addition, hyperglycemia may be associated with further brain damage and should be treated. In general, decisions regarding individualized fluid and electrolyte replacement therapy are based on the extent of intracranial edema, symptoms of increased ICP, central venous pressure levels, laboratory values for electrolytes, and intake and output.

Increased ICP is more likely to occur with hemorrhagic strokes but can occur with ischemic strokes. Increased ICP from cerebral edema usually peaks in 72 hours and may cause brain herniation. Management of increased ICP includes practices that improve venous drainage, such as elevating the head of the bed, maintaining head and neck in alignment, and avoiding hip flexion. Hyperthermia, which is seen commonly following stroke and may be associated with poorer outcome, is avoided. Increased temperature contributes to increased cerebral metabolism. Other measures include pain management, avoidance of hypervolemia, and management of constipation. Cerebrospinal fluid drainage may be used in some patients to reduce ICP. Diuretic drugs, such as mannitol (Osmitrol) and furosemide (Lasix), may be used to decrease cerebral edema. As a last resort in the management of ICP, a bone flap may be removed to allow for cerebral edema without increases in ICP. The bone flap is frozen and replaced later.[31]

Drug therapy. Recombinant tissue plasminogen activator (tPA) is used to reestablish blood flow through a blocked artery to prevent cell death in patients with the acute onset of ischemic stroke symptoms. Thrombolytic drugs, such as tPA, produce localized fibrinolysis by binding to the fibrin in the thrombi. The lytic action of tPA occurs as the plasminogen is converted to plasmin (fibrinolysin), whose enzymatic action digests fibrin and fibrinogen and thus lyses the clot. Because it is clot specific in its activation of the fibrinolytic system, tPA is less likely to cause hemorrhage compared with streptokinase or urokinase. (Thrombolytic therapy is discussed in Chapter 33.)

tPA must be administered within 3 hours of the onset of clinical signs of ischemic stroke. Therefore the single most important factor is timing. Patients are screened carefully before tPA can be given. Screening includes a CT or MRI scan to rule out hemorrhagic stroke, blood tests for coagulation disorders, and screening for recent history of gastrointestinal bleeding, stroke or head trauma within the past 3 months, or major surgery within 14 days. Thrombolytic therapy given within 3 hours of the onset of symptoms reduces disability, but at the expense of an increase in deaths within the first 7 to 10 days and an increase in intracranial hemorrhage.[32]

During infusion of the drug, the patient's vital signs and neurologic status are monitored closely to assess for improvement or for potential deterioration related to intracerebral hemorrhage. Control of blood pressure is critical during treatment and for 24 hours following. No anticoagulant or antiplatelet drugs are given for 24 hours after tPA treatment.

Patients with stroke caused by thrombi and emboli may also be treated with platelet inhibitors and anticoagulants (after the first 24 hours if treated with tPA) to prevent further clot formation. Common anticoagulants include heparin and warfarin (Coumadin, Panwarfin). Platelet inhibitors include aspirin, ticlopidine (Ticlid), clopidogrel (Plavix), and dipyridamole (Persantine). IV heparin or low-molecular-weight heparin may be given in the situation of rapidly evolving strokes or stroke caused by emboli traveling from the heart. IV heparin is administered via continuous infusion, and activated partial thromboplastin time is closely monitored.

Typically, heparin is replaced by oral warfarin for long-term administration. Warfarin dosage is regulated according to the international normalized ratio (INR), a standardized measure of prothrombin time that adjusts for assay variations. The therapeutic range for the INR is two to three times normal. Patients must be monitored closely for hemorrhage at other body sites while using anticoagulants and platelet inhibitors. A patient teaching guide for patients taking long-term warfarin is found in Table 37-14. Subcutaneous heparin may be administered for deep vein thrombosis prophylaxis.

Anticoagulants and platelet inhibitors are contraindicated for patients with hemorrhagic strokes. The calcium channel blocker nimodipine (Nimotop) is given to patients with subarachnoid hemorrhage to decrease the effects of vasospasm and minimize cerebral damage. Although nimodipine is a calcium channel blocker, its exact mechanism of action in reducing vasospasm is not known.[33]

Acetylsalicylic acid (aspirin) is also used to prevent platelet aggregation at the site of atherosclerotic plaque. Complications of aspirin include gastrointestinal bleeding with higher doses. Aspirin administration should be done cautiously if the patient has a history of peptic ulcer disease or is taking other anticoagulants.

Drug therapies to treat hyperthermia include aspirin or acetaminophen (Tylenol). A temperature elevation of even 1° C can increase brain metabolism by 10% and contribute to further brain damage. Cooling blankets may be used to cautiously lower temperature. The nurse must closely monitor the patient's temperature.[34]

Approximately 10% to 15% of patients who experience a stroke will have seizures, usually within 24 hours. An antiseizure drug, such as phenytoin (Dilantin), is given if a seizure occurs. The Stroke Council of the American Heart Association recommends uniform seizure prophylaxis in the acute period after intracerebral and subarachnoid hemorrhages.[35] In these patients, seizure activity may result in further neuronal injury and contribute to coma, although no clinical data support this recommendation. In other types of strokes, prophylactic use of antiseizure drugs is not recommended for patients who have not had a seizure.[35]

Surgical therapy. Surgical interventions for stroke include immediate evacuation of aneurysm-induced hematomas or cerebellar hematomas larger than 3 cm. Subarachnoid hemorrhage is usually caused by a ruptured aneurysm. Approximately 20% of patients will have multiple aneurysms. Treatment of an aneurysm involves clipping, wrapping, or coiling the aneurysm to prevent rebleeding (see Figs. 56-4 and 56-5). Treatment of arteriovenous malformation (AVM) is surgical resection and/or radiosurgery (i.e., gamma knife). Both may be preceded by interventional neuroradiology to embolize the blood vessels that supply the AVM.

Subarachnoid and intracerebral hemorrhage can involve bleeding into the ventricles of the brain. This situation produces hydro-

TABLE 56-7	Nursing Assessment Stroke

Subjective Data

Important Health Information

Past health history: Hypertension; previous stroke, TIA, aneurysm, cardiac disease (including recent myocardial infarction), arrhythmias, congestive heart failure, valvular disease, infective endocarditis, hyperlipidemia, polycythemia, diabetes, gout, family history of hypertension, diabetes, stroke, or coronary artery disease

Medications: Use of oral contraceptives, use of and compliance with antihypertensive and anticoagulant agents

Functional Health Patterns

Health perception–health management: Positive family history; alcohol abuse, smoking

Nutritional-metabolic: Anorexia, nausea, vomiting; dysphagia, disturbances in taste and smell

Elimination: Change in bowel and bladder patterns

Activity-exercise: Loss of movement and sensation; syncope; weakness on one side; generalized weakness, easy fatigability

Cognitive-perceptual: Numbness, tingling of one side of the body; loss of memory; alteration in speech, language, problem-solving ability; pain; headache, possibly sudden and severe (hemorrhage); visual disturbances; denial of illness

Objective Data

General

Emotional lability, lethargy, apathy or combativeness, fever

Respiratory

Loss of cough reflex, labored or irregular respirations, tachypnea, rhonchi (aspiration), airway occlusion (tongue), apnea

Cardiovascular

Hypertension, tachycardia, carotid bruit

Gastrointestinal

Loss of gag reflex, bowel incontinence, decreased or absent bowel sounds, constipation

Urinary

Frequency, urgency, incontinence

Neurologic

Contralateral motor and sensory deficits, including weakness, paresis, paralysis, anesthesia; unequal pupils, hand grasps; akinesia, aphasia (expressive, receptive, global), dysarthria (slurred speech), agnosias, apraxia, visual deficits, perceptual or spatial disturbances, altered level of consciousness (drowsiness to deep coma) and Babinski sign, ↓ followed by ↑ deep tendon reflexes, flaccidity followed by spasticity, amnesia, ataxia, personality change, nuchal rigidity, seizures

Possible Findings

Positive CT, CTA, MRI, MRA, or other neuroimaging scans showing size, location, and type of lesion; positive Doppler ultrasonography and angiography indicating stenosis

CT, Computed tomography; *CTA,* computed tomography angiography; *MRA,* magnetic resonance angiography; *MRI,* magnetic resonance imaging; *TIA,* transient ischemic attack.

cephalus, which further damages brain tissue from increased ICP. Insertion of a ventriculostomy for cerebrospinal fluid drainage can result in dramatic improvement in these situations.

Rehabilitation Care. After the stroke has stabilized for 12 to 24 hours, collaborative care shifts from preserving life to lessening disability and attaining optimal function. The patient may be evaluated by a *physiatrist* (a physician who specializes in physical medicine and rehabilitation). It is important to remember that some aspects of rehabilitation actually begin in the acute care phase as soon as the patient is stabilized. Depending on the patient's status, other medical conditions, rehabilitation potential, and available resources, the patient may be transferred to a rehabilitation unit. Other options for rehabilitation include outpatient therapy and home care–based rehabilitation.

As part of the long-term collaborative care after a stroke, various members of the health care team may be involved in the effort to promote optimal function of the patient and family. The composition of the team depends on patient and family needs and rehabilitation facility resources.

NURSING MANAGEMENT
STROKE

■ Nursing Assessment

Subjective and objective data that should be obtained from a person who has had a stroke are presented in Table 56-7. Primary assessment is focused on cardiac and respiratory status and neurologic assessment. If the patient is stable, the nursing history is obtained as follows: (1) description of the current illness with attention to initial symptoms, including onset and duration, nature (intermittent or continuous), and changes; (2) history of similar symptoms previously experienced; (3) current medications; (4) history of risk factors and other illnesses such as hypertension; and (5) family history of stroke or cardiovascular diseases. This information is gained through an interview of the patient, family members, significant others, or caregiver.

Secondary assessment should include a comprehensive neurologic examination of the patient. This includes (1) level of consciousness (Glasgow Coma Scale), (2) cognition, (3) motor abilities, (4) cranial nerve function, (5) sensation, (6) proprioception, (7) cerebellar function, and (8) deep tendon reflexes. Clear documentation of initial and ongoing neurologic examinations is essential to note changes in patient status.

■ Nursing Diagnoses

Nursing diagnoses for the person with a stroke may include, but are not limited to, those presented in NCP 56-1.

■ Planning

The patient, family, and nurse establish the goals of nursing care in a cooperative manner. Typical goals are that the patient will (1) maintain a stable or improved level of consciousness, (2) attain maximum physical functioning, (3) attain maximum self-care abilities and skills, (4) maintain stable body functions (e.g., bladder control), (5) maximize communication abilities, (6) maintain adequate nutrition, (7) avoid complications of stroke, and (8) maintain effective personal and family coping.

NURSING CARE PLAN 56-1

Patient with Stroke

NURSING DIAGNOSIS **Ineffective tissue perfusion (cerebral)** *related to* decreased cerebral blood flow secondary to thrombus, embolus, hemorrhage, or edema *as manifested by* ICP >15 mm Hg for 15 to 30 seconds or longer, decreasing Glasgow Coma Scale score, and altered respiratory pattern.

OUTCOMES—NOC

Tissue Perfusion: Cerebral (0406)
- Neurologic function _____
- Intracranial pressure WNL _____
- Unexplained anxiety not present _____
- Headache not present _____

_____

Outcome Scale
1 = Extremely compromised
2 = Substantially compromised
3 = Moderately compromised
4 = Mildly compromised
5 = Not compromised

INTERVENTIONS—NIC and *RATIONALES*

Cerebral Perfusion Promotion (2550)
- Assess neurologic status (ICP, LOC) at least hourly initially *to detect changes indicative of worsening or improving condition.*
- Monitor patient's ICP and neurologic response to activities *because ICP can increase with changes in positioning and movement.*
- Plan nursing care activities *to minimize increases in ICP.*
- Avoid neck flexion or extreme hip/knee flexion *to avoid obstruction of arterial and venous blood flow.*
- Monitor respiratory status *to assess changes in neurologic status.*

NURSING DIAGNOSIS **Ineffective airway clearance** *related to* inability to raise secretions *as manifested by* adventitious breath sounds, diminished breath sounds, and ineffective cough.

OUTCOMES—NOC

Respiratory Status: Airway Patency (0410)
- Moves sputum out of airway _____
- Free of adventitious breath sounds _____
- Choking not present _____

_____

Outcome Scale
1 = Extremely compromised
2 = Substantially compromised
3 = Moderately compromised
4 = Mildly compromised
5 = Not compromised

INTERVENTIONS—NIC and *RATIONALES*

Cough Enhancement (3250)
- Assist patient to a sitting position with head slightly flexed, shoulders relaxed, and knees flexed *to provide optimal positioning for generating maximum intrathoracic pressure during cough.*
- Instruct patient to inhale deeply, bend forward slightly, and perform three or four huffs (against an open glottis) *to expel secretions.*
- Encourage use of incentive spirometry *to open collapsed alveoli, promote deep breathing, and prevent atelectasis.*

NURSING DIAGNOSIS **Impaired physical mobility** *related to* generalized weakness, muscle atrophy, or paralyzed extremities *as manifested by* decreased physical activity, limited range of motion, decreased muscle strength or control.

OUTCOMES—NOC

Mobility Level (0208)
- Balance performance _____
- Muscle movement _____
- Joint movement _____
- Ambulation: walking _____

_____

Outcome Scale
1 = Dependent, does not participate
2 = Requires assistive person and device
3 = Requires assistive person
4 = Independent with assistive device
5 = Completely independent

INTERVENTIONS—NIC and *RATIONALES*

Exercise Therapy: Muscle Control (0226)
- Assess and document range of motion, transfer abilities, and positioning ability *to determine extent of problem and plan appropriate interventions.*
- Determine patient's readiness to engage in activity or exercise protocol *to assess expected level of participation.*
- Maintain alignment with support pillows and footboard according to procedures; teach and assist family and patient with positioning techniques *to prevent contractures.*
- Encourage patient to practice exercises independently *to promote patient's sense of control.*
- Provide restful environment for patient after periods of exercise *to facilitate recuperation.*

ICP, Intracranial pressure; *LOC,* level of consciousness; *WNL,* within normal limits.

Continued

NURSING CARE PLAN 56-1

Patient with Stroke—cont'd

NURSING DIAGNOSIS **Impaired verbal communication** *related to* residual aphasia *as manifested by* refusal or inability to speak, word-finding problems, use of inappropriate words, inability to follow verbal directions.

OUTCOMES—NOC	INTERVENTIONS—NIC and *RATIONALES*
Communication: Expressive Ability (0903)	*Communication Enhancement: Speech Deficit (4976)*
▪ Use of spoken language: vocal _____ ▪ Use of written language _____ ▪ Use of sign language _____ ▪ Directs message appropriately _____ _____ **Outcome Scale** 1 = Extremely compromised 2 = Substantially compromised 3 = Moderately compromised 4 = Mildly compromised 5 = Not compromised	▪ Assess communication deficits and strengths *to determine type of communication problem and plan appropriate interventions.* ▪ Listen attentively *to convey the importance of patient's thoughts and to promote a positive environment for learning.* ▪ Provide positive reinforcement and praise *to build self-esteem and confidence.* ▪ Use short, simple questions that elicit "yes" and "no" answers; speak slowly and allow adequate time for response *to avoid overwhelming patient with verbal stimuli.* ▪ Provide verbal prompts and reminders (especially if patient is frustrated) *to assist patient to express self.*

NURSING DIAGNOSIS **Unilateral neglect** *related to* visual field cut and sensory loss on one side of body *as manifested by* consistent inattention to stimuli on affected side.

OUTCOMES—NOC	INTERVENTIONS—NIC and *RATIONALES*
Body Image (1200)	*Unilateral Neglect Management (2760)*
▪ Description of affected body part _____ ▪ Willingness to touch affected body part _____ ▪ Adjustment to changes in body function _____ ▪ Willingness to use strategies to enhance appearance and function _____ _____ **Outcome Scale** 1 = Never positive 2 = Rarely positive 3 = Sometimes positive 4 = Often positive 5 = Consistently positive	▪ Assess and document abnormal responses to three primary types of stimuli: sensory, visual, and auditory *to determine the presence of and degree to which unilateral neglect exists (i.e., inability to see objects on affected side, leaving food on a plate that corresponds to affected side, lack of sensation on affected side).* ▪ Teach patient to turn and look from left to right *to scan the entire environment.* ▪ Early in care, approach patient on unaffected side; place objects in patient's field of vision; give physical and verbal cues to aid in path finding *to compensate for visual field deficits.* ▪ Later in care, approach patient on affected side *to encourage patient to turn head.* ▪ Provide visual stimulation *to promote use of full range of visual capabilities.* ▪ Teach family and patient to stimulate paralyzed limbs using touch and warm and cold stimuli *to promote reintegration with the whole body.* ▪ Encourage patient to use cue cards and mirrors *as reminder to survey his/her whole body for position, cleanliness, and appropriate dress.*

NURSING DIAGNOSIS **Impaired urinary elimination** *related to* impaired impulse to void or inability to reach toilet or manage tasks of voiding *as manifested by* incontinence and flow of urine at unpredictable times.

OUTCOMES—NOC	INTERVENTIONS—NIC and *RATIONALES*
Urinary Continence (0502)	*Urinary Bladder Training (0570)*
▪ Recognizes urge to void _____ ▪ Responds in timely manner to urge _____ ▪ Maintains environment barrier free to independent toileting _____ ▪ Free of urine leakage between voidings _____ _____ **Outcome Scale** 1 = Never demonstrated 2 = Rarely demonstrated 3 = Sometimes demonstrated 4 = Often demonstrated 5 = Consistently demonstrated	▪ Keep a continence record for 3 days, specifically noting intake and output, *to establish voiding pattern and plan appropriate interventions.* ▪ Establish interval of initial toileting schedule based on voiding pattern *to initiate process of improving bladder functioning and increased muscle tone.* ▪ Toilet patient or remind patient to void at prescribed intervals *to assist patient in adapting to new toileting schedule.* ▪ Teach patient to consciously hold urine until the scheduled toileting time *to improve muscle tone.* ▪ Discuss daily record of continence with patient to provide reinforcement and *to allow time to ask questions, make comments, or share concerns.*

NURSING CARE PLAN 56-1

Patient with Stroke—cont'd

NURSING DIAGNOSIS   **Impaired swallowing** *related to* weakness or paralysis of affected muscles *as manifested by* drooling, difficulty in swallowing, choking.

OUTCOMES—NOC	INTERVENTIONS—NIC and *RATIONALES*
Swallowing Status (1010)	*Aspiration Precautions (3200)*
▪ Handles oral secretions _____	*Swallowing Therapy (1860)*
▪ Maintains food in mouth _____	▪ Assess patient *to determine ability to swallow and presence of gag reflex.*
▪ Choking, coughing, or gagging not present _____	▪ Assist patient to sit in an erect position (as close to 90-degree angle as possible) for feeding exercise *to provide optimal position for chewing and swallowing without aspirating.*
▪ Comfort with swallowing _____	▪ Teach patient to take small bites and place in unaffected side of mouth, keep chin down, and stroke throat *to stimulate swallowing.*
	▪ Assist to maintain sitting position for 30 minutes after completing meal *to prevent regurgitation of food.*
	▪ Instruct caregiver on emergency measures for choking *to prevent complications in the home setting.*
Outcome Scale	▪ After patient has eaten, check oral cavity for pocketed food and teach patient and family this technique *to prevent collection and putrefaction of food and resultant risk of infection.*
1 = Extremely compromised	▪ Give oral care after meals *to promote comfort and oral health.*
2 = Substantially compromised	▪ Monitor body weight *to determine adequacy of nutritional intake.*
3 = Moderately compromised	
4 = Mildly compromised	
5 = Not compromised	

NURSING DIAGNOSIS   **Situational low self-esteem** *related to* actual or perceived loss of function *as manifested by* refusal to touch or look at affected body parts, increasing dependence on others, refusal to participate in self-care.

OUTCOMES—NOC	INTERVENTIONS—NIC and *RATIONALES*
Self-Esteem (1205)	*Self-Esteem Enhancement (5400)*
▪ Maintenance of grooming/hygiene _____	▪ Encourage patient to verbalize feelings *to assess effect of stroke sequelae on self-esteem.*
▪ Acceptance of self-limitations _____	▪ Encourage patient to identify strengths *to facilitate patient's recognition of intrinsic value.*
▪ Open communications _____	▪ Establish achievable goals; explain all procedures and involve patient in planning goals; offer praise for every success and step of progress; involve patient as soon as possible in rehabilitation program *to promote sense of satisfaction, independence, and control and to reduce frustrations.*
▪ Description of self _____	▪ Monitor levels of self-esteem over time *to determine stressors or situations that trigger low self-esteem and to teach coping mechanisms.*
	Body Image Enhancement (5220)
Outcome Scale	▪ Monitor whether patient can look at the changed body part *to determine patient's level of acceptance with new image.*
1 = Never positive	▪ Help patient to determine the extent of actual changes in the body *to prevent misperceptions concerning new level of physiologic functioning.*
2 = Rarely positive	
3 = Sometimes positive	
4 = Often positive	
5 = Consistently positive	

▪ Nursing Implementation

Health Promotion. To reduce the incidence of stroke, the nurse should focus teaching efforts toward stroke prevention, particularly for persons with known risk factors (see Table 56-1). In any health care setting and for the population as a whole, nurses can play a major role in the promotion of a healthy lifestyle. An overall program to prevent events such as stroke includes recognizing that people are responsible to some degree for their own health and for the health of future generations.

Another very important aspect of health promotion is teaching patients and families about early symptoms associated with stroke or TIA and when to seek health care for symptoms (Table 56-8).

Acute Intervention

Respiratory system. During the acute phase following a stroke, management of the respiratory system is a nursing priority. Stroke patients are particularly vulnerable to respiratory problems. Advancing age and immobility increase the risk for atelectasis and pneumonia. Risk for aspiration pneumonia may be high because of impaired consciousness or dysphagia. Airway obstruction can occur because of problems with chewing and swallowing, food pocketing (food remaining in the buccal cavity of the mouth), and the tongue falling back. Some stroke patients, especially brainstem or hemorrhagic, may require endotracheal intubation and mechanical ventilation, initially and/or with in-

NURSING RESEARCH
Community Education Regarding Stroke

Citation Becker K et al: Community-based education improves stroke knowledge, *Cerebrovas Dis* 11:34, 2001.

Purpose To test the effectiveness of a community-based education campaign about stroke and the need to call 911.

Methods A pretest-posttest design was used with telephone interviews carried out before and after the community-based education campaign to assess stroke knowledge. The education campaign included public service announcements, television, newspaper, and public stroke screenings. Telephone interviews were completed for 547 individuals before and 511 individuals after the campaign.

Results and Conclusions Before the campaign, 45% of respondents knew that the brain was the organ injured in stroke. This increased to 50% following the campaign. On completion of the education campaign, respondents were 52% more likely to know a stroke risk factor and 35% more likely to know a stroke symptom. Overall, a severe knowledge deficit about stroke was identified, which was greatest among the elderly, the less educated, individuals with lower income, men, and Asian Americans.

Implications for Nursing Practice The general public's knowledge about stroke risk factors, symptoms, and treatment is lacking. This can contribute to greater mortality and morbidity from stroke. Further study is needed to develop strategies that result in translation of knowledge to changes in behavior. Particular efforts must be focused on high-risk groups and those with the greatest knowledge deficits. Nurses can have a key role in these efforts.

Patient & Family Teaching Guide
TABLE 56-8   Warning Signs of Stroke

If someone is having one or more of these signs, do not ignore them. Call 911 and get medical help immediately.
- Sudden weakness, paralysis, or numbness of the face, arm, or leg, especially on one side of the body
- Sudden dimness or loss of vision in one or both eyes
- Sudden loss of speech, confusion, or difficulty speaking or understanding speech
- Unexplained sudden dizziness, unsteadiness, loss of balance or coordination
- Sudden severe headache

creasing cerebral edema and/or ICP. Enteral tube feedings also place the patient at risk for aspiration pneumonia.

Nursing interventions to support adequate respiratory function are individualized to meet the needs of the patient. An oropharyngeal airway may be used in comatose patients to prevent the tongue from falling back and obstructing the airway and to provide access for suctioning. Alternately, a nasopharyngeal airway may be used to provide airway protection and access. When an artificial airway will be required for a prolonged time,

a tracheostomy may be performed. Nursing interventions include frequent assessment of airway patency and function, oxygenation, suctioning, patient mobility, positioning of the patient to prevent aspiration, and encouraging deep breathing. Patients who have an unclipped or uncoiled aneurysm may experience rebleeding and the possibility of further ICP increases with coughing exercises. Interventions related to maintenance of airway function are described in NCP 56-1.

Neurologic system. The patient's neurologic status must be monitored closely to detect changes suggesting extension of the stroke, increased ICP, vasospasm, or recovery from stroke symptoms. Neurologic assessment includes the Glasgow coma scale (a standardized assessment of level of consciousness), mental status, pupillary responses, and extremity movement and strength. (The Glasgow coma scale is shown in Table 55-5.) Vital signs are also closely monitored and documented. A decreasing level of consciousness may indicate increasing ICP. ICP and cerebral perfusion pressure may be monitored as well if the patient is in a critical care environment. Data from the nursing assessment are recorded on flow sheets to communicate evaluation of neurologic status to the interdisciplinary team.

Cardiovascular system. Nursing goals for the cardiovascular system are aimed at maintaining homeostasis. Many patients with stroke have decreased cardiac reserves from the secondary diagnoses of cardiac diseases. Cardiac efficiency may be further compromised by fluid retention, overhydration, dehydration, and blood pressure variations. Fluids are retained if there is increased production of ADH and aldosterone secondary to stress. Fluid retention plus overhydration can result in fluid overload. It can also increase cerebral edema and ICP. At the same time, dehydration can add to the morbidity and mortality associated with stroke, especially in the patient with vasospasm. IV therapy should be carefully regulated. The nurse should closely monitor intake and output. Central venous pressure, pulmonary artery pressure, or hemodynamic monitoring may be used as indicators of fluid balance or cardiac function in the critical care unit.

Nursing interventions include (1) monitoring vital signs frequently; (2) monitoring cardiac rhythms; (3) calculating intake and output, noting imbalances; (4) regulating IV infusions; (5) adjusting fluid intake to the individual needs of the patient; (6) monitoring lung sounds for crackles and rhonchi indicating pulmonary congestion; and (7) monitoring heart sounds for murmurs or for S_3 or S_4 heart sounds. Bedside monitors or telemetry may record cardiac rhythms. Hypertension is sometimes seen following a stroke as the body attempts to increase cerebral blood flow.

After a stroke, the patient is at risk for deep vein thrombosis, especially in the weak or paralyzed lower extremity. This is related to immobility, loss of venous tone, and decreased muscle pumping activity in the leg. The most effective prevention is to keep the patient moving. Active range-of-motion exercises should be taught if the patient has voluntary movement in the affected extremity. For the patient with hemiplegia, passive range-of-motion exercises should be done several times a day. Additional measures to prevent deep vein thrombosis include positioning to minimize the effects of dependent edema and the use of elastic compression gradient stockings or support hose. Intermittent pneumatic compression stockings may be ordered for bedridden patients. Deep vein thrombosis prophylaxis may include low-molecular-weight heparin (e.g., Lovenox). The nursing assessment for deep vein thrombosis includes measuring the calf and thigh daily, observing swelling of the lower extremities, noting unusual warmth of the leg, and asking the patient about pain in the calf.

Musculoskeletal system. The nursing goal for the musculoskeletal system is to maintain optimal function. This is accomplished by the prevention of joint contractures and muscular atrophy. In the acute phase, range-of-motion exercises and positioning are important nursing interventions. Passive range-of-motion exercise is begun on the first day of hospitalization. If the stroke is due to subarachnoid hemorrhage, the movement is limited to the extremities. The patient is taught to actively exercise as soon as possible. Muscle atrophy secondary to lack of innervation and activity can develop within 1 month following stroke.

The paralyzed or weak side needs special attention when the patient is positioned. Each joint should be positioned higher than the joint proximal to it to prevent dependent edema. Specific deformities on the weak or paralyzed side that may be present in patients with stroke include internal rotation of the shoulder; flexion contractures of the hand, wrist, and elbow; external rotation of the hip; and plantar flexion of the foot. Subluxation of the shoulder on the affected side is common. Careful positioning and moving of the affected arm may prevent the development of a painful shoulder condition. Immobilization of the affected upper extremity may precipitate a painful shoulder-hand syndrome.

Nursing interventions to optimize musculoskeletal function include (1) trochanter roll at the hip to prevent external rotation; (2) hand cones (not rolled washcloths) to prevent hand contractures; (3) arm supports with slings and lap boards to prevent shoulder displacement; (4) avoidance of pulling the patient by the arm to avoid shoulder displacement; (5) posterior leg splints, footboards or high-topped tennis shoes to prevent footdrop; and (6) hand splints to reduce spasticity. Use of a footboard for the patient with spasticity is controversial. Rather than preventing plantar flexion (footdrop), the sensory stimulation of a footboard against the bottom of the foot increases plantar flexion. Likewise, there is disagreement on whether hand splints facilitate or diminish spasticity. The decision regarding the use of footboards or hand splints is made on an individual patient basis.

Integumentary system. The skin of the patient with stroke is particularly susceptible to breakdown related to loss of sensation, decreased circulation, and immobility. This is compounded by patient age, poor nutrition, dehydration, edema, and incontinence. The nursing plan for prevention of skin breakdown includes (1) pressure relief by position changes, special mattresses, or wheelchair cushions; (2) good skin hygiene; (3) emollients applied to dry skin; and (4) early mobility. The ideal position change schedule is side-back-side with a maximum duration of 2 hours for any position. Nurses should position the patient on the weak or paralyzed side for only 30 minutes. If an area of redness develops and does not return to normal color within 15 minutes of pressure relief, the epidermis and dermis are damaged. The damaged area should not be massaged because this may cause additional damage. Control of pressure is the single most important factor in both the prevention and treatment of skin breakdown. Pillows can be used under lower extremities to reduce pressure on the heels. Vigilance and good nursing care are required to prevent pressure sores.

Gastrointestinal system. The stress of illness contributes to a catabolic state that can interfere with recovery. Neurologic, car-

diac, and respiratory problems are considered priorities in the acute phase of stroke. However, the nutritional needs of the patient require quick assessment and treatment. The patient may initially receive IV infusions to maintain fluid and electrolyte balance, as well as for administration of drugs. Patients with severe impairment may require enteral or parenteral nutrition support. Depending on the severity of the stroke, individual assessment and planning for nutrition are necessary.

The first oral feeding should be approached carefully because the gag reflex may be impaired. Before initiation of feeding, the gag reflex may be assessed by gently stimulating the back of the throat with a tongue blade. If a gag reflex is present, the patient will gag spontaneously. If it is absent, feeding should be deferred and exercises to stimulate swallowing should be started. The speech therapist or occupational therapist is usually responsible for designing this program. However, the nurse may be called on to develop the program in some clinical settings.

To assess swallowing ability, the nurse should elevate the head of the bed to an upright position (unless contraindicated) and give the patient a small amount of crushed ice or ice water to swallow. If the gag reflex is present and the patient is able to swallow safely, the nurse may proceed with feeding.

After careful assessment of swallowing, chewing, gag reflex, and pocketing, oral feedings can be initiated. Mouth care before feeding helps stimulate sensory awareness and salivation and can facilitate swallowing. The patient should remain in a high-Fowler's position, preferably in a chair with the head flexed forward for the feeding and for 30 minutes following. Various dietary items may be recommended by the speech therapist. Foods should be easy to swallow and provide enough texture, temperature (warm or cold), and flavor to stimulate a swallow reflex. Crushed ice can be used as a stimulant. The patient is instructed to swallow and then swallow again. Pureed foods are not usually the best choice because they are often bland and too smooth. Thin liquids are often difficult to swallow and may promote coughing. Milk products should be avoided because they tend to increase the viscosity of mucus and increase salivation. Food should be placed on the unaffected side of the mouth. The nurse should ensure an unrushed, nonstressful atmosphere. Feedings must be followed by scrupulous oral hygiene because food may collect on the affected side of the mouth.

The most common bowel problem for the patient who has experienced a stroke is constipation. Patients may be prophylactically placed on stool softeners and/or fiber (psyllium [Metamucil]). If the patient does not have a daily or every-other-day bowel movement, the patient should be checked for impaction. The patient who has liquid stools should also be checked for stool impaction. Depending on the patient's fluid balance status and swallowing ability, fluid intake should be 1800 to 2000 ml per day and fiber intake up to 25 g per day. Physical activity also promotes bowel function. Laxatives, suppositories, or additional stool softeners may be ordered if the patient does not respond to increased fluid and fiber. Similarly, enemas are used only if suppositories and digital stimulation are ineffective because they cause vagal stimulation and increase ICP.

Urinary system. In the acute stage of stroke, the primary urinary problem is poor bladder control, resulting in incontinence. Efforts should be made to promote normal bladder function and avoid the use of indwelling catheters. If an indwelling catheter must be used initially, it should be removed as soon as the patient is medically and neurologically stable. Long-term use of an indwelling catheter is associated with urinary tract infections and delayed bladder retraining. An intermittent catheterization program may be used for patients with urinary retention because of the lower incidence of urinary infections. An alternative to intermittent catheterizations is the external catheter for male patients with urinary incontinence. External catheters do not alleviate the problem of urine retention. Overdistention should be avoided.

A bladder retraining program consists of (1) adequate fluid intake with the majority given between 8 AM and 7 PM; (2) scheduled toileting every 2 hours using bedpan, commode, or bathroom; and (3) noting signs of restlessness, which may indicate the need for urination.

Communication. During the acute stage of stroke, the nurse's role in meeting the psychologic needs of the patient is primarily supportive. An alert patient is usually anxious because of lack of understanding about what has happened and because of difficulty with, or inability to, communicate. The patient is assessed both for the ability to speak and the ability to understand. The patient's response to simple questions can give the nurse a guideline for structuring explanations and instructions. If the patient cannot understand words, gestures may be used to support verbal cues. It is helpful to speak slowly and calmly, using simple words or sentences to enhance communication. The nurse must give the patient extra time to comprehend and respond to communication. The stroke patient with aphasia may easily be overwhelmed by verbal stimuli. (Guidelines for communicating with a patient who has aphasia are presented in Table 56-9.) Evaluation and treatment of language and communication deficits are often done by the speech pathologist once the patient has stabilized.

TABLE 56-9   Communication with a Patient with Aphasia

1. Decrease environmental stimuli that may be distracting and disrupting to communication efforts.
2. Treat the patient as an adult.
3. Present one thought or idea at a time.
4. Keep questions simple or ask questions that can be answered with "yes" or "no."
5. Let the person speak. Do not interrupt. Allow time for the individual to complete thoughts.
6. Make use of gestures or demonstration as an acceptable alternative form of communication. Encourage this by saying, "Show me . . ." or "Point to what you want."
7. Do not pretend to understand the person if you do not. Calmly say you do not understand and encourage the use of nonverbal communication, or ask the person to write out what he or she wants.
8. Speak with normal volume and tone.
9. Give the patient time to process information and generate a response before repeating a question or statement.
10. Allow body contact (e.g., the clasp of a hand, touching) as much as possible. Realize that touching may be the only way the patient can express feelings.
11. Organize the patient's day by preparing and following a schedule (the more familiar the routine, the easier it will be).
12. Do not push communication if the person is tired or upset. Aphasia worsens with fatigue and anxiety.

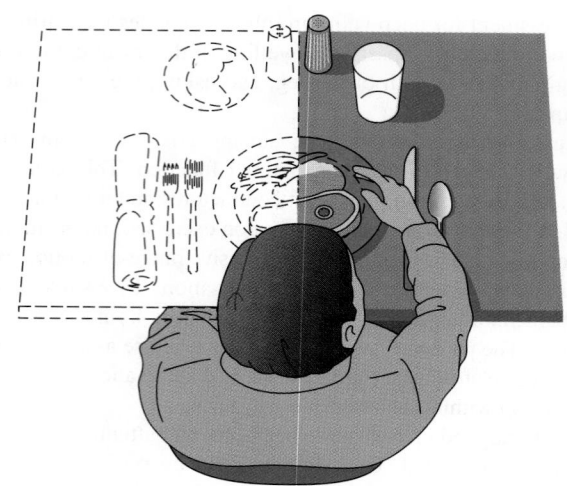

FIG. 56-8 Spatial and perceptual deficits in stroke. Perception of a patient with homonymous hemianopsia shows that food on the left side is not seen and thus is ignored.

Sensory-perceptual alterations. Homonymous hemianopsia (blindness in the same half of each visual field) is a common problem after a stroke (Fig. 56-8). Persistent disregard of objects in part of the visual field should alert the nurse to this possibility. Initially, the nurse helps the patient to compensate by arranging the environment within the patient's perceptual field, such as arranging the food tray so that all foods are on the right side or the left side to accommodate for field of vision (see Fig. 56-8). Later, the patient learns to compensate for the visual defect by consciously attending or scanning the neglected side. The weak or paralyzed extremities are carefully checked for adequacy of dressing, for hygiene, and for trauma.

In the clinical situation it is often difficult to distinguish between a visual field cut and a neglect syndrome. Both problems may occur with strokes affecting either the right or the left side of the brain. A person may be unfortunate enough to have both homonymous hemianopsia and a neglect syndrome, which increases the inattention to the weak or paralyzed side. A neglect syndrome results in decreased safety awareness and places the patient at high risk for injury. Immediately after the stroke, the nurse must anticipate potential safety hazards and provide protection from injury. Safety measures can include close observation of the patient, elevating side rails, lowering the height of the bed, and video monitors. The use of restraints and soft vests is avoided because this may agitate the patient.

Other visual problems may include *diplopia* (double vision), loss of the corneal reflex, and *ptosis* (drooping eyelid), especially if the area of stroke is in the vertebrobasilar distribution. Diplopia is often treated with an eye patch. If the corneal reflex is absent, the patient is at risk for corneal abrasion and should be observed closely and protected against eye injuries. Corneal abrasion can be prevented with artificial tears or gel to keep the eyes moist and an eye shield (especially at night). Ptosis is generally not treated because it usually does not inhibit vision.

Coping. A stroke is usually a sudden, extremely stressful event for the patient, family members, and significant others. A stroke is often a family disease, affecting the family emotionally, socially, and financially, as well as changing roles and responsibilities within the family. An older couple may perceive the stroke as a very real threat to life and to accustomed lifestyle. Reactions to this threat vary considerably but may involve fear, apprehension, denial of the severity of stroke, depression, anger, and sorrow. During the acute phase of caring for the stroke patient and the family, nursing interventions designed to facilitate coping involve providing information and emotional support.

Explanations to the patient about what has happened and about diagnostic and therapeutic procedures should be clear and understandable. It is particularly challenging to keep the aphasic patient adequately informed. Tone, demeanor, and touch may also be used to convey support.

The patient's family should be given a careful, detailed explanation of what has happened to the patient. However, if the family is extremely anxious and upset during the acute phase, explanations may need to be repeated at a later time. Because family members usually have not had time to prepare for the illness, they may need assistance in arranging care for family members or pets and for transportation and finances. A social services referral is often helpful.

Ambulatory and Home Care. The patient is usually discharged from the acute care setting to home, an intermediate or long-term care facility, or a rehabilitation facility. Criteria for transfer to rehabilitation may include the patient's ability to participate in therapies for a minimum number of hours per day. Functional status scales such as the Barthel Index, Modified Rankin Scale, and Functional Independence Measure are used to evaluate the patient.[36] Ideally, discharge planning with the patient and family starts early in the hospitalization and promotes a smooth transition from one care setting to another. The interdisciplinary team provides the guidance for the appropriate care required after discharge. If the patient requires a short- or long-term health care facility, the team can make appropriate referrals that allow time for family selection and arrangement of care. A critical factor in discharge planning is the patient's level of independence in performing ADLs. If the patient is returning home, the team can make referrals for needed equipment and services in preparation for discharge.

Nurses have an excellent opportunity to prepare the patient and family for discharge through education, demonstration and return demonstration, practice, and evaluation of self-care skills before discharge. Total care is considered in discharge planning: medications, nutrition, mobility, exercises, hygiene, and toileting. Follow-up care is carefully planned to permit continuing nursing, physical, occupational, and speech therapy, as well as medical care. Community resources should be identified to provide recreational activities, group support, spiritual assistance, respite care, adult day care, and home assistance based on the individual patient's needs.

Rehabilitation is the process of maximizing the patient's capabilities and resources to promote optimal functioning related to physical, mental, and social well-being. The goals of rehabilitation are to prevent deformity and maintain and improve function. Regardless of the care setting, ongoing rehabilitation is essential to maximize the patient's abilities.

Rehabilitation requires a team approach so the patient and family can benefit from the combined, expert care of an interdisciplinary team. The team must communicate and coordinate care to achieve the patient's and family's goals. The nurse is in a good position to facilitate this process and is often key to successful rehabilitation efforts. The patient's and family's participation in decision making during rehabilitation is essential to goal achievement after a stroke. The interdisciplinary team is composed of many members, including nurses, physicians, psychiatrist, physical therapist, occupational therapist, speech therapist, registered dietitian, respiratory therapist, vocational therapist, recreational therapist, social worker, psychologist, pharmacist, and chaplains. Physical therapy focuses on mobility, progressive ambulation, transfer techniques, and equipment needed for mobility. Occupational therapy emphasizes retraining for skills of daily living such as eating, dressing, hygiene, and cooking. Occupational therapists are also skilled in cognitive and perceptual evaluation and training. Speech therapy focuses on speech, communication, cognition, and eating abilities.

Many of the nursing interventions outlined in the nursing care plan for the patient with a stroke (see NCP 56-1) are initiated in the acute phase of care and continue throughout rehabilitation. Some of the interventions are independent nursing actions, whereas others involve the entire rehabilitation team.

The rehabilitation nurse assesses the patient and family with attention to (1) rehabilitation potential of the patient, (2) physical status of all body systems, (3) presence of complications caused by the stroke or other chronic conditions, (4) cognitive status of the patient, (5) family resources and support, and (6) expectations of the patient and family related to the rehabilitation program.

The goals for rehabilitation of the patient with stroke are mutually set by the patient, family, nurse, and other members of the rehabilitation team. The rehabilitation goals typically include the following:

- Learn techniques to self-monitor and maintain physical wellness
- Demonstrate self-care skills
- Exhibit problem-solving skills with self-care
- Avoid complications associated with stroke
- Establish and maintain a useful communication system
- Maintain nutritional and hydration status
- List community resources for equipment, supplies, and support
- Establish flexible role behaviors to promote family cohesiveness

Musculoskeletal function. The nurse initially emphasizes the musculoskeletal functions of eating, toileting, and walking for the rehabilitation of the patient. Initial assessment consists of determining the stage of recovery of muscle function. If the muscles are still flaccid several weeks after the stroke, the prognosis for regaining function is poor and the focus of care is on preventing additional loss. Most patients begin to show signs of spasticity with exaggerated reflexes within 48 hours following the stroke. Spasticity at this phase of stroke denotes progress toward recovery. As improvement continues, small voluntary movements of the hip or shoulder may be accompanied by involuntary movements in the rest of the extremity (synergy). The final stage of recovery occurs when the patient has voluntary control of isolated muscle groups.

Interventions for musculoskeletal system advance in a manner of progressive activity. Balance training is the initial step and begins with the patient sitting up in bed or dangling on the edge of the bed. The nurse evaluates tolerance by noting dizziness or syncope caused by vasomotor instability. The next step is transferring from bed to chair or wheelchair. The chair is placed beside the bed so that the patient can lead with the stronger arm and leg.

The patient sits on the side of the bed, stands, places the strong hand on the far wheelchair arm, and sits down. The nurse may either supervise the transfer or provide minimal assistance by guiding the patient's strong hand to the wheelchair arm, standing in front of the patient blocking the patient's knees with the nurse's knees to prevent knee buckling, and guiding the patient into a sitting position.

In some rehabilitation units the Bobath approach is used as an approach to mobility. The goal of this approach is to help the patient gain control over patterns of spasticity by inhibiting abnormal reflex patterns. Therapists and nurses use the Bobath approach to encourage normal muscle tone, normal movement, and promotion of bilateral function of the body. An example is to have the patient transfer into the wheelchair using the weak or paralyzed side and the stronger side to facilitate more bilateral functioning.

Another more recent approach to stroke rehabilitation is constraint-induced movement therapy (CIMT). CIMT encourages the patient to use the weakened extremity by restricting movement of the normal extremity. The ability of patients to comply with this approach is challenging and may limit its use.[37]

Supportive or assistive equipment, such as canes, walkers, and leg braces, may be needed on a short-term or long-term basis for mobility. The physical therapist usually selects the most appropriate supportive device(s) to meet individual needs and instructs the patient regarding use. The nurse should incorporate physical therapy activities into the patient's daily routine for additional practice and repetition of rehabilitation efforts.

Nutritional therapy. After the acute phase, a dietitian can assist in determining the appropriate daily caloric intake based on the patient's size, weight, and activity level. If the patient is unable to take in an adequate oral diet, a percutaneous gastrostomy (PEG) may be used for nutritional support if dysphagia persists. Most commercially prepared formulas provide about 1 calorie per milliliter. (Enteral feedings are described in Chapter 39.)

The nurse and speech therapist must assess the ability of the patient to swallow solids and fluids and adjust the diet appropriately. The dietitian plans the diet type, texture, calorie count, and fluids to meet the patient's nutritional needs. The occupational therapist and nurse must evaluate the patient's ability to feed himself or herself and recommend assistive devices to allow for independent eating. Nurses are involved in the daily planning, implementation, and evaluation of the nutritional status of the patient.

The inability to feed oneself can be frustrating and may result in malnutrition and dehydration. Interventions to promote self-feeding include using the unaffected upper extremity to eat; employing assistive devices such as rocker knives, plate guards, and nonslip pads for dishes (Fig. 56-9); removing unnecessary items from the tray or table, which can reduce spills; and providing a nondistracting environment to decrease sensory overload and distraction. The effectiveness of the dietary program is evaluated in terms of maintenance of weight, adequate hydration, and patient satisfaction.

Bowel function. A bowel management program is implemented for problems with bowel control, constipation, or incontinence. A high-fiber diet (see Table 41-9) and adequate fluid intake (2500 to 3000 ml) are usually recommended. Patients with

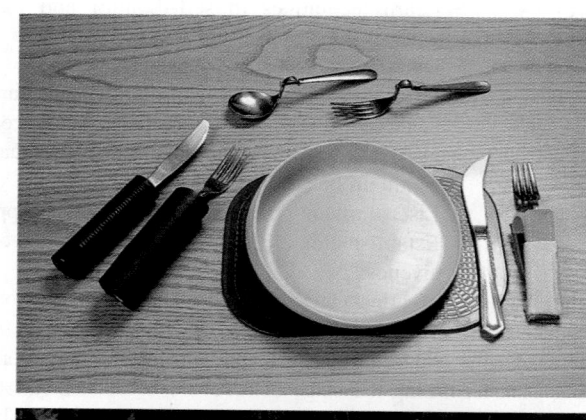
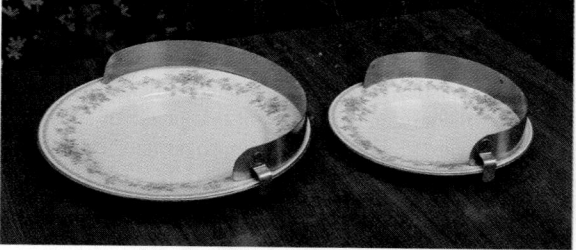
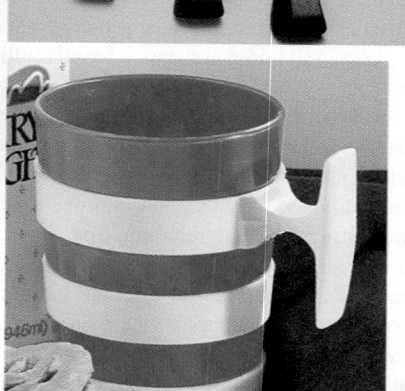
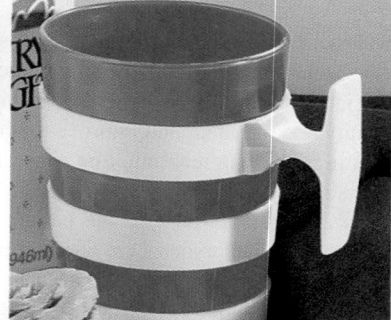

FIG. 56-9 Assistive devices for eating. **A,** The curved fork fits over the hand. The rounded plate helps keep food on the plate. Special grips and swivel handles are helpful for some persons. **B,** Knives with rounded blades are rocked back and forth to cut food. The person does not need a fork in one hand and a knife in the other. **C,** Plate guards help keep food on the plate. **D,** Cup with special handle.

stroke frequently have constipation, which responds to the following dietary management:

- Fluid intake of 2500 to 3000 ml daily unless contraindicated
- Prune juice (120 ml) or stewed prunes daily
- Cooked fruit three times daily
- Cooked vegetables three times daily
- Whole-grain cereal or bread three to five times daily

The bowel management program for incontinence consists of placing the patient on the bedpan or bedside commode or taking the patient to the bathroom at a regular time daily to reestablish bowel regularity. A good time for the bowel program is 30 minutes after breakfast because eating stimulates the gastrocolic reflex and peristalsis. The time can be adjusted for individual bowel habits and preferred timing. Sitting on the commode or toilet promotes bowel elimination through both gravity and increased abdominal pressure. Stool softeners or suppositories may be ordered if the bowel program is ineffective in reestablishing bowel regularity. A glycerin suppository can be inserted 15 to 30 minutes before evacuation time to stimulate the anorectal reflex. The bisacodyl (Dulcolax) suppository is a chemical stimulant to the bowel and is used when other measures are ineffective. Ideally the suppository use is for short-term management.

Bladder function. The nurse often assists the patient with urinary difficulties or incontinence that may follow a stroke. Often the patient with stroke has functional incontinence, which is associated with communication difficulties, mobility problems, and dressing or undressing difficulties. Nursing interventions focused on urinary continence include (1) assessment for bladder distention by palpation; (2) offering the bedpan, urinal, commode, or toilet every 2 hours during waking hours and every 3 to 4 hours at night; (3) focusing the patient on the need to urinate with direct command; (4) assistance with clothing and mobility; (5) scheduling the majority of fluid intake between 7 AM and 7 PM; and (6) encouraging the usual position for urinating (standing for men and sitting for women). Short-term interventions for urinary incontinence may include indwelling catheters, intermittent catheterization, external catheters for men, or incontinence briefs. These are not long-term solutions for urinary incontinence because complications such as urinary infections or skin irritation may occur. A coordinated program by the entire nursing staff is needed to achieve urinary continence.

Sensory-perceptual function. Patients who have had a stroke frequently have perceptual deficits. Patients with a stroke on the right side of the brain usually have difficulty in judging position, distance, and rate of movement. These patients are often impulsive and impatient and tend to deny problems related to strokes. They may fail to correlate spatial-perceptual problems with the inability to perform activities, such as guiding a wheelchair through the doorway. The patient with a right-brain stroke (left hemiplegia) is at higher risk for injury because of mobility difficulties. Directions for activities are best given verbally for comprehension. The task should be broken down to simple steps for ease of understanding. Environmental control such as removing clutter and obstacles, and good lighting, aids in concentration and safer mobility. One-sided neglect is common for people with right-brain stroke, so the nurse may assist or remind the patient to dress the weak or paralyzed side or shave the forgotten side of the face.

Patients with a left brain stroke (right hemiplegia) commonly are slower in organization and performance of tasks. They tend to have impaired spatial discrimination. These patients usually admit to deficits and have a fearful, anxious response to a stroke. Their behaviors are slow and cautious. Nonverbal cues and instructions are helpful for comprehension with patients who have had a left-brain stroke.

Affect. Patients who have had strokes often exhibit emotional responses that are not appropriate or typical for the situation. Patients may appear apathetic, depressed, fearful, anxious, weepy, frustrated, and angry. Some patients exhibit exaggerated mood swings, especially those with a stroke on the left side of the brain (right hemiplegia). The patient may be unable to control emotions and may suddenly burst into tears or laughter. This behavior is out of context and often is unrelated to the underlying emotional state of the patient. Nursing interventions for atypical emotional response are to (1) distract the patient who suddenly becomes emotional, (2) explain to the patient and family the reason for emotional outbursts, (3) maintain a calm environment, and (4) avoid shaming or scolding the patient during emotional outbursts.

Coping. The patient with a stroke may experience many losses, including sensory, intellectual, communicative, functional, role behavior, emotional, social, and vocational losses. The patient and family often go through the process of grief and mourning associated with the losses. Some patients experience long-term depression with symptoms such as anxiety, weight loss, loss of energy, poor appetite, and sleep disturbances. In addition, the time and energy required to perform previously simple tasks can result in anger and frustration.

The patient and family need help with coping with the losses associated with stroke. The nurse may assist the coping by (1) supporting communication between the patient and family; (2) discussing lifestyle changes resulting from stroke deficits; (3) discussing changing roles and responsibilities within the family; (4) being an active listener to allow the expression of fear, frustration, and anxiety; (5) including the family and patient in short- and long-term goal planning and patient care; and (6) supporting family conferences. Maladjusted dependence with inadequate coping occurs when the patient does not maintain optimal functioning for self-care, family responsibilities, decision making, or socialization. This situation can cause resentment from both the patient and family with a negative cycle of interpersonal dependency and control. Maladjusted independence occurs when the patient overestimates personal cognitive or physical capabilities and energy levels. These patients are at risk for injury.

Family members must cope with three aspects of the patient's behavior: (1) recognition of behavioral changes resulting from neurologic deficits that are not changeable, (2) responses to multiple losses both by the patient and the family, and (3) behaviors that may have been reinforced during the early stages of stroke as continued dependency. The patient and family may express feelings of guilt over not living healthy lifestyles or not seeking professional help sooner. Family therapy is a helpful adjunct to rehabilitation. The patient and family need support and reassurance. Open communication, information regarding the total effects of stroke, education regarding stroke treatment, and therapy are helpful. Stroke support groups within rehabilitation facilities and in the community are helpful in terms of mutual sharing, education, coping, and understanding.

Sexual function. A patient who has had a stroke may be concerned about the loss of sexual function. Many patients are comfortable talking about their anxieties and fears regarding sexual function if the nurse is comfortable and open to the topic. The nurse may initiate the topic with the patient and spouse or significant other. Common concerns of sexual activity involving the patient with a stroke are impotence and the occurrence of another stroke during sex. Nursing interventions for sexual activity include education on (1) optional positioning of partners, (2) timing for peak energy times, and (3) patient and partner counseling.

Communication. Speech, comprehension, and language deficits are the most difficult problems for the patient and family. Speech therapists can assess and formulate a plan of care to support communication. The nurse can be a role model for communication with the patient who has aphasia. Nursing interventions that support communication include (1) frequent, meaningful communication; (2) allowing time for the patient to comprehend and answer; (3) using simple, short sentences; (4) using visual cues; (5) structuring conversation so that it permits simple answers by the patient; and (6) praising the patient honestly for improvements with speech.

Community integration. Traditionally, successful community integration following stroke may be difficult for the patient because of persistent problems with cognition, coping, physical deficits, and emotional lability that interfere with functioning. Older patients who have had a stroke often have more severe deficits and frequently experience multiple health problems. Failure to continue the rehabilitation regimen at home may result in deterioration and further complications. Advances in health care have resulted in an increased survival rate for patients with extensive stroke damage. Successful community integration can be redefined by the patient, family, and interdisciplinary health team as successful mobility, achievement of ADLs, and quality of life with family and friends.

Community resources can be an asset to patients and their families. The National Stroke Association provides information, resources, referral services, and quarterly newsletters on stroke. The American Stroke Association, a division of the American Heart Association, has information regarding stroke, hypertension, diet, exercise, and assistive devices. This association sponsors self-help groups in many areas. The Easter Seal Society provides wheelchairs and other assistive devices for stroke patients.

Local groups can offer more daily assistance such as meals and transportation. These resources can be identified by nurse case managers, home health nurses, discharge planners, and clinical nurse specialists. (Resources are listed at the end of the chapter.)

■ Gerontologic Considerations: Stroke

Stroke is a significant cause of death and disability. The highest incidence of stroke occurs among older adults. Stroke can result in a profound disruption in the life of an older person. The magnitude of disability and changes in total function can leave patients wondering if they can ever return to their "old self," and loss of independence may be a major concern. The ability to perform ADLs may require many adaptive changes because of physical, emotional, perceptual, and cognitive deficits. Home management may be a particular challenge if the patient has an elderly spouse caretaker who also has health problems. There may be limited family members (including adult children) living in close proximity to provide help.

The rehabilitative phase and assisting the older patient to deal with the residual deficits of stroke, as well as aging, can provide a challenging nursing experience. Patients may become fearful and depressed because they think they may have another attack or die. The fear can become immobilizing and interfere with effective rehabilitation.

Changes may occur in the patient-spouse relationship. The dependency resulting from a stroke may be threatening. The spouse may also have chronic medical problems that affect the ability to take care of the stroke survivor. The patient may not want anyone other than the spouse to provide care, putting a significant burden on the spouse.

The nurse has the opportunity to assist the patient and family in the transition through acute hospitalization, rehabilitation, long-term care, and home care. The needs of the patient and family require ongoing nursing assessment and adaptation of interventions in response to changing needs to optimize quality of life for both the patient and family. ■

CRITICAL THINKING EXERCISES

Case Study
Stroke

Patient Profile. Suzanne, a 66-year-old white woman, awoke in the middle of the night and fell when she tried to get up and go to the bathroom. She fell because she was not able to control her left leg. Her husband took her to the hospital, where she was diagnosed with an acute ischemic stroke. Because she had awakened with symptoms, the actual time of onset was unknown and she was not a candidate for tPA.

Subjective Data
- Left arm and leg are weak and feel numb
- Feeling depressed and fearful
- Requires help with ADLs
- Concerned regarding having another stroke
- Says she has not taken her drugs for high cholesterol
- History of a brief episode of left-sided weakness and tingling of the face, arm, and hand 3 months earlier, which totally resolved and for which she did not seek treatment

Objective Data
- BP: 180/110
- Left-sided arm weakness (3/5) and leg weakness (4/5)
- Decreased sensation on the left side, particularly the hand
- Left homonymous hemianopsia
- Overweight
- Alert, oriented, and able to answer questions appropriately but mild slowness in responding

CRITICAL THINKING QUESTIONS
1. How does Suzanne's prior health history put her at risk for a stroke?
2. How can the nurse address Suzanne's concerns regarding having another stroke?
3. How can Suzanne and her family address activity issues such as driving after the stroke?
4. What strategies might the home health nurse use to help Suzanne and her family cope with her feeling depressed?

CRITICAL THINKING EXERCISES—cont'd

5. What lifestyle changes should Suzanne make to reduce the likelihood of another stroke?
6. How will homonymous hemianopsia affect Suzanne's hygiene, eating, driving, and community activities?
7. What factors should the nurse assess for related to outpatient rehabilitation for Suzanne?
8. Based on the assessment data provided, write one or more nursing diagnoses. Are there any collaborative problems?

Nursing Research Issues

1. Determine the effectiveness of weight loss and stop-smoking programs in reducing the incidence of stroke.
2. Examine the relationship between functional abilities and level of independence following a stroke.
3. Determine the effectiveness of nursing interventions to promote full-field visualization for patients with homonymous hemianopsia.
4. Examine the spouse-patient relationship and coping styles following a stroke.
5. Examine the impact of stroke on socialization, quality of life, and loneliness.

REVIEW QUESTIONS

The number of the question corresponds to the same-numbered objective at the beginning of the chapter.

1. Of the following patients, the nurse recognizes that the one with the highest risk for a stroke is
   a. an obese 45-year-old Native American.
   b. a 35-year-old Asian American woman who smokes.
   c. a 32-year-old white woman taking oral contraceptives.
   d. a 65-year-old African American man with hypertension.
2. The factor related to cerebral blood flow that most often determines the extent of cerebral damage from a stroke is the
   a. amount of cardiac output.
   b. oxygen content of the blood.
   c. degree of collateral circulation.
   d. level of carbon dioxide in the blood.
3. Information provided by the patient that would help differentiate a hemorrhagic stroke from a thrombotic stroke includes
   a. sensory disturbance.
   b. a history of hypertension.
   c. presence of motor weakness.
   d. sudden onset of severe headache.
4. A patient with right-sided hemiplegia and aphasia resulting from a stroke most likely has involvement of the
   a. brainstem.
   b. vertebral artery.
   c. left middle cerebral artery.
   d. right middle cerebral artery.
5. The nurse explains to the patient with a stroke who is scheduled for angiography that this test is used to determine the
   a. presence of increased ICP.
   b. site and size of the infarction.
   c. presence of blood in the cerebrospinal fluid.
   d. patency of the cerebral blood vessels.

6. A patient experiencing TIAs is scheduled for a carotid endarterectomy. The nurse explains that this procedure is done to
   a. decrease cerebral edema.
   b. reduce the brain damage that occurs during a stroke in evolution.
   c. prevent a stroke by removing atherosclerotic plaques blocking cerebral blood flow.
   d. provide a circulatory bypass around thrombotic plaques obstructing cranial circulation.
7. Nursing management of the patient with hemiplegia during the acute phase of a stroke includes
   a. restricting active movement.
   b. positioning each joint higher than the proximal joint.
   c. performing passive range of motion on all limbs every 4 hours.
   d. maintaining the patient in a recumbent, side-lying position.
8. Bladder training in a male patient who has urinary incontinence after a stroke includes
   a. limiting fluid intake.
   b. keeping a urinal in place at all times.
   c. assisting the patient to stand to void.
   d. catheterizing the patient every 4 hours.
9. The most common response of the stroke patient to the change in body image is
   a. denial.
   b. depression.
   c. disassociation.
   d. intellectualization.

REFERENCES

1. Goldstein et al: Primary prevention of ischemic stroke, *Circulation* 103:163, 2001.
2. Heart and Stroke Foundation of Canada (last updated Sept 19, 2001). General Info–Stroke Statistics. Available at *http://www.heartandstroke.ca/* (accessed Nov 21, 2001).
3. American Heart Association: *2001 Heart and stroke statistical update*, Dallas, 2002, American Heart Association.
4. Helgason CM, Wolf PA: American Heart Association prevention conference IV: prevention and rehabilitation of stroke, *Circulation* 96:701, 1997.
5. The Intercollegiate Working Party for Stroke: National clinical guidelines for stroke: a concise update, *Clin Med* 2:231, 2002.
6. Matchar DB et al: Improving the quality of anticoagulation of patients with atrial fibrillation in managed care organizations: results of the managing anticoagulation services trial, *Am J Med* 113:42, 2002.
7. Desbiens NA: Deciding on anticoagulating the oldest old with atrial fibrillation: insights from cost-effectiveness analysis, *J Am Geriatr Soc* 50:863, 2002.
8. Wolf PA et al: Probability of stroke: a risk profile from the Framingham Study, *Stroke* 22:3, 1991.
9. Kothari V et al: UKPDS 60: risk of stroke in type 2 diabetes estimated by the UK Prospective Diabetes Study risk engine, *Stroke* 33:1776, 2002.
10. Liao JK: Statins and ischemic stroke, *Atheroscler Suppl* 3:21, 2002.
11. Leys D et al: Stroke prevention: management of modifiable vascular risk factors, *J Neurol* 249:507, 2002.
12. Bolego C, Poli A, Paoletti R: Smoking and gender, *Cardiovasc Res* 53:568, 2002.
13. Tuhrim S: Management of stroke and transient ischemic attack, *Mt Sinai J Med* 69:121, 2002.
14. Sacco RL et al: The protective effect of moderate alcohol consumption on ischemic stroke, *JAMA* 281:1, 1999.
15. Rexrode KM et al: A prospective study of body mass index, weight change, and risk of stroke in women, *JAMA* 277:19, 1997.
16. Sacco RL et al: Leisure-time physical activity and ischemic stroke risk: the northern Manhattan stroke study, *Stroke* 29:2, 1998.
17. Petitti DB et al: Stroke and cocaine or amphetamine use, *Epidemiology* 9:6, 1998.
18. Neiman J, Haapaniemi HM, Hillbom M: Neurological complications of drug abuse: pathophysiological mechanisms, *Eur J Neurol* 6:595, 2000.
19. Gillum RF, Mussolino ME, Ingram DD: Physical activity and stroke incidence in women and men. The NHANES I epidemiologic follow-up study, *Am J Epidemiol* 143:9, 1996.
20. Heinemann et al: Thromboembolic stroke in young women: a European case-control study on oral contraceptives, *Contraception* 57:29, 1998.
21. Writing Group for the Women's Health Initiative Investigators: Risks and benefits of estrogen plus progestin in healthy postmenopausal women: principal results from the Women's Health Initiative randomized controlled trial, *JAMA* 288:321, 2002.
22. Hankey GJ et al: Inherited thrombophilia in ischemic stroke and its pathogenic subtypes, *Stroke* 32:1793, 2001.
23. Fisher M, Bogousslavsky J: *Current review of cerebrovascular disease*, ed 4, Philadelphia, 2001, Current Medicine.
24. Barnett HJM et al: *Stroke: pathophysiology, diagnosis, and management*, ed 3, New York, 1998, Churchill Livingstone.
25. Gilroy J: *Basic neurology*, New York, 2000, McGraw-Hill.
26. Broderick et al: Guidelines for the management of spontaneous intracerebral hemorrhage, *Stroke* 30:905, 1999.
27. Greener J, Langhorne P: Systematic reviews in rehabilitation for stroke: issues and approaches to addressing them, *Clin Rehabil* 16:69, 2002.
28. Coull BM et al: Anticoagulants and antiplatelets agents in acute ischemic stroke: report of the Joint Stroke Guideline Development Committee of the American Academy of Neurology and the American Stroke Association, *Stroke* 33:1934, 2002.
29. Bailes JE: Carotid endarterectomy, *Neurosurgery* 50:1290, 2002.
30. Nussbaum ES, Erickson DL: Extracranial-intracranial bypass for ischemic cerebrovascular disease refractory to maximal medical therapy, *Neurosurgery* 46:37, 2000.
31. Csokay A et al: Vascular tunnel creation to improve the efficacy of decompressive craniotomy in post-traumatic cerebral edema and ischemic stroke, *Neurosurgery* 57:126, 2002.
32. Wardlaw JM, del Zoppo G, Yamaguchi T: Thrombolysis for acute ischemic stroke, Cochrane Stroke Group, *Cochrane Database Syst Rev*, Issue 1, 2002.
33. Feigin VL et al: Calcium antagonists for aneurismal subarachnoid hemorrhage, *The Cochrane Library*, Issue 2, Oxford, 2002 Update Software.
34. Mitchell M: *Neuroscience nursing: a nursing diagnosis approach*, Baltimore, 2001, WB Saunders.
35. Broderick J et al: Guidelines for the management of spontaneous intracerebral hemorrhage: a statement for the healthcare professionals from a special writing group of the Stroke Council, American Heart Association, *Stroke* 30:905, 1999.
36. Pettersen R, Dahl T, Wyller TB: Prediction of long-term functional outcome after stroke rehabilitation, *Clin Rehabil* 16:149, 2002.
37. Page SJ et al: Stroke patients' and therapists' opinions of constraint-induced movement therapy, *Clin Rehabil* 16:55, 2002.

RESOURCES

American Association of Neuroscience Nurses (AANN)
4700 West Lake Avenue
Glenview, IL 60025
888-557-2266 or 847-375-4733
Fax: 847-375-6333
www.aann.org

American Stroke Association
National Center
7272 Greenville Avenue
Dallas, TX 75231
888-4-STROKE or 888-478-7653
www.strokeassociation.org

Association of Rehabilitation Nurses (ARN)
4700 West Lake Avenue
Glenview, IL 60025-1485
800-229-7530 or 847-375-4710
Fax: 877-734-9384
www.rehabnurse.org

Canadian Association of Neuroscience Nurses (CANN)
www.cann.ca

Heart and Stroke Foundation of Canada
222 Queen Street, Suite 1402
Ottawa, ON
K1P 5V9 Canada
613-569-4361
Fax: 613-569-3278
http://ww1.heartandstroke.ca

National Institute of Neurological Disorders and Stroke
NIH Neurological Institute
PO Box 5801
Bethesda, MD 20824
800-352-9424
www.ninds.nih.gov

National Stroke Association
9707 East Easter Lane
Englewood, CO 80112
800-STROKES (787-6537) or 303-649-9299
Fax: 303-649-1328
www.stroke.org

Society for Neuroscience
11 Dupont Circle NW, Suite 500
Washington, DC 20036
202-462-6688
Fax: 202-462-9740
www.sfn.org

Stroke Clubs International
805 12th Street
Galveston, TX 77550
409-762-1022
strokeclub@aol.com

For additional Internet resources, see the website for this book at *http://evolve.elsevier.com/Lewis/medsurg/.*

CHAPTER 57

NURSING MANAGEMENT
Chronic Neurologic Problems

Judith M. Ozuna

LEARNING OBJECTIVES

1. Compare and contrast tension-type, migraine, and cluster headaches in terms of etiology, clinical manifestations, collaborative care, and nursing management.
2. Describe the etiology, clinical manifestations, diagnostic studies, collaborative care, and nursing management of seizure disorder, multiple sclerosis, Parkinson's disease, and myasthenia gravis.
3. Describe the clinical manifestations and collaborative care of amyotrophic lateral sclerosis and Huntington's chorea.
4. Explain the potential impact of chronic neurologic disease on physical and psychologic well-being.
5. Outline the major goals of treatment for the patient with a chronic, progressive neurologic disease.

KEY TERMS

absence (petit mal) seizure, p. 1556
amyotrophic lateral sclerosis, p. 1577
atypical absence seizure, p. 1556
aura, p. 1550
cluster headaches, p. 1551
epilepsy, p. 1555
generalized seizures, p. 1556
headache, p. 1549
Huntington's disease, p. 1577

migraine headache, p. 1550
multiple sclerosis, p. 1563
myasthenia gravis, p. 1573
myasthenic crisis, p. 1574
Parkinson's disease, p. 1569
partial seizures, p. 1556
restless legs syndrome, p. 1576
seizure, p. 1555
status epilepticus, p. 1557
tension-type headache, p. 1549
tonic-clonic seizure, p. 1556

Headache

Headache is probably the most common type of pain experienced by humans. The majority of people have functional headaches, such as migraine or tension-type headaches; the remainder have organic headaches caused by intracranial or extracranial disease.

Not all tissues of the cranium are sensitive to pain. The pain-sensitive structures in the head include the venous sinuses, dura, cranial blood vessels, three divisions of the trigeminal nerve (CN V), facial nerve (CN VII), glossopharyngeal nerve (CN IX), vagus nerve (CN X), and first three cervical nerves. Thus headache pain can arise from both intracranial and extracranial sources.

Headaches are classified using the International Headache Society (IHS) diagnostic criteria based on the characteristics of the headache and the facial pain. The primary classifications include tension-type, migraine, and cluster headaches. Characteristics of these headaches are shown in Table 57-1. A patient may have more than one type of headache. The history and neurologic examination are diagnostic keys to determining the type of headache.

TENSION-TYPE HEADACHE

Tension-type headache, the most common type of headache, is characterized by a bilateral feeling of pressure around the head. Tension-type headache has been called muscle-contraction, tension, psychogenic, and rheumatic headache. Tension-type headaches are often subcategorized as acute or episodic and chronic.

Etiology and Pathophysiology

It was originally thought that tension-type headache was the result of sustained and painful contraction of the muscles of the scalp and the neck. Recent evidence, however, does not support this mechanism in all patients with tension-type headaches. It is likely that neurovascular factors similar to those involved in migraine headaches play a role in the development of tension-type headaches.

Clinical Manifestations

There is no *prodrome* (early manifestation of impending disease) in tension-type headache. The IHS classification system defines *tension-type headache* as involving at least two of the following characteristics: pressure or tightness sensation, mild to moderate severity, bilateral location, or worsening with physical activity. The headache does not involve nausea or vomiting but may involve sensitivity to light (*photophobia*) or sound (*phonophobia*). The headaches may occur intermittently for weeks, months, or even years. Many patients can have a combination of migraine and tension-type headaches, with features of both headaches occurring simultaneously. Patients with migraine headaches may experience tension-type headaches between migraine attacks.

Diagnostic Studies

Careful history taking is probably the most important diagnostic tool for tension-type headache. Electromyography (EMG) may be performed. This test may reveal sustained contraction of the neck, scalp, or facial muscles, but many patients may not show increased muscle tension with this test, even when the test

Reviewed by Mary S. Baird, RN, MN, CNRN, ARNP, Nurse Practitioner, Northwest Neuromuscular Association, Olympia, Wash.

1549

TABLE 57-1	**Comparison of Tension-Type, Migraine, and Cluster Headaches**		
PATTERN	**TENSION-TYPE HEADACHE**	**MIGRAINE HEADACHE**	**CLUSTER HEADACHE**
Site	Bilateral, bandlike pressure at base of skull, in face, or in both	Unilateral (in 60%), may switch sides, commonly anterior	Unilateral, radiating up or down from one eye
Quality	Constant, squeezing tightness	Throbbing, synchronous with pulse	Severe, bone-crushing
Frequency	Cycles for several years	Periodic; cycles of several months to years	May have months or years between attacks; attacks occur in clusters: one to three times a day over a period of 4 to 8 weeks
Duration	Intermittent for months or years	Continuous for hours or days	30 to 90 minutes
Time and mode of onset	Not related to time	May be preceded by prodrome; onset after awakening; gets better with sleep	Nocturnal; commonly awakens patient from sleep
Associated symptoms	Palpable neck and shoulder muscles, stiff neck, tenderness	Nausea or vomiting, edema, irritability, sweating, photophobia, phonophobia, prodrome of sensory, motor, or psychic phenomena; family history (in 65%)	Vasomotor symptoms such as facial flushing or pallor, unilateral lacrimation, ptosis, and rhinitis

is done during the actual headache. Conversely, patients with diagnosed migraine headaches may show increased muscle tension on EMG. If tension-type headache is present during physical examination, increased resistance to passive movement of the head and tenderness of the head and neck may be present.

MIGRAINE HEADACHE

Migraine headache is a recurring headache characterized by unilateral or bilateral throbbing pain, a triggering event or factor, strong family history, and manifestations associated with neurologic and autonomic nervous system dysfunction. The onset of migraine usually occurs in childhood or adolescence. A family history of migraine can be found in 65% of patients with migraine. At some point in their lives, 7% to 9% of men and 16% to 25% of women will experience migraine headaches.[1]

Etiology and Pathophysiology

Although the exact cause of migraine headaches is not known, evidence suggests that neurologic, vascular, and chemical factors are involved.[2] The neurogenic model of migraine implies that a stimulus can trigger the trigeminovascular system (trigeminal nerve and its connections to meningeal blood vessels), producing inflammation of the blood vessels and vasodilation. This vasodilation ultimately results in headache. The neurotransmitter serotonin produces cerebrovascular dilation and stimulates afferent pain fiber activation, both of which are important in promoting migraine progression.

In addition to the headache itself, migraines can be preceded by prodrome and aura. The prodrome may precede the headache phase by several hours or several days. The **aura** (sensation of light or warmth) of migraine is associated with "spreading depression," a wave of *oligemia* (diminished cerebral blood flow) beginning in the occipital lobe and spreading forward in the brain at a rate of 2 to 3 mm per minute.

Migraine headaches, in many cases, have no known precipitating events. However, for other patients, the headache may be precipitated or triggered by stress, excitement, bright lights, menstruation, alcohol, or certain foods such as chocolate or cheese.

Clinical Manifestations

Migraines are subdivided by the IHS into those with aura (formerly called classic migraine) and those without aura (formerly called common migraine).

Migraine with aura is defined by IHS as involving at least three of the following: (1) reversible aura involves brain dysfunction; (2) aura symptoms develop gradually over more than 4 minutes, or two or more symptoms occur in succession; (3) no aura lasts more than 60 minutes; and (4) headache follows aura within 60 minutes. Migraine with aura occurs in only 10% of migraine headache episodes. The sharply defined aura may last for 10 to 30 minutes before the start of the headache and may include sensory dysfunction (e.g., visual field defects, tingling or burning sensations, paresthesias), motor dysfunction (e.g., weakness, paralysis), dizziness, confusion, and even loss of consciousness. The classic aura symptom is perception of flashing lights in one quadrant of the visual field, often termed *scintillating scotomata*. Migraine with aura usually peaks in 1 hour and may last several hours.

The IHS classification defines *migraine without aura* as involving at least two of the following characteristics: unilateral location, pulsating quality, moderate to severe intensity, worsening with activity, and at least one of either (1) nausea and vomiting or (2) photophobia and phonophobia. Migraine without aura is the most common type of migraine headache. The headache itself may last several hours or days.

Clinical manifestations that might occur in migraine with and without aura are generalized edema, irritability, pallor, nausea and vomiting, and sweating. In migraine with and without aura, the prodrome is not sharply defined. The prodrome can include psychic disturbances, gastrointestinal upset, and changes in fluid balance.

During the headache phase, some patients with migraine may tend to "hibernate"; that is, they seek shelter from noise, light, odors, people, and problems. The headache is described as a steady, throbbing pain that is synchronous with the pulse. However, the presentation of migraine is varied in its severity. Not all migraine headaches are disabling, and many patients who have migraine headaches do not seek health care treatment for them. Although the headache is usually unilateral, it may switch to the opposite side in another episode.

Diagnostic Studies

There are no specific laboratory or radiologic tests for migraine headache. The diagnosis of migraine headache is usually made from the history. The neurologic and other diagnostic examinations are often normal.

The IHS criteria are used as the clinical basis for migraine diagnosis. If atypical features are present, secondary headaches must be ruled out. Neuroimaging techniques (e.g., head computed tomography [CT], with or without contrast, and magnetic resonance imaging [MRI]) are not recommended for routine evaluation of headache unless abnormal findings are found on the neurologic examination.

CLUSTER HEADACHE

Cluster headaches are characterized by repeated headaches that can occur for weeks to months at a time, followed by periods of remission. It is one of the most severe forms of head pain. Cluster headache occurs less frequently than migraine (the cluster headache to migraine frequency is 1:10) and is more frequent in men than in women by a ratio of 8:1. The onset is usually between 20 and 50 years of age.

Etiology and Pathophysiology

Neither the cause nor the pathophysiologic mechanism of cluster headache is fully known. The vasodilation that occurs in the affected part of the face is extracranial. Similar to migraine headaches, the trigeminal nerve is implicated in the production of pain. Activation of this nerve causes release of substance P and other vasoactive substances that cause vasodilation, stimulation of afferent pain fibers, and neurogenic inflammation with extravasation (movement of fluid out of blood vessels). The periodicity (i.e., regularity in terms of timing) and autonomic symptoms of cluster headache indicate a dysfunction of the biologic clock mechanisms of the hypothalamus.[3] These headaches can also be triggered by alcohol ingestion.

Clinical Manifestations

The IHS classification defines *cluster headache* as involving severe unilateral orbital, supraorbital, or temporal pain and at least one of the following signs present on the pain side: conjunctival injection, lacrimation, nasal congestion, rhinorrhea, forehead and facial swelling, *miosis* (constricted pupil), *ptosis* (eyelid dropping), eyelid edema. The headache has an abrupt onset, usually without a prodrome. It peaks in 5 to 10 minutes and lasts 30 to 90 minutes. It is not uncommon for this type of headache to start at night, awakening the patient after a few hours of sleep. Headaches may recur several times a day over a period of several days, with each cluster lasting 2 to 3 months. It usually affects the upper face, the periorbital region, and the forehead on one side of the face and the head. The headache may not recur for months or years.

The patient may also exhibit conjunctivitis, increased lacrimation (tearing), and nasal congestion on the side of the headache.

Sweating may occur on the forehead of the affected side. A partial *Horner's syndrome* (miosis and ptosis on the affected side) may be seen. The headache is described as deep, steady, and penetrating but not throbbing.

Unlike the patient with migraine, who seeks isolation and quiet, the patient with a cluster headache paces the floor, cries out, and resents being touched. The patient with a cluster headache does not experience the systemic manifestations that accompany a migraine headache, such as nausea or vomiting. As with migraine headaches, there are usually no complications with cluster headaches.

Diagnostic Studies

The diagnosis of cluster headache is primarily based on the history. However, CT scan, MRI, or magnetic resonance angiography (MRA) may be performed to rule out an aneurysm, tumor, or infection.

OTHER TYPES OF HEADACHES

Although tension, migraine, and cluster headaches are by far the most common types of headaches, other types of headaches can also occur. These headaches may be the first symptom of a more serious illness. Headache can accompany subarachnoid hemorrhage; brain tumors; other intracranial masses; arteritis; vascular abnormalities; trigeminal neuralgia (tic douloureux); diseases of the eyes, nose, and teeth; and systemic illness (e.g., bacteremia, carbon monoxide poisoning, mountain sickness, polycythemia vera). The symptoms vary greatly. Because of the variety of causes of headache, clinical evaluation must be thorough. It should include an evaluation of personality, life adjustment, environment, and family situation, as well as a comprehensive evaluation of neurologic and physical status.

Collaborative Care for Headaches

If no systemic underlying disease is found, therapy is directed toward the functional type of headache. Table 57-2 outlines the general workup for a patient with headache to rule out any intracranial or extracranial disease. Table 57-3 summarizes the current therapies for prophylaxis and symptomatic relief of common

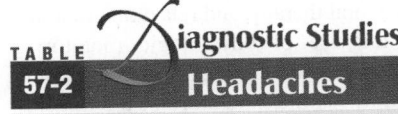

TABLE 57-2	Diagnostic Studies — Headaches

History and physical examination
Neurologic examination (often negative)
   Inspection for local infections
   Palpation for tenderness, bony swellings
   Auscultation for bruits over major arteries
Routine laboratory studies
   CBC
   Electrolytes
   Urinalysis
CT scan of sinuses
Special studies (e.g., CT scan, angiography, EMG, EEG, MRA, MRI)

CBC, Complete blood count; *CT,* computed tomography; *EEG,* electroencephalography; *EMG,* electromyography; *MRA,* magnetic resonance angiography; *MRI,* magnetic resonance imaging.

TABLE 57-3 *Collaborative Care*

Headaches

	TENSION-TYPE HEADACHE	MIGRAINE HEADACHE	CLUSTER HEADACHE
Diagnostic	History of neck and head tenderness, resistance to movement	History*	History
Collaborative Therapy			

Symptomatic	Nonnarcotic analgesics: aspirin, ibuprofen, acetaminophen
	Analgesic combinations: butalbital and aspirin (Fiorinal); butalbital and acetaminophen (Fioricet); dichloralphenazone, acetaminophen, and isometheptene (Midrin)
	Muscle relaxants
		Nonnarcotic analgesics:
		  aspirin, acetaminophen, ibuprofen
		Serotonin receptor agonists:
		  almotriptan (Axert)
		  eletriptan (Relpax)
		  frovatriptan (Frova)
		  naratriptan (Amerge)
		  rizatriptan (Maxalt)
		  sumatriptan (Imitrex)
		  zolmitriptan (Zomig)
		α-Adrenergic blockers:
		  ergotamine tartrate (Ergomar, DHE)
		Analgesic combination:
		  acetaminophen, dichloralphenazone, and isometheptene (Midrin)
		Corticosteroids:
		  dexamethasone (Decadron)
			α-Adrenergic blockers: ergotamine tartrate
			Vasoconstrictors
			Oxygen

Prophylactic	Tricyclic antidepressants:
	  doxepin (Sinequan)
	  amitriptyline (Elavil)
	β-Adrenergic blockers: propranolol (Inderal)
	Biofeedback
	Psychotherapy
	Muscle relaxation training
		β-Adrenergic blockers: propranolol (Inderal)
		Antidepressants: amitriptyline (Elavil)
		  imipramine (Tofranil)
		Calcium channel blockers: verapamil (Isoptin)
		Antiseizure: valproate (Depakene)
		Serotonin antagonist:† methysergide (Sansert)
		Biofeedback
		Relaxation therapy
		Cognitive-behavioral therapy
			α-Adrenergic blockers: ergotamine tartrate
			Serotonin antagonist:
			  methysergide (Sansert)
			Corticosteroids: prednisone
			Calcium channel blockers:
			  verapamil (Isoptin)
			Lithium
			Biofeedback

EMG, Electromyography.
*Magnetic resonance imaging (MRI) should be considered in nonacute headache patients with unexplained abnormal neurologic examination, atypical headache, headache features, or an additional risk factor, such as immune deficiency.
†Only for patients suffering from one or more severe headaches per week.

headaches. These therapies include drugs, meditation, yoga, biofeedback, cognitive-behavioral therapy, and relaxation training.

Biofeedback involves the use of physiologic monitoring equipment to give the patient information regarding muscle tension and peripheral blood flow (skin temperature of the fingers). The patient is trained to relax the muscles and raise the finger temperature and is given reinforcement (operant conditioning) in accomplishing these physiologic alterations.

Cognitive-behavioral therapy and relaxation therapy used alone or in conjunction with drug therapy may be beneficial to some patients. Acupuncture, acupressure, and hypnosis are also therapies that have worked well in some patients with headaches. These therapies are described further in Chapter 7. Treatments for tension-type headache include physical therapy (e.g., massage, hot packs, cervical collar), injection of local anesthetic into spastic muscles, and correction of faulty posture.

Drug Therapy

Tension-type headache. Drug treatment for tension-type headache usually involves a nonnarcotic analgesic (e.g., aspirin, acetaminophen) used alone or in combination with a sedative, mus-

cle relaxant, tranquilizer, or codeine. However, many of these drugs have serious side effects. The patient should be cautioned about the long-term use of aspirin and aspirin-containing drugs because they can cause gastric bleeding and coagulation abnormalities in susceptible patients. Long-term use of Fiorinal should be avoided because in addition to aspirin it contains a barbiturate (butalbital), which may be habit forming. Drugs containing acetaminophen (Tylenol, Phenaphen, Midrin) can cause kidney damage with chronic use and liver damage when combined with alcohol.

Migraine headache. Drug treatment of the acute migraine attack is aimed at terminating or decreasing the symptoms of the attack. Many people with mild or moderate migraine can obtain relief with aspirin or acetaminophen. Ergotamine (Ergomar) is often used when simple analgesics do not relieve headache. Ergotamine inhibits the reuptake of norepinephrine into postganglionic nerve terminals of the sympathetic nervous system. This allows more norepinephrine to attach to α-adrenergic sites on smooth muscle in the artery wall, thereby causing prolonged vasoconstriction of cranial blood vessels. Ergotamine can be administered orally, sublingually, parenterally, rectally, or by inhalation. The usual dosage is 1 to 2 mg (oral or rectal) at the onset of the headache, followed by 2 mg within 1 hour. No more than 6 mg is given for any single attack. Dihydroergotamine mesylate is available as a nasal spray called Migranal.

Drugs that affect selected serotonin receptors, the "triptans," are aimed at treating the pathologic process of migraine. These drugs reduce neurogenic inflammation of the cerebral blood vessels and produce vasoconstriction. They include sumatriptan (Imitrex), naratriptan (Amerge), rizatriptan (Maxalt), almotriptan (Axert), frovatriptan (Frova), zolmitriptan (Zomig), and eletriptan (Relpax). Because these drugs cause constriction of coronary arteries, they are avoided in patients with heart disease. Triptans should be taken at the first symptom of migraine headache. Other drugs that may relieve migraine headache include butalbital with aspirin or acetaminophen (Fiorinal, Fioricet), isometheptene with acetaminophen and dichloralphenazone (Midrin, Migratine), and, in certain cases, narcotics.

A variety of drugs are used to reduce the frequency and severity of tension-type and migraine attacks. They are taken on a daily basis and are usually used when headaches occur more than twice a month. Preventive drugs for migraine headaches include β-adrenergic blockers (e.g., propranolol [Inderal], atenolol [Tenormin]), tricyclic antidepressants (e.g., amitriptyline [Elavil]), selective serotonin reuptake inhibitors (e.g., fluoxetine [Prozac]), calcium channel blockers (e.g., verapamil [Isoptin]), divalproex (Depakote), clonidine (Catapres), and thiazides. Another drug, methysergide (Sansert), competitively blocks serotonin receptors in the central and peripheral nervous systems. However, because of side effects, including retroperitoneal, pulmonary, and cardiac fibrosis, the patient taking methysergide requires regular follow-up. It is recommended that a patient taking methysergide have a break (drug holiday) every 4 to 6 months.

Cluster headache. Because cluster headaches occur suddenly, often at night, and are not long lasting, drug therapy is not as useful as it is for the other types of headaches. Prophylactic drugs may include verapamil, lithium, ergotamine, divalproex, or nonsteroidal antiinflammatory drugs (NSAIDs). Acute treatment of cluster headache is inhalation of 100% oxygen delivered at a rate of 7 to 9 L per minute for 15 to 20 minutes, which may relieve headache by causing vasoconstriction. It can be repeated after a 5-minute rest. However, a drawback to this treatment is that the patient must have continuous access to the oxygen supply. Sumatriptan is also effective in treating acute cluster headache. Methysergide may be used prophylactically when the cluster headache recurs at a known time.

Patients with frequent headaches may overuse analgesic drugs.[4] Such overuse can lead to chronic daily headache, also called *analgesic rebound headache* or drug-induced headache. Drugs known to cause this problem are acetaminophen, aspirin, NSAIDs (e.g., ibuprofen), butalbital, sumatriptan, and narcotics. Treatment involves abrupt withdrawal of the offending drug, except for opioids, which need to be tapered, and initiation of alternative drugs such as amitriptyline.

NURSING MANAGEMENT
HEADACHES

■ Nursing Assessment

Subjective and objective data that should be obtained from a patient with headache are presented in Table 57-4. Because the history provides the key to assessment of headache, it should include specific details of the headache itself, such as the location and type of pain, onset, frequency, duration, relation to events (emotional, psychologic, physical), and time of day of the occurrence. Information about previous illnesses, surgery, trauma, al-

TABLE 57-4	Nursing Assessment — Headaches

Subjective Data

Important Health Information

Past health history: Seizures, cancer, recent fall or trauma, cranial infection, stroke; asthma or allergies; mental illness; relationship of headache to overwork, stress, menstruation, exercise, food, sexual activity, travel, bright lights, or noxious environmental stimuli

Medications: Use of hydralazine, bromides, nitroglycerin, ergotamine (withdrawal), nonsteroidal antiinflammatory drugs (in high daily doses), estrogen preparations, oral contraceptives, over-the-counter or prescription remedies

Surgery or other treatments: Craniotomy, sinus surgery, facial surgery

Functional Health Patterns

Health perception–health management: Positive family history; malaise

Nutritional-metabolic: Ingestion of alcohol, caffeine, cheese, chocolate, monosodium glutamate, aspartame, lunch meats (nitrites in cured meats), sausage, hot dogs, onions, avocados; anorexia, nausea, vomiting (migraine prodrome); unilateral lacrimation (cluster)

Activity-exercise: Vertigo, fatigue, weakness, paralysis, fainting

Sleep-rest: Insomnia

Cognitive-perceptual:

Migraine: aura; unilateral, severe, throbbing (possible switching of side) headache; visual disturbances; photophobia; phonophobia; dizziness; tingling or burning sensations

Cluster: unilateral and severe, nocturnal headache; nasal stuffiness

Tension-type: bilateral, bandlike, dull and persistent, base-of-skull headache, neck tenderness

Self-perception–self-concept: Depression

Coping–stress tolerance: Stress, anxiety, irritability, withdrawal

Objective Data

General

Anxiety, apprehension

Integumentary

Cluster: forehead diaphoresis, pallor, unilateral facial flushing with cheek edema, conjunctivitis

Migraine: generalized edema (prodrome), pallor, diaphoresis

Neurologic

Horner's syndrome, restlessness (cluster), hemiparesis (migraine)

Musculoskeletal

Resistance of head and neck movement, nuchal rigidity (meningeal, tension-type), palpable neck and shoulder muscles (tension-type)

Possible Findings

Possible evidence of disease, deformity, or infection on brain imaging (CT, MRI, MRA), cerebral angiogram, lumbar puncture, EEG, EMG; nonspecific brain imaging or laboratory tests

CT, Computed tomography; *EEG,* electroencephalography; *EMG,* electromyography; *MRA,* magnetic resonance angiography; *MRI,* magnetic resonance imaging.

lergies, family history, and response to medication should also be obtained. The nurse can suggest that the patient keep a diary of headache episodes with specific details. This type of record can be of great help in determining the type of headache and the precipitating events. If the patient has a history of migraine, tension-type, or cluster headaches, it is important to determine if the character, intensity, or location of the headache has changed. This may be an important clue as to the cause of the headache.

■ Nursing Diagnoses

Nursing diagnoses for the patient with headache may include, but are not limited to, those presented in NCP 57-1.

■ Planning

The overall goals are that the patient with a headache will (1) have reduced or no pain, (2) experience increased comfort and decreased anxiety, (3) demonstrate understanding of triggering events and treatment strategies, (4) use positive coping strategies to deal with chronic pain, and (5) experience increased quality of life and decreased disability.

■ Nursing Implementation

Patients with chronic headache present a great challenge to health care providers. Headaches may be related to an inability to cope with daily stresses. The most effective therapy may be to help patients examine their lifestyle, recognize stressful situations, and learn to cope with them more appropriately. Precipitating factors can be identified, and ways of avoiding them can be developed. Daily exercise, relaxation periods, and socializing can be encouraged because each can help decrease the recurrence of headache. The nurse can suggest alternative ways of handling the pain of headache through techniques such as relaxation, meditation, yoga, and self-hypnosis.

In addition to using analgesics and analgesic combination drugs for the symptomatic relief of headache, the patient should be encouraged to use relaxation techniques because they are effective in relieving tension-type and migraine headaches. The migraine sufferer often needs a quiet, dimly lit environment. Massage and moist hot packs to the neck and head can help a patient with tension-type headaches. The patient should learn about the drugs prescribed for prophylactic and symptomatic treatment of headache and should be able to describe the purpose, action, dosage, and side effects of the drug. To prevent accidental overdose, the patient should make a written note of each dose of drug or headache remedy.

For the patient whose headaches are triggered by food, dietary counseling may be provided. The patient is encouraged to eliminate foods that may provoke headaches, such as vinegar, chocolate, onions, alcohol (particularly red wine), excessive caffeine, cheese, fermented or marinated foods, monosodium glutamate,

NURSING CARE PLAN 57-1

Patient with Headache

EXPECTED PATIENT OUTCOMES	NURSING INTERVENTIONS and *RATIONALES*
NURSING DIAGNOSIS	**Acute pain** *related to* headache *as manifested by* complaint of steady, throbbing, or severe crushing pain.
• Reduced pain • Satisfaction with pain relief	• Assess pain intensity, characteristics, location, and duration *to determine appropriate interventions*. • Encourage patient to keep a pain log including associated or precipitating factors *to provide patient some control in identifying and controlling factors that may precipitate headaches*. • Encourage patient to use alternative therapies such as massage, meditation, yoga, biofeedback, and relaxation techniques *to provide sense of control over pain*. • Support patient's use of counseling or psychotherapy *to promote stress reduction*. • Administer drugs as ordered *to reduce pain*.* • Monitor patient following administration of pain medication *to assess drug efficacy and identify adverse drug effects*.
NURSING DIAGNOSIS	**Anxiety** *related to* lack of knowledge about headache's etiology and ways to treat it *as manifested by* ↑ heart rate, insomnia, feeling of helplessness.
• ↑ Psychologic comfort and ↓ anxiety • Effective coping mechanisms to manage anxiety	• Assess level of anxiety *to determine appropriate interventions*. • Encourage patient to verbalize concerns *because this reduces anxiety*. • Explain possible etiology of patient's specific headache type *to reduce patient's fear of unknown*. • Reinforce health care provider's explanation of diagnostic tests and treatment measures *to relieve concerns about cause and seriousness of headache*.
NURSING DIAGNOSIS	**Hopelessness** *related to* chronic pain, alteration of lifestyle, and ineffective treatment modalities *as manifested by* expressions of apathy and listlessness, lack of interest in doing usual activities.
• Expression of confidence in ability to function in spite of headaches	• Assess patient's degree of hopelessness *to enable appropriate planning*. • Explore patient's self-treatment of pain and alterations in lifestyle *to make appropriate adjustments if necessary*. • Promote verbalization of fears and concerns *to convey empathy and correct possible misconceptions*. • Assist patient in identifying support systems that can be used *to bolster hopefulness*.

*See Table 57-3.

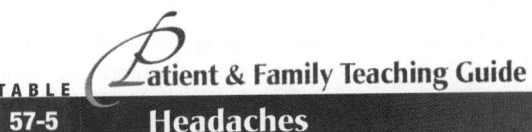

TABLE 57-5	Patient & Family Teaching Guide
	Headaches

1. Keep a diary or calendar of headaches and possible precipitating events
2. Avoid factors that can trigger a headache:
   - Foods containing amines (cheese, chocolate), nitrites (meats such as hot dogs), vinegar, onions, monosodium glutamate
   - Fermented or marinated foods
   - Caffeine
   - Nicotine
   - Ice cream
   - Alcohol (particularly red wine)
   - Emotional stress
   - Fatigue
   - Drugs such as ergot-containing and monoamine oxidase inhibitors
3. Describe the purpose, action, dosage, and side effects of drugs taken
4. Be able to self-administer sumatriptan (Imitrex) subcutaneously if prescribed
5. Use stress-reduction techniques such as relaxation
6. Participate in regular exercise
7. Contact health care provider if the following occur:
   - Symptoms become more severe, last longer than usual, or are resistant to medication
   - Nausea and vomiting (if severe or not typical), change in vision, or fever occur with the headache
   - Problems with drugs

and aspartame. Active challenge and provocative testing with specific foods may be necessary to determine the specific causative agents. However, food triggers may change over time. Patients should avoid smoking and exposure to triggers such as strong perfumes, volatile solvents, and gasoline fumes. Cluster headache attacks may occur at high altitudes with low oxygen levels during air travel. Ergotamine, taken before the plane takes off, may decrease the likelihood of these attacks. A teaching guide for the patient with a headache is presented in Table 57-5.

■ Evaluation

Expected outcomes for the patient with headache are addressed in NCP 57-1.

Chronic Neurologic Disorders

SEIZURE DISORDERS AND EPILEPSY

Seizure is a paroxysmal, uncontrolled electrical discharge of neurons in the brain that interrupts normal function. Seizures are often symptoms of an underlying illness. They may accompany a variety of disorders, or they may occur spontaneously without any apparent cause. Seizures resulting from systemic and metabolic disturbances are not considered epilepsy if the seizures cease when the underlying problem is corrected. In the adult, metabolic disturbances that cause seizures include acidosis, electrolyte imbalances, hypoglycemia, hypoxia, alcohol and barbitu-

rate withdrawal, dehydration, and water intoxication. Extracranial disorders that can cause seizures are heart, lung, liver, or kidney diseases; systemic lupus erythematosus; diabetes mellitus; hypertension; and septicemia.

Epilepsy is a condition in which a person has spontaneously recurring seizures caused by a chronic underlying condition. The prevalence of epilepsy is 5 to 10 per 1000 persons.[5] It is higher in undeveloped countries. The incidence rates are high during the first year of life, decline through childhood and adolescence, plateau in middle age, and rise sharply again among the elderly.

Etiology and Pathophysiology

The most common causes of seizure disorder during the first 6 months of life are severe birth injury, congenital defects involving the central nervous system (CNS), infections, and inborn errors of metabolism. In patients between 2 and 20 years of age, the primary causative factors are birth injury, infection, trauma, and genetic factors. In individuals between 20 and 30 years of age, seizure disorder usually occurs as the result of structural lesions, such as trauma, brain tumors, or vascular disease. After 50 years of age the primary causes of seizure disorders are cerebrovascular lesions and metastatic brain tumors. Although many causes of seizure disorders have been identified, three fourths of all seizure disorder cases cannot be attributed to a specific cause and are considered *idiopathic.*

The role of heredity in the etiology of seizure disorders has been difficult to determine because of the problem of separating hereditary from environmental or acquired influences. In addition, some families carry a predisposition to seizure disorders in the form of an inherently low threshold to seizure-producing stimuli, such as trauma, disease, and high fever. Nevertheless, at least 40 seizure disorder syndromes have been linked to specific genetic defects.[6]

In recurring seizures (epilepsy) a group of abnormal neurons *(seizure focus)* seems to undergo spontaneous firing. This firing spreads by physiologic pathways to involve adjacent or distant areas of the brain. If this activity spreads to involve the whole brain, a generalized seizure occurs. The factor that causes this abnormal firing is not clear. Any stimulus that causes the cell membrane of the neuron to depolarize induces a tendency to spontaneous firing. Often the area of the brain from which the epileptic activity arises is found to have scar tissue *(gliosis).* The scarring is thought to interfere with the normal chemical and structural environment of the brain neurons, making them more likely to fire abnormally.

Repetitive electrical discharges from an epileptic focus in experimental animals can produce long-lasting and possibly permanent changes in neuron excitability, both locally and in distant areas of the brain. This effect is called *kindling,* and it presents an interesting and important implication for epilepsy in humans: seizures can beget more seizures. Clinical experience indicates that the longer a patient goes without good seizure control, the lower the likelihood that the seizures will be controllable. Therefore a vigorous attempt must be made to control recurring seizures.

Clinical Manifestations

The specific clinical manifestations of a seizure are determined by the site of the electrical disturbance. The preferred method of classifying recurring seizures is the International Classification System[7] (Table 57-6). This system is based on the clinical and electroencephalographic manifestations of seizures. In this system, seizures are divided into two major classes: *general-*

TABLE 57-6	International Classification of Seizure Disorders

Generalized Seizures (Bilaterally Symmetric and without Local Onset)
Absence seizures, atypical absence seizures
Myoclonic seizures
Clonic seizures
Tonic seizures
Tonic-clonic seizures
Atonic seizures

Partial Seizures (Local Onset)
Simple partial seizures (no impairment of consciousness)
- With motor symptoms
- With somatosensory or special sensory symptoms
- With autonomic symptoms
- With psychic symptoms
Complex partial seizures (impairment of consciousness)
- Simple partial seizures with progression to impairment of consciousness
    With no other features
    With features of simple partial seizures
    With automatisms
- Impairment of consciousness at onset
    With no other features
    With features of simple partial seizures
    With automatisms

Unclassified Epileptic Seizures (Inadequate or Incomplete Data)

Modified from Commission on Classification and Terminology of the International League against Epilepsy: Proposal for revised clinical and electroencephalographic classification of epileptic seizures, *Epilepsia* 22:489, 1981.

ized and *partial*. Depending on the type, a seizure may progress through several phases, which include (1) the *prodromal* phase with signs or activity, which precede a seizure; (2) the *aural phase* with a sensory warning; (3) the *ictal phase* with full seizure; and (4) the *postictal phase*, which is the period of recovery after the seizure.

Generalized Seizures. **Generalized seizures** are characterized by bilateral synchronous epileptic discharges in the brain from the onset of the seizure. Because the entire brain is affected at the onset of the seizures, there is no warning or aura. In most cases, the patient loses consciousness for a few seconds to several minutes.

Tonic-clonic seizures. The most common generalized seizure is the generalized tonic-clonic, or grand mal, seizure. **Tonic-clonic seizure** is characterized by loss of consciousness and falling to the ground if the patient is upright, followed by stiffening of the body (tonic phase) for 10 to 20 seconds and subsequent jerking of the extremities (clonic phase) for another 30 to 40 seconds. Cyanosis, excessive salivation, tongue or cheek biting, and incontinence may accompany the seizure.

In the postictal phase the patient usually has muscle soreness, is very tired, and may sleep for several hours. Some patients may not feel normal for several hours or days after a seizure. The patient has no memory of the seizure.

Typical absence seizures. The **absence (petit mal) seizure** usually occurs only in children and rarely continues beyond adolescence. This type of seizure may cease altogether as the child matures, or it may evolve into another type of seizure. The typical clinical manifestation is a brief staring spell that lasts only a few seconds, so it often occurs unnoticed. There may be an extremely brief loss of consciousness. When untreated, the seizures may occur up to 100 times a day.

The electroencephalogram (EEG) demonstrates a 3-Hz (cycles per second) spike-and-wave pattern that is unique to this type of seizure. Absence seizures can often be precipitated by hyperventilation and flashing lights.

Atypical absence seizures. Another type of generalized seizure is **atypical absence seizure,** which is characterized by a staring spell accompanied by other signs and symptoms, including brief warnings, peculiar behavior during the seizure, or confusion after the seizure. The EEG demonstrates atypical spike-and-wave patterns, usually greater or less than 3 Hz.

Other types of generalized seizures. Other generalized seizures are myoclonic and akinetic seizures. A *myoclonic seizure* is characterized by a sudden, excessive jerk of the body or extremities. The jerk may be forceful enough to hurl the person to the ground. These seizures are very brief and may occur in clusters.

The terms *akinetic* (arrest of movement), *atonic* (loss of tone), and *astatic* (loss of balance) have been used interchangeably to describe drop attacks or falling spells. This type of seizure involves either a tonic episode or a paroxysmal loss of muscle tone and begins suddenly with the person falling to the ground. Consciousness usually returns by the time the person hits the ground, and normal activity can be resumed immediately. Patients with this type of seizure are at a great risk of head injury and often have to wear protective helmets. A less severe akinetic seizure involves brief loss of muscle tone without falling.

Partial Seizures. **Partial seizures** are the other major class of seizures in the International Classification System. They are also referred to as partial focal seizures. Partial seizures begin in a specific region of the cortex, as indicated by the EEG and usually by the clinical manifestations. For example, if the discharging focus is located in the medial aspect of the postcentral gyrus, the patient may experience paresthesias and tingling or numbness in the leg on the side opposite the focus. If the discharging focus is located in the part of the brain that governs a particular function, sensory, motor, cognitive, or emotional manifestations may occur.

Partial seizures may be confined to one side of the brain and remain partial or focal in nature, or they may spread to involve the entire brain, culminating in a generalized tonic-clonic seizure. Any tonic-clonic seizure that is preceded by an aura or warning is a partial seizure that generalizes secondarily. Many tonic-clonic seizures that appear to be generalized from the outset may actually be secondary generalized seizures, but the preceding partial component may be so brief that it is undetected by the patient, by the observer, or even on the EEG. Unlike the primary generalized tonic-clonic seizure, the secondary generalized seizure may result in a transient residual neurologic deficit postictally. This is called *Todd's paralysis* (focal weakness), which resolves after varying lengths of time.

Partial seizures are further divided into (1) simple partial seizures (those with simple motor or sensory phenomena) and (2) complex partial seizures (those with complex symptoms). *Simple partial seizures* with elementary symptoms do not involve loss of consciousness and rarely last longer than 1 minute. They may involve motor, sensory, or autonomic phenomena or a combination of these. The terms *focal motor, focal sensory,* and *jacksonian* have been used to describe seizures of the simple partial type.

Complex partial seizures can involve a variety of behavioral, emotional, affective, and cognitive functions. The location of the discharging focus is usually in the temporal lobe, hence the term *temporal lobe seizure.* These seizures usually last longer than 1 minute and are frequently followed by a period of postictal confusion. Complex partial seizures are distinct from simple partial (focal motor, focal sensory) seizures in that they involve some alteration in consciousness. The sole manifestation of complex partial seizures may be clouding of consciousness or a confused state without any motor or sensory components. This type of attack is sometimes termed *temporal lobe absence.* There is rarely the complete loss of consciousness that is typical of the generalized absence attack, nor does the patient snap back to the preseizure state as does the patient who has had a generalized absence attack.

The most common complex partial seizure involves lip smacking and *automatisms* (repetitive movements that may not be appropriate). These are often called *psychomotor seizures.* The patient may continue an activity that was initiated before the seizure, such as counting out change or picking items from a grocery shelf, but after the seizure does not remember the activity performed during the seizure. Other automatisms are less organized, such as picking at clothing, fumbling with objects (real or imaginary), or simply walking away.

A variety of psychosensory symptoms may occur during a complex partial seizure, including distortions of visual or auditory sensations and vertigo. There may be alterations in memory, such as a feeling of having experienced an event before *(déjà vu),* or alterations in thought processes. Alterations in sexual functioning can vary from hyposexuality to hypersexuality. Many patients with temporal lobe seizures have decreased sexual drive or erectile dysfunction. However, some may experience sexual sensations during their seizures. This is because the abnormal electrical activity arises from the brain centers responsible for these sensations. Some experience increased sexual drive just after a seizure. In addition, some antiseizure drugs can cause a decrease in sexual drive because of sedation. Others can cause erectile dysfunction.

Complications

Physical. **Status epilepticus** is a state of continuous seizure activity or a condition in which seizures recur in rapid succession without return to consciousness between seizures. It is the most serious complication of epilepsy and is a neurologic emergency. Status epilepticus can involve any type of seizure. During repeated seizures the brain uses more energy than can be supplied. Neurons become exhausted and cease to function. Permanent brain damage may result. Tonic-clonic status epilepticus is the most dangerous because it can cause ventilatory insufficiency, hypoxemia, cardiac arrhythmias, hyperthermia, and systemic acidosis, all of which can be fatal.

Another complication of seizures is severe injury and even death from trauma suffered during a seizure. Patients who lose consciousness during a seizure are at greatest risk. Death can result from head injury incurred in a fall, from drowning in the bathtub, or from severe burns.

Psychosocial. Perhaps the most common complication of seizure disorders is the effect it has on a patient's lifestyle. Although attitudes have improved in recent years, epilepsy still carries a social stigma. It used to be associated with supernatural powers, possession by the devil, and insanity. Today the stigma probably exists because the characteristics of seizures are in direct conflict with modern societal values of self-control, conformity, and independence. The patient with epilepsy may experience discrimination in employment and educational opportunities. Transportation may be difficult because of legal sanctions against driving in most states and Canada. The patient may develop ineffective methods of coping.

Diagnostic Studies

The most useful diagnostic tools are accurate and comprehensive description of the seizures and the patient's health history (Table 57-7). The EEG is a useful diagnostic adjuvant to the history but only if it shows abnormalities. Abnormal findings help determine the type of seizure and help pinpoint the seizure focus. Unfortunately, only a small percentage of patients with seizure disorders have abnormal findings on the EEG the first time the test is done. EEGs may need to be repeated often, or continuous EEG monitoring may be needed to detect abnormalities. Abnormal discharges may not occur during the 30 to 40 minutes of sampling during EEG, and the test may never indicate an abnormality. It is not a definitive test because some patients who do not have seizure disorders have abnormal patterns on their EEGs, whereas many patients with seizure disorders have normal EEGs between

TABLE 57-7 Collaborative Care Seizure Disorders and Epilepsy

Diagnostic
History and Physical Examination
Birth and development history
Significant illnesses and injuries
Family history
Febrile seizures
Comprehensive neurologic assessment
Seizure History
Precipitating factors
Antecedent events
Seizure description (including onset, duration, frequency, postictal state)
Diagnostic Studies
CBC, urinalysis, electrolytes, creatinine, fasting blood glucose
Lumbar puncture
CT, MRI, MRA, MRS, PET scan
Electroencephalography (EEG)

Collaborative Therapy
Antiseizure drugs (see Table 57-9)
Surgery (see Table 57-10)
Vagal nerve stimulation
Psychosocial counseling

CBC, Complete blood count; *CT,* computed tomography; *MRA,* magnetic resonance angiography; *MRI,* magnetic resonance imaging; *MRS,* magnetic resonance spectroscopy; *PET,* positron emission tomography.

seizures. Magnetoencephalography may be done in conjunction with the EEG. This test has greater sensitivity in detecting small magnetic fields generated by neuronal activity.

A complete blood count, serum chemistries, studies of liver and kidney function, and urinalysis should be done to rule out metabolic disorders. A CT or MRI scan should be done in any new-onset seizure to rule out a structural lesion. Cerebral angiography, single-photon emission computed tomography (SPECT), magnetic resonance spectroscopy (MRS), MRA, and positron emission tomography (PET) may be used in selected clinical situations.

Collaborative Care

Most seizures do not require professional emergency medical care because they are self-limiting and rarely cause bodily injury. However, if status epilepticus occurs, if significant bodily harm occurs, or if the event is a first-time seizure, medical care should

be sought immediately. Table 57-8 summarizes emergency care of the patient with a generalized tonic-clonic seizure, the seizure most likely to warrant professional emergency medical care. The diagnostic studies and collaborative care of seizure disorders are summarized in Table 57-7.

Drug Therapy. Seizure disorders are treated primarily with antiseizure drugs (Table 57-9). Therapy is aimed at preventing seizures because cure is not possible. Drugs generally act by stabilizing nerve cell membranes and preventing spread of the epileptic discharge. In about 70% of the patients, seizure disorders are controlled by medication. The primary goal of antiseizure drug therapy is to obtain maximum seizure control with a minimum of toxic side effects. The principle of drug therapy is to begin with a single drug and increase the dosage until seizures are controlled or toxic side effects occur. Serum levels of the drug should be monitored if seizures continue to occur, if seizure fre-

---

TABLE 57-8

*E*mergency Management

Tonic-Clonic Seizures

ETIOLOGY	ASSESSMENT FINDINGS	INTERVENTIONS
Head Trauma Epidural hematoma Subdural hematoma Intracranial hematoma Cerebral contusion Traumatic birth injury **Drug-Related Processes** Overdose Withdrawal of alcohol, opioids, antiseizure drugs Ingestion, inhalation **Infectious Processes** Meningitis Septicemia Encephalitis **Intracranial Events** Brain tumor Subarachnoid hemorrhage Stroke Hypertensive crisis Increased ICP secondary to clogged shunt **Metabolic Imbalances** Fluid and electrolyte imbalance Hypoglycemia **Medical Disorders** Heart, liver, lung, or kidney disease Systemic lupus erythematosus **Other** Cardiac arrest Idiopathic Psychiatric disorders High fever	• Aura—peculiar sensations that precede seizure • Loss of consciousness • Bowel and bladder incontinence • Tachycardia • Diaphoresis • Warm skin • Pallor, flushing, or cyanosis • *Tonic phase:* continuous muscle contractions • *Hypertonic phase:* extreme muscular rigidity lasting 5 to 15 seconds • *Clonic phase:* rigidity and relaxation alternate in rapid succession • *Postictal phase:* lethargy, altered level of consciousness • Confusion and headache • Repeated tonic-clonic seizures for several minutes	**Initial** • Ensure patent airway. • Assist ventilations if patient does not breathe spontaneously after seizure. Anticipate need for intubation if gag reflex absent. • Suction as needed. • Stay with patient until seizure has passed. • Protect patient from injury during seizure. *Do not restrain.* Pad side rails. • Establish IV access. • Anticipate administration of phenobarbital, phenytoin (Dilantin), or benzodiazepines (diazepam [Valium], midazolam [Versed], lorazepam [Ativan]) to control seizures. • Remove or loosen tight clothing. **Ongoing Monitoring** • Monitor vital signs, level of consciousness, oxygen saturation, Glasgow coma scale, pupil size and reactivity. • Reassure and orient the patient after seizure. • Never force an airway between a patient's clenched teeth. • Give dextrose for hypoglycemia.

ICP, Intracranial pressure; *IV,* intravenous.

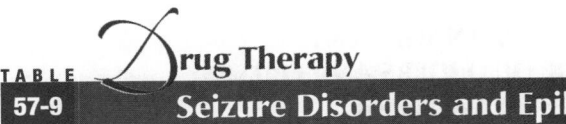

TABLE
57-9

Seizure Disorders and Epilepsy

Generalized Tonic-Clonic and Partial Seizures

carbamazepine (Tegretol)
divalproex (Depakote)
felbamate (Felbatol)
gabapentin (Neurontin)
lamotrigine (Lamictal)
levetiracetam (Keppra)
oxcarbazepine (Trileptal)
phenobarbital
phenytoin (Dilantin)
primidone (Mysoline)
tiagabine (Gabitril)
topiramate (Topamax)
valproic acid (Depakene)
zonisamide (Zonegran)

Absence, Akinetic, and Myoclonic Seizures

clonazepam (Klonopin)
divalproex (Depakote)
ethosuximide (Zarontin)
phenobarbital
valproic acid (Depakene)

quency increases, or if drug compliance is questioned. The therapeutic range for each drug indicates the serum level above which most patients experience toxic side effects and below which most continue to have seizures. Therapeutic ranges are only guides for therapy. If the patient's seizures are well controlled with a sub-therapeutic level, the drug dose need not be increased. Likewise, if a drug level is above the therapeutic range and the patient has good seizure control without toxic side effects, the drug dose need not be decreased. Many of the newer drugs do not require drug level monitoring because the therapeutic range is very large. If seizure control is not achieved with a single drug, the drug may be changed or a second drug may be added.

For many years the primary drugs for treatment of generalized tonic-clonic and partial seizures were phenytoin (Dilantin), carbamazepine (Tegretol), phenobarbital, and divalproex (Depakote). For treatment of absence, akinetic, and myoclonic seizures the drugs included ethosuximide (Zarontin), divalproex (Depakote), and clonazepam (Klonopin).

Recently, many new drugs have become available, including gabapentin (Neurontin), lamotrigine (Lamictal), topiramate (Topamax), tiagabine (Gabitril), levetiracetam (Keppra), and zonisamide (Zonegran). These drugs are effective for partial seizures and for some of the primary generalized seizure disorders as well.

Felbamate (Felbatol) may be used to treat patients whose seizure disorders are refractory to other drugs. However, its use is limited because it can cause aplastic anemia and liver toxicity.

Treatment of status epilepticus requires initiation of a rapid-acting antiseizure drug that can be given intravenously. The drugs most commonly used are lorazepam (Ativan) and diazepam (Valium). Because these are short-acting drugs, they must be followed by administration of long-acting drugs such as phenytoin or phenobarbital.

Current drugs used in seizure management are shown in Table 57-9. Because many of these drugs (e.g., phenytoin, phenobarbital, ethosuximide, lamotrigine, topiramate) have a long half-life, they can be given in once- or twice-daily doses. This increases the patient's compliance with taking the drug by simplifying the drug regimen and avoiding the need to take it at work or school. Antiseizure drugs should not be discontinued abruptly because this can precipitate seizures.

Toxic side effects of antiseizure drugs involve the CNS and include diplopia, drowsiness, ataxia, and mental slowing. Neurologic assessment for dose-related toxicity involves testing the eyes for nystagmus, hand and gait coordination, cognitive functioning, and general alertness.

Idiosyncratic side effects involve organs outside the CNS, including the skin (rashes), gingiva (hyperplasia), bone marrow (blood dyscrasias), liver, and kidneys. Nurses should be knowledgeable about these side effects so that patients can be informed and proper treatment can be instituted. A common side effect of phenytoin is gingival hyperplasia (excessive growth of gingival tissue), especially in children and young adults. This can be limited by good dental hygiene, including regular toothbrushing and flossing. If gingival hyperplasia is extensive, the hyperplastic tissue may have to be surgically removed (gingivectomy), and phenytoin may have to be replaced by another antiseizure drug. Because phenytoin can also cause hirsutism in young people, other drugs are often used first.

Surgical Therapy. A significant number of patients whose epilepsy cannot be controlled with drug therapy are candidates for surgical intervention to remove the epileptic focus or prevent spread of epileptic activity in the brain (Table 57-10). The major types of surgery are removal of one lobe (usually the temporal

TABLE 57-10 Surgical Procedures for Seizure Disorders and Epilepsy		
TYPE OF SEIZURE	**SURGICAL PROCEDURE**	**RESULTS**
Complex partial seizure of temporal lobe origin	Resectioning of epileptogenic tissue	Absence of seizures 5 yr postoperatively in 55%–70% of patients
Partial seizures of frontal lobe origin	Resectioning of epileptogenic tissue (if in resectable area)	Absence of seizures 5 yr postoperatively in 30%–50% of patients
Generalized seizures (Lennox-Gastaut syndrome or drop attacks)	Sectioning of corpus callosum	Persistence of seizures, less violent, less frequent, less disabling events
Intractable unilateral multifocal epilepsy associated with infantile hemiplegia	Hemispherectomy or callosotomy	Reduction in seizure frequency and type, improvement in behavior

lobe), removal of cortex, or separation of the two hemispheres (corpus callosotomy).[8]

The benefits of surgery include cessation or reduction in frequency of the seizures, but not all types of epilepsy benefit from surgery. An extensive preoperative evaluation is important, including continuous EEG monitoring and other specific tests to ensure precise localization of the focal point. Before surgery is performed, three requirements must be met: (1) the diagnosis of epilepsy must be confirmed; (2) there must have been an adequate trial with drug therapy without satisfactory results; and (3) the electroclinical syndrome (type of seizure disorder) must be defined.

Other Therapies. Another treatment for seizure disorders is vagal nerve stimulation. An electrode is surgically placed around the left vagus nerve in the neck. It is connected to a battery placed beneath the skin in the upper chest. The device is programmed to deliver intermittent electrical stimulation to the brain to reduce the frequency and intensity of seizures. The exact mechanism of action is unknown, although the stimulation may interrupt synchronization of epileptic brain-wave activity. This method is currently used in only a small number of patients.

Biofeedback to control seizures is aimed at teaching the patient to maintain a certain brain-wave frequency that is refractory to seizure activity. This method is still in the experimental stage.

NURSING MANAGEMENT
SEIZURE DISORDERS AND EPILEPSY

■ Nursing Assessment

Subjective and objective data that should be obtained from a patient with a seizure disorder are presented in Table 57-11. Data related to a specific seizure episode can be obtained from a witness.

■ Nursing Diagnoses

Nursing diagnoses for the patient with seizure disorders and epilepsy may include, but are not limited to, those presented in NCP 57-2.

■ Planning

The overall goals are that the patient with seizures will (1) be free from injury during a seizure, (2) have optimal mental and physical functioning while taking antiseizure drugs, and (3) have satisfactory psychosocial functioning.

■ Nursing Implementation

Health Promotion. Many cases of seizure disorders can be prevented by promotion of general safety measures, such as the wearing of helmets in situations involving risk of head injury. Improved perinatal, labor, and delivery care have reduced fetal

---

TABLE 57-11 Nursing Assessment
Seizure Disorders and Epilepsy

Subjective Data

Important Health Information

Past health history: Previous seizures, birth defects or injuries, anoxic episodes; CNS trauma, tumors, or infections; stroke; metabolic disorders, alcoholism; exposure to metals and carbon monoxide; hepatic or renal failure; fever; pregnancy, systemic lupus erythematosus

Medications: Compliance with antiseizure medications; barbiturate or alcohol withdrawal; use and overdose of cocaine, amphetamines, lidocaine, theophylline, penicillin, lithium, phenothiazines, tricyclic antidepressants, benzodiazepines

Functional Health Patterns

Health perception–health management: Positive family history

Cognitive-perceptual: Headaches, aura, mood or behavioral changes before seizure; mentation changes; abdominal pain, muscle pain (postictal)

Self-perception–self-concept: Anxiety, depression; loss of self-esteem, social isolation

Sexuality-reproductive: Decreased sexual drive, erectile dysfunction; increased sexual drive (postictal)

Objective Data

General

Precipitating factors, including severe metabolic acidosis or alkalosis, hyperkalemia, hypoglycemia, dehydration, or water intoxication

Integumentary

Bitten tongue, soft-tissue damage, cyanosis, diaphoresis (postictal)

Respiratory

Abnormal respiratory rate, rhythm, or depth; apnea (ictal); absent or abnormal breath sounds, possible airway occlusion

Cardiovascular

Hypertension, tachycardia or bradycardia (ictal)

Gastrointestinal

Bowel incontinence; excessive salivation

Urinary

Incontinence

Neurologic

Generalized

Tonic-clonic: Loss of consciousness, muscle tightening, then jerking; dilated pupils; hyperventilation, then apnea; postictal somnolence

Absence: Altered consciousness (5 to 30 seconds), minor facial motor activity

Partial

Simple: Aura; consciousness; focal sensory, motor, cognitive, or emotional phenomena (focal motor); unilateral "marching" motor seizure (jacksonian)

Complex: Altered consciousness with inappropriate behaviors, automatisms, amnesia of event

Musculoskeletal

Weakness, paralysis, ataxia (postictal)

Possible Findings

Positive toxicology screen or alcohol level; altered serum electrolytes, acidosis or alkalosis, very low blood glucose level, ↑ blood urea nitrogen or serum creatinine, liver function tests, ammonia; abnormal CT scan or MRI of head, abnormal findings from lumbar puncture; abnormal discharges on EEG

CNS, Central nervous system; *CT,* computed tomography; *EEG,* electroencephalogram; *MRI,* magnetic resonance imaging.

trauma and hypoxia and thereby have reduced brain damage leading to seizure disorders.

The patient with a seizure disorder should practice good general health habits (e.g., maintaining a proper diet, getting adequate rest, exercising). The patient should be helped to identify events or situations that precipitate the seizures and should be given suggestions for avoiding them or handling them better. Excessive alcohol intake, fatigue, and loss of sleep should be avoided, and the patient should be helped to handle stress constructively.

Acute Intervention. The nurse caring for a hospitalized patient with a seizure disorder or a patient who has had seizures as a result of metabolic factors involves several responsibilities, including observation and treatment of the seizure, education, and psychosocial intervention.

When a seizure occurs, the nurse should carefully observe and record details of the event because the diagnosis and subsequent treatment often rest solely on the seizure description. All aspects of the seizure should be noted. What events preceded the seizure? When did the seizure occur? How long did each phase (aural [if any], ictal, postictal) last? What occurred during each phase?

Both subjective data (usually the only type of data in the aural phase) and objective data are important. Objective data should

NURSING CARE PLAN 57-2

Patient with Seizure Disorder or Epilepsy

EXPECTED PATIENT OUTCOMES	NURSING INTERVENTIONS and *RATIONALES*
NURSING DIAGNOSIS	**Ineffective breathing pattern** *related to* neuromuscular impairment secondary to prolonged tonic phase of seizure or during postictal period *as manifested by* abnormal respiratory rate, rhythm, or depth.
• Appropriate rate, rhythm, and depth of respirations	• Loosen constricting clothing *to avoid restricting breathing.* • Assess breathing pattern, observing for labored respiration, tachypnea, bradypnea, dyspnea, and apnea *to determine presence and extent of problem and to initiate appropriate interventions.* • Provide manual ventilation or O₂ when necessary; be prepared to assist with endotracheal intubation *to maintain adequate oxygenation and prevent hypoxia.* • Insert oral airway (if indicated) only after seizure activity has ceased *to prevent mouth and teeth injury from forcing airway between clamped teeth.*
NURSING DIAGNOSIS	**Risk for injury** *related to* seizure activity and subsequent impaired physical mobility secondary to postictal weakness or paralysis.
• No injury • Verbalization of knowledge of potential for injury during seizure • Arrangement of environment to minimize risk for injury	• Assess for trauma to mouth, cheek, tongue, lips; abrasions, bruises; broken bones; burns *because these injuries may occur during seizure activity.* • Assess for weakness, paralysis of one side of body, ataxia, fatigue, lethargy *as potential postictal risks for injury to plan appropriate interventions.* • If patient anticipates a seizure may occur, assist to a safe location or position; use seizure precautions as appropriate; remove potentially harmful objects from surrounding area; gently guide arm or leg movements *to prevent injury during a seizure.* • Refrain from moving or restraining patient during a seizure *to prevent bone or soft tissue injury.* • Assist in determining whether operation of a motor vehicle or dangerous machinery is appropriate for patient *to assist patient in making the appropriate choice about driving.*
NURSING DIAGNOSIS	**Ineffective coping** *related to* perceived loss of control and denial of diagnosis *as manifested by* verbalizations about not having epilepsy, lack of truth-telling regarding seizure frequency, noncompliant behavior.
• Acceptance of disorder as evidenced by using the words *seizure disorder* or *epilepsy* to describe illness • Acknowledgment that a seizure has occurred	• Explore reasons for denial *to determine extent of problem and to plan appropriate interventions.* • Implement and individualize teaching plan about causes and mechanisms of seizures, effectiveness of drugs in controlling seizures, inaccuracy of myths about epilepsy, avoidance of precipitating factors, state law regarding driving, pros and cons of medical identification tags, moderation in drinking and eating, exposure to stress, and avoidance of hazardous activities *to promote effective coping by providing correct information.*
NURSING DIAGNOSIS	**Ineffective therapeutic regimen management** *related to* lack of knowledge about management of seizure disorder *as manifested by* verbalization of lack of knowledge, inaccurate perception of health status, noncompliance with prescribed health behavior.
• Therapeutic drug levels of antiseizure medication • Compliance with therapeutic regimen	• Provide teaching to patient and family about seizure activity and therapeutic management including diagnosis, treatment, lifestyle adjustments, and community resources *so that patient and family can make necessary lifestyle modifications to manage a chronic disease.*

include the exact onset of the seizure (which body part was affected first and how); the course and nature of the seizure activity (loss of consciousness, tongue biting, automatisms, stiffening, jerking, total lack of muscle tone); the body parts involved and their sequence of involvement; and the presence of autonomic signs, such as dilated pupils, excessive salivation, altered breathing, cyanosis, flushing, diaphoresis, or incontinence. Assessment of the postictal period should include a detailed description of the level of consciousness, vital signs, memory loss, muscle soreness, speech disorders (aphasia, dysarthria), weakness or paralysis, sleep period, and the duration of each sign or symptom.

During the seizure it is important to maintain a patent airway. This may involve supporting and protecting the head, turning the patient to the side, loosening constrictive clothing, or easing the patient to the floor, if seated. The patient should not be restrained, and no objects should be placed in the mouth. After the seizure the patient may require suctioning, and oxygen may be needed.

A seizure can be a frightening experience for the patient and for others who may witness it. The nurse should assess the level of their understanding and provide information about how and why the event occurred. This is an excellent opportunity for the nurse to dispel many common misconceptions about seizures.

Ambulatory and Home Care. Prevention of recurring seizures is the major goal in the treatment of epilepsy. Because many seizure disorders cannot be cured, drugs must be taken regularly and continuously, often for a lifetime. The nurse should ensure that the patient knows this, as well as the specifics of the drug regimen and what to do if a dose is missed. Usually the dose should be made up if the omission is remembered within 24 hours. The patient should be cautioned not to adjust drug doses without professional guidance because this can increase seizure frequency and even cause status epilepticus. The patient should be encouraged to report any medication side effects and to keep regular appointments with the health care provider.

Nurses play an important role in teaching the patient and the family. Guidelines for teaching are shown in Table 57-12. Nurses should teach family members and significant others the emergency management of tonic-clonic seizures (see Table 57-8). They should be reminded that it is not necessary to call an ambulance or send a person to the hospital after a single seizure unless the seizure is prolonged, another seizure immediately follows, or extensive injury has occurred.

Patients with a seizure disorder also experience concerns or fears related to recurrent seizures, incontinence, or loss of self-control. The nurse provides support for the patient through education and by helping to identify coping mechanisms.

Perhaps the greatest challenge that a seizure disorder presents to the patient is adjusting to the personal limitations imposed by the illness. Discrimination in employment is the most serious problem facing the person with a seizure disorder. For issues relating to job discrimination, patients can be referred to the State Human Rights Commission or the State Department of Vocational Rehabilitation.

A variety of other resources can be offered to the patient with a seizure disorder who has a specific problem. If the nurse believes that associating with others who have a seizure disorder would be beneficial, the patient can be referred to the local chapter of the Epilepsy Foundation (EF), a voluntary agency that offers a variety of services to patients with epilepsy. The

---

TABLE 57-12 Patient & Family Teaching Guide

Seizure Disorders and Epilepsy

The patient should be taught the following:
1. Drugs must be taken as prescribed. Any and all side effects of drugs should be reported to the health care provider. When necessary, blood drawings are done to ensure that therapeutic levels are maintained.
2. Use of nondrug techniques, such as relaxation therapy and biofeedback training, to potentially reduce the number of seizures.
3. Availability of resources in the community.
4. Need to wear a medical alert bracelet, necklace, and identification card.
5. Avoidance of excessive alcohol intake, fatigue, and loss of sleep.
6. Regular meals and snacks in between if feeling shaky, faint, or hungry.

Family members should be taught the following:
1. For first aid treatment of tonic-clonic seizure, it is not necessary to call an ambulance or send the patient to the hospital after a single seizure unless the seizure is prolonged, another seizure immediately follows, or extensive injury has occurred.
2. During an acute seizure, it is important to protect the patient from injury. This may involve supporting and protecting the head, turning the patient to the side, loosening constrictive clothing, and easing the patient to the floor, if seated.

---

patient who is an eligible veteran can be referred to a Department of Veterans Affairs medical center that provides comprehensive care.

The patient should be informed that medical alert bracelets, necklaces, and identification cards are available through the EF, local pharmacies, or companies specializing in identification devices (e.g., Medic Alert). However, the use of these medical identification tags is optional. Some patients have found them beneficial, but others have found them to be more a burden than a help because they prefer not to be identified as having a seizure disorder.

Social workers and welfare agencies can help with financial problems and living arrangements. State services for individuals with developmental disabilities include assistance with job training and placement for patients whose seizures are not well controlled. Sheltered housing and funding for special needs, such as medical and psychologic evaluation and transportation, are also offered. State agencies specializing in vocational rehabilitation services can offer vocational assessment, counseling, funding for training, and assistance with job placement. They can also offer financial assistance for transportation and medical costs that are necessary for vocational rehabilitation or job maintenance. If intensive psychologic counseling is needed, the nurse can refer the patient to a community mental health center.

The patient should be encouraged to learn more about epilepsy through self-education materials. The EF provides several information pamphlets and may facilitate support groups. Many agencies that offer services to epileptic patients, as well as local chapters of EF, have these available as teaching aids.

■ Evaluation

Expected outcomes for the patient with seizures are addressed in NCP 57-2.

MULTIPLE SCLEROSIS

Multiple sclerosis (MS) is a chronic, progressive, degenerative disorder of the CNS characterized by disseminated demyelination of nerve fibers of the brain and spinal cord. It is not known exactly how many people have MS. High prevalence rates (over 30 per 100,000) occur in northern Europe, northern United States, southern Canada, and southern Australia and New Zealand. Low prevalence rates (less than 5 per 100,000) occur in southern Europe, Japan, China, and South America. This difference may be related to climate or racial differences or both. MS is 5 times more prevalent in temperate climates (between 45 and 65 degrees of latitude), such as those found in the northern United States, Canada, and Europe, as compared with tropical regions.[9] MS is considered a disease of young to middle-age adults, with the onset usually being between 15 and 50 years of age. Women are affected more often than men.

Etiology and Pathophysiology

The cause of MS is unknown, although research findings suggest that MS is related to infectious (viral), immunologic, and genetic factors and is perpetuated as a result of intrinsic factors (e.g., faulty immunoregulation). The susceptibility to MS appears to be inherited. First-, second-, and third-degree relatives of patients with MS are at a slightly increased risk. Multiple genes confer susceptibility to MS.

The role of precipitating factors such as exposure to pathogenetic agents in the etiology of MS is controversial. It is possible that their association with MS is random and that there is no cause-and-effect relationship. Possible precipitating factors include infection, physical injury, emotional stress, excessive fatigue, pregnancy, and a poorer state of health.

MS is characterized by chronic inflammation, demyelination, and gliosis (scarring) in the CNS. The primary neuropathologic condition is an autoimmune disease orchestrated by autoreactive T cells (lymphocytes). This process may be initially triggered by a virus in genetically susceptible individuals. The activated T cells in the systemic circulation migrate to the CNS, causing blood-brain barrier disruption. This is likely the initial event in the development of MS. Subsequent antigen-antibody reaction within the CNS results in activation of the inflammatory response and through multiple effector mechanisms leads to demyelination of axons. The disease process consists of loss of myelin, disappearance of oligodendrocytes, and proliferation of astrocytes. These changes result in characteristic plaque formation, or sclerosis, with plaques scattered throughout multiple regions of the CNS.

Initially the myelin sheaths of the neurons in the brain and spinal cord are attacked (Fig. 57-1, *A* and *B*). Early in the disease the myelin sheath is damaged; but the nerve fiber is not affected, and nerve impulses are still transmitted (Fig. 57-1, *C*). At this point the patient may complain of a noticeable impairment of function (e.g., weakness). However, the myelin can regenerate, and the symptoms disappear, resulting in a remission.

In addition to myelin disruption, the axon also becomes involved (Fig. 57-1, *D*). Myelin is replaced by glial scar tissue, which forms hard, sclerotic plaques in multiple regions of the

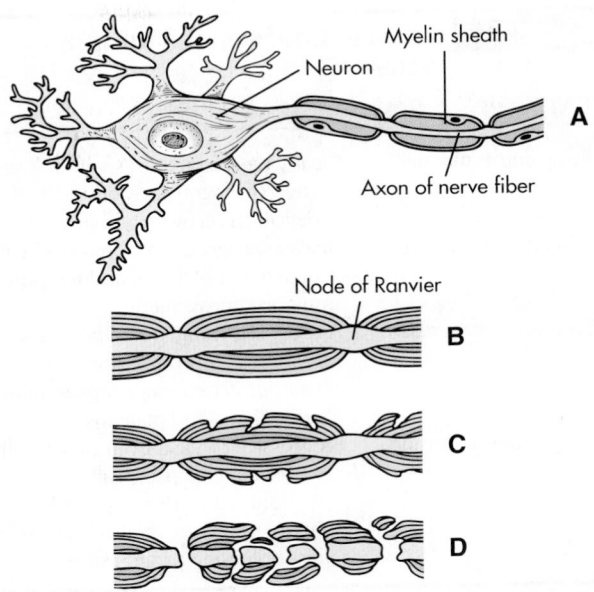

FIG. 57-1 Pathogenesis of multiple sclerosis. **A,** Normal nerve cell with myelin sheath. **B,** Normal axon. **C,** Myelin breakdown. **D,** Myelin totally disrupted; axon not functioning.

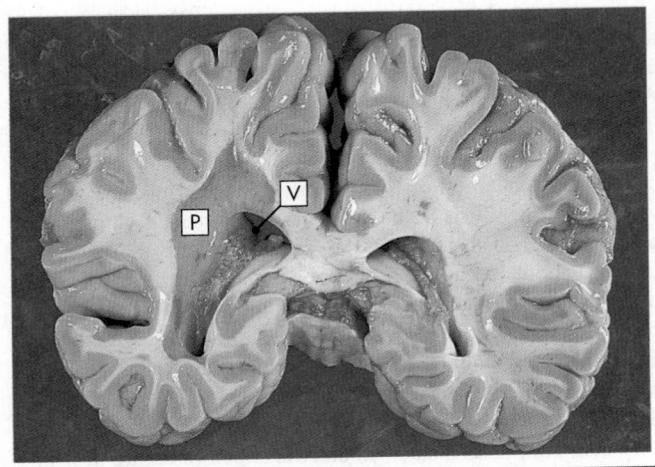

FIG. 57-2 Chronic multiple sclerosis. Demyelination plaque *(P)* at gray–white junction and adjacent partially remyelinated shadow plaque *(V).*

CNS (Fig. 57-2). Without myelin, nerve impulses slow down, and with destruction of nerve axons, impulses are totally blocked, resulting in permanent loss of function. In many chronic lesions, demyelination continues with progressive loss of nerve function.

Clinical Manifestations

Because the onset is often insidious and gradual, with vague symptoms that occur intermittently over months or years, the disease may not be diagnosed until long after the onset of the first symptom. The disease process has a spotty distribution in the CNS, so the signs and symptoms vary over time. The disease is characterized by chronic, progressive deterioration in some persons and by remissions and exacerbations in others. With repeated exacerbations, however, progressive scarring of the myelin sheath occurs, and the overall trend is progressive deterioration in neurologic function.

TABLE 57-13 Clinical Courses of Multiple Sclerosis

CATEGORY	CHARACTERISTICS
Relapsing-remitting	Clearly defined relapses with full recovery or sequelae and residual deficit on recovery
Primary-progressive	Disease progression from onset with occasional plateaus and temporary minor improvements
Secondary-progressive	A relapsing-remitting initial course, followed by progression with or without occasional relapses, minor remissions, and plateaus
Progressive-relapsing	Progressive disease from onset, with clear acute relapses, with or without full recovery; periods between relapses are characterized by continuing progression

The clinical manifestations vary according to the areas of the CNS involved. Some patients have severe, long-lasting symptoms early in the course of the disease. Others may experience only occasional and mild symptoms for several years after onset. A classification scheme that identifies the various courses of MS has been developed[10] (Table 57-13).

Common signs and symptoms of MS include motor, sensory, cerebellar, and emotional problems. Motor symptoms include weakness or paralysis of the limbs, trunk, or head; diplopia; scanning speech; and spasticity of the muscles that are chronically affected. Patients with MS experience a variety of sensory abnormalities, including numbness and tingling and other paresthesias, patchy blindness (scotomas), blurred vision, vertigo, tinnitus, decreased hearing, and chronic neuropathic pain. Radicular (nerve root) pains may be present, particularly in the low thoracic and abdominal regions. Lhermitte's phenomenon is a transient sensory symptom described as an electric shock radiating down the spine or into the limbs with flexion of the neck. Cerebellar signs include nystagmus, ataxia, dysarthria, and dysphagia.

Bowel and bladder function can be affected if the sclerotic plaque is located in areas of the CNS that control elimination. Problems with defecation usually involve constipation rather than fecal incontinence. Urinary problems are variable. A common problem in MS patients is a spastic (uninhibited) bladder. This indicates a lesion above the second sacral nerve, which cuts off suprasegmental inhibiting influences on bladder contractility. As a result, the bladder has a small capacity for urine, and its contractions are unchecked. This is accompanied by urinary urgency and frequency and results in dribbling or incontinence. A flaccid (hypotonic) bladder indicates a lesion in the reflex arc governing bladder function. The bladder has a large capacity for urine because there is no sensation or desire to void, no pressure, and no pain. Generally, there is urinary retention, but urgency and frequency may also occur with this type of lesion. Another urinary problem is a combination of the previous two problems. Urinary problems cannot be adequately diagnosed and treated unless urodynamic studies are done.

Sexual dysfunction occurs in many persons with MS. Physiologic erectile dysfunction may result from spinal cord involvement in men. Women may experience decreased libido, difficulty with orgasmic response, painful intercourse, and decreased vaginal lubrication. Diminished sensation can prevent a normal sexual response in both sexes. The emotional effects of chronic illness and the loss of self-esteem also contribute to loss of sexual response.

MS has no apparent effect on the course of pregnancy, labor, delivery, or lactation. Some women with MS who become pregnant experience remission or an improvement in their symptoms during the gestation period. The hormonal changes associated with pregnancy appear to affect the immune system. However, during the postpartum period, women are at greater risk for exacerbation of the disease.[11]

Although intellectual functioning generally remains intact, emotional stability may be affected. Cognitive sequelae can produce significant disability for some patients with MS. Persons may experience anger, depression, or euphoria. Signs and symptoms of MS are aggravated or triggered by physical and emotional trauma, fatigue, and infection.

The average life expectancy after the onset of symptoms is more than 25 years. Death usually occurs because of infective complications (e.g., pneumonia) of immobility or because of an unrelated disease.

Diagnostic Studies

Because there is no definitive diagnostic test for MS, diagnosis is based primarily on history, clinical manifestations, and the presence of multiple lesions over time as measured by MRI (Table 57-14). Certain laboratory tests are currently used as adjuncts to the clinical examination. In some patients, cerebrospinal fluid (CSF) analysis may show an increase in oligo-

TABLE 57-14 Collaborative Care Multiple Sclerosis

Diagnostic
History and physical examination
CSF analysis
Evoked response testing (also called evoked potential testing, e.g., somatosensory evoked potential [SSEP], auditory evoked potential [AEP], visual evoked potential [VEP])
CT scan
MRI, MRS

Collaborative Therapy
*Drug Therapy**
Corticosteroids
Immunomodulators
Immunosuppressants
Cholinergics
Anticholinergics
Muscle relaxants
Surgical Therapy
Thalamotomy (unmanageable tremor)
Neurectomy, rhizotomy, cordotomy (unmanageable spasticity)

*See Table 57-15.
CSF, Cerebrospinal fluid; CT, computed tomography; MRI, magnetic resonance imaging; MRS, magnetic resonance spectroscopy.

clonal immunoglobulin G. The CSF also contains a high number of lymphocytes and monocytes. Evoked responses are often delayed in persons with MS because of decreased nerve conduction from the eye and the ear to the brain. MRI scan may be helpful because sclerotic plaques as small as 3 to 4 mm in diameter can be detected. Characteristic white-matter lesions scattered through the brain or spinal cord are evident on such a scan. MRS may also be used to evaluate patients with MS.

Collaborative Care

Drug Therapy. Because there is no cure for MS, collaborative care is aimed at treating the disease process and providing symptomatic relief (see Table 57-14). The disease process is treated with drugs (Table 57-15), and the symptoms are controlled with a variety of drugs and other forms of therapy.[12] Adrenocorticotropic hormone, methylprednisolone, and pred-

nisone are helpful in treating acute exacerbations of the disease, probably by reducing edema and acute inflammation at the site of demyelination. Although the dose and route of administration may vary, these drugs are used in patients with all types of MS. However, these drugs do not affect the ultimate outcome or degree of residual neurologic impairment from the exacerbation.

Immunosuppressive drugs, such as azathioprine (Imuran), methotrexate, and cyclophosphamide (Cytoxan), have been shown to produce some beneficial effects in patients with progressive-relapsing, secondary-progressive, and primary-progressive MS. However, the potential benefits of these drugs in patients with MS must be counterbalanced against the potentially serious side effects.

Immunomodulator drugs modify the disease process. Interferon β-1b (Betaseron) is used for ambulatory patients with relapsing-remitting MS. Interferon β-1a (Avonex) is similar to interferon β-1b in efficacy and is used in similar patient groups with

TABLE 57-15 Drug Therapy — Multiple Sclerosis

DRUG	SYMPTOMS RELIEVED	SIDE EFFECTS AND PRECAUTIONS	PATIENT TEACHING
Corticosteroids ACTH, prednisone, methylprednisolone	Exacerbations	Edema, mental changes (euphoria), weight gain, redistribution of body fat*; widespread effects on many metabolic processes; few adverse effects with use for less than 1 month at a time	• Restrict salt intake • Do not abruptly stop therapy • Know drug interactions
Immunomodulators β-interferon (Betaseron, Avonex, Rebif)	Exacerbations	Flulike symptoms, local skin reactions, depression; monitor CBC, blood chemistries, and liver function tests every 3 months	• Perform self-injection techniques • Report side effects
glatiramer acetate (Copaxone)	Exacerbations	Local skin reactions; chest pain, weakness; no laboratory monitoring required	• Perform self-injection techniques • Report side effects
Immunosuppressants mitoxantrone (Novantrone)	Exacerbations	Nausea, vomiting, diarrhea, mucositis, alopecia, hepatotoxicity, myelosuppression; cardiovascular disease; lifetime dose limit because of cardiotoxicity; monitor CBC and liver function every month	• Receive regular monitoring and follow-up • Consult health care provider before getting immunizations • Be aware that urine may turn a blue-green color initially • Maintain adequate fluid intake
Cholinergics bethanechol (Urecholine) neostigmine (Prostigmin)	Urinary retention (flaccid bladder)	Hypotension, diarrhea, diaphoresis, muscle weakness; history of cardiac dysfunction, hypotension, allergies, peptic ulcer disease, asthma	• Consult with health care provider before using other drugs, including over-the-counter drugs
Anticholinergics probanthine (Pro-Banthine) oxybutynin (Ditropan)	Urinary frequency[†] and urgency (spastic bladder)	Dry mouth, blurred vision, constipation, hypertension, flushing, urinary retention (too high of dose); contraindicated with history of glaucoma, prostatic hyperplasia, cardiac dysfunction, intestinal obstruction	• Consult health care provider before using other drugs, especially sleeping aids, antihistamines (possibly leading to potentiated effect)

*See Chapter 48 for effects of long-term corticosteroid therapy.
†Urodynamic studies must be done before initiation of therapy because patients with MS have multiple lesions and type of bladder dysfunction cannot be diagnosed from symptoms alone.
ACTH, Adrenocorticotropic hormone; *CBC,* complete blood count; *CNS,* central nervous system; *MAO,* monoamine oxidase.

Continued

TABLE 57-15 Drug Therapy
Multiple Sclerosis—cont'd

DRUG	SYMPTOMS RELIEVED	SIDE EFFECTS AND PRECAUTIONS	PATIENT TEACHING
Muscle Relaxants			
diazepam (Valium)	Spasticity	Drowsiness, ataxia, fatigue; contraindicated with history of narrow–angle glaucoma	• Avoid driving and similar activities because of CNS depressant effects • Be aware of addictive potential • Avoid long-term use • Avoid concomitant use of barbiturates, MAO inhibitors, antidepressants
baclofen (Lioresal)	Spasticity	Drowsiness, weakness; used cautiously with a history of hypersensitivity and renal damage; possible exacerbation of seizures in patients with seizure disorders	• Do not abruptly stop therapy (possibility of hallucinations) • Avoid driving and similar activities because of sedative effects • Avoid use of other CNS depressants • Take with food or milk
dantrolene (Dantrium)	Spasticity	Drowsiness, dizziness, malaise, fatigue, diarrhea; used cautiously in patients with a history of respiratory or cardiac dysfunction; risk of hepatotoxicity	• Avoid driving when drug is used • Avoid use with tranquilizers and alcohol (possibly causing photosensitivity) • Obtain baseline liver function tests
tizanidine (Zanaflex)	Spasticity	Drowsiness, dry mouth, fatigue, nausea; used cautiously in patients with history of hypersensitivity, liver or renal disease, hypotension, bradycardia	• Avoid driving when drug is used • Avoid use with tranquilizers and alcohol (possibly causing photosensitivity) • Eat small frequent meals to reduce nausea • Change position slowly when going from lying or sitting position to standing

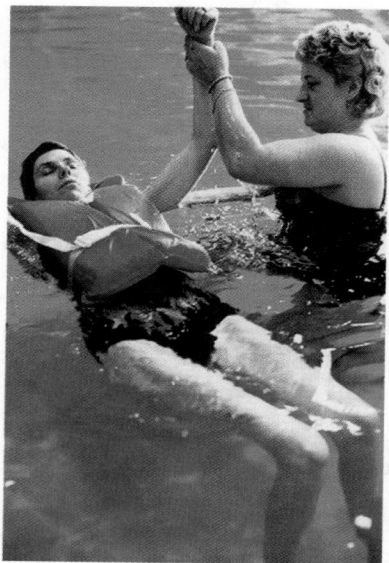

FIG. 57-3 Water therapy provides exercise and recreation for the patient with a chronic neurologic disease.

MS. It is given intramuscularly once a week. Interferon β-1a (Rebif) is administered subcutaneously 3 times weekly. Glatiramer acetate (Copaxone), formerly known as copolymer-1, is unrelated to interferon. It is given subcutaneously every day in patients with relapsing-remitting MS.[12] Natalizumab (Antegren), a recombinant monoclonal antibody to a leukocyte adhesion molecule, is a promising new therapy for MS. It works by inhibiting the migration of lymphocytes, thus decreasing the inflammatory process.

Mitoxantrone (Novantrone) is a new drug for the treatment of primary-progressive and progressive-relapsing MS. It is an immunosuppressant drug that reduces both B and T lymphocytes and impairs antigen presentation. It is given intravenously monthly. Unlike the other disease-modifying drugs, mitoxantrone has a lifetime dose limit because of cardiac toxicity. Therefore it cannot be used for more than 2 to 3 years.

Many other drugs are used to treat the symptoms of MS. Antispasmodics are used for spasticity. Amantadine (Symmetrel) and CNS stimulants (pemoline [Cylert], methylphenidate [Ritalin], and modafinil [Provigil]) are used for fatigue. Anticholinergics are used to treat bladder symptoms. Tricyclic antidepressants and antiseizure drugs are used for chronic pain syndromes.

Other Therapies. Spasticity is primarily treated with antispasmodic drugs. However, surgery (e.g., neurectomy, rhizotomy, cordotomy), dorsal-column electrical stimulation, or intrathecal baclofen (Lioresal) pump may be required. Tremors that become unmanageable with drugs are sometimes treated by thalamotomy or deep brain stimulation.

Neurologic dysfunction sometimes improves with physical therapy and speech therapy. Physical therapy is important in keeping the patient as functionally active as possible. The purpose of therapy is to relieve spasticity, increase coordination, and train the patient to substitute unaffected muscles for impaired ones. An especially beneficial type of physical therapy is water exercise (Fig. 57-3). Water gives buoyancy to the body and allows the patient to perform activities that would normally be impossible. In water, the patient experiences more control over the body.

Nutritional Therapy. Various nutritional measures have been used in the management of MS, including megavitamin therapy (cobalamin [vitamin B_{12}], vitamin C) and diets consisting of low-fat and gluten-free food and raw vegetables. These particular dietary measures have not come into widespread use because of lack of proof of their effectiveness.

A nutritious, well-balanced diet is essential. Although there is no standard prescribed diet, a high-protein diet with supplementary vitamins is often advocated. A diet high in roughage may help relieve the problem of constipation. Vitamins are merely supplemental and not curative.

NURSING MANAGEMENT
MULTIPLE SCLEROSIS

■ Nursing Assessment

Subjective and objective data that should be obtained from a patient with MS are presented in Table 57-16.

■ Nursing Diagnoses

Nursing diagnoses for the patient with MS may include, but are not limited to, those presented in NCP 57-3.

■ Planning

The overall goals are that the patient with MS will (1) maximize neuromuscular function, (2) maintain independence in activities of daily living for as long as possible, (3) optimize psychosocial well-being, (4) adjust to the illness, and (5) reduce factors that precipitate exacerbations.

■ Nursing Implementation

The patient with MS should be aware of triggers that may cause exacerbations or worsening of the disease. Exacerbations of MS are triggered by infection (especially upper respiratory and urinary tract infections), trauma, immunization, delivery after pregnancy, stress, and change in climate. Of these the best documented are upper respiratory infections, postpartum period, and head trauma.[13] Each person responds differently to these triggers. The nurse should help the patient identify particular triggers and develop ways to avoid them or minimize their effects.

The most common reasons for hospitalization of the patient with MS are for a diagnostic workup and treatment of an acute exacerbation. During the diagnostic phase the patient needs reassurance that even though there is a tentative diagnosis of MS, certain diagnostic studies must be done to rule out other neurologic disorders. The nurse should assist the patient in dealing with the anxiety caused by a diagnosis of a disabling illness. The patient with recently diagnosed MS may need assistance with the grieving process.

During an acute exacerbation the patient may be immobile and confined to bed. The focus of nursing intervention at this phase is to prevent major complications of immobility, such as respiratory and urinary tract infections and pressure ulcers.

Patient teaching should focus on building general resistance to illness, including avoiding fatigue, extremes of heat and cold, and exposure to infection. The last measure involves avoiding exposure to cold climates and to people who are sick, as well as

TABLE 57-16	Nursing Assessment Multiple Sclerosis

Subjective Data
Important Health Information
Past health history: Recent or past viral infections or vaccinations, other recent infections, residence in cold or temperate climates, recent physical or emotional stress, pregnancy, exposure to extremes of heat and cold
Medications: Use of and compliance in taking corticosteroids, immunomodulators, immunosuppressants, cholinergics, anticholinergics, antispasmodics

Functional Health Patterns
Health perception–health management: Positive family history; malaise
Nutritional-metabolic: Weight loss; difficulty in chewing, dysphagia
Elimination: Urinary frequency, urgency, dribbling or incontinence, retention; constipation
Activity-exercise: Generalized muscle weakness, muscle fatigue; tingling and numbness, ataxia (clumsiness)
Cognitive-perceptual: Eye, back, leg, joint pain; painful muscle spasms; vertigo; blurred or lost vision; diplopia; tinnitus
Sexuality-reproductive: Impotence, decreased libido
Coping-stress tolerance: Anger, depression, euphoria, social isolation

Objective Data
General
Apathy, inattentiveness
Integumentary
Pressure ulcers
Neurologic
Scanning speech, nystagmus, ataxia, tremor, spasticity, hyperreflexia, decreased hearing
Musculoskeletal
Muscular weakness, paresis, paralysis, spasms, foot dragging, dysarthria
Possible Findings
↓ T-suppressor cells, demyelinating lesions on MRI or MRS scans, increased IgG or oligoclonal banding in cerebrospinal fluid, delayed evoked potential

IgG, Immunoglobulin G; *MRI,* magnetic resonance imaging; *MRS,* magnetic resonance spectroscopy.

vigorous and early treatment of infection when it does occur. It is important to teach the patient to (1) achieve a good balance of exercise and rest, (2) eat nutritious and well-balanced meals, and (3) avoid the hazards of immobility (e.g., contractures, pressure ulcers). Patients should know their treatment regimens, the side effects of drugs and how to watch for them, and drug interactions with over-the-counter medications. The patient should consult a health care provider before taking nonprescription drugs.

Bladder control is a major problem for many patients with MS. Although anticholinergics may be beneficial for some patients to decrease spasticity, other patients may need to be taught self-catheterization (see Chapter 44). Bowel problems, particularly constipation, occur frequently in patients with MS. Increasing the dietary fiber intake may help some patients achieve regularity in bowel habits.

NURSING CARE PLAN 57-3

Patient with Multiple Sclerosis

EXPECTED PATIENT OUTCOMES	NURSING INTERVENTIONS and *RATIONALES*
NURSING DIAGNOSIS	**Impaired physical mobility** *related to* muscle weakness or paralysis and muscle spasticity *as manifested by* inability to ambulate, intermittent muscle spasms, pain associated with muscle spasms.
• Demonstration of use of adaptive devices • Maintenance of or increased strength of limbs • ↓ Muscle spasms	• Use assistive devices as indicated *to decrease fatigue and enhance independence, comfort, and safety.* • Do active range-of-motion exercises at least 2 times per day *to prevent contractures and minimize muscle atrophy.* • Encourage and assist with ambulation and transfer as indicated *to maintain mobility, promote independence, and provide for safety.* • Change position of patient (if bedridden) at least q2hr to prevent circulatory problems and pressure ulcers. • Perform stretching exercises every 6 to 8 hours *to relieve spasms and contracted muscles.*
NURSING DIAGNOSIS	**Dressing/grooming self-care deficit** *related to* muscle spasticity and neuromuscular deficits *as manifested by* inability to perform some or all activities of daily living (ADLs).
• Maximum level of functioning • ADL needs met by self or others	• Assess self-care problems *to plan appropriate interventions to meet care needs.* • Promote use of appropriate assistive devices *so that patient can maximally participate in self-care activities with minimum fatigue.* • Perform or assist with ADLs only as indicated *to promote patient's independence.*
NURSING DIAGNOSIS	**Risk for impaired skin integrity** *related to* immobility, sensorimotor deficits, and inadequate nutrition.
• Intact skin	• Assess skin for redness and breakdown *to monitor changes in skin integrity and make appropriate plan for interventions.* • Use circular massage of unreddened bony prominences with each turning *to improve circulation to these areas.* • Provide high-protein diet *to promote healthy skin resistant to breakdown.*
NURSING DIAGNOSIS	**Impaired urinary elimination pattern** *related to* sensorimotor deficits and/or inadequate fluid intake *as manifested by* posturination residual volume >50 ml, dribbling, bladder distention.
• Residual urine volume <50 ml • Maintenance of urinary continence	• Administer cholinergic drugs as ordered *to improve the muscle tone of bladder and facilitate bladder emptying.* • Follow intermittent catheterization protocol *to prevent distention or dribbling.* • Use Credé maneuver or reflex stimulation (manual stimulation) *as an alternative method of emptying bladder.* • Maintain fluid intake of 3000 ml per day *to dilute urine and reduce risk of urinary tract infection.* • Teach patient signs and symptoms of urinary tract infection *to ensure early identification and treatment.* • Initiate bladder training program *to help restore adequate bladder function.*
NURSING DIAGNOSIS	**Sexual dysfunction** *related to* neuromuscular deficits *as manifested by* impotence, verbalization of problem, decreased libido.
• Verbalization of satisfaction with expression of sexuality	• Initiate sexual counseling if indicated *because not all nurses have the education required for this type of counseling.* • Suggest alternative methods of achieving sexual gratification *because sexual intercourse may not be possible as a result of neuromuscular deficits.*
NURSING DIAGNOSIS	**Interrupted family processes** *related to* changing family roles, potential financial problems, and fluctuating physical condition *as manifested by* strained family relations, ineffective communication, verbalization of financial concerns.
• Open communication between family and patient • Able to seek outside assistance when indicated	• Facilitate open communication among patient and family *to promote better interpersonal relationships.* • Promote problem solving *to enable the family to handle the issues of long-term illness.* • Refer for family and financial counseling (if indicated) *to provide additional help in coping with a chronic debilitating disease.* • Educate family regarding fluctuating nature of disease *because lack of knowledge about MS affects ability to cope with the changes.*

The patient with MS and the family must make many emotional adjustments because of the unpredictability of the disease, the need to change lifestyles, and the challenge of avoiding or decreasing precipitating factors. The National Multiple Sclerosis Society and its local chapters can offer a variety of services to meet the needs of patients with MS.

■ Evaluation

Expected outcomes for the patient with MS are addressed in NCP 57-3.

PARKINSON'S DISEASE

Parkinson's disease (PD) is a disease of the basal ganglia characterized by a slowing down in the initiation and execution of movement (bradykinesia), increased muscle tone (rigidity), tremor at rest, and impaired postural reflexes. It is the most common form of *parkinsonism* (a syndrome characterized by similar symptoms). Parkinson's disease is named after James Parkinson, who, in 1817, wrote a classic essay on "shaking palsy," a disease whose cause is still unknown.

Etiology and Pathophysiology

The prevalence of Parkinson's disease is about 160 per 100,000 and the incidence is about 20 per 100,000. The diagnosis of Parkinson's disease increases with age, with the peak onset in the sixth decade. Onset of Parkinson's disease before age 50 is more likely related to a genetic defect.[14] Parkinson's disease is more common in men by a ratio of 3:2.

There are many forms of parkinsonism other than Parkinson's disease. Encephalitis lethargica, or type A encephalitis, has been clearly associated with the onset of parkinsonism. However, the incidence of postencephalitic parkinsonism has dwindled since the 1920s, when there was a large outbreak of this infectious illness. Parkinsonism-like symptoms have occurred after intoxication with a variety of chemicals, including carbon monoxide and manganese (among copper miners) and the product of meperidine-analog synthesis, MPTP. Drug-induced parkinsonism can follow reserpine (Serpasil), methyldopa (Aldomet), lithium, haloperidol (Haldol), and phenothiazine (Thorazine) therapy. Parkinsonism can also be seen following the use of illicit drugs including amphetamine and methamphetamine. Other causes of parkinsonism include hydrocephalus, hypoxia, infections, stroke, tumor, and trauma.[15]

The pathologic process of Parkinson's disease involves degeneration of the dopamine-producing neurons in the substantia nigra of the midbrain (Figs. 57-4 through 57-6), which in turn disrupts the normal balance between dopamine (DA) and acetylcholine (ACh) in the basal ganglia. DA is a neurotransmitter essential for normal functioning of the extrapyramidal motor system, including control of posture, support, and voluntary motion. Symptoms of Parkinson's disease do not occur until 80% of neurons in the substantia nigra are lost.

Clinical Manifestations

The onset of Parkinson's disease is gradual and insidious, with a gradual progression and a prolonged course. It may involve only one side of the body initially. In the beginning stages, only a mild tremor, a slight limp, or a decreased arm swing may be evident. Later in the disease the patient may have a shuffling, propulsive gait with arms flexed and loss of postural reflexes. In some patients there may be a slight change in speech patterns. None of these alone is sufficient evidence for a diagnosis of the disease.

Tremor. *Tremor,* often the first sign, may be minimal initially, so the patient is the only one who notices it. This tremor can affect handwriting, causing it to trail off, particularly toward the ends of words. Parkinsonian tremor is more prominent at rest and is aggravated by emotional stress or increased concentration.

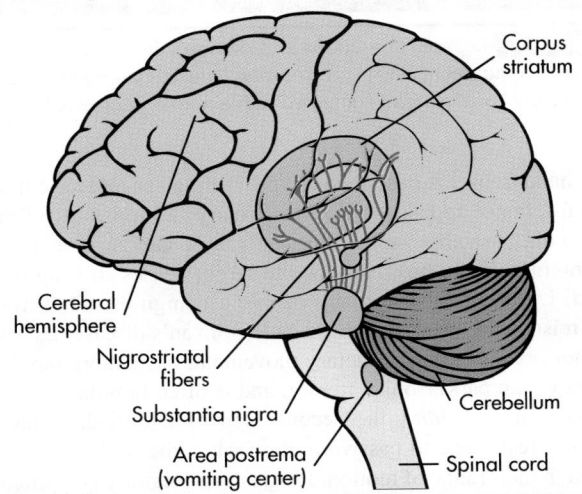

FIG. 57-4 Nigrostriatal disorders produce parkinsonism. Left-sided view of the human brain showing the substantia nigra and the corpus striatum *(shaded area)* lying deep within the cerebral hemisphere. Nerve fibers extend upward from the substantia nigra, divide into many branches, and carry dopamine to all regions of the corpus striatum.

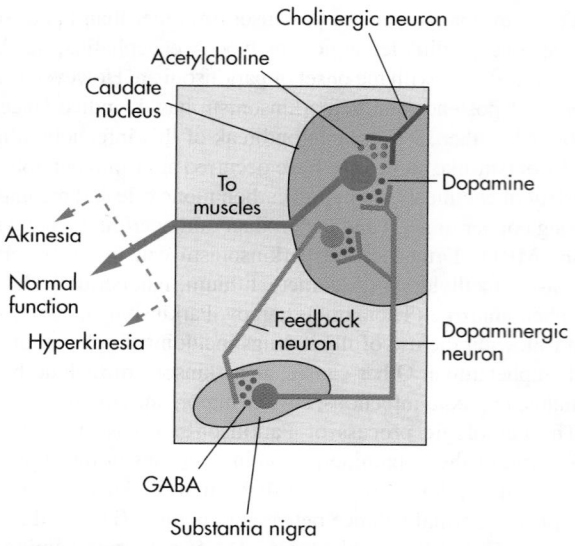

FIG. 57-5 Dopaminergic synaptic activity is mediated by dopamine. Cholinergic synaptic activity is mediated by acetylcholine. A balance between the two kinds of activity produces normal motor function. A relative excess of cholinergic activity produces akinesia and rigidity. A relative excess of dopaminergic activity produces involuntary movements. Neurons in the caudate nucleus contain γ-aminobutyric acid (GABA) and possibly control dopaminergic neurons in the substantia nigra through a feedback pathway.

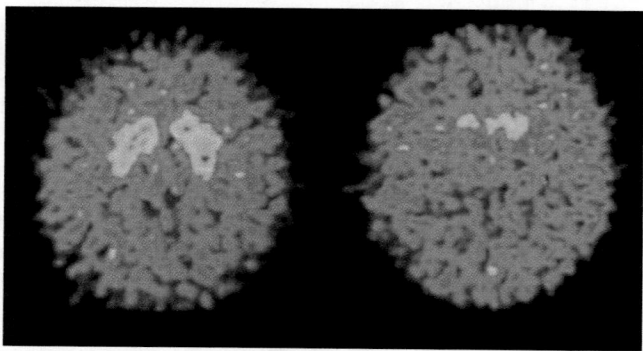

FIG. 57-6 Reduced fluorodopa in Parkinson's disease. Positron emission tomography (PET) scan showing reduced fluorodopa uptake in the basal ganglia (right) compared with a normal control (left).

The hand tremor is described as "pill rolling" because the thumb and forefinger appear to move in a rotary fashion as if rolling a pill, coin, or other small object. Tremor can involve the diaphragm, tongue, lips, and jaw but rarely causes shaking of the head. Unfortunately, in many people a benign essential tremor has mistakenly been diagnosed as Parkinson's disease. Essential tremor occurs during voluntary movement, has a more rapid frequency than parkinsonian tremor, and is often familial.

Rigidity. *Rigidity*, the second sign of the triad, is the increased resistance to passive motion when the limbs are moved through their range of motion. Parkinsonian rigidity is typified by a jerky quality, as if there were intermittent catches in the movement of a cogwheel, when the joint is moved. This is termed *cogwheel rigidity*. The rigidity is caused by sustained muscle contraction and consequently elicits a complaint of muscle sore-

ness; feeling tired and achy; or pain in the head, upper body, spine, or legs. Another consequence of rigidity is slowness of movement because it inhibits the alternating of contraction and relaxation in opposing muscle groups (e.g., biceps and triceps).

Bradykinesia. *Bradykinesia* is particularly evident in the loss of automatic movements, which is secondary to the physical and chemical alteration of the basal ganglia and related structures in the extrapyramidal portion of the CNS. In the unaffected patient, automatic movements are involuntary and occur subconsciously. They include blinking of the eyelids, swinging of the arms while walking, swallowing of saliva, self-expression with facial and hand movements, and minor movement of postural adjustment. The patient with Parkinson's disease does not execute these movements, and there is a lack of spontaneous activity. This accounts for the stooped posture, masked facies (deadpan expression), drooling of saliva, and shuffling gait (festination) that are characteristic of a person with this disease. In addition, there is difficulty in initiating movement.

Complications

Many of the complications of Parkinson's disease are caused by the progressive deterioration and loss of spontaneity of movement. Swallowing may become very difficult (dysphagia) in severe cases, leading to malnutrition or aspiration. General debilitation may lead to pneumonia, urinary tract infections, and skin breakdown. Mobility is greatly decreased. The gait slows, and turning is especially difficult. The gait usually consists of rapid, short, shuffling ministeps. The posture is that of the "old man" image, with the head and trunk bent forward and the legs constantly flexed (Fig. 57-7). The lack of mobility may lead to constipation, ankle edema, and, more seriously, contractures.

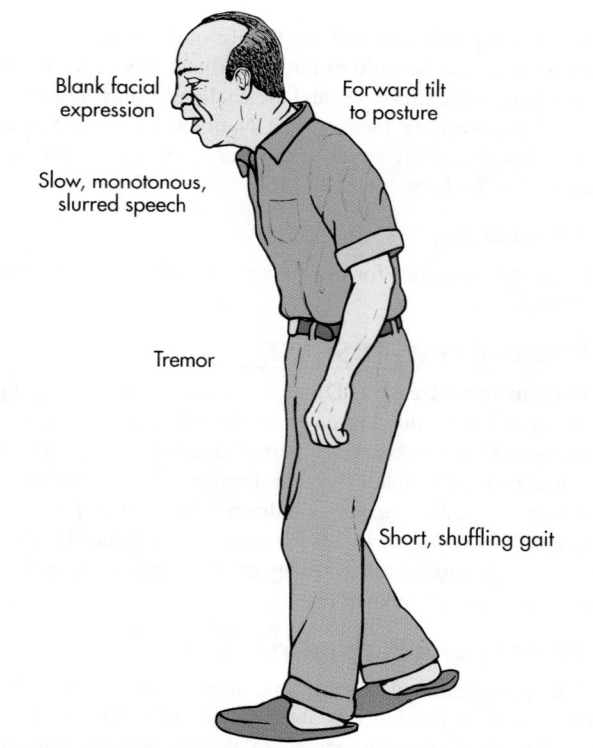

FIG. 57-7 Characteristic appearance of a patient with Parkinson's disease.

Orthostatic hypotension may occur in some patients and, along with loss of postural reflexes, may result in falls or other injury. Bothersome complications include seborrhea (increased oily secretion of the sebaceous glands of the skin), dandruff, excessive sweating, conjunctivitis, difficulty in reading, insomnia, incontinence, and depression.

Many of the apparent complications of Parkinson's disease are the result of side effects of drugs, particularly levodopa. These include *dyskinesias* (e.g., fidgeting movements of limbs), hallucinations, orthostatic hypotension, weakness, and akinesia (total immobility). These complications become apparent after prolonged levodopa (L-dopa) therapy.

Diagnostic Studies

Because there is no specific diagnostic test for Parkinson's disease, the diagnosis is based solely on the history and the clinical features. A firm diagnosis can be made only when at least two of the three characteristic signs of the classic triad are present: tremor, rigidity, and bradykinesia (slow or retarded movement). Dementia occurs in up to 40% of patients with Parkinson's disease.[16] The ultimate confirmation of Parkinson's disease is a positive response to antiparkinsonian drugs.

Collaborative Care

Because there is no cure for Parkinson's disease, collaborative management (Table 57-17) is aimed at relieving the symptoms.

Drug Therapy. Drug therapy for Parkinson's disease is aimed at correcting an imbalance of neurotransmitters within the CNS. Antiparkinsonian drugs either enhance the release or supply of DA (dopaminergic) or antagonize or block the effects of the overactive cholinergic neurons in the striatum (anticholinergic). Levodopa with carbidopa (Sinemet) is often the first drug to be used. Levodopa is a precursor of DA and can cross the blood-brain barrier. It is converted to DA in the basal ganglia. Sinemet is the preferred drug because it also contains carbidopa, an agent that inhibits the enzyme dopa-decarboxylase in the peripheral tissues. This enzyme breaks down levodopa before it reaches the brain. The net result of the combination of levodopa and carbidopa is that more levodopa reaches the brain, and therefore less drug is needed.

Many patients are given Sinemet early in the disease course. However, some health care providers believe that after a few years of therapy, the effectiveness of Sinemet wears off, so they prefer to initiate therapy with a DA receptor agonist instead. These drugs include bromocriptine (Parlodel), pergolide (Permax), ropinirole (Requip), and pramipexole (Mirapex). These drugs directly stimulate DA receptors. When more moderate to severe symptoms are present, levodopa with carbidopa (Sinemet) is added to the drug regimen.

Anticholinergic drugs are also used to manage Parkinson's disease. These drugs act by decreasing the activity of acetylcholine, thus providing balance between cholinergic and dopaminergic actions. Antihistamines (e.g., diphenhydramine [Benadryl]) with anticholinergic properties or a β-adrenergic blocker (e.g., propranolol [Inderal]) are used to manage tremors. The antiviral agent amantadine (Symmetrel) is also an effective antiparkinsonian drug. Although its exact mechanism of action is not known, amantadine promotes the release of DA from neurons.

Selegiline (Eldepryl) is a monoamine oxidase (MAO) inhibitor that is sometimes used in combination with Sinemet. By inhibiting MAO, the degradative enzyme for DA, the levels of DA are increased. Entacapone (Comtan) and tolcapone (Tasmar) block the enzyme catechol-o-methyl transferase (COMT), which breaks down levodopa in the peripheral circulation, thus prolonging the effect of Sinemet. This helps to manage symptoms caused by "wearing off" of Sinemet before the next dose is due.

Table 57-18 summarizes the drugs commonly used in Parkinson's disease, the symptoms they relieve, and their common side effects. The use of only one drug is preferred because there are fewer side effects and the drug dosage is easier to adjust than when several drugs are used. However, as the disease progresses, combination therapy is often required. Excessive amounts of dopaminergic drugs can lead to *paradoxic intoxication* (aggravation rather than relief of symptoms).

Surgical Therapy. Surgical procedures are aimed at relieving symptoms of Parkinson's disease and are usually used in patients who are unresponsive to drug therapy or who have developed severe motor complications. Surgical procedures fall into three categories: ablation (destruction), deep brain stimulation (DBS), and transplantation. *Ablation surgery* involves stereotactic ablation of areas in the thalamus *(thalamotomy),* globus pallidus *(pallidotomy),* and subthalamic nucleus *(subthalamic nucleotomy).* Ablative procedures have been used for Parkinson's disease for over 50 years, but they have been replaced recently by DBS. DBS involves placing an electrode in either the thalamus, globus pallidus, or subthalamic nucleus and connecting it to a generator placed in the upper chest (like a pacemaker). The device is programmed to deliver a specific current to the targeted brain location. Unlike ablation procedures, DBS can be adjusted to control symptoms better and is reversible (the device can be removed). These ablative and DBS procedures work by reducing the increased neuronal activity produced by DA depletion.[17]

Transplantation of fetal neural tissue into the basal ganglia is designed to provide DA-producing cells in the brains of patients with Parkinson's disease. This form of therapy is still in the experimental stages.

Nutritional Therapy. Diet is of major importance to the patient with Parkinson's disease because malnutrition and constipation can be serious consequences of inadequate nutrition. Patients who have dysphagia and bradykinesia need appetizing

TABLE 57-17	*C*ollaborative Care **Parkinson's Disease**

Diagnostic
History and physical examination
Tremor
Rigidity
Bradykinesia
Positive response to antiparkinson drugs*
Rule out side effects of phenothiazines, reserpine, benzodiazepines, haloperidol

Collaborative Therapy
Antiparkinson drugs*
Surgical destruction or deep brain stimulation of ventrolateral nucleus of the thalamus or posteroventral globus pallidus

*See Table 57-18.

TABLE 57-18 Drug Therapy — Parkinson's Disease

DRUG	SYMPTOMS RELIEVED	SIDE EFFECTS AND PRECAUTIONS
Dopaminergic		
levodopa (L-dopa)	Bradykinesia, tremor, rigidity	Nausea, dyskinesia, hypotension, palpitations, arrhythmias; agitation, hallucinations, confusion (in older patient); avoidance of vitamin pills and diet high in vitamin B_6 (reversal of effect of levodopa); contraindicated in narrow–angle glaucoma
levodopa-carbidopa (Sinemet)	Same as above	Less nausea but greater chance of dyskinesia, confusion, hallucinations; periodic check of BUN, AST, WBCs, Hct; contraindicated in melanoma, narrow-angle glaucoma, combination with MAO inhibitors, reserpine, methyldopa, guanethidine, antipsychotics
bromocriptine mesylate (Parlodel)	Same as above	Orthostatic hypotension, nausea, vomiting, toxic psychosis, limb edema, phlebitis, dizziness, headache, insomnia
pergolide (Permax)	Same as above	Same as above
pramipexole (Mirapex)	Same as above	
ropinirole (Requip)	Same as above	
amantadine (Symmetrel)	Rigidity, akinesia	Nervousness, insomnia, confusion, hallucinations, dry mouth, nausea, edema, orthostatic hypotension
Anticholinergic		
trihexyphenidyl (Artane)	Tremor	Dry mouth, blurred vision, constipation, delirium, anxiety, agitation, hallucinations; avoidance of drugs with similar actions, including over-the-counter drugs containing scopolamine or antihistamines (e.g., Sominex), antispasmodics (e.g., Donnatal, Bellergal), tricyclic antidepressants (e.g., imipramine [Tofranil], amitriptyline [Elavil])
cycrimine (Pagitane)		
procyclidine (Kemadrin)		
benztropine (Cogentin)		
biperiden (Akineton)		
Antihistamine		
diphenhydramine (Benadryl)	Tremor, rigidity	Sedation, same precautions as for anticholinergic drugs
orphenadrine (Disipal)		
chlorphenoxamine (Phenoxene)		
phenindamine (Thephorin)		
Monoamine Oxidase Inhibitor		
selegiline (Eldepryl, Carbex)	Bradykinesia, rigidity, tremor	Similar to dopaminergic drugs
Catechol-O-Methyl Transferase (COMT) Inhibitor		
entacapone (Comtan)	By blocking COMT, this drug slows down the breakdown of levodopa, thus prolonging the action of levodopa	Similar to dopaminergic drugs; works only when used in combination with Sinemet
tolcapone (Tasmar)		

AST, Aspartate aminotransferase; *BUN,* blood urea nitrogen; *Hct,* hematocrit; *MAO,* monoamine oxidase; *WBCs,* white blood cells.

foods that are easily chewed and swallowed. The diet should contain adequate roughage and fruit to avoid constipation. Food should be cut into bite-sized pieces before it is served, and it should be served on a warmed plate to preserve its appeal. Eating six small meals a day may be less exhausting than eating three large meals a day. Ample time should be planned for eating to avoid frustration and encourage independence. In addition, absorption of levodopa can be impaired by protein ingestion. Some patients are advised to limit their protein intake to the evening meal to avoid this problem.

NURSING MANAGEMENT PARKINSON'S DISEASE

■ Nursing Assessment

Subjective and objective data that should be obtained from a patient with Parkinson's disease are presented in Table 57-19.

■ Nursing Diagnoses

Nursing diagnoses for the patient with Parkinson's disease may include, but are not limited to, those presented in NCP 57-4.

■ Planning

The overall goals are that the patient with Parkinson's disease will (1) maximize neurologic function, (2) maintain independence in activities of daily living for as long as possible, and (3) optimize psychosocial well-being.

■ Nursing Implementation

Promotion of physical exercise and a well-balanced diet are major concerns for nursing care. Exercise can limit the consequences of decreased mobility, such as muscle atrophy, contractures, and constipation. The American Parkinson Disease

TABLE 57-19	Nursing Assessment Parkinson's Disease

Subjective Data

Important Health Information

Past health history: CNS trauma, cerebrovascular disorders, exposure to metals and carbon monoxide, encephalitis

Medications: Use of major tranquilizers, especially haloperidol (Haldol), and phenothiazines, reserpine, methyldopa, amphetamines

Functional Health Patterns

Health perception–health management: Fatigue

Nutritional-metabolic: Excessive salivation, dysphagia; weight loss

Elimination: Constipation, incontinence; excessive sweating

Activity-exercise: Difficulty in initiating movements; frequent falls; loss of dexterity; micrographia (handwriting deterioration)

Sleep-rest: Insomnia

Cognitive-perceptual: Diffuse pain in head, shoulders, neck, back, legs, and hips; muscle soreness and cramping

Self-perception–self-concept: Depression; mood swings, hallucinations

Objective Data

General

Blank (masked) facies, slow and monotonous speech, infrequent blinking

Integumentary

Seborrhea, dandruff; ankle edema

Cardiovascular

Postural hypotension

Gastrointestinal

Drooling

Neurologic

Tremor at rest, first in hands (pill rolling), later in legs, arms, face, and tongue; aggravation of tremor with anxiety, absence in sleep; poor coordination; subtle dementia, impaired postural reflexes

Musculoskeletal

Cogwheel rigidity, dysarthria, bradykinesia, contractures, stooped posture, shuffling gait

Possible Findings

Lack of specific tests; diagnosis on basis of history and physical findings and ruling out of other diseases

CNS, Central nervous system.

Association (see Resources at the end of this chapter) publishes a series of booklets and videotapes that are helpful in terms of exercise that can be used by family members and health care professionals.

A physical therapist may be consulted to design a personal exercise program aimed at strengthening and stretching specific muscles. Overall muscle tone, as well as specific exercises to strengthen the muscles involved with speaking and swallowing, should be included. Although exercise will not halt the progress of the disease, it will enhance the patient's functional ability.

Because Parkinson's disease is a chronic degenerative disorder with no acute exacerbations, nurses should note that teaching and nursing care are directed toward maintenance of good health, encouragement of independence, and avoidance of complications such as contractures.

Problems secondary to bradykinesia can be alleviated by relatively simple measures. The following are helpful hints for patients who tend to "freeze" while walking: consciously think about stepping over imaginary or real lines on the floor, drop rice kernels and step over them, rock from side to side, lift the toes when stepping, take one step backward and two steps forward. The patient should be assessed for the possibility of levodopa overdose because it is a common cause of akinesia "freezing." A brief period of dyskinesia, usually *athetosis* (slow, writhing, continuous, and involuntary movement) of the neck, should alert the nurse to this possibility.

Getting out of a chair can be facilitated by using an upright chair with arms and placing the back legs on small (2-inch) blocks. Other aspects of the environment can be altered. Rugs and excess furniture can be removed to avoid stumbling. An ottoman can be used to elevate the legs and avoid dependent ankle edema. Clothing can be simplified by the use of slip-on shoes and Velcro hook-and-loop fasteners or zippers on clothing, instead of buttons and hooks. An elevated toilet seat can facilitate getting on and off the toilet. The nurse should work closely with the patient's family in exploring creative adaptations that allow maximum independence and self-care.

■ Evaluation

Expected outcomes for the patient with Parkinson's disease are addressed in NCP 57-4.

MYASTHENIA GRAVIS

Myasthenia gravis (MG) is an autoimmune disease of the neuromuscular junction characterized by the fluctuating weakness of certain skeletal muscle groups. The prevalence rate is 14 per 100,000 in the United States. MG can occur at any age but most commonly occurs between the ages of 10 and 65. The peak age at onset in women is 20 to 30 years. MG is three times more common in women, but at older ages both sexes are equally affected.[18]

Etiology and Pathophysiology

MG is caused by an autoimmune process in which antibodies attack acetylcholine (ACh) receptors, resulting in a decreased number of ACh receptor sites at the neuromuscular junction. This prevents ACh molecules from attaching and stimulating muscle contraction. Anti-ACh receptor antibodies are detectable in the serum of 85% to 90% of patients with generalized MG and in 50% to 60% of patients with ocular myasthenia.[18] Thymic tumors are found in about 15% of patients, and abnormal thymus tissue is found in most others.

Clinical Manifestations and Complications

The primary feature of MG is fluctuating weakness of skeletal muscle. Strength is usually restored after a period of rest. The muscles most often involved are those used for moving the eyes and eyelids, chewing, swallowing, speaking, and breathing. The muscles are generally the strongest in the morning and become exhausted with continued activity. Consequently, by the end of the day, muscle weakness is prominent.

In 90% of cases, the eyelid muscles or extraocular muscles are involved. Facial mobility and expression can be impaired. There may be difficulty in chewing and swallowing food. Speech is affected, and the voice often fades after a long conversation. The muscles of the trunk and limbs are less often affected. Of these, the proximal muscles of the neck, shoulder, and hip are more of-

NURSING CARE PLAN 57-4

Patient with Parkinson's Disease

EXPECTED PATIENT OUTCOMES	NURSING INTERVENTIONS and *RATIONALES*

NURSING DIAGNOSIS | **Impaired physical mobility** *related to* rigidity, bradykinesia, and akinesia *as manifested by* difficulty in initiation of purposeful movements.

- Safe ambulation
- Maintenance of joint mobility

- Assist with ambulation *to assess degree of impairment and to prevent injury.*
- Perform active range-of-motion (ROM) exercises to all extremities *to maintain joint ROM, prevent atrophy, and strengthen muscles.*
- Consult physical therapist or occupational therapist for aids *to facilitate activities of daily living and safe ambulation.*
- Teach techniques to assist with mobility by instructing patient to step over imaginary line, rock from side to side to initiate leg movements *because these are helpful in dealing with "freezing" (akinesia) while walking.*

NURSING DIAGNOSIS | **Impaired verbal communication** *related to* dysarthria and tremor or bradykinesia *as manifested by* decreased amount of communication, slow and slurred speech, inability to move facial muscles, decreased tongue mobility, and micrographia.

- Development of communication method to meet needs

- Allow sufficient time for communication *to reduce patient's frustration.*
- Encourage deep breaths before speaking.
- Consult speech therapist *to provide specialized guidance in care of the patient.*
- Provide alternative communication methods such as picture books or flash cards *because muscle involvement has impaired writing and speaking ability.*
- Massage patient's facial and neck muscles *to foster relaxation that can facilitate speech.*

NURSING DIAGNOSIS | **Imbalanced nutrition: less than body requirements** *related to* dysphagia *as manifested by* difficulty in swallowing and chewing, drooling, decreased gag reflex.

- Maintenance of satisfactory body weight

- Carefully monitor swallowing ability during drug administration and mealtime *to evaluate patient's level of impairment and minimize risk of aspiration.*
- Provide soft-solid and thick-liquid diet *because these consistencies are more easily swallowed.*
- Maintain patient in upright position for all meals *to reduce risk of aspiration.*
- Consult speech therapist and dietitian *because they can provide specific plans to improve swallowing and intake.*
- Have suction available *to remove pooled secretions and prevent choking and aspiration.*

NURSING DIAGNOSIS | **Deficient diversional activity** *related to* inability to perform usual recreational activities *as manifested by* boredom, lack of participation, restlessness, depression, hostility.

- Engagement in satisfying diversional activities
- Expression of acceptance of diminished capabilities

- Assess patient's activity *to determine physical and emotional response to difficulties.*
- Determine preferred diversional activities *so that individual needs are considered.*
- Adapt difficult activities when possible *so that patient is able to continue performing activities.*
- Initiate new activities within patient's capabilities *such as reading to replace activities patient can no longer perform.*
- Encourage patient to discuss emotional response to decreasing capabilities *to provide opportunity to problem-solve and demonstrate a caring attitude.*

---

ten affected than the distal muscles. No other signs of neural disorder accompany MG; there is no sensory loss, reflexes are normal, and muscle atrophy is rare.

The course of this disease is highly variable. Some patients may have short-term remissions, others may stabilize, and others may have severe, progressive involvement. Restricted ocular myasthenia, usually seen only in men, has a good prognosis. Exacerbations of MG can be precipitated by emotional stress, pregnancy, menses, secondary illness, trauma, temperature extremes, and hypokalemia. Ingestion of drugs including aminoglycoside antibiotics, β-adrenergic blockers, procainamide, quinidine, and phenytoin can aggravate MG. Psychotropic drugs (e.g., lithium carbonate, phenothiazines, benzodiazepines, tricyclic antidepressants) have also been associated with worsening of myas-

thenia as have neuromuscular blocking agents (d-tubocurarine, pancuronium, succinylcholine [Anectine]).

Myasthenic crisis is an acute exacerbation of muscle weakness triggered by infection, surgery, emotional distress, or overdose of or inadequate drugs. The major complications of MG result from muscle weakness in areas that affect swallowing and breathing resulting in aspiration, respiratory insufficiency, and respiratory infection.

Diagnostic Studies

The diagnosis of MG can be made on the basis of history and physical examination. However, other tests may be used if the diagnosis is still in doubt. Blood tests show that antibodies to ACh receptors are found in 85% to 90% of patients with generalized MG.

EMG may show a decrementing response to repeated stimulation of the hand muscles, indicative of muscle fatigue. Use of drugs may also aid in the diagnosis. The Tensilon test in a patient with MG reveals improved muscle contractility after intravenous injection of the anticholinesterase agent edrophonium chloride (Tensilon). (Anticholinesterase blocks the enzyme acetylcholinesterase.) This test also aids in the diagnosis of cholinergic crisis (secondary to overdose of anticholinesterase drug). In this condition, Tensilon does not improve muscle weakness but may actually increase it. Atropine, a cholinergic antagonist, should be readily available to counteract Tensilon effects when it is used diagnostically.

Collaborative Care

Drug Therapy. Drug therapy for MG includes anticholinesterase drugs, alternate-day corticosteroids, and immunosuppressants (Table 57-20). Anticholinesterase drugs are aimed at enhancing function of the neuromuscular junction. Acetylcholinesterase is the enzyme that breaks down ACh in the synaptic cleft. Thus inhibition of this enzyme by an anticholinesterase inhibitor will prolong the action of ACh and facilitate transmission of impulses at the neuromuscular junction. Neostigmine (Prostigmin) and pyridostigmine (Mestinon) are the most successful drugs of this group in treating MG. Tailoring the dose to avoid a myasthenic or cholinergic crisis often presents a clinical challenge. Because of the autoimmune nature of the disorder, corticosteroids (specifically prednisone) are used to suppress the immune response. Drugs such as azathioprine (Imuran) and cyclophosphamide (Cytoxan) may also be used for immunosuppression.

Many drugs are contraindicated or must be used with caution in patients with MG. Classes of drug that should be cautiously evaluated before use include anesthetics, antiarrhythmics, antibiotics, quinine, antipsychotics, barbiturates and sedative-hypnotics, cathartics, diuretics, narcotics, muscle relaxants, thyroid preparations, and tranquilizers.

Surgical Therapy. Because the presence of the thymus gland in the patient with MG appears to enhance the production of ACh receptor antibodies, removal of the thymus gland results in improvement in a majority of patients. Thymectomy is indicated for almost all patients with thymoma, for patients with generalized MG between the ages of puberty and about 65 years, and for patients with purely ocular MG.[19]

Other Therapies. Plasmapheresis can yield a short-term improvement in symptoms and is indicated for patients in crisis or in preparation for surgery when corticosteroids must be avoided. (Plasmapheresis is discussed in Chapter 13.) Intravenous immunoglobulin G has been used with some success and is recommended as a second-line treatment for MG.[20]

NURSING MANAGEMENT
MYASTHENIA GRAVIS

■ Nursing Assessment

The nurse can assess the severity of MG by asking the patient about fatigability, what body parts are affected, and how severely they are affected. The patient's coping abilities and understanding of the disorder should also be assessed. Some patients become so fatigued that they are no longer able to work or even ambulate.

Objective data should include respiratory rate and depth, oxygen saturation, arterial blood gas analyses, pulmonary function tests, and evidence of respiratory distress in patients with acute myasthenic crisis. Muscle strength of all face and limb muscles should be assessed, as should swallowing, speech (volume and clarity), and cough and gag reflexes.

■ Nursing Diagnoses

Nursing diagnoses for the patient with MG may include, but are not limited to, the following:
- Ineffective breathing pattern *related to* intercostal muscle weakness
- Ineffective airway clearance *related to* intercostal muscle weakness and impaired cough and gag reflex
- Impaired verbal communication *related to* weakness of the larynx, lips, mouth, pharynx, and jaw
- Imbalanced nutrition: less than body requirements *related to* impaired swallowing
- Disturbed sensory perception (visual) *related to* ptosis, decreased eye movements, and disconjugate gaze
- Activity intolerance *related to* muscle weakness and fatigability
- Disturbed body image *related to* inability to maintain usual lifestyle and role responsibilities

■ Planning

The overall goals are that the patient with MG will (1) have a return of normal muscle endurance, (2) avoid complications, and (3) maintain a quality of life appropriate to disease course.

■ Nursing Implementation

The patient with MG who is admitted to the hospital usually has a respiratory tract infection or is in an acute myasthenic crisis. Nursing care is aimed at maintaining adequate ventilation, continuing drug therapy, and watching for side effects of therapy. The nurse must be able to distinguish cholinergic from myasthenic crisis (Table 57-21) because the causes and treatment of the two conditions differ greatly.

As with other chronic illnesses, care focuses on the neurologic deficits and their impact on daily living. A balanced diet with food that can be chewed and swallowed easily should be prescribed. Semisolid foods may be easier to eat than solids or

TABLE 57-20	Collaborative Care Myasthenia Gravis

Diagnostic
History and physical examination
    Fatigability with prolonged upward gaze (2 to 3 minutes)
    Muscle weakness
EMG
Tensilon test
Acetylcholine receptor antibodies

Collaborative Therapy
Drugs
    Anticholinesterase agents
    Corticosteroids
    Immunosuppressive agents
Surgery (thymectomy)
Plasmapheresis

EMG, Electromyography.

TABLE 57-21 Comparison of Myasthenic Crisis and Cholinergic Crisis

	MYASTHENIC CRISIS	CHOLINERGIC CRISIS
Causes	Exacerbation of myasthenia following precipitating factors or failure to take drug as prescribed or drug dose too low	Overdose of anticholinesterase drugs resulting in increased ACh at the receptor sites, remission (spontaneous or after thymectomy)
Differential diagnosis	Improved strength after IV administration of anticholinesterase drugs; increased weakness of skeletal muscles manifesting as ptosis, bulbar signs (e.g., difficulty in swallowing, difficulty in articulating words), or dyspnea	Weakness within 1 hr after ingestion of anticholinesterase; increased weakness of skeletal muscles manifesting as ptosis, bulbar signs, dyspnea; effects on smooth muscle include pupillary miosis, salivation, diarrhea, nausea or vomiting, abdominal cramps, increased bronchial secretions, sweating, or lacrimation

ACh, Acetylcholine; *IV,* intravenous.

liquids. Scheduling doses of drugs so that peak action is reached at mealtime may make eating less difficult. Diversional activities that require little physical effort and match the interests of the patient should be arranged. Teaching should focus on the importance of following the medical regimen, potential adverse reactions to specific drugs, planning activities of daily living to avoid fatigue, the availability of community resources, and the complications of the disease and therapy (crisis conditions) and what to do about them. Contact with the Myasthenia Gravis Foundation or an MG support group may be helpful and should be explored.

■ Evaluation

The overall expected outcomes are that the patient with MG will

- maintain optimal muscle function
- be free from side effects of drugs
- not experience complications, in particular myasthenic or cholinergic crises, from the disease
- maintain a quality of life appropriate to the disease course

RESTLESS LEGS SYNDROME

Etiology and Pathophysiology

Restless legs syndrome (RLS) is characterized by unpleasant sensory (paresthesias) and motor abnormalities of one or both legs. Prevalence rates vary from 1% to 15%, although the numbers may be higher because the condition is underdiagnosed.[21] Although the exact cause of RLS is not known, probably more than half of all cases are transmitted in an autosomal dominant pattern.[21] RLS can be seen in metabolic abnormalities associated with iron deficiency, renal failure, polyneuropathy associated with diabetes mellitus, rheumatic disorders (e.g., rheumatoid arthritis), or pregnancy. However, the majority of cases are idiopathic.

Idiopathic RLS may be related to nervous system dysfunction. Although the exact cause remains to be determined, several theories include (1) an alteration in dopaminergic transmission in the basal ganglia, (2) axonal neuropathy, or (3) a brainstem disinhibition phenomenon resulting in motor and sensory disturbances.

Clinical Manifestations

The severity of RLS sensory symptoms ranges from infrequent minor discomfort (paresthesias including numbness, tingling, "pins and needles" sensation) to severe pain. Sensory symptoms often appear first and are manifested as an annoying and uncomfortable (but usually not painful) sensation in the legs. The sensation is often compared with the sensation of bugs creeping or crawling on the legs. The leg pain is localized within the calf muscles. Patients can also experience pain in the upper extremities and trunk. The discomfort occurs when the patient is sedentary and usually occurs in the evening or at night.

The pain at night can produce sleep disruptions and is often relieved by physical activity such as walking, stretching, rocking, or kicking. In the most severe cases, patients sleep only a few hours at night, resulting in daytime fatigue and disruption of the daily routine. The motor abnormalities associated with RLS consist of voluntary restlessness and stereotyped, periodic, involuntary movements. The involuntary movements usually occur during sleep. Symptoms are aggravated by fatigue. Over time, RLS advances to more frequent and more severe episodes.

Diagnostic Studies

RLS is a clinical diagnosis and is based in large part on the patient's history or the report of the bed partner related to nighttime activities. The International Restless Legs Study Group proposed four minimum diagnostic criteria.[22] They are (1) desire to move the limbs, (2) motor restlessness, (3) symptoms that are worse or exclusively present at rest with at least partial and temporary relief by activity, and (4) symptoms that are worse in the evening or night. Polysomnography studies during sleep may be performed for the patient with RLS to distinguish the problem from other clinical conditions (e.g., sleep apnea) that can disturb sleep. However, periodic leg movements in sleep are a common feature in RLS patients. The patient's history of diabetes mellitus and its management may provide information to determine whether paresthesias are caused by peripheral neuropathy or RLS.

NURSING *and* COLLABORATIVE MANAGEMENT RESTLESS LEGS SYNDROME

The goal of collaborative management is to reduce patient discomfort and distress and to improve sleep quality. When RLS is secondary to uremia or iron deficiency, correction of these conditions will decrease symptoms. Nonpharmacologic approaches to RLS management include establishing regular sleep habits, encouraging exercise, avoiding activities that cause symptoms, and eliminating aggravating factors such as alcohol, caffeine, and certain drugs (neuroleptics, lithium, antihistamines, and antidepressants).

If nonpharmacologic measures fail to provide symptom relief, drug therapy may be started. The main drugs used in RLS are dopaminergic agents, opioids, and benzodiazepines. Dopaminergic agents such as carbidopa-levodopa (Sinemet) and DA agonists (pergolide [Permax], bromocriptine [Parlodel], pramipexole [Mirapex]) are the drugs of choice in treating RLS. These agents are effective in managing sensory and motor symptoms. Dopaminergic agents have a number of side effects, including hypotension and gastric irritation.

Other agents that may be used include antiseizure drugs such as gabapentin (Neurontin), divalproex (Depakote), lamotrigine (Lamictal), and carbamazepine (Tegretol). Clonidine (Catapres) and propranolol (Inderal) are also effective in some patients. Opioids (e.g., oxycodone) are usually reserved for those patients with severe symptoms who fail to respond to other drug therapies. When used, opioids given in low doses have also been found to be effective in reducing the symptoms associated with RLS. The main side effect of opioids is constipation, so the patient may need to take a stool softener or laxative.

AMYOTROPHIC LATERAL SCLEROSIS

Amyotrophic lateral sclerosis (ALS) is a rare progressive neurologic disorder characterized by loss of motor neurons. ALS usually leads to death within 2 to 6 years after diagnosis. This disease became known as Lou Gehrig's disease when the famous baseball player was stricken with it in the early 1940s. The onset is usually between 40 and 70 years of age. ALS is more common in men than women by a ratio of 2:1.

For unknown reasons, motor neurons in the brainstem and spinal cord gradually degenerate in ALS (Fig. 57-8). Dead motor neurons cannot produce or transport vital signals to muscles. Consequently, electrical and chemical messages originating in the brain do not reach the muscles to activate them.

The typical symptoms are weakness of the upper extremities, dysarthria, and dysphagia. However, weakness may begin in the legs. Muscle wasting and fasciculations result from the denervation of the muscles and lack of stimulation and use. Death usually results from respiratory infection secondary to compromised respiratory function. Unfortunately, there is no cure for ALS. Riluzole (Rilutek) slows the progression of ALS.[23,24] This drug works to decrease the amount of glutamate (an excitatory neurotransmitter) in the brain. In clinical trials, riluzole has been shown to delay the need for tracheostomy and death by a few months.[25]

The illness trajectory for ALS is devastating because the patient remains cognitively intact while wasting away. The challenge of nursing care is to support the patient's cognitive and emotional functions by facilitating communication, reducing risk of aspiration, decreasing pain secondary to muscle weakness, decreasing risk of injury related to falls, providing diversional activities such as reading and human companionship, and helping the person and family with advance care planning and anticipatory grieving related to loss of motor function and ultimately death.

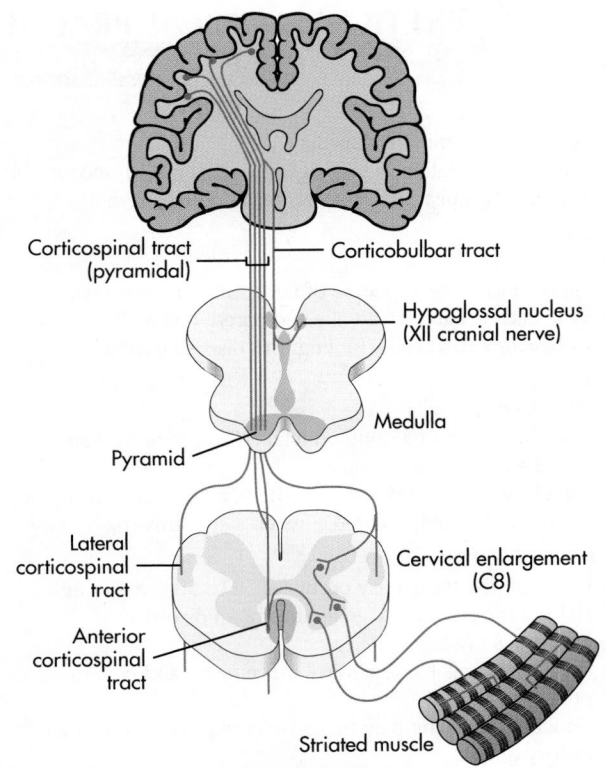

FIG. 57-8 Pathogenesis of amyotrophic lateral sclerosis. This disease is characterized by degeneration of the pyramidal tract and the motor cells in the anterior gray horns. In cases with corticobulbar involvement, the motor nuclei of cranial nerves V, VII, IX, X, XI, and XII also undergo degeneration.

HUNTINGTON'S DISEASE

Huntington's disease (HD) is a genetically transmitted, autosomal dominant disorder that affects both men and women of all races. The offspring of a person with this disease have a 50% risk of inheriting it (see Genetics in Clinical Practice box on p. 1578). The onset of HD is usually between 30 and 50 years of age. Often the diagnosis is made after the affected individual has had children. In the United States the incidence of HD is 1 in 10,000, and there are currently 30,000 Americans with HD.[26] Diagnosis in the past was based on family history and clinical symptoms. However, since the gene for HD has been discovered, one now can be tested for the presence of the gene. People who are asymptomatic but who have a positive family history of HD face the dilemma of whether or not to get tested. If the test is positive, the person will develop HD, but when and to what extent the disease develops cannot be determined.

Like Parkinson's disease, the pathologic process of HD involves the basal ganglia and the extrapyramidal motor system. However, instead of a deficiency of DA, HD involves a deficiency of the neurotransmitters ACh and γ-aminobutyric acid (GABA). The net effect is an excess of DA, which leads to symptoms that are the opposite of those of parkinsonism. The clinical manifestations are characterized by abnormal and excessive involuntary movements *(chorea)*. These are writhing, twisting movements of the face, limbs, and body. The movements get

GENETICS in CLINICAL PRACTICE
Huntington's Disease

Genetic Basis
- Autosomal dominant disorder
- Caused by mutation of single gene located on chromosome 4
- Expression similar in homozygotes and heterozygotes

Incidence
- 1 in 10,000
- Higher incidence in people of European ancestry
- With each pregnancy an affected parent has a 50% chance of having a child with Huntington's disease (HD)

Genetic Testing
- DNA testing is available
- DNA testing can be done on fetal cells obtained by amniocentesis or chorionic biopsy
- Genetic testing can determine whether a person is a carrier
- No test is available to predict when symptoms will develop

Clinical Implications
- Onset of disease usually occurs at 30 to 50 years of age
- HD is a progressive, degenerative brain disorder
- No cure is available
- Drugs are available to control movements and behavioral problems
- Genetic counseling may be considered if there is a family history of HD

worse as the disease progresses. Facial movements involving speech, chewing, and swallowing are affected and may cause aspiration and malnutrition. The gait deteriorates, and ambulation eventually becomes impossible. Perhaps the most devastating deterioration is in mental functions, which include intellectual decline, emotional lability, and psychotic behavior. Death usually occurs 10 to 20 years after the onset of symptoms.

Because there is no cure, collaborative care is palliative. Antipsychotic (e.g., haloperidol [Haldol]), antidepressant (fluoxetine [Prozac], sertraline [Zoloft], nortriptyline [Aventyl]), and antichorea (clonazepam [Klonopin]) drugs are prescribed and have some benefit. However, they do not alter the course of the disease. Transplantation of fetal striatal neural tissues into the striatum (caudate and putamen) of the brain is an experimental treatment that may be effective.[26] HD presents a great challenge to health care professionals. The goal of nursing management is to provide the most comfortable environment possible for the patient and the family by maintaining physical safety, treating the physical symptoms, and providing emotional and psychologic support. Because of the choreic movements, caloric requirements are high. Patients may require as many as 4000 to 5000 calories per day to maintain body weight. As the disease progresses, meeting caloric needs becomes a greater challenge when the patient has difficulty swallowing and holding the head still. Depression and mental deterioration can also compromise nutritional intake.

CRITICAL THINKING EXERCISES

Case Study
Myasthenia Gravis

Patient Profile. Mr. D., a 58-year-old African American, was diagnosed with myasthenia gravis after an episode of double vision and drooping of the left eyelid years ago. He was offered thymectomy but refused it. He has been taking pyridostigmine (Mestinon) and prednisone since then and has had few symptoms until recently. While visiting his daughter, he developed severe weakness in his arms and legs and had breathing problems.

Subjective Data
- Reports difficulty "getting enough air"
- Tires easily
- Reports food "gets stuck in my throat" sometimes
- Reports trouble speaking clearly

Objective Data

Physical Examination
- Jaw muscle weakness
- Generalized weakness
- Tense and anxious
- Shallow respirations

Diagnostic Studies
- Chest CT scan shows large mediastinal mass, likely thymoma
- Pulmonary function tests show decreased expiratory effort

CRITICAL THINKING QUESTIONS
1. What is the pathogenesis of myasthenia gravis?
2. What is this exacerbation called?
3. What is the likely explanation for this exacerbation?
4. What teaching plan should be developed for Mr. D.?
5. What treatment would be appropriate for Mr. D.?
6. Write one or more appropriate nursing diagnoses based on the assessment data presented. Are there any collaborative problems?

Nursing Research Issues
1. What kinds of physical activity can enhance functioning and well-being in patients with multiple sclerosis and Parkinson's disease?
2. What are the most effective ways to assist patients with chronic neurologic problems to maintain a positive self-esteem?
3. What factors influence the quality of life for patients with epilepsy?
4. What can be done to promote self-efficacy in patients with chronic neurologic conditions?

REVIEW QUESTIONS

The number of the question corresponds to the same-numbered objective at the beginning of the chapter.

1. The nurse plans care for the patient with a migraine headache based on the knowledge that during a migraine the patient is most likely to
   a. withdraw from stimuli.
   b. act out with bizarre behavior.
   c. seek out the company of others.
   d. experience painful facial spasms and tearing.

2. The triad of symptoms the nurse would expect to find during assessment of the patient with Parkinson's disease is
   a. spasticity, diplopia, tremor.
   b. tremor, rigidity, bradykinesia.
   c. ataxia, drowsiness, dysarthria.
   d. diplopia, tremor, bradykinesia.

3. During assessment of the patient with ALS, the nurse would expect to find
   a. emotional lability.
   b. mental deterioration.
   c. muscle weakness and wasting.
   d. sensory loss in the extremities.

4. The emotional response of the patient with a chronic neurologic disease is often
   a. symptoms of intellectual deterioration.
   b. absent in patients with cognitive impairment.
   c. a result of physical disability and changes in body image.
   d. reduced in patients who have family members to care for them.

5. A major goal of treatment for the patient with a chronic, progressive neurologic disease is
   a. reversal of pathophysiologic features.
   b. total remission of the disease.
   c. continuation of usual lifestyle.
   d. adaptation by patient and family to the disease.

REFERENCES

1. Rasmussen BK, Stewart WF, Welch KMA: Epidemiology of migraine. In Olesen J, Tfelt-Hansen P, editors: *The headaches,* Philadelphia, 2000, Lippincott Williams & Wilkins.
2. Olesen J, Oadsby PJ: Synthesis of migraine mechanisms. In Olesen J, Tfelt-Hansen P, editors: *The headaches,* Philadelphia, 2000, Lippincott Williams & Wilkins.
3. Raskin N: Migraine and other headaches. In Rowland LP, editor: *Merritt's neurology,* Philadelphia, 2000, Lippincott Williams & Wilkins.
4. Zed P, Loewen P, Robinson G: Medication induced headache: overview and systematic review of therapeutic approaches, *Ann Pharmacother* 33:61, 1999.
5. Shorvon SD: *Handbook of epilepsy treatment,* London, 2000, Blackwell Science.
6. Prasad A et al: Recent advances in the genetics of epilepsy: insights from human and animal studies, *Epilepsia* 40:1329, 1999.
7. Commission on Classification and Terminology of the International League Against Epilepsy: Proposal for the revised clinical and electroencephalographic classification of epileptic seizures, *Epilepsia* 22:249, 1981.
8. Leppik IE: *Contemporary diagnosis and management of the patient with epilepsy,* Newton, Pa, 2000, Handbooks in Health Care.
9. Miller JR: Multiple sclerosis. In Rowland LP, editor: *Merritt's neurology,* Philadelphia, 2000, Lippincott Williams & Wilkins.
10. Lubin FD, Reingold SC: Defining the clinical course of multiple sclerosis, *Neurology* 46:907, 1996.
11. Confavreux C et al: Rates of pregnancy-related relapse in multiple sclerosis, *N Engl J Med* 339:285, 1998.
12. Polman CH, Uitdehaag BM: Drug treatment of multiple sclerosis, *BMJ* 321(7259):490, 2000.
13. Edwards S et al: Clinical relapses and disease activity on magnetic resonance imaging associated with viral upper respiratory infections in multiple sclerosis, *J Neurol Neurosurg Psychiatry* 64:736, 1998.
14. Fahn S, Przedborski S: Parkinsonism. In Rowland LP, editor: *Merritt's neurology,* Philadelphia, 2000, Lippincott Williams & Wilkins.
15. Waters CH: *Diagnosis and management of Parkinson's disease,* Caddo, Okla, 1998, Professional Communications Inc.
16. Glosser G: Neurobehavioral effects of movement disorders, *Neurol Clin* 19:535, 2001.
17. Ahlskog JE: Parkinson's disease: medical and surgical treatment, *Neurol Clin* 19:579, 2001.
18. Penn AS, Rowland LP: Myasthenia gravis. In Rowland LP, editor: *Merritt's neurology,* Philadelphia, 2000, Lippincott Williams & Wilkins.
19. Urschel JD, Grewal RP: Thymectomy for myasthenia gravis, *Postgrad Med J* 74:139, 1998.
20. Bril V et al: IGIV in neurology—evidence and recommendations, *Can J Neurol Sci* 26:139, 1999.
21. Tan E, Ondo W: Restless legs syndrome: clinical features and treatment, *Am J Med Sci* 319:397, 2000.
22. Walters AS: Toward a better definition of restless legs syndrome, *Mov Disord* 10:634, 1995.
23. Miller RG: New approaches to therapy of amyotrophic lateral sclerosis, *West J Med* 168:262, 1998.
24. Riviere M et al: An analysis of extended survival in patients with amyotrophic lateral sclerosis treated with riluzole, *Arch Neurol* 55:526, 1998.
25. Miller RG et al: Riluzole for amyotrophic lateral sclerosis (ALS)/motor neuron disease (MND) (Cochrane Review), *Cochrane Database Syst Rev* 2:CD001447, 2002.
26. Freeman TB et al: Transplanted fetal striatum in Huntington's disease: phenotypic development and lack of pathology, *Proc Natl Acad Sci* 97:13877, 2000.

RESOURCES

ALS Association (ALSA)
27001 Agoura Road, Suite 150
Calabasas Hills, CA 91301-5104
800-782-4747 or 818-880-9007
www.alsa.org

American Association of Neuroscience Nurses (AANN)
4700 West Lake Avenue
Glenview, IL 60025-1485
888-557-2266 or 847-375-4733
Fax: 847-375-6333
www.aann.org

American Council for Headache Education (ACHE)
19 Mantua Road
Mt. Royal, NJ 08061
857-423-0258
Fax: 856-423-0082
www.achenet.org

American Parkinson Disease Association
1250 Hylan Boulevard, Suite 4B
Staten Island, NY 10305-1946
800-223-2732 or 718-981-8001
Fax: 781-981-4399
www.apdaparkinson.com

Association of Rehabilitation Nurses (ARN)
4700 West Lake Avenue
Glenview, IL 60025-1485
800-229-7530 or 847-375-4710
Fax: 877-734-9384
www.rehabnurse.org

Epilepsy Foundation
4351 Garden City Drive
Landover, MD 20785-7223
800-332-1000 or 301-459-3700
www.efa.org

Huntington's Disease Society of America
158 West 29th Street, 7th Floor
New York, NY 10001-5300
800-345-HDSA
Fax: 212-239-3430
www.hdsa.org

Myasthenia Gravis Foundation of America
5841 Cedar Lake Road, Suite 204
Minneapolis, MN 55416
800-541-5454 or 952-545-9438
Fax: 952-545-6073
www.myasthenia.org

National Headache Foundation
428 West St. James Place, 2nd Floor
Chicago, IL 60614-2750
888-NHF-5552
www.headaches.org

National Institute of Neurological Disorders and Stroke
PO Box 5801
Bethesda, MD 20824
800-352-9424 or 301-468-5981
www.ninds.nih.gov

National Multiple Sclerosis Society
733 Third Avenue
New York, NY 10017
800-FIGHT-MS (344-4867)
www.nmss.org

Restless Legs Syndrome Foundation
819 Second Street SW
Rochester, MN 55902-2985
877-463-6757 or 507-287-6465
www.rls.org

For additional Internet resources, see the website for this book at *http://evolve.elsevier.com/Lewis/medsurg/.*

CHAPTER 58

NURSING MANAGEMENT
Alzheimer's Disease and Dementia

Margaret McLean Heitkemper
Lissi Hansen
Sharon Mantik Lewis

LEARNING OBJECTIVES

1. Describe the etiology, pathophysiology, clinical manifestations, diagnostic studies, and collaborative management of delirium.
2. Define dementia and describe its impact on society.
3. Compare and contrast different etiologies of dementia.
4. Describe the clinical manifestations, diagnostic studies, and collaborative management of dementia.
5. Describe the clinical manifestations, diagnostic studies, and collaborative management of Alzheimer's disease.
6. Describe the nursing management of the patient with Alzheimer's disease.
7. Describe other neurodegenerative disorders associated with dementia, including Lewy body disease, Pick's disease, Creutzfeldt-Jakob disease, and normal-pressure hydrocephalus.

KEY TERMS

Alzheimer's disease, p. 1586
Creutzfeldt-Jakob disease, p. 1598
delirium, p. 1581
dementia, p. 1583
familial Alzheimer's disease, p. 1586
frontotemporal dementia, p. 1599
Lewy body disease, p. 1598

mild cognitive impairment, p. 1587
neuritic plaque, p. 1586
neurofibrillary tangles, p. 1586
normal pressure hydrocephalus, p. 1599
Pick's disease, p. 1599
vascular dementia, p. 1584

The three most common cognitive problems in adults are delirium (acute confusion), dementia, and depression. These problems often occur together. It is important to be able to identify the distinguishing characteristics because the treatment for each problem is very different.

DELIRIUM

Delirium, a state of temporary but acute mental confusion, is common in older adults who have a short-term illness such as lung or heart disease, infections, poor nutrition, drug interactions, and metabolic or hormone disorders. Approximately 10% to 40% of patients are delirious when admitted to the hospital, and another 25% to 60% develop delirium during hospitalization. It is also estimated that delirium will complicate the hospitalizations of more than 2.2 million persons each year. Patients who experience delirium are at greater risk for longer hospitalizations, further functional decline, and institutionalization.[1]

Reviewed by Catherine M. Harris, RNCS, PhD, Professor Emeritus, College of Nursing, University of New Mexico, Albuquerque, NM, and Senior Vice President, Dementia Care Design International, San Antonio, Tex.

Etiology and Pathophysiology

The pathophysiologic mechanism of delirium is poorly understood. Neuroimaging studies indicate that both cortical and subcortical structures (thalamus, basal ganglia, and pontine reticular formation) are involved.[1] The finding that subcortical structures are involved may explain the high risk of delirium in patients with Parkinson's disease. The neurotransmitter acetylcholine may be a critical factor in the development of delirium.[2] This is based in part on three observations: (1) anticholinergic drugs can precipitate delirium in older adults; (2) anticholinesterase agents (physostigmine [Antilirium]) can reverse delirium caused by anticholinergic drug use; and (3) other risk factors for delirium, such as hypoglycemia, hypoxia, and thiamine deficiency, decrease the central nervous system (CNS) production of acetylcholine.[3] Other neurotransmitters including γ-aminobutyric acid, norepinephrine, dopamine, and serotonin may also be involved in delirium but are less well studied.

Delirium associated with infection, inflammation, and cancer may be related to the action of specific cytokines such as interleukins and interferons.[4] In addition, patients treated with cytokine therapies (e.g., interferon for hepatitis C) can develop neuropsychiatric side effects including delirium.[5]

Clinically, delirium is rarely caused by a single factor. It is often the result of the interaction of the patient's underlying condition with a precipitating event. Delirium can occur following a relatively minor insult in a vulnerable patient. For example, the patient with underlying health problems such as congestive heart failure, cancer, cognitive impairment, or sensory limitations may develop delirium in response to a relatively minor change (e.g., use of a sleeping medication). In other nonvulnerable patients, it may take a combination of factors (e.g., anesthesia, major surgery, infection, prolonged sleep deprivation) to precipitate delirium.[1] Delirium can also be a symptom of a serious medical illness such as bacterial meningitis.

Understanding factors that can lead to delirium can help to determine effective interventions. Several factors identified as pre-

---

TABLE 58-1   Factors That Can Precipitate Delirium

- Absence of time and place cues (e.g., watch, clock)
- Change in environment
- Chronic illness (e.g., congestive heart failure)
- Dehydration
- Dementia
- Electrolyte imbalances (hyponatremia, hypercalcemia)
- Hospitalization (e.g., intensive care unit)
- Hypercarbia
- Hyperthermia
- Hypoglycemia
- Hypothermia
- Hypoxia
- Immobilization
- Infection
- Liver disease
- Medications (e.g., sedative-hypnotics, narcotics, benzodiazepines)
- Metabolic disorders
- Pain (untreated)
- Renal disease
- Sensory deprivation
- Sensory overload
- Stress
- Trauma

cipitating delirium are shown in Table 58-1. One of the most important risk factors for delirium is preexisting dementia. Many of the conditions that can precipitate delirium are more common in older patients. In addition, older patients have limited compensatory mechanisms to deal with physiologic insults such as hypoxia, hypoglycemia, and dehydration. Older adults are more susceptible to drug-induced delirium, in part because of their increased use of multiple drugs. Medications including sedative-hypnotics, narcotics (especially meperidine [Demerol]), benzodiazepines, and drugs with anticholinergic properties can cause or contribute to delirium, especially in older or vulnerable patients.

Clinical Manifestations

Patients with delirium can present with a variety of manifestations ranging from hypoactivity and lethargy to hyperactivity including agitation and hallucinations.[6] Patients can also have mixed delirium and manifest both hypoactive and hyperactive symptoms. In most patients delirium usually develops over a 2- to 3-day period. The early manifestations often include inability to concentrate, irritability, insomnia, loss of appetite, restlessness, and confusion. Later the manifestations may include agitation, misperception, misinterpretation, and hallucinations. Delirium is an acute problem.

Manifestations of delirium are sometimes confused with dementia and depression. Table 58-2 compares the features of delirium, dementia, and depression. A key distinction between delirium and dementia is that the person who exhibits sudden

---

TABLE 58-2   Comparison of the Clinical Features of Delirium, Dementia, and Depression

FEATURE	DELIRIUM	DEMENTIA	DEPRESSION
Onset	Rapid, often at night	Usually insidious	Coincides with life changes; often abrupt
Course	Fluctuates, worse at night; lucid intervals	Long; symptoms progressive yet relatively stable over time	Diurnal effects, typically worse in the morning; situational fluctuations
Progression	Abrupt	Slow but even	Variable, rapid-slow but uneven
Duration	Hours to less than 1 month	Months to years	At least 2 weeks, but can be several months to years
Awareness	Reduced	Clear	Clear
Alertness	Fluctuates, lethargic or hypervigilant	Generally normal	Normal
Orientation	Fluctuates in severity, generally impaired	Progressive impairment	Selective disorientation resulting from impaired concentration and attention span, which may manifest as memory deficit
Thinking	Disorganized, distorted, fragmented; slow or accelerated incoherent speech	Difficulty with abstraction, thoughts impoverished, judgment impaired, words difficult to find	Intact but with apathy, fatigue; may not want to live; may be at risk for suicide
Perception	Distorted; illusions, delusions, and hallucinations	Misperceptions often present; delusions, illusions, and hallucinations	May deny depression
Psychomotor behavior	Variable; hypokinetic, hyperkinetic, or mixed	Apraxia	Variable; psychomotor retardation or agitation
Sleep-wake cycle	Disturbed, cycle reversed	Frequent awakenings	Disturbed, often early morning awakening
Mental status testing	Distracted from task; poor performance; improves when patient recovers	Frequent "near miss" answers, struggles with test, great effort to find an appropriate reply; consistently poor performances	Frequent "don't know" answers, little effort, frequently gives up, indifferent

cognitive impairment, disorientation, or clouded sensorium is more likely to have delirium rather than dementia.

Diagnostic Studies

A careful medical and psychologic history and physical examination are the first steps in the diagnosis of delirium. This includes careful attention to medications, both prescription and over-the-counter drug use. A variety of cognitive measures can be used, including the Mini-Mental State Examination (see Table 58-5 later in the chapter). The information may have to be obtained from a reliable informant if the patient is unable to provide the information. It is important to distinguish whether the delirium is part of an underlying problem of dementia.

Once delirium has been diagnosed, potential causes of the delirium are explored. These include careful review of the patient's health history and medication record. Laboratory tests include complete blood count, serum electrolytes, blood urea nitrogen and creatinine levels, electrocardiogram, urine analysis, liver function tests, thyroid function, and oxygen saturation level. Drug and alcohol levels may be obtained. If unexplained fever or nuchal rigidity is present and meningitis or encephalitis is suspected, a lumbar puncture may be performed. Cerebrospinal fluid (CSF) is examined for glucose and protein and the presence of bacteria. If the patient's history includes head injury, appropriate x-ray or scans may be ordered. In general, brain imaging studies, computed tomography (CT) or magnetic resonance imaging (MRI), are used only in those situations in which head injury is known or suspected.

NURSING *and* COLLABORATIVE MANAGEMENT
DELIRIUM

Preventing delirium in patients at risk for delirium is important. Patient groups at risk include those with neurologic disorders (e.g., stroke, dementia, CNS infection, Parkinson's disease), sensory impairment, and advanced age. Other risk factors include hospitalization in an intensive care unit, lack of a watch or calendar, and absence of reading glasses.[6,7] Untreated pain may also precipitate delirium.

Care of the patient with delirium is focused on eliminating precipitating factors. If it is drug-induced, medications are discontinued. It is important to keep in mind that delirium can also accompany drug and alcohol withdrawal. Depending on patient history, drug screening may be performed. Fluid and electrolyte imbalances and nutritional deficiencies (e.g., thiamine) are corrected if appropriate. If the problem is related to environmental conditions (e.g., overstimulating or understimulating environment), changes should be made. If delirium is secondary to infection, appropriate antibiotic therapy is started. Similarly, if delirium is secondary to chronic illness such as chronic kidney disease or congestive heart failure, treatment is focused on these conditions.

Care of the patient experiencing delirium includes protecting the patient from harm. Priority is given to creating a calm and safe environment. This may include encouraging family members to stay at the bedside, providing familiar objects, transferring the patient to a private room or one closer to the nurses' station, and planning for consistent staff care if possible. Reorientation and behavioral interventions should be used in all patients with delir-

ium. The patient is provided with reassurance and reorienting information as to place, time, and procedures. Clocks, calendars, and listing the patient's scheduled activities are also useful in reducing confusion. Environmental stimuli including noise and light levels may have to be reduced if possible.

Personal contact through touch and verbal communication can be important reorienting strategies. If the patient uses eyeglasses or a hearing aid, it should be made readily available because sensory deprivation can precipitate delirium. The use of restraints should be avoided. Other interventions, including relaxation techniques, music therapy, and massage, may also be appropriate for some patients with delirium.

Comprehensive, institutional-based programs focused on reducing risk factors for delirium (cognitive impairment, sleep deprivation, immobility, visual impairment, hearing impairment, and dehydration) have been shown to be effective in reducing overall episodes of delirium in hospitalized older patients.[8] An interdisciplinary team approach is needed to reduce polypharmacy, decrease pain, enhance nutritional intake, and reduce incontinence. The patient experiencing delirium is also at risk for the adverse consequences of immobility, including skin breakdown. Attention is given to increasing physical activity or providing range-of-motion exercises, when appropriate, and preventing skin breakdown.

The nurse should also focus on supporting the family and caregivers during episodes of delirium. Family members need to understand factors that may have precipitated the delirium, as well as the potential outcomes.

Drug Therapy. Drug therapy is reserved for those patients with severe agitation, especially in those patients whose agitation interferes with needed medical therapy (e.g., fluid replacement, intubation, dialysis). Agitation can put the patient at risk for falls and injury. Drug therapy is used cautiously because many of the drugs used to manage agitation have psychoactive properties.

Patients are often treated with low-dose antipsychotics (neuroleptics) such as haloperidol (Haldol). Haloperidol can be administered intravenously, intramuscularly, or orally and will produce sedation. In addition to sedation, other side effects include hypotension, extrapyramidal side effects including *tardive dyskinesia* (involuntary muscle movements of the face, trunk, and arms), *athetosis* (involuntary writhing movements of the limbs), muscle tone changes, and anticholinergic effects. Older patients receiving antipsychotic agents need to be carefully monitored. Newer antipsychotics including risperidone (Risperdal), olanzapine (Zyprexa), and quetiapine (Seroquel) can be used to manage agitated behavior in older adults. These drugs have fewer side effects compared with haloperidol.

Short-acting benzodiazepines (e.g., lorazepam [Ativan]) can be used to treat delirium associated with sedative and alcohol withdrawal or in conjunction with antipsychotics to reduce extrapyramidal side effects. However, these drugs may worsen delirium caused by other factors and must be used cautiously.

DEMENTIA

Dementia is a syndrome characterized by dysfunction or loss of memory, orientation, attention, language, and judgment and reasoning and by changes in behavior. Ultimately these problems result in alterations in the individual's ability to work, social and family responsibilities, and activities of daily living.

The World Health Organization has defined *dementia* as a syndrome caused by disease of the brain, usually of a chronic or progressive nature, in which there is disturbance of multiple cortical functions, calculation, learning capacity, language, and judgment. Impairments of cognitive function are commonly ac-

TABLE 58-3	Causes of Dementia
Neurodegenerative disorders	Alzheimer's disease
	Lewy body disease
	Frontal lobe dementia
	Frontal-temporal dementia (e.g., Pick's disease)
	Down syndrome
	Amyotrophic lateral sclerosis (ALS)
	Parkinson's disease
	Huntington's disease
Vascular diseases	Vascular (multiinfarct) dementia
	Cardiac disease producing emboli or decreased perfusion
	Binswanger's disease
	Subarachnoid hemorrhage*
	Chronic subdural hematoma*
Toxic or metabolic diseases	Alcoholism
	Thiamine (vitamin B_1) deficiency*
	Cobalamin (vitamin B_{12}) deficiency*
	Folate deficiency*
	Hyperthyroidism*
	Hypothyroidism*
	Hypoglycemia*
	Hypercalcemia*
Immunologic diseases or infections	Multiple sclerosis
	Chronic fatigue syndrome
	Infections (e.g., Creutzfeldt-Jakob disease)
	Acquired immunodeficiency syndrome (AIDS)
	Meningitis*
	Encephalitis*
	Neurosyphilis*
	Systemic lupus erythematosus*
Systemic diseases	Uremic encephalopathy*
	Dialysis dementia*
	Hepatic encephalopathy*
	Wilson's disease
Trauma	Head injury*
Cancer	Brain tumors (primary)*
	Metastatic tumors*
Ventricular disorders	Hydrocephalus*
Seizure disorders	Epilepsy
Drugs†	Diuretics
	digoxin
	Anticholinergics
	Narcotics
	Hypnotics
	Antihypertensives
	Antiparkinsonian drugs
	Antihistamines

*Potentially reversible.
†These are examples of drugs that may cause cognitive impairment that is potentially reversible.

companied and occasionally preceded by deterioration in emotional control, social behavior, and motivation.[9]

Dementia is a disorder that occurs most often in older adults. As the average life span of humans increases, the number of those affected with dementia is growing and is now a major international public health concern.[10] In the United States half of all patients in long-term care facilities have Alzheimer's disease (AD) or a related dementia. In Canada approximately 60,000 new cases of dementia are identified each year.[11]

Etiology and Pathophysiology

Causes of dementia are due to both treatable and nontreatable conditions (Table 58-3). The two most common causes of dementia are neurodegenerative conditions (e.g., AD) and vascular disorders. Neurodegenerative conditions account for 60% to 80% of all dementias. Advanced age and family history are important risk factors for dementia. Infectious conditions such as bacterial meningitis and viral encephalitis can result in both vascular and neurodegenerative changes that may ultimately result in dementia.

Dementia is sometimes caused by treatable conditions that are potentially reversible (see Table 58-3). Initially these conditions may be reversible. However, with prolonged exposure or disease, irreversible changes may occur.

Vascular causes are the second most common cause of dementia. **Vascular dementia,** also called multiinfarct dementia, is the loss of cognitive function resulting from ischemic, ischemic-hypoxic, or hemorrhagic brain lesions caused by cardiovascular disease. This type of dementia is the result of decreased blood supply from narrowing and blocking of arteries that supply the brain. Vascular dementia may be caused by a single stroke (infarct) or by multiple strokes.

A history of smoking, cardiac arrhythmias (e.g., atrial fibrillation), hypertension, hypercholesterolemia, diabetes mellitus, and coronary artery disease predispose to vascular dementia. Recently, high homocysteine levels have been associated with the development of dementia and AD.[12]

Clinical Manifestations

Depending on the cause of the dementia, the onset of symptoms may be insidious and gradual or somewhat more abrupt. Often dementia associated with neurologic degeneration is gradual and progressive over time. Causes of vascular dementia can result in more abrupt symptoms or symptoms that progress in a more stepwise pattern. However, it is difficult to distinguish the etiology of dementia (vascular versus neurodegenerative) based on symptom progression alone. An acute (days to weeks) or subacute (weeks to months) pattern of change may be indicative of an infectious or metabolic cause including encephalitis, meningitis, hypothyroidism, or drug-related dementia.

Clinical manifestations of dementia are classified as mild, moderate, and severe (Table 58-4). Regardless of the cause of dementia the initial symptoms are related to changes in cognitive functioning. Patients may have complaints of memory loss, mild disorientation, and/or trouble with words and numbers. Often it is a family member, in particular the spouse, who complains to the health care provider about the patient's declining memory. Almost all adults experience some changes with memory related to aging. Normal age-related memory decline

TABLE 58-4   Clinical Manifestations of Dementia

EARLY (MILD)	MIDDLE (MODERATE)	LATE (SEVERE)
• Forgetfulness beyond what is seen in a normal person • Short-term memory impairment, especially for new learning • Difficulty recognizing what numbers mean • Loss of initiative and interests • Decreased judgment • Geographic disorientation	• Impaired ability to recognize close family or friends • Agitation • Wandering, getting lost • Loss of remote memory • Confusion • Impaired comprehension • Forgets how to do simple tasks • Apraxia • Receptive aphasia • Expressive aphasia • Insomnia • Delusions • Illusions, hallucinations • Behavioral problems	• Little memory, unable to process new information • Cannot understand words • Difficulty eating, swallowing • Repetitious words or sounds • Unable to perform self-care activities • Immobility • Incontinence

is characterized as mild changes that do not impact on activities of daily living. In dementia the memory loss is initially for recent events with remote memories still intact. With time and progression of the dementia, memory loss includes both recent and remote memory and ultimately affects the ability to perform self-care.

Diagnostic Studies

The diagnosis of dementia is focused on determining the cause (e.g., reversible versus nonreversible factors). An important first step is a thorough medical, neurologic, and psychologic history. A thorough physical examination is performed to rule out other potential medical conditions. Screening for cobalamin (vitamin B_{12}) deficiency and hypothyroidism are often performed. Based on patient history, testing for neurosyphilis (see Chapter 57) may be performed. The American Academy of Neurology recommends cognitive evaluation and ongoing clinical monitoring of persons with mild cognitive impairment because of their increased risk of developing dementia.[13]

Mental status testing is an important component for the patient evaluation. Patients with mild dementia may be able to compensate, making it difficult to evaluate cognitive function only through conversation. Cognitive testing is focused on evaluating memory, ability to calculate, language, visuospatial skills, and degree of alertness. The Mini-Mental State Examination (Table 58-5) is the most commonly used tool to assess cognitive functioning.

Depression is often mistaken for dementia in older adults, and, conversely, dementia for depression. Manifestations of depression (especially in the older adult) include sadness, difficulty thinking and concentrating, fatigue, apathy, feelings of despair, and inactivity. When the depression is severe, poor concentration and attention may occur, causing memory and functional impairment. When dementia and depression do occur together (which may be in as many as 40% of dementia cases), the intellectual deterioration may be more extreme. Depression, alone or in combination with dementia, is treatable. The challenge is to make an early assessment.

TABLE 58-5   Mini-Mental State Examination (MMSE)

MMSE SAMPLE ITEMS

Orientation to Time
"What is the date?"

Registration
"Listen carefully, I am going to say three words. You say them back after I stop. Ready? Here they are. . .
HOUSE (pause), CAR (pause), LAKE (pause). Now repeat those words back to me." (Repeat up to five times, but score only the first trial.)

Naming
"What is this?" (Point to a pencil or pen.)

Reading
"Please read this and do what it says." (Show examinee the words on the stimulus form.) CLOSE YOUR EYES

Diagnosis of dementia related to vascular causes is based on the presence of cognitive loss, the presence of vascular brain lesions demonstrated by neuroimaging techniques, and the exclusion of other causes of dementia (e.g., AD). The American Academy of Neurology guidelines include the use of structural neuroimaging with CT or MRI in the evaluation of patients with dementia.[14] Although both single photon emission computed tomography (SPECT) and positron emission tomography (PET) scanning techniques can be used to characterize CNS changes in dementia, these tools are not routinely used in the initial diagnosis of dementia. There are no genetic markers or CSF markers that are currently recommended for routine evaluation of patients with dementia.

NURSING and COLLABORATIVE MANAGEMENT
DEMENTIA

Collaborative and nursing management of the patient with dementia is similar to that described for AD (see later in this chapter). Vascular dementia can be prevented. Preventive measures include treatment of risk factors including hypertension, diabetes, smoking, hyperfibrinogenemia, hyperhomocysteinemia, orthostatic hypotension, and cardiac arrhythmias. (Stroke is discussed in Chapter 56.) Cholinesterase inhibitors (e.g., donepezil [Aricept]) that are used for patients with AD are also useful in patients with vascular dementia.

ALZHEIMER'S DISEASE

Alzheimer's disease (AD) is a chronic, progressive, degenerative disease of the brain. It is the most common form of dementia, accounting for approximately 60% to 80% of all cases of dementia. AD is named after Alois Alzheimer, a German physician who in 1906 described changes in the brain tissue of a 51-year-old woman who had died of an unusual mental illness.

Approximately 4 million Americans suffer from AD. It is estimated that 10% of people over age 65 and 50% of those over age 85 have AD. Worldwide it is estimated that more than 22 million individuals will have AD by 2025.[10] The course of the disease can span 5 to 20 years. The economic costs of AD in the United States range from approximately $19,000 annually for the care of the person with early disease to $37,000 annually for the person with late disease.[15] Nationally the annual costs of AD are estimated at $100 billion dollars. The burden on the individual, family, caregivers, and society as a whole is staggering.

The incidence of AD is approximately the same for all ethnic groups although the risk may be slightly higher in African Americans and Hispanic Americans. AD has been associated with lower socioeconomic status and education level and poor access to health care. Therefore additional research is needed to determine whether ethnic differences are related to genetic or environmental risk factors.[15] Women are more likely than men to develop AD primarily because they live longer. Individuals with Down syndrome are at high risk for AD. They may develop clinical signs around the age of 20, and by age 40, 95% of patients with Down syndrome will have evidence of AD based on autopsy findings.[15]

Etiology and Pathophysiology

The exact etiology of AD is unknown. Similar to other forms of dementia, age is the most important risk factor for developing AD. However, AD is not a normal part of aging. AD is a disease that destroys brain cells, which is not a normal part of aging. Only a small percentage of people younger than 60 years old will develop AD. When AD develops in someone less than the age of 60, it is referred to as *early onset AD*. AD that becomes evident in individuals after the age of 60 is called *late onset AD* (see the Genetics in Clinical Practice box on this page).

Persons in whom a clear pattern of inheritance within a family is established are said to have **familial Alzheimer's disease** (FAD). Others in whom no familial connection can be made are termed *sporadic*. FAD is associated with earlier onset (before 60 years of age) and more rapid disease course. In both FAD and sporadic AD, the pathogenesis of AD is similar.

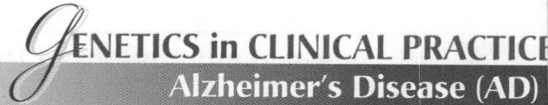

GENETICS in CLINICAL PRACTICE
Alzheimer's Disease (AD)

Genetic Basis

Early Onset (Familial) (<60 years old at onset)
- Autosomal dominant disorder
- Various mutations in the following genes:
  Amyloid precursor protein (APP) gene on chromosome 21
  Presenilin-1 (PSEN1) gene on chromosome 14
  Presenilin-2 (PSEN2) gene on chromosome 1

Late Onset (Sporadic) (>60 years old at onset)
- Genetically more complex than early onset form
- Presence of apolipoprotein E (ApoE)-4 gene on chromosome 19 increases the likelihood of developing AD
- If two ApoE-4 alleles are inherited, there is a higher risk of AD
- Presence of ApoE-2 allele is associated with a lower risk for AD

Incidence

Early Onset
- Rare form of AD accounting for less than 10% of cases
- 50% risk of disease for children of affected parents

Late Onset
- Many ApoE-4 positive people do not develop AD, and many ApoE-4 negative people do.

Genetic Testing

Early Onset
- Genetic screening for mutations on chromosomes 1, 14, and 21

Late Onset
- Blood test to identify presence of ApoE-4 gene
- No consensus on the clinical appropriateness of ApoE testing
- ApoE testing is mainly used for research

Clinical Implications
- AD is the most common cause of dementia.
- Overall the incidence of AD is three times higher among people with one affected parent than in those with no affected parents.
- Genetic testing and counseling for family members of patients with early onset AD may be appropriate.
- If person tests positive for ApoE-4, it does not mean that the person will develop AD.

The characteristic findings in AD are the presence of abnormal clumps (neuritic or senile plaques) and tangled bundles of fibers (neurofibrillary tangles) in the brain (Fig. 58-1). The **neuritic plaque** is a cluster of degenerating axonal and dendritic nerve terminals that contain amyloid-beta protein. **Neurofibrillary tangles** are seen in the cytoplasm of abnormal neurons in those areas of the brain (hippocampus, cerebral cortex) most affected by AD (Fig. 58-2). In the cerebral cortex they are found in those areas of brain associated with cognition, learning, sleep, and memory.

Genetic factors may play a critical role in how the brain processes the amyloid-beta protein.[15] Overproduction of amyloid-beta appears to be an important risk factor for AD. Amyloid-beta (A-beta) is part of a larger protein called amyloid precursor protein (APP) that is involved in cell membrane function and is produced by cells throughout the body. Large amounts of APP are

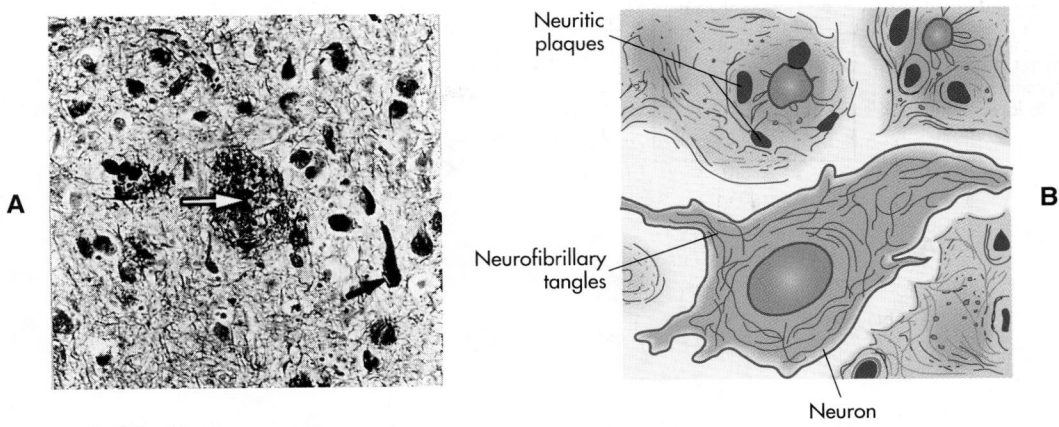

FIG. 58-1 Pathologic changes in Alzheimer's disease. **A,** Senile plaque with central amyloid core *(white arrow)* next to a neurofibrillary tangle *(black arrow)* on the histologic specimen from a brain autopsy. **B,** Schematic representation of neuritic plaque and neurofibrillary tangle.

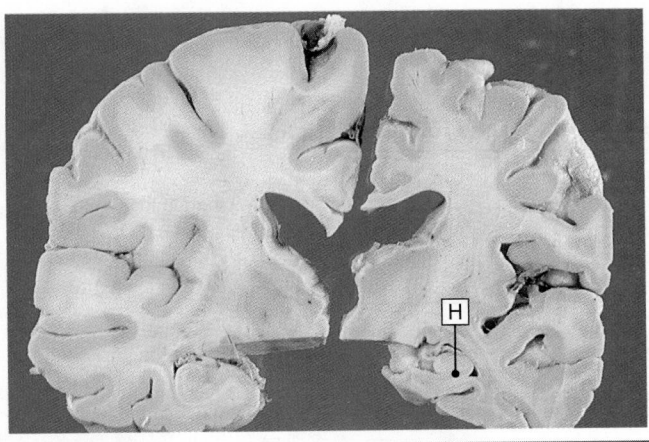

FIG. 58-2 Alzheimer's disease. This shows slices from two brains. On the left is a normal brain from a 70-year-old; on the right is the same region from a 70-year-old with Alzheimer's disease. The diseased brain is atrophic with loss of cortex and white matter, most marked in the hippocampal region *(H).*

produced in the brain. Neuritic plaques are composed of A-beta proteins. Abnormally high levels of A-beta are thought to produce cell damage either directly or through eliciting an inflammatory response and ultimately neuron death (Fig. 58-3, *A*).[16]

Understanding why neurons produce A-beta led researchers to examine the enzymes (and their genes) that are responsible for both the synthesis and processing of APP. In patients with early onset AD, three genes have been identified as important in the etiology of AD (see Genetics in Clinical Practice box on p. 1586). When the presenilin 1 and presenilin 2 genes are mutated, they cause brain cells to overproduce A-beta.

The first gene associated with AD was the epsilon (E) 4 allele of the apolipoprotein E (ApoE) gene on chromosome 19.[15] ApoE comes in several different forms or alleles, but three occur most commonly. People inherit one allele (ApoE-2, ApoE-3, ApoE-4) from each parent. ApoE may play a role in clearing amyloid

plaques. Mutations in this gene result in greater amyloid deposition. The presence of ApoE-4 increases the risk of a person developing late onset AD. However, the presence of the gene alone is not adequate to account for AD because many people with ApoE-4 do not develop AD.

An important part of the neurofibrillary tangle is a protein called tau. *Tau* proteins in the CNS are involved in providing support for intracellular structure through their support of microtubules. Tau proteins hold the microtubules together like railroad ties hold the railroad tracks together. In AD it appears that the tau protein is altered, and as a result, the microtubules twist together in a helical fashion (see Fig. 58-3, *B*). This ultimately forms the neurofibrillary tangles observed in the neurons of persons with AD.

The presence of neuritic plaques and neurofibrillary tangles appears to be related to neuronal death. However, whether they are directly toxic or predispose to cell injury via other mechanisms remains to be determined. For example, examination of autopsied brain tissue from AD patients shows evidence of inflammatory changes. These findings suggest that AD may involve an inflammatory process. This inflammatory response may be elicited by cell damage or death secondary to A-beta or neurofibrillary tangle formation.

Neuritic plaques and neurofibrillary tangles are not unique to patients with AD or dementia. They are also found in the brains of individuals without evidence of cognitive impairment. However, they are more plentiful in the brains of individuals with AD.

Cholinergic neurons are lost in people with AD, particularly in regions essential for memory and cognition. Other neurotransmitter systems, including serotonin and norepinephrine, also show losses over time in patients with AD. Such neurotransmitter changes are the basis of current drug therapies for AD.

Clinical Manifestations

Pathologic changes often precede clinical manifestations of dementia by anywhere from 5 to 20 years. **Mild cognitive impairment** refers to a state of cognition and functional ability between normal aging and early AD (Table 58-6). The Alzheimer's Association has developed a list of warning signs that include common

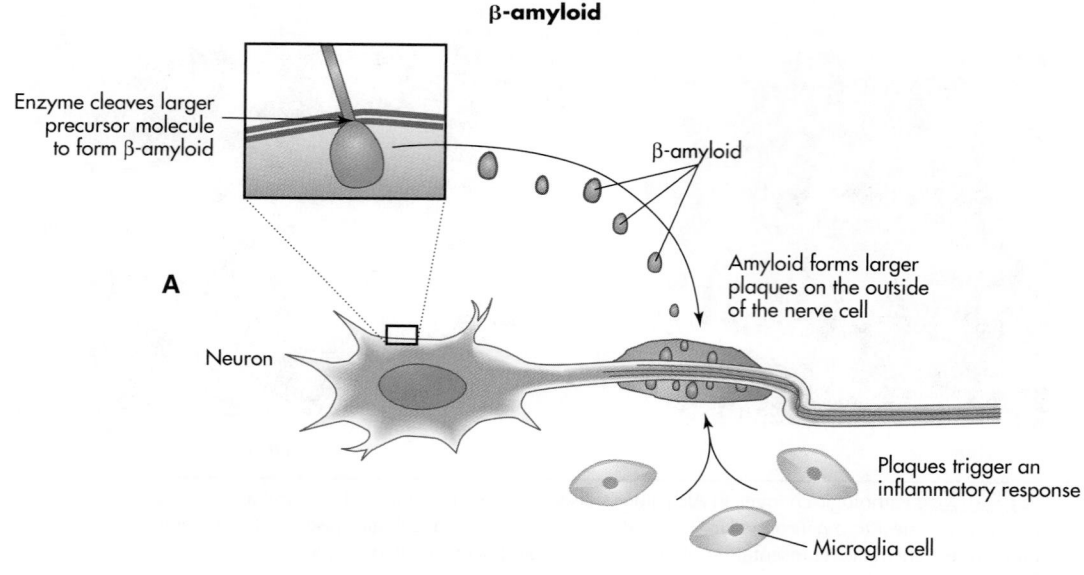

FIG. 58-3 Current etiologic theories for the development of Alzheimer's disease. **A,** Abnormal amounts of amyloid are cleaved and released into the circulation. The amyloid forms plaques that attach to the neuron. This stimulates an inflammatory response. **B,** Tau proteins provide structural support for the neuron microtubules. Chemical changes in the neuron produce structural changes in tau proteins. This results in twisting and tangling (neurofibrillary tangles).

manifestations of AD (Table 58-7). The manifestations of AD can be categorized similar to those for dementia as mild, moderate, and late (see Table 58-4). The rate of progression from mild to late is highly variable from individual to individual and ranges from 3 to 20 years. Some patients may have mild cognitive impairment for years, whereas others, especially those with early onset AD, may progress over a few years from mild to severe impairment.

An initial sign of AD is a subtle deterioration in memory. Inevitably this progresses to more profound memory loss that interferes with the patient's ability to function. As the disease progresses, manifestations are more easily noticed and become serious enough to cause people with AD or their family members to seek medical help. Recent events and new information cannot be recalled. Personal hygiene deteriorates, as does the ability to concentrate and maintain attention. Ongoing loss of neurons in

AD can cause a person to act in altered or unpredictable ways. Behavioral manifestations of AD (e.g., agitation) result from changes that take place within the brain. They are neither intentional nor controllable by the individual with the disease. Some patients develop psychotic manifestations (e.g., delusions, illusions, hallucinations).

With progression of AD, additional cognitive impairments are noted. These include *dysphasia* (difficulty comprehending language and oral communication), *apraxia* (inability to manipulate objects or perform purposeful acts), *visual agnosia* (inability to recognize objects by sight), and *dysgraphia* (difficulty communicating via writing). Eventually long-term memories cannot be recalled, and patients lose the ability to recognize family members and friends. Other problems include aggression and a tendency to wander.

TABLE 58-6	Mild Cognitive Impairment (MCI)
Description	• MCI refers to a state of cognition and functional ability between normal aging and early Alzheimer's disease (AD). • Individuals are memory impaired but otherwise functionally normal. • MCI may be considered a transitional state between aging and AD.
Characteristics	• Memory complaint • Abnormal memory for age • Intact activities of daily living • Normal general cognitive functioning • Not demented
Progression to AD	• More than 80% of patients with MCI develop AD within 10 years at a rate of 10% to 15% of patients per year.
Significance	• It is important to identify and treat patients with MCI. • Treatment strategies must be developed to stop or reverse the decline in cognitive function. • If treated appropriately, the progression to onset of AD may be delayed.

Later in the disease, the ability to communicate and to perform activities of daily living is lost. In the late or final stages of AD, the patient is unresponsive, incontinent, and requires total care.

Diagnostic Studies

The diagnosis of AD is primarily a diagnosis of exclusion. No single clinical test can be used to diagnose AD. In patients with cognitive impairment, there is increased emphasis on early and careful evaluation of the patient. As indicated earlier in this chapter, there are many conditions that can cause manifestations of dementia, some of which are treatable or "reversible" (see Table 58-3).

When all other possible conditions that can cause cognitive impairment have been ruled out, a clinical diagnosis of AD can be made. A comprehensive patient evaluation includes a complete health history, physical examination, neurologic and mental status assessments, and laboratory tests (Table 58-8). Brain imaging tests include CT or MRI. A CT or an MRI scan may show brain atrophy and enlarged ventricles in the later stages of the disease, although this finding occurs in other diseases and can also be seen in persons without cognitive impairment. Newer techniques include SPECT, magnetic resonance spectroscopy (MRS), and PET. These techniques allow for detection of changes early in the disease as well as monitoring of treatment response. Blood levels of ApoE-4 may be obtained (see Genetics in Clinical Practice box on p. 1586). Although neuroimaging, neuropsychologic testing, and examination of genetic markers may provide a diagnosis of possible or probable AD, a definitive diagnosis requires examination of brain tissue and the presence of neurofibrillary tangles and neuritic plaques at autopsy.

Neuropsychologic testing with tools such as the Mini-Mental State Examination (see Table 58-5) can help document the de-

TABLE 58-7	Patient & Family Teaching Guide Early Warning Signs of Alzheimer's Disease

1. *Memory loss that affects job skills.* Frequent forgetfulness or unexplainable confusion at home or in the workplace may signal that something is wrong. This type of memory loss goes beyond forgetting an assignment, colleague's name, deadline, or phone number.
2. *Difficulty performing familiar tasks.* It is not abnormal for most people to become distracted and to forget something (e.g., leave something on the stove too long). People with Alzheimer's disease (AD) may cook a meal but then forget not only to serve it but also that they made it.
3. *Problems with language.* Most people have trouble with finding the "right" word from time to time. Persons with AD may forget simple words or substitute inappropriate words, making their speech difficult to understand.
4. *Disorientation to time and place.* While most individuals occasionally forget the day of the week or what they need from the store, people with AD can become lost on their own street, not knowing where they are, how they got there, or how to get back home.
5. *Poor or decreased judgment.* Many individuals from time to time may choose not to dress appropriately for the weather (e.g., not bringing a coat or sweater on a cold evening). A person with AD may dress inappropriately in more noticeable ways, such as wearing a bathrobe to the store or sweater on a hot day.
6. *Problems with abstract thinking.* For the person with AD this goes beyond challenges such as balancing a checkbook. The person with AD may have difficulty recognizing numbers or doing even basic calculations.
7. *Misplacing things.* For many individuals, temporarily misplacing keys, purses, or wallets is a normal albeit frustrating event. The person with AD may put items in inappropriate places (e.g., eating utensils in clothing drawers) but have no memory of how they got there.
8. *Changes in mood or behavior.* Most individuals experience mood changes. The person with AD tends to exhibit more rapid mood swings for no apparent reason.
9. *Changes in personality.* As most individuals age, they may demonstrate some change in personality (e.g., become less tolerant). The person with AD can change dramatically, either suddenly or over time. For example, someone who is generally easygoing may become angry, suspicious, or fearful.
10. *Loss of initiative.* The person with AD may become and remain uninterested and uninvolved in many or all of his or her usual pursuits.

Adapted from *Early warning signs,* Alzheimer's Association, Chicago, Ill.

gree of cognitive impairment. Neuropsychologic testing is important not only for diagnostic purposes but also to determine a baseline from which changes over time can be evaluated.

A urine test that measures isoprostanes (by-products of fat metabolism associated with free radicals) may provide a mechanism for assessing risk of AD in those with mild cognitive im-

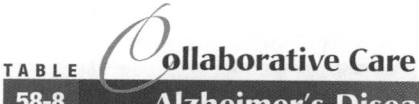

TABLE 58-8 Collaborative Care — Alzheimer's Disease

Diagnostic

History and physical examination, including psychologic evaluation

Neuropsychologic testing including Mini–Mental State Examination (see Table 58-5)

Brain imaging tests: CT, MRI, MRS, SPECT, PET

Complete blood count

Electrocardiogram

Serum glucose, creatinine, BUN

Serum levels of vitamins B_1, B_6, B_{12}

Thyroid function tests

Liver function tests

Screening for depression

Collaborative Therapy

Drug therapy for cognitive problems (see Table 58-9)

Drug therapy for behavioral problems (see Table 58-9)

Behavioral modification

Moderate exercise

Assistance with functional independence

Music, particularly with meals and bathing

Assistance and support for caregiver

BUN, Blood urea nitrogen; *CT,* computed tomography; *MRI,* magnetic resonance imaging; *MRS,* magnetic resonance spectroscopy; *PET,* positron emission tomography; *SPECT,* single photon emission computed tomography.

pairment.[17] However, widespread use of this marker is not currently available.

Collaborative Care

At this time there is no cure for AD. The collaborative management of AD is aimed at improving or controlling decline in cognition and controlling the undesirable manifestations that the patient may exhibit (see Table 58-8).

Drug Therapy. Drug therapy for AD is listed in Table 58-9. Cholinesterase inhibitors are used in the treatment of mild and moderate dementia.[18,19] They block cholinesterase, the enzyme responsible for the breakdown of acetylcholine in the synaptic cleft (Fig. 58-4). Cholinesterase inhibitors include donepezil (Aricept), rivastigmine (Exelon), and galantamine (Reminyl). These drugs have been shown to either improve or stabilize cognitive decline in some people with AD. As a result, they can enhance the patient's functional abilities. However, these drugs do not cure or reverse the progression of the disease. It is not known whether the long-term administration of these drugs will actually delay the progression of the neurologic damage.

Memantine (Ebixa) is a new drug for the treatment of the middle to late stages of AD. Memantine appears to protect the brain's nerve cells against excess amounts of glutamate, which is released in large amounts by cells damaged by AD. The attachment of glutamate to *N*-methyl-D-aspartate (NMDA) receptors permits calcium to flow freely into the cell, which in turn may lead to cell degeneration. Memantine may prevent this destructive sequence by adjusting the activity of glutamate.

Drug therapy is often used for the management of behavioral problems that occur in patients with AD. Conventional antipsychotic drugs (e.g., haloperidol [Haldol]) can be used to manage acute episodes of agitation, aggressive behavior, and psychosis.

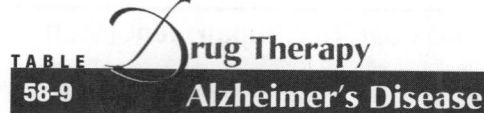

TABLE 58-9 Drug Therapy — Alzheimer's Disease

PROBLEM	DRUGS
Decreased memory and cognition	Cholinesterase inhibitors • donepezil (Aricept) • rivastigmine (Exelon) • galantamine (Reminyl)
Depression	Selective serotonin reuptake inhibitors (SSRIs) • sertraline (Zoloft) • fluvoxamine (Luvox) • citalopram (Celexa) • fluoxetine (Prozac) Tricyclic antidepressants • nortriptyline (Aventyl, Pamelor) • amitriptyline (Elavil) • imipramine (Tofranil) • doxepin (Sinequan) Atypical antidepressant • trazodone (Desyrel)
Behavioral problems (e.g., agitation, disinhibition)	Conventional antipsychotics (neuroleptics) • loxapine (Loxitane) • haloperidol (Haldol) Atypical antipsychotics (neuroleptics) • risperidone (Risperdal) • olanzapine (Zyprexa) • quetiapine (Seroquel) Benzodiazepines • lorazepam (Ativan) • temazepam (Restoril) • oxazepam (Serax)
Sleep disturbances	zolpidem (Ambien)

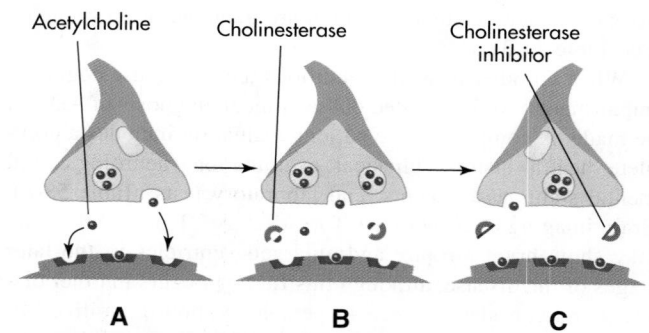

FIG. 58-4 Mechanism of action of cholinesterase inhibitors. Acetylcholine (**A**) is released from the nerve synapses and carries a message across the synapse. Cholinesterase (**B**) breaks down acetylcholine. Cholinesterase inhibitors (**C**) block cholinesterase, thus giving acetylcholine more time to transmit the message.

However, these antipsychotics are often associated with side effects including extrapyramidal symptoms and anticholinergic activity, especially in older adults. Therefore atypical antipsychotics are being used more commonly for behavioral management in AD. These include risperidone (Risperdal), olanzapine (Zyprexa), and quetiapine (Seroquel). They reduce aggression, improve behavior, and usually have fewer side effects.

Treating the depression that is often associated with AD may improve cognitive ability. Depression is often treated with selective serotonin reuptake inhibitors including fluoxetine (Prozac), sertraline (Zoloft), fluvoxamine (Luvox), and citalopram (Celexa). The antidepressant trazodone (Desyrel) may help with problems related to sleep. However, this agent may result in hypotension. Antiseizure drugs (neuroleptics) including valproic acid (Depakene) and carbamazepine (Tegretol) are also used to manage behavioral problems. These drugs tend to act as mood stabilizers.

There has been some debate about the ability of certain drugs, hormones, and herbs (e.g., ginkgo biloba) to prevent or treat AD. Early observational studies indicated that estrogen slowed the progression of AD in those who already had it. However, at this time estrogen is not recommended for the prevention or treatment of AD. Currently, several large studies are exploring the relationship between estrogen and AD. Ginkgo biloba (see the Complementary and Alternative Therapies box on this page) can be used in patients with AD. In Germany ginkgo is considered a form of treatment for AD patients.

Preliminary results from studies investigating the incidence and onset of AD in patients with arthritis who have taken nonsteroidal antiinflammatory drugs (NSAIDs) suggest that NSAIDs may have a protective effect. Although NSAIDs have been shown through epidemiologic studies to be associated with a reduced risk of AD, controlled clinical trials in patients with AD have not demonstrated a clear benefit.[19] When NSAIDs are used in older adults at high doses, there are concerns related to increased potential for upper gastrointestinal bleeding.

Antioxidants may prove to be helpful in slowing the progression of AD. Vitamin C, vitamin E, and selegiline (Eldepryl) are antioxidants and may prevent nerve cell damage by destroying toxic free radicals.[20] *Free radicals* are by-products of normal cell metabolism. Immune cells that are in the brain responding to chronic brain inflammation from AD may release free radicals. Studies of antioxidants and their potential role in prevention or slowing of AD are ongoing.

A number of ongoing clinical drug trials are attempting to find drugs that can limit or decrease the rate of disease progression, as well as manage the signs and symptoms of AD. These new agents will focus on enhancing communications between nerve cells, regulating defective cell processes (reducing A-beta deposition), protecting nerve cells from damage, and repairing nerve cells in the brain.[21]

COMPLEMENTARY & ALTERNATIVE THERAPIES
Ginkgo Biloba

Clinical Uses
Alzheimer's disease and dementia, depression, peripheral arterial vascular disease, tinnitus

Effects
Memory improvement. Increases blood flow to the brain and extremities. Is an antioxidant. Inhibits platelet aggregation.

Nursing Implications
Must be used with caution, or not at all, in people at risk for bleeding or taking anticoagulants. Needs 1 to 3 months to achieve full therapeutic effect. May be of some benefit in treating dementia. There is no evidence that ginkgo will cure or prevent dementia.

NURSING MANAGEMENT
ALZHEIMER'S DISEASE

■ Nursing Assessment

Subjective and objective data that should be obtained from a person with AD are presented in Table 58-10. Useful questions for the patient and informant are, "When did you first notice the memory loss?" and "How has the memory loss progressed since then?"

■ Nursing Diagnoses

Nursing diagnoses for AD may include, but are not limited to, those presented in the NCP 58-1.

■ Planning

The overall goals are that the patient with AD will (1) maintain functional ability for as long as possible, (2) be maintained in a safe environment with a minimum of injuries, (3) have personal care needs met, and (4) have dignity maintained. The over-

TABLE 58-10	*N*ursing Assessment **Alzheimer's Disease**

Subjective Data
Important Health Information
Past health history: Repeated head trauma, stroke, exposure to metals (e.g., mercury, aluminum), previous CNS infection, family history of dementia
Medications: Use of any drug to decrease symptoms (e.g., tranquilizers, hypnotics, antidepressants, antipsychotics)
Functional Health Patterns
Health perception–health management: Positive family history; emotional lability
Nutritional-metabolic: Anorexia, malnutrition, weight loss
Elimination: Incontinence
Activity-exercise: Poor personal hygiene; gait instability, weakness; inability to perform activities of daily living
Sleep-rest: Frequent nighttime awakening, daytime napping
Cognitive-perceptual: Forgetfulness, inability to cope with complex situations, difficulty with problem solving (early signs); depression, withdrawal, suicidal ideation (early)

Objective Data
General
Disheveled appearance, agitation
Neurologic
Early: Loss of recent memory; disorientation to date and time; flat affect; lack of spontaneity; impaired abstraction, cognition, and judgment
Middle: Agitation; impaired ability to recognize close family and friends; loss of remote memory; confusion, apraxia, agnosia, alexia (inability to understand written language); aphasia; inability to do simple tasks
Late: Inability to do self-care; incontinence; immobility; limb rigidity; flexor posturing
Possible Findings
Diagnosis by exclusion, cerebral cortical atrophy on CT scan, poor scores on mental status tests, hippocampal atrophy on MRI scan, abnormal changes on PET, SPECT, and MRS

CNS, Central nervous system; *MRI,* magnetic resonance imaging; *MRS,* magnetic resonance spectroscopy; *PET,* positron emission tomography; *SPECT,* single photon emission computed tomography.

all goals for the caregiver of a patient with AD are to (1) reduce caregiver stress, (2) maintain personal health, and (3) cope with the long-term effects of caregiving.

■ Nursing Implementation

Health Promotion. At this time there is no known method of reducing the risk of AD. Ongoing studies suggest that antioxidants may be beneficial. However, additional data are clearly needed. Because traumatic brain injury may be a risk factor for developing AD, the nurse should promote safety in physical activities and driving. Depression should be recognized and treated early. At this time genetic testing for AD is not performed on a regular basis.

Early recognition and treatment of AD are important. The nurse has a responsibility in terms of informing patients and their families regarding the early signs of AD. The warning signs of

---

NURSING CARE PLAN 58-1

Patient with Alzheimer's Disease

NURSING DIAGNOSIS   **Disturbed thought processes** *related to* effects of dementia *as manifested by* loss of memory and other cognitive deficits.

OUTCOMES—NOC	INTERVENTIONS—NIC and *RATIONALES*
Distorted Thought Control (1403)	*Dementia Management (6460)*
• Behaviors indicate accurate interpretation of environment _____ • Asks for validation of reality _____ • Interacts with others appropriately _____	• Include family members in planning, providing, and evaluating care to the extent desired *to plan appropriate and consistent interventions.* • Determine physical, social, and psychologic history of patient, usual habits, and routines *to maintain familiar routines.* • Prepare for interaction with eye contact and touch as appropriate *to provide respect and acceptance of the patient.* • Give one simple direction at a time *to decrease potential for increasing confusion and frustration.* • Use distraction, rather than confrontation, to manage behavior, *which will decrease anxiety.* • Provide patient a general orientation to the season of the year by using appropriate cues such as calendars, pictures, and seasonal decorations *to promote memory and reduce confusion.* • Refrain from arguing or contradicting the patient.
Outcome Scale 1 = Never demonstrated 2 = Rarely demonstrated 3 = Sometimes demonstrated 4 = Often demonstrated 5 = Consistently demonstrated	*Cognitive Stimulation (4720)* • Stimulate memory by repeating patient's last expressed thought. • Orient to time, place, and person *to promote memory and reduce confusion.*

NURSING DIAGNOSIS   **Self-care deficit (bathing, dressing, toileting)** *related to* memory deficit and neuromuscular impairment *as manifested by* inability to independently and appropriately bathe, dress, or toilet.

OUTCOMES—NOC	INTERVENTIONS—NIC and *RATIONALES*
Self-Care: Activities of Daily Living (0300)	*Self-Care Assistance (1800)*
• Dressing _____ • Bathing _____ • Toileting _____	• Monitor patient's ability for independent self-care *to plan appropriate interventions specific to patient's unique problems.* • Use consistent repetition of daily health routines as a means of establishing them *because memory loss impairs patient's ability to plan and complete specific sequential activities.* • Assist patient in accepting dependency *to ensure that all needs are met.* • Teach family to encourage independence and to intervene only when the patient is unable to perform *to promote independence.*
	Self-Care Assistance: Bathing/Hygiene (1801) • Provide desired personal articles, such as bath soap and hairbrush, *to enhance memory and provide care.* • Facilitate patient's bathing self as appropriate *to facilitate independence and provide appropriate help in hygiene.*
	Self-Care Assistance: Dressing/Grooming (1802) • Provide patient's clothes in accessible area *to facilitate dressing.* • Be available for assistance in dressing as necessary *to facilitate independence and provide appropriate help in dressing.*
Outcome Scale 1 = Dependent, does not participate 2 = Requires assistive person and device 3 = Requires assistive person 4 = Independent with assistive device 5 = Completely independent	*Self-Care Assistance: Toileting (1804)* • Assist patient to toilet at specified intervals *to promote regularity.* • Facilitate toilet hygiene after completion of elimination *to prevent discomfort and skin breakdown.*

NURSING CARE PLAN 58-1

Patient with Alzheimer's Disease—cont'd

NURSING DIAGNOSIS   Risk for injury *related to* impaired judgment, possible gait instability, muscle weakness, and sensory/perceptual alteration.

OUTCOMES—NOC	**INTERVENTIONS—NIC and *RATIONALES***
Safety Behavior: Fall Prevention (1909) ▪ Correct use of assistive devices _____ ▪ Use of restraints as needed _____ ▪ Use of well-fitting tied shoes _____ ▪ Use of vision-correcting devices _____ **Outcome Scale** 1 = Never demonstrated 2 = Rarely demonstrated 3 = Sometimes demonstrated 4 = Often demonstrated 5 = Consistently demonstrated	*Fall Prevention (6490)* ▪ Identify cognitive or physical deficits of the patient that may increase potential of falling in a particular environment *to decrease or prevent occurrence of injury.* ▪ Provide assistive devices, such as walker, *to steady gait and provide ambulation support.* ▪ Ensure that patient wears shoes that fit properly, fasten securely, and have nonskid soles *to provide support during ambulation.* ▪ Instruct patient to wear prescription glasses *to allow for proper vision.*

NURSING DIAGNOSIS   Ineffective coping *related to* depression in response to diagnosis of Alzheimer's disease *as manifested by* depression, withdrawal, fatigue, social isolation.

OUTCOMES—NOC	**INTERVENTIONS—NIC and *RATIONALES***
Coping (1302) ▪ Identifies effective coping patterns _____ ▪ Uses effective coping strategies _____ **Outcome Scale** 1 = Never demonstrated 2 = Rarely demonstrated 3 = Sometimes demonstrated 4 = Often demonstrated 5 = Consistently demonstrated	*Coping Enhancement (5230)* ▪ Appraise the impact of the patient's life situation on roles and relationships *to develop appropriate interventions.* ▪ Encourage social and community activities *to provide pleasurable activities to relieve depression.* ▪ Encourage the use of spiritual resources, if desired, *to allow familiarity and provide a sense of calming to the patient.* ▪ Encourage the family to verbalize feelings about patient and increase communication *to foster mutual understanding among family members.* ▪ Determine the risk of the patient inflicting self-harm *to identify possibility of violent behavior and initiate appropriate nursing plan.*

NURSING DIAGNOSIS   Ineffective therapeutic regimen management *related to* decreasing level of cognitive functioning and memory.

OUTCOMES—NOC	**INTERVENTIONS—NIC and *RATIONALES***
Compliance Behavior (1601) ▪ Performs activities of daily living as prescribed _____ ▪ Reports following prescribed regimen _____ **Outcome Scale** 1 = Never demonstrated 2 = Rarely demonstrated 3 = Sometimes demonstrated 4 = Often demonstrated 5 = Consistently demonstrated	*Anticipatory Guidance (5210)* ▪ Assist the patient to identify possible upcoming situations and the effects on the personal and family life *to establish possible outcomes and identify support systems.* ▪ Provide information on realistic expectations related to the patient's behavior and lifestyle changes such as driving *to prepare for the future needs of daily living.* ▪ Include the family and significant others as appropriate in planning *to ensure agreement* of plans and *to ensure patient's wishes are respected and health care needs are met.*

NURSING DIAGNOSIS   Wandering *related to* disease process *as evidenced by* getting lost numerous times a day and patient's statement of "I don't know where I am."

OUTCOMES—NOC	**INTERVENTIONS—NIC and *RATIONALES***
Safety Behavior: Personal (1911) ▪ Provision of secure environment _____ **Outcome Scale** 1 = Not adequate 2 = Slightly adequate 3 = Moderately adequate 4 = Substantially adequate 5 = Totally adequate	*Area Restriction (6420)* ▪ Provide verbal reminders, as necessary, to remain in designated area *to reorient the patient.* *Surveillance: Safety (6654)* ▪ Monitor environment for potential safety hazards *to prevent injury to patient.* ▪ Monitor patient for alterations in physical or cognitive function that might lead to unsafe behavior *to assess any changes that may occur.* ▪ Provide appropriate level of supervision/surveillance *to monitor patient and to allow for therapeutic actions.* ▪ Provide appropriate activities *as diversion from restlessness associated with wandering.*

AD developed by the Alzheimer's Association are shown in Table 58-7.

Acute Intervention. The diagnosis of AD is traumatic for both the patient and the family. It is not unusual for the patient to respond with depression, denial, anxiety and fear, isolation, and feelings of loss. The nurse is in an important position to assess for depression and suicidal ideation. Antidepressant drugs and counseling may be appropriate interventions to assist the patient. Family members may also be in denial and may not seek medical attention early in the disease. The nurse must assess family members and their abilities to accept and cope with the diagnosis.

Although there is no current treatment for reversing AD, there is a need for ongoing monitoring of both the patient with AD and the patient's caregiver. An important nursing responsibility is to work collaboratively with the patient's caregiver to manage clinical manifestations effectively as they change over time. The nurse is often responsible for teaching the caregiver to perform the many tasks that are required to manage the patient's care. The nurse must consider both the patient with AD and the caregiver as patients with overlapping but unique problems. To aid in identifying the many problems of the caregiver, a nursing care plan for the caregiver of a person with AD is presented (NCP 58-2).

EVIDENCE-BASED PRACTICE
Interventions for Patients with Dementia and Their Caregivers

Clinical Problem

Do pharmacotherapy, educational, or other nonpharmacologic interventions improve outcomes in patients with dementia or for their caregivers?

Best Clinical Practice

- Cholinesterase inhibitors improve outcomes in some patients with Alzheimer's disease.
- Antipsychotics are effective in treating agitation, and antidepressants are effective in treating depression in patients with dementia.
- Educational interventions for family caregivers of patients with Alzheimer's disease improve caregiver and patient outcomes, thus delaying time to institutionalization of the patient.
- Nonpharmacologic interventions, such as behavior modification, are effective for patients with Alzheimer's disease.
- Educating staff in long-term care facilities about Alzheimer's disease minimizes the unnecessary use of antipsychotic drugs.
- Behavior modification, scheduled toileting, and prompted voiding reduce urinary incontinence in people with dementia.

Implications for Nursing Practice

- Effective management of patients with Alzheimer's disease requires a multifaceted approach including drugs specific for the disease, as well as for behavioral problems related to the disease.
- It is essential to consider the needs of the caregiver when planning care for the patient with dementia.

Reference for Evidence

Review: Pharmacologic and nonpharmacologic interventions improve outcomes in patients with dementia and for their caregivers, *ACP Journal Club* 135:94, 2001.

Patients with AD may be hospitalized for other health care problems. Patients with AD are subject to acute and other chronic illnesses and may require surgical interventions. Their inability to communicate symptoms of health problems places the responsibility for assessment and diagnosis on caregivers and health care professionals. Hospitalization of the patient with AD can be a traumatic event for both the patient and the caregiver and can precipitate a worsening of the disease or delirium. Patients with AD hospitalized in the acute care setting will need to be observed more closely because of concerns for safety, frequently oriented to place and time, and given reassurance. The use of the consistent nurses may be helpful in reducing anxiety or disruptive behavior.

Ambulatory and Home Care. Currently, family members and friends care for the majority of individuals who suffer from AD in their homes. Others with AD reside in various facilities, including long-term care and assisted living facilities. Care for these individuals requires further research to identify optimal methods for providing quality of life. A facility that is good for one person may not be suitable for another. Also, what is helpful for a person at one point in the disease process may be completely different from what is best when the disease progresses.

Patients with AD progress through the stages at variable rates. The nursing care needs of the patient with AD change as the disease progresses, emphasizing the need for regular assessment, monitoring, and support. Regardless of the setting, the severity of the problems and the amount of care required intensify over time. The specific manifestations of the disease will depend on the area of the brain involved. Nursing care is focused on decreasing clinical manifestations, preventing harm, and supporting the patient and caregiver through the disease process.

In the mild cognitive impairment phase, memory aids (e.g., calendars) may be beneficial. During this phase depression is likely to occur. Depression is related to the diagnosis of an incurable disorder, as well as the impact of the disease on activities of daily living (e.g., driving, socializing with friends, participating in hobbies or recreational activities). Drug therapy with cholinesterase inhibitors appears to be most effective during the early stages of AD. However, not all patients will show improvement. Drugs must be taken on a regular basis. Because memory is one of the key functions to be altered early in AD, drug compliance may be challenging.

Following the initial diagnosis, patients need to be aware that the progression of the disease is variable. Effective management of the disease can slow the progress of the disease and decrease the burden on the patient, caregiver, and family. However, decisions related to care should be made with the patient, family members, and the health care team early in the disease. The nurse has a role in advising the patient and the caregiver to initiate health care and advanced directives and decisions while the patient still has the capacity to do so. This can ease the burden for the caregiver as the disease progresses.

Adult day care is one of the options available to the person with AD. Although programs vary in size, structure, physical environment, and degree of experience of staff, the common goals of all day care programs are to provide respite for the family and a protective environment for the patient. During the early and middle stages of AD the person can still benefit from stimulating activities that encourage independence and decision making in a protective environment. Graded assistance, practice, and positive

NURSING CARE PLAN 58-2

Caregiver of the Patient with Alzheimer's Disease

EXPECTED PATIENT OUTCOMES	NURSING INTERVENTIONS and *RATIONALES*
NURSING DIAGNOSIS	**Caregiver role strain** *related to* grieving the family member's illness, change in role, and pressure from unrelieved caregiving *as manifested by* statements about stress and inadequate resources to provide care and worry about having to put the family member in a long-term care facility.
• Seeking of appropriate assistance by caregiver • Satisfactory care to the person with Alzheimer's disease	• Assess health status of caregiver *to determine if health planning is needed.* • Refer for medical evaluation when appropriate. • Discuss effects of caregiving with the caregiver *to determine status of caregiver and to enable open discussion of needs.* • Encourage visits and help from other family members *to provide support and relief to caregiver as needed.* • Acknowledge caregiver's fears of being unable to care for family member *to demonstrate empathy and awareness of this fear.* • Provide financial or social service referrals *to assist caregiver with planning for long-term care.* • Counsel and support caregiver if patient is placed in a long-term care facility to *allay guilt and reinforce services the patient now requires.*
NURSING DIAGNOSIS	**Social isolation** *related to* diminishing social relationships, behavioral problems of patient with Alzheimer's disease, and underdeveloped social support system *as manifested by* feelings of abandonment and uselessness, behavior changes, inability to make decisions or concentrate.
• Satisfactory contact with significant others or members of a support group	• Assess past social network and diversional activities *to determine size and scope of network and personal interests.* • Assess social support system of family and willingness and ability to participate in care *to develop care alternatives.* • Assist in planning respite care *to enable caregiver to continue with important activities and social contacts.* • Refer to social services *for realistic appraisal of financial resources for respite care and for linkage to community resources.* • Provide information regarding available support groups (e.g., Alzheimer's Association) *because these groups can meet socialization, recreational, and educational needs of caregiver.*
NURSING DIAGNOSIS	**Anxiety** *related to* uncertain outcome, perceived powerlessness, possible change in role functioning, behavioral problems of the person with Alzheimer's disease, and financial insecurity *as manifested by* apprehension, helplessness, fear, irritability, forgetfulness, inability to concentrate.
• Decreased anxiety • Sense of control of situation	• Assess past roles of patient with Alzheimer's disease and of caregiver *to determine extent of role changes required of caregiver.* • Document changes in role expectations and refer to community resources or provide instruction as needed; assess knowledge of behavioral management techniques and instruct as appropriate; assist caregiver in problem-solving techniques *to ensure that caregiver has skills to manage changing roles and patient status.* • Refer to appropriate agencies as indicated for complete list of community resources and possible sources of financial aid *to relieve anxiety related to financial insecurity.*
NURSING DIAGNOSIS	**Ineffective health maintenance** *related to* unrelieved caregiving responsibilities, fatigue, and chronic stress *as manifested by* failure to care for self.
• Optimal health • Appropriate health practices for age and sex	• Assess physical and emotional health status of caregiver *to determine if problem is present and to plan appropriate interventions.* • Collaborate with caregiver in planning interventions in major identified problem areas *to prevent further deterioration of health.* • Assist with planning of continued care of patient *so that caregiver's personal health needs can be pursued.* • Emphasize need for maintaining own health *to avoid increasing the complexity of the caregiving situation.*

EVIDENCE-BASED PRACTICE
Reality Orientation for Patients with Dementia

Clinical Problem

Is reality orientation effective as a therapy for elderly patients with dementia?

Best Clinical Practice

- Reality orientation (presentations of orientation information such as time, place, person) provides the person with dementia with a greater understanding of his or her surroundings, possibly resulting in an improved sense of control and self-esteem.
- Reality orientation has positive benefits on both cognition and behavior for patients with dementia.

Implications for Nursing Practice

- Nurses can use reality orientation in taking care of patients with dementia.
- Reality orientation can improve the quality of life of confused older adults.
- Continued reinforcement of reality orientation must be ongoing.

Reference for Evidence

Spector A et al: Reality orientation for dementia, *Cochrane Database Syst Rev*, issue 3, 2002.

---

reinforcement can help patients increase their functional independence.[20] The patient returns home tired, content, less frustrated, and ready to be with the family. The respite from the demands of care allows the caregiver to be more responsive to the patient's needs.

Although adult day care may delay the transition, the demands on the caregiver eventually exceed the resources, and the person with AD may be placed in a long-term care facility. Special units to care for persons with AD are becoming increasingly common in long-term care settings. The Alzheimer's unit is designed to be a safer environment for patients with AD. Although there are a variety of these units, many are characterized by spaces that allow the patient to walk freely on the unit yet are closed to prevent patients from wandering.

As the patient with AD progresses to the late stages (severe impairment) of AD, there is increased difficulty with the most basic functions, including walking and talking. Total care is required.

Specific problems relate to the care of the patient with AD across the phases of the disease. These problems are described in the following text.

Behavioral problems. Behavioral disturbances occur in about 90% of patients with AD. Behavioral problems can include repetitiveness (asking the same question repeatedly), delusions (false beliefs), illusions, hallucinations, agitation, aggression, altered sleeping patterns, and wandering. Many times these behaviors are unpredictable and challenge caregivers. Caregivers need to be aware that these behaviors are not intentional and are often difficult to control. Behavioral symptoms often lead to the placement of patients in institutional care settings.

Behaviors do not occur in a vacuum and are often in response to a precipitating factor (e.g., pain, frustration, temperature extremes, anxiety). Controlling the environment to reduce stimuli is the first step in behavior management. This includes identifying factors that can trigger behavior disruptions. Extremes in temperature, as well as excessive noise, may result in behavior change. The use of consistent routines may help to manage behavioral symptoms. Using touch and eye contact when communicating with the patient can have benefit in terms of orienting the patient.

Other strategies can be employed to deal with difficult behavior. These include redirection, distraction, and reassurance. For the patient who is restless or agitated, redirecting would involve having the patient perform activities such as sweeping, raking, or dusting. Examples of strategies to distract the agitated patient might include snacks, car rides, porch swing, rocker, favorite music or videotapes, looking at family photographs, or walking. Repetitive activities, songs, poems, music, massage, aromas, or a favorite object can be soothing to some patients. Reassuring involves letting the patient know that he or she will be protected from danger, harm, or embarrassment.

When nonpharmacologic therapies are ineffective or there is concern about self-injury, disruptive behavior may be treated by medications (see Table 58-9). However, many of these drugs have adverse side effects that can be distressing for the patient and caregiver. Thus the side effects of the drugs are weighed against the distress and potential safety concerns for the patient created by the behavior. As verbal skills decline, the caregiver and nurse may need to rely more on the patient's body language to anticipate care needs.

Safety. The person with AD is at risk for a number of problems related to personal safety. These include injury from falls, injury from ingesting dangerous substances, wandering, injury to others and self with sharp objects, fire or burns, and inability to respond to crisis situations.[22] These concerns require careful attention to the home environment to minimize risk, as well as the need for supervision. As the patient's cognitive function declines over time, the patient may have difficulty navigating physical spaces and interpreting environmental cues. Stairwells must be well lit. Handrails should be graspable with the end of rail shaped differently to alert the patient that it is the end of the stairway. Carpets should have their edges tacked down, and throw rugs should be removed. Polished floor surfaces and linoleum can predispose to falls. Extension cords should be removed because the patient may trip over them. In the bathroom, nonskid mats should be used in the tub or shower, and handrails should be installed in the bath and commode. The nurse can assist the caregiver to evaluate the home environment with safety in mind.

Wandering is a major concern for caregivers. Wandering may be due to loss of memory, side effects of drugs, an expression of a physical or emotional need, restlessness, curiosity, or stimuli that trigger memories of earlier routines.[23] Similar to other behaviors, the nurse should observe for factors or events that may precipitate wandering. For example, the patient may be sensitive to stress and tension in the environment. In such cases, wandering may reflect an attempt to leave the environment. AD patients who tend to wander can be registered with Safe Return, a federally supported program through the Alzheimer's Association. The Safe Return program includes identification products (e.g., wallet cards), a national photo/information database, a 24-hour toll-free emergency crisis line, local chapter support, and wandering behavior education and training for caregivers and families.[10]

Pain management. Because of difficulties with oral and written language associated with AD, patients may have difficulty expressing physical complaints, including pain. The nurse must rely on other clues, including the patient's behavior. Pain can result in alterations in the patient's behavior, such as increased vocalization, agitation, withdrawal, and changes in function. Similar to other patients, pain should be treated with drug therapies and the patient's response monitored.

Eating and swallowing difficulties. Loss of interest in food and decreased ability to feed self *(feeding apraxia)*, as well as comorbid conditions, can result in significant nutritional deficiencies in the patient with AD. In long-term care facilities, inadequate assistance with feeding may further add to the problem.

Pureed foods, thickened liquids, and nutritional supplements can be used when chewing and swallowing become problematic for the patient. Patients may need to be reminded to chew their food and to swallow. Dietary restrictions such as a low-salt diet are eased to increase the patient's appetite. Patients need a quiet and unhurried environment for eating. Distractions at mealtimes, including the television, should be avoided. Low lighting, music, and simulated nature sounds may improve eating behaviors.[19] Easy-grip eating utensils and finger foods may allow the patient to self-feed. Liquids should be offered frequently.

When oral feeding is not possible, alternative routes may be explored. Nasogastric (NG) feeding may be used for short periods. However, for the long term the NG tube is uncomfortable and may add further to the patient's agitation. A percutaneous endoscopic gastrostomy (PEG) tube provides another option. Little long-term benefit including increased longevity or reduced complications has been noted in patients receiving PEG feedings.[24] In addition, patients with AD are particularly vulnerable to aspiration of feeding formula and tube dislodgment. The potential positive outcomes to be gained from nutritional therapies are considered in light of overall outcome goals and potential adverse effects of the specific therapy. Nutritional support therapies are described in Chapter 39.

Oral care. In the late stages of AD, the patient will be unable to perform oral self-care. With decreased tooth brushing and flossing, dental problems are likely to occur. Because of swallowing difficulties, patients may pocket food in the mouth, adding to the potential for tooth decay. Dental caries and tooth abscess can add to patient discomfort or pain and subsequently may increase agitation. The mouth should be inspected regularly and mouth care provided to those patients unable to do self-care.

Infection prevention. Urinary tract infection and pneumonia are the most common infections to occur in patients with AD. Such infections are ultimately the cause of death in many patients with AD. Because of feeding and swallowing problems, the patient with AD is at risk for aspiration pneumonia. Immobility can also predispose to pneumonia. Reduced fluid intake, prostate hyperplasia in men, poor hygiene, and urinary drainage devices (e.g., catheter) can predispose to bladder infection. Manifestations of infection including change in behavior, fever, cough (pneumonia), and pain on urination (bladder) are evaluated and appropriately treated.

Skin care. It is important to monitor the patient's skin over time. Rashes, areas of redness, and skin breakdown should be noted and treated as appropriate. In the late stages, incontinence along with immobility and undernutrition can place the patient at risk for skin breakdown. The skin should be kept dry and clean and the patient's position changed regularly to avoid areas of pressure over bony prominences.

Elimination problems. During the middle and late stages of AD, urinary and fecal incontinence become problems. If possible, habit or behavioral retraining of bladder and bowel function (e.g., scheduled toileting) may help decrease episodes of incontinence. Drug therapy including oxybutynin (Ditropan) may decrease bladder excitability and improve control. For women, estrogen cream may be helpful if atrophic vaginitis is present.

A variety of approaches may be used to help decrease problems with constipation. Constipation may be due to immobility, dietary intake (e.g., reduced fiber intake), and decreased fluid intake. Increasing dietary fiber, fiber supplements, and stool softeners are the first lines of management. The combination of aging, other health problems, and swallowing difficulties may increase the risk of complications associated with the use of mineral oil, stimulants, osmotic agents, and enemas. Management of constipation is discussed in Chapter 41.

Caregiver support. AD is a disease that disrupts all aspects of personal and family life. Persons caring for the person with AD spend significantly more time on caregiving tasks than do people caring for individuals with other illnesses.[15,22] Caregivers of patients with AD also exhibit more adverse consequences in terms of the impact on their employment, mental and physical health, family conflict, and caregiver strain. Caregivers with a history of depression may have greater difficulty in adjusting to the demands placed on them. Suggested caregiver needs based on disease stage are provided in Table 58-11.

As the disease progresses, the relationship of the caregiver to the patient changes. Family roles may be altered or reversed (e.g., son caring for father). A range of decisions must be made including when to tell the patient about the diagnosis, when to have the patient stop driving or doing activities that might be dangerous, when to ask for assistance, and when to place the patient with AD in adult day care or long-term care facility. With early onset AD, the adult is affected during his or her most productive years in terms of career and family. The consequences can be devastating for the individual and the family.

Sexual relations for couples are also seriously affected by AD. As the disease progresses, sexual interest may decline for both the patient and the partner. A number of reasons account for this, including caregiver fatigue, as well as memory impairment and episodes of incontinence in the patient with AD. It is also possible for the patient to become very sexually driven as the disease progresses and the patient becomes more uninhibited.

The nurse should work with the caregiver to determine stressors and strategies to reduce the burden of caregiving. For example, the nurse should ask which behaviors are most disruptive to family life and remember that this is likely to change over time as the disease progresses. Establishing what the caregiver views as most disruptive or distressful can help to establish priorities for care. Risk to the safety of the patient and caregiver is given high priority. It is also important to assess what the caregiver's expectations are regarding the patient's behavior. Are the expectations reasonable given the progression of the disease? Working with the caregiver to identify risk factors for complications including behavioral problems is an important responsibility of the nurse.

Caregivers, most of whom are women, may be older adults themselves. Caregiving stress or burden can have adverse outcomes for their health, especially for those who have chronic health problems. Adult children are often caregivers. The impact

TABLE 58-11 Family & Caregiver Teaching Guide
Alzheimer's Disease

Mild Stage

1. Confirm the diagnosis. Many treatable (and potentially reversible) conditions can mimic Alzheimer's disease (see Table 58-3).
2. Get the person to stop driving. Confusion and poor judgment can impair driving skills and potentially put others at risk.
3. Encourage activities such as visiting with friends and family, listening to music, participating in hobbies, and exercising.
4. Provide cues in the home, establish a routine, and determine specific location where essential items (e.g., glasses) need to be kept.
5. Do not correct misstatements or faulty memory.
6. Register with Safe Return, a program established by the Alzheimer's Association to locate individuals who may wander from their homes.
7. Make plans for the future in terms of care options, financial concerns, and personal preference for care.

Moderate Stage

1. Install door locks for patient safety.
2. Provide protective wear for urinary and fecal incontinence.
3. Ensure that the home has good lighting, install handrails in stairways and bathroom, and remove area rugs or ensure that they are tacked down.
4. Label drawers and faucets (hot and cold) to ensure safety.
5. Develop strategies such as distraction and diversion to cope with behavioral problems. Identify and reduce potential triggers (e.g., reduce stress, extremes in temperature) for disruptive behavior.
6. Provide memory triggers, such as pictures of family and friends.

Late Stage

1. Provide a regular schedule for toileting to reduce incontinence.
2. Provide care to meet needs, including oral care and skin care.
3. Monitor diet and fluid intake to ensure their adequacy.
4. Continue communication through talking and touching.
5. Consider placement in a long-term care facility when providing total care becomes too difficult.

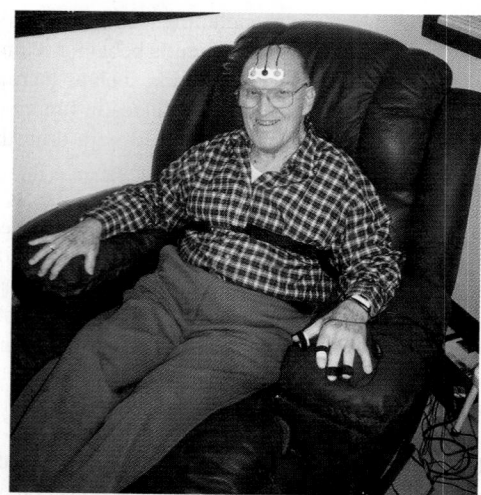

FIG. 58-5 Biofeedback can be used to teach relaxation techniques to caregivers.

■ Evaluation

Expected outcomes for the patient with AD are addressed in the NCP 58-1. Expected outcomes for the caregiver of a patient with AD are addressed in NCP 58-2.

OTHER NEURODEGENERATIVE DISEASES

Parkinson's disease and Huntington's disease are both neurodegenerative diseases (see Chapter 57). Both diseases are chronic, progressive, and incurable. Despite differences in the etiology and pathophysiology of these diseases, both are associated with the development of dementia in the later stages of disease.

Lewy body disease is a condition characterized by the presence of Lewy bodies (intraneural cytoplasmic inclusions) in the brainstem and cortex. The disease has features of both AD and Parkinson's disease. Patients with this form of dementia exhibit disabling mental impairment progressing to dementia, fluctuation in cognitive function, visual hallucinations, and features of Parkinson's disease, especially rigidity. The diagnostic criteria for Lewy body dementia is based on clinical signs and symptoms and confirmed at autopsy by histologic examination of brain tissue.

Creutzfeldt-Jakob disease (CJD) is a rare and fatal brain disorder thought to be caused by a prion protein. A *prion* is a small infectious pathogen containing protein but lacking nucleic acids. Worldwide, sporadic CJD affects one in a million individuals each year.

There are three types of CJD: sporadic CJD, hereditary CJD, and acquired CJD. A variant of CJD (vCJD) was first described in the mid-1980s. The source of this infection appeared to be beef used in baby food preparations obtained from animals contaminated with bovine spongiform encephalopathy, which is also called *mad cow disease*. Worldwide, approximately 110 cases of vCJD have been identified.[25]

The earliest symptom of the disease may be memory impairment and behavior changes. The disease progresses rapidly with mental deterioration, involuntary movements (muscle jerks), weakness in the limbs, blindness, and eventually coma. There is no diagnostic test for CJD. Only autopsy and examination of brain tissue can confirm the diagnosis. There is no treatment for CJD. Emphasis is on reducing the risk of acquiring CJD via food products.

of the caregiving role can be overwhelming for adult children caregivers. They may need to relocate their family or their parent(s), juggle employment and family responsibilities, face financial strain, and realize the "loss" of their own lives.

Support groups for caregivers and family members have been formed throughout the United States and other countries to provide an atmosphere of understanding and to give current information about the disease itself and related topics such as safety, legal, ethical, and financial issues. Nurses often receive personal and professional satisfaction in participating in such support groups. Other strategies related to stress management including relaxation and biofeedback training (Fig. 58-5) are discussed in Chapters 7 and 8.

The Alzheimer's Association has many educational and support systems available to help family caregivers. This organization can provide help in many different ways to caregivers.

Pick's disease, a type of frontotemporal dementia, is a rare brain disorder characterized by disturbances in behavior, sleep, personality, and eventually memory. The major distinguishing characteristic between these disorders and AD is marked symmetric lobar atrophy of the temporal and/or frontal lobes. The disease is relentless in its progression, which may ultimately include language impairment, erratic behavior, and dementia. Because of the strange behavior associated with Pick's disease and frontotemporal dementia, psychiatrists often see these patients first. There is no specific treatment. The diagnosis can be confirmed at autopsy.

Normal Pressure Hydrocephalus

Normal pressure hydrocephalus is an uncommon disorder characterized by an obstruction in the flow of CSF, which causes a buildup of this fluid in the brain. Symptoms of the condition include dementia, urinary incontinence, and difficulty in walking. Meningitis, encephalitis, or head injury may cause the condition. If diagnosed early in the disease, normal-pressure hydrocephalus is treatable by surgery in which a shunt is inserted to divert the fluid away from the brain.

CRITICAL THINKING EXERCISES

Case Study
Alzheimer's Disease

Patient Profile. Mr. Y., an 80-year-old African American man, was diagnosed with AD 3 years ago. Today his 78-year-old wife brings him to the emergency department because he wandered from his home, fell, and injured his left hip.

Subjective Data
- Can state his name
- Confused as to place and time
- Denies memory of wandering or falling
- Agitated, trying to get up
- Denies pain

Objective Data
Physical Examination
- Left leg shorter than right leg
- Tense and anxious

Diagnostic Studies
- X-ray of left hip indicates a fracture
- Mini-Mental State Examination shows cognitive impairment

CRITICAL THINKING QUESTIONS

1. What is the pathogenesis of AD?
2. What precipitating factors may have resulted in Mr. Y's fall?
3. What precautions need to be taken regarding the inpatient care of Mr. Y?
4. What teaching plan should be developed for Mr. Y and his wife?
5. Write one or more appropriate nursing diagnoses based on the assessment data presented. Are there any collaborative problems?

Nursing Research Issues

1. What nursing interventions can be used in long-term care facilities to reduce agitated behaviors in patients with dementia?
2. What specific factors can be used to rate a patient's risk of developing delirium while in the acute care facility?
3. What strategies can be used to reduce burden and enhance coping skills in caregivers of patients with AD?
4. Does early intervention in patients with AD reduce the progression of the disease?

REVIEW QUESTIONS

The number of the question corresponds to the same-numbered objective at the beginning of the chapter.

1. Which of the following patients is most at risk for developing delirium?
   a. A 50-year-old woman with cholecystitis
   b. A 19-year-old man with a fractured femur
   c. A 42-year-old woman having an elective hysterectomy
   d. A 78-year-old man admitted to the medical unit with complications related to congestive heart failure

2. Dementia is defined as a
   a. syndrome that results only in memory loss.
   b. disease associated with abrupt changes in behavior.
   c. disease that is always due to reduced blood flow to the brain.
   d. syndrome characterized by cognitive dysfunction and loss of memory.

3. Vascular dementia is associated with
   a. transient ischemic attacks.
   b. bacterial or viral infection of neuronal tissue.
   c. cognitive changes secondary to cerebral ischemia.
   d. abrupt changes in cognitive function that are irreversible.

4. The clinical diagnosis of dementia is based on
   a. brain biopsy.
   b. electroencephalogram.
   c. patient history and cognitive assessment.
   d. CT or MRS.

5. The early stage of AD is characterized by
   a. no noticeable change in behavior.
   b. memory problems and mild confusion.
   c. increased time spent sleeping or in bed.
   d. incontinence, agitation, and wandering behavior.

6. A major goal of treatment for the patient with AD is to
   a. maintain patient safety.
   b. maintain or increase body weight.
   c. return to a higher level of self-care.
   d. enhance functional ability over time.

7. Creutzfeldt-Jakob disease is characterized by
   a. remissions and exacerbations over many years.
   b. memory impairment, muscle jerks, and blindness.
   c. parkinsonian symptoms including muscle rigidity and tremors at rest.
   d. increased intracranial pressure secondary to decreased CSF drainage.

REFERENCES

1. Inouye SK: Assessment and management of delirium in hospitalized older patients, *Ann Long-Term Care* 8:53, 2000.
2. Burt T: Donepezil and related cholinesterase inhibitors as mood and behavioral controlling agents, *Curr Psychiatry Rep* 2:473, 2000.
3. Tune LE, Egeli S: Acetylcholine and delirium, *Dement Geriatr Cogn Disord* 10:342, 1999.
4. Broadhurst C, Wilson K: Immunology of delirium: new opportunities for treatment and research, *Br J Psychiatry* 179:288, 2001.
5. Hosoda S et al: Psychiatric symptoms related to interferon therapy for chronic hepatitis C: clinical features and prognosis, *Psychiatry Clin Neurosci* 54:565, 2000.
6. Henry M: Descending into delirium, *Am J Nurs* 102:49, 2002.
7. McCusker J et al: Environmental risk factors for delirium in hospitalized older people, *J Am Geriatr Soc* 49:1327, 2001.
8. Inouye SK et al: A multicomponent intervention to prevent delirium in hospitalized older patients, *N Engl J Med* 340:669, 1999.
9. Fleming KD, Adams AC, Petersen RC: Dementia: diagnosis and evaluation, *Mayo Clin Proc* 70:1093, 1995.
10. Alzheimer's Association: About Alzheimer's. Available at *www.alz.org/AboutAD/overview.htm* (accessed August 22, 2002).
11. The Canadian Study of Health and Aging Working Group: The incidence of dementia in Canada, *Neurology* 55:66, 2000.
12. Seshadri S et al: Plasma homocysteine as a risk factor for dementia and Alzheimer's disease, *N Engl J Med* 346:476, 2002.
13. Petersen RC et al: Practice parameter: early detection of dementia: mild cognitive impairment (an evidence-based review), *Neurology* 56:1133, 2001.
14. Knopman DS: Practice parameter: diagnosis of dementia (an evidence-based review), *Neurology* 56:1143, 2001.
15. National Institute on Aging, NIH: 2000 progress report on Alzheimer's disease, NIH Publication No. 00-4859. Available at *www.alzheimers.org/pubs/prog00.htm* (accessed August 22, 2002).
16. Sinha S: The role of beta-amyloid in Alzheimer's disease, *Med Clin North Am* 86:629, 2002.
17. Pratico D et al: Increase of brain oxidative stress in mild cognitive impairment: a possible predictor of Alzheimer disease, *Arch Neurol* 59:972, 2002.
18. Sramek JJ et al: Acetylcholinesterase inhibitors for the treatment of Alzheimer's disease, *Ann Long Term Care* 9:15, 2001.
19. Blais MA et al: The treatment and management of Alzheimer's disease, *Clin Geriatr* 9:58, 2001.
20. Doody RS: Practice parameter: management of dementia (an evidence-based review), *Neurology* 56:1154, 2001.
21. Bonner LT, Peskind ER: Pharmacologic treatments of dementia, *Med Clin North Am* 86:657, 2002.
22. Gitlin LN et al: A randomized, controlled trial of a home environmental intervention: effect on efficacy and upset in caregivers and on daily function of persons with dementia, *Gerontologist* 41:4, 2001.
23. Alzheimer's wandering, Mayo Clinic. Available at *www.mayohealth.org/mayo/9901/htm/wandering.htm* (accessed August 22, 2002).
24. Braun UK et al: Malnutrition in patients with severe dementia: is there a place for PEG tube feeding, *Ann Long Term Care* 9:47, 2001.
25. Taylor DM: Current perspectives on bovine spongiform encephalopathy and variant Creutzfeldt-Jakob disease, *Clin Microbiol Infect* 8:332, 2002.

RESOURCES

Administration on Aging (AoA)
330 Independence Avenue, SW
Washington, DC 20201
202-619-0724
www.aoa.dhhs.gov

Alzheimer's Association
919 North Michigan Avenue, Suite 1100
Chicago, IL 60611-1676
800-272-3900 or 312-335-8700
Fax: 312-335-1110
www.alz.org

Alzheimer's Disease Education and Referral Center
P.O. Box 8250
Silver Spring, MD 20907-8250
800-438-4380
www.alzheimers.org

American Association for Geriatric Psychiatry
7910 Woodmont Avenue, Suite 1050
Bethesda, MD 20814-3004
301-654-7850
Fax: 301-654-4137
www.aagponline.org

American Association of Retired Persons
601 E Street, NW
Washington, DC 20049
800-424-3410
www.aarp.org

National Alliance for Caregiving
4729 Montgomery Lane, Suite 642
Bethesda, MD 20814
www.caregiving.org

National Council on the Aging (NCOA)
409 Third Street SW, Suite 200
Washington, DC 20024
202-479-1200
Fax: 202-479-0735
www.ncoa.org

National Family Caregivers Association (NFCA)
10400 Connecticut Avenue, #500
Kensington, MD 20895-3944
800-896-3650
Fax: 301-942-2302
www.nfcacares.org

National Institute on Aging
Building 31, Room 5C27
31 Center Drive, MSC 2292
Bethesda, MD 20892
800-222-2225 or 301-496-1752
www.nia.nih.gov

National Institute of Mental Health (NIMH)
6001 Executive Boulevard
Room 8184, MSC 9663
Bethesda, MD 20892-9663
800-421-4211 or 301-443-4513
Fax: 301-443-4279
www.nimh.nih.gov

National Institute of Neurological Disorders and Strokes
NIH Neurological Institute
P.O. Box 5801
Bethesda, MD 20824
800-352-9424
www.ninds.nih.gov

National Mental Health Association
1021 Prince Street
2001 North Beauregard Street, 12th Floor
Alexandria, VA 22311
800-969-NMHA (6642) or 703-684-7722
Fax: 703-684-5968
www.nmha.org

For additional Internet resources, see the website for this book at *http://evolve.elsevier.com/Lewis/medsurg.*

CHAPTER 59

NURSING MANAGEMENT
Peripheral Nerve and Spinal Cord Problems

Catherine Warms

LEARNING OBJECTIVES

1. Explain the etiology, clinical manifestations, collaborative care, and nursing management of trigeminal neuralgia and Bell's palsy.
2. Explain the etiology, clinical manifestations, collaborative care, and nursing management of Guillain-Barré syndrome, botulism, tetanus, and neurosyphilis.
3. Describe the classification of spinal cord injuries and associated clinical manifestations.
4. Describe the clinical manifestations, collaborative care, and nursing management of spinal cord shock.
5. Correlate the clinical manifestations of spinal cord injury with the level of disruption and rehabilitation potential.
6. Describe the nursing management of the major physical and psychologic problems of the patient with a spinal cord injury.
7. Describe the effects of spinal cord injury on the older adult population.
8. Explain the types, clinical manifestations, collaborative care, and nursing management of spinal cord tumors.

KEY TERMS

anterior cord syndrome, p. 1612	neurogenic shock, p. 1611
autonomic dysreflexia, p. 1625	neurosyphilis, p. 1610
Bell's palsy, p. 1605	paraplegia, p. 1611
botulism, p. 1608	poikilothermism, p. 1614
Brown-Séquard syndrome, p. 1612	posterior cord syndrome, p. 1612
central cord syndrome, p. 1612	spinal shock, p. 1611
Guillain-Barré syndrome, p. 1606	tetanus, p. 1609
neurogenic bladder, p. 1626	tetraplegia, p. 1610
neurogenic bowel, p. 1627	trigeminal neuralgia, p. 1601

Cranial Nerve Disorders

Cranial nerve disorders are commonly classified as peripheral neuropathies. The 12 pairs of cranial nerves are considered the peripheral nerves of the brain. The disorders usually involve the motor or sensory (or both) branches of a single nerve (*mononeuropathies*). Causes of cranial nerve problems include tumors, trauma, infections, inflammatory processes, and idiopathic (unknown) causes. Two cranial nerve disorders are trigeminal neuralgia (tic douloureux) and acute peripheral facial paralysis (Bell's palsy).

TRIGEMINAL NEURALGIA

Etiology and Pathophysiology

Trigeminal neuralgia *(tic douloureux)* is a relatively uncommon cranial nerve disorder diagnosed in approximately 15,000 Americans each year. However, it is the most commonly diagnosed neuralgic condition. It is seen approximately twice as often in women as in men. The majority of cases (over 90%) are diagnosed

in individuals over the age of 40.[1] The trigeminal nerve is the fifth cranial nerve (CN V) and has both motor and sensory branches. In trigeminal neuralgia the sensory or afferent branches, primarily the maxillary and mandibular branches, are involved (Fig. 59-1).

The pathophysiology of trigeminal neuralgia is not fully understood. One theory is that compression of blood vessels, the superior cerebellar artery in particular, occurs, resulting in chronic irritation of the trigeminal nerve at the root entry zone. This irritation results in increased firing of the afferent or sensory fiber. Other factors that may result in neuralgia include herpesvirus infection, infection of teeth and jaw, and a brainstem infarct. The effectiveness of antiseizure drug therapy in reducing pain may be related to the ability of these drugs to stabilize the neuronal membrane and decrease paroxysmal afferent impulses of the nerve.[1]

Clinical Manifestations

The classic feature of trigeminal neuralgia is an abrupt onset of paroxysms of excruciating pain described as a burning, knifelike, or lightninglike shock in the lips, upper or lower gums, cheek, forehead, or side of the nose. Intense pain, twitching, grimacing, and frequent blinking and tearing of the eye occur during the acute attack (giving rise to the term *tic*). Some patients may experience facial sensory loss as well. The attacks are usually brief, lasting only seconds to 2 or 3 minutes, and are generally unilateral. Recurrences are unpredictable; they may occur several times a day or weeks or months apart. After the refractory (pain-free) period, a phenomenon known as *clustering* can occur. Clustering is characterized by a cycle of pain and refractoriness that continues for hours.

The painful episodes are usually initiated by a triggering mechanism of light cutaneous stimulation at a specific point (*trigger zone*) along the distribution of the nerve branches. Precipitating stimuli include chewing, teeth brushing, a hot or cold blast of air on the face, washing the face, yawning, or even talking. Touch and tickle seem to predominate as causative triggers rather than

Reviewed by Kathleen T. Lucke, RN, PhD, Assistant Professor, School of Nursing, University of Texas Health Science Center, San Antonio, Tex.

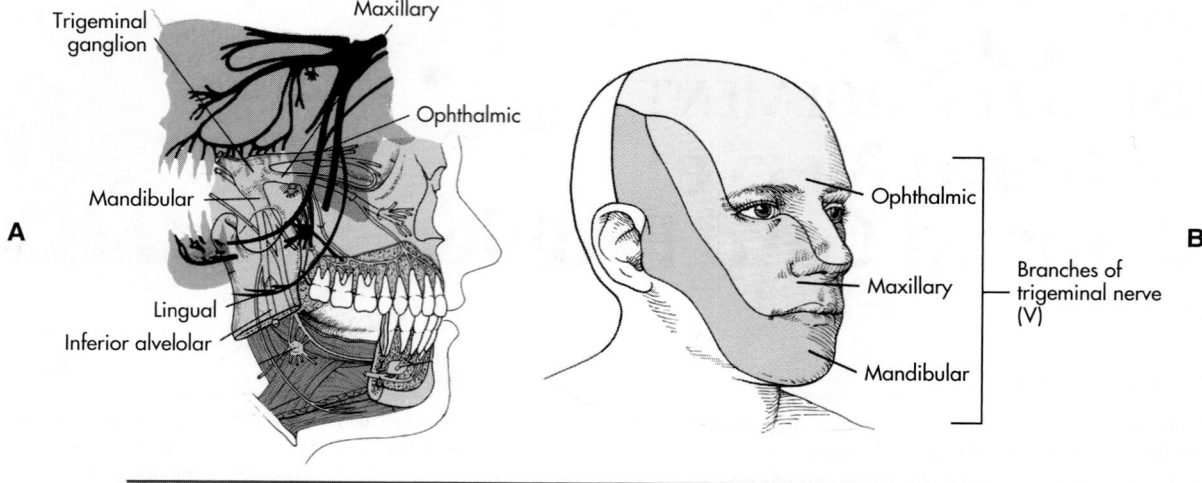

FIG. 59-1 **A,** Trigeminal (fifth cranial nerve and its three main divisions—the ophthalmic, maxillary, and mandibular nerves). **B,** Cutaneous innervation of the head.

pain or changes in temperature. As a result, the patient may eat improperly, neglect hygienic practices, wear a cloth over the face, and withdraw from interaction with other individuals. The patient may sleep excessively as a means of coping with the pain.

Although this condition is considered benign, the severity of the pain and the disruption of lifestyle can result in almost total physical and psychologic dysfunction or even suicide.

Diagnostic Studies

It is important to rule out other problems with similar manifestations, such as other forms of facial and cephalic neuralgias and pain arising from the sinuses, teeth, and jaws. In young adults with bilateral facial pain, a computed tomography (CT) scan is performed to rule out any lesions or vascular abnormalities, and a lumbar puncture and magnetic resonance imaging (MRI) are done to rule out multiple sclerosis. A complete neurologic assessment is done including audiologic evaluation, although results are usually normal. Additional tests used to rule out other pathologic conditions include electromyography (EMG), cerebrospinal fluid (CSF) analysis, arteriography, and myelography. Once the diagnosis is made, the goal of treatment is relief of pain either medically or surgically (Tables 59-1 and 59-2).

Collaborative Care

Drug Therapy. The majority of patients obtain adequate relief through antiseizure drugs such as carbamazepine (Tegretol), phenytoin (Dilantin), and valproate (Depakene). Carbamazepine is considered the first-line therapy for trigeminal neuralgia. By acting on sodium channels, carbamazepine and other antiseizure drugs lengthen the time needed for neuron repolarization, resulting in decreased neuron firing. Side effects of carbamazepine may include bone marrow suppression leading to blood abnormalities. Therefore routine complete blood cell (CBC) counts are required. Newer antiseizure drugs used in the management of trigeminal neuralgia include oxcarbazepine (Trileptal), gabapentin (Neurontin), lamotrigine (Lamictal), and topiramate (Topamax). These antiseizure drugs may prevent an acute attack or promote a remission of symptoms. Because drug therapy may not provide permanent pain relief, some patients may seek continued help by

TABLE **Collaborative Care**
59-1 **Trigeminal Neuralgia**
Diagnostic
History and physical examination
Audiologic evaluation
CT scan
MRI
EMG
CSF analysis
Arteriography
Posterior myelography
Collaborative Therapy
Drug therapy (e.g., phenytoin [Dilantin], carbamazepine [Tegretol], valproate [Depakene], oxcarbazepine [Trileptal], gabapentin [Neurontin], lamotrigine [Lamictal], topiramate [Topamax])
Local nerve blocking
Biofeedback
Surgical intervention (see Table 59-2)

CSF, Cerebrospinal fluid; *CT,* computed tomography; *EMG,* electromyography; *MRI,* magnetic resonance imaging.

numerous visits to otolaryngologists or from therapies such as acupuncture and megavitamins.

Conservative Therapy. Nerve blocking with local anesthetics is another treatment possibility. Local nerve blocking results in complete anesthesia of the area supplied by the injected branches. Relief of pain is temporary, lasting from 6 to 18 months. This treatment is usually tolerated well by older adults.

Biofeedback is another strategy that may be helpful for some patients. In addition to controlling the pain, the patient may experience a strong sense of personal control by mastering the technique and altering certain body functions. (Biofeedback is discussed in Chapter 7.)

Surgical Therapy. If a conservative approach including drug therapy is not effective, surgical therapy is available (see

TABLE 59-2	Surgical Interventions for Trigeminal Neuralgia	
PROCEDURE	**TECHNIQUE**	**BENEFIT**
Peripheral		
Glycerol rhizotomy (injection into one or more branches of the trigeminal nerve)	Chemical ablation	Total pain relief with sparing of touch and corneal reflex
Intracranial		
Percutaneous radiofrequency rhizotomy	Destruction of sensory fibers by low-voltage current	Total pain relief, sparing of touch and corneal reflex (increased risk for sensory changes)
Microvascular decompression (Jannetta procedure)	Lifting of artery pressing on nerve root in posterior fossa with wedge of sponge, leading to removal of pressure at nerve-root entry zone or removing the involved vessel	Pain relief without loss of sensation
Gamma knife radiosurgery	Technique that uses high doses of radiation focused on the trigeminal nerve root using stereotactic localization	Pain relief 1 day to 4 months post-treatment; noninvasive; no loss of sensation
Retrogasserian rhizotomy	Temporal craniotomy (sectioning of sensory root in middle cranial fossa)	Permanent anesthesia
Suboccipital craniotomy	Sectioning of sensory root of posterior fossa	Permanent anesthesia

Table 59-2). Glycerol rhizotomy is a percutaneous procedure. *Glycerol rhizotomy* consists of an injection of glycerol through the foramen ovale into the trigeminal cistern (Fig. 59-2). Glycerol rhizotomy is a more benign procedure with less sensory loss and fewer sensory aberrations than radiofrequency rhizotomy and with comparable or better pain relief. However, for some patients the pain will return over time.[2,3]

Percutaneous radiofrequency rhizotomy (electrocoagulation) and microvascular decompression afford the greatest relief of pain. *Percutaneous radiofrequency rhizotomy* consists of placing a needle into the trigeminal rootlets that are adjacent to the pons and destroying the area by means of a radiofrequency current. This can result in facial numbness (although some degree of sensation may be retained), corneal anesthesia, and trigeminal motor weakness. This procedure is easily performed with minimal risk to the patient and is based on the exchange of pain for numbness. The procedure is usually performed on an outpatient basis with few complications. It is tolerated well by older adults and avoids a major operative procedure in the high-risk patient.[2]

Microvascular decompression of the trigeminal nerve is another commonly used procedure for neuralgia. It is accomplished by displacing and repositioning blood vessels that appear to be compressing the nerve at the root entry zone where it exits the pons. This procedure relieves pain without residual sensory loss, but it is potentially dangerous, as is any surgery near the brainstem. Microvascular decompression has a long-term success rate equal to or superior to percutaneous procedures without the higher rate of permanent neurologic outcomes such as numbness. It is a safe procedure with an almost negligible mortality and low morbidity when performed in younger adults by a skilled surgeon.[2]

Gamma knife radiosurgery is another surgical treatment that is used for trigeminal neuralgia. Radiosurgery using the gamma knife provides precise radiation of the proximal trigeminal nerve identified on high-resolution imaging. This image-guided approach has been useful for both patients with persistent pain after other surgeries and as a primary surgical option.[3] Two other

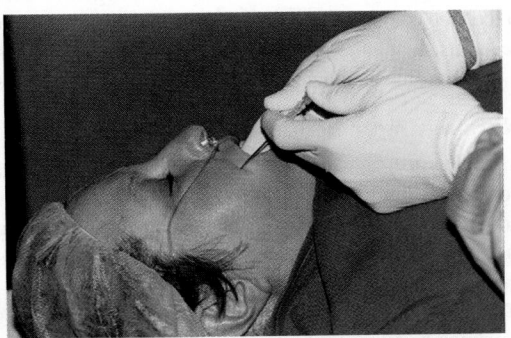
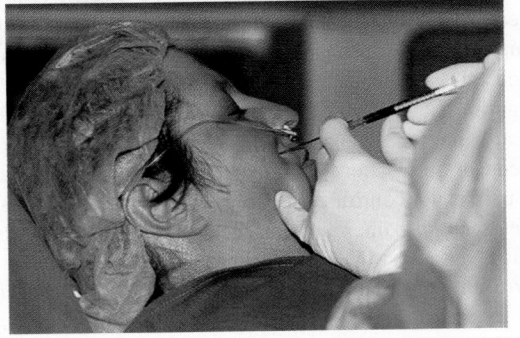

FIG. 59-2 A, Patient with trigeminal neuralgia having needle placed. B, Physician injecting glycerol.

intracranial procedures include the retrogasserian rhizotomy and suboccipital craniotomy (see Table 59-2).

NURSING MANAGEMENT
TRIGEMINAL NEURALGIA

■ Nursing Assessment

Assessment of the attacks, including the triggering factors, characteristics, frequency, and pain management techniques, helps the nurse plan for patient care. The nursing assessment should include the patient's nutritional status, hygiene (especially oral), and behavior (including withdrawal). Evaluation of the degree of pain and its effects on the patient's lifestyle, drug history, emotional state, and suicidal tendencies are other important factors.

■ Nursing Diagnoses

Nursing diagnoses for the patient with trigeminal neuralgia include, but are not limited to, the following:

- Acute pain *related to* inflammation or compression of the trigeminal nerve
- Imbalanced nutrition: less than body requirements *related to* fear of triggering pain by eating or chewing
- Anxiety *related to* uncertainty of timing and initiating event of pain and uncertainty regarding effectiveness of pain-relieving treatments
- Impaired oral mucous membrane *related to* unwillingness to practice oral hygiene measures secondary to potential for initiating pain
- Social isolation *related to* anxiety over pain attacks and desire to maintain nonstimulating environment

■ Planning

The overall goals are that the patient with trigeminal neuralgia will (1) be free of pain, (2) maintain adequate nutritional and oral hygiene status, (3) have minimal to no anxiety, and (4) return to normal or previous socialization and occupational activities.

■ Nursing Implementation

Health Promotion. Because the etiology of trigeminal neuralgia remains unknown, health promotion is directed at reducing recurrent episodes in those who have trigeminal neuralgia. Awareness and reduction of triggering events may be possible in some patients.

Acute Intervention. Patients with trigeminal neuralgia are treated primarily on an outpatient basis. Pain relief is primarily obtained by the administration of the recommended drug therapy. The nurse monitors the patient's response to therapy and notes any side effects. Strong narcotics such as morphine should be used cautiously because of the potential for addiction over time. Alternative pain relief measures, such as biofeedback, should be explored for the patient who is not a surgical candidate and whose pain is not controlled by other therapeutic measures. Careful assessment of pain, including history, pain relief, and drug dependency, can assist in selecting appropriate interventions.

Environmental management is essential during an acute period to lessen triggering stimuli. The room should be kept at an even, moderate temperature and free of drafts. A private room is preferred during an acute period. The nurse must use care to avoid touching the patient's face or jarring the bed. Many patients prefer to carry out their own care, fearing that someone else will inadvertently injure them.

The nurse must teach the patient about the importance of nutrition, hygiene, and oral care and convey understanding if previous oral neglect is apparent. The nurse should provide lukewarm water and soft cloths or cotton saturated with solutions not requiring rinsing for cleansing the face. A small, soft-bristled toothbrush or a warm mouthwash assists in promoting oral care. Hygiene activities are best carried out when analgesia is at its peak.

The patient will probably not engage in extensive conversation during the acute period. Alternative communication methods such as paper and pencil should be provided.

Food should be high in protein and calories and easy to chew. It should be served lukewarm and offered frequently. The diet should be individualized according to personal, cultural, and religious preferences. When oral intake is sharply reduced and the patient's nutritional status is compromised, a nasogastric tube can be inserted on the unaffected side for enteral feedings.

The nurse is responsible for instruction related to diagnostic studies to rule out other problems, such as multiple sclerosis, dental or sinus problems, and neoplasms, and for preoperative teaching if surgery is planned. The nurse may also need to reinforce the surgeon's instructions related to postoperative expectations; Appropriate teaching related to postoperative activities depends on the type of procedure planned (e.g., percutaneous, intracranial). The patient needs to know that he or she will be awake during local procedures so that he or she can cooperate when corneal and ciliary reflexes and facial sensations are checked. Patients are informed about the potential risk of postoperative facial numbness.

After the procedure the patient's pain is compared with the preoperative level. The corneal reflex, extraocular muscles, hearing, sensation, and facial nerve function are evaluated frequently (see Chapter 54). If there is impairment of the corneal reflex, special attention must be paid to eye protection. This includes the use of artificial tears or eye shields. General postoperative nursing care after a craniotomy is appropriate if intracranial surgery is performed. (Nursing care related to craniotomy is discussed in Chapter 55.) Diet and ambulation should be increased according to the patient's progress or specific orders.

After a radiofrequency percutaneous electrocoagulation procedure, an ice pack is applied to the jaw on the operative side for 3 to 5 hours. To avoid injuring the mouth, the patient should not chew on the operative side until sensation has returned.

Ambulatory and Home Care. Regular follow-up care should be planned. The patient needs instruction regarding the dosage and side effects of medications. Although relief of pain may be complete, the patient should be encouraged to keep environmental stimuli to a moderate level and to use stress reduction methods. The patient may have developed protective practices to prevent pain and may need counseling or psychiatric assistance in the readjustment, especially in reestablishing personal relationships. Herpes simplex infection (cold sores) can occur from manipulation of the gasserian ganglion. Treatment consists of antiviral agents such as acyclovir (Zovirax) (see Chapter 23).

Long-term management after surgical intervention depends on the residual effects of the type of procedure. If anesthesia is present or the corneal reflex is altered, the patient should be taught to (1) chew on the unaffected side; (2) avoid hot foods or beverages, which can burn the mucous membranes; (3) check the oral cavity after meals to remove food particles; (4) practice meticulous oral hygiene and continue with semiannual dental visits; (5) protect the face against extremes of temperature; (6) use an electric razor; and (7) wear a protective eye shield.

■ Evaluation

The expected outcomes are that the patient with trigeminal neuralgia will

- have decreased or relief from pain
- appear more comfortable and less anxious
- have normal facial sensation or expected paresthesias and anesthesias
- return to previous socialization and occupational activities

BELL'S PALSY

Etiology and Pathophysiology

Bell's palsy (peripheral facial paralysis, acute benign cranial polyneuritis) is a disorder characterized by a disruption of the motor branches of the facial nerve (CN VII) on one side of the face in the absence of any other disease such as a stroke. Bell's palsy is an acute, peripheral facial paresis of unknown cause. Each year approximately 20 per 100,000 individuals will be diagnosed with Bell's palsy. It can affect any age group, but it is more commonly seen in the 20- to 60-year-old age range. Despite its good prognosis, Bell's palsy leaves more than 8000 people a year in the United States with permanent, potentially disfiguring facial weakness.[4]

Although the exact etiology is not known, there is evidence that reactivated herpes simplex virus (HSV) may be involved in some cases. The reactivation of the HSV causes inflammation, edema, ischemia, and eventual demyelination of the nerve, creating pain and alterations in motor and sensory function.

Bell's palsy is considered benign with full recovery after 6 months in about 85% of patients, especially if treatment is instituted immediately. The remaining 15% of patients continue to be bothered by asymmetric movement of facial muscles.[4]

Clinical Manifestations

The onset of Bell's palsy is often accompanied by an outbreak of herpes vesicles in or around the ear. Patients may complain of pain around and behind the ear. In addition, manifestations may include fever, tinnitus, and hearing deficit. The paralysis of the motor branches of the facial nerve typically results in a flaccidity of the affected side of the face, with drooping of the mouth accompanied by drooling (Fig. 59-3). An inability to close the eyelid, with an upward movement of the eyeball when closure is attempted, is also evident. A widened *palpebral fissure* (the opening between the eyelids); flattening of the nasolabial fold; and inability to smile, frown, or whistle are also common. Unilateral loss of taste is common. Decreased muscle movement may alter chewing ability, and although some patients may experience a loss of tearing, many patients complain of excessive tearing. The muscle weakness causes the lower lid to turn out, allowing overflow of normal tear production. Pain may be present behind the ear on the affected side, especially before the onset of paralysis.

Complications can include psychologic withdrawal because of changes in appearance, malnutrition, dehydration, mucous membrane trauma, corneal abrasions, muscle stretching, and facial spasms and contractures.

Diagnostic Studies

The diagnosis of Bell's palsy is one of exclusion. There is no definitive test. The diagnosis and prognosis are indicated by observation of the typical pattern of onset and signs and the testing of percutaneous nerve excitability by EMG.

Collaborative Care

Methods of treatment for Bell's palsy include moist heat, gentle massage, and electrical stimulation of the nerve and prescribed exercises. Stimulation may maintain muscle tone and prevent atrophy. Care is primarily focused on relief of symptoms, prevention of complications, and protection of the eye on the affected side.

Drug Therapy. Corticosteroids, especially prednisone, are started immediately, and the best results are obtained if corticosteroids are initiated before paralysis is complete.[4] When the patient improves to the point that the corticosteroids are no longer necessary, they should be tapered off over a 2-week period. Usually, the corticosteroid treatment decreases the edema and pain, but mild analgesics can be used if necessary. Because the HSV is implicated in approximately 70% of cases of Bell's palsy, treatment with acyclovir (Zovirax), alone or in conjunction with prednisone, is used.[4] Additional antiviral agents, including valacyclovir (Valtrex) and famciclovir (Famvir), have also been used in the management of Bell's palsy.

NURSING MANAGEMENT
BELL'S PALSY

■ Nursing Assessment

Early recognition of the possibility of Bell's palsy is important. Because HSV is a possible etiologic factor, any person who is prone to herpes simplex should be alerted to seek health care if pain occurs in or around the ear. Assessment of facial muscles for any signs of weakness should also be done. Careful recording of assessment data provides information related to the progress of the syndrome.

■ Nursing Diagnoses

The nursing diagnoses for the patient with Bell's palsy may include, but are not limited to, the following:
- Acute pain *related to* the inflammation of CN VII (facial nerve)
- Imbalanced nutrition: less than body requirements *related to* inability to chew secondary to muscle weakness
- Risk for injury (corneal abrasion) *related to* inability to blink
- Disturbed body image *related to* change in facial appearance secondary to facial muscle weakness

■ Planning

The overall goals are that the patient with Bell's palsy will (1) be pain free or have pain controlled, (2) maintain adequate nutritional status, (3) maintain appropriate oral hygiene, (4) not experience injury to the eye, (5) return to normal or previous

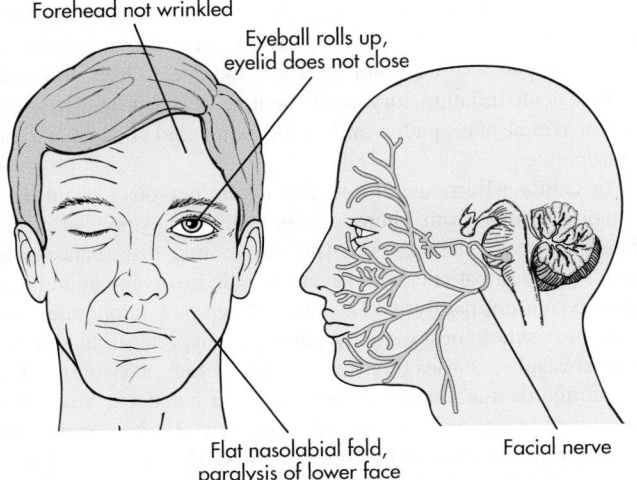

Forehead not wrinkled

Eyeball rolls up, eyelid does not close

Flat nasolabial fold, paralysis of lower face

Facial nerve

FIG. 59-3 Bell's palsy: facial characteristics.

perception of body image, and (6) be optimistic about disease outcome.

■ Nursing Implementation

The patient with Bell's palsy is treated on an outpatient basis. The following interventions are used throughout the course of the disease. Mild analgesics can relieve pain. Hot wet packs can reduce the discomfort of herpetic lesions, aid circulation, and relieve pain. The face should be protected from cold and drafts because trigeminal *hyperesthesia* (extreme sensitivity to pain or touch) may accompany the syndrome. Maintenance of good nutrition is important. The patient should be taught to chew on the unaffected side of the mouth to avoid trapping food and to enjoy the taste of food. Thorough oral hygiene must be carried out after each meal to prevent the development of parotitis, caries, and periodontal disease from accumulated residual food.

Dark glasses may be worn for protective and cosmetic reasons. Artificial tears (methylcellulose) should be instilled frequently during the day to prevent drying of the cornea. The eye should be inspected for the presence of eyelashes. Ointment and an impermeable eye shield can be used at night to retain moisture. In some patients, taping the lids closed at night may be necessary to provide protection. The patient is taught to report ocular pain, drainage, or discharge.

A facial sling may be helpful to support affected muscles, improve lip alignment, and facilitate eating. The facial sling is usually made and fitted by a physical or occupational therapist. Vigorous massage can break down tissues, but gentle upward massage has psychologic benefits even if physical effects other than the maintenance of circulation are questionable. When function begins to return, active facial exercises are performed several times a day.

The change in physical appearance as a result of Bell's palsy can be devastating. The patient must be reassured that a stroke did not occur and that chances for a full recovery are good. The patient's need for privacy should be respected, especially during meals, but the nurse's assistance in the patient's adjustment to the physical changes should not be delayed. Enlisting support from family and friends is important. It is important to share with the patient that most patients recover within about 6 weeks of the onset of symptoms.

■ Evaluation

The expected outcomes are that the patient with Bell's palsy will

- be free of pain
- not experience any complications
- maintain appropriate nutritional intake
- experience minimal side effects associated with corticosteroid treatment
- return to previous perception of body image

Polyneuropathies

GUILLAIN-BARRÉ SYNDROME

Etiology and Pathophysiology

Guillain-Barré syndrome (Landry-Guillain-Barré-Strohl syndrome, postinfectious polyneuropathy, ascending polyneuropathic paralysis) is an acute, rapidly progressing, and potentially fatal form of polyneuritis. It affects the peripheral nervous system and

results in loss of myelin (a segmental demyelination) and edema and inflammation of the affected nerves, causing a loss of neurotransmission to the periphery. The syndrome affects both genders equally and is more commonly seen in adults, although it is observed in all age groups. Worldwide the incidence has varied from 0.4 to 1.7 cases per 100,000 persons per year. Guillain-Barré syndrome has an estimated annual cost of 2 to 3 billion dollars in the United States. With adequate supportive care, 85% of these patients recover completely from this disorder.

The etiology of this disorder is unknown, but it is believed to be a cell-mediated immunologic reaction directed at the peripheral nerves. The syndrome is often preceded by immune system stimulation from a viral infection, trauma, surgery, viral immunizations, human immunodeficiency virus (HIV), or lymphoproliferative neoplasms. *Campylobacter jejuni* is the most recognized organism associated with Guillain-Barré syndrome.[5] *C. jejuni* gastroenteritis is thought to precede Guillain-Barré syndrome in approximately 30% of cases. Other potential pathogens include *Mycoplasma pneumoniae,* cytomegalovirus, Epstein-Barr virus, varicella-zoster virus, and vaccines (rabies, swine influenza). These stimuli are thought to cause an alteration in the immune system, resulting in sensitization of T lymphocytes to the patient's myelin and, ultimately, myelin damage. Demyelination occurs, and the transmission of nerve impulses is stopped or slowed down. The muscles innervated by the damaged peripheral nerves undergo denervation and atrophy. In the recovery phase, remyelination occurs slowly, and neurologic function returns in a proximal to distal pattern.

Clinical Manifestations

Guillain-Barré syndrome is a heterogeneous condition with symptoms ranging from mild to severe. Symptoms of Guillain-Barré syndrome usually develop 1 to 3 weeks after an upper respiratory or gastrointestinal (GI) infection. Weakness of the lower extremities (evolving more or less symmetrically) occurs over hours to days to weeks, usually peaking about the fourteenth day. Distal muscles are more severely affected. *Paresthesia* (numbness and tingling) is frequent, and paralysis usually follows in the extremities. *Hypotonia* (reduced muscle tone) and *areflexia* (lack of reflexes) are common, persistent symptoms. Objective sensory loss is variable, with deep sensitivity more affected than superficial sensations.

Miller Fisher syndrome is a clinical variant of Guillain-Barré syndrome, accounting for 5% to 10% of cases. It is characterized by a triad of symptoms including ataxia, areflexia, and *ophthalmoplegia* (paralysis of motor nerves of the eye).[6] Other subtypes include acute inflammatory demyelinating polyneuropathy, acute motor axonal neuropathy, and acute motor and sensory axonal neuropathy.

In Guillain-Barré syndrome, autonomic nervous system dysfunction results from alterations in both the sympathetic and parasympathetic nervous systems. Autonomic disturbances are usually seen in patients with severe muscle involvement and respiratory muscle paralysis. The most dangerous autonomic dysfunctions include orthostatic hypotension, hypertension, and abnormal vagal responses (bradycardia, heart block, asystole). Other autonomic dysfunctions include bowel and bladder dysfunction, facial flushing, and diaphoresis. Patients may also have syndrome of inappropriate antidiuretic hormone (SIADH) secretion. SIADH is discussed in Chapter 48. Progression of Guillain-Barré syndrome to include the lower brainstem involves the facial, abducens, oculomotor, hypoglossal, trigeminal, and vagus nerves (CNs VII, VI, III, XII, V, and X, respectively). This involvement manifests itself through facial weakness, extraocular eye movement difficulties, dysphagia, and paresthesia of the face.

Pain is a common symptom in the patient with Guillain-Barré syndrome. The pain can be categorized as paresthesias, muscular aches and cramps, and hyperesthesias. Pain appears to be worse at night. Narcotics may be indicated for those experiencing severe pain. Pain may lead to a decrease in appetite and may interfere with sleep.

Complications. The most serious complication of this syndrome is respiratory failure, which occurs as the paralysis progresses to the nerves that innervate the thoracic area. Constant monitoring of the respiratory system by checking respiratory rate, depth, forced vital capacity, and negative inspiratory force provides information about the need for immediate intervention including intubation and mechanical ventilation. Respiratory or urinary tract infections (UTIs) may occur. Fever is generally the first sign of infection, and treatment is directed at the infecting organism. Immobility from the paralysis can cause problems such as paralytic ileus, muscle atrophy, deep vein thrombosis, pulmonary emboli, skin breakdown, orthostatic hypotension, and nutritional deficiencies.

Diagnostic Studies

Diagnosis is based primarily on the patient's history and clinical signs. CSF is normal or has a low protein content initially, but after 7 to 10 days it shows an elevated protein level to 700 mg/dl (7 g/L) (normal protein is 15 to 45 mg/dl [0.15 to 0.45 g/L]) with a normal cell count. Results of EMG and nerve conduction studies are markedly abnormal (reduced nerve conduction velocity) in the affected extremities.

Collaborative Care

Management is aimed at supportive care, particularly ventilatory support, during the acute phase. Plasma exchange is used in the first 2 weeks of Guillain-Barré syndrome. In patients with severe disease who are treated within 2 weeks of onset, there is a distinct reduction in the length of hospital stay, length of time on ventilator, and time required to resume walking. Intravenous (IV) administration of high-dose immunoglobulin (Sandoglobulin) has also shown to be as effective as plasma exchange and has the advantage of immediate availability and greater safety. However, patients receiving high-dose immunoglobulin need to be well hydrated and have adequate renal function. (Plasmapheresis is discussed in Chapter 13.) After 3 weeks of disease onset, plasma exchange and immunoglobulin therapies have little value. Corticosteroids appear to have little effect on the prognosis or duration of the disease.[7]

Nutritional Therapy. Nutritional intake is compromised in the patient with Guillain-Barré syndrome. During the acute phase, the patient may experience difficulty swallowing because of cranial nerve involvement. Mild dysphagia can be managed by placing the patient in an upright position and flexing the head forward during feeding. For more severe dysphagia, tube feedings may be required. Patients who experience paralytic ileus or intestinal obstruction may require total parenteral nutrition. Later in the course of the disease, motor paralysis or weakness continues to affect the ability to self-feed. The patient's nutritional status, including body weight, serum albumin levels, and calorie counts, must be evaluated at regular intervals.

NURSING MANAGEMENT
GUILLAIN-BARRÉ SYNDROME

■ Nursing Assessment

Assessment of the patient is the most important aspect of nursing care during the acute phase. The nurse must monitor the ascending paralysis; assess respiratory function; monitor arterial blood gases (ABGs); and assess the gag, corneal, and swallowing reflexes during the routine assessment. Reflexes are usually decreased or absent.

Monitoring blood pressure and cardiac rate and rhythm is also important during the acute phase because transient cardiac arrhythmias have been reported. Autonomic dysfunction is common and usually takes the form of bradycardia and arrhythmias. Orthostatic hypotension secondary to muscle atony may occur in severe cases. Vasopressor agents and volume expanders may be needed to treat the low blood pressure. However, the presence of SIADH may require fluid restriction.

■ Nursing Diagnoses

Nursing diagnoses for the patient with Guillain-Barré syndrome may include, but are not limited to, the following:

- Impaired spontaneous ventilation *related to* progression of disease process resulting in respiratory muscle paralysis
- Risk for aspiration *related to* dysphagia
- Acute pain *related to* paresthesias, muscle aches and cramps, and hyperesthesias
- Impaired verbal communication *related to* intubation or paralysis of the muscles of speech
- Fear *related to* uncertain outcome and seriousness of the disease
- Self-care deficits *related to* inability to use muscles to accomplish activities of daily living (ADLs)

■ Planning

The overall goals are that the patient with Guillain-Barré syndrome will (1) maintain adequate ventilation, (2) be free from aspiration, (3) be pain free or have pain controlled, (4) maintain an acceptable method of communication, (5) maintain adequate nutritional intake, and (6) return to usual physical functioning.

■ Nursing Implementation

The objective of therapy is to support body systems until the patient recovers. Respiratory failure and infection are serious threats. Monitoring the vital capacity and ABGs is essential. If the vital capacity drops to less than 800 ml (15 ml/kg or two thirds of the patient's normal vital capacity) or the ABGs deteriorate, endotracheal intubation or tracheostomy may be done so that the patient can be mechanically ventilated (see Chapter 66). Meticulous suctioning technique is needed to prevent infection whether the patient has an endotracheal tube or tracheostomy. Thorough bronchial hygiene and chest physiotherapy help clear secretions and prevent respiratory deterioration. If fever develops, sputum cultures should be obtained to identify the pathogen. Appropriate antibiotic therapy is then initiated.

A communication system must be established with the use of the patient's available abilities. This is extremely difficult if the disease progresses to involvement of the cranial nerves. At the peak of a severe episode the patient may be incapable of communicating. The nurse must explain all procedures before doing them and reassure the patient that muscle function will return.

Urinary retention is common for a few days. Intermittent catheterization is preferred to an indwelling catheter to avoid UTIs. However, for the acutely ill patient receiving a large volume of fluids (>2.5 L/day), indwelling catheterization may be safer to reduce overdistention of a temporarily flaccid bladder and to prevent vesicoureteral reflux. Physical therapy is indicated early to help prevent problems related to immobility. Passive range-of-motion exercises and attention to body position help maintain function and prevent contractures. Patients who develop facial paralysis must receive meticulous eye care to avoid corneal irritation or damage (exposure keratitis). Artificial tears should be instilled frequently during the day to prevent drying of the cornea. The eyes should be inspected for the presence of eyelashes. Ointment and an impermeable eye shield can be used at night to retain moisture.

Nutritional needs must be met in spite of possible problems associated with delayed gastric emptying, paralytic ileus, and potential for aspiration if the gag reflex is lost. In addition to checking for the gag reflex, nurses should note drooling and other difficulties with secretions, which may be more indicative of an inadequate gag reflex. Initially, tube feedings or parenteral nutrition may be used to ensure adequate caloric intake. Because of delayed gastric emptying, residual volumes of the feedings should be assessed at regular intervals or before feedings (see Chapter 39). Fluid and electrolyte therapy must be monitored carefully to prevent electrolyte imbalances. A bowel program should be initiated because constipation is a common problem related to diet changes, immobility, and decreased GI motility.

Throughout the course of the illness, the nurse needs to provide support and encouragement to the family and patient. Because residual problems and relapses are uncommon except in the chronic form of the disease, complete recovery can be anticipated although it is generally a slow process that takes months or years if axonal degeneration occurs.

■ Evaluation

The expected outcomes are that the patient with Guillain-Barré syndrome will
- return to usual level of physical functioning
- be free from pain and discomfort
- maintain nutritional status

BOTULISM

Etiology and Pathophysiology

Botulism is the most serious type of food poisoning. It is caused by GI absorption of the neurotoxin produced by *Clostridium botulinum*. This organism is found in the soil, and the spores are difficult to destroy. It can grow in any food contaminated with the spores. Improper home canning of foods is often the cause. In 1999, there were 174 cases of botulism reported to the Centers for Disease Control.[8] It is thought that the neurotoxin destroys or inhibits the neurotransmission of acetylcholine at the myoneural junction, resulting in disturbed muscle innervation.

Clinical Manifestations

Symptoms are usually nausea, vomiting, and abdominal cramps, generally within 6 to 48 hours after consumption of the contaminated food. Neurologic manifestations develop rapidly over 2 to 4 days. They include difficulty in convergence of the eyes, photophobia, ptosis, paralysis of extraocular muscles, blurred vision, diplopia, dry mouth, sore throat, and difficulty in swallowing. Other manifestations include paralytic ileus, mild muscle weakness, seizures, and respiratory symptoms that can rapidly deteriorate to respiratory arrest and/or cardiac arrest. The course of the disease depends on the amount of toxin absorbed from the gut. If only a small amount is absorbed, symptoms are mild and recovery is complete. When large amounts are absorbed, death usually occurs in 4 to 8 days from circulatory failure, respiratory paralysis, or development of pulmonary complications.[8]

Because botulism is a reportable disease, local, state, and federal health agencies, particularly the Centers for Disease Control and Prevention (CDC) in Atlanta, must be notified. Botulism can also be contracted through nasal inhalation, as well as oral ingestion. It has been highlighted as a potential bioterrorism agent and is discussed further in Chapter 67.

Diagnostic Studies and Collaborative Care

Blood and CSF are obtained for studies to rule out other diseases. In the patient with botulism the blood and CSF results are normal.

Drug Therapy. The initial treatment of botulism is IV administration of botulinum antitoxin. Before administration of the antitoxin, an intradermal test dose for sensitivity to horse serum is given. If there are no reactions, the test dose is followed by daily doses of 50,000 units of botulism antitoxin until improvement begins.

The GI tract is purged by laxatives, high colonic enemas, and gastric lavage to decrease the absorption of the toxin. Activated charcoal is most effective if administered within 1 hour of ingestion.

NURSING MANAGEMENT
BOTULISM

■ Nursing Implementation

Primary prevention is the goal of nursing management through educating consumers to be alert to situations that may result in botulism. Particular attention should be given to foods with a low acid content, which support germination and the production of botulin, a deadly poison. These foods include fish, vichyssoise, and peppers. All varieties of spores are destroyed by boiling for 10 minutes or maintaining a temperature of 176° F (80° C) for 30 minutes. Specific suggestions related to the preparation, storage, and use of food include the following:
- In home canning, the equipment manufacturer's directions should be followed. Only fresh fruits and vegetables (with all questionable spots removed) should be used. All containers and utensils must be cleansed, and the seal on the can or jar must be airtight. Canned foods should be stored properly in a cool, dry place.
- A can with a swollen end should never be used; the swelling may be caused by gases from *C. botulinum*.
- If the food is forcefully expelled when a container is opened, it should be discarded immediately and the contents should not be tasted.

- If the contents of a can look or smell bad after opening, the can should be discarded without tasting the contents. Materials may be flushed down the toilet or disposed of in the garbage disposal if a large amount of water is used.

Nursing care during the acute illness is similar to that for Guillain-Barré syndrome. Supportive nursing interventions include rest, activities to maintain respiratory function, adequate nutrition, and prevention of loss of muscle mass. Because the recovery process is slow, the patient may develop problems related to a feeling of helplessness, boredom, and low morale.

TETANUS

Etiology and Pathophysiology

Tetanus (lockjaw) is an extremely severe polyradiculitis and polyneuritis affecting spinal and cranial nerves. It results from the effects of a potent neurotoxin released by the anaerobic bacillus *Clostridium tetani*. The toxin interferes with the function of the reflex arc by blocking inhibitory transmitters at the presynaptic sites in the spinal cord and brainstem. The spores of the bacillus are present in soil, garden mold, and manure. Thus *Clostridium tetani* enters the body through a traumatic or suppurative wound that provides an appropriate low-oxygen environment for the organisms to mature and produce toxin. Other possible sources include dental infection, injections of heroin, human and animal bites, frostbite, compound fractures, and gunshot wounds. The incubation period is usually 7 days but can range from 3 to 21 days, with symptoms frequently appearing after the original wound is healed. In general, the longer the incubation period, the milder the illness and the better the prognosis.

Worldwide the number of cases per year is estimated to be 1 million. In the United States about 100 to 200 cases occur each year and are due to infection of puncture wounds of the extremities by nails or splinters or IV drug use.[9] Of the reported cases the majority of patients are over the age of 59 years. However, the number of individuals under the age of 40 with tetanus is increasing, most likely related to IV drug use. Mortality rates vary according to age, with infants and persons over 50 years of age most seriously affected. Overall mortality rates are declining and are at about 10% in the United States.

Clinical Manifestations

Manifestations of generalized tetanus include a feeling of stiffness in the jaw *(trismus)* or neck, slight fever, and other symptoms of general infection. Generalized tonic spasms occur because of the lack of reciprocal innervation. As the disease progresses, the neck muscles, back, abdomen, and extremities become progressively rigid. In severe forms, continuous tonic convulsions may occur with *opisthotonos* (extreme arching of the back and retraction of the head). Laryngeal and respiratory spasms cause apnea and anoxia. Additional effects are manifested by overstimulation of the sympathetic nervous system, including profuse diaphoresis, labile hypertension, episodic tachycardia, hyperthermia, and arrhythmias. The slightest noise, jarring motion, or bright light can set off the seizure. These seizures are agonizingly painful. Mortality is almost 100% in the severe form. Death is usually attributable to asphyxia or heart failure, the result of constantly recurring spasms. Residual injury, such as vertebral fracture, muscle contracture, and brain damage secondary to hypoxia, may be long-term consequences.

Collaborative Care

Serum electrolytes, CBC count, albumin, clotting factors, glucose, and ABGs are monitored. Cardiac function is monitored by electrocardiogram and auscultation. As increasing numbers of nerve cells become involved, their inhibitory control over muscle activity decreases and symptoms develop.

Drug Therapy. The management of tetanus includes administration of tetanus toxoid booster (Td) and tetanus immune globulin (TIG) before the onset of symptoms to neutralize circulating toxins (see Table 67-6). Control of spasms is essential and is managed by deep sedation, usually with diazepam (Valium), barbiturates, or chlorpromazine (Thorazine). Chlorpromazine is also helpful in reducing hyperthermia. A 10-day course of penicillin is recommended to inhibit further growth of the organism.

Because of laryngospasm, a tracheostomy is usually performed early and the patient is maintained on mechanical ventilation. If sedation does not control seizures, skeletal muscle–paralyzing drugs such as D-tubocurarine (Curare) are used. Pain is relieved by means of codeine or meperidine, often with the addition of promethazine (Phenergan). Any recognized wound should be debrided or an abscess drained. Antibiotics may be given to prevent secondary infections.

Nutrition is maintained through parenteral nutrition or nasogastric feeding. The mortality rate associated with tetanus is declining. However, for those who recover there is a long convalescence that includes extensive physical therapy.

NURSING MANAGEMENT
TETANUS

■ Nursing Implementation

Health teaching is aimed at ensuring tetanus prophylaxis, which is the most important factor influencing the incidence of this disease. Tetanus prevention and immunization protocols are summarized in Table 67-6. The patient should be taught that immediate, thorough cleansing of all wounds with soap and water is important in the prevention of tetanus. If an open wound occurs and the patient has not been immunized within 10 years, the health care provider should be contacted so that a tetanus booster can be given.

If equine tetanus antitoxin is to be used, the patient should be tested for sensitivity. Administration of equine antitoxin is not recommended if sensitivity occurs; anaphylactic shock is potentially life threatening, and desensitization is ineffective. The side effects of routine administration of the antitoxin are mild and include a sore arm, swelling at the site, and itching. Serious side effects rarely occur. Routine administration of a booster shot to an adequately immunized patient can cause arm swelling and lymphadenopathy.

Every patient should receive a written record of immunizations and be encouraged to complete the active immunization schedule. The patient's immunization history should be accurately recorded to protect the patient and health care providers.

The acute nursing management of the patient with tetanus is aimed at supportive care based on the treatment of clinical manifestations. The patient should be placed in a quiet, darkened room that is insulated against noise. Judicious sedation should be given. Nursing care should be administered with the utmost caution to avoid triggering spasms. For example, the nurse should avoid unnecessary touching, use firm touching when necessary, avoid the use of linens to cover the patient, and maintain a slightly higher than normal ambient temperature. Nursing care related to tracheostomy and mechanical ventilation is given as appropriate. An indwelling urinary catheter may be used to prevent bladder distention and urinary reflux in the presence of spasms in the muscles of the pelvic floor. Attention is also given to skin care. The patient needs emotional support during the acute phase because the fear of death is real. The family also needs support and education.

NEUROSYPHILIS

Neurosyphilis (tertiary syphilis) is an infection of any part of the nervous system by the organism *Treponema pallidum*. It is the result of untreated or inadequately treated syphilis (see Chapter 51). The organism can invade the central nervous system within a few months of the original infection. Except for causing some changes in the CSF, including increased white blood cells (WBCs) and protein and positive serologic reaction, the organism lies dormant for years. Untreated neurosyphilis, although not contagious, can be fatal. Penicillin therapy is effective for syphilitic meningitis, but the neurologic deficits remain.

Late neurosyphilis results from degenerative changes in the spinal cord (tabes dorsalis) and brainstem (general paresis). *Tabes dorsalis* (progressive locomotor ataxia) is characterized by vague, sharp pains in the legs; ataxia; "slapping" gait; loss of proprioception and deep tendon reflexes; and zones of hyperesthesia. *Charcot's joints,* which are characterized by enlargement, bone destruction, and hypermobility, also occur as a result of joint effusion and edema. Other manifestations of neurosyphilis include seizures and vision and hearing problems.

Neurologic symptoms associated with neurosyphilis are numerous and many times nonspecific.[10] Neurosyphilis is a differential diagnosis for patients with neurologic and psychiatric symptoms. *Dementia paralytica* is an ongoing spirochetal meningoencephalitis that causes a general dissolution of mental and physical capabilities. It may mimic a number of major or minor psychoses. Management includes treatment with penicillin, symptomatic care, and protection from physical injury.

Spinal Cord Problems

SPINAL CORD TRAUMA

Before World War II, the life expectancy for the person with a spinal cord injury ranged from months to 10 years from the onset of injury. The leading causes of death were renal failure and sepsis. Today, with improved treatment strategies (specifically, intermittent catheterization), even the very young patient with a spinal cord injury can anticipate a long life. The prognosis for life is generally only about 5 years less than for persons of the same age without spinal cord injury. The cause of premature death in the patient with **tetraplegia** (paralysis of both arms and legs), which was formerly called quadriplegia, is usually related to compromised respiratory function.

The potential for disruption of individual growth and development, altered family dynamics, economic loss in terms of absence from work, and the high cost of rehabilitation and long-term health care make spinal cord trauma a major problem. According to estimates from the Centers for Diseases Control

and Prevention (CDC), 11,000 Americans suffer spinal cord injuries each year.[11] The number of persons with spinal cord injuries living in the United States at any one time ranges from 183,000 to 230,000. The cost of spinal cord injury care can be high. The average cost of care for a person with a high cervical injury is $572,178 in the first year and $102,491 in each subsequent year.[12] Although many people with spinal cord injuries can care for themselves independently, those with the highest level of injury may require round-the-clock care at home or in a long-term care facility. Today almost 90% of patients with spinal cord injury are discharged from the hospital to home or another non-institutionalized residence.[12] The remaining 10% are discharged to nursing homes, chronic care facilities, or group homes.

Etiology and Pathophysiology

The segment of the population with the greatest risk for spinal cord injury is young adult men between the ages of 16 and 30 years. Eighty percent of people with spinal cord injury are male, and the most common age at injury is 19.

Causes of spinal cord injury include many types of trauma. Motor vehicle crashes account for 39%; violence, 25%; falls, 22%; sports injuries, 7%; and other miscellaneous causes, 7% of spinal cord injuries.[12] In large urban areas, gunshot wounds have recently surpassed falls as the second most common cause of spinal cord injuries.

There has also been an increase in the number of older adults with spinal cord injuries. People who were at least 61 years of age when injured increased from 4.7% of patients with spinal cord injury in the 1970s to 10% currently. Besides having greater mortality, older adults with traumatic injuries experience more complications than younger ones, and they are hospitalized longer. This trend toward older age at time of injury explains the overall increase in mean age of people with spinal cord injury from 28 years in the 1970s to 35.3 years at this time.[12]

Initial Injury. Spinal cord injury can be due to cord compression by bone displacement, interruption of blood supply to the cord, or traction resulting from pulling on the cord. The spinal cord is wrapped in tough layers of dura and is rarely torn or transected by direct trauma. Penetrating trauma, such as gunshot and stab wounds, can result in tearing and transection. The initial mechanical disruption of axons as a result of stretch or laceration is referred to as the *primary injury. Secondary injury* refers to the ongoing, progressive damage that occurs after the initial injury.[13]

There are several theories on what causes this ongoing damage at the molecular and cellular levels. These include free radical formation, uncontrolled calcium influx, ischemia, and lipid peroxidation. At the molecular level, *apoptosis* (cell death) occurs and may continue sometimes for weeks or months after the initial injury. Thus the complete cord damage (previously thought to be transection) in severe trauma is related to autodestruction of the cord. This is confirmed by observations that shortly after the injury, petechial hemorrhages are noted in the central gray matter of the cord. Hemorrhagic areas in the center of the spinal cord appear within 1 hour, and by 4 hours there may be infarction in the gray matter.[13] This ongoing destructive process makes it critical that the initial care and management of the patient with a spinal cord injury limit further activation of these processes.

Fig. 59-4 illustrates the cascade of events causing secondary injury following traumatic spinal cord injury. The resulting hyp-

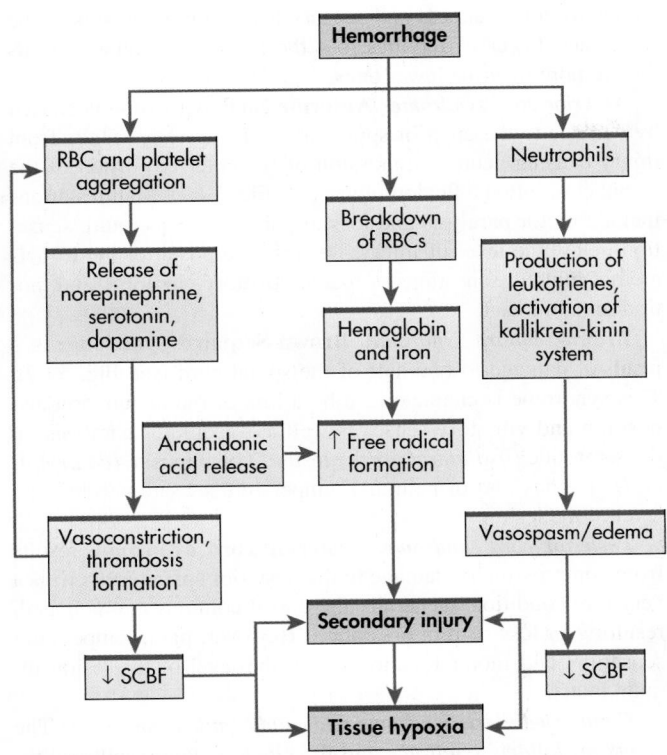

FIG. 59-4 Cascade of metabolic and cellular events that leads to spinal cord ischemia and hypoxia of secondary injury. *SCBF,* Spinal cord blood flow. (Redrawn from Marciano FF et al: *BNI Quarterly* 11:6, 1995.)

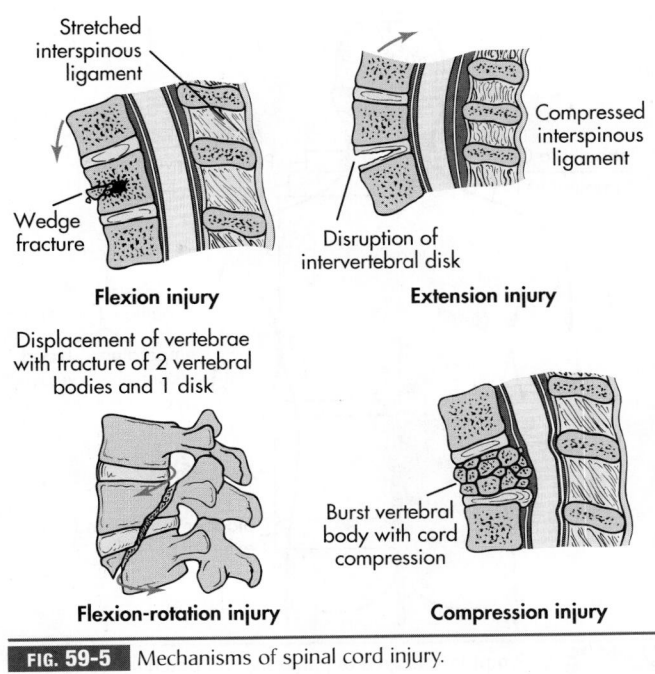

FIG. 59-5 Mechanisms of spinal cord injury.

oxia reduces the oxygen tension below the level that meets the metabolic needs of the spinal cord. Lactate metabolites and an increase in vasoactive substances including norepinephrine, serotonin, and dopamine are noted. At high levels, these vasoactive substances cause vasospasms and hypoxia, leading to subsequent necrosis. Unfortunately, the spinal cord has minimal ability to adapt to vasospasm.

By 24 hours or less, permanent damage may occur because of the development of edema. Edema secondary to the inflammatory response is particularly harmful because of lack of space for tissue expansion. Therefore resultant compression of the cord and extension of edema above and below the injury increase the ischemic damage.

The extent of the neurologic damage caused by a spinal cord injury results from primary injury damage (actual physical disruption of axons) and secondary injury damage (ischemia, hypoxia, microhemorrhage, and edema).[13] Because secondary injury processes occur over time, the extent of injury and prognosis for recovery are most accurately determined at 72 hours or more after injury.[14]

Spinal and neurogenic shock. About 50% of people with acute spinal cord injury experience a temporary neurologic syndrome known as **spinal shock** that is characterized by decreased reflexes, loss of sensation, and flaccid paralysis below the level of the injury.[15] This syndrome lasts days to months and may mask postinjury neurologic function. Active rehabilitation may begin in the presence of spinal shock. **Neurogenic shock,** in contrast, is due to the loss of vasomotor tone caused by injury and is char-

acterized by hypotension, bradycardia, and warm, dry extremities. Loss of sympathetic innervation causes peripheral vasodilation, venous pooling, and a decreased cardiac output. These effects are generally associated with a cervical or high thoracic injury.

Classification of Spinal Cord Injury. Spinal cord injuries are classified by the mechanism of injury, skeletal and neurologic level of injury, and completeness or degree of injury.

Mechanisms of injury. The major mechanisms of injury are flexion, hyperextension, flexion-rotation, extension-rotation, and compression (Fig. 59-5). The flexion-rotation injury is the most unstable of all injuries because the ligamentous structures that stabilize the spine are torn. This injury is most often implicated in severe neurologic deficits.

Level of injury. *Skeletal level* of injury is the vertebral level where there is the most damage to vertebral bones and ligaments. *Neurologic level* is the lowest segment of the spinal cord with normal sensory and motor function on both sides of the body. The level of injury may be cervical, thoracic, or lumbar. Cervical and lumbar injuries are most common because these levels are associated with the greatest flexibility and movement. If the cervical cord is involved, paralysis of all four extremities occurs, resulting in tetraplegia. However, even with a cervical injury the arms are rarely completely paralyzed. If the thoracic or lumbar cord is damaged, the result is **paraplegia** (paralysis and loss of sensation in the legs). Fig. 59-6 shows affected structures and functions at different levels of cord injury.

Degree of injury. The degree of spinal cord involvement may be either complete or incomplete (partial). *Complete cord involvement* results in total loss of sensory and motor function below the level of the lesion (injury). *Incomplete cord involvement* results in a mixed loss of voluntary motor activity and sensation and leaves some tracts intact. The degree of sensory and motor

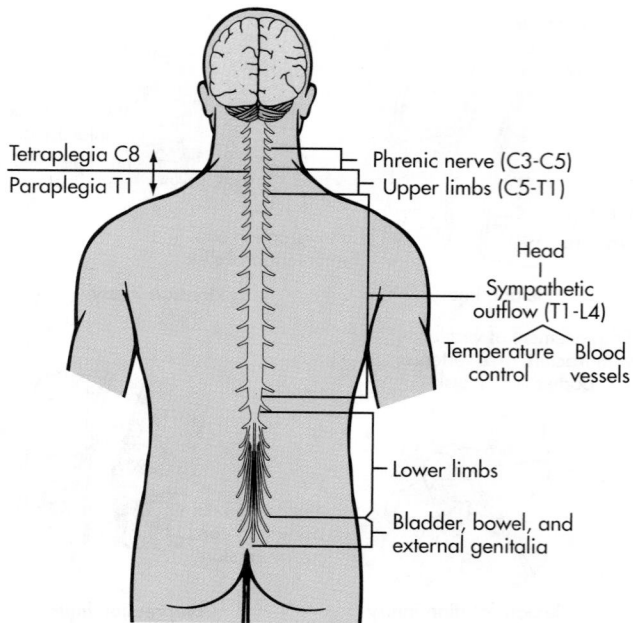

Tetraplegia C8
Paraplegia T1

Phrenic nerve (C3-C5)
Upper limbs (C5-T1)

Head
Sympathetic
outflow (T1-L4)

Temperature   Blood
control   vessels

Lower limbs

Bladder, bowel, and
external genitalia

FIG. 59-6 Symptoms, degree of paralysis, and potential for rehabilitation depend on the level of the lesion.

loss varies depending on the level of the lesion and reflects the specific nerve tracts damaged and those spared. Six syndromes are associated with incomplete lesions: central cord syndrome, anterior cord syndrome, Brown-Séquard syndrome, posterior cord syndrome, cauda equina syndrome, and conus medullaris syndrome.

Central cord syndrome. Damage to the central spinal cord is termed **central cord syndrome** (Fig. 59-7). It occurs most commonly in the cervical cord region and is more common in older adults. Motor weakness and sensory loss are present in both the upper and lower extremities, but the upper extremities are affected more than the lower ones.

Anterior cord syndrome. **Anterior cord syndrome** is caused by damage to the anterior spinal artery. It typically results from injury causing acute compression of the anterior portion of the spinal cord, often a flexion injury (see Fig. 59-7). Manifestations include motor paralysis and loss of pain and temperature sensation below the level of injury. Because the posterior cord tracts are not injured, sensations of touch, position, vibration, and motion remain intact.

Brown-Séquard syndrome. **Brown-Séquard syndrome** is a result of damage to one half of the spinal cord (see Fig. 59-7). This syndrome is characterized by a loss of motor function and position and vibratory sense, as well as vasomotor paralysis on the same side *(ipsilateral)* as the lesion. The opposite *(contralateral)* side has loss of pain and temperature sensation below the level of the lesion.

Posterior cord syndrome. **Posterior cord syndrome** results from compression or damage to the posterior spinal artery. It is a very rare condition. Generally the dorsal columns are damaged, resulting in loss of proprioception. However, pain, temperature sensation, and motor function below the level of the lesion remain intact.

Conus medullaris syndrome and cauda equina syndrome. The *conus medullaris syndrome* and the *cauda equina syndrome* result from damage to the very lowest portion of the spinal cord *(conus)* and the lumbar and sacral nerve roots *(cauda equina)*. Injury to these areas produces flaccid paralysis of the lower limbs and areflexic (flaccid) bladder and bowel.

American Spinal Injury Association (ASIA) Impairment scale. The ASIA Impairment scale is commonly used for classifying the severity of impairment resulting from spinal cord injury. It combines assessments of motor and sensory function to determine neurologic level and completeness of injury (Figs. 59-8 and 59-9).[16] This scale is useful for recording changes in neurologic status and identifying appropriate functional goals for rehabilitation.[14]

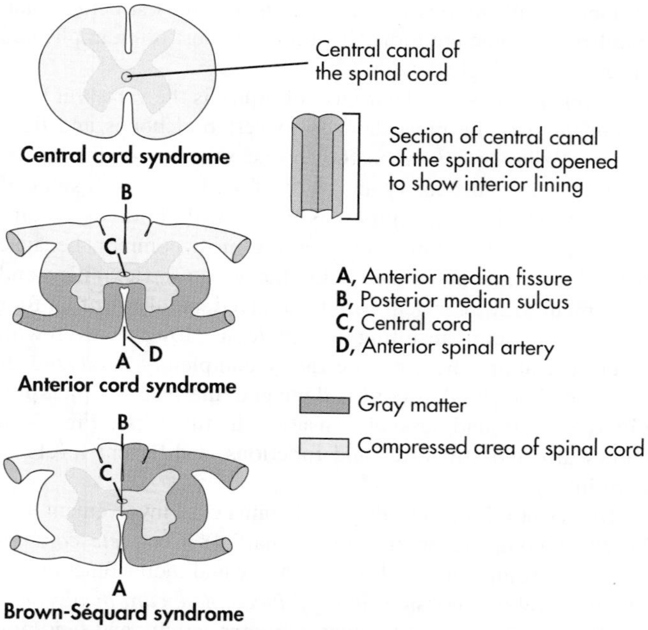

Central canal of
the spinal cord

Central cord syndrome

Section of central canal
of the spinal cord opened
to show interior lining

A, Anterior median fissure
B, Posterior median sulcus
C, Central cord
D, Anterior spinal artery

Anterior cord syndrome

▨ Gray matter
☐ Compressed area of spinal cord

Brown-Séquard syndrome

FIG. 59-7 Syndromes associated with incomplete cord lesions.

American Spinal Injury Association (ASIA) Impairment Scale

☐ **A = Complete:** No motor or sensory function is preserved in the sacral segments S4-S5.

☐ **B = Incomplete:** Sensory but not motor function is preserved below the neurologic level and includes the sacral segments S4-S5.

☐ **C = Incomplete:** Motor function is preserved below the neurologic level, and more than half of key muscles below the neurologic level have a muscle grade less than 3.

☐ **D = Incomplete:** Motor function is preserved below the neurologic level, and at least half of key muscles below the neurologic level have a muscle grade of 3 or more.

☐ **E = Normal:** Motor and sensory function are normal.

FIG. 59-8 The American Spinal Injury Association Impairment scale.

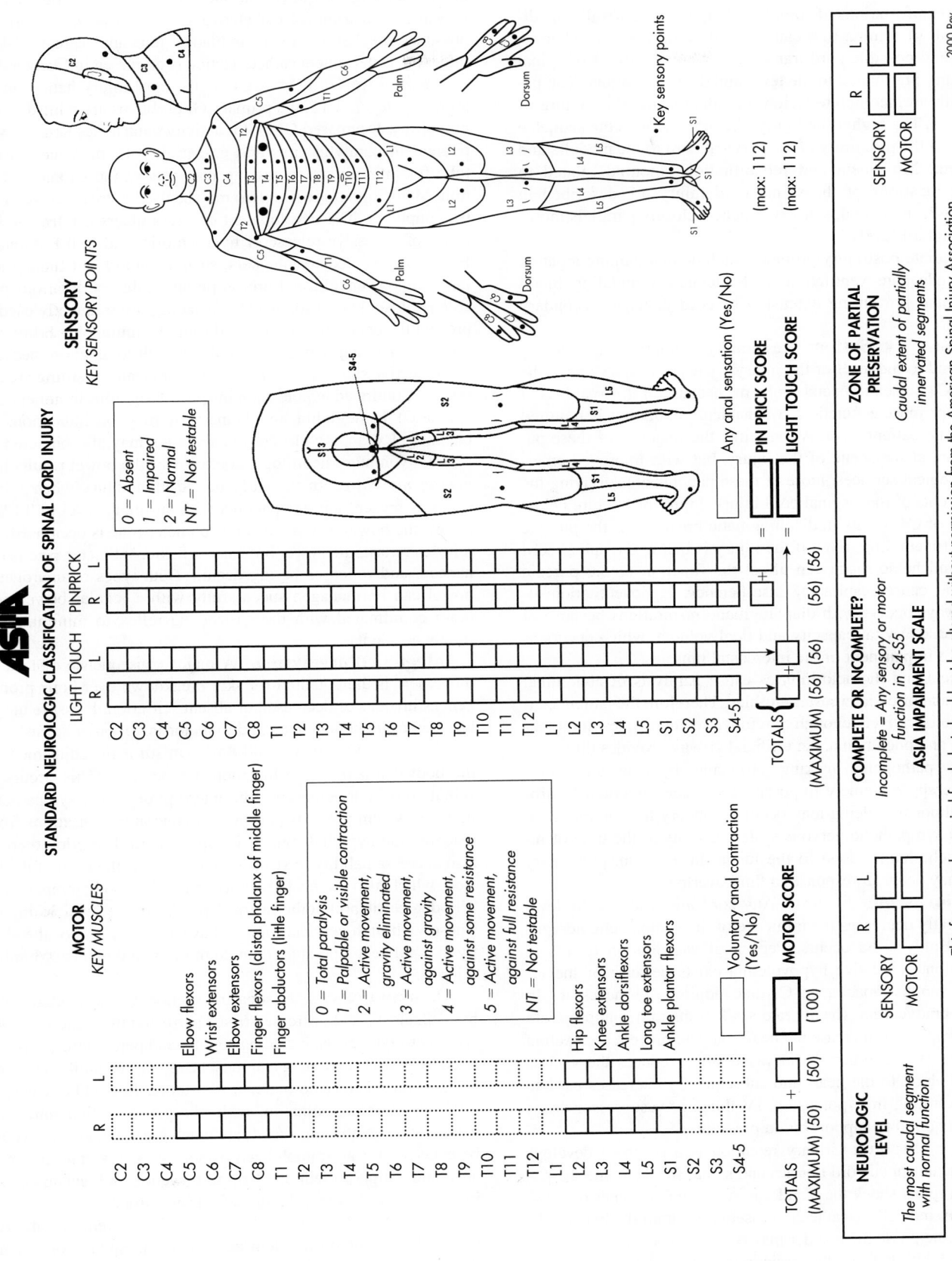

FIG. 59-9 Standard neurologic classification of spinal cord injury.

Clinical Manifestations

The manifestations of spinal cord injury are generally the direct result of trauma that causes cord compression, ischemia, edema, and possible cord transection. Manifestations of spinal cord injury are related to the level and degree of injury. The patient with an incomplete lesion may demonstrate a mixture of symptoms. The higher the injury, the more serious the sequelae because of the proximity of the cervical cord to the medulla and brainstem. Movement and rehabilitation potential related to specific locations of the spinal cord injury are described in Table 59-3. In general, sensory function closely parallels motor function at all levels.

Immediate postinjury problems include maintaining a patent airway, adequate ventilation, and adequate circulating blood volume and preventing extension of cord damage (secondary damage).

Respiratory System. Respiratory complications closely correspond to the level of the injury.[15] Cervical injury above the level of C4 presents special problems because of the total loss of respiratory muscle function. Mechanical ventilation is required to keep the patient alive. At one time the majority of these patients died at the scene of the injury, but with improved emergency medical services, more of these patients are surviving the initial events of their spinal cord injury. Injury or fracture below the level of C4 results in diaphragmatic breathing if the phrenic nerve is functioning. Even if the injury is below C4, spinal cord edema and hemorrhage can affect the function of the phrenic nerve and cause respiratory insufficiency. Hypoventilation almost always occurs with diaphragmatic respirations because of the decrease in vital capacity and tidal volume, which occurs as a result of impairment of the intercostal muscles.

Cervical and thoracic injuries cause paralysis of abdominal muscles and often intercostal muscles. Therefore the patient cannot cough effectively enough to remove secretions, leading to atelectasis and pneumonia. An artificial airway provides direct access for pathogens, making bronchial hygiene and chest physiotherapy extremely important to reduce infection. Neurogenic pulmonary edema may occur secondary to a dramatic increase in sympathetic nervous system activity at the time of injury, which shunts blood to the lungs. In addition, pulmonary edema may occur in response to fluid overload.

Cardiovascular System. Any cord injury above the level of T6 greatly decreases the influence of the sympathetic nervous system. Bradycardia occurs. Peripheral vasodilation results in hypotension. A relative hypovolemia exists because of the increase in venous capacitance. Cardiac monitoring is necessary. In marked bradycardia (heart rate <40 beats/min), appropriate drugs (atropine) to increase the heart rate and prevent hypoxemia are necessary.[15] The peripheral vasodilation reduces the venous return of blood to the heart and subsequently decreases cardiac output, resulting in hypotension. IV fluids or vasopressor drugs may be required to support blood pressure.

Urinary System. Urinary retention is a common development in acute spinal cord injuries and spinal shock. While the patient is in spinal shock the bladder is atonic and becomes overdistended. An indwelling catheter is inserted to drain the bladder. In the postacute phase the bladder may become hyperirritable, with a loss of inhibition from the brain resulting in reflex emptying. Chronic indwelling catheterization increases the risk of infection.

Once the patient is medically stable and large quantities of IV fluids are no longer required, the indwelling catheter should be removed and intermittent catheterization should begin as early as possible. This helps to maintain bladder tone and decrease risk of infection. (Intermittent catheterization is discussed in Chapter 44.)

Gastrointestinal System. If the cord injury has occurred above the level of T5, the primary GI problems are related to hypomotility. Decreased GI motor activity contributes to the development of paralytic ileus and gastric distention. A nasogastric tube for intermittent suctioning may relieve the gastric distention. Metoclopramide (Reglan) may be used to treat delayed gastric emptying. The development of stress ulcers is common because of excessive release of hydrochloric acid in the stomach. Histamine H_2-receptor blockers, such as ranitidine (Zantac) and famotidine (Pepcid), and proton pump inhibitors (e.g., omeprazole [Prilosec] or lansoprazole [Prevacid]) are frequently used to prevent the occurrence of ulcers during the initial phase. Intraabdominal bleeding may occur and is difficult to diagnose because no subjective signs such as pain, tenderness, and guarding are observed. Continued hypotension in spite of vigorous treatment and decreased hemoglobin and hematocrit may be indications of bleeding. Expanding girth of the abdomen may also be noted.

Less voluntary neurologic control over the bowel results in a *neurogenic bowel*. In the early period after injury when spinal shock is present and for patients with an injury level of T12 or below, the bowel is areflexic and sphincter tone is decreased. As reflexes return, the bowel becomes reflexic, sphincter tone is enhanced, and reflex emptying occurs. Both types of neurogenic bowel can be managed successfully with a regular bowel program coordinated with the gastrocolic reflex to minimize untimely accidents.

Integumentary System. A major consequence of lack of movement is the potential for skin breakdown over bony prominences in areas of decreased or absent sensation. Pressure ulcers can occur quickly and can lead to major infection or sepsis.

Thermoregulation. **Poikilothermism** is the adjustment of the body temperature to the room temperature. This occurs in spinal cord injuries because the interruption of the sympathetic nervous system prevents peripheral temperature sensations from reaching the hypothalamus. With spinal cord disruption there is also decreased ability to sweat or shiver below the level of the lesion, which also affects the ability to regulate body temperature. The degree of poikilothermism depends on the level of injury. Those with high cervical injuries have a greater loss of the ability to regulate temperature than do those with thoracic or lumbar injuries.

Metabolic Needs. Nasogastric suctioning may lead to metabolic alkalosis, and decreased tissue perfusion may lead to acidosis. Electrolyte levels, including sodium and potassium, can be altered by gastric suctioning and must be monitored until suctioning is discontinued and a normal diet is resumed. Loss of body weight (10% or more) is common, with nitrogen excretion mirroring weight loss.[15] Nutritional needs are much greater than what would be expected for an immobilized person. A positive nitrogen balance and a high-protein diet help to prevent skin breakdown and infections and decrease the rate of muscle atrophy.

Peripheral Vascular Problems. Deep vein thrombosis (DVT) is a common problem accompanying spinal cord injury during the first 3 months. It is more difficult to detect a DVT in a person with a spinal cord injury because the usual signs and symptoms, such as pain, tenderness, and a positive Homans' sign, will not be present.[17] Pulmonary embolism is one of the leading causes of death in patients with spinal cord injury. Techniques for assessment of DVT include Doppler examination, impedance plethysmography, and measurement of leg and thigh girth.

Diagnostic Studies

Once the patient is immobilized, diagnostic studies can be done. Complete spine films are performed to assess for vertebral fracture. X-rays including visualization of C1 through T1 are

TABLE 59-3	Functional Level of Spinal Cord Injury and Rehabilitation Potential	
LEVEL OF INJURY	**MOVEMENT REMAINING**	**REHABILITATION POTENTIAL**
Tetraplegia		
C1-C3 Often fatal injury, vagus nerve domination of heart, respiration, blood vessels, and all organs below injury	Movement in neck and above, loss of innervation to diaphragm, absence of independent respiratory function	Ability to drive electric wheelchair equipped with portable ventilator by using chin control or mouth stick, headrest to stabilize head; computer use with mouth stick, head wand, or noise control; 24-hour attendant care, able to instruct others
C4 Vagus nerve domination of heart, respirations, and all vessels and organs below injury	Sensation and movement in neck and above; may be able to breathe without a ventilator	Same as C1-C3
C5 Vagus nerve domination of heart, respirations, and all vessels and organs below injury	Full neck, partial shoulder, back, biceps; gross elbow, inability to roll over or use hands; decreased respiratory reserve	Ability to drive electric wheelchair with mobile hand supports; indoor mobility in manual wheelchair; able to feed self with setup and adaptive equipment; attendant care 10 hours per day
C6 Vagus nerve domination of heart, respirations, and all vessels and organs below injury	Shoulder and upper back abduction and rotation at shoulder, full biceps to elbow flexion, wrist extension, weak grasp of thumb, decreased respiratory reserve	Ability to assist with transfer and perform some self-care; feed self with hand devices; push wheelchair on smooth, flat surface; drive adapted van from wheelchair; independent computer use with adaptive equipment; attendant care 6 hours per day
C7-C8 Vagus nerve domination of heart, respirations, and all vessels and organs below injury	All triceps to elbow extension, finger extensors and flexors, good grasp with some decreased strength, decreased respiratory reserve	Ability to transfer self to wheelchair; roll over and sit up in bed; push self on most surfaces; perform most self-care; independent use of wheelchair; ability to drive car with powered hand controls (in some patients); attendant care 0 to 6 hours per day
Paraplegia		
T1-T6 Sympathetic innervation to heart, vagus nerve domination of all vessels and organs below injury	Full innervation of upper extremities, back, essential intrinsic muscles of hand; full strength and dexterity of grasp; decreased trunk stability, decreased respiratory reserve	Full independence in self-care and in wheelchair; ability to drive car with hand controls (in most patients); independent standing in standing frame
T6-T12 Vagus nerve domination only of leg vessels, GI and genitourinary organs	Full, stable thoracic muscles and upper back; functional intercostals, resulting in increased respiratory reserve	Full independent use of wheelchair; ability to stand erect with full leg brace, ambulate on crutches with swing (although gait difficult); inability to climb stairs
L1-L2 Vagus nerve domination of leg vessels	Varying control of legs and pelvis, instability of lower back	Good sitting balance; full use of wheelchair; ambulation with long leg braces
L3-L4 Partial vagus nerve domination of leg vessels, GI and genitourinary organs	Quadriceps and hip flexors, absence of hamstring function, flail ankles	Completely independent ambulation with short leg braces and canes; inability to stand for long periods

GI, Gastrointestinal.

done to document the presence of vertebral injury. A CT scan may be used to assess the stability of the injury, location and degree of bony injury, soft and neural tissue changes, and degree of spinal canal compromise.[17] MRI is used in cases in which there is unexplained neurologic deficit or worsening of neurologic status. A comprehensive neurologic examination is performed along with assessment of head, chest, and abdomen for additional injuries or trauma. Patients with cervical injuries who demonstrate altered mental status may also need vertebral angiography to rule out vertebral artery damage.

Collaborative Care

The initial goals for the patient with a spinal cord injury are to sustain life and prevent further cord damage. Table 59-4 outlines the emergency management of the patient with a spinal cord injury. Systemic and neurogenic shock must be treated to maintain blood pressure. For injury at the cervical level, all body systems must be maintained until the full extent of the damage can be evaluated.

Collaborative care during the acute phase for a patient with a cervical injury is described in Table 59-5. The systemic support required by the patient is less intense for spinal cord injuries of the thoracic and lumbar vertebrae. Respiratory compromise is not as severe, and bradycardia is not a problem. Specific problems are treated symptomatically. After stabilization at the accident scene, the person is transferred to a medical facility. A thorough assessment is done to specifically evaluate the degree of deficit and to establish the level and degree of injury. A history is obtained, with emphasis on how the accident occurred and the extent of injury as perceived by the patient immediately after the accident. Assessment involves testing muscle groups rather than individual muscles. Muscle groups should be tested with and against gravity, alone and against resistance, and on both sides of the body. Spontaneous movement should be noted. The patient should be asked to move legs and then hands, spread fingers, extend wrists, and shrug shoulders. After assessment of motor status, a sensory examination including touch and pain as tested by pinprick should be carried out, starting at the toes and working upward. If time and conditions permit, position sense and vibration can also be assessed.

The types of accidents that cause spinal cord trauma may also result in brain injury. The patient should therefore be assessed for history of unconsciousness, signs of concussion, and increased intracranial pressure (see Chapter 55). In addition, a careful assessment for musculoskeletal injuries and trauma to internal organs should be performed. Because there are no muscle, bone, or visceral sensations, the only clue to internal trauma with hemorrhage may be a rapidly falling hematocrit level. Urinary output is examined for hematuria, which is also indicative of internal injuries.

The patient must be moved in alignment as a unit or moved "as a log" during transfers and when repositioning to prevent further injury. Respiratory, cardiac, urinary, and GI functions should be monitored closely. The patient may go directly to surgery following initial immobilization and stabilization or to the intensive care unit (ICU) for monitoring and management.

Nonoperative Stabilization. Nonoperative treatments are focused on stabilization of the injured spinal segment and decompression, either through traction or realignment. Stabilization methods eliminate damaging motion at the injury site. They

TABLE 59-4	Emergency Management — Spinal Cord Injury		

ETIOLOGY	ASSESSMENT FINDINGS	INTERVENTIONS
Blunt • Compression, flexion, extension, or rotational injuries to spinal column • Motor vehicle accidents • Pedestrian accidents • Falls • Diving **Penetrating** • Stretched, torn, crushed, or lacerated spinal cord • Gunshot • Stab wounds	• Pain, tenderness, deformities, or muscle spasms adjacent to vertebral column • Numbness, paresthesias • Alterations in sensation: temperature, light touch, deep pressure, proprioception • Weakness or heaviness in limbs • Weakness, paralysis, or flaccidity of muscles • Spinal shock • Cuts; bruises; open wounds over head, face, neck, or back • Neurogenic shock: hypotension; bradycardia; dry, flushed skin • Bowel and bladder incontinence • Urinary retention • Difficulty breathing • Priapism • Diminished rectal sphincter tone	**Initial** • Ensure patent airway. • Stabilize cervical spine. • Administer oxygen via nasal cannula or non-rebreather mask. • Establish IV access with two large-bore catheters to infuse normal saline or lactated Ringer's solution as appropriate. • Assess for other injuries. • Control external bleeding. • Obtain cervical spine radiographs or CT scan. • Prepare for stabilization with cranial tongs and traction. • Administer high-dose methylprednisolone. **Ongoing Monitoring** • Monitor vital signs, level of consciousness, oxygen saturation, cardiac rhythm, urine output. • Keep warm. • Monitor for urinary retention, hypertension. • Anticipate need for intubation if gag reflex absent.

CT, Computed tomography; *IV*, intravenous.

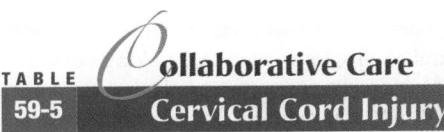

TABLE 59-5	Collaborative Care
	Cervical Cord Injury

Diagnostic

History and physical examination including complete neuro-
logic examination
ABGs
Serial bedside PFTs
Electrolytes, glucose, hemoglobin, and hematocrit levels
Urinalysis
Anteroposterior, lateral, and odontoid spinal x-ray studies
CT scan, MRI
X-ray of vertebral spine
Myelography
EMG to measure evoked potentials
Venous duplex studies

Collaborative Therapy

Acute Care

Immobilization of vertebral column by skeletal traction
Maintenance of heart rate (e.g., atropine) and blood pressure
(e.g., dopamine [Intropin])
Methylprednisolone high-dose therapy
Insertion of nasogastric tube and attachment to suction
Intubation (if indicated by ABGs and PFT)
O$_2$ by high humidity mask
Indwelling urinary catheter
Administration of IV fluids
Stress ulcer prophylaxis
Deep vein thrombosis prophylaxis
Bowel and bladder training

Rehabilitation and Home Care

Physical therapy
Range-of-motion exercises
Mobility training
Muscle strengthening
Occupational therapy (splints, activities of daily living training)
Bowel and bladder training
Autonomic dysreflexia prevention
Pressure ulcer prevention
Recreation therapy

ABGs, Arterial blood gases; *CT;* computed tomography; *EMG,* electromyography;
MRI, magnetic resonance imaging; *PFTs,* pulmonary function tests.

are intended to prevent secondary spinal cord damage caused by
repeated contusion or compression.[15]

Surgical Therapy. The decision to perform surgery on a
patient with a spinal cord injury often depends on the preference
of a particular physician. When cord compression is certain or
the neurologic disorder progresses, benefit may be seen following immediate surgery. Surgery stabilizes the spinal column.
There is some evidence to suggest that early cord decompression
results in reduced secondary injury to the spinal cord and therefore improved outcomes.[18] Other criteria used in the decision for
early surgery include (1) evidence of cord compression, (2) progressive neurologic deficit, (3) compound fracture of the vertebrae, (4) bony fragments (may dislodge and penetrate the cord),
and (5) penetrating wounds of the spinal cord or surrounding
structures.

The more common surgical procedures include decompression laminectomy by anterior cervical and thoracic approaches
with fusion, posterior laminectomy with the use of acrylic wire
mesh and fusion, and insertion of stabilizing rods (e.g., Harring-
ton rods for the correction and stabilization of thoracic deformities). (Specific surgical and nursing interventions for these techniques are discussed in Chapter 61.)

Drug Therapy. The National Acute Spinal Cord Injury
Study II (NASCIS II, 1990) and NASCIS III (1997) showed that
methylprednisolone (MP), when administered early and in a large
dose, resulted in greater recovery of neurologic function.[19-21] MP
(Solu-Medrol) is effective if given within 8 hours of injury. When
the loading dose of 30 mg/kg is given within 3 hours of injury, this
is followed by 24 hours of 5.4 mg/kg IV MP drip (see Evidence-
Based Practice box). If this loading dose is given between 3 and
8 hours postinjury, the IV drip is maintained for 48 hours. Patients
do not benefit from MP if it is given more than 8 hours postinjury
or the injury is penetrating. MP, a blocker of lipid peroxidation
by-products, improves blood flow and reduces edema in the spinal
cord. MP produces a number of effects that may account for the
overall improvement noted in the spinal cord–injured patient, including reduction of posttraumatic spinal cord ischemia, improvement of energy balance, restoration of extracellular calcium,
improvement of nerve impulse conduction, and repression of the
release of free fatty acids from spinal cord tissues. Side effects of
MP include immunosuppression, increased frequency of upper GI
bleeding, and increased risk of infection.[19] Although MP treatment is currently considered to be the standard of care, controversy exists over whether the benefits outweigh the risks.

The NASCIS III also determined tirilazad mesylate (Free-
dox), a potent lipid peroxidation inhibitor, administered for
48 hours postinjury provided motor recovery rates equivalent to
MP. There was an indication of fewer adverse effects in comparison with 48-hour treatment with MP. GM-1 ganglioside
(Sygen), which enhances neuronal conductance and may pre-

EVIDENCE-BASED PRACTICE
Drug Therapy for Spinal Cord Injury

Clinical Problem

Does pharmacologic treatment in the early hours following an
acute spinal cord injury reduce the extent of permanent
paralysis during the rest of the patient's life?

Best Clinical Practice

High-dose methylprednisolone therapy is the only pharmacologic therapy shown to be effective in reducing the extent of
permanent paralysis when it is administered within 8 hours
of injury.
High-dose methylprednisolone has been accepted as standard therapy in many countries.

Implications for Nursing Practice

▪ Assess involved systems before and periodically throughout
the course of high-dose methylprednisolone therapy.
▪ Risk for infections and gastrointestinal bleeding is increased
when this therapy is administered.

Reference for Evidence

Bracken MB: Pharmacological interventions for acute spinal cord injury,
Cochrane Injuries Group, *Cochrane Database Syst Rev,* Issue 1, 2002.

vent postischemic neuronal damage, has also demonstrated safety and efficacy in early clinical trials.[18] Other neuroprotective drugs are being tested, and more treatment options may be available soon.

Vasopressor agents such as dopamine (Intropin) are employed in the acute phase as adjuvants to treatment. These agents are used to maintain the mean arterial pressure at a level greater than 80 to 90 mm Hg so that perfusion to the spinal cord is improved.

Pharmacologic properties and drug metabolism are altered in spinal cord injury. Therefore drug interactions may occur. The differences in drug metabolism correlate with level and completeness of injury, with greater change apparent in people with cervical injury than in those with injury of lower spinal levels.[22]

Pharmacologic agents are used to treat specific autonomic dysfunctions such as GI hypoactivity, bradycardia, orthostatic hypotension, inadequate emptying of the bladder, and autonomic dysreflexia. The nurse must know the intended effects of such agents, observe responses, and provide specific interventions when adverse reactions are seen.

NURSING MANAGEMENT
SPINAL CORD TRAUMA

■ Nursing Assessment

Subjective and objective data that should be obtained from a patient with a recent spinal cord injury are presented in Table 59-6.

■ Nursing Diagnoses

Nursing diagnoses for the patient with a spinal cord injury depend on the severity of the injury and the level of dysfunction. The nursing diagnoses for a patient with a spinal cord injury may include, but are not limited to, those presented in NCP 59-1. The care plan presented is for a patient with a complete cervical cord injury.

■ Planning

The overall goals are that the patient with a spinal cord injury will (1) maintain optimal level of neurologic functioning; (2) have minimal or no complications of immobility; (3) learn new skills, gain new knowledge, and acquire new behaviors to be able to care for self or successfully direct others to do so; and (4) return to home and the community at an optimal level of functioning.

■ Nursing Implementation

Health Promotion. Nursing interventions for injury prevention include identification of risk populations, counseling, and education. Support of local legislation related to seat belt use in cars, helmets for motorcyclists and bicyclists, child safety seats, and tougher penalties for drunk-driving offenses is a professional responsibility.

Roles of nursing in health promotion as it applies to spinal cord injury include injury prevention, counseling and education of people with spinal cord injury regarding health behaviors (e.g., smoking, substance abuse, diet, exercise), and ensuring that ongoing health care after hospital discharge includes appropriate general health screening and health promotion, as well as spinal cord injury care.

After injury, health-promoting behaviors can have a significant impact on the health and well-being of the individual with

spinal cord injury. Nursing interventions include education, counseling, and referral to programs such as smoking cessation classes, recreation and exercise programs, or alcohol treatment programs. Outpatient health care requires that screening and prevention programs be accessible to people with spinal cord injury. Nurses in these settings should facilitate wheelchair-accessible

TABLE 59-6 Nursing Assessment: Spinal Cord Injury

Subjective Data
Important Health Information
Past health history: Motor vehicle accident, sports injury, industrial accident, gunshot or stabbing injury, falls
Functional Health Patterns
Health perception–health management: Use of alcohol or recreational drugs; risk-taking behaviors
Activity-exercise: Loss of strength, movement, and sensation below level of injury; dyspnea, inability to breathe adequately ("air hunger")
Cognitive-perceptual: Presence of tenderness, pain at or above level of injury; numbness, tingling, burning, twitching of extremities
Coping–stress tolerance: Fear, denial, anger, depression

Objective Data
General
Poikilothermism (unable to regulate body heat)
Integumentary
Warm, dry, flushed extremities below level of injury (neurogenic shock)
Respiratory
Lesions at C1 to C3: apnea, inability to cough; lesions at C4: poor cough, diaphragmatic breathing, hypoventilation; lesions at C5 to T6: decreased respiratory reserve
Cardiovascular
Lesions above T5: bradycardia, hypotension, postural hypotension, absence of vasomotor tone
Gastrointestinal
↓ or absent bowel sounds (paralytic ileus in lesions above T5), abdominal distention, constipation, fecal incontinence, fecal impaction
Urinary
Retention (for lesions between T1 and L2); flaccid bladder (acute stages); spasticity with reflex bladder emptying (later stages)
Reproductive
Priapism, loss of sexual function
Neurologic
Complete: Flaccid paralysis and anesthesia below level of injury resulting in tetraplegia (for lesions above C8) or paraplegia (for lesions below C8), hyperactive deep tendon reflexes, bilaterally positive Babinski test (after resolution of spinal shock)
Incomplete: Mixed loss of voluntary motor activity and sensation
Musculoskeletal
Muscle atony (in flaccid state), contractures (in spastic state)
Possible Findings
Location of level and type of bony involvement on spinal x-ray: lesion, edema, compression on CT scan and MRI; positive finding on myelogram

CT, Computed tomography; *MRI,* magnetic resonance imaging.

examination rooms, adjustable height examination tables, and scheduling that allows extra time if needed.

Acute Intervention. High cervical injury caused by flexion-rotation is the most complex spinal cord injury and is discussed in this section. Interventions for this type of injury can be modified for patients with less severe problems.

Immobilization. Proper immobilization of the neck involves the maintenance of a neutral or slight extension position. Sandbags, hard cervical collars, and backboards can be used to stabilize the neck to prevent lateral rotation of the cervical spine. The body should always be correctly aligned, and turning should be performed so that the patient is moved as a unit (e.g., logrolling)

NURSING CARE PLAN 59-1

Patient with a Spinal Cord Injury*

EXPECTED PATIENT OUTCOMES	NURSING INTERVENTIONS and *RATIONALES*
NURSING DIAGNOSIS	**Impaired gas exchange** *related to* diaphragmatic fatigue or paralysis and retained secretions *as manifested by* decreased PaO_2 content, increased $PaCO_2$ concentration, fatigue, diminished breath sounds.
▪ ABGs and PFT within normal limits ▪ Normal chest x-ray ▪ Clear lungs on auscultation ▪ Absence of respiratory distress	▪ Maintain a patent airway *to prevent respiratory arrest.* ▪ Assess all respiratory parameters initially and at least q2hr *to determine extent of problem and plan appropriate interventions.* ▪ Monitor ABGs and PFT *to determine oxygenation and ventilation status.* ▪ Provide aggressive pulmonary toilet, including chest physical therapy and assisted coughing (see Chapter 66, Fig. 66-6) q4hr *to facilitate the raising of secretions.* ▪ Assess strength of cough at least q4hr *to determine adequacy for raising secretions.* ▪ Suction as necessary *to remove accumulated secretions.*
NURSING DIAGNOSIS	**Decreased cardiac output** *related to* venous pooling of blood, bradycardia, and immobility *as manifested by* hypotension, restlessness, oliguria, decreased pulmonary artery pressures.
▪ Adequate cardiac output ▪ Stable blood pressure and pulse ▪ Absence of arrhythmias ▪ No complications such as venous thrombosis or pulmonary emboli	▪ Monitor blood pressure and pulse at least q2hr initially; monitor cardiac rhythm *as indicators of cardiac status.* ▪ Mobilize gradually *to prevent orthostatic hypotension.* ▪ Administer dopamine (Intropin) or other vasopressor agents *to maintain mean blood pressure >80 mm Hg.* ▪ Apply pneumatic compression devices to calves and/or compression gradient stockings *to prevent venous pooling and thromboemboli.* ▪ Perform range-of-motion to all extremities at least q8hr *to cause muscle contractions, which aid in venous return.*
NURSING DIAGNOSIS	**Impaired skin integrity** *related to* immobility and poor tissue perfusion *as manifested by* reddened skin over bony prominences and pin and tong sites.
▪ Intact skin ▪ No pressure ulcers	▪ Inspect all skin areas, especially over bony prominences, at least q2hr; observe area around pins or tongs for signs of breakdown or infection *so that interventions can be initiated promptly if a problem develops.* ▪ Turn patient at least q2hr; use kinetic treatment table (see Fig. 66-11) or other specialty care devices as needed *to prevent development of pressure areas.* ▪ Ensure adequate nutritional intake *to maintain healthy skin resistant to breakdown.* ▪ Wash and dry patient's skin thoroughly *to prevent moisture from predisposing to skin breakdown.* ▪ Teach patient and family to inspect bony prominences *to detect reddened areas* and ways to prevent pressure ulcers (Table 12-25).
NURSING DIAGNOSIS	**Constipation** *related to* neurogenic bowel, inadequate fluid intake, diet low in roughage, and immobility *as manifested by* lack of bowel movement for more than 2 days, decreased bowel sounds, palpable impaction, hard stool or stool incontinence.
▪ Established bowel program ▪ Bowel movement at least every other day	▪ Auscultate bowel sounds at least q4hr; monitor abdominal distention *to determine if peristalsis is present.* ▪ Begin bowel program as soon as bowel sounds return and include suppository every other day and stool softeners *to establish a bowel routine as quickly as possible.* ▪ Teach patient and family the bowel program *to ensure continuity of the program.* ▪ Ensure appropriate food and fluid intake *because bulk, fiber, and fluid are necessary to the success of a bowel program.*

*This care plan is suitable for a patient with a high cervical injury caused by flexion-rotation. It can be modified for patients with less severe problems. *ABGs,* Arterial blood gases; *PFT,* pulmonary function test.

Continued

NURSING CARE PLAN 59-1

Patient with a Spinal Cord Injury—cont'd

EXPECTED PATIENT OUTCOMES	NURSING INTERVENTIONS and *RATIONALES*

NURSING DIAGNOSIS | **Impaired urinary elimination** *related to* spinal injury and limited fluid intake *as manifested by* lack of urine output, bladder distention, involuntary emptying of bladder (after spinal shock).

- No urinary retention or infection
- Able to perform self-catheterization to empty bladder or able to void with adequate emptying

- Palpate bladder *because loss of autonomic and reflex control of bladder and sphincter can cause distention.*
- Insert indwelling catheter during acute phase *to ensure continuous flow of urine to prevent reflux of urine into the kidneys.*
- Begin intermittent catheterization program when appropriate; teach patient and family intermittent catheterization using a clean technique *to avoid long-term use of indwelling catheter with high potential for infection.*
- Maintain accurate intake and output records *to evaluate fluid balance.*
- Encourage fluids (2 to 4 L/day) *to maintain high volume of dilute urine,* which aids in preventing infection with indwelling catheter.
- Encourage fluids (2 L/day) divided into 200 to 250 ml every 2 to 3 hours while awake *to maintain regular bladder volumes (<500 ml) during intermittent catheterization.*
- Monitor bladder volumes regularly using bladder ultrasound for patients who are regaining ability to void *to assess adequacy of emptying and to prevent bladder overdistention.*
- Monitor blood urea nitrogen and creatinine levels, urine cultures, and WBC count *to monitor kidney function and presence of infection.*

NURSING DIAGNOSIS | **Impaired physical mobility** *related to* spinal cord injury, vertebral column instability, or forced immobilization by traction *as manifested by* inability to move purposefully, limited muscle strength, impaired perception of position or presence of body parts.

- No complications of immobility

- Assess motor and sensory function at least q4hr initially *to promptly detect deterioration of neurologic status.*
- Promote good pulmonary function *because pulmonary complications are a common sequelae of immobility.*
- Use specialty bed or turn patient q1-2hr *to prevent prolonged pressure, which can lead to pressure ulcers.*
- Perform full range-of-motion to all extremities several times a day *to promote circulation and prevent contractures.*
- Use splints and foot boards as appropriate *to prevent contractures and promote functional positioning.*

NURSING DIAGNOSIS | **Risk for autonomic dysreflexia** *related to* reflex stimulation of sympathetic nervous system after spinal shock resolves.

- No occurrence of dysreflexia
- Receive immediate and appropriate nursing or medical interventions if dysreflexia occurs

- Assess for hypertension, bradycardia, severe headache, sweating, blurred vision, flushed feeling, nasal congestion *as signs of dysreflexia.*
- Reduce or eliminate noxious stimuli such as fecal impaction, urinary retention, tactile stimulation, and skin lesions by appropriate interventions *to prevent occurrence of dysreflexia.*
- If dysreflexia occurs, check for elevated blood pressure and administer antihypertensive medication as ordered; check for and correct possible sources of irritation such as a distended bladder or bowel; elevate head of bed immediately *to reduce blood pressure by allowing blood to pool in the lower extremities.*
- If nursing interventions do not reverse symptoms, notify physician so that immediate medical interventions can be initiated *to prevent a life-threatening situation from developing.*
- Teach patient and family to recognize and treat dysreflexia *to reverse occurrence and prevent occurrence of status epilepticus, stroke, and possible death.*

NURSING CARE PLAN 59-1

Patient with a Spinal Cord Injury—cont'd

EXPECTED PATIENT OUTCOMES	NURSING INTERVENTIONS and *RATIONALES*
NURSING DIAGNOSIS	**Imbalanced nutrition: less than body requirements** *related to* increased metabolic demand, gastrointestinal hypomotility, and inability to eat independently *as manifested by* weight loss >10% of admission weight, decreased serum albumin or protein.
• Weight loss <10% • Normal values for serum protein and albumin	• Assess weight on admission *to provide baseline for comparison over time.* • Ensure enteral feedings are given as ordered during acute phase *so that nutrient intake is not interrupted.* • When patient is eating, encourage high-protein, high-carbohydrate, high-calorie diet with high bulk *to counteract the severe catabolism that occurs with spinal cord injury.* • Keep a calorie count and weigh patient at least weekly *to evaluate nutritional plan and continue or revise as necessary.*
NURSING DIAGNOSIS	**Risk for ineffective coping** *related to* loss of control over bodily functions and altered lifestyle secondary to paralysis.
• Verbalization of ability to cope with effects of spinal cord injury	• Assess for prolonged use of inappropriate defense mechanisms, inability to accept current status, refusal to use available support services *to determine presence of risk factors for ineffective coping.* • Offer support and acceptance of feelings; assist patient with problem solving *to bolster patient's confidence in ability to cope.* • Foster decision making regarding care *to increase feelings of control.* • Encourage use of support systems *to discuss concerns.* • Provide information *because knowledge of expectations can help patient cope with the future.* • Teach patient healthy coping behaviors such as relaxation techniques to *prevent patient from practicing ineffective behaviors such as smoking, drinking, or angry outbursts.*
NURSING DIAGNOSIS	**Disturbed body image** *related to* paralysis *as manifested by* expression of anger or other negative feelings, refusal to discuss changes in function, participate in social contacts, or look at body.
• Expression of feelings about self • Work through feelings to facilitate adaptation	• Encourage discussion of feelings *to aid patient in venting and clarifying feelings.* • Allow patient to grieve *because spinal cord injury results in a real loss, which requires adjustment through grieving.* • Encourage social interaction *to foster sense of returning normalcy to life.* • Assist family members in supporting patient *to enhance patient's sense of worth and value as a person.* • Make referral for counseling as needed.
NURSING DIAGNOSIS	**Interrupted family processes** *related to* change in function of ill family member *as manifested by* poor communication patterns among family members, use of ineffective coping techniques (e.g., shouting, blaming), inability of family members to meet needs of patient.
• Family will maximize individual and collective strengths and meet patient's needs	• Assess family dynamics related to roles and responsibilities *to determine problematic areas and strengths.* • Encourage open communication among family members regarding long-term planning to meet patient's needs, including financial aspects *so that ideas and concerns of all involved family members are considered.* • Assist family members to understand patient's feelings *to strengthen patient's feeling of worth and support.* • Assist family members to develop an action plan to meet patient's needs *to reduce sense of frustration and helplessness.* • Coordinate an organized team approach *to help the patient and family cope with the complex changes.*

to prevent movement of the spine. For cervical injuries, skeletal traction is usually provided by Crutchfield (Fig. 59-10), Vinke, or Gardner-Wells tongs or other types of skull tongs. Traction is provided by a rope that is extended from the center of the tongs over a pulley and has weights attached at the end. Traction must be maintained at all times. One disadvantage of skull tongs is that the skull pins can be displaced. If this occurs, the head should be held in a neutral or extended position and help should be summoned. Sandbags can be positioned to stabilize the head while the physician reinserts the tongs.

Infection at the sites of tong insertion is another potential problem. Preventive care includes cleansing the sites twice a day with normal saline solution and applying an antibiotic ointment, which acts as a mechanical barrier to the entrance of bacteria. The preventive care of insertion sites may vary depending on individual hospital standards of care.

Special beds are often used in the management of the patient with a spinal cord injury (see Fig. 66-11). Kinetic therapy uses a continual side-to-side slow rotation 62 degrees laterally with the patient in constant motion. The bed allows a frequency of turns greater than 200 times per day. The bed is used to decrease the likelihood of pressure sores and cardiopulmonary complications. However, in some patients the turning can induce motion sickness and fear of falling out of bed when turned to the extremes. (Motion sickness is unlikely when automatic rather than manual turning is used.)

Depending on the type of injury and therapeutic interventions, the tongs and traction may be removed 1 to 4 weeks after injury. In a stable injury for which surgery is not done, halo traction may be applied. The removal of traction and application of a collar brace or halo traction device allow the patient to be more mobile and to begin active rehabilitation. After cervical fusion or other stabilization surgery, a Philadelphia collar or sternal-occipital-mandibular immobilizer brace is worn until the fusion becomes solid (Fig. 59-11).[13] The halo apparatus applies cervical traction by means of a jacketlike arrangement that allows greater mobility and wheelchair activity than other traction systems (Fig. 59-12). Patients with thoracic or lumbar spine injuries are immobilized with a custom thoracolumbar orthosis ("body jacket"), which controls spinal flexion, extension, and rotation, or with a Jewett brace, which restricts forward flexion.

Immobilization of the neck of the patient with a spinal cord injury prevents further injury, but the effects of immobility are profound. Meticulous skin care is critical because decreased sensation and circulation make the patient particularly susceptible to skin breakdown. Patients should be removed from backboards as soon as possible, and cervical collars should be properly fitted or replaced with other forms of immobilization to prevent coccygeal and occipital area skin breakdown. It is important that areas under the halo vest or jacket or under braces or orthoses be inspected to assess skin condition.

Respiratory dysfunction. During the first 48 hours after injury, spinal cord edema may increase the level of dysfunction and respiratory distress may occur. If the injury is at or above C3, or if the patient is exhausted from labored breathing or ABGs deteriorate (indicating inadequate oxygenation or ventilation), endotracheal intubation or tracheostomy and mechanical ventilation should be initiated. Respiratory arrest is a possibility that requires careful monitoring of the respiratory system and prompt action, should it occur. Pneumonia and atelectasis are potential problems because of reduced vital capacity and the loss of intercostal and abdominal muscle function, resulting in diaphragmatic breathing, pooled secretions, and an ineffective cough.[23] The older adult has a more difficult time responding to hypoxia and hypercapnia and is extremely intolerant of hypoxia caused by lack of reserve. Therefore aggressive chest physiotherapy, ad-

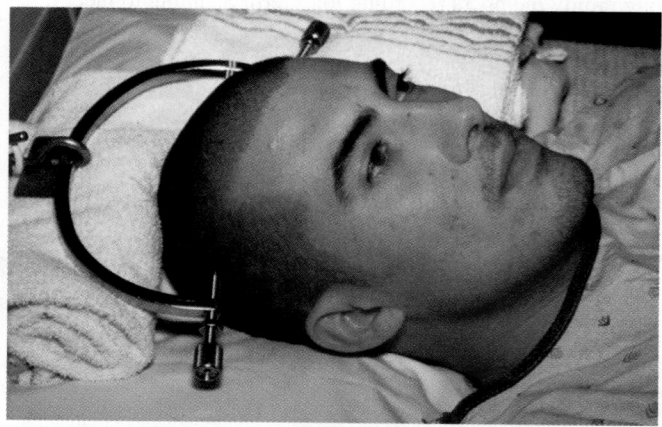

FIG. 59-10 Cervical traction is attached to tongs inserted in the skull.

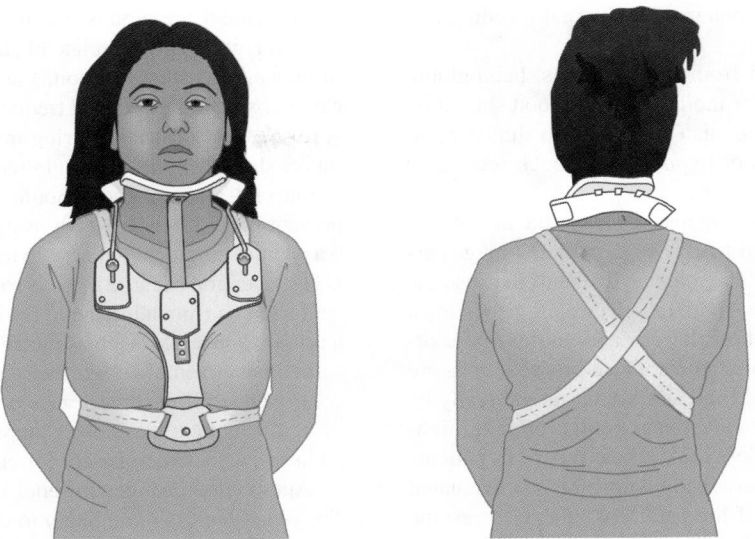

FIG. 59-11 Sternal-occipital-mandibular immobilizer (SOMI) brace.

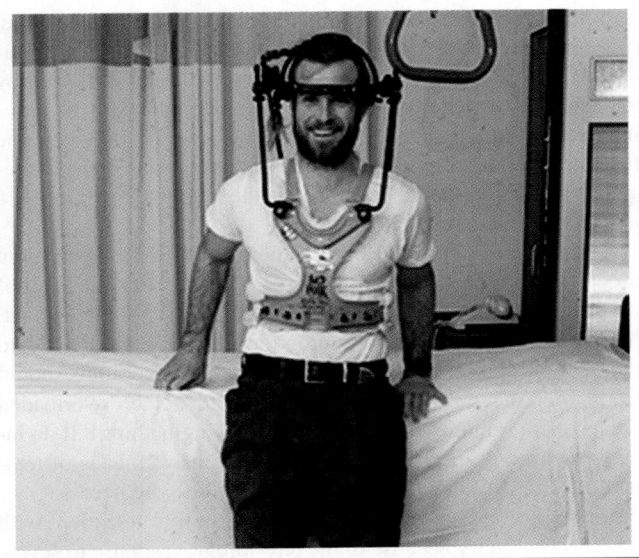

FIG. 59-12 Halo vest, Ace manufacturing design. Note the rigid shoulder straps and encompassing vest. Various vest sizes are available prefabricated. The halo ring, superstructure, and vest are MRI-compatible.

equate oxygenation, and proper pain management are essential to maximize respiratory function and gas exchange. Other problems include nasal stuffiness and bronchospasms.

The nurse needs to regularly assess (1) breath sounds, (2) ABGs, (3) tidal volume, (4) vital capacity, (5) skin color, (6) breathing patterns (especially the use of accessory muscles), (7) subjective comments about the ability to breathe, and (8) the amount and color of sputum. A PaO_2 (partial pressure of oxygen in arterial blood) above 60 mm Hg and a $PaCO_2$ (partial pressure of carbon dioxide in arterial blood) below 45 mm Hg are acceptable values in a patient with uncomplicated tetraplegia. A patient who is unable to count to 10 out loud without taking a breath needs immediate attention.

In addition to monitoring, the nurse can intervene in maintaining ventilation. Oxygen is administered until ABGs stabilize.

Chest physiotherapy and assisted coughing facilitate the raising of secretions. Assisted coughing simulates the action of the ineffective abdominal muscles during the expiratory phase of a cough. The nurse places the heels of both hands just below the xiphoid process and exerts firm upward pressure to the area timed with the patient's efforts to cough (see Fig. 66-6). Tracheal suctioning should be performed if crackles or rhonchi are present. Incentive spirometry is an additional technique that can be used to improve the patient's respiratory status.

Cardiovascular instability. Because of unopposed vagal response, the heart rate is slowed, often to below 60 beats per minute. Any increase in vagal stimulation such as turning or suctioning can result in cardiac arrest. Loss of sympathetic tone in peripheral vessels results in chronic low blood pressure with potential postural hypotension. Lack of muscle tone to aid venous return can result in sluggish blood flow and predispose the patient to DVT.

Vital signs should be assessed frequently. If bradycardia is symptomatic, an anticholinergic drug such as atropine is administered. A temporary pacemaker may be inserted in some instances. Hypotension is managed with a vasopressor agent, such as dopamine (Intropin) or norepinephrine, and fluid replacement.

In the older adult, the prevalence of cardiovascular disease must be considered. The cardiovascular system becomes less able to handle the stress of traumatic injury because heart contractions weaken, and cardiac output is reduced. Maximum heart rate is also reduced.

Compression gradient stockings can be used to prevent thromboemboli and to promote venous return. The stockings must be removed every 8 hours for skin care. The use of pneumatic compression devices for the calves is advocated, and they must be applied as soon as possible after admission and maintained throughout the hospitalization. Venous duplex studies may be performed before applying compression devices. The nurse should also perform range-of-motion exercises and stretching regularly. The thighs and calves of the legs should be assessed every shift for signs of DVT.

Prophylactic use of heparin or low-molecular-weight heparin (e.g., enoxaparin [Lovenox]) may be used to prevent DVT unless contraindicated. Contraindications include internal bleeding and recent surgery.

If blood loss has occurred from other injuries, hemoglobin and hematocrit levels should be monitored and blood should be administered according to protocol. The nurse also should monitor the patient for indications of hypovolemic shock secondary to hemorrhage.

Fluid and nutritional maintenance. During the first 48 to 72 hours after the injury the GI tract may stop functioning (paralytic ileus) and a nasogastric tube must be inserted. Because the patient cannot have oral intake, fluid and electrolyte needs must be carefully monitored. Specific solutions and additives are ordered based on individual requirements. Once bowel sounds are present or flatus is passed, oral food and fluids can gradually be introduced. Because of severe catabolism, a high-protein, high-calorie diet is necessary for energy and tissue repair. In patients with high cervical cord injuries, swallowing must be evaluated before starting oral feedings. If the patient is unable to resume eating, total parenteral nutrition may be started to provide nutritional support.

Some patients experience anorexia, which can be due to psychologic depression, boredom with institutional food, or discomfort at being fed (often by a hurried nurse). Some patients have a normally small appetite. Occasionally, refusal to eat is used as a means of maintaining control over the environment because of diminished or absent body control. If the patient is not eating adequately, the cause should be thoroughly assessed. On the basis of this assessment, a contract may be made with the patient using mutual goal setting regarding the diet. This gives the patient increased control of the situation and often results in improved nutritional intake. General measures such as providing a pleasant eating environment, allowing adequate time to eat (including any self-feeding the patient can achieve), encouraging the family to bring in special foods, and planning social rewards for eating may be useful. A calorie count should be kept, and the patient's daily weight recorded as a means of evaluating progress. If feasible, the patient should participate in recording calorie intake. Increased dietary fiber should be included to promote bowel function. The nurse should avoid allowing the patient's nutritional intake to become a basis for a power struggle.

Bladder and bowel management. Immediately after injury, urine is retained because of the loss of autonomic and reflex control of the bladder and sphincter. Because there is no sensation of fullness, overdistention of the bladder can result in reflux into the kidney with eventual renal failure. Bladder overdistention may even result in rupture of the bladder. Consequently, an indwelling catheter is usually inserted as soon as possible after injury. Its patency must be ensured by frequent inspection and irrigation if necessary. In some institutions a physician's order is required for this procedure. Strict aseptic technique for catheter care is essential to avoid introducing infection.

After the patient is stabilized, the best means of managing long-term urinary function is assessed. Usually the patient is started on an intermittent catheterization program. Intermittent catheterization has been shown to reduce UTIs when compared with an indwelling catheter, and it is the safest method of bladder management for protecting the kidneys.[23] The patient is often maintained on a fluid restriction of 1800 to 2000 ml per day to facilitate a bladder training program. Urinary output is monitored closely.

UTIs are a common problem. The best method for preventing UTIs is regular and complete bladder drainage. During the period of indwelling catheterization, a large fluid intake is required. The catheter should be checked frequently to prevent kinking and ensure free flow of urine. During intermittent catheterization, fluid intake should be moderate and regular (200 to 300 ml every 2 to 3 hours). Catheterization should be done every 3 to 4 hours to prevent bacterial overgrowth resulting from urinary stasis. Cranberry juice and/or cranberry extract tablets may be helpful for UTI prevention because there is some evidence that they may prevent bacteria from adhering to the bladder wall. Ascorbic acid and a urinary antiseptic, such as methenamine hippurate (Hiprex), are sometimes given although their use in preventing UTIs remains controversial. If the appearance or odor of the urine is suspicious or if the patient develops symptoms of a UTI (chills, fever, malaise), a specimen is sent for culture.

Age-related changes in renal function should be considered. The older adult is more likely to develop renal calculi, and older men may have prostatic hyperplasia, which may interfere with urinary flow and complicate urinary management.

Constipation is generally a problem during spinal shock because no voluntary or involuntary (reflex) evacuation of the bowels occurs. A bowel program should be started during acute care. This consists of choosing a rectal stimulant (suppository or minienema) to be inserted daily at a regular time of day followed by gentle digital stimulation or manual evacuation done by the nurse until evacuation is complete. Initially the program may be done in bed in the side-lying position, but as soon as the patient has resumed sitting, it should be done in the upright position on a padded bedside commode chair.[24]

Temperature control. Because there is no vasoconstriction, piloerection, or heat loss through perspiration below the level of injury, temperature control is largely external to the patient. Therefore the nurse must monitor the environment closely to maintain an appropriate temperature. Body temperature should be monitored regularly. The patient should not be overloaded with covers or unduly exposed (such as during bathing). If an infection with high fever develops, more extensive means of temperature control, such as a cooling blanket, may be necessary.

Stress ulcers. Stress ulcers are a problem for the patient with a spinal cord injury because of the physiologic response to severe trauma, psychologic stress, and high-dose corticosteroids. Peak incidence of stress ulcers is 6 to 14 days after injury. Stool and gastric contents are tested daily for blood, and the hematocrit is observed for a slow drop. When corticosteroids are given, they should be accompanied by antacids or food. Histamine H_2-receptor blockers, such as ranitidine (Zantac) and famotidine (Pepcid), or proton pump inhibitors, such as omeprazole (Prilosec), may be given prophylactically to decrease the secretion of hydrochloric acid.

Sensory deprivation. The nurse must compensate for the patient's absent sensations to prevent sensory deprivation. This is done by stimulating the patient above the level of injury. Conversation, music, strong aromas, and interesting flavors should be a part of the nursing care plan. Prism glasses are provided so that the patient can read and watch television. Every effort should be made to prevent the patient from withdrawing from the environment.

Patients with spinal cord injury often report altered sensorium and vivid dreams during the acute phase of their treatment. Whether this is due to drugs used to manage pain and anxiety is not known. Patients may also experience disrupted sleep patterns as a result of the hospital environment or posttraumatic stress disorder.

Reflexes. Once spinal cord shock is resolved, the return of reflexes may complicate rehabilitation. Lacking control from the higher brain centers, reflexes are often hyperactive and produce exaggerated responses. Penile erections can occur from a variety of stimuli, causing embarrassment and discomfort. Spasms ranging from mild twitches to convulsive movements below the level of the lesion may also occur. This reflex activity may be interpreted by the patient or family as a return of function, and the nurse must tactfully explain the reason for the activity. The patient may be informed of the positive use of these reflexes in sexual, bowel, and bladder retraining. Spasms may be controlled with the use of antispasmodic drugs. Most commonly prescribed are baclofen (Lioresal), dantrolene (Dantrium), and tizanidine (Zanaflex). Botulism toxin injections may also be given to treat severe spasticity.[25]

Autonomic dysreflexia. The return of reflexes after the resolution of spinal shock means that patients with an injury level at T6 or higher may develop autonomic dysreflexia. **Autonomic dysreflexia** is a massive uncompensated cardiovascular reaction mediated by the sympathetic nervous system. It occurs in response to visceral stimulation once spinal shock is resolved in patients with spinal cord lesions above T7. The condition is a life-threatening situation that requires immediate resolution. If resolution does not occur, this condition can lead to status epilepticus, stroke, myocardial infarction, and even death.

The most common precipitating cause is a distended bladder or rectum, although any sensory stimulation may cause autonomic dysreflexia. Contraction of the bladder or rectum, stimulation of the skin, or stimulation of the pain receptors may also cause autonomic dysreflexia. Manifestations include hypertension (up to 300 mm Hg systolic), blurred vision, throbbing headache, marked diaphoresis above the level of the lesion, bradycardia (30 to 40 beats per minute), *piloerection* (erection of body hair) as a result of pilomotor spasm, flushing of the skin above the level of the lesion, blurred vision or spots in the visual fields, nasal congestion, anxiety, and nausea. It is important to measure blood pressure when a patient with a spinal cord injury complains of a headache.[26]

The pathology of autonomic dysreflexia involves the stimulation of sensory receptors below the level of the cord lesion. The intact autonomic nervous system below the level of the lesion responds to the stimulation with a reflex arteriolar vasoconstriction that increases blood pressure. Baroreceptors in the carotid sinus and the aorta sense the hypertension and stimulate the parasympathetic system. This results in a decrease in heart rate, but the visceral and peripheral vessels do not dilate because efferent impulses cannot pass through the cord lesion.

Nursing interventions in this serious emergency are elevation of the head of the bed 45 degrees or sitting the patient upright, notification of the physician, and assessment to determine the cause. The most common cause is bladder irritation. Immediate catheterization to relieve bladder distention may be necessary. Lidocaine jelly should be instilled in the urethra before catheterization. If a catheter is already in place, it should be checked for kinks or folds. If plugged, small-volume irrigation should be performed slowly and gently to open a plugged catheter, or a new catheter may be inserted. Stool impaction can also result in auto-

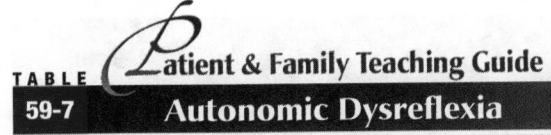

TABLE 59-7	**Patient & Family Teaching Guide** **Autonomic Dysreflexia**

Patient and family members must know the signs and symptoms of autonomic dysreflexia so that timely intervention can occur. These include the following:
- Sudden onset of acute headache
- Elevation in blood pressure and/or reduction in pulse rate
- Flushed face and upper chest (above the level of the lesion) and pale extremities (below the level of the lesion)
- Sweating above the level of the lesion
- Nasal congestion
- Feeling of apprehension

Immediate interventions include the following:
- Raise the person to a sitting position.
- Remove the stimulus (fecal impaction, kinked urinary catheter).
- Call the health care provider if above actions do not relieve the signs and symptoms.

Efforts to decrease the likelihood of autonomic dysreflexia include the following:
- Maintain regular bowel function.
- If manual rectal stimulation is used, local anesthetics may reduce stimulation of autonomic dysreflexia.
- Monitor urine output.
- Wear a medical alert bracelet indicating a history of autonomic dysreflexia.

nomic dysreflexia. A digital rectal examination should be performed only after application of an anesthetic ointment to decrease rectal stimulation and to prevent an increase of symptoms. The nurse should remove all skin stimuli, such as constrictive clothing and tight shoes. Blood pressure should be monitored frequently during the episode. If symptoms persist after the source has been relieved, an α-adrenergic blocker or an arteriolar vasodilator (e.g., nifedipine [Procardia]) is administered. Careful monitoring must continue until the vital signs stabilize.

The patient and family should be taught the causes and symptoms of autonomic dysreflexia (Table 59-7). They must understand the life-threatening nature of this dysfunction and must know how to relieve the cause.

Rehabilitation and Home Care. The physiologic and psychologic rehabilitation of the person with spinal cord injury is complex and involved. With physical and psychologic care and intensive and specialized rehabilitation, the patient with a spinal cord injury learns to function at the highest level of wellness. It is recommended that all patients with a new spinal cord injury receive comprehensive inpatient rehabilitation in a rehabilitation unit or center that specializes in spinal cord rehabilitation.

Many of the problems identified in the acute period become chronic and continue throughout life. Rehabilitation focuses on refined retraining of physiologic processes and extensive patient and family teaching about how to manage the physiologic and life changes resulting from injury (Fig. 59-13).

Rehabilitation is a multidisciplinary endeavor carried out through a team approach. Team members include rehabilitation nurses, physicians, physical therapists, occupational therapists, speech therapists, vocational counselors, psychologists, thera-

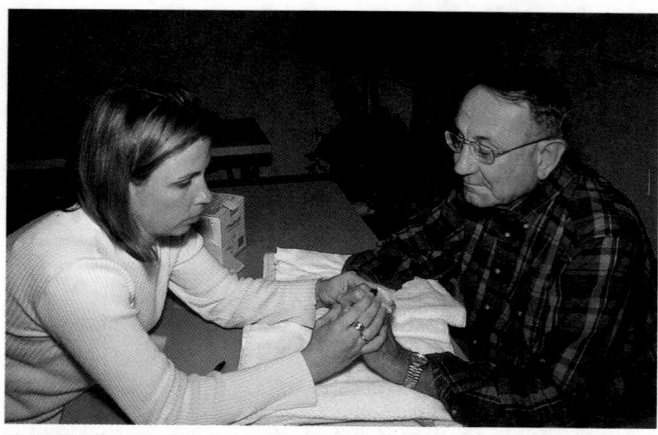

FIG. 59-13 Patient participating in occupational therapy.

peutic recreation specialists, prosthetists, orthotists, and dietitians. Rehabilitation care is organized around the individual patient's goals and needs. During rehabilitation, patients are expected to be involved in therapies and learn self-care for several hours each day. Such intensive work at a time when the patient is dealing with the sudden change in health and functional status can be very stressful. Progress may be slow, and frequent encouragement may be required. The rehabilitation nurse has a pivotal role in providing encouragement, specialized nursing care, patient and family teaching, and helping to coordinate the efforts of the rehabilitation team.

Respiratory rehabilitation. The patient with high cervical spinal cord injury may have greatly increased mobility with phrenic nerve stimulators or electronic diaphragmatic pacemakers. These devices are not appropriate for all ventilator-dependent patients but may be helpful for those with an intact phrenic nerve. Today, ventilators are also reasonably portable, and ventilator-dependent tetraplegic patients can be mobile and somewhat independent. Patients and family members should be taught all aspects of home ventilator care, and referrals should be made to appropriate community agencies. Patients with cervical level injuries who are not ventilator dependent should be taught assisted coughing and regular use of incentive spirometry or deep breathing exercises.

Neurogenic bladder. A **neurogenic bladder** is any type of bladder dysfunction related to abnormal or absent bladder innervation. After spinal cord shock resolves, depending on the completeness of the spinal cord injury, patients usually have some degree of neurogenic bladder. Normal voiding requires nervous system coordination of urethral and pelvic floor relaxation with simultaneous contraction of the detrusor muscle.[27] Depending on the lesion, a neurogenic bladder may have no reflex detrusor contractions (areflexic, flaccid), may have hyperactive reflex detrusor contractions (hyperreflexic, spastic), or may have lack of coordination between detrusor contraction and urethral relaxation *(dyssynergia)*. Common problems with a neurogenic bladder include urgency, frequency, incontinence, inability to void, and high bladder pressures resulting in reflux of urine into the kidneys.

Neurogenic bladder can be classified according to reflex detrusor activity, intravesical filling pressure, and continence function. Types of neurogenic bladder are outlined in Table 59-8. Diagnostic and collaborative care of neurogenic bladder is described in Table 59-9. The patient with a spinal cord injury and a neurogenic bladder requires a comprehensive program to manage bladder function.

After the patient's overall condition is stable and there is evidence of neurologic reflexes, urodynamic testing, an IV pyelogram, and a urine culture are done. The method used for urinary drainage depends on the type of neurogenic bladder dysfunction, the preference of the patient, and availability of a family caregiver, the physician, and the nursing staff. Numerous drainage methods are possible, including bladder reflex retraining if partial voiding control remains, indwelling catheter, intermittent catheterization, and external catheter (condom catheter). Surgical options including sphincterectomy, implantation of a functional electrical stimulation device, and urinary diversion.

Many factors are considered when selecting a bladder management strategy. These include upper extremity function, caregiver burden, and lifestyle choices. The type of bladder dysfunction also defines treatment goals and management options. A

TABLE 59-8 **Types of Neurogenic Bladder**

TYPE	CHARACTERISTICS	CAUSES	CLINICAL MANIFESTATIONS
Reflexic (spastic, uninhibited, upper motor neuron)	No inhibitions influence time and place of voiding; bladder empties in response to stretching of bladder wall	Corticospinal tract lesion; observed in spinal cord injury, stroke, multiple sclerosis, brain tumor, brain trauma	Incontinence, frequency, urgency; voiding is unpredictable and incomplete
Areflexic (autonomous, flaccid, lower motor neuron)	Bladder acts as if there were paralysis of all motor functions, fills without emptying	Lower motor neuron lesion caused by trauma involving S2-S4; lesions of cauda equina, pelvic nerves	If sensory function intact, feels bladder distention and hesitancy; no control of micturition, resulting in overdistention of bladder and overflow incontinence
Sensory	Lack of sensation of need to urinate	Damage to sensory limb of bladder spinal reflex arc; seen in multiple sclerosis, diabetes mellitus	Poor bladder sensation, infrequent voiding, large residual volume

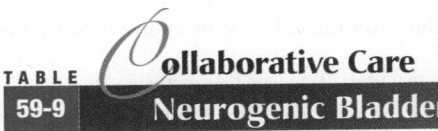

TABLE 59-9	Collaborative Care — Neurogenic Bladder

Diagnostic
History and physical examination including neurologic examination
Urodynamic testing
IV pyelogram
Urine culture

Collaborative Therapy
Drug therapy
Suppress bladder contractions (anticholinergics)
Relaxation of urethral sphincter (α-adrenergic blockers)
Suppress pelvic floor spasticity (baclofen [Lioresal])
Fluid intake of 1800 to 2000 ml/day
Urine drainage
Voluntary or reflex voiding
Intermittent catheterization
Indwelling catheter
Surgery
Sphincterotomy
Electrical stimulation
Urinary diversion

IV, Intravenous.

reflexic bladder with detrusor and sphincter dyssynergia requires interventions to provide low-pressure storage, low-pressure voiding, and adequate emptying. Anticholinergic drugs (oxybutynin [Ditropan], tolterodine [Detrol]) may be used to suppress bladder contraction. α-Adrenergic blockers (e.g., terazosin [Hytrin], doxazosin [Cardura]) may be used to decrease outflow resistance at the bladder neck, and antispasmodic drugs (e.g., baclofen [Lioresal] may be used to decrease spasticity of pelvic floor muscles.

Drainage options include intermittent catheterization, external catheter, or indwelling catheter. A reflexic bladder with detrusor hyperreflexia may be treated with anticholinergic drugs, intravesical capsaicin, or botulinum A toxin. An areflexic bladder is usually managed with intermittent catheterization or indwelling catheter.

The long-term use of an indwelling catheter should be carefully evaluated because of the associated high incidence of UTI, fistula formation, and diverticula. However, there may be patients for whom this is the best option. Adequate fluid intake and patency of the catheter should be ensured. The frequency of routine catheter changes ranges from 1 week to 1 month, depending on the type of catheter used and agency policy.

Intermittent catheterization is the most commonly recommended method of bladder management (see Chapter 44). Nursing assessment is important in selecting the time interval between catheterizations. Initially, catheterization is done every 4 hours. Bladder volume can be assessed before catheterization using the portable bladder ultrasound machine. If less than 200 ml of urine is measured, the time interval may be extended. If 500 ml or more of urine is measured, the time interval is shortened. An overdistended bladder can cause ischemia of the bladder wall, which may predispose tissues to bacterial invasion and infection. Patients often experience diuresis at a regular time during a 24-

hour period. The number of intermittent catheterizations per day is usually five or six.

Urinary diversion surgery may be necessary if the patient has repeated UTIs with renal involvement or repeated stones or if therapeutic intervention has been unsuccessful (see Chapter 44). Surgical treatment of neurogenic bladder includes bladder neck revision (sphincterotomy), bladder augmentation (augmentation cystoplasty), penile prosthesis, artificial sphincter, perineal ureterostomy, cystotomy, vesicotomy, and anterior urethral transplantation.

No matter which bladder management strategy is selected, the nurse must teach the patient and the family or caregivers about how to accomplish successful self-management. Management techniques, how to obtain necessary supplies, care of supplies and equipment, and when to seek health care must be taught. Resources and referrals for supplies and ongoing care must be arranged.

Neurogenic bowel. Careful management of bowel evacuation is necessary in the patient with a spinal cord injury because voluntary control of this function may be lost as a result of a condition called **neurogenic bowel.** The usual measures for preventing constipation include a high-fiber diet and adequate fluid intake (see Table 41-9). Patient and family teaching guidelines related to bowel management are presented in Table 59-10. However, these measures by themselves may not be adequate to stimulate evacuation. In addition, suppositories (bisacodyl [Dulcolax] or glycerin) or small-volume enemas and digital stimulation by the nurse or patient may be necessary. In the patient with an upper motor neuron lesion, digital stimulation is necessary to relax the external sphincter to promote defecation. A stool softener such as docusate sodium (Colace) can be used to regulate stool consistency. Oral stimulant laxatives should be used only if absolutely necessary for a day or two and not on a regular basis.

Valsalva maneuver and manual stimulation are useful in patients with lower motor neuron lesions. The Valsalva maneuver requires intact abdominal muscles, so it is used in those patients with injuries below T12. In general, a bowel movement every other day is considered adequate. However, preinjury patterns should be considered. Incontinence can result from too much stool softener or a fecal impaction.

Careful recording of bowel movements, including amount, time, and consistency, is important to the overall success of the program. Timing of defecation may also be an important factor. If bowel evacuation is planned for 30 to 60 minutes following the first meal of the day, this may enhance success by taking advantage of the gastrocolic reflex induced by eating. Again, patient and family education is required to promote successful independent bowel management.

Neurogenic skin. Prevention of pressure ulcers and other types of injury to insensitive skin are essential for every patient with spinal cord injury. Nurses in rehabilitation are responsible for teaching these skills and providing information about daily skin care. A comprehensive visual and tactile examination of the skin should be done twice daily with special attention given to areas over bony prominences. The areas most vulnerable to breakdown include the ischia, trochanters, heels, and the sacrum. Careful positioning and repositioning should be done initially every 2 hours with gradual increases in the times between turns if there is no redness over bony prominences at the time of turning. Pressure-relieving cushions must be used in wheelchairs, and special

Patient & Family Teaching Guide

TABLE 59-10

Bowel Management after Spinal Cord Injury

The following are teaching guidelines for a patient with a spinal cord injury:

1. Optimal nutritional intake includes:
   Three well-balanced meals each day
   Two servings from the milk group
   Two or more servings from the meat group, including beef, pork, poultry, eggs, fish
   Four or more servings from the vegetable and fruit groups
   Four or more servings from the bread and cereal group
2. Fiber intake should be approximately 20 to 30 g per day. The amount of fiber eaten should be increased gradually over 1 to 2 weeks.
3. Three quarts of fluid per day should be consumed unless contraindicated. Water or fruit juices should be used, and caffeinated beverages such as coffee, tea, and cola should be avoided. Fluid softens hard stools; caffeine stimulates fluid loss through urination.
4. Foods that produce gas (e.g., beans) or upper GI upset (spicy foods) should be avoided.
5. *Timing*: A regular schedule for bowel evacuation should be established. A good time is 30 minutes after the first meal of the day.
6. *Position*: If possible, an upright position with feet flat on the floor or on a stepstool enhances bowel evacuation. Staying on the toilet, commode, or bedpan for longer than 20 to 30 minutes may cause skin breakdown. Based on stability, someone may need to stay with the patient.
7. *Activity*: Exercise is important for bowel function. In addition to improving muscle tone, it also increases GI transit time and increases appetite. Muscles should be exercised. This includes stretching, range-of-motion, position changing, and functional movement.
8. *Drug treatment*: Suppositories may be necessary to stimulate a bowel movement. Manual stimulation of the rectum may also be helpful in initiating defecation. Stool softeners should be used as needed to regulate stool consistency. Oral laxatives should be used only if necessary.

GI, Gastrointestinal.

mattresses may also be needed. Movement during turns and transfers should be done carefully to avoid stretching and folding of soft tissues (shear), as well as friction or abrasion.[27]

Nutritional status should be assessed regularly. Both body weight loss and weight gain can contribute to skin breakdown. Adequate intake of protein is essential for skin health. Measurement of prealbumin, total protein, and albumin can help identify inadequate protein intake. The importance of nutrition to skin health should be stressed to the patient and family.

Protection of the skin also requires avoidance of thermal injury. Burns can be caused by hot food or liquids, bath or shower water that is too warm, radiators, heating pads, and uninsulated plumbing. Thermal injury also can result from extreme cold (frostbite). Injuries may not be noticed until severe damage is done. Anticipatory guidance about potential risks is essential.

Patient and family education related to skin is provided in Tables 59-11 and 59-12.

Sexuality. Knowledge of the level and completeness of injury is needed to understand the male patient's potential for orgasm, erection, and fertility and the patient's capacity for sexual satisfaction (Table 59-13). Sexuality is an important issue regardless of the patient's age or gender. To provide accurate and sensitive counseling and education about sexuality, the nurse must have an awareness and an acceptance of personal sexuality, as well as knowledge of human sexual responses. When discussing sexual potential, the nurse should use scientific terminology rather than slang whenever possible.

Reflex sexual function capability is possible if the patient has an upper motor neuron lesion. The presence of tone in the external rectal sphincter indicates an upper motor lesion. The absence of external rectal sphincter tone, bulbocavernosus reflex, or both indicates that the patient has lower motor neuron involvement and may be capable of psychogenic erection but not reflex erection. If ejaculation occurs, it may be retrograde into the bladder.

The type of lesion determines the physical sexual response. Men with upper motor neuron lesions may have reflexogenic erections that are produced by reflex activity or external stimuli or that occur spontaneously. These spontaneous erections are often short lived and uncontrolled and cannot be maintained or summoned at the time of coitus. Orgasm and ejaculation are usually not possible for men with a complete upper motor neuron lesion.

Most patients with a complete lower motor neuron lesion are unable to have either psychogenic or reflexogenic erections. Patients with incomplete lower motor neuron lesions have the highest possibility of successful psychogenic erection with ejaculation, and up to 10% of these patients are fertile.

Treatments for erectile dysfunction include drugs, vacuum devices, and surgical procedures. Sildenafil (Viagra) has become the treatment of choice since several studies have documented its effectiveness in men with spinal cord injury. Penile injection of vasoactive substances (papaverine, prostaglandin E) is another

Patient & Family Teaching Guide

TABLE 59-11

Skin Care for Patient with Spinal Cord Injury

Skin breakdown is a potential problem after spinal cord injury. The following measures are used to decrease this possibility:

Change Position Frequently
- If in a wheelchair, lift self up and shift weight every 15 to 30 minutes.
- If in bed, a regular turning schedule (at least every 2 hours) that includes sides, back, and abdomen is encouraged to change position.
- Use special mattresses and wheelchair cushions.
- Use pillows to protect bony prominences when in bed.

Monitor Skin Condition
- Inspect skin frequently for areas of redness, swelling, and breakdown.
- Keep fingernails trimmed to avoid scratches and abrasions.
- If a wound develops, follow standard wound care management procedures.

medical treatment. Risks include *priapism* (prolonged penile erection) and scarring, so these substances are often considered only after failure of sildenafil. Vacuum suction devices use negative pressure to encourage blood flow into the penis. Erection is maintained by a constriction band placed at the base of the penis.

TABLE 59-12 Patient & Family Teaching Guide Halo Vest Care

The following are teaching guidelines for a patient with a halo vest:

1. Inspect the pins on the halo traction ring. Report to health care provider if pins are loose or if there are signs of infection including redness, tenderness, swelling, or drainage at the insertion sites.
2. Clean around pin sites carefully with hydrogen peroxide on a cotton swab. Repeat the procedure using water.
3. Use alcohol swabs to cleanse pin sites of any drainage.
4. Apply antibiotic ointment as prescribed.
5. To provide skin care, have the patient lie down on a bed with his or her head resting on a pillow to reduce pressure on the brace. Loosen one side of the vest. Gently wash the skin under the vest with soap and water, rinse it, and then dry it thoroughly. At the same time, check the skin for pressure points, redness, swelling, bruising, or chafing. Close the open side and repeat the procedure on the opposite side.
6. If the vest becomes wet or damp, it can be carefully dried with a blow dryer.
7. An assistive device (e.g., cane, walker) may be used to provide greater balance. Flat shoes should be worn.
8. Turn the entire body, not just the head and neck, when trying to view sideways.
9. In case of an emergency, keep a set of wrenches close to the halo vest at all times.
10. Mark the vest strap such that consistent buckling and fit can be maintained.
11. Avoid grabbing bars or vest to assist patient.
12. Keep sheepskin pad under vest. Change and wash at least weekly.
13. If perspiration or itching is a problem, a cotton T-shirt can be worn under sheepskin. The T-shirt can be modified with Velcro seam closure on one side.

The main surgical option is implantation of a penile prosthesis.[28] (Erectile dysfunction is discussed in Chapter 53.)

Male fertility is affected by spinal cord injury causing poor sperm quality and ejaculatory dysfunction. Recent advances in methods of retrieving sperm (penile vibratory stimulation and electroejaculation) combined with ovulation induction and intrauterine insemination of the female partner have changed the prognosis for men with spinal cord injury to father children from unlikely to a reasonable possibility of successful outcomes.[29]

The effect of spinal cord injury on female sexual response is less clear. Lubrication is similar to erections in males, with reflex and psychogenic components. Women with upper motor neuron injuries may retain the capacity for reflex lubrication, whereas psychogenic lubrication depends on the completeness of injury. Orgasm is reported by about 50% of women with spinal cord injury.[29]

The woman of childbearing age with a spinal cord injury usually remains fertile. The injury does not affect the ability to become pregnant or to deliver normally through the birth canal. Menses may cease for as long as 6 months. If sexual activity is resumed, protection against an unplanned pregnancy is necessary. A normal pregnancy may be complicated by UTIs, anemia, and autonomic dysreflexia. Because uterine contractions are not felt, a precipitous delivery is always a danger.

Sexual rehabilitation for both men and women should begin informally after the acute phase of the injury has passed. Questions such as, "Have you had an erection since your accident?" and "Have your menstrual periods continued since the accident?" are nonthreatening ways to introduce the topic of sexual functioning. The male patient may pose a question such as, "Can I ever be a man again?"

Open discussion with the patient is essential. This important aspect of rehabilitation should be handled by someone specially trained in sexual counseling. A nurse or other rehabilitation professional with such expertise works with the patient and partner to provide support with the emphasis on open communication. The nurse's educational role requires respect for every couple's personal standards of religious and cultural beliefs. Alternative methods of obtaining sexual satisfaction such as oral-genital sex (cunnilingus and fellatio) may be suggested. Explicit films (e.g., *Touching*) may also be used. This film demonstrates the sexual activities of a patient with paraplegia and a nondisabled partner. Graphics should be used cautiously because they may be too lim-

TABLE 59-13 Potential for Sexual Function in Men with Spinal Cord Injury

ERECTION	EJACULATION	ORGASM
Upper Motor Neuron		
Complete		
Frequent (92%), reflexogenic only	Rare (4%)	Rare
Incomplete		
Most frequent (99%) including reflexogenic (80%) and psychogenic (19%)	Less frequent (32%), after reflexogenic erection (74%), after psychogenic erection (26%)	Present (if ejaculation occurs)
Lower Motor Neuron		
Complete		
Infrequent (26%)	Infrequent (18%)	Present (if ejaculation occurs)
Incomplete		
Psychogenic and reflexogenic	Frequent (70%), after psychogenic and reflexogenic erections	Present (if ejaculation occurs)

iting or focus too much on the mechanics of sex rather than on the relationship.

Sexual activities may require more planning and be less spontaneous than before the injury. For example, an attendant may have to undress the patient and remove equipment. A relaxed atmosphere with music and perfume creates an attractive environment. Ample time for caressing, fondling, and kissing is essential. The partners should be encouraged to explore each other's erogenous areas, such as the lips, neck, and ears, which can arouse psychogenic erection or orgasm. Few demands should be made initially.

Care should be taken not to dislodge an indwelling catheter during sexual activity. If an external catheter is used, it should be removed before sexual activity and the patient should refrain from fluids. The bowel program should include evacuation the morning of sexual activity. The partner should be informed that an accident is always possible. The woman may need a water-soluble lubricant to supplement diminished vaginal secretions and facilitate vaginal penetration.

Grief and depression. Patients with spinal cord injuries may feel an overwhelming sense of loss. They may temporarily lose control over everyday life activities and must depend on others for ADLs and for life-sustaining measures. Patients may believe that they are useless and burdens to their families. At a stage when independence is often of the greatest importance, they may be totally dependent on others.

The patient's response and recovery differ in some important aspects from those experiencing loss from amputation or terminal illness. First, regression can and does occur at different stages. Working through grief is a difficult, lifelong process with which the patient needs support and encouragement. With recent advances in rehabilitation, it is usual for the patient to be independent physically and discharged from the rehabilitation center before completion of the grief process. The goal of recovery is related more to adjustment than to acceptance. Adjustment implies the ability to go on with living with certain limitations. Although the patient who is cooperative and accepting is easier to treat, the nurse should expect a wide fluctuation of emotions from a patient with a spinal cord injury. Depression may not be a component of the recovery process. Societal norms allow depression after severe loss and almost impose it on those confronted with death or radical lifestyle changes. However, every patient may not experience depression.

The nurse's role in grief work is to allow mourning as a component of the rehabilitation process. Table 59-14 summarizes the mourning process and appropriate nursing interventions. Maintaining hope is an important strategy during the grieving process and should not be interpreted as denial. During the shock and denial stage the nurse reassures the patient and stresses the expertise of the entire health care team. During the anger stage, the nurse assists the patient in achievement of control over the environment, particularly by allowing the patient's input into the plan of care. The nurse should not respond to anger or manipulation or become involved in a power struggle with the patient. As self-care abilities increase, the patient's independence increases.

The patient's family also requires counseling to avoid promoting dependency in the patient through guilt or misplaced sympathy. The family is also experiencing an intense grieving process. A support group of family members and friends of patients with

TABLE 59-14 Mourning Process and Nursing Interventions in Spinal Cord Injury

PATIENT BEHAVIOR	NURSING INTERVENTION
Shock and Denial Struggle for survival, complete dependence, excessive sleep, withdrawal, fantasies, unrealistic expectations	• Use of meticulous nursing care. • Be honest. • Use simple diagrams to explain injury. • Encourage patient to begin road to recovery. • Establish agreement to use and improve all current abilities while not denying the possibility of future improvement.
Anger Refusal to discuss paralysis, decreased self-esteem, manipulation, hostile and abusive language	• Coordinate care with patient and encourage self-care. • Support family members; prevent alleviation of guilt by supporting dependency. • Use humor liberally. • Allow patient outbursts. • Do not allow fixation on injury.
Depression Sadness, pessimism, anorexia, nightmares, insomnia, agitation, psychomotor retardation, "blues," suicidal preoccupation, refusal to participate in any self-care activities	• Encourage family involvement and resources. • Plan graded steps in rehabilitation to give success with minimal opportunity for frustration. • Give cheerful and willing assistance with activities of daily living. • Avoid sympathy. • Use firm kindness.
Adjustment Planning for future, active participation in therapy, finding of personal meaning in experience and continuation of growth, return to premorbid personality	• Remember that patients have individual personalities. • Balance support systems to encourage independence. • Set goals with patient input. • Emphasize potentials.

spinal cord injury can help increase family members' knowledge and participation in the grieving process, physical difficulties, rehabilitation plan, and the meaning of the disability in society.

During the stage of depression, the nurse must be patient and persistent and maintain a sense of humor. Sympathy is not helpful. The patient should be treated in an adult manner and be involved in decision making about care, but the nurse must insist that the care be performed. A primary nurse relationship is helpful. Staff planning and sessions in which staff members can express their feelings are helpful in providing consistency of care. To achieve the stage of adjustment, the patient needs continual support throughout the rehabilitation process in the forms of acceptance, affection, and caring. The nurse must be attentive when the patient needs to talk and sensitive to needs at the various stages of the grief process.

Although the stage of depression during the grief process usually lasts days to weeks, there are some individuals who may become clinically depressed and require treatment for depression. Evaluation by a psychiatric nurse or psychiatrist is recommended. Treatment may include drugs and psychotherapy.[30]

■ Evaluation

Expected outcomes for the patient with a spinal cord injury are presented in NCP 59-1 on p. 1619.

■ Gerontologic Considerations: Spinal Cord Injury

The demographics of patients living with spinal cord injury are changing. The fact that persons with spinal cord injury now have longer life spans has contributed to the increasing number of older adults living with spinal cord injury. Aging is also associated with an increased likelihood of other chronic illnesses that may have a serious impact on the older adult with a spinal cord injury. As patients with spinal cord injury age, both individual aging changes and duration since injury impact functional ability. For example, bowel and bladder dysfunction can increase with duration and severity of spinal cord injury. Musculoskeletal repetitive trauma injuries are more common.

Health promotion and screening are important for the older patient with a spinal cord injury. Daily skin inspections, UTI prevention measures, and monthly breast exams for women and regular prostate cancer screening for men are recommended. Cardiovascular disease is the most common cause of morbidity and mortality among spinal cord–injured persons. The lack of sensation including angina in those with high level injuries may mask acute myocardial ischemia. Altered autonomic nervous system function and decreases in physical activity can place the patient at risk for cardiovascular problems including hypertension.[31]

At the same time, because of increased work and recreational activities of older adults, more older adults are experiencing spinal cord injury. Health promotion to decrease injury risk includes fall prevention strategies (e.g., using a stepstool or a grab bar to reach high shelves, handrails on stairs). Rehabilitation for the older person who has undergone a spinal cord injury may likely take longer because of other preexisting conditions and poorer health status at the time of the initial injury. ■

SPINAL CORD TUMORS

Etiology and Pathophysiology

Tumors that affect the spinal cord account for 0.5% to 1% of all neoplasms. These tumors are classified as primary (arising from some component of cord, dura, nerves, or vessels) or secondary (from primary growths in the breast, thyroid, lung, kidney, and other sites). Spinal cord tumors are further classified as extradural (outside the spinal cord), intradural extramedullary (within the dura but outside the actual spinal cord), and intradural intramedullary (within the spinal cord itself). These latter tumors are usually astrocytomas or ependy-

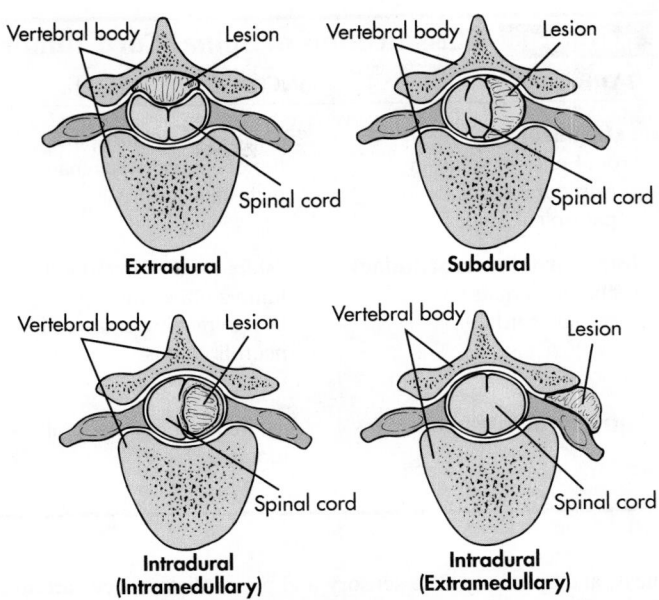

FIG. 59-14 Types of spinal cord tumors.

momas (Fig. 59-14, Table 59-15). Approximately 90% of all spinal tumors are extradural. Extradural tumors are usually metastatic and most often arise in the vertebral bodies. These metastatic lesions can invade intradurally and compress the spinal cord. Spinal intradural-extramedullary tumors account for two thirds of all intraspinal neoplasms and are mainly represented by meningiomas and schwannomas.

Because many of these tumors are slow growing, their symptoms stem from the mechanical effects of slow compression and irritation of nerve roots, displacement of the cord, or gradual obstruction of the vascular supply. The slowness of growth does not cause autodestruction (secondary injury) as in traumatic lesions. Therefore complete functional restoration may be possible when the tumor is removed, except with the intradural-intramedullary tumors.

Most metastatic tumors are extradural lesions. Tumors that commonly metastasize to the spinal epidural space are those that spread to bone, such as carcinomas of the breast, lung, prostate, and kidney.

Clinical Manifestations

Both sensory and motor problems may result with the location and extent of the tumor determining the severity and distribution of the problem. The most common early symptom of a spinal cord tumor outside the cord is pain in the back with radicular pain simulating intercostal neuralgia, angina, or herpes zoster. The location of the pain depends on the level of compression. The pain worsens with activity, coughing, straining, and lying down. Sensory disruption is later manifested by coldness, numbness, and tingling in an extremity or in several extremities, slowly progressing upward until it reaches the level of the lesion. Impaired sensation of pain, temperature, and light touch precedes a deficit in vibration and position sense that may progress to complete anesthesia. Motor weakness accompanies the sensory disturbances and consists of slowly increasing clumsiness, weak-

TABLE 59-15   Classification of Spinal Cord Tumors

TYPE	INCIDENCE	TREATMENT	PROGNOSIS
Extradural From bones of spine, in extradural space, or in paraspinal tissue	20%–50% of all intraspinal tumors, mostly malignant metastatic lesions	Relief of cord pressure by surgical laminectomy, radiation, chemotherapy, or combination approach	Poor
Intradural Extramedullary Within dura mater outside cord	Most frequent of intradural tumors (40%), mostly benign meningiomas and neurofibromas	Complete surgical removal of tumor (if possible), partial removal followed by radiation	Usually very good if lack of damage to cord from compression
Intradural Intramedullary	Least frequent of intradural tumors (5%–10%)	Partial surgical removal, radiation therapy (resulting in only temporary improvement)	Very poor

ness, and spasticity. The sensory and motor disturbances are ipsilateral to the lesion. Bladder disturbances are marked by urgency with difficulty in starting the flow and progressing to retention with overflow incontinence.

Manifestations of intradural spinal tumor develop as progressive damage to the long spinal tracts, producing paralysis, sensory loss, and bladder dysfunction. Pain can be severe as a result of compression of spinal roots or vertebrae.

NURSING *and* COLLABORATIVE MANAGEMENT SPINAL CORD TUMORS

Extradural tumors are seen early on routine spinal x-rays, whereas intradural and intramedullary tumors require MRI or CT scans for detection. CSF analysis may reveal tumor cells. The cord is decompressed after removal of the tumor by a laminectomy. More than 85% of primary neoplasms are benign and can be completely resected; 90% of patients recover without residual problems.

Compression of the spinal cord is an emergency. Relief of the ischemia related to the compression is the goal of therapy. Corticosteroids are generally prescribed immediately to relieve tumor-related edema. Dexamethasone (Decadron) is usually used, often in large doses.

Treatment for nearly all spinal cord tumors is surgical removal. The exception is the metastatic tumor that is sensitive to radiation and that has caused only minimal neurologic deficits in the patient. In general, tumors of the extradural or intradural-extramedullary group can be completely removed surgically. Intramedullary tumors offer a less favorable prognosis; however, exploration and removal are usually attempted.

Radiation therapy after the operation is fairly effective. Maximum permissible tissue dose is given over 6 to 8 weeks. Chemotherapy has also been used in conjunction with radiation therapy.

Relief of pain and return of function are the ultimate goals of treatment. Nurses must be aware of the neurologic status of the patient before and after treatment. Ensuring that the patient receives pain medication as needed is an important nursing responsibility. Depending on the amount of neurologic dysfunction exhibited, the patient may need to be cared for as though recovering from a spinal cord injury. Rehabilitation of patients with spinal cord tumors is similar to spinal cord injury rehabilitation.[32]

CRITICAL THINKING EXERCISES

Case Study
Spinal Cord Injury

Patient Profile. Samuel D., a 25-year-old white man, is admitted to the emergency department with the diagnosis of a cervical spinal cord injury. Samuel was swimming at a neighbor's backyard pool. He dove into the shallow end, striking his head on the bottom of the pool. His friends noticed that he did not resurface. They rescued him and brought him to the side of the pool. They maintained neck immobilization until the rescue crews arrived.

Subjective Data
- Is awake and alert
- Has complaints of neck pain
- Is anxious and asking why he cannot move his legs
- Is asking to see his family

Objective Data
Physical Examination
- Weak biceps movement
- No triceps movement
- Gross elbow movement present
- Decreased sensation from the shoulders down
- No bladder or bowel control
- BP: 90/56; pulse: 56; respirations: 32 and labored

Diagnostic Studies
- X-rays revealed C5 fracture dislocation

Collaborative Care
- Placed in tongs and traction in the emergency department
- Started on methylprednisolone in the emergency department
- Admitted to ICU

CRITICAL THINKING EXERCISES—cont'd

CRITICAL THINKING QUESTIONS

1. What nursing activities would be a priority on Samuel D.'s arrival in the ICU?
2. What physiologic problems are causing Samuel D. to have hypotension and bradycardia?
3. What would the first line of treatment be for Samuel D.'s hypotension and bradycardia?
4. What signs and symptoms would indicate respiratory distress and what physiologic problem would cause respiratory distress in Samuel D.'s injury state?
5. What can the nurse do to decrease Samuel D.'s anxiety?
6. Based on the assessment data provided, write one or more nursing diagnoses. Are there any collaborative problems?

Nursing Research Issues

1. What is the best method of education in the prevention of spinal cord injuries?
2. What type of support or education is best for the families of patients with spinal cord injuries to help them cope with their situation?
3. What nursing interventions enhance self-care in the patient with a spinal cord injury?
4. What is the best method of preventing UTIs in the spinal cord injured patient?
5. What is the relationship between the functional ability of spinal cord injury and quality of life?

REVIEW QUESTIONS

The number of the question corresponds to the same-numbered objective at the beginning of the chapter.

1. During assessment of the patient with trigeminal neuralgia, the nurse should
   a. inspect all aspects of the mouth and teeth.
   b. lightly palpate the affected side of the face for edema.
   c. test for temperature and sensation perception on the face.
   d. ask the patient to describe factors that initiate an episode.

2. During routine assessment of a patient with Guillain-Barré syndrome, the nurse finds the patient to be short of breath. The patient's respiratory distress is caused by
   a. elevated protein levels in the CSF.
   b. immobility resulting from ascending paralysis.
   c. degeneration of motor neurons in the brainstem and spinal cord.
   d. paralysis ascending to the nerves that stimulate the thoracic area.

3. A patient is admitted to the ICU with a C7 spinal cord injury and diagnosed with Brown-Séquard syndrome. On physical examination, the nurse would most likely find
   a. upper extremity weakness only.
   b. complete motor and sensory loss below C7.
   c. loss of position sense and vibration in both lower extremities.
   d. ipsilateral motor loss and contralateral sensory loss below C7.

4. A patient is admitted to the hospital with a spinal cord injury following an automobile accident. The nurse recognizes that the pathophysiology of secondary spinal cord injury involves
   a. initial infarction of the white matter of the cord.
   b. mechanical transection of the cord by the trauma.
   c. necrotic destruction of the cord from hemorrhage and edema.
   d. release of epinephrine leading to massive vasodilation of spinal cord vessels.

5. A rehabilitation goal for the patient with an injury at the C5 level includes
   a. feeding self with hand devices.
   b. driving an electric wheelchair.
   c. assisting with transfer activities.
   d. controlling bowel and bladder functions.

6. A patient with a C7 spinal cord injury undergoing rehabilitation tells the nurse he must have the flu because he has a bad headache and nausea. The initial action of the nurse is to
   a. call the physician.
   b. check the patient's temperature.
   c. take the patient's blood pressure.
   d. elevate the head of the bed to 90 degrees.

7. For a 65-year-old female patient who has lived with a T1 spinal cord injury for 20 years, the nurse would emphasize the following health teaching information:
   a. A mammogram is needed every year.
   b. Bladder function tends to improve with age.
   c. Heart disease is not common in persons with spinal cord injury.
   d. As a person ages, the need to change body position is less important.

8. The most common early symptom of a spinal cord tumor is
   a. urinary incontinence.
   b. back pain that worsens with activity.
   c. paralysis below the level of involvement.
   d. impaired sensation of pain, temperature, and light touch.

REFERENCES

1. Rozen TD: Antiepileptic drugs in the management of cluster headache and trigeminal neuralgia, *Headache* 41:S25, 2001.
2. Peiper DR, Dickerson J, Hassenbusch SJ: Percutaneous retrogasserian glycerol rhizolysis for treatment of chronic intractable cluster headaches: long-term results, *Neurosurgery* 46:363, 2000.
3. Tronnier VM et al: Treatment of idiopathic trigeminal neuralgia: comparison of long-term outcome after radiofrequency rhizotomy and microvascular decompression, *Neurosurgery* 48:1261, 2001.
4. Grogan PM, Gronseth GS: Practice parameter: steroids, acyclovir, and surgery for Bell's palsy (an evidence-based review), *Neurology* 56:830, 2001.
5. Nachamkin I: Chronic effects of *Campylobacter* infection, *Microbes Infect* 4:399, 2002.
6. Willison HJ, O'Hanlon GM: The immunopathogenesis of Miller Fisher syndrome, *J Neuroimmunol* 100:3, 1999.
7. Hughes RA, van det Meche FG: Corticosteroids for treating Guillain-Barre syndrome, *Cochrane Database Syst Rev* 2:CD001446, 2000.
8. Centers for Disease Control and Prevention: Botulism. Available at *http://www.cdc.gov/nip/publications/pink/botulism* (accessed July 29, 2002).
9. Centers for Disease Control and Prevention: Tetanus. Available at *http://www.cdc.gov/nip/publications/pink/tetanus* (accessed July 29, 2002).
10. Hutto B: Syphilis in clinical psychiatry: a review, *Psychosomatics* 42:453, 2001.
11. Centers for Disease Control and Prevention: What you should know about spinal cord injuries. Available at *http://www.cdc.gov/safeusa/home/sci.htm* (accessed June 12, 2002).
12. Spinal cord injury facts and figures, May 2001. Available at *http://www.spinalcord.uab.edu* (accessed June 12, 2002).
13. Atrice MB et al: Traumatic spinal cord injury. In Umphred DA, editor: *Neurological rehabilitation*, ed 4, St Louis, 2001, Mosby.
14. Kirshblum SC, O'Connor KC: Levels of spinal cord injury and predictors of neurologic recovery, *Phys Med Rehabil Clin N Am* 11:1, 2000.
15. Nockels RP: Nonoperative management of acute spinal cord injury, *Spine* 26:531, 2001.
16. American Spinal Injury Association/International Medical Society of Paraplegic (ASIA/IMSOP): *International standards for neurological functional classification of spinal cord injury patients* (revised). Chicago, 2002, American Spinal Injury Association.
17. Kim V, Spandorfer J: Epidemiology of venous thromboembolic disease, *Emerg Med Clin North Am* 19:839, 2001.
18. Papadopoulos SM et al: Immediate spinal cord decompression for cervical spinal cord injury: feasibility and outcome, *J Trauma* 52:323, 2002.
19. Dumont RJ et al: Acute spinal cord injury, part II: contemporary pharmacotherapy. *Clin Neuropharmacol* 24:265, 2001.
20. Bracken MB, Holford TR: Neurological and functional status 1 year after acute spinal cord injury: estimates of functional recovery in National Acute Spinal Cord Injury Study II from results modeled in National Acute Spinal Cord Injury Study III, *J Neurosurg* 96:259, 2002.
21. Bracken MB: Steroids for acute spinal cord injury (Cochrane Review), *Cochrane Database Syst Rev* 3:CD001046, 2002.
22. Segal JL, Pathak MS: Optimal drug therapy and therapeutic drug monitoring after spinal cord injury: a population-specific approach, *Am J Ther* 8:451, 2001.
23. Ball PA: Critical care of spinal cord injury, *Spine* 26:S27, 2001.
24. Consortium for spinal cord medicine: neurogenic bowel management in adults with spinal cord injury, Clinical Practice Guidelines. Washington DC, 1998, Paralyzed Veterans of America.
25. Burchiel KJ, Hsu FPK: Pain and spasticity after spinal cord injury, *Spine* 26: S146, 2001.
26. Consortium for spinal cord medicine: Acute management of autonomic dysreflexia: individuals with spinal cord injury presenting to health-care facilities, *J Spinal Cord Med* 25:S67, 2002.
27. Consortium for spinal cord medicine: pressure ulcer prevention and treatment following spinal cord injury: a clinical practice guideline for health-care professionals, *J Spinal Cord Med* 24:S40, 2001.
28. Burns AS, Rivas DA, Dilunno JF: The management of neurogenic bladder and sexual dysfunction after spinal cord injury, *Spine* 26:S129, 2001.
29. Benevento BT, Sipski ML: Neurogenic bladder, neurogenic bowel, and sexual dysfunction in people with spinal cord injury, *Phys Ther* 82:601, 2001.
30. Consortium for spinal cord medicine: *Depression following spinal cord injury: a clinical practice guideline for primary care physicians,* Washington DC, 1998, Paralyzed Veterans of America.
31. Groah SL et al: Spinal cord injury medicine. 5. Preserving wellness and independence of the aging patient with spinal cord injury: a primary care approach for the rehabilitation medicine specialist, *Arch Phys Med Rehabil* 83:S82, 2002.
32. Kirshblum S et al: Rehabilitation of persons with central nervous system tumors, *Cancer* 92:1029, 2001.

RESOURCES

American Association of Spinal Cord Injury Nurses (AASCIN)
75-20 Astoria Boulevard
Jackson Heights, NY 11370-1177
718-803-3782
Fax: 718-803-0414
www.aascin.org

American Paraplegia Society
75-20 Astoria Boulevard
Jackson Heights, NY 11370
718-803-3782
Fax: 718-803-0414
www.apssci.org

Canadian Paraplegic Association
1101 prom. Prince of Wales Drive, Suite 230
Ottawa, ON
K2C 3W7 Canada
800-720-4933 or 613-723-1033
Fax: 613-723-1060
www.canparaplegic.org

Christopher Reeve Paralysis Foundation
500 Morris Avenue
Springfield, NJ 07081
800-225-0292 or 973-379-2690
Fax: 973-912-9433
www.christopherreeve.org

Guillain-Barré Syndrome Foundation International
P.O. Box 262
Wynnewood, PA 19096
610-667-0131
Fax: 610-667-7036
www.guillain-barre.com

National Institute of Neurological Disorders and Stroke (NINDS)
National Institutes of Health Neurological Institute
P.O. Box 5801
Bethesda, MD 20824
800-352-9424
www.ninds.nih.gov

National Rehabilitation Information Center (NARIC)
4200 Forbes Boulevard, Suite 202
Lanham, MD 20706
800-346-2742 or 301-459-5900
www.naric.com

National Spinal Cord Injury Association
6701 Democracy Boulevard, Suite 300-9
Bethesda, MD 20817
800-962-9629 or 301-588-6959
Fax: 301-588-9414
www.spinalcord.org

Paralyzed Veterans of America
801 18th Street NW
Washington, DC 20006-3517
800-424-8200
www.pva.org

Spinal Cord Society
19051 County Highway 1
Fergus Falls, MN 56537-7609
218-739-5252 or 739-5261
Fax: 218-739-5262
http://members.aol.com/scsweb

For additional Internet resources, see the website for this book at *http://www.evolve.elsevier.com/Lewis/medsurg*.

CHAPTER 60

NURSING ASSESSMENT
Musculoskeletal System

Dottie Roberts

LEARNING OBJECTIVES

1. Describe the gross anatomic and microscopic composition of bone.
2. Explain the classification system of joints and movements at synovial joints.
3. Describe the types and structure of muscle tissue.
4. Describe the functions of cartilage, muscles, ligaments, tendons, fascia, and bursae.
5. Describe age-related changes in the musculoskeletal system and differences in assessment findings.
6. Identify the significant subjective and objective data related to the musculoskeletal system that should be obtained from a patient.
7. Describe the appropriate techniques used in the physical assessment of the musculoskeletal system.
8. Differentiate normal from abnormal findings of a physical assessment of the musculoskeletal system.
9. Describe the purpose, significance of results, and nursing responsibilities related to diagnostic studies of the musculoskeletal system.

KEY TERMS

abduction (Table 60-3), p. 1643	flexion (Table 60-3), p. 1643
adduction (Table 60-3), p. 1643	isometric contractions, p. 1638
ankylosis (Table 60-6), p. 1644	isotonic contractions, p. 1638
arthrocentesis, p. 1648	kyphosis, (Table 60-6), p. 1644
arthroscopy, p. 1648	lordosis, (Table 60-6), p. 1644
atrophy (Table 60-6), p. 1644	motor end plate, p. 1638
contracture (Table 60-6), p. 1644	neuromuscular junction, p. 1638
crepitation (Table 60-6), p. 1644	scoliosis, p. 1644
extension (Table 60-3), p. 1643	x-ray, p. 1644

The unique structures of the musculoskeletal system allow human beings to complete complex movements in their interactions with the environment. The dexterity of the upper extremities enables an individual to perform complicated technical tasks, while stronger lower extremities allow mobility for varied activities. The musculoskeletal system is composed of voluntary muscle and five types of connective tissue: bones, cartilage, ligaments, tendons, and fascia.[1]

Resilient bone and cartilage absorb energy from any impact, minimizing the risk of injury to other body structures. However, this characteristic ability makes the musculoskeletal system itself particularly vulnerable to injury from external forces. Any damage to bone and related soft tissues can cause functional disruption for an individual. Deformity, alteration in body image, alteration in mobility, pain, or permanent disability may result from musculoskeletal injury.

STRUCTURES AND FUNCTIONS OF THE MUSCULOSKELETAL SYSTEM

Bone

Function. The main functions of bone are support, protection of internal organs, voluntary movement, blood cell production, and mineral storage.[2] Bones provide the supporting frame-

work that keeps the body from collapsing and also allow the body to bear weight. Bones also protect underlying vital organs and tissues. For example, the skull encloses the brain, the vertebrae surround the spinal cord, and the rib cage contains the lungs and heart. Bones serve as a point of attachment for muscles, which are connected to bones by tendons. Bones act as a lever for muscles, and movement occurs as a result of muscle contractions applied to these levers. Bones contain hematopoietic tissue for the production of red and white blood cells. Bones also serve as a site for storage of inorganic minerals such as calcium and phosphorus.

Bone was previously considered to be a static, inert substance. In reality, it is a dynamic tissue that continually changes form and composition. It contains both organic material (collagen) and inorganic material (calcium, phosphate). The internal and external growth and remodeling of bone are ongoing processes. Bone is classified according to structure as *cortical* (compact and dense) or *cancellous* (spongy).

Microscopic Structure. Cylinder-shaped structural units (*haversian* systems) fit closely together in compact bone, creating a dense bone structure (Fig. 60-1, *A*). Within the systems, the haversian canals run parallel to the bone's long axis and contain the blood vessels that travel to the bone's interior from the periosteum. Surrounding the haversian canals are concentric rings known as *lamellae*, which characterize mature bone. Smaller canals (*canaliculi*) extend from the haversian canals to the *lacunae*, where mature bone cells are embedded. Cancellous bone lacks the organized structure of cortical (compact) bone. The lamellae are not arranged in concentric rings but rather along the lines of maximum stress placed on the bone. Networks of bone tissue are filled with red or yellow marrow, and blood reaches the bone cells by passing through spaces in the marrow.

The three types of bone cells are osteoblasts, osteocytes, and osteoclasts. *Osteoblasts* synthesize organic bone matrix (collagen) and are the basic bone-forming cells. *Osteocytes* are the mature bone cells. *Osteoclasts* participate in bone remodeling by assisting in the breakdown of bone tissue. *Bone remodeling* is the removal of old bone by osteoclasts (*resorption*) and the deposi-

---

Reviewed by Helen L. Lamothe, RN, BSN, PHN, ONC, Nurse Consultant, Office Practice, Golden, Colo.

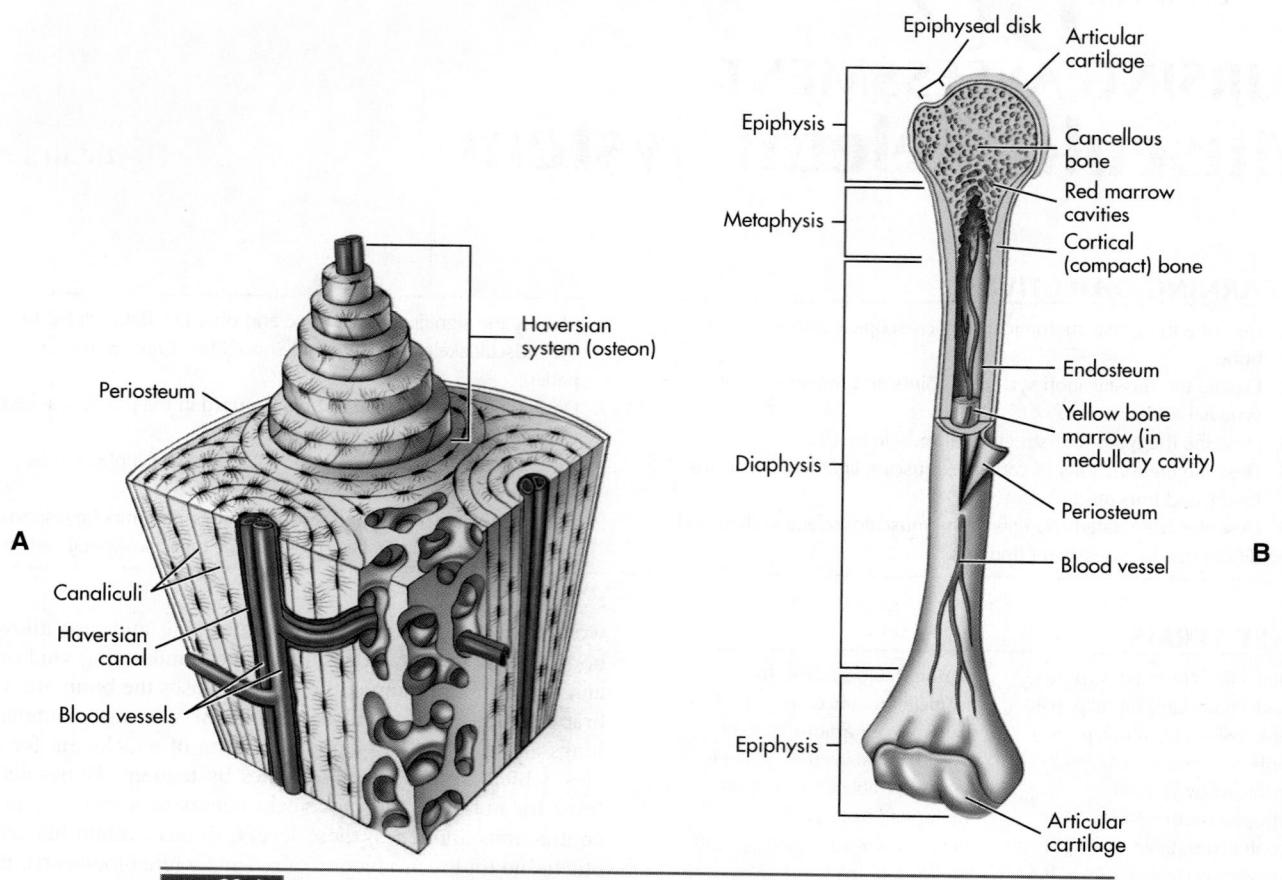

FIG. 60-1 Bone structure. **A**, Cortical (compact) bone showing haversian system. **B**, Anatomy of a long bone (humerus).

tion of new bone by osteoblasts (*ossification*). The inner layer of bone is primarily made up of osteoblasts with a few osteoclasts.

Gross Structure. The anatomic structure of bone is best represented by a typical long bone such as the humerus (see Fig. 60-1, *B*). Each long bone consists of the epiphysis, the diaphysis, and the metaphysis. The *epiphysis,* the widened area found at each end of a long bone, is composed primarily of cancellous bone. The wide epiphysis allows for greater weight distribution and provides stability for the joint. The epiphysis is also the location of muscle attachment. Articular cartilage covers the ends of the epiphysis to provide a smooth surface for joint movement. The *diaphysis* is the main shaft of the bone. It provides structural support and is composed of compact bone. The tubular structure of the diaphysis allows it to more easily withstand bending and twisting forces. The *metaphysis* is the flared area between the epiphysis and the diaphysis. Like the epiphysis, it is composed of cancellous bone. The *epiphyseal plate,* or growth zone, is the cartilaginous area between the epiphysis and metaphysis. It actively produces bone to allow longitudinal growth in children. Injury to the epiphyseal plate in a growing child can lead to a shorter extremity that can cause significant functional problems. In the adult, the metaphysis and epiphysis become joined as this plate hardens to mature bone.

The *periosteum* is composed of fibrous connective tissue that covers the bone. Tiny blood vessels penetrate the periosteum to provide nutrition to underlying bone. Musculotendinous fibers anchor to the outer layer of the periosteum. The inner layer of the periosteum is attached to the bone by bundles of collagen. No periosteum exists on the articular surfaces of long bones. These bone ends are covered by articular cartilage.

The medullary (marrow) cavity is in the center of the diaphysis and contains either red or yellow bone marrow.[3] In the growing child, red bone marrow is actively involved in hematopoiesis. In the adult, the medullary cavity of long bones contains yellow bone marrow, which is mainly adipose tissue. Yellow marrow will only be involved in hematopoiesis in times of great blood cell need. Blood cell production in the adult normally occurs in the red bone marrow of the skull, ribs, sternum, pelvis, vertebrae, and the shoulders.

Types. The skeleton consists of 206 bones, which are classified according to shape as long, short, flat, or irregular.

Long bones are characterized by a central shaft (diaphysis) and two widened ends (epiphyses) (Fig. 60-2). Examples include the femur, humerus, and radius. Short bones are composed of cancellous bone covered by a thin layer of compact bone. Examples include the carpals in the hand and the tarsals in the foot.

Flat bones have two layers of compact bone separated by a layer of cancellous bone. Examples include the ribs, skull, scapula, and sternum. The spaces in the cancellous bone contain

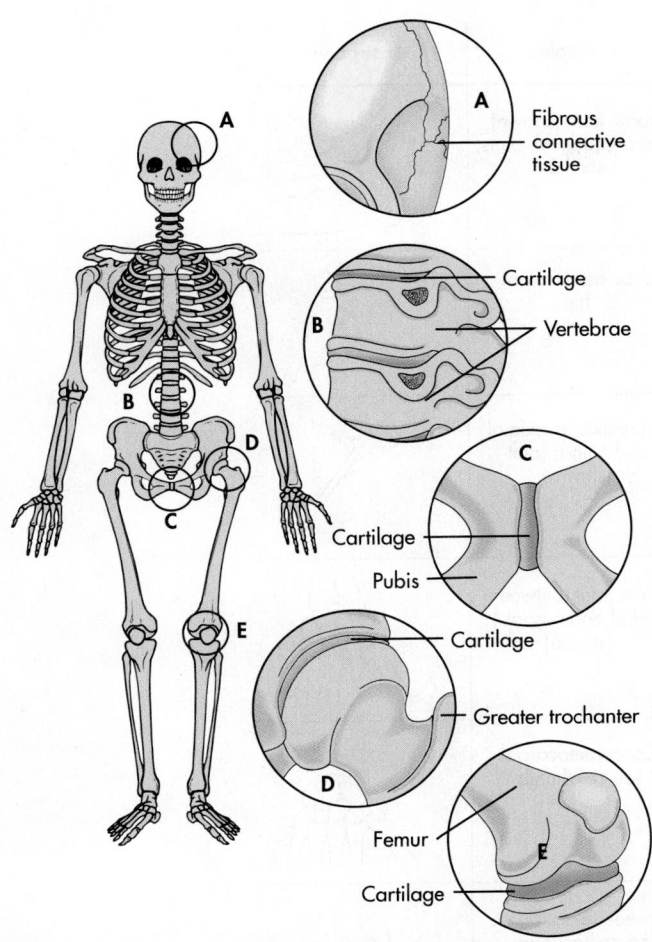

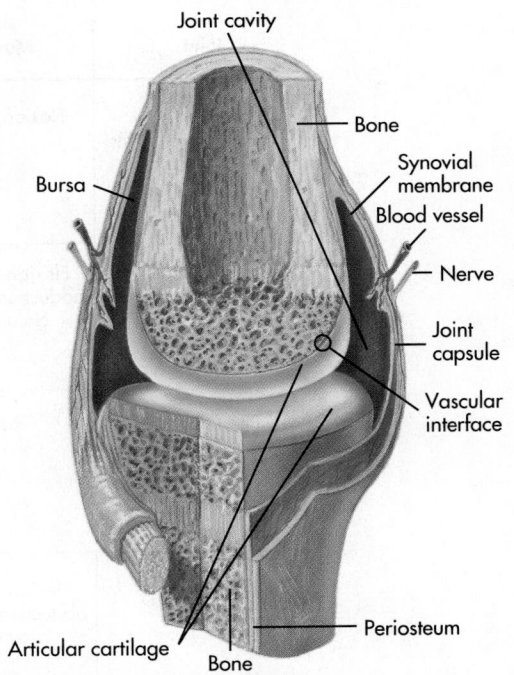

FIG. 60-3 Structure of synovial joint.

bone marrow. Irregular bones appear in a variety of shapes and sizes. Examples include the vertebrae, sacrum, and mandible.

Joints

A *joint* (articulation) is a place where the ends of two bones are in proximity and move in relation to each other. Joints are classified according to the degree of movement that they allow (see Fig. 60-2).

The most common joint is the freely movable *diarthrodial* (synovial) type. Each joint is enclosed in a capsule of fibrous connective tissue, which joins the two bones together to form a cavity (Fig. 60-3). The capsule is lined by a synovial membrane, which secretes a thick synovial fluid to lubricate the joint and reduce friction. The end of each bone is covered with articular (hyaline) cartilage. Supporting structures (e.g., ligaments, tendons) reinforce the joint capsule and provide limits to joint movement.[4] Types of diarthrodial joints are shown in Fig. 60-4.

Cartilage

Cartilage is a rigid connective tissue that serves as a support for soft tissue and provides the articular surface for joint movement. It protects underlying tissues. The cartilage in the epiphyseal plate is also involved in the growth of long bones before

physical maturity is reached. Because articular cartilage is relatively avascular, it must receive nourishment by the diffusion of material from the synovial fluid. The lack of a direct blood supply contributes to the slow metabolism of cartilage cells and explains why cartilage tissue heals slowly.

The three types of cartilage tissue are hyaline, elastic, and fibrous. *Hyaline cartilage,* the most common, contains a moderate amount of collagen fibers. It is found in the trachea, bronchi, nose, epiphyseal plate, and articular surfaces of bones. *Elastic cartilage,* which contains both collagen and elastic fibers, is more flexible than hyaline cartilage. It is found in the ear, epiglottis, and larynx. Fibrous cartilage (fibrocartilage) consists mostly of collagen fibers and is a tough tissue that often functions as a shock absorber. It is found between the vertebral disks and also forms a protective cushion between the bones of the pelvic girdle, knee, and shoulder.

Muscle

Types. The three types of muscle tissue are *cardiac* (striated, involuntary), *smooth* (nonstriated, involuntary), and *skeletal* (striated, voluntary) muscle. Cardiac muscle is found in the heart. Its spontaneous contractions propel blood through the circulatory system. Smooth muscle occurs in the walls of hollow structures such as airways, arteries, gastrointestinal (GI) tract, urinary bladder, and uterus. Smooth muscle contraction is modulated by neuronal and hormonal influences. Skeletal muscle, which requires neuronal stimulation for contraction, accounts for about half of a human being's body weight. It is the focus of the following discussion.

Structure. The structural unit of muscle is the muscle cell or muscle fiber, which is highly specialized for contraction. Skeletal muscle fibers are long, multinucleated cylinders that contain many mitochondria to support their high metabolic activity. Mus-

Joint	Movement	Examples	Illustration
Hinge joint	Flexion, extension	Elbow joint (shown), interphalangeal joints, knee joint	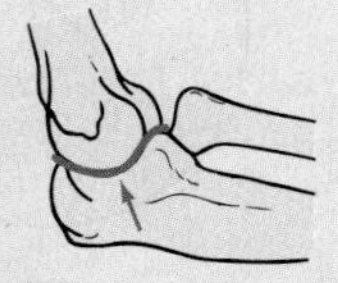
Ball and socket (spheroidal)	Flexion, extension; adduction, abduction; circumduction	Shoulder (shown), hip	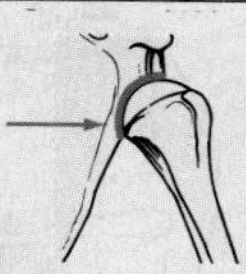
Pivot (rotary)	Rotation	Atlas-axis, proximal radioulnar joint (shown)	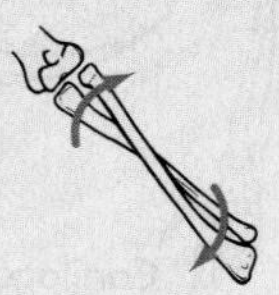
Condyloid	Flexion, extension; abduction, adduction; circumduction	Wrist joint (between radial and carpals) (shown)	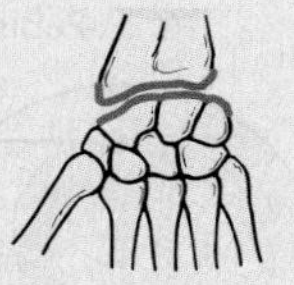
Saddle	Flexion, extension; abduction, adduction; circumduction, thumb-finger opposition	Carpometacarpal joint of thumb	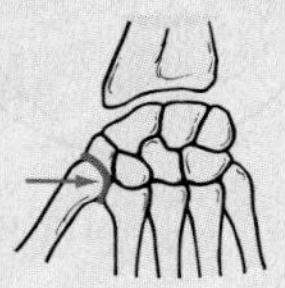
Gliding	One surface moves over another surface	Between tarsal bones, sacroiliac joint, between articular processes of vertebrae, between carpal bones (shown)	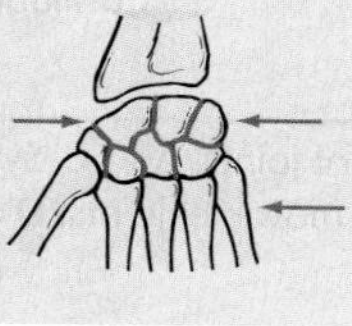

FIG. 60-4 Types of diarthrodial (synovial) joints.

cle fibers are composed of myofibrils, which in turn are made up of contractile filaments.

The *sarcomere* is the contractile unit of the myofibrils.[5] Each sarcomere consists of myosin (thick) filaments and actin (thin) filaments. The arrangement of the thin and thick filaments accounts for the characteristic banding of muscle when it is seen under a microscope. Muscle contraction occurs as thick and thin filaments slide past each other, causing the sarcomeres to shorten.

Contractions. Skeletal muscle contractions allow posture maintenance, movement, and facial expressions. **Isometric contractions** increase the tension within a muscle but do not produce movement. Repeated isometric contractions make muscles grow larger and stronger. **Isotonic contractions** shorten a muscle to produce movement. Most contractions are a combination of tension generation (isometric) and shortening (isotonic). Muscular *atrophy* (decrease in size) occurs with the absence of contraction that results from immobility, whereas increased muscular activity leads to *hypertrophy* (increase in size).

Skeletal muscle fibers are divided into two groups based on the type of activity they demonstrate. Slow-twitch muscle fibers

support prolonged muscle activity such as marathon running. Because they also support the body against gravity, they assist in posture maintenance. Fast-twitch muscle fibers are used for rapid muscle contraction required for activities such as blinking the eye, jumping, or sprinting.

Neuromuscular Junction. Skeletal muscle fibers require a nerve impulse to contract. A nerve fiber and the skeletal muscle fibers it stimulates are called a **motor end plate.** The junction between the axon of the nerve cell and the adjacent muscle cell is called the *myoneural* or **neuromuscular junction** (Fig. 60-5).

Acetylcholine is released from the motor end plate of the neuron and diffuses across the neuromuscular junction to bind with receptors on the muscle fiber. In response to this stimulation, the sarcoplasmic reticulum releases calcium ions into the cytoplasm. The presence of calcium triggers the contraction in the myofibrils.

Energy Source. The direct energy source for muscle fiber contractions is adenosine triphosphate (ATP). ATP is synthesized by cellular oxidative metabolism in numerous mitochondria located close to the myofibrils. It is rapidly depleted through conversion to adenosine diphosphate (ADP) and must be rephos-

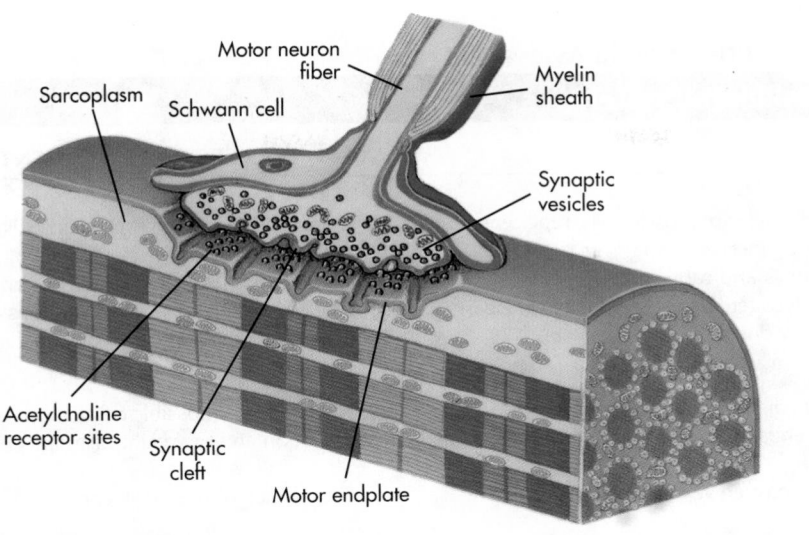

FIG. 60-5 Neuromuscular junction.

phorylated. Phosphocreatine provides a rapid source for the resynthesis of ATP, but it is in turn converted to creatine and must be recharged. Glycolysis can serve as a source of ATP when the oxygen supply is inadequate for the metabolic needs of the muscle tissue. Glucose is broken down to pyruvic acid, which can be further converted to lactic acid to make more oxygen available. An accumulation of lactic acid in tissues leads to fatigue and pain.

Ligaments and Tendons

Ligaments and tendons are both composed of dense, fibrous connective tissue that contains bundles of closely packed collagen fibers arranged in the same plane for additional strength. Tendons attach muscles to bones as an extension of the muscle sheath that adheres to the periosteum. Ligaments connect bones to bones (e.g., tibia to femur at knee joint). They have a higher elastic content than tendons.[6] Ligaments provide stability while permitting controlled movement at the joint.

Ligaments and tendons have a relatively poor blood supply, usually making tissue repair a slow process after injury. For example, the stretching or tearing of ligaments that occurs with a sprain may require a long time to mend.

Fascia

Fascia refers to layers of connective tissue with intermeshed fibers that can withstand limited stretching. Superficial fascia lies immediately under the skin. Deep fascia is a dense, fibrous tissue that surrounds the muscle bundles, nerves, and blood vessels. It also encloses individual muscles, allowing them to act independently and to glide over each other during contraction. In addition, fascia provides strength to muscle tissues.

Bursae

Bursae are small sacs of connective tissue lined with synovial membrane and containing synovial fluid. They are typically located at bony prominences or joints to relieve pressure and prevent friction between moving parts. For example, bursae are found between the patella and the skin (prepatellar bursa), between the olecranon process of the elbow and the skin (olecranon

bursa), between the head of the humerus and the acromion process of the scapula (subacromial bursa), and between the greater trochanter of the proximal femur and the skin (trochanteric bursa). *Bursitis* is an inflammation of a bursa sac.

■ Gerontologic Considerations: Effects of Aging on the Musculoskeletal System

Many of the functional problems experienced by the aging adult are related to changes of the musculoskeletal system. Although some changes begin in early adulthood, obvious signs of musculoskeletal impairment may not appear until later adult years. Alterations may affect the older adult's ability to complete self-care tasks and pursue other customary activities. Effects of musculoskeletal changes may range from mild discomfort and decreased ability to perform activities of daily living to severe, chronic pain and immobility. The risk for falls also increases in the older adult.

The bone remodeling process is altered in the aging adult. Increased bone resorption and decreased bone formation cause a loss of bone density, contributing to development of osteopenia and osteoporosis (see Chapter 62). Muscle mass and strength also decrease with aging. Almost 30% of muscle mass is lost by the eighth decade of life.[7] A loss of motor neurons can cause additional problems with skeletal muscle movement. Tendons and ligaments become less flexible, and movement becomes more rigid. Joints in the aging adult are also more likely to be affected by osteoarthritis (see Chapter 63).

In addition to the usual musculoskeletal assessment with a particular emphasis on exercise practices, the nurse should determine the impact of age-related changes of the musculoskeletal system on the functional status of the older patient. Functional limitations that are accepted by older adults as a normal part of aging can often be halted or reversed with appropriate preventive strategies (see Chapter 61, Table 61-1).

Diseases such as osteoarthritis and osteoporosis are not the normal consequences of growing old. The nurse should carefully differentiate between expected changes and the effects of disease in the aging adult. Symptoms of disease can be treated in many

TABLE 60-1 Gerontologic Differences in Assessment
Musculoskeletal System

CHANGES	DIFFERENCES IN ASSESSMENT FINDINGS
Muscle	
Decreased number and diameter of muscle cells, replacement of muscle cells by fibrous connective tissue	Decreased muscle strength and bulk, abdominal protrusion, flabby muscle
Loss of elasticity in ligaments and cartilage	Decreased fine motor dexterity, decreased agility
Reduced ability to store glycogen; decreased ability to release glycogen as quick energy during stress	Slowed reaction times and reflexes as a result of slowing of impulse conduction along motor units; earlier fatigue with activity
Joints	
Increased risk for cartilage disruption that contributes to direct contact between bone ends and overgrowth of bone around joint margins	Joint stiffness, possible crepitation on movement; pain with motion and/or weight bearing
Loss of water from disks between vertebrae, narrowing of intervertebral spaces	Loss of height from disk compression; posture change
Bone	
Decrease in bone density	Loss of height from vertebral compression, back pain; deformity such as dowager's hump (kyphosis) caused by vertebral compression

cases, helping the older adult to return to a higher functional level. Age-related changes in the musculoskeletal system and differences in assessment findings are presented in Table 60-1. ■

ASSESSMENT OF THE MUSCULOSKELETAL SYSTEM

Correct diagnosis of any complaint depends on a complete patient history and thorough physical examination. Musculoskeletal assessment can focus on a specific body part, or it can be done as part of a general physical examination or as an examination in itself. The nurse uses the patient's complaint as a guide in selecting all or part of the components of the musculoskeletal history and physical examination. For example, accidents may result in multisystem trauma. Because serious or life-threatening injuries do not usually involve the musculoskeletal system, critical information about the patient's condition is obtained to support immediate treatment, and a complete assessment of the musculoskeletal system may be deferred.

The most common symptoms of musculoskeletal impairment include pain, weakness, deformity, limitation of movement, stiffness, and joint crepitation.[8] Information should also be sought about changes in sensation or in the size of a muscle.

Subjective Data

Important Health Information. Appropriate questions to ask during a musculoskeletal assessment are included in Table 60-2.

Past health history. Because certain illnesses are known to affect the musculoskeletal system either directly or indirectly, the nurse should carefully question the patient about past medical problems. These include tuberculosis, poliomyelitis, diabetes mellitus, parathyroid problems, hemophilia, rickets, scurvy, soft tissue infection, and neuromuscular disabilities. In addition, past or developing musculoskeletal problems can affect the patient's overall health. Trauma to the musculoskeletal system is a common reason for seeking medical evaluation. Questions should also focus on symptoms of arthritic and connective tissue diseases (e.g., gout, psoriatic arthritis, systemic lupus erythematosus), osteomalacia, osteomyelitis, and fungal infection of the bones or joints. The patient should also be asked about possible sources of a secondary bacterial infection, such as the ears, tonsils, teeth, sinuses, or genitourinary tract. These infections can enter the bones, resulting in osteomyelitis. A detailed account of the course and treatment of any of these problems should be obtained.

Medications. The nurse should carefully question the patient regarding prescription and over-the-counter drugs and herbal products and nutritional supplements (see Complementary and Alternative Therapies box on p. 34). Detailed information should be obtained about each treatment, including its name, the dose and frequency, length of time it was taken, its effects, and any possible side effects. Specific inquiry should be made about skeletal muscle relaxants, opioids, nonsteroidal antiinflammatory drugs, and systemic and topical corticosteroids. The patient who has taken antiinflammatory drugs should be questioned about GI distress or signs of bleeding.

In addition to drugs taken for treatment of a musculoskeletal problem, the patient should be questioned about drugs that can have detrimental effects on this system. These drugs and their potential side effects include antiseizure drugs (osteomalacia), phenothiazines (gait disturbances), corticosteroids (avascular necrosis, decreased bone and muscle mass), and potassium-depleting diuretics (muscle cramps and weakness). Women should be questioned about their menstrual history. Episodes of amenorrhea can contribute to early development of osteoporosis. Questions about the use of hormone replacement therapy and calcium and vitamin D supplements are important for postmenopausal women.

Surgery or other treatments. Information should be obtained about past hospitalizations from a musculoskeletal problem. The nurse should carefully document the reason for hospitalization, the date and duration, and the treatment. Details of emergency treatment for musculoskeletal injuries should also be sought. Specific information should also be obtained regarding any sur-

TABLE
60-2
Health History
Musculoskeletal System

Health Perception–Health Management Pattern
- Describe your usual daily activities.
- Do you experience any difficulties performing these activities?* Describe what you do if you experience difficulty in dressing, preparing meals and feeding yourself, performing basic hygiene, or maintaining your home.
- Do you use any mechanical assistive devices?*
- Do you have to lift heavy objects? Describe any specialized equipment you use or wear when you work or exercise that helps protect you from injury.
- What other safety precautions do you take?
- Do you take any drugs or herbal products to manage your musculoskeletal problem? If so, what is the name of the drug(s) and what are the expected effects?
- When did you have your last tetanus and polio immunizations? When were you last tested for tuberculosis?

Nutritional-Metabolic Pattern
- Give a 24-hour diet recall.
- What dietary supplements do you take? (Ask specifically about calcium, vitamin D supplements, and herbal products.)
- What is your weight? Describe any recent weight loss or gain. Were your musculoskeletal symptoms affected by the change in your weight?*

Elimination Pattern
- Does your musculoskeletal problem make it difficult for you to reach the toilet in time?*
- Do you need any assistive devices or equipment to achieve satisfactory toileting?*
- Do you experience constipation related to decreased mobility or to drugs taken for your musculoskeletal problem?*

Activity-Exercise Pattern
- Do you require assistance in completing your usual daily activities because of a musculoskeletal problem?*
- Describe your usual exercise pattern. Do you experience musculoskeletal symptoms before, during, or after exercising?*

- Are you able to move all your joints comfortably through full range of motion? Describe any limitations in mobility.
- Do you use any prosthetic or orthotic devices?*

Sleep-Rest Pattern
- Do you experience any difficulty sleeping because of a musculoskeletal problem?* Do you require frequent position changes at night?*
- Do you wake up at night because of musculoskeletal pain?*

Cognitive-Perceptual Pattern
- Describe any musculoskeletal pain you experience. How do you manage your pain? (Ask specifically about adjunctive therapies such as heat and cold or alternative therapies such as acupuncture.)

Self-Perception–Self-Concept Pattern
- Describe how changes in your musculoskeletal system (posture, walking, muscle strength) and decreased ability to do certain things have affected how you feel about yourself. How have these changes affected your lifestyle?

Role-Relationship Pattern
- Do you live alone?
- Describe how family members or others assist you with your musculoskeletal problem.
- Describe the effect of your musculoskeletal problem on your work and on your social relationships.

Sexuality-Reproductive Pattern
- Describe any sexual concerns related to your musculoskeletal problem.

Coping–Stress Tolerance Pattern
- Describe how you deal with problems such as pain or immobility that have resulted from your musculoskeletal problem.

Value-Belief Pattern
- Describe any cultural practices or religious beliefs that may influence the treatment of your musculoskeletal problem.

*If yes, describe.

gical procedure and the postoperative course. If the patient experienced a period of prolonged immobilization, the development of osteoporosis and muscle atrophy should be considered.

Functional Health Patterns. The use of functional health patterns assists the nurse in organizing the data and formulating diagnoses based on information collected about the musculoskeletal system. Table 60-2 summarizes specific questions to ask in relation to functional health patterns.

Health perception–health management pattern. The nurse should ask about the patient's health practices related to the musculoskeletal system, such as maintenance of a normal body weight, avoidance of excessive stress on muscles and joints, and the use of proper body mechanics when lifting objects.[9]

The patient should be specifically questioned about tetanus and polio immunizations. The most current date and reaction to a tuberculin skin test should also be obtained.

Food or contact allergies have little direct relation to musculoskeletal problems, but the general malaise often associated with allergic reactions may manifest in musculoskeletal stiffness

and lethargy. Allergic reactions to drugs used to treat musculoskeletal problems can be significant if they interfere with therapy. An alternative treatment may have to be used if the reaction is severe.

The patient who is a good historian can recount numerous minor and major injuries of the musculoskeletal system. Information should be recorded chronologically and should include the following:

1. Mechanism of the injury (e.g., twist, crush, stretch)
2. Circumstances related to the injury
3. Diagnostic evaluations
4. Methods of treatment
5. Duration of treatment
6. Current status related to the injury
7. Need for assistive devices
8. Interference with activities of daily living

A family history should be obtained related to rheumatoid arthritis, sickle cell disease, osteoarthritis, gout, osteoporosis, and scoliosis because these problems have a familial predisposition.

Safety practices can affect the patient's predisposition for certain injuries and illnesses. Therefore the nurse should ask the patient about safety practices as they relate to work environment, recreation, and exercise. For example, if the patient is a computer programmer, the nurse should ask about ergonomic adaptations in the office that decrease the risk of carpal tunnel syndrome or low back pain. Identification of problems in this area will direct the plan for patient teaching.

Nutritional-metabolic pattern. The patient's description of a typical day's diet provides clues to areas of nutritional concern that can affect the musculoskeletal system. Adequate amounts of vitamins C and D, calcium, and protein are essential for a healthy, intact musculoskeletal system. Abnormal nutritional patterns can predispose individuals to problems such as osteomalacia and osteoporosis. In addition, maintenance of normal weight is an important nutritional goal. Obesity places additional stress on weight-bearing joints such as the knees, hips, and spine, and it predisposes individuals to ligamentous instability.

Elimination pattern. Questions about the patient's mobility may reveal difficulty with ambulating to the toilet. The patient should be asked if an assistive device such as an elevated toilet seat or a grab bar is necessary to accomplish toileting. Decreased mobility secondary to a musculoskeletal problem can lead to constipation. In addition, musculoskeletal problems can contribute to bowel or bladder incontinence.

Activity-exercise pattern. The nurse should obtain a detailed account of the type, duration, and frequency of exercise and recreational activities. Daily, weekend, and seasonal patterns should be compared because occasional or sporadic exercise can be more problematic than regular exercise. Many musculoskeletal problems can affect the patient's activity-exercise pattern. The nurse should question the patient about limitations of movement, pain, weakness, clumsiness, crepitus, or any change in the bones or joints that interferes with daily activities.

Extremes of activity related to occupation can also affect the musculoskeletal system. A sedentary occupation can negatively impact muscle flexibility and strength. Jobs that require extreme effort through heavy lifting or pushing can lead to damage of joints and supporting structures. The nurse should specifically question the patient about work-related injuries to the musculoskeletal system, including treatment and time lost from work.

Sleep-rest pattern. The discomfort caused by musculoskeletal disorders can interfere with a normal sleep pattern. The patient should be questioned about possible alterations in sleep patterns. If the patient describes sleep interference related to a musculoskeletal problem, the nurse should inquire further about the type of bedding and pillows used, sleeping partner, and sleeping positions.

Cognitive-perceptual pattern. Any pain experienced by the patient as a result of a musculoskeletal problem should be fully explored and documented. To provide a baseline for later reassessment, the patient should be asked to describe the intensity of the pain on a scale from 1 to 10 (0 = no pain, 10 = most severe pain imaginable). Reassessments over time will assist in determining the effectiveness of any treatment plan. The patient should also be questioned about measures used at home for pain management and about related problems such as joint swelling or muscle weakness. (Pain is discussed in Chapter 9.)

Self-perception–self-concept pattern. Many chronic musculoskeletal problems lead to deformities that can have a serious negative impact on the patient's body image and sense of personal worth. The nurse should address the patient's feelings about each of these changes.

Role-relationship pattern. Impaired mobility and chronic pain from musculoskeletal problems can negatively affect the patient's ability to perform in roles of spouse, parent, or employee. The ability to pursue and maintain meaningful social and personal relationships can also be affected by musculoskeletal problems. The nurse should carefully question the patient about role performance and relationships.

If the patient lives alone, the current musculoskeletal problem and its rehabilitation may make it difficult or impossible to continue this arrangement. The degree of assistance available from family, friends, and organized caregivers should be determined.

Sexuality-reproductive pattern. The pain of musculoskeletal problems can greatly affect the patient's ability to obtain sexual satisfaction. The nurse should sensitively explore this area, helping the patient feel comfortable in discussing any sexual problems related to pain, movement, and positioning.

Coping–stress tolerance pattern. Mobility limitations and pain, whether acute or chronic, are serious potential stressors that challenge the patient's coping resources. The nurse must recognize the potential for ineffective coping in the patient and family or significant other. Additional questioning will help determine if a musculoskeletal problem is causing coping difficulties.

Objective Data

Physical Examination. Examination involves observation, palpation, motion, and muscular assessment.[10] Although a general overview will be conducted, data obtained in a careful health history will guide the nurse in choosing areas on which to concentrate the local examination. Specific measurements may be taken as indicated by the local examination.

Inspection. Inspection begins during the nurse's initial contact with the patient. The patient's use of an assistive device such as a walker or cane should be noted. The nurse also observes general body build, muscle configuration, and symmetry of joint movement. If the patient is able to move independently, the nurse should assess posture and gait by watching the patient walk, stand, and sit. Musculoskeletal and neurologic problems can result in changes from a normal gait.

A systematic inspection is performed starting at the head and neck and proceeding to the upper extremities, the lower extremities, and the trunk. A specific order is not required, but the regular use of a systematic approach is important to avoid missing important aspects of the examination. The skin is inspected for general color, scars, or other overt signs of previous injury or surgery. The nurse notes any swelling, deformity, nodules or masses, and discrepancies in limb length or muscle size. The patient's opposite body part is used for comparison when an abnormality is suspected.

Palpation. Any area that has aroused concern because of a subjective complaint or appears abnormal on inspection should be carefully palpated. As with inspection, palpation usually proceeds cephalopedally (head to toe) to examine the neck, shoulders, elbows, wrists, hands, back, hips, knees, ankles, and feet. Both superficial and deep palpation are usually performed consecutively.

The nurse's hands should be warm to prevent muscle spasm, which can interfere with identification of essential landmarks or soft tissue structures. Palpation of both muscles and joints allows for evaluation of skin temperature, local tenderness, swelling, and crepitation. The nurse must establish the relationship of adjacent structures and evaluate the general contour, abnormal prominences, and local landmarks.

Motion. When assessing the patient's joint mobility, the nurse must carefully evaluate both passive and active range of joint motion. Measurements should be similar for both active and passive range of motion. *Active range of motion* means the patient takes his or her own joints through all movements without assistance. *Passive range of motion* occurs when someone else moves the patient's joints without his or her participation. The nurse should be cautious in performing passive range of motion because of the risk of injury to underlying structures. Manipulation must cease immediately if pain or resistance is encountered. If deficits in active or passive range of motion are noted, the nurse must also assess functional range of motion to determine if performance of activities of daily living has been affected by joint changes. This is done by asking the patient if activities such as eating and bathing must be performed with assistance or cannot be done at all.

Range of motion is most accurately assessed with a goniometer, which measures the angle of the joint (Fig. 60-6). Specific degrees of range of motion of all joints are usually not measured unless a musculoskeletal problem has been identified. A less exact but valuable assessment method is to compare the range of motion of one extremity with the range of motion on the opposite side. The most common movements that occur at the synovial joints are described in Table 60-3.

Muscle-strength testing. The nurse grades the strength of individual muscles or groups of muscles during contraction (Table 60-4). The patient should be instructed to apply resistance to the force exerted by the nurse. For example, the examiner tries to pull the bent arm down while the patient tries to raise it. Muscle strength should also be compared with the strength of the opposite extremity. Subtle variations in muscle strength may be noted when comparing the patient's dominant side with the nondominant side.

Measurement. When length discrepancies or subjective problems are noted, the nurse will often obtain limb length and circumferential muscle mass measurements. For example, leg length should be measured when gait disorders are observed. The affected limb is measured between two bony prominences and compared with the similar measurement of the opposite extremity. Muscle mass is measured circumferentially at the largest area of the muscle. When recording measurements, the

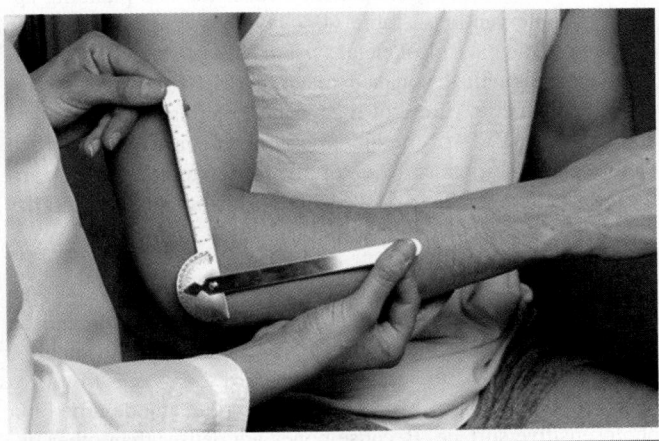

FIG. 60-6 Measurement of joint motion with a goniometer.

TABLE 60-3   Movement at Synovial Joints

MOVEMENT	DESCRIPTION
Abduction	Movement of part away from midline of body
Adduction	Movement of part toward midline of body
Circumduction	Combination of flexion, extension, abduction, and adduction resulting in circular motion of a body part
Eversion	Turning of sole outward away from midline of body
Extension	Straightening of joint that increases angle between two bones
External rotation	Movement along longitudinal axis away from midline of body
Flexion	Bending of joint as a result of muscle contraction that results in decreased angle between two bones
Hyperextension	Extension in which angle exceeds 180 degrees
Internal rotation	Movement along longitudinal axis toward midline of body
Inversion	Turning of sole inward toward midline of body
Pronation	Turning of palm downward
Supination	Turning of palm upward

TABLE 60-4   Muscle Strength Scale

0	No detection of muscular contraction
1	A barely detectable flicker or trace of contraction with observation or palpation
2	Active movement of body part with elimination of gravity
3	Active movement against gravity only and not against resistance
4	Active movement against gravity and some resistance
5	Active movement against full resistance without evident fatigue (normal muscle strength)

TABLE 60-5   Normal Physical Assessment of the Musculoskeletal System

Full range of motion of all joints without pain or laxity
No joint swelling, deformity, or crepitation
Normal spinal curvatures
No tenderness on palpation of spine
No muscle atrophy or asymmetry
Muscle strength of 5

nurse should document the exact location at which the measurements were obtained (e.g., the quadriceps muscle is measured 15 cm above the patella). This informs the next examiner of the exact area to be measured and ensures consistency during reassessment.

Other. Assessment of reflexes is discussed in Chapter 54. Table 60-5 is an example of how to record a normal physical assessment of the musculoskeletal system. Common abnormal as-

TABLE 60-6 Common Assessment Abnormalities — Musculoskeletal System

FINDING	DESCRIPTION	POSSIBLE ETIOLOGY AND SIGNIFICANCE
Ankylosis	Scarring within a joint leading to stiffness or fixation	Chronic joint inflammation
Atrophy	Wasting of muscle, characterized by decreased circumference and flabby appearance leading to decreased function and tone	Muscle denervation, contracture, prolonged disuse as a result of immobilization
Contracture	Resistance of movement of muscle or joint as a result of fibrosis of supporting soft tissues	Shortening of muscle or ligaments, tightness of soft tissue, incorrect positioning of immobilized extremity
Crepitation (crepitus)	Crackling sound or grating sensation as a result of friction or broken bone or cartilage bits in joint	Fracture, dislocation, chronic inflammation, osteoarthritis
Effusion	Fluid in joint possibly with swelling and pain	Trauma, especially to knees; inflammation
Ganglion	Small fluid-filled synovial cyst usually on dorsal surface of wrist or foot	Degeneration of connective tissue close to tendons and joints leading to formation of small cysts
Hypertrophy	Increase in size of muscle as a result of enlargement of existing cells	Exercise or other increased stimulation, increased androgens
Kyphosis (dowager's hump)	Anteroposterior or forward bending of thoracic spine with convexity of curve in posterior direction	Poor posture, tuberculosis, arthritis, osteoporosis, growth disturbance of vertebral epiphyses
Lordosis	Lumbar spinal deformity resulting in anteroposterior curvature with concavity in posterior direction	Secondary to other spinal deformities, muscular dystrophy, obesity, flexion contracture of hip, congenital dislocation of hip
Pes planus	Flatfoot	Congenital condition, muscle paralysis, mild cerebral palsy, early muscular dystrophy
Scoliosis	Deformity resulting in lateral curvature of thoracic spine (see Fig. 60-7)	Idiopathic or congenital condition, fracture or dislocation, osteomalacia
Subluxation	Partial dislocation of joint	Instability of joint capsule and supporting ligaments (e.g., from trauma, arthritis)
Valgus (bow legs)	Angulation of bone away from midline	Alteration in gait, pain, arthritis
Varus (knock-knees)	Angulation of bone toward midline	Alteration in gait, pain, arthritis

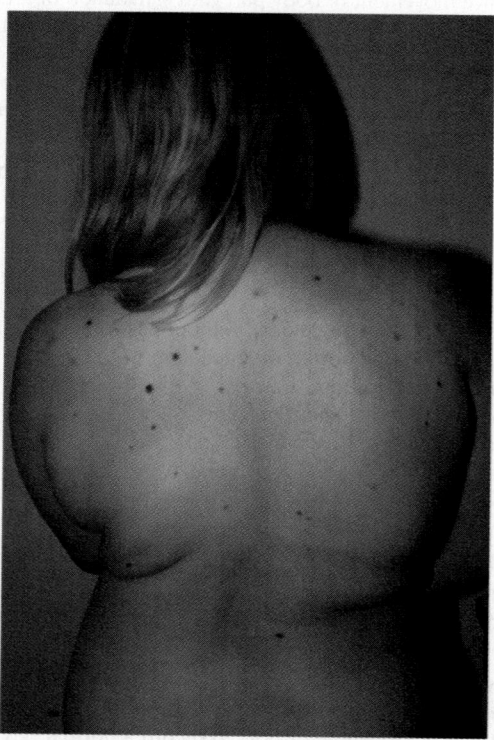

FIG. 60-7 Scoliosis in a standing erect posture.

sessment findings of the musculoskeletal system are presented in Table 60-6. **Scoliosis** is a lateral S-shaped curvature of the thoracic and lumbar spine.[9] Unequal shoulder and scapula height is usually noted (Fig. 60-7). If the deformity is greater than 45 degrees, lung and cardiac function is generally impaired.

DIAGNOSTIC STUDIES OF THE MUSCULOSKELETAL SYSTEM

Diagnostic studies provide important objective data that aid the nurse in monitoring the patient's condition and planning appropriate interventions. Table 60-7 contains diagnostic studies common to the musculoskeletal system. Use of studies such as x-rays and magnetic resonance imaging (MRI) has greatly improved orthopedic care, but diagnostic imaging has resulted in approximately 50% of the increase in health care costs over the last decade.[11] Tests must be carefully chosen to enhance or clarify information gained from the patient's history and physical examination.

X-ray

The **x-ray**, or roentgenogram, is the most common diagnostic study used to assess musculoskeletal problems and to monitor the effectiveness of treatment. A standard x-ray is a film produced by the action of x-rays emitted from a cathode tube on a photosensitive surface. Because bones are denser than other tissues, x-rays do not penetrate them. Dense areas show as white on

TABLE 60-7   Diagnostic Studies

Musculoskeletal System

STUDY	DESCRIPTION AND PURPOSE	NURSING RESPONSIBILITY
Radiologic Studies		
• Standard x-ray	An x-ray is taken to determine density of bone. Study evaluates structural or functional changes of bones and joints. In anteroposterior view, x-ray beam passes from front to back, allowing one-dimensional view; lateral position provides two-dimensional view.	Avoid excessive exposure of patient and self. Before procedure, remove any radiopaque objects that can interfere with results. Explain procedure to patient. Verify patient is not pregnant.
• Arthrogram	Study involves injection of contrast medium or air into joint cavity, which permits visualization of joint structures. Joint movement is followed with series of x-rays.	Assess patient for possible allergy to contrast medium. Explain procedure.
• Diskogram	An x-ray of cervical or lumbar intervertebral disk is done after injection of contrast dye into nucleus pulposus. Study permits visualization of intervertebral disk abnormalities.	Same as for arthrogram.
• Sinogram	An x-ray is taken after injection of contrast dye into sinus tract (deep draining wound). Study visualizes course of sinus and tissues involved.	Same as for arthrogram.
• Computed tomography (CT) scan	An x-ray beam is used with a computer to provide a three-dimensional picture. It is used to identify soft tissue abnormalities, bony abnormalities, and various musculoskeletal trauma.	Inform patient that procedure is painless. Inform patient of importance of remaining still during procedure.
• Magnetic resonance imaging (MRI)	Radio waves and magnetic field are used to view soft tissue. Study is especially useful in the diagnosis of avascular necrosis, disk disease, tumors, osteomyelitis, ligament tears, and cartilage tears. Patient is placed inside scanning chamber. Gadolinium may be injected into a vein to enhance visualization of the structures. Open MRI does not require the patient to be placed inside a chamber.	Inform patient that procedure is painless. Be aware that it is contraindicated in patient with aneurysm clips, metallic implants, pacemakers, electronic devices, hearing aids, shrapnel, and extreme obesity. Ensure that patient has no metal on clothing (e.g., snaps, zippers, jewelry, credit cards). Inform patient of importance of remaining still throughout examination. Inform patients who are claustrophobic that they may experience symptoms during examination. Administer antianxiety agent if indicated and ordered. Open MRI may be indicated for obese patient or patient with large chest and abdominal girth or severe claustrophobia. Open MRI may not be available at all facilities.
Bone Mineral Density (BMD) Measurements		
• Dual energy x-ray absorptiometry (DEXA)	Technique measures bone mass of spine, femur, forearm, and total body. Allows assessment of bone density with minimal radiation exposure; used to diagnose metabolic bone disease and to monitor changes in bone density with treatment.	Inform patient that procedure is painless.
• Quantitative ultrasound (QUS)	Evaluates density, elasticity, and strength of patella and calcaneus using ultrasound rather than radiation.	Inform patient that procedure is painless.
Radioisotope Studies		
• Bone scan	Technique involves injection of radioisotope (usually sodium pertechnetate) that is taken up by bone. Radiation detector (Geiger counter) scans entire body (front and back), and recording is made on paper. Degree of uptake is related to blood flow to bone. Increased uptake is seen in osteomyelitis, osteoporosis, primary and metastatic malignant lesions of bone, and certain fractures. Decreased uptake is seen in areas of avascular necrosis.	Explain that technician gives a calculated dose of radioisotope 2 hr before procedure. Ensure that bladder is emptied before scan. Inform patient that procedure requires 1 hr while patient lies supine and that no pain or harm will result from isotopes. Explain that no follow-up scans are required. Increase fluids after the examination.

Continued

TABLE 60-7 **Diagnostic Studies**

Musculoskeletal System—cont'd

STUDY	DESCRIPTION AND PURPOSE	NURSING RESPONSIBILITY
Endoscopy		
▪ Arthroscopy	Study involves insertion of arthroscope into joint (usually knee) for visualization of structure and contents. It can be used for exploratory surgery (removal of loose bodies and biopsy) and for diagnosis of abnormalities of meniscus, articular cartilage, ligaments, or joint capsule. Other structures that can be visualized through the arthroscope include the shoulder, elbow, wrist, jaw, hip, and ankle.	Inform patient that procedure is performed in operating room with strict asepsis and that either local or general anesthesia is used. After procedure, cover wound with sterile dressing.
Mineral Metabolism		
▪ Alkaline phosphatase	This enzyme, produced by osteoblasts of bone, is needed for mineralization of organic bone matrix. Elevated levels are found in healing fractures, bone cancers, osteoporosis, osteomalacia, and Paget's disease. *Normal:* 20 to 90 U/L (0.3 to 2.7 mmol/L).	Obtain blood samples by venipuncture. Observe venipuncture site for bleeding or hematoma formation. Inform patient that procedure does not require fasting.
▪ Calcium	Bone is primary organ for calcium storage. Calcium provides bone with rigid consistency. Decreased serum level is found in osteomalacia, renal disease, and hypoparathyroidism; increased level is found in hyperparathyroidism, some bone tumors. *Normal:* 9 to 11 mg/dl (2.3 to 2.7 mmol/L).	Same as above.
▪ Phosphorus	Amount present is indirectly related to calcium metabolism. Decreased level is found in osteomalacia; increased level is found in chronic renal disease, healing fractures, osteolytic metastatic tumor. *Normal:* 2.8 to 4.5 mg/dl (0.9 to 1.5 mmol/L).	Same as above.
Serologic Studies		
▪ Rheumatoid factor (RF)	Study assesses presence of autoantibody (rheumatoid factor) in serum. Factor is not specific for rheumatoid arthritis and is seen in other connective tissue diseases, as well as in a small percentage of normal population. *Normal:* negative or titer <1:20.	Same as above.
▪ Erythrocyte sedimentation rate (ESR)	Study is nonspecific index of inflammation. Study measures rapidity with which red blood cells settle out of unclotted blood in 1 hr. Results are influenced by physiologic factors, as well as diseases. Elevated levels are seen with any inflammatory process (especially rheumatoid arthritis, rheumatic fever, osteomyelitis, and respiratory infections). *Normal:* <20 mm/hr. Some gender variation.	Same as above.
▪ Antinuclear antibody (ANA)	Study assesses presence of antibodies capable of destroying nucleus of body's tissue cells. Finding is positive in 95% of patients with systemic lupus erythematosus and may also be positive in individuals with systemic sclerosis (scleroderma) or rheumatoid arthritis and in a small percentage of normal population.	Same as above.
▪ Anti-DNA antibody	Study detects serum antibodies that react with DNA. It is the most specific test for systemic lupus erythematosus.	Same as above.
▪ Complement	Complement, a normal body protein, is essential to both immune and inflammatory reactions. Complement components used up in these reactions are depleted. Complement depletions may be found in patients with rheumatoid arthritis or systemic lupus erythematosus.	Same as above.

TABLE 60-7

*D*iagnostic Studies

Musculoskeletal System—cont'd

STUDY	DESCRIPTION AND PURPOSE	NURSING RESPONSIBILITY
Serologic Studies—cont'd		
• Uric acid	End product of purine metabolism is normally excreted in urine. Although not specific, levels are usually elevated in gout. *Normal:* men, 4.5 to 6.5 mg/dl (268 to 387 μmol/L); women, 2.5 to 5.5 mg/dl (149 to 327 μmol/L).	Obtain blood samples by venipuncture. Observe venipuncture site for bleeding or hematoma formation. Inform patient that procedure does not require fasting.
• C-reactive protein (CRP)	Study is used to diagnose inflammatory diseases, infections, and active widespread malignancy. CRP is synthesized by the liver and is present in large amounts in serum 18 to 24 hr after onset of tissue damage. *Normal:* negative.	Same as above.
• Human leukocyte antigen (HLA)–B27	Antigen present in disorders such as ankylosing spondylitis and rheumatoid arthritis.	Same as above.
Muscle Enzymes		
• Creatine kinase (CK)	Highest concentration is found in skeletal muscle. Increased values are found in progressive muscular dystrophy, polymyositis, and traumatic injuries. *Normal:* men, 5 to 55 U/L (0.1 to 0.9 μkat/L); women, 5 to 35 U/L (0.01 to 7.5 U/L (16.7-125 μkat/L).	Same as above.
• Aldolase	Study is useful in monitoring muscular dystrophy and dermatomyositis. *Normal:* 1 to 7.5 U/L (16.7 to 125 μkat/L).	Same as above.
Invasive Procedures		
• Arthrocentesis	Incision or puncture of joint capsule is done to obtain samples of synovial fluid from within joint cavity or to remove excess fluid. Local anesthesia and aseptic preparation are used before needle is inserted into joint and fluid aspirated. Study is useful in diagnosis of joint inflammation, infection, and subtle fractures.	Inform patient that procedure is usually done at bedside or in examination room. Send samples of synovial fluid to laboratory for examination (if indicated). After procedure apply compression dressing. Observe for leakage of blood or fluid on dressing.
• Electromyogram (EMG)	Study evaluates electrical potential associated with skeletal muscle contraction. Small-gauge needles are inserted into certain muscles. Needle probes are attached to leads that feed information to EMG machine. Recordings of electrical activity of muscle are traced on audiotransmitter, as well as on oscilloscope and recording paper. Study is useful in providing information related to lower motor neuron dysfunction and primary muscle disease.	Inform patient that procedure is usually done in electromyogram laboratory while patient lies supine on special table. Keep patient awake to cooperate with voluntary movement. Inform patient that procedure involves some discomfort from needle insertion. Avoid administration of stimulants including caffeine and sedatives 24 hr before procedure.
Miscellaneous		
• Thermography	Technique uses infrared detector, which measures degree of heat radiating from skin surface. Study is useful in investigation of cause of inflamed joint and in following up patient's response to antiinflammatory drug therapy.	Inform patient that procedure is painless and noninvasive.
• Plethysmography	Study records variations in volume and pressure of blood passing through tissues. Test is nonspecific.	Inform patient that procedure is painless and noninvasive.
• Somatosensory evoked potential (SSEP)	Study evaluates evoked potential of muscle contractions. Electrodes are placed on skin and provide recordings of electrical activity of muscle. Study is useful in identifying subtle dysfunction of lower motor neuron and primary muscle disease. SSEP measures nerve conduction along pathways not accessible by EMG. Transcutaneous or percutaneous electrodes are applied to the skin and help identify neuropathy and myopathy.	Inform patient that procedure is similar to EMG but does not involve needles. Electrodes are applied to the skin.

the standard x-ray. X-rays provide information about bone deformity, joint congruity, bone density, and calcification in soft tissue. Fracture diagnosis and management are the primary indications for x-ray, but it is also useful in the evaluation of hereditary, developmental, infectious, inflammatory, neoplastic, metabolic, and degenerative disorders.

The anteroposterior and lateral views are the most commonly used standard x-ray perspectives. Additional views in combination with other studies can aid in differential diagnosis.

Magnetic Resonance Imaging

MRI is a diagnostic study that shows the hydrogen density of tissues within the body. The body is composed primarily of hydrogen, and hydrogen possesses magnetic properties that make it appropriate as the basis for MRI. In MRI, radio waves and magnetic fields are used to construct soft tissue and bone images. The study is particularly advantageous in identifying soft tissue disorders, including cartilage or ligament tears and herniated disks, but it can also be helpful in diagnosing bone disorders such as avascular necrosis, tumors, and multiple myeloma.

Arthroscopy

A small fiberoptic tube called an arthroscope is used to directly examine the interior of a joint cavity in a procedure known as **arthroscopy.** Arthroscopy is performed under sterile conditions. After anesthesia has been administered, a large-bore needle is inserted into the joint, and the joint is distended with fluid or air (Fig. 60-8). When the arthroscope is inserted, the surgeon is able to perform extensive, accurate visualization of the joint cavity. Photographs or videotapes can be made through the scope, and a biopsy of the synovium or cartilage can be obtained. Torn tissue can be repaired through arthroscopic surgery, eliminating the need for a larger incision and greatly decreasing the recovery time.

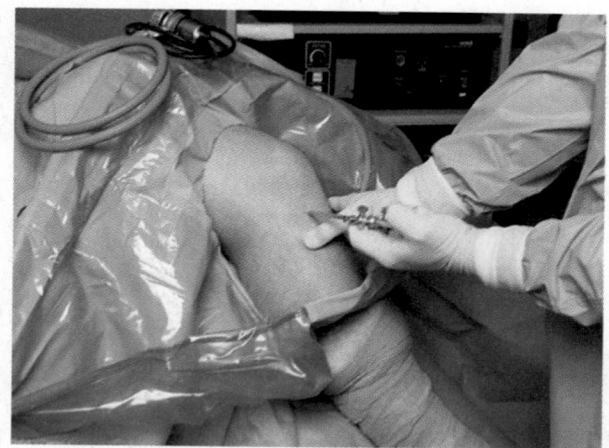

FIG. 60-8 Arthroscopy of a knee.

Typically performed as an outpatient procedure, arthroscopy is a highly cost-effective diagnostic test that is typically done on an ambulatory basis.

Arthrocentesis and Synovial Fluid Analysis

An **arthrocentesis** or joint aspiration is usually performed for a synovial fluid analysis. It may also be used to instill medications for the patient with septic arthritis or to remove fluid from joints to relieve pain. After the skin has been cleaned, a local anesthetic is instilled. An 18-gauge or larger needle is inserted into the joint, and fluid is withdrawn. The appropriate sterile container should be readily available to receive the aspirated fluid, which must be transported immediately to the laboratory. The fluid will be examined grossly for volume, color, clarity, viscosity, and mucin clot formation. Normal synovial fluid is transparent and colorless or straw-colored. It should be scant in amount and of low viscosity. Fluid from an infected joint may be purulent and thick or gray and thin. In gout the fluid may be whitish yellow. Blood may be aspirated if there is hemarthrosis because of injury or a bleeding disorder. The mucin clot test indicates the character of the protein portion of the synovial fluid. Normally a white, ropelike mucin clot is formed. In the presence of an inflammatory process, the clot breaks apart easily and fragments. The fluid is examined grossly for floating fat globules, which indicate bone injury.

The fluid is examined microscopically for cell count and identification. The normal white blood cell (WBC) count is less than 200 cells/μl, with fewer than 25% neutrophils and no bacteria. Infection would be suspected if the cell count reveals more than 25,000 WBC/μl and more than 25% polymorphonuclear cells. Protein content is elevated, and glucose is considerably decreased in septic arthritis. Presence of uric acid crystals suggests a diagnosis of gout. A Gram stain and culture may also be done of the aspirated fluid.

Muscle Enzymes

Muscle enzymes are released from injured or dead muscle cells. Determinations of muscle enzyme values are used to distinguish between muscle weakness that is due to nerve innervation problems and dystrophic disease of the muscle itself. The level of enzymes reflects the progress of the disorder and the effectiveness of treatment. Creatine kinase is a reliable measure of muscle damage.

Serologic Studies

Approximately 80% of people with rheumatoid arthritis and related diseases have an autoantibody known as rheumatoid factor (RF) in their serum. RF is an autoantibody directed against the immunoglobulin IgG. RF titers are higher during periods of increased disease activity. Elevated erythrocyte sedimentation rate and C-reactive protein are nonspecific indicators of active inflammation.

REVIEW QUESTIONS

The number of the question corresponds to the same-numbered objective at the beginning of the chapter.

1. The bone cells that function in the breakdown of bone tissue (resorption) are called
   a. osteoids.
   b. osteocytes.
   c. osteoclasts.
   d. osteoblasts.

2. While performing passive range of motion for a patient, the nurse puts a hinge joint through the movements of
   a. rotation.
   b. flexion and extension.
   c. flexion, extension, abduction, and adduction.
   d. flexion, extension, abduction, adduction, and circumduction.

3. The nurse teaches a patient with a leg immobilized in traction to prevent muscle atrophy in the affected leg by performing
   a. twitch contractions.
   b. tetanic contractions.
   c. isotonic contractions.
   d. isometric contractions.

4. A patient with bursitis of the shoulder asks the nurse what the bursa does. The nurse's response is based on the knowledge that bursae
   a. connect bone to bone.
   b. separate muscle from muscle.
   c. lubricate joints with synovial fluid.
   d. relieve friction between moving parts.

5. The decreased agility found during assessment of the older adult is caused by the age-related change of
   a. decrease in bone mass.
   b. erosion of articular cartilage.
   c. loss of elasticity in ligaments and cartilage.
   d. decrease in number and diameter of muscle cells.

6. While obtaining subjective assessment data related to the musculoskeletal system, it is particularly important for the nurse to ask about family history in the patient with
   a. osteomyelitis.
   b. osteomalacia.
   c. low back pain.
   d. rheumatoid arthritis.

7. When grading muscle strength, the nurse records a score of 2, indicating
   a. active movement against gravity.
   b. a barely detectable flicker of contraction.
   c. active movement with elimination of gravity.
   d. active movement against full resistance without evident fatigue.

8. A normal assessment finding of the musculoskeletal system is
   a. muscle strength of 4.
   b. a lateral curvature of the spine.
   c. angulation of bone toward midline.
   d. simultaneous occurrence of stance and swing phase of gait.

9. A patient is scheduled for an electromyogram. The nurse explains that this diagnostic test involves
   a. placement of thin needles into the muscles.
   b. placement of electrodes on the skin to record electrical activity of muscles.
   c. measurement of the heat of muscle contractions radiating from the skin surface.
   d. administration of a calculated dose of radioisotope 2 hours before the procedure.

REFERENCES

1. Maher AB, Salmond SW, Pellino TA, editors: *Orthopaedic nursing,* ed 3, Philadelphia, 2002, WB Saunders.
2. National Association of Orthopaedic Nurses: *An introduction to orthopaedic nursing,* ed 2, Pitman NJ, 1998, NAON.
3. Thibodeau GA, Patton KT: *The human body in health and disease,* ed 3, St Louis, 2002, Mosby.
4. Schoen DC: *Core curriculum for orthopaedic nursing,* ed 4, Pitman NJ, 2001, NAON.
5. McCance KL, Huether SE, editors: *Pathophysiology: the biologic basis for disease in adults and children,* ed 4, St Louis, 2002, Mosby.
6. Herlihy B, Maebius NK: *The human body in health and illness,* ed 2, Philadelphia, 2003, WB Saunders.
7. Ebersole P, Hess P, editors: *Toward healthy aging,* ed 5, St Louis, 1998, Mosby.
8. Swartz MH: *Textbook of physical diagnosis,* ed 4, Philadelphia, 2002, WB Saunders.
9. Jarvis C: *Physical examination and health assessment,* ed 4, Philadelphia, 2004, WB Saunders.
10. Brinker MR, Miller MD: *Fundamentals of orthopaedics,* Philadelphia, 1999, WB Saunders.
11. Galen B: Diagnostic imaging: an overview, *Prim Care Pract* 3:5, 1999.

RESOURCES

Resources for this chapter are listed after Chapter 61 on page 1691, Chapter 62 on page 1714, and Chapter 63 on page 1755.

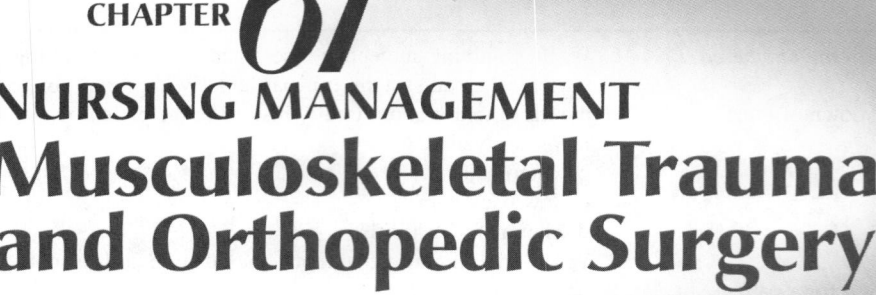

CHAPTER 61

NURSING MANAGEMENT
Musculoskeletal Trauma and Orthopedic Surgery

Cathleen E. Kunkler

LEARNING OBJECTIVES

1. Explain the etiology, pathophysiology, clinical manifestations, and collaborative care of soft tissue injuries, including strains, sprains, dislocations, subluxations, bursitis, repetitive strain injury, carpal tunnel syndrome, rotator cuff injury, meniscus injury, and muscle spasms.
2. Describe the sequential events involved in fracture healing.
3. Differentiate among closed reduction, cast immobilization, open reduction, and traction regarding purpose, complications, and nursing management.
4. Describe the neurovascular assessment of an injured extremity.
5. Explain common complications associated with fracture injury and fracture healing.
6. Describe the collaborative care and nursing management of patients with specific fractures.
7. Describe the indications for and the collaborative care and nursing management of the patient with an amputation.
8. Describe the types of joint replacement surgery associated with arthritis and connective tissue diseases.
9. Identify the preoperative and postoperative management of the patient having joint replacement surgery.

KEY TERMS

arthroplasty, p. 1685	osteotomy, p. 1685
bursitis, p. 1656	phantom limb sensation, p. 1682
carpal tunnel syndrome, p. 1654	repetitive strain injury, p. 1653
compartment syndrome, p. 1671	sprain, p. 1650
debridement, p. 1685	strain, p. 1651
dislocation, p. 1652	subluxation, p. 1652
fat embolism syndrome, p. 1672	synovectomy, p. 1685
fracture, p. 1657	traction, p. 1664

The most common cause of musculoskeletal problems is injury from a traumatic event resulting in fracture, dislocations, and associated soft tissue injuries. Although most of these injuries are not fatal, the cost in terms of pain, disability, medical expense, and lost wages is enormous. For all ages, accidents are exceeded only by heart disease, cancer, and strokes as a cause of death. Accidents are the leading cause of death in children and young adults.

The nurse has an important role in educating the public about the basic principles of safety and accident prevention. The morbidity associated with accidents can be significantly reduced if people are aware of environmental hazards, use existing safety equipment, and apply safety and traffic rules. In the industrial setting, the nurse should teach employees and employers about the use of proper safety equipment and avoidance of hazardous working situations.

In the home environment, falls account for many musculoskeletal injuries. Preventive education should be directed toward the importance of wearing shoes with functional soles and heels, avoidance of wet or slippery surfaces, careful placement of throw rugs, and removal of obstacles from the pathway of high-risk individuals such as persons with gait instability or visual or cognitive impairment. Ways to prevent common musculoskeletal problems in the older adult are listed in Table 61-1.

SOFT TISSUE INJURIES

Soft tissue injuries include sprains, strains, dislocations, and subluxation. These common injuries are usually caused by trauma. The increase in the number of people who have committed themselves to a regular fitness program or participating in sports has contributed to the increased incidence of soft tissue injuries. Common sports-related injuries are summarized in Table 61-2. Most sport injuries result from direct trauma, contusion, or indirect stretch injury.[1]

SPRAINS AND STRAINS

Sprains and strains are the two most common types of injury affecting the musculoskeletal system. These injuries are usually associated with abnormal stretching or twisting forces that may occur during vigorous activities. These injuries tend to occur around joints.

A **sprain** is an injury to ligamentous structures surrounding a joint, usually caused by a wrenching or twisting motion. A sprain is classified according to the amount of ligament fibers torn. A first-degree (mild) sprain involves tears of only a few fibers resulting in mild tenderness and slight swelling. A second-degree (moderate) sprain is partial disruption of the involved tissue with more swelling and tenderness. A third-degree (severe) sprain is a complete tearing of the ligament. A gap in the muscle may be apparent or palpated through the skin if the muscle is torn. Because these areas are rich in nerve endings, the injury can be extremely painful. The most common areas of sprains occur in the ankle and wrist.

Reviewed by Sharon G. Childs, RN, MS, CRNP-CS, ONC, CEN, Adult Nurse Practitioner, Orthopedic Clinical Specialist, Concentra Medical Center, Baltimore, Md.

A **strain** is an excessive stretching of a muscle and its facial sheath. It often also involves the tendon. Strains may also be classified as first-degree (mild or slightly pulled muscle), second-degree (moderate or moderately pulled muscle), and third-degree (severely pulled muscles).[2] The clinical manifestations of sprains and strains are similar and include pain, edema, decrease in function, and bruising. Pain aggravated by continued use is common.

TABLE

*P*atient & Family Teaching Guide

61-1 **Prevention of Musculoskeletal Problems in the Older Adult**

1. Use ramps in buildings and at street corners instead of steps to prevent falls.
2. Eliminate scatter rugs in the home.
3. Treat pain and discomfort from osteoarthritis.
   - Rest in reclining position to decrease discomfort.
   - Use plain or enteric-coated aspirin or nonsteroidal anti-inflammatory drugs to decrease inflammation of joints and reduce pain.
4. Use a walker or cane to help with walking to prevent falls.
5. Eat the amount and kind of foods to prevent excess weight gain because obesity adds stress to joints, which may predispose to osteoarthritis.
6. Get regular and frequent exercise.
   - Activities of daily living provide range-of-motion exercises.
   - Hobbies (e.g., jigsaw puzzles, needlework, model building) exercise finger joints and prevent stiffness.
   - Some weight-bearing exercise daily (e.g., walking) is essential and should be done two or three times daily.
7. Use shoes with good support to provide for safety and promote comfort.
8. Gradually initiate activities to promote optimal coordination. Rise slowly to a standing position to prevent dizziness, falls, and fractures.

Edema develops in the injured area because of tiny hemorrhages within the disrupted tissues and the ensuing inflammatory response. Usually the patient will recount a history of traumatic injury, possibly of a twisting nature, or recent exercise activity.

Minor sprains and strains are usually self-limiting, with full function returning within 3 to 6 weeks. A severe sprain can result in an *avulsion fracture,* in which the ligament pulls loose a fragment of bone. Alternatively, the joint structure may become unstable and result in subluxation or dislocation. At the time of injury, *hemarthrosis* (bleeding into a joint space or cavity) or disruption of the synovial lining may occur. An acute strain may involve partial or complete rupture of a muscle. Third-degree strains occasionally require surgical suturing of the muscle and surrounding fascia.

X-rays of the affected part are usually taken to rule out a fracture or widening of the joint structure. Surgical repair may be necessary if the injury is significant enough to produce severe disruption of ligamentous or muscle structures, fracture, or dislocation.

NURSING MANAGEMENT
SPRAINS AND STRAINS

■ Nursing Implementation

Health Promotion. Stretching and warm-up exercises before vigorous activity significantly reduce sprains and strains. Preconditioning exercise protects an inherently weak joint because slow stretching is tolerated better by tissues than is quick stretching. Warm-up exercises "prelengthen" potentially strained tissues by avoiding the quick stretch often encountered in sports. Warm-up exercises also increase the temperature of muscle, which increases cell metabolism and nerve impulse transmission. The increased metabolism contributes to better oxygenation of muscle fiber during work. Stretching is also thought to improve kinesthetic awareness, thus lessening the chance of uncoordinated movement.

The use of elastic support bandages or adhesive tape wrapping before beginning a vigorous activity is thought to reduce the

TABLE 61-2   Common Sports-Related Injuries

INJURY	DEFINITION	TREATMENT
Impingement syndrome	Entrapment of soft tissue structures under coracoacromial arch of the shoulder	NSAIDs; rest until symptoms decrease and then gradual ROM and strengthening exercises
Rotator cuff tear	Tear within muscle or ligaments of shoulder	If minor tear, rest, NSAIDs, and gradual mobilization with ROM and strengthening exercises If major tear, surgical repair
Shin splints	Inflammation along tibial shaft from tearing away of tendons caused by improper shoes, overuse, or running on hard pavement	Rest, ice, NSAIDs, proper shoes; gradual increase in activity; if pain persists, x-ray should be done to rule out stress fracture of tibia
Tendinitis	Inflammation of tendon in upper or lower extremity as a result of overuse or incorrect use	Rest, ice, NSAIDs; gradual return to sport activity; protective brace (orthosis) may be necessary if symptoms recur
Ligament injury	Tearing or stretching of ligament; usually occurs as a result of direct blow; characterized by sudden pain, swelling, and instability	Rest, ice, NSAIDs; protection of affected extremity by use of brace; if symptoms persist, surgical repair may be necessary
Meniscal injury	Injury to fibrocartilage of the knee characterized by popping, clicking, or tearing sensation, swelling	Rest, ice, NSAIDs; gradual return to regular activities; if symptoms persist, surgical arthroscopy to diagnose and repair meniscal injury may be necessary

NSAIDs, Nonsteroidal antiinflammatory drugs; *ROM,* range of motion.

occurrence of sprains. However, some health care providers do not support preventive wrapping or taping because it may predispose the athlete to injury.

Acute Intervention. If an injury occurs, the immediate care focuses on (1) rest and limitation of movement, (2) application of ice to the injured area, (3) compression of the involved extremity, (4) elevation of the extremity, and (5) analgesia as necessary (Table 61-3). RICE (rest, ice, compression, elevation) has been found to be effective for most injuries of the musculoskeletal system.[3] Movement should be limited and the extremity rested as soon as pain is felt. Unless the injury is severe, prolonged rest is usually not necessary. Cold *(cryotherapy)* in several forms can be used to produce hypothermia to the involved part. Physiologic changes that occur in soft tissue as a result of the use of cold include vasoconstriction and reduction in the transmission of nerve impulses. These changes result in analgesia and anesthesia, reduction of muscle spasm without changes in muscular strength or endurance, reduction of local edema and inflammation, and reduction of local metabolic requirements. Few unwanted side effects accompany the use of cold to treat a soft tissue injury. Cold is most useful when applied immediately after the injury has occurred. Ice applications should not exceed 20 to 30 minutes per application, allowing a "warm-up" time of 10 to 15 minutes between applications.

Compression also helps limit swelling, which, if left uncontrolled, could lengthen healing time. An elastic compression bandage can be wrapped around the injured part. The bandage is too tight if numbness is felt in the area or there is cramping or additional pain or swelling beyond the edge of the bandage. The bandage can be left in place for 30 minutes and then removed for 15 minutes.

The injured part should be elevated above the heart level to help mobilize excess fluid from the area and impede further edema. The injured part should be elevated even during sleep. Mild analgesics such as nonsteroidal antiinflammatory drugs (NSAIDs) may be necessary to manage patient discomfort. The cyclooxygenase-2 (COX-2) inhibitors (celecoxib [Celebrex],

rofecoxib [Vioxx]) may be given to patients if gastrointestinal problems are a concern.[4]

After the acute phase (usually lasting 24 to 48 hours), warm, moist heat can be applied to the affected part to reduce swelling and provide comfort. Heat applications should not exceed 20 to 30 minutes, allowing a "cool-down" time between applications. NSAIDs may be recommended to decrease edema and pain. The patient is encouraged to use the limb, provided that the joint is protected by means of casting, bracing, taping, or splinting. Movement of the joint maintains nutrition to the cartilage, and muscle contraction improves circulation and resolution of the contusion.

Ambulatory and Home Care. With the exception of treatment in the emergency department following the injury, sprains and strains are treated in the outpatient setting. The patient should be instructed in the use of ice and elevation for 24 to 48 hours after the injury to reduce edema. The use of mild analgesics to promote comfort should be encouraged. Use of an elastic wrap may provide additional support during activity. To prevent reinjury, the patient should learn proper measures of prevention.

The physical therapist may help provide pain relief by means of specialized techniques such as ultrasound. The therapist may also teach the patient exercises to perform for flexibility and to strengthen shortened muscles. Referral to a sports medicine clinic may be appropriate to aid the patient in learning stretching and warm-up exercises to prevent future injury.

DISLOCATION AND SUBLUXATION

A **dislocation** is a severe injury of the ligamentous structures that surround a joint. Dislocation results in the complete displacement or separation of the articular surfaces of the joint. A **subluxation** is a partial or incomplete displacement of the joint surface. The clinical manifestations of a subluxation are similar to those of a dislocation but are less severe. Treatment of subluxation is similar to that of a dislocation, but subluxation may require less healing time.

Dislocations characteristically result from overwhelming forces transmitted to the joint that cause a disruption of the soft

TABLE 61-3	Emergency Management	
Acute Soft Tissue Injury		
ETIOLOGY	**ASSESSMENT FINDINGS**	**INTERVENTIONS**
Falls	• Edema	**Initial**
Direct blows	• Ecchymosis	• Ensure airway, breathing, and circulation.
Crush injury	• Pain, tenderness	• Assess neurovascular status of involved limb.
Motor vehicle collisions	• Decreased sensation with severe edema	• Elevate involved limb.
Sports injuries	• Decreased pulse, coolness, and capillary refill	• Apply compression bandage unless dislocation present.
	• Decreased movement	• Apply ice packs to affected area.
	• Pallor	• Immobilize affected extremity in the position found.
	• Shortening or rotation of extremity	• Anticipate x-rays of injured extremity.
	• Inability to bear weight when lower extremity involved	• Give analgesia as necessary.
	• Decreased function with upper-extremity involvement	• Administer tetanus prophylaxis if skin integrity broken.
	• Muscle spasms	**Ongoing Monitoring**
		• Monitor for changes in neurovascular status.
		• Eliminate weight bearing when lower extremity involved.
		• Anticipate compartment pressure monitoring if neurovascular status changes.

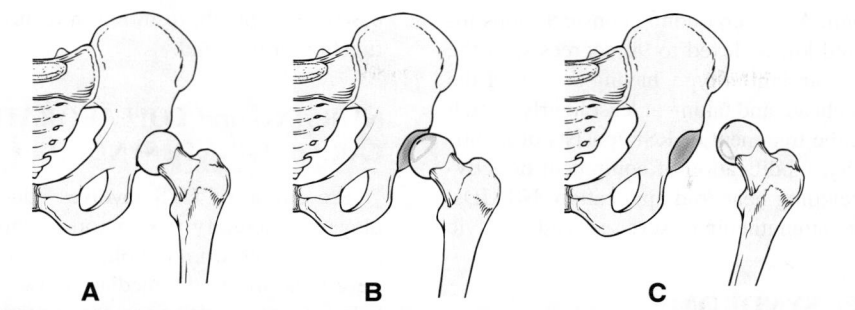

FIG. 61-1 Soft tissue injury of the hip. A, Normal. B, Subluxation (partial dislocation). C, Dislocation.

tissues surrounding the joint. The joints most frequently dislocated in the upper extremity include the thumb, elbow, and shoulder. In the lower extremity, the hip is vulnerable to dislocation occurring as a result of severe trauma, often associated with motor vehicle accidents (Fig. 61-1). The patella may dislocate because of instability of the tendons, ligaments, and muscles surrounding the knee or a severe twisting blow. Dislocations may also be the result of a congenital anomaly or of a pathologic origin.

The most obvious clinical manifestation of a dislocation is asymmetry of the musculoskeletal contour. For example, if a hip is dislocated, the limb is shorter on the affected side. Additional manifestations include local pain, tenderness, loss of function of the injured part, and swelling of the soft tissues in the region of the joint. The major complications of a dislocated joint are open joint injuries, intraarticular fractures, fracture dislocation, *avascular necrosis* (bone cell death as a result of inadequate blood supply), and damage to adjacent neurovascular tissue. Neurovascular assessment is critical.

X-ray studies are performed to determine the extent of shifting of the involved structures. The joint may also be aspirated to determine the presence of blood (hemarthrosis) or fat cells. Fat cells in the aspirate indicate a probable intraarticular fracture.

NURSING *and* COLLABORATIVE MANAGEMENT DISLOCATION

A dislocation requires prompt attention, especially the knee joint. A dislocation is considered an orthopedic emergency.[5] The longer the joint remains unreduced, the greater the possibility of avascular necrosis. The hip joint is particularly susceptible to avascular necrosis. The first goal of management is to realign the dislocated portion of the joint in its original anatomic position. This can be accomplished by a closed reduction, which may be performed under local or general anesthesia or intravenous (IV) conscious sedation. Anesthesia is often necessary to produce muscle relaxation so that the bones can be manipulated. In some situations, surgical open reduction may be necessary. After reduction, the extremity is usually immobilized by taping or using a sling to allow the torn ligaments and capsular tissue time to heal.

Nursing management of subluxation or dislocation is directed toward relief of pain and support and protection of the injured joint. After the joint has been reduced and immobilized, motion is usually restricted. A carefully regulated rehabilitation program can prevent the formation of contractures. Gentle range of motion (ROM) may be started if the joint is stable and the affected joint is well supported. The patient should not stretch the joint beyond its limits because the torn capsule and ligament heal in a shortened position with fibrous scar tissue that is not as strong as the original tissue. An exercise program slowly and methodically restores the joint to its original ROM without causing another dislocation. The patient should gradually return to normal activities.

A patient who has dislocated a joint may be at greater risk for repeated dislocations because the joint has been weakened by shortened ligaments and scar tissue. Activity restrictions of the affected joint may be imposed to decrease the risk of repeatedly dislocating the joint.

REPETITIVE STRAIN INJURY

Repetitive strain injury (RSI) is a cumulative trauma disorder resulting from prolonged, forceful, or awkward movements. RSI is also reported as repetitive trauma disorder, nontraumatic musculoskeletal injury, overuse syndrome (sports medicine), regional musculoskeletal disorder, work-related disorder, and "nintendinitis" (Nintendo games).[6] Repeated movements strain tendons, ligaments, and muscles, causing tiny tears that become inflamed. If the tissues are not given time to heal properly, scarring can occur. Blood vessels of the arms and hands may become constricted, depriving tissues of vital nutrients and causing an accumulation of factors such as lactic acid. Without intervention, tendons and muscles can deteriorate and nerves can become hypersensitive. At this point even the slightest movement can cause pain.

In addition to the repetitive movements, other factors related to RSI include poor posture and positioning, poor work space ergonomics, a badly designed keyboard, and lifting of heavy workloads without sufficient muscle rest. The result may cause chronic dysfunction to the muscles, tendons, and nerves of the neck, shoulder, forearm, and hand. Symptoms of RSI include pain, weakness, numbness, or impairment of motor function. Persons most often affected by RSI include musicians, dancers, electricians, butchers, keyboard operators, cashiers, grocery clerks, packers, postal workers, poultry processors, and vibratory tool workers.

RSI is becoming a serious public health problem for youth. More young people are employed an average of 15 to 20 hours per week; many work in the fast food industry where the equipment has been designed for adult workers. Farm laborers, competitive athletes, and poorly trained athletes may develop RSI. Swimming, overhead throwing (e.g., baseball), weight lifting, gymnastics, dancing, tennis, skiing, soccer (kicking sports), and horseback riding require repetitive motion, and overtraining compounds the effects.

RSI can be prevented through education, ergonomics (consideration of the interaction of humans and their work environment), and appropriate job design. A few ergonomic considerations include keeping the hips and knees flexed to 90 degrees with the feet flat, keeping the wrist straight to type, having the top of the monitor even with the forehead, and taking at least hourly stretch breaks. Once diagnosed, the treatment of RSI consists of identifying precipitating activity, modification of equipment or activity, pain management including heat/cold application, NSAIDs, rest, physical therapy for strengthening exercises, and lifestyle changes.

CARPAL TUNNEL SYNDROME

Carpal tunnel syndrome (CTS) is a condition caused by compression of the median nerve beneath the transverse carpal ligament within the narrow confines of the carpal tunnel located in the wrist (Fig. 61-2). CTS is the most common compression neuropathy. This condition often is due to pressure from trauma or edema caused by inflammation of a tendon (tenosynovitis), neoplasm, rheumatoid synovial disease, or soft tissue masses such as ganglia. Symptoms of CTS are often seen during the premenstrual period, pregnancy, and menopause, in diabetes mellitus and thyroid dysfunction, or in conditions with increased fluid retention.[7] This syndrome is associated with occupations that require continuous wrist movement (e.g., butchers, dentists, seamstresses, machine operators, musicians, hair stylists, secretaries, painters, carpenters, computer operators, bowlers, knitters, guitarists).

The clinical manifestations of CTS are weakness (especially of the thumb), burning pain (causalagia) and numbness, or impaired sensation in the distribution of the median nerve and clumsiness in performing fine hand movements. Numbness and tingling may be present that awaken the patient at night. Holding the wrist in acute flexion for 60 seconds will produce tingling and numbness over the distribution of the median nerve, the palmar surface of the thumb, the index finger, the middle finger, and part of the ring finger. This is known as a positive *Phalen's sign.* Tapping gently over the area of the inflamed median nerve may reproduce the paresthesia. This is known as a positive *Tinel's sign.* In late stages there is atrophy of the thenar muscles around the base of the thumb, resulting in recurrent pain and eventual dysfunction of the hand.

NURSING *and* COLLABORATIVE MANAGEMENT CARPAL TUNNEL SYNDROME

Prevention of CTS involves educating employees and employers to identify risk factors. Adaptive devices such as wrist splints may be worn to hold the wrist in slight dorsiflexion to relieve pressure on the median nerve. Special keyboard pads that help prevent repetitive pressure on the median nerve are available for computer operators to help prevent or reduce CTS by decreasing tension on the carpal tunnel. Other ergonomic changes include workstation modifications, change in body positions, and frequent breaks.

Collaborative care of the patient with CTS is directed toward relieving the underlying cause of the nerve compression. The early symptoms associated with CTS can usually be relieved by stopping the aggravating movement and by placing the hand and wrist at rest by immobilizing them in a hand splint. If the cause is inflammation, injection of a corticosteroid drug directly into the carpal tunnel may provide short-term (up to 6 months) relief. The patient's sensation may be impaired during this time. Therefore the patient should be instructed to avoid hazards such as extreme heat because of the risk of thermal injury. The patient may be required to consider occupational changes because of discomfort and sensory and functional changes.

If the problem continues, the median nerve may have to be surgically decompressed by longitudinal division of the transverse carpal ligament under regional anesthesia (see Fig. 61-2). This surgery is done on an outpatient basis. After surgery, the neurovascular status of the hand should be evaluated before discharge, and the patient should be instructed in the appropriate assessments to perform at home. Endoscopic carpal tunnel release is a surgical procedure in which the decompression is performed through a small incision puncture site with the patient under local anesthesia. Modified open carpal tunnel release procedure is another alternative surgical intervention.

ROTATOR CUFF INJURY

The rotator cuff is a complex of four muscles in the shoulder: supraspinatus, infraspinatus, teres minor, and subscapularis. These muscles act to stabilize the humeral head in the glenoid fossa while assisting with the ROM of the shoulder joint and rotation of the humerus. Degenerative changes of the rotator cuff are associated with normal aging.

A tear in the rotator cuff may occur as a gradual, degenerative process resulting from aging, poor posture, repetitive stress (especially overhead arm motions), or use of an arm to break a fall. The rotator cuff will rupture as a result of sudden adduction forces applied to the cuff while the arm is held in abduction. In sports, repetitive overhead motions, such as in swimming, racquet sports (tennis, racquetball), and baseball (especially pitching), are often activities that initiate injury. A fall to an outstretched hand or a blow to the upper arm, heavy lifting, or repetitive work motions are also causative factors.[8]

Patients with a rotator cuff injury will complain of shoulder pain and inability to initiate or maintain abduction of the arm or shoulder. The weakness and decreased ROM accompany a positive Neer's test and Hawkin's test, which both will yield a positive

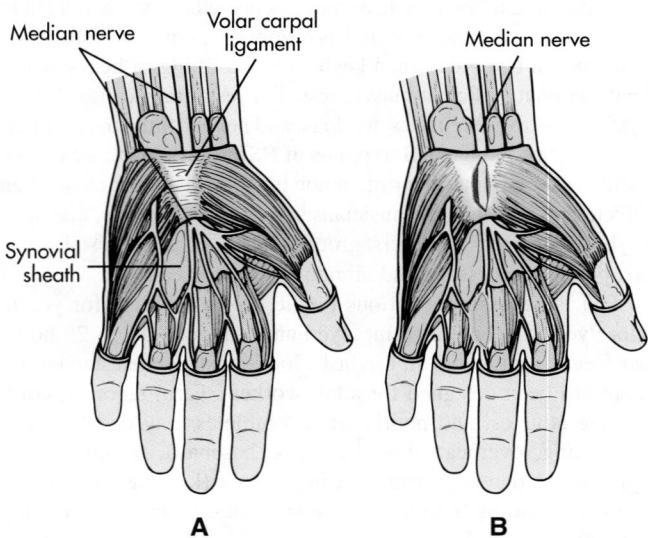

Median nerve

Volar carpal ligament

Median nerve

Synovial sheath

A   **B**

FIG. 61-2   **A,** Wrist structures involved in carpal tunnel syndrome. **B,** Decompression of median nerve.

response to pain. An x-ray alone is usually not beneficial in the diagnosis of a rotator cuff injury. A tear can be confirmed by arthrogram or magnetic resonance imaging (MRI).[9] The Simple Shoulder Test is also diagnostic in evaluating rotator cuff function. In this test patients are evaluated in their ability to place the arm comfortably at the side, ability to sleep with the arm at their side, ability to tuck in a shirt or blouse behind, place hand behind head, place a coin on a shelf, place a pound on a shelf, place 8 lb on a shelf, carry 20 lb, toss underhand, throw overhand, wash the opposite shoulder, and perform their usual work.[10]

The goal of treatment emphasizes maintaining passive ROM and the return of abduction strength. The patient may be treated conservatively with rest, ice and heat, NSAIDs, periodic corticosteroid injections into the joint, and physical therapy. If the patient does not respond to conservative treatment or if a complete tear is present, a surgical repair may be necessary. Surgical repair may be done through the arthroscope. If an extensive tear is present, acromioplasty (surgical removal of part of the acromion to relieve compression of rotator cuff during movement) may be necessary. An immobilization device such as a sling or, more commonly, a shoulder immobilizer may be used immediately after surgery. However, the shoulder should not be immobilized for too long a period because frozen shoulder or arthrofibrosis may occur. Pendulum exercises and physical therapy begin the first postoperative day.

MENISCUS INJURY

The meniscus is the fibrocartilage in the knee and other joints. Meniscus injuries are closely associated with ligament sprains commonly occurring in athletes engaged in sports such as basketball, rugby, football, soccer, and hockey. These activities produce rotational stress when the knee is in varying degrees of flexion and the foot is planted or fixed. A blow to the knee can cause the meniscus to be sheared between the femoral condyles and the tibial plateau, resulting in a torn meniscus. (The knee joint is shown in Fig. 61-3.) Occupations that require persons to work in a squatting or kneeling position may be at higher risk for meniscus injuries.

Meniscus injuries alone do not usually cause chronic edema because cartilage is avascular and aneural. However, a torn meniscus may be suspected when local tenderness or pain is reported. Pain is elicited by abduction or adduction of the leg at the knee. The usual clinical picture is a feeling by the patient that the knee is unstable and a report that the knee may "click, lock, and give away."[11] Quadriceps atrophy is evident if the injury has been present for some time. Traumatic arthritis may occur from repeated meniscal injury and chronic inflammation.

An arthrogram, arthroscopy, or both can diagnose knee problems. MRI is beneficial in confirming the diagnosis before arthroscopy is used. MRI has eliminated the use of an arthrogram as a diagnostic tool in many cases. Surgery may be indicated for a torn meniscus. Degree of knee pain and dysfunction, occupation, sport activities, and age may affect the patient's decision to have or postpone surgery.

NURSING *and* COLLABORATIVE MANAGEMENT
MENISCUS INJURY

Because meniscal injuries are commonly caused by sports-related activity, athletes should be taught to do warm-up activities. Proper stretching may make the patient less prone to meniscal injury when a fall or twisting occurs. Examination of the acutely injured knee should occur within 24 hours of injury. Initial care of this type of injury involves application of ice, immobilization, and partial weight bearing with crutches. Most meniscal injuries are treated in an outpatient setting. The patient should be allowed to ambulate as tolerated. Crutches may be necessary. Use of a knee brace or immobilizer during the first few days after the injury protects the knee and offers some pain relief.

After acute pain has decreased, gradual increases in flexion and muscle strengthening may assist the patient to full functioning. Physical therapy is generally recommended to help the patient to strengthen the quadricep muscles before returning to sport activities. Surgical repair or excision of part of the menis-

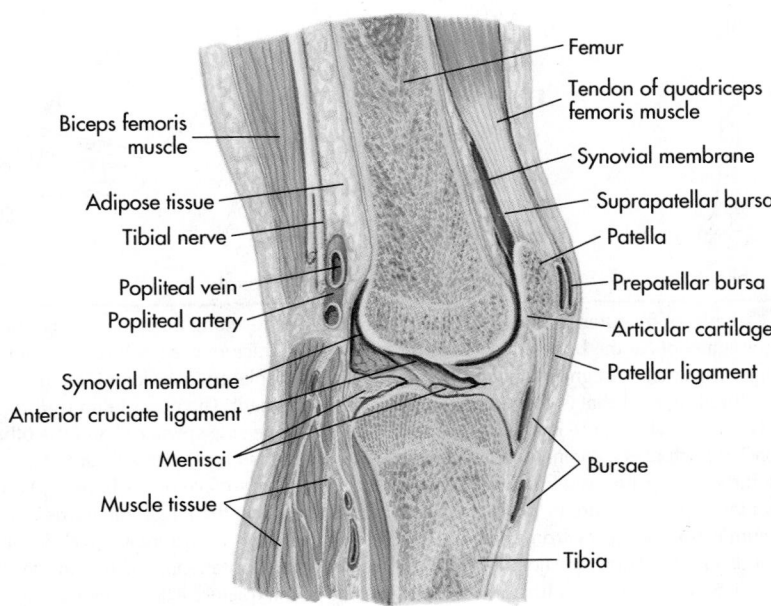

Biceps femoris muscle
Adipose tissue
Tibial nerve
Popliteal vein
Popliteal artery
Synovial membrane
Anterior cruciate ligament
Menisci
Muscle tissue

Femur
Tendon of quadriceps femoris muscle
Synovial membrane
Suprapatellar bursa
Patella
Prepatellar bursa
Articular cartilage
Patellar ligament
Bursae
Tibia

FIG. 61-3   Sagittal section through knee joint.

cus (meniscectomy) may be necessary. Often this can be done by arthroscopy. Pain relief may include NSAIDs, tramadol (Ultram), or a mild combination of drugs such as acetaminophen with hydrocodone. Rehabilitation starts soon after surgery, including ROM and quadricep and hamstring strengthening exercises. When the patient's strength is back to its preinjury level, normal activities may be resumed.

BURSITIS

Bursae are closed sacs that are lined with synovial membrane and contain a small amount of synovial fluid. They are located at sites of friction, such as between tendons and bones and near the joints. **Bursitis** (inflammation of the bursa) results from repeated or excessive trauma or friction, gout, rheumatoid arthritis, or infection. The primary clinical manifestations of bursitis are warmth, pain, swelling, and limited ROM in the affected part. Sites at which bursitis commonly occurs include the hand, knee, greater trochanter of the hip, shoulder, and elbow. Repetitive kneeling (carpet layers, coal miners, and gardeners), jogging in worn-out shoes, and prolonged sitting with crossed legs are common precipitators of injury.[12]

Attempts are made to determine and correct the cause of the bursitis. Rest is often the only treatment needed. Icing the area will decrease pain and may reduce inflammation. The affected part may be immobilized in a compression dressing or plaster splint. NSAIDs may be used to reduce inflammation and pain.[13] Aspiration of the bursal fluid (dark, bloody, cloudy) and injection of a corticosteroid may be necessary. If the bursal wall has become thickened and continues to interfere with normal joint function, surgical excision (bursectomy) may be necessary. For example, subacromial bursal thickening causes pain and loss of ROM on abduction of the shoulder. Septic bursae usually require surgical incision and drainage.

MUSCLE SPASMS

Local muscle spasms are a common condition often associated with sports and excessive everyday activities. Injury to a muscle results in inflammation and edema, which irritates nerve endings, resulting in muscle spasm. The spasms produce additional pain, creating a repetitive cycle. The clinical manifestations of muscle spasm include pain; palpable, tense, firm muscle mass; diminished ROM if a joint is involved; and limitation of daily or occupational activities.

A careful history and physical examination should be performed to rule out central nervous system (CNS) problems. Muscle spasms may be managed with drug therapy, physical therapy, or both. Drugs used for treatment of local muscle spasms include mild analgesics, NSAIDs, and skeletal muscle relaxants. A physical therapy program might include the use of heat or ice, supervised exercise, massage, hydrotherapy, local heat-producing ap-

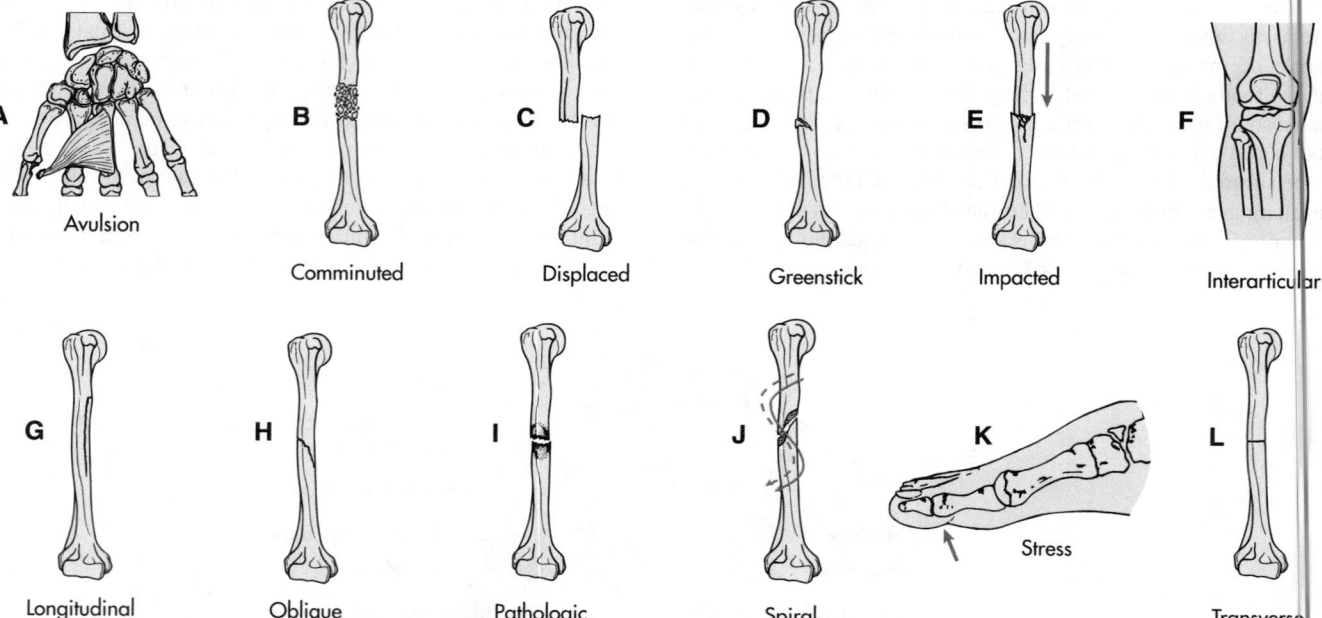

FIG. 61-4 Types of fractures. **A,** Avulsion is a fracture of bone resulting from the strong pulling effect of tendons or ligaments at the bone attachment. **B,** Comminuted fracture is a fracture with more than two fragments. The smaller fragments appear to be floating. **C,** Displaced (overriding) fracture involves a displaced fracture fragment that is overriding the other bone fragment. The periosteum is disrupted on both sides. **D,** Greenstick fracture is an incomplete fracture with one side splintered and the other side bent. **E,** Impacted fracture is a comminuted fracture in which more than two fragments are driven into each other. **F,** Interarticular fracture is a fracture extending to the articular surface of the bone. **G,** Longitudinal fracture is an incomplete fracture in which the fracture line runs along the longitudinal axis of the bone. The periosteum is not torn away from the bone. **H,** Oblique fracture is a fracture in which the line of the fracture extends in an oblique direction. **I,** Pathologic fracture is a spontaneous fracture at the site of a bone disease. **J,** Spiral fracture is a fracture in which the line of the fracture extends in a spiral direction along the shaft of the bone. **K,** Stress fracture is a fracture that occurs in normal or abnormal bone that is subject to repeated stress, such as from jogging or running. **L,** Transverse fracture is a fracture in which the line of the fracture extends across the bone shaft at a right angle to the longitudinal axis.

plications (oil of wintergreen), ultrasound (deep heat), manipulation, and bracing.

Fractures

Classification

A **fracture** is a disruption or break in the continuity of the structure of bone. Traumatic injuries account for the majority of fractures, although some fractures are secondary to a disease process (pathologic fractures). Fractures are described and classified according to (1) type (Fig. 61-4); (2) communication or noncommunication with the external environment (Fig. 61-5); and (3) anatomic location of fracture on the involved bone (Fig. 61-6) as well as the appearance, position, and alignment of the fragments; and classic names.[14]

Fractures are also described as stable or unstable. A *stable fracture* occurs when a piece of the periosteum is intact across the fracture and either external or internal fixation has rendered the fragments stationary. Stable fractures are usually transverse, spiral, or greenstick. An *unstable fracture* is grossly displaced during injury and is a site of poor fixation. Unstable fractures are usually comminuted or oblique.

A fracture can also be classified as closed (simple) or open. An *open fracture* (formerly called compound fracture) involves

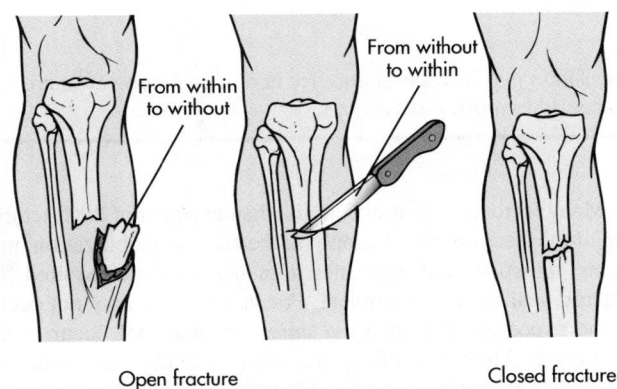

Open fracture   Closed fracture

FIG. 61-5 Fracture classification according to communication.

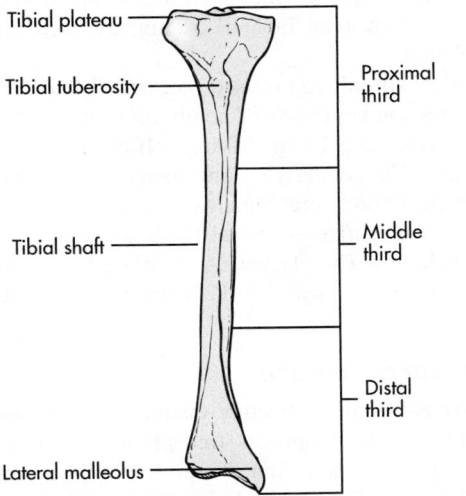

FIG. 61-6 Fracture classification according to location.

communication of the fracture through the skin with the external environment.

Clinical Manifestations

The patient's history indicates a mechanism of injury associated with numerous signs and symptoms, including immediate localized pain, decreased function, and inability to bear weight or use the affected part (Table 61-4). The patient guards and protects the extremity against movement. The fracture may not be accompanied by obvious bone deformity. If a fracture is suspected, the extremity is immobilized in the position in which it is found. Unnecessary movement increases soft-tissue damage and may convert a closed fracture to an open fracture or create further injury to adjacent neurovascular structures.

Fracture Healing

It is important to understand the principles of fracture healing (Fig. 61-7) to provide appropriate therapeutic interventions. Bone goes through a remarkable reparative process of self-healing (termed *union*) that occurs in the following stages:

1. *Fracture hematoma.* When a fracture occurs, bleeding and edema create a hematoma, which surrounds the ends of the fragments. The hematoma is extravasated blood that changes from a liquid to a semisolid clot. This occurs in the initial 72 hours after injury.

2. *Granulation tissue.* During this stage, active phagocytosis absorbs the products of local necrosis. The hematoma converts to granulation tissue. Granulation tissue (consisting of new blood vessels, fibroblasts, and osteoblasts) produces the basis for new bone substance called *osteoid* during days 3 to 14 postinjury.

3. *Callus formation.* As minerals (calcium, phosphorus, and magnesium and new bone matrix) are deposited in the osteoid, an unorganized network of bone is formed that is woven about the fracture parts. *Callus* is primarily composed of cartilage, osteoblasts, calcium, and phosphorus. It usually begins to appear by the end of the second week after injury. Evidence of callus formation can be verified by x-ray.

4. *Ossification.* Ossification of the callus occurs from 3 weeks to 6 months after the fracture and continues until the fracture has healed. Callus ossification is sufficient to prevent movement at the fracture site when the bones are gently stressed. However, the fracture is still evident on x-ray. During this stage of clinical union the patient can be converted from skeletal traction to a cast, or the cast can be removed to allow limited mobility.

5. *Consolidation.* As callus continues to develop, the distance between bone fragments diminishes and eventually closes. This stage is called consolidation, and ossification continues. It can be equated with radiologic union.

6. *Remodeling.* Excess bone tissue is reabsorbed in the final stage of bone healing, and union is completed. Gradual return of the injured bone to its preinjury structural strength and shape occurs. Bone remodels in response to physical stress.[14] Initially, stress is provided through exercise. Weight bearing is gradually introduced. New bone is deposited in sites subjected to stress and resorbed at areas where there is little stress. Radiologic union occurs when there is x-ray evidence of complete bony union. This phase can occur up to a year following injury.

TABLE 61-4	Clinical Manifestations of Fracture
MANIFESTATION	**SIGNIFICANCE**
Edema and Swelling Disruption of soft tissues or bleeding into surrounding tissues	Unchecked edema in closed space can occlude circulation and damage nerves (i.e., there is a risk of compartment syndrome).
Pain and Tenderness Muscle spasm as a result of involuntary reflex action of muscle, direct tissue trauma, increased pressure on sensory nerve, movement of fracture parts	Pain and tenderness encourage splinting of fracture with reduction in motion of injured area.
Muscle Spasm Protective response to injury and fracture	Muscle spasms may displace nondisplaced fracture or prevent it from reducing spontaneously.
Deformity Abnormal position of bone as result of original forces of injury and action of muscles pulling fragment into abnormal position; seen as a loss of normal bony contours	Deformity is cardinal sign of fracture; if uncorrected, it may result in problems with bony union and restoration of function of injured part.
Ecchymosis Discoloration of skin as a result of extravasation of blood in subcutaneous tissues	Ecchymosis may appear immediately after injury and may appear distal to injury. The nurse should reassure patient that process is normal.
Loss of Function Disruption of bone, preventing functional use	Fracture must be managed properly to ensure restoration of function.
Crepitation Grating or crunching together of bony fragments, producing palpable or audible crunching sensation	Crepitation may increase chance for nonunion if bone ends are allowed to move excessively.

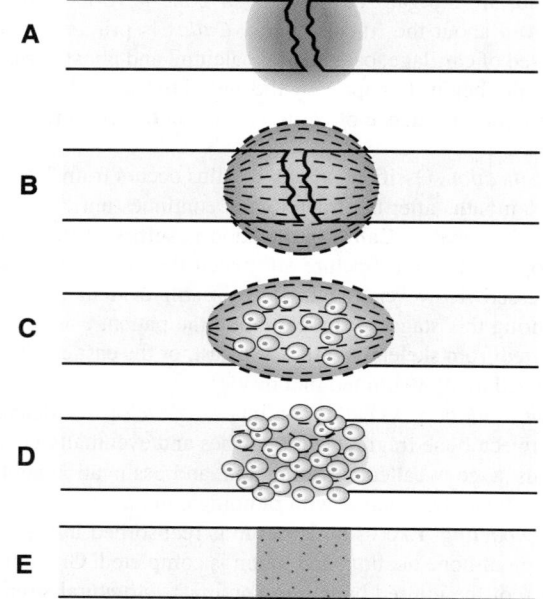

FIG. 61-7 Bone healing (schematic representation). **A,** Bleeding at broken ends of the bone with subsequent hematoma formation. **B,** Organization of hematoma into fibrous network. **C,** Invasion of osteoblasts, lengthening of collagen strands, and deposition of calcium. **D,** Callus formation: new bone is built up as osteoclasts destroy dead bone. **E,** Remodeling is accomplished as excess callus is reabsorbed and trabecular bone is laid down.

Many factors, such as age, initial displacement of the fracture, site of the fracture, blood supply to the area, immobilization, implants, infection, and hormones influence the time required for fracture healing to be complete. Fracture healing may not occur in the expected time *(delayed union)* or may not occur at all *(nonunion)*. The ossification process is arrested by causes such as inadequate reduction and immobilization, excess movement, infection, poor nutrition, and systemic disease. Healing time for fractures increases with age. For example, an uncomplicated midshaft fracture of the femur heals in 3 weeks in a newborn and in 20 weeks in an adult. Table 61-5 summarizes complications of fracture healing.

Electrical stimulation is used successfully to stimulate bone healing in some situations of nonunion or delayed union. The electric current acts by modifying cell behavior causing bone remodeling. The underlying mechanism for electrically induced bone remodeling remains unknown. It is thought to be related to negative electrical fields attracting positive ions such as calcium. The electrodes are placed over the patient's skin or cast and are used 10 to 12 hours each day, usually while sleeping.

Collaborative Care

The overall goals of fracture treatment are (1) anatomic realignment of bone fragments (reduction), (2) immobilization to maintain realignment, and (3) restoration of normal or near-normal function of the injured part. Table 61-6 summarizes the collaborative care of fractures.

TABLE 61-5	**Complications of Fracture Healing**
PROBLEM	**DESCRIPTION**
Delayed union	Fracture healing progresses more slowly than expected; healing eventually occurs.
Nonunion	Fracture fails to heal properly despite treatment, resulting in fibrous union or pseudarthrosis.
Malunion	Fracture heals in expected time but in unsatisfactory position, possibly resulting in deformity or dysfunction.
Angulation	Fracture heals in abnormal position in relation to midline of structure (type of malunion).
Pseudarthrosis	Type of nonunion occurring at fracture site in which false joint is formed on shaft of long bones. It is a fracture site that failed to fuse. Each bone end is covered with fibrous scar tissue.
Refracture	New fracture occurs at original fracture site.
Myositis ossificans	Condition occurring in response to muscle hemorrhage caused by trauma. Hematoma ossifies.

TABLE 61-6	**Collaborative Care** **Fractures**

Diagnostic
History and physical examination
X-ray examination
CT scan, MRI
Collaborative Therapy
Fracture Reduction
Manipulation
Closed reduction
Traction devices
  Skin traction
  Skeletal traction
Open reduction
Fracture Immobilization
Casting
Traction
External fixation
Internal fixation
Open Fractures
Surgical debridement and irrigation
Tetanus immunization
Prophylactic antibiotic therapy
Immobilization

CT, Computed tomography; *MRI*, magnetic resonance imaging.

Fracture Reduction

Closed reduction. *Closed reduction* is a nonsurgical, manual realignment of bone fragments to their previous anatomic position. Traction and countertraction are manually applied to the bone fragments to restore position, length, and alignment. Closed reduction is usually performed with the patient under local or general anesthesia. After reduction, the injured part is immobilized by traction, casting, external fixation, splints, or orthoses (braces) to maintain alignment until healing occurs.

Open reduction. *Open reduction* is the correction of bone alignment through a surgical incision. It often includes internal fixation of the fracture with the use of wire, screws, pins, plates, intramedullary rods, or nails. The type and location of the fracture, age of patient, and concurrent disease, as well as the result of attempted closed reduction by means of traction, may influence the decision to use open reduction. The chief disadvantages of this form of treatment are the possibility of infection and the complications associated with anesthesia.

If open reduction with internal fixation (ORIF) is used for intraarticular fractures (involving joint surfaces), early initiation of ROM of the joint is indicated. Machines that provide continuous passive motion (CPM) to various joints are now available. Use of such machines can result in prevention of intraarticular adhesions, faster reconstruction of the subchondral (beneath cartilage) bone plate, more rapid healing of the articular cartilage, and possibly decreased incidence of later posttraumatic arthritis. ORIF facilitates early ambulation, which decreases the risk of complications related to prolonged immobility, and promotes fracture healing with gradually increasing increments of stress.

Traction. Traction devices apply a pulling force on the fractured extremity to attain realignment while countertraction pulls in the opposite direction. The two most common types of traction are skin traction and skeletal traction. *Skin traction* is generally used for short-term treatment (48 to 72 hours) until skeletal traction or surgery is possible. Tape, boots, or splints are applied directly to the skin to maintain alignment, assist in reduction, and help diminish muscle spasms in the injured extremity. The traction weights are usually limited to 5 to 10 lb (2.3 to 4.5 kg). *Skeletal traction,* generally in place for longer periods, is used to align injured bones and joints or to treat joint contractures and congenital hip dysplasia. It provides a long-term pull that keeps the injured bones and joints aligned. To establish skeletal traction, the physician inserts a pin or wire into the bone, either partially or completely, to align and immobilize the injured body part. Weight for skeletal traction ranges from 5 to 45 lb (2.3 to 20.4 kg).

When traction is used to treat fractures, the forces are usually exerted on the distal fragment to obtain alignment with the proximal fragment. Several types of traction are used for this purpose (Table 61-7). Fracture alignment depends on the correct positioning and alignment of the patient while the traction forces remain constant. For extremity traction to be effective, forces must be pulling in the opposite direction (countertraction) to prevent the patient from sliding to the end or side of the bed. Countertraction is commonly supplied by the patient's body weight or may be augmented by elevating the end of the bed. It is imperative that the nurse maintain the traction constantly and not interrupt the weight applied to the traction.

Fracture Immobilization

Casts. A cast is a temporary circumferential immobilization device. Casting is a common treatment following closed reduction. It allows the patient to perform many normal activities of daily living while providing sufficient immobilization to ensure stability. Cast materials are natural (plaster of paris), synthetic, fiberglass free, latex-free polymer, or a hybrid of materials.[15]

After immersion in water, plaster of paris is wrapped and molded around the affected part. It is composed of anhydrous calcium sulfate embedded in gauze roll. The strength of the cast

TABLE 61-7 **Common Types of Traction**

TYPE	INDICATIONS	NURSING IMPLICATIONS
Skin **Buck's** 	Used for many conditions affecting hip, femur, knee, or back. It is generally used for temporary immobilization and stabilization of fractured hips or fractures of the femoral shaft. It can be unilateral or bilateral. May also be used to correct knee and hip joint contractures.	All assessments should be at least q4hr. Assess for altered neurovascular status caused by original injury or the application of the bandages used in Buck's traction. Especially note decreased peripheral vascular flow and peroneal nerve deficit by assessing for ability to dorsiflex toes and foot, and for changes in sensation in the first webspace between the great and second toes. Pressure from the elastic wrap may result in pressure necrosis, especially over bony prominences and areas prone to pressure (anterior tibial border, fibular head, both malleoli, Achilles tendon, calcaneus, and dorsum of the foot). In addition, assess for an allergic reaction to the adhesive material, rotation of the extremity, and constant traction and countertraction forces.
Russell's 	Used for fractures of femur or hip.	Same as above. An additional area prone to pressure necrosis is the area over the hamstring tendons in the popliteal space.
Bryant's 	Used for fractures of the femur, fractures in small children, and stabilization of hip joints in children under 2 yr or 30 lb (14 kg) in weight.	Be aware that with traction in place, buttocks should just clear the mattress. Check for undue pressure over the outer head and neck of fibula, dorsum of foot, Achilles tendon, scapulae, and shoulders. Check that bandages or boot has not slipped. Be aware that these are usually removed for skin care and assessment q4hr.
Pelvic belt (or girdle) 	Used for sciatica, muscle spasms (low back), and minor fractures of the lower spine.	Check for security of the pelvic belt. Check frequently for skin irritation over iliac crests and in the intergluteal fold. Use measures to prevent skin breakdown. Check and adjust pelvic belt straps so that they are unrestricted and equal in length. Secure the straps with adhesive tape. Use a footboard to prevent footdrop. Maintain the correct angle of pull of the traction. Be aware that the physician orders the type of countertraction.
Pelvic sling traction	Used for pelvic fractures to provide compression for a separated pelvic girdle.	The sling should keep the pelvis just above the surface of the bed. Assess for pressure necrosis and skin irritation q4hr; especially assess for pressure over the iliac crests, intergluteal fold, and greater trochanters. Monitor for soiling of the sling and change as needed; use a fracture bedpan for toileting. Limit use of trapeze because it will reduce compressive force from the sling. Use alternating air pressure mattress or other pressure–dispersing devices; provide frequent back care.

TABLE 61-7	Common Types of Traction—cont'd	
TYPE	**INDICATIONS**	**NURSING IMPLICATIONS**

Skin—cont'd
Head halter

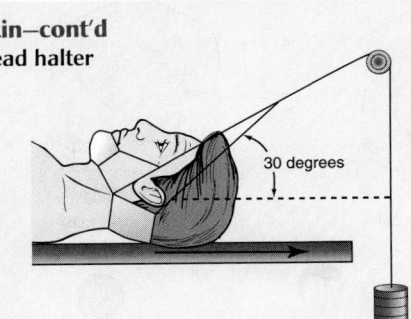

30 degrees

Used for soft tissue disorders and degenerative disk disease of the cervical spine. It is not commonly used for unstable fractures of the cervical spine.

Assess for alignment with trunk, areas of local pressure over the ears and mandibular joints and under the chin and occipital area, and pain or dysfunction in the temporomandibular joint. Patients may be permitted to remove traction for meals; if not, provide a liquid or mechanical soft diet to reduce temporomandibular joint pain. Because this traction is commonly used in the home, ensure patients can demonstrate safe and effective setup, application, and use of the traction before discharge.

Skeletal
Overhead arm (90 degrees–90 degrees)

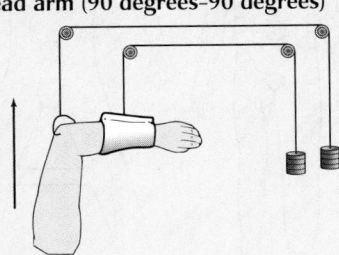

Commonly used for immobilization of fractures and dislocations of the upper arm and shoulder.

Be aware that the shoulder and elbow joint are maintained at 90-degree angles. Assess for pressure necrosis beneath the sling, especially over bony prominences. Assess distal neurovascular status; because of exposure, skin temperature may be cool and thus not indicative of decreased perfusion. Perform assessments q4hr. Inspect the pin site and perform pin site care according to protocol.

Lateral arm

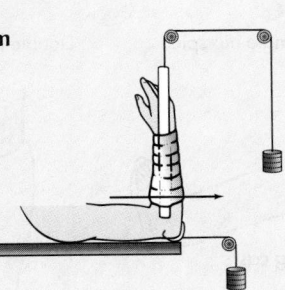

Commonly used in immobilization of fractures and dislocations of the upper arm and shoulder.

Inspect the pin site and perform pin site care according to protocol. Assess neurovascular status.

Balanced suspension traction

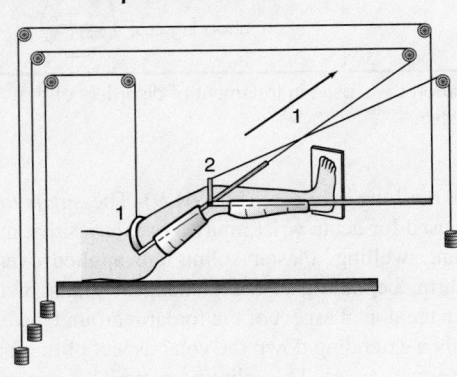

Used for injury or fracture of the femoral shaft of the femur, acetabulum, hip, tibia, or any combination of these.

Be aware that this traction uses half-ring Thomas splint (1) and Pearson attachment (2) and that suspension of the extremity and direct skeletal traction are applied. This allows raising of the buttocks off the bed for bedpan use and skin care without altering the line of traction. Maintain countertraction (e.g., position patient high in bed so that feet do not press on foot of bed; do not elevate the head of the bed >25 degrees if it causes continual movement toward foot of the bed). Encourage self-help in patient's performance of activities of daily living, movement in bed with help of trapeze, and flexion and extension of affected foot to prevent footdrop. Assess for pressure necrosis in areas contacted by the traction, especially the greater trochanter, ischial tuberosity, hamstring tendons, fibular head, and both malleoli. Assess distal neurovascular status q4hr. Inspect the pin site and perform pin site care according to protocol.

is determined by the number of layers of plaster bandage and the technique of application. As the cast dries a thermochemical reaction occurs in which the calcium sulfate recrystallizes and hardens. The patient may experience increased warmth about the fracture site. Increased edema as a result of the improved circulation may occur as a result of heat produced by the drying cast. After the cast is completely dry, it is strong and firm and can withstand stresses. The plaster hardens within 15 minutes, so the patient may move around without difficulty. However, it is not strong enough for weight bearing until about 24 to 72 hours.

A fresh cast should never be covered with a blanket because air cannot circulate and heat builds up in the cast. During the drying period the cast should not be subjected to any wetness, soiling, or abnormal stresses that can cause weakening or a break in the cast. It should be carefully handled by the palms of the hands rather than with the fingertips to avoid indentations that will dry and become potential pressure areas. Once the cast is thoroughly dry, the edges may need to be petaled to avoid skin irritation from rough edges and to prevent plaster of paris debris from falling into the cast and causing irritation or pressure necrosis (Fig. 61-8).

Synthetic casting materials (thermolabile plastic, thermoplastic resins, polyurethane, and fiberglass) are molded to fit the torso or extremity after being activated by submersion in cool or tepid water. Casts made of synthetic materials are frequently used because they are lightweight and relatively waterproof and support immediate mobilization.

Types of casts. Immobilization of an acute fracture or soft tissue injury of the upper extremity is often accomplished by use of (1) the sugar-tong splint, (2) the posterior splint, (3) the short

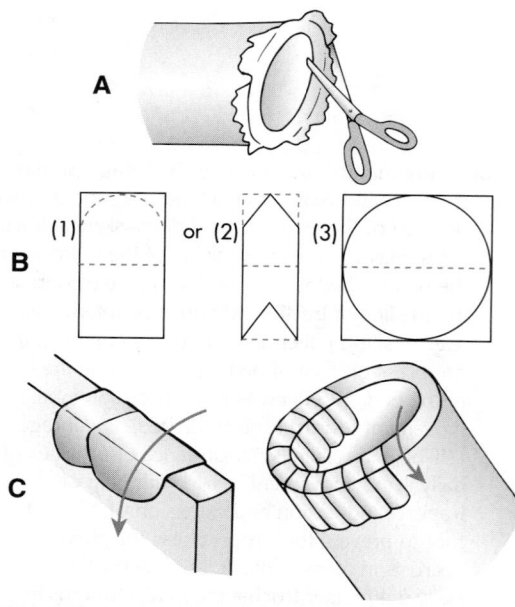

FIG. 61-8 Petaling edges of cast with waterproof adhesive strips. **A,** Cast must be thoroughly dry. The nurse trims the excess sheet wadding and stretches the stockinette over the cast edge (when possible). **B,** Several strips (petals) of waterproof adhesive tape (2-inch-wide strips for wide areas and 1-inch-wide strips for small areas, each 1 inch long) are made in advance. **C,** Uncut end of the tape is placed beneath the cast edge. Each succeeding petal overlaps the previous one by one-half inch, ensuring a smooth cast edge.

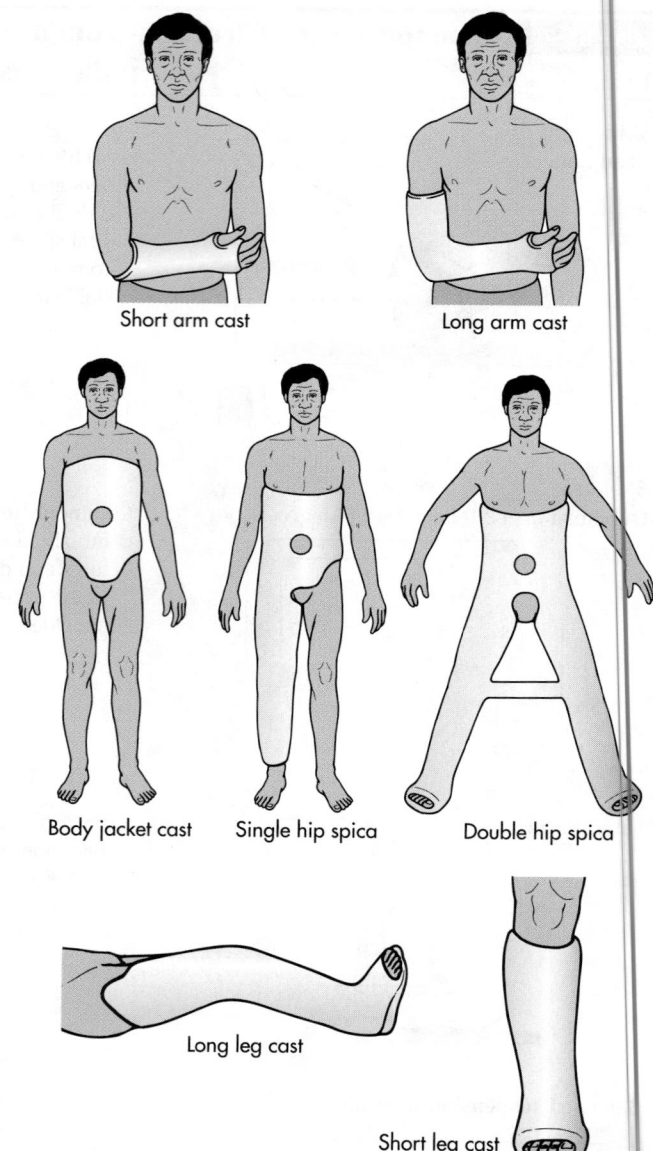

FIG. 61-9 Common casts used in treatment of disorders of the musculoskeletal system.

arm cast, and (4) the long arm cast (Fig. 61-9). The *sugar-tong splint* is typically used for acute wrist injuries or injuries that may result in significant swelling. Plaster splints are applied over a well-padded forearm, beginning at the phalangeal joints of the hand, extending up the dorsal aspect of the forearm around the distal humerus, and then extending down the volar aspect of the forearm to the distal palmar crease. The splinting material is wrapped with either elastic bandage or bias stockinette. The major advantage of the sugar-tong cast and posterior splint is avoidance of the circumferential effects of a nonelastic cylinder cast. The sugar-tong posterior splints accommodate for swelling in the fractured extremity that occurs postinjury.

The *short arm cast* is often used for the treatment of stable wrist or metacarpal fractures. An aluminum finger splint can be fabricated into the short arm cast for concurrent treatment of phalangeal injuries. The short arm cast is a circular cast extending from the distal palmar area to the proximal forearm. This cast provides wrist immobilization and permits unrestricted elbow motion.

The *long arm cast* is commonly used for stable forearm or elbow fractures and unstable wrist fractures. It is similar to the short arm cast but extends to the proximal humerus, restricting motion in the wrist and elbow. Nursing measures should be directed toward supporting the extremity and reducing the effects of edema by maintaining extremity elevation with a sling. However, when a hanging arm cast is used for a proximal humerus fracture, elevation or a supportive sling are contraindicated because hanging provides traction and promotes fracture healing.

When a sling is used, the nurse must ensure that the axillary area is well padded to prevent skin maceration associated with direct skin-to-skin contact. Placement of the sling should not put undue pressure on the posterior neck. Movement of the fingers (unless contraindicated) should be encouraged to enhance the pumping action of vascular and soft tissue structures to decrease edema. The nurse should also encourage the patient to actively move nonimmobilized joints of the upper extremity to prevent stiffness and contractures.

The *body jacket cast* is often used for immobilization and support for stable spine injuries of the thoracic or lumbar spine. This cast is applied around the chest and abdomen and extends from above the nipple line to the pubis. After application of the cast, the nurse must assess the patient for the development of *cast syndrome*. This condition occurs if the body cast is applied too tightly and the cast compresses the superior mesenteric artery against the duodenum. The patient generally complains of abdominal pain, abdominal pressure, nausea, and vomiting. The abdomen should be assessed for decreased bowel sounds (a window may be left over the umbilicus). Treatment includes gastric decompression with a nasogastric (NG) tube and suction. The cast may need to be removed or split. Nursing assessment also includes observation of respiratory status, bowel and bladder function, and areas of pressure over the bony prominences, especially the iliac crest. During the time required for the cast to dry, the nurse should reposition the patient every 2 to 3 hours to promote even cast drying and to relieve pressure and discomfort.

The *hip spica cast* is used for treatment of femoral fractures. The purpose of the hip spica cast is to immobilize the affected extremity and the trunk securely. It includes two casts joined together: (1) the body jacket cast and (2) the long leg cast. The location of the femoral fracture will determine whether the thigh of the unaffected extremity will have to be immobilized to restrict rotation of the pelvis and possible hip motion on the side of the femur fracture. The hip spica cast extends from above the nipple line to the base of the foot (single spica) and may include the opposite extremity up to an area above the knee (spica and a half) or both extremities (double spica).

The nurse should assess the patient with a hip spica cast for the same problems that are associated with the body jacket cast. During the initial drying stage the patient should not be placed in the prone position because the cast may break. The patient should be slightly turned from side to side and supported with pillows. When the patient is repositioned, the support bar joining the thighs must never be used to assist in moving because the bar can break and cause cast disruption. After the cast has dried, the nurse (with assistance) can turn the patient to the prone position and provide pillow support under the chest and immobilized extremity. Skin care around the cast edges (petaling) and the areas not encompassed by plaster is important to prevent any pressure sores. The nurse should instruct the patient in the positioning activities required to get on and off the bedpan. A fracture bedpan may be used to provide comfort and ease the movement of getting on and off the bedpan. After the hip spica cast has dried sufficiently, the patient may be instructed in ambulation techniques by the physical therapist.

Injuries to the lower extremity. Injuries to the lower extremity are often immobilized by a long leg cast, short leg cast, cylinder cast, or a Jones dressing. The usual indications for applying a long leg cast are an unstable ankle fracture, soft tissue injuries, a fractured tibia, and knee injuries. The cast usually extends from the base of the toes to the groin and gluteal crease. The short leg cast can be used for a variety of conditions but is primarily used for stable ankle and foot injuries. A cylinder cast is used for knee injuries or fractures. The cast extends from the groin to the malleoli of the ankle. A Jones dressing is composed of bulky padding materials (absorption dressing and sheet wadding), splints, and an elastic wrap or bias-cut stockinette. The Jones dressing, like the sugar-tong splint, is used for knee fractures or surgery when there is a risk of significant edema. After the application of a lower-extremity cast or dressing, the extremity should be elevated with pillows above the heart level for the first 24 hours. After the initial phase, the casted extremity should not be placed in a dependent position because of the possibility of excessive edema.

Initially, no weight can be put on the injured extremity. Later, a walking heel or cast shoe may be added to the cast if the patient is allowed to bear weight and walk on the affected leg. Following cast application, the nurse should observe for signs of pressure, especially in the regions of the heel, anterior tibial border, fibular head, and malleoli.

External fixation. An external fixator is a metallic device composed of metal pins that are inserted into the bone and attached to external rods to stabilize the fracture while it heals. It can be used to apply traction or to compress fracture fragments and to immobilize reduced fragments when the use of a cast or other traction is not appropriate. The external device holds fracture fragments in place much like surgically implanted internal devices do. The external fixator is attached directly to the bones by percutaneous transfixing pins or wires (Fig. 61-10). External fixation is indicated in simple fractures (either open or closed), complex fractures with extensive soft tissue damage, correction of bony defects (congenital), pseudoarthrosis, and nonunion or malunion and for limb lengthening.

External fixation has many advantages over other fracture management strategies and is often employed to salvage complex mangled extremity fractures that otherwise might be amputated at the time of injury. Because the use of an external device is a long-term process, assessment for pin loosening and infection is critical. Infection signaled by exudate, redness, tenderness, and pain may require removal of the device. Meticulous pin care must be taught to the patient and the support person. Although each physician has a protocol for pin care cleaning, half-strength hydrogen peroxide with normal saline is often used.

Internal fixation. Internal fixation devices (pins, plates, intramedullary rods and screws) are surgically inserted at the time of realignment. Biologically inert metal devices such as stainless steel, Vitallium, or titanium are used to realign and maintain bony

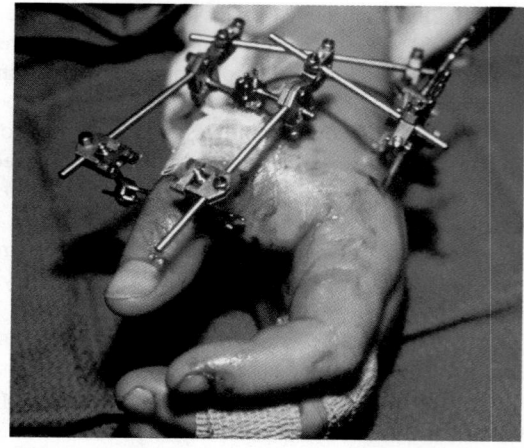

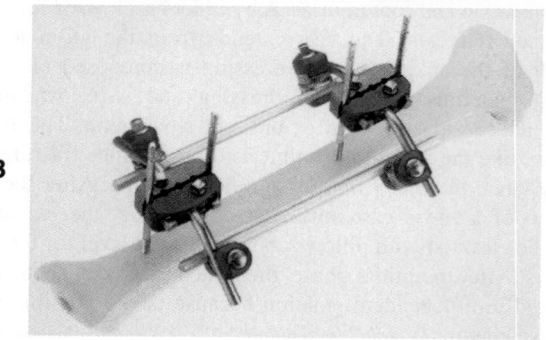

FIG. 61-10 External fixators. **A,** Mini–Hoffman system in use on hand. **B,** Hoffman II on the tibia (standard system).

fragments. Proper alignment is evaluated by x-ray studies at regular intervals.

Traction. Traction is the application of a pulling force to an injured or diseased part of the body or an extremity while countertraction pulls in the opposite direction. The purpose of any traction is to (1) prevent or reduce muscle spasm, (2) immobilize a joint or part of the body, (3) reduce a fracture or dislocation, and (4) treat a joint pathologic condition.[16] Traction is also indicated to (1) provide immobilization to prevent soft tissue damage (2) reduce muscle spasm associated with low back pain or cervical whiplash, (3) expand a joint space during arthroscopic procedures, and (4) expand a joint space before major joint reconstruction. A continuous pulling force can be applied directly to bone with wires and pins (skeletal traction) or can be applied indirectly by weights that are attached to the skin with slings, belts, adhesive straps, or boots (skin traction).

Skin traction is usually applied directly to the extremity by adhesive material that is wrapped circumferentially with a bandage or slings, belts, or a special splint that is attached to a rope with a weight. Skin traction for extremities is applied for a short time and usually consists of not more than 7 to 10 lb (3.2 to 4.5 kg) of traction weight because of skin intolerance to pressure. Pelvic or cervical skin traction may require heavier weights applied intermittently.

Skeletal traction is usually indicated when the traction forces are expected to exceed 10 lb (4.5 kg) or when traction will be used for a long time. Use of too much weight to maintain traction can result in delayed union or nonunion. The major disadvan-

tages of skeletal traction are infection in the area of bone where the skeletal pin has been inserted and the consequences of prolonged immobility necessitated by skeletal traction.

Drug Therapy. Patients with fractures often experience varying degrees of pain associated with muscle spasms. These spasms are caused by involuntary reflexes that result from edema following muscle injury. Muscle relaxants, such as carisoprodol (Soma), cyclobenzaprine (Flexeril), or methocarbamol (Robaxin), may be prescribed for relief of pain associated with muscle spasms.

Common side effects associated with muscle relaxants are drowsiness, lassitude, headache, weakness, fatigue, blurred vision, ataxia, and gastrointestinal upset. Hypersensitivity reactions may include skin rash or pruritus. Ingestion of large doses of muscle relaxants may cause hypotension, tachycardia, or respiratory depression. The possible habituating effects associated with long-term use and the potential for abuse must be carefully considered.

Some physicians do not advocate the use of muscle relaxants for relief of muscle spasms. Their rationale is that the reflex spasm will continue as long as the precipitating pain persists. If the pain is controlled by use of appropriate analgesia, the muscle spasms will cease.

In an open fracture the threat of tetanus occurring can be reduced with tetanus-diphtheria toxoid or immunoglobulin for the patient who has not been previously immunized. A bone-penetrating antibiotic (such as a cephalosporin) is used prophylactically.

Nutritional Therapy. Proper nutrition is an essential component of the reparative process in injured tissue. An adequate energy source is needed to promote muscle strength and tone, build endurance, and enhance ambulation and gait-training skills. The patient's dietary requirements must include ample protein (e.g., 1 g per kilogram of body weight), vitamins (especially D, B, and C), and calcium to ensure optimal soft tissue and bone healing. Low serum protein levels and vitamin C deficiencies interfere with tissue healing. Immobility and callus formation increase calcium needs. Three well-balanced meals a day will usually provide the necessary nutrients. The well-balanced meal should be supplemented by a fluid intake of 2000 to 3000 ml per day to promote optimal bladder and bowel function. Adequate fluid and a high-fiber diet with fruits and vegetables will prevent constipation. If immobilized in a body jacket or hip spica bandage, the patient should be instructed to eat six small meals so as not to overeat and thus avoid abdominal pressure and cramping.

NURSING MANAGEMENT
FRACTURES

■ Nursing Assessment

A brief history of the accident, mechanism of injury, and the position in which the victim was found can be obtained from the patient or witnesses. As soon as possible, the patient should be transported to an emergency department where a thorough assessment and treatment can be initiated (Table 61-8). Subjective and objective data that should be obtained from an individual with a fracture are presented in Table 61-9.

Special emphasis must be focused on the region distal to the site of injury. Clinical findings must be documented before fracture treatment is initiated to avoid doubts about whether a prob-

TABLE 61-8   Emergency Management   Fractured Extremity

ETIOLOGY	ASSESSMENT FINDINGS	INTERVENTIONS

Blunt
Motor vehicle collision
Pedestrian event
Falls
Direct blows
Forced flexion or
  hyperextension
Twisting forces
 	
Penetrating
Gunshot
Blast
 	
Other
Pathologic conditions
Violent muscle
  contractions (seizures)
Crush injury
	▪ Deformity (loss of normal bony contours)
	  or unnatural position of affected limb
	▪ Edema and ecchymosis
	▪ Muscle spasm
	▪ Tenderness and pain
	▪ Loss of function
	▪ Numbness, tingling, loss of distal pulses
	▪ Grating (crepitus)
	▪ Open wound over injured site, exposure
	  of bone
		Initial
		▪ Treat life-threatening injuries first.
		▪ Ensure airway, breathing, and circulation.
		▪ Control external bleeding with direct pressure or sterile
		  pressure dressing.
		▪ Splint joints above and below fracture site.
		▪ Check neurovascular status distal to injury before and
		  after splinting.
		▪ Elevate injured limb if possible.
		▪ Do *not* attempt to straighten fractured or dislocated
		  joints.
		▪ Do *not* manipulate protruding bone ends.
		▪ Apply ice packs to affected area.
		▪ Obtain x-rays of affected limb.
		▪ Administer tetanus prophylaxis if skin integrity is violated.
		▪ Mark location of pulses to facilitate repeat assessment.
		▪ Splint fracture site, including joints above and below frac-
		  ture site.
		
		Ongoing Monitoring
		▪ Monitor vital signs, level of consciousness, oxygen satu-
		  ration, peripheral pulses, and pain.
		▪ Monitor for compartment syndrome characterized by ex-
		  cessive pain, pain with passive stretch, pallor, paresthesia,
		  paralysis, pulselessness.
		▪ Monitor for fat embolism (dyspnea, chest pain).

TABLE 61-9   Nursing Assessment   Fracture

Subjective Data	Objective Data

Important Health Information
Past health history: Traumatic injury; long-term repetitive forces
  (stress fracture); bone or systemic diseases, prolonged immo-
  bility (pathologic fracture), osteopenia, osteoporosis
Medications: Use of corticosteroids (pathologic fractures);
  analgesics
Surgery or other treatments: First aid treatment of fracture
Functional Health Patterns
Health perception–health management: Estrogen replacement
  therapy, calcium supplementation
Activity-exercise: Loss of motion or weakness of affected part;
  muscle spasms
Cognitive-perceptual: Sudden and severe pain in affected area;
  numbness, tingling, loss of sensation distal to injury; chronic
  pain that increases with activity (stress fracture)
	General
	Apprehension, guarding of injured site
	Integumentary
	Skin lacerations, pallor and cool skin or bluish and warm skin
	  distal to injury; ecchymosis, hematoma, edema at site of fracture
	Cardiovascular
	Reduced or absent pulse distal to injury, ↓ skin temperature,
	  delayed capillary refill
	Neurologic
	Paresthesias, ↓ or absent sensation, hypersensation
	Musculoskeletal
	Restricted or lost function of affected part, local bony deformi-
	  ties, abnormal angulation, shortening, rotation, crepitation;
	  muscle weakness
	Possible Findings
	Localization and extent of fractures on x-ray, bone scans, tomo-
	  grams, CT scan, or MRI

CT, Computed tomography; *MRI*, magnetic resonance imaging.

lem discovered later was missed during the original examination or was caused by the treatment.

Neurovascular Assessment. Musculoskeletal injuries have the potential of causing changes in the neurovascular system. The original trauma, application of a cast or constrictive dressing, poor positioning, and the physiologic response to the injury can cause nerve or vascular damage, usually distal to the injury. A thorough neurovascular assessment consists of a peripheral vascular assessment (color, temperature, capillary refill, peripheral pulses, and edema) and a peripheral neurologic assessment (sensation, motor

NURSING CARE PLAN 61-1

Patient with a Fracture

EXPECTED PATIENT OUTCOMES	NURSING INTERVENTIONS and *RATIONALES*

NURSING DIAGNOSIS   **Risk for peripheral neurovascular dysfunction** *related to* nerve compression.

- Has normal neurovascular examination

- Assess for signs and symptoms of peripheral neurovascular dysfunction such as pain in affected extremity that is unrelieved by drugs, paresthesias, pain on passive movement, weakness, cool temperature, pallor, diminished pulses *to ensure early recognition and intervention.*
- Elevate extremity above heart level *to reduce edema by promoting venous return.* (Note: If compartment syndrome is suspected, elevate extremity no higher than heart level.)
- Apply ice compresses as ordered *to reduce edema and provide comfort.* (Note: If compartment syndrome is suspected, remove ice because it may decrease tissue perfusion.)
- Notify physician immediately if patient complains of increasing pain that is unrelieved by drugs *because this may indicate neurovascular impairment, which can result in significant injury if unrelieved.*
- Teach patient the signs of peripheral neurovascular dysfunction *to enable her or his participation in care.*

NURSING DIAGNOSIS   **Acute pain** *related to* edema, movement of bone fragments, and muscle spasms *as manifested by* pain descriptors, guarding, crying.

- Tolerable or no pain
- Satisfaction with plan for pain relief

- Gently and correctly position fractured extremity *to minimize pain and prevent bone displacement.*
- Use a pain scale *to assess pain and evaluate effectiveness of interventions.*
- Give patient analgesics and/or muscle relaxants as indicated *to relieve pain and promote muscle relaxation.*
- Elevate, apply ice (if prescribed), and support affected extremity *to reduce edema and promote comfort.*
- Be alert for pain that is not diminished after analgesic is administered *because this may indicate an impending compartment syndrome.*

NURSING DIAGNOSIS   **Risk for infection** *related to* disruption of skin integrity and presence of environmental pathogens secondary to open fracture, external fixation pins, surgical incision.

- No evidence of wound infection
- Temperature in normal range
- WBC count in normal range

- Assess fracture or pin insertion points for blistering, tenting discoloration, and drainage as indicators of infection.
- Use aseptic technique when providing pin or wound care or when performing dressing change *to prevent cross-contamination and possible introduction of infection.*
- Obtain culture of wound if infection is suspected *to identify infective organism.*
- Administer antibiotics as ordered *to provide prophylaxis or treatment of diagnosed infection.*
- Monitor temperature q2hr *because fever may indicate infection.*
- Monitor WBC count *because elevation may indicate infection.*

NURSING DIAGNOSIS   **Risk for impaired skin integrity** *related to* immobility and presence of cast.

- No evidence of skin breakdown

- Examine potential pressure areas q4hr *to assess condition of skin.*
- Petal cast edges *to prevent skin abrasion or cast crumbs from falling beneath the cast.*
- Assess exposed skin areas of traction sites for signs of infection or irritation *because improper positioning of traction devices can cause localized pressure necrosis.*
- Instruct patient not to insert items (e.g., hangers, forks) into cast to scratch *because these may cause tissue injury.*
- Instruct patient to report areas of warmth, pain, burning, or moisture beneath the cast; foul odor from cast ends; or areas of new or increasing drainage on cast surfaces.

NURSING DIAGNOSIS   **Impaired physical mobility** *related to* ineffective use of crutches *as manifested by* inability to move about independently.

- Crutches correctly used to move about as needed

- Teach gait-training principles to patient (non–weight-bearing gait status unless otherwise ordered by physician); sit with feet over edge of bed, stand with no weight on affected extremity, measure and adjust crutches *to promote mobility according to patient's abilities.*
- Ensure gait is compatible with weight-bearing status *to prevent malalignment.*
- Work with physical therapist regarding exercise and gait-training *to reinforce plan and to provide unified approach to patient.*

NURSING CARE PLAN 61-1

Patient with a Fracture—cont'd

EXPECTED PATIENT OUTCOMES	NURSING INTERVENTIONS and *RATIONALES*
NURSING DIAGNOSIS	**Ineffective therapeutic regimen management** *related to* lack of knowledge regarding muscle atrophy, exercise program, and cast care *as manifested by* questioning of long-term effect of casting and cast care, activity restrictions.
▪ Minimal loss of muscle bulk of affected extremity ▪ Verbalization of confidence in ability to follow the prescribed discharge plan	▪ Instruct patient on home care measures related to exercise, cast care, and prevention of complications *so that patient can carry out prescribed discharge plan.* ▪ Explain factors that contribute to atrophy; emphasize relationship of inactivity to muscle atrophy *so that patient will exercise involved extremity to maximum allowed and will not be alarmed at appearance of extremity when cast is removed.* ▪ Provide written instructions of prescribed exercise plan.

function, and pain).[17] Throughout the neurovascular assessment, both extremities are compared to obtain an accurate assessment.

An extremity's color (pink, pale, cyanotic) and temperature (hot, warm, cool, cold) in the area of the affected extremity are assessed. Cyanosis or a cool/cold extremity below the injury could indicate arterial insufficiency. A warm, bluish extremity could indicate poor venous return. Capillary refill (blanching of the nailbed) is next assessed. The standard for a compressed nailbed to return to its original color is within 3 seconds. Accurate documentation and ongoing assessment of capillary refill are the cornerstones of nursing care for the individual with a musculoskeletal injury.

Pulses on both the unaffected and injured extremity are compared to identify differences in rate or quality. Pulses are described as strong, diminished, audible by Doppler, or absent. A diminished or absent pulse distal to the injury can indicate vascular insufficiency. However, some adults do not have specific pulses, including an absent dorsalis pedis (17% of all ethnic groups) and an absent posterior tibial (9% of African Americans).[18] Peripheral edema is also assessed, and pitting edema may be present with severe injury.

Sensation and motor innervation in the upper extremity are assessed by evaluating the ulnar, median, and radial nerves. Neurovascular status can be assessed by abduction and adduction of the fingers, opposition of the fingers, and supination and pronation of the hand. In the lower extremity, dorsiflexion and plantar flexion assess motor function of the peroneal and tibial nerves. Sensory innervation is evaluated for the peroneal nerve on the dorsal part of the foot between the web space of the great and second toes. Tibial nerve assessment is performed by stroking the volar part (sole) of the foot. Ipsilateral evaluation is critical. Paresthesia (abnormal sensation [e.g., numbness, tingling]), decreased sensation, hypersensation, partial or full loss of sensation [paresis/paralysis] may be reported by the patient. Reduced motion or strength in an injured extremity alerts the nurse to potential limb-threatening complications or disability.

Pain is the final element of the neurovascular assessment. The nurse must carefully assess the location, quality, and intensity of the pain. Current nursing practice is to evaluate the patient's level of pain on a scale of 1 to 10.[17] Pain unrelieved by drugs and out of proportion to the injury is an indication of compartment syndrome or complex regional pain syndrome.[19]

Patients should be instructed to report any changes in their neurovascular status. Patients must verbalize and demonstrate a thorough understanding of all elements before discharge from the emergency department or outpatient setting.

▪ Nursing Diagnoses

Nursing diagnoses for the patient with a fracture may include, but are not limited to, those presented in NCP 61-1.

▪ Planning

The overall goals are that the patient with a fracture will (1) have physiologic healing with no associated complications, (2) obtain satisfactory pain relief, and (3) achieve maximal rehabilitation potential.

▪ Nursing Implementation

Health Promotion. The public should be taught to take appropriate safety precautions to prevent injuries while at home, at work, when driving, or when participating in sports. Nurses should be vocal advocates for personal actions known to reduce injuries such as regular use of seat belts, driving within posted speed limits, stretching before exercise, use of protective athletic equipment (helmets and knee, wrist, and elbow pads), and not combining drinking and driving.

Older adults should be encouraged to participate in moderate exercise to aid in the maintenance of muscle strength and balance. To reduce falls, their living environment should be examined to rule out the use of scatter rugs, to ensure adequate footwear and lighting, and to clear paths to bathrooms for nighttime use. The nurse should also stress the importance of adequate calcium and vitamin D intake.

Acute Intervention. Patients with fractures may be treated in an emergency department or a physician's office and released to home care, or they may require hospitalization for varying

EVIDENCE-BASED PRACTICE

Falls and Osteoporotic Fractures Among Older Adults

Clinical Problem

Is there a relationship between physical activity and the risk of falls and osteoporotic fractures among older adults?

Best Clinical Practice

- Strong evidence shows that a physically active lifestyle reduces the risk of hip fracture.
- Exercise programs can reduce the risk of falls.

Implications for Nursing Practice

- Older adults should be encouraged to participate in exercise programs.
- Future research is necessary to evaluate the types and quantity of physical activity needed for optimal protection from falls and to identify which populations will most benefit from exercise.
- Older adults should be encouraged to maintain a lifestyle that includes regular activity.

Reference for Evidence

Gregg EW, Pereira MA, Caspersen CJ: Physical activity falls and fractures among older adults: a review of the epidemiologic evidence, *J Am Geriatr Soc* 48:883-893, 2000.

amounts of time. Specific nursing measures depend on the type of treatment used and the setting in which patients are placed.

Preoperative management. If surgical intervention is required to treat the fracture, patients will need preoperative preparation. In addition to the usual preoperative nursing measures (see Chapter 17), the nurse should inform patients of the type of immobilization device that will be used and the expected activity limitations. Patients must be assured that their needs will be met by the nursing staff until they can again meet their own needs. Assurance that pain medication will be available, if needed, is often beneficial.

Proper skin preparation is an important part of preoperative preparation. The protocol for skin preparation varies among agencies and may be the responsibility of the nurse. The aim of skin preparation is to clean the skin and remove debris and hair to reduce the possibility of infection. Careful attention to this preoperative treatment can influence the postoperative course.

Postoperative management. In general, postoperative nursing care and management are directed toward monitoring vital signs and applying the general principles of postoperative nursing care (see Chapter 19). Frequent neurovascular assessments of the affected extremity are necessary to detect changes. Any limitations of movement or activity related to turning, positioning, and extremity support should be monitored closely. Pain and discomfort can be minimized through proper alignment and positioning. Dressings or casts should be carefully observed for any overt signs of bleeding or drainage. A significant increase in size of the drainage area should be reported. If a wound drainage system is in place, the patency of the system and the volume of drainage should be regularly assessed. Whenever the contents of a drainage system are measured or emptied, the nurse should use sterile technique to avoid contamination. Additional nursing responsibilities depend on the type of immobilization used. A blood salvage and reinfusion system that allows for recovery and

reinfusion of the patient's own blood may be used. The blood is retrieved from a joint space or cavity, and the patient receives this blood in the form of an autotransfusion. (Autotransfusion is discussed in Chapter 30.)

Other measures. Patients with musculoskeletal injury often have reduced mobility as a result of the fracture. The nurse must plan care to prevent the many complications associated with limited mobility. Constipation can be prevented by activity and maintenance of a high fluid intake (more than 2500 ml per day) and a diet high in bulk and roughage (fresh fruit and vegetables). If these measures are not effective in maintaining the patient's normal bowel pattern, stool softeners, laxatives, or suppositories may be necessary. Maintaining a regular time for elimination aids in promoting regularity.

Renal calculi can develop as a result of bone demineralization. The resulting hypercalcemia causes a rise in urine pH and stone formation resulting from the precipitation of calcium. Unless contraindicated, a fluid intake of 2500 ml per day is recommended. Cranberry juice or ascorbic acid (500 mg per day) may be recommended to acidify the urine and prevent calcium precipitation. (Renal calculi are discussed in Chapter 44.)

Rapid deconditioning of the cardiopulmonary system can occur as a result of prolonged bed rest, resulting in orthostatic hypotension and decreased lung capacity. Unless contraindicated, these effects can be diminished by permitting the patient to sit on the side of the bed, allowing the patient's lower limbs to dangle over the bedside and the patient to perform standing transfers. When the patient is allowed to increase activity, careful evaluation should be made to assess for orthostatic hypotension. Patients must also be assessed for the risk of deep vein thrombosis (DVT) and pulmonary emboli.

Traction. The nurse is responsible for patient comfort and safety while traction is used and for ensuring proper functioning of the traction equipment. The equipment should be regularly examined for frayed ropes, loose knots, ropes out of the groove of the pulley, pulley clamps not fastened firmly to the bed frame, and weights not hanging freely.

When slings are used with traction, the nurse should inspect the skin area that is exposed in and near the sling regularly. Pressure over a bony prominence or a wrinkled area may cause pressure necrosis and can impair blood flow, causing injury to the peripheral neurovascular structures. Skeletal traction pin sites must be observed for signs of infection. Pin site care varies but usually includes regular removal of exudate with half-strength hydrogen peroxide, rinsing pin sites with sterile saline, and drying of the area with sterile gauze.[20]

External rotation of the hip can occur when skin traction is used on the lower extremity. The nurse can correct this position by placing a pillow, sandbag, or rolled-up draw sheet along the greater trochanteric region of the femur. When traction is used, the nurse should ensure that the patient's body is always correctly aligned. Generally, the patient should be in the center of the bed in a supine position. Incorrect alignment can result in increased pain, nonunion, or malunion.

To offset some of the problems associated with prolonged immobility, the nurse should discuss specific patient activity with the health care provider. If exercise is permitted, the nurse should encourage participation by the patient in a simple exercise regimen within activity restrictions. Activities that the patient should participate in include frequent position changes, ROM exercises of unaffected joints, deep breathing exercises, isometric exercises, and use of the trapeze bar (if permitted) to raise oneself off the bed for linen changes and use of the bedpan. These activities should be performed several times each day.

Active exercises that move uninvolved joints through the ROM are the preferred activity, if allowed. Frequent exercise of the trunk and extremities is an excellent stimulus to deep breathing. Active, resistive exercise (isotonic) of uninvolved extremities helps reduce deconditioning from prolonged immobility.

Ambulatory and Home Care

Cast care. Because many fractures are casted in an outpatient setting, the patient often requires only a short hospitalization or none at all. Regardless of the type of material of which it is made, a cast can interfere with circulation and nerve function from being applied too tightly or because of excessive edema after application. Thus frequent neurovascular assessments of the immobilized extremity are critical. The patient must be taught about signs of cast complications so that they can be reported promptly. Elevation of the extremity above the level of the heart to promote venous return and applications of ice to control or prevent edema are measures frequently used during the initial phase. The nurse should instruct the patient to exercise joints above and below the cast. Pulling out cast padding and scratching or placing foreign objects inside the cast is forbidden because it predisposes the patient to skin breakdown and infection.

Patient teaching is an important nursing responsibility to prevent complications. In addition to specific instructions for cast care and recognition of complications, the nurse should encourage the patient to contact the clinic or care provider should questions arise. Table 61-10 summarizes patient and family instructions for cast care. The nurse should validate the patient's and family's understanding of these instructions before discharge from the outpatient setting, emergency department, or hospital. A follow-up phone contact is appropriate, and home care nursing visits are warranted, especially with body or spica casts.

Cast removal is done in the outpatient setting. Patients often fear being cut by the oscillating blade of the cast saw, and the nurse should reassure the patient. More importantly, the nurse should educate the patient as to the possible alteration in the appearance of the skin, which has been beneath the cast. Anxiety will also be present related to weight bearing and continued follow-up care.

Psychosocial problems. Short-term rehabilitative goals are directed toward the transition from dependence to independence in performing simple activities of daily living and preservation or increasing strength and endurance. Long-term rehabilitative goals are aimed at preventing problems associated with musculoskeletal injury (Table 61-11). An important part of nursing care during the rehabilitative phase is assisting the patient to adjust to any problems caused by the injury (e.g., separation from family, financial impact of medical care, loss of income from inability to work, potential for lifetime disability). The nurse must exhibit gentleness, support, and encouragement and should actively listen to the patient's and family's fears.

Ambulation. The nurse must know the overall goals of physical therapy in relation to the patient's abilities, needs, and tolerance. Mobility training and instruction in the use of assistive aids constitute major areas of responsibility of the physical therapist. The patient with lower extremity dysfunction is usually started in mobility training when able to sit in bed and dan-

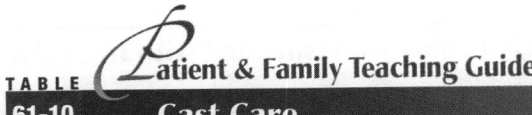

TABLE 61-10	**Patient & Family Teaching Guide**
	Cast Care

Do Not
1. Get plaster cast wet
2. Remove any padding
3. Insert any foreign object inside cast
4. Bear weight on new cast for 48 hr (not all casts are made for weight bearing; check with health care provider when unsure)
5. Cover cast with plastic for prolonged periods

Do
1. Apply ice directly over fracture site for first 24 hr (avoid getting cast wet by keeping ice in plastic bag and protecting cast with cloth)
2. Check with health care provider before getting fiberglass cast wet
3. Dry cast thoroughly after exposure to water
   - Blot dry with towel
   - Use hair dryer on low setting until cast is thoroughly dry
4. Elevate extremity above level of heart for first 48 hr
5. Move joints above and below cast regularly
6. Report signs of possible problems to health care provider
   - Increasing pain
   - Swelling associated with pain and discoloration of toes or fingers
   - Pain during movement
   - Burning or tingling under cast
   - Sores or foul odor under the cast
7. Keep appointment to have fracture and cast checked

EVIDENCE-BASED PRACTICE
Hip Fracture Protectors

Clinical Problem
Do hip protectors reduce the risk of sustaining a fracture in a fall involving the hip in older adults?

Best Clinical Practice
- Hip protectors appear to reduce the risk of hip fracture within a selected population at high risk of sustaining a hip fracture.
- Generalization of the results is unknown beyond high-risk populations.
- User acceptability of the protectors remains a problem because of discomfort and practicality.

Implications for Nursing Practice
- Falls can be prevented in older persons.
- Older adults and their families need to be informed that hip protectors are available.
- The most effective interventions to prevent hip fractures are multifaceted (see Table 61-1) and targeted to individuals in high-risk categories.

References for Evidence
EBM Reviews: Falls can be prevented in older persons, but interventions should be multifaceted and targeted, *ACP Journal Club* 134:100, May/June 2001.
Parker MJ, Gillespie LD, Gillespie WJ: Hip protectors for preventing hip fractures in the elderly, Cochrane Musculoskeletal Injuries Group, *Cochrane Database Syst Rev,* Issue 3, 2002.

TABLE 61-11	Problems Associated with Injury of the Musculoskeletal System	
PROBLEM	**DESCRIPTION**	**NURSING CONSIDERATIONS**
Muscle atrophy	Decreased muscle mass normally occurs as a result of disuse following prolonged immobilization.	An isometric muscle-strengthening exercise regimen within the confines of the immobilization device assists in reducing the amount of atrophy. Muscle atrophy interferes with and prolongs the rehabilitation process.
Contracture	Abnormal condition of joint characterized by flexion and fixation. Caused by atrophy and shortening of muscle fibers or by loss of normal elasticity of skin over a joint.	Can be prevented by frequent position change, correct body alignment, and active-passive range-of-motion exercises several times a day. Intervention requires gradual and progressive stretching of the muscles or ligaments in the region of the joint.
Footdrop	Plantar-flexed position of the foot (footdrop) occurs when the Achilles tendon in the ankle shortens because it has been allowed to assume an unsupported position.	Nursing management of the patient with long-term injuries must include preventive measures by supporting the foot in a neutral position. Once footdrop has developed, ambulation and gait training may be significantly hindered.
Pain	Frequently associated with fractures, edema, and muscle spasm; pain varies in intensity from mild to severe and is usually described as aching, dull, burning, throbbing, sharp, or deep.	Causes of pain include incorrect positioning and alignment of the extremity, incorrect support of the extremity, sudden movement of the extremity, and immobilization device that is applied too tightly or in an incorrect position, constrictive dressings, and motion occurring at the fracture site. Causes of pain should be determined so that corrective nursing action can be taken.
Muscle spasms	Caused by involuntary muscle contraction after fracture and may last as long as several weeks. Pain associated with muscle spasms is often intense and can last from several seconds to several minutes.	Nursing measures to reduce the intensity of the muscle spasms are similar to the corrective actions for pain control. Muscle spasms should not be massaged. Thermotherapy, especially heat, may reduce muscle spasm.

gle the feet over the side. This activity should be done two or three times for 10 to 15 minutes, with the nurse assisting as necessary. Collaboration of the nurse and physical therapist to coordinate pain management and thus increase patient participation at therapy sessions is critical. As endurance increases, the patient is instructed in the techniques of transferring from bed to chair. Progressive ambulation is usually started with parallel bars and progresses to ambulatory assistive devices. When the patient begins to ambulate, the nurse must know the weight bearing allowed for the affected extremity and the correct technique if the patient is using an assistive device. There are different degrees of weight-bearing ambulation: (1) non–weight-bearing (no weight borne) ambulation, (2) touch-down/toe-touch weight-bearing ambulation (contact with floor but no weight borne), (3) partial–weight-bearing ambulation (25% to 50% of patient's weight borne), (4) weight-bearing as tolerated (dictated by patient's pain and tolerance), and (5) full–weight-bearing ambulation (no limitations).[15]

Assistive devices. Devices for ambulation range from a cane, which can relieve up to 40% of the weight normally borne by a lower limb, to a walker or crutches, which may allow for complete non–weight-bearing ambulation. The decision about which device is appropriate for a patient involves weighing the need for maximum stability and safety versus maneuverability, which is required in small spaces such as bathrooms and buses. The decision is made more easily by discussing with patients the requirements of their lifestyles and determining the device with which each patient feels most secure and independent.

The technique for using assistive devices varies. The involved limb is usually advanced at the same time or immediately after the advance of the device. The uninvolved limb is advanced last.

In almost all cases, canes are held in the hand opposite the involved extremity.

The common gait patterns with assistive devices are the two-point gait, the four-point gait, the swing-to gait, and the swing-through gait:

- *Two-point gait.* Crutch on one side advances simultaneously with the opposite foot; this gait is also used with cane ambulation.
- *Four-point gait.* A slower version of the two-point gait, each "point" is advanced separately.
- *Swing-to gait.* Both crutches are advanced together, followed by the lifting of both lower limbs to the same place; this gait is also used with walkers.
- *Swing-through gait.* This gait is similar to the swing-to gait, but the patient swings body past the crutches. An alternate four-point sweep-through gait for patients with concurrent visual and neuromuscular disability provides exploration of upcoming terrain by the crutches before they are placed in the traditional position.[21]

A transfer belt should be placed around the patient's waist to provide stability during the learning stages. The nurse should discourage the patient from reaching for furniture or relying on another person for support. When there is inadequate upper limb strength or poorly fitted crutches, the patient bears weight at the axilla rather than at the hands, endangering the neurovascular bundle that passes across the axilla. If verbal coaching does not correct the problem, the patient should be instructed in another form of ambulation until strength is adequate (e.g., platform crutches, walker).

Patients who must ambulate without weight bearing require sufficient upper limb strength to lift their own weight at each step. Because the muscles of the shoulder girdle are not accustomed to this work, they require vigorous and diligent training in preparation for this task. Push-ups, pull-ups using the overhead trapeze bar, and lifting weights develop the triceps and biceps. Straight-leg raises and quadriceps-setting exercises strengthen the quadriceps.

Counseling and referrals. During the rehabilitative process the patient's family assumes an important role in the provision and follow-through of long-term care plans. The family must be instructed in the techniques of strength and endurance exercises, assistance with mobility training, and promoting activities that enhance the quality of daily living. Sexual counseling should be included in discharge planning. Unless nurses have specific preparation for sexual health counseling, they should remember that wrong answers may be more harmful than no answers. For referral purposes, nurses must know whether weight-bearing status will affect sexual activity and whether any immobilization or support devices are necessary.

Patients also need to be evaluated for posttraumatic stress disorder. This is especially important if significant injury to others or fatalities were associated with the patient's injuries.

■ Evaluation

The expected outcomes for a patient with a fracture are presented in NCP 61-1.

COMPLICATIONS OF FRACTURES

The majority of fractures heal without complications. If death occurs after a fracture, it is usually the result of damage to underlying organs and vascular structures or from complications of the fracture or immobility. Complications of fractures may be either direct or indirect. Direct complications include problems with bone infection, bone union, and avascular necrosis. Indirect complications of fractures are associated with blood vessel and nerve damage resulting in conditions such as compartment syndrome, venous thrombosis, fat embolism, and traumatic or hypovolemic shock.[18] Although most musculoskeletal injuries are not life threatening, open fractures or fractures accompanied by severe blood loss and fractures that damage vital organs (such as the lung, heart, or bladder) are medical emergencies requiring immediate attention.

Infection

Open fractures and soft tissue injuries have a high incidence of infection. An open fracture usually results from the impact of severe external forces. Massive or blunt soft tissue injury often has more serious consequences than the fracture. Devitalized and contaminated tissue is an ideal medium for many common pathogens, including gas-forming (anaerobic) bacilli. Treatment of infections is costly in terms of extended nursing and medical care, time for treatment, and loss of patient income. Osteomyelitis can become chronic (see Chapter 62).

Collaborative Care. Open fractures require aggressive surgical debridement. The wound is initially cleansed by jet pulsed lavage in the operating room. Gross contaminants are irrigated and mechanically removed. Contused, contaminated, and devitalized tissue such as muscle, subcutaneous fat, skin, and fragments of bone are surgically excised (debridement). The extent of the soft tissue damage determines whether the wound will be closed at the time of surgery, whether closed suction drainage

may be necessary, and whether skin grafting will be needed. Depending on the location and extent of the fracture, reduction may be maintained by external fixation or traction. During surgery the open wound may be irrigated with antibiotic solution. Antibiotic impregnated beads may also be placed in the surgical site. During the postoperative phase the patient will have antibiotics administered intravenously for 3 to 7 days. Antibiotics, in conjunction with aggressive surgical management, have greatly reduced the occurrence of infection.

Compartment Syndrome

Compartment syndrome is a condition in which elevated intracompartmental pressure within a confined myofascial compartment compromises the neurovascular function of tissues within that space.[22] Compartment syndrome causes capillary perfusion to be reduced below a level necessary for tissue viability and is classified as acute, chronic/exertional, or crush. Thirty-eight compartments are located in the upper and lower extremities. Two basic etiologies create compartment syndrome, including (1) decreased compartment size resulting from restrictive dressings, splints, casts, excessive traction, or premature closure of fascia and (2) increased compartment content related to bleeding, edema, chemical response to snakebite, or IV infiltration. Depending on the patient's age and body mass index, the expected range of intracompartmental readings is 0 to 8 mm Hg. Readings of 30 to 40 mm Hg indicate compartment syndrome.

Edema is a physiologic response to soft tissue injury in the general region of trauma and may elevate the compartment pressure. This can create sufficient pressure to obstruct circulation and cause venous occlusion, which increases edema. Eventually arterial flow is compromised, resulting in inadequate arterial circulation (ischemia) to the extremity. As ischemia continues, muscle and nerve cells are destroyed over time, and fibrotic tissue replaces the healthy tissue. Contracture, disability, and loss of function can occur. Delay in diagnosis and treatment can result in irreversible muscle and nerve ischemia, resulting in a functionally useless or severely impaired extremity.

Compartment syndrome is associated with fractures, extensive soft tissue damage, crush injury, reperfusion syndrome, severe burns, venomous snakebite, or following knee or leg surgery. Prolonged pressure on a muscle compartment may occur when someone is trapped under a heavy object or a person's limb is trapped beneath the body because of an obtunded state such as drug or alcohol overdose. It has even been known to occur as a result of massive infiltration of IV fluids. Exertional compartment syndrome may occur after intensive exercise. The upper arm and lower leg are the most common sites of compartment syndrome. Fractures of the distal humerus and proximal tibia are the most common fractures associated with compartment syndrome. In the upper extremity this condition is referred to as Volkmann's ischemic contracture (Fig. 61-11) and in the lower extremity as anterior tibial compartment syndrome, although the underlying pathophysiologic mechanism is similar.

Clinical Manifestations. Early recognition and treatment of compartment syndrome are essential to avoid permanent damage to muscles and nerves.[23] Ischemia can occur within 4 to 12 hours after onset. Regular neurovascular assessments should be performed on all patients with fractures, but especially those with injury of the distal humerus or proximal tibia or soft tissue disruption in these areas. Compartment syndrome may occur initially

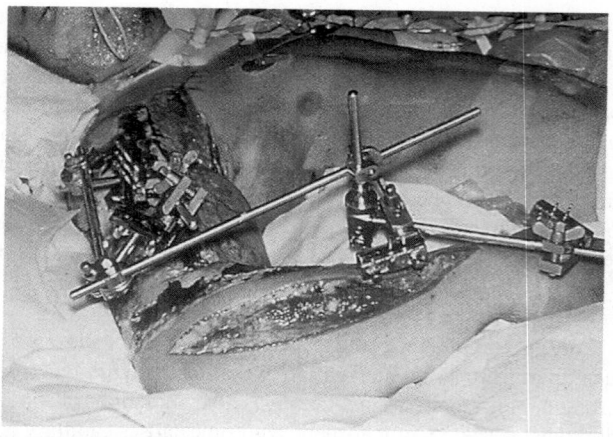

FIG. 61-11 Volkmann's ischemic contracture of the forearm following acute compartment syndrome secondary to a supracondylar fracture of the humerus. Note the incision line of an unsuccessful fasciotomy.

from the physiologic response of the body or may be delayed for several days from the original insult/injury.

The six *P*s are characteristic of an impending compartment syndrome: (1) *paresthesia* (numbness and tingling); (2) *pain* distal to the injury that is not relieved by narcotic analgesics and pain on passive stretch of muscle (positive Homans' sign in lower extremity) traveling through the compartment; (3) *pressure* of the compartment rises; (4) *pallor,* coolness, and loss of normal color of the extremity; (5) *paralysis* or loss of function; and (6) *pulselessness* or diminished/absent peripheral pulses. The patient may present with one or all of the six *P*s. Absence of a peripheral pulse is an ominous late sign that indicates severe disturbance of circulation.[24] Ongoing neurovascular assessment by the nurse must be accurately documented. The health care provider should be notified immediately of the patient's changing condition.

Because of the possibility of muscle damage, urine output must be assessed. Myoglobin, released from damaged muscle cells, can be trapped in renal tubules because of its high molecular weight. Large amounts of myoglobinemia may result in acute tubular necrosis, which precipitates acute renal failure. Common signs of myoglobinuria are (1) dark reddish brown urine and (2) clinical manifestations associated with acute renal failure (see Chapter 45).

Collaborative Care. Prompt, accurate diagnosis of compartment syndrome is critical. Prevention or early recognition is the key. Elevation of the extremity may raise venous pressure and slow arterial perfusion, thus the extremity should not be elevated above heart level. Similarly, the application of cold compresses may result in vasoconstriction and exacerbate compartment syndrome. Elevation and ice should not be used in patients with suspected compartment syndrome. It may also be necessary to remove or loosen the bandage and bivalve the cast. A reduction in traction weight may also decrease external circumferential pressures.

Surgical decompression (e.g., fasciotomy) of the involved compartment may be necessary.[25] The fasciotomy site is left open for several days to ensure adequate soft tissue decompression. Infection resulting from delayed wound closure is a potential problem following a fasciotomy. Severe compartment syndrome may

require amputation to decrease myoglobinemia or to replace a functionally useless extremity with a prosthesis.

Venous Thrombosis

The veins of the lower extremities and pelvis are highly susceptible to thrombus formation after fracture, especially hip fracture. Precipitating factors are venous stasis caused by incorrectly applied casts or traction, local pressure on a vein, or immobility. Venous stasis is aggravated by inactivity of the muscles that normally assist in the pumping action of venous blood returning to the extremities. In addition to wearing compression gradient stockings (antiembolism hose) and using sequential compression devices, the patient should be instructed to move (dorsiflex/plantarflex) the fingers or toes of the affected extremity against resistance and to perform ROM exercises on the unaffected lower extremities.

Because of the high risk of venous thrombosis in the patient with limited mobility, prophylactic anticoagulant drugs such as aspirin, warfarin, or heparin may be ordered.[26] Low-molecular-weight heparin (LMWH) (e.g., enoxaparin [Lovenox]) is frequently used to prevent venous thrombosis. Because LMWH has a predictable dose response, monitoring of prothrombin time is not necessary. A new class of antithrombotic drugs (e.g., fondaparinux [Arixtra]) works by inhibiting factor Xa, a key blood-clotting component. (Assessment and management of venous thrombosis are discussed in Chapter 37.)

Fat Embolism Syndrome

Fat embolism syndrome (FES) is characterized by the presence of fat globules in tissues and organs after a traumatic skeletal injury.[27] FES is a contributory factor in many deaths associated with fractures. The fractures that most often cause FES are those of the long bones, ribs, tibia, and pelvis. FES has also been known to occur following total joint replacement, spinal fusion, liposuction, crush injuries, and bone marrow transplantation. Two theories related to the origin of fat emboli exist: the mechanical theory and the biochemical theory. The mechanical theory suggests that fat is released from the marrow of injured bone. It is driven out by an increase in intramedullary pressure and enters the circulation through draining veins traveling to pulmonary capillaries, where it lodges. Some fat droplets traverse the capillary bed to enter systemic circulation and embolize to other organs such as the brain. The biochemical theory postulates that catecholamines released at the time of trauma mobilize free fatty acids from the adipose tissue, causing loss of chylomicron emulsion stability. The chylomicrons form large fat globules that eventually lodge in the lungs. This is possibly due to some biochemical change initiated by injury. The tissues of the lungs, brain, heart, kidneys, and skin are most often affected.

Clinical Manifestations. Early recognition of FES is crucial in preventing a potentially lethal course. Initial manifestations usually occur 24 to 48 hours after injury. Severe forms have occurred within hours of injury. The fat globules transported to the lungs cause a hemorrhagic interstitial pneumonitis that produces signs and symptoms of acute respiratory distress syndrome (ARDS), such as chest pain, tachypnea, cyanosis, dyspnea, apprehension, tachycardia, and decreased partial pressure of arterial oxygen (PaO$_2$). All of these symptoms are caused by poor oxygen exchange. Because they are frequently the presenting symptoms, changes in the mental status as a result of hypoxemia are important to recognize. Memory loss, restlessness, confusion, elevated temperature, and headache prompt further investigation so that CNS involvement is not mistaken for alcohol withdrawal or acute head injury. The continued change in level of consciousness and petechiae located around the neck, anterior chest wall, axilla, buccal membrane, and conjunctiva of the eye help distinguish fat emboli from other problems. Petechiae result from intravascular thromboses caused by decreased oxygenation.

The clinical course of a fat embolus may be rapid and acute. Frequently the patient expresses a feeling of impending disaster. In a short time, skin color changes from pallor to cyanosis, and the patient may become comatose. No specific laboratory examinations are available to aid in the diagnosis. However, certain diagnostic abnormalities may be present. These include fat cells in the blood, urine, or sputum; a decrease of the PaO_2 to less than 60 mm Hg; ST segment changes on electrocardiogram; a decrease in the platelet count and hematocrit levels; and a prolonged prothrombin time resulting from hemorrhaging into the lungs. A chest x-ray may reveal areas of pulmonary infiltrate or multiple areas of consolidation. This is sometimes referred to as the white-out effect.

Collaborative Care. Treatment for fat embolism is directed at prevention. Careful immobilization of a long bone fracture is probably the most important factor in the prevention of fat embolism. Management of FES is essentially symptom related and supportive, and fluid resuscitation is given to prevent hypovolemic shock, correction of acidosis, and replacement of blood loss. Coughing and deep breathing should be encouraged. The patient should be repositioned as little as possible before fracture immobilization or stabilization because of the danger of dislodging more fat droplets into the general circulation. Use of corticosteroids to prevent or treat fat embolism is controversial. Oxygen is administered to treat hypoxia. Intubation or intermittent positive pressure breathing may be considered if a satisfactory PaO_2 cannot be obtained with supplemental oxygen alone. Some patients may develop pulmonary edema, ARDS, or both, leading to an increased mortality rate. Most survive FES with few sequelae.

Types of Fractures

COLLES' FRACTURE

A *Colles' fracture* is a fracture of the distal radius and is one of the most common fractures in adults. The styloid process of the ulna may be involved as well. The injury usually occurs when the patient attempts to break a fall with an outstretched hand. This type of fracture most often occurs in women over age 50 whose bones are osteoporotic. The clinical manifestations of Colles' fracture are pain in the immediate area of injury, pronounced swelling, and dorsal displacement of the distal fragment (dinner-fork deformity). This may appear as an obvious deformity on the wrist. The major complication associated with a Colles' fracture is vascular insufficiency as a result of edema.

A Colles' fracture is usually managed by closed manipulation of the fracture and immobilization by either a splint or a cast or, if displaced, by external fixation.[28] The elbow must be immobilized to prevent wrist supination and pronation. Nursing management should include measures to prevent or reduce edema and frequent neurovascular assessments. Support and protection of the extremity should be provided, along with encouragement of active movement of the thumb and fingers. This type of movement helps reduce edema and increases venous return. The patient should be instructed to perform active movements of the shoulder to prevent stiffness or contracture.

FRACTURE OF THE HUMERUS

Fractures involving the shaft of the humerus are a common injury among young and middle-aged adults. The prominent clinical manifestations are an obvious displacement of the humerus shaft, shortened extremity, abnormal mobility, and pain (Fig. 61-12). The major complications associated with fracture of the humerus are radial nerve injury and vascular injury to the brachial artery as a result of laceration, transection, or muscle spasm.

The treatment for a fracture of the humerus depends on the location and displacement of the fracture. Nonoperative treatment may include a hanging arm cast, a shoulder immobilizer, or the sling and swathe, which is a type of immobilization that prevents glenohumeral movement. The swathe encircles the trunk and

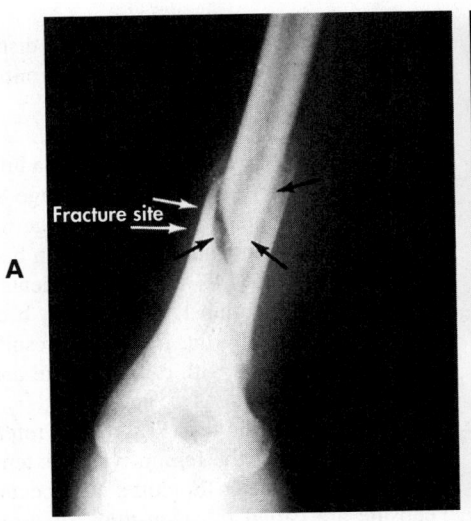
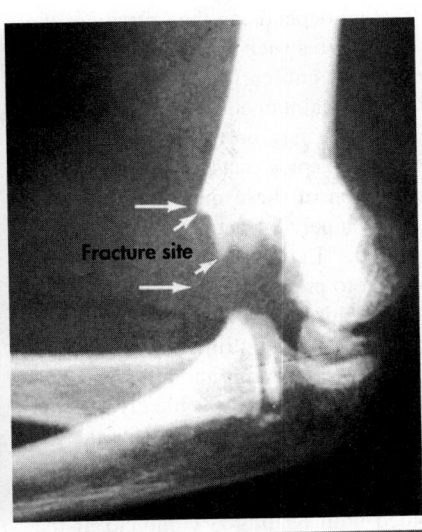

FIG. 61-12 **A,** Supracondylar fracture of the humerus. This type of injury results in the formation of a large hematoma. **B,** Fracture of distal shaft of humerus.

humerus as an additional binder. It is often used for surgical repairs and shoulder dislocation.

When these devices are used, the head of the bed should be elevated to assist gravity in reducing the fracture. The arm should be allowed to hang freely when the patient is sitting and standing. Nursing care should include measures to protect the axilla and prevent skin maceration by placing lightly powdered absorbable dressing pads in the axilla and changing them twice daily or as needed. Skin or skeletal traction may be used for purposes of reduction and immobilization.

During the rehabilitative phase an exercise program geared toward improving strength and motion of the injured extremity is extremely important. This should include assisted motion of the hand and fingers. The shoulder can also be exercised if the fracture is stable. This helps to prevent stiffness secondary to frozen shoulder or arthrofibrosis.

FRACTURE OF THE PELVIS

Pelvic fractures range from benign to life threatening depending on the mechanism of injury and associated vascular insult. High-speed vehicular or motorcycle accidents or skiing accidents can result in open book (anterior-posterior compression) fractures resulting in hemorrhagic life-threatening situations. An *open book fracture* is sustained when the external force pulls the pelvis apart, such as when struck or crushed from the front. A *closed book* (lateral compression) fracture is sustained from lateral force impact, whereas a vertical shear injury is the result of a fall. Although only a small percentage of all fractures are pelvic fractures, this type of injury is associated with the highest mortality rate.[29] Preoccupation with associated injuries at the time of a traumatic event may result in an oversight of pelvic injuries. Pelvic fractures may cause serious intraabdominal injury such as paralytic ileus, hemorrhage, and laceration of the urethra, bladder, or colon. Patients may survive the initial pelvic injury, only to die from sepsis, FES, or DVT complications.

Physical examination demonstrates local swelling, tenderness, deformity, unusual pelvic movement, and ecchymosis on the abdomen. The neurovascular status of the lower extremities and manifestations of associated injuries should be assessed. Pelvic fractures are diagnosed by x-ray study.

Treatment of a pelvic fracture depends on the severity of the injury. Stable, nondisplaced fractures such as those sustained in a fall require limited intervention and early mobilization. Bed rest for stable pelvic fractures is maintained from a few days to 6 weeks. More complex fractures may be treated with pelvic sling traction, skeletal traction, hip spica casts, external fixation, open reduction, or a combination of these methods. Open reduction and internal fixation of a pelvic fracture may be necessary if the fracture is displaced.[30] Extreme care in handling or moving the patient is important to prevent serious injury from a displaced fracture fragment. Because a pelvic fracture can damage other organs, assessment of bowel and urinary tract function and distal neurovascular status are important nursing measures.

The patient should be turned only when specifically ordered by the health care provider. Back care is provided while the patient is raised from the bed either by independent use of the trapeze or with adequate assistance. Weight bearing on the affected side should be avoided until healing is complete. If the pelvic fracture is nondisplaced, the patient is usually allowed to

ambulate using a walker or crutches to distribute the weight bearing between the upper and lower extremities.

FRACTURE OF THE HIP

Hip fractures are common in older adults. More than 200,000 hip fractures occur annually, and by age 80, one in five women will fracture a hip.[31] In adults over age 65, hip fracture occurs more frequently in women than in men because of osteoporosis. It is estimated that 14% to 36% of patients who experience a hip fracture will die within 1 year of injury because of medical complications caused by the fracture or resulting immobility. Only half of older adults with a hip fracture are able to return home and be independent.[32]

A fracture of the hip (Fig. 61-13) refers to a fracture of the proximal third of the femur, which extends up to 5 cm below the lesser trochanter. Fractures that occur within the hip joint capsule are called *intracapsular fractures*. Intracapsular fractures (femoral neck) are further identified by a name derived

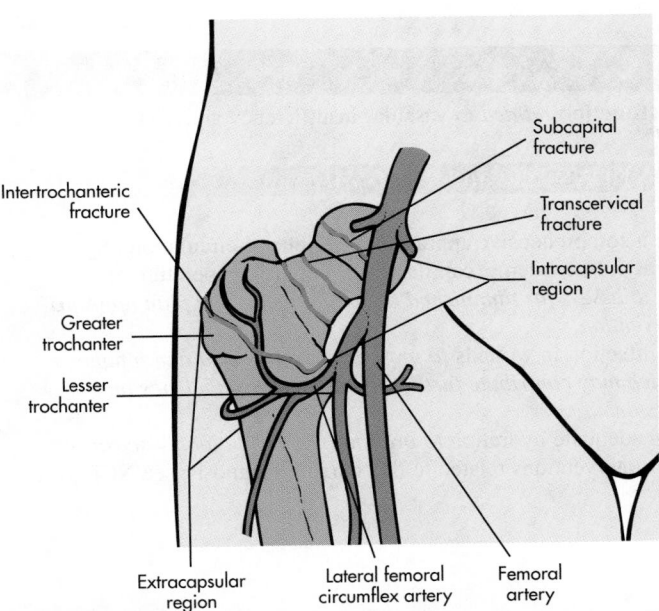

FIG. 61-13 Femur with location of various types of fracture.

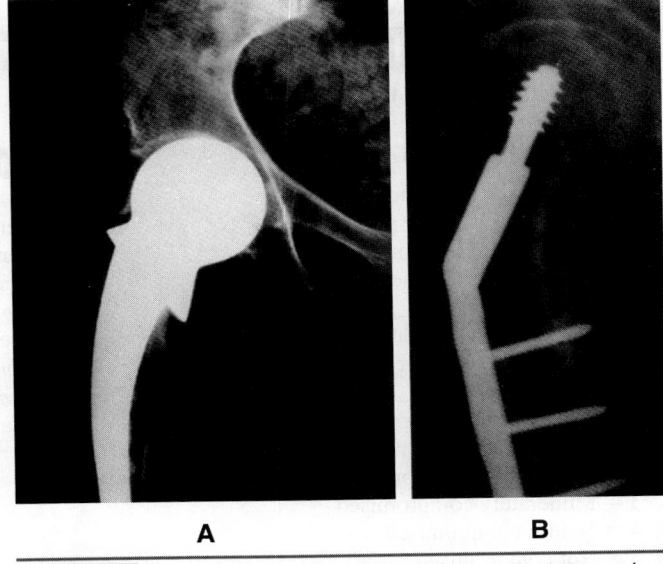

FIG. 61-14 Types of internal fixation for a hip fracture. **A,** Femoral head endoprosthesis. **B,** Type of hip compression screw with side plate.

from specific locations: (1) capital (fracture of the head of the femur), (2) subcapital (fractures just below the head of the femur), and (3) transcervical (fractures of the neck of the femur). These fractures are often associated with osteoporosis and minor trauma. *Extracapsular fractures* occur outside the joint capsule and are termed (1) *intertrochanteric* if they occur in a region between the greater and lesser trochanter or (2) *subtrochanteric* if they occur in the region below the lesser trochanter. Extracapsular fractures are usually caused by severe direct trauma or a fall.

Clinical Manifestations

The clinical manifestations of hip fractures are external rotation, muscle spasm, shortening of the affected extremity, and severe pain and tenderness in the region of the fracture site. Displaced femoral neck fractures cause serious disruption of the blood supply to the femoral head, which can result in avascular necrosis.

Collaborative Care

Surgical repair is the preferred method of managing intracapsular and extracapsular hip fractures. Surgical treatment permits early mobilization of the patient and decreases the risk of major complications. Initially the affected extremity may be temporarily immobilized by Buck's traction until the patient's physical condition is stabilized and surgery can be performed. Buck's traction relieves painful muscle spasms and is used for 24 to 48 hours maximum.

Intracapsular (femoral neck) fractures are usually repaired with the use of an endoprosthesis to replace the femoral head (hemiarthroplasty) (Fig. 61-14, *A*). Extracapsular fractures are repaired using fixed nail plates, sliding nail plates, intramedullary devices, and replacement prostheses (Fig. 61-14, *B*). The principles of patient care for these procedures are similar.

NURSING MANAGEMENT
HIP FRACTURE

■ Nursing Implementation

Preoperative Management. Because older adults are most prone to hip fractures, chronic health problems must often be considered when planning treatment. Diabetes mellitus, hypertension, cardiac decompensation, pulmonary disease, and arthritis are chronic problems that may complicate clinical status. Surgery may be delayed for a brief time until the patient's general health is stabilized.

Before surgery, severe muscle spasms can increase pain. Spasms are managed by appropriate analgesics or muscle relaxants, comfortable positioning unless contraindicated, and properly adjusted traction.

Careful preoperative patient teaching can affect future mobility.[33] Often this is done in the emergency department because quick surgical intervention is the standard of care today. Many patients will not have an overnight preoperative period in which to receive instructions, or the patient may not have the cognitive abilities to retain this important patient education. When possible, the patient can be taught the method and frequency for exercising the unaffected leg and both arms. The patient should also be encouraged to use the overhead trapeze bar and the opposite side rail to assist in changing positions. A physical therapist can begin to teach out-of-bed and chair transfers. The family must also be informed about the patient's weight-bearing status after surgery. Plans for discharge begin as the patient enters the hospital because the length of stay postoperatively will be only a few days.

Postoperative Management. The initial postoperative management of a patient following open reduction with internal fixation (ORIF) of a hip fracture is similar to that for any older surgical patient. The nurse must monitor vital signs, intake, and

NURSING CARE PLAN 61-2

Patient with a Hip Fracture

NURSING DIAGNOSIS **Risk for peripheral neurovascular dysfunction** *related to* vascular insufficiency and nerve compression secondary to edema.

OUTCOMES—NOC	INTERVENTIONS—NIC and *RATIONALES*
Tissue Perfusion: Peripheral (0407)	*Circulatory Precautions (4070)*
▪ Peripheral edema not present _____	▪ Perform a comprehensive appraisal of peripheral circulation (e.g., peripheral pulses, edema, capillary refill, color, temperature of extremity) *to assess for diminished tissue perfusion and plan appropriate intervention.*
▪ Localized extremity pain not present _____	
▪ Distal peripheral pulses strong _____	
▪ Capillary refill brisk _____	
▪ Sensation level normal _____	▪ Prevent infection in wounds *to prevent further edema and inflammation, which may contribute further to vascular insufficiency and nerve compression.*
▪ Extremity temperature warm _____	
	▪ Maintain adequate hydration *to prevent increased blood viscosity.*
Outcome Scale	▪ For other interventions related to this nursing diagnosis, see NCP 61-1.
1 = Extremely compromised	
2 = Substantially compromised	
3 = Moderately compromised	
4 = Mildly compromised	
5 = Not compromised	

NURSING DIAGNOSIS **Acute pain** *related to* tissue trauma, disruption of skin integrity and edema secondary to hip fracture *as manifested by* reluctance to move, guarding of affected area, persistent score of >8 on 10-point pain scale, and facial grimacing.

OUTCOMES—NOC	INTERVENTIONS—NIC and *RATIONALES*
Pain Control (1605)	*Pain Management (1400)*
▪ Recognizes pain onset _____	▪ Align and position extremity and patient correctly *to reduce pressure on nerves and tissue.*
▪ Uses nonanalgesic pain relief measures _____	
▪ Uses analgesics appropriately _____	▪ Encourage patient to monitor own pain and to intervene appropriately *to increase patient's control over pain management.*
▪ Reports pain controlled _____	
	▪ Implement the use of patient-controlled analgesia (PCA) *to give patient control.*
Outcome Scale	▪ Administer medication before an activity *to increase participation in mobility exercises, which will ultimately decrease healing time.*
1 = Never demonstrated	
2 = Rarely demonstrated	
3 = Sometimes demonstrated	▪ Evaluate the effectiveness of the pain control measures used through ongoing assessment of the pain experience *so that pain relief is in accordance with the healing process.*
4 = Often demonstrated	
5 = Consistently demonstrated	

NURSING DIAGNOSIS **Risk for impaired skin integrity** *related to* immobility and shearing forces.

OUTCOMES—NOC	INTERVENTIONS—NIC and *RATIONALES*
Tissue Integrity (1101)	*Pressure Management (3500)*
▪ Skin intactness _____	▪ Elevate injured extremity *to increase venous return and decrease edema.*
▪ Tissue perfusion _____	
▪ Sensation in expected range (IER) _____	▪ Monitor patient's nutritional status *to ensure adequate intake to facilitate bone and wound healing.*
▪ Tissue lesion free _____	
	▪ Monitor for sources of pressure and friction to relieve *pressure and friction in a timely manner.*
Outcome Scale	▪ Monitor skin for areas of redness or breakdown using Braden scale (see Table 12-21) *to assess for signs and symptoms of skin breakdown.*
1 = Extremely compromised	
2 = Substantially compromised	
3 = Moderately compromised	▪ Monitor patient's mobility and activity *to assess for changes in range of motion in affected limb.*
4 = Mildly compromised	
5 = Not compromised	

output; supervise respiratory activities, such as deep breathing and coughing; administer pain medication cautiously; and observe the dressing and incision for signs of bleeding and infection. Specific nursing interventions for the patient with a fracture of the hip are described in NCP 61-2.

In the early postoperative period there is a potential for neurovascular impairment. The nurse assesses the patient's extremity for (1) color, (2) temperature, (3) capillary refill, (4) distal pulses, (5) edema, (6) sensation, (7) motor function, and (8) pain. Edema is alleviated by elevation of the leg whenever the patient is in a chair. The pain resulting from poor alignment of the affected extremity can be reduced by keeping pillows (or an abductor splint) between the knees when the patient is turning to either side. Sandbags and pillows are also used to prevent external

NURSING CARE PLAN 61-2

Patient with a Hip Fracture—cont'd

NURSING DIAGNOSIS   **Impaired physical mobility** *related to* decreased muscle strength, pain, presence of immobilization device *as manifested by* inability to purposefully move, limited joint ROM, inability to bear weight.

OUTCOMES—NOC

Ambulation: Walking (0200)
- Bears weight _____
- Walks at slow pace _____
- Walks with effective gait ____

Mobility Level (0208)
- Body positioning performance ____
- Joint movement ____
- Ambulation: Walking____

Outcome Scale
1 = Dependent, does not participate
2 = Requires assistive person and device
3 = Requires assistive person
4 = Independent with assistive device
5 = Completely independent

INTERVENTIONS—NIC and *RATIONALES*

Exercise Therapy: Joint Mobility (0740)
Exercise Therapy: Ambulation (0221)
- Get patient out of bed and into chair, usually within 24 to 48 hours after surgery *to reduce the complications associated with immobility.*
- Instruct and assist patient with transfer from bed to chair to *prevent accidental falling and improper movements.*
- Collaborate with physical therapist in developing and implementing an exercise program to *maximize patient's progress in rehabilitation.*
- Provide written instructions for exercises for patient to refer to as needed.
- Provide positive reinforcement for performing exercises *to enhance motivation.*
- Encourage family to get involved with exercises *so that they can provide continuity of care.*

---

rotation. If an endoprosthesis was placed, the patient is at risk for hip dislocation. Hip precautions must be demonstrated and explained to the patient.

The physical therapist usually supervises active-assistance exercises for the affected extremity and ambulation when the surgeon permits it. Ambulation usually begins on the first or second postoperative day. The nurse in collaboration with the physical therapist monitors the patient's ambulation status for proper crutch walking or use of the walker. For the patient to be discharged home, the patient must be able to safely demonstrate use of crutches or a walker, the ability to transfer into and from a chair and bed, and the ability to ascend and descend stairs.

Complications associated with femoral neck fracture include nonunion, avascular necrosis, dislocation, and degenerative arthritis. As a result of an intertrochanteric fracture, the affected leg may be shortened. A cane or built-up shoe may be required for safe ambulation.

If the hip fracture has been treated by insertion of a femoral head prosthesis, measures to prevent dislocation must always be used (Table 61-12). The patient and family must be fully aware of positions and activities that predispose the patient to dislocation (greater than 90 degrees of flexion, adduction, or internal rotation). Many daily activities may reproduce these positions, including putting on shoes and socks, crossing the legs or feet while seated, assuming the side-lying position incorrectly, standing up or sitting down while the body is flexed relative to the chair, and sitting on low seats, especially low toilet seats. Until the soft tissue surrounding the hip has healed sufficiently to stabilize the prosthesis, these activities must be avoided, usually for at least 6 weeks. Sudden severe pain, a lump in the buttock, limb shortening, and external rotation indicate prosthesis dislocation. This requires a closed reduction with conscious sedation or open reduction to realign the femoral head in the acetabulum.

In addition to teaching the patient and family how to prevent prosthesis dislocation, the nurse should (1) place a large pillow

between the patient's legs when turning, (2) keep leg abductor splints on the patient except when bathing, (3) avoid extreme hip flexion, and (4) avoid turning the patient on the affected side until approved by the surgeon.

If the hip fracture is treated by pinning, dislocation precautions are not necessary. The patient is out of bed on the first postoperative day. Weight bearing on the involved extremity varies. Weight bearing of especially fragile fractures may be restricted until x-ray examination indicates adequate healing, usually 6 to 12 weeks.

The nurse assists both the patient and the family in adjusting to the restrictions and dependence imposed by the hip fracture. Depression can easily occur, but creative nursing care and awareness of the problem can do much to prevent it. The patient and family may need to be informed about community referral services that can assist in the postdischarge rehabilitation phase. Hospitalization averages 4 days. Patients frequently require care in a subacute unit, at a skilled nursing facility, or in a rehabilitation facility for a few weeks before returning home. Regular follow-up care after discharge including home health nursing should be arranged.

■ Evaluation

The expected outcomes for the patient with fracture of the hip are presented in NCP 61-2.

■ Gerontologic Considerations: Hip Fracture

Factors that contribute to the occurrence of a hip fracture in older adults include a propensity to fall, inability to correct a postural imbalance, orientation of the fall, inadequacy of local tissue shock absorbers (e.g., fat, muscle bulk), and underlying skeletal strength. Several factors have been identified in older persons that increase their risk of falling. These include gait and balance problems, decreased vision and hearing, decreased reflexes, orthostatic hypotension, and medication use. Leading hazards of

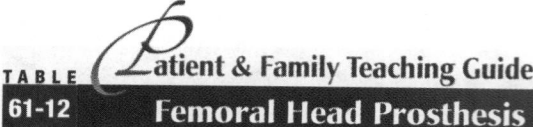

TABLE 61-12

Patient & Family Teaching Guide

Femoral Head Prosthesis

Do Not

- Force hip into greater than 90 degrees of flexion*
- Force hip into adduction
- Force hip into internal rotation
- Cross legs
- Put on own shoes or stockings until 8 wk after surgery without adaptive device (e.g., long-handled shoehorn or stocking-helper)
- Sit on chairs without arms to aid rising to a standing position*

Do

- Use toilet elevator on toilet seat*
- Place chair inside shower or tub and remain seated while washing
- Use pillow between legs for first 8 wk after surgery when lying on "good" side or when supine*
- Keep hip in neutral, straight position when sitting, walking, or lying*
- Notify surgeon if severe pain, deformity, or loss of function occurs*
- Inform dentist of presence of prosthesis before dental work so that prophylactic antibiotics can be given

*These precautions may also apply after a hip pinning.

falls are loose rugs and slippery or uneven surfaces. Many falls are associated with getting in or out of a chair or bed. Falls to the side, the most common type in the frail elderly, are more likely to result in a hip fracture than a forward fall.

Two important factors influencing the amount of force imposed on the hip are the presence of energy-absorbing soft tissue over the greater trochanter and the state of leg muscle contraction at the time of the fall. Because many elderly persons have poor muscle tone, these are important factors in the severity of a fall. Finally, elderly women often have osteoporosis and accompanying low bone density, which increases the risk of hip fracture.[34]

Targeted interventions to reduce hip fractures in the elderly include a variety of strategies. Calcium and vitamin D supplementation, estrogen replacement, and drug therapy have been shown to decrease bone loss or increase bone density and decrease the likelihood of fracture. (Osteoporosis is discussed in Chapter 62.) Nurses must be vigilant in planning interventions for the elderly that are known to reduce the incidence of hip fracture. ■

FEMORAL SHAFT FRACTURE

Femoral shaft fracture is a common injury occurring particularly in young adults. Severe direct force is required to produce this injury because the femur can bend slightly before actual fracture occurs. The force exerted to cause the fracture often causes damage to the adjacent soft tissue structures. These injuries may be more serious than the bone injury. Displacement of the fracture fragments often results in open fracture and increased soft tissue damage. This can result in considerable blood loss (1 to 1.5 L).

The clinical manifestations of a fracture of the femoral shaft are usually obvious. They include marked deformity and angulation, shortening of the extremity, inability to move either the hip

or knee, and pain. The common complications associated with fracture of the femoral shaft include fat embolism, nerve and vascular injury, and problems associated with bone union, open fracture, and soft tissue damage.

Initial management is directed toward stabilization of the patient and immobilization of the fracture. Treatment may consist of skeletal traction via a femoral or tibial pin and balanced suspension traction for 8 to 12 weeks. The nurse must encourage the patient to perform exercises and ROM activities for the uninvolved extremities and joints to discourage deconditioning. The physician determines when active exercise can be instituted on the affected extremity. When there is sufficient clinical evidence of bone union, a hip spica or long leg cast may be applied. Use of prolonged traction is uncommon as the current standard of care.

ORIF has become the preferred method to manage a femoral fracture. It is carried out with an intramedullary rod, compression plate, and screws or side plate with an intercondylar nail. Internal fixation is often the preferred treatment because it reduces hospital stay and the complications associated with prolonged bed rest. Other indications for internal fixation are failure to obtain satisfactory reduction by nonsurgical methods and multiple associated injuries. In some instances the surgically repaired femur may be supported by suspension traction for 3 to 4 days to prevent excessive movement of the extremity and to control rotation; non–weight-bearing gait training is then begun. Fractures associated with extensive soft tissue injury may be treated with external fixation.

Promotion and maintenance of strength in the affected extremity usually include gluteal and quadricep isometric exercises. It is important to ensure performance of ROM and strengthening exercises for all uninvolved extremities in preparation for ambulation. The patient may be immobilized in a hip spica cast and gradually progress to an articulating cast brace or may be allowed to begin non–weight-bearing activities with an ambulatory assistive device. Full weight bearing is usually restricted until there is x-ray evidence of union of the fracture fragments.

FRACTURE OF THE TIBIA

Although the tibia is vulnerable to injury because it lacks anterior muscle covering, strong force is required to produce a fractured tibia. As a result, soft tissue damage, devascularization, and open fracture are frequent. Other complications associated with tibial fractures are compartment syndrome, fat embolism, problems associated with bony union, and possible infection associated with open fracture. Amputation may be required if adequate muscle and tissue coverage is not achieved following muscle and flap grafts.

The recommended management for closed tibial fracture is closed reduction followed by immobilization in a long leg cast. ORIF with intramedullary rods or compression plate or external fixation is indicated for complex fractures and those with extensive soft tissue damage. With either method of reduction, emphasis is placed on maintaining the strength of the quadriceps.

The neurovascular status of the affected extremity must be assessed at least every 2 hours during the first 48 hours. Patients are instructed to perform active ROM exercises with all uninvolved extremities, as well as exercises for the upper extremities, to build the strength required for crutch walking. When the physician has determined that the patient is ready for gait training, the patient is instructed in the principles of crutch walking. The patient may be on non–weight-bearing status for 6 to 12 weeks depending on healing. Patients with external fixation must be taught pin care and dressing changes if extensive tissue has been debrided. Home nursing visits can be initiated to augment outpatient appointments and monitor the patient's progress.

STABLE VERTEBRAL FRACTURES

Stable fractures of the vertebral column are usually caused by motor vehicle accidents, falls, diving, or athletic injuries. A stable fracture is one in which the fracture or the fragment is not likely to move or cause spinal cord damage. This type of injury is frequently confined to the anterior element (vertebral body) of the spinal column in the lumbar region, and involves the cervical and thoracic regions less frequently. The vertebral bodies are usually protected from displacement by the intact spinal ligaments.

Most patients with spinal fractures have stable fractures and experience only brief periods of disability. However, if the ligamentous structures are significantly disrupted, dislocation of the vertebral structures may occur, resulting in instability and injury to the spinal cord (unstable fracture). These injuries generally require surgery. The most serious complication of vertebral fractures is fracture displacement, which can cause damage to the spinal cord (see Chapter 59). Although stable vertebral fractures are not associated with abnormal spinal cord pathologic conditions, all spinal injuries should initially be considered unstable and potentially serious until diagnostic tests are done and the physician determines that the fracture is stable.

The most common injury to the vertebral body is the compression type of fracture caused by excessive vertical loading, such as a severe fall on the buttocks or injury resulting from sudden flexion that forces the spine beyond its normal ROM. The patient usually complains of pain and tenderness in the affected region of the spine. Compression fractures are associated with a "gibbous" deformity (flexion angulation of several vertebrae). This deformity may be noted during the physical examination. In patients with osteoporosis, several vertebral levels may be involved as evidenced by a "dowager's hump" (abnormal backward curvature of thoracic spine). The cervical spine may also be involved. Bowel and bladder dysfunction may be an indication of an interruption of the autonomic nervous system or injury to the spinal cord.

The overall goal in management of stable fractures of a vertebral body is to keep the spine in good alignment until union has been accomplished. Many nursing interventions are aimed at assessing for the possibility of spinal cord trauma. Vital signs and bowel and bladder function should be evaluated regularly, as should the motor and sensory status of the peripheral nerves distal to the injured region. Any deterioration in the patient's neurovascular status should be promptly reported.

Treatment includes support, heat, and traction. The patient is usually placed in a standard hospital bed with firm support from the mattress or a bed board. The aim is to support the spinal column, relax muscles, and release any compression on nerve roots. Heat and traction may be used to relieve muscle spasms resulting from the fracture. Traction may also be used to reduce and immobilize fracture fragments. A trapeze is not usually allowed because its use disrupts spinal alignment. Both an upright position and turning of the torso are prohibited. When turning, the patient should be taught to keep the spine straight by turning shoulders and pelvis together. Nursing assistance is necessary for the patient to learn how to turn in this "logrolling" fashion.[35] Several days after the initial injury, the physician may apply a specially constructed orthotic device (e.g., Milwaukee, Jewett, or Taylor brace), a jacket cast, or a removable corset if there is no evidence of neurologic deficit.

If the fracture is in the cervical spine, a cervical collar may be worn by the patient. Some cervical fractures are immobilized by use of a halo vest (see Fig. 59-12). This consists of a plastic jacket or cast fitted about the chest and attached to a halo that is held in place by skeletal pins inserted into the cranium. These devices immobilize the spine in the fracture area but allow patient mobility. The patient is discharged after (1) regaining ambulation skills, (2) learning care of the cast or orthotic device, and (3) learning how to cope with interferences in safety and security imposed by injury and treatment.

FACIAL FRACTURES

Any bone of the face can be fractured as a result of trauma. Fractures can occur as a result of collision with another person or object, fighting, or blunt trauma. The primary concern after facial injury is to establish and maintain a patent airway and to provide adequate ventilation by removal of foreign material and blood. Suctioning may be necessary. An artificial airway (tracheostomy) may be needed if a patent airway cannot be maintained. Hemorrhage is controlled by pressure packing. Cervical spine injuries are common. All patients with facial injuries should be treated as though they have a cervical injury until proven otherwise by examination and imaging studies (e.g., x-ray). Table 61-13 describes the clinical manifestations of common facial fractures.

Concurrent soft tissue injury often makes assessment of a facial injury difficult. Oral and facial examinations should be performed after the patient has been stabilized and any life-threatening situations have been treated. Careful assessment is made of the ocular muscles and cranial nerve involvement. An x-ray documents the extent of the injury. Computed tomography (CT) imaging helps differentiate between bone and soft tissue and gives a more specific view of the fracture.

Injury to the eye must be suspected when a facial injury occurs, particularly if the injury is near the orbit. If a global rupture is suspected, the examination is stopped and a protective shield is placed over the eye until examined by the ophthalmologist. Signs

TABLE 61-13	Clinical Manifestations of Facial Fractures
FRACTURE	**CLINICAL MANIFESTATION**
Frontal bone	Rapid edema that may mask underlying fractures
Periorbital	Possible frontal sinus involvement, entrapment of ocular muscles
Nasal	Displacement of nasal bones, epistaxis
Zygomatic arch	Depression of zygomatic arch
Maxilla	Segmental motion of maxilla
Mandible	Tooth fractures, bleeding, limited motion of mandible

of global rupture include brown tissue (iris or ciliary body) on the surface of the globe or penetrating through a laceration with an eccentric or teardrop-shaped pupil.[36] Specific treatment of a facial fracture depends on the site and extent of the fracture and the associated soft tissue injury. Immobilization or surgical stabilization may be necessary.

The patient who sustains a facial fracture requires sensitive nursing care because alteration in appearance after the trauma may be drastic. Edema and discoloration subside with time, but concurrent soft tissue injuries may result in permanent scarring. Attention to maintenance of a patent airway and adequate nutrition are ongoing concerns of the nurse throughout the recovery period. Suction should always be available to maintain a patent airway for these patients.

Mandible Fracture

A fracture of the mandible may result from trauma to the face or jaws. Maxillary fractures may also occur, but they are less common than mandibular fractures. The fracture may be simple, with no bone displacement, or it may involve loss of tissue and bone. The fracture may require immediate and sometimes long-term treatment to ensure survival and restore satisfactory appearance and function. Mandibular fracture may also be therapeutically performed to correct an underlying malocclusion problem that cannot be corrected by orthodontic procedures alone. In these conditions, the mandible is resected during surgery and manipulated forward or backward depending on the occlusion problem. For this patient, the procedure is performed on an elective basis.

Surgery consists of immobilization, usually by wiring the jaws (intermaxillary fixation). Internal fixation may be accomplished with screws and plates. In a simple fracture with no loss of teeth, the lower jaw is wired to the upper jaw. First, wires are placed around the teeth; then cross-wires or rubber bands are used to hold the lower jaw tight against the upper jaw (Fig. 61-15). Arch bars may be placed on the maxillary and mandibular arches of the teeth. Vertical wires are placed between the arch bars holding the jaws together. When teeth are missing or if there is bone displacement, other forms of fixation such as metal arch bars in the mouth or insertion of a pin in the bone may be used. The immobilization is usually necessary for only 4 to 6 weeks because the fractures heal rapidly.

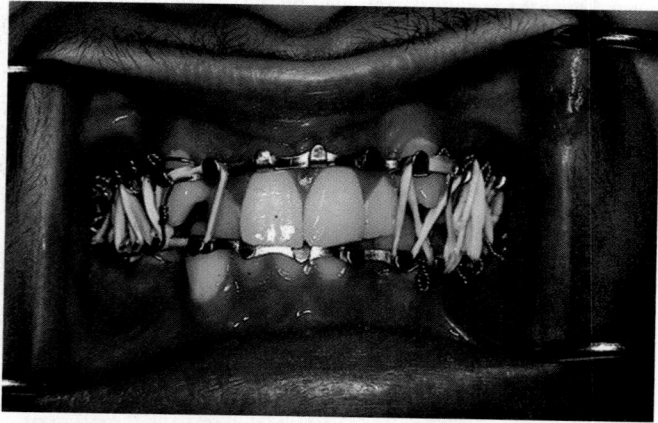

FIG. 61-15 Intermaxillary fixation.

NURSING MANAGEMENT
MANDIBULAR FRACTURE

■ Nursing Implementation

Preoperative Management. The patient should be told preoperatively about the surgical procedure, including what it involves, how the face will look, and alterations the surgery will cause. The patient must be reassured about the ability to breathe normally, speak, and swallow liquids. Usually hospitalization is brief unless there are other injuries or problems.

Postoperative Management. Postoperative care should focus on a patent airway, oral hygiene, communication, and adequate nutrition. Two major potential problems in the immediate postoperative period are airway obstruction and aspiration of vomitus. Because the patient cannot open the jaws, measures to ensure an airway are essential. The nurse must observe for signs of respiratory distress. The patient should be placed on the side with the head slightly elevated immediately after surgery. A wire cutter or scissors (for rubber bands) must be taped to the head of the bed and sent with the patient on all appointments and examinations away from the bedside. These may be used to cut the wires or elastic bands in case of an emergency. The wires should be cut only as a last resort. Once the patient is awake the wires should be cut only in case of cardiac or respiratory arrest.

The physician should explain, by using a picture, the appropriate wire or wires to cut, and this should be included in the care plan. In some cases, cutting the wires may cause the entire facial and upper jaw structure to collapse and worsen the problem. A tracheostomy tray or an endotracheal tray should always be available.

If the patient begins to vomit or choke, the nurse should try to clear the mouth and airway. Suctioning may be necessary and may be done by the nasopharyngeal or oral route, depending on the extent of injury and the type of repair. An NG tube may be used for decompression to remove fluids and gas from the stomach to help prevent aspiration. It also helps prevent vomiting. Antiemetics may also be used. The NG tube can later be used as a feeding tube. The nurse should teach the patient to clear secretions and vomitus.

Oral hygiene is an important part of the nursing care. The mouth should be rinsed frequently, particularly after meals and snacks, to remove food debris. Warm normal saline solution, water, or alkaline mouthwashes may be used. A soft rubber catheter or a Water-Pik is effective for a thorough oral cleansing. The nurse should inspect the mouth several times a day to see that it is clean. A flashlight is necessary, and a tongue depressor is used to retract the cheeks. The lips and corners of the mouth should be kept moist.

Communication may be a problem, particularly in the early postoperative period. An effective way of communication must be established preoperatively (e.g., use of picture board, pad and pencil, small chalkboard). Usually the patient can speak well enough to be understood, especially after the first few postoperative days.

Ingestion of sufficient nutrients poses a challenge because the diet must be liquid. The patient easily tires of sucking through a straw or laboriously using a spoon. The diet must be planned to include adequate calories, protein, and fluids. Liquid protein supplements may be helpful for improving the nutritional status. The nurse works with the dietitian and the patient to ensure adequate nutrition. The low-bulk, high-carbohydrate diet and the intake of air through the straw create a problem with constipation and flatus. Ambulation, prune juice, and bulk-forming laxatives may help relieve these problems.

The patient is usually discharged with the wires in place. The nurse should allow the patient to verbalize feelings about the altered appearance. Discharge teaching should include oral care, techniques of handling secretions, diet, and how and when to use wire cutters.

AMPUTATION

During the past 20 years, major advances have been made in surgical amputation techniques, prosthetic design, and rehabilitation programs. These advances are enabling amputees to return to productive and satisfying social roles. There are an estimated 400,000 amputees in the United States, with an annual increase of 20,000. The middle and older age-groups have the highest incidence of amputation because of the effects of peripheral vascular disease, atherosclerosis, and vascular changes related to diabetes mellitus.

Clinical Indications

The clinical indications for an amputation depend on the underlying disease or trauma. Amputation is required more often in persons engaged in hazardous occupations, with a greater incidence in men. Common indications for amputation include circulatory impairment resulting from a peripheral vascular disorder, traumatic and thermal injuries, malignant tumors, uncontrolled or widespread infection of the extremity (e.g., gas gangrene, osteomyelitis), and congenital disorders. These conditions may manifest as loss of sensation, inadequate circulation, pallor, and local or systemic manifestations of infection. Although pain is often present, it is not usually the primary reason for an amputation. The underlying problem dictates whether the amputation is performed as elective or emergency surgery. Consideration must also be given to the patient's ability to successfully use a prosthetic device.

Diagnostic Studies

The types of diagnostic studies performed depend on the underlying problem that makes the amputation necessary (Table 61-14). An elevated white blood cell (WBC) count may indicate infection. Vascular studies such as arteriography and venography provide information about the circulatory status of the extremity.

Collaborative Care

The potential for revascularization surgery rather than amputation can be assessed on the basis of vascular studies. If amputation is to be considered "elective," the patient's general health is carefully assessed. Chronic illnesses and infection are monitored closely. The patient and family should be helped to understand the need for the amputation and be assured that rehabilitation can result in an active, useful life. If the amputation is done on an emergency basis as a result of trauma, the management is physically and emotionally more complicated.

The goal of amputation surgery is to preserve extremity length and function while removing all infected, pathologic, or ischemic tissue. This improves the possibility of good prosthetic, cosmetic, and functional satisfaction. (Levels of amputation of upper and lower extremities are illustrated in Fig. 61-16.) The type of amputation depends on the reason for the surgery. A

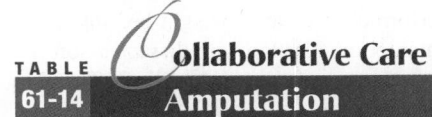

TABLE 61-14	Collaborative Care Amputation

Diagnostic
History and physical examination
   Physical appearance of soft tissues
   Skin temperature
   Sensory function
   Presence of peripheral pulses
Arteriography
Thermography
Plethysmography
Transcutaneous ultrasonic Doppler recordings

Collaborative Therapy
Medical
Appropriate management of underlying disease
Stabilization of trauma victim
Surgical
Appropriate type of amputation, leaving as long a residual
   limb as possible
Residual limb management
   Immediate prosthetic fitting
   Delayed prosthetic fitting
Rehabilitation
Coordination of prosthesis-fitting and gait-training activities
Coordination of muscle-strengthening and physical therapy
   regimens

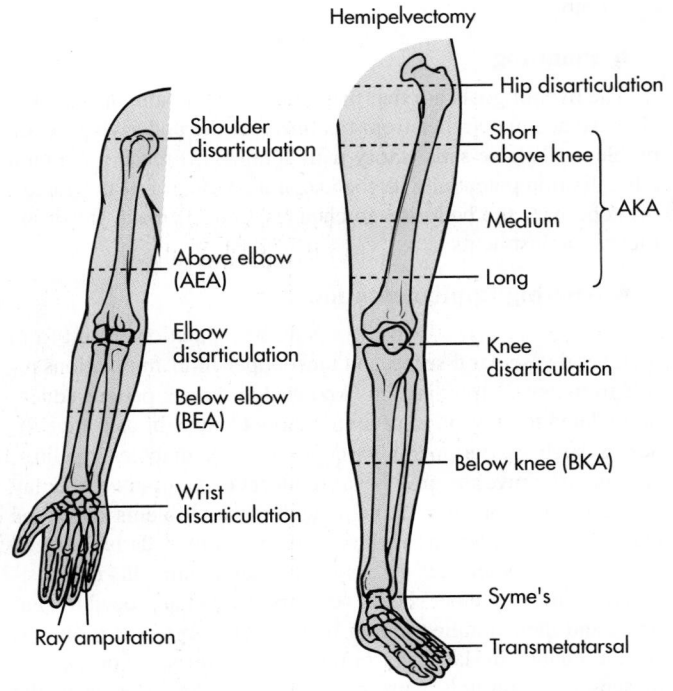

FIG. 61-16 Location and description of amputation sites of the upper and lower extremities. *AKA,* Above the knee amputation.

closed amputation is performed to create a weight-bearing residual limb (or stump). An anterior skin flap with dissected soft tissue padding covers the bony part of the residual limb. The skin flap is sutured posteriorly so that it will not be positioned in a weight-bearing area. Special care is necessary to prevent the accumulation of drainage, which can produce pressure and harbor infection. Disarticulation is an amputation performed through a joint. A Syme's amputation is a form of disarticulation at the ankle. An open amputation leaves a surface on the residual limb that is not covered with skin. This type of surgery is generally indicated for control of actual or potential infection. The wound is usually closed later by a second surgical procedure or closed by skin traction surrounding the residual limb. This type of amputation is often called a "guillotine amputation."

NURSING MANAGEMENT
AMPUTATION

■ Nursing Assessment

Preexisting illnesses must be adequately assessed because most amputations are performed as a result of vascular problems. Assessment of the vascular and neurologic status is an important part of this assessment process (see Chapters 31 and 54).

■ Nursing Diagnoses

Nursing diagnoses for the patient with an amputation may include, but are not limited to, the following:
- Disturbed body image *related to* amputation and impaired mobility
- Impaired skin integrity *related to* immobility and improperly fitted prosthesis
- Chronic pain *related to* phantom limb sensation
- Impaired physical mobility *related to* amputation of lower limb

■ Planning

The overall goals are that the patient with an amputation will (1) have adequate relief from treatment of the underlying health problem, (2) have satisfactory pain control, (3) reach maximum rehabilitation potential with the use of a prosthesis (if indicated), (4) cope with the body image changes, and (5) make satisfying lifestyle adjustments.

■ Nursing Implementation

Health Promotion. Most lower-limb amputations result from peripheral vascular disease, and most upper-limb amputations result from severe trauma. This knowledge directs patient education related to prevention of amputation. Control of causative illnesses such as peripheral vascular disease, diabetes mellitus, chronic osteomyelitis, and pressure ulcers can eliminate or delay the need for amputation. Patients with these problems should be taught to carefully examine their lower extremities daily for signs of potential problems. If the patient cannot assume this responsibility, a family member should be instructed in the procedure. Patients and their families should be instructed to report problems such as change in skin color or temperature, decrease or absence of sensation, tingling, pain, or the presence of a lesion to the health care provider.

Instruction in proper safety precautions in recreation and in the performance of hazardous work is an important nursing responsibility, especially for occupational health nurses. Limb mutilation and subsequent amputation are serious consequences of trauma that can be avoided through such instruction.

Acute Intervention. The nurse must recognize the tremendous psychologic and social implications of an amputation for the patient. The disruption in body image caused by an amputation often causes a patient to go through psychologic stages similar to the grieving process. Allowing the patient to go through a grieving process or period of depression and recognizing it as a normal consequence may do much to aid the patient's acceptance of the amputation. The patient's family must also be helped to work through the process to arrive at a realistic and positive attitude about the future. The reasons for an amputation and the rehabilitation potential depend on age, diagnosis, occupation, personality, resources, and support systems.

Preoperative management. Before surgery, the nurse should reinforce information that the patient and family have received about the reasons for the amputation, the proposed prosthesis, and the mobility training program. In addition to the usual preoperative instructions, the patient undergoing an amputation has special education needs. To meet these needs, the nurse must know the level of amputation, the type of postsurgical dressing to be applied, and the type of prosthesis planned. The patient should receive instruction in the performance of upper-extremity exercises such as push-ups in bed or the wheelchair to promote arm strength. This instruction is essential for later crutch walking and gait training. General postoperative nursing care should be discussed, including positioning, support, and residual limb care. If a compression bandage is to be used after surgery the patient should be instructed about its purpose and how it will be applied. If an immediate prosthesis is planned, the general ambulation program should be discussed.

The patient should be warned that she or he may feel as though the amputated limb is still present after surgery. This phenomenon, termed **phantom limb sensation,** occurs in 80% of amputees and may cause patients grave concern unless they are forewarned. If pain was present in the affected limb preoperatively, the patient may also experience phantom limb pain postoperatively. The patient may have feelings of coldness and heaviness, cramping, shooting, burning, or crushing pain. Often the patient may be extremely anxious about this pain because the patient knows the limb is gone but still feels pain in it. As recovery and ambulation progress, phantom limb sensation and pain usually subside, although the pain can become chronic.[37]

Postoperative management. General postoperative care for the patient who has had an amputation depends largely on the patient's general state of health, the reason for the amputation, and the patient's age. Nursing care must be individualized on the basis of these factors. For example, an older adult patient needs particularly careful monitoring of respiratory status. A victim of a motor vehicle accident may need careful neurologic monitoring. Individuals who undergo amputation as a result of a traumatic injury need to be monitored for posttraumatic stress disorder because they had no time to prepare or perhaps even participate in the decision to have a limb amputated.

Prevention and detection of complications are important nursing responsibilities during the postoperative period. Careful monitoring of the patient's vital signs and dressing can alert the nurse to hemorrhage in the operative area. Careful attention to sterile technique during dressing changes reduces the potential for wound infection and subsequent interruption of rehabilitation.

If an immediate postoperative prosthesis has been applied, the nurse must monitor vital signs carefully because the surgical site is heavily covered and may not be visible. A surgical tourniquet must always be available for emergency use. If hemorrhage occurs, the surgeon should be notified immediately, and efforts to control the hemorrhage should begin at once.

The orthopedic surgeon will decide the type of prosthetic fitting that will be used after surgery. An immediate prosthetic fitting, often called the immediate postsurgical fitting or the immediate postoperative fitting, is done in the operating room after the amputation. A rigid, castlike bandage is applied around the closed residual limb with a prosthetic pylon and an ankle-foot assembly. While the patient is still anesthetized, the prosthetic pylon and ankle-foot assembly are aligned and adjusted to provide a smooth gait and to avoid excessive pressure on the residual limb area. A strap is placed on the proximal anterior surface of the rigid plaster bandage and attached to a waistband to prevent slippage. The main advantages of this device are reduction of edema and the psychologic benefit of early ambulation. A disadvantage is the inability to directly visualize the surgical site.

The delayed prosthetic fitting may be the best choice for certain patients. Patients who have had amputations above the knee or below the elbow, older adults, debilitated individuals, and those with infection usually have delayed prosthetic fittings (Fig. 61-17). The appropriate time for use of a prosthesis depends on satisfactory healing of the residual limb, as well as on the general condition of the patient. A temporary prosthesis may be used for partial weight bearing once the sutures are removed. Barring any problems, patients can bear full weight on permanent prostheses by approximately 3 months after amputation.

Not all patients are candidates for a prosthesis. It is important that the surgeon discuss ambulation possibilities frankly with the patient and family. The seriously ill or debilitated patient may not have the energy required to use a prosthesis. Mobility with a wheelchair may be the most realistic goal for this type of patient.

Collaborative care also includes the direction and coordination of the rehabilitation program for the amputee. Success depends on the physical and emotional health of the patient. Chronic illness and debilitation complicate aggressive rehabilita-

tion efforts. Both physical and occupational therapy must be an integral component of the patient's overall plan of care.

Flexion contractures may delay the rehabilitation process. The most common and debilitating contracture is hip flexion. Hip adduction contracture is rare. Patients should avoid sitting in a chair for more than 1 hour with hips flexed or having pillows under the surgical extremity to prevent flexion contractures. Unless specifically contraindicated, patients should lie on their abdomen for 30 minutes three to four times each day and position the hip in extension while prone.

Proper residual limb bandaging fosters shaping and molding for eventual prosthesis fitting (Fig. 61-18). The physician usually orders a compression bandage to be applied immediately after surgery to support the soft tissues, reduce edema, hasten healing, minimize pain, and promote residual limb shrinkage and maturation. This bandage may be an elastic roll applied to the residual limb or a residual limb shrinker, which is an elastic stocking that fits tightly over the residual limb and lower trunk area.[38]

The compression bandage is initially worn at all times except during physical therapy and bathing. The bandage is taken off and reapplied several times daily, and care is taken so that it is applied snugly but not so tight as to interfere with circulation. Shrinker bandages should be washed and changed daily. It is recommended that the patient have two residual limb shrinker bandages so that one can be worn while the other is being washed. After healing has occurred, the residual limb is bandaged only when the patient is not wearing the prosthesis. The patient should

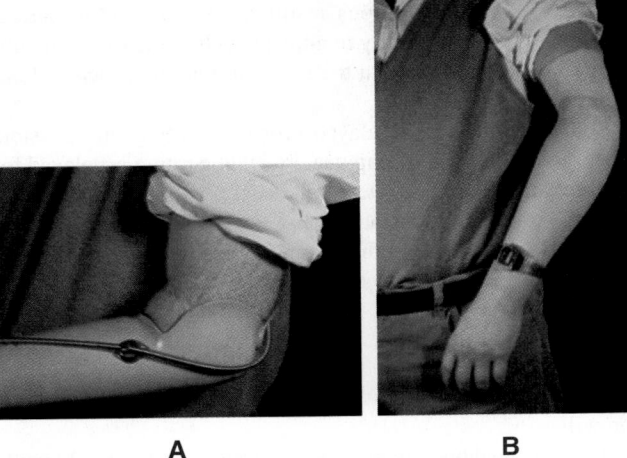

FIG. 61-17 Two types of prosthesis. **A,** Traditional fiberglass. **B,** New materials and techniques have made possible fabrication of prosthetic sockets that are light, soft, flexible, and secure.

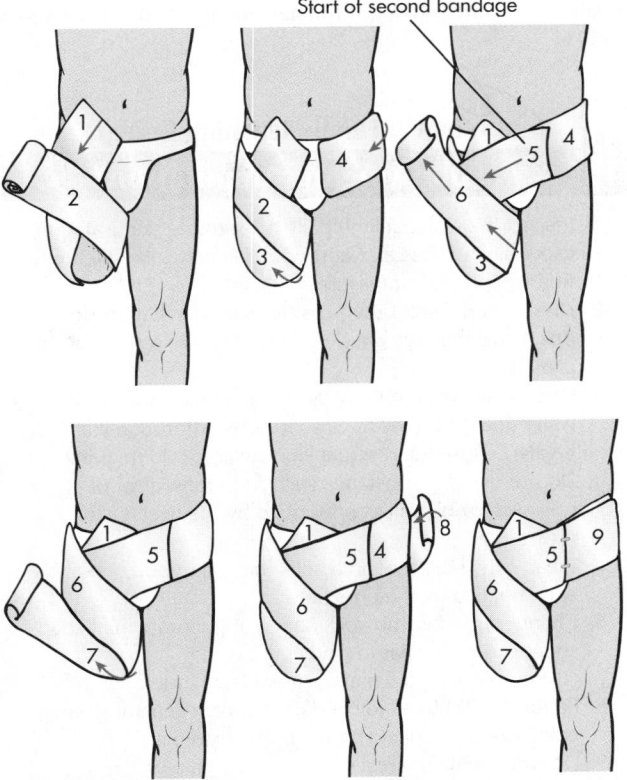

FIG. 61-18 Bandaging for the above-the-knee amputation residual limb. Figure-of-eight style covers progressive areas of the residual limb. Two elastic wraps are required.

be instructed to avoid dangling the residual limb over the bedside to minimize edema formation.

As the patient's overall condition improves, the nurse begins instruction in the principles and techniques of transferring from bed to chair and back. Active exercises and conditioning are essential in developing ambulation skills. The exercise regimen is normally started under the supervision of the physician and the physical therapist. The nurse must have a clear understanding of the exercise regimen to reinforce it and ensure that the exercises are performed correctly. Active ROM exercises of all joints should be started as soon after surgery as the patient's pain level and medical status permit. In preparation for mobility, the patient should increase triceps and shoulder strength and lower limb support and learn balance of the altered body. The loss of the weight of a limb requires adaptation of the patient's proprioceptive mechanisms to prevent falls and frustration.

Crutch walking is started as soon as patients are physically able. If they have had immediate postsurgical fitting, orders related to weight bearing must be carefully followed to avoid disruption of the skin flap and delay of the healing process. Initial periods of ambulation should not exceed 5 minutes to prevent dependent edema.

Before discharge, the patient and family need careful instruction related to residual limb care, ambulation, prevention of contractures, recognition of complications, exercise, and follow-up care. Table 61-15 outlines patient and family teaching following an amputation.

Ambulatory and Home Care. When the healing has occurred satisfactorily and the residual limb is well molded, the patient is ready for fitting a prosthesis. Walking with a below-the-knee prosthesis requires 40% additional energy, and an above-the-knee prosthesis requires 60% more energy. Matching a patient with a suitable prosthesis involves many factors, including age, general health, intelligence, motivation, occupation, and finances. After the physician makes the recommendation, the patient is referred to a prosthetist, who initially makes a mold of the residual limb and measures landmarks for the fabrication of the prosthesis. The molded residual limb socket allows the residual limb to fit snugly into the prosthesis.[39] The residual limb is covered with a residual limb stocking to ensure good fit and prevent skin breakdown. The residual limb may continue to shrink, causing a loose fit, in which case a new socket has to be fabricated. The patient may need to have the prosthesis adjusted to prevent rubbing and friction between the residual limb and the socket. Excessive movement of a loose prosthesis can cause severe skin irritation and breakdown.

The prosthesis is fitted by the prosthetist, who may also train the amputee to use it. It is important for the nurse to be familiar with the training program to encourage and assist the patient. Most often this learning occurs after the patient has been discharged from the inpatient setting. Learning to use a prosthesis is frustrating, and the patient may easily become discouraged. The nurse must continually offer support until the patient is able to manage alone.

Artificial limbs become an integral part of the patient's body image. Proper care ensures their long life and useful functioning. The patient should be instructed to clean the prosthesis socket daily with a mild soap and rinse thoroughly to remove irritants. The leather and metal parts of the prosthesis should not get wet. The patient should be encouraged to have regular maintenance of the prosthesis. Consideration of the condition of the shoe is also necessary. A badly worn shoe alters the gait and may cause damage to the prosthesis.

Referral to a community health nurse can foster optimal physical and emotional adjustment. The family should be instructed on ambulation and transfer techniques and proper residual limb care.

Special Considerations in Upper-Limb Amputation. The emotional implications of an upper-limb amputation are often more devastating than those for lower-limb amputation. The enforced dependency brought about by one-handedness is both frustrating and humiliating to many patients. Because most upper-extremity amputations result from trauma, the patient has not had the opportunity to adjust psychologically to an amputation or to participate in the decision-making process about amputation.

Both immediate and delayed prosthetic fittings are possible for the below-the-elbow amputee. Prosthetic fitting is delayed for the above-the-elbow amputee. The usual functional prosthesis is the arm and hook. A cosmetic hand is available but has limited functional value. As with the lower-limb prosthesis, patient motivation and endurance are major factors contributing to a satisfactory outcome.

■ Evaluation

The expected outcomes are that the patient with an amputation will

- accept changed body image and integrate changes into lifestyle
- have no evidence of skin breakdown
- have reduction or absence of pain
- become mobile within limitations imposed by amputation

TABLE 61-15	*Patient & Family Teaching Guide* **Following an Amputation**

1. Inspect the residual limb daily for signs of skin irritation, especially redness and abrasion. Pay particular attention to areas prone to pressure.
2. Discontinue use of the prosthesis if an irritation develops. Have the area checked before resuming use of the prosthesis.
3. Wash residual limb thoroughly each night with warm water and a bacteriostatic soap. Rinse thoroughly and dry gently. Expose the residual limb to air for 20 minutes.
4. Do not use any substance such as lotions, alcohol, powders, or oil unless prescribed by the health care provider.
5. Wear only a residual limb sock that is in good condition and supplied by the prosthetist.
6. Change residual limb sock daily. Launder in a mild soap, squeeze, and lay flat to dry.
7. Use prescribed pain management techniques.
8. Perform ROM to all joints daily. Perform general strengthening exercises including the upper extremities daily.
9. Do not elevate the residual limb on a pillow.
10. Lay prone with hip extension for 30 minutes three to four times daily.

ROM, Range of motion.

■ Gerontologic Considerations: Amputation

If a lower-limb amputation has been performed on an older adult, the patient's previous ability to ambulate may affect the extent of recovery. Use of a prosthesis requires a significant amount of energy for ambulation. Older adults whose general health is weakened by disorders such as cardiac or pulmonary problems may not be candidates for prosthesis use. This patient's ability to ambulate will be limited. If possible, this should be discussed with the patient and family before surgery so that realistic expectations can be set. ■

Common Joint Surgical Procedures

Surgery plays an important role in the treatment and rehabilitation of patients with various forms of arthritis, conditions related to trauma, and other painful conditions resulting in functional disability. Joint replacement surgery is the most common orthopedic operation performed on older adults. Significant advances in the field of reconstructive surgery have resulted in improvements in prosthetic design, materials, and surgical techniques that provide significant relief of pain and deformity and improve function and joint motion for patients with arthritis.

Indications for Joint Surgery

Surgery is aimed at relieving pain, improving joint motion, correcting deformity and malalignment, reducing vertical loads and shear stresses, and removing intraarticular causes of erosion. Debilitating joint pain is one of the primary reasons for arthroplasty. In addition to the effects of chronic pain on the physical and emotional well-being of the patient, any movement of the painful joint is often avoided. If this decreased functional ability is not corrected, contraction with permanent limitation of motion often occurs. Limitation of motion at any joint can be demonstrated on physical examination and by joint-space narrowing on radiologic examination.

There may also be a slow loss of cartilage in affected joints, which may be related to loss of motion. Synovitis can cause tendon damage, resulting in rupture or subluxation of the joint and subsequent loss of function. Continuing disease activity may cause loss of cartilage and bony surface and result in mechanical barriers to movement requiring surgical intervention.

Additional indications for hip or knee arthroplasty include failed prior procedures, sepsis, tumors, Paget's disease, congenital hip dysplasia, severe varus or valgus deformity, and spondyloarthropathies.[40]

TYPES OF JOINT SURGERIES

Synovectomy

Synovectomy (removal of synovial membrane) is used as a prophylactic measure and as a palliative treatment of rheumatoid arthritis (RA). Removal of synovial membrane, thought to be the location of the basic pathologic changes in joint destruction, helps prevent further progression of joint damage. A synovectomy is best performed early in the disease process to prevent serious destruction of joint surfaces. Removal of the thickened synovium prevents extension of the inflammatory process into the adjacent cartilage, ligaments, and tendons.

It is impossible to surgically remove all the synovium in a joint. The underlying disease process is still present and will again affect the regenerating synovium. However, the disease appears to be milder after synovectomy, and definite improvement in pain, weight bearing, and ROM can be expected. Common sites for this surgery include the elbow, wrist, and fingers. Synovectomy in the knee is done less frequently because knee joint replacement techniques are usually used.

Osteotomy

An **osteotomy** is performed by removing or adding a wedge or slice of bone to change its alignment and shift weight bearing, thereby correcting deformity and relieving pain. Cervical osteotomy may be used to correct deformity in some patients with ankylosing spondylitis. A halo and body jacket are worn until fusion occurs (3 or 4 months). Subtrochanteric or femoral osteotomy may provide some relief of pain and improve motion in selected patients with hip osteoarthritis. Osteotomy has proven ineffective in patients with inflammatory joint disease. Osteotomy of the knee provides relief of pain in selected patients, but advanced joint destruction is usually corrected by joint replacement surgery. The postoperative care is similar to the treatment of an internal fixation of a fracture at a comparable site (see p. 1668). The osteotomy is usually fixed by internal wires, screws and plates, bone grafts, or an external fixator.

Debridement

Debridement is the removal of degenerative debris such as loose bodies, osteophytes, joint debris, and degenerated menisci from a joint. This procedure is usually performed on the knee or the shoulder using a fiberoptic arthroscope. The procedure is usually done on an outpatient basis. A compression dressing is applied postoperatively. Weight bearing is permitted following knee arthroscopy. Patient education includes monitoring for signs of infection, managing pain, and restricting excessive activity for 24 to 48 hours.

Arthroplasty

Arthroplasty is the reconstruction or replacement of a joint. This surgical procedure is performed to relieve pain, improve or maintain ROM, and correct deformity. The most common uses of arthroplasty are for patients with osteoarthritis (OA), RA, avascular necrosis, congenital deformities or dislocations, and other systemic problems. There are several types of arthroplasty, including replacement of part of a joint (hemiarthroplasty), surgical reshaping of the bones of the joints, and total joint replacement. Replacement arthroplasty is available for the elbow, shoulder, phalangeal joint of the finger, hip, knee, ankle, and foot.[41]

Hip Arthroplasty. Total hip arthroplasty (THA) has provided significant relief of pain and improvement of function for patients with OA and RA. Implants are often "cemented" in place with polymethylmethacrylate, which bonds to the bone. With time, a significant number of femoral components loosen and require revision surgery. Because of this risk, cemented THAs are recommended for less active, older adults with compromised bone strength. Younger individuals receive "cementless" arthroplasties in an effort to prolong the lifetime of the prosthesis. Cementless THAs provide long-term implant stability by facilitating biologic ingrowth of new bone tissue into the porous surface

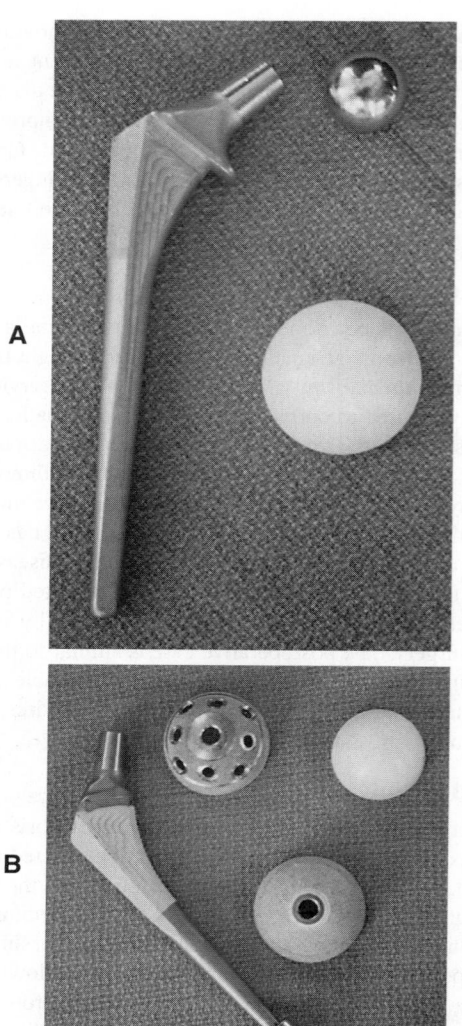

FIG. 61-19 Total hip replacements. A, Coated cemented components. B, Porous cementless components.

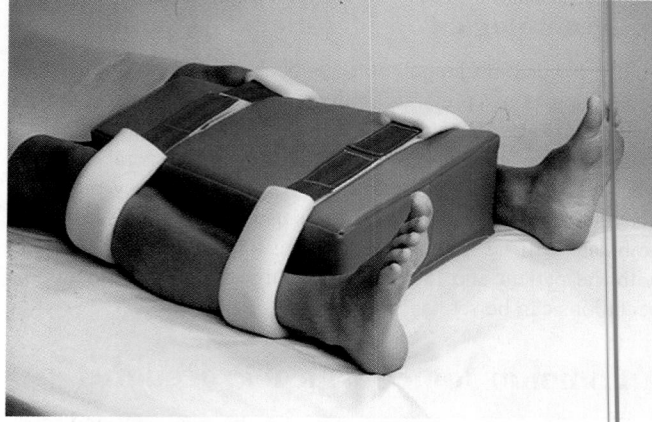

FIG. 61-20 Maintaining postoperative abduction following total hip replacement.

coating of the prosthesis. A patient with a high activity potential and a life expectancy of 25 years or more is an excellent candidate for a cementless prosthesis. Total hip replacements are shown in Fig. 61-19.

In both types of arthroplasties, extremes of internal rotation, adduction, and 90-degree flexion of the hip must be avoided for 4 to 6 weeks postoperatively. A foam abduction pillow is sometimes placed between the legs to prevent dislocation of the new joint (Fig. 61-20). Following surgery, patients must not allow their hips to be lower than their knees, and elevated toilet seats and chair alterations at home are necessary. Tub baths and driving a car are not allowed for 4 to 6 weeks. An occupational therapist may teach the patient to use assistive devices, such as reach bars ("reachers") to avoid bending over to pick something off the floor, long-handled shoehorns, or sock pullers. The knees must be kept apart; the patient must never cross the legs or twist to reach behind. Physical therapy is initiated the first postoperative day with ambulation and weight bearing with a walker for patients with a cemented prosthesis and weight bearing on the operative side for those with an uncemented prosthesis.

Exercises are designed to restore strength and muscle tone in the hip muscles essential to improved function and ROM. These include quadriceps setting, gluteal muscle setting, leg raises in supine and prone positions, and abduction exercises (swinging the leg out but never crossing midline) from supine and standing positions. The patient will continue these for many months after discharge, and the family should be well acquainted with the exercise program to offer encouragement at home.

Home care considerations include ongoing assessment of pain management, monitoring for infection, and prevention of DVT. Not all patients will qualify for home nursing visits. The incision may be closed with metal staples, which are removed at the surgeon's office. Because of the high risk for DVT, prothrombin times will be drawn weekly and anticoagulation adjusted accordingly if warfarin is used. Enoxaparin (Lovenox), a LMWH, is administered subcutaneously and can be given at home by the patient or family member. An advantage of enoxaparin is that it does not require monitoring of the patient's coagulation status. The patient should be instructed to use prophylactic antibiotics before dental appointments or procedures that might put the patient at risk for bacteremia.

A physical therapist will assess ROM, ambulation, and compliance with the exercise regimen. The patient will gradually increase the number of repetitions of exercises, add weights to ankles, swim, and may eventually use a stationary bicycle to tone quadriceps and improve cardiovascular fitness. High-impact exercises and sports, such as jogging and tennis, may loosen the implant and should be avoided. The elderly adult may require rehabilitation at a subacute or extended care facility until able to function independently.[42]

Knee Arthroplasty. Unremitting pain and instability as a result of severe destructive deterioration of the knee joint is the main indication for total knee arthroplasty (TKA). The presence of osteoporosis may necessitate bone grafting to augment defects and to correct bone deficiencies. Either part or all of the knee joint may be replaced with a metal and plastic prosthetic device. A compression dressing is used to immobilize the knee in extension immediately after the operation. This is removed before discharge and may be replaced with a knee immobilizer or posterior plastic shell, which maintains extension during ambulation and at rest for about 4 weeks.

Great emphasis is placed on postoperative exercising, and dislocation is not typical with TKA. Isometric quadriceps setting begins the first day after surgery. The patient progresses to straight-leg raises and gentle ROM to increase muscle strength and obtain 90-degree knee flexion. Active flexion exercises through the use of a CPM machine postoperatively promotes joint mobility.[43] Full weight bearing is begun before discharge. An active home exercise program involves progressive ROM, muscle strengthening, and stationary bicycle exercising.

Finger Joint Arthroplasty. A silicone rubber arthroplastic device is used to help restore function in the fingers of the patient with RA. The goal of hand surgery is primarily to restore function related to grasp, pinch, stability, and strength rather than to correct cosmetic deformity. The metacarpophalangeal and proximal interphalangeal joints take longer to heal.[44] Ulnar deviation is often present, which results in severe functional limitations of the hand. Before surgery the patient is instructed in hand exercises, including flexion, extension, abduction, and adduction of the fingers. Postoperatively, the hand is kept elevated with a bulky dressing in place. Neurovascular assessment is conducted postoperatively, and the nurse assesses for signs of infection. The success of the surgery depends largely on the postoperative treatment plan, which is often carried out under the direction of an occupational therapist. Once the dressing is removed, a guided splinting program is initiated. The patient is discharged with splints to use while sleeping and hand exercises to perform for 10 to 12 weeks at least three to four times a day. The patient is also instructed to avoid lifting heavy objects.

Elbow and Shoulder Arthroplasty. Although available, total replacement of elbow and shoulder joints is not as common as other forms of arthroplasty. Shoulder replacements are used in patients with severe pain because of RA, OA, avascular necrosis, or an old trauma. The shoulder replacement is usually considered if the patient has adequate surrounding muscle strength and bone stock. If joint replacement is necessary for both elbow and shoulder, the elbow is usually done first because a severely painful elbow interferes with the shoulder rehabilitation program.

Significant pain relief has been achieved following arthroplasty, with 90% of patients having no pain at rest or minimal pain with activity. Functional improvements have resulted in better hygiene and increased ability to perform activities of daily living in most patients. Rehabilitation is longer and more difficult than with other joint surgeries.

Ankle Arthroplasty. Total ankle arthroplasty (TAA) is indicated for RA, OA, and avascular necrosis. Ankle fusion is often selected over arthroplasty because the result is more durable. However, the patient is left with a stiff foot and the inability to change heel height. TAA is advantageous because a more normal gait pattern can be achieved. Postoperatively, the patient may not weight-bear for 6 weeks, must elevate the extremity to reduce and prevent edema, be extremely careful to prevent postoperative infection, and maintain immobilization as directed by the physician. Although the use of TAA is not widespread, it is becoming a viable alternative to fusion for the treatment of severe ankle arthritis in selected patients.

Arthrodesis

Arthrodesis is the surgical fusion of a joint. This procedure is indicated only if articular surfaces are too severely damaged or infected to allow joint replacement or for reconstructive surgery

failures. Arthrodesis relieves pain and provides a stable but immobile joint. The fusion is usually accomplished by removal of the articular hyaline cartilage and the addition of bone grafts across the joint surface. The affected joint must be immobilized until bone healing has occurred. Common areas of fusion are the wrist, ankle, cervical spine, lumbar spine, and the metatarsophalangeal joint of the great toe.

Complications of Joint Surgery

Infection is a serious complication of joint surgery, particularly joint replacement surgery. The most common causative organisms are gram-positive aerobic streptococci and staphylococci. Infection almost always leads to pain and loosening of the prosthesis, generally requiring extensive surgery. Efforts to reduce the incidence of infection include the use of specially designed hypersterile operating rooms with laminar airflow and prophylactic antibiotic administration.

DVT is another potentially serious complication after joint surgeries, particularly those involving the lower extremities. Prophylactic measures such as aspirin, warfarin, low-molecular-weight heparin (LMWH), and pneumatic compression of the legs are usually instituted. Patients may be followed postoperatively with venous Doppler ultrasound to detect DVT, the source of most pulmonary emboli. FES may also occur after total hip arthroplasty.

Collaborative Care

Preoperative Management. As surgical techniques and care improve, more patients with chronic diseases such as RA are being considered as surgical candidates. Over 250,000 persons annually undergo total joint arthroplasty. The primary goal of preoperative assessment is to identify risk factors associated with postoperative complications so that nursing strategies can be implemented to promote optimal positive outcomes. A careful history will include previous medical diagnosis and complications such as diabetes and thrombophlebitis, pain tolerance and management preferences, current functional status and expectations following surgery, and level of social support and home care needs after discharge. The patient should be free from evidence of infection and acute joint inflammation.

If lower-extremity surgery is planned, upper-extremity muscle strength and joint function are assessed to determine the type of assistive devices needed postoperatively for ambulation and activities of daily living. Preoperative teaching informs the patient and family of the expected hospital course and postoperative management at home. In addition, it prepares them to maximize the usefulness and longevity of the prosthesis. Research has shown that preoperative education alone is not sufficient to ensure successful joint replacement; the patient must have a sense of self-efficacy for an optimal outcome to be achieved.[45] Patients also need to realize that recovery is "not going to happen overnight." Both patients and their families or significant others need to speak with individuals who have had a total joint arthroplasty to better understand the reality of dealing with a joint replacement.

Postoperative Management. Postoperatively, neurovascular assessment is performed to assess nerve function and circulatory status. Anticoagulation therapy, analgesia, and parenteral antibiotics are administered. In general, the affected joint is exercised, and ambulation is encouraged as early as possible to prevent complications of immobility. Specific protocols vary ac-

NURSING CARE PLAN 61-3

Patient with Joint Replacement Surgery

EXPECTED PATIENT OUTCOMES	NURSING INTERVENTIONS and *RATIONALES*
NURSING DIAGNOSIS	**Impaired physical mobility** *related to* pain, stiffness, and surgical procedure *as manifested by* difficulty in ambulating, inability to participate in physical rehabilitation, guarded movement.
▪ Functional ROM of joint	▪ Assess effect of surgery on patient's mobility *to plan appropriate interventions.* ▪ Maintain proper positioning *to prevent dislocation or other complications.* ▪ Begin exercise program as directed *to minimize mobility impairment and stiffness.* ▪ Collaborate with physical and occupational therapist *to increase patient compliance and promote continuity of exercise.* ▪ Give pain medication before exercise *to decrease discomfort from exercise and increase patient participation.*
NURSING DIAGNOSIS	**Self-care deficit** *related to* restrictions imposed by joint surgery, pain, weakness *as manifested by* inability to perform part or all activities of daily living.
▪ Activities of daily living (ADLs) met satisfactorily by patient or caregivers	▪ Assess patient's ability to perform ADLs *to plan appropriate assistance.* ▪ Work with physical therapy and patient in learning to use assistive devices *to ensure independence.* ▪ Assure patient that self-care abilities will be resumed with time *to decrease anxiety over dependency.* ▪ Teach family how to assist with care.
NURSING DIAGNOSIS	**Risk for peripheral neurovascular dysfunction** *related to* edema and dislocated prosthesis.
▪ Palpable peripheral pulses ▪ Warm extremities	▪ Assess nerve and circulatory status q1hr for first 24 hours, then every 2 to 4 hours *to determine if problem is present so that treatment can be initiated promptly.* ▪ Notify surgeon immediately if abnormalities are noted *so that interventions are started without delay.* ▪ Initiate measures such as cold packs and elevation of affected part *to minimize edema.* ▪ Carry out measures to prevent dislocation *because this can be a cause of neurovascular dysfunction.* ▪ Teach patient to report signs of neurovascular dysfunction such as paresthesia, coldness, pallor, excessive pain, swelling of affected extremity or body area *so that treatment is not delayed.*
NURSING DIAGNOSIS	**Ineffective therapeutic regimen management** *related to* lack of knowledge of follow-up care *as manifested by* expression of concern with ability to care for self after discharge, frequent questioning about follow-up care, lack of plan for follow-up care.
▪ Confidence in ability to manage self-care after discharge and to make necessary lifestyle changes	▪ Instruct patient on usual follow-up protocol, including activity limitations, drugs, follow-up visits, signs of infection, dislocation *to prepare patient for self-care and decision making.* ▪ Assist patient to identify activities that require modification *so that appropriate changes can be made.* ▪ Initiate a nurse referral *to monitor the long-term exercise program at home.*

COLLABORATIVE PROBLEM

NURSING GOALS	NURSING INTERVENTIONS AND *RATIONALES*
POTENTIAL COMPLICATION	**Deep vein thrombophlebitis** *related to* surgery and immobilization.
▪ Monitor and report signs of thrombosis ▪ Carry out appropriate medical and nursing interventions	▪ Monitor for redness, swelling, and tenderness or pain of the extremity *to recognize and report signs of thrombophlebitis.* ▪ Apply elastic compression stockings and instruct patient to perform isotonic exercises such as quadriceps setting, ankle rolling, and pushing on footboard *to promote circulation and prevent clot formation.* ▪ Provide adequate parenteral and oral fluids *to prevent dehydration and thrombus formation.* ▪ Instruct the patient in the importance of home exercise *to prevent venous stasis.* ▪ Instruct the patient and caregivers in the proper administration and follow-up of anticoagulation drug therapy (e.g., low-molecular-weight heparin, warfarin) *to prevent side effects* (see Table 37-4).

cording to patient, type of prosthesis, and surgeon preference. Pain management postoperatively may use epidural analgesia, patient-controlled analgesia, IV injections, and oral narcotics or NSAIDs.[46]

The hospital stay after arthroplasty is 3 to 5 days depending on the patient's course and need for physical therapy. Physical therapy and ambulation enhance mobility, build muscle strength, and reduce the risk of thrombus formation. If the patient is taking warfarin, therapy starts on the day of surgery and continues for 3 weeks with a prothrombin time done on a regular basis. For those taking LMWH (e.g., enoxaparin), therapy starts 24 to 36 hours after surgery and continues for 2 weeks postoperatively. Daily monitoring of the patient's coagulation status is not necessary with LMWH. The decision to use warfarin or LMWH depends on many factors, including the patient's age and overall state of health.

NURSING MANAGEMENT
JOINT SURGERY

The nursing management of the patient undergoing joint surgery begins with preoperative teaching and realistic goal setting. It is important that the patient understands and accepts the limitations of the proposed surgery and realizes that it will not remove the underlying disease process. Postoperative procedures such as turning, deep breathing, use of bedpan and bedside com-

mode, and use of abductor pillows should be explained and opportunities for practice provided. The patient should be reassured that pain relief will be available. Patient-controlled analgesia can be helpful. A preoperative visit from a physical therapist allows practice of postoperative exercises and measurement for crutches or other assistive devices.

Discharge planning begins immediately. The duration of the hospital stay and the expected postoperative events should be discussed because the patient and family must prepare ahead. The home environment must be assessed for safety (e.g., presence of scatter rugs and electrical cords) and accessibility. Are the bathroom and bedroom on the first floor? Are door frames wide enough to accommodate a walker? Social support must also be assessed. Is a friend or family member available to assist the patient in the home? Will the patient require homemaker or meal services? The elderly patient may need the rehabilitation services of a subacute or extended care facility for a few weeks postoperatively to progressively develop independent living skills. Specific nursing interventions related to joint surgery are summarized in NCP 61-3.

Patient teaching includes instructions on reporting complications, including infection (e.g., fever, increased pain, drainage) and dislocation of the prosthesis (e.g., pain, loss of function, shortening or malalignment of an extremity). The home care nurse acts as the liaison between the patient and the surgeon, monitoring for postoperative complications, assessing comfort and ROM, and facilitating improvements in functional performance.

CRITICAL THINKING EXERCISES

Case Study
Lower Extremity Fracture
Patient Profile. Brad Hamil, a 32-year-old white construction worker, was admitted into the emergency department. A load of lumber fell from the forklift and crushed his legs. His legs were crushed for approximately 30 minutes before the weight could be relieved. He has a bone protruding from his left femur and his right leg is mangled. It appears he sustained an open fracture with massive internal bleeding into the left thigh muscle and lower extremity.

Subjective Data
- Complains of severe, excruciating pain involving both legs
- Complains of thirst and dizziness

Objective Data

Physical Examination
- Blood pressure: 90/60
- Diaphoretic and pale skin
- Pain not relieved by narcotic analgesic
- Moderately profuse bleeding from left femur wound
- Popliteal and posterior tibial pulses absent in both legs by Doppler auscultation
- Compartment pressures: left femur, 68 mm Hg; left proximal tibial region, 52 mm Hg

Diagnostic Studies
- X-rays of his left leg revealed an open comminuted, oblique fracture of the left femur and fractures of the proximal tibia, distal tibia, and fibula. No fractures are present in his right leg.
- Hematocrit 25%; hemoglobin 13 g/dl; WBC 15,000/μl (15 × 10^9/L); urine negative for myoglobin; chemistry panel within expected ranges

Collaborative Care
- Surgical reduction and fixation of fractures
- cefazolin (Ancef) 1 g intravenously every 8 hours
- Intake and output for 48 hours postoperatively
- morphine sulfate per patient-controlled analgesia pump

CRITICAL THINKING QUESTIONS
1. How do the pathophysiologic features of Brad's fracture predispose him to compartment syndrome?
2. What other complications of severe musculoskeletal trauma is Brad at high risk for developing?
3. What are the preoperative and postoperative priorities of nursing care for Brad?
4. What nursing interventions might help Brad cope with his long-term rehabilitation?
5. Based on the data presented, write one or more appropriate nursing diagnoses. Are there any collaborative problems?

Nursing Research Issues
1. What body image and self-concept issues does a patient who has undergone an amputation experience?
2. Are casual and weekend athletes using proper protective gear to prevent injury?
3. What is the most effective technique of providing pin care for a patient in skeletal traction?
4. Do nurses recognize the signs and symptoms of deep vein thrombosis and fat embolism syndrome?
5. What home health nursing interventions are most effective for increasing mobility in the patient recovering from a hip fracture?

REVIEW QUESTIONS

The number of the question corresponds to the same-numbered objective at the beginning of the chapter.

1. The nurse suspects an ankle sprain when a patient at the urgent care center
   a. is hit by another soccer player on the field.
   b. has ankle pain after running a 10-mile race.
   c. drops a 10-lb weight on his lower leg at the health club.
   d. has a twisting injury while running bases during a baseball game.

2. The nurse explains to a patient with a distal tibial fracture returning for a 3-week checkup that healing is indicated by
   a. callus formation.
   b. complete union of bone.
   c. presence of granulation tissue.
   d. formation of a hematoma at the fracture site.

3. A patient with a comminuted fracture of the femur is to have an open reduction with internal fixation (ORIF) of the fracture. The nurse explains that ORIF is indicated when
   a. a cast would be too large to provide normal mobility.
   b. the patient is able to tolerate long-term immobilization.
   c. adequate alignment cannot be obtained by other methods.
   d. the patient cannot tolerate the discomfort of a closed reduction.

4. An indication of a neurovascular problem noted during assessment of the patient with a fracture is
   a. exaggeration of extremity movement.
   b. petechiae on the head and upper thorax.
   c. decreased sensation distal to the fracture site.
   d. purulent drainage at the site of an open fracture.

5. A patient with a stable, closed fracture of the humerus caused by trauma to the arm has a temporary splint with bulky padding applied with an elastic bandage. The nurse suspects compartment syndrome and notifies the physician when the patient experiences
   a. pain at the fracture site.
   b. increasing edema of the limb.
   c. muscle spasms of the lower arm.
   d. pain when the nurse passively extends the fingers.

6. A patient with symphysis pubis and pelvic rami fractures should be monitored for
   a. sudden thirst.
   b. changes in urinary output.
   c. a palpable lump in the buttock.
   d. sudden decrease in blood pressure.

7. During the postoperative period, the patient with an above-the-knee amputation should be instructed that the residual limb should not be routinely elevated because
   a. this position reduces the development of phantom pain.
   b. the flexed position can promote hip flexion contracture.
   c. this position promotes clot formation at the incision site and thigh.
   d. unnecessary movement of the extremity can cause wound dehiscence.

8. A patient with rheumatoid arthritis is scheduled for an arthroplasty. The nurse explains that the purpose of this procedure is to
   a. fuse a joint and reduce pain.
   b. prevent further joint damage.
   c. assess the extent of joint damage.
   d. replace the joint and improve function.

9. The nurse teaches a patient recovering from a total hip replacement that it is important to avoid
   a. sleeping on the abdomen.
   b. sitting with the legs crossed.
   c. abduction exercises of the affected leg.
   d. bearing weight on the affected leg for 6 weeks.

REFERENCES

1. Schoen D: *Adult orthopaedic nursing,* Philadelphia, 2000, Lippincott.
2. Maher A: Trauma. In Schoen D, editor: *Core curriculum for orthopaedic nursing,* ed 4, Pitman, NJ, 2001, Jannetti.
3. Childs S: Nursing care for hand and wrist problems. In Schoen D, editor: *Core curriculum for orthopaedic nursing,* ed 4, Pitman, NJ, 2001, Jannetti.
4. Barry M: Ankle sprains, *AJN* 101:38, 2001.
5. Perron A, Brady W, Sing R: Orthopedic pitfalls in the ED: vascular injury associated with knee dislocation, *Am J Emerg Med* 19:583, 2001.
6. Bagwell-Crum C: The shoulder. In Schoen D, editor: *Core curriculum for orthopaedic nursing,* ed 4, Pitman, NJ, 2001, Jannetti.
7. Ferry S et al: Carpal tunnel syndrome: a nested case-control study of risk factors in women, *Am J Epidemiol* 151:6, 2000.
8. Litaker D et al: Returning to the bedside: using the history and physical examination to identify rotator cuff tears, *J Am Geriatr Soc* 48:2, 2000.
9. Skinner H et al: Identifying structural hip and knee problems, *Postgrad Med* 106:7, 1999.
10. Breuninger C et al: *Diseases,* ed 3, Springhouse, Pa, 2001, Springhouse Corporation.
11. Kunkler C: Fractures. In Maher AB, Salmond SW, Pellino TA, editors: *Orthopaedic nursing,* ed 3, St Louis, 2002, Mosby.
12. Ruda S: Fracture biomechanics and healing. In Williamson V, editor: *Management of lower extremity fractures,* Pitman, NJ, 1998, Jannetti.
13. Sanchez Y, Bush T: Bursitis and tendonitis: injection therapy basics, *J Musculoskeletal Med* 19:21, 2002.
14. Kunkler C: Therapeutic modalities. In Schoen D, editor: *Core curriculum for orthopaedic nursing,* ed 4, Pitman, NJ, 2001, Jannetti.
15. Ceccio C: Key concepts in the care of patients in traction. In Schoenly L, editor: *An introduction to orthopaedic nursing,* ed 2, Pitman, NJ, 1999, Jannetti.
16. Kunkler C: Neurovascular assessment. In Schoenly L, editor: *An introduction to orthopaedic nursing,* ed 2, Pitman, NJ, 1999, Jannetti.
17. Kunkler C: Care of the casted lower extremity. In Williamson V, editor: *Management of lower extremity fractures,* Pitman, NJ, 1998, Jannetti.

18. Childs S, Holmes S: *Guidelines for orthopaedic nursing: adult trauma,* National Association of Orthopaedic Nurses, 1998, Jannetti.

19. Astifidia R: Reflex sympathetic dystrophy complex regional pain syndrome of the upper extremity. In Childs S, editor: *The upper extremity: traumatic injuries and conditions,* Pitman, NJ, 1999, Jannetti.

20. McKenzie L: In search of a standard for pin care, *Orthop Nurs* 18:73, 1999.

21. Pellino T et al: Complications of orthopaedic disorders and orthopaedic surgery. In Maher AB, Salmond SW, Pellino TA, editors: *Orthopaedic nursing,* ed 3, St Louis, 2002, Mosby.

22. Harvey C: Compartment syndrome: when it is least expected, *Orthop Nur* 20:3, 2001.

23. Perrin A, Brady W, Keats T: Orthopedic pitfalls in the ED: acute compartment syndrome, *Am J Emerg Med* 19:413, 2001.

24. Ross D: Complications of lower extremity trauma. In Williamson V, editor: *Management of lower extremity fractures,* Pitman, NJ, 1998, Jannetti.

25. Tumbarello C: Acute extremity compartment syndrome, *J Trauma Nurs* 7:30, 2000.

26. Crowther C: *Primary orthopedic care,* St Louis, 1999, Mosby.

27. Choi H: Management of post-traumatic fat embolism in the emergency department, *Aust Emerg Nurs J* 2:10, 1999.

28. Newport M: Colles fracture: managing a common upper extremity injury, *J Musculoskeletal Med* 17:292, 2000.

29. Rose D, Rowen D: AANA Journal Course I: update for nurse anesthetists: perioperative considerations in major orthopedic trauma: pelvic and long bone fractures, *AANA J* 70:131, 2002.

30. Korovessis P et al: Medium and long-term results of open reduction and internal fixation for unstable pelvic ring fractures, *Orthopedics* 23:1165, 2000.

31. Yarnold B: Hip fracture, *AJN* 99:36, 1999.

32. Gallagher B et al: A fall prevention program for the home environment, *Home Care Provid* 6:157, 2001.

33. Richmind J, Zuckerman J, Koval K: Geriatric hip fractures, *J Musculosketal Med* 17:626, 2000.

34. Kamel H et al: Hormone replacement therapy and fractures in older adults, *J Am Geriatr Soc* 49:179, 2001.

35. Groeneveld A et al: Logrolling: establishing consistent practice, *Orthop Nurs* 20:2, 2001.

36. Beers M, Berkow R, editors: Eye injuries. In *Merck manual of diagnosis and therapy,* ed 17 [electronic version], Whitehouse Station, NJ, 1999, Merck and Co.

37. Dillingham T et al: Use and satisfaction with prosthetic devices among persons with trauma related amputations: a long-term outcome study, *Am J Phys Rehabil* 80:563, 2001.

38. Bryant G: Stump care, *AJN* 101:2, 2001.

39. Kapp S: Transfemoral socket design and suspension options, *Phys Med Rehabil Clin North Am* 11:569, 2000.

40. Roberts D: Degenerative disorders. In Maher AB, Salmond SW, Pellino TA, editors: *Orthopaedic nursing,* ed 3, St Louis, 2002, Mosby.

*41. Kelly M et al: Total joint arthroplasty: a comparison of post-acute settings on patient functional outcomes, *Orthop Nurs* 18:5, 1999.

*42. Ridge R et al: The relationship between multidisciplinary discharge outcomes and functional status after total hip replacement, *Orthop Nurs* 19:1, 2000.

43. O'Driscoll S, Giori N: Continuous passive motion (CPM): theory and principles of clinical application, *J Rehabil Res Dev* 37:179, 2000.

44. Childs S: Finger injury, *Lippincotts Prim Care Pract* 3:397, 1999.

*45. Moon LB et al: Relationships among self-efficacy, outcome expectancy, and postoperative behaviors in total joint replacement patients, *Orthop Nurs* 19:2, 2000.

46. Curtiss C: JCAHO: meeting the standards for pain management, *Orthop Nurs* 20:2, 2001.

---

*Nursing research–based reference.

RESOURCES

American Academy of Orthopedic Surgeons (AAOS)
6300 North River Road
Rosemont, IL 60018-4262
800-346-AAOS or 847-823-7186
Fax: 847-823-8125
www.aaos.org

American College of Sports Medicine (ACSM)
P.O. Box 1440
401 West Michigan Street
Indianapolis, IN 46202
317-637-9200
Fax: 317-634-7817
www.acsm.org

Amputees in Motion
P.O. Box 2703
Escondido, CA 92033
619-454-9300

National Amputation Foundation
38-40 Church Street
Malverne, NY 11565
516-887-3600
Fax: 516-887-3667
www.nationalamputation.org

National Arthritis/Musculoskeletal and Skin Diseases Information Clearinghouse
9000 Rockville Pike
Bethesda, MD 20892-2350
800-283-7800
www.nih.gov/niams

National Association of Orthopaedic Nurses, Inc. (NAON)
East Holly Avenue, Box 56
Pitman, NJ 08071-0056
800-289-NAON (6266) or 856-256-2310
Fax: 856-589-7463
www.orthonurse.org

National Easter Seal Society
230 West Monroe Street, Suite 1800
Chicago, IL 60606
800-221-6827 or 312-726-6200
Fax: 312-726-1494
www.easter-seals.org

Older Women's League
666 11th Street NW, Suite 700
Washington, DC 20001
800-825-3695 or 202-783-6686
Fax: 202-638-2356
www.owl-national.org

For additional Internet resources, see the website for this book at *http://www.evolve.elsevier.com/Lewis/medsurg.*

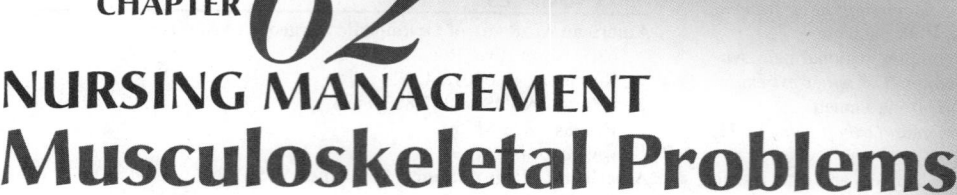

CHAPTER 62
NURSING MANAGEMENT
Musculoskeletal Problems

Cathleen E. Kunkler

LEARNING OBJECTIVES

1. Describe the pathophysiology, clinical manifestations, collaborative care, and nursing management of osteomyelitis.
2. Describe the types, pathophysiology, clinical manifestations, and collaborative care of bone cancer.
3. Differentiate between the causes and characteristics of acute and chronic low back pain.
4. Describe the conservative and surgical therapy of herniated intervertebral disk.
5. Describe the postoperative nursing management of a patient who has undergone spinal surgery.
6. Explain the etiology and nursing management of common foot disorders.
7. Describe the etiology, pathophysiology, clinical manifestations, and collaborative and nursing management of osteomalacia, osteoporosis, and Paget's disease.

KEY TERMS

Ewing's sarcoma, p. 1697
herniated intervertebral disk, p. 1702
low back pain, p. 1699
multiple myeloma, p. 1696
muscular dystrophy, p. 1698

osteoclastoma, p. 1696
osteogenic sarcoma, p. 1696
osteomalacia, p. 1707
osteomyelitis, p. 1692
osteoporosis, p. 1708
Paget's disease, p. 1711

OSTEOMYELITIS

Etiology and Pathophysiology

Osteomyelitis is a severe infection of the bone, bone marrow, and surrounding soft tissue. The most common infecting microorganism is *Staphylococcus aureus*. A variety of microorganisms can cause osteomyelitis, including *Escherichia coli, Salmonella, Neisseria gonorrhoeae, Staphylococcus epidermidis,* and *Pseudomonas aeruginosa*[1,2] (Table 62-1). Aerobic gram-negative bacteria alone or mixed with gram-positive organisms are often found. The widespread use of antibiotics in conjunction with surgical treatment has significantly reduced the mortality rate and complications associated with osteomyelitis.

The infecting microorganisms can invade by indirect or direct entry. The *indirect entry (hematogenous)* of microorganisms in osteomyelitis most frequently affects growing bone in boys less than 12 years old, and is associated with their higher incidence of blunt trauma. The most common sites of indirect entry in children are the distal femur, proximal tibia, humerus, and radius.[3] Adults with vascular insufficiency disorders (e.g., diabetes mellitus) and genitourinary and respiratory infections are at higher risk for a primary infection to spread via the blood to the bone. The pelvis and vertebrae, which are vascular-rich sites of bone, are the most common sites of infection.

Direct entry osteomyelitis can occur at any age when there is an open wound (e.g., penetrating wounds, fractures) and microorganisms gain entry to the body. Osteomyelitis may also occur in the presence of a foreign body such as an implant or an orthopedic prosthetic device (e.g., plate, total joint prosthesis). After gaining entrance to the bone by way of the blood, the microorganisms then lodge in an area of bone in which circulation slows, usually the metaphysis. The microorganisms grow, resulting in an increase in pressure because of the nonexpanding nature of most bone. This increasing pressure eventually leads to ischemia and vascular compromise of the periosteum. Eventually the infection passes through the bone cortex and marrow cavity, ultimately resulting in cortical devascularization and necrosis. Once ischemia occurs, the bone dies. The area of devitalized bone eventually separates from the surrounding living bone, forming *sequestra*. The part of the periosteum that continues to have a blood supply forms new bone called *involucrum* (Fig. 62-1).

TABLE 62-1	Causative Organisms in Osteomyelitis
ORGANISM	**POSSIBLE PREDISPOSING PROBLEM**
Staphylococcus aureus	Pressure ulcer, penetrating wound, open fracture, orthopedic surgery, abscessed tooth, vascular insufficiency disorders (e.g., diabetes, atherosclerosis)
Staphylococcus epidermidis	Indwelling prosthetic devices (e.g., joint replacements, fractured fixation devices)
Escherichia coli	Urinary tract infection
Mycobacterium tuberculosis	Tuberculosis
Neisseria gonorrhoeae	Gonorrhea
Pseudomonas	Puncture wounds, intravenous drug use
Salmonella	Sickle cell disease
Fungi, mycobacteria	Immunocompromised host

Reviewed by Brenda Elliff, RN, MPA, ONC, CCM, LNCC, Nurse Consultant, Elliff Legal and Medical Services, Coeur d'Alene, Idaho.

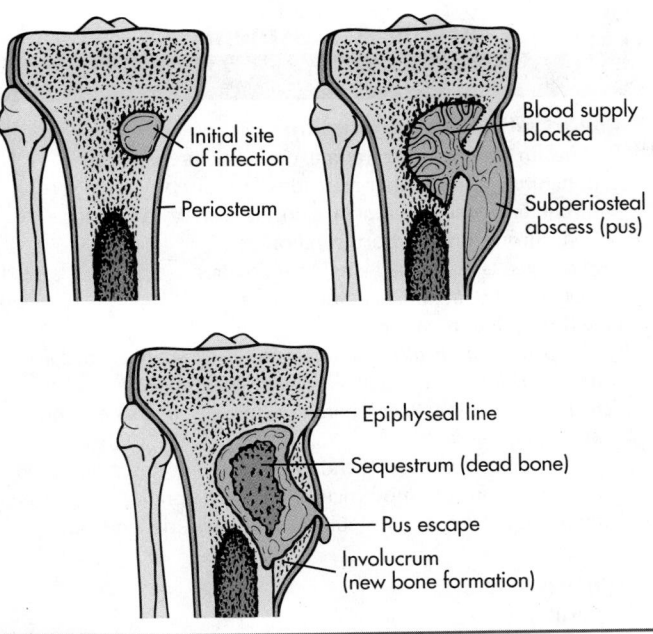

FIG. 62-1 Development of osteomyelitis infection with involucrum and sequestrum.

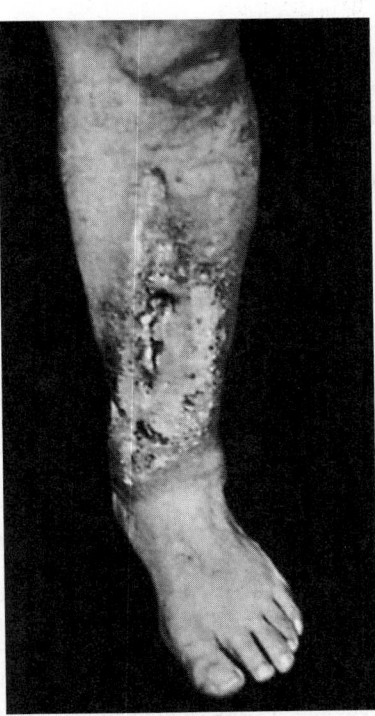

FIG. 62-2 Chronic osteomyelitis of the tibia. Marked skin scarring and draining sinuses are evident.

Once formed, a sequestrum continues to be an infected island of bone, surrounded by pus and difficult to reach by blood-borne antibiotics or white blood cells (WBCs). Sequestrum may enlarge and serve as a site for microorganisms that spread to other sites, including the lungs and brain. The sequestrum can move out of the bone and into the soft tissue. Once outside the bone, the sequestrum may revascularize and then undergo removal by normal immune processes. Another possibility is that the sequestrum can be surgically removed through debridement of the necrotic bone. If the necrotic sequestrum is not resolved naturally or surgically, it may develop a sinus tract, resulting in a chronic, purulent cutaneous drainage (Fig. 62-2).

Chronic osteomyelitis is either a continuous, persistent problem (a result of inadequate acute treatment) or a process of exacerbations and remission. Over time, granulation tissue turns to scar tissue. This avascular scar tissue provides an ideal site for continued microorganism growth and is impenetrable to antibiotics.

Clinical Manifestations

Acute osteomyelitis refers to the initial infection or an infection of less than 1 month in duration. The clinical manifestations of acute osteomyelitis are both systemic and local. Systemic manifestations include fever, night sweats, chills, restlessness, nausea, and malaise. Local manifestations include constant bone pain that is unrelieved by rest and worsens with activity; swelling, tenderness, and warmth at the infection site; and restricted movement of the affected part. Later signs include drainage from sinus tracts to the skin and/or the fracture site.

Chronic osteomyelitis refers to a bone infection that persists for longer than 1 month or an infection that has failed to respond to the initial course of antibiotic therapy. Systemic signs may be diminished, with local signs of infection more common, including constant bone pain and swelling, tenderness, and warmth at the infection site.

Diagnostic Studies

A bone or soft tissue biopsy is the definitive way to determine the causative microorganism. The patient's blood and/or wound cultures are frequently positive for the presence of microorganisms. An elevated WBC and erythrocyte sedimentation rate (ESR) may also be found. Radiologic signs suggestive of osteomyelitis usually do not appear until 10 days to weeks after the appearance of clinical symptoms, by which time the disease will have progressed. Radionuclide bone scans (gallium and indium) are helpful in diagnosis and are usually positive in the area of infection. Magnetic resonance imaging (MRI) and computed tomography (CT) scans may be used to help identify the extent of the infection including soft tissue involvement.[4]

Collaborative Care

Vigorous and prolonged intravenous (IV) antibiotic therapy is the treatment of choice for acute osteomyelitis, as long as bone ischemia has not yet occurred. Cultures or a bone biopsy should be done if possible before drug therapy is initiated. If antibiotic therapy is delayed, surgical debridement and decompression are often necessary.

Treatment for osteomyelitis previously involved an extended hospital stay for IV antibiotic treatment. Today patients are often discharged to home care with IV antibiotics delivered via a central venous catheter or peripherally inserted central catheter. IV antibiotic therapy may initially be started in the hospital and continued in the home for 4 to 6 weeks or as long as 3 to 6 months. A variety of antibiotics may be prescribed depending on the microorganism. These drugs include penicillin, nafcillin (Nafcil), neomycin, cephalexin (Keflex), cefazolin (Ancef), cefoxitin (Mefoxin), gentamicin (Garamycin), and tobramycin (Nebcin).

In adults with chronic osteomyelitis, oral therapy with a fluoroquinolone (ciprofloxacin [Cipro]) for 6 to 8 weeks may be prescribed instead of IV antibiotics. Oral antibiotic therapy may also be given after acute IV therapy is complete to ensure resolution of the infection. The patient's response to drug therapy is monitored through bone scans and ESR tests.

Surgical treatment for chronic osteomyelitis includes removal of the poorly vascularized tissue and dead bone and the extended use of antibiotics.[5] Antibiotic-impregnated polymethylmethacrylate bead chains may also be implanted at this time to aid in combating the infection.[6] After debridement of the devitalized and infected tissue, the wound may be closed, and a suction irrigation system is inserted. Intermittent or constant irrigation of the affected bone with antibiotics may also be initiated. Protection of the limb or surgical site with casts or braces is frequently done.

Hyperbaric oxygen therapy of 100% oxygen may be administered in chronic osteomyelitis. This therapy is thought to promote antibiotic activity and stimulate circulation and healing in the infected tissue. Orthopedic prosthetic devices (if a source of chronic infection) may have to be removed. Myocutaneous flaps or skin and bone grafting may be necessary if destruction is extensive. Amputation of the extremity may then be necessary to preserve life and improve the quality of life.

Long-term and mostly rare complications of osteomyelitis include septicemia, septic arthritis, pathologic fractures, squamous cell carcinoma, and amyloidosis.

NURSING MANAGEMENT
OSTEOMYELITIS

■ Nursing Assessment

Subjective and objective data that should be obtained from an individual with osteomyelitis are presented in Table 62-2.

■ Nursing Diagnoses

Nursing diagnoses for the patient with osteomyelitis may include, but are not limited to, those presented in NCP 62-1.

■ Planning

The overall goals are that the patient with osteomyelitis will (1) have satisfactory pain and fever control, (2) not experience any complications associated with osteomyelitis, (3) cooperate with the treatment plan, and (4) maintain a positive outlook on the outcome of the disease.

■ Nursing Implementation

Health Promotion. The control of infections already in the body (e.g., urinary, respiratory tract) is important in preventing osteomyelitis. Adults who are immunocompromised, have orthopedic prosthetic devices, and/or have vascular insufficiencies are especially susceptible. These patients should be instructed regarding the local and systemic manifestations of osteomyelitis. Families should also be aware of their role in monitoring the patient's health. Symptoms of bone pain, fever, swelling, and restricted limb movement should be reported immediately to the health care provider.

Acute Intervention. Some immobilization of the affected limb (e.g., splint, traction) is usually indicated to decrease pain. The involved limb should be handled carefully to avoid excessive manipulation, which increases pain and may cause pathologic

TABLE 62-2	Nursing Assessment Osteomyelitis

Important Health Information

Past health history: Bone trauma, open fracture, open or puncture wounds, other infections (e.g., streptococcal sore throat, bacterial pneumonia, sinusitis, skin or tooth infection, chronic urinary tract infection)
Medications: Use of analgesics or antibiotics
Surgery or other treatments: Bone surgery

Functional Health Patterns

Health perception–health management: IV drug abuse; malaise
Nutritional-metabolic: Anorexia, weight loss; chills
Activity-exercise: Weakness, paralysis, muscle spasms around affected bone
Cognitive-perceptual: Local tenderness over affected area, increase in pain with movement of affected bone
Coping–stress tolerance: Irritability, withdrawal, dependency, anger

Objective Data

General
Restlessness; high, spiking temperature; night sweats
Integumentary
Diaphoresis; erythema, warmth, edema at infected bone
Musculoskeletal
Restricted movement; wound drainage; spontaneous fractures
Possible Findings
Leukocytosis, positive blood and/or wound cultures, ↑ erythrocyte sedimentation rate; presence of sequestrum and involucrum on x-rays, radionuclide bone scans, CT, and MRI

CT, Computed tomography; *IV,* intravenous; *MRI,* magnetic resonance imaging.

fracture. An important nursing responsibility is to assess the patient's pain. Minor to severe pain may be experienced with muscle spasms. Nonsteroidal antiinflammatory drugs (NSAIDs), narcotic analgesics, and muscle relaxants may be prescribed to provide patient comfort. Nonpharmacologic (e.g., guided imagery, hypnosis) approaches to pain should be encouraged by the nurse (see Chapters 7 and 9).

Dressings are used to absorb the exudate from draining wounds and to debride devitalized tissue from the wound site when removed. Types of dressings used include dry, sterile dressings; dressings saturated in saline or antibiotic solution; and wet-to-dry dressings. Soiled dressings should be handled carefully to prevent cross-contamination of the wound or spread of the infection to other patients. When the dressing is changed, sterile technique is essential.

The patient is frequently on bed rest in the early stages of the acute infection. Good body alignment and frequent position changes prevent complications associated with immobility and promote comfort. Flexion contracture, especially of the hip or knee, is a common sequela of osteomyelitis of the lower extremity because the patient frequently positions the affected extremity in a flexed position to promote comfort. The contracture may then progress to a deformity. Footdrop can develop quickly in the lower extremity if the foot is not correctly supported by a splint. The patient should be instructed to avoid any activities such as exercise or heat application that increase circulation and serve as

NURSING CARE PLAN 62-1

Patient with Osteomyelitis

EXPECTED PATIENT OUTCOMES	NURSING INTERVENTIONS and *RATIONALES*
NURSING DIAGNOSIS	**Acute pain** *related to* inflammatory process secondary to infection *as manifested by* guarding, moaning, crying, restlessness, altered muscle tone, decreased activity, rated pain as >4 on a 10-point rating scale.
▪ Decrease in or absence of pain ▪ Satisfaction with pain relief	▪ Assess location and severity of pain and previous pain-relieving measures *to plan appropriate interventions.* ▪ Use a pain scale *to assess pain and evaluate effectiveness of interventions.* ▪ Give analgesics as indicated *to relieve pain.* ▪ Instruct patient to request analgesia *before pain becomes severe.* ▪ Use gentle handling and support when moving extremity *to reduce pain and prevent pathologic fractures.* ▪ Use the prescribed immobilization device and maintain patient's body in correct alignment and positioning *to prevent unusual position or muscle stretching from increasing pain.* ▪ Restrict ambulation or teach patient to use assistive device (e.g., crutches) *to prevent pathologic fracture, pain, and increased stress on bone.* ▪ Elevate extremity *to reduce swelling and provide comfort.* ▪ Instruct patient in nonpharmacologic methods of pain control such as distraction, relaxation breathing, guided imagery *to reduce the need for analgesics.*
NURSING DIAGNOSIS	**Impaired physical mobility** *related to* pain, immobilization devices, and weight-bearing limitations *as manifested by* inability or unwillingness to move.
▪ Consistent increase in mobility and range of motion with minimal pain or discomfort	▪ Assist patient as needed *to reduce patient's frustration with impaired mobility and prevent injury.* ▪ Explain the rationale for immobilization *to foster the patient's cooperation.* ▪ Increase mobility as ordered and tolerated *to maintain muscle function and strength.* ▪ Provide assistive devices (e.g., pick-up stick, long-handled shoehorn, stocking helpers) *to increase independence in activities of daily living.*
NURSING DIAGNOSIS	**Ineffective therapeutic regimen management** *related to* lack of knowledge regarding long-term management of osteomyelitis *as manifested by* verbalization of concern and uncertainty about procedures and skills needed for home care.
▪ Verbalization of confidence in self or caregiver's ability to carry out home management routine	▪ Provide information and instruction regarding wound care, aseptic technique, and dressing disposal *to reduce risk of cross-contamination and encourage wound healing.* ▪ Review drug regimen including schedule, name, dosage, purpose, and side effects *because long-term antibiotic therapy is required.* ▪ Stress importance of proper diet, rest, follow-up, and physical rehabilitation *to facilitate wound healing and reduce risk of chronic osteomyelitis.* ▪ Provide written instructions about the preceding information along with a phone number to call with any questions.

stimuli to the spread of infection. Uninvolved joints and muscles should continue to be exercised.

The patient should also be taught the potential adverse and toxic reactions associated with prolonged and high-dose antibiotic therapy. These reactions include hearing deficit, fluid retention, and neurotoxicity, which can occur with the aminoglycosides (e.g., tobramycin, neomycin), and jaundice, colitis, and photosensitivity from the extended use of the cephalosporins (e.g., cefazolin). Peak and trough blood levels of most antibiotics must be carefully monitored throughout the course of therapy to avoid these adverse effects. Lengthy antibiotic therapy can also result in an overgrowth of *Candida albicans* in the genitourinary and oral cavities, especially in immunosuppressed and older patients. The nurse should instruct the patient to report any whitish, yellow, curdlike lesions to the health care provider.

The patient and family are often frightened and discouraged because of the serious nature of the disease, uncertainty of the outcome, and the lengthy cost and course of treatment. Continued psychologic and emotional support is an integral part of nursing management.

Ambulatory and Home Care. With the introduction of various intermittent venous access devices, IV antibiotics can be administered to the patient in a long-term care or home setting. If at home, the patient and family must be instructed on the proper care and management of the venous access device. They must also be taught how to administer the antibiotic when scheduled and the need for follow-up laboratory testing. The importance of continuing to take antibiotics after the symptoms have subsided should be stressed. Periodic home nursing visits provide the family with support, which helps to reduce anxiety. If there is an open wound, dressing changes are often necessary. The patient and family may require supplies and instruction in the technique. Family members also need to understand that the infection is not contagious.

If the osteomyelitis becomes chronic, patients need physical and psychologic support for a prolonged period. They may become suspicious and hostile toward the health care providers when treatment plans do not result in a cure. Well-informed patients are better able to participate in decisions and cooperate in treatment plans.

■ Evaluation

The expected outcomes for the patient with osteomyelitis are presented in NCP 62-1.

Bone Cancer

Primary malignant bone neoplasms are rare in adults. In 2002, 2400 new cases of bone cancer occurred in the United States with an estimated 1300 deaths.[7] Primary neoplasms occur most often during childhood through young adulthood. They are characterized by their rapid metastasis and bone destruction.

MULTIPLE MYELOMA

In adults, multiple myeloma (plasma cell myeloma) is the most frequently occurring primary tumor arising in bone. **Multiple myeloma** is a malignant neoplasm of plasma cells causing widespread infiltration and destruction of bone marrow and cortex, which produces osteolytic lesions throughout the skeletal system. The most commonly involved bones are those with active marrow, such as the axial skeleton, sternum, ribs, spine, clavicles, skull, pelvis, and long bones. Recurrent infection, anorexia, fatigue, weight loss, back pain, anemia, thrombocytopenia, and bleeding tendencies are common presenting manifestations. The diagnosis of multiple myeloma is confirmed by bone marrow biopsy and x-rays indicating lytic lesions.

Patients with multiple myeloma generally have a poor prognosis because by the time a diagnosis has been confirmed, the disease has usually invaded the axial skeleton. Chemotherapeutic treatment of multiple myeloma is directed toward suppressing plasma cell growth and includes melphalan (Alkeran), vincristine (Oncovin), or doxorubicin (Adriamycin).[8] Corticosteroid therapy is commonly used in conjunction with chemotherapy drugs. Radiation therapy may be helpful in reducing pain. Early aggressive cell therapy with autologous stem cell transplantation may prolong survival. Myeloma in the spinal cord may require decompression. (Multiple myeloma is discussed in further detail in Chapter 30.)

OSTEOGENIC SARCOMA

Osteogenic sarcoma (osteosarcoma) is a primary neoplasm of bone that is extremely malignant and is characterized by rapid growth and metastasis. It usually occurs in the metaphyseal region of the long bones of the extremities, particularly in the regions of the distal femur, proximal tibia, and proximal humerus, as well as the pelvis (Fig. 62-3). Osteogenic sarcoma is the most common malignant bone tumor affecting children and young adults; the highest incidence is in males in the 10- to 25-year-old age-group. Secondary osteosarcoma is known to occur in adults over age 60 and is most commonly associated with Paget's disease.

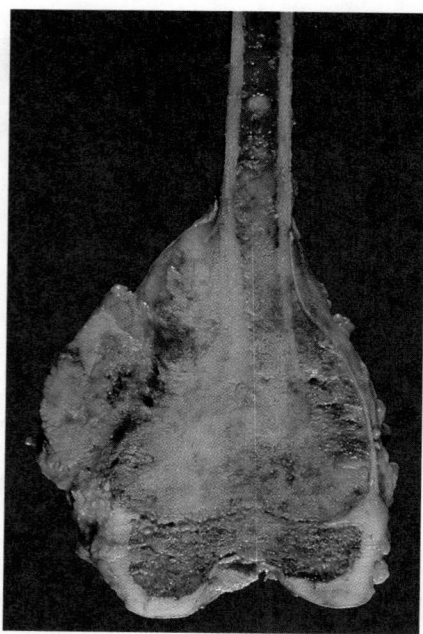

FIG. 62-3 Osteogenic sarcoma in the femur. Bone cortex has been destroyed.

Clinical manifestations of osteogenic sarcoma are usually associated with a gradual onset of pain and swelling, especially around the knee. A minor injury does not cause the neoplasm but may bring the preexisting condition to medical attention. The neoplasm grows rapidly and can restrict joint motion if the tumor is close to a joint structure. The diagnosis is confirmed from biopsied tissue specimens; elevation of serum alkaline phosphatase and calcium levels; and findings on x-ray, CT or positron emission tomogram (PET) scans, and MRI. Metastasis is present in 10% to 20% of individuals on diagnosis, with the lung being the most frequent site.

Major advances continue to be made in the treatment of osteosarcoma. Preoperative (neoadjuvant) chemotherapy is used to decrease tumor size. As a result, limb-salvage procedures, including a wide surgical resection of the tumor, are being used more often. Limb-salvage procedures are considered when there is a clear 6- to 7-cm margin surrounding the lesion. Limb salvage is contraindicated if there is major neurovascular involvement, pathologic fracture, infection, skeletal immaturity, or extensive muscle involvement.[9] Quality-of-life considerations also factor in the decision of limb salvage compared with amputation. Current use of adjunct chemotherapy following amputation has increased the projected 5-year survival rate to 60%.[10] Chemotherapeutic agents include methotrexate, doxorubicin (Adriamycin), cisplatin (Platinol), cyclophosphamide (Cytoxan), bleomycin (Blenoxane), dactinomycin (Cosmegen), and ifosfamide (Ifex).

OSTEOCLASTOMA

Osteoclastoma (*giant cell tumor*) is a destructive tumor that arises in the cancellous ends of long bones in young adults. Most (98%) of these variant giant cell tumors are benign, but they can be locally aggressive and spread to the lungs. Giant cell tumors most commonly occur in females between the ages of 20 and 35. Common tumor sites are in the distal ends of the femur, tibia, and radius.[11] Clinical manifestations are usually swelling, local pain,

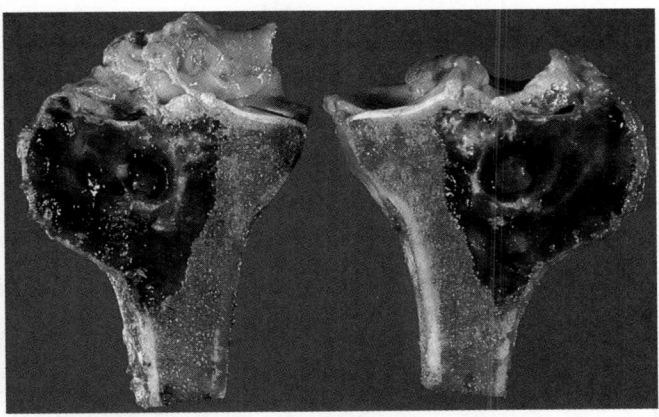

FIG. 62-4 Osteoclastoma (giant cell tumor) in a long bone.

and some disturbances in joint function. X-ray evidence of giant cell tumor is variable but usually reveals local areas of bone destruction and eventual expansion of the bone ends (Fig. 62-4).

Biopsy is used to establish the diagnosis. After diagnosis, surgical curettage of the tumor is usually done, followed by bone grafting. Cryosurgery aids to preserve joint motion and reduce the need for amputation. Complications from cryosurgery include future pathologic fracture and delayed union. After treatment there is a greater than 50% chance of recurrence. Recurrent giant cell tumors may have to be treated with amputation.

EWING'S SARCOMA

Ewing's sarcoma is one of the most common primary malignant neoplasms of bone and soft tissue. It occurs more often in males during periods of rapid bone growth (5 to 15 years of age). This neoplasm is characterized by rapid growth within the medullary cavity of long bone, especially the femur, humerus, pelvis, and tibia. Metastasis occurs early, and the most frequent site is the lungs. Common manifestations are progressive local pain, swelling, palpable soft tissue mass, noticeable increase in size of the affected part, fever, and leukocytosis. Initially, x-rays, CT, and MRI show periosteal bone destruction. Bone biopsy confirms the diagnosis. Treatment usually involves radiation therapy and wide surgical resection of the tumor or amputation. Multidrug chemotherapy has improved survival rates. Chemotherapeutic agents commonly used are cyclophosphamide (Cytoxan), vincristine (Oncovin), ifosfamide (Ifex), doxorubicin (Adriamycin), etoposide (VePesid), and dactinomycin (Cosmegen). These drugs are also used in treating metastatic Ewing's sarcoma.[12] Surgical resection of the tumor has helped decrease the rate of recurrence. The use of radiation, surgical resection, and chemotherapy has increased the 5-year survival rate to 60%.[13]

METASTATIC BONE DISEASE

The most common type of malignant bone tumor occurs as a result of metastasis from a primary tumor. Common sites for the primary tumor include the breast, prostate, gastrointestinal tract, lungs, kidney, ovary, and thyroid.[14] Metastatic cancer cells travel to other sites from the primary tumor via the lymph and blood. The metastatic bone lesion is commonly found in the vertebrae, pelvis, femur, humerus, or ribs. Pathologic fractures at the site of metastasis are common because of weakening of the involved bone.

Once a primary lesion has been identified, radionuclide bone scans are often done to detect the presence of metastatic lesions before they are visible on x-ray. It is important to note that metastatic bone lesions may occur at any time (even years later) following diagnosis and treatment of the primary tumor. Metastasis to the bone should be suspected in any patient who has local bone pain and a past history of cancer. Treatment may be palliative and consists of pain management and radiation. Surgical stabilization of the fracture may be indicated if there is a fracture or pending fracture. Prognosis depends on the extent of metastasis and location.

NURSING MANAGEMENT
BONE CANCER

■ Nursing Assessment

The patient with bone cancer should be assessed for the location and severity of pain. Weakness caused by anemia and decreased mobility may also be noted. Swelling at the involved site and decreased joint function, depending on the tumor site, should also be monitored.

■ Nursing Diagnoses

Nursing diagnoses for the patient with bone cancer may include, but are not limited to, the following:

- Acute pain *related to* the disease process or inadequate pain medication or comfort measures
- Impaired physical mobility *related to* disease process, pain, weakness, and debility
- Disturbed body image *related to* possible amputation, deformity, swelling, and effects of chemotherapy
- Anticipatory grieving *related to* poor prognosis of the disease
- Risk for injury *related to* disease process, possible pathologic fracture, or inadequate handling or positioning of affected body part
- Impaired home maintenance *related to* lack of knowledge about care needed at home or how to perform the necessary skills

■ Planning

The overall goals are that the patient with bone cancer will (1) have satisfactory pain relief; (2) maintain preferred activities as long as possible; (3) demonstrate acceptance of body image changes resulting from chemotherapy, radiation, and surgery; (4) e free from injury; and (5) verbalize a realistic idea of disease progression and prognosis.

■ Nursing Implementation

Health Promotion. The nurse should teach the public to recognize the warning signs of bone cancer, including swelling, bone pain of unexplained origin, limitation of joint function, and changes in skin temperature. As with all forms of cancer, health promotion should stress the importance of periodic screening and health examinations.

Acute Intervention. Nursing care of the patient with a malignant bone neoplasm does not differ significantly from the care given to the patient with a malignant disease of any other body system (see Chapter 15). However, special attention is required to reduce the complications associated with prolonged bed rest and to prevent falls and pathologic fractures. Careful handling and support of the affected extremity and logrolling for those on bed rest is important to prevent pathologic fractures.[15] The patient is often reluctant to participate in therapeutic activities because of weakness from the disease and treatment and fear of pain. Regular rest periods should be provided between activities.

Ambulatory and Home Care. The nurse must be able to assist the patient and family in accepting the guarded prognosis associated with bone neoplasms. Inability to accomplish age-specific developmental tasks can increase the frustrations with this condition. General principles related to cancer nursing are applicable (see Chapter 15). Special attention is necessary for the problems of pain and disability, chemotherapy, and specific surgery such as spinal cord decompression or amputation.

■ Evaluation

The expected outcomes are that the patient with bone cancer will

- have minimal to no pain
- have no falls
- have no pathologic fractures
- accept changes in body image
- retain dignity and active participation in treatment decisions
- have maximal functional ability

Muscular Dystrophy

Muscular dystrophy (MD) is a group of genetically transmitted diseases characterized by progressive symmetric wasting of skeletal muscle without evidence of neurologic involvement. In all forms of MD an insidious loss of strength occurs with increasing disability and deformity. The types of MD differ in the groups of muscles affected, age of onset, rate of progression, and mode of genetic inheritance.[16] Types of MD are presented in Table 62-3.

Duchenne and Becker MD are sex-linked recessive disorders usually seen only in males. In these disorders there is a genetic mutation of the dystrophin gene. Dystrophin in normal muscle cells helps to attach skeletal muscle fibers to the basement membrane. Abnormalities in dystrophin can lead to defects in the plasma membrane of muscle fiber with subsequent muscle fiber degeneration.

Diagnostic studies for MD include muscle serum enzymes (especially creatine kinase), electromyogram (EMG) testing, muscle fiber biopsy, electrocardiogram abnormalities reflective of cardiomyopathy, and genetic pedigree (see Chapter 13). Mus-

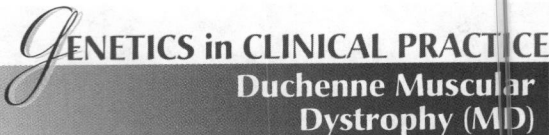

GENETICS in CLINICAL PRACTICE
Duchenne Muscular Dystrophy (MD)

Genetic Basis
- Sex-linked recessive disorder

Incidence
- About 30 in 100,000 males

Genetic Testing
- DNA testing for mutation in dystrophin gene

Clinical Implications
- Duchenne MD is present at birth but does not usually become clinically apparent until at least age 3.
- Very few individuals with the disease live to adulthood.
- Genetic testing and counseling should be considered in individuals with a family history of Duchenne MD.
- Because there are many types of MD with different genetic bases, establishing the type of MD is important to determine treatment and possible genetic counseling recommendations.

cle biopsy confirms the diagnosis with classic findings of fat and connective tissue deposits, degeneration and necrosis of muscle fibers, and a deficiency of the muscle protein dystrophin.[17]

Presently, no definitive therapy is available to stop the progressive wasting of MD. Corticosteroid therapy may significantly halt the disease progression for up to 3 years. The goal of treatment is to preserve mobility and independence through exercise, physical therapy, and orthopedic appliances. The nurse should encourage communication among family members (and parents) to cope with the emotional and physical strains of MD. An emphasis should be placed on teaching the patient and family range-of-motion exercises, nutrition, and signs of progression. Genetic testing and counseling may be recommended for individuals with a family history of MD.

Nursing care should focus on keeping the patient active as long as possible. Prolonged bed rest should be avoided because immobility can lead to further muscle wasting. As the disease progresses, the focus will shift to teaching the patient to limit sedentary periods when skin integrity or respiratory complications could develop. Ongoing medical and nursing care will be required throughout the individual's lifetime.

TABLE 62-3	Types of Muscular Dystrophy	
TYPE	**GENETIC BASIS**	**CLINICAL MANIFESTATIONS**
Duchenne (pseudohypertrophic)	X-linked Mutation of dystrophin gene	Onset before age 5; progressive weakness of pelvic and shoulder muscles; unable to walk after age 12; cardiomyopathy; respiratory failure in second or third decade; mental impairment
Becker (benign pseudohypertrophic)	X-linked Mutation of dystrophin gene	Onset between 5 and 15 years; slower course of pelvic and shoulder muscle wasting than Duchenne; cardiomyopathy; respiratory failure; may survive into fourth or fifth decade
Landouzy-Dejerine (facioscapulohumeral)	Autosomal dominant deletion of chromosome 4q35	Onset before age 20; slowly progressive weakness of face, shoulder muscles, and foot dorsiflexion; deafness
Erb (limb-girdle)	Autosomal recessive or autosomal dominant	Onset ranges from early childhood to early adulthood; slow progressive weakness of shoulder and hip muscles

Low Back Pain

Etiology and Pathophysiology

Low back pain is common and has probably affected about 80% of adults in the United States at least once during their lifetime. Backache is second only to headache as the most common pain complaint.[18] Low back pain in persons under age 45 is responsible for more lost working hours than any other medical condition and represents one of the nation's most costly health problems.[19] Low back pain is a common problem because the lumbar region (1) bears most of the weight of the body, (2) is the most flexible region of the spinal column, (3) contains nerve roots that are vulnerable to injury or disease, and (4) has an inherently poor biomechanical structure.

Several risk factors are associated with low back pain, including lack of muscle tone and excess body weight, poor posture, cigarette smoking, and stress. Jobs that require repetitive heavy lifting, vibration (such as a jackhammer operator), and prolonged periods of sitting are also associated with low back pain.

Low back pain is most often due to a musculoskeletal problem. The causes of low back pain of musculoskeletal origin include (1) acute lumbosacral strain, (2) instability of lumbosacral bony mechanism, (3) osteoarthritis of the lumbosacral vertebrae, (4) intervertebral disk degeneration, and (5) herniation of the intervertebral disk. Of these, the most common cause is mechanical strain of paravertebral muscles. Herniation of the nucleus pulposus is another common cause of low back pain. Other causes include metabolic, circulatory, gynecologic, urologic, or psychologic problems.

ACUTE LOW BACK PAIN

Acute low back pain lasts 4 weeks or less. Acute low back pain is usually associated with some type of activity that causes undue stress (often hyperflexion) on the tissues of the lower back. Often symptoms do not appear at the time of injury but develop later because of a gradual increase in paravertebral muscle spasms. Few definitive diagnostic abnormalities are present with paravertebral muscle strain. One test is the straight-leg raise, which may produce pain in the lumbar area without radiation along the sciatic nerve. MRI and CT scans are generally not done unless trauma or systemic disease (e.g., cancer, spinal infection) is suspected.

Collaborative Care

If the acute muscle spasms and accompanying pain are not severe and debilitating, the patient may be treated on an outpatient basis with a combination of the following: (1) analgesics, such as NSAIDs; (2) muscle relaxants (e.g., cyclobenzaprine [Flexeril]); (3) massage and back manipulation; and (4) the daytime use of a corset. Severe pain may require a brief course of narcotic analgesics. A corset prevents rotation, flexion, and extension of the lower back.

A brief period (1 to 2 days) of rest at home may be necessary for some persons, whereas others do better with a continuation of regular activities.[18] The effectiveness of invasive treatments, such as epidural corticosteroid injections and implanted devices that deliver pain medication, remains controversial.[20] All patients during this time should avoid activities that aggravate the pain, including lifting, bending, twisting, and prolonged sitting. Most cases spontaneously improve within 2 weeks.

NURSING MANAGEMENT
ACUTE LOW BACK PAIN

■ Nursing Assessment

Subjective and objective data that should be obtained from the patient with low back pain are summarized in Table 62-4.

■ Nursing Diagnoses

Nursing diagnoses for the patient with low back pain may include, but are not limited to, those presented in NCP 62-2.

■ Planning

The overall goals are that the patient with low back pain will (1) have satisfactory pain relief, (2) avoid constipation secondary to medication and immobility, (3) learn back-sparing practices, and (4) return to previous level of activity within prescribed restrictions.

TABLE 62-4	Nursing Assessment — Low Back Pain

Subjective Data
Important Health Information
Past health history: Acute or chronic lumbosacral strain, osteoarthritis, degenerative disk disease, obesity
Medications: Use of analgesics, muscle relaxants, nonsteroidal antiinflammatory drugs, corticosteroids, over-the-counter remedies including herbal products and nutritional supplements
Surgery or other treatments: Previous back surgery, epidural corticosteroid injections
Functional Health Patterns
Health perception–health management: Smoking, lack of exercise
Nutritional-metabolic: Obesity
Activity-exercise: Poor posture, muscle spasms; activity intolerance
Elimination: Constipation
Sleep-rest: Interrupted sleep
Cognitive-perceptual: Pain in back, buttocks, or leg associated with walking, turning, straining, coughing, leg raising; numbness or tingling of legs, feet, toes
Role-relationship: Occupation requiring heavy lifting, vibrations, or extended driving

Objective Data
General
Guarded movement
Neurologic
Depressed or absent Achilles tendon reflex; positive straight-leg raise test
Musculoskeletal
Tense, tight paravertebral muscles on palpation, decreased range of motion of spine
Possible Findings
Localization of site of lesion or disorder on myelogram, CT scan, or MRI; determination of nerve irritation on electromyography

CT, Computed tomography; *MRI,* magnetic resonance imaging.

NURSING CARE PLAN 62–2

Patient with Low Back Pain

ACUTE MANAGEMENT

EXPECTED PATIENT OUTCOMES	NURSING INTERVENTIONS and *RATIONALES*
NURSING DIAGNOSIS	**Acute pain** *related to* herniated nucleus pulposus, muscle spasms, and ineffective comfort measures *as manifested by* verbalization of back pain on movement, guarded movements, palpable muscle spasm, decreased physical activity, rating pain as >4 on a 10-point pain scale.
• Reduction or absence of pain and muscle spasms • Expression of satisfaction with pain relief (rates pain as <4 on pain scale of 10)	• Assess location, severity, and characteristics of pain *to plan appropriate interventions.* • Use a pain scale and evaluate pain relief interventions *to assess pain and treatment measures.* • Enforce decreased activity *to reduce paravertebral muscle spasms and resulting pain.* • Keep head of bed elevated 20 degrees and knee of bed flexed *to promote comfort by reducing stress on lower back muscles.* • Apply moist heat or ice to lower back *to reduce pain and muscle spasm.* • Administer analgesics, nonsteroidal antiinflammatory drugs, and/or muscle relaxants as ordered; document effect *to promote comfort and evaluate effectiveness.*
NURSING DIAGNOSIS	**Impaired physical mobility** *related to* pain *as manifested by* limited active joint range of motion (ROM), movement restrictions, muscle spasms.
• Unrestricted gait • Ambulation within normal limits • Resumption of previous level of mobility • Performance of prescribed exercises	• Have patient perform ROM and muscle-strengthening exercises daily *to strengthen the supporting muscles and maintain all joints in normal ROM.* • Start ambulation program and progress with assistance *to promote gradual and progressive return to previous mobility level.* • Avoid having patient bend, sit, or lift *to prevent back strain and increased pain.* • Provide written instructions that describe each exercise and activity and a phone number to call with any questions.

CHRONIC MANAGEMENT

EXPECTED PATIENT OUTCOMES	NURSING INTERVENTIONS and *RATIONALES*
NURSING DIAGNOSIS	**Chronic pain** *related to* progression of problem *as manifested by* verbal report or evidence of pain longer than 6 months in duration.
• Development of effective methods of managing pain • Expression of satisfaction with pain control measures	• Assess variety and effectiveness of pain management techniques *to determine extent of problem and develop appropriate interventions.* • Use a pain scale *to assess pain and to evaluate pain control interventions.* • Instruct patient and family about home care and alternative methods of pain control, including use of heat, transcutaneous electrical nerve stimulation *to provide information about supplementary methods of pain management.* • Assist in identifying activities that exacerbate pain *to make adjustments so that pain is reduced.*
NURSING DIAGNOSIS	**Ineffective coping** *related to* effects of chronic pain *as manifested by* verbalization of inability to cope, irritability, tension, inability to meet role expectations, altered participation in social events, ineffective or inappropriate use of defense mechanisms.
• Return to previous levels of work and lifestyle or successfully adapt to lifestyle changes	• Explain factors that may contribute to development of maladaptive coping behavior *to communicate information and a caring attitude.* • Discuss how to develop therapeutic coping skills that enhance self-esteem and social interaction *to foster effective coping behaviors and adjustment to chronic pain.*
NURSING DIAGNOSIS	**Ineffective therapeutic regimen management** *related to* lack of knowledge regarding posture, exercises, body mechanics, and weight reduction *as manifested by* lack of necessary knowledge to participate in treatment plan, inadequate understanding, or inaccurate follow-through of previous instructions.
• Use of proper body mechanics at all times • Maintenance of weight within normal limits • Maintenance of activity and ambulation appropriate to age and state of health	• Assess body mechanics *to identify incorrect techniques and intervene appropriately.* • Instruct patient on proper body mechanics and use of firm mattress or bed board *to reduce risk of reinjury, provide back support, and maintain proper body alignment.* • Assess for decreasing muscle strength *to identify complications and modify care plan.* • Refer to physical therapist for low back exercises *to develop abdominal and paravertebral muscle strength to provide increased support.* • Encourage activity and ambulation within limitations *to maintain physical mobility.* • Teach about weight reduction and/or refer to dietitian if indicated *because increased abdominal weight puts strain on low back.*

■ Nursing Implementation

Health Promotion. The nurse is a significant role model and teacher for patients with low back problems. As a role model, the nurse should use proper body mechanics at all times. This should be a primary consideration when teaching patients and health care providers transfer and turning techniques. The nurse should assess the patient's use of body mechanics and offer advice when activities that could produce back strain are used (Table 62-5).

Some health care providers refer patients with back pain to a program called "Back School." It is a formal program usually taught by health professionals such as physicians, nurses, and physical therapists. It is designed to teach the patient how to minimize back pain and avoid repeat episodes of low back pain. Tips for prevention of back injury are listed in Table 62-5. Exercises to strengthen the back are presented in Table 62-6.

Patients are also advised to maintain appropriate body weight. Excess body weight places extra stress on the lower back and weakens the abdominal muscles that support the lower back.

The position assumed while sleeping is also important in preventing low back pain. Sleeping in a prone position should be avoided because it produces excessive lumbar lordosis, placing excessive stress on the lower back. A firm mattress is recommended. The patient should sleep in either a supine or side-lying position with the knees and hips flexed to prevent unnecessary pressure on support muscles, ligamentous structures, and lumbosacral joints. Patients should be educated about the necessity to avoid or cease smoking. Nicotine has been shown to decrease circulation to the vertebral disks, and a causal relationship exists between smoking and some types of low back pain.[21]

Acute Intervention. The primary nursing responsibilities in acute low back pain are to assist the patient to maintain activity limitations, promote comfort, and educate the patient about the health problem and appropriate exercises. Other nursing interventions are summarized in NCP 62-2. Use of analgesics, NSAIDs, thermotherapy (ice and heat), and muscle relaxants to promote comfort is incorporated into the plan of care.

Muscle stretching and strengthening exercises may be part of the management plan. Although the actual exercises are often taught by the physical therapist, it is the nurse's responsibility to ensure that the patient understands the type and frequency of exercise prescribed, as well as the rationale for the program.

Ambulatory and Home Care. The goal of management is to make an episode of acute low back pain an isolated incident. If the lumbosacral mechanism is unstable, repeated episodes can be anticipated. The lumbosacral spine may be unable to meet the demands placed on it without strain because of factors such as obesity, poor posture, poor muscular support, advancing age, or local trauma. Intervention is aimed at strengthening the supporting muscles by exercise. The use of a corset limits extremes of movement. In addition, weight reduction decreases the mechanical demands on the lower back.

Persistent use of poor body mechanics may result in repeated episodes of low back pain. If the strain is work related, occupa-

---

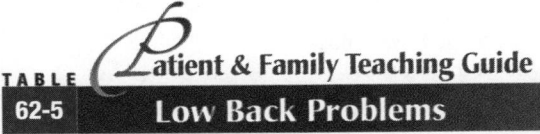

TABLE 62-5

*P*atient & Family Teaching Guide
Low Back Problems

Do Not

- Lean forward without bending knees
- Lift anything above level of elbows
- Stand in one position for prolonged time
- Sleep on abdomen or on back or side with legs out straight
- Exercise without consulting health care provider if having severe pain
- Exceed prescribed amount and type of exercises without consulting health care provider

Do

- Prevent lower back from straining forward by placing a foot on a step or stool during prolonged standing
- Sleep in a side-lying position with knees and hips bent
- Sleep on back with a lift under knees and legs or on back with 10-inch-high pillow under knees to flex hips and knees
- Sit in a chair with knees higher than hips and support arms on chair or knees
- Exercise 15 min in the morning and 15 min in the evening regularly; begin exercises with a 2- or 3-min warm-up period by moving arms and legs, by alternately relaxing and tightening muscles; exercise slowly with smooth movements as directed by a physical therapist
- Avoid chilling during and after exercising
- Maintain appropriate body weight
- Use local heat and cold application
- Use a lumbar roll or pillow for sitting

---

*E*VIDENCE-BASED PRACTICE
Nonspecific Low Back Pain

Clinical Problem

Are back schools and/or massage effective for patients with nonspecific low back pain?

Best Clinical Practice

- Evidence exists that back schools have better short-term effects than other treatments for chronic low back pain.
- Evidence exists that back schools in an occupational setting are more effective than placebo or wait-list control groups.
- Insufficient evidence exists to recommend massage as a stand-alone treatment for nonspecific low back pain.

Implications for Nursing Practice

- Back schools usually involve information-giving interventions where patients are taught about anatomy and function of the back, mechanical strain, and posture. Isometric exercises for abdominal muscles and physical activity programs are also taught.
- Back schools may be effective for patients with recurrent and chronic low back pain, especially in occupational settings. Little is known about the cost-effectiveness of back schools.
- Additional high-quality controlled trials are needed to evaluate the effects of massage for nonspecific low back pain.

References for Evidence

Furlan AD et al: Massage for low back pain, Cochrane Back Review Group, *Cochrane Database Syst Rev,* issue 1, 2002.

Tulder MW et al: Back schools for non-specific low back pain, Cochrane Back Review Group, *Cochrane Database Syst Rev,* issue 1, 2002.

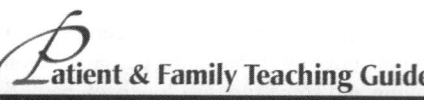

TABLE
62-6

Patient & Family Teaching Guide

Back Exercises

Knee-to-chest lift (to stretch hip, buttocks, lower back muscles)
- Lie on back on the floor with knees bent and feet flat on floor.
- Draw both knees up to chest.
- Place both hands around knees and pull them firmly against chest. Hold for 30 seconds.
- Lower legs and return to starting position.
- Repeat 5-10 times.

Simple leg lift
- Lie flat on back on floor with left knee bent and left foot flat on floor.
- Raise right leg as high as comfortably possible.
- Hold for 5 counts.
- Slowly return leg to floor.
- Bend right knee and put right foot flat on floor.
- Raise left leg and hold for 5 counts.
- Repeat 5-10 times for each leg.

Double leg lift
- Lie flat on back.
- Slowly lift legs until feet are 12 inches from the floor.
- Keep legs straight and hold this position for 10 counts.
- Lower legs to floor.
- Repeat 5 times.

Pelvic tilt
- Lie flat on back on floor with knees bent and feet flat on the floor.
- Firmly tighten your buttock muscles.
- Hold for 5 counts.
- Relax buttocks.
- Repeat 5-10 times.
- Be sure to keep lower back flat against floor.

Half sit-ups (to strengthen abdominal muscles)
- Lie flat on floor on back with knees bent, feet flat on floor, and hands on chest.
- Slowly raise head and neck to top of chest.
- Reach both hands forward and place them on knees.
- Hold for 5 counts.
- Return to starting position.
- Repeat 5-10 times.

Elbow props (to extend lower back)
- Lie face down with your arms beside your body and your head turned to one side.
- Stay in this position for 2-5 minutes, making sure that you relax completely.
- Remain face down and prop yourself on your elbows.
- Hold this position for 2-3 minutes.
- Return to starting position and relax for 1 minute.
- Repeat 5-10 times.

Hip tilts
- Lie flat on back with knees bent.
- Slowly bend legs and hips to one side as far as possible.
- Bend to other side.
- Repeat 5 times.

Toe touches
- Stand straight and relaxed.
- Lower head and body and try to touch floor with fingertips.
- Keep knees straight.
- Do not jerk or lunge toward floor.
- Bend only as far as you can.
- Repeat 5 times.

From Canobbio MM: *Mosby's handbook of patient teaching*, ed 2, St Louis, 2000, Mosby.

tional counseling may be necessary. The frustration, pain, and disability imposed on the patient with low back pain require emotional support and understanding care by the nurse.

■ Evaluation

The expected outcomes for the patient with low back pain are presented in NCP 62-2.

CHRONIC LOW BACK PAIN

Chronic back pain lasts more than 3 months or is a repeated incapacitating episode. The causes of chronic low back pain include degenerative disk disease, lack of physical exercise, prior injury, obesity, structural and postural abnormalities, and systemic disease. Osteoarthritis (OA) of the lumbar spine is found in patients over 50, whereas chronic back pain in younger patients with OA usually involves the thoracic or lumbar spine.[2] Periods of inactivity, particularly on awakening or after long periods of sitting, increase the discomfort.

Treatment regimens are much the same as acute low back pain: a reduction in the pain associated with daily activities, a formal back pain program, and ongoing medical care. Cold, damp weather aggravates the back pain but can be relieved with rest and local heat application. Relief of pain and stiffness by the use of mild analgesics, such as NSAIDs, is integral to the daily comfort of the individual with chronic low back pain. Weight reduction, sufficient rest periods, local heat or cold application, and exercise and activity throughout the day help to keep the muscles and joints mobilized.

Surgery may be indicated in patients with severe chronic low back pain who do not respond to conservative care and/or have continued neurologic deficits.[22] (Surgery for low back pain is discussed on p. 1704.)

HERNIATED INTERVERTEBRAL DISK

Etiology and Pathophysiology

An intervertebral disk is interposed between the adjacent surfaces of vertebral bodies from the cervical axis to the sacrum. An acute **herniated intervertebral disk** (slipped disk) can be the result of natural degeneration with age or repeated stress and trauma to the spine. The nucleus pulposus (gelatinous center of the disk) may rupture to cause acute injury and back pain. The most common sites of rupture are the lumbosacral disks, specifically L4-5 and L5-S1. Disk herniation may also occur at C5-6 and C6-7.

COMPLEMENTARY &ALTERNATIVE THERAPIES
Acupuncture

Acupuncture is a traditional Chinese medical practice of inserting very fine needles into the skin to stimulate specific anatomic points in the body (called acupoints) for therapeutic purposes. Used to regulate the flow of Qi (life force or energy), the acupuncture needles unblock the obstruction of Qi through the meridians (see Chapter 7).

Clinical Uses

Lower back pain and other types of pain. Postoperative and chemotherapy-associated nausea and vomiting. Addiction, stroke rehabilitation, menstrual cramps, fibromyalgia, and myofascial pain. Table 7-2 on p. 98 lists other conditions that may benefit from acupuncture.

Effects

Release of endorphins, activation of the hypothalamus and pituitary gland, and alterations in the levels of neurotransmitters.

Nursing Implications

Acupuncture is considered a safe therapy when (1) the practitioner has been appropriately trained and (2) the practitioner uses sterilized or disposable needles. Acupuncture should be used with caution with those who have a history of seizures; are carriers of hepatitis B or have chronic hepatitis C; or have human immunodeficiency viral infection, bleeding disorders, thrombocytopenia, or skin infections.

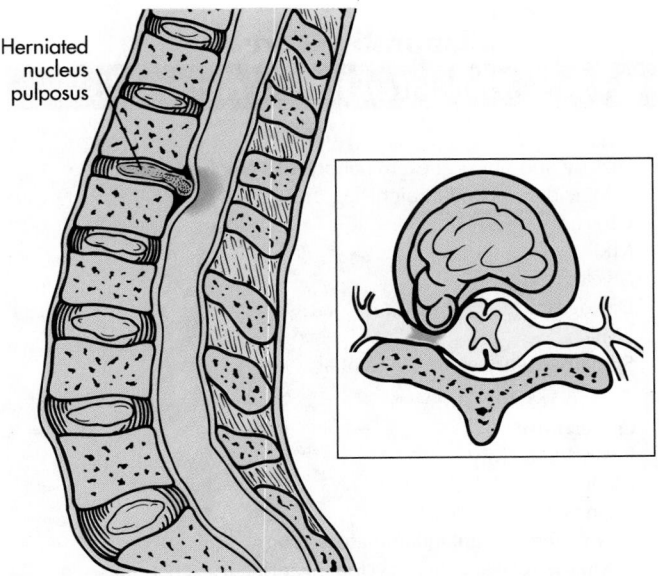

FIG. 62-5   Compression of spinal cord caused by herniation of nucleus pulposus into spinal cord. *Inset,* Pressure on nerves as they leave the spinal canal.

Herniated nucleus pulposus

Structural degeneration of the intervertebral disk is a result of degenerative disk disease. The degeneration results in intervertebral narrowing and a lessening of the efficiency of the intervertebral disks in acting as shock absorbers. As stress on the degenerated disk continues and eventually exceeds the strength of the disk, herniation of the intervertebral disk may result. Compression of the nerve roots and cord may then occur (Fig. 62-5).

Clinical Manifestations

The most common feature of a lumbar herniated disk is low back pain, radiating down the buttock and below the knee, along the distribution of the sciatic nerve *(radiculopathy)*. (Specific manifestations based on the level of lumbar disk herniation are summarized in Table 62-7.) The straight-leg raise test may be positive, indicating nerve root irritation. Back or leg pain may be reproduced by raising the leg and flexing the foot at 90 degrees. Low back pain from other causes may not be accompanied by leg pain. Reflexes may be depressed or absent, depending on the spinal nerve root involved. Paresthesia or muscle weakness in the legs, feet, or toes may be reported by the patient. Multiple nerve root (cauda equina) compression may be manifested as bowel and bladder incontinence or impotence.

Diagnostic Studies

X-rays are done to note any structural defects. A myelogram, MRI, or CT scan is helpful in localizing the site of herniation. An epidural venogram or diskogram may be necessary if other methods of diagnosis are unsuccessful. An EMG of the extremities can be performed to determine the severity of nerve irritation caused by herniation or to rule out other pathologic conditions such as peripheral neuropathy.

Collaborative Care

The patient with a suspected disk herniation is usually managed first with conservative therapy (Table 62-8). This includes limitation of extremes of spinal movement (brace, corset, or belt), local heat or ice, ultrasound and massage, traction, and

TABLE 62-7	**Neurologic Assessment of Herniated Intervertebral Disk***			
INTERVERTEBRAL LEVEL	**SUBJECTIVE PAIN**	**AFFECTED REFLEX**	**MOTOR FUNCTION**	**SENSATION**
L3-L4	Back to buttocks to posterior thigh to inner calf	Patellar	Quadriceps, anterior tibialis	Inner aspect of lower leg, anterior part of thigh
L4-L5	Back to buttocks to dorsum of foot and big toe	None	Anterior tibialis, extensor hallucis longus, gluteus medius	Dorsum of foot and big toe
L5-S1	Back to buttocks to sole of foot and heel	Achilles	Gastrocnemius, hamstring, gluteus maximus	Heel and lateral foot

*A disk herniation can involve pressure on more than one nerve root.

TABLE 62-8 Collaborative Care
Herniated Intervertebral Disk

Diagnostic
History and physical examination with emphasis on neuro-
   logic deficits and straight-leg raising
CT scan
MRI
Myelogram
Diskogram
EMG
Somatosensory evoked potential

Collaborative Therapy
Conservative
Restricted activity
Medication
   Analgesics
   Nonsteroidal antiinflammatory drugs
   Muscle relaxants (e.g., cyclobenzaprine [Flexeril])
Local ice or heat
Physical therapy
Surgical
Laminectomy with or without spinal fusion
Diskectomy
Percutaneous laser diskectomy
Spinal fusion with or without instrumentation

CT, Computed tomography; *EMG,* electromyogram; *MRI,* magnetic resonance imaging.

transcutaneous electrical nerve stimulation. Drug therapy includes NSAIDs, short-term narcotic opioids, and muscle relaxants. Conservative treatment can result in a healing over of the herniated area with a concomitant decrease in pain. Once the symptoms subside, back strengthening exercises are begun twice a day and are encouraged for a lifetime. The patient should be taught the principles of good body mechanics. Extremes of flexion and torsion are strongly discouraged.

Most patients with a herniated disk recover with a conservative treatment plan. However, if conservative treatment is unsuccessful, *radiculopathy* (nerve root pain) becomes progressively worse, or loss of bowel or bladder control (cauda equina) is documented, surgery may then be indicated.

Surgical Therapy. Surgery for disk disease is generally indicated when diagnostic tests point out a herniation not responding to conservative treatment, consistent pain, and/or a persistent neurologic deficit.[23]

The traditional and most common procedure for lumbar disk disease is a *laminectomy.* It involves the surgical excision of part of the posterior arch of the vertebra (referred to as the lamina) to gain access to part or all of the protruding disk to remove it.

A *diskectomy* is another common type of surgical procedure that may be performed to decompress the nerve root. Microsurgical diskectomy is a version of the standard diskectomy in which the surgeon uses a microscope to allow better visualization of the disk and disk space during surgery to aid in the removal of the herniated portion.

A *percutaneous laser diskectomy* is an outpatient surgical procedure using a tube that is passed through the retroperitoneal soft tissues to the lateral border of the disk with local anesthesia and the aid of fluoroscopy. A laser is then used on the herniated portion of the disk. Small stab wounds are used, and minimal blood loss occurs during the procedure. The procedure is effective and safe and has been shown to decrease rehabilitation time.[24]

A *spinal fusion* may be performed if an unstable bony mechanism is present. The spine is stabilized by creating an ankylosis (fusion) of contiguous vertebrae with a bone graft from the patient's fibula or iliac crest or from a donated cadaver bone. Metal fixation with rods, plates, or screws may be implanted at the time of spinal surgery to provide more stability and decrease vertebral motion. A posterior lumbar interbody fusion may be performed in patients to provide extra support for bone grafting or a prosthetic device. A new device, the InFuse Bone Graft/LT-CAGE, is being used to eliminate the need to use bone from the patient in grafting. The device contains genetically engineered protein that stimulates the body to grow new bone at the spinal fusion site.[25]

NURSING MANAGEMENT
SPINAL SURGERY

Postoperative nursing interventions focus on maintaining proper alignment of the spine at all times until healing has occurred. Flat bed rest may be maintained for 1 to 2 days depending on the extent of surgery. Log rolling patients when turning is essential to maintain proper body alignment. Pillows can be used under the thighs of each leg when supine and between the legs when in the side-lying positions to provide comfort and ensure alignment. The patient often fears turning or any movement that increases pain by straining the surgical area. The nurse must offer reassurance to the patient that the proper technique is being used to maintain body alignment. Sufficient staff should be available to move the patient without undue pain or strain on staff members or the patient.

Postoperatively, most patients will require narcotic opioids such as morphine intravenously for 24 to 48 hours. Patient-controlled analgesia allows for optimal analgesic levels and is the preferred method of continued pain management during this time. Once fluids are being taken, the patient may be switched to oral drugs such as acetaminophen with codeine, hydrocodone (Vicodin), or oxycodone (Percocet). Diazepam (Valium) may be prescribed for muscle relaxation. The nurse should monitor pain management and its effectiveness for at least 3 weeks after the surgery.

Because the spinal canal may be entered during surgery, there is potential for cerebrospinal fluid (CSF) leakage. Severe headache or leakage of CSF on the dressing should be reported immediately. CSF appears as clear or slightly yellow drainage on the dressing. It has a high glucose concentration and will be positive for glucose when a dipstick test is done. The amount and characteristics of drainage should be noted.

Frequent monitoring of peripheral neurologic signs of the extremities is a routine postoperative nursing responsibility after spinal surgery. Movement of the arms and legs and assessment of sensation should be unchanged when compared with the preoperative status. Table 62-9 summarizes a lumbar laminectomy assessment appropriate for the patient who has undergone back

TABLE 62-9	Postoperative Assessment Following Lumbar Surgery

Sensation*
Assess sensation of extremities for paresthesia in all appropriate dermatomes.

Movement*
Assess ability to move all extremities.

Muscle Strength*
Assess for any weakness of the extremities.

Wound
Assess dressing for drainage and note amount, color, characteristics.

Pain
Document location of the pain.
Ask patient to rate the pain on a scale of 1 to 10, with 1 being no pain and 10 being worst pain.
Evaluate pain after analgesia has been administered.

*Postoperative findings should be compared with preoperative assessments. It is not unusual for the patient to continue to experience these symptoms after surgery. Symptoms gradually decrease over several months.

surgery. These assessments are repeated every 2 to 4 hours during the first 48 hours after surgery, and findings are compared with the preoperative assessment. Paresthesias, such as numbness and tingling, may not be relieved immediately after surgery. Any new muscle weakness or paresthesias should be documented and reported to the surgeon immediately.

Paralytic ileus and interference with bowel function may occur for several days and may manifest as nausea, abdominal distention, and constipation. The nurse should assess whether the patient is passing flatus, has bowel sounds in all quadrants, and has a flat, soft abdomen. Stool softeners (e.g., docusate [Colace]) may aid in relieving and preventing constipation.

Adequate bladder emptying may be altered because of activity restrictions, narcotics, or anesthesia. If allowed by the surgeon, men should be encouraged to dangle or stand to urinate. Patients should use the commode or ambulate to the bathroom when allowed to promote adequate emptying of the bladder. The nurse should ensure that privacy is maintained. It is necessary to clarify whether the patient can be allowed up to the bathroom without the corset or brace. Intermittent catheterization or an indwelling catheter may be necessary for patients who have difficulty urinating.

Loss of sphincter tone or bladder tone may indicate nerve damage. Incontinence or difficulty evacuating the bowel or bladder must be monitored closely and reported to the surgeon.

Activity prescriptions vary with surgeons, but the patient who has had spinal surgery usually ambulates early in the postoperative period. It is a nursing responsibility to know the specific orders related to activity for any patient.

In addition to the nursing care appropriate for a patient who has had a laminectomy, there are other nursing responsibilities if the patient has also had a spinal fusion. Because a bone graft is usually involved, the postoperative healing time is prolonged compared with that of a laminectomy. Immobilization over an extended time may

be necessary. A rigid orthosis (thoracic-lumbar-sacral orthosis or chairback brace) is often used during the period of immobilization. Some surgeons require that the patient be taught to put it on and take it off by log rolling in bed, whereas others allow their patients to apply the brace in a sitting or standing position. The nurse should verify the preferred method before initiating this activity. The extended immobilization required by a spinal fusion carries with it all the potential problems related to immobility.

In addition to the primary surgical site, the donor site for the bone graft must be regularly assessed. The posterior iliac crest is the most commonly used donor site, although the fibula may also be used. The donor site usually causes greater postoperative pain than the fused area. The donor site is bandaged with a pressure dressing to prevent excessive bleeding. If the donor site is the fibula, neurovascular assessments of the extremity are a postoperative nursing responsibility.

As the bone graft heals, the patient must adjust to the permanent immobility at the graft or fusion site. Instruction in proper body mechanics is essential and should be evaluated during the hospital stay.

The patient should be instructed to avoid sitting or standing for prolonged periods. Activities that should be encouraged include walking, lying down, and shifting weight from one foot to the other when standing. The patient should learn to mentally think through an activity before starting any potentially injurious task such as bending, lifting, or stooping. Any twisting movement of the spine is contraindicated. The thighs and knees, rather than the back, should be used to absorb the shock of activity and movement. A firm mattress or bed board is essential.

NECK PAIN

Cervical neck sprains and strains occur from hyperflexion and hyperextension injury. Patients have symptoms of stiffness and neck pain and possible pain radiating into the arm and hand. Pain may also radiate into the head, anterior chest, thoracic spine region, and shoulders. Cervical nerve root compression from degenerative disk disease or herniation may be indicated by weakness or paresthesia of the arm and hand. Diagnosing the cause of neck pain is done by history, physical examination, x-ray, MRI, CT scan, and myelogram. An EMG of the upper extremities is done to diagnose cervical radiculopathy.

Nonoperative treatment options for neck pain include head support via cervical collars, heat applications, massage, physical therapy, ultrasound, and NSAIDs. Surgical intervention on the cervical spine is similar to that performed on the lower back, including a diskectomy, laminectomy, and spinal fusion. If surgery is done on the cervical spine, the nurse must be alert for symptoms of spinal cord edema such as respiratory distress and a worsening neurologic status of the upper extremities. After surgery, the patient's neck is immobilized in either a soft or hard cervical collar.

FOOT DISORDERS

The foot is the platform that provides support for the weight of the body and absorbs considerable shock in ambulation. It is a complicated structure composed of bony structures, muscles, tendons, and ligaments. It can be affected by (1) congenital conditions, (2) structural weakness, (3) traumatic injuries, and (4) systemic conditions such as diabetes mellitus and rheumatoid arthritis. Abnormalities of the foot affect over 80 million persons in the United States. Much of the pain, deformity, and disability associated with foot disorders can be directly attributed to or accentuated by improperly fitting shoes, which cause crowding and angulation of the toes and inhibition of the normal movement of foot muscles. The purposes of footwear are to (1) provide support, foot stability, protection, shock absorption, and a foundation for orthoses; (2) increase friction with the walking surface; and (3) treat foot abnormalities. (Table 62-10 summarizes common foot disorders.) One of the most common forefoot disorders

TABLE 62-10   Common Foot Disorders

DISORDER	DESCRIPTION	TREATMENT
Forefoot		
Hallux valgus (bunion)	Painful deformity of great toe consisting of lateral angulation of great toe toward second toe, bony enlargement of medial side of first metatarsal head, and formation of bursa or callus over bony enlargement (see Fig. 62-6)	Conservative treatment includes wearing shoes with wide forefoot or "bunion pocket" and use of bunion pads to relieve pressure on bursal sac. Surgical treatment is removal of bursal sac and bony enlargement and correction of lateral angulation of great toe; may include temporary or permanent internal fixation.
Hallux rigidus	Painful stiffness of first metatarsophalangeal joint caused by osteoarthritis or local trauma	Conservative treatment includes intraarticular corticosteroids and passive manual stretching of first metatarsophalangeal joint. A shoe with a stiff sole decreases pain in the joint during walking. Surgical treatment is joint fusion or arthroplasty with silicone rubber implant.
Hammertoe	Deformity of second through fifth toes, including dorsiflexion of metatarsophalangeal joint, plantar flexion of proximal interphalangeal joint, and callus on dorsum of proximal interphalangeal joint and end of involved toe; complaints related to hammertoe include burning on bottom of foot and pain and difficulty in walking when wearing shoes	Conservative treatment consists of passive manual stretching of proximal interphalangeal joint and use of metatarsal arch support. Surgical correction consists of resection of base of middle phalanx and head of proximal phalanx and bringing raw bone ends together. Kirschner wire maintains straight position.
Morton's neuroma (Morton's toe or plantar neuroma)	Neuroma in web space between third and fourth metatarsal heads, causing sharp, sudden attacks of pain and burning sensations	Surgical excision is the usual treatment.
Midfoot		
Pes planus (flatfoot)	Loss of metatarsal arch causing pain in foot or leg	Symptoms are relieved by use of resilient longitudinal arch supports. Surgical treatment consists of triple arthrodesis or fusion of subtalar joint.
Pes cavus	Elevation of longitudinal arch of foot resulting from contracture of plantar fascia or bony deformity of arch	Treatment is manipulation and casting (in patients <6 yr of age); surgical correction is necessary if it interferes with ambulation (in patients >6 yr of age).
Hindfoot		
Painful heels	Complaint of heel pain with weight bearing; common cause of plantar bursitis or calcaneal spur in adult	Corticosteroids are injected locally into inflamed bursa and sponge rubber heel cushion is used; surgical excision of bursa or spur is performed.
Local Problems		
Corn	Localized thickening of skin caused by continual pressure over bony prominences, especially metatarsal head, frequently causing localized pain	Corn is softened with warm water or preparations containing salicylic acid and trimmed with razor blade or scalpel. Pressure on bony prominences caused by shoes is relieved.
Soft corn	Painful lesion caused by bony prominence of one toe pressing against adjacent toe; usual location in web space between toes; softness caused by secretions keeping web space relatively moist	Pain is relieved by placing cotton between toes to separate them. Surgical treatment is excision of projecting bone spur (if present).
Callus	Similar formation to corn but covering of wider area and usual location on weight-bearing part of foot	Same as for corn.
Plantar wart	Painful papillomatous growth caused by virus that may occur on any part of skin on sole of foot	Excision with electrocoagulation or surgical removal is done; ultrasound may also be used.

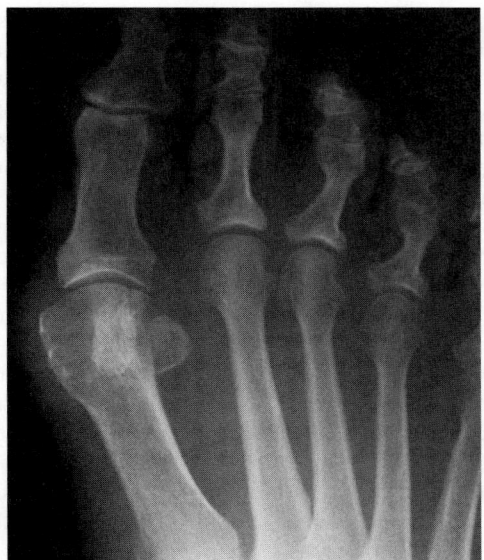

FIG. 62-6 Hallux valgus, with bunion of the great toe.

is a bunion (Fig. 62-6). A lateral deviation of the great toe, termed *hallux valgus*, occurs with a bunion.[26]

NURSING MANAGEMENT
FOOT DISORDERS

■ Nursing Implementation

Health Promotion. Well-constructed and properly fitted shoes are essential for healthy, pain-free feet. Fashion styles, especially for women, often influence selection of footwear instead of considerations of comfort and support. Patient teaching should stress the importance of having a shoe that conforms to the foot rather than to current fashion trends. The shoe must be long enough and wide enough to prevent crowding of the toes and forcing of the great toe into a position of hallux valgus. At the metatarsal head, the width of the shoe should be sufficient to allow free movement of the foot muscles and permit bending of the toes. The shank (narrow part of sole under the instep) of the shoe should be rigid enough to give optimal support. The height of the heel should be realistic in relation to the purpose for which the shoe is worn. Ideally, the heel of the shoe should not rise more than 1 inch higher than the forefoot support.

Acute Intervention. Many foot problems require referral to a podiatrist. Depending on the problem, conservative therapy is usually tried first (Table 62-10). These therapies include NSAIDs, shock-wave therapy, icing, physical therapy, alterations in foot wear, stretching, warm soaks, ultrasound, and corticosteroid injections. If these methods do not offer relief, surgery may then be recommended.

When surgery is performed, the foot is usually immobilized by a bulky dressing, short leg cast, slipper (plaster) cast, or a platform "shoe" that fits over the dressing and has a rigid sole (known as a bunion boot). The foot should be elevated with the heel off the bed to help reduce discomfort and prevent edema. The neurovascular status should be assessed frequently during the immediate postoperative period. Depending on the type of surgery, pins or wires may extend through the toes, or a protec-

tive splint that extends over the end of the foot may be in place. Care must be taken not to jar these devices and cause pain. The devices may interfere with or preclude assessment for movement. The nurse should be aware that sensation may be difficult to evaluate because postoperative pain can interfere with the patient's ability to differentiate pain caused by the surgical procedure from pain resulting from nerve pressure or circulatory impairment.

The type and extent of surgery determine the degree of ambulation allowed. Crutches or canes may be necessary. The patient may experience pain or a throbbing sensation when starting ambulation. The nurse should reinforce instructions given by the physical therapist and ensure that the patient does not develop a faulty gait pattern such as walking on the heels in an attempt to avoid excessive pain or pressure. The nurse must reinforce the importance of walking with an erect posture and with proper weight distribution. Dysfunction of gait or continued pain should be reported to the physician. The nurse should instruct the patient on the importance of frequent rest periods with the foot elevated.

Ambulatory and Home Care. Foot care should include daily hygienic care and the wearing of clean stockings. Stockings should be long enough to avoid wrinkling and the development of pressure areas. Trimming toenails straight across helps prevent ingrown toenails and reduces the possibility of infection. Persons with impaired circulation or diabetes mellitus require detailed instruction to prevent serious complications associated with blisters, pressure areas, and infections. (See Table 47-21 for guidelines for foot care.)

■ Gerontologic Considerations: Foot Problems

The older adult is prone to developing foot problems because of poor circulation, atherosclerosis, and decreased sensation in the lower extremities. This is especially a problem for older patients with diabetes mellitus. A patient may develop an open wound but not feel it because of altered sensation. This may be the result of peripheral vascular disease or diabetic neuropathy. Older adults should be instructed to inspect their feet daily and report any open wounds or breaks in the skin to their physician. If left untreated, wounds may become infected, lead to osteomyelitis, and require surgical debridement. If the infection becomes widespread, lower limb amputation may be necessary.[27] ■

Metabolic Bone Diseases

Normal bone metabolism is affected by hormones, nutrition, and hereditary factors. When there is dysfunction in any of these factors, a generalized reduction in bone mass and strength may result. Metabolic bone diseases include osteomalacia, osteoporosis, and Paget's disease.

OSTEOMALACIA

Osteomalacia is a rare condition of adult bone associated with vitamin D deficiency, resulting in decalcification and softening of bone. This disease is the same as rickets in children except that the epiphyseal growth plates are closed in the adult. Vitamin D with its complex actions and method of synthesis is required for the absorption of calcium from the intestine. Insufficient vitamin D intake can interfere with the normal mineralization of bone, causing failure or insufficient calcification of bone, which results in bone softening. Etiologic factors in the development of osteomalacia include lack of exposure to ultraviolet rays (which is needed for vitamin D synthesis), gastrointestinal malabsorption, extensive burns, chronic diarrhea, pregnancy, kidney disease, and drugs such as phenytoin (Dilantin).

The most common clinical feature of osteomalacia is persistent skeletal pain, especially during weight bearing. Other clinical manifestations include low back and bone pain; progressive muscular weakness, especially in the pelvic girdle; weight loss; and progressive deformities of the spine (kyphosis) or extremities. Fractures are common and demonstrate delayed healing when they occur. Mineralization may take 2 to 3 months as opposed to the normal 6 to 10 days.[28]

Laboratory findings commonly associated with osteomalacia are decreased serum calcium or phosphorus levels, decreased 25-hydroxyvitamin D, and elevated serum alkaline phosphatase. X-rays may demonstrate the effects of generalized bone demineralization, especially loss of calcium in the bones of the pelvis and the presence of associated bone deformity. Looser's transformation zones (ribbons of decalcification in bone found on x-ray) are diagnostic of osteomalacia. However, significant osteomalacia may exist without demonstrable x-ray changes.

Collaborative care of osteomalacia is directed toward correction of the vitamin D deficiency. Vitamin D_3 (cholecalciferol) and vitamin D_2 (ergocalciferol) can be supplemented, and the patient often shows a dramatic response. Calcium salts or phosphorus supplements may also be prescribed. Dietary ingestion of eggs, low-fat milk, fish, and vegetables is encouraged. Exposure to sunlight (and ultraviolet rays) is also valuable, along with weight-bearing exercise.

OSTEOPOROSIS

Osteoporosis, or porous bone (fragile bone disease), is a chronic, progressive metabolic bone disease characterized by low bone mass and structural deterioration of bone tissue, leading to increased bone fragility (Fig. 62-7). At least 28 million persons in the United States have some degree of osteoporosis, and with the projected increase in life expectancy, this number is expected to grow. One in two women and one in eight men over the age of 50 will sustain an osteoporosis-related fracture during their lifetime. In the United States, the total cost of osteoporosis in terms of medical care, nursing home fees, and loss of income is estimated to exceed $13 billion. Osteoporosis is known as the "silent thief" because it slowly and insidiously over many years robs the skeleton of its banked resources. Bones can eventually become so fragile that they cannot withstand normal mechanical stress.[29]

Osteoporosis is 8 times more common in women than in men for several reasons: (1) women tend to have lower calcium intake than men throughout their lives (men between 15 and 50 years of age consume twice as much calcium as women); (2) women have less bone mass because of their generally smaller frame; (3) bone resorption begins at an earlier age in women and is accelerated at menopause; (4) pregnancy and breastfeeding deplete a woman's skeletal reserve unless calcium intake is adequate; and (5) longevity increases the likelihood of osteoporosis, and women live longer than men. Although osteoporosis is more common in women than men, it is important to realize that men can also develop osteoporosis.[30]

Etiology and Pathophysiology

Risk factors for osteoporosis are female gender, increasing age, family history of osteoporosis, white (European descent) or Asian race, small stature, early menopause, anorexia, oophorectomy, sedentary lifestyle, and insufficient dietary calcium. In-

CULTURAL & ETHNIC CONSIDERATIONS
Osteoporosis

- White and Asian American women have a higher incidence of osteoporosis than African American women.
- African American women have 10% more bone mass than non–African American women.
- Hispanic women have a lower incidence of osteoporosis than white women.
- Postmenopausal women are at the highest risk for osteoporosis regardless of ethnic group.

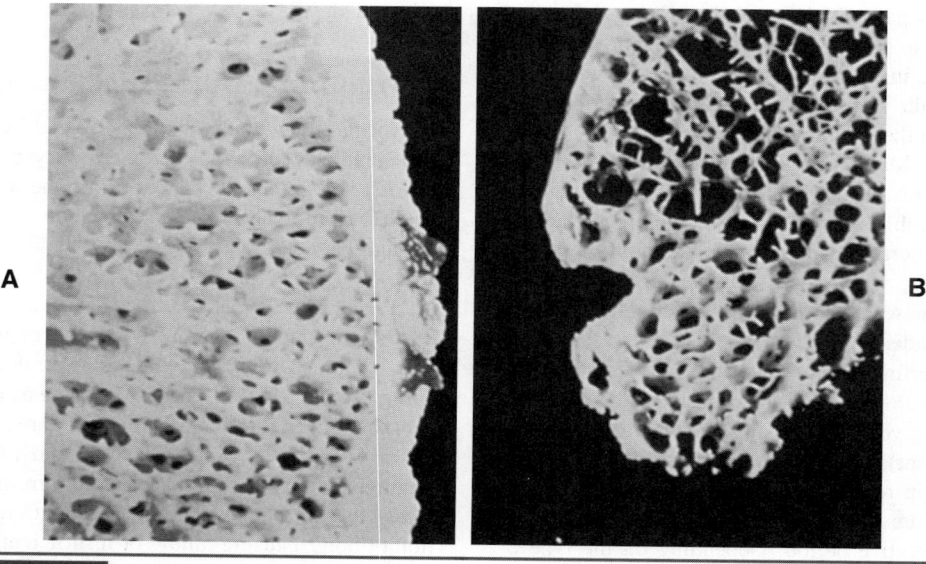

FIG. 62-7 A, Normal bone. B, Osteoporotic bone.

TABLE 62-11   Risk Factors for Osteoporosis

- Female gender
- Thin, small framed
- Family history of osteoporosis
- Diet low in calcium
- White or Asian ethnicity
- Excessive use of alcohol
- Cigarette smoking
- Inactive lifestyle
- Long-term use of corticosteroids, thyroid replacements, or antiseizure medications
- Postmenopausal, including early or surgically induced menopause
- History of anorexia nervosa or bulimia, chronic liver disease, or malabsorption

From National Osteoporosis Foundation: *Position paper: current perspectives on diagnosis, prevention, and treatment of osteoporosis,* Washington, DC, 1998, The Foundation.

creased risk is associated with cigarette smoking and alcoholism, and decreased risk is associated with regular weight-bearing exercise and fluoride and vitamin D ingestion.[31] Risk factors for osteoporosis are listed in Table 62-11. Low testosterone levels is a major risk factor in men.[30]

Peak bone mass (maximum bone tissue) is mainly achieved before age 20. It is determined by a combination of four major factors: hereditary, nutrition, exercise, and hormone function. Heredity may be responsible for up to 70% of a person's peak bone mass. Bone loss from midlife (age 35 to 40 years) onward is inevitable, but the rate of loss varies. At menopause, women experience rapid bone loss when the decline in estrogen production is the sharpest. This rate of loss then slows, and eventually matches the rate of bone lost by men 65 to 70 years old.

Bone is continually being deposited by osteoblasts and resorbed by osteoclasts, a process called remodeling. Normally the rates of bone deposition and resorption are equal to each other so that the total bone mass remains constant. In osteoporosis, bone resorption exceeds bone deposition. Although resorption affects the entire skeletal system, osteoporosis occurs most commonly in the bones of the spine, hips, and wrists. Over time, wedging and fractures of the vertebrae produce gradual loss of height and a humped back known as *"dowager's hump,"* or *kyphosis.* The usual first signs are back pain or spontaneous fractures.[32] The loss of bone substance causes the bone to become mechanically weakened and prone to either spontaneous fractures or fractures from minimal trauma.

Specific diseases associated with osteoporosis include intestinal malabsorption, kidney disease, rheumatoid arthritis, hyperthyroidism, advanced alcoholism, cirrhosis of the liver, hypogonadism, and diabetes mellitus.

Many drugs can interfere with bone metabolism, including corticosteroids, antiseizure drugs (e.g., valproate [Depakote], phenytoin [Dilantin]), aluminum-containing antacids, heparin, certain cancer treatments, and excessive thyroid hormones. At the time a drug is prescribed, the patient should be informed of this possible side effect.[33] Long-term corticosteroid use is a major contributor to osteoporosis. When a corticosteroid is taken, there is a disproportionate loss of bone resulting from the inhibition of new bone formation.

Clinical Manifestations

Osteoporosis is often called the "silent disease" because bone loss occurs without symptoms. People may not know they have osteoporosis until their bones become so weak that a sudden strain, bump, or fall causes a hip, vertebral, or wrist fracture. Collapsed vertebrae may initially be manifested as back pain, loss of height, or spinal deformities such as kyphosis or severely stooped posture.

Diagnostic Studies

Osteoporosis often goes unnoticed because it cannot be detected by conventional x-ray until more than 25% to 40% of calcium in the bone is lost. Serum calcium, phosphorus, and alkaline phosphatase levels usually are normal, although alkaline phosphatase may be elevated after a fracture. Bone mineral density (BMD) measurements are typically used to measure the bone density. BMD assesses the mass of bone per unit volume, or how tightly the bone is packed. (BMD measurements are presented in Table 60-7.) Quantitative ultrasound measures bone density with sound waves in the heel, kneecap, or shin.[34] One of the most common BMD studies is dual-energy x-ray absorptiometry (DEXA), which measures bone density in the spine, hips, and forearm (the most common sites of fractures resulting from osteoporosis). DEXA studies are also useful to evaluate changes in bone density over time and to assess the effectiveness of treatment. Bone biopsy is effective to differentiate the diagnosis of osteoporosis from osteomalacia.

NURSING and COLLABORATIVE MANAGEMENT OSTEOPOROSIS

Collaborative care of osteoporosis focuses on proper nutrition, calcium supplementation, exercise, prevention of fractures, and drugs (Table 62-12). Prevention and treatment of osteoporosis focuses on adequate calcium intake (1000 mg per day in pre-

TABLE 62-12   Collaborative Care   Osteoporosis

Diagnostic
History and physical examination
Serum calcium, phosphorus, and alkaline phosphatase levels
Bone mineral densitometry
Dual energy x-ray absorptiometry (DEXA)
Quantitative ultrasound

Collaborative Therapy
Calcium supplements (see Table 62-14)
Diet high in calcium (see Table 62-13)
Vitamin D supplements
Exercise program
Estrogen replacement therapy
Bisphosphonates
  etidronate (Didronel)
  alendronate (Fosamax)
  raloxifene (Evista)
  calcitonin (Calcimar)

menopausal women and postmenopausal women taking estrogen and 1500 mg per day in postmenopausal women who are not receiving supplemental estrogen). If dietary intake of calcium is inadequate, supplemental calcium should be taken.[35] Foods that are high in calcium content include whole and skim milk, yogurt, turnip greens, cottage cheese, ice cream, sardines, and spinach

TABLE 62-13	Nutritional Therapy — Sources of Calcium	
FOOD	**CALCIUM (MG)**
1 cup milk	
Buttermilk	285
Chocolate	284
Whole	291
Low-fat	300
Skim	302
Half and half	254
Evaporated, canned	657
Egg nog	330
1 oz cheese	
American	174
Blue	150
Brie	52
Camembert	110
Cheddar	130
Cottage	130
Mozzarella	207
Parmesan	390
Swiss	272
8 oz yogurt	415
1 cup ice cream	176
Soft serve	272
3 oz seafood	
Salmon	167
Sardines with bones	372
Shrimp	98
Oysters	113
1 med stalk cooked broccoli	158
1 cup cooked spinach	200
1 cup cooked mustard greens	193
1 cup turnip greens	252
1 cup cooked collard greens with stems	289
1 cup bok choy	250
1 cup kale	206
Bonus Sources	
1 cup almonds	304
1 cup hazelnuts	240
1 tbs blackstrap molasses	137
Poor Sources	
Egg	28
1 cup cabbage	44
1 oz cream cheese	23
3 oz beef, pork, poultry	10
Apple, banana	10
½ grapefruit	20
1 med potato	14
1 med carrot	14
¼ head lettuce	27

TABLE 62-14	Elemental Calcium Content of Various Oral Calcium Preparations	
CALCIUM PREPARATION	**ELEMENTAL CALCIUM CONTENT**
Calcium carbonate (Tums 500)	500 mg/tablet
Calcium carbonate + 5 μg vitamin D_2 (Os-Cal 250)	250 mg/tablet
Calcium gluconate	40 mg/500 mg
Calcium carbonate	400 mg/g
Calcium lactate	80 mg/600 mg
Calcium citrate	40 mg/300 mg

(Table 62-13). The amount of elemental calcium varies in different calcium preparations (Table 62-14). Calcium supplementation inhibits age-related bone loss; however, no new bone is formed.

Vitamin D is important in calcium absorption and function and may have a role in bone formation. Most people get enough vitamin D from the diet or naturally through synthesis in the skin from exposure to sunlight. However, supplemental vitamin D (400 to 800 IU) may be recommended for older adults, those who are homebound, and those who get minimal sun exposure.

Moderate amounts of exercise are important to build up and maintain bone mass. Exercise also increases muscle strength, coordination, and balance. The best exercises are weight-bearing exercises that force an individual to work against gravity. These exercises include walking, hiking, weight training, stair climbing, tennis, and dancing. Walking is preferred to high-impact aerobics or running, both of which may put too much stress on the bones of patients with osteoporosis. Walking 30 minutes, three times a week, is recommended.

Cigarette smoking and excess alcohol intake are risk factors for osteoporosis. Regular consumption of 2 to 3 ounces of alcohol a day may increase the degree of osteoporosis, even in young men and women. Patients should be instructed to quit smoking and cut down on alcohol intake to decrease the likelihood of losing bone mass.

Although loss of bone cannot be significantly reversed, further loss can be prevented if the patient follows a regimen of calcium and vitamin D supplementation, exercise, estrogen replacement, and alendronate (Fosamax) or raloxifene (Evista), if indicated. Efforts should be made to keep patients with osteoporosis ambulatory to prevent further loss of bone substance as a result of immobility. Treatment also involves protecting areas of potential pathologic fractures; for example, a corset can be used to prevent vertebral collapse.

■ **Drug Therapy**

Estrogen replacement therapy after menopause is used to prevent osteoporosis. Although the exact mechanism for the protective function of estrogen is not known, it is believed that estrogen inhibits osteoclast activity, leading to decreased bone resorption and preventing both cortical and trabecular bone loss. Estrogen replacement therapy is most effective when combined with calcium (see Table 62-14). The greatest benefit of estrogen is probably in the first 10 years after menopause. Transdermal estrogen treatment has been shown to be effective in the treatment of postmenopausal

EVIDENCE-BASED PRACTICE
Osteoporosis

Clinical Problem
In postmenopausal women with osteoporosis, what is the effectiveness of parathyroid hormone (PTH) in decreasing fracture rates and increasing bone mineral density (BMD)?

Best Clinical Practice
- In postmenopausal women with osteoporosis, PTH decreases the development of new fractures and increases BMD.

Implications for Nursing Practice
- PTH stimulates the growth of new bone
- PTH therapy offers a different approach from other osteoporosis treatments currently available.
- Serum calcium levels and bone density should be periodically assessed during therapy with PTH.

Reference for Evidence
EBM Reviews: Parathyroid hormone decreased fracture rates and increased bone mineral density in postmenopausal women, *ACP Journal Club* 135:95, November/December 2001.

women with established osteoporosis. (See Chapter 52 for further discussion of estrogen replacement therapy.)

Calcitonin is secreted by the thyroid gland and inhibits osteoclastic bone resorption by directly interacting with active osteoclasts. Calcitonin (Calcimar) is available in intramuscular, subcutaneous, and intranasal forms. The nasal form is easy to administer, and patients should be taught to alternate nostrils daily. Nasal dryness and irritation are the most frequent side effects. Administration of the intramuscular or subcutaneous form of the drug at night has been shown to decrease the side effects of nausea and facial flushing. Nausea does not occur with the nasal spray. When calcitonin is used, calcium supplementation is necessary to prevent secondary hyperparathyroidism.[36]

Bisphosphonates inhibit osteoclast-mediated bone resorption, thereby increasing BMD and total bone mass. This group of drugs includes etidronate (Didronel), alendronate (Fosamax), pamidronate (Aredia), risedronate (Actonel), clodronate (Bonefos), tiludronate (Skelid), and ibandronate (Boniva). Common side effects are anorexia, weight loss, and gastritis. The most commonly used bisphosphonate drug in treating osteoporosis is alendronate. Patients should be instructed on the proper administration of alendronate to aid in its absorption.[36] It should be taken after rising in the morning with a full glass of water. The patient should not eat or drink anything for 30 minutes after taking it. The patient should also be instructed not to lie down after taking the drug. These precautions have shown to decrease gastrointestinal side effects (especially esophageal irritation) and increase absorption. Alendronate is available as a once-per-week oral tablet.

Another type of drug used in treating osteoporosis is selective estrogen receptor modulators, such as raloxifene (Evista). These drugs mimic the effect of estrogen on bone by reducing bone resorption without stimulating the tissues of the breast or uterus. Raloxifene in postmenopausal women significantly increases BMD.[37] The most commonly reported side effects are leg cramps and hot flashes.

Teriparatide (Forteo) is used for the treatment of osteoporosis in men and postmenopausal women who are at high risk for having a fracture. Teriparatide is a portion of human parathyroid hormone (PTH) and works by increasing the action of osteoblasts. Teriparatide is the first drug approved for the treatment of osteoporosis that stimulates new bone formation. Most drugs used to treat osteoporosis prevent further bone loss. Teriparatide is administered by subcutaneous injection once a day.

Medical management of patients receiving corticosteroids includes prescribing the lowest possible dose of the drug, as well as calcium and vitamin D supplementation. If osteopenia is evident on bone densitometry, treatment with bisphosphonate agents, such as alendronate (Fosamax), should be considered.

PAGET'S DISEASE

Paget's disease *(osteitis deformans)* is a skeletal bone disorder in which there is excessive bone resorption followed by replacement of normal marrow by vascular, fibrous connective tissue. The new bone is larger, disorganized, and structurally weaker. The regions of the skeleton commonly affected are the pelvis, long bones, spine, ribs, sternum, and cranium. The etiology of Paget's disease is unknown, although a viral cause has been proposed.[38] Up to 40% of all patients with Paget's disease have at least one relative with the disorder. Men are affected 2:1 over women, and Paget's disease is rarely seen in persons under 40 years of age.

In milder forms of Paget's disease, patients may remain free of symptoms, and the disease may be discovered incidentally on x-ray or serum chemistry. The initial clinical manifestations are usually insidious development of bone pain (which may progress to severe intractable pain), complaints of fatigue, and progressive development of a waddling gait. Patients may complain that they are becoming shorter or that their heads are becoming larger. Headaches, dementia, visual deficits, and loss of hearing can result with an enlarged, thickened skull. Increased bone volume in the spine can cause spinal cord or nerve root compression. Pathologic fracture is the most common complication of Paget's disease and may be the first indication of the disease. Other complications include malignant osteosarcoma, fibrosarcoma, and osteoclastoma (giant cell) tumors.

Serum alkaline phosphatase levels are markedly elevated (indicating high bone turnover) in advanced forms of the disease. X-rays may demonstrate that the normal contour of the affected bone is curved and the bone cortex is thickened and irregular, especially the weight-bearing bones and cranium. Bone scans using a radiolabeled biphosphate demonstrate increased uptake in the skeletal areas affected.

Collaborative care of Paget's disease is usually limited to symptomatic and supportive care and correction of secondary deformities by either surgical intervention or braces. Bone resorption, relief of acute symptoms, and lowering the serum alkaline phosphatase levels may be significantly influenced by the administration of calcitonin (Cibacalcin), which inhibits osteoclastic activity. Response to calcitonin therapy is not permanent and often stops when therapy is discontinued. Bisphosphonate drugs including risedronate (Actonel), etidronate (Didronel), pamidronate (Aredia), tiludronate (Skelid), and alendronate (Fosamax) are also used to retard bone resorption.[39] Calcium and vitamin D are often given to decrease hypocalcemia, a common side effect with these drugs. Drug effectiveness may be monitored by serum alkaline phosphatase levels. Salmon calcitonin (Calcimar) is recommended for patients who cannot tolerate bisphosphonate drugs.

Pain is usually managed by NSAIDs (acetaminophen), and the COX-2 inhibitor drugs (e.g., celecoxib [Celebrex]). Orthopedic surgery for fractures, hip and knee replacements, and knee realignment may be necessary.

A firm mattress should be used to provide back support and to relieve pain. The patient may be required to wear a corset or light brace to relieve back pain and provide support when in the upright position. The patient should be proficient in the correct application of such devices and know how to regularly examine areas of the skin for friction damage. Activities such as lifting and twisting should be discouraged. Physical therapy may increase muscle strength. Good body mechanics are essential. A properly balanced nutritional program is important in the management of metabolic disorders of bone, especially pertaining to vitamin D, calcium, and protein, which are necessary to ensure the availability of the components for bone formation. Prevention measures such as patient education, use of an assistive device, and environmental changes should be actively pursued to prevent falls and subsequent fractures.

■ Gerontologic Considerations: Metabolic Bone Diseases

Osteoporosis and Paget's disease are common in older adults. Patients should be instructed in proper nutritional management to prevent further bone loss such as that occurring from osteoporosis.

Because metabolic bone disorders increase the possibility of pathologic fractures, the nurse must use extreme caution when the patient is turned or moved. It is important to keep the patient as active as possible to retard demineralization of bone resulting from disuse or extended immobilization. A supervised exercise program is an essential part of the treatment program. If the patient's condition permits, ambulation without causing fatigue must be encouraged. ■

CRITICAL THINKING EXERCISES

Case Study
Osteoporosis

Patient Profile. Rose Tan is a 56-year-old Asian American librarian who had a total hysterectomy and salpingo-oophorectomy for removal of a benign ovarian cyst 4 years ago.

Subjective Data
- Experiences chronic, mild lumbar pain and tenderness that radiates to her right hip and the lateral thigh
- Regular walking offers some relief
- Had a stress fracture in wrist 6 months ago
- Reports no noticeable loss of height
- Has maternal history of osteoporosis
- Has been taking corticosteroids for past 6 years for Addison's disease
- Drinks socially—two alcoholic beverages per day
- Dislikes dairy products

Objective Data
- 5 feet 6 inches tall, 116 lb

Diagnostic Studies
- Bone mass/density tests show decreased bone mineral density at spine and hip
- Laboratory tests reveal normal serum calcium, phosphorus, and alkaline phosphatase levels

Collaborative Care
- Premarin 0.625 mg PO daily
- Alendronate (Fosamax) 70 mg once/wk
- Calcium supplements 1200 mg PO daily
- High-calcium diet
- Reduce alcohol intake
- Maintain regular exercise program

CRITICAL THINKING QUESTIONS

1. What risk factors made Rose prone to develop osteoporosis?
2. Why does regular exercise help Rose's symptoms?
3. What is the purpose of prescribing estrogen replacement for Rose?
4. What teaching should the nurse provide to Rose regarding alendronate?
5. How might the nurse assist Rose in increasing her intake of calcium?
6. Based on the assessment data presented, write one or more nursing diagnoses. Are there any collaborative problems?

Nursing Research Issues

1. What factors are important for the nurse to address in helping an adolescent female increase her calcium intake?
2. What are the differences in pain management in the adolescent patient with Ewing's sarcoma compared with the adult patient with osteosarcoma?
3. How does patient teaching regarding back care and exercise affect the long-tern outcomes for chronic low back pain?
4. What are the risks of postoperative complications on laminectomy patients who are hospitalized versus those who have same-day procedures?
5. How can nurses best influence the footwear purchase of urban and rural young adult women related to heel height and toe box configuration?

REVIEW QUESTIONS

The number of the question corresponds to the same-numbered objective at the beginning of the chapter.

1. A patient with osteomyelitis is treated with surgical debridement followed by continuous irrigation of the affected bone with antibiotics. In responding to the patient who asks why oral or IV antibiotics cannot be used alone, the nurse explains that
   a. the irrigation is necessary to wash out dead tissue and pus from the infected area.
   b. the ischemia and bone death associated with osteomyelitis are frequently impenetrable to most blood-borne antibiotics.
   c. there are no effective oral or IV antibiotics to treat *S. aureus,* the most common cause of osteomyelitis.
   d. an irrigation can penetrate involucrum created by the infection and prevent bacterial spreading to other tissue.

2. A patient with an osteogenic sarcoma of the left femur has a nursing diagnosis of risk for injury (pathologic fracture) related to bone tissue changes. The nursing management of this patient is primarily directed toward
   a. preventing pain.
   b. relieving edema.
   c. increasing physical mobility.
   d. supporting and positioning the leg.

3. In identifying people at risk for back injuries, the nurse recognizes that the person at greatest risk for low back pain is a(n)
   a. long-distance truck driver.
   b. 62-year-old widow who walks daily.
   c. aerobics instructor who weighs 100 lb.
   d. 25-year-old nurse who works in a newborn nursery.

4. The primary nursing responsibility in caring for a patient with acute low back pain associated with severe pain and muscle spasms is
   a. teaching exercises such as straight-leg raises to decrease pain.
   b. positioning the patient on the abdomen with the legs extended.
   c. providing pain medication to promote exercise and ambulation.
   d. assisting the patient to maintain activity restrictions with a gradual increase in activity.

5. In caring for the patient after a spinal fusion, the nurse recognizes that interventions for this surgery differ from a simple laminectomy in that
   a. body alignment is maintained by the fusion procedure.
   b. earlier ambulation is permitted because the spine is more stabilized.
   c. the donor site for the bone graft may be more painful than the spinal incision.
   d. teaching regarding body mechanics and prevention of future back injuries is not as critical.

6. Before discharge from the same-day surgery unit, the nurse instructs the patient who has had a surgical correction of bilateral hallux valgus to
   a. rest frequently with the feet elevated.
   b. soak the feet in warm water several times a day.
   c. walk primarily on the heels to relieve pressure on the toes.
   d. expect the feet to be numb for several days postoperatively.

7. The nurse advises the patient with early osteoporosis to
   a. lose weight.
   b. stop smoking.
   c. eat a high-protein diet.
   d. start swimming for exercise.

REFERENCES

1. Breuninger C, Wittig P, editors: *Disease,* ed 3, Springhouse, Pa, 2001, Springhouse.
2. Schoen D: *Adult orthopaedic nursing,* Philadelphia, 2000, JB Lippincott.
3. Darville T, Jacobs R: Acute osteomyelitis in children: intervening for early control, *J Musculoskeletal Med* 16:49, 1999.
4. Tehranzadeh J et al: Imaging of osteomyelitis in the mature skeleton, *Radiol Clin North Am* 39:223, 2001.
5. DiPasquale D: Chronic osteomyelitis in adults: aggressive management required, *J Musculoskeletal Med* 17:250, 2000.
6. Roeder B et al: Antibiotic beads in the treatment of diabetic pedal osteomyelitis, *J Foot Ankle Surgery* 39:124, 2000.
7. Jemal A et al: Cancer statistics 2002, *CA Cancer J Clinicians* 52:23, 2002.
8. Barrick M, Mitchell S: Multiple myeloma, *AJN* 11(suppl):4, 2001.
9. Bridge J et al: Sarcomas of bone. In Abeloff M, Lichter A, Niederhuber J, editors: *Clinical oncology,* ed 2, New York, 2000, Livingstone.
10. Kelley C, Thomas R: Osteogenic sarcoma. In Miaskowski C, Buchsel P, editors: *Oncology nursing: assessment and clinical care,* St Louis, 1999, Mosby.
11. Haynes K: Tumors of the musculoskeletal system. In Schoen, D. editor: *Core curriculum for orthopaedic nursing,* ed 4, Pitman, NJ, 2001, Jannetti.
12. Pinkerton C et al: Treatment strategies for metastatic Ewing's sarcoma, *Eur J Cancer* 37:1338, 2001.
13. Ruyman F, Grovas A: Progress in the diagnosis and treatment of rhabdomyosarcoma and related soft tissue sarcomas, *Cancer Invest* 18:223, 2000.
14. Coleman R et al: Bone metastases. In Abeloff M, Lichter A, Niederhuber J, editors: *Clinical oncology,* ed 2, New York, 2000, Livingstone.
15. Hayes K: Neoplasms of the musculoskeletal system. In Maher AB, Salmond SW, Pellino TA, editors: *Orthopaedic nursing,* ed 3, Philadelphia, 2002, WB Saunders.
16. Mason K: Pediatric and congenital disorders. In Schoen D, editor: *Core curriculum for orthopaedic nursing,* ed 4, Pitman, NJ, 2001, Jannetti.
17. Alexander M: Congenital and developmental disorders. In Maher AB, Salmond SW, Pellino TA, editors: *Orthopedic nursing,* ed 3, Philadelphia, 2002, WB Saunders.
18. Deyo R, Weinstein J: Low back pain, *N Engl J Med* 344:363, 2001.
19. Andersson G: Epidemiologic features of chronic low back pain, *Lancet* 354:581, 1999.
20. Katz J: Controlling pain: getting the low down on back pain, *Nursing 2001* 31:24, 2001.
21. Stein R: An overview of the lumbar spine. In *An introduction to orthopaedic nursing,* ed 2, Pitman, NJ, 1999, Jannetti.
22. Dawson E, Bernbeck J: The surgical management of low back pain, *Phys Med Rehabil Clin North Am* 9:489, 1999.
23. Hellmann D, Stone J: Arthritis and musculoskeletal disorders. In Tierney L et al, editors: *Current medical diagnosis and treatment 2001,* ed 40, New York, 2001, Lange/McGraw-Hill.

24. Choy D: Percutaneous laser disc decompression: twelve years' experience with 752 procedures in 518 patients, *J Clin Laser Surg* 16:325, 1998.

25. Food and Drug Administration: FDA approves first device to utilize genetically engineered protein to treat degenerative disc disease. FDA Talk Paper [on-line]. Available at *www.fda.gov/bbs/topics* (accessed Aug 8, 2002).

26. Chou L: Disorders of the metatarsophalangeal joint: diagnosis of great-toe pain, *Physician Sportsmed* 28:32, 2000.

27. Findlow A et al: The management of diabetic foot ulcers, *Diabetic Foot* 4:112, 2001.

28. Pacala J: Osteoporosis and osteomalacia, *Clin Geriat* 8:13, 2000.

29. Turner L et al: Osteoporosis diagnosis and fracture, *Orthop Nurs* 18:5, 1999.

30. Tsitouras P et al: Equal time for the older male, *Annals Long-Term Care* 9:15, 2001.

31. Curry L, Hogstel M: Osteoporosis, *AJN* 102:26, 2002.

32. Burke S: Boning up on osteoporosis, *Nursing* 31:36, 2001.

33. Field-Munves E: Evidence-based decisions for the treatment of osteoporosis, *Annals Long-Term Care* 9:3, 2001.

34. Overdorf J et al: Osteoporosis: there's so much we can do, *RN* 64:30, 2001.

35. Taft L et al: Osteoporosis: a disease management opportunity, *Orthop Nurs* 19:2, 2000.

36. Capriotti T: Pharmacologic prevention and treatment of osteoporosis in women, *Med Surg Nurs* 9:2, 2000.

37. McCoy PW: Pharmacologic management of osteoporosis, *Topics Geriatr Rehabil* 17:38, 2001.

38. Helfrich MH et al: A negative search for a paramyxoviral etiology of Paget's disease of bone: molecular, immunological, and ultrastructural studies in UK patients, *J Bone Miner Res* 15:2315, 2000.

39. Vasikaran S: Biphosphates: an overview with special reference to alendronate, *Ann Clin Biochem* 38:608, 2001.

RESOURCES

American Academy of Orthopedic Surgeons (AAOS)
6300 North River Road
Rosemont, IL 60018-4262
800-346-AAOS or 847-823-7186
Fax: 847-823-8125
www.aaos.org

American Cancer Society
1599 Clifton Road, NE
Atlanta, GA 30329-4251
800-ACS-2345
www.cancer.org

American College of Foot and Ankle Surgeons
515 Busse Highway
Park Ridge, IL 60068
847-292-2237 or 800-421-2237
www.acfas.org

American College of Sports Medicine
P.O. Box 1440
401 W Michigan Street
Indianapolis, IN 46202
317-637-9200
Fax: 317-634-7817
www.acsm.org

American Orthopedic Foot and Ankle Society
2517 Eastlake Avenue East
Seattle, WA 98102
206-223-1120
Fax: 206-223-1178
www.aofas.org

American Podiatric Medical Association
9312 Old Georgetown Road
Bethesda, MD 20814
800-ASK-APMA or 301-571-9200
Fax: 301-530-2752
www.apma.org

Calcium Information Center
Oregon Health Sciences University
1221 SW Yamwill, Suite 303
Portland, OR 97205
800-321-2681

Cancer Survivors Network
800-333-HOPE (4673)
www.acscsn.org

Muscular Dystrophy Association
National Headquarters
3300 East Sunrise Drive
Tucson, AZ 85718
800-572-1717
www.mdausa.org

National Arthritis and Musculoskeletal and Skin Diseases
Information Clearinghouse, National Institutes of Health
1 AMS Circle
Bethesda, MD 20892-3675
877-22-NIAMS or 301-495-4484
Fax: 301-718-6366
www.nih.gov/niams

National Association of Orthopaedic Nurses (NAON)
Box 56
Pitman, NJ 08071
856-256-2310
Fax: 856-589-7463
http://naon.inurse.com

National Easter Seal Society
230 West Monroe Street, Suite 1800
Chicago, IL 60606
800-221-6827 or 312-726-6200
Fax: 312-726-1494
www.easter-seals.org

National Institutes of Health, Osteoporosis, and Related Bone Diseases—National Resource Center
1232 22nd Street NW
Washington, DC 20037-1292
800-624-BONE or 202-223-0644
Fax: 202-293-2356
www.osteo.org

National Osteoporosis Foundation
1232 22nd Street NW
Washington, DC 20037-1292
800-223-9994 or 202-223-2226
www.nof.org

Older Women's League
666 Eleventh Street SW, Suite 700
Washington, DC 20001
800-TAKE-OWL or 202-783-6686
Fax: 202-638-2356
www.owl-national.org

Osteoporosis Society of Canada
33 Laird Drive
Toronto, ON
M4G 3S9 Canada
416-696-2663
Fax: 416-696-2673
www.osteoporosis.ca

The Paget Foundation for Paget's Disease of Bone and Related Disorders
120 Wall Street, Suite 1602
New York, NY 10005-4001
800-23-PAGET or 212-509-5335
Fax: 212-509-8492
www.paget.org

For additional Internet resources, see the website for this book at *http://www.evolve.elsevier.com/Lewis/medsurg/.*

CHAPTER 63
NURSING MANAGEMENT
Arthritis and Connective Tissue Diseases

Dottie Roberts

LEARNING OBJECTIVES

1. Compare and contrast the sequence of events leading to joint destruction in osteoarthritis and rheumatoid arthritis.
2. Describe the clinical manifestations, collaborative care, and nursing management of osteoarthritis and rheumatoid arthritis.
3. Compare and contrast the pathophysiology, clinical manifestations, collaborative care, and nursing management of ankylosing spondylitis, psoriatic arthritis, and Reiter syndrome.
4. Describe the pathophysiology, clinical manifestations, and collaborative care of septic arthritis, Lyme disease, and gout.
5. Describe the pathophysiology, clinical manifestations, collaborative care, and nursing management of systemic lupus erythematosus, polymyositis, dermatomyositis, and Sjögren syndrome.
6. Describe the drug therapy and related nursing management associated with arthritis and connective tissue diseases.
7. Compare and contrast the possible etiologies, clinical manifestations, and collaborative and nursing management of myofascial pain syndrome, fibromyalgia syndrome, and chronic fatigue syndrome.

KEY TERMS

ankylosing spondylitis, p. 1734
chronic fatigue syndrome, p. 1751
CREST syndrome, p. 1745
dermatomyositis, p. 1746
fibromyalgia syndrome, p. 1749
gout, p. 1737
Lyme disease, p. 1736
myofascial pain syndrome, p. 1748
osteoarthritis, p. 1715

polymyositis, p. 1746
Raynaud's phenomenon, p. 1745
Reiter syndrome, p. 1735
rheumatoid arthritis, p. 1724
septic arthritis, p. 1735
Sjögren syndrome, p. 1748
spondyloarthropathies, p. 1733
systemic lupus erythematosus, p. 1739
systemic sclerosis, p. 1744

OSTEOARTHRITIS

Osteoarthritis (OA), the most common form of joint (articular) disease in North America, is a slowly progressive noninflammatory disorder of the diarthrodial (synovial) joints. Previously identified as *degenerative joint disease*, it is now known to involve the formation of new joint tissue in response to cartilage destruction.[1]

Although OA is no longer considered to be a normal part of the aging process, growing older continues to be the most consistently identified risk factor for disease development.[2] Cartilage destruction can actually begin between ages 20 and 30, and more than 90% of adults are affected by age 40. Few patients experience symptoms until after age 60, but as many as 60% of those over 65 years of age have symptomatic disease. Before the age of 50, men are more often affected than women. However, the incidence of OA after age 50 is twice as great in women as in men.[3]

Etiology and Pathophysiology

OA may occur as an idiopathic (formerly primary) or secondary disorder.[4] The cause of idiopathic OA is unknown. Secondary OA, on the other hand, is caused by a known event or condition that directly damages cartilage or causes joint instability (Table 63-1).

TABLE 63-1	Causes of Secondary Osteoarthritis	
CAUSE	**EFFECTS ON JOINT CARTILAGE**
Trauma	Dislocations or fractures may lead to avascular necrosis or uneven stress on cartilage.
Mechanical stress	Repetitive physical activities (e.g., sports activities) cause cartilage deterioration.
Inflammation	Release of enzymes in response to local inflammation can affect cartilage integrity.
Joint instability	Damage to supporting structures causes instability, placing uneven stress on articular cartilage.
Neurologic disorders	Pain and loss of reflexes from neurologic disorders, such as diabetic neuropathy, and Charcot joint cause abnormal movements that contribute to cartilage deterioration.
Skeletal deformities	Congenital or acquired conditions such as Legg-Calvé-Perthes disease or dislocated hip contribute to cartilage deterioration.
Hematologic/ endocrine disorders	Chronic hemarthrosis (e.g., hemophilia) can contribute to cartilage deterioration.
Use of selected drugs	Drugs such as indomethacin (Indocin), colchicine, and corticosteroids can stimulate collagen-digesting enzymes in joint synovium.

Reviewed by Sharon G. Childs, RN, MS, CRNP-CS, ONC, CEN, Adult Nurse Practitioner, Orthopedic Clinical Specialist, Concentra Medical Center, Baltimore, Md.

Researchers have been unable to identify a single cause for OA, but a number of factors have been linked to disease development. The increased incidence of OA in aging women is believed to be due to estrogen reduction at menopause. Genetic factors also appear to play a significant role in the occurrence of OA. Modifiable risk factors have been identified, including obesity, which contributes to knee OA. Regular moderate exercise, which also helps with weight control, has been shown to decrease the likelihood of disease development and progression. On the other hand, strenuous exercise through activities such as football and soccer has been linked to an increased risk of OA.

OA results from cartilage damage that triggers a metabolic response at the level of the chondrocytes (Fig. 63-1). Progression of OA causes the normally smooth, white, translucent articular cartilage to become dull, yellow, and granular. Affected cartilage gradually becomes softer, less elastic, and less able to resist wear with heavy use. The body's attempts at cartilage repair cannot keep up with the destruction that is occurring. Continued changes in the collagen structure of the cartilage lead to fissuring, fibrillation, and erosion of the articular surfaces. As the central cartilage becomes thinner, cartilage and bony growth (osteophytes) increase at the joint margins. The resulting incongruity in joint surfaces creates an uneven distribution of stress across the joint and contributes to a reduction in motion.

While inflammation is not characteristic of OA, a secondary synovitis may result when phagocytic cells try to rid the joint of small pieces of cartilage torn from the joint surface. These inflammatory changes contribute to the early pain and stiffness of OA. The pain of later disease results from contact between exposed bony joint surfaces after the articular cartilage has completely deteriorated.

Clinical Manifestations

Systemic. Systemic manifestations, such as fatigue or fever, are not present in OA. Organ involvement is also absent, marking an important distinction between OA and inflammatory joint disorders such as rheumatoid arthritis.

Joints. Manifestations of OA range from mild discomfort to significant disability. Joint pain is the predominant symptom of OA and the typical reason that the patient seeks medical attention. Pain generally worsens with joint use. In the early stages of OA, joint pain is relieved by rest. In advanced disease, however, the patient may complain of pain with rest or experience sleep disruptions caused by increasing joint discomfort. Pain may also become worse as barometric pressures fall before inclement weather. As OA progresses, increasing pain can contribute significantly to disability and loss of function. The pain of OA may be referred to the groin, buttock, or medial side of the thigh or

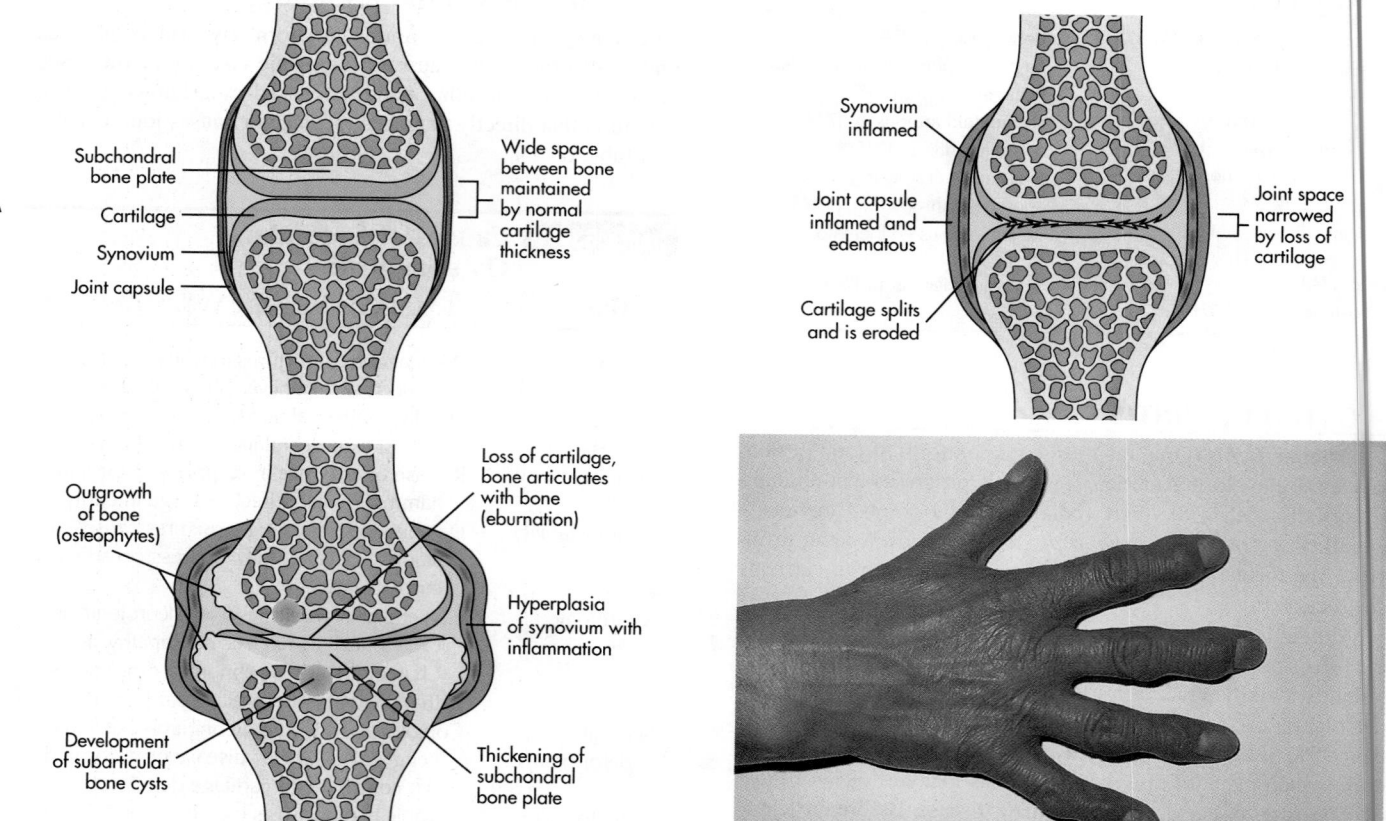

FIG. 63-1 Pathologic changes in osteoarthritis. **A,** Normal synovial joint. **B,** Early change in osteoarthritis is destruction of articular cartilage and narrowing of the joint space on x-ray. There is inflammation and thickening of the joint capsule and synovium. **C,** With time, there is thickening of subarticular bone caused by constant friction of the two bone surfaces, leading to a highly polished bony articular surface. Osteophytes form around the periphery of the joint by irregular outgrowths of bone. **D,** In osteoarthritis of the hands, osteophytes on the interphalangeal joints of the fingers are termed Heberden's nodes and appear as small nodules.

knee. Sitting down becomes difficult, as does rising from a chair when the hips are lower than the knees. As OA develops in the intervertebral (apophyseal) joints of the spine, localized pain and stiffness are common.

Unlike pain, which is typically provoked by activity, joint stiffness occurs after periods of rest or static position. Early morning stiffness is common but generally resolves within 30 minutes, a factor distinguishing OA from inflammatory arthritic disorders. Overactivity can cause a mild joint effusion that temporarily increases stiffness. *Crepitation,* a grating sensation caused by loose particles of cartilage in the joint cavity, can also contribute to stiffness. Crepitation indicates the loss of cartilage integrity and is present in more than 90% of patients with knee OA.

OA usually affect joints asymmetrically. The most commonly involved joints are the distal interphalangeal (DIP) and proximal interphalangeal (PIP) joints of the fingers, the carpometacarpal joint of the thumb, weight-bearing joints (hips, knees), the metatarsophalangeal (MTP) joint of the foot, and the cervical and lower lumbar vertebrae (Fig. 63-2).

Deformity. Deformity or instability associated with OA is specific to the involved joint. For example, *Heberden's nodes* occur on the DIP joints as an indication of osteophyte formation and loss of joint space (see Fig. 63-1). They can appear in the OA patient as early as age 40 and tend to be seen in family members. *Bouchard's nodes* on the PIP joints indicate similar disease involvement. Heberden's and Bouchard's nodes are often red, swollen, and tender. Although these bony enlargements do not

usually cause significant loss of function, the patient may be distressed by the visible disfigurement.

Knee OA often leads to joint malalignment as a result of cartilage loss in the medial compartment. The patient has a characteristic bow-legged appearance and may develop an altered gait in response to the obvious deformity. In advanced hip OA, one of the patient's legs may become shorter from a loss of joint space.

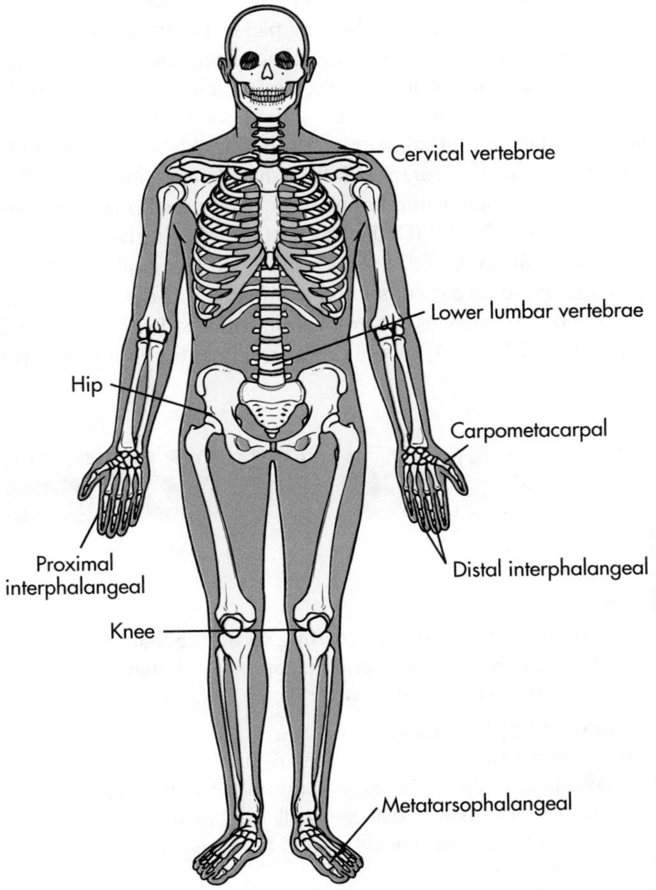

Diagnostic Studies

A bone scan, computed tomography scan, or magnetic resonance imaging may be useful in early OA because of the sensitivity of these tests to joint changes. X-rays are helpful in confirming disease and monitoring the effectiveness of treatment. As OA progresses, x-rays typically show joint space narrowing, bony sclerosis, and osteophyte formation. However, these changes do not always correlate with the degree of pain experienced by the patient. Despite significant radiologic indications of disease, the patient may be relatively free of symptoms. Conversely, another patient may have severe pain with only minimal x-ray changes.

No laboratory abnormalities are a specific diagnostic indicator of OA. The erythrocyte sedimentation rate (ESR) is normal except in instances of acute synovitis, when minimal elevations may be noted. Other routine blood tests (e.g., complete blood count [CBC], renal and liver function tests) are useful only in screening for related conditions or for establishing baseline values before the initiation of therapy. Synovial fluid analysis allows differentiation between OA and other forms of inflammatory arthritis. In the presence of OA, the fluid remains clear yellow with little or no sign of inflammation.

Collaborative Care

Because there is no cure for OA, collaborative care focuses on managing pain and inflammation, preventing disability, and maintaining and improving joint function (Table 63-2). Nonpharmacologic interventions are the foundation for OA management and

FIG. 63-2 Joints most frequently involved in osteoarthritis.

| Cervical vertebrae |
| Lower lumbar vertebrae |
| Hip |
| Carpometacarpal |
| Proximal interphalangeal |
| Distal interphalangeal |
| Knee |
| Metatarsophalangeal |

TABLE 63-2   Collaborative Care

Osteoarthritis

Diagnostic
History and physical examination
Radiologic studies of involved joints
Synovial fluid analysis

Collaborative Therapy
Nutritional counseling
Rest and joint protection, use of assistive devices
Therapeutic exercise
Heat and cold
Complementary and alternative therapies
  Herbal products
  Movement therapies
  Nutritional supplements
Drug therapy*
  Acetaminophen
  Nonsteroidal antiinflammatory drugs
  Intraarticular hyaluronic acid
Reconstructive surgery

*See Table 63-3.

should be maintained throughout the patient's treatment period. Drug therapy serves as an adjunct to nonpharmacologic treatments. Symptoms of disease are often managed conservatively for many years, but the patient's loss of joint function, unrelieved pain, and diminished ability to independently perform self-care may prompt a recommendation for surgery. Reconstructive surgical procedures are discussed in Chapter 61. In general, arthroscopic surgery for debridement is usually not recommended for OA. However, arthroscopic surgery to repair cartilage or ligament tears or remove bone bits or cartilage is effective.[5]

Rest and Joint Protection. The OA patient must understand the importance of a balance of rest and activity. The affected joint should be rested during any periods of acute inflammation and maintained in a functional position with splints or braces if necessary. However, immobilization should not exceed 1 week because of the risk of joint stiffness with inactivity. The patient may need to modify his or her usual activities to decrease stress on affected joints. For example, the patient with knee OA should avoid prolonged periods of standing, kneeling, or squatting. Using an assistive device such as a cane, walker, or crutches can also help decrease stress on arthritic joints.

Heat and Cold Applications. Applications of heat and cold may help reduce complaints of pain and stiffness. Although ice is not used as often as heat in the treatment of OA, it can be appropriate if the patient experiences acute inflammation. Heat therapy is especially helpful for stiffness, including hot packs, whirlpool baths, ultrasound, and paraffin wax baths.

Nutritional Therapy and Exercise. If the patient is overweight, a weight-reduction program is a critical part of the total treatment plan. The nurse should help the patient evaluate the current diet to make appropriate changes. (Chapter 39 discusses ways to assist the patient in attaining and maintaining a healthy body weight.) Because the load on the joints and the degree of joint mobilization are essential to the preservation of articular cartilage integrity, the American College of Rheumatology has identified exercise as a fundamental part of OA management.[5] Aerobic conditioning and specific programs for muscle strengthening have led to a modest reduction in pain and disability for some patients with knee OA.

Complementary and Alternative Therapies. Complementary and alternative therapies for symptom management of arthritis have become increasingly popular with patients who have failed to find relief through traditional medical care. Acupuncture, for example, has been found to be a safe and effective method for arthritis pain management[6] (see the Evidence-Based Practice box below). Other therapies include the use of yoga, massage, guided imagery, and therapeutic touch (see Chapter 7). In particular, the use of nutritional supplements such as glucosamine and chondroitin sulfate for relieving arthritis pain and improving joint mobility have shown promising results[7] (see the Complementary and Alternative Therapies box below).

Drug Therapy. Drug therapy is based on the severity of the patient's symptoms (Table 63-3). The patient with mild-to-moderate joint pain may receive relief from acetaminophen (Tylenol). The patient may receive up to 1000 mg every 6 hours, with the daily dose not to exceed 4 g. A topical agent such as capsaicin cream may also be beneficial, either alone or in conjunction with acetaminophen. Capsaicin comes from cayenne red pepper. It blocks pain by locally interfering with substance P, which is responsible for the transmission of pain impulses. The cream can be applied to affected joints four times daily. A concentrated product is available by prescription, but creams of 0.025% to 0.075% capsaicin are sold over the counter (OTC). The patient should be told that a local burning sensation may accompany initial use. The cream should not be used with an external heat source such as a heating pad or hot water bottle.

For the patient who fails to obtain adequate pain management with acetaminophen or for the patient with moderate to severe OA pain, nonacetylated salicylates (e.g., aspirin) or a nonsteroidal antiinflammatory drug (NSAID) may provide greater relief. Ibuprofen (Motrin) has been shown to offer greater relief than acetaminophen in patients with severe knee pain from OA.[8] NSAID therapy is typically initiated in low-dose OTC strengths (200 mg up to four times daily), with the dose increased as patient symptoms indicate. If the patient is at risk for or experiences gastrointestinal (GI) side effects with a conventional NSAID, supplemental treatment with a protective

EVIDENCE-BASED PRACTICE
Acupuncture for Osteoarthritis

Clinical Problem
Is acupuncture effective in relieving pain related to osteoarthritis?

Best Clinical Practice
- Acupuncture is becoming a common therapeutic modality for pain relief.
- Acupuncture is more effective for symptomatic treatment of osteoarthritis of the hip than advice and exercise.

Implications of Nursing Practice
- The nurse should become knowledgeable about acupuncture and what problems can be treated with it. (Acupuncture is discussed in Chapter 7.)
- In addition to teaching patients with osteoarthritis about exercise, diet, and other measures to manage osteoarthritis (see Table 63-4), the nurse should inform the patient about acupuncture as a potential treatment modality.

Reference for Evidence
Haslam R: A comparison of acupuncture with advice and exercises on the symptomatic treatment of osteoarthritis of the hip—a randomized controlled trial, *Acupunct Med* 9:19, 2001.

COMPLEMENTARY & ALTERNATIVE THERAPIES
Glucosamine

Clinical Uses
Osteoarthritis

Effects
Glucosamine is a naturally occurring substance that is found in mucopolysaccharides and mucoproteins. It may have a role in the synthesis of new cartilage.

Nursing Implications
Few adverse effects have been seen with the use of glucosamine. It should be taken with food. It should not be used in patients with diabetes mellitus. It may enhance the effects of hypoglycemic drugs and thus lower blood glucose levels.

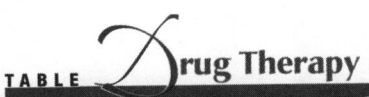

TABLE
63-3
Drug Therapy
Arthritis and Connective Tissue Disorders

DRUG	MECHANISM OF ACTION	SIDE EFFECTS	NURSING CONSIDERATIONS
Salicylates aspirin, salsalate (Disalcid, Asaphen) choline salicylate (Arthropan) choline magnesium trisalicylate (Trilisate)	Antiinflammatory Analgesic Antipyretic Act by inhibiting synthesis of prostaglandins	GI irritation (dyspepsia, nausea, ulcer, hemorrhage) Prolonged bleeding time Exacerbation of asthma (aspirin-sensitive asthma) Tinnitus, dizziness with repeated large doses	Administer drug with food, milk, antacids as prescribed, or full glass of water; may use enteric-coated aspirin. Report signs of bleeding (e.g., tarry stools, bruising, petechiae, nosebleeds).
Nonsteroidal Antiinflammatory Drugs ibuprofen (Motrin, Advil, Novoprofen) naproxen (Naprosyn, Anaprox, Aleve, Rhodiaprox, Synflex) ketoprofen (Orudis, Actron, Orafen) piroxicam (Feldene, Fexicam, Novopirocam) indomethacin (Indocin, Indocid) sulindac (Clinoril, Apo-Sulin, Novo-Sundac) tolmetin (Tolectin) diclofenac (Voltaren, Diclo SR) meclofenamate (Meclomen) oxaprozin (Daypro) meloxicam (Mobic) celecoxib (Celebrex) rofecoxib (Vioxx) valdecoxib (Bextra)	Antiinflammatory Analgesic Antipyretic Act by inhibiting synthesis of prostaglandins	GI irritation (dyspepsia, nausea, ulcer, hemorrhage) Prolonged bleeding time Headache, tinnitus Rash Acute renal insufficiency and other renal medullary changes Exacerbation of asthma (cross-reactivity with aspirin)	Administer drug with food, milk, or antacids as prescribed. Report signs of bleeding (e.g., tarry stools, bruising, petechiae, nosebleeds), edema, skin rashes, persistent headaches, visual disturbances. Monitor BP for elevations related to fluid retention. Needs to be used regularly for maximal effect.
Nonopioid Analgesics acetaminophen (Tylenol, Abenol) capsaicin cream (Zostrix)	Analgesic Antipyretic Topical analgesic Depletes substance P from nerve endings, interrupting pain signals to the brain	Rash, urticaria Hepatotoxicity (especially in presence of alcohol abuse) Leukopenia Localized burning sensation, erythema	Advise patient that concomitant use of alcohol may cause liver damage. Teach patient not to exceed recommended dosage. Must be used regularly over time for maximal effect. Aloe vera cream may moderate burning sensation. Advise patient not to use cream with external heat source (heating pad) because of risk of burns. Available in OTC and prescriptive strengths.
tramadol (Ultram)	Analgesic Centrally acting, binds to opioid receptors	GI irritation (dyspepsia, nausea, ulcer, hemorrhage) Dizziness, headache Somnolence Pruritus	Not recommended with concomitant MAO inhibitors or CNS depressants. May potentiate seizure risk with MAO inhibitors or neuroleptics. Advise patient to make position changes slowly because orthostatic hypotension may occur.

BP, Blood pressure; *CNS,* central nervous system; *GI,* gastrointestinal; *MAO,* monoamine oxidase; *OTC,* over-the-counter.

Continued

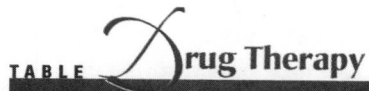

TABLE 63-3 — Drug Therapy
Arthritis and Connective Tissue Disorders—cont'd

DRUG	MECHANISM OF ACTION	SIDE EFFECTS	NURSING CONSIDERATIONS
Opioid Analgesics propoxyphene with acet-aminophen or aspirin (Darvocet, Darvon, Darvon-N) codeine with acetamino-phen or aspirin (Tylenol #3 or #4, Empirin #3 or #4) hydrocodone (Hycodan, Robidone); with acetamino-phen or aspirin (Lortab, Vicodin, Lortab ASA) oxycodone (OxyContin); with acetaminophen or aspirin (Percodan, Percocet, Tylox, Supeudol)	Analgesic	GI irritation (dyspepsia, nausea/vomiting, constipation) Dizziness, headache, orthostatic hypotension Sedation, respiratory depression	Advise patient regarding potential for constipation; encourage fluids and fiber if not con-traindicated. Administer with antiemetic if nausea occurs. Report signs of bleeding with aspirin-containing products. Monitor CBC and liver function tests. Teach patient and family to report any CNS or respira-tory changes.
Corticosteroids **Intraarticular Injections** methylprednisolone acetate (Depo-Medrol) triamcinolone (Aristospan)	Antiinflammatory Analgesic Act by inhibiting synthesis and/or release of mediators of inflammation	Local osteoporosis, tendon rupture, neuropathic arthropa-thy from frequent injection Dermal/subdermal changes leading to depression at injec-tion site Possibility of local infection	Use strict aseptic technique for joint fluid aspiration or corticosteroid injection. Inform patient that joint may feel worse immediately after injection. Inform patient that im-provement lasts weeks to months after injection. Advise patient to avoid overusing af-fected joint after injection.
Systemic hydrocortisone sodium succinate (Solu-Cortef) methylprednisolone sodium succinate (Solu-Medrol) dexamethasone (Decadron) prednisone triamcinolone (Aristocort, Triaderm)		Cushing syndrome (including fluid retention), GI irritation, osteo-porosis, insomnia, hyperten-sion, steroid psychosis, diabetes mellitus, acne, menstrual irregu-larities, hirsutism, risk of antibiotic-resistant infection, bruising	Use only in life-threatening exacer-bation or when symptoms persist after treatment with less potent antiinflammatory drugs. Administer for limited time only, tapering dose slowly. Be aware that exacerbation of symptoms occurs with abrupt withdrawal of drug. Monitor BP, weight, CBC, and potassium level. Limit sodium intake. Report signs of infection. Instruct patient to report corticosteroid use to surgeon or dentist to avoid post-operative adrenal insufficiency.
Disease-Modifying Antirheumatic Drugs (DMARDs) methotrexate (Rheumatrex)	Antimetabolite Antirheumatic Inhibits DNA, RNA, protein synthesis	Hepatotoxicity occurs more often with frequent small doses than with large intermittent doses. Smaller dose and different ad-ministration schedule for RA make it less likely that patient will develop symptoms related to drug's antineoplastic activity (e.g., GI and skin toxicity, bone marrow depression, nephropathy).	Monitor CBC and hepatic and renal function. Advise patient to report signs of anemia (fatigue, weakness). Keep patient well hydrated. Teratogenic potential cautions against use for chil-dren or women of childbearing age. Inform patient that contra-ception should be used during and 3 mo after treatment.

CBC, Complete blood count.

TABLE 63-3   Drug Therapy
Arthritis and Connective Tissue Disorders—cont'd

DRUG	MECHANISM OF ACTION	SIDE EFFECTS	NURSING CONSIDERATIONS
Disease–Modifying Antirheumatic Drugs (DMARDs)			
sulfasalazine (Azulfidine, Salazopyrin)	Sulfonamide Antiinflammatory Blocks prostaglandin synthesis	GI effects (anorexia, nausea/vomiting) Bleeding, bruising, jaundice Headache Rash, urticaria, pruritus	Advise patient that drug may cause orange-yellow discoloration of urine or skin. Space doses evenly around the clock, taking drug after food with 8 oz water. Treatment may be continued even after symptoms are relieved. Monitor CBC.
leflunomide (Arava)	Antiinflammatory Antirheumatic Immunomodulatory agent that inhibits proliferation of lymphocytes	Nausea, diarrhea Respiratory tract infection Alopecia Rash	Evaluate for relief of pain, swelling, stiffness; increase in joint mobility. Advise patient that medication can be taken without regard to food. Advise patient that improvement may take >8 wk.
penicillamine	Antiinflammatory Exact mechanism of action in RA unknown but may decrease cell-mediated immune response	GI irritation (nausea/vomiting, anorexia, diarrhea), reduced/altered taste Rash Proteinuria, hematuria Iron deficiency (especially in menstruating women)	Monitor WBC, platelets, urinalysis. Advise patient to take medication 1 hr before or 2 hr after meals or at least 1 hr from any other drug, food, or milk. Advise women of childbearing age to avoid pregnancy.
Gold Compounds			
Parenteral (gold sodium thiomalate [Myochrysine], aurothioglucose [Solganall]) Oral (auranofin [Ridaura])	Alters immune responses, suppressing synovitis of active RA Antirheumatic	Decreased hemoglobin, leukopenia, thrombycytopenia Proteinuria, hematuria Stomatitis	Rule out pregnancy before beginning treatment. Monitor CBC, urinalysis, and hepatic and renal function. Advise patient that therapeutic response may not occur for 3 to 6 mo. Advise patient to immediately report pruritus, rash, sore mouth, indigestion, or metallic taste.
Antimalarials			
hydroxychloroquine (Plaquenil)	Antirheumatic action unknown but may suppress formation of antigens	Ocular toxicity (retinopathy) may progress even after drug is discontinued Ototoxicity Peripheral neuritis, neuromyopathy, hypotension, electrocardiogram changes with prolonged therapy	Monitor CBC and hepatic function. Advise patient that therapeutic response may not occur for up to 6 mo. Advise patient to immediately report visual difficulties, muscular weakness, and decreased hearing/tinnitus.
Immunosuppressants			
azathioprine (Imuran) cyclophosphamide (Cytoxan)	Inhibits DNA, RNA, protein synthesis	GI irritation (nausea/vomiting; anorexia with large doses) Rash	Evaluate for relief of pain, swelling, stiffness; increase in joint mobility. Advise patient to immediately report unusual bleeding or bruising. Advise patient that therapeutic response may take up to 12 wk. Advise women of childbearing age to avoid pregnancy.

RA, Rheumatoid arthritis.

Continued

TABLE 63-3 Drug Therapy
Arthritis and Connective Tissue Disorders—cont'd

DRUG	MECHANISM OF ACTION	SIDE EFFECTS	NURSING CONSIDERATIONS
Biologic Therapy			
etanercept (Enbrel)	Binds TNF, blocking its inter-action with cell surface receptors to decrease inflammatory and immune responses	Injection site reaction including erythema, pain, itching, swelling Abdominal pain, vomiting Dizziness, headache Rhinitis, pharyngitis, cough	Evaluate for relief of pain, swelling, stiffness; increase in joint mobility. Advise patient that injection site reaction gen-erally occurs in first month of treatment and decreases with continued therapy. Advise patient to not receive live vac-cines during treatment.
infliximab (Remicade) adalimumab (Humira)	Monoclonal antibody that binds to TNF; reduces infil-tration of inflammatory cells	Abdominal pain, nausea/vomiting Dizziness, headache Rhinitis, cough, sinusitis, pharyngitis	Evaluate for relief of pain, swelling, stiffness; increase in joint mobility.
anakinra (Kineret)	Blocks the action of inter-leukin-1, thus decreases the inflammatory response	Injection site reaction Leukopenia, headache Abdominal pain, rash	Evaluate for relief of pain, swelling, stiffness; increase in joint mobility. Advise patient that injection site reaction gen-erally occurs in first month of treatment and decreases with continued therapy. Evaluate renal function. Monitor for in-fection. Do not take drug with other biologic therapy.
Antibiotics			
minocycline (Minocin) (antirheumatic use needs additional validation in clinical studies)	Antirheumatic effect possibly related to immunomodula-tory/antiinflammatory properties	GI effects (nausea/vomiting, diar-rhea, stomach cramps) Dizziness Photosensitivity (severe)	May be reasonable alternative for patient with mild disease but probably not appropriate in severe destructive disease.

TNF, Tumor necrosis factor.

agent such as misoprostol (Cytotec) may be indicated. Arthrotec, a combination of misoprostol and the NSAID diclofenac (Voltaren), is also available.

Because traditional NSAIDs block the production of prosta-glandins from arachidonic acid by inhibiting the production of cyclooxygenase-1 (COX-1) and cyclooxygenase-2 (COX-2) (see Fig. 12-7), the risk for GI erosion and bleeding is in-creased. Traditional NSAIDs affect platelet aggregation, lead-ing to a prolonged bleeding time. Concerns have also been raised regarding the possible negative effects of long-term NSAID treatment on cartilage metabolism, particularly in older patients who may already have diminished cartilage integrity. As an alternative to traditional NSAIDs, treatment with the newer, selective COX-2 inhibitors may be considered, includ-ing celecoxib (Celebrex), valdecoxib (Bextra), and rofecoxib (Vioxx). These drugs inhibit production of COX-2 without af-fecting COX-1, an enzyme that primarily protects the stomach

lining. Research continues to focus on the potential side effects of these drugs.[9]

When given in equivalent antiinflammatory dosages, all NSAIDs are considered comparable in efficacy but vary widely in cost. Individual responses to the NSAIDs are also variable. As-pirin is no longer a common treatment, and it should not be used in combination with NSAIDs because both inhibit platelet func-tion and prolong bleeding time.

Intraarticular injections of corticosteroids may be appropri-ate for the elderly patient with local inflammation and effu-sion. Four or more injections without relief should suggest the need for additional intervention. Systemic use of corticos-teroids is not indicated and can actually accelerate the disease process.

Another treatment for OA is hyaluronic acid (HA). HA con-tributes to both the viscosity and elasticity of synovial fluid, and its degradation can result in joint damage. Intraarticular HA injections have been shown to be safe and effective in treating the pain and functional impairment of knee OA.[10] Synthetic and naturally occurring HA derivatives (Orthovisc, Synvisc, Artz, and Hyalgan) are administered in three weekly injections. Although the exact mechanism of action is unknown, these compounds appear to have antiinflammatory benefits and a short-term lubricant effect. In addition, an analgesic effect may occur through the direct buffering effect of HA on synovial nerve endings.

NURSING MANAGEMENT
OSTEOARTHRITIS

■ Nursing Assessment

The nurse should carefully assess and document the type, location, severity, frequency, and duration of the patient's joint pain and stiffness. The patient should also be questioned about the extent to which these symptoms affect his or her ability to perform activities of daily living. Pain-relieving practices should be noted, and the patient should be questioned about the duration and success of treatment for each intervention. Physical examination of the affected joint or joints includes assessment of tenderness, swelling, limitation of movement, and crepitation. An involved joint should be compared with the contralateral joint if it is not affected.

■ Nursing Diagnoses

Nursing diagnoses for the patient with OA may include, but are not limited to, the following:

- Acute and chronic pain *related to* physical activity and lack of knowledge of pain self-management techniques
- Disturbed sleep pattern *related to* pain
- Impaired physical mobility *related to* weakness, stiffness, or pain on ambulation
- Self-care deficits *related to* joint deformity and pain with activity
- Imbalanced nutrition: more than body requirements *related to* intake in excess of energy output
- Chronic low self-esteem *related to* changing physical appearance and social and work roles

■ Planning

The overall goals are that the patient with OA will (1) maintain or improve joint function through a balance of rest and activity, (2) use joint protection measures (Table 63-4) to improve activity tolerance, (3) achieve independence in self-care and maintain optimal role function, and (4) use pharmacologic and nonpharmacologic strategies to manage pain satisfactorily.

■ Nursing Implementation

Health Promotion. Prevention of primary OA is not possible. However, community education should focus on the elimination of modifiable risk factors through weight loss and the reduction of occupational and recreational hazards. Athletic instruction and physical fitness programs should include safety measures that protect and reduce trauma to the joint structures. Congenital conditions, such as Legg-Calvé-Perthes disease, that are known to predispose a patient to the development of OA should be treated promptly.

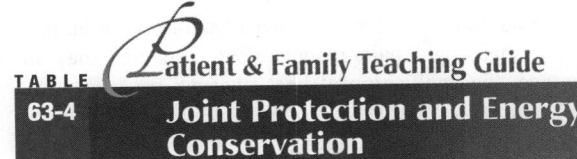

TABLE 63-4	**Patient & Family Teaching Guide** **Joint Protection and Energy Conservation**

- Lose or maintain weight.
- Use assistive devices, if indicated.
- Avoid forceful repetitive movements.
- Avoid positions of joint deviation and stress.
- Use good posture and proper body mechanics.
- Seek assistance with necessary tasks that may cause pain.
- Develop organizing and pacing techniques for routine tasks.
- Modify home and work environment to create less stressful ways to perform tasks.

Acute Intervention. The person with OA most often complains of pain, stiffness, limitation of function, and the frustration of coping with these physical difficulties on a daily basis. The older adult may believe that OA is an inevitable part of the aging process and that nothing can be done to ease the discomfort and related disability.

The OA patient is usually treated on an outpatient basis, often by an interdisciplinary team of health care providers that includes a rheumatologist, a nurse, an occupational therapist, and a physical therapist. Health assessment questionnaires are often used to pinpoint areas of difficulty for the patient with arthritis. Questionnaires are updated at regular intervals to document disease and treatment progression. Treatment goals can be developed based on data from the questionnaires and the physical examination, with specific interventions to target identified problems. The patient is usually hospitalized only if joint surgery is planned (see Chapter 61).

EVIDENCE-BASED PRACTICE
Exercise in Osteoarthritis of the Knee

Clinical Problem
How effective is physical therapy and exercise in patients with osteoarthritis of the knee?

Best Clinical Practice
- In patients with osteoarthritis of the knee, physical therapy and exercise decrease pain and stiffness and increase function and ability to walk.

Implications for Nursing Practice
- Assessment of patients with osteoarthritis should include careful documentation of the nature, location, severity, and frequency of joint pain and stiffness.
- Overall goals for the patient with osteoarthritis of the knee are to balance rest and exercise and use joint protection measures.

Reference for Evidence
EMB Reviews: Manual physical therapy and exercise improve function in osteoarthritis of the knee, *ACP Journal Club* 133:57, 2000.

Drugs are administered for the relief of pain and inflammation. Nonpharmacologic pain management strategies may include massage, the application of heat (thermal packs) or cold (ice packs), relaxation, and guided imagery. Splints may be prescribed to rest and stabilize painful or inflamed joints. Once an acute flare has subsided, a physical therapist can provide valuable assistance in planning an exercise program. Therapists may often recommend Tai Chi as a low-impact form of exercise. Tai Chi can be performed by patients of all ages and may be done in a wheelchair. The nurse should emphasize the importance of warming up before practice to prevent stretch injuries.

Patient and family teaching related to OA is an important nursing responsibility in any care setting and is the foundation of successful disease management. Teaching should include information about the nature and treatment of the disease, pain management, correct posture and body mechanics, correct use of assistive devices such as a cane or walker, principles of joint protection and energy conservation (see Table 63-4), nutritional choices and weight management, stress management, and a therapeutic exercise program. The patient should be assured that OA is a localized disease and that severe deforming arthritis is not the usual course. The patient can also gain support and understanding of the disease process through community resources such as the Arthritis Foundation's Self-Help Course.

Ambulatory and Home Care. Chronic pain and a loss of function of the affected joints continue to be a primary concern. Home management goals must be individualized to meet the patient's needs, and family members or significant others should be included in goal setting and teaching. Home and work environment modification is essential for patient safety.[11] Measures include removing scatter rugs, providing rails at the stairs and bathtub, using night-lights, and wearing well-fitting supportive shoes. Assistive devices such as canes, walkers, elevated toilet seats, and grab bars also reduce the load on the joint and promote safety. The nurse should urge the patient to continue all prescribed pharmacologic and nonpharmacologic therapies at home and also be open to the discussion of new approaches to symptom management.

Sexual counseling may help the patient and significant other to enjoy physical closeness by introducing the idea of alternate positions and timing for intercourse. Discussion also increases awareness of each partner's needs. The nurse should encourage the patient to take analgesics or a warm bath to decrease joint stiffness before sexual activity.

■ Evaluation

The expected outcomes are that the patient with OA will

- experience adequate amounts of rest and activity
- achieve satisfactory pain management
- maintain joint flexibility and muscle strength through joint protection and therapeutic exercise
- verbalize acceptance of OA as a chronic disease, collaborating with health care providers in disease management

RHEUMATOID ARTHRITIS

Rheumatoid arthritis (RA) is a chronic, systemic disease characterized by inflammation of connective tissue in the diarthrodial (synovial) joints, typically with periods of remission and exacerbation. RA is frequently accompanied by extraarticular manifestations.

RA occurs globally, affecting all ethnic groups. It can occur at any time of life, but the incidence increases with age, peaking between the fourth and sixth decades. Women are affected by RA two to three times more frequently than men.[12] Smoking appears to be linked to both disease development and severity.[13]

Etiology and Pathophysiology

The cause of RA is unknown. Despite past theories, no infectious agent has been cultured from blood and synovial tissue or fluid with enough reproducibility to suggest an infectious cause for the disease. An autoimmune etiology is currently the most widely accepted.

1. *Autoimmunity.* The autoimmune theory suggests that changes associated with RA begin when a susceptible host experiences an initial immune response to an antigen. The antigen, which is probably not the same in all patients, triggers the formation of an abnormal immunoglobulin G (IgG). RA is characterized by the presence of autoantibodies against this abnormal IgG. The autoantibodies are known as *rheumatoid factor* (RF), and they combine with IgG to form immune complexes that initially deposit on synovial membranes or superficial articular cartilage in the joints. Immune complex formation leads to the activation of complement, and an inflammatory response results. (Complement activation is discussed in Chapter 12, and immune complex formation is discussed in Chapter 13.) Neutrophils are attracted to the site of inflammation, where they release proteolytic enzymes that can damage articular cartilage and cause the synovial lining to thicken (Fig. 63-3). Other inflammatory cells include T helper (CD4) cells, which are the primary orchestrators of cell-mediated immune responses. Activated CD4 cells stimulate monocytes, macrophages, and synovial fibroblasts to secrete the proinflammatory cytokines interleukin-1 (IL-1), interleukin-6 (IL-6), and tumor necrosis factor (TNF). These cytokines are the primary factors that drive the inflammatory response in RA.

Joint changes from chronic inflammation begin when the hypertrophied synovial membrane invades the surrounding cartilage, ligaments, tendons, and joint capsule. *Pannus* (highly vascular granulation tissue) forms within the joint. It eventually covers and erodes the entire surface of the articular cartilage. The production of inflammatory cytokines at the pannus-cartilage junction further contributes to cartilage destruction. The pannus also scars and shortens supporting structures such as

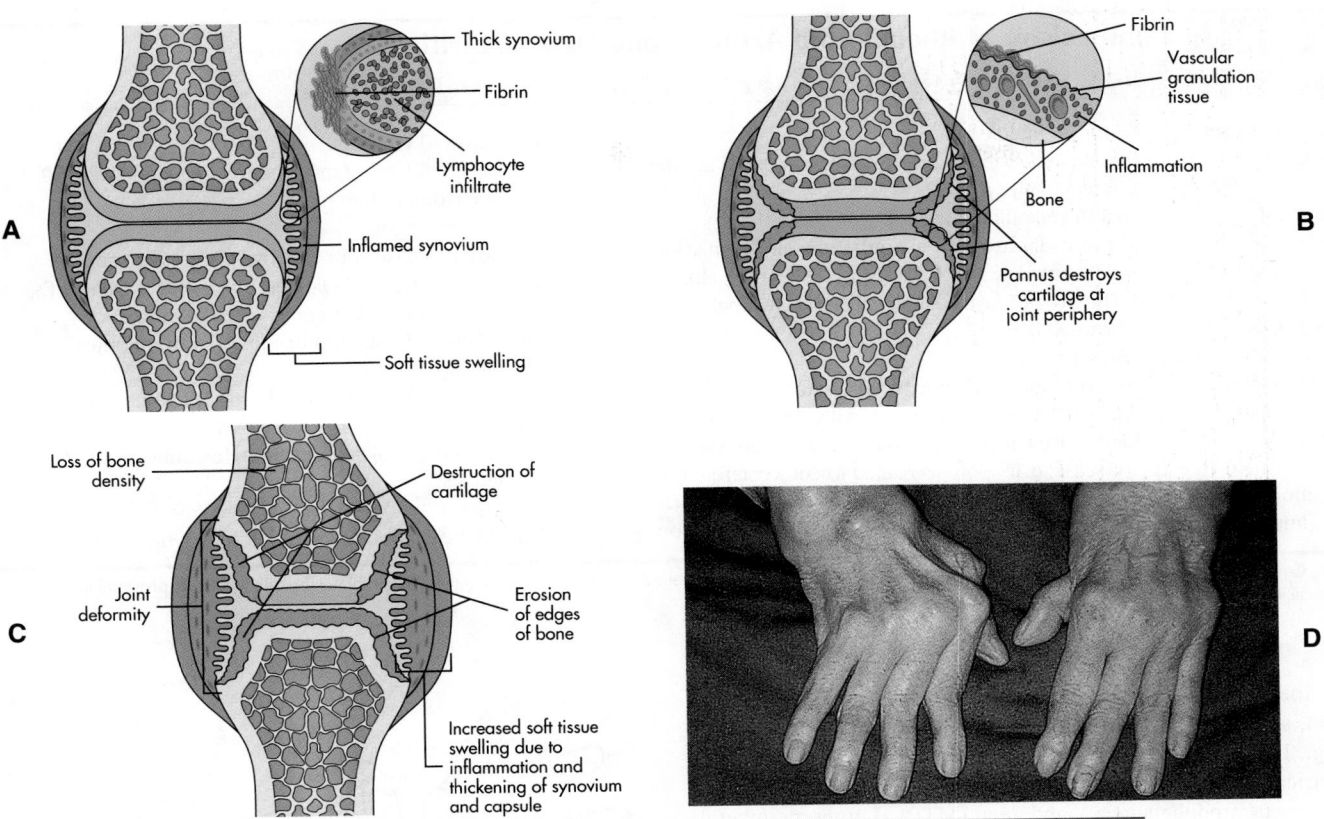

FIG. 63-3 Rheumatoid arthritis. **A,** Early pathologic change in rheumatoid arthritis is rheumatoid synovitis. The synovium is inflamed. There is a great increase in lymphocytes. **B,** With time, there is articular cartilage destruction; vascular granulation tissue grows across the surface of the cartilage (pannus) from the edges of the joint, and the articular surface shows loss of cartilage beneath the extending pannus, most marked at the joint margins. **C,** Inflammatory pannus causes focal destruction of bone. At the edges of the joint there is osteolytic destruction of bone, responsible for erosions seen on x-rays. This phase is associated with joint deformity. **D,** Characteristic deformity and soft tissue swelling associated with long-standing rheumatoid disease of the hands.

tendons and ligaments, ultimately causing joint laxity, subluxation, and contracture.

2. *Genetic factors.* Genetic predisposition appears to be important in the development of RA. For example, a higher occurrence of the disease has been noted in identical rather than fraternal twins. The strongest evidence for a familial influence is the increased occurrence of a human leukocyte antigen (HLA) known as HLA-DR4 in white RA patients. Other HLA variants have also been identified in patients from other ethnic groups. (HLA is discussed in Chapter 13.)

The pathogenesis of RA is more clearly understood than its etiology. If unarrested, the disease progresses through four stages, which are identified in Table 63-5.

Clinical Manifestations

Joints. The onset of RA is typically insidious. Nonspecific manifestations such as fatigue, anorexia, weight loss, and generalized stiffness may precede the onset of arthritic complaints. The stiffness becomes more localized in the following weeks to months. Some patients report a history of a precipitating stressful event such as infection, work stress, physical exertion, childbirth, surgery, or emotional upset. However, research has been unable to correlate such events directly with the onset of RA.

TABLE 63-5 **Anatomic Stages of Rheumatoid Arthritis**

Stage I—Early
No destructive changes on x-ray, possible x-ray evidence of osteoporosis

Stage II—Moderate
X-ray evidence of osteoporosis, with or without slight bone or cartilage destruction, no joint deformities (although possibly limited joint mobility), adjacent muscle atrophy, possible presence of extraarticular soft tissue lesions (e.g., nodules, tenosynovitis)

Stage III—Severe
X-ray evidence of cartilage and bone destruction in addition to osteoporosis; joint deformity, such as subluxation, ulnar deviation, or hyperextension, without fibrous or bony ankylosis; extensive muscle atrophy; possible presence of extraarticular soft tissue lesions (e.g., nodules, tenosynovitis)

Stage IV—Terminal
Fibrous or bony ankylosis, criteria of stage III

Data from Kirwan JR: Using the Larsen Index to assess radiographic progression in rheumatoid arthritis, *J Rheumatology* 27:264, 2000.

TABLE 63-6   Comparison of Rheumatoid Arthritis and Osteoarthritis

PARAMETER	RHEUMATOID ARTHRITIS	OSTEOARTHRITIS
Age at onset	Young to middle age	Usually >40 yr of age
Gender	Female/male ratio is 2:1 or 3:1; less marked gender difference after age 60	Before age 50, more men than women; after age 50, more women than men
Weight	Lost or maintained weight	Often overweight
Disease	Systemic disease with exacerbations and remissions	Localized disease with variable, progressive course
Affected joints	Small joints first (PIPs, MCPs, MTPs), wrists, elbows, shoulders, knees; usually bilateral, symmetric	Weight-bearing joints (knees, hips), MCPs, DIPs, PIPs, cervical and lumbar spine; often asymmetric
Stiffness	1 hr to all day	On arising but usually subsides after 30 minutes
Effusions	Common	Uncommon
Nodules	Present, especially on extensor surfaces	Heberden's (DIPs) and Bouchard's (PIPs) nodes
Synovial fluid	WBC count >2000/μl with mostly neutrophils	WBC <2000/μl (mild leukocytosis)
X-rays	Joint space narrowing, erosion, subluxation with advanced disease; osteoporosis related to corticosteroid use	Joint space narrowing, osteophytes, subchondral cysts, sclerosis
Laboratory findings	RF positive in 80% of patients Elevated ESR, CRP indicative of active inflammation	RF negative Transient elevation in ESR related to synovitis

CRP, C-reactive protein; *DIP*, distal interphalangeal; *ESR*, erythrocyte sedimentation rate; *MCP*, metacarpophalangeal; *MTP*, metatarsophalangeal; *PIP*, proximal interphalangeal; *RF*, rheumatoid factor.

Specific articular involvement is manifested clinically by pain, stiffness, limitation of motion, and signs of inflammation (e.g., heat, swelling, tenderness).[14] Joint symptoms occur symmetrically and frequently affect the small joints of the hands (PIP and metacarpophalangeal) and feet (MTP). Larger peripheral joints such as the wrists, elbows, shoulders, knees, hips, ankles, and jaw may also be involved. The cervical spine may be affected, but the axial spine is generally spared. Table 63-6 compares the manifestations of RA and OA.

The patient characteristically experiences joint stiffness after periods of inactivity. Morning stiffness may last from 60 minutes to several hours or more, depending on disease activity. Metacarpal and PIP joints are typically swollen. In early disease, the fingers may become spindle shaped from synovial hypertrophy and thickening of the joint capsule (see Fig. 63-3). Joints become tender, painful, and warm to the touch. Joint pain increases with motion, varies in intensity, and may not be proportional to the degree of inflammation. Tenosynovitis frequently affects the extensor and flexor tendons around the wrists, producing manifestations of carpal tunnel syndrome and making it difficult for the patient to grasp objects.

As disease activity progresses, inflammation and fibrosis of the joint capsule and supporting structures may lead to deformity and disability. Atrophy of muscles and destruction of tendons around the joint cause one articular surface to slip past the other (*subluxation*). Typical distortions of the hand include ulnar drift ("zig zag deformity"), swan-neck, and boutonnière deformities (Fig. 63-4). Metatarsal-head subluxation and hallux valgus (bunion) in the feet may cause pain and walking disability.

Extraarticular Manifestations. RA can affect nearly every system in the body. Extraarticular manifestations of RA are depicted in Fig. 63-5. The three most common are rheumatoid nodules, Sjögren syndrome, and Felty syndrome.

Rheumatoid nodules develop in up to 25% of all patients with RA. Those affected with nodules usually have high titers of RF. Rheumatoid nodules appear subcutaneously as firm, nontender, granuloma-type masses and are usually over the extensor sur-

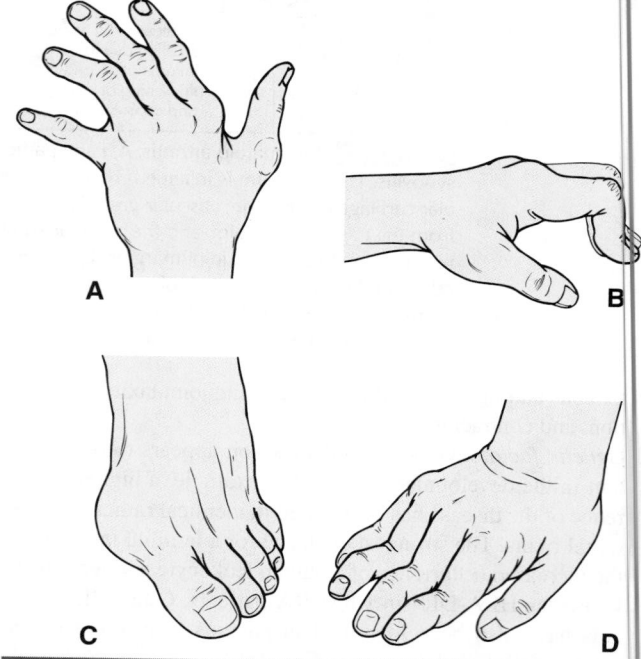

FIG. 63-4 Typical deformities of rheumatoid arthritis. **A,** Ulnar drift. **B,** Boutonnière deformity. **C,** Hallux valgus. **D,** Swan-neck deformity.

faces of joints such as fingers and elbows. Nodules at the base of the spine and back of the head are common in older adults. Nodules develop insidiously and can persist or regress spontaneously. They are usually not removed because of the high probability of recurrence, but they can easily break down or become infected. Nodules may also appear on the sclera or lungs; these indicate active disease and a poorer prognosis.

Sjögren syndrome is seen in 10% to 15% of patients with RA. Sjögren syndrome can occur as a disease by itself or in conjunction with other arthritic disorders such as RA and systemic lupus

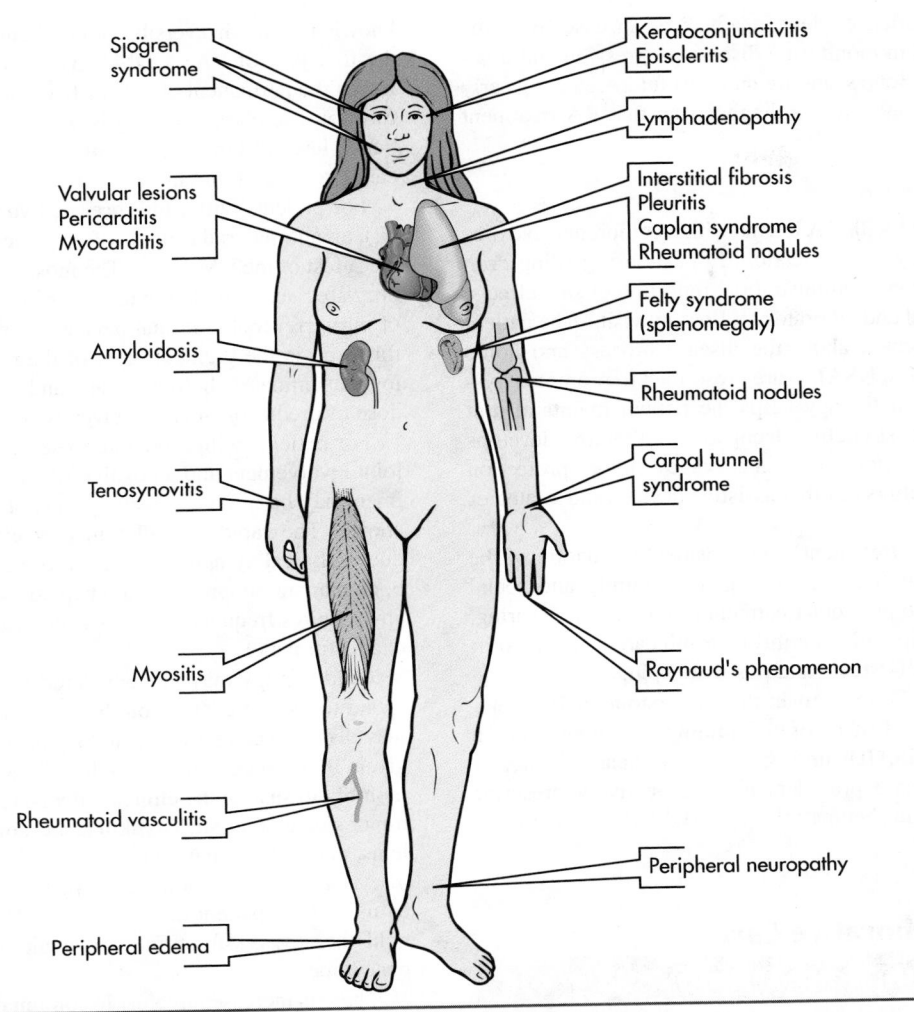

Sjögren syndrome

Keratoconjunctivitis
Episcleritis

Lymphadenopathy

Valvular lesions
Pericarditis
Myocarditis

Interstitial fibrosis
Pleuritis
Caplan syndrome
Rheumatoid nodules

Felty syndrome
(splenomegaly)

Amyloidosis

Rheumatoid nodules

Carpal tunnel
syndrome

Tenosynovitis

Myositis

Raynaud's phenomenon

Rheumatoid vasculitis

Peripheral neuropathy

Peripheral edema

FIG. 63-5   Extraarticular manifestations of rheumatoid arthritis.

erythematosus (SLE). Affected patients have diminished lacrimal and salivary gland secretion, leading to complaints of burning, gritty, itchy eyes. They experience decreased tearing and photosensitivity (see p. 1748).

Felty syndrome occurs most commonly in patients with severe, nodule-forming RA. It is characterized by inflammatory eye disorders, splenomegaly, lymphadenopathy, pulmonary disease, and blood dyscrasias (anemia, thrombocytopenia, granulocytopenia).

Complications

Without treatment, joint destruction begins as early as the first year of the disease. Flexion contractures and hand deformities cause diminished grasp strength and affect the patient's ability to perform self-care tasks. Nodular myositis and muscle fiber degeneration can lead to pain similar to that of vascular insufficiency. Cataract development and loss of vision can result from scleral nodules. Complications can also result from rheumatoid nodules. On the skin, these nodules can ulcerate, similar to pressure sores. Nodules on the vocal cords lead to progressive hoarseness, and nodules in the vertebral bodies can cause bone destruction. In later disease, cardiopulmonary effects are not uncommon. These may include pleurisy, pleural effusion, peri-

carditis, pericardial effusion, and cardiomyopathy. Carpal tunnel syndrome results from neuromuscular involvement.

Diagnostic Studies

An accurate diagnosis is essential to the initiation of appropriate treatment and the prevention of unnecessary disability. A diagnosis is often made based on history and physical findings, but some laboratory tests are useful for confirmation and to monitor disease progression (Table 63-6). Positive RF occurs in approximately 80% of patients, and titers rise during active disease. ESR and C-reactive protein (CRP) are general indicators of active inflammation. Antinuclear antibody (ANA) titers are also seen in some RA patients.

Synovial fluid analysis in early disease often shows a straw-colored fluid with many fibrin flecks. The white blood cell (WBC) count of synovial fluid is elevated (up to 25,000/μl). Inflammatory changes in the synovium can be confirmed by tissue biopsy.

X-rays are not specifically diagnostic of RA. They may be inconclusive during early stages of the disease, revealing only soft tissue swelling and possible bone demineralization. In later disease, narrowing of the joint space, destruction of articular cartilage, erosion, subluxation, and deformity are seen. Malalignment and ankylosis are often evident in advanced disease. Baseline films may be useful in monitoring disease progression and treatment effectiveness. Bone scans are more useful in detecting early joint changes and confirming a diagnosis so that RA treatment can be initiated.

Collaborative Care

Care of the patient with RA begins with a comprehensive program of drug therapy and education. Education regarding drug therapy includes correct administration, reporting of side effects, and frequent medical and laboratory follow-up visits. The patient and family are educated about the disease process and home management strategies. NSAIDs are prescribed to promote physical comfort. Physical therapy helps the patient maintain joint motion and muscle strength. Occupational therapy develops upper-extremity function and encourages joint protection through the use of splints or other assistive devices and strategies for activity pacing.

An individualized treatment plan considers the nature of the disease activity, joint function, age, gender, family and social roles, and response to previous treatment (Table 63-7). A caring, long-term relationship with an arthritis health care team can promote the patient's self-esteem and positive coping.

Drug Therapy. Drugs remain the cornerstone of RA treatment (see Table 63-3). Instead of maintaining the patient on high doses of aspirin or NSAIDs until x-rays show clear evidence of the disease, health care providers now aggressively prescribe disease-modifying antirheumatic drugs (DMARDs) with the

knowledge that irreversible joint changes can occur as early as the first year of RA. A DMARD is a drug with the potential to lessen the permanent effects of RA, such as joint erosion and deformity. The choice of drug is based on disease activity, the patient's level of function, and lifestyle considerations, such as the desire to bear children.

For patients with mild disease, hydroxychloroquine (Plaquenil), an antimalarial drug, is often prescribed initially. It is one of the safest of the DMARDs. The most common side effects of this drug are nausea, abdominal discomfort, and rash. The possibility of rare, irreversible retinal degeneration caused by deposition of this drug in the pigment layer of the retina requires ophthalmologic examination before therapy and at 6-month intervals. A low dose of prednisone may be given with hydroxychloroquine.

For patients with moderate to severe disease with symmetric joint involvement and a positive RF, a more aggressive drug regimen may be initiated. Usually methotrexate is the first drug of choice. The rapid antiinflammatory effect of methotrexate reduces clinical symptoms in days to weeks. Side effects include bone marrow suppression and hepatotoxicity. Methotrexate therapy requires frequent laboratory monitoring, including CBC and chemistry panel.

Gold therapy may be considered for patients who do not respond to methotrexate. Gold has an antiinflammatory action and may decrease phagocytosis and lysosomal activity.[15] It is usually given in a weekly injection for 5 months, then biweekly or monthly to sustain the clinical effects. Gold therapy often causes minor side effects, such as skin rashes, mouth sores, and GI problems, particularly diarrhea.

Azathioprine (Imuran) or D-penicillamine (Cuprimine) may be used if the patient does not respond to either methotrexate or gold therapy. Azathioprine and penicillamine may cause mild pancytopenia.

There is increased interest in combination therapy to treat RA. Possible combinations include methotrexate plus sulfasalazine (Azulfidine) and hydroxychloroquine plus sulfasalazine. Multiple agents may provide a synergistic effect and more adequately control symptoms.[16]

The newer-generation NSAIDs, COX-2 inhibitors, are effective in RA, as well as OA. These include celecoxib (Celebrex), rofecoxib (Vioxx), and valdecoxib (Bextra) (see Table 63-3).

Biologic therapy using TNF inhibitors is a new class of drugs used to slow disease progression in RA.[17] These drugs include etanercept (Enbrel), infliximab (Remicade), adalimumab (Humira), and anakinra (Kineret). These drugs can be used to treat patients with moderate to severe disease who have not responded to DMARDs.

Etanercept is a biologically engineered copy (using recombinant DNA technology) of the TNF cell receptor. This soluble TNF receptor binds to TNF in circulation before TNF can bind to the cell surface receptor. By inhibiting binding of TNF, etanercept inhibits the inflammatory response. This drug is given two times per week as a subcutaneous injection.

Infliximab and adalimumab are monoclonal antibodies against TNF. They bind to TNF, thus preventing it from binding to TNF receptors on cells. Infliximab is given IV on a weekly basis. Adalimumab is given subcutaneously every other week.

Anakinra (Kineret) is a recombinant version of IL-1 receptor antagonist (IL-1Ra). It blocks the biologic activity of IL-1 by competitively inhibiting IL-1 binding to the IL-1 receptor. It is given as

TABLE 63-7	Collaborative Care Rheumatoid Arthritis

Diagnostic
History and physical examination
Laboratory studies
    Complete blood cell count (CBC)
    Erythrocyte sedimentation rate (ESR)
    Rheumatoid factor (RF)
    Antinuclear antibody (ANA)
    C-reactive protein (CRP)
Radiologic studies of involved joints
Synovial fluid analysis

Collaborative Therapy
Nutritional counseling
Therapeutic exercise
Rest and joint protection, use of assistive devices
Heat and cold
Complementary and alternative therapies
    Herbal products
    Movement therapies
Drug therapy*
    Disease-modifying antirheumatic drugs (DMARDs)
    Intraarticular or systemic corticosteroids
Biologic therapy
Orthopedic surgery
    Implants
    Arthroplasty

*See Table 63–3.

a subcutaneous injection. Anakinra is used to reduce the pain and swelling associated with moderate to severe RA.[18] Side effects are minor, including redness and swelling at the injection site. It can be used in combination with DMARDs but not with TNF inhibitors. Concurrent use of these agents can cause serious infection and neutropenia.

Corticosteroid therapy can be used to aid in symptom control. Intraarticular injections may temporarily relieve the pain and inflammation associated with disease flare-ups. Long-term use of oral corticosteroids should not be a mainstay of RA treatment because of the risk of osteoporosis and avascular necrosis. However, low-dose prednisone may be used for a limited time in select patients to decrease disease activity until a DMARD effect is seen.

Various NSAIDs and salicylates continue to be included in the drug regimen to treat arthritis pain and inflammation. Aspirin is often used in high dosages of 4 to 6 g per day (10 to 18 tablets). Because enteric-coated aspirin is absorbed in the small intestine, it can be prescribed in higher doses than regular tablets. The ability to obtain serum salicylate levels is helpful in developing and evaluating individualized treatment plans.

NSAIDs have antiinflammatory, analgesic, and antipyretic properties. Although many NSAIDs are potent inhibitors of inflammation, they do not appear to alter the natural history of RA. Some relief may be noted within days of the start of treatment with NSAIDs, but full effectiveness may take 2 to 3 weeks. NSAIDs may be used when the patient cannot tolerate high doses of aspirin. Those antiinflammatory drugs that are taken only once or twice a day may improve the patient's ability to follow the treatment regimen (see Table 63-3).

Antibiotics may be used in treatment of RA. The antirheumatic effect of minocycline (Minocin) may be due to its immunomodulatory and antiinflammatory properties. The drug is usually given for mild cases because of its only moderate effect on the disease. Dosage is typically 200 mg daily.

Apheresis. A blood filtration device used in apheresis called the Prosorba column is now being used to treat severe RA in patients who are not responding to other treatments. RF is removed from the patient's blood as it passes through the column. Patients are treated once a week for 12 weeks. Limited data have shown a decrease in RA signs and symptoms in most patients treated.[19] (Apheresis is discussed in Chapter 13.)

Nutritional Therapy. Although there is no special diet for RA, balanced nutrition is important. Fatigue, pain, depression, limited endurance, and mobility deficits often accompany RA and may cause a loss of appetite or interfere with the patient's ability to shop for and prepare food. Weight loss may result. The occupational therapist may help the patient to modify the home environment and to use assistive devices to make food preparation easier.

Corticosteroid therapy or immobility secondary to pain may result in unwanted weight gain. A sensible weight loss program consisting of balanced nutrition and exercise reduces stress on arthritic joints. Corticosteroids also increase the appetite, resulting in a higher caloric intake. In addition, the patient may become distressed as signs and symptoms of Cushing syndrome, including moon face and the redistribution of fatty tissue to the trunk, change one's physical appearance. The patient must be encouraged to continue a balanced diet and not to alter the corticosteroid dose or stop therapy abruptly. Weight slowly adjusts to normal several months after cessation of therapy.

NURSING MANAGEMENT
RHEUMATOID ARTHRITIS

■ Nursing Assessment

Subjective and objective data that should be obtained from the patient with RA are presented in Table 63-8.

■ Nursing Diagnoses

Nursing diagnoses for the patient with RA may include, but are not limited to, those presented in NCP 63-1.

TABLE 63-8	Nursing Assessment Rheumatoid Arthritis

Subjective Data

Important Health Information

Past health history: Recent infections; presence of precipitating factors such as emotional upset, infections, overwork, childbirth, surgery; pattern of remissions and exacerbations

Medications: Use of aspirin, NSAIDs, corticosteroids, DMARDs

Surgery or other treatments: Any joint surgery

Health Patterns

Health perception–health management: Positive family history for rheumatoid arthritis, malaise, ability to participate in therapeutic regimen

Nutritional-metabolic: Anorexia, weight loss; dry mucous membranes of mouth and pharynx

Activity-exercise: Stiffness and joint swelling, muscle weakness, difficulty walking, fatigue

Cognitive-perceptual: Paresthesias of hands and feet; numbness, tingling, loss of sensation; symmetric joint pain and aching that increases with motion or stress on joint

Objective Data

General

Lymphadenopathy, fever

Integumentary

Keratoconjunctivitis; subcutaneous rheumatoid nodules on forearm, elbows; skin ulcers; shiny, taut skin over involved joints; peripheral edema

Cardiovascular

Symmetric pallor and cyanosis of fingers (Raynaud's phenomenon); distant heart sounds, murmurs, arrhythmias

Respiratory

Chronic bronchitis, tuberculosis, histoplasmosis, fibrosing alveolitis

Gastrointestinal

Splenomegaly (Felty syndrome)

Musculoskeletal

Symmetric joint involvement with swelling, erythema, heat, tenderness, and deformities; enlargement of proximal phalangeal and metacarpophalangeal joints; limitation of joint movement; muscle contractures, muscle atrophy

Possible Findings

Positive rheumatoid factor, ↑ ESR, anemia; ↑ WBC in synovial fluid; evidence of joint space narrowing, and bony erosion and deformity on x-ray (osteoporosis with advanced disease)

DMARDs, Disease-modifying antirheumatic drugs; *ESR,* erythrocyte sedimentation rate; *NSAIDs,* nonsteroidal antiinflammatory drugs; *WBC,* white blood cells.

■ Planning

The overall goals are that patient with RA will (1) have satisfactory pain relief, (2) have minimal loss of functional ability of the affected joints, (3) participate in planning and carrying out the therapeutic regimen, (4) maintain a positive self-image, and (5) perform self-care to the maximum amount possible.

■ Nursing Implementation

Health Promotion. Prevention of RA is not possible at this time. However, community education programs should focus on symptom recognition to promote early diagnosis and treatment of RA. The Arthritis Foundation offers many publications, classes, and support activities (see the Resources at end of this chapter).

Acute Intervention. The primary goals in the management of RA are reduction of inflammation, management of pain, maintenance of joint function, and prevention or correction of joint deformity. Goals may be met through a comprehensive program of drug therapy, rest, joint protection, heat and cold applications, exercise, and patient and family teaching. The nurse is an integral member of the health team, working closely with the health care provider, physical and occupational therapists, and social worker to restore function and to help the patient make appropriate lifestyle adjustments to chronic illness.

NURSING CARE PLAN 63-1

Patient with Rheumatoid Arthritis

NURSING DIAGNOSIS   **Chronic pain** *related to* joint inflammation, overuse of joint, and ineffective pain and/or comfort measures *as manifested by* communication of pain descriptors, guarding behavior, and limited joint function; hot, swollen, painful joints.

OUTCOMES–NOC

Pain Control (1605)
- Recognizes causal factors _____
- Uses preventive measures _____
- Uses nonanalgesic relief measures _____
- Uses analgesics appropriately _____

_____

Outcome Scale
1 = Never demonstrated
2 = Rarely demonstrated
3 = Sometimes demonstrated
4 = Often demonstrated
5 = Consistently demonstrated

Comfort Level (2100)
- Expressed satisfaction with pain control _____
- Reported satisfaction with symptom control _____

_____

Outcome Scale
1 = None
2 = Limited
3 = Moderate
4 = Substantial
5 = Extensive

INTERVENTIONS–NIC and *RATIONALES*

Pain Management (1400)
- Perform a comprehensive pain assessment to include location, characteristics, onset/duration, frequency, quality, intensity or severity of pain, and precipitating factors *to establish a pattern and baseline assessment and to plan appropriate interventions.*
- Evaluate with the patient, family, and the health care team the effectiveness of past pain control measures that have been used *to assess what has helped and not helped in the past.*
- Reduce or eliminate factors that precipitate or increase the pain experience such as fear, fatigue, and lack of knowledge *to minimize negative stimuli that may increase pain.*
- Teach the use of nonpharmacologic techniques, such as relaxation, distraction, warm applications and massage, before pain occurs or increases *to promote muscle relaxation and decrease tension.*
- Provide the patient with optimal pain relief with prescribed analgesics as appropriate *to help decrease pain and inflammation.*

NURSING DIAGNOSIS   **Impaired physical mobility** *related to* joint pain, stiffness, and deformity *as manifested by* limitation of joint motion, strength, and endurance; inability to perform routine activities of daily living.

OUTCOMES–NOC

Mobility Level (0208)
- Joint movement _____
- Body positioning performance _____

_____

Outcome Scale
1 = Dependent, does not participate
2 = Requires assistive person and device
3 = Requires assistive device
4 = Independent with assistive device
5 = Completely independent

INTERVENTIONS–NIC and *RATIONALES*

Exercise Therapy: Joint Mobility (0224)
- Determine limitations of joint movement and effect on function *to establish baseline for plan of care.*
- Collaborate with physical therapy in developing and executing an exercise program *to maintain and improve joint function.*
- Explain to patient and family the purpose and plan for joint exercises *to provide information and support for the patient.*
- Apply moist heat to affected joints (e.g., hot packs, warm shower) *to relieve stiffness and increase mobility.*
- Instruct patient on correct application of resting splints, selection of properly fitting footwear, maintenance of proper posture and body alignment, and selection and use of assistive devices *to prevent or limit joint deformity.*

NURSING CARE PLAN 63-1

Patient with Rheumatoid Arthritis—cont'd

NURSING DIAGNOSIS   **Disturbed body image** *related to* chronic disease activity, long-term treatment, deformities, stiffness, and inability to perform usual activities *as manifested by* social withdrawal, flat affect, altered self-concept, and reduced sexual interest.

OUTCOMES—NOC

Psychosocial Adjustment: Life Changes (1305)
- Maintenance of self-esteem _____
- Expressions of productivity _____
- Expressions of feeling socially engaged _____

Outcome Scale
1 = None
2 = Limited
3 = Moderate
4 = Substantial
5 = Extensive

INTERVENTIONS—NIC and *RATIONALES*

Body Image Enhancement (5220)
- Identify the significance of the patient's culture, religion, race, sex, and age on body image *to determine extent of problems and plan appropriate interventions.*
- Assist patient to discuss changes caused by illness *to identify problems and plan appropriate interventions.*
- Assist patient to separate physical appearance from feelings of personal worth *so that a positive body image is fostered in spite of physical manifestations.*
- Facilitate contact with individuals with similar changes in body image *to promote sharing and socialization for patient.*

Sexual Counseling (5248)
- Provide referral/consultation with other members of the health care team, such as a sex therapist, *because sexual problems and concerns can have a serious impact on body image.*
- Include the spouse/sexual partner in the counseling as much as possible *to encourage communication.*

NURSING DIAGNOSIS   **Ineffective therapeutic regimen management** *related to* complexity of chronic health problem, pain, and fatigue *as manifested by* questioning management plan, self-doubt about ability to manage disease, ability to perform activities for only short periods.

OUTCOMES—NOC

Participation: Health Care Decisions (1606)
- Seeks information _____
- Demonstrates self-direction in decision making _____
- States intent to act on decision _____
- Seeks services to meet desired outcomes _____

Outcome Scale
1 = Never demonstrated
2 = Rarely demonstrated
3 = Sometimes demonstrated
4 = Often demonstrated
5 = Consistently demonstrated

INTERVENTIONS—NIC and *RATIONALES*

Anticipatory Guidance (5210)
- Assess patient's knowledge of disease *to plan appropriate interventions.*
- Determine the patient's usual method of problem solving *to identify where interventions should focus.*
- Provide information on realistic expectations related to the patient's behavior and illness *to ensure correct understanding of disease management.*
- Refer the patient to community agencies, such as Meals on Wheels or the Arthritis Foundation, as appropriate *to allow the patient to meet desired outcomes.*
- Include the family/significant others in disease management *to increase their sense of control and to increase patient's sense of support.*
- Discuss patient's problems of pain and fatigue *because these are major deterrents to successful disease management and must be addressed.*

NURSING DIAGNOSIS   **Self-care deficit (total)** *related to* disease progression, weakness, and contracture *as manifested by* inability to perform activities of daily living.

OUTCOMES—NOC

Self-Care: Activities of Daily Living (ADL) (0300)
- Eating _____
- Dressing _____
- Toileting _____
- Bathing _____
- Grooming _____

Outcome Scale
1 = Dependent, does not participate
2 = Requires assistive person and device
3 = Requires assistive person
4 = Independent with assistive device
5 = Completely independent

INTERVENTIONS—NIC and *RATIONALES*

Self-Care Assistance (1800)
- Monitor patient's ability for independent self-care *to plan appropriate interventions.*
- Monitor patient's need for adaptive devices for personal hygiene, dressing, grooming, toileting, and eating *to compensate for contractures and weakness so that patient can perform as many self-care activities as possible.*
- Establish a routine for self-care activities with rest periods *to foster maximum independence with minimal fatigue.*
- Assist patient in accepting dependency needs *to ensure all needs are met.*
- Teach family to encourage independence and to intervene only when the patient is unable to perform *to promote independence.*

The newly diagnosed RA patient is usually treated on an outpatient basis, although hospitalization may be necessary for patients with extraarticular complications or advancing disease requiring reconstructive surgery for disabling deformities. Nursing intervention begins with a careful physical assessment (e.g., joint pain, swelling, range of motion [ROM], and general health status). The nurse must also evaluate psychosocial needs (e.g., family support, sexual satisfaction, emotional stress, financial constraints, vocation and career limitations) and environmental concerns (e.g., transportation, home or work modifications). After problem identification, a carefully planned program for rehabilitation and education can be coordinated by the nurse for the interdisciplinary health care team.

Suppression of inflammation is most effectively achieved through the administration of NSAIDs and DMARDs. Careful attention to timing is critical to sustain a therapeutic drug level and reduce early morning stiffness. The nurse should discuss the action and side effects of each prescribed drug and the importance of necessary laboratory monitoring. Many patients with RA will take several different drugs, and the nurse must make the drug regimen as understandable as possible.

Nonpharmacologic relief of pain may include the use of therapeutic heat and cold, rest, relaxation techniques, joint protection (see Tables 63-4 and 63-9), biofeedback (see Chapter 7), transcutaneous electrical nerve stimulation (see Chapter 9), and hypnosis. Assessment for individual differences and preference allows the nurse to help the patient and family choose therapies that promote optimal comfort within the parameters of their lifestyle.

Lightweight splints may be prescribed to rest an inflamed joint and prevent deformity from muscle spasms and contractures. The occupational therapist may help to identify additional self-help devices that can assist in activities of daily living. Splints should be removed at regular intervals to give skin care and perform ROM exercises. After assessment has been completed and supportive care has been given, the splints should be reapplied as prescribed.

Morning care and procedures should be planned around the patient's morning stiffness. Sitting or standing in a warm shower, sitting in a tub with warm towels around the shoulders, or simply soaking the hands in a basin of warm water may help relieve joint stiffness and allow the patient to more comfortably perform activities of daily living. Careful skin care should be offered, particularly if the patient is confined to bed.

Ambulatory and Home Care

Rest. Alternating scheduled rest periods with activity throughout the day helps relieve fatigue and pain. The amount of rest needed varies according to the severity of the disease and the patient's limitations. The patient should rest before becoming exhausted. Total bed rest is rarely necessary and should be avoided to prevent stiffness and immobility. However, even a patient with mild disease may require daytime rest in addition to 8 to 10 hours of sleep at night. The nurse should help the patient identify ways to modify daily activities to avoid overexertion that can lead to fatigue and an exacerbation of disease activity. For example, the patient may tolerate meal preparation more easily if the patient sits on a high stool in front of the sink. The nurse should assist the patient to pace activities and set priorities on the basis of realistic goals.

Good body alignment while resting can be maintained through use of a firm mattress or bed board. Positions of extension should be encouraged, and positions of flexion should be avoided. Splints and casts may be helpful in maintaining proper alignment and promoting rest, especially when joint inflammation is present. Lying prone for half an hour twice daily is also recommended. Pillows should never be placed under the knees. A small, flat pillow may be used under the head and shoulders.

Joint protection. Protecting joints from stress is important. The nurse can help the patient to identify ways to modify tasks to put less stress on joints during routine activities (see Table 63-9). Energy conservation requires careful planning. The emphasis is on work simplification techniques. Work should be done in short periods with scheduled rest breaks to avoid fatigue (pacing). Work should be spread throughout the week rather than attempted at one time (e.g., all cleaning should not be done on the weekend). Activities should be carefully organized to avoid going up and down stairs repeatedly. Carts should be used to carry supplies, or materials that are used often can be stored in a convenient, easily reached area. Time-saving joint protective devices (e.g., electric can opener) should be used whenever possible. Tasks can also be delegated to other family members.

Patient independence may be increased by occupational therapy training with assistive devices that help simplify tasks, such as built-up utensils, buttonhooks, modified drawer handles, lightweight plastic dishes, and raised toilet seats.[20] Wearing shoes with Velcro fasteners and clothing with buttons or a zipper down the front instead of the back makes dressing easier. A cane or a walker offers support and relief of pain when walking. A platform-wheeled walker further minimizes strain on the small joints of the hands and wrists. The Arthritis Foundation offers many programs to assist people and is an excellent resource for additional suggestions related to self-care.

TABLE 63-9

Patient & Family Teaching Guide
Protection of Small Joints

1. Maintain joint in neutral position to minimize deformity.
   - Press water from a sponge instead of wringing.
2. Use strongest joint available for any task.
   - When rising from chair, push with palms rather than fingers.
   - Carry laundry basket in both arms rather than with fingers.
3. Distribute weight over many joints instead of stressing a few.
   - Slide objects instead of lifting them.
   - Hold packages close to body for support.
4. Change positions frequently.
   - Do not hold book or grip steering wheel for long periods without resting.
   - Avoid grasping pencil or cutting vegetables with knife for extended periods.
5. Avoid repetitious movements.
   - Do not knit for long periods.
   - Rest between rooms when vacuuming.
6. Modify chores to avoid stress on joints.
   - Avoid heavy tasks.
   - Sit on stool instead of standing during meal preparation.

Heat and cold therapy and exercise. Heat and cold applications can help relieve stiffness, pain, and muscle spasm. Application of ice is especially beneficial during periods of disease exacerbation, whereas moist heat appears to offer better relief of chronic stiffness. The treatment modality should be selected according to disease severity, ease of application, and cost. Superficial heat sources such as heating pads, moist hot packs, paraffin baths, whirlpool baths, and warm baths or showers can relieve stiffness to allow participation in therapeutic exercises. Plastic bags of frozen vegetables (peas or corn), which can easily mold around the shoulder, wrists, or knees, are an easy home treatment. The patient can also use ice cubes or small paper cups of frozen water to massage proximally or distally to a painful joint. Heat and cold can be used as often as desired; however, the heat application should not exceed 20 minutes at one time, and the cold application should not exceed 10 to 15 minutes at one time. The nurse should alert the patient to the possibility of a burn, especially if a heat-producing cream (e.g., capsaicin) is used together with another external heat device.

Individualized exercise is an integral part of the treatment plan.[21] A therapeutic exercise program is usually developed by a physical therapist and includes exercises to improve flexibility, strength, and endurance. The nurse should reinforce program participation and ensure that the exercises are being done correctly. Inadequate joint movement can result in progressive joint immobility and muscle weakness, and overaggressive exercise can result in increased pain, inflammation, and joint damage.

Gentle ROM exercises are usually done daily to keep the joints functional. The patient should have the opportunity to practice the exercises with supervision. The nurse should emphasize that usual daily activities do not provide adequate exercise to maintain joint motion. Careful adherence to the prescribed exercise program should be a prime goal of the teaching program. Aquatic exercises in warm water (78° to 86° F [25° to 30° C]) allow easier joint movement because of the buoyancy of the water. At the same time, although movement seems easier, water provides two-way resistance that makes muscles work harder than they would on land. Aerobic conditioning programs have been shown to improve the physical fitness levels of patients with arthritis. During acute inflammation, exercise should be limited to one or two repetitions.

Psychologic support. Self-management and adherence to an individualized home treatment program can only be accomplished if the patient has a thorough understanding of RA, the nature and course of the disease, and the goals of therapy. In addition, the patient's value system and perception of the disease must be considered. The patient is constantly threatened by problems of limited function and fatigue, loss of self-esteem, altered body image, and fear of disability and deformity. Alterations in sexuality should be discussed. Chronic pain or loss of function may make the patient vulnerable to unproven or even dangerous remedies through the claims of false advertising. The nurse can help the patient recognize fears and concerns that are faced by all people who live with chronic illness.

Evaluation of the family support system is important. Financial planning may be necessary.[22] Community resources such as a home care nurse, homemaker services, and vocational rehabilitation may be considered. Self-help groups are beneficial for some patients.

■ Gerontologic Considerations: Arthritis

The prevalence of arthritis in older adults is high, and the disease is accompanied by problems unique to this age group. The most problematic areas related to rheumatic disease in older adults include the following:

1. The high incidence of OA expected in older adults often keeps the health care provider from considering the presence of other types of arthritis.
2. Age alone causes changes in serologic profiles, making interpretation of laboratory values such as RF and ESR more difficult.
3. Polypharmacy in the older adult can result in iatrogenic arthritis.
4. Nonorganic musculoskeletal pain syndromes and weakness may be related to depressive reactions and physical inactivity.
5. Diseases such as SLE, which commonly occurs in younger adults, can develop in a milder form in older adults.

Aging brings many physical and metabolic changes that may increase the older patient's sensitivity to both the therapeutic and toxic effects of some drugs. The use of NSAIDs with a shorter half-life may require more frequent dosing but may also produce fewer side effects in the older patient with altered drug metabolism. The older adult who takes NSAIDs has an increased risk for side effects, particularly GI bleeding and renal toxicity. The common occurrence of polypharmacy makes the use of additional drugs in RA treatment particularly problematic in the older adult because of the increased likelihood of untoward drug interactions. The frequency of taking drugs and the complexity of the drug regimen should be simplified as much as possible to increase compliance in the older adult, particularly for the patient without regular assistance.

A major concern of treatment in the older patient relates to the use of corticosteroid therapy. Corticosteroid-induced osteopenia adds to the problem of age-related and inactivity-related loss of bone density and can increase the occurrence of pathologic fractures, especially compression fractures of vertebrae. Corticosteroid-induced myopathy can be minimized or prevented by an age-appropriate exercise program. Although important for all age-groups, an adequate support system for the older adult is a critical factor in the ability to follow a treatment regimen that includes nutritional planning, exercise, general health maintenance, and appropriate pharmacotherapy. ■

Spondyloarthropathies

The **spondyloarthropathies** are a group of interrelated multisystem inflammatory disorders that affect the spine, peripheral joints, and periarticular structures. These disorders are all negative for RF, thus they are often referred to as seronegative arthropathies. Inheritance of HLA-B27 is strongly associated with occurrence of these diseases. Both genetic and environmental factors play a role in the development of this group of diseases, which includes ankylosing spondylitis, psoriatic arthritis, and Reiter syndrome. (HLAs and their relationship to autoimmune diseases are discussed in Chapter 13.) The spondyloarthropathies share clinical and laboratory characteristics that make it difficult to distinguish among them in early disease. According to the European Spondyloarthropathy Study Group criteria, a diagnosis is made when inflammatory spinal pain or asymmetric synovitis is accompanied by one or more of the following: (1) episodes of alternating buttock pain; (2) radiographic evidence of sacroiliitis; (3) heel enthesopathy (e.g., plantar fasciitis, Achilles tendinitis); (4) positive family history of spondyloarthropathy in first-degree relative; (5) current psoriasis or documented history of psoriasis; (6) current chronic inflammatory bowel disease or documented history of disease; and (7) urethritis, cervicitis, or acute diarrhea that occurred within the month preceding onset of arthritic symptoms.[23]

ANKYLOSING SPONDYLITIS

Ankylosing spondylitis (AS) is a chronic inflammatory disease that primarily affects the axial skeleton, including the sacroiliac joints, intervertebral disk spaces, and costovertebral articulations. The HLA-B27 antigen is found in approximately 90% of whites and 50% of African Americans with AS. Although the usual age of onset is 15 to 35 years of age, the highest incidence of the disease is in persons 25 to 34 years of age. Men are three to four times more likely to develop AS than women.[24] The disease may go undetected in women because of a milder course.

Etiology and Pathophysiology

The cause of AS is unknown. Genetic predisposition appears to play an important role in the disease pathogenesis, but the precise mechanisms are unknown. Aseptic synovial inflammation in joints and adjacent tissue causes the formation of granulation tissue (pannus) and the development of dense fibrous scars that lead to fusion of articular tissues. Extraarticular inflammation can affect the eyes, lungs, heart, kidneys, and peripheral nervous system.

𝒢ENETICS in CLINICAL PRACTICE
Ankylosing Spondylitis

Genetic Basis
- Inheritance of HLA-B27 antigen

Incidence
- More than 90% of white patients with ankylosing spondylitis (AS) have HLA-B27 antigen.
- Only 2% of people with HLA-B27 have clinically detectable disease.
- AS is three times more common in men than women.
- It occurs more often in whites.
- It affects 7 in 100,000 people.

Genetic Testing
- HLA testing for B27

Clinical Implications
- AS usually occurs in the second and third decades of life.
- AS has a strong association with inflammatory bowel disease (IBD).
- About 50% to 70% of patients with both AS and IBD are HLA-27 positive.
- It is a systemic disease often affecting the eyes and heart.
- Genetic and environmental factors play a role in pathogenesis of disease.

Clinical Manifestations and Complications

AS is characterized by symmetric sacroiliitis and progressive inflammatory arthritis of the axial skeleton. Symptoms of inflammatory spine pain are the first clues to a diagnosis of AS. The patient typically complains of low back pain, stiffness, and limitation of motion that is worse during the night and in the morning but improves with mild activity. In women, early symptoms of disease may present as pain and stiffness in the neck rather than the lower back. General symptoms such as fever, fatigue, anorexia, and weight loss are rarely present. Iritis is the most common nonskeletal symptom. It can appear as an initial presentation of the disease years before arthritic symptoms develop. AS patients may also experience chest pain that mimics the pain of angina or pleurisy.[25]

Severe postural abnormalities and deformity can lead to significant disability for the patient with AS. Impaired spinal ROM and fixed kyphosis contribute to altered visual function, raising concerns about safe ambulation. Aortic insufficiency and pulmonary fibrosis are frequent complications. Cauda equina syndrome can also result, contributing to lower-extremity weakness and bladder dysfunction. In addition, the patient is at risk for spinal fracture because of osteoporosis.

Diagnostic Studies

X-rays are essential for the diagnosis of AS. Spinal views are seldom useful in initial diagnosis. Instead, pelvic x-rays demonstrate characteristic changes of sacroiliitis that range from subtle erosion to completely fused joints in which joint spaces have been obliterated. Changes on later spinal films include the appearance of "bamboo spine," which is due to calcifications (syndesmophytes) that bridge from one vertebra to another. Laboratory testing is not specific, but an elevated ESR and mild anemia may be seen. HLA-B27 testing is often done, but because the antigen can occur in unaffected individuals, it is of little diagnostic value. The test can be used to exclude the disease if negative.[25]

Collaborative Care

Prevention of AS is not possible. However, families with other diagnosed HLA-B27–positive rheumatic diseases should be alert to signs of low back pain for early identification and treatment of AS.

Care of the AS patient is aimed at maintaining maximal skeletal mobility while decreasing pain and inflammation. Heat applications can help in the relief of local symptoms. NSAIDs and salicylates are commonly prescribed. Intractable pain may respond to DMARDs including sulfasalazine (Azulfidine) or methotrexate. Etanercept (Enbrel) (see Table 63-3) can be used to treat patients with active AS. The use of infliximab (Remicade), which is also used in the treatment of RA, shows promise for treating AS.[26]

Once pain and stiffness are managed, exercise is essential. Postural control is important to minimize spinal deformity. The exercise regimen should include back, neck, and chest stretches. Hydrotherapy has also been shown to decrease pain and facilitate spinal extension. Surgery may be indicated for severe deformity and mobility impairment. Spinal osteotomy and total joint replacement are the most commonly performed procedures (see Chapter 61).

NURSING MANAGEMENT
ANKYLOSING SPONDYLITIS

The key nursing responsibility for the patient with AS is education about the disease and principles of therapy. The home management program should include regular exercise and attention to posture, local moist heat applications, and knowledgeable use of drugs.

Baseline ROM assessment by the nurse should include chest expansion (using breathing exercises). Smoking cessation should be encouraged to decrease the risk for lung complications in those with reduced chest expansion. Ongoing physical therapy should include gentle, graded stretching and strengthening exercises to preserve ROM and improve thoracolumbar flexion and extension. Excessive physical exertion during periods of active flare-up of the disease should be discouraged. Proper positioning at rest is essential. The mattress should be firm, and the patient should sleep on the back with a flat pillow, avoiding positions that encourage flexion deformity. Postural training emphasizes avoiding spinal flexion (e.g., leaning over a desk); heavy lifting; and prolonged walking, standing, or sitting. Sports that facilitate natural stretching, such as swimming and racquet games, should be encouraged. Family counseling and vocational rehabilitation are important.

PSORIATIC ARTHRITIS

Psoriasis is a common benign, inflammatory skin disorder that appears to have a genetic predisposition (see Chapter 23). Approximately 10% of the 3 million people with psoriasis develop psoriatic arthritis (PsA). PsA is now recognized as a progressive inflammatory disease that can cause significant disability. The exact cause of PsA is unknown, but a combination of immune, genetic, and environmental factors is suspected.[27] PsA can occur in five forms:

Arthritis involving primarily the small joints of the hands and feet
Asymmetric arthritis involving joints of the extremities
Symmetric polyarthritis resembling RA
Arthritis of the sacroiliac joints and spine (psoriatic spondylitis)
Arthritis mutilans, a rare but very deforming and destructive disease[28]

On x-ray, the cartilage loss and erosion resemble that of RA. Advanced cases of PsA often reveal widened joint spaces, and a "pencil in cup" deformity is common at the DIP joints.[29] Elevated ESR, mild anemia, and elevated blood uric acid levels can be seen in some patients; gout must be excluded. Treatment includes splinting, joint protection, and physical therapy. Although intramuscular gold therapy has been used with some success in the treatment of PsA, methotrexate continues to be one of the most effective agents for both cutaneous and articular manifestations. Sulfasalazine (Azulfidine) has been successfully used in treating PsA.

REITER SYNDROME

Reiter syndrome *(reactive arthritis)* more commonly occurs in young men and is associated with a symptom complex that includes urethritis or cervicitis, conjunctivitis, and mucocutaneous lesions.[30] Although the exact etiology is unknown, Reiter syndrome appears to occur after a genitourinary infection or gas-troenteritis. *Chlamydia trachomatis* is most often implicated in sexually transmitted Reiter syndrome. Men and women appear to have equal risk for developing dysenteric Reiter syndrome, which typically occurs within days or weeks after infection with *Shigella, Salmonella, Campylobacter,* or *Yersinia.*[31] Most affected individuals have inherited HLA-B27.

Urethritis develops within 1 to 2 weeks after sexual contact or dysentery. Low-grade fever, conjunctivitis, and arthritis may occur over the next several weeks. The arthritis of Reiter syndrome tends to be asymmetric, frequently involving the large joints of the lower extremities and the toes. Lower back pain may occur with severe disease. Mucocutaneous lesions commonly occur as small, painless, superficial ulcerations on the tongue, oral mucosa, and glans penis. Soft tissue manifestations commonly include enthesopathies such as Achilles tendinitis or plantar fasciitis. Few laboratory abnormalities occur, although the ESR may be elevated.

Prognosis is favorable, with most patients recovering after 2 to 16 weeks. Because Reiter syndrome is often associated with *C. trachomatis* infection, treatment of patients and their sexual partners with tetracycline (Doxycycline) 100 mg twice daily for up to 3 months is widely recommended. Conjunctivitis and lesions require no treatment, but topical ophthalmic corticosteroids are typically prescribed for treatment of iritis. Physical therapy may be helpful during disease recovery.

Joints heal completely, and many patients have complete remission with full joint function. Up to 50% may develop chronic or recurring disease, which can result in major disability. X-ray changes in chronic disease closely resemble those of AS. Treatment of chronic Reiter syndrome is symptomatic.

SEPTIC ARTHRITIS

Septic arthritis (infectious or bacterial arthritis) is an invasion of the joint cavity with microorganisms. Bacteria can travel through the bloodstream from another site of active infection, resulting in hematogenous seeding of the joint. Organisms can also be introduced directly through trauma or surgical incision. Any bacteria can cause the infection. In the immunocompromised patient, even nonpathogenic bacteria can be responsible for development of septic arthritis. *Staphylococcus aureus* is the most common causative organism. *Streptococcus hemolyticus* is also seen. *Neisseria gonorrhoeae* is the most common cause in sexually active young adults. Septic arthritis occurs twice as often as does osteomyelitis.[32] Factors that increase the risk of infection include diseases where there is decreased host resistance, such as leukemia and diabetes mellitus; treatment with corticosteroids or immunosuppressive drugs; and debilitating chronic illness.

Large joints such as the knee and hip are most frequently involved. Inflammation of the joint cavity causes severe pain, erythema, and swelling. Because infection has often spread from a primary site elsewhere in the body, fever or shaking chills often accompany articular manifestations. Precise diagnosis is made by aspiration of the joint (arthrocentesis) and culture of the synovial fluid. Blood cultures for aerobic and anaerobic organisms should also be obtained.

Septic arthritis is a medical emergency that requires prompt diagnosis and treatment to prevent joint destruction. Based on identification of the causative organism, parenteral antibiotics are prescribed and administered until there are no clinical signs of active synovitis or inflammation in the joint fluid. Infections may respond to treatment within 2 weeks or may take as long as 4 to 8 weeks, depending on the causative organism. Open surgical drainage may be required. If diagnosis and treatment are delayed, destruction of articular cartilage can occur, followed by loss of joint function. Chronic infection can develop. Septic arthritis of the hip can also contribute to development of avascular necrosis.

Nursing intervention includes assessment and monitoring of joint inflammation, pain, and fever. Immobilization of affected joints to control pain can be achieved by use of resting splints or traction. Gentle ROM exercises should be performed on a regular schedule. Strict aseptic technique should be used during assistance with joint aspiration procedures. The nurse should explain the need for antibiotics and the importance of their continued use until the infection is resolved. Support should be offered to the patient who requires arthrocentesis or operative drainage.

LYME DISEASE

Lyme disease is a spirochetal infection caused by *Borrelia burgdorferi* and transmitted by the bite of an infected deer tick.[33] It was first identified in 1975 in Lyme, Connecticut, after an unusual clustering of arthritis in children and is now the most common vector-borne disease in the United States. The tick typically feeds on mice, dogs, cats, cows, horses, deer, and humans. Wild animals do not exhibit the illness, but clinical Lyme disease does occur in domestic animals. Person-to-person transmission does not occur. The peak season for human infection is during the summer months. Most U.S. cases occur in three endemic areas: along the northeastern coast from Maryland to Massachusetts; in the midwestern states of Wisconsin and Minnesota; and along the northwestern coast of northern California and Oregon. The reported incidence of Lyme disease has doubled in the last 10 years to 16,700 cases annually.[34]

Lyme disease is often called the "great imitator" because its symptoms can mimic other diseases such as multiple sclerosis, mononucleosis, and meningitis. The most characteristic clinical symptom of early localized disease is erythema migrans (EM), a skin lesion that occurs at the site of the tick bite within 2 to 30 days after exposure (Fig. 63-6). The lesion begins as a red macule or papule that slowly expands to form a large round lesion with a bright red border and central clearing. The EM lesion is often accompanied by acute viral-like symptoms, such as fever, chills, headache, stiff neck, fatigue, swollen lymph nodes, and migratory joint and muscle pain.

If not treated, symptoms of Lyme disease can progress within several weeks or months to include nervous system problems such as severe headaches, temporary facial paralysis (e.g., Bell's palsy), or poor motor coordination. In late disease, which can occur from months to years after the initial infection, arthritis pain and swelling may occur in a few large joints. Arthritic symptoms are often temporary, but about 10% of people with Lyme disease will develop chronic Lyme arthritis if untreated. Neurologic disorders can also occur at this stage, including one condition known as tertiary neuroborreliosis that results in confusion and forgetfulness.

A diagnosis of Lyme disease is often based on clinical manifestations, in particular, the EM lesion, and a history of exposure in an endemic area. Routine laboratory tests play only a minor

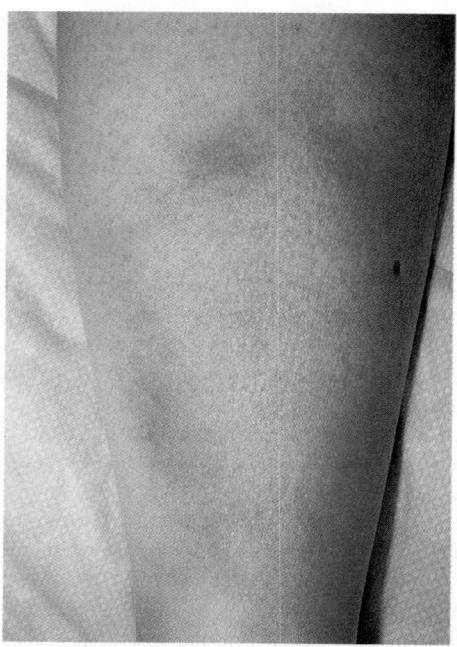

FIG. 63-6 Erythema migrans. Early skin lesion in Lyme disease.

role in diagnosis. CBC and ESR results are usually normal. Lyme serology tests for antibodies are not usually positive initially because it takes many weeks to get clinical detectable levels of circulating antibodies.[34] Cerebrospinal fluid should be examined in individuals with neurologic involvement.

Active lesions can be treated with antibiotic therapy. Oral doxycycline (Vibramycin) or amoxicillin is often effective in early stage infection and in prevention of later stages of the disease. Doxycycline has also proven to be very effective in preventing Lyme disease when given within 3 days after the bite of a deer tick. Short-term therapy of 2 to 3 weeks is usually effective for solitary EM, but long-standing infection may require extended parenteral antibiotic therapy. Intravenous ceftriaxone (Rocephin) is prescribed for cardiac or neurologic abnormalities. LYMErix, a vaccine, is given optimally in three doses over a 2-month period and is 76% effective against the disease.[35] The vaccine is recommended for individuals whose occupations or recreational activities place them at risk for *B. burgdorferi* exposure. However, the manufacturer recently discontinued the commercial availability of the vaccine. New vaccines are currently being investigated. Patient and family teaching for the prevention of Lyme disease in endemic areas is outlined in Table 63-10.

HUMAN IMMUNODEFICIENCY VIRUS–ASSOCIATED RHEUMATIC DISEASE

A group of inflammatory musculoskeletal disorders develop in the course of human immunodeficiency virus (HIV) infection.[36] The cause of these disorders in HIV-infected persons is not clearly known. However, it appears that an autoimmune process and an inflammatory response are occurring at the same time in the patient who is immunosuppressed.[37] Up to 70% of HIV-infected patients may develop a rheumatic disease. Rheumatic diseases associated with HLA-B27 appear to be more severe in HIV-infected patients. Conditions typically associated with HIV

TABLE 63-10	Patient & Family Teaching Guide
	Prevention of Lyme Disease (Endemic Areas)

- Avoid walking through tall grasses and low brush.
- Mow grass and remove brush along paths, and around buildings and campsites.
- Move woodpiles and bird feeders away from house.
- Wear long pants or nylon tights of tightly woven, light-colored fabric so that ticks can be easily seen.
- Tuck pants into boots or long socks, tuck long-sleeved shirts into pants, and wear closed shoes when hiking.
- Check often for ticks crawling from legs to open skin.
- Thoroughly inspect and wash clothes.
- Spray insect repellant containing DEET on skin or permethrin on clothes, especially on lower extremities.
- Have pets wear tick collars, inspect them often, and do not allow them on furniture or beds.
- Remove attached ticks with tweezers (not fingers). Grasp tick's mouth parts as close to skin as possible and gently pull straight out. Do not twist or jerk.
- Dispose of tick in alcohol or flush down toilet. Do not crush with fingers.
- Wash bitten area with soap and water and apply antiseptic. Wash hands.
- See a doctor immediately if flulike symptoms or "bull's-eye" rash appears within a 2 to 30 days after removal of tick.

DEET, N,N–diethyl-M-toluamide.

TABLE 63-11	Conditions That Can Cause Hyperuricemia

Acidosis or ketosis
Alcoholism
Atherosclerosis
Chemotherapeutic drugs
Diabetes mellitus
Drug-induced renal impairment
Hyperlipidemia
Hypertension
Malignant disease
Myeloproliferative disorders
Obesity or starvation
Renal disease
Sickle cell anemia
Use of certain common drugs (salicylates, diuretics)

Etiology and Pathophysiology

Uric acid is the major end product of purine catabolism and is primarily excreted by the kidneys. Hyperuricemia may be the result of increased purine synthesis, decreased renal excretion, or both. A high dietary intake of purine alone has relatively little effect on uric acid levels. Hyperuricemia may result from prolonged fasting or excessive alcohol drinking because of the increased production of keto acids, which then inhibit uric acid excretion.

Clinical Manifestations and Complications

In the acute phase, gouty arthritis may occur in one or more joints but usually less than four. Affected joints may appear dusky or cyanotic and are extremely tender. Inflammation of the great toe *(podagra)* is the most common initial problem. Other affected joints may include the midtarsal area of the foot, ankle, knee, and wrist. Olecranon bursae may also be involved. Acute gouty arthritis is usually precipitated by events such as trauma, surgery, alcohol ingestion, or systemic infection. Onset of symptoms is typically rapid, with swelling and pain peaking within several hours, often accompanied by low-grade fever. Individual attacks usually subside, treated or untreated, in 2 to 10 days. The affected joint returns entirely to normal, and patients are often free of symptoms between attacks.

Chronic gout is characterized by multiple joint involvement and visible deposits of sodium urate crystals called *tophi.* These are typically noted in the synovium, subchondral bone, olecranon bursae, and vertebrae; along tendons; and in the skin and cartilage (Fig. 63-7). Tophi are rarely present at the time of the initial attack and are generally noted only many years after the onset of disease.

The severity of gouty arthritis is variable. The clinical course may consist of infrequent mild attacks or multiple severe episodes associated with a slowly progressive disability. In general, the higher the serum uric acid level, the earlier the appearance of tophi and the greater the tendency toward more frequent, severe episodes of acute gout. Chronic inflammation may result in joint deformity, and cartilage destruction may predispose the joint to secondary OA. Large and unsightly tophaceous deposits

infection include SLE, Reiter syndrome, PsA, Sjögren syndrome, polymyositis, and vasculitis. The knees and ankles are generally the most affected joints. Most patients improve with conventional arthritis treatments such as NSAIDs, but patients with Reiter syndrome or PsA may not respond as well and develop progressive deformities. As with other patients, appropriate physical therapy is recommended.

GOUT

Gout is caused by an increase in uric acid production, underexcretion of uric acid by the kidneys, or increased intake of foods containing purines, which are metabolized to uric acid by the body. Characteristic deposits of monosodium urate crystals occur in articular, periarticular, and subcutaneous tissues. Joint involvement includes recurrent attacks of acute arthritis.

Gout may be classified as primary or secondary.[38] In *primary gout,* a hereditary error of purine metabolism leads to the overproduction or retention of uric acid. *Secondary gout* may be related to another acquired disorder (Table 63-11) or may be the result of drugs known to inhibit uric acid excretion. Secondary gout may also be caused by drugs that increase the rate of cell death, such as the chemotherapeutic agents used in treating leukemia. Primary gout, which accounts for 90% of cases, occurs predominantly in middle-aged men, with almost no incidence in premenopausal women. Hyperuricemia may also develop in patients taking thiazide diuretics, postmenopausal women, and in organ transplant recipients who are receiving immunosuppressive agents.

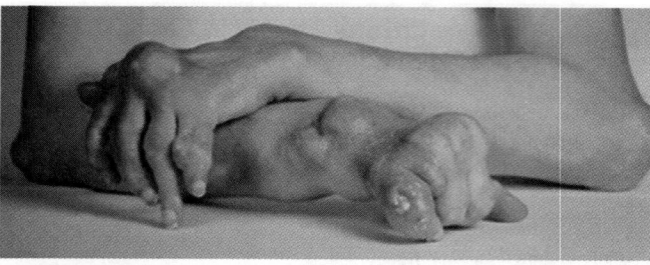

FIG. 63-7   Tophaceous gout.

may perforate overlying skin, producing draining sinuses that often become secondarily infected. Excessive uric acid excretion may lead to kidney or urinary tract stone formation. Pyelonephritis associated with intrarenal sodium urate deposits and obstruction may contribute to renal disease.

Diagnostic Studies

Serum uric acid levels are almost always elevated to 8 mg/dl. However, hyperuricemia is not specifically diagnostic of gout because increased levels may be related to a variety of drugs or may exist as a totally asymptomatic abnormality in the general population. Specimens for 24-hour urine acid levels may be obtained to determine if the disease is caused by decreased renal excretion or overproduction of uric acid. Synovial fluid aspiration is a potentially controversial part of patient evaluation because an accurate diagnosis of gout is possible in 80% of patients based on clinical symptoms alone. However, aspiration may have therapeutic value by decompressing a swollen joint capsule. Joint aspiration is also the only reliable method to distinguish gout from septic arthritis and pseudogout. Affected fluid characteristically contains needlelike crystals of sodium urate.

Collaborative Care

Goals for care of the patient with gout (Table 63-12) include termination of an acute attack through use of an antiinflammatory agent such as colchicine, with NSAIDs prescribed adjunctively for pain management. Future attacks are prevented by a maintenance dose of allopurinol (Zyloprim) in combination with weight reduction, as needed, and possible avoidance of alcohol and food high in purine (red and organ meats). Treatment is also aimed at preventing the formation of uric acid kidney stones and the development of associated conditions such as hypertriglyceridemia and hypertension.

Drug Therapy. Acute gouty arthritis is treated with colchicine and NSAIDs. Colchicine has known antiinflammatory effects but no analgesic properties, so an NSAID is added to the treatment regimen primarily for pain management. Oral administration of colchicine generally produces dramatic pain relief within 24 to 48 hours. Colchicine also has diagnostic merit in that a good response to treatment gives further evidence for the diagnosis of gout. As another possible therapy, intraarticular injection of corticosteroids can be helpful in monoarthritic gout. Systemic corticosteroids may be used only if routine therapies are contraindicated or ineffective. Adrenocorticotropic hormone (ACTH) may also be used for treating acute gout.[39]

For many years the standard therapy for hyperuricemia caused by urate underexcretion has been uricosuric drugs such as

TABLE 63-12	Collaborative Care — Gout

Diagnostic
History and physical examination
Family history of gout
Presence of monosodium urate monohydrate crystals in synovial fluid
Elevated serum uric acid levels
Elevated 24 hr urine for uric acid levels

Collaborative Therapy
Joint immobilization
Local application of heat or cold
Joint aspiration and intraarticular corticosteroids
Drug therapy
   Nonsteroidal antiinflammatory drugs
   colchicine
   probenecid (Benemid)
   allopurinol (Zyloprim)
Dietary avoidance of food/fluids with high purine content (e.g., anchovies, liver, wine/beer)

probenecid (Benemid), which inhibit renal tubular reabsorption of urates. However, this class of drugs is ineffective when creatinine clearance is reduced, as can occur in patients over the age of 60. Aspirin inactivates the effect of uricosurics, resulting in urate retention, and should be avoided while patients are taking uricosuric drugs. Acetaminophen can be used safely if analgesia is required.

Adequate urine volume with normal renal function (2 to 3 L per day) must be maintained to prevent precipitation of uric acid in the renal tubules. Allopurinol (Zyloprim), which blocks the production of uric acid, is particularly useful in patients with uric acid stones or renal impairment in whom uricosuric drugs may be ineffective or dangerous. For patients who cannot tolerate allopurinol because of minor reactions, oxypurinol can be prescribed. Oxypurinol is the active metabolite of allopurinol. The angiotensin II receptor antagonist losartan (Cozaar) may be especially useful for treatment of elderly patients with both gout and hypertension. Losartan given 50 mg daily will promote urate diuresis and may normalize serum urate levels. Combination therapy with losartan and allopurinol may also be given. Regardless of which drugs are prescribed, serum uric acid levels must be checked regularly to monitor treatment effectiveness.

Nutritional Therapy. Traditional dietary restrictions include limiting the use of alcohol and the consumption of foods high in purine (see Table 44-12). However, drugs can often control gout without necessitating these changes. Obese patients should be instructed in a carefully planned weight-reduction program.

NURSING MANAGEMENT
GOUT

Nursing intervention for the patient with acute gouty arthritis includes supportive care of the inflamed joints. Special care is taken to avoid causing pain to an inflamed joint by careless handling. Bed rest may be appropriate, with affected joints properly immobilized. Involvement of a lower extremity may require use of a cradle or foot board to protect the painful area from the weight of bed clothes. The limitation of motion and degree of pain should be assessed, and treatment effectiveness should be documented.

The nurse should help the patient and the family to understand that hyperuricemia and gouty arthritis are chronic problems that can be controlled with careful adherence to a treatment program. Thorough explanations should be given concerning the importance of drug therapy and the need for periodic determination of serum uric acid levels. The patient should be able to demonstrate knowledge of precipitating factors that may cause an attack, including excessive caloric intake or overindulgence in purine-containing foods and alcohol; starvation (fasting); drug use (e.g., aspirin, diuretics); and major medical events (e.g., surgery, myocardial infarction).

SYSTEMIC LUPUS ERYTHEMATOSUS

Systemic lupus erythematosus (SLE) is a chronic multisystem inflammatory disease associated with abnormalities of the immune system. It typically affects the skin, joints, and serous membranes (pleura, pericardium), along with the renal, hematologic, and neurologic systems. The overall incidence of SLE in the United States is 2 to 8 per 100,000. Most cases of SLE occur in women in their childbearing years.[40] African Americans, Asian Americans, and Native Americans are approximately three times more likely to develop SLE than whites. SLE is characterized by variability within and among persons, and its chronic unpredictable course is marked by alternating periods of exacerbations and remissions.

Etiology and Pathophysiology

The etiology of SLE is unknown.[41] Based on the high prevalence of SLE among family members, a genetic influence has long been suspected. Multiple susceptibility genes from the HLA complex show associations with SLE. Hormones are also known to play a role in the etiology of SLE. Onset or exacerbation of disease symptoms sometimes occurs after the onset of menarche, with the use of oral contraceptives, and during and after pregnancy. The disease tends to worsen in the immediate postpartum period.

Environmental factors are believed to contribute to the occurrence of SLE, with sun exposure and burns as the most significant environmental triggers. Infectious agents could serve as a stimulus for immune hyperactivity. SLE may also be precipitated or aggravated by certain drugs such as procainamide (Pronestyl), hydralazine (Apresoline), and a number of antiseizure drugs.

SLE is a disorder of immunoregulation. Autoimmune reactions are directed against constituents of the cell nucleus, particularly DNA. The overaggressive antibody response is related to B and T cell hyperactivity.[42] When autoantibodies bind to their specific antigens, complement activation occurs, and immune complexes are deposited in the basement membranes of capillaries in the kidneys, heart, skin, brain, and joints. The specific manifestations of SLE depend on which cell types or organs are involved.

Clinical Manifestations and Complications

SLE is extremely variable in its severity, ranging from a relatively mild disorder to a rapidly progressive one affecting many organ systems (Fig. 63-8). No characteristic pattern occurs in the progressive organ involvement of SLE. Theoretically, any organ can be affected by an accumulation of circulating immune complexes. The most commonly affected tissues are the skin and muscle, the lining of the lungs, the heart, nervous tissue, and the kidneys. Generalized complaints such as fever, weight loss, arthralgia, and excessive fatigue may precede an exacerbation of disease activity.

Dermatologic Manifestations. Cutaneous vascular lesions can appear in any location but are most likely to develop in sun-exposed areas. Severe skin reactions can occur in persons who are photosensitive. The classic butterfly rash over the cheeks and bridge of the nose occurs in 50% of patients with SLE (Fig. 63-9). A small number of patients have persistent lesions, photosensitivity, and mild systemic disease in a syndrome referred to as *subacute cutaneous lupus*.

Ulcers of the oral or nasopharyngeal membranes occur in up to one third of patients with SLE. Transient diffuse or patchy hair loss (alopecia) is also common, with or without underlying scalp lesions. The hair may grow back during remission, but hair loss may be permanent over lesions. The scalp becomes dry, scaly, and atrophied.

Musculoskeletal Problems. Polyarthralgia with morning stiffness is often the patient's first complaint and may precede the onset of multisystem disease by many years. Arthritis occurs in more than 90% of patients with SLE. Diffuse swelling is accompanied by joint and muscle pain, and some stiffness may be experienced. Lupus-related arthritis is generally nonerosive, but it may cause deformities such as swan-neck appearance of the fingers (see Fig. 63-4), ulnar deviation, and subluxation with hyperlaxity of the joints.

Cardiopulmonary Problems. Tachypnea and cough in patients with SLE are suggestive of restrictive lung disease. Pleurisy with or without pleural effusion is also possible. Cardiac involvement may include arrhythmias resulting from fibrosis of the sinoatrial and atrioventricular nodes. This occurrence is an ominous sign of advanced disease, contributing significantly to the morbidity and mortality seen in SLE. Clinical factors such as hypertension and hypercholesterolemia require aggressive therapy and careful monitoring. SLE accelerates coronary artery disease (CAD), and the risk of developing CAD also increases.[43]

Renal Problems. Lupus nephritis (LN) occurs in about 50% of patients within 1 year of diagnosis with SLE. Manifestations of LN vary from mild proteinuria to rapid, progressive glomerulonephritis. Nearly all patients with SLE show renal histologic abnormalities in renal biopsy studies or autopsy results.

The primary goal in treating LN is to slow the progression of nephropathy and preserve renal function by managing the underlying disease. The importance of obtaining a renal biopsy is controversial, but findings can help to guide treatment, which typically includes corticosteroids, cytotoxic agents (cyclophosphamide [Cytoxan]), and immunosuppressive agents (azathioprine [Imuran], cyclosporine [Sandimmune]). Cyclophosphamide is the most effective cytotoxic therapy, but azathioprine is considered to be less toxic. Oral prednisone or pulsed intravenous methylprednisolone may also be used as an intervention for LN, especially in the initial treatment period when cytotoxic agents have not had time to take effect.

Nervous System Problems. Along with renal involvement, neurologic effects are the most prevalent in SLE. Generalized or focal seizures are the most common manifestation in-

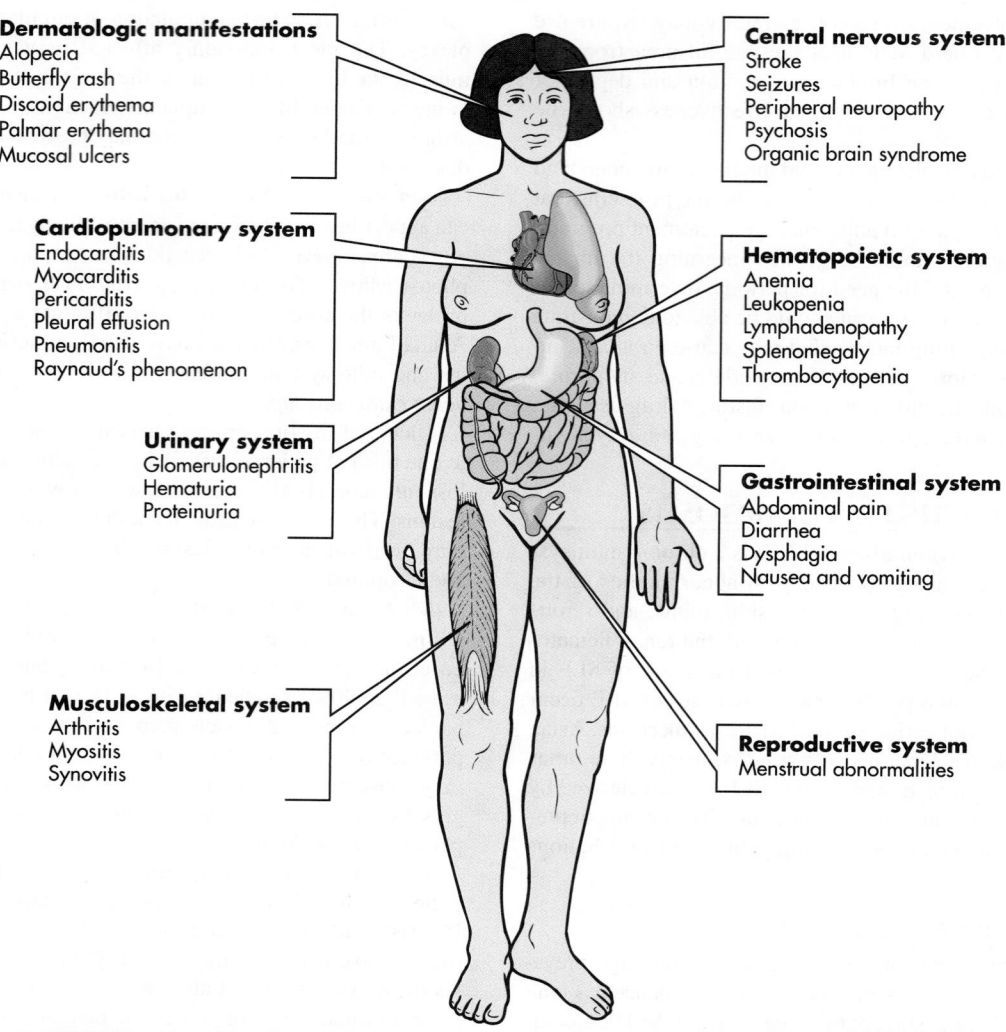

Dermatologic manifestations
Alopecia
Butterfly rash
Discoid erythema
Palmar erythema
Mucosal ulcers

Central nervous system
Stroke
Seizures
Peripheral neuropathy
Psychosis
Organic brain syndrome

Cardiopulmonary system
Endocarditis
Myocarditis
Pericarditis
Pleural effusion
Pneumonitis
Raynaud's phenomenon

Hematopoietic system
Anemia
Leukopenia
Lymphadenopathy
Splenomegaly
Thrombocytopenia

Urinary system
Glomerulonephritis
Hematuria
Proteinuria

Gastrointestinal system
Abdominal pain
Diarrhea
Dysphagia
Nausea and vomiting

Musculoskeletal system
Arthritis
Myositis
Synovitis

Reproductive system
Menstrual abnormalities

FIG. 63-8   Multisystem involvement in systemic lupus erythematosus.

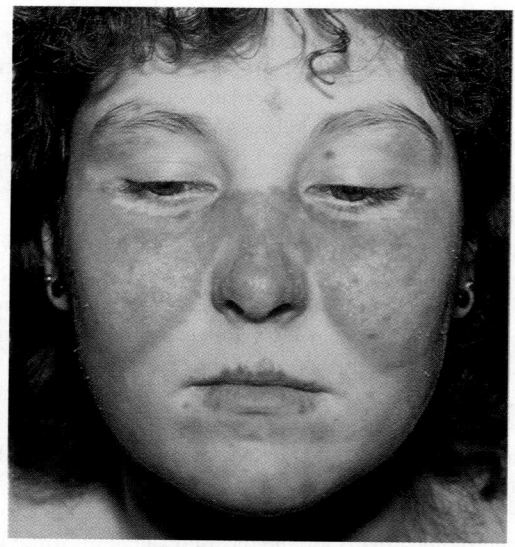

FIG. 63-9   Butterfly rash of systemic lupus erythematosus.

volving the central nervous system (CNS), and occur in as many as 15% of patients with SLE by the time of diagnosis. Seizures are generally controlled by corticosteroids or antiseizure drugs. Peripheral neuropathy can also occur, leading to sensory and motor deficits.

Organic brain syndrome, recognized as a CNS manifestation of SLE, may result from the deposition of immune complexes within brain tissue. It is characterized by disordered thought processes, disorientation, memory deficits, and psychiatric symptoms such as severe depression and psychosis. Recovery from organic brain disease is expected, although some residual impairment may result. Occasionally a stroke or aseptic meningitis may be attributable to SLE. It is difficult to differentiate neuropsychiatric SLE from non-SLE neurologic problems.

Hematologic Problems. The formation of antibodies against blood cells, such as erythrocytes, leukocytes, thrombocytes, and coagulation factors, is also a common feature of SLE. Anemia, mild leukopenia, and thrombocytopenia are often present in SLE. Some patients develop a tendency toward coagulopathy involving either excessive bleeding or blood clot development. A manifestation of antiphospholipid antibody syndrome is a common cause of hypercoagulability in SLE patients, many of whom benefit from high-intensity treatment with warfarin sodium (Coumadin).

Infection. Patients with SLE appear to have increased susceptibility to infections, possibly related to defects in their ability to phagocytize invading bacteria, deficiencies in production of antibodies, and the immunosuppressive effect of many antiinflammatory drugs. Infection is a major cause of death, with pneumonia being the most common infection. Fever should be considered serious because it may indicate an underlying infectious process rather than lupus activity alone. Vaccinations are generally safe for patients with SLE. The exception is avoidance of live-virus vaccines with patients who are being treated with corticosteroids or cytotoxic agents.

Diagnostic Studies

The diagnosis of SLE is based on the presence of distinct criteria revealed through patient history, physical examination, and laboratory findings (Table 63-13). No specific test is diagnostic for SLE, but a variety of abnormalities may be present in the blood. SLE is characterized by the presence of ANA. Other antibodies include anti-DNA, antineuronal, anticoagulant, anti-WBC, anti–red blood cell (RBC), antiplatelet, and anti–basement membrane. The tests that are most specific for SLE include the anti–double-stranded DNA and the anti-Smith (Sm). High levels of anti-DNA are rarely found in any condition other than SLE, and anti-Sm seems to be found almost exclusively in SLE. The lupus erythematosus (LE) cell prep test is a nonspecific test for SLE and is positive in other rheumatic diseases. ESR and CRP levels are not diagnostic of SLE but may be used to monitor disease activity.

Collaborative Care

A major challenge in treatment of SLE is to manage the active phase of the disease while preventing complications of treatments that cause long-term tissue damage. An improving prognosis of SLE may be the result of earlier diagnosis, prompt recognition of serious organ involvement, and better therapeutic regimens. Survival is influenced by several factors, including age, race, gender, socioeconomic status, accompanying morbid conditions, and severity of disease.

Drug Therapy. NSAIDs continue to be an important intervention, especially for patients with mild polyarthralgias or polyarthritis. Because prolonged therapy is likely, careful patient monitoring must include the potential for GI effects from NSAID use. Antimalarial agents such as hydroxychloroquine (Plaquenil) are also often used to treat polyarthritis. Retinopathy can develop with use of these agents, but it generally reverses when they are discontinued. If the patient cannot tolerate an antimalarial agent, an antileprosy drug such as dapsone may be used.

Corticosteroid exposure should be limited, but tapering doses of intravenous methylprednisolone may be useful in controlling severe exacerbations of polyarthritis. Steroid-sparing drugs such as methotrexate can serve as an alternate treatment and are prescribed in combination with folic acid to decrease minor side effects. However, high doses of corticosteroids may be especially appropriate for the patient with very severe cutaneous SLE. Immunosuppressive drugs such as azathioprine (Imuran) and cyclophosphamide (Cytoxan) may be prescribed to reduce the need for long-term corticosteroid therapy. Close monitoring is necessary to minimize drug toxicity and side effects.[44]

Disease management is most appropriately monitored by serial anti-DNA titers (Table 63-14). Simpler and less costly tests such as ESR or CRP may also help in monitoring treatment effectiveness.

TABLE 63-13   Criteria for Diagnosis of Systemic Lupus Erythematosus*

Malar rash
Discoid rash
Photosensitivity
Oral ulcers
Arthritis: nonerosive, involvement of two or more joints characterized by tenderness, swelling, and effusion
Serositis: pleuritis or pericarditis
Renal disorder: persistent proteinuria or cellular casts in urine
Neurologic disorder: seizures or psychosis
Hematologic disorder: hemolytic anemia, leukopenia, lymphopenia, or thrombocytopenia
Immunologic disorder: positive LE preparation; anti-DNA antibody or antibody to Sm nuclear antigen; or false-positive serologic tests for syphilis
Antinuclear antibodies

Data from American College of Rheumatology [on-line]. Available at *www.rheumatology.org/research/classification/sle/html.*
*A person is classified as having SLE if four or more of the criteria are present, serially or simultaneously, during any interval of observation. Revised criteria by a subcommittee of the American College of Rheumatology are used for the purpose of *classification* in population surveys, *not* for the diagnosis of individual patients.
Sm, Smith.

TABLE 63-14   Collaborative Care — Systemic Lupus Erythematosus

Diagnostic
History and physical examination
Antibodies
  Anti-DNA antibody
  Anti-Sm antibody
  Antinuclear antibody (ANA)
Complete blood cell count
LE cell prep
Urinalysis
X-ray of affected joints
Chest x-ray
ECG to determine extraarticular involvement
Collaborative Therapy
NSAIDs
Steroid-sparing drugs (e.g., methotrexate)
Antimalarials (e.g., hydroxychloroquine [Plaquenil])
Corticosteroids for exacerbations and severe disease
Immunosuppressive drugs
  cyclophosphamide (Cytoxan)
  azathioprine (Imuran)

LE, Lupus erythematosus; *NSAIDs,* nonsteroidal antiinflammatory drugs; *Sm antibody,* Smith antibody.

Patient teaching related to prescribed drugs must include their indications for use, proper administration, and possible side effects (see Chapter 48). The patient should understand that abrupt cessation may precipitate exacerbation of disease activity.

NURSING MANAGEMENT
SYSTEMIC LUPUS ERYTHEMATOSUS

■ Nursing Assessment

As in the majority of rheumatic diseases, the chronic and unpredictable nature of SLE presents many challenges to the patient and family. The physical, psychologic, and sociocultural problems associated with the long-term management of SLE require the varied approaches and skills of the multidisciplinary health care team.

Subjective and objective data that should be obtained from the patient with SLE are presented in Table 63-15. In particular, the extent to which pain and fatigue influence activities of daily living must be evaluated. A developmental approach focuses on age-appropriate education and counseling on issues such as personal relationships, family planning, occupational responsibilities, and recreational activities.

■ Nursing Diagnoses

Nursing diagnoses for the patient with SLE may include, but are not limited to, those presented in NCP 63-2.

■ Planning

As overall disease management goals, the patient with SLE will (1) have satisfactory pain relief, (2) comply with therapeutic regimen to achieve maximum symptom management, (3) demonstrate awareness of and avoid activities that cause disease exacerbation, and (4) maintain optimal role function and a positive self-image.

■ Nursing Implementation

Health Promotion. Prevention of SLE is not possible at this time. However, education of health professionals and the community should promote a clear understanding of the disease and the need for earlier diagnosis and treatment.

Acute Intervention. During an exacerbation of SLE, the patient may become abruptly and dramatically ill. Nursing interventions include accurately recording the severity of symptoms and documenting the response to therapy. Fever pattern, joint inflammation, limitation of motion, location and degree of discomfort, and fatigability should be specifically assessed. The patient's weight and fluid intake and output should be monitored if corticosteroids are prescribed because of the fluid-retention effect of these drugs and the possibility of renal failure. Collection of 24-hour urine samples for protein and creatinine clearance may be ordered. The nurse should observe for signs of bleeding that result from drug therapy, such as pallor, skin bruising, petechiae, or tarry stools.

TABLE 63-15	Nursing Assessment
	Systemic Lupus Erythematosus

Subjective Data	Objective Data
Important Health Information	**General**
Past health history: Exposure to ultraviolet radiation, drugs, chemicals, viral infections; physical or psychologic stress; states of increased estrogen activity, including early onset of menarche, pregnancy, and postpartum period; pattern of remissions and exacerbations	Fever, lymphadenopathy, periorbital edema
	Integumentary
Medications: Use of oral contraceptives, procainamide (Pronestyl), hydralazine (Apresoline), isoniazid (INH), antiseizure drugs, antibiotics (possibly precipitating symptoms of SLE); corticosteroids, NSAIDs	Alopecia; dry, scaly scalp; keratoconjunctivitis, malar "butterfly" rash, palmar or discoid erythema, urticaria, periungual erythema, purpura, or petechiae; leg ulcers
Functional Health Patterns	**Respiratory**
	Pleural friction rub, decreased breath sounds
Health perception–health management: Family history of autoimmune disorders; frequent infections; malaise	**Cardiovascular**
Nutritional-metabolic: Weight loss, oral and nasal ulcers; nausea and vomiting; xerostomia (salivary gland dryness), dysphagia; photosensitivity with rash; frequent infections	Vasculitis; pericardial friction rub; hypertension, edema, arrhythmias, murmurs; bilateral, symmetric pallor and cyanosis of fingers (Raynaud's phenomenon)
	Gastrointestinal
Elimination: Decreased urine output; diarrhea or constipation	Oral and pharyngeal ulcers; splenomegaly
Activity-exercise: Morning stiffness; joint swelling and deformity; shortness of breath, dyspnea; excessive fatigue	**Neurologic**
	Facial weakness, peripheral neuropathies, papilledema, dysarthria, confusion, hallucination, disorientation, psychosis, seizures, aphasia, hemiparesis
Sleep-rest: Insomnia	**Musculoskeletal**
Cognitive-perceptual: Visual disturbances; vertigo; headache; polyarthralgia; chest pain (pericardial, pleuritic); abdominal pain; joint pain; pain, throbbing, coldness of fingers with numbness and tingling	Myopathy, myositis, arthritis
	Urinary
	Proteinuria
Sexuality-reproductive: Amenorrhea, irregular menstrual periods	**Possible Findings**
Coping–stress tolerance: Depression, withdrawal	Presence of anti-DNA, Sm, and antinuclear antibodies; anemia, leukopenia, thrombocytopenia; ↑ erythrocyte sedimentation rate (ESR); positive LE cell prep; ↑ serum creatinine; microscopic hematuria, cellular casts in urine; pericarditis or pleural effusion evident on chest x-ray

ANA, Antinuclear antibody; *NSAIDs,* nonsteroidal antiinflammatory drugs.

NURSING CARE PLAN 63-2

Patient with Systemic Lupus Erythematosus

EXPECTED PATIENT OUTCOMES	NURSING INTERVENTIONS and *RATIONALES*
NURSING DIAGNOSIS	**Fatigue** *related to* disease process *as manifested by* lack of energy, inability to maintain usual routine.
▪ Completion of priority activities ▪ Pacing of activities ▪ Verbalization of having more energy	▪ Analyze energy level patterns *to plan daily activities.* ▪ Assist patient to prioritize activities *to establish preferred daily routine.* ▪ Teach energy conservation techniques, such as sitting at kitchen sink, enlisting aid of others *to accomplish as much as possible with minimum energy expended.** ▪ Include family in planning *to increase patient's support and family's understanding of disease and related problems.* ▪ Teach techniques such as meditation and yoga *to provide patient with stress-reducing strategies.* ▪ Encourage patient to rest regularly and as needed *to temporarily reverse effect of fatigue.*
NURSING DIAGNOSIS	**Acute pain** *related to* disease process and inadequate comfort measures *as manifested by* complaints of joint pain, lack of relief from pain-relieving measures; reduction of activity to avoid exacerbating pain.
▪ Expression of satisfaction with pain relief measures ▪ Performance of activities of daily living without pain	▪ Assess pain location and severity *to plan appropriate interventions.* ▪ Administer analgesia as ordered and monitor effect, teach joint protection measures; apply heat or cold as determined *to relieve pain.* ▪ Use nonpharmacologic pain interventions such as relaxation and imagery *to replace or supplement analgesics.*
NURSING DIAGNOSIS	**Impaired skin integrity** *related to* photosensitivity, skin rash, and alopecia *as manifested by* rash anywhere on body, butterfly rash on face, hair loss, areas of ulceration on fingertips, complaints of urticaria and photosensitivity.
▪ Limitation of direct exposure to sun and use of sunscreens ▪ No open skin lesions ▪ Strategies to cope with alopecia	▪ Assess and monitor location and progression of rash *to plan appropriate interventions.* ▪ Administer drugs and apply ointments as ordered *to control skin manifestations.* ▪ Keep skin clean and dry *to avoid secondary infections.* ▪ Discuss need to limit direct sun exposure and use of sunscreens and sun protective clothing when outdoors *because sun exacerbates manifestations.*
NURSING DIAGNOSIS	**Activity intolerance** *related to* arthralgia, weakness, and fatigue *as manifested by* inability or unwillingness to ambulate or engage in physical activity, abnormal response to activity (e.g., increased pulse, respiratory rate).
▪ Expression of satisfaction with activity pattern ▪ Pacing of activities to match level of tolerance	▪ Teach patient to pace activities and allow periods of rest between activities *to promote recuperation and to foster maximum participation in activities.* ▪ Encourage patient to assist in setting activity schedule *to allow patient a sense of control and foster cooperation with the plan.* ▪ Provide rest during exacerbation *to conserve energy for vital activities.* ▪ Encourage use of assistive devices *to minimize energy expenditure.*
NURSING DIAGNOSIS	**Ineffective therapeutic regimen management** *related to* lack of knowledge of long-term management of disease *as manifested by* questions about SLE or incorrect answers to questions by patient or family, use of unproven remedies.
▪ Expression of confidence in ability to manage SLE over time and in home environment	▪ Teach patient about disease process, including chronic management *to increase probability of successful long-term management.* ▪ Include family in teaching *to provide support during exacerbation and increase their sense of involvement.* ▪ Discuss need to wear medical alert bracelet *to alert health care providers in time of emergency.* ▪ Teach patient to report signs and symptoms of complications of disease such as fever, edema, decreased urine output, chest pain, and dyspnea *to ensure early intervention.* ▪ Inform patient of availability of assistance from Lupus Foundation and Arthritis Foundation *to provide additional sources of information and support.*

*See Tables 63-4 and 63-9.

Careful assessment of neurologic status includes observation for visual disturbances, headaches, personality changes, seizures, and forgetfulness. Psychosis may indicate CNS disease or may be the effect of corticosteroid therapy. Irritation of the nerves of the extremities (peripheral neuropathy) may produce numbness, tingling, and weakness of the hands and feet.

The nurse must explain the nature of the disease, modes of therapy, and all diagnostic procedures. Emotional support for the patient and family is essential.

Ambulatory and Home Care. Nursing interventions must emphasize health teaching and the importance of patient cooperation for successful home management. The patient must understand that even perfect adherence to the treatment plan is not a guarantee against exacerbation because the course of the disease is unpredictable. However, a variety of factors may increase disease activity, such as fatigue, sun exposure, emotional stress, infection, drugs, and surgery. Nursing interventions should be directed toward assisting the patient and family to eliminate or minimize exposure to precipitating factors (Table 63-16).

Lupus and pregnancy. Because SLE is most common in women of childbearing age, treatment during pregnancy must be considered. The women's primary physician (or rheumatologist) and obstetrician should thoroughly discuss with the woman her desire to become pregnant. Infertility may have already resulted from renal involvement and the use of high-dose corticosteroid therapy. The SLE patient should understand that spontaneous abortion, stillbirth, and intrauterine growth retardation are common problems with pregnancy. They occur because of deposits of immune complexes in the placenta and because of inflammatory responses in the placental blood vessels. Renal, cardiovascular, pulmonary, and central nervous systems may be especially affected during pregnancy. Women who already demonstrate serious SLE involvement in these systems should be counseled against pregnancy. For the best outcome, pregnancy should be planned at a point when the disease activity is minimal. Exacerbation is common during the postpartum period. Therapeutic abortion offers the same risk of postdelivery exacerbation as carrying the fetus to term.

Neonatal lupus erythematosus (NLE) may occur in infants born of women with SLE. A risk for congenital heart block is correlated with high antibody titers.[45] A characteristic skin rash is seen in more than 30% of the cases of NLE.

Psychosocial issues. The patient with SLE confronts many psychosocial issues.[46] Disease onset may be vague, and SLE may be undiagnosed for long periods. Supportive therapies may become as important as medical treatment. The nurse should counsel the patient and family that SLE has a good prognosis for the majority of persons. Families are anxious about hereditary aspects and want to know whether their children will also have SLE. Many couples require pregnancy and sexual counseling. Individuals making decisions about marriage and careers worry about how SLE will interfere with their plans. The nurse may have to educate teachers, employers, and coworkers.

The obvious physical effects of skin rashes, discoid lesions, and alopecia may cause social isolation for the patient with SLE, affecting the individual's self-esteem and body image. However, pain and fatigue are cited most frequently as interfering with quality of life. Friends and relatives are confused by the patient's complaints of transient joint pain and overwhelming fatigue. Pacing techniques and relaxation therapy can help the patient remain involved in day-to-day activities. The nurse should stress the importance of planning both recreational and occupational activities. Young adults find sun restrictions and physical limitations particularly difficult to follow. Nursing interventions should assist the patient in developing and accomplishing reasonable goals for improving or maintaining mobility, energy levels, and self-esteem.

■ Evaluation

The expected outcomes for the patient with SLE are presented in NCP 63-2.

SYSTEMIC SCLEROSIS

Systemic sclerosis (SS), or *scleroderma,* is a disorder of connective tissue characterized by fibrotic, degenerative, and occasionally inflammatory changes in the skin, blood vessels, synovium, skeletal muscle, and internal organs. Skin thickening and tightening are the cardinal features.[47] The disease course of SS is variable. A localized or limited form of the disease, which is more common in children, is characterized by fewer symptoms mostly on the skin or in the muscles. Rarely does this localized sclerosis develop into systemic disease.[48]

SS affects women four times more often than men. SS has been reported in all ethnic groups but is more common in African Americans than whites. Although symptoms may begin at any time, the usual age at onset is between 30 and 50 years. Overall incidence increases with age. SS affects approximately 300,000 people in the United States.

Etiology and Pathophysiology

The exact cause of SS remains unknown. Immunologic dysfunction and vascular abnormalities are believed to play a role in development of widespread systemic disease. Other risk factors associated with skin thickening include environmental occupational exposure to coal, plastics, and silica dust. Collagen, the protein that gives normal skin its strength and elasticity, is overproduced (Fig. 63-10). Disruption of the cell is followed by platelet aggregation and fibrosis. Proliferation of collagen dis-

---

TABLE 63-16

Patient & Family Teaching Guide
Systemic Lupus Erythematosus

Teaching related to the disease and appropriate management should include:
1. Disease process
2. Names of drugs, actions, side effects, dosage, administration
3. Pain management strategies
4. Energy conservation and pacing techniques
5. Therapeutic exercise, use of heat therapy (for arthralgia)
6. Avoidance of physical and emotional stress
7. Avoidance of exposure to individuals with infection
8. Avoidance of drying soaps, powders, household chemicals
9. Use of sunscreen protection (at least SPF 15), with minimal sun exposure from 11 AM to 3 PM
10. Regular medical and laboratory follow-up
11. Marital and pregnancy counseling as needed
12. Community resources and health care agencies

SPF, Sun protection factor.

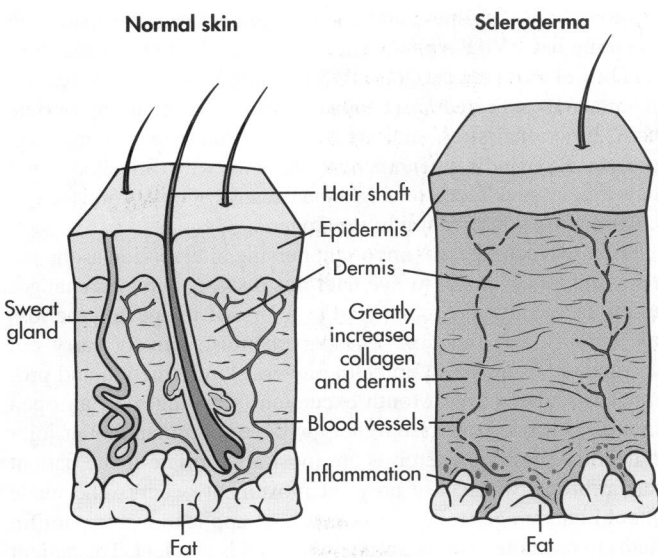

FIG. 63-10 Scleroderma skin changes.

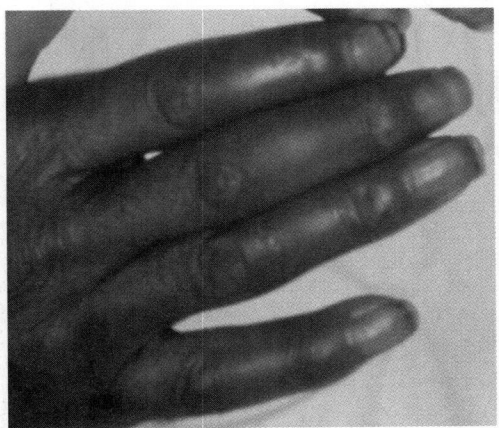

FIG. 63-11 Hand of a patient with systemic sclerosis showing sclerodactyly.

rupts the normal functioning of internal organs, such as the lungs, kidney, heart, and GI tract.

Clinical Manifestations

Manifestations of SS range from a diffuse cutaneous thickening with rapidly progressive and fatal visceral involvement to a more benign variant called CREST syndrome. **CREST syndrome** is characterized by the following five symptoms[49]:

Calcinosis—painful deposits of calcium in the skin
Raynaud's phenomenon—abnormal blood flow in response to cold or stress (Raynaud's phenomenon is explained in Chapter 37.)
Esophageal dysfunction—difficulty with swallowing caused by internal scarring
Sclerodactyly—tightening of the skin on the fingers and toes
Telangiectasia—red spots on the hands, forearms, palms, face and lips

Raynaud's Phenomenon. **Raynaud's phenomenon** (paroxysmal vasospasm of the digits) is the most common initial complaint in CREST syndrome. Patients have diminished blood flow to the fingers and toes on exposure to cold (blanching or white phase), followed by cyanosis as hemoglobin releases oxygen to the tissues (blue phase) and then erythema during rewarming (red phase). The color changes are often accompanied by numbness and tingling. Raynaud's phenomenon may precede the onset of systemic disease by months, years, or even decades.

Skin and Joint Changes. Symmetric painless swelling or thickening of the skin of the fingers and hands may progress to diffuse scleroderma of the trunk. In CREST syndrome, skin thickening is generally limited to the fingers and face. The skin loses elasticity and becomes taut and shiny, producing the typical expressionless facies with tightly pursed lips. Skin changes in the face may also contribute to reduced ROM in the temporomandibular joint. The hands may be affected by *sclerodactyly* in which the fingers are in a semiflexed position, with tightened skin to the wrist (Fig. 63-11). Reduced peripheral joint function may occur as an early symptom of polyarthritis.

Internal Organ Involvement. Esophageal fibrosis causes dysphagia and frequent reflux of gastric acid. If swallowing becomes difficult, the patient often decreases food intake and loses weight. GI effects include constipation resulting from colonic hypomotility and diarrhea caused by malabsorption from bacterial overgrowth.

Lung involvement includes pleural thickening, pulmonary fibrosis, and pulmonary function abnormalities. The patient develops a cough and dyspnea.

Primary heart disease consists of pericarditis, pericardial effusion, and cardiac arrhythmias. Myocardial fibrosis resulting in congestive heart failure occurs most frequently in patients with diffuse SS.

Renal disease is a major cause of death in SS. Malignant hypertension associated with rapidly progressive and irreversible renal insufficiency is often present. Recent improvements in dialysis, bilateral nephrectomy in patients with uncontrollable hypertension, and kidney transplantation have offered some hope to patients with renal failure.

Diagnostic Studies

Laboratory findings are relatively normal. Blood studies may reveal a mildly elevated ESR and mild hemolytic anemia as a result of RBC damage from diseased small vessels. The scleroderma antibody SCL-70 is found in about 35% of patients with systemic disease, and serum RF is found in 30% of affected patients. An anticentromere antibody is seen in many patients with CREST syndrome. If renal involvement is present, urinalysis may show proteinuria, microscopic hematuria, and casts. X-ray evidence of subcutaneous calcification, distal esophageal hypomotility, or bilateral pulmonary fibrosis is diagnostic of SS. Pulmonary function studies reveal decreased vital capacity and lung compliance.

Collaborative Care

The collaborative care of SS (Table 63-17) offers no specific treatment with long-term effects. Care is directed toward attempts to prevent or treat secondary complications of involved organs. Various drugs such as antiinflammatory agents, D-penicillamine (Cuprimine), minocycline (Minocin), and colchicine have been used with varying degrees of success.

TABLE 63-17 Collaborative Care — Systemic Sclerosis

Diagnostic
History and physical examination
Antinuclear antibody titers
Anticentromere antibody
Nailbed capillary microscopy
X-rays of chest and hands
Skin or visceral biopsy
Urinalysis (proteinuria, hematuria, casts)

Collaborative Therapy
Vasoactive agents
Calcium channel blockers (diltiazem [Cardizem])
reserpine (Serpasil)
Nonsteroidal antiinflammatory drugs
penicillamine (Cuprimine)
Corticosteroids
Physical therapy

Physical therapy helps maintain joint mobility and preserve muscle strength. Occupational therapy assists the patient in maintaining functional abilities. Gastroesophageal reflux disease (GERD) may be treated by antacids and periodic dilation of the esophagus. (GERD is discussed in Chapter 40.)

Drug Therapy. No specific drugs or combination of drugs has been proven effective for the treatment of SS. Treatment is directed at symptoms and the prevention of complications. Vasoactive agents are often prescribed in early disease, and calcium channel blockers (nifedipine [Adalat, Procardia] and diltiazem [Cardizem]) are now a common treatment choice for Raynaud's phenomenon. Reserpine (Serpasil), an adrenergic blocking agent, increases blood flow to the fingers.

Corticosteroids are generally reserved for patients with significant joint or muscle involvement or severe skin disease with ulcerations. D-penicillamine increases the solubility of dermal collagen and may cause thinning of the skin. However, it is not accepted as a treatment option by all health care providers because of its possible toxic side effects, including myasthenia gravis and blood and liver dyscrasias. Topical agents may provide some relief from joint pain. Capsaicin cream may be useful not only as a local analgesic but also as a vasodilator. Other therapies are prescribed to address specific systemic problems, such as tetracycline for diarrhea caused by bacterial overgrowth, an H_2 histamine receptor blocker (e.g., cimetidine [Tagamet]) and proton pump inhibitor (e.g., omeprazole [Prilosec]) for esophageal symptoms, and an antihypertensive agent (e.g., captopril [Capoten], propranolol [Inderal], methyldopa [Aldomet]) for hypertension with renal involvement.

NURSING MANAGEMENT
SYSTEMIC SCLEROSIS

Because prevention is not possible, nursing intervention often begins during a hospitalization for diagnostic purposes. Diagnostic studies should be thoroughly explained. The nurse can help the patient resolve feelings of helplessness by providing information about the illness and encouraging active participation in planning care. Vital signs, weight, intake and output, respiratory and bowel function, and joint ROM should be assessed at regular intervals as indicated by specific symptoms to plan appropriate care. Emotional stress and cold ambient temperatures may aggravate Raynaud's phenomenon. Patients with SS should not have finger-stick blood testing done because of compromised circulation and poor healing of the fingers.

Health teaching is an important nursing intervention as the patient and family begin to live with this disease. Obvious changes in the face and hands often lead to poor self-image and the loss of mobility and function. The patient must actively carry out therapeutic exercises at home to prevent skin retraction and promote vascularization. Mouth excursion (yawning with an open mouth) is a good exercise to help with temporomandibular joint function. Isometric exercises are most appropriate if the patient has arthropathy because no joint movement occurs. The nurse should encourage the use of moist heat applications or paraffin baths to promote skin flexibility in the hands and feet. The patient should use assistive devices as appropriate and organize activities to preserve strength and reduce disability.

Hands and feet should be protected from cold exposure and possible burns or cuts that might heal slowly. Smoking should be avoided because of its vasoconstricting effect. Signs of infection should be promptly reported. Lotions may help alleviate skin dryness and cracking, but they must be rubbed in for an unusually long time because of the thickness of the skin.

Dysphagia may be reduced by eating small, frequent meals; chewing carefully and slowly; and drinking fluids. Heartburn may be minimized by using antacids 45 to 60 minutes after each meal and by sitting upright for at least 2 hours after eating. Using additional pillows or raising the head of the bed on blocks may help reduce nocturnal gastroesophageal reflux.

Job modifications are often necessary because stair climbing, typing, writing, and cold exposure may pose particular problems. The patient may become socially withdrawn as skin tightening alters the appearance of the face and hands. Dining out may become a socially embarrassing event because the patient's small mouth, difficulty swallowing, and reflux make eating less enjoyable. Some individuals with SS wear gloves to protect fingertip ulcers and to provide extra warmth. Sensitive areas on fingertips resulting from ulcers or calcinosis may require padded utensils or special assistive devices to reduce discomfort. Daily oral hygiene must be emphasized, or neglect may lead to increased tooth and gingival problems. The patient needs a dentist who is familiar with SS and can deal with a small oral aperture. Psychologic support reduces stress and may positively influence peripheral motor response. Biofeedback training and relaxation techniques can reduce tension, improve sleeping habits, and raise the temperature of the fingers and toes.

Sexual dysfunction resulting from body changes, pain, muscular weakness, limited mobility, decreased self-esteem, erectile dysfunction, and decreased vaginal secretions may require sensitive counseling by the nurse. Specific suggestions based on individual patient assessment should be offered.

POLYMYOSITIS AND DERMATOMYOSITIS

Polymyositis (PM) and **dermatomyositis** (DM) are diffuse, idiopathic, inflammatory myopathies of striated muscle, producing bilateral weakness usually most severe in the proximal or limb-girdle muscles. These disorders, which are relatively rare, occur twice as often in women as in men. In a bimodal distribution, children ages 5 to 14 years and adults ages 45 to 65 years are most often affected by PM and DM.[50] Some cases of DM are associated with concurrent malignant disease.[51]

Etiology and Pathophysiology

The exact cause of PM and DM is unknown. Theories include an infectious agent, neoplasms, drugs or vaccinations, and stress. Because disease severity is not well correlated with altered immune complexes, it is unclear if the complexes occur as primary or secondary phenomena. Because cytotoxic T cells and macrophages have been found near the damaged muscle fibers of PM, the disease is believed to be caused by cell-mediated injury.

Clinical Manifestations and Complications

Muscular. Over several months, the patient experiences weight loss and increasing fatigue. Gradually developing weakness of the muscles leads to difficulty in performing routine activities. The most commonly affected muscles are those of the shoulders, legs, arms, and pelvic girdle. The patient may have difficulty rising from a chair or bathtub, climbing stairs, combing the hair, or reaching into a high cupboard. Neck muscles may become so weak that the patient is unable to raise the head from the pillow. Muscle discomfort or tenderness is uncommon. Muscle examination reveals an inability to move against resistance or even gravity. Weak pharyngeal muscles may produce dysphagia and dysphonia (nasal or hoarse voice).

Dermal. Skin changes include the classic violet-colored, cyanotic, or erythematous symmetric rash (heliotrope) with edema around the eyelids. Reddened, smooth, or scaly patches appear at the PIP joints (Gottron's sign) and can be confused with psoriasis or seborrheic dermatitis. Violet-colored or erythematous papules and small plaques can also develop on the knuckles (Gottron's papules).[52] On the back and on the extensor surfaces of the forearms, an erythematous scaling rash may develop (poikiloderma). Hyperemia and telangiectasias are often present at the nailbeds. Calcium nodules (calcinosis cutis), which can develop throughout the skin, are especially common in long-standing DM.

Other Manifestations. Joint redness, pain, and inflammation often occur and contribute to limitations in joint ROM. Contractures and muscle atrophy may occur with advanced disease. Weakened pharyngeal muscles can lead to a poor cough effort, difficulty swallowing, and increased risk for aspiration pneumonia. "Cotton-wool" patches can occur in the retina. Childhood DM appears to have a more progressive, crippling course.

Diagnostic Studies

Diagnosis of PM or DM is confirmed after excluding other neuromuscular diseases. The most important laboratory finding is an elevation of the enzyme creatine kinase (CK). Increased levels of CK indicate muscle damage. Because test results change with disease activity, serum CK levels can also be valuable in determining the patient's response to treatment. Elevation of ESR is also expected with active disease. An electromyogram suggestive of PM will show bizarre high-frequency discharges and spontaneous fibrillation, with positive spikes at rest. Muscle biopsy reveals necrosis, degeneration, regeneration, and fibrosis. Complete pulmonary function testing is necessary to determine the extent of lung involvement.

Collaborative Care

PM and DM are initially treated with high-dose corticosteroids. Improvement is generally achieved if corticosteroid therapy is promptly instituted, and the dosage can typically be reduced as improvement is noted. Relapses are common. If corticosteroids prove ineffective or lead to myopathy, immunosuppressive drugs may be administered (methotrexate, azathioprine [Imuran] or cyclophosphamide [Cytoxan]) using oral or intermittent intravenous dosing. Topical corticosteroids may also be prescribed to treat the skin rash.

Physical therapy can be helpful and should be tailored to the activity of the disease. Massage and passive movement are appropriate during active disease. More aggressive exercises should be reserved for periods when disease activity is minimal, as evidenced by low serum enzyme levels.

A careful search for possible malignant lesions should be undertaken for the patient more than 40 years of age.[53] If malignant disease is found, it should be treated appropriately. Complete remission of DM may occur if the malignant lesion is removed.

NURSING MANAGEMENT
POLYMYOSITIS AND DERMATOMYOSITIS

Prevention is not possible. However, improved ability to discriminate PM from other muscular disorders may favorably influence prognosis by more rapid diagnosis and institution of therapy.

Nursing interventions should include a thorough explanation of the nature of the disease, the prescribed therapies, all diagnostic tests, and the importance of regular medical care. Assessment of muscular weakness and limitation of motion should be performed. It is important for the patient to understand that the benefits of therapy are often delayed. For example, weakness may increase during the first few weeks of corticosteroid therapy. The nurse should maintain the patient on bed rest and assist the patient with activities of daily living when extreme weakness is present. Special attention is paid to patient safety. To prevent aspiration, the patient should be encouraged to rest before meals, maintain an upright position when eating, and choose a diet of easily swallowed foods. Use of assistive devices should be encouraged as a fall prevention strategy.

The nurse should assist the patient to organize activities and use pacing techniques to conserve energy. Daily ROM exercises are encouraged to prevent contractures. When active inflammation is not evident, muscle-strengthening (repetitive) exercises may be started. Home care will be necessary during the acute phase of PM because profound muscle weakness renders the patient unable to carry out activities of daily living. Homemaker services, visiting nurses, and family caregivers are needed to assist the patient in routine hygiene, meal preparation and eating, and ambulation.

OVERLAPPING FORMS OF CONNECTIVE TISSUE DISEASE

Patients having a combination of clinical features of several rheumatic diseases are described as having *overlapping* or *mixed connective tissue disease*. Although this combination was originally believed to be a distinct clinical disorder, follow-up revealed an evolution primarily from SLE or SS. This early undifferentiated or transitional form of connective tissue disease has a typical serologic pattern, including high titers of a speckled pattern of ANA, high levels of antibody to ribonuclease-sensitive extractable nuclear antibody, and autoantibodies to ribonucleoprotein.

SJÖGREN SYNDROME

Sjögren syndrome is an autoimmune disease that targets moisture-producing glands, leading to the common symptoms of *xerostomia* (dry mouth) and keratoconjunctivitis *sicca* (dry eyes). The nose, throat, airways, and skin can also become dry. The disease can affect other glands as well, including those in the stomach, pancreas, and intestines (extraglandular involvement). The disease is usually diagnosed in women over age 40.[54]

In primary Sjögren syndrome, symptoms can be traced to problems with the lacrimal and salivary glands. The patient with primary disease is likely to have antibodies against the cytoplasmic antigens SS-A and SS-B, as well as ANA. The patient with secondary Sjögren syndrome typically has had another autoimmune disease (e.g., RA, SLE) before Sjögren develops.

Sjögren syndrome appears to be caused by genetic and environmental factors. Several genes seem to be involved. One gene predisposes whites to the disease, whereas other genes are linked to the disease in people of Japanese, Chinese, and African American heritage. The trigger may be a viral or bacterial infection that adversely stimulates the immune system. In Sjögren syndrome, lymphocytes attack and damage the lacrimal and salivary glands.

Dry eyes and dry mouth are the main symptoms. Decreased tearing leads to a "gritty" sensation in the eyes, burning, blurred vision, and photosensitivity. Dry mouth produces buccal membrane fissures, altered sense of taste, dysphagia, and increased frequency of mouth infections or dental caries. Dry skin and rashes, joint and muscle pain, and thyroid problems may also be present. Other exocrine glands can be affected. For example, vaginal dryness may lead to dyspareunia (painful intercourse). Autoimmune thyroid disorders are common with Sjögren syndrome, including Graves' disease or Hashimoto's thyroiditis. Histologic study reveals lymphocyte infiltration of salivary and lacrimal glands. The disease may become more generalized and involve the lymph nodes, bone marrow, and visceral organs (pseudolymphoma). Lymphoma develops in about 5% of patients with Sjögren syndrome.

Ophthalmologic examination (Schirmer test), salivary flow rates, and lower lip biopsy of minor salivary glands confirm the diagnosis.[55] The treatment is symptomatic, including (1) instillation of artificial tears as often as necessary to maintain adequate hydration and lubrication, (2) surgical punctual occlusion, and (3) increased fluids with meals. Dental hygiene is important. Pilocarpine (Salagen) and cevimeline (Evoxac) can be used to treat symptoms of dry mouth.[56] Increased humidity at home may reduce respiratory infections. Vaginal lubrication with a water-soluble product such as K-Y jelly may increase comfort during intercourse. Corticosteroids and immunosuppressive drugs are indicated for treatment of pseudolymphoma.

Soft Tissue Rheumatic Syndromes

Myofascial pain syndrome, fibromyalgia syndrome (FMS), and chronic fatigue syndrome (CFS) are three soft tissue disease syndromes that have many commonalities and may be related.

Ongoing research continues to explore links among these three syndromes. A multidisciplinary team approach consisting of a rheumatologist, nurse, mental health professional, and physical therapist may be especially helpful for patients with these syndromes whose disease course may be chronic.

MYOFASCIAL PAIN SYNDROME

Myofascial pain syndrome is characterized by musculoskeletal pain and tenderness in one anatomic region of the body. The pain has been shown to originate in anterior and posterior trigger points that have resulted from muscle trauma and/or chronically strained muscles (e.g., desk or computer work). Regions of pain are often within the taut bands and fascia of skeletal muscles. When activated by pressure, trigger points are thought to activate a characteristic pattern of pain. The incidence and the age groups and gender that are most affected are not known.

Patients complain of the pain as deep and aching accompanied by a sensation of burning, stinging, and stiffness.[57] The muscles frequently involved are located in the chest, neck, lower back, and shoulders. Referred pain from these muscle groups can also travel to the buttock, hand, and the head, causing severe headaches. Additional systemic manifestations have not been reported.

A test used to diagnose myofascial pain syndrome is the palpation of trigger points. On physical examination of the patient, palpation reveals induration and frequently a muscle twitch in the area of a trigger point. Once a trigger point is palpated, pain is then referred to a region often at some distance away.[58] These findings have also been noted to occur in normal healthy persons and in persons with FMS. Similarities in myofascial pain syndrome with FMS have led to the suggestion that myofascial pain may be a form of or evolve into FMS. A comparison of the two syndromes is shown in Table 63-18.

The active management of myofascial pain can often result in relief of the patient's pain. Positive results have been seen by locally injecting the trigger points with a local anesthetic (e.g., 1% lidocaine), passive muscle stretching and manipulation, and spraying the trigger point with a cold agent such as ethyl chloride. Massage, acupuncture, biofeedback, and ultrasound therapy have also shown to benefit some patients.

Patient and family teaching is an important nursing responsibility. Instruction should focus on the prevention of muscle tension in work and leisure activities. Good posture and resting and sleeping positions should also be reviewed. Most patients with

TABLE 63-18	Comparison of Fibromyalgia and Myofascial Pain Syndromes	
VARIABLE	**FIBROMYALGIA**	**MYOFASCIAL PAIN**
Location	Generalized	Regional
Examination	Tender points	Trigger points
Response to local therapy	Not sustained	Curative
Gender	Female/male ratio: 10:1	Equal or unknown
Systemic features	Characteristic	Unknown

From McCance KL, Huether SE: *Pathophysiology: the biologic basis for disease in adults and children,* ed 4, St Louis, 2002, Mosby.

myofascial pain syndrome are able to lead a normal and active lifestyle.

FIBROMYALGIA SYNDROME

Fibromyalgia syndrome (FMS) is a chronic disorder characterized by widespread, nonarticular musculoskeletal pain and fatigue with multiple tender points. People with FMS also typically experience nonrestorative sleep, morning stiffness, irritable bowel syndrome, and anxiety. The former name for this disorder, fibrositis, implied inflammation of the muscles and soft tissues. However, FMS is now known to be nondegenerative, nonprogressive, and noninflammatory.

Fibromyalgia is a commonly diagnosed musculoskeletal disorder and a major cause of disability. FMS affects over 6 million Americans, typically occurring in women 20 to 55 years old.[59,60] FMS and CFS share many commonalities (Table 63-19).

Etiology and Pathophysiology

Research continues to focus on identifying the underlying causes and pathophysiologic mechanisms of FMS. Currently multiple theories exist regarding the etiology of FMS. One possible factor may involve the CNS. Neurotransmitters in the CNS including serotonin, substance P, and norepinephrine are at abnormal levels in patients with FMS.[61] These neurotransmitters regulate mood, sleep, and pain perception. Sleep disturbances, depression, and widespread soft tissue pain are common in FMS.

A hyperfunctioning of the hypothalamic-pituitary-adrenal (HPA) axis, which plays a major role in the stress response, may also exist. Changes in the HPA axis can negatively affect a person's physical and mental state. An increase in cortisol levels, with a concomitant decrease in ACTH levels, has been noted in persons with FMS.[62,63] These findings can be linked to depression and a decreased response to stress. It is not known if depression is a cause or an effect of the disease.

A dysfunction in the autonomic nervous system may cause changes in the vascular system leading to orthostatic hypotension and decreased heart rate variability. A recent viral illness or Lyme disease may serve as an infectious trigger in susceptible persons. A noted decrease in growth hormone may be responsible for the muscle pain.

Clinical Manifestations and Complications

Clinical manifestations of FMS overlap with those of CFS.[64] The patient complains of a widespread burning pain that worsens and improves through the course of a day. It is often difficult for the patient to discriminate if pain occurs in the muscles, joints, or soft tissues. Head or facial pain often results from stiff or painful neck and shoulder muscles. It can accompany temporomandibular joint dysfunction, which affects an estimated one third of FMS patients. Nonrestorative sleep and resulting fatigue are typical. Physical examination characteristically reveals point tenderness at 11 or more of 18 identified sites[65] (Fig. 63-12). Patients with FMS are sensitive to painful stimuli throughout the body and not merely at the identified tender sites. In addition, point tenderness can vary from day to day. On some occasions, the FMS patient may respond to fewer than 11 tender points; at other times, palpation of all sites may elicit pain.

Cognitive effects range from difficulty concentrating to memory lapses and a feeling of being overwhelmed when dealing with multiple tasks. Many individuals report migraine headaches. Depression and anxiety often occur and may require drugs. Numbness or tingling in the hands or feet (paresthesia) often accompanies FMS. Restless legs syndrome is also typical, with the patient describing an irresistible urge to move the legs when at rest or lying down.

Irritable bowel syndrome with manifestations of digestive disturbances, abdominal pain, and bloating is common. FMS patients may also experience difficulty swallowing, perhaps because of abnormalities in esophageal smooth muscle function. Increased frequency of urination and urinary urgency, in the absence of a bladder infection, are typical complaints. Women with FMS may experience more difficult menstruation, with a worsening of disease symptoms during this time.

Diagnostic Studies

A definitive diagnosis of FMS is often difficult to establish. Laboratory results in most cases serve to rule out other suspected disorders based on the patient's history and physical examination. Occasionally a low ANA titer is seen, but it is not considered diagnostic. Muscle biopsy may reveal a nonspecific moth-eaten appearance or fiber atrophy. The American College of Rheumatology classifies an individual as having FMS if two criteria are met: (1) pain is experienced in 11 of the 18 tender points on palpation (see Fig. 63-12) and (2) a history of widespread pain is noted for at least 3 months. Widespread pain is defined as occurring on both sides of the body and above and below the waist. Up to 70% all patients with FMS will also meet the criteria for a diagnosis of CFS.[61]

Collaborative Care

The treatment of FMS is symptomatic and requires a high level of patient motivation. The nurse can play a key role in teaching the patient to be an active participant in the therapeutic

TABLE 63-19	Commonalities Between Fibromyalgia Syndrome and Chronic Fatigue Syndrome
Occurrence	Previously healthy, young, and middle-aged women
Etiology (theories)	Infectious trigger, dysfunction in HPA axis, alteration in CNS
Clinical manifestations	Malaise and fatigue, cognitive dysfunction, headaches, sleep disturbances, depression, anxiety, fever, generalized musculoskeletal pain
Course of disease	Variable-intensity of symptoms fluctuate over time
Diagnosis	No definitive laboratory tests or joint and muscle examinations, mainly a diagnosis of exclusion
Collaborative care	Treatment is symptomatic and may include antidepressant drugs such as amitriptyline (Elavil) and fluoxetine (Prozac). Other measures are heat, massage, regular stretching, biofeedback, stress management, and relaxation training. Patient and family teaching is essential.

CNS, Central nervous system; *HPA,* hypothalamic-pituitary-adrenal.

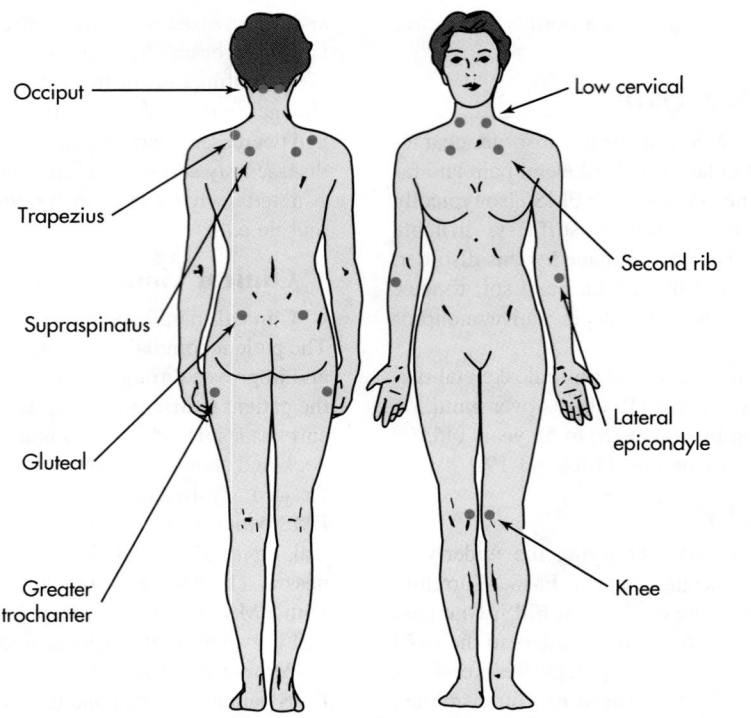

FIG. 63-12 Tender points in fibromyalgia syndrome.

Labels: Occiput, Trapezius, Supraspinatus, Gluteal, Greater trochanter, Low cervical, Second rib, Lateral epicondyle, Knee

regimen. Pain, aching, and tenderness can be helped by rest. Analgesics such as acetaminophen (Tylenol), and NSAIDs (e.g., tramadol [Ultram]) are effective for some patients. Stress, fatigue, and sleep disturbances can be helped by taking a low-dose tricyclic antidepressant such as amitriptyline (Elavil), which has undergone extensive clinical testing for use in the treatment of FMS (see the Evidence-Based Practice box). The skeletal muscle relaxant cyclobenzaprine (Flexeril) is also commonly used to treat sleep disturbances. Both drugs have sedative effects that can help in improving nighttime rest for the patient with FMS. If amitriptyline is not well tolerated, other similar drugs can be substituted (e.g., doxepin [Sinequan], imipramine [Tofranil], or trazodone [Desyrel]). Selective serotonin reuptake inhibitor (SSRI) antidepressants (e.g., sertraline [Zoloft] or paroxetine [Paxil]) tend to be reserved for FMS patients who also have depression. SSRIs are often prescribed at low doses during the day and sometimes combined with a tricyclic antidepressant at bedtime.

Benzodiazepines (e.g., diazepam [Valium], alprazolam [Xanax], clonazepam [Klonopin]) are often prescribed with low doses of ibuprofen (Motrin, Advil) to treat anxiety, as well as the muscle spasms that affect many FMS patients. The drug zolpidem tartrate (Ambien) is sometimes prescribed for short-term intervention in patients with severe sleep disturbances.

EVIDENCE-BASED PRACTICE
Antidepressants for Fibromyalgia

Clinical Problem
Are antidepressants effective in the treatment of fibromyalgia?

Best Clinical Practice
- Antidepressants improve overall symptoms related to fibromyalgia.
- Antidepressants improve individual symptoms of fatigue, sleep, and pain in patients with fibromyalgia.

Implications for Nursing Practice
- Fibromyalgia can be a devastating disease and significantly affect quality of life.
- Patients with fibromyalgia should be offered antidepressants as a form of treatment to decrease their symptoms.

Reference for Evidence
EMB Reviews: Antidepressants improve symptoms of fibromyalgia, *ACP Journal Club* 134:85, 2001.

NURSING MANAGEMENT
FIBROMYALGIA SYNDROME

Because of the chronic nature of FMS and the necessity of maintaining an ongoing rehabilitation program, the patient with FMS needs consistent support from the nurse and other members of the health care team. Massage is often combined with ultrasound or the application of alternating heat and cold packs to soothe tense, sore muscles and increase blood circulation. Gentle stretching can be performed by a physical therapist or practiced by the FMS patient at home to relieve muscle tension and spasm. Yoga and Tai Chi are often appropriate choices. Low-impact aerobic exercise such as walking can help prevent muscle atrophy. A cardinal rule for the FMS patient is to start slowly and build up exercise tolerance in increments.[66]

Dietitians often urge FMS patients to limit their consumption of sugar, caffeine, and alcohol because these substances have been shown to be muscle irritants. Vitamin and mineral supplements may be appropriate to combat stress, correct deficiencies, and support the immune system. However, unproven "miracle diets" or supplements should be carefully investigated by the FMS patient and discussed with the health care provider before using them. The patient should understand that some foods and supplements may cause serious or even dangerous side effects when mixed with certain drugs.

Pain and the related symptoms of FMS can cause significant stress. There is also some indication that FMS patients simply do not process stress well. Effective relaxation strategies include biofeedback, guided imagery, and autogenic training. Patients need to receive initial training for these interventions, but they can then continue to practice in their own homes. Psychologic counseling (individual or group) may also prove beneficial for the FMS patient.

CHRONIC FATIGUE SYNDROME

Chronic fatigue syndrome (CFS), also called chronic fatigue and immune dysfunction syndrome, is a disorder characterized by debilitating fatigue and a variety of associated complaints. Immune abnormalities are also frequently present. CFS is three times more common in women than in men. Its onset typically occurs between the ages of 25 and 45. The prevalence of CFS is difficult to determine. It is estimated that 500,000 people in the United States have a CFS-like condition.[67] CFS is a poorly understood condition and can have a devastating impact on the lives of patients and their families. CFS and FMS share some common features (see Table 63-19).

Etiology and Pathophysiology

Despite numerous attempts to determine the etiology and pathology of CFS, the precise mechanisms remain unknown. However, there are many theories about the cause of CFS.[68] It was once thought that CFS was postinfectious and followed a viral infection. Several microorganisms have been investigated as etiologic agents, including herpesviruses (e.g., Epstein Barr [EBV], cytomegalovirus [CMV]), retroviruses, enteroviruses, *Candida albicans,* and mycoplasma. Antibody titers to many infectious agents are elevated in patients with CFS. However, studies have shown no causal relationships between these specific viral agents and CFS. It is known that viruses can precipitate the syndrome. In addition, EBV and CMV infections may contribute to the fatigue and exhaustion experienced in CFS.

Abnormal immune function appears to be a central event in CFS. These abnormalities include decreased immunoglobulin production, reduced NK cell activity, altered cytokine production, decreased lymphocyte proliferation, altered CD4/CD8 ratio, and an increased percentage of activated T cells. If the mechanism of CFS involves a continuing immune response to an initial viral infection, the symptoms may be due in part to the production of cytokines. These immune mediators can cause muscle and CNS manifestations, including fatigue. However, immune alterations do not occur in all patients.

Dysfunctioning of the HPA axis may exist, causing neuroendocrine regulation alterations.[69,70] Changes in the HPA axis can alter the immune system, cause a decrease in energy, and affect mood states in patients with CFS. Because of the activation of the HPA axis, there is a reduced production of corticotropin-releasing hormone in the hypothalamus. Serum cortisol levels are low, and ACTH levels are correspondingly high.

Alterations in the CNS are thought to play a role in CFS. Patients often manifest cognitive deficits including problems with memory, attention, and concentration. A disturbance in the regulation of blood pressure and pulse is commonly found in patients with CFS.

Because mild to moderate depression occurs in many of these patients, it has been proposed that CFS is a psychiatric disorder. However, it is difficult to determine if depression is a cause or an effect of debilitating chronic fatigue.

Clinical Manifestations

It is often difficult to distinguish between CFS and FMS because many clinical features are similar (see Table 63-19). In about half of the cases, CFS develops insidiously, or the patient may have intermittent episodes that gradually become chronic. Incapacitating fatigue is the most common symptom of CFS and is the problem that causes the patient to seek health care. Associated symptoms (Table 63-20) may fluctuate in intensity over time. In other situations, CFS arises suddenly in a previously active, healthy individual. An unremarkable flulike illness or other acute stress is often identified as a triggering event.

The patient may become angry and frustrated with the inability of health care providers to diagnose a problem. The disorder may have a major impact on work and family responsibilities. Some individuals may even need help with activities of daily living.

Diagnostic Studies

Physical examination and diagnostic studies can be used to rule out other possible causes of the patient's symptoms. No laboratory test can diagnose CFS or measure its severity. The Centers for Disease Control and Prevention have developed diagnostic criteria based on the patient's symptoms (see Table 63-20). In general, it remains a diagnosis of exclusion.[71]

TABLE 63-20	**Diagnostic Criteria for Chronic Fatigue Syndrome***

Major Criteria
- Unexplained, persistent, or relapsing chronic fatigue is of new and definite onset (not lifelong).
- Fatigue is not due to ongoing exertion.
- Fatigue is not substantially alleviated by rest.
- Fatigue results in substantial reduction in occupational, educational, social, or personal activities.

Minor Criteria
- Substantial impairment in short-term memory or concentration
- Sore throat
- Tender cervical or axillary lymph nodes
- Muscle pain
- Multijoint pain without joint swelling or tenderness
- Headaches of a new type, pattern, or severity
- Unrefreshing sleep
- Postexertional malaise lasting more than 24 hours

Adapted from Fukuda K et al (International Chronic Fatigue Syndrome Study Group): The chronic fatigue syndrome: a comprehensive approach to its definition and study, *Ann Intern Med* 121:953, 1994.
*For a diagnosis to be made, the patient must fulfill all the major criteria, plus four or more of the minor criteria. Each minor criterion must have persisted or recurred during 6 or more consecutive months of illness and must not have predated the fatigue. These criteria were prepared by the Centers for Disease Control and Prevention, National Institutes of Health, and International Chronic Fatigue Syndrome Study Group.

NURSING *and* COLLABORATIVE MANAGEMENT
CHRONIC FATIGUE SYNDROME

Because there is no definitive treatment for CFS, supportive management is essential. The patient should be informed about what is known about the disease, and all complaints should be taken seriously. NSAIDs can be used to treat headaches, muscle and joint aches, and fever. Because many patients with CFS also have allergies and sinusitis, antihistamines and decongestants can be used to treat allergic symptoms. Tricyclic antidepressants (e.g., doxepin [Sinequan], amitriptyline [Elavil]) and SSRIs (e.g., fluoxetine [Prozac], paroxetine [Paxil]) can improve mood and sleep problems. Clonazepam (Klonopin) can also be used to treat sleep disturbances and panic disorders. The use of low-dose hydrocortisone is being studied to decrease fatigue and disability.

Total rest is not advised because it can potentiate the self-image of being an invalid. On the other hand, strenuous exertion can exacerbate the exhaustion. Therefore it is important to plan a carefully graduated exercise program. A well-balanced diet including fiber and fresh dark-colored fruits and vegetables for antioxidant action is essential in treatment. Behavioral therapy may be used to promote a positive outlook, as well as improve overall disability, fatigue, and other symptoms.[72,73]

One of the major problems facing many CFS patients is financial instability. When the illness strikes, they cannot work or must decrease the amount of time working. Loss of a job often leads to loss of medical insurance. Obtaining disability benefits can be frustrating because of the difficulty of establishing a diagnosis of CFS.

CFS does not appear to progress. Although most patients recover or at least gradually improve over time, some never show substantial improvement. Recovery is more common in individuals with a sudden onset of CFS. Patients with CFS suffer from substantial occupational and psychosocial impairments and loss, including the social pressure and isolation from being characterized as lazy or "crazy."

CRITICAL THINKING EXERCISES

Case Study
Systemic Lupus Erythematosus

Patient Profile. Grace Anderson, a 30-year-old married African American woman, is seen at the rheumatology clinic following a recent vacation to Hawaii.

Subjective Data
- Works in a flower shop
- Complains of joint pain, photosensitivity, fatigue, and a facial rash
- Is 4 months pregnant
- Has Raynaud's phenomenon when she works in the refrigerator room stocking flowers
- Fears something is horribly wrong with her
- Is afraid to take drugs because of pregnancy

Objective Data

Physical Examination
- Malar rash
- Swelling of third and fourth metacarpophalangeal joints of both hands
- Dry, scaly scalp
- Pain on motion of both wrists, shoulders, and knees with no obvious swelling

Diagnostic Studies
- WBC count 4000/μl (4 × 10^9/L)
- Platelets 100,000/μl (150 × 10^9/L)
- Complement (C3) 60 mg/dl (0.6 g/L)
- Positive ANA and Sm antibodies

Collaborative Care
- Diagnosed with SLE
- Started on prednisone 10 mg daily

CRITICAL THINKING QUESTIONS

1. How might the nurse explain the pathophysiology of SLE to Grace?
2. How might the vacation have influenced the symptoms that she is currently experiencing?
3. What are some home and work modifications that the nurse can suggest to Grace that will reduce her symptoms?
4. Discuss the types of prenatal and postpartum considerations essential in caring for Grace.
5. What other sources of information regarding SLE might the nurse suggest to Grace and her family?
6. Based on the assessment data presented, write one or more nursing diagnoses. Are there any collaborative problems?

Nursing Research Issues

1. What is the relationship between social support systems and quality of life for people with rheumatoid arthritis?
2. What are the needs of the family when the patient is diagnosed with SLE?
3. Are gender and age of the patient related to use of alternative therapies with arthritic pain?
4. What are effective measures that the nurse can institute to improve patient compliance with arthritis home management programs?
5. Does regular well-tolerated exercise by a patient with arthritis or connective tissue disease improve quality of life?

REVIEW QUESTIONS

The number of the question corresponds to the same-numbered objective at the beginning of the chapter.

1. In assessing the joints of a patient with rheumatoid arthritis, the nurse understands that the joints are damaged by
   a. the development of Heberden's nodes in the joint capsule.
   b. the deterioration of cartilage by the enzyme hyaluronidase.
   c. invasion of pannus into the joint capsule and subchondral bone.
   d. bony ankylosis following inflammation of the joints in HLA-B27–positive individuals.

2. Assessment data noted by the nurse in the patient with osteoarthritis commonly include
   a. elevated ESR.
   b. evening but no morning stiffness.
   c. progressive joint pain with activity.
   d. symmetric swelling of metacarpophalangeal joints.

3. An important nursing intervention in caring for the patient with ankylosing spondylitis is to teach the patient
   a. thoracic stretching and ROM exercises to prevent deformity.
   b. to sleep on the side with the legs flexed and supported with pillows.
   c. to prevent enteric and venereal infections that precipitate recurring attacks.
   d. that continuous therapeutic blood levels of NSAIDs can limit the progression of the disease.

4. When teaching the patient with gout, the nurse should instruct the patient to
   a. avoid foods high in fat and calories.
   b. drink plenty of fluids on a daily basis.
   c. apply ice packs to decrease joint pain.
   d. have CBC and WBC levels monitored regularly.

5. In teaching a patient with SLE about the disorder, the nurse uses the knowledge that the pathophysiology of SLE includes
   a. production of autoantibodies directed against constituents of cellular DNA.
   b. an autoimmune reaction resulting in degeneration, necrosis, and fibrosis of muscle fibers.
   c. deposition in tissues of immune complexes formed from IgG autoantibodies reacting with IgG.
   d. chronic inflammation and cytokine activity, which results in synovial proliferation and cartilage and bone damage.

6. The nurse planning teaching for the patient with rheumatoid arthritis who is receiving multiple drug therapy includes information related to the need to
   a. use aspirin only on an as-needed basis for pain relief.
   b. use birth control during and 3 months following gold therapy.
   c. have frequent laboratory monitoring while taking methotrexate.
   d. stop taking any corticosteroids as soon as symptoms are relieved.

7. In teaching a patient with fibromyalgia (FMS) about this disorder, the nurse understands that
   a. more men than women are affected.
   b. trigger points are a definitive diagnostic test.
   c. many symptoms are similar to chronic fatigue syndrome.
   d. FMS is characterized by progression of worsening inflammation.

REFERENCES

1. Roberts D: Arthritis and connective tissue disorders. In Schoen D, editor: *NAON core curriculum for orthopaedic nursing,* ed 4, Pitman, NJ, 2001, Jannetti.
2. Ling SM, Bathon JM: Osteoarthritis in older adults, *Am Geriatr Soc* 46:215-225, 1998.
3. Kee CC: Osteoarthritis: manageable scourge of aging, *Nurs Clin North Am* 35:1, 2000.
4. Roberts D: Degenerative disease. In Maher AB, Salmond SW, Pellino TA, editors: *Orthopaedic nursing,* ed 3, Philadelphia, 2002, Saunders.
5. Moseley JB et al: A controlled trial of arthroscopic surgery for osteoarthritis of the knee, *N Engl J Med* 347:81, 2002.
6. Horstman J: *The Arthritis Foundation's guide to alternative therapies,* Atlanta, 1999, Arthritis Foundation.
7. University of California, Berkeley: *Wellness Letter* 17:8, 2001, School of Public Health. Available at *www.WellnessLetter.com.*
8. Altman RD, IAP Study Group: Ibuprofen, acetaminophen and placebo in osteoarthritis of the knee: a six-day double-blind study, *Arthritis Rheum* 42:S9, 1999.
9. Food and Drug Administration: Labeling Changes for Celebrex [online]. Available at *www.fda.gov/bbs/topics/answers/2002* (accessed June 7, 2002).
10. Goorman SD et al: Functional outcome in knee osteoarthritis after treatment with Hylan G-F 20: A prospective study, *Arch Phys Med Rehab* 81:2000.
11. Mann W et al: Changes in health, functional and psychosocial status and coping strategies of home based older persons with arthritis over three years, *Occup Therapy Research* 19:126, 1999.
12. McDonald PA: Autoimmune and inflammatory disorders. In Maher AB, Salmond SW, Pellino TA, editors: *Orthopaedic nursing,* ed 3, Philadelphia, 2002, Saunders.

13. Dunkin MA, Morgan P: AT research spotlight: smoking linked to RA, *Arthritis Today* 15:3, 2001.

14. Wilson S, Giddens J: *Health assessment for nursing practice,* ed 2, St. Louis, 2001, Mosby.

15. Edmunds M, Mayhew M, editors: *Pharmacology for the primary care provider,* St Louis, 2000, Mosby.

16. O'Dell et al: Treatment of rheumatoid arthritis with methotrexate and hydroxychloroquine, methotrexate and sulfasalazine, or a combination of the three medications: results of a two-year, randomized, double-blind, placebo-controlled trial, *Arthritis Rheum* 46:1164, 2002.

17. Kassimos D et al: Biological response modifiers in rheumatoid arthritis, *Lancet* 359:352, 2002.

18. Dayer J, Bresnihan B: Targeting interleukin-1 in the treatment of rheumatoid arthritis, *Arthritis Rheum* 43:1001, 2000.

19. Food and Drug Administration: Prosorba column, summary of safety and effectiveness data [on-line]. Available at *www.fda.gov/cdrh* (accessed June 17, 2002).

20. Eckloff S, Thorntin B: Prescribing assistive devices for patients with rheumatoid arthritis: careful selection of equipment helps patients perform daily functions, *J Musculoskeletal Med* 19:27, 2002.

21. Westby M: A health professional's guide to exercise prescription for people with arthritis: a review of aerobic fitness activities, *Arthritis Care Res* 45:50, 2001.

22. Escalante A, Del Rincon I: The disablement process in rheumatoid arthritis, *Arthritis Care Res* 47:333, 2002.

23. Glaser V: Recognizing the spondyloarthropathies, Patient Care [on-line]. Available at *http://pc.pdr.net/pc/content/journals/p/data/1999/p4a/p4a/183.html* (accessed 1999).

24. Harvard Medical School, Boston: *Harvard Health Letter Special Report-Arthritis,* 1999, Health Publications Group, Boston, Mass.

25. Spondylitis Association of America: What is AS? [on-line]. Available at *www.spondylitis.org* (accessed 2002).

26. Stone M et al: Clinical and imaging correlates of response to treatment with infliximab in patients with ankylosing spondylitis, *J Rheumatology* 28:1605, 2001.

27. American College of Rheumatology: Psoriatic arthritis [on-line]. Available at *www.rheumatology.org/patients/factsheet/psoriati.html* (accessed 2002).

28. Danning C: Psoriatic arthritis: diagnosis and management of a diverse disease, *J Musculoskeletal Med* 17:169, 2000.

29. Psoriatic arthritis. *Wheeless' textbook of orthopaedics* [on-line]. Available at *www.medmedia.com/oa4/62.htm* (accessed 2002).

30. The Merck manual: Reiter's syndrome [on-line]. Available at *www.merck.com/pubs/mmanual/section5/chapter51/51b.htm* (accessed 2002).

31. Stone M, Inman R: Recognizing and managing reaction arthritis: the physician must search for the inciting event, *J Musculoskeletal Med* 19:37, 2002.

32. Zorn KE: Infections. In Schoen D, editor: *NAON core curriculum for orthopaedic nursing,* ed 4, Pitman, NJ, 2001, National Association of Orthopaedic Nurses.

33. Centers for Disease Control and Prevention: CDC Lyme disease home page [on-line]. Available at *www.cdc.gov/ncidod/diseases* (accessed June 10, 2002).

34. Centers for Disease Control and Prevention: Lyme disease-United States 2000, *MMWR* 51:29, 2002.

35. Eppes S: Lyme disease: current therapies and prevention, *Infect Med* 18:388, 2001.

36. American College of Rheumatology: HIV-associated rheumatic disease syndromes [on-line]. Available at *www.rheumatology.org/patients/factsheet/hiv.html* (accessed 2002).

37. Dequeker J (International League of Associations for Rheumatology): HIV infection and arthritis [on-line]. Available at *www.rheuma21st.com/archives/cutting_dequeker-hiv.html* (accessed 2001).

38. Crowther C: *Primary orthopedic care,* St Louis, 1999, Mosby.

39. Terkeltaub R: Pathogenesis and treatment of crystal-induced inflammation. In Koopman W, editor: *Arthritis and allied conditions,* ed 14, Philadelphia, 2001, JB Lippincott.

40. Kammer G et al: Abnormal T cell signal transduction in systemic lupus erythematosus, *Arthritis Rheum* 46:1139, 2002.

41. Centers for Disease Control and Prevention: Trends in deaths from systemic lupus erythematosus-United States 1979-1998, *MMWR* 51:371, 2002.

42. Lipsky P: Systemic lupus erythematosus: an autoimmune disease of B cell hyperactivity, *Nat Immunol* 2:764, 2002.

43. Maddison P et al: The rate and pattern of organ damage in late onset systemic lupus erythematosus, *J Rheumatoid* 29:913, 2002.

44. Godfrey T, Ryan P: Systemic lupus erythematosus: current management, *Med J Aust* 175:125, 2001.

45. Salomonsson S et al: A serologic marker for fetal risk of congenital heart block, *Arthritis Rheum* 46:1223, 2002.

46. Dobkin P et al: Psychosocial contributors to mental and physical health in patients with systemic lupus erythematosus, *Arthritis Care Res* 11:23, 1998.

47. Sabir S, Werth V: Cutaneous manifestation of sclerosing conditions, *J Musculoskeletal Med* 17:207, 2000.

48. Scleroderma Foundation: Scleroderma fact sheet [on-line]. Available at *www.scleroderma.org/fact.html* (accessed 2002).

49. Scleroderma Research Foundation: Scleroderma facts [on-line]. Available at *www.srfcure.org* (accessed 2002).

50. O'Rourke K: Myopathies in the elderly, *Rheum Dis Clin North Am* 26:647, 2000.

51. Paget S: Atypical rheumatic diseases, *Postgrad Med* 111:71, 2002.

52. Brown C, Marschall S: Connective tissue update: focus on dermatomyositis, *Consultant* 39:2876, 1999.

53. Yazici Y, Kagen L: The association of malignancy with myositis, *Curr Opin Rheum* 12:498, 2000.

54. National Institute of Arthritis and Musculoskeletal and Skin Disease: Questions and answers about Sjögren's syndrome [on-line]. Available at *www.niams.nih.gov/topics/sjogrens/index.htm* (accessed 2001).

55. Manthorpe R: How should we interpret the lower lip biopsy findings in patients investigated for Sjögren's syndrome? [on-line] Available at *www3.interscience.wiley.com/* (accessed April 5, 2002).

56. Hashimi I: The management of Sjögren's syndrome in dental practice, *J Am Dental Assoc* 132:1409, 2001.

57. Sheon R: Overview of soft-tissue rheumatic diseases [on-line]. Available at *www.uptodateonline.com* (accessed July 1, 2002).

58. Graff-Radford SB: Regional myofascial pain syndrome and headache: principles of diagnosis and treatment, *Curr Pain Headache Rep* 5:376, 2001.

59. Leslie M: Fibromyalgia syndrome: a comprehensive approach to identification and management, *Clin Excellence Nurse Pract* 3:165, 1999.

60. American College of Rheumatology: Criteria for classification of fibromyalgia [on-line]. Available at *www.nfra.net* (accessed July 23, 2002).

61. Goldenberg D: Pathogenesis and treatment of fibromyalgia [on-line]. Available at *www.uptodateonline.com* (accessed July 1, 2002).

62. Deuschle M et al: Effects of major depression, aging and gender upon calculated diurnal free plasma cortisol concentrations: a re-evaluation study, *Stress* 2:21, 1998.

63. Adler G et al: Reduced hypothalamic-pituitary and sympathoadrenal responses to hypoglycemia in women with fibromyalgia syndrome, *Am J Med* 106:534, 1999.

64. Goldenberg D: Differential diagnosis of fibromyalgia [on-line]. Available at *www.uptodateonline.com* (accessed July 1, 2002).

65. Russell I: Fibromyalgia syndrome: formulating a strategy for relief, *J Musculoskeletal Med* 15:4, 1998.

66. Coward B: Fibromyalgia, *AJN* 99:42, 1999.

67. Centers for Disease Control and Prevention: Chronic fatigue syndrome-demographics [on-line]. Available at *www.cdc.gov.ncidod.diseases* (accessed July 20, 2002).

68. Straus SE: Chronic fatigue syndrome. In Braunwald E et al, editors: *Harrison's principles of internal medicine,* ed 5, New York, 2001, McGraw-Hill.

69. Buskila D, Press J: Neuroendocrine mechanisms in fibromyalgia-chronic fatigue, *Best Pract Res Clin Rheumatol* 15:747, 2001.

70. Parker AJ, Wessely S, Cleare AJ: The neuroendocrinology of chronic fatigue syndrome and fibromyalgia, *Psychol Med* 31:1331, 2001.

71. Craig T, Kakumanu S: Chronic fatigue syndrome: evaluation and treatment, *Am Fam Physician* 65:6, 2002.

72. Kinsella P: Review: behavioural interventions show the most promise for chronic fatigue syndrome, *Evid Based Nurs* 5:46, 2002.

73. Smith RC: Review: behavioral interventions show the most promise for the chronic fatigue syndrome, *ACP J Club* 136:61, 2002.

RESOURCES

American Association for Chronic Fatigue Syndrome
515 Minor Avenue, Suite 8
Seattle, WA 98104
206-781-3544
Fax: 206-749-9052
www.aacfs.org

American College of Rheumatology
1800 Century Place, Suite 250
Atlanta, GA 30345
404-633-3777
Fax: 404-633-1870
www.rheumatology.org

Arthritis Foundation
P.O. Box 7669
Atlanta, GA 30309-0669
800-283-7800
www.arthritis.org

Lupus Foundation of America, Inc.
1300 Piccard Drive, Suite 200
Rockville, MD 20850-4303
800-558-0121 or 301-670-9292
Fax: 301-670-9486
www.lupus.org

National Fibromyalgia Research Association
P.O. Box 500
Salem, OR 97302
www.nfra.net

National Institute of Arthritis and Musculoskeletal and Skin Diseases
Information Clearinghouse, National Institutes of Health
1 AMS Circle
Bethesda, MD 20892-3675
877-22-NIAMS (226-4267) or 301-495-4484
Fax: 301-718-6366
www.niams.nih.gov

National Institute of Neurological Disorders and Stroke
NIH Neurological Institute
P.O. Box 5801
Bethesda, MD 20824
800-352-9424
www.ninds.nih.gov

National Organization for Rare Disorders (NORD)
55 Kenosia Avenue
P.O. Box 1968
Danbury, CT 06813-1968
800-999-6673 or 203-744-0100
Fax: 203-798-2291
www.rarediseases.org

National Psoriasis Foundation
6600 SW 92nd Avenue, Suite 300
Portland, OR 97223-7195
800-723-9166 or 503-244-7404
Fax: 503-245-0626
www.psoriasis.org

Scleroderma Foundation
12 Kent Way, Suite 101
Byfield, MA 01922
978-463-5843
Info line: 800-722-HOPE (4673)
Fax: 978-463-5809
www.scleroderma.org

Scleroderma Research Foundation
2320 Bath Street, Suite 315
Santa Barbara, CA 93105
800-441-CURE or 805-563-9133
www.srfcure.org

Spondylitis Association of America
14827 Ventura Boulevard, # 222
Sherman Oaks, CA 91403
800-777-8189 or 818-981-1616
www.spondylitis.org

For additional Internet resources, see the website for this book at
http://www.evolve.elsevier.com/Lewis/medsurg.

Nursing Care in Specialized Settings

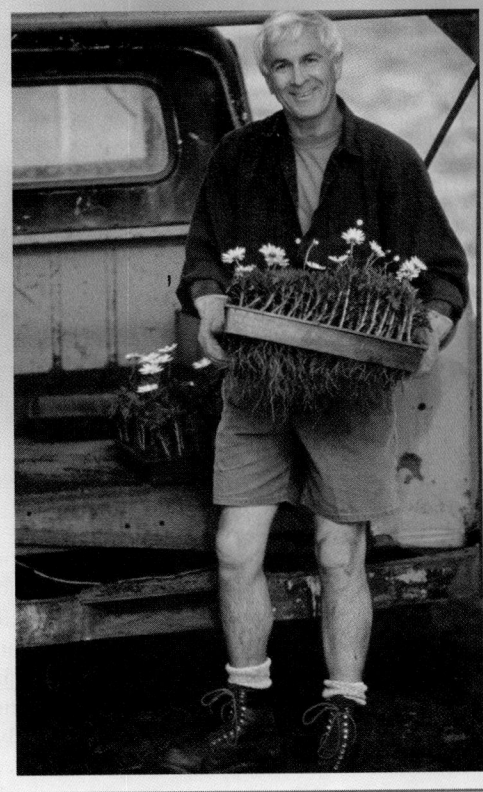

CHAPTER *64*

NURSING MANAGEMENT
Critical Care Environment

Linda Bucher

LEARNING OBJECTIVES

1. Differentiate the certification roles of the critical care nurse: CCRN, CCNS, and ACNP.
2. Select appropriate nursing interventions to manage common problems and needs of critically ill patients.
3. Develop effective strategies to manage issues related to the families of critically ill patients.
4. Discuss the principles of hemodynamic monitoring and related collaborative care of critically ill patients.
5. Describe the purpose, indications, and function of circulatory assist devices and related collaborative care.
6. Select appropriate nursing interventions to manage the care of an intubated patient.
7. Differentiate the indications for and modes of mechanical ventilation.
8. Describe the principles of mechanical ventilation and related collaborative care of critically ill patients.

KEY TERMS

assist-control ventilation, p. 1783
bag-valve-mask, p. 1777
circulatory assist devices, p. 1772
closed-suction technique, p. 1778
continuous positive airway pressure, p. 1785
controlled mandatory ventilation, p. 1783
endotracheal intubation, p. 1776
extubation, p. 1780
hemodynamic monitoring, p. 1762
high-frequency ventilation, p. 1785
impedance cardiography, p. 1770
intraaortic balloon pump, p. 1772
mechanical ventilation, p. 1781

negative pressure ventilation, p. 1781
open-suction technique, p. 1778
partial liquid ventilation, p. 1785
phlebostatic axis, p. 1764
positive end-expiratory pressure, p. 1785
positive pressure ventilation, p. 1781
pressure support ventilation, p. 1784
pressure ventilators, p. 1782
synchronized intermittent mandatory ventilation, p. 1783
ventricular assist device, p. 1775
volume ventilators, p. 1782
weaning, p. 1788

CRITICAL CARE NURSING

Critical Care Units

Critical care units (CCUs) or intensive care units (ICUs) are designed to meet the special needs of acutely and critically ill patients. Florence Nightingale forwarded the concept of clustering the most acutely ill patients as far back as the 1800s.[1] During poliomyelitis and tuberculosis pandemics in the middle of the twentieth century, special units were established, equipped with technical equipment to manage the airway and ventilate the patient, and staffed by specialized care providers. Finally, lessons learned from World War II and the Korean War solidified the concepts of triage and specialty nursing units, and by the late 1950s, these concepts were being incorporated into hospital systems.[2]

In the 1960s technologic developments allowed for more accessible monitoring of the electrocardiogram (ECG), arterial and central venous pressures, and arterial blood gases (ABGs). Coronary care units were developed for patients with acute myocardial infarction. In these units patients were continually monitored for cardiac arrhythmias. Nurses followed protocols to aggressively manage arrhythmias. By the 1970s the ICU was a standard unit in most general hospitals worldwide. Since that time, technical advances have continued at a rapid pace, bringing improved monitoring capabilities and new strategies to manage life-threatening problems.

The term *critical care nursing* is often used interchangeably with the term *intensive care nursing*, but it is not exclusively restricted to that specialty area. The critical care nurse is responsible for assessing life-threatening conditions, instituting appropriate interventions, and evaluating the outcomes of the interventions. The biotechnology available in the ICU is extensive and continually evolving. The capability exists to continuously monitor ECG, blood pressure, oxygenation saturation, ventilation, intracranial pressure, and temperature. More advanced monitoring devices allow for the measurement of cardiac index, stroke volume, ejection fraction, end-tidal carbon dioxide (CO_2), and tissue oxygen consumption. (See Table 64-1 for common abbreviations used in critical care nursing.) Patients may be receiving continual support from mechanical ventilators, intraaortic balloon pumps, or dialysis machines. A typical CCU is illustrated in Fig. 64-1.

Critical Care Nurse

The critical care nurse cares for patients and the families of patients with acute and unstable physiologic problems in an environment equipped for technically advanced methods of assessing and managing patient problems. The American Association of Critical Care Nurses (AACN) defines critical care nursing as that specialty dealing with human responses to life-threatening problems. Critical care nursing requires in-depth knowledge of anatomy, physiology, pathophysiology, pharmacology, and advanced assessment skills, as well as the ability to use advanced biotechnology. The critical care nurse provides ongoing assessment and early recognition and management of complications

Reviewed by Elisabeth G. Bradley, RN, APN, CCRN, Cardiac Clinical Nurse Specialist, Christiana Care Health Systems, Newark, Del.; and Michelle Kelly, RN, BSc, MN, Faculty of Nursing, Midwifery, and Health, University of Technology, Sydney, New South Wales, Australia.

ABBREVIATION	TERM
CI	Cardiac index
CO	Cardiac output
CVP	Central venous pressure
FIO_2	Fraction of inspired oxygen
IABP	Intraaortic balloon pump
MAP	Mean arterial pressure
PA	Pulmonary artery
PAS, PAD	PA systolic (pressure), PA diastolic (pressure)
PAWP	Pulmonary artery wedge pressure
PVR	Pulmonary vascular resistance
SpO_2	Percent oxygen saturation of hemoglobin measured by pulse oximetry
SvO_2	Percent oxygen saturation of hemoglobin in mixed venous blood (e.g., in the PA)
SVI	Stroke volume index
SV	Stroke volume
SVR	Systemic vascular resistance
VAD	Ventricular assist device

TABLE 64-1   Abbreviations Commonly Used in the Intensive Care Unit

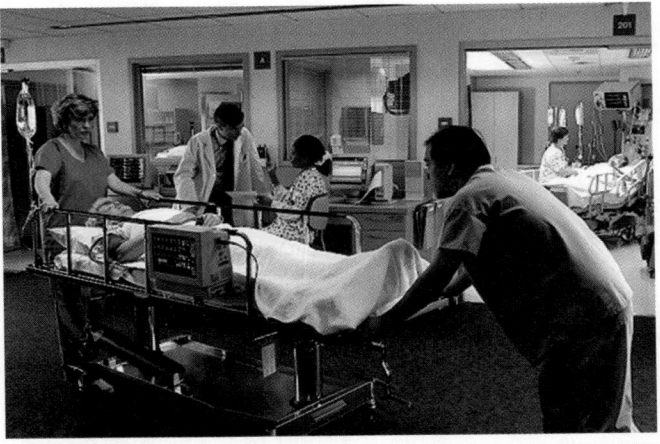

FIG. 64-1 Typical intensive care unit.

while fostering healing and recovery. Appropriate actions by an astute nurse can prevent many complications. The nurse must also be able to provide psychologic support to the patient and the family. To be effective, the critical care nurse must be able to communicate and collaborate effectively with all health team providers (e.g., physician, dietitian, respiratory therapist, occupational therapist).

Nursing practice in the ICU often follows a primary care model with the patient cared for by a limited group of nurses who become thoroughly familiar with the patient's condition and the needs of the patient and the family. The ICU nurse spends most working hours near the patient's bedside. Specialization in ICU nursing usually requires formal, in-service education combined with a preceptored clinical orientation.

The AACN Certification Corporation offers critical care certification (CCRN) in adult, pediatric, and neonatal critical care nursing. The designation requires registered nurse licensure, practice experience in critical care nursing, and successful completion of a written test. Continued critical care practice and retesting or continuing education is required for recertification. CCRN certification validates knowledge of critical care nursing; it is not the same as advanced practice.

Advanced practice critical care nurses have a graduate (master's or doctorate) degree. These nurses are employed in a variety of roles: patient and staff educators, consultants, administrators, researchers, or expert practitioners. The advanced practice critical care nurse who is a clinical nurse specialist (CNS) typically functions in one or more of these roles. Certification for the CNS in acute and critical care (CCNS) is available through the AACN Certification Corporation. Another advanced practice role is the acute care nurse practitioner (ACNP). This advanced practice nurse provides comprehensive care to select critically ill patients and their families. The ACNP conducts comprehensive assessments, orders and interprets diagnostic tests, manages health

problems and disease-related symptoms, prescribes treatments, and coordinates care during transitions in settings. The ACNP may practice independently (e.g., providing comprehensive care to the chronically critically ill) or collaboratively (e.g., providing symptom management in conjunction with physicians). Certification as an ACNP is available through the AACN Certification Corporation and the American Nurses Credentialing Center. Prescriptive authority regulations for advanced practice nurses vary by state.

Critical Care Patient

A patient is generally admitted to the ICU for one of three reasons. First, the patient may be physiologically unstable, requiring advanced and sophisticated clinical judgments by the nurse or physician. Second, the patient may be at risk for serious complications and require frequent and often invasive assessments. Third, the patient may require intensive and complicated nursing support related to the use of intravenous polypharmacy (e.g., neuromuscular blockade, thrombolytics, drugs requiring titration) and advanced biotechnology (e.g., ventricular assist devices, mechanical ventilation, intracranial pressure monitoring, continuous renal replacement therapy, hemodynamic monitoring).

ICU patients can be clustered by disease condition (e.g., neurology, pulmonary) or age-group (e.g., neonatal, pediatrics). ICU patients are sometimes clustered by acuity (e.g., acute and unstable versus technology dependent but stable). Patients commonly treated in the ICU include those with respiratory distress, myocardial ischemia or infarction, or acute neurologic impairment or those receiving care after cardiac surgery or major organ transplantation. The care of the critically injured patient is provided in trauma and burn ICUs. The patient with a medical emergency (e.g., sepsis, diabetic ketoacidosis, drug overdoses, or poisonings or thyroid, adrenal, or hematologic crises) is often treated in a medical ICU. The patient with multiple comorbidities may be monitored in the ICU while receiving care for unrelated conditions. The patient who is not expected to recover from an illness is usually not admitted to an ICU. For example, the ICU should not be used to manage the patient in a persistent coma, nor should ICU care be used to prolong the natural process of death.

Despite the emphasis on caring for the patient who can survive, death is common in ICU patients. It is reported that 10% of patients admitted to ICUs will die, and another 20% may leave the ICU but will not survive to discharge. This suggests a need for caution and coordination of care when transferring patients from ICUs to general care units. In general, nonsurvivors were older, had preexisting health problems, and experienced longer ICU stays.[3,4]

Progressive care units (PCUs), also called high-dependency units or stepdown units, have been established as intermediate units between the ICU and the general care unit. Generally, patients in PCUs are at risk for serious complications, but their risk is lower than that of ICU patients. Examples of patients found in PCUs include patients scheduled for interventional cardiac procedures (e.g., stent placement, pacemaker implantation), awaiting heart transplant, receiving vasoactive intravenous drugs (e.g., diltiazem [Cardizem]), or being weaned from prolonged mechanical ventilation. Patients in these units can be monitored for cardiac rhythm, arterial blood pressure, oxygen saturation, and end-tidal CO_2.[5] The use of PCUs provides specialized nursing care for an at-risk patient population in a more cost-effective environment.

Common Problems of Critical Care Patients. The patient admitted to the ICU is at risk for numerous complications and special problems. Critically ill patients are usually immobile and at risk for skin problems (see Chapter 23). The use of multiple, invasive devices predisposes the patient to iatrogenic infections. Sepsis and multiple organ dysfunction syndrome (MODS) may follow (see Chapter 65). Adequate nourishment for the critically ill patient is paramount but frequently overlooked. Other special problems for ICU patients relate to anxiety, pain, impaired communication, sensory-perceptual problems, and sleep difficulties.

Nutrition. Patients are often admitted to ICUs with conditions that result in either hypermetabolic states (e.g., burns, trauma, sepsis) or catabolic states (e.g., acute renal failure). Other times, patients may be admitted in severely malnourished states, such as those that occur with wasting syndrome and chronic liver disease. In general, malnutrition has been linked to increases in mortality and morbidity. Determining who to feed, what to feed, when to feed, and how to feed (e.g., route of administration) are crucial questions that must be asked when caring for a critically ill patient.[6] The critical care nurse must collaborate with the physician and the dietitian to determine how best to meet the nutritional needs of ICU patients.

The primary goal of nutritional support is to prevent or correct nutritional deficiencies. This is usually accomplished by the provision of enteral nutrition (i.e., delivery of calories via the gastrointestinal [GI] tract) or parenteral nutrition (i.e., delivery of calories intravenously). Enteral nutrition is thought to preserve the structure and function of the gut mucosa and help to prevent translocation of gut bacteria, a major trigger of MODS (see Chapter 65).[5,6] In addition, enteral nutrition is associated with fewer complications and is less expensive when compared with parenteral nutrition.[6] (See Evidence-Based Practice box on nutritional support on this page.) (Enteral and parenteral nutrition are discussed in Chapter 39.)

Parenteral nutrition should be considered only when the enteral route is unsuccessful in providing adequate nutrition or contraindicated. Examples of these conditions are paralytic ileus, diffuse peritonitis, intestinal obstruction, pancreatitis, GI ischemia, intractable vomiting, and severe diarrhea.[6]

EVIDENCE-BASED PRACTICE
Nutritional Support in Critically Ill Patients

Clinical Problem

What is the relationship between nutritional support and outcomes for critical care patients?

Best Clinical Practice

- When nutrition support is indicated, enteral nutrition should be preferentially used over parenteral nutrition.
- Parenteral nutrition is not recommended for critically ill patients with an intact gastrointestinal tract.
- In adult surgical patients, the early use of enteral nutrition is associated with a reduction in complications and shorter hospital stay.
- Early use of enteral nutrition is recommended in critically ill surgical patients and should be considered for other critically ill patients.
- Further studies are needed to determine the optimal timing and composition of parenteral nutrition in patients not tolerating enteral nutrition.

Implications for Nursing Practice

- Nurses have a very important role in assessing the nutritional status of critically ill patients.
- Providing nutritional support should be a standard of practice for critically ill patients.

References for Evidence

Heyland DK: Nutritional support in the critically ill patient: a critical review of the evidence, *Database of Abstracts of Reviews of Effectiveness* 2:2002.

Heyland DK: Parenteral nutrition in the critically ill patient: more harm than good? *Proc Nutr Soc* 59:457, 2000.

Heyland DK: Enteral and parenteral nutrition in the seriously ill, hospitalized patient: a critical review of the evidence, *J Nutr Health Aging* 4:31, 2000.

Anxiety. It has been reported that as many as 70% to 80% of ICU patients experience some degree of anxiety.[7] The primary sources of anxiety for patients include the perceived or anticipated threat to physical health and the seemingly hostile environment. Many patients and families feel uncomfortable in the ICU environment with its complex equipment, high noise and light levels, isolation from family, and intense pace of activity. Pain and sleeplessness enhance anxiety as do immobilization, loss of control, and impaired communication.[7]

In one study of over 700 critical care nurses, 71% reported that assessing patients for anxiety was very important. The nurses also identified agitation, increased blood pressure, increased heart rate, patient verbalization of anxiety, and restlessness as the five most important clinical indicators of anxiety.[7] To help reduce anxiety, the nurse should encourage patients and families to express concerns, ask questions, and state their needs. The nurse should include the patient and family in all conversations and explain the purpose of equipment and procedures. The nurse should also structure the patient's surrounding environment in a way that may decrease anxiety. For example, family members can be encouraged to bring in photographs and personal items. Judicious use of antianxiety drugs (e.g., lorazepam [Ativan]) and complementary therapies (e.g., imagery, music, massage) may reduce the stress response that can be triggered by anxiety and should be considered.[8,9]

Pain. The control of pain in the ICU patient is paramount. It is reported that as many as 70% of ICU patients recount having moderate to severe unrelieved pain.[10] Inadequate pain control is often linked with agitation and anxiety and is known to contribute to the stress response. ICU patients at high risk for pain include patients (1) who have medical conditions that include ischemic, infectious, or inflammatory processes; (2) who are immobilized; (3) who have invasive monitoring devices; (4) and who are scheduled for any invasive or noninvasive procedures.[10]

For some critically ill patients, continuous intravenous sedation (e.g., propofol [Diprivan]) is a practical and effective strategy for pain control. However, patients receiving deep sedation are unresponsive, and this prevents the nurse and other health care providers from properly assessing the patient's neurologic status. To address this limitation, policies that include a daily, scheduled interruption of sedation have been developed. Daily, sedative interruption allows the patient to awaken and the health care provider to conduct a neurologic examination.[8] In one study, patients who had interrupted sedation were extubated faster and discharged sooner from the ICU than patients who did not have their sedation interrupted.[11] (Chapter 9 has more detailed information on pain management.)

Impaired communication. Inability to communicate can be a distressing problem for the patient who may be unable to speak because of the use of paralyzing drugs or an endotracheal tube. As part of any procedure the nurse should explain what will happen or is happening to the patient. When the patient cannot speak, the nurse should explore alternative methods of communication, including the use of devices such as picture boards, notepads, magic slates, or computer keyboards. When speaking with the patient, the nurse should look directly at the patient and use hand gestures when appropriate. For patients who do not speak English, the use of a medical interpreter is strongly recommended (see Chapter 2).

Nonverbal communication is important. High levels of procedure-related touch and decreased levels of affection-related or comfort-related touch characterize the ICU. Patients have different levels of tolerance for being touched, usually related to cultural background and personal history. It may be appropriate to provide comforting touch with ongoing evaluation of the patient's response. Often the ICU nurse encourages the family to touch and talk with the patient.

Sensory-perceptual problems. Acute and reversible sensory-perceptual changes are common in ICU patients. The combination of alterations in mentation (e.g., delusions, short attention span, loss of recent memory), psychomotor behavior (e.g., restlessness, lethargy), and sleep-wake cycle (e.g., daytime sleepiness, nighttime agitation) has been inappropriately labeled *ICU psychosis.* The patient experiencing these alterations is not psychotic but is suffering from delirium. It is estimated that the prevalence of delirium in ICU patients ranges from 15% to 40%.[12] Demographic factors predisposing the patient to delirium include advanced age, preexisting cerebral illnesses (e.g., dementia), and a history of drug or alcohol abuse. Environmental factors that can contribute to delirium include sleep deprivation, anxiety, sensory overload, and immobilization. Physical conditions such as hemodynamic instability, hypoxemia, electrolyte disturbances, and severe infections can precipitate delirium. Last, certain drugs (e.g., sedatives [benzodiazepines], furosemide [Lasix], antimicrobials [aminoglycosides]) have been associated with the development of delirium.[12] (Delirium is discussed in Chapter 58.)

The task of the ICU nurse is to identify all predisposing factors and attempt to improve the patient's mental clarity and cooperation with therapy. It is imperative that physiologic factors be addressed (e.g., correction of oxygenation, perfusion, and electrolyte problems). The use of clocks and calendars may help the patient remain oriented. If the patient demonstrates unsafe behavior, hyperactivity, insomnia, or delusions, symptoms may be managed pharmacologically with neuroleptic drugs (e.g., haloperidol [Haldol]).[12] In addition, the presence of family members may help reorient the patient and reduce agitation.

Sensory overload can also result in patient distress and anxiety. Environmental noise levels are particularly high in the ICU.[13,14] The nurse can limit noise and assist the patient in understanding noises that cannot be prevented. Conversation is a particularly stressful noise, especially when the discussion concerns the patient and is conducted in the presence of, but without participation from, the patient. The nurse can eliminate this source of stress by identifying suitable places for patient-related discussions and, whenever possible, by including the patient in the discussion. The nurse can also limit noise levels directly by muting phones, setting alarms appropriate to the patient's condition, and eliminating unnecessary alarms. For example, the nurse should silence the blood pressure alarms while manipulating invasive lines and then reactivate the alarms when the procedures are complete. Similarly, ventilator alarms should be transiently silenced during endotracheal suctioning. Overhead paging and other unnecessary noise should be limited in patient care areas.

Sleep problems. Nearly all ICU patients experience sleep disturbances. Patients may have difficulty falling asleep or have disrupted sleep because of noise, anxiety, pain, frequent monitoring, or treatment procedures.[14] Drugs such as sedatives and hypnotics may result in disturbed sleep patterns, including reductions in slow wave and rapid eye movement (REM) sleep.[15] Sleep disturbance is a significant stressor in the ICU, contributing to delirium and possibly affecting recovery. The ICU nurse can structure the environment to promote the patient's sleep-wake cycle. Strategies include clustering activities, scheduling rest periods, dimming lights at nighttime, opening curtains during the daytime, obtaining physiologic measurements without disrupting the patient, limiting noise, and providing comfort measures (e.g., massage, evening care).

Issues Related to Families

When someone becomes critically ill, care must be extended beyond the patient to the patient's family because they are intimately connected. Family members play a valuable role in the patient's recovery and should be considered members of the health care team. They can contribute to the patient's well-being by:

1. Providing a link to the patient's personal life (e.g., news of friends, family, and job)
2. Advising the patient in health care decisions or functioning as the decision maker when the patient cannot
3. Helping with activities of daily living (e.g., bathing, oral suctioning)
4. Providing positive, loving, and caring support

To be effective in caring for their loved one, family members need guidance and support from the nurse. The experience of having a friend or family member in the ICU is physically and emotionally difficult. Anxiety regarding the patient's condition and prognosis and concerns regarding the patient's pain and other discomforts are some of the issues families confront. They may question the quality of care that the patient is receiving. In addition, it is common for families to experience anxiety regarding the financial issues related to the provision of care in the recovery phase of the illness.

The family will typically be experiencing disruption of their daily routines to support the patient. They may be far from their own home and supportive friends and family members. Ultimately, families of the critically ill are considered in crisis, and family-centered care is imperative.[16,17] To provide family-centered care effectively, the nurse must be skilled in crisis intervention. The nurse should conduct a family assessment and intervene as necessary. Interventions can include active listening, reduction of anxiety, and support of those who become upset or angry.[17] The family's feelings should be acknowledged and accepted and their decisions supported. Other health team members, such as chaplains, social workers, and psychologists, may be helpful in assisting the family to adjust and should be consulted as necessary. The extent to which family-centered care is provided will, in turn, affect the patient's clinical course in the ICU.

The major needs of families of critically ill patients have been categorized as informational needs, reassurance needs, and convenience needs.[16] Lack of information is a major source of anxiety for the family. The nurse should assess the family's understanding of the patient's status, treatment plan, and prognosis and provide information as appropriate. The nurse should also provide information to the family when the patient's condition changes. It is recommended that a spokesperson for the family be identified so that information between the health care team and the family can be coordinated.

The family needs reassurance regarding the way in which the patient's care is managed and decisions are made. The family should have the opportunity to be involved in decision making. If the patient has an advance directive or living will, the family will need to see that the patient's wishes are understood and respected. When patients are incapable of making their own health care decisions, they may have designated a durable power of attorney, and this person should be involved in the patient's plan of care.[18] The family should also be invited to meet the health care team members, including physicians, dietitian, respiratory therapist, social worker, physical therapist, and chaplain. The nurse should evaluate the appropriateness of including family members in multidisciplinary care conferences. It helps family members to accept and cope with problems if they observe that health care providers are hopeful, caring, and competent; decisions are deliberate; and they have the opportunity to help shape the course of care.

Research has demonstrated that families of critically ill patients need the convenience of access to the patient and that limiting family visitation does not protect that patient from adverse physiologic consequences.[16] Rigid visitation policies in ICUs should be abolished, and a move toward less restrictive, individualized visiting policies is strongly recommended by the AACN.[17] This can be accomplished by assessing the patient's and family members' needs and preferences and incorporating these into the plan of care. The first time family members visit, it is important for the nurse to prepare them for the experience by briefly describing the patient's appearance and the physical environment (e.g., equipment, noise). It is helpful if the nurse can accompany the family members as they enter the room. They should be encouraged to participate in the patient's care if they desire. The nurse should observe the responses of both the patient and family. In some ICUs, visitation has been expanded to include the family pet visitation or animal-assisted therapy. The positive benefits of pet visitation (e.g., decreases in blood pressure and anxiety) far outweigh the risks (e.g., transmission of infection from pet to patient) and should be considered as part of the visitation policy.[16,19]

■ Culturally Competent Care: Critical Care Patients

Providing culturally competent care to critically ill patients and families is challenging. Often, the nurse is focused on meeting the physiologic needs of the patient and may not appreciate the influence of the patient's culture on the illness experience. Minimally, the cultural dimensions of the meaning of sickness and health, pain, dying and death, and grief should be explored when caring for critically ill patients and their families. (See Chapter 2 for discussions on cultural issues related to sickness, health, and pain.)

Cultural perspectives on dying and death are complex. Telling some patients that they are dying as a way of letting them prepare for death is considered an infringement on the role of the family.[20] Others view a discussion about advance directives as a legal device to deny care. One study of African American patients found that most would opt to extend life even at the expense of the quality of life.[20] Similarly, customs surrounding dying and death vary widely, from leaving a window open to allow the spirit of the deceased to leave to providing the final bath for the deceased.[21] The nurse caring for the dying patient must make every attempt to understand and accommodate the family's cultural traditions. The expressions of grief that follow the loss of a loved one are highly individualized and influenced by several variables. These include the relationship between the grieving person and the person lost, whether the loss is sudden or anticipated, the support systems available to the grieving person, past experiences with loss, and the person's religious and cultural beliefs.[21] It is of utmost importance that the critical care nurse proceeds cautiously when approaching patients facing death and their families. Asking patients, "What do you want to know?" and "Who do you want with you when discussing options?" is a good starting point.[20] (See Chapter 10 for additional information on end-of-life care.) ■

HEMODYNAMIC MONITORING

Hemodynamic monitoring refers to measurement of pressure, flow, and oxygenation within the cardiovascular system. Both invasive (internally placed devices) and noninvasive (external devices) hemodynamic measurements are made in the ICU. Values commonly measured include systemic and pulmonary arterial pressures, central venous pressure (CVP), pulmonary artery wedge pressure (PAWP), cardiac output/index, stroke volume/index, and oxygen saturation of the hemoglobin of arterial blood (SaO_2) and mixed venous blood (SvO_2). From these measurements the clinician calculates several values, including the resistance of the systemic and pulmonary arterial vasculature and oxygen content, delivery, and consumption. When these data are integrated with clinical assessment data, the nurse can derive a picture of the patient's hemodynamic status and the effect of therapy. It is important that all measures be made with attention to technical accuracy. False or inaccurate data are potentially misleading and thus dangerous.

Hemodynamic Terminology

Cardiac Output and Cardiac Index. *Cardiac output* (CO) is the volume of blood pumped by the heart in 1 minute. *Cardiac index* (CI) is the measurement of the CO adjusted for body size and it is a more precise measurement of the efficiency of the pumping action of the heart. Although minor beat-to-beat changes may occur, generally the left and right ventricles pump the same volume. The volume pumped with each heartbeat is the stroke volume (SV). Like CI, stroke volume index (SVI) is the measurement of SV adjusted for body size. CO and the forces opposing blood flow determine blood pressure, the force exerted by blood on the vessel wall. The opposition to blood flow offered by the vessels is called systemic vascular resistance (SVR) or pulmonary vascular resistance (PVR). Preload, afterload, and contractility (see Chapter 31) determine SV (and thus CO and blood pressure). Understanding these concepts and relationships is essential for the critical care nurse. In addition, the nurse must understand the effects of manipulation of each of these variables. The formulas and normal values for common hemodynamic parameters are given in Table 64-2.

Preload. *Preload* is the volume within a cardiac chamber at the end of diastole. Unfortunately, chamber volume measurements are difficult to obtain. Instead, various pressures are used to estimate volume. Left ventricular preload is called left ventricular end-diastolic pressure. PAWP, a measure of pulmonary capillary pressure, reflects left ventricular end-diastolic pressure under normal conditions (i.e., when there is no mitral valve pathologic condition, intracardiac defect, or arrhythmia). CVP, measured in the right atrium or in the vena cava close to the heart, is the right ventricular preload or right ventricular end-diastolic pressure when there is no tricuspid valve pathologic condition, intracardiac defect, or arrhythmia.

The effects of preload are explained by *Starling's law,* which states that the more a myocardial fiber is stretched during filling, the more it shortens during systole and the greater the force of the contraction. As preload increases, force generated in the following contraction increases, thus SV and CO increase. The greater the preload, the greater the myocardial (heart muscle) stretch and the greater the oxygen requirement of the myocardium. Hence, increases in CO via increased preload require increased delivery of oxygen to the myocardium. It should be remembered that the change in SV with preload comes about because of stretching of the heart muscle. However, the clinical measurement made is not a direct measurement of the muscle length; the measurement made is pressure at the time of the peak stretch (end diastole) (see Table 64-2). This pressure indirectly indicates the amount of stretch and the volume. This pressure is also important because it indicates pressure in the blood vessels of the lung or in the blood returning to the heart. Preload can be increased by fluid administration and decreased by diuresis.

Afterload. *Afterload* refers to the forces opposing ventricular ejection. These forces include systemic arterial pressure, the resistance offered by the aortic valve, and the mass and density of the blood to be moved. Clinically, although the measures fail to include all the components of afterload, SVR and arterial pressure are indices of left ventricular afterload. Similarly, PVR and pulmonary arterial pressure are indices of right ventricular after-

---

TABLE 64-2   Hemodynamic Parameters at Rest

INDICATORS	NORMAL RANGE
Preload	
Right atrial pressure (RAP) or central venous pressure (CVP)	2–8 mm Hg
Pulmonary artery wedge pressure (PAWP) or left atrial pressure (LAP)	6–12 mm Hg
Pulmonary artery diastolic pressure (PADP)	4–12 mm Hg
Afterload	
Pulmonary vascular resistance (PVR) = $\dfrac{(\text{Pulmonary artery mean pressure [PAMP]} - \text{PAWP}) \times 80}{\text{Cardiac output (CO)}}$	<250 dynes/sec/cm^{-5}
Pulmonary vascular resistance index (PVRI) = (PAMP – PAWP) × 80/Cardiac index (CI)	160–380 dynes/sec/cm^{-5}/m^2
Systemic vascular resistance (SVR) = (Mean arterial pressure [MAP] – CVP) × 80/CO	800–1200 dynes/sec/cm^{-5}
Systemic vascular resistance index (SVRI) = (MAP – CVP) × 80/CI	1970–2390 dynes/sec/cm^{-5}/m^2
Mean arterial pressure (MAP) = $\dfrac{\text{Systolic blood pressure} + 2(\text{Diastolic blood pressure})}{3*}$	70–105 mm Hg
Pulmonary artery mean pressure (PAMP) = $\dfrac{\text{Pulmonary artery systolic pressure (PASP)} + 2\text{PADP}}{3*}$	10–20 mm Hg
Other	
Stroke volume (SV) = CO/Heart rate	60–150 ml/beat
Stroke volume index (SVI) = CI/Heart rate	30–65 ml/beat/m^2
Heart rate (HR)	60–100 beats/min
CO = SV × HR	4–8 L/min
Cardiac index (CI) = CO/Body surface area (BSA)	2.2–4 L/min/m^2
Arterial hemoglobin oxygen saturation	95%–99%
Mixed venous hemoglobin oxygen saturation	60%–80%

*This formula is an approximation because it does not take into consideration the heart rate. The monitor looks at the area under the pressure curve, as well as the heart rate, to calculate MAP and PAMP.

load. Increased afterload often results in a decreased CO. CO can be restored by decreasing afterload (i.e., decreasing forces opposing contraction). When afterload is reduced, myocardial oxygen needs are decreased. Thus CO is increased, and myocardial oxygen requirements are decreased. Drug therapy directed at reducing afterload (e.g., milrinone [Primacor]) is often used in the management of heart failure (see Chapter 34).

Vascular Resistance. *Systemic vascular resistance* (SVR) is the resistance of the systemic vascular bed. *Pulmonary vascular resistance* (PVR) is the resistance of the pulmonary vascular bed. Both of these measures reflect afterload as described earlier and can be adjusted for body size (see Table 64-2).

Contractility. *Contractility* describes the strength of contraction. Contractility is said to increase when preload is not changed yet the heart contracts more forcefully. Epinephrine, norepinephrine, isoproterenol (Isuprel), dopamine, dobutamine, digitalis-like drugs, calcium, and milrinone (Primacor) increase contractility. These agents are termed *positive inotropes.* Contractility is diminished by *negative inotropes,* such as acidosis and certain drugs (e.g., barbiturates, alcohol, procainamide [Pronestyl], calcium channel blockers, β-adrenergic blockers). Increased contractility results in increased SV and increased myocardial oxygen requirements. There are no direct clinical measures of cardiac contractility. To indirectly determine contractility, the nurse measures the patient's preload (PAWP) and CO and graphs the results. If preload, heart rate, and afterload remain constant yet CO changes, contractility is altered. Contractility is diminished in the failing heart.

Principles of Invasive Pressure Monitoring

Invasive lines are commonly used in the ICU to measure systemic and pulmonary blood pressures. Components of a typical invasive arterial pressure monitoring system are illustrated in Fig. 64-2. Catheter, pressure tubing, flush system, and usually the transducer are disposable.

To accurately measure pressure, equipment must be referenced and zero balanced and dynamic response characteristics optimized. *Referencing* means positioning the transducer so that the zero reference point is at the level of the atria of the heart.[22] The stopcock nearest the transducer is usually the zero reference for the transducer. To place this level with the atria, the nurse uses an external landmark, the phlebostatic axis. To identify the **phlebostatic axis,** two imaginary lines are drawn with the patient supine (Fig. 64-3, *A*). The first line, a horizontal line, is drawn through the midchest, halfway between the outermost anterior and posterior surfaces. The second line, a vertical line, is drawn through the fourth intercostal space at the sternum. The phlebostatic axis is the intersection of the two imaginary lines. Once the phlebostatic axis is identified, it should be marked on the patient's chest with a permanent marker. The port of the stopcock nearest the transducer must be positioned level with the phlebostatic axis. It is recommended that the transducer be taped to the patient's chest at the phlebostatic axis or mounted on a bedside pole.[22]

Zeroing confirms that when pressure within the system is zero, the equipment reads zero. This is accomplished by opening the reference stopcock to room air and observing the monitor for a reading of zero. Most transducers in current use are disposable and have little zero drift. Zeroing the transducer is recommended during initial setup, immediately after insertion of the arterial

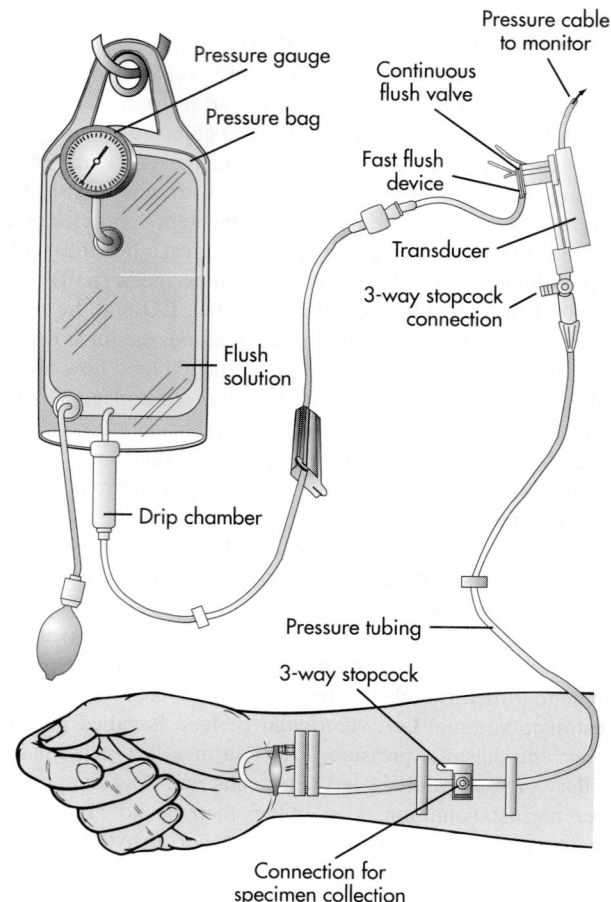

FIG. 64-2 Components of a pressure monitoring system. The cannula, shown entering the radial artery, is connected via pressure (nondistensible) tubing to the transducer. The transducer converts the pressure wave into an electronic signal. The transducer is wired to the electronic monitoring system, which amplifies, conditions, displays, and records the signal. Stopcocks are inserted into the line for specimen withdrawal and for referencing and zero-balancing procedures. A flush system, consisting of a pressurized bag of intravenous fluid, tubing, and a flush device, is inserted into the line. The flush system provides continuous slow (approximately 3 ml/hr) flushing and provides a mechanism for fast flushing of lines. All items except the electronic monitoring system are commonly disposable equipment.

line, when the transducer has been disconnected from the pressure cable or the pressure cable has been disconnected from the monitor, and when the accuracy of the measurements is questioned, and it should be done according to the manufacturer's guidelines.[22,23]

Optimizing dynamic response characteristics involves checking that the equipment reproduces without distortion a signal that changes rapidly. A *dynamic response test (square wave test)* is performed every 8 to 12 hours and when the system is opened to air or the accuracy of the measurements is questioned. It involves checking that the equipment reproduces a distortion-free signal (Fig. 64-4).[24]

Steps in obtaining blood pressure measurements with an invasive line are given in Table 64-3. Pressure measurements can be obtained from both digital and printed analog outputs, but accurate readings are best obtained from a printed pressure tracing

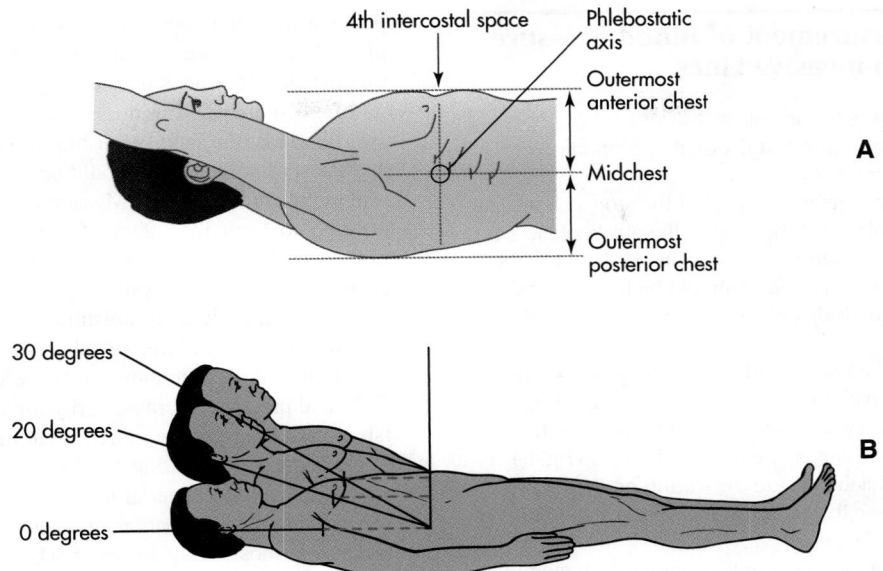

FIG. 64-3 Identification of phlebostatic axis. **A,** Phlebostatic axis is an external landmark used to identify the level of the atria in the supine patient. The phlebostatic axis is defined as the intersection of two imaginary lines: one drawn vertically through the fourth intercostal space at the sternum and another drawn horizontally through the midchest, halfway between the outermost anterior and outermost posterior points of the chest. **B,** As the backrest of the supine patient is elevated, the phlebostatic axis remains at the same anatomic location, becoming progressively elevated from the floor. The zero reference point must be repositioned with changes in backrest elevation to keep it at the phlebostatic level.

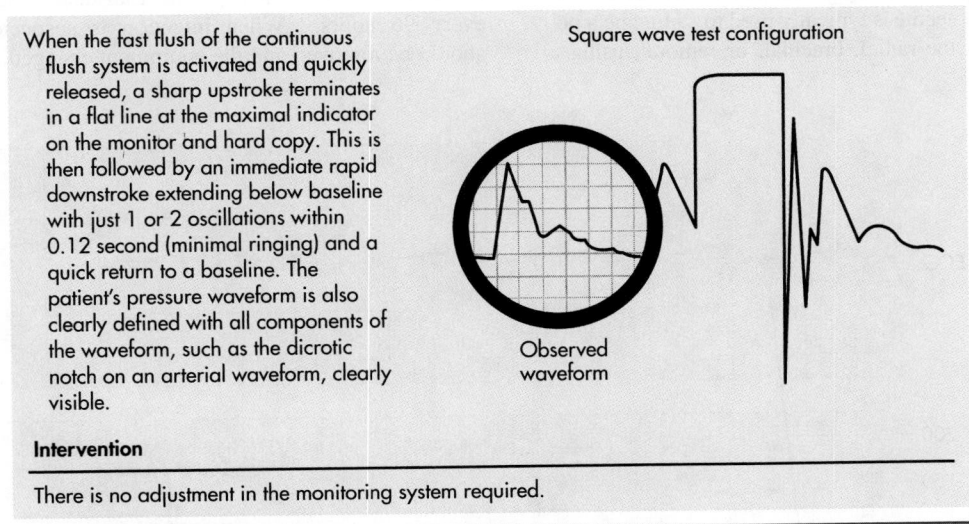

When the fast flush of the continuous flush system is activated and quickly released, a sharp upstroke terminates in a flat line at the maximal indicator on the monitor and hard copy. This is then followed by an immediate rapid downstroke extending below baseline with just 1 or 2 oscillations within 0.12 second (minimal ringing) and a quick return to a baseline. The patient's pressure waveform is also clearly defined with all components of the waveform, such as the dicrotic notch on an arterial waveform, clearly visible.

Intervention

There is no adjustment in the monitoring system required.

FIG. 64-4 Optimally damped system. Dynamic response test (square wave test) using the fast flush system: normal response.

at the end of expiration. Initial readings are made with the patient flat. Unless the patient's blood pressure is extremely sensitive to orthostatic changes, values at modest degrees of backrest elevation (up to 45 degrees) are generally equivalent to measurements with the patient flat. Studies have not demonstrated the accuracy of readings obtained for patients in the lateral position.[22] It is not necessary to reposition the patient for each pressure reading. However, it is necessary to move the zero reference stopcock to keep it positioned at the phlebostatic axis (see Fig. 64-3, *B*).

TABLE 64-3 **Measurement of Blood Pressure with Invasive Lines**

1. Explain the procedure to the patient.
2. Position the patient supine and flat or, if appropriate, elevated up to 45 degrees.
3. Confirm that the zero reference (port of the stopcock nearest the transducer) is placed at the level of the phlebostatic axis (see Fig. 64-3). If the reference stopcock is not taped to the patient's chest, a carpenter's level should be used to position the stopcock on a bedside pole at the point level with the phlebostatic axis.
4. Observe the monitor tracing and assess the quality of the tracing. Perform a dynamic response test (see Fig. 64-4).
5. Obtain an analog printout, if available, and measure the systolic and diastolic pressures at end expiration (see Fig. 64-5). If no printout is available, freeze the tracing on the oscilloscope screen and use the cursor to measure the pressures at end expiration.
6. Record the pressure measurements promptly, including (if available) the printout marked to identify the points read.

Types of Invasive Pressure Monitoring

Arterial Blood Pressure. Continuous arterial pressure monitoring is indicated for patients in many situations, including acute hypertension and hypotension, respiratory failure, shock, neurologic injury, coronary interventional procedures, continuous infusion of vasoactive drugs (sodium nitroprusside [Nipride]), and frequent ABG sampling. A 20-gauge, 2-inch (5.1 cm) nontapered Teflon cannula-over-the needle is typically used to cannulate a peripheral artery, such as the radial, brachial, or femoral, using a percutaneous approach. After insertion, the catheter is sutured in place.[25] It is important that the insertion site be immobilized so that the catheter line is not dislodged and lines are not kinked.

Measurements. The nurse can use the arterial line to obtain systolic, diastolic, and mean blood pressures (Fig. 64-5). High- and low-pressure alarms should be set based on the patient's current status and activated. Measurements are obtained at end expiration to limit the effect of the respiratory cycle on arterial pressure.[24] In heart failure, the systolic upstroke may be slower. In volume depletion, systolic pressure varies greatly with mechanical ventilation, diminishing during inspiration. In severe congestive heart failure, systolic amplitude does not vary with ventilation. With arrhythmias it is useful to observe simultaneous ECG and pressure tracings. Arrhythmias that significantly diminish arterial pressure are more urgent than those that cause only a slight decrease in systolic amplitude.

Complications. Arterial lines carry the risk of hemorrhage, infection, thrombus formation, and neurovascular impairment. Hemorrhage is most likely to occur when the catheter becomes dislodged or the line becomes disconnected. To avoid this serious complication, the nurse uses Luer-Lok connections and always checks the arterial waveform and that the alarms are activated. If the pressure in the line falls (e.g., when the line is disconnected), the low-pressure alarm sounds immediately, allowing prompt correction of the problem. Pressure is always monitored when an arterial line is in place, even if the line was placed for ABG sampling.

Infection is a risk with any invasive line. The nurse should inspect the insertion site for local signs of inflammation and monitor the patient for signs of systemic infection. To limit the risk of contamination and catheter-related infection, the catheter site, pressure tubing, flush bag, and transducer should be changed every 96 hours.[24] When infection is suspected, the catheter should be removed and the equipment changed.

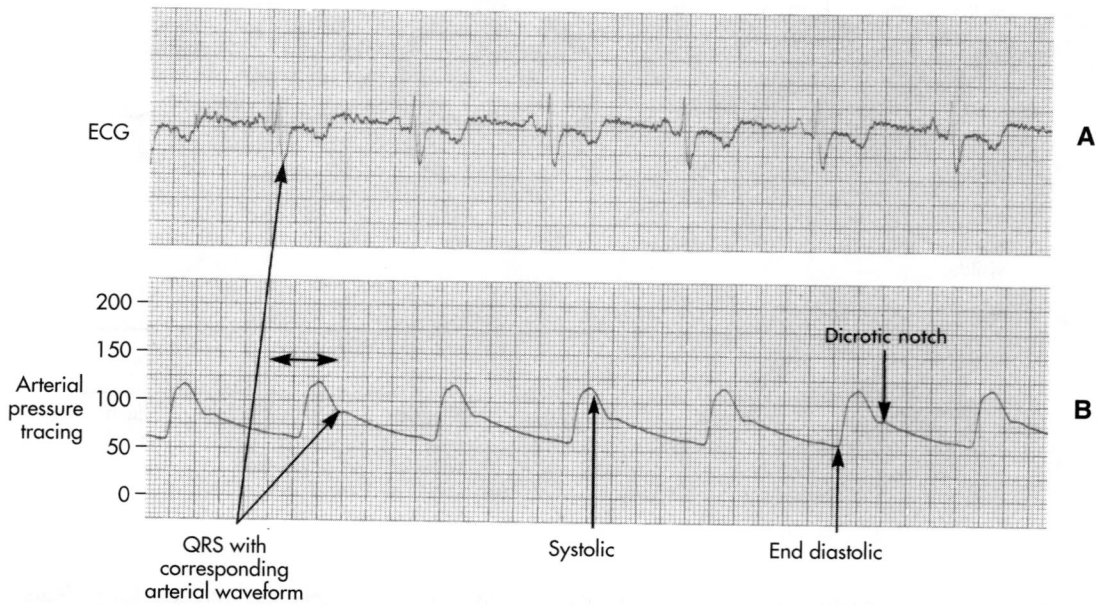

FIG. 64-5 **A,** Simultaneously recorded electrocardiogram (ECG) tracing and, **B,** systemic arterial pressure tracing. Systolic pressure is the peak pressure. The dicrotic notch indicates aortic valve closure. Diastolic pressure is the lowest value before contraction. Mean pressure is the average pressure over time calculated by the monitoring equipment.

Circulatory impairment can result from formation of a thrombus around the catheter, release of an embolus, spasm, or occlusion of the circulation by the catheter. Before inserting a line into the radial artery, an Allen test should be performed to confirm that ulnar circulation is sufficient to sustain the hand. In this test, pressure is applied to the radial and ulnar arteries simultaneously. The patient is instructed to open and close the hand repeatedly. The hand should blanch. The nurse then releases the pressure on the ulnar artery while compressing the radial artery. If pinkness fails to return within 6 seconds, the ulnar artery is insufficient, indicating that the radial artery should not be used for line insertion.

To help maintain line patency and limit thrombus formation, the nurse should assess the continuous flush irrigation system every 1 to 4 hours to determine that the pressure bag is inflated to 300 mm Hg, the flush bag contains fluid, and the system is delivering 1 to 3 ml per hour. It is recommended that a solution of heparinized saline (e.g., 1 to 4 U/ml) be used for the flush solution unless contraindicated.[24]

Once the catheter is inserted, the nurse should evaluate the neurovascular status distal to the arterial insertion site hourly. The limb with compromised arterial flow will appear cool and pale, with capillary refill greater than 3 seconds. There may be symptoms of neurologic impairment, such as tingling or paresthesia. Neurovascular impairment can result in loss of a limb and is an emergency.

Pulmonary Artery Flow-Directed Catheter. Pulmonary artery (PA) pressure monitoring is used to guide acute-phase management of patients with complicated cardiac, pulmonary, and intravascular volume problems (Table 64-4). PA diastolic (PAD) pressure and PAWP are sensitive indicators of fluid volume status and cardiac function. PAD pressure and PAWP are increased in fluid volume overload and heart failure. They are decreased with volume deficit. Fluid therapy based on PA pressure allows restoration of fluid balance while avoiding overcorrection of the problem. Monitoring PA pressures can allow precise therapeutic manipulation of preload, which allows CO to be maintained without placing the patient at risk for pulmonary edema.

A PA flow-directed catheter (e.g., Swan-Ganz) is used to measure PA pressures, including PAWP. The standard PA catheter is number 7.5 French, 43 inches (110 cm) long, with four or five lu-

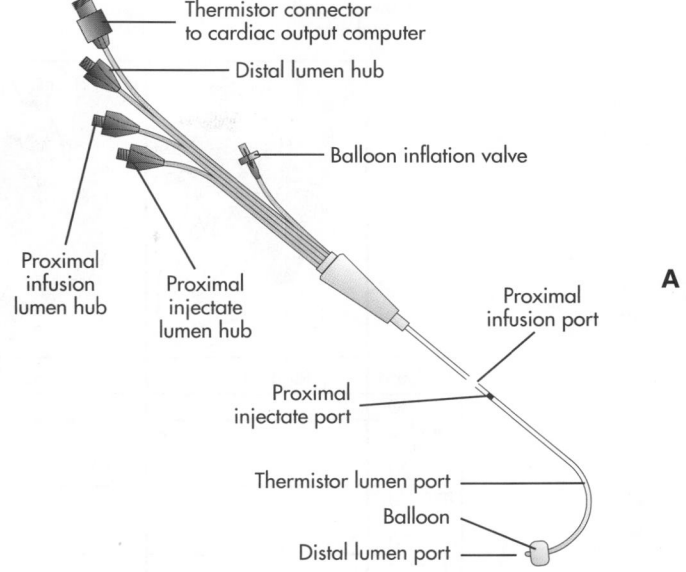

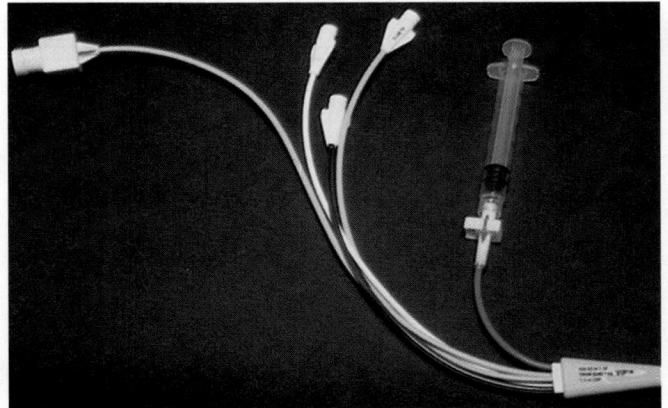

FIG. 64-6 Pulmonary artery (PA) catheter. **A,** Illustrated catheter has five lumens. When properly positioned, the distal lumen port is in the PA, and the proximal lumen ports are in the right atrium and right ventricle. The distal and one of the proximal ports are used to measure PA and central venous pressures, respectively. A balloon surrounds the catheter near the distal end. The balloon inflation valve is used to inflate the balloon with air to allow reading of the pulmonary artery wedge pressure. A thermistor located near the distal tip senses PA temperature and is used to measure thermodilution cardiac output when solution cooler than body temperature is injected into a proximal port. **B,** Photo of an actual catheter.

TABLE 64-4 **Clinical Indications for Pulmonary Artery Catheterization**

Acute respiratory distress syndrome
Acute respiratory failure in patients with chronic obstructive pulmonary disease
Cardiac tamponade
Complex fluid imbalance (e.g., trauma, burns, sepsis)
Evaluation of circulatory syndromes (e.g., heart failure, mitral valve regurgitation, intraventricular shunts)
Intraaortic balloon pump therapy
Myocardial infarction with complications (e.g., left ventricular failure, cardiogenic shock, ventricular septal rupture)
Perioperative fluid imbalance in high-risk patients (e.g., cardiac history)
Shock states (e.g., cardiogenic, septic, hypovolemic)
Vasoactive drug therapy support

---

mens (Fig. 64-6). When properly positioned, the distal lumen port (catheter tip) is within the PA (Fig. 64-7). This port is used to monitor PA pressures and withdraw mixed venous blood specimens (e.g., to evaluate oxygen saturation). A balloon connected to an external valve via the second lumen surrounds the distal lumen port. Balloon inflation has two purposes: (1) to allow moving blood to float the catheter forward and (2) to allow PAWP measurement. There will be one or two proximal lumens, with exit ports in the right atrium (if only one) or right atrium and right ventricle (if two). The right atrium port is used for measurement of CVP, injection of fluid for CO determination, and withdrawal of

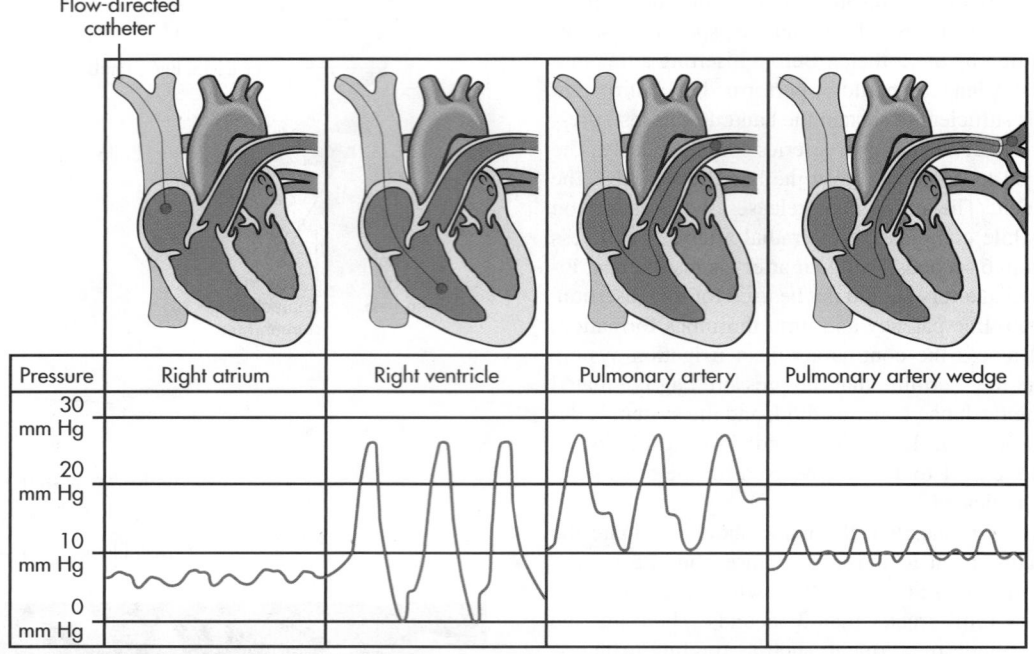

Flow-directed
catheter

Pressure	Right atrium	Right ventricle	Pulmonary artery	Pulmonary artery wedge
30 mm Hg				
20 mm Hg				
10 mm Hg				
0 mm Hg				

FIG. 64-7   Position of the pulmonary artery flow-directed catheter during progressive stages of insertion with corresponding pressure waveforms.

blood specimens. If a second proximal port is available, it is used for infusion of fluids and drugs or blood sampling. A thermistor lumen port located near the distal tip is wired to an external connector. This port is used for monitoring blood or core temperature and in the thermodilution method of measuring CO.

In addition to these relatively standard and common features of the PA flow-directed catheter, catheters with other features are available. One modification is the inclusion of an atrial electrode, useful in recording the atrial ECG or pacing the heart. Another common modification is inclusion of a fiberoptic sensor in the distal tip that detects mixed venous oxygen saturation. Another type of catheter provides continuous measurement of right ventricular volume and ejection fraction, while another catheter provides continuous CO monitoring.[26] The PA catheter sheath usually has a side port that serves as another intravenous line. Most catheters also have a plastic "sleeve" connected to the sheath, which permits manipulation of the catheter while maintaining sterility.

Pulmonary artery catheter insertion. Before PA catheter insertion, the nurse notes the patient's electrolyte, acid-base, oxygenation, and coagulation status. Imbalances such as hypokalemia, hypomagnesemia, hypoxemia, or acidosis can make the heart more irritable and increase the risk of ventricular arrhythmia during catheter insertion. Coagulopathy increases the risk of hemorrhage. The nurse prepares for the procedure by arranging the monitor, cables, and flush and infusion solutions. The system is zero referenced to the phlebostatic axis. The procedure is explained to the patient, and informed consent is obtained. The patient is positioned supine with the head of the bed flat.[27] The PA catheter is inserted through a sheath percutaneously into the internal jugular, subclavian, antecubital, or femoral vein using surgical asepsis. Venous cut-down is rarely required. The line is then advanced through the venous system to the right side of the heart.

Catheter insertion is guided by continuously observing the characteristic waveforms on the monitor as the catheter is advanced through the heart to the PA (see Fig. 64-7). When the tip reaches the right atrium, the balloon is inflated.[27] Inflation of the balloon should not exceed the balloon's capacity (usually 1 to 1.5 ml of air). The catheter is then floated through the tricuspid valve into the right ventricle and then through the pulmonic valve and into the PA. Once a typical PAWP tracing is observed, the balloon is deflated, and the PA waveform should return on the monitor. Following insertion, a chest x-ray is obtained to confirm the position. To maintain the catheter in its proper position, the catheter is then secured at its point of entry into the skin. The measurement at the exit point should be noted and recorded. An occlusive dressing is applied and changed according to unit protocol. It is necessary to monitor the ECG continuously during insertion because of the risk for arrhythmias, particularly when the catheter reaches the right ventricle.

Pulmonary artery pressure measurements. Systolic, diastolic, and mean pressures are routinely monitored. PA systolic is the peak pressure and PA diastolic is the lowest pressure point on the PA waveform. Mean PA pressure is the time-weighted average. Because PA ports are in the chest, intrathoracic pressures alter PA pressure. To produce accurate data, PA measurements are obtained at the end of expiration.[27,28]

The measurement of PAWP is obtained by slowly inflating the balloon with air (not to exceed balloon capacity) until the PA waveform changes to a PAWP waveform (Fig. 64-8). Before inflation the PA pressure tracing on the monitor looks like an arterial tracing, with a systolic peak, dicrotic notch, and then the diastolic low point. As the waveform becomes "wedged," the tracing changes shape and amplitude. Generally, the PAWP waveform is characterized by two small positive waves, the *a* and *v* waves. The *a wave* indicates atrial contraction, and it is followed by the

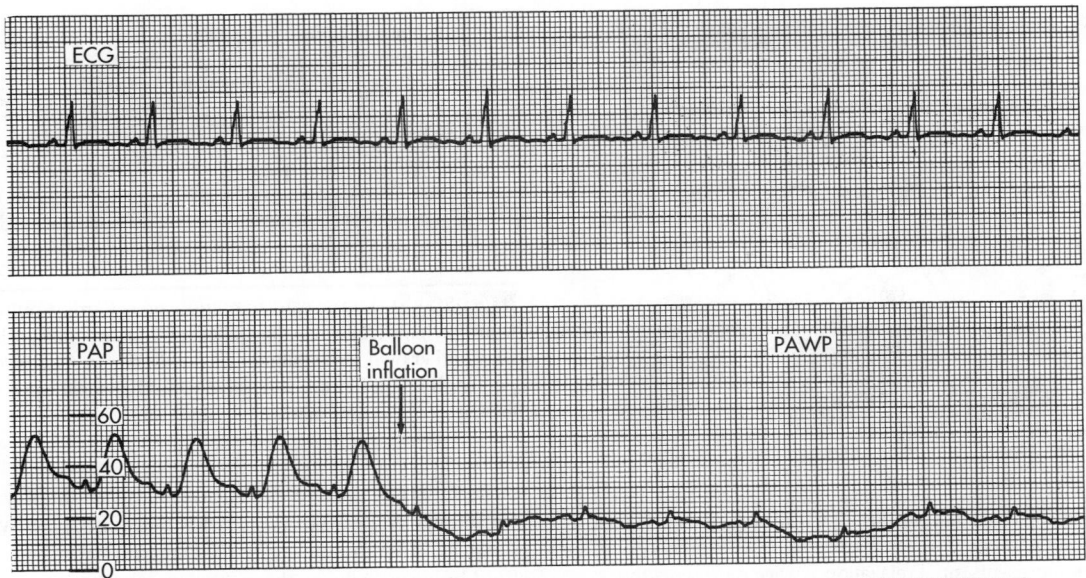

FIG. 64-8 Change in pulmonary artery pressure *(PAP)* waveform to pulmonary artery wedge pressure *(PAWP)* waveform with balloon inflation. The balloon is inflated while observing the bedside monitor for change in the waveform. Balloon inflation *(arrow)* in patient with a normal PAWP.

x descent, indicating atrial relaxation. At times, a *c wave* may be seen following the *a* wave and indicates closure of the mitral valve. The *v wave* is seen during the interval between the T and P waves of the ECG. The *v* wave indicates inflow into the left atrium when the mitral valve is closed and the ventricle is contracting. The *v* wave is followed by the *y descent,* indicating the emptying of the left atrium when the mitral valve opens and the ventricle fills.[28]

When measuring the PAWP, the balloon should be inflated for no more than four respiratory cycles or 8 to 15 seconds.[26,27] There

is danger of rupture of the PA if the catheter migrates distally into a smaller vessel or if the balloon is overinflated. This is suspected when less than 1 ml is needed to wedge the tracing or an "overwedge" tracing is obtained (Fig. 64-9). Readings should be acquired from an analog strip pressure recording, and the strip should be placed into the patient's record. If a printout of the tracing is not available, the readings can be taken from the monitor using the cursor.

Central venous or right atrial pressure measurement. CVP is a measurement of right ventricular preload. It can be measured

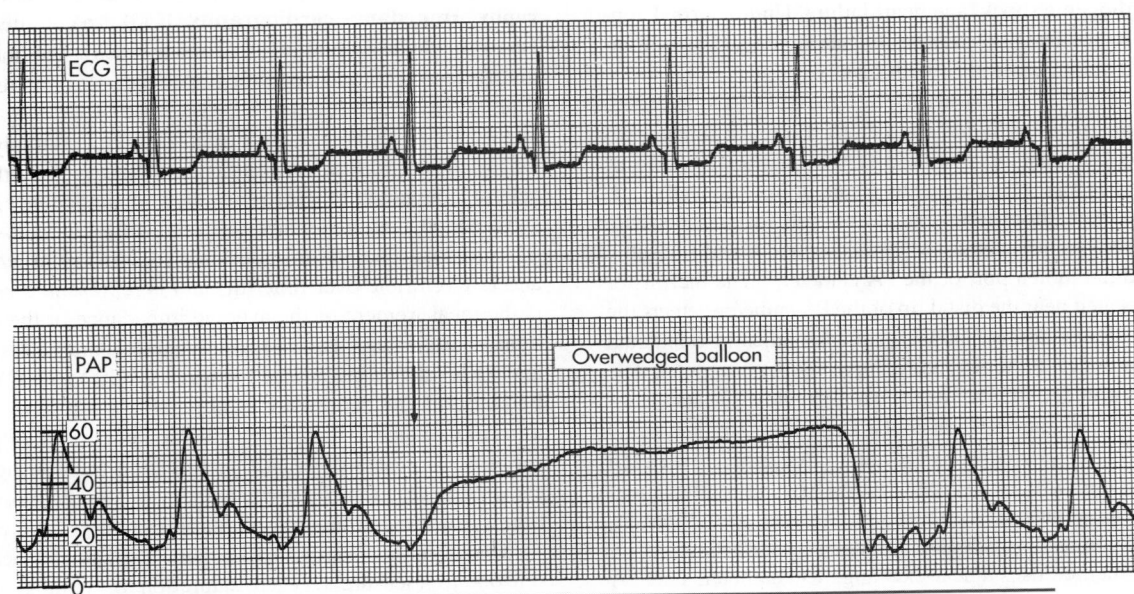

FIG. 64-9 Balloon inflation *(arrow)* in patient with elevated wedge pressure. Overwedging of balloon (balloon has been overinflated). The danger of overinflating the balloon is that the pulmonary artery *(PA)* vessel may rupture from the pressure of the balloon. *PAP,* Pulmonary artery pressure.

Schematic of waveform and cardiac cycle events

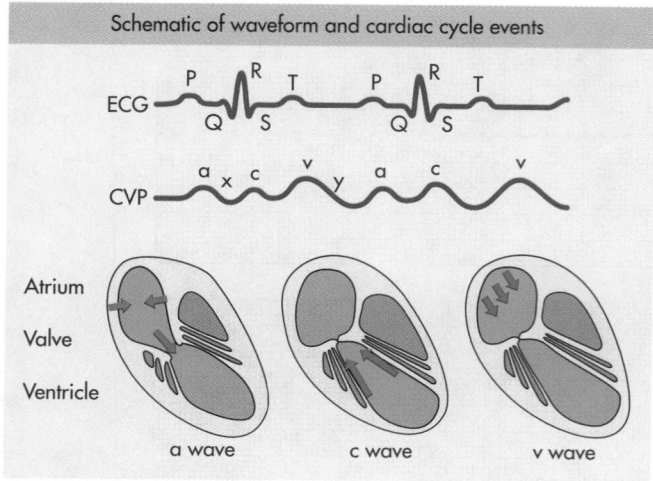

FIG. 64-10 Cardiac events that produce the central venous pressure (CVP) waveform with *a*, *c*, and *v* waves. *a* wave represents atrial contraction. *x* descent represents atrial relaxation. *c* wave represents the bulging of the closed tricuspid valve into the right atrium during ventricular systole. *v* wave represents atrial filling. *y* descent represents opening of the tricuspid valve and filling of the ventricle.

with a PA catheter using one of the proximal lumens or with a central venous catheter placed in the internal jugular or subclavian vein. CVP is measured as a mean pressure at the end of expiration. CVP waveforms (Fig. 64-10) are similar to PAWP waveforms. Although the PA diastolic pressure and PAWP are more sensitive indicators of fluid volume status, CVP also reflects fluid volume problems. An elevated CVP indicates right ventricular failure or volume overload. A low CVP indicates hypovolemia.

Invasive cardiac output measurement techniques. CO is frequently monitored in patients with hemodynamic instability. Normal resting CO is 4 to 8 L per minute and varies with body size. CI accounts for variations in body size and is normally 2.2 to 4 L/min/m². CO is decreased in conditions such as hypovolemia, cardiogenic shock, and heart failure. Under normal conditions, CO increases with exercise. Increases in CO at rest indicate a hyperdynamic state seen with fever or sepsis.

The PA catheter is commonly used to measure CO via the intermittent bolus *thermodilution* CO (TDCO) method or the *continuous* CO (CCO) method. With the TDCO method, a fixed volume (5 to 10 ml) of 5% dextrose solution (or saline, if contraindicated) of room temperature (or iced for patients with low or high COs) is injected rapidly (≤4 seconds) and smoothly into the proximal lumen port of the PA catheter.[29] The thermistor lumen port located near the distal tip of the PA catheter detects the drop in blood temperature. The CO is mathematically calculated from the area under the temperature curve by the computer. The larger the area under the curve, the smaller the CO, and, conversely, the smaller the area under the curve, the larger the CO (Fig. 64-11).[29] This procedure is repeated three times, with each measurement 1 to 2 minutes apart. Any CO measurement that does not have a normal curve is discarded. An average of three acceptable measurements is calculated to determine the CO.

The CCO method uses a heat-exchange CO catheter. This PA catheter contains a thermal filament that is located in the right atrium. This filament emits a pulsed signal every 30 to 60 seconds that allows for the mixing of blood with heat as it passes through the right ventricle. The thermistor lumen port detects the

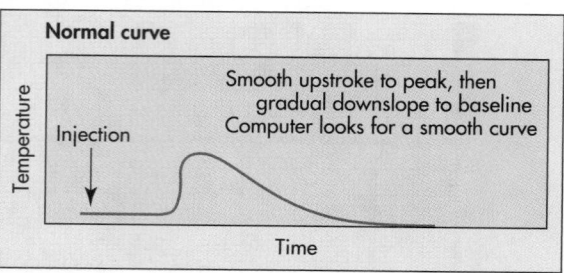

FIG. 64-11 Normal cardiac output curve. Cardiac output is calculated from the temperature change in the pulmonary artery when a fixed volume and known temperature of a solution is injected into the proximal port in the right atrium. The nurse should observe the curve during injection to make sure that it is smooth.

change in temperature. A bedside computer displays digital measurements every 30 to 60 seconds that reflect the average CO for the past 3 to 6 minutes. The CCO method eliminates the need for fluid boluses, reduces the risk of contamination, and permits ongoing evaluation (or trending) of the CO. Comparisons of the TDCO method with the CCO method have shown the CCO method to be reliable.[29]

SVR, SVR index (SVRI), SV, and SV index (SVI) can be calculated each time that CO is measured. The formulas for calculating these parameters are shown in Table 64-2. Increased SVR (>1200 dynes/sec/cm⁻⁵) indicates vasoconstriction from shock, increased release or administration of epinephrine or norepinephrine, or left ventricular failure. A low SVR (<800 dynes/sec/cm⁻⁵) indicates vasodilation, which may occur during sepsis, septic shock, or neurogenic shock or with drugs that reduce afterload. Changes in SV are rapidly becoming more important indicators of the pumping status of the heart. A high SV may be seen in bradycardia and exercise and with the use of positive inotropes (e.g., milrinone). Low SV is seen with tachyarrhythmias, extreme vasodilation, and cardiac tamponade.

Noninvasive hemodynamic monitoring: impedance cardiography. **Impedance cardiography** (ICG) is a continuous, noninvasive method of obtaining CO and assessing thoracic fluid status. Based on the concepts of impedance (the resistance to the flow of electrical current [Z]), ICG uses four sets of external electrodes to deliver a high-frequency, low-amplitude current that is similar to that used in apnea monitors.[30] Blood is an excellent conductor of electricity (lowers impedance), and pulsatile blood flow generates electrical impedance changes. ICG measures the change in impedance (dZ) in the ascending aorta and left ventricle over time (dt) and is represented as dZ/dt. Zo is the measurement of the average impedance of the fluid in the thorax. Impedance-based hemodynamic parameters (CO, SV, and SVR) can be calculated from Zo, dZ/dt, MAP, CVP, and the ECG. Some indications for ICG include early signs and symptoms of cardiac dysfunction, evaluation of cardiac or pulmonary cause of shortness of breath, justification for insertion of a PA catheter, evaluation of pharmacotherapy, and diagnosis of rejection following cardiac transplantation.[30]

Mixed venous oxygen saturation. PA catheters can include sensors to measure oxygen saturation of hemoglobin of PA blood. This value is the *mixed venous oxygen saturation* (SvO₂), and it is useful in determining the adequacy of tissue oxygenation. SvO₂ reflects the dynamic balance between oxygenation of the arterial blood, tissue perfusion, and tissue oxygen consump-

TABLE 64-5   Clinical Interpretation of SvO₂ Measurements

SvO₂ MEASUREMENT	PHYSIOLOGIC BASIS FOR CHANGE IN SvO₂	CLINICAL DIAGNOSIS AND RATIONALE
High SvO₂ (80%–95%)	Increased oxygen supply Decreased oxygen demand	Patient receiving more oxygen than required by clinical condition Anesthesia, which causes sedation and decreased muscle movement Hypothermia, which lowers metabolic demand (e.g., with cardiopulmonary bypass) Sepsis caused by decreased ability of tissues to use oxygen at the cellular level False high positive because pulmonary artery catheter is wedged in a pulmonary capillary
Normal SvO₂ (60%–80%)	Normal oxygen supply and metabolic demand	Balanced oxygen supply and demand
Low SvO₂ (<60%)	Decreased oxygen supply caused by: Low hemoglobin Low arterial saturation (SaO₂) Low cardiac output Increased oxygen consumption (VO₂)	 Anemia or bleeding with compromised cardiopulmonary system Hypoxemia resulting from decreased oxygen supply or lung disease Cardiogenic shock caused by left ventricular pump failure Metabolic demand exceeds oxygen supply in conditions and increases metabolic rate, including physiologic states such as shivering, seizures, and hyperthermia and nursing interventions such as obtaining bed scale weight and repositioning that increase muscle movement

From Urden LD, Stacy KM, Lough ME: *Thelan's critical care nursing: diagnosis and management*, ed 4, St Louis, 2002, Mosby.

tion (VO_2). SvO_2, when considered in conjunction with the arterial oxygen saturation, is useful in analyzing hemodynamic status and response to treatments or activities (Table 64-5). Normal SvO_2 at rest is 60% to 80%.

Sustained decreases and increases in SvO_2 must be analyzed carefully. Decreased SvO_2 may indicate decreased arterial oxygenation, low CO, low hemoglobin, or increased oxygen consumption. If the SvO_2 falls, the nurse determines which of these four factors has changed. The nurse observes for changes in arterial oxygenation by monitoring pulse oximetry or ABGs. By noting any changes in level of consciousness, strength and quality of peripheral pulses, urine output, and skin color and temperature, the nurse can grossly assess CO and tissue perfusion. If arterial oxygenation, CO, and hemoglobin are unchanged, a fall in SvO_2 indicates increased oxygen consumption, which could result from an increased metabolic rate, pain, movement, or fever. If oxygen consumption increases without a comparable increase in oxygen delivery, more oxygen is extracted from the blood, and SvO_2 will continue to fall.

Increased SvO_2 is also clinically significant and may indicate a clinical improvement (e.g., increased arterial oxygen saturation, improved perfusion, decreased metabolic rate) or problems (e.g., sepsis, ventricular septal defect). In sepsis, oxygen may not be extracted properly at the tissue level, resulting in increased mixed venous oxygen saturation.

Nursing interventions may be guided by changes in SvO_2. The nurse might note that the patient's heart rate increased moderately during repositioning but that the SvO_2 remained stable. In this case the nurse might conclude that the position change was tolerated. If the SvO_2 had dropped, this would be an indication to stop the activity until the SvO_2 returns to the previous level.

In many cases as activity or metabolism increases, heart rate and CO increase, and SvO_2 remains constant or varies slightly. However, it is not uncommon for critically ill patients to have conditions that prevent substantial increases in CO. For example, this could occur in the patient with heart failure, shock, arrhythmias, or cardiac transplantation. In these cases, SvO_2 can provide a useful indicator of the balance between oxygen delivery and consumption.

Complications with PA catheters. Infection and sepsis are serious problems associated with PA catheters. Careful surgical asepsis for insertion and maintenance of the catheter and tubing line is mandatory to prevent infection. The skin is cleaned according to unit procedure, usually with an iodine preparation. The insertion site is covered with a sterile occlusive dressing. The nurse should monitor the patient for local and systemic signs of infection (e.g., redness and exudate at the insertion site, fever, increased white blood cell count). The PA catheter must be removed if there are local or systemic signs of infection. To reduce the risk of infection, the flush bag, pressure tubing, transducer, and stopcock should be changed every 72 hours, and the PA catheter should be removed once hemodynamic monitoring is no longer needed.[22]

Air embolus is another risk associated with PA catheters. Air embolus can be caused by injection of air into the lumen of a ruptured balloon or by balloon rupture. The nurse decreases the risk of air embolus by first aspirating to check for the absence or presence of blood and by injecting only the prescribed volume of air into the balloon before obtaining the PAWP. Catheters are also checked for balloon leak before insertion; defective catheters are not used. If the nurse aspirates blood from the balloon port or observes that injected air does not flow back into the syringe, the catheter should be so labeled and the physician notified. Air can also be introduced into the system if connections are not tight, and Luer-Lok connections should be used on all pressure lines. In addition, the low-pressure alarm is activated for all pressure lines to signal any substantial drop in the pressure. Any time the line needs to be disconnected to change the apparatus, the nurse closes the line to the patient via clamping or stopcocks.

The patient with a PA catheter is at risk for pulmonary infarction or PA rupture from the following causes: (1) the balloon may rupture, releasing fragments that could embolize; (2) prolonged balloon inflation may obstruct blood flow; (3) the catheter may advance into a wedge position, obstructing blood flow; and (4) a thrombus could form and embolize. To reduce the risk of pulmonary infarction and rupture, the balloon must never be inflated beyond the balloon's capacity (usually 1 to 1.5 ml of air). The balloon must not be left inflated for more than four breaths (except during insertion) or 15 seconds.[26,27] PA pressure waveforms are monitored continuously for evidence of catheter occlusion, dislocation, or spontaneous wedging. The pressure tracing will be blunted if the catheter starts to be occluded. The pressure tracing will appear wedged if the PA catheter advances and becomes spontaneously wedged. In each of these cases, the catheter must be immediately repositioned. To reduce the risk of thrombus and embolus formation, the PA catheter is continuously flushed with a slow infusion of heparinized (unless contraindicated) saline solution to prevent thrombus formation.[22]

Ventricular arrhythmias can occur during PA catheter insertion or removal or if the tip migrates back from the PA to the right ventricle and irritates the ventricular wall. In addition, the nurse may observe that the PA catheter cannot be wedged. In these situations, the catheter may need to be repositioned by the physician or a qualified nurse.

Noninvasive Arterial Oxygenation Monitoring. *Pulse oximetry* is a noninvasive and continuous method of determining arterial oxygenation (SpO_2), and monitoring SpO_2 may reduce the frequency of ABG sampling (see Chapter 25). SpO_2 is normally 95% to 100%. A common use for pulse oximetry is to evaluate the effectiveness of oxygen therapy. Decreased SpO_2 indicates inadequate oxygenation of the blood in the pulmonary capillaries. This may be corrected by increasing the fraction of inspired oxygen (FIO_2) and evaluating the patient's response. Similarly, the nurse uses SpO_2 to monitor how the patient tolerates decreases in FIO_2 and responds to changes in position and treatments. For example, the nurse might note that SpO_2 falls when the patient is positioned in a left lateral recumbent position. The nurse could then plan position changes that pose less risk for the patient.

Accurate SpO_2 measurements may be difficult to obtain on patients who are hypothermic, receiving intravenous vasopressor therapy (e.g., norepinephrine [Levophed]), or experiencing hypoperfusion (e.g., shock). Alternate locations for placement of the pulse oximetry probe may need to be considered (e.g., forehead, earlobe).

NURSING MANAGEMENT
HEMODYNAMIC MONITORING

Assessment of hemodynamic status requires integration of data from many sources and comparison of the data over time. Thorough, basic nursing observations provide important clues about the patient's hemodynamic status. The nurse should begin by obtaining baseline data regarding the patient's general appearance, level of consciousness, skin color and temperature, vital signs, peripheral pulses, and urine output. Does the patient appear tired, weak, exhausted? There may be too little cardiac reserve to sustain even minimum activity. Pallor, cool skin, and diminished pulses may indicate decreased CO. Changes in mental clarity may reflect problems with cerebral perfusion or oxygenation. Monitoring urine output reflects the adequacy of perfusion to the kidneys. The patient with diminished perfusion to the GI tract may develop hypoactive or absent bowel sounds. If the patient is bleeding and developing shock, blood pressure might initially be relatively stable, yet the patient may become increasingly pale and cool from peripheral vasoconstriction. Conversely, the patient experiencing septic shock may remain warm and pink yet develops tachycardia and blood pressure instability. Although heart rates of 100 beats per minute are common among stressed, compromised, critically ill patients, sustained tachycardia greatly increases myocardial oxygen demand and may result in diminished CO.

The astute critical care nurse correlates observational data with data obtained from biotechnology (e.g., ECG; arterial, PA, PAWP pressures; SvO_2). Single hemodynamic values are rarely significant. The nurse must evaluate the whole clinical picture with the goals of recognizing early clues and intervening before problems escalate.

CIRCULATORY ASSIST DEVICES

Mechanical **circulatory assist devices** (CADs), such as the intraaortic balloon pump (IABP) and left ventricular assist device (VAD), are used to decrease cardiac work and improve organ perfusion in patients with heart failure when conventional drug therapy is no longer adequate. The type of device used depends on the extent and nature of the myocardial problem and the capabilities of the institution and staff. CADs provide interim support in three types of situations: (1) the left ventricle requires support while recovering from acute injury; (2) the heart requires surgical repair (e.g., a ruptured septum), but the patient must be stabilized; and (3) the heart has failed, and the patient is awaiting cardiac transplantation. All CADs decrease left ventricular workload, increase myocardial perfusion, and augment circulation. The most commonly used CAD is the IABP. Several types of VADs are available, and additional devices are under development.

Intraaortic Balloon Pump

The **intraaortic balloon pump** (IABP) provides temporary circulatory assistance to the compromised heart by reducing afterload (via reduction in systolic pressure) and augmenting the aortic diastolic pressure. Table 64-6 lists clinical conditions for which the IABP is used. The IABP consists of a sausage-shaped balloon, a pump that inflates and deflates the balloon, control devices for synchronizing the balloon inflation to the cardiac cycle, and fail-safe devices (Fig. 64-12). The balloon is inserted percutaneously or surgically, under strict aseptic technique, into the femoral artery, advanced toward the heart, and positioned in the descending thoracic aorta just below the left subclavian artery (Fig. 64-13). Following placement, the position is confirmed by x-ray. A pneumatic device cyclically fills the balloon with helium at the start of diastole (immediately after aortic valve closure) and deflates it just before systole. The ECG is the primary trigger used to initiate the deflation on the R wave (of the QRS) and inflation on the T wave, and the dicrotic notch of the arterial pressure tracing is used to refine timing (Fig. 64-14, *A*). IABP support is referred to as *counterpulsation* because the timing of balloon inflation is opposite to ventricular contraction. The IAPB assist ratio is 1:1 in the acute phase of treatment, that is, one IABP cycle of inflation and deflation for every heartbeat.[31]

TABLE 64-6 Indications and Contraindications for the Intraaortic Balloon Pump

Indications

Refractory unstable angina (when drugs have failed)

Short-term bridge to cardiac transplantation

Acute myocardial infarction with any of the following:*
  Ventricular aneurysm accompanied by ventricular arrhythmias
  Acute ventricular septal defect
  Acute mitral valve dysfunction
  Cardiogenic shock
  Recurrent chest pain with or without ventricular arrhythmias

Preoperative, intraoperative, and postoperative cardiac surgery (e.g., prophylaxis before surgery, failure to wean from cardiopulmonary bypass, left ventricular failure after cardiopulmonary bypass)

High-risk interventional cardiology procedures

Contraindications

Irreversible brain damage

Terminal or untreatable diseases of any major organ system

Abdominal aortic and thoracic aneurysms

Moderate to severe aortic insufficiency

Generalized peripheral vascular disease†

*Allows time for emergent angiography and corrective cardiac surgery to be performed.

†May inhibit placement of balloon and is considered a relative contraindication; sheathless insertion may be used.

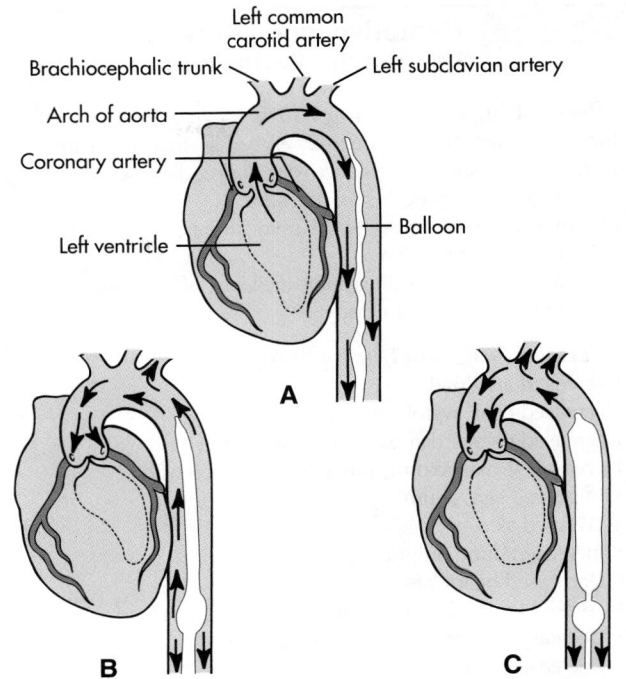

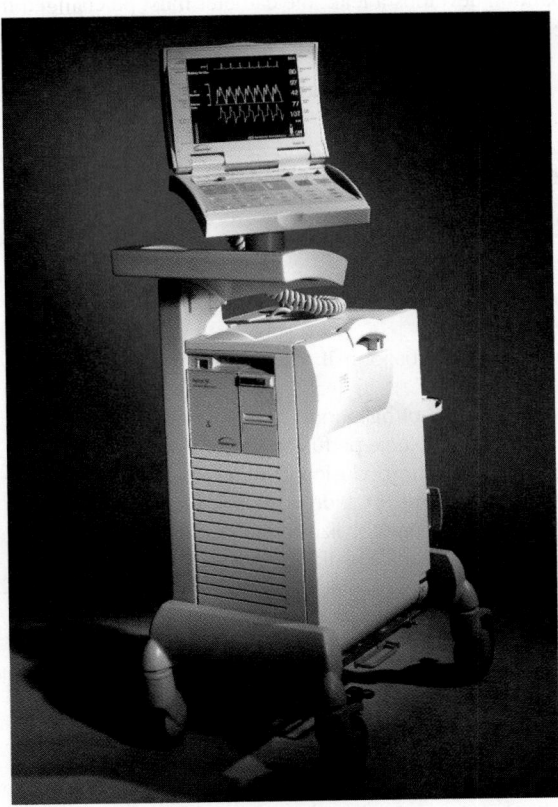

FIG. 64-12 Intraaortic balloon pump machine.

FIG. 64-13 Intraaortic balloon pump. **A**, During systole the balloon is deflated, which facilitates ejection of the blood into the periphery. **B**, In early diastole, the balloon begins to inflate. **C**, In late diastole, the balloon is totally inflated, which augments aortic pressure and increases the coronary perfusion pressure with the end result of increased coronary and cerebral blood flow.

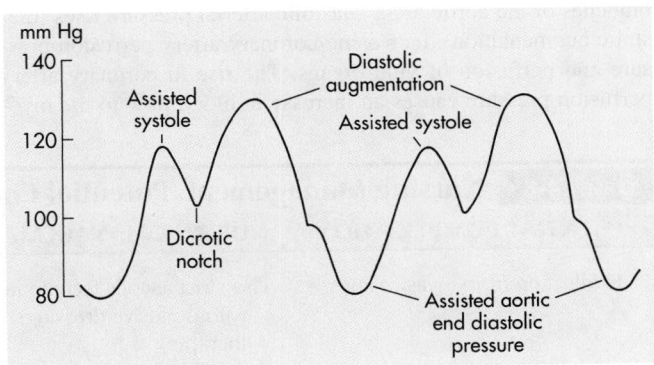

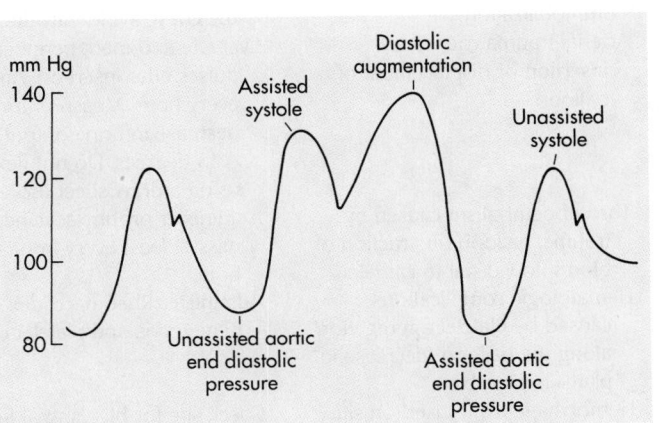

FIG. 64-14 **A**, Correct 1:1 intraaortic balloon pump frequency. **B**, Correct 1:2 intraaortic balloon pump frequency.

TABLE 64-7 Hemodynamic Effects of Intraaortic Balloon Pumps

Effects of Inflation During Diastole
Increased diastolic pressure (may exceed systolic pressure)
Increased pressure in the aortic root during diastole
Increased coronary perfusion pressure
Improved oxygen delivery to the myocardium
- Decreased angina pain
- Decreased electrocardiographic evidence of ischemia
- Decreased ventricular ectopy

Effects of Deflation During Systole
Decreased afterload
Decreased peak systolic pressure
Decreased myocardial oxygen consumption
Increased stroke volume, possibly associated with:
- Improved sensorium
- Warmed skin
- Increased urine output
- Decreased heart rate
Increased forward flow of blood, decreasing preload
- Decreased PA pressures, including PAWP
- Decreased crackles

PA, Pulmonary artery; *PAWP,* PA wedge pressure.

Effects of Counterpulsation. In late diastole when the balloon is totally inflated, blood is forcibly displaced distally to the extremities and proximally to the coronary arteries and main branches of the aortic arch. Diastolic arterial pressure rises (diastolic augmentation), increasing coronary artery perfusion pressure and perfusion of vital organs. The rise in coronary artery perfusion pressure causes an increase in blood flow to the myo-

cardium. The balloon is rapidly deflated just before systole. The suddenly created vacuum causes aortic pressure to drop. With aortic resistance to left ventricular ejection reduced (reduced afterload), the left ventricle empties more easily and completely. As with other types of afterload reduction, the SV increases, yet the myocardial oxygen consumption decreases.[31] Hemodynamic effects of the IABP are summarized in Table 64-7.

Complications with Intraaortic Balloon Pumps. Complications are common with the IABP (Table 64-8). Vascular injuries such as dislodging of plaque, aortic dissection, and compromised distal circulation are common, occurring in 3% to 65% of cases. Thrombus and embolus formation add to the risk of circulatory compromise to the extremity. Peripheral nerve damage can occur, particularly when a cut-down is performed for insertion.[32,33] To reduce these risks, cardiovascular, neurovascular, and hemodynamic assessments are necessary every 15 to 60 minutes depending on the patient's status.[31] The action of the balloon pump can cause physical destruction of platelets, and thrombocytopenia is common. Coagulation profiles must be monitored, and the patient must be assessed for evidence of systemic bleeding. Displacement of the balloon can occlude the left subclavian, renal, or mesenteric arteries and can result in diminished or absent radial pulse, decreased urine output, and diminished or absent bowels sounds. Patients receiving IABP therapy are prone to infection, and local or systemic signs of infection necessitate catheter removal.[31]

Mechanical complications are rare but may occur. Improper timing of balloon inflation may cause increased afterload, decreased CO, myocardial ischemia, and increased myocardial oxygen use and must be immediately recognized by the nurse. If the balloon develops a leak, the catheter must be changed immediately to avoid a helium gas embolus. Signs of a leak include less effective augmentation, repeated alarms for gas loss, and blood backing up into the catheter. A malfunction of the balloon

---

TABLE 64-8 Nursing Management: Potential Complications of the Intraaortic Balloon Pump

POTENTIAL COMPLICATION	NURSING MANAGEMENT
Site infection from invasive lines	Use strict aseptic technique for insertion and dressing changes for all lines. Cover all insertion sites with occlusive dressings. Administer prescribed prophylactic antibiotic for entire course of therapy.
Pneumonia associated with immobilization	Reposition patient q2hr, being careful not to displace balloon. If patient requires physical therapy of the chest, avoid introducing an ECG artifact.
Arterial trauma caused by insertion or displacement of balloon	Evaluate and mark peripheral pulses before insertion of balloon to use as baseline for assessing pulses after insertion. After insertion of balloon, evaluate perfusion to both extremities at least every hour. Measure urine output at least every hour (occlusion of renal arteries causes severe decrease in urine output). Observe arterial waveforms for sudden changes. Keep head of bed <45 degrees. Do not flex cannulated leg at the hip. Immobilize cannulated leg to prevent flexion using a draw sheet tucked under the mattress, soft ankle restraint, or knee immobilizer.
Thromboembolism caused by trauma, balloon obstruction of blood flow distal to catheter	Administer prophylactic heparin if ordered. Evaluate pulses, urine output, and level of consciousness at least every hour. Check circulation, sensation, and movement in both legs at least every hour.
Hematologic complications caused by platelet aggregation along the balloon (decrease in platelets possible)	Administer Rheomacrodex (low-molecular-weight dextran) if ordered. Monitor coagulation profiles, hematocrit, and platelet count.
Hemorrhage from insertion site	Check site for bleeding at least every hour. Observe vital signs for hypovolemia with each vital sign check.

ECG, Electrocardiogram.

or console triggers fail-safe alarms and automatic shutdown of the unit.

The patient with an IABP is relatively immobile, limited to side-lying or supine positions with the head of the bed elevated less than 45 degrees.[31] The leg in which the catheter is inserted must not be flexed at the hip. The patient may be receiving ventilatory support and will likely have multiple invasive lines that increase the challenge of comfortable positioning. The patient may experience sleeplessness and anxiety. Adequate sedation, pain relief, skin care, and comfort measures are required.

IABP therapy is weaned as the patient improves; that is, circulatory support provided by the IABP is gradually reduced. Weaning involves reducing the IABP assist ratio from 1:1 to 1:2 and assessing the patient's response (see Fig. 64-14, *B*). If hemodynamic parameters remain stable, the ratio can be changed from 1:3 to 1:8 until the IABP catheter is removed. Even if the patient is stable without IABP, pumping is continued until the line is removed.[31] This reduces the risk of thrombus formation around the catheter. Frequent hemodynamic assessment continues to be required during the weaning phase.

Ventricular Assist Devices

The **ventricular assist device** (VAD) provides longer-term support for the failing heart (usually months) and allows more mobility than the IABP. VADs are inserted into the path of flowing blood to augment or replace the action of the ventricle. Some VADs are implanted (e.g., peritoneum), and others are positioned externally. A typical VAD would shunt the blood from the left atrium or ventricle to the device and then to the aorta (Fig. 64-15). Some VADs provide biventricular support.

Failure to wean from cardiopulmonary bypass (CPB) after surgery has been the primary indicator for VAD support. Increasingly the VAD is used to support patients with ventricular failure caused by myocardial infarction and patients awaiting cardiac transplantation. A VAD is a temporary device with the capability to partially or totally support circulation until the heart recovers or a donor heart can be obtained. Cannula sites depend on the type of device used. For support of the right side of the heart, the right atrium and PA are cannulated. The left ventricular apex can be cannulated for left VADs. Direct cannulation of the atria and great vessels occurs in the operating room through a sternotomy.

Patient selection for VAD therapy is critical. Indications for VAD therapy include (1) extension of CPB for failure to wean or postcardiotomy cardiogenic shock, (2) bridge to recovery or cardiac transplantation, and (3) patients with New York Heart Association Classification IV (See Table 34-4) who have failed medical therapy. Relative contraindications for VAD therapy include (1) body surface area <1.3 m^2, (2) renal or liver failure unrelated to cardiac incident, and (3) untreatable metastatic cancer.[34]

Implantable Artificial Heart

Every year in the United States approximately 2000 patients receive donor hearts, yet the demand for these hearts far exceeds the supply. Research on mechanical CADs has led to the development of a fully implantable artificial heart that can sustain the body's circulatory system. This device is designed not only to extend life but also to provide a satisfactory quality of life for the thousands of patients with irreversible heart disease who never receive a donor heart. One major anticipated advantage of the artificial heart compared with heart transplantation is decreased costs for implantation and drug therapies. Patients will not require immunosuppression therapy, nor will they experience the inevitable, long-term effects of this therapy.[35]

NURSING MANAGEMENT CIRCULATORY ASSIST DEVICES

The patient with an IABP requires highly skilled nursing care. Detailed cardiovascular assessment, including measurement of hemodynamic parameters (e.g., PA and arterial pressures, CO, CI, SVR, SV), cardiac and thoracic auscultation; and evaluation of the ECG (e.g., rate, rhythm), is performed frequently. Assessment of adequate tissue perfusion (e.g., skin color and temperature, mentation, peripheral pulses, urine output, bowel sounds) is also performed at regular intervals.[31] It is expected that with IABP therapy these parameters should improve.

Nursing care of the patient with a VAD is similar to that of the patient with an IABP. The patient is observed for bleeding, cardiac tamponade, ventricular failure, infection, arrhythmias, renal failure, hemolysis, and thromboembolism. Unlike the patient with an IABP, who must remain in bed with limited position change, the patient with VAD may be mobile and require an activity plan.[34] In some cases, patients with VADs may go home. Preparation for discharge is complex and requires in-depth teaching about the device. Patients must have a competent caregiver present at all times.

Ideally, patients with CADs will recover through ventricular improvement, heart transplantation, or artificial heart implantation. However, many patients die, or the decision to terminate the device is made and death follows. Both the patient and family re-

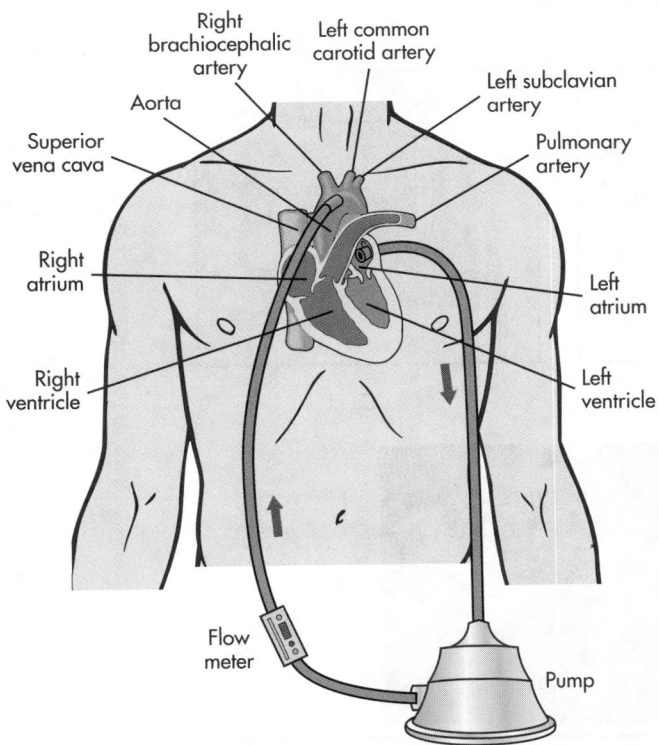

FIG. 64-15 Schematic diagram of a left ventricular assist device.

quire psychologic support. Nursing care should include the family as much as possible. Other members of the health care team, such as social workers or clergy, should be consulted as needed.

ARTIFICIAL AIRWAYS

The patient in the ICU often requires mechanical assistance to maintain airway patency. Inserting a tube into the trachea, bypassing upper airway and laryngeal structures, creates an artificial airway. The tube is placed into the trachea via the mouth or nose past the larynx (**endotracheal [ET] intubation**) or through a stoma in the neck *(tracheostomy).* ET intubation is more common in ICU patients. It can be performed quickly and safely at the bedside. Indications for ET intubation include (1) upper airway obstruction (e.g., secondary to trauma, tumor, bleeding), (2) high risk of aspiration, (3) ineffective clearance of secretions, and (4) respiratory distress.[36] ET tubes are illustrated in Fig. 64-16.

A *tracheotomy* is a surgical procedure that is performed when the need for an artificial airway is long term. There is ongoing debate regarding the timing of a tracheotomy in the patient with an ET tube. The situation varies with the patient, physician, and institution. Some institutions use ET intubation in patients for up to 6 weeks without harmful sequelae. Tracheostomy tubes and related nursing management are discussed in Chapter 26.

Endotracheal Tubes

In *oral intubation* the ET tube is passed through the mouth and vocal cords and into the trachea with the aid of a laryngoscope or bronchoscope. In nasal intubation, the ET tube is manipulated through the nose, nasopharynx, and vocal cords. Oral ET intubation is the procedure of choice for most emergencies because the airway can be secured rapidly. Compared with the nasal route, a larger-diameter tube can be used for oral intubation. With a larger-bore ET tube, work of breathing is reduced because there is less airway resistance. It is easier to remove secretions and perform fiberoptic bronchoscopy if needed.

There are disadvantages of oral ET intubation. It is difficult to place an oral tube if head and neck mobility are limited (e.g., suspected spinal cord injury). Teeth can be chipped or inadvertently dislodged during the procedure. Salivation is increased, and swallowing is difficult. Often a patient will obstruct the ET tube by biting down on it. A bite block or oropharyngeal airway can be used to avoid this. The ET tube and bite block (if used) should be secured (separately) to the face. Mouth care is a challenge. Finally, the larger tubes used in oral intubation are associated with laryngeal trauma and subglottic stenosis, particularly in smaller individuals.

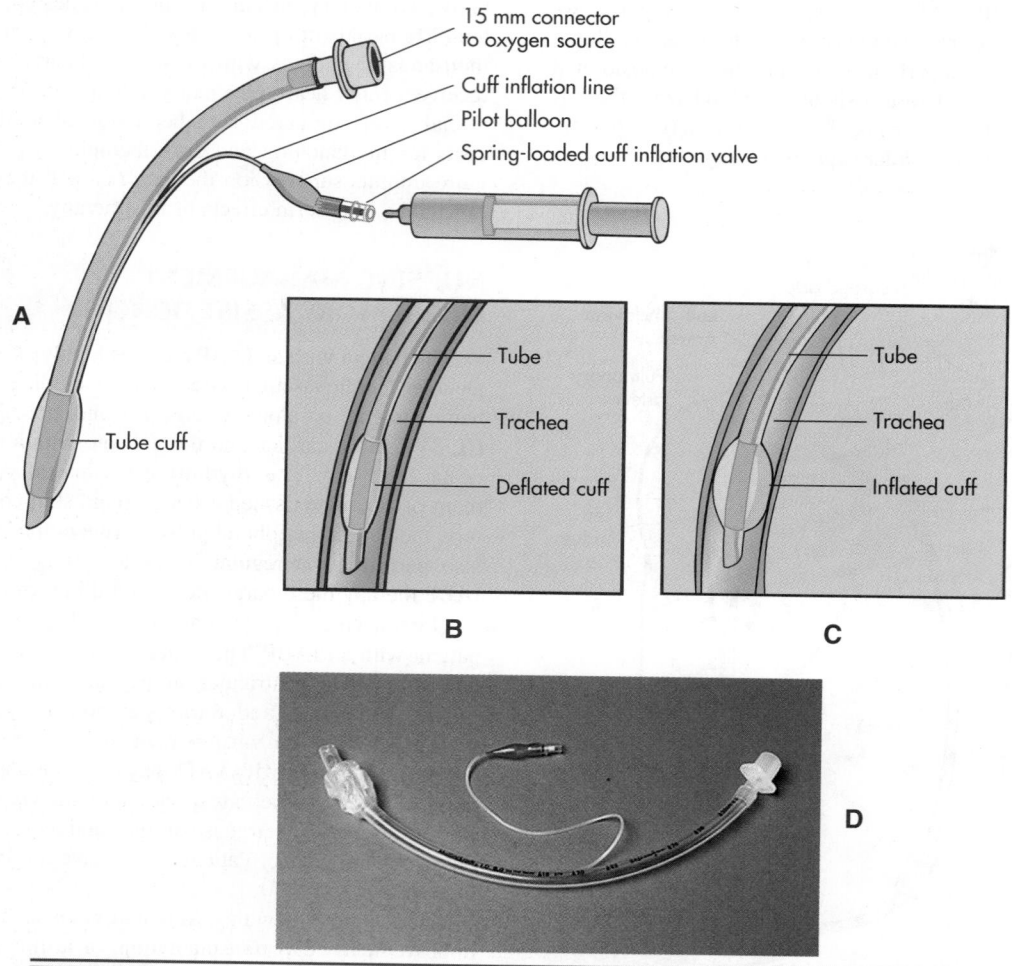

FIG. 64-16 Endotracheal tube. **A,** Parts of an endotracheal tube. **B,** Tube in place with cuff deflated. **C,** Tube in place with the cuff inflated. **D,** Photo of tube before placement.

Nasal ET intubation is sometimes preferred because it is more stable than the oral tube and more difficult to dislodge. It is placed "blindly," that is, without visualizing the larynx, and is indicated when head and neck manipulation is risky. The nasal tube may be uncomfortable for some patients because it presses on the septum, whereas others may prefer it because there is no need for a bite block and mouth care is more easily accomplished. However, nasal ET tubes are more subject to kinking than oral tubes; the work of breathing is greater because the longer, narrower tube offers more airflow resistance; and suctioning and secretion removal are more difficult. Nasal tubes have been linked with increased incidence of sinus infections, which may be a source of sepsis.[37]

Endotracheal Intubation Procedure

Before the procedure, the patient and family should be told the reason for ET intubation, the steps that will occur in the procedure, and the patient's role in the procedure (if indicated). It is also important to explain that while intubated, the patient will not be able to speak, but that other means of communication will be provided, and that the patient's hands may be immobilized for safety purposes.[38]

All patients undergoing intubation and receiving mechanical ventilation need to have a self-inflating **bag-valve-mask** (BVM) device (e.g., *Ambu bag*) attached to oxygen and suctioning equipment ready and available at the bedside. The BVM device should contain a reservoir to sequester oxygen so that oxygen concentrations of 90% to 95% can be delivered. The slower the bag is deflated and inflated, the higher the oxygen concentration that will be delivered. The nurse assembles and checks the equipment to be used, removes the patient's dentures and/or partial plates (for oral intubation), and administers drugs as ordered. Premedication varies, depending on the patient's level of consciousness (e.g., awake, obtunded) and the nature of the procedure (e.g., emergent, nonemergent). A sedative-hypnotic-amnesic (e.g., midazolam [Versed]) is used if the patient is agitated, disoriented, or combative. A rapid-onset narcotic such as fentanyl (Sublimaze) may be used to blunt the pain of laryngoscopy and intubation. A paralytic drug such as succinylcholine (Anectine) may be used to produce skeletal muscle paralysis. Atropine may be used to limit secretions. Pulse oximetry is used during the procedure to assess oxygenation.

For oral intubation, the patient is placed supine with the head extended and the neck flexed *("sniffing position")*. This position allows for visualization of the vocal cords by aligning the axes of the mouth, pharynx, and trachea.[38] For nasal intubation it may be helpful to have the patient extrude the tongue. Before intubation is attempted, the patient is preoxygenated using a self-inflating BVM device with 100% O_2 for 3 to 5 minutes. Each intubation attempt is limited to 30 seconds. If unsuccessful, the patient is ventilated between successive attempts using the BVM device with 100% O_2.[36,38]

Following intubation, the cuff is inflated, and the placement of the ET tube is confirmed while manually ventilating the patient with 100% O_2. A disposable CO_2 detector is placed between the BVM device and the ET tube and observed for a color change (indicating the presence of CO_2). The lung bases and apices are auscultated for bilateral breath sounds, and the chest is observed for symmetric chest wall movement. In addition, SpO_2 should be >95%.[36] If the evidence supports proper ET tube placement, the tube is connected to an O_2 source and secured in place per insti-

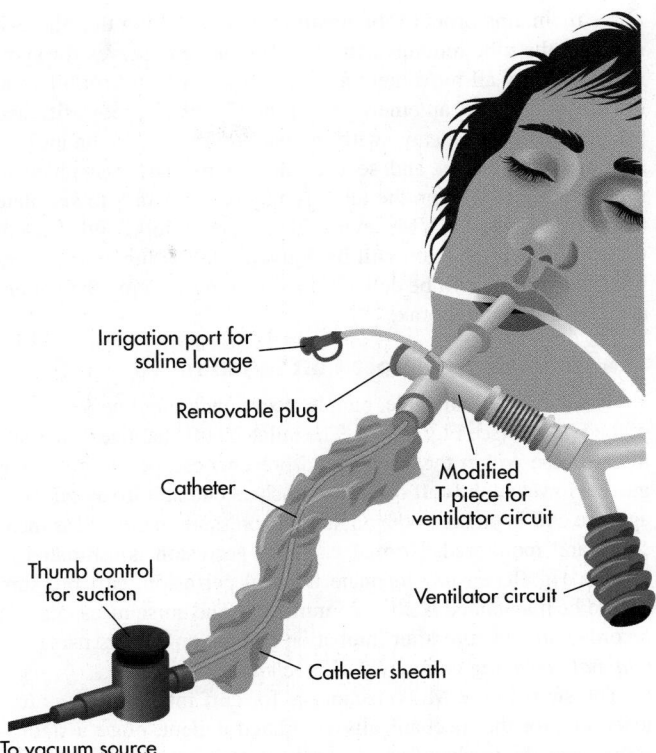

FIG. 64-17 Closed tracheal suction system.

tutional policy (Fig. 64-17). A bite block is inserted as needed. The ET tube and the pharynx should be suctioned as needed. A chest x-ray is immediately obtained to confirm tube placement (3 to 5 cm above the carina in the adult). This position allows the patient to move the neck without dislodging the tube or causing it to enter the right mainstem bronchus. Once proper positioning is confirmed with x-ray, the position of the tube at the teeth (usually 21 cm for women and 23 cm for men) or nose ("exit mark") is recorded and marked.[36] Excess tubing is cut to reduce dead space.

The ET tube is connected either to humidified air, O_2, or a mechanical ventilator. ABGs should be obtained 10 to 20 minutes after intubation to determine oxygenation and ventilation status. ABG values are reviewed and used to guide oxygenation and ventilation changes. Pulse oximetry provides useful continuous monitoring of arterial oxygenation.

NURSING MANAGEMENT
ARTIFICIAL AIRWAY

Nursing responsibilities for the patient with an artificial airway include (1) maintaining correct tube placement, (2) maintaining proper cuff inflation, (3) monitoring oxygenation and ventilation, (4) maintaining tube patency, (5) assessing for complications, (6) providing oral care and maintaining skin integrity, and (7) fostering comfort and communication (see NCP 64-1 on p. 1790).

■ Maintaining Correct Tube Placement

The nurse must monitor the patient with an ET tube for proper placement at least every 2 to 4 hours.[38] If the tube is dislodged, it could terminate in the pharynx or enter the esophagus or the right mainstem bronchus (thus ventilating only the right lung). The nurse maintains proper tube position by confirming that the exit mark on the tube remains constant. The nurse observes for symmetric chest wall movement and auscultates to confirm bilateral breath sounds. It is an emergency if the ET tube is not positioned properly. The nurse stays with the patient, maintains the airway, supports ventilation, and secures the appropriate assistance to immediately reposition the tube. It may be necessary to ventilate the patient with a BVM device. If a malpositioned tube is not repositioned, no oxygen will be delivered to the lungs or the entire tidal volume will be delivered to one lung, placing the patient at risk for pneumothorax.

■ Maintaining Proper Cuff Inflation

The cuff is an inflatable, pliable sleeve encircling the outer wall of the ET tube (see Fig. 64-16). The inflated cuff stabilizes and seals the ET tube within the trachea and prevents escape of ventilating gases. However, the cuff can cause tracheal damage. To avoid damage, the cuff is inflated with air, and the pressure in the cuff is measured and monitored. Normal capillary perfusion is estimated at 30 mm Hg. To ensure adequate tracheal perfusion, cuff pressure should be maintained at 20 to 25 mm Hg.[38] The nurse measures and records cuff pressure after intubation and every 8 hours using the *minimal occluding volume (MOV) technique.*

The steps in the MOV technique for cuff inflation are as follows: (1) for the mechanically ventilated patient, place a stethoscope over the trachea and inflate the cuff to MOV by adding air until no air leak is heard at peak inspiratory pressure (end of ventilator inspiration); (2) for the spontaneously breathing patient, inflate until no sound is heard after a deep breath or after inhalation with an BVM; (3) use a manometer to verify that cuff pressure is between 20 and 25 mm Hg; and (4) record cuff pressure in the chart. If adequate cuff pressure cannot be maintained or larger volumes of air are needed to keep the cuff inflated, the cuff could be leaking or there could be tracheal dilation at the cuff site. In these situations the ET tube should be changed within 24 hours or sooner if the patient decompensates.

■ Monitoring Oxygenation and Ventilation

The patient with an ET tube is vigilantly monitored for adequate oxygenation by assessing clinical findings, ABGs, SpO_2, and SvO_2. The nurse must assess for clinical signs of hypoxemia such as confusion, anxiety, dusky skin, and arrhythmias. Periodic ABGs (specifically PaO_2) and continuous SpO_2 provide objective data regarding oxygenation. Lower values are expected in patients with obstructive pulmonary disease. PA catheters with SvO_2 capability can give an indirect indication about the patient's oxygenation status (see Table 64-5).

Indicators of ventilation include assessment of clinical findings, $PaCO_2$, and partial pressure of end-tidal CO_2 ($PETCO_2$). The patient's respirations should be assessed for rate and rhythm and use of accessory muscles. The patient who is hyperventilating will be breathing rapidly and deeply and may experience circumoral and peripheral numbness and tingling. The patient who is hypoventilating will be breathing shallowly or slowly and may appear dusky. $PaCO_2$ is the best indicator of alveolar hyperventilation (e.g., decreased $PaCO_2$, increased pH indicate respiratory alkalosis) or hypoventilation (e.g., increased $PaCO_2$, decreased pH indicate respiratory acidosis).

$PETCO_2$ monitoring is done by analyzing exhaled gas directly at the patient-ventilator circuit *(mainstream sampling)* or by transporting a sample of gas via a small-bore tubing to a bedside monitor *(sidestream sampling).*[39] Continuous $PETCO_2$ monitoring can be used to assess the patency of the airway and the presence of breathing. In addition, gradual changes in $PETCO_2$ values may accompany an increase in CO_2 production (e.g., sepsis, hypoventilation, neuromuscular blockade) or decrease in CO_2 production (e.g., hypothermia, decreased CO, metabolic acidosis). In patients with normal ventilation-to-perfusion ratios (see Chapter 66), $PETCO_2$ can be used as an estimate of $PaCO_2$, with $PETCO_2$ generally 1 to 5 mm Hg lower than $PaCO_2$. However, in patients with unusually large dead space or serious mismatch between ventilation and perfusion, $PETCO_2$ is not a reliable estimate of $PaCO_2$.[39]

■ Maintaining Tube Patency

The patient should be assessed routinely to determine a need for suctioning, but the patient should not receive suctioning routinely. Indications for suctioning include (1) visible secretions in the ET tube, (2) sudden onset of respiratory distress, (3) suspected aspiration of secretions, (4) increase in peak airway pressures, (5) auscultation of adventitious breath sounds over the trachea and/or bronchi, (6) increase in respiratory rate and/or sustained coughing, and (7) sudden or gradual decrease in PaO_2 and/or SpO_2.[39]

When the presence of secretions is confirmed, the nurse encourages the patient to cough to expel the secretions through the ET tube. If the patient cannot expel the secretions, suctioning is indicated. Two recommended suctioning methods, the **closed-suction technique** (CST) and the **open-suction technique** (OST), are described in Table 64-9. The CST uses a suction catheter that is enclosed in a plastic sleeve connected directly to the patient-ventilator circuit (see Fig. 64-17). With the CST, oxygenation and ventilation are maintained during suctioning and exposure to the patient's secretions is reduced. The CST should be considered for patients who require high levels of positive end-expiratory pressure (PEEP) (>10 cm H_2O) and/or FIO_2 (>80%), who have bloody pulmonary secretions and/or active tuberculosis, and who experience hemodynamic instability with the OST.[40]

Potential complications associated with suctioning include hypoxemia, bronchospasm, increased intracranial pressure, arrhythmias, mucosal damage, pulmonary bleeding, and infection.[40] The nurse must closely assess the patient before, during, and after the suctioning procedure. If the patient does not tolerate suctioning (e.g., decreased SpO_2, increased blood pressure, sustained coughing, development of arrhythmias), the procedure is halted, and the patient is manually ventilated with 100% oxygen or placed back on the ventilator until equilibration occurs and before another suction pass is attempted. Hypoxemia is prevented by hyperoxygenating the patient before and after each suctioning pass and limiting each suctioning pass to 10 seconds or less (see Table 64-9). There are only limited data that support the effectiveness of ventilator-delivered hyperoxygenation in increasing arterial oxygen levels over other methods.[40] If SvO_2 and/or SpO_2 are used, trends should be assessed throughout the suctioning procedure. Spontaneously breathing patients with chronic hypercapnia (e.g., patients with chronic obstructive pulmonary disease [COPD]) should be hyperoxygenated with FIO_2 ≤60%. Spontaneous respirations should be confirmed after the suctioning procedure to rule out oxygen-induced apnea.

TABLE 64-9   Suctioning Procedures for a Patient on a Mechanical Ventilator

General Measures

1. Gather all equipment.
2. Wash hands and don personal protective equipment.
3. Explain procedure and anticipated sensations to patient.
4. Monitor patient's cardiopulmonary status (e.g., vital signs, SpO_2, SvO_2, ECG, level of consciousness) before, during, and after the procedure.
5. Turn on suction and set vacuum to 100 to 120 mm Hg.
6. Pause ventilator alarms.

Open-Suction Technique

1. Open sterile catheter package using the inside of the package as a sterile field. Note: Suction catheter should be no wider than half the diameter of the ET tube (e.g., for a 7-mm ET tube, select a 10-French suction catheter).
2. Fill the sterile solution container with sterile normal saline or water.
3. Don sterile gloves.
4. Pick up sterile suction catheter with dominant hand. Using nondominant hand, secure the connecting tube (to suction) to the suction catheter.
5. Check equipment for proper functioning by suctioning a small volume of sterile saline solution from the container. (Go to Step 7.)

Closed-Suction Technique

6. Connect the suction tubing to the closed suction port.
7. Hyperoxygenate the patient for 30 seconds using one of the following methods:
   - Activate the suction hyperoxygenation setting on the ventilator using nondominant hand.
   - Increase FIO_2 to 100%. For patients with chronic hypercapnia who are breathing spontaneously, use FIO_2 of ≤60%.

Note: FIO_2 must be returned to baseline level at the completion of the procedure.
   - Disconnect the ventilator tubing from the ET tube and manually ventilate the patient with 100% O_2 using a BVM device. Administer 5 to 6 breaths over 30 seconds. Note: Use of a second person to deliver the manual breaths will significantly increase the tidal volume delivered.

8. With suction off, gently and quickly insert the catheter using the dominant hand. When resistance is met, pull back 1 to 2 cm.
9. Apply continuous or intermittent suction using the nondominant thumb. Rotate the catheter between the dominant thumb and forefinger and withdraw the catheter over 10 seconds or less.
10. Hyperoxygenate for 30 seconds as described in Step 7.
11. If secretions remain and the patient has tolerated the procedure, two to three suction passes may be performed as described in Steps 8 and 9. Note: Rinse the suction catheter with sterile saline solution between suctioning passes as needed.
12. Reconnect patient to ventilator (open-suction technique).
13. At the completion of ET tube suctioning, rinse the catheter and connecting tubing with the sterile saline solution.
14. Suction nasal and/or oral pharynx. Note: A separate catheter must be used for this step when using the closed-suction technique.
15. Discard the suction catheter and rinse the connecting tubing with the sterile saline solution (open-suction technique).
16. Reset FIO_2 (if necessary) and ventilator alarms.
17. Reassess patient for signs of effective suctioning.

Adapted from Chulay M: Endotracheal or tracheostomy tube suctioning. In Lynn-McHale DJ, Carlson KK, editors: *AACN procedure manual for critical care,* ed 4, Philadelphia, 2001, WB Saunders.
BVM, Bag-valve-mask; *ECG,* electrocardiogram; *ET,* endotracheal.

Causes of arrhythmias during suctioning include hypoxemia resulting in myocardial hypoxia; vagal stimulation caused by tracheal irritation; and sympathetic nervous system stimulation caused by anxiety, discomfort, or pain. Arrhythmias include tachycardia, bradycardia, premature beats, and asystole. Suctioning should be halted if any new arrhythmias develop. Excessive suctioning should be avoided in patients with severe hypoxemia or bradycardia.

Tracheal mucosal damage may occur because of excessive suction pressures, overly vigorous catheter insertion, and the characteristics of the suction catheter itself. The presence of blood streaks or tissue shreds in aspirated secretions indicates that mucosal damage has occurred. Mucosal damage increases the risk of infection and bleeding.[40] Trauma to the mucosa can be prevented by following the steps described in Table 64-9.

Secretions may be thick and difficult to suction because of inadequate hydration, inadequate humidification, infection, or inaccessibility of the left mainstem bronchus or lower airways. Adequately hydrating the patient (e.g., oral or intravenous fluids) and providing supplemental humidification of inspired gases may assist in thinning secretions. Instillation of normal saline into the ET tube, a common practice thought to facilitate the removal of secre-

tions with suctioning, is to be discouraged. It is not effective and may cause decreases in arterial oxygenation. If infection is the cause of thick secretions, the patient should be given appropriate antibiotics. Postural drainage, percussion, and turning the patient every 2 hours may help move secretions into larger airways.[40]

■ Providing Oral Care and Maintaining Skin Integrity

When an oral ET tube is in place, the patient's mouth is always open, and the lips and mouth should be moistened with saline or water swabs to prevent mucosal drying. Oral care, including cleaning of teeth, tongue, and gums, should be performed every 2 to 4 hours and as needed to provide comfort and to prevent injury to the gums and plaque accumulation. If excessive nasal or oral secretions are noted, naso-oropharyngeal suctioning should be performed.

Meticulous care is required to prevent skin breakdown on the face, lips, tongue, and/or nares as a result of pressure from the ET tube and/or bite block or from the method used to secure the ET tube to the patient's face. The ET tube should be retaped or secured every 24 hours and as needed.[37] If the patient is nasally intubated, the nurse should remove the old tape or ties and clean the

FIG. 64-18 Methods for securing adhesive tape. Example of protocol for securing endotracheal tube using adhesive tape:

1. Clean the patient's skin with mild soap and water.
2. Remove oil from the skin with alcohol and allow to dry.
3. Apply a skin adhesive product to enhance tape adherence. (When tape is removed, an adhesive remover will be necessary.)
4. Place a hydrocolloid membrane over the cheeks to protect friable skin.
5. Secure with adhesive tape as shown here..

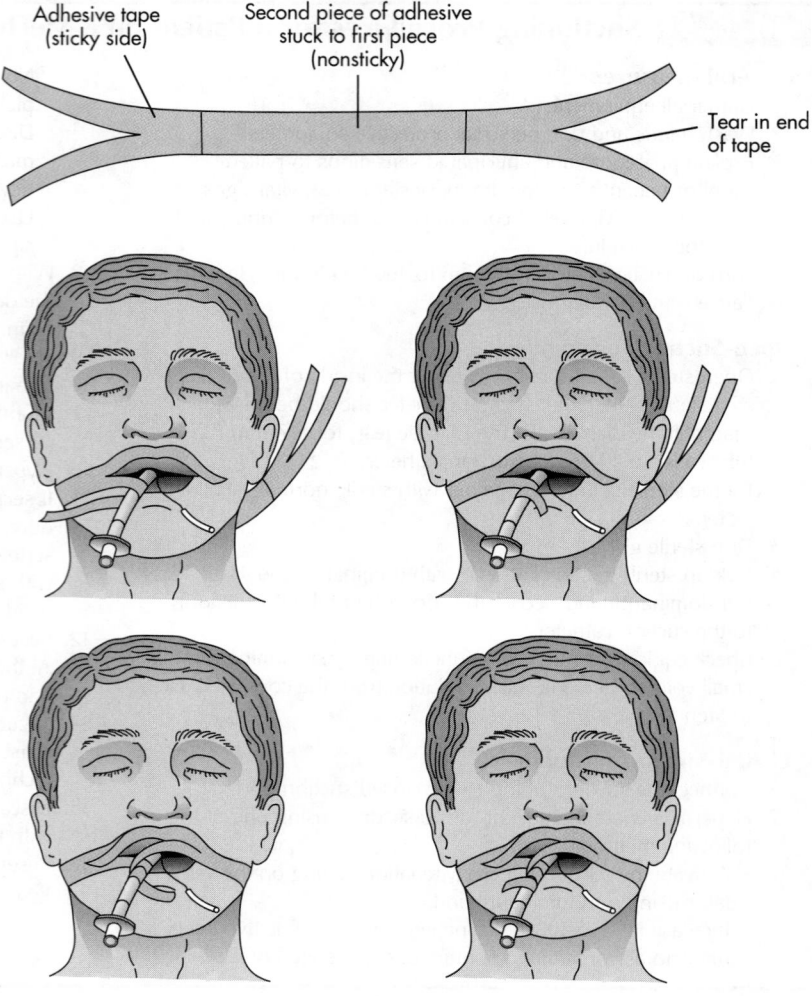

skin around the ET tube with saline-soaked gauze or cotton swabs. If the patient is orally intubated, the nurse should remove the bite block (if present) and the old tape or ties. Oral hygiene should be provided, and the ET tube should be repositioned to the opposite side of the mouth. The nurse replaces the bite block (if appropriate) and reconfirms proper cuff inflation and tube placement.[37] The ET tube is resecured per institutional policy (Fig. 64-18). If a manufactured tube holder is used, the straps can be loosened, the area under the straps massaged, and the straps reapplied. If the patient is anxious or uncooperative, it is recommended that two caregivers perform the repositioning procedure to prevent accidental dislodgment. The patient should be monitored for any signs of respiratory distress throughout the procedure.

■ Fostering Comfort and Communication

Patients have reported that intubation is a major stressor in the ICU.[41] The intubated patient may experience anxiety because of the inability to communicate and not knowing what to expect. Communicating with the intubated patient can be a frustrating experience for the patient, family, and the nurse. To communicate more effectively, the nurse should employ a variety of methods (see earlier section, Common Problems of Critically Care Patients).

The physical discomfort associated with ET intubation and mechanical ventilation often necessitates sedating the patient or administering an analgesic until the ET tube is no longer required. The patient may require morphine, lorazepam (Ativan), or other sedatives to blunt the anxiety and discomfort related to intubation. The nurse should evaluate the effectiveness of the drugs used to achieve an acceptable level of patient comfort. In addition, the nurse should consider initiating alternative therapies (e.g., music therapy) to complement drug therapy.[9]

Complications of Endotracheal Intubation

Two major complications of ET intubation are inadvertent extubation and aspiration. Inadvertent (unplanned) **extubation** (removal of the ET tube from the trachea) can be a catastrophic event and usually complicates the patient's recovery. Usually the inadvertent extubation is obvious (the patient is holding the ET tube). Other times, the tip of ET tube is in the hypopharynx or esophagus and the extubation is not so obvious. Signs of inadvertent extubation may include patient vocalization, activation of the low-pressure ventilator alarm, diminished or absent breath sounds, respiratory distress, and gastric distention.[42] The nurse is responsible for preventing inadvertent extubation by immobilizing the patient's hands through the use of soft wrist restraints (per institutional policy) and/or sedation. The nurse should reinforce the purpose of the restraints to the patient and family. In one study of elderly ICU patients, being intubated and not being able to breathe were more distressing and memorable than being restrained.[41]

Should an accidental extubation occur, the nurse should stay with the patient. Interventions are directed at maintaining the patient's airway, supporting ventilation (usually by manually ventilating the patient with 100% oxygen), and securing the appropriate assistance to immediately reintubate the patient (if necessary).

Aspiration is a potential hazard for the patient with an ET tube. The ET tube passes through the epiglottis, splinting it in an open position. Thus the intubated patient cannot protect the airway from aspiration. The cuff cannot totally prevent the trickle of oral or gastric secretions into the trachea. Furthermore, secretions accumulate above the cuff. When the cuff is deflated, those secretions move into the lungs. Oral intubation increases salivation, yet swallowing is difficult, so the mouth must be suctioned frequently. The posterior pharynx should always be suctioned before cuff deflation. This may be performed with a Yankauer (tonsil-tip) suction catheter by the patient. Other contributing factors to aspiration include improper cuff inflation and tracheoesophageal fistula. The patient with an ET tube is at risk for aspiration of gastric contents. Even when the cuff is properly inflated, the nurse must take precautions to avoid emesis, which can lead to aspiration. Frequently, a nasogastric (NG) tube is inserted and connected to low, intermittent suction when a patient is intubated. If the patient is receiving enteral feedings through an NG tube, the head of the bed should be elevated.

MECHANICAL VENTILATION

Mechanical ventilation is the process by which room air or oxygen-enriched air is moved into and out of the lungs mechanically. Mechanical ventilation is not curative. It is a means of supporting patients until they recover the ability to breathe independently or a decision is made to withdraw ventilatory support. Indications for mechanical ventilation are listed in Table 64-10.

Patients with chronic pulmonary disease and their families should be given the opportunity to decide the issue of mechanical ventilation before terminal respiratory disease develops. Other patients with chronic illnesses should also be encouraged to discuss the subject. It is much easier for the health care team, patient, and family to decide not to institute ventilatory support initially than it is to remove the support once it has been initiated. The decision to use mechanical ventilation must be made carefully, respecting the informed wishes of the patient and family.

Types of Mechanical Ventilation

The two major types of mechanical ventilation are negative pressure and positive pressure ventilation.

Negative Pressure Ventilation. **Negative pressure ventilation** involves the use of chambers that encase the chest or body and surround it with intermittent subatmospheric or negative pressure. Intermittent negative pressure around the chest wall causes the chest to be pulled outward. This reduces intrathoracic pressure. Air rushes in via the upper airway, which is outside the sealed chamber. Expiration is passive; the machine cycles off, allowing chest retraction. This type of ventilation is similar to normal ventilation in that decreased intrathoracic pressures produce inspiration and expiration is passive. An artificial airway is not required.

New developments in negative pressure ventilation enable both control and assist-control ventilation modes. Lightweight, portable negative pressure ventilators are used in the home for patients with neuromuscular diseases, central nervous system disorders, diseases and injuries of the spinal cord, and severe COPD (Fig. 64-19). Negative pressure ventilators are not used extensively for acutely ill patients.

Positive Pressure Ventilation. **Positive pressure ventilation** (PPV) is the primary method used with acutely ill patients (Figs. 64-20 and 64-21). During inspiration the ventilator pushes

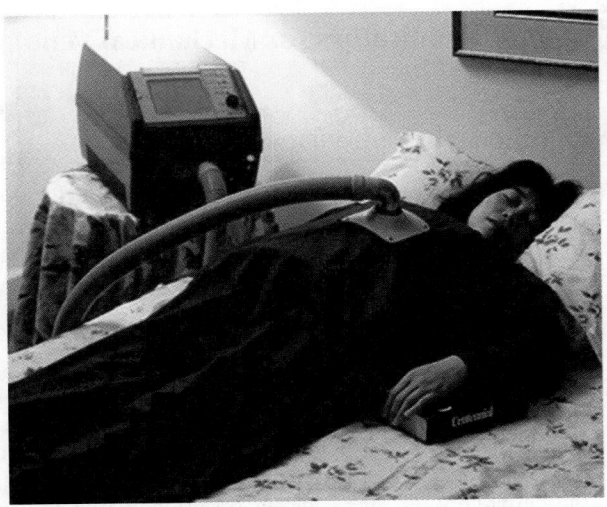
FIG. 64-19 Negative pressure ventilator.

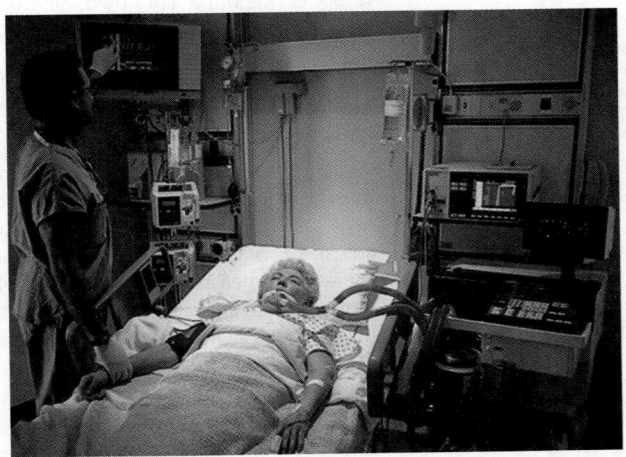
FIG. 64-20 Patient receiving mechanical ventilation.

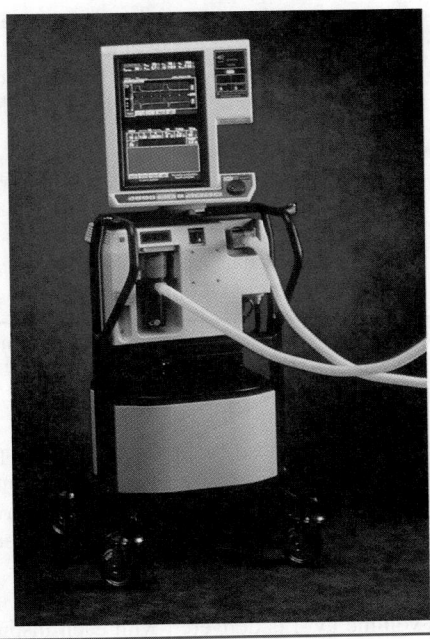
FIG. 64-21 Typical positive pressure ventilator.

TABLE 64-10   Indicators for Mechanical Ventilation and Weaning

MEASUREMENT	SIGNIFICANCE	NORMAL VALUES*	MECHANICAL VENTILATION INDICATED*	WEANING FEASIBLE*
Tests of Ventilatory Reserve or Mechanical Ability				
Spontaneous tidal volume (SV$_T$)	Amount of air exchanged during normal breathing at rest; measure of muscle endurance	7-9 ml/kg	<5 ml/kg	≥5 ml/kg
Spontaneous respiratory rate (fx)		12-20	<10 or >35	12-20
Vital capacity (VC)	Maximal inspiration and then measurement of air during maximal forced expiration; measure of respiratory muscle endurance or reserve or both; requires patient cooperation	65-75 ml/kg	<10-15 ml/kg	≥15 ml/kg
Positive expiratory pressure (PEP) or force (PEF)	After complete occlusion of expiratory valve, pressure manometer attached to airway or mouth for 10-20 seconds while positive expiratory efforts of patient noted; measure of expiratory muscle strength and ability to cough; requires patient cooperation	60-85 cm H_2O	<30 cm H_2O	≥30 cm H_2O
Maximal inspiratory pressure (MIP) or negative inspiratory pressure (NIP)	After complete occlusion of inspiratory valve, pressure manometer attached to airway or mouth for 10-20 seconds while negative inspiratory efforts of patient noted; measure of inspiratory muscle strength; measurement is effort independent (patient does not have to actively cooperate); most reliable of the weaning criteria	−75 to −100 cm H_2O	>−20 cm H_2O	≤−20 cm H_2O
Forced expiratory volume in 1 sec (FEV$_1$)	Volume of air measured in first second of exhalation of forced vital capacity maneuver; used in patients with COPD to determine degree of obstruction	50-60 ml/kg	<10 ml/kg	>16 ml/kg
Resting minute ventilation	Multiplication of tidal volume by respiratory rate for 1 min, general indication of patient's total ventilation	5-10 L/min	>10 L/min	≤10 L/min
Dead space to tidal volume ratio (V$_D$/V$_T$)	Estimation from V$_T$; accurate calculation requiring PaCO$_2$ and partial pressure of CO_2 in mixed expired gas; measurement of portion of V$_T$ that does not participate in gas exchange; indication of lungs' efficiency in removing CO_2	0.25-0.40	>0.6	<0.6
PaCO$_2$	Indication of lungs' efficiency in removing CO_2 and reflection of body's acid-base status	35-45 mm Hg	>55 mm Hg (acute)	<45 mm Hg
Tests of Oxygenation Capability				
FIO$_2$	Fraction (percent) of inspired O$_2$ needed to maintain adequate PaO$_2$	21% (room air)	>50%	≤50%
PaO$_2$/FIO$_2$	Provision of evidence of lung's ability to oxygenate arterial blood; couples PO$_2$ with amount of oxygen given	350-400	<200	>300

*These parameters are only guidelines and must be related to the individual patient's status (e.g., patients with severe COPD may have a normal PaCO$_2$ of 60 mm Hg and values lower than normal for FEV$_1$).
COPD, Chronic obstructive pulmonary disease.

air into the lungs under positive pressure. Unlike spontaneous ventilation, intrathoracic pressure is raised during lung inflation rather than lowered. Expiration occurs passively as in normal expiration. Positive pressure ventilators are categorized into volume and pressure ventilators.

Volume ventilators. With **volume ventilators,** a predetermined tidal volume (V$_T$) is delivered with each inspiration, and

the amount of pressure needed to deliver the breath varies based on the compliance and resistance factors of the patient-ventilator system. Consequently, the V$_T$ is consistent from breath to breath, but airway pressures will vary.[42,43]

Pressure ventilators. With **pressure ventilators,** the peak inspiratory pressure is predetermined, and the V$_T$ delivered to the patient varies based on the selected pressure and the compliance and resistance factors of the patient-ventilator system.[42,43] With this understanding, careful attention must be given to the V_T to prevent unplanned hyperventilation or hypoventilation. For example, when the patient breathes out of synchrony with the ventilator, the pressure limit may be reached quickly, and the volume of gas delivered may be small. Initially, pressure ventilation was used only in stable patients being weaned from the ventilator. Today, pressure ventilation is frequently selected to treat critically ill patients.[42]

Settings of Mechanical Ventilators

Mechanical ventilator settings regulate the rate, depth, and other characteristics of ventilation (Table 64-11). Settings are based on the patient's status (ABGs, body weight, level of consciousness, muscle strength). The ventilator is tuned as finely as possible to match the patient's ventilatory pattern. Settings are evaluated and adjusted frequently until the patient achieves optimal ventilation. Some settings serve as a fail-safe mechanism, alerting staff to problems with ventilation. It is important that the nurse ensure and document that all ventilator alarms are on at all times. Alarms sense potentially dangerous situations such as mechanical malfunction, apnea, or patient asynchrony with the ventilator. On many ventilators the alarms can be temporarily suspended or silenced for up to 2 minutes for suctioning or testing. After that period of time, the alarm system automatically becomes functional again.

Modes of Volume Ventilation

The variable methods by which the patient and the ventilator interact to deliver effective ventilation are called modes. The *ventilator mode* selected is based on how much work of breathing (WOB) the patient ought to or can perform and is determined by the patient's ventilatory status, respiratory drive, and ABGs. Generally, ventilator modes are controlled or assisted. With controlled ventilatory support, the ventilator does all of the work of breathing, and with assisted ventilatory support, the ventilator and the patient share the work of breathing.[43] Modes are further categorized as volume modes and pressure modes. For the past 25 years, volume modes such as controlled mandatory ventilation (CMV), assist-control ventilation (ACV), and synchronized intermittent mandatory ventilation (SIMV) have been used to treat critically ill patients. Over the last decade, pressure modes such as pressure support ventilation (PSV) and pressure-controlled inverse ratio ventilation (PC-IRV) have become more widespread.[43] These modes are described in Table 64-12.

Controlled Mandatory Ventilation. With **controlled mandatory ventilation** (CMV), breaths are delivered at a set rate per minute and V_T, which are independent of the patient's ventilatory efforts. Although CMV is used infrequently, it is used when the patient has no drive to breathe (e.g., the anesthetized patient) or is unable to breathe spontaneously (e.g., the paralyzed patient). The patient performs no WOB in this mode and cannot adjust respirations to changing demands.

Assist-Control Mechanical Ventilation. With **assist-control ventilation** (ACV), the ventilator delivers a preset V_T at a preset frequency, and when the patient initiates a spontaneous breath, a full V_T is delivered. The ventilator senses a decrease in intrathoracic pressure and then delivers the preset V_T. The patient can breathe faster than the preset rate but not slower. This mode has the advantage of allowing the patient some control over ventilation while providing some assistance. ACV is used in patients with a variety of conditions, including neuromuscular disorders (e.g., Guillain-Barré syndrome), pulmonary edema, and acute respiratory failure. The patient with ACV mode has the potential for hypoventilation and hyperventilation. The spontaneously breathing patient can easily be overventilated, resulting in hyperventilation. If the volume or minimum rate is set low and the patient is apneic or weak, the patient will be hypoventilated. Thus these patients require vigilant assessment and monitoring of ventilatory status, including respiratory rate, ABGs, SpO_2, and SvO_2. It is important that the amount of negative pressure required to initiate a breath is appropriate to the patient's condition. For example, if it is too difficult to initiate a breath, the WOB is increased and the patient may tire.

Synchronized Intermittent Mandatory Ventilation. With **synchronized intermittent mandatory ventilation** (SIMV), the ventilator delivers a preset V_T at a preset frequency in synchrony with the patient's spontaneous breathing. Between ventilator-delivered breaths, the patient is able to breathe spon-

TABLE 64-11	Settings of Mechanical Ventilation
PARAMETER	**DESCRIPTION**
Respiratory rate (f)	Number of breaths the ventilator delivers per minute; usual setting is 4-20 breaths/min
Tidal volume (V_T)	Volume of gas delivered to patient during each ventilator breath; usual volume is 5-15 ml/kg
Oxygen concentration (FIO_2)	Fraction of inspired oxygen delivered to patient; may be set between 21% (essentially room air) and 100%; usually adjusted to maintain PaO_2 level >60 mm Hg or SaO_2 level >90%
I:E ratio	Duration of inspiration (I) to duration of expiration (E); usual setting is 1:2 to 1:1.5 unless IRV is desired
Flow rate	Speed with which the V_T is delivered; usual setting is 40-100 L/min
Sensitivity/trigger	Determines the amount of effort the patient must generate to initiate a ventilator breath; it may be set for pressure triggering or flow triggering; usual setting for a pressure trigger is 0.5-1.5 cm H_2O below baseline pressure and for a flow trigger is 1-3 L/min below baseline flow
Pressure limit	Regulates the maximal pressure the ventilator can generate to deliver the V_T; when the pressure is reached, the ventilator terminates the breath and spills the undelivered volume into the atmosphere; usual setting is 10-20 cm H_2O above peak inspiratory pressure

From Urden LD, Stacy KM, Lough ME: *Thelan's critical care nursing: diagnosis and management*, ed 4, St Louis, 2002, Mosby.
IRV, Inverse ratio ventilation.

TABLE 64-12   Modes of Mechanical Ventilation

Volume Modes

Control Ventilation (CV) or Controlled Mandatory Ventilation (CMV)

With this mode, the ventilator provides all of the patient's minute ventilation. The clinician sets the rate, V_T, inspiratory time, and positive end-expiratory pressure (PEEP). Generally, this term is used to describe those situations in which the patient is chemically relaxed or is paralyzed from a spinal cord or neuromuscular disease and is therefore unable to initiate spontaneous breaths. The ventilator mode setting may be set on CMV, assist-control (AC), or synchronized intermittent mandatory ventilation (SIMV) because all these options provide volume breaths at the clinician-selected rate.

Assist-Control (AC) or Assisted Mandatory Ventilation (AMV)

This option requires that a rate, V_T, inspiratory time, and PEEP be set for the patient. The ventilator sensitivity is also set, and when the patient initiates a spontaneous breath, a full volume breath is delivered.

Intermittent Mandatory Ventilation (IMV) and Synchronized Intermittent Mandatory Ventilation (SIMV)

This mode requires that rate, V_T, inspiratory time, sensitivity, and PEEP are set by the clinician. In between "mandatory breaths," patients can spontaneously breathe at their own rates and V_T. With SIMV, the ventilator synchronizes the mandatory breaths with the patient's own inspirations.

Pressure Modes

Pressure Support Ventilation (PSV)

This mode provides an augmented inspiration to a spontaneously breathing patient. The clinician selects an inspiratory pressure level, PEEP, and sensitivity. When the patient initiates a breath, a high flow of gas is delivered to the preselected pressure level and pressure is maintained throughout inspiration. The patient determines the parameters of V_T, rate, and inspiratory time.

Pressure-Controlled Inverse Ratio Ventilation (PC-IRV)

This mode combines pressure-limited ventilation with an inverse ratio of inspiration to expiration. The clinician selects the pressure level, rate, inspiratory time (1:1, 2:1, 3:1, 4:1), and the PEEP level. With the prolonged inspiratory times, auto-PEEP may result. The auto-PEEP may be a desirable outcome of the inverse ratios. Some clinicians use PC without IRV. Conventional inspiratory times are used and rate, pressure level, and PEEP are selected.

Positive End-Expiratory Pressure (PEEP) and Continuous Positive Airway Pressure (CPAP)

PEEP

This ventilatory option creates positive pressure at end exhalation. PEEP restores functional residual capacity (FRC). The term PEEP is used when end-expiratory pressure is provided during ventilator positive pressure breaths.

Continuous Positive Airway Pressure (CPAP)

Similar to PEEP, CPAP restores functional residual capacity. However, this pressure is continuous during spontaneous breathing; no positive pressure breaths are present.

From Burns SM: Ventilatory management: volume and pressure modes. In Lynn-McHale DJ, Carlson KK, editors: *AACN procedure manual for critical care*, ed 4, Philadelphia, 2001, WB Saunders.

taneously through the ventilator circuit. Thus the patient receives the preset FIO_2 concentration during the spontaneous breaths but self-regulates the rate and depth of those breaths. This mode of ventilation differs from ACV, in which all breaths are of the same preset volume. SIMV is the most common mode of ventilatory support. It is used during continuous ventilation and during weaning from the ventilator. Potential benefits of SIMV include improved patient-ventilator synchrony (the patient "fights" the ventilator less), lower mean airway pressure, and prevention of muscle atrophy as the patient takes on more of the WOB.[43]

SIMV has advantages over other modes with respect to cardiovascular effects. Spontaneous inspiration decreases intrathoracic pressure, reduces mean intrathoracic pressure, and enhances venous blood return to the heart. Thus the patient with an extracellular fluid volume deficit is better able to maintain CO. Because of the lower mean intrathoracic pressure, higher levels of PEEP may be used with SIMV than with other modes of volume ventilation.

There are disadvantages with SIMV. If spontaneous breathing decreases when the preset rate is low, ventilation might not be adequately supported. Low-rate SIMV should be used only in patients with regular, spontaneous breathing. Weaning with SIMV demands close monitoring and may take longer because the rate of breathing is gradually reduced. Patients being weaned with SIMV may become fatigued, especially during the night.

Pressure Support Ventilation. With **pressure support ventilation** (PSV), positive pressure is applied to the airway only during inspiration and is used in conjunction with the patient's spontaneous respirations. A preset level of positive airway pressure is selected so that the gas flow rate is greater than the patient's inspiratory flow rate. As the patient initiates a breath, the machine senses the spontaneous effort and supplies a rapid flow of gas at the initiation of the breath and variable flow throughout the breath. With PSV the patient determines inspiratory length, V_T, and respiratory rate.[42,43] V_T depends on the pressure level and airway compliance. PSV is used with continuous ventilation and is especially helpful in combination with SIMV during weaning. PSV is not used as a sole ventilatory support during acute respiratory failure because of the risk of hypoventilation. Advantages to PSV include increased patient comfort, decreased WOB (because inspiratory efforts are augmented), decreased oxygen consumption (because inspiratory work is reduced), and increased endurance conditioning (because the patient is exercising respiratory muscles).[42,43]

Pressure-Controlled Inverse Ratio Ventilation. *Pressure-controlled inverse ratio ventilation* (PC-IRV) combines pressure-limited ventilation with an inverse ratio of inspiration (I) to expiration (E). The I/E ratio is the ratio of duration of inspiration (I) to the duration of expiration (E). This value is normally <1. With IRV the I/E ratio approaches 1. With IRV a prolonged positive pressure is applied, increasing inspiratory time. IRV progressively expands collapsed alveoli. The short expiratory time has a PEEP-like effect, preventing alveolar collapse. Because IRV imposes a nonphysiologic breathing pattern, the patient requires sedation or paralysis. IRV is indicated for patients with acute respiratory distress syndrome (ARDS) who continue to have refractory hypoxemia despite high levels of PEEP. Not all patients with poor oxygenation respond to IRV.

Other Ventilatory Maneuvers

Positive End-Expiratory Pressure. **Positive end-expiratory pressure** (PEEP) is a ventilatory maneuver in which positive pressure is applied to the airway during exhalation. Normally during exhalation, airway pressure drops to zero, and exhalation occurs passively. With PEEP, exhalation remains passive, but pressure falls to a preset level greater than zero, often 3 to 20 cm H_2O. With PEEP, lung volume during expiration and between breaths is greater than normal. Thus PEEP increases functional residual capacity (FRC), and this often improves oxygenation. The mechanisms by which PEEP increases FRC and oxygenation include increased aeration of patent alveoli, aeration of previously collapsed alveoli, and prevention of alveolar collapse throughout the respiratory cycle.[43]

PEEP is prescribed in increments of 2 to 5 cm H_2O and is titrated to the point that oxygenation improves without compromising hemodynamics.[43] This is termed best or optimal PEEP. Often 5 cm H_2O PEEP (referred to as *physiologic PEEP*) is used prophylactically to replace the glottic mechanism, help maintain a normal FRC, and prevent alveolar collapse. PEEP of 5 cm H_2O is also used for patients with a history of alveolar collapse during weaning. PEEP has demonstrated improvements in gas exchange, vital capacity, and inspiratory force when used during weaning.

In general, the major purpose of PEEP is to maintain or improve oxygenation while limiting risk of oxygen toxicity. FIO_2 can often be reduced when PEEP is used. PEEP is thought to be useful in pulmonary edema, providing a counterpressure opposing fluid extravasation. PEEP is indicated in lungs with diffuse disease, severe hypoxemia unresponsive to FIO_2 >50%, and loss of compliance or stiffness. The classic indication for PEEP therapy is ARDS (see Chapter 66). PEEP is generally contraindicated or used with extreme caution in patients with highly compliant lungs (e.g., COPD), unilateral or nonuniform disease, hypovolemia, and low CO. In these situations the adverse effects of PEEP may outweigh any benefits.

Continuous Positive Airway Pressure. **Continuous positive airway pressure** (CPAP) restores FRC and is similar to PEEP. However, the pressure in CPAP is delivered continuously during spontaneous breathing, thus preventing the patient's airway pressure from falling to zero. For example, if CPAP is 5 cm H_2O, airway pressure during expiration is 5 cm H_2O. During inspiration, 1 to 2 cm H_2O of negative pressure is generated, thus reducing airway pressure to 3 or 4 cm H_2O. The patient receiving SIMV with PEEP receives CPAP when breathing spontaneously. CPAP is commonly used in the treatment of obstructive sleep apnea. CPAP can be administered by a tight-fitting mask or an ET or tracheal tube. CPAP increases work of breathing because the patient must forcibly exhale against the CPAP and so must be used with caution in patients with myocardial compromise.

High-Frequency Ventilation. **High-frequency ventilation** (HFV) involves delivery of a small tidal volume (usually 1 to 5 ml per kg of body weight) at rapid respiratory rates (100 to 300 breaths per minute) in an effort to recruit and maintain lung volume and reduce intrapulmonary shunting (see Chapter 66). One benefit of HFV may be the ability to support gas exchange while minimizing the risk of barotrauma. HFV has been widely accepted in neonatal and pediatric ICUs, but its use in adults is still considered investigational and limited to patients with ARDS.[44]

There are three types of HFV. *High-frequency jet ventilation (HFJV)* delivers humidified gas from a high pressure source through a small-bore cannula positioned in the airway. With HFJV, precise V_T is difficult to predict and is a function of numerous variables. *High-frequency percussive ventilation (HFPV)* attempts to combine the positive effects of both HFV and conventional mechanical ventilation. A piston mechanism positioned at the end of the ET tube is driven by a high-pressure gas supply at a rate of 200 to 900 beats per minute. These high-frequency beats are superimposed on a conventional pressure-controlled ventilator mode.[44] *High-frequency oscillatory ventilation (HFOV)* uses a diaphragm or a piston in the ventilator to generate vibrations (or oscillations) of subphysiologic volumes of gas. HFOV can produce respiratory frequencies in excess of 3000 breaths per minute.[44] Patients receiving HFV must be paralyzed to suppress spontaneous respiration. In addition, patients must receive concurrent sedation and analgesia as necessary adjuncts when inducing paralysis (see Chapter 66).

Partial Liquid Ventilation. Currently, clinical trials are investigating the use of perflubron (LiquiVent) in **partial liquid ventilation** (PLV) for patients with ARDS. Perflubron is an inert, biocompatible, clear, odorless liquid derived from organic compounds that has an affinity for both oxygen and carbon dioxide and surfactant-like qualities.[45] Perflubron is trickled down a specially designed ET tube through a side port into the lungs of a mechanically ventilated patient. The amount used is usually equivalent to a patient's FRC. Perflubron evaporates quickly and must be replaced to maintain a constant level during the therapy (usually 3 to 5 days). Patients receiving PLV need close observation. Frequent assessment of vital signs, ABGs, and continuous SpO_2 and SvO_2 monitoring are required before, during, and after PLV. PLV has demonstrated few detrimental effects on hemodynamics and may evolve as an important adjunct in the management of ARDS.[45]

Complications of Positive Pressure Ventilation

Although mechanical ventilation may be essential to maintain ventilation and oxygenation, it can cause adverse effects. It is often difficult to distinguish complications of mechanical ventilation from the underlying disease.

Cardiovascular System. PPV can affect circulation because of the transmission of increased mean airway pressure to the thoracic cavity. With increased intrathoracic pressure, thoracic vessels are compressed. This results in decreased venous return to the heart, decreased left ventricular end-diastolic volume (preload), decreased CO, and hypotension. Mean airway pressure is further increased if titrating PEEP to improve oxygenation.

If the lungs are noncompliant (as in ARDS), airway pressures are not as easily transmitted to the heart and blood vessels. Thus effects of PPV on CO are reduced. Conversely, with compliant lungs (e.g., emphysema), there is increased danger of transmission of high airway pressures and negative effects on hemodynamics.

Compromise of venous return by PPV is exaggerated by hypovolemia (e.g., hemorrhage, multiple trauma) and decreased venous tone (e.g., sepsis, spinal shock). Restoration and maintenance of the circulating blood volume are important in minimizing cardiovascular complications.

Pulmonary System

Barotrauma. As lung inflation pressures increase, risk of *barotrauma* increases. Patients with compliant lungs (e.g., COPD) are at greater risk for barotrauma because the increased airway pressure readily distends the lungs and may rupture alveoli or emphysematous blebs. Patients with stiff lungs (e.g., ARDS) who are given high inspiratory pressures and high levels of PEEP and patients with suppurative lung abscesses resulting from necrotizing organisms (e.g., staphylococci) are also susceptible to barotrauma.

Air can escape into the pleural space from alveoli or interstitium, accumulate, and become trapped. Pleural pressure increases and collapses the lung, causing pneumothorax. (Clinical manifestations of pneumothorax are discussed in Chapter 27.) The lung receives air during inspiration but cannot expel it during expiration. Respiratory bronchioles are larger on inspiration than expiration. They may close on expiration, and air becomes trapped. With PPV, a simple pneumothorax can become a life-threatening tension pneumothorax. With tension pneumothorax, the mediastinum and contralateral lung are compressed, compromising CO. Immediate treatment of the pneumothorax is required.

Pneumomediastinum usually begins with rupture of alveoli into the lung interstitium; progressive air movement then occurs into the mediastinum and subcutaneous neck tissue. This is commonly followed by pneumothorax. Occurrence of new, unexplained subcutaneous emphysema is an indication for immediate chest x-ray. Pneumomediastinum and subcutaneous emphysema in the neck may be too small to be detected radiographically or clinically before the development of a pneumothorax.

Volu-pressure trauma. The concept of *volu-pressure trauma* in PPV relates to the lung injury that occurs when large tidal volumes are used to ventilate noncompliant lungs (e.g., ARDS). Volu-pressure trauma results in alveolar fractures and movement of fluids and proteins into the alveolar spaces. To limit this complication, it is recommended that smaller tidal volumes or pressure ventilation be used in patients with stiff lungs. A recent development in ventilator technology is a *volume-assured pressure mode*. This mode combines the advantages of pressure ventilation while ensuring a preset tidal volume on a breath-to-breath basis.[42]

Alveolar hypoventilation. *Hypoventilation* can be caused by inappropriate ventilator settings, leakage of air from the ventilator tubing or around the ET tube or tracheostomy cuff, lung secretions or obstruction, and low ventilation/perfusion ratio. Low V_T or respiratory rate decreases minute ventilation, causing hypoventilation. A leaking cuff or tubing that is not secured may cause air leakage, lowering the delivered V_T. Too low a SIMV rate in a patient who is unable to produce adequate spontaneous respirations causes hypoventilation, respiratory acidosis, and additional problems related to acidosis such as cardiac arrhythmias. Excess lung secretions can cause hypoventilation. Turning the patient every 1 to 2 hours, providing chest physical therapy to lung areas with increased secretions, encouraging deep breathing and coughing, and suctioning as needed can alleviate this. Atelectasis may develop. Increasing the V_T, adding small increments of PEEP, and adding a preset number of sighs to the ventilator settings lessen the likelihood of atelectasis.

Alveolar hyperventilation. Respiratory alkalosis can occur if the respiratory rate or V_T is set too high (*mechanical overventilation*) or if the patient receiving assisted ventilation is *hyperventilating*. It is easy to overventilate a patient on PPV. Particularly at risk are patients with chronic alveolar hypoventilation and CO_2 retention (e.g., patients with COPD). The patient with COPD may have a chronic $PaCO_2$ elevation (acidosis) and compensatory bicarbonate retention by the kidneys. When the patient is ventilated, the patient's "normal baseline" rather than the standard normal values should be the therapeutic goal. If the COPD patient is returned to a standard normal $PaCO_2$, the patient will develop alkalosis because of the retained bicarbonate. Such a patient could move from compensated respiratory acidosis to serious metabolic alkalosis. The presence of alkalosis makes weaning from the ventilator difficult. Alkalosis, especially if the onset is abrupt, can have additional serious consequences, including hypokalemia, hypocalcemia, and arrhythmias. Neuromuscular irritability, seizures, coma, and death can occur. Usually the patient with COPD who is supported on the ventilator does better with a short inspiratory and longer expiratory time.

If hyperventilation is spontaneous, it is important to determine the cause and treat it. Causes might include hypoxemia, pain, fear, anxiety, or compensation for metabolic acidosis. Patients who fight the ventilator or breathe out of synchrony may be anxious or in pain. If the patient is anxious and fearful, sitting with the patient and verbally coaching the patient to breathe with the ventilator may help. If these measures fail, manually ventilating the patient slowly with 100% oxygen source may slow breathing enough to bring it in synchrony with the ventilator.

Ventilator-associated pneumonia. The risk for iatrogenic pneumonia is highest in patients requiring PPV because the ET or tracheostomy tube bypasses normal upper airway defenses. In addition, poor nutritional state, immobility, and the underlying disease process (e.g., immunosuppression, organ failure) make the patient more prone to infection. The prevalence of *ventilator-associated pneumonia (VAP)* has been reported to range from 5.6 to 21.1 cases per 1000 ventilator days. In addition, patients who develop VAP have significantly longer hospital stays and higher mortality rates than those who do not develop VAP.[46]

In patients receiving prolonged PPV, sputum cultures often grow gram-negative bacteria such as *Pseudomonas*, *Serratia*, and *Klebsiella*. These are abundant in the hospital environment and the patient's GI tract. Organisms can spread in a number of ways, including contaminated respiratory equipment, inadequate hand washing, adverse environmental factors such as poor room ventilation and high traffic flow, and decreased patient ability to cough and clear secretions. Colonization of the oropharynx tract by gram-negative organisms is a predisposing factor in the development of gram-negative pneumonia.

Clinical evidence suggesting VAP includes fever, elevated white blood cell count, purulent sputum, odorous sputum, crackles or rhonchi on auscultation, and pulmonary infiltrates noted on chest x-ray. The patient is treated with antibiotics after appropriate cultures are taken by tracheal suctioning or bronchoscopy and when infection is evident.

Infection can be minimized by using strict aseptic technique while suctioning or handling the artificial airway (see earlier section, Nursing Management: Artificial Airway on p. 1777). Frequent hand washing is imperative. The nurse should wear latex or other impermeable gloves when in contact with the patient or equipment and change gloves between activities (e.g., bathing the patient, administering an intravenous drug). Finally, condensation that collects in the ventilator tubing should be drained away from the patient as it collects.

Sodium and Water Imbalance. Progressive fluid retention often occurs after 48 to 72 hours of PPV. PPV, especially with PEEP, is associated with decreased urinary output and increased sodium retention. Fluid balance changes may be due to decreased CO, which in turn results in diminished renal perfusion. Consequently, renin release is stimulated with subsequent production of angiotensin and aldosterone (Fig. 43-4). This results in sodium and water retention. It is also possible that pressure changes within the thorax are associated with decreased release of atrial natriuretic peptide, also causing sodium retention. Mild water retention is also associated with PPV. There is less insensible water loss via the airway because ventilated delivered gases are humidified with body temperature water. In addition, as a part of the stress response, release of antidiuretic hormone and cortisol may be increased, contributing to sodium and water retention.

Neurologic System. In patients with head injury, PPV, especially with PEEP, can impair cerebral blood flow. This is related to increased intrathoracic positive pressure impeding venous drainage from the head, as evidenced by jugular venous distention. As a result of the impaired venous return and increase in cerebral volume, the patient may exhibit increases in intracranial pressure. Elevating the head of the bed and keeping the patient's head in alignment may decrease the deleterious effects of PPV on intracranial pressure.

Gastrointestinal System. Patients receiving PPV are often stressed because of serious illness, immobility, and discomforts associated with the ventilator. Thus the ventilated patient is at risk for developing stress ulcers and GI bleeding. Patients with a preexisting ulcer or those receiving corticosteroid therapy are at an especially increased risk. Any kind of circulatory compromise, including reduction of CO caused by PPV, may contribute to ischemia of the gastric and intestinal mucosa and possibly increase the risk of translocation of GI bacteria.[6]

Prophylactic administration of histamine H$_2$-receptor blockers (e.g., ranitidine [Zantac]) or proton pump inhibitors (e.g., omeprazole [Prilosec]) decrease gastric acidity and diminish the risk of stress ulcer and hemorrhage. Target gastric pH is >5. Specially designed feeding tubes with a pH-sensitive probe allow for the measurement of gastric pH. Other methods of assessment include checking the pH of gastric aspirates.

Gastric and bowel dilation may occur as a result of gas accumulation in the GI tract from swallowed air. The irritation of an artificial airway may cause excessive air swallowing and subsequent gastric dilation. Gastric or bowel dilation may put pressure on the vena cava, decrease CO, and prohibit adequate diaphragmatic excursion during spontaneous breathing. Elevation of the diaphragm as a result of paralytic ileus or bowel dilation leads to compression of the lower lobes of the lungs, which may cause atelectasis and compromise respiratory function. Decompression of the stomach can be accomplished by the insertion of an NG tube.

Immobility, sedation, circulatory impairment, decreased oral intake, use of opioid pain medications, and stress contribute to decreased peristalsis. The patient's inability to exhale against a closed glottis may make defecation difficult. As a result, the ventilated patient could be predisposed to constipation. With the early use of enteral nutrition, constipation is usually not a problem.

Musculoskeletal System. Maintenance of muscle strength and prevention of the problems associated with immobility are important. Exercise tolerance is enhanced by adequate analgesia and adequate nutrition. Progressive ambulation of patients receiving long-term PPV can be attained without interruption of mechanical ventilation. The ventilator can be pushed around the room, or the patient can be manually ventilated with a BVM device while ambulating. Passive and active exercises, consisting of movements to maintain muscle tone in the upper and lower extremities, should be done in bed. Simple maneuvers such as leg lifts, knee bends, quadriceps setting, or arm circles are appropriate. Prevention of contractures, pressure ulcers, footdrop, and external rotation of the hip and legs by proper positioning is important.

Psychosocial Needs. The patient receiving mechanical ventilation may experience physical and emotional stress. In addition to the problems related to critical care patients discussed at the beginning of this chapter, the patient supported by a mechanical ventilator is unable to speak, eat, move, or breathe normally. Tubes and machines may cause pain, fear, and anxiety. Ordinary activities of daily living such as eating, elimination, and coughing are extremely complicated.

In studying the psychosocial needs of ICU patients, one researcher discovered that feeling safe was an overpowering need of ICU patients. In addition, four related needs were the need to know (information), the need to regain control, the need to hope, and the need to trust. Patients reported that when these needs were met, they felt safe.[47] The nurse should work to strengthen the various factors that affect feeling safe. Communication must be creative in the case of the intubated patient and information must be forthright. Patients should be involved in decision making as much as possible. The nurse should encourage hope and build trusting relationships with the patient and family.[47]

Patients receiving PPV usually require some type of sedation (e.g., propofol [Diprivan]) and/or analgesia (e.g., fentanyl) to facilitate optimal ventilation. Before initiating sedation and/or analgesia in the mechanically ventilated patient who is agitated or anxious, it is important to assess for the cause of distress. Common problems that can result in patient agitation or anxiety include PPV, nutritional deficits, pain, hypoxemia, hypercapnia, drugs, and environmental stressors (e.g., sleep deprivation).[48]

At times the decision is made to paralyze the patient with a neuromuscular blocking agent (e.g., pancuronium [Pavulon]) to provide more effective synchrony with the ventilator and increased oxygenation. If the patient is paralyzed, the nurse should remember that the patient can hear, see, smell, think, and feel. Intravenous sedation and analgesia must always be administered concurrently when the patient is paralyzed. Many patients have few memories of their time in the ICU, whereas others remember vivid details.[47] Although appearing to be asleep, sedated, or paralyzed, patients may be aware of their surroundings and should always be addressed as though awake and alert.

Machine Disconnection or Malfunction. Mechanical ventilators may become disconnected or malfunction. When turned on and operative, alarms alert the nurse to problems. Most deaths from accidental ventilator disconnection occur while the alarm is turned off, and most accidental disconnections in critical care settings are discovered by low-pressure alarm activation. The most frequent site for disconnection is between the tracheal tube and the adapter. Connections should be pushed together and then twisted to secure more tightly. The nurse should ascertain that alarms are set at all times and should chart that this is the case. Alarms can be paused (not inactivated) during suctioning or removal from the ventilator.

Ventilator malfunction may also occur and may be related to several factors. Although most institutions have emergency generators in the event of a power failure, the nurse should always consider the possibility that power may fail and have a plan for manually ventilating all the patients who are dependent on a ventilator. If, at any time, the nurse determines that the ventilator is malfunctioning (e.g., failure of oxygen supply), the patient should be disconnected from the machine and manually ventilated with 100% oxygen until the ventilator is fixed or replaced.

Nutritional Therapy: Patient Receiving Positive Pressure Ventilation

PPV and the hypermetabolism associated with critical illness can contribute to inadequate nutrition. Presence of an ET tube eliminates the normal route for eating. Although patients who are nasotracheally intubated may be allowed liquid and semiliquid feedings orally, it is difficult to ingest sufficient calories, protein, and fat. A patient with a tracheostomy can eat normally once the stoma has healed. When a tracheostomy tube is present, the patient should tilt the head slightly forward to facilitate swallowing and to prevent aspiration. Often, soft foods (e.g., puddings, ice cream) are more easily swallowed than liquids.

Patients likely to be without food for 3 to 5 days should have a nutritional program initiated. Inadequate nutrition makes the patient receiving prolonged mechanical ventilation more prone to poor oxygen transport secondary to anemia and to poor tolerance of minimal exercise. Poor nutrition and the disuse of respiratory muscles contribute to decreased respiratory muscle strength. In addition, the hypermetabolism associated with critical illness, trauma, and surgery and the presence of anxiety, pain, and increased WOB greatly increase caloric expenditure. Serum protein levels (e.g., albumin, prealbumin, transferrin, total protein) are usually decreased. Inadequate nutrition can delay weaning, decrease resistance to infection, and decrease the speed of recovery.[49] Enteral feeding via a small-bore feeding tube is the preferred method to meet caloric needs of ventilated patients (see Chapter 39 for discussion of enteral feeding).

A concern regarding the nutritional support of patients receiving PPV is the carbohydrate content of the diet. Metabolism of carbohydrates can contribute to an increase in serum CO_2 levels. The resulting CO_2 load results in a higher required minute ventilation. This, in turn, can cause an increase in WOB. Limiting carbohydrate content in the diet may lower CO_2 production. Preparations such as Pulmocare, which are high in protein and fat but low in carbohydrate content, may be beneficial to ventilated patients. The dietitian can provide useful consultation for the ventilated patient.

Weaning from Positive Pressure Ventilation and Extubation

The process of reducing ventilator support and resuming spontaneous ventilation is termed **weaning.** The weaning process differs for patients requiring short-term ventilation (≤ 3 days) versus long-term ventilation (>3 days). Patients requiring short-term ventilation (e.g., after cardiac surgery) will experience a linear weaning process. Patients likely to require prolonged PPV (e.g., patients with COPD who develop respiratory failure) will most likely experience a weaning process that consists of peaks and valleys.[50] Conceptually, preparation for weaning should begin when PPV is initiated and should involve a team approach (e.g., nurse, physician, patient, family, respiratory therapist, dietitian, physical therapist).[51]

Weaning can be viewed as consisting of three phases: the *preweaning phase,* the *weaning process,* and the *outcome phase.* The preweaning or assessment phase determines the patient's ability to breathe spontaneously. Assessment in this phase depends on a combination of respiratory (see Table 64-10) and nonrespiratory factors. Standard respiratory weaning criteria assess muscle strength (negative inspiratory pressure [NIP] and positive expiratory pressure [PEP]) and endurance (spontaneous tidal volume [SV_T] and vital capacity [VC]).[50,52] In addition, the patient's lungs should be reasonably clear on auscultation and chest x-ray. Nonrespiratory factors include the assessment of the patient's neurologic status, hemodynamics, fluid and electrolytes/acid-base balance, nutrition, and hemoglobin.[51] It is important to have an alert, well-rested, and well-informed patient relatively free from pain who can cooperate with the weaning plan. This does not mean complete withdrawal from sedatives or analgesics. Instead, drugs should be titrated to achieve comfort without causing excessive drowsiness.

A variety of weaning modes is available, and no single method is superior. All methods can be delivered with the patient remaining connected to the ventilator circuit. The patient receiving SIMV can have the ventilator breaths gradually reduced as the patient's ventilatory status permits. CPAP or PSV can be added to SIMV. Another method involves PSV, CPAP, or both delivered without SIMV. PSV is thought to provide gentle, slow respiratory muscle conditioning and may be especially beneficial for patients who are deconditioned or have cardiac problems. Some patients may be weaned by simply providing humidified oxygen (T-piece or flow-by method).[50]

Weaning is usually carried out during the day, with the patient ventilated at night. Regardless of the weaning mode selected, all team members should be familiar with the weaning plan. For example, a weaning plan using CPAP might involve placing the patient on CPAP at 0 cm H_2O for up to 2 hours (as tolerated). CPAP trials may be scheduled twice a day, with the second trial scheduled 6 hours after the first. Extubation is considered once the patient can tolerate 2 hours of CPAP.[50] Regardless of the method used, it is important to permit the patient's respiratory muscles to rest between weaning trials. Once the respiratory muscles become fatigued, they may require 12 to 24 hours to recover.

The patient being weaned and the family should be provided continuing psychologic support. The weaning process should be explained, and the patient and family informed of progress. The patient should be placed in a sitting or semirecumbent position and made comfortable. Baseline vital signs and respiratory parameters are measured (V_T, NIP, PEP, VC, SpO_2). During the weaning trial, the patient must be monitored closely for noninvasive criteria that may signal intolerance and result in cessation of the trial (e.g., tachypnea, dyspnea, tachycardia, arrhythmias, sustained desaturation [SpO_2 <91%], hypertension or hypotension, agitation, diaphoresis, anxiety, sustained V_T <5 ml/kg, changes in level of consciousness).[50] Documentation of the patient's tolerance throughout the weaning process is important and should include statements regarding the patient and family's perceptions.

The weaning outcome phase refers to the period when weaning stops and the patient is extubated or weaning is stopped because no further progress is being made. The patient who is ready for *extubation* (tube removal) should receive hyperoxygenation and suctioning (e.g., oropharynx, ET tube). The patient should be instructed to take a deep breath, and at the peak of inspiration, the cuff should be deflated and the tube removed in one motion.[53] After removal, the patient should be encouraged to deep breathe and cough, and the pharynx should be suctioned as needed. Supplemental oxygen should be applied and naso-oral care provided. The nurse must carefully monitor the patient's vital signs, respiratory status, and oxygenation immediately following extubation, within 1 hour, and per institutional policy.[53] If the patient cannot tolerate extubation, immediate reintubation may be necessary.

Home Mechanical Ventilation

Mechanical ventilators are no longer limited to the ICU but are now a part of home care.[54] In some instances, terminally ill, ventilated patients may be discharged to hospice.[55] In either case, the emphasis on controlling hospital health care costs has increased the early discharge of patients and the need to provide highly technical care such as mechanical ventilation in home settings.[56] The success of home mechanical ventilation will depend, in part, on careful predischarge assessment and planning.

Both negative pressure and positive pressure ventilators can be used in the home. Negative pressure ventilators are often the ventilator of choice because they do not require an artificial airway and are less complicated to use. Several types of small, portable (battery-powered) positive pressure ventilators are available and can be attached to a wheelchair or placed on a bedside table. Settings and alarms on these ventilators are similar to the standard ventilators used in ICUs.[56]

Home mechanical ventilation has advantages and disadvantages. Having the patient in the home eliminates the strain that the hospital setting may impose on family dynamics. The feeling of helplessness by family members when they first hear about the necessity for long-term mechanical ventilation is frequently countered by the ability of the family to participate fully in the patient's care in the home setting. At home the patient may be able to participate more in activities of daily living around a more individualized schedule and, because of the smaller size of the home ventilator, be more mobile.[54] Another advantage of home

mechanical ventilation is the reduction in the patient's risk of nosocomial infection.

Disadvantages of home mechanical ventilation include problems related to reimbursement, equipment, caregiver stress, and the complex needs of these patients. Ventilated patients are usually dependent, requiring extensive nursing care, at least initially. Disposable products may be nonreimbursable. Financial resources must be carefully assessed when arranging home mechanical ventilation, and a consultation with a social worker should be initiated. Another disadvantage of home mechanical ventilation is its potential impact on the family. Family members may seem enthusiastic about caring for their loved one in the home but may be motivated by numerous, complex factors. They may lack understanding of the potential sacrifices they may have to make financially and in personal time and commitment. Families should be encouraged to consider respite care to periodically relieve caregiver stress and strain.[56]

NURSING MANAGEMENT
MECHANICAL VENTILATION

Nursing management of the patient receiving mechanical ventilation is presented in NCP 64-1.

OTHER CRITICAL CARE CONTENT

Table 64-13 lists additional critical care content presented in other chapters of this book.

TABLE 64-13	Cross-References to Other Critical Care Content
TOPIC	**DISCUSSED IN CHAPTER**
Acute congestive heart failure	34
Acute respiratory distress syndrome	66
Acute respiratory failure	66
Advanced cardiac life support	35
Burns	24
Cardiac arrhythmias	35
Cardiac pacemakers	35
Cardiac surgery	34
Cardiopulmonary resuscitation	35
Emergencies	67
Enteral nutrition	39
Head injury, including ICP monitoring	55
Myocardial infarction	33
Multiple organ dysfunction syndrome	65
Oxygen delivery	28
Pulmonary edema	34
Renal dialysis, including renal replacement therapy	45
Shock	65
Systemic inflammatory response syndrome	65
Total parenteral nutrition	39
Tracheostomy	26
Trauma	67

ICP, Intracranial pressure.

NURSING CARE PLAN 64-1

Patient Receiving Mechanical Ventilation

EXPECTED PATIENT OUTCOMES	NURSING INTERVENTIONS and *RATIONALES*

NURSING DIAGNOSIS

Risk for injury *related to* artificial airway, possible machine malfunction, accidental disconnection or extubation, inability to breathe unassisted, asynchrony with ventilator, and settings ineffective in maintaining adequate oxygenation.

- ABGs within normal range for patient
- Early detection of signs and symptoms of ↓ PaO$_2$ and ↑ PaCO$_2$
- Synchronous breathing with ventilator
- Early detection, correction, or prevention of complications associated with mechanical malfunction or disconnection
- Properly placed and patent artificial airway with appropriate cuff pressure

- Monitor for risk factors such as hypoxemia, hypercapnia, tachycardia, tachypnea, ↑ BP, agitation, confusion, pain, lethargy, cyanosis; respiratory pattern asynchronous with machine's pattern of ventilation; machine malfunction or disconnection *to determine presence of risk factors and plan for appropriate intervention.*
- Begin mechanical ventilation slowly (especially in patients with COPD); lower PaCO$_2$ only to patient's baseline level *to prevent alkalosis, especially in patient with compensated respiratory acidosis.*
- Assess patient for possible causes of hyperventilation such as retained secretions, hypoxemia, pain, fear, and anxiety *in order to treat appropriately.*
- Check ventilator settings (FIO$_2$, respiratory rate, V$_T$, O$_2$ flow rate, PEEP, airway pressure, thermistor temperature, and I:E ratio) *to determine if appropriate to clinical situation.*
- Keep BVM device connected to O$_2$ source at bedside *for use in case of an emergency.*
- If patient is fighting ventilation, slowly bag for three to six breaths and verbally coach patient to breathe *to help synchronize patient with ventilator.*
- If asynchrony persists, consider chemical paralysis and sedation and analgesia *to facilitate effective ventilation.*
- Turn all alarms on; pause, but do not turn off alarms during suctioning and disconnections *to prevent unnoticed ventilator malfunction.*
- Respond immediately to all alarms *because potentially dangerous situations of mechanical malfunction, accidental disconnection or extubation, or patient asynchrony with the ventilator may be present.*
- Check ET tube for proper placement and cuff for proper pressure and/or leaks *to prevent loss of ventilation gas and aspiration of oral secretions and to avoid inadvertent dislodgment of the ET tube.*
- Monitor ventilator tubing q1-2hr for condensed water and drain *to prevent aspiration of accumulated fluid.*
- Immobilize patient's hands with soft wrist restraints if needed *to prevent inadvertent extubation by the patient.*
- Use bite block or oral airway *to keep patient from biting and obstructing the ET tube opening.*

NURSING DIAGNOSIS

Decreased cardiac output *related to* impeded venous return by PPV *as manifested by* ↓ BP, ↓ SV and PAWP, ↑ heart rate, decreased urine output, presence of arrhythmias, mental confusion.

- BP and CO within normal range or patient's normal baseline
- Adequate urinary output

- Monitor vital signs and level of consciousness q1-4hr *to track trends.*
- Observe and monitor for clinical manifestations of ↓ CO *to identify decreased venous return to the heart, decreased left ventricular end-diastolic volume, and lowered BP.*
- Monitor hemodynamic parameters, especially when >10 cm H$_2$O of PEEP is used *to anticipate need for plasma expanders, vasopressors, and intravenous fluids as ordered because hemodynamic complications of decreased venous return induced by PPV are exaggerated by hypovolemia.*

NURSING DIAGNOSIS

Ineffective airway clearance *related to* presence of artificial airway, problems with positioning, accumulation of secretions, and immobility *as manifested by* presence of abnormal breath sounds, absent cough, presence of thick or copious secretions.

- Normal breath sounds
- Thin and easily removed secretions

- Change patient's position q2hr and perform postural drainage, vibration, and percussion maneuvers when indicated *to prevent pooling of secretions in the lungs.*
- Have patient cough and, if feasible, deep breathe q2hr *to remove secretions and to prevent hypoventilation.*
- Suction oropharynx q1-2hr and as needed *to remove pooled secretions.*
- Perform tracheobronchial suctioning *to remove retained secretions and improve oxygenation* (see Table 64-9).
- Assess breath sounds and other respiratory parameters (e.g., SpO$_2$, SvO$_2$, V$_T$, respiratory rate) q2-4hr *to monitor trends and effectiveness of interventions.*
- Assess for adequate systemic hydration and provide supplemental humidification of ventilator-delivered gases *because these will assist with the thinning of secretions.*

V_T, Tidal volume.

NURSING CARE PLAN 64-1

Patient Receiving Mechanical Ventilation—cont'd

EXPECTED PATIENT OUTCOMES	NURSING INTERVENTIONS and *RATIONALES*
NURSING DIAGNOSIS	**Impaired physical mobility** *related to* restricted movement *as manifested by* inability to perform active range-of-motion exercises, inability to get out of bed.
• Normal range of motion of joints • Absence of contractures, footdrop, pressure ulcer	• Perform active and passive range-of-motion exercises (e.g., leg lifts, knee bends, quadriceps setting, arm circles) *to maintain patient's joint and muscle functioning and improve circulation.* • Position patient properly *to prevent contractures and other musculoskeletal complications (e.g., external rotation of hips).* • Use footboard, high-top sneakers, and frequent foot flexion *to prevent foot drop.* • Change patient's position q2hr and assess skin *to maintain skin integrity and prevent the development of pressure ulcers.* • Get patient out of bed unless contraindicated *to improve circulation and oxygenation and facilitate exercises.* • Provide progressive ambulation for patients receiving long-term ventilation *to prevent complications of immobility.*
NURSING DIAGNOSIS	**Anxiety** *related to* clinical condition, pain, inability to communicate, and fear of death, suffocation, choking, and ICU environment *as manifested by* expression of feelings of anxiety, anxious appearance, agitation, rigid body posture.
• Effective communication of needs • Absent or manageable anxiety level	• Give simple, honest explanations regarding care and progress *to foster a realistic understanding of activities and to help patient make informed decisions and feel safe.* • When possible, allow patient to make decisions regarding all aspects of care *to help patient regain and maintain a sense of control.* • Provide patient with an appropriate means of communication (e.g., alphabet board) *to reduce anxiety associated with inability to speak and to provide means for patient to communicate anxieties.* • Provide for diversion (e.g., music therapy, pet therapy, occupational therapy) as desired and tolerated by the patient *to relieve anxiety.* • Keep call bell accessible to patient *to enable patient to call for assistance.* • Refer to psychiatric clinical nurse specialist, psychiatrist, and/or hospital chaplain when appropriate *to offer additional counseling and support.* • Be available to family; offer support and help *to lessen their anxiety and increase their cooperation.* • Administer and evaluate effectiveness of antianxiety medications and/or analgesics *to chemically manage patient's anxiety and/or pain.*
NURSING DIAGNOSIS	**Dysfunctional ventilatory weaning response** *related to* too-rapid pacing of weaning plan, insufficient knowledge of the weaning plan, and anxiety *as manifested by* restlessness, tachypnea, dyspnea, cyanosis, pallor, fatigue, ↑ or ↓ BP, use of accessory muscles, tachycardia, oxygen desaturation.
• Achievement of progressive weaning goals • Communication of increased comfort during weaning • Less tired from WOB • Remain extubated	• Assess respiratory parameters (e.g., negative inspiratory pressure, positive expiratory pressure, spontaneous tidal volume and vital capacity) *to determine patient's weaning ability.* • Explain the weaning process so that patient understands what is expected *to decrease anxiety and facilitate cooperation.* • Jointly negotiate progressive weaning goals *to provide patient a level of control in establishing the plan.* • Adopt a weaning pace that will ensure success and minimize setbacks *to maintain patient confidence.* • Monitor patient's tolerance during weaning trials (e.g., SpO_2, respirations, ECG, level of consciousness, ABGs) *to evaluate patient's weaning progress.* • Monitor for respiratory distress and place patient back on ventilator if observed *to ensure adequate ventilation.* • If the weaning process is discontinued, explain rationale and revised plan to patient *to minimize frustration and disappointment and enhance cooperation.*

Continued

NURSING CARE PLAN 64-1

Patient Receiving Mechanical Ventilation—cont'd

EXPECTED PATIENT OUTCOMES	NURSING INTERVENTIONS and *RATIONALES*
NURSING DIAGNOSIS	**Risk for infection** *related to* exposure to pathogens and loss of normal protective barrier to infection.
▪ No evidence of infection ▪ Negative sputum cultures	▪ Monitor for global signs of infection: change in color, quantity, odor, and viscosity of sputum; difficulty in suctioning secretions; increase in cough; fever; chills; diaphoresis; abnormal breath sounds (e.g., crackles, wheezing); tachycardia; deterioration of ABGs; flushing of skin; elevated white blood cell count; evidence of infiltrate or atelectasis on chest x-ray; positive sputum cultures *to determine if infection is present or developing.* ▪ Obtain sputum culture and order sensitivity test if secretions become purulent or tenacious, change color, or become odorous and/or obtain blood cultures if patient develops fever *to diagnose infectious agent.* ▪ Keep head of bed elevated (especially if receiving enteral nutrition) *to prevent aspiration.* ▪ Keep ventilator tubing cleared of condensed water *to eliminate source of infection.* ▪ Use sterile technique with suctioning (see Table 64-9) *to reduce the risk of infection.* ▪ Administer antiinfectives as ordered and monitor effectiveness (e.g., decrease in secretions, decrease in fever) *to determine efficacy of the drugs.*
NURSING DIAGNOSIS	**Imbalanced nutrition: less than body requirements** *related to* inability to take in adequate nourishment orally and increased caloric demands secondary to clinical condition and need for PPV *as manifested by* loss of 10% of body weight.*

COLLABORATIVE PROBLEMS

NURSING GOALS	NURSING INTERVENTIONS and *RATIONALES*
POTENTIAL COMPLICATION	**Barotrauma, volu-pressure trauma** *related to* PPV.
▪ Monitor for signs of pneumothorax, pneumomediastinum, subcutaneous emphysema ▪ Monitor for changes in breath sounds ▪ Report positive findings ▪ Carry out appropriate emergency interventions as needed	▪ Record level of peak inspiratory pressure *to establish baseline data to evaluate changes in lung compliance.* ▪ Observe for sudden increase (by 5 cm H_2O or more) in peak inspiratory pressure, sudden patient agitation or coughing, frequent activation of high-pressure alarm, decrease in compliance, palpable subcutaneous emphysema over neck and anterior chest areas, deterioration in ABGs and BP, decrease or absence of breath sounds, hyperresonance on percussion; pneumothorax on chest x-ray *to detect consequences of barotrauma.* ▪ Determine minimal tidal volume needed for adequate ventilation *to limit risk of volu-pressure trauma.* ▪ Ventilate with a BVM with 100% O_2 *to reduce airway pressures until a chest tube can be inserted.* ▪ Notify physician and set up for chest tube insertion immediately *because pneumothorax can convert to a life-threatening tension pneumothorax.* ▪ Check and record ventilator settings q2hr *to maintain accuracy.*
POTENTIAL COMPLICATION	**Gastric distention** *related to* improper ET tube placement, GI bleeding, or ileus.
▪ Perform abdominal assessment q4hr ▪ Report deviations from expected findings	▪ Assess for abdominal distention, tympany, and bowel sounds and measure abdominal girth *to detect signs of bowel dilation and/or ileus.* ▪ Test stools and gastric drainage for occult blood *because the patient is at risk of developing stress ulcers and GI bleeding.* ▪ Check for gastric air on chest x-ray *to confirm or eliminate suspicions.* ▪ Administer H_2-receptor blocker, proton pump inhibitor, and tube feedings as ordered *to reduce the occurrence of GI bleeding and to decrease the acidity of gastric secretions.* ▪ If abdominal distention is present, elevate head of bed *to allow for optimal diaphragmatic excursion.* ▪ Obtain order and place NG tube or, if present, confirm patency by irrigating *to relieve gastric tension.* ▪ Confirm correct position of NG tube *to prevent aspiration and the accumulation of GI fluids.*

*Interventions for this nursing diagnosis are presented in the nursing care plan for the patient with acute respiratory failure (NCP 66-1) on pp. 1832-1833.

CRITICAL THINKING EXERCISES

Case Study
Critical Care and Mechanical Ventilation

Patient Profile. An older man was found lying on the street by the police. He had no identification on him. He was unconscious on admission and remains unconscious. He has an ET tube in place and is receiving mechanical ventilation. He weighs 198 lb. An arterial line was placed for blood pressure monitoring. The nurses in the ICU call him Mr. R.

Subjective Data
None; patient is unresponsive to painful stimuli

Objective Data
Physical Examination
- Arterial blood pressure is 100/75; heart rate is 120 (uncontrolled atrial fibrillation); temperature is 102° F (38.8° C); SpO_2 is 98%
- Purulent secretions from ET tube
- Breath sounds: rhonchi bilaterally, decreased breath sounds on the right

Diagnostic Studies
- Chest x-ray reveals right lower lung consolidation
- ABGs: pH, 7.48; PaO_2, 94 mm Hg; $PaCO_2$, 30 mm Hg; HCO_3, 34 mEq/L

Collaborative Care
- Positive pressure ventilation settings: assist-control mode at 16 breaths per minute; tidal volume, 900 ml; FIO_2, 60%
- Enteral nutrition at 25 ml/hr via small-bore feeding tube
- Indwelling urinary catheter to bedside drainage
- Change position every 2 hours
- Perform chest physical therapy every 2 to 4 hours
- gentamycin (Garamycin) 80 mg IV q8hr
- ceftriaxone (Rocephin) 1 g IV q12hr
- D_5NS with KCl 20 mEq/L at 100 ml/hr

CRITICAL THINKING QUESTIONS

1. Identify two reasons for intubating and providing mechanical ventilation for Mr. R.
2. What do Mr. R.'s ABGs indicate, and which ventilator setting(s) should be changed?
3. What is his PaO_2/FIO_2 ratio, and what does it signify?
4. Mr. R.'s blood pressure drops to 80 mm Hg, and he remains in atrial fibrillation with a ventricular rate of 138. A PA catheter is inserted for hemodynamic monitoring. What would be the purpose of hemodynamic monitoring in this patient? Identify two major nursing considerations for a patient with a PA catheter.
5. Mr. R.'s initial PAWP is 14 mm Hg, CI is 2 L/min/m^2, and SVRI is 2667 dynes/sec/cm^{-5}/m^2. How would you interpret these values? What medical interventions might be considered?
6. Mr. R.'s pulmonary condition deteriorates. PaO_2 drops to 70 mm Hg, and SpO_2 is 89%. PEEP is added to the ventilator settings. What implications does this have for Mr. R. given his hemodynamic status?
7. Based on the data presented, identify two priority nursing diagnoses. Are there any collaborative problems?
8. After 6 days, Mr. R. remains unresponsive and is developing renal failure. The physician believes the situation is hopeless and wishes to discuss termination of life support. What approach should the nurse take in locating Mr. R.'s next of kin?
9. Based on the assessment data provided, write one or more nursing diagnoses. Are there any collaborative problems?

Nursing Research Issues

1. Are hemodynamic parameters obtained when patients are in a lateral (side-lying) position accurate?
2. How can communication be best facilitated in the mechanically ventilated patient?
3. What interventions can reduce the incidence of ventilator-associated pneumonia?
4. How can pet therapy be initiated safely and effectively in a critical care unit?

REVIEW QUESTIONS

The number of the question corresponds to the same-numbered objective at the beginning of the chapter.

1. Certification in critical care nursing by the American Association of Critical Care Nurses indicates that a nurse
   a. has earned a master's degree in the field of providing advanced critical care nursing.
   b. is an advanced practice nurse in the care of acutely ill patients.
   c. may practice independently to provide symptom management for the critically ill.
   d. has practiced in critical care and successfully completed a test of critical care knowledge.

2. An appropriate nursing intervention for the patient with delirium in the ICU is to
   a. use tranquilizers to establish normal sleep patterns.
   b. identify the factors contributing to the patient's confusion and irritability.
   c. silence all alarms, overhead paging, and conversations around the patient.
   d. sedate the patient with psychotropic drugs to protect the patient from harmful behaviors.

Continued

REVIEW QUESTIONS—cont'd

3. The critical care nurse recognizes that an ideal plan for family involvement includes
   a. a family member at the bedside at all times.
   b. allowing family at the bedside at preset, brief intervals.
   c. an individually devised plan with family involved with care and comfort measures.
   d. restriction of visiting in the ICU because the environment is overwhelming to visitors.

4. To establish hemodynamic monitoring for a patient, the nurse zeros the
   a. cardiac output monitoring system to the level of the left ventricle.
   b. pressure monitoring system to the level of the catheter tip located in the patient.
   c. pressure monitoring system to the level of the atrium, identified as the midaxillary line.
   d. pressure monitoring system to the level of the atrium, identified as the phlebostatic axis.

5. The hemodynamic changes the nurse expects to find after successful initiation of an intraaortic balloon pump in a patient in cardiogenic shock include
   a. decreased PAWP and increased CO.
   b. decreased SVR and decreased SV.
   c. increased diastolic BP and decreased systolic BP.
   d. decreased CVP and increased right atrial pressure.

6. The nursing management of a patient with an artificial airway includes
   a. routine suctioning of the tube at least every 2 hours.
   b. observing for cardiac arrhythmias during suctioning.
   c. maintaining ET tube cuff pressure at 30 cm H_2O.
   d. preventing tube dislodgment by limiting mouth care to lubrication of the lips.

7. The purpose of adding PEEP to positive pressure ventilation is to
   a. increase functional residual capacity and improve oxygenation.
   b. increase FIO_2 in an attempt to wean the patient and avoid oxygen toxicity.
   c. determine if the patient is able to be weaned and avoid the risk of pneumomediastinum.
   d. determine if the patient is in synchrony with the ventilator or needs to be paralyzed.

8. The nurse monitors the patient with positive pressure mechanical ventilation for
   a. paralytic ileus because pressure on the abdominal contents affects bowel motility.
   b. diuresis and sodium depletion because of increased release of atrial natriuretic peptide.
   c. signs of cardiovascular insufficiency because pressure in the chest impedes venous return.
   d. respiratory acidosis in a patient with COPD because of alveolar hyperventilation and increased PaO_2 levels.

REFERENCES

1. Nightingale F: *Notes on hospitals,* ed 3, London, 1863, Longman, Roberts, & Green.
*2. Lynaugh JE, Fairman J: *Critical care nursing: a history,* Philadelphia, 1998, University of Pennsylvania Press.
3. Goldhill DR, Summer A: Outcome of intensive care patients in a group of British intensive care units, *Crit Care Med* 26:1337, 1998.
4. Miller PA, Forbes S, Boyle DK: End-of-life care in the intensive care unit: a challenge for nurses, *Am J Crit Care* 10:230, 2001.
5. Bucher L, Melander S: Critical care across the health care continuum. In Bucher L, Melander S, editors: *Critical care nursing,* Philadelphia, 1999, Saunders.
6. Trujillo EB, Robinson MK, Jacobs DO: Feeding critically ill patients: current concepts, *Crit Care Nurse* 21:60, 2001.
*7. Frazier SK et al: Critical care nurses' assessment of patients' anxiety: reliance on physiological and behavioral parameters, *Am J Crit Care* 11:57, 2002.
8. White SK et al: A renaissance in critical care nursing: technological advances and sedation strategies, *Crit Care Nurse* 21(suppl):1, 2001.
*9. Keegan L: Alternative and complementary modalities for managing stress and anxiety in acute and critical care. In Chulay M, Molter NC, editors: *Protocols for practice: creating a healing environment,* Aliso Viejo, Calif, 1998, AACN.
*10. Stanik-Hutt J: Pain management in the acutely ill. In Chulay M, Molter NC, editors: *Protocols for practice: creating a healing environment,* Aliso Viejo, Calif, 1998, AACN.
*11. Kress JP et al: Daily interruption of sedative infusions in critically ill patients undergoing mechanical ventilation, *N Engl J Med* 342:1471, 2000.
12. Roberts BL: Managing delirium in adult intensive care patients, *Crit Care Nurse* 21:48, 2001.

13. Kahn DM et al: Identification and modification of environmental noise in an ICU setting, *Chest* 114:535, 1998.
*14. Richards KC et al: Promoting sleep in acute and critical care. In Chulay M, Molter NC, editors: *Protocols for practice: creating a healing environment,* Aliso Viejo, Calif, 1998, AACN.
15. Grozinger M et al: Effects of lorazepam on the automatic online evaluation of sleep EEG data in healthy volunteers, *Pharmacopsychiatry* 31:55, 1998.
16. Doherty MH et al: Impact of critical illness on the patient and family. In Bucher L, Melander S, editors: *Critical care nursing,* Philadelphia, 1999, WB Saunders.
*17. Titler MG: Family visitation and partnership in the critical care unit. In Chulay M, Molter NC, editors: *Protocols for practice: creating a healing environment,* Aliso Viejo, Calif, 1997, AACN.
18. Green ML: Legal and ethical issues in critical care nursing. In Bucher L, Melander S, editors: *Critical care nursing,* Philadelphia, 1999, WB Saunders.
*19. Titler MG, Drahozal R: Family pet visiting, animal-assisted activities, and animal-assisted therapy in critical care. In Chulay M, Molter NC, editors: *Protocols for practice: creating a healing environment,* Aliso Viejo, Calif, 1997, AACN.
20. Mitty EL: Ethnicity and end-of-life decision-making, *Reflec Nurs Leadersh* 27:28-31, 2001.
21. Germain C: Cultural issues in critical care nursing. In Bucher L, Melander S, editors: *Critical care nursing,* Philadelphia, 1999, WB Saunders.
*22. Arnone M: Single and multiple pressure transducer system. In Lynn-McHale DJ, Carlson KK, editors: *AACN procedure manual for critical care,* ed 4, Philadelphia, 2001, WB Saunders.
*23. Imperial-Perez F, McRae M: Arterial pressure monitoring. In Chulay M, Gawlinski A, editors: *Protocols for practice: hemodynamic monitoring,* Aliso Viejo, Calif, 1998, AACN.

*Nursing research–based reference.

*24. Shaffer RB: Arterial catheter insertion (assist), care, and removal. In Lynn-McHale DJ, Carlson KK, editors: *AACN procedure manual for critical care,* ed 4, Philadelphia, 2001, WB Saunders.

*25. Becker DE: Arterial catheter insertion (perform). In Lynn-McHale DJ, Carlson KK, editors: *AACN procedure manual for critical care,* ed 4, Philadelphia, 2001, WB Saunders.

*26. Keckeisen M: Pulmonary artery pressure monitoring. In Chulay M, Gawlinski A, editors: *Protocols for practice: hemodynamic monitoring,* Aliso Viejo, Calif, 1998, AACN.

*27. Lynn-McHale DJ, Preuss T: Pulmonary artery catheter insertion (assist) and pressure monitoring. In Lynn-McHale DJ, Carlson KK, editors: *AACN procedure manual for critical care,* ed 4, Philadelphia, 2001, WB Saunders.

28. Bridges EJ: Monitoring pulmonary artery pressures: just the facts, *Crit Care Nurse* 20:59, 2000.

*29. Gould KA, Hartigan C, Keane SF: Cardiac output measurement techniques (invasive). In Lynn-McHale DJ, Carlson KK, editors: *AACN procedure manual for critical care,* ed 4, Philadelphia, 2001, WB Saunders.

*30. Von Rueden KT: Noninvasive hemodynamic monitoring: impedance cardiography. In Lynn-McHale DJ, Carlson KK, editors: *AACN procedure manual for critical care,* ed 4, Philadelphia, 2001, WB Saunders.

*31. Lynn-McHale DJ: Intra-aortic balloon pump management. In Lynn-McHale DJ, Carlson KK, editors: *AACN procedure manual for critical care,* ed 4, Philadelphia, 2001, WB Saunders.

32. Davidson J et al: Intra-aortic balloon pump: indications and complications, *J Natl Med Assoc* 90:137, 1998.

33. Busch T et al: Vascular complications related to intraaortic balloon counterpulsation: an analysis of ten years experience, *Thorac Cardiovasc Surg* 45:55, 1997.

*34. Ruess LA: Ventricular assist devices. In Lynn-McHale DJ, Carlson KK, editors: *AACN procedure manual for critical care,* ed 4, Philadelphia, 2001, Saunders.

35. Berger EE: Abiomed: AbioCor frequently asked questions. AbioCor clinical trial information. Available at *www.abiomed.com/abiocor/faq.html* (accessed Feb 26, 2002).

*36. Goodrich C: Performing endotracheal intubation. In Lynn-McHale DJ, Carlson KK, editors: *AACN procedure manual for critical care,* ed 4, Philadelphia, 2001, WB Saunders.

*37. Deutsch JM: Endotracheal tube care. In Lynn-McHale DJ, Carlson KK, editors: *AACN procedure manual for critical care,* ed 4, Philadelphia, 2001, WB Saunders.

*38. Deutsch JM: Assisting with endotracheal intubation. In Lynn-McHale DJ, Carlson KK, editors: *AACN procedure manual for critical care,* ed 4, Philadelphia, 2001, WB Saunders.

*39. Good VS: Continuous end-tidal carbon dioxide monitoring. In Lynn-McHale DJ, Carlson KK, editors: *AACN procedure manual for critical care,* ed 4, Philadelphia, 2001, WB Saunders.

*40. Chulay M: Endotracheal or tracheostomy tube suctioning. In Lynn-McHale DJ, Carlson KK, editors: *AACN procedure manual for critical care,* ed 4, Philadelphia, 2001, WB Saunders.

*41. Minnick A, Leipzig RM, Johnson ME: Elderly patients' reports of physical restraint experiences in intensive care units, *Am J Crit Care* 10:168, 2001.

*42. Burns SM: Ventilatory management—volume and pressure modes. In Lynn-McHale DJ, Carlson KK, editors: *AACN procedure manual for critical care,* ed 4, Philadelphia, 2001, WB Saunders.

*43. Pierce LNB: Traditional and nontraditional modes of mechanical ventilation. In Chulay M, Burns SM, editors: *Protocols for practice: care of the mechanically ventilated patient,* Aliso Viejo, Calif, 1998, AACN.

44. Hynes-Gay P, MacDonald R: Using high-frequency oscillatory ventilation to treat adults with acute respiratory distress syndrome, *Crit Care Nurse* 21:38, 2001.

45. Schlicher ML: Using liquid ventilation to treat patients with acute respiratory distress syndrome: a guide to a breath of fresh liquid, *Crit Care Nurse* 21:55, 2001.

*46. Byers JF, Sole ML: Analysis of factors related to the development of ventilator-associated pneumonia: use of existing databases, *Am J Crit Care* 9:344, 2000.

*47. Hupcey JE: Feeling safe: the psychosocial needs of ICU patients, *J Nurs Scholarsh* 32:361, 2000.

48. Arbour R: Sedation and pain management in critically ill adults, *Crit Care Nurse* 21:39, 2000.

*49. Stamps DC: Enteral nutrition. In Lynn-McHale DJ, Carlson KK, editors: *AACN procedure manual for critical care,* ed 4, Philadelphia, 2001, WB Saunders.

*50. Burns SM: Weaning procedure. In Lynn-McHale DJ, Carlson KK, editors: *AACN procedure manual for critical care,* ed 4, Philadelphia, 2001, WB Saunders.

51. Henneman EA: Liberating patients from mechanical ventilation—a team approach, *Crit Care Nurse* 21:25, 2001.

*52. Burns SM: Standard weaning criteria: negative inspiratory pressure, positive expiratory pressure, spontaneous tidal volume, and vital capacity. In Lynn-McHale DJ, Carlson KK, editors: *AACN procedure manual for critical care,* ed 4, Philadelphia, 2001, WB Saunders.

*53. Greenlee KK: Performing extubation and decannulation. In Lynn-McHale DJ, Carlson KK, editors: *AACN procedure manual for critical care,* ed 4, Philadelphia, 2001, WB Saunders.

*54. Glass CA: Home care management of ventilator-assisted patients. In Chulay M, Burns SM, editors: *Protocols for practice: care of the mechanically ventilated patient,* Aliso Viejo, Calif, 1998, AACN.

55. Creechan T: Combining mechanical ventilation with hospice care in the home: death with dignity, *Crit Care Nurse* 20:49, 2000.

56. McNeal GJ: *AACN guide to acute care procedures in the home,* Philadelphia, 2000, Lippincott.

RESOURCES

American Association of Critical Care Nurses (AACN)
101 Columbia
Aliso Viejo, CA 92656-4109
800-899-2226 or 949-362-2000
Fax: 949-362-2020
www.aacn.org

Australian College of Critical Care Nurses
P.O. Box 219
South Carlton
Victoria, Australia 3053
www.acccn.com.au

Canadian Association of Critical Care Nurses (CACCN)
P.O. Box 25322
London, ON N6C 6B1
519-649-5284
Fax: 519-649-1458
www.caccn.ca

Society of Critical Care Medicine (SCCM)
701 Lee Street, Suite 200
Des Plaines, IL 60016
847-827-6869
Fax: 847-827-6886
www.sccm.org

For additional Internet resources, see the website for this book at *http://evolve.elsevier.com/Lewis/medsurg/.*

CHAPTER 65

NURSING MANAGEMENT
Shock and Multiple Organ Dysfunction Syndrome

JoAnne K. Phillips

LEARNING OBJECTIVES

1. Define *shock*.
2. Differentiate the two major classifications of shock: low blood flow and maldistribution of blood flow.
3. Describe the pathophysiology and clinical manifestations of shock.
4. Compare and contrast the effects of sepsis, systemic inflammatory response syndrome, shock, and multiple organ dysfunction syndrome on the major body systems.

5. Compare the collaborative care, drug therapy, and nursing management of patients with different types of shock.
6. Describe the nursing management of a patient experiencing multiple organ dysfunction syndrome.

KEY TERMS

absolute hypovolemia, p. 1798	relative hypovolemia, p. 1798
anaphylactic shock, p. 1802	sepsis, p. 1802
cardiogenic shock, p. 1796	septic shock, p. 1802
hypovolemic shock, p. 1798	shock, p. 1796
multiple organ dysfunction syndrome, p. 1819	systemic inflammatory response syndrome, p. 1818
neurogenic shock, p. 1801	

Shock, systemic inflammatory response syndrome (SIRS), and multiple organ dysfunction syndrome (MODS) are serious and interrelated problems. Fig. 65-1 shows the relationship among shock, SIRS, and MODS. Shock is a complex process that often leads to the development of SIRS and MODS. This chapter provides an overview of shock, SIRS, and MODS.

SHOCK

Shock is a syndrome characterized by decreased tissue perfusion and impaired cellular metabolism. This results in an imbalance between the supply of and demand for oxygen and nutrients. The exchange of oxygen and nutrients at the cellular level is essential to life. When a cell experiences a state of hypoperfusion, the demand for oxygen and nutrients exceeds the supply.

Classification of Shock

Although the cause and initial presentation of various types of shock differ, the physiologic responses of the cell to hypoperfusion are similar. In addition, the management strategies for each type of shock vary widely. For the purposes of discussion, shock will be classified as *low blood flow* (cardiogenic and hypovolemic shock) or *maldistribution of blood flow* (septic, anaphylactic, and neurogenic shock)[1,2] (Table 65-1).

Low Blood Flow Shock

Cardiogenic shock. Cardiogenic shock occurs when either systolic or diastolic dysfunction of the myocardium results in compromised cardiac output. The heart's inability to pump the blood forward is classified as *systolic dysfunction*. Systolic dysfunction primarily affects the left ventricle, because systolic pressure and tension are greater on the left side of the heart. When systolic dysfunction affects the right side of the heart, blood flow through the pulmonary circulation is compromised. Precipitating causes of systolic dysfunction include myocardial infarction (MI), cardiomyopathies, severe systemic or pulmonary hypertension, blunt cardiac injury, and myocardial depression from sepsis. From 5% to 10% of patients who experience an acute MI will develop cardiogenic shock, most within 48 hours of the initial insult.[3]

Diastolic dysfunction is an impaired ability of the right or left ventricle to fill during diastole. Decreased filling of the ventricle will result in decreased stroke volume (amount of blood ejected from the heart with each contraction).

Fig. 65-2 describes the pathophysiology of cardiogenic shock. Whether the initiating event is an MI, a structural problem (e.g., valvular abnormality, papillary muscle dysfunction, acute ventricular septal defect), or arrhythmias, the physiologic responses are similar. The patient experiences impaired tissue perfusion and impaired cellular metabolism as a result of cardiogenic shock.[4]

The early clinical presentation of a patient with cardiogenic shock is similar to that of a patient with acute heart failure (see Chapter 34). The patient will have tachycardia, hypotension, and a narrowed pulse pressure. An increase in systemic vascular resistance (SVR) increases the workload of the heart, thus increasing the myocardial oxygen consumption.[5] The heart's inability to pump blood forward will result in a low cardiac index (less than 2.1 L/min/m^2). On examination, the patient will be tachypneic and pulmonary congestion will be evident by the presence of crackles. The hemodynamic profile will demonstrate an increase in the pulmonary artery wedge pressure (PAWP) and pulmonary

Reviewed by Joseph J. Napolitano, RN, MPH, MSN, APRN, Program Officer, Dorothy Rider Pool Health Care Trust, Allentown, Pa.

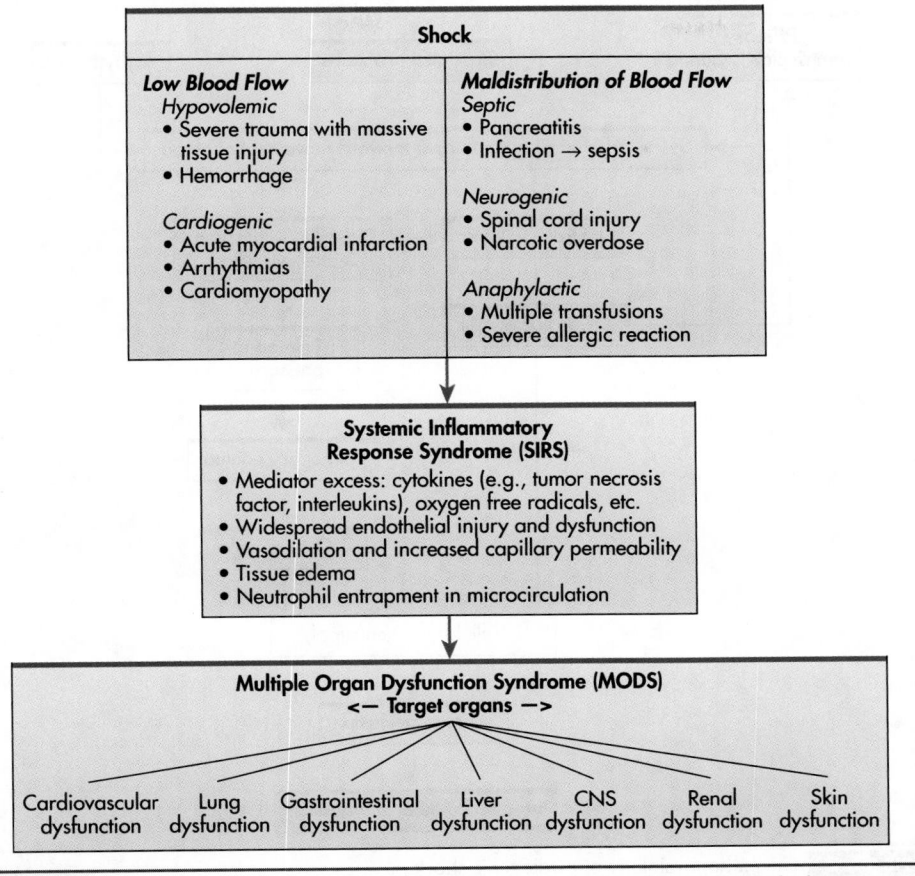

FIG. 65-1 Relationship of shock, systemic inflammatory response syndrome, and multiple organ dysfunction syndrome. *CNS*, Central nervous system.

TABLE 65-1   Classification and Precipitating Factors of Shock

LOW BLOW FLOW	MALDISTRIBUTION OF BLOOD FLOW
Cardiogenic Shock ▪ Systolic dysfunction: inability of the heart to pump blood forward (e.g., myocardial infarction, cardiomyopathy) ▪ Diastolic dysfunction: inability of the heart to fill during diastole (e.g., cardiac tamponade) ▪ Arrhythmias (e.g., bradycardia, tachycardia) ▪ Structural factors: valvular abnormality (e.g., stenosis or regurgitation), papillary muscle dysfunction, acute ventricular septal defect **Hypovolemic Shock** **Absolute hypovolemia** ▪ Loss of whole blood (e.g., hemorrhage from trauma, surgery, GI bleeding) ▪ Loss of plasma (e.g., burn injuries) ▪ Loss of other body fluids (e.g., vomiting, diarrhea, excessive diuresis, diaphoresis, diabetes insipidus, diabetes mellitus) **Relative hypovolemia** ▪ Pooling of blood or fluids (e.g., ascites, peritonitis, bowel obstruction) ▪ Internal bleeding (e.g., fracture of long bones, ruptured spleen, hemothorax, severe pancreatitis) ▪ Massive vasodilation (e.g., sepsis)	**Neurogenic Shock** ▪ Hemodynamic consequence of injury and/or disease to the spinal cord at or above T5 ▪ Spinal anesthesia ▪ Vasomotor center depression (e.g., severe pain, drugs, hypoglycemia, injury) **Septic Shock** ▪ Infection (e.g., urinary tract, respiratory tract, invasive procedure, indwelling lines and catheters) ▪ At risk patients: older adults, patients with chronic diseases (e.g., diabetes mellitus, chronic renal failure, congestive heart failure), patients receiving immunosuppressive therapy or who are malnourished or debilitated ▪ Gram-negative bacteria most common; also gram-positive bacteria, viruses, fungi, and parasites **Anaphylactic Shock** ▪ Contrast media, blood/blood products, drugs, insect bites, anesthetic agents, food/food additives, vaccines, environmental agents, latex

GI, Gastrointestinal.

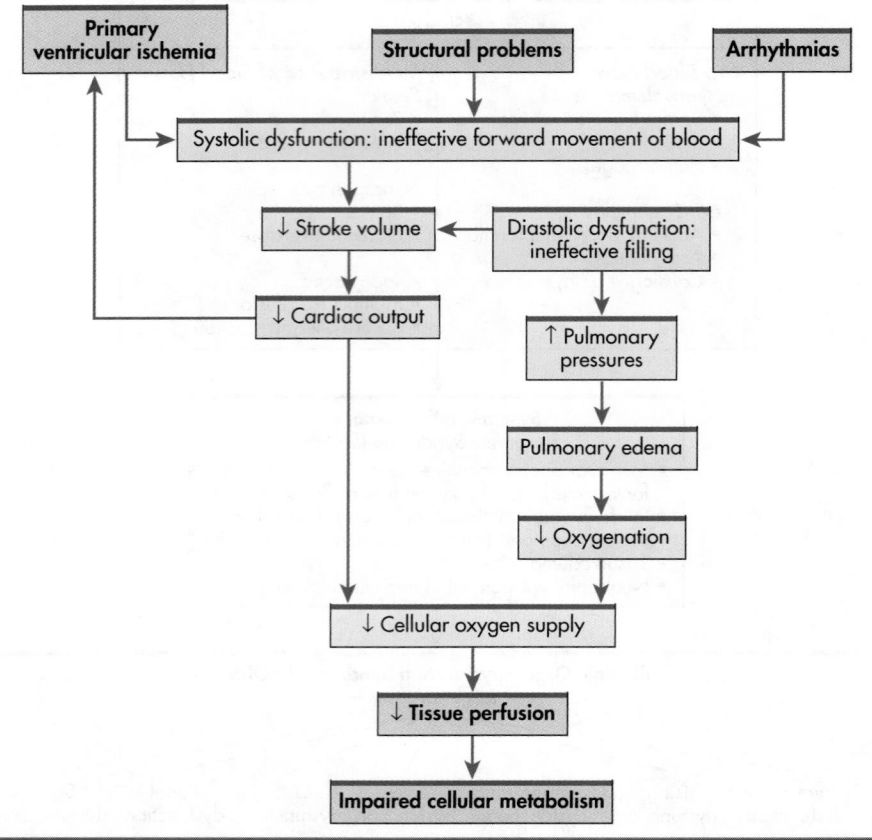

FIG. 65-2   The pathophysiology of cardiogenic shock.

TABLE 65-2   Effects of Shock, Systemic Inflammatory Response Syndrome, and Multiple Organ Dysfunction Syndrome on Hemodynamic Parameters

TYPE	HR	PULSE PRESSURE	BP	SVR	PVR	CVP	PAP	PAWP	CO	SvO₂
Cardiogenic shock	↑	↓	↓	↑	↑	≈↑	↑	↑	↓	↓
Hypovolemic shock	↑	↓	↓	↑	↑	↓	↓	↓	↓	↓
Anaphylactic shock	↑	↓	↓	↓	≈↑	↓	↓	↓	↓	↓
Neurogenic shock	↓	↓	↓	↓	≈	↓	↓	↓	↓	↓
Septic shock	↑	↓	↓	↓	≈↑	↓	↑≈↓	↓	↑	↑≈↓
SIRS	↑	≈	≈	↓	≈↑	↓	↑≈↓	↓	↑	↑≈↓
MODS	↑	≈	≈	↓	↑	↓	↑≈↓	↓≈↑	↓	↑

NOTE: Hemodynamic effects in some illnesses are highly variable. The hemodynamic findings in MODS depend on the system failing.
KEY: ↓, decrease; ↑, increase; ≈, no change.
BP, Blood pressure; *CO*, cardiac output; *CVP*, central venous pressure; *HR*, heart rate; *MODS*, multiple organ dysfunction syndrome; *PAP*, pulmonary artery pressure; *PAWP*, pulmonary artery wedge pressure; *PVR*, pulmonary vascular resistance; *SIRS*, systemic inflammatory response syndrome; *SvO₂*, mixed venous oxygen saturation; *SVR*, systemic vascular resistance.

vascular resistance (Table 65-2). Signs of peripheral hypoperfusion (e.g., cyanosis, pallor, cool and clammy skin, decreased capillary refill time) will be apparent. Decreased renal blood flow will result in sodium and water retention and decreased urine output. Anxiety and delirium may develop as cerebral perfusion is impaired. Studies that may be helpful in diagnosing cardiogenic shock include laboratory studies (e.g., cardiac enzymes, troponin levels) (Table 65-3), electrocardiogram (ECG), chest x-ray, and echocardiogram. The overall clinical presentation of a patient with cardiogenic shock is presented in Table 65-4.

Hypovolemic shock. The second type of low blood flow shock is hypovolemic shock. **Hypovolemic shock** occurs when there is a loss of intravascular fluid volume. In hypovolemic shock, the volume is inadequate to fill the vascular space. The volume loss may be either an absolute or relative volume loss. **Absolute hypovolemia** results when fluid is lost through hemorrhage, gastrointestinal (GI) loss (e.g., vomiting, diarrhea), fistula drainage, diabetes insipidus, or diuresis. In **relative hypovolemia**, fluid volume moves out of the vascular space into extravascular space (e.g., interstitial or intracavitary space). This type of

TABLE
65-3

Diagnostic Studies
Laboratory Abnormalities in Shock

LABORATORY STUDY	FINDING	SIGNIFICANCE OF FINDING
Blood		
Red blood cell count, hematocrit, hemoglobin	Normal	• Remains within normal limits in shock because of relative hypovolemia and pump failure and in hemorrhagic shock before fluid restoration
	Decreased	• Decreases in hemorrhagic shock after fluid resuscitation when fluids other than blood are used
	Increased	• Increases in nonhemorrhagic shock due to actual hypovolemia because fluid lost does not contain erythrocytes
DIC screen		
Fibrin split products (FSP)	Increased	• Acute DIC can develop within hours to days after an initial assault on the body (e.g., shock)
Fibrinogen level	Decreased	
Platelet count	Decreased	
PTT and PT	Prolonged	
Thrombin time	Increased	
D-Dimer	Increased	
Creatine kinase	Increased	• Increases in trauma, myocardial infarction in response to cellular damage and/or hypoxia
Troponin	Increased	• Increases in myocardial infarction
BUN	Increased	• Indicates impaired kidney function due to hypoperfusion as a result of severe vasoconstriction or occurs secondary to catabolism of cells (e.g., trauma, infection)
Creatinine	Increased	• Indicates impaired kidney function due to hypoperfusion as a result of severe vasoconstriction; is more sensitive indicator of renal function than BUN
Glucose	Increased	• Found in early shock because of release of liver glycogen stores in response to sympathetic nervous system stimulation and cortisol; insulin insensitivity develops
	Decreased	• Occurs because of depleted glycogen stores with hepatocellular dysfunction possible as shock progresses
Serum electrolytes		
Sodium	Increased	• Found in early shock because of increased secretion of aldosterone, causing renal retention of sodium
	Decreased	• May occur iatrogenically when excess hypotonic fluid is administered after fluid loss
Potassium	Increased	• Results when cellular death liberates intracellular potassium; also occurs in acute renal failure and in the presence of acidosis
	Decreased	• Found in early shock because of increased secretion of aldosterone, causing renal excretion of potassium
Arterial blood gases	Respiratory alkalosis	• Found in early shock secondary to hyperventilation
	Metabolic acidosis	• Occurs later in shock when organic acids, such as lactic acid, accumulate in blood from anaerobic metabolism
Base deficit	>−6	• Indicates acid production secondary to hypoxia
Blood cultures	Growth of organisms	• May grow organisms in patients who are in septic shock
Lactate	Increased	• Usually increases once significant hypoperfusion and impaired oxygen utilization at the cellular level have occurred; by-product of anaerobic metabolism
Liver enzymes (ALT, AST, GGT)	Increased	• Elevations indicate liver cell destruction in progressive stage of shock
Urine		
Specific gravity	Increased	• Occurs secondary to the action of ADH
	Fixed at 1.010	• Occurs in renal failure

ADH, Antidiuretic hormone; *ALT,* alanine aminotransferase; *AST,* aspartate aminotransferase; *BUN,* blood urea nitrogen; *DIC,* disseminated intravascular coagulation; *GGT,* gamma-glutamyl transferase; *PT,* prothrombin time; *PTT,* partial thromboplastin time.

TABLE 65-4	Clinical Presentation of the Major Types of Shock				
	CARDIOGENIC SHOCK	**HYPOVOLEMIC SHOCK**	**NEUROGENIC SHOCK**	**ANAPHYLACTIC SHOCK**	**SEPTIC SHOCK**
Cardiovascular (see Table 65-2 for hemodynamic profile)	↓ Capillary refill time ↑ MVO_2 Cardiac index <2.1 L/min/m² PAWP >20 mm Hg Chest pain may or may not be present	↓ Preload ↓ Stroke volume ↓ Capillary refill time	↓/↑ Temperature	Chest pain Third spacing of fluid	**Early** ↓/↑ Temperature ↑ HR ↓ SVR, ↑ CO ↓ BP Biventricular dilation: ↓ ejection fraction ↑ SvO_2 **Late** ↓/↑ Temperature ↓ CO/↑ SVR ↓ SvO_2
Pulmonary	Tachypnea Cyanosis Crackles Rhonchi	Tachypnea → bradypnea (late)	Dysfunction related to level of injury	Swelling of lips and tongue Shortness of breath Edema of larynx and epiglottis Wheezing Rhinitis Stridor	Hyperventilation Respiratory alkalosis → respiratory acidosis Hypoxemia Respiratory failure ARDS Pulmonary hypertension Crackles ↓ Urine output
Renal	↑ Na^+ and H_2O retention ↓ Renal blood flow ↓ Urine output	↓ Urine output			
Skin	Pallor Cool, clammy	Pallor Cool, clammy	↓ Skin perfusion Cool or warm Dry	Flushing Pruritus Urticaria Angioedema	**Early** Warm and flushed **Late** Cool and mottled
Neurologic	↓ Cerebral perfusion: anxiety, confusion, agitation	Anxiety Confusion Agitation	Flaccid paralysis below the level of the lesion Loss of reflex activity, bowel and bladder function	Anxiety Feeling of impending doom Confusion ↓ LOC Metallic taste	**Early** Alteration in mental status Agitation **Late** Coma
Gastrointestinal	↓ Bowel sounds Nausea/vomiting	Absent bowel sounds		Cramping Abdominal pain Nausea Vomiting Diarrhea	GI bleeding Paralytic ileus
Diagnostic findings (also see Table 65-3)	↑ Cardiac markers ↑ Blood glucose ↑ BUN ECG (e.g., arrhythmias) Echocardiogram (e.g., left ventricular dysfunction) Chest x-ray (e.g., pulmonary infiltrates)	↓ Hematocrit ↑ Lactate ↑ Urine specific gravity Changes in electrolytes		Sudden onset History of allergies Exposure to contrast media	↑/↓ WBC ↓ Platelets ↑ Lactate ↑ Urine specific gravity ↓ Urine Na^+ Positive blood cultures

BP, Blood pressure; *BUN,* blood urea nitrogen; *ECG,* electrocardiogram; *GI,* gastrointestinal; *LOC,* level of consciousness; *MVO₂,* myocardial oxygen consumption; *PAWP,* pulmonary artery wedge pressure; *SvO₂,* mixed venous oxygen saturation; *SVR,* systemic vascular resistance; *WBC,* white blood cell.

fluid shift is called *third spacing*. One example of relative volume loss is leakage of fluid from the vascular space to the interstitial space from increased capillary permeability, as seen in sepsis. Other examples include sequestration of fluid into the colon from a bowel obstruction, loss of blood volume into a fracture site (e.g., pelvic fracture), burns (Chapter 24), and ascites (see Table 65-1).

In hypovolemic shock, the size of the vascular compartment remains unchanged while the volume of blood or plasma decreases. Whether the loss of intravascular volume is absolute or relative, the physiologic consequences are similar. A reduction in intravascular volume results in a decreased venous return to the heart, decreased preload, decreased stroke volume, and decreased cardiac output (see Table 65-2). A cascade of events results in decreased tissue perfusion and impaired cellular metabolism, the hallmarks of shock (Fig. 65-3).

The patient's response to acute volume loss is dependent on a number of factors, including extent of injury or insult, age, and general state of health (see Table 65-4). An overall assessment of physiologic reserve may indicate the patient's ability to compensate. A healthy young adult can compensate for a sudden loss of up to 15% of the total blood volume (or approximately 750 ml out of the average 5 L total blood volume in a 70 kg person).[6] Further loss of volume (15% to 30%) will result in a sympathetic nervous system (SNS)–mediated response. This response results in an increase in heart rate, cardiac output, and respiratory rate and depth. The stroke volume and PAWP are decreased because of the decreased circulating blood volume. The patient may appear anxious and urine output will begin to decrease. If hypovolemia is corrected at this time, tissue dysfunction is generally reversible. If volume loss is greater than 30%, blood volume must be replaced aggressively with blood or blood products, as the compensatory mechanisms become overwhelmed. Loss of more than 40% of the total blood volume is characterized by loss of autoregulation in the microcirculation and results in irreversible tissue destruction.[7,8] Laboratory studies that may be done include measurements of serial hemoglobin and hematocrit levels, urine specific gravity, serum electrolytes, and lactic acid (see Table 65-3).

Maldistribution of Blood Flow Shock

Neurogenic shock. Neurogenic shock is a hemodynamic phenomenon that occurs after a spinal cord injury at the fifth thoracic (T5) vertebra or above.[9] The injury results in a massive vasodilation without compensation as a consequence of the loss of SNS vasoconstrictor tone. This massive vasodilation leads to a pooling of blood in the blood vessels. The most important clinical manifestations are hypotension (from the massive vasodilation) and bradycardia. The unopposed activation of the parasympathetic nervous system leads to bradycardia.

The patient in neurogenic shock also characteristically has hypothalamic dysfunction, which may result in temperature dysregulation. The patient will often have *poikilothermia* (taking on the temperature of the environment), which, combined with massive vasodilation, promotes heat loss, often resulting in hypothermia. With poikilothermia, the skin could be cool or warm depending on the ambient temperature. In either case, the skin will usually be dry. Initially, the skin will be warm due to the massive dilation without compensation. As the heat dissipates, the skin loses heat and the patient is at risk for hypothermia.

The pathophysiology of neurogenic shock is described in Fig. 65-4. Hypoperfusion associated with neurogenic shock also results in impaired tissue perfusion. Onset of neurogenic shock

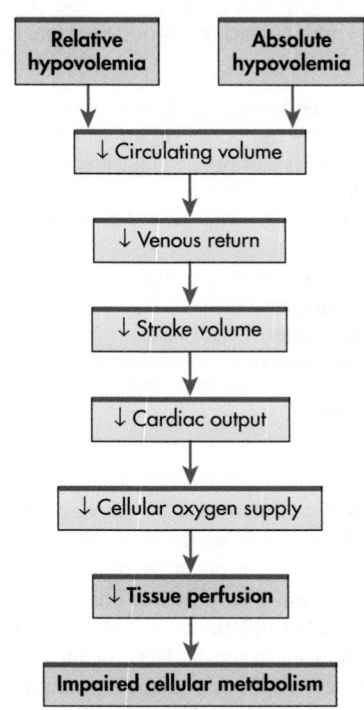

FIG. 65-3 The pathophysiology of hypovolemic shock.

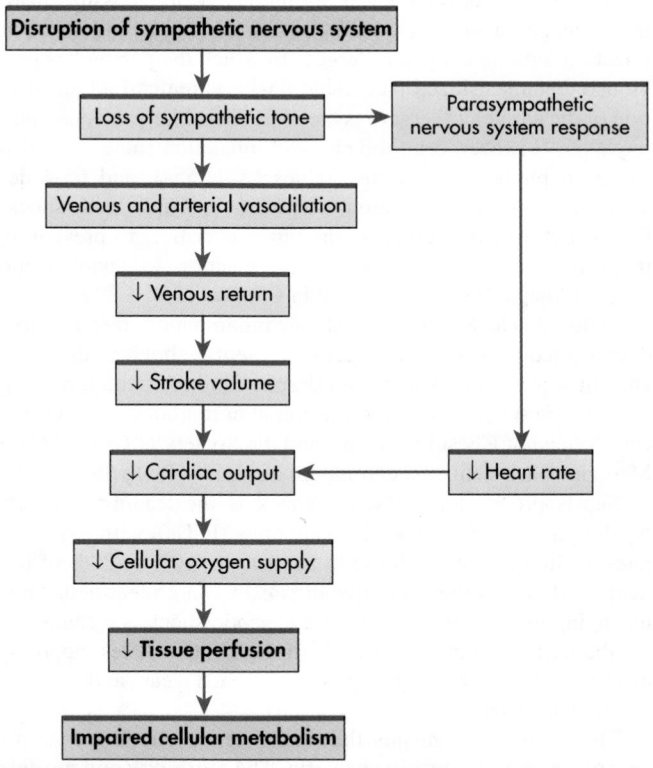

FIG. 65-4 The pathophysiology of neurogenic shock.

can begin as soon as 30 minutes after the injury, and may last from days to weeks following spinal cord injury.

Table 65-1 lists the causes of neurogenic shock. In addition to spinal cord injury, spinal anesthesia can also block transmission of impulses from the SNS. Depression of the vasomotor center of the medulla as a result of drugs (e.g., benzodiazepines, narcotics) can also result in decreased vasoconstrictor tone of the peripheral blood vessels, resulting in neurogenic shock. Tables 65-2, 65-3, and 65-4 further describe the clinical presentation of a patient with neurogenic shock.

Although spinal shock and neurogenic shock often occur in the same patient, they are not the same disorder. *Spinal shock* is a phenomenon that is present after an acute spinal cord injury (see Chapter 59). The patient with spinal shock will experience the absence of all voluntary and reflex neurologic activity below the level of the injury.[9]

Anaphylactic shock. **Anaphylactic shock** is an acute and life-threatening hypersensitivity (allergic) reaction to a sensitizing substance (e.g., drug, chemical, vaccine, food, or insect venom). It is an immediate reaction that causes massive vasodilation, release of vasoactive mediators, and an increase in capillary permeability. As capillary permeability increases, fluid leaks from the vascular space into the interstitial space. Anaphylactic shock can lead to respiratory distress, as a result of laryngeal edema or severe bronchospasm, and circulatory failure, as a result of massive vasodilation.[10] The patient experiences a sudden onset of symptoms, including hypotension, chest pain, swelling of the lips and tongue, wheezing, and stridor. Skin changes include flushing, pruritus, urticaria, and angioedema. In addition, the patient may feel an impending sense of doom and become very anxious and confused.

A patient can develop a severe allergic reaction, possibly leading to anaphylactic shock, after contact, inhalation, ingestion, or injection with an antigen (allergen) to which the person has previously been sensitized (see Table 65-1). Parenteral administration of the antigen (allergen) is the route most likely to cause anaphylaxis. However, oral, topical, and inhalation routes can also cause anaphylactic reactions. Tables 65-2, 65-3, and 65-4 describe the clinical presentation of a patient in anaphylactic shock. Quick and decisive action by the nurse is critical to preventing the progression of an anaphylactic reaction to anaphylactic shock. (Anaphylaxis is discussed in Chapter 13.)

Septic shock. **Sepsis** is a systemic inflammatory response to a documented or suspected infection.[11] **Septic shock** is the presence of sepsis with hypotension despite fluid resuscitation along with the presence of tissue perfusion abnormalities. The American College of Chest Physicians and the Society of Critical Care Medicine have defined a continuum of sepsis (Table 65-5).

Sepsis progressing to septic shock is the leading cause of death in noncoronary intensive care units (ICUs), with mortality rates as high as 40% to 60%. In as many as 10% to 30% of patients with sepsis, the causative organism is not identified. Thus managing the patient with sepsis and septic shock is a challenge for the entire health care team.[12] In the United States, approximately 750,000 cases of sepsis occur each year, and at least 225,000 are fatal.

The primary organisms that cause septic shock are gram-negative and gram-positive bacteria. The morbidity and mortality rates from infections with gram-negative organisms are greater than those from gram-positive organisms.[12] Parasites,

| TABLE 65-5 | Definitions of Sepsis, Severe Sepsis, Septic Shock, and Multiple Organ Dysfunction Syndrome* |

Infection
- Disease caused by an invasion of the body by pathogenic organisms

Bacteremia
- Presence of viable bacteria in the blood; demonstrated by positive blood cultures

Systemic Inflammatory Response Syndrome (SIRS)
- Systemic inflammatory response to a variety of insults, including infection, ischemia, infarct, injury; manifested by two or more of the following:
  1. Temperature >100.4° F (38° C) or <97.0° F (36° C)
  2. Heart rate >90 beats/min
  3. Respiratory rate >20 breaths/min or $PaCO_2$ <32 mm Hg
  4. White blood cell count >12,000 cells/μl or <4000 cells/μl or >10% immature neutrophils (bands)

Sepsis
- A systemic inflammatory response to a documented or suspected infection

Severe Sepsis
- Sepsis associated with organ dysfunction, hypoperfusion, or hypotension

Septic Shock
- Sepsis with hypotension despite adequate fluid resuscitation along with the presence of tissue perfusion abnormalities (e.g., lactic acidosis, oliguria, alteration in mental status)

Hypotension
- A systolic BP of <90 mm Hg or a reduction of >40 mm Hg from baseline and in which BP is not adequate for normal perfusion

Multiple Organ Dysfunction Syndrome (MODS)
- Failure of more than one organ in an acutely ill patient such that homeostasis cannot be maintained without intervention

Primary MODS
- Occurs early and results from well-defined illness or injury

Secondary MODS
- Results from uncontrolled systemic inflammation with resultant organ dysfunction
- Develops latently after several insults

*These definitions are from the American College of Chest Physicians and Society of Critical Care Medicine.
BP, Blood pressure.

fungi, and viruses can also lead to the development of septic shock. The pathogenesis of septic shock is complex (Fig. 65-5).

The cell walls of gram-negative organisms contain a substance called *endotoxin.* The release of endotoxin into circulation stimulates a cascade of inflammatory responses that produce the detrimental effects seen in sepsis. The cascade begins with the release of several key mediators, including tumor necrosis factor (TNF) and interleukin 1 (IL-1). These mediators stimulate the release of other inflammatory mediators, such as platelet activating factor, thromboxanes, leukotrienes, prostaglandins, and inter-

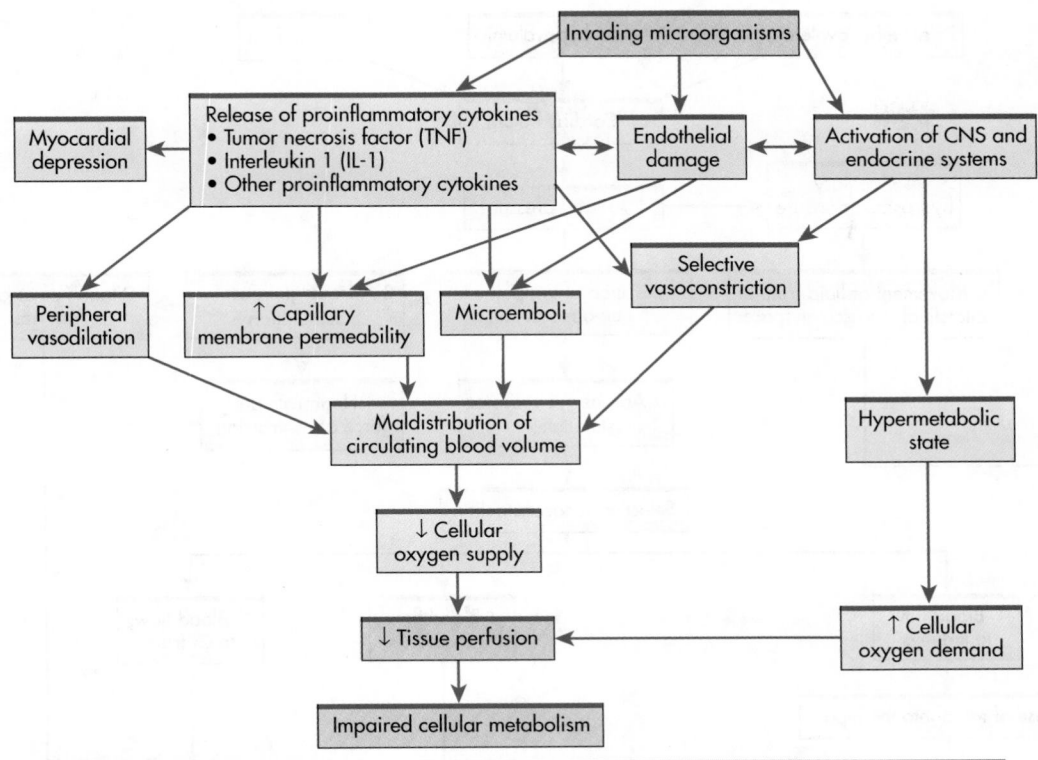

FIG. 65-5 The pathophysiology of septic shock. *CNS,* Central nervous system.

leukin 6 (IL-6) and interleukin 8 (IL-8).[13] (See Chapters 12 and 13 for discussion of the inflammatory response.) The combined effects of the mediators result in damage to the endothelium, vasodilation, increased capillary permeability, and neutrophil and platelet aggregation and adhesion to the endothelium.

In septic shock there is an increase in coagulation and inflammation and a decrease in fibrinolysis. The release of platelet activating factor results in the formation of microthrombi and obstruction of the microvasculature.

The clinical presentation of sepsis includes decreased SVR with a compensatory increase in cardiac output, hypotension, tachypnea, and temperature dysregulation (high or low). Tables 65-2 and 65-4 further delineate the clinical presentation of a patient with septic shock.

The combination of TNF and IL-1 is thought to have a role in sepsis-induced myocardial dysfunction. The ejection fraction is decreased for the first few days after the initial insult. Because of a decreased ejection fraction, the ventricles will dilate in order to maintain the stroke volume. The ejection fraction typically improves and the ventricular dilation resolves over 7 to 10 days. Persistence of a high cardiac output and a low SVR beyond 24 hours is an ominous finding and is often associated with an increased development of hypotension and MODS. Coronary perfusion and myocardial oxygen metabolism are normal in septic shock.[13]

In addition to the cardiovascular dysfunction that accompanies sepsis, respiratory failure is common. The patient will initially hyperventilate as a compensatory mechanism, resulting in respiratory alkalosis. Once the patient can no longer compensate, respiratory acidosis will develop. Respiratory failure will develop in 85% of patients with sepsis, and 40% will develop acute respiratory distress syndrome (ARDS). Other clinical signs of septic shock include decreased urine output, alteration in neuro-

logic status, and GI dysfunction, such as GI bleeding and paralytic ileus (see Table 65-4).

Stages of Shock

In addition to understanding the underlying pathogenesis of the type of shock the patient is experiencing, monitoring and management are also guided by knowing where the patient is on the shock "continuum." This continuum begins with the initial stage of shock, followed by the compensatory and progressive stages. If tissue perfusion is not restored, and the progression of the shock is not halted, the patient will deteriorate to the refractory (final) stage of shock, from which recovery is unlikely. Although there are no clear-cut divisions between the stages, they provide a framework for discussing shock.

Initial Stage. The *initial stage* of shock may not be clinically apparent. The patient will have no outward signs of decreased tissue perfusion despite the fact that the body begins to respond to the imbalance of oxygen supply and demand at the cellular level. Metabolism changes from aerobic to anaerobic, and as a result, lactic acid, which is harmful to cells, begins to accumulate as a waste product. The lactic acid must be removed by the blood and broken down by the liver. This process also requires oxygen, which is unavailable at the cellular level in shock.[14]

Compensatory Stage. The next stage of shock is the *compensatory stage.* In this stage, the body activates several compensatory mechanisms in an attempt to overcome the increasing consequences of anaerobic metabolism and to maintain homeostasis (Fig. 65-6). There are neural, hormonal, and biochemical compensatory mechanisms. The patient's clinical presentation begins to reflect the body's responses to the imbalance in oxygen supply and demand (Table 65-6).

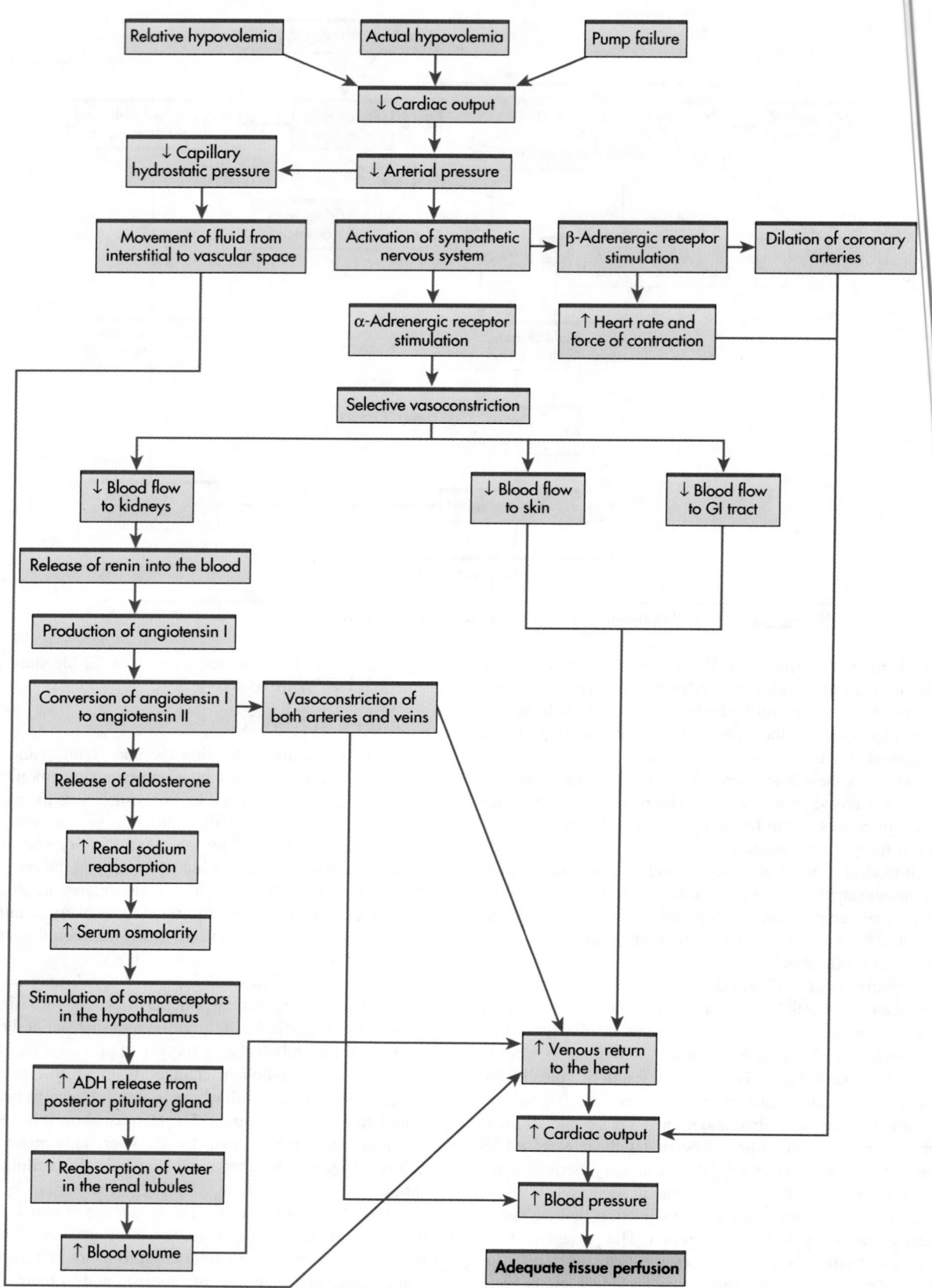

FIG. 65-6 Compensated stage: reversible stage during which compensatory mechanisms are effective and homeostasis is maintained.

TABLE 65-6	**Clinical Manifestations of the Stages of Shock**		
SYSTEM	**COMPENSATORY STAGE**	**PROGRESSIVE STAGE**	**REFRACTORY STAGE**
Neurologic	Oriented to person, place, time Restless, agitated, apprehensive Change in level of consciousness	↓ Cerebral perfusion pressure ↓ Cerebral blood flow Listless or agitated ↓ Responsiveness to stimuli	Unresponsive Areflexia (loss of reflexes) Pupils unreactive and dilated
Cardiovascular	Sympathetic nervous system response: Release of epinephrine/norepinephrine, which promotes vasoconstriction ↑ MVO_2 ↑ Contractility ↑ HR Coronary artery dilation BP adequate to perfuse vital organs (heart, brain)	Loss of autoregulation in microcirculation ↑ Capillary permeability → systemic interstitial edema ↓ Cardiac output → ↓ BP and ↑ HR MAP <60 mm Hg (or 40 mm Hg drop in BP from baseline) ↓ Coronary perfusion → • Arrhythmias • Myocardial ischemia • Myocardial infarction • Myocardial dysfunction → impaired cardiac output ↓ Peripheral perfusion → ischemia of distal extremities, diminished pulses, ↓ Capillary refill	Profound hypotension ↓ Cardiac output Bradycardia; irregular rhythm ↓ BP inadequate to perfuse vital organs
Respiratory	↓ Blood flow to the lungs • ↑ Physiologic dead space • ↑ Ventilation–perfusion mismatch • Hyperventilation • ↑ Minute ventilation (VE)	Noncardiogenic pulmonary edema (ARDS) • ↑ Capillary permeability • Pulmonary vasoconstriction • Pulmonary interstitial edema • Alveolar edema • Diffuse infiltrates • ↑ Respiratory rate • ↓ Compliance Moist crackles	Severe refractory hypoxemia Respiratory failure
Gastrointestinal	↓ Blood supply Hypoactive bowel sounds	Vasoconstriction and ↓ perfusion → ischemic gut (e.g., stomach, small and large intestines, gall bladder, pancreas) • Erosive ulcers • GI bleeding • Translocation of GI bacteria • Impaired absorption of nutrients	Ischemic gut
Renal	↓ Renal blood flow ↑ Renin resulting in release of angiotensin (vasoconstrictor) ↑ Aldosterone resulting in Na^+ and H_2O reabsorption ↑ Antidiuretic hormone resulting in H_2O reabsorption	Renal tubules become ischemic → acute tubular necrosis ↓ Urine output ↑ BUN/creatinine ratio ↑ Urine sodium ↓ Urine osmolarity and specific gravity ↓ Urine potassium Metabolic acidosis	Anuria
Hepatic		Failure to metabolize drugs and waste products Jaundice (decreased clearance of bilirubin) ↑ NH_3 and lactate	Metabolic changes from accumulation of waste products (e.g., NH_3, lactate, CO_2)
Hematologic		DIC • Thrombin clots in microcirculation • Consumption of clots in microcirculation	DIC
Temperature	Normal or abnormal	Hypothermia Sepsis: hypothermia or hyperthermia	Hypothermia
Skin	Pale and cool Warm and flushed (early stage of septic shock)	Cold and clammy	Mottled, cyanotic
Key Laboratory Findings	↑ Blood glucose ↑ pH ↓ PaO_2 ↓ $PaCO_2$	↑ Liver enzymes: ALT, AST, GGT ↑ Bleeding times Thrombocytopenia	↓ Blood glucose ↑ NH_3, lactate, and K^+ Metabolic acidosis

ALT, Alanine aminotransferase; *ARDS,* acute respiratory distress syndrome; *AST,* aspartate aminotransferase; *BUN,* Blood urea nitrogen; *DIC,* disseminated intravascular coagulation; *GGT,* gamma-glutamyl transferase; *GI,* gastrointestinal; *HR,* heart rate; *MAP,* mean arterial pressure; *MVO₂,* myocardial oxygen consumption.

One of the first clinical signs of shock may be a fall in BP, which occurs as a result of a decrease in cardiac output. The baroreceptors in the carotid and aortic bodies immediately respond by activating the SNS. The SNS stimulates vasoconstriction and the release of epinephrine and norepinephrine, both of which are potent vasoconstrictors. Blood flow to the most essential (vital) organs, the heart and the brain, is maintained, while blood flow to the nonvital organs, such as the kidneys, GI tract, skin, and lungs, is diverted or shunted.

Decreased blood flow to the kidneys activates the renin-angiotensin system. Renin is released, which activates angiotensinogen to produce angiotensin I, which is then converted to angiotensin II (see Chapter 43, Fig. 43-4). Angiotensin II is a potent vasoconstrictor, which causes both arterial and venous vasoconstriction. The net result is an increase in venous return to the heart and an increase in blood pressure. Angiotensin II also stimulates the adrenal cortex to release aldosterone, which results in sodium that water reabsorption and potassium excretion by the kidneys. The increase in sodium reabsorption raises the serum osmolality and stimulates the release of antidiuretic hormone (ADH) from the posterior pituitary gland. ADH works by increasing water reabsorption by the kidneys, thus further increasing blood volume. The increase in total circulating volume results in an increase in cardiac output and BP.

The shunting of blood from other organ systems also results in clinically important changes. The decrease in blood flow to the GI tract results in impaired motility and a slowing of peristalsis, thus increasing the risk for the development of a paralytic ileus. Decreased blood flow to the skin results in the patient feeling cool and clammy. The exception is the patient in early septic shock who will feel warm and flushed.

Shunting blood away from the lungs has an important clinical effect in the patient in shock. Decreased blood flow to the lungs increases the patient's physiologic dead space. *Physiologic dead space* is the anatomic dead space (the amount of air that will not reach gas-exchanging units) plus any inspired air that cannot participate in gas exchange. The clinical result of an increase in dead space ventilation is a ventilation-perfusion mismatch. There will be areas of the lungs participating in ventilation that will not be perfused because of the decreased blood flow to the lungs. Arterial oxygen levels will decrease, and the patient will have a compensatory increase in the rate and depth of respirations.[14]

The myocardium responds to the SNS stimulation and the increase in oxygen demand by increasing the heart rate and contractility. However, increased contractility also increases myocardial oxygen consumption (MVO_2). The coronary arteries dilate in an attempt to meet the increased oxygen demands of the myocardium.

A multisystem response to decreasing tissue perfusion is initiated in the compensatory stage of shock. At this stage, the body is able to compensate for the changes in tissue perfusion, whatever the cause. If the perfusion deficit (the cause of the shock) is corrected, the patient will recover with little or no residual sequelae. If the perfusion deficit is not corrected and the body is unable to compensate, the patient enters the progressive stage of shock.

Progressive Stage. The *progressive stage* of shock begins as compensatory mechanisms fail (Fig. 65-7). In this stage of shock, aggressive interventions are necessary to prevent the development of MODS. The hallmarks of this stage of shock are decreased cellular perfusion and altered capillary permeability. The altered capillary permeability allows leakage of fluid and protein out of the vascular space into the surrounding interstitial space. In addition to the decrease in circulating volume, there is an increase in systemic interstitial edema. The patient may have *anasarca,* or diffuse profound edema. Fluid leakage from the vascular space affects the solid organs (e.g., liver, spleen, GI tract, lungs), as well as the peripheral tissues.

The pulmonary system is often the first system to display signs of critical dysfunction. During the compensatory stage, blood flow to the lungs is already reduced. In response to the decreased blood flow and the SNS stimulation, the pulmonary arterioles constrict, resulting in increased pulmonary artery pressure. As the pressure within the pulmonary vasculature increases, blood flow to the pulmonary capillaries decreases, and ventilation-perfusion mismatch worsens. Another key response in the lungs is the movement of fluid from the pulmonary vasculature into the interstitium. As capillary permeability increases, the movement of fluid from the pulmonary vasculature to the interstitium results in interstitial edema, bronchoconstriction, and a decrease in functional residual capacity. With further increases in capillary permeability the fluid moves to the alveoli, with resultant alveolar edema and a decrease in surfactant production. The combined effects of pulmonary vasoconstriction and bronchoconstriction are impaired gas exchange, decreased compliance, and worsening ventilation-perfusion mismatch. Clinically, the patient has tachypnea, crackles, and an overall increased work of breathing.

The cardiovascular system is profoundly affected in the progressive stage of shock. Cardiac output begins to fall, with a resultant decrease in BP and peripheral perfusion, including a decrease in coronary artery perfusion. Capillary permeability continues to increase, enhancing the movement of fluid from the vascular space into the interstitial space. Sustained hypoperfusion results in weak peripheral pulses, and ischemia of the distal extremities eventually occurs. Myocardial dysfunction from decreased perfusion results in arrhythmias, myocardial ischemia, and potentially MI. The end result is a complete deterioration of the cardiovascular system.

The effect of prolonged hypoperfusion on the kidneys is renal tubular ischemia. The resulting acute tubular necrosis (ATN) may lead to the development of acute renal failure, which can be worsened by nephrotoxic drugs, including certain antibiotics, anesthetics, and diuretics (see Chapter 45). Renal function is markedly impaired during the progressive stage of shock. The patient will have a decreased urine output and an elevated blood urea nitrogen (BUN) and serum creatinine. Metabolic acidosis occurs from an inability to excrete acids and reabsorb bicarbonate.

The GI system is also affected by prolonged decreased tissue perfusion. As the blood supply to the GI tract is decreased, the normally protective mucosal barrier becomes ischemic. This ischemia predisposes the patient to erosive ulcers and GI bleeding and increases the risk for translocation of bacteria from the GI tract to the blood. The decreased perfusion also leads to a decreased ability to absorb nutrients from the GI system.[13]

Other systems are also affected by the sustained hypoperfusion in the progressive stage of shock. The loss of the functional ability of the liver leads to a failure of the liver to metabolize drugs and waste products such as ammonia and lactate. Jaundice results from an accumulation of bilirubin. As the liver cells die,

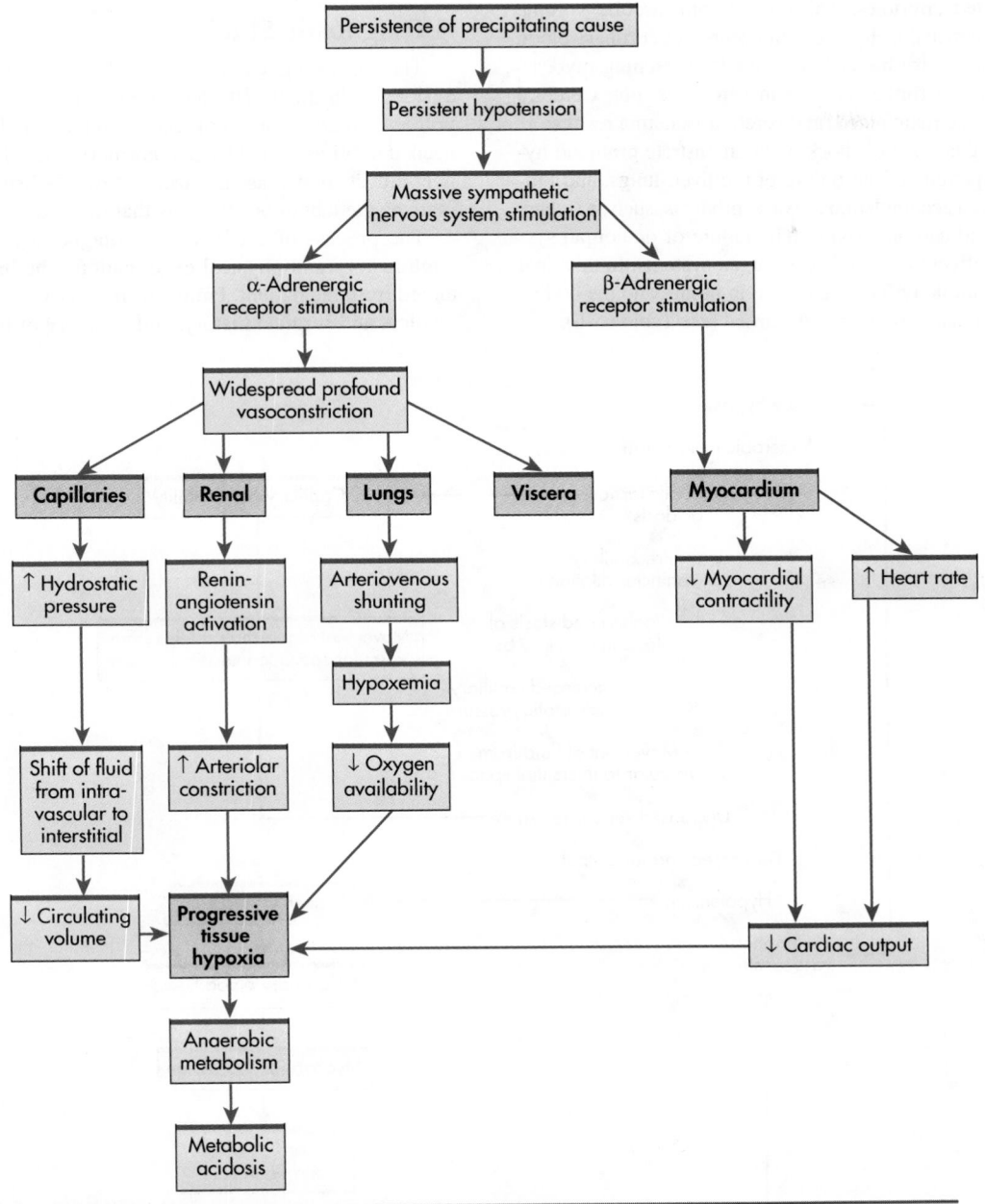

FIG. 65-7 Progressive stage: compensatory mechanisms are becoming ineffective and fail to maintain perfusion to vital organs.

enzymes become elevated, in particular alanine aminotransferase (ALT), aspartate aminotransferase (AST), and γ-glutamyl transferase (GGT). The liver also loses its ability to function as an immune organ. The bacteria that have translocated from the GI system are unable to be scavenged by the Kupffer cells. Instead, they are released into the bloodstream, thus increasing the possibility of the development of bacteremia.

Dysfunction of the hematologic system adds to the complexity of the clinical picture. The patient is at risk for the development of disseminated intravascular coagulation (DIC). In DIC, there is a consumption of the platelets and clotting factors with secondary fibrinolysis. This results in clinically significant bleeding from many orifices, including, but not limited to, the

GI tract, lungs, and puncture sites (see Chapter 30). Altered laboratory values in DIC include decreased platelets, prolonged prothrombin time, prolonged partial thromboplastin time, decreased fibrinogen, and increased fibrin split products (see Tables 65-3 and 65-6).

Refractory Stage. In the final stage of shock, the *refractory stage,* decreased perfusion from peripheral vasoconstriction and decreased cardiac output exacerbate anaerobic metabolism (Fig. 65-8). The accumulation of lactic acid contributes to an increased capillary permeability and dilation of the capillaries. Increased capillary permeability allows fluid and plasma proteins to leave the vascular space and move to the interstitial space. Blood pools in the capillary beds secondary to the constricted venules and dilated arterioles. The loss of intravascular volume worsens hypotension and tachycardia and decreases coronary blood flow. Decreased coronary blood flow leads to worsening myocardial depression and a further decline in cardiac output. Cerebral blood flow cannot be maintained, and cerebral ischemia results.

The patient in this stage of shock will demonstrate profound hypotension and hypoxemia. The failure of the liver, lungs, and kidneys will result in an accumulation of waste products, such as lactate, urea, ammonia, and carbon dioxide. The failure of one organ system will have an effect on several other organ systems. In this final stage, recovery is unlikely. The organs are in failure and the body's compensatory mechanisms are overwhelmed (see Table 65-6).

Diagnostic Studies

There is no single diagnostic study to determine whether or not a patient is in shock. The decreased tissue perfusion seen in shock will lead to an elevation of lactate and a base deficit (the amount needed to bring the pH back to normal). These laboratory changes may reflect an increase in anaerobic metabolism. Table 65-3 summarizes the laboratory findings that may be seen in shock.

The process of establishing a diagnosis begins with a thorough history and physical examination. The history may be obtained from the patient, family, or friends. Obtaining the patient's medical and surgical history, and a history of recent events (e.g.,

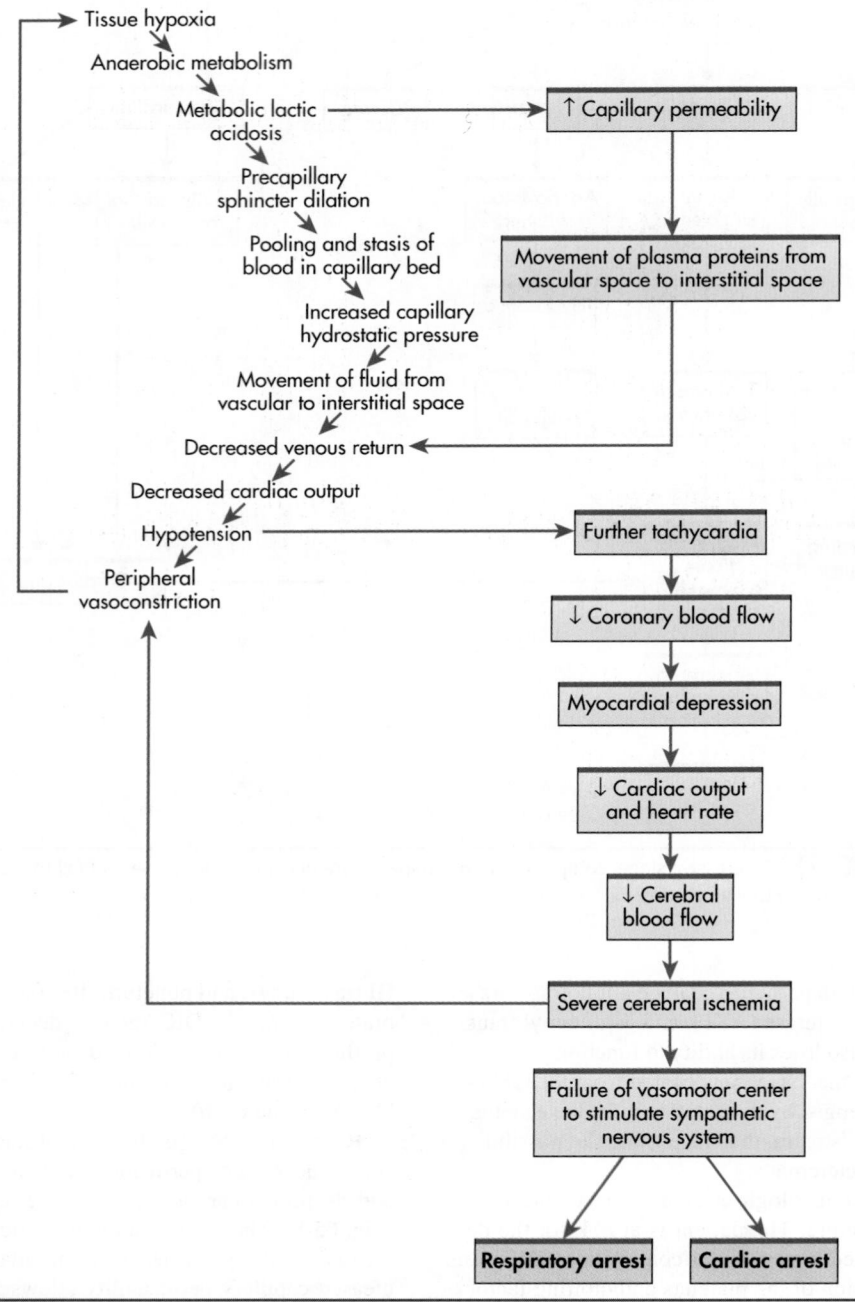

FIG. 65-8 Irreversible or refractory stage: compensatory mechanisms are not functioning or are totally ineffective, leading to multiple organ dysfunction syndrome.

upper respiratory tract infection, surgery, chest pain), will provide valuable data. Important diagnostic studies include a 12-lead ECG, continuous cardiac monitoring, chest x-ray, hemodynamic monitoring (e.g., arterial pressure monitoring, pulmonary artery pressure monitoring), and continuous pulse oximetry (see Chapter 64).

Collaborative Care: General Measures

Critical factors in the successful management of a patient experiencing shock relate to the early recognition and treatment of the shock state. Prompt intervention in the early stages of shock (initial and compensatory stages) may prevent the decline to the progressive or refractory stage. Successful management of the patient in shock includes the following:

1. Identification of patients at risk for the development of shock
2. Integration of the patient's history, physical examination, and clinical findings to establish a diagnosis
3. Interventions to control or eliminate the cause of the decreased perfusion
4. Protection of target and distal organs from dysfunction
5. Provision of multisystem supportive care

Table 65-7 provides an overview of the initial assessment findings and interventions for the emergency care of patients in shock. General management strategies for a patient in shock begin with ensuring that the patient has a patent airway. Once the airway is established, either with a natural airway or an endotracheal tube, oxygen delivery must be optimized. Mechanical ventilation may be necessary to support the delivery of oxygen to maintain an arterial oxygen saturation of 90% or greater (PaO_2 >60 mm Hg) to avoid hypoxemia (see Chapter 64). The mean arterial pressure and circulating blood volume are optimized with fluid replacement and drug therapy.

Oxygen and Ventilation. Oxygen delivery is dependent on cardiac output (CO), available hemoglobin, and arterial oxygen saturation (SaO_2). Methods to optimize oxygen delivery are directed at increasing supply and decreasing demand. Supply can be increased by (1) optimizing the CO with drug therapy or fluid replacement, (2) increasing the hemoglobin by the transfusion of blood or packed red blood cells (RBCs), and/or (3) increasing the arterial oxygen saturation with supplemental oxygen and mechanical ventilation.

Care must be planned so as not to disrupt the balance of oxygen supply and demand. The nurse must evaluate interventions that increase the patient's oxygen demand and appropriately space those interventions so that the patient's supply and demand balance is not disrupted. The use of a pulmonary artery (PA) catheter that includes a sensor to measure the mixed venous oxygen saturation (SvO_2) may be useful in determining the adequacy of tissue oxygenation. SvO_2 reflects the dynamic balance between oxygenation of the arterial blood, tissue perfusion, and tissue oxygen consumption. SvO_2, when considered in conjunction with the arterial oxygen saturation, is useful in analyzing the patient's hemodynamic status and response to treatments or activities (see Chapter 64).

TABLE 65-7   Emergency Management
Shock

ETIOLOGY*	ASSESSMENT FINDINGS	INTERVENTIONS
Surgical • Postoperative bleeding • Ruptured organ/vessel • Gastrointestinal bleeding • Aortic dissection • Vaginal bleeding • Ruptured ectopic pregnancy or ovarian cyst **Medical** • Myocardial infarction • Dehydration • Addisonian crisis • Diabetes insipidus • Sepsis • Diabetes mellitus • Pulmonary embolus **Trauma** • Ruptured or lacerated vessel or organ (e.g., spleen) • Fractures • Multisystem or multiorgan injury	• Decreased level of consciousness • Restlessness • Anxiety • Weakness • Rapid, weak, thready pulses • Arrhythmias • Hypotension • Narrowed pulse pressure • Cool, clammy skin (warm skin in early stage of septic shock) • Tachypnea, dyspnea, or shallow, irregular respirations • Decreased O_2 saturation • Extreme thirst • Nausea and vomiting • Chills • Feeling of impending doom • Pallor • Cyanosis • Obvious hemorrhage or injury • Temperature dysregulation	**Initial** • Establish and maintain patent airway. • Administer high-flow oxygen (100%) by non-rebreather mask or bag-valve–mask. • Anticipate need for intubation. • Stabilize cervical spine as appropriate. • Establish IV access with two large-bore catheters (14–16 gauge) and begin fluid resuscitation with crystalloids (e.g., normal saline solution, lactated Ringer's solution). • Control any external bleeding with direct pressure or pressure dressing. • Assess for life-threatening injuries (e.g., cardiac tamponade, liver laceration, tension pneumothorax). • Consider vasopressor therapy only after hypovolemia has been corrected. • Insert an indwelling bladder catheter and nasogastric tube. • Treat arrhythmias. **Ongoing Monitoring** • Vital signs, including pulse oximetry, peripheral pulses, capillary refill • Level of consciousness • Cardiac rhythm • Urine output

*See Table 65-1 for additional etiologies of shock.

Fluid Replacement. Except for cardiogenic shock, all other classifications of shock involve decreased circulating blood volume. The cornerstone of therapy for septic, hypovolemic, neurogenic, and anaphylactic shock is volume expansion with the administration of the appropriate fluid. Before beginning fluid resuscitation, two large-bore (e.g., 14 to 16 gauge) IV catheters must be inserted, preferably into the antecubital veins.

Both crystalloids (e.g., normal saline solution) and colloids (e.g., albumin) have a role in fluid resuscitation (Table 65-8). The choice of fluid for resuscitation remains controversial. Currently, it is generally accepted that isotonic crystalloids, such as normal saline, are used in the initial resuscitation of shock, even though approximately two thirds of the crystalloid volume will diffuse out of the vascular space and into the interstitial space. Lactated Ringer's solution should be used cautiously in all shock situations because the failing liver cannot convert lactate to bicarbonate, thus increasing the serum lactate levels. Colloids are effective volume expanders because the size of their molecules keeps them in the vascular space for a longer period of time. Despite this fact, no definitive studies demonstrate that using colloids for resuscitation improves patient outcomes.[15]

The choice of fluid for resuscitation must also be based on the type and volume of fluid lost and the patient's clinical status. If the patient does not respond to 2 L of crystalloids, blood administration and central venous monitoring may be instituted. Serial blood pressures with an automatic BP cuff or an indwelling arterial catheter can be used to monitor the patient's status. An indwelling bladder catheter will also assist in monitoring the patient's fluid status.

When large amounts of fluid replacement are required, the patient must be protected against complications. Two major complications are hypothermia and coagulopathy. The patient can be protected from hypothermia by warming both crystalloid and colloid solutions used during massive fluid resuscitation. If the patient is receiving large volumes of packed RBCs, it is important to remember that they do not contain clotting factors. Therefore clotting factors will need to be replaced. Generally, 1 to 2 U of fresh frozen plasma are administered for every 5 U of packed RBCs.[16]

If the patient does not respond to volume replacement, a PA catheter may be considered to assist in evaluating the status of the intravascular volume. A PA catheter allows the measurement and/or computation of cardiac output (CO), preload, afterload, and SvO_2. If the patient has persistent hypotension after adequate volume resuscitation, a vasopressor agent, such as dopamine (Intropin), may be added. The goal for resuscitation remains the restoration of tissue perfusion. Thus decisions on which vasopressor or inotrope to use should be based on the physiologic goal. Although BP helps determine whether the patient's CO is adequate, an assessment of end-organ perfusion (e.g., urine output, neurologic function, peripheral pulses) provides more relevant information.

Drug Therapy. The primary goal of drug therapy for shock is the correction of decreased tissue perfusion. Medications used to improve perfusion in shock are administered intravenously via an infusion pump and often via a central venous line. One of the key reasons for administration of these medications via a central line is that many of the medications that have vasoconstrictor properties may have deleterious effects if administered peripherally and the drug extravasates (Table 65-9).[17]

TABLE 65-8	Fluid Therapy in Shock		
FLUID TYPE	**MECHANISM OF ACTION**	**TYPE OF SHOCK**	**NURSING IMPLICATIONS**
Crystalloids **Isotonic** • 0.9% NaCl (NSS) • Lactated Ringer's (LR)	Fluid primarily remains in the intravascular space, increasing intravascular volume	Used for initial volume replacement in most types of shock	Monitor patient closely for circulatory overload. LR should not be used in patients with liver failure.
Blood/Blood Products • Whole blood/packed red blood cells	Replaces blood loss, increases oxygen-carrying capability	All types of shock if hemoglobin is <12 g/dl (120 g/L) or if the patient does not respond to crystalloids	Same precautions as any blood administration (see Chapter 30).
Colloids • Hetastarch (Hespan)	Made from starch and acts as volume expander; is at least as effective as albumin; can exert osmotic effect for up to 36 hours	All types of shock	May be 50% less costly than albumin. Use cautiously in patients with congestive heart failure, renal failure, or bleeding disorders (due to anticoagulant effect).
• Human serum albumin (5%, 25%), plasma protein fraction (5% albumin in 500 ml NSS)	Can increase plasma colloid osmotic pressure; rapid volume expansion	All types of shock except cardiogenic	Monitor for circulatory overload. Mild side effects of chills, fever, and urticaria may develop. More expensive than other colloids.
• dextran dextran 40 dextran 70	Hyperosmotic glucose polymer; has similar degrees of volume expansion with dextran 40 and dextran 70; longer duration of action with dextran 70	Limited use because of side effects including reducing platelet adhesion, diluting clotting factors	Increases risk of bleeding. Important to monitor patient for allergic reactions and acute renal failure.

NSS, Normal saline solution.

TABLE 65-9	*D*rug Therapy — Shock			
DRUG*	**MECHANISM OF ACTION**	**HEMODYNAMIC EFFECTS**	**TYPE OF SHOCK**	**NURSING IMPLICATIONS**
dobutamine (Dobutrex)	↑ Myocardial contractility ↓ Ventricular filling pressures	↓ SVR/PAWP ↑ CO/stroke volume/ CVP ↑↓ HR	Used in cardiogenic shock with severe systolic dysfunction Used in septic shock with normal CO that is not meeting ↑ metabolic demands	Correct hypovolemia. Do not administer in same line with NaHCO₃. Administration via central line recommended. Monitor HR. Monitor for arrhythmias.
dopamine (Intropin)	Precursor to epinephrine and norepinephrine Hemodynamic effects from release of norepinephrine Positive inotropic effects: ↑ Myocardial contractility ↑ Automaticity ↑ Atrioventricular conduction Low doses: ↑ blood flow to renal, mesenteric, and cerebral circulation High doses: can cause progressive vasoconstriction	↑ HR ↑ CO ↑ BP	Cardiogenic shock: ↑ Mean arterial pressure ↑ HR ↑ MVO₂	Correct hypovolemia. Administer via central line. Do not administer with NaHCO₃. Monitor for peripheral vasoconstriction at moderate to high doses. Monitor for tachyarrhythmias.
epinephrine (Adrenalin)	Low doses: β-adrenergic agonist (cardiac stimulation, bronchial dilation, peripheral vasodilation) High doses: α-adrenergic agonist (peripheral vasoconstriction)	↑ HR/contractility/ CO ↓ SVR ↑ Stroke volume ↑ Systolic/↓ diastolic BP, widened pulse pressure ↑ CVP/PAWP	Cardiogenic shock combined with afterload reduction Anaphylactic shock Cardiac arrest, pulseless ventricular tachycardia, ventricular fibrillation, asystole	Correct hypovolemia if appropriate. Monitor for HR >110. Monitor for dyspnea, pulmonary edema. Monitor for chest pain, arrhythmias secondary to ↑ MVO₂. Monitor for renal failure secondary to ischemia.
norepinephrine (Levophed)	β₁-adrenergic agonist (cardiac stimulation) α-adrenergic agonist (peripheral vasoconstriction) Renal/splanchnic vasoconstriction	↑ BP, MAP ↑ CVP/PAWP ↑ SVR ↑↓ CO	Cardiogenic shock after myocardial infarction Septic shock: works by increasing vascular tone	Used for hypotension unresponsive to adequate fluid resuscitation. Administer via a central line (infiltration leads to tissue sloughing). Monitor for arrhythmias secondary to ↑ MVO₂ requirements.
phenylephrine (Neo-Synephrine)	α-adrenergic agonist Vasoconstriction: renal, mesenteric, splanchnic, cutaneous, and pulmonary vessels	↑ HR ↑ BP ↑ SVR ↑↓ CO	Neurogenic shock	Monitor for reflex bradycardia, headache, restlessness. Monitor for renal failure secondary to ↓ renal blood flow. Infiltration leads to tissue sloughing.
nitroglycerin (Tridil)	Venodilation Dilates coronary arteries ↓ Preload ↓ MVO₂	↓ SVR ↓ BP ↓ CVP/PAWP ↓↑ CO	Cardiogenic shock	Monitor for postural hypotension; reflex tachycardia. Use glass bottles for storage.
sodium nitroprusside (Nipride)	Arterial and venous vasodilation ↓ Preload/afterload	↓ BP ↓ CO	Cardiogenic shock with ↑ SVR	Continuously monitor BP. Protect solution from light; wrap infusion bottle with opaque covering. Administer with D₅W only. Monitor for cyanide toxicity (e.g., tinnitus, hyperreflexia, confusion, seizures).

*Consult individual facility's guidelines, pharmacist, pharmacology references, and drug manufacturer's administration materials for additional information and exact dosing.
BP, Blood pressure; *CO,* cardiac output; *CVP,* central venous pressure; *HR,* heart rate; *MVO₂,* myocardial oxygen consumption; *PAWP,* pulmonary artery wedge pressure; *SVR,* systemic vascular resistance.

Sympathomimetic drugs. Many of the drugs used in the treatment of shock have an effect on the SNS. Drugs that mimic the action of the SNS are termed *sympathomimetic*. The effects of these drugs are mediated through their binding to α-adrenergic or β-adrenergic receptors. The various drugs differ in their relative α-adrenergic and β-adrenergic effects. (See Chapter 32, Table 32-1, for a discussion of adrenergic receptors.)

Many of the sympathomimetic drugs cause peripheral vasoconstriction and are referred to as vasopressor drugs (e.g., epinephrine [Adrenalin], norepinephrine [Levophed]). At high doses these vasopressor drugs have the potential to cause severe peripheral vasoconstriction and further jeopardize tissue perfusion, either directly or indirectly. The increased SVR increases the workload of the heart and can be detrimental to a patient in cardiogenic shock by causing further myocardial damage. Use of vasopressor drugs is generally reserved for patients who have been unresponsive to other therapies. Adequate volume replacement must be administered before the use of any vasopressor because peripheral vasoconstrictor effects in patients with low blood volume will cause further reduction in tissue perfusion.

The goals of vasopressor therapy are to achieve and maintain a mean arterial pressure (MAP) of at least 60 mm Hg. The nurse must continuously monitor end-organ perfusion (e.g., urine output, neurologic function) to ensure that the BP is providing adequate perfusion.

Vasodilator drugs. Some patients in shock show evidence of excessive vasoconstriction and poor tissue perfusion in spite of volume replacement and normal or even high systemic BP. This is especially true of patients in cardiogenic shock. Although generalized sympathetic vasoconstriction is a useful compensatory mechanism for maintaining systemic pressure, excessive constriction can reduce tissue blood flow and increase the workload of the heart. The rationale for using vasodilator therapy for a patient in shock is to break the deleterious cycle in which widespread vasoconstriction causes a decrease in CO and BP, resulting in further sympathetic-induced vasoconstriction.

The goal of vasodilator therapy, as in vasopressor therapy, is to maintain MAP at 60 mm Hg or greater. It is also important to closely monitor PA pressures along with MAP so that fluid administration can be increased or the dose of the vasodilator decreased if a serious fall in BP occurs. The vasodilator agent most often used for the patient in cardiogenic shock is nitroglycerin (Tridil). Vasodilation may be enhanced with nitroprusside (Nipride) in noncardiogenic shock.

Nutritional Therapy. Protein-calorie malnutrition is one of the primary manifestations of hypermetabolism in shock. Nutrition is vital to decreasing morbidity. Some type of nutrition should be implemented within the first 24 hours. Generally, parenteral feeding is used only if enteral feedings have failed, are contraindicated, or fail to meet the patient's caloric requirements. (Total parenteral nutrition and enteral tube feedings are discussed in Chapter 39.) The patient is started on continuous drip of very small amounts of enteral feedings. Early enteral feedings are thought to enhance perfusion of the GI tract and prevent translocation of gut bacteria.

A patient in shock should be weighed daily on the same scale at the same time of day. If the patient experiences a significant weight loss, dehydration should be ruled out before additional calories are provided parenterally. Large weight gains are common because of third spacing of fluids. Therefore daily weights may function as an indicator of fluid status rather than caloric needs and balance. Serum protein, nitrogen balance, BUN, serum glucose, and serum electrolytes are all used to assess nutritional status.

Collaborative Care: Specific Measures

Cardiogenic Shock. For a patient in cardiogenic shock, the overall goal is to restore blood flow to the myocardium by restoring the balance between oxygen supply and demand. Definitive measures to restore blood flow include thrombolytic therapy, angioplasty with stenting, and emergency revascularization (see Chapter 33). Cardiac catheterization should be performed as soon as possible after the initial insult. Coronary angioplasty with or without stenting may be performed during the cardiac catheterization. Until these interventions can be performed, the heart must be supported to optimize stroke volume and CO in an effort to facilitate optimal perfusion (Tables 65-9 and 65-10).

Hemodynamic management of a patient in cardiogenic shock is geared toward reducing the workload of the heart through drug therapy or mechanical interventions. Drug selection is based on the clinical goal and a thorough understanding of the pharmacodynamics of each drug. Drugs can be used to decrease the workload of the heart by dilating coronary arteries (e.g., nitrates), reducing preload (e.g., diuretics), reducing afterload (e.g., angiotensin-converting enzyme [ACE] inhibitors), and reducing heart rate and contractility (e.g., β-adrenergic blockers).

The patient may also benefit from a circulatory assist device such as an intraaortic balloon pump (IABP) or a ventricular assist device (VAD) (see Chapter 64). The IABP is a circulatory assist device that is inserted into the femoral artery and placed in the aorta just distal to the aortic arch. The goal of this intervention is to decrease the SVR and thus left ventricular workload. Another type of circulatory assist device, the VAD, may also be used on a temporary basis for the patient in cardiogenic shock and/or awaiting cardiac transplantation. Cardiac transplantation is an option for a small and select group of patients with cardiogenic shock.

Hypovolemic Shock. The underlying principles of managing patients with hypovolemic shock focus on stopping the loss of fluid and restoring the circulating volume. Table 65-8 delineates the different types of fluid used for volume resuscitation, the mechanisms of action, and specific nursing implications for each fluid type.

Septic Shock. Patients in septic shock require large amounts of fluid replacement, sometimes as much as 6 to 10 L of isotonic crystalloids and 2 to 4 L of colloids.[18] Predetermined end points of resuscitation are suggested in Table 65-10. To optimize and evaluate large-volume resuscitation, hemodynamic monitoring with a PA catheter and continuous BP monitoring with an arterial catheter may be necessary. The overall goal of fluid resuscitation is to restore perfusion. If that cannot be accomplished with intravenous fluids, vasopressor drug therapy may be added. Vasodilation and low cardiac index, or vasodilation alone, can cause low blood pressure in spite of adequate volume resuscitation. The addition of a vasopressor drug may increase BP but may also result in a decrease in stroke volume. An inotropic agent is often added to offset the decrease in stroke volume (see Table 65-9).

In an attempt to meet the increasing tissue demands coupled with a low SVR, the patient may demonstrate a high CO. If the

TABLE

*C*ollaborative Care

65-10   **Specific Measures for the Treatment of Shock**

CARDIOGENIC SHOCK	HYPOVOLEMIC SHOCK	SEPTIC SHOCK	NEUROGENIC SHOCK	ANAPHYLACTIC SHOCK

▪ Improve O₂ delivery by ↓ demand
▪ Reestablish blood flow with thrombolytics, angioplasty, emergency revascularization
▪ ↑ O₂ supply by providing supplemental O₂
▪ Drug therapy:
  ▪ Dilate coronary arteries (e.g., nitrates)
  ▪ Improve contractility (e.g., inotropes)
  ▪ Reduce preload (e.g., nitrates, morphine, diuretics, ACE inhibitors)
  ▪ Reduce afterload (e.g., ACE inhibitors, phosphodiesterase inhibitors, β-adrenergic agonists, vasodilators)
  ▪ Reduce heart rate (e.g., β-adrenergic blockers, calcium channel blockers)
  ▪ Reduce contractility (e.g., β-adrenergic blockers [contraindicated with ↓ ejection fraction])
▪ Correct arrhythmias
▪ Circulatory assist devices: IABP, VAD
	▪ Optimize oxygenation
	▪ Correct the cause (e.g., stop bleeding, GI losses)
	▪ Volume replacement (e.g., blood/blood products, crystalloids, colloids)
	▪ Rapid fluid replacement with two large-bore (14-16 gauge) peripheral IVs
	▪ Use warmed fluids
	▪ Endpoints of resuscitation:
	  ▪ CVP 15 mm Hg
	  ▪ PAWP 10-12 mm Hg
	  ▪ CI >3 L/min/m²
	  ▪ Blood lactate <4 mmol/L
	  ▪ Base deficit −3 to +3 mmol/L
		▪ Optimize oxygen delivery by ↑ supply/↓ demand
		▪ Fluid resuscitation
		▪ Optimize cardiac output:
		  ▪ Volume
		  ▪ Vasopressors
		  ▪ Vasopressors and inotropes (e.g., dobutamine)
		▪ Vasopressors (↑ BP) (e.g., dopamine, norepinephrine, phenylephrine)
		▪ Correct acidosis
		▪ Obtain culture before beginning antibiotics
		▪ Antibiotics as ordered
			▪ Treat according to the cause (see Table 65-1)
			▪ Minimize spinal cord trauma with stabilization
			▪ Careful administration of fluids
			▪ Drug therapy:
			  ▪ Dopamine for hypotension and bradycardia
			  ▪ Administration of phenylephrine or norepinephrine to increase SVR
			▪ Monitor for hypothermia
				▪ Prevention via avoidance of known allergens
				▪ Premedication with history of prior sensitivity (e.g., contrast media)
				▪ Identify and remove offending cause
				▪ Maintain patent airway
				▪ Intubation/mechanical ventilation
				▪ Drug therapy:
				  ▪ Epinephrine subcutaneous, IV, nebulized
				  ▪ Bronchodilators: nebulized, IV
				  ▪ Antihistamines
				  ▪ Corticosteroids (if hypotension persists)
				▪ Fluid resuscitation with colloids

ACE, Angiotensin–converting enzyme; *BP,* blood pressure; *CI,* cardiac index; *CVP,* central venous pressure; *GI,* gastrointestinal; *IABP,* intraaortic balloon pump; *PAWP,* pulmonary artery wedge pressure; *VAD,* ventricular assist device.

patient is unable to achieve and maintain an adequate CO and has unmet tissue oxygen demands, the CO may need to be increased using drug therapy (e.g., dobutamine [Dobutrex]). The adequacy of the CO can be determined using the mixed venous oxygen saturation (SvO₂). The SvO₂ (normal, 60% to 80%) is a reflection of the balance between oxygen delivery and consumption (see Chapter 64). If the balance is maintained, the tissue demands will be met and CO will be adequate.

Septic shock is always associated with a documented or suspected infection (see Table 65-5), and antibiotics are an important component of therapy. Before beginning definitive treatment for the infection, the cause of the infection must first be identified. Cultures (e.g., blood, wound exudate, urine, stool, sputum) are obtained before antibiotics are started. Broad-spectrum antibiotics are given initially, followed by more specific antibiotics once the organism has been identified.

Mortality rates from septic shock remain high, and until recently research efforts had not helped to improve outcomes for patients with septic shock. Drotrecogin (Xigris), a recombinant form of activated protein C, has demonstrated promise in treating patients with severe sepsis. Activated protein C is a naturally occurring substance whose exact mechanism of action is unknown. It is thought to produce an antiinflammatory effect by inhibiting TNF production and limiting inflammation. Activated protein C is found in subnormal levels in patients with sepsis. Drotrecogin interrupts the body's response to severe sepsis, including bleeding, clotting abnormalities, and cardiovascular and renal failure. The use of drotrecogin has resulted in a significant decrease in mortality rate when it is used for patients with severe sepsis.[19] Bleeding is the most common serious adverse effect associated with its use.

Neurogenic Shock. The specific treatment of neurogenic shock is dependent on the cause. If the cause is spinal cord injury, general measures to promote spinal stability (e.g., spinal precautions, cervical stabilization with a collar) are initially used. Once the spine is stabilized, definitive treatment of the hypotension and bradycardia is essential to prevent further spinal cord damage. Hypotension, which occurs as a result of a loss of sympathetic tone, is associated with peripheral vasodilation and decreased venous return. If the venous return is not optimized by volume, the addition of an α-adrenergic agonist (e.g., phenylephrine [Neo-Synephrine]) may be indicated (see Table 65-9).

The patient with a spinal cord injury will also need to be monitored for hypothermia due to hypothalamic dysfunction (see Table 65-10). Although corticosteroids do not have an effect in neurogenic shock, methylprednisolone (Solu-Medrol) is used for patients with a spinal cord injury to prevent secondary spinal cord damage caused by the release of chemical mediators (see Chapter 59).

Anaphylactic Shock. The first strategy in managing patients at risk for anaphylactic shock is prevention. A thorough history is key in avoiding the risk factors for anaphylaxis (see Table 65-1). The clinical presentation of anaphylactic shock is dramatic, and immediate intervention is required. Epinephrine is the drug of choice to treat anaphylactic shock.[15] It causes peripheral vasoconstriction and bronchodilation and opposes the effect of histamine. Diphenhydramine (Benadryl) is administered to block the massive release of histamine from the allergic reaction.

Maintaining a patent airway is important, because the patient can quickly develop airway compromise from laryngeal edema or bronchoconstriction. Nebulized bronchodilators are highly effective. Aerosolized epinephrine can also be used to treat laryngeal edema. Endotracheal intubation or cricothyroidotomy may be necessary to secure and maintain a patent airway.

Hypotension results from leakage of fluid out of the intravascular space into the interstitial space as a result of increased vascular permeability and vasodilation. Aggressive fluid replacement, predominantly with colloids, is necessary. Intravenous corticosteroids may be helpful in anaphylactic shock if significant hypotension persists after 1 to 2 hours of aggressive therapy (see Tables 65-9 and 65-10).

NURSING MANAGEMENT
SHOCK

■ Nursing Assessment

The role of the nurse is vital in caring for patients who are at risk for developing shock or are in a state of shock. The initial assessment should be geared toward the ABCs: airway, breathing, and circulation. Further assessment should focus on the assessment of tissue perfusion and includes evaluation of vital signs, peripheral pulses, level of consciousness, capillary refill, skin (e.g., temperature, color, moisture), and urine output. As shock progresses, the patient's skin will become cooler and mottled, urine output will decrease, and neurologic status will continue to deteriorate.

To understand the complexity of the patient's clinical status, the nurse must integrate all of the assessment data. As care is initiated (see Tables 65-7 and 65-10), it is essential for the nurse to obtain a brief history from the patient or other knowledgeable person. This information should include a description of the events leading to the shock condition, time of onset and duration of symptoms, and a health history (e.g., medications, allergies, date of last tetanus vaccination). In addition, details regarding any care that the patient received before hospitalization are also important.

■ Nursing Diagnoses

Nursing diagnoses for the patient with shock may include, but are not limited to, those presented in NCP 65-1.

■ Planning

The overall goals for caring for a patient in shock include (1) assurance of adequate tissue perfusion, (2) restoration of normal BP, (3) return/recovery of organ function, and (4) avoidance of complications from prolonged states of hypoperfusion.

■ Nursing Implementation

Health Promotion. It is important for nurses to become involved in the prevention of shock. To prevent shock, the nurse needs to identify patients at risk. In general, patients who are older, those with debilitating illnesses, and those who are immunocompromised are at an increased risk. Any person who sustains surgical or accidental trauma is at high risk for shock resulting from hemorrhage, spinal cord injury, and other conditions (see Table 65-1). Any patient who is at risk for decreased oxygen delivery or tissue hypoxia is also at risk for the development of shock.

Planning is essential to help prevent shock after a susceptible individual has been identified. For example, a person with an acute MI, especially an anterior wall MI, is at risk for cardiogenic shock. The primary goal for the patient with an acute MI is to limit the size of the infarction. The infarct size can be limited by restoring coronary blood flow through thrombolytic therapy, percutaneous coronary intervention (PCI), or surgical revascularization. Rest, analgesics, sedation, and judicious use of paralytic agents (if the patient is intubated) can reduce the myocardial demand for oxygen. The nurse can modify the patient's environment to provide care at intervals that will not increase the patient's oxygen demand. For example, if the patient becomes anxious with bathing, that activity can be planned at a time so as not to interfere with x-rays or other activities that may also increase oxygen demand.

A person with a severe allergy to such substances as drugs, shellfish, and insect bites is at increased risk to develop anaphylactic shock. The risk of anaphylactic shock can be decreased if the patient is carefully questioned about allergies before administering a new drug (even if the patient has received this drug in the past) or before undergoing diagnostic procedures involving the use of contrast media. Patients with severe allergies should wear a Medic Alert tag and report their allergies to their health care providers. These patients should also be instructed about the availability of special kits that contain equipment and medication (e.g., epinephrine [EpiPen]) for the treatment of acute hypersensitivity reactions. If a patient's condition warrants receiving a medication to which he or she is at high risk for an allergic reaction (e.g., contrast media), the patient should receive a premedication such as diphenhydramine or methylprednisolone.

Careful monitoring of fluid balance can help to prevent hypovolemic shock. Ongoing monitoring of intake and output and daily weights are important. In addition, monitoring of the patient's clinical status is essential because trends in clinical findings are more meaningful than any single piece of clinical information.

All patients must be carefully monitored for the development of infection. Progression from an infection to sepsis and septic shock is dependent on the patient's host defense mechanisms. Pa-

NURSING CARE PLAN 65-1

Patient in Shock

EXPECTED PATIENT OUTCOMES	NURSING INTERVENTIONS and *RATIONALES*

NURSING DIAGNOSIS

Decreased cardiac output *related to* shock state *as manifested by* increased diastolic BP, decreased systolic BP; postural hypotension; tachycardia; weak, thready pulses; flat neck veins; low CVP and PAWP; thirst and dry mucous membranes; urinary output <0.5 ml/kg/hr; altered mentation; arrhythmias; tachypnea; hypoxemia; pallor or cyanosis; cool, clammy skin.

- Normal or baseline BP (for patient)
- HR 60-100 beats/min and regular
- Strong peripheral pulses
- Normal CVP (1-8 mm Hg) and PAWP (6-12 mm Hg)
- Warm, dry skin
- Urinary output >0.5 ml/kg/hr
- Normal mentation
- Respiratory rate >12 and <20 breaths/min
- SaO$_2$ ≥90%

- Monitor vital signs, CVP, pulmonary artery pressures every 15 min to 1 hr *to monitor patient's status and detect fluid deficits or excesses, and to assess patient's response to treatment.*
- Administer crystalloids, colloids, and/or blood *to restore blood and fluid volume to maintain perfusion of vital organs.*
- Titrate drug therapy (as indicated) to support BP *to maintain perfusion.*
- Record accurate intake and output; daily weights *to monitor fluid balance status.*
- Monitor laboratory and x-ray findings *to evaluate patient's response to treatment.*
- Keep patient at normal body temperature *to prevent an increase in metabolic need for O$_2$ and increased CO$_2$ production.*
- Administer oxygen *to keep SaO$_2$ ≥90%.*

NURSING DIAGNOSIS

Fear and anxiety *related to* severity of condition *as manifested by* verbalization of anxiety about condition and fear of death, or withdrawal with no communication; restlessness; sleeplessness; increase in heart and respiratory rate.

- Verbalization of anxieties and/or fears
- Verbalization of reduced anxiety and/or fear

- Acknowledge expressed fear and anxiety *to validate patient's feelings.*
- Demonstrate concern and respect for patient.
- Provide time to listen to patient and to draw out patient if withdrawn *to encourage verbalization and discussion of fears.*
- Seek out significant other's perception of situation *to enlist help.*
- Maintain calm and reassuring demeanor and environment *to reduce patient's anxieties and oxygen need.*
- Explain interventions, patient status, and equipment simply and honestly *to reduce patient's fear of the unknown and assist patient in making informed decisions.*

COLLABORATIVE PROBLEMS

NURSING GOALS	NURSING INTERVENTIONS and *RATIONALES*

POTENTIAL COMPLICATION

Organ ischemia/dysfunction *related to* decreased tissue perfusion.

Neurologic Ischemia/Dysfunction
- Monitor for signs of neurologic ischemia
- Report deviations from acceptable parameters
- Carry out medical and nursing interventions

- Perform neurologic assessment every hour, including assessment of changes in mentation or level of consciousness, *to provide information regarding status of cerebral blood flow.*
- Record and report any changes *to guide selection of appropriate interventions.*
- Closely observe and protect confused patient *to prevent injury.*
- Take measures to minimize noise *to control sensory input and allow for rest.*

Renal Ischemia/Dysfunction
- Monitor for signs of renal ischemia
- Report deviations from acceptable parameters
- Carry out medical and nursing interventions

- Monitor for urine output <0.5 ml/kg/hr, increase in urine specific gravity, elevation in serum BUN and creatinine, abnormal serum electrolytes, low urine sodium, protein and blood in urine, metabolic acidosis *to assess renal function.*
- Insert bladder catheter *to accurately measure urinary output.*
- Perform daily weights *to monitor fluid status and evaluate renal function.*
- Administer fluids and drug therapy as ordered and assess results *to maintain adequate renal perfusion.*
- Monitor signs and symptoms of fluid overload *to identify a possible complication of overtreatment.*

BP, Blood pressure; *BUN,* blood urea nitrogen; *CVP,* central venous pressure; *HR,* heart rate; *PAWP,* pulmonary artery wedge pressure.

Continued

NURSING CARE PLAN 65-1

Patient in Shock—cont'd

COLLABORATIVE PROBLEMS

NURSING GOALS	NURSING INTERVENTIONS and *RATIONALES*
POTENTIAL COMPLICATION—cont'd	**Organ ischemia/dysfunction** *related to* decreased tissue perfusion.

Gastrointestinal Ischemia/Dysfunction

• Monitor for signs of GI ischemia • Report deviations from acceptable parameters • Carry out medical and nursing interventions	• Monitor for presence of abdominal pain, distention, nausea, vomiting, anorexia, diarrhea, thirst; auscultate bowel sounds every 4 hr *to assess GI status.* • Measure intake and output and daily weight *to determine fluid balance.* • Initiate enteral or parenteral nutrition as soon as possible (if ordered) *to provide adequate calories to meet metabolic demands.*

Peripheral Vascular Ischemia/Dysfunction

• Monitor for signs of peripheral vascular ischemia • Report deviations from acceptable parameters • Carry out appropriate medical and nursing interventions	• Monitor for presence of cool, pale, or cyanotic extremities; diminished or absent peripheral pulses; pain, tingling, or numbness in extremities; necrotic or gangrenous extremities; poor capillary refill *as indicators of peripheral vascular ischemia.* • Report any changes in peripheral perfusion *so treatment can be initiated promptly.* • Initiate proper skin care measures *to maintain skin integrity and prevent pressure ulcers because they can develop quickly when immobility is combined with tissue ischemia.* • Keep patient warm and dry *to promote comfort and prevent vasoconstriction.*

Respiratory Ischemia/Dysfunction

• Monitor for signs of respiratory distress • Report deviations from acceptable parameters • Carry out appropriate medical and nursing interventions	• Monitor for the following: altered respiratory rate and depth, dyspnea, use of accessory muscles, cyanosis, adventitious breath sounds, cough, abnormal chest x-ray *to assess for respiratory distress.* • Initiate oxygen and maintain $SaO_2 \geq 90\%$ *to ensure adequate oxygenation.* • Monitor ABGs *to evaluate gas exchange in the lungs and acid-base balance.* • Auscultate and record breath sounds every 1-2 hr to determine presence of crackles, wheezes, and decreased or unequal breath sounds *as indicators of impaired respirations.* • Assist patient to deep breathe *to open up alveoli and improve gas exchange.* • Suction as needed *to remove secretions patient cannot remove independently.* • Maintain patent airway and prepare for possible intubation and mechanical ventilation.

ABGs, Arterial blood gases; *GI,* gastrointestinal.

---

tients who are immunocompromised or immunosuppressed are at especially high risk to develop an opportunistic infection. Interventions to decrease the risk of infection for hospitalized patients include decreasing the number of indwelling catheters (e.g., central lines, indwelling urinary catheters), using aseptic technique during invasive procedures, and strict attention to hand washing. In addition, all equipment must be changed according to institutional policy, or thoroughly cleaned or discarded (if disposable) between patient use.

Acute Intervention. The role of the nurse in shock involves (1) monitoring the patient's ongoing physical and emotional status to detect subtle changes in the patient's condition, (2) planning and implementing nursing interventions and therapy, (3) evaluating the patient's response to therapy, (4) providing emotional support to the patient and family, and (5) collaborating with other members of the health team when warranted by the patient's condition (see NCP 65-1).

Neurologic status. Neurologic status, including orientation and level of consciousness, should be assessed at least every hour. The patient's neurologic status is the best indicator of cerebral blood flow. The nurse should be aware of the clinical manifestations that may indicate neurologic involvement, such as changes

in behavior, restlessness, hyperalertness, blurred vision, confusion, and paresthesias. The astute nurse must also be alert to any subtle changes in the neurologic status (e.g., mild agitation).

Attempts should be made to orient the patient to time, place, person, and events. If the patient is in an ICU, orientation to the environment is particularly important. Measures such as minimizing noise and light levels should be taken to control sensory input. A day-night cycle of activity and rest should be maintained as much as possible. Sensory overload and disruption of the patient's diurnal cycle may contribute to delirium.

Cardiovascular status. Much of the therapy for shock is based on information about the patient's cardiovascular status. If the patient is unstable, the heart rate, blood pressure (BP), central venous pressure (CVP), and PA pressures (if available) should be determined at least every 15 minutes. PAWP should be measured every 1 to 2 hours. (Hemodynamic monitoring is discussed in Chapter 64.) Once the patient is stable, the PAWP should be obtained only as often as needed to avoid complications associated with balloon inflation. If the pulmonary artery diastolic pressure and the PAWP correlate, the pulmonary artery diastolic pressure may be used to estimate the PAWP. The PAWP most accurately reflects left ventricular function, especially in the presence of lung problems (e.g., pulmonary embolism, chronic lung disease), when the PA pressure is often elevated. Monitoring trends in PA pressure and other hemodynamic parameters yields more important information than individual numbers. Integration of hemodynamic data with physical assessment data is essential in planning strategies to manage the patient with shock.

The patient's ECG should be continuously monitored to detect arrhythmias that may result from the cardiovascular and metabolic derangements associated with shock. Heart sounds should be assessed for the presence of an S_3 or S_4 sound or new murmurs. The presence of an S_3 sound in an adult usually indicates heart failure. The frequency of this monitoring is decreased as the patient's condition improves.

In addition to monitoring the patient's cardiovascular status, the nurse must administer the prescribed therapy that is designed to correct the dysfunctions of the cardiovascular system. The response to fluid and medication administration must be assessed at least every 15 minutes. Appropriate adjustments should be made as needed. Once tissue perfusion is restored, medications that are being used to support blood pressure and tissue perfusion are slowly weaned after the patient becomes stabilized.

Respiratory status. The respiratory status of the patient in shock must be frequently assessed to ensure adequate oxygenation, detect complications early, and provide data regarding the patient's acid-base status. The rate, depth, and rhythm of respirations are initially monitored every 15 to 30 minutes. Increased rate and depth provide information regarding the patient's attempts to correct metabolic acidosis. Breath sounds should be assessed every 4 hours for any changes, which may indicate fluid overload or accumulation of secretions.

Pulse oximetry is used to continuously monitor oxygen saturation. Pulse oximetry using a patient's finger or toe may not be accurate in an advanced shock state because of poor peripheral circulation. In this situation, the probe should be attached to the nose, ear, or forehead (according to the manufacturer's guidelines) to increase accuracy. Arterial blood gases (ABGs) provide definitive information on oxygenation status and acid-base balance. Initial interpretation of ABGs is often the nurse's responsibility. A PaO_2 below 60 mm Hg (in the absence of chronic lung disease) indicates the presence of hypoxemia and the need for the administration of higher oxygen concentrations or for a different mode of oxygen administration. A low $PaCO_2$ in the presence of a low pH and low bicarbonate level may indicate that the patient is hyperventilating in an attempt to compensate for the metabolic acidosis. A rising $PaCO_2$ in the presence of a persistently low pH and PaO_2 may indicate the need for intubation and mechanical ventilation.

Most patients in shock will be intubated and on mechanical ventilation. Maintaining a patent airway and monitoring for ventilator-related complications are critical. (Artificial airways and mechanical ventilation are discussed in Chapter 64.)

Renal status. Hourly measurements of urinary output are essential in assessment of the adequacy of renal perfusion. An indwelling bladder catheter is inserted to facilitate measurements. Urine output of less than 0.5 ml/kg per hour may indicate inadequate perfusion of the kidneys. BUN and serum creatinine values are additional indicators used to assess renal function. Serum creatinine is a better indicator of renal function because BUN levels can be influenced by the catabolic state of the patient.

Body temperature and skin changes. In the presence of an elevated or subnormal temperature, tympanic or pulmonary arterial temperatures should be obtained hourly. If normal, the temperature should be monitored only every 4 hours. The patient should be kept comfortably warm with the use of light covers and the control of environmental temperature. If the patient's temperature rises above 101.5° F (38.6° C) and the patient becomes uncomfortable or experiences cardiovascular compromise, the fever may be managed with nonsteroidal antiinflammatory drugs (NSAIDs) (e.g., ibuprofen), with acetaminophen, or by removing some of the patient's covers.

The patient's skin should be monitored for pallor, flushing, cyanosis, diaphoresis, or piloerection. In addition, the rapidity of capillary refill should be monitored as an indicator of peripheral perfusion.

Gastrointestinal status. Bowel sounds should be auscultated at least every 4 hours, and abdominal distention should be assessed. If a nasogastric tube is used, the drainage should be measured as part of the fluid output and tested for occult blood. If the patient has a bowel movement, the stool should be checked for occult blood.

Personal hygiene. Hygiene is especially important to the patient in shock because impaired tissue perfusion predisposes the patient to skin breakdown and infection. However, bathing and other nursing measures must be carried out judiciously because a patient in shock is experiencing problems with oxygen delivery to tissues. The nurse must use clinical judgment in determining priorities of care in order to limit the demands for increased oxygen.

Oral care for the patient in shock is essential because mucous membranes may become dry and fragile in the volume-depleted patient. In addition, the intubated patient usually has difficulty swallowing, resulting in pooled secretions in the mouth. A water-soluble lubricant applied to the lips prevents drying and cracking. Moist swabbing of the tongue and oral mucosa with saline solution or diluted mouthwash is also beneficial. Lemon glycerin swabs should not be used because they can cause further drying of the mucosa.

Passive range of motion should be performed three to four times per day to maintain joint mobility. The patient should be turned at least every 1 to 2 hours and positioned in good body alignment to help prevent pressure ulcers. Use of a pressure-relieving mattress or a specialty bed may also be needed. If possible, oxygen consumption (SvO_2) should be monitored during all nursing interventions to monitor the patient's tolerance to activity.

Emotional support and comfort. The effects of anxiety and fear in the face of a critical, life-threatening situation on the patient and family are frequently overlooked or underestimated. Anxiety, fear, and pain may aggravate respiratory distress and increase the release of catecholamines. When implementing care, the nurse should assess and monitor the patient's anxiety and pain. Medication to decrease anxiety and pain are common modes of therapy. Continuous infusions of a benzodiazepine (e.g., lorazepam [Ativan]), a narcotic (e.g., morphine), and occasionally a neuromuscular blocking agent (e.g., pancuronium [Pavulon]) are extremely helpful in decreasing anxiety, pain, and oxygen utilization.

The nurse should talk to the patient, even if the patient is intubated, sedated, and paralyzed or appears comatose. Hearing is often the last sense to be diminished, and even if the patient cannot respond, he or she may still be able to hear. If the intubated patient is capable of writing, a "magic slate" or a pencil and pa-

NURSING RESEARCH
Effects of Positioning Critically Ill Patients on Measures of Tissue Oxygenation

Citation
Banasik JL, Emerson RJ: Effect of lateral positions on tissue oxygenation in the critically ill, *Heart Lung* 30:269, 2001.

Purpose
To determine the effects of lateral positions on tissue oxygenation in adult critical care patients.

Methods
A prospective, quasi-experimental design was used. Critically ill patients ($n = 12$) who required hemodynamic monitoring, including arterial pressure monitoring, and who were mechanically ventilated were included in the study. All patients had impaired arterial oxygenation ($PaO_2 \leq 70$ mm Hg) and/or cardiac index ≤ 2.0 L/min/m². Patients were passively turned to each of three positions (supine, 45 degrees right lateral, and 45 degrees left lateral) using a randomized positioning schedule. Data on dependent variables (heart rate, cardiac output, arterial and venous blood gases, oxygen consumption, arterial oxygen content, and serum lactate) were collected 15 minutes after each position change.

Results and Conclusions
Analysis of variance for repeated measures revealed no differences in the dependent variables among the various positions. These findings suggest that positioning patients who are hypoxemic and/or had low cardiac outputs does not further impair tissue oxygenation.

Implications for Nursing Practice
Repositioning critically ill patients to prevent or limit the complications of immobility is essential. Evidence exists that some patients with impaired oxygenation tolerate repositioning without any untoward effects. Nurses should continue to monitor patient responses (i.e., physiologic data) to position changes when caring for them.

per should be provided. Alphabet boards or signboards with common requests (e.g., turn, fan, lights) are also useful. The patient should also receive simple explanations of procedures before they are carried out, as well as information regarding the current plan of care and its rationale. If the patient asks questions about progress and prognosis, simple and honest answers should be given.

Many patients desire a visit from a priest, rabbi, or minister. One way to provide support is to offer to call a member of the clergy rather than wait for the patient or family to express a wish for spiritual counseling.

Family and significant others can have a therapeutic effect on the patient. To perform this role, they need to be supportive and comforting. Family and significant others (1) link the patient to the outside world, (2) facilitate decision making and advise the patient, (3) assist with activities of daily living, (4) act as liaisons to advise the health care team of the patient's wishes for care, and (5) provide safe, caring, familiar relationships for the patient.[20] The fam-

ily primarily needs to be kept informed of the patient's condition. If possible, the same nurses should continuously care for the patient to decrease anxiety, limit contradictory information, and increase trust. Should the prognosis become increasingly grave, the patient's family should be given support when making difficult decisions regarding continuation of life support. The nursing staff must support the family's decisions and facilitate realistic expectations and outcomes. It is important for the nurse to remember that compassionate understanding is as essential as scientific and technical expertise in the total care of a patient and family.

Family time with the patient should be facilitated, provided this time is perceived as comforting by the patient. The nurse should explain in simple terms the purpose of tubes and equipment surrounding the patient, and the family should be informed of what they may and may not touch. If possible, the patient's hands and arms can be kept outside the sheets to encourage therapeutic touch. If desired, the family may be encouraged to perform simple comfort measures. Privacy should be provided as much as possible, but the patient and family should be assured that assistance is readily available should it be required. The call bell should be in reach at all times.

Ambulatory and Home Care. Rehabilitation of the patient who has experienced critical illness necessitates correction of the precipitating cause and prevention or early treatment of complications. The nurse should continue to monitor the patient for indications of complications throughout the recovery period. Complications may include decreased range of motion, decreased physical endurance, chronic renal failure following acute tubular necrosis, and the development of fibrotic lung disease as a result of ARDS (see Chapters 45 and 66). Thus patients recovering from shock may require diverse services on discharge. These can include admission to transitional care units (e.g., for weaning), rehabilitation centers (inpatient or outpatient), or home health care agencies. The nurse should begin to anticipate and facilitate a safe transition from the hospital to home on admission.

■ Evaluation

Expected outcomes for the patient with shock are addressed in NCP 65-1.

SYSTEMIC INFLAMMATORY RESPONSE SYNDROME AND MULTIPLE ORGAN DYSFUNCTION SYNDROME

Etiology and Pathophysiology

Systemic inflammatory response syndrome (SIRS) is a systemic inflammatory response to a variety of insults, including infection, ischemia, infarct, and injury (see Table 65-5). SIRS is characterized by generalized inflammation in organs remote from the initial insult. Normally, the inflammatory process is contained within a confined environment.

A systemic inflammatory response can be triggered by many mechanisms (see Fig. 65-1). Examples include the following:

- Mechanical tissue trauma: burns, crush injuries, surgical procedures
- Abscess formation: intraabdominal, extremities
- Ischemic or necrotic tissue: pancreatitis, vascular disease, myocardial infarction
- Microbial invasion: bacteria, viruses, fungi, parasites

- Endotoxin release: gram-negative bacteria
- Global perfusion deficits: post–cardiac resuscitation
- Regional perfusion deficits: distal perfusion deficits

Multiple organ dysfunction syndrome (MODS) is the failure of more than one organ system in an acutely ill patient such that homeostasis cannot be maintained without intervention (see Table 65-5 and Fig. 65-1). MODS results from SIRS. These two entities represent a continuum, and transition from SIRS to MODS does not occur in a clear-cut manner.[21]

MODS can develop as a result of a primary injury (primary MODS) or a secondary injury (secondary MODS). Primary MODS occurs early and results from a well-defined illness or injury (e.g., pulmonary contusion, aspiration, inhalation injury). Secondary MODS results from uncontrolled systemic inflammation with resultant organ dysfunction. It develops latently, often after many insults.[22]

Organ and Metabolic Dysfunction. When the inflammatory response is not controlled, consequences occur. These include activation of inflammatory cells and release of mediators, direct damage to the endothelium, and hypermetabolism. Vasodilation becomes excessive and leads to decreased SVR and hypotension. In addition, there is also an increase in vascular permeability that allows mediators and protein to leak out of the endothelium and into the interstitial space. The white blood cells begin to phagocytize the foreign debris, and the coagulation cascade is activated (see Chapter 29). Organ perfusion may be compromised because of hypotension, decreased perfusion, microemboli, and redistributed or shunted blood flow.

The respiratory system is often the first system to show signs of dysfunction in SIRS and MODS. Inflammatory mediators have a direct effect on the pulmonary vasculature. The endothelial damage from the release of inflammatory mediators results in an increase in capillary permeability and facilitates movement of proteinaceous fluid from the pulmonary vasculature into the pulmonary interstitial spaces. The fluid then moves to the alveoli, causing alveolar edema. Type I pneumocytes (alveolar cells) are destroyed. Type II pneumocytes become dysfunctional, and there is a decrease in surfactant production. The alveoli collapse, creating an increase in *shunt* (blood flow to the lungs that does not participate in gas exchange) and a worsening of the ventilation-perfusion mismatch. The end result is ARDS. Patients with ARDS require aggressive pulmonary management with mechanical ventilation. (See Chapter 66 for a complete discussion of ARDS.)

Cardiovascular changes include myocardial depression and massive vasodilation in response to increasing tissue demands. Vasodilation results in decreased SVR (decreased afterload) and decreased blood pressure. The baroreceptor reflex causes release of *inotropic* (increasing force of contraction) and *chronotropic* (increasing heart rate) factors that enhance cardiac output. To compensate for hypotension, CO increases by an increase in heart rate and stroke volume. Increases in capillary permeability cause a shift of albumin and fluid out of the vascular space, further diminishing venous return and thus preload. The patient becomes warm and tachycardic with a high CO and a low SVR. Other signs include poor capillary refill, skin mottling, increased CVP and PAWP, and arrhythmias. SvO_2 may be abnormally high because the patient is perfusing areas not consuming much oxygen (e.g., skin, nonworking muscle) while other areas may have blood shunted away from them. Eventually, either perfusion of vital organs becomes insufficient or the cells are unable to use oxygen and their function is compromised. As MODS progresses, myocardial dysfunction worsens.[23] The effects of SIRS and MODS on hemodynamic parameters are summarized in Table 65-2.

Neurologic dysfunction commonly manifests as mental status changes with SIRS and MODS. Acute alteration in mental status can be an early sign of MODS. The patient may become confused and agitated, combative, disoriented, lethargic, or comatose. These changes may be due to hypoxemia, the direct effect of the inflammatory mediators, or impaired perfusion. Mediators may damage neuronal tissue directly or indirectly via capillary leakage and related tissue damage. This in turn may produce cerebral edema, resulting in increased intracranial pressure.[24]

Acute renal failure (ARF) is frequently seen in SIRS and MODS. ARF can be caused not only by hypoperfusion but also by the effects of the mediators. When there is decreased perfusion to the kidneys, the SNS and the renin-angiotensin system are activated. The stimulation of the renin-angiotensin system results in systemic vasoconstriction and aldosterone-mediated sodium and water reabsorption. Another risk factor for the development of ARF is the use of nephrotoxic drugs. Antibiotics commonly used to treat gram-negative bacteria, such as aminoglycosides, can also be nephrotoxic. Careful monitoring of drug levels is essential to avoid the nephrotoxic effects.

The GI tract also plays a key role in the development of MODS. In the early stages of SIRS and MODS, the highly vascular GI mucosa has blood shunted away, making it highly vulnerable to ischemic injury. Decreased perfusion leads to a breakdown of this normally protective mucosal barrier, thus increasing the risk for ulceration and GI bleeding. With the breakdown of the mucosal barrier of the gut, bacteria translocate from the GI tract into circulation, resulting in the development of bacteremia. Gastrointestinal motility is also decreased in critical illness, causing abdominal distention and paralytic ileus.

Metabolic changes are pronounced in SIRS and MODS. Both syndromes trigger a hypermetabolic response. Glycogen stores are rapidly converted to glucose (glycogenolysis). Once glycogen is depleted, amino acids are converted to glucose (gluconeogenesis), reducing protein stores. Fatty acids are mobilized for fuel. Catecholamines and glucocorticoids are released and result in hyperglycemia and insulin resistance. The net result is a catabolic state, and lean body mass (muscle) is lost.

The hypermetabolism that is associated with SIRS and MODS may last for several days and results in liver dysfunction. Liver dysfunction in MODS may exist long before clinical evidence is present. Protein synthesis is impaired. The liver is unable to synthesize albumin, one of the key proteins that has an essential role in maintaining plasma oncotic pressure. Consequently, plasma oncotic pressure is altered and fluid and protein leak from the vascular spaces to the interstitial space. Administration of albumin does not normalize oncotic pressure in these patients.

As the state of hypermetabolism persists, the patient is unable to convert lactate to glucose, and lactate accumulates (lactic acidosis). Despite increases in glycogenolysis and gluconeogenesis, eventually the liver is unable to maintain a glucose level and the patient becomes hypoglycemic.

TABLE 65-11   Multiple Organ Dysfunction Syndrome: Clinical Manifestations and Management

SYSTEM	CLINICAL MANIFESTATIONS OF ORGAN FAILURE	MANAGEMENT
Respiratory	Development of ARDS (see Chapter 66): • Severe dyspnea • PaO_2/FIO_2 ratio <200 • Bilateral fluffy infiltrates on chest x-ray • PAWP <18 mm Hg • Ventilation-perfusion $(\dot{V}/\dot{Q})$ mismatch • Pulmonary hypertension • Increased minute ventilation • Increased respiratory rate • Decreased compliance • Refractory hypoxemia	Prevention Optimize oxygen delivery/minimize oxygen consumption Mechanical ventilation (see Chapter 64) • Positive end-expiratory pressure • Pressure control inverse ratio ventilation • Permissive hypercapnia Positioning (e.g., continuous lateral rotation therapy, prone positioning)
Renal	Prerenal: renal hypoperfusion • BUN/creatinine ratio >20:1 • ↓ Urine Na^+ <20 mEq/L • ↑ Urine specific gravity >1.020 • ↑ Urine osmolality Intrarenal: acute tubular necrosis • BUN/creatinine ratio <10:1-15:1 • ↑ Urine Na^+ >20 mEq/L • ↓ Urine osmolality • Urine specific gravity (~1.010)	Diuretics • Loop diuretics (e.g., furosemide [Lasix]) • May need to increase dose due to ↓ glomerular filtration rate Dopamine (Intropin) • Enhances renal blood flow • Improves renal perfusion • Increases urine output (if volume resuscitated) • May work synergistically with diuretics Renal replacement therapy (see Chapter 45)
Hepatic	Bilirubin >2 mg/dl (34 μmol/L) ↑ Liver enzymes (ALT, AST, GGT) ↑ Serum NH_3 ↓ Serum albumin, prealbumin, transferrin Jaundice Hepatic encephalopathy	Maintain adequate tissue perfusion Provide nutritional support (e.g., enteral feedings) Judicious use of hepatically metabolized drugs
Gastrointestinal	Mucosal ischemia • ↓ Intramucosal pH • Gut "leakiness" → translocation of gut bacteria Hypoperfusion → ↓ peristalsis, paralytic ileus Mucosal ulceration on endoscopy GI bleeding	Stress ulcer prophylaxis • Antacids (e.g., Maalox) • Histamine H_2 receptor blockers (e.g., cimetidine [Tagamet]) • Proton pump inhibitors (e.g., omeprazole [Prilosec]) • Sucralfate (Carafate) Enteral feedings • Stimulate mucosal activity • Provide nutrients
Central Nervous	Acute change in neurologic status Fever Hepatic encephalopathy Seizures Confusion/disorientation Failure to wean/prolonged rehabilitation	Evaluate for hepatic/metabolic encephalopathy Optimize cerebral blood flow ↓ Cerebral oxygen requirements Prevent secondary tissue ischemia • Calcium channel blockers (reduce cerebral vasospasm) Prevent further compromise
Cardiovascular	Myocardial depression Biventricular failure Systolic/diastolic dysfunction ↑ HR/CO/SVR ↓ Stroke volume ↓ MAP ↓ Ejection fraction/contractility	Volume management • PA catheter for hemodynamic monitoring • ↑ preload via volume replacement • Maximize myocardial function • Maintain CO • Maintain MAP >60 mm Hg Vasopressors Balance O_2 supply and demand Continuous ECG monitoring Circulatory assist devices • Intraaortic balloon pump • Ventricular assist device

ALT, Alanine aminotransferase; *ARDS*, acute respiratory distress syndrome; *AST*, aspartate aminotransferase; *BUN*, blood urea nitrogen; *CO*, cardiac output; *ECG*, electrocardiogram; *GGT*, gamma–glutamyl transferase; *GI*, gastrointestinal; *MAP*, mean arterial pressure; *PA*, pulmonary artery; *PAWP*, pulmonary artery wedge pressure; *SVR*, systemic vascular resistance.

TABLE 65-11	Multiple Organ Dysfunction Syndrome: Clinical Manifestations and Management—cont'd	
SYSTEM	**CLINICAL MANIFESTATIONS OF ORGAN FAILURE**	**MANAGEMENT**
Hematologic	↑ Bleeding times, ↑ PT, ↑ PTT ↓ Platelet count (thrombocytopenia) ↑ Fibrin split products ↑ D-dimer test	Observe for bleeding from obvious and/or occult sites Replace factors being lost (e.g., platelets) Minimize traumatic interventions (e.g., intramuscular injections, multiple venipunctures)

PT, prothrombin time; *PTT*, partial thromboplastin time.

Failure of the coagulation system manifests as DIC. DIC results in simultaneous microvascular clotting and bleeding because of the depletion of clotting factors and platelets and excessive fibrinolysis. (DIC is discussed in Chapter 30.)

Electrolyte imbalances, which are common, are related to hormonal and metabolic changes and fluid shifts. These changes exacerbate mental status changes, neuromuscular dysfunction, and arrhythmias. The release of antidiuretic hormone and aldosterone results in sodium and water retention. Aldosterone increases urinary potassium loss, and catecholamines cause potassium to move into the cell, resulting in hypokalemia. Hypokalemia is associated with arrhythmias and muscle weakness. Metabolic acidosis results from impaired tissue perfusion, hypoxia, and a shift to anaerobic metabolism with a resultant increase in hydrogen ion production. Progressive renal dysfunction also contributes to metabolic acidosis. Hypocalcemia, hypomagnesemia, and hypophosphatemia are common.

Clinical Manifestations of SIRS and MODS

The defining manifestations of SIRS and MODS are delineated in Table 65-5. The clinical manifestations of MODS are presented in Table 65-11.

NURSING *and* COLLABORATIVE MANAGEMENT SIRS AND MODS

The prognosis for the patient with MODS is poor, with estimated mortality rates at 90% to 95% when three or more organ systems fail.[24] Therefore the most important goal is to prevent the progression of SIRS to MODS. A critical component of the nursing role is vigilant assessment and ongoing monitoring to detect early signs of deterioration or organ dysfunction.

Collaborative care for patients with MODS focuses on (1) prevention and treatment of infection, (2) maintenance of tissue oxygenation, (3) nutritional and metabolic support, and (4) appropriate support of individual failing organs. Table 65-11 summarizes the management for patients with MODS.

■ Prevention and Treatment of Infection

Aggressive infection control strategies are essential to decrease the risk for nosocomial infections. Despite aggressive strategies, host dysfunction may lead to the development of an infection. Once an infection is suspected, interventions to control the source must be instituted. Appropriate cultures should be sent, and broad-spectrum antibiotic therapy should be initiated. Early, aggressive surgery is recommended to remove necrotic tissue (e.g., early de-

bridement of burn tissue) that may provide a culture medium for microorganisms. Once a specific organism is identified, therapy should be modified. Aggressive pulmonary management, including early ambulation, can reduce the risk of infection. Strict asepsis can decrease infections related to intraarterial lines, endotracheal tubes, urinary catheters, IV lines, and other invasive devices or procedures.

■ Maintenance of Tissue Oxygenation

Hypoxemia frequently occurs in patients with SIRS or MODS. These patients have greater oxygen needs and decreased oxygen supply to the tissues. Interventions that decrease oxygen demand and increase oxygen delivery are essential. Sedation, mechanical ventilation, analgesia, paralysis, and rest may decrease oxygen demand and should be considered. Oxygen delivery may be increased by maintaining normal levels of hemoglobin (e.g., transfusion of packed RBCs) and PaO_2 (80 to 100 mm Hg), using positive end-expiratory pressure (PEEP), increasing preload or myocardial contractility to enhance cardiac output, or reducing afterload to increase cardiac output.

■ Nutritional and Metabolic Needs

Hypermetabolism in SIRS or MODS can result in profound weight loss, cachexia, and further organ failure. Protein-calorie malnutrition is one of the primary manifestations of hypermetabolism and MODS. Total energy expenditure is often increased 1.5 to 2.0 times the normal metabolic rate. Because of their relatively short half-life, plasma transferrin and prealbumin levels are monitored to assess hepatic protein synthesis.

The goal of nutritional support is to preserve organ function. Providing adequate nutrition decreases morbidity and mortality rates in patients with SIRS and MODS. The use of the enteral route is preferable to parenteral nutrition and may limit translocation of gut bacteria. If the enteral route cannot be used, parenteral nutrition should be initiated. (Enteral and parenteral nutrition are discussed in Chapter 39.)

■ Support of Failing Organs

Support of any failing organ is a primary goal of therapy. For example, the patient with ARDS requires aggressive oxygen therapy and mechanical ventilation (see Chapter 64). DIC should be treated appropriately (e.g., blood products) (see Chapter 30). Renal failure may require renal replacement therapy. Continuous renal replacement therapy is better tolerated than hemodialysis, especially in a patient with hemodynamic instability (see Chapter 45).

CRITICAL THINKING EXERCISES

Case Study
Shock

Patient Profile. Mr. S., a 25-year-old Korean American, was an unrestrained driver involved in a motor vehicle crash. He was found face down 15 feet from his car. There were no passengers. The windshield was broken and the car was found up against a tree. Mr. S. was found conscious and moaning. He was taken to the emergency department (ED).

Subjective Data
- States, "I can't breathe."
- Cries out when abdomen is palpated.

Objective Data
Physical Examination
- Cardiovascular: BP 84/70; apical pulse 120 but no radial or brachial pulses palpable; carotid pulse present but weak
- Lungs: respiratory rate 35/min; labored breathing with severe respiratory distress; asymmetric chest wall movement; absence of breath sounds on left side
- Abdomen: slightly distended and painful on palpation

Diagnostic Studies
- Chest x-ray: hemopneumothorax and rib fractures on left side
- Hematocrit: 28%

Collaborative Care
- In the ED, placement of chest tube, which drained bright red blood

Surgical Procedure
- Splenectomy
- Repair of torn thoracic artery

CRITICAL THINKING QUESTIONS
1. What type of shock was present in Mr. S.? What clinical manifestations did he display?
2. What were the causes of Mr. S.'s shock? What are other causes of this type of shock?
3. What are the initial nursing responsibilities for Mr. S.?
4. What continual nursing assessment parameters are essential for this patient?
5. Based on the assessment data presented, write one or more nursing diagnoses. Are there any collaborative problems?

Nursing Research Issues
1. What nursing measures can be implemented to conserve oxygen and decrease oxygen utilization in patients with shock or MODS?
2. Which patient positions maximize oxygenation and circulatory status in patients with different types of shock?
3. Is there a difference in the accuracy of the following BP monitoring devices used to detect BP changes in shock: invasive arterial monitoring versus noninvasive devices?

REVIEW QUESTIONS

The number of the question corresponds to the same-numbered objective at the beginning of the chapter.

1. Shock is best defined as
   a. cardiovascular collapse.
   b. loss of sympathetic tone.
   c. inadequate tissue perfusion.
   d. blood pressure less than 90 mm Hg systolic.

2. A patient has a spinal cord injury at T4. Vital signs include a falling blood pressure with bradycardia. The nurse recognizes that the patient is experiencing
   a. a relative hypervolemia.
   b. an absolute hypovolemia.
   c. neurogenic shock from low blood flow.
   d. neurogenic shock from a maldistribution of blood flow.

3. The effect that shock has on the body includes
   a. sympathetic nervous system activation that results in stimulation of adrenergic receptors.
   b. massive vasoconstriction in the heart and brain that causes stimulation of the renin-angiotensin system.
   c. heart rate that is usually slow and irregular in the compensatory stage because of parasympathetic nervous stimulation.
   d. decreased tissue perfusion that causes the cells to undergo aerobic metabolism, leading to the development of lactic acidosis.

4. A 78-year-old man has confusion and temperature of 104° F (40° C). He is a diabetic with purulent drainage from his right great toe. His hemodynamic findings are BP 84/40; heart rate 110; respiratory rate 42 and shallow; CO 8 L/min; and PAWP 4 mm Hg. This patient's symptoms are most likely indicative of
   a. sepsis.
   b. septic shock.
   c. multiple organ dysfunction syndrome.
   d. systemic inflammatory response syndrome.

5. Appropriate treatment modalities for the management of cardiogenic shock include
   a. dopamine to increase myocardial contractility.
   b. vasopressors to increase systemic vascular resistance.
   c. corticosteroids to stabilize the cell wall in the infarcted myocardium.
   d. plasma volume expanders such as albumin to decrease an elevated preload.

6. The most accurate assessment parameters for the nurse to use to determine adequate tissue perfusion in the patient with MODS are
   a. blood pressure, pulse, and respirations.
   b. breath sounds, blood pressure, and body temperature.
   c. pulse pressure, level of consciousness, and pupillary response.
   d. level of consciousness, urine output, and skin color and temperature.

REFERENCES

1. Rice V: *Shock, a clinical syndrome,* ed 2, Aliso Viejo, Calif, 1997, American Association of Critical Care Nurses.
2. Edwards S: Shock: types, classifications and explorations of their physiological effects, *Emergency Nurse* 9:29, 2001.
3. Silvestry FE, Herling IM: Cardiogenic shock and other pump failure states. In Lanken PE, Hanson CW, Manaker S, editors: *Intensive care manual,* Philadelphia, 2001, WB Saunders.
4. Prieto A, Eisenberg J, Thakur RK: Nonarrhythmic complications of acute myocardial infarction, *Emerg Med Clin North Am* 19:397, 2001.
5. Hand H: Myocardial infarction, part II, *Nursing Standard* 15:45, 2001.
6. Mower-Wade DM et al: Shock: do you know how to respond? *Nursing* 30:34, 2000.
7. DoNofrio D, Loh E: Cardiogenic pulmonary edema. In Lanken PE, Hanson CW, Manaker S, editors: *Intensive care manual,* Philadelphia, 2001, WB Saunders.
8. Schiller HJ, Anderson HL: Hemorrhagic shock and other low preload states. In Lanken PE, Hanson CW, Manaker S, editors: *Intensive care manual,* Philadelphia, 2001, WB Saunders.
9. Marcotte P, Freese A: Spinal injury. In Lanken PE, Hanson CW, Manaker S, editors: *Intensive care manual,* Philadelphia, 2001, WB Saunders.
10. Jurewicz MA: Anaphylaxis: when the body over reacts, *Nursing* 30:58, 2000.
11. Balk RA: Severe sepsis and septic shock: definitions, epidemiology, and clinical manifestations, *Crit Care Clin* 16:179, 2000.
12. Lent M, Hirshberg P, Margolis G: Systemic toxins: signs, symptoms and management of patients in septic shock, *JEMS* 26:54, 2001.
13. Manaker S: Septic shock and other low afterload states. In Lanken PE, Hanson CW, Manaker S, editors: *Intensive care manual,* Philadelphia, 2001, WB Saunders.
14. Collins T: Understanding shock, *Nursing Standard* 14:35, 2000.
15. McQuillan KA: Initial management of traumatic shock. In McQuillan K et al: *Trauma nursing from resuscitation through rehabilitation,* ed 3, Philadelphia, 2002, WB Saunders.
16. DeJong MJ, Karch AM: *Lippincott's critical care drug guide,* Philadelphia, 2000, Lippincott.
17. Jindal N, Hollenberg SM, Dellinger RP: Pharmacologic issues in the management of septic shock, *Crit Care Clin* 16:233, 2000.
*18. Hollenberg SM et al: Practice parameters for hemodynamic support of sepsis in adult patients in sepsis, *Crit Care Med* 27:639, 1999.
19. Bernard GR et al: Efficacy and safety to recombinant human activated protein C for sever sepsis, *N Engl J Med* 344:699, 2001.
*20. Eichhorn DJ et al: Family presence during invasive procedures and resuscitation: hearing the voice of the patient, *Am J Nurs* 101:48, 2001.
21. Cryer HG et al: Multiple organ failure: by the time you predict it, it's already there, *J Trauma* 46:597, 1999.
22. Evans TW, Smithies M: ABCs of intensive care: organ dysfunction, *Br J Med* 318:1606, 1999.
23. Marshall JC: Inflammation, coagulopathy, and the pathogenesis of multiple organ dysfunction syndrome, *Crit Care Med* 29:S99, 2001.
24. Johnson D, Mayers I: Multiple organ dysfunction syndrome: a narrative review, *Can J Anaesth* 48:502, 2001.

RESOURCES

Resources for this chapter are listed after Chapter 64 on page 1795 and Chapter 67 on page 1868.

---

*Nursing research–based reference.

CHAPTER *66*

NURSING MANAGEMENT
Respiratory Failure and Acute Respiratory Distress Syndrome

Richard B. Arbour

LEARNING OBJECTIVES

1. Compare the pathophysiologic mechanisms that result in hypoxemic and hypercapnic respiratory failure.
2. Differentiate between early and late clinical manifestations of acute respiratory failure.
3. Describe the nursing and collaborative management of the patient with hypoxemic or hypercapnic respiratory failure.
4. Relate the pathophysiologic mechanisms that result in acute respiratory distress syndrome (ARDS) to the clinical manifestations.
5. Describe the nursing and collaborative management of the patient with ARDS.
6. Identify complications that may result from acute respiratory failure or ARDS and measures to prevent or reverse these complications.

KEY TERMS

acute respiratory distress syndrome, p. 1837
alveolar hypoventilation, p. 1827
diffusion limitation, p. 1827
hypercapnia, p. 1824
hypercapnic respiratory failure, p. 1825

hypoxemia, p. 1824
hypoxemic respiratory failure, p. 1824
hypoxia, p. 1829
refractory hypoxemia, p. 1839
shunt, p. 1827

ACUTE RESPIRATORY FAILURE

The major function of the respiratory system is gas exchange, which involves the transfer of oxygen (O_2) and carbon dioxide (CO_2) between the atmosphere and the blood (Fig. 66-1).[1] *Respiratory failure* results when one or both of these gas-exchanging functions are inadequate. For example, insufficient O_2 is transferred to the blood or inadequate CO_2 is removed from the lungs. Clinical states that interfere with adequate O_2 transfer result in **hypoxemia,** which is manifested by a decrease in arterial O_2 tension (PaO_2) and a decrease in arterial O_2 saturation (SaO_2). Insufficient CO_2 removal results in **hypercapnia,** which is manifested by an increase in arterial CO_2 tension ($PaCO_2$).[2] Arterial blood gases (ABGs) can be used to assess changes in pH, PaO_2, $PaCO_2$, and SaO_2, and pulse oximetry can be used to intermittently or continuously assess arterial oxygen saturation (SpO_2). Data should be interpreted within the context of the clinical assessment findings, as well as the patient's baseline. For example, an individual with chronic lung disease may have a baseline $PaCO_2$ higher than what is considered the "normal" range.

Respiratory failure is not a disease; it is a condition that occurs as a result of one or more diseases involving the lungs or other body systems (Tables 66-1 and 66-2). Respiratory failure can be classified as hypoxemic or hypercapnic (Fig. 66-2). Hypoxemic respiratory failure is also referred to as *oxygenation failure* because the primary problem is inadequate O_2 transfer between the alveoli and the pulmonary capillary bed.[2,3] Although no universal definition exists, **hypoxemic respiratory failure** is commonly defined as a PaO_2 of 60 mm Hg or less when the patient is receiving an inspired O_2 concentration of 60% or greater. This definition incorporates two important concepts: (1) the PaO_2 is at a level that indicates inadequate O_2 saturation of hemoglo-

Glossary of Abbreviations

Arterial Blood Monitoring

ABGs	Arterial blood gases
pH	Negative log of the free hydrogen ion [H^+]
PaO_2	Partial pressure of oxygen in arterial blood
$PaCO_2$	Partial pressure of carbon dioxide in arterial blood
SaO_2	Oxygen saturation in arterial blood measured by ABGs
SpO_2	Oxygen saturation in arterial blood measured by pulse oximetry

Oxygen and Lung Function Monitoring

FIO_2	Fraction of inspired oxygen concentration
FRC	Functional residual capacity (volume of air in lung at end of expiration)
PEEP	Positive end-expiratory pressure (pressure in lungs at end of expiration)
PEFR	Peak expiratory flow rate (maximum airflow during a forced expiration)
$\dot{V}/\dot{Q}$	Ventilation/perfusion ratio (relationship of ventilation to perfusion in the lungs)
V_E	Minute ventilation (product of tidal volume times respiratory rate)
V_T	Tidal volume (volume of air inspired with each breath)

Reviewed by John J. Gallagher, RN, MSN, CCNS, CCRN, CEN, RRT, Clinical Nurse Specialist for Critical Care, Crozer Chester Medical Center, Upland, Pa.

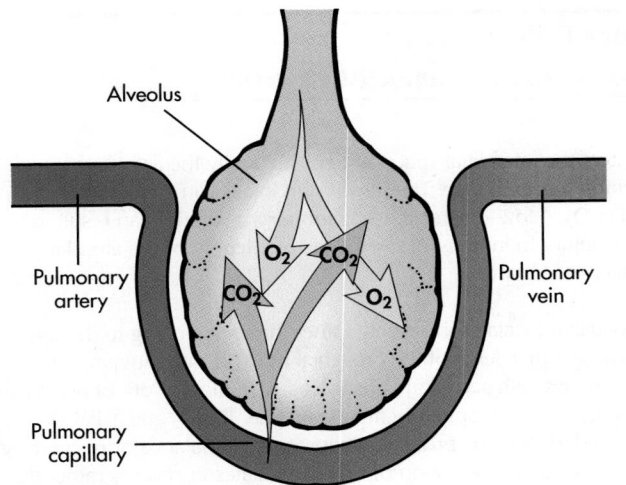

FIG. 66-1 Normal gas exchange unit in the lung.

bin; and (2) this PaO$_2$ level exists despite administration of supplemental O$_2$ at a percentage (60%) that is about three times that in room air (21%). Disorders that interfere with O$_2$ transfer into the blood include pneumonia, pulmonary edema, pulmonary emboli, and alveolar injury related to inhalation of toxic gases (e.g., smoke inhalation). In addition, low-cardiac-output states (e.g., congestive heart failure, shock) can also cause hypoxemic respiratory failure.[1]

Hypercapnic respiratory failure is also referred to as *ventilatory failure* because the primary problem is insufficient CO$_2$ removal. **Hypercapnic respiratory failure** is commonly defined as a PaCO$_2$ above normal (greater than 45 mm Hg) in combination with acidemia (arterial pH less than 7.35). This definition incorporates three important concepts: (1) the PaCO$_2$ is higher than normal; (2) there is evidence of the body's inability to compensate for this increase (acidemia); and (3) the pH is at a level where a further decrease may lead to severe acid-base imbalance. (See Chapter 16 for a discussion of acid-base balance.) Disorders that compromise lung ventilation and subsequent CO$_2$ removal include drug overdoses with central nervous system (CNS) depressants, neuromuscular diseases (e.g., myasthenia gravis), and trauma or diseases involving the spinal cord and its role in lung ventilation. Many patients experience both hypoxemic and hypercapnic respiratory failure.

Etiology and Pathophysiology

Hypoxemic Respiratory Failure. Common diseases and conditions that cause hypoxemic respiratory failure are listed in Table 66-1. Four physiologic mechanisms may cause hypoxemia and subsequent hypoxemic respiratory failure: (1) mismatch between ventilation ($\dot{V}$) and perfusion ($\dot{Q}$), commonly referred to as $\dot{V}/\dot{Q}$ mismatch; (2) shunt; (3) diffusion limitation; and (4) hypoventilation. The most common causes are $\dot{V}/\dot{Q}$ mismatch and shunt.[1-3]

Ventilation-perfusion ($\dot{V}/\dot{Q}$) mismatch. In the normal lung, the volume of blood perfusing the lungs each minute (4 to 5 L) is approximately equal to the amount of fresh gas that reaches the alveoli each minute (4 to 5 L). In a perfectly matched system, each portion of the lung would receive about 1 ml of air for each 1 ml of blood flow. This match of ventilation and perfusion

TABLE 66-1	Types of Respiratory Failure and Common Causes
HYPOXEMIC RESPIRATORY FAILURE*	**HYPERCAPNIC RESPIRATORY FAILURE***
Respiratory System Acute respiratory distress syndrome Pneumonia Toxic inhalation (smoke inhalation) Hepatopulmonary syndrome (low-resistance flow state, $\dot{V}/\dot{Q}$ mismatch) Massive pulmonary embolism (e.g., thrombus emboli, fat emboli) **Cardiac System** Anatomic shunt (ventricular septal defect) Cardiogenic pulmonary edema Shock (decreasing blood flow through pulmonary vasculature)	**Respiratory System** Asthma COPD Cystic fibrosis **Central Nervous System** Brainstem infarction Sedative and narcotic overdose Spinal cord injury Severe head injury **Chest Wall** Thoracic trauma (e.g., flail chest) Kyphoscoliosis Pain Massive obesity **Neuromuscular System** Myasthenia gravis Critical illness polyneuropathy Acute myopathy Toxic ingestion (tree tobacco) Amyotrophic lateral sclerosis Phrenic nerve injury Guillain-Barré syndrome Poliomyelitis Muscular dystrophy Multiple sclerosis

*This list is not all-inclusive.
COPD, Chronic obstructive pulmonary disease.

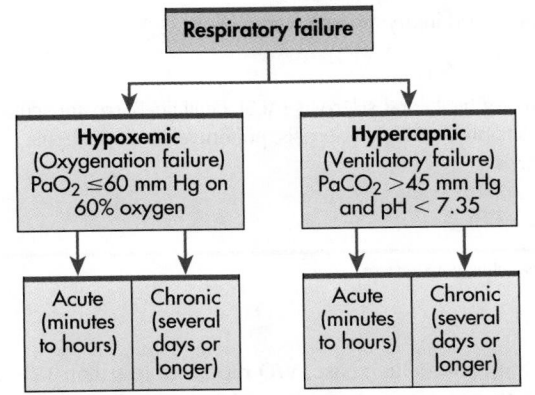

FIG. 66-2 Classification of respiratory failure.

would result in a $\dot{V}/\dot{Q}$ ratio of 1:1 (e.g., 1 ml of air per 1 ml of blood), which is expressed as $\dot{V}/\dot{Q}$ = 1. Ventilation is ideally matched with perfusion.

Although this example implies that ventilation and perfusion are ideally matched in all areas of the lung, this situation does not normally exist. In reality, there is some regional mismatch. At the lung apex, $\dot{V}/\dot{Q}$ ratios are greater than 1 (more ventilation than

TABLE 66-2 **Predisposing Factors for Acute Respiratory Failure**

PREDISPOSING FACTORS	MECHANISMS OF RESPIRATORY FAILURE
Airways and Alveoli	
Acute respiratory distress syndrome	Fluid enters the interstitial space and subsequently the alveoli, markedly impairing gas exchange. The result is an initial ↓ in PaO_2 and later an ↑ in $PaCO_2$. A low-flow state to pulmonary capillaries can result in ischemic injury to lung tissues with loss of integrity of the alveolar-capillary membrane.
Direct lung injury: aspiration; severe, disseminated pulmonary infection; near-drowning; toxic gas inhalation; or airway contusion	
Indirect lung injury: sepsis/septic shock, severe nonthoracic trauma, cardiopulmonary bypass	
Asthma	Bronchospasm escalates in severity rather than responding to therapy. Bronchospasm, edema of the bronchial mucosa, and plugging of small airways with secretions greatly reduce airflow. Work of breathing increases, causing respiratory muscle fatigue. ↓ PaO_2 and ↑ $PaCO_2$.
Chronic obstructive pulmonary disease (COPD)	Alveoli are destroyed by protease-antiprotease imbalance or respiratory infection, or an exacerbation of COPD escalates in severity rather than responding to therapy. Secretions obstruct airflow. Work of breathing increases and causes respiratory muscle fatigue. ↓ PaO_2 and ↑ $PaCO_2$.
Cystic fibrosis	Abnormal Na^+ and Cl^- transport produces secretions that are viscous, poorly cleared, and therefore foci for infection. Over time the airways become clogged with copious, purulent, often greenish colored sputum. Secretions obstruct airflow. Repeated infections destroy alveoli. Work of breathing increases, causing respiratory muscle fatigue. ↓ PaO_2 and ↑ $PaCO_2$.
Central Nervous System	
Narcotic or other drug overdose with CNS depressant	Respirations slowed by drug effect. Insufficient CO_2 is excreted, resulting in ↑ $PaCO_2$.
Brainstem infarction, head injury	Medulla cannot alter respiratory rate in response to changes in $PaCO_2$.
Chest Wall	
Severe soft tissue injury, flail chest, rib fracture, pain	Prevent normal rib cage expansion resulting in inadequate gas exchange.
Kyphoscoliosis	Change in spinal configuration compresses the lungs and prevents normal expansion of the chest wall.
Massive obesity	Weight of the chest and abdominal contents prevents normal rib cage movement.
Neuromuscular Conditions	
Cervical cord injury, phrenic nerve injury	Neural control is lost, preventing use of the diaphragm, the major muscle of respiration. As a consequence, the patient inspires a smaller tidal volume, which predisposes to an ↑ in $PaCO_2$.
Amyotrophic lateral sclerosis (ALS), Guillain-Barré, muscular dystrophy, multiple sclerosis, poliomyelitis, myasthenia gravis	Respiratory muscle weakness or paralysis occurs, preventing normal CO_2 excretion. Dysfunction may be slowly progressive (muscular dystrophy, multiple sclerosis), progressive with no potential of recovery (ALS), rapid with good expectation of recovery (Guillain-Barré), or stable for extended periods of time (poliomyelitis, myasthenia gravis).

CNS, Central nervous system.

perfusion). At the lung base, $\dot{V}/\dot{Q}$ ratios are less than 1 (less ventilation than perfusion). Because changes at the lung apex balance changes at the base, the net effect is a close overall match (Fig. 66-3).

Many diseases and conditions alter overall $\dot{V}/\dot{Q}$ matching and thus cause $\dot{V}/\dot{Q}$ *mismatch* (Fig. 66-4). The most common are those in which increased secretions are present in the airways (e.g., chronic obstructive pulmonary disease [COPD]), alveoli (e.g., pneumonia), and when bronchospasm is present (e.g., asthma). $\dot{V}/\dot{Q}$ mismatch may also result from alveolar collapse (atelectasis) or as a result of pain. Unrelieved or inadequately relieved pain interferes with chest and abdominal wall movement,

compromising lung ventilation. Additionally, pain increases muscle and motor tension, producing generalized muscle rigidity; causes systemic vasoconstriction and activation of the stress response; and increases O_2 consumption and CO_2 production.[4,5] All of these conditions result in limited airflow (ventilation) to alveoli but have no effect on blood flow (perfusion) to the gas exchange units.[4] The consequence is $\dot{V}/\dot{Q}$ mismatch. A pulmonary embolus affects the perfusion portion of the $\dot{V}/\dot{Q}$ relationship. The embolus limits blood flow but has no effect on airflow to the alveoli, again causing $\dot{V}/\dot{Q}$ mismatch (see Fig. 66-4).

O_2 therapy is an appropriate first step to reverse hypoxemia caused by $\dot{V}/\dot{Q}$ mismatch because not all gas exchange units are

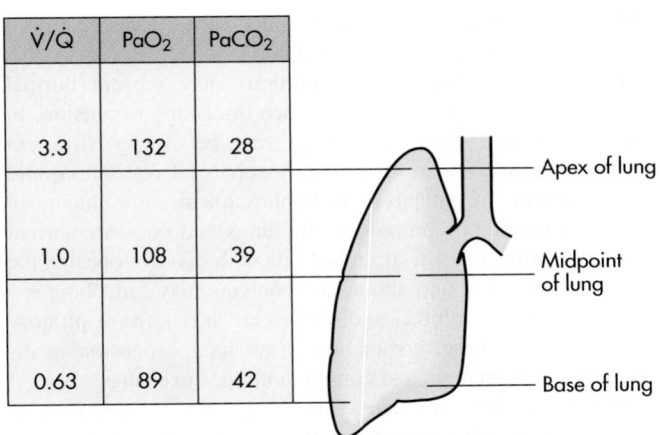

V̇/Q̇	PaO₂	PaCO₂
3.3	132	28
1.0	108	39
0.63	89	42

Apex of lung

Midpoint of lung

Base of lung

FIG. 66-3 Regional $\dot{V}/\dot{Q}$ differences in the normal lung. At the lung apex, the $\dot{V}/\dot{Q}$ ratio is 3.3, at the midpoint 1.0, and at the base 0.63. This difference causes the PaO_2 to be higher at the apex of the lung and lower at the base. Values for $PaCO_2$ are the opposite (i.e., lower at the apex and higher at the base). Blood that exits the lung is a mixture of these values.

affected. O_2 therapy increases the PaO_2 in blood leaving normal gas exchange units, thus causing a higher than normal PaO_2. The well-oxygenated blood mixes with poorly oxygenated blood, raising the overall PaO_2 of blood leaving the lungs. Ultimately, the optimal approach to hypoxemia caused by a $\dot{V}/\dot{Q}$ mismatch is one directed at the cause.

Shunt. **Shunt** occurs when blood exits the heart without having participated in gas exchange. A shunt can be viewed as an extreme $\dot{V}/\dot{Q}$ mismatch (see Fig. 66-4). There are two types of shunt: anatomic and intrapulmonary. An *anatomic shunt* occurs when blood passes through an anatomic channel in the heart (e.g., a ventricular septal defect) and therefore does not pass through the lungs. An *intrapulmonary shunt* occurs when blood flows through the pulmonary capillaries without participating in gas exchange. Intrapulmonary shunt is seen in conditions in which the alveoli fill with fluid (e.g., acute respiratory distress syndrome [ARDS], pneumonia, pulmonary edema). O_2 therapy alone may be ineffective in increasing the PaO_2 if hypoxemia is due to shunt because (1) blood passes from the right to the left side of the heart without passing through the lungs (anatomic shunt); or (2) the alveoli are filled with fluid, which prevents gas exchange (intrapulmonary shunt). Patients with shunt are usually more hypoxemic than patients with $\dot{V}/\dot{Q}$ mismatch, and they may require mechanical ventilation and a high fraction of inspired oxygen (FIO_2) to improve gas exchange.

Diffusion limitation. **Diffusion limitation** occurs when gas exchange across the alveolar-capillary membrane is compromised by a process that thickens or destroys the membrane (Fig. 66-5). Diffusion limitation can also be worsened by conditions that affect the pulmonary vascular bed such as severe emphysema or recurrent pulmonary emboli. Some diseases cause the alveolar-capillary membrane to become thicker (fibrotic), which slows gas transport. These diseases include pulmonary fibrosis, interstitial lung disease, and ARDS. Diffusion limitation is more likely to cause hypoxemia during exercise than at rest. During exercise, blood moves more rapidly through the lungs. Because transit time is increased, red blood cells are in the lungs for a shorter time, de-

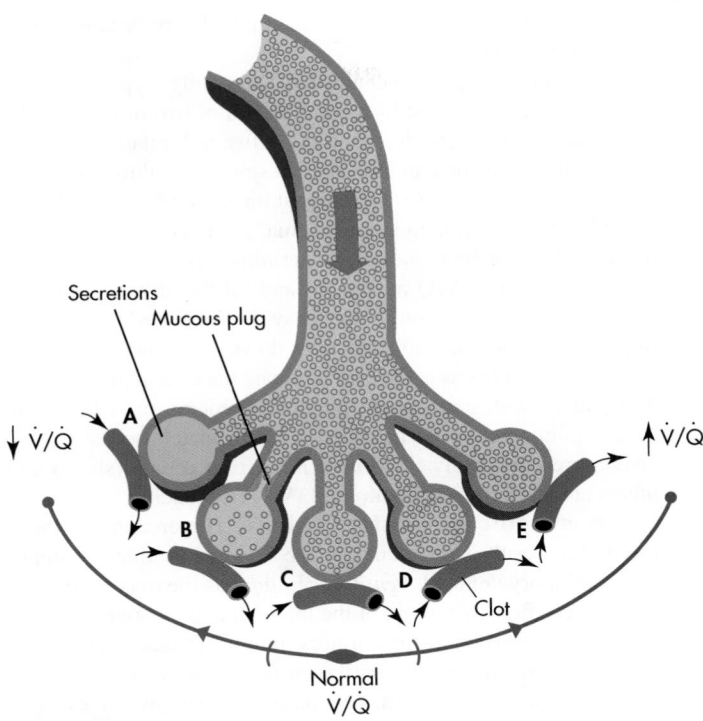

Secretions
Mucous plug
$\downarrow \dot{V}/\dot{Q}$
A
B
C
D
E
Clot
$\uparrow \dot{V}/\dot{Q}$
Normal
$\dot{V}/\dot{Q}$

FIG. 66-4 Range of ventilation to perfusion ($\dot{V}/\dot{Q}$) relationships. **A,** Absolute shunt, no ventilation due to fluid filling the alveoli. **B,** $\dot{V}/\dot{Q}$ mismatch, ventilation partially compromised by secretions in the airway. **C,** Normal lung unit. **D,** $\dot{V}/\dot{Q}$ mismatch, perfusion partially compromised by emboli obstructing blood flow. **E,** Dead space, no perfusion due to obstruction of the pulmonary capillary.

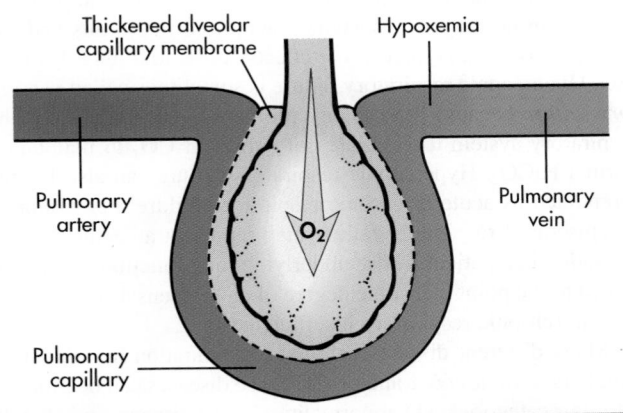

Thickened alveolar capillary membrane
Hypoxemia
Pulmonary artery
Pulmonary vein
O_2
Pulmonary capillary

FIG. 66-5 Diffusion limitation. Exchange of CO_2 and O_2 cannot occur because of the thickened alveolar-capillary membrane.

creasing the time for diffusion of O_2 across the alveolar-capillary membrane. The classical sign of diffusion limitation is hypoxemia that is present during exercise but not at rest.

Alveolar hypoventilation. **Alveolar hypoventilation** is a generalized decrease in ventilation that results in an increase in the $PaCO_2$ and a consequent decrease in PaO_2. Alveolar hypoventilation may be the result of restrictive lung disease, CNS disease, chest wall dysfunction, or neuromuscular disease. Although alveolar hypoventilation is primarily a mechanism of hypercapnic respiratory failure, it is mentioned here because it can also cause hypoxemia.

Interrelationship of mechanisms. Frequently, hypoxemic respiratory failure is caused by a combination of two or more of the following: $\dot{V}/\dot{Q}$ mismatch, shunting, diffusion limitation, and hypoventilation. The patient with acute respiratory failure secondary to pneumonia may have a combination of $\dot{V}/\dot{Q}$ mismatch and shunt because the inflammation, edema, and hypersecretion of exudate within the bronchioles and terminal respiratory units obstruct the airways ($\dot{V}/\dot{Q}$ mismatch) and fill the alveoli with exudate (shunt). In addition, shunt may be increased because of improper positioning (affected lung down) and endogenous vasodilator mediators as is the case with pneumococcal pneumonia.[6] The patient with cardiogenic pulmonary edema or ARDS may have a combination of shunt and $\dot{V}/\dot{Q}$ mismatch because some alveoli are completely filled with fluid from edema (shunt) and others are partially filled with fluid ($\dot{V}/\dot{Q}$ mismatch).

Hypercapnic Respiratory Failure. Hypercapnic respiratory failure results from an imbalance between ventilatory supply and ventilatory demand. *Ventilatory supply* is the maximum ventilation (gas flow in and out of the lungs) that the patient can sustain without developing respiratory muscle fatigue. *Ventilatory demand* is the amount of ventilation needed to keep the $PaCO_2$ within normal limits. Normally, ventilatory supply far exceeds ventilatory demand. As a consequence, individuals with normal lung function can engage in strenuous exercise, which greatly increases CO_2 production without an elevation in $PaCO_2$. Patients with preexisting lung disease such as severe emphysema do not have this advantage and cannot effectively increase lung ventilation in response to exercise or metabolic demands. However, considerable dysfunction is typically present before ventilatory demand exceeds ventilatory supply.

When ventilatory demand does exceed ventilatory supply, the $PaCO_2$ can no longer be sustained within normal limits and hypercapnia occurs. Hypercapnia reflects substantial lung dysfunction. Hypercapnic respiratory failure is sometimes called *ventilatory failure* because the primary problem is the inability of the respiratory system to ventilate out sufficient CO_2 to maintain a normal $PaCO_2$. Hypercapnic respiratory failure can also be differentiated as acute or chronic respiratory failure. For example, an episode of respiratory failure may represent an acute decompensation in a patient whose underlying lung function has deteriorated to the point that some degree of decompensation is always present (chronic respiratory insufficiency).

Many different diseases can cause a limitation in ventilatory supply (see Tables 66-1 and 66-2). These diseases can be grouped into four categories: (1) abnormalities of the airways and alveoli, (2) abnormalities of the CNS, (3) abnormalities of the chest wall, and (4) neuromuscular conditions.

Airways and alveoli. Patients with asthma, emphysema, chronic bronchitis, and cystic fibrosis are at high risk for hypercapnic respiratory failure because the underlying pathophysiology of these conditions results in airflow obstruction and air trapping.

Central nervous system. A variety of problems may suppress the drive to breathe. A common example is an overdose of a narcotic or other respiratory depressant drug. A brainstem infarction or severe head injury may also interfere with normal function of the respiratory center in the medulla. Patients with these conditions are at risk for respiratory failure because the medulla does not alter the respiratory rate in response to a change in $PaCO_2$.

CNS dysfunction may also include spinal cord injuries that limit innervation to the respiratory muscles.

Chest wall. A variety of conditions may prevent normal movement of the chest wall and hence limit lung expansion. In patients with flail chest, fractures prevent the rib cage from expanding normally because of pain, mechanical restriction, and muscle spasm. In patients with kyphoscoliosis, the change in spinal configuration compresses the lungs and prevents normal expansion of the chest wall. In patients with massive obesity, the weight of the chest and abdominal contents may limit lung expansion. Patients with these conditions are at risk for respiratory failure because these dysfunctions limit lung expansion or diaphragmatic movement and consequently gas exchange.

Neuromuscular conditions. Various types of neuromuscular diseases may result in respiratory muscle weakness or paralysis (see Table 66-1). For example, patients with Guillain-Barré syndrome, muscular dystrophy, or multiple sclerosis are at risk for respiratory failure because the respiratory muscles are weakened or paralyzed as a consequence of the underlying neuromuscular condition. Therefore they are unable to maintain normal $PaCO_2$ levels.

In summary, respiratory failure may occur in three of these categories (CNS, chest wall, neuromuscular conditions) despite the presence of normal lungs. Respiratory failure occurs because the medulla, chest wall, peripheral nerves, or respiratory muscles are not functioning normally. The patient may have no damage to lung tissue but may be unable to inspire a tidal volume sufficient to expel CO_2 from the lungs.

Tissue Oxygen Needs. It is important to remember that even though PaO_2 and $PaCO_2$ determine the definition of respiratory failure, the major threat of respiratory failure is the inability of the lungs to meet the oxygen demands of the tissues. This inability may occur as a result of inadequate tissue O_2 delivery or because the tissues are unable to use the O_2 delivered to them. It may also occur as a result of the stress response and dramatic increases in tissue oxygen consumption.[5] Tissue O_2 delivery is determined by the amount of O_2 carried in the hemoglobin, as well as cardiac output. Therefore respiratory failure places the patient at greater risk if there are coexisting cardiac problems or anemia. Failure of O_2 utilization most commonly occurs as a result of septic shock. In this situation, adequate O_2 may be delivered to the tissues, but an abnormally high amount of O_2 returns in the venous blood, indicating that it is not being extracted and used at the tissue level. (Shock is discussed in Chapter 65.)

Clinical Manifestations

Respiratory failure may develop suddenly (minutes or hours) or gradually (several days or longer). A sudden decrease in PaO_2 or a rapid rise in $PaCO_2$ implies a serious condition, which can rapidly become a life-threatening emergency. An example is the patient with asthma who develops severe bronchospasm and a marked decrease in airflow, resulting in respiratory arrest. A more gradual change in PaO_2 and $PaCO_2$ is better tolerated because compensation can occur. An example is the patient with COPD who develops a progressive increase in $PaCO_2$ over several days following the onset of a respiratory infection. Because the change occurred over several days, there is time for renal compensation (e.g., retention of bicarbonate), which will minimize the change in arterial pH. The patient has compensated respiratory acidosis.[3,7] (See Chapter 16 for a discussion of renal compensation for acid-base disorders.)

Manifestations of respiratory failure are related to the extent of change in PaO_2 or $PaCO_2$, the rapidity of change (acute versus chronic), and the ability to compensate to overcome this change. When the patient's compensatory mechanisms fail, respiratory failure occurs. Because clinical manifestations are variable, it is important to monitor trends in ABGs and/or pulse oximetry to evaluate the extent of change. These measurements cannot substitute for clinical assessment and should be interpreted within the context of clinical assessment findings. Frequently, the initial indication of respiratory failure is a change in the patient's mental status. Because the cerebral cortex is so sensitive to variations in oxygenation and acid-base balance, mental status changes will occur early and frequently before ABG results are obtained. Restlessness, confusion, agitation, and combative behavior suggest inadequate delivery of O_2 to the brain and should be fully investigated.

The nurse may detect manifestations of respiratory failure that are specific (arise from the respiratory system) or nonspecific (arise from other body systems) (Table 66-3). An understanding of the significance of these manifestations is critical to the ability to detect the onset of respiratory failure and effectiveness of treatment.

Tachycardia and mild hypertension can also be early signs of respiratory failure. Such changes may indicate an attempt by the heart to compensate for decreased O_2 delivery. A severe morning headache may suggest that hypercapnia may have occurred during the night, increasing cerebral blood flow by vasodilation and causing a morning headache. At night the respiratory rate is slower and the lungs of patients at risk for respiratory failure may remove less $PaCO_2$. Rapid, shallow breaths suggest that the tidal volume may be inadequate to remove CO_2 from the lungs. Cyanosis is an unreliable indicator of hypoxemia and is a late sign of respiratory failure because it does not occur until hypoxemia is severe ($PaO_2 \leq 45$ mm Hg).

Consequences of Hypoxemia and Hypoxia. *Hypoxemia* occurs when the amount of O_2 in arterial blood is less than the normal value (see Chapter 25 for normal values). **Hypoxia** occurs when the PaO_2 has fallen sufficiently to cause signs and symptoms of inadequate oxygenation (see Table 66-3). Hypoxemia can lead to hypoxia if not corrected. If hypoxia or hypoxemia is severe, the cells shift from aerobic to anaerobic metabolism. Anaerobic metabolism uses more fuel and produces less energy and is less efficient than aerobic metabolism. The waste product of anaerobic metabolism, lactic acid, is more difficult to remove from the body than CO_2 because lactic acid has to be buffered with sodium bicarbonate. When the body does not have adequate amounts of sodium bicarbonate to buffer the lactic acid produced by anaerobic metabolism, metabolic acidosis results and cell death may occur.

Hypoxia and metabolic acidosis have adverse effects on the vital organs, especially the heart and CNS. The heart tries to compensate for the decreased O_2 level in the blood by increasing the heart rate and cardiac output. As the PaO_2 decreases and acidosis increases, the heart muscle may become dysfunctional and cardiac output may decrease. In addition, angina and arrhythmias may occur. All of these consequences result in a further decrease in oxygen delivery. Permanent brain damage may occur because of O_2 deprivation. Renal function may also be impaired, and sodium retention, edema formation, acute tubular necrosis, and uremia may occur. Gastrointestinal (GI) system alterations include tissue ischemia, increased permeability of the intestinal wall, and possible translocation of bacteria from the GI tract into circulation.

Specific Clinical Manifestations. The patient in respiratory failure may have several clinical findings indicating distress. The patient may have a rapid, shallow breathing pattern or a respiratory rate that is slower than normal. Both changes predispose to insufficient CO_2 removal. The patient may increase the respiratory rate in an effort to blow off accumulated CO_2. This breathing pattern requires a substantial amount of work and predisposes to respiratory muscle fatigue. A change from a rapid rate to a slower rate in a patient in acute respiratory distress suggests extreme fatigue and the possibility of an impending respiratory arrest.

The position that the patient assumes is an indication of the effort associated with breathing. The patient may be able to lie

TABLE 66-3	Clinical Manifestations of Hypoxemia and Hypercapnia*	
SPECIFIC	**NONSPECIFIC**	
Hypoxemia		
Respiratory	**Cerebral**	
Dyspnea	Agitation	
Tachypnea	Disorientation	
Prolonged expiration (I:E = 1:3, 1:4)	Delirium	
Intercostal muscle retraction	Restless, combative behavior	
Use of accessory muscles in respiration	Confusion	
$\downarrow SpO_2$ (<80%)	$\downarrow$ Level of consciousness	
Paradoxic chest/abdominal wall movement with respiratory cycle (late)	Coma (late)	
Cyanosis (late)	**Cardiac**	
	Tachycardia	
	Hypertension	
	Skin cool, clammy, and diaphoretic	
	Arrhythmias (late)	
	Hypotension (late)	
	Other	
	Fatigue	
	Unable to speak without pausing to breathe	
Hypercapnia		
Respiratory	**Cerebral**	
Dyspnea	Morning headache	
$\downarrow$ Respiratory rate or $\uparrow$ rapid rate with shallow respirations	Disorientation	
	Progressive somnolence	
$\downarrow$ Tidal volume	Coma (late)	
$\downarrow$ Minute ventilation	**Cardiac**	
	Arrhythmias	
	Hypertension	
	Tachycardia	
	Bounding pulse	
	Neuromuscular	
	Muscle weakness	
	$\downarrow$ Deep tendon reflexes	
	Tremor, seizures (late)	
	Other	
	Pursed-lip breathing	
	Use of tripod position	

*List is not all-inclusive.

down (mild distress), be able to lie down but prefer to sit (moderate distress), or be unable to breathe unless sitting upright (severe distress). A common position is to sit with the arms propped on the overbed table. This position, called the tripod position, helps decrease the work of breathing because propping the arms increases the anterior-posterior diameter of the chest and changes pressure in the thorax. Pursed-lip breathing may be used. This strategy causes an increase in SaO_2 because it slows respirations, allows more time for expiration, and prevents the small bronchioles from collapsing, thus facilitating air exchange. (Pursed-lip breathing is discussed in Chapter 28.) Another assessment parameter is the number of pillows the patient requires to breathe comfortably when resting. This is termed *orthopnea* and may be documented as one-, two-, three-, or four-pillow orthopnea.

The person who is experiencing dyspnea is working hard to breathe and may be able to speak only a few words at a time between breaths. The ability of the patient to speak without pausing to breathe is an indication of the severity of dyspnea. The patient may speak in sentences (mild or no distress), phrases (moderate distress), or words (severe distress). The number of words is also a clue (e.g., how many words can the patient say without pausing to breathe?). The patient may have "two-word" or "three-word" dyspnea, signifying that only two or three words can be said before pausing to breathe. There may also be earlier onset of fatigue with walking. An additional assessment parameter is how far the patient is able to walk without stopping to rest.

There may be a change in the *inspiratory (I) to expiratory (E) (I:E) ratio*. Normally, the I:E ratio is 1:2, which means that expiration is twice as long as inspiration. In patients in respiratory distress, the ratio may increase to 1:3 or 1:4. This change signifies airflow obstruction and that more time is required to empty the lungs.

The nurse may observe *retraction* (inward movement) of the intercostal spaces or the supraclavicular area and use of the accessory muscles during inspiration or expiration. Use of the accessory muscles signifies moderate distress. Paradoxic breathing indicates severe distress. Normally, the thorax and abdomen move outward on inspiration and inward on exhalation. During *paradoxic breathing*, the abdomen and chest move in the opposite manner—outward during exhalation and inward during inspiration. Paradoxic breathing results from maximal use of the accessory muscles of respiration. The patient may also be diaphoretic from the work associated with breathing.

Auscultation should be performed in order to assess the patient's baseline breath sounds, as well as any changes from baseline. The nurse should note the presence and location of any adventitious breath sounds. Crackles and rhonchi may indicate pulmonary edema or emphysema. Absent or diminished breath sounds may indicate atelectasis or pleural effusion. The presence of bronchial breath sounds over the lung periphery often results from lung consolidation that is seen with pneumonia. A pleural friction rub may also be heard in the presence of pneumonia that has involved the pleura.

A thorough nursing assessment may result in early detection of manifestations associated with respiratory insufficiency, allowing therapy to be instituted before the patient experiences respiratory failure. Patients with end-stage (severe) chronic lung disease may have low PaO_2 values or elevated $PaCO_2$ levels and crackles as their "normal" baseline. It is especially important to monitor specific and nonspecific signs of respiratory failure in patients with COPD because a small change can cause significant decompensation (see Table 66-3). Any deterioration in mental status, such as agitation, combative behavior, confusion, or decreased level of consciousness, should be reported immediately because this change may indicate the onset of rapid deterioration in clinical status and the need for mechanical ventilation.

Diagnostic Studies

After physical assessment, the most common diagnostic study used to determine respiratory failure is ABG analysis. ABGs are used to determine the levels of $PaCO_2$, PaO_2, and pH. An indwelling catheter may be inserted into a peripheral artery for monitoring systemic blood pressure and obtaining blood for ABGs. Pulse oximetry is frequently used for monitoring oxygenation status, but tells little regarding lung ventilation. In respiratory failure, ABGs are necessary to obtain both oxygenation (PaO_2) and ventilation ($PaCO_2$) status, as well as information related to acid-base balance.

Other diagnostic studies that may be done include a chest x-ray, complete blood cell count, serum electrolytes, urinalysis, and electrocardiogram (ECG). Cultures of the sputum and blood are obtained as necessary to determine sources of possible infection. If pulmonary embolus is suspected, a ventilation/perfusion ($\dot{V}/\dot{Q}$) lung scan or pulmonary angiography may be done. Although not commonly done in acute situations, pulmonary function tests may be performed. For the patient in severe respiratory failure requiring endotracheal intubation, end-tidal CO_2 ($EtCO_2$) may be used to assess tube placement within the trachea immediately following intubation. $EtCO_2$ may also be used during ventilator management to assess trends in lung ventilation as determined by expired CO_2.

In severe respiratory failure, a pulmonary artery catheter may be inserted to measure heart pressures and cardiac output, as well as mixed venous oxygen saturation. This information is helpful in determining the adequacy of tissue perfusion and the patient's response to treatment measures. Pulmonary artery, pulmonary artery wedge, and left atrial pressures are monitored to determine whether the accumulation of fluid in the lungs is the result of cardiac or pulmonary problems. These parameters are also monitored to determine the response of the lung and heart to hypoxemia and the patient's response to therapy. Pulmonary arterial pressure monitoring can also provide feedback on the physiologic effects of mechanical ventilation on hemodynamic status. (Hemodynamic monitoring is discussed in detail in Chapter 64.)

NURSING *and* COLLABORATIVE MANAGEMENT ACUTE RESPIRATORY FAILURE

Because many different problems cause respiratory failure, specific care of these patients varies. This section discusses general assessment and collaborative care measures that apply to patients with acute respiratory failure. In acute care settings there is often an overlap of function between nursing and other members of the health care team.

■ Nursing Assessment

Subjective and objective data that should be obtained from the patient with acute respiratory failure are presented in Table 66-4.

TABLE 66-4	Nursing Assessment
	Acute Respiratory Failure

Subjective Data

Important Health Information

Past health history: Chronic lung disease; potential occupational exposures to lung toxins; smoking (pack-years); previous hospitalizations related to lung disease; thoracic or spinal cord trauma; extreme obesity; altered consciousness; age (physiologic and chronologic); use/abuse of alcohol, other drugs

Medications: Use of oxygen, inhalers (bronchodilators), home nebulization, over-the-counter medications; immunosuppressant (corticosteroid) therapy, CNS depressants

Surgery or other treatments: Previous intubation and mechanical ventilation; recent thoracic or abdominal surgery

Functional Health Patterns

Health perception–health management: Exercise, self-care activities; immunizations (flu, pneumonia, hepatitis)

Nutritional-metabolic: Anorexia, bloatedness, heartburn; weight gain or loss; decreased appetite; diaphoresis, eating habits, vitamin/herbal supplements

Activity-exercise: Fatigue, dizziness; dyspnea at rest or with activity, wheezing, cough (productive or nonproductive); sputum (volume, color, viscosity); palpitations, swollen feet

Sleep-rest: Changes in sleep pattern

Cognitive-perceptual: Headache, chest pain or tightness

Coping–stress tolerance: Anxiety, depression

Objective Data

General

Restlessness, agitation

Integumentary

Pale, cool, clammy skin or warm flushed skin; peripheral and central cyanosis; peripheral dependent edema

Respiratory

Shallow, increased respiratory rate progressing to decreased rate; use of accessory muscles with evidence of retractions, altered I:E ratio; increased diaphragmatic excursion or asymmetric chest expansion; asynchronous respirations; tactile fremitus, crepitus, or deviated trachea on palpation; resonant, hyperresonant, or dull percussion note; absent, diminished, or adventitious breath sounds; bronchial or bronchovesicular sounds heard in other than normal location, inspiratory stridor, pleural friction rub

Cardiovascular

Tachycardia progressing to bradycardia, arrhythmias, extra heart sounds (S_3, S_4); bounding pulse; hypertension progressing to hypotension; pulsus paradoxus; jugular vein distention; pedal edema

Gastrointestinal

Abdominal distention with tympany; ascites, epigastric tenderness, hepatojugular reflex

Neurologic

Somnolence, confusion, slurred speech, restlessness, delirium, agitation, tremors, seizures, coma; asterixis, decreased deep tendon reflexes; papilledema

Possible Laboratory Findings

↑/↓ pH, ↑/↓ $PaCO_2$, ↓ PaO_2, ↓ SaO_2, ↓ PEFR, ↓ tidal volume, ↓ forced vital capacity, ↓ minute ventilation, ↓ negative inspiratory force; altered values of serum electrolytes, hemoglobin, and hematocrit; abnormal findings on chest x-ray; abnormal pulmonary artery and pulmonary artery wedge pressures

CNS, Central nervous system; *I:E,* inspiratory:expiratory; *PEFR,* peak expiratory flow rate.

■ Nursing Diagnoses

Nursing diagnoses for the patient with acute respiratory failure include, but are not limited to, those presented in NCP 66-1.

■ Planning

The overall goals are that the patient in acute respiratory failure will have (1) ABG values within the patient's baseline, (2) breath sounds within the patient's baseline, (3) no dyspnea or breathing patterns within the patient's baseline, and (4) effective cough and ability to clear secretions.

■ Prevention

As part of the plan of care for any patient who may be at risk for respiratory failure, prevention and early recognition of respiratory distress is important. Prevention involves a thorough physical assessment and history to identify the patient at risk for respiratory failure and, then, the initiation of appropriate nursing interventions. For example, a patient at risk for respiratory failure should receive appropriate patient teaching regarding coughing, deep breathing, incentive spirometry, and ambulation as appropriate. Prevention of atelectasis, pneumonia, and complications of immobility, as well as optimizing hydration and nutrition, can po-

tentially decrease the risk of respiratory failure in the acutely or critically ill patient.

■ Respiratory Therapy

The major goals of care for acute respiratory failure include maintaining adequate oxygenation and ventilation. This goal is accomplished by collaboration among the nursing, medical, and respiratory care teams. The interventions used include O_2 therapy, mobilization of secretions, and positive pressure ventilation (Table 66-5).

Oxygen Therapy. The primary goal of O_2 therapy is to correct hypoxemia. If hypoxemia is secondary to $\dot{V}/\dot{Q}$ mismatch, supplemental O_2 administered at 1 to 3 L/min by nasal cannula or 24% to 32% by simple face mask or Venturi mask should improve the PaO_2 and SaO_2. Hypoxemia secondary to an intrapulmonary shunt is usually not responsive to high O_2 concentrations, and the patient will usually require positive pressure ventilation (PPV). PPV offers a means of providing O_2 therapy and humidification, decreasing the work of breathing, and reducing respiratory muscle fatigue. In addition, the positive pressure may assist in opening collapsed airways and decreasing shunt. PPV may be provided via an endotracheal tube (most frequently) or noninva-

NURSING CARE PLAN 66-1

Patient with Acute Respiratory Failure*

EXPECTED PATIENT OUTCOMES	NURSING INTERVENTIONS and *RATIONALES*
NURSING DIAGNOSIS	**Ineffective airway clearance** *related to* excessive secretions, ↓ level of consciousness, presence of an artificial airway, neuromuscular dysfunction, and pain *as manifested by* difficulty in expectorating sputum, presence of rhonchi or crackles, ineffective or absent cough.
• No abnormal breath sounds (e.g., rhonchi, crackles) • Normal baseline breath sounds • Presence of effective cough • Effective expectoration of sputum	• Assess patient's ability to cough *to determine need for assistance in secretion removal.* • Implement deep breathing/coughing exercises, assistive coughing strategies, and incentive spirometry *to promote secretion removal.* • Position patient with head of bed elevated at least 45 degrees or in the tripod position *to promote maximal chest expansion and cough efforts.* • Humidify O₂ if over 3 L/min *to prevent drying of the mucosa.* • Perform tracheobronchial suctioning if cough is ineffective or if artificial airway is present *to remove secretions and improve oxygenation.* • Perform chest physical therapy *to enhance removal of secretions.* • Splint any abdominal or chest incision with pillow *to reduce pain and allow for improved inspiratory efforts.* • Turn every 2 hours *to prevent stasis of secretions and promote optimal ventilation.* • Ensure adequate fluid intake of 2-3 L/day *to liquefy secretions.* • Administer prescribed routine and as needed bronchodilator and mucolytic medications *to promote better airflow and secretion removal.*
NURSING DIAGNOSIS	**Ineffective breathing pattern** *related to* neuromuscular impairment of respirations, pain, anxiety, ↓ level of consciousness, respiratory muscle fatigue, and bronchospasm *as manifested by* respiratory rate <12 or >24 breaths/min, altered I:E ratio, irregular breathing pattern, use of accessory muscles, asynchronous thoracoabdominal movement, wheezing, apnea.
• Respiratory rate, depth, and rhythm within normal limits for patient • Synchronous thoraco-abdominal movement • Use of accessory muscles appropriate for level of activity	• Monitor for ↑ or ↓ respiratory rate, periods of apnea, and ↓ inspiratory depth between chest and abdomen *to assess for presence of inability to sustain ventilation.* • Position patient with head of bed elevated at least 45 degrees or in a tripod position *to promote diaphragmatic excursion.* • Place oral or nasal airway and Ambu bag at the bedside *because airway support may be needed in the event of severely impaired ventilation or apnea.* • Provide comfort measures (e.g., analgesics, positioning) *to reduce anxiety and promote patient cooperation.* • Anticipate the need for possible application of NIPPV or intubation with mechanical ventilation *to maintain adequate oxygenation and ventilation.*
NURSING DIAGNOSIS	**Risk for imbalanced fluid volume** *related to* ↑ in peripheral or pulmonary fluid.
• Normal breath sounds • ↓ or absent peripheral edema • Normal pulmonary artery or pulmonary artery wedge pressures	• Assess for manifestations of fluid volume excess such as abnormal breath sounds (crackles), dyspnea, weight gain, jugular venous distention, peripheral or sacral edema *to identify if problem is present.* • Monitor fluid status by intake and output measurements, daily weights, pulmonary artery or pulmonary artery wedge pressures, and central venous pressure *to monitor for changes in systemic fluid volume.* • Restrict fluid intake and administer diuretics as ordered *to prevent or reduce fluid overload.*
NURSING DIAGNOSIS	**Anxiety** *related to* dyspnea, intubation, severity of illness, loss of personal control, and uncertain outcome *as manifested by* ↑ heart rate, respiratory rate, and blood pressure; agitation, restlessness; verbalization of anxiety.
• ↓ Anxiety • Relaxed demeanor • ↑ Sense of personal control • Verbalization of positive attitude toward outcome	• Perform interventions in a calm, assured manner *to ↓ patient's anxiety.* • Reassure patient of competence of caregivers *to encourage patient relaxation.* • Answer questions simply and honestly *to provide patient with needed information for decision making.* • Teach and demonstrate relaxation techniques of slow pursed-lip breathing, progressive relaxation, and guided imagery *to promote restoration of control over breathing.* • Administer and evaluate patient's response to any prescribed antianxiety medication *to determine therapeutic efficacy.*

*The nursing care for the patient on mechanical ventilation is presented in NCP 64-1 and discussed in Chapter 64.
I:E, Inspiratory:expiratory; *NIPPV,* noninvasive positive pressure ventilation.

NURSING CARE PLAN 66-1

Patient with Acute Respiratory Failure—cont'd

EXPECTED PATIENT OUTCOMES	NURSING INTERVENTIONS and *RATIONALES*
NURSING DIAGNOSIS	**Impaired gas exchange** *related to* alveolar hypoventilation, intrapulmonary shunting, $\dot{V}/\dot{Q}$ mismatch, and diffusion impairment *as manifested by* hypoxemia or hypercapnia.
▪ PaO$_2$ and PaCO$_2$ within normal ranges for patient ▪ Normal breath sounds	▪ Monitor for clinical manifestations of hypoxemia and hypercapnia *to detect systemic manifestations of $\downarrow$ O$_2$ and $\uparrow$ CO$_2$.* ▪ Administer O$_2$ as ordered *to $\uparrow$ PaO$_2$ and SaO$_2$ levels.* ▪ Monitor ABGs for PaO$_2$ below 60 mm Hg, SaO$_2$ below 90%, and PaCO$_2$ above 50 mm Hg *to assess pulmonary gas exchange.* ▪ Place the patient on continuous pulse oximetry *to assess for $\uparrow$ or $\downarrow$ in blood O$_2$ levels.* ▪ Monitor apical-radial heart rate for irregular rhythm, tachycardia, bradycardia, and cardiac arrhythmias on the cardiac monitor *because hypoxemia may precipitate cardiac arrhythmias.* ▪ Teach and encourage pursed-lip breathing *to improve gas exchange.* ▪ Anticipate the need for ventilatory support *to improve oxygenation and ventilation status.* ▪ Withhold sedative drugs unless discussed with physician *because they can depress respirations.*
NURSING DIAGNOSIS	**Imbalanced nutrition: less than body requirements** *related to* poor appetite, shortness of breath, presence of artificial airway, $\downarrow$ energy level, and $\uparrow$ caloric requirements *as manifested by* weight loss, weakness, muscle wasting, dehydration, poor muscle tone, poor skin integrity.
▪ Maintenance of weight or weight gain ▪ Serum albumin and protein within normal ranges	▪ Provide high-protein, high-calorie, enteral or parenteral nutrition as ordered *to meet $\uparrow$ nutritional requirements.* ▪ If able to take nutrition orally, provide six small meals per day *to $\downarrow$ O$_2$ energy expenditure during digestion.* ▪ Provide between-meal nutritional supplements *to maintain adequate caloric intake.* ▪ Maintain the ordered O$_2$ delivery device during meals *to prevent shortness of breath and blood oxygen desaturation while eating.* ▪ Monitor for signs of $\uparrow$ CO$_2$ with parenteral nutrition *because carbohydrates may $\uparrow$ CO$_2$ levels in patients with hypercapnia.*

sively by means of a tight-fitting mask.[8] (Mechanical ventilation is discussed in detail in Chapter 64.)

The type of O$_2$ delivery system chosen for the patient in acute respiratory failure should (1) be tolerated by the patient, because anxiety caused by feelings of claustrophobia related to the face mask or dyspnea may prompt the patient to remove the O$_2$ device; and (2) maintain PaO$_2$ at 55 to 60 mm Hg or more and SaO$_2$ at 90% or more at the lowest O$_2$ concentration possible. High O$_2$ concentrations replace the nitrogen gas normally present in the alveoli, causing instability and atelectasis. In intubated patients, exposure to 60% or greater O$_2$ for longer than 48 hours poses a significant risk for O$_2$ toxicity. In nonintubated patients, the risk is less clear. The effects of prolonged exposure to high levels of O$_2$ include increased pulmonary microvascular permeability, decreased surfactant production and surfactant inactivation, and fibrotic changes in the alveoli. (O$_2$ delivery devices are discussed in Chapter 28.)

Additional risks of O$_2$ therapy are specific to the patient with chronic hypercapnia such as the patient with COPD. Chronic hypercapnia may blunt the response of chemoreceptors in the medulla, a condition termed *CO$_2$ narcosis*. In this situation, respirations are stimulated by hypoxia. If the PaO$_2$ is suddenly increased, the patient will no longer be hypoxemic, will have a decreased stimulus to breathe, and may experience a respiratory arrest. Patients with chronic hypercapnia should receive O$_2$ through a low-flow device such as a nasal cannula at 1 to 2 L/min or a Venturi mask at 24% to 28%. They should be closely monitored for changes in mental status and respiratory rate and ABG results until their PaO$_2$ level has reached their baseline normal value.

Mobilization of Secretions. Retained pulmonary secretions may cause or exacerbate acute respiratory failure by blocking movement of O$_2$ into the alveoli and pulmonary capillary blood and removal of CO$_2$ during the respiratory cycle. Secretions can be mobilized through effective coughing, adequate hydration and humidification, chest physical therapy, and tracheal suctioning.

Effective coughing and positioning. If secretions are obstructing the airway, the patient should be encouraged to cough. The patient with a neuromuscular weakness from a disease or exhaustion may not be able to generate sufficient airway pressures to produce an effective cough. *Augmented coughing (quad coughing)* may be of benefit to these patients. Augmented cough-

TABLE	Collaborative Care
66-5	**Acute Respiratory Failure**

Diagnostic
History and physical examination
Arterial blood gases
Pulse oximetry
Chest x-ray
CBC
Serum electrolytes and urinalysis
ECG
Blood and sputum cultures (if indicated)
PAP, PAWP, LAP

Collaborative Therapy

Respiratory Therapy
O_2 therapy
Mobilization of secretions
▪ Effective coughing
▪ Incentive spirometry
▪ Hydration/humidification
▪ Chest physical therapy
▪ Airway suctioning
Positive pressure ventilation
▪ Noninvasive positive pressure ventilation
▪ Intubation with mechanical ventilation

Drug Therapy
Relief of bronchospasm (e.g., albuterol [Proventil])
Reduction of airway inflammation (corticosteroids)
Reduction of pulmonary congestion (e.g., furosemide [Lasix])
Treatment of pulmonary infections (e.g., antibiotics)
Reduction of severe anxiety and restlessness (e.g., lorazepam [Ativan])

Medical Supportive Therapy
Management of the underlying cause of respiratory failure
Maintenance of adequate cardiac output
Maintenance of adequate hemoglobin concentration

Nutritional Therapy
Parenteral nutrition support
Enteral nutrition support

CBC, Complete blood count; *ECG,* electrocardiogram; *LAP,* left atrial pressure; *PAP,* pulmonary artery pressure; *PAWP,* pulmonary artery wedge pressure.

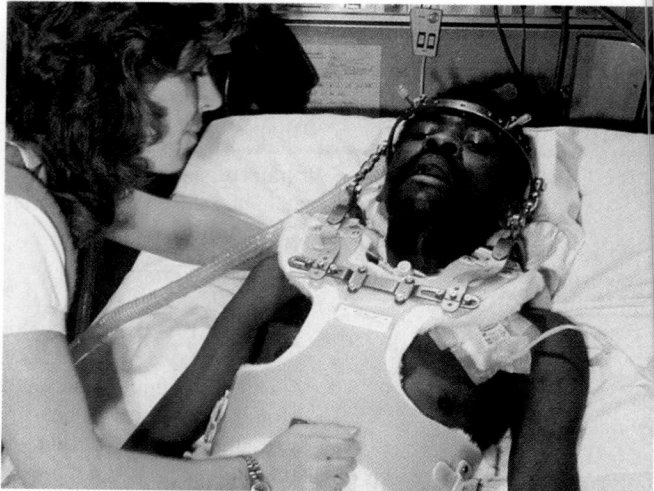

FIG. 66-6 Augmented cough. Augmented coughing is performed by placing the palm of the hand on the abdominal musculature below the xiphoid process. As the patient ends a deep inspiration and begins the expiration, the hand should be moved forcefully downward, increasing abdominal pressure, resulting in a forceful cough.

ing is performed by placing the palm of the hand or hands on the abdomen below the xiphoid process (Fig. 66-6). As the patient ends a deep inspiration and begins the expiration, the hands should be moved forcefully downward, increasing abdominal pressure and facilitating the cough. This measure helps increase expiratory flow and thereby facilitate secretion clearance.

Some patients may benefit from therapeutic cough techniques. *Huff coughing* is a series of coughs performed while saying the word "huff." This technique prevents the glottis from closing during the cough. Patients with COPD generate higher flow rates with a huff cough than is possible with a normal cough. The huff cough is effective in clearing only the central airways, but it may assist in moving secretions upward. The staged cough also assists secretion mobilization. To perform the *staged cough,* the patient sits in a chair, breathes three or four times in

and out through the mouth, and coughs while bending forward and pressing a pillow inward against the diaphragm.

Positioning the patient either by elevating the head of the bed at least 45 degrees or by using a reclining chair or chair bed may help maximize thoracic expansion, thereby decreasing dyspnea and improving secretion mobilization. A sitting position improves pulmonary function and assists in venous pooling in dependent body areas such as the lower extremities. When lungs are upright, ventilation and perfusion are best in the lung bases. Lateral or side-lying positioning may be used in patients with disease involving only one lung. This position, termed *down with the good lung,* allows for improved $\dot{V}/\dot{Q}$ matching in the affected lung. Pulmonary blood flow and ventilation are optimal in dependent lung areas. This positioning also allows for secretions to drain out of the affected lung to the point where they may be removed by suctioning. For example, in patients with a significant right middle lobe pneumonia, optimal positioning would be to place them on their left side to maximize ventilation and perfusion in the "good" lung and facilitate secretion removal from the affected lung (postural drainage). All patients should be side lying if there is any possibility that the tongue will obstruct the airway or that aspiration may occur. An oral or nasal airway should be kept at the bedside for use if necessary.

Hydration and humidification. Thick and viscous secretions are difficult to raise and should be thinned. Adequate fluid intake (2 to 3 L per day) is necessary to keep secretions thin and easy to expel. If the patient is unable to take sufficient fluids orally, intravenous (IV) hydration will be used. Thorough assessment of the patient's cardiac and renal status is paramount to determine whether he or she can tolerate the intravascular volume and avoid congestive heart failure (CHF) and pulmonary edema. Assessment for signs of fluid overload (e.g., crackles, dyspnea, and increased central venous pressure) at regular intervals is paramount. These considerations would also apply to the patient with renal dysfunction. An appropriate humidification device is an adjunct in secretion management. Aerosols of sterile normal saline, administered by a nebulizer, may be used to liquefy secretions. Oxygen may also be administered by aerosol mask to thin secretions and facilitate their removal. Aerosol therapy may induce bronchospasm and severe coughing, causing a decreased PaO_2. As such, frequent assessment of patient tolerance to therapy is paramount.[9] Mucolytic agents such as nebulized acetylcysteine (Mucomyst) mixed with a bronchodilator may be used to thin secretions but, as a side effect, may also cause airway erythema and bronchospasm. Therefore it is used only in special situations (e.g., during bronchoscopy to remove thick, copious secretions).

Chest physical therapy. Chest physical therapy is indicated in patients who produce more more than 30 ml of sputum per day or have evidence of severe atelectasis or pulmonary infiltrates. If tolerated, postural drainage, percussion, and vibration to the affected lung segments may assist in moving secretions to the larger airways where they may be removed by coughing or suctioning. Because positioning may affect oxygenation, patients may not tolerate head-down or lateral positioning because of extreme dyspnea or hypoxemia caused by $\dot{V}/\dot{Q}$ mismatch. (Chest physical therapy is discussed in Chapter 28.)

Airway suctioning. If the patient is unable to expectorate secretions, nasopharyngeal, oropharyngeal, or nasotracheal suctioning (blind suctioning without a tracheal tube in place) is indicated. Suctioning through an artificial airway, such as endotracheal or tracheostomy tubes, may also be performed (see Chapters 26 and 64). A mini-tracheostomy (or mini-trach) may be used to suction patients who have difficulty mobilizing secretions and when blind suctioning is difficult or ineffective. The *mini-trach* is a 4 mm indwelling plastic cuffless cannula inserted through the cricothyroid membrane. It is used to instill sterile normal saline solution to elicit a cough and to perform suctioning using a size 10 or less French catheter. Contraindications for a mini-trach include an absent gag reflex, history of aspiration, and the need for long-term mechanical ventilation.

Positive Pressure Ventilation. If intensive measures fail to improve ventilation and oxygenation and the patient continues to exhibit manifestations of acute respiratory failure, ventilatory assistance may be initiated. Positive pressure ventilation (PPV) may be provided invasively through endotracheal or nasotracheal intubation or noninvasively through a nasal or face mask. Patients who require PPV are typically cared for in a critical care unit. (See Chapter 64 for a discussion of artificial airways and mechanical ventilation.)

Noninvasive positive pressure ventilation (NIPPV) may be used as a treatment for patients with acute or chronic respiratory failure. During NIPPV a mask is placed over the patient's nose or nose and mouth and the patient breathes spontaneously while PPV is delivered (Fig. 66-7). With NIPPV it is possible to decrease the work of breathing without the need for endotracheal intubation. Bilevel positive airway pressure (BiPAP ventilatory support system) is a form of NIPPV in which different positive pressure levels are set for inspiration and expiration (Fig. 66-7). Continuous positive airway pressure (CPAP) is another form of NIPPV in which a constant positive pressure is delivered to the airway during inspiration and expiration.[8,10]

NIPPV is most useful in managing chronic respiratory failure in patients with chest wall and neuromuscular disease (see

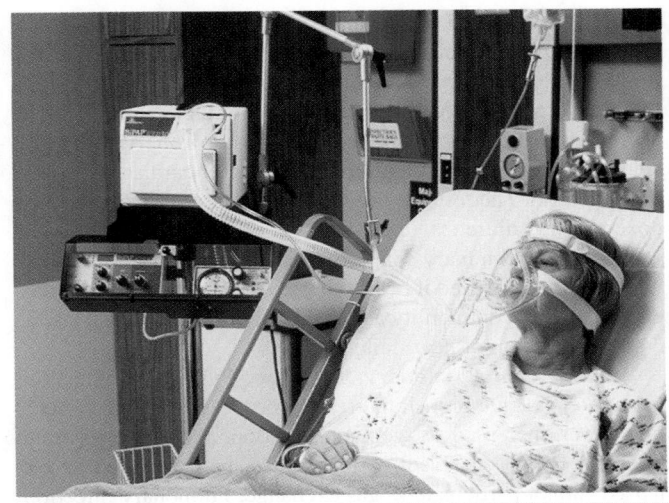

FIG. 66-7   Noninvasive bilevel positive pressure ventilation. A mask is placed over the nose or nose and mouth. Positive pressure from a mechanical ventilator assists the patient's breathing efforts, decreasing the work of breathing.

Table 66-1). NIPPV has been used in patients with hypoxemic respiratory failure (e.g., ARDS, cardiogenic pulmonary edema), but with less success. NIPPV may also be used for patients who refuse endotracheal intubation but still desire some palliative ventilatory support (e.g., patients with end-stage COPD). NIPPV is not appropriate for the patient who has absent respirations, excessive secretions, decreased level of consciousness, high O_2 requirements, facial trauma, or hemodynamic instability.[8,10-12]

■ Drug Therapy

Goals of drug therapy for patients in acute respiratory failure include relief of bronchospasm, reduction of airway inflammation and pulmonary congestion, treatment of pulmonary infection, and reduction of severe anxiety and restlessness.

Relief of Bronchospasm. Alveolar ventilation will be increased with relief of bronchospasm. Short-acting *bronchodilators,* such as metaproterenol (Alupent) and albuterol (Ventolin), are frequently administered to reverse bronchospasm using either a handheld nebulizer or a metered-dose inhaler with a spacer.[8] In acute bronchospasm these drugs may be given at 30- to 60-minute intervals until it can be determined that a response is occurring. If severe bronchospasm continues, IV aminophylline may be administered. The bronchodilator effects of all of these medications can sometimes cause a worsening of arterial hypoxemia by redistributing the inspired gas to areas of decreased perfusion. Administering the bronchodilator with an O_2-enriched gas mixture usually alleviates this effect.[1] (See Chapter 28 for nursing management related to bronchodilators.)

Reduction of Airway Inflammation. Corticosteroids (e.g., methylprednisolone [Solu-Medrol]) may be used in conjunction with bronchodilating agents when bronchospasm and inflammation are present. When administered intravenously, corticosteroids have an immediate onset of action. Inhaled corticosteroids are not used for acute respiratory failure, because they require 4 to 5 days before optimum therapeutic effects are seen.[13]

Reduction of Pulmonary Congestion. Pulmonary interstitial fluid can occur as a consequence of direct or indirect injury to the alveolar capillary membrane (e.g., ARDS) or from right- or left-sided heart failure, and therefore can be either cardiac or noncardiac in origin. The result is decreased alveolar ventilation and hypoxemia. IV diuretics (e.g., furosemide [Lasix]) are used to decrease the pulmonary congestion caused by heart failure. Digitalis may also be used if heart failure or atrial fibrillation is present to increase contractility and decrease heart rate. (See Chapter 34 for discussion of heart failure.)

Treatment of Pulmonary Infections. Pulmonary infections (pneumonia, acute bronchitis) result in excessive mucus production, fever, increased oxygen consumption, and inflamed, fluid-filled, or collapsed alveoli. Alveoli that are fluid filled or collapsed cannot participate in gas exchange. Pulmonary infections can either cause or exacerbate acute respiratory failure. IV antibiotics, such as vancomycin (Vancocin, Lyphocin) or ceftriaxone (Rocephin), are frequently administered to inhibit bacterial growth. Chest x-rays are performed to determine the location and extent of a suspected infectious process. Sputum cultures are used to determine the type of organisms causing the infection and their sensitivity to antimicrobial medications.

Reduction of Severe Anxiety, Pain, and Agitation. Anxiety, restlessness, and agitation result from cerebral hypoxia. In addition, fear caused by the inability to breathe and a sense of loss of control may exacerbate anxiety. Anxiety, pain, and agitation increase O_2 consumption, which may worsen the degree of hypoxemia. Anxiety, pain, and agitation also increase CO_2 production, affect ventilator management, and increase morbidity.[14,15] Several nursing strategies can assist the patient in reducing the level of anxiety and pain (see NCP 66-1).

Sedation and analgesia with drug therapy such as benzodiazepines (e.g., lorazepam [Ativan], midazolam [Versed]) and narcotics (e.g., morphine, fentanyl [Sublimaze]) may be used to decrease anxiety, agitation, and pain. Continued agitation will increase the patient's work of breathing, O_2 consumption, CO_2 production, and risk of injury (e.g., accidental extubation). When receiving any sedative or analgesic agent, patients must be monitored closely for cardiovascular and respiratory depression.[14,15] In the critical care setting, sedation and analgesia are commonly used for severely restless, anxious, and agitated patients who may be experiencing pain and are in acute respiratory failure.

Patients who breathe asynchronously with mechanical ventilation may also benefit from titration of ventilator flow rates and other settings, as well as addressing treatable causes of agitation such as hypoxemia, pain, or hypercapnia. Patients who remain asynchronous with mechanical ventilation may require neuromuscular blockade with agents such as vecuronium (Norcuron) or cisatracurium (Nimbex) to produce skeletal muscle relaxation and synchrony with mechanical ventilation. Neuromuscular blockade may also decrease the patient's risk of lung injury related to excessive inspiratory/intrathoracic pressures. In this way, the ventilator can then provide optimal respiratory support. Patients receiving neuromuscular blockade should receive sedation and analgesia to the point of unconsciousness for patient comfort, to eliminate patient awareness and to avoid the terrifying experience of being awake and in pain while paralyzed (see Nursing Research box).[14-16]

NURSING RESEARCH
Sedation Practices in Critical Care

Citation
Weinert CR, Chlan L, Gross C: Sedating critically ill patients: factors affecting nurses' delivery of sedative therapy, *Am J Crit Care* 10:156, 2001.

Purpose
To explore the beliefs and attitudes of nurses toward critical illness and sedation practices, and to identify processes that nurses use to assess patients' need for sedation.

Methods
A qualitative design was used to interview 34 experienced critical care nurses in focus group settings. All interviews were audiotaped and transcribed.

Results and Conclusions
Five themes were extracted from the data and validated by four of the study participants and two experienced critical care nurses who did not participate. It was discovered that patients' family members and the nurses' workload influence nurses' sedation practices. Conflicts with physicians were reported when sedation goals for the patient were not shared. Nurses believed that the goals of sedation were to provide for patient comfort, amnesia, and safety. Finally, nurses used a variety of patient cues to determine level of sedation and reported mixed feelings about the efficacy of sedation protocols.

Implications for Nursing Practice
Several nonpatient factors (e.g., social, personal) were reported to influence the sedation practices of nurses. Ideally, these factors should be limited. Sedation goals should reflect the individual patient's needs. The use of sedation protocols could achieve this directive and should be studied.

■ Medical Supportive Therapy

Therapeutic goals and interventions to maximize O_2 delivery and treat the underlying cause of the respiratory failure are essential to improving the patient's oxygenation and ventilation status. The primary goal is to treat the underlying cause of the respiratory failure. Other goals include maintaining an adequate cardiac output and hemoglobin concentration.

Treating the Underlying Cause. Interventions are directed toward reversing the disease process that resulted in the development of acute respiratory failure. Patients with hypoventilation can be diagnosed and treated rapidly. Patients with $\dot{V}/\dot{Q}$ mismatch, shunting, or diffusion limitation are managed differently depending on the underlying cause. In all patient situations, monitoring treatment effects, including trends in ABGs and changes in respiratory status, is a continuous process.

Maintaining Adequate Cardiac Output. Cardiac output reflects the blood flow reaching the tissues. Blood pressure is an important indicator of the adequacy of cardiac output. Usually a systolic blood pressure of at least 90 mm Hg is adequate to maintain perfusion to the vital organs. If the systolic blood pressure is at least 90 mm Hg, changes in mental status may be attributed to the level of O_2 and CO_2 rather than decreased cerebral perfusion. Decreased cardiac output is treated by administration of IV fluids, medications, or both. (See Chapter 65 for a discussion of drugs used to treat decreased cardiac output and shock.) Cardiac output may also be decreased by changes in intrathoracic or intrapulmonary pressures from positive pressure ventilation. Consequently, clinical indicators of adequate cardiac output and tissue perfusion should be monitored closely with initiation or titration of mechanical ventilation by mask or endotracheal intubation.

Maintaining Adequate Hemoglobin Concentration. Hemoglobin is the primary carrier when delivering O_2 to the tissues. If the patient is anemic, tissue O_2 delivery will be compromised. A hemoglobin concentration of 9 to 10 g/dl (90 to 100 g/L) or greater typically ensures adequate O_2 saturation of the hemoglobin. The patient should be monitored for sites of blood loss and transfused with packed red blood cells if an adequate hemoglobin concentration cannot be maintained.

■ Nutritional Therapy

Maintenance of protein and energy stores is especially important in patients who experience acute respiratory failure because nutritional depletion causes a loss of muscle mass, including the respiratory muscles, and may prolong recovery. During the acute manifestations of respiratory failure, the risk of aspiration typically prevents oral nutritional intake. Therefore enteral or parenteral nutrition may be administered. When the acute manifestations subside, the patient may resume oral intake as tolerated. A multitude of nutritional supplements are available for this patient population. A high-carbohydrate diet may need to be avoided in the patient who retains CO_2 because carbohydrates metabolize into CO_2 and increase the CO_2 load of the patient. However, research is currently being done in this area, and it remains controversial.

■ Evaluation

The expected outcomes for the patient with acute respiratory failure are presented in NCP 66-1.

■ Gerontologic Considerations
Respiratory Failure

The elderly population is the fastest growing age-group in North America, a trend that is increasingly reflected within the patient populations in acute care and critical care settings. Multiple factors contribute to an increased risk of respiratory failure in older adults. They are at higher risk of developing respiratory failure because of the reduction in ventilatory capacity that accompanies aging, especially if other risk factors are present. Physiologic aging of the lung may produce alveolar dilation, larger air spaces, and loss of surface area. Diminished elastic recoil within the airways, decreased chest wall compliance, and decreased respiratory muscle strength also occur. In older adults, the PaO_2 falls further and the $PaCO_2$ rises to a higher level before the respiratory system is stimulated to alter the rate and depth of breathing. This delayed response can contribute to the development of respiratory failure. In addition, a history of smoking is a risk factor. Lifelong smoking can accelerate age-related respiratory changes. Poor nutritional status and less available physiologic reserve in cardiovascular, respiratory, and autonomic nervous systems increase the risk of additional disease states such as pneumonia and cardiac disease

that may compromise respiratory function and precipitate respiratory failure.[17,18]

Assessment parameters must also be adjusted for age. For example, heart rate and blood pressure generally increase with age and related changes in the cardiovascular system. Therefore determination of the patient's baseline vital signs and using them as a basis for comparison of physical assessment findings is most appropriate in evaluating changes in cardiopulmonary function in the older adult. ■

ACUTE RESPIRATORY DISTRESS SYNDROME

Acute respiratory distress syndrome (ARDS) is a sudden and progressive form of acute respiratory failure in which the alveolar capillary membrane becomes damaged and more permeable to intravascular fluid (Fig. 66-8). The alveoli fill with fluid, resulting in severe dyspnea, hypoxemia refractory to supplemental O_2, reduced lung compliance, and diffuse pulmonary infiltrates.[19-22]

The incidence of ARDS in the United States is estimated at more than 150,000 cases annually. Despite supportive therapy, the mortality rate from ARDS is approximately 50%. Patients who have both gram-negative septic shock and ARDS have a mortality rate of 70% to 90%.[20]

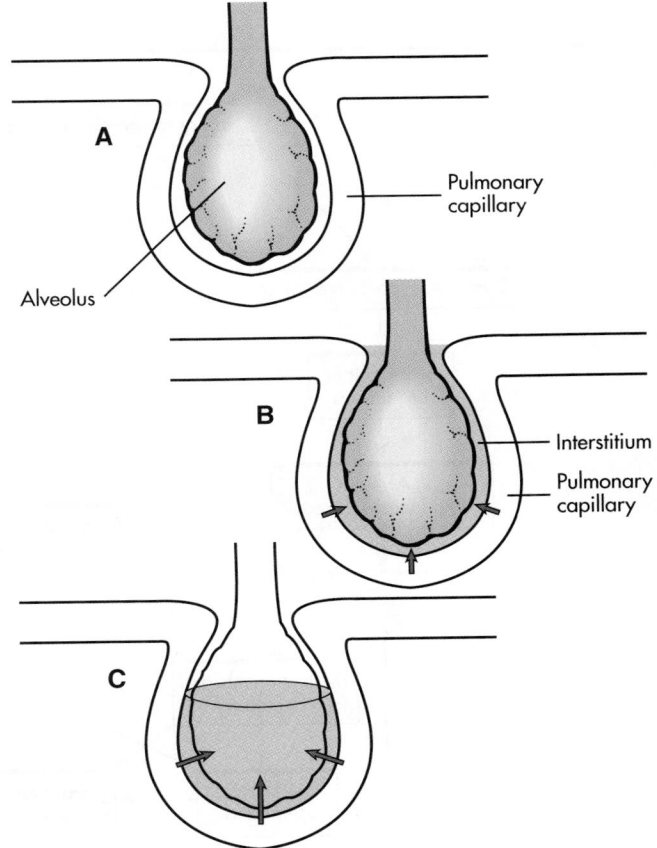

FIG. 66-8 Stages of edema formation in acute respiratory distress syndrome. **A,** Normal alveolus and pulmonary capillary. **B,** Interstitial edema occurs with increased flow of fluid into the interstitial space. **C,** Alveolar edema occurs when the fluid crosses the blood–gas barrier.

TABLE 66-6	Conditions Predisposing to Acute Respiratory Distress Syndrome

Direct Lung Injury

Common Causes
Aspiration of gastric contents or other substances
Viral/bacterial pneumonia

Less Common Causes
Chest trauma
Embolism: fat, air, amniotic fluid
Inhalation of toxic substances
Near-drowning
O_2 toxicity
Radiation pneumonitis

Indirect Lung Injury

Common Causes
Sepsis (especially gram-negative infection)
Severe massive trauma

Less Common Causes
Acute pancreatitis
Anaphylaxis
Cardiopulmonary bypass
Disseminated intravascular coagulation
Multiple blood transfusions
Narcotic drug overdose (e.g., heroin)
Nonpulmonary systemic diseases
Severe head injury
Shock states

Etiology and Pathophysiology

Table 66-6 lists conditions that predispose patients to the development of ARDS. The most common cause of ARDS is sepsis. Patients with multiple risk factors are three to four times more likely to develop ARDS.

Direct lung injury may cause ARDS (Fig. 66-9), or ARDS may develop as a consequence of the systemic inflammatory response syndrome (SIRS) (see Chapter 65, Fig. 65-1). SIRS may have an infectious or a noninfectious etiology and is characterized by widespread inflammation or clinical responses to inflammation following a variety of physiologic insults, including severe trauma, gut ischemia, lung injury, and sepsis.[22] ARDS may also develop as a consequence of multiple organ dysfunction syndrome (MODS). MODS results from organ system dysfunction that progressively increases in severity and ultimately results in multisystem organ failure. (SIRS and MODS are discussed in Chapter 65.)

An exact cause for the damage to the alveolar-capillary membrane is not known. However, the pathophysiologic changes of ARDS are thought to be due to stimulation of the inflammatory and immune systems, which causes an attraction of neutrophils to the pulmonary interstitium.[10] The neutrophils cause a release of biochemical, humoral, and cellular mediators (Table 66-7) that produce changes in the lung, including increased pulmonary capillary membrane permeability, destruction of elastin and collagen, formation of pulmonary microemboli, and pulmonary artery vasoconstriction (see Fig. 66-9).[20-22] (These mediators are discussed in Chapters 12 and 13.)

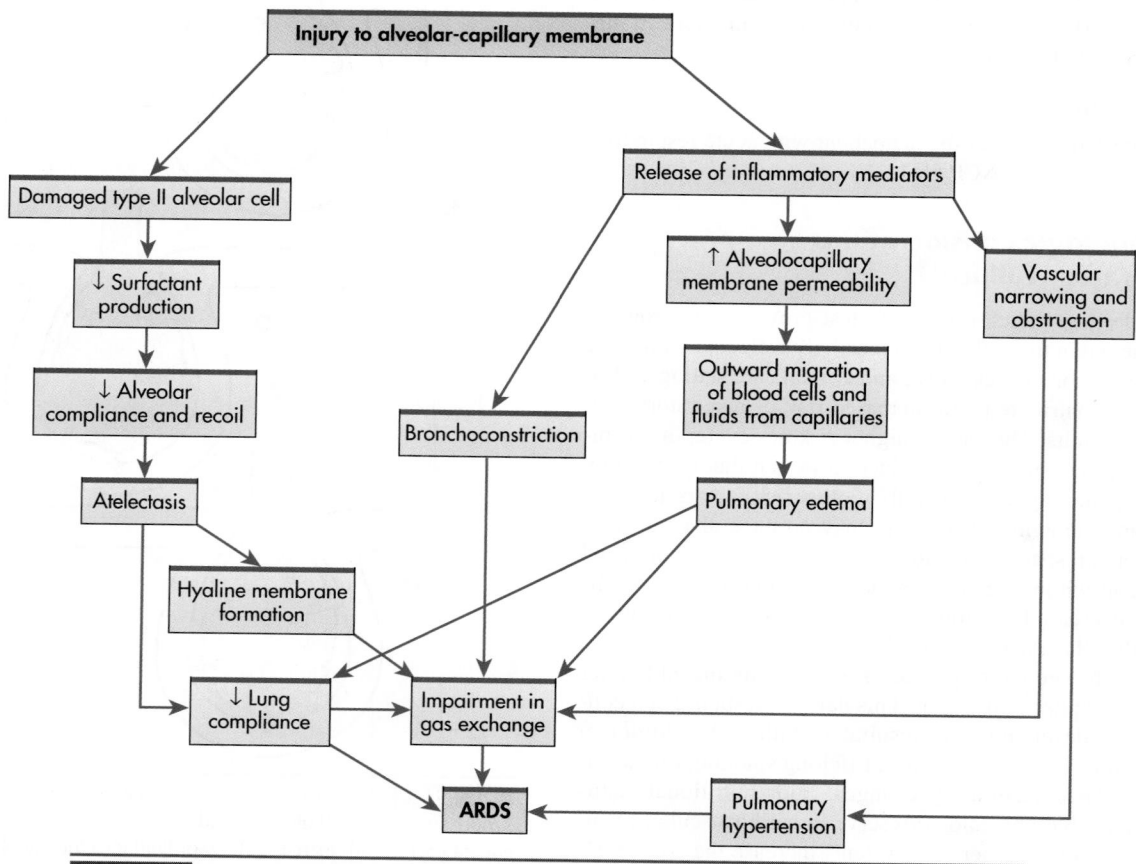

FIG. 66-9 Pathophysiology of acute respiratory distress syndrome (ARDS).

TABLE 66-7	Mediators of Acute Lung Injury

Complement component C5a
Neutrophil products, including proteases and O_2 radicals
Monocyte and macrophage products, including tumor necrosis factor, interleukin-1, and colony-stimulating factor
Arachidonic acid metabolites, including prostaglandins and leukotrienes
Coagulation products, including kallikreins, kinins, fibrin degradation products, and plasminogen-activating factor
Histamine
Serotonin
Endotoxin
Elastase
Collagenase

The pathophysiologic changes in ARDS are divided into three phases: (1) injury or exudative phase, (2) reparative or proliferative phase, and (3) fibrotic phase.

Injury or Exudative Phase. The *injury or exudative phase* occurs approximately 1 to 7 days (usually 24 to 48 hours) after the initial direct lung injury or host insult. Neutrophils adhere to the pulmonary microcirculation, causing damage to the vascular endothelium and increased capillary permeability. In the earliest phase of injury, there is engorgement of the peribronchial and perivascular interstitial space, which produces interstitial edema. Next, fluid from the interstitial space crosses the alveolar epithelium and enters the alveolar space. Intrapulmonary shunt develops because the alveoli fill with fluid, and blood passing through them cannot be oxygenated (see Figs. 66-4 and 66-8).

Alveolar type I and type II cells (which produce surfactant) are damaged by the changes caused by ARDS. This damage, in addition to further fluid and protein accumulation, results in surfactant dysfunction. The function of *surfactant* is to maintain alveolar stability by decreasing alveolar surface tension and preventing alveolar collapse. Decreased synthesis of surfactant and inactivation of existing surfactant cause the alveoli to become unstable and collapse (atelectasis). Widespread atelectasis further decreases lung compliance, compromises gas exchange, and contributes to hypoxemia.[21,22]

Also during this stage, hyaline membranes begin to line the alveoli. The hyaline membrane is composed of necrotic cells, protein, and fibrin and lies adjacent to the alveoli wall. These hyaline membranes are thought to result from the exudation of high-molecular-weight substances (particularly fibrinogen) in the edema fluid. Hyaline membranes contribute to the development of fibrosis and atelectasis, leading to a decrease in gas exchange capability and lung compliance.

The primary pathophysiologic changes that characterize the *injury or exudative phase* of ARDS are interstitial and alveolar edema (noncardiogenic pulmonary edema) and atelectasis.[23] Severe $\dot{V}/\dot{Q}$ mismatch and shunting of pulmonary capillary blood result in hypoxemia unresponsive to increasing concentrations of O_2 (termed **refractory hypoxemia**). Diffusion limitation, caused by hyaline membrane formation, further contributes to the severity of the hypoxemia. As the lungs become less compliant because of decreased surfactant, pulmonary edema, and atelectasis, the patient must generate higher airway pressures to inflate "stiff" lungs. Reduced lung compliance greatly increases the patient's work of breathing.

Hypoxemia and the stimulation of juxtacapillary receptors in the stiff lung parenchyma (J reflex) initially cause an increase in respiratory rate and decrease in tidal volume. This breathing pattern increases CO_2 removal, producing respiratory alkalosis. Cardiac output increases in response to hypoxemia, a compensatory effort to increase pulmonary blood flow. However, as atelectasis, pulmonary edema, and pulmonary shunt increase, compensation fails, and hypoventilation, decreased cardiac output, and decreased tissue O_2 perfusion eventually occur.

Reparative or Proliferative Phase. The *reparative or proliferative phase* of ARDS begins 1 to 2 weeks after the initial lung injury. During this phase, there is an influx of neutrophils, monocytes, and lymphocytes and fibroblast proliferation as part of the inflammatory response. The injured lung has an immense regenerative capacity after acute lung injury. The proliferative phase is complete when the diseased lung becomes characterized by dense, fibrous tissue. Increased pulmonary vascular resistance and pulmonary hypertension may occur in this stage because fibroblasts and inflammatory cells destroy the pulmonary vasculature. Lung compliance continues to decrease as a result of interstitial fibrosis. Hypoxemia worsens because of the thickened alveolar membrane, causing diffusion limitation and shunting. If the reparative phase persists, widespread fibrosis results. If the reparative phase is arrested, the lesions resolve.[19,21]

Fibrotic Phase. The *fibrotic phase* of ARDS occurs approximately 2 to 3 weeks after the initial lung injury. This phase is also called the *chronic or late phase* of ARDS. By this time, the lung is completely remodeled by sparsely collagenous and fibrous tissues. There is diffuse scarring and fibrosis, resulting in decreased lung compliance. In addition, the surface area for gas exchange is significantly reduced because the interstitium is fibrotic, and therefore hypoxemia continues. Pulmonary hypertension results from pulmonary vascular destruction and fibrosis.

Clinical Progression

Progression of ARDS varies among patients. Some persons survive the acute phase of lung injury; pulmonary edema resolves and complete recovery occurs in a few days. The chance for survival is poor in patients who enter the fibrotic (chronic or late) stage, which requires long-term mechanical ventilation. It is not known why injured lungs repair and recover in some patients, and in others ARDS progresses. Several factors seem to be important in determining the course of ARDS, including the nature of the initial injury, extent and severity of coexisting diseases, and pulmonary complications.[1,20,21]

Clinical Manifestations

The initial presentation of ARDS is often insidious. At the time of the initial injury, and for several hours to 1 to 2 days afterward, the patient may not experience respiratory symptoms, or the patient may exhibit only dyspnea, tachypnea, cough, and restlessness. Chest auscultation may be normal or reveal fine, scattered crackles. ABGs usually indicate mild hypoxemia and respiratory alkalosis caused by hyperventilation. Respiratory alkalosis results from hypoxemia and the stimulation of juxtacapillary receptors. The chest x-ray may be normal or exhibit evidence of minimal scattered interstitial infiltrates. Edema may not show on the x-ray until there is a 30% increase in fluid content in the lung.[20,21]

As ARDS progresses, symptoms worsen because of increased fluid accumulation and decreased lung compliance. Respiratory discomfort becomes evident as the work of breathing increases. Tachypnea and intercostal and suprasternal retractions may be present. Pulmonary function tests in ARDS reveal decreased compliance and decreased lung volumes, particularly a decreased functional residual capacity (FRC). Tachycardia, diaphoresis, changes in sensorium with decreased mentation, cyanosis, and pallor may be present. Chest auscultation usually reveals scattered to diffuse crackles and rhonchi. The chest x-ray demonstrates diffuse and extensive bilateral interstitial and alveolar infiltrates. A pulmonary artery catheter may be inserted. Pulmonary artery wedge pressure does not increase in ARDS because the cause is noncardiogenic (not related to cardiac function).

Hypoxemia and a PaO_2/FIO_2 ratio below 200 despite increased FIO_2 by mask, cannula, or endotracheal tube are hallmarks of ARDS. ABGs may initially demonstrate a normal or decreased $PaCO_2$ despite severe dyspnea and hypoxemia. Hypercapnia signifies that hypoventilation is occurring, and the patient is no longer able to maintain the level of ventilation needed to provide optimum gas exchange.

As ARDS progresses it is associated with profound respiratory distress requiring endotracheal intubation and positive pressure ventilation (PPV). The chest x-ray is often termed *whiteout* or *white lung*, because consolidation and coalescing infiltrates are widespread throughout the lungs, leaving few recognizable air spaces. Pleural effusions may also be present. Severe hypoxemia, hypercapnia, and metabolic acidosis, with symptoms of target organ or tissue hypoxia, may ensue if prompt therapy is not instituted.

In summary, no precise criteria define ARDS. ARDS is considered to be present if the patient has (1) refractory hypoxemia, (2) a chest x-ray with new bilateral interstitial or alveolar infiltrates, (3) a pulmonary artery wedge pressure of 18 mm Hg or less and no evidence of heart failure, and (4) a predisposing condition for ARDS within 48 hours of clinical manifestations (Table 66-8).

Complications

Complications may develop as a result of ARDS itself or its treatment. (Table 66-9 lists the common complications of ARDS.) The major cause of death in ARDS is MODS, often accompanied by sepsis. The vital organs most commonly involved are the kidneys, liver, and heart. The organ systems most often involved are the CNS, hematologic system, and gastrointestinal system.

Nosocomial Pneumonia. A frequent complication of ARDS is nosocomial pneumonia, occurring in as many as 68%

TABLE 66-8	Diagnostic Findings in Acute Respiratory Distress Syndrome

Refractory Hypoxemia
PaO_2 <50 mm Hg on FIO_2 >40% with PEEP >5 cm H_2O
PaO_2/FIO_2 ratio <200

Chest X-ray
New bilateral interstitial and alveolar infiltrates

Pulmonary Artery Wedge Pressure
≤18 mm Hg and no evidence of heart failure

Predisposing Condition
Identification of a predisposing condition for ARDS within 48 hours of clinical manifestations

ARDS, Acute respiratory distress syndrome; *PEEP,* positive end-expiratory pressure.

TABLE 66-9	Complications Associated with Acute Respiratory Distress Syndrome

Infection Catheter-related infection Nosocomial pneumonia Sepsis (bacteremia)	**Renal Complications** Acute renal failure

Respiratory Complications
O_2 toxicity
Pulmonary barotrauma (e.g.,
  pneumothorax, pneumo-
  mediastinum, subcutaneous
  emphysema)
Pulmonary emboli
Pulmonary fibrosis
	Cardiac Complications
	Arrhythmias
	Decreased cardiac output
	
	Hematologic Complications
	Anemia
	Disseminated intravascular
	  coagulation
	Thrombocytopenia

Gastrointestinal Complications Paralytic ileus Pneumoperitoneum Stress ulceration and hemorrhage	**ET Intubation Complications** Laryngeal ulceration Tracheal malacia Tracheal stenosis Tracheal ulceration

ET, Endotracheal tube.

of patients with ARDS. Risk factors include impaired host defenses, contaminated medical equipment, invasive monitoring devices, aspiration of gastrointestinal contents, and prolonged mechanical ventilation, as well as colonization of the respiratory tract. Strategies to prevent nosocomial pneumonia include infection control measures (e.g., strict hand washing and sterile technique during endotracheal suctioning) and elevating the head of the bed 45 degrees or more to prevent aspiration.[24] (See Chapter 27 for discussion of pneumonia.)

Barotrauma. *Barotrauma* may result from rupture of overdistended alveoli during mechanical ventilation. The high peak airway pressures that may be required in patients with ARDS predispose to this complication. Barotrauma results in the presence of alveolar air in locations where it is not usually found. This can lead to pulmonary interstitial emphysema, pneumothorax, subcutaneous emphysema, pneumoperitoneum, pneumomediastinum, and tension pneumothorax. (See Chapter 27 for discussion of pneumothorax.) To avoid barotrauma, the patient with ARDS is sometimes ventilated with smaller tidal volumes, resulting in higher $PaCO_2$. This method of mechanical ventilation is termed *permissive hypercapnia* because the $PaCO_2$ is allowed (permitted) to rise above normal limits.[9]

Volu-pressure Trauma. *Volu-pressure trauma* can occur in patients with ARDS when large tidal volumes are used to ventilate noncompliant lungs. Volu-pressure trauma results in alveolar fractures and movement of fluids and proteins into the alveolar spaces. To limit this complication, it is recommended that smaller tidal volumes or pressure ventilation be used in patients with ARDS (see Chapter 64).[25]

Stress Ulcers. Critically ill patients with acute respiratory failure are at high risk for stress ulcers. Bleeding from stress ulcers occurs in 30% of patients with ARDS who require PPV, a higher incidence than other causes of acute respiratory failure. Management strategies include correction of predisposing conditions such as hypotension, shock, and acidosis. Prophylactic management includes antiulcer agents (e.g., famotidine [Pepcid], omeprazole [Prilosec], sucralfate [Carafate]) and early initiation of enteral nutrition (see Chapters 39 and 64).

Renal Failure. Renal failure can occur from decreased renal tissue oxygenation as a result of hypotension, hypoxemia, or hypercapnia. Renal failure may also be caused by administration of nephrotoxic drugs (e.g., aminoglycosides), which are used to treat infections associated with ARDS.

NURSING and COLLABORATIVE MANAGEMENT
ACUTE RESPIRATORY DISTRESS SYNDROME

The collaborative care for acute respiratory failure (see Table 66-5) is applicable to ARDS. The following section discusses additional collaborative care measures for the patient with ARDS (Table 66-10). Patients with ARDS are commonly cared for in critical care units. The nursing care plan for acute respiratory failure (see NCP 66-1) is applicable to patients with ARDS.

■ Nursing Assessment

Because ARDS causes acute respiratory failure, the subjective and objective data that should be obtained from a person with ARDS are the same as that for acute respiratory failure (see Table 66-4). Abnormal findings on physical examination are indications that ARDS has progressed beyond the initial stages.

■ Nursing Diagnoses

Nursing diagnoses for the patient with ARDS may include, but are not limited to, those described for acute respiratory failure (see NCP 66-1).

■ Planning

With appropriate therapy, the overall goals for the patient with ARDS are a PaO_2 of at least 60 mm Hg and adequate lung ventilation to maintain normal pH. The patient following recovery from ARDS will have (1) PaO_2 within normal limits for age or baseline values on room air (FIO_2 of 21%), (2) SaO_2 greater than 90%, (3) patent airway, and (4) clear lungs on auscultation.

TABLE 66-10   Collaborative Care: Acute Respiratory Distress Syndrome

Diagnostic
See Table 66-8.
Collaborative Therapy
Respiratory Therapy
O_2 administration
Prone positioning
Lateral rotation therapy
Mechanical ventilation with PEEP
Supportive Therapy
Identification and treatment of underlying cause
Hemodynamic monitoring
Inotropic/vasopressor medications
  Dopamine (Intropin)
  Dobutamine (Dobutrex)
Diuretics
IV fluid administration

PEEP, Positive end-expiratory pressure.

■ Respiratory Therapy

Oxygen Administration. The primary goal of O_2 therapy is to correct hypoxemia. O_2 administered via a simple face mask or nasal cannula is usually inadequate to treat refractory hypoxemia that is associated with ARDS. Masks with high-flow systems that deliver higher O_2 concentrations are initially used to maximize O_2 delivery. Pulse oximetry (SpO_2) is continuously monitored to assess the effectiveness of O_2 therapy. The general standard for O_2 administration is to give the patient the lowest concentration that results in a PaO_2 of 60 mm Hg or greater. When the FIO_2 exceeds 60% for more than 48 hours, the risk for O_2 toxicity increases. Patients with ARDS commonly need intubation with mechanical ventilation because the PaO_2 cannot otherwise be maintained at acceptable levels.

Mechanical Ventilation. Endotracheal intubation and mechanical ventilation provide additional respiratory support. However, even with these interventions it may be necessary to maintain the FIO_2 at 60% or greater to maintain the PaO_2 at 60 mm Hg or greater. During mechanical ventilation, it is common to apply positive end-expiratory pressure (PEEP) at 5 cm H_2O to compensate for loss of glottic function caused by the presence of the endotracheal tube. In patients with ARDS, higher levels of PEEP (e.g., 10 to 20 cm H_2O) may be used. The mechanism of action of PEEP is related to its ability to increase FRC and recruit (open up) collapsed alveoli. PEEP is typically applied in 3 to 5 cm H_2O increments until oxygenation is adequate with FIO_2 of 60% or less. PEEP may improve $\dot{V}/\dot{Q}$ in respiratory units that collapse at low airway pressures, thus allowing the FIO_2 to be lowered.

However, PEEP is not a benign therapy. The additional intrathoracic and intrapulmonic pressures can compromise venous return to the right side of the heart, thereby decreasing preload, cardiac output, and blood pressure. PEEP can also cause hyperinflation of the alveoli, compression of the pulmonary capillary bed, a reduction in blood return to the left side of the heart, and a dramatic reduction in blood pressure. In addition, PEEP or excessive inspiratory pressures can result in barotrauma and volupressure trauma.[25]

If hypoxemic failure persists in spite of high levels of PEEP, alternative modes and therapies may be used. These include pressure support ventilation, pressure release ventilation, pressure control ventilation, inverse ratio ventilation, high-frequency ventilation, and permissive hypercapnia (low tidal volumes that allow $PaCO_2$ to increase slowly, maintaining normal pH and low airway pressures).[26,27] Additional information on mechanical ventilation and PEEP is provided in Chapter 64.

Extracorporeal membrane oxygenation (ECMO) and extracorporeal CO_2 removal ($ECCO_2R$) pass blood across a gas-exchanging membrane outside the body and then return oxygenated blood back to the body. $ECCO_2R$ with low-frequency PPV allows the lung to heal while the lung is not functional.[19,28]

Positioning Strategies. Some patients with ARDS demonstrate a marked improvement in PaO_2 when turned from the supine to prone position (e.g., PaO_2 70 mm Hg supine, PaO_2 90 mm Hg prone) with no change in inspired O_2 concentration (Fig. 66-10). The response may be sufficient to allow a reduction in inspired O_2 concentration or PEEP.

In the early phases of ARDS, fluid moves freely throughout the lung. Because of gravity, this fluid pools in dependent regions of the lung. As a consequence, some alveoli are fluid filled (dependent areas), whereas others are air filled (nondependent areas). In

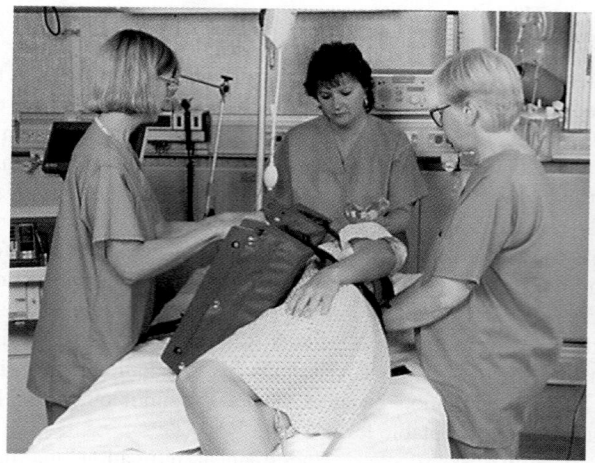
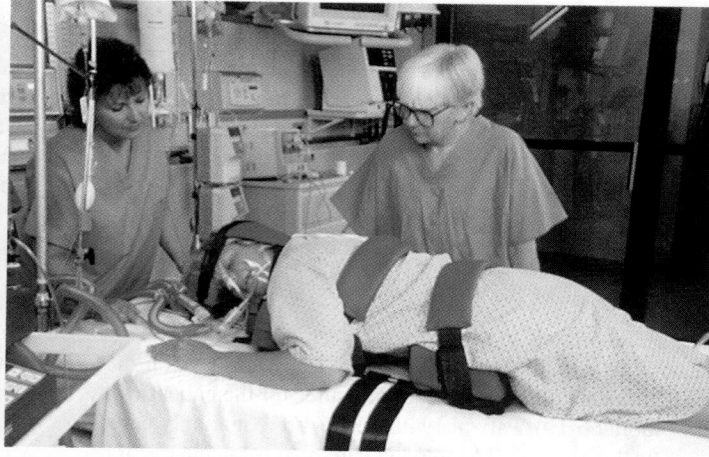

FIG. 66-10 A, Turning patient prone on Vollman Prone Positioner. B, Patient lying prone on Vollman Prone Positioner. (© 2001 Hill-Rom Services, Inc. REPRINTED WITH PERMISSION. ALL RIGHTS RESERVED.)

addition, when the patient is supine the heart and mediastinal contents place more pressure on the lungs than in the prone position, which changes pleural pressure and predisposes to atelectasis. If the patient is turned from supine to prone, air-filled, nonatelectic alveoli in the ventral (anterior) portion of the lung become dependent. Perfusion may be better matched to ventilation, causing less $\dot{V}/\dot{Q}$ mismatch. Not all patients respond to prone positioning with an increase in PaO_2, and there is no reliable way of predicting who will respond. Prone positioning is typically reserved for patients with refractory hypoxemia who do not respond to other strategies to increase PaO_2. When this positioning strategy is used, there must be a plan in place for immediate repositioning for cardiopulmonary resuscitation in the event of a cardiac arrest.[26,29-31]

Another positioning strategy that can be considered for patients with ARDS is lateral rotation therapy. The purpose of this therapy is to provide continuous, slow, side-to-side turning of the patient by rotating the actual bed frame (Fig. 66-11). The lateral movement of the bed is maintained for 18 of every 24 hours to simulate postural drainage and to help mobilize pulmonary secretions. In addition, the bed may also contain a vibrator pack that can provide chest physical therapy to further assist with secretion mobilization and removal. Baseline assessment of the patient's pulmonary status (e.g., respiratory rate and rhythm, breath sounds, ABGs, SpO_2) should be obtained before the initiation of the therapy and continued throughout the use of the therapy.[32]

■ Medical Supportive Therapy

Maintenance of Cardiac Output and Tissue Perfusion. Patients on PPV and PEEP frequently experience decreased cardiac output. One cause is decreased venous return, which results from the PEEP-induced increase in intrathoracic pressure. Cardiac output may also be decreased by impaired contractility and decreased preload. Continuous hemodynamic monitoring is essential to detect these changes and titrate therapy. An arterial catheter is inserted to permit continuous monitoring of blood pressure and sampling of blood for ABGs. A pulmonary artery catheter is normally inserted to allow monitoring of pulmonary artery pressure and pulmonary artery wedge pressures (which indicate the fluid status of the left side of the heart) and cardiac output. If the cardiac output falls, it may be necessary to administer

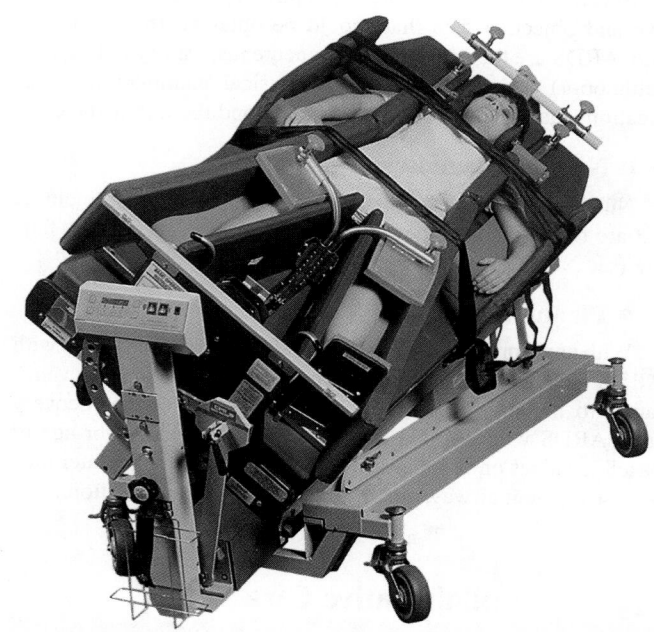

FIG. 66-11 Lateral rotation therapy bed.

crystalloid fluids or colloid solutions or to lower PEEP. Use of inotropic drugs such as dobutamine (Dobutrex) or dopamine (Intropin) may also be necessary. (See Chapter 64 for discussion of hemodynamic monitoring.)

The hemoglobin level is usually kept at levels of more than 9 to 10 g/dl (90 to 100 g/L) with an oxygen saturation of 90% or greater (when PaO_2 is more than 60 mm Hg). Packed red blood cells may be administered to increase hemoglobin and thus the O_2-carrying capacity of the blood.

Maintenance of Fluid Balance. Maintenance of fluid balance is challenging in the patient with ARDS. Increasing pulmonary capillary permeability results in fluid in the lungs and causes pulmonary edema. At the same time, the patient may be volume depleted and therefore prone to hypotension and decreased cardiac output from mechanical ventilation and PEEP.

Pulmonary artery wedge pressures, daily weights, and intake and output are monitored to assess the patient's fluid status. Controversy exists as to the benefits of fluid replacement with crystalloids versus colloids. Critics of colloid replacement believe that proteins in colloid fluid may leak into the pulmonary interstitium, exacerbating the movement of proteinaceous fluid into the alveoli. Advocates of colloid replacement believe that colloids help keep fluid from leaking into the alveoli. The pulmonary artery wedge pressure is kept as low as possible without impairing cardiac output in order to limit pulmonary edema. The patient is usually placed on mild fluid restriction, and diuretics are used as necessary.[33]

■ Evaluation

The expected outcomes for the patient with ARDS are similar to those for a patient with acute respiratory failure and are presented in NCP 66-1.

SEVERE ACUTE RESPIRATORY SYNDROME

Severe acute respiratory syndrome (SARS) is a serious, acute respiratory infection caused by a coronavirus. The virus spreads by close contact between people. SARS is most likely spread via droplets in the air. It is possible that SARS may also be spread more broadly through the air or from touching objects that have become contaminated.

In general, SARS begins with a fever greater than 100.4° F (>38.0° C). Other manifestations may include headache, an overall feeling of discomfort, and muscle aches. Some people also experience mild respiratory symptoms. After 2 to 7 days, SARS patients may develop a dry cough and have trouble breathing.

Because the disease is severe, treatment needs to be started based on the symptoms and before the cause of the illness is confirmed. First, people who are suspected of having SARS should be placed in isolation to protect other patients and health care workers. Although there is no definitive treatment, antiviral medications (such as ribavirin), antibiotics, and corticosteroids may be used. Although antibiotics will not help with SARS (because it is believed to be caused by a virus), they may be used in cases where the person also has a bacterial infection.

About 80% to 90% of infected people start to recover after 6 to 7 days. However, 10% to 20% go on to develop very severe breathing problems and may need mechanical ventilation to breathe. The risk of death is higher for this group, and appears to be linked to the person's preexisting health conditions. People over age 40 are more likely to develop severe breathing problems.[34]

CRITICAL THINKING EXERCISES

Case Study
Acute Respiratory Distress Syndrome

Patient Profile. Mr. J. is a 55-year-old African American man who was admitted 72 hours ago to a general surgical unit after surgery for a bowel obstruction. The surgical procedure involved extensive abdominal surgery to repair a perforated colon, irrigate the abdominal cavity, and provide hemostasis. During surgery his systolic blood pressure dropped to 70 mm Hg. Seven units of packed red blood cells and 4 L of normal saline were administered intravenously to restore blood loss and circulating volume. He is receiving 60% O_2 through an aerosol face mask. He is being monitored with a cardiac monitor and pulse oximeter. He has a central intravenous catheter in place and is receiving 0.9% normal saline intravenously at 125 ml per hour. A urinary catheter is in place.

Subjective Data
- Complains of shortness of breath, inability to lie flat, and diffuse abdominal pain

Objective Data
Physical Assessment
- General: alert, well-nourished man who appears restless and anxious; head of bed elevated 45 degrees; skin cool with moderate diaphoresis.
- Respiratory: no accessory muscle use, retractions, or paradoxic breathing; respiratory rate 28 breaths/min; SpO_2 88%; fine crackles at lung bases.
- Cardiovascular: BP 100/60 mm Hg; cardiac monitor shows sinus tachycardia at 120 beats/min, with equal apical-radial pulse; temperature 101° F (38° C) orally.
- Gastrointestinal: surgical dressing dry and intact; sharp pain on palpation over incisional area.
- Urologic: urinary catheter draining concentrated urine, less than 30 ml per hour.

Diagnostic Findings
- ABG results: pH 7.35, PaO_2 59 mm Hg, $PaCO_2$ 27 mm Hg, bicarbonate 16 mEq/L, O_2 sat 89%.
- Chest x-ray shows new scattered interstitial infiltrates compatible with an ARDS pattern as interpreted by the radiologist.

CRITICAL THINKING QUESTIONS

1. How does the pathophysiology of ARDS predispose to the development of refractory hypoxemia?
2. What clinical manifestations does Mr. J. exhibit that support a diagnosis of ARDS?
3. What are the possible causes of ARDS in Mr. J.?
4. What are the possible complications that Mr. J. is at risk for developing secondary to ARDS?
5. What respiratory care interventions might be implemented to improve Mr. J's hypoxemia?
6. Based on the assessment data presented, write one or more appropriate nursing diagnoses.
7. Discuss any collaborative problems that might apply to this patient.

Nursing Research Issues

1. What should be the key components of an assessment tool to predict patients at risk for acute respiratory failure?
2. Compare the efficacy of prone positioning and continuous lateral rotation therapy in patients with ARDS.
3. What are the effects of a nurse-implemented sedation protocol for patients requiring mechanical ventilation on patient and family comfort and satisfaction with care?

REVIEW QUESTIONS

The number of the question corresponds to the same-numbered objective at the beginning of the chapter.

1. Hypercapnic respiratory failure can be caused by
   a. ARDS.
   b. asthma.
   c. pneumonia.
   d. pulmonary emboli.

2. An early sign of acute respiratory failure is
   a. coma.
   b. cyanosis.
   c. restlessness.
   d. paradoxic breathing.

3. The oxygen delivery system chosen for the patient in acute respiratory failure should
   a. always be a low-flow device, such as a nasal cannula.
   b. correct the PaO_2 to a normal level as quickly as possible.
   c. administer positive pressure ventilation to prevent CO_2 narcosis.
   d. maintain the PaO_2 at 60 mm Hg or greater at the lowest O_2 concentration possible.

4. The most common early clinical manifestations of ARDS that the nurse may observe are
   a. dyspnea and tachypnea.
   b. cyanosis and apprehension.
   c. hypotension and tachycardia.
   d. respiratory distress and frothy sputum.

5. Maintenance of fluid balance in the patient with ARDS involves
   a. hydration using colloids.
   b. administration of surfactant.
   c. mild fluid restriction and diuretics as necessary.
   d. keeping the hemoglobin at levels of 15 to 16 g/dl (150 to 160 g/L).

6. Which of the following interventions is designed to prevent or limit barotrauma in the patient with ARDS who is mechanically ventilated?
   a. increasing PEEP
   b. increasing the tidal volume
   c. use of permissive hypercapnia
   d. use of pressure support ventilation

REFERENCES

1. Murray JF et al, editors: *Textbook of respiratory medicine,* ed 3, New York, 2000, WB Saunders.
2. Grippi MA: Respiratory failure: an overview. In Fishman AP et al, editors: *Fishman's pulmonary diseases and disorders,* ed 3, New York, 1998, McGraw-Hill.
3. Hornick DB: An approach to the analysis of arterial blood gases and acid-base disorders. University of Iowa Health Care. Available at *www.int-med.uiowa.edu/education/abg.htm* (accessed Nov 13, 2001).
4. Desai PM: Pain management and pulmonary dysfunction, *Crit Care Clin* 15:151, 1999.
5. Epstein J, Breslow MJ: The stress response of critical illness, *Crit Care Clin* 15:17, 1999.
6. Light RB: Pulmonary pathophysiology of pneumococcal pneumonia, *Semin Respir Infect* 14:218, 1999.
7. Panettiere RA, Murray RK: Chronic obstructive pulmonary disease. In Foshman AP, editor: *Pulmonary diseases and disorders: companion handbook,* ed 3, New York, 1998, McGraw-Hill.
8. Mehta S, Hill NS: State of the art: noninvasive ventilation, *Am J Respir Crit Care Med* 163:540, 2001.
9. Vines DL, Shelledy DC, Peters J: Current respiratory care: oxygen therapy, oximetry, bronchial hygiene, *J Crit Illn* 15:507, 2000.
10. Moore MJ, Schmidt GA: Keys to effective noninvasive ventilation: initial steps, *J Crit Illn* 16:64, 2001.
11. Crawshaw L, Pennock BE: Noninvasive ventilatory support: who benefits. SpringNet-Nursing Community. Available at *www.springnet.com/criticalcare/noninvas.htm* (accessed Nov 13, 2001).
12. Hill NS, Meyer TJ: Lesson 3, volume 9: noninvasive positive pressure ventilation. Available at *www.chestnet.org/education/pccu/best/lesson03-09.html* (accessed Nov 13, 2001).
13. Que LG, Huang YCT: Pharmacological adjuncts during mechanical ventilation, *Semin Respir Crit Care Med* 21. Available at *http://respiratorycare.medscape.com/thieme/SRCCM/2000/v21.n03/r...pnt-rcm2103.02que.htm* (accessed Sept 9, 2001).
14. Lowson SM, Sawh S: Adjuncts to analgesia: sedation and neuromuscular blockade, *Crit Care Clin* 15:119, 1999.
15. Arbour R: Sedation and pain management in critically ill adults, *Crit Care Nurse* 20:39, 2000.
16. Arbour R: Mastering neuromuscular blockade, *DCCN* 19:4, 2000.
17. Janssens JP, Pache JC, Nicod LP: Physiological changes in respiratory function associated with aging, *Eur Respir J* 13:197, 1999.
18. Sue DS: Acute respiratory failure in the elderly patient, *Clin Geriatr* 8:37, 2000.
19. Zwischenberger JB: ARDS and mechanical ventilation, *J Respir Care Pract* 13:47, 2000.
20. Steinberg KS, Hudson LD: Acute lung injury and acute respiratory distress syndrome—the clinical syndrome, *Clin Chest Med* 21:401, 2000.
21. Soeren MH et al: Pathophysiology and implications for treatment of acute respiratory distress syndrome, *AACN Clin Issues* 11:179, 2000.
22. Davies P: Guarding your patient against ARDS, *Nursing* 32:36, 2002.
23. Urden LD, Stacy KM, Lough ME: *Thelan's critical care nursing: diagnosis and management,* ed 3, St Louis, 1998, Mosby.
24. Mayer J, Campbell D: ATS recommendations for treatment of adults with hospital-acquired pneumonia. Available at *www.medscape.com/SCP/IIM/1996/v13.n12/m1991.mayer/m1991.mayer.html* (accessed July 20, 2002).
*25. Burns SM: Ventilatory management—volume and pressure modes. In Lynn-McHale DJ, Carlson KK, editors: *AACN procedure manual for critical care,* ed 4, Philadelphia, 2001, WB Saunders.
26. Hirvela ER: Advances in the management of acute respiratory distress syndrome, *Arch Surg* 135:126, 2000.
27. Houston P: An approach to ventilation in acute respiratory distress syndrome, *Can J Surg* 43:263, 2000.
28. Bartlett RH: Extracorporeal life support in the management of severe respiratory failure, *Clin Chest Med* 21:555, 2000.
*29. Breilburg AN et al: Efficacy and safety of prone positioning for patients with acute respiratory distress syndrome, *J Adv Nurs* 32:922, 2000.
30. Ball C et al: Clinical guidelines for the use of the prone position in acute respiratory distress syndrome, *Intensive Crit Care Nurs* 17:94, 2001.
31. Marion BS: A turn for the better: "prone positioning" of patients with ARDS, *Am J Nurs* 101:26, 2001.
*32. Tomaselli NL, Goldberg MT, Wind S: Pressure-reducing devices: lateral rotation therapy. In Lynn-McHale DJ, Carlson KK, editors: *AACN procedure manual for critical care,* ed 4, Philadelphia, 2001, WB Saunders.
33. Sadikot RT, Christman JW: ARDS: what's new in management, *J Respir Dis* 20:499, 1999.
34. http://www.cdc.gov/ncidod/sars/

RESOURCES

Resources for this chapter are listed after Chapter 64 on page 1795.

---

*Nursing research–based references.

CHAPTER 67

NURSING MANAGEMENT
Emergency Care Situations

Linda Bucher

LEARNING OBJECTIVES

1. Apply the sequential steps in the primary and secondary survey to a patient in an emergency situation.
2. Describe the pathophysiology, assessment, and collaborative care of select environmental emergencies, including hyperthermia, hypothermia, submersion injury, and animal bites.
3. Discuss the pathophysiology, assessment, and collaborative care of select toxicologic emergencies.
4. Differentiate between the various types and victims of violence.
5. Describe the difference between emergency and disaster preparedness from the perspective of the emergency department.
6. Identify the agents most likely to be used in a terrorist attack.

KEY TERMS

bioterrorism, p. 1862
disaster, p. 1866
domestic violence, p. 1862
emergency, p. 1866
frostbite, p. 1854
heat cramps, p. 1852
heat exhaustion, p. 1852
heat stroke, p. 1852
hypothermia, p. 1854
jaw-thrust maneuver, p. 1847

pneumatic antishock garment, p. 1848
primary survey, p. 1847
rapid-sequence intubation, p. 1847
secondary survey, p. 1848
submersion injury, p. 1856
triage, p. 1847
violence, p. 1862

Most patients with life-threatening or potentially life-threatening problems arrive at the hospital through the emergency department (ED). Many more patients report to the ED for less urgent conditions. Visits to the ED have increased significantly because of the lack of health insurance or a primary care provider, increased violence, and inability to access a health care provider.[1] Emergency nurses care for patients of all ages and with a variety of problems. However, some EDs specialize in certain patient populations or conditions, such as pediatric ED or trauma ED.

The Emergency Nurses Association (ENA) is the largest specialty nursing organization aimed at advancing emergency nursing practice. The ENA provides standards of care for nurses working in the ED, as well as a certification process that allows nurses to become a certified emergency nurse (CEN). This certification validates the knowledge that a nurse needs to provide competent care in emergency settings.[2]

Specific emergency management of patients with various medical, surgical, and traumatic emergencies is presented throughout this book where the disorders are discussed. Tables that highlight emergency management of specific problems are presented throughout the book. Table 67-1 lists each emergency management table by title, number, and page. This chapter focuses on initial assessment and management of the trauma patient and emergency conditions not addressed elsewhere in this book, including heat- and cold-related emergencies, submersion injuries, bites, stings, and poisonings. In addition, a brief overview of issues related to violence and emergency and disaster preparedness is presented.

TABLE 67-1 Emergency Management — Emergency Management Tables

TITLE	CHAPTER	PAGE
Abdominal trauma	41	1065
Acute abdominal pain	41	1061
Acute soft tissue injury	61	1652
Anaphylactic shock	13	251
Arrhythmias	35	867
Chemical burns	24	520
Chest pain	33	818
Chest trauma	27	619
Cocaine and amphetamine toxicity	11	182
Depressant drugs, overdose of	11	186
Diabetic ketoacidosis	47	1293
Electrical burns	24	521
Eye injury	21	445
Fractured extremity	61	1665
Head injury	55	1510
Hyperthermia	67	1853
Hypothermia	67	1855
Inhalation injury	24	521
Sexual assault	52	1413
Shock	65	1809
Spinal cord injury	59	1616
Stroke	56	1534
Submersion injuries	67	1857
Surface skin wound	23	495
Thermal burns	24	522
Thoracic injuries	27	620
Tonic-clonic seizures	57	1558

Reviewed by Linda Laskowski-Jones, RN, MS, CS, CCRN, CEN, Director of Trauma, Emergency, and Aeromedical Services, Christiana Care Health System, Newark, Del.

TABLE 67-2	Triage Acuity Systems		
	EMERGENT	**URGENT**	**NONURGENT**
Colors	Red	Yellow	Green
Numbers	Priority I	Priority II	Priority III
Urgency	Life, limb, eye threatening; needs immediate attention	Needs treatment in 20 minutes to 2 hours	Can wait hours or days
Recommended reevaluation	Continuous	Every 30-60 min	Every 1-2 hr
Examples	Trauma, chest pain, cardiac arrest, severe respiratory distress, chemicals in the eyes, limb amputation, acute neurologic deficits	Fever >104° F (40° C), diastolic blood pressure >130 mm Hg, kidney stone, simple fracture, abdominal pain, asthma/no respiratory distress	Sprain, minor laceration, cold symptoms, rash, simple headache

TABLE 67-3	Primary Survey of an Emergency Patient
ASSESSMENT	**INTERVENTIONS**

Airway with Simultaneous Cervical Spine Stabilization and/or Immobilization

ASSESSMENT	INTERVENTIONS
- Clear and open airway - Assess for obstructed airway - Assess for respiratory distress - Check for loose teeth or foreign objects - Assess for bleeding, vomitus, or edema	- Suction - Jaw thrust - Nasal or oral airway, endotracheal tube, cricothyroidotomy - Cervical spine immobilization using collar, backboard, soft rolls; tape forehead

Breathing

ASSESSMENT	INTERVENTIONS

- Assess ventilation
  - Look for paradoxic movement of the chest wall during inspiration and expiration
  - Note use of accessory muscles or abdominal muscles
  - Listen for air being expired through nose and mouth
  - Feel for air being expelled
- Observe and count respiratory rate
- Note color of nail beds, mucous membranes, skin
- Auscultate lungs
- Assess for jugular venous distention and position of trachea
	- Ventilate with bag-valve-mask with 100% O_2
	- Prepare to intubate if respiratory arrest
	- Have suction available
	- Give supplemental O_2 via appropriate delivery system
	- If absent breath sounds, prepare for needle thoracostomy and chest tube insertion

Circulation

ASSESSMENT	INTERVENTIONS
- Check carotid or femoral pulse - Palpate pulse for quality and rate - Assess color, temperature, and moisture of skin - Check capillary refill - Assess for external bleeding - Auscultate blood pressure	- If absent pulse, initiate cardiopulmonary resuscitation and advanced life support measures - If shock symptoms or hypotensive, start two large-bore (14- to 16-gauge) IVs and initiate infusions of normal saline or lactated Ringer's solution - Administer blood products if ordered - Consider autotransfusion if isolated chest trauma - Consider use of a pneumatic antishock garment in the presence of pelvic fracture - Obtain blood samples for type and crossmatch - Control bleeding with direct pressure

Disability—Brief Neurologic Assessment

ASSESSMENT	INTERVENTIONS
- Assess level of consciousness by determining response to verbal and/or painful stimuli - Assess pupils for size, shape, equality, and response to light	- Periodically reassess level of consciousness - Consider hyperventilation if signs of brain herniation (e.g., motor posturing)

IVs, Intravenous lines.

CARE OF THE EMERGENCY PATIENT

Recognition of life-threatening illness or injury is one of the most important aspects of emergency care. Before a diagnosis can be made, recognition of dangerous clinical signs and symptoms with initiation of interventions to reverse or prevent a crisis is essential. This process begins with the first patient contact. The emergency nurse is usually confronted with multiple patients who have a variety of problems. Prompt identification of patients requiring immediate treatment and determination of appropriate treatment area are essential in a busy ED.[3]

A *triage system* identifies and categorizes patients so that the most critical are treated first. **Triage** is a French word meaning "to sort."[4] The process is based on the premise that patients who have a threat to life, vision, or limb should be treated before other patients. When patients call the ED with health-related questions, triage is conducted over the telephone.[5] The ED uses a system of words, color coding, or numbers for determining triage decisions (Table 67-2).

The emergency nurse must complete an initial assessment to determine the presence of actual or potential threats to life and then rapidly initiate interventions appropriate for the patient's condition.[6] A history is obtained simultaneously. A systematic approach to the initial patient assessment decreases the time required to identify potential threats and minimizes the risk of missing a life-threatening condition. Two systematic approaches, a primary survey and a secondary survey, were initially developed for use with the trauma patient, but these can be easily applied to assessment of any emergency patient.

Primary Survey

The **primary survey** (Table 67-3) focuses on airway, breathing, circulation, and disability and serves to identify life-threatening conditions so that appropriate interventions can be initiated. Life-threatening conditions related to airway, breathing, circulation, and disability (Table 67-4) may be identified at any point during the primary survey. When this occurs, interventions are started immediately and before proceeding to the next step of the survey.

A = Airway with Cervical Spine Stabilization and/or Immobilization. Nearly all immediate trauma deaths occur because of airway obstruction. Saliva, bloody secretions, vomitus, laryngeal trauma, facial trauma, fractures, and the tongue can obstruct the airway. Medical patients at risk for airway compromise include those who have seizures, near-drowning, anaphylaxis, foreign body obstruction, or cardiopulmonary arrest. If an airway is not maintained, obstruction of airflow occurs and hypoxia, acidosis, and death result.

Primary signs and symptoms in a patient with a compromised airway include dyspnea, inability to vocalize, presence of foreign body in the airway, and trauma to the face or neck. Airway maintenance should progress rapidly from the least to the most invasive method. Treatment includes opening the airway using the **jaw-thrust maneuver** (avoiding hyperextension of the neck) (Fig. 67-1), suctioning and/or removal of foreign body, insertion of a nasopharyngeal or oropharyngeal airway (will cause gag if patient is conscious), and endotracheal intubation. If unable to intubate because of airway obstruction, an emergency cricothyroidotomy or tracheotomy should be performed (see

| TABLE 67-4 | Causes of Life-Threatening Conditions Identified during the Primary Survey* |

Airway
- Inhalation injury
- Obstruction, partial or complete, from foreign bodies, debris (e.g., vomitus), or the tongue
- Penetrating wounds and/or blunt trauma to the upper airway structures

Breathing
- Anaphylaxis
- Flail chest with pulmonary contusion
- Hemothorax
- Open pneumothorax
- Tension pneumothorax

Circulation
- Direct cardiac injury (e.g., myocardial infarction, trauma)
- Pericardial tamponade
- Shock (e.g., massive burns)
- Uncontrolled external hemorrhage

Disability
- Head injury
- Stroke

*List is not all-inclusive.

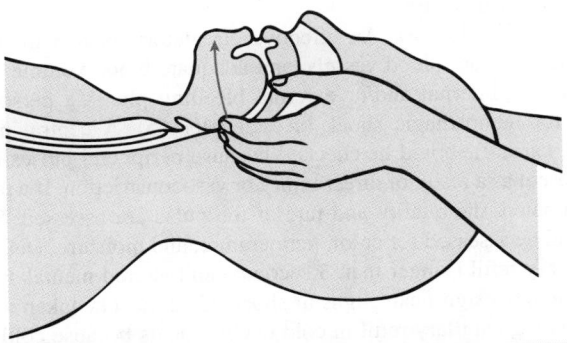

FIG. 67-1 Jaw-thrust maneuver is the only widely recommended procedure for use on an unconscious patient with possible neck or spinal injuries. The patient should be lying supine with the rescuer kneeling at the top of the head. The rescuer should carefully reach forward and gently place one hand on each side of the patient's chin at the lateral angles of the lower jaw. The patient's head should be stabilized with the rescuer's forearms, then the jaw pushed forward while pressure is applied with the index fingers.

Chapter 26). Patients should be ventilated with 100% oxygen using a bag-valve-mask (BVM) device before intubation or cricothyroidotomy.[7]

Rapid-sequence intubation is the preferred procedure for securing an unprotected airway in the ED. It involves the use of sedation (e.g., etomidate [Amidate]) and paralysis (e.g., succinylcholine [Anectine]) to facilitate intubation while minimizing the risk of aspiration and airway trauma.[8,9]

Any patient with significant upper torso injuries or face, head, or neck trauma should always be suspected of cervical spine trauma. The cervical spine must be stabilized (head maintained in a neutral position) and/or immobilized during assessment of the airway. At the scene of the injury, the cervical spine is immobilized with a rigid cervical collar or a cervical immobilization device (CID) (also known as "head blocks"), and towel rolls are taped to a backboard on either side of the head. Finally, the patient's forehead is taped to the backboard. Sandbags should not be used because the weight of the bags could move the head if the patient must be logrolled.

B = Breathing. Adequate airflow through the upper airway does not ensure adequate ventilation. Breathing alterations are caused by many conditions, including fractured ribs, pneumothorax, penetrating injury, allergic reactions, pulmonary emboli, and asthma attacks. Patients with these conditions may experience a variety of signs and symptoms, including dyspnea (e.g., due to pulmonary emboli), paradoxic or asymmetric chest wall movement (e.g., flail chest), decreased or absent breath sounds on the affected side (e.g., pneumothorax), visible wound to chest wall (e.g., penetrating injury), cyanosis (e.g., due to asthma), tachycardia, and hypotension.

Every critically injured or ill patient has an increased metabolic and oxygen demand and should have supplemental oxygen. High-flow oxygen (100%) via a non-rebreather mask should be administered and the patient's response monitored. Life-threatening conditions, such as tension pneumothorax and flail chest, can severely compromise ventilation. Interventions in these situations include BVM ventilation with 100% oxygen, intubation, and treatment of the underlying cause.

C = Circulation. An effective circulatory system includes the heart, intact blood vessels, and adequate blood volume. Uncontrolled internal and/or external bleeding places a person at risk for hemorrhagic shock (see Chapter 65). A central pulse (e.g., carotid) should be checked because peripheral pulses may be absent as a result of direct injury or vasoconstriction. If a pulse is palpated, the quality and rate of the pulse are assessed. Skin should be assessed for color, temperature, and moisture. Delayed capillary refill (longer than 3 seconds) and altered mental status are the most significant signs of shock. Care must be taken when evaluating capillary refill in cold environments because cold delays refill.

Intravenous (IV) lines are inserted into veins in the upper extremities unless contraindicated, such as in a massive fracture or an injury that affects limb circulation. Two large-bore (14- to 16-gauge) IV catheters should be inserted and aggressive fluid resuscitation initiated using lactated Ringer's solution or normal saline. Direct pressure with a sterile dressing should be applied to obvious bleeding sites. Blood samples are obtained for typing to determine ABO and Rh group. Type-specific packed red blood cells should be administered if needed. In an emergency (life-threatening) situation, uncrossmatched blood may be given if immediate transfusion is warranted.

The use of the **pneumatic antishock garment** (PASG) is a temporary strategy that can be considered for pelvic fracture bleeding with hypotension. The PASG is a three-chambered suit that is applied to the patient's legs and abdomen and is inflated with a foot pump. Physiologically, the PASG increases peripheral resistance in the patient's lower extremities, thus elevating blood pressure, and works to control pelvic fracture bleeding.[10]

D = Disability. A brief neurologic examination completes the primary survey. The degree of disability is measured by the patient's level of consciousness. Determining the patient's response to verbal and/or painful stimuli is one approach to assessing level of consciousness. A simple mnemonic to remember is AVPU: A = alert, V = responsive to voice, P = responsive to pain, and U = unresponsive. In addition, the Glasgow Coma Scale (GCS) is used to further assess the arousal aspect of the patient's consciousness (see Chapter 55). Finally, pupils should be also assessed for size, shape, equality, and response to light.

Secondary Survey

After each step of the primary survey is addressed and any lifesaving interventions are initiated, the secondary survey begins. The **secondary survey** is a brief, systematic process that is aimed at identifying *all* injuries (Table 67-5).

E = Exposure/Environmental Control. All trauma patients should have their clothes removed so that a thorough physical assessment can be performed. Once the patient is exposed, it is important to limit heat loss and prevent hypothermia by using warming blankets, overhead warmers, and warmed IV fluids.

F = Full Set of Vital Signs/Five Interventions/Facilitate Family Presence. A complete set of vital signs, including blood pressure, heart rate, respiratory rate, and temperature, should be obtained after the patient is exposed. Blood pressure should be obtained in both arms if the patient has sustained or is suspected of having sustained chest trauma.

At this point, it must be determined whether to proceed with the secondary survey or to perform additional interventions. The availability of other team members often influences this decision. For patients who have sustained significant trauma and/or have required lifesaving interventions during the primary survey, the following five interventions should be performed at this time.

First, the patient should be monitored by electrocardiogram (ECG) for heart rate and rhythm. Second, pulse oximetry should be initiated and oxygen saturation (SpO_2) monitored. Third, an indwelling catheter should be inserted to monitor urine output and to check for hematuria. An indwelling catheter should not be inserted if a urethral tear is suspected. Patients with pelvic injuries or blood at the meatus, and men with a high-riding prostate gland on digital rectal examination, are at risk for a urethral tear or transection. A urethrogram should be obtained before a catheter is inserted. Fourth, an orogastric or a nasogastric tube should be inserted to provide gastric decompression and emptying to reduce the risk of aspiration and to test the contents for blood. A nasogastric tube should not be placed in the nares in a patient suspected of having facial fractures or a basilar skull fracture because the tube could enter the brain through the cribriform plate; rather, it should be placed orally. Fifth, laboratory studies for typing and crossmatching, hematocrit, hemoglobin, blood urea nitrogen, creatinine, blood alcohol, toxicology screening, arterial blood gases, electrolytes, coagulation profile, liver enzymes, cardiac enzymes, and pregnancy should be facilitated.

Facilitating *family presence* (FP) completes this step of the secondary survey. Research supports the positive benefits of FP during invasive procedures (IPs) and cardiopulmonary resuscitation (CPR) to patients, families, and staff.[11,12] Patients reported that having family members present comforted them, served as an advocate for them, and helped to remind the health care team of their "personhood."[11] Family members who wished to be pre-

TABLE 67-5	Secondary Survey of an Emergency Patient
PARAMETER	**ASSESSMENT**
Exposure and Environmental Control	Remove clothing for adequate examination. Keep patient warm with blankets, warmed IV fluids, overhead lights.
Full Set of Vital Signs	Obtain vital signs: temperature, heart rate, respiratory rate, blood pressure bilaterally.
Five Interventions	Heart rhythm, O_2 saturation, insertion of a urinary catheter (if not contraindicated), insertion of gastric tube, blood for laboratory studies.
Facilitate Family Presence	Determine family's desire to be present during invasive procedures or cardiopulmonary resuscitation.
Give Comfort Measures	Level of pain, anxiety.
History and Head-to-Toe Assessment History	Details of the incident/illness, mechanism and pattern of injury, length of time since incident occurred, injuries suspected, treatment provided and patient's response, level of consciousness. Allergies. Medication history. Past health history (e.g., preexisting medical conditions, last menstrual period). Last meal. Events/environment preceding illness or injury. Note general appearance, including skin color.
Head, neck, face	Examine face and scalp for lacerations, bone or soft tissue deformity, tenderness, bleeding, and foreign bodies. Examine eyes, ears, nose, and mouth for bleeding, foreign bodies, drainage, pain, deformity, ecchymosis, lacerations. Examine head for depressions of cranial or facial bones, contusions, hematomas, areas of softness, bony crepitus. Examine neck for stiffness, pain in cervical vertebrae, tracheal deviation, distended neck veins, bleeding, edema, difficulty swallowing, bruising, subcutaneous emphysema, bony crepitus.
Chest	Observe rate, depth, and effort of breathing, including chest wall movement. Palpate for bony crepitus, subcutaneous emphysema. Use of accessory muscles. Auscultate breath sounds. Obtain ECG. External signs of injury: petechiae, bleeding, cyanosis, bruises, abrasions, lacerations, old scars.
Abdomen and flanks	Symmetry of external abdominal wall and bony structures. External signs of injury: bruising, abrasions, lacerations, punctures. Assess for masses, guarding, femoral pulses. Type and location of pain, rigidity, or distention of abdomen. Assess bowel sounds.
Pelvis and perineum Extremities	Assess genitalia for blood at the meatus, priapism, ecchymosis, rectal bleeding, anal sphincter tone. Signs of external injury: deformity, ecchymosis, abrasions, lacerations, swelling. Pain. Movement and strength in arms and legs. Sensation in each limb. Color of skin. Presence and quality of peripheral pulses.
Inspect posterior surfaces	Logroll and inspect and palpate back for deformity, bleeding, lacerations, bruising.

ECG, Electrocardiogram; *IV,* intravenous.

sent during IPs and CPR viewed themselves as active participants in the care process. They also believed that they provided comfort to the patient and that it was their right to be with the patient.[12] Staff nurses reported that family members who participated in FP functioned as "patient helpers" (e.g., providing support) and "staff helpers" (e.g., acting as a translator) and reinforced that FP helped to convey the sense of the patient's personhood.[12] Should a family member request FP, it is essential that

a member of the team explain care delivered and be available to answer questions.

G = Give Comfort Measures. Provision of comfort measures is of paramount importance when caring for patients in the ED. It has been reported that as many as 78% of all patients who come to the ED are in pain.[13] Pain management strategies should include a combination of pharmacologic (e.g., IV narcotics) and nonpharmacologic (e.g., imagery) measures.[14,15] Emergency nurses play a pivotal role in pain management because of their frequent contact with patients. However, emergency nurses have reported knowledge deficits regarding pain management principles (e.g., pharmacology; differentiating physical dependence, addiction, and tolerance).[13,14] General comfort measures such as verbal reassurance, listening, reducing stimuli (e.g., dimming lights), and developing a trusting relationship with the patient and family should be provided to all patients in the ED.

H = History and Head-to-Toe Assessment. The history of the incident, injury, or illness provides clues to the cause of the crisis and suggests specific assessment and intervention needs. The patient may be unable to give a history. However, family, friends, witnesses, and prehospital personnel can frequently provide important information. Prehospital information should focus on the mechanism and pattern of injury, injuries suspected, vital signs, and treatment initiated and patient responses.

Details of the incident are extremely important because the mechanism of injury and injury patterns can predict specific injuries. For example, a front-seat passenger with a seat belt may have a head injury from hitting the steering wheel; knee, femur, or hip fractures or dislocation from striking the dashboard; and an abdominal injury from the seat belt. If other victims were dead at the scene, the patient has a high chance of significant injury.

Patients who jump from buildings or bridges may have bilateral calcaneal (heel) fractures, bilateral wrist fractures, and lumbar spine compression fractures, and they may be at risk for aortic tears. Older patients who have climbed ladders and fallen may have had a stroke or myocardial infarction that led to the fall.

Prehospital personnel will often provide a detailed description of the patient's general condition, level of consciousness, and apparent injuries. An experienced ED team can complete a history within 5 minutes of the patient's arrival. If the patient is emergently ill, a thorough history is obtained from family or friends after the patient is taken to the treatment area. The history should include the following questions:

1. What is the chief complaint? What caused the patient to seek attention?
2. What are the patient's subjective complaints?
3. What is the patient's description of pain (e.g., location, duration, quality, character)?
4. What are witnesses' (if any) descriptions of the patient's behavior since the onset?
5. What is the patient's health care history? The mnemonic *AMPLE* assists the nurse in remembering to ask about the following:

A   Allergies
M   Medication history
P   Past health history (e.g., preexisting medical conditions, previous hospitalizations/surgeries, smoking history, recent use of drugs/alcohol, tetanus immunization, last menstrual period)
L   Last meal
E   Events/environment preceding illness or injury

Head, neck, and face. The patient should be assessed for general appearance, skin color, and temperature. The eyes should be evaluated for extraocular movements. A disconjugate gaze is an indication of neurologic damage. "Raccoon eyes," or periorbital ecchymosis, is usually caused by a basilar skull fracture. The tympanic membranes and external canal are checked for blood and cerebrospinal fluid (see Chapter 55). Clear drainage from the ear or nose should not be stopped.

The airway is assessed for foreign bodies, bleeding, edema, and loose or missing teeth. Assess for difficulty swallowing, movement of the palate, and ability to open the mouth. The neck should be examined for bruising, edema, bleeding, or distended neck veins. The trachea is palpated and visualized to determine whether it is in the midline. A deviated trachea may signal a life-threatening tension pneumothorax. Subcutaneous emphysema may indicate laryngotracheal disruption. A stiff or painful cervical spine area may signify a fracture of a cervical vertebra. The cervical spine must be protected using a rigid collar and supine positioning. Patients must be logrolled when movement is necessary.

Chest. The chest is examined for paradoxic chest movements and large sucking chest wounds. The sternum, clavicles, and ribs are palpated for deformity and point tenderness. The chest is assessed for pain on palpation, respiratory distress, decreased breath sounds, distant heart sounds, and distended neck veins. In addition to tension pneumothorax and open pneumothorax, the patient should be evaluated for rib fractures, pulmonary contusion, blunt cardiac injury, and simple pneumothorax. A 12-lead ECG should be obtained, particularly on an older patient or a patient with suspected heart disease. The ECG should be done to detect arrhythmias and evidence of ischemia or infarction.

Abdomen and flanks. The abdomen and flanks are more difficult to assess. Frequent evaluation for subtle changes in the abdominal examination is essential. Motor vehicle collisions and assaults can cause blunt trauma. Penetrating trauma tends to injure specific organs. Decreased bowel sounds may indicate a temporary paralytic ileus. Bowel sounds in the chest may indicate a diaphragmatic rupture. The abdomen is percussed for distention (e.g., tympany [excessive air], dullness [excessive fluid]) and palpated for peritoneal irritation.

If intraabdominal hemorrhage is suspected, a diagnostic peritoneal lavage (DPL) may be performed to determine the presence of blood in the peritoneal space (hemoperitoneum). Before the procedure, a gastric tube and a bladder catheter must be inserted to decompress these organs and reduce the possibility of perforation. An alternative to DPL that is gaining support is an ultrasonography procedure called a *focused abdominal sonography for trauma* (FAST). This procedure is noninvasive and can be performed quickly.[10]

Pelvis and perineum. The pelvis is gently palpated. If pain is elicited, it may indicate a pelvic fracture. The genitalia are inspected for bleeding and obvious injuries. A rectal examination is performed to check for blood, a high-riding prostate gland, and loss of sphincter tone. Assess for bladder distention, hematuria, dysuria, or the inability to void.

Extremities. The upper and lower extremities are assessed. Injured extremities are splinted above and below the injury to decrease further soft tissue injury and pain. Grossly deformed, pulseless extremities should be realigned and splinted. Pulses are checked before and after movement or splinting of an extremity. A pulseless extremity represents a time-critical vascular or orthopedic emergency.

The extremities are palpated for point tenderness, crepitus, and abnormal movements. Injured extremities should be elevated and ice packs applied. Prophylactic antibiotics are administered for open fractures. Patients with fractures should receive IV analgesia.[14]

I = Inspect the Posterior Surfaces. The trauma patient should always be turned (using spinal precautions) to inspect the patient's posterior surfaces. The back is inspected for ecchymosis, abrasions, puncture wounds, cuts, and obvious deformities. The entire spine is palpated for misalignment, deformity, and pain.

Intervention and Evaluation

Once the secondary survey is complete, all findings are recorded. All patients should be evaluated to determine their need for tetanus prophylaxis. Information about the patient's past vaccination history and the condition of any wounds is needed in order to make an appropriate decision (Table 67-6).

Regardless of the patient's chief complaint, ongoing patient monitoring and evaluation of interventions are critical in an emergency situation. The nurse is responsible for providing appropriate interventions and assessing the patient's response. The evaluation of airway patency and the effectiveness of breathing will always assume highest priority. The nurse will monitor O_2 saturation and arterial blood gases (ABGs) to help determine the patient's progress in these areas. Level of consciousness, vital signs, quality of peripheral pulses, urine output, and skin temperature, color, and moisture provide key information about circulation and perfusion and are also monitored.

Depending on the patient's injuries and/or illness, the patient may be (1) transported for diagnostic tests such as a computed tomography (CT) scan, x-ray, or magnetic resonance imaging (MRI); (2) admitted to a general or intensive care unit; or (3) transferred to another facility. The emergency nurse is responsible for monitoring the patient during transport and notifying the team should the patient's condition change from baseline. Nurses accompanying critically ill patients on intrafacility or interfacility transports must be competent in advanced life support measures.

Death in the Emergency Department

Unfortunately, there are a number of emergency patients who do not benefit from the skill, expertise, and technology available in the ED. It is important for the emergency nurse to be able to deal with feelings about sudden death so that the nurse can help families and significant others begin the grieving process.[16]

The emergency nurse should recognize the importance of certain hospital rituals in preparing the bereaved to grieve, such as collecting the belongings, arranging for an autopsy, viewing the body, and making mortuary arrangements. The death must seem real so that the significant others can begin to grieve and accept the death. The emergency nurse plays a significant role in providing comfort to the surviving loved ones after a death in the ED.

Many patients who die in the ED could potentially be a candidate for *non–heart beating donation* (NHBD). Certain tissues and organs such as corneas, heart valves, bone, and kidneys can be harvested from patients after death. Approaching families about donation after an unexpected death is distressing to both the staff and the family. For many families, however, the act of donation may be the first positive step in the grieving process.[17] *Organ procurement agencies* (OPAs) are available to assist in the process of screening potential donors, counseling donor families, obtaining informed consent, and harvesting organs from patients who have died in the ED.

■ Gerontologic Considerations: Emergency Care

The proportion of the population over age 65 is growing, with most leading active lives. Regardless of a patient's age, aggressive interventions are warranted for all injuries or illnesses unless the patient is known to have a preexisting terminal illness, an extremely low probability of survival, or an advance directive indicating a different course of action.[18]

The elderly population is at high risk for injury due to many of the anatomic and physiologic changes that occur with aging (e.g., reduced visual acuity, limited neck rotation, slower gait, reduced reaction time). Of the injury-related admissions for people age 65 or older, approximately 52% are for fractures, with many of these resulting from falls. The three most common causes of falls in the elderly are generalized weakness, environmental hazards (e.g., loose mats, furniture), and orthostatic hypotension (e.g., side effect of medications).[18] When assessing a patient who has experienced a fall, it is important to determine whether the physical findings may have actually caused the fall or may be due to the fall itself. For example, a patient may exhibit acute confusion. The confusion may be due to an acute myocardial infarction that caused the patient to lose consciousness and fall, or the patient may have suffered a head injury as a result of a fall from tripping.

Knowledge of the concepts of aging will improve the care delivered to the elderly in the ED (see Chapter 5). Unfortunately, many older adults dismiss symptoms as simply "normal for their age." Any complaint by an older adult must be fully investigated. ■

Environmental Emergencies

Increased interest in outdoor activities such as running, hiking, cycling, skiing, sailing, and swimming has increased the number of environmental emergencies seen in the ED. Illness or injury may be caused by the activity, exposure to weather, or at-

---

TABLE 67-6   Prophylaxis against Tetanus in Wound Management

| | TYPE OF WOUND | | | |
| | TETANUS-PRONE WOUND | | NON–TETANUS-PRONE WOUND | |
HISTORY OF TETANUS TOXOID (DOSES)	Td	TIG*	Td	TIG
Unknown to fewer than three	Yes	Yes	Yes	No
Three or more†	No‡	No	No§	No

*When TIG and Td are administered concurrently, separate sites and syringes must be used.
†If only three doses of fluid toxoid have been received, a fourth dose of toxoid, preferably absorbed toxoid, should be given.
‡Yes, if more than 5 years since last dose. More frequent boosters are not needed and can accentuate side effects.
§Yes, if more than 10 years since last dose.
Td, Tetanus-diphtheria toxoid absorbed (for adult use); *TIG*, tetanus immune globulin (human).

tack from various animals or humans. Specific environmental emergencies discussed in this section include heat-related emergencies, cold-related emergencies, submersion injuries, bites, and stings.

HEAT-RELATED EMERGENCIES

Brief exposure to intense heat or prolonged exposure to less intense heat leads to heat stress when thermoregulatory mechanisms such as sweating, vasodilation, and increased respirations cannot compensate for exposure to increased ambient temperatures.[19] Ambient temperature is a product of environmental temperature and humidity. Strenuous activities in hot or humid environments, clothing that interferes with perspiration, high fevers, and preexisting illnesses predispose individuals to heat stress (Table 67-7). Effects can be mild (heat rash and heat edema) or severe (heat exhaustion and heat stroke). The management of heat-related emergencies is summarized in Table 67-8.

Heat rash (miliaria or prickly heat) is a fine, red, papular rash that occurs on the torso, neck, and skinfolds. The rash occurs when sweat ducts are obstructed and become inflamed so that sweat excretion does not occur. The rash usually occurs in warm weather, but has also been reported in cold weather as a result of clothing.

Heat syncope is associated with prolonged standing and heat exposure. Manifestations include dizziness, orthostatic hypotension, and syncope. Inadequate vasomotor tone associated with aging places the elderly at greater risk for heat syncope.

Heat edema is characterized by swelling of the hands, feet, and ankles, usually in nonacclimatized individuals as a result of prolonged standing or sitting. Swelling usually resolves in days with rest, elevation, and support hose. Diuretics are not recommended because this condition is self-limiting and requires no additional treatment.

Heat Cramps

Heat cramps are severe cramps in large muscle groups fatigued by heavy work. Cramps are brief, intense, and tend to occur during rest after exercise or heavy labor. Nausea, tachycardia, pallor, weakness, and profuse diaphoresis are often present. The condition is seen most often in healthy, acclimated athletes with inadequate fluid intake. Cramps resolve rapidly with rest and oral or parenteral replacement of sodium and water. Elevation, gentle massage, and analgesia minimize pain associated with heat cramps. The patient should avoid strenuous activity for at least 12 hours after the development of heat cramps. Education should emphasize salt replacement during strenuous exercise in hot, humid environments. Commercially prepared electrolyte solutions (e.g., sports drinks) are recommended.

Heat Exhaustion

Prolonged exposure to heat over hours or days leads to **heat exhaustion,** a clinical syndrome characterized by fatigue, lightheadedness, nausea, vomiting, diarrhea, and feelings of impending doom (see Table 67-8). Tachypnea, hypotension, tachycardia, elevated body temperature, dilated pupils, mild confusion, ashen color, and profuse diaphoresis are also present. Hypotension and mild to severe temperature elevation (99.6° to 104° F [37.5° to 40° C]) are due to dehydration.[19] Heat exhaustion usually occurs in individuals engaged in strenuous activity in hot, humid weather, but it also occurs in sedentary individuals.

Treatment begins with placement of the patient in a cool area and removal of constrictive clothing. The patient is monitored for airway, breathing, and circulation (ABCs), including cardiac arrhythmias (due to electrolyte imbalances). Oral fluid and electrolyte replacement is initiated unless the patient is nauseated. Salt tablets are not recommended because of potential gastric irritation and hypernatremia. A 0.9% normal saline solution is initiated intravenously when oral solutions are not tolerated. An initial fluid bolus may be used to correct hypotension. However, fluid replacement should be correlated to clinical and laboratory parameters. A moist sheet placed over the patient decreases core temperature through evaporative heat loss. Hospital admission is considered for the elderly, the chronically ill, or those who do not improve within 3 to 4 hours.

Heat Stroke

Heat stroke, the most serious form of heat stress, results from failure of the central thermoregulatory mechanisms and is considered a medical emergency. Table 67-7 lists risk factors for

---

TABLE 67-7	Risk Factors for Heat-Related Emergencies

Age
Elderly
Infants

Environmental Conditions
High environmental temperature
High relative humidity
Low wind

Preexisting Illness
Cardiovascular disease
Cystic fibrosis
Diabetes
Obesity
Previous stroke or other central nervous system lesion
Skin disorders (e.g., large burn scars)

Prescription Drugs
Anticholinergics
Antihistamines
Antiparkinsonian drugs
Antispasmodics
β-Adrenergic blockers
Butyrophenones
Diuretics
Phenothiazines
Tricyclic antidepressants

Street Drugs
Amphetamines
Jimsonweed
Lysergic acid diethylamide (LSD)
Phencyclidine (PCP)

Alcohol

From Emergency Nurses Association, Newberry L, editor: *Sheehy's emergency nursing: principles and practice,* ed 5, St Louis, 2003, Mosby.

TABLE 67-8 Emergency Management — Hyperthermia

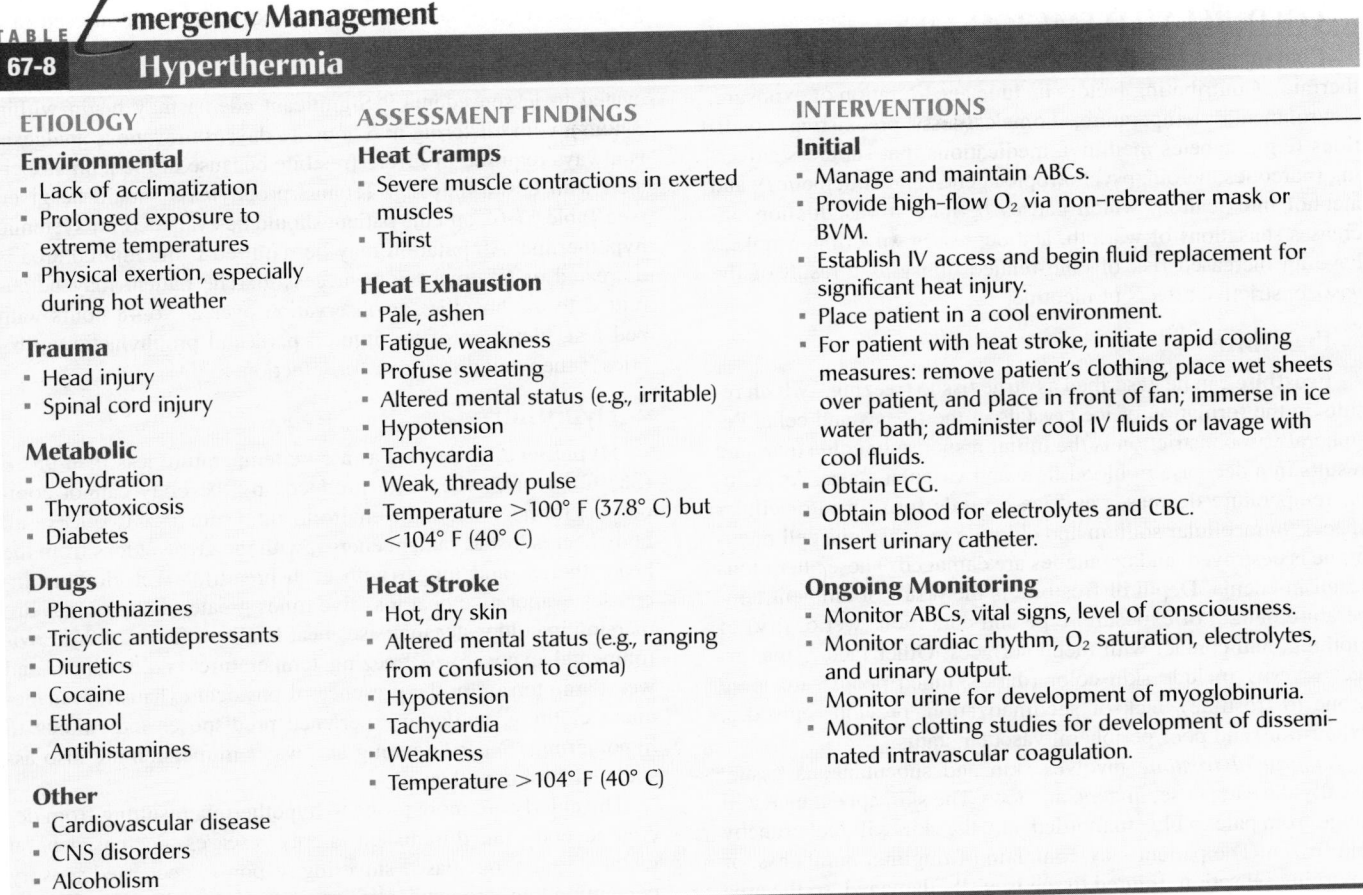

ETIOLOGY	ASSESSMENT FINDINGS	INTERVENTIONS
Environmental • Lack of acclimatization • Prolonged exposure to extreme temperatures • Physical exertion, especially during hot weather **Trauma** • Head injury • Spinal cord injury **Metabolic** • Dehydration • Thyrotoxicosis • Diabetes **Drugs** • Phenothiazines • Tricyclic antidepressants • Diuretics • Cocaine • Ethanol • Antihistamines **Other** • Cardiovascular disease • CNS disorders • Alcoholism	**Heat Cramps** • Severe muscle contractions in exerted muscles • Thirst **Heat Exhaustion** • Pale, ashen • Fatigue, weakness • Profuse sweating • Altered mental status (e.g., irritable) • Hypotension • Tachycardia • Weak, thready pulse • Temperature >100° F (37.8° C) but <104° F (40° C) **Heat Stroke** • Hot, dry skin • Altered mental status (e.g., ranging from confusion to coma) • Hypotension • Tachycardia • Weakness • Temperature >104° F (40° C)	**Initial** • Manage and maintain ABCs. • Provide high-flow O_2 via non-rebreather mask or BVM. • Establish IV access and begin fluid replacement for significant heat injury. • Place patient in a cool environment. • For patient with heat stroke, initiate rapid cooling measures: remove patient's clothing, place wet sheets over patient, and place in front of fan; immerse in ice water bath; administer cool IV fluids or lavage with cool fluids. • Obtain ECG. • Obtain blood for electrolytes and CBC. • Insert urinary catheter. **Ongoing Monitoring** • Monitor ABCs, vital signs, level of consciousness. • Monitor cardiac rhythm, O_2 saturation, electrolytes, and urinary output. • Monitor urine for development of myoglobinuria. • Monitor clotting studies for development of disseminated intravascular coagulation.

ABCs, Airway, breathing, circulation; *BVM*, bag-valve-mask; *CBC*, complete blood count; *CNS*, central nervous system; *ECG*, electrocardiogram; *IV*, intravenous.

heat-related emergencies, especially heat stroke. Increased sweating, vasodilation, and increased respiratory rate (the body's attempt to lower temperature) deplete fluids and electrolytes. Eventually, sweat glands stop functioning, so core temperature increases rapidly. The patient has core temperature greater than 104° F (40° C), altered mentation, absence of perspiration, and circulatory collapse. The skin is hot, dry, and ashen. Because the brain is extremely sensitive to thermal injuries, a range of neurologic symptoms occur, such as hallucinations, loss of muscle coordination, and combativeness. Cerebral edema and hemorrhage may occur as a result of direct thermal injury to the brain and decreased cerebral blood flow.

The development of heat stroke is directly related to the amount of time that the patient's body temperature remains elevated.[19] Prognosis is related to age, baseline health status, and length of exposure. Older adults and individuals with diabetes mellitus, chronic renal disease, cardiovascular disease, pulmonary disease, or other physiologic compromise are particularly vulnerable.

Collaborative Care. Treatment of heat stroke focuses on stabilizing the patient's ABCs and rapidly reducing the core temperature. Administration of 100% O_2 compensates for the patient's hypermetabolic state. Ventilation with a BVM or intubation and mechanical ventilation may be required. Fluid and electrolyte imbalances are corrected, and continuous cardiac monitoring for arrhythmias is initiated.

Various cooling methods are available, such as removal of clothing, covering with wet sheets, and placing the patient in front of a large fan (evaporative cooling); providing an ice water bath (conductive cooling); and administering cool fluids or lavaging with cool fluids.[20] Whatever method is selected, the nurse is responsible for closely monitoring the patient's temperature and controlling shivering. Shivering increases core temperature (due to the associated heat generated by muscle activity) and complicates cooling efforts. Chlorpromazine (Thorazine) IV is the drug of choice to suppress shivering. Aggressive temperature reduction should continue until core temperature reaches 102° F (38.9° C).[20] Antipyretics are not recommended.

The patient is also monitored for signs of *rhabdomyolysis* (a fatal disease characterized by breakdown of skeletal muscle). The muscle breakdown leads to myoglobinuria, which places the kidneys at risk for acute failure. Therefore urine should be carefully monitored for color, amount, pH, and myoglobin. Finally, clotting studies are performed to monitor the patient for signs of disseminated intravascular coagulation (DIC) (see Chapter 30).

Patient and family teaching focuses on how to avoid future problems. Essential information regarding proper hydration during hot weather and physical exercise is imperative. Patients should also be instructed on the early signs of and interventions for heat-related stress.

COLD-RELATED EMERGENCIES

Cold injuries may be localized (frostbite) or systemic (hypothermia). Contributing factors include age, duration of exposure, environmental temperature, homelessness, preexisting conditions (e.g., diabetes mellitus), medications that suppress shivering (narcotics, heroin, psychotropic agents, and antiemetics), and alcohol intoxication, which causes peripheral vasodilation, increases sensations of warmth, and depresses shivering. Smokers have an increased risk of cold-related injury as a result of the vasoconstrictive effects of nicotine.

Frostbite

Frostbite can be described as "true tissue freezing," which results in the formation of ice crystals in the tissues and cells. Peripheral vasoconstriction is the initial response to cold stress and results in a decrease in blood flow and vascular stasis. As cellular temperature decreases and ice crystals form in intracellular spaces, intracellular sodium and chloride increase, the cell membrane is destroyed, and organelles are damaged. These alterations result in edema. Depth of frostbite is the result of ambient temperature, length of exposure, type and condition (wet or dry) of clothing, and contact with metal surfaces. Other factors that affect severity include skin color (dark-skinned people are more prone to frostbite), lack of acclimatization, previous episodes, exhaustion, and poor peripheral vascular status.

Superficial frostbite involves skin and subcutaneous tissue, usually the ears, nose, fingers, and toes. The skin appearance will range from pale to blue to mottled, and the skin will feel crunchy and frozen. The patient may complain of tingling, numbness, or a burning sensation. Injured tissue is easily damaged, so the area should be handled carefully and never squeezed, massaged, or scrubbed. Clothing and jewelry should be removed because they may constrict the extremity and decrease circulation. The affected area should be immersed in a water bath (102° to 108° F) [38.9° to 42.2° C]).[21] Warm soaks may be used for the face. The patient often experiences a warm, stinging sensation as tissue thaws. Blisters form within a few hours (Fig. 67-2). The blisters should be debrided and a sterile dressing applied. Heavy blankets and clothing should be avoided because friction and weight can lead to sloughing of damaged tissue. Rewarming is extremely painful. Residual pain may last weeks or even years. Analgesia should be administered and tetanus prophylaxis should be given as appropriate (see Table 67-6). The patient should be evaluated for systemic hypothermia.

Deep frostbite involves muscle, bone, and tendon. The skin is white, hard, and insensitive to touch. The area has the appearance of deep thermal injury with mottling gradually progressing to gangrene (Fig. 67-3). The affected extremity is submersed in a circulating water bath (102° to 108° F [38.9° to 42.2° C]) until distal flush occurs. After rewarming, the extremity should be elevated to lessen edema.[21] Significant edema may begin within 3 hours, with blistering in 6 hours to days. Intravenous analgesia is always required in severe frostbite because of the pain associated with tissue thawing. Tetanus prophylaxis should be given (see Table 67-6), and the patient should be evaluated for systemic hypothermia. Amputation may be required if the injured area is untreated or treatment is unsuccessful. The patient may be admitted to the hospital for observation over 24 to 48 hours with bed rest, elevation of the injured part, and prophylactic antibiotics if the wound is at risk for infection.

Hypothermia

Hypothermia, defined as a core temperature less than 95° F (35° C), occurs when heat produced by the body cannot compensate for heat lost to the environment. From 55% to 60% of all body heat is lost as radiant energy, with the greatest loss from the head, thorax, and lungs (with each breath).[19] Wet clothing increases evaporative heat loss five times greater than normal; immersion in cold water increases heat loss by a factor of 25. Environmental exposure to freezing temperatures, cold winds, and wet, damp terrain in the presence of physical exhaustion, inadequate clothing, and/or inexperience predisposes individuals to hypothermia.[6] Near-drowning and water immersion are also associated with hypothermia.

The elderly are more prone to hypothermia resulting from decreased body fat, diminished energy reserves, decreased basal metabolic rate, decreased shivering response, decreased sensory perception, chronic medical conditions, and medications that alter body defenses. In addition, certain drugs, alcohol, and diabetes are considered risk factors for hypothermia.

Hypothermia mimics cerebral or metabolic disturbances causing ataxia, confusion, and withdrawal, so the patient may be misdiagnosed. Peripheral vasoconstriction is the body's first attempt to conserve heat. As cold temperatures persist, shivering and movement are the body's only mechanisms for producing heat. Death usually occurs when core temperature falls below 78° F (25.6° C).

Core temperature below 87° F (30.6° C) is severe and potentially life threatening. Assessment findings in hypothermia are variable and dependent on core temperature (Table 67-9). Patients with *mild hypothermia* (90° to 95° F [32.2° to 35° C]) have

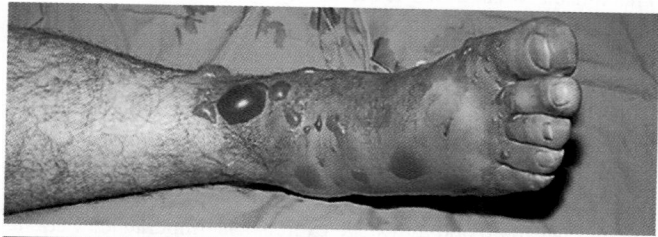

FIG. 67-2 Edema and blister formation 24 hours after frostbite injury occurring in an area covered by a tightly fitted boot.

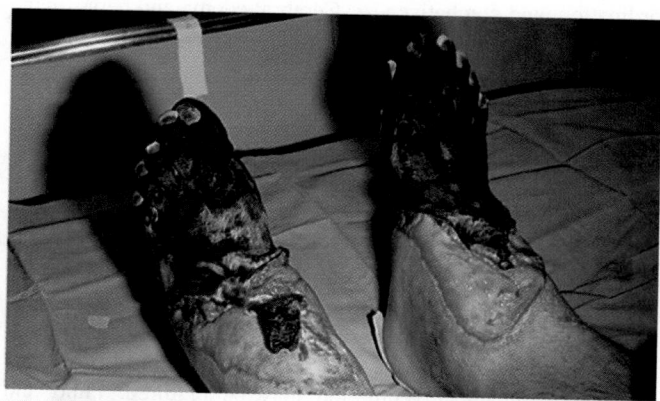

FIG. 67-3 Gangrenous necrosis 6 weeks after the frostbite injury shown in Fig. 67-2.

| TABLE 67-9 Emergency Management Hypothermia |

Emergency Management
Hypothermia

ETIOLOGY	ASSESSMENT FINDINGS	INTERVENTIONS
Environmental • Prolonged exposure to cold • Prolonged submersion • Inadequate clothing for environmental temperature **Metabolic** • Hypoglycemia • Hypothyroidism **Iatrogenic** • Cold IV fluids • Blood administration • Inadequate warming or rewarming in the ED or surgery • Administration of neuromuscular blocking agents **Other** • Phenothiazines • Barbiturates • Alcohol • Trauma • Shock	• Core body temperature: Mild hypothermia: 90°-95° F (32.2°-35° C) Moderate hypothermia: 87°-90° F (30.6°-32.2° C) Profound hypothermia: <87° F (30.6° C) • Shivering (diminished or absent at core body temperature ≤ 92° F) (33.3° C) • Hypoventilation • Hypotension • Altered mental status (ranging from confusion to coma) • Areflexia (absence of reflexes) • Pale, cyanotic skin • Blue, white, or frozen extremities • Arrhythmias: bradycardia, atrial fibrillation, ventricular fibrillation, asystole • Fixed, dilated pupils	**Initial** • Remove patient from cold environment. • Manage and maintain ABCs. • Provide high-flow O_2 via non-rebreather mask or BVM. • Anticipate intubation for diminished or absent gag reflex. • Rewarm patient: *Passive:* remove wet clothing, apply dry clothing and warm blankets, administer warm fluids. *Active external:* use body-to-body contact, apply heating devices (e.g., air-filled warming blankets) or radiant lights. *Active core warming:* administer warmed IV fluids; heated, humidified O_2; peritoneal, gastric, or colonic lavage with warmed fluids. • Anticipate the need for hemodialysis or cardiopulmonary bypass. • Warm central trunk first in patients with profound hypothermia to avoid aftershock. • Establish IV access with two large-bore catheters for fluid resuscitation. • Assess for other injuries. • Keep patient's head covered with warm, dry towels, or stocking cap, to limit loss of heat. • Treat patient gently to avoid increased cardiac irritability. **Ongoing Monitoring** • Monitor ABCs, level of consciousness, temperature, vital signs. • Monitor O_2 saturation, cardiac rhythm. • Monitor electrolytes, glucose.

ABCs, Airway, breathing, circulation; *BVM,* bag-valve-mask; *ED,* emergency department; *IV,* intravenous.

---

shivering, lethargy, confusion, rational to irrational behavior, and minor heart rate changes. Shivering disappears at temperatures less than 92° F (33.3° C). *Moderate hypothermia* (87° to 90° F [30.6° to 32.2° C]) causes rigidity, bradycardia, slowed respiratory rate, blood pressure obtainable only by Doppler, metabolic and respiratory acidosis, and hypovolemia.

As core temperature drops, basal metabolic rate decreases two or three times. The cold myocardium is extremely irritable, so any movement can precipitate ventricular fibrillation. Decreased renal blood flow decreases glomerular filtration rate, which impairs water reabsorption and leads to dehydration. The hematocrit increases as intravascular volume decreases. Cold blood becomes thick and acts as a thrombus, placing the patient at risk for stroke, myocardial infarction, pulmonary emboli, acute tubular necrosis, and renal failure. Decreased blood flow leads to lactic acid accumulation from anaerobic metabolism and subsequent metabolic acidosis.

Profound hypothermia (less than 87° F [30.6° C]) makes the person appear dead. Metabolic rate, heart rate, and respirations are so slow that they may be difficult to detect. Reflexes are absent and the pupils fixed and dilated. Profound bradycardia, asystole, or ventricular fibrillation may be present. Every effort is made to warm the patient to at least 90° F (32.2° C) before the

person is pronounced dead. The cause of death is usually refractory ventricular fibrillation.

Collaborative Care. Treatment of hypothermia focuses on managing and maintaining ABCs, rewarming the patient, correcting dehydration and acidosis, and treating cardiac arrhythmias (see Table 67-9). Passive or active external rewarming is used for mild hypothermia. *Passive external rewarming* involves moving the patient to a warm, dry place, removing damp clothing, and placing warm blankets on the patient. Gentle handling is essential to prevent stimulation of the cold myocardium. *Active external rewarming* involves body-to-body contact, fluid- or air-filled warming blankets, or radiant heat lamps. The patient should be closely monitored for marked vasodilation and hypotension during rewarming.

Active core rewarming is used for moderate to profound hypothermia and refers to heat applied directly to the core. Techniques include heated (105° to 115° F [40.6° to 46.1° C]), humidified oxygen; warmed intravenous fluids; and peritoneal, gastric, or colonic lavage with warmed fluids. Hemodialysis or cardiopulmonary bypass may also be considered in profound hypothermia.[19,20]

Core temperature should be carefully monitored during rewarming procedures. Warming places the patient at risk for *afterdrop*, a further drop in core temperature, which occurs when cold peripheral blood returns to the central circulation. Aftershock can produce hypotension and arrhythmias. Thus patients with moderate to profound hypothermia should have the core warmed before the extremities. Rewarming should be discontinued once the core temperature reaches 93° F (33.9° C).[19,21]

Patient teaching should focus on how to avoid future cold-related problems. Essential information includes dressing in layers for cold weather, covering the head, carrying high-carbohydrate foods for extra calories, and developing a plan for survival should an injury occur.

SUBMERSION INJURIES

Submersion injury results when a person becomes hypoxic due to submersion in a substance, usually water. Approximately 8000 deaths occur from submersion injuries annually in the United States. Forty percent of these victims are children under 5 years of age. The primary risk factors for submersion injury include inability to swim, use of alcohol or drugs, trauma, seizures, hypothermia, and stroke.

Drowning is death from suffocation after submersion in water or other fluid medium. *Near-drowning* is defined as survival from potential drowning. *Immersion syndrome* occurs with immersion in cold water, which leads to stimulation of the vagus nerve and potentially fatal arrhythmias (e.g., bradycardia).

Death from a submersion injury is caused by hypoxia secondary to aspiration and swallowing of fluid, usually water. Swallowed water may cause vomiting and additional aspiration. The majority of all drowning victims aspirate water into the pulmonary tree and develop pulmonary edema. Victims who do not aspirate fluid develop intense bronchospasm and airway obstruction, the cause of death in "dry drowning." Regardless of what fluid is aspirated into the pulmonary tree, the ultimate result is pulmonary edema. The osmotic gradient caused by aspirated fluid causes fluid imbalances in the body. Hypotonic fresh water is rapidly absorbed into the circulatory system through the alveoli. Fresh water may be contaminated with chlorine, mud, and algae, causing the breakdown of lung surfactant, fluid seepage, and pulmonary edema. Hypertonic salt water draws protein-rich fluid from the vascular space into the alveoli, impairing alveolar ventilation and resulting in hypoxia. Fig. 67-4 shows the pulmonary effects of saltwater and freshwater aspiration.

The body attempts to compensate for hypoxia by shunting blood to the lungs. This results in increased pulmonary pressures and deteriorating respiratory status. More and more blood is shunted through the alveoli. However, the blood is not adequately oxygenated, so the hypoxemia worsens. Anaerobic metabolism occurs, which leads to lactic acidosis.

The assessment findings of a patient with a submersion injury are listed in Table 67-10. Aggressive resuscitation efforts and the mammalian diving reflex improve survival of near-drowning victims even after submersion in cold water for long periods of time.[20,22] Cold water lowers the body's metabolic rate and oxygen demand. The mammalian diving reflex causes apnea, bradycardia, and peripheral vasoconstriction and further decreases metabolic rate. Blood flow is redistributed to the most vital organs (i.e., heart, lungs, and brain).

Collaborative Care

Treatment of submersion injuries focuses on correcting hypoxia, acid-base imbalances, and fluid imbalances; supporting basic physiologic functions; and rewarming when hypothermia is

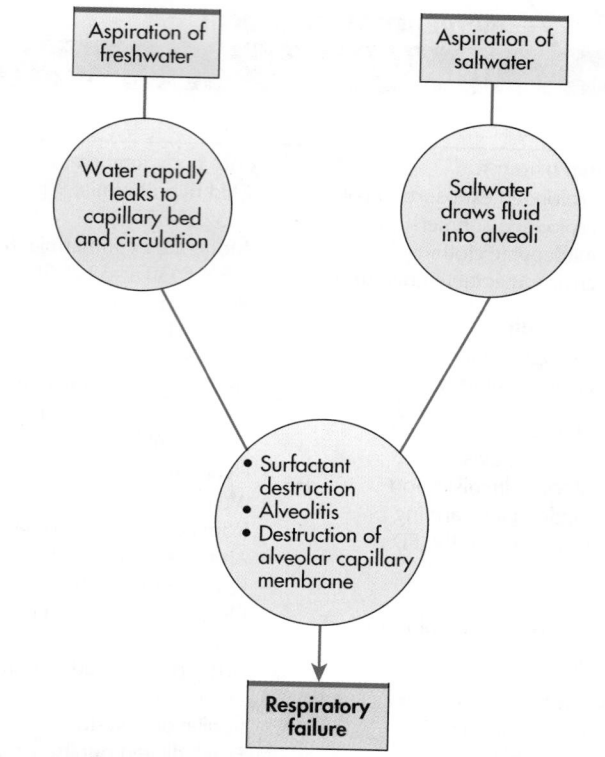

FIG. 67-4   Pulmonary effects of water aspiration.

present. Initial evaluation involves assessment of airway, cervical spine, breathing, and circulation. Other interventions are listed in Table 67-10.

Mechanical ventilation with positive end-expiratory pressure or continuous positive airway pressure may be used to improve gas exchange across the alveolar-capillary membrane when significant pulmonary edema is present. Ventilation and oxygenation are the primary techniques used to treat acidosis. Mannitol or furosemide (Lasix) may be given to decrease free water and treat cerebral edema.

Deterioration in neurologic status suggests cerebral edema, increased hypoxia, or profound acidosis. Near-drowning victims may also have head injuries that cause prolonged alterations in level of consciousness. All victims of near-drowning should be observed in a hospital for a minimum of 4 to 6 hours. Delayed pulmonary edema (also called *secondary drowning*), pneumonia, and cerebral edema have been reported in patients who were essentially free of symptoms immediately after the near-drowning episode but later developed problems.

Teaching should focus on water safety and minimizing the risks for drowning. Swimming pool gates should be locked; life jackets should be used on all water craft, including inner tubes and rafts; and water survival skills (i.e., swimming lessons) should be a priority. The dangers of combining alcohol and drugs with swimming and other water sports should be emphasized.[20]

BITES AND STINGS

Animals, spiders, and insects cause injury and even death by biting or stinging. Morbidity is a result of either direct tissue damage or lethal toxins. Direct tissue damage is a product of an-

TABLE 67-10 Emergency Management: Submersion Injuries

ETIOLOGY	ASSESSMENT FINDINGS	INTERVENTIONS
• Inability to swim or exhaustion while swimming • Entrapment or entanglement with objects in water • Loss of ability to move secondary to trauma, stroke, hypothermia, acute myocardial infarction • Poor judgment due to alcohol or drugs • Seizure while in water	**Pulmonary** • Ineffective breathing • Dyspnea • Respiratory distress • Respiratory arrest • Crackles, rhonchi • Cough with pink-frothy sputum • Cyanosis **Cardiac** • Tachycardia • Bradycardia • Arrhythmia • Hypotension • Cardiac arrest **Other** • Panic • Exhaustion • Coma • Coexisting illness (e.g., acute MI) or injury (e.g., cervical spine injury) • Core temperature slightly elevated or below normal depending on water temperature and length of submersion	**Initial** • Manage and maintain ABCs. • Assume cervical spine injury in all drowning victims and stabilize and/or immobilize cervical spine. • Provide 100% O_2 via non-rebreather mask or BVM. • Anticipate need for intubation if gag reflex is absent. • Establish IV access with two large-bore catheters for fluid resuscitation and infuse warmed fluids if appropriate. • Assess for other injuries. • Remove wet clothing and cover with warm blankets. • Obtain temperature and begin rewarming if needed. • Obtain cervical spine and chest x-rays. • Insert gastric tube. **Ongoing Monitoring** • Monitor ABCs, vital signs, level of consciousness. • Monitor O_2 saturation, cardiac rhythm. • Monitor temperature and maintain normothermia. • Monitor for signs of acute respiratory failure.

ABCs, Airway, breathing, circulation; *BVM,* bag-valve mask; *IV,* intravenous; *MI,* myocardial infarction.

imal size, characteristics of the animal's teeth, and strength of the jaw. Tissue may be lacerated, crushed, or chewed while toxins released through teeth, fangs, stingers, spines, or tentacles have local or systemic effects. Death associated with animal bites is due to blood loss, allergic reactions, or lethal toxins. Injuries caused by insects, spiders, scorpions, ticks, snakes, dogs, cats, rodents, and humans are described below.

Hymenopteran Stings

The *Hymenoptera* family includes bees, yellow jackets, hornets, and wasps. Stings can cause mild discomfort or life-threatening anaphylaxis (see Chapters 13 and 65). Venom may be cytotoxic, hemolytic, allergenic, or vasoactive. Symptoms may begin immediately or be delayed up to 48 hours. Reactions are more severe with multiple stings. Most hymenopterans sting repeatedly. However, the honeybee stings only once, usually leaving the stinger in the skin so that release of venom continues. A scraping motion with a fingernail, knife, or needle is recommended for removing the stinger. Tweezers squeeze the stinger and may cause more venom release. However, the fastest method of removing the stinger is ultimately the best, so if tweezers are available, they can be used.

Manifestations vary from stinging, burning, swelling, and itching to edema, headache, fever, syncope, malaise, nausea, vomiting, wheezing, bronchospasm, laryngeal edema, and hypotension. Treatment depends on the severity of the reaction. Mild reactions are treated with elevation, cool compresses, antipruritic lotions, and oral antihistamines. Rings, watches, and restrictive clothing are removed. More severe reactions require intramuscular or intravenous antihistamines (diphenhydramine [Benadryl]), subcutaneous epinephrine, and corticosteroids. Allergic reactions and anaphylaxis are discussed in Chapter 13.

Spider Bites (Arachnid)

Although there are 20,000 species of venomous spiders in the world, only 50 species cause illness. Two venomous spiders found in the United States are the black widow spider and the brown recluse spider.[19] Their venom can cause a localized reaction or systemic anaphylaxis. Tarantulas appear more dangerous than they actually are because their bite causes only localized stinging and pain. Other types of spiders release venom when they bite and may cause allergic reactions in some individuals, but they are not considered poisonous.

Black Widow Spiders. Black widow spiders are the most feared of all spiders. The female's venom is especially poisonous to people. Both the female and male are black in color (Fig. 67-5). The female rarely leaves the web, biting defensively if disturbed. Black widow spiders are found among fallen branches, among firewood, and under objects of many kinds, including furniture, outhouse seats, and trash.

The black widow spider venom is neurotoxic. When bitten, the patient will feel a pinprick-like sensation and a tiny, red bite mark will appear. Approximately 15 to 60 minutes later, the patient will report severe pain that will increase over the next 12 to 48 hours. Systemic symptoms will develop 30 minutes after *envenomation* (the introduction of poisonous venoms into the body by a bite or a sting). These can include nausea, vomiting, abdominal cramping,

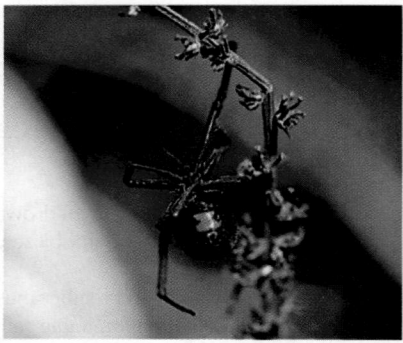

FIG. 67-5 Female black widow spider. The fully grown female is about 1.2 cm (0.5 in) long and is jet black, with an hourglass-shaped red mark on the underside of the abdomen. The female's sting is poisonous to humans. Males are only about half as long and usually have four pairs of red dots along the sides of the abdomen. Males are rarely seen and are harmless.

hypertension, dyspnea, paresthesias, and tachycardia. Symptoms usually peak 2 to 3 hours after onset; however, muscle spasms and hypertension can recur for 12 to 24 hours. Chest and abdominal pain, seizures, and shock can also occur. Bites on the lower body cause abdominal rigidity, whereas bites on the upper body lead to chest, back, and shoulder rigidity. A black widow spider bite is not prominent and can be easily missed. Patients not aware of the bite can be misdiagnosed, because symptoms mimic a perforated ulcer, appendicitis, pancreatitis, or other abdominal emergency.

Treatment includes cooling the area to slow the action of the neurotoxin. IV access should be established and oxygen administered as needed. The wound should be cleaned and tetanus prophylaxis given as appropriate. Muscle spasms are treated with calcium gluconate, methocarbamol (Robaxin), or diazepam (Valium). Severe pain may require narcotic analgesia. Although antivenin is rarely used, it can be used for severe reactions, young children, or adults with hypertension or cardiac disease.[19]

Brown Recluse Spiders. Brown recluse spiders are usually found in dark areas such as garages, closets, and boxes. The spider, common in the southeastern, south-central, and southwestern United States, is a light brown color with a characteristic dark brown fiddle shape that extends from the eyes down the back. The venom is cytotoxic, so local tissue effects can be dramatic. Initially, the bite is insignificant, with a local reaction beginning in 2 to 8 hours. A painful, purple purpura develops in a ring around the bite, and eventually may progress to a necrotic ulcerating wound by 7 to 14 days. The wound can extend deep into tissue and may persist for weeks. Occasionally, systemic manifestations of envenomation occur and can include fever, chills, joint pain, malaise, nausea, and vomiting.[19]

Treatment depends on severity of the reaction. Treatment is necessary when there is bleb or bulla formation, intense pain, and signs of rapidly progressive ischemia and necrosis. Initial interventions include cleansing the bite with mild antiseptic soap, providing cool compresses, and elevating the affected extremity. Analgesia, tetanus prophylaxis, antihistamines, corticosteroids, and antibiotics for prevention of secondary infection may also be required. Surgical debridement with grafting is necessary for some patients. Hyperbaric oxygen therapy may also be considered to enhance tissue healing. Dapsone (Avlosulfon), a polymorphonuclear leukocyte inhibitor, has been used for patients

with deep crater wounds. Patients with systemic manifestations are hospitalized and monitored for hemolysis, disseminated intravascular coagulation, and acute renal failure.

Tick Bites

Ticks are found in various parts of the United States, but they are most common in the Rocky Mountain region and the Northwest. Emergencies associated with tick bites include Rocky Mountain spotted fever, Lyme disease, and tick paralysis. Disease is caused by an infected tick or by the release of neurotoxin. Ticks release a neurotoxic venom as long as the tick head is attached to the body. Therefore removal of the attached tick is essential for effective treatment. Forceps may be used to safely remove the tick by grasping at the point of entry and pulling upward in a steady motion. Covering the tick with alcohol, mineral oil, petroleum jelly, or ether causes the tick to release from the skin. These methods work because the tick breathes through the skin in which it is embedded.

Rocky Mountain spotted fever caused by *Rickettsia rickettsii* has an incubation period of 2 to 14 days. A pink, macular rash appears on the palms, wrists, soles, feet, and ankles within 10 days of exposure. Other symptoms include fever, chills, malaise, myalgias, and headache. Treatment is antibiotic therapy.

Lyme disease is the most common arthropod-borne disease in the United States. Symptoms appear within 4 to 20 days of a bite from the *Ixodes* tick and result from exposure to the spirochete *Borrelia burgdorferi* that is found on the tick. The initial stage of this disease is characterized by nonspecific flulike symptoms (e.g., headache, stiff neck, fatigue) and a characteristic bull's-eye rash—an expanding circular area of redness of 5 cm diameter or more. Symptoms will disappear in 2 weeks if not treated. Monoarticular arthritis, meningitis, and neuropathies occur days or weeks after the initial symptoms. Chronic arthritis and myocarditis characterize the later stage of the disease, which can develop several months to 2 years after the initial skin lesion. Treatment includes antibiotic therapy; however, controversy exists over what the most effective regimen should be. (Lyme disease is discussed in Chapter 63.)

Tick paralysis occurs 5 to 7 days after exposure to the wood tick or dog tick. Classic symptoms are flaccid ascending paralysis, which develops over 1 to 2 days. Without tick removal, the patient dies as respiratory muscles become paralyzed. Tick removal leads to return of muscle movement, usually within 48 to 72 hours.

Snakebite

Only 375 of the 3000 species of snakes in the world are poisonous. Poisonous snakes indigenous to the United States are members of the Crotalidae and Elapidae family. Crotalidae, or pit vipers, include rattlesnakes, copperheads, and water moccasins. Coral snakes belong to the Elapidae family. Other poisonous snakes in the Elapidae family not indigenous to the United States are the highly venomous cobras, kraits, mambas, and sea snakes. Coral snakes do not exhibit the triangular head of pit vipers but are recognized by their bright colors. Coral snakes always have a blunt black snout and red, yellow, and black rings that completely encircle the body (Fig. 67-6). There is a yellow ring on both sides of every red ring. The beauty of this snake represents a true danger because small children may readily pick it up, thus providing an opportunity for a bite from this otherwise docile reptile. Other poisonous snakes in

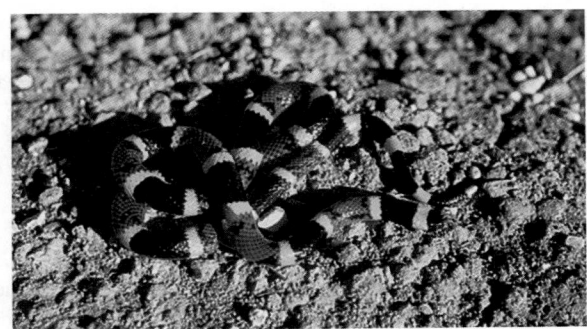

FIG. 67-6 Western coral snake. The venom from this snake is neurotoxic.

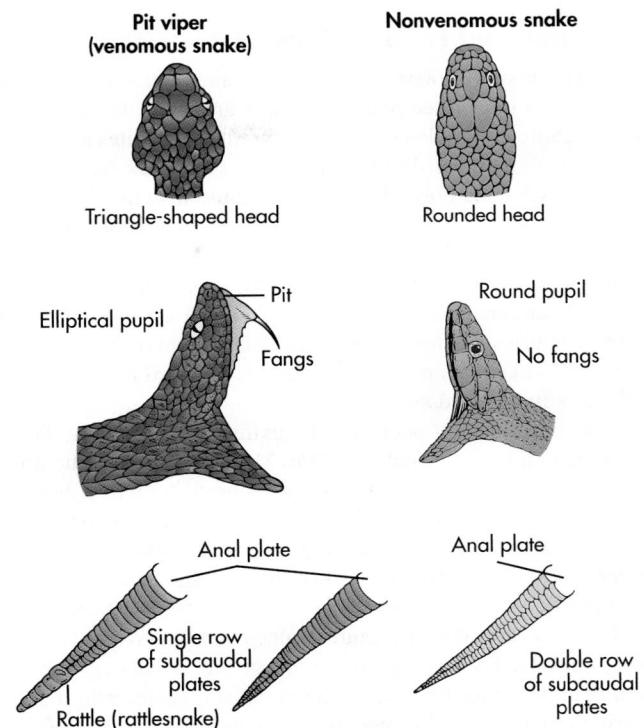

FIG. 67-7 Comparison of pit viper (a type of venomous snake) and nonvenomous snake.

the Elapidae family not indigenous to the United States are the cobra and the mamba. Fig. 67-7 highlights differences between the pit viper (a poisonous snake) and a nonpoisonous snake.

Venom from the pit viper is hemolytic, whereas coral snake venom is neurotoxic. Envenomation occurs in approximately 75% to 80% of all snakebites. If swelling does not occur within 30 minutes after the bite, envenomation is unlikely. Local reaction is characterized by one or two fang marks associated with pain, bruising, and edema within 36 hours of injury, petechiae, ecchymosis, and erythema. Loss of function and necrosis of the affected limb may occur 16 to 36 hours after the bite. Systemic reactions include nausea and vomiting, dizziness, tachycardia, muscle fasciculations, gastrointestinal bleeding, and respiratory problems. The patient may experience a metallic or rubber taste. Neurologic symptoms such as constricted pupils, drowsiness, weakness, fasciculations, muscle weakness, and seizures occur with neurotoxic venom. Life-threatening problems associated with systemic envenomation include severe hemorrhage, renal failure, and hypovolemic shock.

Treatment focuses on preventing the spread of venom. Rings, watches, and restrictive clothing should be removed, and then the affected limb should be immobilized at the level of the heart. Ice and tourniquets are not recommended. Incision of the wound is controversial. If done within 3 minutes of injury with the appropriate device (e.g., Sawyer extractor), 25% to 30% of the venom may be removed. Caffeine, alcohol, and smoking increase the spread of venom and should be avoided.

ED management includes vascular access with a large-bore (14- to 16-gauge) catheter and administration of crystalloids to maintain blood pressure. Diagnostic tests include complete blood count, urinalysis, coagulation studies, blood urea nitrogen, creatinine, creatine kinase, and electrolytes. Other measures include assessment of extremity swelling, usually through documentation of circumference every 30 to 60 minutes. Pain should be treated with acetaminophen. Aspirin and nonsteroidal antiinflammatory drugs should be avoided because they may exacerbate bleeding; narcotics may cause respiratory depression. Tetanus prophylaxis should be administered as needed (see Table 67-6). Secondary infection caused by microorganisms in the snake's mouth or other contaminants may require antibiotic therapy. Debridement or fasciotomy (see Chapter 24) is necessary in some patients. Antivenin (polyvalent Crotalidae antivenin ovine Fab [Cro-Fab]) therapy is used in mild to moderate reactions; the amount of antivenin required depends on the timing, type, and severity of envenomation (Table 67-11). Incomplete dosage is the most common cause of treatment failure.

TABLE 67-11	Antivenin* Snakebite Treatment	
ENVENOMATION	**SIGNS AND SYMPTOMS**	**NUMBER OF VIALS OF ANTIVENIN†**
None	Fang marks, no local swelling, hemorrhage, or paresthesia	No antivenin, tetanus prophylaxis, observation
Mild to moderate	*Mild:* Fang marks, local swelling of hands or feet, pain, no systemic reactions *Moderate:* Fang marks, progressive swelling beyond bite, mild systemic reaction (e.g., nausea, vomiting, paresthesias, hypotension)	*Initial dose:* 4–6 vials (3000–4500 mg) infused over 1 hour; infusion should be initiated slowly for the first 10 minutes to detect any allergic reactions; if initial control of symptoms is not achieved, dose may be repeated once *Additional regimen:* 2 vials every 6 hours for 18 hours

*Polyvalent Crotalidae antivenin ovine Fab (Cro-Fab).
†For Crotalidae envenomation (e.g., rattlesnakes, copperheads).

Animal and Human Bites

Approximately 500,000 to 2 million animal bites are reported each year in the United States. Children are at greatest risk. The most significant problems associated with animal bites are infection and mechanical destruction of the skin, muscle, tendons, blood vessels, and bone. The bite may cause a simple laceration or be associated with crush injury, puncture wound, or tearing or avulsion of tissue. The severity of injury depends on animal size, victim size, and anatomic location of the bite. Animal bites from cats and dogs are common, with dog bites accounting for 90% of the bite injuries that are treated in the ED.[19] Wild or domestic rodents are ranked behind cats and dogs as the third most frequent offenders in reported animal bites.

Dog bites usually occur on the extremities; however, facial bites are common in small children. Most victims own the dogs that bite them. Dog bites may involve significant tissue damage with fatalities reported, usually in children. Skull fractures with intracranial injury and death may occur in children less than 2 years old. Disfiguring wounds of the face should be evaluated by a plastic surgeon.

Cat bites cause deep puncture wounds that can involve tendons and joint capsules. Cat bites result in a greater incidence of infection than dog bites because of the organism, *Pasteurella,* that is carried in the mouths of most healthy cats.[19] Septic arthritis, osteomyelitis, and tenosynovitis have been reported in cat bites.

Humans bites also cause puncture wounds or lacerations and carry a high risk of infection from oral bacterial flora, most commonly *Staphylococcus aureus* and streptococci, and hepatitis virus. Hands, fingers, ears, nose, vagina, and penis are the most common sites of human bites and are frequently a result of violence or sexual activity. Boxer's fracture, fracture of the fifth metacarpal, is often associated with an open wound when the knuckles strike teeth. The human jaw has great crushing ability, causing laceration, puncture, crush injury, soft tissue tearing, and even amputation. More than 40 potential pathogens found in the human mouth account for an infection rate of approximately 50% in cases where victims did not seek medical intervention within 24 hours of injury.

Collaborative Care. Initial treatment for animal and human bites includes cleaning with copious irrigation, debridement, tetanus prophylaxis, and analgesics as needed. Prophylactic antibiotics are used for animal and human bites at risk for infection such as wounds over joints, those greater than 6 to 12 hours old, puncture wounds, and bites of the hand or foot. Individuals at greatest risk of infection are infants, older adults, immunosuppressed patients, alcoholics, diabetics, and people taking corticosteroids.

Puncture wounds are left open, whereas lacerations are loosely sutured. Wounds over joints are splinted. However, initial closure is reserved only for facial wounds. The patient is admitted for IV antibiotic therapy when an infection is present. There is an increased incidence of cellulitis, osteomyelitis, and septic arthritis in these patients. Human bites must be reported to the police in some states.

Consideration of rabies prophylaxis is an essential component in management of animal bites. A neurotoxic virus found in the saliva of some mammals causes rabies. If untreated, the condition is fatal in humans. Rabies exposure should be considered if an animal attack was not provoked, involved a wild animal, or involved a domestic animal not immunized against rabies. Rabies prophylaxis is always given when the animal cannot be found or a carnivorous wild animal causes the bite. An initial injection of rabies immune globulin (RIG) to provide passive immunity starts the prophylaxis regimen. This is followed by a series of five injections of human diploid cell vaccine (HDCV) on days 0, 3, 7, 14, and 28 to provide active immunity. Dosage is based on the patient's weight.

POISONINGS

A poison is any chemical that harms the body. In 2000, more than 2 million cases of human poison exposure were reported in the United States.[23] Poisonings can be accidental, occupational, recreational, or intentional. Natural or manufactured toxins can be ingested, inhaled, injected, splashed in the eye, or absorbed through the skin. Common poisons are reviewed in Table 67-12. Other poisonings related to the use of illegal drugs such as amphetamines, narcotics, and hallucinogens are discussed in Chapter 11. Poisoning may also be due to toxic plants or contaminated foods. (Food poisoning is discussed in Chapter 40.)

Severity of the poisoning depends on type, concentration, and route of exposure. Toxins can affect every tissue of the body, so symptoms can be seen in any body system. Specific management of toxins involves decreasing absorption, enhancing elimination, and implementation of toxin-specific interventions. The local poison control center is available 24 hours a day and should be consulted for the most current treatment protocols for specific poisons.

Options for decreasing absorption of poisons include emesis, gastric lavage, activated charcoal, dermal cleansing, and eye irrigation. Ipecac syrup (15 to 45 ml for adults) followed by 250 to 500 ml of water is used to induce emesis. This process is most effective if used within 30 minutes of ingestion. Use of ipecac has lost favor over the past decade for a variety of reasons. Onset of action is delayed and unpredictable, overall rate of drug return is low, and ipecac syrup is not effective with drugs that are rapidly absorbed, such as alcohol.[24] Ipecac is also potentially cardiotoxic if emesis does not occur or if a large dose is given. Other problems associated with induced emesis include fluid losses, electrolyte abnormalities, and acid-base disturbances secondary to protracted vomiting.

Gastric lavage involves oral insertion of a large-diameter (36 to 40 French) gastric tube for installation of copious amounts of saline. The head of the bed should be elevated or the patient placed on the side to prevent aspiration. Patients with an altered level of consciousness or diminished gag reflex are intubated before lavage. Lavage is contraindicated in patients who ingested caustic agents, coingested sharp objects, or ingested nontoxic substances.[25] Problems associated with lavage include epistaxis, esophageal perforation, and aspiration.

The most effective intervention for management of poisonings is administration of activated charcoal orally or via a gastric tube. Toxins adhere to charcoal and are excreted through the gastrointestinal (GI) tract rather than absorbed into the portal circulation. Adults receive 50 to 100 g of charcoal. Activated charcoal can absorb a number of poisons from the GI tract, but it does not absorb ethanol, alkali, iron, boric acid, lithium, methanol, or cyanide. For some toxins (e.g., phenobarbital) multiple-dose charcoal may be required.[25] Contraindications to charcoal administration are diminished bowel sounds, ileus, ingestion of a substance poorly absorbed by charcoal, or previous administration of *N*-acetylcysteine (NAC [Mucomyst]). Charcoal inactivates NAC, the antidote used for acetaminophen toxicity.

TABLE 67-12	**Common Poisons**	
POISON	**MANIFESTATIONS**	**TREATMENT**
• Acetaminophen (Tylenol)	*Phase 1:* within 24 hours of ingestion: malaise, diaphoresis, nausea and vomiting *Phase 2:* 24-28 hours: right upper quadrant pain, decreased urine output, diminished nausea, LFTs rise *Phase 3:* 72-96 hours: nausea and vomiting, malaise, jaundice, hypoglycemia, enlarged liver, possible coagulopathies, including DIC *Phase 4:* 7-8 days after ingestion: recovery, resolution of symptoms, LFTs return to normal	Activated charcoal, *N*-acetylcysteine (oral form may cause vomiting, IV form available on experimental basis).
• Acids and alkalis *Acids:* toilet bowel cleaners, antirust compounds *Alkalis:* drain cleaners, dishwashing detergents, ammonia	Excess salivation, dysphagia, epigastric pain, pneumonitis; burns of mouth, esophagus, and stomach	Immediate dilution (water, milk), corticosteroids (for alkali burns), induced vomiting is contraindicated.
• Aspirin and aspirin-containing medications	Tachypnea, tachycardia, hyperthermia, seizures, pulmonary edema, occult bleeding/hemorrhage, metabolic acidosis	Gastric lavage, activated charcoal with or without cathartic, urine alkalinization, hemodialysis for severe acute ingestion, intubation and mechanical ventilation, supportive care.
• Bleaches	Irritation of lips, mouth, and eyes, superficial injury to esophagus; chemical pneumonia and pulmonary edema	Washing of exposed skin and eyes, dilution with water and milk, gastric lavage, prevention of vomiting and aspiration.
• Carbon monoxide	Dyspnea, headache, tachypnea, confusion, impaired judgment, cyanosis, respiratory depression	Removal from source, administration of 100% O_2 via non-rebreather mask, BVM, or intubation and mechanical ventilation; consider hyperbaric oxygen therapy.
• Cyanide	Almond odor to breath, headache, dizziness, nausea, confusion, hypertension, bradycardia followed by hypotension and tachycardia, tachypnea followed by bradypnea and respiratory arrest	Amyl nitrate (nasally), IV sodium nitrate, IV sodium thiosulfate, supportive care.
• Ethylene glycol	Sweet aromatic odor to breath, nausea and vomiting, slurred speech, ataxia, lethargy, respiratory depression	Gastric lavage, activated charcoal, supportive care.
• Iron	Vomiting (often bloody), diarrhea (often bloody), fever, hyperglycemia, lethargy, hypotension, seizures, coma	Gastric lavage, chelation therapy (deferoxamine [Desferal]).
• Nonsteroidal antiinflammatory drugs	Gastroenteritis, abdominal pain, drowsiness, nystagmus, hepatic and renal damage	Gastric lavage, activated charcoal, cathartics, supportive care.
• Tricyclic antidepressants (e.g., amitriptyline [Elavil])	In low doses: anticholinergic effects, agitation, hypertension, tachycardia; in high doses: central nervous system depression, arrhythmias, hypotension, respiratory depression	Multidose activated charcoal, gastric lavage, serum alkalinization with sodium bicarbonate, intubation and mechanical ventilation, supportive care; never induce vomiting.
• Alcohol, barbiturates, benzodiazepines, cocaine, hallucinogens, stimulants	See Chapter 11	See Chapter 11

LFTs, Liver function tests; *BVM,* bag-valve-mask; *DIC,* disseminated intravascular coagulation; *IV,* intravenous.

Skin and ocular decontamination involves removal of toxins from eyes and skin using copious amounts of water or saline. With the exception of mustard gas, most toxins can be safely removed with water or saline.[25] Water mixes with mustard gas and releases chlorine gas. As a general rule, dry substances should be brushed from the skin and clothing before water is used. Powdered lime should not be removed with water; it should just be brushed off. Personal protective equipment (gloves, gowns, goggles, and respirators) should be worn for decontamination to prevent secondary exposure. Decontamination procedures are usually done by those specially trained in hazardous material decontamination before the patient arrives at the hospital. Decontamination takes priority over all interventions except basic life support techniques.

Elimination of poisons is increased through administration of cathartics, whole-bowel irrigation, hemodialysis, hemoperfusion, urine alkalinization, chelating agents, and antidotes. Cathartics such as sorbitol, magnesium citrate, or magnesium sulfate are given together with activated charcoal to stimulate intestinal motility and increase elimination. Multiple doses of cathartics should be avoided because of potentially fatal electrolyte abnormalities. Whole bowel irrigation is controversial and involves administration of a nonabsorbable bowel evacuant solution (e.g., GoLYTELY). The solution is administered every 4 to 6 hours until stools are clear. This process can be effective for swallowed objects such as cocaine-filled balloons or condoms. There is a high risk of electrolyte imbalance due to fluid and electrolyte losses with this procedure.[25]

Hemodialysis and hemoperfusion are reserved for patients who develop severe acidosis from ingestion of toxic substances (e.g., aspirin). Other interventions include alkalinization and chelation therapy. Sodium bicarbonate administration raises the pH (greater than 7.5), which is particularly effective for phenobarbital and salicylate poisoning. Vitamin C may be added to IV fluids to enhance excretion of amphetamines and quinidine. Chelation therapy may be considered for heavy metal poisoning (e.g., edetate calcium disodium [EDTA] for lead poisoning). A limited number of true antidotes are available, and many of these agents are themselves toxic.[25]

Education for toxic emergencies focuses on how the poisoning occurred. Patients who experience poisoning because of a suicide attempt or related to substance abuse should be evaluated by a mental health counselor and then referred for alcohol or drug detoxification or scheduled for follow-up with a mental health professional. The Occupational Safety and Health Administration should evaluate all poisoning related to an occupational hazard.

VIOLENCE

Violence is the acting out of the emotions of fear or anger to cause harm to someone or something. It may be the result of organic disease (e.g., temporal lobe epilepsy), psychosis (e.g., schizophrenia), or antisocial behavior (e.g., homicide).[26] The patient cared for in the ED may be the victim of violence or the perpetrator of violence. Violence can take place in a variety of settings, including the home, workplace, and community.

Domestic violence is a pattern of coercive behavior in a relationship that involves fear, humiliation, intimidation, neglect, and/or intentional physical, emotional, financial, or sexual injury (see Chapter 52 for information on sexual assault). It is found in all professions, cultures, socioeconomic groups, ages, and genders. Although men can be victims of domestic violence, most victims are women, children, and the elderly. It has been estimated that 20% to 50% of women treated at EDs have been *battered* (assaulted) by spouses, significant others, or individuals known to them.[27,28]

ED nurses are well situated to conduct domestic violence screening, yet research indicates that this is not always done (see Nursing Research box). Barriers to conducting effective screening include limited privacy for screening, lack of time, and lack of knowledge about how to inquire about domestic violence. The development and implementation of specific policies, procedures, and staff education programs can improve the domestic violence screening practices of ED staff.[27-30] For any patient who is found to be a victim of abuse, appropriate interventions such as making referrals, providing emotional support, and informing victims about their options (e.g., safe house, legal rights) should be initiated.[27] See Resources at the end of this chapter for additional information on domestic violence.

NURSING RESEARCH
Caring for Battered Women in the Emergency Department

Citation
Yam M: Seen but not heard: battered women's perceptions of the emergency department (ED) experience, *J Emerg Nurs* 26:464, 2000.

Purpose
To describe the experiences of battered women seen in the ED.

Methods
A phenomenologic approach was used to allow women to express themselves in their own words. Five women were interviewed individually, and all interviews were audiotaped and transcribed.

Results and Conclusions
Five categories emerged from the data and were confirmed by an expert consultant in the phenomenologic method. The women reported a multitude of emotions during their visit (e.g., fear of their partner, loneliness, concern for children) and a belief that the ED staff does not understand abuse and may even blame the victim. The women did report a satisfaction with the care that they received for their physical injuries but dissatisfaction with how the issue of abuse was managed. All women found it difficult to discuss the abuse with the staff. Reasons for this difficulty included fear (of the abuser), embarrassment, and lack of resources and/or support. Finally, the women requested that caregivers display compassion and take time to talk to them privately about their injuries and options.

Implications for Nursing Practice
These findings provide important insights into the perceptions of abused women seen in the ED. The dissatisfaction reported by this sample is similar to findings from previous studies. Nurses need to evaluate their practice and care models that provide for the physical, emotional, and safety needs of victims of abuse. It is extremely important for nurses to focus on the emotional needs of women who have been abused.

AGENTS OF TERRORISM

The threat of terrorism has emerged as a growing concern. Terrorism involves overt actions such as the dispensing of disease pathogens (e.g., **bioterrorism**) or other agents (e.g., chemical, radiologic) as weapons for the expressed purpose of causing harm. Prompt recognition and identification of potential health hazards are essential in the preparedness of health care professionals.

Table 67-13 summarizes general information regarding biologic agents of terrorism. The pathogens most likely to be used in a bioterrorist attack are anthrax, smallpox, botulism, plague, tularemia, and hemorrhagic fever.

Among the agents considered likely to be biologic weapons, those that cause anthrax, plague, and tularemia could be treated effectively with commercially available antibiotics if sufficient supplies were available and the organisms were not resistant. Smallpox can be prevented or ameliorated by vaccination even when first given after exposure. Botulism can be treated with antitoxin. There is no established treatment for viruses that cause hemorrhagic fever.[31]

TABLE 67-13 Agents of Bioterrorism			
PATHOGEN AND DESCRIPTION	**CLINICAL MANIFESTATIONS**	**TRANSMISSIBILITY**	**TREATMENT**
Anthrax *Bacillus anthracis* **Inhalation** <ul><li>Bacterial spores multiply in the alveoli</li><li>Toxins cause hemorrhage and destruction of lung tissue</li><li>High mortality rate</li></ul>	<ul><li>Incubation period: 1-2 days to 6 weeks</li><li>Abrupt onset</li><li>Dyspnea</li><li>Diaphoresis</li><li>Fever</li><li>Cough</li><li>Chest pain</li><li>Septicemia</li><li>Shock</li><li>Meningitis</li><li>Respiratory failure</li><li>Widened mediastinum (seen on chest x-ray)</li><li>Incubation period: up to 12 days</li></ul>	<ul><li>No person-to-person spread</li><li>Found in nature and most commonly infects wild and domestic hoofed animals</li><li>Spread through direct contact with bacteria and its spores</li><li>Spores are dormant, encapsulated bacteria that become active when they enter a living host</li></ul>	<ul><li>Antibiotics prevent systemic manifestations</li><li>Effective only if treated early</li><li>Ciprofloxacin (Cipro) is the treatment of choice</li><li>Penicillin</li><li>Doxycycline</li><li>Postexposure prophylaxis for 30 days (if vaccine available) or 60 days (if vaccine not available)</li><li>Vaccine has limited availability</li></ul>
Cutaneous <ul><li>95% of anthrax infections</li><li>Least lethal form</li><li>Spores enter skin through cuts or abrasions</li><li>Handling of contaminated animal skin products</li><li>Toxins destroy surrounding tissue</li></ul>	<ul><li>Small papule resembles an insect bite</li><li>Advances to a depressed, black ulcer</li><li>Swollen lymph nodes in adjacent areas</li><li>Edema</li></ul>		
Gastrointestinal <ul><li>Ingestion of contaminated, undercooked meat</li><li>Intestinal lesions in ileum or cecum</li><li>Acute inflammation of intestines</li></ul>	<ul><li>Nausea</li><li>Vomiting</li><li>Anorexia</li><li>Hematemesis</li><li>Diarrhea</li><li>Abdominal pain</li><li>Ascites</li><li>Sepsis</li></ul>		
Smallpox Variola major and minor viruses <ul><li>United States ended routine vaccination in 1971</li><li>Global eradication declared in 1980</li></ul>	<ul><li>Incubation period: 7-17 days</li><li>Sudden onset of symptoms</li><li>Fever</li><li>Headache</li><li>Myalgia</li><li>Lesions that progress from macules to papules to pustular vesicles</li><li>Malaise</li><li>Back pain</li></ul>	<ul><li>Highly contagious</li><li>Direct person-to-person spread</li><li>Transmitted in air droplets</li><li>Transmitted by handling contaminated materials</li></ul>	<ul><li>No known care</li><li>Cidofovir (Vistide) under testing</li><li>Isolation for containment</li><li>Vaccine available for those exposed</li><li>Vaccinia immune globulin (VIG) available</li></ul>
Botulism *Clostridium botulinum* <ul><li>Spore-forming anaerobe</li><li>Found in soil</li><li>Seven different toxins</li><li>Lethal bacterial neurotoxin</li><li>Can die within 24 hours</li></ul>	<ul><li>Incubation period: 12-72 hr</li><li>Abdominal cramps</li><li>Diarrhea</li><li>Nausea</li><li>Vomiting</li><li>Cranial nerve palsies (diplopia, dysarthria, dysphonia, dysphagia)</li><li>Skeletal muscle paralysis</li><li>Respiratory failure</li></ul>	<ul><li>Spread through air or food</li><li>No person-to-person spread</li><li>Improperly canned foods</li><li>Contaminated wound</li></ul>	<ul><li>Induce vomiting</li><li>Enemas</li><li>Antitoxin</li><li>Mechanical ventilation</li><li>Penicillin</li><li>No vaccine available</li><li>Toxin can be inactivated by heating food or drink to 85° C for at least 5 minutes</li></ul>

Continued

TABLE 67-13 **Agents of Bioterrorism—cont'd**

PATHOGEN AND DESCRIPTION	CLINICAL MANIFESTATIONS	TRANSMISSIBILITY	TREATMENT
Plague *Yersinia pestis* • Bacteria found in rodents and fleas **Forms** • Bubonic (most common) • Pneumonic • Septicemic (most deadly)	• Incubation period: 2-4 days • Hemoptysis • Cough • High fever • Chills • Myalgia • Headache • Respiratory failure • Lymph node swelling	• Direct person-to-person spread • Transmitted through flea bites • Ingestion of contaminated meat	• Antibiotics only effective if administered immediately • Drug of choice: strepto-mycin or gentamicin • Vaccine under development • Hospitalization • Isolation for containment
Tularemia *Francisella tularensis* • Bacterial infectious disease of animals • Mortality rate about 35% without treatment	• Incubation period: 3-10 days • Sudden onset • Fever • Swollen lymph nodes • Fatigue • Sore throat • Weight loss • Pneumonia • Pleural effusion • Ulcerated sore from tick bite	• No person-to-person spread • Aerosol or intradermal route • Spread by rabbits and ticks • Contaminated food, air, water	• Gentamicin treatment of choice • Streptomycin, doxycycline, and ciprofloxacin are alter-natives • Vaccine in developmental stage
Hemorrhagic Fever • Caused by several viruses, including Marburg, Lassa, Junin, and Ebola • Ebola virus is life threatening	• Fever • Conjunctivitis • Headache • Malaise • Prostration • Hemorrhage of tissues and organs • Nausea • Vomiting • Hypotension • Organ failure	• Carried by rodents and mosquitoes • Direct person-to-person spread by body fluids • Virus can be aerosolized	• No intramuscular injections • No antiplatelet drugs • Isolation for containment • Ribavirin (Virazole) effective in some cases • No known treatment available

TABLE 67-14 **Chemical Agents of Terrorism by Target Organ or Effect**

NERVE	BLOOD	PULMONARY	BLISTER/VESICANTS
Sarin (isopropyl methylphosphanofluoridate) Tabun (ethyl *N,N*-dimethylphosphoramido-cyanidate) Soman (pinacolyl methyl phosphonofluoridate) GF (cyclohexylmethylphosphonofluoridate) VX (O-ethyl S-[2-diisopropylaminoethyl] methylphosphonothiolate)	Hydrogen cyanide Cyanogen chloride	Phosgene Chlorine Vinyl chloride	Nitrogen and sulfur mustards Lewisite (an aliphatic arsenic com-pound, 2-chlorovinyldichloroarsine) Phosgene oxime

Chemicals may also be used as agents of terrorism and are categorized according to their target organ or effect (Table 67-14).[32] For example, sarin is a highly toxic nerve gas that can cause death within minutes of exposure. It enters the body through the eyes and skin and acts by paralyzing the respiratory muscles. Phosgene is a colorless gas normally used in chemical manufacturing. If inhaled at high concentrations for a long enough period, it causes severe respiratory distress, pulmonary edema, and death. Mustard gas is yellow to brown in color and has a garlic-like odor. The gas irritates the eyes and causes skin burns and blisters. Protocols to treat victims of chemical exposure are varied and relate to the specific agent.[33]

Ionizing radiation, such as that from a nuclear bomb or damage to a nuclear reactor, represents another major agent of terrorism. Exposure to radiation may or may not include skin contamination with radioactive material. If external radioactive contaminants are present, decontamination procedures must be initiated. Acute radiation syndrome develops after a substantial exposure to radiation and follows a predictable pattern (Table 67-15).[34]

TABLE 67-15   Acute Radiation Syndrome

		WHOLE BODY RADIATION FROM EXTERNAL RADIATION OR INTERNAL ABSORPTION					
		SUBCLINICAL RANGE		SUBLETHAL RANGE		LETHAL RANGE	
PHASE OF SYNDROME	FEATURE	0-100 RAD	100-200 RAD	200-600 RAD	600-800 RAD	600-3000 RAD	>3000 RAD
Initial or prodromal	Nausea, vomiting	None	5%-50%	50%-100%	75%-100%	90%-100%	100%
	Time of onset		3-6 hr	2-4 hr	1-2 hr	<1 hr	<1 hr
	Duration		<24 hr	<24 hr	<48 hr	<48 hr	<48 hr
	Lymphocyte count/μl			<1000 at 24 hr	<500 at 24 hr		
	CNS function	No impairment	No impairment	Routine task performance; cognitive impairment for 6-20 hr	Simple and routine task performance; cognitive impairment for >24 hr	Progressive incapacitation occurs	Progressive incapacitation occurs
"Manifest illness" (obvious illness)	Signs and symptoms	None	Moderate leukopenia	Severe leukopenia, purpura, hemorrhage Pneumonia Hair loss after 300 rad	Severe leukopenia, purpura, hemorrhage	Diarrhea Fever Electrolyte disturbance	Convulsions, ataxia, tremor, lethargy
	Time of onset		>2 wk	2 days-2 wk	2 days-2 wk	2-3 days	2-3 days
	Critical period		None	4-6 wk	4-6 wk	5-14 days	1-48 hr
	Organ system			Hematopoietic and respiratory (mucosal) systems	Hematopoietic and respiratory (mucosal) systems	GI tract Mucosal systems	CNS
	%						
Hospitalization		0	<5%	90%	100%	100%	100%
Fatality		0%	0%	0%-80%	90%-100%	90%-100%	90%-100%
Time to death				3 wk-3 mo	3 wk-3 mo	1-2 wk	1-2 days

From Armed Forces Radiobiology Research Institute: *Pocket guide for responders to ionizing radiation terrorism.* Available at *www.afrri.usuhs.mil/www/outreach/pocketguide.htm* (accessed July 25, 2002).
CNS, Central nervous system; *GI,* gastrointestinal.

EMERGENCY AND DISASTER PREPAREDNESS

The term **emergency** usually refers to any extraordinary event (e.g., multivictim train crash) that requires a rapid and skilled response and that can be managed by a community's existing resources.[35] An *emergency* is differentiated from a *disaster* in that a **disaster** is a manmade (e.g., biologic warfare) or natural (e.g., hurricane) event that overwhelms a community's ability to respond with existing resources.[36] Disasters result in mass casualties (more than 100 victims), physical and emotional suffering, and permanent changes within a community. In addition, disasters require assistance from people and resources outside the affected community (Fig. 67-8).[35]

The ED nurse has an important role in emergency and disaster management. Knowledge of the agency's *emergency response plan,* including individual roles and responsibilities of the members of the response team, and participation in emergency/disaster preparedness drills are necessary. See Resources at the end of this chapter for additional information on emergency and disaster preparedness.

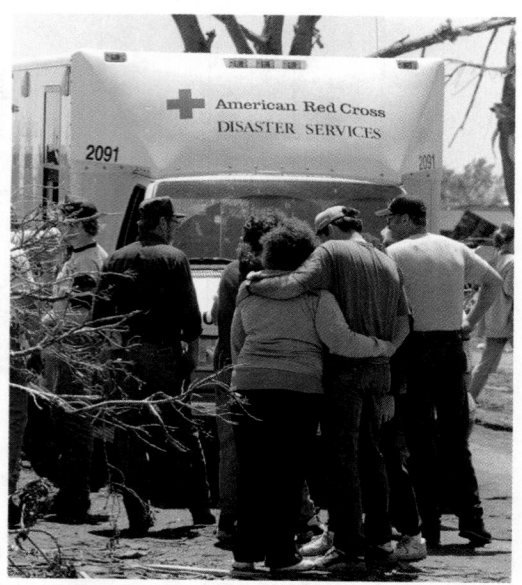

FIG. 67-8 American Red Cross.

CRITICAL THINKING EXERCISES

Case Study

Trauma

Patient Profile. A 20-year-old Hispanic female trauma patient is brought to the ED in an ambulance. She was the driver in a motor vehicle collision and was not wearing a seat belt. Two children in the car were pronounced dead at the scene. The paramedics stated that there was significant damage to the car on the driver's side.

Subjective Data
- Patient asks, "What happened? Where are the children?"
- Complains of shortness of breath and abdominal pain

Objective Data

Physical Examination
- 4 cm head laceration
- Badly deformed right lower leg with a pedal pulse by Doppler only
- Glasgow Coma Score = 14; unequal pupils
- Decreased breath sounds on left side of chest
- Asymmetric chest movement
- Vital signs: blood pressure 90/40, heart rate 130 beats/min, respiratory rate 36 breaths/min
- O_2 saturation 82%

CRITICAL THINKING QUESTIONS

1. What life-threatening injury does this patient probably have?
2. What is the priority of care?
3. What interventions are needed immediately?
4. What other interventions should the nurse consider?
5. Several family members have arrived in the ED, including the mother of one of the children who died. The second child who died was the patient's child. How should the nurse approach the family?
6. Based on assessment data presented, write one or more nursing diagnoses. Are there any collaborative problems?

Nursing Research Issues

1. Can the use of complementary therapies in the ED help patients manage pain?
2. What are the most effective teaching strategies for patients and their families following discharge from the ED?
3. Can the use of a screening tool for domestic violence increase the number of appropriate referrals?
4. What are the most effective strategies for helping family members in an ED setting?

REVIEW QUESTIONS

The number of the question corresponds to the same-numbered objective at the beginning of the chapter.

1. An elderly man arrives at the ED disoriented and breathing rapidly. He has hot, dry skin. The priority for treatment at this point is to
   a. assess his airway, breathing, and circulation.
   b. obtain a detailed medical history from his family.
   c. determine the kind of insurance he has before treating him.
   d. start oxygen administration and have the ED physician see him.

2. A patient has a core temperature of 90° F (32.2 °C). The most appropriate rewarming technique would be
   a. passive rewarming with body-to-body contact.
   b. active core rewarming using warmed IV fluids.
   c. passive rewarming using air-filled warming blankets.
   d. active external rewarming by submersing in a warm bath.

3. The most effective intervention in decreasing absorption of an ingested poison is
   a. ipecac syrup.
   b. milk dilution.
   c. gastric lavage.
   d. activated charcoal.

4. An elderly patient arrives in the ED with his son. The older man is in no apparent distress, although his clothes are soiled with urine and feces and he is tearful. The nurse should consider
   a. cancer.
   b. stroke.
   c. neglect.
   d. depression.

5. A chemical spill has occurred in a nearby industrial site. The first responders report that approximately 20 victims need to be transported to the ED after decontamination at the site. This is an example of
   a. an emergency.
   b. a natural disaster.
   c. a manmade disaster.
   d. an emergency response plan.

6. Which of the following biologic agents of bioterrorism has no effective treatment?
   a. anthrax
   b. botulism
   c. smallpox
   d. hemorrhagic fever

REFERENCES

*1. MacLean SL et al: The LUNAR project: a description of individuals who seek health care at emergency departments, *J Emerg Nurs* 25:269, 1999.

2. Emergency Nurses Association: ENA position statement on specialty certification in emergency nursing. Available at *www.ena.org/services/posistate/statements/Specialty/Certification.htm* (accessed Feb 20, 2002).

*3. Gerdtz MF, Bucknall TK: Triage nurses' clinical decision making: an observational study of urgency assessment, *J Adv Nurs* 35:550, 2001.

4. Rund DA, Rausch TS: *Triage,* St Louis, 1981, Mosby.

5. Rutenberg CD: Telephone triage, *Am J Nurs* 100:77, 2000.

6. Emergency Nurses Association, Newberry L, editor: *Sheehy's emergency nursing: principles and practice,* ed 5, St Louis, 2003, Mosby.

7. Jacobs BB, Hoyt KS, editors: *Trauma nursing core course,* ed 5, Des Plaines, Ill., 2000, Emergency Nurses Association.

*8. Li J et al: Complications of emergency intubation with and without paralysis, *Am J Emerg Med* 17:141, 1999.

*9. Sakles JC et al: Airway management in the emergency department: a one-year study of 610 tracheal intubations, *Ann Emerg Med* 33:325, 1998.

10. Laskowski-Jones L: Trauma. In Bucher L, Melander S, editors: *Critical care nursing,* Philadelphia, 1999, WB Saunders.

*11. Eichhorn DJ et al: Family presence during invasive procedures and resuscitation: hearing the voice of the patient, *Am J Nurs* 101:48, 2001.

*12. Meyers TA et al: Family presence during invasive procedures and resuscitation, *Am J Nurs* 100:32, 2000.

*13. Tanabe P, Buschmann M: Emergency nurses' knowledge of pain management principles, *J Emerg Nurs* 26:299, 2000.

*14. Kelly AM: A process approach to improving pain management in the emergency department: development and evaluation, *J Accid Emerg Med* 17:185, 1999.

*15. Tanabe P et al: The effect of standard care, ibuprofen, and music on pain relief and patient satisfaction in adults with musculoskeletal trauma, *J Emerg Nurs* 27:124, 2001.

*16. Socorro LL, Tolson D, Fleming V: Exploring Spanish emergency nurses' lived experience of the care provided for suddenly bereaved families, *J Adv Nurs* 35:562, 2001.

*17. Boulstridge HPM: Tissue donation after death in the accident and emergency department: an opportunity wasted? *J Accid Emerg Med* 16:117, 1999.

18. Linder JE, Fleming AW: Trauma in the elderly, *Clin Geriatr* 9:52, 2001.

19. Semonin-Holleran R: Environmental emergencies. In Jordan KS, editor: *Emergency nursing core curriculum,* ed 5, Philadelphia, 2000, WB Saunders.

20. Laskowski-Jones L: Responding to summer emergencies, *DCCN* 19:2, 2000.

21. Laskowski-Jones L: Responding to winter emergencies, *DCCN* 18:13, 1999.

22. DeBoer SL: Neurologic outcomes after near drowning, *Crit Care Nurse* 17:4, 1997.

*Nursing research–based reference.

23. Litovitz TL et al: 2000 Annual report of the American Association of Poison Control Centers toxic exposure surveillance system, *Am J Emerg Med* 19:337, 2001.

24. Emergency Nurses Association, Newberry L, editor: *Sheehy's emergency nursing: principles and practice,* ed 5, St Louis, 2003, Mosby.

25. McDeed-Breault C: Toxicological emergencies. In Jordan KS, editor: *Emergency nursing core curriculum,* ed 5, Philadelphia, 2000, WB Saunders.

26. Polli GE, Lazear SE: Mental health emergencies. In Jordan KS, editor: *Emergency nursing core curriculum,* ed 5, Philadelphia, 2000, WB Saunders.

*27. Ellis JM: Barriers to effective screening for domestic violence by registered nurses in the emergency department, *Crit Care Nurs Q* 22:27, 1999.

28. Emergency Nurses Association: ENA position statement on domestic violence. Available at *www.ena.org/services/posistate/data/domvio.htm* (accessed Feb 2, 2002).

*29. Brymer C et al: The effect of a geriatric education program on emergency nurses, *J Emerg Nurs* 27:27, 2001.

*30. Fulmer T et al: Elder neglect assessment in the emergency department, *J Emerg Nurs* 26:436, 2000.

31. On drugs and therapeutics, *Med Lett* 43:87, 2001.

32. Centers for Disease Control and Prevention: Biological and chemical terrorism: strategic plan for preparedness and response, October 2001. Available at *www.cdc.gov/mmwr/preview/mmwrhtml/rr4904a1.htm* (accessed July 23, 2002).

33. National Center for Environmental Health: Demilitarization of chemical weapons: emergency room procedures in chemical hazard emergencies—a job aid. Last reviewed May 4, 2002. Available at *www.cdc.gov/nceh/demil/articles/initialtreat.htm* (accessed July 23, 2002).

34. Armed Forces Radiobiology Research Institute: Pocket guide for responders to ionizing radiation terrorism. Last update June 25, 2002. Available at *www.afrri.usuhs.mil/www/outreach/pocketguide.htm* (accessed July 23, 2002).

35. Gebbie KM, Qureshi K: Emergency and disaster preparedness: core competencies for nurses, *Am J Nurs* 102:46, 2002.

36. Klein J: Disaster preparedness/disaster management. In Jordan KS, editor: *Emergency nursing core curriculum,* ed 5, Philadelphia, 2000, WB Saunders.

RESOURCES

American College of Emergency Physicians
1125 Executive Circle
Irving, TX 75038-2522
800-798-1822 or 972-550-0911
Fax: 972-580-2816
www.acep.org

American Nurses Association
Bioterrorism and Disaster Response Website
www.nursingworld.org/news/disaster

American Red Cross
P.O. Box 37243
Washington, DC 20013
800-HELP-NOW
www.redcross.org

American Trauma Society
8903 Presidential Parkway, Suite 512
Upper Marlboro, MD 20772
800-556-7890 or 301-420-4189
www.amtrauma.org

Association of Emergency Physicians (AEP)
127 Branchaw Boulevard
New Lenox, IL 60451
800-449-4237
Fax: 815-463-9230
www.aep.org

CDC Public Health Awareness and Response Website
Bioterrorism Preparedness and Response Planning
Centers for Disease Control and Prevention
Mailstop C-18
1600 Clifton Road
Atlanta, GA 30333
888-246-2675
www.bt.cdc.gov

Center for the Prevention of Sexual and Domestic Violence
2400 North 45th Street, #10
Seattle, WA 98103
206-634-1903
Fax: 206-634-0115
www.cpsdv.org

Emergency Nurses Association (ENA)
915 Lee Street
Des Plaines, IL 60016-6569
800-243-8362
www.ena.org

Federal Emergency Management Agency
500 C Street, SW
Washington, DC 20472
202-566-1600
www.fema.gov

National Coalition Against Domestic Violence
P.O. Box 18749
Denver, CO 80218
National Domestic Violence Hotline: 800-799-SAFE (7233)
303-839-1852
Fax: 303-831-9251
www.ncadv.org

National Domestic Violence Hotline
P.O. Box 16180
Austin, TX 78716
800-799-SAFE
Fax: 512-453-8541
www.ndvh.org

National Response Center
c/o United States Coast Guard (G-OPF)
2100 2nd Street, SW, Room 2611
Washington, DC 20593-0001
800-424-8802 or 202-267-2675
Fax: 202-267-2165
www.nrc.uscg.mil/index.htm

U.S. Department of Health and Human Services, Office of Emergency Preparedness
National Disaster Medical System
12300 Twinbrook Parkway, Suite 360
Rockville, MD 20857
301-443-1167 or 800-USA-NDMS
Fax: 301-443-5146 or 800-USA-KWIK
www.ndms.dhhs.gov/index.html

Wilderness Medicine Institute
National Outdoor Leadership School
284 Lincoln Street
Lander, WY 82520
307-332-7800
http://wmi.nols.edu

For additional Internet resources, see the website for this book at *http://evolve.elsevier.com/Lewis/medsurg/*.

APPENDIX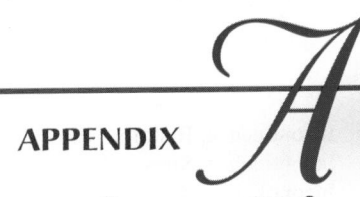

Nursing Diagnoses

ALPHABETICAL LISTING

Activity Intolerance
Activity Intolerance, Risk for
Adjustment, Impaired
Airway Clearance, Ineffective
Allergy Response, Latex
Allergy Response, Risk for Latex
Anxiety
Anxiety, Death
Aspiration, Risk for
Attachment, Risk for Impaired
   Parent/Infant/Child
Autonomic Dysreflexia
Autonomic Dysreflexia, Risk for
Body Image, Disturbed
Body Temperature, Risk for Imbalanced
Bowel Incontinence
Breastfeeding, Effective
Breastfeeding, Ineffective
Breastfeeding, Interrupted
Breathing Pattern, Ineffective
Cardiac Output, Decreased
Caregiver Role Strain
Caregiver Role Strain, Risk for
Communication, Impaired Verbal
Communication, Readiness for
   Enhanced
Conflict, Decisional
Conflict, Parental Role
Confusion, Acute
Confusion, Chronic
Constipation
Constipation, Perceived
Constipation, Risk for
Coping, Ineffective
Coping, Ineffective Community
Coping, Readiness for Enhanced
Coping, Readiness for Enhanced
   Community
Coping, Defensive
Coping, Compromised Family
Coping, Disabled Family
Coping, Readiness for Enhanced Family

Denial, Ineffective
Dentition, Impaired
Development, Risk for Delayed
Diarrhea
Disuse Syndrome, Risk for
Diversional Activity, Deficient
Energy Field, Disturbed
Environmental Interpretation Syndrome,
   Impaired
Failure to Thrive, Adult
Falls, Risk for
Family Processes, Dysfunctional:
   Alcoholism
Family Processes, Interrupted
Family Processes, Readiness for
   Enhanced
Fatigue
Fear
Fluid Balance, Readiness for Enhanced
Fluid Volume, Deficient
Fluid Volume, Excess
Fluid Volume, Risk for Deficient
Fluid Volume, Risk for Imbalanced
Gas Exchange, Impaired
Grieving, Anticipatory
Grieving, Dysfunctional
Growth and Development, Delayed
Growth, Risk for Disproportionate
Health Maintenance, Ineffective
Health-Seeking Behaviors
Home Maintenance, Impaired
Hopelessness
Hyperthermia
Hypothermia
Identity, Disturbed Personal
Incontinence, Functional Urinary
Incontinence, Reflex Urinary
Incontinence, Stress Urinary
Incontinence, Total Urinary
Incontinence, Urge Urinary
Incontinence, Risk for Urinary Urge
Infant Behavior, Disorganized
Infant Behavior, Risk for Disorganized
Infant Behavior, Readiness for
   Enhanced Organized
Infant Feeding Pattern, Ineffective
Infection, Risk for
Injury, Risk for
Injury, Risk for Perioperative-Positioning

Intracranial Adaptive Capacity,
   Decreased
Knowledge, Deficient
Knowledge, Readiness for Enhanced
Loneliness, Risk for
Memory, Impaired
Mobility, Impaired Bed
Mobility, Impaired Physical
Mobility, Impaired Wheelchair
Nausea
Neglect, Unilateral
Noncompliance
Nutrition, Imbalanced: Less than Body
   Requirements
Nutrition, Imbalanced: More than Body
   Requirements
Nutrition, Readiness for Enhanced
Nutrition, Risk for Imbalanced: More
   than Body Requirements
Oral Mucous Membrane, Impaired
Pain, Acute
Pain, Chronic
Parenting, Impaired
Parenting, Readiness for Enhanced
Parenting, Risk for Impaired
Peripheral Neurovascular Dysfunction,
   Risk for
Poisoning, Risk for
Post-Trauma Syndrome
Post-Trauma Syndrome, Risk for
Powerlessness
Powerlessness, Risk for
Protection, Ineffective
Rape-Trauma Syndrome
Rape-Trauma Syndrome: Compound
   Reaction
Rape-Trauma Syndrome: Silent Reaction
Relocation Stress Syndrome
Relocation Stress Syndrome, Risk for
Role Performance, Ineffective
Self-Care Deficit, Bathing/Hygiene
Self-Care Deficit, Dressing/Grooming
Self-Care Deficit, Feeding
Self-Care Deficit, Toileting
Self-Concept, Readiness for Enhanced
Self-Esteem, Chronic Low
Self-Esteem, Situational Low
Self-Esteem, Risk for Situational Low
Self-Mutilation

Modified from NANDA International (2002).
*NANDA Nursing Diagnoses: Definitions and
Classification 2003-2004.* Philadelphia: NANDA;
and Gordon M: *Manual of nursing diagnosis,*
ed 10, St. Louis, 2002, Mosby.

Self-Mutilation, Risk for
Sensory Perception, Disturbed
Sexual Dysfunction
Sexuality Patterns, Ineffective
Skin Integrity, Impaired
Skin Integrity, Risk for Impaired
Sleep Deprivation
Sleep Pattern, Disturbed
Sleep, Readiness for Enhanced
Social Interaction, Impaired
Social Isolation
Sorrow, Chronic
Spiritual Distress
Spiritual Distress, Risk for
Spiritual Well-Being, Readiness for
    Enhanced
Sudden Infant Death Syndrome, Risk for
Suffocation, Risk for
Suicide, Risk for
Surgical Recovery, Delayed
Swallowing, Impaired
Therapeutic Regimen Management,
    Effective
Therapeutic Regimen Management,
    Ineffective
Therapeutic Regimen Management,
    Ineffective Community
Therapeutic Regimen Management,
    Ineffective Family
Therapeutic Regimen Management,
    Readiness for Enhanced
Thermoregulation, Ineffective
Thought Processes, Disturbed
Tissue Integrity, Impaired
Tissue Perfusion, Ineffective
Transfer Ability, Impaired
Trauma, Risk for
Urinary Elimination, Impaired
Urinary Elimination, Readiness for
    Enhanced
Urinary Retention
Ventilation, Impaired Spontaneous
Ventilatory Weaning Response,
    Dysfunctional
Violence, Risk for Other-Directed
Violence, Risk for Self-Directed
Walking, Impaired
Wandering

GROUPED BY FUNCTIONAL HEALTH PATTERNS

Health Perception–Health Management Pattern

Energy Field, Disturbed
Falls, Risk for
Health Maintenance, Ineffective
Health-Seeking Behaviors
Infection, Risk for

Injury, Risk for
Injury, Risk for Perioperative-
    Positioning
Noncompliance
Poisoning, Risk for
Protection, Ineffective
Suffocation, Risk for
Therapeutic Regimen Management,
    Effective
Therapeutic Regimen Management,
    Ineffective
Therapeutic Regimen Management,
    Ineffective Family
Therapeutic Regimen Management,
    Ineffective Community
Therapeutic Regimen Management,
    Readiness for Enhanced
Trauma, Risk for

Nutritional-Metabolic Pattern

Allergy Response, Latex
Allergy Response, Risk for Latex
Aspiration, Risk for
Body Temperature, Risk for Imbalanced
Breastfeeding, Effective
Breastfeeding, Ineffective
Breastfeeding, Interrupted
Dentition, Impaired
Failure to Thrive, Adult
Fluid Volume, Deficient
Fluid Volume, Risk for Deficient
Fluid Volume, Excess
Fluid Volume, Risk for Imbalanced
Fluid Volume, Readiness for Enhanced
Hyperthermia
Hypothermia
Infant Feeding Pattern, Ineffective
Nausea
Nutrition, Imbalanced: Less than Body
    Requirements
Nutrition, Imbalanced: More than Body
    Requirements
Nutrition, Risk for Imbalanced: More
    than Body Requirements
Nutrition, Readiness for Enhanced
Oral Mucous Membrane, Impaired
Skin Integrity, Impaired
Skin Integrity, Risk for Impaired
Swallowing, Impaired
Thermoregulation, Ineffective
Tissue Integrity, Impaired

Elimination Pattern

Constipation
Constipation, Perceived
Constipation, Risk for
Diarrhea
Incontinence, Bowel
Incontinence, Functional Urinary
Incontinence, Reflex Urinary

Incontinence, Risk for Urinary Urge
Incontinence, Stress
Incontinence, Total
Incontinence, Urge
Urinary Elimination, Impaired
Urinary Elimination, Readiness for
    Enhanced
Urinary Retention

Activity-Exercise Pattern

Activity Intolerance
Activity Intolerance, Risk for
Airway Clearance, Ineffective
Autonomic Dysreflexia
Autonomic Dysreflexia, Risk for
Breathing Pattern, Ineffective
Cardiac Output, Decreased
Development, Risk for Delayed
Disuse Syndrome, Risk for
Diversional Activity, Deficient
Fatigue
Gas Exchange, Impaired
Growth and Development, Delayed
Growth, Risk for Disproportionate
Home Maintenance, Impaired
Infant Behavior, Disorganized
Infant Behavior, Readiness for
    Enhanced Organized
Infant Behavior, Risk for Disorganized
Intracranial Adaptive Capacity,
    Decreased
Mobility, Impaired Bed
Mobility, Impaired Physical
Mobility, Impaired Wheelchair
Peripheral Neurovascular Dysfunction,
    Risk for
Self Care Deficit, Bathing/Hygiene
Self Care Deficit, Dressing/Grooming
Self Care Deficit, Feeding
Self Care Deficit, Toileting
Surgical Recovery, Delayed
Tissue Perfusion, Ineffective
Transfer Ability, Impaired
Ventilation, Impaired Spontaneous
Ventilatory Weaning Response,
    Dysfunctional
Walking, Impaired
Wandering

Sleep-Rest Pattern

Sleep Deprivation
Sleep Pattern, Disturbed
Sleep, Readiness for Enhanced

Cognitive-Perceptual Pattern

Confusion, Acute
Confusion, Chronic
Conflict, Decisional
Environmental Interpretation Syndrome,
    Impaired

Knowledge, Deficient
Knowledge, Readiness for Enhanced
Memory, Impaired
Neglect, Unilateral
Pain, Acute
Pain, Chronic
Thought Processes, Disturbed

Self-Perception–Self-Concept Pattern

Anxiety
Anxiety, Death
Body Image, Disturbed
Fear
Hopelessness
Identity, Disturbed Personal
Loneliness, Risk for
Powerlessness
Powerlessness, Risk for
Self-Concept, Readiness for
   Enhanced
Self-Esteem, Chronic Low
Self-Esteem, Risk for Situational Low
Self-Esteem, Situational Low
Violence, Risk for Self-Directed

Role–Relationship Pattern

Attachment, Risk for Impaired Parent/
   Infant/Child

Caregiver Role Strain
Caregiver Role Strain, Risk for
Communication, Impaired Verbal
Communication, Readiness for
   Enhanced
Conflict, Parental Role
Family Processes, Dysfunctional:
   Alcoholism
Family Processes, Interrupted
Family Processes, Readiness for
   Enhanced
Grieving, Anticipatory
Grieving, Dysfunctional
Parenting, Impaired
Parenting, Risk for Impaired
Parenting, Readiness for Enhanced
Relocation Stress Syndrome
Relocation Stress Syndrome, Risk for
Role Performance, Ineffective
Social Interaction, Impaired
Social Isolation
Sorrow, Chronic
Violence, Risk for Other-Directed

Sexuality–Reproductive Pattern

Rape-Trauma Syndrome
Rape-Trauma Syndrome: Compound
   Reaction

Rape-Trauma Syndrome: Silent
   Reaction
Sexual Dysfunction
Sexuality Patterns, Ineffective

Coping–Stress Tolerance Pattern

Adjustment, Impaired
Coping, Ineffective
Coping, Ineffective Community
Coping, Readiness for Enhanced
Coping, Readiness for Enhanced
   Community
Coping, Defensive
Coping, Compromised Family
Coping, Disabled Family
Coping, Readiness for Enhanced Family
Denial, Ineffective
Post-Trauma Syndrome
Post-Trauma Syndrome, Risk for
Self-Mutilation
Self-Mutilation, Risk for
Suicide, Risk for

Value–Belief Pattern

Spiritual Distress
Spiritual Distress, Risk for
Spiritual Well-Being, Readiness for
   Enhanced

APPENDIX

B

Laboratory Values

The tables in this appendix list some of the most common tests, their normal values, and possible etiologies of abnormal values. Laboratory values may vary with different techniques or different laboratories. Possible etiologies are presented in alphabetic order. Abbreviations appearing in the tables are defined as follows:

<	=	less than
>	=	greater than
L	=	liter
mEq	=	milliequivalent
ml	=	milliliter
dl	=	deciliter
mm Hg	=	millimeter of mercury
fl	=	femtoliter
mm	=	millimeter

g	=	gram
mg	=	milligram (10^{-3})
μg	=	microgram (one millionth of a gram) (10^{-6})
ng	=	nanogram (one billionth of a gram) (10^{-9})
pg	=	picogram (one trillionth of a gram) (10^{-12})
μU	=	microunit
μl	=	microliter
IU	=	international unit
mOsm	=	milliosmole
U	=	unit
mmol	=	millimole
μmol	=	micromole
nmol	=	nanomole
pmol	=	picomole
kPa	=	kilopascal
μkat	=	microkatal

TABLE B-1	Serum, Plasma, and Whole Blood Chemistries			

| | NORMAL VALUES | | POSSIBLE ETIOLOGY | |
| | CONVENTIONAL | | | |
TEST	UNITS	SI UNITS	HIGHER	LOWER
Acetone			Diabetic ketoacidosis, high-fat diet, low-carbohydrate diet, starvation	
Quantitative	0.3-2.0 mg/dl	52-344 μmol/L		
Qualitative	Negative	Negative		
Albumin	3.5-5.0 g/dl	35-50 g/L	Dehydration	Chronic liver disease, malabsorption, malnutrition, nephrotic syndrome, pregnancy
Aldolase	1.0-7.5 U/L	0.02-0.13 μkat/L	Skeletal muscle disease	Renal disease
α_1-Antitrypsin	78-200 mg/dl	0.78-2.0 g/L	Acute and chronic inflammation, arthritis, stress syndrome	Chronic lung disease (early onset), malnutrition, nephrotic syndrome
α_1-Fetoprotein	<15 ng/ml	<15 μg/L	Cancer of testes and ovaries, carcinoma of liver	
Ammonia	30-70 μg/dl	17.6-41.1 μmol/L	Severe liver disease	
Amylase	0-130 U/L (method dependent)	0-2.17 μkat/L	Acute and chronic pancreatitis, mumps (salivary gland disease), perforated ulcers	Acute alcoholism, cirrhosis of liver, extensive destruction of pancreas
Ascorbic acid	0.4-1.5 mg/dl	23-85 μmol/L	Excessive ingestion of vitamin C	Connective tissue disorders, hepatic disease, renal disease, rheumatic fever, vitamin C deficiency
Bicarbonate	22-26 mEq/L	22-26 mmol/L	Compensated respiratory acidosis, metabolic alkalosis	Compensated respiratory alkalosis, metabolic acidosis
Bilirubin			Biliary obstruction, impaired liver function, hemolytic anemia, pernicious anemia, prolonged fasting	
Total	0.2-1.3 mg/dl	3.4-22.0 μmol/L		
Indirect	0.1-1.0 mg/dl	1.7-17.0 μmol/L		
Direct	0.1-0.3 mg/dl	1.7-5.1 μmol/L		
Blood gases*				
Arterial pH	7.35-7.45	Same as conventional units	Alkalosis	Acidosis
Venous pH	7.35-7.45	Same as conventional units		
Arterial PCO$_2$	35-45 mm Hg	4.67-6.00 kPa	Compensated metabolic alkalosis	Compensated metabolic acidosis
Venous PCO$_2$	42-52 mm Hg	5.60-6.93 kPa	Respiratory acidosis	Respiratory alkalosis
Arterial PO$_2$	75-100 mm Hg	10.0-13.33 kPa	Administration of high concentration of oxygen	Chronic lung disease, decreased cardiac output
Venous PO$_2$	30-50 mm Hg	4.0-6.67 kPa		
Calcium	9-11 mg/dl (4.5-5.5 mEq/L)	2.25-2.74 mmol/L	Acute osteoporosis, hyperparathyroidism, vitamin D intoxication, multiple myeloma	Acute pancreatitis, hypoparathyroidism, liver disease, malabsorption syndrome, renal failure, vitamin D deficiency
Calcium, ionized	4-4.6 mg/dl (2-2.3 mEq/L	1.0-1.15 mmol/L		
Carbon dioxide (CO$_2$ content)	20-30 mEq/L	20-30 mmol/L	Same as bicarbonate	
Carotene	10-85 μg/dl	0.19-1.58 μmol/L	Cystic fibrosis, hypothyroidism, pancreatic insufficiency	Dietary deficiency, malabsorption disorders
Chloride	95-105 mEq/L	95-105 mmol/L	Metabolic acidosis, respiratory alkalosis, corticosteroid therapy, uremia	Addison's disease, diarrhea, metabolic alkalosis, respiratory acidosis, vomiting

*Because arterial blood gases are influenced by altitude, the value for PO$_2$ decreases as altitude increases. The lower value is normal for an altitude of 1 mile.

Continued

TABLE B-1	Serum, Plasma, and Whole Blood Chemistries—cont'd			
	NORMAL VALUES		POSSIBLE ETIOLOGY	
TEST	CONVENTIONAL UNITS	SI UNITS	HIGHER	LOWER
Cholesterol	140-200 mg/dl (age dependent)	3.6-5.2 mmol/L	Biliary obstruction, hypothyroidism, idiopathic hypercholesterolemia, renal disease, uncontrolled diabetes	Extensive liver disease, hyperthyroidism, malnutrition, corticosteroid therapy
HDL (high-density lipoproteins)				
Male	>45 mg/dl	>1.2 mmol/L		
Female	>55 mg/dl	>1.4 mmol/L		
LDL (low-density lipoproteins)	<130 mg/dl	<3.4 mmol/L		
Cholinesterase (RBC)	0.65-1.00 pH	Same as conventional units	Exercise	Acute infections, insecticide intoxication, liver disease, muscular dystrophy
Pseudocholinesterase (plasma)	5-12 U/ml	Same as conventional units		
Copper	80-150 μg/dl	12.6-23.6 μmol/L	Cirrhosis, female on contraceptives	Wilson's disease
Cortisol	8 AM: 5-25 μg/dl 8 PM: <10 μg/dl	0.14-0.69 μmol/L <0.28 μmol/L	Cushing syndrome, pancreatitis, stress	Adrenal insufficiency, panhypopituitary states
Creatine	0.2-1.0 mg/dl	15.3-76.3 μmol/L	Active rheumatoid arthritis, biliary obstruction, hyperthyroidism, renal disorders, severe muscle disease	Diabetes mellitus
Creatine kinase (CK)			Musculoskeletal injury or disease, myocardial infarction, severe myocarditis, exercise, numerous intramuscular injections, brain damage	
Male	15-105 U/L	0.26-1.79 μkat/L		
Female	10-80 U/L	0.17-1.36 μkat/L		
CK-MB (CK-2)	0-9 U/L	<0.1 μkat/L	Acute myocardial infarction	
Creatinine	0.5-1.5 mg/dl	44-133 μmol/L	Severe renal disease	
Ferritin (serum)			Sideroblastic anemia, anemia of chronic disease (infection, inflammation, liver disease)	Iron-deficiency anemia
Male	20-300 ng/ml	20-300 μg/L		
Female	10-120 ng/ml	10-120 μg/L		
Folic acid (folate)	3-25 ng/ml	7-57 nmol/L	Hypothyroidism	Alcoholism, hemolytic anemia, inadequate diet, malabsorption syndrome, megaloblastic anemia
Gamma-glutamyl transpeptidase (GGT)	0-30 U/L	0-0.5 μkat/L		Liver disease, infectious mononucleosis
Glucose, fasting	70-120 mg/dl	3.89-6.66 mmol/L	Acute stress, cerebral lesions, Cushing's disease, diabetes mellitus, hyperthyroidism, pancreatic insufficiency	Addison's disease, hepatic disease, hypothyroidism, insulin overdosage, pancreatic tumor, pituitary hypofunction, postgastrectomy dumping syndrome
Glucose tolerance (GTT)			Diabetes mellitus	Hyperinsulinism
Fasting	70-120 mg/dl	3.89-6.66 mmol/L		
30 min	30-60 mg/dl above fasting	1.67-3.33 mmol/L		
60 min	20-50 mg/dl above fasting	1.11-2.78 mmol/L		
120 min	5-15 mg/dl above fasting	0.28-0.83 mmol/L		
180 min	Fasting level or lower	Fasting level or lower		

RBC, Red blood cell.

TABLE B-1	Serum, Plasma, and Whole Blood Chemistries—cont'd			
	NORMAL VALUES		**POSSIBLE ETIOLOGY**	
TEST	**CONVENTIONAL UNITS**	**SI UNITS**	**HIGHER**	**LOWER**
Haptoglobin	26–185 mg/dl	260–1850 mg/L	Infectious and inflammatory processes, malignant neoplasms	Hemolytic anemia, mononucleosis, toxoplasmosis, chronic liver disease
Insulin	4–24 μU/ml	29–172 pmol/L	Acromegaly, adenoma of islet cells, untreated mild case of type 2 diabetes	Diabetes mellitus, obesity
Iron, total	50–150 μg/dl	9.0–26.9 μmol/L	Excessive RBC destruction	Iron-deficiency anemia, anemia of chronic disease
Iron-binding capacity	250–410 μg/dl	45–73 μmol/L	Iron-deficient state, oral contraceptive use, polycythemia	Cancer, chronic infections, pernicious anemia, uremia
Lactic acid	5–20 μg/dl	0.56–2.2 mmol/L	Acidosis, congestive heart failure, shock	
Lactic dehydrogenase (LDH)	50–150 U/L	0.83–2.5 μkat/L	Congestive heart failure, hemolytic disorders, hepatitis, metastatic cancer of liver, myocardial infarction, pernicious anemia, pulmonary embolus, skeletal muscle damage	
Lactic dehydrogenase isoenzymes				
LDH$_1$	20%–35%	0.20–0.35	Myocardial infarction, pernicious anemia	
LDH$_2$	30%–40%	0.30–0.40	Pulmonary embolus, sickle cell crisis	
LDH$_3$	15%–25%	0.15–0.25	Malignant lymphoma, pulmonary embolus	
LDH$_4$	0%–10%	0–0.10	Lupus erythematosus, pulmonary infarction	
LDH$_5$	4%–12%	0.04–0.12	Congestive heart failure, hepatitis, pulmonary embolus and infarction, skeletal muscle damage	
Lipase	0–160 U/L	0–2.66 μkat/L	Acute pancreatitis, hepatic disorders, perforated peptic ulcer	
Magnesium	1.5–2.5 mEq/L	0.62–1.03 mmol/L	Addison's disease, hypothyroidism, renal failure	Chronic alcoholism, hyperparathyroidism, hyperthyroidism, hypoparathyroidism, severe malabsorption
Osmolality	285–295 mOsm/kg	285–295 mmol/kg	Chronic renal disease, diabetes mellitus	Addison's disease, diuretic therapy
Oxygen saturation (arterial)	95%–98%	0.95–0.98 saturated	Polycythemia	Anemia, cardiac decompensation, respiratory disorders
pH	See blood gases			
Phenylalanine	0–2 mg/dl	0–121 μmol/L	Phenylketonuria	
Phosphatase, acid	0–0.6 U/L	0–90 μkat/L	Advanced Paget's disease, cancer of prostate, hyperparathyroidism	
Phosphatase, alkaline	30–120 U/L	0.5–2.0 μkat/L	Bone diseases, marked hyperparathyroidism, obstruction of biliary system, rickets	Excessive vitamin D ingestion, hypothyroidism, milk-alkali syndrome
Phosphorus, inorganic	2.8–4.5 mg/dl	0.90–1.45 mmol/L	Healing fractures, hypoparathyroidism, renal disease, vitamin D intoxication	Diabetes mellitus, hyperparathyroidism, vitamin D deficiency

Continued

| TABLE B-1 | Serum, Plasma, and Whole Blood Chemistries—cont'd | | | |

| | NORMAL VALUES | | POSSIBLE ETIOLOGY | |
TEST	CONVENTIONAL UNITS	SI UNITS	HIGHER	LOWER
Potassium	3.5–5.5 mEq/L	3.5–5.5 mmol/L	Addison's disease, diabetic ketosis, massive tissue destruction, renal failure	Cushing syndrome, diarrhea (severe), diuretic therapy, gastrointestinal fistula, pyloric obstruction, starvation, vomiting
Prostate-specific antigen (PSA)	<4 ng/mL	<4 µg/L	Prostate cancer	
Proteins			Burns, cirrhosis (globulin fraction), dehydration	Congenital agammaglobulinemia, liver disease, malabsorption
Total	6.0–8.0 g/dl	60–80 g/L		
Albumin	3.5–5.0 g/dl	35–50 g/L		
Globulin	2.0–3.5 g/dl	20–35 g/L		
Albumin/globulin ratio	1.5:1–2.5:1	Same as conventional units	Multiple myeloma (globulin fraction), shock, vomiting	Malnutrition, nephrotic syndrome, proteinuria, renal disease, severe burns
Renin			Renal hypertension, volume decrease (e.g., hemorrhage)	Increased salt intake, primary aldosteronism
Supine position	1.4–2.9 ng/ml/hr	0.39–0.81 ng/L·sec		
Upright position	0.4–4.5 ng/ml/hr	0.11–1.25 ng/L·sec		
Sodium	135–145 mEq/L	135–145 mmol/L	Dehydration, impaired renal function, primary aldosteronism, corticosteroid therapy	Addison's disease, diabetic ketoacidosis, diuretic therapy, excessive loss from gastrointestinal tract, excessive perspiration, water intoxication
Testosterone				Hypofunction of testes
Male	300–1200 ng/dl	10.4–41.6 nmol/L		
Female	25–90 ng/dl	0.87–3.1 nmol/L	Polycystic ovary, virilizing tumors	
T_4 (thyroxine), total	5–12 µg/dl	64–154 nmol/L	Hyperthyroidism, thyroiditis	Cretinism, hypothyroidism, myxedema
T_4 (thyroxine), free	0.8–2.3 ng/dl	10–30 pmol/L		
T_3 uptake	25%–35%	0.25–0.35	Hyperthyroidism, metastatic neoplasms	Hypothyroidism, pregnancy
T_3 (triiodothyronine)	110–230 ng/dl	1.7–3.5 nmol/L	Hyperthyroidism	Hypothyroidism
Thyroid-stimulating hormone (TSH)	0.3–5.4 µU/ml	0.3–5.4 mU/L	Myxedema, primary hypothyroidism, Graves' disease	Secondary hypothyroidism
Transaminases				
Serum glutamic oxaloacetic (SGOT) or aspartate aminotransferase (AST)	7–40 U/L	0.12–0.67 µkat/L	Liver disease, myocardial infarction, pulmonary infarction, acute hepatitis	
Serum glutamate pyruvate (SGPT) or alanine aminotransferase (ALT)	5–36 U/L	0.08–0.6 µkat/L	Liver disease, shock	
Triglycerides	40–150 mg/dl	0.45–1.69 mmol/L	Diabetes mellitus, hyperlipidemia, hypothyroidism, liver disease	Malnutrition
Urea nitrogen (BUN)	10–30 mg/dl	1.8–7.1 mmol/L	Increase in protein catabolism (fever, stress), renal disease, urinary tract infection	Malnutrition, severe liver damage

TABLE B-1	Serum, Plasma, and Whole Blood Chemistries—cont'd			
	NORMAL VALUES		**POSSIBLE ETIOLOGY**	
TEST	**CONVENTIONAL UNITS**	**SI UNITS**	**HIGHER**	**LOWER**
Uric acid			Gout, gross tissue destruction, high-protein weight reduction diet, leukemia, renal failure, eclampsia	Administration of uricosuric drugs
Male	4.5-6.5 mg/dl	149-327 μmol/L		
Female	2.5-5.5 mg/dl	268-387 μmol/L		
Vitamin A	15-60 μg/dl	0.52-2.09 μmol/L	Excess ingestion of vitamin A	Vitamin A deficiency
Vitamin B$_{12}$	200-1000 pg/ml	148-738 pmol/L	Chronic myeloid leukemia	Strict vegetarianism, malabsorption syndrome, pernicious anemia, total or partial gastrectomy
Zinc	50-150 μg/dl	7.6-22.9 μmol/L		Alcoholic cirrhosis

TABLE B-2	Hematology			
	NORMAL VALUES		**POSSIBLE ETIOLOGY**	
TEST	**CONVENTIONAL UNITS**	**SI UNITS**	**HIGHER**	**LOWER**
Bleeding time (Simplate)	3.0-9.5 min	180-570 sec	Defective platelet function, thrombocytopenia, von Willebrand's disease, aspirin ingestion, vascular disease	
Activated partial thromboplastin time (APTT)	24-36 sec*	Same as conventional units	Deficiency of factors I, II, V, VIII, IX and X, XI, XII; hemophilia; liver disease; heparin therapy	
Prothrombin time (Protime, PT)	10-14 sec*	Same as conventional units	Warfarin therapy; deficiency of factors I, II, V, VII, and X; vitamin K deficiency; liver disease	
Fibrinogen	200-400 mg/dl	2.0-4.0 g/L	Burns (after first 36 hr), inflammatory disease	Burns (during first 36 hr), DIC, severe liver disease
Fibrin split (degradation) products	<10 μg/ml	Same as conventional units	Acute DIC, massive hemorrhage, primary fibrinolysis	
D-Dimer	Negative	Negative	DIC, myocardial infarction, deep vein thrombosis, unstable angina	
Erythrocyte count† (altitude dependent)			Dehydration, high altitudes, polycythemia vera, severe diarrhea	Anemia, leukemia, posthemorrhage
Male	4.5-6.0 × 10^6/μL	4.5-6.0 × 10^{12}/L		
Female	4.0-5.0 × 10^6/μL	4.0-5.0 × 10^{12}/L		
Mean corpuscular volume (MCV)	82-98 fl	Same as conventional units	Macrocytic anemia	Microcytic anemia
Mean corpuscular hemoglobin (MCH)	27-33 pg	Same as conventional units	Macrocytic anemia	Microcytic anemia
Mean corpuscular hemoglobin concentration (MCHC)	32%-36%	0.32-0.36	Spherocytosis	Hypochromic anemia

*Values depend on reagent and instrumentation used.
†Components of complete blood count (CBC).
COPD, Chronic obstructive pulmonary disease; *DIC,* disseminated intravascular coagulation; *WBC,* white blood cell.

Continued

TABLE B-2	Hematology—cont'd			
	NORMAL VALUES		**POSSIBLE ETIOLOGY**	
TEST	**CONVENTIONAL UNITS**	**SI UNITS**	**HIGHER**	**LOWER**
Erythrocyte sedimentation rate (ESR), Westergren			*Moderate increase:* acute hepatitis, myocardial infarction; rheumatoid arthritis	Malaria, severe liver disease, sickle cell anemia
Male <50 yr	<15 mm/hr	Same as conventional units	*Marked increase:* acute and severe bacterial infections, malignancies, pelvic inflammatory disease	
>50 yr	<20 mm/hr			
Female <50 yr	<20 mm/hr	Same as conventional units		
>50 yr	<30 mm/hr			
Hematocrit (altitude dependent)†			Dehydration, high altitudes, polycythemia	Anemia, hemorrhage, overhydration
Male	40%-54%	0.40-0.54		
Female	38%-47%	0.38-0.47		
Hemoglobin (altitude dependent)†			COPD, high altitudes, polycythemia	Anemia, hemorrhage
Male	13.5-18.0 g/dl	135-180 g/L		
Female	12.0-16.0 g/dl	120-160 g/L		
Hemoglobin, glycosylated	4.0%-6.0%	Same as conventional units	Poorly controlled diabetes mellitus	Sickle cell anemia, chronic renal failure, pregnancy
Red cell distribution width (RDW)	10.2%-14.5%	Same as conventional therapy		Anisocytosis, macrocytic anemia, microcytic anemia
Platelet count (thrombocytes)	150-400 × 10³/μl	150-400 × 10⁹/L	Acute infections, chronic granulocytic leukemia, chronic pancreatitis, cirrhosis, collagen disorders, polycythemia, postsplenectomy	Acute leukemia, DIC, thrombocytopenic purpura
Reticulocyte count (manual)	0.5%-1.5% of RBC	Same	Hemolytic anemia, polycythemia vera	Hypoproliferative anemia, macrocytic anemia, microcytic anemia
White blood cell count†	4.0-11.0 × 10³/μl	4.0-11.0 × 10⁹/L	Inflammatory and infectious processes, leukemia	Aplastic anemia, side effects of chemotherapy and irradiation
WBC differential				
Segmented neutrophils	50%-70%	0.50-0.70	Bacterial infections, collagen diseases, Hodgkin's disease	Aplastic anemia, viral infections
Band neutrophils	0%-8%	0-0.08	Acute infections	
Lymphocytes	20%-40%	0.20-0.40	Chronic infections, lymphocytic leukemia, mononucleosis, viral infections	Corticosteroid therapy, whole body irradiation
Monocytes	4%-8%	0.04-0.08	Chronic inflammatory disorders, malaria, monocytic leukemia, acute infections, Hodgkin's disease	
Eosinophils	0%-4%	0-0.04	Allergic reactions, eosinophilic and chronic granulocytic leukemia, parasitic disorders, Hodgkin's disease	Corticosteroid therapy
Basophils	0%-2%	0-0.02	Hypothyroidism, ulcerative colitis, myeloproliferative diseases	Hyperthyroidism, stress
Sickle cell solubility test	Negative	Negative	Sickle cell anemia	

TABLE B-3   **Serology-Immunology**

TEST	NORMAL VALUES CONVENTIONAL UNITS	SI UNITS	POSSIBLE ETIOLOGY HIGHER	LOWER
Antinuclear antibody (ANA)	Negative or titer <1:10	Same as conventional units	Chronic hepatitis, rheumatoid arthritis, scleroderma, systemic lupus erythematosus	
Anti-DNA antibody	Negative or titer <1:10 or <20% binding	Same as conventional units	Systemic lupus erythematosus	
Anti-RNP	Negative	Negative	Mixed connective-tissue disease, rheumatoid arthritis, systemic lupus erythematosus, Sjögren syndrome, scleroderma	
Anti-Sm (Smith)	Negative	Negative	Systemic lupus erythematosus	
Antistreptolysin-O (ASO)	≤166 Todd units or ≤1:85	Same as conventional units	Acute glomerulonephritis, rheumatic fever, streptococcal infection	
C-reactive protein (CRP)	Negative or ≤1.2 mg/dl	Same as conventional units	Acute infections, any inflammatory condition, widespread malignancy	
Carcinoembryonic antigen (CEA)	≤2.5 ng/ml	≤2.5 μg/L	Carcinoma of colon, liver, pancreas; chronic cigarette smoking; inflammatory bowel disease; other cancers	
Complement components				Acute glomerulonephritis, systemic lupus erythematosus, rheumatoid arthritis, subacute bacterial endocarditis, serum sickness
C1q	11-21 mg/dl	0.11-0.21 g/L		
C3	80-180 mg/dl	0.8-1.8 g/L		
C4	15-50 mg/dl	0.15-0.5 g/L		
Direct antihuman globulin test (DAT) or direct Coombs	Negative	Negative	Acquired hemolytic anemia, hemolytic disease of the newborn, drug reactions, transfusion reactions	
Fluorescent treponemal antibody absorption (FTAAbs)	Nonreactive	Negative	Syphilis	
Hepatitis A antibody	Negative	Negative	Hepatitis A	
Hepatitis B surface antigen (HBₛAg)	Negative	Negative	Hepatitis B	
Hepatitis C antibody	Negative	Negative	Hepatitis C	
Immunoglobulins				
IgA	90-400 mg/dl	0.9-4.0 g/L	IgA myeloma, chronic liver disease, chronic infection, rheumatoid arthritis, autoimmune disorders	Burns, hereditary telangiectasia, malabsorption syndromes
IgD	0.5-12.0 mg/dl	5-120 mg/L	Chronic infection, connective tissue disease	
IgE	<1.0 mg/dl	<10 mg/L	Anaphylactic shock, atopic disease (allergies), parasite infections	
IgG	650-1800 mg/dl	6.5-18.0 g/L	Infections—acute and chronic, hepatitis, IgG monoclonal gammopathy, systemic lupus erythematosus	Congenital deficiencies, acquired deficiencies, nephrotic syndromes, burns, immunosuppression
IgM	55-300 mg/dl	0.5-3.0 g/L	Acute infections, rheumatoid arthritis, liver disease	Congenital and acquired antibody deficiencies, lymphocytic leukemia, protein-losing enteropathies

Continued

TABLE B-3	Serology-Immunology—cont'd			
	NORMAL VALUES		POSSIBLE ETIOLOGY	
TEST	CONVENTIONAL UNITS	SI UNITS	HIGHER	LOWER
Monospot or monotest	Negative	Negative	Infectious mononucleosis	
Rheumatoid factor (RA factor)	Negative or titer <1:20	Same as conventional units	Rheumatoid arthritis, Sjögren syndrome, systemic lupus erythematosus	
RPR	Nonreactive	Same as conventional units	Syphilis, systemic lupus erythematosus, rheumatoid arthritis, leprosy, malaria, febrile diseases, IV drug abuse	
VDRL	Nonreactive	Same as conventional units	Syphilis	
Thyroid antibodies	≤1:10 titer	Same as conventional units	Hashimoto's thyroiditis, thyroid carcinoma, early hypothyroidism, pernicious anemia, systemic lupus erythematosus, Graves' disease	

CSF, Colony-stimulating factor; *RNP*, ribonuclear protein; *RPR*, rapid plasma reagin test; *VDRL*, Venereal Disease Research Laboratory test.

TABLE B-4	Urine Chemistry				
		NORMAL VALUES		POSSIBLE ETIOLOGY	
TEST	SPECIMEN	CONVENTIONAL UNITS	SI UNITS	HIGHER	LOWER
Acetone	Random	Negative	Negative	Diabetes mellitus, high-fat and low-carbohydrate diets, starvation states	
Aldosterone	24 hr	1-80 µg/day (depends on urinary sodium)	2.7-222 nmol/day	*Primary aldosteronism:* adrenocortical tumors *Secondary aldosteronism:* cardiac failure, cirrhosis, large dose of ACTH, salt depletion	ACTH deficiency, Addison's disease, corticosteroid therapy
Amylase	24 hr	1-17 U/hr	Same as conventional units	Acute pancreatitis	
Bence Jones protein	Random	Negative	Negative	Multiple myeloma, biliary duct obstruction	
Bilirubin	Random	Negative	Negative	Hepatitis	
Calcium	24 hr	100-250 mg/day	2.5-6.3 mmol/day	Bone tumor, hyperparathyroidism, milk-alkali syndrome	Hypoparathyroidism, malabsorption of calcium and vitamin D
Catecholamines Epinephrine Norepinephrine	24 hr	<20 µg/day <100 µg/day	<118 nmol/day <591 nmol/day	Pheochromocytoma, progressive muscular dystrophy, heart failure	
Chloride	24 hr	110-250 mEq/day	110-250 mmol/day	Addison's disease	Burns, excess perspiration, vomiting, diarrhea, menstruation
Copper	24 hr	<30 µg/day	<0.5 µmol/day	Cirrhosis, Wilson's disease	

TABLE B-4	Urine Chemistry—cont'd				

| | | NORMAL VALUES | | POSSIBLE ETIOLOGY | |
| | | CONVENTIONAL UNITS | SI UNITS | HIGHER | LOWER |
TEST	SPECIMEN				
Coproporphyrin	24 hr	50–200 μg/day	76–305 nmol/day	Lead poisoning, oral contraceptive use, poliomyelitis	
Creatine	24 hr	<100 mg/day	<763 μmol/day	Carcinoma of liver, hyperthyroidism, diabetes, Addison's disease, infections, burns, muscular dystrophy, skeletal muscle atrophy	Hypothyroidism
Creatinine	24 hr	0.8–2.0 g/day	7.1–17.7 mmol/day	Anemia, leukemia, muscular atrophy, salmonellae	Renal disease
Creatinine clearance	24 hr	85–135 ml/min	1.42–2.25 ml/sec		Renal disease
Estrogens	24 hr			Gonadal or adrenal tumor	Agenesis of ovaries, endocrine disturbance, ovarian dysfunction, menopause
Female					
Ovulation peak		28–100 μg/day	104–370 nmol/day		
Luteal peak		22–80 μg/day	81–296 nmol/day		
Pregnancy		Up to 45,000 μg/day	Up to 166,455 nmol/day		
Menopause		1.4–19.6 μg/day	5.2–72.5 nmol/day		
Male		5–18 μg/day	18–67 nmol/day		
Glucose	Random	Negative	Negative	Diabetes mellitus, low renal threshold for glucose resorption, physiologic stress, pituitary disorders	
Hemoglobin	Random	Negative	Negative	Extensive burns, glomerulonephritis, hemolytic anemias, hemolytic transfusion reaction	
5-Hydroxyindole-acetic acid (5-HIAA)	24 hr	2–9 mg/day	10.5–47.1 μmol/day	Malignant carcinoid syndrome	
Ketone bodies	24 hr	20–50 mg/day	0.34–0.86 mmol/day	Marked ketonuria	
Lead	24 hr	<100 μg/day	<0.48 μmol/day	Lead poisoning	
Metanephrine	24 hr	<1.3 mg/day	<7.1 μmol/day	Pheochromocytoma	
Myoglobin	Random	Negative	Negative	Crushing injuries, electric injuries, extreme physical exertion	
pH	Random	4.0–8.0	Same as conventional units	Chronic renal failure, compensatory phase of alkalosis, salicylate intoxication, vegetarian diet	Compensatory phase of acidosis, dehydration, emphysema
Phenylpyruvic acid	Random	Negative	Negative	Phenylketonuria	
Phosphorus, inorganic	24 hr	0.9–1.3 g/day	29–42 mmol/day	Fever, hypoparathyroidism, nervous exhaustion, rickets, tuberculosis	Acute infections, nephritis

Continued

| TABLE B-4 | Urine Chemistry—cont'd |

TEST	SPECIMEN	NORMAL VALUES CONVENTIONAL UNITS	NORMAL VALUES SI UNITS	POSSIBLE ETIOLOGY HIGHER	POSSIBLE ETIOLOGY LOWER
Porphobilinogen	Random 24 hr	Negative <2.0 mg/day	Negative <9 μmol/day	Acute intermittent porphyria, liver disorders	
Protein (dipstick)	Random	Negative	Negative	Congestive heart failure, nephritis, nephrosis, physiologic stress	
Protein (quantitative)	24 hr	<150 mg/day	<0.15 g/day	Cardiac failure, inflammatory processes of urinary tract, nephritis, nephrosis, toxemia of pregnancy	
Sodium	24 hr	40-250 mEq/day	40-250 mmol/day	Acute tubular necrosis	Hyponatremia
Specific gravity	Random	1.003-1.030	Same as conventional units	Albuminuria, dehydration, glycosuria	Diabetes insipidus
Titratable acidity	24 hr	20-50 mEq/day	Same as conventional units	Metabolic acidosis	Metabolic alkalosis
Uric acid	24 hr	250-750 mg/day	1.5-4.5 mmol/day	Gout, leukemia	Nephritis
Urobilinogen	24 hr	0.5-4.0 EU/day	Same as conventional units	Hemolytic disease, hepatic parenchymal cell damage, liver disease	Complete obstruction of bile duct
	Random	<1.0 Erhlich unit	Same as conventional units		
Uroporphyrins	Random	Random	Same as conventional units	Porphyria	
Vanillylmandelic acid	24 hr	1-8 mg/day 1.5-7.0 μg/mg creatine	5-40 μmol/day	Pheochromocytoma	

ACTH, Adrenocorticotropic hormone; *EU,* Ehrlich unit.

| TABLE B-5 | Gastric Analysis |

TEST	NORMAL VALUES CONVENTIONAL UNITS	NORMAL VALUES SI UNITS	POSSIBLE ETIOLOGY HIGHER	POSSIBLE ETIOLOGY LOWER
Basal				
Free hydrochloric acid	0.30 mEq/L	Same as conventional units	Hypermotility of stomach	Pernicious anemia
Total acidity	15-45 mEq/L	Same as conventional units	Gastric and duodenal ulcers, Zollinger-Ellison syndrome	Gastric carcinoma, severe gastritis
Poststimulation				
Free hydrochloric acid	10-130 mEq/L	Same as conventional units		
Total acidity	20-150 mEq/L	Same as conventional units		

TABLE B-6	**Fecal Analysis**			
	NORMAL VALUES		**POSSIBLE ETIOLOGY**	
TEST	**CONVENTIONAL UNITS**	**SI UNITS**	**HIGHER**	**LOWER**
Fecal fat	<6 g/24 hr	Same as conventional units	Chronic pancreatic disease, obstruction of common bile duct, malabsorption syndrome	
Urobilinogen	30-220 mg/100 g of stool	51-372 μmol/100 g of stool	Hemolytic anemias	Complete biliary obstruction
Mucus	Negative	Negative	Mucous colitis, spastic constipation	
Pus	Negative	Negative	Chronic bacillary dysentery, chronic ulcerative colitis, localized abscesses	
Blood*	Negative	Negative	Anal fissures, hemorrhoids, malignant tumor, peptic ulcer, inflammatory bowel disease	
Color				
Brown			Various color depending on diet	
Clay			Biliary obstruction or presence of barium sulfate	
Tarry			More than 100 ml of blood in gastrointestinal tract	
Red			Blood in large intestine	
Black			Blood in upper gastrointestinal tract or iron medication	

*Ingestion of meat may produce false-positive results. Patient may be placed on a meat-free diet for 3 days before the test.

TABLE B-7	**Cerebrospinal Fluid Analysis**			
	NORMAL VALUES		**POSSIBLE ETIOLOGY**	
TEST	**CONVENTIONAL UNITS**	**SI UNITS**	**HIGHER**	**LOWER**
Pressure	60-150 mm H_2O	Same as conventional units	Hemorrhage, intracranial tumor, meningitis	Head injury, spinal tumor, subdural hematoma
Blood	Negative	Negative	Intracranial hemorrhage	
Cell count (age dependent)				
WBC	0-5 cells/μl	0.5×10^6/L	Inflammation or infections of CNS	
RBC	0	0×10^6/L		
Chloride	100-130 mEq/L	100-130 mmol/L	Uremia	Bacterial infections of CNS (meningitis, encephalitis)
Glucose	40-75 mg/dl	2.5-4.2 mmol/L	Diabetes mellitus, viral infections of CNS	Bacterial infections and tuberculosis of CNS
Protein				
Lumbar	15-45 mg/dl	0.15-0.45 g/L	Guillain-Barré syndrome, poliomyelitis, traumatic tap	
Cisternal	15-25 mg/dl	0.15-0.25 g/L	Syphilis of CNS	
Ventricular	5-15 mg/dl	0.05-0.15 g/L	Acute meningitis, brain tumor, chronic CNS infections, multiple sclerosis	

CNS, Central nervous system.

| TABLE B-8 | Toxicology of Common Drugs | | | |

DRUG	THERAPEUTIC LEVEL		TOXIC LEVEL	
	CONVENTIONAL UNITS	SI UNITS	CONVENTIONAL UNITS	SI UNITS
acetaminophen (Tylenol)	0.2–0.6 mg/dl	13–40 μmol/L	>5 mg/dl	>330 μmol/L
Barbiturates				
Short acting	1–2 mg/dl	Dependent on composition of mixture	>5 mg/dl	
Intermediate acting	1–5 mg/dl		>10 mg/dl	
Long acting	15–35 mg/dl		>40 mg/dl	
Carbon monoxide (carboxyhemoglobin)				
Normal values	<5% saturation of hemoglobin	<0.05	Symptoms with >20% saturation	>0.20
Urban nonsmokers	<5% saturation of hemoglobin	<0.05		
Rural nonsmokers	0.5%–2.0% saturation of hemoglobin	0.005–0.02		
Smokers	5%–9% saturation of hemoglobin	0.05–0.09		
Heavy smokers	>9% saturation of hemoglobin	>0.09		
chlordiazepoxide (Librium)	0.05–5.0 mg/L	2–17 μmol/L	>10 mg/L	>33 μmol/L
chlorpromazine (Thorazine)	0.5 μg/ml	1.6 μmol/L	>2.0 μg/ml	>6.3 μmol/L
diazepam (Valium)	0.10–0.25 mg/L	0.35–0.88 μmol/L	>1.0 mg/L ≥2.0 mg/L (lethal)	>3.5 μmol/L
Digitalis preparations				
digoxin	0.8–2.4 ng/ml	1.0–3.1 nmol/L	>2.5 ng/ml	>2.6 nmol/L
digitoxin	14–30 ng/ml	18–39 nmol/L	>30 ng/ml	>39 nmol/L
Dilantin	10–20 mg/L	40–80 μmol/L	>30 mg/L	>120 μmol/L
gentamicin (Garamycin)				
Peak	4–10 mg/L	9–22 μmol/L	>10 mg/L	>22 μmol/L
Trough	<2 mg/L	<4 mmol/L	>2 mg/L	>4 μmol/L
propranolol (Inderal)	50–100 ng/ml	192–386 nmol/L	>200 ng/ml	>771 nmol/L
Salicylates	10–20 mg/dl	0.724–1.45 mmol/L	>20 mg/dl	>1.45 mmol/L
Alcohol (ethanol)*			>60 mg/dl (lethal)	>4.34 mmol/L

*See Table 10-10.

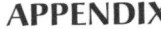

APPENDIX C

Answer Key to Review Questions

Chapter 1
1. d
2. c
3. a
4. c
5. c
6. d
7. c
8. c
9. b
10. d
11. c

Chapter 2
1. d
2. d
3. a
4. b
5. b
6. c
7. a

Chapter 3
1. d
2. a
3. a
4. a
5. c
6. b

Chapter 4
1. d
2. c
3. a
4. a
5. b
6. a
7. b
8. d
9. b
10. a

Chapter 5
1. a
2. c
3. c
4. c
5. d
6. d
7. c
8. c
9. a
10. b
11. a
12. c

Chapter 6
1. d
2. c

3. d
4. d

Chapter 7
1. a
2. b
3. d
4. a
5. b
6. d
7. c
8. b
9. c

Chapter 8
1. b
2. b
3. a
4. c
5. d
6. b
7. a
8. a
9. d

Chapter 9
1. b
2. d
3. d
4. c
5. c
6. b
7. b
8. c
9. d
10. d

Chapter 10
1. b
2. a
3. d
4. c
5. c
6. d
7. d
8. a
9. c

Chapter 11
1. d
2. c
3. a
4. b
5. d
6. b
7. b
8. d
9. b
10. b

Chapter 12
1. b
2. a
3. b
4. d
5. b
6. b
7. d
8. d
9. a
10. b
11. a
12. b
13. c

Chapter 13
1. d
2. c
3. d
4. c
5. a
6. d
7. a
8. d
9. c
10. d
11. a
12. c
13. a

Chapter 14
1. a
2. b
3. d
4. a
5. c
6. c
7. c
8. a
9. a
10. c

Chapter 15
1. d
2. d
3. d
4. a
5. d
6. b
7. c
8. b
9. d
10. c
11. a
12. c
13. a
14. d
15. a

Chapter 16
1. b
2. a
3a. a
3b. a
3c. c
3d. c
3e. c
3f. a
4. a
5. d
6. b

Chapter 17
1. d
2. c
3. c
4. a
5. b
6. c
7. a
8. d

Chapter 18
1. b
2. c
3. c
4. c
5. a
6. d
7. d
8. c
9. c
10. b

Chapter 19
1. d
2. b
3. d
4. a
5. c
6. a

Chapter 20
1. c
2. d
3. c
4. a
5. b
6. d
7. a

Chapter 21
1. b
2. d
3. c
4. b
5. d
6. b

7. a
8. a
9. b
10. a
11. d

Chapter 22
1. b
2. b
3. d
4. c
5. d
6. c
7. d
8. a
9. b

Chapter 23
1. b
2. b
3. d
4. a
5. b
6. a
7. c
8. b
9. a
10. a

Chapter 24
1. c
2. a
3. c
4. d
5. c
6. c
7. b
8. b
9. a
10. b
11. b

Chapter 25
1. c
2. d
3. a
4. a
5. c
6. b
7. d
8. a
9. a
10. a
11. a

Chapter 26
1. d
2. d
3. a
4. c
5. b
6. d
7. a
8. c

Chapter 27
1. a
2. d
3. d
4. a
5. c
6. d

7. c
8. c
9. a
10. c
11. d
12. c
13. b

Chapter 28
1. a
2. a
3. b
4. d
5. d
6. c
7. d

Chapter 29
1. b
2. c
3. b
4. a
5. a
6. c
7. a
8. b

Chapter 30
1. a
2. b
3. d
4. c
5. a
6. a
7. d
8. c
9. d
10. d
11. c
12. c
13. b
14. c
15. d
16. d

Chapter 31
1. c
2. c
3. c
4. d
5. c
6. d
7. b
8. a
9. c
10. a
11. b

Chapter 32
1. d
2. b
3. d
4. b
5. d
6. d
7. a
8. b

Chapter 33
1. c
2. a
3. a

4. d
5. c
6. c
7. c
8. b
9. c

Chapter 34
1. b
2. c
3. a
4. a
5. c
6. a

Chapter 35
1. d
2. b
3. d
4. a
5. b
6. c
7. d
8. d

Chapter 36
1. a
2. b
3. a
4. a
5. c
6. c
7. b
8. c
9. c
10. c

Chapter 37
1. c
2. c
3. b
4. d
5. c
6. b
7. a
8. d
9. b
10. c
11. b
12. d
13. c
14. d

Chapter 38
1. d
2. b
3. b
4. a
5. b
6. c
7. b
8. a
9. b

Chapter 39
1. c
2. d
3. a
4. c
5. b
6. a
7. d

8. d
9. c

Chapter 40
1. b
2. d
3. c
4. d
5. c
6. c
7. a
8. d
9. d
10. b

Chapter 41
1. a
2. d
3. b
4. c
5. a
6. c
7. a
8. b
9. d
10. a
11. d

Chapter 42
1. a
2. b
3. b
4. b
5. d
6. a
7. d
8. d
9. c
10. a
11. b

Chapter 43
1. d
2. b
3. d
4. b
5. a
6. a
7. b
8. d

Chapter 44
1. d
2. a
3. b
4. a
5. d
6. a
7. d
8. d
9. b
10. a
11. b
12. d

Chapter 45
1. a
2. b
3. b
4. c
5. d
6. c

7. d
8. c
9. a
10. d
11. b

Chapter 46
1. b
2. c
3. a
4. d
5. a
6. c
7. a
8. c
9. a

Chapter 47
1. b
2. d
3. d
4. d
5. d
6. c
7. c
8. a

Chapter 48
1. b
2. b
3. c
4. a
5. d
6. d
7. a
8. c

Chapter 49
1. c
2. c
3. d
4. c
5. c
6. a
7. a
8. d

Chapter 50
1. d
2. d
3. d
4. a
5. c
6. c
7. d
8. a

Chapter 51
1. b
2. a
3. c
4. d
5. c
6. c
7. a

Chapter 52
1. b
2. d
3. d
4. d
5. c
6. a
7. b
8. c
9. d
10. b
11. b
12. c
13. a

Chapter 53
1. b
2. d
3. c
4. a
5. c
6. c
7. c

Chapter 54
1. c
2. d
3. d
4. c
5. b
6. b
7. d
8. a
9. c
10. a
11. b

Chapter 55
1. b
2. d
3. b
4. c
5. a
6. a
7. c
8. d
9. b

Chapter 56
1. d
2. c
3. d
4. c
5. d
6. c
7. b
8. c
9. b

Chapter 57
1. a
2. b
3. c
4. c
5. d

Chapter 58
1. d
2. d
3. c
4. c
5. b
6. a
7. b

Chapter 59
1. d
2. d
3. d
4. c
5. b
6. c
7. a
8. b

Chapter 60
1. c
2. b
3. d
4. d
5. c
6. d
7. c
8. d
9. a

Chapter 61
1. d
2. a
3. c
4. c
5. d
6. b

7. b
8. d
9. b

Chapter 62
1. b
2. d
3. a
4. d
5. c
6. a
7. b

Chapter 63
1. c
2. c
3. a
4. b
5. a
6. c
7. c

Chapter 64
1. d
2. b
3. c
4. d
5. a
6. b
7. a
8. c

Chapter 65
1. c
2. d
3. a
4. b
5. a
6. d

Chapter 66
1. b
2. c
3. d
4. a
5. c
6. c

Chapter 67
1. a
2. b
3. d
4. c
5. a
6. d

Illustration Credits

Chapter 1
1-1, From Potter PA, Perry AG: *Fundamentals of nursing: concepts, process, and practice,* ed 4, St Louis, 1997, Mosby; **1-4, 1-5,** from Rick Brady, Riva, MD.

Chapter 2
2-1, 2-2, 2-3, 2-4, From Rick Brady, Riva, MD.

Chapter 3
3-1, From Wilson SF, Giddens JF: *Health assessment for nursing practice,* ed 2, St Louis, 2001, Mosby.

Chapter 4
4-2, Reprinted from *Patient Educ Couns,* vol. 27, Boise L et al: Facing chronic illness: the family support model and its benefits, p. 76, 1996, with permission from Elsevier Science; **4-3, 4-5,** From Rick Brady, Riva, MD; **4-6,** from Wilson SF, Giddens JF: *Health assessment for nursing practice,* ed 2, St Louis, 2001, Mosby.

Chapter 5
5-1, From US Bureau of Census; **5-2, 5-3, 5-4, 5-6, 5-7, 5-8,** from Rick Brady, Riva, MD; **5-5,** redrawn from Benzon J: Approaching drug regimens with a therapeutic dose of suspicion, *Geriatr Nurs* 12(4):1813, 1991.

Chapter 6
6-1, From Potter PA, Perry AG: *Basic nursing: a critical thinking approach,* ed 4, St Louis, 1999, Mosby; **6-2, 6-3,** from Potter PA, Perry AG: *Fundamentals of nursing: concepts, process, and practice,* ed 4, St Louis, 1997, Mosby; **6-4,** from Rick Brady, Riva, MD.

Chapter 7
7-1, 7-2, 7-3, 7-5, 7-8, From Rick Brady, Riva, MD; **7-7,** from Blake S: *Alternative remedies CD-ROM,* St Louis, 1999, Mosby.

Chapter 8
8-7, From Rick Brady, Riva, MD.

Chapter 9
9-2, Developed by McCaffery M, Pasero C, Paice JA. From McCaffery M, Pasero C: *Pain: clinical manual,* ed 2, St Louis, 1999, Mosby; **9-6,** from McCaffery M, Pasero C: *Pain: clinical manual,* ed 2, St Louis, 1999, Mosby; **9-7,** from Acute Pain Management Guideline Panel, 1992; **9-12,** from Salerno E, Willens J: *Pain management handbook,* St Louis, 1996, Mosby; **9-14,** from Rick Brady, Riva, MD.

Chapter 10
10-1, 10-5, 10-6, Courtesy Kathleen A. Pollard, RN, MSN, CHPN, Phoenix, Ariz; **10-2, 10-4, 10-7,** from Rick Brady, Riva, MD; **10-3,** from Potter PA, Perry AG: *Fundamentals of nursing: concepts, process, and practice,* ed 4, St Louis, 1997, Mosby.

Chapter 11
11-1, 11-2, From Rick Brady, Riva, MD.

Chapter 12
12-2, Courtesy Cameron Bangs, MD. From Auerbach PS, Donner HJ, Weiss EA: *Field guide to wilderness medicine,* St Louis, 1999, Mosby;

12-10, courtesy Molnlyche Health Care, Eddystone, Pa. In Potter PA, Perry AG: *Fundamentals of nursing,* ed 5, St Louis, 2001, Mosby; **12-11A,** from Habif TP: *Clinical dermatology: a color guide to diagnosis and therapy,* ed 2, St Louis, 1992, Mosby; **12-11B,** from Lemmi FO, Lemmi CAE: *Physical assessment findings CD-ROM,* Philadelphia, 2000, Saunders; **12-12,** from Potter PA, Perry AG: *Fundamentals of nursing,* ed 5, St Louis, 2001, Mosby.

Chapter 13
13-1, From Thibodeau GA, Patton KT: *The human body in health and disease,* ed 3, St Louis, 2002, Mosby; **13-12,** from Cerio R, Jackson WF: *A colour atlas of allergic skin disorders,* London, 1992, Wolfe Publishing.

Chapter 14
14-6, 14-7, From Grimes DE, Grimes RM: *AIDS and HIV infection,* St Louis, 1994, Mosby; **14-8,** from the Centers for Disease Control and Prevention. Courtesy Jonathan WM Gold, MD, New York, NY; **14-9,** from Seidel HM et al: *Mosby's guide to physical examination,* ed 5, St Louis, 2003, Mosby. Courtesy Douglas A. Jabs, MD, the Wilmer Ophthalmological Institute, The Johns Hopkins University and Hospital, Baltimore.

Chapter 15
15-4, From Stevens A, Lowe J: *Pathology: illustrated review in color,* ed 2, London, 2000, Mosby; **15-5,** adapted from DeVita VT, Helman S, Rosenberg SA, editors: *Cancer: principles and practice of oncology,* Philadelphia, 1997, Lippincott-Raven; **15-9,** modified from Krakoff IH: Systemic treatment of cancer, *CA Cancer J Clin* 46:134, 1996; **15-18A,** courtesy Pharmacia Deltec, Inc, St Paul, Minn; **15-19,** courtesy Strato/Infusaid, Inc, Norwood, Mass; **15-20,** data from The World Health Organization, 1990.

Chapter 16
16-14, From McCance KL, Huether SE: *Pathophysiology: the biologic basis for disease in adults and children,* ed 4, St Louis, 2002, Mosby.

Chapter 17
17-1, Courtesy St Joseph Hospital, Albuquerque.

Chapter 18
18-1, Courtesy Greg McVicar; **18-2,** courtesy Joseph T. Rothrock, III. From Meeker MH, Rothrock JC: *Alexander's care of the patient in surgery,* ed 11, St Louis, 1999, Mosby; **18-4,** courtesy of The Methodist Hospital, Houston, Tex. Photograph by Donna Dahms, RN, CNOR; **18-5,** from Meeker MH, Rothrock JC: *Alexander's care of the patient in surgery,* ed 11, St Louis, 1999, Mosby.

Chapter 20
20-1, 20-8, From Thibodeau GA, Patton KT: *The human body in health and disease,* ed 3, St Louis, 2002, Mosby; **20-3,** from Thibodeau GA, Patton KT: *Anatomy and physiology,* ed 5, St Louis, 2003, Mosby; **20-7,** courtesy Eye Institute, Department of Ophthalmology and Visual Sciences, University of Iowa Health Care, Iowa City, Iowa; **20-9,** from Seidel HM et al: *Mosby's guide to physical examination,* ed 5, St Louis, 2003, Mosby.

Chapter 21
21-9, From Lemmi FO, Lemmi CAE: *Physical assessment findings CD-ROM,* Philadelphia, 2000, Saunders; **21-10,** courtesy Siemens Hearing Solutions, Piscataway, NJ; **21-11,** courtesy Advanced Bionics Corp., Valencia, Calif.

Chapter 22

Photos in **Table 22-4** (macule, papule, vesicle, plaque, wheal, pustule, fissure, ulcer, atrophy, excoriation), from Thibodeau GA, Patton KT: *The human body in health and disease,* ed 3, St Louis, 2002, Mosby; photos in **Table 22-4** (scale, scar, and atrophy), from Thompson JM, Wilson SF: *Health assessment for nursing practice,* St Louis, 1996, Mosby; **22-1,** from Jarvis C: *Physical examination and health assessment,* ed 4, Philadelphia, 2003, Saunders; **22-3, 22-4,** from Habif TP: *Clinical dermatology: a color guide to diagnosis and therapy,* ed 3, St Louis, 1996, Mosby.

Chapter 23

23-1, From Hooper BJ, Goldman NP: *Primary dermatologic care,* St Louis, 1999, Mosby; **23-2,** from Goldstein BG, Goldstein AO: *Practical dermatology,* ed 2, St Louis, 1997, Mosby. Courtesy Department of Dermatology, Medical College of Georgia, Augusta, Ga; **23-3, 23-4, 23-6, 23-7, 23-10, 23-11,** from Habif TP: *Clinical dermatology: a color guide to diagnosis and therapy,* ed 3, St Louis, 1996, Mosby; **23-5, 23-12,** from Lemmi FO, Lemmi CAE: *Physical assessment findings CD-ROM,* Philadelphia, 2000, Saunders; **23-8,** from Cox N, Lawrence C: *Diagnostic problems in dermatology,* St Louis, 1998, Mosby; **23-13, 23-14,** from Fortunato N, McCullough SM: *Plastic and reconstructive surgery,* St Louis, 1998, Mosby.

Chapter 25

21-1, Redrawn from Price SA, Wilson LM: *Pathophysiology: clinical concepts of disease processes,* ed 6, St Louis, 2003, Mosby; **25-2, 25-3,** from Thompson JM et al: *Mosby's clinical nursing,* ed 5, St Louis, 2002, Mosby; **25-4A,** from Bone RC et al, editors: *Pulmonary and critical care medicine,* vol 1, St Louis, 1993, Mosby; **25-4B,** from Staub NC, Albertine KH: *Anatomy of the lungs.* In Murray JF, Nadel JA, editors: *Textbook of respiratory medicine,* ed 2, Philadelphia, 1994, Saunders; **25-8A,** redrawn from *Principles of pulse oximetry,* Nellcor, Inc, Haywood, Calif; **25-8B,** from Potter PA, Perry AG: *Fundamentals of nursing: concepts, process, and practice,* ed 4, St Louis, 1997, Mosby; **25-10,** redrawn from Wilkins RL et al: *Clinical assessment in respiratory care,* ed 3, St Louis, 1995, Mosby; **25-12, 25-13,** modified from Thompson JM et al: *Mosby's clinical nursing,* ed 5, St Louis, 2002, Mosby; **25-14,** from Beare PG, Myers JL: *Adult health nursing,* ed 3, St Louis, 1998, Mosby; **25-15A,** courtesy Olympus America, Melville, NY; **25-15B,** from Meduri GU et al: Protected bronchoalveolar lavage, *Am Respir Dis* 143:855, 1991; **25-16,** redrawn from Du Bois RM, Clarke SW: *Fiberoptic bronchoscopy in diagnosis and management,* Orlando, Fla, 1987, Grune & Stratton.

Chapter 26

26-4, Courtesy Robert Margulies, Miami. From Smolley LA: How to help patients with obstructive sleep apnea, *J Respir Dis* 11:723, 1990; **26-5,** courtesy Respironics, Inc, Murrysville, Pa; **26-11,** courtesy Passy-Muir, Inc, Irvine, Calif; **26-13,** from the American Cancer Society; **26-16,** courtesy CLG Photographics, Inc, St Louis.

Chapter 27

27-4, From Damjanov I, Linder J: *Anderson's pathology,* ed 10, St Louis, 1996, Mosby; **27-10,** courtesy of Deknatel, Inc, Fall River, Mass.

Chapter 28

28-3, Redrawn from Price SA, Wilson LM: *Pathophysiology: clinical concepts of disease processes,* ed 6, St Louis, 2003, Mosby; **28-5,** from Togger DA, Breener PS: Metered dose inhalers, *Am J Nurs* 101(10):26-32, 2001; **28-11,** from Potter PA, Perry AG: *Fundamentals of nursing,* ed 5, St Louis, 2001, Mosby; **28-14,** courtesy Nellcor Puritan Bennett, Inc; **28-17,** courtesy Axcan Scandipharm, Inc., Birmingham, Ala.

Chapter 29

29-2, From Thibodeau GA, Patton KT: *The human body in health and disease,* ed 3, St Louis, 2002, Mosby; **29-3,** copyright Dennis Kunkel Microscopy, Inc., Kailua, Hawaii; **29-6,** from Seidel HM et al: *Mosby's guide to physical examination,* ed 5, St Louis, 2003, Mosby; **29-8,** from Herlihy B, Maebius N: *The human body in health and illness,* ed 2, Philadelphia, 2003, Saunders.

Chapter 30

30-2, Redrawn from Raven PH, Johnson GB: *Biology,* ed 2, St Louis, 1991, Mosby; **30-3,** redrawn from McCance KL, Huether SE: *Pathophysiology: the biologic basis for disease in adults and children,* ed 4, St Louis, 2002, Mosby; **30-6,** from Bingham BJG, Hawke M, Kwok P: *Atlas of clinical otolaryngology,* St Louis, 1992, Mosby; **30-10, 30-11, 30-14,** from Skarin AT: *Atlas of diagnostic oncology,* ed 2, London, 1996, Mosby-Wolfe; **30-13,** from Cotran RS, Kumar V, Collins T: *Robbins pathologic basis of disease,* ed 6, Philadelphia, 1999, Saunders.

Chapter 31

31-1, 31-3, Modified from Price SA, Wilson LM: *Pathophysiology: clinical concepts of disease processes,* ed 6, St Louis, 2003, Mosby; **31-5, 31-9, 31-12,** modified from Kinney M et al: *Comprehensive cardiac care,* ed 8, St Louis, 1996, Mosby; **31-14,** modified from Kinney M et al: *Comprehensive cardiac care,* ed 7, St Louis, 1991, Mosby.

Chapter 32

32-1, Redrawn from West JB: *Physiological basis of medical practice,* ed 12, Baltimore, 1991, Williams & Wilkins; **32-3,** from Kissane JM: *Anderson's pathology,* ed 9, St Louis, 1990, Mosby; **32-4, 32-5,** from US Department of Health and Human Services: *The sixth report of the Joint National Committee on Detection, Evaluation, and Treatment of High Blood Pressure (JNC-VI),* Washington, DC, 1997, National Institutes of Health.

Chapter 33

33-1, 33-2, From *2002 Heart and stroke statistical update,* American Heart Association; **33-9,** modified and reprinted with permission from Matrisciano L, Alspach JG: Unstable angina: an overview, *Critical Care Nurses* 12:31, 1992; **33-10, 33-11,** courtesy of Mayo Clinic, Rochester, Minn; **33-17,** from *Heart Disease and Stroke* 2:201, 1993, copyright American Heart Association.

Chapter 34

34-1, Redrawn from McCance KL, Huether SE: *Pathophysiology: the biologic basis for disease in adults and children,* ed 4, St Louis, 2002, Mosby; **34-2, 34-4,** redrawn from Urden LD, Stacy KM, Lough ME: *Thelan's critical care nursing: diagnosis and management,* ed 4, St Louis, 2002, Mosby; **34-3, 34-5,** from Cotran RS, Kumar V, Collins T: *Robbins pathologic basis of disease,* ed 6, Philadelphia, 1999, Saunders.

Chapter 35

35-1, 35-5, 35-6, 35-7, 35-8, 35-9, 35-11, 35-12, 35-13, 35-14, 35-15, 35-16, 35-17, 35-18, 35-19, From Huszar RJ: *Basic dysrhythmias: interpretation and management,* ed 3, St Louis, 2002, Mosby; **35-2,** from Goldberger AL, Goldberger E: *Clinical electrocardiography: a simplified approach,* ed 6, St Louis, 1999, Mosby; **35-4, 35-10,** from Urden LD, Stacy KM, Lough ME: *Thelan's critical care nursing: diagnosis and management,* ed 4, St Louis, 2002, Mosby; **35-20, 35-26,** courtesy Medtronic Physio-Control, Redmond, Wash; **35-22A, 35-23A, 35-24,** courtesy Medtronic, Inc., Minneapolis.

Chapter 36

36-2, From Kissane JM: *Anderson's pathology,* ed 9, St Louis, 1990, Mosby; **36-4,** from Cotran RS, Kumar V, Collins T: *Robbins pathologic basis of disease,* ed 6, Philadelphia, 1999, Saunders; **36-5,** from Guzetta CE, Dossey BM: *Cardiovascular nursing: holistic practice,* St Louis, 1992, Mosby; **36-6,** redrawn from Lorell BH, Braunwald E: *Pericardial disease in heart disease: a textbook of cardiovascular medicine,* ed 3, Philadelphia, 1998, Saunders; **36-7, 36-10, 36-11B,** from Stevens A, Lowe J: *Pathology: illustrated review in color,* ed 2, St Louis, 2000, Mosby; **36-9, 36-11A,** from McCance KL, Huether SE: *Pathophysiology: the biologic basis for disease in adults and children,* ed 4, St Louis, 2002, Mosby; **36-12,** redrawn from Block PC: Balloon valvuloplasty, *Cardiol Consult* 9:4, 1988; **36-13A,** courtesy St Jude Medical, Inc, St Paul. All rights reserved; **36-13B,** courtesy Medtronic, Inc, Minneapolis; **35-13C,** courtesy American Red Cross Tissue Services and Baxter Healthcare Corporation, CardioVascular Group, Santa Ana, Calif.

Chapter 37

37-2, Courtesy Jo Menzoian, Boston, Mass; **37-5,** from Damjanov I, Linder J: *Anderson's pathology,* ed 10, St Louis, 1996, Mosby; **37-6,** courtesy FW LoGerfo, Boston; **37-7, 37-8, 37-12,** from Kamal A, Brockelhurst JC: *Color atlas of geriatric medicine,* ed 2, 1991, Mosby–Year Book–Europe; **37-10,** from Lofgren KA: Varicose veins. In Haimovici H, editor: *Vascular surgery: principles and techniques,* New York, 1976, McGraw-Hill.

Chapter 38

38-1, 38-3, From Thibodeau GA, Patton KT: *Anatomy and physiology,* ed 4, St Louis, 1999, Mosby; **38-9,** from Doughty DB, Jackson DB: *Gastrointestinal disorders,* St Louis, 1993, Mosby.

Chapter 39

39-1A, From *Human nutrition information service: making health food choices,* Washington, DC, 1993, US Department of Agriculture; **39-1B,** courtesy The Health Connection, Hagerstown, Md; **39-2,** from Morgan SL, Weiniser RL: *Fundamentals of clinical nutrition,* ed 2, St Louis, 1998, Mosby; **39-3,** redrawn from Mahan LK, Arlin M: *Krause's food, nutrition, and diet therapy,* ed 4, 1992, Saunders; **39-7,** copyright 1978, George A. Bray, MD.

Chapter 40

40-1, From McKenry LM, Salerno E: *Mosby's pharmacology in nursing,* ed 21, St Louis, 2001, Mosby; **40-2,** courtesy University of Washington, Division of Gastroenterology; **40-3,** from Doughty DB, Jackson DB: *Gastrointestinal disorders,* St Louis, 1993, Mosby; **40-5,** from Curon Medical, Inc., Sunnyvale, Calif; **40-6, 40-8, 40-11, 40-15,** redrawn from Price SA, Wilson LM: *Pathophysiology: clinical concepts of disease processes,* ed 6, St Louis, 2003, Mosby; **40-10,** from Stevens A, Lowe J: *Pathology: illustrated review in color,* ed 2, London, 2000, Mosby; **40-12,** from Damjanov I, Linder J: *Anderson's pathology,* ed 10, St Louis, 1996, Mosby.

Chapter 41

41-2, From Damjanov I, Linder J: *Anderson's pathology,* ed 10, St Louis, 1996, Mosby; **41-5, 41-15,** from Stevens A, Lowe J: *Pathology: illustrated review in color,* ed 2, London, 2000, Mosby; **41-8,** from McCance KL, Huether SE: *Pathophysiology: the biologic basis for disease in adults and children,* ed 4, St Louis, 2002, Mosby. Courtesy David Bjorkman, MD, University of Utah School of Medicine, Department of Gastroenterology; **41-10,** from McCance KL, Huether SE: *Pathophysiology: the biologic basis for disease in adults and children,* ed 4, St Louis, 2002, Mosby; **41-12,** redrawn from Meeker MH, Rothrock JC: *Alexander's care of the patient in surgery,* ed 9, St Louis, 1991, Mosby; **41-13,** redrawn from Hampton BG, Bryant RA: *Ostomies and continent diversions,* St Louis, 1992, Mosby; **41-17B,** from Swartz MH: *Textbook of physical diagnosis: history and examination,* ed 4, Philadelphia, 2002, Saunders.

Chapter 42

42-1, From Kamal A, Brockelhurst JC: *Color atlas of geriatric medicine,* ed 2, St Louis, 1991, Mosby–Year Book–Europe; **42-4,** from Damjanov I, Linder J: *Anderson's pathology,* ed 10, St Louis, 1996, Mosby; **42-6,** adapted from Doughty DB, Jackson DB: *Gastrointestinal disorders,* St Louis, 1993, Mosby; **42-10,** from LaBerge JM et al: Transjugular intrahepatic portosystemic shunts: preliminary results in 25 patients, *J Vasc Surg* 16:258, 1992; **42-12, 42-14, 42-16,** from Stevens A, Lowe J: *Pathology: illustrated review in color,* ed 2, London, 2000, Mosby.

Chapter 43

43-1A, 43-2, 43-3, 43-5, From Thibodeau GA, Patton KT: *Anatomy and physiology,* ed 4, St Louis, 1999, Mosby; **43-4,** adapted from Herlihy B, Maebius N: *The human body in health and illness,* ed 2, Philadelphia, 2003, Saunders; **43-6,** from Brundage DJ: *Renal disorders,* St Louis, 1992, Mosby; **43-7,** from Price S, Wilson L: *Pathophysiology: clinical concepts of disease processes,* ed 6, St Louis, 2003, Mosby; **43-9,** courtesy Circon Corp, Santa Barbara, Calif.

Chapter 44

44-4A, From Stevens A, Lowe J: *Pathology: illustrated review in color,* ed 2, London, 2000, Mosby; **44-6,** from Brundage DJ: *Renal disorders,* St Louis, 1992, Mosby; **44-7,** from Lemmi FO, Lemmi CAE: *Physical assessment findings CD-ROM,* Philadelphia, 2000, Saunders; **44-10, 44-12, 44-13,** courtesy Lynda Brubacher, Virginia Mason Hospital, Seattle.

Chapter 45

45-2, From United States Renal Data System, Minneapolis; **45-7, 45-10,** copyright 1994 Baxter Healthcare Corp; **45-12A,** courtesy Quinton Instrument Co, Seattle.

Chapter 46

46-2, Modified from Thibodeau GA, Patton KT: *Anatomy and physiology,* ed 5, St Louis, 2003, Mosby; **46-3, 46-4,** from Herlihy B, Maebius N: *The human body in health and illness,* ed 2, Philadelphia, 2003, Saunders; **46-6,** from McCance KL, Huether SE: *Pathophysiology: the biologic basis for disease in adults and children,* ed 4, St Louis, 2002, Mosby; **46-8, 46-9, 46-10,** from Thibodeau GA, Patton KT: *The human body in health and disease,* ed 3, St Louis, 2002, Mosby; **46-11,** from Thompson JM, Wilson SF: *Health assessment for nursing practice,* St Louis, 1996, Mosby.

Chapter 47

47-6, Courtesy Novo Nordisk Pharmaceuticals, Inc., Princeton, NJ; **47-7,** courtesy Medtronic MiniMed, Northridge, Calif; **47-8, 47-11,** redrawn from McCance KL, Huether SE: *Pathophysiology: the biologic basis for disease in adults and children,* ed 4, St Louis, 2002, Mosby; **47-12,** from Urden LD, Stacy KM, Lough ME: *Thelan's critical care nursing: diagnosis and management,* ed 4, St Louis, 2002, Mosby.

Chapter 48

48-1, Courtesy Linda Haas, Seattle; **48-3, 48-4,** redrawn from Urden LD, Stacy KM, Lough ME: *Thelan's critical care nursing: diagnosis and management,* ed 4, St Louis, 2002, Mosby; **48-5,** from Lemmi FO, Lemmi CAE: *Physical assessment findings CD-ROM,* Philadelphia, 2000, Saunders; **48-6,** courtesy Paul W. Ladenson, MD, The Johns Hopkins University and Hospital, Baltimore. From Seidel HM et al: *Mosby's guide to physical examination,* ed 5, St Louis, 2003, Mosby; **48-7,** from Seidel HM et al: *Mosby's guide to physical examination,* ed 5, St Louis, 2003, Mosby.

Chapter 49

49-1, 49-2, 49-9, From Thibodeau GA, Patton KT: *The human body in health and disease,* ed 3, St Louis, 2002, Mosby; **49-3, 49-4,** from Seidel HM et al: *Mosby's guide to physical examination,* ed 5, St Louis, 2003, Mosby; **49-5,** from Thibodeau GA, Patton KT: *Anatomy and physiology,* ed 4, St Louis, 1999, Mosby; **49-6,** modified from Thibodeau GA, Patton KT: *Anatomy and physiology,* ed 5, St Louis, 2003, Mosby.

Chapter 50

50-2, From Powell DE, Stelling CB: *The diagnosis and detection of breast diseases,* St Louis, 1993, Mosby; **50-3,** from Evans A et al: *Atlas of breast disease management,* Philadelphia, 1998, Saunders; **50-5,** courtesy Proxima Therapeutics, Inc., Alpharetta, Ga; **50-7, 50-8B,** from Fortunato N, McCullough SM: *Plastic and reconstructive surgery,* St Louis, 1998, Mosby. Courtesy Brian W. Davies, MD; **50-8A,** from Cameron J: *Current surgical therapy,* ed 5, St Louis, 1995, Mosby; **50-9,** modified from Beare PG, Myers JL: *Adult health nursing,* ed 3, St Louis, 1998, Mosby, and Fortunato N, McCullough SM: *Plastic and reconstructive surgery,* St Louis, 1998, Mosby.

Chapter 51

51-1, 51-2, 51-3, 51-6, 51-7, 51-9, From Morse S, Moreland A, Holmes K, editors: *Atlas of sexually transmitted diseases and AIDS,* London, 1996, Mosby-Wolfe; **51-4,** courtesy US Public Health Service, Washington, DC; **51-5,** from Habif T: *Clinical dermatology: a color guide to diagnosis and therapy,* ed 3, St Louis, 1996, Mosby; **51-8, 51-10,** reproduced with permission of GlaxoSmithKline, Research Triangle Park, NC.

Chapter 52

52-2, Courtesy Ethicon, Inc., Cornelia, Ga; **52-3,** from Seidel HM et al: *Mosby's guide to physical examination,* ed 5, St Louis, 2003, Mosby; **52-4,** from Lowdermilk DL, Perry SE, Bobak IM: *Maternity and women's health care,* ed 7, St Louis, 2000, Mosby; **52-6,** from Mishell DR et al: *Comprehensive gynecology,* ed 3, St Louis, 1997, Mosby; **52-7,** redrawn from Novak ER, Woodruff JD, editors: *Novak's gynecologic and obstetric pathology,* ed 6, Philadelphia, 1967, Saunders. In McCance KL, Huether SE: *Pathophysiology: the biologic basis for disease in adults and children,* ed 4, St Louis, 2002, Mosby; **52-8, 52-9,** from Symonds EM, MacPherson MBA: *Color atlas of obstetrics and gynecology,* London, 1994, Mosby-Wolfe. **52-10,** from Phipps WJ, Sands JK, Marek JF: *Medical-surgical nursing: concepts and clinical practice,* ed 6, St Louis, 1999, Mosby; **52-12,** redrawn from Seidel HM et al: *Mosby's guide to physical examination,* ed 5, St Louis, 2003, Mosby; **52-13,** from Seidel HM et al: *Mosby's guide to physical examination,* ed 4, St Louis, 1999, Mosby.

Chapter 53

53-5, From Iwamoto RR, Maher KE: Radiation therapy for prostate cancer, *Semin Oncol Nurs* 17(2):90-100, 2001; **53-7, 53-8,** from Swartz MH: *Textbook of physical diagnosis: history and examination,* ed 4, Philadelphia, 2002, Saunders; **53-9,** from Seidel HM et al: *Mosby's guide to physical examination,* ed 5, St Louis, 2003, Mosby.

Chapter 54

54-1, 54-10, 54-11, 54-13, 54-14, 54-15, 54-20, From Thibodeau GA, Patton KT: *Anatomy and physiology,* ed 5, St Louis, 2003, Mosby; **54-4,** from Herlihy B, Maebius N: *The human body in health and illness,* ed 2, Philadelphia, 2003, Saunders; **54-5, 54-6,** adapted from Thibodeau GA, Patton KT:

Anatomy and physiology, ed 5, St Louis, 2003; **54-12,** from McCance KL, Huether SE: *Pathophysiology: the biologic basis for disease in adults and children,* ed 4, St Louis, 2002, Mosby; **54-19A,** courtesy Hitachi Medical Systems America, Inc., Twinsburg, Ohio; **54-19B,** from Chipps E, Clanin N, Campbell V: *Neurologic disorders,* St Louis, 1992, Mosby.

Chapter 55
55-4, Redrawn from McCance KL, Huether SE: *Pathophysiology: the biologic basis for disease in adults and children,* ed 4, St Louis, 2002, Mosby; **55-6,** redrawn from Urden LD, Stacy KM, Lough ME: *Thelan's critical care nursing: diagnosis and management,* ed 4, St Louis, 2002, Mosby; **55-7,** from Clochesy JM et al: *Critical care nursing,* ed 2, Philadelphia, 1996, Saunders; **55-9,** redrawn from Barker E: *Neuroscience nursing: a spectrum of care,* ed 2, St Louis, 2002, Mosby; **55-10,** from Wong J, Wong S, Dempster JK: Care of the unconscious patient: a problem-oriented approach, *Am Assoc Neurosci Nurses* 16:145, 1984; **55-13,** from Bingham BJG, Hawke M, Kwok P: *Clinical atlas of otolaryngology,* St Louis, 1992, Mosby; **55-14,** redrawn from Barker E: *Neuroscience nursing: a spectrum of care,* ed 2, St Louis, 2002, Mosby; **55-15,** from Price SA, Wilson LM: *Pathophysiology: clinical concepts of disease processes,* ed 6, St Louis, 2003, Mosby; **55-16,** from Stevens A, Lowe J: *Pathology: illustrated review in color,* ed 2, London, 2000, Mosby; **55-18,** courtesy Department of Neurological Surgery, Vanderbilt University Medical Center, Nashville, TN.

Chapter 56
56-5, Courtesy Joseph C. Maroon, MD; **56-8,** modified from Hoeman SP: *Rehabilitation nursing,* ed 2, St Louis, 1995, Mosby; **56-9,** courtesy Sammons Preston, Bolingbrook, Ill.

Chapter 57
57-2, From Stevens A, Lowe J: *Pathology: illustrated review in color,* ed 2, London, 2000, Mosby; **57-5,** from McCance KL, Huether SE: *Pathophysiology: the biologic basis for disease in adults and children,* ed 4, St Louis, 2002, Mosby; **57-6,** from Perkin DG: *Mosby's color atlas and text of neurology,* London, 1998, Mosby-Wolfe; **57-7,** redrawn from Rudy E: *Advanced neurological and neurosurgical nursing,* St Louis, 1984, Mosby; **56-8,** redrawn from Barker E: *Neuroscience nursing: a spectrum of care,* ed 2, St Louis, 2002, Mosby.

Chapter 58
58-1A, From Damjanov I, Linder J: *Anderson's pathology,* ed 10, St Louis, 1996, Mosby; **58-2,** from Stevens A, Lowe J: *Pathology: illustrated review in color,* ed 2, London, 2000, Mosby.

Chapter 59
59-1, From Thibodeau GA, Patton KT: *Anatomy and physiology,* ed 5, St Louis, 2003, Mosby; **59-2,** courtesy Joe Rothrock, Media, Pa; 59-3, redrawn from Chipps E, Clanin N, Campbell V: *Neurologic disorders,* St Louis, 1992, Mosby; **59-4,** redrawn from Marciano FF et al: *BNI Quarterly* 11(2):6, 1995. In McCance KL, Huether SE: *Pathophysiology: the biologic basis for disease in adults and children,* ed 4, St Louis, 2002, Mosby; **59-8, 59-9,** from American Spinal Injury Association/International Medical Society of Paraplegic (ASIA/IMOSP): *International standards for neurological functional classification of spinal cord injury patients* (revised), Chicago, 2002, American Spinal Cord Injury Assn; **59-10, 59-13,** courtesy Michael S Clement, MD, Mesa, Ariz; **59-12,** courtesy Acromed Corp, Cleveland; **59-14,** from Barker E: *Neuroscience nursing: a spectrum of care,* ed 2, St Louis, 2002, Mosby.

Chapter 60
60-1, From Herlihy B, Maebius N: *The human body in health and illness,* ed 2, Philadelphia, 2003, Saunders; **60-3, 60-5,** from Thibodeau GA, Patton KT: *Anatomy and physiology,* ed 5, St Louis, 2003, Mosby; **60-6, 60-8,** from Mourad LA: *Orthopedic disorders,* St Louis, 1991, Mosby; **60-7,** from Lemmi FO, Lemmi CAE: *Physical assessment findings CD-ROM,* Philadelphia, 2000, Saunders.

Chapter 61
61-1, Redrawn from Price SA, Wilson LM: *Pathophysiology: clinical concepts of disease processes,* ed 6, St Louis, 2003, Mosby; **61-2,** from Thompson JM et al: *Mosby's clinical nursing,* ed 5, St Louis, 2002, Mosby; **61-3,** from Thibodeau GA, Patton KT: *Anatomy and physiology,* ed 5, St Louis, 2003, Mosby; **61-7,** redrawn from Long BC, Phipps WJ, Cassmeyer VL: *Medical-surgical nursing: a nursing process approach,* St Louis, 1993, Mosby;

61-10, courtesy Howmedica, Inc; **61-11,** from Ryan DW, Park GR: *Color atlas of critical and intensive care: diagnosis and investigation,* London, 1995, Mosby-Wolfe; **61-14,** from Thompson JM et al: *Mosby's clinical nursing,* ed 4, St. Louis, 1998, Mosby; **61-15,** courtesy RA Weinstein, Denver, Colo; **61-17,** from Macklin EJ et al: *Hunter, Macklin, and Callahan's rehabilitation of the hand and upper extremity,* vol. 2, ed 5, St Louis, 2002, Mosby; **61-19,** from Maher A, Salmond S, Pellino T: *Orthopedic nursing,* ed 3, Philadelphia, 2002, Saunders; **61-20,** courtesy Zimmer, Inc., Warsaw, Ind.

Chapter 62
62-1, Redrawn from Mourad L: *Orthopedic disorders,* St Louis, 1992, Mosby; **62-2,** from Gartland J: *Fundamentals of orthopaedics,* Philadelphia, 1987, Saunders; **62-3, 62-4,** from Damjanov I, Linder J: *Anderson's pathology,* ed 10, St Louis, 1996, Mosby; **62-6,** from Mercier LR: *Practical orthopedics,* ed 4, St Louis, 1996, Mosby; **62-7,** from Maher A et al: *Orthopedic nursing,* ed 3, Philadelphia, 2002, Saunders.

Chapter 63
63-1, 63-3, From Stevens A, Lowe J: *Pathology: illustrated review in color,* ed 2, London, 2000, Mosby; **63-6, 63-9,** from Habif TP: *Clinical dermatology: a color guide to diagnosis and therapy,* ed 3, St Louis, 1996, Mosby; **63-7,** reprinted from the Clinical Slide Collection on the Rheumatic Diseases, copyright 1991, 1995, 1997. Used by permission of the American College of Rheumatology; **63-11,** from Zitelli BJ, Davis HW: *Atlas of pediatric physical diagnosis,* ed 4, St Louis, 2002, Mosby; **63-12,** redrawn from Freundlich B, Leventhal L: The fibromyalgia syndrome. In Schumacher HR Jr, Klippel JH, Koopman WJ, editors: *Primer on the rheumatic diseases,* ed 11, Atlanta, 1997, Arthritis Foundation. Reprinted with permission from The Arthritis Foundation, 1330 W. Peachtree St., Atlanta, GA 30309.

Chapter 64
64-1, 64-20, Courtesy Spacelabs Medical, Redmond, Wash; **64-2,** redrawn from Gardner PE: *Hemodynamic pressure monitoring,* Redmond, Wash, 1994, Spacelabs Medical; **64-3,** redrawn from Flynn JBM, Bruce NP: *Introduction to critical care skills,* St Louis, 1993, Mosby; **64-4,** from Darovic GO: *Hemodynamic monitoring,* ed 2, Philadelphia, 1995, Saunders; **64-5, 64-7, 64-10,** from Urden LD, Stacy KM, Lough ME: *Thelan's critical care nursing: diagnosis and management,* ed 4, St Louis, 2002, Mosby; **64-6,** courtesy Edwards Critical Care Division, Baxter Healthcare Corporation, Santa Ana, Calif; **64-8, 64-9,** from Lynn-McHale DJ, Carlson KK: *AACN procedure manual for critical care,* ed 4, Philadelphia, 2001, Saunders; **64-12, 64-14,** courtesy Datascope Corporation, Montvale, NJ; **64-15,** redrawn from Thelan LA et al: *Critical care nursing: diagnosis and management,* ed 3, St Louis, 1998, Mosby; **64-16A,** from Beare PG, Myers JL: *Adult health nursing,* ed 3, St Louis, 1998, Mosby; **64-17,** from Sills JR: *Respiratory care certification guide: the complete review resource for the entry level exam,* ed 3, St Louis, 1998, Mosby. In Urden LD, Stacy KM, Lough ME: *Thelan's critical care nursing: diagnosis and management,* ed 4, St Louis, 2002, Mosby; **64-18,** from Henneman E, Ellstrom K, St. John RE: *AACN protocols for practice: care of the mechanically ventilated patient series,* Aliso Viejo, Calif, 1999, American Association of Critical Care Nurses; **64-19,** courtesy Lifecare, Westminster, Colo; **64-21,** courtesy Mallinckrodt, Inc, Carlsbad, Calif.

Chapter 65
65-2, 65-3, 65-4, 65-5, From Urden LD, Stacy KM, Lough ME: *Thelan's critical care nursing: diagnosis and management,* ed 4, St Louis, 2002, Mosby.

Chapter 66
66-6, From Richmond TS: A critical care challenge: the patient with a cervical spinal cord injury, *Focus Crit Care* 12:27, 1985; **66-7,** courtesy Respironics, Inc, Pittsburgh; **66-10,** courtesy Hill-Rom, Inc, Batesville, Ind; **66-11,** courtesy Kinetic Concepts, Inc, San Antonio, Tex.

Chapter 67
67-2, 67-3, Courtesy Cameron Bangs, MD. From Auerbach PS, Donner HJ, Weiss EA: *Field guide to wilderness medicine,* St Louis, 1999, Mosby; **67-5,** from Auerbach PS, Donner HJ, Weiss EA: *Field guide to wilderness medicine,* St Louis, 1999, Mosby; **67-6,** courtesy Sherman Minton, MD. From Auerbach PS, Donner HJ, Weiss EA: *Field guide to wilderness medicine,* St Louis, 1999, Mosby; **67-7,** redrawn from Rosen P et al: *Emergency medicine,* vol 1, ed 2, St Louis, 1988, Mosby; **67-8,** photo used with the permission of the American Red Cross.

Index

Note: Disorder names are in **bold face.** Entries in **bold face** indicate main discussions. Page numbers followed by *f, t,* and *b* indicate figures, tables, or boxed material, respectively.

Note: Disorder names are in **bold** face. Entries in **bold**
face indicate main discussions. Page numbers followed
by *f*, *t*, and *b* indicate figures, tables, or boxed material,
respectively.

Note: Disorder names are in **bold face.** Entries in **bold face** indicate main discussions. Page numbers followed by *f, t,* and *b* indicate figures, tables, or boxed material, respectively.

Note: Disorder names are in **bold face.** Entries in **bold
face** indicate main discussions. Page numbers followed
by *f, t,* and *b* indicate figures, tables, or boxed material,
respectively.

Note: Disorder names are in **bold face**. Entries in bold face indicate main discussions. Page numbers followed by f, t, and b indicate figures, tables, or boxed material, respectively.

Note: Disorder names are in **bold face.** Entries in **bold face** indicate main discussions. Page numbers followed by *f, t,* and *b* indicate figures, tables, or boxed material, respectively.

Note: Disorder names are in **bold face.** Entries in **bold face** indicate main discussions. Page numbers followed by *f, t,* and *b* indicate figures, tables, or boxed material, respectively.

Note: Disorder names are in **bold face.** Entries in **bold face** indicate main discussions. Page numbers followed by *f, t,* and *b* indicate figures, tables, or boxed material, respectively.

Note: Disorder names are in **bold face.** Entries in **bold face** indicate main discussions. Page numbers followed by *f, t,* and *b* indicate figures, tables, or boxed material, respectively.

Note: Disorder names are in **bold face.** Entries in **bold
face** indicate main discussions. Page numbers followed
by *f*, *t*, and *b* indicate figures, tables, or boxed material,
respectively.

Note: Disorder names are in **bold face.** Entries in **bold face** indicate main discussions. Page numbers followed by *f, t,* and *b* indicate figures, tables, or boxed material, respectively.

Note: Disorder names are in **bold face.** Entries in **bold face** indicate main discussions. Page numbers followed by *f, t,* and *b* indicate figures, tables, or boxed material, respectively.

Note: Disorder names are in **bold face**. Entries in **bold face** indicate main discussions. Page numbers followed by *f*, *t*, and *b* indicate figures, tables, or boxed material, respectively.

Note: Disorder names are in **bold** face. Entries in **bold face** indicate main discussions. Page numbers followed by *f*, *t*, and *b* indicate figures, tables, or boxed material, respectively.

Note: Disorder names are in **bold face.** Entries in **bold face** indicate main discussions. Page numbers followed by *f*, *t*, and *b* indicate figures, tables, or boxed material, respectively.

Note: Disorder names are in **bold** face. Entries in **bold**
face indicate main discussions. Page numbers followed
by *f, t,* and *b* indicate figures, tables, or boxed material,
respectively.

Note: Disorder names are in **bold face.** Entries in **bold face** indicate main discussions. Page numbers followed by *f, t,* and *b* indicate figures, tables, or boxed material, respectively.

Note: Disorder names are in bold face. Entries in bold
face indicate main discussions. Page numbers followed
by f, t, and b indicate figures, tables, or boxed material,
respectively.

Note: Disorder names are in **bold face.** Entries in **bold face** indicate main discussions. Page numbers followed by *f, t,* and *b* indicate figures, tables, or boxed material, respectively.

Note: Disorder names are in **bold face.** Entries in **bold face** indicate main discussions. Page numbers followed by *f, t,* and *b* indicate figures, tables, or boxed material, respectively.

Note: Disorder names are in bold face. Entries in bold
face indicate main discussions. Page numbers followed
by f, t, and b indicate figures, tables, or boxed material,
respectively.

Note: Disorder names are in **bold face.** Entries in **bold face** indicate main discussions. Page numbers followed by *f, t,* and *b* indicate figures, tables, or boxed material, respectively.

Note: Disorder names are in **bold face**. Entries in **bold face** indicate main discussions. Page numbers followed by *f*, *t*, and *b* indicate figures, tables, or boxed material, respectively.